(Continued inside back cover)

CECIL
TEXTBOOK
OF
MEDICINE

The Consulting Editors

20TH EDITION
VOLUME 2

CECIL
TEXTBOOK
OF
MEDICINE

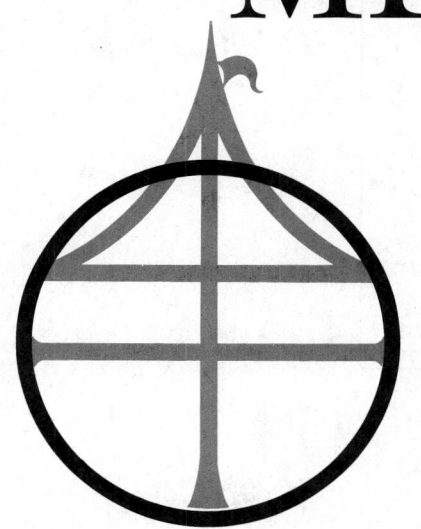

Edited by

J. CLAUDE BENNETT, M.D.

President, University of Alabama at Birmingham
Birmingham, Alabama;
Formerly Spencer Professor of Medicine
and Chairman, Department of Medicine
University of Alabama School of Medicine
Birmingham, Alabama

FRED PLUM, M.D.

Anne Parrish Titzell Professor of Neurology and Neuroscience
Chairman, Department of Neurology and Neuroscience
Cornell University Medical College;
Neurologist-in-Chief
The New York Hospital-Cornell Medical Center
New York, New York

W.B. SAUNDERS COMPANY

A Division of Harcourt Brace & Company

PHILADELPHIA • LONDON • TORONTO • MONTREAL • SYDNEY • TOKYO

W. B. SAUNDERS COMPANY
A Division of Harcourt Brace & Company

The Curtis Center
Independence Square West
Philadelphia, PA 19106

Library of Congress Cataloging-in-Publication Data

Cecil textbook of medicine / edited by J. Claude Bennett, Fred Plum.—20th ed.

    p.   cm.

   Includes bibliographical references and index.

   ISBN 0-7216-3561-X (single v.).—ISBN 0-7216-3574-1 (v. 1).—ISBN 0-7216-3575-X (v. 2).—
ISBN 0-7216-3573-3 (set)

   1. Internal medicine. I. Cecil, Russell L. (Russell La Fayette), 1881-1965. II. Bennett, J. Claude.
III. Plum, Fred, IV. Title: Textbook of medicine.
   [DNLM: 1.   Medicine. WB 100 C3888 1996]
RC46.C423   1996
616—dc20

DNLM/DLC   94-43773

ISBN 0-7216-3574-1   Volume 1
ISBN 0-7216-3575-X   Volume 2
ISBN 0-7216-3573-3   Set (Vols 1 & 2)
ISBN 0-7216-3561-X   Single volume

CECIL TEXTBOOK OF MEDICINE

Last digit is the print number: 9   8   7   6   5   4   3   2

CONTENTS

(Detailed Table of Contents begins on the following page)

COLOR PLATES

HIGHLIGHTED TABLES

The tables listed below contain important information about administering medications, their possible interactions, and necessary precautions as well as immunization information. Highlighted tables are indicated in the text by a check mark.

PART XV

METABOLIC DISEASES

168 APPROACH TO THE PATIENT WITH METABOLIC DISEASE

Louis J. Elsas II

In this chapter we approach the principles of screening, diagnosing, and treating inherited metabolic diseases, many of which are detailed in subsequent chapters. In Ch. 24, inborn errors of metabolism are defined in terms of the function and location of proteins and the pathophysiologic consequences to the human organism when they are impaired. Here we invoke the predictive power of a genetic approach in identifying and preventing irreversible damage from an inborn error of metabolism. The goal is to diagnose the disorder and intervene to prevent damage by a return to metabolic homeostasis before disease is irreversible. Genetic screening is used to accomplish this objective. Once the disorder is detected, if its pathophysiology is understood, intervention can restore metabolic homeostasis and prevent progressive disease.

Genetic screening is a process by which a small population of high-risk individuals is selected from a much larger group. From the smaller population, a diagnosis, preferably presymptomatic, is made. Screening is performed in at least five categories of heritable risk, age, or reproductive condition.

Nonselected screening at a population base is performed to identify the homozygously affected individual and to prevent death, mental retardation, and other irreversible clinical manifestations. Certain principles are used to determine which diseases would be ethically, legally, and socially acceptable for such a public health activity (Table 168–1) (see Ch. 2). At present this type of screening is limited to the newborn owing to this population's accessibility, the rapidity of progression, and the lifelong burden of disease processes. Disorders currently being screened for in various combinations include phenylketonuria, maple syrup urine disease, galactosemia, homocystinuria, tyrosinemia, sickle cell disease, congenital adrenal hyperplasia, biotinidase deficiency, hypothyroidism, and cystic fibrosis.

Selective screening of newborns, children, and adults is performed to identify inherited disorders that may not be preventable. The objectives are to provide amelioratory treatment; determine the genetic component of the disorder; provide genetic counseling to patients, parents, and relatives; provide new information about the disorder's pathophysiology; and develop prevalence data. The laboratory diagnostic methods used in selective screening are different from those used in nonselective mass screening, and clinical judgment is the primary criterion for entry into this type of genetic screening. The preventive aspects of genetic screening of the symptomatic patient are important, particularly in disorders in which the onset of irreversible manifestations requires time for full expression. Given a specific diagnosis, genetic counseling may alter reproductive or life-planning behavior. Examples of heritable disorders amenable to selective screening are peroxisomal disorders, Wilson's disease, cystinuria, familial hypercholesterolemia, various organic acidemias, mucopolysaccharidosis and other lysosomal disorders, cystinosis, Duchenne's muscular dystrophy, disorders of mitochondrial function, and disorders of connective tissue.

Selective and nonselective genetic screening in pregnant women is achieved by fetal sonography, chorionic villus biopsy, or amniocentesis coupled with biochemical, chromosomal, or molecular analyses of cultured fetal cells. Maternal blood is a useful screening source for the fetal disorders Down syndrome and spina bifida. If maternal blood concentrations of α-fetoprotein, chorionic gonadotropin, or estriol vary above or below mean values of normal at a specific age of gestation, further fetal studies by sonography and amniocentesis are indicated. Considerable research is in progress to isolate fetal cells from maternal blood to avoid invasion of the amniotic cavity in prenatal screening.

Screening selected populations at risk for environmental hazards is generally applied to the adult population. Pharmacogenetic disorders fall into this category and include screening plasma pseudocholinesterase concentrations preoperatively to detect *pseudocholinesterase deficiency* and prevent death from succinyldicholine, and determining α-antitrypsin genotypes in individuals exposed to dust to prevent occupation-related, early-onset emphysema from α_1-antitrypsin deficiency.

Screening for asymptomatic heterozygotes in a "high-risk" population is another preventive approach to inborn errors of metabolism. The objective is to provide genetic counseling and reproductive alternatives in high-risk mating. An example is screening for *Tay-Sachs disease* carriers in the Ashkenazi Jewish population (see Ch. 24). Implementing newborn screening for sickle cell hemoglobin detects not only the homozygously affected infant, but also the SA heterozygote. The data from either genotype could be used to develop pedigrees and provide genetic counseling to at-risk family members.

THERAPY OF INHERITED DISEASE

Because the metabolic diseases considered in this section have in common that they are inherited and caused by single genes of large effect, a general approach to their treatment is appropriate. These approaches are outlined in Table 168–2. The level at which therapy is rendered depends on the level of understanding of the pathophysiologic mechanisms producing disease and the interventional methods available. Thus genetic counseling is used for diseases whose mechanisms are not yet understood, whereas engineered enzyme is replaced in *Gaucher disease, type I* by recurrent intravenous infusion.

Genetic counseling is a unique and fundamental aspect of management in inherited metabolic diseases. Patients and relatives usually ask the following questions: Why did this disease occur? Will this disease happen in me or my children? Can it be cured or prevented? Genetic counseling tries to answer these questions through complex processes involving several elements (see Ch. 29). One cannot overemphasize the importance of an accurate diagnosis before entering into formal genetic counseling.

TABLE 168–1. PRINCIPLES FOR NONSELECTIVE GENETIC SCREENING

The disorder should produce a high burden to the affected individual yet be preventable.

Methods for screening, retrieval, diagnosis, and management must be practical and available to the target population as a whole.

Inheritance and pathogenesis of the disease should be understood and genetic counseling available.

Benefit-to-cost ratio of the program should be greater than 1.

Patients' rights should be protected (voluntariness, informed consent, confidentiality).

Sensitivity and specificity should be high for the methods used.

TABLE 168–2. GENETIC APPROACHES TO THERAPY OF INHERITED DISEASE

Genetic Counseling: Prospective therapy
  Diagnosis, risk assessment, informational transfer, support for resource allocation

Reproductive Alternatives: Contraception, abstinence, artificial insemination, *in vitro* fertilization, risk-taking with or without prenatal monitoring

Environmental Engineering
  Avoiding offending agent
  Supplemental physical, speech, developmental therapy
  Nutritional management
    Limit toxic precursor
    Provide deficient product
    Detoxify through alternate metabolic route
    Provide feedback inhibitor
    Provide supraphysiologic amounts of vitamin precursor
    Induce protein (enzyme) production

Protein and Enzyme Replacement
  Infuse protected pure enzyme
  Provide clotting factors and peptide hormones
  Transplantation (prospective)
    Organ transplant
    Bone marrow transplant

Genetic Engineering
  Somatic gene therapy
    Random insertion
    Homologous recombination (site specific)
  Germ line therapy

cycle, protein intake is limited to reduce ammonia accumulation. Arginine is supplemented to provide deficient product of the blocked reaction and alternate pathways are induced for nitrogen excretion. The latter therapy is made possible by a ubiquitous enzyme N-glycine-acylase, which forms adducts with benzoic acid and glycine to produce hippuric acid that is excreted, thus ridding the body of one nitrogen molecule. *Orotic aciduria* is caused by mutations in the bifunctional enzyme orotate phosphoribosyl transferase-orotidine-5′-monophosphate decarboxylase. The disease process, which includes severe anemia and immune deficiency, is caused by deficient end-product, uridine, and is treated by replacing 100 to 200 mg per kilogram per day of uridine (orally). Feedback inhibition is important in treating *congenital adrenal hypertrophy* with replacement doses of hydrocortisone to prevent virilization from testosterone overproduction. Glucose decreases overproduction of the precursors δ-aminolevulinic acid and porphobilinogen in *acute intermittent porphyria* caused by porphobilinogen deaminase deficiency. Using supraphysiologic amounts of a specific vitamin is important if it is the precursor for coenzyme in a genetically impaired holoenzyme. There are many vitamin-dependent metabolic disorders such as pyridoxine (vitamin B_6)–dependent *homocystinuria,* and vitamin C–dependent *Ehlers-Danlos syndrome type VI.* In vitamin B_6–dependent homocystinuria mutant cystathionine synthase is stabilized to biologic degradation when saturated with pyridoxal phosphate. Others include vitamin B_{12}-dependent methylmalonic aciduria, thiamine-dependent maple syrup urine disease, and biotin-dependent propionic aciduria. Some blocked metabolic reactions can be augmented by inducing transcription of their gene. For example, phenobarbital and several other drugs induce hepatic UDP–glucuronyl transferase gene expression and reduce the accumulation of unconjugated bilirubin in *Gilbert syndrome.*

If the specific protein or enzyme has been purified and engineered to function in its specified organ or subcellular organelle, it can be used to treat an inherited metabolic disease. One good example is glucocerebrosidase, which has been purified in large quantities from placenta and biochemically engineered to contain the mannose recognition site for cellular uptake into lysosomal compartments. It has been used successfully to prevent and reverse the pancytopenia and bone disease of *type I Gaucher disease* (see Ch. 174.2). Many proteins are now made through recombinant techniques to treat metabolic disease and bypass the risks of AIDS and hepatitis attendant on using human-derived biologicals. These include Factor VIII for *hemophilia type A,* and growth hormone for *growth hormone deficiency.* Several other engineered proteins used to treat inherited metabolic disease include 1-deamino-8-D-arginine vasopressin to treat *X-linked recessive diabetes insipidus,* and recombinant α_1-antitrypsin made stable by inactivating methionine 385 in the treatment of α_1-antitrypsin deficiency. Some enzymes such as adenosine deaminase have been modified with polyethylene glycol to reduce immunogenicity and prolong biological half-life in the blood. It is used to treat *severe combined immunodeficiency (SCID).*

For metabolic disorders that are lethal and have no other available therapy, organ transplantation may be life-saving. Transplantation with histocompatible organs has become clinically important due to advances in immunology which not only allow for better tissue typing but also enable chronic immunosuppression with such drugs as cyclosporine, azathioprine, and prednisone to prevent rejection.

Several principles are required for successful treatment of an inherited metabolic disorder by organ transplant: (1) The normal enzyme, protein, or function must be provided by the transplanted organ. (2) Usually the affected organ must be removed. (3) The host must be immunologically tolerant to the gene product being introduced in addition to the transplanted organ itself. These principles are particularly relevant when displacement bone marrow transplantation is used. In the latter, normal donor stem cells differentiate and provide their enzymes to the recipient's reticuloendothelial system. Diseases associated with accumulation of products in the central nervous system are not yet ameliorated by bone marrow transplantation, although accumulation in bone, liver, and spleen is reduced. One group of metabolic diseases uses stem cell bone marrow transplantation to prevent leukemia caused by syndromes that include defective DNA repair, such as *Fanconi's anemia, Bloom*

Surgical intervention may be a useful adjunct for treating heritable disorders. For example, stabilizing hypoplastic cervical vertebrae may prevent quadriparesis or death in a variety of *chondrodysplasias* and *mucopolysaccharidoses,* accompanied by hypoplasia of the odontoid process. In *Marfan syndrome,* careful monitoring of aortic root diameter with surgical removal and prosthesis may prevent a lethal aortic dissection. Similarly, evaluation of polyps and early colectomy may prevent disseminated adenocarcinoma in families with the autosomal dominant forms of *familial polyposis coli.* Preventing heritable cancer by early surgical excision is therapeutic for thyroid carcinoma in *medullary thyroid carcinoma, Wilms' tumors,* and neurofibromas of *von Recklinghausen's disease.* Other examples of the benefit of preventive surgery for inborn errors include splenectomy for hemolytic anemias associated with spherocytosis and pyloroplasty in pyloric stenosis.

Environmental engineering is the most commonly used approach to preventing disease in patients affected by inherited metabolic disease. The environment (nutritional intake, exposure to toxins, sun, stress, climatic variation, and drug therapy) may produce a disease state in individuals who have inherited single genes or polygenic susceptibility to the environmental stress. Pharmacogenetic disorders exemplify the simple treatment of *avoidance* once the genetic susceptibility is identified. Health then can be viewed as a continual adaptation between the individual and the environment. Environmental engineering is a form of genetic therapy in which individual genetic susceptibility is identified and the environment is altered to provide optimal health for that individual's unique genetic constitution. The frequency of diseases caused by genetic susceptibility to the environment varies from rare to 100%. All humans develop *scurvy* unless ascorbate is provided in the diet because we are all homozygously deficient for the ability to convert glucuronic acid to glucuronolactone and ascorbate. Humans and primates lost this anabolic pathway during evolution. By contrast, humans readily synthesize tetrahydrobiopterin (BH_4), a cofactor in many hydroxylase reactions including phenylalanine hydroxylase. There are rare diseases (about 1 in 500,000) of increased blood phenylalanine and severe progressive neurodegeneration in which biopterin (BH_2) is not synthesized. BH_2 replacement may treat defects in biosynthesis and exemplifies a group of metabolic disorders known as *vitamin-dependency disorders.*

Nutritional management involves correcting the metabolic block and returning the patient to homeostasis through diet manipulation and drug therapy. Many of the diseases listed in this section are amenable to this approach and use the pathophysiologic mechanisms listed in Table 24–2. For example, in disorders of the urea *syndrome,* and *ataxia-telangiectasia.* Organ transplantation of liver or kidney can reverse growth and developmental delay in type I glycogen storage disease, cystinosis, acute intermittent porphyria, type I tyrosinemia, Fabry's disease, oxalosis, and non-neuronotrophic lysosomal storage diseases. Lung transplantation has been successful in cystic fibrosis and α_1-antitrypsin deficiency, and prophylactic aortic transplantation has prevented aortic dissection in Marfan syndrome.

In the past decade somatic cell gene therapy to treat patients afflicted with genetic disease has entered the arena of clinical research. Numerous laboratories throughout the world are actively designing strategies by which exogenous DNA can be incorporated in the genomic DNA of patients to provide a missing gene function. It is not overly optimistic to assume that some form of *gene therapy* for a number of inherited metabolic diseases will be routinely available by the end of the century (see Ch. 25).

Desnick RJ: Treatment of Genetic Diseases. New York, Churchill Livingstone, 1991. *A multiauthored review of various approaches to metabolic disease therapy.*

Elsas LJ: Newborn screening. *In* Rudolph AM (ed.): Pediatrics. 20th ed. New York, Appleton-Century-Crofts, 1994. *Approaches to genetic screening.*

Elsas LJ, Acosta PB: Nutrition support of inherited metabolic disease. *In* Shils ME, Olson JA, Shike M (eds.): Modern Nutrition in Health and Disease. 8th ed, Philadelphia, Lea & Febiger, 1993. *Complete discussion of how to manage metabolic disease by diet.*

Disorders of Carbohydrate Metabolism

169 GALACTOSEMIA
Stanton Segal

The galactosemias are toxicity syndromes exhibited by patients with an inherited inability to metabolize the sugar galactose, a constituent of the disaccharide lactose found in milk and milk products. There are three disorders, each resulting from a deficiency of one of the enzymes that catalyze the normal conversion of galactose to glucose. Uridyltransferase deficiency is the most prevalent and is commonly referred to as classic galactosemia (Table 169–1). For all three disorders, the elevations of the level of galactose and its metabolites in blood, urine, and tissues can be diminished and acute neonatal clinical manifestations alleviated by omitting dietary galactose.

ETIOLOGY. Galactokinase, galactose-1-phosphate (P) uridyltransferase, and uridine diphosphate-4-epimerase deficiencies are all autosomal recessive genetic disorders. The individual human genes have been located on chromosomes 17, 9, and 1, respectively. The tissues of obligate heterozygotes contain about 50% of the normal enzyme activity, whereas homozygotes exhibit absence or very little activity of enzymes. Immunoelectrophoretic analysis has shown that patients with transferase deficiency produce a protein similar to the normal, but with severely reduced or no enzyme activity. Sequence analysis of the cloned uridyltransferase gene reveals several mutations responsible for single amino acid substitutions. The most common is the replacement of an arginine for glutamine at amino acid 188 near the active site of the enzyme, which results in a protein with no catalytic activity. More than 70% of Caucasian patients are either homozygous or heterozygous for this mutation.

PREVALENCE. Uridyltransferase deficiency has a prevalence of 1 per 40,000 births and a carrier rate of about 1% in the United States population. A gene known as the Duarte variant is allelic to the normal transferase and codes for a protein that is electrophoretically different and enzymatically less active. The gene frequency of the Duarte variant is about 0.05%, and homozygotes for the Duarte variant have about 50% of normal transferase activity in their red blood cells (RBC's). With widespread neonatal screening, a number of babies have been detected with low red cell transferase activity who are compound heterozygotes with one gene for defective transferase and another for the Duarte variant. Such infants have only 10 to 25% of red cell enzyme activity but rarely have impaired galactose utilization that requires treatment.

Galactokinase deficiency is quite rare, having a prevalence of 1 in 500,000 to 1 in 1 million births. Epimerase deficiency is also rare. The benign type has mainly been described in Swiss and Japanese populations, whereas only a few cases of symptomatic epimerase deficiency have been detected.

PATHOGENESIS. Galactose is converted to glucose by a unique series of three enzyme reactions (Fig. 169–1). Normally this pathway functions efficiently. Galactose rapidly disappears from blood after intravenous infusion, even faster than a comparable amount of glucose. In normal individuals liver extraction of galactose results in a rise in the level of blood glucose.

In each of the three forms of galactosemia, diminished enzyme activity produces an accumulation of the substrates proximal to the metabolic block (Fig. 169–1). When galactose is increased, alternative pathways form large amounts of otherwise trace metabolites. In one reaction galactose is reduced to form the sugar alcohol galactitol, whereas in another galactose is oxidized to galactonic acid. These metabolites accumulate in tissues and are excreted in considerable amounts in the urine.

Identification of accumulated metabolites and the elucidation of alternative pathways have provided insights into the relationship of biochemical toxicity and clinical manifestations of the disorders. Cataract formation appears to be due to the galactitol formed by lens aldose reductase. Galactitol, which cannot be further metabolized, accumulates in the lens and produces osmotic changes with inhibition of fluid, lens swelling, and protein precipitation. The exact biochemical alterations in other target organs affected by transferase deficiency have not been defined. No specific structural alterations of the brain are associated with mental retardation in cases of transferase deficiency, although white matter changes have been seen on magnetic resonance imaging and cerebellar atrophy noted on computed tomography scans. Liver dysfunction may be accompanied by altered architecture of liver characterized by pseudoacinar formation of hepatic cells.

There are several possibilities for the pathogenesis of the long-term complications of mental retardation, speech abnormalities, ataxia, and hypogonadism in women affected with transferase-deficient galactosemia despite strictly eliminating galactose from the diet. (1) There is *in utero* damage. Elevated levels of galactitol are

TABLE 169–1. GALACTOSEMIA ENZYME DEFICIENCIES

Enzyme Defect	Accumulated Metabolite(s)	Effects
Galactokinase	Galactose	Cataracts early in life; no multiple organ involvement
Galactose-1-P uridyltransferase	Galactose Galactose-1-P	Syndrome of nutritional failure, liver disease, abnormal renal tubule function, cataracts, mental retardation, ovarian abnormalities
Uridine diphosphate-4-epimerase	Galactose Galactose-1-P UDP galactose	Resembles transferase deficiency, but may occur in a benign form

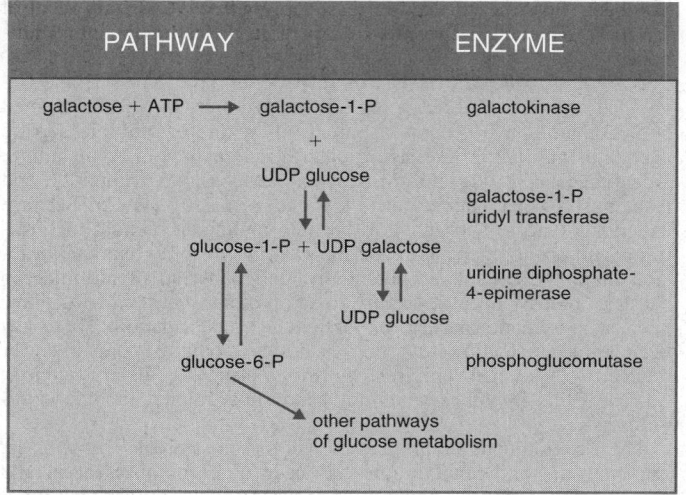

FIGURE 169-1. Normal enzymatic pathway that converts galactose to glucose.

found in affected fetuses and galactose-1-P is increased in cord RBC's. Indeed, cataractous change can be found in the embryonal and fetal lens, and the ovaries of females with hypergonadotropic gonadism may be small, fibrotic, or streaked, consistent with a developmental abnormality. (2) There is continuous self-intoxication, a concept based on the constantly elevated red cell galactose-1-P and urinary galactitol in patients on galactose-restricted diets. This could occur from galactose liberated by the turnover of complex carbohydrates or from galactose-1-P resulting from pyrophosphorylatic cleavage of UDP galactose derived from UDP glucose. (3) There may be depletion of essential metabolites. Tissue inositol levels are low in the galactose toxic state and a decrease in red cell UDP galactose levels has been reported in some patients. (4) There may be hidden sources of galactose in the diet even when extreme care has been taken to eliminate known sources. Tomatoes and watermelon are now known to be rich in free galactose.

CLINICAL MANIFESTATIONS. Cataracts are the principal finding in patients with galactokinase deficiency, who otherwise are healthy. The cataracts are usually discovered in infants and children examined for other medical reasons. Pseudotumor cerebri has been described in some galactokinase-deficient patients as well as those with transferase deficiency. Cataracts have been observed in some heterozygous carriers, and patients younger than 40 with cataracts frequently have lower than normal red cell galactokinase levels.

Uridyltransferase deficiency usually manifests itself shortly after birth or within the first few weeks of life with growth failure, vomiting, diarrhea, hepatomegaly, ascites, jaundice, hemolytic anemia, hypoglycemia, proteinuria, and a renal Fanconi's syndrome. Cataracts may not be easily observed with an ophthalmoscope in young infants but are found on slit-lamp examination. Infants with this disease may die in the first few days of life from overwhelming *Escherichia coli* sepsis before other manifestations are evident. Without eliminating galactose from the diet, severely affected infants die of inanition and liver failure. Occasionally, because of vomiting, the infant's formula is changed to one that is galactose-free, with subsequent cessation of the toxicity syndrome. Later in childhood these patients with undetectable red cell transferase activity have severe mental retardation and cataracts after milk is reintroduced into the diet.

Black patients with transferase deficiency may have a milder toxicity syndrome and in some cases have no symptoms. This has been called the Negro variant. Such patients have been found to metabolize some galactose because of the presence of 10% of normal transferase activity in liver and intestinal mucosa. A toxicity syndrome resembling transferase deficiency can occur in some cases of epimerase deficiency.

DIAGNOSIS. Suspect galactokinase deficiency in any infant or child with cataracts, and confirm the diagnosis by assaying RBC or cultured fibroblast galactokinase. A presumptive diagnosis is possible by detecting reducing sugar in urine that is glucose oxidase negative (galactose) or by chromatographic analysis for galactitol in the urine. These urinary findings also obtain in transferase deficiency, whose definitive diagnosis requires assaying RBC transferase activity. Because severely affected babies may be given blood transfusions before a diagnosis of galactosemia is considered, red cell transferase assay should be delayed until transfused blood has been replaced by the infant's own cells. However, an assay of transferase of parents' red cells with 50% of normal activity found in both may be helpful in making presumptive diagnosis in such infants or in those who may have died before specimens for assay were obtained.

Besides the quantitative assay of RBC transferase, starch gel electrophoresis or isoelectric focusing to determine isoenzyme banding may be useful in distinguishing the carrier for classic galactosemia, the homozygous Duarte variant whose RBC enzyme activity is comparable to that of carriers for the classic disease, and mixed Duarte-classic galactosemia carriers who have 10 to 25% of normal activity.

In the differential diagnosis, hereditary fructose intolerance with hepatomegaly, liver dysfunction, hypoglycemia, renal Fanconi's syndrome, and nonglucose reducing substance in the urine should be considered. Lactosuria, a common finding in a variety of gastrointestinal disorders, also causes a positive test result for reducing substance. However, many laboratories use glucose oxidase–based tests for determining blood and urinary sugar, and in such instances, galactosemia and galactosuria would go undetected. The greatest confusion in differential diagnosis is the distinction between transferase deficiency and primary liver disease. Because the liver is the major organ metabolizing galactose, any disruption of hepatocellular function may result in galactosemia and galactosuria. Red cell transferase assay should make the distinction. Patients with clinical findings resembling classic transferase deficiency galactosemia who have normal red cell transferase activity should also be tested for red cell epimerase activity.

Many cases are currently diagnosed as a result of neonatal screening. More than 40 U.S. states and several foreign countries test all newborns by analyzing heel-stick blood spots on filter paper. All positive test results require confirmation by quantitative assay of the individual enzymes and isoelectric focusing analysis. Such screening has resulted in delineation of the benign form of epimerase deficiency in which galactose-1-phosphate appears to accumulate only in RBC's. Subsequent studies have indicated that the epimerase in such cases is unstable because of increased requirement for cofactor NAD, which can be supplied by other cells but not by RBC's.

TREATMENT. A galactose-free diet is the cornerstone of treatment. Eliminating galactose early in classic galactosemia may cause cataracts to regress, liver dysfunction and renal tubule abnormalities to disappear, and early growth and development to be normal. Besides banning milk and all milk products, care should be taken to eliminate foods in which milk is used in cooking and baking or lactose has been added. Attention should be paid to fruits and vegetables (watermelon and tomatoes). There is no indication that the ability to metabolize galactose increases with age, so dietary restrictions should not be relaxed in older children. Despite cessation of postnatal galactose toxicity with an early-instituted lactose-free diet, there are later manifestations of slow mental development, speech abnormalities called verbal dyspraxia, ataxia, and ovarian failure with hypogonadotropic hypogonadism in affected females.

PROGNOSIS. Dietary galactose restriction does not ensure a normal outcome. Despite excellent treatment from birth, many patients with transferase deficiency have below-average mental development with learning defects, diminished attention span, and visual perceptual difficulties. More than 60% have speech abnormalities and 80% of affected females have hypergonadotropic hypogonadism. The outcome does not differ in patients without neonatal symptoms treated at birth from those recognized within the first several weeks of life on the basis of the acute galactose toxicity syndrome due to ingesting galactose-containing feeds. Untreated infants, however, may not survive. Older patients may develop an ataxic neurologic syndrome while on galactose-restricted diets.

PREVENTION. Prenatal diagnosis can be performed by assaying transferase of a chorionic villus biopsy or cultured amniotic cells or by determining galactitol in amniotic fluid. Galactose restriction during pregnancy in which the fetus is at risk has not altered the prognosis.

Elsas LJ, Fridovich-Kiel JL, Leslie N: Galactosemia: A molecular approach to the enigma. Int Pediatr 8:101, 1993. *Presents the structure of the human uridyltransferase gene and the frequency of mutations, demonstrating the high incidence of the arginine substitution for glutamine at position 188 (Q188R) in the amino acid sequence.*

Segal S, Berry G: Disorders of galactose metabolism. *In* Scriver CH, Beaudet AL, Sly WS, et al. (eds.): The Metabolic and Molecular Bases of Inherited Disease. 7th ed, New York, McGraw-Hill, 1995. *A monograph and molecular bases on all aspects of galactose metabolism, galactosemia, and the pathophysiology of galactose intoxication.*

170 GLYCOGEN STORAGE DISEASES

Harry L. Greene

Glycogen is the storage form of glucose and is present in varying amounts in virtually all cells, although the liver is the primary organ for storage and subsequent release of glucose into the circulation. Glycogen is synthesized from glucose and glucose hydrolized and released from glycogen; this highly regulated process helps maintain normal blood glucose concentrations during fasting. At least eight enzymes involved in glycogen synthesis and the hydrolysis to glucose are utilized in this control.

Glycogen storage diseases are characterized by an abnormal tissue concentration (> 70 mg per gram of liver or > 15 mg per gram of muscle) and/or an abnormal structure of the glycogen molecule. During the past 40 years, patients who have deficient activity in virtually every enzyme important in the normal synthesis or degradation of glycogen have been identified. With the exception of phosphorylase kinase deficiency, all are inherited in an autosomal recessive manner. Although the enzyme deficiency may vary among patients, the clinical expression of the disease can usually be traced to either the liver or the muscle.

HEPATIC FORMS OF GLYCOGENESIS

The various hepatic enzymatic deficiencies are expressed primarily as hypoglycemia and hepatomegaly, and three defects (branching enzyme, glycogen synthetase, and debranching enzyme) result in the accumulation of abnormally structured glycogen and may cause progressive hepatic cirrhosis and associated splenomegaly. Conversely, the accumulation of normally structured glycogen, as seen with deficiency of phosphorylase, phosphorylase b kinase, acid alpha-glucosidase, or glucose-6-phosphatase, is usually not associated with hepatic fibrosis and splenomegaly. Figure 170–1 summarizes the general location of enzymatic defects resulting in the hepatic forms of glycogenesis. With the exception of lysosomal acid glucosidase deficiency, hypoglycemia is a common presenting feature. Clinical and biochemical expressions of the various types of glycogen storage diseases are summarized in Table 170–1, and the more commonly diagnosed types are discussed below.

GLUCOSE-6-PHOSPHATASE DEFICIENCY (TYPE I GLYCOGEN STORAGE DISEASE). This disorder has been subcategorized into types a, b, or c, with type a the most common; but all types have similar clinical features. As noted in Figure 170–1, all other enzymatic defects directly affect the formation or degradation of glycogen, with the exception of glucose-6-phosphatase. Similarly, the clinical expression of this defect is distinctly different from that of the other forms of glycogenosis. For example, fasting-induced hypoglycemia may be extreme, and lactic acidosis, hyperlipidemia, and hyperuricemia may be unique to patients with type I. The mechanism for the striking abnormalities in lipid and purine metabolism as well as carbohydrate metabolism results primarily from overproduction of substrate in response to a decline in blood glucose, as indicated in Figure 170–1. The documented reversal of these abnormalities by treatment that maintains the blood glucose level between 80 and 90 mg per deciliter supports the postulate that these changes are the result of hormonal responses to the hypoglycemia. Therapeutic intervention has been evaluated more extensively in patients with this defect than any other. As a result, it

has been possible to devise reasonably effective dietary control for these patients that results in favorable development into adulthood.

Late Complications. As more patients have survived and developed into active, functioning adults, two subsequent, unexpected complications have become apparent: (1) single or multiple hepatic adenomas and (2) progressive glomerulosclerosis with renal failure. Adenomas usually develop in patients between ages 16 and 22, and it is unusual for a patient not to have adenomas by age 25. Because adenomas tend to subsequently become malignant, annual monitoring by ultrasonography is recommended. Any rapidly expanding lesion should be considered potentially malignant and should undergo surgical biopsy because serum α-fetoprotein measurements have been an unreliable marker for malignant transformation. There has been some indication that the adenomas could be prevented or reduced in younger children by more stringent dietary control; however, this hypothesis has not been substantiated in older individuals.

The development of progressive glomerulosclerosis, proteinuria, hypertension, and renal failure has been a recent observation and usually occurs in older patients (> 18 years) who are less well managed and exhibit recurrent hypoglycemic episodes, chronic hypertriglyceridemia, and lactic acidosis. The mechanism causing the renal lesion is not defined, although some improvement in proteinuria has been seen following treatment with angiotensin-converting enzyme inhibitors.

DEBRANCHING ENZYME DEFICIENCY (TYPE III GLYCOGEN STORAGE DISEASE). This disease most often affects only the liver but may affect muscle as well. When muscles are involved, the serum creatine phosphokinase (CPK) level is elevated, and patients are usually classified as having type IIIb disease. Some patients may not show elevated CPK levels during early life, and so evaluation during later childhood or adolescence should be performed. Hypoglycemia with fasting is less severe (usually 40 to 50 mg per deciliter) than in patients with type I, although hepatic enlargement may be substantially greater. Serum aspartate aminotransferase (AST) and alanine aminotransaminase (ALT) concentrations are commonly above 500 units per milliliter. Correspondingly, hepatic fibrosis of varying degrees is usually present during childhood and may be progressive. At least two adult patients (ages 43 and 55) presenting with "cryptogenic cirrhosis" and bleeding esophageal varices have been diagnosed as having debrancher enzyme deficiency.

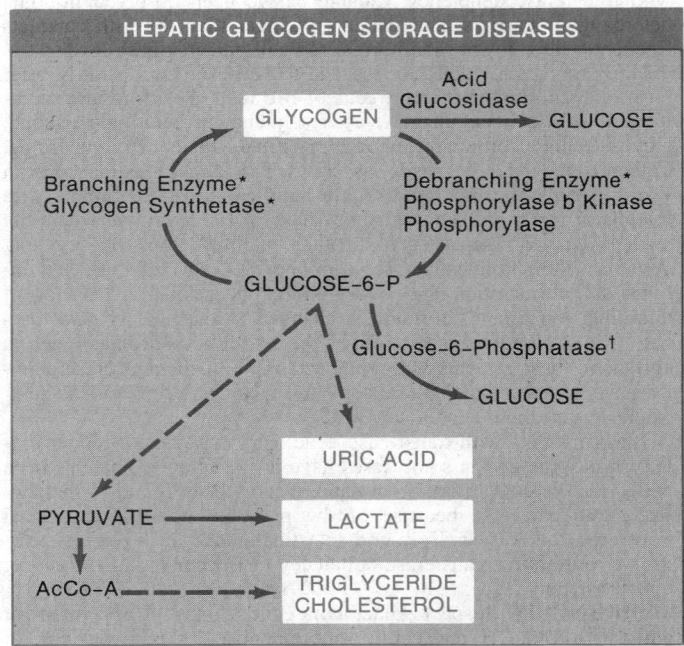

FIGURE 170–1. Mechanism for abnormalities in lipid, purine, and carbohydrate metabolism in type I (glucose-6-phosphatase deficiency) glycogen storage disease. * = associated with hepatic cirrhosis. † = associated with elevated serum uric acid, lactate, and lipid levels and with hepatic adenoma.

TABLE 170–1. CLASSIFICATION OF GLYCOGEN STORAGE DISEASES

Type	Enzyme Affected	Primary Organ Involved	Manifestations
O	Glycogen synthetase	Liver	Hypoglycemia, hyperketonia, FFT, early death
Ia	Glucose-6-phosphatase	Liver	Enlarged liver and kidney growth failure, fasting hypoglycemia, acidosis, thrombocyte dysfunction
Ib	Microsomal membrane G-6-P translocase	Liver	As in Ia; in addition, recurrent neutropenia, bacterial infections
Ic	Microsomal membrane P-transporter	Liver	As in Ia
II	Lysosomal acid glucosidase	Skeletal and cardiac muscle	*Infantile form:* early-onset, progressive muscle hypotonia, cardiac failure, death before 2 years *Juvenile form:* late-onset myopathy and variable cardiac involvement *Adult form:* limb-girdle muscular dystrophy-like feature
III	Amylo-1,6-glucosidase (debrancher enzyme)	Liver, skeletal muscle, heart	Fasting hypoglycemia, hepatomegaly in infancy; some have myopathic features, rarely clinical cardiac features
IV	Amylo-1,4-1,6-transglucosidase (brancher enzyme)	Liver, muscle	Hepatosplenomegaly, cirrhosis; may have late-onset myopathy
V	Muscle phosphorylase	Skeletal muscle	Exercise-induced muscular pain, cramps, and progressive weakness, sometimes with myoglobinuria; symptoms usually begin during adolescence or early adulthood
VI	Liver phosphorylase	Liver	Hepatomegaly, mild hypoglycemia, good prognosis
VII	Phosphofructokinase	Muscle, red blood cells	As in V; in addition, mild hemolytic anemia
Formerly VIb, VIII, or IX	Phosphorylase b kinase	Liver, leukocytes, (?) muscle	As in VI; X-linked inheritance
X	Cyclic AMP-dependent kinase	Liver, muscle	Hepatomegaly, mild hypoglycemia

Treating these patients has not been advocated because the natural course of the disease has been thought to be benign. However, because growth retardation and cirrhosis may be serious complications, several patients have been treated with frequent feedings and raw cornstarch to maintain blood glucose levels between 75 and 100 mg per deciliter. Treated patients often show a significant reduction in serum transaminase levels and improvements in growth, and they may demonstrate improved muscle strength, although serum CPK activities remain elevated.

Clinical and laboratory features of the other, more unusual forms of hepatic glycogenesis are presented in Table 170–1.

MUSCULAR FORMS OF GLYCOGEN STORAGE

ACID ALPHA-GLUCOSIDASE DEFICIENCY (POMPE'S DISEASE, TYPE II GLYCOGEN STORAGE DISEASE). In this condition, virtually all tissues have an increased glycogen content. However, presenting clinical manifestations of the illness are cardiac enlargement, myocardial failure, and generalized muscle hypotonia without muscle wasting. The classic infantile form manifests during the first months of life, and few survive past the first year. The juvenile variant presents in later infancy or early childhood and progresses more slowly, with death in the second or third decade. The adult type manifests as a slowly developing adult-onset myopathy. In each case, the diagnosis is dependent on finding deficient activity of acid α-1, 4-glucosidase in muscle specimens or cultured fibroblasts. No treatment, including bone marrow transplantation and systemic enzyme infusion, has proved to be of long-term benefit to these patients.

MYOPHOSPHORYLASE DEFICIENCY (TYPE V GLYCOGEN STORAGE DISEASE, McARDLE'S DISEASE). Most of these patients are asymptomatic during early childhood and escape diagnosis until the second or third decade of life. A history of muscle pain and cramps after exercise, signs of myoglobinuria, and painful cramping on an ischemic exercise test are characteristic. The diagnosis is suggested by an elevation in serum muscle CPK isoenzyme activity and by failure to elevate the serum lactate level with exercise. The diagnosis is established by documenting elevated muscle glycogen in the sarcolemmal regions and reduced muscle phosphorylase activity. Glucose or fructose ingestion prior to exercise is said to reduce the symptoms.

MUSCLE PHOSPHOFRUCTOKINASE DEFICIENCY (MUSCLE PHOSPHOGLYCERATE MUTASE DEFICIENCY, LACTATE DEHYDROGENASE [LDH-M] SUBUNIT DEFICIENCY, TYPE VII GLYCOGEN STORAGE DISEASE). These muscle glycogenoses are rare and clinically similar to myophosphorylase deficiency. Patients with phosphofructokinase deficiency may also show a mild hemolytic anemia. Diagnosis depends on muscle enzyme analysis. Treatment is aimed at avoiding strenuous exercise.

DIAGNOSIS AND PRENATAL DIAGNOSIS OF GLYCOGEN STORAGE DISEASE

Diagnostic enzyme analysis on hepatic or muscle tissue for most types of glycogen storage diseases is currently funded at Duke Medical Center, Division of Genetics. Prenatal diagnosis of three types of glycogen storage diseases (types II, III, and IV) is also possible and is performed on cultured amniotic cells in this laboratory.

Chen YT, Cornblath M, Sidbury JB: Cornstarch therapy in type I glycogen storage disease. N Engl J Med 310:171, 1984. *The usefulness of dietary raw cornstarch to maintain blood glucose concentrations is demonstrated.*

Ding JH, deBarsy T, Brown B, et al.: Immunoblot analyses of glycogen debranching enzyme in different subtypes of glycogen storage disease type III. J Pediatr 116:95, 1990. *Provides newer insights into the molecular basis of type III glycogenoses.*

Ghishan FK, Greene HL: Inborn errors of metabolism that lead to permanent liver injury. *In* Zakim D, Boyer TD (eds.): Hepatology: A Textbook of Liver Disease. 2nd ed. Philadelphia, WB Saunders, 1990. *An extensively referenced review that focuses on the altered metabolism, treatment, and outcome of the hepatic forms of glycogenesis.*

Hers HG, Van Hoof F, deBarsy T: The glycogen storage diseases. *In* Scriver CR, Brandet AL, Sly WS, Valle D (eds.): The Metabolic Basis of Inherited Disease, 6th ed. New York, McGraw-Hill, 1989. *This extensively referenced article provides information on the clinical and biochemical aspects of the glycogen storage diseases.*

Parker PH, Ballew M, Greene HL: Nutritional management of glycogen storage disease. Annu Rev Nutr 13:83, 1993. *Combines the biochemical abnormalities of the glycogenoses and associated research findings with a practical guide to dietary management of children and adults.*

171 FRUCTOSE INTOLERANCE

Harry L. Greene

Fructose, a normal dietary constituent of fruits, vegetables, honey, and the disaccharide sucrose (table sugar), is present at a level of 50 to 100 grams per day in the average Western diet. At this level of intake, it is rapidly absorbed in the proximal small intestine by a specific transport mechanism and is extracted on the first pass from the portal vein. Because fructose malabsorption has been described in some individuals, the relative tolerance of dietary fructose in normal children was evaluated by feeding 31 children 2 grams of fructose per kilogram of body weight. Four children developed gastrointestinal symptoms and 71% developed abnormal breath hydrogen excretion, suggesting that a significant increase in dietary fructose can result in malabsorption in some individuals.

Initial metabolism of fructose primarily involves three enzymes: fructokinase, aldolase B, and triokinase (Fig. 171–1), although hexokinase phosphorylates some of the fructose. Five enzymatic defects involving fructose metabolism have been identified: (1) fructokinase deficiency, (2) aldolase A deficiency, (3) aldolase B deficiency, (4) fructose-1, 6-diphosphatase deficiency, and (5) D-glycerate kinase deficiency. The enzymatic defects in fructose metabolism are illustrated in Figure 171–1, and each of the defects is discussed below.

FRUCTOKINASE DEFICIENCY (Essential Fructosuria)

Fructokinase deficiency is a rare (about 1 in 130,000 births), asymptomatic, autosomal-recessive condition caused by deficient activity of fructokinase, the first enzyme in fructose utilization. Because no pathologic condition results from this defect, the primary concern relates to the fact that fructose is a reducing sugar. Thus, a positive reaction with urinary Clinitest tablets may result in the erroneous suggestion of diabetes unless glucose oxidase is determined with a dipstick. The precise nature of the enzymatic defect is not known because the gene for fructokinase has not yet been identified.

ALDOLASE DEFICIENCY

Three aldolases (A, B, and C) are responsible for the conversion of fructose-1, 6-diphosphate into glyceraldehyde-3-phosphate and dihydroxyacetone phosphase. Embryonic tissue produces aldolase A; adult liver, kidney, and intestine expresses aldolase B; and nervous tissue expresses aldolase C. Although all three aldolases are tetramers of identical 40-kDa subunits, each is coded for different genes on different chromosomes: aldolase A on chromosome 16,16q22-q24, aldolase B on chromosome 9,9q13-q32, and aldolase C on chromosome 17,17 cen-q 21.

ALDOLASE A DEFICIENCY. Aldolase A deficiency may be detrimental because of its pivotal role in glycolysis. This is apparently of special relevance to the developing embryo, which ex-

presses only aldolase A. Only a few patients with this deficit have been described, and not all symptoms are expressed to the same degree. Potential symptoms include mental retardation, short stature, hemolytic anemia, and abnormal facial appearance. Because aldolase B becomes normal at birth, patients do not show fructosuria; thus, restricting dietary fructose is of no benefit.

ALDOLASE B DEFICIENCY (HEREDITARY FRUCTOSE INTOLERANCE, HFI). Aldolase B deficiency (prevalence about 1 in 20,000 births) is a potentially life-threatening autosomal-recessive disorder than can be effectively treated by eliminating dietary fructose. This disorder is due to deficiency of fructose-1-phosphate aldolase (aldolase B). Aldolase B is normally present in large amounts in the liver, intestine, and renal cortex; thus, excessive fructose intake by patients with HFI adversely affects each of these organs.

Symptoms do not become manifested until the patient ingests fructose or fructose-containing foods. Because lactose is the carbohydrate source in mammalian milk, infants do not develop symptoms until the introduction of dietary fruits or other fructose-containing foods or medication, i.e., fruits, fruit juices, medicinal syrups, sucrose-containing infant formulas, and so forth. The primary presentation is vomiting and other features hypoglycemia within 20 to 30 minutes after fructose ingestion. These acute manifestations may not be apparent following lower chronic intakes, for example with fructose-containing infant formulas. In these instances, failure to thrive, hepatomegaly, and cirrhosis may represent the dominant presenting features. Concomitant laboratory findings include an acute decrease in serum glucose and phosphate concentrations and an elevated uric acid concentration. With continued exposure to fructose, hyperbilirubinemia, lactic acidosis, hepatosplenomegaly, and liver failure develop in conjunction with renal tubular dysfunction (bicarbonaturia, aminoaciduria, phosphaturia). At this stage, liver biopsy shows fatty infiltration of hepatocytes with cellular necrosis and mild bile duct proliferation with fibrosis. If exposure to fructose continues, progressive fibrosis, cirrhosis, and death from liver failure follow. The brain may also show diminished neurons.

The diagnosis is suggested by the presence of urinary reducing sugar detectable by Clinitest tablets and not by urinary dipstick,

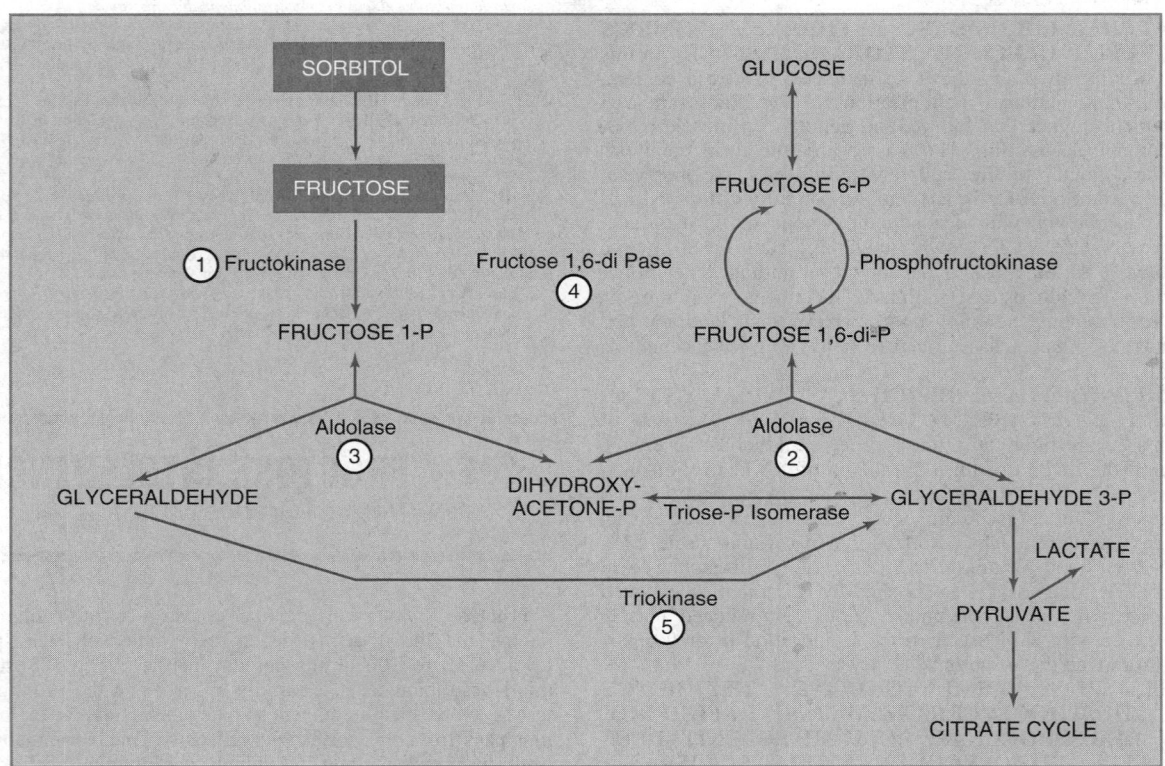

FIGURE 171–1. The major pathway for fructose metabolism in the liver, showing the five defects discussed in the text. Aldolase deficiency consists primarily of defects in aldolase B(③). Aldolase A deficiency(②) is extremely rare and is expressed primarily during embryogenesis.

which measures glucose oxidase. Because similar clinical features may be present with galactosemia or tyrosinemia, diagnosis can be confirmed by measuring fructose-1-phosphate aldolase activity in liver or intestinal biopsy specimens. An intravenous fructose tolerance test (0.2 to 0.3 gram per kilogram in adults or 3 grams per square meter in children) after restriction of dietary fructose for several weeks has been used to confirm the illness, but this procedure may cause hypoglycemia. Patients should be monitored closely to prevent complications during fructose tolerance tests. Fructose loading cannot detect heterozygotes; for this purpose, ^{31}P magnetic resonance spectroscopy applied to fructose metabolism is necessary.

Five mutations have been identified in the aldolase B gene: two large deletions of 1.65 and 1.4 kb and three small deletions of 7 and 4 bp. In addition, six point mutations have been identified: (1) a single $G \rightarrow C$ mutation changing alanine to proline at position 149 of the protein subunit; (2) a change of alanine to aspartate at position 174; (3) a change of asparagine to lysine at position 334; (4) a change of alanine to valine at position 337; (5) a stop codon at position 288, the consequence of a deletion of cytosine of the leucine codon; and (6) a stop codon at position 297, shortening the carboxy terminus by 67 residues.

In spite of recurrent bouts of hypoglycemia and substantial liver disease, restriction of dietary fructose usually results in almost complete recovery during a 3- to 5-week period, and affected adults have normal intelligence. Older children and adults are protected from large dietary intakes of fructose by an aversion to sweets, although small amounts taken chronically may result in isolated, often reversible, somatic growth retardation.

FRUCTOSE-1, 6-DIPHOSPHATASE (FDPase) DEFICIENCY

This rare disorder was first described in 1970. Patients usually present before age 6 months with fasting-induced lactic acidosis, hypoglycemia, and hepatomegaly. The reaction to glycerol is similar to that from fructose ingestion but is less severe than that of patients with HFI. The condition is due to a defect of hepatic fructose-1, 6-diphosphatase, a gluconeogenic enzyme (Fig. 171–1). Thus, when hepatic glycogen stores are depleted, fasting hypoglycemia develops. During fasting, urinary organic acids are similar to those of tyrosinemia type I but with an absence of succinyl acetate. In addition, starvation leads to increased excretion of glycerol.

The human gene for FDPase has not been isolated, so prenatal diagnosis is unlikely. The enzyme is a tetramer for identical 36 kD. The diagnosis is suspected when, after about 12 to 16 hours of fasting, the blood sugar concentration falls and is not restored when glucagon is administered, and acidosis (lactate) is present. Loading tests with fructose or glycerol may be dangerous because they lead to hypoglycemia and lactic acidosis. Diagnosis is confirmed by measuring the enzyme in hepatic biopsy material. Treatment consists of avoiding fasting and restricting dietary fructose and glycerol.

D-GLYCERATE KINASE DEFICIENCY (D-GLYCERIC ACIDURIA)

This is a rare (10 patients described), clinically variable disorder resulting in either no symptoms, metabolic acidosis and failure to thrive, or profound psychomotor retardation and seizures. The variable phenotypic expression has not been fully explained on the basis of the enzymatic defect, but all patients who show a substantial increase in D-glycerate excretion after fructose ingestion should avoid dietary fructose.

Baker L, Winegrad AI: Fasting hypoglycemia and metabolic acidosis associated with deficiency of hepatic fructose-1, 6-diphosphatase activity. Lancet 2:13, 1970. *The first description of a patient with deficient fructose-1, 6-diphosphatase activity.*

Ghishan FK, Greene HL: Inborn errors of metabolism that lead to permanent liver injury. *In* Zakim D, Boyer TD (eds.): Hepatology: A Textbook of Liver Disease. 2nd ed. Philadelphia, WB Saunders, 1990. *An extensively referenced review that focuses on the altered metabolism, treatment, and outcome of fructose intolerance.*

Hommes FA: Inborn errors of fructose metabolism. Am J Clin Nutr 58(Suppl):788, 1993. *A recent correlation between the genotype and phenotype of the five various defects in fructose metabolism.*

Odievre M, Gentil C, Gautier M, et al.: Hereditary fructose intolerance in childhood. Am J Dis Child 132:605, 1978. *This article is an excellent presentation of the clinical, hepatic, and biochemical changes that can be expected in children with HFI.*

Schulte MJ, Lenz W: Fatal sorbitol infusion in a patient with fructose-sorbitol intolerance. Lancet 2:188, 1977. *This paper illustrates the need to restrict sorbitol as well as fructose in patients with HFI.*

172 PRIMARY HYPEROXALURIA
Richard E. Hillman

Primary hyperoxaluria refers to two different peroxisomal enzyme deficiencies that are characterized by massive synthesis and urinary excretion of oxalic acid. Oxalate is also deposited in the heart, the eye, the skin, and other organs, leading to a variety of clinical pictures. Particularly in type I disease, the clinical manifestations present early in childhood with nephrolithiasis or nephrocalinosis and lead to renal failure within the first decade of life. However, the ready availability of oxalate assays in the last few years has led to the description of milder cases, mostly type II, which are either asymptomatic or present only with water deprivation. Both types are inherited as autosomal recessive traits and must be distinguished from secondary hyperoxalurias due to increased absorption of oxalate by the gut. These secondary causes include inflammatory bowel disease and fat malabsorption, which may tie up calcium and convert insoluble calcium oxalate to more absorbable salts. Although most adult patients with calcium oxalate nephrolithiasis excrete normal amounts of oxalate, it is now clear that hyperoxaluria must be considered in the differential diagnosis.

Primary hyperoxaluria type I (glycolic aciduria) is caused by a defect in the peroxisomal enzyme alanine:glyoxylate aminotransferase. This enzyme normally converts glycolic acid to the amino acid glycine. In its absence, glycolic acid leaves the peroxisome and is converted to oxalic acid by lactic dehydrogenase (LDH). Both glycolic and oxalic acids are excreted in large amounts, usually > 60 mg per 1.73 meters^2 per 24 hours. In most cases, this concentration exceeds the solubility of oxalic acid. This enzyme has been cloned, and multiple defects have been demonstrated.

Primary hyperoxaluria type II (glyceric aciduria) is due to one of two defects. Until recently it was believed that the defect lay in the enzyme D-glyceric dehydrogenase. This enzyme leads to the accumulation of hydroxypyruvic acid, which is reduced in the cytoplasm to L-glyceric acid. It had been unclear why this defect caused hyperoxaluria. Recently, it was suggested that this enzyme may be the same as glyoxalate reductase, which leads to accumulation of glyoxalate and production of oxalate by LDH. Type II is a much milder disease in most cases than type I. Asymptomatic cases or cases with only a single attack of oxaluria have been reported. Two recent cases only became symptomatic following severe water deprivation, one while sailing, one while running in hot weather.

Some patients with type I disease respond to large doses of pyridoxine (20 to 200 mg per day). This vitamin is the cofactor for the enzyme. It appears to act by stabilizing the remaining activity and is effective only in patients with some enzyme, in general the milder cases. Dilute urine should be maintained by high fluid intake, and some reports suggest that diuretics may help. Attempts to form more soluble salts of oxalate, particularly with magnesium, have met with some success. The only "cure" for this disease has been a combined renal and liver transplant. Renal transplants alone have failed due to the accumulation of oxalate from other organs. Type II patients are very variable. Pyridoxine has no effect. Other measures that maintain a dilute urine seem to be enough in the milder cases.

Danpure CJ, Purdue PE, Fryer P, et al.: Enzymological and mutational analysis of a complex primary hyperoxaluria type I phenotype. Am J Hum Genet 53:417, 1993. *The latest data on type I enzyme deficiencies, including variability.*

Hillman RE: Primary hyperoxalurias. *In* Scriver CR, Beaudet AL, Sly WS, et al. (eds.): The Metabolic Basis of Inherited Disease. 6th ed. New York, McGraw-Hill, 1989, p 933. *A general review of the biochemistry of primary oxalosis and related secondary disorders.*

Seageant LE, de Groot GW, Dilling LA, et al.: Primary oxaluria type 2 (L-glyceric aciduria): A rare cause of nephrolithiasis in children. J Pediatr 118:912, 1991. *A review of clinical information on type II disease.*

Disorders of Lipid Metabolism

173 THE HYPERLIPOPROTEINEMIAS
Joseph L. Witztum and Daniel Steinberg

Hyperlipidemia, abnormal elevation of plasma cholesterol and/or triglyceride levels, is one of the most common clinical problems that confront the physician in daily practice. Much attention has been focused on these disorders because there is a strong association of hyperlipidemia—especially hypercholesterolemia—with development of atherosclerosis, and of hypertriglyceridemia with pancreatitis. Hyperlipidemia may occur because of a primary genetic disorder or as a result of environmental influences secondary to other medical conditions, or any combination of these factors. Because lipids are transported in plasma as components of lipoprotein complexes, understanding lipoprotein physiology is necessary for informed diagnosis and therapeutic planning.

PHYSIOLOGY OF LIPOPROTEIN TRANSPORT

Lipoproteins are complex macromolecules that transport nonpolar lipids through the aqueous environment of plasma. The more nonpolar lipids—triglycerides and cholesteryl esters—are carried almost exclusively in the central core of the spherical lipoprotein particles. The more polar lipids (such as phospholipids and free cholesterol), together with amphipathic apolipoproteins, form a surface monolayer that serves to "solubilize" the particles and allows them to remain in stable solution in the aqueous plasma.

Each lipoprotein particle contains on its surface one or more apolipoproteins that have a variety of functional and structural roles. Some apolipoproteins provide structural stability to the lipoprotein, serve as ligands for cellular lipoprotein receptors that help determine the metabolic fate of individual particles and act as cofactors for plasma enzymes involved in plasma lipid and lipoprotein metabolism. Other apolipoproteins play several roles, e.g., apolipoprotein B (apo B) is the major structural apolipoprotein of the triglyceride-rich lipoproteins secreted by the liver (very low-density lipoproteins [VLDL]), but it also serves as the ligand for binding of low-density lipoproteins (LDL) (formed from VLDL) to cellular LDL receptors. Table 173–1 lists major apoproteins,

lipoproteins on which they reside, and known or postulated functions.

The most widely used classification of lipoproteins is based on their different densities, which determine their behavior during preparative equilibrium ultracentrifugation. The fact that lipoprotein particles exist as relatively discrete species when separated this way led to the currently used density classification system outlined in Table 173–2. A second classification system originally proposed many years ago assigns priority to the apoprotein content of the lipoproteins. For example, in the high-density lipoprotein (HDL) density class there are lipoprotein particles that contain mainly apo A-I and others that contain both apo A-I and apo A-II; these are designated LpA-I and LpA-I, A-II, respectively. Current research suggests that it is primarily LpA-I that confers the antiatherogenic properties of HDL. Thus, in the future, full evaluation may include this type of analysis, but for now more research is needed to determine its clinical value.

An older classification system of the lipoproteins, based on their electrophoretic patterns (lipoprotein pattern typing), while important historically for the development of our understanding of lipid transport disorders, is not used commonly today. However, for the sake of completeness, the electrophoretic mobility of each lipoprotein class is also given in Table 173–1.

SYNTHESIS AND TRANSPORT OF ENDOGENOUS LIPIDS. The endogenous lipid transport system can be divided into two major classes: the apo B-100 lipoprotein system (VLDL, IDL [intermediate-density lipoprotein], and LDL) and the apo A-I lipoprotein system (HDL).

Metabolism of Very Low-Density Lipoproteins (VLDL). Between meals, free fatty acids are mobilized from the adipose tissue and serve as a major source for hepatic triglyceride synthesis. Lipogenesis, the synthesis of fatty acids *de novo* from carbohydrate or protein, also can occur in the liver. Fatty acids can either enter mitochondria (where beta oxidation occurs) or they can undergo esterification to form triglycerides in the cytosol. Control of triglyceride synthesis is a complex process that appears to be regulated in part by changes in insulin and glucagon that occur with feeding. Glucagon enhances fatty acid oxidation, whereas insulin prevents it. In addition, insulin may induce lipogenic enzymes in the liver. Triglycerides, together with cholesterol synthesized *de novo* in the liver or delivered to the liver by chylomicron remnants, are packaged together with apo B and phospholipids and form a nascent VLDL (Fig. 173–1). Plasma VLDL also contain other apolipoproteins, including the C apoproteins, and apo E. Apo B is found as a full-length protein termed apo B-100 (or apo B), which is made by the liver, or as a shortened form termed apo B-48, which is made in humans only by the intestine. Apo B is an obligatory component for nascent VLDL assembly and secretion from the hepatocyte; other apoproteins are added to VLDL after their entry into plasma. The size of the VLDL particle released depends on the availability of triglycerides in the liver. Very large triglyceride-rich VLDL are secreted when excess hepatic triglyceride synthesis is occurring, as in obesity, non–insulin dependent diabetes, and excess alcohol consumption. In contrast, small VLDL are secreted when availability of triglyceride, but not cholesterol, is decreased. Each VLDL particle contains one molecule of apo B, yet under ordinary circumstances the rate of apo B synthesis is not rate limiting for VLDL secretion. Although enhanced triglyceride synthesis can lead to enhanced triglyceride output, the *number* of VLDL particles released is not necessarily increased. Instead, *larger* individual VLDL particles containing more triglyceride are released. Understanding the processes regulating VLDL assembly and release by the hepatocytes is necessary to understand the etiology of clinically important disorders, such as familial combined hyperlipidemia (FCH) or hyperapobetalipoproteinemia, which are characterized by increased rates of secretion of VLDL particles from the liver. Other lipoprotein disorders (familial hypertriglyceridemia) are caused by hepatic secretion of a normal number of VLDL particles but ones that are enriched with triglycerides. The half-life of VLDL is about 1 hour or less.

TABLE 173–1. APOLIPOPROTEIN CHARACTERISTICS

Apoprotein	Lipoproteins	Function
Apo B-100	VLDL, IDL, LDL	Secretion of VLDL from liver. Structural protein of VLDL, IDL, and LDL. Ligand for the LDL receptor
Apo B-48	Chylomicrons, remnants	Secretion of chylomicrons from intestine
Apo E	Chylomicrons, VLDL, IDL, HDL	Ligand for binding of IDL and remnants to LDL receptor and LRP
Apo A-I	HDL, Chylomicrons	Structural protein of HDL Activator of LCAT
Apo A-II	HDL, Chylomicrons	Unknown
Apo C-II	Chylomicrons, VLDL, IDL, HDL	Activator of LPL
Apo C-III	Chylomicrons, VLDL, IDL, HDL	Inhibitor of LPL (*in vitro*)

TABLE 173-2. CHARACTERISTICS OF MAJOR LIPOPROTEIN CLASSES

Lipoprotein Class	Density (gm/ml)	Diameter (nm)	Major Lipid	Electrophoretic Mobility
Chylomicron and remnants	<< 1.006	5000–800	Dietary triglycerides	Remains at origin
VLDL	< 1.006	800–300	Endogenous triglycerides	Pre-β
IDL	1.006–1.019	350–250	Cholesteryl esters, triglycerides	Slow pre-β
LDL	1.019–1.063	250–180	Cholesteryl esters	β
HDL	1.063–1.210	50–120	Cholesteryl esters, phospholipids	α
Lp(a)	1.055–1.085	300	Cholesteryl esters	Slow pre-β

The primary function of lipoprotein particles is to transport lipids from one site to another. Triglyceride-rich lipoproteins serve to transport endogenously synthesized triglyceride to adipose tissue for storage in the fed state or to muscle for utilization in the fasting state. The enzyme that catalyzes peripheral triglyceride uptake is lipoprotein lipase (LPL). This enzyme is synthesized in adipose tissue and skeletal muscle cells, secreted, and transported across the capillary endothelial cell, where it binds to glycoproteins on the endothelial luminal surface. When VLDL bind to LPL, the LPL is activated by apo C-II present on the surface of the VLDL particle. This leads to triglyceride hydrolysis and release of fatty acids, which are then transported into the fat (or muscle) cell where they are re-esterified with glycerol and stored as intracellular triglyceride. The vast majority of triglyceride in adipose tissue is acquired by this mechanism because essentially no lipogenesis occurs *de novo* from glucose in human adipose tissue. The activity of LPL in adipose tissue is increased in the fed state, effectively providing for triglyceride storage. Insulin is required to maintain adequate LPL levels in adipose tissue. It appears to do so by maintaining synthesis and release, but it does not acutely affect changes in LPL levels. This is in contrast to "hormone-sensitive lipase" (HSL), an enzyme that hydrolyzes intracellular triglycerides, releasing fatty acids to plasma for uptake by the liver. HSL is acutely inhibited by insulin, while glucagon increases its activity. Thus, following a meal, high insulin levels serve to promote storage of fatty acids in the

adipocyte as triglyceride, while in the fasting state hydrolysis is promoted, providing fatty acids for uptake by muscle and liver.

As noted above, the action of LPL requires the cofactor, apo C-II. Shortly after VLDL enters into plasma, apo C-II is transferred to VLDL from a reservoir on circulating HDL. After hydrolysis of triglyceride in VLDL, the apo C-II is released and presumably picked up again by HDL. The importance of apo C-II is demonstrated by individuals with genetic deficiency of C-II, which leads to impaired LPL activity and massive hypertriglyceridemia. Other apolipoproteins, such as C-III, are also transferred between VLDL and HDL. *In vitro*, apo C-III can inhibit LPL-mediated hydrolysis, but its physiologic role *in vivo* is still unclear.

Hydrolysis of triglycerides in VLDL profoundly alters the structure of the VLDL with collapse of the core. The excess surface components, including cholesterol, phospholipids, and the non-apoB apoproteins, are transferred to HDL. The triglyceride-depleted VLDL, with its associated loss of other lipids and apoproteins, now becomes an IDL, cholesterol-enriched and containing only apo B and apo E. Under normal conditions this particle is rapidly removed from plasma by the liver through a complex interaction with several hepatic receptors, including the LDL receptor, which recognizes apo B and apo E, and with another receptor, termed the remnant receptor, which is specific for apoprotein E. This latter receptor is thought to be the LDL-receptor–related protein (LRP). While the majority of IDL particles are normally removed from plasma by

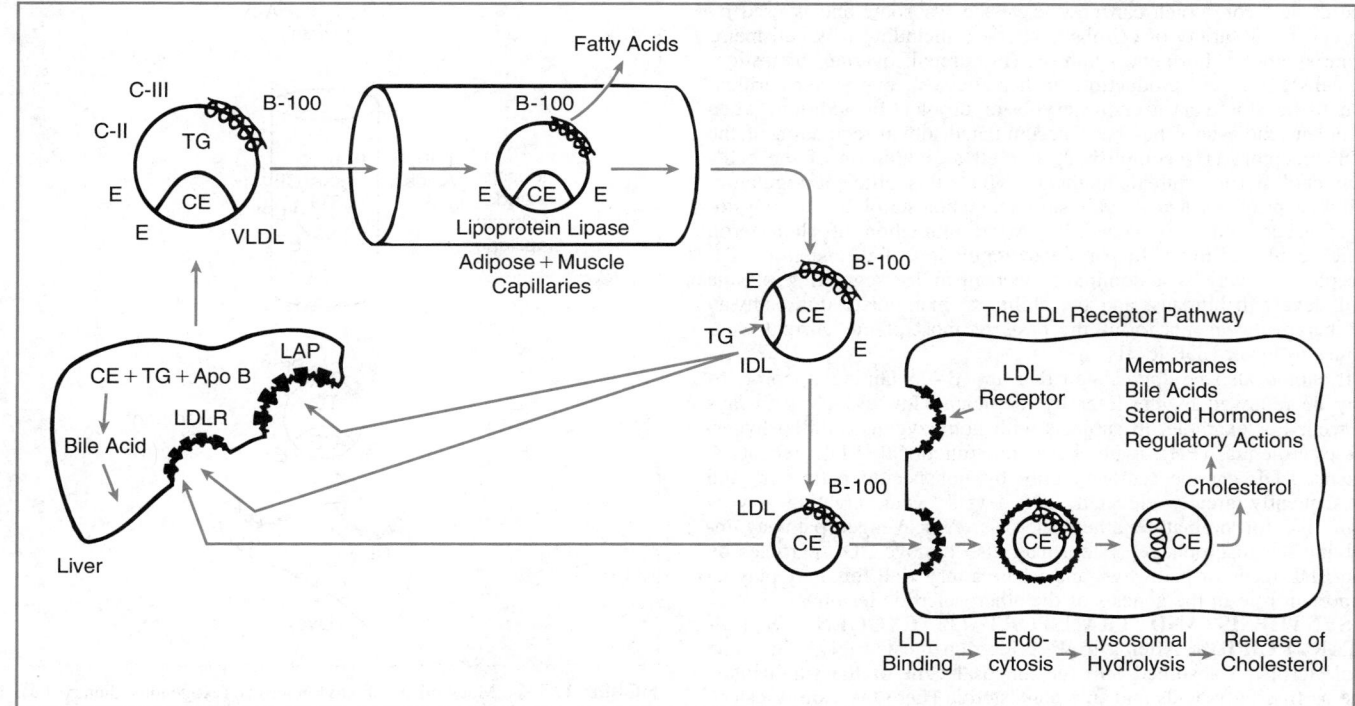

FIGURE 173-1. Simplified scheme of metabolism of apo B-containing lipoproteins. In the liver, triglyceride *(TG)*, cholesteryl esters *(CE)*, and apolipoprotein B-100 *(B-100)* are packaged and released into plasma as very low-density lipoproteins *(VLDL)*. In capillary beds, lipoprotein lipase hydrolyzes TG to release free fatty acids. The TG-depleted particle is termed an intermediate-density lipoprotein *(IDL)*. The particle is further metabolized to CE-rich low-density lipoprotein *(LDL)*. A major fraction of IDL particles is removed from plasma by hepatic receptors, both by LDL receptors *(LDLR)* and LDL receptor-related protein *(LRP)*. A portion of IDL is converted to LDL, which is then removed from plasma by LDLR on liver and peripheral cells. Uptake of LDL via the LDLR pathway leads to regulation of cholesterol synthesis and LDLR synthesis as explained in text. (Modified from Witztum, JL: Current approaches to drug therapy for the hypercholesterolemic patient. Circulation 80:1101, 1989. By permission of the American Heart Association, Inc.).

this process in other species, in humans a significant fraction is converted into LDL. By the time the cholesterol-rich LDL has been formed, most of the triglyceride has been removed and apo B is now the sole apoprotein remaining from the original VLDL particle. Under normal circumstances, most of the cholesterol found in plasma is present in the form of LDL particles, and only minute amounts of IDL are present.

Apo E, which acts as a ligand for both the LDL receptor and the LRP, appears to be crucial for both the direct removal of IDL and conversion of IDL particles to LDL. Patients who either lack apo E or are homozygous for apo E isoforms (E_2) that bind less efficiently to these receptors may have excess plasma accumulation of IDL particles (and chylomicron remnants) and are both hypercholesterolemic and hypertriglyceridemic, a condition known as dysbetalipoproteinemia.

Metabolism of LDL. Each LDL particle is derived from VLDL via IDL and contains one copy of apo B. All other apolipoproteins have now been removed, together with much of the phospholipid and triglyceride and some of the cholesterol. Although only a small percentage of VLDL particles ultimately end up as LDL, the bulk of plasma cholesterol is accounted for by LDL particles because of the relatively slow rate of clearance of LDL from plasma (half-life of 2 to 3 days). Because LDL particles contain only apo B, their efficient clearance can occur only by way of the LDL receptor pathway. In normal humans, approximately 75% of LDL particles are cleared by the LDL receptor pathway and approximately two thirds of LDL particles are removed by the liver. Nobel prize winners Brown and Goldstein elucidated the LDL receptor pathway, one of the major achievements of modern medical science. The rate of LDL removal via this pathway is the primary determinant of LDL levels. The LDL receptor, which binds apo B with high affinity and leads to internalization of the LDL particle via the LDL receptor pathway, is found on virtually every mammalian cell. As shown in the right side of Figure 173–1, the LDL particle binds to the receptor on the surface of the cell, and subsequently the receptor and the bound LDL particle are internalized. LDL is then delivered to the lysosome, but the receptor recycles to the surface of the cell. Within the lysosome, the protein component, apo B, is degraded to amino acids or oligopeptides. The cholesteryl ester is hydrolyzed to free cholesterol, which can now leave the lysosome and is used by the cell for a variety of cellular processes, including new cell membrane synthesis, hormone synthesis (in adrenal, ovarian, or testicular cells), bile acid production (in hepatocytes), or for re-esterification to be stored as a cholesteryl-ester droplet. In addition, when sufficient cholesterol has been accumulated, down-regulation of the LDL receptors is accomplished, as well as inhibition of the cell's own cholesterol synthetic pathway. Thus, this efficient regulatory pathway provides a cell with sufficient cholesterol for its physiologic needs, but it prevents the overaccumulation of cholesterol, which could be toxic. In particular, regulation of the *hepatic* LDL receptor pathway is a dominant mechanism for regulating plasma LDL levels in humans, and the ability to manipulate this pathway by therapeutic agents forms the basis of most of our current techniques to lower LDL levels.

It should also be appreciated that apo B–containing lipoproteins may be removed by the liver by inefficient, low-affinity pathways as well. For example, in subjects with homozygous familial hypercholesterolemia (FH), who have no functional LDL receptors, plasma LDL can be removed only by nonspecific pathways, and consequently greatly elevated LDL levels occur, creating a very high risk for premature atherosclerosis. A scavenger pathway involving the macrophage system may also remove LDL particles by non-LDL receptor pathways, and in the artery wall this may play an important role in the genesis of the atherosclerotic lesion.

SYNTHESIS AND TRANSPORT OF EXOGENOUS (DIETARY) LIPIDS.

After a triglyceride-rich meal, triglycerides and cholesterol are absorbed into the mucosal cells of the small intestine as free fatty acids and free cholesterol. There they are re-esterified to triglyceride and cholesteryl esters and incorporated into the core of a nascent lipoprotein, the chylomicron. The surface coat of the chylomicron is composed of phospholipid and apoproteins A-I, A-II, and A-IV. Apo B-48 is a crucial component of chylomicrons and is a product of the same gene that codes for apoprotein B-100. Apo B-48 is so named because it is identical to the first 48% (the

amino terminal portion) of apo B-100. In humans, the intact, full-length apo B-100 is made only in the liver, while apo B-48 is made only in the intestine. Apo B-48 appears to be required for the small intestine to produce chylomicrons, as individuals with abetalipoproteinemia, who are incapable of secreting apo B from intestinal (or hepatic) cells, cannot assemble chylomicron particles. Apo B-48 is transcribed from the apo B-100 gene, but the mRNA is first edited by a cytosine-to-uracil change creating a stop-codon. The domain of intact apo B-100 that binds to the LDL receptor is contained in the carboxy terminal end. Because apo B-48 lacks this domain it is unable to bind to LDL receptors. Thus, once the chylomicron has been secreted by the intestine, apo B-48 functions primarily as a structural component.

Triglycerides constitute >90% by weight of the chylomicron particle, and consequently the density of this lipoprotein is the lowest of any in plasma. When plasma is left overnight in the refrigerator, if chylomicrons are present, they will float to the top and appear as a layer of "cream" on top, which is the basis for the chylomicron test. In normal individuals, this test is always negative after an 8- to 12-hour fast, as chylomicrons have a short half-life in plasma. The presence of a positive chylomicron test in a 12-hour fasting sample is abnormal and indicative of marked delay in chylomicron clearance.

Chylomicrons are delivered to the plasma via the thoracic duct (Fig. 173–2). While in the lymph and after entering plasma, chylomicrons acquire apo C-II, C-III, and apo E by transfer. After having acquired sufficient apo C-II, which is absolutely required for LPL activity, the chylomicron can interact with LPL in a manner

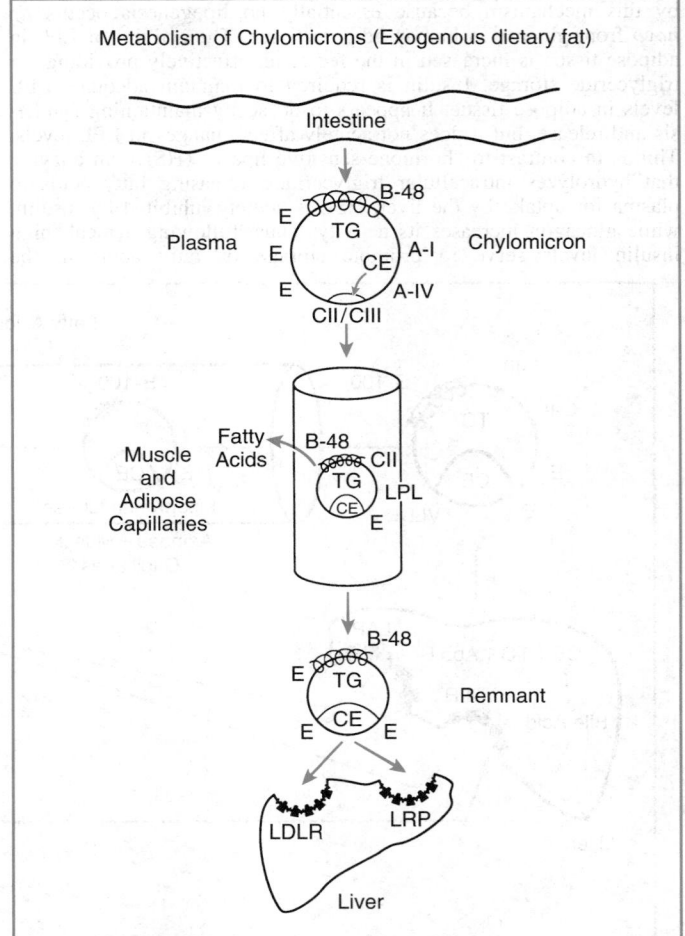

FIGURE 173–2. Metabolism of chylomicrons (exogenous dietary fat). In the intestine, triglyceride (TG) and small amounts of cholesteryl esters (CE) are packaged with apo B-48, apo A-I, and apo A-IV and released into lymph. The chylomicron particle acquires apo E and apo C-II/C-III in lymph and plasma. In capillary beds, TG is hydrolyzed by lipoprotein lipase (LPL). The remnant particle is then removed primarily by liver, mediated by binding to LRP and LDLR as well as to surface proteoglycans. Chylomicron remnants are not a source of LDL.

analogous to that of VLDL. After sufficient triglyceride hydrolysis has occurred, the remaining chylomicron particle, now termed a remnant, has a markedly reduced core volume and its excess surface components, including apoproteins such as C-II, C-III, and some of the apo E, are transferred to HDL as described for VLDL. The remnant particle is still relatively cholesteryl-ester–rich. In part, this cholesterol comes from dietary sources, but a significant amount is also transferred into the particle from HDL mediated by cholesterol ester transfer protein (CETP). In addition, because it is still a relatively large particle, it contains many copies of apo E on its surface, and it is believed that this represents the ligand that leads to rapid interaction with remnant receptors in the liver and efficient removal from the circulation. The exact pathway for uptake of chylomicron remnants by the liver is still being investigated but probably includes the LRP, the LDL receptor itself, as well as cell-surface glycosaminoglycans that can also bind apo E. Apo E is central to the process of remnant removal, just as it is for IDL uptake. Individuals who either lack apo E or synthesize only apo E isoforms that bind poorly to receptors can accumulate chylomicron remnants in plasma.

HDL-CONTAINING LIPOPROTEINS. When chylomicrons and VLDL are hydrolyzed by LPL to release fatty acids for peripheral use, their surface coat of unesterified cholesterol, phospholipid, and various apoproteins forms excess surface material that must be disposed of. HDL play a principal role in this by acting as an acceptor or "sink" for this excess surface material (Fig. 173–3). Nascent HDL particles are synthesized by the liver and the intestine and are composed primarily of phospholipid and two major structural proteins, apoproteins A-I and A-II. HDL accepts the phospholipid (mainly lecithin) and unesterified cholesterol from the excess surface of triglyceride-rich lipoproteins as they are catabolized. An enzyme associated with HDL—lecithin-cholesterol acyl transferase (LCAT)—removes a fatty acid from lecithin and transfers it to cholesterol, producing cholesteryl ester and lysolecithin. The esterified cholesterol moves into the core of the HDL particle, making it possible to accept another free cholesterol molecule onto the surface of the HDL particle. In turn, the cholesteryl esters are then transported back to the liver (reverse cholesterol transport) either directly or by transfer to other lipoproteins, such as VLDL, IDL, or LDL via CETP. The uptake of these cholesteryl-ester–enriched lipoproteins by the liver results in net removal from plasma of cholesteryl esters. This HDL/LCAT/CETP system plays a pivotal role in removing excess cellular cholesterol, facilitating its transfer back to the liver for excretion. The removal of excess cholesterol from arterial wall cells by such a mechanism could play a crucial role in minimizing cholesterol accumulation in the artery wall and thus inhibiting atherogenesis (see Ch. 40). Thus, HDL may be viewed as playing a vital role in transporting excess cholesterol from extrahepatic tissues back to the liver where it is excreted in the bile. In addition to its role in reverse cholesterol transport, HDL may also serve as the reservoir for apoproteins such as C-II, C-III, and E as they shuttle back and forth from triglyceride-rich lipoproteins while being catabolized.

BILE ACID PRODUCTION (see Ch. 126). Nearly all cells of the body have the capacity to synthesize cholesterol *de novo*, but none has the ability to degrade it completely. However, hepatocytes have the capacity to convert cholesterol into bile acids, which can then be secreted into the bile along with free cholesterol and phospholipids. Nearly 95% of secreted bile acids are reabsorbed in the distal ileum and enter the enterohepatic circulation, i.e., they are taken up by the liver and recycled. Cholesterol delivered to the liver in the form of chylomicrons or other lipoproteins could be recycled and secreted as VLDL or converted to bile acids for secretion into the bile.

DISORDERS OF LIPOPROTEIN METABOLISM

Disorders of lipoprotein metabolism can lead to hypercholesterolemia or hypertriglyceridemia or both. While these disorders appear to be common in the general population, the molecular events responsible for them are only currently being elucidated. For purposes of organization the hyperlipoproteinemias are grouped into disorders leading primarily to hypercholesterolemia (due to elevations of LDL levels) or to hypertriglyceridemia (due to elevations of VLDL or chylomicrons) or to combined elevations of both triglycerides and cholesterol. Several monogenic disorders have been defined that lead to each type of hyperlipidemia, but for many cases the etiology is likely to be polygenic. These disorders affect plasma lipoprotein levels by overproduction of lipoproteins and/or decreased clearance.

Hyperlipoproteinemia Resulting Primarily in Hypercholesterolemia

FAMILIAL HYPERCHOLESTEROLEMIA AND FAMILIAL DEFECTIVE APOLIPOPROTEIN B. *Familial hypercholesterolemia* (FH) is a common autosomal dominant disorder due to absence of or defective LDL receptors resulting in decreased capacity to remove plasma LDL. Familial defective apolipoprotein B is an autosomal dominant disorder in which the ligand binding region of apo B is defective, also leading to delayed plasma LDL clearance. In both disorders LDL cholesterol levels are strikingly increased, frequently associated with characteristic xanthomas in the Achilles tendons, the patellar tendons, the extensor tendons of the hands, and by the presence of xanthelasma. It is frequently associated with early coronary artery disease (CAD). In heterozygous FH, estimated to be present in 1 in 500 individuals, there is one abnormal allele for the LDL receptor. The abnormal allele may produce no receptors or produce abnormal LDL receptors that are largely nonfunctional. In the heterozygote a 50% decrease exists in hepatic LDL receptor number, a corresponding decrease in LDL catabolism, and an approximately twofold to threefold increase in plasma LDL levels. In the rare homozygous FH patient (only 1 in 1,000,000 people) almost no functional LDL receptors are found, and plasma LDL levels may be increased sixfold to tenfold. In this situation, LDL can be removed from plasma only by low-affinity pathways. In familial defective apolipoprotein B, the ligand-binding domain of apo B is defective because of a missense mutation at amino acid 3500. This mutation leads to impaired binding of LDL to the LDL receptor and clinical consequences similar to those seen in FH. It is likely that other mutations in apo B affecting its ability to bind to the LDL receptor also occur.

These disorders are characterized by greatly elevated concentrations of LDL cholesterol. If untreated, patients with FH have premature CAD, as well as other clinical manifestations of atherosclerosis (see Ch. 41). Peripheral vascular disease and cerebral vascular disease are also increased, although not as much as CAD. Tendon xanthomas are seen only in FH and in patients with familial defective apo B. Bilateral, irregular, firm and nodular thickenings in the Achilles tendons or extensor tendons of the hands or knees are usually present and can be so large as to interfere with normal functions, such as wearing shoes. Xanthelasma typically occurs in this

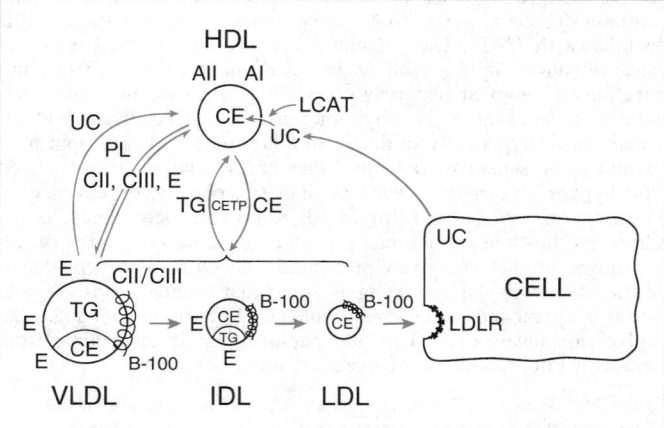

FIGURE 173–3. Interactions of high-density lipoproteins *(HDL)* and apo B-containing lipoproteins. HDL has particles containing apo A-I and particles containing apo A-I, A-II. Nascent HDL, made primarily by liver and intestine, accepts unesterified cholesterol *(UC)* from VLDL and from membranes of cells. The enzyme lecithin-cholesterol-acyltransferase *(LCAT)*, which is associated with HDL, esterifies the cholesterol to form cholesteryl esters *(CE)*, which then form the core of the HDL. The enzyme cholesterol ester transfer protein *(CETP)* transfers CE from HDL into apo B-containing lipoproteins in exchange for TG. HDL also serves as a "sink" for apoproteins C-II/C-III and E, which shuttle back and forth from the HDL to VLDL and IDL.

setting, and corneal arcus is frequently seen as well, although this latter is seen in other lipoprotein disorders and can be seen in elderly, normolipidemic patients as well.

Plasma cholesterol levels in heterozygous FH exceed the upper 1% of levels seen in the general population and are generally in the range of 300 to 500 mg per deciliter. In rare patients, homozygous for FH, plasma cholesterol levels can exceed 800 to 1000 mg per deciliter. Triglyceride levels are usually normal, but in 10% of subjects may be mildly elevated. Patients with defective remnant removal or with marked chylomicronemia may also have markedly elevated cholesterol levels, but they will have very high triglyceride levels as well. In addition, their plasma will appear turbid or creamy, in contrast to plasma in FH patients, which is always clear.

Because myocardial infarction can occur in men with heterozygous FH when they are in their early 40's, these subjects deserve vigorous therapy to lower LDL levels and to decrease other risk factors as well. Women with FH also have an accelerated risk for CAD, although the absolute risk is less than that of men and the CAD occurs at a later age. For both men and women the risk of atherosclerosis is greatly accelerated by the presence of other risk factors such as smoking, hypertension, diabetes, low HDL cholesterol levels, and high Lp(a) levels. A diet low in saturated fat and cholesterol should be initiated in all affected individuals with this disorder, although frequently only modest reductions in LDL levels occur. Effective therapy can be achieved using a bile acid-binding resin, frequently combined with high-dose nicotinic acid (niacin) given with meals. HMG-CoA reductase inhibitors, a class of compounds termed *statins,* are increasingly being used as first-line therapy as they effectively lower LDL cholesterol levels by 20 to 40% and infrequently have side effects. When these statins are combined with a bile acid–binding resin, decreases of LDL levels by 50 to 60% can frequently be achieved. In some individuals, triple therapy with a statin, a bile acid-binding resin, and niacin may be necessary to normalize LDL levels. Unfortunately, subjects homozygous for FH will usually not respond to these measures, which work in large part by increasing the LDL receptor activity. For such individuals heroic measures are required, such as repeated plasmapheresis or a more specialized procedure, termed LDL apheresis, in which apo B-containing lipoproteins are removed from blood as it passes extracorporeally through a column that binds apo B. In selected individuals, liver transplantation has been used. In the future it is hoped that gene therapy may lead to correction of the primary genetic defect.

POLYGENIC HYPERCHOLESTEROLEMIA. Irrespective of one's definition of hypercholesterolemia, it is clear that a large number of individuals in the general population have elevated LDL-cholesterol levels (see Table 173–4). If one uses the conventional definition that the top 5% of the general population have hypercholesterolemia, then on average only 1 of 25 of such hypercholesterolemic individuals will have FH, and only 2 will have familial combined hyperlipidemia (FCH) (described below). The large majority have hypercholesterolemia due to a complex interaction of multiple genetic factors and environmental factors, i.e., polygenic hypercholesterolemia. The cause of the hypercholesterolemia is unknown, but it is likely due to the convergence of several subtle alterations that affect regulation of LDL levels. Differences may exist in dietary responsiveness to cholesterol and saturated fat, differences in regulation of cholesterol and/or bile acid biosynthesis, and/or differences in regulation of LDL receptor activity and in the secretion and intravascular catabolism of apo B-containing lipoproteins.

FAMILIAL HYPERALPHALIPOPROTEINEMIA. Occasionally, patients are seen who have mildly elevated total cholesterol levels due to elevated HDL cholesterol. They usually have normal levels of LDL and VLDL. In these individuals the elevated HDL cholesterol level is genetic, and in some families it is inherited as an autosomal dominant trait. In other families the etiology appears to be polygenic. High levels of HDL can also be seen with chronic alcoholism, in response to estrogen administration, and after exposure to chlorinated hydrocarbon pesticides. In some families a genetic deficiency of CETP is associated with strikingly elevated HDL cholesterol levels, especially in Japanese populations. Individuals with hyperalphalipoproteinemia do not have any unusual clinical features, and they have been reported to have slightly increased longevity due to a decreased incidence of CAD.

Hyperlipoproteinemias Resulting Primarily in Hypertriglyceridemia

LIPOPROTEIN LIPASE DEFICIENCY AND APO C-II DEFICIENCY. LPL deficiency is a rare autosomal recessive trait that is characterized by the absence of active LPL in all tissues, leading to massive hypertriglyceridemia from birth and the clinical consequences of eruptive xanthoma and episodes of pancreatitis. This same clinical syndrome may also occur with deficiency of apo C-II, an obligatory activator of LPL, though clinical manifestations tend to occur later in life.

In infants and young children with LPL deficiency, the hypertriglyceridemia results primarily from chylomicron accumulation, while impairment of VLDL triglyceride removal becomes more important in later life. Homozygosity for LPL deficiency or for apo C-II deficiency is necessary for this disorder to occur. Heterozygosity for LPL deficiency may lead to moderate hypertriglyceridemia and may be one factor in the etiology of FCH. Infants with homozygous LPL deficiency have massive hypertriglyceridemia and grossly lipemic serum. They frequently fail to thrive and have severe abdominal pain and pancreatitis as a consequence of their marked hyperchylomicronemia. Eruptive xanthomas can occur on the extensor surfaces, notably on the elbows, knees, back, and buttocks but can occur elsewhere, and when seen are pathognomonic for chylomicronemia. Hepatomegaly is frequent, as is splenomegaly, which occurs because of the accumulation of lipid-laden foam cells. LPL activity can be measured by assaying plasma after injection of heparin, which releases LPL into plasma. Apo C-II levels can be assayed by immunoassay. The clinical manifestations will rapidly disappear with elimination of fat from the diet, which leads to elimination of the chylomicronemia. With effective fat restriction, plasma triglyceride levels can usually be maintained between 500 and 800 mg per deciliter or lower, and at this level, episodes of eruptive xanthoma, abdominal pain, and pancreatitis can usually be avoided. Substances that increase endogenous VLDL output, such as alcohol and glucocorticoids, must be avoided. With effective attention to diet, individuals can grow and easily reach adulthood without difficulty. There is no indication that any increased risk for atherosclerosis exists in this disorder.

FAMILIAL HYPERTRIGLYCERIDEMIA. Individuals with this condition have marked hypertriglyceridemia, normal to low LDL levels, and marked decreases in HDL cholesterol levels. When studied in detail, the number of VLDL particles is relatively normal, but they are triglyceride enriched. LPL-related triglyceride removal and remnant removal appears to be normal. HDL particle number is also relatively normal, but the triglyceride content in the HDL, which is normally very low, is considerably increased at the expense of cholesterol. The underlying defect in this disorder is postulated to be enhanced hepatic triglyceride synthesis. This disorder has been defined as an autosomal dominant trait that is quite common. There is some controversy about the association of this disorder with CAD. These patients are usually detected only because of routine lipid screening, or occasionally as a result of complications of marked hypertriglyceridemia. They do not have xanthomas unless there is chylomicronemia. Affected individuals usually have hypertriglyceridemia in adulthood, and they appear to be unusually sensitive to factors that are known to be associated with hypertriglyceridemia such as diabetes, obesity, excess alcohol consumption, or use of estrogen, diuretics, glucocorticoids, or β-adrenergic blockers, which can greatly exaggerate the degree of hypertriglyceridemia and even precipitate the chylomicronemia syndrome. Although the reasoning is somewhat circular, most experts would not treat individuals with isolated hypertriglyceridemia, e.g., triglyceride levels of 250 to 500 per deciliter, if they come from families without evidence of increased atherosclerosis.

Hyperlipoproteinemias Resulting in Mixed or Combined Hyperlipidemia

DYSBETALIPOPROTEINEMIA. Dysbetalipoproteinemia, also known as broad-beta or type III hyperlipoproteinemia, is a condition in which there is abnormal accumulation of cholesterol-rich IDL-type particles, commonly termed β-VLDL. This disorder is due to interaction of (1) an autosomal recessive defect in apo E that leads to abnormal remnant catabolism and (2) an independent aggravating environmental factor (e.g., obesity, diabetes, pregnancy) or genetic factor (FCH) leading to overproduction of apo B-containing lipoproteins. The combination of these two factors leads to accumulation of IDL-like particles (resulting from impaired VLDL catabolism) and remnants (resulting from impaired chylomicron metabolism) that lead to xanthomas, peripheral vascular disease, and CAD.

There are three major alleles for apo E, differing from each other by a single amino acid substitution at one or two sites. These are termed E_2, E_3, and E_4. An individual can be homozygous for any of these alleles, or heterozygous for any combination. The apo E encoded by the E_2 allele has sharply reduced ability to bind to lipoprotein receptors. Individuals homozygous for this allele (i.e., E_2/E_2 homozygotes), who compose about 2% of the population, have a relative defect in IDL and remnant catabolism. This can lead to relative accumulation in plasma of cholesteryl-ester–rich IDL and chylomicron remnant particles (β-VLDL) and corresponding decrease in LDL levels because of defective conversion of VLDL to LDL (see Fig. 173–1). Yet, in the absence of aggravating factors, total plasma cholesterol levels are actually low in such individuals and triglyceride levels are normal. However, in an estimated 1 of 100 individuals with E_2/E_2 homozygosity, there is also an associated condition leading to overproduction of VLDL. This combination results in the absolute accumulation of β-VLDL particles, which are atherogenic when present in excess. This is expressed as marked hypertriglyceridemia and hypercholesterolemia. Normally, VLDL particles have "pre-β" mobility on agarose gel electrophoresis, but the VLDL remnants in dysbetalipoproteinemia are much closer to LDL in composition and therefore have "β" mobility ("β-VLDL"). Hence, the designation dysbetalipoproteinemia. Because individuals who are homozygous for the E_2 allele will have low levels of such qualitatively abnormal VLDL present in plasma even when total lipids are normal (or even low), some experts use the term dysbetalipoproteinemia to refer to the condition of homozygosity for E_2, while the term type III hyperlipoproteinemia or broad-beta syndrome is reserved for those individuals with associated hyperlipidemia. The type III hyperlipoproteinemia phenotype can also be caused by total absence of apo E, which has been observed in rare families.

If VLDL is not overproduced, there are no clinical manifestations. However, when overproduction of VLDL occurs, marked hyperlipidemia appears, and this disorder may present as premature clinical atherosclerosis with peripheral vascular disease and/or CAD. The presence of hypothyroidism has been noted frequently in individuals with clinical symptoms. These patients frequently have highly characteristic planar xanthomas in the creases of the palms as well as tuberous or tuberoeruptive xanthomas on the elbows or knees that are virtually diagnostic for this disorder. Occasionally these manifestations can be seen with obstructive liver disease. Although the apo E abnormality is present from birth, it is unusual to see hyperlipidemia in a male younger than age 30 and in a female before menopause. The presence of hypertriglyceridemia accompanied by unusual degrees of hypercholesterolemia when associated with palmar or tuberous xanthomas is highly suggestive of this disorder. Liver disease and hypothyroidism need to be excluded. Electrophoresis of a VLDL fraction of plasma will reveal particles of beta mobility, rather than the typical pre-β mobility. The E_2 isoforms can be identified by isoelectric focusing in specialty laboratories, and genotyping is also available. The concentration of LDL is typically low even in hyperlipidemic patients, and a normal or elevated LDL level should make one consider an alternative diagnosis. HDL levels are normal or slightly decreased, depending on the degree of hypertriglyceridemia.

In many E_2/E_2 adults with clinical manifestations of hyperlipidemia, there is associated obesity, and weight reduction is of primary importance. In postmenopausal women, low-dose estrogen replacement frequently normalizes the abnormal lipoprotein profile and corrects the hyperlipidemia. All patients should be checked for mild degrees of hypothyroidism using sensitive TSH assays; if hypothyroidism is present, treatment may frequently completely normalize the lipoprotein profile. Gemfibrozil is frequently effective in decreasing lipid levels in these individuals; high-dose nicotinic acid may also be useful. Use of an HMG-CoA reductase inhibitor has been found to be quite successful in reducing the hypercholesterolemia and, when combined with low-dose gemfibrozil, has frequently normalized triglyceride levels in severe cases.

FAMILIAL COMBINED HYPERLIPIDEMIA. Among patients with myocardial infarction, a significant number have an apparently dominantly inherited pattern of hyperlipoproteinemia that is expressed by a variable lipoprotein phenotype. Thus, individuals may have increased levels of VLDL, or LDL, or both lipoproteins.

Some first-degree relatives have elevated VLDL levels, some have elevated LDL, and some have both. This entity appears to be monogenic and inherited in an autosomal dominant manner and has been termed familial combined hyperlipidemia (FCH) or familial multiple lipoprotein-type hyperlipidemia. The lipoprotein phenotype is not stable over time. A person can have VLDL elevations noted on one visit but marked increases in LDL, or both VLDL and LDL, at another visit. While there remains much uncertainty about classification of this disorder, all clinicians seeing patients with premature CAD recognize the frequency of this pattern. A characteristic of this disorder is increased accumulation of small LDL particles, which are cholesterol depleted. Thus, patients may have a relatively normal "LDL cholesterol" level, yet the number of LDL particles is increased and therefore the LDL-apo B level is increased. Some investigators have termed this condition familial hyperapobetalipoproteinemia. Most evidence suggests that the underlying defect is increased hepatic secretion of VLDL. These VLDL appear to be smaller than normal, with less triglyceride per particle. Undoubtedly this disorder represents several different genetic traits interacting with the basic defect–overproduction of VDL. For example, overproduction of VLDL may become manifested primarily as elevations in VLDL if a relative or absolute defect in VLDL catabolism occurs in addition, as for example, with relative deficiency in LPL activity. Recently, a number of cases of heterozygous LPL deficiency have been found in association with this phenotype. Conversely, in the face of appropriate VLDL and IDL catabolism, LDL may accumulate because of the increased rate of generation of LDL and/or functional disturbances in LDL catabolic mechanisms. These individuals also typically have low levels of HDL with decreases in both HDL cholesterol and apo A-I.

This phenotype is associated with a clinical constellation that includes mild abdominal obesity, insulin resistance, mild hypertension, elevated VLDL levels, the presence of an excess number of small dense LDL, and decreased HDL. This syndrome has been referred to as the insulin-resistance syndrome or syndrome X (see Ch. 205). This disorder is more typically seen in men and is associated with a strikingly high rate of premature CAD. The effect of other risk factors appears to be greatly exaggerated in these individuals, and a history of smoking is frequently found in those with early CAD. Patients do not have any characteristic xanthomas, and the diagnosis is made by a characteristic family history that is unusually positive for early CAD, by documentation of the variable lipoprotein phenotype, and, if possible, by lipoprotein phenotyping of first-degree relatives. Women may also be affected by this phenotype, although the clinical manifestations of CAD appear to be expressed later in life. Because this disorder is associated with a high risk of premature CAD, vigorous efforts should be made to lower lipoprotein levels of affected individuals. Nicotinic acid may be quite efficacious in some individuals in lowering VLDL and raising HDL levels. Other regimens include the use of an HMG-CoA reductase inhibitor alone or in combination with gemfibrozil. The use of gemfibrozil alone to lower VLDL levels will often be highly effective but is almost always associated with significant rises in LDL.

OTHER FORMS OF HYPERTRIGLYCERIDEMIA. Mild hypertriglyceridemia is one of the most commonly encountered hyperlipidemias. Although many patients with hypertriglyceridemia will fit into one of the categories noted above, there are many other patients with triglyceride levels of 400 to 2000 mg per deciliter who do not seem to fall into any of those categories. They may have a family history of hypertriglyceridemia and/or quite commonly have one of the secondary forms of hypertriglyceridemia, such as that due to excess alcohol use or diabetes mellitus. Frequently, treating the underlying cause will ameliorate the hypertriglyceridemia, but often a milder form remains, probably indicative of an underlying as yet undefined genetic defect.

ACQUIRED DISORDERS OF LIPOPROTEIN METABOLISM

Many medical conditions are associated with mild or even severe hyperlipidemia in the absence of underlying genetic hyperlipoproteinemia. With underlying genetic hyperlipidemia, acquired disorders can lead to greatly exaggerated effects on lipoprotein levels. Table 173–3 lists disorders commonly associated with changes in lipoprotein levels.

TABLE 173-3. ACQUIRED DISORDERS OF LIPOPROTEIN METABOLISM

Hypercholesterolemia
Nephrotic syndrome
Hypothyroidism
Dysgammaglobulinemia
Acute intermittent porphyria
Obstructive liver disease
Combined Hyperlipidemia
Nephrotic syndrome
Hypothyroidism
Glucocorticoid excess/Cushing's disease
Diuretics
Uncontrolled diabetes
Hypertriglyceridemia
Diabetes mellitus
Uremia
Sepsis
Obesity
Systemic lupus erythematosus
Dysgammaglobulinemia
Glycogen storage disease, type I
Lipodystrophy
Drugs
    Alcohol
    Estrogens
    β-Adrenergic blocking agents
    Isotretinoin (13-cis-retinoic acid)

DIABETES MELLITUS (see Ch. 205). Persons with untreated insulin-dependent diabetes, as well as uncontrolled non–insulin-dependent diabetes, frequently have hypertriglyceridemia, low HDL levels, and associated small dense LDL particles. These individuals appear to have low adipose tissue or muscle LPL activity that leads to relative impairment in VLDL clearance. Although LDL levels are not absolutely elevated in these individuals as a rule, for the degree of hypertriglyceridemia, the LDL levels are higher than expected. In part, this may be due to nonenzymatic glycosylation of the LDL particle caused by hyperglycemia as well as by down-regulation of LDL receptors because of insulin lack.

CHRONIC UREMIA AND DIALYSIS (see Ch. 78.1). Many individuals with chronic uremia have elevated VLDL levels with associated hypertriglyceridemia and low HDL cholesterol levels. This condition persists even after initiation of maintenance hemodialysis or peritoneal dialysis. These lipoprotein abnormalities are related to defects in LPL-mediated triglyceride removal and/or associated overproduction.

ALCOHOL AND OTHER DRUGS. Among the many associated factors that cause mild degrees of hypertriglyceridemia, alcohol consumption is probably the most common; it increases triglyceride levels in most individuals. This occurs because both fatty acid synthesis and VLDL output are stimulated, and LPL activity is inhibited. In individuals with normal baseline VLDL levels this is not usually a problem, but in those in whom there is excess VLDL secretion or some other additional basis for impairment in VLDL clearance, marked hypertriglyceridemia ensues with alcohol use. Diuretic agents and β-adrenergic blocking agents are also frequently associated with mild increases in triglyceride levels in patients with no underlying abnormality in lipoprotein metabolism but with quite marked increases in those with underlying hypertriglyceridemia. In individuals with genetic hypertriglyceridemia or FCH, estrogen use may also lead to marked increases in VLDL levels. Hypertriglyceridemia occurs in 25% of people given isotretinoin (13-cis-retinoic acid) for cystic acne.

HYPOTHYROIDISM (see Ch. 203). Thyroid hormone is crucial in many steps of lipoprotein metabolism. LDL receptor activity is particularly sensitive to thyroxine levels, and in hypothyroidism LDL levels are elevated because of down-regulation of LDL receptor number. In addition, LPL activity is low, leading to elevated VLDL levels and even, rarely, chylomicronemia, especially in subjects with dysbetalipoproteinemia.

NEPHROTIC SYNDROME (see Ch. 79). With massive proteinuria and with hypoalbuminemia, a compensatory increase occurs in overall hepatic protein synthesis, and in particular there is

marked increase in VLDL output. An associated defect in VLDL catabolism is also seen, in part due to depressed LPL activity.

HYPERLIPOPROTEINEMIA AND ATHEROSCLEROSIS

The etiology of atherosclerosis is multifactorial; a more general discussion of its pathogenesis can be found in Ch. 40. However, the cause-and-effect relationship between hypercholesterolemia and atherosclerosis has been proved in a large number of animal model studies and by large randomized, double-blind clinical intervention trials. Reducing plasma LDL cholesterol levels sharply reduces the risk of subsequent clinical CAD in both patients with pre-existing CAD and in patients free of CAD at the beginning of the study. In studies extending over 5 to 7 years, morbidity and mortality from new coronary events have been reduced by as much as 20 to 40%. A statistically significant decrease in *total* mortality was also seen in two large studies, the Coronary Drug Project (in the group of men treated with nicotinic acid) and in a recent Scandinavian trial using an HMG-CoA reductase inhibitor to lower plasma cholesterol levels. Angiographic studies have documented that intensive cholesterol-lowering regimens slow progression of coronary lesions: In some cases there has even been significant regression of lesions. Plasma triglyceride levels also correlate very significantly with risk of CAD, but the interpretation of this correlation is less clear, as elevation of triglyceride levels is frequently associated with other factors that may be more immediately relevant to the increase in CAD risk. The atherogenicity of individual lipoprotein classes is discussed below.

CHYLOMICRONS AND VLDL. Almost no evidence exists that chylomicrons are proatherogenic, and they are probably too large to penetrate into the artery. VLDL may also be too large, but CAD risk correlates with hypertriglyceridemia almost as well as it does with hypercholesterolemia in the fasting state and most of the triglycerides in plasma are carried in VLDL. This correlation may be explained by the frequent association of hypertriglyceridemia with obesity, low HDL levels, small, dense LDL, and diabetes mellitus. More likely is the possibility that the catabolic products of VLDL, the IDL, are atherogenic. Indeed, in hyperlipidemic patients with dysbetalipoproteinemia, the lipoprotein that accumulates is a type of IDL—so-called β-VLDL. Such patients are at increased risk of atherosclerosis and its complications. Moreover, the lipoprotein class that accumulates in experimental animals fed a high-fat, high-cholesterol diet is predominantly the same sort of β-VLDL.

LDL. There is no doubt about the atherogenicity of LDL. Patients with FH have strikingly premature atherosclerosis. However, in addition to greatly increased LDL, they also have some increase in IDL. Yet patients with a mutation of apo B that reduces its affinity for the LDL receptor accumulate *only* LDL, and their risk of premature CAD at any given plasma cholesterol level appears to be just as great as that of patients with LDL receptor deficiency. Increasing evidence suggests that oxidative modification of LDL within the artery is important, if not obligatory, for mediating the atherogenicity of LDL. Much evidence has been obtained that oxidized LDL is formed in the artery wall. Products of oxidized LDL may contribute to atherogenesis by many mechanisms, including attracting monocytes to the lesion and facilitating their conversion into macrophages. In turn, macrophages express scavenger receptors that take up oxidized LDL, leading to foam cells and the fatty streak lesion. In addition, products of oxidized LDL are toxic, producing endothelial damage and initiation of thrombosis. Treatment with antioxidants has been shown to slow the progress of atherosclerosis in several animal models, but similar data are not yet available in humans.

HDL. A wealth of epidemiologic evidence establishes that a high level of plasma HDL is associated with a lower risk of CHD. Until recently it was not certain whether the protective effect of a high HDL level was referable to a direct effect of the HDL or whether it represented a "marker" for some other factor. Studies in transgenic mice have now shown that increasing HDL reduces the susceptibility of these mice to atherosclerosis. It is widely believed that HDL protects against atherosclerosis by facilitating reverse cholesterol transport, i.e., the ability of HDL to accept excess cholesterol from tissues and return it to the liver, either directly or via other lipoproteins, but this has not been explicitly proved.

Lp(a). An increased risk for CAD has been found in many populations in association with increased levels of Lp(a), in particular when elevated levels of LDL are also present. However, Lp(a) appears to be an independent risk factor. Lp(a) is an LDL particle to which an additional large protein, termed apo (a), is attached via a disulfide bond. There are many different allelic forms of apo (a) protein, varying widely in molecular size and determined in large part by genetic factors. Apo (a) has high homology to plasminogen, but lacks the catalytically active site. Speculation has centered on the possibility that it interferes with plasminogen binding to its receptors and thus inhibits plasmin formation and thrombolysis. Alternatively, Lp(a) may have increased binding to the extracellular matrix of the artery, leading to greater deposition of the associated LDL. To date, no effective therapy has been found to lower elevated Lp(a) levels.

PRACTICAL MANAGEMENT OF HYPERLIPIDEMIA

TREATMENT OF HYPERCHOLESTEROLEMIA. Irrespective of the cause of elevated LDL levels, patients are usually managed similarly. In almost all cases, lowering LDL levels is achieved first by dietary intervention and then, if necessary, by adding drug therapy. Because the LDL receptor plays such an important role in regulating plasma LDL levels, therapy is aimed at achieving maximal expression of hepatic LDL receptor activity. Dietary cholesterol and saturated fat both lead to suppression of hepatic LDL receptor activity, and therefore reduction of these dietary components leads to up-regulation of hepatic LDL receptors and lowered plasma cholesterol levels. Individuals heterozygous for FH are more restricted in their response, and generally even stringent diets lower their LDL levels by no more than 5 to 10% below baseline levels. However, all individuals should be instructed in these diets, because some are unusually responsive.

Regulation of hepatic LDL receptor activity also appears to underlie mechanisms by which many commonly used hyperlipidemic drugs affect plasma cholesterol levels. As shown in Figure 173–4, the hepatocyte is the primary site of cholesterol synthesis. The cholesterol made by this cell is either excreted into plasma in the form of VLDL or is converted into bile acids, which are released into the intestine in response to meals. Normally, >95% of bile acids are reabsorbed and transported to the liver via the enterohepatic circulation and recycled through the liver up to six to seven times per day. Bile acid–binding resins work by binding bile acids in the intestine and promoting their subsequent loss in the stool. This prevents reabsorption and results in depletion of hepatic bile acid pools. In response, the hepatocyte actually increases cholesterol (and triglyceride) synthesis, as well as compensatory bile acid synthesis to replete the depleted bile acid pool. Despite this enhanced cholesterol synthesis, it is not sufficient to compensate for depletion of some crucial intracellular sterol pool, and the hepatocyte responds by also increasing LDL receptor expression. In turn, this directly removes LDL particles (or their precursors) from circulation. In this way, a nonsystemic agent leads to enhanced removal of plasma LDL particles and lowered plasma cholesterol levels. Very likely the soluble dietary fibers, such as oat bran, also lower plasma cholesterol by binding bile acids in a similar manner. For many individuals, this degree of plasma cholesterol lowering is sufficient.

However, in others the enhanced cholesterol (and triglyceride) synthesis leads to enhanced VLDL synthesis and release, and in effect, negates in part the cholesterol-lowering effect. In fact, many patients develop a transient or even permanent increase of plasma triglycerides (VLDL) in response to bile sequestrant therapy, even as LDL levels are lowered. This enhanced production of VLDL leads to generation of more LDL, which offsets in part the enhanced LDL removal, leading to suboptimal lowering of LDL levels. For this reason, a second agent, in combination with a bile sequestrant, is frequently used and leads to synergistic lowering of LDL levels. For example, nicotinic acid, which effectively inhibits release of lipoproteins from the liver, is quite effective when combined with a bile acid–binding resin. Even more effective is the use of an HMG-CoA reductase inhibitor. This class of drugs, which have been termed statins, directly inhibits cholesterol biosynthesis and as a result not only inhibits the production of new lipoproteins but also, by apparently depleting still further specific hepatic sterol pools, leads to maximal expression of hepatic LDL receptor activity (see Fig. 173–4). This effect is greatly enhanced when used in combination with a bile acid–binding resin and can lower LDL levels by >50%. If these two drugs are combined with nicotinic acid as a third agent, LDL levels can be lowered by as much as 70% or more.

WHOM TO TREAT. The definition of hypercholesterolemia has been undergoing marked changes in recent years as it has become clear that "ideal" or "optimal" cholesterol levels are quite different from "normal" levels, which have been arbitrarily defined as values below the 90th or 95th percentile of the bell-shaped curve of the general population. The expert panel of the National Cholesterol Education Program (NCEP) has recommended specific desirable blood cholesterol levels for the population as a whole (Table 173–4). Many experts have argued that any plasma cholesterol level above 160 to 180 mg per deciliter is above *ideal* values, such as those found in the Japanese, for example, who have a low incidence of CAD. Unfortunately the vast majority of people in the United States have plasma cholesterol levels that are far above this ideal. For this reason, there is an intensive ongoing effort to educate the general public as to appropriate dietary guidelines to lower plasma cholesterol levels.

It should be appreciated that these cutoff points are appropriate for the population as a whole, but assessment of appropriate cholesterol levels for any given patient must take into account the presence of other risk factors. Although many individuals with very high plasma cholesterol levels clearly are at increased risk for CAD (see Ch. 41), most patients who develop CAD actually have total and LDL cholesterol levels that would place them in the borderline or, not infrequently, even below the borderline category. Thus, individuals with hypertension, smoking history, obesity, or diabetes are clearly at increased risk at any given plasma cholesterol level. Individuals with low levels of HDL (i.e., <35 mg per deciliter) are also at significantly increased risk. A strong family history of heart disease is highly predictive of those individuals who are at increased risk. Finally, for patients who have existing CAD and, in particular, for those who have already undergone coronary artery bypass graft or other types of intervention, the cholesterol levels listed above are probably still too high. Achievement of ideal plasma cholesterol levels (i.e., 160 mg per deciliter) is probably more appropriate. Studies in experimental animals and data from clinical trials show that the greater the reduction in plasma cholesterol levels, the greater the clinical benefit achieved.

The NCEP has devised a protocol for screening and management of blood cholesterol in the general population. It is recommended that plasma total cholesterol levels should be measured in all adults over age 20 at least once every 5 years. HDL cholesterol should be measured at the same time whenever possible. These measurements may be made in the nonfasting state. In individuals free of CAD,

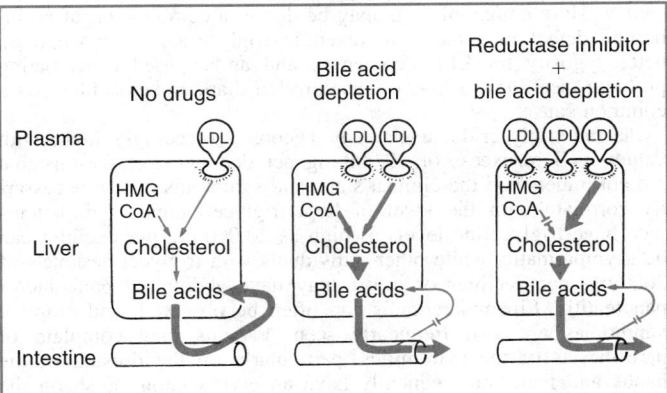

FIGURE 173–4. Mechanisms by which a bile acid–binding resin and an HMG CoA-reductase inhibitor lower plasma LDL levels (From Brown MS, Goldstein JL: A receptor-mediated pathway for cholesterol homeostasis. Science 232:34, 1986. Copyright 1986 by the American Association for the Advancement of Science.)

TABLE 173–4. BLOOD CHOLESTEROL LEVELS

(mg per dl)	Desirable	Borderline	High
Total blood cholesterol	<200	200–239 (borderline high)	>240
LDL	<130	130–159	>160

total cholesterol levels are classified into desirable, borderline, and high levels. It should be appreciated that the cutoff point that defines high blood cholesterol, 240 mg per deciliter, is a value that represents the top 20th percentile of the U.S. adult population and corresponds to a value at which risk for CHD rises more steeply. Similarly, an HDL-cholesterol level < 35 mg per deciliter is defined as low and represents an independent risk factor. For individuals with desirable blood cholesterol levels (< 200 mg per deciliter) the level of HDL cholesterol determines the appropriate follow-up. Those with HDL cholesterol levels >35 mg per deciliter are advised about dietary modification, physical activity, and other risk-reduction activities and to have repeat determinations of total and HDL cholesterol levels in 5 years. Those with HDL cholesterol levels < 35 and/or those who have two or more risk factors should have a formal lipoprotein analysis in the fasting state. These risk factors include man >45 years, woman >55 years or premature menopause not taking estrogen, a positive family history of premature CAD, history of smoking, hypertension, diabetes, obesity, and an HDL cholesterol level below 35 mg per deciliter. The lipoprotein analysis includes measurement of fasting levels of total cholesterol, total triglyceride, and HDL cholesterol. From these values, LDL cholesterol is calculated as follows:

$$\text{LDL cholesterol} = \text{Total cholesterol} - \text{HDL cholesterol} - (\text{triglycerides}/5).$$

Further classification is based on LDL values: LDL cholesterol levels < 130 mg per deciliter are defined as desirable; those 130 to 159 mg per deciliter as borderline high-risk; and those >160 mg per deciliter as high-risk LDL cholesterol levels. Patients with desirable LDL cholesterol levels can be provided education about general dietary habits and risk factor modification. Patients with borderline elevated levels and with fewer than two risk factors can similarly be given dietary instruction with re-evaluation annually. Patients with borderline LDL elevations and two or more risk factors should undergo thorough evaluation, receive dietary therapy, and be considered for drug therapy if they fail to respond. Finally, individuals with high-risk LDL cholesterol levels, >160 mg per deciliter, should have a thorough evaluation to rule out any secondary causes and the presence of a familial lipoprotein disorder and then should begin dietary therapy. Presently the American Heart Association step I or step II diets, which restrict dietary saturated fat and cholesterol, should be prescribed to all individuals with greater than desirable cholesterol levels. This diet is safe for a wide spectrum of individuals, from those as young as age 2 years to the elderly, and usually works best when followed by the whole family.

The NCEP guidelines suggest that all patients with existing CAD have a formal lipoprotein analysis. If LDL cholesterol levels are < 100 mg per deciliter, patients should receive individual instruction on diet and risk-factor reduction. If LDL cholesterol levels are > 100 mg per deciliter, patients should be instructed on an appropriate diet and be considered for drug therapy. The therapeutic goal for treatment of hypercholesterolemia is listed in Table 173–5. The decision to initiate drug therapy for elevated LDL cholesterol levels should be considered in most patients only after the individual has been on a diet for 3 to 6 months. In general, a young or middle-aged adult who has been on such a diet, yet continues to have LDL cholesterol levels >190 mg per deciliter is a candidate for drug therapy even in the absence of other risk factors. Individuals with existing CAD or those who have high LDL cholesterol levels of 160 to 190 mg per deciliter and other risk factors are also candidates for drug therapy, including an HMG-CoA reductase inhibitor, bile acid–binding resins, and nicotinic acid.

The statin class of drugs, which are being used increasingly as primary therapy, lower LDL levels by 25 to 35%. Combinations of a statin and a bile acid–binding resin are also highly efficacious, and LDL lowering of > 50% can frequently be achieved. They have now been in use for more than 10 years with practically no serious side effects. A myositis-like picture has been rarely associated with their use, particularly when combined with nicotinic acid, gemfibrozil, or rarely, with erythromycin. This appears as muscle pain and is associated with increases in muscle creatine kinase (creatine phosphokinase; [CPK]). Rarely, frank rhabdomyolysis has occurred. This side effect has been seen particularly in transplant patients treated with cyclosporine. Abnormalities in liver function tests oc-

TABLE 173–5. THERAPEUTIC GOAL FOR TREATMENT OF HYPERCHOLESTEROLEMIA

Therapeutic Goal LDL cholesterol (mg per dl)	Patient Categories
< 130	Moderate risk for CAD
	Patients with no family history of CAD and no other CAD risk factors
	Young adults with familial hypercholesterolemia
	Adults with familial hypercholesterolemia and no other risk factors
< 100	High risk for CAD
	With family history of CAD or two or more CAD risk factors
	Adult familial hypercholesterolemia patients with family history of CAD or one or more risk factors
	Individual with existing CAD
	Individual after CABG
	Individual with low HDL cholesterol and family history of CAD

LDL = low-density lipoprotein; HDL = high-density lipoprotein; CAD = coronary artery disease; CABG = coronary artery bypass graft surgery.

cur occasionally, but frequently when this occurs there is associated excess alcohol use. CPK levels should be measured prior to the start of statin therapy to obtain baseline levels, at bimonthly intervals during initial use of therapy, and semiannually after that.

TREATMENT OF MILD HYPERTRIGLYCERIDEMIA. The NCEP guidelines do not directly address the issue of hypertriglyceridemia. As noted above, the link between triglycerides and CAD is complex and may be explained by associations between high triglyceride and low HDL levels and atherogenic forms of LDL. Patients with milder degrees of hypertriglyceridemia should be treated initially with nonpharmacologic therapy. This should include weight reduction in overweight patients, increased physical activity, and low-fat diets. Alcohol should be restricted. Gemfibrozil lowers VLDL levels, but frequently there is an associated rise in LDL levels. Niacin has been used to both decrease VLDL and increase HDL. Many experts now use a statin as initial therapy for treating patients with familial combined hyperlipidemia. VLDL levels are lowered, HDL increases, and there is no increase in LDL. In some patients the combined use of gemfibrozil and a statin has been useful, but this combination may increase slightly the risk of myositis.

RECOGNITION AND TREATMENT OF MARKED HYPERTRIGLYCERIDEMIA: THE CHYLOMICRONEMIA SYNDROME. Marked chylomicronemia with plasma triglyceride levels >1000 mg per deciliter is associated with a combination of signs and symptoms that has been termed the *chylomicronemia syndrome*. Prompt and effective therapy is indicated to prevent severe medical complications, including pancreatitis. This syndrome occurs whenever there is excess accumulation of chylomicrons. Rarely this occurs as a result of homozygous LPL deficiency, or apo C-II deficiency. More commonly this may be due to a combination of an inherited defect in a factor involved in triglyceride clearance (e.g., heterozygosity for LPL deficiency) and an acquired exacerbating problem (see Table 173–3). Uncontrolled diabetic ketoacidosis is a common cause.

Plasma triglyceride levels may become exceedingly high, with values well in excess of 20,000 mg per deciliter. For reasons that are not understood the clinical signs and symptoms do not necessarily correlate with the level of hypertriglyceridemia, and patients who have triglyceride levels as high as 20,000 mg per deciliter can be asymptomatic, while other individuals with triglyceride levels of 3000 mg per deciliter or lower may have abdominal pain and/or pancreatitis. Lipemia retinalis can often be observed, and eruptive xanthomas are also frequently seen. Patients may complain of paresthesias of the extremities, particularly on the dorsum of the hands and feet, and frequently have an erythematous flush on the face and chest. With marked hyperchylomicronemia, impairment of recent memory has been noted. Patients also may complain of symmetric arthralgia, although physical findings or joint involvement is not found. In diabetics, this syndrome may be associated with marked insulin resistance, marked hyperglycemia, and frequently diabetic ketoacidosis. Because of the marked hyperchylomicrone-mia, an increased proportion of the total blood volume is occupied by fat, and many routine laboratory tests will be invalid because fat is sampled as well as the water space. For example, hyponatremia is frequently seen in samples from hyperchylomicronemic subjects, but this is a "pseudo hyponatremia" that occurs because of inclusion of lipid in the aliquot of blood sampled, and lipid does not contain sodium. Simple removal of chylomicrons from plasma by a brief centrifugation step before laboratory tests can eliminate such artifacts. Frequently a false-negative test for amylase occurs in lipemic plasma, apparently due to an inhibitor of amylase activity.

The diagnosis is made by the presence of chylomicrons in fasting plasma, which will always appear milky. Plasma will usually appear turbid when plasma triglycerides are > 350 mg per deciliter, because of the excess accumulation of VLDL, and will appear grossly lipemic when triglycerides are > 1000 mg per deciliter. With extreme degrees of hypertriglyceridemia the whole blood takes on the appearance of cream of tomato soup, and plasma allowed to sit in a refrigerator overnight will develop a thick layer of chylomicrons on top. Since the major cause of hyperchylomicronemia is accumulation of dietary-induced fat, the treatment is absolute elimination of fat from the diet until triglyceride levels have fallen to a safe level. With associated pancreatitis, patients usually receive nothing orally, and in this setting plasma triglyceride levels will usually fall by 50% every 2 to 3 days. When refeeding begins, fat (of all kinds) must be totally avoided initially and then replaced very gradually.

RARE DISORDERS OF LIPOPROTEIN METABOLISM

There are a number of inherited disorders of lipoprotein metabolism that are rare but that have taught us a great deal about lipoprotein function. Patients with *hypobetalipoproteinemia* have mutations in one or both apo B alleles that lead to truncated apo B proteins. Because of defective synthesis and/or enhanced intravascular catabolism, there are markedly reduced levels of apo B−containing lipoproteins in plasma. Heterozygotes may have LDL cholesterol levels of ≤ 50 mg per deciliter, and rare compound heterozygotes may have LDL cholesterol levels of ≤ 5 mg per deciliter. Usually these patients are asymptomatic and long lived. Patients with the rare autosomal recessive disorder of *abetalipoproteinemia* have total inability to release apo B-48 from intestinal cells or apo B-100 from liver. They have a normal apo B gene, but lack a lipid transfer protein required for assembly of lipoproteins. Because they cannot make chylomicrons, they malabsorb fat and fat-soluble vitamins. They manifest ataxia, neuropathy, and retinitis pigmentosa and are responsive to high doses of vitamin E. Patients with *Tangier disease* have virtually no HDL in plasma, apparently because of abnormally rapid removal of HDL from plasma. This leads to generation of abnormal chylomicron remnants, which are stored as cholesteryl esters in phagocytic cells. Patients typically have enlarged, orange tonsils and develop corneal opacities and polyneuropathy. Premature atherosclerosis does not seem to occur. No therapy is indicated.

Patients with mutations in *cholesterol ester transfer protein* (CETP) have also recently been described, particularly in Japanese populations, and this is associated with cholesteryl ester enrichment of HDL and greatly elevated HDL cholesterol values, frequently > 100 mg per deciliter. Although not proven, it is generally believed that this mutation is associated with protection from CAD. In contrast, in patients with deficiency of *lecithin cholesterol acyltransferase* (LCAT), unesterified cholesterol accumulates in plasma and tissues, and patients may develop premature CAD. In addition, they have corneal opacities, hemolytic anemia, and early renal failure. Therapy consists of renal transplantation and fat-restricted diets. Two rare disorders leading to accumulation of abnormal sterols have also been described. Patients with *cerebrotendinous xanthomatosis* have defective bile acid synthesis with associated oversynthesis and accumulation of cholestanol and cholesterol in brain, tendons, and other tissues. They can have neurologic symptoms (including cerebellar ataxia and dementia), tendon xanthomas, atherosclerosis, and cataracts. Finally, patients may have large tendon xanthomas due to abnormal accumulation of plant sterols, chiefly β-sitosterol. Normally, plant sterols are not absorbed, but in patients with *sitosterolemia* there is unexplained intestinal absorption and accumulation of β-sitosterol in plasma and tendons. Treatment consists of diets low in plant sterols and cholesterol and the use of cholestyramine to promote gastrointestinal loss.

Breslow J: Familial disorders of high-density lipoprotein metabolism. *In* Scriver CR, Baudet AL, Sly WS, Valle D (eds.): The Metabolic and Molecular Basis of Inherited Disease. New York, McGraw-Hill, 1995, p. 2031. *Comprehensive overview of HDL metabolism.*

Brown MS, Goldstein JL: A receptor-mediated pathway for cholesterol homeostasis. Science 232:34, 1986. *Classic citation describing the LDL receptor pathway—this was the lecture delivered on the occasion of receipt of the Nobel Prize.*

Brunzell JD: Familial lipoprotein lipase deficiency and other causes of the chylomicronemia syndrome. *In* Scriver CR, Baudet AL, Sly WS, Valle D (eds.): The Metabolic and Molecular Basis of Inherited Disease. New York, McGraw-Hill, 1995, p. 1913. *Comprehensive description of disorders leading to accumulation of chylomicrons.*

Goldstein JL, Hobbs HH, Brown MS: Familial hypercholesterolemia. *In* Scriver CR, Baudet AL, Sly WS, Valle D (eds.): The Metabolic and Molecular Basis of Inherited Disease. New York, McGraw Hill, 1995, p. 1981. *Comprehensive description of pathogenesis and clinical description of this important cause of hypercholesterolemia.*

Havel RJ, Kane JP: Introduction: Structure and metabolism of plasma lipoproteins. *In* Scriver CR, Baudet AL, Sly WS, Valle D (eds.): The Metabolic and Molecular Basis of Inherited Disease. New York, McGraw-Hill, 1995, p. 1841. *Excellent overview of lipoprotein metabolism.*

Kane JP, Havel RJ: Disorders of the biogenesis and secretion of lipoproteins containing the B-apolipoproteins. *In* Scriver CR, Baudet AL, Sly WS, Valle D (eds.): The Metabolic and Molecular Basis of Inherited Disease. New York, McGraw-Hill, 1995, p. 1853. *Comprehensive and current concepts of metabolism of apo B-containing lipoproteins.*

Mahley RW, Rall SC: Type III hyperlipoproteinemia (dysbetalipoproteinemia): The role of apolipoprotein E in normal and abnormal lipoprotein metabolism. *In* Scriver CR, Baudet AL, Sly WS, Valle D (eds.): The Metabolic and Molecular Basis of Inherited Disease. New York, McGraw-Hill, 1995, p. 1953. *Most comprehensive and up-to-date discussion of role of apo E in lipoprotein metabolism.*

Steinberg D, Olefsky JM: Hypercholesterolemia and Atherosclerosis: Pathogenesis and Prevention. New York, Churchill Livingstone, 1987. *Easy-to-read book covering both basic research and clinical aspects of lipoprotein metabolism and their relationship to atherosclerosis.*

Witztum JL, Steinberg D: The role of oxidized LDL in atherogenesis. J Clin Invest 88:1785, 1991. *Overview of hypothesis that oxidation of lipoproteins contributes to their atherogenicity.*

174 LYSOSOMAL STORAGE DISEASES

Margaret M. McGovern and Robert J. Desnick

The lysosomal storage diseases are a family of more than 30 disorders resulting from different defects in lysosomal function. Although most of these disorders are caused by the deficiency of a specific hydrolytic enzyme, others are due to impaired receptors or deficiencies of crucial cofactors or protective proteins. Prevalent among these disorders are Fabry's disease, Gaucher's disease, and Niemann-Pick disease, lipid storage diseases that result from mutations in specific genes that encode lipid-degrading enzymes. The respective enzymatic defects lead to the storage in lysosomes of specific lipids and their metabolites. All three of these disorders have later-onset forms that can present in adult life. In addition, Gaucher's disease and Niemann-Pick disease have severe, fatal infantile forms that are described briefly.

FABRY'S DISEASE

DEFINITION. Fabry's disease is an X-linked inborn error of glycosphingolipid metabolism characterized by angiokeratomas (telangiectatic skin lesions), hypohidrosis, corneal and lenticular opacities, acroparesthesias, and vascular disease of the kidney, heart, and/or brain. The disease has an estimated incidence of 1 in 40,000 males.

ETIOLOGY AND PATHOGENESIS. Fabry's disease is an X-linked recessive trait that is manifested in affected hemizygous males. Atypical hemizygous males with residual α-galactosidase A activity may be asymptomatic or have late-onset, mild disease manifestations primarily limited to the heart. Heterozygous females are usually asymptomatic or exhibit mild manifestations. The disease results from the deficient activity of a lysosomal hydrolase (Table 174–1). The course of the disease is more severe in affected males with blood group B or AB, since the blood group B substance also

TABLE 174-1. BIOCHEMICAL AND PHENOTYPIC CHARACTERISTICS OF LYSOSOMAL STORAGE DISEASES

	Deficiency	Accumulation	Accumulation Site	Resultant Complications
Fabry's	α-Galactosidase A	Primarily globotriaosylceramide	Lysosomes of vascular endothelial and smooth muscle cells	Ischemia, infarction
Gaucher's				
Type 1	Acid β-glucosidase	Primarily glucosylceramide	Macrophage-monocyte system	Infiltration of bone marrow, progressive hepatosplenomegaly, skeletal complications
Type 2	Acid β-glucosidase	Primarily glucosylceramide	Macrophage-monocyte system; CNS	Infiltration of bone marrow, progressive hepatosplenomegaly, skeletal complications, neurodegeneration
Type 3	Acid β-glucosidase	Primarily glucosylceramide	Macrophage-monocyte system; CNS	Progressive neurodegeneration
Niemann-Pick				
Type A	Acid sphingomyelinase	Sphingomyelin	Monocyte-macrophage system; CNS	Hepatosplenomegaly, no neurologic disease
Type B	Acid sphingomyelinase	Sphingomyelin	Monocyte-macrophage system	Progressive hepatosplenomegaly, infiltrative lung disease

accumulates as it is normally degraded by α-galactosidase A. The molecular basis of Fabry's disease has been identified for a number of patients (Table 174–2).

PATHOLOGY. Fabry's disease is characterized by marked deposition of globotriaosylceramide and related glycosphingolipids with terminal α-galactosyl moieties primarily in the plasma and in the lysosomes of endothelial, perithelial, and smooth muscle cells of blood vessels. These glycosphingolipid deposits also are prominent in epithelial cells of the cornea, in glomeruli and tubules of the kidney, in muscle fibers of the heart, and in ganglion cells of the dorsal roots and autonomic nervous system. The skin lesions are telangiectases. Capillaries, venules, and arterioles show pathologic lipid storage, and there is marked dilatation of the capillaries of the dermal papillae just below the epidermis. The larger lesions are usually located in the upper dermis, where they may produce elevation, flattening, or hypertrophy of the epithelium, with keratosis—hence the term angiokeratoma. Ultrastructurally the glycosphingolipid inclusions in lysosomes have a concentrically arranged lamellar or myelin-like structure.

CLINICAL MANIFESTATIONS. The angiokeratomas usually occur in childhood, which may lead to early diagnosis. They increase in size and number with age and range from barely visible to several millimeters in diameter. The lesions are punctate, dark red to blue-black, and flat or slightly raised. They do not blanch with pressure, and the larger ones may show slight hyperkeratosis. Characteristically the lesions are most dense between the umbilicus and knees, in the "bathing trunk area," but may occur anywhere, including the oral mucosa. The hips, thighs, buttocks, umbilicus, lower abdomen, scrotum, and glans penis are common sites, and there is a tendency toward bilateral symmetry. Variants without skin lesions have been described. Sweating is usually decreased or absent. Corneal opacities and characteristic lenticular lesions, observed in slit-lamp examination, are present in affected males as well as in about 70% of asymptomatic heterozygotes. Conjunctival and retinal vascular tortuosity are common and result from the systemic vascular involvement.

Pain is the most debilitating symptom in childhood and adolescence. Fabry crises, lasting from minutes to several days, consist of agonizing, burning pain in the hands and feet and proximal extremities and are usually associated with exercise, fatigue, and/or fever. These painful acroparesthesias usually become less frequent in the third and fourth decades of life, although in some men they may become more frequent and severe. Attacks of abdominal or flank pain may simulate appendicitis or renal colic.

With increasing age, the major morbid symptoms result from the progressive involvement of the vascular system. Early in the course of the disease, casts, red cells, and lipid inclusions with characteristic birefringent "Maltese crosses" appear in the urinary sediment. Proteinuria, isothenuria, and gradual deterioration of renal function and development of azotemia occur in the second to fourth decades of life. Cardiovascular findings may include hypertension, left ventricular hypertrophy, anginal chest pain, myocardial ischemia or infarction, and congestive heart failure. Mitral insufficiency is the most common valvular lesion. Abnormal electrocardiographic and echocardiographic findings are common. Cerebrovascular manifestations result primarily from multifocal small vessel involvement. Other features may include chronic bronchitis and dyspnea, lymphedema of the legs without hypoproteinemia, episodic diarrhea, osteoporosis, retarded growth, and delayed puberty. Death most often results from uremia or vascular disease of the heart or brain. Prior to hemodialysis or renal transplantation, the mean age at death for affected men was 41 years. Atypical male variants with residual α-galactosidase A activity who are asymptomatic or mildly affected have been described, and more recently, several patients with late-onset isolated cardiac or cardiopulmonary disease have been reported. These patients do not have the early classic manifestations. These "cardiac variants" have cardiomegaly, usually involving the left ventricular wall and interventricular septum, and electrocardiographic abnormalities consistent with cardiomyopathy. Others have had hypertrophic cardiomyopathy and/or myocardial infarctions.

DIAGNOSIS. The diagnosis in classically affected males is most readily made from the history of painful acroparesthesias, hypo-

TABLE 174-2. MOLECULAR GENETICS OF FABRY'S, GAUCHER'S, AND NIEMANN-PICK DISEASES

	Chromosome Assignment	Molecular Characteristics	Comments
Fabry's	Xq22	cDNA, entire genomic sequences, > 50 mutant alleles known	Many mutations responsible for disease include amino acid substitutions, gene rearrangements, mRNA splicing defects
Gaucher's	1q21	cDNA, functional and pseudogenomic sequences, > 35 mutant alleles known	4 mutations (N370S, L444P, 84insG, IVS2^{+1}) account for 90–95% of mutant alleles in Ashkenazi Jewish patients
Niemann-Pick			
Types A and B	11p15.1 to p15.4	cDNA, entire genomic sequence, > 30 mutant alleles known	3 mutations account for > 90% of mutant alleles in Ashkenazi Jewish patients with type A disease
Type C	Chromosome 18	—	Specific gene and nature of cholesterol defect unknown

cDNA = complimentary DNA; mRNA = messenger RNA.

hidrosis, the presence of characteristic skin lesions, and the observation of the characteristic corneal opacities and lenticular lesions. The disorder is often misdiagnosed as rheumatic fever, erythromelalgia, or neurosis. The skin lesions must be differentiated from the benign angiokeratomas of the scrotum (Fordyce's disease) or from angiokeratoma circumscriptum. Angiokeratomas identical to those of Fabry's disease have been reported in fucosidosis, aspartylglycosaminuria, late-onset GM_1 gangliosidosis, galactosialidosis, α-N-acetylgalactosaminidase deficiency, and sialidosis. The diagnosis of the mild cardiac variants should be considered in individuals with left ventricular hypertrophy and/or cardiomyopathy. The diagnosis of classic and variant cases is confirmed biochemically by markedly decreased α-galactosidase A activity in plasma, isolated leukocytes, or cultured fibroblasts or lymphoblasts.

Heterozygous females may have corneal opacities, isolated skin lesions, and intermediate activities of α-galactosidase A in plasma or cell sources. Rare female heterozygotes may have manifestations as severe as those in affected males. However, in asymptomatic at-risk females in families affected by Fabry's disease, optimal diagnosis should be by direct analysis of their family's specific mutation. Prenatal detection of affected males can be accomplished by demonstrating deficient α-galactosidase A activity or by detecting the family's specific gene mutation in chorionic villi obtained in the first trimester of pregnancy or in cultured amniocytes obtained by amniocentesis in the second trimester.

TREATMENT. Phenytoin and carbamazepine have been shown to decrease the frequency and severity of the chronic acroparesthesias and the periodic crises of excruciating pain. Otherwise, treatment of the disease complications is supportive and nonspecific. Renal transplantation and long-term hemodialysis have become life-saving procedures. Replacement therapy using partially purified human enzyme has proved to be biochemically effective in pilot trials; however, sufficient enzyme has not been available to evaluate the clinical effectiveness of long-term replacement therapy. The recent availability of the cDNA encoding human α-galactosidase A should permit the future expression of sufficient quantities of recombinantly produced, active enzyme for further trials of enzyme replacement therapy and future trials of gene therapy.

Desnick RJ, Ioannou YA, Eng CM: Fabry disease: α-Galactosidase deficiency and Schindler disease: α-N-acetylgalactosaminidase deficiency. *In* Scriver CR, Beaudet AL, Sly WS, Valle D (eds.): The Metabolic and Molecular Bases of Inherited Disease, 7th ed. New York, McGraw-Hill, 1995. *Definitive chapter describing clinical, pathologic, biochemical, and molecular manifestations of Fabry's disease with more than 400 references.*
Eng CM, Desnick RJ: Molecular basis of Fabry disease: Mutations and polymorphisms in the human α-galactosidase A gene. Hum Mutation 3:103, 1994. *Description of mutations in classic and variant cases.*

GAUCHER'S DISEASE

DEFINITION. Gaucher's disease is a lipid storage disease characterized by deposition of glucocerebroside in cells of the macrophage-monocyte system. There are three clinical subtypes delineated by the absence or presence and progression of neurologic involvement: Type 1 or the adult, non-neuronopathic form; type 2, the infantile or acute neuronopathic form; and type 3, the juvenile or Norrbotten form. All three subtypes are inherited as autosomal recessive traits. Type 1 disease is the most common lysosomal storage disease and the most prevalent genetic disorder among Ashkenazi Jewish individuals, with an incidence of about 1 in 1000 and a carrier frequency of about 1 in 16 to 18.

ETIOLOGY AND PATHOGENESIS. All three subtypes of Gaucher's disease result from deficient activity of a lysosomal hydrolase (Table 174–1). The molecular basis of Gaucher's disease has been identified for 90 to 95% of Ashkenazi Jewish patients (Table 174–2). Genotype/phenotype correlations have been noted for the different subtypes and may provide the molecular basis for the remarkable clinical variation in type 1 Gaucher's disease. Presumably the amount of residual enzymatic activity determines disease subtype and severity. For example, type 1 patients homozygous for the milder N370S mutation tend to have a later onset and milder course than patients with one N370S allele and another mutant allele. However, the wide variability in clinical presentation among Gaucher's disease patients cannot be fully explained by the underlying acid β-glucosidase mutations. The lesions causing the severe type 2 (infantile) disease express little, if any, enzymatic activity *in vitro*.

PATHOLOGY. The pathologic hallmark is the presence of the Gaucher cell in the macrophage-monocyte system, particularly in the bone marrow. These cells, which are 20 to 100 μm in diameter, have a characteristic wrinkled-paper appearance resulting from intracytoplasmic substrate deposition. These cells stain strongly positive with periodic acid–Schiff, and their presence in bone marrow and/or other tissues suggests the diagnosis (Fig. 174–1). The accumulated glycolipid, glucosylceramide, is derived primarily from the phagocytosis and degradation of senescent leukocytes and to a lesser extent erythrocyte membranes. Glycolipid storage results in organomegaly and pulmonary infiltration. Neuronal cell loss in patients with types 2 and 3 disease presumably results from accumulation of the cytotoxic glycolipid, glucosphingosine, in the brain due to the severe deficiency of acid β-glucosidase activity. Glucosylceramide accumulation in the bone marrow, liver, spleen, lungs, and kidney leads to pancytopenia, massive hepatosplenomegaly, diffuse infiltrative pulmonary disease, and nephropathy or glomerulonephritis. The progressive infiltration of Gaucher cells in the bone marrow causes thinning of the cortex, pathologic fractures, bone pain, bony infarcts, and osteopenia. Central nervous system (CNS) involvement occurs only in patients with types 2 and 3 disease.

CLINICAL MANIFESTATIONS. There is a broad spectrum of clinical expression among patients with type 1 disease, in part due to a combination of different mutant alleles. Onset of clinical manifestations occurs from early childhood to late adulthood with most seen by adolescence. At presentation, patients may have easy bruisability due to thrombocytopenia, chronic fatigue secondary to anemia, hepatomegaly with or without elevated liver function tests, splenomegaly, and bone pain or pathologic fractures. Occasional patients have pulmonary involvement. Patients whose disease is diagnosed in the first 5 years of life are frequently non-Jewish and typically have a more malignant disease course. Patients with milder disease are discovered later in life during evaluations for hemato-

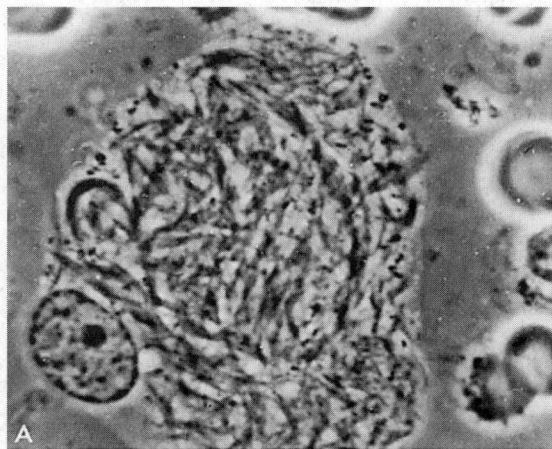

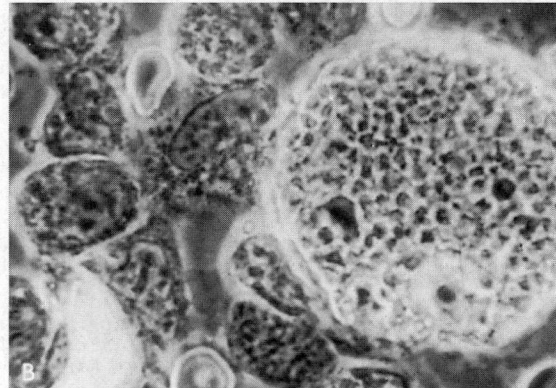

FIGURE 174–1. Typical Gaucher cell *(A)* and a foam cell seen in Niemann-Pick disease *(B)*. Both are viewed under phase microscopy in unstained smears of aspirated bone marrow. Magnification can be estimated from adjacent red cells.

logic or skeletal problems or are found to have splenomegaly on routine examinations. In symptomatic patients, splenomegaly is progressive and can become massive. Clinically apparent bony involvement, which occurs in >20% of patients, can present as bone pain or pathologic fractures. Most patients have radiologic evidence of skeletal involvement, including an Erlenmeyer flask deformity of the distal femur, which is an early skeletal change. In patients with symptomatic bone disease, lytic lesions can develop in the long bones, ribs, and pelvis, and osteosclerosis may be evident at an early age. Bone crises with severe pain and swelling can occur. Bleeding secondary to thrombocytopenia may manifest as epistaxis and bruising and is frequently overlooked until other symptoms become apparent. Children with massive splenomegaly are short of stature because of energy expenditure required by the enlarged organ.

Type 2 disease, which is rare and panethnic in distribution, is characterized by a rapid neurodegenerative course with extensive visceral involvement and death within the first 2 years of life. The disease occurs in infancy with increased tone, strabismus, and organomegaly. Failure to thrive and stridor due to laryngospasm are typical. The progressive psychomotor degeneration leads to death, usually due to respiratory compromise.

Type 3 disease is noted in infancy or childhood. In addition to the organomegaly and bony involvement, neurologic involvement is present. There is a high frequency of type 3 disease in Sweden (1 in 50,000), which has been traced to a common founder in the 17th century. Type 3 has been further classified as type 3a and 3b based on the extent of neurologic involvement and whether there is progressive myotonia and dementia (type 3a) or isolated supranuclear gaze palsy (type 3b).

DIAGNOSIS. Gaucher's disease should be considered in the differential diagnosis of patients with unexplained organomegaly, easy bruisability, and/or bone pain. Bone marrow examination usually reveals the presence of Gaucher cells; however, all suspect diagnoses should be confirmed by demonstrating deficient acid β-glucosidase activity in isolated leukocytes or cultured fibroblasts. For possible genotype/phenotype correlations, the specific acid β-glucosidase mutation may be determined, particularly inAshkenazi Jewish patients. Carrier identification can be achieved by enzymatic assay confirmed with DNA testing in most Jewish families. Testing should be offered to all family members, but it should be kept in mind that heterogeneity even among members of the same kindred can be so great that cases may be diagnosed in asymptomatic affected individuals during such testing. Prenatal diagnosis is available by determining enzymatic activity or specific mutations in chorionic villi or cultured amniotic fluid cells.

TREATMENT. In the past, management of patients with type 1 disease was primarily symptomatic, including blood transfusions for anemia, partial or total splenectomy for severe mechanical cardiopulmonary compromise or hypersplenism, analgesics for bone pain, and orthopedic procedures for joint replacement. A small number of patients also have undergone bone marrow transplantation, which, if successful, is curative. However, a matched donor is required, and there are significant morbidity and mortality due to the procedure. There is no effective treatment for the neurologic involvement in types 2 and 3 disease. More recently, the safety and efficacy of enzyme replacement with purified placental or recombinant acid β-glucosidase has been demonstrated in type 1 disease. Clinical trials have demonstrated that most extraskeletal symptoms are reversed by initial debulking doses of enzyme (30 to 60 IU per kilogram) administered by intravenous infusion every other week. The effectiveness of enzyme replacement in reversing and preventing bony manifestations is still under study; however, early data indicate that it may be efficacious. Efforts are also under way to develop gene therapy for type 1 disease.

Beutler E, Grabowski G: Gaucher disease. *In* Scriver CR, Beaudet AL, Sly WS, Valle D (eds.): The Metabolic and Molecular Bases of Inherited Disease, 7th ed. New York, McGraw-Hill, 1995. *Comprehensive review of the clinical, biochemical, and molecular features of Gaucher's disease.*

Pastores GM, Sibille AR, Grabowski GA: Enzyme therapy in Gaucher disease type 1: Dosage efficacy and adverse events in 33 patients treated for 6 to 24 months. Blood 82:408, 1991. *Description of initial experience with enzyme replacement therapy.*

NIEMANN-PICK DISEASE

DEFINITION. The four major subtypes of Niemann-Pick disease (NPD) are characterized by accumulation of sphingomyelin and cholesterol in lysosomes of cells of the macrophage-monocyte system. Type A disease is a fatal disorder of infancy, whereas type B disease is a non-neuronopathic form in which most affected individuals live into adulthood and suffer primarily from hepatic and pulmonary involvement. Types C and D disease are neurodegenerative disorders with onset in early or late childhood. All four subtypes are inherited as autosomal recessive traits and display variable clinical features.

ETIOLOGY AND PATHOGENESIS. Types A and B NPD result from deficient activity of a lysosomal hydrolase (Table 174–1). In Types C and D NPD the genetic defect(s) involve the defective transport of cholesterol from the lysosome to the cytosol. The gene encoding the defect in type C disease has been localized (Table 174–2), but the specific gene and nature of the cholesterol transport defect remain unknown.

PATHOLOGY. The pathologic hallmark in types A and B NPD is the histochemically characteristic lipid-laden foam cell, often referred to as the Niemann-Pick cell. These cells, which can be readily distinguished from Gaucher cells by their histologic and histochemical characteristics, are not pathognomic for NPD, since histologically similar cells are found in patients with Wolman's disease, cholesterol ester storage disease, lipoprotein lipase deficiency, and in some patients with GM$_1$ gangliosidosis, type 2. Sphingomyelin is the major lipid that accumulates in the cells and tissues of patients with types A and B NPD. In most normal tissues, sphingomyelin constitutes 5 to 20% of the total cellular phospholipid content; however, in patients with types A and B NPD the sphingomyelin levels may be elevated up to 50-fold, constituting about 70% of the total phospholipid fraction. Lysosomal sphingomyelin accumulation in brain, liver, kidney, and lungs have been documented with organs from patients with types A and B NPD which contain about the same amount of sphingomyelin, with the notable exception that patients with type B NPD have little or no lipid storage in their CNS. In general, patients with type A disease have less than 5% of normal acid sphingomyelinase activity when determined in cultured fibroblasts and/or lymphocytes, whereas cells from type B patients typically have 10 to 20% of normal activity that presumably prevents development of the neurologic symptoms.

CLINICAL MANIFESTATIONS. The clinical presentation and course of type A NPD is relatively uniform and is characterized by normal appearance at birth, although the newborn period is sometimes complicated by prolonged jaundice. Hepatosplenomegaly, moderate lymphadenopathy, and psychomotor retardation are evident by 6 months of life and are followed by rapid neurodegeneration. The loss of motor function and deterioration of intellectual capabilities are progressive. In later stages, spasticity and rigidity are evident with affected infants experiencing complete loss of contact with their environment.

In contrast to the stereotyped type A phenotype, the clinical presentation and course in patients with type B disease are more variable. Most cases are diagnosed in infancy or childhood when enlargement of the liver and/or spleen is detected during a routine physical examination. At diagnosis, type B patients also have evidence of mild pulmonary involvement, usually detected as a diffuse reticular or finely nodular infiltration on chest roentenogram. In most patients, hepatosplenomegaly is particularly prominent in childhood, but with increasing linear growth the abdominal protuberance decreases and becomes less conspicuous. In mildly affected patients the splenomegaly may not be noted until adulthood, and there may be minimal disease manifestations. In most patients with type B disease, decreased pulmonary diffusion due to alveolar infiltration becomes evident in childhood and progresses with age. Severely affected individuals may experience significant pulmonary compromise by age 15 to 20. Such patients have low PO$_2$ values and dyspnea on exertion. Life-threatening bronchopneumonia may occur and cor pulmonale has been described. Severely affected patients also may have liver involvement leading to life-threatening cirrhosis, portal hypertension, and ascites. Clinically significant pancytopenia due to secondary hypersplenism may necessitate partial or total splenectomy. Typically, patients with type B disease do not have neurologic involvement and are intellectually intact.

Patients with type C disease often have prolonged neonatal jaundice, appear normal for 1 to 2 years, and then experience a slowly progressive and variable neurodegenerative course. Their hepatosplenomegaly is less severe than in patients with types A or B disease, and they may survive into adulthood. Patients with type D NPD develop neurologic symptoms later in childhood and have a slower neurodegenerative course than patients with type C. Most patients with type D disease share a common ancestry traceable to the Acadians from Yarmouth County, Nova Scotia. It appears that these patients also have an abnormality in cholesterol metabolism and that the defect may be allelic with that causing type C disease.

DIAGNOSIS. Type A disease is diagnosed in the patient's first year of life with failure to thrive, organomegaly, and severe psychomotor retardation. In type B NPD, splenomegaly is usually noted early in childhood; however, in very mild cases, the enlargement may be subtle and detection may be delayed until adolescence or adulthood. The presence of the characteristic Niemann-Pick cells in the bone marrow supports the diagnosis. However, patients with types C and D disease also have extensive infiltration of these cells in the bone marrow. Thus, all suspect cases should be evaluated enzymatically to confirm the clinical diagnosis by measuring the sphingomyelinase activity level in peripheral leukocytes, cultured fibroblasts, and/or lymphoblasts. Patients with type A and B disease will have markedly decreased levels of enzymatic activity (1 to 10% of normal), whereas patients with types C and D disease may have slightly decreased sphingomyelinase activity (50 to 75% of normal), and patients with Gaucher's disease and other storage disorders presenting with hepatosplenomegaly and/or neurologic involvement will have normal or near-normal levels. Types C and D disease can be biochemically documented by demonstrating the cholesterol transport defect in cultured fibroblasts. The enzymatic identification of type A and B carriers is problematic. However, in families in which the specific molecular lesion has been identified, family members can be accurately tested for heterozygote status by DNA analysis. Heterozygote identification for types C and D disease is unavailable. Prenatal diagnosis of types A and B disease may be reliably made by measuring acid sphingomyelinase activity in cultured amniocytes or chorionic villi. In families in which the specific molecular lesions are known, the prenatal diagnosis can be made by DNA analysis of the fetal cells.

TREATMENT. At present there is no specific treatment available for any of the NPD subtypes. Orthotopic liver transplantation in an infant with type A disease and amniotic cell transplantation in several patients with type B disease have been attempted with little or no success. Bone marrow transplantation in a type B patient was successful in reducing the spleen and liver volumes, the sphingomyelin content of the liver, the number of Niemann-Pick cells in the marrow, and the radiologic infiltration of the lungs. However, no long-term information is available as this patient died 3 months after transplantation. To date, lung transplantation has not been performed in any severely compromised patient with type B disease. Future prospects for treatment of type B disease include enzyme replacement and gene therapy. Treatment of types A, C, and D disease are presently precluded by the severe neurologic involvement.

Schuchman EH, Desnick RJ: Types A and B Niemann-Pick Disease. *In* Scriver CR, Beaudet AL, Sly WS, Valle D (eds.): The Metabolic and Molecular Bases of Inherited Disease, 7th ed. New York, McGraw-Hill, 1994. *The most up-to-date description of the clinical, metabolic, and molecular nature of Niemann-Pick types A and B.*

Inborn Errors of Amino Acid Metabolism

175 HYPERAMINOACIDURIA
(With a Classification of the Inborn and Developmental Errors of Amino Acid Metabolism)
Charles R. Scriver

Study of inborn errors has improved our knowledge of amino acid metabolism, as well as the diagnosis and treatment of associated diseases. The inborn errors of renal amino acid transport affect either a carrier or a metabolic process coupled to the transcellular flux that achieves normal reabsorption.

L-Aminoaciduria, representing less than 2 to 3% of the total urinary nitrogen, is a normal phenomenon. More than 95% of the filtered amino acid load is reabsorbed by the proximal portion of the renal tubule; the remainder is excreted in the urine. Efficiency of renal tubular transport of an amino acid is related to its chemical and steric structure, the amount in the glomerular filtrate, and the gender, age, and physiologic state of the subject. Abnormal aminoaciduria (hyperaminoaciduria) is a result of acquired or hereditary disturbances of cellular metabolism or transport. Table 175-1 shows the known hyperaminoacidurias. (The table includes several disorders of amino acid metabolism that do not show hyperaminoaciduria but affect organic acid and fatty acid derivatives; they can be detected in urine by gas chromatography.)

The hyperaminoacidurias are explained by several mechanisms acting on net reabsorption in the proximal tubule (Fig. 175-1):

1. *Saturation:* The concentration of amino acid in filtrate approaches or exceeds the capacity of the tubular system to reabsorb it (overflow or prerenal aminoaciduria).
2. *Competition:* One amino acid at elevated concentration competes with another sharing the same transporter ("combined" aminoaciduria).
3. *Modification of transporter:* The amino acid is not transported efficiently because its carrier is altered (renal aminoaciduria).
4. *Inhibition of substrate transfer:* The coupling of energy to the transporter is altered, and flux is impaired (renal aminoaciduria).

Renal transporters show preferences for either single free amino acids or specific groups of them. The transport systems identified in Table 175-1 (group III) were revealed through loss of function in the variant (mutant or developmental) state. Oligopeptides are transported on carriers different from those used by free amino acids.

Scriver CR, Beaudet A, Sly W, Valle D (eds.): The Metabolic and Molecular Bases of Inherited Disease. 7th ed. New York, McGraw-Hill, 1995. *The mendelian disorders of amino acid metabolism (catabolism or transport) are described, chapter by chapter, in detail.*

Scriver CR, Tenenhouse HS: Mendelian phenotypes as "probes" of renal transport systems for amino acids and phosphate. *In* Windhager E (ed.): Handbook of Physiology: Renal Physiology. New York, Oxford University Press, Section 8, Vol. II, pp. 1977–2016, 1992. *A review of the inborn errors of renal amino acid transport and associated transport systems.*

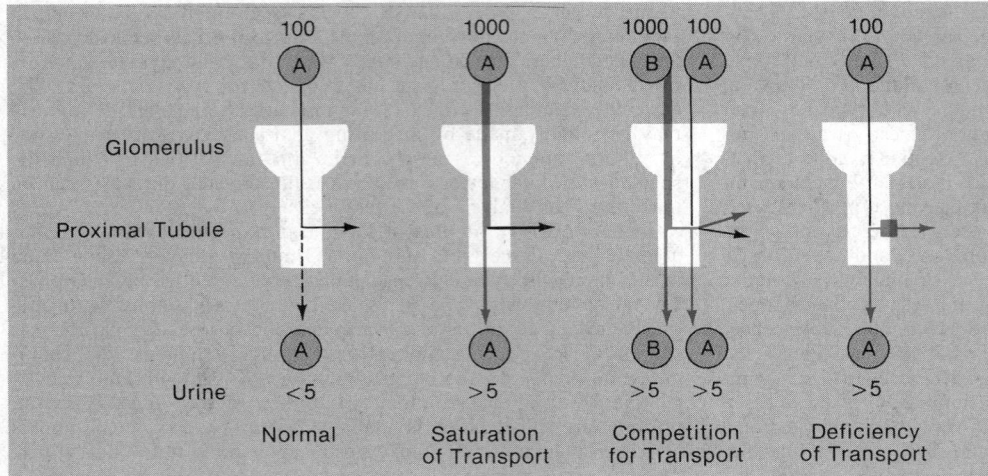

FIGURE 175–1. Mechanism of hyperaminoaciduria. *Panel 1:* Normal reabsorption reclaims >95% of filtered amino acid molecules. Hyperaminoaciduria can occur if *(Panel 2)* filtered load increases (10× increase shown) and transport mechanism is saturated, if *(Panel 3)* amino acid (B) (in excess) competes with another (A) on a shared carrier, or if *(Panel 4)* carrier itself or coupling of energy to carrier is impaired.

TABLE 175–1. HEREDITARY AND ACQUIRED AMINOACIDOPATHIES

The aminoacidurias presented in this table are divided into acquired and inherited types. Disturbances related to perinatal adaptive phenomena of multifactorial origin are included. The classification recognizes physiologic factors affecting amino acid distribution between plasma and urine, and whether the disorder primarily affects catabolism or membrane transport of the amino acid(s).

Thus the disorders are grouped according to mechanism and preferred fluid for detection. The data refer to those conditions associated with perturbation of the normal content of ninhydrin-reactive metabolites in plasma or urine; some exceptions have been made to include ninhydrin-negative metabolites where it is relevant.

GROUP IA

The primary defect is in catabolism. There is a low renal clearance of amino acid but a hyperaminoaciduria by saturation of transepithelial transport. Detection in the plasma is preferable unless otherwise indicated, but using urine for screening (or diagnosis) is not precluded; assignment to this group implies primarily that diagnosis (or screening) of the condition is feasible by virtue of significant metabolite accumulation in blood (or plasma).

Amino Acid Affected:
↓ = decreased; ↑ = increased. Source of enzyme number is *Enzyme Commission.* IP = apparent inheritance pattern; AR = autosomal recessive; AD = autosomal dominant; (AR) = probably autosomal recessive; XL = X-linked. *Remarks:* CNS = central nervous system; CoA = coenzyme A; CSF = cerebrospinal fluid.

Condition or Disease	Amino Acid Affected	Enzyme Affected (Synonym) In Group A	IP	Remarks
Common Perinatal (Adaptive) Traits*				
Neonatal hyperphenylalaninemia	Phenylalanine	? Phenylalanine 4-mono-oxygenase (phenylalanine-hydroxylating system) [1.14.16.1]	—	Benign; may respond to folic acid; often occurs with tyrosinemia
Neonatal tyrosinemia	Tyrosine	4-Hydroxyphenylpyruvate dioxygenase (p-hydroxyphenyl pyruvic acid hydroxylase) [1.13.11.27]	—	Benign; responds to ascorbic acid and reduced protein intake
Hypermethioninemia	Methionine	Methionine adenosyltransferase (ATP: L-methionine S-adenosyltransferase) [2.5.1.6]; hepatic isoenzyme	—	Benign; usually found with high protein intake
Hyperhistidinemia	Histidine	? L-Histidine ammonia-lyase [4.3.1.3]	—	Benign; related to high protein intake
Inherited Traits				
Hyperphenylalaninemia				
Classic phenylketonuria	Phenylalanine	Phenylalanine 4-mono-oxygenase (L-phenylalanine, tetrahydropteridine:oxygen oxidoreductase [4-hydroxylating]) [1.14.16.1]	AR	Plasma phenylalanine >1 mM; causes mental retardation when untreated; L-phenylalanine tolerance in diet is 250–500 mg/day
"Mild" phenylketonuria	Phenylalanine	Same	AR	Plasma phenylalanine >1 mM; similar to entry above, but dietary tolerance for L-phenylalanine is >500 mg/day
Transient "hyperphenylalaninemia"	Phenylalanine	Pterin-4α-carbinolamine hydratase	AR	Plasma phenylalanine elevated; change in status to that of next entry or normal, several months (or years) after birth
Non-PKU hyperphenylalaninemia	Phenylalanine	Phenylalanine 4-mono-oxygenase	AR	Plasma phenylalanine <1 mM on normal diet; less effect on IQ
Dihydropteridine reductase deficiency	Phenylalanine	Dihydropteridine reductase [1.6.99.7]	AR	Deficient tetrahydrobiopterin cofactor recycling also impairs biosynthesis of L-dopa and 5-hydroxytryptamine (5-HT) in CNS; low-phenylalanine diet does not correct this

TABLE 175–1. HEREDITARY AND ACQUIRED AMINOACIDOPATHIES *Continued*

Condition or Disease	Amino Acid Affected	Enzyme Affected (Synonym) *In Group A*	IP	Remarks
Inherited Traits (Continued)				
Biopterin synthesis defects	Phenylalanine	GTP-cyclohydrolase [3.5.4.16] or 6-pyruvoyltetrahydropterin synthase [4.6.1.10] in pathway for tetrahydrobiopterin synthesis	AR	Deficient cofactor synthesis; see preceding entry for effect
Hypertyrosinemia				
Tyrosinosis (Medes)	Tyrosine	? Tyrosine aminotransferase (L-tyrosine:α-ketoglutarate aminotransferase) [2.6.1.5]	(AR)	One case known; myasthenia gravis probably incidental finding
Hypertyrosinemia I	Tyrosine (and methionine in acute stage)	Fumarylacetoacetate hydrolase [3.7.1.2]	AR	Hepatic cirrhosis and renal tubular failure; usually fatal in absence of effective treatment
Hypertyrosinemia II	Tyrosine	Soluble (cytosol) tyrosine aminotransferase [2.6.1.5]	AR	Can be associated with developmental retardation; Richner-Hanhart syndrome in most patients
Hawkinsinuria	Tyrosine	4-Hydroxyphenylpyruvate dioxygenase [1.13.11.27]	AD	Disease signs are variable and include failure to thrive; reflect formation of epoxides and adducts of glutathione
Hyperhistidinemia†				
Classic form	Histidine (alanine high in some cases)	L-Histidine ammonia-lyase [4.3.1.3]; liver, epidermis	AR	Harmless condition in majority
Branched-chain hyperaminoacidemia‡ Maple syrup urine disease (classic)	Leucine, isoleucine, valine, alloisoleucine	Branched-chain α-keto acid lipoate oxidoreductase (probably decarboxylase component) [1.2.4.3(4)]	AR	Clinical variants from: postnatal collapse and mental retardation in survivors (diet therapy can be effective); to intermittent symptoms (development may be otherwise normal); to unremittent (milder than classic form).
Thiamine-responsive form	Same	Same	AR	Mild form; responsive to thiamine (vitamin B₁)
Multiple dehydrogenase form; E₃ deficiency	Same (plus pyruvate and α-ketoglutarate)	Dihydrolipoamide dehydrogenase [1.8.1.4]	AR	Congenital lactic acidosis plus branched-chain amino-keto acid disorder
Hypervalinemia	Valine	Branched-chain amino-acid aminotransferase (valine aminotransferase) [2.6.1.66]	AR	Retarded development and vomiting; responds to diet
Hyperlysinemia and related disorders Hyperlysinemia	Lysine (and saccharopine); (secondary pipecolic acidemia)	Deficient "α-aminoadipic semialdehyde synthase" (bifunctional enzyme with lysine-ketoglutarate reductase [1.5.1.8] + saccharopine reductase [1.5.1.9] activities)	AR	Probably benign
Saccharopinuria variant	Saccharopine (and lysine)	Only saccharopine reductase activity of bifunctional enzyme is deficient	AR	Same as above
α-Aminoadipic aciduria	α-Aminoadipic acid	? Mitochondrial α-aminoadipate amino transferase [2.6.1.39]	(AR)	Variable clinical features
α-Ketoadipic aciduria	α-Aminoadipic and α-ketoadipic acids	? α-Ketoadipic decarboxylase	(AR)	Mental retardation
2-Hydroxyglutaric aciduria	Hyperlysinemia (in some patients)	? Glutaryl CoA dehydrogenase [1.3.99.7]	AR	Progressive ataxia, mental retardation, leukoencephalopathy, cerebellar atrophy
Pipecolic acidemia (primary form)	Pipecolic acid	L-Pipecolate dehydrogenase (pipecolate oxidase) [1.5.99.3]		A peroxisomal disease with hepatomegaly and mental retardation (variant of Zellweger syndrome and adrenoleukodystrophy)
Hypermethioninemia	Methionine	Hepatic ATP: L-methionine S-adenosyltransferase [2.5.1.6]	AR	Variable associations, probably benign
Homocyst(e)inemia/uria Classic form	Methionine high; homocyst(e)ine high	Cystathionine β-synthase [L-serine hydrolase (adding homocysteine)] [4.2.1.22]	AR	Risk factor for occlusive vascular disease in heterozygotes. Homozygotes have dislocated optic lens and osteoporosis and may have impaired mental development
Tetrahydrofolate-deficient form	Methionine low; homocyst(e)ine high	5,10-Methylene tetrahydrofolate reductase [1.7.99.5]		Variable manifestations: developmental delay to severe psychomotor retardation. Heterozygotes for thermolabile variant putatively at elevated risk for coronary artery disease

Table continued on following page

TABLE 175–1. HEREDITARY AND ACQUIRED AMINOACIDOPATHIES *Continued*

Condition or Disease	Amino Acid Affected	Enzyme Affected (Synonym) *In Group A*	IP	Remarks
Inherited Traits (Continued)				
Homocyst(e)inuria (with methylmalonic aciduria)	Homocyst(e)ine (high), methionine (low): methylmalonate (high)	Defective cobalamin coenzyme biosynthesis Defective cobalamin transport (lysosomal)	AR (AR)	Defective remethylation of homocysteine and impaired methylmalonyl-CoA mutase (MMA mutase) activity; developmental delay
Cystathioninuria†	Cystathionine	Cystathionine γ-lyase [4.4.1.1]	AR	Probably benign trait; vitamin B_6 corrects biochemical trait in most patients
Hyperglycinemia				
Ketotic form	Glycine and other glucogenic amino acids	Propionyl-CoA carboxylase [6.4.1.3]	AR	Ketosis, neutropenia, mental retardation; often fatal
Ibid.	Ibid.	Methylmalonyl-CoA mutase [5.4.99.2]	AR	Symptoms are those of methylmalonic aciduria with acidosis (some mutase-affected patients are responsive to vitamin B_{12})
Ibid.	Ibid.	Acetyl-CoA acyltransferase (β-ketothiolase) [2.3.1.16] deficiency¶	AR	Signs are those of α-methyl-β-hydroxybutyric aciduria (with or without tiglic aciduria) and acidosis
Nonketotic form	Glycine	Glycine cleavage reaction (CO_2, NH_3, and hydroxymethyltetrahydrofolate formed) [2.1.2.10] P, H, T, & L proteins in complex; P is deficient in 80% of cases	AR	Severe CNS depression; high CSF: plasma glycine ratio. Benzoate and dextromethorphan (NMDA blocker) for therapy
Sarcosinemia				
Sarcosinemia (classic form)†	Sarcosine	Sarcosine oxidase (sarcosine:oxygen oxidoreductase [demethylating]) [1.5.3.1]	AR	Benign trait
"Sarcosinemia" (glutaric aciduria, type II)	Sarcosine (glutaric acid and multiple fatty acids)	Electron transfer flavoprotein (affecting multiple aryl-CoA dehydrogenases) [1.3.99.2–3]	AR	Postnatal lethargy, vomiting, coma, and acidosis; odor; multiple abnormalities of fatty acid oxidation
Hyperprolinemia				
Type I	Proline	L-Proline dehydrogenase (oxidase) [1.5.99.8]	AR	Benign trait
Type II	Proline	1-Pyrroline dehydrogenase (Δ¹-nicotinamide-pyrroline-5-carboxylate: adenine dinucleotide [NAD⁺] oxidoreductase) [1.5.1.12]	AR	Δ¹-pyrroline-5-carboxylate and 3-hydroxy-1-pyrroline-5-carboxylate excreted in urine. Proline concentration higher in type II than type I; seizures
Hyperhydroxyprolinemia	Hydroxyproline	4-Hydroxy-L-proline dehydrogenase (oxidase) [1.1.1.104]	AR	Benign trait
Hydroxylysinemia	Free hydroxylysine	? Hydroxylysine kinase [2.7.1.81]	(AR)	Mental retardation
Tryptophanemia	Tryptophan (with indoleketonuria)	? Formamidase [3.5.1.9]	(AR)	Variable, probably benign
Hyperammonemia				
Carbamoyl phosphate synthetase (CPS) deficiency	Glycine, glutamine	Carbamate kinase (ATP carbamate phosphotransferase) [2.7.2.2]	AR	Ammonia intoxication, protein intolerance, hepatomegaly, vomiting
Ornithine transcarbamoylase (OTC) deficiency	Glutamine	Ornithine carbamoyltransferase (carbamoylphosphate:L-ornithine carbamoyltransferase) [2.1.3.3]	XL	Same as above
Citrullinemia	Citrulline	Argininosuccinate synthetase (L-citrulline:L-aspartate ligase (adenosine monophosphate [AMP]-forming)) [6.3.4.5]	AR	Same as above
Argininosuccinicaciduria†	Argininosuccinic acid	Argininosuccinate lyase (L-argininosuccinate arginine-lyase) [4.3.2.1]	AR	Same as above; also has trichorrhexis nodosa
Hyperargininemia	Arginine	Argininase (L-arginine amidinohydrolase) [3.5.3.1]	AR	Deterioration of CNS function and IQ in childhood; hyperammonemia (inconstant) aggravated by protein
Hyperornithinemia	Ornithine	Unknown (mitochondrial ornithine transport system?)	AR	Associated with hyperammonemia and homocitrullinemia (HHH syndrome)
Hyperornithinemia (without hyperammonemia)	Ornithine	L-Ornithine; 2-oxoacid aminotransferase [2.6.1.13]	AR	Associated with gyrate atrophy of choroid and retina but no hyperammonemia

TABLE 175–1. HEREDITARY AND ACQUIRED AMINOACIDOPATHIES *Continued*

Condition or Disease	Amino Acid Affected	Enzyme Affected (Synonym) *In Group A*	IP	Remarks
Inherited Traits (Continued)				
Hyperalaninemia	Alanine	Pyruvate dehydrogenase (lipoate) (pyruvate dehydrogenase) [1.2.4.1] deficiency, pyruvate carboxylase [6.4.1.1] deficiency, and other defects	AR	Lactic acidosis, various other manifestations
Aspartylglucosaminuria	Glycoasparagine	Aspartylglucosylaminase (2-acetamido-1[β^1-L-aspartamidol]-1,2-dideoxyglucose amidohydrolase) [3.5.1.26]	AR	Lysosomal disease; mental retardation
Glutathionemia†	Glutathione or related peptides	γ-Glutamyltransferase (γ-glutamyltranspeptidase) [2.3.2.2]	AR	Mental retardation?
Hyperthreoninemia	Threonine	Unknown	(AR)	Seizures
Other Conditions That May Affect Amino Acids in Plasma				
Protein-calorie malnutrition	Tryptophan/leucine/isoleucine/ valine ↓; tyrosine/glycine/ proline ↑	—	—	Severity of change related to severity of malnutrition
Prolonged fasting	Alanine ↓; threonine, glycine ↑	—	—	Early fasting does not show same pattern
Obesity	Leucine/isoleucine/valine/ phenylalanine/tyrosine ↑; glycine ↓	—	—	Reflects insulin insensitivity
Hepatitis	Methionine/tyrosine ↑	—	—	Reflects severity of liver disease

* These conditions have been detected by screening methods applied in the newborn period of life. They should not be misdiagnosed as permanent disorders of amino acid metabolism also identifiable by screening.

† Urine screening is as efficient as, or even more reliable than, blood screening in these conditions.

‡ A number of disorders of branched-chain amino acid catabolism cause accumulation of substances that are ninhydrin negative. These compounds can usually be detected by gas-liquid chromatographic methods (see Goodman SI: Am J Hum Genet 32:781, 1980).

§ Partial activity; >2% of normal.

¶ Hyperglycemia observed only in some patients with this enzyme deficiency.

GROUP IB

The primary defect is in catabolism. There is a high renal clearance of amino acid and a hyperaminoaciduria by saturation of transepithelial transport. Detection in the urine is preferable.

Source of enzyme number is *Enzyme Commission.* IP = apparent inheritance pattern; AR = autosomal recessive; (AR) = probably autosomal recessive; AD = autosomal dominant.

Condition or Disease	Substance Affected (Synonym)	Enzyme Affected (Synonym) [Enzyme Commission No.]	IP	Remarks
Hypophosphatasia	Phosphoethanolamine	Deficiency of alkaline phosphatase (tissue nonspecific (liver, body, kidney) isoenzyme) [3.1.3.1]	AR	"Rickets" unresponsive to vitamin D; craniosynostosis; hypercalcemia, elevated pyridoxal phosphate (blood marker)
Pseudohypophosphatasia	Phosphoethanolamine	Same as above; activity present but altered	AR	Same as above
β-Aminoisobutyricaciduria	β-Aminoisobutyric acid	Hepatic R-β-aminoisobutyrate-pyruvate transaminase [2.6.1.40]	AD/AR	Benign metabolic polymorphic trait

Condition or Disease	Substance Affected (Synonym)	Enzyme Affected (Synonym) *In Group A*	IP	Remarks
4-Hydroxybutyricaciduria (γ-aminobutyrate pathway)	γ-OH butyrate	Succinic semialdehyde dehydrogenase [1.2.1.24]	AR	Mental retardation, hypotonia; detectable by gas chromatographic analysis of urine, plasma, CSF
Hyper-β-alaninemia	β-Alanine	? β-Alanine-pyruvate aminotransferase (β-alanine transaminase) [2.6.1.18]		Seizures; somnolence; mental retardation
Carnosinemia	Carnosine	Serum aminoacyl-histidine dipeptidase (carnosinase) [3.4.13.3]	AR	Benign (most cases)
Pyroglutamic aciduria*	L-Pyroglutamic acid (5-oxo-L-proline; pyrrolidone-2-carboxylic acid)	Glutathione synthetase [6.3.2.3]	AR	L-Pyroglutamic acid formed via modified γ-glutamyl cycle. Associated metabolic acidosis

GROUP II

There is a primary defect in catabolism and a secondary defect in transport. Hyperaminoaciduria is of combined origin—saturation and competition.

Detection is possible in both plasma and urine.

Disease	Amino Acids		Remarks
	Affected in Plasma	*Present in Urine*	
Hyperprolinemia, types I and II	Proline	Proline, + hydroxyproline and glycine	See entries in group 1A; competition occurs on iminoglycine transport system (see group III)
Hyper-β-alaninemia	β-Alanine	β-Alanine, + β-aminoisobutyric acid and taurine	See entry in Hyper-β-alaninemia in group IB; competition occurs on β-amino transport system

Table continued on following page

TABLE 175–1. HEREDITARY AND ACQUIRED AMINOACIDOPATHIES *Continued*

Disease	Amino Acids		Remarks
	Affected in Plasma	**Present in Urine**	
Hyperlysinemia	Lysine	Lysine, + ornithine and arginine	See entries in group IA; competition occurs on "dibasic" transport system (see group III)
Hyperargininemia	Arginine	Ornithine and lysine and sometimes generalized hyperaminoaciduria	See entry in group IA; competition occurs on "dibasic" transport system (see group III); pathogenesis of generalized aminoaciduria unknown

* Urine screening is as efficient as, or even more reliable than, blood screening in these conditions.

GROUP III

The primary defect is in the renal membrane transport site. There is a high renal clearance of amino acid, and detection is possible only in the urine. *Activity Affected:* Presumed gene product activity affected by mutant gene. IP = apparent inheritance pattern; AD = autosomal dominant; (AD) = probably autosomal dominant; AR = autosomal recessive; (AR) = probably autosomal recessive; XL = X-linked. *Remarks:* PTH = parathyroid hormone.

Trait	Substance Affected	Activity Affected	Other Tissues Affected	IP	Remarks
Common Perinatal (Adaptive) Trait					
Neonatal iminoglycinuria	Proline, hydroxyproline, glycine	Specific proline and specific glycine transport (probably)	—	—	Benign adaptive trait; prolinuria subsides at ~100 days, glycinuria at ~200 days after full-term birth
Neonatal cystine-lysinuria	Cystine and dibasic amino acids (lysine, ornithine, and arginine)	Specific dibasic transport system	—	—	Reflects heterozygosity for cystinuria (see below) plus ontogeny
Inherited Hyperaminoacidurias					
Selective					
Hyperdibasic aminoaciduria type 2 (Lysinuric-protein intolerance)	Lysine, ornithine, arginine ("dibasic" group)	Shared "dibasic" amino acid transport system in basolateral membrane	Intestine (basolateral membrane, efflux defect); fibroblasts (plasma membrane; efflux defect on y^+ system)	AR	Associated with protein intolerance, failure to thrive, hyperammonemia
Hyperdibasic aminoaciduria type I	Lysine, ornithine, arginine	Shared "dibasic" amino acid transport system (brush-border membrane)	Intestine	AR	Associated with mental retardation in one reported patient; heterozygotes have hyperdibasic aminoaciduria
Isolated hyperlysinuria	Lysine	Lysine-specific system (brush border)	Intestine	AR	One proband reported
Classic cystinuria	Lysine, ornithine, arginine, and cystine	Shared system in brush border membrane	Intestine	AR	"Negative" reabsorption of affected amino acid can occur; three alleles (? same locus), each causing different phenotypes: in type I carrier (vs. types II and III) no excess of amino acids in urine ("silent"); in type III patient, intestinal transport intact (or partial defect)
Hypercystinuria	Cyst(e)ine	Specific system for cyst(e)ine	?	(AR)	One pedigree only
Iminoglycinuria	Proline; hydroxyproline; glycine	Shared system for imino acids, glycine (and sarcosine)	Intestine	AR	Benign; 4 alleles (? same locus); I and II are silent carriers; III and IV are hyperglycinuric carriers; I associated with intestinal defect; IV with K_m mutant
Hartnup disorder	Neutral amino acids (excluding imino acids, glycine, cyst(e)ine, and β-amino acids)	Shared system for large neutral amino acid group (luminal membrane)	Intestine	AR	Usually benign; 3 alleles (? same locus); I, intestine affected; II, intestine normal; III, kidney normal; carrier "silent" in all
Hyperhistidinuria	Histidine	Specific system for histidine	Intestine	AR	Associated with mental retardation in siblings
Hyperdicarboxylic aminoaciduria (glutamate-aspartate transport defect)	Glutamic acid, aspartic acid	Shared dicarboxylic amino acid transport system (brush border membrane)	Intestine ±	AR	Benign
Idiopathic (primary genetic) Fanconi's syndrome	Generalized effect on all solutes and water	? Mitochondrial defect disrupted ATP energized ion pump (basolateral membrane); impaired sodium-coupled transporter (apical membrane)	Secondary to renal phenotype	AR (and AD)	Adult-onset and infantile-childhood forms are differentiated

TABLE 175–1. HEREDITARY AND ACQUIRED AMINOACIDOPATHIES *Continued*

Trait	Substance Affected	Activity Affected	Other Tissues Affected	IP	Remarks
		*Inherited Hyperaminoacidurias* (Continued)			
Secondary genetic forms of renal Fanconi's syndrome					
Cystinosis; type I, type II	Same as above (secondary response)	Cystine storage (lysosomal defect), with secondary damage to tubule and glomerulus (later)	Organ damage from cystine storage (thyroid, retina, CNS)	AR*	Several alleles; infantile (type I) and adolescent (type II) forms have differing rates for onset of nephropathy; "adult" form (type III) has no nephropathy
Hereditary fructose intolerance	Same as above, + fructose	Fructose-1-phosphate aldolase (fructose biphosphate aldolase) (with secondary effects on cellular ATP)	Secondary to renal phenotype (hepatic cirrhosis)	AR	Nephropathy dependent on intact PTH-cAMP axis in kidney; responds to fructose withdrawal
Galactosemia	Same as above, + galactose	Galactose-1-phosphate uridyltransferase (with secondary effects on cellular ATP)	Secondary to renal phenotype (cataracts, CNS effects)	AR	Fanconi's syndrome responds to galactose withdrawal; "galactosemia" due to galactokinase deficiency does *not* have Fanconi's syndrome
Hereditary tyrosinemia	Same as above, + tyrosine metabolites	Fumarylacetoacetate hydrolase	Secondary to renal phenotype (hepatic cirrhosis)	AR	Fanconi's syndrome responds to tyrosine restriction
Wilson's disease	Same as above, with proximal and distal renal tubular acidosis	WND protein, in P-type ATPase family of cation transporters	Hepatolenticular degeneration	AR	Fanconi's syndrome responds to depletion of copper burden
Lowe's oculocerebrorenal syndrome	Generalized dysfunction with defective urinary NH_3 production	? In OCRL-1 protein (strong homology with inositol polyphosphate-5-phosphatase)	An oculo-cerebro-intestinal-renal syndrome	XL†	Treatment does not improve mental retardation or the cataracts and hydrophthalmia
Vitamin D dependency (pseudodeficiency rickets)	Generalized defect (secondary response)	Type I: 25-Hydroxyvitamin D-1-α-hydroxylase Type II: defective binding of hormone	Impaired receptor synthesis or ligand binding affects intestinal absorption of calcium and initiates PTH response	AR	Nephropathy dependent on PTH excess and hypocalcemia (phenocopy occurs in vitamin D deficiency)

* For each type.
† Recessive.

Data from Benson PF, Fensom AH: Genetic Biochemical Disorders. Oxford Monographs on the Medical Genetics No. 12. Oxford, Oxford University Press, 1985. *A "handbook," leaner than* The Metabolic and Molecular Bases of Inherited Disease *(the standard "encyclopedia"), that covers, in short essays, nearly all entries in Table 175–1.* Scriver CT, Tenenhouse HS: Mendelian phenotypes as "probes" of renal transport systems for amino acids and phosphate. Handbook of Physiology (Renal Section, 1987). *A review of the amino acid transport systems (in kidney and other tissues) delineated by mutations in humans and of their relative importance in metabolic homeostasis.* Wellner D, Meister A: A survey of inborn errors of amino acid metabolism and transport in man. Annu Rev Biochem 50:911, 1981. *A crisp review of events in a field that now moves more slowly than it once did.*

176 THE HYPERPHENYLALANINEMIAS AND ALKAPTONURIA

Charles R. Scriver

A widely accepted medical model of disease attributes manifestations (signs and symptoms) to a deviant underlying process (pathogenesis) that has its origins in both proximate and ultimate causes. According to this model, phenylketonuria, the best known form of hyperphenylalaninemia, is no longer a disease, although it continues to be a risk factor, because its principal manifestations (mental retardation, pigment dilution, mousy odor, neurotransmitter deficiency) occur only in rare cases escaping early diagnosis. This satisfactory turn of events came about because pathogenesis from hyperphenylalaninemia (the risk factor) is offset by treatment. Genetic forms of hyperphenylalaninemia are described here; they are all autosomal recessive disorders. About 0.01% of live births are affected. Physicians for adult-age patients must be aware of maternal hyperphenylalaninemia (see below).

PHENYLALANINE METABOLISM. Phenylalanine is an essential amino acid. The normal concentration in plasma is < 125 μmole per liter (1 μmole = 165 μg). The balance between intake and utilization is largely controlled by a hydroxylation reaction (Fig. 176–1A). Impaired hydroxylation is the chief explanation for

hyperphenylalaninemia. The reaction requires the apoenzyme *phenylalanine hydroxylase,* molecular oxygen, and *tetrahydrobiopterin* cofactor; the last-named is consumed in stoichiometric amounts to form tyrosine, the reaction product. The catalytic property of phenylalanine hydroxylase requires both moment-to-moment regeneration of tetrahydrobiopterin from dihydrobiopterin, a by-product of the hydroxylating reaction, and long-term renewal of the tetrahydrobiopterin pool by synthesis from precursors. The former is achieved by the enzyme *dihydropteridine reductase,* the latter by a *synthesis pathway* in which several enzymes act in sequence (Fig. 176–1B). Accordingly, there are several ways to impair phenylalanine hydroxylation. Failure to recognize the biologic heterogeneity of hyperphenylalaninemia may lead to erroneous counseling and ineffective (or unnecessary) treatment; all of its forms require special management of women during the reproductive years.

DISORDERS OF PHENYLALANINE HYDROXYLASE INTEGRITY. The phenylalanine hydroxylase enzyme is multimeric and homopolymeric. The polypeptide is encoded by a gene on chromosome 12, region q24.1, which is expressed only in liver in humans. Mutations at this locus cause either phenylketonuria (with plasma phenylalanine values > 1 mM on a normal diet) or nonphenylketonuric hyperphenylalaninemia (values < 1 mM, but > 0.125 mM). Phenylketonuria is typically associated with mental retardation in the untreated patient; the other form is not. The incidence of the phenylketonuric form (about 1 per 10,000 births) varies widely by population.

The hydroxylation reaction accounts for about three quarters of the moment-by-moment outflow of phenylalanine; incorporation into protein is the other important route (Fig. 176–1A). If there is deficient hydroxylating activity, and dietary intake is not curtailed, phenylalanine accumulates in body fluids. Overflow into the alternative pathways generates excessive amounts of metabolites derived from phenylalanine, such as the pyruvic (causing phenylketonuria), lactic, and acetic acid derivatives (Fig. 176–1A). Overburden of phenylalanine and its by-products impairs brain development in ways still not fully understood.

Phenylketonuria was first described as a clinical entity in 1934 by Asjborn Fölling, who surmised that the disorder was autosomal recessive and an inborn error of metabolism. In the following three decades, phenylketonuria was seen as a paradigm for the biochemical basis of mental disease, of disease that could be prevented by deliberately restoring normal metabolism, and of chemical individuality that could be used as the basis for a screening test and early diagnosis. Newborn screening for hyperphenylalaninemia is now one of the most widely applied "genetic" tests. The incidence of the risk factor has not changed, but the frequency of the associated disease is now trivial in screened populations. The practical issues for physicians are interpretation of a positive screening test result, accuracy of the test, and maternal hyperphenylalaninemia (all discussed below).

TETRAHYDROBIOPTERIN-DEFICIENT FORMS OF HYPERPHENYLALANINEMIA.

Not every case of persistent hyperphenylalaninemia is explained by a primary hydroxylase deficiency. Tetrahydrobiopterin insufficiency impairs function of three hydroxylases (for phenylalanine, tryptophan, and tyrosine) and synthesis of their products, notably 5-hydroxytryptophan (the precursor of serotonin) and L-dopa (the precursor of catecholamines) (Fig. 176–1B). The products function as neurotransmitters in the brain, and a deficiency of them gives rise to central nervous system disease (including retarded psychomotor development, basal ganglion dysfunction, and unstable body temperature). Regeneration of tetrahydrobiopterin is necessary to maintain catalytic function of the three hydroxylases. *Deficient activity of quininoid dihydropteridine reductase* (gene on chromosome 4, region p15.3) or of *4α-carbinolamine dehydratase* (gene on chromosome 10q22) impairs recycling of dihydrobiopterin. *Deficient activity of guanosine triphosphate cyclohydrolase I or 6-pyruvoyl tetrahydropterin synthase* (gene on chromosome 11q22.3-q23.4) impairs synthesis of tetrahydrobiopterin.

SCREENING AND DIAGNOSIS. Screening newborn infants for hyperphenylalaninemia is public policy. Capillary blood collected on filter paper from heel puncture is analyzed by the bacterial inhibition (Guthrie) assay, fluorimetric analysis, or other quantitative methods. Blood phenylalanine values >2 mg per deciliter (125μM) on the first day of life or thereafter are considered abnormal and require further investigation. The screening test is not infallible, and false-negative results do occur, some for biologic reasons. Urine screening for "phenylketones" is not reliable.

Every infant with persistent hyperphenylalaninemia is investigated to rule out disorders of tetrahydrobiopterin homeostasis. Urine pterin metabolites or blood cofactor levels are measured under special conditions; there are distinctive urine profiles as well as low blood levels in the disorders of tetrahydrobiopterin synthesis. The tests are done at established centers and require experienced interpretation. Measures of phenylalanine hydroxylase require liver biopsy and are seldom done. Dihydropteridine reductase can be measured in blood spots, fibroblasts, and amniocytes, the cyclohydrolase in phytohemagglutinin-stimulated leukocytes, and the synthase in erythrocytes.

After excluding disorders of tetrahydrobiopterin metabolism, hyperphenylalaninemia is classified as follows. About one half of cases with primary phenylalanine hydroxylase deficiency have "phenylketonuria," a generic term for severe hyperphenylalaninemia (>1 mM), low phenylalanine tolerance (<500 mg per day), and high risk of mental retardation in the absence of treatment. The remainder have nonphenylketonuric hyperphenylalaninemia with lower blood phenylalanine values (<1 mM), higher tolerance for dietary phenylalanine (>500 mg per day), and no elevated risk for mental retardation if not treated. There is a correlation between level of hepatic hydroxylase activity and clinical form; in broad terms, activity is <1% of normal in phenylketonuria and >1% of normal in nonphenylketonuric hyperphenylalaninemia.

DNA analysis identifies mutations at the hydroxylase (Fig. 176–2) and other cloned loci. Interpretation of phenotype by mutation analysis is clinically relevant. Prenatal diagnosis by analysis of

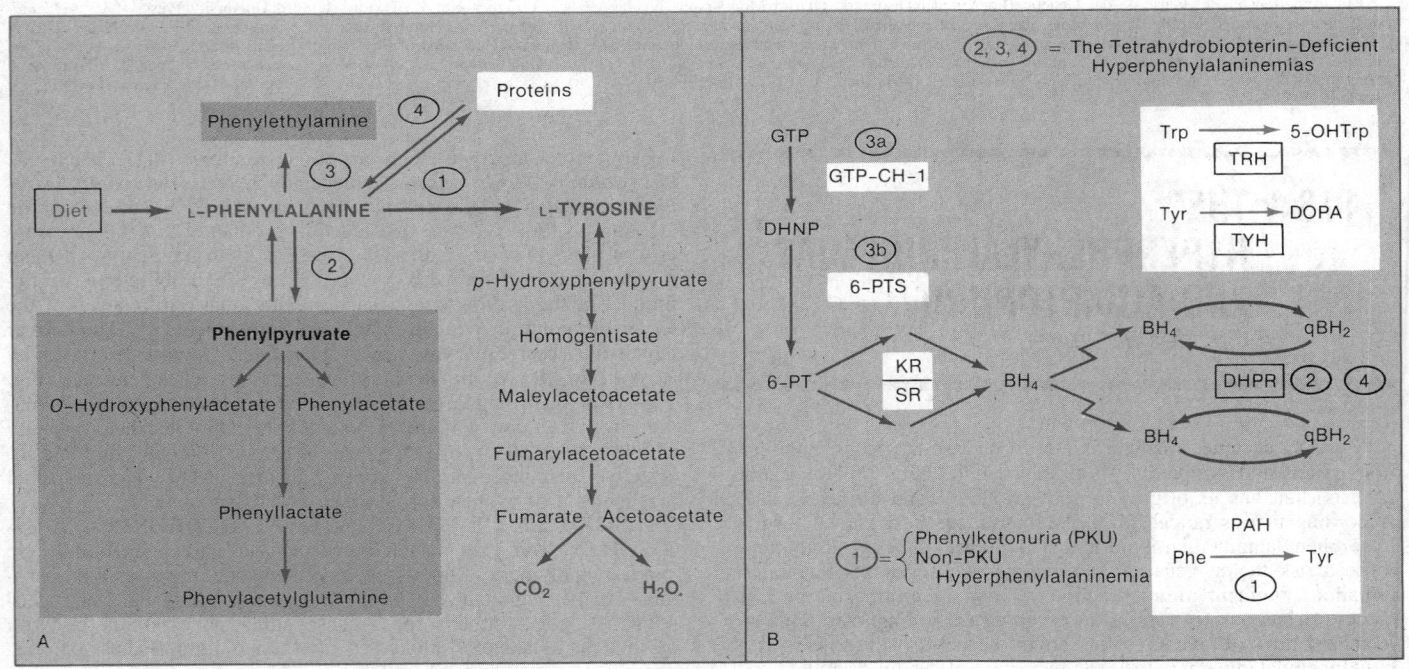

FIGURE 176–1. *A*, Intake of phenylalanine (an essential amino acid supplied only by diet) and its disposal by hydroxylation (1) (representing three quarters of normal runout), transamination (2), decarboxylation (3), and incorporation into proteins (4) (representing under a quarter of runout). *B*, Interrelations between phenylalanine hydroxylase (PAH), dihydropteridine reductase (DHPR), and the tetrahydrobiopterin (BH₄) biosynthesis pathway serving aromatic amino acid hydroxylation reactions. Mutations at the relevant chromosomal loci impair the hydroxylation reactions with effects on PAH activity only (1); DHPR activity (2); GTP-cyclohydrolase 1 (GTP-CH-1) activity (3a); 6-pyruvoyltetrahydropterin synthase activity (6-PTS) (3b); and 4α-carbinolamine dehydratase (4). Disorders 2, 3a, 3b, and 4 can impair function of three hydroxylases: PAH, tyrosine hydroxylase (TYH), and tryptophan hydroxylase (TRH). GTP = guanosine triphosphate; DHNP = dihydroneopterin triphosphate; 6-PT = 6-pyruvoyltetrahydropterin; KR = 2′-ketotetrahydropterin reductase; SR = sepiapterin reductase; qBH₂ = quinonoid dihydrobiopterin.

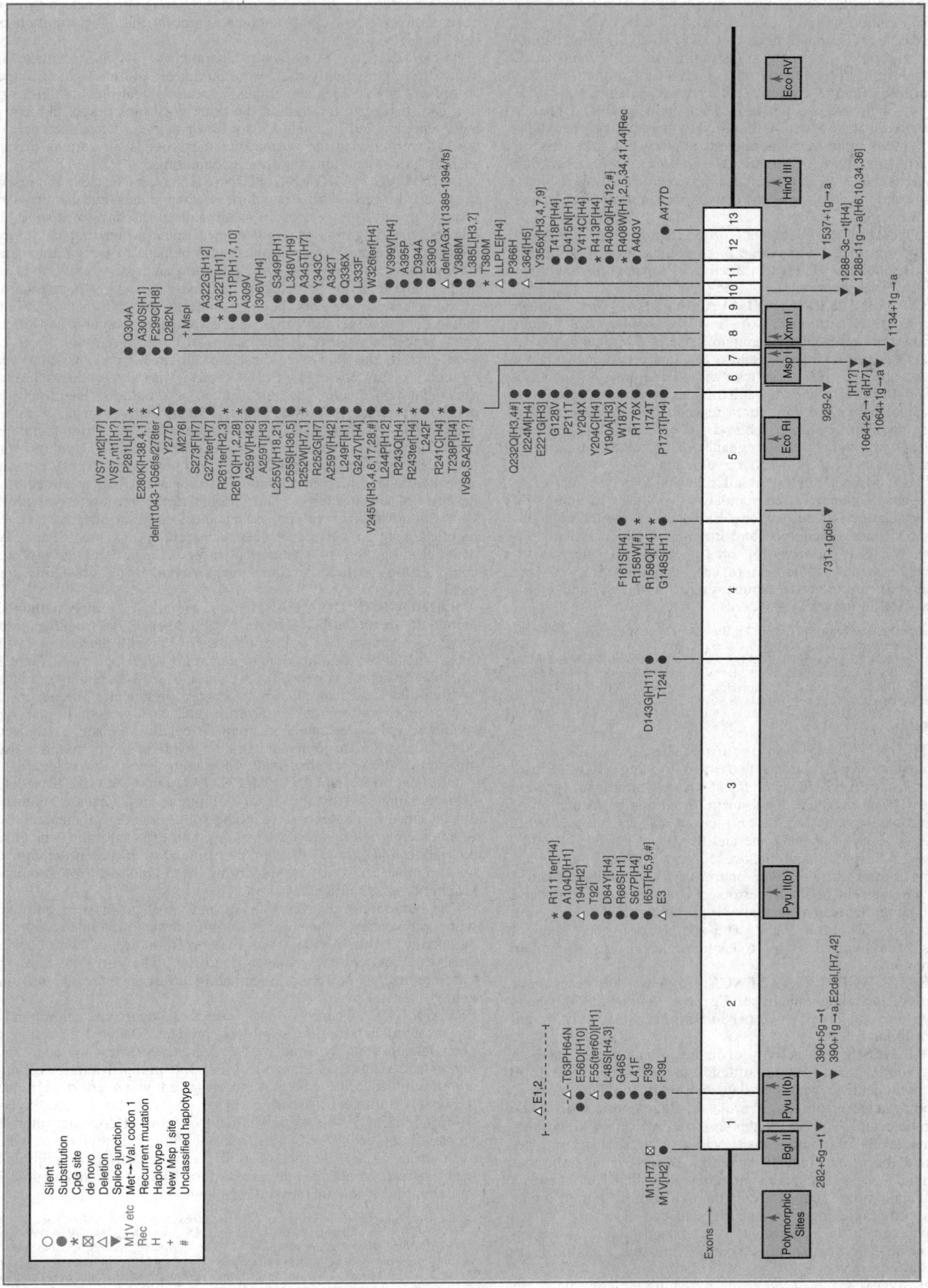

FIGURE 176–2. Diagram of the phenylalanine hydroxylase (PAH) gene (≈ 90 kb, chromosome 12q24.1), showing exons (*vertical bars*), polymorphic restriction sites (*arrows*), and regions of some associated with phenylketonuria. The code (e.g., MIV) indicates normal residue, position in the PAH polypeptide, and replacement residue. Several mutations involve hypermutable CpG dinucleotides; some are "recurrent." Over 200 mutations were known before this edition went to press.

DNA in chorionic villus samples or amniocytes is now feasible for most ($\approx 85\%$) couples at risk.

TREATMENT. The main treatment for primary phenylalanine hydroxylase deficiency is dietary restriction of the amino acid. There are several semisynthetic diet products ("orphan foods") for this purpose. Phenylketonuric patients can tolerate only 250 to 500 mg of phenylalanine per day to maintain the blood phenylalanine level well below 1 mM. Intake, blood levels of phenylalanine, and growth rate are monitored at frequent intervals to avoid undertreatment or overtreatment. *Treatment into adult life is now recommended to maintain normal neuropsychologic function.* Well-treated patients have normal or near-normal intellectual development.

The tetrahydrobiopterin-deficient forms require continuous replacement therapy of cofactor alone or in combination with neurotransmitter precursors. Whether effective postnatal treatment of these disorders is feasible remains to be seen.

MATERNAL HYPERPHENYLALANINEMIA. *This problem is relevant to all practitioners who counsel women about pregnancy.* Intrauterine hyperphenylalaninemia places the fetus at risk of microcephaly, mental retardation, and organ malformations (notably cardiac). Accordingly, all females with hyperphenylalaninemia should be identified, followed (registries exist for this purpose), counseled about risk when they attain reproductive age, and treated with diet to maintain near-normal blood phenylalanine levels before conception and throughout the pregnancy. This treatment prevents harm to the fetus, but it is still under evaluation.

GENETICS. Mutant alleles (at all relevant loci) are recessive. Their aggregate frequency in the population is ≈ 0.01, meaning that 2% of the population is heterozygous. Explanations for the high frequency of this "rare" phenotype and its genes include founder effects and genetic drift (observed in some populations), selective advantage in the heterozygote (unproved), hypermutability at the locus (observed), reproductive compensation (unlikely), and multiple loci involved in the trait (observed).

Levy HL: Maternal phenylketonuria. Prog Clin Biol 281:227, 1988. *A good discussion of a major problem (maternal hyperphenylalaninemia).*

Scriver CR, Kaufman S, Woo SLC: The hyperphenylalaninemias. *In* Scriver CR, Beaudet AL, Sly WS, et al. (eds.): The Metabolic and Molecular Bases of Inherited Disease. 7th ed. New York, McGraw-Hill, 1995. *A reference covering all major issues concerning the hyperphenylalaninemias.*

ALKAPTONURIA*

DEFINITION. Alkaptonuria is a rare hereditary disease in which homogentisic acid oxidase activity is missing. Homogentisic acid produced during the metabolism of phenylalanine and tyrosine accumulates and is excreted in the urine. It causes pigmentation of cartilage and other connective tissue (ochronosis) and in later years a degenerative arthritis of the spine and the larger peripheral joints. The disease has historical significance, for it was chiefly on the basis of study of families with alkaptonuria that Sir Archibald Garrod developed the concept of inborn errors of metabolism. The disease is inherited as an autosomal recessive trait. No method of detection of heterozygotes has been found. The alkaptonuria gene (symbol AKU) has been mapped to a 16 centimorgan region on human chromosome 3q2.

INCIDENCE AND PREVALENCE. At least 600 cases have been reported, including one in an Egyptian mummy 3500 years old. A prevalence of three to five per million individuals was found in Northern Ireland.

PATHOGENESIS. The activity of homogentisic acid oxidase in the normal adult human liver is sufficient to metabolize over 1600 grams of homogentisic acid per day. Normally, no homogentisic acid can be detected in plasma or urine. In alkaptonuric individuals there is no detectable activity of this enzyme in liver or kidney tissue. Plasma levels of homogentisic acid rise to about 3 mg per deciliter, and the urinary excretion ranges from 4 to 8 grams per day. Mammalian tissue contains an enzyme called homogentisic acid polyphenoloxidase that catalyzes the oxidation of homogentisic acid to an ochronotic pigment, but pigment can also be produced nonenzymatically in the presence of oxygen and alkali, as, for example, in urine. The homogentisic acid polymer has a high affinity

for cartilage and connective tissue macromolecules. The stained tissue is fragile and eventually may break down, leading to degenerative intervertebral disc or joint disease. Homogentisic acid may also have a direct effect upon collagen synthesis through inhibition of lysyl hydroxylase.

PATHOLOGY. In an adult alkaptonuric patient, cartilage in many areas, particularly the costal, laryngeal, and tracheal cartilage, is densely pigmented, sometimes appearing coal-black. Pigmentation is also present throughout the body in fibrous tissue, fibrocartilage, tendons, and ligaments. To a lesser degree, it is also found in the endocardium, in the intima of larger vessels, in various organs such as kidney and lung, and in the epidermis.

CLINICAL MANIFESTATIONS. Homogentisic acid is present in urine from birth. Urine is colorless when passed but darker when alkaline or after long exposure to air. Before the days of disposable diapers, the diagnosis was sometimes made when diapers turned brown in alkaline soaps. Pigment may appear in perspiration and stain clothing in the axillary and genital regions. Generally, the earliest change that can be detected externally is a slight pigmentation of the sclerae or the ears, beginning at age 20 to 30. The cartilage of the ears may be slate blue or gray and feel irregular and thickened. Sometimes dusky discolorations of underlying tendons can be seen through the skin over the hands. In many patients, however, pigment is scarcely evident. The arthritis usually produces limitation of motion of the hips, knee joints, or shoulders. There may be periods of acute inflammation, and later there is usually rather marked limitation of motion and ankylosis in the lumbosacral region. The arthritic complications are often severe and painful and may lead to extensive crippling. In addition, alkaptonuric patients appear to have a high incidence of cardiovascular disease, including generalized arteriosclerosis and chronic mitral and aortic valvulitis, with calcification of valves and annulus. At least one degenerated pigmented aortic valve has been replaced with a prosthesis. Myocardial infarction is a common cause of death. Other reported complications include ruptured intervertebral discs, prostatitis, and renal stones.

RADIOGRAPHIC CHANGES. These may be almost pathognomonic of alkaptonuria. The vertebral bodies of the lumbar spine show degeneration of the intervertebral discs with narrowing of the space and dense calcification of remaining disc material. There is variable fusion of vertebral bodies, but little osteophyte formation and minimal calcification of intervertebral ligaments. The degenerative changes of ochronotic arthritis are most severe in the hip, shoulder, and knee, and there may be calcific deposits in the tendons. The sacroiliac joints and smaller joints of the extremities usually show little or no abnormality. Ear cartilage may be calcified.

DIAGNOSIS AND DIFFERENTIAL DIAGNOSIS. The diagnosis is suggested by the history of pigmentary changes of urine, the presence of nonglucose reducing substance, the pigmentation of sclerae or cartilage, arthritic episodes, and especially the typical radiographic changes of the lumbar spine. Specific identification of homogentisic acid in urine can be accomplished by chromatographic or enzymatic assays.

The ochronotic changes of skin and cartilage may be confused with pigmentary changes resulting from prolonged use of quinacrine hydrochloride (Atabrine) or from use of carbolic acid dressings for chronic cutaneous ulcers. The arthritis must be differentiated chiefly from rheumatoid arthritis, osteoarthritis, and gout.

TREATMENT. There is no effective treatment although a low protein diet for life would be prudent. Dietary restriction of phenylalanine and tyrosine of the degree necessary to reduce homogentisic aciduria is impractical and potentially deleterious. Large amounts of ascorbic acid have been given in an effort to reduce pigment formation. Ascorbic acid protects lysyl hydroxylase from inhibition by homogentisic acid *in vitro*. It does not alter the metabolic defect. NTBC (2-(2-nitro-4-trifluoromethylbenzoyl)-1,3-cyclohexanedione), the potent inhibitor of p-hydroxyphenylpyruvic acid oxidase, would prevent excess formation of homogentisic acid and could be a new therapy in alkaptonuria.

La Du BN: Alkaptonuria. *In* Scriver CR, Beaudet AL, Sly WS, Valle D (eds.): The Metabolic and Molecular Bases of Inherited Disease. 7th ed. New York, McGraw-Hill, 1995. *A detailed discussion of the history, clinical features, and biochemical derangements of alkaptonuria and ochronosis.*

Pollak M, Chou Y-H W, Cerda JJ, et al.: Homozygosity mapping of the gene for alkaptonuria to chromosome 3q2. Nature Genetics 5:201, 1993. *A significant step in the history of this classic disease.*

---

*James B. Wyngaarden, M.D., wrote this section for the 19th edition. His text is used here with minor revisions; there is some new material.

177 THE HYPERPROLINEMIAS AND HYDROXYPROLINEMIA
James M. Phang

There are three autosomal recessive genetic disorders in the degradative pathways for proline and hydroxyproline. Although these rare disorders are generally benign, the resulting metabolic abnormalities, at least for one, is associated with neurologic manifestations in childhood.

The α-nitrogen of the imino acids proline and hydroxyproline is incorporated within a pyrrolidine ring. This feature confers structural and functional properties to proteins. Owing to the ring structure, the metabolism of proline, including biosynthesis from glutamate and ornithine and degradation back to glutamate, is catalyzed by a specific set of enzymes. Both synthetic and degradative pathways share Δ^1-pyrroline-5-carboxylate as an intermediate. The cycling of proline may mediate the transfer of reducing-oxidizing potential to regulate metabolic pathways. Preformed hydroxyproline is not incorporated into proteins. Instead, hydroxyproline is formed from peptide-linked proline primarily in collagen.

HYPERPROLINEMIAS. The two genetic disorders in proline metabolism are characterized by hyperprolinemia and iminoglycinuria, but they are due to different enzyme deficiencies; type II hyperprolinemia can be diagnosed directly. This disorder is due to a deficiency of Δ^1-pyrroline-5-carboxylate dehydrogenase, which catalyzes the second step in the degradative pathway for proline (Fig. 177–1); the deficiency in enzyme activity can be determined in extracts of circulating leukocytes or cultured fibroblasts. Hyperprolinemia in type II is more marked than in type I, but the distinguishing feature of type II is the accumulation of Δ^1-pyrroline-5-carboxylate in plasma and its excretion in urine. The hyperprolinemia in type I is due to a deficiency of the first enzyme in the pathway, proline oxidase. Although plasma proline is generally lower than in type II, the diagnosis of type I is one of exclusion, i.e., hyperprolinemia unaccompanied by Δ^1-pyrroline-5-carboxylate in urine or plasma.

Clinical manifestations have been described with the hyperprolinemias, but the association may be due to chance because in most cases hyperprolinemia was identified fortuitously in patients presenting with clinical abnormalities (biased ascertainment). This is true especially for type I hyperprolinemia: Renal disease and mental retardation found in some pedigrees were shown to segregate independently of hyperprolinemia. For type II hyperprolinemia, however, clinical associations untainted by biased ascertainment have been identified. Screening of a large pedigree in Ireland identified 14 new cases confirmed by elevated plasma Δ^1-pyrroline-5-carboxylate and undetectable enzyme activity in leukocytes. Nine of these 14 new subjects had a history of recurrent childhood febrile seizures requiring hospitalization and treatment with anticonvulsants. Thus, the association of type II hyperprolinemia with a predisposition to seizures appears convincing. Adults in this pedigree were fertile and otherwise normal. Although the mechanism for this association remains unclear, the recent cloning of a high-affinity proline transporter in rat brain suggests that proline or its metabolites may have a neuromodulatory function.

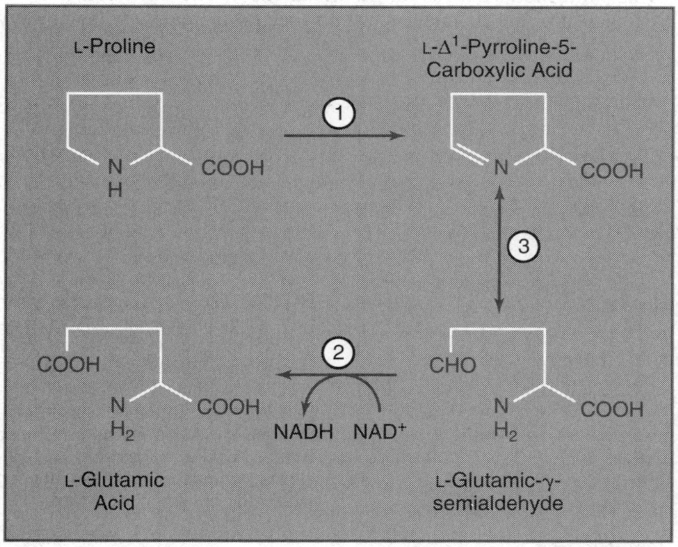

HYDROXYPROLINEMIA. Hydroxyprolinemia with hydroxyprolinuria, but without hyperprolinemia or hyperprolinuria, has been described in members of several families. Although the degradation of hydroxyproline parallels that of proline, the pathway enzymes are distinct except that the second degradation step is catalyzed by a common enzyme that dehydrogenates both Δ^1-pyrroline-5-carboxylate (see above) and 3-OH-Δ^1-pyrroline-5-carboxylate. The first step in the degradation, however, is catalyzed by distinct oxidases. The absence of urinary Δ^1-pyrroline-5-carboxylate or its hydroxylated congener leads to the conclusion that this autosomal recessive disorder is due to a deficiency of hydroxyproline oxidase. In this disorder there are no clinical manifestations related to abnormalities in collagen metabolism or central nervous system function, and therapy is not indicated.

Flynn MP, Martin MC, Moore PT, et al.: Type II hyperprolinaemia in a pedigree of Irish travellers (nomads). Arch Dis Child 64:1699, 1989.
Fremeau RT Jr, Caron MG, Blakely RD: Molecular cloning and expression of a high affinity L-proline transporter expressed in putative glutamatergic pathways of rat brain. Neuron 8:915, 1992.
Phang JM, Scriver CR: Disorders of proline and hydroxyproline metabolism. In Scriver CR, Beaudet AL, Sly WS, et al. (eds.): The Metabolic Basis of Inherited Disease. 6th ed. New York; McGraw-Hill, 1989, p 577.

178 DISEASES OF THE UREA CYCLE
Stephen D. Cederbaum

Ammonia is a highly toxic metabolic product, which, when present at levels no more than two times the upper limits of normal (10 to 25 μM), may cause symptoms. The urea cycle is a five-step metabolic pathway in which two ammonia molecules and one bicarbonate molecule are converted to the relatively easily excreted and nontoxic urea. It is the only major pathway to remove waste nitrogen derived from ingested protein or from normal or augmented protein turnover in the body. The urea cycle occurs predominantly or possibly exclusively in the liver.

In children, the vast majority of cases of hyperammonemia are the result of inborn errors of metabolism, primarily of the urea cycle. In adults, a larger proportion are due to liver failure and less frequently to toxic ingestion. Nevertheless, with the wider availability of blood ammonia tests, the increased recognition of urea cycle disorders, and more successful treatment modalities, the inherited disorders of ammonia metabolism are being recognized with greater frequency in adolescents and adults with acute or intermittent organic brain syndrome. Hyperammonemia appears to be better tolerated in infants and young children, in part because the cranium is more compliant. Ammonia levels that leave minimal residual damage in infants may be deadly in adults. Ammonia itself appears to be the metabolite toxic to the central nervous system; however, there is some speculation that the accumulation of glutamine, a compound in equilibrium with ammonia, may be involved as well. The primary toxic effect appears to be the uptake of fluid into as-

FIGURE 177–1. Schematic of the degradative pathway for proline. Reaction 1 is catalyzed by proline oxidase (EC number unassigned); reaction 2 is catalyzed by Δ^1-pyrroline-5-carboxylic acid dehydrogenase (EC 1.5.1.12) and reaction 3 is spontaneous. Type I hyperprolinemia is due to blockade at reaction 1 (deficiency of proline oxidase), and type II hyperprolinemia is due to blockade at reaction 2 (deficiency of Δ^1-pyrroline-5-carboxylic acid dehydrogenase).

trocytes causing cerebral edema. Death is caused acutely by herniation of the brain through the foramen magnum with consequent cerebral ischemia, but survivors may have various degrees of brain damage.

The urea cycle is shown in Figure 178–1. The five enzymes generally associated with it are carbamoylphosphate synthetase 1 (CPS-1) and ornithine transcarbamoylase (OTC), found in the mitochondrion; and argininosuccinate synthetase (ASAS), argininosuccinate lyase (ASAL), and arginase 1 (ARG-1) found in the cytoplasm. N-Acetylglutamate synthetase catalyzes the synthesis of N-acetylglutamate, which activates CPS-1 and modulates urea cycle function, and the ornithine transporter recycles ornithine to the mitochondrion. Deficiency of these latter enzymes has been associated with symptomatic hyperammonia, the former only in infants.

The normal urea cycle can increase its ureagenic capacity greatly in response to ammonia challenge. The genes for all five enzymes have been cloned and are available for defining mutations, prenatal diagnosis, and population studies.

Disorders of the urea cycle are estimated to occur in 1 in 25,000 births. It is probable that 2 to 4% of the population is heterozygous for a urea cycle defect, although only women who are carriers of ornithine transcarbamoylase deficiency are known to be prone to disease. It is unclear whether patients receiving intensive chemotherapy for leukemia, in whom hyperammonemia occurs rarely, or patients receiving valproate anticonvulsant therapy, in whom it occurs more mildly, are heterozygotes for one or another of these enzyme deficiencies.

Complete deficiency of any of the first four enzymes in the cycle usually leads to severe hyperammonemia in the first 2 to 4 days of life. The patients have irritability, lethargy, and poor feeding that progress rapidly to stupor, seizures, coma, respirator dependence, and death. The plasma ammonia level often exceeds 1000 μM, and urea levels are extremely low. Episodic hyperammonemia occurs in association with periods of endogenous protein catabolism and severely affects patients, such as those with severe OTC deficiency; they almost certainly die or suffer severe neurologic impairment during one of these episodes. Patients with partial deficiency of urea cycle enzymes or those who avoid hyperammonemia in the neonatal period may present at any time later in life, from infancy to adulthood. Older patients have irritability, vomiting, and disorientation, which may progress (as in the infants) to stupor, seizures, coma, and death. These episodes are often precipitated by severe infection, excessive protein intake, parturition, or rarely by menstruation, or they may have no apparent cause.

Some general genetic characteristics of defects in the urea cycle are presented in Table 178–1.

TABLE 178–1. GENETIC CHARACTERISTICS OF DISORDERS OF THE UREA CYCLE

Enzyme Defect	Inheritance Pattern	Heterozygote Detection	Heterozygote Symptoms	Prenatal Diagnosis*
Carbamoyl phosphate synthetase	AR†	No‡	No	Yes
Ornithine transcarbamoylase	X-linked	Yes, in most instances*	Yes	Yes
Argininosuccinate synthetase	AR	No‡	No	Yes
Argininosuccinate lyase	AR	Yes	No	Yes
Arginase I	AR	Yes	No	Yes

* With varying degrees of ease.
† AR = Autosomal recessive.
‡ Heterozygotes for all disorders can be detected, if the specific base change in the gene has been ascertained. This is not practical at this time outside of the research laboratory.

ENZYME DEFICIENCIES

DEFICIENCY OF CARBAMOYL PHOSPHATE SYNTHETASE. This, the first enzyme in the urea cycle, constitutes up to 25% of the mitochondrial matrix protein in liver, and ordinarily all of the carbamyl phosphate synthesized from ammonium and bicarbonate by CPS-1 is used to produce urea. Orotic acid and pyrimidine are products of carbamoylphosphate as well, which is synthesized by a second, independently regulated cytoplasmic enzyme. Patients with both the neonatal and later-onset forms have been described. Diagnosis may be inferred from hyperammonemia, low to absent levels of citrulline in the plasma amino acid profile, and normal or elevated bicarbonate levels. During acute hyperammonemia there is usually a generalized hyperaminoacidemia with particular prominence of glutamine. Liver transplantation alone offers definitive treatment. Restricting dietary protein, supplementing essential amino acids and citrulline, hospitalizing for "catabolic crises," hemodialysis or peritoneal dialysis, and administering phenylacetate (or phenylbutyrate) and benzoate to divert ammonia to phenylacetylglutamine and benzoylglycine (hippurate) are used to control symptoms and treat crises (Fig. 178–2). Patients with this and other urea cycle defects are prone to develop severe hyperammonemia with valproate anticonvulsant therapy.

DEFICIENCY OF ORNITHINE TRANSCARBAMOYLASE. This mitochondrial enzyme catalyzes the reaction of carbamyl phosphate with ornithine to form citrulline, which is then transported out of the mitochondrion for further metabolism. The acute form of this X-linked enzyme deficiency usually occurs in males. Uncommonly

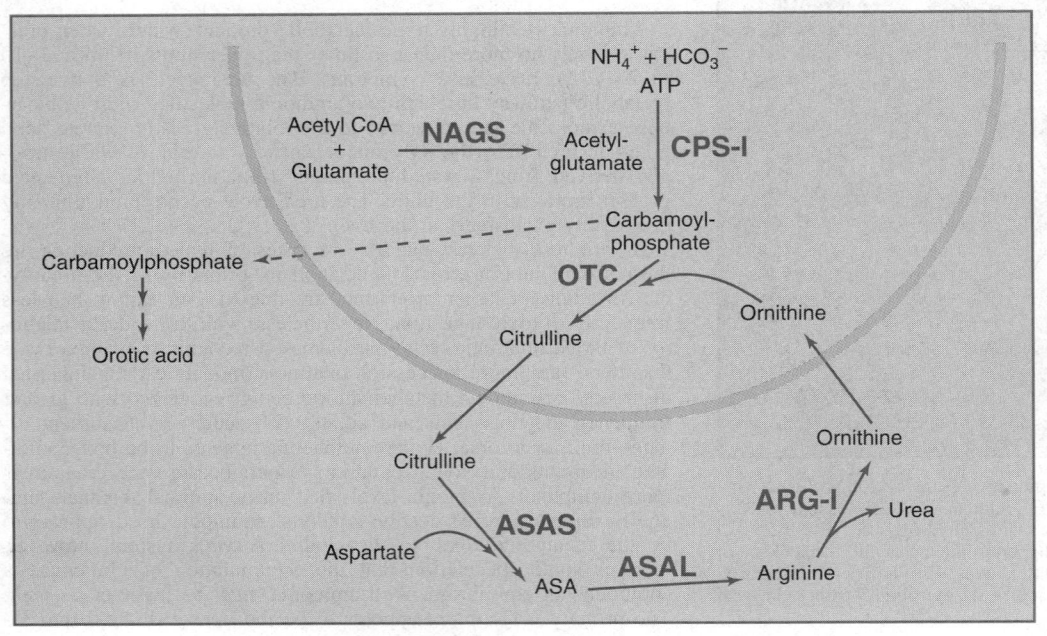

FIGURE 178–1. Abbreviated pathway for the urea cycle. NAGS = N-acetylglutamate synthetase; CPS-1 = carbamoylphosphate synthetase 1; OTC = ornithine transcarbamoylase; ASAS = argininosuccinate synthetase; ASAL = argininosuccinate lyase; ARG-1 = arginase 1. Enzymes within the bold line function within the mitochondrial matrix.

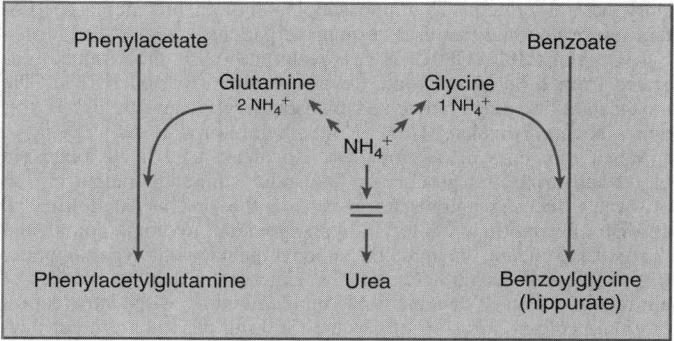

FIGURE 178–2. Mechanisms of ammonia diversion from the urea cycle with administration of sodium phenylacetate and sodium benzoate.

a newborn female may be severely affected, thought to be due to random X-chromosome inactivation. Female carriers of this co-dominant trait usually escape obvious symptoms, but those who have them usually present later in life or at parturition with hyper-ammonemic crises, some of which may be severe enough to be fatal. A smaller number of males with partial enzyme deficiency may present later as well. Patients with this "later-onset" form of the disease may suffer from severe and otherwise inexplicable protein intolerance. The amino and organic acid profiles resemble those of CPS-1 deficiency. OTC deficiency is distinguished by extraordinarily high levels of orotic acid in the urine, formed when the excess carbamoyl phosphate accumulating in the mitochondrion leaks into the cytoplasm and is channelled into the pyrimidine biosynthetic pathway (see Fig. 178–1). Orotic acid levels may be normal when ammonia has been controlled. Because of this typical clinical biochemical picture, liver biopsy to confirm enzymes is less frequently undertaken than in CPS-1 deficiency. An allopurinol challenge may be necessary to detect carrier females, a test with <100% accuracy. The treatment is identical to that described for CPS-1 deficiency.

DEFICIENCY OF ARGININOSUCCINATE SYNTHETASE (CITRULLINEMIA). This cytoplasmic enzyme condenses the citrulline synthesized by OTC with aspartate to form argininosuccinate in a reaction that introduces the second ammonia nitrogen for excretion as urea. ASAS deficiency leads to hyperammonemia, greatly increased blood citrulline levels, and excretion of excessive amounts of citrulline and orotic acid in the urine. Here, too, neonatal, later-onset, or symptomless deficiency of the enzyme has been reported. Genetic heterogeneity at the ASAS locus has been demonstrated by residual enzyme activity or by study of the gene and its mRNA.

Treatment is similar to that for CPS-1 and OTC deficiencies except that arginine is supplemented instead of citrulline. Citrulline excretion is more complete than that of ammonia, and managing this condition is somewhat easier.

DEFICIENCY OF ARGININOSUCCINATE LYASE (AR-GININOSUCCINIC ACIDURIA). ASA is cleaved into two smaller product molecules, arginine and fumarate, in a reaction catalyzed by ASA lyase. This enzyme deficiency results in massive accumulation and excretion of ASA. Variable onset or lack of symptoms characterizes this enzyme deficiency as well. ASA is actively secreted by the renal tubules and its synthesis can be stimulated by stoichiometric amounts of arginine as a source of ornithine to drive the urea cycle. By this means, ammonia levels are rapidly reduced and can be controlled more reliably than in any other urea cycle disorder.

DEFICIENCY OF ARGINASE 1 (HYPERARGININEMIA). Arginase, the final enzyme in the urea cycle, catalyzes the hydrolysis of arginine to urea and ornithine, the latter returned to the mitochondrion to participate in another cycle of ammonia detoxification (see Fig. 178–1). Clinical symptoms of hyperargininemia, the rarest of the urea cycle defects, are of later onset, are more gradual and relentless in progression, and are less frequently or seriously punctuated by apparent episodes of acute hyperammonemia and organic brain syndrome. Rather typically, normal patients begin to develop gait abnormalities and spasticity at age 2 to 3, and cortical and pyramidal tract dysfunction progresses slowly. More than 80% of the reported patients are still alive, some at age 30 or older. The di-

agnosis is often suspected when arginine levels are found to be elevated in blood or urine. Excess arginine excretion in urine along with secondary cystinuria pattern is more variable and less reliable as a screening method. Hyperammonemia is usually seen only during acute catabolic episodes.

Although most patients have been moderately to severely retarded at detection, treatment by limiting protein and diverting ammonia reverses many of the most severe manifestations of the disease, and presymptomatic treatment has allowed two patients to reach the age of 20 or older without apparent clinical manifestations.

FUTURE TREATMENT

Urea cycle defects, originally considered a pediatric problem, are moving into the realm of internal medicine. Internists must cast aside the lactulose used for hyperammonemia of liver failure and gastrointestinal bleeding in favor of diversion therapy and hemodialysis. Soon liver replacement, the artificial liver, and gene therapy will be more widely used. As breakthroughs in gene technology allow us to dissect the pathobiology of the acute catabolic process, efforts to control this process rather than control its consequences will become increasingly important.

Bachmann C: Urea cycle disorders. *In* Fernandes J, Saudubray J-M, Tada K (eds.): Inborn Metabolic Diseases. New York, Springer-Verlag, 1990, p 211. *A practical clinical chapter on urea cycle disorders reflecting a transatlantic perspective.*

Brusilow SW, Horwich AL: Urea cycle enzymes. *In* Scriver CR, Beaudet AL, Sly WS, Valle, D (eds.): The Metabolic and Molecular Bases of Inherited Disease. 7th ed. New York, McGraw-Hill, 1995. *The definitive clinical and molecular discussion of these inborn errors.*

Elsas III LJ, Acosta PB: Nutritional support of inherited metabolic diseases. *In* Shils ME, Olson JA, Shike M (eds.): Modern Nutrition in Health and Disease. 8th ed. Malvern, PA, Lea & Febiger, 1994, p 1147. *A practical guide to the nutritional aspects of treating this and other metabolic disorders.*

179 BRANCHED-CHAIN AMINOACIDURIAS
Louis J. Elsas

Leucine, isoleucine, and valine are essential amino acids that share branching, aliphatic chains.

MAPLE SYRUP URINE DISEASE (MSUD). This disorder, also called branched-chain α-ketoaciduria, derives its name from the burnt-sugar smell of affected infants. MSUD is caused by impaired branched chain α-ketoacid dehydrogenase, which catalyzes decarboxylation of the α-ketoacid derivatives of all three of these amino acids. Isovaleric acidemia affects only the next step of leucine catabolism and is caused by defects in isovaleryl CoA dehydrogenase. Both disorders conform to autosomal recessive patterns of inheritance. The affected homozygote exhibits impaired activity in the branched-chain α-ketoacid dehydrogenase (BCKD) multienzyme complex. This enzyme catalyzes oxidative decarboxylation and transacylation of α-ketoisocaproate, α-keto-β-methylvalerate, and α-ketoisovalerate, which are derived from deamination of leucine, isoleucine, and valine, respectively. The blocked reaction is

$$\text{Branched chain}-\overset{\displaystyle O}{\overset{\|}{C}}-\text{COOH} + \text{CoASH} + \text{NAD}^+ \longrightarrow$$

$$\text{Branched chain}-\overset{\displaystyle O}{\overset{\|}{C}}-\text{CoA} + CO_2 + \text{NADH} + H^+$$

If impaired, branched chain α-ketoacids and amino acids accumulate throughout the body and produce neurotoxicity by poorly defined mechanisms.

The disease is caused by mutations in one of six genes, which code for the six different proteins that make up the branched chain α-ketoacid dehydrogenase multienzyme complex. A wide range of mutations is defined, along with the consequent severity of impaired enzyme and clinical manifestations (Table 179–1).

TABLE 179-1. GENES, PROTEINS, AND MUTATIONS IN THE HUMAN BRANCHED-CHAIN α-KETOACID DEHYDROGENASE COMPLEX

Name (Function)	Chromosome Locus	Gene Size (kb)	Mature Protein (kd)	Mutation
E1α (decarboxylase)	19q13.1-q13.2	55	47	Y393N (Mennonite missense mutation)
E1β (stabilizes decarboxylase)	6p21-p22	100	37	11bp deletion (frameshift with premature STOP)
E2 (acyltransferase)	1p31	68	52	E163STOP F215C (exonic and intronic insertions, deletions, and transitions)
E3 (dehydrogenase)	7	?	55	Affects other substrate-specific dehydrogenases (α-ketoglutarate and pyruvate)
E1α kinase (inactivates)	?	?	43	?
E1α phosphatase (activates)	?	?	?	?

These proteins are encoded in the nuclear genome. Once translated in the cytosol, they are guided to the mitochondria by amino terminal leader sequences, transmigrate through outer and inner membrane, and assemble in the mitochondrial matrix. The six proteins are (1) a dimeric E1 or branched-chain α-ketoacid decarboxylases (E1α and E1β); (2) a branched-chain dihydrolipoamide acyltransferase (E2); (3) lipoamide oxidoreductase (E3); (4) E1 α kinase; and (5) E1 α phosphatase.

Several cofactors are involved in the overall reaction, including thiamin pyrophosphate, lipoamide covalently bound to E2, coenzyme A, and nicotinamide adenine dinucleotide. Many patients respond to pharmacologic excesses of thiamine supplement (8 mg per kilogram per day). The presumed mechanism is that by saturating binding sites for thiamine pyrophosphate on E1α, the multienzyme complex is stabilized to biologic degradation.

Diagnosis. In typical MSUD, feeding difficulties and apnea develop in a newborn who was normal at birth. Convulsions and decorticate rigidity may develop, and, before newborn screening, affected infants died or were severely damaged. With newborn screening, retrieval, diagnosis, and diet intervention before age 2 weeks, these children not only survive but have reached adulthood and can reproduce.

In surveyed populations the frequency of MSUD varies from 1 in 760 (in Mennonites) to an average United States figure of 1 in 200,000 newborns. Atypical cases with less severe clinical manifestations may be missed in newborn screening and appear with intermittent ataxia in later childhood or early adulthood. The diagnosis should be suspected clinically by the patient's intermittent symptoms related to protein ingestion and sweet smell to the earwax. A positive dinitrophenylhydrazine reaction is seen in urine, and the diagnosis is confirmed by the abnormal excesses of branched-chain amino acids and ketoacids in blood and urine. The enzyme defect is demonstrable in leukocytes and fibroblasts, and prenatal monitoring has been accomplished both biochemically and through DNA analysis.

Treatment. Treatment is aimed at limiting intake of branched-chain amino acids to prevent accumulation of neurotoxic branched-chain α-ketoacids. However, these essential amino acids must be ingested in large enough quantities to enable new protein synthesis and normal growth. Commercial formulas are available to accomplish this goal. In infancy and early childhood, anabolism is encouraged by providing excess calories and maintaining total protein intake at the recommended daily allowance. Treatment is monitored clinically by growth and development and biochemically by analyzing plasma amino acid concentrations. Because leucine residues are more frequent than isoleucine and valine in natural proteins, care must be given not to overrestrict isoleucine and valine while attempting to lower blood concentrations of leucine by restricting dietary natural protein. Thiamine supplements enable increased protein intake in some thiamine-responsive patients.

ISOVALERIC ACIDEMIA. Isovaleryl CoA is the product generated from α-ketoisocaproate (leucine's derivative) by BCKD. The next catabolic step is catalyzed by isovaleryl CoA dehydrogenase, which coverts isovaleryl CoA to β-methylcrotonyl CoA.

When this enzyme is impaired, isovaleric acid accumulates in blood and urine and produces a foul odor similar to rancid cheese or sweaty feet. Symptoms are severe in the first week of life and consist of vomiting, acidosis, hypoglycemia, tremors, coma, and death. Leukopenia, anemia, thrombocytopenia, and hyperammonemia may occur during acute attacks. Emergency therapy consists of eliminating dietary leucine and supplementing with intravenous, oral, and colonic infusion of glycine (300 mg per kilogram per day) to provide an alternate excretory pathway for the nontoxic adduct, isovaleryl glycine. Carnitine (100 mg per kilogram) may provide nontoxic adducts of isovaleryl carnitine. Both adducts are excreted in the urine. As patients mature, they have less frequent attacks and are developmentally normal. "Attacks" are caused by excess leucine ingestion, starvation, infections, or other causes of catabolism. Chronic intermittent forms of this disorder have not been differentiated from acute infantile forms at the biochemical or molecular level of enzyme or gene analysis and may result from epigenetic phenomena.

Diagnosis. The diagnosis is suspected from the clinical presentation and associated odor and is established by demonstrating excess isovaleric acid and its adducts in the urine by gas-liquid chromatography. The gene has been cloned and sequenced and some mutations have been defined.

Treatment. Chronic therapy includes reduced intake of leucine. Unlike MSUD, valine and isoleucine are normally catabolized and are required as essential nutrients in normal amounts in the diet. Supplements of glycine (90 to 100 mg per kilogram per day) and carnitine (10 mg per kilogram per day) are used as part of chronic dietary management. Outcome is excellent in both infantile and later-onset forms of isovaleric acidemia diseases if the acute, irreversible effects of the neonatal disease are prevented.

Danner DJ, Elsas LJ: Disorders of branched chain amino and keto acid metabolism. *In* Scriver CR, Beaudet A, Sly W, Valle D (eds.): The Metabolic and Molecular Bases of Inherited Disease. 7th ed. New York, McGraw-Hill, 1995. *Sophisticated discussion of clinical, biochemical, and pathophysiologic characteristics of these diseases (268 references).*
Elsas LJ, Acosta PB: Nutrition support of inherited metabolic disease. *In* Shils ME, Olson JE, Shike M (eds.): Modern Nutrition in Health and Disease. 8th ed. Malvern, PA, Lea & Febiger, 1994, p 1147. *A complete approach to dietary therapy of these diseases.*

180 HOMOCYSTINURIA
Bruce A. Barshop

Homocystinuria *per se* refers to abnormal urinary excretion of the disulfide form of homocysteine, and excessive blood homocysteine or homocystine, that is, homocyst(e)inemia, is a sign of a small number of specific metabolic disorders. Cardinal signs of the homocyst(e)inemia sequence include ocular lens dislocation, mental retardation, skeletal abnormalities, and thromboembolic complications. Cystathionine β-synthase deficiency is the most common cause. Rarer causes are disorders of homocysteine remethylation due to methylenetetrahydrofolate reductase deficiency or a variety of disorders of vitamin B_{12} distribution or metabolism to the active methylcobalamin cofactor for methionine synthase. Homocystinuria may also arise pharmacologically, as with triacetyl-azauridine, possibly related to pyridoxine depletion.

BIOCHEMISTRY

Homocysteine is a nonprotein amino acid that is the transmethylation product of methionine (Fig. 180-1). Homocysteine may be remethylated to methionine or may participate in a transulfuration sequence. The proportion of remethylation to transulfuration is regulated in humans, varying with availability of methionine and cysteine.

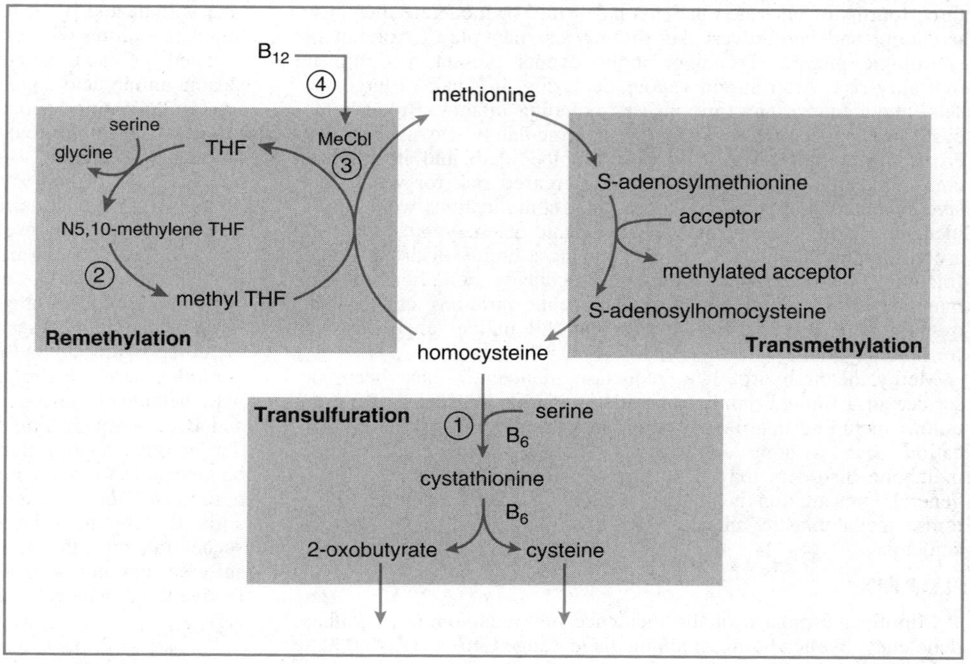

FIGURE 180–1. Pathways of homocysteine metabolism. The systems of transmethylation, remethylation, and transulfuration are marked. Steps discussed are numbered: (1) cystathionine β-synthase; (2) methylenetetrahydrofolate reductase; (3) methionine synthase; (4) systems of cobalamin absorption, distribution, and reduction: THF = tetrahydrofolate; MeCbl = methylcobalamin; B_{12} = cyanocobalamin/hydroxocobalamin; B_6 = pyridoxine.

Deficiency of cystathionine β-synthase results from a range of structural enzyme mutations, with heterogeneity in severity, most notably with respect to responsiveness of the biochemical abnormalities to pyridoxine. Approximately half of reported patients are pyridoxine responsive, and in these patients the course is generally less severe. While there is intrafamilial as well as interfamilial variability in clinical expression, there is complete concordance at the extremes of pyridoxine unresponsiveness or absence of immunoreactive material. Defects in homocysteine remethylation arise from deficiency of methylenetetrahydrofolate reductase or disorders of cobalamin metabolism, due to either impaired cellular accumulation in both adenosylcobalamin and methylcobalamin (Cbl C and D defects), defective cobalamin reduction on methionine synthase (Cbl E and G), or decreased lysosomal cobalamin entry or efflux (transcobalamin II deficiency or Cbl F, respectively). All of these inborn conditions are inherited in an autosomal recessive manner.

Cystathionine β-synthase maps to chromosome 21q22, a region associated with the Down syndrome phenotype. Transcobalamin II maps to chromosome 22q11-q13.1, and the remaining disorders are not mapped.

CLINICAL FEATURES

Cystathionine β-synthase deficiency is pleiotropic, with effects in eye, skeleton, and central nervous and vascular systems (Table 180–1). Nontraumatic dislocation of the ocular lens can be a presenting finding. Almost all untreated patients develop some abnormality of the skeletal system. Eye and skeletal system changes resemble those in Marfan syndrome, which is due to a defect in the fibrillin gene. Fibrillin, present in high concentration in the zonular fibers and the matrix of the periosteum and perichondrium, is extremely rich in cysteine; fibrillin structure may be affected either by cysteine limitation or homocysteinylation. Between one third and

TABLE 180–1. HOMOCYSTINURIA

Class	Cause	Biochemical Features			Clinical Features	
		hcys	met	MMA	System	Signs
Homocysteine transulfuration defect	Cystathionine β-synthase deficiency	↑	↑	—	Ocular	Ectopia lentis, myopia, glaucoma, optic atrophy, retinal detachment
					Skeletal	Elongated and thinned bones, arachnodactyly, genu valgum, pectus malformation, scoliosis
					Vascular	Thromboembolic events (arterial or venous)
					Neurologic	Mental retardation often in untreated cases Cerebrovascular thromboses, seizures Psychiatric disorders, personality disorder
Homocysteine remethylation defect	Methylenetetrahydrofolate reductase deficiency	↑	↓	—	Ocular	Ectopia lentis
					Vascular	Thromboses
					Neurologic	Variable—psychiatric to severe neurologic
	Cobalamin metabolic defects B_{12} uptake/distribution					
	Transcobalamin II deficiency	—/↑	—/↓	+/—	Hematologic	Pancytopenia, macrocytosis
	Cbl F (lysosomal B_{12} efflux defect)				Pansystemic	Methylmalonic acidemia, ketoacidosis
	B_{12} reduction/synthesis of adenosyl-cobalamin and methylcobalamin				Pansystemic	Methylmalonic acidemia, ketoacidosis
	Cbl C, Cbl D	—/↑	—/↓	+	Hematologic	Pancytopenia
					Neurologic	Mental retardation
	B_{12} reduction/fixation of methyl-cobalamin to methionine synthetase					
	Cbl E, Cbl G	↑	—/↓	—	Vascular	Vaso-occlusive phenomena

Hcys = homocyst(e)inemia/homocystinuria; met = elevated plasma methionine; MMA = methylmalonic acidemia three fourths of untreated patients have mild or moderate mental retardation, and cerebrovascular thrombosis may play a role in the neurologic picture. Thromboembolic events present a significant mortality risk. Arterial and venous occlusion, in small or large vessels, may occur at any time in life, including infancy. Blood homocyst(e)ine concentrations may be intermediately elevated in heterozygotes, particularly after a methionine load, and it has been considered that heterozygotes are at increased risk for vaso-occlusive events. Although increased vascular complications were not evident in a large outcome survey of obligate heterozygotes, there are a considerable number of studies showing a highly disproportionate fraction of patients with various vaso-occlusive complications who manifest either blood homocyst(e)ine concentrations or fibroblast cystathionine β-synthase activities that fall in the range observed for heterozygotes.

Methylenetetrahydrofolate reductase deficiency has been described in a limited number of patients, with a spectrum of presentations including neurologic symptoms, thromboses, and lens dislocation, but without conspicuous skeletal changes. Cobalamin metabolic disorders may have clinical features in common, but in general, presentation is in early childhood with neurologic symptoms, megaloblastic anemia, and in some cases, methylmalonic acidemia.

PREVALENCE

Minimum estimates of the incidence of cystathionine β-synthase deficiency by newborn screening have ranged from 1:300,000 to 1:60,000 live births, varying with population and method. Estimates for incidence have been in the range of 1:40,000 in Europe, corresponding to a carrier frequency of about 1%. The incidence of homocysteine remethylation defects appears to be < 1:800,000.

DIAGNOSIS

Urine metabolic screening generally reveals a positive reaction with cyanide-nitroprusside, but this is neither specific nor particularly sensitive. Quantitative amino acid analysis is superior. Urine, which normally has no measurable homocysteine or homocystine, may have up to 700 μmol homocysteine per day in affected individuals. Diagnosis also requires measuring plasma amino acids, since artifactual homocystinuria (e.g., bacterial contamination of cystathioninuric urine) can be excluded, and since various causes of homocystinuria may be distinguished (Table 180–1). In cystathionine β-synthase deficiency, methionine (normally below 30 μM) may be up to 2000 μM in the plasma, whereas in methylenetetrahydrofolate reductase deficiency or cobalamin metabolic defects that affect methionine synthase, the concentrations of methionine are decreased or normal. In urinary organic acid analysis, the presence of methylmalonic acid (and associated propionate metabolites) in addition to homocystinuria and/or homocysteinemia is characteristic of the defects of cobalamin metabolism. Anemia and macrocytosis are characteristic of the cobalamin metabolism defects, but not of uncomplicated cystathionine β-synthase or methylenetetrahydrofolate reductase deficiency. Associated immunodeficiency is also unique to the cobalamin metabolic defects among these disorders. Methionine loads have been used diagnostically. An oral bolus of methionine (typically 100 mg per kilogram) can distinguish heterozygotes and homozygotes on the basis of peak blood homocysteine concentration at around 4 hours, but overlap with the normal range is considerable for heterozygotes. Assay of cultured cells or biopsy tissue may confirm the diagnosis. Cystathionine β-synthase deficiency can be assayed in liver biopsy specimens, lymphocyte preparations, or fibroblasts; heterozygotes can be distinguished, but there is considerable overlap with normal values. Methylenetetrahydrofolate reductase can be assayed in fibroblasts or liver biopsy specimens, and the cobalamin defects can be distinguished by complementation or uptake studies in cultured fibroblasts.

TREATMENT

In *cystathionine β-synthase deficiency* it is important to determine initially whether a patient is responsive to pyridoxine. Doses of 100 to 500 mg or greater are given per day, and levels of plasma and urinary amino acids should be followed over the course of a few weeks. Folic acid repletion should precede the trial of pyridox-

ine. If the patient responds, pyridoxine supplementation should be continued indefinitely. Dietary management with low methionine intake is indicated if the response to pyridoxine is less than complete. Supplementation with cysteine may be beneficial. The diet must be adjusted in each patient individually so as to approach normal plasma amino acid concentrations. The incidence of certain progressive complications appears to be reduced with dietary therapy, and certainly the intellectual outcome is improved with early institution of dietary treatment. Betaine (*N,N,N*-trimethylglycine) allows for remethylation of homocysteine by an alternate pathway and may be useful in pyridoxine-unresponsive patients. Dipyridamole and low-dose aspirin may be useful adjuvants, and avoiding agents that can promote thromboembolism, such as oral contraceptives, is probably prudent. Surgery is not contraindicated, but requires special caution; surgical procedures are without thromboembolic complication in more than 95% of cases in which appropriate precautions are taken, including hydration and possibly perioperative pyridoxine treatment.

Methylenetetrahydrofolate reductase deficiency can be treated with betaine, folinic acid, methionine, and additional vitamins B$_6$ and B$_{12}$, although, *uniformly,* results have been less than complete. On the other hand, milder variants may occur in adulthood and may be amenable to treatment aimed at decreasing homocysteine. *Cobalamin metabolic disorders* may be treated with large amounts of vitamin B$_{12}$ (up to 1 mg daily). The response may be dramatically successful, but may be incomplete, and neurologic damage already suffered may not be reversible. Hydroxocobalamin may be more effective than cyanocobalamin.

Mudd SH, Skovby F, Levy HL, et al.: The natural history of homocystinuria due to cystathionine β-synthase deficiency. Am J Hum Genet 37:1, 1985. *The course of the untreated disease is defined in this international questionnaire study covering more than 600 patients, and some effects of treatment are analyzed statistically.*
Pyeritz RE: Homocystinuria. *In* Beighton P (ed.): McKusick's Heritable Disorders of Connective Tissue. St. Louis, CV Mosby, 1993, pp 137–178. *Complete discussion of clinical and metabolic features of homocystinuria with insights into possible effects on fibrillin structure.*

181 DISORDERS OF PURINE AND PYRIMIDINE METABOLISM

*Beverly S. Mitchell and
Michael S. Hershfield*

PURINE ENZYME DEFICIENCIES AND DISORDERS OF IMMUNE FUNCTION

ADENOSINE DEAMINASE DEFICIENCY. Adenosine deaminase (ADA) deficiency in its usual severe form causes the syndrome of severe combined immunodeficiency disease (SCID) with absence of both T- and B-lymphocyte function. Less complete ADA deficiency is associated with T-cell dysfunction and more variable loss of B-cell function. It is now recognized that ADA deficiency can result in slowly progressive immune dysfunction presenting in adolescents or adults. ADA deficiency accounts for approximately 20% of all SCID's and for one third to one half of those with autosomal recessive inheritance. Several hundred families with ADA deficiency have been identified to date. The frequency of ADA deficiency has been estimated at 1 in 200,000 to 1 in 1 million births.

Etiology and Pathogenesis. The gene for ADA is located on chromosome 20q. More than 25 single base changes within the coding region, as well as several deletions and splicing mutations leading to loss of enzymatic activity, have been identified. The majority of affected individuals are compound heterozygotes for two different molecular defects. A so-called partial deficiency of ADA activity resulting from mutations that cause a less severe loss of enzymatic activity in the absence of clinical manifestations has been identified in population screening programs.

ADA catalyzes the irreversible deamination of adenosine to inosine, and of 2′-deoxyadenosine to 2′-deoxyinosine (Fig. 181–1). In the absence of ADA activity, increased plasma levels of both adenosine and 2′-deoxyadenosine in the range of 0.5 to 10 μM occur; high levels of 2′-deoxyadenosine, but not adenosine, are excreted in

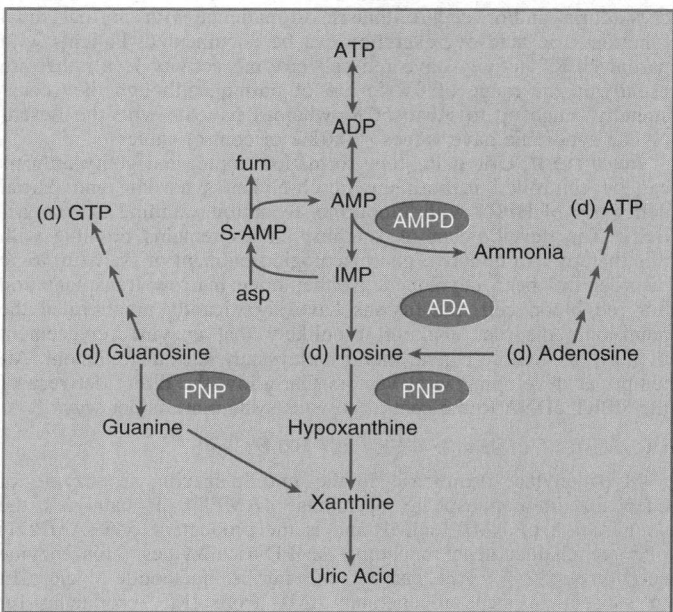

FIGURE 181-1. Schema of purine metabolism demonstrating metabolic reactions catalyzed by adenosine deaminase (ADA), purine nucleoside phosphorylase (PNP), and AMP deaminase (AMPD). asp = aspartate; fum = fumarate.

the urine. The pathogenesis of this disorder and its selectivity for cells of the immune system are not completely understood. The major pathogenic mechanism involves the accumulation of 2'-deoxy ATP derived from 2'-deoxyadenosine in lymphocyte progenitors and the toxicity of this metabolite for lymphoid cells. Deoxy ATP pool expansion inhibits ribonucleotide reductase, thus inhibiting DNA replication. In addition, 2'-deoxyadenosine inactivates the enzyme S-adenosylhomocysteine hydrolase, which may result in the accumulation of S-adenosylhomocysteine, an inhibitor of transmethylation reactions mediated by S-adenosylmethionine.

Clinical Manifestations. ADA deficiency is most frequently diagnosed in children with signs of immunodeficiency manifested by lymphopenia, failure to thrive, and recurrent infections with both ordinary pathogens and opportunistic organisms. *Pneumocystis carinii* infections and candidiasis are commonly observed, as well as cytomegalovirus, varicella, and other viral pneumonias and infections. Vaccination with live organisms may be fatal, and an increased incidence of B-cell lymphomas has been reported. Although the diagnosis has most commonly been made in very young children, there is increasing recognition of less severe forms of ADA deficiency presenting over the first two decades of life with milder forms of immunodeficiency. Chronic respiratory infections may lead to pulmonary insufficiency in older individuals. Physical findings are unremarkable with the exception of an absence of lymph nodes and tonsillar tissue and the presence in some affected infants of very prominent costochondral junctions. Neurologic abnormalities have been reported in occasional cases, as have autoimmune abnormalities such as hypothyroidism, hemolytic anemia, and immune thrombocytopenic purpura. Chest radiography reveals the absence of a thymus and peripheral blood examination usually demonstrates an absolute lymphopenia of <500 per microliter with a marked reduction in mature T cells and a more variable decrease in B cells associated with hypogammaglobulinemia and lack of specific antibody response to immunization. *In vitro* tests of lymphocyte function, including proliferative responses to mitogens and antigen, are abnormal.

Diagnosis. The disorder should be looked for in individuals with recurrent infections associated with unexplained lymphopenia. The diagnosis is made by measuring ADA activity in the hemolysates of untransfused patients. Determining the degree of elevation of 2'-deoxy ATP and the reduction of S-adenosylhomocysteine hydrolase activity in erythrocytes is useful to gauge the severity of ADA deficiency. In kindreds in which the mutations in

the ADA gene have been identified because of a previously affected sibling, the diagnosis can be made at the molecular level by amplifying specific regions of the gene using the polymerase chain reaction (PCR) and DNA sequencing. Prenatal diagnosis can be accomplished by ADA activity assay of cultured amniotic or chorionic villus cells, as well as by DNA analysis when the mutations are known.

Treatment. Specific antibiotic treatment for infections is essential. In addition, patients should receive prophylaxis for *Pneumocystis carinii* and fungal infections and should not receive live virus vaccines or unirradiated blood products. Most patients are also treated with intravenous immunoglobulin. Once the diagnosis is established, the patient is a candidate for either bone marrow transplantation from an HLA-identical or haploidentical donor or enzyme replacement therapy with polyethylene glycol (PEG)–conjugated bovine ADA. The long-term survival with engraftment for second siblings (who are less ill at diagnosis) with HLA-identical transplants is >90%, and this remains the treatment of choice if a donor is available. Haploidentical transplants with T-cell–depleted marrow have been less successful, with the probability of long-term survival ranging from 28 to 67%. Enzyme replacement with PEG-conjugated ADA (PEG-ADA), which maintains high levels of ADA activity in plasma, is uniformly effective in correcting metabolic abnormalities caused by ADA deficiency. Improving lymphocyte counts and function by restoring the thymus has occurred within weeks to a few months of intramuscular treatment with PEG-ADA given once or twice weekly. Although lymphocyte counts do not return to normal, the majority of patients have a major reduction in infectious episodes and have resumed growth and normal activities. Experimental somatic cell gene therapy (see Ch. 25) has been used in several patients who have been treated concomitantly with PEG-ADA. Retroviral vector–mediated transduction of ADA cDNA into the patients' interleukin-2–activated peripheral blood T cells has increased ADA activity that has persisted for several months. This disorder has been considered a prime target for gene therapy directed at lymphohematopoietic stem cells derived from bone marrow, and umbilical cord blood in prenatally diagnosed patients and clinical trials using this approach are in progress.

PURINE NUCLEOSIDE PHOSPHORYLASE DEFICIENCY. Purine nucleoside phosphorylase (PNP) catalyzes the reversible phosphorolysis of the nucleosides inosine and 2'-deoxyinosine to the base hypoxanthine and guanosine and 2'-deoxyguanosine to guanine (Fig. 181-1). Deficiency of PNP has been reported in approximately 30 families, and mutations in the PNP gene located on chromosome 14q have been identified in several individuals. Lack of PNP activity is associated primarily with T-cell depletion and cellular immune dysfunction, although either B-cell dysfunction or B-cell hyperactivity associated with autoimmune disorders also occurs in about one third of patients. Neurologic abnormalities including spasticity, ataxia, behavioral abnormalities, hypertonia, and hypotonia have been seen in >50% of affected individuals. Patients generally present in childhood with recurrent infections associated with markedly reduced lymphocyte counts with specific loss of T cells and are found to lack a thymus gland. Absence or marked reduction of PNP activity in erythrocytes is diagnostic. Supportive laboratory tests consist of a marked decrease in uric acid due to the inability to convert PNP substrates to hypoxanthine and guanine. Serum and urinary levels of all four nucleoside substrates of PNP are increased. The metabolite of 2'-deoxyguanosine, 2'-deoxy GTP, is found in erythrocytes and is thought to be causally associated with the T-cell depletion because it accumulates in T-cell precursors leading to a block in DNA replication. Treating this disorder with either red cell transfusions or with infusions of deoxycytidine aimed at restoring DNA replication has not resulted in any consistent therapeutic response. The efficacy of bone marrow transplantation to date remains poor. PEG-conjugated PNP and gene therapy remain developmental, and the small number of affected patients makes clinical research on this disorder difficult.

LESCH-NYHAN SYNDROME

The Lesch-Nyhan syndrome is an X-linked disorder caused by absence or severe deficiency of the enzyme hypoxanthine-guanine phosphoribosyltransferase (HPRT). It is manifested as a devastating neurologic disorder consisting of compulsive self-mutilation, choreoathetosis, spasticity, and often mental retardation. The syndrome occurs with a frequency of 1 in 100,000 births and is associated with a marked overproduction of purines, resulting in hyperuricemia and gout (see Ch. 251). Partial deficiency of the enzyme also causes hyperuricemia, but without severe neurologic deficits, and accounts for < 1% of patients with gout.

Etiology and Pathogenesis. The molecular basis of HPRT deficiency has been studied in detail, and a large number of point mutations, splicing defects, and deletions have been identified. HPRT catalyzes the reaction whereby the purine bases hypoxanthine and guanine are condensed with ribose-5-PO$_4$ derived from PP-ribose-P to form the corresponding nucleotides, inosine and guanosine monophosphate, thus salvaging the purine bases for nucleotide metabolism. In the absence of HPRT activity, hypoxanthine and guanine can be catabolized only through xanthine to uric acid, causing hyperuricemia and markedly increased uric aciduria. In addition, an increase in the intracellular concentration of PP-ribose-P and reduced formation of inosine monophosphate (IMP) and guanosine monophosphate (GMP) leads to a marked increase in the overall rate of *de novo* synthesis of purine nucleotides, further increasing the generation of uric acid. The clinical sequelae of hyperuricemia and increased uric acid excretion are the juvenile onset of uric acid stone formation and gouty arthritis. The pathogenesis of the neurologic defects is not well understood but could involve guanine nucleotide deficiency as a result of decreased guanine salvage in neurons that depend on the salvage pathway for purine nucleotide synthesis. Positron emission tomography has demonstrated a selective decrease in glucose metabolism in the caudate nucleus, but anatomic studies of the brains of affected individuals have not revealed any structural lesions.

Clinical Manifestations. The Lesch-Nyhan syndrome is manifested in affected males during the first year of life by an initial delay in motor development, followed by extrapyramidal signs leading to choreoathetosis and, at approximately age 1, by pyramidal tract involvement with hyperreflexia, clonus, and scissoring of the legs. Compulsive self-destructive behavior appears sometime between early childhood and adolescence and constitutes a behavior pattern unique to this disorder. Affected individuals bite their fingers, lips, and buccal mucosa, necessitating restraints and in some cases edentulation. Repeated attempts at self-injury, such as placing extremities in dangerous areas and self-inflicted head trauma, are common. Mental and growth retardation also occur in the majority of cases. Uric acid crystalluria may be noted as orange crystals in the diaper during the first weeks of life and, if untreated, may lead to nephrolithiasis, obstructive uropathy, and azotemia. Hyperuricemia is usually present and may attain levels of 18 mg per deciliter. Gout may develop later in the course of the disease, but generally not before puberty. Death usually occurs in the second or third decade from infection or renal failure.

Patients with partial deficiency of HPRT develop uric acid crystalluria and renal calculi in childhood, and gouty arthritis often occurs before age 20. Neurologic manifestations, including mental retardation, mild spastic quadriplegia, dysarthria, cerebellar ataxia, and seizures, are noted in 20% of patients, but self-mutilation does not develop. Patients with partial HPRT deficiency may seek medical attention due to passing a renal calculus or an attack of gouty arthritis. Life expectancy is normal.

Diagnosis. The clinical diagnosis of the Lesch-Nyhan syndrome is strongly suggested by the self-mutilation and characteristic choreoathetosis; mental retardation of other origins is very rarely accompanied by the induction of self-injury, especially in the presence of intact sensation. The presence of hyperuricemia supports the diagnosis. The definitive diagnosis is made by demonstrating a lack of HPRT enzymatic activity in red cells or other tissues. The molecular defect has been established in many patients. Female carriers cannot be definitively identified by HPRT activity assay of peripheral blood cells but may be detected using cultured skin fibroblasts or by DNA analysis if the nature of the mutation in an affected male relative has been defined.

Partial deficiency of HPRT is manifested by the early onset of gouty arthritis in male patients or by the early onset of uric acid crystalluria and/or nephrolithiasis. In patients with normal renal function, uric acid overexcretion can be documented. Patients with partial HPRT activity have red cell enzyme activity levels that are usually in the range of 0.2 to 5% of normal, although they occasionally range up to 30 to 50%, whereas patients with the Lesch-Nyhan syndrome have values <0.01% of control values.

Treatment. Uric acid stone formation, tophi, and gouty arthritis can be controlled in both the Lesch-Nyhan syndrome and partial deficiency of HPRT with allopurinol to inhibit xanthine oxidase activity. The development of xanthine stones remains possible with this therapy. No effective pharmacologic treatment of the neurologic disorder has been developed. Neither bone marrow transplantation nor red blood cell transfusions have significantly ameliorated the neurologic disorder, making it unlikely that enzyme replacement therapy or stem cell gene therapy plays any role in treatment. Attempts at developing viral vectors that allow the direct delivery of the HPRT cDNA to the central nervous system are under way.

MYOADENYLATE DEAMINASE DEFICIENCY AND MYOPATHY

Myoadenylate deaminase is the muscle-specific isoenzyme of adenosine monophosphate deaminase (AMPD). It catalyzes the deamination of AMP to IMP and is the product of one (AMPD1) of three distinct genes encoding AMPD isoenzymes. This enzyme activity is an integral part of the purine nucleotide cycle that in subsequent steps regenerates AMP from IMP, producing fumarate (Fig. 181–1), and appears to play a major role in energy production in skeletal tissue. Deficiency of AMPD1 has been documented in 2% of all muscle biopsies submitted for histologic examination. Inherited deficiency of myoadenylate deaminase is associated with exercise-related cramps and myalgias. An acquired deficiency of AMPD1 is associated with a number of primary muscle disorders.

ETIOLOGY AND PATHOGENESIS. The AMPD1 gene is located on chromosome 1 and is expressed predominantly in skeletal muscle, whereas AMPD2 and 3 are expressed in other tissues. The normal expression of AMPD1 is associated with an alternatively spliced 12 bp second exon of the gene, so that 0.6 to 2% of the mRNA in human skeletal muscle lacks exon 2 and encodes a protein of four fewer amino acids. A single nonsense mutation within this second exon has been identified at frequencies ranging from 0.13 to 0.19 in the general population and is associated in its homozygous form with a marked reduction in AMPD1 protein. To date, no other mutations have been identified as causing this enzyme deficiency state. Acquired AMPD1 deficiency is associated with decreased AMPD1 mRNA levels that may be due to a regulatory defect in gene expression in a variety of muscle disorders.

AMPD1 protein has been shown to bind to myosin heavy chain in skeletal muscle. During contraction, the activity of AMPD1 increases markedly. Operation of the next two steps in the purine nucleotide cycle regenerates AMP and produces fumarate, an intermediate in the citric acid cycle, as a by-product. Patients deficient in AMPD1 do not generate IMP, NH3, or fumarate in skeletal muscle during exercise.

CLINICAL MANIFESTATIONS. Individuals with the inherited form of AMPD deficiency may develop fatigue, cramps, or myalgias following vigorous exercise; myoglobinuria has been reported occasionally. The majority of these patients have presented between childhood and early adulthood. The disorder has been documented in > 200 individuals. With the high frequency of the nonsense mutation in the general population, it is apparent that a large number of homozygous mutant individuals must exist who do not have clinical symptoms severe enough to warrant medical evaluation. It has been postulated that the low level of normal alternative splicing that eliminates the exon containing the nonsense codon results in production of a protein product with some enzymatic activity in many homozygous individuals. Acquired deficiency of AMPD1 is found in a number of muscle diseases, including neurogenic disorders, divergent myopathies, and collagen vascular disorders. The clinical symptoms of these individuals are dictated by the primary muscle disease. Whether the clinical heterogeneity of this disorder relates to the expression of the spliced variant of the enzyme and/or to the expression of other AMPD's in muscle tissue or indeed whether the enzyme deficiency state is causally associated with symptoms is under investigation.

DIAGNOSIS. Individuals with AMPD1 deficiency do not produce NH_3 on ischemic exercise of the forearm and may have an elevated CPK in 50% of cases. Histochemical stains and enzyme activity determinations demonstrate an absence of AMPD1 enzyme in muscle biopsies. The genetic abnormality may be detected by an altered restriction enzyme digestion site in genomic DNA.

TREATMENT. No treatment has been demonstrated to be highly effective. Oral ribose has been administered in an attempt to enhance the synthesis of purine nucleotides with variable subjective improvement.

2,8-DIHYDROXYADENINE RENAL STONES

Deficiency of the enzyme adenine phosphoribosyltransferase (APRT) leads to an accumulation of its substrate—adenine—which in turn is oxidized, although inefficiently, by xanthine oxidase to 2,8-dihydroxyadenine. Because of the insolubility of this product, patients with the autosomal recessive form of this disorder are predisposed to develop radiolucent renal calculi composed of 2,8-dihydroxyadenine. Renal stones may develop within the first months of life or present as late as the fifth decade, although many APRT-deficient individuals never develop stones. The diagnosis may be made by analyzing the stones with ultraviolet, infrared, or mass spectrometry or x-ray crystallography. Definitive diagnosis requires demonstrating the absence of APRT activity in erythrocyte lysates. No other biochemical or clinical abnormalities have been reported in individuals homozygous for this enzyme deficiency; heterozygous individuals have no clinical abnormalities. Mutations at the APRT locus are particularly common in individuals of Japanese ancestry, and investigation of the molecular basis of this defect reveals a single base mutation at codon 136 in 68% of the defective alleles, with two other mutations accounting for 28% of defects. Analysis of both germline and somatic cell mutations in non-Japanese subjects has revealed clustering of the mutations at the intron 4 splice donor site and at codon 87. Thus, the molecular basis of this disorder appears to result from relatively few mutations. Therapy for individuals with 2,8-dihydroxyadenine calculi consists of restricting dietary purines, high fluid intake, and treatment with allopurinol to prevent the oxidation of adenine by xanthine oxidase.

XANTHINURIA

Classic xanthinuria results from deficiency of the enzyme xanthine oxidase. As a consequence, xanthine and hypoxanthine produced by the catabolism of purines cannot be oxidized to uric acid, resulting in very low serum urate and urinary uric acid excretion values. Serum oxypurine (xanthine and hypoxanthine) concentrations and urinary oxypurine excretion are increased. This disorder has been identified in > 60 individuals, with approximately one third of these developing radiolucent renal calculi composed of xanthine. Crystalline deposits of xanthine and hypoxanthine in muscle have been described in a few individuals with muscle cramps following exercise and may also be associated with polyarthritis. The diagnosis is strongly suggested by the presence of low serum and urinary uric acid levels in conjunction with elevated serum and urinary oxypurine concentrations. Deficiency of xanthine oxidase activity can be confirmed by direct enzymatic assay. Therapy for xanthine calculi consists primarily of increasing fluid intake.

A combination of xanthine oxidase deficiency and sulfite oxidase deficiency may also result in xanthinuria and has been attributed to an absence of the molybdenum cofactor for catalytic activity required for both enzymes to be active. The few reported patients with this disorder have presented in infancy with a severe neurologic disorder characterized by seizures, nystagmus, enophthalmos, ocular lens dislocation, and Brushfield spots characteristic of sulfite oxidase deficiency.

DISORDERS OF PYRIMIDINE METABOLISM

Hereditary orotic aciduria is a rare genetic disorder of pyrimidine metabolism that is characterized by megaloblastic anemia, leukopenia, retarded growth and development, and high levels of urinary orotic acid excretion, frequently associated with crystal or stone formation. The disorder is inherited as an autosomal recessive defect and results from deficiency of activity of the bifunctional enzyme uridine monophosphate (UMP) synthase that in two steps catalyzes the conversion of orotic acid to UMP. This enzyme is, therefore, essential for the *de novo* synthesis of pyrimidine nucleotides. The gene encoding this enzyme has been localized to the long arm of chromosome 3 and two point mutations in the cDNA encoding the enzyme have been described that result in loss of its activity and the clinical syndrome. Administering uridine (2 to 4 grams per day) has been demonstrated to ameliorate the clinical sequelae of this enzymatic defect because uridine can be directly phosphorylated to UMP.

Pyrimidine 5'-nucleotidase deficiency is an autosomal recessive disorder that results in hereditary hemolytic anemia associated with prominent basophilic stippling of red blood cells. Erythrocytes contain high levels of cytidine and uridine monophosphates that are substrates for the enzyme, as well as a number of pyrimidine conjugates, including cytidine diphosphate (CDP)-choline and CDP-ethanolamine and uridine diphosphate-glucose. Acquired pyrimidine 5'-nucleotidase activity is found associated with lead toxicity and also with the induction of basophilic stippling due to undegraded ribosomal nucleoprotein and with accumulation of pyrimidine nucleotides. Diagnosis of the hereditary disorder is made by measuring erythrocyte pyrimidine 5'-nucleotidase enzymatic activity or by demonstrating elevated pyrimidine nucleotides by UV absorption spectra in red cell lysates.

Dihydropyrimidine dehydrogenase deficiency is a rare autosomal recessive disorder characterized by deficiency of the enzymatic activity responsible for degrading the pyrimidine bases uracil and thymidine. High excretion levels of these metabolites are found in the urine and may be detected when screening for organic aciduria. Although no clinical symptoms have been associated with this defect, administering fluoropyrimidines (5-fluorouracil; 5-fluorodeoxyuridine) to enzyme-deficient patients with malignancy can result in severe and prolonged drug-related toxicity.

Diasio RB, Beavers TL, Carpenter JT: Familial deficiency of dihydropyrimidine dehydrogenase: Biochemical basis for familial pyrimidinemia and severe 5-fluorouracil-induced toxicity. J Clin Invest 81:47, 1988. *This study documents the lack of dihydropyrimidine dehydrogenase activity as a causal factor in 5-FU toxicity.*

Hershfield MS, Mitchell BS: Immunodeficiency diseases caused by adenosine deaminase deficiency and purine nucleoside phosphorylase deficiency. *In* Scriver CR, Beaudet AL, Sly WS, Valle D (eds.): The Molecular and Metabolic Bases of Inherited Disease. 7th ed. New York, McGraw-Hill, 1995. *Highly detailed discussion of clinical, metabolic, and molecular aspects of ADA and PNP deficiency states.*

Kamatani N, Hakoda M, Otsuka S, et al.: Only three mutations account for almost all defective alleles causing adenine phosphoribosyltransferase deficiency in Japanese patients. J Clin Invest 90:130, 1992. *Analyzes 141 defective APRT alleles from 71 Japanese families to document that the number of mutations underlying the defect in the Japanese population is limited.*

Markert ML: Purine nucleoside phosphorylase deficiency. Immun Def Rev 3:45, 1991. *An excellent, comprehensive clinical review of patients with PNP deficiency.*

Sabina RL, Holmes EW: Myoadenylate deaminase deficiency. *In* Scriver CR, Beaudet AL, Sly WS, Valle D (eds.): The Molecular and Metabolic Bases of Inherited Disease. 7th ed. New York, McGraw-Hill, 1995. *In-depth description of the clinical and biochemical abnormalities associated with myoadenylate deficiency states.*

Sculley DG, Dawson PA, Emmerson BT, et al.: A review of the molecular basis of hypoxanthine-guanine phosphoribosyltransferase (HPRT) deficiency. Hum Genet 90:195, 1992. *A general review of the Lesch-Nyhan syndrome, HPRT gene structure, and HPRT mutations.*

Webster D, Becroft DMO, Suttle DP: Hereditary orotic aciduria and other deficiencies of pyrimidine metabolism. *In* Scriver CR, Beaudet AL, Sly WS, Valle D (eds.): The Molecular and Metabolic Bases of Inherited Disease. 7th ed. New York, McGraw-Hill, 1995. *An excellent review describing the clinical syndrome and the biochemistry of the enzyme deficiency state in great detail.*

Inherited Disorders of Connective Tissue

182 THE MUCOPOLYSACCHARIDOSES

Hans C. Andersson and Emmanuel Shapira

The mucopolysaccharidoses (MPS's) are a heterogeneous group of inherited lysosomal storage disorders. The common feature of these disorders is intracellular storage and urinary excretion of glycosaminoglycans (GAG's), previously termed acidic mucopolysaccharides. The GAG's result from proteolytic cleavage of large macromolecules—the proteoglycans. They are highly glycosylated and sulfated molecules that are normally degraded in a stepwise manner in the lysosome by specific enzymes that either cleave terminal sulfate or glycosyl groups or acetylate the GAG to facilitate further degradation. The MPS's result from the deficient activity of one of these lysosomal enzymes. This deficiency arrests further degradation of GAG's and leads to their storage in various tissues. The storage causes progressive disruption of cellular function and leads to physical deformation of various tissues.

The group of MPS disorders demonstrates two principles of human genetics—heterogeneity and variability. Heterogeneity refers to the observation that mutations in different enzymes located at different loci can lead to clinically indistinguishable phenotypes. This phenomenon is exemplified by the four types of MPS III (Sanfilippo). Within each type of MPS, a considerable clinical variability exists as to the age of onset, the rate of progression, and the extent to which various organs are involved. Typically, they manifest within a spectrum of severity from early, severe childhood forms to milder, late childhood or adolescent forms. This clinical variability can sometimes be explained by the biochemical and molecular observation of particular mutations with varying degrees of residual enzyme activity. Many of the genes coding for enzymes involved in the MPS diseases have been cloned, making possible mutation analysis in individual patients. The more severely affected patients have a mutation resulting in the complete absence of detectable enzyme protein in their tissues, whereas mildly affected patients have point mutations leading to an amino acid substitution with detectable enzyme protein but with markedly decreased residual activity. Other factors in addition to the specific gene mutation may also be involved in modifying the patient's clinical presentation.

CLINICAL FEATURES

Most patients with MPS diseases appear normal at birth and gradually develop pathologic findings in the first 2 years of life. The various MPS's share multiple organ system involvement, organomegaly, dysostosis multiplex, and facial coarsening. Dysostosis multiplex refers to the collective bony abnormalities, including thickened calvarium, J-shaped sella, anterior vertebral hypoplasia leading to kyphoscoliosis, impaired long bone growth with irregular metaphyses, poorly formed pelvis, and oar-shaped ribs that invariably lead to short stature. MPS I, II, III, and VII are usually also characterized by central nervous system (CNS) storage, resulting in progressive mental retardation. MPS IV (Morquio) spares the CNS but has unusually severe skeletal abnormalities, including odontoid hypoplasia that may become life-threatening. In many of the MPS's, sensorineural and conductive hearing loss and vision defects (corneal and retinal) may also contribute to poor intellectual development. Cardiac disease from GAG stored in valve leaflets, endocardium, myocardium, and coronary arteries is a common feature in middle childhood and is often the cause of death.

The MPS's are inherited as autosomal recessive disorders, with the exception of MPS II, which has an X-linked mode of inheritance. The incidence of each of the various MPS's is relatively rare, in the range of 1 in 40,000 to 1 in 100,000 live births. Table 182–1 summarizes some of the distinguishing clinical and biochemical features of the MPS's.

DIAGNOSIS

Whenever the diagnosis of MPS is suspected, a urine-screening test for GAG's should be performed. The most commonly used screening test is the toluidine blue spot test; it is relatively sensitive but has a significant false-positive rate owing to reactivity with chondroitin sulfate, which is a normal finding in the urine. In some MPS III and IV patients, the spot test can be falsely negative. In patients with a positive spot test and those suspected of being falsely negative, the various GAG's in the urine should be identified by either thin-layer chromatography or electrophoresis. Based on the clinical presentation and the pattern of urinary GAG's, the diagnosis should be established by demonstration of the specific enzyme deficiency in leukocytes, fibroblasts, or other tissues (Table 182–1). Mutation analysis is available for most MPS disorders, and a genotype-phenotype correlation has been established for some mutations.

MANAGEMENT AND TREATMENT

SUPPORTIVE CARE. In managing families with an MPS-affected member, proper counseling is one of the most important and difficult tasks (see Ch. 29). The basic explanation of the pathophysiology of the disease, emphasizing that nothing that the parents did or did not do led to the disorder, can alleviate the guilt and anger that parents of newly diagnosed MPS patients experience. The risk for other unaffected family members should be provided, including the option of prenatal diagnosis in future pregnancies in all family members with an increased risk for having affected offspring.

Treatment for patients with MPS is mainly symptomatic because treatments for the primary defect are few and variably effective. Supportive treatment should be aimed at the following complications:

1. Orthopedic: Because of the generalized and progressive nature of the skeletal involvement, a conservative orthopedic approach is most appropriate, minimizing surgical treatment. Surgical intervention is critical in patients with spinal cord compression and atlantoaxial instability. Orthopedic shoes and ankle braces can be used to maintain mobility in the early stages of the disease. In some patients, elongating the Achilles tendon may be helpful. Surgery is advised for carpal tunnel syndrome when progressive median nerve compression is documented.

2. Cardiorespiratory: Early alveolar involvement is relatively common in some of the MPS's. Small airway obstruction by accumulated storage material, thickened mucosal secretions, hypertrophy of tonsils/adenoids, and the associated macroglossia all contribute to the respiratory problems. Sleep apnea should be considered and treated in the early stages of the disease, whereas tracheostomy might be considered in the very advanced stages of the disorder. Managing a tracheostomy can be difficult owing to tenacious secretions. Cardiac insufficiency may be palliated by medical therapy, but valvular dysfunction is more difficult to correct, especially because these are very high-risk anesthesia patients.

3. Hernias: Inguinal and umbilical hernias are relatively common and often require surgical correction.

4. Neurologic: Only the relatively rare complication of hydrocephalus can be treated by ventriculoperitoneal shunting. Anticipatory diagnostic studies should attempt to ascertain those patients at risk for atlantoaxial dislocation.

5. Anesthesia: Patients with MPS should be considered at high risk whenever general anesthesia is considered. This is due to the associated respiratory complications, temporomandibular ankylosis, and atlantoaxial instability. General anesthesia should be restricted to mandatory surgical procedures that cannot be performed under local anesthesia.

TABLE 182–1. THE MUCOPOLYSACCHARIDOSES

MPS Type	Eponym	Enzyme Deficiency	Urinary GAG	Clinical Presentation
I				
I-H	Hurler	α-L-Iduronidase	DS HS	Onset < 2 yrs, early corneal clouding and organomegaly, coarse facies, MR; later onset of cardiorespiratory failure
I-S	Scheie	α-L-Iduronidase	DS	Later onset (> 5 yrs), similar to I-H but with normal intellect, milder skeletal involvement, and slower progression
II	Hunter	Iduronate sulfatase	DS HS	Onset < 4 yrs, early skeletal involvement, organomegaly, but no corneal clouding; X-linked inheritance, MR usually severe; mild form with normal intelligence and slower progression
III	Sanfilippo			Same for all types (A–D)
IIIA		Heparan-N-sulfatase	HS	Onset > 2 yrs, rapidly progressive neurologic/intellectual regression; late mild visceral and skeletal involvement
IIIB		α-N-Acetylglucosaminidase		
IIIC		N-Acetyl-CoA : α-glucosaminide acetyltransferase		
IIID		N-Acetylglucosamine-6-sulfatase		
IV	Morquio			
IVA		N-Acetyl-galactosamine-6-sulfatase	KS	Onset < 4 yrs, mainly skeletal involvement, rapidly progressive kyphoscoliosis, short stature, odontoid hypoplasia, late corneal clouding, and normal intellect
IVB		β-Galactosidase	KS	Same as IVA, but may develop MR
VI	Maroteaux-Lamy	Arylsulfatase B	DS	Onset < 4 yrs, phenotype as in MPS I-H, but with normal intellect; rare adult form with slower progression
VII	Sly	β-Glucuronidase	HS DS ChS	Variable age of onset, MR and skeletal involvement; few patients present as hydrops fetalis

DS = dermatan sulfate; HS = heparan sulfate; KS = keratan sulfate; ChS = chondroitin sulfate; MR = mental retardation.

6. Dental care: Dental care is a relatively common problem in patients with MPS's owing to the decreased mouth opening, gingival hypertrophy, and poor dental hygiene in patients with mental retardation. Awareness of the need for continuous dental care should be maintained.

ENZYME AND GENE THERAPY. Attempts to treat patients with MPS types I and II by high-volume plasma transfusions were made nearly 25 years ago. The amount of enzyme that could be provided with the maximal plasma transfusion led to some decreased urinary excretion of the GAG's but no meaningful phenotypic improvement. Attempts to purify large quantities of enzymes from human tissues (placental) or by genetic engineering are currently under way in several laboratories. Thus far, the amount of purified enzyme required for clinical trials is not available for MPS therapy (see Ch. 25). The additional problem of targeting enzyme to the affected tissue, especially the brain, must still be overcome.

Enzyme replacement by bone marrow transplantation has been attempted in a limited number of patients. Some of the patients with MPS VI who have received a bone marrow transplant had significant clinical improvement with complete or nearly complete arrest of the progressive disorder. Bone marrow transplantation did not prevent the severe skeletal deformities in MPS IV nor the severe neurologic regression in patients with MPS III. The clinical indications for bone marrow transplantation in patients with MPS I-H and MPS II are not established owing to the lack of consistent improvement in the neurologic sequelae. As this transplantation can only arrest the progression but not reverse the symptoms, attempts were made to provide this treatment to patients within the early stages of the disease. It is not clear whether the few patients who appeared to benefit from bone marrow transplantation had mutations with residual activity and therefore had better outcomes. The correlation of genotype with phenotype that is becoming available might enable a conclusive answer to this question. A national collaborative study is being done to evaluate the possible role of bone marrow transplantation in patients with certain MPS's.

Gene therapy (see Ch. 25) for MPS's by providing the normal gene carried by one vector or another to the desirable tissue remains a desirable goal for the future. Major hurdles that need to be overcome include choosing vector, establishing stable incorporation of the normal gene, and targeting the gene to the affected tissue.

Gieselmann V: Lysosomal storage diseases. Biochem Biophys Acta 1270:1, 1995. *An excellent review of the molecular understanding of lysosomal enzymes and their mutations, with an emphasis on genotype-phenotype correlation.*

Neufeld EF, Muenzer J: The mucopolysaccharide storage diseases. *In* Scriver CR, Beaudet AL, Sly WS, Valle D (eds.): The Metabolic and Molecular Bases of In-

herited Disease. 7th ed. New York, McGraw-Hill, 1995. *The most comprehensive review of MPS's available in the definitive reference text for metabolic diseases. This discussion of basic science and clinical issues related to lysosomal storage diseases offers a biochemical understanding of these diseases.*

Whitley CB: The mucopolysaccharidoses. *In* Beighton P (ed.): McKusick's Heritable Disorders of Connective Tissue. 5th ed. St. Louis, Mosby-Year Book, 1993. *An extremely readable clinical summary of MPS's with many illustrative graphs and clinical photographs. Gives the nongeneticist a concise overview of the MPS's.*

183 THE MARFAN SYNDROME
Peter H. Byers

DEFINITION. The Marfan syndrome is a dominantly inherited connective tissue disorder characterized by musculoskeletal abnormalities (arachnodactyly, tall stature, scoliosis, pectus deformities, and ligamentous laxity), cardiovascular abnormalities (mitral valve prolapse [MVP] and regurgitation, aortic valve insufficiency, and aortic dilatation, aneurysm, and dissection), lens dislocation, and myopia.

ETIOLOGY AND PATHOGENESIS. The Marfan syndrome results from mutations in the gene (FIBN1) that encodes fibrillin I, located on chromosome 15q21. Fibrillin is a 350-kDa glycoprotein that contains 43 repeats of a calcium binding EGF-precursor–like motif and other cysteine-rich motifs. This protein is ubiquitously distributed in the extracellular matrix and is a major constituent of microfibrils of elastic tissue and of the zonular fibrils of the lens. Many different mutations in the gene have now been identified and have been shown to interfere with the synthesis, secretion, or accumulation in the extracellular matrix of the normal protein. Genetic linkage studies suggest that most, if not all, individuals with typical Marfan syndrome have mutations in the FIBN1 gene.

PREVALENCE. The Marfan syndrome affects about 1 in 15,000 individuals without racial or ethnic predilection. About 60 to 70% of affected individuals have an affected parent; the remainder have new mutations.

PATHOLOGY. The mitral and aortic valves are characterized by "myxomatous degeneration" or the appearance of large pools of nonfibrous material that separates the normal cells of the valves. The valves may be thickened. In the absence of dissection, metachromatic material accumulates in the aortic media and the normal elastic laminae are disrupted. Aortic dissection characteristically begins in the ascending aorta and may proceed in both directions. Death frequently results from cardiac tamponade due to hemopericardium, coronary occlusion, occlusion of the arteries to the brain, or loss of perfusion of multiple abdominal organs.

CLINICAL MANIFESTATIONS. The Marfan syndrome is highly variable in its clinical manifestations, and affected members within the same family may differ in the manner in which they express the mutation. The differences between families may be explained, in part, by different mutations in the FIBN1 gene. The diagnosis of the Marfan syndrome requires that criteria in two or more major areas be met (family history, cardiac, musculoskeletal, or ocular findings) with a family history, and an additional criterion if there is a new mutation. The diagnosis can be made occasionally in newborns because of lens dislocation, MVP, scoliosis, and tall stature with arachnodactyly; in addition, there is a particularly severe newborn variant of the condition. More commonly, diagnosis is made during childhood or adolescence because of tall stature, MVP, lens dislocation, and arachnodactyly. Aortic root diameter is generally within the normal range during childhood, although it tends to be in the upper range. Scoliosis may progress rapidly during the adolescent growth spurt. More than half the individuals with the Marfan syndrome have lens subluxation, usually in the superior direction. Lens subluxation is generally not progressive after adolescence but if the position of the lens interferes with vision, replacing it with an artificial lens is often beneficial. Cataracts and glaucoma are occasional complications of ectopia lentis.

The major life-threatening complication of the Marfan syndrome is aortic dissection and rupture, and most deaths result from cardiovascular disease when the aorta is untreated. The risk of dissection is correlated with aortic diameter. Commonly aortic diameters do not exceed the normal adult range (20 to 37 mm) until the third decade and then enlarge slowly, although the rate varies with individuals. Aortic dissection in the Marfan syndrome is occasionally asymptomatic, but usually there is prolonged, severe substernal chest pain of a tearing or searing quality, often with radiation into the neck, back, and arms. It is often accompanied by diaphoresis, hypotension, and shock. Blood pressure in the two arms may differ. Rarely, pregnancy is complicated by aortic dissection.

DIFFERENTIAL DIAGNOSIS. *Isolated ectopia lentis,* a dominantly inherited disorder, also results from mutation in the FIBN1 gene but is not accompanied by significant aortic dilatation or dissection. *Congenital contractural arachnodactyly (CCA)* is a dominantly inherited disorder characterized by arachnodactyly, joint contractures, small cup-shaped ears, pectus deformity, mild scoliosis, and MVP, but lens dislocation is absent and aortic dilatation is not a complication. CCA has been linked to the FIBN2 gene on chromosome 5. *Homocystinuria* (see Ch. 180) is characterized by autosomal recessive inheritance, tight joints, peripheral vascular disease, thrombosis of arterial vessels, lens dislocation, osteoporosis, and, in some, mild mental retardation. The diagnosis is confirmed by detecting excessive homocysteine in the urine. Because of MVP, tall stature, and some of the skeletal features, the *mitral valve prolapse syndrome* is commonly mistaken for the Marfan syndrome. The disorder is dominantly inherited but quite variable; the absence of lens dislocation and lack of aortic root dilation distinguish the MVP syndrome from the Marfan syndrome. Individuals with the *Stickler syndrome* may have a marfanoid habitus, degenerative arthritis of multiple joints, cleft palate, and vitreal degeneration. In most families, the condition results from mutations in the COL2A1 gene that encodes the chains of type II collagen. The marfanoid habitus may be found in some people with sickle cell disease, the Klinefelter syndrome (the 47,XXY karyotype), and multiple endocrine adenomatosis type IIB (see Ch. 210.1).

TREATMENT AND CARE. The major objective of treating people with the Marfan syndrome is to prevent or treat aneurysm and dissection. Because aortic dissection is the principal cause of death, efforts to slow the rate of increase of aortic diameter hold promise to delay major complications. Recent studies suggest that aortic enlargement may slow in some people treated with β-blockers. It is not clear if some physical or molecular features identify those who respond. Blood pressure should always be maintained in the normal range. Advances in surgical technique have made replacing aneurysmal portions of the aorta a routine treatment that increases life expectancy. Replacement should be considered when aortic root diameter reaches approximately 55 to 60 mm and before

decompensation of the left ventricle from aortic valvular insufficiency. Yearly echocardiographic examination permits a sound basis for following aortic enlargement. A family history of aortic dissection at smaller diameters may be considered in timing the replacement. Either a human cadaver homograft that includes the aortic valve or a composite graft that contains a prosthetic valve is now used. Replacing the proximal aorta leaves the remainder of the vessel at risk, and follow-up by imaging of the remaining vessel is important in planning further surgery. Routine care consists of yearly echocardiography with referral to the cardiac surgeon when the aortic diameter reaches 50 to 55 mm, regular ophthalmologic evaluation, and continuing follow-up by a physician familiar with the syndrome.

There may be an increased risk for the mother with Marfan syndrome during pregnancy if the aortic diameter is greater than normal. There is a 50% risk of transmitting the gene for Marfan syndrome with each pregnancy, and molecular diagnosis of affected status of the fetus may be available in some families. Genetic counseling is important to determine if others are affected and to provide detailed information about the condition (see Ch. 29).

Dietz HC, Cutting GR, Pyeritz RE, et al.: Marfan syndrome caused by a recurrent de novo missense mutation in the fibrillin gene. Nature 352:337, 1991. *The demonstration that mutations in fibrillin produce the Marfan syndrome.*
Pyeritz RE: The Marfan syndrome. *In* Royce PM, Steinmann B (eds.): Connective Tissue and Its Heritable Disorders: Molecular, Genetic, and Medical Aspects. New York, Wiley-Liss, 1993, p 437. *The most recent, comprehensive review of the Marfan syndrome in all its aspects.*
Shores J, Berger KR, Murphy EA, et al.: Progression of aortic dilation and the benefit of long-term β-adrenergic blockade in Marfan's syndrome. N Engl J Med 330:1335, 1994. *The only published controlled trial of treatment with β blocker.*

184 EHLERS-DANLOS SYNDROME
Peter H. Byers

DEFINITION. Ehlers-Danlos syndrome (EDS) is a group of more than 10 inherited connective tissue disorders characterized by abnormalities of the skin, ligaments, and internal organs. The clinical manifestations include skin fragility, abnormal scar formation, excessive bruising, joint laxity, and, in one variety, rupture of viscera and arteries (Table 184–1).

ETIOLOGY. Some forms of EDS result from defects in the synthesis and processing of types I and III collagens, the major proteins of skin, ligaments, tendons, blood vessels, and viscera. The known defects include mutations affecting the structure, synthesis, processing, or stability of type III collagen (EDS type IV); deficient hydroxylation of lysyl residues in type I and type III collagen (EDS type VI); defective conversion of type I procollagen to collagen (EDS type VII); defective collagen cross-linking and abnormal cellular utilization of copper (EDS type IX); and a functional defect in fibronectin (EDS type X). The molecular bases of EDS types I, II, III, V, and VIII are not known.

PREVALENCE. The prevalence of EDS is estimated at about 1 in 5000 births. EDS type III, benign familial hypermobility, accounts for most patients identified as having EDS; some forms are uncommon (EDS types IV, VI, VII, and VIII); others have been found in only a few families (EDS types IX and X). There is no racial or ethnic predisposition for any of the common types of EDS.

PATHOLOGY AND PATHOGENESIS. Dermal collagen fibrils in patients with EDS types I, II, III, and VI are larger than normal and irregular in outline when viewed by electron microscopy. In EDS type IV, skin is thin and collagen fibril diameter is frequently smaller than normal. Arterial wall thickness is usually less than normal, and tensile strength is diminished. Fibroblastic cells in dermis frequently have marked dilatation of the rough endoplasmic reticulum as a result of defective secretion of type III procollagen. There are no specific pathologic features of the other types of EDS.

CLINICAL MANIFESTATIONS. The clinical manifestations of each type of EDS are different (Table 184–1); it is important to identify patients with EDS type IV because of the grave consequences of the disease and to identify those with EDS types V, VI, and IX because of the risk of recurrence in their families.

EDS types I and II are characterized by marked joint laxity; soft, velvety, and hyperextensible skin; easy bruising; and "cigarette-paper" scars in areas of trauma. They differ in severity. Prematurity is common in EDS type I but rare in EDS type II. The major complications of both are recurrent joint dislocations, skin fragility, and early-onset osteoarthritis. The manifestations of joint laxity are more severe in childhood and decrease following puberty. At present the diagnosis depends on recognizing the appropriate clinical findings; electron microscopic studies of dermis may be confirmatory but are not specific. Patients with EDS type III are commonly seen by rheumatologists because of the joint discomfort and early onset of degenerative joint disease.

EDS type IV, the most severe form, results from dominant mutations in the genes of type III collagen. The diagnosis is confirmed by finding decreased amounts of type III collagen in skin, by identifying a defect in the structure, synthesis, or secretion of type III procollagen by cultured dermal fibroblasts, or by identifying a defect in gene structure. In the newborn period some infants already have bruising, but most affected infants are difficult to identify. By adolescence the veins are readily visible on the trunk and extremities, and bruising is common. Vascular or bowel rupture is rare during childhood. Arterial fragility may manifest as sudden death, stroke, shock from retroperitoneal or intra-abdominal bleeding, or compartmental syndromes, depending on the site of vessel rupture. Prompt surgical intervention may be lifesaving, although tissue friability may make repairs difficult. Pregnancy may be complicated by arterial or uterine rupture, either of which is often fatal. Recurrent abdominal pain may result from repeated mural hemorrhage in the small intestine. Sigmoid rupture is common. Survival beyond the fifth decade is rare.

EDS type VI is an autosomal recessive disorder characterized by a marfanoid habitus, skin and joint findings similar to those in EDS type II, ocular fragility, and scoliosis. The diagnosis is made by finding decreased amounts of hydroxylysine in skin and confirmed by low levels of lysyl hydroxylase measured in cultured dermal fibroblasts. Mutations have been identified in lysyl hydroxylase. Late complications may include vascular rupture, as well as blindness from retinal detachment or globe rupture.

EDS type VII is often detected in the newborn period, because of bilateral congenital hip dislocation and marked joint laxity. The hips are often difficult to stabilize, and recurrent dislocation may continue at the hips and other joints. When suspected clinically the diagnosis can be confirmed in some patients by identifying intermediates in the conversion of type I procollagen to collagen in skin and confirming the defect in cultured dermal fibroblasts. The most common defect recognized is an abnormal structure of the proα2(I) chain caused by exon 6 skipping in the COL1A2 gene. Similar mutations in the COL1A1 gene produce a somewhat more severe phenotype. Both these disorders result from loss of the cleavage site for the N-terminal procollagen proteinase. A recessively inherited deficiency of the proteinase itself results in the clinical picture of dermatosparaxis (EDS type VIIC), a very rare disorder characterized by extreme joint laxity and skin fragility and laxity.

EDS type VIII is characterized by the combination of noninflammatory gingival loss (often leading to loss of teeth) and the cutaneous and joint signs of the EDS type II phenotype.

EDS type IX is noted in childhood with skin hyperextensibility and laxity, drooping facies, and minor skeletal anomalies. Evidence of bladder dysfunction may be present by age 6, and diverticula of the bladder and hydronephrosis may occur. Mild chronic diarrhea, orthostatic hypotension, short upper arms with limited pronation and supination, and the occipital inferior horns become apparent during adolescence. Intelligence is usually in the normal range; inheritance is X-linked recessive. The diagnosis is made by the low serum copper and ceruloplasmin levels and confirmed by low lysyl oxidase levels in cultured dermal fibroblasts. The disease is allelic to Menkes' syndrome, a defect of copper metabolism. Maintaining normal urinary drainage is important to prevent renal failure, and continuing bladder drainage may be essential to prevent rupture. There is some variation in severity among families.

DIFFERENTIAL DIAGNOSIS. The differential diagnosis is generally limited to the varieties of EDS, although some individuals with the Marfan syndrome have marked joint laxity and others with forms of osteogenesis imperfecta have joint laxity and easy bruising. Patients with EDS type IV and EDS types I and II are often investigated for a bleeding diathesis before the correct diagnosis is made. Because of joint instability and laxity many patients with EDS types I, II, III, VI, and VII are investigated for developmental delay before it is recognized that they have a form of EDS.

TREATMENT. The gaping skin wounds that occur in some forms of EDS should be approximated carefully, and the removable sutures should be left in place for twice the usual time. Recurrent dislocations can often be repaired surgically, although further recurrence is more common than in unaffected individuals. Arterial rupture in patients with EDS type IV needs to be treated surgically unless bleeding is controlled by compartmental limitation (e.g., some

TABLE 184–1. CLINICAL FEATURES, MODE OF INHERITANCE, AND BIOCHEMICAL DISORDERS OF THE EHLERS-DANLOS SYNDROME

Type	Clinical Features	Inheritance	Molecular Defect
I: Gravis	Soft, velvety, hyperextensible skin; easy bruising; "cigarette paper" scars; hypermobile joints; varicose veins; prematurity	AD	Not known
II: Mitis	Similar to EDS type I but less severe	AD (AR, rare)	Not known COL1A2 null alleles
III: Familial hypermobility	Soft skin, no scarring, marked large and small joint hypermobility	AD	Not known
IV: Arterial	Thin, translucent skin with visible veins; marked bruising; skin and joints have normal extensibility; arterial, bowel, and uterine rupture	AD	Mutations in the COL3A1 gene that alter type III collagen synthesis, secretion, and structure
V: X-linked	Similar to EDS type II	XLR	Not known
VI: Ocular	Soft, velvety, hyperextensible skin; hypermobile joints; scoliosis; ocular fragility and keratoconus	AR	Lysyl hydroxylase deficiency due to mutations in the LOH gene
VII: A and B: Arthrochalasis multiplex congenita	Congenital hip dislocation; joint hypermobility; soft skin with normal scarring	AD	A: COL1A1 exon 6 skipping mutation that deletes N-proteinase cleavage site B: COL1A2 exon 6 skipping mutation that deletes N-proteinase cleavage site
C: Dermatosparaxis	Very soft, fragile, bruisable skin; marked joint hypermobility	AR	Procollagen N-proteinase deficiency
VIII: Periodontal	Generalized periodontitis; skin similar to EDS type II	AD	Not known
IX: X-linked cutis laxa; occipital horn syndrome	Soft, extensible, lax skin; bladder diverticula and rupture; short arms, limited pronation and supination; broad clavicles, occipital horns	XLR	Abnormal intracellular copper utilization with defect in lysyl oxidase; allelic to Menkes' syndrome
X: Fibronectin defect	Similar to EDS type II	AR	Defect in fibronectin

AD = Autosomal dominant; AR = Autosomal recessive; XLR = X-linked recessive.

retroperitoneal bleeding). The repair of affected arteries is often difficult because of extreme friability. If colon rupture recurs, the colon can be excised to prevent further episodes. Rupture of the small bowel is very rare. Some patients with EDS type VI respond to ascorbic acid (1 to 4 grams per day) with some symptomatic improvement and increased excretion of hydroxylysine in the urine. There is no metabolic treatment for other forms of EDS, and management is largely symptomatic.

PROGNOSIS. The prognosis in EDS depends on the specific type with which the patient is affected. Life expectancy is considerably shortened in EDS type IV because of organ and vessel rupture and may be decreased in EDS type VI; in all others, life expectancy is normal. With the exception of EDS type VI, no specific therapy is available that affects the natural history of the condition.

Prevention by prenatal diagnosis is feasible for some types of EDS. Heterozygosity for the EDS type VI mutation has been recognized by examination of amniotic fluid cells in a family at risk for recurrence. The structural mutations in EDS type VII and in EDS type IV should be recognizable by studies of collagens synthesized by chorionic villus cells in culture or by analysis of the specific mutation. Analysis of copper uptake and distribution by amniotic fluid cells should facilitate prenatal diagnosis of EDS type IX. All families should have access to genetic counseling once a proband is identified.

McKusick VA: Heritable Disorders of Connective Tissue. 4th ed. St Louis, CV Mosby, 1972, p 292. *Although the classification is not up to date, the richness of clinical detail is unsurpassed. A delight to read because of the many case histories and the personal touch.*
Steinmann B, Royce PM, Superti-Furga A: The Ehlers-Danlos syndrome. *In* Royce PM, Steinmann B (eds.): Connective Tissue and Its Heritable Disorders: Molecular, Genetic, and Medical Aspects. New York, Wiley-Liss, 1992, p 351. *The most comprehensive recent review of the clinical, biochemical, and molecular genetic aspects of EDS.*

185 OSTEOGENESIS IMPERFECTA
Peter H. Byers

DEFINITION. Osteogenesis imperfecta (OI) is a heterogeneous group of disorders characterized by bone fragility and associated connective tissue involvement. The clinical picture depends on the nature of the mutation and ranges from a form that is lethal in the perinatal period to a mild phenotype in which stature is normal and bone fractures are only slightly more common than usual.

ETIOLOGY AND PATHOGENESIS. In virtually all instances, OI results from mutations in one of the two genes, COL1A1 and COL1A2, that encode the proα1(I) and proα2(I) of type I collagen,

respectively. Type I collagen is the major structural protein of bone and of many other connective tissues (tendon, skin, sclera, ligament). The protein contains three chains—two α1(I) chains and a single α2(I) chain in a triple helix—that require glycine in every third position of each chain. OI phenotypes result from mutations that substitute for virtually any of the third position glycine residues, splice junction mutations, and short genomic deletions or duplications. The severity of the OI reflects the nature of the mutation, the location, and the gene in which the mutation occurred and the effect of the mutations on the protein. OI type I, the mildest form, results from synthesis of about half the normal amount of type I collagen, whereas the other forms (Table 185–1) result from mutations that alter the protein's structure. These mutations alter the ability of the molecules to be secreted, to form extracellular fibrils, and to be mineralized. The deficit of normal collagen in bone leads to fracture and deformity, the extent of which depends on the nature of the protein abnormality.

PREVALENCE. The incidence of OI is thought to be approximately 1 in 15,000 to 20,000 births. The mild dominant form, OI type I, is most prevalent. The incidence of the lethal perinatal form is approximately 1 in 50,000 to 60,000.

CLINICAL MANIFESTATIONS (Table 185–1).

OI Type I. Fracture rate is highest during childhood, decreases at puberty, and may increase in the postmenopausal period for women. Adult-onset hearing loss is common.

OI Type II. Affected infants have very marked bone deformity and diminished mineralization of bone. Death is usually the consequence of pulmonary insufficiency due to a very small thorax.

OI Type III. This form is characterized by marked short stature, progressive limb deformity, scoliosis, and thin bones that are susceptible to fracture. People with this form of OI frequently use a wheelchair for most of their activities and may be among the shortest adults an internist encounters, with some less than 3 feet tall. Progressive pulmonary and cardiac insufficiency may decrease life span. Basilar impression, compression of the brain stem due to settling of the skull on the vertebral column, may lead to neurologic impairment, tussive headache, neurologic compromise, sleep apnea, and death. Life expectancy is shortened, although some individuals with this form of OI live an average span.

OI Type IV. Severity is between OI type III and OI type I. Stature is decreased but generally above 4 feet for males.

DIFFERENTIAL DIAGNOSIS. In the perinatal period, OI needs to be distinguished from forms of *hypophosphatasia* and *severe chondrodysplasia (e.g., spondyloepiphyseal dysplasia, achondrogenesis, and hypochondrogenesis), and Menkes' syndrome.* Radiographs and serum levels of alkaline phosphatase and of copper distinguish among these conditions. During early childhood, *nonaccidental trauma* may be confused with OI in some children; the characteristic radiographic features of trauma may be helpful in the diagnosis. During adolescence, *idiopathic juvenile osteoporosis* may be confused with OI, and biochemical studies of cultured dermal fibroblasts may help to distinguish the two. Other forms of brittle bone disorders, including sclerosing bone disease such as *pykno-*

TABLE 185–1. OSTEOGENESIS IMPERFECTA

Type	Clinical Features	Inheritance	Biochemical and Genetic Abnormalities
I	Normal stature, little or no deformity; blue sclerae; hearing loss in 50%; dentinogenesis imperfecta is rare and may distinguish a subset	AD	*Common:* "Nonfunctional" COL1A1 allele
II	Lethal in the perinatal period; minimal calvarial mineralization; beaded ribs; compressed femurs; marked longbone deformity; platyspondyly	AD (new)	*Common:* Substitutions for glycyl residues in the triple-helical domains of both chains of type I collagen *Rare:* Rearrangement in the COL1A1 and COL1A2 genes; exon deletions in triple-helical domain of COL1A1 and COL1A2
		AR (rare)	Small deletion in COL1A2 on the background of null allele
III	Progressively deforming bones, usually with moderate deformity at birth; sclerae variable in hue, often lighten with age; dentinogenesis common; hearing loss common; stature very short	AD AR (uncommon)	Point mutations in the COL1A1 and COL1A2 gene Frame-shift (4 bp deletion) in COL1A2 that prevents incorporation of chains into molecules
IV	Normal sclerae; mild to moderate bone deformity and variable short stature; dentinogenesis is common and hearing loss occurs in some	AD	Point mutations in COL1A1 and COL1A2 gene; exon skipping mutations in COL1A2

AD = autosomal dominant; AR = autosomal recessive.

dysostosis and *osteopetrosis* are rarely confused with OI. In adult life, OI may be thought to be *osteoporosis*.

TREATMENT AND CARE. Currently no medical therapies have been demonstrated to alter growth or decrease fracture rate in any form of OI. As a consequence, treatment is largely mechanical and directed toward preservation of function and, especially for those who depend on wheelchairs for mobility, ensuring independence in adult life. The mainstays of care are active physical therapy and habilitation and appropriate orthopedic intervention. Recurrent fracture of long bones may lead to periods of inactivity which, in turn, may decrease bone mineralization and predispose to further fracture. Placing intramedullary rods in the bones of the legs can short-circuit this cycle and lead to ambulation in some who fracture readily. Monitoring hearing, particularly in the adult, is important, and awareness of the symptoms of basilar impression in people with OI type III and OI type IV may reduce complications if intervention is necessary.

Prenatal diagnosis by ultrasonography is available for OI type II (14 to 16 weeks' gestation) and OI type III (15 to 19 weeks' gestation). Biochemical studies of chorionic villus cells can identify a fetus that synthesizes abnormal type I collagen molecules (OI types II, III, and IV), if the abnormality is known from study of an affected individual. In appropriate families, linked DNA markers can identify the affected allele and can be used for presymptomatic and prenatal diagnosis.

Byers PH: Osteogenesis imperfecta. *In* Royce PM, Steinmann B (eds.): Connective Tissue and Its Heritable Disorders: Molecular, Genetic, and Medical Aspects. New York, Wiley-Liss, 1993, p 317. *A detailed review of biochemical, molecular, genetic, and clinical abnormalities in OI.*

186 PSEUDOXANTHOMA ELASTICUM

Jouni Uitto

Pseudoxanthoma elasticum (PXE) (synonyms: Grönblad-Strandberg syndrome, systemic elastorrhexis) is a generalized progressive connective tissue disorder primarily affecting the elastic fibers. Clinically, PXE manifests as characteristic cutaneous lesions, ocular changes, and widespread vascular abnormalities. The relative severity of these changes results in a variety of clinical pictures. The on-

set of the disease may be in early childhood, and in most cases the cutaneous changes are evident before age 30. The exact incidence of PXE is not known, although estimates are about 1 in 160,000 persons. The male-female ratio is probably 1:1.

CLINICAL MANIFESTATIONS. *Skin*. The primary cutaneous lesions are relatively small (1 to 3 mm) yellowish papules that give the affected area a pebbly, "plucked chicken skin" appearance. The primary lesions tend to coalesce into larger plaques, and the skin of the involved areas becomes thickened and leathery (Fig. 186–1). Gradually, the affected skin becomes redundant, lax, and inelastic. The predilection sites are the face, neck, axillary folds, lower abdomen, and thighs. The nasolabial folds and chin creases may be strikingly accentuated. Yellowish lesions similar to those noted on the skin can also be seen on the mucous membranes.

***Eye*.** The ocular changes are characterized by angioid streaks, i.e., grayish or brownish-red, poorly defined streaks radiating across the fundus of the eye. Their development usually starts later than that of the cutaneous lesions, often during the third or fourth decade. The ocular changes are commonly bilateral and include hemorrhages and exudates in Bruch's membrane, an elastin-rich structure located between the retina and the choroid. The degenerative changes of the eye frequently lead to impaired vision, and complete blindness, although rare, is one of the major complications of PXE. Angioid streaks may be present without noticeable cutaneous changes, but other accompanying observations, such as vascular changes, may lead to correct diagnosis of PXE. Angioid streaks can also be associated with other diseases—for example, Paget's disease of bone, sickle cell anemia, tumoral calcinosis, lead poisoning, and idiopathic thrombocytopenia.

***Vascular Manifestations*.** The early manifestations of arterial involvement include hypertension, weak peripheral pulses, and, occasionally, intermittent claudication. The most devastating complications develop as a result of coronary occlusion or cerebral hemorrhage; the most frequent complication is recurrent bleeding from the gastrointestinal tract. A common site of the gastrointestinal bleeding is the gastric mucosa, where the elastic fibers of the arteries are particularly affected. Bleeding from the urinary tract can also occur.

INHERITANCE. Most cases of PXE are inherited as an autosomal recessive disease. However, autosomal dominant inheritance has been documented in some families, although delayed onset, incomplete expression, and lack of carrier detection complicate the genetic analysis. In addition to the inherited forms, several cases with cutaneous findings consistent with PXE but without family history and without vascular or ocular involvement have been re-

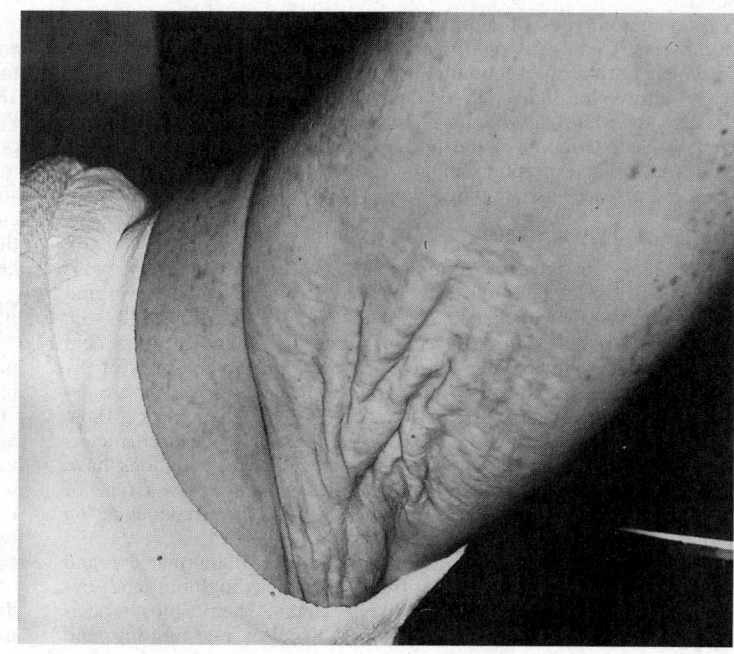

FIGURE 186–1. Typical cutaneous manifestations of pseudoxanthoma elasticum. The lesion demonstrates redundant and inelastic skin in the axillary fold.

ported. Periumbilical perforating PXE appears to be a distinct acquired form of the disease.

PATHOLOGY. Histopathologic examination of the involved skin demonstrates an accumulation of structures in the middle or lower dermis that stain positively with stains specific for elastic fibers, e.g., Verhoeff's stain. In contrast to the elastic fibers in normal skin, the elastic material in PXE appears irregularly clumped and fragmented. The accumulation of elastic fibers has also been quantitated by computerized morphometric analyses and by assay of desmosine, an elastin-specific crosslink compound. Characteristically, the fragmented elastic fibers contain calcium that appears bluish on routine hematoxylin-eosin stain and that can be demonstrated by calcium-specific stains. Electron microscopy of affected skin demonstrates that the amorphous elastin component has been replaced by bundles of granular material with staining properties different from those of normal elastin. Also, foci containing calcium hydroxyapatite crystals can be detected in the elastic fibers. These morphologic findings thus provide evidence for derangement in the organization of the elastic structures in PXE. Biochemical proof of the exact molecular defect in the structure or metabolism of elastin is, however, lacking, and it is unclear whether the calcification of elastic fibers is a primary or secondary event.

THERAPY. No specific treatment is available, and the primary prevention entails genetic counseling (see Ch. 29). Although treatment with vitamin E, vitamin C, or a low-calcium diet has been advocated in isolated case reports, there is no clinical proof of their efficacy. In selected cases, plastic surgery may be helpful to improve the skin's cosmetic appearance.

Christiano AM, Uitto J: Molecular pathology of the elastic fibers. J Invest Dermatol 103:53S, 1994. *A review of the molecular defects of elastin in heritable connective tissue diseases, including PXE.*

Lebwohl M, et al.: Classification of pseudoxanthoma elasticum. J Am Acad Dermatol 30:103, 1994. *Report of a consensus conference on PXE.*

Neldner KH: Pseudoxanthoma elasticum. Clin Dermatol 6:1, 1988. *Extremely useful clinical account of PXE, based on the author's data on 100 patients followed over a 10-year period.*

Neldner KH, Martinez-Hernandez A: Localized acquired cutaneous pseudoxanthoma elasticum. J Am Acad Dermatol 1:523, 1979. *Clinical description of a distinct acquired form of pseudoxanthoma elasticum.*

Disorders of Porphyrins and Metals

187 THE PORPHYRIAS
Karl E. Anderson

Porphyrias are due to deficiencies of specific enzymes of the heme biosynthetic pathway and, when clinically expressed, are associated with striking accumulations of heme pathway intermediates. These conditions are more prevalent, and more often manifested, in adults than are most well-characterized metabolic diseases, and are likely to be encountered by physicians in many disciplines. The three most common porphyrias differ considerably from each other and are managed very differently. Most porphyrias are inherited, but other factors are important in determining their severity.

Two major types of clinical manifestations are characteristic of porphyrias. *Cutaneous photosensitivity* occurs in types of porphyria in which porphyrins accumulate. Porphyrins are activated by long-wave ultraviolet light (UV-B) and generate oxygen radicals that damage the skin. *Neurologic effects* occur in porphyrias characterized by accumulation of the porphyrin precursors δ-aminolevulinic acid (ALA) and porphobilinogen (PBG). (Standard abbreviations for these diseases are shown in Table 187–1.)

THE HEME BIOSYNTHETIC PATHWAY AND THE PORPHYRIAS

The genes for most of the eight enzymes of this important pathway have been cloned and characterized at the molecular level and their chromosomal locations identified (Fig. 187–1; Table 187–1). Mutations of the erythroid-specific form of δ-aminolevulinic acid synthase, the first enzyme, have been found in some cases of X-linked sideroblastic anemia. Porphyrias and related disorders are associated with deficiencies of the other seven enzymes (Table 187–1). Mutations in genes for these enzymes have been characterized in detail in five types of porphyria. Different mutations have generally been found in unrelated families with any given type of porphyria. Thus these diseases are probably all heterogeneous at the molecular level.

Heme is synthesized in largest amounts in bone marrow and liver, where it is used primarily to make hemoglobin and cytochrome P-450 enzymes, respectively. Hepatic heme biosynthesis is regulated primarily by ALA synthase, which is rate-limiting, and under sensitive feedback control by cellular free heme content. Hepatic ALA synthase is induced by many of the same drugs and steroids that induce P-450 enzymes. Additional pathway enzymes and cellular uptake of iron are important in regulating heme synthesis in erythroid cells.

Most heme pathway intermediates are conserved and excreted only in small amounts. ALA and PBG are normally excreted in much larger amounts than porphyrins. Porphyrinogens (hexahydroporphyrins) undergo auto-oxidation outside cells and are excreted primarily as porphyrins. ALA, PBG, and porphyrinogens are colorless and nonfluorescent. Porphyrins are reddish and fluoresce when exposed to long-wave UV light. ALA, PBG, uroporphyrin, and hepta-, hexa-, and pentacarboxyl porphyrins are excreted mostly in urine, coproporphyrin (a tetracarboxyl porphyrin) in urine and bile, and harderoporphyrin (a tricarboxyl porphyrin) and protoporphyrin (a dicarboxyl porphyrin) in bile and feces.

CLASSIFICATION

Traditionally, porphyrias have been divided into erythropoietic and hepatic types, based on whether the excess production of intermediates takes place primarily in bone marrow or liver (Table 187–1). Some porphyrias have both erythroid and hepatic features. Porphyrias with neurovisceral symptoms are also termed "acute porphyrias." They share many clinical features and are similarly managed. Several "cutaneous porphyrias" manifest similar skin lesions but differ considerably in their treatment and prognosis. The cutaneous features of erythropoietic protoporphyria (EPP) are distinct. Now that these disorders are better characterized, they are best classified in terms of their specific enzyme deficiencies.

THE MOST COMMON PORPHYRIAS

It is important to appreciate that the three most common types of porphyria, which are likely to be encountered periodically by any physician, differ markedly from each other with regard to major clinical manifestations, exacerbating factors, tests important for diagnosis, and effective therapies (Table 187–2). Because their features are so distinct, a feature learned about one of these porphyrias will not apply to the others. On the other hand, these three conditions are prototypic: They share some important features with the other less common porphyrias. This should be evident from the brief descriptions of each of the porphyrias that follow.

ALA DEHYDRATASE DEFICIENT–PORPHYRIA (ADP). In this very rare autosomal recessive disorder, ALA dehydratase is markedly reduced (1 to 2% of normal). Symptoms resemble acute

TABLE 187–1. ENZYMES OF THE HEME BIOSYNTHETIC PATHWAY AND CLASSIFICATION AND INHERITANCE OF DISEASES ASSOCIATED WITH THEIR DEFICIENCIES*

Enzyme	Chromosomal Location	Disease	Inheritance	Classifications of Porphyrias			
				Hepatic	*Erythropoietic*	*Acute*	*Cutaneous*
ALA synthase							
Erythroid	Xp11.21	Sideroblastic anemia	X-linked recessive				
Nonerythroid	3p21	None known					
ALA dehydratase	9q34	δ-Aminolevulinic acid dehydratase–deficient porphyria (ADP)	Autosomal recessive	?X		X	
Porphobilinogen deaminase†	11q24.1 -> q24.2	Acute intermittent porphyria (AIP)	Autosomal dominant	X		X	
Uroporphyrinogen III cosynthase	10q25.2 -> q26.3	Congenital erythropoietic porphyria (CEP)	Autosomal recessive		X		X
Uroporphyrinogen decarboxylase	1p34	Porphyria cutanea tarda (PCT)‡	Autosomal dominant	X			X
		Hepatoerythropoietic porphyria (HEP)	Autosomal recessive	X	X		X
Coproporphyrinogen oxidase	9	Hereditary coproporphyria (HCP)	Autosomal dominant	X		X	X
Protoporphyrinogen oxidase	?14	Variegate porphyria (VP)	Autosomal dominant	X		X	X
Ferrochelatase	18q21.3 or 22	Erythropoietic protoporphyria (EPP)	Autosomal dominant		X		X

* The most precise classification is according to the specific enzyme deficiencies. Other classifications based on the major tissue site of overproduction of heme pathway intermediates (hepatic versus erythropoietic) or the type of major symptoms (acute neurovisceral versus cutaneous) are useful but not precise or mutually exclusive.
† This enzyme is also known as hydroxymethylbilane synthase and formerly as uroporphyrinogen I synthase.
‡ PCT is primarily acquired. Inherited deficiency of uroporphyrinogen decarboxylase is partially responsible for familial (type II) PCT.

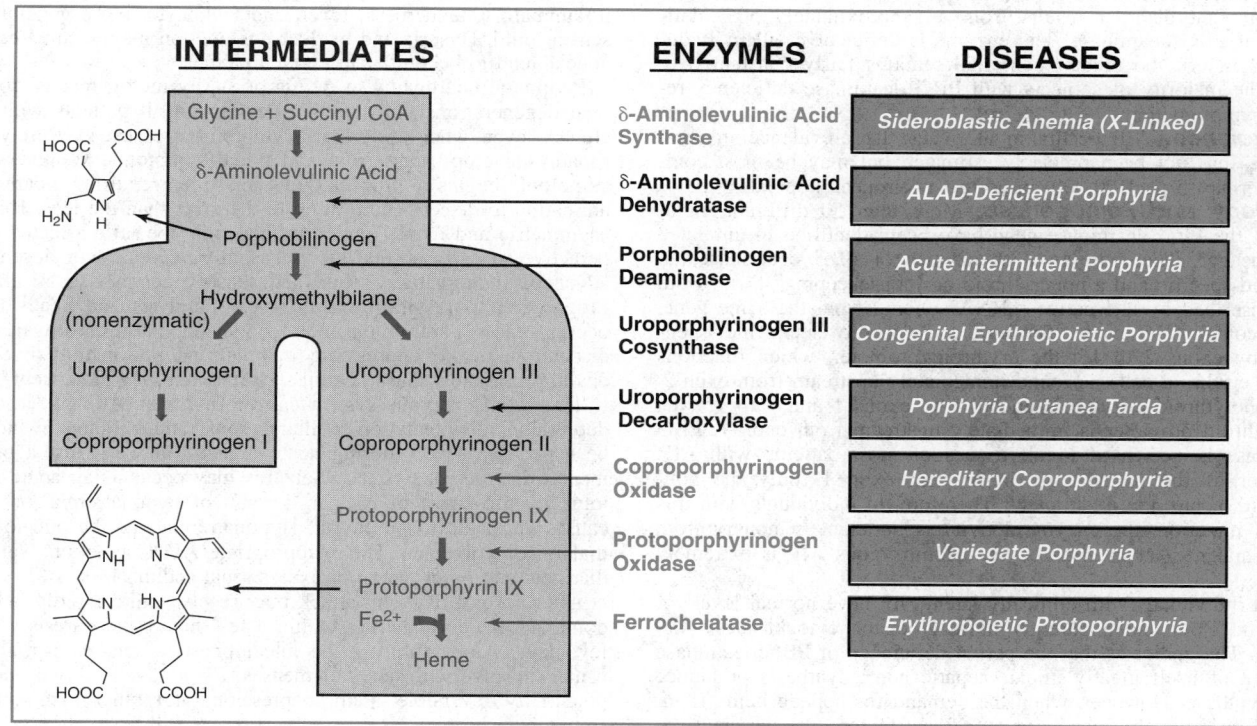

FIGURE 187–1. Intermediates and enzymes of the heme biosynthetic pathway and the major diseases of porphyrin metabolism that have been associated with deficiencies of specific enzymes. The initial and last three enzymes (in red) are mitochondrial and the other four (in black) are cytosolic. Heme is synthesized from glycine and succinyl CoA. Intermediates in the pathway include δ-aminolevulinic acid (an amino acid), porphobilinogen (a pyrrole), and hydroxymethylbilane (a linear tetrapyrrole). Uroporphyrinogen III cosynthase catalyzes closure of hydroxymethylbilane, with inversion of one of the pyrroles, to form a porphyrin macrocycle, uroporphyrinogen III. (Nonenzymatic closure occurs without inversion of this pyrrole, forming uroporphyrinogen I, which is not metabolized beyond coproporphyrinogen I.) The next two enzymes result in decarboxylation of six of the eight side chains of uroporphyrinogen III, with sequential formation of 7-, 6-, and 5-carboxylate porphyrinogens, coproporphyrinogen III, 3-carboxylate porphyrinogen, and protoporphyrinogen IX. The final two enzymes catalyze oxidation of protoporphyrinogen IX to protoporphyrin IX and insertion of ferrous iron into the porphyrin macrocycle to form heme (iron protoporphyrin IX). With the exception of protoporphyrin IX, all porphyrin intermediates are in their reduced forms (hexahydroporphyrins or porphyrinogens). Chemical structures of two intermediates are shown.

TABLE 187–2. THREE MOST COMMON HUMAN PORPHYRIAS AND THEIR MAJOR DISTINGUISHING FEATURES

	Presenting Symptoms	Exacerbating Factors	Most Important Screening Tests	Treatment
Acute intermittent porphyria (AIP)	Neurovisceral (acute)	Drugs (mostly P-450 inducers); progesterone; dietary restriction	Urinary porphobilinogen	Heme; glucose
Porphyria cutanea tarda (PCT)	Blistering skin lesions (chronic)	Iron; alcohol; estrogens; hepatitis C virus; halogenated hydrocarbons	Plasma (or urine) porphyrins	Phlebotomy; low-dose chloroquine
Erythropoietic protoporphyria (EPP)	Painful skin and swelling (mostly acute)		Plasma (or erythrocyte) porphyrins	β-Carotene

intermittent porphyria (AIP) but may begin in childhood. Hemolysis is sometimes present. Urinary ALA and coproporphyrin III and erythrocyte zinc protoporphyrin are increased. In this and other disorders in which ALA accumulates, coproporphyrin III may originate from excess ALA that is metabolized to coproporphyrinogen III in tissues other than the tissue of origin of the excess ALA.

Several other conditions are associated with ALA dehydratase deficiency and increased ALA. *Lead poisoning* and *hereditary tyrosinemia* can present with symptoms (abdominal pain, ileus, and motor neuropathy) that are strikingly similar to those of the acute porphyrias. Lead concentrates in erythroid cells and also inhibits ferrochelatase, leading to excess erythrocyte zinc protoporphyrin. Urinary coproporphyrin excretion is also increased. Deficient erythrocyte ALA dehydratase in lead poisoning can be restored to normal with dithiothreitol *in vitro*. In hereditary tyrosinemia, a deficiency of fumarylacetoacetase leads to accumulation of succinylacetone (2,3-dioxoheptanoic acid). This structural analogue of ALA is a potent inhibitor of ALA dehydratase. Other heavy metals or styrene exposure can also inhibit ALA dehydratase.

ACUTE INTERMITTENT PORPHYRIA (AIP). This autosomal dominant disorder results from an approximately 50% deficiency of PBG deaminase. The enzyme is deficient in all individuals who inherit the mutant gene and remains fairly constant over time. The majority of subjects with PBG deaminase deficiency remain asymptomatic.

Prevalence. AIP occurs in all races. Its prevalence in most countries has not been precisely estimated but may be most common (perhaps 5 per 100,000) in northern European populations.

Etiology and Pathogenesis. More than 50 different mutations of the PBG deaminase gene have been identified in unrelated AIP lineages. There are two isoenzymes of PBG deaminase, an erythroid-specific and a nonerythroid or "housekeeping" form. Both are transcribed by alternative mRNA splicing from the same gene, which contains 15 exons. The erythroid-specific isoenzyme is encoded by exons 2 to 15; the erythroid promoter, which functions only in erythroid cells, is found immediately upstream from exon 2. The nonerythroid enzyme is encoded by exons 1 and 3 to 15; the nonerythroid promoter is immediately upstream from exon 1. PBG deaminase is decreased in all tissues of most patients with AIP. However, if the mutation is in or near exon 1, only the nonerythroid isoenzyme is deficient. Therefore, in individuals with this type of mutation, the enzyme activity is deficient in nonerythroid tissues and normal in erythrocytes. Homozygous AIP is extremely rare.

Most individuals with clinically latent AIP have normal levels of ALA and PBG and apparently normal hepatic cytochrome P-450 content. This indicates that the partial deficiency of PBG deaminase does not of itself greatly impair hepatic heme synthesis or induce ALA synthase. However, when the demand for hepatic heme is increased by drugs, hormones, or nutritional factors, the deficient enzyme can become limiting for heme synthesis, induction of hepatic ALA synthase is accentuated, and ALA and PBG accumulate in liver and increase in plasma and urine. Excess porphyrins originate nonenzymatically from PBG or enzymatically from ALA transported to tissues other than the liver.

Most drugs that are harmful in AIP induce hepatic ALA synthase and cytochrome P-450 enzymes. Sulfonamide antibiotics are not inducers and may inhibit PBG deaminase. Reduced caloric and carbohydrate intakes enhance induction of ALA synthase in animals and in AIP can increase ALA and PBG and precipitate symptoms. Administering carbohydrate can reduce hepatic ALA synthase and P-450 enzymes.

The mechanism of neural damage in AIP is unknown. Porphyrias and related disorders associated with increased ALA have similar neurologic manifestations. ALA is structurally analogous to γ-aminobutyric acid (GABA) and can interact with GABA receptors. However, ALA and other products of the heme pathway have not been convincingly shown to be neurotoxic. The suggestion that heme deficiency may occur in nervous tissue in these disorders is also unproven.

Clinical Manifestations. Symptoms rarely occur before puberty and seldom if ever recur throughout adult life. Characteristically, attacks last for several days or longer, often require hospitalization, and are followed by complete recovery. Abdominal pain is the most common symptom; it is usually steady and poorly localized but may be cramping. Tachycardia, hypertension, restlessness, fine tremors, and excess sweating may be due to sympathetic overactivity. Other manifestations include nausea; vomiting; constipation; pain in the limbs, head, neck, or chest; muscle weakness; and sensory loss. Ileus, with distention and decreased bowel sounds, is common. However, increased bowel sounds and diarrhea may be seen. Because the abdominal symptoms are neurologic rather than inflammatory, tenderness, fever, and leukocytosis are generally absent or mild. Dysuria and bladder dysfunction may occur. Recurrent attacks tend to be similar in a given patient.

Peripheral neuropathy in AIP is primarily motor, results from axonal degeneration, and does not develop in all patients with acute attacks, even when abdominal symptoms are severe. Rarely, neuropathy develops apart from abdominal symptoms. Weakness most commonly begins in proximal muscles (often requiring a careful examination to detect), more often in the arms than the legs. It can be asymmetric and focal. Tendon reflexes may be little affected or hyperactive in early stages but are usually decreased or absent with advanced neuropathy. Cranial and sensory nerves can be affected. Progression to respiratory and bulbar paralysis and death seldom occurs unless porphyria is not recognized, harmful drugs are not discontinued, and appropriate treatment is not instituted. Sudden death, presumably due to cardiac arrhythmia, may also occur.

The central nervous system can be involved. Anxiety, insomnia, depression, disorientation, hallucinations, and paranoia, which can be especially severe during acute attacks, may suggest a primary mental disorder or hysteria. Seizures may occur as an acute neurologic manifestation of AIP, as a result of hyponatremia, or due to causes unrelated to porphyria. Hyponatremia may be due to hypothalamic involvement and inappropriate ADH secretion; vomiting, diarrhea, and poor intake; or excess renal sodium loss.

After several days, an attack may resolve quite rapidly, with abdominal pain disappearing within a few hours and paresis within a few days. Attacks during the luteal phase of the menstrual cycle usually resolve with onset of menses. Even advanced neuropathy is potentially reversible. Pain, depression, and other symptoms are sometimes chronic.

Chronic hepatic abnormalities are common in AIP, and there is an increased risk of hepatocellular carcinoma (apparently not associated with hepatitis B or C). AIP may predispose to chronic hypertension and be associated with impaired renal function. The mechanisms of these associations are unknown.

Precipitating Factors. Recognition of precipitating factors is important for management. Endogenous steroid hormones are probably most important. This is indicated by rarity of symptoms and excess ALA and PBG before puberty, more frequent clinical expression in women, premenstrual attacks in some women, and exacerbations after use of sex steroid preparations. Some patients manifest increased proportions of 5β-H steroid metabolites that are potent inducers of hepatic ALA synthase. Recurrent cyclic attacks are troublesome in some women and occur when progesterone levels are highest; progesterone and its metabolites are potent inducers of ALA synthase, whereas estrogens are not. Pregnancy is usually well tolerated despite high progesterone levels. Some women are more prone to attacks during pregnancy, possibly due in part to hyperemesis gravidarum and reduced caloric intake.

Drugs remain important as causes of AIP attacks. The major drugs known to be harmful or safe in the acute porphyrias are listed in Table 187-3. Barbiturates and sulfonamides are most notorious. Benzodiazepines are much less hazardous. Published information is insufficient to allow most drugs to be classified as definitely harmful or safe. Advice can be sought from a center with experience in porphyria with regard to unpublished information.

Reduced caloric intake, usually instituted in an effort to lose weight, is a common cause of attacks. Attacks are also provoked by intercurrent infections, major surgery, and other conditions. Attacks are almost always due to two or more factors acting in an additive fashion. Probably for this reason (a) drugs may produce attacks in adults but are rarely reported to do so in children with PBG deaminase deficiency; (b) anticonvulsants do not produce attacks in some PBG deaminase–deficient subjects; and (c) barbiturate anesthetics more frequently exacerbate porphyria if symptoms were present prior to anesthetic exposure.

Diagnosis and Differential Diagnosis. AIP and other acute porphyrias are uncommon, their symptoms are nonspecific, and physical findings are minimal. Therefore, a high index of suspicion is necessary for diagnosis. The diagnosis is established by demonstrating a marked increase in urinary PBG, using a quantitative method (see later discussion of laboratory methods). During an acute attack, PBG excretion generally is in the range of 50 to 200 mg per day (reference range 0 to 4 mg per day), and ALA excretion 20 to 100 mg per day (reference range 0 to 7 mg per day). Such increases virtually assure a diagnosis of AIP, variegate porphyria (VP), or hereditary coproporphyria (HCP). ALA and PBG excretion generally decrease with clinical improvement. Such decreases are particularly dramatic (but transient) after heme therapy. After an attack of AIP it is distinctly unusual for ALA and PBG to decrease to persistently normal levels, except after prolonged periods of latency. In HCP and VP, excretion of ALA and PBG may decrease to normal levels more readily. Fecal porphyrins are usually

TABLE 187-3. DRUGS CONSIDERED UNSAFE AND SAFE IN AIP, HCP, AND VP

Unsafe	Safe
Barbiturates*	Narcotic analgesics
Sulfonamide antibiotics*	Aspirin
Meprobamate*	Acetaminophen
Carisoprodol*	Phenothiazines
Glutethimide*	Penicillin and derivatives
Methyprylon	Streptomycin
Ethchlorvynol*	Glucocorticoids
Phenytoin*	Bromides
Mephenytoin	Insulin
Succinimides (ethosuximide, methsuximide)	Atropine
Carbamazepine*	Cimetidine
Clonazepam	Ranitidine*·†
Primidone*	?Estrogens*·‡
Valproic acid*	
Pyrazolones (aminopyrine, antipyrine)	
Griseofulvin*	
Ergots	
Metoclopramide*	
Rifampin*	
Pyrazinamide*	
Diclofenac*	
Progesterone and synthetic progestins*	
Danazol*	
Alcohol	

* Porphyria is listed as a contraindication, warning, precaution, or adverse effect in US labeling for these drugs.

† Although porphyria is listed as a precaution in US labeling for this drug, it is regarded as safe by other sources.

‡ There is little evidence that estrogens alone are harmful in acute porphyrias. They have been implicated as harmful based mostly on experience with estrogen-progestin combinations and because they can exacerbate PCT.

normal or minimally increased, which distinguishes AIP from HCP and VP. Urinary uroporphyrin and coproporphyrin and erythrocyte protoporphyrin may be increased, but these are not specific findings.

Decreased PBG deaminase (most conveniently measured in erythrocytes) confirms the diagnosis of AIP. However, as already noted, some mutations of the PBG deaminase gene reduce only the nonerythroid enzyme. Furthermore, erythrocyte PBG deaminase has a wide normal range (up to threefold) that somewhat overlaps the AIP range and is increased by inapparent concurrent conditions that stimulate erythropoiesis. The enzyme is not reduced in HCP and VP, which is also important to consider when acute porphyria is suspected. For these reasons, measurement of erythrocyte PBG deaminase is not useful in acutely ill patients. On the other hand, its measurement is highly useful to analyze pedigrees of known AIP patients, if it is established that the propositus has a low value. In screening family members, urinary PBG should also be measured. Diagnosis of AIP *in utero* is possible but is seldom indicated in view of the favorable outlook for most PBG deaminase–deficient subjects.

No single laboratory test fully excludes AIP, HCP, and VP. However, a normal result of a quantitative test for urinary PBG virtually excludes these disorders as a cause of current symptoms. Attempting to provoke increases in ALA and PBG for diagnostic purposes by glycine loading or administering phenobarbital may be dangerous and is not definitive.

Treatment. Acute attacks usually require hospitalization for treatment of severe pain, nausea, and vomiting and for administration of intravenous glucose and heme. Hospitalization also facilitates observation for neurologic complications, electrolyte imbalances, and nutritional status and investigation of precipitating factors. Symptomatic therapy includes narcotic analgesics, which are usually required for abdominal pain, and small to moderate doses of a phenothiazine for nausea, vomiting, anxiety, and restlessness. Chloral hydrate can be used for insomnia. Diazepam in low doses is probably safe if a minor tranquilizer is required. Bladder distention may require catheterization. After recovery, continued treatment with a phenothiazine is seldom indicated.

Heme therapy and carbohydrate loading are specific therapies because they repress hepatic ALA synthase and overproduction of ALA and PBG. Heme therapy is most effective in this regard and should be initiated early, but only after the diagnosis of a porphyric attack is confirmed by a marked increase in urinary PBG. Diagnosis is more difficult after heme therapy, which can at least transiently normalize ALA and PBG.

The standard regimen for heme therapy is 3 mg heme per kilogram of body weight, infused intravenously once daily for 4 days. A longer course of treatment is seldom necessary if treatment is started early. Efficacy is reduced and recovery is less rapid when treatment is delayed and neuronal damage is more advanced. It is not effective for chronic symptoms of AIP. A lyophilized hematin (hydroxy-heme) preparation is available in the United States. The manufacturer recommends reconstitution with sterile water. However, the product is unstable and degradation products adhere to endothelial cells, platelets, and coagulation factors, causing a transient anticoagulant effect and phlebitis at the site of infusion. Reconstitution with human albumin enhances the stability of hematin and prevents these side effects. Heme arginate, which is available in Europe and South Africa, is much more stable than hematin and also does not have these side effects. It is an investigational drug in the United States.

Carbohydrate loading may suffice for mild attacks and can be given orally as sucrose, glucose polymers, or carbohydrate-rich foods. If oral intake is poorly tolerated or is contraindicated by distention and ileus, glucose administered intravenously (at least 300 grams daily) is usually indicated. A central venous line facilitates more complete parenteral nutritional support and avoids excess fluid volumes. Parenteral nutritional support may be indicated in some patients who require heme therapy.

Treatment of seizures is problematic because virtually all antiseizure drugs (except bromides) can exacerbate AIP. β-Adrenergic blocking agents may control tachycardia and hypertension in acute attacks of porphyria but may be hazardous in patients with hypovolemia, in whom increased catecholamine secretion may be an important compensatory mechanism. Numerous other therapies have been tried in this disease but have not been consistently useful.

Prognosis. In the past 20 years, attacks of porphyria have rarely been fatal. If acute attacks are treated appropriately, inciting factors removed, and precautions taken to prevent further attacks, the outlook for patients with AIP is usually excellent. Recurrent attacks of porphyria occur in some patients and can be disabling but do not occur throughout adult life. The great majority of relatives with PBG deaminase deficiency never develop symptoms, especially if they have normal urinary porphyrin precursors. Although such individuals are less sensitive to inducing drugs than are patients with prior porphyric symptoms, they should follow the same precautions as AIP patients. Latent AIP should never be construed as a health risk that limits availability of health insurance.

Prevention. Some specific measures are helpful in preventing clinical expression of AIP. (1) Family members should be screened to detect latent cases. (2) Harmful drugs should be avoided. (3) "Crash diets" for weight reduction and even brief periods of starvation (e.g., during postoperative periods or intercurrent illnesses) should be avoided. Diet regimens for obesity should provide for gradual weight loss during periods of clinical remission of porphyria. (4) Investigational approaches for preventing frequent attacks include use of gonadotropin-releasing hormone analogues (for women with frequent cyclic attacks) or periodic heme infusions. Oophorectomy is not an acceptable option for preventing cyclic attacks.

CONGENITAL ERYTHROPOIETIC PORPHYRIA (CEP). This autosomal recessive disorder is due to a deficiency of uroporphyrinogen III cosynthase. Less than 200 cases have been reported. CEP occurs in several animal species (including all fox squirrels).

Etiology and Pathogenesis. At least six different mutations of the uroporphyrinogen III cosynthase gene have been identified in CEP. Most patients have unrelated parents and have inherited a different mutation from each parent. Severity of the disease is variable and relates to the degree of enzyme deficiency caused by the particular mutations. Intramedullary hemolysis and shortened survival of circulating erythrocytes are caused by porphyrins produced and accumulated in bone marrow erythroid cells that are actively synthesizing hemoglobin. Even in the most severe cases there is some residual cosynthase activity, and heme production is actually increased in response to hemolysis. Increased heme production occurs at the expense of a considerable accumulation of hydroxymethylbilane (the substrate of the deficient enzyme), which is converted nonenzymatically to uroporphyrinogen I. Excretion of type III porphyrin isomers is also increased. Splenomegaly can contribute to anemia and cause leukopenia and thrombocytopenia. Sunlight, other sources of UV light, and minor trauma to friable skin are other determinants of clinical expression. Drugs, steroids, and nutrition have little influence.

Clinical Manifestations. In most cases, reddish urine and severe cutaneous photosensitivity are noted in early infancy. Recently, patients with very severe cases have presented as nonimmune hydrops, received intrauterine transfusions, and soon after birth developed marked photosensitivity when phototherapy was initiated for neonatal jaundice. In at least five cases symptoms began in adult life. Cutaneous features resemble those in porphyria cutanea tarda (PCT) but are usually more severe. Lesions on sun-exposed skin include bullae and vesicles, which are prone to rupture and become infected, hypopigmented or hyperpigmented areas, and hypertrichosis. Loss of digits and facial features and corneal scarring can be severe. Porphyrins are deposited in the teeth (producing a reddish-brown color termed *erythrodontia*) and in bone. Bone demineralization can be substantial. There are no neurologic manifestations. Hemolysis and splenomegaly are almost always present. Life expectancy is often shortened by infections or hematologic complications.

Diagnosis and Differential Diagnosis. Porphyrin excretion and porphyrin levels in red cells and plasma are generally much greater than in other forms of porphyria. Porphyrins in urine are primarily uroporphyrin and coproporphyrin, and in feces mostly coproporphyrin. ALA and PBG are normal. In most cases uroporphyrin I predominates in erythrocytes. A predominance of protoporphyrin in red cells has been described in some cases and is characteristic of bovine CEP. Stimulating erythropoiesis increases

uroporphyrin and coproporphyrin in erythrocytes in this condition. CEP is readily distinguished from EPP clinically but may resemble HEP and homozygous cases of AIP, VP, and HCP.

Treatment. Protection of the skin from sunlight and minor trauma and prompt treatment of secondary bacterial infections help prevent scarring and mutilation. Blood transfusions sufficient to suppress erythropoiesis may be the most effective treatment. Improvement may occur after splenectomy. Oral charcoal may be helpful by increasing fecal excretion of porphyrins.

Prevention. In affected families heterozygotes with intermediate deficiencies of the cosynthase can be detected, and CEP can be diagnosed *in utero*. Therefore, there are options for preventing genetic transmission.

PORPHYRIA CUTANEA TARDA (PCT). This, the most common and readily treated form of porphyria, is caused by a deficiency of uroporphyrinogen decarboxylase in the liver. It is most common in men but has become more frequent in women, associated with alcohol and estrogen use.

Etiology and Pathogenesis. PCT is fundamentally an acquired disorder, although in some cases an inherited deficiency of uroporphyrinogen decarboxylase is a predisposing factor. Currently, PCT is classified into three types. In the "sporadic" form (type I), which constitutes the majority of cases, the enzyme is deficient in liver but not in erythrocytes and other tissues, and there are no mutations at the uroporphyrinogen decarboxylase locus. Moreover, the amount of hepatic uroporphyrinogen decarboxylase protein, as measured immunochemically, is normal, suggesting that an acquired process has inactivated the enzyme. With treatment and remission of the disease, the enzyme activity gradually increases to normal. Familial (type II) PCT is distinguished from type I by an approximately 50% deficiency of the decarboxylase in nonhepatic tissues, such as erythrocytes, and mutations in the uroporphyrinogen decarboxylase gene. The mutant alleles do not express detectable enzyme protein. The inherited autosomal dominant trait is not associated with overt disease unless the product of the normal allele is inactivated by the same acquired factors that are important in type I PCT. In type III PCT, the enzyme is deficient in liver but not other tissues, as in type I. However, unlike type I, more than one family member is affected. All three types are clinically similar and difficult to distinguish, and they respond to the same therapies.

Examples of *toxic porphyria* have resembled PCT. Most notably, an extensive outbreak of porphyria occurred in eastern Turkey in the late 1950's after seed wheat containing the fungicide hexachlorobenzene was used for food. Di- and trichlorophenols and 2,3,7,8-tetrachlorodibenzo-*p*-dioxin (TCDD, dioxin) have been implicated in smaller outbreaks and single cases in humans. When administered to animals, these chemicals decrease uroporphyrinogen decarboxylase (only in liver) and induce a pattern of excess porphyrins resembling PCT. There is seldom a history of exposure to such chemicals in sporadic (type I) PCT.

A notable feature of PCT is massive accumulation of porphyrins in liver, which may develop over many months. This precedes the appearance of excess porphyrins in plasma and urine. Hepatic ALA synthase may be little increased because amounts of porphyrins produced in PCT are small relative to rates of hepatic heme formation. By contrast, during attacks of the acute porphyrias much larger amounts of intermediates are excreted (as porphyrin precursors) and ALA synthase is substantially induced. Worsening of PCT by factors (other than alcohol) that induce heme synthesis is seldom reported.

The pattern of porphyrins that accumulate in PCT is complex and characteristic. The enzyme-catalyzed decarboxylation of uroporphyrinogen occurs in four sequential steps. Therefore, when the enzyme is markedly deficient, uroporphyrin and the hepta-, hexa-, and pentacarboxyl porphyrins (type I and III isomers, and derived from the corresponding porphyrinogens) accumulate. In addition, pentacarboxyl porphyrinogen can be metabolized by coproporphyrinogen oxidase to a series of tetracarboxyl porphyrins termed isocoproporphyrins. These are excreted primarily in bile and feces and are diagnostic of uroporphyrinogen decarboxylase deficiency.

Acquired factors may contribute to inactivation of hepatic uroporphyrinogen decarboxylase as follows: (1) A normal or increased amount of hepatic iron seems essential in this disease. One or more mechanisms may be involved. Ferrous iron may directly inhibit the enzyme. Iron may catalyze the formation of free radicals that damage the enzyme protein or oxidize its porphyrinogen substrates to porphyrins. (2) Cytochrome P-450 enzymes may also be involved in the oxidation of porphyrinogen substrates. (3) Alcohol intake may promote iron absorption, stimulate hepatic heme and porphyrin synthesis, or generate free radicals that damage the decarboxylase. (4) Estrogens, but apparently not other steroids, can exacerbate PCT, perhaps by an unknown oxidative mechanism. (5) The strong association with chronic hepatitis C virus infection suggests that hepatocellular damage induced by this virus, which appears to be accentuated by iron, can involve specific cellular proteins including uroporphyrinogen decarboxylase.

Clinical Manifestations. Most PCT patients have a history of moderate or heavy alcohol intake. The disease may develop in men treated with estrogens for prostate cancer and women taking oral contraceptives or replacement estrogens. Cutaneous photosensitivity is the major clinical feature. Vesicles and bullae develop on the face, dorsa of the hands and feet, forearms, and legs. Sun-exposed skin becomes friable, and minor trauma may precede the formation of bullae or cause denudation of the skin. Small white plaques ("milia") may precede or follow vesicle formation. Involved skin tends to heal slowly. Hypertrichosis and hyperpigmentation sometimes present even in the absence of vesicles. Thickening, scarring, and calcification of affected skin ("pseudoscleroderma") may be striking. Neurologic effects are not observed.

Liver histopathology is usually not diagnostic of alcoholic liver disease. Cirrhosis and hepatocellular carcinomas are most common in older patients and at autopsy. In many locations as many as 80% of PCT patients are chronically infected with hepatitis C virus. This strong association may explain much of the chronic liver damage and many of the hepatocellular carcinomas that have been observed in PCT. The disease is also associated with systemic lupus erythematosus and the acquired immunodeficiency syndrome (AIDS).

PCT sometimes occurs in patients with advanced renal disease. Skin lesions may be more severe and plasma porphyrin levels much higher in this setting because urinary excretion of porphyrins is not possible, and they are poorly dialyzed.

Very rarely, hepatic tumors themselves contain and presumably produce excess porphyrins. Some of these cases have resembled PCT.

Diagnosis and Differential Diagnosis. Skin lesions in PCT, VP, and HCP are indistinguishable clinically and histologically. It is important to differentiate these conditions by laboratory testing before starting therapy. A predominance of uroporphyrin and 7-carboxylate porphyrin in urine and increased isocoproporphyrin in feces are diagnostic of PCT. In PCT, urinary ALA may be slightly increased; PBG is normal. Total fecal porphyrins are usually less increased in PCT than in other types of porphyria with photosensitivity. Plasma porphyrins are always increased in patients with skin lesions due to any type of porphyria; the fluorescence spectrum of plasma can distinguish VP and EPP from PCT (see below).

Treatment. A course of phlebotomies is the preferred treatment and almost always produces a remission. Patients are also advised to discontinue alcohol, estrogens, iron supplements, or other contributing factors. Because iron stores in PCT are seldom markedly increased and may be normal, removal of only 5 to 6 units of blood at 1- to 2-week intervals is usually sufficient. Plasma (or serum) ferritin and porphyrin levels should be followed. Ferritin decreases before porphyrins. Phlebotomies should be stopped when the ferritin is near the lower limit of normal. Further iron depletion is of no additional benefit and may cause anemia and associated symptoms. Remission may be prolonged even if the ferritin level later returns to normal. In some cases relapses occur and respond to another course of phlebotomies. Deferoxamine, an iron chelator, may be effective in PCT but is much less efficient.

A course of low-dose chloroquine (e.g., 125 mg twice weekly for several months or as needed) or hydroxychloroquine is usually effective when repeated phlebotomies are contraindicated. The mechanism of their effects in PCT is not established. One hypothesis is that chloroquine forms complexes with porphyrins and promotes their removal from the liver. Chloroquine given in usual doses to PCT patients can cause marked increases in photosensitivity and porphyrin levels in plasma and urine, and nausea, malaise, fever, and hepatocellular damage. Although these adverse effects are generally transient and are followed by complete remission, it is prudent to avoid them by using a low-dose regimen.

Therapy is more difficult when PCT occurs with advanced renal disease because phlebotomy is usually contraindicated by anemia (usually due to erythropoietin deficiency). Recent studies indicate that genetic recombinant erythropoietin can mobilize excess iron, support phlebotomy, and lead to remission of PCT in these patients.

HEPATOERYTHROPOIETIC PORPHYRIA (HEP). This rare, recently recognized autosomal recessive disease is clinically similar to CEP but is distinguished by excess isocoproporphyrin in feces and urine and decreased uroporphyrinogen decarboxylase activity in erythrocytes (and other tissues). The mutations in the uroporphyrinogen decarboxylase gene found in this disease are associated with some residual enzyme activity, unlike those in familial PCT. Therefore, strictly speaking, HEP is not the homozygous form of familial PCT. Increased erythrocyte protoporphyrin probably reflects an earlier accumulation of uroporphyrinogen in erythroblasts, which after completion of hemoglobin synthesis is metabolized to protoporphyrin. A similar explanation can account for increased erythrocyte protoporphyrin in other homozygous forms of porphyria.

HEREDITARY COPROPORPHYRIA (HCP) AND VARIEGATE PORPHYRIA (VP). These autosomal dominant acute hepatic porphyrias are clinically similar to AIP but are much less common in most countries. However, VP is quite prevalent in South Africa, where most cases have been traced to a couple who immigrated from Holland in the late 1600's. Unlike AIP, these disorders can cause cutaneous photosensitivity.

Etiology and Pathogenesis. HCP and VP are due to approximately 50% deficiencies of coproporphyrinogen oxidase and protoporphyrinogen oxidase, respectively. As in AIP, ALA and PBG are increased during acute attacks. This reflects induction of hepatic ALA synthase by factors such as endogenous steroids, drugs, and nutritional alterations, and the fact that PBG deaminase activity is almost as low as ALA synthase even in normal liver. When coproporphyrinogen III accumulates in HCP and coproporphyrinogen III and protoporphyrinogen IX in VP, they are auto-oxidized to the corresponding porphyrins. Coproporphyrinogen III may accumulate in VP because there is a functional association between coproporphyrinogen oxidase and the deficient protoporphyrinogen oxidase in mitochondria. Furthermore, coproporphyrinogen is more readily lost from the liver than are other porphyrinogens, and its loss increases further when heme synthesis is stimulated. In one form of HCP, termed *harderoporphyria,* a structurally altered coproporphyrinogen oxidase with reduced substrate affinity results in accumulation of harderoporphyrin as well as coproporphyrin. A few homozygous cases of HCP and VP have been described.

Clinical Manifestations. Drugs, steroids, and nutritional factors that are detrimental in AIP also exacerbate HCP and VP. Neurologic manifestations are identical to those in AIP. Skin manifestations are similar to those of PCT and usually occur apart from the neurovisceral symptoms. Impaired biliary excretion by concurrent liver diseases or drugs such as contraceptive steroids can cause porphyrin retention and worsen photosensitivity.

Diagnosis and Differential Diagnosis. Urinary ALA, PBG, and uroporphyrin are increased during acute attacks. When symptoms resolve, these normalize more readily than in AIP. Urinary coproporphyrin is markedly increased in both HCP and VP. A marked, isolated increase in fecal coproporphyrin is distinctive for HCP. Fecal coproporphyrin and protoporphyrin are about equally increased in VP. The fluorescence spectrum of plasma porphyrins (at neutral pH) is characteristic and very useful for rapidly distinguishing VP from the other porphyrias. This test is probably the most sensitive method for detecting VP, including latent cases, at least in adults.

Treatment and Prognosis. Acute attacks of VP are treated as in AIP. Striking decreases in attacks and deaths from VP in South Africa are attributed to identifying latent cases, avoiding harmful drugs, and providing better treatment during acute attacks. Measures that protect the skin from sunlight are helpful for photosensitivity. Phlebotomies and chloroquine are not effective. Cholestyramine may decrease photosensitivity occurring with liver dysfunction.

ERYTHROPOIETIC PROTOPORPHYRIA (EPP). This is an autosomal dominant condition due to a deficiency of ferrochelatase.

Etiology and Pathogenesis. At least 10 different point mutations in the ferrochelatase gene have been identified in various EPP families. Ferrochelatase is deficient in all tissues in EPP but becomes rate-limiting for protoporphyrin metabolism primarily in bone marrow. Some obligate carriers have little or no increase in red cell protoporphyrin. Increases in plasma and fecal protoporphyrin are also variable. This marked variation in clinical expression is evident within individual kindreds and is not well explained.

Individuals with clinically expressed EPP accumulate excess protoporphyrin in erythroid cells, plasma, bile, and feces. Bone marrow reticulocytes are the primary source of the excess protoporphyrin. Circulating erythrocytes and the liver contribute smaller amounts. Protoporphyrin in erythrocytes in EPP is not complexed with zinc and compared with zinc protoporphyrin (found in lead poisoning, iron deficiency, and homozygous forms of porphyria) diffuses more readily into plasma. Zinc protoporphyrin dissociates less readily from hemoglobin binding sites and persists in the red cell as long as it circulates. Disposition of the excess protoporphyrin in EPP depends on hepatic uptake, biliary excretion, and degree of enterohepatic circulation. These processes are impaired by liver damage.

Clinical Manifestations. Cutaneous manifestations usually begin in childhood and are distinctly different from those of other porphyrias. Burning, itching, erythema, and swelling can occur within minutes of sun exposure. Diffuse edema of sun-exposed areas may resemble angioneurotic edema. Other characteristic skin changes include lichenification, leathery pseudovesicles, labial grooving, and nail changes. Scarring is rarely severe or deforming. Vesicles, pigment changes, friability, and hirsutism are unusual. There is no fluorescence of the teeth and no neuropathic manifestations. Drugs that exacerbate hepatic porphyrias are not known to worsen EPP, although they are generally avoided as a precaution.

Hemolysis is uncommon or very mild in uncomplicated cases. Erythropoiesis and iron metabolism are generally normal. Mild anemia with hypochromia and microcytosis is noted in some cases and is unexplained. Patients with EPP may develop gallstones containing protoporphyrin.

Liver function is usually normal in EPP. A minority of patients with EPP develop liver disease, which can progress rapidly to death from liver failure. Excess protoporphyrin itself may have cholestatic effects and damage hepatocytes. Intercurrent factors such as viral hepatitis, alcohol, iron deficiency, fasting, and oral contraceptive steroids have played a role in some patients.

Diagnosis and Differential Diagnosis. Protoporphyrin is increased in bone marrow, erythrocytes, plasma, bile, and feces of EPP patients. Urinary porphyrins and porphyrin precursors are normal. Hepatic complications of EPP are often preceded by increasing levels of erythrocyte and plasma protoporphyrin, abnormal liver function tests, marked deposition of protoporphyrin in liver cells and bile canaliculi, and increased photosensitivity.

Treatment and Prognosis. β-Carotene was developed primarily for treating EPP. Its clinical benefits have been substantiated in large series of patients. No side effects other than a mild and dose-related skin discoloration due to carotenemia have been noted. Its mechanism of action may involve quenching of singlet oxygen or free radicals. Cholestyramine may reduce protoporphyrin levels by interrupting its enterohepatic circulation. Iron deficiency, caloric restriction, and drugs or hormone preparations that impair hepatic excretory function should be avoided.

Hepatic complications may resolve spontaneously if a reversible cause of liver dysfunction, such as viral hepatitis or alcohol, is contributing. Transfusions or heme therapy may suppress erythroid and hepatic protoporphyrin production. Splenectomy, correction of iron deficiency, and use of cholestyramine or activated charcoal may be beneficial. Liver transplantation is sometimes required.

DUAL PORPHYRIA. This term refers to patients with porphyria and deficiencies of more than one enzyme of the heme biosynthetic pathway. Examples include double heterozygotes with both VP and familial PCT, deficiencies of both porphobilinogen deaminase and uroporphyrinogen decarboxylase (with symptoms of AIP, PCT, or both), and deficiencies of both coproporphyrinogen oxidase and uroporphyrinogen III cosynthase.

LABORATORY DIAGNOSIS OF PORPHYRIAS

Appropriate laboratory testing for these disorders is both specific and sensitive. An array of tests for porphyria is available, but some are subject to overuse and misinterpretation. Porphyrias can be readily detected and misdiagnoses avoided by relying primarily on

TABLE 187–4. FIRST-LINE LABORATORY TESTS FOR SCREENING FOR PORPHYRIAS AND SECOND-LINE TESTS FOR FURTHER EVALUATION WHEN INITIAL TESTING IS POSITIVE

Testing	Symptoms Suggesting Porphyria	
	Acute Neurovisceral Symptoms	*Cutaneous Photosensitivity*
First-line	Urinary ALA and PBG (quantitative; random urine)	Total plasma porphyrins†
Second-line	Urinary ALA, PBG, and total porphyrins* (quantitative; 24-hour urine)	Erythrocyte porphyrins
		Urinary ALA, PBG, and total porphyrins* (quantitative, 24-hour urine)
	Total fecal porphyrins*	
	Erythrocyte PBG deaminase	
	Total plasma porphyrins†	Total fecal porphyrins*

* Urinary and fecal porphyrins are fractionated only if the total is increased.
† The preferred method is by direct fluorescent spectrophotometry.
Abbreviations: ALA = δ-aminolevulinic acid; PBG = porphobilinogen.

a few first-line tests. The preferred approach for screening, as outlined in Table 187–4, is to rely on measurement of *urinary porphyrin precursors (ALA and PBG)* in patients with neurovisceral symptoms and a fluorometric measurement of *total plasma porphyrins* when it is suspected that skin photosensitivity may be due to porphyria.

In acutely ill patients, it is important to identify or exclude acute porphyria promptly. Urinary PBG is always markedly increased during acute attacks of AIP, HCP, and VP. A normal level effectively excludes these disorders as a cause of current symptoms. Because PBG is so strikingly increased during an attack, quantitation on a spot sample is highly informative. Assays for PBG use Ehrlich's aldehyde (p-dimethylaminobenzaldehyde), which forms reddish-purple chromogens with PBG, urobilinogen, and other substances in urine. Qualitative methods (e.g., Watson-Schwartz and Hoesch tests) are still widely used to screen for increased PBG. They are subject to misinterpretation and false-positive readings, do not quantitate PBG, and are less sensitive and only slightly more rapid than quantitative methods, which separate PBG from interfering substances by ion-exchange chromatography. If a qualitative test for PBG is used for screening, positive samples should be retested by a quantitative method. Urinary ALA and coproporphyrin, but not PBG, are increased in ADP.

Total plasma porphyrins are always increased in patients with active skin lesions. Normal plasma porphyrin levels exclude porphyria as a cause of cutaneous symptoms if the measurement is carried out by a simple and direct fluorometric method. Plasma porphyrins in VP are mostly covalently bound to plasma porphyrins and may not be detected by other methods.

The interpretation of urine, fecal, and erythrocyte porphyrin levels is often problematic, for the following reasons: (1) In contrast to plasma porphyrins, these measurements do not individually detect all cutaneous porphyrias. (2) Urine and erythrocyte porphyrins can be increased in many conditions other than porphyria, whereas an increased plasma porphyrin concentration is much more specific for porphyria. (3) Fecal porphyrin determinations are semiquantitative and subject to interference by diet and other factors.

More extensive testing is required if an initial screening test for porphyria is positive or may also be necessary initially if subclinical porphyria is suspected. Laboratory testing of relatives is not appropriate until test results have firmly established a diagnosis of porphyria in the propositus. Results of testing the propositus guide the choice of tests for relatives. Consultation with a physician and laboratory with experience in testing for porphyrias is done in these situations. Incorrect diagnoses of porphyria are not uncommon in patients with symptoms due to other diseases. Therefore, the laboratory data that were the basis for an original diagnosis of porphyria should remain available for future reference.

Anderson KE: The porphyrias. *In* Zakim D, Boyer T (eds.): Hepatology. Philadelphia, WB Saunders, in press. *One of several recent and detailed reviews on the genetic, biochemical, and clinical aspects of the porphyrias.*

Bonkovsky HL, Healey BS, Lourie AN, et al.: Intravenous heme-albumin in acute intermittent porphyria: Evidence for repletion of hepatic hemoproteins and regulatory heme pools. Am J Gastroenterol 86:1050, 1991. *This article describes a method for reconstituting and stabilizing lyophilized hematin with human albumin to prevent phlebitis and other side effects.*

Herrero C, Vicente A, Bruguera M, et al.: Is hepatitis C virus infection a trigger of porphyria cutanea tarda? Lancet 341:788, 1993. *Discussion of the recently described strong association of PCT with hepatitis C infection.*

Kauppinen R, Mustajoki P: Prognosis of acute porphyria: Occurrence of acute attacks, precipitating factors, and associated diseases. Medicine 71:1, 1992. *A recent review of clinical aspects of the acute porphyrias, emphasizing new developments.*

Long S, Smyth SJ, Woolf J, et al.: Detection of latent variegate porphyria by fluorescence emission spectroscopy of plasma. Br J Dermatol 129:9, 1993. *Measurement of total plasma porphyrins is an underutilized laboratory method that is useful for diagnosis, differential diagnosis, and assessing treatment of cutaneous porphyrias. This article demonstrates its usefulness in detecting latent as well as overt VP.*

Mustajoki P, Nordmann Y: Early administration of heme arginate for acute porphyric attacks. Arch Intern Med 153:2004, 1993. *A large series of patients treated with intravenous heme, emphasizing the importance of early treatment.*

Ratnaike S, Blake D, Campbell D, et al.: Plasma ferritin levels as a guide to the treatment of porphyria cutanea tarda by venesection. Australas J Dermatol 29:3, 1988. *Experience showing that plasma ferritin and total plasma porphyrins are the best predictors of response of PCT during treatment by phlebotomy.*

Verstraeten L, Van Regemorter N, Pardou A, et al.: Biochemical diagnosis of a fatal case of Gunther's disease in a newborn with hydrops-fetalis. Eur J Clin Chem Clin Biochem 31:121, 1993. *A case report describing recent developments in molecular and clinical aspects of CEP, and presentation of severe disease in utero.*

188 WILSON'S DISEASE
Andrew Deiss

DEFINITION. Wilson's disease (hepatolenticular degeneration) is a hereditary disorder characterized by the accumulation of copper in the body, especially in the liver, brain, kidneys, and corneas. The excess copper leads to tissue injury and ultimately, if effective treatment is not instituted, to death.

ETIOLOGY AND PREVALENCE. Wilson's disease is inherited as an autosomal recessive trait. The gene has been mapped to chromosome 13q14.3. It probably codes for a copper-transporting ATPase. The prevalence of the disease is approximately 30 per million.

PATHOGENESIS. Normally, loss of copper from the body occurs primarily through the bile. Much of biliary copper is secreted in a poorly absorbable form and thus is lost in the feces. Copper balance is normally maintained by this mechanism. In Wilson's disease biliary excretion of copper is impaired, and as a consequence nearly total body copper is progressively increased. The specific nature of the metabolic abnormality that causes this defect is not known.

Positive copper balance begins in infancy in Wilson's disease and continues thereafter unless appropriate therapy is given. However, the distribution of copper changes as the disease progresses. Liver copper is actually greater in presymptomatic homozygotes than in symptomatic ones. Thus not only does net deposition of liver copper cease, but also a portion of previously deposited copper is lost from the liver and deposited elsewhere. This copper redistribution probably takes place when liver injury occurs. If this injury occurs abruptly in many hepatocytes, liver disease may be clinically manifested, and a large amount of copper may be released over a short period, creating the potential for acute erythrocyte injury and hemolytic anemia as well. However, if hepatocyte injury is more gradual, acute liver disease does not occur and the patient remains asymptomatic as the important site of copper deposition shifts to the brain. With the latter course, most patients later develop neurologic or psychiatric symptoms, usually with clinically inapparent cirrhosis.

The serum concentration of the copper-containing protein ceruloplasmin is low in 95% of patients with Wilson's disease. The hypoceruloplasminemia is probably due in part to a decrease in ceruloplasmin gene transcription.

PATHOLOGY. The diagnosis cannot be made on the basis of histologic sections of the liver. Fatty change and glycogen-filled nuclei are present early, followed later by piecemeal necrosis, lymphocytic infiltration, erosion of limiting plates, parenchymal collapse, and fibrosis. Ultimately, these abnormalities evolve into postnecrotic cirrhosis. Stains for copper are unreliable, being negative most frequently during the early stages of the disease, when diagnostic help is most needed.

In the brain, abnormal astrocytes and neuronal necrosis are widely distributed, and there is atrophy or cavitation of the basal ganglia and occasionally the cerebral cortex.

CLINICAL MANIFESTATIONS. Wilson's disease is a disorder of young persons. Although the disease may occur at any time from the age of 5 into the sixth decade, two thirds of patients seek medical attention between the ages of 8 and 20. The physician should suspect the disorder in young people with signs of chronic or recurrent hepatic dysfunction or with characteristic neurologic abnormalities.

The hepatic symptoms are quite diverse. Commonly, a brief illness characterized by malaise, anorexia, jaundice, and increased aminotransferases is mistaken for viral hepatitis. Similar episodes may recur at intervals of months or years, or a latent period may occur during which the patient is asymptomatic until neurologic symptoms begin. If clinically overt hepatocyte injury persists over a longer period, a syndrome resembling chronic active hepatitis results. Occasionally, liver injury occurs precipitously. The need for prompt diagnosis is urgent because without rapid institution of appropriate treatment, death is likely in these patients. More commonly, however, hepatocyte injury is gradual and is not accompanied by symptoms of liver disease; nevertheless, cirrhosis develops ultimately in all patients. This liver injury may not be recognized until neurologic disease is evaluated.

Episodes of hemolytic anemia occur when massive release of copper from the liver takes place. Thus hemolysis is usually accompanied by overt liver disease; it occurs regularly in patients with fulminant hepatic failure. Hemolysis usually lasts only a short period and disappears spontaneously.

Neurologic disease may begin with a variety of motor symptoms, including involuntary movement, such as tremor or chorea, or decreased movement. The tremor is primarily proximal, often characterized by a "wing-beating" rhythmic oscillating tremor of the upper extremities that may eventually extend to the trunk. Dystonic signs include slowness of movement or speech, unsteady gait, dystonic posturing, and dystonic facies in which the upper lip is drawn tightly over the teeth. Frequently, loss of coordination of fine movements, such as those required for handwriting, is the earliest neurologic sign. As the disease progresses, patients may develop combinations of these abnormalities. Dysarthria, rigidity, drooling, and titubation are late features. Seizures are infrequent and sensory abnormalities absent. The Kayser-Fleischer (K-F) ring, described below, is definitively diagnostic in the neurologic variety and nearly so in the hepatic form of the disease.

Psychological symptoms of Wilson's disease are prominent and consist of early development of intellectual deterioration, personality changes, and unstable behavior. Children begin to fail at school, and young adults may show difficulty in performing jobs once considered routine. Schizophreniform symptoms and other forms of bizarre behavior may appear, but the mental status examination always shows signs of organic dementia. Effectively removing excess copper often improves but usually fails to eliminate these symptoms completely.

K-F rings are golden brown or greenish rings or arcs in Descemet's membrane at the limbus of the cornea. They are composed of copper-containing granules and develop primarily after redistribution of liver copper. They may be visible with the unaided eye, but slit-lamp examination should always be obtained. K-F rings are present in all or nearly all patients in the neurologic or psychiatric stage of the disease but are not present in about one third of those with hepatic symptoms.

Rare symptoms ascribable to Wilson's disease include cholelithiasis, sunflower cataracts, arthropathy, renal calculi, heart disease, and Fanconi's syndrome.

DIAGNOSIS. The classic diagnostic features are K-F rings, low serum ceruloplasmin concentration (< 20 mg per deciliter), and increased amounts of liver and urinary copper (> 250 μg per gram of dry weight and > 100 μg per 24 hours, respectively). Computed tomography or preferably magnetic resonance scans may show atrophy or cavitation even in patients with no neurologic abnormalities, but they may be entirely normal. The role of genetic diagnosis is not established, but it is likely to be complicated by the reported great allelic heterogeneity.

The classic diagnostic signs are present in nearly all patients with fully evolved neurologic Wilson's disease but only in about two thirds of those presenting with liver disease. In these patients, K-F rings often have not yet formed, and the serum ceruloplasmin concentration may be difficult to interpret. Even in Wilson's disease, serum ceruloplasmin increases during inflammation, estrogen administration, and pregnancy and may decrease during liver failure. Measurement of the copper content of the liver should resolve the problem. Hepatic copper is often greater than normal (50 μg per gram of dry weight) in a variety of chronic liver diseases, but it seldom reaches the concentration seen in most patients with Wilson's disease (> 250 μg per gram of dry weight). In a patient with a disease clinically suggestive of Wilson's disease, hepatic copper of this magnitude is essentially diagnostic. If the diagnosis is still in doubt, incorporation of radioactive copper into ceruloplasmin can be measured; incorporation is negligible in Wilson's disease, normal in other liver disease, even with copper loading, and intermediate in 75% of heterozygotes, but there is much overlap between groups. All measurements of copper metabolism should be entrusted only to laboratories experienced with their determination, and the normal values of that laboratory should be used. In patients with fulminant hepatic failure, it has been proposed that the ratios of alkaline phosphatase (IU per liter) to total bilirubin (mg per deciliter) and of AST (IU per liter) to ALT (IU per liter) of < 2.0 and > 4.0, respectively, identify patients with Wilson's disease, but the specificity has been questioned.

In primary biliary cirrhosis and chronic cholestasis, diseases with acquired abnormalities of copper excretion, liver copper may be greatly increased and K-F rings occur rarely. The age, symptoms, and laboratory abnormalities of patients with these diseases help distinguish them from those with Wilson's disease.

Early during the hemolytic anemia the urinary copper excretion is very great. The Coombs test result is negative. When hemolysis and acute liver disease occur concurrently in a young person, Wilson's disease is the most probable cause.

Examination of all siblings of patients with Wilson's disease is mandatory to identify presymptomatic homozygotes. K-F rings are usually absent. Serum ceruloplasmin concentration is reduced in 95% of homozygotes and 20% of heterozygotes. If it is low, liver copper content should be measured. Hepatic copper is slightly increased in most heterozygotes. If the copper is > 250 μg per gram of dry weight, Wilson's disease is present, and it should be treated as in symptomatic patients. Heterozygotes never become symptomatic and should not be treated. Some homozygotes are missed by this evaluation, so continued follow-up is necessary.

TREATMENT. Without effective lifetime therapy, Wilson's disease is inevitably fatal. If treatment is begun early enough, symptomatic recovery usually is complete, and a life of normal length and quality can be expected. If treatment is begun too late, death may not be prevented, or recovery will be only partial.

Effective therapy depends on establishing negative copper balance, thereby preventing deposition of more copper and mobilizing for excretion excess copper already deposited. Three agents are available that seem to be equally efficacious.

D-Penicillamine remains the drug of choice, at least until there is substantially more experience with the other agents. The usual dosage is 1 gram per day, given in divided doses 1 hour before meals and at bedtime. Pyridoxine, 25 mg per day, is also given. Response typically is quite slow, occurring over months, but it may occur more rapidly. A year or more is often required to obtain maximum improvement. At least 10% of patients experience a worsening of neurologic symptoms during the first month or two of treatment, and this phenomenon should not suggest that the diagnosis is in error. Compliance and the effectiveness of therapy must be monitored at 1- to 2-month intervals for the first year and twice yearly thereafter; monitoring consists of measurements of urinary copper, serum ceruloplasmin, and serum nonceruloplasmin copper (total serum copper minus ceruloplasmin copper). Nonceruloplasmin copper should decrease early and ceruloplasmin more gradually if treatment is adequate. Urinary copper levels increase at once to 1 to 5 mg per 24 hours during the first few months and then gradually decline as the excess of copper decreases.

Toxic effects are frequent. Rash, fever, adenopathy, neutropenia, or thrombocytopenia often occurs during the first 2 weeks of treatment. In such circumstances, penicillamine should be discontinued; when the symptoms have cleared, prednisone should be begun at a dose of 40 mg per day and penicillamine resumed at 250 mg per day and gradually increased to full dose over a period of a few weeks. The steroids can then be tapered and stopped. Side effects that occur later after penicillamine is begun include proteinuria, nephrotic syndrome, systemic lupus erythematosus, Goodpasture's syndrome, and a variety of chronic skin diseases. These side effects can often be reversed by temporarily stopping penicillamine and resuming it after the symptoms have abated, sometimes adding steroids. Treatment should never be suspended for more than a few months.

If penicillamine toxicity is not manageable, either trientine (250 mg 1 hour before meals and at bedtime) or zinc (50 mg of elemental zinc 1 hour before meals, preferably as the acetate) is an effective alternative. Experience is not extensive with either, but side effects have been minimal.

Some patients, especially those with fulminant hepatic failure, are so severely ill that the benefits of medical treatment cannot occur rapidly enough to prevent death. In these patients, liver transplantation, if successful, is curative.

Brewer GJ, Yazbasiyan-Gurkan V: Wilson disease. Medicine 71:139, 1992. *A good review, with emphasis on zinc treatment, by the authors who developed it.*

Cartwright GE: Diagnosis of treatable Wilson's disease. N Engl J Med 298:1347, 1978. *An excellent description of the protean and often confusing clinical presentations of Wilson's disease and a few illustrations of what happens when the diagnosis is missed.*

Scheinberg IH, Sternlieb I: Wilson's Disease. Philadelphia, WB Saunders, 1984. *The authoritative monograph based on the authors' extensive experience with all aspects of Wilson's disease.*

Walshe JM: Diagnosis and treatment of presymptomatic Wilson's disease. Lancet 2:435, 1988. *Criteria for identifying asymptomatic homozygotes in families of patients with Wilson's disease. Liver biopsies should be obtained for confirmation as the author recommends, and therefore more frequently than he has actually done.*

189 IRON OVERLOAD (Hemochromatosis)

Virgil F. Fairbanks and
William P. Baldus

DEFINITION. Hemochromatosis is a state of total body iron overload due to increased iron absorption that results in parenchymal tissue damage. In persons of European descent, the disorder arises most often as the genetic disorder known as *hereditary* or *primary hemochromatosis*. *Secondary hemochromatosis* occurs in a variety of chronic anemias caused by ineffective erythropoiesis, the most common being homozygous β-thalassemia; multiple transfusions; and less frequent conditions listed in Table 189–1.

PREVALENCE, GENETICS, AND ETIOLOGY. Hereditary hemochromatosis, transmitted by an autosomal recessive gene, is the most common single gene disorder of people of Caucasian descent. Approximately 3 to 5 persons per 1000 are homozygous for the disease in the United States, Canada, France, Sweden, the

TABLE 189–1. DISORDERS ASSOCIATED WITH IRON OVERLOAD

Hereditary hemochromatosis
Chronic anemias
  Thalassemia major
  Sideroblastic anemia
    Hereditary sideroblastic anemia
    Refractory anemia with ringed sideroblasts
  Congenital dyserythropoietic anemia
Exogenous iron overload
  Transfusion-dependent anemia
  Chronic oral iron ingestion (in absence of iron deficiency)
African (Bantu) hemochromatosis
Porphyria cutanea tarda
Portacaval shunt
Juvenile hemochromatosis
Neonatal hemochromatosis
Congenital transferrinemia

United Kingdom, Australia, New Zealand, and South Africa. Heterozygotes are approximately 10% of the Caucasian population of these countries. Northern Portugal has the highest incidence, with an estimated 24% of the population being heterozygous and 2% homozygous. African-Americans have a lower prevalence of homozygous hemochromatosis, but it is thought to be about 0.3 to 0.5 per thousand. Hemochromatosis is rare in Asians. The paradoxical occurrence of clinical hemochromatosis in successive generations of kindreds carrying a recessive gene is best explained by homozygotes marrying heterozygotes. Statistically, this must occur in 10% of matings, reflecting the high heterozygote frequency in Caucasians.

The hemochromatosis gene is in linkage disequilibrium with the HLA-A and HLA-B genes. Seventy percent of persons with hemochromatosis have HLA-A3 antigens, compared with 28% in the general population. They also exhibit increased frequencies of HLA-B7 and B14 antigens. In the course of numerous generations, the effect of normal meiotic recombination should be to render the HLA allele frequencies in hemochromatosis similar to those of the general population. The most likely explanation for the high frequencies of certain HLA alleles is that the mutation is relatively recent, although it occurred and became widely prevalent before Europeans colonized North America, Australia, New Zealand, and South Africa.

Hereditary hemochromatosis is due to a mutation in a gene on the short arm of chromosome 6. The exact site of the mutation remains unknown. The gene product also remains unknown. Preliminary laboratory studies show that in persons with hereditary hemochromatosis there is increase in a membrane iron-binding protein that is normally present on the surface of intestinal mucosal cells and hepatocytes.

Normal adult men absorb approximately 1 mg of iron daily from the intestinal tract in order to balance iron loss. Normal women, during the reproductive years, absorb approximately 2 mg of iron each day, the greater need reflecting menstrual iron loss. Persons homozygous for hereditary hemochromatosis absorb from their intestinal tracts only a few milligrams of iron each day in excess of need. Clinical signs and symptoms, when they appear, reflect an iron accumulation of 15 to 40 grams. Manifestations can begin even before age 20. Not all homozygotes develop overt disease, however, because clinical manifestations also depend on cofactors of age, gender, iron content of the diet, alcohol, and other unknown factors. Women, for example, regularly lose iron during menses and childbirth. Therefore, despite an equal frequency of homozygosity, they express the disease one-tenth as often as do men. Ethanol abuse or hepatitis accelerates liver and pancreatic disease in hereditary hemochromatosis. Either ethanol abuse or hepatitis may increase serum iron concentration due to marked ferritinemia that results from hepatocyte injury. Alcohol abuse occurs in as many as one third of patients with hemochromatosis. The frequency of serum antibodies to hepatitis C also is higher than in the normal population.

METABOLIC AND TISSUE EFFECTS. Iron accumulates over decades, as ferritin and hemosiderin, in nearly all cells of the body. Tissue damage that leads to morbidity occurs in liver, thyroid, hypothalamus, heart, pancreas, gonads, and joints. This leads to cirrhosis of the liver, hypothyroidism, hypothalamic hypogonadotropic hypogonadism, cardiomyopathy, diabetes mellitus, arthralgias, and deforming arthritis. There is pigment deposition in skin, principally melanin. Cardiac deposition of ferritin and hemosiderin causes cardiac arrhythmias and impaired contractility of cardiac muscle.

The liver is a target organ because iron absorbed from the intestinal tract enters the portal circulation and passes through the liver before it enters any other organ. Iron that exceeds the binding capacity of transferrin is deposited in the liver. In hereditary hemochromatosis, excess iron is deposited initially as hemosiderin granules in hepatocytes, in a periportal pattern, i.e., the heaviest deposition is at the periphery of the lobule. Marked deposition of hemosiderin also occurs in the epithelial cells of the biliary canaliculi. As iron overloading progresses, hemosiderin deposition occurs in Kupffer cells. Signs of hepatocellular injury are also first apparent and most pronounced in the periphery of the lobule. These changes consist of cytoplasmic ballooning and fatty change. As the disease progresses, filaments of fibrous tissue begin to traverse the lobule and periportal fibrosis occurs. The other changes of severe cirrhosis follow. Similar histologic changes occur in the pancreas, heart, and other organs.

In secondary hemochromatosis, as in that which may follow numerous transfusions for chronic anemia, hemosiderin deposition is initially more marked in the Kupffer cells. Ultimately, however, the histologic pattern becomes indistinguishable from that of hereditary hemochromatosis. Furthermore, other histologic changes may be indistinguishable between late-stage hemochromatosis and alcoholic cirrhosis, except for the marked hemosiderosis in the former.

CLINICAL MANIFESTATIONS. Although many people with hemochromatosis are asymptomatic, all are at risk for developing severe dysfunction of the heart, liver, pancreas, pituitary, gonads, or joints, as well as for fatal peritonitis or sepsis.

Clinical manifestations are more common in men older than 20 and in postmenopausal women. Rare cases may involve adolescent children and young women. Table 189–2 lists the potential symptoms, signs, and laboratory abnormalities of hemochromatosis. The most common symptoms are fatigue, that may be overwhelming; arthralgias; abdominal discomfort; impotence; amenorrhea; and palpitations. Cardiac arrhythmia is a common presenting sign and may be either atrial or ventricular. Suntan-like hyperpigmentation of the skin can affect both exposed and nonexposed areas as well as scars. In advanced cases, the skin may be slate gray. Hepatosplenomegaly, ascites, pleural effusion, or arthritis may develop early or late. The arthritis may affect any joint but most commonly involves the second and third metacarpophalangeal joints, knees, and hips. The affected joints may be deformed, with or without inflammatory signs. Signs of hypothyroidism and testicular atrophy often appear. There may be loss of hair on body and extremities. Mild abdominal pain is common. Infrequently, there may be an abrupt onset of abdominal pain followed by prostration, shock, and death. In some cases of fatal acute peritonitis or septicemia, *Yersinia enterocolitica* or *Vibrio vulnificus* have been incriminated.

Hemochromatosis, because of its associated asthenia and cardiac, hypogonadal, or multiple-organ pathology, may bring patients initially to seek the attention of general physicians, cardiologists, pediatricians, urologists, endocrinologists, neurologists, or psychiatrists. Its features should be understood by all physicians because concentrating on a particular organ system—like one of the six blind men of Hindustan describing an elephant—may preclude early diagnosis and preventive treatment, which crucially influence prognosis.

LABORATORY ABNORMALITIES AND DIAGNOSIS. The most useful laboratory test to ascertain hemochromatosis is measuring serum iron concentration, total iron-binding capacity, and transferrin saturation. These should be done together. The transferrin saturation is calculated from $100 \times$ serum iron concentration divided by total iron-binding capacity. Characteristically, the transferrin saturation is $>60\%$ and may approach 100% in hemochromatosis, whereas normally it is 20 to 50%. Other conditions may

TABLE 189–2. CLINICAL AND LABORATORY MANIFESTATIONS OF HEMOCHROMATOSIS

Symptoms	Signs	Laboratory Abnormalities
None (common)	Alopecia	Increased serum iron concentration
Fatigue	Hyperpigmentation	
Weakness	Tender, swollen joints	Serum transferrin saturation $>60\%$
Arthralgia	Cardiac arrhythmia	
Abdominal pain	Cardiomegaly	Increased serum ALT or AST transaminases
Impotence	Hepatomegaly	
Amenorrhea	Splenomegaly	Increased blood glucose
Dyspnea	Pleural effusion	Abnormal glucose tolerance
Abdominal swelling	Ascites	Low serum testosterone
Weight loss	"Spider" telangiectasia	Low serum estrogen and progesterone
	Signs of hypothyroidism	Low FSH and LH
	Testicular atrophy	Low serum T_4, high TSH
		Azoospermia
		Thrombocytopenia
		Macrocytosis
		Electrocardiographic abnormalities
		Echocardiographic abnormalities
		Roentgenographic and imaging abnormalities

also elevate serum iron concentration and transferrin saturation, particularly the recent ingestion of medicinal iron, iron-fortified vitamin preparations, or oral contraceptives (Table 189–3). Therefore, if the transferrin saturation is elevated, the test should be repeated after eliminating such confounding variables. If it is still elevated, serum ferritin assay should be performed. When iron overload is marked, as in advanced hemochromatosis, the serum ferritin concentration commonly exceeds 500 μg per liter and may be > 5000 μg per liter. However, because serum ferritin is an acute phase reactant, elevated values may result from chronic disease, such as inflammation (as in rheumatoid arthritis), or from malignancies. Liver injury from hepatitis or alcohol abuse also elevates the serum ferritin concentration. Elevated concentration of serum ferritin may be observed in Gaucher's disease. Therefore, elevated values of serum ferritin concentration must be interpreted in the context of the presence or absence of these other conditions.

Among other frequent laboratory abnormalities are elevated blood glucose concentration, abnormal glucose tolerance test results, elevated serum AST or ALT activity, low serum thyroxine, elevated serum thyroid-stimulating hormone, low serum values for pituitary gonadotropins, and thrombocytopenia (reflecting liver disease). Hemoglobin concentration, hematocrit, erythrocyte count, erythrocyte indices, leukocyte count, and differential are usually normal, although chronic liver disease may be reflected in macrocytosis. Bone marrow examination with iron stain variably shows increase in hemosiderin; hence, it is not reliable for diagnosis of iron overload.

Roentgenographic examinations of affected joints show soft tissue swelling, narrowing of joint spaces, irregular articular surfaces, osteoporosis, and subcapsular cysts. There may be chondrocalcinosis or calcification of periarticular ligaments. Synovial fluid often contains calcium pyrophosphate and apatite crystals. Distinction from either degenerative arthritis or rheumatoid arthritis may be difficult.

Electrocardiography may reveal atrial or ventricular arrhythmia, low QRS amplitude, and repolarization abnormalities of ST segment and T waves. Echocardiography and cinecardiography may

TABLE 189–3. PHENOMENA KNOWN TO AFFECT SERUM IRON CONCENTRATION, TOTAL IRON-BINDING CAPACITY, AND TRANSFERRIN SATURATION

Phenomenon	Effect
Menstrual cycle	Premenstrually, elevated values (SI increased by 10–30%); at menstruation, low values (SI decreased by 10–30%)
Pregnancy	May elevate SI due to increased progesterone; may lower SI due to Fe deficiency
Ingestion of iron (including iron-fortified vitamins)	High values (SI may rise by 300+ μg/dL and transferrin saturation to 75%)
Iron contamination of Vacutainer tube or other glassware (phenomenon may be rare, sporadic, very difficult to prove)	High values (SI 200–300 μg/dL, transferrin saturation of 75–100%)
Iron dextran injection	Very high values (SI may be > 500 μg/dL, transferrin saturation 100%, probably from circulating iron dextran; effect may persist for several weeks)
Hepatitis (including steatohepatitis)	Very high values (SI may exceed 1000 μg/dL due to hyperferritinemia from hepatocyte injury)
Acute inflammation (respiratory infection), abscess, immunization, myocardial infarction	Low or normal SI; normal or low Tsat
Chronic inflammation or malignancy	Low or normal SI; normal or low Tsat
Iron deficiency	Low or normal SI; increased TIBC; low or normal Tsat
Iron overload (hemochromatosis)	High SI, high Tsat

Abbreviations: SI = serum iron; TIBC = total iron binding capacity; Tsat = transferrin saturation (in %).

show dilated, or, less commonly, restrictive cardiomyopathy. There may be radiographic evidence of pulmonary vascular congestion or pleural effusion.

Definitive diagnosis usually requires liver biopsy. This also permits evaluation of the severity of liver injury and thus the prognosis. In addition to hematoxylin and eosin stain, the biopsy specimen should be stained for iron by Perls' Prussian blue method. In the absence of iron overload, the stainable iron is 0 to 1+. In heterozygotes or those with alcoholic cirrhosis, it may be 1 to 2+; in those with homozygous hemochromatosis, it is usually 3 to 4+. These semiquantitative estimates from iron stain correlate with quantitative measurements of hepatic iron concentration. The hepatic iron concentration can be measured in the liver biopsy specimen. Normal hepatic iron concentrations are < 40 (men) and < 33 (women) μmol per gram of tissue (dry weight). In alcoholic cirrhosis and in heterozygotes for hemochromatosis, the hepatic iron concentration is < 100 μmol per gram of tissue. In homozygous hemochromatosis, the hepatic iron concentration usually exceeds 200 μmol per gram of tissue. A useful index is obtained by dividing the hepatic iron concentration in μmol per gram by the patient's age in years. This "hepatic iron index" is usually > 1.9 in homozygous hemochromatosis.

Imaging methods, such as computed tomography or magnetic resonance imaging, have led to the correct diagnosis of hemochromatosis in many instances. However, compared with conventional laboratory methods, imaging procedures are both too insensitive and too expensive to be used in the screening of patients for hemochromatosis.

HLA typing has almost no role in diagnosis of hemochromatosis. Of persons whose leukocytes have the HLA-A3 antigen, only about 1 in 90 are found to have hemochromatosis. Such persons are more likely to be normal or to have alcoholic cirrhosis than hereditary hemochromatosis. As a screening test, HLA typing would yield unacceptably high frequencies of both false-positive and false-negative results. It may be used, however, to help identify affected siblings of a known patient. When so used, it does not matter what the HLA type is: Within a sibship, anyone whose HLA genotype is identical with that of a sibling who has proven disease is also presumed to have homozygous hemochromatosis.

Physicians must examine other members of a sibship for hemochromatosis because within any hemochromatosis sibship, on average 25% of sibs are homozygous for hemochromatosis. Measuring transferrin saturation and serum ferritin concentration is sufficient to identify other affected sibs.

TREATMENT. The treatment of hemochromatosis is repeated phlebotomy, the most efficient, least inconvenient, and least expensive way to remove excess iron from the body. Chelating therapy or dietary manipulation has no place in treating hereditary hemochromatosis. Because iron stores may be 25 to 40 grams of iron, and each half-liter of blood removed contains approximately 200 mg of iron, phlebotomies can be sustained at the rate of one to two times per week for 1 to 3 years or longer before the iron stores become depleted. Patients should be advised that they may need to have 50 to 100 or more phlebotomies before their iron stores are reduced to normal. This is usually done at the rate of one to two phlebotomies per week until the venous hemoglobin concentration or hematocrit begins to decline and does not return to normal (Fig. 189–1). Then, serum ferritin assay determines whether additional phlebotomies are required. The objective is to lower the serum ferritin concentration to < 20 μg per liter before reducing the rate of phlebotomy. After that, most patients require four to six phlebotomies annually to keep the serum ferritin concentration in the normal range. Because the transferrin saturation is often high irrespective of the state of iron stores, the measurement of serum iron, total iron-binding capacity, and transferrin saturation is less reliable for determining when additional phlebotomies are needed.

People with hemochromatosis should abstain from handling or eating uncooked shellfish or marine fish because they are susceptible to fatal septicemia from the marine bacterium *V. vulnificus* (see Ch. 109). No other dietary restrictions should be imposed. However, complete abstinence from use of alcohol must be observed.

In addition to measures directed toward removing iron from the body, treating cardiac dysfunction may require cardiac glycosides or diuretics, diabetes may require insulin, hypothyroidism requires thyroid replacement, impotence may be relieved with androgens, and

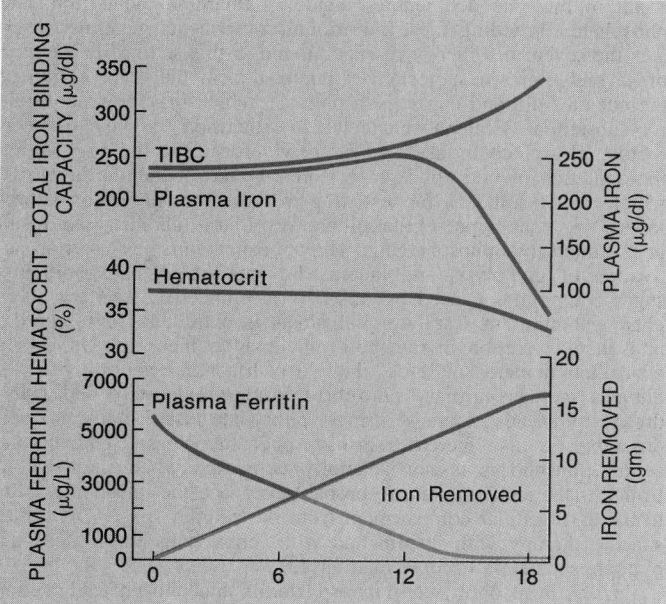

FIGURE 189–1. Serial changes in the hematocrit, plasma iron concentration, total iron-binding capacity, and plasma ferritin concentration in a subject with idiopathic hemochromatosis on repeated venesection therapy. Plasma iron = serum iron, plasma ferritin = serum ferritin. (N.B.: Plasma from EDTA-anticoagulated specimen will have spuriously low plasma iron due to chelation of iron by EDTA. Therefore, *only serum specimens are tested.*) (From Bothwell TH, Charlton RW, Cook JD, et al.: Idiopathic haemochromatosis. *In* Iron Metabolism in Man. Oxford, Blackwell Scientific, 1979.)

painful joints may require salicylates or nonsteroidal anti-inflammatory agents. In advanced cases, liver transplant may be required. Early diagnosis and vigorous treatment should prevent the need for these drastic and costly measures that have high morbidity and uncertain outcomes.

PROGNOSIS. Historically, the median survival was about 2 years from diagnosis. A greatly improved prognosis results from early diagnosis and treatment. When the diagnosis precedes onset of signs and symptoms, and in the absence of hepatic cirrhosis or diabetes, survival is the same as for the age- and gender-matched cohort of the general population. When cirrhosis or diabetes is already present at the time of diagnosis, the outlook is poorer. Cirrhosis rarely disappears as a result of phlebotomy therapy. Patients may die of hepatic or cardiac failure or may exsanguinate from ruptured esophageal varices. They are at risk of death from infections, such as peritonitis. Patients with cirrhosis have a 30% probability of developing hepatocellular carcinoma, even after iron stores are depleted by phlebotomy. Diabetes is not improved by removing iron, although it may not progress as rapidly. Arthritis is not improved by iron removal and, unfortunately, may first appear after adequate removal of excess iron. However, cardiac dysfunction is often substantially improved. Impotence requires continued androgen therapy. Azoospermia is not alleviated. Amenorrhea may rarely be alleviated. Osteoporosis that follows premature menopause requires estrogen therapy. The risk of sudden death from sepsis or peritonitis is diminished.

It is tragic whenever this easily diagnosed and easily treated disorder is permitted to evolve unrecognized and untreated. Patients for whom the diagnosis is not made in a timely manner may develop cirrhosis, severe cardiac dysfunction, or both. A few dozen such patients, who could not otherwise be salvaged, have had liver or heart transplantation or both. Such procedures may be warranted, although extremely costly and attended by long-term morbidity even when successful. The long-term survival of patients who have had these transplants is still unknown, although a few have survived as long as 5 years following liver transplant.

Balan V, Baldus WP, Fairbanks VF, et al.: Screening for hemochromatosis. A cost-effectiveness study based on 12,258 patients. Gastroenterology, 107:453, 1994.

Edwards CQ, Kushner JP: Screening for hemochromatosis. N Engl J Med 328:1616, 1993. *These two references extensively analyze all considerations in screening for hemochromatosis, follow-up tests, and examinations. A reasonable cost estimate of screening and the potential for salvaging years of life is approximately $2000 per year of life saved per person who is homozygous for hereditary hemochromatosis. Even when morbidity and productivity loss that attend hemochromatosis are not considered, cost-benefit relationship is favorable.*
Fargion S, Mandelli C, Piperno A, et al.: Survival and prognostic factors in 212 Italian patients with genetic hemochromatosis. Hepatology 15:655, 1992. *Patients adequately treated by phlebotomy before developing cirrhosis had normal survival; for cirrhotic patients, median survival was 8 years. Hepatocellular cancer occurred in 17% of cirrhotic patients and was the most common cause of death. Other prognostic variables are considered.*
Summers KM, Halliday JW, Powell LW: Identification of homozygous hemochromatosis subjects by measurement of hepatic iron index. Hepatology 12:20, 1990. *The hepatic iron index, obtained by dividing hepatic iron concentration, in μmol per gram by patient's age, provides the best criterion for identifying homozygotes with iron overload.*

190 PHOSPHORUS DEFICIENCY AND HYPOPHOSPHATEMIA
Wadi N. Suki

Phosphorus is an integral constituent of all body tissues. It is a component of hydroxyapatite, the main crystalline structure of bone, and of the phospholipids in all cell membranes. It is a component of nucleotides and furnishes the backbone of DNA. It is also a component of the second messengers, cyclic adenosine monophosphate (cAMP) and cyclic guanosine monophosphate (cGMP). It combines with a number of proteins, under the influence of various kinases, to activate their enzyme activity. As a component of 2,3-diphosphoglycerate (2,3-DPG), it facilitates the release to tissues of oxygen from oxyhemoglobin. In ATP and creatine phosphate, it serves as an energy store, and when excreted in the urine, it serves as an important buffer to facilitate excretion of urinary acid. When all the functions of phosphate are taken into consideration, it becomes evident why severe deficiency of this anion can lead to disordered function of a large number of systems.

NORMAL PHOSPHORUS METABOLISM. More than 700 grams (22 moles) of phosphorus are present in an average-sized adult: 80% of the total phosphorus is present in bone, 10% is present in skeletal muscle. In muscle cells and in other cells, phosphate in the form of phospholipids, phosphoproteins, and phosphosugars represents the major intracellular anion and is present in a concentration of approximately 100 mmol per liter of cell water.

In the extracellular fluid, phosphorus is present in a concentration of 4.0 to 7.0 mg per 100 ml in children and 2.7 to 4.5 mg per 100 ml in adults. Phosphate in blood is mostly free (only 10% is protein bound) and is present in two ionic forms, dibasic (HPO_4^{-}) and monobasic ($H_2PO_4^{-}$), the relative amounts of which vary with the blood pH, being present in a ratio of 4:1 at pH 7.4. Therefore, phosphate concentration in blood should be considered in terms of millimoles (0.9 to 1.5 mmol per liter in adults and 1.4 to 2.2 mmol per liter in children) rather than milliequivalents (which would vary with blood pH).

Depending on the composition of the diet, the average adult in the United States consumes 800 to 1500 mg of phosphorus daily, derived primarily from dairy products and meat. Most of the ingested phosphorus is absorbed, and, except in growing children, most is excreted in the urine. Urinary excretion depends on glomerular filtration and tubular reabsorption, with only 12% of the filtered load being excreted in the urine. Intestinal absorption of phosphate is augmented by the active metabolites of vitamin D, whereas tubular absorption is inhibited by parathyroid hormone acting through its second-messenger cAMP.

HYPOPHOSPHATEMIA. Moderate or severe hypophosphatemia is seen in approximately 2% of hospitalized patients.

Etiology. (Table 190–1). Hypophosphatemia may result from a shift into cells, in which case body phosphorus stores are normal.

TABLE 190-1. CLASSIFICATION OF HYPOPHOSPHATEMIA

Transient hypophosphatemia with normal body stores
  Ingestion of carbohydrates
  Respiratory alkalosis
Sustained hypophosphatemia with reduced body stores
  Moderate hypophosphatemia
    Depressed tubular absorption
      Hyperparathyroidism
      Expanded ECF volume
      Alkali administration
      Glucocorticoids
      Magnesium depletion
      Fanconi's syndrome
      Familial hypophosphatemic rickets
    Reduced intestinal absorption
      Reduced intake
      Malabsorption
      Vitamin D deficiency
      Phosphate-binding antacids
    Extracorporeal losses—dialysis
  Severe hypophosphatemia
    Prolonged use of phosphate-binding antacids
    Parenteral alimentation
    Nutritional recovery syndrome
    Recovery phase of severe burns
    Severe respiratory alkalosis
    Poorly controlled diabetes mellitus
    Alcoholism and alcohol withdrawal

On the other hand, hypophosphatemia may be associated with depleted total body stores, resulting from poor dietary intake, reduced gastrointestinal absorption, or increased renal losses.

Hypophosphatemia may be sustained or may be transient, as seen after ingestion of carbohydrates due to the phosphorylation of sugars before they enter the body cells, or in respiratory alkalosis, wherein alkalinization of the cytosol activates intracellular glycolysis and increases the formation of phosphorylated sugars.

Moderate Hypophosphatemia. In addition to carbohydrate administration and respiratory alkalosis, which cause transient hypophosphatemia, a number of other disorders can result in moderate hypophosphatemia (serum phosphorus 1 to 2.5 mg per deciliter). These disorders may be classified into those that increase renal losses of phosphate, decrease intestinal absorption of phosphate, or increase extracorporeal loss of phosphate such as in hemodialysis against a phosphate-free dialysate. Renal losses of phosphate are increased when tubular absorption is depressed, as seen in hyperparathyroidism (see Ch. 214), in expansion of the extracellular fluid volume, in administration of alkali or glucocorticoids, in hypomagnesemia and magnesium depletion, and in renal tubular defects such as Fanconi's syndrome (see Ch. 82) or familial hypophosphatemic rickets (see Ch. 213).

Reduced intestinal absorption may be caused by drastically reduced intake, malabsorption, vitamin D deficiency, and the use of phosphate-binding antacids. Moderate hypophosphatemia causes only osteomalacia.

Severe Hypophosphatemia (serum phosphorus < 1 mg per deciliter). This causes serious systemic manifestations that demand prompt attention and correction. The most common causes of this disorder are prolonged use of phosphate-binding antacids, hyperalimentation, nutritional recovery syndrome and recovery from severe burns, severe respiratory alkalosis, poorly controlled diabetes mellitus, and alcoholism and alcohol withdrawal syndrome. Phosphate-binding compounds, such as aluminum and magnesium oxides, bind phosphate in the intestinal lumen and impair its absorption. The excessive use of these compounds by patients with peptic ulcer disease or by patients with chronic renal failure who are treated with these compounds to prevent the development of hyperphosphatemia, results in phosphate depletion. Enteral and parenteral alimentation, if not accompanied by phosphate, can also result in phosphate depletion. Phosphate excretion in the urine is increased by administering glucose and amino acids. Furthermore, glucose and amino acids entering into cells and their incorporation into intracellular compounds consume phosphate and deplete body stores. Overzealous refeeding of severely malnourished subjects also may

result in multiple deficiencies including thiamine, potassium, and phosphate. Providing these nutritional components generally obviates the severe disorder once encountered in this setting. In the case of severely burned subjects, healing results in the reabsorption of the edema fluid and consequent diuresis, which may be responsible for substantial renal phosphate loss. Furthermore, as new tissue is rebuilt, phosphate is taken up by newly formed cells, aggravating the depletion of body phosphate stores. Unlike metabolic alkalosis, which may result in a modest drop in the serum phosphorus, prolonged vigorous hyperventilation and respiratory alkalosis can result in profound hypophosphatemia. Hypophosphatemia results from activation of glycolysis and increased formation of phosphorylated sugar compounds caused by raised intracellular pH. Urinary phosphate excretion in respiratory alkalosis is extremely low, whereas phosphate excretion in metabolic alkalosis is increased. In poorly controlled diabetes mellitus, the glucosuria and resulting osmotic diuresis increase urinary phosphate loss. Acetoacetate and β-hydroxybutyrate also increase urinary phosphate loss. Finally, the acidosis *per se* also increases urinary phosphate loss. However, the serum phosphorus is not generally depressed when poorly controlled diabetics first present, probably because the phosphate shifts to the extracellular compartment from the cellular space. Only after starting therapy with insulin and with intravenous fluids does the hypophosphatemia become manifested.

Finally, in alcoholics hypophosphatemia and phosphate depletion are caused by multiple factors: the phosphaturic effect of ethanol, the phosphaturia resulting from magnesium depletion, poor dietary intake, and ketoacidosis. Other contributing factors can be vomiting, diarrhea, and the use of phosphate-binding antacids.

MANIFESTATIONS (Table 190-2). Severe hypophosphatemia alters cell membrane composition and function, depletes intracellular phosphorylated compounds, such as ATP and 2,3-DPG, and increases intracellular calcium. This constellation of disorders results in disturbed function of multiple body systems.

MANAGEMENT (Table 190-3). When total body phosphorus stores are normal, phosphate supplementation is unnecessary. When body phosphate stores are reduced, urinary losses need to be mini-

TABLE 190-2. MANIFESTATIONS OF HYPOPHOSPHATEMIA

Symptoms and Signs	Comments
Central nervous system	
Symptoms and signs of metabolic encephalopathy	Irritability, malaise, ataxia, seizures, coma
Neuromuscular	
Generalized muscle weakness or paralysis	Ventilatory insufficiency, respiratory failure
Rhabdomyolysis	Increased creatine kinase; large muscle tenderness; may mask underlying hypophosphatemia
Cardiac muscle dysfunction	Congestive cardiomyopathy
Hematologic	
Altered red cell function	Depleted 2,3-DPG shifts oxyhemoglobin dissociation curve to the left and impairs tissue oxygen delivery. Depleted ATP, increases intracellular calcium causing hemolysis
Impaired leukocyte function	Impaired leukotaxis, phagocytosis, and bactericidal activity, susceptibility to infection
Impaired platelet aggregation	Bleeding tendency from lips and oral mucosa
Bone	
Bone resorption, osteomalacia, increased 1α-hydroxylation of vitamin D	Increased calcium absorption, mild increase of serum calcium, depressed PTH secretion, and marked renal hypercalciuria
Renal	
Impaired tubular function	Increased urine calcium and magnesium, renal glucosuria, decreased ammoniagenesis and metabolic acidosis
Liver	
Transient hyperbilirubinemia	
Metabolism	
Hypoglycemia	

TABLE 190-3. MANAGEMENT OF HYPOPHOSPHATEMIA

	Treatment	Dose
Normal body phosphorus stores		
Transient hydrophosphatemia	Treat underlying disorder	No phosphate replacement
Reduced body phosphorus stores		
Moderate hypophosphatemia	Minimize urinary losses, reduce sodium diuresis, enhance gastrointestinal absorption, discontinue phosphate binders	
	If patient capable of oral intake:	
	High-phosphate foods	e.g., skimmed cow's milk (contains 1 mg P/ml)
	Oral supplements:	
	Sodium salt	Phospho-Soda 750 mg P per 5 ml
	Potassium salt (potassium not contraindicated/desirable)	Neutra-Phos 250 mg P/capsule with 7 mEq of K; Neutra-Phos K; 250 mg P/capsule with 14 mEq of K; K Phos 150 mg P/tablet with 3.65 mEq K; or K-Phos Neutral 250 mg P with 2 mEq K
Severe hypophosphatemia		
Patient incapable of oral/enteral intake, or with organ manifestations of P depletion	Parenteral P	P 2.5–5 mg/kg body weight (0.08–0.16 mmol/kg) infused over 6 hrs, repeated every 6 hrs until serum P is 2.0–2.5 mg/dl
Hypocalcemic patient, renal failure		Lower dose than above

mized, gastrointestinal absorption needs to be enhanced, and phosphate supplements may be necessary. To replete body phosphorus stores, 1000 to 2000 mg of phosphorus may need to be supplemented daily for up to 2 weeks. Whenever phosphate replacement is given, the serum calcium, magnesium, phosphorus, and electrolytes should be monitored closely. The complications of administering phosphate include diarrhea (after oral administration), hypocalcemia, metastatic calcification, hypotension, hyperkalemia and/or hypernatremia, and metabolic acidosis.

Stoff JS: Phosphate homeostasis and hypophosphatemia. Am J Med 72:489, 1982. *A concise review of the physiology of hypophosphatemia, its manifestations, and treatment.*

191 DISORDERS OF MAGNESIUM METABOLISM

Allen C. Alfrey

Magnesium is the second most common intracellular cation, with only three other cations—potassium, calcium, and sodium—occurring with greater abundance in the body. It plays a crucial role in storing and using energy, as all enzymatic reactions involving ATP frequently require magnesium. Because magnesium is also an essential element for plants, being a constituent of chlorophyll, it is present in virtually all food sources. Despite this wide distribution, the average dietary intake of magnesium is about 25 mEq per day, which only marginally meets recommended daily requirements for this element. Fractional absorption of magnesium varies from 80% on a magnesium-restricted diet to $< 10\%$ when large oral loads of magnesium are consumed. Renal magnesium reabsorption occurs in multiple nephron segments, and a tubular maximum (TM) mechanism can be described for the whole kidney. The normal tubular reabsorption for magnesium is very close to the TM_{Mg} glomerular filtration rate (GFR). Therefore, small changes in the serum magnesium are accompanied by rather rapid increases or decreases in urinary magnesium excretion. This intrinsic TM phenomenon, which is not directly controlled hormonally, allows the kidney to be the major determinant of plasma magnesium levels.

MAGNESIUM DEPLETION

The prevalence of hypomagnesemia in a general hospital setting has been estimated to range from 6.9 to 12%, being as high as 20% in patients in an ICU. Clinical findings of severe hypomagnesemia are confined mainly to the neuromuscular system and consist of muscle fasciculations and tremors, positive Chvostek's and Trousseau's signs, overt tetany, weakness, anorexia, apathy, and rarely seizures. The biochemical findings of symptomatic hypomagnesemia are serum magnesium levels usually < 1 mEq per liter associated with hypokalemia and hypocalcemia.

MECHANISMS. Magnesium depletion can result from either gastrointestinal or renal causes (Table 191–1). When serum magnesium falls only slightly, and if the kidneys respond normally, urine magnesium excretion falls to < 12 mg (1 mEq) per day. Therefore, urine magnesium is low if magnesium depletion results from gastrointestinal causes; however, it is in the normal range (120 to 160 mg per day) if depletion results from a renal leak.

Magnesium depletion has been found in 35% of patients with steatorrheic states. Fecal magnesium content correlates with the amount of stool fat, suggesting that magnesium malabsorption is a result of magnesium forming an insoluble complex with fat in the gastrointestinal tract. Any severe diarrheal state such as ulcerative colitis, amebic colitis, and intestinal resection can also deplete magnesium. Another gastrointestinal cause of magnesium depletion is an isolated defect in magnesium absorption that usually occurs in infants.

Renal magnesium wasting (Table 191–1) can result from either an intrinsic disorder of the renal tubule or from extrinsic or reversible factors. The three major intrinsic causes of renal magnesium wasting are familial or sporadic renal magnesium wasting, Bartter's syndrome, and drug nephrotoxicity. Familial or sporadic renal magnesium wasting can severely deplete magnesium.

TABLE 191-1. CAUSES OF HYPOMAGNESEMIA

Gastrointestinal
    Steatorrheic states
    Severe diarrhea
    Familial magnesium malabsorption
Renal
    Intrinsic
        Familial or sporadic renal magnesium wasting
        Bartter's syndrome
        Nephrotoxic agents
    Extrinsic (intrarenal)
        Volume expansion
        Hypercalciuria
        Diabetic ketoacidosis
        Diuretics
Miscellaneous
    Alcoholism
    Thyrotoxicosis
    Burns
    Parathyroidectomy
    Lactation

Although hypomagnesemia is common in Bartter's syndrome, it rarely, if ever, is severe enough to cause symptoms. Drugs that most commonly cause this complication are the aminoglycosides, cyclosporine, and *cis*-diamminodichloride platinum (*cis*-DDP). *Cis*-DDP commonly causes renal magnesium wasting that can persist for months after the drug has been discontinued. A number of extrinsic or intrarenal factors, including virtually all diuretics, volume expansion, diabetic ketoacidosis, and hypercalciuria, can cause mild to moderate renal magnesium wasting. There are several miscellaneous causes of magnesium depletion, including alcoholism, thyrotoxicosis, pancreatitis, lactation, parathyroidectomy, and burns. Alcoholism is the most important. Magnesium depletion in this condition results from a number of causes, including poor dietary intake and some enhanced renal excretion of this cation. Hypomagnesemia, which correlates with the severity of the hyperthyroid state, is a result of redistribution rather than deficiency of this element. Hypomagnesemia can also result from redistribution following parathyroidectomy, which results from magnesium being incorporated into bone, along with calcium salts, during the rapid healing that follows parathyroid surgery.

EFFECT OF MAGNESIUM ON CALCIUM METABOLISM. Magnesium depletion is the most common cause of hypocalcemia in a general hospital population. Parathyroid hormone (PTH) levels have been shown to be either low or inappropriately normal when the patient has hypomagnesemia-induced hypocalcemia. This is a problem of release rather than synthesis of PTH in that PTH levels rapidly increase within minutes of giving magnesium replacement. Besides affecting PTH secretion, with more severe magnesium depletion there is also bone resistance to PTH, as manifested by a lack of calcemic response.

INTERRELATIONSHIP BETWEEN MAGNESIUM AND POTASSIUM. Approximately 40% of hypomagnesemic patients have coexisting hypokalemia. In muscle and myocardium, when either intracellular magnesium or potassium falls, there is a corresponding decrease in the other cation. Conversely in primary potassium depletion there is intracellular muscle magnesium depletion without hypomagnesemia. The interrelationship between intracellular potassium and magnesium is further demonstrated by the fact that repletion of potassium frequently cannot be accomplished without concomitantly administering magnesium. The term "refractory potassium repletion states" has been used to describe this condition. Intracellular depletion of magnesium has been suggested as responsible for causing a variety of cardiovascular alterations, including increased sensitivity to digitalis toxicity, cardiac arrhythmias such as premature ventricular contractions, and torsades de pointes. However, it is unclear whether these cardiovascular alterations are a direct result of magnesium depletion or a consequence of the associated intracellular potassium depletion.

DIAGNOSIS AND MANAGEMENT OF MAGNESIUM DEPLETION. Magnesium depletion is usually readily diagnosed by measuring the serum magnesium level. Mild asymptomatic magnesium depletion requires no treatment if the patient is able to eat a normal diet. Patients with symptomatic hypomagnesemia usually require parenteral magnesium replacement. As a rule, the magnesium deficit can be roughly calculated by assuming that the space of distribution is the extracellular volume. Because half the administered magnesium is excreted in the urine, replacement is approximately twice the calculated deficit. Although an occasional patient may require intravenous replacement, the intramuscular route is safer and the preferred method of administering magnesium. Suggested magnesium replacement for hypomagnesemic states is given in Table 191–2. It has been suggested that intravenous magnesium should be routinely given to patients with acute myocardial infarction to replace depleted intracellular magnesium, partially based on the finding of reduced muscle magnesium and potassium levels, especially in patients on diuretics. This has been suggested to enhance tissue potassium repletion, decrease death rates, and reduce the number of episodes of arrhythmias in this patient population. The evidence is good that magnesium replacement can enhance intracellular potassium replacement and under certain conditions is necessary for potassium repletion. However, there is continuing controversy about what if any other benefit magnesium therapy affords patients with acute myocardial infarction.

TABLE 191–2. MANAGEMENT OF HYPOMAGNESEMIA

Severe hypomagnesemia (serum Mg < 1 mEq/L)
Intramuscular replacement
  4 ml of 50% $MgSO_4 \cdot 7(H_2O)$ (magnesium sulfate heptahydrate), 16.3 mEq (196 mg/Mg) IM every 4 hours for the first 24 hours.
  Subsequent replacement as required for persistent hypomagnesemia should be 2 ml 50% $MgSO_4 \cdot 7(H_2O)$ IM every 6 hours.
Intravenous replacement
  Initially 12 ml of 50% $MgSO_4 \cdot 7(H_2O)$ (49 mEq Mg) in 1000-ml solution in 5% dextrose infused over 3 hours.
  Additional 2 liters containing 12 ml of 50% $MgSO_4 \cdot 7(H_2O)$ administered over the remainder of the first 24-hour period.
  Over the next 3 to 4 days, 49 mEq Mg per day may be given intravenously.
Symptomatic hypomagnesemia (tetany or seizures)
  4 ml (16.3 mEq) of a 50% $MgSO_4 \cdot 7(H_2O)$ solution diluted to 100 ml and infused over a 10-minute period.
Chronic oral replacement therapy (steatorrheic states and renal magnesium wasting)
  Magnesium oxide (550 mg Mg/gram), 250 to 500 mg four times daily as tolerated without developing diarrhea.

HYPERMAGNESEMIA

Mild hypermagnesemia is seen in hypothyroidism, adrenal insufficiency, and advanced renal failure. The majority of cases of symptomatic hypermagnesemia have resulted from administering large oral loads of magnesium, in the form of laxatives or antacids, to patients with advanced renal insufficiency. In patients with normal renal function, life-threatening hypermagnesemia has been described in only a few unusual circumstances. Several fatalities in children have resulted from accidentally ingesting Epsom salts (magnesium sulfate). Normal subjects receiving 800 to 1600 mEq of magnesium sulfate per rectum have been found to have serum magnesium levels of 6 to 16 mEq per liter. Administering hypertonic magnesium solutions poses an additional risk of producing magnesium intoxication in patients with normal renal function. With hypertonic magnesium solutions, i.e., 50% $MgSO_4$, fluid moves from the extracellular space into the gastrointestinal tract. This decreases effective blood volume and reduces renal perfusion, which compromises the ability to excrete the magnesium absorbed from the large gastrointestinal load. This combination of increased absorption and decreased ability to excrete magnesium can cause life-threatening hypermagnesemia.

SYMPTOMS. Usually no symptoms are noted until the serum magnesium is >4 mEq per liter, at which time deep tendon reflexes may be slightly depressed. When serum magnesium increases to 10 to 15 mEq per liter, deep tendon reflexes are absent and the patient may also develop a flaccid quadriplegia. Other symptoms include lethargy, nausea, dilated pupils, respiratory depression, hypotension, bradycardia, and rarely complete heart block and cardiac arrest.

TREATMENT OF ACUTE HYPERMAGNESEMIA. Severe hypermagnesemia requires emergency management because patients can die of respiratory failure or cardiac arrest. Calcium is a direct antagonist to magnesium, and as little as 5 to 10 mEq of calcium administered intravenously can readily reverse these potentially lethal complications. This should be followed by methods to reduce the serum magnesium concentration. In patients with reasonable renal function, the combination of furosemide and 0.5N saline to replace urine volume and maintain diuresis can augment magnesium excretion. The most effective way of reducing plasma magnesium levels is hemodialysis using a magnesium-free dialysate.

Millane TA, Ward DE, Camm AJ: Electrophysiology, pacing and arrhythmia. Clin Cardiol 15:103, 1992. *An excellent, well-referenced review on the interrelationship between magnesium and potassium and cardiac arrhythmias.*
Rude RK: Magnesium metabolism and deficiency. Endocrinol Metab Clin North Am 22:377, 1993. *A recent review with 142 articles referenced.*
Whang R, Whang DD, Ryan MP: Refractory potassium repletion. A consequence of magnesium deficiency. Arch Intern Med 152:40, 1992. *Emphasizes the need for combined replacement with potassium and magnesium in certain conditions.*
Woods KL, Fletcher S, Roffe C, et al.: Intravenous magnesium sulphate in suspected acute myocardial infarction: Results of the second Leicester intravenous magnesium intervention trial (LIMIT-2). Lancet 1:1553, 1992. *A double-blind study supporting the benefits of magnesium replacement in acute myocardial infarction.*

192 NUTRITION'S INTERFACE WITH HEALTH AND DISEASE

192.1 Introduction
Douglas C. Heimburger

OLD AND NEW PARADIGMS

Nutrition science has been characterized by two major phases in the twentieth century. During the first, nutrition scientists discovered, characterized, and synthesized the various vitamins and described their deficiency syndromes in detail. The dietary requirements for these nutrients were determined and have been periodically updated by the National Academy of Sciences as the *Recommended Dietary Allowances* (RDA's, Table 192–1). These are estimated with a margin of error designed to prevent classic deficiencies in practically all persons and do not represent minimum requirements. For nutrients for which too little information exists to estimate recommended intakes, the Academy has published *Estimated Safe and Adequate Daily Dietary Intakes* (Table 192–2).

The second phase of modern nutrition science has focused on the relationships of diet and nutritional status to the diseases that plague western societies, such as coronary heart disease, cancer, and the other leading causes of death. Particularly during the last decade, this has led to expansion of the perspectives of nutrition scientists and the evolution of a new paradigm for understanding nutrition, which is contrasted with the older paradigm in Table 192–3. It is likely that this development will produce exciting changes in the way nutrition and health are understood during the next decade. Specifics of the new paradigm are detailed in Ch. 192.2.

NUTRITION'S INFLUENCE ON MORTALITY AND MORBIDITY

The causal connections between diet and chronic disease are difficult to tease out of the complex network of other risk factors, including social and behavioral variables, so a wide variety of studies must be relied on to establish them with reasonable certainty. The first links between diet and disease are often derived from epidemiologic studies, but these are unable to infer causal relationships and may be confounded by variables that have not been examined. Epidemiologic studies are also challenged by the difficulty of accurately assessing the diets of free-living individuals. Animal and *in vitro* studies can overcome some of these drawbacks, but may be confounded by experimental conditions that differ from those encountered by humans. A large number of prospective, randomized human intervention trials have been undertaken to test the effects of dietary change on the risk for disease. However, even these will not always be conclusive because of pitfalls associated with selecting study populations and isolating individual dietary factors.

Nevertheless, taken together, epidemiologic, animal, *in vitro*, and intervention studies are proving that human dietary habits contribute importantly to the pathogenesis of most of the major causes of death in developed countries. The 10 leading causes of death in the United States are listed in Table 9–4. Table 192–4 lists those causes as well as several other morbid conditions that have well-established dietary links.

Nutritional influences on the most common cause of death in the United States, coronary heart disease (CHD), have been the subject of a great deal of productive research. The overall US mortality rate from CHD peaked in the 1960's and, in a trend that surprised medical science, has declined steadily ever since. While the causes of the decline are not firmly established, it is apparent that changes in lifestyle, including diet, are probably more responsible than is high-tech care of patients with established CHD. Elevated plasma low-density lipoprotein cholesterol (LDL-C) levels are a major risk factor for CHD and peripheral atherosclerosis correlating strongly with dietary saturated fat intake and less strongly with cholesterol intake. Both of these in the United States derive largely from foods of animal origin such as meats, dairy products, and eggs. Attempts to produce less atherogenic substitutes for some of these foods have not always proven beneficial. For instance, hydrogenation of vegetable oils to create margarine and shortening results in the formation of *trans* fatty acids that affect serum cholesterol levels in a manner similar to the saturated fatty acids found in butter and lard. LDL-C levels can be lowered modestly by increasing the intake of soluble fibers from legumes, fruits, and vegetables. LDL must be oxidized before it induces injury to arterial wall epithelial cells; adequate dietary levels of the antioxidant vitamins C and E, and β-carotene, have been shown to inhibit LDL oxidation.

Epidemiologic evidence suggests that fish consumption may reduce CHD risk, perhaps through the action of ω-3 fatty acids. Evidence also indicates that moderate consumption of alcohol, especially wine, is associated with decreased risk for CHD, possibly through increasing high-density lipoprotein cholesterol (HDL-C) levels or preventing oxidation of LDL. Circulating levels of the amino acid homocysteine, which are asymptomatically elevated in 20 to 25% of Americans, have been strongly correlated with risk for CHD. Homocysteine levels can be reduced by increasing the intake of folic acid (mainly from legumes and vegetables) and decreasing the intake of methionine (principally from animal protein). A conservative estimate suggests that moderate dietary modification by the US population, consisting mainly of replacing saturated fats with complex carbohydrates, fiber, monounsaturated fats, and fish, should lead to a 10% reduction in serum cholesterol levels and a 20% reduction in CHD mortality compared to 1987 levels.

Nutrients, non-nutritive dietary constituents, and nutritional status can influence the risk for cancer in a variety of ways. Nutrition interacts with each step of carcinogenesis (carcinogen activation and tumor initiation, promotion, and progression). Humans are exposed to countless potential carcinogens, but to many anticarcinogens as well, each day through dietary and other means. Excess caloric intake may favor the generation of free radicals and reduce the body's ability to detoxify carcinogens. By contrast, antioxidant nutrients scavenge free radicals and other (pre)carcinogens, inhibiting their activation and/or their ability to initiate mutations. Folic acid may improve a cell's ability to preserve or repair its DNA, either preventing or reversing the tendency to mutation. Obesity, excess dietary fat intake, and excess alcohol appear to promote tumor growth.

Much evidence indicates that the number one cancer killer, lung cancer, is strongly influenced by diet. While the most important causal factor is cigarette smoking, the consumption of fruits and vegetables and of one of their major micronutrient constituents, β-carotene, associates inversely with lung cancer risk in both smokers and nonsmokers. This is also true of plasma levels of β-carotene. It is probable that other nutrients in fruits and vegetables, such as folic acid, as well as non-nutritive components, are partly responsi-

TABLE 192–1. FOOD AND NUTRITION BOARD, NATIONAL ACADEMY OF SCIENCES—NATIONAL RESEARCH COUNCIL RECOMMENDED DIETARY ALLOWANCES,[a] REVISED 1989

Designed for the maintenance of good nutrition of practically all healthy people in the United States

Category	Age (years) or Condition	Weight[b] (kg)	(lb)	Height[b] (cm)	(in)	Protein (g)	Fat-Soluble Vitamins Vitamin A (μg RE)[c]	Vitamin D (μg)[d]	Vitamin E (mg α-TE)[e]	Vitamin K (μg)	Water-Soluble Vitamins Vitamin C (mg)	Thiamine (mg)	Riboflavin (mg)	Niacin (mg NE)[f]	Vitamin B6 (mg)	Folate (μg)	Vitamin B12 (μg)	Minerals Calcium (mg)	Phosphorus (mg)	Magnesium (mg)	Iron (mg)	Zinc (mg)	Iodine (μg)	Selenium (μg)
Infants	0.0–0.5	6	13	60	24	13	375	7.5	3	5	30	0.3	0.4	5	0.3	25	0.3	400	300	40	6	5	40	10
	0.5–1.0	9	20	71	28	14	375	10	4	10	35	0.4	0.5	6	0.6	35	0.5	600	500	60	10	5	50	15
Children	1–3	13	29	90	35	16	400	10	6	15	40	0.7	0.8	9	1.0	50	0.7	800	800	80	10	10	70	20
	4–6	20	44	112	44	24	500	10	7	20	45	0.9	1.1	12	1.1	75	1.0	800	800	120	10	10	90	20
	7–10	28	62	132	52	28	700	10	7	30	45	1.0	1.2	13	1.4	100	1.4	800	800	170	10	10	120	30
Males	11–14	45	99	157	62	45	1,000	10	10	45	50	1.3	1.5	17	1.7	150	2.0	1,200	1,200	270	12	15	150	40
	15–18	66	145	176	69	59	1,000	10	10	65	60	1.5	1.8	20	2.0	200	2.0	1,200	1,200	400	12	15	150	50
	19–24	72	160	177	70	58	1,000	10	10	70	60	1.5	1.7	19	2.0	200	2.0	1,200	1,200	350	10	15	150	70
	25–50	79	174	176	70	63	1,000	5	10	80	60	1.5	1.7	19	2.0	200	2.0	800	800	350	10	15	150	70
	51+	77	170	173	68	63	1,000	5	10	80	60	1.2	1.4	15	2.0	200	2.0	800	800	350	10	15	150	70
Females	11–14	46	101	157	62	46	800	10	8	45	50	1.1	1.3	15	1.4	150	2.0	1,200	1,200	280	15	12	150	45
	15–18	55	120	163	64	44	800	10	8	55	60	1.1	1.3	15	1.5	180	2.0	1,200	1,200	300	15	12	150	50
	19–24	58	128	164	65	46	800	10	8	60	60	1.1	1.3	15	1.6	180	2.0	1,200	1,200	280	15	12	150	55
	25–50	63	138	163	64	50	800	5	8	65	60	1.1	1.3	15	1.6	180	2.0	800	800	280	15	12	150	55
	51+	65	143	160	63	50	800	5	8	65	60	1.0	1.2	13	1.6	180	2.0	800	800	280	10	12	150	55
Pregnant						60	800	10	10	65	70	1.5	1.6	17	2.2	400	2.2	1,200	1,200	320	30	15	175	65
Lactating	1st 6 months					65	1,300	10	12	65	95	1.6	1.8	20	2.1	280	2.6	1,200	1,200	355	15	19	200	75
	2nd 6 months					62	1,200	10	11	65	90	1.6	1.7	20	2.1	260	2.6	1,200	1,200	340	15	16	200	75

[a] The allowances, expressed as average daily intakes over time, are intended to provide for individual variations among most normal persons as they live in the United States under usual environmental stresses. Diets should be based on a variety of common foods in order to provide other nutrients for which human requirements have been less well defined.

[b] Weights and heights of Reference Adults are actual medians for the designated age, as reported by NHANES II. The use of these figures does not imply that the height-to-weight ratios are ideal.

[c] Retinol equivalents. 1 retinol equivalent = 1 μg retinol or 6 μg β-carotene.

[d] As cholecalciferol: 10 μg cholecalciferol = 400 IU of vitamin D.

[e] α-Tocopherol equivalents; 1 mg D-α-tocopherol = 1 α-TE.

[f] 1 NE (niacin equivalent) is equal to 1 mg of niacin or 60 mg of dietary tryptophan.

TABLE 192–2. ESTIMATED SAFE AND ADEQUATE DAILY DIETARY INTAKES OF SELECTED VITAMINS AND MINERALS[a]

Category	Age (years)	Vitamins			Trace Elements[b]				
		Biotin (µg)	Pantothenic Acid (mg)	Copper (mg)	Manganese (mg)	Fluoride (mg)	Chromium (µg)	Molybdenum (µg)
Infants	0–0.5	10	2	0.4–0.6	0.3–0.6	0.1–0.5	10–40	15–30
	0.5–1	15	3	0.6–0.7	0.6–1.0	0.2–1.0	20–60	20–40
Children and adolescents	1–3	20	3	0.7–1.0	1.0–1.5	0.5–1.5	20–80	25–50
	4–6	25	3–4	1.0–1.5	1.5–2.0	1.0–2.5	30–120	30–75
	7–10	30	4–5	1.0–2.0	2.0–3.0	1.5–2.5	50–200	50–150
	11 +	30–100	4–7	1.5–2.5	2.0–5.0	1.5–2.5	50–200	75–250
Adults		30–100	4–7	1.5–3.0	2.0–5.0	1.5–4.0	50–200	75–250

[a] Because there is less information on which to base allowances, these figures are not given in Table 192–1 and are provided here in the form of ranges of recommended intakes.
[b] Since the toxic levels for many trace elements may be only several times usual intakes, the upper levels for the trace elements given in this table should not be habitually exceeded.

From the National Research Council: Recommended Dietary Allowances, 10th ed. Washington, DC, National Academy Press, 1989.

ble for the protective effects. This argues against relying on antioxidant supplements to reduce disease risk. It is noteworthy that the plasma levels of antioxidant nutrients (β-carotene and vitamins C and E) and folic acid are lower in smokers than nonsmokers and intermediate in persons passively exposed to smoke. Probably caused in large part by oxidants in cigarette smoke, this is an example of an interaction between nutritional factors and environmental exposures that explains more of the variation in cancer incidence than does either factor alone.

The second largest cause of cancer deaths in women, breast cancer, associates positively with dietary fat intake and obesity, especially when the latter affects predominantly the abdomen. Because of the inconsistencies between ecologic and cohort studies noted earlier, however, it is unclear whether dietary fat per se, total calorie intake, or other factors are responsible for the associations. Epidemiologic evidence suggests that alcohol intake may also be a risk factor for this disease. Colorectal cancer is the second highest cause of cancer mortality in men and the third in women. Its risk correlates positively with dietary fat intake in both ecologic and cohort studies and inversely with intake of dietary fiber, calcium, and folic acid. Other malignant diseases for which dietary fat intake appears to increase risk include prostate and ovarian cancers.

The interaction of all these influences is powerful enough to indicate that diet contributes to about 35% of cancer deaths in western countries. Even though the independent influences of potentially protective nutrients such as carotenoids, vitamins C and E, folic acid, and fiber are not known because they are all present in vegetables and fruits, the evidence that a liberal intake of fruits and vegetables reduces cancer risk is overwhelming, supported by 128 of 156 epidemiologic studies reviewed in 1992.

Hypertension is a major risk factor for stroke, CHD, congestive heart failure, peripheral vascular disease, and renal disease. It often associates with obesity, especially abdominal obesity, and weight reduction in obese hypertensives usually leads to improvements in blood pressure. Sodium restriction also usually reduces blood pressure levels. In addition to these well-known effects, blood pressure levels have correlated inversely with the intake of potassium, calcium, and magnesium and are sometimes reduced when these nutrients are supplemented. Because alcohol intake elevates blood pressures, its use should be minimized in hypertensive patients.

Type II diabetes mellitus is strongly associated with obesity (see Ch. 205). This is especially true for abdominal obesity and less so for peripheral obesity. Sugar consumption does not lead to diabetes except to the extent that it may promote weight gain. Past recommendations to restrict total carbohydrate intake in diabetics have been abandoned, so that 55 to 60% of a diabetic's energy intake should come from carbohydrate, preferably unrefined carbohydrates that include fiber. Because higher fat diets tend to promote both obesity and CHD, for which diabetics are at high risk, dietary fat intake should be kept low. Alcohol can cause hypoglycemia, hyperglycemia, and increased triglyceride levels in diabetics, and its use should be minimized. In both diabetics and nondiabetics, excess alcohol intake is responsible for many deaths, particularly from accidents and liver disease, and is a factor in some suicidal deaths.

Osteoporosis is influenced by several dietary factors. Inadequate calcium intake during adolescence may result in suboptimal peak bone mass in early adulthood, and during later life it may lead to more rapid bone loss, thereby increasing the risk for osteoporosis. Other nutrients that influence bone mass have received much less attention. Sodium, phosphorus, and protein, all of which are consumed by Americans in greater quantities than required, may promote excess bone loss. Vitamin D and magnesium assist in maintaining optimal bone mass.

The causes and health effects of obesity, one of the most prevalent nutritional disorders in the United States, are reviewed in Ch. 196. Low dietary fiber intake causes constipation, and although not conclusively established, it is thought to be a cause of intestinal diverticular disease. Inadequate maternal folic acid intake has been conclusively proven to be a major risk factor for congenital neural tube defects such as spina bifida and myelomeningocele.

TRANSLATING EVIDENCE INTO DIETARY CHANGE

Thus there is strong evidence that dietary habits can influence the incidence and severity of many potentially incapacitating or lethal diseases in the United States. No justification exists for the belief that modification of the "usual" American diet is unnecessary or futile. The only questions are whether it is feasible and what is re-

TABLE 192–3. OLD AND NEW PARADIGMS IN NUTRITION

Old Paradigm	New Paradigm
Major nutritional problems = classic deficiency syndromes	Major nutritional problems = chronic diseases
Micronutrients (vitamins, minerals, trace elements) function primarily as cofactors in biochemical reactions	Micronutrients also function as antioxidants, regulators of genes and cell-cell communications, hormones, and pharmacologic agents
Nutrient needs (Recommended Dietary Allowances) determined by amounts required to prevent classic deficiency syndromes	Nutrient needs (not yet distilled into consensus recommendations) determined by amounts required to provide optimal function and health and prevent chronic disease; amounts are affected by individual's genetic makeup and environmental exposures
Micronutrient deficiencies are global, affecting whole body	Micronutrient deficiencies may be localized, and affect the functions of specific tissues
General effects of nutrients	Specific effects of nutrient subtypes, e.g., individual fatty acids, amino acids, and particular forms of micronutrients
All benefits of food are derived from nutrients; many can be obtained from supplements	Many non-nutritive components of foods, e.g., fiber, pigments, protease inhibitors, flavonoids, and others have important effects; even if some become available through supplements, many undetected ones may exist in foods

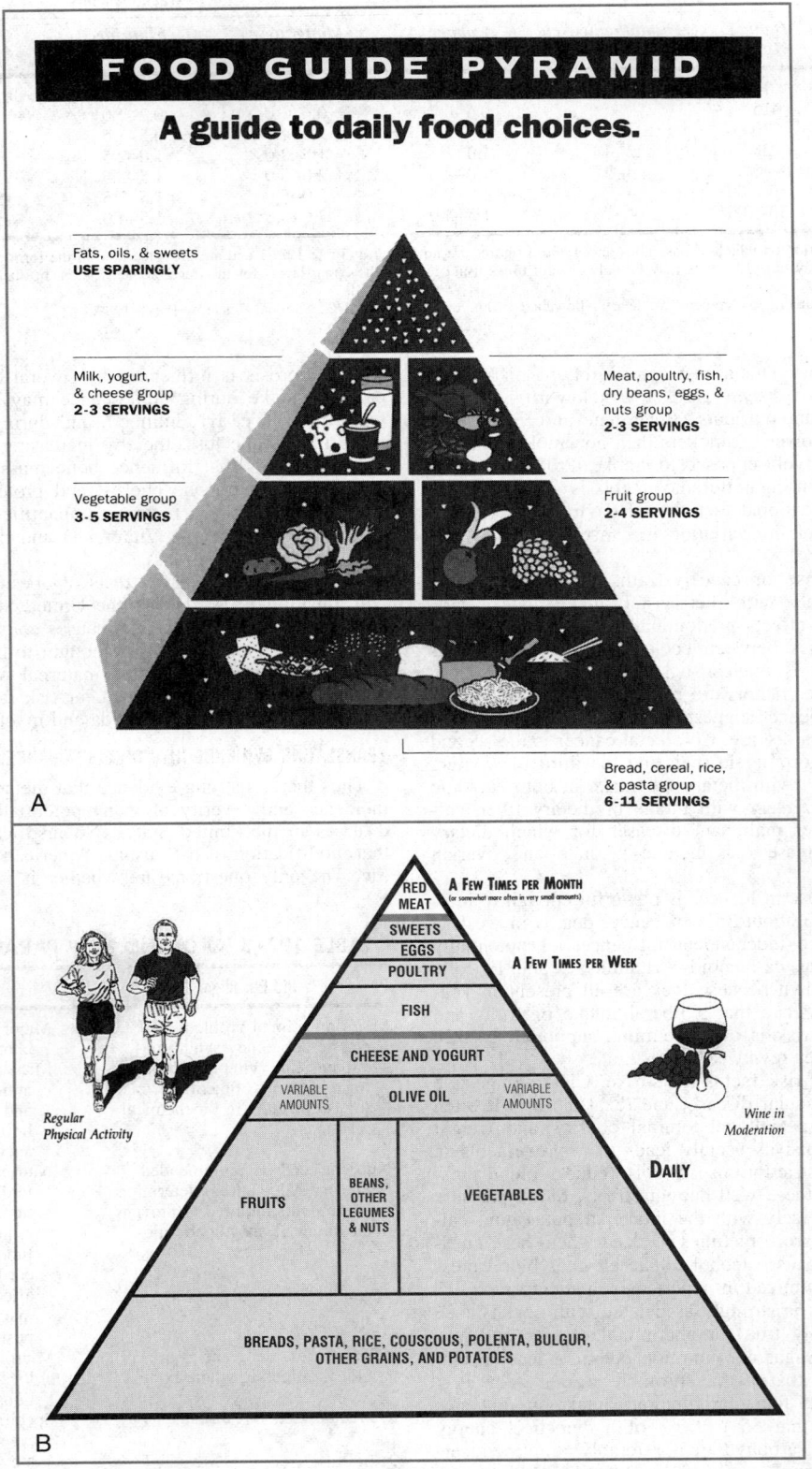

FIGURE 192.1–1. *A,* USDA/DHHS Food Guide Pyramid. *B,* Traditional healthy Mediterranean diet pyramid. (*A,* From USDA/DDHS. *B,* Copyright 1994, Oldways Preservation & Exchange Trust and The President and Fellows of Harvard College. Used by permission.)

TABLE 192–4. DIETARY INFLUENCES ON MAJOR CAUSES OF DEATH AND MORBIDITY IN UNITED STATES

	Possible Beneficial Influences	Possible Deleterious Influences
Cause of Death		
Coronary heart disease	Complex carbohydrates, particular fatty acids (e.g., mono-unsaturated, polyunsaturated, and ω-3 fatty acids from fish), soluble fiber, antioxidants (vitamins E, C; β-carotene, selenium), folic acid, moderate alcohol	Saturated fat, cholesterol; excess calories, sodium, animal protein; abdominal distribution of body fat
Cancer	Fruits and vegetables (for β-carotene, vitamins A, C, D, E, folic acid, calcium, selenium, phytochemicals), fiber	Excess calories, fat, alcohol, red meat, salt- and nitrite-preserved meats, possibly grilled meats; abdominal distribution of body fat
Stroke	Potassium, calcium, ω-3 fatty acids	Sodium, alcohol (as with hypertension)
Accidents		Alcohol
Diabetes mellitus	Fiber	Excess calories, fat, alcohol; abdominal distribution of body fat
Suicide		Alcohol
Chronic liver disease		Alcohol
Atherosclerosis (peripheral)	Particular fatty acids (e.g., monounsaturated and ω-3 fatty acids), soluble fiber, antioxidant vitamins	Saturated fat, cholesterol
Cause of Morbidity		
Obesity		Excess calories and fat
Hypertension	Potassium, calcium, ω-3 fatty acids	Sodium, alcohol, excess calories; abdominal distribution of body fat
Osteoporosis	Calcium, vitamin D	Sodium, phosphorus, protein
Diverticular disease, constipation		Fiber
Neural tube defects	Folic acid	

quired to effect change. Various health agencies and the US government have used public education, particularly the publication of dietary goals, as their primary means. The US Departments of Agriculture (USDA) and Health and Human Services (USDHHS) developed the food guide pyramid to replace the traditional basic four food groups in educating the public (Fig. 192–1A). It indicates that a healthy diet should be founded on ample servings of the complex carbohydrates present in breads, cereals, rice, and pasta. Vegetables and fruits should be a prominent component as well. Foods of animal origin, such as meat, eggs, and dairy products, should form a less central part of the diet, and fats, oils, and sweets should be used sparingly.

Even these recommendations do not typify an ideal diet based on the available evidence, but reflect a consensus on what can be realistically expected of the American public. A potentially more "ideal" pyramid, based on observations of low rates of chronic disease and high adult life expectancies in the Mediterranean region in 1960, has been promulgated by the Department of Nutrition at Harvard University (Fig. 192–1B). In this pyramid, sources of monounsaturated fatty acids, such as olive oil and nuts, are given a more prominent place in the diet, as are beans and other legumes. Fish and poultry are preferable over red meat. Moderate consumption of wine (normally with meals) is recommended as optional, unless it would put the individual or others at risk.

Beginning in May 1994, the US Food and Drug Administration and USDA initiated a major public education effort by requiring substantial changes in the listing of nutrient contents and health claims on food labels. Issues that were previously left to the discretion of food manufacturers, such as the serving sizes and particular nutrients listed, are now stipulated. Labels must delineate total calories and percentage of calories from fat, amounts of total fat, saturated fat, cholesterol, sodium, total carbohydrates, dietary fiber, sugars, protein, vitamins A and C, calcium, and iron. Labels also must indicate how a food's contents of these nutrients conform to recommended intakes, based on a reference 2000 calorie diet. Definitions for "low," "high," "light," "reduced," "free," and "healthy" have been standardized (Table 192–5). Further, only the particular health claims listed in Table 192–6 are permitted on food labels. As further evidence accumulates on the relationships between diet and disease, the approved claims will undoubtedly be revised.

For more details on the rationale for and methods of implementing the recommended dietary changes, please see Ch. 9.2. Physicians can importantly influence their patients' health by encouraging them to optimize their dietary habits and providing them with instructional materials and assistance from dietitians that can help them make needed changes.

National Academy of Sciences; Diet and Health: Washington, DC, 1989. *Comprehensive and easily readable analysis of the scientific evidence on the role of diet in the etiology and prevention of chronic disease in the United States, prepared by a committee of experts.*

Shils ME, Olson JA, Shike M (eds.): Modern Nutrition in Health and Disease, 8th ed. Malvern, PA, Lea & Febiger, 1994. *Comprehensive and detailed source for information on all aspects of human nutrition.*

US DHHS. Washington, DC, DHHS, 1989. Promoting Health/Preventing Disease: Year 2000 Objectives for the Nation. *Health promotion/disease prevention priorities and goals for the nation in nutrition and other areas.*

TABLE 192–5. DEFINITIONS OF TERMS USED ON FOOD LABELS

Low fat	≤ 3 grams per serving
Low saturated fat	≤ 1 gram per serving, ≤15% of calories
Low calorie	≤ 40 calories per serving
High	≥ 20% of desired daily value per serving
Light	Half the fat or one-third the calories of the regular product
Reduced	≤ 75% of content of regular product
Free	None, or insignificant amount (e.g., < 1 gram fat or < ½ gram sugar per serving)
Healthy	Low total and saturated fat, sodium, and cholesterol; ≥ 10% daily value for vitamin A, vitamin C, iron, calcium, protein, or fiber

From USDHHS, FDA, USDA,

TABLE 192–6. PERMISSIBLE HEALTH CLAIMS FOR FOOD LABELS

Calcium	May lower risk for osteoporosis
Fat	May increase risk for cancer
Saturated fat and cholesterol	Increase risk for coronary heart disease
Fiber-containing grain products, fruits, and vegetables	May reduce risk for coronary heart disease and cancer
Sodium	May increase risk for high blood pressure
Folic acid supplementation	Reduces risk for neural tube defects

From USDHHS, FDA, USDA.

192.2 Consequences of Altered Micronutrient Status

Joel B. Mason

Micronutrients are a highly diverse array of dietary components necessary to sustain health. The physiologic roles of micronutrients are as varied as their composition: Some are used in enzymes as either coenzymes or prosthetic groups; others, as biochemical substrates or hormones; and in some instances, the functions are not well defined. Under normal circumstances, the average daily dietary intake for each micronutrient required to sustain normal physiologic operations is measured in milligram or smaller quantities. This quantification distinguishes micronutrients from macronutrients, the latter category encompassing carbohydrates, fats, and proteins, as well as the macrominerals calcium, magnesium, and phosphorus.

For homeostasis to proceed properly, most dietary nutrients must be ingested in quantities that are neither too small nor too great. Disorders may arise when this "physiologic window" is either not met or is exceeded. The size of the window varies for each micronutrient and should be kept in mind, particularly in present-day circumstances when the administration of large quantities of certain micronutrients is being increasingly explored for possible therapeutic implications. Many factors determine the dietary requirement for a particular micronutrient, only one of which is the amount needed to sustain those physiologic functions for which it is used (Table 192–7). The *US Recommended Daily Allowances* (RDAs) provides dietary guidelines that indicate how much of each nutrient is "adequate to meet the known nutrient needs of practically all healthy persons"; the RDAs are listed in Table 192–1. Adequate intake, which is the amount necessary to prevent a deficiency state, is not necessarily synonymous with optimal intake, an issue this chapter discusses in more detail.

SALIENT FEATURES OF VITAMINS AND TRACE ELEMENTS: TRADITIONAL PERSPECTIVES

VITAMINS (Table 192–8). Vitamins have long been categorized as either fat soluble (A,D,E,K) or water soluble (all the others). This remains a physiologically meaningful manner of categorization. None of the fat-soluble vitamins appears to serve as a coenzyme. Their absorption is primarily through a micellar route, and pathophysiologic conditions associated with fat malabsorption frequently are associated with selective deficiencies of the fat-soluble vitamins. In contrast, most water-soluble vitamins function as coenzymes. Furthermore, the water-soluble vitamins are not absorbed through the lipophilic phase in the intestine.

TRACE ELEMENTS (Table 192–9). Fifteen trace elements have been identified as essential for health in animal studies: iron, zinc, copper, chromium, selenium, iodine, fluorine, manganese, molybdenum, cobalt, nickel, tin, silicon, vanadium, and arsenic. Nevertheless, only for the first 10 of these is there compelling evidence of essentialness in humans. Cobalt seems to be essential solely as a component of vitamin B_{12}; an isolated deficiency state has never been described. Deficiency syndromes for several of the other essential trace elements were not recognized until recently because of their exceedingly small requirements and their ubiquitous nature in foodstuffs. Only under exceptional circumstances, such as long-term dependence on total parenteral nutrition (TPN) that lacked the elements (a situation that has since been corrected), have some of the deficiency syndromes been observed.

The biochemical functions of trace elements have not been as well characterized as those for the vitamins, but most of their functions appear to be as components of prosthetic groups or as cofactors for a number of enzymes. Determination of essential trace element status is problematic except for iron, selenium, and iodine. The vanishingly low concentrations of these elements in bodily fluids and tissues, the fact that blood levels frequently do not correlate well with levels in the target tissues, and the fact that functional tests cannot be devised until biochemical functions are better understood, preclude an accurate and convenient laboratory method of assessment for most of the trace elements.

CONDITIONS THAT INCREASE THE REQUIRED DIETARY INTAKE FOR VITAMINS AND MINERALS

Many physiologic, pathophysiologic, and pharmacologic factors increase the dietary requirements for micronutrients (Table 192–7), and these factors when compounded enhance the risk of developing a deficiency state.

PHYSIOLOGIC FACTORS. Stages of the life cycle have an important impact on the requirements of certain nutrients. Phases of rapid growth and development, such as in utero development, infancy, adolescence, and pregnancy, are associated with remarkable increases in the utilization of certain micronutrients on a per-kilogram basis. Requirements for most micronutrients increase in pregnancy; those for iron and folate are particularly increased, because of the rapid proliferation of placental and fetal tissues. Periods of lactation are similarly associated with remarkable increases in requirements. A lactating woman experiences disproportionately large increases in her requirements for zinc and vitamins A, E, and C, in addition to the needs for pregnancy, to meet the metabolic demands incurred by milk production.

Infancy carries with it particular vulnerabilities to specific micronutrient inadequacies: Healthy infants in the United States are typically supplemented with vitamin K at birth and with iron and vitamin D during the course of the first year because of their particular susceptibility to deficiencies of these nutrients.

The ability to maintain adequate iron status from menarche through menopause is compromised in women by the additional losses incurred by menstruation, pregnancy, and lactation. As a result, the highest rate of iron deficiency affects women of childbearing age.

Specific dietary recommendations for the elderly have not yet been formally adopted, but these will inevitably appear because aging also affects the requirements for certain micronutrients. Vitamin B_{12} status, for instance, declines significantly with aging because of the high prevalence of atrophic gastritis and its associated impairment in protein-bound B_{12} absorption. The average decline is big enough to put a measurable proportion of the elderly population at risk of clinically important B_{12} deficiency and thus warrants an increase in B_{12} intake in this age group. Elderly persons, particularly those institutionalized for a long time, are also susceptible to vitamin D deficiency; increased intake is therefore indicated. The causes include diminished cutaneous synthesis of vitamin D by senile skin and decreased sun exposure, as well as in many instances to smaller dietary intakes.

PATHOPHYSIOLOGIC AND PHARMACOLOGIC FACTORS. Intestinal malabsorptive and maldigestive states predispose to multiple micronutrient deficiencies. Both fat-soluble and water-soluble micronutrients are absorbed predominantly in the proximal small intestine, the only exception being vitamin B_{12}. Diffuse mucosal diseases, therefore, that affect the proximal portion of the gastrointestinal tract are very likely to result in deficiencies. Even in the absence of mucosal disease of the proximal small intestine, however, extensive ileal disease, small bowel bacterial overgrowth, and chronic cholestasis can each interfere with the maintenance of adequate intraluminal conjugated bile acid concentrations and thereby impair absorption of fat-soluble vitamins. Maldigestion is usually the result of chronic pancreatitis. Untreated, it frequently

TABLE 192–7. FACTORS THAT DETERMINE THE DIETARY REQUIREMENT FOR A MICRONUTRIENT

Physiologic Factors
1. *Bioavailability:* the proportion of an ingested micronutrient that can be assimilated and utilized for physiologic purposes
2. Quantity required to fulfill physiologic roles
3. Extent to which the body can reutilize the micronutrient
4. Distribution of nutrient in the body: storage compartments, etc.
5. Influence of gender
6. Stage of life cycle: intrauterine development, childhood, adulthood, elder adulthood, pregnancy, lactation

Pathophysiologic and Pharmacologic Factors
1. Inborn errors of metabolism that variously affect assimilation, utilization, or excretion of micronutrients
2. Acquired disease states that alter the amounts required to sustain homeostasis (e.g., malabsorption, maldigestion, states that increase utilization)
3. Lifestyle habits, e.g., smoking, ethanol consumption
4. Drugs: may alter bioavailability and/or utilization

TABLE 192–8. VITAMINS AND THEIR FUNCTIONS

Fat-Soluble Vitamins

	Biochemistry and Physiology	Deficiency	Toxicity	Assessment of Status
Vitamin A	A subset of the retinoid compounds with biologic activity qualitatively similar to retinol. Carotenoids are structurally related to retinoids. Some carotenoids, most notably β-carotene, are metabolized into compounds with vitamin A activity and are considered to be provitamin A compounds. Vitamin A is an integral component of rhodopsin and iodopsins, light-sensitive proteins in retinal rod and cone cells.	Follicular hyperkeratosis and night blindness are early indicators. Conjunctival xerosis, degeneration of the cornea (*keratomalacia*), and de-differentiation of rapidly proliferating epithelia indicate more severe deficiency. *Bitot spots* (focal areas of the conjunctiva or cornea with foamy appearance) are an indication of xerosis. Blindness, due to corneal destruction and retinal dysfunction, ensues if left uncorrected. Increased susceptibility to infection also a consequence.	> 500,000 IU may cause *acute* toxicity: intracranial hypertension, skin exfoliation and hepatocellular necrosis. *Chronic* toxicity may occur with habitual daily intake of > 33,000 IU: alopecia, ataxia, dermatitis, cheilitis, pseudotumor cerebri, hepatocellular necrosis, and hyperlipidemia. Daily ingestion of > 25,000 IU during early pregnancy can be teratogenic. Excessive intake of most carotenoids causes a benign, yellowish discoloration of the skin. Large doses of canthaxanthin, a carotenoid, can induce retinopathy.	Retinol concentration in the plasma as well as vitamin A concentrations in the milk and tears are reasonably accurate measures. Toxicity best assessed by elevated levels of retinyl esters in plasma. A quantitative measure of dark adaptation for night vision or an electroretinogram are useful functional tests.
Vitamin D	A group of sterol compounds whose parent structure is cholecalciferol (vitamin D_3). Cholecalciferol is formed in the skin from 7-dehydrocholesterol by exposure to UV-B radiation. A plant sterol, ergocalciferol, can be similarly converted into vitamin D_2, and has similar vitamin D activity. Maintains intracellular and extracellular concentrations of calcium and phosphate by enhancing intestinal absorption of the two ions and, in conjunction with parathormone, promoting their mobilization from bone mineral.	Deficiency results in *rickets* in childhood and *osteomalacia* in adults. Expansion of the epiphyseal growth plates and replacement of normal bone with unmineralized bone matrix are the cardinal features. Deformity of bone and pathologic fractures occur. Serum concentrations of calcium and phosphate may decline.	Excess amounts result in abnormally high serum concentrations of calcium and phosphate: metastatic calcifications, renal damage, and altered mentation may ensue.	The serum concentration of the major circulating metabolite, 25-hydroxy vitamin D, indicates systemic status except in chronic renal failure, in which the impairment of renal 1-hydroxylation results in disassociation of the monohydroxy and dihydroxy vitamin concentrations. Measuring the serum concentration of 1,25-dihydroxy vitamin D is then necessary.
Vitamin E	A group of at least 8 naturally occurring compounds that share a spectrum of biologic activities. Some are tocopherols and some tocotrienols. The most biologically active of the vitameric forms is α-tocopherol. Acts as an antioxidant and free radical scavenger in lipophilic environments, most notably in cell membranes. Acts in conjunction with other antioxidants such as selenium.	Deficiency due to dietary inadequacy rare in developed countries. Usually affects premature infants, individuals with fat malabsorption, and persons with abetalipoproteinemia. Red blood cell fragility can produce hemolytic anemia. Neuronal degeneration produces peripheral neuropathies, ophthalmoplegia, and destruction of posterior columns of spinal cord. Neurologic disease frequently irreversible if deficiency is not corrected early enough. May contribute to hemolytic anemia and retrolental fibroplasia in premature infants.	Depressed levels of vitamin K-dependent procoagulants and potentiation of oral anticoagulants has been reported, as has impaired leukocyte function. Doses of 800 IU/d may increase the incidence of hemorrhagic stroke.	Plasma or serum concentration of α-tocopherol is most commonly used. Additional accuracy is obtained by expressing this value per mg of total plasma lipid. Red blood cell peroxide hemolysis test is not entirely specific, but is a useful functional measure of antioxidant potential of cell membranes.
Vitamin K	A family of naphthoquinone compounds with similar biologic activity. Phylloquinone (vitamin K_1) is derived from plants; a variety of menaquinones (vitamin K_2) are derived from bacterial sources. Serves as an essential cofactor in the post-translational α- or gamma-carboxylation of glutamic acid residues in many proteins. These proteins include several circulating procoagulants and anticoagulants as well as proteins in the bone matrix and renal epithelium.	Deficiency syndrome uncommon except in (1) breast-fed newborns, in whom it may cause "hemorrhagic disease of the newborn"; (2) adults with fat malabsorption or who are taking drugs that interfere with vitamin K metabolism (e.g., coumarin, phenytoin, broad-spectrum antibiotics); and (3) individuals taking large doses of vitamin E and anticoagulant drugs. Excessive hemorrhage is usual manifestation.	Rapid intravenous infusion of K_1 has been associated with dyspnea, flushing and cardiovascular collapse, probably related to dispersing agents in the solution. Supplementation may interfere with coumarin-based anticoagulation. Pregnant women taking large amounts of the provitamin menadione may deliver infants with hemolytic anemia, hyperbilirubinemia and kernicterus.	The prothrombin time is typically used as a measure of functional K status; it is neither sensitive nor specific for vitamin K deficiency. Determination of undercarboxylated prothrombin in the plasma is more accurate but less widely available.

Table continued on following page

causes malabsorption and deficiencies of fat-soluble vitamins. Vitamin B_{12} malabsorption often can be demonstrated in this setting, a result of inadequate R-protein digestion, but clinical B_{12} deficiency is rarely reported in patients with pancreatitis.

A myriad of rare inborn errors of metabolism has been described that impair an individual's ability to assimilate, utilize, or retain a particular vitamin or mineral. Such defects are usually partial and can often be overcome, at least in part, by administering doses of the nutrient that are several degrees of magnitude greater than is usually required. Suspicion for such defects should be entertained if: (1) a known defect exists in the family, (2) a deficiency syndrome arises at birth or during infancy, and (3) the deficiency syndrome is present despite adequate dietary intake and the absence of any disease that would impair the ability to assimilate the nutrient.

The long-term administration of many drugs may adversely affect micronutrient status and may either induce an overt deficiency syn-

TABLE 192–8. VITAMINS AND THEIR FUNCTIONS *(Continued)*

Water-Soluble Vitamins

	Biochemistry and Physiology	Deficiency	Toxicity	Assessment of Status
Thiamine (vitamin B_1)	A water-soluble compound containing substituted pyrimidine and thiazole rings and a hydroxyethyl side chain. The coenzyme form is thiamine pyrophosphate (TPP). Serves as a coenzyme in many -keto acid decarboxylation and transketolation reactions. Inadequate thiamine availability leads to impairments of above reactions, resulting in inadequate ATP synthesis and abnormal carbohydrate metabolism. May have an additional role in neuronal conduction independent of above mentioned actions.	Classic deficiency syndrome ("beriberi") described in Asian populations consuming polished rice diet. Alcoholism and chronic renal dialysis are also common precipitants. High carbohydrate intake increases need for B_1. Deficiency produces various combinations of peripheral neuropathy, cardiovascular and cerebral dysfunction. Cardiovascular involvement ("wet beriberi") includes congestive heart failure and low peripheral vascular resistance. See Ch. 406 for neurologic changes. Deficiency syndrome responds to parenteral thiamine, but is at least partially irreversible after a certain stage.	Excess intake is largely excreted in the urine although parenteral doses of > 400 mg/d are reported to cause lethargy, ataxia, and reduced tone of the gastrointestinal tract.	The most effective measure of B_1 status is the erythrocyte transketolase activity coefficient, which measures enzyme activity before and after addition of exogenous TPP: Red cells from a deficient individual express a substantial increase in enzyme activity with addition of TPP. Thiamine concentrations in the blood or urine are also used.
Riboflavin (vitamin B_2)	A compound consisting of a substituted isoalloxazine ring with a ribitol side chain. Serves as a coenzyme for diverse biochemical reactions. The primary coenzymatic forms are flavin mononucleotide (FMN) and flavin adenine dinucleotide (FAD). Riboflavin holoenzymes participate in oxidation-reduction reactions in myriad metabolic pathways.	Deficiency is usually found in conjunction with deficiencies of other B vitamins. Isolated deficiency of riboflavin produces hyperemia and edema of nasopharyngeal mucosa, cheilosis, angular stomatitis, glossitis, seborrheic dermatitis and a normochromic, normocytic anemia.	Toxicity not reported in humans.	The most common assessment is determining the activity coefficient of glutathione reductase in red blood cells (the test is invalid for individuals with glucose-6-phosphate dehydrogenase deficiency). Measurements of blood and urine concentrations are less desirable methods.
Niacin (vitamin B_3)	Refers to nicotinic acid and the corresponding amide, nicotinamide. The active coenzymatic forms are composed of nicotinamide affixed to adenine dinucleotide, forming NAD or NADP. Over 200 apoenzymes use these coenzymes as electron acceptors or hydrogen donors. The essential amino acid, tryptophan, is utilized as a precursor of niacin; 60 mg of dietary tryptophan yields approximately 1 mg of niacin. Dietary requirements depend partly on tryptophan content of diet.	*Pellagra* is the classic deficiency syndrome and often affects populations where corn is the major source of energy. Still endemic in parts of China, Africa, and India. Diarrhea, dementia (or associated symptoms of anxiety or insomnia) and pigmented dermatitis that develops in sun-exposed areas are typical. Glossitis, stomatitis, vaginitis, vertigo, and burning dysesthesias are early signs. Seen also in carcinoid syndrome, which diverts tryptophan to other synthetic pathways.	Human toxicity known largely through studies examining hypolipidemic effects. Includes vasomotor phenomenon (flushing), hyperglycemia, parenchymal liver damage, and hyperuricemia.	Assessment is problematic: Blood levels of vitamin not reliable. Measurement of urinary excretion of the niacin metabolites, N-methylnicotinamide and 2-pyridone are thought to be the most effective means of assessment at present.
Vitamin B_6	Refers to several derivatives of pyridine, including pyridoxine (PN), pyridoxal (PL), and pyridoxamine (PM). The coenzymatic forms are pyridoxal-5-phosphate (PLP) and pyridoxamine-5-phosphate (PMP). As a coenzyme, B_6 is involved in many transamination reactions (and thereby in gluconeogenesis), in the synthesis of niacin from tryptophan, of several neurotransmitters, and of ∂-aminolevulinic acid (and therefore in heme synthesis).	Deficiency usually seen in conjunction with other water-soluble vitamin deficiencies. Stomatitis, angular cheilosis, glossitis, irritability, depression and confusion occur in moderate to severe depletion; normochromic, normocytic anemia has been reported in severe deficiency. Abnormal EEG's and, in infants, convulsions have been observed. Some sideroblastic anemias respond to B_6 administration. Isoniazid, cycloserine, penicillamine, ethanol, and theophylline can inhibit B_6 metabolism.	Chronic use with doses exceeding 200 mg/d (in adults) may cause peripheral neuropathies and photosensitivity.	Many laboratory methods of assessment exist. The plasma or erythrocyte PLP levels are most common. Urinary excretion of xanthurenic acid after an oral tryptophan load or activity indices of RBC alanine or aspartic acid transaminases (ALT and AST, respectively) all are functional measures of B_6-dependent enzyme activity.

drome or predispose to one. The manner in which drug-nutrient interactions occur varies; some of the more common mechanisms are outlined in Table 192–10. Some drugs exert their therapeutic effects by specifically inhibiting the actions of a micronutrient. Examples include coumarin, which inhibits gamma-carboxylation reactions mediated by vitamin K, and methotrexate, which binds tightly to dihydrofolate reductase, thereby inhibiting folate metabolism.

Tobacco smoking alters the metabolism of several micronutrients, including folate, β-carotene, and vitamins C and E. In large surveys, diminished plasma levels of folate and ascorbic acid have been observed in long-time smokers. Smoking is also associated with diminished levels of folate in cells of the oral mucosa, diminished ascorbic acid levels in leukocytes, and decreased concentrations of vitamin E in lung alveolar fluid.

NEW FRONTIERS IN MARGINAL DEFICIENCY STATES

REDEFINING THE CONCEPT OF NUTRIENT DEFICIENCY. An important evolution in the understanding of micronutrient requirements has occurred over the past century: As nutritional science has expanded its appreciation for additional

TABLE 192–8. VITAMINS AND THEIR FUNCTIONS *(Continued)*

Water-Soluble Vitamins

	Biochemistry and Physiology	Deficiency	Toxicity	Assessment of Status
Folate	A group of over 35 related pterin compounds. The fully oxidized form, folic acid, is not found in nature but is the pharmacologic form of the vitamin. All folate functions relate to their ability to transfer one-carbon groups. The step is essential in the *de novo* synthesis of nucleotides, in the metabolism of several amino acids, and is an integral component for the regeneration of the "universal" methyl donor, S-adenosylmethionine. Inhibition of bacterial and cancer cell folate metabolism is the basis for the sulfonamide antibiotics and chemotherapeutic agents such as methotrexate and 5-fluorouracil.	Women of childbearing age are the most likely individuals to develop deficiency. The "classical" deficiency syndrome is megaloblastic anemia. The hemopoietic cells in the bone marrow develop megaloblastic features, reflecting ineffective DNA synthesis. The peripheral blood smear demonstrates macroovalocytes and polymorphonuclear leukocytes with an average of more than 3.5 nuclear lobes. Megaloblastic changes in the oral and gastrointestinal epithelia often occur, producing glossitis and diarrhea, respectively. Sulfasalazine and phenytoin inhibit absorption and predispose to deficiency.	Doses $> 400 \mu g/d$ may partially correct the anemia of B_{12} deficiency and mask (and perhaps exacerbate) the associated neuropathy. Doses $> 400 \mu g$ also reported to lower seizure threshold in individuals prone to seizures. Rarely parenteral administration is reported to cause allergic phenomena, but are probably due to dispersion agents.	Serum folate measures short-term folate balance, whereas RBC folate better reflects tissue status. Serum homocysteine rises early in deficiency but is nonspecific since B_{12} deficiency or renal insufficiency also may cause elevations.
Vitamin C (ascorbic and dehydro-ascorbic acid)	Ascorbic acid readily oxidizes to dehydroascorbic acid. Since the latter can be reduced *in vivo*, it possesses vitamin C activity. Total vitamin C is therefore measured as the sum of ascorbic and dehydroascorbic acid concentrations. Because of its reductant properties, it serves primarily as a biologic antioxidant and free radical scavenger in aqueous environments. The biosyntheses of collagen, carnitine, bile acids, and norepinephrine, as well as proper functioning of the hepatic mixed-function oxygenase system, all depend on these properties. Vitamin C in foodstuffs increases the intestinal absorption of non-heme iron.	Overt deficiency is uncommonly observed in developed countries. The classic deficiency syndrome is *scurvy*, characterized by fatigue, depression, and widespread abnormalities in connective tissues such as inflamed gingivae, petechiae, perifollicular hemorrhages, impaired wound healing, coiled hairs, hyperkeratosis, bleeding into body cavities. In infants, defects in ossification and bone growth may occur. Tobacco smoking lowers plasma and leukocyte vitamin C levels.	Quantities exceeding 500 mg/d (in adults) sometimes cause nausea and diarrhea. Acidification of the urine with supplementation, and the potential for enhanced oxalate synthesis, have raised concerns regarding nephrolithiasis, but this has yet to be demonstrated. Supplementation may interfere with laboratory tests based on redox potential (e.g., fecal occult blood testing, serum cholesterol and glucose). Withdrawal from chronic ingestion of high doses of vitamin C supplements should occur gradually over a month since accommodation does occur, raising a concern of "rebound scurvy."	Plasma ascorbic acid concentration reflects recent dietary intake whereas leukocyte levels more closely reflect tissue stores. Women's plasma levels are approximately 20% higher than men's for any given dietary intake.
Vitamin B_{12}	A group of closely related cobalamin compounds composed of a corrin ring (with a cobalt atom in its center) connected to a ribonucleotide via an aminopropanol bridge. Microorganisms are the ultimate source of all naturally occurring B_{12}. The two active coenzyme forms are desoxyadenosylcobalamin and methylcobalamin. Both are needed for the synthesis of succinyl CoA, which is essential in lipid and carbohydrate metabolism, as well as the synthesis of methionine. The latter reaction is essential for amino acid metabolism, for purine and pyrimidine synthesis, for many methylation reactions, and for the intracellular retention of folates.	Dietary inadequacy rarely causes deficiency except in strict vegetarians. Most deficiencies reflect loss of intestinal absorption: this may result from pernicious anemia, pancreatic insufficiency, atrophic gastritis, small bowel bacterial overgrowth, or ileal disease. Megaloblastic anemia and megaloblastic changes in other epithelia (see Folate) are the result of sustained depletion. Details of the hematologic (see Ch. 133) and neurologic (see Ch. 406) complications are described elsewhere. Hematologic and neurologic complication may occur independently.	A few allergic reactions have been reported to crystalline B_{12} preparations and are probably due to impurities, not the vitamin.	Serum, or plasma, concentrations are generally accurate. Subtle deficiency with neurologic complications, as described in the Deficiency column, can best be confirmed by measuring the concentration of serum methylmalonic acid, which is a sensitive indicator of cellular deficiency.
Biotin	A bi-cyclic compound consisting of a ureido ring fused to a substituted tetrahydrothiophene ring. Most dietary biotin is linked to lysine, a compound called biotinyl lysine, or biocytin. The lysine must be hydrolyzed by an intestinal enzyme called biotinidase before intestinal absorption occurs. Acts primarily as a co-enzyme for several carboxylases; each holoenzyme catalyzes an ATP-dependent CO_2 transfer. The carboxylases are critical enzymes in carbohydrate and lipid metabolism.	Isolated deficiency is rare. Deficiency in humans has been produced experimentally, by prolonged diets lacking the vitamin, and by ingestion of large quantities of raw egg white, which contains avidin, a protein which binds biotin with extremely high affinity. Alterations in mental status, myalgias, hyperesthesias, and anorexia occur. Later, a seborrheic dermatitis and alopecia develop. Biotin deficiency is usually accompanied by lactic acidosis and organic aciduria.	Toxicity has not been reported in humans with doses as high as 60 mg/d in children.	Plasma and urine concentrations of biotin are diminished in the deficient state. Elevated urine concentrations of methyl citrate, 3-methylcrotonylglycine and 3-hydroxyisovalerate are observed in deficiency.

Table continued on following page

TABLE 192-8. VITAMINS AND THEIR FUNCTIONS (Continued)

Water-Soluble Vitamins

	Biochemistry and Physiology	Deficiency	Toxicity	Assessment of Status
Pantothenic acid	Consists of pantoic acid linked to β-alanine through an amide bond. Pantothenate serves as an essential precursor of coenzyme A(CoA). CoA is essential for the synthesis and β-oxidation of fatty acids, and the synthesis of cholesterol, steroid hormones, vitamins A and D, and other isoprenoid derivatives. CoA is also involved in the synthesis of several amino acids and ∂-aminolevulinic acid, a precursor for the corrin ring of vitamin B_{12}, the porphyrin ring of heme, and of cytochromes. CoA is also necessary for the acetylation and fatty acid acylation of a variety of proteins.	Usually seen in conjunction with other water-soluble vitamin deficiencies. Experimental, isolated deficiency in humans produces fatigue, abdominal pain and vomiting, insomnia, and paresthesias of the extremities.	Doses exceeding 10 g/d may induce diarrhea.	Whole blood and urine concentrations of pantothenate are indicators of status; serum levels are not accurate.

TABLE 192-9. NUTRITIONAL TRACE ELEMENTS AND THEIR CLINICAL IMPLICATIONS

Trace Elements

	Biochemistry and Physiology	Deficiency	Toxicity	Assessment of Status
Chromium	Dietary chromium consists of both inorganic and organic forms. Its primary function in humans is to potentiate insulin action. It accomplishes this as a circulating dinicotino-glutathione complex called glucose tolerance factor. It thereby impacts on carbohydrate, fat, and protein metabolism.	Deficiency in humans described only in long-term TPN patients receiving insufficient chromium. Hyperglycemia, or impaired glucose intolerance, is uniformly observed. Elevated plasma free fatty acid concentrations, neuropathy, encephalopathy, and abnormalities in nitrogen metabolism are also reported. Whether supplemental chromium may improve glucose tolerance in mildly glucose intolerant but otherwise healthy individuals remains controversial.	Toxicity after oral ingestion is uncommon and seems confined to gastric irritation. Airborne exposure may cause contact dermatitis, eczema, skin ulcers, and bronchogenic carcinoma.	Plasma or serum concentration of chromium is a crude indicator of chromium status; it appears to be meaningful when the value is markedly above or below the normal range.
Copper	Copper is absorbed by a specific intestinal transport mechanism. It is carried to the liver where it is bound to ceruloplasmin, which circulates systemically and delivers copper to target tissues in the body. Excretion of copper is largely through bile into feces. Absorptive and excretory processes vary with the levels of dietary copper, providing a means of copper homeostasis. Copper serves as a component of many enzymes, including amine oxidases, ferroxidases, cytochrome c oxidase, dopamine β-hydroxylase, superoxide dismutase, and tyrosinase.	Dietary deficiency is rare; it has been observed in premature and low birth weight infants fed exclusively a cow's milk diet and in individuals receiving long-term TPN lacking copper. The clinical manifestations include depigmentation of skin and hair, neurologic disturbances, leukopenia, hypochromic microcytic anemia, and skeletal abnormalities. The anemia arises from impaired utilization of iron and is therefore a conditioned form of iron deficiency anemia. The deficiency syndrome, except for the anemia and leukopenia, is also observed in Mencke's disease, a rare inherited condition associated with impaired copper utilization.	Acute copper toxicity has been described after excessive oral intake and with absorption of copper salts applied to burned skin. Milder manifestations include nausea, vomiting, epigastric pain and diarrhea; coma and hepatic necrosis may ensue in severe cases. Toxicity may be seen with doses as low as 70 μg/kg/d. Chronic toxicity is also described. Wilson's disease is a rare, inherited disease associated with abnormally low ceruloplasmin levels and accumulation of copper in the liver and brain, eventually leading to damage to these two organs (see Ch. 188).	Practical methods for detecting marginal deficiency are not available. Marked deficiency is reliably detected by diminished serum copper and ceruloplasmin concentrations as well as low erythrocyte superoxide dismutase activity.
Fluorine	Known more commonly by its ionic form, fluoride. It is incorporated into the crystalline structure of bone, thereby altering its physical characteristics.	An intake of < 0.1 mg/d in infants, and < 0.5 in children is associated with a decreased incidence of dental caries. Optimal intake in adults is between 1.5 and 4 mg/d.	Acute ingestion of > 30 mg/kg body weight fluoride is likely to cause death. Excessive chronic intake (> 0.1 mg/kg/d) leads to mottling of the teeth (dental fluorosis), calcification of tendons and ligaments, exostoses, and may increase the brittleness of bones.	Estimates of intake or clinical assessment are used since no good laboratory test exists.

TABLE 192–9. NUTRITIONAL TRACE ELEMENTS AND THEIR CLINICAL IMPLICATIONS *(Continued)*

	Trace Elements			
	Biochemistry and Physiology	**Deficiency**	**Toxicity**	**Assessment of Status**
Iodine	Readily absorbed from the diet, concentrated in the thyroid, and integrated into the thyroid hormones, thyroxine (T_4), and triiodothyronine (T_3). The hormones circulate largely bound to thyroxine-binding globulin. They modulate resting energy expenditure and, in the developing human, growth and development.	In the absence of supplementation, populations relying primarily on food from soils with low iodine content have endemic iodine deficiency. Maternal iodine deficiency leads to fetal deficiency, which produces spontaneous abortions, stillbirths, hypothyroidism, cretinism, and dwarfism. Permanent cognitive deficits may also be induced by iodine deficiency during infancy and childhood. In the adult, compensatory hypertrophy of the thyroid (goiter) occurs along with varying degrees of hypothyroidism.	Large doses (> 2 mg/d in adults) may induce hypothyroidism by blocking thyroid hormone synthesis. Supplementation with > 100 μg per day to an individual who was formerly deficient occasionally induces hyperthyroidism.	Iodine status of a population can be estimated by the prevalence of goiter. Urinary excretion of iodine is an effective laboratory means of assessment. The TSH (thyroid-stimulating hormone) level in the blood is an indirect, and therefore not an entirely specific, means of assessment.
Iron	Participates in redox reactions in a number of metalloproteins such as hemoglobin, myoglobin, and the cytochrome enzymes. Primary storage form is ferritin. Intestinal absorption is 15–20% for "heme" iron and 1–8% for the iron contained in vegetables. Absorption of the latter form is enhanced by the ascorbic acid in foodstuffs, by poultry, fish, or beef and by an iron-deficient state; it is decreased by phytate and tannins.	The most common micronutrient deficiency in the world. Women of childbearing age constitute the highest risk group because of menstrual blood losses, pregnancy, and lactation. The classic deficiency syndrome is hypochromic, microcytic anemia. Glossitis and koilonychia (spoon nails) are also observed. Easy fatigability often develops as an early symptom. In children, mild deficiency insufficient to cause anemia is associated with behavioral disturbances and poor school performance.	Iron overload occurs when habitual dietary intake is extremely high, intestinal absorption is excessive, or repeated parenteral administration occurs. Excessive iron stores usually accumulate in reticuloendothelial tissues and cause little damage (hemosiderosis). If overload continues, iron eventually begins to accumulate in tissues such as the liver, pancreas, heart, and synovium; the result is hemochromatosis (see Ch. 189). Hereditary hemochromatosis arises as a result of homozygosity of a common, recessive trait. Excessive intestinal absorption of iron is observed in homozygotes.	Negative iron balance initially leads to depletion of iron stores in the bone marrow and an associated decrease in serum ferritin. As the severity of deficiency proceeds, serum iron (SI) decreases and total iron-binding capacity (TIBC) increases. An iron saturation (=SI/TIBC) of $< 16\%$ suggests iron deficiency (see Ch. 132).
Manganese	A component of several metalloenzymes. Most manganese is in mitochondria, where it is a component of manganese superoxide dismutase.	Manganese deficiency in the human has not been conclusively demonstrated. It is said to cause hypocholesterolemia, weight loss, hair and nail changes, dermatitis, and impaired synthesis of vitamin K-dependent proteins.	Toxicity by oral ingestion unknown in humans. Toxic inhalation causes hallucinations, other alterations in mentation, and extrapyramidal movement disorders.	Until the deficiency syndrome is better defined, an appropriate measure of status will be difficult to develop.
Molybdenum	A cofactor in several enzymes, most prominently xanthine oxidase and sulfite oxidase.	A probable case of human deficiency is described secondary to parenteral administration of sulfite. This resulted in hyperoxypurinemia, hypouricemia, and low sulfate excretion.	Toxicity not well described in the human although it may interfere with copper metabolism at high doses.	Laboratory means of assessment not meaningful until deficiency syndrome is better defined.

Table continued on following page

physiologic functions of micronutrients, an ever increasing need to redefine the concept of deficiency has ensued. The original means by which the necessary intake of these nutrients was defined was typically based on a disease entity that occurred as a result of a flagrant deficiency of the nutrient, the so-called classic deficiency syndrome. In retrospect, this was naive, since it is now evident that most, if not all, micronutrients serve important functions in a wide variety of distinct biochemical systems. As the science of nutrition has come to appreciate this diversity in function, new deficiency syndromes are being defined.

Nevertheless, the redefinition of micronutrient deficiencies and the re-examination of recommended daily intakes have proven difficult for several reasons. In some instances there continues to be less than definitive evidence for the role of a particular micronutrient in a new function that has been proposed. Furthermore, even if a novel biochemical or physiologic role is well demonstrated for a nutrient, an appropriate question is whether optimization of such function translates into optimization of health. For example, providing supplemental vitamin E to elderly individuals who are vitamin E replete enhances T lymphocyte responsiveness to mitogens. Nevertheless, it is unclear whether this diminishes infection rates among the elderly. Another difficult problem pertains

to the use of micronutrients in supraphysiologic quantities, i.e., intakes that greatly exceed all conventional concepts of what is necessary for health. When taken in large quantities, some micronutrients affect physiologic functions beneficially (e.g., gram quantities of niacin to reduce low density lipoprotein [LDL] cholesterol). Such physiologic effects are not observed at more conventional levels of intake and are therefore usually considered to be "pharmacologic" effects of the nutrient. Nevertheless, if the dietary requirement of a nutrient is strictly defined as the minimal dose necessary for the maintenance of optimal health, as has been suggested, then supraphysiologic doses may have to be considered as the dietary requirement in such instances. Thus, the determination of "optimal" nutrient intake depends considerably on which physiologic effect is sought. Furthermore, if only a segment of the population will benefit from supraphysiologic quantities of a nutrient, should dietary guidelines for the entirety be established according to this effect?

Determining an adequate level of intake implies the existence of a means of measuring nutrient status. In seeking such indices, the diversity of function often makes it difficult to decide the most germane measurement. Tobacco smoking, for example, appears to diminish vitamin E levels in alveolar fluid but not in the serum. The

TABLE 192–9. NUTRITIONAL TRACE ELEMENTS AND THEIR CLINICAL IMPLICATIONS (Continued)

Trace Elements

	Biochemistry and Physiology	Deficiency	Toxicity	Assessment of Status
Selenium	Selenium is a component of several enzymes, most notably glutathione peroxidase and superoxide dismutase. These enzymes appear to prevent oxidative and free radical damage of various cell structures. Evidence suggests that the antioxidant protection conveyed by selenium operates in conjunction with vitamin E, since deficiency of one seems to enhance damage induced by a deficiency of the other. Selenium also participates in the enzymatic conversion of thyroxine to its more active metabolite, tri-iodothyronine.	Deficiency is rare in North America except in individuals receiving long-term total parenteral nutrition (TPN) lacking selenium. Such individuals have myalgias and/or cardiomyopathies. Populations in some regions of the world, most notably some parts of China, have marginal intake of selenium. In these regions, *Keshan's disease*, a condition characterized by cardiomyopathy, is endemic. The disease can be prevented (but not treated) by selenium supplementation.	Toxicity is associated with nausea, diarrhea, alterations in mental status, peripheral neuropathy, loss of hair and nails; such symptoms were observed in adults who inadvertently consumed between 27 and 2400 mg.	Erythrocyte glutathione peroxidase activity and plasma, or whole blood, selenium concentrations are moderately accurate indicators of status.
Zinc	Intestinal absorption occurs by a specific process that is enhanced by pregnancy and corticosteroids and diminished by coingestion of phytates, phosphates, iron, copper, lead, or calcium. Diminished intake of zinc leads to increased efficiency of absorption and decreased fecal excretion, providing a means of zinc homeostasis. Zinc is a component of over 100 enzymes; among these are DNA polymerase, RNA polymerase and tRNA synthetase.	Mild deficiency causes growth retardation in children. More severe deficiency is associated with growth arrest, teratogenicity, hypogonadism and infertility, dysgeusia, poor wound healing, diarrhea, a dermatitis on the extremities and around orifices, glossitis, alopecia, corneal clouding, loss of dark adaptation and behavioral changes. Impaired cellular immunity is observed. Excessive loss of gastrointestinal secretions through chronic diarrhea, fistulas, etc., may precipitate deficiency. *Acrodermatitis enteropathica* is a rare, recessively inherited disease in which intestinal absorption of zinc is impaired.	Acute zinc toxicity can usually be induced by ingestion of >200 mg of zinc in a single day (in adults). It is manifested by epigastric pain, nausea, vomiting, and diarrhea. Hyperpnea, diaphoresis, and weakness may follow inhalation of zinc fumes. Copper and zinc compete for intestinal absorption: chronic ingestion of >25 mg/d of zinc may lead to copper deficiency. Chronic ingestion of >150 mg/d has been reported to cause gastric erosions, low HDL cholesterol levels, and impaired cellular immunity.	There are no accurate indicators of zinc status available for routine clinical use. Plasma, erythrocyte, and hair zinc concentrations are frequently misleading. Acute illness, in particular, is known to diminish plasma zinc levels, in part by inducing a shift of zinc out of the plasma compartment and into the liver. Functional tests that determine dark adaptation, taste acuity, and rate of wound healing lack specificity.

concepts of "localized" nutrient deficiencies and tissue-specific requirements add a level of complexity to the determination of nutrient status.

The following examples illustrate how advances in nutritional science are prompting the redefinition of micronutrient requirements.

Folate. Guidelines regarding the necessary intake of folate were based, until recently, on the prevention of megaloblastic anemia. Measurements of serum and erythrocyte folate concentrations have been the most common means of assessing status; maintaining such levels within accepted normative ranges provides good assurance that folate status is adequate to prevent anemia.

It has become increasingly evident, however, that low folate levels that are insufficiently severe to cause anemia may still disturb normal biochemical and physiologic homeostasis. This is evidenced in part by an increase in serum homocysteine, an amino acid that is normally metabolized by a folate-dependent pathway. Some nutritional surveys identify elevated serum homocysteine levels in certain individuals whose habitual intake of folate is at or just above the US RDA (see Table 192–1), as well as in those whose serum folate levels are marginally above the conventional thresholds of deficiency. This elevation reflects less than optimal disposal of homocysteine, which is now believed to enhance the development of occlusive vascular disease. Vitamins B_6 and B_{12} are also important components of the biochemical pathways by which the body disposes of homocysteine, although their responsibility for hyperhomocysteinemia in the population is less evident.

The ingestion of folate in quantities considerably above the present recommended allowances appears to have other health benefits. Women taking folate supplements at the time of conception have a significantly lower risk of delivering a baby with a neural tube defect compared to women who do not take folate supplements but whose dietary intake or serum folate levels fall within conventionally accepted ranges. A more controversial observation is the inverse relationship that exists between the ingestion of folate and the incidence of epithelial neoplasia of the uterine cervix, the colorectum, and the bronchopulmonary tree; the inverse relationship is observed even when folate status (or dietary intake) falls within the range of conventionally accepted norms.

These observations suggest that the ingestion of folate in quantities above what is presently regarded as adequate may contribute to the optimization of health. Substantial increases in the suggested intake of any micronutrient must be tempered, however, by the consideration of toxicity: with folate, this is primarily related to its ability to mask B_{12} deficiency when taken in doses exceeding 400 μg per day.

TABLE 192–10. EXAMPLES OF DRUG-MEDIATED EFFECTS ON MICRONUTRIENT STATUS

Drug(s)	Nutrient	Mechanism of Interaction
Dextroamphetamine, fenfluramine, levodopa	Potentially all micronutrients	Induce anorexia
Cholestyramine	Vitamin D, folate	Adsorbs nutrient, decreases absorption
Omeprazole	Vitamin B_{12}	Induces modest bacterial overgrowth; decreases gastric acid, impairing absorption
Sulfasalazine, methotrexate	Folate	Impair absorption and/or inhibit folate-dependent enzymes
Isoniazid	Pyridoxine	Impairs utilization of B_6
Nonsteroidal anti-inflammatory agents	Iron	Gastrointestinal blood loss
Penicillamine	Zinc	Increases renal excretion

Antioxidant and Free-Radical Scavenging Vitamins/Provitamins. Vitamins A, C, and E, as well as many of the carotenoids, are effective antioxidants. In addition, vitamins C and E and some of the carotenoids can scavenge free radicals when taken in adequate quantities. Such properties have long been appreciated, but it is only recently that oxidation and free radical damage have been thought to play important roles in common degenerative illnesses such as atherosclerosis, cancer, cataracts, retinal degeneration, and neurodegenerative disorders.

Growing evidence indicates that LDL can undergo oxidation in vivo and that LDL thus transformed is particularly atherogenic. Prevention of LDL oxidation, at least in animal models, retards the process of atherogenesis. Supplementation in human subjects with severalfold the RDA of vitamin E, and perhaps some of the other antioxidant micronutrients, is an effective means of preventing LDL oxidation. Such intervention, however, remains unproved as a way to confer beneficial effects on human atherogenesis. Some evidence suggests that large doses of β-carotene may protect against the recurrence of coronary heart disease. If so, it is not yet clear whether this possible effect is mediated through the prevention of LDL oxidation.

Many epidemiologic studies indicate that the occurrence of cancers of the oral cavity, lung, esophagus, stomach, and perhaps colorectum is inversely related to dietary intake of fresh vegetables and fruits. Careful dissection of dietary data suggests that β-carotene and vitamin E content are the most protective components of these foodstuffs. High doses of vitamin A and some of its synthetic analogues (e.g., 13-cis-retinoic acid) can effectively reduce the recurrence of head and neck cancers, although hepatic toxicity is sometimes a limiting factor. Similarly, when taken in large doses, these agents as well as β-carotene or vitamin E have been shown to promote the regression of oral leukoplakia, a premalignant lesion. Daily supplementation with one to three times the US RDA of β-carotene, selenium, and vitamin E has been found to reduce the incidence of gastric adenocarcinoma in a disease-prevalent region of China. Contrarily, an intervention trial in Finland showed, if anything, an increase in lung cancer in smokers with daily supplementation of β-carotene. Further investigation is necessary to define any circumstances under which antioxidant nutrients can effectively prevent cancer.

Epidemiologic associations also suggest an inverse relationship between lens cataracts, macular degeneration, and the intake of vitamins C, E, and β-carotene. Considerable experimental evidence indicates that photo-oxidation can contribute to both of these common degenerative conditions of the eye. In animal models these degenerative processes have been retarded by supraphysiologic supplementation with vitamin C or E. Individuals who ingest vitamin C in excess of the US RDA have a lower incidence of cataract than those ingesting the RDA, suggesting a preventive role for larger than conventionally recommended doses of these nutrients. Nevertheless, insufficient prospective data exist at the present time to conclude that antioxidants specifically prevent cataracts and macular degeneration.

Vitamin B₁₂ and Neuropsychiatric Disease. Plasma B_{12} concentrations are considered to be an accurate indication of B_{12} status. The normal range for a healthy population has typically been considered 150 to 900 pg per milliliter; values above 150 or 200 pg per milliliter were felt to exclude B_{12} deficiency as a cause of neurologic or psychiatric syndromes. Some observations, still controversial, suggest that 7 to 10% of individuals who have plasma B_{12} values between 150 and 400 pg per milliliter may develop neuropsychiatric complications of B_{12} deficiency in the absence of megaloblastic anemia. Such persons can be identified by an elevated level of methylmalonic acid in the blood that decreases to normal after parenteral B_{12} administration. An elevation in serum methylmalonic acid is both a sensitive and specific indication of cellular B_{12} deficiency. Awareness of this phenomenon is particularly important, since it is now clear that atrophic gastritis, an asymptomatic condition that affects approximately 30% of the elderly population, frequently produces a modest decrease in B_{12} absorption.

Table 192–11 lists several examples of biochemical functions of vitamins that have only recently been identified. As nutritional science proceeds with defining the clinical significance of each of these new roles, and determines what quantities of each vitamin are necessary to optimize such functions, redefinition of the desirable range of vitamin status may well occur.

TABLE 192–11. NEWLY IDENTIFIED ROLES FOR VITAMINS

Vitamin or Provitamin	Classic Role(s)	New Role(s)
β-Carotene	Provitamin A	Antioxidant, free radical scavenger, cell-cell gap junction modulation
Niacin	NAD/NADP coenzyme	Reduction of LDL, and elevation of HDL, cholesterol
Folate	Hemopoietic factor	Diminishes homocysteinemia, incidence of neural tube defects
Vitamin A	Transduction of visual input in retina	Induction and maintenance of epithelial differentiation, maintenance of cell-mediated immunity, morphogenetic signal in embryogenesis
Vitamin D	Regulator of calcium, phosphate metabolism	Modulates epithelial proliferation and promotes differentiation
Vitamin B₆	Coenzyme for transamination	Modulation of steroid activity
Vitamin C	Hydroxylation coenzyme	Antioxidant

Sauberlich H, Machlin L (eds.): Beyond Deficiency: New Views on the Function and Health Effects of Vitamins. Ann NY Acad Sci 1992, vol. 669. *Excellent collection of discussions pertaining to new perspectives on functions of vitamins and how these perspectives impact on the definition of deficiency.*

Shils M, Olson J, Shike M (eds.): Modern Nutrition in Health and Disease, 8th ed. Malvern, Pa, Lea & Febiger, 1994, vol. 1. *Comprehensive, up-to-date reviews of biochemistry, physiology, and nutrition of each micronutrient.*

193 NUTRITIONAL ASSESSMENT
Bruce R. Bistrian

Nutritional assessment in clinical medicine has three primary goals: to identify the presence and type of malnutrition, to define health-threatening obesity, and to devise suitable diets as prophylaxis against disease later in life. The focus of this chapter is on the diagnosis of protein energy malnutrition (PEM) because of its wide prevalence and major impact on disease outcome. Other deficiency diseases are of much less relevance, since most occur in conjunction with PEM or with specific disease states such as thiamine deficiency with alcoholic liver disease, or fat-soluble vitamin deficiency with malabsorptive states. The classic deficiency diseases, either primary or secondary, are considered elsewhere in this volume. The widespread availability of parenteral and enteral therapeutic measures over the past decade that can provide adequate feeding regimens in virtually any disease condition make a rudimentary knowledge of the pathophysiology of PEM and its nutritional assessment essential for all primary care practitioners. (See Ch. 194.)

CLINICAL NUTRITIONAL ASSESSMENT

The clinical assessment of protein nutritional status is based principally on clinical history, simple anthropometry, and measurements of the levels of several secretory proteins. Although detailed dietary assessment can at times be helpful, in most circumstances physicians can safely limit their diet questions to whether patients have been following a prescribed diet and how much alcohol they drink. In ambulatory patients the ability to maintain usual and adequate weight generally indicates that serious micronutrient deficiency is not likely due to dietary inadequacy. Isolated vitamin deficiencies in the absence of weight loss or symptoms are rare, except perhaps for folate and B_{12}. Although nutritional anemias do exist, the role of dietary deficiency in folic acid or vitamin B_{12}-related anemias is minimal in the absence of underlying disease or weight loss. Only iron deficiency is a reasonable cause as a dietary anemia. By contrast, full dietary assessment and diet prescriptions are likely to help conditions such as fat malabsorption accompanied by weight loss, cramps, or diarrhea. Such evaluations are most effectively carried out by dietitians. Thus, detailed nutritional assessment of PEM with secondary assessment of vitamin and mineral deficiencies usually is needed only when PEM or a specific disorder known to interfere with nutrient metabolism, such as celiac disease, pernicious anemia, or nutrient-drug interactions, coexists. Even then the assessment should emphasize the likely deficiencies. For fat malabsorption, one should check levels of the fat-soluble vitamins, A, D, E, and K as well as important divalent and trivalent cations (Ca^{tt}, Zn^{tt}, Mg^{tt}, Fe^{ttt}). When ileal resection has occurred, serum B_{12} levels should be measured. Weight loss due to short gut syndrome should prompt assessment of the fat-soluble vitamins, folic acid, vitamin B_{12}, calcium, magnesium, zinc, and iron. Measurements of body water status (BUN, creatinine, serum sodium) and acid-base balance (CO_2 combining power, chloride, potassium, urine, and arterial pH) should be obtained if the diarrhea is profuse.

Clinically obvious marasmus and hypoalbuminemic malnutrition affect 25 to 50% of patients hospitalized for acute care. Many of these patients can benefit from nutritional support and require a thorough clinical nutritional assessment, including dietary history, physical examination, and laboratory tests that serve to confirm clinical impressions. The history should list information about the timing and amount of weight loss, medical illnesses, medications, gastrointestinal symptoms (abdominal pain, diarrhea, dysphagia), diet habits (eating fewer than two meals a day, alcohol consumption, dental status), social habits (eats alone, needs assistance in self-care), economic status (enough money for food), and mental status, particularly the presence of depressive symptoms. A special focus should be reserved for the elderly in whom PEM due to these last factors is more common.

WEIGHT LOSS

A recent unintended weight loss of 10 pounds should prompt efforts to diagnose the underlying disorder or social circumstance. Weight loss alone does not distinguish the composition of tissue loss, which can range from 25 to 30% lean tissue in semistarvation to 50% lean tissue loss following starvation plus injury. Therefore, unintentional weight loss of more than 10 pounds indicates a need for thorough nutritional assessment. Weight loss in excess of 10% of usual weight should be considered to represent PEM that will impair physiologic function, particularly muscle strength and endurance. Weight loss in excess of 20% should be considered severe PEM that will substantially impair most organ systems. If major elective surgery is planned, such individuals would likely benefit from adequate feeding preoperatively. If palliative or curative radiotherapy or systemic chemotherapy is planned, adequate feeding during therapy by use of supplemental formulas, tube feeding, or parenteral nutrition (in that order) is indicated. However, if the weight loss represents end-stage systemic illness (e.g., cancer, end-stage liver disease, AIDS) for which no primary therapy is planned or effective, invasive nutritional support is rarely indicated.

PHYSICAL EXAMINATION

Although the patient's external appearance and a check of his or her skin, eyes, mouth, hair, and nails often provide a clue to the presence of nutritional abnormalities (Table 193–1), the physical findings of deficiency syndromes of vitamins, essential fatty acids, and trace metals are relatively insensitive and nonspecific. With respect to PEM, only the marasmic form of semistarvation is evident at examination. Loss of subcutaneous fat and skeletal muscle is manifested by sunken temples, thin extremities, wasting of the muscles of the hand, and rarely edema. While kwashiorkor in children is characterized by severe edema, and a pot-belly appearance due to hepatomegaly and ascites, one rarely encounters these clinical signs in hypoalbuminemic malnutrition.

The most useful element in the physical examination is body weight, which is expressed as a relative value to evaluate the patient in relation to the healthy population. Weight and height are easily obtained and there are established standards for comparison (Table 193–2). Although newer standards are available, they reflect the increasing prevalence of obesity in the U.S. population. Use of the 1959 standards allows the same tables to be used to diagnose significant PEM (less than 85% desirable weight, which approximates the 5th percentile) and significant obesity defined as incurring excessive mortality risk (greater than 130% desirable weight). Although severe PEM will often occur at levels greater than 85% desirable weight, this generally will be detected by percent weight loss or upper arm anthropometry. Height can be measured in the reclining patient by using a tape measure, and in certain situations patient history may be relied upon. The major confounding variable that limits the value of weight and height as an index of PEM is the tendency for water retention with disease, and thus weight gain may not reflect an increase in lean body mass or protein content. Fluid retention is particularly a problem with hypoalbuminemic malnutrition because of the effects of aldosterone, antidiuretic hormone, and insulin stimulated by the stress response to cause sodium and fluid retention. Fluid retention, however, is not common on presentation to the physician's office or initially to the hospital except in diseases such as cardiac failure, end-stage liver disease, and severe renal disease.

TABLE 193–1. DESIRABLE WEIGHT IN POUNDS IN RELATION TO HEIGHT FOR ADULT MEN AND WOMEN, 25 YEARS OR OLDER*

Men Medium Frame				Women Medium Frame			
Height Ft.	In.	Range	Midpoint	Height Ft.	In.	Range	Midpoint
				4	8	93–104	98.5
				4	9	95–107	101
				4	10	98–110	104
				4	11	101–113	107
				5	0	104–116	110
5	1	113–124	118.5	5	1	107–119	113
5	2	116–128	122	5	2	110–123	116.5
5	3	119–131	125	5	3	113–127	120
5	4	122–134	128	5	4	117–132	124.5
5	5	125–138	131.5	5	5	121–136	128.5
5	6	129–142	135.5	5	6	125–140	132.5
5	7	133–147	140	5	7	129–144	136.5
5	8	137–151	144	5	8	133–148	140.5
5	9	141–155	148	5	9	137–152	144.5
5	10	145–160	153	5	10	141–156	148.5
5	11	149–165	157				
6	0	153–170	161.5				
6	1	157–175	166				
6	2	162–180	171				
6	3	167–185	176				

Adapted from the Metropolitan Life Insurance Company Statistical Bulletin 40:1, 1959.
* Corrected to nude weights and heights by assuming 1-inch heel for men, 2-inch heel for women, and indoor clothing weight of 5 and 3 pounds for men and women, respectively.

TABLE 193-2. CLINICAL SIGNS AND SYMPTOMS OF NUTRITIONAL INADEQUACY IN ADULT PATIENTS

	Clinical Sign or Symptom	Nutrient
General	Wasted, skinny	Calorie
	Loss of appetite	Protein-energy
Skin	Psoriasiform rash, eczematous scaling	Zinc, vitamin A, EFA
	Pallor	Folate, iron, vitamin B_{12}, copper
	Follicular hyperkeratosis	Vitamin A, vitamin C
	Perifollicular petechiae	Vitamin C
	Flaking dermatitis	Protein-energy, niacin, riboflavin, zinc
	Bruising	Vitamin C, vitamin K
	Pigmentation changes	Niacin, protein-energy
	Scrotal dermatosis	Riboflavin
	Thickening and dryness of skin	Linoleic acid
Head	Temporal muscle wasting	Protein-energy
Hair	Sparse and thin, dyspigmentation	Protein
	Easy to pull out	Protein
	Corkscrew hairs	Vitamin C
Eyes	History of night blindness (also impaired visual recovery after glare)	Vitamin A, zinc
	Photophobia, blurring, conjunctival inflammation	Riboflavin, vitamin A
	Corneal vascularization	Riboflavin
	Xerosis, Bitot spots, keratomalacia	Vitamin A
Mouth	Glossitis	Riboflavin, niacin, folic acid, vitamin B_{12}, pyridoxine
	Bleeding gums	Vitamin C, riboflavin
	Cheilosis	Riboflavin, pyridoxine, niacin
	Angular stomatitis	Riboflavin, pyridoxine, niacin
	Hypogeusia	Zinc
	Tongue fissuring	Niacin
	Tongue atrophy	Riboflavin, niacin, iron
	Nasolabial seborrhea	Pyridoxine
Neck	Goiter	Iodine
	Parotid enlargement	Protein
Thorax	Thoracic rosary	Vitamin D
Abdomen	Diarrhea	Niacin, folate, vitamin B_{12}
	Distention	Protein-energy
	Hepatomegaly	Protein-energy
Extremities	Edema	Protein, thiamine
	Softening of bone	Vitamin D, calcium, phosphorus
	Bone tenderness	Vitamin D
	Bone ache, joint pain	Vitamin C
	Muscle wasting and weakness	Protein, calorie, vitamin D, selenium, sodium chloride
	Muscle tenderness, muscle pain	Thiamine
Nails	Spooning	Iron
	Transverse lines	Protein
Neurologic	Tetany	Calcium, magnesium
	Paresthesias	Thiamine, vitamin B_{12}
	Loss of reflexes, wrist drop, foot drop	Thiamine
	Loss of vibratory and position sense	Vitamin B_{12}
	Ataxia	Vitamin B_{12}
	Dementia, disorientation	Niacin
Blood	Anemia	Vitamin B_{12}, folate, iron, pyridoxine
	Hemolysis	Phosphorus, vitamin E

Modified from Russel RM: Nutritional assessment. *In* Wyngaarten JB, Smith LH Jr, Bennett JC: Cecil Textbook of Medicine, 19th ed. Philadelphia, 1992, WB Saunders, pp 1151–1155.

The body mass index (BMI), which is the weight in kilograms divided by the height in meters squared, has recently gained favor as a nutritional measure because of two valuable attributes. The measure is relatively independent of height, and the same standards apply to males and females. Normal nutrition is defined as a BMI of 18 to 25 with significant obesity defined as a BMI > 28. Evidence from less developed countries suggests the BMI is better correlated with outcome than weight/height.

UPPER ARM ANTHROPOMETRY

Approximately 50% of body fat is subcutaneous. The use of skinfold calipers to define the triceps skinfold is the most practical technique to estimate body fat. Standards for skinfold measurements are available from the Health and Nutrition Examination Survey (HANES I and II), which were derived from a probability sample of the U.S. population. Generally less than the 5th percentile is used to define abnormality (Table 193-3). The principal value of the triceps skinfold (TSF) is to determine the arm muscle circumference (AMC) or arm muscle area.

$$AMC(cm) = \text{Arm Circumference} - \frac{(\pi)\,(\text{TSF in mm})}{10}$$

The arm muscle circumference is a specific measure of PEM if the 5th or 10th percentile is chosen as the cutoff point and is particularly valuable in edematous states or in amputees in whom weights are inaccurate or insensitive. The triceps skinfold and arm muscle circumference measurements are most useful in initial defining of marasmic-type malnutrition or the mixed disorder. Nearly all dietitians are skilled in upper arm anthropometry.

SERUM PROTEINS

Despite many concerns, the serum albumin level remains the traditional standard for nutritional assessment by virtue of its extensive history and its continued use to separate the two principal forms of PEM. Hypoalbuminemia is a strong predictor of risk for morbidity and mortality in both hospitalized and ambulatory patients. In almost all cases, except perhaps for hereditary analbuminemia, excessive loss due to nephrosis, and occasionally in protein-losing enteropathy, hypoalbuminemia identifies the injury response and thus the presence of an illness with the accompanying effects of anorexia and depression of immune function. Given the half-life for albumin of 18 to 20 days and the fractional replacement rate of about 10% per day, the return of serum albumin to normal takes about 2 weeks of feeding when the stress response remits. Levels of other proteins such as transferrin, prealbumin, and

TABLE 193-3. 5TH, 10TH, AND 50TH PERCENTILE FOR TRICEPS SKINFOLD (TSF) AND MID UPPER ARM MUSCLE CIRCUMFERENCE (MUAMC) OF AMERICAN MEN AND WOMEN FROM THE NHANES I SURVEY

Age Group	MUAMC (cm) Percentile			TSF (mm) Percentile		
	5TH	10TH	50TH	5TH	10TH	50TH
Male						
18–24	23.8	24.8	27.9	4.5	6.0	11.0
18–24	23.5	24.4	27.2	4.0	5.0	9.5
25–34	24.2	25.3	28.0	4.5	5.5	12.0
35–44	25.0	25.6	28.7	5.0	6.0	12.0
45–54	26.0	26.9	28.1	5.0	6.0	11.0
55–64	22.8	26.4	27.9	5.0	6.0	11.0
65–74	22.5	23.7	26.9	4.5	5.5	11.0
Female						
18–24	13.4	19.0	21.8	11.0	13.0	22.0
18–24	17.7	18.5	20.6	9.4	11.0	18.0
25–34	18.3	18.9	21.4	10.5	12.0	21.0
35–44	18.5	19.2	22.0	12.0	14.0	23.0
45–54	18.8	19.5	22.2	13.0	15.0	25.0
55–64	18.6	19.5	22.6	11.0	14.0	25.0
65–74	18.6	19.5	22.5	11.5	14.0	23.0

From Bishop CW, Bowen PE, Ritchey SJ: Norms for nutritional assessment of American adults by upper arm anthropometry. Am J. Clin. Nutr. 34:2530, 1981.

retinol-binding protein with respective half-lives of 7 days, 2 days, and ½ day also fall acutely with injury and respond more quickly when stress remits. However, serum transferrin also varies with iron status, and prealbumin and retinol-binding protein vary with dietary carbohydrate and renal function. As a result, these proteins do not identify the presence and severity of the stress response any better than albumin.

NUTRITIONAL THERAPY AND ITS ASSESSMENT

The same indices that are used in the baseline nutritional assessment can be used to assess response to therapy, provided certain points are kept in mind. In the stressed, hospitalized patient receiving nutrition, day-to-day weight changes generally reflect shifts in fluid balance rather than energy balance. In the ambulatory setting, weight increases or decreases are most likely to reflect changes in protein nutritional status and body fat, because the underlying illness is usually less severe. Even the most sensitive research methods for assessing changes in lean body mass, however, do not offer major improvements in diagnosis in the more seriously ill. Techniques that measure total body water such as isotope dilution and underwater weighing, from which lean tissue is extrapolated, fail to account for the distortion in hydration of lean tissue with illness. Surrogate measures of total body protein to estimate lean tissues such as total body potassium measurement do not adjust for differing potassium/nitrogen ratios with disease. A newer method, multifrequency body impedance, does show promise as a simple, accurate, noninvasive method that may allow distinction between intracellular and extracellular water, with the former used to estimate lean tissue.

In the unstressed patient with marasmus, appropriate protein and calorie intake should cause a positive nitrogen balance of 2 to 6 grams per day (60 to 180 grams lean tissue) and slow weight gain depending on the positive energy balance. For instance, a 300 kilocalorie excess of intake over expenditure would provide approximately 120 grams of lean tissue (100 kilocalorie equivalent) plus 200 kilocalories (22 grams) as fat for a total of 140 grams or about ⅓ pound of weight per day. Weight gains in excess of this probably reflect sodium and water retention due to the insulin stimulated by dietary carbohydrate. Such overhydration can be improved by reducing salt and limiting fluid intake. In patients with hypoalbuminemic malnutrition who are no longer stressed, a similar nutritional regimen will lead to a comparable gain of tissue, but weight change may vary as edema becomes mobilized, with normalization in serum albumin in 2 to 4 weeks. In stressed patients with hypoalbuminemic malnutrition, appropriate nutritional support will often not restore lean tissue but will improve other important functions such as wound healing and immune competence. Both the stress response and the limited activity level reduce the efficiency of skeletal muscle repletion, which represents 30% of body weight and 75% of actively metabolizing lean tissue. Functional testing of muscle strength and endurance such as hand dynamometry may prove useful as assessment tools in the future. Similarly, any reduction of other physiologic function or impairment in performing the usual activities of daily living will accentuate PEM.

Although caloric expenditure can now be reliably and easily measured with portable indirect calorimeters, estimated energy expenditures are sufficient in most clinical situations. The three components of total energy expenditure (TEE) are basal energy expenditure (about 55 to 65% of TEE), thermal effect of feeding (about 10% of TEE), and activity energy expenditure (the remainder). An energy intake of 30 to 35 kilocalories per kilogram of body weight will maintain most sedentary ambulatory patients, with adjustments upward or downward in 200- to 300-kilocalorie increments as prompted by biweekly changes in weight. Although young, severely burned or traumatized patients may require 35 to 40 kilocalories per kilogram in the acute phase to meet TEE, most postoperative patients who require invasive nutritional support for mechanical or infectious complications need no more than 30 kilocalories per kilogram because of their older age and reduced activity energy expenditure. Overfeeding should be avoided in such patients.

Daley BJ, Bistrian BR: Nutritional assessment. *In* Zaloga G (ed.): Nutrition in Critical Care. St Louis, CV Mosby, 1993, pp 9–33. *Discusses etiologic factors in development of protein-caloric malnutrition (PCM) and nutritional assessment methods.*

Functional tests of PCM and indirect calorimetry are adjunctive measures of nutritional status.

Hill G: Body composition research: Implications for the practice of clinical nutrition. JPEN 16:197, 1992. *Superb presentation of clinical nutritional assessment in critically ill patients evaluated in terms of functional indices, protein kinetic studies, and basic body composition techniques of in vivo neutron activation analysis and labeled water.*

McMahon MM, Bistrian BR: Anthropometric assessment of nutritional status in hospitalized patients. *In* Himes JH (ed.): Anthropometric Assessment of Nutritional Status. New York, Wiley-Liss, 1991, pp 365–381. *Discusses in detail the value of upper arm anthropometry and creatinine excretion in nutritional assessment.*

194 PROTEIN-ENERGY MALNUTRITION
Robert B. Baron

Protein-energy malnutrition (PEM) occurs when inadequate protein and/or calories are ingested to meet an individual's nutritional requirements. PEM may be primary, as a result of inadequate food intake, or secondary, as a result of illness. In developing nations, PEM is most often primary and affects predominantly infants and children. It is the most important nutritional disorder and one of the developing world's most important health problems. In industrialized nations, PEM is most often secondary to other diseases and affects both children and adults. In North America and Europe, 28 to 80% of hospitalized patients have been reported to have secondary PEM. This chapter emphasizes clinical features of secondary PEM as seen in industrialized nations.

Pathogenesis

Secondary PEM is caused by decreased intake of calories and protein, increased nutrient losses, or increased nutrient requirements (Table 194–1). It can develop slowly owing to chronic illness or chronic semistarvation or rapidly owing to acute illness.

In uncomplicated starvation and semistarvation, metabolism adapts to reduce the breakdown of lean body mass. Fat and fat-derived fuels gradually replace glucose as the major energy source. During the initial phase of a complete fast, glucose requirements for the brain, bone marrow, renal medulla, and peripheral nerves are provided by glycogen. Glycogen stores, however, last for only 12 to 24 hours. As glucose levels decline, insulin levels also decline and glucagon levels increase. Amino acids, particularly alanine, are released by muscle. Hepatic gluconeogenesis from amino acids provides glucose for the central nervous system and other glycolytic tissues. The changes in insulin and glucagon also favor lipolysis. Mobilized fatty acids provide the fuel for the remaining tissues. By the second week of a complete fast, fatty acids are less completely oxidized and more of them form ketone bodies. Ketones become the primary energy source for the brain and reduce the need for glucose. The muscles catabolize less protein and release less alanine, thus conserving their protein content.

TABLE 194–1. CAUSES OF PROTEIN-ENERGY MALNUTRITION IN HOSPITALIZED PATIENTS

Decreased Oral Intake	
Anorexia	Poverty
Nausea	Old age
Dysphagia	Social isolation
Pain	Substance abuse
Gastrointestinal obstruction	Depression
Poor dentition	
Increased Nutrient Losses	
Malabsorption	Nephrosis
Diarrhea	Fistula drainage
Bleeding	Protein-losing enteropathy
Glycosuria	
Increased Nutrient Requirements	
Fever	Trauma
Infection	Burns
Neoplasms	Medications
Surgery	

Adaptation also decreases the body's total energy requirement, by as much as 40% in severe chronic undernutrition. Absolute requirements decrease as body weight diminishes owing to a decrease in body mass. More importantly, however, energy requirements also decrease per unit of body mass. Both ingested food and circulating endogenous substrates are utilized more efficiently. More endogenous amino acids, for example, are utilized for protein synthesis than for oxidation. In addition, virtually all of the body's biochemical and physiologic processes are curtailed. Less energy is expended for the sodium-potassium pump, protein turnover, temperature regulation, the inflammatory response, and the function of most body organs during chronic undernutrition.

During a severe acute illness, hormonal and inflammatory responses prevent this adaptation to starvation and result in changes in protein and energy metabolism that can rapidly lead to PEM (Table 194–2). Circulating levels of the catecholamines, glucocorticoids, glucagon, and growth hormone are all increased. Although necessary to mediate the body's response to physical stress, these hormonal and inflammatory changes result in marked increases in energy expenditure, nitrogen loss, gluconeogenesis, and the failure of ketoadaptation. In this manner, changes in body composition, including depletion of protein and fat stores, may occur rapidly. Several other compounds mediate the systemic response to inflammation, including cytokines such as tumor necrosis factor, interleukin (IL)-1, IL-2, IL-6, interferon-γ, and lipid mediators such as platelet-activating factor, thromboxane A_2, leukotriene B_4 and prostaglandin E_2. Complex interconnections relate hormones, cytokines, and lipid mediators and are only partially understood. Rather than a simple cascade, mediators may respond variably to different stimuli; some with overlapping effects may be initiated simultaneously, whereas others may be interconnected by amplification and feedback loops.

The resting metabolic expenditure (RME) may increase significantly during the response to illness. In burns involving greater than 40% of the body surface area, for example, the RME may double. In other critical illnesses such as trauma or sepsis, the RME typically increases by 20 to 50%. Nitrogen losses also typically increase by 20 to 100%. During the response to illness, skeletal muscles release amino acids at an accelerated rate. These can then be metabolized for energy or shifted to the liver or other visceral organs, where their need for protein synthesis is more immediate. During prolonged illness and continued energy and protein deficiency, however, depletion of visceral protein also occurs and can lead to functional impairment of body organs.

Physiologic Consequences

Virtually every organ and organ system of the body can undergo marked morphologic and functional changes during protein-energy malnutrition.

BODY WEIGHT. The most obvious manifestation of chronic PEM is loss of body weight. Most patients can tolerate a loss of 5% to 10% without significant consequences, but losses greater than 40% below ideal weight are almost always fatal. Both adipose tissue and the lean body mass are depleted, but losses of adipose tissue are greater. Extracellular water remains nearly constant, resulting in its relative increase. In severe PEM, the body's visceral organs also decrease in size. In experimental animals, for example, a 7-day fast results in a 40% decrease in liver mass, 28% decrease in the gastrointestinal tract, 20% decrease in the kidneys, and 17% decrease in cardiac mass. During acute PEM caused by critical illness, changes in body weight and adipose stores may be less marked despite changes in organ morphology and function. Many patients may actually gain weight owing to retention of sodium and body water.

HEART. Severe PEM results in both quantitative and qualitative changes in the heart. In the "Minnesota Experiment," in which 32 male volunteers were semistarved for 6 months, a 24% decrease in body weight was associated with an 18% decrease in cardiac stroke volume and a 38% decrease in cardiac index. Animal studies have demonstrated similar findings, as well as decreases in left ventricular contractility and compliance, decreased myocardial glycogen, myofibrillar atrophy, and interstitial edema. These changes are reversed with nutritional repletion.

LUNG. The lung parenchyma is minimally affected during PEM, but marked changes in pulmonary function can occur as a result of the loss of mass and strength of the muscles of breathing. In the Minnesota Experiment, vital capacity, tidal volume, and minute volume declined by 8%, 19%, and 30%, respectively, after 24 weeks of semistarvation. The ventilatory response to hypoxia is also decreased during semistarvation, but the clinical significance of this is unclear.

GASTROINTESTINAL TRACT. During severe PEM, gastric motility slows and gastric acid secretion decreases. The most significant effects of PEM on the luminal gastrointestinal tract affect the small intestine. Total small bowel mass decreases, primarily owing to mucosal atrophy and loss of villi. Lymphocytic infiltration of surface epithelial cells can occur, and epithelial cell renewal slows down. Both disaccharidase enzyme activity and the rate of absorption of amino acids decline. Although pancreatic endocrine activity is spared, exocrine insufficiency can accompany severe PEM. Similar changes in the gastrointestinal tract are observed in individuals fed exclusively with parenteral nutrition, suggesting that stimulation of the gut by intraluminal nutrients is necessary for normal structure and function.

LIVER. In typical secondary PEM, liver mass decreases but its histology remains normal. Fat, protein, and glycogen are depleted, but the number of hepatocytes is preserved. In contrast, children with severe, primary protein deficiency resulting in kwashiorkor have enlarged livers with fatty infiltration and excess glycogen. In both instances, serum levels of albumin and other serum transport proteins commonly go down owing to diminished hepatic synthesis.

KIDNEY. Renal mass decreases during PEM, but histology remains normal. Renal function is well preserved except for an impaired concentrating ability due to a lowering of the medullary osmotic gradient.

ENDOCRINE. The endocrine response to PEM is complex and affected by the extent of concurrent illnesses, as discussed above. Serum thyroxine typically falls to the lower limits of normal or slightly below. Peripheral conversion of thyroxine (T_4) to triiodothyronine (T_3) is commonly decreased, favoring the conversion to reverse triiodothyronine. Serum TSH and the TSH response to TRH remain unaltered. Gonadal hormones are also affected. In men, testosterone levels are decreased and LH and FSH levels are appropriately increased. In women, gonadotropin release is depressed despite low levels of circulating estrogens.

IMMUNOLOGIC FUNCTION. Severe PEM importantly affects the immune system. Virtually all components of the immune system are adversely affected in rough proportion to the degree of nutritional impairment. Peripheral blood lymphocyte counts commonly decline to values often < 1200 per cubic millimeter. Both the percentage of T cells and T-cell functions are depressed. Skin tests for delayed hypersensitivity reactions often become nonreactive, and lymphocyte responses weaken to phytohemagglutinin and poke weed mitogens.

Humoral immunity is affected in a more variable fashion. Specific antibody responses are depressed in some instances and preserved in others. For example, antibody production following administration of poliovirus, tetanus, diphtheria, measles, and pneumococcal polysaccharide antigens remains normal, whereas impaired responses follow the administration of yellow fever and

TABLE 194–2. PHYSIOLOGIC COMPARISON OF UNCOMPLICATED STARVATION AND SEVERE CATABOLIC ILLNESS

Physiologic Characteristics	Uncomplicated Starvation	Catabolic Illness
Catecholamines	Decreased	Increased
Glucagon	Decreased	Increased
Cortisol	Decreased	Increased
Insulin	Decreased	Increased
Cytokines	Variable	Increased
Metabolic rate	Decreased	Increased
Proteolysis	Decreased	Increased
Gluconeogenesis	Decreased	Increased
Nitrogen excretion	Decreased	Increased
Fatty acid utilization	Increased	Increased
Adaptation to starvation	Present	Absent

Adapted from Weinsier RD, Heimburger DC, Butterworth CE: Handbook of Clinical Nutrition. 2nd ed. St. Louis, CV Mosby, 1989.

influenza A vaccines. In some instances, the affinities and binding capacity of antibodies are reduced.

Slight neutropenia may occur during PEM but the usual concurrent bacterial infections cause leukocytosis. Neutrophils are normal morphologically, but some measures of neutrophil function, including chemotaxis and bacterial killing, are abnormal. Phagocytosis is usually normal.

Levels of individual complement components, other than C4, and total serum hemolytic complement activity are commonly decreased. Other nonspecific host defense mechanisms, including interferon production, opsonization, and plasma lysozyme production, may also be adversely affected by protein-calorie undernutrition. Acute phase reactants such as C-reactive proteins, α_2-macroglobulin, α_1-antitrypsin, and haptoglobin tend to be elevated. Changes in the body's anatomic barriers to infection, including atrophy of the skin and gastrointestinal mucosa, may contribute to an increased risk of infection.

It is not possible to define the exact mechanisms of enhanced susceptibility to infections observed with PEM. Each of the abnormalities of the immune response probably contributes in part. Micronutrient deficiencies may occur concurrently with PEM and can also cause significant abnormalities in the immune response.

WOUND HEALING. Almost all aspects of wound healing are adversely affected in patients with severe PEM. Neovascularization, fibroblast proliferation, collagen synthesis, and wound remodeling are delayed. Local factors, such as edema associated with hypoalbuminemia and micronutrient deficiencies, may contribute to poor wound healing in undernourished patients. In mild PEM, however, wound healing is relatively well-preserved despite negative nitrogen balance. Even during complete starvation, endogenous substrates can be effectively utilized for collagen synthesis during the early phases of wound healing.

Clinical Manifestations

The diverse clinical manifestations of PEM range from mild growth retardation and weight loss to several distinct clinical syndromes. This diversity reflects differences in the relative degree of protein and energy deficiency, the cause of the deficiency, the severity and duration of the deficiency, the age of the patient, and the association of other illnesses or nutritional deficiencies. In children in the developing world with severe PEM, for example, the classic syndromes of kwashiorkor (predominant protein deficiency) and marasmus (predominant energy deficiency) may develop. Marasmic kwashiorkor and intermediate syndrome may be seen when protein deficiency develops in combination with chronic energy deficiency.

KWASHIORKOR. Children with severe kwashiorkor commonly have a decreased blood pressure, bradycardia, and hypothermia. Body weight is usually low but may be normal owing to edema and anasarca. Affected children are characteristically apathetic, lethargic, and anorectic. They may move about little, or not at all. Their skins develop a "flaky paint" dermatitis with dry, hyperpigmented, hyperkeratotic lesions over the face, extremities, and perineum. The hair is typically sparse, dry, and brittle and may be reddish or yellowish. The abdomen is distended owing to hepatomegaly and ascites. The extremities are commonly wasted and edematous. Clinical signs of concurrent micronutrient deficiency may also be present (see Ch. 192.2).

The serum albumin typically falls below 2.8 grams per deciliter with a lymphocyte count less than 1200 cells per cubic millimeter. A mild anemia is common; it is usually normochromic and normocytic unless other deficiencies coexist. The serum transferrin usually declines but may be normal or slightly elevated if iron deficiency coexists. Other serum transport proteins, including prealbumin and retinol-binding protein, decrease. Serum glucose and lipids likewise go down. Serum levels of liver enzymes most often remain normal and may be low. Blood urea nitrogen and urinary urea nitrogen are low. Fluid and electrolyte disorders are common, particularly hypokalemia, hypophosphatemia, and a hyperchloremic metabolic acidosis.

MARASMUS. Children with marasmus have less characteristic manifestations. Although their pulse, blood pressure, and body temperature may be low, they tend to be less apathetic and lethargic and to have a good appetite. Growth is retarded and the weight low. Muscle wasting is obvious, as is loss of body fat. Such children look emaciated, but have no edema. The skin is dry and loose with decreased turgor. The dermatitis of kwashiorkor is usually absent. The hair is thin, dry, and dull. The abdomen is thin without signs of hepatomegaly or edema. Typically, there are fewer laboratory abnormalities than in children with kwashiorkor. Serum albumin and other transport proteins are often normal. A mild anemia is common. Any of the other laboratory abnormalities of kwashiorkor may exist but usually are absent.

SECONDARY PROTEIN-ENERGY MALNUTRITION. The clinical manifestations of secondary PEM also vary considerably, in large part reflecting the associated illness that has caused the malnutrition, the nutritional status of the patient prior to the illness, and the rate at which it develops (Table 194–3). Marasmus-like secondary PEM typically results from chronic indolent diseases such as chronic obstructive pulmonary disease or cancer. Most patients experience a gradual wasting process that begins with weight loss and proceeds through stages of mild, moderate, and severe cachexia. In its most severe form, virtually all body fat stores disappear and muscle mass wastes away, most noticeably in the temporal and interosseous muscles. Laboratory studies may be relatively unremarkable. Serum albumin, for example, may be normal or slightly decreased, rarely decreasing to <2.8 grams per deciliter.

In contrast, kwashiorkor-like secondary PEM occurs primarily in association with acute life-threatening illnesses such as trauma, burns, and sepsis. Owing to the rapidity of onset, subcutaneous fat and muscle mass reflect the patient's baseline nutritional status and are typically normal or, if the patient is obese, increased. Serum proteins, however, typically decline with serum albumin <2.8 grams per deciliter. Dependent edema, ascites, and anasarca may be present and the hair may be easily pluckable. As with primary PEM, combinations of marasmus-like secondary PEM and kwashiorkor-like secondary PEM can occur simultaneously, typically in patients with indolent chronic diseases who develop a superimposed acute illness.

Diagnosis

The absence of distinct clinical manifestations can make the diagnosis of PEM difficult. A high index of suspicion based on the patient's risk factors for malnutrition, the overall clinical setting, and close observation is often necessary.

BODY WEIGHT. The most sensitive diagnostic measure is a documented history of weight loss, quantified as a percent of origi-

TABLE 194–3. COMPARISON OF SEVERE MARASMUS-LIKE AND KWASHIORKOR-LIKE SECONDARY PROTEIN-ENERGY MALNUTRITION

Syndrome	Clinical Setting	Time Course	Clinical Features	Laboratory Findings	Prognosis
Marasmus-like PEM	Chronic illness	Months	History of weight loss Muscle wasting Absent subcutaneous fat	Normal or mildly reduced serum proteins	Variable; depends on underlying disease
Kwashiorkor-like PEM	Acute, catabolic illness	Weeks	Normal fat and muscle Edema Easily pluckable hair	Serum albumin <2.8 g/dl	Poor

Adapted from Weinsier RL, Heimburger DC, Butterworth CE: Handbook of Clinical Nutrition. 2nd ed. St. Louis, CV Mosby, 1989.

nal body weight. Weight changes, however, may be obscured by edema. Some patients, particularly those with a severe acute illness such as sepsis, burns, or multiple trauma, can develop severe protein depletion rapidly without undergoing much weight loss. Nevertheless, most authors consider a 10% loss of body weight occurring during an acute illness to be clinically significant.

LABORATORY TESTS. Each of the clinical abnormalities affecting patients with severe PEM can be used as a diagnostic test to detect undernutrition. Most valuable are the serum albumin, other serum transport proteins such as transferrin, prealbumin, and retinol-binding protein, anergy to skin test antigens, total lymphocyte count, blood urea nitrogen, urinary excretion of creatinine, and anthropometric measures of body composition such as skinfold thickness and mid-arm muscle circumference. Each of these tests when abnormal has been shown to predict poor clinical outcomes in patients in a variety of clinical settings. It remains unclear whether the poor outcomes predicted by excessive weight loss or by abnormalities in these tests reflect the consequences of PEM or the severity of the underlying illness.

CLINICAL ASSESSMENT. A thorough, nutritionally focused history and physical examination can predict outcomes as well as can any of the above tests and indices. The history should examine recent reduction in dietary intake, changes in body weight, gastrointestinal symptoms, the underlying illness, and the patient's functional status. The physical examination should emphasize loss of subcutaneous fat, muscle wasting, volume status, and signs of micronutrient deficiencies (see Ch. 192.2). The initial clinical assessment is often equivocal; that is, the presence of clinically meaningful undernutrition is uncertain. In such cases, serial evaluations of the clinical examination, body weight, and laboratory parameters, as well as close observation of the patient's nutrient intake as a function of estimated requirements, are necessary to make the diagnosis of PEM.

Treatment

The goals of treatment of PEM are to provide adequate energy, protein, and micronutrients to restore body composition to normal and treat the underlying process that caused the deficiency.

STRATEGY. Treatment should proceed in two stages. In severe PEM, the first priority should be to correct fluid and electrolyte abnormalities and treat acute medical problems, especially infections. Although any combination of electrolyte and acid-base abnormalities can occur, most common are hypokalemia, hypocalcemia, hypophosphatemia, hypomagnesemia, and a hyperchloremic metabolic acidosis.

In the second phase one must provide adequate nutritional substrate to begin repletion. Nutrients should be provided gradually to prevent complications of overfeeding. In most adult patients no more than 0.8 gram of protein per kilogram and 30 Kcal per kilogram of actual body weight should be provided per day. As the patient's condition stabilizes, protein and energy intake can be increased to 35 to 40 Kcal per kilogram and 1.0 to 1.5 grams of protein per kilogram per day. Adequate micronutrients must be simultaneously provided. Patients with severe, life-threatening PEM should be fed even more cautiously.

ROUTE OF THERAPY. Nutrients can be provided either enterally or parenterally. Patients whose gastrointestinal tract is functioning and who can protect their airway should be fed enterally, either by mouth, feeding tube, or tube enterostomy. Patients with contraindications to enteral feeding can be given required nutrients parenterally via either peripheral or central veins (see Ch. 198). An algorithm for selecting the most appropriate method of nutritional support is shown in Figure 194–1.

REHABILITATION. Treating patients with PEM requires more than the provision of nutrients. Physical therapy and other measures to improve functional status are effective adjuncts to nutrition. Physical therapy may result in greater repletion of muscle mass and smaller adipose tissue stores than nutritional repletion without muscle contraction.

The most important non-nutritional factor in treatment is the resolution of the disease or social process that caused the PEM. In most instances, if the underlying process cannot be effectively treated, little benefit is derived from treating the patient's nutritional deficiencies. In particular, patients with terminal illnesses who become progressively malnourished as they near death will obtain little benefit from aggressive nutritional treatment. In these instances,

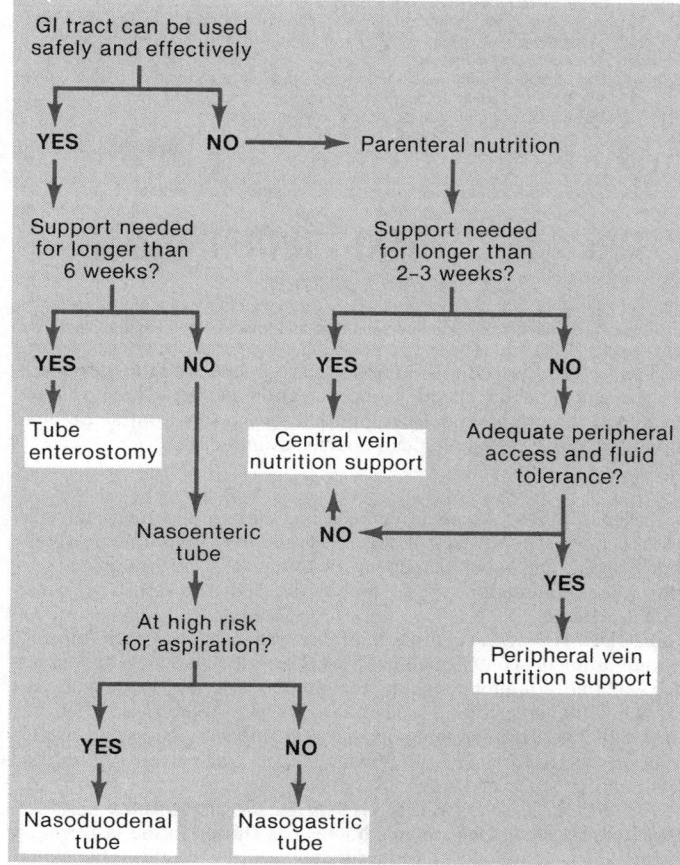

FIGURE 194–1. Decision tree concerning method of nutritional support.

such therapy can be withheld using the same criteria as for other life-sustaining treatments.

Prevention

In industrialized societies protein-calorie undernutrition is best prevented by the early identification of high-risk patients during admission to the hospital. Each such patient should be screened for predisposing risk factors (see Table 194–1). Patients at risk should receive more formal assessment of their nutritional status. Those identified early in the course of their illness, while PEM is still mild, can often be treated with noninvasive nutritional support, preventing the consequences of PEM and the complications of nutritional support. Patients who require prolonged hospitalization, including those in chronic care facilities, should be regularly re-evaluated for the development of new evidence of PEM.

The prevention of primary PEM in the developing world is much more complex and difficult. Poverty and underdevelopment are the primary causes of undernutrition in those areas. Although the direct transfer of food during periods of famine can be lifesaving, the development of agricultural techniques, food distribution systems, and other public health improvements is more important for the long-term prevention of PEM. The identification and early treatment of individual cases of protein-calorie undernutrition among children are also of great importance. Programs that monitor growth and development, that provide nutritional information and supplements to pregnant and lactating women, infants, and children, and that provide family planning and prenatal care are important measures. It is particularly important to abolish programs that distribute infant formulas and discourage traditional breast feeding practices.

Detsky AS, Smalley PS, Chang J: Is this patient malnourished? JAMA 271:54, 1994. *A systemic clinical approach for identifying patients with PEM.*
Hardin TC: Cytokine mediators of malnutrition: Clinical implications. Nutrition Clin Pract 8:55, 1993. *Practical review of current data suggesting that cytokines are important mediators of the metabolic changes associated with critical illness.*

Torun B, Chew F: Protein energy malnutrition. *In* Shils ME, Olson JA, Shike M (eds.): Modern Nutrition in Health and Disease. 8th ed. Malvern, PA, Lea & Febiger, 1994. *Comprehensive review of PEM with emphasis on prevention, pathophysiology, diagnosis, and treatment.*

Wilmore DW: Catabolic illness: Strategies for enhancing recovery. N Engl J Med 325:695, 1991. *Excellent discussion of the metabolic and nutritional events of critical illness and potential strategies for modifying them.*

195 THE EATING DISORDERS
Douglas A. Drossman

The eating disorders—anorexia nervosa and bulimia nervosa—attract much public attention and scientific inquiry. Diagnosis and treatment require an understanding that they result from a combination of biologic, psychological, and social influences.

ANOREXIA NERVOSA

DEFINITION. Anorexia nervosa is a chronic disorder characterized behaviorally by self-induced weight loss, psychologically by body-image and other perceptual disturbances, and biologically by physiologic alterations (e.g., amenorrhea) that result from nutritional depletion.

EPIDEMIOLOGY. Anorexia nervosa afflicts predominantly young, affluent white females (95%). The incidence may be increasing. In one community study the number of new cases per year over a 10-year period rose from 0.55 per 100,000 to 3.26 per 100,000. The disorder is associated with higher social class, occurring in up to 1 in 250 adolescent students in private school and with an incidence of 1%.

ETIOLOGY AND PATHOGENESIS. Sociocultural Factors. The cultural ideal for women's bodies has shifted in the last century from that of plumpness (formerly representing wealth, abundance, maternalism, and fertility) to a slimmer female image (representing independence, assertiveness, and success). Thinner women predominate on prime-time television and among beauty pageant contestants and high-fashion models. Social pressures from peers, particularly during adolescence, seem to influence young women and girls to engage in anorectic behaviors. These factors are probably not sufficient for the disorder to develop, but may create the proper environment for its expression in the predisposed individual. Recent studies also report an association of childhood sexual abuse history among patients with anorexia nervosa.

Psychological Factors. It is believed that anorectics have an incompletely developed personal identity and struggle to maintain a sense of control over their environment. Psychiatric interviews suggest that the patient develops within a family that values outward appearance, proper behavior, and achievement more than self-actualization. In response to parental expectations, the pre-anorectic child learns to be hard working, eager to please, and attentive to family needs. In turn, the parents support and indulge in the behaviors of their model child ("best little girl in the world"). Therefore, these actions are mutually reinforced, leading to interdependence among the family members (enmeshment). However, the high standards within the family are rarely achieved by the child, who obsessively struggles for parental approval.

It follows that "negative" childhood behaviors (e.g., assertiveness, rebellion) are not permitted. These behaviors are believed necessary for the development of individual identity. As a result, the pre-anorectic child comes to rely on externally imposed ideal values to maintain self-esteem, but at the expense of self-actualization and a sense of autonomy.

It is not surprising that a distressing period for the pre-anorectic child occurs during or soon after puberty, when physical, social, and psychological events (menarche, growth spurt, school, and adolescent peer pressure) encourage separation from the family and individuation. Over 80% of anorectic patients develop the disorder within 7 years of menarche. The compounded life events at this time are experienced with feelings of helplessness and ineffectiveness. The decision to diet, while not fully understood, may be a desperate attempt for control of one's body, at least, in a distressing new environment.

Biologic Factors. There is increased risk of anorexia nervosa among siblings (6%), with a four- to five-fold difference in concordance rates for monozygotic twins, suggesting a predisposing role for genetic factors. Also, there are more perinatal complications reported among anorexia nervosa patients. The higher birth weight and the increased prevalence of obesity preceding the onset of illness suggest that premorbid obesity is an influencing factor. Abnormalities in satiety, temperature regulation, and endocrine function suggest that a hypothalamic abnormality exists, although no specific lesion has been identified. It is more likely that the hypothalamus serves a modulating role. In the predisposed individual, the biologic and psychosocial events around the time of adolescence may produce neurotransmitter, endocrine, or immune changes via the hypothalamus, leading to the physiologic and behavioral changes characteristic of the disorder.

CLINICAL MANIFESTATIONS. There are no characteristic pathologic or physiologic findings, and no consistent psychiatric diagnosis is found. The consistency of the medical and behavioral features, however, argues for classifying the disorder as a clinical entity.

Psychological and Behavioral Features. **Pursuit of Thinness.** Patients are not truly anorectic, but struggle against hunger to achieve an unrealistic degree of weight loss. Interestingly, they are preoccupied with food and exhibit bizarre food preferences or elaborately prepare food for others. For most anorectics, weight loss is accomplished through dietary restriction and exercise (restrictor subgroup), although up to 50% will also self-induce vomiting or take purgatives (bulimic subgroup).

Perceptual Disturbances. Anorectics overestimate their body width, insisting they are too fat despite profound weight loss. Their assessment of the body habitus of others is not affected. Anorectics may also exhibit abnormalities in the perception of enteroceptive stimuli. They distort hunger awareness, deny fatigue, and fail to recognize emotional states such as anger and depression.

Sense of Ineffectiveness. Patients feel as though they are controlled by their environment and seem unable to function separately from family or other relationships. They gauge their responses to the expectations of others.

Cognitive Deficits. Patients may exhibit deficits in conceptual thought and abstract reasoning. They may be unable to view situations in anything but extremes, and they interpret events in a rigid and highly personalized form.

Medical Features. Most of the physical, metabolic, and endocrine abnormalities of anorexia nervosa are also seen in starvation secondary to the other conditions. The severity of the findings correlates with the nutritional state.

Physical Signs. Patients may have severe loss of subcutaneous fat and exhibit bony prominences. Core temperature, blood pressure, and pulse are decreased. Examination of the skin may reveal acrocyanosis, downy hair (lanugo), and yellow discoloration (hypercarotenemia). Elevated serum carotene and vitamin A levels are due either to excess intake of dietary carotenoids or to an acquired defect in the utilization or metabolism of these compounds. Secondary sexual features remain absent when anorexia develops before puberty.

Endocrine Abnormalities. *Gonadal.* The endocrine hallmark is gonadal dysfunction. Females develop amenorrhea, have decreased follicle-stimulating (FSH) and luteinizing hormone (LH), and do not exhibit secretory bursts of LH throughout the day in response to endogenous luteinizing hormone releasing factor (LH-RF). Normal menses usually recur with weight gain, when body fat content reaches 22%. Male anorectics lose libido and are infertile.

Thyroid. Clinical features, such as decreased vital signs, dry skin, constipation, cold intolerance, and a delayed ankle jerk, suggest hypothyroidism. T_3 levels tend to be low, with a corresponding increase in reverse T_3, the relatively inactive isomer of T_3. Under the stress of malnutrition, the liver preferentially deiodinates T_4 to rT_3. The clinical findings of mild hypothyroidism may arise from decreased availability of the more active T_3 isomer, which preferentially binds to the thyroid receptor. Free thyroxine, total T_4 levels, and the TSH response to TRH are normal. Clinically significant hypothyroidism does not occur, and treatment with exogenous thyroid is not indicated.

Adrenal. Anorectic patients usually have normal or slightly elevated plasma cortisol levels with decreased urinary excretion of 17-hydroxycorticosteroids. This is due to a decrease in the metabolic clearance of cortisol from plasma with an increase in cortisol-binding capacity. The 24-hour cortisol production rate and basal ACTH secretion are normal. The response to ACTH stimulation may be increased, and the response to metyrapone stimulation is normal. Decreased libido and delayed virilization in males may reflect a shift of androgen metabolism from the 5α-reductase enzyme system (yielding testosterone and its congeners) to the 5β-reductase system, producing the weaker androgen etiocholanolone.

Growth Hormone. Human growth hormone (hGH) levels are normal or slightly elevated. Concurrently there is a decrease in somatomedin levels. This growth-promoting peptide is produced by the liver and other tissues under the influence of hGH. Somatomedin mediates the anabolic effects of hGH but not its lipolytic effects. Thus, anorectic patients and other malnourished individuals maintain their adipose tissue breakdown (increased hGH) without growth effects.

Cardiovascular Abnormalities. Cardiovascular function deteriorates with decreased cardiac O_2 consumption, left ventricular wall thickness, cardiac chamber size, and blood pressure. These are adaptive responses to malnutrition and decreased catecholamine levels. Electrocardiographic changes include bradycardia, decreased QRS amplitude, prolonged QT interval, nonspecific ST segment changes, and U waves. Patients may also develop arrhythmias (tachycardia, sinus arrest, and ectopic atrial, junctional, or ventricular rhythms) due either to the primary disorder or to metabolic disturbances secondary to purgation. Sudden death has been reported among severely emaciated patients.

Hematologic Findings. Leukopenia and decreased white cell function, anemia, thrombocytopenia, and hypocomplementemia may occur. Anorectic patients do not seem to have a greater susceptibility to infection, however.

Gastrointestinal Findings. Changes in gastrointestinal function from malnutrition underlie the common complaints of early satiety, bloating, belching, vomiting, and constipation. Generally, transit times throughout the gastrointestinal tract are increased, so constipation and delayed gastric emptying are common. Pancreatic fibrosis and jejunal dilatation may occur. Malabsorptive diarrhea and acute gastric dilatation may develop with rapid refeeding.

DIAGNOSIS. Social and cultural factors promote and maintain anorectic behaviors, making medical diagnosis difficult. Within some population groups (e.g., high-fashion models, ballerinas) low body weight is an economic necessity, and the associated anorectic behaviors are accepted. The use of criteria such as those proposed by the American Psychiatric Association (Table 195–1) is recommended for clinical diagnosis. The diagnosis is confirmed by identifying the described behavioral features and by excluding any treatable medical disorders.

The differential diagnosis in this young population includes primary endocrine disorders (panhypopituitarism, Addison's disease, hyperthyroidism, diabetes mellitus), gastrointestinal disease (Crohn's disease, celiac sprue), chronic infection (tuberculosis), neoplastic disorders (lymphoma), AIDS, and, rarely, CNS disorders (hypothalamic tumor, vascular malformation).

All patients should receive a nutritional assessment to determine the severity of the malnutrition and to establish a baseline for follow-up. Height and weight are usually sufficient. Other nutritional measures (serum transferrin, albumin, measurement of triceps skin fold thickness, skin test reactivity to *Candida* antigen) should be obtained in patients with marked weight loss to gauge the approach to nutritional treatment.

TREATMENT. There are two goals in the treatment of patients with anorexia nervosa: nutritional restitution with alleviation of medical complications, and modification of the psychological and environmental factors that promote anorectic behavior. No single treatment is superior, and a multidisciplinary approach involving medical, psychiatric/psychological, and nutritional (dietitians, pharmacists) personnel is needed.

General Medical Care. The medical physician performs the initial clinical assessment, is responsible for the medical and nutritional care of the patient, and provides psychological support. The general approach should include (1) fostering a sense of autonomy in the patient by encouraging her to take personal responsibility in the treatment plan, (2) remaining objective, consistent, and honest to maintain the patient's trust, (3) involving the family as part of the treatment program, (4) serving as liaison and patient advocate with the various consultants and counselors.

Nutritional Care. With mild degrees of weight loss (e.g., weight 80% of ideal or better), nutritional and psychological counseling is sufficient. The physician's role includes personal support, education about adolescent body development and its relationship to diet, and scheduling of periodic visits to observe for clinical deterioration. With moderate malnutrition (weight 65 to 80% of ideal) nutritional supplements may be necessary, but hospitalization usually is not required. Oral replacement with a palatable, nutritionally complete formulation (e.g., Ensure Plus) may help, with the goal being intake of 250 to 500 calories above daily energy requirement. In some cases, cisapride, metoclopramide, or bethanechol may be used to improve gastric emptying and the patient's tolerance of larger meals. With severe malnutrition (weight less than 65% of ideal), hospitalization is usually required. Oral replacement may be attempted, but if the patient is unable or unwilling to comply, tube feeding into the duodenum may be necessary. The patient can receive 400 to 600 calories above daily caloric need, with the goal being no more than 1 to 2 kg weight gain per week.

Severely malnourished patients who tolerate feeding tubes poorly or refuse to eat, must be nourished parenterally. The peripheral venous route is preferred, since central hyperalimentation is more expensive and is associated with a greater frequency of complications. If a central venous route is chosen, it should be supervised by an experienced hyperalimentation team. Caloric delivery should begin with one half of the daily requirement, progressing to full requirement by day three or four. Electrolytes, serum chemistry, and hepatic and renal function must be monitored.

The goal of enteral or parenteral supplementation is to *slowly* get the patient to a body weight out of the range of medical risk. Rapid refeeding produces excess water stores and edema, secondary metabolic disturbances, and possibly cardiac failure. Continued nutritional intervention beyond achieving a "dry weight" of 80% of ideal is not recommended because it is psychologically invasive and minimizes the patient's involvement in the treatment. Supplements interfere with appetite and with attempts to re-establish normal eating patterns.

Pharmacotherapy. No pharmacologic agent is of proven value. Chlorpromazine, amitriptyline, lithium carbonate, and cyproheptadine have been reported effective in small, short-term inpatient treatment trials. Their use should be ancillary to the long-term nutritional and behavioral approaches.

Psychotherapy. Psychotherapy is used to help the patient modify the aberrant eating behavior and to improve psychosocial function. Behavior modification is an effective means of achieving short-term weight gain. Family therapy offers the best potential for long-term benefit, since treatment is directed toward modifying the family interactions that maintain the anorectic behavior. Insight therapy may occasionally help the motivated patient.

TABLE 195–1. DIAGNOSTIC CRITERIA FOR ANOREXIA NERVOSA*

A. Refusal to maintain body weight over a minimal normal weight for age and height (e.g., weight loss leading to maintenance of body weight 15% below that expected) or failure to make expected weight gain during period of growth, leading to body weight 15% below that expected.

B. Intense fear of gaining weight or becoming fat, even though underweight.

C. Disturbance in the way in which one's body weight, size, or shape is experienced (e.g., claiming to "feel fat" even when emaciated or belief that one area of the body is "too fat" even when obviously underweight).

D. In females, absence of at least three consecutive menstrual cycles when otherwise expected to occur (primary or secondary amenorrhea; a woman is considered to have amenorrhea if her periods occur only following hormone [e.g., estrogen] administration).

* Used by permission from the American Psychiatric Association Diagnostic and Statistical Manual of Mental Disorders (DSM-IIIR), 4th ed. Washington, D.C., American Psychiatric Association, 1987.

PROGNOSIS. The short-term prognosis is generally favorable; over 75% of patients will attain a body weight above 75% of ideal. Menses will resume in at least half; however, less than one third of patients will resume normal eating patterns. The long-term prognosis varies, and relapses requiring hospitalization occur in about half of the patients. The mortality rate among hospitalized patients averages 6%, with the main causes of death being inanition and severe electrolyte disturbances; suicide occurs in 1%. A poorer prognosis is associated with a late age of onset, self-induced vomiting or laxative abuse, long duration of illness, male sex, and the presence of associated psychiatric disturbance. A better prognosis is associated with the patient's ability to achieve a degree of social integration (e.g., with parent, spouse, and friends). Whatever the immediate outcome, anorexia nervosa is a lifelong behavioral disorder with periodic exacerbations requiring medical, psychological, and nutritional intervention.

BULIMIA NERVOSA

DEFINITION. Bulimia, derived from the Greek meaning "ox-eating," is a behavioral disorder characterized by episodes of overeating (binging), usually followed by acts to "undo" the threatened weight gain with self-induced vomiting, cathartic or diuretic abuse (purging), fasting, or excessive physical activity. Bulimia nervosa particularly describes patients who binge *and* purge. Compared to anorectics, bulimics have normal body weight and tend to have less distortion of body image. Bulimics are more aware that their behavior, although secretive, is aberrant, and they may therefore be more accepting of treatment.

EPIDEMIOLOGY. Binge eating, at least once, occurs in half of the population, and weekly binge eating is reported by up to 15%. Self-induced vomiting or laxative/diuretic abuse associated with binge eating occurs in up to 20% of college students, and 4% report this type of behavior at least weekly. Bulimia is almost exclusively diagnosed in young (< 30 years) women (> 95%). Most bulimics carry on their activity secretly; less than one third discuss their behavior with physicians. In one survey only 2.5% were under medical care.

ETIOLOGY AND PATHOGENESIS. Affected persons commonly report obesity during childhood or adolescence, and the onset of bulimia in association with a conscious decision to diet. At some point they lose control of their compulsion to eat large amounts of "forbidden foods" and binge. Self-induced vomiting is discovered as a convenient method of re-establishing weight control. Thus, a binge-purge cycle becomes established.

As with anorexia nervosa, societal influences seem to play a prominent role in the desire not to be fat. The ancient Romans ate lavishly and then induced vomiting at feasts. Socialites who must attend many dinner parties sometimes induce vomiting. Bulimics report coming from families that emphasize hearty eating and use food to celebrate happy times and to console during sad times: Eating takes on greater meaning than simply to achieve nutritional benefit, and this may help to explain the emotional and behavioral investment present in food and eating.

These behaviors appear to have biochemical correlates. Neurotransmitters, including serotonin (5-HT), dopamine, norepinephrine, opioids, and cholecystokinin (CCK), modulate hunger and regulation of food intake. All have been implicated as contributing to clinical expression of this disorder. For example, 5-HT has a satiety-promoting effect, and reduced brain levels in animals lead to carbohydrate binges similar to those affecting bulimics. Bulimic women, compared to normal persons, have blunted meal-induced secretion of CCK, and this correlates with satiety.

These and other data suggest that the behavioral features of bulimia may relate to dysregulation of CNS neurotransmitter systems. This would support the association of this disorder with its psychological features and with the potential therapeutic role for psychopharmacologic agents.

CLINICAL MANIFESTATIONS. *Psychological and Behavioral Features.* The characteristic behavioral feature is the binge-purge cycle: an eating compulsion associated with failure to achieve or to respond to normal satiety. The episodes occur secretly and are often associated with feelings of frustration, loneliness, or the sight of tempting foods. Binges are usually planned, and the preparation is associated with anxiety and excitement. The binge is usually terminated when feelings of guilt or physical discomfort such as nausea, abdominal pain, or headache occur. At this point patients self-induce vomiting and/or take cathartics or laxatives. Bulimics generally look healthy, and their behaviors go unnoticed by friends and family. They are more outgoing than their anorectic counterparts. Some patients may exhibit impulsive or antisocial behaviors such as drug abuse, kleptomania, and sexual promiscuity. The patient who seeks help does so because of feelings of guilt, anxiety, or depression, or when he or she is no longer able to continue the habit and still function in daily activities.

Medical Features. The medical findings of bulimia derive from the vomiting and laxative abuse. The physical examination may reveal parotid or salivary gland swelling due to vomiting, bruising of the knuckles from their rubbing against the upper incisors during the induction of vomiting ("Russell's" sign), pharyngitis and dental erosions from reflux of gastric acid, or conjunctival hemorrhages from retching.

Frequent vomiting may be complicated by esophagitis, Mallory-Weiss tears, or aspiration pneumonitis. Hypokalemic hypochloremic metabolic alkalosis due to loss of H^+, Cl^-, and K^+ is the most common metabolic complication, and this may lead to cardiac arrhythmias or renal injury. Secondary metabolic disturbances may produce weakness, tetany, and seizures. Emetics such as ipecac may produce cardiac conduction defects and arrhythmias. The use of stimulant laxatives can produce a "cathartic colon" with degeneration of Auerbach's plexus.

Most bulimic patients are clinically depressed by the time they request medical help, and 5% sooner or later attempt suicide. A large proportion of bulimic patients have first-degree relatives with major affective disorders.

DIAGNOSIS. The diagnosis is based on recognition of the binge eating pattern and the exclusion of other medical diseases that might explain the behavior. The differential diagnosis, which is limited in this young population group, would include schizophrenia, use of oral contraceptives, seizures, and rare neurologic disorders. The latter may include *Klüver-Bucy syndrome,* a disorder of bilateral temporal lobe damage associated with indiscriminate sexual behavior, hyperphagia, and pica, and *Kleine-Levin syndrome,* a sleep disorder associated with hypersomnia and overeating.

TREATMENT. The goal of treatment is to help the patient overcome the urge to overeat. Bulimic patients recognize their behaviors as maladaptive. Compared to anorectics, they are more aware of associated psychological difficulties and are more willing to work with physicians and counselors in a treatment plan.

The currently most favored psychotherapeutic approach consists of cognitive-behavioral treatment in which the patient identifies the abnormal behaviors and then uses behavioral techniques to extinguish them, thereby accomplishing greater self-control. The treatment is safe and probably effective.

Antidepressants have been reported to be successful in decreasing the binge activity and in increasing the patient's sense of well-being. They appear effective regardless of whether symptoms of clinical depression exist. One recent study also indicates that combined treatment using cognitive-behavior and antidepressant therapy is superior to antidepressant treatment alone.

Agras WS, Rossiter EM, Arnow B, et al.: Pharmacologic and cognitive-behavioral treatment for bulimia nervosa: A controlled comparison. Am J Psychiatry 149:82, 1992. *Well-controlled study shows that both cognitive-behavioral and antidepressant treatment can be helpful for bulimia nervosa. Cognitive-behavioral therapy more effective in preventing relapse; combined treatment approach may have additional advantages.*

Bemporad JR, Beresin E, Ratey JJ, et al.: A psychoanalytic study of eating disorders: I. A developmental profile of 67 index cases. J Am Acad Psychoanal 20:509, 1992. *Supports idea that clinical expression of the disorder results from disturbances in early relationships leading to impaired feelings of security and interpersonal difficulties.*

Drossman DA: Approach to unexplained weight loss and the eating disorders. *In* Yamada T (ed.): Textbook of Gastroenterology, 2nd ed. Philadelphia, JB Lippincott, 1994. *Comprehensively reviews epidemiology, pathophysiology, medical and psychosocial characteristics, diagnosis, and treatment of major eating disorders.*

Freund KM, Graham SM, Lesky LG, Moskowitz MA: Detection of bulimia in a primary care setting. J Gen Intern Med 8:236, 1993. *Offers simple questions that can be used to identify patients with bulimia.*

Kennedy SH, Garfinkel PE: Advances in diagnosis and treatment of anorexia nervosa and bulimia nervosa. Can J Psychiatry 37:309, 1992. *Reviews treatment approach and outcome of patients having anorexia nervosa and bulimia nervosa.*

196 OBESITY
F. Xavier Pi-Sunyer

Obesity is a frustrating condition for patient and physician alike. Its underlying cause is rarely clear, and its treatment is fraught with difficulty and failure. Management of obesity therefore requires much understanding and persistence.

About 34 million adult Americans (26% of those aged 20 to 75 years) are overweight, 12.4 million severely so. The percentage of adult women who are overweight (27.1%) is somewhat greater than that of men (24.2%).

DEFINITION

Visual inspection of a patient can give a subjective but fairly accurate estimate of the degree of obesity. More objective measures are height-weight tables, weight-related indices, and other anthropometric measurements.

The three most commonly used indices are (1) tables of average weights by height and age; (2) tables of desirable weights for height associated with lowest mortalities in insured populations; and (3) indices derived from height and weight, of which the body mass index is the most useful.

TABLES OF AVERAGE WEIGHTS. National Health and Nutrition Examination Surveys (NHANES) are periodically conducted on a representative United States population and then compiled in percentile tables as weights for height for gender. These cross-sectional data can be used for defining obesity, with a commonly made arbitrary decision that a weight above the 85th percentile for a young adult population is "overweight" for everyone. This comparison to a reference population makes no statement as to health risk involved at any weight level. The biggest problem is finding an appropriate reference population, particularly for minorities.

IDEAL WEIGHT TABLES. The Metropolitan Life Insurance Company Tables of Heights and Weights indicate the weight at which longevity is greatest, based on those insured. The 1983 tables were derived from the pooled data of 25 insurance companies in the United States and Canada, including about 4.2 million policies issued between 1950 and 1971. People with major diseases were screened out. The tables show weights based on lowest mortality for men and women at ages 25 to 59 by height and body frame.

The Metropolitan tables have been criticized as being inaccurate because (1) insured subjects do not represent a random sample of the population; (2) insured subjects are screened for illness and so are healthier than average; (3) no actual body frame measurements were taken when data were gathered so that the division into three frame categories (small, medium, and large) was a *post hoc* manipulation of the data; (4) about 20% of the subjects used in the tables reported their heights and weights but were not actually measured (the bias being that women tend to under-report their weight and men to over-report their height); (5) the tables do not distinguish between obesity and overweight.

BODY MASS INDEX (BMI). A third way to classify overweight is by computing the BMI:

$$BMI = kg/(ht\ in\ meters)^2$$
$$or\ BMI = lb/(ht\ in\ inches)^2 \times 703.1$$

This simple measurement correlates well with other estimates of fatness, although some very muscular individuals may be classified as obese when they are not. It is also a somewhat more accurate index of fatness for males than for females.

The mean BMI (weighted for the height distribution of the US population) taken from the mid-point of the medium frame of the 1983 Metropolitan tables is 22.4 kg per square meter for men and 22.5 kg per square meter for women. Patients can be divided for degree of obesity as shown in Figure 196-1. Health risks increase as BMI increases above 25.

Aging is a fattening process, so that a young and old person of comparable body weight are not comparably obese (Fig. 196-2). This has led to controversy concerning whether it is the total weight of an individual that should stay constant from 25 years to 70 years or the fat-free mass, that is, the working cellular mass of

the body plus the skeleton. The average weight data from the US population show a gradually increasing weight with age, more pronounced and sustained for women than for men (Fig. 196-3).

Whereas many studies suggest that an increase from one's weight at 25 years old may increase mortality, a number have suggested that for the lowest mortality, the pattern of body weight should be leanness in the twenties followed by a very moderate weight gain as one gets older. The minimal mortality points in relation to BMI for each age-gender grouping have been calculated. The regression lines, computed separately for men and women, are presented in Figure 196-4. Clearly, age strongly affects the BMI associated with the lowest mortality in this study. Also, the regression lines for men and women are nearly the same. The "best" BMI gradually increases with age in both genders, with no consistent difference between men and women. As a result, a single set of weight goal tables (Table 196-1) can be constructed which are applicable for both men and women. The goals, which are somewhat more liberal for certain age groups than are the Metropolitan tables, are given by decade of age, with generally higher allowable weights as persons get older. Until the issue is further clarified, these goals seem to be reasonable for a physician to utilize in counseling patients in preventive medicine. Two caveats must be added. First, these tables have been derived from and are applicable primarily to white men and women in the United States. Second, the tables have been derived from populations without known risk factors. Patients with significant risk factors such as coronary artery disease, hypertension, and diabetes mellitus are better counseled on stricter tables, such as the Metropolitan Life Tables of 1983 (see Ch. 193).

OTHER METHODS. Over half of the fat in the body is deposited under the skin. Its thickness can be measured at various sites using standard skin calipers. It is not difficult to become adept in the use of the calipers, and a running record of a patient's estimated body fat can be easily kept. The most useful and accurate tables are based on the measurement of four skinfold thicknesses—biceps, triceps, subscapular, and suprailiac. For such tables, see the *British Journal of Nutrition* 2:77, 1974.

Other methods of defining obesity are more difficult and expensive and therefore are used mostly for research purposes: (1) Total body water can be measured by dilution with tritiated or deuterated water. Water is then assumed to be a fixed proportion of fat-free

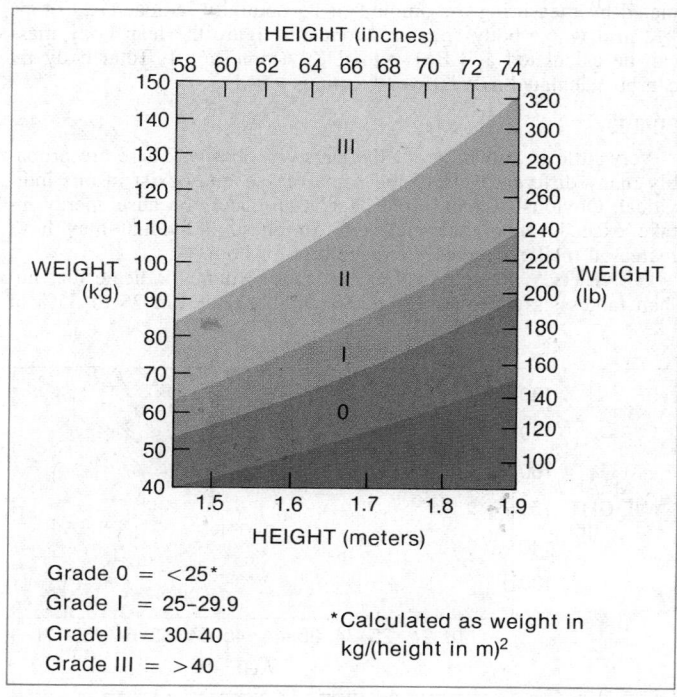

Grade 0 = <25*
Grade I = 25–29.9
Grade II = 30–40
Grade III = >40

*Calculated as weight in kg/(height in m)²

FIGURE 196–1. Grades of obesity as defined by body mass index. (From Garrow JS: Obesity and Related Diseases. New York, Churchill Livingstone, 1988.)

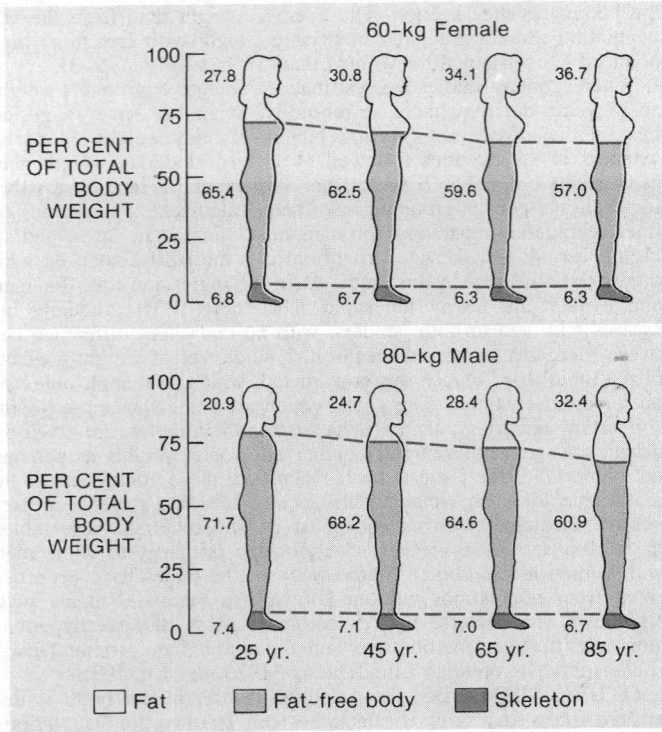

FIGURE 196-2. Body composition change with aging of representative normal adults. (Adapted from Moore FD, Olesen KH, McMurrey JE, et al.: The Body Cell Mass and Its Supporting Environment. Philadelphia, WB Saunders, 1963.)

mass (FFM = water mass/0.73), and FFM is subtracted from total body weight to obtain total body fat. (2) Body density can be measured by underwater weighing (with accurate correction for lung and abdominal air) and the amount of fat-free mass and body fat can be calculated. (3) The amount of body potassium can be estimated by measuring the amount of its naturally radioactive isotope ^{40}K in a whole-body counter. From this figure the lean body mass can be calculated as LBM = total K^+ (mmol)/68.1. Total body fat can be calculated as total weight minus LBM.

ETIOLOGY

Very little is known about the cause of obesity. There are probably many different causes, and some may even coexist in one individual. Obviously excess lipid deposition occurs because energy intake exceeds energy expenditure. An obese individual may have increased intake, decreased expenditure, or both.

GENETICS. Recent twin and adoption studies indicate that human fatness is under strong genetic influence. From 25 to 35% of

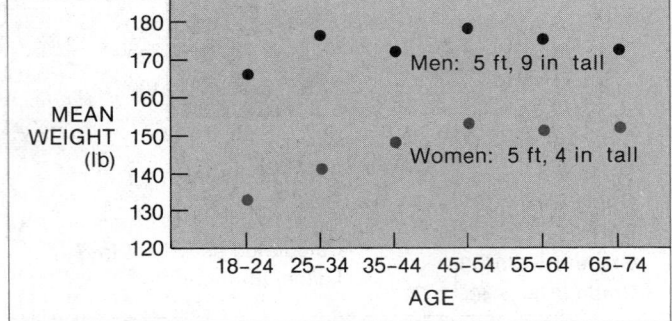

FIGURE 196-3. Weight change with aging for men and women. (Adapted from National Center for Health Statistics: Weight by height and age for adults 18–74 years, United States, 1971–1974. DHEW Publication No. [PHS] 79-1656, Series 11, No. 208, 1979.)

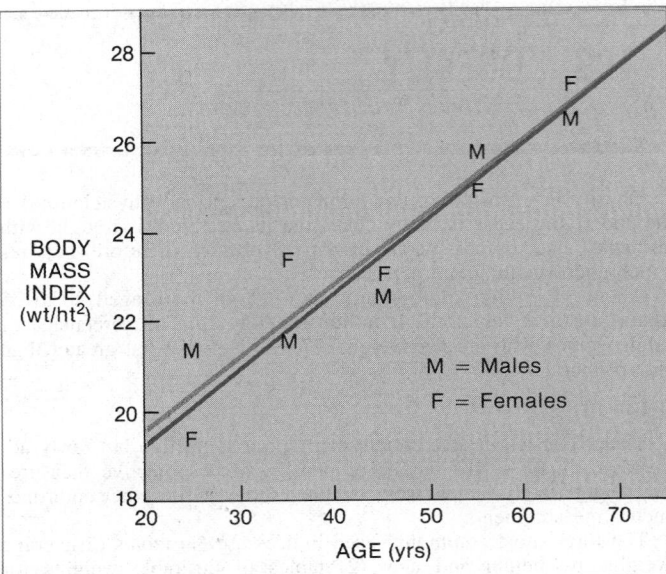

FIGURE 196-4. The effect of age on the body mass index (BMI) associated with lowest mortality. Minimal mortality points were computed for each age-gender group. The regression lines were computed separately for men (dark red line) and for women (light red line). Note that there is a strong effect of age on the BMI associated with lowest mortality and that the regression lines for men and women are nearly identical. (From The Build Study, 1979. Adapted by Andres R: In Andres R, Bierman EL, Hazzard WR, Blass JP [eds.]: Principles of Geriatric Medicine. Copyright © 1990 by McGraw-Hill, Inc. Used by permission of McGraw-Hill Book Company.)

the variance in skinfold thickness, body mass index, and relative weight has been attributed to genetic factors. The studies that have shown this degree of variance describe the genetic influences found in persons living under particular environmental conditions, namely those of Western society. Because the environment in which heritable characteristics are expressed affects the expression, these variance ranges may not apply to all societies. Not only is there a strong genetic component to fatness, but there is also a similarly strong genetic component to regional fat distribution. Thus, a person's genotype is an important determinant of how adaptation to excess energy intake occurs. Environment is also clearly important, and the interrelation of genetics to particular environments needs to be further investigated.

A number of rare genetic diseases are associated with obesity, but through unknown mechanisms: the Prader-Willi syndrome, the Laurence-Moon-Biedl syndrome, the Alstrom syndrome, the Cohen syndrome, the Carpenter syndrome, and Blount's disease. The reader is referred to textbooks on genetic disorders for further descriptions of these entities.

ENERGY INTAKE. Hyperphagia is the striking cause of obesity in a number of animal models (both genetic and brain-lesioned). The cause of human obesity is much less straightforward. Obesity has been regarded as an eating disorder for centuries, but the presumed abnormality has been difficult to document. Measuring food intake in a free-living environment is subject to large errors. Most studies have suggested that obese persons do overeat (at least in their weight-gaining phases). Many reports describe individuals who categorically deny overeating but lose weight when brought into a metabolic ward and placed on a calculated weight-maintaining diet for their height and age.

Possibly obese persons are unduly attracted by the hedonic aspects of food, or they have impaired feedback signals registering satiety, or they have insensitive brain receptor centers for the feedback signals. It has also been suggested that feeding behavior is learned and that satiety is a conditioned response. Maladaptive conditioning is said to occur in obese persons. None of these theories has been scientifically validated.

ENERGY EXPENDITURE. *Resting Metabolic Expenditure.* Obese individuals may gain weight because they are "thrifty"; i.e., less ingested nutrient is spent as heat and thus more is available for storage. Impaired thermogenesis exists in certain animal

TABLE 196-1. AGE-SPECIFIC WEIGHT-FOR-HEIGHT TABLES* (GERONTOLOGY RESEARCH CENTER)

Height (ft–in)	Weight Range (lbs) for Men and Women by Age (Years)†				
	25	35	45	55	65
4–10	84–111	92–119	99–127	107–135	115–142
4–11	87–115	95–123	103–131	111–139	119–147
5–0	90–119	98–127	106–135	114–143	123–152
5–1	93–123	101–131	110–140	118–148	127–157
5–2	96–127	105–136	113–144	122–153	131–163
5–3	99–131	108–140	117–149	126–158	135–168
5–4	102–135	112–145	121–154	130–163	140–173
5–5	106–140	115–149	125–159	134–168	144–179
5–6	109–144	119–154	129–164	138–174	148–184
5–7	112–148	122–159	133–169	143–179	153–190
5–8	116–153	126–163	137–174	147–184	158–196
5–9	119–157	130–168	141–179	151–190	162–201
5–10	122–162	134–173	145–184	156–195	167–207
5–11	126–167	137–178	149–190	160–201	172–213
6–0	129–171	141–183	153–195	165–207	177–219
6–1	133–176	145–188	157–200	169–213	182–225
6–2	137–181	149–194	162–206	174–219	187–232
6–3	141–186	153–199	166–212	179–225	192–238
6–4	144–191	157–205	171–218	184–231	197–244

* Values in this table are for height without shoes and weight without clothes. To convert inches to centimeters, multiply by 2.54; to convert pounds to kilograms, multiply by 0.455.

† Data from Andres R: Gerontology Research Center, National Institute of Aging, Baltimore, MD.

models of obesity. Although it has been more difficult to document in humans, recent studies in both adults and infants have reported that a low rate of energy expenditure may predispose to obesity.

Thermogenesis can be divided into three components—resting metabolic rate (RMR), thermic effect of food (TEF), and thermic effect of exercise or activity (TEE).

RMR is the energy expended in the postabsorptive state to drive basic life-supporting processes under thermoneutral conditions. RMR, expressed as total amount of energy spent per unit time, is higher in obese persons than in lean ones. RMR can be well correlated with total weight but can be better correlated with lean body mass (LBM). This explains why men have higher RMR's than women and why RMR's decrease with age.

Obese individuals have a higher LBM than those who are lean because they require an extra amount of sustaining cell mass to maintain the extra fat. When RMR is expressed as kilocalories per kilogram of LBM, obese persons have values equivalent to the lean. It is only when RMR is expressed as kilocalories per kilogram of body weight that they have values below those who are lean. This is because per unit of weight they have a relatively lower amount of metabolizing cell mass and a larger amount of stored fat, which is relatively inert in energy utilization. In terms of basal or resting energetics, therefore, the obese once they are obese do not have impaired RMR's and are not more "efficient" than lean persons.

The RMR varies as much as ± 15% from individual to individual, even when they are matched for age, gender, and surface area. If a difference in metabolic rate between individuals can be as great as one third, it is clear that at a given caloric intake one individual may gain weight and another may lose it. Energy balance depends on matching intake to expenditure. It is not surprising that different individuals maintain weight on widely differing caloric intakes.

Expenditure in Activity. The obese expend more energy during physical activity because an obese person is moving a greater load through space, whether walking, running, or climbing stairs. This is true, although less so, even when body weight is supported, as in cycle ergometer exercise, because of the higher cost of moving the larger leg mass. Thus, more kilowatts of energy are expended.

Studies of obese persons show most of them to be less active, both in engaging in physical activities and in moving about once engaged. The amount of energy expended over 24 hours in physical activity varies considerably from individual to individual, however, and it is difficult to generalize.

Expenditure After Food. Food is an important thermogenic stimulant because it generates heat as it is metabolized. Because of

this, a fed person has a higher metabolic rate than a fasting one. This elevation of postcibal metabolic rate above basal has been called the thermic effect of food (TEF). With a mixed diet, about 10% of the metabolizable energy ingested is lost as heat.

Obese persons may have equivalent or somewhat depressed TEF responses compared with lean persons. The impaired response appears to be related to insulin resistance, which leads to a slower glucose disposal. The impaired utilization of glucose by the cells of the body slows down heat production. This impaired thermogenic effect can be normalized by giving insulin, so that a thermic response equivalent to that of insulin-sensitive persons occurs. Therefore, it seems likely that a thermogenic defect relating to carbohydrate disposal is found in obese patients who are insulin resistant and not found in those who are equivalently obese but insulin sensitive. Thus, there is evidence for an overall somewhat diminished thermic effect of food in obese compared with lean individuals. However, even insulin-resistant obese persons with a decreased TEF have a total energy expenditure greater than do lean persons for the 3- to 4-hour period after the meal, because the slight decrease in TEF is less than the inherent elevation in their RMR.

In summary, although hypometabolism may predispose to obesity in some cases, RMR is higher once obesity is present. Thermogenic responses to ordinary stimuli (food, stress, cold) are small *per se,* and differences between lean and obese persons are small to nonexistent. The net result is that 24-hour energy expenditure in the typical obese person is greater than that of the typical sedentary lean person.

Expenditure After Overfeeding. Small rodents can waste rather than store much of excess ingested calories. This seems to be mediated through the sympathetic nervous system, which activates and causes hypertrophy of brown adipose tissue (BAT), a tissue that is specialized to generate heat. A deficient ability to burn off excess calories in this fashion has been documented in a number of genetically obese rodents. Little evidence suggests that humans have an adequate amount of brown fat to mount a similar excess of heat production.

In lean humans, significant overfeeding (of the order of 2000 extra calories per day) for about 10 days or more may lead to energy wastage. In the few studies of overfeeding done in obese volunteers, no evidence of similar energy wastage was found, but few long-term studies are available.

Do obese people lack a protective mechanism, i.e., heat dissipation, that lean people possess if they overeat? There is not much convincing experimental evidence to date, although it is a tempting hypothesis that needs to be further investigated.

PATHOPHYSIOLOGY

FAT CELLS. Fat cells (adipocytes) form a reservoir of energy that expands or contracts according to the energy balance of the organism. Fat cells develop from precursor preadipocytes to accommodate excess nutrient calories. Adipocytes gradually increase in volume to about 1 μg of mass, at which point little further enlargement seems to be possible. With continuing positive energy balance, new adipocytes form from precursor cells and the total cell number increases. Adipocytes can increase in number in an unlimited fashion, so that fat mass can reach huge dimensions through hyperplasia.

Once fat cells are formed, it is difficult to dedifferentiate them. This has been termed the "ratchet effect," because a ratchet turns in only one direction. Even though weight may be lost, fat cell numbers remain fixed. As a result, fat cell size reverts toward normal and with sustained weight loss may actually go below normal.

What the stimulus is for the differentiation of preadipocytes into adipocytes is unknown. Adipose tissue lipoprotein lipase (LPL) may be involved. LPL acts to break down triglyceride to glycerophosphate and free fatty acids (FFA). Whereas LPL activity seems to rise with weight loss and is thought to be important in the accelerated weight regain of many patients, it seems to drop after the maintenance of weight loss for a time, suggesting that its elevation in the obese patient may be secondary rather than primary.

REGIONAL DISTRIBUTION OF ADIPOSE TISSUE. Fat mass is distributed differently in men and women. The android, or male, pattern is characterized by fat distributed predominantly in the upper body above the waist, whereas the gynecoid, or female, pattern shows fat predominantly in the lower body, that is, lower abdomen, buttocks, hips, and thighs. Upper body fat has a significantly worse prognosis for morbidity and mortality than does lower body fat. Evidence suggests that the intra-abdominal or visceral component of fat rather than the subcutaneous abdominal component is responsible. The regional distribution can be measured in a variety of ways. The easiest, most common, and very useful way is by measuring body circumference at the waist and at the hips and calculating a waist:hip ratio. A ratio of greater than 0.85 in women and greater than 1.0 in men can be considered abnormally high.

Fat cells from the upper body seem to be functionally different from fat cells in the lower body. They are more sensitive to catecholamines and insulin. It is likely that the greater lipolytic and lipogenic potential of the upper body cells is related to an underlying difference in sex-hormone response of the two tissues. Thus, testosterone and estrogen influences may be important and may act differently on upper and lower body fat cells.

Abdominal or android fatness carries a greater risk for hypertension, cardiovascular disease, hyperinsulinemia, diabetes mellitus, gallbladder disease, stroke, and cancer of the breast and endometrium. It also carries a greater risk of overall mortality. Because more men than women have the android distribution, they are more at risk for most of these conditions. Also, women who deposit their excess fat in a more android manner have a greater risk than women whose fat distribution is more gynecoid. Upper body fat deposition tends to occur primarily by hypertrophy of the existing cells, whereas lower body fat deposition is by differentiation of new fat cells, i.e., hyperplasia. Reducing a normal number of enlarged fat cells to normal size is easier than reducing large numbers of the cells in the lower body hyperplastic depot to normal or below normal size. This may explain the weight loss difficulties of many women with lower body obesity.

Thus, three components of body fat are associated with health risk: percent body fat, subcutaneous truncal or abdominal fat, and visceral fat in the abdominal cavity. While partly correlated with each other, they do show independence of expression.

SET POINT. The concept of a "set point" of body weight suggests that each person has a control system that "sets" how much weight, or alternatively how much fat, he or she should have. How the control system is regulated, that is, where the feedback signals from "weight" or "fat" originate and how they might be transmitted (humoral, neural, both?) to the hypothalamic feeding and satiety areas are totally unknown.

This set-point theory suggests that people possess a given weight because they are "set" there. That is, one's set point is the weight one normally maintains. Although this is circular thinking, set-point theory has been used to suggest that weight loss programs are misguided and that the effort to lose weight is inevitably fraught with failure because set point will bring individuals up to their preweightloss weight.

The set-point theory has been used to suggest that exercise and some drugs lower set point and most palatable foods raise it. Once these statements have been made, however, no closer understanding of the regulation of body weight and of food intake has been attained. Certainly, if there is a "set point," it is a very movable one that seems to change easily under the influence of a number of environmental conditions.

CLINICAL MANIFESTATIONS

INSULIN RESISTANCE. Obesity induces an insulin-resistant state in man, one that is associated with both basal and stimulated hyperinsulinemia. This results from a change in β-cell insulin release rather than in the threshold to glucose stimulation. The enlarged fat cell is less sensitive to the antilipolytic and lipogenic actions of insulin. Although a decreased number of insulin receptors contributes to the insulin resistance, the resistance is generally much greater than would be predicted from the magnitude of this decrease. A "postreceptor" defect therefore occurs as well. This defect in glucose utilization occurs also in other insulin-sensitive tissues, particularly muscle. The liver is also less responsive to insulin. As the insulin resistance becomes more profound, glucose uptake in peripheral tissues is impaired and hepatic glucose output increases.

DIABETES MELLITUS. In a certain number of obese individuals, diabetes mellitus occurs, as the non–insulin-dependent (NIDDM) type (see Ch. 205). The prevalence of diabetes is approximately three times higher in overweight than in nonoverweight persons. In the United States about 85% of patients with NIDDM are obese. Clinically manifest diabetes develops only with the appropriate genetic legacy, but obesity, by enhancing insulin resistance, increases the demand on the pancreatic islets and tends to unmask and exacerbate an underlying genetic propensity.

HYPERTENSION. The prevalence of hypertension (blood pressure greater than 140/90 mm Hg) is approximately three times higher for the obese than for the nonobese. In the Framingham Study, high blood pressure developed 10 times more often in persons who were 20% or more overweight than in those of normal weight.

The mechanism by which obesity contributes to high blood pressure is not clear. Hyperinsulinemia leading to increased tubular reabsorption of sodium may be a factor; increased sympathetic tone may be another. Whatever the mechanism, weight loss from dieting leads to a fall in arterial pressure, even when salt intake is not restricted.

CARDIOVASCULAR DISEASE. In obesity, increased blood volume, stroke volume, left ventricular end-diastolic volume, and filling pressure result in a high cardiac output. This can lead to predominantly left ventricular hypertrophy and dilatation. Hypertension also contributes to left ventricular hypertrophy. Thus, obese hypertensive patients are at greater risk for congestive heart failure and sudden death.

BLOOD LIPIDS. Obese people seem to have an adverse pattern of plasma lipoproteins. This is manifested particularly by a low concentration of high density lipoprotein (HDL) cholesterol. LDL cholesterol may be elevated. Hypertriglyceridemia is more prevalent in obese persons, possibly because the insulin resistance and hyperinsulinemia of obesity lead to increased hepatic production of triglycerides. The hypertriglyceridemia generally improves with weight loss, but if a true genetic lipoprotein disorder coexists, more intensive therapy specific for the lipoprotein abnormality may be required (see Ch. 173).

RESPIRATORY PROBLEMS. Severe obesity can lead to chronic hypoxia with cyanosis and hypercapnia. Associated with this are an increased demand for ventilation, an increased breathing workload, respiratory muscle inefficiency, and decreased functional reserve capacity and expiratory reserve volume. Peripheral lung units can close, resulting in a ventilation-perfusion mismatch.

The end-stage associated with severe obesity is the pickwickian syndrome, in which hypoventilation is so marked that hypoxia leads to long periods of somnolence. In these patients, pulmonary hypertension occurs and cardiac failure may supervene.

SLEEP APNEA. Sleep apnea is common in severely obese patients (see Ch. 65). The relationship between obesity and sleep apnea is unclear because the most obese individuals are not necessarily the most severely affected. Apnea can be obstructive or central in nature; both forms are more prevalent in obese persons. In obese persons the upper airways may be obstructed by the large local accumulation of fat tissue, often in combination with micrognathia and enlarged tonsils and adenoids. The obstruction leads to hypoventilation and hypoxia, which somehow trigger apneic episodes that then worsen the hypoxia and hypercapnia. Affected patients benefit from weight loss and sometimes from surgical removal of some of the obstructive tissues. Central apnea is characterized by a cessation of ventilatory drive from brain centers, so that diaphragmatic excursions stop for periods of 10 to 30 seconds. The reason obese persons are prone to this condition is unknown. Pharmacotherapy sometimes helps. Daytime somnolence is common in obese patients with apnea, partly from hypoxia and partly from the continual disturbance of sleep at night, because they tend to awaken after each apneic episode.

VENOUS CIRCULATORY DISEASE. Severely obese individuals often have varicose veins and venous stasis. Congestive heart failure may add to dependent edema, with the further complications of trophic changes of the skin and an increased propensity for thrombophlebitis and thromboembolism. Pulmonary embolism is much more common in the obese than in those of normal weight (see Ch. 59).

CANCER. Endometrial cancer is two to three times more common in obese than in lean women. Risk of breast cancer increases with increasing BMI in postmenopausal women. It has been speculated that this increased risk is due to the stimulatory effect of increased levels of estrogen in the postmenopausal period. Obese women also have a higher incidence of cancer of the gallbladder and of the biliary system. Obese men have a higher mortality from cancer of the colon, rectum, and prostate for reasons that are unknown.

GASTROINTESTINAL DISEASE. Cholesterol gallstones are more prevalent in obesity. The pathogenetic sequence is presumed to be that of greater cholesterol production in the increased body fat depots, greater biliary excretion of cholesterol, and a resulting supersaturation of the cholesterol in bile. The gallstones can lead to cholecystitis (see Ch. 126) and the need for cholecystectomy. The obese carry a greater risk for complications and mortality from such abdominal surgery.

Many obese patients have fatty livers with modest abnormalities of liver function tests, but hepatic diseases in general are not more common in obese than in lean persons.

ARTHRITIS. As the severity of obesity increases, joint symptoms related to osteoarthritis become common. Excess stress is particularly placed on joints of the lower extremities and the lower back.

Body weight and serum uric acid level often correlate. With obesity, urate clearance is decreased and urate production increased. Because hypertension and diabetes mellitus also correlate with elevated uric acid levels, the relationship between hyperuricemia and obesity is multifactorial.

SKIN. Skin problems are common in obesity, particularly intertrigo in redundant folds of skin. Fungal and yeast infections of skin are common. Acanthosis nigricans occurs in a minority of morbidly obese patients. These patients can manifest a syndrome that includes severe insulin resistance.

PSYCHOLOGICAL MANIFESTATIONS

The psychological toll of severe obesity is large. Poor self-image and impaired social relationships are common. Obese individuals are often discriminated against in educational and professional settings, engendering anxiety, anger, and self-doubt. There is no evidence, however, of any particular neurotic or psychotic character in obese individuals. The depression and anxiety seem to be situational rather than endogenous; they often improve if the obesity can be ameliorated.

MORTALITY

Obesity is associated with increased mortality. The effect of obesity on cardiovascular mortality generally occurs through linkage with other risk factors such as hypertension, diabetes, and dyslipidemia. Obesity, however, can also make independent contribution to mortality. In the Framingham Study, for every 10% rise in relative weight, systolic blood pressure rose 6.5 mm Hg, plasma cholesterol 12 mg per deciliter, and fasting blood glucose 2 mg per deciliter. The causes of increased mortality for those 20% or more overweight include coronary heart disease, stroke, diabetes, digestive diseases, and cancer (Table 196–2). The risk of mortality is higher for those with upper body obesity than those with lower body obesity. A number of prospective studies have now described this, particularly as it relates to cardiovascular disease risk.

OBESITY AND THE ENDOCRINE SYSTEM

Although obesity has often been described as an "endocrine" disease, <1% of obese patients have any measurable endocrine dysfunction. Hypothalamic, pituitary, thyroid, adrenal, ovarian, and possibly pancreatic endocrine syndromes have been related to obesity.

HYPOTHALAMIC DISEASE. In this type of obesity, the appetite systems or tracts located in the hypothalamus are affected. Bilateral damage in the ventromedial hypothalamus produces hyperphagic obesity in the rat; conversely, bilateral damage in the extreme lateral portion of the hypothalamus causes aphagia. Rather than a single balance of a "feeding center" and a "satiety center," however, it is now clear that diffuse excitatory and inhibitory neuronal systems controlling feeding course through the limbic system and the whole brain. Following trauma, inflammation, or a tumor (particularly craniopharyngioma) involving the hypothalamus, a few patients develop hyperphagic obesity, most of them after surgery for hypothalamic tumors. The diagnosis is usually based on history, physical findings, and brain imaging studies.

PITUITARY AND ADRENAL DYSFUNCTION. Cushing's disease is the most common form of pituitary dysfunction leading to obesity (see Ch. 207). ACTH is excessively produced, which leads to excess production of cortisol by the adrenal cortex. Cushing's syndrome can also have a variety of other causes, including exogenous glucocorticoids, primary disorders of the adrenal, and paraneoplastic syndromes of excess ACTH production. The hypercortisolism causes adipocytes located primarily at the center of the body to expand, while those at the extremities do so much less. With this central obesity comes hypertension and diabetes.

THYROID DISEASE. Obesity is often ascribed to "hypometabolism" caused by underactivity of the thyroid gland, but this is in fact seldom true. Severe hypothyroidism can lead to some increased fat, but most of the excess weight is actually edema, which is lost with the institution of thyroid hormone replacement.

POLYCYSTIC OVARIAN SYNDROME. Mild hirsutism, irregular menses or amenorrhea, and obesity have been linked in the "polycystic ovarian syndrome." In this disorder the ovaries have atretic follicles, the patient is anovulatory, and menstrual disturbance (long-term amenorrhea to oligomenorrhea) is the rule. The ovaries overproduce androgens. Although hirsutism is common, virilization is not. The relation of obesity to the polycystic ovarian syndrome is not clear, but the two conditions often coexist.

ENDOCRINE CONSEQUENCES OF OBESITY. One of the pathophysiologic consequences of obesity may be certain endocrine abnormalities. The sex-hormone abnormalities associated with obesity are different in males and females. Whereas mildly obese men have no detectable abnormalities, severely obese men have mild hypogonadotropic hypogonadism, with less than two thirds the normal mean plasma levels of total testosterone, free testosterone, and follicle-stimulating hormone. Gonadotropic hormones are suppressed by elevated plasma estrogens derived from increased aromatization of adrenal steroids in the excessive body fat. Obesity may be associated with increased metabolic clearance rates of testosterone, caused partly by decreased sex hormone-binding globulin (SHBG). Spermatogenesis, libido, and potency, however, are normal.

Estrogens are not elevated in obese premenopausal women, probably because the amount of estrone conversion by the adipose tissue is small in comparison with regular ovarian estradiol production. Estrogens are elevated, however, in postmenopausal obese women, most likely owing to increased peripheral conversion of the prehormone androstenedione to estrone. This may be a partial explanation as to why there is less osteoporosis in obese women.

There are differences in the androgen-estrogen environment in persons with upper (UBO) and lower (LBO) body obesity. This is more clearly defined in women. Women with UBO have higher androgen production rates and higher concentrations of testosterone and estradiol levels than those with LBO. They also have decreased levels of SHBG, so that free testosterone concentrations are higher. Women with LBO have increased estrone from peripheral aromatization of circulating androgens.

In obesity, insulin resistance develops and hyperinsulinemia results. Whether impaired glucose tolerance or frank diabetes ensues depends on the degree of insulin resistance and the underlying genetic make-up of the individual. Triiodothyronine (T_3) may be elevated to high normal in conditions of high caloric intake with adequate carbohydrate, while thyroxine levels and TSH levels are normal. Slightly low blood cortisol levels may be present in obe-

TABLE 196–2. PATTERN OF EXCESS MORTALITY VARIATION WITH EXCESS WEIGHT (MEN AGES 15–34 YRS AT ENTRY)

Weight Relative to Average Weight (Percent)	Mortality Ratio
105–115	110
115–125	127
125–135	134
135–145	141
145–155	211
155–165	227

Adapted from Society of Actuaries and Association of Life Insurance Medical Directors of America: *Build Study 1979.* Chicago, Society of Actuaries, March 1980, p 82.

sity, probably because of enhanced turnover rates of cortisol. The circadian rhythm of cortisol secretion is usually normal in obesity. Urinary free cortisol levels are normal if related to the lean body mass or urinary creatinine. Also, obese patients usually suppress normally with dexamethasone (see Ch. 207).

Pseudotumor cerebri (benign intracranial hypertension) occurs most commonly in obese young women. No intracranial pathology has been found, although headache, blurred vision, and papilledema occur. Why obesity affects so many of these patients is unclear.

Hypothalamic control of prolactin and growth hormone is often defective in obesity, with poor responses to insulin hypoglycemia. These abnormalities generally revert to normal with weight loss, but not always. Whether these pituitary abnormalities reflect altered hypothalamic control due to obesity or abet the obesity in some way is unclear.

TREATMENT

Obesity is very difficult to treat, because the primary emphasis must be on active patient self-control rather than on passive drug therapy. The responsibility of the physician is to be as supportive and helpful as possible. The three approaches to weight control are diet, exercise, and drugs.

DIET. A truly motivated individual will generally stay on a diet for a long time, initially for weight loss and then for weight maintenance. Crash diets for a few days or weeks are ineffective. Because of the long-term requirement for a diet, it must be tailored to a person's tastes and habits.

The diet must be nutritionally adequate. It is not possible to calculate a diet under 1100 calories that contains adequate amounts of vitamins and minerals. If the diet is lower in calories than this, vitamin and mineral supplements are necessary. The goal of weight loss is to lose as much fat as possible while losing as little lean body mass as possible. A mixed, balanced diet is a sensible approach to long-term weight reduction. A diet that contains at least 0.8 to 1.2 grams of protein per kilogram of desirable body weight will minimize nitrogen losses. The protein should be of high quality, so that essential amino acids can be utilized to maintain lean body mass.

A useful strategy to induce and maintain weight reduction is to educate the obese patient appropriately with regard to the caloric content of foods. Particularly important is to emphasize the high caloric density of some foods, especially those high in fat. An attempt should be made to get the fat content of the diet below 30% of total calories. The lower the fat content, the lower the caloric content of the diet is likely to be. Foods high in fiber should be used liberally because of their low caloric density. Refined sugars should be reduced because these provide calories without any useful vitamins or minerals.

Very Low Calorie Diets. Very low calorie diets (VLCD) severely limit daily intake to 300 to 700 calories. Some diets are strictly limited to protein and have been called protein-supplemented modified fasts (PSMF). Others allow both protein and carbohydrate. The concept of protein-supplemented fasting arose because the regimen improves nitrogen balance over fasting programs. There is little evidence, however, that at equicaloric levels protein alone is better than protein with carbohydrate. The extra weight lost early in the diet when protein alone is given is that of water. With this water diuresis there is electrolyte loss as well. The calories can be given either in liquid formula form or as natural foods. High-quality protein must be given. It is also imperative that adequate supplements of vitamins and minerals be taken. These very severe diets have been given for extensive periods of time, but it is unwise to allow them to last longer than 16 weeks. The heavier the patient, the safer the diet seems to be. The lighter the patient, the more LBM is lost per unit of weight loss, so that more caution, more liberal calories, and a shorter time period of dieting should be followed. These diets, especially those relying on liquid formulas, have been popular because of their relative ease and because, since they are so hypocaloric, the weight loss is more rapid. However, they can have serious side effects.

Side effects of these severe diets include orthostatic hypotension (secondary to both sodium loss and impaired norepinephrine secretion), fatigue, cold intolerance, dry skin, hair loss, and menstrual irregularities. Cholelithiasis, cholecystitis, and rarely pancreatitis occur. Unfortunately, most individuals rapidly regain weight after being on these crash programs, perhaps in large measure because the very low caloric content and the liquid form of the diet do not educate the patient to make the adjustments in lifestyle and eating behavior necessary to maintain the weight loss.

Behavior Modification. Psychoanalysis and psychotherapy have not been very helpful in weight control. An extended change in eating behavior requires a great change in lifestyle, however, so behavior modification programs have proliferated. Behavior therapy is a fundamental departure from the traditional "dietary" training of the past, in which a list of foods, the allowable quantities, and specific menus were supplied. In behavior modification the patient is first made aware of what and how much he or she eats as a background for changing that behavior. Many persons eat quite unconsciously, with little thought of how much they eat and with little or no knowledge of its caloric content. Initially, in the education process, careful food intake diaries are kept. Patients record not only what and how much was eaten, but where, with whom, how, their feelings, and their degree of hunger. These diaries are analyzed, and nutrient densities of foods are discussed. New modes of eating are suggested, including not eating between meals, eating always at table, eating only three times per day, watching the portions of food eaten, not doing other activities while eating, and eating slowly with concentration. Behavior modification also strives at stimulus control and environmental management. The aim is to break learned associations between environmental cues and food intake. Particular situations that trigger eating are avoided or controlled. Behavior modification therapy is usually done in groups, with continued dialogue between the trained group leader (psychologist, nutritionist, physician), the other group members, and the patient.

EXERCISE. Obesity is a consequence of greater energy intake than energy expenditure. To lose weight, the imbalance must be tipped the other way, with expenditure becoming greater than intake. This is done not only by hypocaloric dieting, but also by increasing activity. Obese persons tend to be inactive; it is therefore important to increase caloric utilization. Patients should be taught the approximate number of calories being expended over basal level in individual activities. Most are surprised at how much exercise it takes to expend just a few calories (Table 196–3).

Moderate exercise only transiently increases the metabolic rate. The calories expended are the calories of work done. In the obese, moderate exercise does not actually lower food intake, but intake does not increase to keep pace with the extra expenditure, as it does in lean persons. This is helpful in inducing weight loss.

DRUG THERAPY. Drugs in weight control have been used as short-term adjunctive therapy to diet and exercise. Over the long term the use of drugs has been disappointing, owing to small effects on weight loss or adverse side effects. In general, drugs affect appetite modestly. Anorectic drugs act centrally through brain catecholamine, dopaminergic, or serotoninergic pathways. For example, amphetamine and its derivatives seem to produce anorexia through stimulating the central hypothalamic neurochemical pathways in which norepinephrine and/or dopamine is the principal neurotransmitter.

Amphetamine not only decreases appetite; it also elevates mood and increases arousal, probably mediated through making norepinephrine and dopamine more abundant at synapses. In contrast, fenfluramine is thought to increase brain serotonin. Mazindol probably works through a dopaminergic mechanism. It therefore appears that increasing the activity of norepinephrine, dopamine, and/or serotonin at certain central nervous system sites can lead to anorexia and weight loss.

All of the drugs mentioned have a greater effect on appetite control than do placebos. Problems arise, however, from abuse potential and side effects. Amphetamine has clearly addictive properties. Amphetamine and phenmetrazine may have disturbing side effects, such as sleep disturbances, agitation, and psychosis. Irritability and insomnia have been reported with diethylpropion, mazindol, and phentermine. Fenfluramine may cause depression, sedation, and diarrhea. Contraindications include severe hypertension, coronary artery disease, glaucoma, and a history of drug abuse.

These drugs are generally prescribed for short periods of time, in an effort to help patients over difficult weight "plateaus" or crisis periods. Some experts suggest that certain of the drugs lower "set point" of weight and should be given chronically. This is not generally accepted practice.

TABLE 196-3. APPROXIMATE ENERGY EXPENDITURE IN SELECTED ACTIVITIES FOR PEOPLE OF DIFFERENT WEIGHTS (CALORIES PER 30 MINUTES)*

Activity	Weight (Pounds)					
	110	130	150	170	190	210
Aerobic dancing						
"walking pace"	99	114	132	150	168	186
"jogging pace"	159	186	213	243	270	300
"running pace"	204	240	276	315	351	387
Basketball	207	243	282	318	357	396
Canoeing—leisure	66	78	90	102	114	126
Canoeing—racing	156	183	210	237	267	294
Carpentry	78	93	105	120	135	147
Cycling—5.5 mph	96	114	132	147	165	183
Cycling—9.4 mph	150	177	204	231	258	285
Dancing—ballroom	78	90	105	117	132	144
Dancing—disco	156	183	210	237	267	294
Gardening	150	177	204	231	258	285
Golf	129	150	174	195	219	243
Judo	294	345	399	450	504	558
Lying or sitting down	33	39	45	51	57	63
Mopping floor	96	105	120	138	153	171
Running						
11.5 minutes per mile	204	240	276	315	351	387
9 minutes per mile	291	342	393	447	498	552
7 minutes per mile	366	417	468	522	573	624
5.5 minutes per mile	435	513	591	669	747	828
Skiing, cross-country	216	252	291	330	369	408
Standing quietly	39	45	51	57	66	72
Swimming						
backstroke	255	300	345	390	435	486
crawl	192	228	261	297	330	366
Table tennis	102	120	138	156	174	195
Tennis	165	192	222	252	282	312
Walking						
3 mph	102	114	126	138	153	165
4 mph	120	141	162	186	207	228

* Adapted from The High Energy Factor, by Bernard Gutin. Copyright © 1983 by Bernard Gutin and Gail Kessler. Reprinted by permission of Random House, Inc.

GOALS. Very often patients, and sometimes physicians, have unrealistic goals of what can be accomplished. One pound of fat is equivalent to 4000 kilocalories. With a deficit of 400 kilocalories per day, losing one pound takes 10 days. The more accurate the knowledge of daily energy expenditure and energy intake is, the closer a physician can predict the rate of weight loss. This may prevent unrealistic goals and disappointment by both patient and therapist. The initial goal for weight loss should be modest, with an effort made to lose 10 to 15% of weight rather than to strive for an "ideal" or "normal" weight. With even this amount of loss, detectable improvement can occur in co-morbid conditions. If such weight loss can be maintained for a period of months, a further effort can be attempted.

SURGERY. Certain patients have severe obesity (greater than 100% over desirable weight), have tried weight control programs without success, and often have complications such as sleep apnea, heart failure, phlebitis, and arthritis. Their life expectancy is much lower than normal. These patients may be candidates for surgery because nonoperative management rarely leads to permanent weight reduction.

Surgery for obesity should be considered experimental, as there is no one accepted procedure and all carry significant risks and complications. Because of the severe side effects of previously done intestinal surgery, gastric surgical procedures have become popular. A small fundic pouch or reservoir is created so that individuals are severely limited in the amount of food that they can eat. The distal stoma created for the pouch has variably been designed to empty into the rest of the stomach or into a loop of jejunum, with the rest of the stomach and duodenum becoming a blind loop. Alternatively, in vertical banded gastroplasty, as opposed to horizontal banding, only a small tubular reservoir remains for food entering from the esophagus. Side effects include gastric distress, vomiting, and electrolyte disturbances. Also, some patients do not lose much weight, because many eat "around" the small reservoir with frequent servings of liquid or semisolid foods. A mean weight loss of two thirds

of excess weight has been reported, but failure is not uncommon. Dilatation of the gastric pouch, stomal dilation, stomal obstruction, and gastric dehiscence can occur as complications.

Surgery is still unsatisfactory and experimental, but it may be advisable in some cases. Because life-long follow-up and vitamin and mineral supplementation are necessary, a responsible and cooperative patient and an experienced surgeon are a requisite duo.

WEIGHT REGAIN

The most difficult problem in the treatment of obesity is the maintenance of a reduced body weight. The ability to maintain weight loss may depend on the severity of obesity and the amount of hypercellularity of the adipocytes in a given individual.

A person who is modestly overweight with enlarged adipocytes but little proliferation of extra adipocytes can more easily maintain weight loss. The adipocyte hyperplasia of greater obesity is likely to create a much greater problem in maintenance of weight loss. The degree of filling of adipocytes is very likely a regulated factor in energy balance. Obese persons with adipocyte hyperplasia begin to decrease the mass of each adipocyte as they lose weight. If the adipocyte mass drops below a normal lower level of about 0.5 μg per cell, individuals seem to have greater difficulty in maintaining weight reduction. Adipocyte mass seems to be a regulated factor with a feedback effect on energy intake, so that the reduced obese seem to experience strong food intake cues that they have trouble resisting.

Lipogenic enzyme activities increase when a hypocaloric diet is liberalized as a patient goes from a weight-loss to a weight-maintenance period. This is consequent to an increase in caloric intake rather than being primarily caused by the reduction in weight. Reduced obese individuals have been reported to require about 25% fewer calories per square meter of surface area to maintain their body weight than do either normal persons or obese individuals who have not dieted and lost weight. This is because, as obese persons reduce, the energy expended in general activity decreases owing to the smaller mass they carry. Their RMR is appropriate to the new lean body mass, but their thermic effect of activity drops unless they can greatly increase their activity pattern over the previous one. Therefore, exercise is very important in the weight maintenance phase.

PREVENTION

The propensity toward obesity is partially inherited, but a large component is also environmental. Obesity leads to an increased morbidity and mortality from a number of diseases, especially for those who are under 45 years old. Being overweight in early adult life is more dangerous than it is at older ages.

It is incumbent on physicians to make their patients aware of these risks and try to keep patients at a body mass index of grade 0 to grade 1 (see Fig. 196–1). This is particularly true for those patients who already have, or have a family history of, the diseases that are precipitated and abetted by obesity.

Atkinson R, Dietz W, Foreyt J, et al. (NIH Task Force on Obesity): Very low calorie diets. JAMA 270:967, 1993. *A review of very low and low calorie diets, their risks and benefits.*

Bjorntorp P: The associations between obesity, adipose tissue distribution and disease. Acta Med Scand (Suppl)723:121, 1988. *A review of the impact of upper body obesity on morbidity and mortality.*

Bouchard C: Genetic factors in obesity. Med Clin North Am 73:67, 1989. *The role of biologic inheritance in human body fat variation is reviewed.*

Danford D, Fletcher SW (eds.): Methods for voluntary weight loss and control. Ann Intern Med 119:641, 1993. *Report of an NIH Consensus Conference. A very useful summary of the papers detailing the present knowledge of weight loss and weight maintenance strategies, including benefits and risks.*

Garrison RJ, Castelli WP: Weight and 30 year mortality of men in the Framingham Study. Ann Intern Med 103:1006, 1985. *A report of the degree of obesity and mortality in a prospective study of men.*

Lew EA, Garfinkel L: Variations in mortality by weight among 750,000 men and women. J Chron Dis 32:563, 1979. *A description of the mortality experience of men and women in a long-term prospective study by the American Cancer Society, documenting that individuals 30 to 40% heavier than average had a mortality rate 50% higher than those of average weight. Mortality comparisons as a function of weight for all common diseases are included.*

Manson JE, Colditz GA, Stampfer MJ, et al.: A prospective study of obesity and risk of coronary heart disease in women. N Engl J Med 322:882, 1990. *A prospective study in women, specifically targeted to coronary heart disease but also following all-cause mortality.*

Pi-Sunyer FX: Health implications of obesity. Am J Clin Nutr 53:1595S, 1991. *A review of the clinical side effects of obesity.*

Ravussin E, Lillioja MB, Knowler WC, et al.: Reduced rate of energy expenditure as a risk factor for body-weight gain. N Engl J Med 318(8):467, 1988. *A report of hypometabolism as a predisposing cause of obesity.*
Segal KR, Pi-Sunyer FX: Exercise, resting metabolic rate, and thermogenesis. Diabetes/Metab Rev 2:19, 1986. *A review of the differences in thermogenic response to food and to exercise in lean and obese persons.*
Stunkard AJ, Sorensen TIA, Harris C, et al.: An adoption study of human obesity. N Engl J Med 314:193, 1986. *A study of the contributions of genetic factors and the family environment to human fatness, concluding that genetic influences have an important role in determining human fatness in adults.*

197 ENTERAL NUTRITION
John L. Rombeau

Enteral nutrition is the provision of liquid formula diets into the gastrointestinal (GI) tract. When compared with total parenteral nutrition (TPN), enteral nutrition measurably increases intestinal mucosal growth and function and is less costly. Because of these acknowledged benefits, enteral nutrition is being used with increasing frequency in medical patients. It is therefore incumbent upon physicians to be familiar with the rationale, indications, administration, and prevention of complications of enteral nutrition.

RATIONALE FOR PROVISION OF ENTERAL NUTRIENTS

EFFECTS ON INTESTINAL GROWTH AND FUNCTION. The most important stimulus for gut growth and function is the presence of nutrients within the GI tract. Enteral nutrients mediate such effects both directly and indirectly. The presence of nutrients within the intestinal lumen directly increases epithelial desquamation and enhances mucosal cell renewal. In the absence of luminal stimuli or intestinal nutrients, the small and large bowel atrophy, not only in the absorptive cells and brush-border enzymes, but in the mucus-secreting cells and the gut-associated lymphoid tissue. These are important protective components of the intestinal barrier against bacteria, endotoxins, and other antigenic macromolecules and may provide a rationale for using small volumes (e.g., 10 ml per hour) of continuous enteral feeding in critically ill patients even if they cannot tolerate larger volumes and must be fed parenterally as well.

Enteral nutrients mediate many of their indirect enterotrophic effects by stimulating gut hormones such as gastrin, neurotensin, bombesin, and enteroglucagon. Gastrin exerts trophic effects on the stomach, duodenum, and possibly the colon. Enteral nutrients given to animal models increase production of additional enterotrophic hormones. Furthermore, because of reduced manufacturing costs of its nutrient components, enteral feeding is less costly than TPN and may be more cost-effective than hand-feeding disabled or debilitated patients.

INDICATIONS

General indications for enteral nutrition include the following: (1) the presence of protein-energy malnutrition (see Ch. 194), (2) a GI tract that can safely tolerate the agents, and (3) anticipated inadequate oral intake for at least 7 days. Safe usage of the GI tract is possible in the absence of obstruction, severe intractable diarrhea, or massive bleeding. The anticipated duration of inadequate oral intake is based solely upon the clinical judgment of the primary physician. Table 197–1 indicates examples of specific medical indications for enteral nutrition. Figure 197–1 gives an algorithm for determining the method of feeding.

DIETARY FORMULAS

Commercial enteral formulas have proliferated rapidly. Table 197–2 outlines the nutrient composition of some of these agents, including polymeric-balanced diets, modified formulas, and modular supplements.

POLYMERIC-BALANCED FORMULAS. Polymeric formulas are "complete" balanced, isotonic diets containing 100% of the

Recommended Daily Allowance (RDA) for substrates, vitamins, and minerals when prescribed in recommended amounts. These formulas are palatable and are the first choice for oral supplementation or tube feeding when digestion and absorption are reasonably normal. The nitrogen source consists of an intact or partially hydrolyzed natural protein (e.g., soy, egg, lactoalbumin), requiring the patient's ability to digest protein, in addition to carbohydrate and fat. The caloric density of these formulas is usually 1 kcal per milliliter, but it can be as high as 1.5 to 2 kcal per milliliter. Calorie-dense formulas are reasonable choices for patients who have unusually high caloric requirements, can tolerate only limited feeding volumes, or require fluid restriction. Most importantly, polymeric-balanced formulas are less expensive than the other formulas. Their major disadvantage is a fixed nutrient composition.

MODIFIED FORMULAS. Conventional modified diets are also "complete" diets. Composed primarily of predigested or "elemental" nutrients, they require minimal digestion and are almost completely absorbed. Although the protein source can be crystalline amino acids, some pancreatic function is required to digest carbohydrates (oligosaccharides and disaccharides) and fats (up to 30% of which are provided as medium-chain triglycerides). In addition, absorption of glucose, sodium, amino acids, fat, vitamins, and trace elements requires intact mucosal transport systems.

Unlike the polymeric-balanced diets, modified diets are hyperosmolar, unpalatable, and relatively expensive, costing between 3 and 10 times as much per calorie as polymeric-balanced formulas. They may produce osmotic diarrhea if administered too rapidly and require flavoring supplements for oral use. Modified diets may be indicated in conditions of digestive or absorptive insufficiency, in which polymeric diets are not well tolerated. Examples of such limiting conditions include chronic pancreatitis, short bowel syndrome, and prolonged ileus.

Disease-Specific. Certain modified formulas are designed for patients with specific nutritional needs. Formulas that contain only essential amino acids as the protein source are designed for patients with renal failure. Formulas that have a protein source high in branched-chain amino acids (BCAA) and low in aromatic amino acids have been formulated for patients with hepatic encephalopathy, severe trauma, and sepsis. Formulas that are high in fat content (~55% of calories) and low in carbohydrate content (~28% of calories) have been recommended for patients with respiratory insufficiency because their oxidation produces less carbon dioxide. The high fat content of these formulas may produce diarrhea in critically ill patients. Little objective evidence justifies the use of any of these expensive, disease-specific formulas; their use should be restricted to patients with specific nutrient needs who cannot tolerate polymeric and conventional modified diets.

MODULAR SUPPLEMENTS. Modular supplements, which consist of single or multiple nutrients, can be added to existing "fixed-ratio" diets without affecting the quality or quantity of other nutrients. They are designed for patients for whom standard fixed-ratio formulas are suboptimal. Commercially available modules include carbohydrate, fat, protein, mineral, electrolyte, and vitamin formulations.

ENTERAL NUTRITION ADMINISTRATION

ACCESS. Selection of the access site for delivery of enteral nutrients is based upon the anticipated duration of forced feeding and the potential risk of aspiration. Ideally, enteral nutrition is given by the oral route in alert patients with intact gag reflexes who require nutritional supplementation only with meals. For patients who cannot tolerate oral nutrition, other access techniques include nasogastric tube, nasoenteric tube, and tube enterostomy.

Nasogastric or nasoenteric tubes are ideal for patients who require short-term (less than 4 weeks) enteral nutrition. To use these

TABLE 197–1. INDICATIONS FOR THE USE OF ENTERAL NUTRITION IN THE ADULT MEDICAL PATIENT

Protein-energy malnutrition with anticipated significantly decreased oral intake for at least 7 days
Anticipated significantly decreased oral intake for 10 days
Severe dysphagia
Massive small bowel resection (used in combination with TPN)
Low output (< 500 ml per day) enterocutaneous fistula

TABLE 197–2. COMMONLY USED COMMERCIAL ENTERAL FEEDING FORMULAS*

Category	1.0 kcal/ml	1.5 kcal/ml	2.0 kcal/ml
Polymeric Balanced			
≤16% protein	Ensure, Resource, Isocal, Osmolite, Nutren 1.0	Nutren 1.5, Ensure Plus, Resource Plus, Sustacal HC	Nutren 2.0, Deliver, Magnacal
17–20% protein	Osmolite HN, Isocal HN, Ensure HN, Ultracal, Jevity	Ensure Plus HN	TwoCal HN
≥20% protein	Sustacal, Replete, Promote	TraumaCal	
Modified-conventional			
≤16% protein	Peptamen, Reabilan, Vivonex Plus, Criticare HN		
17–20% protein	Vital HN, Reabilan HN, AlitraQ		
Modified-disease Specific (% protein)†			
Critical Care	Impact (22%)	Perative (20%)	
Glucose Intolerance	Glucerna (17%)		
Hepatic	Travasorb Hepatic (11%), Hepatic-Aid (15%)		
Malabsorption		Lipisorb (17%)	
Renal		Travasorb Renal (7%)	Nepro (14%), Suplena (6%), Amin-Aid (4%)
Pulmonary		Pulmocare (17%), NutriVent (18%)	
Modular supplements			
Protein	Propac, Casec, ProMod, Nutrisource		
Carbohydrate	Moducal, Polycose, Sumacal, Nutrisource		
Fat	Microlipid, MCT Oil, Nutrisource		

* This table includes only a partial listing of commercial products.

† Manufacturers market these products as disease specific. The author's use of this designation is intended neither to endorse the manufacturers' claims of special efficacy in the diseases specified nor to deny that some of the polymeric-balanced or modified-conventional formulas might be appropriate, or even superior, in these conditions.

access routes safely, patients must have intact gag reflexes and competent lower esophageal sphincters. Ideal candidates are those with poor oral intake such as occurs with cancer of the head and neck and the lung. The stomach is the preferred site of delivery, but the nasoenteric tube should be advanced into the jejunum in patients with gastroparesis and a high risk of aspiration.

Permanent access through tube enterostomies is the preferred route of delivery for long-term enteral nutrition (more than 4 weeks). Tube enterostomies are inserted either endoscopically, laparoscopically, or operatively into the pharynx, stomach, and jejunum.

The percutaneous endoscopic approach (PEG) is the preferred method for gastrostomy placement. It has the advantage of decreased procedure time, local anesthesia, absence of an incision, and avoidance of ileus. The speed, simplicity, low cost, and low complication rate of PEG have resulted in its replacement of surgical gastrostomy in most hospitals. Surgical gastrostomy for feeding is indicated for patients unable to tolerate PEG, or in individuals undergoing concomitant GI surgery.

Jejunostomy is indicated for patients who need long-term enteral nutrition and have chronic aspiration, gastric outlet obstruction, stomach or duodenal cancer, or have had a gastrectomy.

DELIVERY. Formulas are delivered intermittently or continuously. Intermittent feeding is preferred for delivery into the stomach because it is more physiologic and "frees" the patient from the feeding equipment. Feedings of polymeric diets in a volume of 240 to 400 ml every 4 hours are well tolerated. The disadvantages of intermittent feedings consist of an initial requirement for nursing supervision, such as monitoring for gastric residuals, and a higher risk of aspiration if delayed gastric emptying exists. Slow administration of small volumes into the stomach (25 to 40 ml per hour) is well tolerated and avoids the abdominal discomfort often caused by the increased rate and volume of intermittent feedings.

Continuous feeding, administered by infusion pump over 18 to 24 hours, requires less nursing supervision and results in smaller residual volumes as well as a lower risk of aspiration than intermittent feeding. When feeding into the duodenum or jejunum, continuous feeding is required to avoid distention of the bowel, fluid and electrolyte shifts, and diarrhea, all of which can occur with intermittent feeding. Feedings into the small bowel usually employ isotonic polymeric solutions, initially at a rate of 30 ml per hour. The rate is increased approximately 25 ml per hour per day until the desired volume is achieved to meet the patient's nutrient requirements. Infusions should be initiated at very low rates (10 ml per hour) in critically ill patients. Disadvantages of continuous feeding include

the expense of the volumetric infusion pump and the limitation it places on the ambulatory patient.

MONITORING. Patients receiving enteral feedings require the same careful monitoring as do those who receive parenteral nutrition. This is especially true in critically ill ones. Routine monitoring is best accomplished by following a protocol that ensures complete and detailed surveillance, reducing the possibility of error in formula choice and nutrient administration, and assessing progress toward nutritional goals (Table 197–3).

Special attention must be paid to the GI tolerance to the formula. The patient's condition should be evaluated daily for diarrhea, constipation, nausea, cramping, vomiting, and abdominal distention. One must give close attention to the patient's metabolic status and fluid and electrolyte balance. In many instances, potential complications can be avoided by simple maneuvers such as changing the infusion rate, caloric density, or formulation.

Periodic nutritional assessment is required to evaluate the adequacy of the nutritional support. Nitrogen balance, body weight change, and serum protein status should be monitored and the nutrient prescription amended when indicated. Because of frequent disruptions in feeding attempts, it is not uncommon for hospitalized patients to receive as little as 70% of the enteral calories ordered on a daily basis. These considerations may make it necessary to increase the infusion rate or to supplement infusions with parenteral feeding until satisfactory enteral intake is achieved.

COMPLICATIONS

Clinically significant complications of enteral feeding, although few, should be promptly recognized and treated aggressively. As noted, a standardized monitoring protocol helps to prevent and detect possible problems. Complications of enteral feeding are grouped into four major categories: gastrointestinal, metabolic, infectious, and mechanical.

GASTROINTESTINAL. Diarrhea, defined as stool weight (or volume) of more than 200 grams (or milliliters) per 24 hours, the most common complication of enteral nutrition, occurs in 10 to 20% of patients. Its possible causes are listed in Table 197–4. Tube feeding–related factors that have been suggested to predispose to diarrhea but not documented by controlled studies, include formula hyperosmolality, lactose in the presence of relative lactase deficiency, and bacterial contamination of the enteral products and delivery systems. Although contamination has not been documented as a cause for diarrhea, formula containers and administration tubing should be changed daily to avoid this complication. High-fat formulas may cause diarrhea when patients suffer from fat

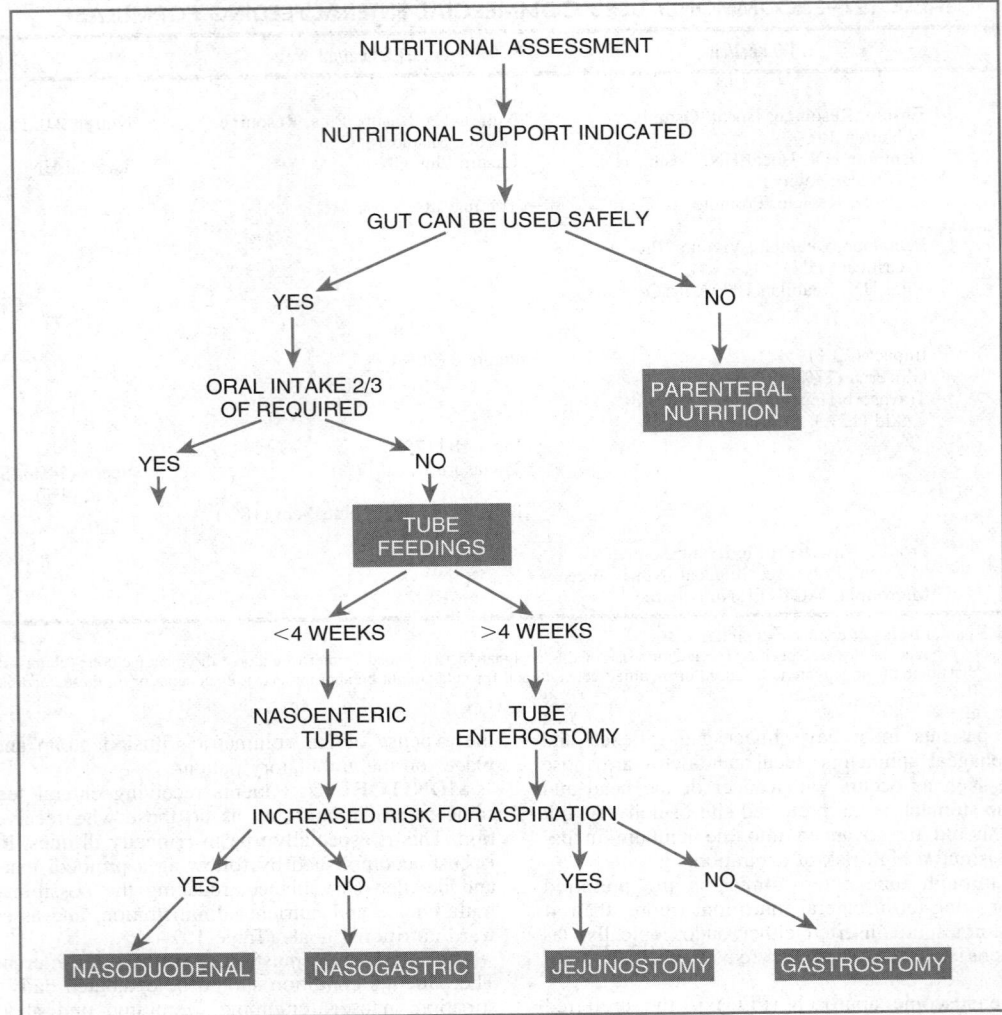

FIGURE 197–1. Decision approach for type and route of nutritional support.

malabsorption (as with pancreatic exocrine insufficiency, biliary obstruction, ileectomy, or ileitis). Enterally administered medications, including antibiotics, hyperosmolar drug solutions such as sorbitol-containing elixirs, and magnesium-containing antacids, can cause diarrhea. Many elixir medications contain substantial amounts (up to 65%) of sorbitol, although the agent is listed in alphabetical order in the drug information insert only as an "inactive" ingredient. For this reason, all elixir medications must be considered potential causes for diarrhea in tube-fed patients, and it is often prudent to discontinue them or change them to tablet or intravenous forms to determine their responsibility.

Treatment of diarrhea is directed at the underlying cause; however, several therapeutic options are available when there is no clearly identifiable cause. Decreasing the feeding flow rate may alleviate diarrhea by allowing time for intestinal mucosal adaptation to occur when the GI tract has not been used for extended periods (i.e., in starvation and TPN-induced intestinal atrophy). The flow rate is then slowly increased over several days. Parenteral feeding may be necessary to meet full nutrient requirements during this in-

TABLE 197–3. STANDARD ORDER FORM FOR PATIENTS RECEIVING ENTERAL NUTRITION

Obtain abdominal radiograph to confirm tube location before feeding.
Elevate head of bed 30 degrees when feeding into the stomach.
Record name, volume, and strength of formula, and duration and rate (ml/hr) of feeding.
Do not allow formula to hang for more than 8 hours.
Check gastric residual every 4 hours in patients receiving gastric feedings. Withhold feedings for 4 hours if residual is 50% greater than ordered volume. Notify physician if two consecutive measurements detect excessive residual.
Weigh patient on Monday, Wednesday, and Friday. Record weight on graph.
Record input and output daily. Every 8 hours, chart volume of formula administered separately from water or other oral intake.
Change administration tubing and cleanse feeding bag daily.
Irrigate feeding tube with 20 ml of water at the completion of each intermittent feeding, when tube is disconnected, after the delivery of crushed medications, or if feeding is stopped for any reason.
When patient is ingesting oral nutrients, request calorie counts daily for 5 days, then weekly thereafter.
Obtain complete blood count with red blood cell indices, SMA 12, serum iron, and serum magnesium every Monday.
Obtain SMA 6 every Thursday.
Collect urine for 24 hours, starting at 8 A.M., and analyze for urea nitrogen and creatinine each week.

TABLE 197–4. CAUSES OF DIARRHEA IN TUBE-FED PATIENTS

Common Causes Unrelated to Tube Feeding
  Elixir medications containing sorbitol
  Magnesium-containing antacids
  Antibiotic-induced sterile gut
  Pseudomembranous colitis
Possible Causes Related to Tube Feeding
  Inadequate fiber to form stool bulk
  High fat content of formula (in presence of fat malabsorption syndrome)
  Bacterial contamination of enteral products and delivery systems (causal association with diarrhea not documented)
  Rapid advancement of rate (after GI tract is unused for prolonged periods)
Unlikely Causes Related to Tube Feeding
  Formula hyperosmolality (proven not to be a cause for diarrhea)
  Lactose (absent from nearly all enteral feeding formulas)

terval. Nonspecific treatment with antidiarrheal agents can also be tried cautiously. Supplementation of formulas with pectin may help solidify the stool and slow transit time in patients not receiving broad-spectrum antibiotics. The fiber contained in some commercial formulas (usually soy polysaccharide) has not been shown to reduce the incidence of diarrhea.

METABOLIC. Metabolic complications include abnormalities of fluid and electrolyte balance, hyperglycemia, trace element deficiencies, vitamin K deficiency, and abnormalities in protein tolerance.

Overhydration occurs in 20 to 25% of patients receiving enteral nutrition. Cardiac failure and renal insufficiency aggravate the problem and complicate its management. Slowing of the infusion rate or substitution of a 1.5 to 2 kcal per milliliter formula usually provides adequate treatment, and diuretics are rarely necessary for acute control. Although uncommon, hypertonic dehydration also can occur in patients fed calorie-dense formulas, especially when they cannot communicate their thirst.

Hyperglycemia occurs in 10 to 30% of tube-fed patients. High-caloric enteral diets may unmask adult-onset diabetes mellitus. Hyperglycemia is corrected by decreasing the formula flow rate or administering insulin or implementing both of these measures. Because hyperglycemia can cause osmotic diuresis, the patient's fluid status must be carefully monitored.

Abnormalities of most electrolytes and trace elements have been reported. Routine screening of these substances permits early detection before clinical manifestations are apparent. This is especially important in patients with renal, cardiac, or hepatic insufficiency.

INFECTIOUS. The most common infectious complication of enteral nutrition is aspiration pneumonia, which is potentially fatal. Its incidence varies from 1 to 44%, depending on how it is defined. Aspiration can occur subtly, without witnessed episodes of vomiting, and it should be suspected with new onset of tachycardia, tachypnea, fever, hypoxemia, or chest radiographic changes. Patients fed nasogastrically appear to have a higher likelihood of aspiration than patients fed by gastrostomy or jejunostomy. Those with an endotracheal tube or a tracheostomy have an especially high risk. Feeding beyond the pylorus probably lowers the incidence of aspiration, although no conclusive evidence supports this premise.

Preventive measures include elevating the head of the bed to 30 degrees, periodic measuring of gastric residuals, and inflating endotracheal tube cuffs. Correct techniques to insert the soft feeding tubes and careful observation of the tube's position may prevent potentially lethal bronchopleural complications. A chest radiograph should be obtained prior to initiating feeding in every patient with a newly inserted nasogastric or nasoenteric tube. Methods for detecting the "silent" aspiration of enteral formulas in intubated patients include checking tracheal aspirates for the presence of glucose with the use of oxidant reagent strips or placing methylene blue dye in the formula, as a potential marker in tracheal aspirates.

MECHANICAL. Mechanical complications associated with enteral nutrition generally relate to the tube itself or to its anatomic position. Nasoenteric tubes can cause nasopharyngeal erosions and discomfort, sinusitis, otitis media, gagging, esophagitis, esophageal reflux, tracheoesophageal fistulas, and rupture of esophageal varices. Feeding tubes can become knotted or clogged. Gastrostomy or jejunostomy tubes can cause mechanical obstruction of the pylorus or small bowel. Additional complications of percutaneous tubes include leakage around the tube, dislodgment to an intraperitoneal position, and occlusion, especially of small-bore needle-catheter jejunostomies.

Guenther PA, Settle RG, Perlmutter S, et al.: Tube feeding–related diarrhea in acutely ill patients. J Parenter Enter Nutr 15:277, 1991. *Review of the causes and potential treatments for diarrhea in patients receiving enteral nutrition.*

Moore FA, Feliciano DV, Andrassy RJ, et al.: Early enteral feeding, compared with parenteral, reduces postoperative septic complications: The results of a meta-analysis. Ann Surg 216:172, 1992. *Review of published clinical trials of enteral nutrition versus TPN. Significant increases in infectious complications were noted in patients receiving TPN.*

Rombeau JL, Caldwell MD (eds.): Clinical Nutrition: Enteral and Tube Feeding, 2nd ed. Philadelphia, W.B. Saunders, 1990. *Detailed and extensively illustrated text includes scientific principles and practical clinical aspects of enteral nutrition.*

The Veterans Affairs Total Parenteral Nutrition Cooperative Study Group: Perioperative total parenteral nutrition in surgical patients. N Engl J Med 325:525, 1991. *Largest published prospective, controlled, clinical trial of TPN. Significant increases in infectious complications were noted in patients receiving TPN.*

198 PARENTERAL NUTRITION
M. Molly McMahon

It was first appreciated in 1968 that patients could receive all of their nutritional requirements intravenously. This advance was a landmark for the field of nutrition and clinical medicine. While parenteral nutrition can be essential, or even lifesaving, its substantial cost and potential for complications necessitate that it be used judiciously.

DEFINITION. The term *parenteral nutrition* (PN) should be used in place of intravenous hyperalimentation. The latter was coined at a time when provision of an excess of calories was believed to be beneficial; it is now accepted that overfeeding should be avoided. PN provides amino acids (nitrogen), dextrose (carbohydrate), fat, electrolytes, minerals, trace elements, vitamins, and water by central vein (central parenteral nutrition, CPN) or by peripheral vein (peripheral parenteral nutrition, PPN). The enteral route should always be selected for the provision of nutrition in malnourished patients with a functional gastrointestinal tract because the bowel atrophies when nutrients are provided exclusively by vein.

NUTRITIONAL CONTENT

PROTEIN. An essential component of PN is nitrogen. All currently manufactured PN solutions use crystalline amino acids as the source of nitrogen for protein synthesis. Each gram of protein provides 4.0 kilocalories. The protein solutions are available with or without added electrolytes and minerals. For the well-nourished healthy subject without stress, the recommended dietary allowance of protein is 0.8 gram per kilogram per day provided that total caloric intake is adequate. Protein is a metabolic fuel although its structural functions are as important as its fuel functions. At steady-state, amino acid oxidation equals protein intake. Therefore, caloric requirements should be estimated as total calories rather than as nonprotein calories.

Protein breakdown and synthesis are dynamic processes. During severe stress, protein catabolism exceeds protein synthesis, resulting in a net loss of body protein. Body protein stores are minimal, and because all amino acids exist as structural protein, net protein loss results in a loss of tissue function. The increase in proteolysis is caused by the actions of hormones and cytokines. Additional protein losses may occur with specific disease states. Diminished protein synthesis results from bed rest and decreased food intake. Most hospitalized patients receiving PN should receive between 1.0 and 1.5 grams of protein per kilogram of body weight per day. Stressed patients should receive the higher end of the protein range. For most patients, provision of greater amounts of protein does not provide benefit, and the excess protein results in ureagenesis. The provision of nutrition support to critically ill, immobilized patients can decrease but not prevent the loss of body protein.

Modified amino acid solutions have been formulated for use in specific disease states. For example, the use of branched-chain enriched amino acid solutions (providing up to 50% of the amino acids as leucine, isoleucine, and valine) has been suggested for patients with hepatic encephalopathy. These patients have decreased plasma levels of branched-chain amino acids and increased levels of the aromatic amino acids. Branched-chain amino acids are uniquely oxidized in skeletal muscle and adipose tissue rather than the liver. Several studies indicate that patients prone to encephalopathy can be given more protein using branched-chain enriched solutions (compared with standard solution) without worsening the encephalopathy. The clinical effectiveness of formulas with high levels of branched-chain amino acids is controversial, however, as few prospective randomized trials have compared results of this treatment with standard therapy. Once the encephalopathy resolves, the less costly standard amino acid solution should be used. Patients with liver disease without encephalopathy can also tolerate the less costly standard amino acid solutions. Insufficient data support the use of branched-chain amino acid solutions in patients with renal failure or severe stress.

Another example of a modified amino acid formulation is a more concentrated (15%) amino acid base solution. Use of this product enables higher caloric and protein provision in less volume for patients with excess total body water and salt. Again, the disadvantages of this product are its expense and the lack of prospective, randomized trials confirming efficacy. PN supplementation with the amino acid glutamine is undergoing investigation. Currently, glutamine is not present in commercially available PN solutions in the United States, because it has a shorter shelf life than the more commonly used amino acids and has been considered a nonessential amino acid. During critical illness, however, glutamine appears to be a conditionally essential amino acid for the intestinal tract. For patients undergoing bone marrow transplantation, use of glutamine-supplemented PN (compared with standard amino acid solution) improved clinical outcome with fewer infections and shortened hospital stay. Additional prospective randomized trials of these modified formulas are needed.

CARBOHYDRATE. Parenteral carbohydrate is provided in the form of dextrose. Solutions of dextrose in concentrations of 10 to 70% are mixed with the appropriate amount of amino acids to obtain the desired solution. The dextrose is hydrated, and each gram of dextrose monohydrate provides 3.4 kilocalories. Body carbohydrate stores are limited. The minimum daily glucose requirement is the amount necessary to meet brain glucose needs (100 to 150 grams per day). In healthy subjects, dextrose infusion suppresses hepatic glucose release (decrease in need for protein-derived gluconeogenic precursors) and stimulates glucose oxidation (decrease in requirement for amino acid oxidation as an energy source). In addition, dextrose infusion stimulates insulin, which is a strong inhibitor of protein breakdown. The beneficial effects of dextrose as a substrate in PN are attributed to the provision of calories with a nitrogen-sparing effect.

INTRAVENOUS FAT EMULSION. Currently available intravenous fat emulsions consist of 10% (1.1 kcal per milliliter) or 20% (2.0 kcal per milliliter) emulsions of long-chain fatty acids derived from safflower and/or soybean oil, egg yolk phospholipid, and an emulsifying agent (glycerin) to render it isotonic. Parenteral fat is calorically dense, isotonic, protein sparing, and can prevent essential fatty acid deficiency. In addition, provision of a portion of calories as fat allows lower rates of dextrose infusion and results in less hyperglycemia and hyperinsulinemia, as well as a lower incidence of abnormalities in liver function tests. The fat can be administered intravenously either by piggyback infusion or as a 3-in-1 admixture of fat, dextrose, and protein in one container. The fat emulsion is hydrolyzed by lipoprotein lipase to free fatty acids and glycerol. When fatty acids are oxidized for fuel, the respiratory quotient and therefore carbon dioxide production rates are lower than those observed if carbohydrate or protein is oxidized; this may be advantageous in certain clinical situations (e.g., severe pulmonary disease).

Adverse effects, including hypoxemia, hepatic dysfunction, and impaired immune function due to uptake of fat by the reticuloendothelial system, have been reported with intravenous fat administration. However, all of the effects have been demonstrated at the higher infusion rates achieved during 8- to 12-hour infusions rather than during 24-hour infusions. At very high infusion rates, enzymatic removal systems for free fatty acids become saturated, a step that can lead to hypertriglyceridemia. No data suggest that intravenous administration of long-chain triglyceride emulsions at rates of 30 to 50 mg per kilogram per hour (for 70-kg patient, approximately 50 to 85 grams per day) to normolipemic patients results in any adverse effects. Thus, continuous lipid infusion is preferable to discontinuous lipid infusion. If the plasma triglyceride concentration exceeds 400 mg per deciliter, the lipid infusion rate should be reduced or the infusion discontinued. The optimal percentage of calories that should be infused as fat is not known. Essential fatty acid deficiency can be prevented if approximately 5% of total calories is given as fat, and provision of 30% of total calories as fat is generally recommended for stressed patients receiving PN. The role of lipid extends beyond that of energy substrate alone, as substitution of different lipid sources has been reported to beneficially modify the host's response to illness. There is active investigation to determine the optimal type (e.g., medium-chain triglycerides, short-chain triglycerides, structured triglycerides, omega-3 fatty acids) and quantity of fat to be provided in PN solutions.

ELECTROLYTES, MINERALS, TRACE ELEMENTS, AND MULTIVITAMINS. Electrolytes and minerals required for health are sodium, potassium, chloride, calcium, phosphorus, magnesium, and sulfur. The electrolytes are supplied as salts, e.g., calcium gluconate, magnesium sulfate, potassium chloride, sodium chloride, and potassium phosphate. Most sodium and potassium cations are added to the PN solution as chloride or acetate salts after the phosphate requirement is met. Acetate is further metabolized by the liver to bicarbonate, providing an alkaline buffer.

The composition of intravenous multivitamin products has been formulated according to the guidelines of the American Medical Association Nutrition Advisory Group. One adult and one pediatric multivitamin formulation are commercially available. The adult formulation provides the daily maintenance for three fat-soluble and nine water-soluble vitamins (Table 198–1). For patients requiring short-term nutrition, vitamin K often is not routinely added to PN solutions. Accordingly, the prothrombin time should be monitored to determine whether vitamin K supplementation is needed. The daily multivitamin dose may be increased for patients with suspected or documented vitamin deficiencies. Serious consequences can result if standard replacement amounts for vitamins are not provided. During a recent nationwide shortage of intravenous multivitamin preparations, three patients receiving thiamine-deficient PN died with refractory lactic acidosis and a clinical course suggestive of beriberi. Autopsy of the brain of two of these patients revealed lesions diagnostic of acute thiamine deficiency.

Trace elements are available commercially as combination products or as single-item injections; 1 ml of the multiple trace element injection contains zinc, copper, manganese, and chromium in amounts that are suggested for medically stable adult patients (Table 198–2). This amount may be adjusted as needed for individual patients. Since iron, iodine, and selenium are not routinely added to PN solutions for patients requiring short-term nutrition support, monitoring of levels and supplementation of these elements may be required for patients receiving long-term PN.

INDICATIONS FOR NUTRITION SUPPORT

MALNUTRITION. Protein catabolism (with eventual depletion of body protein leading to protein-calorie malnutrition) can be a consequence of starvation, severe illness, or a combination. Malnutrition is difficult to define and inevitably arbitrary. It reflects the timing and extent of recent (previous 3- to 6-month interval) unintentional weight loss; the presence or absence of clinical markers of stress; and the anticipated time that the patient will be unable to meet nutritional requirements orally that determine the need for nutritional support. Nutritional support should be provided promptly for severely stressed patients because the metabolic response to illness affects the malnourished individual more seriously than the nourished person. Studies that have demonstrated a beneficial influence of nutritional support on clinical outcome have provided nutrition for a minimum of 1 week. Currently there is no evidence that suggests that nutrition support of briefer duration is beneficial. Additional research is needed to develop clinical markers for malnutrition and identify patients who will benefit from nutrition support.

DELIVERY OF PN

INDICATIONS. Once it has been determined that nutritional support should be initiated, the route for nutrient delivery should be selected. Parenteral nutrition should be used whenever nutrition

TABLE 198–1. STANDARD ADULT MULTIVITAMIN INJECTION

Vitamin	Amount per Dose per Day
A (retinol)	3300 IU
D (ergocalciferol)	200 IU
E (dl-alpha tocopheryl acetate)	10 IU
C (ascorbic acid)	100 mg
B_1 (thiamine)	3 mg
B_2 (riboflavin)	3.6 mg
B_6 (pyridoxine)	4 mg
B_{12} (cyanocobalamin)	5 μg
Folic acid	400 μg
Niacinamide	40 mg
Dexpanthenol	15 mg
Biotin	60 μg

TABLE 198–2. STANDARD ADULT TRACE ELEMENT INJECTION

Trace Element	Amount / Dose / Day
Zinc	4 mg
Copper	1 mg
Manganese	500 μg
Chromium	10 μg

support is indicated in a patient with a nonfunctioning gastrointestinal tract. In particular, PN should be considered for malnourished patients who have persistent bowel obstruction, gastrointestinal motility disorders (other than isolated gastroparesis), malabsorption, short bowel syndrome with insufficient intestinal adaptation to maintain nutritional status using the enteral route, prolonged postoperative ileus, hypotension, severe pancreatitis, and in patients in whom a feeding tube cannot be placed in the desired location. PN can be added supplementally for patients who tolerate tube feeding at a low rate but not at a rate sufficient to meet caloric requirements. While it is difficult to establish absolute criteria for the use of PN, the American Society for Parenteral and Enteral Nutrition has published guidelines for the general use of PN as well as recommendations for its use in selected disease states. Once the decision has been made that PN is indicated, the clinician is faced with the challenge of selecting CPN or PPN as the preferred form of nutrition.

CENTRAL VS. PERIPHERAL PN: INDICATIONS, ADVANTAGES, AND LIMITATIONS. Peripheral parenteral nutrition (PPN) should be considered in medically stable patients requiring short-term (e.g., 7 to 10 days) parenteral support, because it avoids the risks of central venous catheterization. Central parenteral nutrition (CPN) is necessary to provide adequate nutrition to patients who are moderately or severely stressed or who are anticipated to require longer use of parenteral support. It is not possible to administer by PPN the high osmolarity solutions used in CPN because a high incidence of infiltration and phlebitis follows administration of such solutions via peripheral veins. For this reason the osmolarity of PPN solutions should not exceed 1000 mOsm per liter. The addition of isotonic lipid to dextrose and amino acids is believed to enhance vein tolerance to PPN solutions. There are limitations to the use of PPN. The cost is similar to that of CPN solutions. Further, critically ill patients will often not tolerate the high volume rates required to meet nutrition needs.

Parenteral nutrition is an essential form of nutrition for malnourished patients with nonfunctioning gastrointestinal tracts. An understanding of the indications for use, appreciation of the significant cost and potential complications, and the ability to design a nutrition program and monitoring plan are important to effective use of this therapy. Future prospective randomized trials are needed to establish outcome data in appropriate patient groups. Evidence that

the use of alternate fuel sources may beneficially modify the body's response to illness is stimulating research that may expand the role of nutritional support.

Vascular Access. Selection of the site for catheter insertion should be individualized for each patient. Cannulation of a high-flow central vessel permits infusion of hyperosmolar nutrient solutions that are not tolerated by smaller low-flow peripheral veins. In general, the preferred site of central catheter insertion is the subclavian vein, both for patient comfort and ease of management. Central vein cannulation for PN should never be considered an emergency procedure. Coagulation studies should be checked prior to catheterization, and patients should be adequately hydrated. Sterile technique during catheter insertion is mandatory. While placement of double- or triple-lumen catheters is appropriate in patients who require multiple infusions or hemodynamic monitoring in addition to PN, medically stable patients should receive nutrition via a single-lumen catheter. Prior to initiation of CPN, a chest radiograph should be obtained to confirm catheter tip location in the distal superior vena cava.

The peripherally inserted central (PIC) catheter, which has long been used successfully in children, may also be used effectively in selected adult patients. These radiopaque catheters, inserted in the basilic or cephalic vein via the antecubital fossa and advanced to the distal superior vena cava for infusion of CPN, provide reliable venous access for medically stable patients requiring from 1 week to as much as 6 months of CPN. Early reports noted a high incidence of phlebitis with PIC catheter use, but more recent reports have had more favorable results. The use of PIC catheters preserves existing peripheral vasculature, eliminates many of the risks associated with central venous catheter insertion, and is time and cost efficient.

ESTIMATION OF DAILY CALORIC REQUIREMENTS. The daily caloric requirement of patients can be estimated by use of a formula, such as the Harris-Benedict equation, or measured by indirect calorimetry (Table 198–3). For many years it was believed that patients requiring nutritional support had elevated caloric requirements, especially when stressed by surgery, trauma, or sepsis. Over the last decade, however, numerous studies have shown that the majority of hospitalized patients have surprisingly normal energy expenditure, usually between 100% and 120% of predicted caloric expenditure. Overfeeding is poorly tolerated by stressed patients. Excess calories can increase oxygen consumption, carbon dioxide production, minute ventilation, and the work of breathing, which can fatigue patients with impaired lung function. Overfeeding also can cause hyperglycemia, which may adversely affect leukocyte and complement function. Finally, excessive calories can cause abnormal liver test results. To design a specific PN program, the clinician should first determine the appropriate volume for the individual patient, then estimate the caloric requirement, and finally estimate the protein and fat requirements (approximately one third of total calories), providing the remaining calories as carbohydrate.

TABLE 198–3. GUIDELINES FOR ESTIMATING DAILY CALORIC, PROTEIN, AND LIPID REQUIREMENTS OF HOSPITALIZED PATIENTS

Requirements	Moderately to severely stressed patient in intensive care unit*	Mildly to moderately stressed patient in hospital ward*
Calories†	Basal Harris-Benedict	Basal Harris-Benedict to Harris-Benedict plus 20%
Protein‡	1.5 g/kg body weight	1.0–1.5 g/kg of body weight
Lipid	30% of total calories during 24	30% of total calories during 24

Modified from McMahon M, Farnell M, Murray M: Nutritional support of critically ill patients. Mayo Clin Proc 68:911–920, 1993.

Harris-Benedict equation
  Females: 655 + (9.6 × weight, kg) + (1.7 × height, cm) − (4.7 × age, yr)
  Males: 66 + (13.7 × weight, kg) + (5.0 × height, cm) − (6.8 × age, yr).
* If patient weight ≥ 120% of ideal body weight, basal Harris-Benedict estimate of caloric needs (based on current weight) and 1.5 grams of protein per kilogram (based on ideal weight) are adequate. Ideal body weight can be estimated by the following method: females, 45.4 kg for 1.5 meters and 2.3 kg per additional 2.5 cm; males, 48.1 kg for 1.5 meters and 2.7 kg per additional 2.5 cm.
† An indirect calorimetric measurement of daily caloric needs is particularly helpful in the following groups of patients: severely stressed patients (e.g., following closed-head injury, multiple trauma, severe burn), volume-overloaded patients in whom the "dry weight" estimate is uncertain, nutritionally supported patients in whom weaning from mechanical ventilation is difficult, morbidly obese patients, or severely malnourished patients.
‡ Assumes normal or near-normal hepatic and renal function.

MONITORING PN. After initiation of PN, one must carefully monitor the patient's vital signs and laboratory values. The presence of fever should always be explained in a patient with a central catheter. Hemodynamic data, fluid balance, creatinine, urea, and sodium should be reviewed to help determine the appropriate PN volume. Daily weight should be interpreted in light of the fluid balance; weight increases exceeding 0.25 kg over a 24-hour period usually reflect fluid gain. Biochemical monitoring should include a complete blood count, electrolytes, glucose, creatinine, urea nitrogen, amino transferase, bilirubin, alkaline phosphatase, phosphorus, calcium, and albumin. Plasma magnesium, zinc, and copper levels should be measured in patients with impaired absorption or increased gastrointestinal (zinc, copper) or renal (magnesium) output. The calcium, magnesium, and zinc values should be interpreted with knowledge of the albumin level, as they are albumin-bound. For patients receiving fat emulsion, triglyceride levels should be checked prior to and following initiation of PN. The extent and frequency of biochemical monitoring following initiation of PN should be individualized; at a minimum, plasma glucose, electrolytes, and phosphorus levels should be checked until stable. During short-term hospitalization, a serum glucose goal range of 100 to 200 mg per deciliter is appropriate. If glucose values exceed 180 to 200 mg per deciliter, regular insulin may be added to the PN admixture. Initiation of a subcutaneous regular insulin algorithm or a variable intravenous insulin infusion should be considered if glycemic control is not adequate using PN insulin alone.

PN should not constitute the sole treatment for acute abnormalities in volume or electrolyte disturbances, but it is an effective vehicle to replace chronic losses. Knowledge of the volume of gastrointestinal and renal losses allows estimation of electrolyte and mineral losses and appropriate PN supplementation. A daily review of the medication profile is important in an attempt to anticipate and manage metabolic changes (e.g., amphotericin: hypokalemia, hypomagnesemia, renal tubular acidosis; corticosteroids: hyperglycemia, hypokalemia; insulin: hypokalemia, hypophosphatemia, hypomagnesemia; diuretics: hypokalemia, hypomagnesemia, metabolic alkalosis; propofol: this anesthetic agent is in a 10% fat emulsion, and its administration may temporarily eliminate or decrease the requirement for additional fat. The acetate and chloride content of the PN admixture should be adjusted for acid-base disturbances. The acetate and chloride balance should be based on the blood gases (arterial or venous), electrolytes, and the source and volume of gastrointestinal or renal losses. The acetate content may be increased and the chloride content decreased in metabolic acidosis; the converse is true for metabolic alkalosis. Although the extent of the daily examination must be individualized, the catheter site, heart, and lungs should always be examined, and the possible development of peripheral edema assessed. Use of a clinical monitoring record that combines information about the PN composition with biochemical data facilitates prompt recognition of metabolic abnormalities. The daily goal is to determine whether the PN program (volume or composition) needs modification in light of the patient's current condition. Once the gastrointestinal tract regains function, the enteral route should always be used for nutrition. Although sudden discontinuation of PN has been reported to precipitate hypoglycemia, these results occurred when excessive calories were received which could lead to exaggerated insulin responses. In the absence of overfeeding, a 50% decrease in the PN infusion rate for 1 hour prior to discontinuation appears safe and should not cause hypoglycemia.

Volume-Restricted PN. Patients with excess total body water and salt following major surgery or illness are often those most in need of nutrition support. The ability to concentrate CPN solutions may allow earlier and more adequate nutrition support. By use of concentrated commercial solutions of 10% amino acids and 70% dextrose, 1 liter can, for example, provide 70 grams of protein and 200 grams of dextrose (960 total calories). Fat should be added when a larger volume can be tolerated. To further restrict volume the PN admixture may be used as a vehicle for drugs with a stable dose requirement, provided therapeutic efficacy has been documented for continuous drug infusion. Medications commonly added to the PN admixture include histamine receptor antagonists and insulin.

COMPLICATIONS

The complications associated with PN can be categorized into catheter related (mechanical, infectious, and thrombotic), metabolic, and gastrointestinal. Studies have demonstrated that the use of organized interdisciplinary nutrition support teams reduces complications.

Pneumothorax, the most common mechanical complication, is most often related to improper central vein cannulation technique. Anatomic factors (such as cachexia, barrel chest deformity, kyphosis, and morbid obesity) can increase the risk even with satisfactory technique. An important predictor of complications associated with central catheter insertion is the physician's experience in catheter insertion.

Catheter malposition is generally not serious if recognized early. Misdirection most often involves a subclavian catheter traveling up the ipsilateral internal jugular vein. The catheter usually can be repositioned, employing either the catheter guide wire technique or fluoroscopic manipulation. Other uncommon complications related to catheter placement include air embolism, subclavian or internal carotid artery puncture, hemothorax, hemomediastinum, catheter embolism, thoracic duct injury, and brachial plexus injury.

Bacteremia and fungemia are serious complications, and the catheter should always be evaluated as a potential source of infection. Most catheter-related septicemias begin with focal infections of the catheter wound; organisms from the patient's own cutaneous flora invade the intracutaneous tract when the catheter is inserted and thereafter. Hub contamination may also cause catheter-related septicemia. In addition, hematogenous seeding of the fibrin sheath on the catheter tip can occur during an episode of bacteremia or fungemia. Sterile technique and the use of effective antiseptics during catheter insertion are the most important measures to prevent catheter sepsis.

The two types of infection that occur most are catheter infection and catheter-related septicemia. Quantitative cultures of the external surface of the catheter differentiate infection from contamination more reliably than the broth-culture method. Infection is diagnosed when the culture of the catheter grows > 15 colony-forming units. Catheter-related septicemia is diagnosed by semiquantitative catheter cultures and blood cultures that are positive for the same species. The most common organisms that cause catheter-related sepsis are coagulase-negative staphylococci, *Staphylococcus aureus,* and yeast. In selected circumstances (unexplained fever or leukocytosis), replacement of the catheter by guide wire exchange technique is appropriate. Catheters should always be removed immediately if patients appear septic. Blood (peripheral and central) and catheter cultures should always be obtained; if applicable, the catheter site should also be cultured. New types of catheters and cuffs are being developed to reduce the risk of device-related infection.

While subclinical venous thrombosis commonly occurs in patients receiving CPN, clinically important thrombosis is uncommon during short-term nutrition use. The incidence, however, is higher in patients receiving long-term PN. The diagnosis should always be considered when a patient develops swelling in the arm and neck ipsilateral to the catheter and develops swollen veins in the neck. The use of very low doses of heparin (5000 to 6000 U in PN per day) or warfarin (approximately 1 mg per day) can reduce the incidence of central vein thrombosis without causing adverse hemorrhagic effects and should be considered for patients requiring long-term PN.

Profound metabolic consequences can result from several causes, including providing parenteral calories in excess of needs, the exclusive use of dextrose as the caloric source, or either an excess or deficiency of nutrients. Serious and life-threatening complications have been recognized since the advent of PN therapy. The risks increase when chronically malnourished patients are too rapidly refed, principally as a result of fluid and electrolyte abnormalities. Sudden refeeding results in an acute increase in plasma insulin concentration, which can affect salt and water balance and electrolyte homeostasis. Hyperinsulinemia promotes renal tubular reabsorption of sodium, which can expand extracellular fluid and provoke cardiac decompensation in extremely malnourished patients with decreased left ventricular mass. Hyperinsulinemia also can cause a decrease in the plasma concentrations of potassium, phosphorus, and magnesium. Hyperinsulinemia promotes the passage of potassium from the extracellular space into the intracellular space and results in hypokalemia. Glucose- and insulin-stimulated glycolysis enhance cellular uptake and use of phosphorus for the phosphorylation of glycolytic intermediates and for adenosine triphosphate synthesis. Hyperinsulinemia can increase tissue uptake of magnesium, resulting in hypomagnesemia. The adverse sequelae resulting from hypokalemia, hypophosphatemia, and hypomagnesemia are discussed in Chs. 75.3, 190, 191. Patients receiving long-term PN suffer an increased risk of developing metabolic bone disease.

Hepatic abnormalities are the most common gastrointestinal complications associated with PN. The spectrum reflects not only a complication of the therapy itself, but also relates to the patient's underlying medical status and use of medication. In adults, PN-related hepatic abnormalities are common and are generally benign and temporary. Some patients requiring long-term PN, however, have persisting abnormalities in liver function tests associated with fibrotic and/or cholestatic damage. Complications may be biochemical (elevation of serum aminotransferase, alkaline phosphatase, or bilirubin) or histologic (steatosis, portal triaditis). Transaminase elevations generally occur early in therapy (1 to 2 weeks after initiation of PN) and often resolve without change in the PN program. Bilirubin and alkaline phosphatase elevations usually appear slightly later (2 to 3 weeks into therapy). While the etiology of PN-related hepatic abnormalities has not been clearly elucidated, many factors have been proposed, including the PN solution (excessive dextrose or total calories, or fat-free PN), nutritional deficiencies (carnitine, taurine, essential fatty acid deficiency), and cholestasis. Biliary complications associated with PN include acalculous cholecystitis, gallbladder sludge, and cholelithiasis. Sludge, the most common of these, occurs when the gastrointestinal tract is not used.

Abnormalities of the liver function test should not automatically lead to stopping or altering the PN solution, since abnormal liver function tests may not represent true liver dysfunction. Other causes of abnormal hepatic function, such as extrahepatic obstruction, medications, or infection, should be excluded. The nutrition program should be reviewed to be certain that the caloric intake is not excessive and that a mixed-fuel system (i.e., dextrose, protein, and fat) is being infused.

ASPEN: Guidelines for the use of parenteral and enteral nutrition in adult and pediatric patients. JPEN 17S:1SA, 1993. *Provides concise guidelines (and recent references) for the use of PN.*

Driscoll DF, Baptista RJ, Mitrano FP, et al.: Parenteral nutrient admixtures as drug vehicles: Theory and practice in the critical care setting. Ann Pharmacother 25:276, 1991. *Important resource for pharmaceutical information regarding PN admixtures.*

McMahon M, Farnell MB, Murray MJ: Nutritional support of critically ill patients. Mayo Clin Proc 68:911, 1993. *Discusses metabolic response to illness, hormonal and cytokine effects on nutritional assessment, and design of nutritional programs for hospitalized patients.*

Rose BD: Clinical Physiology of Acid-Base and Electrolyte Disorders. New York, McGraw-Hill, 1989. *Superb resource on electrolyte and acid-base metabolism.*

Solomon S, Kirby DF: The refeeding syndrome: A review. JPEN 14:90, 1990. *Discusses pathophysiology of the refeeding syndrome.*

Subcommittee on the Tenth Edition of the RDA's: Recommended Dietary Allowances. National Academy Press, 1989. *A valuable and concise resource on clinical deficiencies and recommended allowances for macronutrients, vitamins, minerals, trace elements, and electrolytes.*

PART XVII

ENDOCRINE AND
REPRODUCTIVE DISEASES

199 PRINCIPLES
OF ENDOCRINOLOGY
Gordon N. Gill

Communication is essential for all life processes. Accurate sensing of the environment and appropriate coordinated responses depend on the nervous and endocrine systems, which are tightly interwoven. Nervous system functions are mediated by hormones and the endocrine system is centrally controlled by the nervous system. Communication between cells is necessary for development from a single fertilized egg to a mature adult, for an orderly reproductive cycle, and for homeostatic adjustments to a constantly changing environment. Hormones, distinct chemical messengers, transmit information from one cell to another to coordinate homeostatic adaptations, growth, development, and reproduction. *Hormones,* a word derived from Greek meaning "excite" or "set in motion," bind with high affinity and specificity to receptors, which are allosteric proteins. Receptor proteins have two essential functional characteristics: a recognition site, which binds hormones with high specificity and affinity, and an activity site, which transduces the information received into a biochemical message. Allosteric receptor proteins adopt various conformational states; binding of the hormone ligand results in the active conformation. The initial event in hormone action is thus a bimolecular reaction dependent on the concentration of hormone, the concentration of receptor, and the affinity of receptor for hormone.

$$\underset{\text{Inactive}}{[\text{Hormone}] + [\text{Receptor}]} \underset{k_{-1}}{\overset{k_1}{\rightleftharpoons}} \underset{\text{Active}}{[\text{Hormone-Receptor}]}$$

Factors that control the concentration of both hormone and receptor determine biologic responses of cells, of organs, and of the whole organism.

Classic endocrinology dealt with the glands that produce hormones and the concentration of hormone to which cells expressing receptors are exposed. Biosynthesis, secretion, transport of hormone to target cells, and metabolic inactivation determine the effective hormone concentration. Diseases of endocrine glands that impair hormone production result in deficiency states, whereas diseases that cause excessive production result in hormone excess states. Expression of receptor is equally important in forming the active hormone-receptor complex. Genetic and acquired diseases that impair receptors result in deficiency states even though hormone concentrations are compensatorily increased. Increased receptor expression results in an excess state, an event that occurs with growth factor receptors in malignant transformation.

Hormones are produced not only by the glands of internal secretion but by a variety of cells throughout the body. Neurohormones, produced in the hypothalamus, are also produced in cells throughout the nervous system to modulate neuronal function. Gastrointestinal hormones are produced within the nervous system. Hormones that regulate production and maturation of cells of the hematopoietic and immune systems are made in cells of these lineages and in endothelial and mesenchymal cells. Growth-promoting and -inhibiting hormones (growth factors and growth inhibitors) are produced by macrophages and mesenchymal cells. Many of these signaling molecules do not travel long distances through the blood to reach target cells as do classic hormones (endocrine) but act on target cells in the vicinity of the producer cell (paracrine) or even on the producer cell itself (autocrine). During development, cell surface hormones may act on the cell surface receptor of a neighbor cell as a cell-cell communication system. Regardless of signaling distance, the same principles of hormone-receptor interactions operate.

HOW HORMONES WORK

Two classes of hormones operate via two types of receptors (Fig. 199–1). Peptide hormones are synthesized as parts of larger protein molecules and processed as secretory proteins. They act via receptors located in the cell membrane with the recognition/binding site exposed on the cell surface and the activity domain facing the inside of the cell. Activated cell surface receptors use a variety of strategies to transduce signal information, often activating second messengers, which amplify and distribute the molecular information. Many peptide hormones ultimately signal via regulation of protein phosphorylation. In this most common process through which proteins are covalently modified, a phosphate group is do-

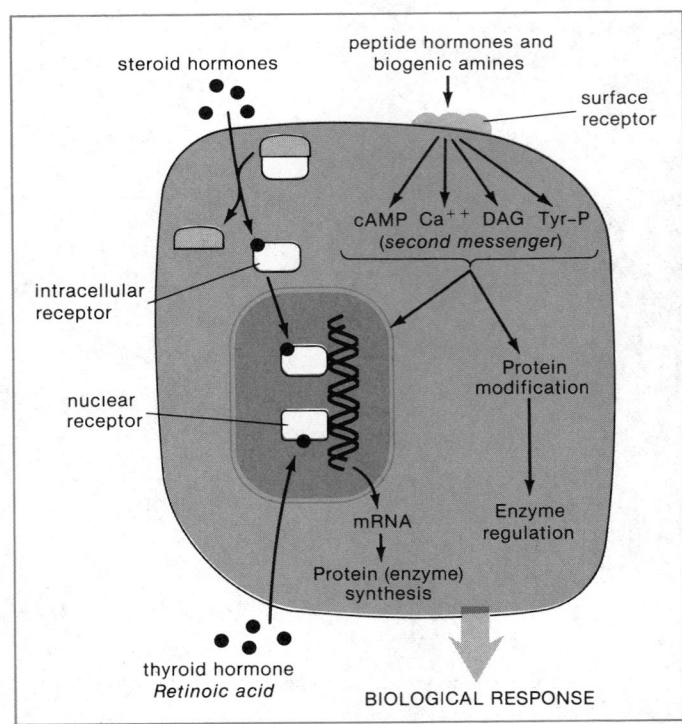

FIGURE 199–1. Mechanisms by which peptide and steroid hormones signal.

nated to the protein by adenosine triphosphate. This allows peptide hormones to change rapidly the conformation and thus the function of existing cell enzymes. It also allows somewhat slower changes in gene transcription to regulate the concentration of enzyme proteins. Biogenic amines function like peptide hormones.

Steroid hormones are synthesized from precursor cholesterol. Thyroid hormone, retinoic acid (vitamin A), and vitamin D are synthesized via separate pathways but act through the same family of receptors and mechanisms as do steroid hormones. This group of hormones acts via structurally related receptors that bind to DNA recognition sites to regulate transcription of target genes. They change the concentration of cell proteins, primarily enzymes, and thus the metabolic activity underlying the physiologic response.

Peptide Hormones Act Via Cell Surface Receptors

HORMONE BINDING AND SIGNAL TRANSDUCTION. Peptide hormone receptors have one of three general structures (Fig. 199–2): (1) a seven-membrane spanning structure in which the recognition site is formed by exterior sequences between membrane-spanning helices and the activity site is formed by interhelical regions inside the cell, (2) a single membrane-spanning helical structure separating the recognition domain from the cytoplasmic domain, which contains an intrinsic enzyme activity, and (3) a single membrane-spanning helix that separates the recognition domain from an intracellular domain that couples to second messenger systems, as do the seven-membrane spanning receptors. The protein coupled may be an intracellular tyrosine kinase or other enzyme.

Hormone ligands and receptors bind with high affinities (equilibrium dissociation constants $[K_D]$ of nanomolar to picomolar), thus providing the specificity necessary for cells to decode the information provided by the low concentration of hormone present among the many other circulating and extracellular proteins. The conformational change resulting from peptide hormone binding activates receptors to signal from the cell surface. Removal of receptors from the cell surface results in down-regulation and attenuation of the response. Binding affinities and dose-response curves for the initial event in cell signaling are the same. Biologic responses consequent to these initial events occur via a series of amplifications, each with its own affinity. The result is a dose-response curve for biologic activities which is more sensitive than that for binding and activation of the initial response. Full biologic responses may thus occur at a low concentration of hormone, resulting in occupancy of only 10% or less of receptors. This provides high sensitivity to small changes in hormone concentration. It also provides significant reserve. Hormone-induced down-regulation may remove 90% of receptors from the cell surface. This renders the cell refractory to the initial hormone concentration, but if the need is great enough, hormone concentrations can increase 10-fold and fully activate the residual 10%

of receptors to give full biologic responses. Such a response system provides high initial sensitivity, buffering via down-regulation against excessive hormone responses, but reserve that can operate when the signal strength is strong enough.

Receptors are mobile in the plane of the membrane. Ligand binding not only transduces signals but also induces down-regulation by removing receptors from the cell surface. Ligand binding may induce sequestration of receptors and their retention inside the cell via interactions with cell proteins, as occurs with rhodopsin and adrenergic receptors. Ligand binding may induce endocytosis via clatharin-coated pits with ultimate degradation via lysosomal enzymes, as occurs with insulin and epidermal growth factor receptors. The concentration of cell surface receptors is regulated by interaction with hormone ligand and by other signals that regulate its synthesis and affinity. The concentration of receptors determines the cells' responsiveness. Antagonists occupy receptors but in general do not induce desensitization. When antagonists are removed, receptor concentrations are high and cells are very responsive to hormone exposure. Effects on receptor concentration are seen clinically as up-regulation (e.g., as excessive adrenergic responses when β blockers are rapidly withdrawn) and as down-regulation (e.g., insulin resistance in type II diabetes). Regulation of receptor synthesis is an important mechanism by which one hormone regulates responsiveness to another to coordinate biologic effects.

A class of cell surface receptors serves a nutrient delivery rather than an informational function. These molecules include the low density lipoprotein (LDL) receptor, the transferrin receptor, and the asialoglycoprotein receptor. LDL and transferrin receptors, which are clustered in coated pits, internalize, deliver LDL (cholesterol) and iron to the cell interior, and then recycle to the cell surface. Such receptors do not down-regulate but undergo repeated rounds of recycling to provide the cell with essential nutrients.

INTRACELLULAR SECOND MESSENGERS. *Cyclic AMP and Cyclic GMP.* The concept of second messengers was established by Earl Sutherland, who discovered cAMP, an intracellular allosteric effector that mediates the action of many peptide hormones. Hormone receptors are coupled to catalytic adenylate cyclase via guanosine nucleotide binding (G) proteins, the β-adrenergic receptor being a paradigm for this signaling pathway (Fig. 199–3). This receptor belongs to the seven-membrane spanning class. On ligand binding, the receptor interacts with a G protein trimer consisting of α, β, and γ subunits. Because G proteins bind GDP with higher affinity than GTP, guanine nucleotide exchange is triggered by proteins that facilitate exchange of GTP for GDP; activity is reversed by hydrolysis of GTP to GDP. Binding of hormones to receptors that operate through the cAMP second messen-

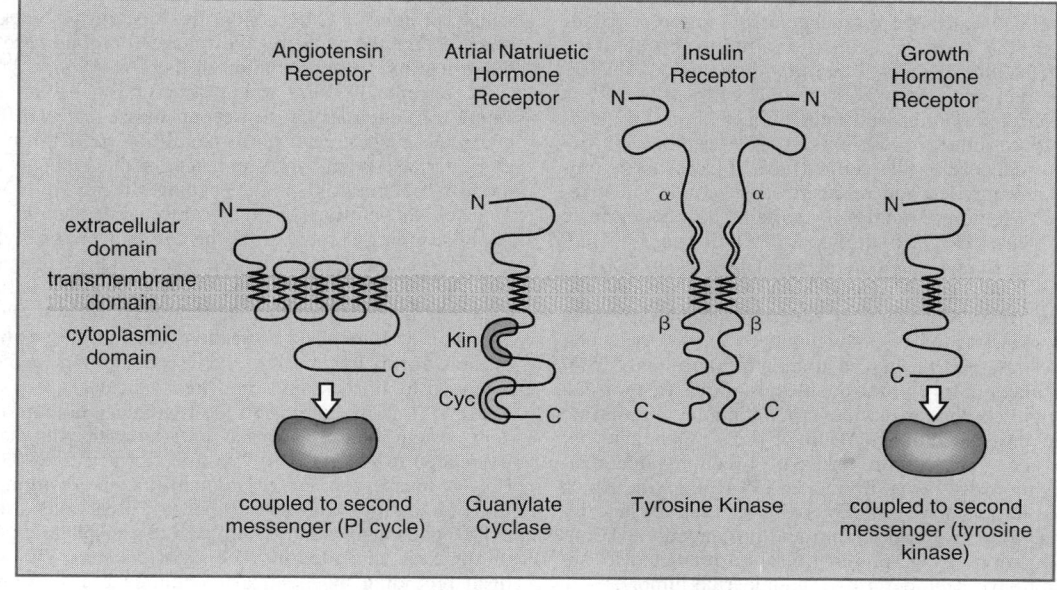

FIGURE 199–2. Structures of peptide hormone receptors.

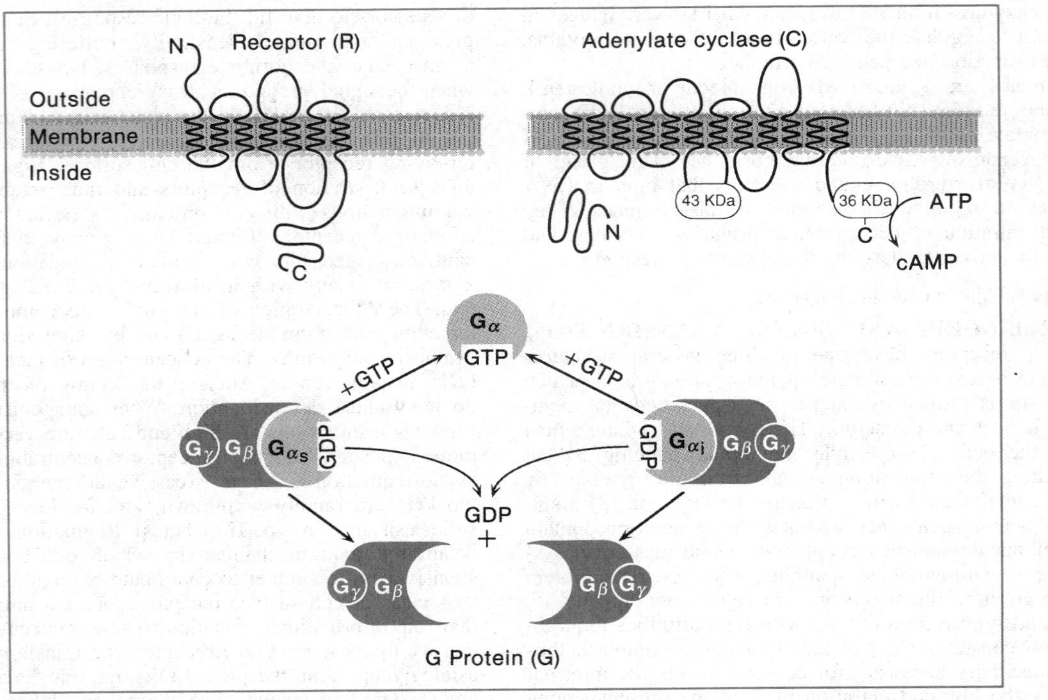

FIGURE 199-3. Hormone-regulated adenylate cyclase.

ger system results in a conformational change causing receptors to bind to G proteins. Ligand-activated receptors facilitate exchange of GTP for GDP so that the activated $G_\alpha s$ (stimulating α GTP binding subunit) dissociates from the β and γ subunits. The [ligand · hormone receptor] · $[G_\alpha s \cdot GTP]$ complex activates adenylate cyclase to catalyze formation of cAMP from ATP. Each hormone ligand induces formation of multiple cAMP molecules via this mechanism. Inhibitory G proteins operate in a similar manner to decrease cAMP formation. In both cases ligand-activated receptors act to exchange GTP for GDP, analogous to proteins that catalyze this process to regulate protein synthesis.

Adenylate cyclase is a large complex molecule with a 12-membrane spanning structure. The two large cytoplasmic domains have internal sequence similarities and are related to sequences in guanylate cyclase. Eight adenylate cyclases have been identified, and their channel-like structure suggests that they may function as transporters in addition to catalyzing formation of cAMP.

Activation of adenylate cyclase is buffered and terminated by several mechanisms: (1) Hormone dissociates from receptor. Binding of $G_\alpha \cdot GTP$ to the receptor decreases affinity for hormone about one order of magnitude to facilitate this dissociation. (2) Receptors desensitize and are removed from the cell surface by a process involving phosphorylation and interaction with cell proteins termed *arrestins*. If hormone exposure is short, receptors are dephosphorylated and reappear on the cell surface; if exposure is prolonged, receptors are degraded and resensitization requires new receptor synthesis. (3) Most importantly, G_α proteins possess intrinsic GTPase activity so that GTP is hydrolyzed to GDP and, on GDP binding, G_α is inactivated and reassociates with the β/γ subunits.

There are many consequences when this mechanism of signal transduction is perturbed. Mutations in seven-membrane spanning receptors may inactivate so that signaling is defective; some mutations, such as those observed in thyroid-stimulating hormone (TSH) receptors in hyperfunctioning thyroid nodules, may activate so that receptors signal in the absence of hormone. Continuous exposure to hormone results in desensitization or tachyphylaxis. Deficiency of G protein, which occurs in certain forms of pseudohypoparathyroidism, results in insensitivity to hormone. Cholera toxin, which activates ADP ribosylation of $G_\alpha s$, inhibits GTPase activity and interferes with reversibility so that profound and prolonged elevations in cAMP occur. Mutations in G_α proteins that are predicted to impair GTPase activity have been described in endocrine tumors.

cAMP, an intracellular allosteric effector, binds to the regulatory subunit of cAMP-dependent protein kinase. A-kinase is a tetrameric protein consisting of two regulatory and two catalytic subunits. Binding of cAMP dissociates the inhibitory regulatory subunits as a dimer from the two catalytic subunits. The latter then catalyze the transfer of the γ phosphate of ATP to serine and threonine residues in proteins. This covalent modification by phosphorylation causes an allosteric conformational change in the substrate protein which results in a change in its activity. The hormonal signal is transduced into an alteration in enzyme activity and thus in cell function. Phosphorylation of cytoplasmic proteins results in alterations such as glycolysis; the activated catalytic kinase subunit also migrates to the nucleus to phosphorylate and activate transcription factors such as the cAMP response element binding protein (CREB).

cAMP actions are reversed by hydrolysis of cAMP by phosphodiesterase to 5' AMP, and protein phosphorylation is reversed by the action of phosphatases. Phosphodiesterases are regulated and are a frequent target of inhibitor drugs such as methylxanthines, which prolong cAMP action by blocking its degradation. Phosphatases are regulated by phosphatase-inhibitor proteins, which are fine tuned by phosphorylation of these molecules.

A conceptually similar but structurally distinct system provides signal transduction via the second messenger cGMP. Two forms of guanylate cyclase catalyze formation of cGMP from GTP. The best-characterized mammalian enzyme is the receptor for atrial natriuretic hormone (ANH). The binding site for ANH is located on the extracellular portion of its receptor separated by a single membrane-spanning domain from the cytoplasmic guanylate cyclase (see Fig. 199–2). In contrast to adenylate cyclase, receptor and catalytic activities reside in the same molecule. Activity is regulated primarily by ligand binding but also depends on phosphorylation of the enzyme, with dephosphorylation causing desensitization. A cytoplasmic form of guanylate cyclase contains a heme moiety and is activated by nitrous oxide and free radicals.

cGMP acts by binding to the regulatory domain of cGMP-dependent protein kinase. G-kinase, a dimeric enzyme that is evolutionarily related to A-kinase, is allosterically activated on cGMP binding. Like A-kinase, it catalyzes protein phosphorylation to alter enzyme function and physiologic responses. Reactions are terminated by cGMP phosphodiesterase and protein phosphatases. cGMP phosphodiesterase is activated by binding of calcium · calmodulin, a mechanism providing biochemical communication between two signaling systems.

Calcium and Diacylglycerol. Hormone receptors that activate the phosphatidylinositol (PI) cycle transmit information to the interior of the cell via two second messengers: calcium (Ca^{2+}) and diacylglycerol (DAG) (Fig. 199–4). The cycle of PI metabolism consists of synthesis of this phospholipid, its breakdown, and its resynthesis. PI is composed of a 3-carbon glycerol backbone with long-chain fatty acids esterified at carbons 1 and 2 and an inositol ring esterified via a phosphoester bond at carbon 3. Distinct kinase enzymes catalyze phosphorylation of the inositol ring at positions 3, 4, and 5. Quantitatively the principal phosphorylations occur sequentially at positions 4 and then 5. The principal function of activated hormone receptors is to stimulate phosphoinositidase (phospholipase C), which releases the phosphorylated inositol to generate inositol trisphosphate (IP_3, inositol 1,4,5 P_3) and DAG (the glycerol backbone with fatty acids attached at carbons 1 and 2). IP_3 increases the concentration of cytoplasmic $[Ca^{2+}]$. It mobilizes stored intracellular Ca^{2+} by binding to specific receptors on intracellular membranes and by facilitating opening of calcium channels. The concentration of basal cytoplasmic Ca^{2+} is at least 1000-fold less than that in storage sites and outside the cell. The release from intracellular stores or entry of Ca^{2+} into the cell rapidly increases cytoplasmic $[Ca^{2+}]$.

Ca^{2+} plays a regulatory role in muscle contraction, in neuromuscular transmission, and in hormone signaling. Ca^{2+} binds to calmodulin and alters its conformation, causing the $Ca^{2+} \cdot$ calmodulin complex to bind to a variety of enzymes to regulate their activities. $Ca^{2+} \cdot$ calmodulin regulates protein kinases, including myosin light chain kinase involved in smooth muscle contraction, phosphorylase kinase involved in breakdown of glycogen, and calmodulin-dependent protein kinase important in synaptic transmission. $Ca^{2+} \cdot$ calmodulin regulates cyclic nucleotide phosphodiesterase and adenylate and guanylate cyclases to influence cAMP and cGMP concentrations, and it is involved in microtubule assembly and disassembly. $Ca^{2+} \cdot$ calmodulin is thus able to bind to a variety of other proteins and to alter their activity in response to information provided by the cytoplasmic Ca^{2+} concentration.

DAG acts as a second messenger by binding to protein kinase C to activate this important regulatory enzyme. Protein kinase C also requires Ca^{2+} for activation, so both second messengers of this pathway cooperate to increase the activity of this enzyme. Tumor promoters, such as active phorbol esters, are DAG analogues and act via protein kinase C.

The components of this second messenger system are diverse and complex. There are multiple isoenzyme forms of protein kinase C and of phosphoinositidase. Although one isoenzyme form of phosphoinositidase is activated via receptor-coupled G proteins, another is activated by binding to receptor tyrosine kinases and undergoing tyrosine phosphorylation. Additional kinases phosphorylate alternate positions on the inositol ring; PI 3-kinase is activated by certain tyrosine kinases to yield unique PI metabolites with functions distinct from Ca^{2+} mobilization. Sphingosine, a component of glycosphingolipid metabolism, inhibits protein kinase C, which provides dual regulation of this protein. Specific phosphatases remove the phosphate groups from the inositol ring to terminate its activity; lithium blocks the activity of one of these phosphatases to enhance accumulation of the biologically active inositol phosphates. Like other information pathways, this one is diffused to generate coordinated cellular responses and is buffered and ultimately turned off when the signal strength decreases.

Protein Tyrosine Kinases. A group of peptide hormone receptors contains intrinsic protein tyrosine kinase activity. Ligand binding to the extracellular domain results in an allosteric change that is transmitted across the single membrane-spanning segment to activate the cytoplasmic kinase domain (see Fig. 199–2). In a second structural motif a transmembrane receptor is coupled to a distinct cytoplasmic tyrosine kinase subunit. The lymphocyte receptor CD4 and cellular p56[lck] belong to this second class.

Within the cell the great majority of protein-bound phosphate is attached to serine and threonine residues, with only a small fraction being attached to tyrosine. Numerous kinases, however, covalently modify tyrosine residues in proteins as a central regulatory function in cell proliferation, developmental processes, and differentiated function. The extracellular ligand-binding domains of receptors of this class contain cysteine-rich regions that create the binding sites either as monomers (epidermal growth factor [EGF] receptor) or as dimers (insulin receptor) or contain immunoglobulin-like structures (platelet-derived growth factor [PDGF] and fibroblast growth factor [FGF] receptors). The cytoplasmic protein tyrosine kinase domains are highly homologous, containing ATP and substrate-binding sites, but different receptors recognize distinct substrates to give specific biologic responses. For example, insulin stimulates glucose uptake while EGF stimulates cell proliferation. The tyrosine kinases contain variable domains on both sides of the tyrosine kinase core as well as inserts within the kinase domain

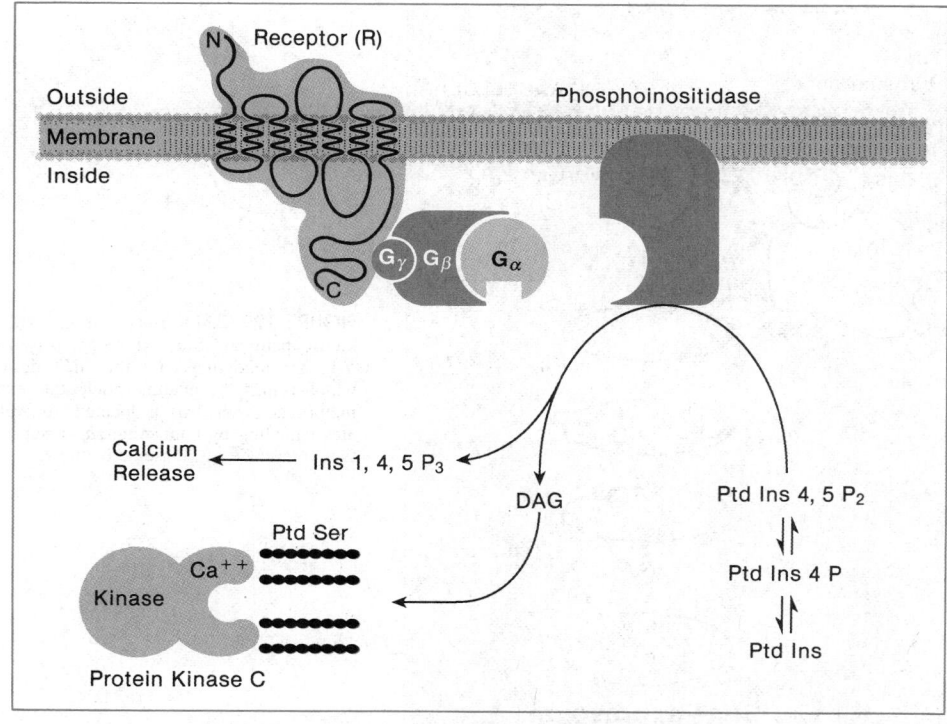

FIGURE 199–4. The phosphatidylinositol signaling pathway.

which provide regulatory sites that modulate ligand-activated tyrosine kinase activity.

Information received by a cell surface tyrosine kinase receptor is transmitted via a signal transduction pathway that begins with direct physical coupling of two proteins and proceeds via the GTP-binding protein *ras* (Fig. 199–5). In response to ligand binding, receptor tyrosine kinases either self-phosphorylate or phosphorylate a linker substrate. Proteins that contain a 100 amino acid domain homologous to a region in *src*, SH2, bind tightly to these sites of tyrosine phosphorylation. The growth factor receptor binding protein 2 *(Grb2)* is a molecular coupler containing an SH2 domain that plugs into a tyrosine phosphorylation site. *Shc* is another molecule coupler frequently used. *Grb2* also contains two SH3 domains that act as a receptacle for proline-rich domains of the guanine nucleotide exchange protein *SOS*. These high-affinity protein-to-protein interactions bring *SOS* to the cell membrane, where *ras* is present in its inactive GDP-bound form. Activated GTP-bound *ras* then couples to a serine/threonine protein kinase cascade involving first *raf*-1, then MEK and MAP (mitogen-activated protein) kinases. Information is thus relayed, expanded, and diffused to ultimately control gene expression and cell division. Operative mechanisms for this, as for other hormone-signaling pathways, include ligand or protein-protein interactions, activated GTP-bound G proteins, and protein phosphorylation. Receptor tyrosine kinases also couple to additional signaling pathways via SH2 domains in other proteins and via tyrosine phosphorylation of these proteins including phospholipase C-γ, a transcription control protein STAT 91, and PI 3-kinase.

Increased tyrosine kinase activity is reversed by four principal mechanisms: (1) ligand-induced endocytosis and down-regulation of surface receptors, (2) tyrosine phosphatases, which specifically remove phosphate from tyrosine residues, (3) reversal of the kinase reaction to transfer the phosphate from tyrosine residues in protein to ADP, and (4) hydrolysis of *ras*-bound GTP to GDP.

Regulation and reversibility of ligand-activated tyrosine kinases are important. Mutations involving these proteins occur frequently in cells transformed from normal to cancerous patterns of growth. Mutations may bypass regulatory features so that the kinases are constitutively active. The kinases may be overexpressed, most frequently owing to gene amplification but also owing to enhanced transcription, or the ligand may be constitutively expressed to activate receptors continuously. Mutant *ras* proteins may be constitutively active owing to decreased GTPase activity or to a defect in a protein that stimulates the GTPase activity of *ras*. Any of these changes converts a normal regulatory protein into an oncoprotein, one capable of causing neoplastic transformation.

Steroid Hormones Act Via Nuclear Receptors

THE SUPERFAMILY OF STEROID HORMONE RECEPTORS. All steroid hormone receptors share structural similarities indicative of a common ancestral molecule. The most conserved structural feature is the DNA-binding domain that contains zinc "fingers" (Fig. 199–6). The diagnostic spacing of cysteine residues creates a structure coordinated to a Zn^{2+} atom and an α helix that binds to the major groove of DNA. Because the energy of protein-DNA interaction depends on the area of contact, most proteins bind DNA as complexes. Steroid hormone receptors of the glucocorticoid receptor subfamily bind to DNA as homodimers; receptors of the thyroid hormone receptor subfamily may bind as homodimers but more commonly bind as heterodimers with a common partner, the retinoid X receptor (RXR).

The DNA recognition element consists of two half-sites of six base pairs, each half binding one monomer surface of the dimeric receptor protein. The half-sites are arranged as direct, inverted, or everted repeats. Receptors of the glucocorticoid receptor subfamily most often bind to palindromic sites, whereas receptors of the thyroid hormone receptor subfamily most often bind to sites made up of directly repeated DNA sequences. Small variations in the DNA-binding domain and in the DNA recognition element provide specificity for hormone action. One important determinant for receptor binding and activity is the spacing between the two half-sites for dimeric receptor binding. The spacing rules for DNA recognition elements that are arranged as direct repeats (DR) indicate that a spacing of 1 (DR + 1) directs RXR homodimer binding and 9-*cis*-retinoic acid responses, DR + 3 directs vitamin D receptor · RXR binding and vitamin D responses, DR + 4 directs thyroid hormone receptor · RXR binding and thyroid hormone responses, and DR + 5 directs retinoic acid receptor · RXR binding and all-*trans*-retinoic acid responses. RXR binds to the upstream half and the hormone-specific receptor binds to the downstream half of these DNA response elements to mediate hormone-dependent changes in transcription. Spacing between half-sites is crucial for binding homodimeric receptors of the glucocorticoid receptor class, but the

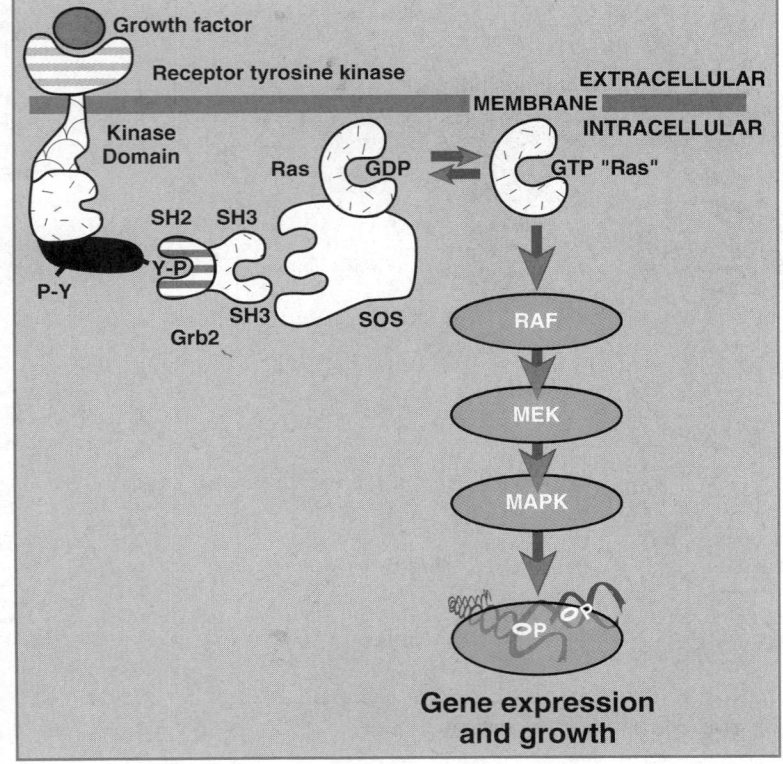

FIGURE 199–5. Information transfer through a receptor tyrosine kinase pathway. Sites of receptor tyrosine self-phosphorylation, Y-P, are recognized by the SH2 domain of the linker *Grb2*, which brings the guanine nucleotide exchange factor *SOS* to the membrane where *ras* is located. Activated GTP-bound *ras* initiates signaling by contacting *raf,* a serine/threonine kinase, to initiate a cascade of kinase activations.

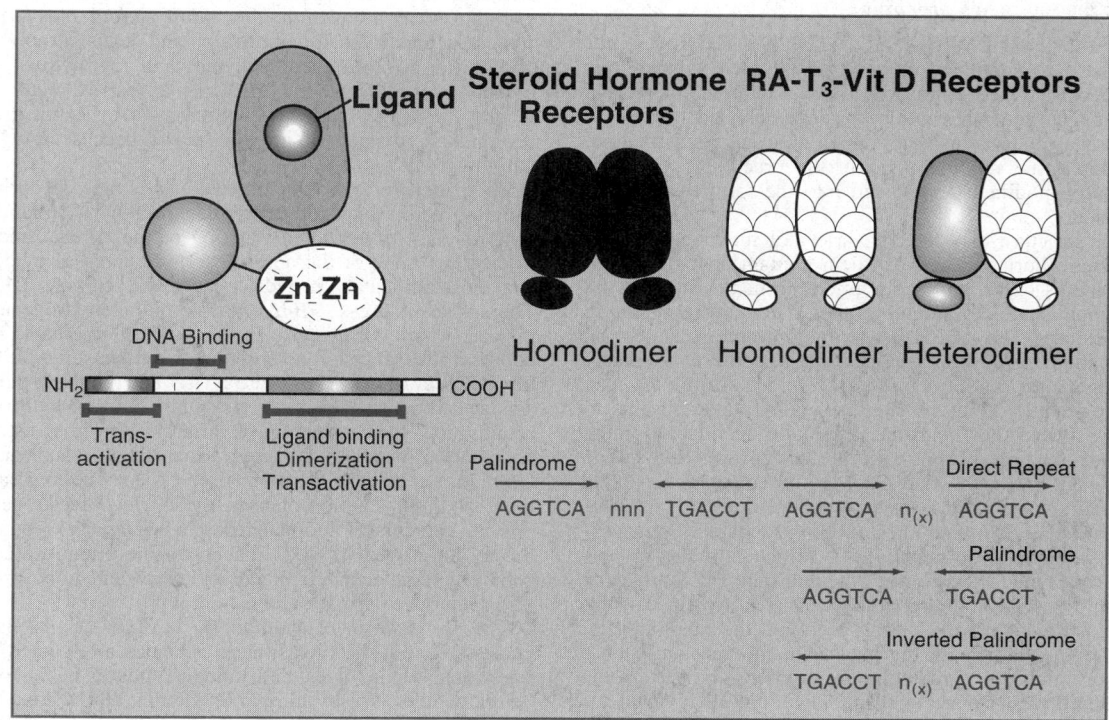

FIGURE 199–6. Structural features of steroid hormone receptors. *Left,* The DNA-binding domain, which consists of two zinc finger structures, is flanked by N′ terminal activation sequences and by C′ terminal ligand binding, dimerization, and activation sequences. *Right,* Glucocorticoid receptor family members bind as homodimers to palindromes. Thyroid hormone receptor family members bind primarily as heterodimers with retinoid X receptor to direct repeat motifs separated by varying numbers of base pairs.

sequence of the half-site provides an essential discriminant. Specificity is quantitative, not absolute. For example, progesterone receptors bind to glucocorticoid response elements, and retinoic acid receptors bind to thyroid hormone receptor DNA response elements. Specificity is sufficient for generating hormone-specific responses but may permit overlapping functions as in ligand-activated progesterone receptor induction of glucocorticoid-regulated genes.

Hormone binding activates the biologic function of the receptor. Cortisol receptors exist in inactive complexes with other proteins; cortisol binding induces an allosteric change that facilitates dissociation, allowing the ligand-bound receptor to bind to DNA. Thyroid hormone and retinoic acid receptors exist bound to DNA rather than complexed to protein; hormone binding results in an allosteric change that activates the receptor, so it interacts with other components of the transcription machinery.

The steroid hormone receptor family is a large one that includes subfamilies of receptors: at least four for retinoic acid, two for thyroid hormone, several for $1,25(OH)_2$ vitamin D and for fatty acids or metabolites causing perixosome proliferation, and a group of "orphans" whose ligands remain to be identified. The general structural motif is an important one, which, in evolution, has diverged to specify responses to many hormonal signals and to control expression of numerous genes.

REGULATION OF GENE TRANSCRIPTION. Hormone-activated receptor proteins bound to their DNA response element targets act as *cis*-active enhancers. They act from various positions relative to the start of transcription and in various combinations with other regulatory proteins to control the rate of initiation of gene transcription. Gene promoters lie upstream of the site where eukaryotic RNA polymerase II initiates transcription of messenger RNA. The best characterized promoter contains a TATA box that binds a protein, transcription factor II D (TF II-D), which directs accurate transcription by RNA polymerase II ~ 30 base pairs downstream. Seven proteins (TATA-associated factors or TAF's) associate with TF II-D in a specific complex that provides a molecular surface for interaction with the transcription-regulatory proteins, which are bound elsewhere to DNA. Other promoter motifs include a basal initiator and GC-rich regions in which multiple transcription start sites exist. Gene expression is induced by increasing the rate

of transcription. The gene must contain a DNA response/binding element for the receptor to generate a response; multiple binding sites give greater enhancement. The DNA-binding elements position the steroid hormone receptors so that other regions of the protein can interact with proteins in the transcription initiation complex. Adaptor proteins may connect the proteins bound at enhancer sites to the proteins of the basal transcription complex bound at the promoter.

Hormone-activated receptors can also repress transcription. Negative feedback loops operate through this process. Activated cortisol receptors repress transcription of the gene encoding the ACTH precursor; activated thyroid hormone receptors inhibit transcription of both α- and β-TSH subunit genes. The principle of ligand-activated receptors binding to specific DNA target sequences in the regulated gene is the same as that required for inductive responses. The receptor may inhibit transcription by displacing positive enhancers, by blocking RNA polymerase engagement, or by silencing transcription through interactions with the core transcriptional machinery, analogous to protein-protein interactions that enhance transcription.

Many other proteins regulate initiation of transcription, both as inducers and as inhibitors. These bind to DNA via specific sequences, as do steroid receptors, or they may interact with proteins which do. These proteins may be modified in response to hormonal signals initiated at the cell surface. Such alterations account for the changes in gene transcription due to hormones acting via surface receptors. Two general and cooperative mechanisms exist: phosphorylation and translocation of transcription factors from cytoplasm to nucleus. Genes regulated by cAMP contain DNA sequences that specify binding of a specific nuclear transcription regulator (CREB). CREB, which undergoes changes in activity upon phosphorylation, is a required final mediator of gene induction by peptide hormones that act at the cell surface to activate adenylate cyclase and cAMP-dependent protein kinase. STAT-91 and related proteins are phosphorylated on tyrosine residues and, when phosphorylated, enter the nucleus to activate transcription of specific genes. This chain of effects alters transcription of mRNA's and cell protein concentrations to dictate changes in cell function and organ physiology.

BIOSYNTHESIS OF HORMONES AND RECEPTORS

SYNTHESIS AND DELIVERY OF PEPTIDE HORMONES. Peptide hormones are small secretory proteins; their biosynthesis and secretion occur via the same processes as other nonhormonal secretory proteins. In general, peptide hormones are synthesized as part of larger precursor proteins that contain additional information. Within the endoplasmic reticulum space, the precursor protein is cleaved, covalently modified, and folded into the form that will be ultimately secreted.

The precursor structure may have a variety of functions. Precursors for antidiuretic hormone and oxytocin contain specific neurophysins that serve as carriers of the peptides from the site of synthesis in the hypothalamus to storage granules in axon terminals in the posterior pituitary. The ACTH precursor, pro-opiomelanocortin, contains information for several peptides that may be coordinately involved in stress responses. Structures in the precursor protein may serve to fold the peptide correctly. The connecting peptide in the insulin precursor between the β and the α subunits facilitates folding for formation of mature insulin with correctly formed disulfide bonds between and within the two chains. The connecting peptide is then excised and removed from mature α-β insulin.

Within the endoplasmic reticulum and Golgi apparatus, glycosylation of TSH, luteinizing hormone (LH), follicle-stimulating hormone (FSH), and human chorionic gonadotropin (hCG) occurs. Secretory granules containing highly concentrated hormone accumulate in the unstimulated cell. During secretion the membrane of the secretory granule fuses with the plasma membrane, and stored hormone is discharged into the circulation, a process termed *exocytosis*. Rapid release of hormone in response to stimuli reflects discharge of secretory granules, whereas prolonged secretion reflects release of newly synthesized hormone.

Peptide hormones may also be derived from precursors with receptor-like structures or from circulating forms. EGF and transforming growth factor-α (TGF-α) are made as a part of the surface domain of a transmembrane protein with a receptor-like structure. These are released by proteolysis, although they may act on adjacent cells without processing to provide cell-to-cell communication. Renin, an enzyme released from juxtaglomerular cells, acts on angiotensinogen secreted from liver. Active angiotensin is synthesized by progressive proteolysis of a precursor outside of cells: renin to yield angiotensin I and angiotensin-converting enzyme to yield angiotensin II.

Secreted peptide hormones have a short half-life of about 3 to 7 minutes in the circulation. Glycoprotein hormones have longer half-lives of 1 to 4 hours. The short circulating half-life and peptide degradation by gastric acid and intestinal enzymes have precluded oral use of this class of hormones. Several attempts to prolong half-lives have met with partial success: Complexing with Zn^{2+} and protamine creates a slowly absorbed and longer-acting form of injectable insulin; removing the amino group from the N' terminal amino acid and substituting a D-arginine creates a longer-acting ADH, which can be absorbed from nasal mucous membranes. At present direct use of peptide hormones is limited to injectable forms. Prolonged action results in receptor desensitization, so recapitulation of normal cyclic secretion typical of endogenous production presents a second difficulty. Use of GnRH must be both by parental routes and pulsatile in nature to induce ovulation and successful pregnancy.

SYNTHESIS AND TRANSPORT OF STEROID HORMONES. Steroid hormones are derived from cholesterol provided by *de novo* cellular synthesis from acetate or by uptake of circulating cholesterol made in the liver and delivered to cells via low density lipoprotein (LDL) particles. Synthesized steroid hormones are not stored, so secretory rates directly reflect production rates. In adrenal and gonadal tissues the rate-limiting step for increased steroid hormone biosynthesis is transfer of substrate cholesterol to the side chain cleavage enzyme located in the inner mitochondrial membrane. Cleavage of the side chain of cholesterol is catalyzed by a cytochrome P-450 enzyme that resembles other steroid hydroxylases. These enzymes progressively modify the cholesterol nucleus by the sequential addition of hydroxyl groups to specific sites. The rate-limiting step is stimulated in target cells by ACTH, LH, and FSH to result in rapid increases in steroid hormone biosynthesis. The trophic stimulatory hormones also maintain the structure of the target glands and induce each of the enzymes involved in hormone biosynthesis. With hypophysectomy or feedback inhibition of pituitary hormone production, the entire steroid biosynthetic pathway decreases and the adrenal, ovary, and testis atrophy. Addition of trophic hormones induces enzymes and regrowth of target glands. Induction of biosynthetic enzymes appears directly mediated via second messenger pathways, primarily cAMP, but growth requires coordinate provision of growth factors because cAMP, in general, inhibits growth.

The pattern of biosynthetic enzymes expressed during cell differentiation determines which steroid hormone is produced and is the basis of the differentiated function of the adrenal and gonads. The fascicularis zone of the adrenal cortex expresses cytochrome P-450 enzymes that catalyze hydroxylations at carbons 21, 17, and 11. They also express 3β-hydroxysteroid dehydrogenase, $\Delta^{4,5}$ isomerase, which forms cortisol. The zona glomerulosa of the adrenal cortex makes aldosterone through a similar series of reactions, but the pathway lacks 17α-hydroxylase and contains an activity that acts at carbon 18. The testis lacks 21- and 11β-hydroxylases, so reactants flow to testosterone. Ovarian synthesis of estradiol requires cooperation between adjacent theca interna and granulosa cells. Granulosa cells express aromatase, the enzyme that catalyzes placement of three double bonds in the A ring of estrogens but cannot provide precursor androstenedione, which is synthesized in the theca interna cell located adjacent to the granulosa cell. Granulosa cells efficiently convert precursor androstenedione provided by the theca interna to estrone and estradiol.

The active form of vitamin D, $1,25(OH)_2D$, is also made from cholesterol, but the biosynthetic enzymes are located in three separate organs: skin, liver, and kidney. Vitamin D_3 is formed from 7-dehydrocholesterol by ultraviolet irradiation of skin. D_3 is then hydroxylated at carbon 25 in the liver to yield $25(OH)D$. This is converted by 1α-hydroxylase to $1,25(OH)_2D$ in proximal tubule cells of the kidney. In this unique endocrine system, the major site for regulation is the final 1α-hydroxylation in renal proximal tubule cells, a step controlled by parathyroid hormone and phosphate.

In contrast to peptide hormones, steroid hormones have longer circulating half-lives and may be active when administered orally. Following secretion into the circulation, steroid hormones are bound to transport glycoproteins made in the liver. The transport proteins, which have a binding but not an activity site, provide a reservoir of hormone, protected from metabolism and renal clearance, which can be released to cells. Three transport proteins have been characterized: corticosteroid-binding globulin (CBG), which binds cortisol and progesterone, sex steroid hormone–binding globulin (SHBG), which binds testosterone with greater affinity than estradiol, and vitamin D–binding protein, which binds precursor $25(OH)D$ with greater affinity than $1,25(OH)_2D$. Thyroid-binding globulin (TBG) binds L-thyroxine to provide its uniquely long half-life of 7 days. Estrogens induce and androgens inhibit synthesis of these transport proteins. Albumin provides a large carrier system that weakly binds hormones.

Free steroid hormone, which is in equilibrium with that bound to transport protein, enters cells to bind intracellular receptors and generate biologic responses. The free fraction is also the active one in feedback regulation, so it is the concentration of free hormone that is altered in homeostatic responses. The free fraction is very small compared with the bound fraction, but total hormone concentrations from both fractions are measured in most clinical assays. Conditions such as pregnancy, which alter binding protein concentrations, alter total measured hormone but not the biologically relevant free hormone concentration. In special clinical situations measurement of binding protein concentration and of free hormone may be required for accurate assessment.

Steroid hormones are metabolized principally in the liver to inactive water-soluble metabolites. Cortisol is inactivated by reduction of the double bond in the A ring and conjugation to glucuronide or sulfate at carbon 3 to make it water-soluble for renal excretion. However, not all peripheral metabolic alterations are inactivating. 5α-Reductase converts testosterone to 5α-dihydrotestosterone, which is the biologically active species in male reproductive tract and skin. Androstenedione produced in ovary and adrenal can be converted to testosterone in peripheral tissues. Significant quantities of estradiol are produced by conversion of circulating precursors.

Like their hormonal ligands, receptor synthesis is highly regulated to control cellular responses and sensitivity to hormones. Receptor synthesis is increased in response to environmental or developmental need or is repressed in negative feedback loops and during stages of development. Receptor concentration is as important as hormone concentration in determining cell responses. Regulation of receptor synthesis is therefore central to providing coordinated and appropriate endocrine responses.

INTEGRATION OF ENDOCRINE RESPONSES

FEEDBACK LOOPS. Multiple hormones cooperate to coordinate development, reproduction, and homeostasis. When a hormone has elicited an appropriate response, the signal must be terminated. In addition to the buffering that occurs in target cells, feedback control is the principal mechanism through which this occurs (Fig. 199–7). Feedback loops are especially important for communication between organs that are spatially separated. The hormonal products of peripheral endocrine glands such as thyroid, adrenal cortex, ovary, and testis exert negative feedback control over the synthesis and secretion of the stimulatory pituitary hormone. Feedback, which occurs at the level of the pituitary cell and in the hypothalamus, operates via control of several essential steps. The neurohormone thyrotropin-releasing hormone (TRH) stimulates thyrotropes of the anterior pituitary to synthesize and secrete TSH, which in turn increases synthesis and secretion of thyroid hormone. Increased production of thyroid hormone induces appropriate metabolic responses in target organs; it also inhibits production of TSH to return the system to baseline. The prohormone L-thyroxine (T_4) is converted in the pituitary thyrotrope to active T_3, and T_3 binds to nuclear T_3 receptors to inhibit transcription of both α and β TSH subunit genes. T_3-bound receptors also decrease synthesis of TRH receptors, rendering cells less responsive to stimulatory TRH. In addition, T_3 inhibits hypothalamic production of TRH. Conversely, when thyroid hormone concentrations are low, feedback inhibition is relieved and TRH stimulates increased production of TSH, which increases production of T_4 and thus re-establishes homeostasis. Feedback principles provide an exquisitely sensitive system for

making appropriate changes and then returning to the homeostatic set point.

Feedback operates not only via steroid and thyroid hormones but also through peptides and ions. Pituitary FSH production is feedback regulated by the ovarian steroid hormone estrogen and by the ovarian peptide hormone inhibin. Parathyroid hormone (PTH) regulates serum Ca^{2+} concentrations; with hypocalcemia PTH increases and re-establishes normocalcemia. The increase in serum $[Ca^{2+}]$ feedback inhibits PTH synthesis and secretion to re-establish serum PTH concentrations appropriate to normocalcemia. With mutations in the $[Ca^{2+}]$ receptor on parathyroid cell membranes, feedback sensing is impaired and excessive PTH is made.

RECRUITMENT OF COORDINATE RESPONSES. Physiologic responses result from many different cell types and organs acting in concert. The necessary coordination is provided both by a hormone acting at multiple sites and by each hormone eliciting multiple responses, which sum to give the overall effect. Integrated responses require that one hormone regulate the synthesis or action of another; the nervous system is integrated into the overall response. Paradigms of such coordinated responses include stress, fasting, and reproduction.

A major stress, such as trauma with pain and hypovolemia, initiates a central nervous system response that includes synthesis and secretion of corticotropin-releasing hormone (CRH) and antidiuretic hormone. CRH is the major stimulus to increase pituitary secretion of ACTH, which increases adrenal cortisol production. Cortisol maintains not only blood glucose but also vascular responsiveness to epinephrine and norepinephrine. It limits excessive inflammatory responses to prevent further volume loss and tissue damage. CRH acts, in the central nervous system, to stimulate the peripheral sympathetic nervous system. Increased sympathetic nervous system activity mediates adaptive cardiovascular responses, including increased blood pressure and pulse rate. It also induces appropriate

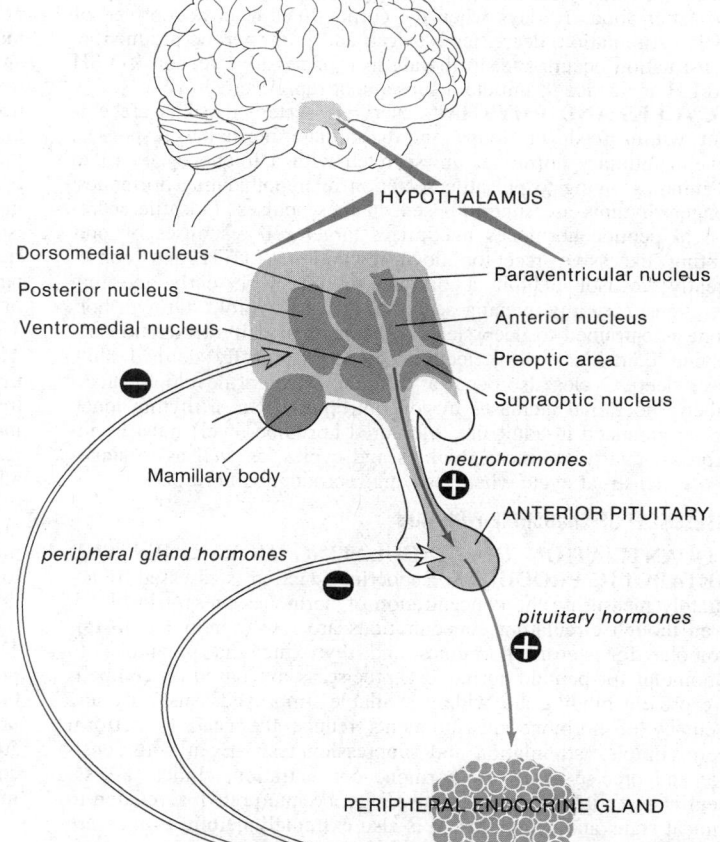

FIGURE 199–7. Forward regulation and negative feedback.

behavioral responses. ADH increases permeability of the collecting duct of the distal nephron to conserve water and intravascular volume. It facilitates CRH-stimulated ACTH secretion. With hypovolemia the renin-angiotensin-aldosterone system is also activated to enhance vasoconstriction and to conserve sodium and intravascular volume. These responses of the hypothalamus, pituitary, and adrenal cortex together facilitate survival from stresses.

With fasting, blood glucose concentrations are maintained for 12 to 24 hours by glucagon- and epinephrine-mediated release of glucose from glycogen stores. With more prolonged fasting cortisol-stimulated gluconeogenesis is the major mechanism that sustains blood glucose. Insulin secretion is suppressed. Metabolic demands are decreased by inhibition of $5'$-deiodinase to decrease conversion of T_4 to active T_3 in peripheral tissues. Growth-promoting hormones, such as insulin-like growth factor I, are also suppressed under conditions of substrate lack. With starvation, gonadotropin secretion decreases and reproductive capacity is diminished.

Female reproductive cycles result from coordinated signaling by hypothalamic, pituitary, and ovarian hormones. Pulsatile secretion of gonadotropin-releasing hormone stimulates pituitary production of LH and FSH. During the follicular phase of the menstrual cycle these peptide hormones regulate ovarian secretion of estrogen and direct maturation of follicles, one of which increases 1000-fold in diameter and becomes dominant for ovulation. FSH induces LH receptors in ovarian granulosa cells, and both LH and FSH induce aromatase as part of the mechanism that enhances estrogen production. LH and FSH increase during the follicular phase and, with follicle development, estrogen secretion rises. Positive feedback effects of estrogen result in the mid-cycle surge of LH and FSH, which induces ovulation. The remaining granulosa and theca cells reorganize to form the corpus luteum, which produces progesterone as well as estrogen. Concentrations of these hormones negatively inhibit FSH and LH production and induce additional uterine changes necessary for implantation. Ovarian inhibin also inhibits FSH production. If fertilization and implantation occur, the corpus luteum is regulated by hCG until placental steroidogenesis is established. If fertilization does not occur, negative feedback of estrogen and progesterone inhibits LH and FSH, and the luteal phase of the menstrual cycle ends after about 10 days when the corpus luteum, now deprived of trophic stimulation, decreases estrogen and progesterone production. Menstruation occurs and, in the absence of negative feedback, FSH and LH again rise to initiate a subsequent reproductive cycle.

CYCLES AND RHYTHMS. Nervous system rhythms are evident within feedback loops and coordinate hormonal responses. Several pituitary hormones are secreted with a frequency of 15 to 60 minutes owing to pulsatile secretion of hypothalamic hormones. Longer rhythms are superimposed on these pulses. Pulsatile secretion of peptide hormones maximizes target cell responses by preventing excessive receptor down-regulation. ACTH and consequently cortisol exhibit a diurnal rhythm with early morning secretion exceeding evening secretion at least twofold. Growth hormone is entrained to deep sleep with maximal daily production occurring coincident with electroencephalographically defined slow wave sleep. Cycles also occur at different stages of development. At puberty nocturnal increases in gonadotropins occur, a rhythm much less pronounced in adult life. Measured hormone levels must be interpreted relative to these rhythms and cycles, as well as to stages of the menstrual cycle when assaying reproductive hormones.

ASSESSMENT OF ENDOCRINE FUNCTION

QUANTITATION OF CIRCULATING HORMONES AND METABOLIC PRODUCTS. Endocrine function is assessed by accurately measuring the concentration of hormones present in blood. Even though circulating concentrations are low (nanomolar to micromolar for steroid hormones and thyroxine and picomolar to nanomolar for peptide hormones), precise assays based on competitive protein binding are widely available. Improved sensitivity and accuracy of hormone measurements reduce the need to perform more complex stimulation and suppression tests. Even with sensitive and precise assays of hormone concentration, clinical assessment is essential. Measured values must be interpreted in relation to clinical signs and symptoms. It is also extremely helpful to measure both arms of a feedback loop. Most hormone concentrations exhibit a gaussian distribution of normal values, so an individual measurement at either end of the normal range may be normal or abnormal

for that individual. Coincident measurement of TSH and T_4, LH and testosterone, ACTH and cortisol, PTH and Ca^{2+} gives greater information than either alone. A T_4 at the lower end of the normal range with an elevated TSH indicates thyroid gland failure, whereas the same T_4 with a normal TSH likely indicates a euthyroid state. An elevated cortisol with suppressed ACTH indicates autonomous production of cortisol by an adrenal tumor. Cycles and rhythms of hormone secretion must also be considered. Evening cortisol concentrations are half or less of peak morning values. Coincident measurement of ACTH clarifies whether a low cortisol represents diurnal rhythm or adrenal insufficiency; an elevated ACTH when cortisol is low suggests adrenal insufficiency. Measurement of gonadotropins, estradiol, and progesterone must be related to normal values for follicular and luteal phases of the menstrual cycle.

Steroid and thyroid hormones are bound to carrier proteins. In pregnancy, in which estrogen increases hepatic production of carrier proteins, total cortisol and T_4 values are elevated but ACTH and TSH are normal. On occasion, however, it is necessary to measure the free, active hormone concentration. Because the free fraction is very small relative to the total amount, careful separation of bound from free fractions without the use of organic solvents is necessary, and very sensitive detection systems are required. Assays for free T_4 and for ionized Ca^{2+} are available for specialized clinical circumstances. One can assess the amount of binding globulin directly, or indirectly measure unoccupied binding sites (T_3 resin uptake test).

Measurement of urinary excretion of some hormones provides an integrated value for daily production rates. Measurement of urinary free cortisol is particularly useful because cortisol-binding globulin, which binds 1 cortisol molecule per molecule of protein, is approximately saturated at the peak morning cortisol concentration. Free unbound cortisol that exceeds binding capacity is filtered at the glomerulus, so an elevated 24-hour urine free cortisol provides an accurate assessment in cortisol excess syndromes.

Measurement of metabolic effects is an essential component of endocrine evaluation. Insulin function is assessed by measuring plasma and urine glucose concentrations, PTH by measuring serum $[Ca^{2+}]$, aldosterone by measuring serum $[K^+]$, and ADH by measuring serum and urine osmolalities.

STIMULATION AND SUPPRESSION TESTS. Measurement of both arms of a feedback loop provides sufficient laboratory information in most endocrine deficiency or excess states. Additional diagnostic information can be gained, however, by perturbing the feedback system through administration of hormones. For stimulation tests a hormone is administered and the ability of the target gland to respond is assessed by measuring its product. This provides an estimate of the ability of the target gland to synthesize hormone, of its trophic maintenance, and its exposure to feedback inhibition. Baseline measurements are made before hormone administration and at the established normal time of peak target gland response. Ranges of normal responses have been established for comparison. Examples include TRH stimulation tests, in which levels of pituitary-produced TSH are measured. In hypopituitarism, serum TSH fails to rise in response to a standard intravenous injection of TRH. In primary hypothyroidism, in which feedback inhibition by thyroid hormone is small, TSH rises excessively, whereas in hyperthyroidism excessive feedback inhibition results in minimal or no increases in TSH. For ACTH stimulation tests, $ACTH_{1-24}$ is administered as an intravenous injection to assess the ability of the adrenal cortex to produce cortisol. A low baseline cortisol that fails to rise indicates adrenal insufficiency. Interpretation requires integration of clinical information because failure to respond to ACTH may also occur when the adrenal cortex has been suppressed owing to treatment with synthetic glucocorticoids. A variation of stimulation tests involves interruption of the feedback loop by metabolic inhibitors of hormone biosynthesis. Metyrapone, an inhibitor of 11β-hydroxylase, decreases serum cortisol, relieving feedback suppression of ACTH production. The resulting increase in ACTH can be measured directly, or ACTH-stimulated 11-desoxycortisol, the precursor of cortisol, can be measured as an indicator of increased ACTH. The metyrapone test provides an assessment of pituitary corticotrope function and reserve. Stimulation tests are most useful in suspected endocrine deficiency states.

Suppression tests, which measure the ability of administered hormone to provide feedback inhibition, are most useful in evaluating hormone excesses. Dexamethasone, a potent synthetic glucocorticoid, is administered to inhibit ACTH production. Because dexamethasone is not detected in cortisol assays, more easily measured cortisol rather than ACTH can be used as an endpoint. In Cushing's syndrome, the source of cortisol excess can be deduced using dexamethasone suppression. Pituitary tumors that produce excess ACTH frequently retain susceptibility to feedback inhibition. These tumors are resistant to doses of dexamethasone that suppress normal corticotrope ACTH production but are inhibited by higher doses of dexamethasone. In contrast, adrenal gland tumors and tumors that ectopically produce ACTH are resistant to even high doses of dexamethasone.

ANATOMIC ASSESSMENT. Imaging of endocrine glands is important, especially when considering surgical therapy. The high sensitivity and precision of computed tomography and nuclear magnetic resonance imaging allow detection of even small endocrine tumors such as pituitary, parathyroid, and adrenal adenomas. Sonographic techniques are also useful for imaging the thyroid gland, ovaries, testes, and pancreas. Radionuclide imaging may also be useful. Radioactive isotopes of iodine (^{123}I, ^{131}I) or compounds that are concentrated by the thyroid gland similar to iodine, such ^{99}Tc, are used to determine anatomy and imply function of the thyroid gland.

Measurement of hormone concentrations in venous effluent of glands may be useful in specialized circumstances to localize the source of abnormal production. Measurement of ACTH in petrosal sinus blood may be useful in localizing pituitary tumors, of PTH in neck and chest veins in localizing unusually located parathyroid adenomas, and of insulin in mesenteric venous drainage in localizing pancreatic insulinomas.

Cytologic and immunocytochemical techniques are important. Fine-needle aspiration of thyroid nodules with cytologic examinations analogous to those used in Papanicolaou smears has become the procedure of choice to distinguish benign and malignant thyroid nodules. Staining of surgical tissues with antihormone antibodies provides proof of hormone production and a guide to future therapy.

Receptors are not routinely measured but can be quantitated using immunologic techniques. Recombinant DNA technologies can be used to define inherited defects in receptors. When oncogenes are identified in specific endocrine neoplasms, these can be measured and mutations identified using DNA hybridization techniques. Autoimmune endocrine diseases can be documented by quantitating antibodies directed against specific organs (thyroid-stimulating immunoglobulin, anti–islet cell antibodies, antiadrenal antibodies).

ABERRATIONS IN DISEASE

DEFICIENCY STATES. The most prevalent endocrine disorders result from hormone deficiencies. A variety of disease states impair or destroy endocrine glands: defects in organ development, genetic defects in biosynthetic enzymes, immune-mediated destruction, neoplasia, infections, hemorrhage, nutritional deficits, and vascular insufficiency. Endocrine gland failure may be acute with rapid development of symptoms or chronic with slower development of symptoms but more pronounced physical changes. Defects in a gland such as the thyroid may result in a multisystem disorder due to failure to produce a single hormone, whereas defects in the hypothalamus or pituitary may result in a multisystem disorder, including thyroid deficiency, due to failure to produce many hormones. Multiple endocrine gland deficiencies may also result from autoimmune-mediated mechanisms in the polyglandular autoimmune deficiency syndromes. Because hormones participate in coordinated responses, secondary changes in other endocrine responses often result from deficiency of a single hormone.

Deficiency states also result from defects in hormone receptors and in signaling mechanisms. Defects may be inherited or acquired. Genetic abnormalities in androgen receptors result in unresponsiveness to androgens and an XY male with a female phenotype; defects in vitamin D receptors result in vitamin D–resistant rickets; defects in thyroid hormone receptors result in the resistance to thyroid hormone of Refetoff's syndrome; defects in growth hormone receptors result in ateliotic dwarfism of Laron's syndrome. Acquired receptor defects most often result from immunologic mechanisms where antibodies bind to receptors, blocking ligand access.

Postreceptor defects may occur. A defect in $G_{\alpha}s$ results in pseudohypoparathyroidism, in which unresponsiveness to PTH occurs. Such patients fail to respond normally to other hormones whose receptors couple to adenylate cyclase (TSH, glucagon, LH). Type II diabetes mellitus, which is inherited, is characterized by in-

sulin resistance. The molecular defect has not yet been characterized, but understanding this pathophysiology underlies therapeutic approaches directed at reducing resistance to and augmenting secretion of insulin. Because receptor and postreceptor defects are characterized by hormone resistance, feedback does not occur and producer glands enlarge and circulating hormone concentrations are high despite clinical evidence for deficiency.

EXCESS STATES. Excessive production of hormone and clinical evidence of such excess implies failure of normal feedback mechanisms. This occurs most commonly with neoplasia and with autoimmunity, in which antireceptor antibodies act as hormone agonists. Tumors of endocrine glands characteristically produce excessive amounts of the hormone made by the cell of origin but are no longer subject to normal feedback controls. Some tumors, such as pituitary adenomas that produce ACTH, retain feedback but require higher concentrations of cortisol to suppress ACTH. Prolactinomas retain dopamine suppression, and both their function and growth can be inhibited by dopamine agonists. Tumors arising in peripheral endocrine glands that are under pituitary trophic hormone regulation are autonomous because they are not normally subject to negative feedback. More undifferentiated tumors may also be insensitive to feedback regulation.

Hormones may be produced in excess by tumors arising from cells that do not normally produce the hormone. Ectopic production of peptide hormones is common in a variety of neoplasms, and symptoms due to the hormone excess may contribute significantly to morbidity. Because steroid hormones are made via a multienzyme pathway, excesses of these hormones occur only with tumors arising in the producer gland or with excessive production of the trophic peptide hormone. Cortisol excess may result from adrenocortical tumors or from excessive stimulation by ACTH produced by pituitary or ectopic neoplasms.

The most prevalent disease due to agonistic antibodies is Graves' disease, in which antibodies are produced that activate the TSH receptor. Because many hormones are available as therapeutic agents, some patients take excessive amounts and present with an endocrine excess syndrome.

GENETIC DETERMINANTS OF DISEASE. Many endocrine diseases result from genetic mutations. Genetic defects in biosynthetic enzymes may result in deficiency states: Hypothyroidism may result from thyroid peroxidase or deiodinase enzyme defects; adrenal insufficiency may result from 21-hydroxylase deficiency or a defect in other steroid biosynthetic enzymes; a form of male hypogonadism may result from 5α-reductase deficiency. Receptor defects are thought to be uncommon, but methods to define these have only recently become available. Type II diabetes, the most common endocrine abnormality, is inherited but its molecular basis is not yet known. Autoimmune endocrine disease also has a genetic basis involving an inherited defect in immune surveillance. Multiple endocrine neoplasia syndromes are due to activating mutations in the *ret* tyrosine kinase receptor so that cell growth and function are constitutively stimulated without ligand.

In the future, methods using nucleic acid probes can be used to make precise diagnoses in disease states and to provide predictive information before overt disease develops. Because genetic defects are present in all DNA, peripheral blood cells or skin fibroblasts provide a ready source of material for assay. Acquired mutations can be assessed by assay of material obtained by biopsy.

Darnell J, Lodish H, Baltimore D (eds.): Cell to cell signaling: Hormones and receptors. *In* Molecular Cell Biology. New York, WH Freeman, 1990. *Good overview of principles of mechanisms of hormone signaling.*

Egan SE, Weinberg RA: The pathway to signal achievement. Nature 365:781, 1993. *Overview of the central mitogenic pathway important for normal growth, which is often deranged in cancer.*

Fantl WJ, Johnson DE, Williams LT: Signalling by receptor tyrosine kinases. Annu Rev Biochem 65:453, 1993. *Review of structure and signaling by an essential class of peptide hormone receptors.*

Goodrich JA, Tjian R: TBP/TAF complexes: Selectivity factors for eukaryotic transcription. Curr Opin Cell Biol 6:403, 1994. *A thoughtful discussion of the way by which regulatory proteins contact the transcriptional machinery.*

Lazar MA: Thyroid hormone receptors: Multiple forms, multiple possibilities. Endocrinol Rev 14:184, 1993. *Review with primary references of how thyroid hormone and related receptors work.*

Mulligan LM, Kwok JBJ, Healey CS, et al.: Germ-line mutations of the RET protooncogene in multiple endocrine neoplasia type 2A. Nature 363:458, 1993. *First demonstration of an inherited mutation that activates a receptor, resulting in neoplasia.*

Tang W-J, Gilman AG: Adenylyl cyclases. Cell 70:869, 1992. *Minireview of the prototypic signal-transducing molecule.*

200 ENDORPHINS/OPIOID PEPTIDES, PROSTAGLANDINS, AND NATRIURETIC HORMONES

200.1 The Endorphin Family of Opioid Peptides: Biochemistry, Anatomy, and Physiology

Stanley J. Watson

Many central and peripheral nervous system structures contain cells that secrete endogenous neuropeptides capable of mimicking opiate alkaloids, such as morphine and heroin. These peptides have a common pentapeptide sequence at their amino terminus [Tyr-Gly-Gly-Phe-Met (or-Leu)], which is important for their opiate activity. Such *endogenous opioid peptides* carry the generic name of endorphins and are divided into three main families: (1) *Pro-Opio-Melano-Cortin* (or POMC), (2) Pro-Enkephalin, and (3) Pro-Dynorphin/Neo-Endorphin (Fig. 200–1). POMC produces one opiate peptide, β-endorphin, and several nonopioid products, e.g., ACTH and α-, β-, and γ-melanocyte-stimulating hormones (MSH). In contrast, pro-enkephalin has seven repeated opioid sequences, and pro-dynorphin has three.

The structural pharmacology of the opiate alkaloids includes active and inactive stereoisomers of both opiate agonists and antagonists. Radiolabeling of the active alkaloids in the 1970's made it possible to identify opiate receptors in brain. A search for their natural ligands followed, and more than 20 active peptide fragments were extracted. Among these are β-endorphin, met- and leu-enkephalin, and dynorphin. Gene and mRNA information has radi-

cally improved our knowledge of the sequences of the endorphins within their precursors and provided better understanding of their relationships with their nonopiate fragments.

Members of all endorphin families are widely distributed in brain, heart, lung, adrenal, ovary, pituitary, testes, and gut. POMC is found in the corticotrophs of the anterior lobe of the pituitary, in the arcuate nucleus in the base of the hypothalamus, and in the nucleus tractus solitarius in the brain stem. POMC fibers project through limbic, autonomic, and pain systems. The dynorphin system is more widespread both within the brain and in the periphery and also resides in testes, ovary, gut wall, adrenal cortex, and LH and FSH cells of anterior pituitary. In brain the dynorphin system is linked to sympathetic tone, pain systems, motor systems, endocrine control, limbic system, and cortical functions. The enkephalin system, even more widespread than dynorphin and POMC, is found with the catecholamine cells of the adrenal medulla. It also resides in heart, lung, gut wall, sympathetic ganglia, pituitary, and many brain fiber systems. Although enkephalin cells are widely distributed in brain, few linking circuits have as yet been identified. The most obvious systems involved by enkephalins are motor, pain, endocrine, autonomic, limbic (reward), cortex, and hippocampus.

Several different endocrine and neural tissues process endorphin peptides. The most obvious example is found with POMC in the pituitary of the rat. In the anterior lobe the corticotrophs produce, among other peptides, the stress hormone ACTH (1-39). In contrast, in the intermediate lobe (found in most species, but in humans present only in pregnant women and fetuses) that same molecule is further processed to make α-melanocyte-stimulating hormone [or N-acetyl ACTH 1-13 amide and ACTH (18-39)]. Similar tissue-specific processing patterns are found for other POMC peptides, such as β-endorphin, as well as for pro-dynorphin– and pro-enkephalin–produced peptides. For example, pro-enkephalin in adrenal is cleaved into larger fragments, whereas in brain it is actively processed to much smaller peptides. In the last 5 years many of the enzymes capable of participating in the cleavage and amidation of peptide precursors and their products have been cloned and studied.

Several principles have emerged about the above processing. A given precursor can give rise to one set of products in one tissue and a different set in another tissue. General processing differences reflect the chosen cleavage site, indicated by the presence of a dibasic peptide bond (e.g., lysine-argenine). In a second type of processing variant, other chemical moieties are added to a given site in a peptide sequence, e.g., amidation, acetylation, sulfation, or phos-

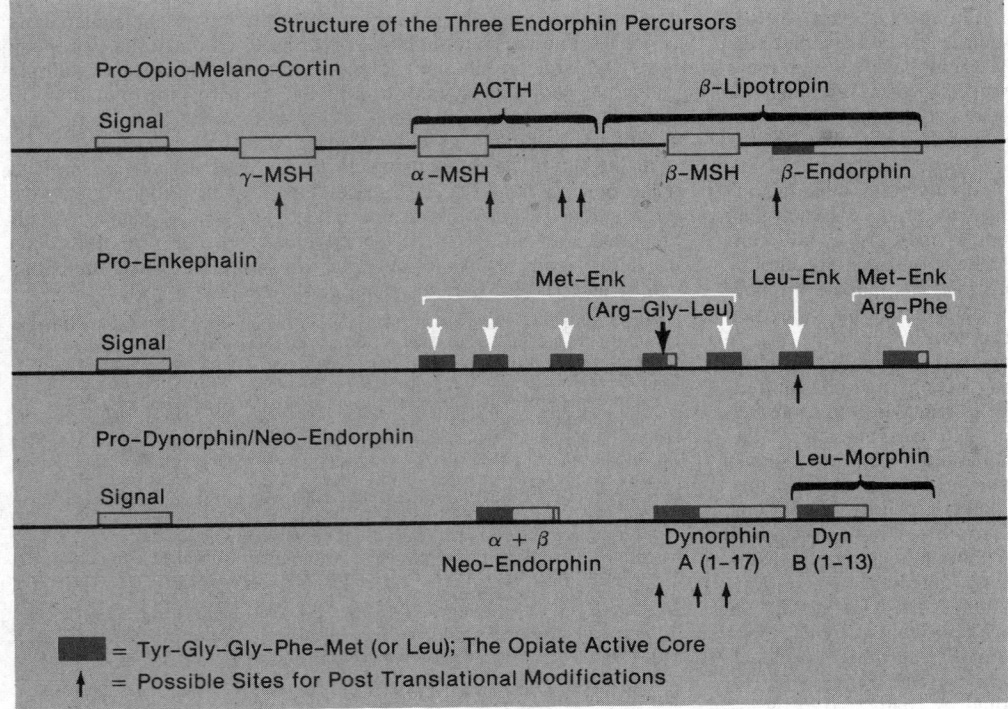

FIGURE 200–1. Simplified schematic of the precursors for all three endorphin families. Note the many peptides produced from each precursor, their similar size, and in the case of pro-enkephalin and pro-dynorphin, the multiple copies of opioid peptides produced by each.

phorylation. Both types of processing choices can alter the nature and potency of these molecules. For example, the addition of an acetyl group to the amino terminal tyrosine of β-endorphin decreases its opiate activity by more than 1000-fold. Thus, two of the largest problems in peptidergic systems, especially in brain, lie in understanding the precursor-processing pathways and the final structure of the peptides produced by each precursor in tissues of interest. Figure 200–1 provides a simplified version of the information.

Peptidergic cells have a range of control over the materials they secrete. To add further complexity, several peptides arise from each of the three endorphin precursors, and nonopioid peptides can be co-produced and co-secreted along with the endorphins (e.g., ACTH and β-endorphin from anterior lobe).

Three main opiate receptor subclasses, each with a different distribution pattern in brain, gut, pituitary, adrenal, and reproductive tissues, have been described (μ, κ, δ).

The μ receptor is very sensitive to morphine; the δ receptor seems to prefer enkephalin-like peptides; the κ receptor was characterized by the action of dynorphin-like peptides. All three opiate receptors have now been cloned, expressed, and localized and are under structural analysis. They are all members of the seven transmembrane G protein-linked receptor class. The selectivity of the receptors is not absolute. For example, dynorphin, while κ preferring, is also a potent μ agonist, and enkephalins, while δ preferring, can interact with the μ site. There is not a one-to-one anatomic link between κ receptors and dynorphin-producing cells and fibers; nor is there one for the δ receptor and pro-enkephalin systems. Rather, one tends to see two or even three opiate receptor subtypes associated with the terminal systems of the peptidergic neurons. Possibly the processing choices of a cell, by altering the peptide products, can alter the receptor preference of the materials secreted. If so, the cell may modulate its products to act on different receptor subtypes at the synapse. Such a system would be extremely flexible in modulating synaptic transmission.

With a multiplicity of peptides and receptors occupying a variety of tissues, it is clear that endorphins do not have a single physiologic role. Furthermore, multiple active transmitters and modulators may exist in the same cell. A particularly clear example of "co-transmission" can be found with the pro-dynorphin peptides in the hypothalamus. Pro-dynorphin peptides (and mRNA) are found in the same cells that produce vasopressin. Consistent with this finding, arginine vasopressin (AVP) and dynorphin are co-released from the posterior pituitary with the same stimuli. It is hypothesized that dynorphin provides local feedback inhibition on further AVP secretion. Other examples of co-transmission among the endorphins include enkephalin and catecholamines in the adrenal medulla, enkephalin and catecholamines in the sympathetic nervous system, and dynorphin and LH/FSH in the anterior pituitary.

Table 200–1 summarizes the main physiologic changes observed with the endorphins. The endorphins have been classically associated with modulation of stress and pain. The neuronal and endocrine systems involved in these responses are the hypothalamic-pituitary-adrenal system and the limbic system. In fact, each major component of the stress-response system contains endorphins. For example, the hippocampus, a main site of corticosteroid feedback, contains enkephalin and dynorphin neurons; the hypothalamus contains all three opioid families; the anterior pituitary contains POMC and enkephalin; the adrenal medulla produces enkephalin; and the adrenal cortex, dynorphin. A similar pattern accompanies pain-modulatory systems in the spinal cord, periaqueductal central gray, thalamus, and the limbic system.

Table 200–1 outlines several patterns effected by the endorphins: (1) These peptides are implicated in a wide variety of physiologic events. (2) Many of these events correlate with their anatomic locus. For example, all three endorphins are found in the nucleus tractus solitarius and are implicated in cardiovascular regulation; gut motility is controlled from the brain and gut opiatergic loci; respiration is regulated partially by the parabrachial nucleus, an area with both opiate peptides and receptors; and motor integration actively involves the nigrostriatal system, rich in opioid anatomy. (3) The functions associated with the endorphins are basic, homeostatic, limbic, "core" activities; they express affective or "drive"-related activities, rather than cognitive ones. (4) There are a few "unexpected" physiologic links, such as appetite modulation, drinking, and thermoregulation.

Coming years undoubtedly will see consolidation and organization of the great wealth of biologic data on these important systems.

TABLE 200–1. PROPOSED FUNCTIONS AND KNOWN ANATOMIC LOCALIZATIONS OF THE ENDOGENOUS OPIOID SYSTEMS

Function	Anatomic Localization
Appetite modulation and eating behavior	Limbic system, including hypothalamus and amygdala
Cardiovascular regulation	NTS, parabrachial nucleus
Drinking and water balance	Subfornical organ, magnocellular hypothalamic-pituitary system
Endocrine responses	Hypothalamic-pituitary-peripheral axis
Stimulatory effects on Growth hormone Melanocyte-stimulating hormone Prolactin	Hypothalamus and anterior lobe
Inhibitory effects on Follicle-stimulating hormone Luteinizing hormone Thyroid-stimulating hormone	Hypothalamus and anterior lobe
Inhibition of release of vasopressin and oxytocin	Hypothalamus and posterior lobe
Gastrointestinal motility	NTS, area postrema, and GI nervous plexuses
Pain inhibition	Thalamus, periaqueductal gray, substantia gelatinosa, NTS, spinal cord
Respiration	Parabrachial nucleus, NTS
Response to stress	Hypothalamic-pituitary-adrenal axis
Sensory-motor integration	Nigrostriatal system, globus pallidus, inferior and superior colliculi
Thermoregulation	Hypothalamus

NTS = Nucleus tractus solitarius.

One of the main foci will be a clearer view of the physiology-peptide-receptor interface; the other will be increased understanding of the genetic regulation of these systems. With the increasing clarity will come improved appreciation of the regulation of a whole series of crucial basic brain functions.

Akil H, Bronstein D, Mansour A: Overview of the endogenous opioid systems. *In* Rodgers RJ, Cooper SJ (eds.): Endorphins, Opiates and Behavioral Processes. Chichester, John Wiley and Sons Limited, 1988, pp 1–23. *General overview of biochemistry, anatomy, and physiology of endorphins.*

Fowler CJ, Fraser GL: μ-, δ-, κ-opioid receptors and their subtypes. A critical review with emphasis on radioligand binding experiments. Neurochem Int 24:401, 1994.

Herbert E, Seasholtz A, Comb M, et al.: Study of the regulation of expression of neuropeptide genes by gene transfer methods. *In* Psychopharmacology: The Third Generation of Progress. New York, Raven Press, 1987, pp 373–384. *Summary of the gene structure and promoter elements of several peptide genes.*

Mansour A, Watson SJ: Anatomical distribution of opioid receptors in mammalians: An overview. *In* Herz A (ed): Opioids I. Handbook of Experimental Pharmacology. Vol. 104/I. New York, Springer-Verlag, 1993, pp 79–105. *Comprehensive overview of opioid peptide producing and ligand binding structure in brain.*

Mansour A, Fox CA, Akil H, Watson SJ: Opioid receptor mRNA expression in the rat CNS: Anatomical and functional implications. Trends Neurosc 18:22, 1995.

Pasternak GW: Review: Pharmacological mechanisms of opioid analgesics. Clin Neuropsychopharmacol 16:1, 1993.

Reisine T, Bell GI: Molecular Biology of Opioid Receptors. Trends Neurosc 16:56, 1993. *Overview of structure and pharmacology of all three opioid receptors.*

200.2 Prostaglandins and Related Compounds

Garret A. FitzGerald

Arachidonic acid, derived from dietary sources, is transported in plasma in both esterified and nonesterified forms, primarily bound to lipoproteins and albumin, respectively. The relative importance of these two sources for cellular delivery is poorly understood. Esterified arachidonic acid in low density lipoproteins is taken up by cells by a process dependent on the low density lipoprotein receptor. The fatty acid is compartmentalized in the phospholipid domain

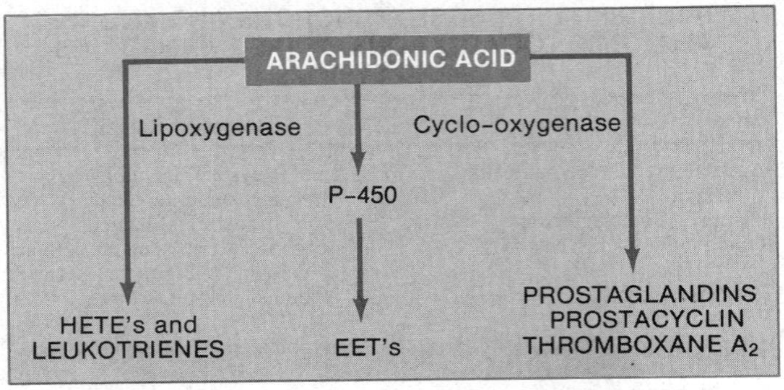

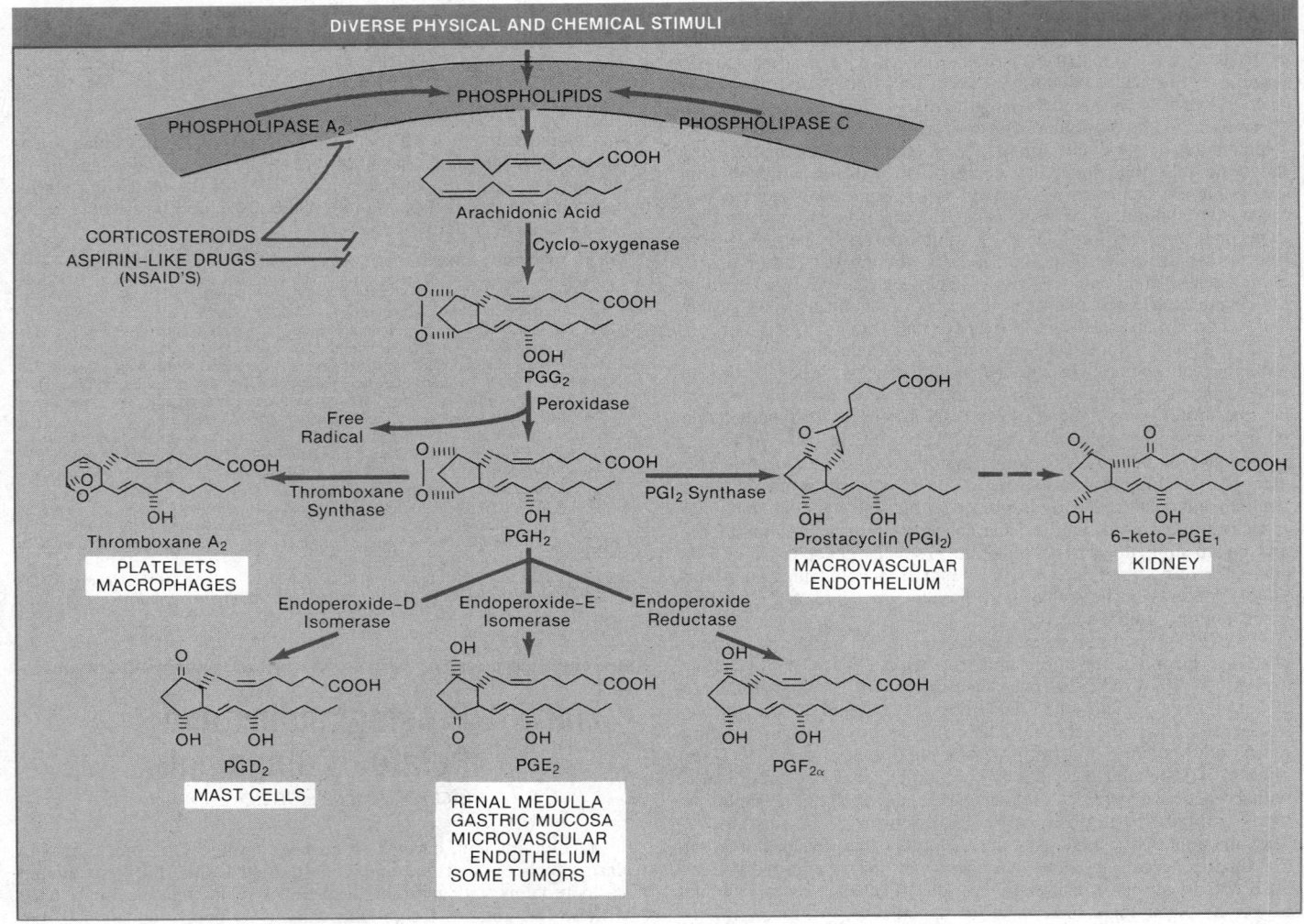

FIGURE 200–2. Major pathways of metabolism of arachidonic acid.

of cell membranes. This localization appears relevant to the availability of arachidonate for release. A cytosolic phospholipase (PL) A$_2$ with high affinity for arachidonic acid is thought to be central to this process. Phosphorylation by mitogen-activated kinase and protein kinase C permits its calcium-dependent translocation to the cell membrane. Other PL's may also participate in arachidonate release. Subsequent oxygenation by either cyclo-oxygenase or lipoxygenase gives rise to biologically active compounds. A third pathway of metabolism via cytochrome P450 also exists (Fig. 200–2).

All cells can release arachidonic acid, but the predominant enzymatic products that are formed are highly cell specific. Because

they are derived from a polyunsaturated eicosanoic (C$_{20}$) fatty acid, these compounds—thromboxane A$_2$, the prostaglandins (PG's), epoxygenases, leukotrienes, and lipoxins—are collectively known as eicosanoids. Because of their diverse biologic properties and rapid metabolism to inactive products, the eicosanoids have been implicated as local mediators of receptor-dependent events in a range of physiologic processes and in diverse human diseases, including bronchial asthma, inflammation, and unstable coronary disease. Arachidonic acid itself and its metabolites may also function as intracellular second messengers, particularly in the modulation of ion channels, ras activity, and perhaps gene expression.

THE CYCLO-OXYGENASE PATHWAY (Fig. 200–3).

The biotransformation of arachidonic acid into thromboxane (Tx)A$_2$, prostacyclin (PGI$_2$), PGE$_2$, PGF$_{2\alpha}$, and PGD$_2$ is catalyzed by a common enzyme, the fatty acid cyclo-oxygenase (COX). The product of the COX reaction is an unstable endoperoxide, PGG. A second oxygen molecule is then introduced at C$_{15}$; this results in the 15-hydroperoxy endoperoxide PGH, and liberates a free radical. There are two COX genes; a constitutive form (COX-1), which is expressed ubiquitously and has recently been crystalized. Although COX-1 is inducible in certain constrained circumstances (e.g., by certain cytokines in bone marrow-derived mast cells or by male sex hormones in ram seminal vesicle), COX-2, which is expressed in a more limited repertoire of cells, is induced by cytokines, tumor promoters, growth factors, and gonadotropins. Consequently, it is presumed to be the COX of predominant importance in the generation of prostaglandins in inflammation and, perhaps, cancer.

FIGURE 200–3. Metabolism of arachidonic acid by fatty acid cyclo-oxygenase. The major tissues of origin of the eicosanoids are shown.

PGH is metabolized by cell-specific enzymes to form either the "classic" prostaglandins of the D, E, and F series, PGI_2, or TxA_2. Arachidonic acid contains four double bonds ($\Delta^{5,8,11,14}$). It is apparent from the sequence of biosynthesis (Fig. 200–3) that two double bonds remain in its (bisenoic) COX products. This is denoted by the subscript 2, as in TxA_2 and PGE_2. Analogous metabolism of other fatty acid substrates gives rise to monoenoic or trienoic prostaglandins and thromboxanes (Fig. 200–4). For example, metabolites of eicosatrienoic acid ($C_{20:3}$n-6) contain only one (Δ^{13}) double bond. Eicosapentaenoic acid (EPA) ($C_{20:5}$n-3), which is prevalent in certain fish and aquatic mammals, is transformed by COX to metabolites with three ($\Delta^{5,13,17}$) double bonds, such as PGI_3 and TxA_3. Structurally, prostaglandins of the D, E, and F series possess a cyclopentane ring and differ only in their substituent groups. The F series prostaglandins are referred to as $PGF_{1\alpha}$, $PGF_{2\alpha}$, and $PGF_{3\alpha}$.

THROMBOXANE A_2. TxA_2, the predominant COX product formed by platelets, stimulates aggregation of these cells and constricts vascular and bronchial smooth muscle. These biologic properties are shared by the PG endoperoxides. A single thromboxane (Tx) receptor gene encodes a member of the G protein–coupled receptor superfamily. Distinct placental and endothelial isoforms have been cloned. Tissue-specific splice variants may differ in their preferential linkage to intracellular effector molecules and in aspects of their desensitization. Although the Tx receptor is phosphorylated, the molecular events that underlie eicosanoid receptor desensitization are poorly understood. Expression of the receptor appears to be transcriptionally regulated by certain growth factors and male sex steroids. Recently, a mutation in the first intracellular loop of the Tx receptor has been linked to a bleeding disorder characterized by a selective defect in the aggregability of platelets *ex vivo* by Tx agonists.

PROSTACYCLIN. Prostacyclin (PGI_2), the predominant COX product of arachidonic acid formed by vascular endothelium and also by subendothelium, both inhibits the aggregation of platelets by all recognized agonists and disaggregates previously aggregated platelets. PGI_2 inhibits the adherence of platelets and neutrophils to foreign surfaces and damaged endothelium and dilates both bronchial and vascular smooth muscle. A PGI receptor has recently been cloned and exhibits about 30 to 40% homology with other eicosanoid receptors. Another potentially important property of PGI_2 is the modulation of cholesterol efflux from arterial walls. Nanomolar quantities of PGI_2 stimulate the activity of both the lysosomal and cytoplasmic cholesterol ester hydrolases when added experimentally to vascular smooth muscle cells but have no effect on the microsomal acyl-CoA cholesterol acyl transferase (ACAT), which re-esterifies free cholesterol. Both PGI and TxA synthase enzymes have been cloned. Although the sequence homology between them is less than 40%, they are both P450 enzymes.

PGI_2 biosynthesis is increased in several human diseases in which evidence of platelet activation is present, including severe peripheral arterial disease and unstable coronary disease. Although this implies a homeostatic role for this eicosanoid, its biologic importance remains ill defined in the absence of pharmacologic antagonists. Recently, local vascular delivery of the COX-1 gene has been reported to limit platelet-dependent vascular occlusive events in a canine model, perhaps by enhancing vascular PGI formation.

PROSTAGLANDIN D_2. Prostaglandin D_2, the principal COX product of the mast cell, is released, together with histamine and other mediators, by IgE-dependent and other stimuli. Infusion of PGD_2 in humans results in nasal stuffiness, systemic hypotension, and flushing. PGD_2 is increased in bronchoalveolar lavage fluid following antigen challenge in atopic individuals, suggesting that it may contribute to the bronchomotor response in allergic asthma. PGD_2 is a minor product of the platelet COX. Both PGD_2 and its 9α, 11β-PGF metabolite inhibit platelet aggregation by stimulating adenylate cyclase, thereby increasing intraplatelet cyclic AMP. In experimental animals, central administration of PGD_2 induces sleep, an event that is countered by infusion of PGE_2. Two forms of the PGD synthase exist—one in brain, which has been cloned, and the other in blood cells. The former is highly expressed in rat leptomeninges and choroid plexus, where it may increase PGD levels in the CSF. Elevated CSF levels of PGD have been reported in patients with African sleeping sickness. Selective knock-out of the PGD synthases and/or the recently cloned PGD receptor may clarify the role of this eicosanoid in sleep regulation and immune function.

PROSTAGLANDIN E_2. The formation of PGE_2 from PGH_2 is catalyzed by a PGE_2 isomerase that is present in renal medulla, gastric mucosa, and platelets. PGE_2 rather than PGI_2 may be the predominant prostaglandin formed by microvascular endothelium. In the kidney, PGE_2 can act both as a vasodilator and as an inhibitor of tubular sodium absorption. It helps maintain renal blood flow, together with PGI, during activation of the renin-angiotensin and sympathoadrenal systems. Three E prostaglandin receptor genes (EP_1, EP_2, and EP_3) have been cloned. Analogous to the Tx receptor, tissue-specific carboxyl terminal splice variants of the EP receptor couple with differing preference for discrete effector pathways in expression systems.

PGE_2 is the predominant COX product of arachidonic acid formed in gastric mucosa. It participates in the regulation of gastric blood flow and limits the effects of diverse physical and chemical

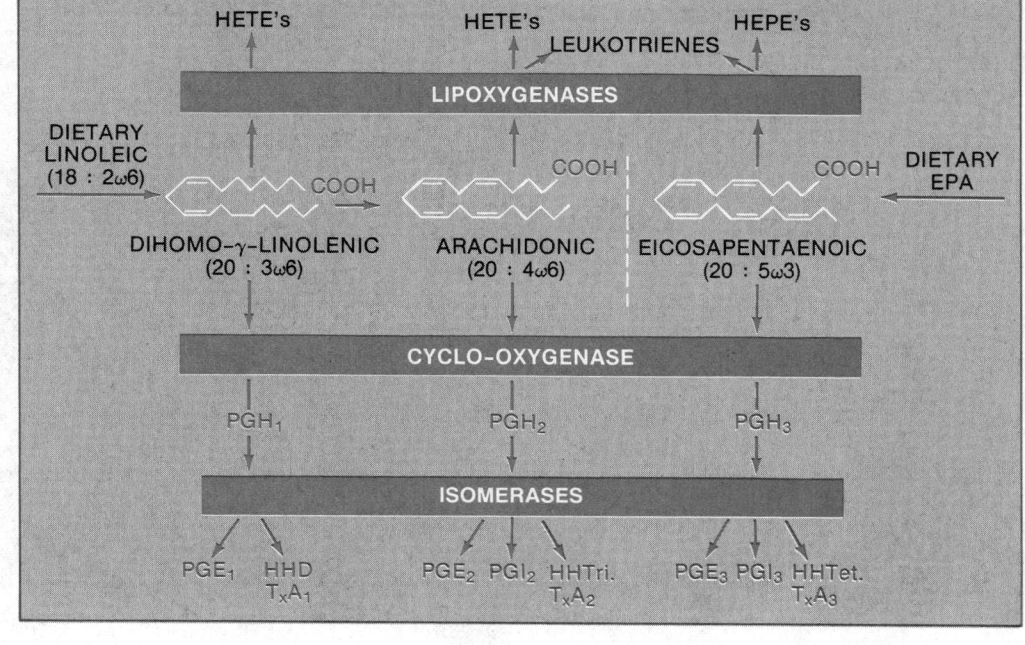

FIGURE 200–4. Analogous formation of mono-, bis-, and trienoic prostaglandins. (Reproduced with permission from FitzGerald GA, Price P, Knapp HR: Biochemical and functional effects of dietary substrate modification in man. *In* Simopoulos AP, Kifer RR, Martin RE [eds.]: Health Effects of Polyunsaturated Fatty Acids in Seafoods. Orlando, FL, Academic Press, 1986, pp 61–80.)

insults to the gastric mucosa. This "cytoprotective" property is shared by PGI_2, but the mechanism by which this protection occurs is unknown. Other biologic properties of PGE_2 include relaxation of bronchial smooth muscle, contraction of uterine smooth muscle (19-hydroxylated E prostaglandins are the major arachidonic acid products in human semen), and modulation of lymphocyte function. PGE_2 modulates neurotransmission via presynaptic receptors on adrenergic neurons in vitro and appears to be important in the sleep/wakefulness cycle.

In a minority of patients with solid tumors, PGE_2 production by the tumor causes hypercalcemia via stimulation of osteoclast activity (see Ch. 159). In such cases, suppression of PGE_2 biosynthesis lowers the level of serum calcium. When metastases to bone occur, however, local mechanisms for hypercalcemia supervene.

PROSTAGLANDIN $F_{2\alpha}$. $PGF_{2\alpha}$, formed from PGH_2 by the action of an endoperoxide reductase, contracts bronchial and uterine smooth muscle and vasoconstricts some uterine beds. Although increases in $PGF_{2\alpha}$ metabolites have been described during dysmenorrhea and allergen-evoked bronchospasm, a unique site for formation of this prostaglandin and its role in pathophysiology remain to be determined. High concentrations of $PEF_{2\alpha}$ and Tx receptor mRNA are found in myometrium.

THE LIPOXYGENASE PATHWAY (Fig. 200–5)

Arachidonic acid is also widely subject to lipoxygenation reactions (Fig. 200–5). In neutrophils, insertion of an oxygen molecule adjacent to one of the double bonds yields the hydroperoxy derivative, 5-hydroperoxyeicosatetraenoic acid (5-HPETE). This can undergo further metabolism to either a 5-hydroxyeicosatetraenoic acid (5-HETE) or to an unstable 5,6-epoxide intermediate, leukotriene (LT)A_4. This compound can be hydrolyzed to 5,12-dihydroxy-eicosatetraenoic acids, one of which is LTB_4. The subscript 4 refers to the number of double bonds. Thus, analogous to the nomenclature for COX products, substitution of eicosapentaenoic acid for arachidonic acid as a substrate would result in formation of LTB_5. The site of the initial lipoxygenation reaction tends to vary with cell type. Thus, 12-HETE is formed predominantly in platelets, 5-HETE by polymorphonuclear leukocytes, and 5-HETE, 11-HETE, and 15-HETE by endothelial cells as measured in culture.

The 5-lipoxygenase (5-LO) of human neutrophils, a cytosolic enzyme, is translocated to the membrane for metabolism of arachidonic acid. It requires an 18K protein, termed the five lipoxygenase activating protein (FLAP), to achieve full activation. Analogous activating proteins do not appear necessary for expression of 12- and 15-lipoxygenase activity. The primary structures of two distinct 12-lipoxygenases have been reported. One, in porcine leukocytes, is immunologically identical to that in porcine brain and human tracheal cells. It is closely related to the 15-lipoxygenase. The human platelet 12-lipoxygenase is a distinct gene product. The role of 12-HETE in platelets is unknown. Platelet 12-lipoxygenase is translocated from the cytosol to the membrane in a calcium-dependent manner, and 12-HETE inhibits the mobilization of a glycoprotein IIb/IIIa complex in tumor cell lines. This complex is analogous to that which serves as a receptor for adhesive macromolecules, such as fibrinogen, in activated platelets. 12-Lipoxygenase products regulate potassium channel flux in Aplysia. Formation of 15-HETE is reportedly increased in atherosclerotic blood vessels, and in situ hybridization studies suggest that expression of the enzyme is increased and co-localized with oxidized low density lipoproteins in human atherosclerotic plaques.

LTA_4 is conjugated enzymatically with glutathione to yield LTC_4. This compound is metabolized to LTD_4 and LTE_4 by successive elimination of a γ-glutamyl residue and glycine. The cysteinyl-containing leukotrienes are powerful bronchoconstrictors and vasoconstrictors. These compounds also dilate microvessels, increase vascular permeability, and stimulate mucus secretion. LTC_4 causes pulmonary bronchoconstriction, an effect that is partially blocked by COX inhibitors. This implies that LTC_4 may mediate this effect via the release of a bronchoconstrictor prostaglandin, such as thromboxane A_2. LTC_4 may cooperate with luteinizing hormone-releasing hormone (LHRH) in the control of LH release by cells of the anterior pituitary, judged by in vitro studies.

LTB_4 stimulates adhesion, migration, aggregation, enzyme release, and generation of superoxide by polymorphonuclear leukocytes. These biologic properties strongly suggest a role for lipoxygenase products in both inflammation and antigen-evoked bronchoconstriction.

Embryonic stem cell knock-out of the 5-LO gene results in a normal phenotype. However, the lethal effects of intravenous injection of platelet-activating factor and the local inflammatory response to topical application of arachidonic acid are modified by gene disruption. It is likely that imminent information from the inactivation and/or overexpression of other enzymes and receptors will clarify further the biologic role of eicosanoids.

DiHETE's can be formed via transcellular metabolism, at least in vitro. Examples include 12,20-DiHETE formed by a mixed suspen-

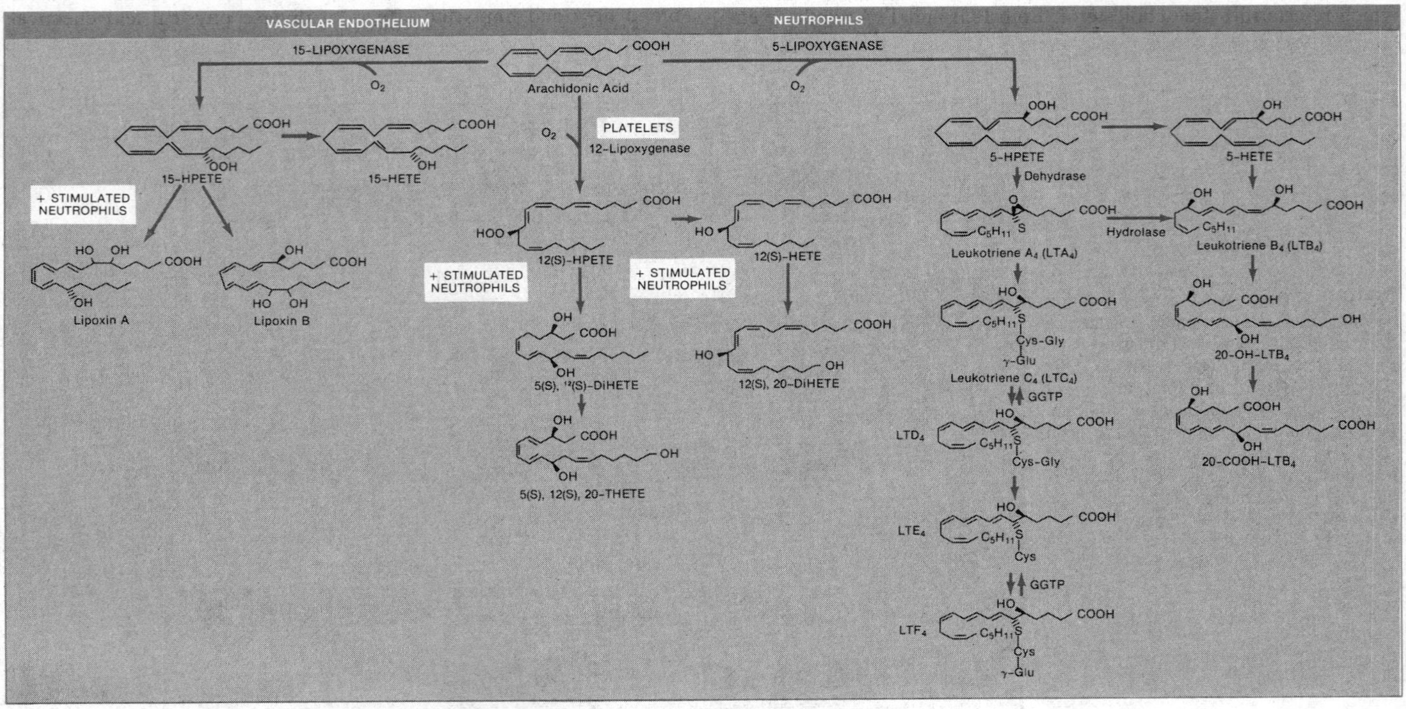

FIGURE 200–5. Metabolism of arachidonic acid by lipoxygenase enzymes.

sion of platelets and polymorphonuclear leukocytes. Leukocytes can utilize erythrocyte LTA_4 to generate LTB_4 and endothelial cells can utilize platelet-derived PGH_2 to generate PGI_2.

Stimulated human leukocytes can convert 15-HPETE to products termed lipoxins (LX) containing a characteristic tetraenoic structure (Fig. 200–5). The two major products are identified as LXA and LXB. LXA is a potent stimulus to superoxide generation by neutrophils and contracts pulmonary tissue. Both LXA and LXB inhibit natural killer cell cytotoxicity *in vitro,* by a mechanism distinct from that of PGE_2, which decreases the binding between target and effector cells. Another series of compounds with potent biologic properties *in vitro* are the hepoxilins, formed by an intramolecular rearrangement of 12-HETE. Glutathione conjugates of hepoxilin A_3 cause hyperpolarization of rat brain neurons at nanomolar concentrations.

THE EPOXYGENASE PATHWAY (Fig. 200–6)

In addition to metabolism by COX and lipoxygenase enzymes, arachidonic acid is subject to ω and ω-1 oxidation by cytochrome P450 enzymes in microsomal preparations. A specific P450 enzyme with high affinity for arachidonic acid has been cloned. This results in the formation of 19-OH and 19-oxo-eicosatetraenoic acid (by ω-1-oxidation) and 20-OH-eicosatetraenoic and eicosatetraene-1,20-dioic acids (by ω oxidation). In addition, a series of epoxides 14(15)-epoxy-, 11(12)-epoxy-, 8(9)-epoxy-, and 5(6)-epoxy-eicosatrienoic acids (EET's) can be formed by this enzyme from arachidonic acid. These compounds can then be further transformed to vicinyl diols by epoxide hydrolases. One such compound, 11,12-dihydroxyeicosatrienoic acid, inhibits the Na^+-K^+-ATPase enzyme in vascular smooth muscle. 5(6)-EET inhibits sodium absorption and potassium secretion by the rabbit cortical collecting duct, and synthetic 5(6)-EET stimulates the release of LH and somatostatin by pituitary cells in culture. Interestingly, 8,9-EET and 14,15-EET stereospecifically inhibit human platelet COX. By contrast, all EET's studied inhibit platelet aggregation *in vitro* by a nonspecific mechanism, independent of an effect on Tx formation. EET's weakly inhibit monocyte and platelet adherence to endothelial cells. Finally, 5(6)-EET is metabolized to epoxides of PGG_1, PGH_1, and PGE_1 and to the 5S, 6S and 5R, 6R isomers of 5-hydroxy-PGI_1. The biosynthesis of EET's has recently been confirmed *in vivo.* Urinary excretion of their vicinyl diols (DHET's) is increased in normal pregnancy, and further increments, particularly of 14(15)-

DHET, are observed in patients with pregnancy-induced hypertension. 5(6)-EET biosynthesis is increased in syndromes of salt and water retention.

THE ISOPROSTANES. Free radicals may catalyze the formation of prostaglandin and leukotriene isomers from arachidonic acid in the sn-2 position of phospholipids. These isoprostanes are potentially susceptible to cleavage by PLA's and may function as either intracellular mediators of oxidant stress and/or as autacoids. Indeed, two such compounds, 8-epi $PGF_{2\alpha}$ and 8-epi PGE are vasoconstrictors—an effect prevented by Tx receptor antagonists. Isoprostane excretion in urine is elevated in clinical conditions putatively associated with oxidant stress, such as reperfusion, certain poisonings, and in apparently healthy cigarette smokers, perhaps due to neutrophil activation.

PHARMACOLOGIC AND DIETARY REGULATION OF BIOSYNTHESIS

With the exception of P450-derived metabolites, and the isoprostanes, none of the oxygenated products of arachidonic acid have the potential for storage in significant quantities for subsequent release by cells. Release is equivalent to biosynthesis. Arachidonate release may occur by several mechanisms. Phosphatidylinositol (PI) may be hydrolyzed by a PI-specific PLC, yielding diacylglycerol (DAG) and inositol phosphate. DAG is then further hydrolyzed, yielding free arachidonic acid and other fatty acids. Alternatively, phosphatidylcholine (PC) may be hydrolyzed by phospholipase A_2(PLA_2), yielding arachidonic acid from the sn-2 position. PLA_2 may also liberate arachidonic acid from phosphatidylethanolamine. Selectivity of phospholipid compartmentalization and phospholipase action permits some HETE's and EET's to modulate second messenger formation. Thus, 15-HETE incubated with endothelial cells is selectively incorporated into PI, and agonist-evoked activation of PLC results in release of a 1-stearoyl-2(15-HETE)-DAG. 15-HETE enrichment of lipidic second messengers modifies β-adrenergic receptor sensitivity in cardiomyocytes. PLD-catalyzed formation of a modified phosphatidic acid has also been demonstrated.

CORTICOSTEROIDS. The effects of steroids on eicosanoid biosynthesis are complex. It is thought that they induce formation of a phospholipase-inhibitory protein, variously named lipocortin, macrocortin, lipomodulin, and renomodulin (see Fig. 200–3). It is

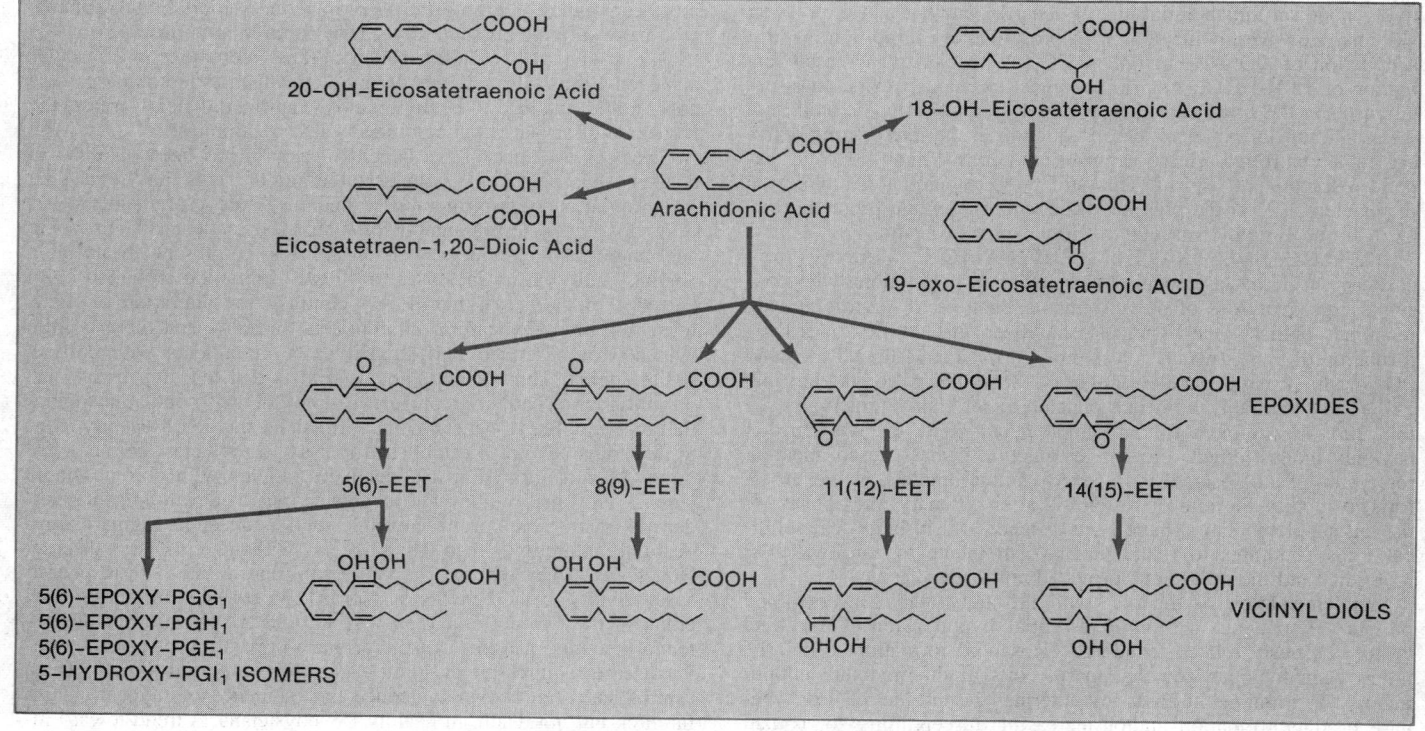

FIGURE 200–6. Metabolism of arachidonic acid by cytochrome P450.

hypothesized that initially steroids bind to specific cytosolic receptors and that the complex is then transferred to the nucleus where steroids regulate the expression of genes and subsequently the synthesis of a PLA_2-inhibitory protein (see Ch. 199). The lipocortin family is derived from a monomeric 40K protein, phosphorylation of which by protein kinases results in its activation as an inhibitor. Interestingly, there is a striking sequence homology between this protein and the 40K protein that is phosphorylated following the binding of epidermal growth factor to its receptor. The amino acid sequence of one member of the family, lipocortin III, is identical to that of inositol 1,2-cyclic phosphate 2 phosphohydrolase. Such a role for lipocortin has been disputed, however, especially as lipocortins bind nonspecifically to phospholipids.

More recently, steroids have been shown to down regulate induction of COX-2 and several PLA's. Regulation of other inducible enzymes, such as nitric oxide synthase, is also of likely relevance to the anti-inflammatory properties of these compounds.

COX INHIBITORS. Nonsteroidal anti-inflammatory drugs (NSAID's) prevent the formation of prostaglandins by inhibiting COX. This group of drugs includes aspirin, salicylates, indomethacin, ibuprofen, piroxicam, fenoprofen, paracetamol, phenylbutazone, oxyphenbutazone, bolmetin, sulfinpyrazone, and sulindac. Paracetamol (acetaminophen) is a considerably less potent inhibitor than the other compounds, except perhaps in the brain. Aspirin is also unlike the other compounds in that it acetylates a serine residue at position 529, close to the active site of the platelet PGG/H synthase, and inhibits the enzyme irreversibly. This accounts for the unique effects of aspirin on the platelet COX-1. Whereas other cells have the capacity for *de novo* protein synthesis, the anucleate platelet does not; thus inhibition of TxA_2 formation by aspirin persists for the lifetime of the platelet. By contrast, the effects of aspirin on eicosanoid formation by other cells (e.g., prostacyclin biosynthesis by vascular endothelium), which expresses both COX-1 and COX-2 are not so prolonged owing to their capacity to generate new enzymes. The irreversible actions of aspirin on platelet COX also account for the cumulative inhibition of platelet TxA_2 formation by the repeated administration of low dosages of aspirin (20 to 40 mg per day; a regular aspirin tablet contains 325 mg). This results in partial inhibition of platelet COX after single-dose administration. Even though low doses of aspirin tend to depress PGI_2 formation, its effect is more pronounced on platelet TxA_2 biosynthesis during long-term therapy. The serine target for aspirin acetylation is conserved in COX-2, and aspirin is a relatively nondiscriminant inhibitor of the two enzymes in expression systems. However, coincident with prostaglandin inhibition, aspirin acetylation of COX-2, but not of COX-1, results in increased formation of 15-R-HETE. Aspirin is subject to extensive first-pass metabolism by the liver, and its deacylated product, salicylic acid, is a weak inhibitor of platelet COX. Reduction in the rate of drug delivery in a controlled-release preparation permits more efficient hepatic extraction of aspirin. This still permits cumulative inhibition of platelet COX in the presystemic circulation, while protecting the COX in the systemic vasculature from aspirin exposure.

DIETARY SUBSTRATE MODIFICATION. Mortality from coronary heart disease seems to be lower in populations who consume large quantities of n-3 fatty acids, such as EPA, from aquatic mammals or fish. One hypothesis has been that a shift toward the formation of TxA_3 (which is less biologically active than TxA_2) and PGI_3 (which is a platelet-inhibitory, vasodilator compound like PGI_2) may favorably influence platelet-vessel wall interactions (see Fig. 200–4). Although fish oil supplementation of the western diet has only modest effects on platelet function, it has caused apparent regression of atherosclerosis in several animal models. However, efforts to modify the rate of restenosis after coronary angioplasty by fish oil supplementation have been unsuccessful in large-scale clinical trials. Attempts to relate dietary fish intake to cardiovascular morbidity and mortality have provided conflicting results.

Supplementation of the diet with n-3 fatty acids lowers blood pressure in patients with mild essential hypertension. This effect is not obviously related to altered eicosanoid formation. Similarly, it has been hypothesized that marine oils might modulate inflammatory or immune diseases by altering the profile of lipoxygenase product formation and/or increasing susceptibility to oxidant injury.

LIPOXYGENASE INHIBITORS AND ANTAGONISTS. Recent clinical studies have demonstrated the efficacy of 5-LO inhibitors and sulfidopeptide receptor antagonists in asthma. They appear to be additive to the effects of β-adrenoreceptor agonists.

FUNCTIONS OF ARACHIDONIC ACID METABOLITES *IN VIVO*

The evidence implicating arachidonate metabolites in mechanisms of some human diseases includes measurements of their biosynthesis and the effects of drugs that prevent their formation or antagonize their actions. Because of the evanescence of the primary compounds, estimates of in vivo synthesis have largely been based upon measurement of long-lived but biologically inactive metabolites. Quantitative assays for the major urinary metabolites of primary prostaglandins, PGI_2 and TxA_2, have been useful in identifying potential targets for drugs designed to modulate their actions. Similar methodology is now available to explore lipoxygenase and epoxygenase product formation in vivo. The capacity of tissues to generate arachidonic acid metabolites greatly exceeds the actual production rates in vivo. Thus, artifacts related to sample collection (for example, platelet activation ex vivo during blood sampling, catheter-induced vascular trauma, or formation of free radical-catalyzed derivatives during sample storage) can seriously confound attempts to measure these compounds in the bloodstream. Measurement of metabolite excretion in urine has been favored as a noninvasive, albeit indirect, approach. The most specific and sensitive method for measurement of eicosanoid metabolites is gas chromatography-mass spectrometry, which has been used to validate radioimmunoassays and enzyme immunoassays for selected compounds.

THE CARDIOVASCULAR SYSTEM. TxA_2 is one of many platelet agonists generated in vivo. While aspirin inhibits Tx-dependent aggregation, other agonists, such as thrombin and high doses of collagen, can induce aggregation in vitro despite the presence of aspirin. In view of these properties, it is superficially surprising that aspirin has been shown to influence clinical outcome in a variety of trials in cardiovascular disease, presumably because of its effects on TxA_2 formation. This may reflect the importance of TxA_2 as an amplifying signal for other platelet agonists.

Aspirin reduces significantly the incidence of stroke in patients suffering transient ischemic attacks or with nonvalvular atrial fibrillation. It also reduces the incidence of thrombotic occlusion following coronary artery bypass graft implantations and the incidence of myocardial infarction and death in patients with unstable coronary disease. The drug reduces the risk of a combined endpoint of myocardial infarction, stroke, and vascular death by about 25%. The most convincing evidence that aspirin reduces mortality in patients who have suffered an acute myocardial infarction is provided by the ISIS-2 study of >17,000 patients. The reduction in mortality achieved by aspirin and the thrombolytic agent streptokinase were comparable and additive. Importantly, aspirin did not increase the incidence of stroke when combined with streptokinase.

Clear-cut evidence of the benefit of aspirin has been obtained in smaller trials of patients with unstable angina. This may reflect the early initiation of aspirin therapy and the more prominent role of thrombosis in determining outcome in these patients. Angioscopic and angiographic evidence of thrombosis is present in unstable angina, and phasic increases of TxA_2 formation coincide with episodes of cardiac ischemia. By contrast, the alteration of TxA_2 formation after myocardial infarction is transient, and there is little evidence of sustained platelet activation in patients with chronic stable angina. Thus, if entry to the trial is delayed after a myocardial infarction, patients represent a more "dilute" population potentially susceptible to benefit from antiplatelet therapy. Recently, controlled trials have also established that aspirin reduces the incidence of myocardial infarction and death in patients with chronic stable angina. Presumably, they are at greater risk of developing platelet-dependent unstable coronary events, such as unstable angina or myocardial infarction, then their peers without coronary disease. Nonetheless, they represent a population more dilute with respect to susceptibility to the benefits of aspirin than patients presenting with either of the two aforementioned conditions. Exploration of the potential benefits of aspirin in the primary prevention of cardiovascular disease requires larger studies than those reported to date. Thus, aspirin has been shown to reduce the incidence of myocardial infarction, but not death, in healthy US physicians. A trend toward increased hemorrhagic stroke in the aspirin group did not attain statistical significance. Although aspirin has been used in combination with dipyridamole in many of these studies, there is little evidence that this latter drug contributes to the antithrombotic efficacy of aspirin in humans. The lowest dose of aspirin that has been shown to be effective in unstable angina has been 75 mg per day.

THE RESPIRATORY SYSTEM. Although TxA_2 as well as LT biosynthesis is increased coincident with the bronchoconstrictor response to inhaled allergen, experiments with aspirin and throboxane antagonists suggest that its functional importance is marginal. A minority of asthmatics, perhaps 10%, exhibit bronchoconstrictive, hypersensitivity reactions to aspirin. This appears to reflect a role for prostaglandins, TxA_2, or leukotrienes, as these attacks are provoked by a range of structurally distinct inhibitors of COX but rarely by salicylate, which resembles aspirin but is a weak inhibitor of that enzyme. No evidence currently supports an allergic basis for this condition. Drug-induced reactions in such patients may be quite severe and often feature profuse rhinorrhea and flushing in addition to bronchospasm. Whether such attacks are mediated by differential inhibition of bronchoconstrictor versus bronchodilator prostaglandins, by a shunting of the arachidonate substrate toward lipoxygenation and the formation of bronchoconstrictor leukotrienes, or by reduced formation of a prostaglandin that normally inhibits release of other mediators of bronchoconstriction is unknown.

Aspirin may also trigger a hypersensitivity response in which alterations in blood pressure, flushing, tachycardia, and diarrhea predominate over bronchospasm. Some of these patients have systemic mastocytosis (see Ch. 231).

THE GASTROINTESTINAL SYSTEM. Both PGI_2 and PGE_2 are cytoprotective of gastric mucosa *in vitro* and are thought to contribute to the regulation of mucosal blood flow. The dose-related gastrointestinal side effects of NSAID's are thought to reflect increased susceptibility to local injury (e.g., H^+ backdiffusion) due to inhibition of these prostaglandins. Interestingly, COX-1 but not COX-2 appears to be expressed in the normal gastrointestinal (GI) tract. Thus, recently developed highly selective COX-2 inhibitors may provide a potent anti-inflammatory effect devoid of GI side effects. An alternative approach has been to combine dimethyl PGE analogues as an adjunct to NSAID therapy. The watery diarrhea associated with multiple endocrine neoplasia often responds to treatment with prostaglandin inhibitors. Excessive formation of LTB_4 has been demonstrated in colonic mucosa and rectal dialysates obtained from patients with inflammatory bowel disease.

Recent epidemiologic data have suggested the possibility that aspirin intake may be inversely associated with the incidence of colon cancer. Controlled trials suggest that a preferential COX-1 inhibitor, sulindac, may cause regression of familial polyposis coli. Although preliminary reports suggest expression of COX-2 in such lesions and in colonic cancers, the clinical potential of COX inhibitors in these disorders remains to be explored.

RENIN RELEASE AND RENAL FUNCTION. Although sympathoadrenal activity is the principal regulator of renin release, it appears to be via a COX metabolite of arachidonic acid. PGI_2 is the most potent of the prostaglandins as a renin secretagogue. Inhibition of COX by NSAID's has implications for the diagnostic application of renin measurements. The associated reduction in aldosterone production may be deleterious for patients with hyperkalemia.

Metabolites of arachidonic acid contribute little to the regulation of renal blood flow under physiologic circumstances. Under conditions of increased vasoconstrictor tone, however, preservation of renal blood flow becomes increasingly dependent upon the generation of vasodilator prostaglandins. This is particularly so in patients with chronic glomerulonephritis, Bartter's syndrome, the nephropathy of systemic lupus erythematosus, congestive heart failure, or combined hepatic and renal dysfunction. It has been proposed that the decline in renal function in such patients following administration of NSAID's is less likely to occur with sulindac as a result of retroconversion of the sulfide to the sulfone. It is important to determine if elaboration of vasodilator prostaglandins in these circumstances is dependent on induction of COX-2. Physiologic stress has been shown to induce spatially selective expression of COX-2 in the central nervous system. Should this mechanism operate in the renal vasculature, it would have serious implications for the clinical development of selective inhibitors of COX-2.

The kidney possesses the capacity to generate TxA_2 in addition to vasodilator prostaglandins. Renal biosynthesis of TxA_2 is increased in some patients with severe nephropathy in association with systemic lupus erythematosus, and infusion of a PGH_2-TxA_2 receptor antagonist improves indices of renal function in such patients. Increased TxA_2 biosynthesis by the kidney has been demonstrated in animal models in response to ureteric obstruction, renal vein thrombosis, and development of hypertension following partial renal ablation and coincident with the development of cyclosporine-induced nephrotoxicity. Increased TxA_2 formation during renal allograft rejection has been reported in humans; however, it is unknown whether this is an epiphenomenon or of primary importance in the rejection process. 16,16-Dimethyl PGE_2 delays renal allograft rejection in man, although the mechanism is unknown.

PGE_2 is the major product formed from arachidonic acid in the renal medulla, where it appears to inhibit sodium reabsorption in the distal tubule. EP receptor subtypes are spatially segregated within the kidney as determined by *in situ* hybridization. The consequent sodium retention caused by administration of a COX inhibitor persists only for a day or two, after which sodium balance is reversed despite continued treatment. Prostaglandins may also influence free water clearance. Indomethacin diminishes the excessive water elimination in nephrogenic and lithium-induced diabetes insipidus. Interestingly, disruption of the COX-2 gene results in marked polydipsia and polyuria in surviving animals.

Although P450-catalyzed metabolism of arachidonate occurs in renal tissue and several of the compounds influence tubular ion flux, glomerular filtration rate, and vascular tone, their precise role in renal physiology and pathology remains to be established.

THE REPRODUCTIVE SYSTEM. Both PGE_2 and $PGF_{2\alpha}$ are potent stimulants of myometrial contraction. Both they and their methylated analogues have been utilized as abortifacients and in the induction of labor, usually as an adjunct to low amniotomy. COX inhibitors are currently being evaluated in the treatment of premature labor. A potential hazard of this approach has been premature closure of the ductus arteriosus, although the incidence of the complication is unknown. Closure of a persistent ductus arteriosus can be achieved with indomethacin in the neonatal period. This implies that a COX metabolite contributes to ductal patency. Infusion of PGE_1 has been used to maintain an open ductus in infants with pulmonary atresia until corrective surgery is performed.

Biosynthesis of the prostaglandins increases during pregnancy, particularly during labor. This may reflect induction of COX-2, which is regulated by gonadotropic hormones. Efforts to create COX-2 knock-outs (many of the homozygotes were lethal) have emphasized the likely importance of this enzyme in developmental biology. COX-2 inhibitors may have potential as "morning after" birth control pills. In the case of PGI_2, biosynthesis is increased markedly from as early as the first trimester. Interestingly, this increment is less pronounced in patients with pregnancy-induced hypertension (PIH). Indeed, diminished PGI_2 biosynthesis is apparent prior to the rise in blood pressure. Studies of TxA_2 biosynthesis indicate that platelet activation is present in normal pregnancy and is further increased in patients with severe PIH. TxA_2 is a potent vasoconstrictor in the placental bed and may contribute to the depressed placental blood flow that is a hallmark of PIH. Multicenter trials have been performed to determine if aspirin will reduce the incidence of PIH in women at risk of developing the disease. They have yielded equivocal results. It has been difficult to document a teratogenic risk from maternal consumption of aspirin in the first trimester.

FEVER AND INFLAMMATION. COX inhibitors share antipyretic, analgesic, and anti-inflammatory actions. Paracetamol differs from the other compounds in being an efficient antipyretic despite weak anti-inflammatory properties in the periphery. The prostaglandins that mediate fever are unknown. Vasodilator prostaglandins seem to act in concert with other mediators to augment the inflammatory response. Among these may be the leukotrienes, which enhance capillary permeability and function as chemoattractants and leukocyte activators. Cross-overs of COX and LO knock-out mice may elucidate the interactive role of these families of eicosanoids in inflammatory disease.

Chen X-S, Sheller JR, Johnson EN, Funk CD: Role of leukotrienes revealed by targeted disruption of the 5-lipoxygenase gene. Nature 372:179, 1994. *The first embryonic stem cell knock-out of a gene encoding an eicosanoid-related protein.*

Lecomte M, Laneuville O, Ji C, et al.: Acetylation of human prostaglandin endoperoxide synthase-2 (cyclooxygenase-2) by aspirin. J Biol Chem 269:13207, 1994. *Inhibition of prostaglandin formation by the inducible COX.*

Morrow JD, Hill KE, Burk RF, et al.: A series of prostaglandin F₂-like compounds are produced *in vivo* in humans by a non-cyclooxygenase, free radical-catalyzed mechanism. Proc Natl Acad Sci 87:9383, 1990. *The first description of isoprostanes in human plasma and urine.*

Namba T, Sugimoto Y, Negishi M, et al.: Alternative splicing of C-terminal tail of prostaglandin E receptor subtype EP3 determines G-protein specificity. Nature 365:166, 1993. *Differential linkage of receptor splice variants to intracellular signals.*

Patrono C: Aspirin as an antiplatelet drug. N Engl J Med 330:1287, 1994. *A comprehensive review of the prototypic prostaglandin inhibitor.*

Picot D, Loll PJ, Garavito RM: The x-ray crystal structure of the membrane protein prostaglandin H₂ synthase-1. Nature 367:243, 1994. *The first crystal structure of an eicosanoid-related protein.*

Samuelsson B: Leukotrienes: Mediators of immediate hypersensitivity and inflammation. Science 220:568, 1983. *A review that concentrates on the biosynthesis and metabolism of these compounds and their role in inflammation.*

200.3 Natriuretic Hormones
Dennis A. Ausiello

In the last decade, considerable interest has focused on endogenous factors that play a role in the regulation of water and electrolyte balance. The isolation and cloning of the cardiac-derived atrial natriuretic peptide (ANP) has led to a rapid definition of its biosynthesis, storage, release response, and action. Although there are still some uncertainties, a picture of its role in physiology and pathophysiology and as a possible therapeutic agent has been developed. A second compound (or compounds), called natriuretic hormone (NH), whose presumed structure and function are distinct from those of ANP, has not yet been completely characterized. Therefore, its physiology, pathophysiology, and therapeutic potential are still unclear.

NATRIURETIC HORMONE (NH)

Experimental observations led to the concept of the existence of an endogenous regulator of mammalian Na⁺-K⁺-ATPase (the Na⁺ pump) more than 25 years ago. At that time intravascular expansion with saline in dogs produced a brisk natriuresis with no change in renal perfusion pressure, glomerular filtration rate, or mineralocorticoid activity. The natriuretic effects of extracellular fluid volume expansion in one animal also occurred in a second animal cross-circulated with the blood of the first. The presumption was that the natriuresis was due to a circulating substance that exerted its effects directly on the renal tubular Na⁺ reabsorptive process without affecting renal hemodynamics. Further experiments confirmed that active extracts from plasma, urine, and tissue sources that were natriuretic *in vivo* had a direct effect on transepithelial sodium transport. These substances have digitalis-like characteristics, although there was no reason to assume a structural identity between the postulated endogenous Na⁺-K⁺-ATPase inhibitor and the cardiac glycosides. Digitalis is a potent inhibitor of Na⁺-K⁺-ATPase and causes both natriuresis and an increase in vascular resistance, although these are not its major pharmacologic effects. Using the digoxin radioimmunoassay, digitalis-like immunoactivity has been found in the urine and plasma of sodium-loaded normal human subjects and in uremic and hypertensive subjects. Whether NH and digitalis-like compounds are the same endogenous Na⁺-K⁺-ATPase inhibitors remains to be defined.

BIOLOGIC ACTIVITIES. The biologic effects that have been claimed for the putative NH include (a) natriuresis *in vivo*, (b) inhibition of sodium transport *in vitro*, (c) Na⁺-K⁺-ATPase inhibition, (d) positive cardiac inotropism, and (e) increased vascular reactivity.

BIOCHEMICAL CHARACTERIZATION. Recently, the chemical structure of the endogenous Na⁺-K⁺-ATPase inhibitor from hypothalamus was chemically characterized as an isomer of the plant-derived cardiac glycoside, ouabain. This mammalian molecule inhibits active sodium transport in renal tubular cells and has positive inotropic and vasoconstrictive properties consistent with the NH/hypertension hypothesis.

SITE OF ORIGIN. The site of origin of the NH also remains uncertain, but the brain has been favored because the natriuretic effects of extracellular fluid volume expansion appear to depend on an intact central nervous system. An ouabain-like compound has been isolated from human cerebrospinal fluid. The hypothalamus represents an enriched source of an endogenous inhibitor of Na⁺-K⁺-ATPase, if not the site of its production.

NH AND THE PATHOPHYSIOLOGY OF ESSENTIAL HYPERTENSION. NH may play a role in normal volume regulation and in the pathophysiology of hypertension and secondary edema states. NH may have an extrarenal action leading to enhanced vascular reactivity. The hypothesis proposed is that in hereditary forms of hypertension, there is a persistent tendency toward renal retention of sodium. This may be due to increased Na⁺-K⁺ cotransport or Na⁺-H⁺ exchange in the proximal tubule, occurring as a manifestation of a generalized genetic defect in Na⁺-Na⁺ (Na⁺-Li⁺) countertransport. This defect exists in the erythrocytes of some patients with essential hypertension and in their first-degree normotensive relatives. The renal sodium retention leads to a transient increase in extracellular fluid volume, which serves as a stimulus for the release of a Na⁺-K⁺-ATPase inhibitor. The sodium pump inhibitor acts on the renal tubule to promote sodium excretion, thus restoring extracellular fluid volume to normal levels. It has similar inhibitory effects on Na⁺-K⁺-ATPase in vascular smooth muscle cells, resulting in a tonic increase in vascular tone, increased total peripheral resistance, and hypertension. It is assumed that Na⁺-K⁺-ATPase inhibition in vascular smooth muscle results in an increase in cytosolic free calcium concentration, which must occur to produce the arterial vasoconstriction. How this occurs is unclear. One of the hypotheses is that altered Na⁺-Ca²⁺ exchange resulting from partial sodium-pump inhibition may account for an increase in intracellular free Ca²⁺ concentration. At this time, this hypothesis remains attractive but unproven.

ATRIAL NATRIURETIC PEPTIDE (ANP)

ANP, a peptide hormone, is secreted primarily by the cardiac atria and produces natriuresis, diuresis, smooth muscle relaxation, and inhibition of renin and aldosterone secretion. Its major sites of action include the cardiovascular, renal, and endocrine systems. Although the exact mechanisms triggering the release of ANP are not clear, stretching of the atria appears to be the principal stimulus.

It has been known for several decades that membrane-bound secretory granules exist in the cardiac atria. In 1981 in a pioneering report, DeBold and his colleagues observed that bolus injection of crude extracts of rat atria, but not ventricles, produced a rapid, massive, and short-lasting diuresis and natriuresis and a modest kaliuresis. This suggested the existence of a natriuretic hormone in the atrial granules. Subsequently, this unique hormonal system has been thoroughly studied. The amino acid sequence of the active circulating peptide and its prehormone forms have been defined together with their gene structure, target tissue receptors, and signal transduction pathways.

STRUCTURE, BIOSYNTHESIS, AND SECRETION. The atrium first produces a pre-pro ANP (151 amino acids), the final 126 amino acids of which is pro ANP. The pro ANP, the principal storage form of the hormone in the atrial granules, is the immediate precursor of the biologically active 28 amino acid ANP, the predominant circulatory peptide. Circulatory ANP has a cysteine-cysteine disulfide crosslink that is essential for its activity.

The human gene for pre-pro ANP is located on the short arm of chromosome 1. Transcription of the pre-pro ANP gene proceeds at a high rate in the cardiac atria, estimated to be 1 to 3% of all mRNA in the atrial cardiocytes. ANP gene expression is transcriptionally regulated by dexamethasone and thyroid hormone. ANP is also expressed at very low levels in other tissues, such as brain, anterior pituitary, adrenal medulla, lung, kidney, thyroid, and submandibular gland. The major site of ANP synthesis is the monocytes of the right cardiac atrium, with lesser production in the left atrium. Pro ANP is cleaved by a specific atrial protease, probably at the time of exocytotic fusion of atrial granules with the plasma membrane and possibly even soon after secretion from the myocyte, resulting in ANP as the predominant form entering the coronary sinus blood.

STIMULI FOR RELEASE. Atrial stretch, measured as atrial transmural pressure, is the principal stimulus for ANP secretion into the circulation. Atrial pressure is also correlated with release of ANP. During infusion of isotonic saline in humans, plasma ANP increases in parallel with the increase of right atrial pressure. This results from rapid conversion of pro ANP to ANP and/or release of ANP. With cardiovascular or pulmonary disease, a significant correlation exists between circulating ANP levels and the right and left atrial pressures.

Mineralocorticoids, as well as glucocorticoids administered in high doses, increase mRNA encoding for pre-pro ANP and circulating ANP levels, indicating an increase in ANP production and release. In addition, adrenalectomized rats do not respond to increased atrial pressure with increased atrial and circulating ANP levels in the absence of glucocorticoid or mineralocorticoid replacement. Thus these hormones may play a permissive role in the volume response mediating ANP release as well as inducing ANP secretion directly.

BIOLOGIC AND PLASMA HALF-LIFE. A sensitive radioimmunoassay, generally specific for the mid to C-terminal peptides of ANP, will detect levels of 1 to 10 pg of the peptide in plasma. In subjects on varied sodium diets, the plasma ANP levels range from 10 to 40 pg per milliliter.

After release from the atrium or after intravenous administration, ANP is rapidly cleared with a plasma half-life between 2 and 4 minutes in humans. Biologic activity of ANP critically depends on the intact ring structure and carboxy-terminal residues. The rank order of tissue degradative potency appears to be kidney > liver > lung > plasma > heart.

ANP RECEPTORS. ANP receptors are localized on the cell surface of target tissues, including most notably adrenal, kidney, and the vasculature. They are also found, to a lesser extent, in the central nervous system, hepatocytes, colonic smooth muscle, and lung. In kidney, ANP binding sites are most prevalent in large vessels, glomeruli, and the renal medulla. In the adrenal, ANP binding is limited primarily to the zona glomerulosa.

Molecular cloning has defined three ANP receptors. The first is the ANP-C (or ANP-R2) clearance receptor, which is not coupled to cGMP production, the signal transduction pathway involved in ANP action. Clearance receptors do not mediate any known physiologic effect. The receptors for ANP in the kidney and vascular smooth muscle are predominantly clearance receptors. Their abundance accounts for the short half-life of circulatory ANP. It seems

probable that the atrial peptide system has a novel receptor-mediated sequestration and clearance mechanism that is responsible, at least in part, for maintaining plasma levels of the hormone. The other ANP receptors are two structurally similar plasma membrane receptors, ANP-R1 and ANP-R3, the biologically active receptor forms. ANP binding to the extracellular domain of R1 or R3 activates the cytoplasmic domain of the receptor, which is a guanylate cyclase responsible for the generation of the second messenger, cGMP.

CELLULAR ACTION. The most apparent action of ANP is to increase intracellular cGMP concentration. ANP is a unique peptide hormone in its use of cGMP as a second messenger, which mediates most of the physiologic actions of the hormone. ANP also influences intracellular calcium homeostasis, which may be responsible for some of its biologic effects.

The physiologic responses to ANP include (1) relaxation of vascular and other smooth muscles, (2) increase in glomerular filtration rate and inhibition of tubular water and sodium transport in the kidney, and (3) inhibition of hormone secretion (Fig. 200–7).

KIDNEY ACTION. The kidney is the primary target organ for ANP. ANP causes natriuresis and diuresis by a concerted action at several nephron segments. The primary sites of action of ANP are the glomerulus, the renal vasculature, and the inner medullary collecting duct, although other nephron segments may be involved in the response to ANP. ANP can increase glomerular filtration rate by raising the glomerular hydraulic pressure gradient from capillary lumen to Bowman's space through differential effects on afferent and efferent arteriole tone. By relaxing glomerular mesangial cells, ANP also increases the glomerular ultrafiltration coefficient, Kf. The combined effects result in an increased filtration pressure and thus an increased filtration fraction, with a higher load of salt and water being delivered to the tubules for excretion.

The increased quantity of sodium filtered is not completely reabsorbed. There is an increased delivery of sodium to the distal tubule and collecting duct, where ANP reduces sodium reabsorption and vasopressin-induced water reabsorption, leading to a profound natriuresis. In addition, redistribution of blood flow from the cortex to inner medulla, which dilutes the papillary interstitium, results in an increase in sodium and water excretion.

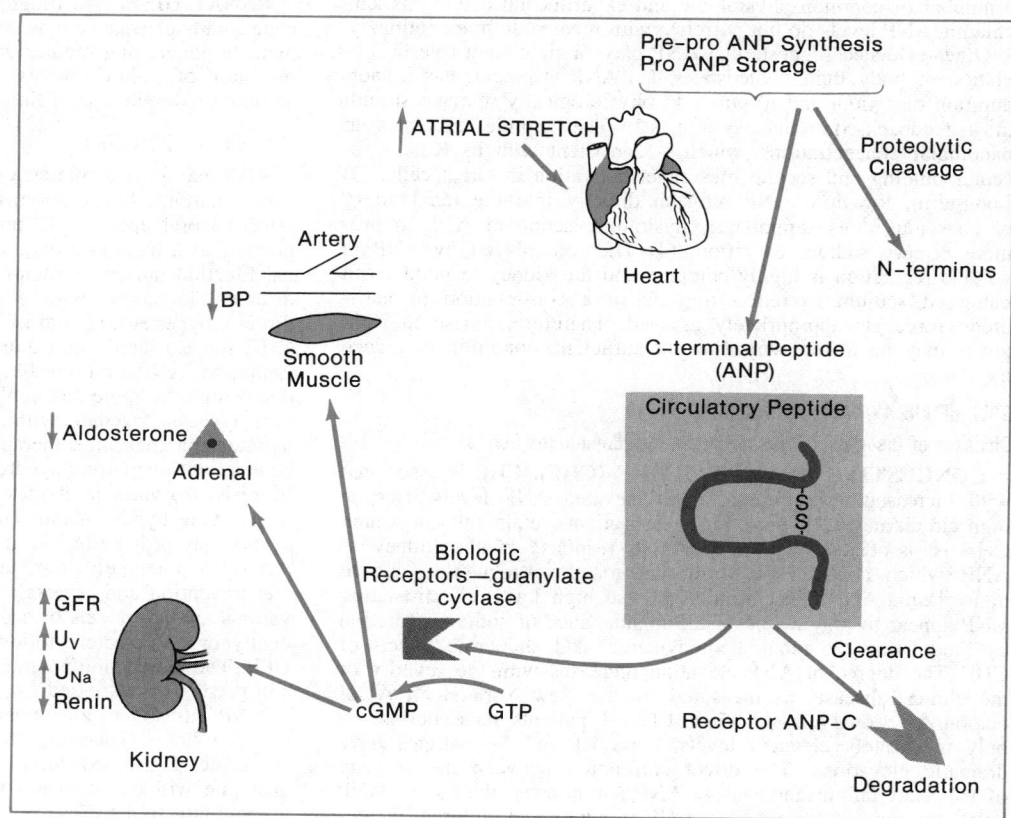

FIGURE 200–7. Major target organs and actions of atrial natriuretic peptide (ANP).

CARDIOVASCULAR ACTION. ANP directly relaxes arterial vascular smooth muscle through the action of its second messenger, cGMP. This ANP-induced vasorelaxation occurs independent of the presence of endothelium. ANP most effectively relaxes large-caliber arteries, such as the aorta and renal and iliac arteries. The more peripheral vascular segments of the arterial tree are less sensitive to the hormone. ANP causes vasorelaxation of aorta constricted with norepinephrine or angiotensin II, compatible with its role as one of the most potent vasodilators known and as a functional antagonist of a variety of vasoconstrictors.

ANP at pharmacologic concentrations reduces mean arterial pressure in man by reducing peripheral vascular resistance and decreasing intravascular volume. This is followed by a decrease in cardiac output attributed to (1) a shift of volume from the intravascular to extravascular space, probably due to alteration in capillary permeability or an increase in resistance to venous return at the site of postcapillary circulation. Hemoconcentration, secondary to a decreased plasma volume, may occur in humans in response to ANP. (2) Preload reduction due to relaxation of venous smooth muscle, leading to an augmentation of venous capacitance and a reduction of venous return.

ENDOCRINE ACTION. ANP modulates renin-angiotensin-aldosterone secretion. Administration of ANP causes a prompt decline in circulatory renin and aldosterone levels. ANP blocks both basal and agonist-stimulated (angiotensin II, ACTH, K^+) secretion of aldosterone in isolated adrenal zona glomerulosa cells. This appears to be a direct action of ANP on these cells. In addition, ANP decreases the biosynthesis and release of vasopressin. The decrease in vasopressin may potentiate a decrease in vascular tone and augment the diuresis and natriuresis induced by ANP.

SIGNIFICANCE OF ANP IN BODY FLUID HOMEOSTASIS

It is not yet possible to describe definitively the physiologic relevance of ANP. Some evidence suggests that ANP exerts a trivial influence on the normal regulation of body fluid homeostasis: (1) Infusion of ANP into conscious animals and normal human subjects results in plasma concentrations slightly above the physiologic range but produces only a slowly developing and relatively modest natriuresis. (2) Ingestion of food containing salt does not increase plasma ANP, yet a natriuresis routinely occurs postprandially. (3) In a number of common physiologic and experimental conditions, circulating ANP levels do not correlate with renal sodium excretion.

Other evidence suggests that ANP plays a significant role in regulation of body fluid homeostasis: (1) ANP is potent, has a short duration of action, and responds to physiologically relevant stimuli in a feedback-controlled system. (2) The peptide circulates at nanomolar concentrations, which is consistent with its Kd for receptor binding and second messenger activation in target cells. (3) Long-term, low-dose ANP infusion directly into the renal artery of conscious dogs supports a physiologic action of ANP to promote urinary sodium excretion. (4) The role played by ANP in volume regulation is highly complex and the kidney responds with increased sodium excretion only when a constellation of natriuretic forces is appropriately assayed. Therefore, a rise in ANP levels may be a necessary, but not sufficient, condition to induce natriuresis.

ROLE OF ANP IN PATHOPHYSIOLOGY

Diseases of Disordered Volume Regulation (Edematous States)

CONGESTIVE HEART FAILURE (CHF). CHF is associated with increased atrial pressure and elevated ANP levels. Despite high circulating ANP, however, these patients retain salt and water. CHF is associated with a decreased response of the kidney to ANP, which could result from receptor down-regulation due to high plasma ANP concentrations. These high levels of circulating ANP appear to play a role in the maintenance of sodium excretion by modulating the renal, hemodynamic, and endocrine effects of CHF. The degree of ANP elevation increases with the severity of the clinical disease, as measured by the New York Heart Association functional classification. Class I patients have normal or only moderately elevated levels; class III and IV patients have dramatic elevations. The direct correlation between the severity of the heart failure and plasma ANP has allowed the use of ANP levels to serve as a marker for CHF in adults and children, including those with congenital heart disease. ANP levels correlate directly with right atrial pressure, pulmonary capillary wedge pressure, and pulmonary artery pressure and inversely with cardiac output and cardiac index.

CIRRHOSIS. Progressive cirrhosis of the liver is accompanied by renal sodium and water retention with the development of ascites and edema. This state is usually accompanied by elevated plasma ANP levels, consistent with the "overflow" theory of ascites formation. As in CHF, raised ANP plasma concentrations in the presence of total body volume expansion implies a "refractory" or "reset" response to ANP. This hyporesponsiveness to ANP in cirrhosis is supported by the observation that ANP levels can be stimulated to increase further by water immersion, peritoneovenous shunting, and acute volume expansion with a resultant natriuresis in some patients. It is probable that a complex balance between ANP and antinatriuretic factors is responsible for renal sodium retention in early and late cirrhosis. In the former, hepatic venous outflow obstruction results in renal salt retention and intravascular volume expansion (overflow hypothesis). This in turn leads to an elevation in ANP levels counterbalanced by antinatriuretic factors such that the net effect is ascites formation. In late cirrhosis, with loss of intravascular volume into the peritoneal compartment (underfill hypothesis), there is a reduced stimulus for ANP secretion such that ANP plasma levels no longer offset antinatriuretic processes.

NEPHROTIC SYNDROME. Why edema forms in the nephrotic syndrome is not completely understood. Traditionally it has been suggested that renal sodium and water retention is a consequence of the lower plasma oncotic pressure from hypoalbuminemia and the resultant reduction in plasma volume. Consistent with this hypothesis, nephrotic syndrome is found to be associated with normal or diminished circulatory levels of ANP that can be stimulated to rise after intravascular volume expansion. Head-out water immersion conducted on patients with nephrotic syndrome demonstrated that ANP levels increased, but renal salt and water excretion was blunted. There thus appears to be an impaired renal response to ANP in the nephrotic syndrome.

ESSENTIAL HYPERTENSION. Patients with essential hypertension have a wide range of plasma ANP concentrations, suggesting that the contribution of ANP may vary in the heterogeneous population of patients with this disease. This finding precludes the use of ANP levels to differentiate among the various causes of hypertension.

RENAL DISEASE. Progressive renal disease is frequently associated with plasma volume expansion and elevated ANP levels. In patients undergoing regular dialysis, ANP levels can be used as an indicator of volume status. Decreased levels correlate with the amount of weight loss of fluid removal in dialysis patients.

THERAPEUTIC POTENTIAL

ANP may have a role as a therapeutic agent, especially in critical care situations. Intervention, in general, is limited by a lack of an effective oral agent. ANP must be administered intravenously. Its potency as a pharmacologic agent in altering cardiovascular and renal function makes it potentially attractive in treating patients with diseases associated with edema (CHF, cirrhosis, nephrotic syndrome), hypertension, and ischemic renal injury: (a) In patients with CHF, the natriuretic and diuretic effects of pharmacologic concentrations of ANP are often limited, but the effect on augmenting cardiac output is quite favorable; (b) in cirrhosis, the renal hyporesponsiveness together with a relatively increased sensitivity to hypotension make the therapeutic use of ANP problematic; (c) in patients with nephrotic syndrome, ANP infusion may result in a natriuresis; (d) variable short-term benefits have been reported in patients with hypertension. The use of low-dose ANP with other agents may prove effective if a satisfactory oral agent is developed; and (e) a potentially important therapeutic action of ANP may be the prevention and reversal of acute renal failure (see Ch. 76). In various animal models of acute renal failure, ANP given prophylactically or immediately following the hemodynamic insult restores GFR. The therapeutic potential of ANP in human acute renal failure still needs to be assessed.

ANP infusion in all human studies has not exceeded a duration of a few hours. Therefore all reported responses to ANP in humans are acute. Prolonged administration of ANP with a nonparenteral analogue will be necessary to evaluate its therapeutic potential in chronic human diseases.

Blaine EH: Atrial natriuretic factor plays a significant role in body fluid homeostasis. Hypertension 15:2, 1990. *Debate on the role ANP plays in body fluid homeostasis.*

Brenner BM, Ballermann BY, Gunning ME, et al.: Diverse biological actions of atrial natriuretic peptide. Physiol Rev 70:665, 1990. *Comprehensive review of the current understanding of the structure of ANP, its synthesis, secretion, cellular and target organ action, and its role in various pathophysiologic states.*

Floras JS: Sympathoinhibitory effects of atrial natriuretic factor in normal humans. Circulation 81:1860, 1990. *Integrative cardiovascular responses to ANP in normal humans.*

Goetz KL: Evidence that atriopeptin is not a physiological regulator of sodium excretion. Hypertension 15:9, 1990. *Debate on the role ANP plays in body fluid homeostasis.*

Haupert GT: Structure and biological activity of the Na$^+$-K$^+$-ATPase inhibitor isolated from bovine hypothalamus: Difference from ouabain. In Bamberg, E, Schoner, W (eds.): The Sodium Pump. New York; Steinkopff Darmstadt Springer, 1994, pp 732–742. *Review of current knowledge of the hypothalamic ouabain-like factor.*

ACKNOWLEDGMENT: I would like to thank Eliezer Holtzman for his invaluable help in preparing this chapter.

201 NEUROENDOCRINOLOGY

201.1 The Neuroendocrine System

Mark E. Molitch

NEUROENDOCRINE REGULATION

Neuroendocrinology refers to the general area of endocrinology in which the nervous system interacts with the endocrine system, serving to link aspects of cognitive and noncognitive neural activity with metabolic and hormonal homeostatic activity. Neural cells that can secrete hormones, i.e., *neurosecretory* cells, serve as the final common pathway linking the brain with the endocrine system. The *neurohypophyseal* neurons originate from the paraventricular and supraoptic nuclei, traverse the hypothalamic-pituitary stalk, and release vasopressin and oxytocin from nerve endings in the posterior pituitary. The *hypophysiotropic* neurons, localized in specific hypothalamic nuclei, project their axons to the median eminence to secrete their peptide and bioamine release and inhibiting hormones into the proximal end of the hypothalamic-pituitary portal vessels (Fig. 201–1). Neurons from other nuclei within the hypothalamus and other parts of the brain influence pituitary hormone secretion by interacting with these specific neurons. The median eminence receives its blood supply from the superior hypophyseal artery, which arborizes into a rich capillary bed. The capillary loops extend into the median eminence and coalesce to form the long portal veins that traverse the pituitary stalk and end in the pituitary. The capillary walls are "fenestrated," allowing entry of peptides secreted by the axon terminals. At the pituitary end of the stalk, the portal vessels again branch to form an extensive capillary plexus.

The neuroendocrine system operates through a series of feedback loops that control central pituitary and target organ hormone levels precisely. Target organ hormones feed back at both the hypothalamic and pituitary levels to complete the loop, and efferent controller factors from the hypothalamus include both stimulatory and inhibitory substances. The feedback loops can be perturbed, resulting in temporary or prolonged alterations of set points by such factors as length of day (circadian periodicity), stress, nutritional status, and systemic illness. The suprachiasmatic nuclei, located just above the optic chiasm, are important in regulating circadian rhythms of the body.

HYPOPHYSIOTROPIC HORMONES

The regulation of pituitary hormones by hypophysiotropic hormones is quite complex, in part because of the multiplicity of substances present in the hypothalamus that can affect pituitary hormone secretion and in part because of the redundancy and overlapping nature of the feedback loops. In addition, some hypophysiotropic hormones exert effects on more than one pituitary

hormone (Fig. 201–2). Some of the hypophysiotropic hormones are also found elsewhere in the body, particularly the gastrointestinal tract and placenta, in which they may have significant physiologic functions. All of the hypophysiotropic hormones are also present in extrahypothalamic brain and function as neurotransmitters. Several hormones can occur in the same hypothalamic nucleus. In each instance, the action of the hypophysiotropic hormone is mediated first by binding to specific receptors and then by alteration of intracellular transduction mechanisms.

THYROTROPIN-RELEASING HORMONE (TRH). TRH is a tripeptide whose secretion is stimulated by norepinephrine and dopamine and inhibited by serotonin. The primary neuroendocrine functions of TRH are to stimulate the synthesis and release of thyroid-stimulating hormone (TSH) and prolactin (PRL). It has been estimated that a single molecule of TRH, through its TSH-releasing effect, induces the release of >100,000 molecules of thyroxine from the thyroid. In hypothyroidism, TRH synthesis and binding to the pituitary are increased, resulting in increased basal and TRH-stimulated TSH and PRL levels. Correction of the hypothyroidism with thyroid hormones decreases the elevated TSH and PRL levels. Conversely, in hyperthyroidism, basal and TRH-stimulated TSH levels are markedly suppressed; basal PRL levels are not low, but the PRL response to TRH is markedly blunted and returns to normal with correction of the hyperthyroidism. The feedback effects of

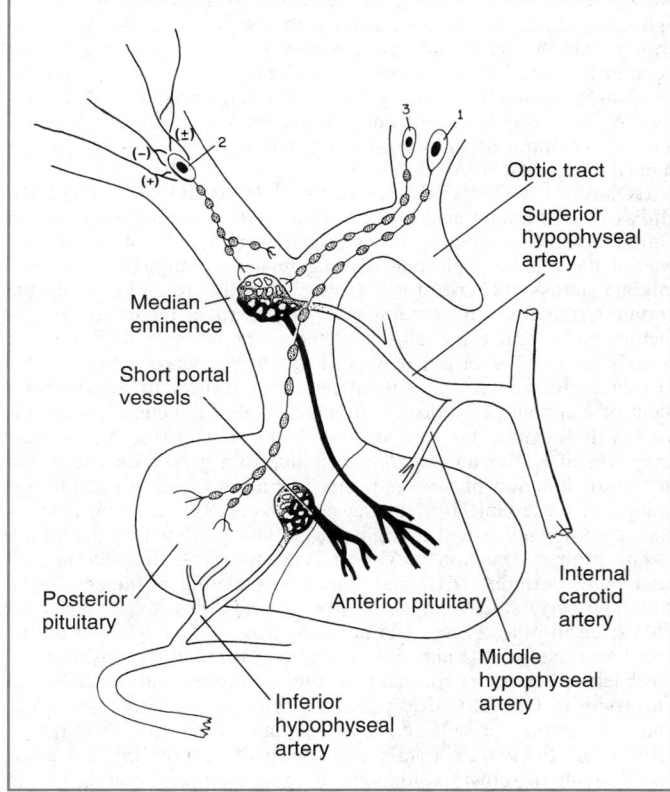

FIGURE 201–1. Neuroendocrine organization of the hypothalamus and pituitary gland. The posterior pituitary is fed by the inferior hypophyseal artery and the hypothalamus by the superior hypophyseal artery, both branches of the internal carotid artery. Most of the blood supply to the anterior pituitary is venous by way of the long portal vessels, which connect the portal capillary beds in the median eminence to the venous sinusoids in the anterior pituitary. Hypophysiotropic neurons (2) terminate in the median eminence on portal capillaries. These neurons of the tuberoinfundibular system secrete hypothalamic hormones into the portal veins for conveyance to the anterior pituitary gland. Multiple inputs to such neurons can be stimulatory, inhibitory, or neuromodulatory. Neuron 1 represents a peptidergic neuron originating in the magnocellular nuclei and projecting directly to the posterior pituitary by way of the hypothalamic-neurohypophyseal tract. Neuron 3 represents a vasopressinergic neuron projecting to the median eminence. (Modified from Lechan RM: Neuroendocrinology of pituitary hormone regulation. Endocrinol Metab Clinic North Am 16:475, 1987.)

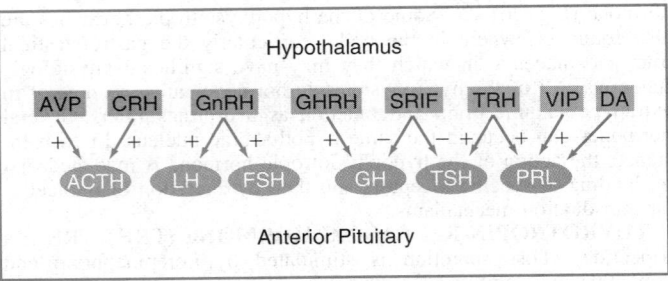

FIGURE 201–2. Interrelationships between hypothalamic and pituitary hormones. (+) indicates stimulatory effect and (−) indicates inhibitory effect. (See text for abbreviations.)

thyroid hormones, therefore, while occurring primarily at the pituitary, also occur at the hypothalamus.

Although TRH is the major regulator of TSH synthesis and secretion, the role of TRH as a physiologic PRL-releasing factor remains questionable. TRH can also stimulate growth hormone (GH) secretion in acromegaly, and in several states in which there is decreased insulin-like growth factor-1 (IGF-1) feedback on GH secretion, such as cirrhosis, renal insufficiency, anorexia nervosa, poorly controlled insulin-dependent diabetes mellitus, and malnutrition. Such responses are also seen in patients with depression and schizophrenia, which may be associated with disordered central bioaminergic regulation. TRH can also stimulate FSH secretion in some patients with gonadotroph adenomas but not in normal individuals. Obviously, somatotroph and gonadotroph cells must have TRH receptors, but "activation" of such receptors, which may involve alteration of intracellular transduction mechanisms, occurs only in special circumstances.

GONADOTROPIN-RELEASING HORMONE (GnRH). GnRH is a 10-amino acid peptide. Embryologic studies suggest that GnRH neurons originally develop in the epithelium of the medial part of the olfactory placode. During fetal development these cells migrate across the cribriform plate, enter the forebrain with the nervus terminalis and vomeronasal nerves, travel medial to the olfactory bulbs, and eventually enter the septal-preoptic region of the hypothalamus. The origin of GnRH-producing neurons from olfactory epithelium is of clinical interest with respect to the development of Kallmann's syndrome, in which GnRH deficiency is associated with anosmia due to agenesis of the olfactory bulbs. At least one form of Kallmann's syndrome is due to a gene defect resulting in loss of function of a protein that facilitates the embryologic migration of these GnRH-producing neurons. GnRH secretion is stimulated by dopamine and norepinephrine and inhibited by serotonin.

The primary function of GnRH is to stimulate the secretion of luteinizing hormone (LH) and follicle-stimulating hormone (FSH). Although early studies suggested the presence of separate LH- and FSH-releasing factors, there is only one identified GnRH and differential secretion of LH and FSH is due to variations in sensitivity of feedback effects of steroid and peptide hormones and variations in sensitivity to GnRH. GnRH pulsatile secretion also directly up-regulates its own receptors; i.e., it causes an increase in GnRH receptor number. In contrast, continuous administration of GnRH is associated with a down-regulation of gonadotropin synthesis and secretion due to decreased receptor numbers as well as postreceptor mechanisms.

In women, positive and negative steroid hormone feedback regulation of the hypothalamic-pituitary-gonadal axis occurs at both the pituitary and hypothalamic levels, the hypothalamic effects being the alteration of GnRH pulse amplitude and frequency and the pituitary effects being the modulation of the gonadotropin response to GnRH. In the follicular phase of the menstrual cycle estrogen feeds back negatively on gonadotropin secretion. At mid-cycle, estrogen feedback becomes positive and rising estrogen levels from the developing follicle stimulate the ovulatory surge of LH and FSH. Following ovulation, the feedback again becomes negative, and the estrogen and progesterone produced by the corpus luteum result in decreasing levels of LH and FSH. In the male, testosterone decreases GnRH pulsatile secretion with resultant decreased go-

nadotropin pulse amplitude and frequency as well as the gonadotropin response to exogenous GnRH.

The negative feedback effects of inhibin, a peptide produced by testicular Sertoli cells and ovarian granulosa cells, are predominantly on FSH at the pituitary. Inhibin causes a dose-related decrease in the sensitivity of gonadotrophs to GnRH, but there may also be a hypothalamic site of action. The related ovarian protein, activin, stimulates FSH synthesis and release from the pituitary. Another gonadal peptide, follistatin, also inhibits the oophorectomy- and GnRH-induced rises in FSH selectively, primarily by binding to activin. These ovarian peptides are also found in the pituitary and therefore may have additional local effects on gonadotropin secretion.

The hormone levels and feedback loops mentioned are primarily those of mature adults. In children, gonadotropin and gonadal steroid levels are very low. At puberty, negative feedback of steroid hormones decreases and gonadotropin and steroid levels gradually rise. During this pubertal development, in females the variation in negative and positive estrogen feedback develops, eventually resulting in the ovulatory menstrual cycle. At menopause, ovarian estrogen production ceases, gonadotropin levels rise markedly, and the symptoms associated with estrogen deficiency develop. In men, aging sometimes produces a decrease in testosterone production with a modest rise in gonadotropins, but there is no clinical syndrome similar to menopause.

GnRH has been successfully administered in a pulsatile manner to individuals with hypogonadotropic hypogonadism due to GnRH deficiency, resulting in restoration of normal sexual function and fertility. Long-acting GnRH agonists have been used to down-regulate GnRH receptors and gonadotropin secretion in a variety of conditions, including precocious puberty, prostate cancer, breast cancer, uterine fibroids, and endometriosis. Direct GnRH antagonists that competitively compete for the GnRH receptor are being explored for similar conditions.

SOMATOSTATIN. Somatostatin (also known as somatotropin release-inhibiting factor [SRIF]) is a tetradecapeptide; a 28-amino acid precursor also has GH inhibitory properties. Somatostatin blocks the rise in GH that occurs with all stimuli in a dose-dependent manner. The interaction of somatostatin and growth hormone–releasing hormone (GHRH) on GH secretion is complex. GH secretory episodes are associated with increased GHRH secretion often accompanied by low somatostatin levels; the basal or trough GH levels are associated with low GHRH levels and more elevated somatostatin levels. Somatostatin also inhibits basal and stimulated TSH secretion. However, dose-response studies in humans using somatostatin infusions have shown that GH is about 10-fold more sensitive to inhibition by somatostatin than is TSH. This suggests that the physiologic role of somatostatin in inhibiting TSH secretion is limited.

Somatostatin is also present in the D cells of the pancreatic islets and the gut mucosa as well as the myenteric neural plexus. Via paracrine and endocrine actions it suppresses the secretion of insulin, glucagon, cholecystokinin, gastrin, secretin, vasoactive intestinal polypeptide (VIP), and other gastrointestinal hormones, as well as such functions as gastric acid secretion, gastric emptying, gallbladder contraction, and splanchnic blood flow. Recently, analogues of somatostatin have been found to be effective in the treatment of acromegaly, carcinoid tumors, VIP-secreting tumors, TSH-secreting pituitary tumors, islet-cell tumors, and diarrhea of a number of causes.

CORTICOTROPIN-RELEASING HORMONE (CRH). CRH releases ACTH, β-endorphin, β-lipotropin, melanocyte-stimulating hormone (MSH), and other peptides generated from pro-opiomelanocortin (POMC) in equimolar amounts. CRH mediates 75% of the ACTH response to stress, and the remaining 25% is due to vasopressin. CRH and vasopressin have synergistic effects on ACTH release. In fact, CRH and vasopressin coexist in about half of the CRH-containing paraventricular neurons and even in the same neurosecretory granules. CRH and vasopressin are not always released coordinately, however, and stress has been shown to selectively activate the vasopressin-containing subset of CRH neurons.

Cortisol feeds back to decrease ACTH secretion at both the hypothalamic and pituitary levels. ACTH and β-endorphin also feed back negatively to decrease CRH release by the hypothalamus. Morphine suppresses the ACTH response to CRH in humans, acting presumably through opioid μ receptors. Central bioamines and peptides also influence CRH secretion. Acetylcholine, dopamine, norepinephrine, and epinephrine stimulate and GABA inhibits hypothalamic CRH secretion. Norepinephrine and epinephrine also stimulate pituitary ACTH secretion directly and are additive to the stimulatory effect of CRH.

Monokines released by inflammatory tissue, such as interleukin-1 and tumor necrosis factor-α stimulate the synthesis and release of CRH and vasopressin from the hypothalamus and the release of ACTH by the pituitary. The consequent increase of cortisol then reduces the intensity of the inflammatory response and release of these monokines, completing the feedback loop. Thus, this neuroendocrine-immune loop serves to modulate the inflammatory response.

Both ovine and human CRH have been given to humans in a variety of experimental paradigms, although CRH has not yet been approved by the U.S. Food and Drug Administration for commercial use. These preparations have been found to be of some use in stimulating ACTH secretion during petrosal sinus sampling in the differential diagnosis of Cushing's disease versus ectopic ACTH syndrome.

GROWTH HORMONE–RELEASING HORMONE (GHRH). GHRH dose-dependently stimulates GH secretion, and in some individuals GHRH is capable of eliciting a small increase in PRL as well. With repetitive administration every 3 hours, GHRH can cause the release of sufficient GH in children with GHRH deficiency to result in an increase in IGF-I levels and an acceleration of growth. Both IGF-I and GH itself feed back negatively on GH secretion, mediated by both a decrease in GHRH and an increase in somatostatin. This feedback effect of IGF-I is clinically relevant, as documented by the high circulating GH levels that occur in IGF-I–deficient states, such as renal insufficiency and cirrhosis. In children with mutations of the GH receptor resulting in their not being responsive to GH (GH insensitivity syndrome, also known as Laron-type dwarfism), IGF-I levels are very low and GH levels are correspondingly elevated. α_2-Adrenergic receptors and serotonin activate GHRH and GH secretion, but γ-aminobutyric acid (GABA) is inhibitory to GHRH secretion.

PROLACTIN-INHIBITORY FACTOR (PIF). The inhibitory component of hypothalamic regulation of PRL secretion predominates over the stimulatory component. Dopamine (DA) is the predominant, physiologic PIF, and the concentration of DA found in the pituitary stalk plasma is sufficient to decrease PRL levels. It is likely that in most physiologic circumstances that cause a PRL rise, such as lactation, there is a simultaneous fall in DA along with a rise in a PRL-releasing factor (PRF), such as vasoactive intestinal peptide (VIP). Blockade of endogenous DA receptors by a variety of drugs, such as the neuroleptics, causes a rise in PRL. Lesions that interrupt the basal hypothalamic neuronal pathways carrying dopamine to the median eminence or that interrupt portal blood flow result in decreased dopamine reaching the pituitary and hyperprolactinemia.

PROLACTIN-RELEASING FACTOR (PRF). A number of hypothalamic peptides other than TRH have also been shown to have PRF activity. VIP stimulates PRL synthesis and release at concentrations found in hypothalamic-pituitary portal blood. Within the VIP precursor is another similarly sized peptide known as peptide histidine methionine (PHM), which also has PRF activity. Complicating the role of VIP as a PRF is the finding that VIP is also synthesized by anterior pituitary tissue. The precise roles of VIP versus PHM and hypothalamic VIP versus pituitary VIP still are not clear.

ENDOGENOUS OPIOID PEPTIDES. The endogenous opioid peptides have only a minor role in neuroendocrine regulation. There are three major opioid peptide receptors and three major groups of opioid peptides, but the correspondence is not one for one. The μ receptor mediates most of the endocrine effects and analgesia; morphine is its prototypic agonist and naloxone is its prototypic antagonist; the primary peptide ligand for the μ receptor is β-endorphin. The δ receptor mediates behavioral, analgesic, and some endocrine effects and has as its primary peptide ligands met- and leu-enkephalins, which are derived from proenkephalin A. The κ receptor mediates sedation and ataxia and binds primarily dynorphin and the neoendorphins, which are derived from proenkephalin B (prodynorphin). All neuronal perikarya containing POMC-derived peptides are located in the arcuate nucleus, from which β-endorphin- and α-MSH–containing fibers project to the median eminence,

other parts of the hypothalamus, and other areas of the brain. Anterior pituitary β-endorphin is secreted with ACTH with CRH and vasopressin stimulation.

Various opioid peptides are linked to a number of bodily functions, including stress, mental illness, narcotic tolerance and dependence, eating, drinking, gastrointestinal function, learning, memory, reward, cardiovascular responses, respiration, thermoregulation, seizures, brain electrical activity, locomotor activity, pregnancy, and neuroimmune activity. The anterior pituitary itself is poor in opioid receptors, but the hypothalamus is quite rich. It has been suggested that the effects of opioid peptides on anterior pituitary hormone secretion occur via modulation of hypothalamic bioamines and hypophysiotropic factors. In general, endogenous opioids have an inhibitory influence on gonadotropin secretion through action on GnRH secretion, probably by inhibition of noradrenergic neuronal input. Opioids feed back negatively on ACTH and β-endorphin secretion and naloxone can increase basal and stimulated ACTH levels. Endogenous opioids have minimal effects on GH, PRL, and TSH secretion.

CNS RHYTHMS AND NEUROENDOCRINE FUNCTION

Pituitary hormones are secreted in a pulsatile fashion with a number of rhythms superimposed. The pulse amplitude of a pituitary hormone reflects the amount of releasing hormone as well as factors that may alter sensitivity to that releasing hormone. Thus, the amplitude can be altered by inhibitory factors (e.g., GHRH versus somatostatin), nutritional factors, feedback effects of target organ hormones, and prior stimulation that depletes a readily releasable pool of hormone. The frequency is generally governed by the frequency of release of the hypophysiotropic factor, regulated by the hypothalamic pulse generator system.

The pituitary has an intrinsic rhythm of small amplitude with a frequency of every 2 to 10 minutes. Superimposed upon this intrinsic rhythm is that from the pulsatile release of hypophysiotropic releasing factors, with or without the withdrawal of a corresponding inhibitory factor. Rhythms that are shorter than a day are referred to as *ultradian* rhythms. The next layer of rhythmicity is the *circadian* rhythm, i.e., rhythms with approximately 24-hour periodicity. These rhythms are usually synchronized with the 24-hour period by a periodic environmental cue, such as the dark-light cycle. The suprachiasmatic nucleus functions as a circadian pacemaker and receives light-induced electrical impulses from the retina via the retinohypothalamic tract, finally transmitting those impulses to the pineal, where they are converted to hormonal signals. Signals for a rhythm with a periodicity longer than 24 hours, i.e., an *infradian* rhythm, include the gravitational influence of the moon, giving rise to the menstrual cycle.

A number of factors may influence circadian and infradian rhythms. One of the most important is the sleep-wake cycle. GH, TSH, PRL, ACTH, and pubertal LH secretion are all entrained more to the sleep-wake cycle than the dark-light cycle. Each has an increase and maximal level that occur following sleep onset. The profound diurnal variation of cortisol and ACTH is often used as an index of "normality" of the system. Loss of this diurnal rhythm occurs with disordered regulation by CRH, which may be due to endogenous depression or excessive alcohol intake, as well as autonomous secretion of ACTH in Cushing's disease. Loss of diurnal rhythm of cortisol has been used as a diagnostic test for Cushing's syndrome.

Interesting changes occur in gonadotropin secretion as the child passes through puberty into adulthood. Early in puberty the amplitude of pulses increases during sleep at night, especially for LH, but in adulthood this nocturnal rise is lost. In patients with anorexia nervosa, the pattern of gonadotropin secretion often reverts to this pubertal pattern, only to lose this pattern again with weight gain. This suggests that body composition may in some way affect the regulation of the pulsatile secretion of the gonadotropins. In fact, the percentage of body composition that is fat has been proposed as being important in the timing of the onset of puberty.

Endocrine rhythms appear to reflect a rather primitive organizing influence that helps the animal to adapt to the environment. The circadian synchronization with the light-dark cycle and sleep and the infradian synchronization with seasonal changes are present very early phylogenetically. However, because humans are able to alter the light-dark cycles, they are less tied to environmental changes. This has led to new, modern problems with these rhythms such as jet-lag, which involves the rapid resynchronization of the rhythms with several hour time-zone displacements. Because not all rhythms resynchronize at the same rates, some of the disorientation and other symptoms associated with jet-lag may be due to abnormal phase relationships of various body rhythms to each other and to the dark-light cycle.

Frohman LA, Downs TR, Chomczynski P: Regulation of growth hormone secretion. Front Neuroendocrinol 14:344, 1992. *A thorough, molecularly oriented review of the regulation of GH secretion.*

Lechan RM: Neuroendocrinology of pituitary hormone regulation. Endocrinol Metab Clinic North Am 16:475, 1987. *An excellent discussion of the anatomic features of neuroendocrine regulation. MRI scans and accompanying diagrams clarify hypothalamic structural anatomy.*

Orth DN: Corticotropin-releasing hormone in humans. Endocr Rev 13:164, 1992. *A thorough review of CRH: its tissue distribution, blood levels, responses to its administration in normals and patients, its diagnostic use, and its secretion ectopically.*

Reichlin S: Neuroendocrine-immune interactions. N Engl J Med 329:1246, 1993. *A critical review of the various interactions between the endocrine and the immune systems, including possible psychological influences. It asks more questions than it answers in this exciting new field.*

Schwanzel-Fukuda M, Jorgenson KL, Bergen HT, et al.: Biology of normal luteinizing hormone–releasing hormone neurons during and after their migration from olfactory placode. Endocrine Rev 13:623, 1992. *Reviews the fascinating unfolding story regarding the migration of GnRH neurons from the olfactory placode to the hypothalamus. Defects in this migration result in Kallmann's syndrome.*

Van Cauter E: Diurnal and ultradian rhythms in human endocrine function: A mini-review. Horm Res 34:45, 1990. *Reviews the physiology and clinical relevance of the rhythms characterizing hormone secretion.*

NEUROENDOCRINE DISEASE

DISEASES OF THE HYPOTHALAMUS. Diseases may affect the hypothalamus by being localized to the hypothalamus, by being part of more generalized central nervous system (CNS) disease, such as neurosarcoidosis, or by indirect means, such as by causing hydrocephalus (Table 201–1). Furthermore, hormonal changes may occur in a variety of psychiatric disorders, mediated by functional alterations in hypothalamic regulation.

The axons projecting to the median eminence that contain the various hypophysiotropic factors are concentrated in the basal portion of the hypothalamus. Thus, lesions located within this final common pathway might be expected to cause significant decreases in the secretion for some or all of the pituitary hormones except PRL, which may increase because of the elimination of the tonic inhibition by dopamine. Diabetes insipidus may also occur. Other functions of the hypothalamus are more diffusely located, such as the regulation of temperature, food intake, and blood pressure.

Symptoms due to hypothalamic dysfunction are related to size of the lesion and consequently to the area of the hypothalamus involved, as well as to the rapidity of increase in lesion size. Slowly growing lesions tend to cause problems of hormone dysregulation rather than dramatic symptoms. Large, slowly growing lesions can cause more acute problems, however, when a slight increment in growth eliminates remaining vestiges of vasopressin or ACTH secretion or completely occludes the aqueduct of Sylvius, causing hydrocephalus.

The best way of discerning lesions affecting the hypothalamus is by magnetic resonance imaging (MRI) with gadolinium enhancement, although computed tomographic (CT) scanning with intravenous contrast is also quite good. Formal visual field testing may discern impingement of the optic nerves and chiasm by hypothalamic lesions, including the suprasellar extension of pituitary tumors. Detailed testing of hypothalamic-pituitary function may reveal evidence of functional hypothalamic disruption with great sensitivity.

Congenital Embryopathic Disorders. The most common embryopathic disorders to affect the hypothalamus are the midline cleft syndromes, which cause varying degrees of defects of midline structures, especially the optic and olfactory tracts, the septum pellucidum, the corpus callosum, the anterior commissure, the hypothalamus, and the pituitary. The clinical presentation of patients with midline cleft defects varies in severity from cyclopia to cleft lip and from isolated hypothalamic hormone defects to panhypopituitarism. The combination of absent septum pellucidum associated with optic nerve hypoplasia is referred to as *septo-optic dysplasia* and is associated with abnormalities of hypothalamic and other di-

TABLE 201–1. ETIOLOGY OF HYPOTHALAMIC DISEASE

Neonates

Intraventricular hemorrhage
Meningitis: bacterial
Tumors: glioma, hemangioma
Trauma
Hydrocephalus, hydranencephaly, kernicterus

1 Month–2 Years

Tumors: glioma, especially optic glioma, histiocytosis X, hemangiomas
Hydrocephalus, meningitis
"Familial" disorders: Laurence-Moon-Bardet-Biedl, Prader-Labhart-Willi

2–10 Years

Tumors: craniopharyngioma, glioma, dysgerminoma, hamartoma, histiocytosis X, leukemia, ganglioneuroma, ependymoma, medulloblastoma
Meningitis: bacterial, tuberculous
Encephalitis: viral and demyelinating, various viral encephalitides and exanthematous demyelinating encephalitides, disseminated encephalomyelitis
"Familial" disorders: diabetes insipidus, etc.
Damage from nasopharyngeal radiation therapy

10–25 Years

Tumors: craniopharyngioma, pituitary tumors, glioma, hamartoma, dysgerminoma, histiocytosis X, leukemia, dermoid, lipoma, neuroblastoma
Trauma
Subarachnoid hemorrhage, vascular aneurysm, arteriovenous malformation
Inflammatory diseases: meningitis, encephalitis, sarcoidosis, tuberculosis
Disease associated with midline brain defects: agenesis of corpus callosum
Chronic hydrocephalus or increased intracranial pressure

25–50 Years

Nutritional: Wernicke's disease
Tumors: glioma, lymphoma, meningioma, craniopharyngioma, pituitary tumors, angioma, plasmacytoma, colloid cysts, ependymoma, sarcoma, histiocytosis X
Inflammatory: sarcoidosis, tuberculosis, viral encephalitis
Subarachnoid hemorrhage, vascular aneurysms, arteriovenous malformation
Damage from pituitary radiation therapy

50 Years and Older

Nutritional: Wernicke's disease
Tumors: sarcoma, glioblastoma, lymphoma, meningioma, colloid cysts, ependymoma, pituitary tumors
Vascular: infarct, subarachnoid hemorrhage, pituitary apoplexy
Infectious: encephalitis, sarcoidosis, meningitis

Adapted from Plum F, Van Uitert R: Non-endocrine diseases of the hypothalamus. *In* Reichlin S, Baldessarini RJ, Martin JB (eds.): The Hypothalamus. New York, Raven Press, 1978, p 415.

encephalic structures. Some patients with septo-optic dysplasia and hypothalamic hypopituitarism have sexual precocity, presumably due to lack of inhibitory influences from other parts of the hypothalamus and intact GnRH-producing structures. Children with very mild midline cleft defects consisting of cleft lip or palate or both have been found to have a markedly increased risk of having GH and other pituitary hormone deficiencies. A recent evaluation with MR scanning of patients with "idiopathic" GH deficiency showed absence of the infundibulum in 43%.

Kallmann's syndrome is an autosomal dominant condition characterized by anosmia or hyposmia and hypogonadotropic hypogonadism. It is due to a gene defect resulting in loss of function of a protein that facilitates the embryologic migration of GnRH-producing neurons. The pituitary is usually intact, and treatment with pulsatile GnRH therapy or gonadotropins results in spermatogenesis and normal gonadal function. In some patients, other neurologic abnormalities may be present, including cerebellar ataxia, nerve deafness, color blindness, cleft lip and palate, mental retardation, and disordered thirst.

Tumors. The most common tumors affecting the hypothalamus are *pituitary adenomas* that have significant suprasellar extension. These tumors can cause varying degrees of hypopituitarism, diabetes insipidus, and hyperprolactinemia by either compressing the normal pituitary or, more commonly, affecting the pituitary stalk and mediobasal hypothalamus. Evidence that hypopituitarism is from pituitary compression includes a low serum PRL level and a lack of TSH response to TRH; pituitary function in such cases usually does not improve after treatment. In patients with normal or elevated PRL levels, pituitary function often returns following therapy.

Craniopharyngiomas are the next most common tumors affecting the hypothalamus. Microscopically, craniopharyngiomas consist of cysts alternating with stratified squamous epithelium. The cyst fluid is usually thick and dark and the material is often calcified. They arise from remnants of Rathke's pouch. A closely related, less common lesion is *Rathke's cleft cyst,* which develops from the space between the anterior and rudimentary intermediate lobes. Rathke's cleft cysts are lined with cuboidal as opposed to squamous epithelium, and the cyst fluid is usually white and mucoid. Craniopharyngiomas sometimes recur postoperatively whereas Rathke's cleft cysts rarely recur. Craniopharyngiomas most commonly present during childhood, but they also may occur in adults and even the elderly. These tumors present because of mass effects, including headache, vomiting, visual disturbance, seizures, hypopituitarism, and polyuria. Some patients present with galactorrhea, amenorrhea, and hyperprolactinemia, suggestive of a prolactinoma. Careful endocrine testing reveals varying degrees of hypopituitarism in 50 to 75% and modest hyperprolactinemia in 25 to 50%. Surgical extirpation of craniopharyngiomas commonly causes a worsening of pituitary function, often resulting in complete panhypopituitarism and diabetes insipidus because of stalk section. Irradiation may also be helpful, especially in children.

Suprasellar dysgerminomas arise from primitive germ cells that have migrated to the CNS during fetal life and structurally are identical to germ cell tumors of the gonads. They most commonly occur in children, where they cause decreased growth because of hypopituitarism, diabetes insipidus, and visual problems. Hyperprolactinemia occurs in >50%, and 10% have precocious puberty due to the production of chorionic gonadotropin by the tumor. As opposed to craniopharyngiomas, these tumors are very radiosensitive, and radiation therapy is the preferred treatment.

A hypothalamic *hamartoma* is a nodule of growth of hypothalamic neurons attached by a pedicle to the hypothalamus between the tuber cinereum and the mammillary bodies and extending into the basal cistern. Asymptomatic hamartomas may be present in up to 20% of random autopsies; rarely, these lesions may enlarge, causing disruption of hypothalamic function because of compression of adjacent tissue. A variant of the hamartoma consisting of similar tissue within the anterior pituitary but without a neural attachment to the hypothalamus is called a choristoma or gangliocytoma. These neuronal tumors are of particular endocrine interest because they can produce hypophysiotropic hormones. A number of cases associated with precocious puberty have been reported in which the hamartomas produce GnRH. Successful treatment has been reported with surgery and with the administration of a long-acting GnRH analogue, which suppresses gonadotropin secretion but does not affect the tumor itself. Medical therapy with the GnRH analogue may be the best choice, as surgery can be noncurative or even fatal, if the hamartoma does not cause other problems from mass effects. Some gangliocytomas have been reported which produce GHRH and acromegaly and CRH and Cushing's syndrome.

Other tumors and space-occupying lesions occurring in the suprasellar area include arachnoid cysts, meningiomas, gliomas, astrocytomas, chordomas, infundibulomas, cholesteatomas, neurofibromas, lipomas, and metastatic cancer (particularly breast and lung). Any such lesion may present with varying degrees of hypopituitarism, diabetes insipidus, and hyperprolactinemia, and surgical therapy often worsens the hormonal deficit.

Inflammatory Disorders. CNS involvement in *sarcoidosis* occurs in 1 to 5% of patients, as determined on clinical grounds, and in up to 16% of cases at autopsy. Isolated CNS sarcoidosis is quite uncommon, however. When sarcoidosis does involve the CNS, the hypothalamus is involved in 10 to 20%. Sarcoid granulomas can involve the hypothalamic stalk or pituitary and may be infiltrative or present as a mass lesion. The most common endocrine findings are varying degrees of hypopituitarism, diabetes insipidus, and hyperprolactinemia. Obesity due to hypothalamic involvement by sarcoidosis has also been reported. In patients with isolated CNS sarcoidosis, the diagnosis may be extremely difficult. Examination of the CSF usually shows elevated protein levels, low glucose levels, a pleocytosis, and variable elevations of angiotensin-converting enzyme. However, biopsy is often necessary. Although corticosteroid therapy has been reported to at least partially reverse the thirst dis-

orders, anterior pituitary hormone deficits usually do not respond. *Langerhans cell histiocytosis* or eosinophilic granulomatous infiltration of the hypothalamus may cause diabetes insipidus, varying degrees of hypopituitarism, and hyperprolactinemia. It is the most common cause of diabetes insipidus in children. Usually this infiltration appears as a thickening of the pituitary stalk, but it may also appear as a mass lesion of the hypothalamus or the pituitary. Osteolytic lesions may be present in the jaw or mastoid and radiographs of the jaw are a worthwhile part of the diagnostic evaluation of an unknown suprasellar mass or diabetes insipidus for this reason. Therapy consists of local surgery, focal irradiation, or chemotherapy with alkylating agents and high-dose corticosteroids.

Vascular Disease. An enlarging aneurysm may present as a mass lesion of the hypothalamic-pituitary area and may cause hypopituitarism and visual field defects. Obviously, the distinction must be made before surgery. Tumors and aneurysms may also coexist, and careful radiologic evaluation with MRI is necessary to discern this. Hypothalamic disease due to vascular infarction is extremely rare.

Trauma. Head trauma can cause defects ranging from isolated ACTH deficiency to panhypopituitarism with diabetes insipidus. Within the first 72 hours of trauma, GH, LH, ACTH, TSH, and PRL levels may actually be elevated in blood, perhaps due to acute release. These levels subsequently fall, and patients either return to normal or develop hypopituitarism. In patients dying of head injury, anterior pituitary infarction has been found in 16% of cases, posterior pituitary hemorrhages in 34%, and hypothalamic hemorrhages or infarction in 42% of cases. The paraventricular and supraoptic nuclei and median eminence are particularly involved with microhemorrhages, resulting in the high frequency of panhypopituitarism with diabetes insipidus. With frontal injuries, the brain travels backward but the pituitary cannot move, resulting in the pituitary stalk becoming avulsed, with interruption of the portal vessels. Most patients with head injury are hyperprolactinemic, confirming clinically that the hypothalamus and/or stalk is the primary site of injury.

Irradiation. Whole brain irradiation for intracranial neoplasms frequently results in hypothalamic dysfunction, as evidenced by endocrine abnormalities and behavioral changes. The most common endocrine abnormality is hyperprolactinemia, but hypopituitarism can also occur. When the radiation therapy is targeted to the hypothalamic area, as in patients with tumors in that area or nasopharyngeal carcinomas, hypopituitarism occurs even more frequently. The frequencies of loss of pituitary function are so high that all patients who have had their pituitary and hypothalamic areas irradiated must be followed closely to detect these deficits when they occur.

EFFECTS OF HYPOTHALAMIC DISEASE ON PITUITARY FUNCTION. Hypothalamic disease can cause both pituitary hyperfunction and hypofunction in varying degrees of severity. Although severe disease can cause absolute deficiencies of the various hormones, milder disease may cause a subtle alteration of feedback loops and timing such that, for example, the integration of signals necessary for menstrual cycling is lost, resulting in "hypothalamic" amenorrhea. Furthermore, the hypothalamic defects may be interrelated, so that the rather common finding of hyperprolactinemia occurring with hypothalamic dysfunction causes a hypogonadotropic hypogonadism that is reversible when the elevated PRL levels are brought down to normal. In many cases no structural lesion can be found on MRI, and a functional defect due to altered neurotransmitter regulation is invoked.

Growth Hormone. Loss of normal GH secretion is the most common hormonal defect occurring with structural hypothalamic disease. Congenital idiopathic GH deficiency (IGHD) is a heterogeneous disorder consisting of hypothalamic and pituitary defects. The diagnosis is usually made between 1 and 3 years of age because of impaired growth. Between 5 and 30% of IGHD subjects have an affected relative, and thus their defect is thought to have a genetic basis; some have been associated with a deletion of the GH gene. In about three-quarters of cases there is a normal GH response to exogenous GHRH, suggesting that the defect is likely disordered hypothalamic regulation. Children with IGHD should be treated with biosynthetic GH, although experimental studies suggest that GHRH treatment is also often successful. Other hormonal defects that may be present also must be treated simultaneously, although therapy with gonadal steroids should be delayed to prevent epiphyseal closure before the final desired height is achieved. A reversible form of IGHD due to inadequate parental care and affection is referred to as the *emotional deprivation syndrome* or *psychosocial dwarfism*. Restoration of a proper social environment for such a child results in prompt normalization of GH secretion and growth. It has been hypothesized that the disordered GH regulation is due to a psychogenic alteration of the neurotransmitter balance necessary for normal GHRH and somatostatin secretion.

Gonadotropins. Hypothalamic Hypogonadism. The primary defect in this group of disorders involves secretion of GnRH, with resultant impairment in pituitary gonadotropin secretion and gonadal function. The disorders causing these conditions may be primary, i.e., congenital defects, or acquired. Depending upon the time of onset, they present either as delayed puberty, interruption of pubertal progression, or loss of adult gonadal function. The lesions causing these disorders may cause loss of other hormones or may be isolated to GnRH. Loss of gonadotropin secretion as the result of hypothalamic structural damage is the second most common defect after GH deficiency. However, a substantial portion of these defects is due to hyperprolactinemia and is reversible with correction of the hyperprolactinemia.

Lesions presenting prepubertally result in the failure of onset of puberty or incomplete progression of puberty if the defect is partial. If the disorder is limited to GnRH and the gonadotropins, prior growth and development are normal. However, the growth spurt occurring at puberty is lost. The most common congenital lesion causing prepubertal GnRH deficiency is Kallmann's syndrome, comprising 50% of males and 37% of females presenting with isolated gonadotropin deficiency. In patients with idiopathic GnRH deficiency, the GnRH gene appears to be normal. However, indirect measures of functional GnRH secretion show that there may be disorders of pulse amplitude and/or frequency. When hyperprolactinemia occurs before puberty, it can prevent the onset of puberty and must always be looked for in this setting.

The ideal therapy for patients with GnRH deficiency is the replacement of GnRH via subcutaneous administration every 2 hours using a portable pump. This causes a rapid rise in the LH and FSH responses to the GnRH and a rise in testosterone to normal, as well as development of normal spermatogenesis. Similar studies in women result in ovulatory cycles in 80%. In men, comparable results can be obtained with exogenous gonadotropins given three times per week. Replacement with testosterone alone causes adequate androgenization but does not result in an increase in testicular size or in spermatogenesis.

Loss of formerly normal GnRH secretion in adults may be due to structural hypothalamic damage such as a tumor, a functional change unassociated with a detectable lesion, or hyperprolactinemia. Structural disease must be excluded in such patients by CT or MR scanning. Most but not all functional hypogonadotropic hypogonadism occurs in women, the most common causes being weight loss, excessive exercise, or psychogenic stress. In some the exercise results in a loss of body fat not detected with total body weight measures and it is unclear whether the hypogonadism is directly due to the loss of body fat or to the exercise *per se*. Studies of pulsatile gonadotropin secretion in such patients reveal absent pulses. Usually there is a normal gonadotropin response to injected GnRH. Regain of weight and stopping of the exercise result in resumption of normal gonadal function. Hyperprolactinemia occurring postpubertally can also decrease GnRH and the pulsatile secretion of LH and FSH, resulting in anovulation with oligo/amenorrhea in women and impotence and infertility in men.

Therapy should be directed at the underlying process, if possible. Efforts at weight gain and restricting exercise should be made when appropriate. In idiopathic, functional hypogonadotropic amenorrhea there are two goals: (1) restoration of a normal estrogen status to promote well-being and to prevent osteoporosis and (2) facilitation of ovulation for fertility. The former can generally be achieved with cyclic estrogen and progesterone, whereas the latter may require clomiphene, GnRH, or gonadotropin therapy.

Hypothalamic Hypergonadism (Precocious Puberty). Precocious puberty is defined as the onset of puberty before the ages of 8 in girls and 9 in boys. "Pseudo"-precocious puberty is that due to peripheral (gonadal or adrenal) causes. Central, "true," or GnRH-dependent precocious puberty is characterized by hormonal changes

similar to those that occur at the time of normal puberty, i.e., an increase in the pulsatile release of LH, an increase in the gonadotropin response to GnRH, and an increase in gonadal steroid secretion. GnRH-dependent precocious puberty therefore represents a premature activation of this GnRH pulse generator by a variety of lesions, or it may also be idiopathic. Less than one-quarter of cases of central precocious puberty occur in boys, but they tend to have more serious underlying disease. In boys with central, GnRH-dependent precocious puberty, hypothalamic hamartomas account for 38% of cases, other CNS lesions represent 31%, familial disease accounts for 23%, and idiopathic disease accounts for only 8%. The picture is quite different in girls, however, as hypothalamic hamartomas account for only 15% of cases, other CNS lesions represent 14%, the McCune-Albright syndrome (polyostotic fibrous dysplasia) accounts for 6%, and fully 65% are idiopathic. Dysgerminomas in the suprasellar or pineal region can produce hCG, which acts like LH in its stimulation of gonadal function. Usually such tumors cause increased sex steroid formation but fail to cause ovulation.

Therapy of central GnRH-dependent precocious puberty consists of surgical removal of the tumor or medical therapy with a long-acting GnRH analogue. The latter can suppress gonadotropin and sex steroid hormone levels and cause a stabilization or even regression of secondary sex characteristics and a slowing of growth and bone maturation in most cases. When therapy is discontinued at the normal time of puberty, sex steroid levels increase, secondary sexual characteristics again develop, growth increases, and regular menses develop spontaneously. For those patients who do not respond to the GnRH analogues, treatment with medroxyprogesterone acetate or testolactone, an aromatase inhibitor, is indicated.

Prolactin. Hypothalamic Hyperprolactinemia. Structural or infiltrative lesions of the hypothalamus, such as those discussed above, can decrease the amount of dopamine reaching the lactotrophs, causing modest hyperprolactinemia. PRL elevations due to such lesions rarely exceed 150 ng per milliliter and usually are less than 100 ng per milliliter. Similar elevations are also seen in patients with an empty sella. Because their therapy is quite different, it is very important to differentiate nonsecreting pituitary adenomas with extensive suprasellar extension causing PRL elevations in this range from PRL-secreting adenomas which, when of such a large size, usually cause PRL elevations 5 to 50 times higher. A number of medications can cause hyperprolactinemia, primarily by interfering with central catecholamines, dopamine in particular (Table 201–2).

Therapy is generally directed at the underlying cause. The hyperprolactinemia itself may impair gonadal function so that efforts may also be made to lower PRL levels with bromocriptine or other dopamine agonists. PRL levels usually fall quite readily in such pa-

TABLE 201–2. CAUSES OF HYPERPROLACTINEMIA

Pituitary Disease	Neurogenic	Medications
Prolactinomas	Chest wall lesions	Phenothiazines
Acromegaly	Spinal cord lesions	Haloperidol
"Empty sella syndrome"	Breast stimulation	Monoamine-oxidase inhibitors
Lymphocytic hypophysitis		Tricyclic antidepressants
Cushing's disease		Reserpine
Pituitary stalk section		Methyldopa
		Metoclopramide
		Amoxepin
		Cocaine
		Verapamil

Hypothalamic Disease	Other
Craniopharyngiomas	Pregnancy
Meningiomas	Hypothyroidism
Dysgerminomas	Chronic renal failure
Nonsecreting pituitary adenomas	Cirrhosis
Other tumors	Pseudocyesis
Sarcoidosis	Adrenal insufficiency
Eosinophilic granuloma	Idiopathic
Neuraxis irradiation	
Vascular	

Modified from Molitch ME: Management of prolactinomas. Annu Rev Med 40:225, 1989.

tients. Restoration of gonadal function is not automatic, however, as the primary hypothalamic lesion may also directly impair release of GnRH. In that circumstance both bromocriptine and sex steroid replacement may be necessary. When psychotropic medications that cause the hyperprolactinemia cannot be stopped, dopamine agonists may be used but may exacerbate the psychosis. In such cases and others in which fertility is not an issue, treatment with cyclic estrogen/progestin replacement can be carried out safely.

Idiopathic Hyperprolactinemia. Idiopathic hyperprolactinemia is a diagnosis of exclusion. PRL levels in this condition are usually < 100 ng per milliliter. In such cases, small pituitary or hypothalamic tumors could exist that are beyond the resolution of current imaging techniques, but when such patients are followed for many years, it is very uncommon for tumors to later be visualized. Idiopathic hyperprolactinemia can cause amenorrhea, galactorrhea, impotence, infertility, and loss of libido, just as occurs with hyperprolactinemia of other causes, and therefore may need to be treated. Premature osteoporosis related to the estrogen deficiency may also occur. The only possible treatment is bromocriptine or another dopamine agonist, and these are successful in >90% of cases. Alternatively, cyclic estrogen/progesterone replacement may be given, but fertility will not be restored.

TSH. *Hypothalamic hypothyroidism,* also referred to as tertiary hypothyroidism, is due to a central lesion that impairs the secretion of TRH, usually along with loss of other hormones. It occurs considerably less commonly than hypothalamic GH and gonadotropin deficiency. TSH levels in this syndrome generally are normal or even slightly elevated, and the response to TRH is delayed, peaking at 60 to 120 minutes rather than at 20 to 30 minutes. TSH in these patients is biologically less active than normal and binds to the TSH receptor less well owing to altered glycosylation as a result of the TRH deficiency. Treatment is with L-thyroxine.

ACTH. *Hypothalamic ACTH deficiency* due to hypothalamic lesions is uncommon. It may occur with loss of other hormones but may also appear as an isolated deficiency. In the absence of CNS lesions or a history of trauma, most cases of isolated ACTH deficiency appear to be a pituitary autoimmune disorder. However, in patients with hypothalamic disease as the cause, basal ACTH levels are low and the ACTH response to injected CRH may be prolonged and exaggerated, much as is the TSH response to TRH. The best test remains the comparison of the ACTH responses to hypoglycemia, which is clearly mediated by the hypothalamus, and to CRH. The ACTH response is low in response to hypoglycemia but increased and delayed in response to CRH in most patients with hypothalamic CRH deficiency. Treatment is with glucocorticoids, and mineralocorticoids are not needed.

Vasopressin (see Ch. 75). Diabetes insipidus can develop as a result of destructive lesions in the supraoptic and paraventricular nuclei or in the mediobasal hypothalamus in the path of the neural fibers containing vasopressin that are passing on to the posterior pituitary. Irritative lesions can trigger the release of vasopressin in an unregulated fashion, resulting in the syndrome of inappropriate ADH (vasopressin) secretion (SIADH).

EFFECTS OF HYPOTHALAMIC DISEASE ON OTHER NEUROMETABOLIC FUNCTIONS. A number of functions that affect the internal milieu, in addition to anterior and posterior pituitary function, are regulated, at least in part, by the hypothalamus, including temperature control, behavior, consciousness, memory, sleep, food intake, and carbohydrate metabolism.

Alterations in Food Intake. Body weight is kept relatively constant in nonobese individuals through an integration of a number of factors relating to the intake of nutrients and the output of energy, which are affected by hormonal, environmental, and genetic factors. As with the regulation of hormone secretion, the regulation of food intake can be conceptually regarded as an adjustment of food intake and energy expenditure around "set-points," which may be different for body weight, total body fat, and lean body mass. A number of areas of the hypothalamus are involved in the regulation of energy balance.

Hypothalamic Obesity. Destruction of the mediobasal hypothalamus sometimes inhibits satiety and may result in hyperphagia and hypothalamic obesity. The hyperphagia is due to destruction of noradrenergic fibers originating in the paraventricular nucleus that pass through the mediobasal hypothalamus. Because of their location, such lesions usually also produce hypopituitarism and diabetes insipidus. There are a number of rare syndromes in which obesity is a major part for which a hypothalamic cause has been postulated. Prader-Willi is the most common of these syndromes, occurring in 1 in 25,000 births. It is characterized by hypotonia, obesity, short stature, mental deficiency, hypogonadism, and small hands and feet. About half have a chromosome 15 deletion. In the few cases studied at autopsy, no discernible hypothalamic lesions were detected. In the other syndromes (Laurence-Moon-Biedl-Bardet, Altrom-Hallgren), no specific hypothalamic lesions have been found.

Hypothalamic Anorexia. Lesions of the lateral hypothalamus, which destroy nigrostriatal dopaminergic fibers that pass through this area, produce hypophagia along with an increase in peripheral norepinephrine turnover and metabolic rate. This syndrome is very rare, probably owing to the requirement of bilateral lesions. The hormonal changes that occur in anorexia nervosa appear to be all secondary to the weight loss, and there is no evidence for a primary hypothalamic disorder in this syndrome.

Hyperglycemia. Hypothalamic activation as part of the generalized response to stress can cause a release of GH, PRL, and ACTH, which serve as counterregulatory hormones with respect to insulin. Of more importance in the acute response to stress, this hypothalamic response results in sympathetic activation with release of catecholamines that inhibit insulin secretion and stimulate glycogenolysis. In rare circumstances of acute hypothalamic injury from trauma, stroke, or infection, severe hyperglycemia can occur which is similar to the hyperglycemia seen in animals when the floor of the fourth ventricle is pricked with a needle, a phenomenon referred to as "piqûre" diabetes by Claude Bernard.

Temperature Regulation. The anterior hypothalamus and preoptic area contain temperature-sensitive neurons that respond to internal temperature changes by initiating certain thermoregulatory responses necessary to maintain a constant temperature. Measures that dissipate heat include cutaneous vasodilation, sweating, panting, and behavioral changes that result in attempts to alter the environment. Measures that increase body heat include increasing metabolic heat production, shivering, cutaneous vasoconstriction, and similar behavioral changes. In humans, much of the increase in metabolic heat production occurs via sympathetic activation. The thermosensitive neurons are affected by endogenous pyrogens and drugs that alter thermoregulation as well as input from thermoreceptors in the skin and spinal cord.

Rare patients have been reported with anterior hypothalamic lesions that caused sustained hypothermia due to failure of heat generation by shivering and vasoconstriction but who had intact heat dissipation or downward resetting of the temperature set point. Paroxysmal hypothermia lasting for minutes to days due to the sudden onset of sweating, vasodilation, and a fall in core temperature has been reported in a number of patients in association with demonstrated lesions such as tumors and agenesis of the corpus callosum. Some of these patients had evidence of other hypothalamic dysfunction, including diabetes insipidus, hypogonadism, and precocious puberty.

Fever as a manifestation of hypothalamic disease is uncommon but has been reported in relation to trauma or bleeding into the region of the anterior hypothalamus. Such fevers rarely persist more than two weeks. Paroxysmal hyperthermia due to hypothalamic dysfunction also occurs. Some cases of paroxysmal hypothermia and hyperthermia respond to anticonvulsant medications, suggesting that the neuronal discharge causing the temperature changes is seizure-like.

Poikilothermia results from the inability to dissipate or generate heat to keep the body temperature constant in the face of varying ambient temperatures. This condition results from bilateral lesions in the posterior hypothalamus and rostral mesencephalon, which are the areas responsible for the final integration of thermoregulatory neural efferents. Patients with this condition do not feel discomfort with temperature changes and are unaware of having a problem. Depending upon the ambient temperature, they may present with life-threatening hypothermia or hyperthermia. Poikilothermia is normally present in infants and frequently occurs in elderly individuals.

Abrahams JJ, Trefelner E, Boulware SD: Idiopathic growth hormone deficiency: MR findings in 35 patients. AJNR 12:155, 1991. *In this series of children with idiopathic GH deficiency, a high proportion were found to have structural abnormalities of the pituitary stalk, making these disorders of midline embryologic development. As imaging techniques improve, more and more "idiopathic" disorders may be found to have structural causes.*

Chapelon C, Ziza JM, Piette JC, et al.: Neurosarcoidosis: Signs, course and treatment in 35 confirmed cases. Medicine 69:261, 1990. *Features of neurosarcoidosis are reviewed and the hypothalamic dysfunction that may occur is described.*

Constine LS, Woolf PD, Cann D, et al.: Hypothalamic-pituitary dysfunction after radiation for brain tumors. N Engl J Med 328:87, 1993. *In this series of 32 patients, more than two thirds had some hormonal dysfunction 2 to 13 years following cranial irradiation. Studies like this point out the need for endocrine evaluation of all patients undergoing cranial irradiation.*

Loes DJ, Barloon TJ, Yuh WTC, et al.: MR anatomy and pathology of the hypothalamus. AJR 156:579, 1991. *This article shows what can be achieved with modern imaging techniques. Hypothalamic anatomy and pathology are shown with great clarity.*

Molitch ME: Pathologic hyperprolactinemia. Endocrinol Metab Clin North Am 21:877, 1992. *Covers current knowledge of regulation of prolactin secretion, various causes of hyperprolactinemia, and therapies available.*

Stein DT: New developments in the diagnosis and treatment of sexual precocity. Am J Med Sci 303:53, 1992. *This review carefully delineates the pathophysiology of sexual precocity, diagnostic maneuvers necessary to establish a precise diagnosis, and various treatment modalities.*

201.2   The Pineal Gland

Alfred J. Lewy

The mammalian pineal is located in the "center" of the brain (above the quadrigeminal plate, just behind the posterior commissure) but is actually outside of the blood-brain barrier. Postganglionic neurons from the superior cervical ganglia release norepinephrine that stimulates β_1-adrenergic receptors on the pinealocytes (Fig. 201–3). This results in the synthesis and release into the CSF and venous circulation of melatonin, the principal putative hormone of the pineal gland. The (paired) suprachiasmatic nuclei are the source of an approximately 24-hour rhythm in melatonin production that persists in conditions of constant darkness or blindness. Photic input, conveyed to the suprachiasmatic nuclei (SCN) via the retino-hypothalamic tracts, synchronizes (entrains) the SCN and its output circadian rhythms to the 24-hour light-dark cycle. Between the SCN and the cell bodies of the preganglionic sympathetic neurons in the spinal cord, there are synapses in the paraventricular nuclei.

Melatonin production by the human pineal is decreased by β-blockers and α_2 agonists and is increased by certain tricyclic antidepressants that block reuptake of norepinephrine. Melatonin production is also increased by extreme physical exercise, norepinephrine, and psoralen. In general, diet and activity have no effect. Increased melatonin in manic states and decreased melatonin in depression probably occur but most likely represent epiphenomena following changes in adrenergic activity.

FUNCTION OF MELATONIN

The function of melatonin in humans remains elusive. In some fish and reptiles melatonin coalesces melanin-containing melanosomes and in this way causes blanching, but this effect has been lost in most animals. Melatonin may possibly have this effect on the mammalian retinal pigmented epithelium. The association of pineal tumors with disorders of puberty is most likely explained by compression of the hypothalamus, since no melatonin-secreting tumor has yet been found. Furthermore, it now appears that the main effect of melatonin on the reproductive system lies in its ability to communicate the time of the year to animals that are seasonal breeders. In such animals it can have either anti- or progonadal activity depending on whether the species is a spring or fall breeder, respectively. Reproductive and endocrine effects of exogenous melatonin administration, not to mention endogenous melatonin secretion, have not been well documented in humans, with the possible exception that melatonin at certain doses can increase prolactin levels in humans.

CHRONOBIOLOGY OF MELATONIN

Melatonin is produced only during nighttime darkness in both diurnal and nocturnal animals with an approximately 12-hour "on" phase and 12-hour "off" phase. Many blind people with a complete absence of light perception have free-running endogenous circadian rhythms. When these individuals' melatonin rhythms are out of phase with their sleep-wake cycles (which have remained more or less synchronized to clock time), they are prone to develop nocturnal insomnia and daytime sleepiness. A pattern of insomnia that recurs every few weeks is almost pathognomonic for free-running circadian rhythms in totally blind individuals.

Although darkness does not induce melatonin production, in sighted people exposure to sufficiently bright light during the night immediately suppresses melatonin production. Two models have been proposed to explain how the nightly melatonin profile is shaped. In the *two-pacemaker model,* it is hypothesized that separate endogenous pacemakers control the onset and offset of melatonin production, cued primarily to dusk and dawn, respectively. In the *"clock-gate" model,* the suppressant effect of light (unique to melatonin) participates in the shortening of the duration of nighttime melatonin production during long photoperiods. Both models attempt to explain the shorter duration of melatonin secretion during the briefer summer nights compared to the longer winter nights.

The changing duration of nighttime melatonin secretion during the calendar year seems to be responsible for the reproductive effects of the light-dark cycle in seasonal breeders. Seasonal rhythms have not been well documented in humans, but it is clear that humans have most, if not all, of the circadian rhythms found in other higher animals. Whereas seasonal rhythms respond to the duration of the photoperiod or scotoperiod, circadian rhythms respond to the 24-hour light-dark cycle. In animals, the light-dark cycle's phase-shifting effects on circadian rhythms can be described by a phase response curve (PRC). This appears to be the case in humans as well. The PRC can be explained as follows: Delay responses (shifts to a later time) result when exposure to light occurs during the first part of the night; advance responses (shifts to an earlier time) result when exposure occurs during the latter part of the night. These phase shifts are greatest in magnitude in the middle of the night and are least during the middle of the day.

Although the suppressant effect of light is unique to melatonin, phase-shifting by light affects the endogenous circadian pacemaker (SCN) and all of its driven rhythms. In fact, the timing of the SCN's circadian rhythms is best measured by the circulating levels of melatonin. In some species injections of exogenous melatonin

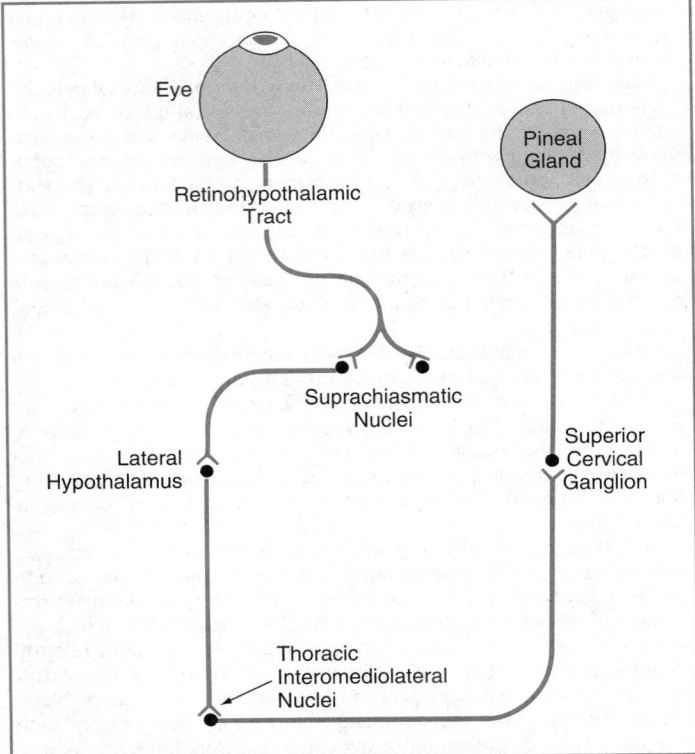

FIGURE 201–3. Schematic diagram for the neuroanatomic regulation of the timing of mammalian melatonin production (see text). (Adapted by permission of the publisher from "Biochemistry and regulation of mammalian melatonin production" by AJ Lewy, in The Pineal Gland, edited by RM Relkin, pp 77–128. Copyright 1983 by Elsevier Science Publishing Co., Inc.)

are capable of causing phase shifts and/or entrainment. In lizards, a PRC for melatonin has been described that is about 12 hours out of phase with the PRC for light; that is, the melatonin PRC resembles a dark-pulse PRC. In humans, exogenous melatonin appears to have circadian phase-shifting effects, which can be described by a PRC that resembles a dark-pulse PRC. Thus, melatonin—which is produced only during the night—may be the chemical messenger of darkness. Therefore, human melatonin production may normally have a role, however small, in the entrainment of the SCN's circadian rhythms. Not being seasonal breeders, perhaps humans have retained the suppressant effect of light in order to use endogenous melatonin to more effectively augment entrainment and phase-shifting effects of the light-dark cycle. The melatonin PRC may also provide the rationale for precise scheduling of exogenous melatonin administration for therapeutic purposes, such as to treat chronobiologic sleep and mood disorders and to facilitate adaptation to shift work and air travel.

PINEAL TUMORS

Three main types of tumors that usually arise in the pineal are (1) pineoblastomas or pineocytomas, the term used depending on the degree of differentiation of this tumor of the pineal parenchyma; (2) germ cell tumors, including germinomas and embryonal carcinomas; and (3) glial tumors. Symptomatic enlargement of pineal by cysts has also been reported, but these are almost always asymptomatic. Destruction of pineal tissue can reduce or even ablate melatonin production, but pineocytomas have rarely been associated with increased circulating levels of melatonin. Melatonin production decreases with age, but this does not seem to be related to pineal calcification. By occluding the cerebral aqueduct, pineal tumors can produce symptoms associated with increased intracranial pressure, sometimes necessitating a shunt. Through pressure on the quadrigeminal plate, pineal tumors can produce Parinaud's syndrome, which includes paresis of upward conjugate gaze. Some germinomas and embryonal carcinomas secrete human chorionic gonadotropin, which has been implicated in cases of delayed onset of puberty. Treatment modalities include surgical extirpation, radiation, and chemotherapy, depending on tumor type and location and the absence or degree of metastases.

Lewy AJ, Sack RL, Singer CM, et al.: Winter depression and the phase shift hypothesis for bright light's therapeutic effects: History, theory and experimental evidence. J Biol Rhythms 3:121, 1988.
Lewy AJ, Wehr TA, Goodwin FK, et al.: Light suppresses melatonin secretion in humans. Science 210:1267, 1980.
Lewy AJ, Ahmed S, Jackson JML, Sack RL: Melatonin shifts circadian rhythms according to a phase-response curve. Chronobiol Int 9:380, 1995.
Neuwelt EA (ed.): Diagnosis and Treatment of Pineal Region Tumors. Baltimore, Williams & Wilkins, 1984.

202 THE PITUITARY

202.1 Anterior Pituitary
J. Larry Jameson

ANATOMY AND EMBRYOLOGY

The pituitary is a relatively small gland located in the sella turcica at the base of the brain. It has a bilobed shape and weighs about 0.6 gram (range 0.4 to 0.9 gram), being somewhat larger in women than in men. The pituitary is divided into anterior and posterior lobes, with the anterior lobe comprising about 80% of the gland. The posterior pituitary, or neurohypophysis, consists of the pituitary stalk as well as the posterior lobe (see Ch. 202.2). Superiorly, the pituitary is covered by the diaphragma sellae, a reflection of the dura mater that forms the roof of the sella and is attached to the clinoid processes. The diaphragma sellae has a central opening that is penetrated by the pituitary stalk and its blood vessels. Importantly, the optic chiasm, formed by the union of the optic nerves, is positioned directly above the pituitary gland and below the third ventricle. The exact position of the chiasm is variable, and the de-

gree to which it is tethered may affect the pattern of visual field changes experienced by patients with pituitary tumors that expand into the suprasellar region. The lateral boundaries of the sella are formed by the cavernous sinuses, which contain the internal carotid artery and branches of cranial nerves III, IV, V, and VI.

The blood supply to the pituitary gland is derived from the superior and inferior hypophyseal arteries, which are connected by a portal system of small vessels and capillaries. Specialized vascular structures, referred to as gomitoli, are located in the median eminence of the hypothalamus and consist of short terminal arterioles draining into portal veins that course down the pituitary stalk to join the sinusoidal capillaries of the anterior lobe. Hypothalamic hormones enter fenestrations in the perigomitolar capillaries to flow from the hypothalamus to the anterior pituitary. Venous drainage from the anterior lobe enters the posterior pituitary capillary bed before draining into the cavernous sinus.

The six major pituitary cell types include somatotropes (growth hormone [GH]–producing), lactotropes (prolactin [Prl]–producing), corticotropes (adrenocorticotropic hormone [ACTH]–producing), thyrotropes (thyroid-stimulating hormone [TSH]–producing), gonadotropes (follicle-stimulating hormone [FSH]– and luteinizing hormone [LH]–producing), and folliculostellate cells, which do not produce the classic pituitary hormones but may have paracrine functions. The biochemical characteristics of the major anterior pituitary hormones are summarized in Table 202–1.

The pituitary is formed early in embryonic life from the fusion of Rathke's pouch (which gives rise to the anterior pituitary) and a portion of the ventral diencephalon (which gives rise to the posterior pituitary). Rathke's pouch is an ectodermal evagination in the roof of the primitive oropharynx. The ontogeny of hormone production during anterior pituitary development has been characterized in detail. The pituitary anlage expresses the glycoprotein hormone α gene even as the progenitor cells are arising from Rathke's pouch. Subsequently, proopiomelanocortin-producing cells can be seen in the hypothalamus and in the pituitary. An evanescent group of TSH-producing cells appear but then fade away, to be followed later by a distinct population of TSH cells in a different location in the pituitary. After gonadotropes develop, GH- and Prl-producing cells appear and later form distinct populations of somatotropes and lactotropes. The transcription factor, Pit-1, a member of the Pou-Homeo domain family, is produced in somatotropes, lactotropes, and thyrotropes. Mutations in Pit-1 prevent the development of these cells and cause hormone deficiencies. This lineage relationship probably accounts for the observation that some GH-producing tumors also secrete Prl and about one third of TSH-producing tumors cosecrete GH.

Anterior pituitary hormone production is largely established by the ninth week of gestation, and the anatomic and biosynthetic mechanisms that comprise an active hypothalamic-pituitary system are functional by 12 to 17 weeks of gestation. In anencephaly, all anterior pituitary cell types, with the exception of corticotropes, are capable of hormone synthesis and secretion, indicating that the embryonic pituitary develops relatively normally in the absence of hypothalamic stimulation.

Somatotropes, which constitute 40 to 50% of anterior pituitary cells, are located predominantly in the lateral aspects of the anterior pituitary. Lactotropes comprise 15 to 25% of cells and are scattered throughout the anterior pituitary. Corticotropes constitute 10 to 20% of anterior pituitary cells and are located mainly in the central region of the anterior pituitary. Gonadotropes, which account for about 10% of pituitary cells, produce both FSH and LH, although a small fraction of gonadotropes appear to selectively secrete only one of the hormones. Only 5% of pituitary cells are thyrotropes. The folliculostellate cells have long, irregular processes that extend between the hormone-producing cells. They do not contain secretory granules but have been shown to produce growth factors such as basic fibroblast growth factor, vascular endothelial growth factor, and follistatin, among others.

Horvath E, Kovacs K: Morphology of adenohypophyseal cells and pituitary tumors. In Imura H (ed.): The Pituitary Gland, 2nd ed. New York, Raven Press, 1994, p. 29. A definitive summary of pituitary pathology.
Voss JW, Rosenfeld MG: Anterior pituitary development: Short tales from dwarf mice. Cell 70:527, 1992. A review of a remarkable series of studies that define pituitary cell lineages.

TABLE 202–1. FEATURES OF THE MAJOR ANTERIOR PITUITARY HORMONES

Hormone	Amino Acids		MW	Serum Half-life	Cell Type	Target Gland
Growth hormone (GH)	191		22 kD	20 min	Somatotrope	Multiple
Prolactin (Prl)	198		23 kD	20 min	Lactotrope	Breast
Adrenocorticotropic hormone (ACTH)	39		4.5 kD	8 min	Corticotrope	Adrenal
Thyroid-stimulating hormone (TSH)	α-subunit, 92 aa	14 kD		50 min	Thyrotrope	Thyroid
	β-subunit, 118 aa	17 kD				
Luteinizing hormone (LH)	α-subunit, 92 aa	14 kD		50 min	Gonadotrope	Gonad
	β-subunit, 121 aa	18 kD				
Follicle-stimulating hormone (FSH)	α-subunit, 92 aa	14 kD		220 min	Gonadotrope	Gonad
	β-subunit, 111 aa	18 kD				

The amino acid lengths are based upon the cloned cDNA's and the molecular weights (MW) include the contributions of the carbohydrates in the case of the glycoprotein hormones (TSH, LH, FSH). The serum half-lives assume single-compartment monoexponential decay.

RADIOLOGY OF THE PITUITARY

Currently, radiologic imaging of the pituitary gland primarily involves computed tomography (CT) and magnetic resonance imaging (MRI). CT scans are performed using high-resolution (1.5-mm), contrast-enhanced procedures with direct coronal sections. Although CT provides excellent resolution, problems include artifacts from metallic objects and dental fillings, and some patients have difficulty assuming the position required for coronal sections. Pituitary tumors typically enhance with contrast on CT, and cystic components are hypodense.

Overall, MRI is the technique of choice for evaluating the sellar region. MRI scans provide multiplanar imaging and excellent resolution of the pituitary and surrounding cerebrovascular fluid (CSF), vascular, and central nervous system structures. There is less radiation exposure with MRI than with CT, allowing repeated imaging as required for evaluation and follow-up. However, bone structures are not well-defined by MRI. The normal anterior pituitary appears isointense with brain white matter, whereas the posterior pituitary exhibits high signal intensity. The optic chiasm can be readily identified superior to the pituitary gland because it is surrounded by hypodense structures. MRI scans detect pituitary microadenomas in nearly all patients with surgically proven tumors. Pituitary adenomas typically appear hypointense on T1-weighted images and show less gadolinium contrast enhancement than surrounding normal tissue. Focal hypodense areas are also seen in about a quarter of normal individuals, which may correspond to cysts or small adenomas that have been described in autopsy series, emphasizing the importance of endocrine evaluation in making the diagnosis of pituitary tumors.

Elster AD: Modern imaging of the pituitary. Radiology 187:1, 1993. *A review focused on MRI of the sellar region.*
Tindall GT: Disorders of the Pituitary. St. Louis, CV Mosby, 1986. *This book reviews multiple pituitary disorders and has particularly good chapters on anatomy, radiology, and transsphenoidal surgery.*

REGULATION OF THE PITUITARY AXIS

The concept of positive and negative feedback control represents a fundamental tenet of endocrinology. The pituitary gland integrates the influences of an array of positive and negative signals to modulate hormone secretion within a narrow range (Table 202–2). The major hypothalamic–pituitary–target gland axes include TRH–TSH–thyroid hormone, CRH–ACTH–cortisol axis, GnRH–LH/FSH–gonads, and GRF–GH–IGF-1. Prolactin is the only major pituitary hormone that is not subject to feedback inhibition by hormones produced in target tissues. However, it is controlled by positive and negative input from the hypothalamus.

The principles of feedback regulation are well-illustrated by the hypothalamic–pituitary–thyroid axis (see Fig. 203–1). Hypothalamic TRH stimulates TSH secretion from the pituitary. TSH increases thyroid hormone secretion, which in turn suppresses hypothalamic TRH as well as pituitary TSH. A typical regulatory loop therefore has both positive (TRH,TSH) and negative (T_4,T_3) components, allowing a high degree of control of hormone levels. In this case, the pituitary gland integrates positive TRH signals and the negative effects of thyroid hormone. The concept of feedback regulation is important not only for understanding pituitary physiology, but because it provides the basis for analyzing pituitary gland function using stimulation and suppression tests.

Feedback regulatory systems are superimposed upon hormonal rhythms that are used for adaptation to the environment. Seasonal changes, the daily occurrence of the light-dark cycles, and stress are but a few of many environmental events that have major impacts on the secretion of pituitary hormones. Some hormonal pathways, such as ACTH secretion, are entrained to the light-dark cycle, causing characteristic peaks of ACTH and cortisol production in the early morning, with a nadir in the late afternoon and evening. The secretion of other hormones, such as GH, is altered by sleep, stress, and meals. The early pubertal surges of LH occur at night and usually in association with sleep. The menstrual cycle provides an example of a pituitary rhythm that occurs on a much longer time scale (approximately 28 days). The pattern of the menstrual cycle is coupled to cycles of follicular development in the ovary. As follicular development progresses, levels of gonadal steroids and inhibin feed back upon the hypothalamus and pituitary to modulate LH and FSH secretion.

Because many hormones are released in a pulsatile manner and in a rhythmic fashion, it is important to be aware of these characteristics of secretion when attempting to relate serum measurements to normal values. Although it is possible to characterize pulsatile patterns of hormone secretion using frequent blood sampling (every 10 min) over several hours, this is not practical in a clinical setting. Alternative approaches include stimulation and suppression tests or the use of "integrated" measurements of hormone production, such as 24-hour urine free cortisol as an index of ACTH secretion or IGF-1 as a biologic marker of GH action.

Crowley WF Jr, Filicori M, Spratt DI, et al.: The physiology of gonadotropin-releasing hormone (GnRH) secretion in men and women. Recent Prog Horm Res 41:473, 1985. *Summary of neuroendocrine control of reproduction with emphasis on the importance of pulsatile secretion.*

HYPOPITUITARISM

Hypopituitarism implies diminished production of one or more anterior pituitary hormones. Although the recognition of complete or panhypopituitarism is usually straightforward, the detection of partial or selective hormone deficiencies is more challenging. Pituitary hormone deficiencies can be caused by loss of hypothalamic stimulation (tertiary hormone deficiency) or by direct loss of pituitary function (secondary hormone deficiency). The distinction between hypothalamic and pituitary causes of hypopituitarism is important for establishing the correct diagnosis and for applying and

TABLE 202–2. FACTORS THAT REGULATE PITUITARY HORMONE SECRETION

Hormone	Releasing Factors	Inhibiting Factors
Growth hormone (GH)	GRF	SMS, IGF-1
Prolactin (Prl)	TRH, VIP, E_2	Dopamine
Adrenocorticotropic hormone (ACTH)	CRH, vasopressin	Cortisol
Thyroid-stimulating hormone (TSH)	TRH	T_4, T_3, SMS, dopamine
Luteinizing hormone (LH)	GnRH	E_2, testosterone
Follicle-stimulating hormone (FSH)	GnRH, activin	Inhibin, E_2, testosterone

GRF, growth hormone–releasing factor; SMS, somatostatin; IGF-1, insulin-like growth factor-1; TRH, thyrotropin-releasing hormone; VIP, vasoactive intestinal peptide; E_2, estradiol; CRH, corticotropin-releasing hormone; T_4, thyroxine; T_3, triiodothyronine. The gonadal steroids, E_2 and testosterone, exert much of their inhibitory effects on gonadotropin secretion at the hypothalamic level.

interpreting the relevant diagnostic endocrine tests. With improved procedures for testing the hypothalamic-pituitary axis, it is apparent that hypothalamic causes of hypopituitarism are more common than previously appreciated (see Ch. 201.1). When hypopituitarism is accompanied by diabetes insipidus, one should particularly consider hypothalamic causes of pituitary dysfunction.

CAUSES OF HYPOPITUITARISM. A variety of congenital causes of hypopituitarism have been described (Table 202–3). Sporadic and familial forms of panhypopituitarism occur, but the underlying genetic or developmental defects have not been elucidated. Congenital combined deficiencies of GH, Prl, and TSH are caused by mutations in the gene encoding Pit-1, a pituitary-specific transcription factor that is involved in the development of somatotrope, lactotrope, and thyrotrope cell lineages. Different types of Pit-1 mutations are inherited in an autosomal dominant or recessive pattern. Congenital GH deficiency can be caused by a heterogeneous group of mutations in the GH gene. These include large deletions of the GH gene that are inherited in an autosomal recessive manner and involve genetic recombination between related DNA sequences in the duplicated GH gene cluster. Point mutations have also been described in the GH gene, and some of these can be inherited in an autosomal dominant manner, apparently because the mutant hormone impairs GH biosynthesis and normal function of the somatotrope cell. Mutations have also been described in the LH-β, FSH-β, and TSH-β genes that cause autosomal recessive forms of selective hormone deficiencies.

Neoplastic lesions, particularly pituitary adenomas, are the most common cause of acquired hypopituitarism. Pituitary adenomas cause hypopituitarism in several different manners. In some cases, there is direct destruction or compression of the normal pituitary. Compression of the pituitary stalk can impair blood supply to the pituitary as well as decrease input from hypothalamic hormones. Hemorrhage into tumors can lead to pituitary infarction. When tested carefully, most patients with macroadenomas have partial deficiencies of one or more pituitary hormones, most often involving GH and gonadotropins. A mild degree of hyperprolactinemia is characteristic of disorders that cause stalk compression, and hyperprolactinemia further impairs gonadotropin secretion. A variety of other neoplasms that occur near the sella, such as craniopharyngiomas, can also cause hypopituitarism (Table 202–3).

Pituitary apoplexy is usually caused by hemorrhage into a tumor with associated infarction. In the absence of a tumor, predispositions to apoplexy include trauma, pregnancy, anticoagulation, sickle cell anemia, and diabetes mellitus. Pituitary infarction in the peripartum period is referred to as Sheehan's syndrome and is usually associated with significant hemorrhage and hypovolemia. It is often heralded by the inability to lactate, amenorrhea, and symptoms of adrenal insufficiency. Sheehan's syndrome is now infrequent owing to improvements in obstetrical care.

Radiation causes hypopituitarism primarily because of its effects on hypothalamic function, although high-dose radiation (e.g., proton beam) can also cause direct pituitary damage. The sellar region is subjected to radiation in the treatment of pituitary adenomas, craniopharyngiomas, clivus chordomas, optic gliomas, meningiomas, dysgerminomas, and other neoplasms. Importantly, the effects of radiation can be delayed as much as several years, and patients at high risk should be evaluated at yearly intervals for radiation-induced hypopituitarism. Although GH and gonadotropin deficiencies develop first in most patients, ACTH or TSH deficiencies occasionally occur first, emphasizing the need to evaluate each of the major axes.

Empty sella syndrome can occur as a primary or an acquired condition. It is caused by defects in the diaphragma sellae which allow herniation of the arachnoid membrane into the hypophyseal fossa. In longstanding cases, sellar enlargement occurs, probably because of persistent transduction of intracranial pressure. With appropriate imaging studies, the pituitary gland can be seen as a flattened rim of tissue along the floor of the sella. Primary empty sella occurs most commonly in women and may be associated with features of benign intracranial hypertension. Pituitary function in patients with primary empty sella syndrome is usually normal, although 15% have mild hyperprolactinemia, probably because of stretching of the pituitary stalk. Acquired forms may occur as a result of surgery, radiation, or pituitary infarction (usually of an adenoma).

DIAGNOSIS AND TREATMENT. The diagnosis of hypopituitarism rests upon the stimulation tests summarized in Table 202–4. The therapy of hypopituitarism depends upon the nature and severity of the hormone deficiencies as well as the desired clinical endpoint. The goal is to replace hormones in a physiologic manner, with efforts to avoid the consequences of overreplacement. In patients with acquired forms of hypopituitarism (e.g., pituitary tumors, radiation treatment), it is not uncommon to encounter a mixture of partial hormone deficiencies. It is generally prudent to provide hormone replacement if partial deficiency is suspected, as patients may experience symptoms over a number of years before an unequivocal diagnosis of hormone deficiency is made. Examples of hormonal replacement paradigms are provided in Table 202–5.

TABLE 202–3. HYPOTHALAMIC AND PITUITARY CAUSES OF HYPOPITUITARISM

Congenital
  Panhypopituitarism, pituitary aplasia
  Combined deficiency of GH, Prl, TSH
  Kallmann syndrome (selective GnRH deficiency with anosmia)
  Isolated GHRH, CRH, TRH deficiencies
  Isolated deficiencies of GH, Prl, ACTH, LH, FSH, or TSH
Neoplastic
  Pituitary adenomas
  Craniopharyngioma
  Metastatic tumors
  Teratomas, dysgerminomas, chordomas, gliomas, meningiomas
  Leukemia/lymphoma
  Hypothalamic hamartoma
  Third ventricular cysts, Rathke's pouch and other cysts
Inflammatory/infiltrative
  Sarcoidosis
  Tuberculosis, syphilis, eosinophilic granulomas, other granulomatous diseases
  Autoimmune lymphocytic hypophysitis
  Histiocytosis X, Hand-Schuller-Christian disease
Vascular
  Neonatal intraventricular hemorrhage
  Pituitary apoplexy
  Sheehan syndrome (postpartum necrosis)
  Internal carotid aneurysm
  Diabetic necrosis
  Sickle cell anemia
  Vasculitis
  Subarachnoid hemorrhage
  Trauma associated with stalk section or necrosis
Metabolic/neurogenic
  Anorexia nervosa
  Hemochromatosis
  Amyloidosis
  Critical illness
  Psychosocial dwarfism
Iatrogenic
  Radiation
  Post-surgical

Phillips JA, Cogan JD: Genetic basis of endocrine disease. 6. Molecular basis of familial human growth hormone deficiency. J Clin Endocrinol Metab 78:11, 1994. *Overview of the heterogeneous types of growth hormone gene mutations.*
Radovick S, Nations M, Du Y, et al.: A mutation in the POU-homeodomain of Pit-1 responsible for combined pituitary hormone deficiency. Science 257:1115, 1992. *One of several reports of Pit-1 mutations in humans.*
Vance ML: Hypopituitarism. N Engl J Med 330:1651, 1994. *A review of causes, diagnosis, and management of hypopituitarism.*
Wakai S, Fukushima T, Teramoto A, et al.: Pituitary apoplexy: Its incidence and clinical significance. J Neurosurg 55:187, 1981. *A summary of clinical features associated with 93 cases of pituitary apoplexy occurring in a series of 563 patients.*

PITUITARY TUMORS

CLASSIFICATION. Pituitary tumors are classified according to the hormones that they produce. The approximate prevalence of the different types of pituitary adenomas is summarized in Table 202–6. Histologically, pituitary tumors are also classified according to their tinctoral staining characteristics (acidophilic, eosinophilic, chromophobe adenomas), but these analyses correlate only loosely with type of hormone produced. In recent years, immunohistochemical studies, using antibodies specific for each of the major pituitary hormones, have been used to define tumor phenotype. Electron microscopy can provide additional ultrastructural information but is

TABLE 202–4. TESTS OF PITUITARY INSUFFICIENCY

Hormone	Test	Interpretation
Growth hormone	*Insulin tolerance test:* Regular insulin (0.05–0.15U/kg) is given IV and blood is drawn at −30, 0, 30, 45, 60, and 90 min for measurement of glucose and GH.	If hypoglycemia occurs (glucose < 40 mg/dL), GH should increase > 10 µg/L. Careful supervision is required during testing.
	L-Dopa test: 10 mg/kg PO with GH measurements at 0, 30, 60, and 120 min.	Normal response is GH > 7 µg/L.
	L-Arginine test: 0.5 gm/kg IV over 30 min with GH measurements at 0, 30, 60, and 120 min.	Normal response is GH > 7 µg/L.
Prolactin	*TRH test:* 200–500 µg IV with measurements of TSH and Prl at 0, 20, and 60 min.	Normal prolactin is > 2 µg/L and > 200% increase after TRH
ACTH	*Insulin tolerance test:* Regular insulin (0.05–0.15 U/kg) is given IV and blood is drawn at −30, 0, 30, 45, 60, and 90 min for measurement of glucose and cortisol.	If hypoglycemia occurs (glucose < 40 mg/dL), cortisol should increase by > 7 µg/dL or to > 20 µg/dL. Careful supervision is required during testing.
	CRH test: 1 µg/kg ovine CRH IV at 8 AM with blood samples drawn at 0, 15, 30, 60, 90, 120 min for measurement of ACTH and cortisol.	In most normals, the basal ACTH increases 2- to 4-fold and reaches a peak (20–100 pg/mL). ACTH responses may be delayed in cases of hypothalamic dysfunction. Cortiso levels usually reach 20–25 µg/dL.
	Metyrapone test: Metyrapone (30 mg/kg) at midnight with measurements of plasma 11-deoxycortisol and cortisol at 8 AM. ACTH can also be measured. A 3-day test is also available.	A normal response is 11-deoxycortisol > 7.5 µg/dL or ACTH > 75 pg/mL. Plasma cortisol should fall below 4 µg/dL to ensure an adequate response.
	ACTH stimulation test: ACTH 1-24 (cosyntropin), 0.25 mg IM or IV. Cortisol and aldosterone are measured at 0, 30, and 60 min. A 3-day ACTH stimulation test consists of 0.25 mg ACTH 1-24 given IV over 8 h each day.	A normal response is cortisol > 18 µg/dL and aldosterone response of > 4 ng/dL above baseline. In suspected hypothalamic-pituitary deficiency, 3-day ACTH test should result in 17-OH steroids of > 25 mg/24h.
TSH	*Basal thyroid function tests:* T_4, T_3, THBI, TSH.	Low free thyroid hormone levels in the setting of TSH levels that are not appropriately increased.
	TRH test: 200–500 µg IV with measurements of TSH and Prl at 0, 20, and 60 min.	TSH should increase by > 5 mU/L unless thyroid hormone levels are increased.
LH, FSH	*Basal levels of LH, FSH, testosterone, estrogen*	Basal LH and FSH should be increased in postmenopausal women. Low testosterone levels in conjunction with low or low-normal LH and FSH are consistent with gonadotropin deficiency.
	GnRH test: GnRH (100 µg) IV with measurements of serum LH and FSH at 0, 30, 60 min.	In most normals, LH should increase by 10 IU/L and FSH by 2 IU/L. Normal responses are variable and repeated stimulation may be required.
	Clomiphene test: Clomiphene citrate (100 mg) is given orally for 5 days. Serum LH and FSH are measured on days 0, 5, 7, 10, and 13.	A 50% increase should occur in LH and FSH, usually by day 5.
Multiple hormones	*Combined anterior pituitary test:* GHRH (1 µg/kg), CRH (1 µg/kg), GnRH (100 µg), TRH (200 µg) are given sequentially IV. Blood samples are drawn at −30, 15, 30, 60, 90, and 120 min for measurements of GH, ACTH, LH, FSH, and TSH.	Combined or individual releasing hormone responses must be evaluated in the context of basal hormone values and may not be diagnostic.

TABLE 202–5. HORMONAL REPLACEMENT THERAPY IN HYPOPITUITARISM

Pituitary Axis	Hormonal Replacements
Growth hormone	In children, GH (0.06–0.1 mg/kg) SC 3×/week or daily.
Prolactin	None
ACTH-cortisol	Prednisone (5 mg PO qAM; 2.5 mg PO qPM) or cortisone acetate (25 mg PO qAM; 12.5 mg PO qPM) or hydrocortisone (20 mg PO qAM; 10 mg PO qPM). Fluorohydrocortisone (0.05–0.1 mg PO qd) is rarely required for secondary adrenal insufficiency.
TSH-thyroid	L-Thyroxine (0.1–0.15 mg) PO qd
Gonadotropins-gonads	Pulsatile GnRH (via pump) can be used for GnRH-deficient subjects, or FSH and LH (or hCG) can be used to induce ovulation in women. hCG alone, or FSH and LH can be used to induce spermatogenesis in men. In men, testosterone enanthate (100–200 mg) IM q1–3 weeks or testosterone cyclopentylpropionate (100–250 mg) IM q1–3 weeks. In women, conjugated estrogens (0.625–1.25 mg) or mestranol (35 µg) PO days 1–25 each month cycled with medroxyprogesterone acetate (5–10 mg) PO qd days 15–25 each month. Low-dose contraceptive pills may also be used.
Posterior pituitary	Desmopressin (DDAVP), 0.05–0.2 ml (5–20 µg) intranasally once or twice daily, or 1/10th this dose can be given SC.

Replacement therapy is dictated by the types of hormone deficiencies and by the clinical circumstances. In each case, the recommended preparations and doses are representative but need to be adjusted for individual patients. Other hormonal preparations are also available.

not used routinely. Tumor grade is not particularly useful for predicting invasiveness, and pituitary adenomas are rarely malignant. Radiologic or clinical evidence of tumor size, impingement, or invasion of local structures surrounding the sella, or evidence of metastasis (usually within the CNS) can provide more practical indices of the biologic behavior of the tumor.

THEORIES OF PITUITARY TUMORIGENESIS. A longstanding controversy exists concerning the clonality of pituitary tumors. Monoclonal tumors arise from a single progenitor cell, presumably because of a somatic mutation to create an oncogene or to inactivate a tumor suppressor gene. Polyclonal tumors, on the other hand, reflect hyperplasia caused by exogenous stimulation of a group of cells by a growth factor or hypothalamic-releasing hormone. Using recombinant DNA techniques to track X-chromosome inactivation as an index of cell lineage, it has been shown that the vast majority of pituitary tumors are monoclonal in origin. This finding does not exclude a role for hormonal stimulation as a predisposing factor for somatic mutations, and the hormonal environment may also affect the rate of tumor growth (e.g., Nelson's syndrome).

Supporting the concept that somatic mutations lead to pituitary tumorigenesis, a subset (35 to 40%) of somatotrope adenomas has mutations in two different amino acids (Arg 201 and Gln 227) which result in activation of the $Gs\alpha$ subunit. Either mutation prevents GTP hydrolysis, causing the $Gs\alpha$ subunit to stimulate adenylyl cyclase in a constitutive manner. The elevated intracellular cAMP levels lead to increased cell growth as well as GH production. Mutations in other oncogenes, such as *ras,* Rb, and p53, are uncommon in pituitary tumors. Thus, the nature of the somatic defects in most pituitary tumors remains unknown.

Two types of inherited predispositions to pituitary tumors are recognized. Patients with McCune-Albright syndrome occasionally de-

TABLE 202-6. PREVALENCE OF DIFFERENT TYPES OF PITUITARY ADENOMAS

Type of Pituitary Adenoma	Disorder	Hormone Produced	Prevalence (%)*
Somatotrope	Acromegaly/gigantism	GH	10–15
Lactotrope (prolactinoma)	Hypogonadism, mass effects	Prolactin	25–40
Corticotrope	Cushing's disease	ACTH	10–15
Gonadotrope	Mass effects, hypopituitarism	FSH and/or LH	10–15
α-subunit	Mass effects, hypopituitarism	Free α-subunit	5
Thyrotrope	Hyperthyroidism	TSH	<3
Nonfunctioning/null cell	Mass effects, hypopituitarism	None	10–25

* The prevalence rates represent ranges described in several different large series. Mixed tumors (e.g., GH and prolactin) and plurihormonal adenomas are not shown. Prolactinomas were underestimated in most recent pathologic series because they are largely managed medically. Most glycoprotein hormone–producing pituitary tumors were classified as nonfunctioning adenomas until the application of immunohistochemical studies.

velop pituitary adenomas as well as characteristic abnormalities in other tissues, particularly the ovary, bone, and thyroid. Interestingly, McCune-Albright syndrome is also caused by mutations in the Gsα subunit. However, the somatic mutations in McCune-Albright syndrome occur early during development, rather than only in the pituitary gland, so that multiple tissues are affected. In multiple endocrine neoplasia type 1 (MEN-1), the predisposition to pituitary tumors is inherited in an autosomal dominant manner and occurs in conjunction with tumors of the parathyroid and pancreas. The MEN-1 gene has been localized on the long arm of chromosome 11 (11q13). Individuals with MEN-1 are thought to inherit one mutant allele, with tumorigenesis occurring after a "second hit" mutates or deletes the normal MEN-1 gene. Deletions of portions of chromosome 11 have also been described in sporadic pituitary tumors. Deletions of other chromosomal regions (loss of heterozygosity) suggest that several different tumor suppressor genes may play a role in the development of pituitary tumors.

Alexander JM, Biller BM, Bikkal H, et al.: Clinically nonfunctioning pituitary tumors are monoclonal in origin. J Clin Invest 86:336, 1990. *One of several studies using X-chromosome inactivation to demonstrate that pituitary tumors are monoclonal in origin.*

Landis CA, Masters SB, Spada A, et al.: GTPase inhibiting mutations activate the alpha chain of Gs and stimulate adenylyl cyclase in human pituitary tumours. Nature 340:692, 1989. *A classic study showing that mutations in the Gsα subunit cause constitutive activation of adenylyl cyclase, leading to somatotrope neoplasia.*

MASS EFFECTS OF PITUITARY ADENOMAS. Many of the clinical manifestations of pituitary adenomas are related to the hypersecretion of hormones. However, the mass effects of the enlarging tumor can also lead to specific signs and symptoms. Particularly in the case of nonfunctioning tumors or those that produce gonadotropins, the primary clinical manifestations are related to effects of the tumor on surrounding structures.

Headaches are common in patients with macroadenomas and appear to be caused by expansion of the diaphragma sellae or by invasion of bone. Headaches may be retro-orbital or referred to the top of the skull, but the location is variable. Severe headache associated with nausea, vomiting, and altered consciousness can also be caused by infarction of a pituitary adenoma. In severe cases, pituitary apoplexy can occur and may require urgent surgical decompression.

The effects of pituitary tumors on the visual fields are well-explained by the relationship of the optic chiasm to the sella turcica. Expansion of macroadenomas into the suprasellar region exerts pressure on the optic chiasm, usually in the central region where nerves emanating from the inferior and medial part of the retina (superior temporal visual fields) cross. Consequently, bitemporal hemianopsia is the most common visual field abnormality associated with pituitary adenomas. However, the exact pattern of visual field loss is variable and is affected by the location and flexibility of the chiasm as well as the direction and extent of tumor growth. Large tumors may grow asymmetrically and invade the cavernous sinus or surround an optic nerve, leading to other patterns of visual field changes or loss of visual acuity. It is essential for all patients with pituitary tumors to undergo high-resolution radiologic imaging to evaluate the size and location of the tumor. Formal visual field testing by an ophthalmologist is required to detect subtle visual field changes and should be performed in all patients with suprasellar extension. Longstanding visual field changes may not be reversed by surgical decompression, but dramatic improvements can occur if visual loss is recent.

The normal pituitary is often compressed into a thin rim of tissue by large pituitary adenomas. Hypopituitarism probably results more from compression of the hypothalamic-pituitary stalk than from direct replacement or pressure on the normal pituitary. GH deficiency and hypogonadotropic hypogonadism are particularly common. Slightly elevated prolactin levels (generally < 100 ng per milliliter) occur in cases of stalk compression because of diminished inhibition by dopamine. It is important not to mistake such tumors for prolactinomas, as they will not decrease in size in response to medical therapy with bromocriptine. Preoperative hypopituitarism caused by a large pituitary mass is reversible in up to half of patients after surgical decompression. Diabetes insipidus (vasopressin deficiency) is rarely caused by pituitary tumors and should raise the suspicion of a craniopharyngioma or other disorders likely to cause hypothalamic dysfunction.

Arafah BM: Reversible hypopituitarism in patients with large nonfunctioning pituitary adenomas. J Clin Endocrinol Metab 62:1173, 1986. *This study of 26 patients with macroadenomas illustrates how pituitary tumors can cause hypopituitarism by compression of the pituitary stalk.*

THERAPY OF PITUITARY ADENOMAS. *Surgical Treatment.* Except for prolactinomas, surgery is the primary mode of therapy for most pituitary tumors that warrant intervention. Indications for surgery include reduction in hormone levels and decompression to relieve mass effects or to prevent further tumor expansion. Currently, the transsphenoidal route is used almost exclusively for decompression or extirpation of pituitary tumors. Because of substantially greater morbidity, transfrontal craniotomy is reserved for patients with tumors that require extensive exploration of the suprasellar region and surrounding structures, including invasion into the third ventricle. The transsphenoidal approach usually involves a sublabial incision, allowing ready access to the sphenoid sinus, which leads to the floor of the sella. After the sella is entered, the tumor is identified and resected in fragments under microscopy. Decompression of the sellar contents can allow tumor in the suprasellar region to drop into the surgical field to allow further resection. In experienced hands, transsphenoidal surgery is effective and complications are uncommon (< 5% complication rate), but include CSF leak, hemorrhage, optic nerve injury, hypopituitarism, and sinusitis. Transient diabetes insipidus occurs in about 5% of patients following surgery but rarely persists long-term. Mortality rates are < 1%.

Surgical cure rates are largely a function of the size and location of the pituitary mass. When stringent hormonal criteria are used to assess surgical success rates, < 30% of macroadenomas are cured by transsphenoidal surgery, although considerable improvements in hormone levels or mass effects can be achieved. On the other hand, hormone hypersecretion by microadenomas (< 1 cm in size) can be corrected completely in up to 80 to 90% of patients, although the cure rates vary considerably at different institutions.

Radiation Therapy. Radiation therapy has been used as a primary mode of treatment of pituitary adenomas and as adjunctive therapy following surgery or in combination with medical therapy. Radiation therapy is typically administered over 4 to 5 weeks at a dose of 45 Gy using ^{60}Co or a linear accelerator. Proton beam therapy has also been used and delivers very high doses of radiation within a localized region, but it is limited to intrasellar lesions and is not widely available. Because response rates are slow (several years) and complete remission is rarely achieved, primary radiation therapy is generally reserved for patients who cannot or choose not to undergo surgery. Radiation therapy is more commonly used as adjunctive therapy following incomplete transsphenoidal resection. The decision regarding adjunctive radiation therapy involves a number of issues, including hormone levels, amount and location of residual tumor, rate of tumor growth, and degree of invasiveness. Because the time to recurrence for most macroadenomas is 5 to 10 years, it is often reasonable to follow patients with imaging techniques, reserving radiation therapy for those with evidence of recurrence. Complications of radiation therapy are dose-related but can also be idiosyncratic. Partial or complete hypopituitarism occurs in 50 to 70% of patients and is primarily due to hypothalamic injury. Less common complications include optic nerve damage, brain necrosis, vascular damage, and predisposition to sarcomas.

Medical Therapy. The emergence of medical therapies for pituitary tumors has dramatically impacted patient management. Dopamine agonists, which include the ergot derivatives (bromocriptine, lisuride, pergolide) and a D_2 selective agonist (CV205-502), have a primary role in the management of prolactinomas. They induce a rapid fall in prolactin levels and, importantly, decrease tumor size. Dopamine agonists are also used in the management of acromegaly, although the GH responses and effects on tumor size are generally much less pronounced than in prolactinomas. Somatostatin analogues, such as octreotide, act to suppress the secretion of a number of hormones, including GH and TSH. Octreotide has been used to treat acromegaly and TSH-producing tumors. Long-acting GnRH agonists and antagonists have been studied in gonadotropin-producing tumors. Unlike the situation in normal individuals, the long-acting agonists do not cause desensitization and suppression of gonadotropins in most pituitary tumors. GnRH antagonists are more effective, reducing FSH in the majority of patients examined, but these agents have little effect on tumor growth. Medical therapy of Cushing's disease is primarily directed toward inhibition of steroid biosynthesis. Therapeutic drugs include ketoconazole, metyrapone, aminoglutethimide, and o′,p′, DDD (mitotane). Because of substantial side effects and because patients with Cushing's disease tend to respond to these drugs by producing more ACTH, medical therapy is used primarily as an adjunctive treatment or to reduce cortisol levels preoperatively.

Halberg FE, Sheline GE: Radiotherapy of pituitary tumors. Endocrinol Metab Clin 16:667, 1987. *A good summary of the use of radiation therapy in multimodality management of pituitary tumors.*

Klibanski A, Zervas NT: Diagnosis and management of hormone-secreting pituitary adenomas. N Engl J Med 324:8221, 1991. *A concise review of the diagnosis and managment of pituitary adenomas.*

GROWTH HORMONE

The pituitary gland contains a large amount of stored GH (5 to 10 mg), a 191 amino acid, single-chain protein that contains two intramolecular disulfide bonds (see Table 202–1). The GH gene is located on chromosome 17 and is part of a five-member gene cluster that includes a GH variant gene, two placental lactogen (hPL) genes that are also referred to as chorionic somatomammotropin (hCS) genes, and an hPL pseudogene that is not expressed. Highly repetitive sequences within the gene cluster appear to account for the propensity for recombination and deletions of the GH gene, causing one form of GH deficiency.

The predominant circulating form of GH is a 22-kD protein. However, a splicing variant creates a 20-kD form that constitutes about 10 to 15% of circulating GH and appears to be biologically active. GH also forms high molecular weight oligomers and is complexed in the circulation to two different binding proteins. The high-affinity binding protein has been identified as a circulating form of the extracellular domain of the GH receptor. In addition to greatly reducing the clearance of GH, this binding protein may also modulate GH action.

GH production is controlled by a complex interplay of hypothalamic stimulatory and inhibitory peptides, neurotransmitters, growth factors, sex steroids, and nutritional conditions. The most important regulators of GH are the hypothalamic factors; GH-releasing factor (GRF), which is stimulatory; and somatostatin, which is inhibitory. GH increases the production of IGF-1 (also known as somatomedin C), which in turn inhibits GH production. GRF acts by a G protein–coupled receptor that is structurally related to receptors in the VIP, glucagon, and secretin family. GRF stimulates cAMP, activates phospholipase C, and causes an increase in intracellular calcium. GRF causes somatotrope hyperplasia and stimulates GH biosynthesis and secretion. The Gsα subunit, which is coupled to the GRF receptor, is one of the targets for activating mutations that lead to somatotrope adenomas. Somatostatin binds to receptors that inhibit adenylate cyclase and thereby lower cAMP levels. As a result, GRF and somatostatin act antagonistically at the level of signal transduction. When both hormones are added concomitantly, somatostatin appears to act dominantly and GH secretion is inhibited.

IGF-1 also inhibits GH secretion and acts at both the pituitary and hypothalamic levels. In addition to reflecting GH action (primarily at the liver), serum IGF-1 is also sensitive to nutritional and metabolic changes. In starvation and anorexia nervosa, IGF-1 levels are low, resulting in increased levels of GH. In obesity, GH levels are low and GRF responses are blunted. Stress, exercise, and a variety of neurogenic stimuli also increase GH secretion. Estrogens stimulate GH secretion, but its effects are less pronounced than for prolactin.

Large bursts of GH secretion characteristically occur at night in association with slow-wave sleep. GH levels tend to be greatest during puberty and decline gradually in adulthood. The amplitude of GH pulses is greater in women than in men, likely reflecting the effects of estrogens. Spontaneous GH pulses can reach 50 ng per milliliter and are cleared rapidly with a half-life of about 20 minutes. Consequently, random GH levels can be very low or high. In addition, GH responses to GRF are highly variable even within an individual, probably reflecting variations in endogenous somatostatin tone.

GH acts through a single transmembrane receptor that is structurally related to prolactin and cytokine receptors (e.g., erythropoietin and colony-stimulating factors). This group of receptors associates with adaptor tyrosine kinases, one of which is referred to as JAK2 (Janus associated kinase 2). After GH stimulation, JAK2 is phosphorylated and initiates a signaling cascade. The GH molecule has two distinguishable receptor-binding domains that allow it to contact two separate receptor molecules to induce receptor dimerization. Mutations in the GH receptor cause GH resistance and severe growth retardation, a condition referred to as Laron-type dwarfism. GH levels are elevated and IGF-1 levels are low, reflecting the inability of the mutant receptor to transduce the GH signal.

Many of the growth and metabolic effects of GH are transmitted indirectly through the actions of IGF-1. GH stimulates IGF-1 production in most tissues, where it then exerts autocrine or paracrine effects. Circulating IGF-1 is derived predominantly from the liver and is a useful marker of GH action because it has a longer half-life and integrates the effects of GH pulses. Although IGF-1 levels are used in the diagnosis of acromegaly and to assess the integrity of the GH axis, it must be remembered that factors other than GH (e.g., malnutrition) can alter IGF-1 levels. IGF-1 acts via widely distributed receptors that are structurally related to insulin receptors. In addition to its growth-promoting and anabolic effects, IGF-1 also stimulates mitogenesis in many tissues.

GH has its major effects on linear growth but also influences a variety of metabolic pathways. Some of these effects are mediated by GH directly, whereas others are conferred by IGF-1. Although the relative roles of GH and IGF-1 are debated, their actions are cooperative in many cases. The effects of GH on linear growth appear to be mediated largely by IGF-1, which has been used to stimulate growth in patients with GH insensitivity syndrome. Linear growth in the fetus and neonate is not GH-dependent, as illustrated by the fact that GH-deficient babies have normal birth lengths. In contrast, normal postnatal linear growth requires GH, as illustrated by the clinical manifestations of GH deficiency. GH and IGF-1 act together to markedly accelerate linear growth, particularly at the time of puberty when sex steroids enhance GH and IGF-1 levels.

GH also induces lipolysis and stimulates anabolic activity, including amino acid uptake and protein synthesis. As a result, it reduces body fat, increases lean body mass, and leads to positive nitrogen balance. These properties of GH are most striking in GH-deficient children who have undergone replacement. GH opposes many of the actions of insulin and can be considered diabetogenic. In diabetics, nocturnal GH secretion accounts in part for the dawn phenomenon in which there is a decrease in glucose utilization, causing a tendency towards hyperglycemia.

GROWTH HORMONE DEFICIENCY (see also Ch. 201.1).
Causes of GH deficiency include hypothalamic disorders, GH gene mutations, combined pituitary hormone deficiencies, radiation, and psychosocial dwarfism (see Table 202–3). The clinical manifestations of GH deficiency depend upon the time of onset and the severity of hormone deficiency. Children with complete GH deficiency have slow linear growth rates (approximately 3 cm per

year), and they rapidly fall below normal on standardized growth charts. GH-deficient children have normal skeletal proportions, and many have a pudgy, youthful appearance because of decreased lipolysis. Particularly in the setting of cortisol deficiency, there is a predisposition to hypoglycemia.

Basal GH does not provide a reliable measure of GH reserve, whereas low IGF-1 levels are consistent with GH deficiency. GH deficiency is most frequently assessed using insulin-induced hypoglycemia, which activates CNS pathways, leading to stimulation of both GH and ACTH secretion (see Table 202–4). The insulin tolerance test requires careful monitoring for symptoms of severe hypoglycemia, such as confusion or depressed consciousness. This test should be avoided in patients with seizure disorders or coronary artery disease. Insulin doses (approximately 0.1 U per kilogram) may need to be decreased if glucocorticoid deficiency is suspected, or increased in conditions of insulin resistance (e.g., obesity). Alternatives to the insulin tolerance test for evaluation of GH include stimulation by L-dopa or arginine. Stimulation tests with GRF have not been well-standardized and appear to show substantial variation even within an individual, perhaps because of changing somatostatin tone.

In children with well-documented GH deficiency, GH replacement is effective and is essential to increase final adult height. In a typical regimen, recombinant GH (0.06 to 0.1 mg per kilogram) is given three times a week or daily as subcutaneous injections. The efficacy of GH treatment depends upon when it is initiated as well as replacement of other hormone deficiencies, if they coexist. In the setting of multiple hormone deficiencies, replacement of thyroid hormone and cortisol is necessary for effective GH action. On the other hand, sex steroids (estrogen in particular) lead to epiphyseal closure and limit linear growth. Consequently, GH is more effective before puberty; if exogenous sex steroids are given, low doses should be used. For unclear reasons, the effects of GH appear to wane after about 1 year of treatment. The potential role of GH replacement in adults is debated. Short-term studies show that it can increase lean body mass and improve the sense of well-being in adults with documented GH deficiency, but safety data for long-term GH administration are still lacking.

GROWTH HORMONE EXCESS: ACROMEGALY AND GIGANTISM. *Etiology and Pathogenesis.* GH-producing pituitary tumors involve the neoplastic proliferation of somatotrope cells and account for about 10 to 15% of pituitary tumors (see Table 202–6). GH-producing tumors are frequently mixed tumors that secrete more than one hormone. Prolactin is produced in the majority of somatotrope adenomas when evaluated by immunohistochemistry, and elevated serum levels of prolactin occur in about 25% of cases. A subset of these tumors are categorized morphologically as mammosomatotrope adenomas. Cosecretion of prolactin may predict a greater likelihood of response to treatment with bromocriptine. GH-producing tumors can also cosecrete glycoprotein hormones, most frequently the common α-subunit (approximately 10 to 30%), or rarely, TSH.

Considerable progress has been made concerning the cause of GH-producing pituitary tumors. Ectopic production of GRF (usually carcinoid or pancreatic islets) is a well-documented but rare (<1%) cause of acromegaly which can result in somatotrope hyperplasia. Gsα mutations occur in 35 to 40% of somatotrope adenomas. Molecular defects in the remaining 60 to 65% of somatotrope adenomas remain to be identified.

Clinical Features. GH-secreting tumors cause acromegaly in adults and gigantism in children in whom GH excess occurs before epiphyseal closure. The annual incidence of acromegaly has been estimated at about 3 per million. It affects men and women with equal frequency and is most often recognized when patients are in their 30's or 40's, usually after a decade of GH excess. The clinical features of acromegaly are summarized in Table 202–7. The most striking features of acromegaly usually involve the face, hands, and feet. The diagnosis is often suspected because of changes in facial appearance, including enlargement of the lower jaw (prognathism), the nose and lips, and the sinuses (causing frontal bossing) (Fig. 202–1). Oral cavity changes, including malocclusion, increased spacing between the teeth, and enlargement of the tongue, may lead to recognition of the disorder by dentists. A hollow, resonant voice is caused by changes in the vocal cords and the soft tissues of the hypopharynx. Sleep apnea can occur in patients with soft tissue obstruction of the pharynx. Few acromegalics wear rings because they

TABLE 202–7. CLINICAL FEATURES OF ACROMEGALY

Musculoskeletal
Acral enlargement of hands and feet
Prognathism
Frontal bossing
Arthritis/arthralgias
Carpal tunnel syndrome
Muscle weakness
Cutaneous
Increased skin folds (e.g., forehead)
Increased soft tissue thickness
Skin tags
Oily skin
Increased sweating
Acanthosis nigricans
Oral/dental (adjectival, as at)
Malocclusion
Increased spacing between teeth
Enlargement of tongue
Enlargement of lips
Reproductive
Decreased libido/impotence
Oligomenorrhea
Galactorrhea in women
Neuropsychiatric
Headaches
Visual field defects
Somnolence
Metabolic
Glucose intolerance or diabetes mellitus
Hypercalciuria
Hyperphosphatemia
Cardiopulmonary
Hypertension
Cardiac enlargement
Sleep apnea
Other
Goiter
Colonic polyps
Deep, resonant voice
Sinusitis
Generalized visceromegaly

have long since outgrown them, and they usually have a history of progressive increase in shoe size and width. In addition to bony enlargement, there is a marked increase in the soft tissue of the hands and feet. A moist, doughy, enveloping handshake is characteristic of acromegaly. Heel pad thickness (which can be assessed radiographically) correlates well with IGF-1 levels and other clinical features of the disease. Arthralgias (hands, feet, hips, knees) are common (approximately 75%) and are caused by cartilage and synovial overgrowth. Some degree of carpal tunnel syndrome is seen in about half of patients. Skin changes include increased skinfolds, particularly over the brow and forehead. The skin is usually oily owing to increased sebaceous activity and sweating. Skin tags are common, and the incidence of colonic polyps is increased. Galactorrhea may be seen in women and reproductive dysfunction occurs in both women and men. Headaches, visual field defects, and other neurologic symptoms depend upon the location and extent of tumor growth.

Acromegaly causes as much as a two- to three-fold increase in mortality. Most of the increased mortality can be attributed to cardiovascular and cerebrovascular diseases and may be related in part to the increased prevalence of hypertension (25 to 35%) and diabetes mellitus (10 to 25%) in acromegaly. There is evidence for cardiac hypertrophy in the majority of acromegalics, and symptomatic heart disease, consisting of coronary ischemia and/or congestive heart failure, occurs in 15 to 20% of patients. Sleep apnea may predispose patients to cardiac dysrhythmias. There is an increased risk of premalignant polyps and colon cancer in acromegaly, and screening with colonoscopy is generally recommended. The disfigurement, metabolic complications, and increased mortality associated with acromegaly emphasize the importance of early diagnosis and implementation of appropriate therapy to lower the GH levels into the normal range.

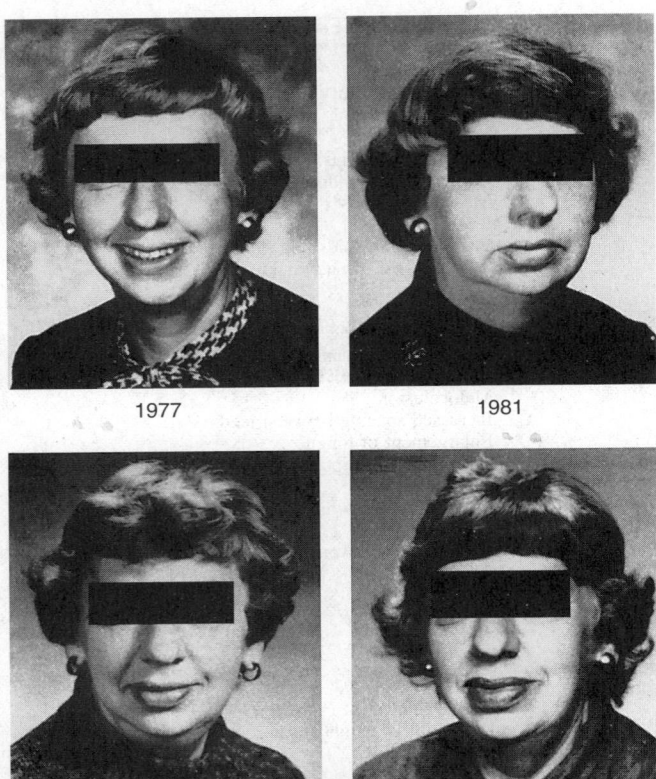

1977   1981

1983   1988

FIGURE 202–1. Clinical features of acromegaly. Serial photographs of a 64-year-old woman with acromegaly. Over an 11-year period, there is a progressive worsening of facial features, including enlargement of the nose and lips and development of prognathism. She also experienced hypertension, arthropathy, and enlargement of the hands. (Courtesy of Dr. Mark E. Molitch. Reprinted with permission from Molitch ME: Clinical manifestations of acromegaly. Endocrinol Metab Clin North Am 21:597,1992.)

Diagnosis. Because GH is secreted in a pulsatile manner and because the amplitude of GH pulses can be large (> 50 ng per milliliter), random GH levels are not very useful in making the diagnosis of acromegaly. IGF-1 levels provide an integrated index of GH production and provide a better screening test for acromegaly. IGF-1 levels are normally elevated during puberty and pregnancy and are suppressed during starvation. Otherwise, they correlate well with 24-hour GH production rates and with disease activity. The most reliable test for acromegaly is the glucose tolerance test (Table 202–8). In acromegaly, increased glucose levels fail to suppress GH below 2 ng per milliliter or cause a paradoxical increase in GH. More than half of patients with acromegaly exhibit a paradoxical stimulation of GH in response to TRH. Cosecretion of prolactin should be evaluated, and the common α-subunit of the glycoprotein hormones may provide an additional marker of tumor activity. After the diagnosis of acromegaly, radiologic studies, preferably using MRI, should be used to evaluate the extent of tumor growth. Unlike Cushing's disease and prolactinomas, the majority of patients with acromegaly have macroadenomas. In the absence of an apparent pituitary tumor, the possibility of ectopic GRF secretion causing somatotrope cell hyperplasia should be considered.

Therapy. The goals of therapy in acromegaly are to reverse or prevent tumor mass effects and to reduce the long-term morbidity and mortality that result from excess GH production. Correction of the disorder prevents further physical disfigurement and can result in substantial resolution of soft tissue changes and improvements in metabolic derangements. Although reductions in GH levels are associated with improvements in symptoms, the ultimate goal is to achieve normal GH and IGF-1 levels and to prevent tumor recurrence without incurring hypopituitarism.

Transsphenoidal surgery results in GH levels < 5 ng per milliliter in about 60% of patients with microadenomas. Not all of these patients are cured of their tumor when assessed by more stringent criteria, such as GH suppression below 2 ng per milliliter during an oral glucose tolerance test. Patients with macroadenomas are rarely cured by surgery (< 30%) but usually have reductions in GH levels.

Medical therapies for acromegaly include the somatostatin analogue octreotide and dopamine agonists such as bromocriptine. Responsiveness to both of these agents depends upon the presence and density of receptors on tumor cells. Octreotide reduces GH and IGF-1 levels in most patients and reduces tumor size in about half. Octreotide is useful as adjunctive therapy in patients who are not cured by surgery and/or radiation. There are also reports that preoperative treatment with octreotide can reduce tumor size and alter tumor consistency, thereby facilitating transsphenoidal resection. Although octreotide has a much longer half-life than somatostatin, it must be given in doses of 100 to 200 μg every 8 hours by subcutaneous injection to maintain GH suppression. Side effects include diarrhea and increased risk of cholelithiasis. Although bromocriptine was used extensively in early studies of medical therapy of acromegaly, it is less effective than octreotide in most patients and can require relatively high doses (up to 30 mg per day). However, some patients respond to bromocriptine but not octreotide, and it is also possible to combine the treatments.

Radiation is not recommended as primary therapy for acromegaly because of the length of time (5 to 10 years) required for reductions in GH levels and the high incidence of hypopituitarism. Adjunctive radiation therapy may be required for patients with macroadenomas when GH levels or mass effects persist after transsphenoidal surgery and medical therapy.

Ezzat S, Snyder PJ, Young WF, et al.: Octreotide treatment of acromegaly. A randomized, multicenter study. Ann Intern Med 117:711, 1992. *This large study shows that octreotide effectively decreases GH and IGF-1 concentrations in 53% and 68% of patients, respectively.*
Fahlbusch R, Honegger J, Buchfelder M: Surgical management of acromegaly. Endocrinol Metab Clin North Am 21:669, 1992. *Role of surgery in acromegaly.*
Melmed S: Acromegaly. N Engl J Med 322:966, 1990. *A review of the diagnosis and clinical management of acromegaly.*

PROLACTIN

Prolactin and GH are derived from a common ancestral gene, accounting for the similarities in structures and some overlap in functional properties. The prolactin gene is located on chromosome 6 and encodes a 198 amino acid protein (23-kD) that is produced in the lactotrope cells. Prolactin contains three intramolecular disulfide bonds, and high molecular variants are reported which may represent dimers or protein aggregates. Although the larger molecular weight forms of prolactin react in radioimmunoassays, they have diminished biologic potency. Prolactin is glycosylated to a small extent, but the role of the sugar chains is unclear. Estrogen stimulates lactotrope proliferation, and their number is consequently greater in women than in men and during pregnancy (approximately 70% of pituitary cells).

Prolactin secretion is controlled by tonic inhibition by dopamine, which acts through D_2-type receptors on lactotropes. Prolactin biosynthesis and secretion are stimulated by the hypothalamic peptides TRH and VIP. Hypothyroidism causes increased TRH output and can result in hyperprolactinemia. VIP, which acts via receptors that increase cAMP, may be responsible for prolactin increases associated with suckling. VIP is also found in the pituitary, where it may act as an autocrine or paracrine regulator of prolactin production. On balance, dopamine inhibition is the dominant influence for prolactin secretion. Prolactin is the one pituitary hormone that increases after pituitary stalk section. A variety of pharmacologic agents can stimulate prolactin secretion, in many cases by impairing dopamine secretion or action (Table 202–9).

Prolactin secretion is pulsatile and increases with sleep, stress, chest wall stimulation, and pregnancy. Prolactin levels are usually less than 15 to 20 ng per milliliter in women and 10 to 15 ng per milliliter in men. The primary function of prolactin is to induce and sustain lactation. However, prolactin binds to specific receptors that are located in several tissues, including breast, gonads, lymphoid cells, and liver. There are several different forms of prolactin receptors, which, like the GH receptor, are members of a cytokine family of receptors. During pregnancy, prolactin levels increase, and, in conjunction with other hormones (estrogens, progesterone, thyroid hormone, cortisol, and insulin), breast epithelium is stimu-

TABLE 202–8. SELECTED TESTS OF EXCESS PITUITARY FUNCTION

Hormone	Test	Interpretation
Growth hormone	*Basal IGF-1*	Elevated IGF-1 levels are consistent with acromegaly when interpreted in the context of age and nutritional status.
	Oral glucose suppression test: After 75-gm glucose load, GH is measured at −30, 0, 30, 60, 90, 120 min.	GH should be suppressed to <2 μg/L in normals. GH may paradoxically increase in acromegaly.
	TRH test: TRH (200 μg) is given IV with serum GH measurements at 0, 20, 60 min.	GH is not stimulated by TRH in most normals. A GH increase of 10 μg/L or $>50\%$ of baseline is consistent with acromegaly but can also occur in other disorders. The test is most useful for evaluating surgical cure.
Prolactin	*Basal prolactin levels*	Elevated prolactin (>200 μg/L) is consistent with a prolactinoma. When prolactin levels are between 20 and 100 μg/L, other causes of hyperprolactinemia should be considered.
ACTH	*Measurement of 24-hour urine free cortisol*	Elevated urine free cortisol is suggestive of Cushing's syndrome, but has several other causes as well.
	Overnight dexamethasone suppression test: Dexamethasone (1 mg) PO at midnight followed by 8 AM plasma cortisol.	AM cortisol should be suppressed to <5 μg/dL in normals. Normal dexamethasone suppression excludes Cushing's syndrome. Several other disorders can cause failure to suppress normally.
	Low-dose dexamethasone suppression test: Dexamethasone (0.5 mg) q6h for 8 doses with basal and end-of-treatment measurements that may include 24-hour urine collections for free cortisol or 17-hydroxysteroids and AM plasma cortisol and ACTH.	17-OH steroids should be suppressed to <4 mg/24h; urine free cortisol should be <20 μg/24h; serum cortisol should be suppressed to <6 μg/dl. Failure to suppress cortisol production is consistent with the diagnosis of Cushing's syndrome.
	High-dose dexamethasone suppression test: Dexamethasone (2 mg) q6h for 8 doses with basal and end-of-treatment measurements that may include 24-hour urine collections for free cortisol or 17-hydroxysteroids and AM plasma cortisol and ACTH.	The high-dose test is intended to distinguish Cushing's disease (pituitary adenoma), ectopic ACTH production, and adrenal adenoma. 50% suppression of 17-OH steroids or 90% suppression of urine free cortisol production is suggestive of Cushing's disease. Less than 50% suppression suggests ectopic ACTH or adrenal adenoma. Low ACTH levels are consistent with adrenal adenoma.
	CRH test: Ovine CRH (1 μg/kg) is administered IV, and ACTH and cortisol are drawn at −15, 0, 15, 30, 60, 90, and 120 min.	In Cushing's disease, there is usually a 50% increase in ACTH and 20% increase in cortisol. Adrenal adenoma is associated with suppressed ACTH. Ectopic ACTH is associated with high basal ACTH and cortisol levels that are not affected by CRH.
	Petrosal sinus ACTH sampling: The inferior petrosal sinus is catheterized, ideally bilaterally, and plasma ACTH is compared with simultaneous peripheral samples. The sampling can be done in conjunction with CRH stimulation.	In Cushing's disease, the ratio of ACTH in the petrosal sinus/periphery is at least 2. In ectopic ACTH, the ratio of petrosal sinus/peripheral level is <1.5.
TSH	*Basal thyroid function tests*	An inappropriately normal or elevated TSH in the setting of increased free thyroid hormone levels is consistent with a TSH-producing tumor or other causes of inappropriate TSH secretion.
	Free α-subunit level	Elevated free α-subunit levels associated with inappropriately elevated TSH are suggestive of a TSH-producing tumor.
FSH, LH	*Basal FSH, LH, testosterone*	Increased LH and testosterone levels in males are consistent with LH-secreting tumors. Elevated FSH and low-normal testosterone are suggestive of an FSH producing tumor if primary gonadal failure is not present. In females, assessment of excess hormone secretion is difficult because of changes during the menstrual cycle and at menopause.
	TRH test: TRH (200 μg) is given IV with measurements of serum FSH, LH, FSH β, and LH β subunits at 0, 20, 60 min.	Stimulation of LH, FSH, or their free β-subunits is suggestive of a gonadotropin-producing adenoma.

lated to proliferate and milk synthesis is induced. High levels of estrogen and progesterone inhibit lactation during pregnancy. The rapid decline in these steroids in the postpartum period permits lactation to occur. Neural pathways leading to the secretion of oxytocin provide the "let-down" reflex that induces lactation in response to suckling. Early in the postpartum period, prolactin secretion is stimulated by suckling, but this response becomes damped with time. Prolactin also suppresses gonadotropins, probably by a direct action on GnRH-secreting neurons. As a result, breastfeeding can suppress ovulation. The role of prolactin in other tissues is not well understood. High levels of prolactin are present in amniotic fluid, and it is produced in the decidual layer of the placenta.

PROLACTIN DEFICIENCY. Prolactin deficiency is rare and occurs primarily in the setting of combined hormone deficiencies. Prolactin levels at or below the limits of detection of radioimmunoassays and failure of prolactin to rise after TRH stimulation are consistent with the diagnosis. The only recognized consequence of prolactin deficiency is the absence of postpartum lactation. No effects on breast development or other tissues have been described in prolactin deficiency.

HYPERPROLACTINEMIA. *Etiology and Pathogenesis.* Hyperprolactinemia can occur as a consequence of pharmacologic alterations in the pathways that control prolactin secretion or of physiologic or metabolic effects on prolactin production and clearance or as a neoplastic condition (Table 202–9). Prolactinomas are neoplastic growths of lactotrope cells and are the most common type of pituitary adenoma (approximately 25 to 40%). Theories concerning the causes of prolactinomas have centered on hormonal stimuli that influence lactotrope growth and prolactin secretion. Estrogen is a potent stimulus for lactotrope proliferation. In rats, chronic estrogen exposure induces lactotrope hyperplasia and prolactinomas, but no clear association exists between estrogens (e.g., oral contraceptive use) and the incidence of prolactinomas in humans. It is possible that estrogen stimulates the growth of pre-existing prolactinomas, and this may account for the fact that some tumors appear to increase in size during pregnancy. Diminished dopamine tone results in increased prolactin but has not been

TABLE 202-9. DIFFERENTIAL DIAGNOSIS OF HYPERPROLACTINEMIA

Hypothalamic-pituitary disease
  Prolactinomas
  Acromegaly (somatomammotrope tumors)
  Pituitary tumors causing stalk compression
  Craniopharyngiomas and other hypothalamic neoplasms
  Metastatic tumors
  Infiltrative and inflammatory disorders
  Post-irradiation
  Empty sella syndrome
Drugs
  Dopamine antagonists (e.g., phenothiazines, butyrophenones, pimozide, domperidone, sulpiride, metoclopramide)
  Tricyclic antidepressants (e.g., imipramine, amitriptyline)
  Monoamine antihypertensives (e.g., methyldopa, reserpine)
  Verapamil
  Estrogens
  Opiates
  H_2 blockers (e.g., cimetidine)
Physiologic/metabolic
  Pregnancy
  Hypothyroidism
  Pseudocyesis
  Renal failure
  Cirrhosis
  Spinal cord lesions
  Chest wall or nipple stimulation
  Exercise, stress, sleep, sexual intercourse
Idiopathic

shown to cause prolactinomas. Prolactin secretory dynamics are generally restored to normal upon resection of prolactinomas, suggesting that an underlying hypothalamic abnormality is not present. Analyses of tumor DNA from a relatively small number of prolactinomas are consistent with a monoclonal origin, but molecular defects in prolactinomas have not been readily identified. Mutations in the *ras* oncogenes have been found in case reports but are not found in most prolactinomas.

Microprolactinomas constitute the great majority of tumors in premenopausal women. In contrast, macroadenomas are more commonly seen in men and postmenopausal women. The predominance of smaller tumors in premenopausal women may be accounted for by a bias of ascertainment, as elevated prolactin levels in this group lead to clinical manifestations (amenorrhea, galactorrhea, or infertility). Subclinical prolactinomas likely exist in men and many older women, as about 10% of individuals have prolactin-positive microadenomas in autopsy series.

Clinical Features. Hyperprolactinemia causes galactorrhea and oligomenorrhea in premenopausal women. Estrogen facilitates prolactin-induced galactorrhea, explaining why it is less common in postmenopausal women or in women with prolonged hypogonadism. Amenorrhea is primarily a consequence of prolactin suppression of GnRH, although prolactin may also have inhibitory effects at the level of the pituitary and the gonad. Amenorrhea is associated with infertility, and prolactin levels should be a routine part of the hormonal evaluation of infertility. Estrogen deficiency can cause decreased libido, vaginal dryness, and dyspareunia. Long-standing estrogen deficiency also leads to osteopenia in some women. A subset of patients have hirsutism and can exhibit elevations of adrenal androgens. Oral contraceptives may mask prolactin-induced oligomenorrhea that becomes apparent upon their discontinuation. In postmenopausal women, prolactinomas are often identified because of mass effects rather than because of their hormonal effects.

In men, hyperprolactinemia causes hypogonadism with suppressed LH and FSH levels and low testosterone levels. Hypogonadism causes diminished libido, impotence, and rarely gynecomastia or galactorrhea. Diminished libido may also reflect suppression of GnRH, as testosterone replacement is not as effective as suppression of hyperprolactinemia. Hyperprolactinemia is found in up to 5% of men being evaluated for sexual dysfunction.

Diagnosis. The four primary causes of hyperprolactinemia must be distinguished if the correct therapy is to be instituted: (1) physi-

ologic hyperprolactinemia; (2) pharmacologic hyperprolactinemia; (3) hypothalamic or pituitary stalk compression; and (4) prolactinoma (Table 202-9). With the exception of pregnancy and renal failure, physiologic causes of increased prolactin (e.g., transient pulses) result in minor elevations in prolactin (usually < 50 ng per milliliter) which may not be present upon repeat testing. Primary hypothyroidism should also be excluded as a cause of mild hyperprolactinemia. A careful drug history should be obtained in all patients with hyperprolactinemia because of the large number of agents that can stimulate prolactin secretion. Psychotropic medications, in particular, can increase prolactin either by reducing dopamine production or by blocking its action. In most cases, the degree of hyperprolactinemia caused by drugs is less than 100 ng per milliliter. A variety of suprasellar and parasellar mass lesions cause hyperprolactinemia (generally between 20 and 100 ng per milliliter) because of compression of the hypothalamus or pituitary stalk. Unless evidence is very good for physiologic or drug-induced hyperprolactinemia, patients with mild hyperprolactinemia should be evaluated with CT or MRI scans to distinguish between microprolactinomas and other large mass lesions that cause stalk compression. To a first approximation, prolactin levels correlate with tumor size. When no pituitary lesions are seen by radiographic studies and physiologic and pharmacologic causes of hyperprolactinemia cannot be identified, the diagnosis of idiopathic hyperprolactinemia is made. Idiopathic hyperprolactinemia may represent small microprolactinomas or altered hypothalamic regulation of prolactin secretion. Whether such patients should be treated depends upon the clinical effects of hyperprolactinemia. Like patients with microprolactinomas, few of these patients develop large tumors.

Therapy. The natural history of prolactinomas has been evaluated in several series. Although large prolactinomas clearly must evolve from smaller lesions, it is uncommon for microprolactinomas to progress to macroadenomas. When patients with microadenomas are followed without treatment over 3 to 5 years, prolactin levels decrease in 10 to 20% and increase in < 10% of patients. Decreased prolactin may occur because of spontaneous tumor infarction. Because of the slow rate of growth, it is reasonable to monitor patients with microprolactinomas without treatment unless the hyperprolactinemia is causing symptoms that warrant therapy.

When hyperprolactinemia causes hypogonadism, osteopenia, or infertility, a dopamine agonist such as bromocriptine is the therapy of choice. Dopamine agonists normalize prolactin levels and correct amenorrhea-galactorrhea in the majority of patients. They also reduce tumor size. Bromocriptine is usually started as a half tablet (1.25 mg) given at bedtime with a snack to avoid side effects (nausea, dizziness, somnolence, and nasal stuffiness). After adaptation to the drug, the dose can be increased gradually over several weeks. A typical final dose is 2.5 mg, two or three times a day with meals, but up to 30 mg per day may be required. The lowest effective dose should be used after achieving adequate suppression of prolactin levels. Unless spontaneous infarction of the tumor occurs, it is uncommon to be able to stop bromocriptine without recurrence of hyperprolactinemia. Some patients who cannot tolerate the side effects of bromocriptine may be able to take other dopamine agonists (e.g., pergolide). In some cases, prolactinomas appear resistant to bromocriptine, but it is important to ensure compliance and to be certain that the underlying lesion is a prolactinoma and not some other cause of hyperprolactinemia. In cases unresponsive to dopamine agonists, transsphenoidal surgery is the treatment of choice. Although initial remission rates (60 to 90%) for transsphenoidal surgery of microprolactinomas are good, long-term recurrence is seen in up to 50% of patients. Radiation therapy is not recommended for microprolactinomas because responses are slow and often incomplete and there is a high incidence of hypopituitarism.

Bromocriptine therapy for infertility or when there is a possibility of pregnancy deserves special consideration. Bromocriptine can induce ovulation in 80 to 90% of patients with hyperprolactinemia. Although bromocriptine has not been associated with congenital malformations or complications during pregnancy, most physicians and patients prefer to avoid its use during pregnancy if possible. A form of barrier contraception is usually recommended until two to three regular menstrual cycles have occurred. Subsequently, pregnancy can be confirmed if a menstrual period is missed, allowing discontinuation of bromocriptine. Less than 2% of patients with microadenomas but 15% of patients with macroadenomas develop symptoms of tumor enlargement (headaches, visual field defects) during pregnancy. If symptoms develop, radiologic studies should be performed. If there is evidence of visual field compromise or tumor growth, bromocriptine therapy should be restarted. Prolactin levels are not very useful because they are normally increased in pregnancy, and prolactin production by an enlarging tumor may not increase substantially. Because problems of tumor growth occur most often in patients with macroadenomas, consideration should be given to the option of transsphenoidal decompression before pregnancy in women with large tumors, as long as fertility can be preserved.

Macroprolactinomas also respond well to dopamine agonists. However, because the tumors are larger and produce greater amounts of prolactin, a longer period of treatment may be required for reduction of prolactin levels. Reversal of hypogonadism can require 3 to 6 months. Visual field defects are a very sensitive index of tumor size, and improvements can be seen in about 90% of patients. A significant reduction in tumor size (approximately 50%) is seen in about half of patients assessed by radiologic studies. Thus, it is reasonable to use bromocriptine as a first-line therapy even in patients with visual field defects as long as visual acuity is not threatened by rapid progression or recent tumor hemorrhage. Bromocriptine doses should be advanced (up to 20 to 30 mg per day) until prolactin levels reach the normal range or a plateau. After prolonged treatment, it is usually possible to reduce the dose of bromocriptine. However, discontinuation of bromocriptine is not recommended for macroadenomas because rapid regrowth of the tumor can occur. Surgery results in remission of macroprolactinomas in <40% of patients and should be reserved for those who do not respond to dopamine agonists. Radiation therapy can be used as an adjunctive measure in patients with large, aggressive tumors that are inadequately controlled by treatment with dopamine agonists and surgical decompression.

Klibanski A, Biller BM, Rosenthal DI, et al.: Effects of prolactin and estrogen deficiency in amenorrheic bone loss. J Clin Endocrinol Metab 67:124, 1988. *This study suggests that estrogen deficiency and amenorrhea associated with hyperprolactinemia reflect a greater risk of developing osteopenia.*
Molitch ME: Management of prolactinomas. Annu Rev Med 40:225, 1989. *A concise and practical summary of the management of prolactinomas.*
Molitch ME: Pregnancy and the hyperprolactinemic woman. N Engl J Med 312:1364, 1985. *A balanced and well-referenced review of issues pertaining to hyperprolactinemia and pregnancy.*
Schlechte J, Dolan K, Sherman B, et al.: The natural history of untreated hyperprolactinemia: A prospective analysis. J Clin Endocrinol Metab 68:412, 1989. *A long-term prospective study of the natural history of hyperprolactinemia in 30 women.*

ACTH (see also Ch. 204)

ACTH is a 39 amino acid peptide that is derived from a precursor polypeptide, pro-opiomelanocortin (POMC). In the anterior pituitary, POMC (241 aa) encodes several peptides, including an aminoterminal peptide, joining peptide, ACTH, and β-lipotropin. The functional roles of the POMC-encoded peptides other than ACTH have not been fully defined. β-lipotropin, in addition to ACTH, may stimulate melanocytes and contribute to hyperpigmentation in conditions of POMC stimulation. β-lipotropin can be processed further to yield γ-lipotropin and β-endorphin. The biologically active portion of ACTH resides within the first 18 of its 39 amino acids. However, because a synthetic peptide (cosyntropin) that includes the first 24 amino acids has a longer half-life, it is used clinically to assess adrenocortical function.

The half-life of ACTH is relatively short (< 10 min), and pulses of ACTH secretion are discrete. Levels of precursor peptides, such as β-LPH, do not always parallel those of ACTH because of their slower clearance rates. β-LPH, but not ACTH, is also elevated in renal failure. In neoplastic conditions, particularly ectopic production of ACTH, the levels of precursor peptides or their processed products may be elevated. The POMC gene can also be expressed from alternate transcription start sites, giving rise to aberrant POMC transcripts in ectopic tumors.

The primary effect of ACTH is to stimulate the adrenal gland to produce cortisol. It also stimulates secretion of adrenal androgens and mineralocorticoids, although production of mineralocorticoids is controlled primarily through non–ACTH-dependent mechanisms (see Ch. 204). Consequently, mineralocorticoid function is preserved in ACTH deficiency, in contrast to primary adrenal insufficiency, which is characterized by loss of glucocorticoid and mineralocorticoid function.

ACTH binds to a high-affinity receptor that is a member of the seven-transmembrane class of receptors that are coupled to G pro-

teins. ACTH acts as a trophic hormone and stimulates the immediate secretion of cortisol and other adrenal steroids. Long-term stimulation by ACTH causes adrenal hyperplasia and enlargement. On the other hand, ACTH deficiency leads to adrenal atrophy, and several days of ACTH stimulation are required before steroid synthesis returns to normal.

The secretion of ACTH is regulated by the hypothalamic-pituitary-adrenal (HPA) axis. Hypothalamic corticotropin-releasing hormone (CRH) is the most important stimulator of ACTH secretion. CRH is a 41 amino acid peptide that is produced in the paraventricular nucleus of the hypothalamus and in other sites in the nervous system and peripheral tissues (see Ch. 201.1). The CRH receptor is structurally related to the calcitonin/VIP/GRF subfamily of seven-membrane spanning, G protein–coupled receptors. CRH stimulates cAMP production and increases POMC gene transcription as well as ACTH secretion. Chronic stimulation by CRH also causes corticotrope cell hyperplasia, which can be seen in cases of ectopic CRH production.

Arginine vasopressin (AVP) weakly stimulates ACTH when given alone, but it acts synergistically when administered with CRH. Several other hypothalamic factors (angiotensin II, VIP, gastrin-releasing peptide, catecholamines) also enhance ACTH secretion, either by stimulating CRH or by acting at the level of the pituitary gland.

ACTH secretion is inhibited by glucocorticoids, which act at both the hypothalamic and pituitary levels. Cortisol inhibits POMC gene transcription by binding to glucocorticoid receptors that interact with negative glucocorticoid response elements (nGREs) in the POMC promoter. Cortisol also inhibits ACTH secretion and blunts the ACTH response to CRH. Consequently, ACTH responses to CRH stimulation tests depend upon ambient concentrations of cortisol and are most robust at night when cortisol levels are low. Cortisol inhibits CRH production and may also act at higher CNS levels. After prolonged glucocorticoid suppression of the HPA axis, the amount of endogenous CRH secretion appears to be rate-limiting and can require several months to recover.

Plasma ACTH is secreted in discrete pulses (10 to 80 pg per milliliter) that occur about once an hour. Because of the marked variation in ACTH levels, random measurements are of little value, and most clinical tests are therefore based upon cortisol or its metabolites, which tend to integrate the effects of ACTH. ACTH secretion exhibits a marked diurnal rhythm, being greatest at night several hours after the initiation of sleep. Cortisol levels are greatest in the early morning and reach a nadir in the late afternoon and evening. Patients with Cushing's disease lose or exhibit a blunted diurnal rhythm of ACTH secretion. ACTH secretion can be stimulated by a variety of different forms of stress, including psychological stimuli such as fright, anticipation of athletic competition, or surgery. Depression is associated with activation of the HPA axis and impairs dexamethasone suppressibility. Hypoglycemia induces ACTH secretion, probably through a central mechanism. The resulting increase in cortisol secretion represents one of several counterregulatory mechanisms that increase glucose production. Insulin-induced hypoglycemia provides a mechanism for testing the integrity of the HPA axis (see Table 202–4). Serious trauma and infection activate an array of cytokines that stimulate CRH and ACTH secretion. Because cortisol levels are often increased up to 10-fold in these circumstances, similar adjustments in cortisol replacement doses may be required in seriously ill patients with adrenal insufficiency.

ACTH DEFICIENCY: SECONDARY HYPOCORTISOLISM. Secondary hypocortisolism causes symptoms of glucocorticoid deficiency, including nausea, vomiting, weakness, fatigue, fever, and hypotension. In addition to reduced levels of cortisol, laboratory tests can detect hyponatremia, hypoglycemia, and eosinophilia. Depending upon its cause, the severity of cortisol deficiency in secondary adrenal insufficiency is often not as marked as in primary adrenal insufficiency. In addition, mineralocorticoid function is preserved in secondary adrenal deficiency. Consequently, the clinical manifestations of volume depletion are less pronounced and hyperkalemia is not a feature of ACTH deficiency. Because ACTH levels are low in secondary adrenal insufficiency, hyperpigmentation is not seen as in primary adrenal insufficiency. In women, reduced adrenal androgens can decrease libido and cause loss of axillary and pubic hair.

The most common cause of ACTH deficiency is treatment with exogenous glucocorticoids, which cause suppression of the HPA axis. Sudden withdrawal of glucocorticoids or an increased requirement induced by the superimposition of severe illness can elicit symptoms of glucocorticoid deficiency. Congenital forms of ACTH deficiency are rare and usually occur in combination with the loss of other pituitary hormones.

ACTH reserve is most often evaluated using CRH or the insulin tolerance test. Caution should be exercised before inducing hypoglycemia in patients with suspected adrenal insufficiency. Insulin-induced hypoglycemia stimulates central responses to neuroglycopenia and mimics some, but not all, stresses that activate ACTH secretion. CRH testing (ovine CRH, 1 μg per kilogram IV) is also useful for distinguishing hypothalamic and pituitary causes of ACTH deficiency, as it still induces an ACTH response in patients with hypothalamic dysfunction and blunted responses to hypoglycemia. The metyrapone test provides an alternative to the insulin tolerance test. Metyrapone inhibits cortisol production, resulting in stimulation of ACTH secretion and an increase in precursor adrenal steroids (e.g., 11-deoxycortisol). Patients should be monitored closely for evidence of adrenal insufficiency. The "short" and "long" ACTH stimulation tests have largely been replaced by more direct measurements of ACTH but can be used to demonstrate improvement in cortisol secretion with repeated infusions of ACTH. Incomplete or normal cortisol responses to the initial ACTH infusion do not exclude ACTH deficiency, as the adrenal may remain ACTH-responsive if ACTH deficiency is recent or incomplete.

ACTH deficiency is treated by replacement with glucocorticoids (see Table 202–5). Doses need to be individualized and are based largely on clinical criteria in which symptoms of glucocorticoid deficiency are balanced against features of glucocorticoid excess. Patients should wear MedicAlert tags and be instructed in the warning signs of cortisol deficiency, including nausea, vomiting, abdominal pain, low-grade fever, fatigue, and postural dizziness. Stress doses of steroids should be used during times of illness. Mineralocorticoid replacement is not usually required in patients with ACTH deficiency.

CUSHING'S DISEASE (see also Ch. 204). *Etiology and Pathogenesis.* Cushing's *disease* results from a pituitary neoplasm that causes excess production of ACTH. It is to be distinguished from a variety of other causes of Cushing's *syndrome* (glucocorticoid excess), which include adrenal causes of cortisol excess, ectopic production of ACTH, and physiologic states that result in overproduction of cortisol. Cushing's disease accounts for about 60 to 70% of cases of Cushing's syndrome. Approximately 10 to 15% of pituitary tumors secrete ACTH. For unknown reasons, Cushing's disease occurs about eight times more often in women than in men.

The cause of Cushing's disease has been the subject of a long-standing controversy. The observations that CRH stimulates corticotrope hyperplasia and that some patients with Cushing's disease have corticotrope hyperplasia when the pituitary is subjected to pathologic evaluation support the idea of a hypothalamic cause of Cushing's disease. This concept has been used to explain the frequent recurrence of Cushing's disease after apparent cure following transsphenoidal surgery. On the other hand, most ACTH-producing pituitary neoplasms, like other pituitary tumors, are monoclonal in origin. A primary defect in corticotrope cells is also supported by several clinical observations. First, most patients who undergo successful removal of a corticotrope adenoma exhibit suppression of the HPA axis after surgery, suggesting that CRH is low rather than high. Second, many patients with Cushing's disease respond to exogenous CRH, suggesting that endogenous CRH levels are not high. On balance, the great majority of cases of Cushing's disease likely arise from a primary defect at the level of the pituitary, with rare cases being caused by a hypothalamic disorder.

In contrast to other pituitary tumors, the great majority (80 to 90%) of ACTH-secreting tumors are microadenomas at the time of diagnosis. The clinical features of cortisol excess may allow detection of corticotrope adenomas before they have grown to a larger size. High levels of cortisol may also restrain tumor growth. ACTH-secreting macroadenomas tend to be locally invasive.

Clinical Features. The clinical features of Cushing's disease are caused by the effects of excess glucocorticoids and by the hypersecretion of ACTH and other POMC peptide products. The severity of the features of Cushing's disease varies greatly and ap-

pears to reflect not only the level of free cortisol, but also the duration of the disease and perhaps the sensitivity to glucocorticoid action. In florid cases of Cushing's disease (Fig. 202–2), the constellation of symptoms and physical features is readily recognized. However, early in the disease or in mild cases, it can be extremely challenging to distinguish the clinical features of Cushing's disease from similar traits that are seen in the normal population. Clinical suspicion is of paramount importance because it establishes the first screening test before embarking upon laboratory studies. On the

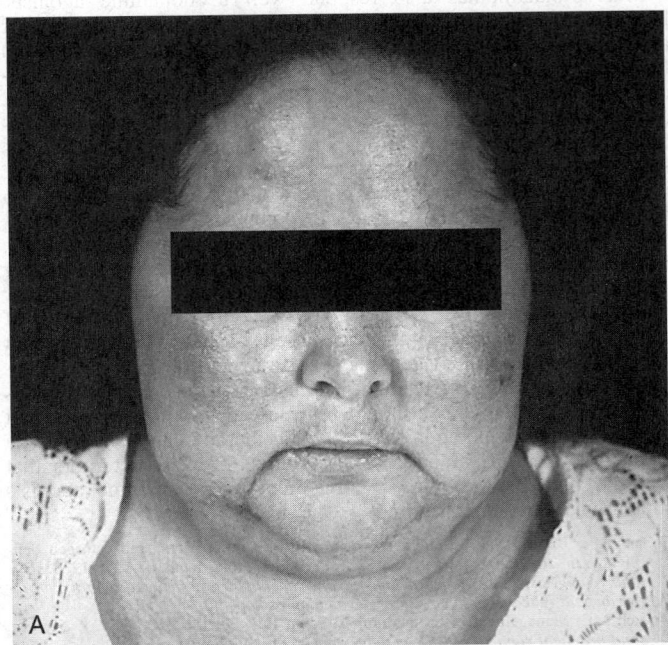

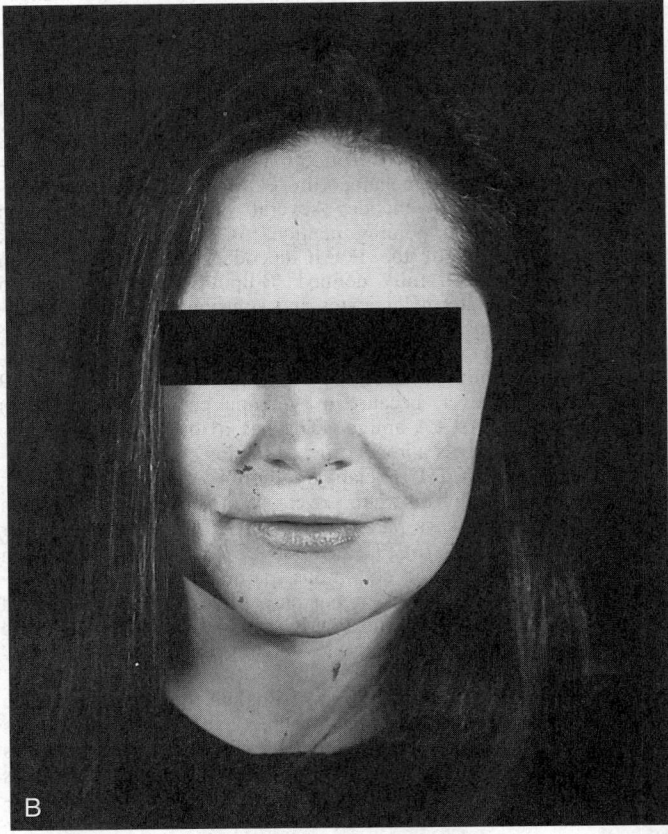

FIGURE 202–2. Clinical features of Cushing's disease. A 25-year-old woman with severe Cushing's disease. *A,* Facial features of Cushing's syndrome, including plethora, moon facies, and hirsutism, are evident. *B,* Dramatic resolution of the manifestations of cortisol excess after successful transsphenoidal surgery. (Courtesy of Dr. Beverly M. K. Biller.)

TABLE 202–10. CLINICAL FEATURES OF CUSHING'S DISEASE

General
- Obesity (centripetal distribution)
- "Moon facies" and mild proptosis
- Increased supraclavicular fat and "buffalo hump"
- Hypertension

Skin
- Hyperpigmentation
- Facial plethora
- Hirsutism
- Violaceous striae and thin skin
- Capillary fragility and easy bruising
- Acne
- Edema

Musculoskeletal
- Muscle weakness (proximal)
- Osteoporosis and back pain

Reproductive
- Decreased libido
- Oligomenorrhea

Neuropsychiatric
- Depression
- Irritability and emotional lability
- Psychosis

Metabolic
- Hypokalemia and alkalosis
- Hypercalciuria and renal stones
- Glucose intolerance or diabetes mellitus
- Impaired wound healing
- Impaired resistance to infection
- Granulocytosis and lymphopenia

Tumor mass effects
- Headache
- Visual field loss
- Hypopituitarism

other hand, one must be discriminating and not formally evaluate everyone with obesity, hypertension, and glucose intolerance. Of the many features listed in Table 202–10, some are relatively specific for Cushing's disease. For example, the centripetal distribution of fat with the characteristic "buffalo hump," "moon facies," and deposition in the supraclavicular area, with minimal fat in the extremities, is much more specific than generalized obesity. Striae that are wide (>1 cm) and purple in color reflect steroid-induced thinning of the dermis and can be distinguished from the more common "stretch marks." Numerous spontaneous ecchymoses also occur because of thinning of the skin and capillary fragility. Proximal muscle weakness represents another relatively specific manifestation of glucocorticoid excess. Osteopenia and hypokalemia, when present, provide objective evidence consistent with ACTH excess. Hypokalemia results from the effects of ACTH on mineralocorticoid production and from the ability of high levels of cortisol to saturate 11β-dehydrogenase, an enzyme in the kidney that inactivates cortisol. As a result, cortisol can "spill over" and act on mineralocorticoid receptors in the distal tubule. The hyperpigmentation associated with Cushing's disease is not as striking as that in Addison's disease or ectopic ACTH syndrome, but in association with other findings, it should raise the suspicion of Cushing's disease and helps to distinguish it from adrenal causes of hypercortisolemia. Hirsutism and acne are caused by the increased production of adrenal androgens and are more prominent in Cushing's disease than in hypercortisolism caused by adrenal adenomas, in which glucocorticoids tend to be the predominant product. Oligomenorrhea probably has several causes, including androgen effects on the reproductive axis and glucocorticoid inhibition of GnRH, which may

also account for diminished libido. Hypertension and glucose intolerance are caused by glucocorticoid excess. Immune suppression, opportunistic infections, and impaired wound healing can lead to considerable morbidity. Neuropsychiatric symptoms, including depression, can be prominent effects of Cushing's disease. Suicide occurs with increased frequency in untreated Cushing's disease.

Diagnosis. The screening tests and differential diagnosis of Cushing's syndrome represent one of the greatest diagnostic challenges in endocrinology (see Ch. 204). In most cases, the complete evaluation of Cushing's syndrome can take place in the outpatient setting. The first step is to determine whether a patient truly has cortisol excess. After confirmation of Cushing's syndrome, one must distinguish among (1) adrenal causes of cortisol excess, (2) pituitary causes of ACTH excess (Cushing's disease), and (3) ectopic sources of ACTH (Table 202–11).

In screening for hypercortisolism, random cortisol levels are not useful because of diurnal variation of the hormone. The overnight dexamethasone test is the most widely used screening test (see Table 202–8). A normal dexamethasone test essentially excludes Cushing's syndrome. It should be noted, however, that abnormal overnight dexamethasone suppression can be seen in up to 30% of hospitalized patients and in many patients with depression. An elevated 24-hour urine free cortisol (UFC) provides an alternative or additional screening test for hypercortisolism. Often, two sequential specimens are collected because of day-to-day variations in hormone production. The sensitivity and specificity of UFC measurements are greater than those of the overnight dexamethasone suppression test, particularly in hospitalized patients.

After demonstrating that cortisol excess is present, the next step is to determine the source of excess ACTH or cortisol. The classic approach is to perform a low-dose, followed by a high-dose dexamethasone suppression test (see Tables 202–8 and 202–11). The low-dose dexamethasone test excludes or confirms the presence of Cushing's syndrome. On the second day of the test, normal individuals suppress plasma cortisol to <5 μg per deciliter and reduce the 17-hydroxysteroids to <2.5 mg per 24 hours or UFC to <20 μg per 24 hours. All forms of Cushing's syndrome fail to suppress according to these criteria.

The high-dose dexamethasone test is one of several means to distinguish ACTH-independent and ACTH-dependent causes of Cushing's syndrome and to discriminate between pituitary and ectopic causes of ACTH-dependent Cushing's syndrome (Table 202–11). Because adrenal sources of cortisol excess are autonomous and ACTH-independent, plasma and urinary cortisol levels are not affected by dexamethasone suppression, even at high doses. In addition, plasma ACTH levels are low in adrenal causes of Cushing's syndrome because the hypothalamic-pituitary axis is suppressed. Pituitary and ectopic causes of Cushing's syndrome are both ACTH-dependent but respond differently to high-dose dexamethasone. Pituitary adenomas have an altered set point for glucocorticoid inhibition but retain a partial ability to respond to high-dose dexamethasone. The exact criteria for dexamethasone suppression in the high-dose test are debated. In most cases of ACTH-producing pituitary adenomas, 17-hydroxysteroids are suppressed to $<50\%$ of baseline, and UFC is suppressed below 90% of baseline during the high-dose dexamethasone test.

The ectopic ACTH syndrome should be suspected in patients with known malignancies, particularly oat cell carcinoma, bronchial, thymic, or gastrointestinal carcinoids, islet cell tumors, medullary carcinoma of the thyroid, and others. Plasma ACTH levels are often very high (>200 pg per milliliter) and can be associated with hyperpigmentation. Clinical features of Cushing's syn-

TABLE 202–11. TESTS USED IN THE DIFFERENTIAL DIAGNOSIS OF CUSHING'S SYNDROME

Etiology	Overnight Dex test	Plasma ACTH	Low-dose Dex	High-dose Dex	CRH stimulation of ACTH	Petrosal/Peripheral ACTH Ratio
Normal	Suppression	Normal	Suppression		Normal	
Pituitary	No suppression	Normal or high	No suppression	Suppression	Normal or increased	>2
Ectopic	No suppression	High or normal	No suppression	No suppression	No response	<1.5
Adrenal	No suppression	Low	No suppression	No suppression	No response	<1.5

Classic responses are indicated. Certain cases of ectopic ACTH production are suppressed by high-dose dexamethasone (Dex) or are stimulated by CRH. In these cases, petrosal sinus sampling is the most reliable method for distinguishing pituitary and ectopic sources of ACTH.

drome may be altered by the rapid onset of extreme hypercortisolemia. Pronounced weakness, fluid retention, glucose intolerance, and poor skin integrity are often seen and can exacerbate problems associated with underlying tumors. Hypokalemia is more common than in other forms of Cushing's syndrome.

Ectopic ACTH syndrome is readily recognized in its classic form. However, a subset of tumors, particularly carcinoids, exhibit dexamethasone suppression similar to that seen with pituitary adenomas. When suspected, carcinoids can sometimes be detected by CT or MRI, but many are too small to be seen even with these techniques. Because of these exceptions to the high-dose dexamethasone test, a variety of procedures have been devised in an attempt to further distinguish ectopic and pituitary-dependent sources of ACTH. The metyrapone test takes advantage of the fact that inhibition of 11β-hydroxylase blocks cortisol production. As a result, negative feedback is reduced and pituitary-dependent sources of ACTH typically exhibit an increase in ACTH, which stimulates the production of precursor adrenal steroids (e.g., 11-deoxycortisol) (see Table 202–4). Although most ectopic causes of ACTH exhibit a blunted response to the decreased cortisol levels, the subset of ectopic tumors that respond atypically to dexamethasone are most likely to give a positive response in the metyrapone test.

In recent years, inferior petrosal sinus sampling has been used to distinguish pituitary and ectopic sources of ACTH when the source of ACTH is not obvious based upon the clinical circumstances or imaging studies. This test requires an experienced radiologist for safe and effective catheterization of the petrosal sinus (which drains the pituitary venous effluent). Blood samples are taken simultaneously from the left and right petrosal sinuses and from the periphery. In the case of ACTH-producing pituitary adenomas, there is a gradient in ACTH levels between the central and peripheral blood specimens. Administration of CRH stimulates ACTH and tends to enhance the gradient. A gradient of 2:1 (central:peripheral) on either the left or the right is consistent with a pituitary source of ACTH. After clinical or biochemical studies suggest the presence of a pituitary adenoma, pituitary imaging should be performed using CT or MRI. Most ACTH-secreting pituitary adenomas are small, and scans are normal in more than half of patients.

Therapy. The efficacy of transsphenoidal surgery for Cushing's disease is greatly aided by making the correct diagnosis preoperatively. In experienced hands, surgical cures of ACTH-producing microadenomas occur in about 75 to 95% of patients undergoing a first operation. As with other pituitary tumors, complete remissions with macroadenomas are much less common. In the event of surgical remission or cure, postoperative hypocortisolism is common because of suppression of the hypothalamic-pituitary axis. After coverage for steroid withdrawal in the postoperative period, cortisol replacement should be minimized to allow recovery of the HPA axis.

If transsphenoidal surgery is unsuccessful, reoperation may be indicated and can result in remission in up to 50% of patients. If transsphenoidal surgery cannot be performed or has failed, alternative forms of therapy should be used to prevent the long-term consequences of hypercortisolism. Pituitary irradiation is usually the second line of treatment for Cushing's disease. It is more efficacious in children and younger patients, but it has a slow therapeutic response, often requiring concomitant medical therapy. Bilateral adrenalectomy represents another alternative for patients with severe hypercortisolism following transsphenoidal surgery. It rapidly and effectively lowers cortisol levels but is associated with relatively high morbidity and mortality (as high as 5%) because of the associated metabolic and immune system alterations caused by hypercortisolism. After adrenalectomy, patients must be maintained on glucocorticoids and mineralocorticoids and are at risk for the development of Nelson's syndrome.

Medical therapy of Cushing's disease has its primary role in preparation for surgery or for control of hypercortisolism during the interval when radiation therapy is taking effect. Because most pituitary adenomas are responsive to changes in cortisol levels, they have a tendency to "escape" from adrenal blockade by producing higher levels of ACTH. Medical therapies include ketoconazole, metyrapone, aminoglutethimide, and mitotane (o,p'-DDD). Whether the glucocorticoid receptor antagonist RU486 has a role in the management of Cushing's syndrome remains to be established.

NELSON'S SYNDROME. Nelson's syndrome was initially described as the appearance of a pituitary adenoma after bilateral adrenalectomy. In addition to an enlarging pituitary mass, the syndrome is characterized by very high ACTH levels and hyperpigmentation. It is caused by a pre-existing ACTH-producing tumor that grows in the absence of feedback inhibition by high levels of glucocorticoids. The incidence of clinically significant Nelson's syndrome after adrenalectomy for Cushing's disease varies from 10 to 50% in different series. Patients with Cushing's disease who have undergone adrenalectomy should be followed with imaging studies and plasma ACTH levels, as tumors that cause Nelson's syndrome can be very aggressive. When there is evidence of mass effects or rapid growth, transsphenoidal surgery should be performed. Postoperative radiation therapy may provide additional benefit, although it appears to be less efficacious than in other ACTH-producing adenomas.

Kaye TB, Crapo L: The Cushing syndrome: An update on diagnostic tests. Ann Intern Med 112:434, 1990. *A critical review of the advantages and shortcomings of various tests used in the differential diagnosis of Cushing's syndrome.*

Mampalam TJ, Tyrrell JB, Wilson CB: Transsphenoidal microsurgery for Cushing disease. A report of 216 cases. Ann Intern Med 109:487, 1988. *A representative study of surgical results from a center with extensive experience.*

Oldfield EH, Doppman JL, Nieman LK, et al.: Petrosal sinus sampling with and without corticotropin-releasing hormone for the differential diagnosis of Cushing's syndrome. N Engl J Med 325:897, 1991. *This classic study shows that simultaneous bilateral sampling of plasma from the inferior petrosal sinuses, with the adjunctive use of CRH, distinguishes patients with Cushing's disease from those with ectopic adrenocorticotropin secretion.*

Schteingart DE: Cushing's syndrome. Endocrinol Metab Clin North Am 18:311, 1989. *This review emphasizes the therapeutic options for Cushing's disease.*

GONADOTROPINS (FSH AND LH)

The pituitary glycoprotein hormones include FSH, LH, and TSH. Chorionic gonadotropin (CG), which is structurally very similar to LH, is made in the placenta. Each of the glycoprotein hormones has a specific β-subunit that forms a noncovalent dimer with the common α-subunit. The α- and individual β-subunits are encoded by separate genes. The β-subunit genes are evolutionarily related and share a common gene structure as well as nucleotide and amino acid sequence homology. Similarities in the structures of the β-subunits account for their ability to form noncovalent dimers with the common α-subunit. The α- and β-subunits each undergo glycosylation, which is important for correct hormone folding, intracellular transport, and secretion. Glycosylation is also required for biologic activity, presumably because of effects on the tertiary structure of the hormones.

The half-life of LH (approximately 50 min) is shorter than that of FSH (approximately 220 min), accounting for the more rapid secretory dynamics of LH, even though both hormones are secreted together. Differences in FSH and LH sequences between the conserved cysteines provide distinct "determinant loops" that allow the hormones to bind to specific receptors. Receptor contacts are made by both the α- and β-subunits. The receptors for FSH and LH are also structurally related and are members of the G protein–coupled seven-transmembrane family. After binding to their receptors, LH and FSH stimulate cAMP production, phosphotidylinositol turnover, and mobilization of calcium.

The gonadotropins are involved in sexual differentiation, sex steroid production, and gametogenesis. The regulation and physiologic roles of gonadotropins are quite different in males and females. In males, receptors for FSH are located on Sertoli cells and seminiferous tubules, whereas LH receptors are located on Leydig cells in the testis. LH stimulates androgen production by the Leydig cells. FSH is involved primarily in sperm maturation in the seminiferous tubules. Thus, FSH and LH act together to induce spermatogenesis (see Ch. 209).

In females, ovarian FSH receptors are located on granulosa cells, where they induce enzymes involved in estrogen biosynthesis. LH receptors are located predominantly on thecal cells in the ovary and stimulate the production of ovarian androgens and steroid precursors that are transported to granulosa cells for aromatization to estrogens. The pattern of FSH and LH secretion during the menstrual cycle results in follicular recruitment and maturation (largely FSH-mediated), followed by ovulation (largely LH-mediated) and steroid production by the corpus luteum.

Gonadotropin secretion is regulated primarily by the hypothalamic decapeptide gonadotropin-releasing hormone (GnRH). The receptor for GnRH is a member of the G protein–coupled seven-transmembrane family of receptors. GnRH stimulates an immediate release of intracellular calcium, followed by a second phase of extracellular calcium influx. GnRH also activates phosphotidylinositol turnover, resulting in production of diacylglycerol (DAG) and inositol triphosphate (IP_3), which act together to stimulate the protein kinase C pathway. The gonadotrope cell is exquisitely sensitive to the pattern of GnRH stimulation. Continuous rather than pulsatile exposure to GnRH causes gonadotrope desensitization and suppression of LH and FSH. Gonadotrope sensitivity to GnRH is modulated by sex steroids and probably other hypothalamic peptides such as neuropeptide Y (NPY). Increased GnRH secretion in combination with a higher density of GnRH receptors and rising estradiol concentrations accounts in part for the dramatic release of gonadotropins that induces ovulation.

The hypothalamic-pituitary-gonadal (HPG) axis is activated during fetal development. However, during the first 2 years of life, LH and FSH levels fall and remain suppressed until puberty. The physiologic basis for gonadotropin suppression during early childhood is not well-understood but involves tonic inhibition of the GnRH pulse generator by the CNS, as the pituitary gland is still responsive to exogenous GnRH. Most theories hold that the onset of puberty reflects disinhibition of the pulse generator. Puberty occurs between ages 8 and 13 in girls and between ages 9 and 14 in boys. In the peripubertal period, sleep-associated bursts of LH secretion can first be detected at night. Subsequently, a gradual increase occurs in LH pulse frequency and amplitude, such that LH pulses are detected during the day and night.

In women, the pattern of GnRH pulse frequency varies across the menstrual cycle. The combination of GnRH stimulation with ovarian feedback regulation results in a complex orchestration of positive and negative hormonal signals that converge at the gonadotrope to regulate LH and FSH secretion. The typical 28-day menstrual cycle is divided into follicular and luteal phases that are separated by ovulation on day 14. Unlike chronic exposure to low concentrations of estrogens, which exert negative feedback regulation and inhibit GnRH, the increasing concentration of estrogen prior to the LH surge exerts positive feedback regulation that results in increased GnRH pulse frequency. Increased GnRH, in combination with increased gonadotrope sensitivity to GnRH, results in the LH/FSH surge. During the luteal phase, the gonadotropin pulse frequency is reduced. In addition to feedback regulation by steroids, ovarian peptides such as inhibin also play a role in control of the reproductive axis. Inhibin causes selective suppression of FSH without affecting LH secretion. A homodimer of inhibin β-subunits, referred to as activin, has opposite actions and selectively stimulates FSH. Circulating inhibin provides one of the negative feedback inputs that lead to FSH suppression as the follicle develops.

The perimenopause is characterized by a gradual cessation of ovarian function. After several years of menstrual cycles that are sometimes anovulatory or irregular, menses cease, thereby defining the menopause. Although there is considerable variation, menopause usually occurs at about age 50. At this point, ovarian follicles have been depleted, and the production of sex steroids changes such that there is minimal production of estrogen and progesterone, but ovarian androgens continue to be made, primarily by stromal cells. The chronic decline in estrogen and progesterone causes loss of feedback inhibition and a marked increase in LH and FSH levels.

In males, the regulation of the HPG axis is relatively constant. After early puberty, LH and FSH pulses occur about once an hour during the night and day. It is notable that there is considerable variation in LH pulse frequency among normal individuals. Because each pulse of LH stimulates testosterone secretion, one also observes pulses of testosterone following LH, although these pulses are muted somewhat by the presence of serum-binding proteins that delay clearance. Nevertheless, testosterone levels can drop below the "normal" range in individuals with slow LH pulse frequencies. Testosterone inhibits the hypothalamic-pituitary axis, although its actions are thought to be mediated, in part, by aromatization to estrogens. Much of the inhibition by gonadal steroids occurs at the hypothalamic level, but there is also evidence for weak inhibition of the gonadotrope at the level of the pituitary gland. The HPG axis in men, unlike that in women, remains intact with aging. However, a gradual decline in testosterone levels is associated with an increase in LH and FSH with aging.

HYPOGONADOTROPIC HYPOGONADISM. Clinical features of hypogonadotropic hypogonadism in women are due primar-

ily to estrogen deficiency and include breast atrophy, vaginal dryness, and diminished libido. Hot flushes are uncommon, in contrast to postmenopausal estrogen deficiency. In premenopausal women, normal menstrual cycles provide evidence for an intact HPG axis. LH and FSH levels should be increased in postmenopausal women. Hypogonadism in men causes decreased libido and sexual function. In men, low testosterone without elevation of LH and FSH is consistent with impaired hypothalamic-pituitary reserve. Because of the variability in circulating testosterone and gonadotropins, it is often necessary to evaluate these hormones on several occasions and at different times of the day. GnRH stimulation can distinguish hypothalamic and pituitary deficiency but may require multiple injections to prime the pituitary, if GnRH deficiency is longstanding.

In premenopausal women, preparations of estrogen and progestins should be used for hormonal replacement and to allow cyclical growth of the endometrium. Pulsatile GnRH (for GnRH-deficient subjects) or gonadotropins can be given to induce ovulation and fertility when desired. Testosterone can be replaced in men using intramuscular injections that are given at 2- to 4-week intervals. Doses and the intervals between injections should be adjusted on an individual basis, using libido and testosterone levels before the next injection as a guide. Oral preparations of androgens should be avoided because of hepatotoxicity. Transdermal preparations are also available, but there is less experience with their long-term acceptance and efficacy. Induction of spermatogenesis requires pulsatile GnRH (for GnRH-deficient subjects) or injections of gonadotropins.

A congenital form of hypogonadotropic hypogonadism is caused by deficiency of GnRH, which in turn causes deficiencies of LH and FSH. When associated with anosmia (absent sense of smell), the condition is referred to as Kallmann's syndrome. A gene defect that causes Kallmann's syndrome has been defined. The so-called KAL gene is located on the tip of the short arm of the X-chromosome and encodes a protein that is proposed to play a critical role in migration of the GnRH-producing neurons during development. Pulsatile GnRH has been used to induce puberty and fertility in both males and females with Kallmann's syndrome.

Secondary hypogonadotropic hypogonadism is relatively common. In most cases it is reversible and is caused by weight loss, anorexia nervosa, stress, heavy exercise, or severe illness. Reversible forms of secondary hypogonadotropic hypogonadism are caused by GnRH deficiency and are more common in women than men. The condition is ideally treated by correcting the underlying cause. Many women have a discrete threshold for weight or exercise level that causes loss of menstrual periods. When it is not possible to correct the underlying abnormality, hormonal replacement can be used in women for protection against osteopenia and to cycle the endometrium.

A variety of pathologic conditions can cause secondary hypogonadotropic hypogonadism, often in association with deficiencies of other pituitary hormones (see Table 202–3). These include hypothalamic lesions or CNS radiation therapy. Pituitary tumors can suppress gonadotropins because of stalk compression and disruption of pulsatile GnRH input as well as by direct destruction of normal pituitary tissue. Hyperprolactinemia can suppress GnRH and lead to reduced gonadotropin levels. In contrast to the aforementioned causes of hypogonadotropic hypogonadism, which result from GnRH deficiency, primary deficiencies of LH and FSH are uncommon. An acquired form of isolated gonadotrope deficiency is rarely encountered and may have an autoimmune basis. Mutations in the LH-β or FSH-β genes have been described in case reports and cause selective loss of individual gonadotropins.

FSH- AND LH-PRODUCING TUMORS. *Etiology and Pathogenesis.* Although most early series suggested that gonadotropin-producing adenomas were relatively uncommon, recent studies using sensitive techniques to characterize tumor phenotype show a prevalence (10 to 15%) that is similar to that of corticotrope or somatotrope adenomas (see Table 202–6). The majority (70 to 80%) of pituitary tumors classified previously as nonfunctioning adenomas can be shown to produce low levels of intact glycoprotein hormones or their uncombined α- or β-subunits. Biosynthetic defects in the tumor cells account for relatively inefficient hormone secretion as well as the propensity to produce uncombined subunits.

FSH is produced more commonly than LH. Elevated levels of free α-subunits are seen more often than increased free β-subunits.

Clinical Features. Gonadotropin-producing tumors are somewhat more common in men than women and increase in prevalence with age. FSH- and LH-producing tumors do not usually cause a characteristic hormone excess syndrome. The tumors are typically large macroadenomas and present as clinically nonfunctioning tumors with symptoms and signs related to local mass effects. Visual field loss due to suprasellar extension and compression of the optic chiasm is found in >70% of patients. Many of these tumors are detected incidentally by CT and MRI scans performed for unrelated indications. Symptoms of hypopituitarism, including hypogonadism with loss of libido, are also common. Men with predominantly FSH-secreting tumors can paradoxically present with hypogonadal features that are related to low levels of testosterone. These patients must be distinguished from those with primary hypogonadism who have testicular dysfunction. Tumors that primarily secrete LH are rare but can cause increased testosterone levels. Premenopausal women with gonadotropin-producing tumors may experience menstrual irregularity or secondary hypogonadism. Postmenopausal women often show reduced gonadotropin levels because the mass effects of the gonadotropin-producing tumors cause stalk compression, impairing GnRH stimulation of gonadotropins from both normal and pituitary tumor cells.

Diagnosis. Because of the absence of a clinical syndrome in most patients, the preoperative diagnosis of gonadotropin-producing pituitary tumors has relied on imaging studies and laboratory tests. Unfortunately, the laboratory diagnosis of gonadotropin-producing tumors is less than satisfactory. First, the tumors synthesize gonadotropins inefficiently, and hormone levels are usually not markedly elevated. Second, because the secretion of gonadotropins is pulsatile, random LH and FSH values are difficult to interpret. Furthermore, gonadotropin levels vary widely and are normally elevated in postmenopausal women. GnRH stimulation tests also do not clearly distinguish patients with gonadotropin-producing tumors from normals, and suppression tests have not proven useful. However, paradoxical responses to TRH have helped to identify gonadotropin-secreting tumors. In contrast to its effect in normals, TRH stimulates secretion of intact gonadotropins or the uncombined FSH and LH β-subunits in most patients with gonadotropin tumors. Once identified, the uncombined α- or β-subunits can serve as tumor markers and can be useful for monitoring responses to therapy.

Men with proven gonadotropin-producing tumors typically have high-normal or elevated FSH levels but low levels of testosterone. Elevated prolactin levels are commonly seen and are caused by tumor mass effects. It is important to distinguish this group from patients with true prolactinomas. As noted above, many women, including those in the postmenopausal group, have paradoxically low gonadotropin levels. Thus, the absence of elevated gonadotropins does not exclude the diagnosis of a gonadotropin-producing tumor.

The postoperative diagnosis of gonadotropin-producing tumors can be made based upon immunohistochemical analyses or using more sophisticated studies of gonadotropin gene expression. These types of analyses confirm that the great majority of clinically nonfunctioning tumors are composed of gonadotropin-producing cell types.

Treatment. Because the major symptoms of the gonadotropin-producing tumors are due to extrasellar extension and local mass effects, the main aim of treatment is reduction in the size of the tumor. Complete or partial reversal of visual field defects and hypopituitarism can be accomplished by surgery unless these have been longstanding. However, transsphenoidal surgery is rarely curative of this group of macroadenomas. Patients with significant residual tumor may benefit from radiation therapy, although there are no large series in which patients have been randomly allocated to treatment groups. Because most tumors are slow growing, one approach is to monitor tumor recurrence using visual fields and CT or MRI. If tumor markers such as free α- or β-subunit levels are available, they can be used alone or in conjunction with TRH testing to monitor tumor function. When follow-up studies show rapid tumor growth, repeat surgery and/or radiation therapy is indicated.

There has been great interest in medical therapies that might be useful as adjuncts to surgery or even as primary therapies in pa-

tients not requiring immediate decompression. The success of bromocriptine and somatostatin analogues in treating hormone over-secretion and tumor mass in prolactinomas and acromegaly has not been seen in most patients with gonadotropin-producing tumors, although exceptions have been described in selected patients. The efficacy of long-acting GnRH agonists or antagonists, which suppress LH and FSH in normal individuals, has also been examined. The GnRH agonists stimulate gonadotropin secretion from tumors without apparent desensitization and have not been useful. GnRH antagonists have been shown to suppress FSH levels in small series of patients, but it is not clear whether these agents will be useful for reducing tumor size, and this treatment remains experimental.

Daneshdoost L, Pavlou SN, Molitch ME, et al.: Inhibition of follicle-stimulating hormone secretion from gonadotroph adenomas by repetitive administration of a gonadotropin-releasing hormone antagonist. J Clin Endocrinol Metab 71:92, 1990. *Repetitive administration of Nal-Glu GnRH antagonist decreased FSH secretion by gonadotroph adenomas in four of five patients.*

Jameson JL, Klibanski A, Black PM, et al.: Glycoprotein hormone genes are expressed in clinically nonfunctioning pituitary adenomas. J Clin Invest 80:1472, 1987. *This study used measurements of mRNA expression to demonstrate that most clinically nonfunctioning pituitary tumors are derived from gonadotrope cells.*

Snyder PJ: Gonadotroph adenomas of the pituitary. Endocrinol Rev 6:552, 1985. *A good summary of the diagnosis and management of FSH- and LH-producing tumors.*

THYROID-STIMULATING HORMONE

Like the other glycoprotein hormones, TSH is a heterodimer composed of the common α-subunit and the unique TSH β-subunit. Both subunits are glycosylated, and the composition of carbohydrates is thought to alter the biologic activity of the hormone. TSH is produced in thyrotrope cells, which account for about 5% of pituitary cell types. TSH is measured by highly sensitive immunoradiometric assays that use antisera directed toward the TSH β-subunit. Normal levels of TSH range from 0.5 to 5.0 μU per milliliter. The detection limit for current TSH assays is <0.01 μU per milliliter, allowing measurement of suppressed TSH levels in hyperthyroidism.

TSH controls thyroid hormone (T_4 and T_3) synthesis and secretion from the thyroid gland. TSH receptors are members of the G protein–coupled seven-transmembrane family and are structurally related to LH and FSH receptors. TSH stimulates cAMP production, acts as a trophic hormone, and stimulates hormone biosynthesis in the thyroid. TSH secretion from the pituitary gland is regulated by the hypothalamic-pituitary-thyroid (HPT) axis. Hypothalamic thyrotropin-releasing hormone (TRH) is a tripeptide that stimulates TSH synthesis and secretion. TRH, acting through its G protein–coupled receptor, elicits phosphoinositol turnover and induces release of intracellular calcium followed by an influx of extracellular calcium. TSH secretion appears to be modulated by alterations in calcium flux, whereas biosynthesis may be controlled by activation of other pathways, such as protein kinase C. A variety of other hypothalamic hormones, including somatostatin and dopamine, can inhibit TSH secretion, but their role in normal physiology has not been clearly elucidated.

Thyroid hormones have an inhibitory effect on the production of TRH and TSH and comprise a powerful negative feedback loop in the HPT axis. The direct effects of thyroid hormone at the level of the pituitary gland are well-illustrated by TSH responses to TRH stimulation tests. In hypothyroidism, TSH responses to exogenous TRH are exaggerated. In hyperthyroidism, TSH responses to TRH are blunted or flat, indicating that the inhibitory effects of thyroid hormone override the stimulatory effects of TRH. Thyroid hormones act via nuclear receptors that function at the transcriptional level to suppress expression of the TRH gene as well as the α- and β-subunit genes of TSH. In hypothyroidism, expression of the TSH α and β genes is stimulated and hormone production is markedly enhanced.

TSH secretion is pulsatile, but the amplitude of the pulses is relatively small and does not create the difficulties that are encountered with measurements of other pituitary hormones. TSH levels are elevated in infants in the immediate postpartum period. Thereafter, thyroid function tests remain remarkably constant throughout life. There is a diurnal rhythm of TSH secretion with a small increase at night. Because of the integrated nature of the HPT axis, thyroid function tests are best interpreted when concentrations of TSH, free T_4, and free T_3 levels are known. Except in conditions of secondary hypothyroidism or TSH-secreting pituitary tumors, TSH levels provide an excellent screening test for thyroid dysfunction. In primary hypothyroidism, TSH levels are elevated, as TSH increases logarithmically in response to falling thyroid hormone levels (see Ch. 203). In hyperthyroidism, TSH is suppressed to levels below or near the detection limits of most sensitive assays.

CENTRAL HYPOTHYROIDISM. Central forms of hypothyroidism include secondary hypothyroidism, which is caused by TSH deficiency, and tertiary hypothyroidism, which is caused by TRH deficiency. Two different types of congenital TSH deficiency are caused by genetic mutations. One type involves the TSH β gene, in which several different types of have been described. The other involves mutations in Pit-1, which cause combined deficiencies of GH, Prl, and TSH. Central forms of hypothyroidism are often associated with other pituitary hormone deficiencies and usually there is no goiter because of low TSH levels. Suspicion of central hypothyroidism should prompt measurements of T_4, T_3, and TSH as well as other pituitary hormones. When TSH deficiency is documented, thyroid hormone is replaced using daily doses of L-thyroxine (0.05 to 0.15 mg per day). Because TSH cannot be used as an endpoint, one monitors serum levels of free T_4 and T_3.

Tests for TSH deficiency are best performed by analyzing free thyroxine levels in combination with TSH. Low free T_4 without elevated TSH is consistent with central hypothyroidism. Free T_4 measurements should be used rather than total T_4 to avoid confusion caused by TBG deficiency (which is suggested by high T_3 resin uptake tests). In some patients with hypothalamic disease, the TSH level is partially elevated in the presence of low free T_4, but the bioactivity of the TSH is reduced. Central forms of hypothyroidism must be distinguished from the sick-euthyroid condition (see Ch. 203). Laboratory tests in the sick-euthyroid syndrome progress through several phases but can include prolonged periods when both TSH and free thyroid hormone levels are low. It can be very difficult in these patients to unequivocally exclude central hypothyroidism. In addition to the clinical setting in which thyroid function tests are measured, the presence of normal thyroid function tests prior to the illness and the absence of known hypothalamic or pituitary disease make true central hypothyroidism unlikely. Increased levels of reverse T_3 are suggestive of sick-euthyroidism, and free T_4 and T_3 may be in the normal or low normal range in sick-euthyroid patients.

TSH-SECRETING TUMORS. *Etiology and Pathogenesis.* TSH-secreting tumors are rare and account for between 1 and 3% of pituitary tumors. Like gonadotropin-producing tumors, a subset of tumors classified as clinically nonfunctioning can be shown to produce TSH, often at subclinical levels. However, because TSH overproduction can cause hyperthyroidism, TSH-secreting tumors are more readily detected than FSH- and LH-producing tumors. As many as 30% of TSH-producing tumors are plurihormonal. Growth hormone and prolactin are co-secreted most often, perhaps reflecting a common cellular lineage for thyrotropes, somatotropes, and lactotropes. Longstanding severe hypothyroidism can cause thyrotrope hyperplasia and pituitary enlargement. However, these hyperplastic masses regress upon thyroid hormone replacement. Most true TSH-producing tumors are relatively autonomous and respond weakly, if at all, to TRH stimulation or thyroid hormone suppression.

Clinical Features. TSH-secreting tumors are usually macroadenomas by the time a diagnosis has been made. Consequently, many patients exhibit mass effects of the tumor as well as hyperthyroidism. The clinical features of TSH-secreting tumors resemble those of Graves' disease except that features of autoimmunity such as ophthalmopathy are absent. Circulating levels of T_4 and T_3 range widely but can be elevated as much as two- to threefold. Diffuse goiter is present in the majority of patients with TSH-producing tumors, and the 24-hour uptake of radioiodine is elevated.

Diagnosis. Because feedback inhibition of TSH is impaired in TSH-producing tumors, TSH levels are inappropriately elevated in the presence of high levels of T_4 and T_3. TSH levels produced by tumors range from the low-normal range to as high as 500 μU per milliliter, but most are minimally elevated. Using ultrasensitive TSH assays, it is now possible to detect nonsuppressed TSH levels without the need for TRH testing. Free α-subunit measurements can be very helpful in confirming the diagnosis of a TSH-secreting tumor. Most TSH-producing tumors (>80%) secrete excess free α-subunit. Thus, the diagnosis of a TSH-secreting tumor can usually be made by demonstrating that a hyperthyroid patient has a detectable serum TSH associated with excess secretion of the free α-

subunit and/or GH. The finding of a mass lesion on CT or MRI scan confirms the diagnosis. Several other causes of inappropriate TSH secretion should be considered, including resistance to thyroid hormone and familial dysalbuminemic hyperthyroxinemia and other disorders that alter serum thyroid hormone binding proteins.

Treatment. The goals are to treat the underlying TSH-secreting tumor and to correct the hyperthyroidism. Transsphenoidal surgery alone is rarely curative because of the large size of most tumors, but it can alleviate mass effects and lower TSH levels. As with other large pituitary tumors, adjunctive radiation therapy may be required to control tumor growth. Somatostatin analogues (e.g., octreotide) have been used as adjunctive medical therapy and decrease TSH and α-subunit levels in about 80% patients with TSH-secreting tumors, but consistent effects on tumor growth have not been demonstrated. Hyperthyroidism caused by TSH-secreting tumors can also be treated using antithyroid drugs or radioiodine.

Comi RJ, Gesundheit N, Murray L, et al.: Response of thyrotropin-secreting pituitary adenomas to a long-acting somatostatin analogue. N Engl J Med 317:12, 1987. *This study of five patients with TSH-secreting tumors shows that the somatostatin analogue SMS 201-995 can reduce hypersecretion of TSH.*

NULL CELL PITUITARY TUMORS. Null cell adenomas, or clinically nonfunctioning tumors, are variably defined depending upon the criteria used to analyze tumor cell phenotype. As noted above, the majority of clinically nonfunctioning adenomas can be shown to produce low levels of the free α-subunit, FSH, and, to a lesser degree, LH when analyzed by immunocytochemistry or for mRNA expression. A smaller fraction can be shown to produce low levels of other pituitary hormones, particularly ACTH or GH, that escaped detection by routine endocrine testing. Even with detailed analyses of hormone production, a subset (10 to 20%) of nonfunctioning adenomas do not appear to produce one of the major pituitary hormones.

The clinical features and management of null cell tumors are similar to those for gonadotropin-producing tumors. The major signs and symptoms result from tumor mass effects that cause visual field defects, headache and other neurologic symptoms, and hypopituitarism. Transsphenoidal surgery is the primary mode of treatment, with a goal of debulking the tumor to relieve mass effects. Because there are no serum tumor markers, patients must be followed by CT or MRI scans in conjunction with visual field tests.

202.2 Posterior Pituitary
Alan G. Robinson

ANATOMY AND HORMONE SYNTHESIS. The hormones of the posterior pituitary, vasopressin and oxytocin, are synthesized in specialized neurons, the magnocellular neurons, that are noted for their large size. In the hypothalamus the magnocellular neurons are clustered in the paired paraventricular nuclei and the paired supraoptic nuclei (Fig. 202–3). Vasopressin and oxytocin are also synthesized in parvicellular (small cell) neurons of the paraventricular nuclei, and vasopressin (but not oxytocin) is synthesized in the suprachiasmatic nucleus. Transcription of vasopressin and oxytocin mRNA and translation of vasopressin and oxytocin prohormone occur entirely in the cell bodies of hormone-specific neurons. The preprohormones are cleaved from the signal peptide in the endoplasmic reticulum, and the prohormones, pro-pressophysin and pro-oxyphysin, are packaged with processing enzymes into neurosecretory granules. In the magnocellular neurons the neurosecretory granules are transported via microtubules down the long axons that form the supraopticohypophyseal tract to terminate in axon terminals in the posterior pituitary. During transport the processing enzymes cleave pro-pressophysin to vasopressin (8 a.a.), vasopressin neurophysin (95 a.a.), and vasopressin glycopeptide (39 a.a.) (Fig. 202–4). Pro-oxyphysin is similarly cleaved to oxytocin and oxytocin neurophysin, but not glycopeptide. Within the neurosecretory granules, neurophysins form neurophysin/hormone complexes that stabilize the hormones. Crystallography demonstrates that tetramers of neurophysin form specific binding sites for five molecules of

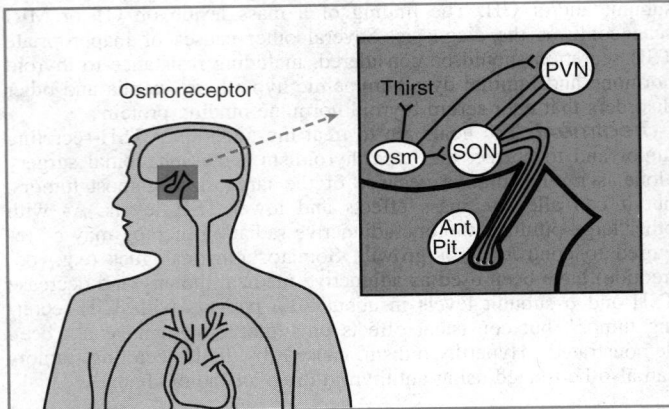

FIGURE 202–3. Sagittal view of the head demonstrating the position of the neurohypophysis. The magnocellular neurons are clustered in two paraventricular nuclei (PVN) and two supraoptic nuclei (SON). Only one nucleus of each pair is illustrated. The supraoptic nuclei are located lateral to the edge of the optic chiasm, while the paraventricular nuclei are central in the wall of the third ventricle. The osmostat and thirst center are located in the hypothalamus anterior to the third ventricle. The axons of the four nuclei combine to form the supraopticohypophyseal tract as they course through the pituitary stalk to their storage terminals in the posterior pituitary. (From Buonocore CM, Robinson AG: Diagnosis and management of diabetes insipidus during medical emergencies. Endocrinol Metab Clin North Am 22:411, 1993.)

hormone. Stimulatory (e.g., cholinergic and angiotensin) neurotransmitter terminals and inhibitory (e.g., γ-aminobutyric acid [GABA], noradrenergic, atrial natriuretic peptide [ANP]) neurotransmitter terminals control release of vasopressin by the activity of contacts on the cell body. Physiologic release of vasopressin and oxytocin into the general circulation is at the level of the posterior pituitary where, in response to an action potential, intracellular calcium is increased to cause the neurosecretory granules to fuse with the axon membrane to release (via exocytosis into the pericapillary) the entire contents of the granule. Once released, there is no further association of vasopressin with neurophysin, and each of the peptide products can be independently detected in the general circulation. Factors that stimulate the release of vasopressin also stimulate synthesis; however, whereas release is instantaneous, synthesis requires a longer time. This may explain the physiologic advantage of the large store of hormone in the posterior pituitary. In most species sufficient hormone is stored in the posterior pituitary to support maximum antidiuresis for several days and baseline levels of antidiuresis for weeks without synthesis of new hormone.

The axons of the parvicellular neurons of the paraventricular nuclei terminate in the median eminence of the basal hypothalamus where, similar to other hypothalamic releasing factors, the hormones are secreted into the portal capillary system and serve as regulators of secretion of adrenocorticotropic hormone (ACTH). Yet other axons secrete hormone into the cerebrospinal fluid of the third ventricle, where the function is unknown.

SECRETION. *Vasopressin and Regulation of Osmolality.* The primary physiologic action of vasopressin is its function as a water-retaining hormone. The central sensing system (osmostat) for control of release of vasopressin is located in a small area of the hypothalamus just anterior to the third ventricle (Fig. 202–3). The osmostat controls release of vasopressin to cause water retention and acts also in stimulation of thirst to cause water repletion. Osmotic regulation of vasopressin release and osmotic regulation of thirst are usually tightly coupled, but experimental lesions and some pathologic situations in humans demonstrate that the regulation can be independent. The primary extracellular osmolyte to which the osmoreceptor responds is sodium. Glucose and urea under normal physiologic conditions readily traverse neuron membranes and do not affect the release of vasopressin. Although the osmolality among normal subjects is between 278 and 294 mOsm per kilogram of water, for each person extracellular fluid osmolality is maintained in a narrow range. An increase in plasma osmolality as little as 1% will stimulate the osmoreceptors to cause release of vaso-

pressin. Basal levels of vasopressin are 0.5 to 2 pg per milliliter, which will maintain urine osmolality above plasma osmolality and urine volume at less than 2 liters per day. With increases in plasma osmolality, there is a linear increase in plasma vasopressin and a linear increase in urine osmolality as illustrated in Figure 202–5. At plasma osmolality of about 294 mOsm per kilogram of water, urine osmolality is maximally concentrated at about 1200 mOsm per kilogram. Thus the entire physiologic range of urine osmolality is accomplished by changes in plasma vasopressin of 0.5 to 5 pg per milliliter.

Water must be not just conserved but consumed as well, in order to replace obligate insensible water loss and obligate urine output. In animals, drinking behavior increases linearly with increases in osmolality similar to the release of vasopressin. In humans, thirst has been less well studied than vasopressin secretion, but it is thought that thirst is not stimulated until a somewhat higher osmolality than the threshold for release of vasopressin. Most humans get sufficient water from catabolism of food or fluids taken daily so that marked thirst is almost never sensed.

Vasopressin acts on V_2, antidiuretic, receptors in the kidney to cause water retention by stimulating cyclic AMP production in the luminal cell membranes of the collecting duct. This opens channels for water transport from the collecting duct to the hypertonic medullary interstitium, and maximum concentration of the final urine is isotonic with the inner medulla of the kidney (see Ch. 74). While the increase in urine osmolality is linear with increases in plasma vasopressin, the changes in urine volume are geometric. This is illustrated in Figure 202–5. Urine volume is maintained at less than 4 liters per day until plasma vasopressin is nearly absent; when maximum urine osmolality decreases to less than 50 mOsm per kilogram, urine volume increases rapidly to 18 to 20 liters per day.

Vasopressin and Pressure and Volume Regulation. In contrast to the osmoregulatory system, volume regulation is anatomically diffuse. High-pressure (baro) receptors are located in the aorta and carotid sinus, and low-pressure volume receptors are located in the left atrium. Stimuli for pressure and volume receptors pass via the glossopharyngeal, ninth, and vagal, tenth, cranial nerves to the brain stem and through the nucleus tractus solitarius to finally converge on the magnocellular neurons, where the predominant action is inhibitory. Decreases in blood pressure or vascular volume stimulate vasopressin release, whereas maneuvers that increase volume or left atrial pressure (e.g., negative pressure breathing) decrease secretion of vasopressin. The release of vasopressin in response to changes in volume or pressure is less sensitive than the release in response to osmoreceptors, and reduction of 10 to 15% in blood volume or pressure is needed to stimulate re-

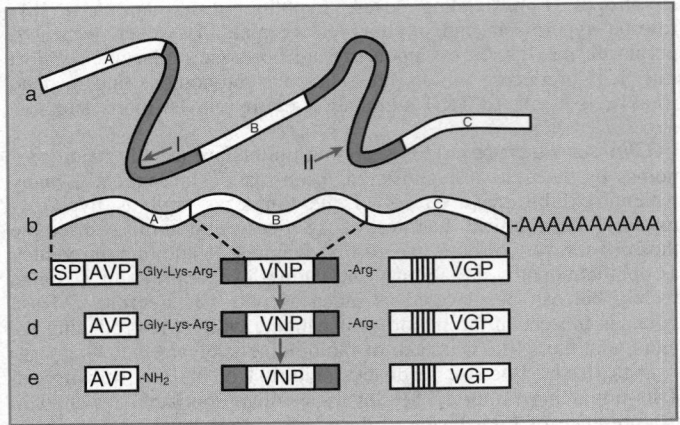

FIGURE 202–4. Synthesis of vasopressin is via: *a,* three exons *(A,B,C)* with intervening intronic sequences. *b,* The introns are cut out to form mature cytoplasmic RNA. *c,* The preprohormone is synthesized, and signal peptide is cleaved in the endoplasmic reticulum. *d,* The intact precursor is packaged into neurosecretory granules. *e,* The prohormone is subsequently cleaved to the final products: vasopressin, vasopressin neurophysin, and vasopressin glycopeptide. The colored regions of vasopressin precursor are hormone specific. (From Robinson AG, Fitzsimmons MD: Diabetes insipidus. Advances in Endocrinology and Metabolism. Chicago, Mosby-Yearbook, Inc., 1994.)

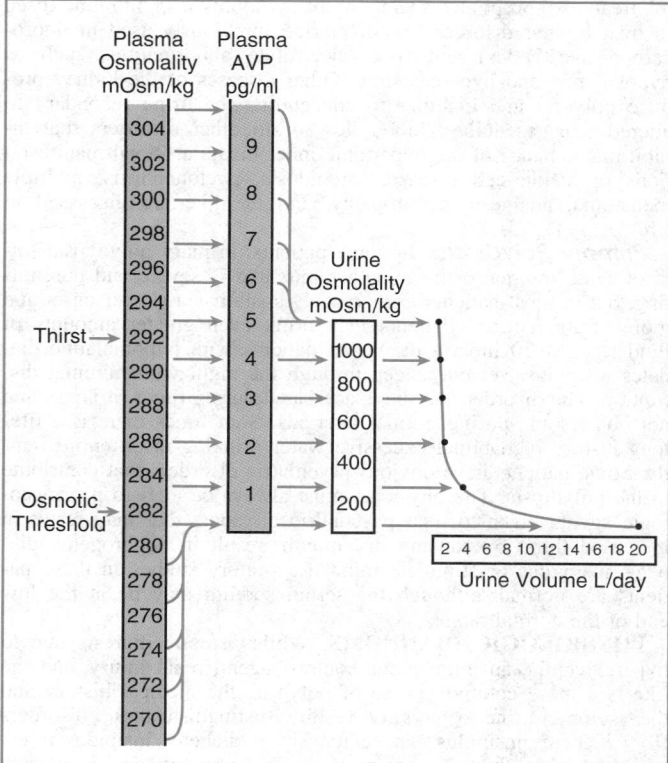

FIGURE 202–5. Idealized schematic of the normal physiologic relationships among plasma osmolality, plasma vasopressin, urine osmolality, and urine volume. The entire physiologic range of urine osmolality occurs with 0 to 5 pg per milliliter of vasopressin. Increases of plasma osmolality above approximately 294 result in increases in plasma vasopressin, but no further concentration of the urine, which is limited by the concentration of the renal inner medulla. Decreases in plasma osmolality below approximately 282 cause no further decrease in vasopressin or increase in urine volume. Note that urine volume is plotted on a horizontal scale to emphasize the geometric relationship between urine volume and urine osmolality. (Adapted from Robinson AG: Disorders of antidiuretic hormone secretion. Clin Endocrinol Metab 14:55, 1985.)

lease of vasopressin. However, once vasopressin is stimulated the increase in response to baroreceptors is logarithmic, and levels of vasopressin achieved are markedly above those achieved by osmotic stimulation. Other nonosmotic stimuli such as nausea and intestinal traction probably act through similar neural pathways to release vasopressin. The effector of the pressor component is the V_1 receptor located on vascular smooth muscle. For V_1 receptors the mechanism of action of vasopressin is to increase intracellular calcium rather than to stimulate adenylate cyclase. In intact animals, pressor activity of vasopressin is weak because of compensatory vasodilatory systems that tend to modulate the action. An action of vasopressin to regulate blood pressure is prominent only when other endocrine systems are deficient (e.g., in autonomic neuropathy).

Interaction of Osmotic and Volume Regulation. In physiologic regulation of water balance, osmotic regulation and volume regulation are usually synergistic. Dehydration causes an increase in osmolality and a decrease in volume, both of which stimulate release of vasopressin. Similarly, excess administration of fluid causes both expansion of volume and decrease in osmolality to inhibit vasopressin secretion. In pathologic situations there may be hyponatremia with inadequate volume, as with diuretic use, or a sense of inadequate volume, as with cardiac failure or cirrhosis. In these situations, volume regulation is predominant and vasopressin levels are high. ANP, described in detail in Ch. 200.3, may affect the osmotic release and action of vasopressin. With volume expansion, ANP is released from atrial myocytes and acts at the kidney to induce natriuresis. ANP is also synthesized in the hypothalamus where it may act to decrease vasopressin secretion.

Physiology of Oxytocin. Oxytocin has similar concentrations in the posterior pituitary of men and women, but a physiologic function for oxytocin has been described only in women. Stimulation of the nipple during suckling causes release of oxytocin to induce myocontraction of ductile smooth muscle in the breast to eject milk. At parturition the uterus becomes increasingly sensitive to oxytocin, and pulses of oxytocin enhance uterine tone at term and delivery. The greatest release of oxytocin occurs with delivery of the infant, probably secondary to stretching of the vaginal wall. Oxytocin may be more important for its effect of inducing uterine contraction that inhibits blood loss after delivery than for its role in initiating parturition. In animal studies, administration of oxytocin to males increases sperm transport, but this has not been documented in humans.

There are no defined syndromes of increased or decreased secretion of oxytocin. Women with diabetes insipidus secondary to traumatic damage of the magnocellular neurons and presumed absence of oxytocin may have normal pregnancy and delivery and breastfeed their infants. Excessive administration of oxytocin to induce labor can stimulate V_2 receptors of the kidney and cause abnormal water retention and hyponatremia.

DIABETES INSIPIDUS

DEFINITION. Diabetes insipidus is the excretion of a large volume of hypotonic, insipid (tasteless) urine, usually accompanied by excessive polydipsia. There are three pathophysiologic mechanisms in the differential diagnosis of diabetes insipidus: (1) *Hypothalamic diabetes insipidus* is the inability to secrete (and usually to synthesize) vasopressin in response to increased osmolality. There is no concentration of the dilute filtrate in the renal collecting duct, and a large volume of urine is excreted. This produces an increase in serum osmolality with stimulation of thirst and secondary polydipsia. Levels of vasopressin in plasma are unmeasurable or low. (2) *Nephrogenic diabetes insipidus* is a disorder in which the otherwise normal kidney is unable to respond to vasopressin. As in hypothalamic diabetes insipidus, the dilute filtrate entering the collecting duct is excreted as a large volume of hypotonic urine. There is a rise in serum osmolality that stimulates thirst and produces polydipsia. Unlike hypothalamic diabetes insipidus, however, measured levels of vasopressin in plasma will be high. (3) *Primary polydipsia* is a primary disorder of thirst stimulation. Ingested water produces a mild decrease in serum osmolality that turns off secretion of vasopressin. In the absence of vasopressin action on the kidney, there is lack of concentration of urine and excretion of a large volume. Measured vasopressin in plasma is low. While the pathophysiologic mechanisms for the three disorders are distinct, patients in each category usually have polyuria, polydipsia, and normal serum sodium. This is because the normal thirst mechanism is sufficiently sensitive to maintain fluid balance in the first two disorders, and the kidney is normally sufficiently responsive to excrete the water load in the third.

CLINICAL PRESENTATION. *Hypothalamic Diabetes Insipidus.* The sudden appearance of hypotonic polyuria after transcranial surgery in the area of the hypothalamus or after head trauma with basal skull fracture and hypothalamic damage obviously suggests the diagnosis of hypothalamic diabetes insipidus. In these situations if the patient is unconscious and unable to recognize thirst, hypernatremia is a common accompaniment. However, even in patients with more insidious progression of a specific disease or in patients with idiopathic hypothalamic diabetes insipidus, the onset of polyuria is often relatively abrupt, occurring over a few days. The presenting problem is the volume of urine and polydipsia, not the decrease in urine osmolality. Most patients do not complain of polyuria until urine volume exceeds 4 liters per day, and, as illustrated in Figure 202–5, urine volume is exponentially related to urine osmolality and to plasma vasopressin. Thus, urine volume does not exceed 4 liters per day until the ability to concentrate the urine is severely limited and plasma vasopressin is nearly absent. This same relationship has been observed in dogs with experimental lesions of the hypothalamus. In such dogs there is little increase in urine volume until only 10% of the vasopressin cells remain, and then loss of the remaining 10% produces rapid and marked increase in urine volume to 10 to 15 times normal. Urine volume seldom exceeds the amount of dilute fluid delivered to the collecting duct (about 18 liters in humans), and in many cases is less because patients voluntarily restrict fluid intake, causing some mild volume contraction and increased proximal tubular reabsorption of fluid. Patients often express a preference for cold liquids, which are probably more effective in assuaging thirst. Both thirst and urine output persist through the night. In patients with partial diabetes insipidus there is some ability to secrete vasopressin, but this secretion is markedly attenuated at normal levels of plasma osmolality. Therefore, these patients have symptoms and urine volume only moderately different from patients with complete diabetes insipidus. As most patients with hypothalamic diabetes insipidus have sufficient thirst to drink fluid to match urine output, there are few laboratory abnormalities at the time of presentation. Serum sodium may be in the high normal range, while blood urea nitrogen (BUN) and uric acid may be low secondary to large urine volume.

A variant of hypothalamic diabetes insipidus is the syndrome of absent osmostat with intact volume receptors. This syndrome is referred to as essential hypernatremia because the patients have increased sodium and absence of thirst. Physiologic maneuvers demonstrate that when the patients are euvolemic, an increase in plasma osmolality produces neither secretion of vasopressin nor sensation of thirst. However, vasopressin is synthesized by the hypothalamus and stored in the posterior pituitary because stimulation of baroreceptors results in prompt secretion of vasopressin, and the kidney is responsive because vasopressin release by volume receptor stimulation causes urinary concentration. Because patients lack thirst, they are chronically dehydrated with increased serum sodium. The amount of urine output depends on the degree of dehydration-induced secretion of vasopressin. Given sufficient fluid replacement to return extracellular volume to normal, patients become markedly polyuric and manifest the underlying diabetes insipidus.

Rarely, hypothalamic diabetes insipidus occurs as an autosomal dominant pattern of inherited disease. In reported families, the disorders are due to single nucleotide substitution or deletion in the vasopressin gene. Interestingly, in an animal model of hereditary diabetes insipidus (the Brattleboro rat), which is also due to a single nucleotide deletion, the diabetes insipidus is autosomal recessive. Diabetes insipidus is expressed only in the homozygote rat because both alleles of the gene are expressed, and 50% expression of vasopressin is adequate to allow normal water balance. In the human disorder, diabetes insipidus is not present at birth, which suggests normal synthesis of vasopressin. But, by an as-yet-undetermined mechanism, the abnormal vasopressin translation product synthesized by the mutant allele causes destruction of vasopressinergic neurons. Cell death produces diabetes insipidus later in childhood or early in adult years.

Diabetes insipidus with onset during pregnancy may be due to rapid catabolism of vasopressin. The placenta produces a cystine-aminopeptidase (oxytocinase or vasopressinase) that enzymatically destroys vasopressin and thus increases the metabolic clearance rate of vasopressin. Polyuria most often becomes manifest in patients who have some underlying decreased ability to secrete vasopressin or to respond to vasopressin action, e.g., partial hypothalamic diabetes insipidus or compensated nephrogenic diabetes insipidus. Treatment may be required only during the pregnancy, and the patient may return to her previous baseline function without need for therapy when the pregnancy ends. In some patients, hypothalamic diabetes insipidus due to any cause first becomes symptomatic during pregnancy and then persists with the usual course.

Myxedema and adrenal insufficiency both impair the ability to excrete free water by renal mechanisms. The simultaneous occurrence of either of these diseases with diabetes insipidus (as may occur with a tumor of the hypothalamus or pituitary) may decrease the large urine output of diabetes insipidus. Replacement treatment for the anterior pituitary deficiency, especially glucocorticoids, may cause sudden and massive excretion of dilute urine. Similarly, the onset of either hypothyroidism or adrenal insufficiency during the course of diabetes insipidus may decrease the need for vasopressin replacement and even cause hyponatremia.

Nephrogenic Diabetes Insipidus. The gene for the V_2 receptor has been localized to the Xq 28 region of the X chromosome. In familial nephrogenic diabetes insipidus, symptoms are noted only in patients homozygous for the disorder, and affected males have excessive polyuria and dehydration from birth.

Nephrogenic diabetes insipidus may also be acquired during treatment with certain drugs such as demeclocycline (which is used to treat inappropriate secretion of vasopressin), lithium (used to treat bipolar disorders), and fluoride (previously used in fluorocarbon anesthetics) and from electrolyte abnormalities such as hypokalemia and hypercalcemia. Other diseases of the kidney produce polyuria and inability to concentrate the urine secondary to altered renal medullary blood flow or to other disorders that inhibit maintenance of the hypertonic inner medulla. Renal manifestations of sickle cell disease, sarcoidosis, pyelonephritis, multiple melanoma, analgesic nephropathy, and the like are discussed in Ch. 77.

Primary Polydipsia. In some patients, primary polydypsia follows acute trauma to the hypothalamus and is severe and unremitting, but in most patients primary polydipsia has a slower onset and more erratic course. Patients may drink even greater amounts of fluid (e.g., > 20 liters a day) than patients with hypothalamic diabetes insipidus, yet may sleep through the night with minimal disruption. The disorder may be exacerbated during times of stress and not bothersome during normal intervals. Sometimes there is a lifelong history of habitual excessive water drinking in an entire family. Some patients have obvious psychiatric disorders that contribute to the polydipsia. The physician must always be alert to pharmacologic agents given to treat psychiatric disorders that may result in increased thirst by causing dry mouth, result in nephrogenic diabetes insipidus, or stimulate thirst. Laboratory studies in these patients are normal, although the serum sodium may be at the low end of the normal range.

PHYSIOLOGIC DIAGNOSIS. While osmotic diuresis due to hyperglycemia, an intravenous contrast agent, renal injury, and the like is a more common cause of polyuria, the medical history and the isotonic urine osmolality readily distinguish these disorders from diabetes insipidus. The diagnosis of diabetes insipidus is established when there is absence of or low concentration of plasma vasopressin and inappropriately low urine osmolality in the presence of elevated serum osmolality due to increased serum sodium. These criteria may be met at presentation, especially in acute diabetes insipidus occurring after trauma or after surgery in which there has not been adequate fluid replacement. In a patient with hypernatremia and hypotonic urine osmolality with normal renal function, diabetes insipidus is diagnosed. One need only administer a vasopressin agonist and document a renal response with decreased urine volume and increased urine osmolality to confirm the diagnosis of hypothalamic diabetes insipidus. Sometimes in the postoperative state there is water diuresis secondary to water retention during the surgical procedure. Vasopressin is normally secreted in response to surgical stress, and intravenously administered fluid may be retained. During recovery, when vasopressin levels fall, there is diuresis of the retained fluid. If further fluid is administered to match the urine output, persistent polyuria might be mistaken for diabetes insipidus. In this situation the physician should decrease the rate of fluid administered and observe the urine output and the serum sodium. If the serum sodium rises above the normal range and the urine is still hypotonic, the response to a vasopressin agonist will document the diagnosis of diabetes insipidus.

Most outpatients will have polyuria, polydipsia, and normal sodium. In these patients it is necessary to perform a test to increase serum osmolality and to measure urinary response. The best described and easiest to administer is the dehydration test and subsequent response to vasopressin (Fig. 202–6). The test should be carried out under controlled observation in the hospital or an appropriately equipped outpatient area. The timing of test administration depends on the symptoms of the patient. If the patient has marked polyuria during the night, it is best to begin the test during the day because the patient readily may become dehydrated. If the patient has only two or three episodes of nocturia per night, it may be best to begin the test in the evening so the major part of the dehydration takes place when the patient is asleep. In either case, the patient is weighed at the beginning of the test and the volume and osmolality (usually determined by freezing point depression) of all excreted urine are measured. The patient is weighed after output of each liter of urine. When two consecutive urine samples have osmolality differing by no more than 10% and the patient has lost 2% of body weight, a blood sample is obtained for measurement of serum osmolality, sodium, and plasma vasopressin. The patient is then given 2 μg of desmopressin intravenously or intramuscularly (or 5 units of aqueous vasopressin). Patients with normal levels of vasopressin have < 5% increase in urine osmolality in response to the administered desmopressin. Patients with complete hypothalamic diabetes

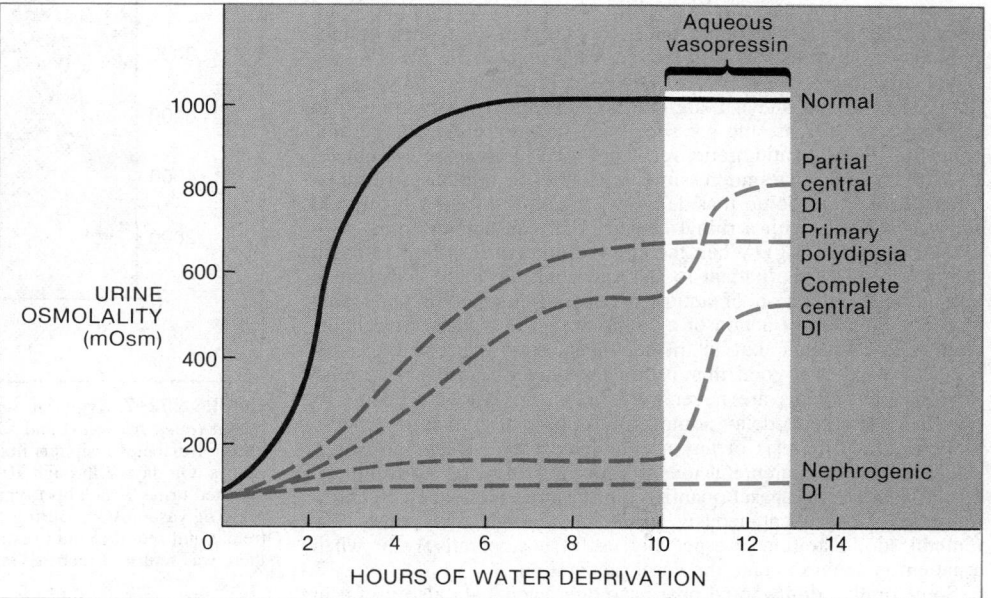

FIGURE 202-6. Responses to the dehydration test described by Miller et al., Annals of Internal Medicine (1970), to differentiate various types of diabetes insipidus and primary polydipsia. The response to dehydration shows a plateau, and the subsequent change in urine osmolality in response to administered vasopressin is illustrated. See discussion in text. *DI* = diabetes insipidus. (From Dennis VW: Investigations of renal function. *In* Wyngaarden JB, Smith LH, Jr, Bennett JC [eds.]: Cecil's Textbook of Medicine, 19th ed. Philadelphia, WB Saunders, 1992, p 495.)

insipidus have minimal concentration of the urine with dehydration and marked increase in urine osmolality in response to administered desmopressin (usually greater than 50%).

In patients with nephrogenic diabetes insipidus there usually is no urine concentration in response to administered vasopressin, although in some cases of acquired nephrogenic diabetes insipidus some urinary concentration may result. Nephrogenic diabetes insipidus is unequivocally distinguished from hypothalamic diabetes insipidus by measure of vasopressin in plasma by radioimmunoassay. Vasopressin levels are usually elevated in nephrogenic diabetes insipidus.

In patients with partial hypothalamic diabetes insipidus and patients with primary polydipsia, the urine is somewhat concentrated in response to dehydration, but it cannot be expected to be concentrated to the maximum of a normal person because the large urine volume, regardless of cause, washes out the medullary osmotic gradient that determines the maximum urine concentration. When vasopressin is administered, patients with partial hypothalamic diabetes insipidus have a further increase (usually greater than 10%) in urine osmolality, whereas patients with primary polydipsia have no further increase. There is controversy about the reliability of distinguishing these last two disorders. Some patients with primary polydipsia may not become sufficiently dehydrated with the test to secrete maximum vasopressin and hence will have an increase in urine osmolality in response to administered desmopressin. Alternatively, some patients with partial diabetes insipidus may become sufficiently dehydrated so there is maximal concentration of urine during the test and no further response to administered desmopressin. When plasma vasopressin assays become sufficiently sensitive, reliable, and available, plasma vasopressin levels at the end of dehydration may better distinguish these two disorders. In the meantime, it is important to have adequate follow-up of patients with partial diabetes insipidus to ensure that during treatment with vasopressin a good therapeutic response is obtained, as would be expected, and that hyponatremia does not occur, as might be expected if the patient had primary polydipsia.

ETIOLOGIC DIAGNOSIS. The dehydration test will confirm that absence of vasopressin is responsible for the polyuria, but the cause of the lack of vasopressin must then be determined. As noted above, vasopressin is synthesized in paired paraventricular nuclei high on the walls of the third ventricle and paired supraoptic nuclei lateral to and above the optic chiasm (see Fig. 202-3). As diabetes insipidus is symptomatic only when 80 to 90% of the vasopressin cells are destroyed, a lesion must be quite large or strategically located where the paths from the four nuclear groups converge into the pituitary stalk just above the diaphragma sellae. Such lesions can be recognized by nuclear magnetic resonance (NMR) scans of the brain. In about 80% of normal subjects, NMR shows a high intense signal (bright spot) in the posterior pituitary on T_1-weighted

images. Commonly in diabetes insipidus, there is loss of the hyperintense signal of the posterior pituitary, which is thought to be due to depletion of stored hormone. It is not known exactly what component of the hormone precursor store is responsible for the hyperintense signal.

Tumors that cause diabetes insipidus are most often benign primary intracranial tumors such as craniopharyngioma, ependymoma (suprasellar germinoma), or pinealoma that arises in the third ventricle. Primary tumors of the anterior pituitary cause diabetes insipidus only when there is suprasellar extension. Metastasis to the hypothalamus from lung, breast, melanoma, and the like may lodge in the portal capillaries of the median eminence and destroy the supraopticohypophyseal tract to cause diabetes insipidus. Granulomatous diseases, such as Langerhans' cell histiocytosis, sarcoidosis, or tuberculosis, may destroy vasopressin cells in the hypothalamus. Leukemic infiltrates of the hypothalamus may cause diabetes insipidus. In diseases with peripheral manifestations the diagnosis is usually suspected on the basis of general medical findings. Idiopathic diabetes insipidus is probably an autoimmune disease, and other autoimmune diseases are recognized in affected patients. When CNS disease is suspected but not diagnosed by NMR or general physical examination, cerebrospinal fluid obtained by lumbar puncture may be helpful in identifying tumor cells or tumor markers. Widening of the posterior pituitary stalk is observed on NMR with a variety of infiltrative diseases of the neurohypophysis, including idiopathic diabetes insipidus, Langherans' cell histiocytosis, suprasellar germinoma, sarcoidosis, tuberculosis, and metastatic disease. An NMR study with a widened pituitary stalk and absence of the hyperintense signal of the posterior pituitary on T_1 is especially suggestive of a granulomatous or inflammatory disease and should prompt the search for evidence of granulomatous disease elsewhere in the body.

Rarely, if patients with diabetes insipidus are unable to drink or are given a hypertonic solution, they develop severe acute hypernatremia. Osmotic equilibrium with intracellular water of neurons and glia produces shrinking of the brain. The brain is in a closed vault (skull), and when the brain shrinks there is engorgement of vasculature of the CNS. Rupture of vessels may produce subarachnoid hemorrhage, gross intracerebral hemorrhage, or intracerebral petechial hemorrhages producing permanent brain damage. If, however, the hypernatremia persists over a longer time, accommodation of the neurons occurs by production of "idiogenic osmoles," which decreases the amount of brain neuron shrinkage. These events, which also occur in nonketotic hyperosmolar coma, will affect treatment recommendations.

TREATMENT. Water diuresis is the primary manifestation of diabetes insipidus and water replacement in adequate quantities avoids metabolic complications. The aim of therapy is to reduce the amount of polyuria and polydipsia to a tolerable level while avoiding overtreatment that might produce water retention and hyponatremia. The best therapeutic agent is the vasopressin agonist desmopressin. Desmopressin is different from vasopressin in that the terminal amino group of cystine has been removed to prolong the duration of action and a D-arginine is substituted for L-arginine in position 8 to decrease the pressor effect. In therapeutic dosage, this agent acts on V_2, antidiuretic, receptors with minimal action on V_1, pressor, receptors. Desmopressin is available for intranasal administration in a spray bottle that delivers a fixed dose of 10 μg in 100 μl or in a bottle with a rhinal catheter that can deliver from 25 to 200 μl (2.5 to 20 μg). When therapy is initiated, it is best to begin at night to allow the patient to sleep through the night and then to determine the duration of action by quantifying polyuria the next day. The duration of action of a single dose varies between patients from 6 to 24 hours, but in most patients a dosage can be determined that gives a good therapeutic response on an every-12-hour schedule. If patients are never polyuric on a 12-hour schedule, it may be advisable to delay administration of a dose once or twice a week to allow diuresis of any accumulated water. Desmopressin is also available for parenteral use in 2 ml vials of 4 μg per milliliter; 5 to 10% of an intranasal quantity administered intravenously, intramuscularly, or subcutaneously gives an equivalent response. Parenteral administration is especially useful postoperatively or when a patient is unable to take the nasal preparation.

Some orally administered pharmacologic agents are also useful in treating diabetes insipidus. Chlorpropamide in doses of 100 to 500 mg daily enhances the effect of vasopressin at the renal tubule and is especially useful in patients with partial hypothalamic diabetes insipidus. Maximum antidiuresis is achieved after 4 days of administration. Carbamazepine (Tegretol) in doses of 200 to 600 mg per day causes release of vasopressin. Clofibrate also stimulates the release of endogenous vasopressin in doses of 500 mg every 6 hours. Thiazide diuretics cause sodium depletion and volume contraction and decrease urine volume by increasing proximal tubular reabsorption of glomerular filtrate. Ibuprofen blocks the normal inhibitory action of prostaglandin E on vasopressin action on the kidney. While ibuprofen is not a primary treatment, it may alter the antidiuretic response of other agents. For each of these pharmacologic agents the prescribing physician should be careful of potential toxicity and side effects.

Some situations require special attention in therapy. If the patient has been chronically hypernatremic and the brain has had time to adapt with production of idiogenic osmoles as described above, therapy should not be overly zealous. Too rapid lowering of osmolality in the extracellular fluid will produce a shift of water into the brain and cause cerebral edema. In this situation, desmopressin can be administered, but the amount of water should be regulated to decrease osmolality by no more than about 1 mEq every 2 hours. Postoperatively or after head trauma, diabetes insipidus may be transient (see prognosis below), and long-term maintenance therapy cannot be reliably established. Pregnant patients with diabetes insipidus can be treated with desmopressin, which has a normal duration of action because it is not destroyed by vasopressinase. It has the additional advantage of having very little action on the oxytocin receptors of the uterus. However, during pregnancy normal plasma osmolality decreases by 10 mOsm per kilogram because of changes in serum sodium. Patients with diabetes insipidus treated during pregnancy require sufficient desmopressin to maintain serum sodium at this lower level.

COURSE AND PROGNOSIS. The prognosis of properly treated diabetes insipidus is excellent. Historical complications of bladder hypertrophy and hydroureter secondary to voluntarily decreasing urine frequency are largely unseen with modern therapy. When the diabetes insipidus is secondary to a recognized disease process, it is that disease that determines the ultimate prognosis. There are some specific clinical situations in which the course is different and characteristic. Postoperative or post-traumatic diabetes insipidus is often due to rupture of the pituitary stalk and can follow a course referred to as "triphasic" (Fig. 202–7). The first phase is diabetes insipidus due to axon shock and lack of release of vasopressin. This lasts for 5 to 10 days. This is followed by a second phase of antidiuresis, which is thought to be produced by uncontrolled release of vasopressin from the large storage pool in the axon terminals of the posterior pituitary. This store is sufficient to

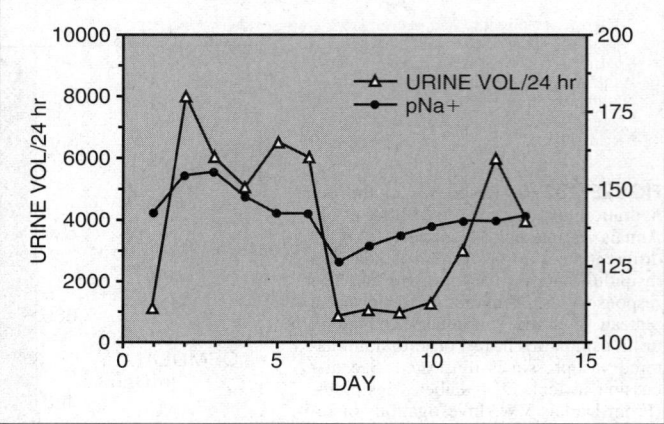

FIGURE 202–7. Triphasic response to trauma of the pituitary stalk. Urine output (*open triangles*) and serum Na+ (*solid dots*) are illustrated. Note the onset of diabetes insipidus immediately after the head trauma and lasting for 6 days. On days 7 through 10 there was a marked decrease in diuresis (with elevated urine osmolality) typical of the second phase with inappropriate release of vasopressin. During this time the patient actually became hyponatremic and required fluid restriction to treat the hyponatremia. After day 10 there was return of diabetes insipidus.

produce constant antidiuresis for an additional 5 to 10 days. The possibility of this course developing is one reason for closely following desmopressin therapy in the postoperative or post-traumatic patient. Continued administration of desmopressin and especially continued forcing of fluids either orally or parenterally will produce profound hyponatremia during the second phase. Hyponatremia is often heralded by nausea or vomiting, and severe hyponatremia may cause cerebral edema and serious neurologic sequelae. Thus, fluids may need to be restricted during this period, as they are in therapy of inappropriate secretion of antidiuretic hormone. The third or final phase is the return of diabetes insipidus after the pool of stored vasopressin has been exhausted. This may be permanent or transient. Eventually there may be return of sufficient vasopressin function to allow a lessening in intensity or discontinuation of treatment. This usually occurs within the first year of diabetes insipidus, but has occurred as long as 10 years after the initiating event. Potential return of function is another reason for occasionally withholding therapy during long-term treatment. Interestingly, the second phase of excess vasopressin and hyponatremia has been reported without preceding or subsequent diabetes insipidus. This is reported as postoperative syndrome of inappropriate secretion of antidiuretic hormone. It is probably due to trauma to only some vasopressin axons. There are sufficient functioning vasopressin neurons to prevent the diabetes insipidus of the first and third phase, but sufficient leakage of vasopressin to cause the second phase. It is only the setting and timing that identify this as an isolated second phase of the triphasic response.

Diabetes insipidus should not be considered idiopathic until after 4 years of follow-up. Over this interval, annual CT or NMR scans are indicated to test for the appearance of a tumor or infiltrative process that may not have been detected at the initial examination.

SYNDROME OF INAPPROPRIATE SECRETION OF ANTIDIURETIC HORMONE

Excess secretion of vasopressin can be caused by abnormal secretion from the posterior pituitary or by ectopic synthesis and secretion of vasopressin by a tumor. The excess vasopressin causes water retention, volume expansion, and natriuresis producing hyponatremia. This disorder is discussed in Ch. 75.

Holtzman EJ, Harris HW, Kolakowski LF, et al.: A molecular defect in the vasopressin V2-receptor gene causing nephrogenic diabetes insipidus. N Engl J Med 328:1534, 1993. *Molecular cause of hereditary nephrogenic diabetes insipidus.*

Ito M, Oiso Y, Murase T, et al.: Possible involvement of inefficient cleavage of preprovasopressin by signal peptidase as a cause for familial central diabetes insipidus. J Clin Invest 91:2565, 1993. *Identity of a genetic defect producing familial central diabetes insipidus.*

Iwasaki Y, Oiso Y, Kondo K, et al.: Aggravation of subclinical diabetes insipidus during pregnancy. N Engl J Med 324:522, 1991. *Compensated partial hypothalamic diabetes insipidus and compensated nephrogenic diabetes insipidus may both become symptomatic during pregnancy.*

Maghnie M, Villa A, Arico M, et al.: Correlation between magnetic resonance imaging of posterior pituitary and neurohypophyseal function in children with diabetes insipidus. J Clin Endocrinol Metab 74:795, 1992. *Describes characteristic hyperintense signal of posterior pituitary on T_1-weighted images with MRI and describes thickened pituitary stalk that may be seen in diabetes insipidus.*

Merendino JJ, Spiegel AM, Crawford JD, et al.: A mutation in the vasopressin V2-receptor gene in a kindred with X-linked nephrogenic diabetes insipidus. N Engl J Med 328:1538, 1993. *Molecular cause of hereditary nephrogenic diabetes insipidus.*

Miller M, Dalakos T, Moses AM, et al.: Recognition of partial defects in antidiuretic hormone secretion. Ann Intern Med 73:721, 1970. *Guide to performing and interpreting dehydration test, which is the "standard" for differential diagnosis of diabetes insipidus.*

Reeves WB, Andreoli TE: The posterior pituitary and water metabolism. *In* Wilson JD, Foster DW (eds.): Williams Textbook of Endocrinology, 8th ed. Philadelphia, WB Saunders, 1992, pp 311–356. *Extensively referenced chapter with detailed description of anatomy of neurohypophysis and physiology of vasopressin and oxytocin.*

Robinson AG, Verbalis JG: Diabetes insipidus. *In* Bardin CW (ed.): Current Therapy in Endocrinology and Metabolism, 5th ed. St. Louis, C.V. Mosby, 1994, pp 1–6. *Concise guide to various acute and chronic treatments of diabetes insipidus.*

203 THE THYROID
Wolfgang H. Dillmann

Anatomy and Physiology

The thyroid, the largest endocrine gland in the body, weighs about 20 grams, the right lobe usually being larger than the left. Adult size is reached at age 15. The two lateral lobes lie anterior to the thyroid cartilage and are connected by a small isthmus located just below the cricoid cartilage. The lobes have a pointed superior pole and a rounded inferior pole with a thickness of about 2 cm, a length of 4 to 5 cm, and a width of 2 to 3 cm. The lobes are divided by fibrous septae into pseudolobes composed of spherical structures called follicles. A dense capillary network surrounds the follicles, which are richly innervated by sympathetic and parasympathetic nerve endings. The follicles consist of a single layer of epithelial cells surrounding a lumen filled with a proteinaceous colloid material consisting of over 75% thyroglobulin. Thyroglobulin is formed by the epithelial thyroid cells, which both synthesize and store the hormone.

A feedback loop involving the hypothalamus, pituitary, and thyroid gland regulates the glandular secretion of thyroid hormone (Fig. 203–1). The hypothalamus generates thyroid-releasing hormone (TRH) to energize pituitary thyroid-stimulating hormone (TSH). TSH, in turn, stimulates thyroid hormonal output, which feeds back on both hypothalamus and pituitary to complete the regulatory circle.

Thyroid Hormone Formation

Thyroxine (T_4) is the major secretory product of the thyroid, with a daily production rate of 80 to 100 μg. T_4 is produced only by the thyroid gland. In contrast, only 20% of the daily production rate of triiodothyronine (T_3) is derived from thyroid secretion and 80% from peripheral T_4 conversion (Fig. 203–2). The daily production rate of T_3 is 30 to 40 μg. Normal thyroid hormone formation requires normal levels of TSH and an adequate but not excessive supply of iodine. Optimal iodine intake is about 150 to 300 μg per day. In some mountainous areas of the world, daily iodine supplies can be as low as 20 to 30 μg. The United States population, however, has a high iodine intake, with a daily supply of 600 to 700 μg, much of which derives from food additives such as iodized salt and flour. Iodine is reduced to iodide (I^-) in the gastrointestinal tract and readily absorbed. Iodide is removed from the bloodstream by uptake and concentration in the thyroid gland and excretion in the urine. Under normal conditions, the kidney clears iodide from plasma at about 30 ml per minute, whereas thyroid clearance is 8 ml per minute, so that only 25% of intake enters the thyroid under normal conditions. Excess iodine intake levels the percentage of uptake; reduced intake raises it. Thyroid uptake of iodide varies from 5 to 30%. Other organs such as the salivary glands, mammary glands, gastric mucosa, and choroid plexus also can take up iodine but cannot form thyroid hormone. The ability of the thyroid to actively accumulate iodine through an iodide transporter localized in

the cell membrane leads to a 20 to 40:1 concentration gradient of cell to plasma. The iodide in the thyroid cells is rapidly oxidized and enzymatically incorporated via thyroid peroxidase into tyrosine molecules of thyroglobulin by a process called organification. Thyroid peroxidase requires activation by H_2O_2. A flavoprotein enzyme, presumably an NAPDH cytochrome C reductase, generates H_2O_2, but the precise identity of the H_2O_2-generating system is uncertain. Antithyroid medications such as propylthiouracil (PTU) and methimazole inhibit thyroid peroxidase, thereby decreasing thyroid hormone formation. Thyroid hormone formation occurs on thyroglobulin, a 660-kD glycoprotein, with 25% of its tyrosine residues accessible to iodination. The monoiodinated tyrosine (MIT) and the deiodinated tyrosine (DIT) are coupled by the thyroid peroxidase enzyme to form T_4 by linking two DIT's or, for T_3 formation, linking one MIT and one DIT molecule. Thyroglobulin contains only 3 or 4 T_4 and 0.2 to 0.3 T_3 residues. The organification and coupling reactions on thyroglobulin occur at the luminal border of the thyrocyte, which then exocytoses and stores it as colloid. Thyroid hormone secretion starts with endocytosis of a colloid droplet by the luminal cell membrane of the thyrocyte. The colloid droplet then combines with lysosomes to form phagolysosomes with thyroglobulin proteolysis and release of T_4 and T_3 at the basal border into the capillaries. Iodotyrosine and especially MIT and DIT, which are liberated from thyroglobulin, are deiodinated by a specific deiodinase. Iodide thus liberated mixes with iodide entering from the blood and is reused for organification. Decreased levels of this deiodinase rarely may cause goiter and hypothyroidism.

REGULATION OF THYROID HORMONE SYNTHESIS

Thyroid hormone synthesis is influenced by intrathyroidal factors, primarily the amount of iodide in the thyroid cell; by extrathyroidal factors, especially peptide hormones, which can occupy the TSH receptor especially under normal conditions; and by the thyroid-stimulating immunoglobulin (TSI) in Graves' disease. Under conditions of very low iodine intake, T_3 preferentially is formed instead of T_4. Iodide excess in the thyroid leads to a short-term inhibition of thyroid hormone formation. After about 48 hours, however, the iodide transporter system decreases and thyroid hormone formation returns to normal in spite of elevated circulating iodide levels. Excess iodide also inhibits thyroid hormone release. Increased iodination of thyroglobulin increases its resistance to proteolytic degradation, thereby freeing less T_4 and T_3. Paradoxically, excess iodide can also increase thyroid hormone formation, especially in abnormal

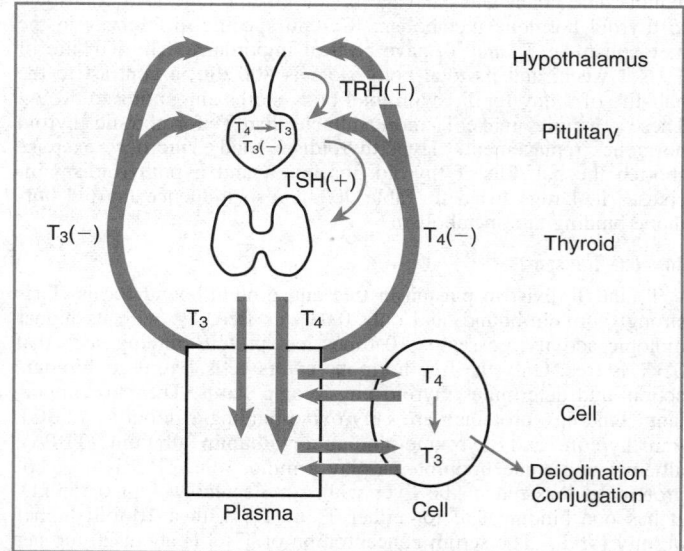

FIGURE 203–1. Hypothalamic-pituitary-thyroid interrelationship. TRH exerts a positive stimulatory effect on TSH secretion, which stimulates thyroid hormone formation. T_4 is the primary thyroid secretory product which is converted in the cells of specific organs, such as kidney and liver, to T_3. T_3 is the most biologically active thyroid hormone and is inactivated by further deiodination or conjugation and biliary excretion.

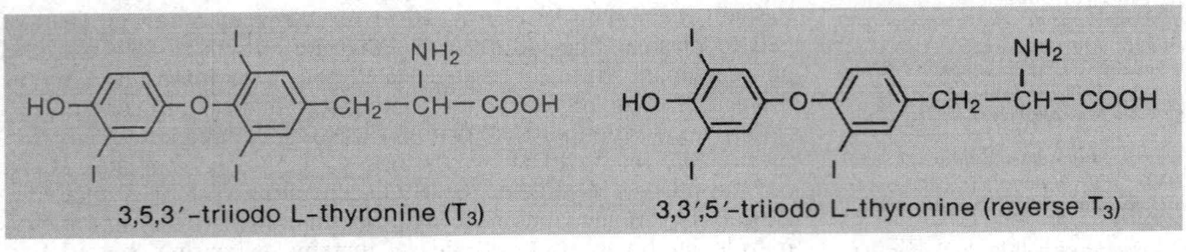

FIGURE 203–2. Structure of the thyroid hormones.

thyroid glands. For these reasons, iodine should not be used to treat thyroid diseases except under special conditions. In addition to iodide, TSH influences thyroid function by stimulating all steps of thyroid hormone formation. TSH binding to TSH receptors stimulates cAMP formation and subsequently protein kinase A activity. Such binding also stimulates the phospholipase C–based signaling system and the *ras* proto-oncogene kinase pathway. In addition to the marked influences that are exerted on thyroid hormone formation by iodide and TSH, IGF-1, EGF, prostaglandins, and cytokines such as interleukins and catecholamines modify thyroid function.

EXTRATHYROIDAL HORMONE PRODUCTION AND TURNOVER

Most T_3 is produced by extrathyroidal $5'$ deiodination of T_4, which allows for alteration in T_3 production independent of changes in thyroid function. Because T_3 is three to four times as biologically active as T_4, extrathyroidal regulation of T_3 levels has important consequences reflected by the nonthyroidal illness syndrome discussed below. The conversion of T_4 to T_3 is performed by two forms of $5'$ deiodinases. Type I $5'$ deiodinase contains the rarely used amino acid selenocysteine and is most active in liver and kidney. The activity of Type I $5'$ deiodinase declines with hypothyroidism and is inhibited by propylthiouracil and glucocorticoids. Type II $5'$ deiodinase is active in the central nervous system (CNS), pituitary, brown adipose tissue, and placenta. It resists inhibition by PTU and increases with hypothyroidism, resulting in near-normal CNS T_3 levels. A third deiodinase, termed 5 deiodinase or Type III 5 deiodinase, removes the inner ring iodide to form the biologically inactive reverse T_3 from T_4 and metabolizes T_3 to diiodothyronine (T_2). The thyroid hormone derivatives, including reverse T_3 and the di- and monothyronine compounds, have no currently recognized biologic importance.

In addition to deiodination, by which 80% of T_4 is metabolized, thyroid hormones are metabolized by transfer of glucoronyl and sulfate residues to the phenolic hydroxyl group of thyroid hormone and by biliary excretion. Deamination and decarboxylation of the alanine side chain and cleavage of the ether bridge also contribute to thyroid hormone metabolism. Certain specific differences in the metabolism of T_4 and T_3 have clinical importance. The half-life of T_4 is 1 week, and its total body store is 800 μg, in contrast to the half-life of 1 day for T_3, with total body stores amounting to 50 μg. These principles make T_4 more suitable than T_3 for chronic thyroid hormone replacement. Hyperthyroidism and vigorous exercise shorten the half-life of thyroid hormones, and hypothyroidism increases it. Drugs listed in Table 203–1 also influence thyroid hormone binding and metabolism.

Hormone Transport

T_4 and T_3 exist in plasma in free and protein-bound forms. T_4 is strongly protein-bound, and only 0.03% is free. T_3, with its higher biologic activity, possesses 10 times less protein binding such that 0.3% is free. Only the free hormone enters cells, exerts its biologic action, and determines thyroid physiologic status. The most important binding proteins are thyroxine-binding globulin (TBG), transthyretin, and thyroxine-binding prealbumin albumin (TBPA); albumin and some lipoproteins play a minor role. TBG is a glycoprotein synthesized in the liver with a molecular weight of 55 kD. It has one binding site for either T_4 or T_3, with a 10-fold higher affinity for T_4. The serum concentration of TBG is about 20 mg per liter to allow for binding of 20 μg of T_4 per deciliter. Transthyretin has two binding sites for T_4, but with an affinity 100-fold lower than that of TBG. T_3 binds weakly to transthyretin. The total binding capacity of transthyretin for T_4 is very large at 200 μg of T_4 per deciliter. Albumin has one binding site for T_4 or T_3, with a 50-fold lower affinity compared to TBG. In normal plasma, the T_4-binding distribution is 80% of T_4 binding to TBG, 15% to transthyretin, and 5% to albumin and lipoproteins. For T_3, the distribution is 90% bound to TBG and the rest to albumin and lipoproteins, with little binding to transthyretin. Table 203–1 lists conditions leading to alterations in TBG. Changes in total T_4 or T_3 resulting from such alterations may be confused with conditions leading to thyroid hormone excess or deficiency due to hyperthyroidism or hypothyroidism. Elevated or decreased total T_4 or T_3 levels caused by abnormalities in binding proteins are always accompanied by normal free T_4 and free T_3 concentrations and a euthyroid state. Elevated levels of TBG as they occur, for example, in pregnant patients or patients with acute hepatitis lead to increased levels of total T_4 and T_3. Because more T_4 is bound, less T_4 is able to enter the tissue to be metabolized and inhibit TSH secretion. Slightly higher TSH levels result in increased thyroid hormone formation and a new steady state accompanied by normal free thyroid hormone concentrations. Specific drugs also can lower thyroid hormone concentrations without lowering thyroid hormone–binding proteins (Table 203–1). For example, salicylic acid or phenytoin competes with thyroid hormone for binding to TBG. The effects of phenytoin are more complex in that they reduce both total serum T_4 levels and slightly lower free T_4 concentrations. TSH concentrations remain normal under such circumstances, and the patients are not hypothyroid. In contrast to alterations in binding proteins, increases or decreases in thyroid hormone production lead to abnormalities in both total and free hormone concentrations.

THYROID HORMONE ACTION

Most thyroid hormone effects are mediated by the binding of T_3 to nuclear thyroid hormone receptor proteins. T_3 has a 10-fold higher affinity for this nuclear receptor than T_4, accounting for the higher biologic activity of T_3. T_3 nuclear receptors belong to the c erbA proto-oncogene family and are encoded by the genes c erbA α and c erbA β. Each gene has several splice variants, only some of which bind T_3. The T_3 nuclear receptor is a T_3-activated transcription factor that binds to specific nucleotide sequences located upstream or downstream of the transcription start site of T_3-responsive genes. Many T_3-responsive genes show an increase in transcription upon T_3 binding to the nuclear T_3 receptor protein. This leads to increased formation of specific mRNA's and proteins such as those coding for growth hormone, malic enzyme, myosin heavy chain α and the calcium pump of the sarcoplasmic reticulum. T_3 suppresses transcription of other genes such as the gene coding for the TSH-α and TSH-β subunits. In this scenario, specific mutations of the c erbA β receptor lead to the generalized thyroid hor-

TABLE 203–1. FACTORS INFLUENCING THYROID HORMONE BINDING TO TBG

Increased TBG concentration
  Congenital abnormality
  Hyperestrogenic state
    Pregnancy, estrogen therapy
  Disease related
    Hepatitis, biliary cirrhosis, acute intermittent porphyria
  Drugs
    Tamoxifen, perphenazine, clofibrate
Decreased TBG concentration
  Congenital abnormality
  Drugs
    Glucocorticoids (large doses), androgenic steroids, asparaginase
  Severe systemic illness
    Nephrotic syndrome, chronic liver disease, protein malnutrition
Drugs interfering with binding to normal TBG
  Salicylates, diazepam, phenytoin, furosemide, high levels of free fatty acids

mone resistant syndrome: The mutant $T_3\beta$ receptor interferes with the action of normal T_3 receptor proteins. In addition to its effects on transcription, T_3 influences the half-life of mRNA and proteins and affects the translation of mRNA, a step that may lead to rapid changes in ion transport.

Braverman LE, Utiger RD (eds.): Werner and Ingbar's The Thyroid, 6th ed., Philadelphia, JB Lippincott, 1991. *A basic text.*

Lazar MA: Thyroid hormone receptors: Multiple forms, multiple possibilities. Endocrinol Rev 14:184, 1993.

Refetoff S, Weiss RE, Usala SJ: The syndromes of resistance to thyroid hormone. Endocrinol Rev 14:348, 1993.

Vassart G, Dumont JE: The thyrotropin receptor and the regulation of thyrocyte function and growth. Endocrinol Rev 13:596, 1992. *The titles of the above articles are self-explanatory.*

EVALUATION OF PATIENTS WITH THYROID DISEASE

The evaluation of patients with thyroid disease includes a physical examination of the thyroid, laboratory tests for thyroid function and, when indicated, specific other procedures including ultrasonography, radioactive iodine uptake and scan, and fine-needle aspiration.

Physical Examination

Palpation of the thyroid gland is an important part of the general physical examination, and abnormalities in size, consistency, and contour of the gland are a common finding. For example, 6% of women have thyroid nodules. An enlargement of the thyroid, however, may be a first clue for Graves' disease; or a firm thyroid nodule can represent thyroid cancer. Examination of the thyroid begins by having the patient swallow while observing the contour of the neck from the side. Thyroid enlargements and irregularities, like a nodule, moving up from the substernal area can be identified. Palpation of the thyroid can be performed by standing behind the patient and using the fingers of both hands to identify the isthmus lying just below the cricoid cartilage. Moving laterally, the second, third, and fourth fingers can palpate both thyroid lobes. By exerting gentle pressure during swallowing, the surface of the thyroid moving past the fingers reveals enlargement or the presence of thyroid nodules. A thyroid examination should always include palpation of lateral and submandibular lymph nodes. The size of thyroid nodules can be recorded by measuring their two largest diameters.

Measurement of Thyroid Hormone Values

Techniques employed for measurement of T_4, free T_4, T_3, and TSH by radioimmunoassays or enzyme-coupled immunoassays are rapidly changing. The newer assays provide for increased assay sensitivity. Radioimmunoassays are progressively being replaced by enzyme-linked immunoabsorption assays, and new chemoluminescent compounds are available for supersensitive TSH assays. Serum thyroid hormone concentrations for T_4, free T_4, T_3, and TSH in normals and patients with thyroid disease are given in Table 203–2. These measurements accurately define thyroid function in most persons, making more specialized tests rarely needed.

TOTAL AND FREE T_4. Total T_4 values (4.5 to 12.5 μg per deciliter) are altered by changes in thyroid function or changes in the concentration affinities of thyroid hormone–binding proteins. Determination of free T_4 levels (non–protein-bound) corrects for these abnormalities. Current laboratory capacities involve quantitation of non–protein-bound T_4 by a two-step fluorometric enzyme immunoassay or by equilibrium dialysis. Normal values range from 0.9 to 2 ng per deciliter. Some of these assays occasionally falsely identify too high free T_4 values in patients with dysalbuminic hyperthyroxemia, but non–protein-bound T_4 measurement by the two-step immunoassay approach gives a good approximation of free T_4. This free T_4 index is constructed by multiplying the total T_4 by an estimated protein binding (usually the T_3 uptake test). The T_4 index does not adequately reflect the thyroid status in patients with the nonthyroidal illness syndrome, as discussed below.

Measurement of total T_3 levels by enzyme-coupled immunoassays has a normal range of 80 to 220 ng per deciliter and is also influenced by alterations in binding proteins, but to a lesser extent. The total T_3 assay should not be confused with the T_3 uptake or T_3 resin test, which is used to calculate the free thyroxine index.

SERUM REVERSE T_3. Reverse T_3 (rT_3) (normal range 20 to 40 ng per deciliter) should be determined only in special situations. Its level is elevated (40 to 120 ng per deciliter) in patients with various systemic illnesses, leading to the nonthyroidal illness syndrome (NTI). Because of decreased T_4, free T_4, and T_3 levels in some of these patients, its determination can help to distinguish NTI from hypothyroidism. In hypothyroid patients, reverse T_3 levels are decreased.

The levels of the thyroxine hormone–binding proteins, TBG, transthyretin, and albumin, can be directly measured by immunoassays. During pregnancy and with estrogen treatment, TBG levels are elevated 2- to 3-fold owing to a decreased metabolic clearance of TBG molecules which have an increase in glycosylation. An albumin variant with increased affinity for T_4 exists in the familial dysalbuminic syndrome and leads to elevated T_4 levels with normal T_3 values and uptake. A transthyretin variant with similar effects on T_4 binding has also been described. Table 203–3 lists causes of increased T_4 levels.

SERUM THYROGLOBULIN. Thyroglobulin is produced only by thyroid tissue. Normal persons have low but detectable thyroglobulin levels. Total surgical removal of thyroid tissue for cancer should result in undetectable thyroglobulin levels. Determination of thyroglobulin levels by immunoassays has its most useful application following thyroid cancer surgery. The upper normal limit of thyroglobulin is 20 to 25 ng per deciliter, and levels above that range may indicate a return of thyroid cancer. Thyroglobulin levels also increase when patients become hypothyroid, as occurs, for example, in preparation for radioactive iodine scanning and treatment. Determination of thyroglobulin levels at that time is strongly recommended. Normal thyroglobulin levels do not completely exclude the return of thyroid cancer because in about 10% of patients with thyroid cancer, thyroglobulin is normal in spite of the return of thyroid cancer. Intake of thyroid hormones leads to a decrease of thyroid tissue and thus lowers thyroglobulin levels. Patients with thyrotoxicosis factitia have, therefore, low thyroglobulin levels, in contrast to patients with thyroiditis. In both of these conditions, radioactive iodine uptake is low and thyroglobulin levels can help distinguish between these two conditions. In the presence of antithyroglobulin antibodies, accurate determination of thyroglobulin by immunoassays is not possible.

THYROID-STIMULATING HORMONE. Serum TSH levels correlate inversely with active thyroid hormone concentrations and represent the best single index to the presence of primary hyperthyroidism or primary hypothyroidism. In hypothyroidism with low thyroid hormone concentrations, TSH levels rise above the upper normal limit of 6 μU per milliliter. In hyperthyroidism with elevated thyroid hormone levels, TSH levels fall below the lower normal limit of 0.3 μU per milliliter. TSH levels as currently measured fall below the lower limit of normal in patients with hyperthyroidism, whatever the cause. Suppressed TSH levels also can accompany other conditions, including pituitary or hypothalamic disease; nonthyroidal illness; treatment with dopamine, glucocorticoids, and other drugs; and psychiatric illness or recent recovery from hyperthyroidism. In secondary hypothyroidism due to pituitary failure (<5% of all hypothyroidism), the formation and secretion of thyroid hormone is low but TSH levels fail to rise. Similarly, in hypothalamic disease leading to decreased TRH formation, TSH levels are not elevated in spite of decreased T_4 and T_3 concentrations. Elevated TSH levels rarely occur in the absence of hypothyroidism. TSH-producing pituitary tumors rarely cause hyperthyroidism. In the generalized thyroid hormone resistance syndrome, however, TSH levels are inappropriately elevated in proportion to the markedly elevated T_4 and T_3 levels. In hypothyroidism, markedly elevated TSH levels decline only slowly after thyroxine therapy achieves normal T_4 and T_3 concentrations. Hypothyroidism leads to an increase in the number of TSH-producing thyrotrophs, which de-

TABLE 203–2. SERUM THYROID HORMONE VALUES IN NORMAL PERSONS AND PATIENTS WITH THYROID DISEASE

	Normal	Hyperthyroid	Hypothyroid
T_4 μg/dl	4.5–12.5	>12.5	<4.5
free T_4 (ng/dl)	0.9–2	>2	<0.9
T_3 (ng/dl)	80–220	>220	<80
TSH (μU/ml)	0.3–6	<0.3	>6

TABLE 203-3. CAUSES OF INCREASED SERUM TOTAL T_4 CONCENTRATION

Thyroid State Condition	T_4	Free T_4	T_3	TSH	Comments
Hyperthyroid state	H	H	H or N	L	High T_4 combined with hypermetabolic state and hyperthyroidism
Euthyroid state					
Binding abnormalities					
TBG levels increased	H	N	H	N	Autosomal dominant
T_4 binding to albumin increased (familial dysalbuminemic hyperthyroxinemia)	H	N,H*	N	N	*Same "free T_4" methods lead to erroneous results
T_4 binding by transthyretin increased (familial)	H	N	N	N	
T_4 antibodies present	H	N,H	N,L,*H*	N	*Method based, anti-T_3 antibody may also be present
Drug effects					
Inhibitors of 5′ deiodinase					
Oral cholecystographic contrast agents (ipodate, iopanoate)	H	H	L	H	Inhibition of T_3 formation
Amiodarone	H	H	L	L,N	
Propranolol	H	N	L,N	N,H	Only with large doses
Heparin	H	N,H	N	N	Temporary after IV doses
T_4 administration	H	H	N	L	Mild hyperthyroxinemia in patients on T_4 replacement
Various disorders					
Nonthyroidal illness syndrome	H,N	N,L	L	N,L,H	See text for detail
Hyperemesis gravidarum	H	H,N	N	L	During early part of pregnancy; remits
Acute psychiatric illness	H,N	H,N	N	L	During acute phase; remits without treatment
Extrathyroidal deiodinase defect	H	H	N	N	A few case reports but not completely documented
Thyroid hormone resistance syndrome (pituitary and generalized)	H	H	H	H	In generalized resistance syndrome, hypothyroid features can be present, especially related to CNS development. If only pituitary resistance, thyrotoxic symptoms

H = high; N = normal; L = low.
Sequence indicates frequency of occurrence, e.g., free T_4 = HN—more frequently free T_4 is high, but normal levels can also be encountered.

cline only slowly after euthyroidism returns. Accordingly, 4 to 6 weeks should be allowed before increasing replacement doses of thyroxine above average on the basis of TSH levels. Severe longstanding hypothyroidism can lead to pituitary enlargement, mimicking pituitary tumors. The availability of sensitive TSH levels allows adequate assessment of pituitary reserves under such circumstances and makes TRH tests less useful.

ANTITHYROID ANTIBODIES. Antibody formation can occur against the thyroid peroxidase enzyme, thyroglobulin, and the TSH receptors T_4 and T_3. These antibodies can be present in serum. The most frequently occurring is the antimicrosomal antibody for which the thyroid peroxidase enzyme is the antigen. In Hashimoto's disease, elevated antibodies occur in >80% of patients with no specific therapeutic requirements resulting from high antiperoxidase antibody titers. Antithyroglobulin antibodies are positive in 60% of Hashimoto's disease. Occurrence of antithyroglobulin antibodies precludes using thyroglobulin levels to follow patients after thyroid cancer surgery or radioactive iodine treatment. Different types of TSH receptor antibodies occur, some of which stimulate thyroid hormone formation, whereas others only stimulate DNA synthesis or block TSH action. The TSI is a TSH receptor antibody that stimulates thyroid hormone formation and accompanies >90% of cases of Graves' disease. The TSI is related to, but not the same as, the long-acting thyroid-stimulating antibody (LATS), a previously used assay. In patients in whom the diagnosis of Graves' disease cannot be made clinically, determination of the TSI may be helpful, but routine TSI determination is not recommended. Persistent high levels of TSI in patients with Graves' disease on long-term antithyroid medication suggests but does not guarantee that stopping the antithyroid medication will not be followed by continuous euthyroidism. Anti-TSH antibodies can cross the placenta and produce neonatal Graves' disease or hypothyroidism. Circulating antibodies to T_4 and T_3 can interfere with the accurate determination of these hormones.

Evaluation of the Thyroid by Radioisotope Tests

RADIOACTIVE IODINE (RAI) UPTAKE. The epithelial cells of the thyroid actively transport iodide (I^-) and molecules of similar charge and configuration such as $^{99m}TcO^-_4$ pertechnetate and ^{201}Th. Only iodide is permanently retained in the thyroid cell by organification. Two separate tests use radioactive iodine: total radioactive uptake and thyroid scanning. Both are contraindicated during pregnancy. The radioactive iodine uptake only roughly indicates thyroid function. The 24-hour uptake ranges widely from 5 to 20%, and this, along with the marked decreased uptake in the presence of increased amounts of bodily cold iodine, makes it an unreliable indicator of thyroid function. Patients with subacute thyroiditis have a markedly reduced or absent uptake, whereas patients with active Graves' disease have a normal or increased uptake. Accordingly, the radioactive iodine uptake may be useful in diagnosing subacute thyroiditis. Its routine use for the diagnosis of Graves' disease is not recommended.

THYROID SCAN. Thyroid scans give graphic representations of the distribution of radioactive iodine in the gland. They are useful in identifying whether thyroid nodules show decreased ("cold") or increased ("hot") accumulation of radioactive iodine compared with normal paranodular tissue. Uptake also identifies thyroid tissue outside the gland. The isotopes ^{123}I, ^{131}I, and ^{99m}Tc can be used. ^{123}I is preferred because it provides a much smaller radiation dose to the thyroid than ^{131}I. With a ^{99m}Tc scan, good quality images can be obtained about 30 minutes after administration. Some thyroid nodules have a normal iodine transporter but lose the ability to organify iodine. Such nodules (about 10%) are not cold on ^{99m}Tc scans, a significant disadvantage of the technique. The ^{131}I isotope is sometimes preferred for identifying thyroid cancer metastases because it has a higher energy gamma ray and better penetrates the tissue. Scans in some patients fail to colocalize palpable nodules adjacent to areas of increased or decreased radioactive iodine retention. Such nodules may be autonomously either hot or cold. Because thyroid cancers exists in <1% of hot nodules compared with 20% of cold ones, the radioactive iodine uptake of thyroid nodules can be useful. In special cases, a suppression scan may be useful. After placing the patient on 150 to 200 μg of T_4 per day for 4 to 6 weeks, one repeats the thyroid scan. Thyroid hormone and TSH values should be normal before thyroxine is started. Autonomous nodules continue to show an increased iodine uptake (hot), whereas other nodules lose their radioactive iodine retention, becoming cold. Cold nodules need to be further evaluated with fine-needle aspiration, but this is not required for hot ones.

THYROID ULTRASONOGRAPHY. Ultrasonography gives a high-resolution image of the thyroid and can identify nodules 1 to 3 mm in diameter. Such small nodules are, however, not clinically relevant. Ultrasonography can distinguish solid from cystic lesions and determine changes in the size of the nodule in response to thyroid hormone suppression therapy. Ultrasound-guided fine-needle aspiration helps in obtaining cytologic material from nodules that are difficult to identify by palpation. Ultrasonography cannot distinguish between benign and malignant thyroid nodules, nor can the technique identify substernal extensions of the thyroid or spread of metastatic disease to this region. For the latter purpose, magnetic resonance imaging (MRI) or computed tomography (CT) can be useful.

Fine-Needle Aspiration of Thyroid Nodules

Aspiration of thyroid nodules with a fine needle (22 to 27 gauge) to obtain material for cytologic examination provides good diagnostic accuracy with minimal side effects. Bleeding into the aspirated nodule is the only unwanted effect and usually has no clinical consequence. Results obtained with this procedure are listed in Table 203–4. Seeding of malignant cells along the needle track does not present a clinical problem with fine-needle aspiration. An experienced cytopathologist is crucial for the successful use of this procedure. Since the advent and wide use of fine-needle aspiration, surgical removal of benign nodules has substantially decreased.

Bayer MF: Effective laboratory evaluation of thyroid status. Med Clin North Am 75:1, 1991. *Provides a succinct guide to modern testing.*
Nicoloff JT, Spencer CA: The use and misuse of sensitive thyrotropin assays. J Clin Endocrinol Metab 71:493, 1990. *A valuable paper on the do's and don'ts of the subject.*
Stocklig JR: Serum thyrotropin and thyroid hormone measurements and assessment of thyroid hormone transport. *In* Braverman LF, Utiger RD (eds.): The Thyroid, 6th ed. Philadelphia, JB Lippincott, 1991, p. 463. *Comprehensively discusses the subject.*

NONTHYROIDAL ILLNESS SYNDROME (NTI)

Severe systemic illness, physical trauma, and psychiatric disturbances can substantially alter thyroid hormone levels in patients without intrinsic thyroid disease. Various terms have been used for this condition, including the nonthyroidal illness syndrome, sick euthyroid syndrome, and low T_3 syndrome. The severity of the illness correlates roughly with the extent of thyroid hormone changes. A decreased serum T_3 concentration is the critical component of the syndrome. The frequent alterations of thyroid hormone levels in severe illness probably make NTI a more common cause of abnormal thyroid hormone values than intrinsic thyroid disease. NTI represents one end of a spectrum of endocrine responses to severe illness which include increases in ACTH and cortisol levels. Increases in cytokines, especially tumor necrosis factor and interleukins-1 and -6, also occur. The consequences, if any, of NTI for total body metabolism and the functional status of specific organs are unclear and therapy is not recommended. Diagnosing the simultaneous occurrence of hypothyroidism or hyperthyroidism in patients with NTI is a difficult diagnostic challenge. Different variants of NTI occur.

LOW T_3, NORMAL T_4 VARIANT. A marked decrease in serum total T_3 and free T_3 concentrations accompanied by normal serum T_4 and TSH levels is the most frequently encountered combination of thyroid hormone values in NTI. A rough correlation exists between the severity of the systemic illness and the decrease in T_3 levels. Decreased T_3 levels are most likely caused by an impairment of extrathyroidal T_4 to T_3 conversion. The decline is accompanied by an increase in rT_3 levels. Diminished 5' deiodinase activity accounts for this reciprocal change, with T_3 no longer being formed from T_4 and reverse T_3 not being metabolized to rT_2. The decrease in T_3 levels may decrease protein turnover and exert a sparing effect on body proteins, but the overall impact on metabolic and organ function is unclear. Because of normal T_4 and TSH levels, this variant of NTI can be clearly distinguished from hypothyroidism.

LOW T_3, LOW T_4 VARIANT. In addition to low T_3 levels, T_4 levels also decline in patients with more severe illness. Several changes contribute: (1) decreases in thyroxine-binding proteins (TBG and transthyretin); (2) displacement of thyroxine from proteins by fatty acids; and (3) decreased thyroid hormone production because of lowered TSH levels. The degree of lowered T_4 levels correlates with disease severity: Mortality increases in patients with T_4 levels below 4 μg per deciliter and approaches 80% in patients with T_4 levels below 2 μg per deciliter. T_4 administration does not influence outcome, and the low levels reflect the severity of the underlying illness but appear not to contribute directly to mortality. In addition to low T_3 and T_4 levels, T_4 indexes are low but dialysis-measured free T_4 levels remain normal or only minimally lowered. TSH levels are low but may be slightly elevated during recovery from severe illness. TSH levels above 20 μU per milliliter are not compatible with NTI and point to hypothyroidism.

Unusual Variants of Nonthyroidal Illness

Elevated T_4 levels with initially normal T_3 levels that subsequently decline occur with liver disease, especially acute hepatitis. Increased synthesis and release of TBG most likely accounts for the increased T_4 levels. A delayed fall in T_3 levels can affect patients with AIDS, indicating a poor prognosis; rT_3 levels are not elevated. In psychiatric illness, especially manic depressive disease, elevated T_4 levels occur during the initial disease phase, T_3 levels are normal, and TSH results vary. Elderly patients frequently show low T_3 levels; possible causes include chronic illness, medication intake, or an adjustment to increasing age. T_3 levels remain normal in selected healthy elderly individuals.

Diagnostic Considerations

The diagnosis of hypothyroidism or hyperthyroidism in severely ill patients with nonthyroidal illness can be difficult. Signs indicating the prior existence of thyroid disease such as a goiter, a thyroidectomy surgical scar, exophthalmos, or pretibial myxedema should be sought. Organ manifestations such as marked bradycardia for hypothyroidism or tachycardia and fine tremor for hyperthyroidism may provide important clues, especially if no other reason for these signs can be identified. As described above, NTI-induced alterations in thyroid function tests suppress the standard indices of hypothyroidism or hyperthyroidism, but certain guidelines can help. A TSH level above 20 μU per milliliter in an NTI patient makes a diagnosis of hypothyroidism highly likely, and thyroxine therapy is indicated. Similarly, TSH levels below 0.03 μU per milliliter and only moderately elevated T_3 and T_4 levels make hyperthyroidism likely. As systemic illness improves, T_3 and T_4 levels rise further and hyperthyroidism becomes evident. If Graves' disease causes the hyperthyroidism, a TSI determination can be helpful. The preferred treatment for such hyperthyroidism is by medical therapy using PTU or methimazole.

THYROTOXICOSIS

Thyrotoxicosis occurs when tissues are exposed to excess amounts of thyroid hormone, resulting in specific metabolic changes and pathophysiologic alterations in organ function. A distinction can be made between thyrotoxicosis and hyperthyroidism. Hyperthyroidism denotes increased formation and release of thyroid hormone from the thyroid gland, whereas thyrotoxicosis describes

TABLE 203–4. RESULTS OBTAINED BY FINE-NEEDLE ASPIRATION OF THYROID NODULES

	Percent of Patients
Adequate tissue obtained	90
Benign tumor	74
Malignant tumor	4
Suspicious or indeterminate	12
Correct diagnosis	<90
False negative	4
False positive	1

One fifth of these nodules are malignant after surgery by final pathology.

the clinical syndrome that results. Excess intake of exogenous thyroid hormone would lead to thyrotoxicosis but by the definition given above, such a patient would not be hyperthyroid. The terms, however, are frequently used interchangeably. Table 203–5 lists causes for thyrotoxicosis. The major ones are (1) increased occupancy of TSH receptors by TSI, TSH, or human chorionic gonadotropin (hCG); (2) autonomous overproduction of thyroid hormone by thyroid nodules; (3) increased release of thyroid hormone during specific phases of thyroiditis; (4) excessive thyroid hormone intake or ectopic thyroid hormone formation. The most frequent cause of thyrotoxicosis is Graves' disease, accounting for 60 to 90% of cases and occurring among women with a frequency of 1.9%. Men experience one tenth of the occurrence in women. Other causes in decreasing order of frequency include toxic thyroid nodules, thyroiditis, factitious thyrotoxicosis, iodine-induced thyrotoxicosis, and hCG- and TSH-induced hyperthyroidism.

Graves' Disease

Graves' disease, also termed Basedow's or Parry's disease, carries the hallmarks of excess formation and secretion of thyroid hormone and diffuse goiter. Additional characteristics include exophthalmos, dermopathy (especially pretibial myxedema), and rarely thyroid acropachy. These supplementary manifestations seldom appear together and often run a divergent time course.

ETIOLOGY AND PATHOGENESIS. Graves' disease is most likely an autoimmune disorder with B lymphocytes producing immunoglobulins, some of which bind to and activate the TSH receptor, stimulating excess thyroid growth and hormone secretion. For these antibodies the TSH receptor appears to represent the antigenic site, and they act like TSH and are termed thyroid-stimulating immunoglobulins (TSI). Other antibodies occur in Graves' and other autoimmune diseases such as Hashimoto's disease. These antibodies bind to the TSH receptor but stimulate only thyroid growth without increasing thyroid hormone secretion. Some antibodies bind to the TSH receptor but block TSH action and lead to thyroid atrophy. A diversity of TSH antibodies occurs in autoimmune thyroid diseases, generating a spectrum of illnesses with Graves' disease and hyperthyroidism at one end and Hashimoto's disease and thyroid atrophy leading to hypothyroidism at the other. The role that specific antibodies play in causing the ophthalmopathy that occurs in 20 to 40% of patients with Graves' disease is less clear. Specific antibodies directed against non-TSH retro-orbital antigens localized on retro-orbital fibroblasts and muscle cells as well as antibodies directed at TSH-like antigens have been described. Retro-orbital fibroblasts appear to express a TSH receptor–like protein. Anti-TSH antibodies occur at a low frequency in Hashimoto's disease and in euthyroid relatives of patients with Graves' disease. The simultaneous occurrence of blocking TSH antibodies may prevent hyperthyroidism in such patients.

The precise sequence of events leading to TSH receptor antibody production and factors that initiate antibody formation have not been clearly identified. A genetically mediated antigen-specific defect in T lymphocyte suppressor function has been proposed. Such a defect in immune surveillance would allow T helper cell clones, which mistake part of the TSH receptor as a foreign antigen, to arise and persist. Such clones would then stimulate B cells to produce anti-TSH receptor antibodies. Alternatively, thyroid cells stimulated by specific cytokines produced in response to a viral infection may express on their cell surface Class II molecules of specific HLA-DR types which present fragments of the TSH receptor to T lymphocytes; these then would stimulate B lymphocytes to produce TSH receptor antibodies. The two mechanisms are not mutually exclusive and both could contribute to TSH receptor–directed antibody formation. The autoimmune response may be promoted by poorly defined factors including the following: (1) iodide excess; for example, the incidence of Graves' disease increases after iodine supplementation in deficient areas; (2) viral or bacterial infection; for example, outbreaks of Graves' disease can follow *Yersinia enterocolitica* infection; (3) glucocorticoid withdrawal or stress; the stress induction has been questioned and may relate to a worsening of symptoms by the combined occurrence of hyperthyroidism and physical or emotional stress which brings the patients to medical attention; (4) parturition: A state of relative immune tolerance develops during pregnancy and reverses after delivery; (5) lithium therapy; this may modify immune responses.

PATHOLOGY. The thyroid gland in Graves' disease enlarges diffusely and contains increased vascularity. The parenchyma exhibits hypertrophy and hyperplasia, with follicular cells showing increased height, surrounding a lumen containing a decreased amount of colloid. Infiltration by lymphocytes indicates the autoimmune nature of the disease. These cells probably generate a considerable amount of TSH receptor antibody. Iodide administration increases the colloid accumulation and decreases vascularity, making the gland firmer. A gland that increases in size in patients receiving antithyroid medication indicates either excess medication, inducing hypothyroidism, or too low a dose, providing inadequate receptor blockade and continued thyroid hormone formation and growth. Severe thyrotoxicosis can lead to muscle atrophy with muscle fiber degeneration, cardiac hypertrophy, focal hepatic necrosis with lymphocyte infiltration, a decrease in bone density, and hair loss. In patients with Graves' disease ophthalmopathy, an increase in retro-orbital contents leads to protrusion of the globe. The retro-orbital tissues show marked infiltration by lymphocytes, mast cells, and plasma cells along with increased amounts of mucopolysaccharide, especially hyaluronic acid. Extraocular muscles show edema, round cell infiltration, and mucopolysaccharide deposition eventually resulting in muscle fibrosis. In patients with pretibial myxedema, the skin shows prominent lymphocyte infiltration and mucopolysaccharide deposition.

CLINICAL FEATURES. Excess thyroid hormone action due to any of the causes listed in Table 203–5 can lead to an increased metabolic rate and changes in the function of several organs. In addition, patients with Graves' disease have specific clinical manifestations resulting from the underlying autoimmune process. The thyrotoxicosis and autoimmune-related manifestations can show independent variations in intensity and time course, causing diagnostic difficulties.

Features of Thyrotoxicosis. Table 203–6 lists common signs and symptoms of thyrotoxicosis. The typical patient with Graves' disease is a woman in her mid-20's to 30's experiencing recent onset of nervousness, difficulty in controlling emotions, and a state of agitated tiredness made worse by sleep disturbances. She speaks rapidly and cannot sit still. Problems of recent onset in interaction with others at home or at work are frequently reported. Questioning brings out feelings of intolerance with excess sweating, palpitations, muscle weakness, frequent bowel movements, and weight loss in spite of good appetite. Sometimes weight gain ensues because the increased appetite and caloric intake exceed the enhanced caloric consumption. Oligomenorrhea and amenorrhea occur in premenopausal women. On physical examination, the skin is warm and moist and has a fine velvety texture. The hair is fine and when combed, sheds substantial amounts, leading to thinning of the hair. Onycholysis with separation of the nail from the fingertip is fre-

---

TABLE 203–5. CAUSES OF THYROTOXICOSIS

Dependent on increased thyroid hormone production
  Dependent on increased occupancy of the TSH receptor by:
    Thyroid-stimulating immunoglobulin (TSI)
      Graves' disease
      Hashitoxicosis
    Human chorionic gonadotropin (hCG)
      Hydatiform mole
      Choriocarcinoma
    Thyroid-stimulating hormone (TSH)
      TSH-producing pituitary tumor
  Autonomous overproduction of thyroid hormone (independent of TSH)
    Toxic adenoma (TSH receptor mutant)
    Toxic multinodular goiter
    Follicular cancer (rare)
  Jodbasedow effect (excess iodine-induced hyperthyroidism)
Independent of increased thyroid hormone production
  Increased thyroid hormone release
    Subacute granulomatous thyroiditis (painful)
    Subacute lymphocytic thyroiditis (painless)
  Nonthyroidal source of thyroid hormone
    Thyrotoxicosis factitia
    "Hamburger" thyrotoxicosis
  Ectopic production by:
    Ovarian teratoma (struma ovarii)
    Metastasis of follicular cancer

TABLE 203–6. TISSUE-SPECIFIC SIGNS AND SYMPTOMS OF THYROTOXICOSIS

Tissue	Symptoms and Signs
Central nervous system	Nervousness and emotional lability Fine tremor of hands
Cardiovascular	Palpitations, tachycardia, atrial fibrillation, increased difference between systolic and diastolic blood pressure
Gastrointestinal (GI)	Hyperdefecation, GI hypermotility, diarrhea
Muscle	Proximal muscle weakness, muscle atrophy, hyperreflexia
Skin	Warm moist smooth skin, onycholysis, fine hair, hair loss, excessive perspiration
Metabolic	Heat intolerance, weight loss usually with increased appetite
Thyroid	Enlargement or nodule(s)

quent. Gynecomastia can occur in men because of increased estrogen production. Fine tremor is noted on the stretched-out hands, and tendon reflexes become hyperactive. The eye signs of thyrotoxicosis are most likely mediated by an increased sympathetic tone and include a widened distance between the upper and lower lid, lid lag on upward gaze, and frequent blinking. These signs do not indicate Graves' ophthalmopathy and are not accompanied by protrusion of the eyes. Cardiovascular manifestations can be marked, characterized by sinus tachycardia, a widened pulse pressure, and an often elevated systolic blood pressure. True hypertension is not frequent in hyperthyroidism but does occur in hypothyroidism. The heart beat is vigorous with a hyperactive pericardium. On auscultation the first sound is increased and a third sound and frequently a systolic murmur are audible. A harsh to-and-fro sound can be audible and is most likely caused by the pleural and pericardial surfaces rubbing each other. Cardiac arrhythmia, especially atrial fibrillation, can contribute to the development of heart failure. Muscle atrophy and weakness develop, and hypokalemic periodic paralysis has a measurable incidence in males of Asian extraction. Bone turnover can be increased, leading to hypercalcemia of as much as 12 mg per deciliter. Unusual blood-detected abnormalities ($<10\%$ of patients) include elevated alkaline phosphatase levels, increased direct bilirubin, mild anemia, and moderate neutropenia. Renal tubular acidosis can occur, and immune complex nephritis has been reported.

In older patients, the manifestations of thyrotoxicosis can be considerably modified. Affected patients frequently appear apathetic rather than nervous. Cardiovascular signs, general muscle weakness, and marked weight loss are more prominent. Cardiac arrhythmias that are refractory to conventional treatment, unexplained heart failure, or the recent onset or marked worsening of pre-existing angina pectoris should lead to a determination of thyroid hormone values.

Features Specific for Graves' Disease.
Autoimmune processes mediate the enlargement of the thyroid gland, infiltrative ophthalmopathy, dermopathy, and acropachy, thereby distinguishing Graves' disease from other causes of thyrotoxicosis. Palpation most frequently reveals diffuse and symmetric thyroid enlargement (two to six times normal). Thyroid nodules can occur and should be biopsied because, although unusual, thyroid cancer can coincide with Graves' disease. Auscultation of the thyroid frequently reveals a thyroid bruit, reflecting the increased blood supply. In a small number of patients, the thyroid remains of normal size. A hallmark finding of Graves' disease is infiltrative ophthalmopathy. Clinically detectable eye disease occurs in 20 to 40% of patients with Graves' disease, but severe ophthalmopathy requiring aggressive treatment affects only about 5%. Affected persons complain of easy tearing, photophobia, a feeling of sand in the eyes, diplopia, and decreased visual acuity. Ophthalmopathy affects the anterior soft tissue structures of the eye and with progressive severity involves more posterior structures as well. Periorbital edema and chemosis occur early and result from impaired drainage of the orbital veins. The swollen and fibrotic muscles cause lid retraction and restrict ocular movement, leading to diplopia. Upward gaze is most frequently impaired; with limitations of lateral gaze occurring less frequently. Tissue edema and accumulation of hydroscopic hyaluronic acid lead to engorgement of extraocular muscles and swelling of retro-orbital connective tissue, pushing the globe forward and resulting in prop-

tosis and further restriction of eye movement. Proptosis and lid retraction prevent complete closure of the eyes, resulting in exposure keratitis and corneal ulceration. Adequate care to prevent drying and infection of the cornea is important. Compression of the optic nerve at the posterior apex by enlarged muscles may lead to blurring and impaired visual acuity, visual field defects, impairment of color vision, and papilledema. Optic nerve compression can occur in the absence of proptosis. Graves' ophthalmopathy that is clinically apparent in only one eye occurs in 5 to 14% of patients. Sensitive imaging techniques like CT, however, show that most of these patients have bilateral orbital disease. Most patients with Graves' ophthalmopathy are hyperthyroid, but dissociation can occur, with ophthalmopathy appearing in patients of euthyroid or hypothyroid status. More unusual manifestations include coexisting myasthenia gravis with Graves' disease. Other cases may include diffuse lymphadenopathy and splenomegaly. Rarely, other autoimmune disorders occur in patients with Graves' disease.

DIAGNOSIS AND DIFFERENTIAL DIAGNOSIS. In patients with severe Graves' disease showing typical signs of thyrotoxicosis and autoimmune-mediated manifestations such as ophthalmopathy, the diagnosis is not difficult (Table 203–6). Gauging the degree of thyroid hormone overproduction guides subsequent therapy. Measurement of free T_4, T_3, and TSH levels constitutes a sufficient laboratory workup. In all patients with Graves' disease, T_3 levels are markedly elevated, and in most such patients free T_4 levels are elevated as well. In some patients, however, the marked stimulation of TSH receptors leads to higher hormone production rates of T_3 so that serum T_3 levels rise markedly while T_4 levels remain normal. This combination of laboratory values is termed T_3 toxicosis and is most frequently found during the initial phases or a relapse of Graves' disease. TSH levels are undetectable and serve to exclude TSH-producing tumors or thyroid hormone resistance as causes for the elevated thyroid hormone levels. In typical Graves' disease, radioactive iodine–based tests and a determination of the TSI are unnecessary. The clinical diagnosis becomes more difficult in patients with milder disease, in older patients manifesting apathetic thyrotoxicosis, and in patients with coexisting illnesses. Determination of free T_4, T_3, and TSH levels adequately establish the degree of thyrotoxicosis in patients with mild disease and older patients with an apathetic picture. Undetectable TSH levels using an ultrasensitive TSH assay are especially helpful in establishing that the body contains an excess amount of thyroid hormone. Intercurrent illness modifies thyroid hormone values by lowering T_3 levels and in some patients T_4 levels. Elevated reverse T_3 levels further implicate an intercurrent illness as a modifier of thyroid hormone values. Obtaining TSI values can be helpful in these patients because their elevation confirms the diagnosis of Graves' disease. Palpation of the thyroid revealing a nodule, a somewhat painful thyroid, or no palpable thyroid tissue is unusual and requires additional diagnostic procedures. A radioactive iodine scan is especially helpful in identifying a cold thyroid nodule surrounded by high uptake in surrounding tissue, a combination compatible with Graves' disease with a cold nodule requiring biopsy. Alternatively, the nodule may be hot, with surrounding areas showing decreased or absent uptake, which makes it more likely that the patient has a toxic adenoma. Very low uptake in patients who experience pain on palpation of the thyroid area indicates thyroiditis. In patients with no palpable thyroid tissue and absent thyroid uptake, ectopic production of thyroid hormone or factitious intake should be suspected. Thyroglobulin levels are very low in such patients.

Discrepancies between the degree of thyrotoxicosis and the extent of autoimmune abnormalities can complicate the diagnosis of Graves' disease. Some patients can exhibit marked bilateral or unilateral ophthalmopathy with minimal or no signs of thyrotoxicosis. In such instances, T_4 and T_3 levels are in the upper normal range and TSH levels are in the low normal or decreased range. The condition has been termed euthyroid ophthalmopathy or euthyroid Graves' disease. Thyrotoxicosis is mimicked by few clinical syndromes, and thyroid hormone values are normal in most of these. Pheochromocytomas can lead to heat intolerance, profuse sweating, palpitations, tachycardia, elevated glucose levels, and a state of anxiety. Anxiety states by themselves also lead to irritability, tremor, weakness, tachycardia, and weight loss. Thyroid hormone values are normal in these conditions.

TREATMENT OF GRAVES' DISEASE. The ophthalmopathy and dermopathy of Graves' disease require separate therapeutic approaches. The therapy of thyrotoxicosis is aimed at decreasing thyroid hormone formation and secretion. Three different therapeutic approaches are used: (1) antithyroid drugs that inhibit the thyroid peroxidase enzyme involved in thyroid hormone formation, (2) radioactive iodine, and (3) surgery. Both of the latter treatments decrease the amount of functional thyroid tissue. The most frequently used treatment modalities are antithyroid drugs or radioactive iodine, and the choice between them depends on the phase and severity of the disease, the specific situation of the patient, and the preference and experience of the physician. Spontaneously occurring increases and decreases of the underlying autoimmune abnormality lead to cycles of worsening and improvement of the thyrotoxic symptoms, making variable the natural history of Graves' disease. Consequently, life-long follow-up is recommended. About 10 to 20% of patients with Graves' disease remit spontaneously, and about half become hypothyroid after 20 to 30 years in the absence of therapy, most likely due to continued autoimmune destruction of the thyroid. Not treating patients and awaiting a spontaneous remission is not recommended. Therapy directed against the autoimmune process is currently not available.

TREATMENT OF THYROTOXICOSIS. *Antithyroid Drug Therapy.* Amelioration of thyrotoxic symptoms by decreasing thyroid hormone formation and release is the initial task in severe thyrotoxicosis. The thionamide derivatives, propylthiouracil (PTU) and methimazole (MMI), are the preferred initial treatment options in Graves' disease in the absence of contraindications. Radioactive iodine can lead to increased release of thyroid hormone and, infrequently, worsen the thyrotoxic symptoms to the point of inducing thyroid storm. Thyroid surgery is contraindicated in severely hyperthyroid patients. PTU and MMI, as well as carbimazole, which is used in Great Britain and is metabolized to methimazole, interfere with organification and iodotyrosine coupling by inhibiting the peroxidase enzyme. Both compounds may exert a mild immunosuppressive effect; a decrease in the level of TSI occurs after the drugs are started. This could be due to a mild immunosuppressive effect but also could result from decreased thyroid hormone secretion. Both drugs are rapidly absorbed from the gastrointestinal tract and concentrated in the thyroid. PTU inhibits peripheral conversion of T_4 to T_3, contributing 10 to 20% to the decrease in T_3 levels. This effect does not occur with MMI. MMI, however, is at least 10 times more potent than PTU and has a longer intrathyroidal residence time. MMI administered once a day is effective, whereas PTU must be given every 6 to 8 hours to exert its full effect. Both PTU and MMI cross the placenta; given in high doses they can interfere with fetal thyroid function. The choice between PTU and MMI and particular dosing schemes vary considerably between different centers. PTU is most useful for patients with severe thyrotoxicosis; those with moderate thyrotoxicosis are started on MMI, which comes in 5- and 10-mg tablets. Starting doses of 20 to 30 mg once daily are used. Improvement of thyrotoxic symptoms, in general, takes 2 to 3 weeks and can lag behind the normalization of thyroid hormone values. Euthyroidism can be achieved in 4 to 6 weeks. Thyroid hormone values are checked 4 weeks after the start of therapy and if no decrease in values occurs in spite of compliance, the dose may be increased to 30 to 40 mg a day. Once thyroid hormone levels normalize, the dose is decreased. A decrease in dose which is accompanied by an increase in free T_4 or T_3 levels and symptoms suggesting disease reactivation requires maintenance at higher dose levels for a longer time. Most patients can be maintained on low doses of 2.5 to 5 mg of MMI for 12 to 24 months.

A few patients with severe hyperthyroidism are started on PTU (100 to 150 mg every 8 hours). The choice is based on the faster decrease in T_3 levels with PTU than MMI. In some patients, higher doses of 200 to 300 mg every 6 hours are required. PTU comes in 50-mg tablets and, when taken in doses of two or three tablets three times a day, can lead to compliance problems. With improvement, the physician can progressively lower PTU doses and switch to once-a-day MMI. Most patients are then maintained on the lower MMI dose (2.5 to 5 mg per day) for 12 to 24 months. It appears that longer duration of antithyroid therapy bodes well for patients staying euthyroid after the medication is stopped. Most relapses occur within the first 3 to 6 months after discontinuation of antithyroid therapy. In young adults, a second course of antithyroid drug therapy can be tried, but the chance of permanent remission declines.

Undesired occurrences during PTU and MMI therapy include an increase in thyroid size, which may result from overtreatment, shown by low T_4 levels and elevated TSH levels, or undertreatment and reactivation of disease. Unfavorable indicators of disease activity are a requirement for higher PTU and MMI doses and T_3 levels that increase excessively compared with T_4 levels. Favorable prognostic signs are continued normalization of thyroid hormone levels, especially a normal T_4 to T_3 ratio in spite of using lower PTU and MMI doses, and decreasing thyroid size and TSI levels. Routine monitoring of TSI is not recommended. A recent report suggests a different treatment protocol. Patients are treated initially with MMI until euthyroid. Subsequently a combination of MMI (10 to 20 mg) plus thyroxine (0.1 mg T_4 per day) is used for another 12 to 24 months, at which time all signs of active Graves' disease have disappeared. MMI is discontinued and the patient is continued on 0.1 mg T_4 for 1 more year. Long-term remissions have been reported to occur in >90% of patients treated with this regimen. Before such a protocol is adopted for routine use, however, confirmation of results in patients of a different ethnic background and iodine exposure should be obtained.

Table 203–7 lists side effects of thionamide compounds. These occur most frequently during the initial 3 to 6 months after the therapy is started. The most frequent complications are allergic in nature, and skin rashes occur in 2 to 3% of patients. The major toxic reaction is agranulocytosis, which develops suddenly and occurs in 0.2 to 0.5% of patients. Routine monitoring of leukocyte counts is not recommended, but a leukocyte count should be obtained before starting therapy. Patients need to be instructed to discontinue their medication and contact their physician when a fever occurs or infections develop, especially in the oropharynx. A white blood count below 0.5×10^9 per liter indicates agranulocytosis and requires both discontinuation of antithyroid drugs and administration of broad-spectrum antibiotics as well as supportive therapy. Other treatment modalities such as radioactive iodine should be chosen for further treatment.

Radioactive Iodine (RAI). RAI therapy (^{131}I) is used most frequently to treat hyperthyroidism in adults in the United States, in contrast to Europe and Japan, where antithyroid medication is the preferred approach. In either event, antithyroid drugs are the preferred initial therapy for thyrotoxicosis. RAI therapy is preferred for older patients with moderate hyperthyroidism and thyroid enlargement, for patients with a prior allergic or toxic reaction to the antithyroid medication, and when frequent medication intake cannot be guaranteed. ^{131}I is also used after a course of antithyroid medication has failed to induce a long-term euthyroid state. RAI treatment is contraindicated during pregnancy; the fetal thyroid becomes able to accumulate iodine at 10 to 12 weeks of gestation. RAI can induce a thyroiditis with glandular swelling leading to potential air-

TABLE 203–7. SIDE EFFECTS OF ANTITHYROID DRUGS

Severe
  Agranulocytosis (0.2–0.5%)
  Only rare cases reported
    Hepatitis (can result in hepatic failure)
    Cholestatic jaundice
    Thrombocytopenia
    Hypoprothrombinemia
    Aplastic anemia
    Lupus-like syndrome with vasculitis
    Hypoglycemia (insulin antibodies)
Less severe
  Most frequent (1–5%)
    Rash
    Urticaria
    Arthralgia
    Decreased leukocyte level (drop in white cell counts by $2-3 \times 10^3$)
    Fever
  Less frequent
    Arthritis
    Diarrhea
    Decreased sense of taste

way obstruction in patients with large retrosternal goiters. A very low RAI uptake caused by excessive iodine exposure also precludes ^{131}I use.

Before ^{131}I administration, antithyroid drugs should be stopped for 3 or 4 days. Different dosing methods have been proposed for ^{131}I application. One approach is to aim at delivering 80 μCi ^{131}I per gram of thyroid tissue. The 80 μCi is then multiplied by the estimated weight of the gland and corrected for ^{131}I uptake. This delivers 6000 to 8000 rad to the thyroid and most frequently requires doses of 5 to 10 mCi. In patients with low uptake, large glands, and severe thyrotoxicosis leading to rapid intrathyroidal iodine turnover, larger doses often are chosen. Improvement in thyrotoxicosis occurs after 4 to 5 weeks, and 40 to 70% of patients regain normal thyroid functions within 6 to 8 weeks. Almost 80% of patients are cured with one dose. The remaining need a second dose, which should not be undertaken before 6 months have elapsed. After giving radioactive iodine, antithyroid drugs can be added at day 5 to reach a euthyroid state more quickly. In addition, β-sympathetic blockade is used to relieve associated symptoms. RAI can induce a painful thyroiditis and lead to acute thyroid hormone release and worsening of thyrotoxicosis. Severe thyroiditis can be treated with anti-inflammatory agents such as aspirin; rarely glucocorticoids are required. RAI treatment–induced worsening of Graves' ophthalmopathy has been reported in some studies but not in others. Administration of glucocorticoids concurrently with RAI treatment may be beneficial, but such treatment is not well enough established to be recommended for routine use. Steroids, however, may be useful for patients with prominent eye disease in whom RAI therapy is the approach of choice. No increase of thyroid cancer, other malignancies, or malformations in subsequent pregnancies have been documented after RAI therapy. It is recommended, however, that pregnancy not occur for 6 to 12 months after RAI treatment. Hypothyroidism is a consequence of RAI treatment. More than 50% of patients become hypothyroid during the first year after therapy, with an additional 2 to 3% during each subsequent year. Unless otherwise treated, transient hypothyroidism occurs 2 to 3 months after radioactive iodine treatment, with subsequent spontaneous normalization of thyroid hormone values. Patients should be informed of this risk and be followed after the acute phase of treatment every 4 to 6 months and subsequently at least once a year.

Surgical Therapy. Surgical removal of a large part of the thyroid (subtotal thyroidectomy) is indicated in patients with large obstructing glands or glands containing nodules that are identified as malignant or equivocal on fine-needle aspiration. Pregnant women with severe hyperthyroidism, which is difficult to control with antithyroid drugs, can be treated with thyroidectomy during the second trimester. In addition, young patients who are difficult to control on antithyroid drugs, patients with toxic reactions to antithyroid drugs, and patients who are not candidates for antithyroid drugs and refuse radioactive iodine are treated by surgery. Nevertheless, patients must be euthyroid before surgery is undertaken. This is achieved by using PTU or MMI for approximately 6 weeks. In patients on PTU or MMI, a saturated solution of potassium iodide (1 drop 3 times a day) can be administered daily for 10 days prior to surgery to reduce the vascularity of the gland. Subtotal thyroidectomy should be performed by an experienced thyroid surgeon. Complications including hypoparathyroidism, recurrent laryngeal nerve paralysis, and hemorrhage should occur in less than 1 to 2% of patients. In addition, transient hypocalcemia, wound infection, and keloid formation leading to unsightly scars may occur. Hypothyroidism occurs to a somewhat lower extent than after RAI, but its frequency may be underestimated. Recurrent hyperthyroidism occurs in about 10% of patients.

ALTERNATIVE AND SUPPORTIVE THERAPIES. In a small number of patients with Graves' disease, the conventional therapies listed above cannot be used. In some, toxic reactions preclude the use of antithyroid drugs and ^{131}I cannot be employed because a very low uptake occurs due to excess iodine exposure or because of pregnancy. Also, some patients may present a high surgical risk because of underlying medical problems. In such cases, the oral cholecystographic agent iopanoic acid or sodium iopodate (Oragrafin), administered at 1 gram per day, inhibits T_4 to T_3 conversion and leads to rapid lowering of T_3 levels. In addition, because of release of iodine from the compound, T_4 levels fall. These compounds should be used for only 2 to 3 months because escape from their antithyroid effect occurs. The perchlorate ion (ClO_4^-) of

$KClO_4$ is a competitive inhibitor of thyroidal iodide transport. In doses limited to 1 gram per day, serious toxic effects such as anaplastic anemia and gastric ulcers can be avoided. The compound is especially effective in iodine-induced hyperthyroidism (Jodbasedow) as occurs, for example, in patients treated with the antiarrhythmic compound amiodarone. Potassium perchlorate should be used for only a short duration and with careful supervision. The isolated use of iodine to treat thyrotoxicosis is ill advised because its inhibitory effects on thyroid hormone secretion often fail. Iodine should be used only in patients who are on antithyroid medication and are prepared for thyroid surgery or in the treatment of thyroid storm (see below).

β-Adrenergic blocking agents such as propranolol, 60 to 120 mg per day in three or four divided doses, help to provide relief of symptoms such as tachycardia, tremor, anxiety, and heat intolerance. The rationale for their use is based on an increased sensitivity of the β-sympathetic system in thyrotoxicosis and on a small inhibitory effect of T_4 to T_3 conversion. Patients with a history of asthma or congestive heart failure should not receive propranolol because it constricts bronchial smooth muscle and has a negative inotropic effect. Propranolol should not be used as a sole agent to treat hyperthyroidism because it neither directly inhibits thyroid hormone action nor induces a euthyroid state. Multivitamin supplementation is advisable in patients with severe thyrotoxicosis, especially if nutrition is not well balanced and adequate.

TREATMENT OF OPHTHALMOPATHY AND DERMOPATHY. Clinically apparent ophthalmopathy affects 20 to 40% of patients with Graves' disease, but severe symptoms occur in only a minority. For most patients with mild eye signs, only general supportive measures are needed. These include elevation of the head at night and wearing of tinted glasses to protect the eyes from sunlight and foreign bodies. Application of 1% methylcellulose drops to the eyes and taking a diuretic to decrease periorbital swelling provide further relief. Patients with more severe ophthalmopathy should be managed in close consultation between an endocrinologist and an ophthalmologist. Severe inflammatory reactions are treated with 60 to 100 mg of prednisone in divided doses for 2 to 4 weeks, with subsequent tapering of the dose over 8 to 12 weeks. Combinations of prednisone and cyclosporine have also been used. External x-ray therapy to the retro-orbital area may be helpful but is less well established as desirable therapy. The total dose is 20 Gy (2000 rad) given in 10 fractions over 2 to 3 weeks. Signs of optic nerve compression such as papillary edema, decreased color vision, and decreased visual acuity require surgical decompression, for which a transantral approach is frequently favored. After the active inflammatory process subsides, corrective surgical procedures may be beneficial. Retro-orbital muscle surgery may correct for eyeball misalignment and double vision. Eyelid surgery aimed at protecting the cornea, relieving discomfort, and cosmetic improvement should be the last surgical step.

Other Causes of Thyrotoxicosis

TOXIC ADENOMA AND TOXIC MULTINODULAR GOITER. Increased formation and secretion of T_3 and T_4 can occur in a single nodule or in multiple thyroid nodules. The latter condition is also termed Plummer's disease. Single nodules need to be larger than 2 to 3 cm in diameter to engender hyperthyroidism. Histologically, these nodules are follicular adenomas. Frequently a large nodule is palpable on one side of the thyroid, with atrophy of the other side. In contrast, patients with toxic multinodular goiter may undergo general nodular enlargement. Such persons frequently are older and have had a goiter for a long time before autonomous overproduction of thyroid hormone ensues. The thyrotoxicosis can be precipitated by excess iodine intake (Jodbasedow effect) and appears to occur particularly frequently in autonomous thyroid tissue, which functions independently of TSH stimulation. On physical examination, multinodular goiters range from small to large with possible substernal extension. Laboratory values show suppressed TSH levels and marked elevation of T_3 levels, with T_4 levels showing a lesser increase. Antibodies against the TSH receptor (TSI) and thyroid peroxidase (anti-TPO) are absent, in contrast to patients with Graves' disease. On RAI scan two patterns can be distinguished. Some patients show an irregular and patchy distribution of increased RAI uptake. In others, one or more distinct hot·nodules occur with marked, localized increased RAI accumulation and no uptake between the hot nodules. Both patterns are compatible with toxic goiter. Clinically affected patients may be difficult to diagnose because the disease affects elderly patients, who tend to present with apathetic hyperthyroidism. As noted earlier, typical thyrotoxic signs can be minimal in such patients, who often show apathy, lethargy, a depressed mood, weight loss, and cardiac abnormalities.

RAI is the treatment of choice for most patients with one toxic adenoma or multinodular toxic goiter. Severely thyrotoxic patients may need a course of antithyroid medication several weeks before they receive RAI to forestall acute worsening and decompensation after ^{131}I administration. The ^{131}I dose is 150 μCi per gram of tissue, twice that used for Graves' disease. Permanent hypothyroidism infrequently develops because remaining thyroid tissue resumes thyroid hormone secretion after ablation of toxic adenomas. Surgery can remove isolated adenomas, especially in younger patients.

RARE CAUSES. Thyrotoxicosis can be caused by TSH-producing pituitary tumors as well as by excess formation of hCG by hydatiform moles or choriocarcinoma. Surgical therapy is appropriate for both pituitary tumors and moles. Choriocarcinoma is treated by appropriate chemotherapy, and persistent thyrotoxicosis may require antithyroid drugs. Ectopic production of thyroid hormone by ovarian teratoma leads to mild thyrotoxicosis. Body scans detect RAI uptake in the location of the ovaries. Surgical removal is corrective. Follicular carcinoma of the thyroid with functioning metastases rarely leads to hyperthyroidism. Therapy is discussed in the section on thyroid cancer. Subacute or chronic thyroiditis can release high amounts of T_4 and T_3 and induce hyperthyroidism lasting for several weeks or months. RAI uptake is very low in such lesions. *Thyrotoxicosis factitia* results from inadvertent or planned ingestion of large amounts of thyroid hormone. It most frequently accompanies efforts at weight loss or occurs in patients with psychiatric problems. Many of these patients have easy access to thyroid hormone because they took it in the past, have relatives or acquaintances who are taking thyroid hormone, or are medical personnel. Ingestion of ground meat products prepared from neck trim containing thyroid tissue has also been reported (hamburger thyrotoxicosis). Patients with thyrotoxic symptoms, suppressed TSH levels, increased T_4 and T_3 levels, low RAI uptake, and suppressed thyroglobulin levels meet the diagnostic criteria for thyrotoxicosis factitia. Patients taking T_3 preparations have elevated T_3 levels but suppressed T_4 levels. Stopping thyroid hormone intake usually suffices. Additive β-sympathetic blockade or agents like ipodate to inhibit T_4 to T_3 conversion are rarely needed.

The term *Jodbasedow effect,* as noted before, designates iodine-induced hyperthyroidism. It occurs most frequently in patients with toxic nodular goiter exposed to excess amounts of iodine but has also been reported in Graves' disease. Problems with the autoregulation of thyroid hormone formation usually exist before iodine exposure; however, some patients have been reported who exhibited completely normal thyroid function after iodine was withheld. The Jodbasedow effect typically occurs in iodine-deficient areas after iodine supplementation is provided. Exposure to iodinated radiographic contrast media and iodinated drugs presents a frequent triggering event for the Jodbasedow effect in the United States. The antiarrhythmic agent amiodarone, which contains 37% iodine, can induce the Jodbasedow effect. The developing hyperthyroidism can worsen arrhythmias and lead to difficult management problems. In milder cases, antithyroid drugs like MMI are used. Potassium perchlorate prevents further iodine uptake and inhibits thyroid hormone formation. The usual dose is 200 mg four times a day.

Special Therapeutic Problems

THYROID STORM. Thyroid storm or thyrotoxic crisis is a life-threatening form of decompensated hyperthyroidism. Thyroid storm occurs most frequently in patients with severe thyrotoxicosis who develop an intercurrent severe illness such as an infection or sepsis or undergo a major surgical procedure. The distinction between severe thyrotoxicosis with an additional intercurrent illness and thyroid storm cannot be clearly drawn. Patients with severe thyrotoxicosis developing an intercurrent illness should be aggressively treated by the approach outlined in Table 203–8 because the illness can quickly decompensate into thyrotoxic crisis. Thyrotoxic crisis

TABLE 203–8. MANAGEMENT OF THYROID STORM

Inhibition of thyroid hormone formation and secretion
PTU, 400 mg q8h PO or by nasogastric tube
Sodium iodide, 1 gram IV in 24 hours, or saturated solution of KI, 5 drops q8h
Sympathetic blockade
Propranolol, 20–40 mg q4-6h, or 1 mg IV slowly (repeat doses until heart rate slows); not indicated in patients with asthma or congestive heart failure that is not rate-related
Glucocorticoid therapy
Hydrocortisone, 50–100 mg IV q6h
Supportive therapy
Intravenous fluids (depending on indication: glucose, electrolytes, multivitamins)
Temperature control (cooling blankets, acetaminophen; avoid salicylates)
O₂ if required
Digitalis for congestive failure and to slow ventricular response; pentobarbital for sedation
Treatment of precipitating event (e.g., infection)

requires no acute increase in thyroid hormone values, and it cannot be identified by laboratory tests. An acute increase in tissue availability of free thyroid hormones caused by a decrease in plasma-binding proteins may cause it, but equally likely are coincident increases in cytokines such as TNF-α and IL-6. Clinical signs compatible with thyrotoxic crisis are fever in excess of the temperature elevation expected from the intercurrent illness, with temperatures of 41°C (105°F) and even higher. In addition, marked tachycardia, extreme restlessness, agitation, and tremor occur. Patients may deteriorate mentally and become delirious, psychotic, obtunded, and even comatose. Hypotension with congestive heart failure and signs of an acute abdomen can develop. Table 203–8 outlines therapy, which includes high doses of antithyroid medication and iodine after starting antithyroid drugs. Cortisol turnover increases markedly, inducing enhanced formation of 11-keto compounds (cortisone), which are less metabolically active. Administration of 300 mg of hydrocortisone in divided doses is therefore indicated. Propranolol provides effective sympathetic blockade that has a favorable effect on rapid heart rate and induced cardiac failure. The compound, however, has a negative inotropic effect and should be used cautiously in patients with congestive heart failure. A history of asthma attacks precludes the use of β-sympathetic blockers. Treatment of precipitating events and supportive therapy must be started immediately.

THYROTOXICOSIS AND PREGNANCY. The most frequent cause of thyrotoxicosis during pregnancy is Graves' disease, but hyperthyroidism can result from toxic multinodular goiter and more rarely an excess of hCG production by hydatiform moles or choriocarcinoma. Hyperthyroidism may be difficult to recognize because pregnancy itself can lead to a hyperdynamic cardiovascular state and heat intolerance. Total T_4 and T_3 levels are increased owing to elevated thyroid hormone–binding protein levels, but T_4 values above 15 μg per deciliter strongly suggest hyperthyroidism. Hyperemesis gravidarum leads to elevated T_4 levels (hyperthyroxinemia), with normal T_3 values. In addition to medical problems of the mother resulting from severe thyrotoxicosis, slight increases in neonatal mortality rate and low birth weight in newborns have been reported. Antithyroid drugs are the initial therapy of choice. RAI is contraindicated, and the patient needs to be euthyroid before surgery can be considered. Because PTU inhibits T_4 to T_3 conversion, crosses the placenta less readily, and is concentrated to a lower extent in mothers milk than MMI, PTU is preferred over MMI in pregnant patients. Isolated cases of aplastica cutis induced by MMI have been reported. At high doses, PTU can induce fetal hypothyroidism and goiter because it crosses the placenta. In contrast, thyroid hormone minimally crosses the placenta. PTU doses are therefore limited to 200 to 300 mg per day; the addition of thyroxine confers no advantage. PTU administered in this way during pregnancy is relatively safe and does not negatively affect either fetal development or the outcome of pregnancy. If adequate control of hyperthyroidism is not possible, subtotal thyroidectomy should be considered, which is best performed during the second trimester. Long-term treatment with propranolol is not recommended because low birth weight can result. In addition, postnatal bradycardia and poor responses to hypoxia have been noted in newborns of mothers treated with propranolol. During the postpartum period, the mother risks developing new Graves' disease, a recurrence of previously quiescent Graves' disease, or postpartum thyroiditis. A state of relative immunosuppression during pregnancy which disappears with delivery has been implicated. Newborns delivered by mothers with Graves' disease can have a state of transient hyperthyroidism due to placental passage of TSI or less frequently long-term Graves' disease because of a genetic propensity. Mild neonatal thyrotoxicosis requires no therapy because the disease is self-limiting. In severe and more long-term thyrotoxicosis, PTU at doses of 10 to 25 mg every 8 hours is given. Nursing mothers with thyrotoxicosis can safely receive PTU in doses of 200 to 300 mg per day; these doses do not lead to levels in the milk that impair a newborn's thyroid function. MMI is concentrated in the milk at higher levels and should not be used.

Cardiac Disease

Thyrotoxicosis in patients with pre-existing cardiac disease can worsen symptoms and induce cardiac decompensation. Rarely, however, does severe hyperthyroidism induce cardiac symptoms in patients without underlying cardiac disease. Nevertheless, angina pectoris or high output failure has been reported after resumption of a euthyroid state in patients with severe thyrotoxicosis without prior evidence of cardiac disease. An increased association exists between Graves' disease and mitral valve prolapse. Most patients with cardiac problems due to hyperthyroidism are elderly, and many have toxic multinodular goiter. It is important to restore a euthyroid state promptly in these patients. This is best achieved by adequate doses of PTU (300 to 600 mg per day). Atrial fibrillation occurs in 10 to 15%; signs of congestive heart failure may be due to the rapid ventricular response and the absence of atrial contraction. Prompt slowing of the ventricular heart rate with digitalis and inducing β-sympathetic blockade with propranolol or atenolol are important. Digitalis must be prescribed with care because thyrotoxic patients are somewhat digitalis resistant, and a narrow margin separates therapeutic and toxic doses. Similarly, β-sympathetic blockers with negative inotropic effects should be used with caution in patients with congestive heart failure. The presence of atrial fibrillation usually requires anticoagulant therapy with aspirin or warfarin sodium. Increased vitamin K metabolism, however, may require lower warfarin doses. Spontaneous reversion from atrial fibrillation to regular sinus rhythm occurs frequently as successfully treated patients achieve a euthyroid state. If sinus rhythm has not returned after a euthyroid period of 4 months, cardioversion should be considered. Angina pectoris can worsen sufficiently in hyperthyroid patients that preinfarction angina becomes a concern. In markedly hyperthyroid patients, interventional procedures such as coronary angioplasty or bypass surgery should not be undertaken without prior treatment with antithyroid drugs because of the danger of thyrotoxic crisis. Calcium channel blockers like diltiazem are useful in patients with contraindications to propranolol. Angiographic procedures using iodinated contrast agents can markedly worsen the thyrotoxicosis because of the induction of the Jodbasedow effect, which especially endangers patients with toxic multinodular goiter. The antiarrhythmic compound amiodarone also can induce the Jodbasedow effect, as described above.

Becks GP, Burrow GN: Thyroid disease and pregnancy. Med Clin North Am 75:121, 1991. *A useful article for physicians caring for pregnant women.*

Burch AB, Wartofsky L: Graves' ophthalmopathy: Current concepts regarding pathogenesis and management. Endocrine Rev 14:747; 1993. *A thorough exploration of this difficult clinical problem.*

Gavin LA: Thyroid crisis. Med Clin North Am 75:179; 1991. *Provides a clinically detailed consideration of the problem.*

McDougall R: Graves' disease. Med Clin North Am 75:79, 1991. *A longer review of the subject.*

HYPOTHYROIDISM

Hypothyroidism is the clinical syndrome that results from decreased secretion of thyroid hormone from the thyroid gland. It most frequently reflects a disease of the gland itself (primary hypothyroidism) but can also be caused by pituitary disease (secondary hypothyroidism) or hypothalamic disease (tertiary hypothyroidism). Hypothyroidism leads to a slowing of metabolic processes and in its most severe form to the accumulation of mucopolysaccharides in the skin, causing a nonpitting edema termed myxedema. The term *myxedema* is reserved by some for a severe form of hypothyroidism, whereas others use the terms interchangeably. The term *cretinism* is reserved for hypothyroidism dating from birth and leading to abnormalities of intellectual and physical development. The generalized thyroid hormone resistance syndrome (GTRS) results from an abnormality in the amino acid sequence of the β form of the nuclear thyroid hormone receptor, leading to decreased T_3 binding. Impairment of thyroid hormone effects in GTRS is partly overcome by increased thyroid hormone levels, thereby preventing significant hypothyroid symptoms in most patients. The condition is rare.

INCIDENCE, ETIOLOGY, AND PATHOGENESIS. The incidence of hypothyroidism varies somewhat with the geographic area. In areas of adequate iodine supply, like the United States, 0.8 to 1.0% of the population are hypothyroid. In iodine-deficient areas of the world, the incidence is 10- to 20-fold higher. Neonatal hypothyroidism occurs with a frequency of 0.02% in the Caucasian population, whereas among African Americans it falls to 0.003%. Table 203–9 lists the causes of hypothyroidism.

Primary hypothyroidism accounts for about 90 to 95% of all cases, the remainder being of pituitary or hypothalamic origin. Most patients with primary hypothyroidism develop thyroid hormone deficiency during adulthood. Only a minority of patients have congenital hypothyroidism resulting from defects in enzymes required for thyroid hormone synthesis, thyroid agenesis, dysgenesis, or ectopic thyroid tissue. Temporary congenital hypothyroidism can be induced by maternal iodine or antithyroid drug administration. Primary hypothyroidism can be of a thyroprivic form, with markedly reduced or absent thyroid tissue, or a goitrous form, with an enlarged thyroid. The most frequent cause of hypothyroidism in adults is autoimmune disease, with goitrous or thyroprivic Hashimoto's disease being the prime example. In autoimmune-based hypothyroidism, antibodies are directed against thyroperoxidase, thyroglobulin, and the TSH receptor. Antithyroglobulin and antiperoxidase antibodies probably serve only as markers of autoimmunity, but anti-TSH antibodies cause disease. TSH receptor antibodies can block TSH action and thus contribute to decreased thyroid hormone formation. In addition to antithyroid antibodies, antibodies can be directed against the proteins of other endocrine organs such as the pancreas, adrenals, parathyroids, and gonads. Affected patients suffer from polyglandular endocrine deficiency states (see Ch. 210.1). A strong family history can be identified in most of these conditions.

Thyroid autoimmune disease also has an increased association with nonendocrine abnormalities such as pernicious anemia, lupus

TABLE 203–9. CAUSES OF HYPOTHYROIDISM

Primary hypothyroidism
Insufficient amount of thyroid tissue
  Destruction of tissue by autoimmune process
    Hashimoto's thyroiditis (atrophic and goitrous forms)
    Graves' disease—end-stage
  Destruction of tissue by iatrogenic procedures
    ^{131}I therapy
    Surgical thyroidectomy
    External radiation
  Destruction of tissue by infiltrative processes
    Amyloidosis, lymphoma, scleroderma
Defects of thyroid hormone biosynthesis
  Congenital enzyme defects
  Congenital mutations in TSH receptor
  Iodine deficiency or excess
  Drug-induced: thionamides, lithium, sulfonamides, interleukins, tumor necrosis factor, and others
Secondary hypothyroidism
Pituitary
  Panhypopituitarism, e.g., neoplasm, radiation, surgery, Sheehan's syndrome
  Isolated TSH deficiency
Hypothalamic
  Congenital
  Infection
  Infiltration (sarcoidosis, granulomas)
Transient hypothyroidism
  Silent and subacute thyroiditis
  Thyroxine withdrawal
Generalized resistance to thyroid hormone

erythematosus, rheumatoid arthritis, Sjögren's syndrome, chronic hepatitis, and myasthenia gravis. Thyroprivic hypothyroidism due to iatrogenic destruction of thyroid tissue by RAI, external beam radiation, or surgery is second only to autoimmune disease in causing hypothyroidism in the United States. Worldwide, hypothyroidism due to iodine deficiencies and goitrogens predominates. Goitrous hypothyroidism develops because TSH hypersecretion results in excessive thyroid growth. Iodine excess also can lead to goitrous hypothyroidism through iodine-induced inhibition of thyroid hormone formation (Wolff-Chaikoff effect). This occurs especially in patients with underlying thyroid disease. The thyroid is unable to reduce iodide uptake in spite of increased iodide stores, and the inability to escape from the Wolff-Chaikoff effect leads to goitrous hypothyroidism.

Secondary hypothyroidism is due to destruction of pituitary thyrotrophs by pituitary or adjacent tumors or by necrosis, as in Sheehan's syndrome. Mutations in the TSH β-subunit can lead to biologically inactive TSH, resulting in secondary hypothyroidism. In addition, mutations in the TSH receptor leading to hypothyroidism are described. Hypothalamic hypothyroidism is due to decreased TRH secretion, resulting in diminished TSH synthesis. TSH produced in the absence of a TRH stimulus does not show normal glycosylation and has decreased biologic activity. In addition to permanent hypothyroidism, transient hypothyroidism affects patients with subacute or painless thyroiditis, including the postpartum variety. Withdrawal of long-time thyroid hormone replacement leads to several weeks of hypothyroidism until the pituitary thyrotroph population is replenished and normal thyroid-pituitary feedback resumes.

Pathologic changes in hypothyroidism depend on the cause. In patients with thyroprivic hypothyroidism, the thyroid atrophies and is replaced by fatty and fibrous tissue. By contrast, in iodine deficiency–induced goitrous hypothyroidism, the gland appears hyperplastic with tall columnar epithelium. Extrathyroidal pathology is more uniform and independent of the cause of hypothyroidism. It is characterized by increased accumulation of glycosaminoglycans in interstitial tissue, giving the skin a waxy appearance. Glycosaminoglycan accumulation occurs because of decreased removal of the substance. With severe longstanding hypothyroidism, increased capillary permeability leads to proteinaceous fluid accumulation which may involve the pericardium.

CLINICAL MANIFESTATIONS. The different causes of hypothyroidism lead to similar symptoms, the most common of which are listed in Table 203–10. The slow and progressive onset in most patients can make clinical diagnosis difficult. This is especially true in elderly patients exhibiting changes like dry skin, reduced body and scalp hair, and memory difficulties, all of which could be due to the aging process in the absence of hypothyroidism. Typical complaints in hypothyroid patients include increased tiredness and sleep requirement with a depressed mood, feeling cold, gaining weight on the same diet, constipation, increased forgetfulness and increased time needed to fulfill a task, and decreased exercise tolerance associated with muscle cramps on strenuous exercises. Affected patients relate these complaints in a low-pitched, hoarse voice with a slow speech pattern. Frequently the changes are only fully appreciated by the patient after thyroid hormone replacement

and return to a euthyroid state. The facial appearance is frequently dull and apathetic with puffiness around the eyes and loss of lateral eyebrows. The skin takes on a yellow complexion due to carotene accumulation and becomes cold, dry, and rough with nonpitting edema (myxedema). The thyroid may be normal, enlarged, or absent, depending on the cause of hypothyroidism. Cardiovascular changes can include bradycardia and an enlarged cardiac silhouette primarily due to pericardial effusion. Hypertension occurs in 10% of hypothyroid patients and resolves after thyroid hormone replacement. Because of the increased occurrence of hypercholesterolemia and hypertension, hypothyroid patients have more coronary artery disease. Angina pectoris sometimes develops only after starting thyroid hormone replacement. Anemias of different causes accompany hypothyroidism and can contribute to angina symptoms. Iron deficiency anemia results from decreased iron absorption. Absorption of folic acid is decreased. Pernicious anemia results from gastric mucosa atrophy with antibodies directed against the gastric mucosa. The decreased oxygen consumption in the hypothyroid state leads to diminished erythropoietin production, resulting in a mild anemia that can be thought of as an adaptive state. Pulmonary function is characterized by shallow and slow breathing and a decreased respiratory response to hypercapnia and hypoxia. Patients are very sensitive to sedatives that can depress the respiratory drive and lead to CO_2 retention and coma. Gastrointestinal motility decreases markedly and can lead to paralytic ileus and the megacolon of myxedema. The kidneys not only have an impaired ability to excrete a free water load, but an inappropriate ADH syndrome (SIADH) can develop and intensify hyponatremia. Because of physical resistance in associated tissues, slow Achilles tendon reflexes are a hallmark of hypothyroidism. Similarly, severe hypothyroidism can lead to cerebellar ataxia and peripheral neuropathy. Endocrine and metabolic abnormalities include hyperprolactinemia leading to galactorrhea, heavy menstrual bleeding, menorrhagia, hypoglycemia, and SIADH. Longstanding and severe hypothyroidism can induce marked thyrotroph hyperplasia, resulting rarely in increased pituitary size and sella enlargement suggesting a pituitary tumor. Hypothyroidism in newborns needs to be treated immediately with thyroxine replacement; otherwise severe retardation of mental development, short stature, and deaf mutism can develop.

DIAGNOSIS. Figure 203–3 gives an approach to the diagnosis of hypothyroidism. An elevated TSH combined with a below-normal free T_4 is diagnostic of primary hypothyroidism. T_3 levels are not useful in the diagnosis of hypothyroidism because they are frequently normal in mild hypothyroidism and are markedly lowered by the NTI syndrome. In pituitary or hypothalamic hypothyroidism, the TSH level is normal or decreased, and only below-normal T_4 or free T_4 levels are diagnostic. With third-generation sensitive TSH assays, the TRH stimulation test provides little additional information. Using the TRH stimulation test, an absent response of TSH indicates secondary hypothyroidism, whereas a partial or delayed TSH response indicates partial pituitary deficiency or hypothalamic disease. Patients with pituitary hypothyroidism frequently show other signs of pituitary deficiency, including low FSH and LH lev-

TABLE 203–10. TISSUE-SPECIFIC SIGNS AND SYMPTOMS OF HYPOTHYROIDISM

Tissue	Signs and Symptoms
Central nervous system	Forgetfulness, stoic appearance, myxedematous dementia, cerebellar ataxia
Cardiovascular	Bradycardia, pericardial effusion, hypertension
Respiratory	Depressed ventilatory drive, pleural effusion, sleep apnea
Gastrointestinal	Constipation, hypomotility
Muscle	Delayed tendon reflexes, muscle stiffness and cramps, increased muscle volume, weakness
Skin	Dry, rough, hyperkeratosis; nonpitting puffiness due to mucopolysaccharide deposits
Metabolic	Basal metabolic rate decreased, cold intolerance, decreased T_4 and drug turnover, weight gain

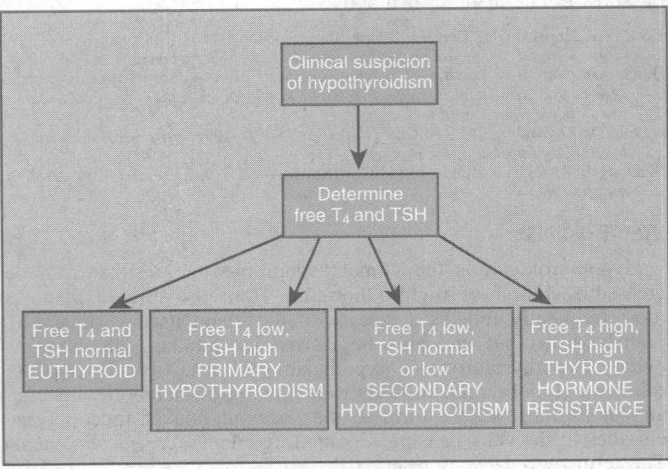

FIGURE 203–3. Diagnostic approach to hypothyroidism.

els in the face of low sex hormone levels. It is especially important to identify deficient ACTH secretion and resulting secondary adrenal insufficiency. When present, thyroid hormone replacement cannot be started before initiating cortisol replacement. Low TSH levels can also be found in patients who recently became hypothyroid after a prolonged period of hyperthyroidism which led to a decrease in the pituitary thyrotroph population. Other laboratory manifestations of hypothyroidism include elevated cholesterol, CPK, LDH, and aspartate transaminase levels.

The presence of antithyroid antibodies is compatible with Hashimoto's disease and presents a risk factor for developing hypothyroidism. During early phases of hypothyroidism, T_4 and free T_4 lie just below the lower normal range. T_3 is normal and TSH is barely elevated. This condition has been termed subclinical hypothyroidism, or the failing gland syndrome. Patients show minimal or no signs of hypothyroidism because a normal T_3 level maintains their metabolic status. Many such patients later develop clinical hypothyroidism with a further increase in TSH levels and a decrease in T_4 and free T_4 levels. In patients with Hashimoto's disease or after RAI treatment of Graves' disease, this pattern occurs frequently. Transient hypothyroidism frequently occurs in postpartum patients, with subacute thyroiditis, or after RAI treatment for Graves' disease. Changes in TSH levels lag behind alterations in T_4 and T_3 levels; careful follow-up is required to determine if permanent hypothyroidism ensues.

DIFFERENTIAL DIAGNOSIS. Fully developed hypothyroidism presents a distinct clinical picture with few imitations. Patients with renal disease resulting in a nephrotic syndrome and hypoalbuminemia can develop a puffy face, peripheral edema, a pale downy skin, anemia, and hypercholesterolemia. Goiter and thyroid nodules occur with increased frequency in patients with renal disease. Lowering of TBG levels leads to a decrease in total T_4 values. In contrast to hypothyroidism, however, free T_4 is not decreased and TSH is not increased. In children, Down syndrome can mimic hypothyroidism. Differential diagnosis is further complicated by an increased incidence of Hashimoto's thyroiditis and resultant hypothyroidism in patients with Down syndrome, but thyroid hormone values are normal in Down's patients without thyroid disease.

TREATMENT. Hypothyroidism is preferentially treated with levothyroxine (T_4), with doses ranging from 0.05 to 0.2 mg per day and an average replacement dose of 1.6 μg per kilogram per day. T_3 is formed from T_4 by intracellular conversion so that both T_4 and T_3 exist in the body. Synthetic T_4 has a long shelf life and uniform potency. Eighty percent is absorbed, and once a day intake leads to stable T_4, T_3, and TSH levels. Accordingly, thyroxine represents the preferred thyroid hormone preparation for chronic replacement. Patients should be informed that replacement probably is needed for the rest of their lives and that periodic evaluation is required. In young healthy adults without coronary artery disease, a starting dose of 75 to 100 μg per day can be used and then adjusted after 2- to 3-week intervals to reach the final replacement level. In elderly patients and those with coronary artery disease, the initial dose should be 12.5 to 25 μg per day and increased by 25 to 50 μg every 4 to 6 weeks to allow a slow increase in metabolic rates, avoiding a mismatch between coronary blood supply and metabolic demand. The aim is to achieve a euthyroid status with TSH, T_4, and T_3 levels in the normal range. Because in the complete absence of functioning thyroid tissue all T_3 is formed from the thyroxine medication and the 20% of thyroidal contribution to T_3 levels is missing, T_3 levels are frequently in the mid-normal range and T_4 levels are in the upper range of normal. A slight increase in T_4 levels occurs 2 to 6 hours after thyroxine intake so that blood for thyroid hormone determination should be drawn 20 to 24 hours later. The average replacement dose for thyroxine varies with age and to a lesser degree with the cause of hypothyroidism and the level of physical activity. Children (5 to 10 years), for example, require average replacement doses of 3 to 4 μg per kilogram. Required replacement doses in elderly persons, by contrast, are 20 to 30% lower (1.4 μg per kilogram per day) than those needed in middle-aged adults. Patients with malabsorption or those taking aluminum preparations (antacids), cholestyramine, lovastatin, ferrous sulfate, and rifampin need higher replacement doses. During pregnancy, especially in the third trimester, thyroxine replacement needs increase by 30 to 50%. After delivery, thyroxine replacement is decreased to standard levels.

The ease of approach, virtual absence of side effects, and observance of a revitalized patient make thyroxine treatment of hypothyroid patients a satisfying therapeutic experience. Thyroxine and T_3 levels normalize within 2 to 3 weeks. TSH levels lag behind for 3 to 4 weeks or more because of the increased number of thyrotrophs in the pituitary after longstanding hypothyroidism. Clinical improvement begins 2 to 3 weeks after therapy, but complete resumption of a euthyroid state can take several months.

Patients receiving chronic T_4 replacement should be evaluated by physical examination and free T_4, T_3, and TSH determination once or twice a year. The TSH level is a good indicator of adequate replacement. In patients with primary hypothyroidism, TSH levels below the normal range indicate overreplacement and levels above the upper normal range indicate underreplacement. Chronic overreplacement with thyroxine can increase bone turnover, which is a special concern in women; however, no evidence currently exists for an increased bone fracture rate. Chronic T_4 overreplacement also can lead to cardiovascular abnormalities, especially arrhythmias and cardiac hypertrophy. The treatment of subclinical hypothyroidism is controversial. Enlargement of the thyroid gland, elevated cholesterol levels—especially with LDL:HDL ratios above 3, or signs of decreased exercise tolerance and mild congestive heart failure warrant treatment.

In addition to thyroxine, triiodothyronine (T_3), combinations of T_4 and T_3, desiccated thyroid, and thyroxine plus iodine in one tablet are available. Only the use of T_3 is recommended in special situations. T_3 is useful for short-term treatment of patients with thyroid cancer after thyroid surgery and before RAI administration, because of its short half-life of 1 day versus the half-life of T_4 of 7 days (see section on thyroid cancer). Parenteral T_3 can be used to treat myxedema coma. In patients with the rare condition of 5' deiodinase deficiency, T_3 preparations are also useful. Other thyroid preparations have no advantage over thyroxine and are not recommended.

Special Clinical Conditions

ANGINA PECTORIS, CARDIAC SURGERY, AND THYROID HORMONE REPLACEMENT. Coronary artery disease occurs with increased frequency in hypothyroid patients. The complaint of angina pectoris most often arises with thyroid hormone replacement, which increases cardiac demand and O_2 consumption. Adequate thyroid hormone replacement is strongly recommended in these patients because in addition to the general benefit of a euthyroid state, cholesterol levels may decrease and blood pressure may normalize. Frequently, worsening of the angina precludes adequate thyroid hormone replacement. Treatment with β-sympathetic blockers such as propranolol (20 to 40 mg three times a day) can sometimes ameliorate the problem but may lead to significant bradycardia. Also, β-blockade fails to solve the basic dilemma between inadequate thyroid hormone replacement and angina production. In such patients with persistent mild to moderate hypothyroidism, percutaneous coronary transluminal angioplasty or coronary bypass surgery can be undertaken. Several studies have shown no deleterious consequences of a mild to moderate hypothyroid state on clinical outcome.

TREATMENT OF MYXEDEMA COMA. Patients with severe myxedema, either spontaneously or suffering from cold exposure, intake of analgesics or sedatives, or infection, may become progressively obtunded and lapse into coma. Myxedema coma is rare but presents a life-threatening emergency with a 20 to 50% mortality which is best treated in an intensive care unit. Treatment should be instituted immediately and if T_4 and TSH levels cannot be readily obtained, therapy may be started on clinical suspicion. Increasing obtundation and elevated PCO_2 levels especially indicate the need for thyroid hormone administration. Assessment of adrenal function should also be undertaken because giving hydrocortisone can disturb pituitary-adrenal feedback and make subsequent diagnosis difficult. Vigorous thyroid hormone replacement is required. Thyroxine can be given as a single 300 μg T_4 bolus followed by daily 50 to 100 μg intravenous T_4 maintenance doses. A T_3 replacement schedule using 10 μg T_3 intravenously every 4 hours until the patient greatly improves and oral therapy can be resumed has recently been advocated. T_3 administration offers the potential advantage that no conversion of T_4 to T_3 is required, a step that may be impaired in severely ill patients. The treatment of myxedema coma is outlined in Table 203–11.

Arlot S, Debussche X, Lalau JD, et al.: Myxedema coma: Response of thyroid hormone with oral and intravenous high-dose L-thyroxine treatment. Intensive Care Med 17:16, 1991.

Becker C: Hypothyroidism and atherosclerotic heart disease: Pathogenesis, medical management, and the role of coronary artery bypass surgery. Endocrinol Rev 6:432, 1985.

Fisher DA: Management of congenital hypothyroidism. Clinical Rev 19. J Clin Endocrinol Metab 72:523, 1991.

Mandel SJ, Larsen PR, Seeley EW, Brent GA: Increased need for thyroxine during pregnancy in women with primary hypothyroidism. N Engl J Med 323:91, 1990.

Mitchell JM: Thyroid disease in the emergency department. Thyroid function tests and hypothyroidism and myxedema coma. Emerg Med Clin North Am 7:885, 1989.

Roti E, Minelli R, Gardini E, et al.: The use and misuse of thyroid hormone. Endocrinol Rev 14:401, 1993.

THYROIDITIS

Thyroiditis includes infectious and autoimmune inflammatory diseases of the thyroid. Thyroiditis is divided into acute (suppurative), subacute painful (granulomatous), subacute painless (lymphocytic), chronic lymphocytic (Hashimoto's), and chronic fibrous (Riedel's) thyroiditis. Postpartum thyroiditis is classified as a variant of subacute painless lymphocytic thyroiditis.

Acute (Suppurative) Thyroiditis

Acute suppurative thyroiditis consists of a rare infection of the gland by bacteria, fungi, *Pneumocystis carinii,* or other organisms. Symptoms include tender swelling, sometimes with fluctuation and an erythematous skin overlying the area. Fever with leukocytosis frequently occurs. Identification of the microbial agent may require fine-needle aspiration of the lesion. Appropriate antibiotics and sometimes drainage of the abscess are required. Long-term sequelae are rare, but when a large part of the thyroid gland is involved, hypothyroidism may occur.

Subacute Painful (Granulomatous) Thyroiditis

INCIDENCE, ETIOLOGY, AND PATHOLOGY. Subacute painful thyroiditis, also termed de Quervain's thyroiditis, giant cell thyroiditis, subacute nonsuppurative thyroiditis, or granulomatous thyroiditis, is the most frequent cause of severe thyroid pain and tenderness. Subacute painful thyroiditis is not rare, resulting in 5% of all medical consultations for thyroid disease. It is most common in women 40 to 50 years old and shows an association with HLA-B35. The disease frequently follows a viral infection, and elevated titers to mumps, adeno-, entro-, echo-, influenza, coxsackie-, measles and other viruses have been found. Increased thyroid antibody titers (antimicrosomal, antithyroglobulin, anti-TSH receptor) occur in 10 to 20% of patients during the subacute phase and disappear as the disease fades. Such antibodies are polyclonal and most likely arise secondary to thyroid damage caused by viral infection. The thyroid is enlarged and edematous with destruction of follicular architecture and the presence of histocytes that coalesce into giant cells.

MANIFESTATIONS, DIAGNOSIS, AND TREATMENT. The disease frequently follows by 1 to 3 weeks the occurrence of viral pharyngitis, mumps, measles, or other viral syndromes. Severe pain develops over the thyroid area, radiates to the ear, and is enhanced by swallowing. A feeling of general malaise with muscle aches, pain, anorexia, and fever is present. On palpation, the thyroid is very tender and may be generally enlarged but can contain unilat-

eral painful areas. Cervical lymphadenopathy rarely occurs. Characteristic laboratory findings are an elevated sedimentation rate, often above 100 mm per hour Westergren, and a markedly decreased RAI uptake (< 2% at 24 hours). The level of free T_4 and TSH depend on the phase of the disease, with high T_4 levels occurring during the early stage owing to follicle disruption and hormone release. At later stages, transient hypothyroidism may follow, with elevated TSH levels. Rarely, permanent hypothyroidism ensues. Thyroglobulin levels are elevated during the acute phase.

Subacute thyroiditis is an inflammatory, self-limiting disorder that at most requires symptomatic therapy. In mild cases, no therapy or analgesics such as aspirin (2 to 3 grams per day) are sufficient. Prednisone, 40 to 60 mg daily, can suppress more severe symptoms and bring relief. Within 8 to 10 days symptoms markedly decrease, and the dose can be tapered and completely stopped after 4 weeks. Sometimes symptoms flare up again and the prednisone taper needs to be reversed. In some patients, more than one attack may occur, leading to an increased risk of permanent hypothyroidism. During the initial phase, the patient may be thyrotoxic and need treatment with β-sympathetic blocking agents such as propranolol. Rarely hepatitis develops, requiring careful follow-up.

Subacute Painless (Lymphocytic) Thyroiditis with Transient Hyperthyroidism

INCIDENCE, ETIOLOGY, AND PATHOLOGY. Subacute painless thyroiditis with transient hyperthyroidism is also called subacute lymphocytic thyroiditis with spontaneously revolving hyperthyroidism and silent thyroiditis. The hallmark of the disorder is a self-limiting episode of thyrotoxicosis and a histologic picture of lymphocytic infiltration which differs from the changes found in Hashimoto's disease. Both postpartum thyroiditis and the sporadic disease occurring in the general population are forms of subacute lymphocytic thyroiditis. The incidence of sporadic subacute painless thyroiditis shows some geographic variability, with the sporadic form occurring more frequently in previously iodine-deficient areas which are now iodine replete, like the Great Lakes area of the United States, where the disease may account for 5 to 15% of all thyroiditis. Postpartum thyroiditis occurs in 2 to 6% of all pregnant women in the United States. The incidence is even higher in Sweden and Japan, reaching 7 to 12%. Eighty percent of cases of the sporadic form affect women between the ages of 30 and 40 years. The disease is most likely autoimmune in origin and independent of a preceding viral illness. Subacute lymphatic thyroiditis is distinguished from chronic lymphocytic thyroiditis (Hashimoto's disease) by a self-limiting course and a lower extent of lymphocyte infiltration with the absence of germinal centers.

MANIFESTATIONS, DIAGNOSIS, AND TREATMENT. Typical are an abrupt onset with signs of thyrotoxicosis such as nervousness, heat intolerance, tachycardia, and weight loss. A small, firm, but painless goiter is noted in about half the patients. Some may present in a hypothyroid state after the initial hyperthyroid phase was unnoticed. Postpartum thyroiditis usually occurs 3 to 6 months after delivery, with an initial transient hyperthyroid phase followed by hypothyroidism. The latter lasts 1 to 3 months, and most patients make a spontaneous recovery. During the initial hyperthyroid phase, which can last 2 to 4 months, T_4 and T_3 are elevated, with relatively higher T_4 levels due to thyroid hormone release from damaged follicles. Thyroid antibodies, especially antiperoxidase, are frequently positive but at low titers. Sedimentation rate is normal or only slightly elevated, in contrast to the marked elevation occurring in subacute painful thyroiditis. The RAI uptake is suppressed. Signs of Graves' disease, such as ophthalmopathy and pretibial myxedema, are absent, and the level of TSI, which is the hallmark of Graves' disease, is normal. Thyroid biopsy shows a typical histologic picture with abundant lymphocyte infiltration, but the procedure is not required for routine diagnosis. Treatment aims at sympathetic blockade using, for example, propranolol to alleviate symptoms during the thyrotoxic phase. Glucocorticoids are not needed. Prolonged hypothyroid episodes may be treated with thyroxine replacement, but with subsequent tapering of the dose and final withdrawal because most patients regain euthyroid status. Increased incidences of goiter and persistent hypothyroidism have been noted in patients who continue to show antiperoxidase antibodies. Similarly, the recurrence of postpartum thyroiditis has been noted in some patients with continued presence of antiperoxidase antibodies after the initial phase of the disease.

TABLE 203–11. TREATMENT OF MYXEDEMA COMA

Thyroid hormone administration
300 μg T_4 over 5–10 minutes initially, followed by 100 μg T_4 IV q24h until oral T_4 therapy can be started
Alternatively, 10 μg T_3 IV q4h until oral T_4 therapy can be started
Glucocorticoid administration
Hydrocortisone, 100 mg IV bolus followed by 25 mg q6h by IV drip
Cover to conserve heat
Intravenous fluids, electrolytes, and glucose to correct electrolyte abnormalities and hypoglycemia
Tracheal intubation and mechanical ventilation as required
Treat precipitating conditions (infection)
Avoid sedatives, narcotics, and overhydration

Chronic Lymphocytic Thyroiditis (Hashimoto's Thyroiditis)

Chronic lymphocytic thyroiditis is the most prevalent form of thyroid autoimmune disease, affecting about 3 to 4% of the population in the United States. It is three times more common in women and most frequently diagnosed between the third and fifth decade of life. A genetic propensity for the disease is demonstrated by an increased familial incidence and an association with major histocompatibility antigens such as HLA-B8. The goitrous variant of Hashimoto's thyroiditis occurs more frequently in patients positive for HLA-DR5, whereas the atrophic variant is associated with HLA-DR3. The presence of antiperoxidase and antithyroglobulin antibodies indicates the autoimmune nature of the disease. Very high levels of thyroid antibodies distinguish Hashimoto's thyroiditis from other forms. In addition, anti-TSH receptor antibodies can occur which are frequently of the blocking variety, impairing TSH action. Rarely, TSI's are present, leading to hyperthyroidism and the combined occurrence of Graves' disease and Hashimoto's disease called Hashitoxicosis. Thyroid pathology is dominated by heavy lymphocyte infiltration destroying the normal follicular architecture. Lymph follicles and germinal centers can be identified. The presence of copious lymphocytes is a hallmark of the disease that distinguishes it from other forms of autoimmune thyroiditis. Differential diagnosis between the abundant lymphocyte infiltrates of Hashimoto's disease and the occurrence of a primary thyroid lymphoma is sometimes difficult. Thyroid lymphomas occur with an increased frequency in Hashimoto's disease but overall are rare. Also, the pathology of the thyroid gland in Hashimoto's disease is characterized by extensive fibrosis throughout the gland. Different manifestations of Hashimoto's disease can be distinguished. The occurrence of a goitrous versus an atrophic variant may be explained by the prevailing autoimmune antibodies. For example, in patients with atrophic thyroiditis, high titers of TSH receptor–blocking antibodies are found. In other patients with Hashimoto's disease, a goiter and features of Graves' disease occur which results from the TSI presence.

CLINICAL MANIFESTATIONS AND DIAGNOSIS. In Hashimoto's thyroiditis, thyroid enlargement is the most frequent manifestation, with 75% of patients having a euthyroid goiter; the remainder have the atrophic variety and may not have a palpable gland. Hypothyroidism occurs as an initial manifestation in 20% of patients. Hyperthyroidism occurs in < 5% of patients and can be either self-limiting or longstanding, representing Hashitoxicosis. The principal abnormalities in the immune system discussed for Graves' disease also apply to Hashimoto's disease. The prevalence of specific forms of TSH receptor antibodies with a predominance of the TSI in Graves' disease versus the occurrence of TSH receptor–blocking antibodies in Hashimoto's disease distinguishes the two autoimmune diseases. In addition, lymphocyte infiltration is much more destructive to the architecture of the normal gland than in Graves' disease. Other autoimmune diseases occur with increased frequency in Hashimoto's patients, including autoimmune diseases of the endocrine system with adrenal, parathyroid, pituitary, and gonad destruction and damage to β cells of the pancreas. Furthermore, an association occurs with pernicious anemia, Sjögren's syndrome, lupus erythematosus, and idiopathic thrombocytopenic purpura. Graves' disease can occur in conjunction with the same illnesses.

On physical examination, a painless symmetrically enlarged thyroid gland is noted which feels firm and rubbery with an irregular surface. The gland can reach a size and firmness that leads to pressure symptoms, impairing swallowing and resulting in inlet obstruction with tracheal compression. Sometimes only one firm lobe or a single firm thyroid nodule may be palpable, representing the only remnant, with other parts of the gland destroyed by the autoimmune process. On laboratory examination, 90% of patients have positive antiperoxidase antibodies and 50% have antithyroglobulin antibodies. T_4 and TSH levels can be normal. In patients with the hypothyroid form, TSH levels are elevated and T_4 and free T_4 levels are decreased. RAI scans are not required for routine workup and are not diagnostic. They can show normal, increased, or decreased overall uptake with local patchy areas of increased and decreased iodine accumulation. Fine-needle aspiration is not routinely used but can be helpful in differentiating a firm nodule as a thyroid remnant in Hashimoto's disease versus a benign thyroid adenoma or thyroid cancer. The incidence of thyroid cancer is not increased in Hashimoto's disease except for the increased occurrence of lymphomas, a rare event.

TREATMENT. The autoimmune abnormality underlying Hashimoto's disease is currently not amenable to therapy. Therapy is directed at achieving a euthyroid state and dealing with mechanical problems resulting from the goiter. Thyroxine replacement is initiated when T_4 levels are low and TSH levels are high. In some patients, only the TSH is slightly elevated and the T_4 is low-normal, with signs of hypothyroidism being absent. These patients can be treated with thyroxine replacement to forestall further thyroid gland enlargement and future clinical hypothyroidism. In some patients, thyroxine therapy cannot decrease the goiter size and obstructive symptoms may require surgery for relief. During the early phases of Hashimoto's disease, transient hyperthyroidism can occur and requires only symptomatic treatment with sympathetic β-blockers. Hyperthyroidism developing in well-established Hashimoto's disease is treated like Graves' disease, with antithyroid medication as the treatment of choice.

Fibrous Thyroiditis (Riedel's Thyroiditis)

In fibrous thyroiditis, thyroid tissue is replaced by dense, chronically inflamed fibrous tissue. The thyroid is rock hard on palpation, a finding that can be compatible with thyroid cancer. Thyroid aspiration can clarify the diagnosis. Tracheal obstruction can occur and may require surgery. Sclerosing mediastinitis, retroperitoneal fibrosis, sclerosis of the biliary tract, and pseudotumors of the orbit have been described in such patients. When hypothyroidism exists, thyroxine replacement is required.

Rapoport B: Pathophysiology of Hashimoto's thyroiditis and hypothyroidism. Ann Rev Med 42:91, 1991. *A thorough review of the subject.*
Singer PA: Thyroiditis. Acute, subacute, and chronic. Med Clin North Am 75:61, 1991. *Provides a thorough discussion of the condition.*

NONTOXIC DIFFUSE AND NODULAR GOITER

The term *nontoxic* or *simple goiter* indicates an increase in the mass of the thyroid gland resulting from excessive replication of benign thyroid epithelial cells. In patients with nontoxic goiter, thyroid hormone values usually are normal. The increase in thyroid size is a slow process evolving over many years, starting with a diffuse initial enlargement, which frequently becomes multinodular with time. Nontoxic goiter is the most common thyroid disease in America, affecting about 5% of the population. Its incidence increases with age and affects women three to five times more frequently than men. Goiters have been classified according to the epidemiologic pattern in which they occur as endemic or sporadic goiters. Thyroid enlargement occurring in > 10% of a population is termed *endemic goiter* and is presumed to result from environmental factors, such as iodine deficiency or the presence of goitrogens in the food chain which inhibit thyroid hormone formation. *Sporadic goiter* indicates thyroid enlargement in a small fraction of the population. The cause of sporadic goiter varies, with thyroid growth most frequently stimulated by extrathyroidal growth factors. TSH is the most frequent stimulator. The observation that goiters also occur in patients with adequate thyroid hormone levels and normal or low TSH levels indicates either that the sensitivity of thyroid cells to TSH can increase markedly or that other factors drive thyroid cell growth. Stimulatory effects of IGF-1 and EGF on thyroid cell growth have been reported. In addition, TSH receptor-directed antibodies that have only a growth-stimulating effect have been described. Different thyroid cells also have a varying propensity to grow and enter the mitotic cycle independent of stimulation by growth factors. Specific thyroid cells and their descendants that possess an increased noncancerous propensity to divide and grow can form new thyroid follicles. These different factors that contribute to goiter formation explain why not all goiters shrink or stop growing on thyroxine supplementation and resultant TSH suppression.

The pathology of the goitrous thyroid varies, depending on the stage and cause of the goiter. Initially, hypertrophic follicles with hypervascularity are prevalent throughout the gland. With increasing duration follicle size varies. Some follicles become involuted whereas others enlarge with colloid accumulation. Fibrotic areas sometimes separate hypertrophic from atrophic and involuted areas. This mixed pattern of follicle activity is reflected in RAI scans with patchy areas of increased and decreased uptake.

MANIFESTATIONS. Patients with nontoxic simple goiter can be asymptomatic or present with symptoms due to mechanical pressure exerted by the enlarged thyroid gland. Structures exposed to pressure are the trachea, esophagus, recurrent laryngeal nerve, and large cervical veins. Substernal goiters are most frequently responsible for tracheal pressure symptoms leading to deviation, narrowing, and chondromalacia. The trachea must be narrowed to 20 to 30% of its normal diameter to produce respiratory symptoms, especially inspiratory stridor. Pull and pressure on the laryngeal nerve leading to hoarseness can occur with benign goiters but should raise the suspicion of malignancy. The presence of a substernal goiter is made evident when patients raise both arms above the head, which pulls the goiter upward into the thoracic inlet. The resultant impediment of jugular venous return leads to a livid suffusion of the face and discomfort for the patient (Pemberton's sign). An acute painful enlargement of an area of the thyroid frequently reflects sudden bleeding into a thyroid nodule; symptoms improve as resorption of the hemorrhage occurs. In a slow and progressively developing dominant nodule, thyroid cancer must be excluded by cytologic examination of a fine-needle aspirate.

Congenital goiter in endemic areas results most frequently from insufficient thyroid hormone formation due to iodine deficiency or the presence of goitrogens and resultant TSH stimulation of the gland. Sporadic congenital goiter is often due to biosynthetic abnormalities in thyroid hormone formation resulting from defects in (1) iodide transport into the thyroid, (2) deficient peroxidase activity, (3) deficient iodotyrosine coupling, (4) formation of abnormal thyroglobulin, (5) impaired thyroglobulin proteolysis, or (6) deiodinases being deficient or absent and not allowing for intrathyroidal iodide conservation. These defects are rare and account for 10% of all congenital hypothyroidism. If these patients are left untreated, goiter and cretinism can result. In other patients, nontoxic goiter with mild hypothyroidism develops. The combination of congenital hypothyroidism and eighth nerve deafness has been termed Pendred's syndrome.

DIAGNOSTIC PROCEDURES. The most sensitive index to evaluate thyroid status in patients with goiter is the TSH level. TSH can be elevated in the face of normal or low-normal T_4 levels and mid-normal T_3 values. Most such patients benefit from thyroxine replacement, with TSH decreasing into the normal range and removing the thyroid growth stimulus. The thyroid status of patients with nontoxic goiter needs to be evaluated once or twice a year because some thyroid nodules develop autonomy over time, and toxic adenomas with resulting thyrotoxicosis can develop. In addition, ingestion of excess iodine can induce thyrotoxicosis due to the Jodbasedow effect. With progressive involution of the goiter, TSH values increase progressively and hypothyroidism develops. The presence of pressure symptoms requires evaluation for substernal extension of the thyroid gland which is best performed by CT scan or MRI. In the absence of such imaging, radiography reveals tracheal deviation, and pulmonary function tests can document inspiratory impairment. In patients with endemic goiter, especially due to iodine deficiency, laboratory values show a low T_4, normal T_3, and elevated TSH level stimulating the thyroid gland for further compensatory growth. The amount of iodine intake can be documented by determining iodide excretion in the urine which is correspondingly low in iodine-deficiency regions.

TREATMENT. The aim of therapy is to decrease the size of the thyroid, relieve pressure-induced symptoms, and achieve a euthyroid state. The approach to the patient with a goiter is outlined in Figure 203–4. In patients with sporadic goiter and elevated TSH levels, a clear rationale for thyroxine therapy is given. Thyroxine is started at 100 µg per day with subsequent dose adjustments to bring TSH into the low-normal but not the undetectable range. In patients with large, nontoxic diffuse goiters and normal T_4 and TSH levels, the same approach is chosen. The efficiency of this approach is indicated by a 20% decrease in thyroid volume after 1 year of treatment. In patients showing a response to therapy, treatment may be indefinite.

Treatment of multinodular goiter, especially in older patients, provides a more difficult problem. The TSH level must be determined, and if it is suppressed or in the low-normal range, thyroxine therapy should not be started. Thyroxine therapy also can be guided by results of an RAI scan and the suppression test, as described above. Identification of autonomous areas excludes thyroxine therapy. In patients with multinodular goiter without autonomous areas

and high-normal or elevated TSH levels, a trial of thyroxine therapy can be undertaken. In older patients, the initial dose of thyroxine should not be higher than 50 µg, and dose increases should be staggered at 25-µg steps at 4- to 6-week intervals. The results of thyroxine suppression therapy in patients with longstanding multinodular goiter are frequently disappointing, with little or no decrease in goiter size. Because thyroid tissue between nodules can decrease considerably, however, the nodules may appear more prominent. If no discernible decrease in size of multinodular goiter occurs after 6 to 12 months, thyroxine therapy should be stopped. In such patients, symptoms of temporary hypothyroidism can occur 1 month after stopping the medication and last for an additional month.

Endemic goiter is best treated by iodine supplementation, providing approximately 200 µg of iodine per day, or by the removal of identifiable goitrogens. Iodine supplementation can induce thyrotoxicosis due to the Jodbasedow effect. Surgical therapy of a goiter should be undertaken only if significant obstructive symptoms occur and goiter size cannot be reduced by thyroxine therapy. After partial thyroidectomy, thyroxine at 1.6 µg per kilogram per day should be supplied to prevent regenerative hyperplasia. RAI therapy for large goiters has been tried with modest success. ^{131}I can induce a thyroiditis and thyroid swelling, leading to an acute increase in obstructive symptoms, and should therefore be performed only in carefully observed patients.

Greenspan FS: The problem of the nodular goiter. Med Clin North Am 75:195, 1991. *Provides a detailed analysis of the problem.*
Studer H, Peter JH, Gerber H: Natural heterogeneity of thyroid cells: The basis for understanding thyroid function and nodular goiter growth. Endocrinol Rev 10:125, 1989. *An excellent explanatory treatise.*

BENIGN AND MALIGNANT THYROID NODULES

A thyroid nodule is a single palpable abnormality in the thyroid gland which can be a benign adenoma or thyroid cancer. Thyroid nodules are frequent and occur in about 5% of the population. In contrast, thyroid cancer is much less frequent, and among 100 patients with thyroid nodules only 4 have thyroid cancer. Distinguishing between benign and malignant lesions is an important task that is best accomplished by sampling cells from the lesions by fine-needle aspiration. This distinction is required to perform selective surgery.

Solitary Thyroid Nodules

INCIDENCE, ETIOLOGY, AND PATHOLOGY. Thyroid nodules must be at least 1 cm in diameter to be palpable. Such clinically detectable nodules occur in 6% of women and about 1.5% of men. The prevalence rises to 40 to 50% if smaller nodules are included which are discovered by autopsy or high-resolution ultrasonography. Ultrasound studies also reveal that abnormalities which appear as single nodules on palpation often represent conglomerates of multiple nodules. A solitary thyroid nodule identified on palpation is, therefore, a rather nonspecific finding. The most common benign lesion forming a single thyroid nodule is a thyroid adenoma. Most likely such adenomas result from clones of follicular cells which progress more quickly through the cell cycle but show benign growth characteristics. An adenoma is defined as a solitary encapsulated nodule composed of follicular cells arranged in an architecture that differs from that of the adjacent gland. The definition distinguishes adenomas from adenomatous nodules, which represent the early stage of a multinodular goiter. Adenomatous nodules lack a well-defined capsule or an architecture similar to the surrounding gland; clinically, adenomatous nodules and thyroid adenomas have a similar appearance. Adenomas vary in size, cell architecture, and appearance of follicular cells. Cell architecture nearly always follows a follicular pattern, with papillary adenomas being very rare. Follicular adenomas are classified into microfollicular or macrofollicular lesions and an embryonal variant containing almost no collagen. Hürthle cell adenomas are made up of follicular cells containing a large amount of mitochondria and have an eosinophilic staining pattern. No clear correlation between functional behavior or a propensity for malignant degeneration has been established for these different types of adenomas, and they are not precursors of thyroid cancer. Because adenomas are often hypercellular and contain mitotic figures, differentiation of a benign follicular adenoma from a follicular carcinoma on cytologic material obtained by aspiration is frequently not possible. Capsular invasion and vessel infil-

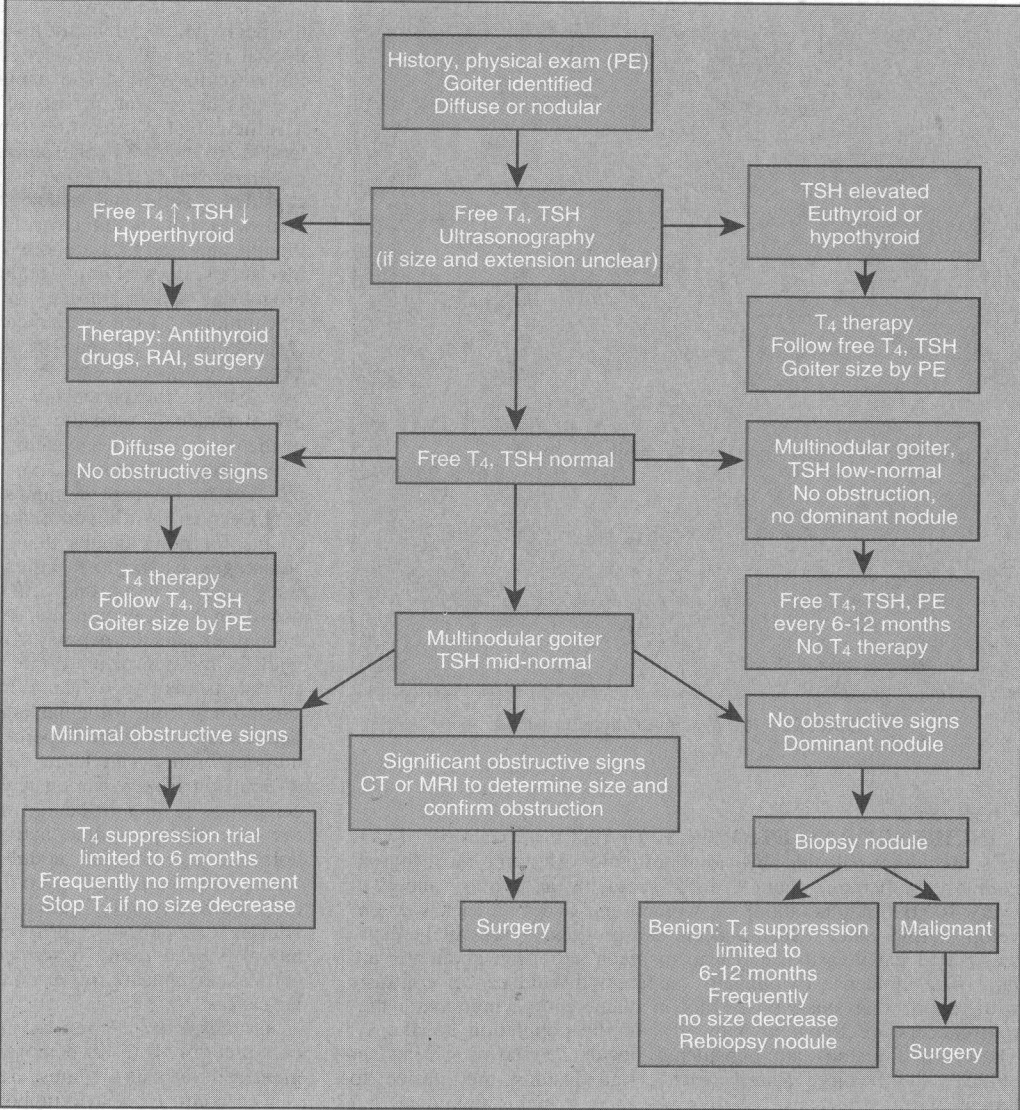

FIGURE 203–4. Evaluation and management of patients with non-toxic diffuse and nodular goiter and undetermined thyroid status.

tration are hallmarks of a malignant lesion, and these can be assessed only by histologic examination of the entire nodule. Frequently nodules outgrow their blood supply and undergo cystic degeneration. Ultimate pathologic evaluation of follicular neoplasms identifies benign adenomas in 85% and carcinomas in 15%.

MANIFESTATIONS, DIAGNOSIS, AND TREATMENT. Most thyroid nodules are discovered on routine physical examination. A systematic approach to thyroid nodules is outlined in Figure 203–5. Only rarely do solitary nodules become large enough or extend below the sternum to cause pressure symptoms. Bleeding into a nodule can lead to acute pain and enlargement. Most patients with thyroid nodules are euthyroid because 85 to 90% of the adenomas concentrate iodine very poorly and do not actively form thyroid hormone. The evaluation of a thyroid nodule includes a history, especially inquiries about the occurrence of specific risk factors such as radiation to the head and neck area. Examination reveals the presence of the nodule and should evaluate lymph nodes in the head and neck area as well as the clinical thyroid status of the patient. Blood determinations of free T_4 and TSH should be obtained to confirm the thyroid status. Fine-needle aspiration of the thyroid nodule to provide material for evaluation by a cytopathologist provides the most accurate assessment. Results to be expected from fine-needle aspiration are listed in Table 203–4. Identification of a nodule as a papillary carcinoma requires thyroid surgery. If a suspicious result is obtained and cannot distinguish between a follicular adenoma and a carcinoma, an RAI scan can be performed: 85 to 90% of thyroid nodules are nonfunctional or "cold" and 20% of such nodules contain a malignancy. Identification of a nodule with a

suspicious cytologic result as nonfunctional on RAI scan should result in surgical removal. About 10 to 15% of thyroid nodules are functional or "hot"; the incidence of thyroid cancer is <1% in such lesions. A recent report indicates that a mutant TSH receptor, which always stimulates thyroid hormone formation even when it is not occupied by TSH, is expressed in functional adenomas. If such patients are euthyroid, they can be followed with careful evaluation of thyroid size and functional status. Sooner or later 25% of these patients become hyperthyroid. Nodules in such patients are surgically removed after the patient is made euthyroid by treatment with PTU or MMI. In older patients or in patients with a high surgical risk, such nodules can be ablated with RAI.

In about 75% of patients, a thyroid nodule aspirate indicates a benign thyroid nodule. Most such patients have few or no pressure symptoms. In patients with a normal TSH level, thyroxine should be given, starting at 100 μg per day but choosing lower doses in elderly patients and those having cardiovascular symptoms, as discussed above. Approximately a one-fifth reduction in the size of these nodules occurs in a majority of patients within 6 to 12 months. If no response to thyroxine occurs, the medication can be stopped. The size of the nodule should then be followed carefully, and a growing nodule should be reaspirated at 1- to 2-year intervals. Rapid growth of a nodule, especially in a patient on thyroxine, requires reaspiration. Increase in nodule size can be due to the accumulation of fluid in a cystic lesion. Although the cyst can be aspirated, fluid frequently reaccumulates and the nodule progressively enlarges. Benign enlarging nodules can be removed surgically.

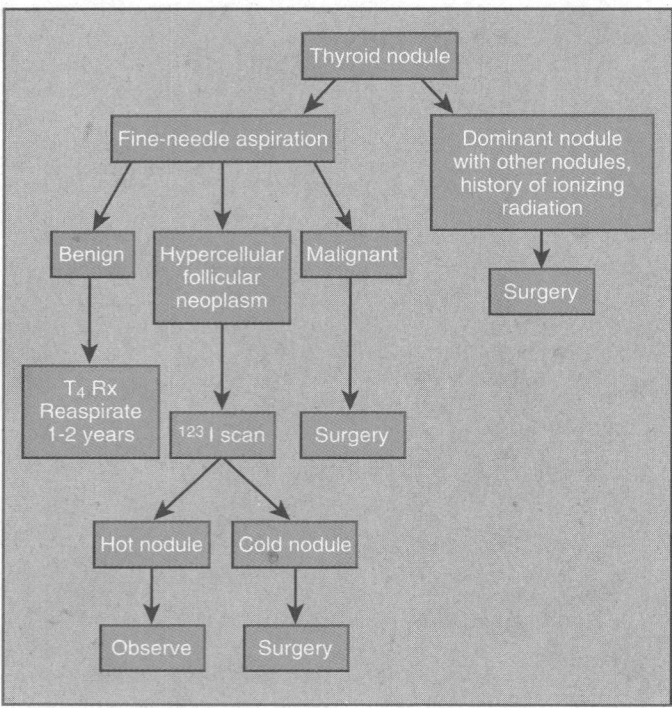

FIGURE 203–5. Workup of thyroid nodules.

Thyroid Cancer

INCIDENCE AND ETIOLOGY. Thyroid cancer almost always presents with a palpable thyroid abnormality. Although most thyroid nodules are benign, about 1 in 25 contains a thyroid cancer. In every 100,000 adults, about six women and two men each year develop thyroid cancer. Such cancers can progress aggressively, especially by local invasion, and lead to much suffering; about 9% are fatal. The incidence of clinically apparent thyroid cancer contrasts with reports that small (< 10 mm in diameter), asymptomatic thyroid cancers are found in 5 to 10% of the population at autopsy. These small lesions are considered occult neoplasms of unclear clinical significance. Rarely such small lesions metastasize to lymph nodes. The cause of thyroid cancer remains unknown, but activation of kinase genes *ret* and *trk* have been reported. In follicular cancer, mutations of the *ras* kinase gene occur in papillary cancer. Anaplastic cancer shows inactivating mutations of the p53 repressor gene. Despite these beginnings, however, a conclusive relationship between specific gene alterations and particular forms of thyroid cancer has not been established. Certain risk factors for thyroid cancer can be identified. Radiation to the head and neck area, especially during early childhood, leads to a 30-fold increase in thyroid cancer with radiation doses up to 1500 rad. Higher radiation doses of 5000 rad or more, as they are delivered to the thyroid by ^{131}I therapy for Graves' disease, do not lead to an increased incidence of thyroid cancer. Other risk factors are primarily genetic and include familial forms of papillary cancer, Gardner's and Cowden's syndrome for papillary cancer, and the multiple endocrine neoplasia (MEA) type II syndrome for medullary cancer. Most thyroid cancers are of follicular epithelial cell origin; chronic TSH stimulation appears to play a permissive but not causative role in differentiated papillary and follicular thyroid cancers. Papillary cancer is the least aggressive malignancy and represents about 70% of all thyroid cancer, with follicular cancers representing 15%. The rest are made up of medullary cancer, anaplastic cancer, lymphomas, and other rare tumors. Metastases to the thyroid occur primarily from malignant melanomas and cancers of breast, lung, and kidney.

PATHOLOGY. Papillary cancer is the most common thyroid cancer in the United States, being two to three times more common in women and relatively more common in young patients. The absolute incidence is higher in the fourth to seventh decades. Papillary cancers occur most frequently in parts of the world where iodine supply is adequate. Papillary cancers generally are not encapsulated, and they grow slowly by infiltrative local spread, initially affecting other parts of the thyroid and extending to regional lymph nodes in the neck. Microscopically, papillary cancer is characterized by epithelial cells with large, irregular, frequently clear nuclei covering fibrovascular stalks. The papillae, which give the tumor its name, may not be present in parts of the tumor, and some parts may have a follicular structure. About half of papillary carcinomas contain laminated, calcified spherules called psammoma bodies. Variants of papillary cancer with good prognosis include the micropapillary encapsulated, solid, and follicular variants. A poor prognosis is associated with tall, columnar cells and diffuse sclerosis variants. Although one study has reported a higher mortality with lymph node metastases, local lymph node invasion is not necessarily a bad prognostic sign in papillary cancer because it occurs even with occult tumors < 1 cm in diameter, which have a favorable prognosis. In patients past 50 years of age, papillary cancers undergo a more aggressive local spread, leading to death from local invasions in over half of the patients. Distant metastases are uncommon (2 to 3% of patients), with the lung more frequently involved than bone or the central nervous system.

Follicular carcinoma develops more frequently with increasing age, but its incidence remains only one fifth that of papillary cancer. Despite this lower incidence, however, follicular cancer accounts for more deaths than papillary cancer because of its early hematogenous spread to lung, bone, brain, and liver. Distant metastases occur in about one fifth of patients. Lymph node involvement occurs in < 1% of patients. Follicular cancer presents as an encapsulated, expansible neoplasm with a microfollicular pattern. Its hallmark is invasion of the tumor capsule and extension into blood vessels at its periphery. These invasive features distinguish follicular carcinomas from follicular adenomas. Aspirates obtained from follicular carcinomas are hypercellular, containing cells with numerous mitotic figures with large nuclei. The diagnosis, however, can be difficult on frozen section. Cyst formation occurs in follicular cancer just as it does in benign thyroid nodules. Rarely follicular cancer concentrates iodine actively and generates sufficient thyroid hormone to create hot nodules leading to thyrotoxicosis. In some forms of differentiated thyroid cancer, epithelial cells called Hürthle cells show oxyphilic staining and contain numerous mitochondria. Hürthle cell cancer is primarily a variant of follicular cancer but has also been rarely described with a papillary structure. Hürthle cell cancer appears to be more aggressive than papillary or follicular cancer.

Anaplastic cancer represents about 5% of thyroid cancer and occurs predominantly in persons older than 70 years. The spindle and giant cell variants are most frequent, and the rare small cell variant can be confused with lymphomas or medullary cancer. Almost one third of anaplastic cancers arise in pre-existing differentiated cancers. The prognosis is dismal, with a mean survival of 7 to 12 months. Death most commonly results from aggressive local invasion causing progressive tracheal obstruction or massive hemorrhage. Distant metastases occur, but the local spread is so rapid that metastatic foci have little clinical importance.

Medullary carcinoma is a malignant tumor of calcitonin-secreting C cells which accounts for 2 to 3% of all thyroid cancer. The tumor produces calcitonin, calcitonin-related peptide, chromogranin A, ACTH, prostaglandins, and carcinoembryonic antigen. Densely packed cells form solid masses separated by hyalinized tumor stroma. Amyloid deposits occur frequently. Several variants of the tumor have been described, with the sporadically occurring form accounting for 80% and genetic or familial variants making up the remainder. The familial variants can be subdivided into those occurring with multiple endocrine neoplasia (MEN)2a, MEN2b, and a familial non-MEN variant. In MEN2a the medullary cancer occurs together with pheochromocytomas and parathyroid adenomas; in MEN2b pheochromocytomas and ganglioneuromas occur. In the familial form, the tumor is multicentric in origin and C cell hyperplasia precedes cancer development. The tumor metastasizes via the lymphatic route and the bloodstream. The peak incidence of the sporadic form is in the sixth and seventh decades. At the time of diagnosis, lymphatic spread has frequently developed. Medullary carcinoma is quite aggressive and less than half its carriers survive for 10 years.

Thyroid lymphoma most frequently consists of the diffuse B-cell variant and occurs most frequently in patients with Hashimoto's disease. Such lymphomas present as rapidly growing masses replacing thyroid tissue and extending through the capsule into adjacent soft tissue. Secondary involvement of the thyroid by malignant lymphoma arising elsewhere occurs in about one fifth of patients with advanced generalized lymphoma.

MANIFESTATIONS, DIAGNOSIS, AND TREATMENT. Thyroid nodules are frequent, but only about 1 in 20 contains a thyroid cancer. Figure 203–5 outlines the approach to such lesions. The task is to identify the cancerous lesion in order to perform selective surgery. Specific features in the patient's history and symptoms and signs can point to the occurrence of cancer but are not conclusive. Thyroid cancer is more likely in a nodule developing in a child or a patient over age 60, especially males. A single hard nodule showing rapid, painless growth is more likely to be a cancerous lesion. A history of radiation to the head and neck area during childhood, a family history of thyroid cancer, Gardner's syndrome, Cowden's syndrome, and MEN2 syndrome all represent strong risk factors. A single hard nodule noted on palpation which is fixed to surrounding tissue and the identification of firm, poorly mobile lateral lymph nodes may indicate cancer spread.

Laboratory tests offer little in the diagnosis of thyroid cancer. In most patients with thyroid nodules, thyroid hormone values are normal. Elevated thyroid hormone levels indicate a follicular carcinoma markedly overproducing thyroid hormone. In the rare patients with medullary cancer, calcitonin-related peptides and calcitonin levels are elevated. The evaluation of patients with MEN2 is discussed in Ch. 210. Fine-needle aspiration of thyroid nodules and examination of the obtained material by a cytopathologist provide the highest diagnostic yield. The procedure is easy to perform and, aside from occasional bleeding in the thyroid nodule, is without serious risk. Results obtained by fine-needle aspiration are listed in Table 203–4. When a trained cytopathologist is not available, the evaluation needs to be modified. A ^{123}I scan is performed to determine if the thyroid nodule is cold. Because 20% of cold nodules coming to attention in a referral center contain thyroid cancer, such nodules are surgically removed. Thyroid ultrasonography can provide further detail, especially related to the presence of fluid and cystic lesions. Most fluid accumulation in thyroid nodules represents cystic degeneration of thyroid nodules, and the incidence of cancer in such lesions is not markedly different from that in solid nodules.

Thyroid surgery should be performed by an experienced thyroid surgeon. Some diversity of opinion exists related to the extent of the operation. For example, some thyroid surgeons treat a 1.5- to 2.0-cm papillary cancer only with a lobectomy, whereas others prefer a near-total thyroidectomy. The author prefers the removal of such lesions by near-total thyroidectomy. In the hands of an experienced surgeon, complications from permanent hypoparathyroidism (2%) or vocal cord paralysis (2%) are no greater for a near-total thyroidectomy than for a lobectomy. A near-total thyroidectomy has the advantage that only small remnants of thyroid tissue remain which can be ablated with RAI. Because normal thyroid tissue accumulates RAI much more avidly than any thyroid cancer, it is not possible to treat thyroid cancer successfully by ^{131}I therapy in the presence of a large amount of normal thyroid tissue. In addition, after near-total thyroidectomy the patient can be followed with thyroglobulin levels. Increases in the level of thyroglobulin indicate a return of thyroid cancer.

^{131}I ablation is used in patients who undergo near-total thyroidectomy, especially if the primary lesion is a papillary cancer >2 cm in diameter or a follicular cancer. The regimen goes as follows: One day after surgery, patients are started on triiodothyronine (Cytomel 25 μg every day or twice a day) and maintained on this dose of T$_3$ for 4 to 6 weeks. T$_3$ has a half-life of 1 day and the patient becomes hypothyroid much more quickly than with thyroxine treatment. When medication is stopped at the end of the 4- to 6-week healing period, the patient becomes markedly hypothyroid, documented by an elevated TSH level. After the TSH has attained levels of at least 40 μU per milliliter, a scanning dose of 3 mCi of ^{123}I is administered. If a small remnant of thyroid tissue is left in the bed of the thyroid, an ablative dose of 29 mCi of ^{131}I is administered. Identification of a larger amount of thyroid tissue or lymph node metastases leads to the administration of a higher dose of ^{131}I, ranging from 75 to 125 mCi according to the amount of remaining tissue. Seven to 10 days after treatment, a second RAI scan can be performed. This post-treatment scan identifies areas of ^{131}I uptake

that were not detected by the initial lower dose diagnostic scan. In the future, administration of human recombinant TSH will induce high TSH levels and stimulate ^{131}I uptake. This step will eliminate the need to achieve hypothyroidism before RAI is administered.

When patients become hypothyroid for RAI scanning, it is important to obtain a thyroglobulin level: Elevated levels indicate that a sizable mass of thyroid tissue was left after surgery. Patients who had considerable thyroid tissue left or tumor spread to lymph nodes should be rescanned 6 months after the initial scan to ensure that the initial RAI treatment ablated all thyroid tissue. Patients who had only a small amount of tissue left can be rescanned within 1 year. Patients whose thyroglobulin levels remain normal should be rescanned 3 years after surgery. If no evidence of RAI accumulation occurs, no subsequent rescanning is necessary and patients can be followed with thyroglobulin values. In about 10% of patients, thyroid cancer can dedifferentiate, resulting in a discrepancy between a positive RAI scan and undetectable thyroglobulin levels. Similarly, patients with elevated thyroglobulin level and minimal or absent RAI uptake on scans have been identified. Such individuals need to be followed carefully and may require additional RAI treatment because the elevated thyroglobulin level can indicate the presence of thyroid cancer. The best initial treatment of patients with near-total thyroidectomy for papillary cancer consists of giving sufficient thyroxine to suppress TSH into the low-normal range combined with RAI therapy. This regimen markedly decreases the late recurrence of papillary cancer. Follicular carcinoma is more aggressive and should be treated more vigorously than papillary cancer. Medullary cancer does not respond to RAI therapy and must be treated with surgery plus external radiation and chemotherapy, especially if bone metastases occur. Anaplastic cancer has a poor prognosis; attempts to increase survival time by treatment with chemotherapy and external radiation therapy have been unsuccessful, although palliative external radiation can especially alleviate obstruction.

Clark OH, Duh Q-Y: Thyroid cancer. Med Clin North Am 75:211, 1991.
Mazzaferri EL: Papillary thyroid carcinoma: Factors influencing prognosis and current therapy. Semin Oncol 14:315, 1987.
Ridgeway EC: Clinician's evaluation of a solitary thyroid nodule. J Clin Endocrinol Metab 74:231, 1992.
Robbins J, Merino MJ, Boice JD Jr, et al.: Thyroid cancer: a lethal endocrine neoplasm. Ann Intern Med 115:133, 1991.

204 THE ADRENAL GLAND

204.1 Adrenal Cortex
D. Lynn Loriaux

The two adrenal glands lie either on top of or next to each kidney (Fig. 204–1). Each gland, between 6 and 8 grams in weight, is composed of a cortex and medulla. The cortex makes steroid hormones, and the medulla, in essence a sympathetic ganglion, makes catecholamines. The cortex includes three histologic zones in the adult: zona glomerulosa, zona fasciculata, and zona reticularis (Fig. 204–2). Each zone can be thought of as an independent organ. The outermost zona glomerulosa produces aldosterone, the primary mineralocorticoid in humans. The zona fasciculata produces primarily cortisol, the primary glucocorticoid in humans, and the zona reticularis produces the "adrenal androgens." The adrenal androgens are, in fact, androgen and estrogen precursors, the parent compound being dehydroepiandrosterone (DHA) and its sulfate conjugate. The biologic actions of these steroid hormones are effected via intracellular receptors, cytoplasmic or nuclear in location, that regulate gene transcription upon binding with the appropriate ligand. DHA has no known receptor. The distribution of these receptors defines the responsive tissues for each hormone. Aldosterone regulates sodium balance, acting primarily on the distal tubule of the nephron. Cortisol maintains physiologic integrity in ways that re-

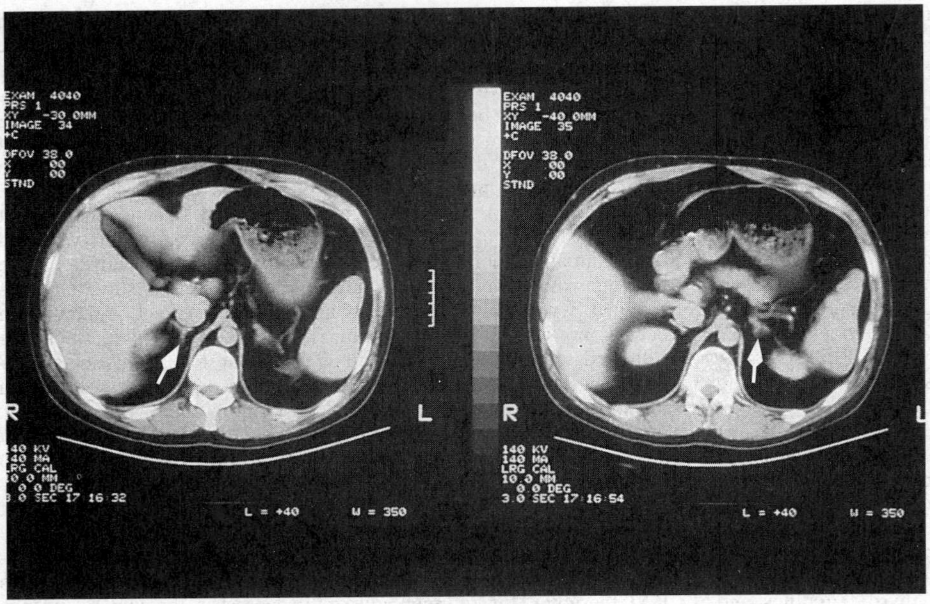

FIGURE 204–1. MRI of abdomen showing the position and relative size of the normal adrenal glands.

main poorly understood, and its receptors are found in virtually every cell in the body. DHA has no identifiable biologic action. The synthesis and secretion of each of these hormones are regulated, in the main, by a separate "feedback" system. The major trophic hormone for aldosterone secretion is renin, for cortisol adrenocorticotropic hormone (ACTH), and for DHA cortical androgen–stimulating hormone (CASH), which is not yet fully characterized. Thus,

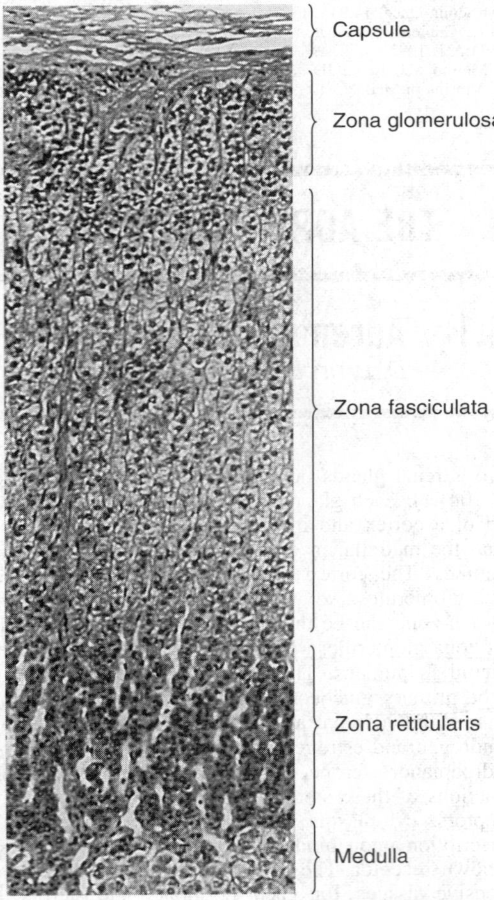

FIGURE 204–2. Histologic section through a normal adult adrenal gland showing the progression, outside in, of the zona glomerulosa, zona fasciculata, and zona reticularis.

in the case of the zona glomerulosa and the zona fasciculata, the functional status of each can be assessed by measuring two hormones: aldosterone and plasma renin, and cortisol and ACTH, respectively.

The adrenal medulla, in essence a sympathetic ganglion, produces catecholamines in response to neural input. Disorders of the adrenal medulla are discussed in Ch. 204.2.

DISORDERS OF ADRENOCORTICAL FUNCTION

Disorders of adrenocortical function can be thought of as disorders of overproduction or underproduction of the four classes of steroid hormones produced by the adrenal gland: cortisol, aldosterone, androgen, and estrogen. In addition, "mixed" disorders, the congenital adrenal hyperplasias, are characterized by a clinical picture of combined hormone excess and deficiency. These disorders are considered separately.

The diagnosis of disorders of adrenocortical function, like that of other endocrine syndromes, requires a compatible clinical picture with biochemical confirmation of the associated underlying abnormality. In years past, the tests used in the diagnosis of adrenal disease were both confusing and many. Fortunately, the last several years have brought order and simplification to the process.

Tests of Adrenocortical Function

THE PORTER-SILBER CHROMOGENS. The 3-carbon side chain of cortisol reacts with meta-dinitrobenzene to form a colored adduct with an absorption maximum at 410 μm. Other adrenal steroids having this configuration in the side chain include cortisone, 11-deoxycortisol, tetrahydrocortisone, tetrahydro-11-deoxycortisol, and tetrahydrocortisol (Fig. 204–3). This reaction, called the Porter-Silber chromogen reaction, was the basis of the first test to provide some measure of cortisol production. It is still in widespread use. Because urinary metabolites are, for the most part, conjugated to glucuronic acid and sulfuric acid, the measurement of Porter-Silber chromogens first involves an acid hydrolysis to cleave these conjugates. This is followed by a lipid extraction with a solvent such as dichloromethane. The Porter-Silber reaction is performed on the steroids in the lipid extract. The absorption maximum is quantitated spectrophotometrically. The normal range for Porter-Silber excretion is 2 to 12 mg per day. The excretion of these steroids is markedly affected by body size, and the normal range is considerably narrowed by normalizing the measurement against urinary creatinine excretion. With this correction, the normal range is the same for all ages, 4.5 $\pm$ 1(SD) mg per gram of creatinine per day. The normal range includes the extinction point for the assay, which means that values below the normal range cannot be measured reliably with this assay.

URINE FREE CORTISOL. Urine free cortisol is that fraction of urinary cortisol that is neither conjugated to glucuronic or sul-

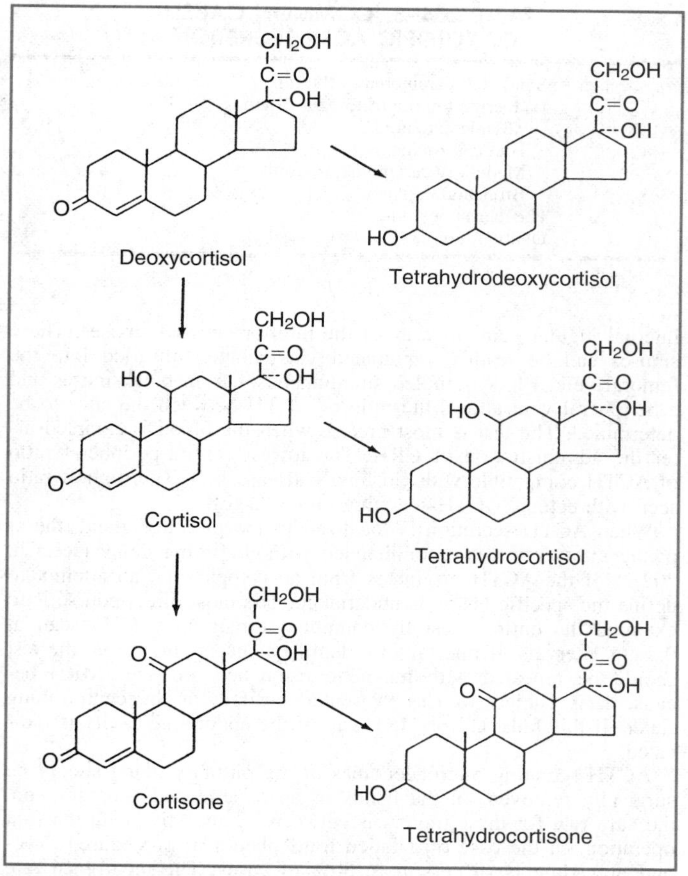

FIGURE 204–3. The family of steroids known as the Porter-Silber chromogens, commonly referred to as the 17-hydroxysteroids.

furic acid nor bound to a protein. Accordingly it is filtered by the renal glomerulus and can be extracted directly from urine with a lipid solvent. The detection limit of this assay also lies in the normal range of cortisol excretion and, hence, is not a reliable test for adrenal insufficiency.

PLASMA CORTISOL. Intuitively, the measurement of circulating plasma cortisol should provide the most direct assessment of adrenal cortisol secretion. The secretion of cortisol is pulsatile, with a steady frequency of about one pulse per hour in adults. The amplitude of these pulses, however, varies markedly, with 8 to 10 high-amplitude pulses clustering in the early morning hours. This pattern creates a diurnal secretory rhythm in plasma cortisol concentration. Cortisol circulates predominantly bound to a glycosylated 59-kD α_2-globulin, cortisol-binding globulin (transcortin [CBG]). This binding protects circulating cortisol from hepatic clearance and gives cortisol a relatively long plasma half-life of 60 to 80 minutes. Normal plasma cortisol concentrations range between 5 and 20 μg per deciliter. At some time each day, normal subjects have plasma cortisol concentrations that cannot be differentiated from zero. These biologic complexities make hazardous the interpretation of isolated plasma cortisol determinations. If cortisol is measured at frequent intervals (30 minutes) over a 24-hour period and the values are averaged, the mean plasma cortisol concentration amounts to 7.5 ± 1 μg per deci-liter. To work within this narrow confidence interval, however, requires the measurement of a large number of plasma cortisol concentrations, which is prohibitive except in extraordinary circumstances.

PLASMA ACTH CONCENTRATION. The development of the two-site immunoradiometric assay (IRMA) for ACTH simplified considerably the differential diagnosis of adrenal disease. The normal range of plasma ACTH extends up to 100 pg per milliliter.

Three provocative tests of adrenal function are in common use. The *ACTH stimulation test* is the most reliable screening test for adrenal hypofunction. It is also the standard method by which suspected enzymatic deficiencies in adrenal steroidogenesis are examined. The test is performed by administering 250 μg of synthetic ACTH (Cortrosyn) intravenously and measuring the serum steroids of interest 45 and 60 minutes later. The normal adrenal gland pro-

duces plasma cortisol concentrations >20 μg per deciliter in response to this challenge. *Corticotropin-releasing hormone (CRH),* the 41-amino acid hypothalamic secretagogue for ACTH, is a useful test for separating ACTH-dependent from ACTH-independent hypercortisolism and is an essential component of the inferior petrosal sinus sampling procedure (IPSS) for localizing the site of ACTH secretion (see Ch. 204.2). The test is performed by infusing CRH, 1 μg per kilogram, intravenously over 1 minute and measuring the ACTH response between 3 and 30 minutes thereafter.

The *dexamethasone suppression test* is widely used to screen for adrenal hyperfunction. The test has so many false-positive and false-negative results (sensitivity and specificity of about 0.8), however, that it is superseded by the tests mentioned above. The test retains some value in the differential diagnosis of mineralocorticoid excess. Many iterations of this test are available, the simplest being 0.5 mg dexamethasone administered by mouth every 6 hours for 2 days.

Plasma and urine aldosterone and plasma renin activity are important tests to evaluate states of apparent mineralocorticoid excess and deficiency.

The differential diagnosis of congenital adrenal hyperplasia requires the measurement of specific steroid biosynthetic intermediates that accumulate proximal to the responsible enzymic deficiencies in the steroid biosynthetic cascade. The most commonly measured are 17-hydroxyprogesterone (21-hydroxylase deficiency) and 11-deoxycortisol (11-hydroxylase deficiency). These steroids are most reliably measured in the context of an ACTH stimulation test, as described above.

Adrenal Hyperfunction

There are four syndromes of adrenal hyperfunction: Cushing's syndrome, hypokalemic metabolic alkalosis, masculinization, and feminization. These result from the excessive secretion of cortisol, mineralocorticoid, androgen, and estrogen, respectively. These disorders can occur in isolation or, more commonly, in combination with one or more of the others.

GLUCOCORTICOID EXCESS—CUSHING'S SYNDROME. *Diagnosis.* Cushing's syndrome is caused by glucocorticoid excess. The "classic" syndrome is defined clinically: weight gain, plethora, striae, hypertension, and proximal muscle weakness (Table 204–1). The weight gain is predominantly truncal, with increased fat deposited in a yokelike pattern around the neck, leading to the well-known dorsocervical fat pad (buffalo hump) and filling in of the supraclavicular fossae. Plethora is evident as a ruddy complexion. The striae of Cushing's syndrome are characteristically violaceous in appearance and occur in thin skin. Proximal muscle weakness is best assessed by testing the ability of the patient to rise unassisted from a squatting position. The biochemical diagnosis depends on the demonstration of an elevated plasma concentration of "bioactive" cortisol, which is best reflected in the excretion of urine free cortisol. If the clinical picture is "strong," urine free cortisol concentrations above the normal range are adequate for the diagno-

TABLE 204–1. CLINICAL FEATURES OF GLUCOCORTICOID EXCESS

	Frequency (%)
Weight gain	90
"Moon facies"	75
Hypertension	75
Violaceous striae	65
Hirsutism	65
Glucose intolerance	65
Proximal muscle weakness	60
Plethora	60
Menstrual dysfunction	60
Acne	40
Easy bruising	40
Osteopenia	40
Dependent edema	40
Hyperpigmentation	20
Hypokalemic metabolic alkalosis	15

sis. If the clinical picture is "weak," urine free cortisol excretion must be above the levels found in "physiologic" causes of adrenal activation, such as stress and depression. This level is generally taken to be 250 μg per day. This approach to the diagnosis of Cushing's syndrome occasionally identifies patients with an "atypical" picture. At one extreme are patients with minimal clinical manifestations of Cushing's syndrome but very high levels of free cortisol excretion. This constellation of findings is characteristic of Cushing's syndrome associated with systemic malignancy, typically a small cell carcinoma of the lung. The clinical picture is dominated by the "cachexia" of malignancy, and the typical "anabolic" features of Cushing's syndrome such as weight gain and dorsocervical fat distribution fail to develop. At the other extreme are patients with well-established clinical signs of Cushing's syndrome but without sufficient urine free cortisol excretion to confirm the diagnosis. This situation is usually the result of iatrogenic or surreptitious exogenous glucocorticoid administration. A careful history and review of systems usually reveal the source of the glucocorticoid. In the rare cases of surreptitious glucocorticoid abuse, measurement of the commonly prescribed synthetic glucocorticoids in randomly obtained serum samples is necessary for the diagnosis. Rarely, naturally occurring Cushing's syndrome can be cyclic or even intermittent. In this case, repeated measures of urine free cortisol at frequent intervals of 3 to 5 days are necessary to establish the diagnosis.

Differential Diagnosis and Treatment. The causes of Cushing's syndrome are shown in Table 204–2. They can be conveniently divided into ACTH-dependent and ACTH-independent causes. This differentiation is made on the basis of the plasma ACTH concentration following the administration of CRH. Values > 10 pg per milliliter indicate ACTH-dependent disease; values ≤ 10 pg per milliliter indicate ACTH-independent disease.

The causes of ACTH-dependent Cushing's syndrome include *Cushing's disease* caused by an ACTH-secreting pituitary tumor and the *ectopic secretion of ACTH* from a neoplasm not of pituitary origin. Cushing's disease is the most common cause of Cushing's syndrome, accounting for 70 to 80% of all noniatrogenic cases (see Ch. 202.1). The ectopic secretion of ACTH by a nonpituitary neoplasm accounts for about 10% of cases. The common causes of ectopic ACTH secretion are listed in Table 204–3. More than 90% of these tumors are found in the chest. The most common cause is small cell cancer of the lung. Other neoplasms include bronchial carcinoid tumors, medullary cancer of the thyroid, islet cell tumors of the pancreas, and pheochromocytoma.

There are two forms of the ectopic ACTH syndrome. In the first, Cushing's syndrome occurs as classically described by Harvey Cushing. It can be thought of as the *anabolic form* of ectopic ACTH secretion because it is associated with weight gain and the characteristic central obesity of the disorder. It is usually caused by slow-growing benign tumors such as bronchial carcinoid tumors. The second form, *the catabolic form,* has none of the anabolic features associated with "classic" Cushing's syndrome. Weight loss, hypertension, edema, and hypokalemia dominate the clinical picture. This form of the disease is commonly associated with advanced and widely metastatic tumors that impair caloric intake and prevent weight gain and the development of central obesity.

Differentiating the two ACTH-dependent forms of Cushing's syndrome from each other depends on localizing the source of the ACTH secretion. The most effective method of doing this is by sampling inferior petrosal sinus blood for the measurement of ACTH levels (IPSS). Pituitary venous blood drains into the cavernous sinuses on either side of the sella turcica and thence into the

TABLE 204–2. CAUSES OF CUSHING'S SYNDROME

ACTH-dependent causes
ACTH-secreting pituitary tumor (Cushing's disease)
Nonpituitary ACTH-secreting neoplasm (ectopic ACTH syndrome)
ACTH-independent causes
Adrenal adenoma
Adrenal carcinoma
Micronodular adrenal disease
Factitious or surreptitious glucocorticoid administration

TABLE 204–3. COMMON CAUSES OF ECTOPIC ACTH SECRETION

Small cell carcinoma of the lung	50%
Endocrine tumors of foregut origin	35%
Thymic carcinoid	
Islet cell tumor	
Medullary carcinoma, thyroid	
Bronchial carcinoid	
Pheochromocytoma	5%
Ovarian tumors	2%

internal jugular veins by way of the inferior petrosal sinuses. These sinuses can be readily cannulated via catheters inserted into the femoral vein. Blood sampled simultaneously from both sinuses and a peripheral vein allows the ratio of ACTH between the sites to be determined. The test is most precise when the blood is sampled after the administration of CRH. The lowest central-peripheral ratio of ACTH compatible with Cushing's disease is 3. The highest ratio seen with ectopic ACTH-secreting tumors is 1.8.

When ACTH secretion is localized to the pituitary gland, therapeutic intervention is recommended without further delay (see Ch. 202.1). If the ACTH originates from an ectopic site, an attempt to define the specific lesion is undertaken. The most direct course is to examine the entire chest by computed tomography (CT) scan at 0.5-cm intervals. If this fails to identify a suspicious lesion, the test should be repeated with magnetic resonance imaging (MRI) because it is subject to less "vascular" artifact in the central lung fields. If this fails, CT or MRI scan of the abdominal cavity is indicated.

ACTH-secreting microadenomas of the pituitary gland should be surgically removed. In the hands of an experienced neurosurgeon, the cure rate for these tumors is between 90 and 95% with the first operation. In the case of a failed transsphenoidal procedure, a second procedure is successful in 50% of cases. The recurrence rate appears to be < 5%. Ectopic tumors should be removed if found. If the tumor cannot be found or is found to be widely metastatic, adrenal blockade with ketoconazole, up to 1200 mg by mouth in divided doses, is an effective treatment for the associated glucocorticoid excess. Ultimately, if the process appears to be headed to a protracted course, bilateral adrenalectomy via flank incision or laparoscopy is a useful adjunct to management.

The causes of ACTH-independent Cushing's syndrome, if iatrogenic and factitious disease are excluded, are adrenal in origin: adrenal adenoma, adrenal cancer, and micronodular adrenal dysplasia. They account for 10 to 20% of naturally occurring cases of Cushing's syndrome. Adrenal adenomas are the most common, accounting for about 15% of cases of Cushing's syndrome. The tumors are typically unilateral, are < 4 cm in diameter, and produce only a single steroid hormone, in this case, cortisol. Adrenal cancers are rare, having an incidence of 1 in 600,000 per year. They are generally unilateral and large at the time of discovery, usually > 6 cm in diameter. Adrenal cancers typically produce more than one steroid hormone, the most common combinations being glucocorticoid and mineralocorticoid, or glucocorticoid and androgen. The differentiation of an adenoma from a carcinoma is made clinically; histologic examination of the tissue is of little value. The most important indicators of malignancy are size at the time of diagnosis, the number of steroid hormones clinically apparent, and any evidence of spread at the time of surgical intervention. Micronodular adrenal dysplasia is characterized by normal or small adrenal glands that show scattered 1- to 3-mm hyperplastic nodules separated by atrophic adrenal cortex. This disease can be sporadic or part of a larger syndrome, Carney's complex, in which the adrenal disease is associated with pigmented lentigines, atrial myxoma, and germ cell tumors (see references).

The differential diagnosis of ACTH-independent Cushing's syndrome depends almost exclusively on the findings produced by CT or MRI scan. Small unilateral lesions with no evidence of metastasis should be removed by a unilateral flank excision or by a laparoscopic procedure. Large lesions should be removed via a transabdominal approach so that the abdominal organs can be carefully examined and the liver biopsied at the time of operation. The treatment for micronodular adrenal dysplasia is bilateral adrenalectomy.

Metastases should be surgically excised until no longer feasible. The only known chemotherapy effective against this cancer is *ortho, para'*-DDD (OP'DDD). It is given orally to tolerance, usually a dose between 6 and 10 grams per day. Side effects are neuropsychiatric and gastrointestinal, with somnolence, ataxia, reduced attention span, nausea, and diarrhea predominating. One-fourth of patients have an objective remission, and the remissions average 7 months in duration. No-one has been cured of metastatic adrenocortical carcinoma.

MINERALOCORTICOID EXCESS. Diagnosis. There are no reliable symptoms of mineralocorticoid excess. Signs include arterial hypertension and dependent edema. Laboratory findings are more specific. The mineralocorticoid effect on the distal nephron is sodium retention at the expense of potassium and hydrogen excretion. Excess mineralocorticoid produces an expanded vascular volume in association with hypokalemia and metabolic alkalosis. Mineralocorticoid excess can be renin-angiotensin–independent or –dependent. Aldosterone-secreting tumors are examples of renin-angiotensin–independent disease. In renin-angiotensin–dependent disease, the mineralocorticoid is produced in response to the renin-angiotensin trophic signal. This is commonly encountered in states of contracted arterial volume such as congestive heart failure or cirrhosis with ascites. The two forms of mineralocorticoid excess can be differentiated on the basis of the plasma renin activity. If resting plasma renin activity is high, the mineralocorticoid excess is renin-angiotensin–dependent. If plasma renin activity is low and cannot be stimulated by 4 hours of upright posture, the mineralocorticoid excess is renin-angiotensin–independent.

Renin-Angiotensin–Independent Mineralocorticoid Excess. **Differential Diagnosis and Treatment.** Table 204–4 lists the causes of renin-angiotensin–independent mineralocorticoid excess. Aldosterone is the offending mineralocorticoid in most but not all of these disorders. The first task is to differentiate cases caused by aldosterone excess from those caused by another mineralocorticoid. Urine and plasma aldosterone measurements provide the answers for this differentiation. If the aldosterone concentration is normal or above, aldosterone is the causative agent. If the aldosterone concentration is below the normal range or undetectable, the disorder is caused by a mineralocorticoid other than aldosterone.

There are two common causes of aldosterone-mediated renin-angiotensin–independent mineralocorticoid excess: aldosterone-producing adenoma and bilateral hyperplasia of aldosterone-secreting cells. Dexamethasone-suppressible hyperaldosteronism is a rare cause of aldosterone-mediated renin-angiotensin–independent mineralocorticoid excess. It can be excluded by finding normal or high levels of circulating aldosterone after 2 days of giving dexamethasone, 2 mg per day by mouth in divided doses. The remaining causes of renin-angiotensin–independent aldosterone excess must be separated from one another to guide the appropriate therapeutic intervention. Aldosterone-secreting adenomas respond well to surgical removal, whereas bilateral hyperplasia does not. The most direct approach to this differentiation is to measure cortisol-aldosterone ratios in adrenal venous blood sampled simultaneously from both glands following the administration of ACTH. The diagnostic accuracy of this test approaches 100%. Aldosterone-secreting adenomas are characterized by high levels of aldosterone from one side and none from the other, the secretion from the nonaffected side being suppressed by the volume-expanded state. Bilateral hyperplasia is characterized by comparable aldosterone levels from each gland, making cortisol-aldosterone ratios in effluent adrenal blood roughly equal on the two sides.

Unilateral adrenal adenomas should be surgically excised. In the hands of an experienced surgeon, the cure rate is very high. Bilateral hyperplasia does not respond well to surgery and is best treated with spironolactone to dampen the metabolic sequelae of mineralocorticoid excess and with antihypertensive medications if spironolactone inadequately controls blood pressure.

The causes of non–aldosterone-mediated renin-angiotensin–independent mineralocorticoid excess are rare (Table 204–5). The first task is to exclude adrenocortical carcinoma. This is best done by imaging the adrenal glands with CT or MRI scan. Failure to find adrenal asymmetry with a dominant mass, usually >4 cm in diameter, essentially excludes the diagnosis. Symmetrically enlarged adrenal glands of moderate degree suggest congenital adrenal hyperplasia. The two congenital adrenal hyperplasias that lead to hypertension are 11-hydroxylase deficiency and 17-hydroxylase deficiency. The first can be diagnosed by measuring the circulating concentration of 11-deoxycortisol. Normally, this steroid does not circulate in plasma. 17-Hydroxylase deficiency is best diagnosed by a unique clinical picture (hypertension, pubertal delay, and genital ambiguity) coupled with an inappropriately elevated plasma progesterone concentration.

The enzyme 11β-hydroxysteroid dehydrogenase (HSD) catalyzes the conversion of cortisol to cortisone. Cortisol interacts with the mineralocorticoid receptor as an agonist; cortisone does not. Because the circulating concentrations of cortisol are 1000 times those of aldosterone, cortisol can have considerable mineralocorticoid activity in humans. This is prevented by the action of 11β-HSD, which converts cortisol to its inactive metabolite, cortisone. If the activity of this enzyme is impaired, cortisol assumes the role of aldosterone. Because cortisol secretion is not regulated by the renin-angiotensin system, a state of mineralocorticoid excess at normal plasma cortisol concentrations results. The appropriate treatment is to suppress cortisol secretion with an exogenous glucocorticoid having little or no mineralocorticoid activity, such as dexamethasone or prednisone.

The active ingredient in licorice, glycyrrhizic acid, is a competitive inhibitor of 11β-HSD. Thus, licorice intoxication can cause hypertension by the same mechanism as spontaneously occurring 11β-HSD deficiency. Licorice intoxication usually can be excluded by history. The most common source of licorice in the United States is chewing tobacco.

All causes of non–aldosterone-mediated renin-angiotensin–independent mineralocorticoid excess except for malignancy should "respond" to adrenal suppression with dexamethasone, 2 mg per day. If this fails, especially in the presence of an adrenal mass, adrenal malignancy is suggested. When adrenal suppression is successful, hydrocortisone, 12 to 15 mg per square meter per day, should be used for long-term treatment.

Adrenal Hypofunction

GLUCOCORTICOID DEFICIENCY (Table 204–6). **Diagnosis.** A broad spectrum of signs and symptoms can herald the presence of glucocorticoid deficiency. At one extreme is the *"chronic syndrome,"* characterized by symptoms of malaise, anorexia, and orthostatic hypotension. Occasionally, vague abdominal pain can occur. Signs include weight loss, hypotension with an orthostatic component, and, in certain cases, a melanin-based hyperpigmentation of the skin. The routine laboratory picture reveals a normochromic normocytic anemia, relative lymphocytosis often with

---

TABLE 204–4. COMMON CAUSES OF RENIN-ANGIOTENSIN–INDEPENDENT MINERALOCORTICOID EXCESS

Aldosterone-secreting adenoma
Adrenal cancer
Congenital adrenal hyperplasia
   11-hydroxylase deficiency
   17-hydroxylase deficiency
11β-hydroxysteroid dehydrogenase deficiency
Licorice intoxication
Glucocorticoid-suppressible hyperaldosteronism

TABLE 204–5. COMMON CAUSES OF RENIN-ANGIOTENSIN–DEPENDENT MINERALOCORTICOID EXCESS

Vomiting
Diuretics
Edematous disorders
   Congestive heart failure
   Hepatic cirrhosis
   Nephrotic syndrome
Renal ischemia
Bartter's syndrome
Renin-secreting tumors

TABLE 204–6. CAUSES OF GLUCOCORTICOID DEFICIENCY

ACTH-independent causes
  Tuberculosis
  Autoimmune (idiopathic)
  Other rare causes
    Fungal infection
    Adrenal hemorrhage
    Metastases
    Sarcoidosis
    Amyloidosis
    Adrenoleukodystrophy
    Adrenomyeloneuropathy
    HIV infection
    Congenital adrenal hyperplasia
    Medications (ketoconazole, OP'DDD)
ACTH-dependent causes
  Hypothalamic-pituitary-adrenal suppression
    Exogenous
      Glucocorticoid
      ACTH
    Endogenous—cure of Cushing's syndrome
  Hypothalamic-pituitary lesions
    Neoplasm
      Primary pituitary tumor
      Metastatic tumor
    Craniopharyngioma
    Infection
      Tuberculosis
      Actinomycosis
      Nocardiosis
  Sarcoid
  Head trauma
  Isolated ACTH deficiency

an unexplained eosinophilia, mild prerenal azotemia, and hyponatremia. If aldosterone secretion is impaired by the process, hyperkalemia also can be observed. At the other extreme is the *"acute syndrome,"* characterized by rapidly evolving agitation, confusion, fever, and abdominal pain, all associated with arterial hypotension. As the hypotension evolves into shock, it is relatively unresponsive to volume replacement and pressor agents, imitating the hemodynamic characteristics of "pump" failure in association with increased vascular volume. The laboratory findings are the same as those found in the chronic syndrome. Untreated, the acute syndrome quickly leads to coma and death. When first seen, the symptoms and signs of most patients with adrenal insufficiency lie somewhere on the continuum between these two extremes.

The diagnosis of glucocorticoid deficiency is confirmed by the inability of the adrenal glands to respond normally to an ACTH challenge. Synthetic ACTH, 250 μg, is administered intravenously, and plasma cortisol is determined 45 and 60 minutes later. The normal adrenal gland produces plasma cortisol concentrations of 20 μg per deciliter or more. Any value < 20 μg per deciliter implies a degree of adrenal compromise. Because the differential diagnosis of adrenal insufficiency relies on the plasma concentration of ACTH, it is prudent to draw a blood sample for ACTH prior to the administration of ACTH and to "hold" the sample in the laboratory pending the results of the plasma cortisol determination.

Differential Diagnosis and Treatment. The first task in the differential diagnosis of glucocorticoid deficiency is to define whether or not the process is ACTH-dependent. ACTH-dependent glucocorticoid deficiency implies disordered function of the hypothalamus and/or pituitary gland leading to ACTH deficiency, whereas ACTH-independent glucocorticoid deficiency is caused by disordered adrenal function, such as destruction of the gland by an infectious process like tuberculosis. This distinction is best made on the basis of plasma ACTH concentration measured at the time of glucocorticoid deficiency (i.e., before treatment with glucocorticoid has been initiated). ACTH concentrations in or below the normal range imply an ACTH-dependent process. ACTH concentrations above the normal range imply an ACTH-independent process.

Glucocorticoid Deficiency Related to Adrenal Suppression. The most common cause of ACTH-dependent glucocorticoid deficiency is hypothalamic-pituitary-adrenal "suppression" by exoge-nously administered glucocorticoids, either iatrogenic or factitious. Whether or not a patient develops adrenal suppression as a result of exogenous glucocorticoid administration depends upon three variables: the dose of the glucocorticoid administered, the duration of administration, and the schedule of administration. It is unusual to develop clinically manifest adrenal suppression with doses of glucocorticoid equal to or less than the daily replacement dose of the preparation employed—20 mg per day of hydrocortisone, 5 mg per day of prednisone or prednisolone, and 0.5 mg per day of dexamethasone. Given doses that exceed these limits, it is unusual to develop clinically manifest glucocorticoid deficiency if the duration of administration is < 3 weeks. Finally, the dosage schedule can affect the rapidity with which the final state of adrenal suppression is reached. Glucocorticoids given as a single dose first thing in the morning are the least suppressive; glucocorticoids given in divided doses throughout the day are the most suppressive. Thus, at one extreme are patients given decreasing doses of prednisone for 14 days to treat an acute inflammatory process such as poison ivy. Signs and symptoms of glucocorticoid deficiency following cessation of the medication are extremely unlikely. At the other extreme are patients treated with large doses of glucocorticoids given in divided doses for long periods of time for the treatment of disorders such as chronic obstructive pulmonary disease. These patients develop many of the stigmata of Cushing's syndrome and manifest signs and symptoms of glucocorticoid deficiency within 48 hours if the glucocorticoid is stopped for any reason. The clinical manifestations of this deficiency can range from the "chronic" syndrome at one extreme to the "acute" syndrome at the other.

Glucocorticoid Deficiency Due to Hypothalamic-Pituitary Disease. Destructive lesions of the hypothalamus and pituitary gland are a rare cause of ACTH-dependent glucocorticoid deficiency. Although it is uncommon, diagnosis is imperative because early therapeutic intervention can prevent many of the serious sequelae of these tumors, including blindness. Examples include pituitary tumor, metastatic tumors to the region, sarcoid, amyloid, craniopharyngioma, and Rathke's pouch cyst. Pituitary infections such as actinomycosis and nocardiosis and vascular accidents such as Sheehan's syndrome also can lead to adrenal insufficiency. The most direct approach to the diagnosis of these lesions is imaging with CT scan using contrast enhancement or with MRI following gadolinium administration. A rare cause of ACTH-dependent glucocorticoid deficiency is *autoimmune lymphocytic hypophysitis.*

The treatment of chronic ACTH-dependent glucocorticoid insufficiency consists of replacing the missing hormone. Glucocorticoid should be replaced in the form of hydrocortisone, the naturally occurring glucocorticoid in humans, at a rate of 12 to 15 mg per square meter per day. Cortisol is secreted in bursts, between 7 and 10 per day, clustering in the morning hours. To reproduce this pattern with replacement steroid is impossible with currently available methods. Empirically, however, it has been found that patients do as well with a single morning dose of cortisol as with divided doses, and compliance is simplified with this regimen. Clinical measures best monitor the adequacy of replacement: Anorexia, weight loss, and hyponatremia suggest underreplacement; weight gain, plethora, and supraclavicular fat deposition suggest overreplacement. The current standard of practice is to increase cortisol dose in the context of "stress," actual or anticipated. The dose of cortisol is doubled for the duration of the stress and returned to replacement levels immediately upon cessation of the stress. Typical stresses include febrile illness; nausea and vomiting; trauma such as lacerations, contusions, and fractures; and surgical procedures, including dental extraction. Acute glucocorticoid deficiency is treated with large doses of cortisol given intravenously, 100 mg every 6 hours, coupled with emergency support of blood pressure plus volume expansion and pressors when indicated.

Primary Adrenal Insufficiency. The most common cause of primary adrenal insufficiency worldwide is tuberculosis. Tuberculosis causes adrenal insufficiency by destroying the adrenal cortex and replacing it with caseating granulomas. The most common cause of adrenal insufficiency in the industrialized west is an autoimmune process, usually as part of the polyglandular deficiency syndrome. In this disorder, an autoimmune "adrenalitis" leads to destruction of the adrenal cortex. This disease has two forms, types I and II. The relative features of the two forms are detailed in Table 204–7. Type I is a disease of childhood with a mean age of onset of 12 years.

TABLE 204–7. POLYENDOCRINE DEFICIENCY SYNDROMES

	Type I	Type II
Age of onset	12 yrs	24 yrs
Adrenal insufficiency	+	+
Diabetes mellitus	−	+
Autoimmune thyroid disease	−	+
Hypoparathyroidism	+	−
Mucocutaneous candidiasis	+	−
Hypogonadism	+	+/−
Chronic active hepatitis	+	−
Pernicious anemia	+	−
Vitiligo	+	+

Type II begins at an average age of 24 years. The dominant features of type I disease are adrenal insufficiency, hypoparathyroidism, and mucocutaneous candidiasis. The dominant features of type II disease are adrenal insufficiency, autoimmune thyroid disease, and insulin-dependent diabetes mellitus. Other important differences include the patterns of inheritance. Type I is transmitted as an autosomal recessive trait, occurring across sibships, whereas type II has a "dominant" pattern of inheritance, appearing in multiple generations of an affected family. Also, type I disease has no HLA association, whereas type II is associated with the DR3/DR4 haplotypes. Both disorders appear to be mediated by an autoimmune process. For example, circulating antibodies to one or more endocrine organs are found in most patients, and defects in T lymphocyte function such as a decrease in "suppressor" activity are described.

All of the clinically important fungi except *Monilia* can cause adrenal destruction. The most common cause is histoplasmosis, which is due to an organism particularly prominent in the Ohio and Tennessee valleys and along the Piedmont Plateau of the Middle Atlantic states. South American blastomycosis is the next most common fungal cause of adrenal insufficiency, followed by North American blastomycosis, coccidioidomycosis, and cryptococcosis. The pathophysiology of fungal adrenalitis is much like that of tuberculosis—destruction leading to adrenal enlargement with caseating granuloma formation. If healing occurs, the adrenal glands can shrink in size, sometimes resuming a relatively normal volume. The healing process is often accompanied by calcification.

The advent of CT scan has revealed adrenal hemorrhage as a more frequent cause of adrenal insufficiency than had been recognized previously. The usual setting is a stressed individual receiving long-term anticoagulation for the prevention of pulmonary or cardiac emboli or other thrombotic phenomena. Typically, affected patients complain of back pain followed, in a few days, by the onset of the first signs and symptoms of adrenal insufficiency.

Metastases to the adrenal gland are common, with a frequency as high as 70% in patients with disseminated breast or lung cancer. Adrenal insufficiency as a result of metastases, however, is uncommon, although moderate abnormalities in adrenal function often can be detected in patients with bilateral adrenal metastases. Tumors commonly associated with adrenal insufficiency are cancers of the breast, lung, stomach, and colon; melanoma; and some lymphomas.

The syndrome of acquired immunodeficiency (AIDS) can be associated with adrenal insufficiency in its late stages. Cytomegalovirus infection of the adrenal glands commonly accompanies this condition, as does infection with *Mycobacterium avium-intracellulare* and the various fungi that can colonize and destroy the adrenal glands. The plasma cortisol response to ACTH administration is abnormal in 10 to 15% of patients with AIDS and its advanced complications.

Adrenoleukodystrophy is an inborn abnormality of long-chain fatty acids causing adrenal insufficiency in association with several neurologically impaired phenotypes. Newborn adrenoleukodystrophy is transmitted as an autosomal recessive trait. Adrenoleukodystrophy, also known as brown Schilder's disease (brown being an adjective describing the hyperpigmentation of the skin) or sudanophilic leukodystrophy, is transmitted as an X-linked disease of children characterized by rapidly progressive central demyelination eventuating in seizures, dementia, cortical blindness, coma, and death. Death usually occurs before puberty is complete. X-linked

adrenomyeloneuropathy is a disease of young adults characterized by a slowly progressive mixed upper and lower motor and sensory neuropathy leading to an ascending spastic paraparesis. Signs and symptoms of spinocerebellar degeneration appear in some cases. Both forms of the disease are associated with progressive failure of all steroid-secreting cells, leading to adrenal and gonadal failure. The metabolic marker for these diseases is an elevated circulating level of very long chain fatty acids (VLCFA's), C-26 and greater in length. The cause of this abnormality seems to be an abnormal peroxisomal transporter protein that prevents the appropriate metabolism of the VLCFA's. Several treatments have been tried, but only autologous bone marrow transplantation appears to be successful.

Other rare causes of primary adrenal insufficiency include amyloidosis, congenital unresponsiveness to ACTH, congenital adrenal hypoplasia, and familial glucocorticoid insufficiency.

The treatment of ACTH-independent glucocorticoid deficiency is the same as that outlined for ACTH-dependent glucocorticoid deficiency except that the addition of a mineralocorticoid is usually required. This is because adrenal cortical destruction impairs both cortisol and aldosterone secretion. The available orally active mineralocorticoid is fludrocortisone acetate (Florinef). It is equipotent with aldosterone. The secretion rate of aldosterone in salt-replete humans is about 100 μg per day. Thus, fludrocortisone, 100 μg per day, is the appropriate replacement dose. The drug has a wide therapeutic window, and no specific monitoring for treatment effect other than an occasional plasma potassium concentration is necessary.

MINERALOCORTICOID DEFICIENCY. *Diagnosis.* The major clinical manifestations of mineralocorticoid deficiency are hyponatremia, hyperkalemia, and mild metabolic acidosis. These can lead to profound muscle weakness and cardiac arrhythmias. Combined glucocorticoid and mineralocorticoid deficiency is a common cause of this picture and should first be excluded with an ACTH stimulation test. If that test is normal, the diagnosis of isolated hypoaldosteronism depends upon the demonstration of an inappropriately low circulating aldosterone level. The causes of isolated hypoaldosteronism are listed in Table 204–8.

Differential Diagnosis and Treatment. Selective hypoaldosteronism was, until recently, believed to be rare. Recent studies, however, show that it accounts for as many as 10% of cases of unexplained hyperkalemia. The causes of hypoaldosteronism can be divided into renin-angiotensin–dependent (hyporeninemic) and renin-angiotensin–independent (hyper-reninemic) causes. The differentiation is made on the basis of the plasma renin activity. The usual test is a measurement of plasma renin activity following 4 hours of upright posture. Levels in the normal or low range identify cases that are renin-angiotensin–dependent, whereas high levels identify cases that are renin-angiotensin–independent.

Renin deficiency, overall, is the most common cause of selective aldosterone deficiency. It is usually found in elderly subjects with mild, nonoliguric renal disease. Many such patients have insulin-dependent diabetes, and diabetic nephropathy is thought to be an important contributing abnormality. Other causes of renin-angiotensin–dependent hypoaldosteronism include autonomic dysfunction associated with prolonged bed rest and, rarely, treatment with prostaglandin synthesis inhibitors such as indomethacin.

TABLE 204–8. CAUSES OF ISOLATED HYPOALDOSTERONISM

Renin-angiotensin–dependent
  Hyporeninemic hypoaldosteronism
  Autonomic neuropathy
  Prostaglandin synthesis inhibitors
Renin-angiotensin–independent
  Inhibition of aldosterone synthesis
    Heparin
    Cyclosporine
    Calcium channel blockers
  Following resection of an aldosterone-secreting adenoma
  18-hydroxylase deficiency
  Aldosterone resistance (pseudohypoaldosteronism)

The causes of renin-angiotensin–independent hypoaldosteronism include all causes of ACTH-independent adrenal insufficiency listed in Table 204–6. In this setting, selective hypoaldosteronism can result if treatment is confined to glucocorticoid replacement. The other causes of this disorder center on alterations in the synthesis and secretion of aldosterone. These include long-term heparin administration and the "salt-wasting" forms of congenital adrenal hyperplasia (21-hydroxylase deficiency, 3β-hydroxysteroid dehydrogenase deficiency, and 17-hydroxylase deficiency). Again, treating these disorders with glucocorticoid alone is a common cause of selective hypoaldosteronism. Finally, any defect in the conversion of corticosterone to aldosterone, such as 18-hydroxylase deficiency, leads to selective hypoaldosteronism.

Treating selective hypoaldosteronism of any cause is straightforward. Aldosterone deficiency does not produce clinical symptoms unless the subject is "salt deprived." This is unlikely to occur at levels of salt intake greater than 10 mEq per kilogram per day. For adults, this equals about 4 grams of sodium chloride per day, which is routinely ingested in the average American diet. Thus, a simple way to treat selective hypoaldosteronism is to ensure adequate dietary salt intake which, in the United States, is not a problem in young and otherwise healthy subjects. This approach, however, fails in patients with "fetish" diets or those who cannot maintain an adequate oral intake of salt for any reason. Important in this regard are the dietary restrictions that frequently accompany old age and those often imposed upon infants and toddlers. In these cases, it is advisable to supply exogenous mineralocorticoid. Fludrocortisone is the only available preparation of orally active mineralocorticoid. It is equipotent with aldosterone and is given in doses that approximate the daily production rate of aldosterone in the salt-replete individual, 100 μg per day. The preparation can be given as a single daily dose with the morning meal. The drug's therapeutic window is wide, so overtreatment is unlikely. Thus, an occasional serum potassium concentration measurement is adequate to monitor efficacy of treatment.

Disorders of Combined Insufficiency and Excess

THE CONGENITAL ADRENAL HYPERPLASIAS. Defects in the synthesis of cortisol lead to compensatory stimulation of adrenal steroidogenesis to maintain normal plasma cortisol concentrations. This inevitably leads to an accumulation of the steroid biosynthetic intermediate immediately before the enzymic defect in the biosynthetic cascade. Clinically, the result is expressed as glucocorticoid deficiency (which can be so mild as to be inapparent or so severe as to be life threatening) in association with mineralocorticoid excess or deficiency and androgen excess or deficiency. These disorders are usually classified as "salt-wasting," "hypertensive," "virilizing," or "feminizing," depending upon the combination of hormone excess and deficiency. They are presented in detail in Ch. 207. Only the attenuated or "nonclassic" form of 21-hydroxylase deficiency is presented here.

21-Hydroxylase deficiency is one of the most prevalent autosomal recessive disorders, with a heterozygote frequency that may be as high as one in five. Although congenital in nature, the disorder usually makes its first appearance with the onset of puberty. Hirsutism, oligomenorrhea, and cystic acne are the most common clinical manifestations. The disorder is identical in presentation to idiopathic hirsutism–polycystic ovarian disease and cannot be differentiated from this disorder without specifically examining adrenal steroidogenesis looking for the 21-hydroxylase block. This is best done in the context of an ACTH stimulation test performed in the usual way, with measurements of 17-hydroxyprogesterone made at 45 and 60 minutes after administration of the ACTH. Normal subjects do not exceed 17-hydroxyprogesterone levels of 350 ng per deciliter, but patients with the disorder attain plasma levels > 1500 ng per deciliter. The incidence of this disorder in young hirsute patients varies between 1 and 30%, depending on ethnic background, averaging about 5% for the population as a whole.

As with the other congenital adrenal hyperplasias, treatment consists of exogenous glucocorticoid replacement to circumvent the deficiency in cortisol biosynthesis. The usual approach is to administer cortisol (Cortef), 12 to 15 mg per square meter per day as a single morning dose. Care should be taken that the adrenal gland is not completely suppressed by the replacement regimen chosen. This can be assessed by an ACTH stimulation test 3 to 6 months following the initiation of treatment.

DISORDERS OF TISSUE RESPONSIVENESS: THE STEROID RESISTANCE SYNDROMES

Two disorders of end-organ resistance are relevant to a discussion of disorders of adrenal function: glucocorticoid resistance and mineralocorticoid resistance.

Glucocorticoid resistance is rare; only 17 separate probands have been described to date. The disease is characterized by markedly elevated indices of cortisol production (increased urine free cortisol excretion) in the absence of any of the clinical stigmata of Cushing's syndrome. Occasionally, signs and symptoms of mineralocorticoid and androgen excess are responsible for bringing the patient to medical attention. Like the situation in congenital adrenal hyperplasia, androgens and mineralocorticoids are elevated in this syndrome as a by-product of the increased adrenal steroidogenesis necessary to produce enough cortisol to maintain life. The cause of the disease, which has not been proved in all cases, is a defect in the ligand-binding domain of the glucocorticoid receptor. The disease is transmitted as an autosomal recessive trait, with heterozygote subjects sometimes manifesting attenuated forms of the disorder.

The diagnosis is suggested by finding elevated rates of urine free cortisol excretion in a subject with none of the stigmata of Cushing's syndrome. The diagnosis is confirmed by demonstrating abnormal binding characteristics of the glucocorticoid receptor, usually in mononuclear leukocytes. Treatment should be reserved for persons manifesting signs and symptoms of androgen or mineralocorticoid excess and consists of the exogenous administration of a synthetic glucocorticoid, usually dexamethasone, in doses sufficient to bring the urine free cortisol excretion into the normal range. This is usually accompanied by remission of the associated steroid excess syndromes.

Mineralocorticoid resistance is characterized by elevated levels of aldosterone and increased plasma renin activity in association with signs and symptoms of mineralocorticoid deficiency. The disorder is generally referred to as pseudohypoaldosteronism. It is commonly divided into two subtypes, but only type 1 appears to fulfill the usual criteria for receptor-mediated end-organ resistance.

Type 1 pseudohypoaldosteronism is a rare inherited disorder presenting with salt loss and failure to thrive in infancy, most commonly between 5 and 7 days of age. The cause appears to be an abnormal mineralocorticoid receptor, with decreased binding affinity and decreased receptor number both described. Hyponatremia, hyperkalemia, and metabolic acidosis in association with elevated plasma and urine aldosterone and an elevated plasma renin activity make the diagnosis. The treatment is to replace dietary salt at a rate of 10 to 40 mEq per kilogram per day.

Aubourg P, Blanche S, Jambaque' I: Reversal of early neurologic and neuroradiologic manifestations of X-linked adrenoleukodystrophy by bone marrow transplantation. N Engl J Med 322:1860, 1990. *Describes a successful outcome from a previously always progressive and often fatal disease.*

Carney JA, Young WF: Primary pigmented nodular adrenocortical disease and its associated conditions. Endocrinologist 2:6, 1992. *Describes an associated complex of abnormalities.*

Donovan DS, Dluhy RG: AIDS and its effect on the adrenal gland. Endocrinologist 1:227, 1991. *The title says it all in this informative review.*

Friedman RB, Oldfield EH, Nieman LK: Repeat transsphenoidal surgery for Cushing's disease. J Neurosurg 71:520, 1989. *Describes the surgical approach when transnasal hypophysectomy fails to remove the tumor.*

Gill JR: Primary hyperaldosteronism: Strategies for diagnosis and treatment. Endocrinologist 1:365, 1991. *The title is self-explanatory.*

Javier E, Reardon GE, Malchoff CD: Glucocorticoid resistance and its clinical presentations. Endocrinologist 1:141, 1991. *A helpful discussion of a rare disorder.*

Miller J, Crapo L: The biochemical analysis of hypercortisolism. Endocrinologist 4:7, 1994. *Brings order and simplification to the subject.*

Muir A, Maclaren NK: Autoimmune diseases of the adrenal glands, parathyroid glands, gonads, and hypothalamic-pituitary axis. Endocrinol Metab Clin North Am 20:619, 1991. *A detailed coverage of the mechanisms and treatment of the autoimmune syndrome.*

Schteingart DE: Treating adrenal cancer. Endocrinologist 2:149, 1992. *Describes treatment and outcome in greater detail.*

Speiser PW, DuPont B, Rubenstein P: High frequency of non-classical steroid 21-hydroxylase deficiency. Am J Hum Genet 37:650, 1985. *Discusses the adult form of the syndrome.*

Urbanic RC: Cushing's disease—18 years' experience. Medicine 60:14, 1981.

Veldhuis JD, Melby JC: Isolated aldosterone deficiency in man: Acquired and inborn errors in the biosynthesis of action of aldosterone. Endocrinol Rev 2:495, 1986. *A clearly stated description of the problem.*

204.2 ADRENAL MEDULLA
Daniel T. O'Connor

The catecholamines (norepinephrine, epinephrine, and dopamine) serve as neurotransmitters and circulating hormones. Catecholamines acquire their name by the catechol (3,4-dihydroxyphenyl) modification of their aromatic (phenyl) rings. *Norepinephrine* is the amine neurotransmitter released from terminals of postganglionic axons of the sympathetic nervous system, as well as from central nervous system noradrenergic axons. Adrenal medullary chromaffin cells store both epinephrine and norepinephrine in catecholamine secretory vesicles.

Chromaffin cells derive embryologically from neuroectoderm. Precursor cells differentiate in the center of the adrenal gland in response to cortisol; the precursors then differentiate into sympathetic neurons in response to nerve growth factor. A few such cells also migrate to form paraganglia, collections of chromaffin cells on both sides of the aorta. The largest such periaortic cluster, often found near the level of the inferior mesenteric artery, is referred to as the organ of Zuckerkandl. Both chromaffin cells and postganglionic sympathetic axons are part of the effector limb of the sympathetic branch of the autonomic nervous system and are innervated by thoracolumbar preganglionic axons emerging from the spinal cord.

Catecholamines are released from the adrenal medulla into the circulation through the adrenal vein. Norepinephrine from sympathetic neurons is released presynaptically and acts as a cell-to-cell neurotransmitter. Circulating plasma norepinephrine influences blood pressure and heart rate under only the most extreme circumstances of sympathetic activation. Relatively selective adrenal catecholamine release occurs during syncope and insulin-evoked hypoglycemia, whereas active, dynamic exercise selectively stimulates sympathetic neuronal norepinephrine release.

CATECHOLAMINE BIOSYNTHESIS AND METABOLISM

Catecholamine biosynthesis starts with the essential dietary amino acid phenylalanine, which is converted to tyrosine by phenylalanine hydroxlase. Tyrosine is hydroxylated to dihydroxyphenylalanine (DOPA) by the action of tyrosine hydroxylase (TH), the rate-limiting enzymatic step in catecholamine biosynthesis. DOPA decarboxylase then converts DOPA to dopamine, which is carried by the vesicular monoamine transporter (VMT) from cytosol into the catecholamine storage vesicle, where dopamine-β-hydroxylase (DβH) converts it to norepinephrine. In sympathetic axons and in 15 to 20% of chromaffin cells, norepinephrine is the final catecholamine product. In 80 to 85% of chromaffin cells a further enzymatic step occurs: phenylethanolamine-*N*-methyltransferase (PNMT), a cytosolic enzyme, catalyzes the *N*-methylation of norepinephrine to epinephrine.

Catecholamines in noradrenergic axons and chromaffin cells are sequestered from the cytosol in membrane-limited organelles: catecholamine storage vesicles (or chromaffin granules, in chromaffin cells). Chromaffin granule cores contain not only catecholamines but also soluble proteins such as DβH and chromogranin A.

The process of catecholamine discharge from chromaffin cells and sympathetic axons is *exocytosis,* wherein all soluble components of the granule are co-released and ultimately make their way to the circulation.

Neuronal uptake ("reuptake") is the major route of norepinephrine removal from synaptic clefts (Fig. 204–4). Characteristics of this process are its location at the presynaptic axonal membrane, high-affinity, stereoselectivity, saturability, dependence on extracellular sodium, and specific pharmacologic inhibition by agents such as tricyclic antidepressants (e.g., desipramine) and cocaine. After neuronal uptake, cytosolic catecholamines can be either retransported into storage vesicles or deaminated by the enzyme monoamine oxidase (MAO), yielding the catecholamine metabolite dihydroxymandelic acid (DHMA). The enzyme catecholamine-O-methyltransferase (COMT), which acts on both catecholamines and DHMA, is present mainly in the cytosol of liver and kidney cells. COMT adds a methyl group to one of the hydroxyl oxygens on the catecholamines' dihydroxyphenyl rings, yielding either metanephrine (or methoxyepinephrine; from epinephrine), normetanephrine (or methoxynorepinephrine; from norepinephrine), or methoxytyramine (from dopamine). The metanephrines can then be deaminated by MAO to yield vanillylmandelic acid (VMA), while deamination of methoxytyramine by MAO yields homovanillic acid (HVA). DHMA is also a substrate for COMT, yielding VMA. Thus, complete enzymatic degradation of catecholamines to VMA (from epinephrine or norepinephrine) or HVA (from dopamine) involves the sequential action of two enzymes (MAO and COMT), either of which may initiate the process. In the bloodstream, catecholamines have a very short half-life, 1 to 2 minutes. They are cleared from the circulation largely by neuronal uptake but are also subject to direct renal excretion or sulfoconjugation of a ring hydroxyl group.

CATECHOLAMINE ACTION

Catecholamine receptors are specific for ligands and are classified as subtypes of the α ($\alpha_{1a,b,c}$, $\alpha_{2a,b,c}$) and β ($\beta_{1,2,3}$) classes. The hemodynamic effects of circulating norepinephrine require extreme concentrations. Whereas plasma norepinephrine may vary normally over a range of 200 to 1000 pg per milliliter during physiologic stimulation of sympathetic neuronal activity, far higher concentrations of infused norepinephrine (in excess of 1000 to 2000 pg per milliliter) are required to substantially affect blood pressure or heart rate. At β receptors, norepinephrine is a strong agonist at β_1 (cardiac, inotropic, and chronotropic) sites, although a relatively weak agonist at β_2 (vascular, vasodilatory) sites. At α receptors, norepinephrine is an effective agonist at both α_1 (vascular, vasoconstrictive) and α_2 (neuronal and vascular) sites. Infused norepinephrine acutely raises both systolic and diastolic blood pressure by actions on both β_1 and α adrenergic receptors, with vasoconstriction accompanied by reflex bradycardia. The hemodynamic effects of circulating epinephrine (50 to 500 pg per milliliter) differ from those

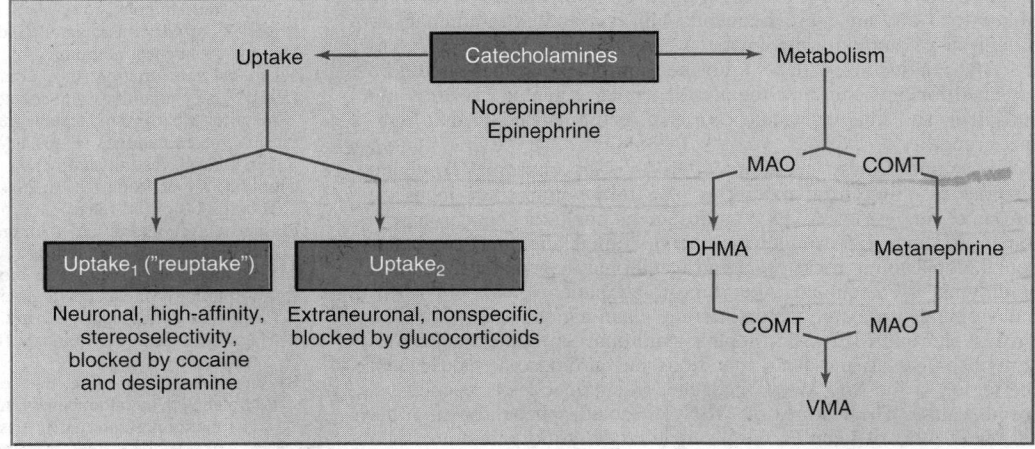

FIGURE 204–4. Catecholamine disposition and metabolism. MAO = monoamine oxidase; COMT = catechol-O-methyltransferase; VMA = vanillylmandelic acid; DHMA = dihydroxymandelic acid.

of norepinephrine. At β receptors, epinephrine is an agonist at both β_1 and β_2 sites. It is also a more potent agonist than norepinephrine at both α_1 and α_2 sites. During acute infusion, it increases systolic blood pressure, heart rate, and cardiac output, with a fall in diastolic blood pressure and systemic resistance, the latter effects resulting from actions at β_2 adrenergic receptors.

With chronic excess of circulating catecholamines, the hemodynamic profile may change substantially, in part as a consequence of desensitization of catecholamine target organs, resulting from adaptive changes in both receptor and postreceptor responses.

PHEOCHROMOCYTOMA

Pheochromocytoma is a chromaffin cell neoplasm that typically causes symptoms and signs of episodic catecholamine release, including paroxysmal hypertension. The tumor is an unusual cause of hypertension, accounting for at most 0.1 to 0.2% of cases of high blood pressure. In population-based cancer studies, its frequency was about two cases per million population. The diagnosis of pheochromocytoma is typically made in young to middle-aged adults, most commonly in the fourth or fifth decade of life; about 10% of diagnoses are made in children (usually male). Autopsy series indicate that the incidence of pheochromocytoma increases progressively with age. In adults, there is no gender difference in incidence.

About 90% of pheochromocytomas exist as solitary, unilateral, encapsulated adrenal medullary tumors. About 10% are bilateral, more commonly among several members of a family in which 40 to 70% may have bilateral tumors. The tumors are vascular, and large ones often contain internal hemorrhagic or cystic areas. Reported sizes have ranged from < 1 gram to several kilograms; the average is about 40 grams. About 10% of tumors are extra-adrenal (paragangliomas), and 90% of these are intra-abdominal, most commonly arising from chromaffin cells near the aortic bifurcation in the organ of Zuckerkandl or near the kidney. Other sites include the paravertebral sympathetic ganglia, the urinary bladder, other autonomic ganglia (celiac, superior or inferior mesenteric), the thorax (including the posterior mediastinum, the heart, and paracardiac regions), and the neck (in sympathetic ganglia, carotid body, cranial nerves, or glomus jugulare). Bilateral and extra-adrenal tumors are more common in children. Histologically, oval groups of cells, in clusters or "nests," stain for chromogranin A; a less frequently used stain identifies neuron-specific enolase. Less than 10% of the tumors are malignant; malignancy occurs more frequently in extra-adrenal tumors and is evidenced by local invasion or distant metastases but cannot be judged reliably from histologic appearance. Local invasion commonly involves adjacent vascular structures, such as the inferior vena cava. Distant metastatic sites include bone, lung, lymph nodes, and liver. Bilateral adrenal medullary hyperplasia has been reported in gene carriers from kindreds with multiple endocrine neoplasia type 2 (MEN-2). This hyperplasia may be a precursor of pheochromocytoma.

The "rule of 10's" is useful to recall approximate frequencies of pheochromocytoma that vary from the usual: 10% bilateral, 10% extra-adrenal, 10% extra-abdominal, 10% malignant, 10% familial, 10% pediatric, and 10% without blood pressure elevation.

ETIOLOGY. *Familial* pheochromocytomas constitute 5 to 10% of the total and are more frequently bilateral and extra-adrenal, although less commonly malignant. A careful family history is essential, and relatives of patients with the familial syndromes should be screened for pheochromocytoma; biochemical screening is often not sufficient, and imaging studies are also recommended in this high-risk group.

Von Hippel-Lindau syndrome (VHLS) is an autosomal dominant disorder resulting from mutations at a tumor-suppressor locus on chromosome 3p25-p26. Its manifestations include pheochromocytoma (in about 14% of gene carriers), retinal angioma, cerebellar hemangioblastoma, renal cysts and carcinoma, pancreatic cysts, and epididymal cystadenoma. Accordingly, all patients with pheochromocytoma deserve careful funduscopic examination.

MEN-2A and MEN-2B (Sipple's syndrome) are autosomal dominant disorders arising from mutations on chromosome 10q11.2 in the region of the *RET* proto-oncogene, which encodes a receptor tyrosine kinase. The features of MEN-2A include pheochromocytoma (in about 40% of gene carriers), medullary thyroid carcinoma, and

primary hyperparathyroidism (adenoma or hyperplasia). Because of this syndrome, it is wise to screen all pheochromocytoma patients for medullary thyroid carcinoma with serum calcitonin. MEN-2B features include pheochromocytoma, medullary thyroid carcinoma, multiple mucosal neuromas (of lips, tongue, buccal mucosa, eyelids, conjunctivae, corneas, and gastrointestinal tract), and marfanoid body habitus (but without lens or aortic abnormalities).

Hereditary neurofibromatosis (von Recklinghausen's disease), an autosomal dominant disorder resulting from mutations at the NF1 (neurofibromin) locus on chromosome 17q11.2, presents with neurofibromas and café-au-lait spots; about 1% of neurofibromatosis patients have pheochromocytoma. Familial pheochromocytoma may also occur in isolation; whether such families represent disease processes etiologically distinct from VHLS or MEN is not clear.

In the 90 to 95% of pheochromocytomas which are *sporadic*, the cause of the neoplastic process remains obscure, although loss of heterozygosity on chromosomes 1p, 3p, 17p, and 22q suggests somatic cell deletion mutation of one autosomal allele at as-yet-uncharacterized tumor suppressor loci.

DIAGNOSIS. Because pheochromocytoma is a potentially curable form of hypertension, the diagnosis is worth considering in each new case of hypertension. However, because hypertension is so commonly encountered in clinical practice (~ 20 to 25% of the adult population), and pheochromocytoma is so distinctly unusual (~ 0.1 to 0.2% of patients with hypertension), laboratory evaluation should be selective and guided by the degree of clinical suspicion, based on criteria outlined below (Table 204–9).

Symptoms and Signs. Paroxysmal symptoms (such as the triad of episodic palpitations, diaphoresis, and headache) are the classic features of pheochromocytoma. These paroxysmal "attacks" characteristically begin abruptly, may last for minutes to hours, and subside gradually, with a frequency varying from many times daily to one or more per week (most commonly) or even every few months. Less common symptoms include apprehension or anxiety, tremulousness, pain in the chest or abdomen, weakness, or weight loss. In some series, > 90% of patients have experienced paroxysmal symptoms of one or more of the classic triad. Autopsy series indicate that as many as 50 to 75% of pheochromocytomas may be undiagnosed during life, suggesting that many pheochromocytomas do not give rise to these classic symptomatic features. Patients over the age of 60 years with pheochromocytoma are especially likely to report minor or no symptoms.

Other features in the history may suggest pheochromocytoma. Affected patients may report an increase in blood pressure after re-

TABLE 204–9. DIAGNOSTIC APPROACH TO PHEOCHROMOCYTOMA

Clinical clues or "tipoffs"
  History
    Paroxysmal symptoms (classic triad is headache, diaphoresis, palpitations)
    History of extraordinarily labile or refractory hypertension
    Family history of pheochromocytoma, von Hippel-Lindau syndrome (VHLS), or multiple endocrine neoplasia (MEN)
    Incidental adrenal abnormality on abdominal imaging test (rarely)
  Physical examination
    Labile, refractory hypertension
    Orthostatic hypotension
    VHLS- or MEN-associated findings (retinal angiomas, thyroid enlargement, mucosal neuromas)
Biochemical confirmation (only after clue or tipoff; begin with urinary tests)
  Urinary catecholamines and metabolites (24-hour sample, or 2-hour sample after a paroxysm; metanephrines, the first screening test)
  Plasma catecholamines (if urinary values are equivocal; take care to obtain a basal, resting sample)
  Clonidine suppression test (if plasma catecholamines are in the equivocal 1000–2000 pg/ml range)
  Plasma chromogranin A (storage vesicle protein released with catecholamines; also elevated by renal failure)
Anatomic localization (only after biochemical confirmation)
  By morphology (most sensitive, less specific)
    Computed tomography (the imaging test most frequently obtained)
    Magnetic resonance imaging (may have advantages for extra-adrenal tumors)
  By function (most specific, less sensitive)
    Radiolabeled metaiodobenzylguanidine (MIBG) scanning (accumulates in functioning chromaffin tissue)

ceiving certain antihypertensive drugs, especially β-adrenergic antagonists and guanethidine, or they may experience a remarkable fall in blood pressure after receiving α_1-adrenergic antagonists such as prazosin. Hypertension in such patients is relatively refractory to medical management. A history of extreme blood pressure lability during intubation, surgery, or induction of general anesthesia also suggests possible pheochromocytoma. A family history of pheochromocytoma, VHLS, or MEN should prompt an evaluation for pheochromocytoma. Paroxysmal symptoms on micturition or bladder distention or painless, gross hematuria may suggest pheochromocytoma of the bladder; the diagnosis is confirmed by cystoscopy.

Hypertension (usually severe and refractory to antihypertensive medications) is the cardinal sign of pheochromocytoma, although it is nonspecific and may be insensitive. In about half of patients, hypertension is sustained, with intermittent blood pressure surges in half or more of these; in about 40%, hypertension is paroxysmal, with relatively normal blood pressure between surges. Hypertensive surges may be precipitated by abdominal manipulation, but generally no antecedent is noted. The heart rate is usually elevated during blood pressure surges but may decline as a result of physiologic reflex bradycardia. Orthostatic hypotension is variably observed. As many as 15 to 20% of patients may have cholesterol gallstones.

Laboratory Diagnosis. Because hypertension is so common and pheochromocytoma so rare, further biochemical evaluation for pheochromocytoma in hypertensives should be selective and focused on subjects who display some relevant clue to pheochromocytoma on history, physical examination, or screening laboratory evaluation. If interpretation of urinary measurements is not clearcut, evaluation should proceed to plasma measurements, which require more careful sampling technique. The number and diversity of biochemical tests obtained should parallel the clinical index of suspicion. If suspicion is low, a single screening test may suffice, usually 24-hour urinary metanephrine excretion. If suspicion is high, multiple tests, both urine and plasma, are in order. Because anatomic or imaging studies may detect nonspecific adrenal abnormalities in up to 2% of the population, such studies should not be undertaken unless biochemical tests are positive.

Routine Tests. Results of routine screening tests obtained for other purposes (such as general health maintenance) may provide tipoffs. Hyperglycemia is common, and about half of pheochromocytoma patients manifest carbohydrate intolerance; frank diabetes requiring insulin is unusual. Lactic acidosis occurs rarely, even without shock. Serum lactic dehydrogenase activity may be elevated from adrenal isoenzyme 3. Rarely, pheochromocytoma may be an incidental finding on computed tomographic or magnetic resonance imaging of the abdomen undertaken for other indications.

Urine Tests. Widely available tests measure urinary free (unconjugated) catecholamines and catecholamine metabolites: the metanephrines and VMA. A 24-hour urine sample is collected, and creatinine is measured in the same sample as an index of adequacy and completeness of collection. Of the available tests, increased urinary metanephrines have the highest diagnostic sensitivity and specificity for pheochromocytoma. The urinary excretions of metanephrines and VMA remain normal until the very end stage of renal disease, so elevated levels validly diagnose pheochromocytoma.

Artifactual false-positive assay results have been greatly minimized in recent years with the introduction of more specific assay methods based on separation of catecholamines and metabolites in urine by high-pressure liquid chromatography. False-positive increases in free catecholamines may result from exogenous sources, such as catecholamines (which may be administered surreptitiously), α-methyldopa (but VMA excretion is characteristically normal), L-DOPA, labetalol, sympathomimetic amines (which release endogenous catecholamines from their stores), and fluorescent drugs such as tetracycline. Misleading elevations of endogenous catecholamines may occur as a consequence of the sympathoadrenal responses to shock, hypoglycemia, physical exertion, increased intracranial pressure, or withdrawal of central α_2 agonists such as clonidine. False-positive metanephrine elevations may result from excessive catecholamines (exogenous or endogenous) or the use of monoamine oxidase inhibitors or propranolol (which interferes with the spectrophotometric assay). False-positive VMA elevations may occur after ingesting carbidopa (a peripheral DOPA decarboxylase inhibitor) or monoamine oxidase inhibitors.

Blood Tests. Biochemical tests on blood samples offer the advantage of patient convenience but the disadvantage that even minor physical or mental stress can result in false-positive elevations. Plasma catecholamines are best sampled from a supine, resting patient in whom an indwelling antecubital venous cannula has been in place for at least 15 minutes. Plasma assay methods provide generally reliable results, with usual normal resting norepinephrine of 200 to 400 pg per milliliter and normal resting epinephrine of 20 to 60 pg per milliliter. Most patients with pheochromocytoma have markedly elevated (>2000 pg per milliliter) resting plasma catecholamines (norepinephrine plus epinephrine); plasma concentrations elevated beyond this point strongly suggest pheochromocytoma. The upper limit of normal (norepinephrine plus epinephrine) is <1000 pg per milliliter. Values between 1000 and 2000 pg per milliliter are equivocal and may represent either pheochromocytoma or sympathoadrenal activation by physical or mental stress. In these subjects the clonidine suppression test discussed below is of particular value.

False-positive plasma catecholamine elevations may result from the same factors that produce false-positive urinary elevations but are a more severe problem because measurements are made at only one time point. These factors include physical stress, such as trauma, surgery, upright posture, acute venipuncture, hypoglycemia, hypovolemia, hypotension, cold, sodium depletion, or mental stress, such as anxiety or pain. Drugs that increase plasma catecholamines include sympathomimetic amines which release catecholamines from their stores, cocaine which blocks catecholamine reuptake, and abrupt clonidine withdrawal. Illnesses known to elevate plasma catecholamines include both acute (e.g., myocardial infarction, diabetic ketoacidosis, or sepsis) and chronic conditions (e.g., congestive heart failure, anemia, respiratory failure, or hypothyroidism). Factors that diminish plasma catecholamines include drugs (clonidine, reserpine, and α-methylparatyrosine), autonomic neuropathy, and congenital deficiency of DβH activity.

As with urine biochemical tests, plasma catecholamine sampling during a paroxysmal attack of hypertension is of value. A finding of normal plasma catecholamines when blood pressure is elevated is quite a useful negative result. Because only extreme elevations of plasma norepinephrine perturb blood pressure, the finding of normal plasma catecholamines while blood pressure is elevated argues strongly against pheochromocytoma as the cause.

Other components of the catecholamine storage vesicle core are released into the bloodstream by pheochromocytomas. The plasma concentration of chromogranin A is elevated in patients with pheochromocytoma, with a diagnostic sensitivity of 83% and specificity of 96%. It is not substantially elevated by acute venipuncture, nor is it affected by drugs used in treatment or diagnosis of pheochromocytoma. Because chromogranin A is released by a variety of neuroendocrine secretory vesicles, its plasma concentration is also elevated in other neuroendocrine neoplasias. Chromogranin A values are also elevated in renal insufficiency because of retained immunoreactive fragments of the protein.

Pharmacologic Diagnostic Tests: Suppressive and Provocative. Pharmacologic tests for pheochromocytoma are generally not necessary because the diagnosis can usually be confirmed by urine and plasma biochemical measurements at rest or during spontaneous blood pressure surges.

The *clonidine suppression test* is of value if plasma catecholamine elevations in a patient with suspected pheochromocytoma are equivocal (that is, from 1000 to 2000 pg per milliliter). The rationale for the test is that pheochromocytoma chromaffin cells, unlike normal adrenal medullary chromaffin cells, are not innervated; hence, catecholamine release from pheochromocytoma chromaffin cells is autonomous and not susceptible to manipulation by drugs that decrease efferent sympathetic outflow, such as the central α_2 agonist clonidine. Blood is obtained for plasma catecholamines before and 3 hours after a single oral dose of 0.3 mg clonidine. In a subject without pheochromocytoma, plasma norepinephrine should fall to <500 pg per milliliter after clonidine. A positive test (failure of catecholamines to decline after clonidine) is sensitive but may not be entirely specific for pheochromocytoma. Although catecholamines do not fall after clonidine in pheochromocytoma, the blood pressure fall is comparable to that seen in essential hypertensives. To prevent inordinate falls in blood pressure during the test, prior volume depletion should be avoided; the test is most safely done in subjects whose diastolic blood pressure prior to clonidine is ≥ 100 mm Hg. Because beta blockers such as propranolol diminish circulating norepinephrine clearance (and hence plasma norepinephrine responses to clonidine), they should be discontinued 48 hours prior to and during the test. The test remains valid during α blockade.

Catecholamine provocative tests (such as the glucagon test) are used in only a few centers because of the potential hazard posed by inordinate catecholamine release.

Anatomic Localization. Tumor location must be known in order to plan the proper surgical route. Ninety-five per cent of pheochromocytomas are in the abdomen, and the great majority of these can be visualized by one of three modalities: computed tomographic (CT) scan, magnetic resonance imaging (MRI), or metaiodobenzylguanidine (MIBG) scintigraphy. CT and MRI are highly sensitive, although nonspecific, because they visualize any mass lesion, not just pheochromocytomas. MIBG scanning is highly specific for chromaffin tissue, although somewhat less sensitive than CT or MRI.

MIBG, a radiolabeled analogue of guanethidine, is transported into chromaffin cells by the reuptake cell membrane catecholamine carrier. Because it accumulates in chromaffin cells, an MIBG abnormality is extraordinarily specific (about 98%) for pheochromocytoma, although somewhat less sensitive (85 to 90%). MIBG imaging is especially useful for metastatic, recurrent, or extra-adrenal tumors. Abdominal ultrasonography is a safe imaging tool but is less sensitive than CT or MRI. Plain abdominal radiographs, intravenous urograms (pyelograms), air insufflation retroperitoneal pneumography, arteriography, and venography are no longer done to localize pheochromocytoma. Indeed, arteriography or venography of the tumor may trigger hypertensive crises.

Differential Diagnosis. Because many conditions can mimic the diagnostic features of pheochromocytoma, as many as 90% of patients who present with some feature of the tumor turn out not to have one after diagnostic testing. Examples include certain drugs, such as surreptitiously self-administered epinephrine or isoproterenol. Abrupt withdrawal from clonidine can provoke a sympathoadrenal discharge with "rebound" blood pressure elevation. Subjects treated with monoamine oxidase inhibitors for depression may develop hypertensive crises if they inadvertently ingest foods rich in tyramine.

Disease states causing or simulating catecholamine excess and hypertension include thyrotoxicosis, acute intracranial disturbances such as subarachnoid hemorrhage or posterior fossa masses, hypertensive crisis of paraplegia which can be initiated by visceral manipulation or bladder distention, and hypoglycemia especially in the presence of β blockade. Damage to carotid sinus baroreceptors by surgery or tumor may result in baroreflex failure, with episodic blood pressure and plasma catecholamine surges; clonidine is the drug of choice. Episodic surges in plasma dopamine have been described in some patients with episodic blood pressure elevation but without pheochromocytoma; the mechanism has not been established.

PATHOPHYSIOLOGY AND COMPLICATIONS. Although circulating catecholamine excess is the ultimate cause of hypertension in pheochromocytoma, the correlation of blood pressure with plasma catecholamines is modest. Desensitization to catecholamine effects may contribute to underdiagnosis of the tumor in the elderly. Pheochromocytomas also release a number of potentially vasoactive substances in addition to catecholamines, which may modify blood pressure. Hemodynamic studies suggest that elevations in systemic vascular resistance rather than cardiac output account for the blood pressure rise.

Acute norepinephrine infusion leads to plasma volume contraction, and a past mainstay of pheochromocytoma management has been an effort to re-expand plasma volume, either spontaneously after therapeutic α blockade, or with preoperative saline infusion. However, recent careful measurements of plasma volume indicate that, on average, it is not as contracted as once believed. Orthostatic hypotension is variably observed in pheochromocytoma. It cannot be clearly attributed to plasma volume contraction and likely reflects catecholamine desensitization, the effects of vasodilator peptides and catecholamines, and dysautonomia.

The major catecholamine secreted by most pheochromocytomas is norepinephrine. Small intra-adrenal tumors (especially early in the course of MEN-2) may secrete predominantly epinephrine. Pure epinephrine secretion by pheochromocytomas is rare.

Cardiomyopathy (myocarditis) occurs in a minority of pheochromocytoma patients, presumably as a consequence of catecholamine excess. This process is generally reversible after tumor removal, and congestive heart failure responds to preoperative α-adrenergic blockade. In most patients, however, the degree of myocardial left ventricular hypertrophy on cardiac ultrasonography is no different from that seen in essential hypertension.

MANAGEMENT. *Preoperative Preparation and Drug Treatment.* Once pheochromocytoma has been diagnosed, the patient is prepared for surgery with adrenergic blockade for a period of 1 to 4 weeks. During α blockade, any catecholamine-induced plasma volume contraction is allowed to correct itself. α Blockade is usually accomplished with oral phenoxybenzamine, an irreversible, noncompetitive antagonist that acts predominantly at α_1 receptors. The drug is begun at 5 mg twice daily, and the dose is adjusted gradually upward by increments of 10 mg every 1 to 4 days to a maximum of 50 to 100 mg twice daily. The usual dose range required is 30 to 80 mg per day. Treatment goals are to normalize blood pressure ($\leq 160/ \leq 90$ mm Hg), prevent paroxysmal hypertension, and abolish tachyarrhythmias (ventricular extrasystoles < 1 to 5 per minute), without inducing intolerable orthostatic hypotension (i.e., orthostatic falls of $> 85/> 45$ mm Hg). Side effects of adequate phenoxybenzamine dosage include orthostatic hypotension, tachycardia, nasal congestion, dry mouth, diplopia, and ejaculatory dysfunction. In patients intolerant of phenoxybenzamine, one can use the α_1-selective antagonist prazosin, in a dose range of 0.5 to 16 mg per day, given orally two to four times daily.

If blood pressure or tachyarrhythmias including sinus tachycardia are not fully controlled by α blockade, β blockade is instituted with oral propranolol, 10 to 40 mg four times daily. β blockade must not be undertaken before α blockade has been instituted; after blockade of vasodilatory vascular β_2-adrenergic receptors, catecholamines' continued access to vasoconstrictive α_1 receptors may induce unopposed vasoconstriction and exacerbation of hypertension. β Blockade may be especially useful for predominant epinephrine-secreting tumors. Metoprolol or labetalol are alternatives to propranolol. In subjects with contraindications to β blockade, lidocaine or amiodarone can be used for tachyarrhythmias.

If combined management with α- plus β-adrenergic antagonists is not fully effective, the tyrosine hydroxylase inhibitor α-methylparatyrosine is added, at an oral dose of 0.25 to 1.0 gram four times daily. Its use may be complicated by sedation, fatigue, anxiety, diarrhea, or extrapyramidal reactions.

For acute management of severe hypertensive crises, intravenous nitroprusside is effective. Intravenous nonselective α_1/α_2 blockade with phentolamine (1 mg bolus, then by continuous infusion) is also useful. Calcium channel blockade with sublingual nifedipine (10 mg broken under the tongue) has also been used.

Avoid opiates (narcotic analgesics), narcotic antagonists (such as naloxone), histamine, ACTH, saralasin, glucagon, or indirect sympathomimetic amines (such as phenylpropanolamine or tyramine). All of these agents may provoke hypertensive surges by releasing catecholamines from the tumor. Drugs that block catecholamine reuptake, such as tricyclic antidepressants (e.g., desipramine), cocaine, or guanethidine, may worsen hypertension. β-Adrenergic antagonists, by blocking vasodilatory vascular β_2 receptors, may cause unopposed α-mediated vasoconstriction by circulating catecholamines, resulting in severe hypertension, unless α blockade is first instituted. Dopaminergic antagonists (such as metoclopramide or sulpiride) may result in hypertension. All should be avoided.

Operative and Perioperative Management. Autopsy series of pheochromocytoma indicate that even clinically unsuspected cases can be lethal. At least 90% of pheochromocytomas are benign, and surgical resection provides a cure, although up to 25% of patients may retain some lesser degree of hypertension. Residual tumor may be diagnosed by urinary catecholamine measurement 1 to 2 weeks postoperatively. The operative mortality of pheochromocytoma resection should not exceed 2 to 3%. In malignant pheochromocytoma, the individual course is highly variable, but long-term 50% survival is < 5 years.

Several surgical approaches are feasible, depending on the particular pheochromocytoma presentation; the experience of the surgeon is crucial. The entire adrenal gland harboring a pheochromocytoma is usually excised. Anesthetic management is guided by selection of agents that do not cause catecholamine release or potentiate catecholamines' dysrhythmic effects. Intravenous glucose replacement (5% dextrose in water or saline) should be given to prevent hypoglycemia, a frequent occurrence after tumor removal. Times at which hypertensive surges are likely to occur include anesthetic induction, intubation, tumor palpation, and ligation of tumor veins. If intraoperative hypotension occurs, the initial treatment should be saline infusion to expand intravascular volume. Only after plasma volume expansion to euvolemia is norepinephrine infusion appropriate.

For intraoperative blood pressure surges, intravenous nitroprusside is often employed. Alternatively, α blockade can be accomplished with intravenous phentolamine (an α_1 and α_2 antagonist), starting with a 1-mg dose and proceeding to infusion. The calcium channel antagonist nicardipine has also been used.

In the postoperative period, several problems occur with some frequency:

1. Hypotension. Most commonly this results from hypovolemia and responds to saline infusion; several liters may be required, often with the guidance of central pressure measurements. After volume repletion, norepinephrine can be infused if needed.

2. Hypertension. Plasma catecholamines remain elevated for several days after complete pheochromocytoma resection. Even 2 weeks postoperatively, up to one fourth of patients still have hypertension. At this time, the differential diagnosis includes residual unresected tumor, essential hypertension, or hypertension secondary to renal damage caused by prior hypertension. A urine collection for catecholamines, obtained at least 1 to 2 weeks after tumor resection, will clarify matters.

3. Hypoglycemia. After correction of catecholamine excess, insulin release may be increased and end-organ responsiveness to insulin augmented, resulting in hypoglycemia. Hypoglycemia may masquerade as refractory hypotension. Infusion of glucose (5% dextrose in water or saline) during the intraoperative and immediate postoperative period is useful.

MALIGNANT PHEOCHROMOCYTOMA. Although most pheochromocytomas are well-encapsulated, localized growths, approximately 5 to 10% are malignant. Malignancy is diagnosed by the biologic behavior of the tumor, in the form of adjacent tissue invasion or distant metastatic spread. Extra-adrenal tumors are more likely to metastasize than are primary adrenal ones. Catecholamine biosynthesis tends to be especially deranged in malignant tumors, with secretion of substantial amounts of DOPA and dopamine (metabolized to HVA, which can be detected in the urine). Increased plasma DOPA in pheochromocytoma suggests malignancy.

In patients with malignant pheochromocytoma, α- and β-adrenergic blockade with phenoxybenzamine and propranolol remain the mainstay of management of symptoms and signs of catecholamine excess. If catecholamine effects are not controlled, the tyrosine hydroxylase inhibitor α-methylparatyrosine can be effective, from 0.25 to 1.0 gram four times daily.

Metastases tend to be slow growing, and the natural history of malignant pheochromocytoma is variable; the 5-year survival is <50%. Common sites of metastasis are the retroperitoneum, skeleton (bone), lymph nodes, and liver. Periodic surgical debulking may help to control symptoms. The response to chemotherapy has been generally disappointing, but the combination of vincristine, cyclophosphamide, and dacarbazine shows promise in many patients. Skeletal metastases show some response to irradiation, although the neoplasm is not particularly susceptible to radiation therapy. High-dose (300 mCi) radiation therapy with intravenous ^{125}I-MIBG remains experimental but is of value in some patients.

CATECHOLAMINE DEFICIENCY DISEASE STATES

Loss of even both adrenal glands seldom produces a catecholamine deficiency state. In diabetics receiving insulin, the usual counterregulatory response to hypoglycemia involves the actions of epinephrine and glucagon to trigger hepatic glycogenolysis. In diabetics who also have autonomic neuropathy, deficient epinephrine release during hypoglycemia, coupled with deficient glucagon responses, may result in impairment of the usual counterregulatory response to hypoglycemia, prolonging its duration.

Several individuals have been described with an apparent congenital deficiency of DβH; such individuals have greatly diminished or undetectable norepinephrine and epinephrine in blood, urine, and cerebrospinal fluid. Presenting features of this lifelong syndrome include severe orthostatic hypotension, ptosis, nasal stuffiness, hyperextensible joints, and retrograde ejaculation. The diagnosis is made in patients with severe orthostatic hypotension, a plasma norepinephrine/dopamine ratio of <1, and undetectable plasma DβH activity. During sympathoadrenal activation in these subjects, increments in efferent sympathetic nerve traffic occur, but sympathetic axons release the precursor dopamine instead of norepinephrine, perhaps compounding the hypotension.

THE INCIDENTAL ADRENAL MASS (OR "INCIDENTALOMA")

Up to 2% of all abdominal CT scans, as well as 9% of autopsies, incidentally discover minimal adrenal gland abnormalities. Rarely do these lesions require further attention.

Occasionally the appearance of an adrenal mass on CT or MRI is sufficiently characteristic for a firm diagnosis; an example is adrenal myelolipoma, a benign accumulation of bone marrow elements in an otherwise normally functioning adrenal, with a characteristic fat-density image on CT or MRI. Myelolipoma requires no treatment.

If an adrenal mass is >4 to 6 cm in span, its chance of malignancy (especially adrenocortical carcinoma) increases, and such masses should be resected unless they have a clearly benign appearance (such as myelolipoma) on CT or MRI. In smaller lesions, adrenal carcinoma is unlikely unless other signs or symptoms of adrenocortical hormone excess are apparent. Incidental masses <4 to 6 cm in span are followed by periodic CT scanning. In subjects with known metastatic carcinoma, adrenal abnormalities are likely to be adrenal metastases. In subjects with recent major abdominal trauma, adrenal abnormalities likely represent hemorrhage and should resolve with time.

Because not all pheochromocytomas manifest hypertension at all times, all patients with incidental adrenal masses should be screened for pheochromocytoma with a 24-hour urine collection for catecholamine metabolites.

Virtually all patients with aldosterone-producing adrenal adenoma have hypertension and hypokalemia. If blood pressure and serum potassium are normal on a diet of >200 mEq sodium per day and <100 mEq potassium per day (confirmed by 24-hour urine), no further evaluation is needed.

Cushing's disease is likely only if other signs or symptoms are suggestive. The diagnosis is made by giving 1 mg of oral dexamethasone at 11 P.M. and sampling serum cortisol the next morning at 8 A.M.

Cryer PE: Pheochromocytoma. West J Med 156:399, 1992. *A comprehensive review contrasting the diagnostic value of plasma versus urinary catecholamines.*

Grossman E, Goldstein DS, Hoffman A, et al.: Glucagon and clonidine testing in the diagnosis of pheochromocytoma. Hypertension 17:733, 1991. *A large series evaluating the sensitivity and specificity of these provocation and suppression tests of catecholamine release.*

Hsiao RJ, Parmer RJ, Takiyyuddin MA, et al.: Chromogranin A storage and secretion: Sensitivity and specificity for the diagnosis of pheochromocytoma. Medicine 70:33, 1991. *The chromaffin storage vesicle protein chromogranin A, co-released by exocytosis with catecholamines, is a sensitive and specific plasma marker of pheochromocytoma in hypertension patients.*

Jovenich JJ: Anesthesia in adrenal surgery. Urol Clin North Am 16:583, 1989. *Practical suggestions on anesthetics to use or avoid.*

Kailasam MT, O'Connor DT, Parmer RJ: The regulation and role of catecholamines in hypertension and pheochromocytoma. Curr Opinion Endocrinol Diabetes 1:135, 1994. *A review emphasizing recent diagnostic developments.*

Malone MJ, Libertino JA, Tsapatsaris NP, et al.: Preoperative and surgical management of pheochromocytoma. Urol Clin North Am 16:567, 1989. *Rationale for selection from several possible surgical approaches.*

Neumann HPH, Berger DP, Sigmund G, et al.: Pheochromocytomas, multiple endocrine neoplasia type 2, and von Hippel-Lindau disease. N Engl J Med 329:1531, 1993. *This large series highlights the importance and yield of screening patients with pheochromocytoma for familial syndromes.*

Ross NS, Aron DC: Hormonal evaluation of the patient with an incidentally discovered adrenal mass. N Engl J Med 323:1401, 1991. *A sensible approach to this increasingly frequent and vexing clinical problem.*

205 DIABETES MELLITUS
Robert S. Sherwin

OVERVIEW

Diabetes mellitus is a chronic disorder characterized by impaired metabolism of glucose and other energy-yielding fuels, as well as the late development of vascular and neuropathic complications. Diabetes mellitus consists of a group of disorders involving distinct pathogenic mechanisms with hyperglycemia as the common denominator. Regardless of cause, the disease is associated with insulin deficiency, which may be total, partial, or relative when viewed in the context of coexisting insulin resistance. Lack of insulin plays a primary role in the metabolic derangements linked to diabetes, and hyperglycemia, in turn, plays a key role in the complications of the disease.

In the United States diabetes mellitus is the fourth most common reason for patient contact with a physician and is a major cause of premature disability and mortality. It is the leading cause of blindness among working-age people, of end-stage renal disease, and of nontraumatic limb amputations. It increases the risk of cardiac, cerebral, and peripheral vascular disease two- to seven-fold and is a major cause of neonatal morbidity and mortality. On the bright side, recent data indicate that most of the debilitating complications of the disease can be prevented or delayed by prospective treatment of hyperglycemia and cardiovascular risk factors.

CLASSIFICATION

Diabetes mellitus can be divided into three subclasses (Table 205–1): (1) type I, or insulin-dependent diabetes mellitus; (2) type II, or non–insulin-dependent diabetes mellitus; and (3) secondary diabetes linked to another identifiable condition or syndrome. In addition, two conditions—impaired glucose tolerance and gestational diabetes—significantly increase the later risk of developing diabetes mellitus and may, in some instances, be part of its natural history.

TYPE I DIABETES MELLITUS. Patients with this disorder have little or no insulin secretory capacity and depend on exogenous insulin to prevent metabolic decompensation (e.g., ketoacidosis) and death. Commonly in previously healthy nonobese children or young adults diabetes appears abruptly over days or weeks, whereas in older age groups it may have a more gradual onset. At the time of initial presentation the patient appears ill, has marked symptoms (e.g., polyuria, polydipsia, polyphagia, and weight loss), and may demonstrate ketoacidosis. Type I diabetes is believed to

TABLE 205–1. CLASSIFICATION OF DIABETES

I. Clinical Diabetes
1. Type I or insulin-dependent diabetes (IDDM). Formerly called juvenile-onset diabetes.
2. Type II or non–insulin-dependent diabetes (NIDDM). Formerly called maturity- or adult-onset diabetes.
   A. Obese (~ 80–85%)
   B. Nonobese (~ 15–20%)
   C. Maturity-onset diabetes of the young (MODY)
3. Secondary diabetes
   A. Pancreatic disease (e.g., chronic pancreatitis, hemochromatosis, cystic fibrosis, pancreatic carcinoma)
   B. Endocrine disease (e.g., acromegaly, Cushing's syndrome, glucagonoma, polycystic ovary syndrome, pheochromocytoma)
   C. Drugs (e.g., thiazide diuretics, glucocorticoids, beta-adrenergic blockers, pentamidine, oral contraceptives, phenytoin)
   D. Genetic syndromes (e.g., Turner's syndrome, myotonic dystrophy, Huntington's disease, lipodystrophy, ataxia-telangiectasia)
   E. Insulin receptor abnormalities (due to defective insulin receptors or to antibodies directed toward the insulin receptor)
   F. Malnutrition-related diabetes

II. Risk Categories
1. Impaired glucose tolerance
2. Gestational diabetes

have a long asymptomatic preclinical stage, often lasting years, during which pancreatic beta cells are gradually destroyed by an autoimmune attack (Fig. 205–1). An acute illness may speed the transition from the preclinical to the clinical stage. Initially insulin therapy is essential to restore metabolism toward normal. A "honeymoon period" may follow, lasting weeks or months, during which time smaller doses of insulin are required due to partial recovery of beta cell function and reversal of insulin resistance caused by acute illness. Thereafter, insulin secretory capacity is gradually lost. This syndrome accounts for about 10% of diabetes in the United States.

TYPE II DIABETES MELLITUS. This is, by far, the most common form of the disease, comprising 85 to 90% of the diabetic population and taking heterogeneous forms. Affected patients retain some endogenous insulin secretory capacity, but insulin levels are low relative to the magnitude of insulin resistance and ambient glucose levels. They do not depend on insulin for immediate survival and rarely develop ketosis, except under conditions of great physical stress. Nevertheless, they may require insulin therapy to control hyperglycemia. Type II diabetes characteristically appears after the age of 40 years, has a high rate of genetic penetrance unrelated to HLA genes, and is associated with obesity. The clinical presentation is much more insidious. The classic symptoms of diabetes may be mild and tolerated for a long time before the patient seeks medical attention. Moreover, if hyperglycemia is asymptomatic, the disease may become evident only after complications develop.

SECONDARY DIABETES. A variety of diabetic syndromes can be attributed to a specific disease, drug, or condition. These include (1) pancreatic disease, (2) endocrine disease, (3) drugs, (4) genetic syndromes, (5) insulin receptor abnormalities, and (6) malnutrition. Severe illness (e.g., burns, trauma, sepsis) may provoke hyperglycemia due to hypersecretion of insulin antagonistic hormones. Although on some occasions this may reflect underlying diabetes, the metabolic disturbance is often self-limited and should not be classified as diabetes until the precipitating illness has resolved.

Most diabetes mellitus can be classified on clinical grounds. A small subgroup of patients differ and display features common to both type I and II diabetes. They are commonly nonobese and have diminished insulin secretion that is not sufficient to make them ketosis prone. Many initially respond to oral agents, but, with time, require insulin. Some may have a slowly evolving form of type I diabetes. Others defy easy categorization.

IMPAIRED GLUCOSE TOLERANCE. The term applies to the finding of glucose levels that are higher than normal but lower than those diagnostic of diabetes mellitus. Impaired glucose tolerance produces neither the symptoms nor the serious complications associated with diabetes. About 25%, however, eventually go on to develop typical type II diabetes.

GESTATIONAL DIABETES. The term categorizes increased glucose levels that are first detected during pregnancy. It excludes known diabetes preexisting conception. Gestational diabetes occurs in about 2% of pregnancies and usually appears in the second or third trimester at the time when pregnancy-associated insulin antagonistic hormones peak. After delivery, glucose tolerance usually reverts to normal. Nevertheless, within 5 to 10 years 30 to 40% develop type II diabetes. Occasionally, pregnancy may precipitate type I diabetes. Although gestational diabetes generally causes only mild, asymptomatic hyperglycemia, rigorous treatment, often with insulin, is required to protect against fetal morbidity and mortality.

DIAGNOSIS

The diagnosis is usually straightforward when diabetes presents with classic symptoms, and a random plasma glucose measurement that is 200 mg per deciliter or greater. Further diagnostic testing is unwarranted and delays treatment. Although glycosuria strongly suggests diabetes, urine testing should never be used exclusively because some persons have a low renal threshold for glucose. If diabetes is suspected but not confirmed by a random glucose determination, the screening test of choice is an overnight fasting plasma glucose level; it varies less from day to day and is more resistant to factors that nonspecifically alter glucose metabolism. Diagnosis is established if glucose equals or exceeds 140 mg per deciliter on at least two separate occasions. Fasting glucose levels < 115 mg per deciliter generally do not warrant further testing; values between 115 mg and 140 mg per deciliter, although not diagnostic, should arouse suspicion. Because such individuals may show postprandial

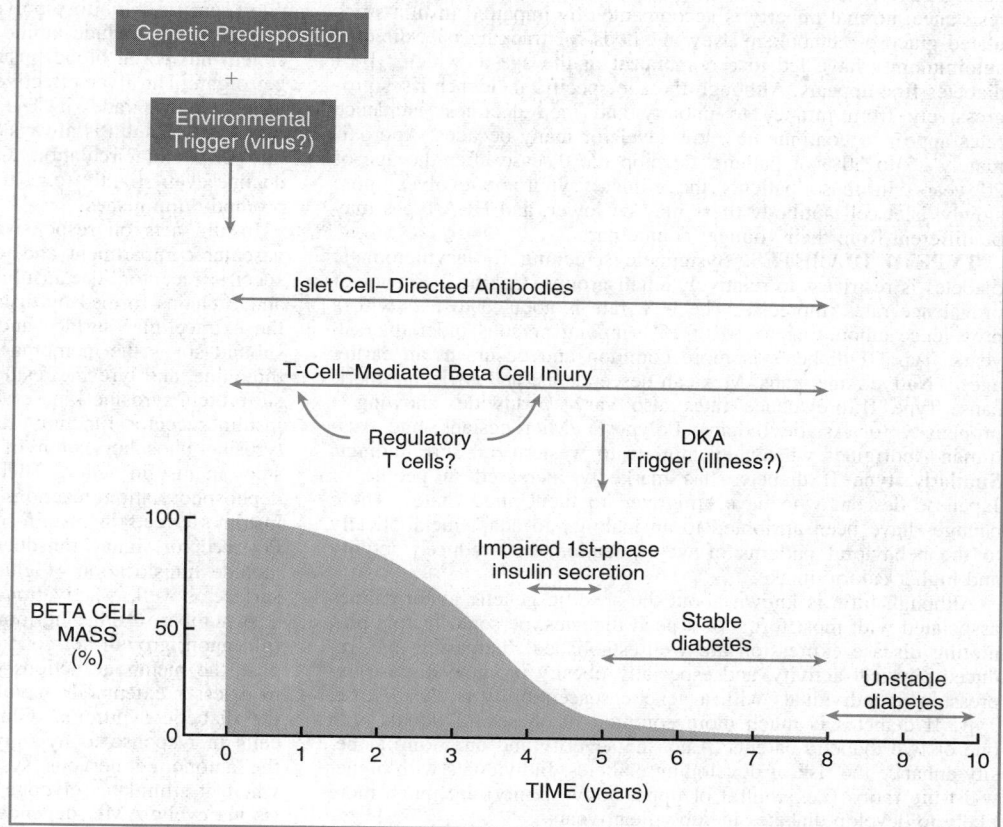

FIGURE 205–1. A summary of the sequence of events that lead to beta cell loss and ultimately to the clinical appearance of type I diabetes.

hyperglycemia, some experts recommend further testing using the oral glucose tolerance test (OGTT). The OGTT has the advantage of detecting diabetes at its earliest stage, when treatment is most effective. The disadvantage is that the test may lead to overdiagnosis unless the clinician recognizes its pitfalls. Common factors that nonspecifically impair glucose tolerance include (1) carbohydrate restriction (<150 grams for 3 days), (2) bed rest (days) or severe inactivity (weeks), (3) medical or surgical stress, (4) drugs (e.g., thiazides, beta-blockers, glucocorticoids, or phenytoin), and (5) smoking during the test or anxiety from needle sticks.

The clinician has several choices when faced with a fasting glucose in the indeterminate range (115 to 140 mg per deciliter). Although the OGTT is the "gold standard" for diagnosing diabetes when fasting glucose is below 140 mg per deciliter and has proved useful as a research tool, its value in the clinical setting is questionable because of its high variability. When the OGTT is employed, some individuals neither meet the diagnostic criteria for diabetes (i.e., a 2-hour OGTT level >200 mg per deciliter) nor show a normal glucose profile. They are classified as having impaired glucose tolerance (IGT) if (a) fasting glucose is less than 140 mg per deciliter, (b) the 2-hour OGTT level is between 140 and 200 mg per deciliter, and (c) an intervening glucose is 200 mg per deciliter or greater. Because no diagnostic markers distinguish those individuals (about 25%) who will become diabetic, they should be tested annually using a fasting glucose measurement. It is also prudent to prescribe the same lifestyle changes suggested to overt diabetic patients, because IGT (like diabetes mellitus) is associated with a higher risk of premature cardiovascular disease.

Because many patients with type II diabetes have the disease years before symptoms are appreciated, it is important to screen (using a fasting glucose measurement) high-risk individuals (Table 205–2). Because mild glucose elevations may have adverse effects on the fetus, a more aggressive approach is recommended for pregnant women. Pregnant women should receive a screening 50-gram OGTT between 24 and 28 weeks of gestation. If fasting glucose is 105 mg per deciliter or the 1-hour OGTT value is >150 mg per deciliter, an extended 100-gram OGTT should be performed. Gesta-

tional diabetes is diagnosed if two values equal or exceed the upper limits of normal: fasting, 105 mg per deciliter; 1 hour, 190 mg per deciliter; 2 hour, 165 mg per deciliter; and 3 hour, 145 mg per deciliter.

PREVALENCE/EPIDEMIOLOGY

TYPE I DIABETES. Prevalence rates for type I diabetes are relatively accurate because patients invariably become symptomatic. Estimates for the United States are about 0.30%. Type I diabetes is more prevalent in Finland, Scandinavia, Scotland, and Sardinia, less prevalent in Southern Europe and the Mid-East, and rare in Asian countries such as Japan. The annual incidence in Northern Europe appears to have risen in the last half century, implying the introduction of an unidentified environmental factor. Prevalence rates are strikingly different among different ethnic groups living in the same geographic environment. Caucasian children living in Allegheny County, Pennsylvania, or in Colorado are about 50 to 70% more likely to develop type I diabetes than nonwhites living in the same area, observations most likely explained by genetic differences in susceptibility.

The recognition that type I diabetes has a protracted preclinical phase has placed some epidemiologic characteristics of the disease in a new light. Its increased incidence in the winter months and its association with specific viral epidemics may be explained by the superimposition of illness-provoked insulin resistance in a patient with marginal beta cell function. Similarly, its common appearance

TABLE 205–2. CANDIDATES FOR DIABETES SCREENING

1. Presence of suggestive symptoms
2. Obesity (especially if centrally distributed)
3. Positive family history
4. Women with a morbid obstetric history or with large babies
5. Recurrent skin or genital infections
6. High-risk populations (African-Americans, Latinos, Native Americans)
7. The elderly (>60 years)
8. Presence of other risk factors for atherosclerosis

during puberty may also be attributed to the appearance of insulin resistance; normal puberty is accompanied by impaired insulin-stimulated glucose metabolism. New methods for tracking islet-directed autoimmunity have led to a reappraisal of the age at which type I diabetes first appears. Although the age-specific incidence rises progressively from infancy to puberty and then declines, incidence rates appear to continue at a low level for many decades. Approximately 25 to 30% of patients develop the disease after the age of 20 years. In these patients the clinical syndrome evolves more slowly, islet cell antibody titers may be lower, and HLA types may be different from their younger counterparts.

TYPE II DIABETES. Systematic screening for asymptomatic diabetes is restricted to relatively small groups, making estimates of prevalence rates imprecise. The U.S. rate is about 3 to 5%, with a prevalence amounting to 10 to 15% among persons older than 50 years. Type II diabetes is more common and occurs at an earlier age in Native Americans, Mexican descendants, and African-Americans. Type II prevalence rates also vary worldwide, showing a propensity for Asiatic Indians, Polynesian/Micronesians, and Australian Aborigines when they migrate to westernized surroundings. Similarly, type II diabetes has markedly increased in people of Japanese descent who have emigrated to the United States. These changes have been attributed to an inability to adapt metabolically to the behavioral patterns of westernization, i.e., reduced activity and higher caloric intake.

Although little is known about the specific genetic abnormalities associated with most forms of type II diabetes, personal factors promoting disease expression are well-established. Increasing age, reduced physical activity, and especially obesity promote disease expression in individuals with a genetic susceptibility to the disease. Type II diabetes is much more common in obese individuals with one or two diabetic parents. Also, the severity and duration of obesity enhance the risk of developing diabetes. Individuals with higher waist-hip ratios (i.e., central or upper-body obesity) are much more likely to develop diabetes in subsequent years.

MALNUTRITION-RELATED DIABETES. This is a disorder of tropical underdeveloped countries occurring in nutritionally deprived adolescents or young adults and characterized by diminished insulin secretion and hyperglycemia, usually without ketosis. It has been divided on clinical grounds into two subclasses, fibrocalculous and protein-deficient pancreatic diabetes, but it is uncertain that these subclasses represent distinct disease entities. Patients with the fibrocalculous form are underweight and have recurrent attacks of abdominal pain in association with pancreatic duct stones and fibrosis. Exocrine pancreatic insufficiency is common. The disease may be linked to the consumption of cassava root, which contains toxic cyanogenic glycosides. The protein-deficient form is characterized by more pronounced wasting, without pancreatic calcifications and fibrosis or abdominal pain. The reduced beta cell function may be secondary to nutritional deficiency.

PATHOPHYSIOLOGY

INSULIN SECRETION AND ACTION. Insulin is initially synthesized in the pancreatic beta cells as a large single-chain polypeptide, proinsulin, which is cleaved, resulting in removal of a connecting strand (C-peptide) and the appearance of the smaller, double-chain insulin molecule (51 amino acid residues). Insulin and the C-peptide remnant are packaged in membrane-bounded storage granules; stimulation of insulin secretion results in the discharge of equimolar amounts of insulin and C-peptide and a small amount of unconverted proinsulin into the portal circulation. Because, unlike insulin, C-peptide escapes hepatic metabolism, its concentration provides a more precise marker of endogenous insulin secretion. The concentration of glucose is the key regulator of insulin secretion. For glucose to activate secretion, it must first be transported by a protein (GLUT 2) into the beta cell, phosphorylated by the enzyme glucokinase, and metabolized. The immediate triggering process is poorly understood but likely involves the activation of signal transduction pathways, closure of ATP-sensitive potassium channels, and the entry of calcium into the beta cell. Normally, when blood glucose rises even slightly above the fasting level of 75 to 100 mg per deciliter, beta cells secrete insulin, initially from preformed stored insulin and later from the synthesis of new insulin. The route of glucose entry as well as its concentration determines the magnitude of the response. Higher insulin levels are produced when glucose is given orally than when given intravenously owing to the simultaneous release of gut peptides (e.g., glucagon-like peptide I, gastric inhibitory polypeptide, cholecystokinin). Other insulin secretagogues include amino acids and vagal stimulation. Once secreted into portal blood, insulin encounters the liver as its first target organ. The liver effectively removes approximately 50% of the insulin and degrades it. The consequence of this uptake is that the portal vein insulin is always at least two- to four-fold higher than in the peripheral circulation. Conversely, when blood glucose levels decline even slightly (e.g., to 70 mg per deciliter), insulin secretion promptly diminishes.

Insulin acts on responsive tissues by first passing through the vascular compartment and, upon reaching its target, binding to its specific receptor. The insulin receptor is a heterodimer with two α and β chains formed by disulfide bridges. The α subunit resides on the extracellular surface and is the site of insulin binding. The β subunit spans the membrane and can be phosphorylated on serine, threonine, and tyrosine residues on the cytoplasmic face. The intrinsic protein tyrosine kinase activity of the β subunit is essential for insulin receptor function. Rapid receptor autophosphorylation and tyrosine phosphorylation of cellular substrates are essential early steps in insulin action. Thereafter, a series of phosphorylation and dephosphorylation reactions are triggered that ultimately produce insulin's effects in insulin-sensitive tissues (liver, muscle, and fat). Postreceptor signal transduction pathways leading to insulin action include translocation of glucose transporters (GLUT 4) to the cell surface as well as activation of MAP and PI3-kinases.

A number of other hormones, termed counterregulatory hormones (glucagon, growth hormone [GH], catecholamines, and cortisol) oppose the metabolic actions of insulin. Among these, glucagon and to a lesser extent GH have important roles in the development of the diabetic syndrome. Glucagon is secreted by pancreatic alpha cells in response to hypoglycemia, amino acids, and activation of the autonomic nervous system. Its major effect is on the liver, where it stimulates glycogenolysis, gluconeogenesis, and ketogenesis via cyclic AMP–dependent mechanisms. It is normally inhibited by hyperglycemia but is absolutely or relatively increased in both type I and type II diabetes despite the presence of hyperglycemia. GH secretion by the anterior pituitary is also inappropriately increased in type I diabetes owing, at least in part, to an attempt to overcome a defect in insulin-like growth factor-1 generation caused by insulin deficiency. The major metabolic actions of GH are on peripheral tissues, where it acts to promote lipolysis and inhibit glucose consumption. In type I diabetic patients with reduced portal vein insulin levels, GH is also capable of stimulating hepatic glucose production.

METABOLIC EFFECTS OF INSULIN. Insulin's pivotal role in diabetes is best appreciated by first examining the extent to which it participates in fuel homeostasis in healthy subjects.

Fasted State. After an overnight fast, low basal levels of insulin diminish glucose uptake in peripheral insulin-sensitive tissues (muscle and fat). Most glucose uptake occurs in non–insulin-sensitive tissues, primarily the brain, which, because of its inability to use free fatty acids (FFA), is critically dependent on glucose for oxidative metabolism. Maintenance of stable blood glucose levels is achieved by release of glucose by the liver at rates (7 to 10 grams per hour) matching those of consuming tissues. The hepatic processes involved consist of glycogenolysis and gluconeogenesis, with gluconeogenesis contributing 25 to 60% and glycogenolysis contributing the remainder. Both play a significant role, and both depend on the balance of insulin and glucagon in the portal circulation. Reduced insulin levels decrease glycogen synthesis, allowing glucagon's effect on glycogenolysis to prevail. Glucagon also stimulates gluconeogenesis, whereas the lowered insulin promotes peripheral mobilization of glucose precursors (amino acids, lactate, pyruvate, glycerol) and fuels (FFA) for gluconeogenesis.

Fed State. Ingestion of a large glucose load triggers multiple homeostatic mechanisms that minimize glucose excursions and restore normoglycemia. These include (1) suppression of hepatic glucose production, (2) stimulation of hepatic glucose uptake, and (3) acceleration of glucose uptake by peripheral tissues, predominantly muscle. Each depends on insulin. In the liver, the increase in portal insulin rapidly suppresses glucose production, limiting glucose entry into the circulation at a time when it is flooded by exogenous glucose. In addition, about 30% of ingested glucose is deposited in the liver. The net effect is substantial hepatic retention of glucose as glycogen. The uptake of glucose by peripheral tissues is mediated predominantly by insulin and to a more limited extent by the mass effect of hyperglycemia itself. Insulin-stimulated glucose transport across the plasmalemma of both adipose and muscle tissue is attributable to the recruitment of glucose-transporting proteins (i.e., GLUT 4) from a cytosolic compartment to the plasma membrane. In muscle, glucose may be used for glycogen synthesis or undergo oxidative or nonoxidative metabolism. In adipose tissue, glucose is utilized for the formation of alpha-glycerophosphate, which is necessary for esterification of FFA to form triglycerides. Intracellular metabolic processes are also facilitated by the action of insulin. Insulin promotes glycogen formation by stimulating glycogen synthase and glucose oxidation by activating pyruvate dehydrogenase and decreasing lipolysis (FFA compete with glucose for oxidative metabolism).

Ingestion of large quantities of glucose is not representative of conditions during ingestion of ordinary meals. If the quantity of carbohydrate consumed and the resultant insulin response are small, glucose homeostasis is maintained largely by a reduction in hepatic glucose production rather than an increase in glucose uptake. This is because glucose production is much more sensitive than glucose uptake to the effects of small changes in insulin secretion. The rise in insulin that accompanies consumption of mixed meals also facilitates protein and fat storage. Because muscle is in negative nitrogen balance in the fasting state, repletion of muscle nitrogen depends on a net uptake of amino acids in response to protein feeding. In muscle, insulin acts to promote positive nitrogen balance by inhibiting the breakdown of protein and stimulating the synthesis of new proteins. Similarly, in adipose tissue insulin accelerates triglyceride uptake by stimulating lipoprotein lipase, while simultaneously inhibiting hormone-sensitive lipase that catalyzes the hydrolysis of stored triglycerides.

Metabolic Defects in Diabetes.
In type II diabetes, fasting hyperglycemia is accompanied by an inappropriate increase in hepatic glucose production that is generally proportionate to the blood glucose elevation. In type I diabetes, portal insulin deficiency is invariably present and thus hepatic glucose production is consistently elevated. In addition, insulin deficiency leads to hypersecretion of glucagon and GH, which further accentuate glucose overproduction. Because basal glucose uptake occurs largely in non–insulin-sensitive tissues, total body glucose uptake tends to be increased owing to the mass action of hyperglycemia. This underscores the crucial role the liver plays in determining the fasting glucose level in diabetes. The increase in glucose production in both types of diabetes is due to an acceleration of gluconeogenesis. The loss of the restraining effect of insulin leads to a relative increase in portal glucagon and, in turn, an increase in the uptake and conversion of glycogenic substrates to glucose within the liver. In the extreme situation of total insulin lack, an excessive release of a variety of counterregulatory hormones causes gluconeogenesis to increase further and blocks compensatory increases in glucose disposal. The clinical correlate is profound hyperglycemia (Fig. 205–2). Fasting levels of FFA are also frequently elevated owing to accelerated mobilization of fat stores. In type II diabetes, FFA elevations occur in the presence of normal or increased insulin, suggesting resistance to insulin's inhibitory effect on lipolysis. Although FFA are not directly converted to glucose, they promote hyperglycemia by providing the liver with factors to support gluconeogenesis and by interfering with glucose consumption in muscle. Endogenous insulin secretion in type II diabetes provides sufficient levels of insulin in portal blood to suppress conversion of FFA to ketones in the liver. In type I diabetes, however, mobilized FFA are more readily converted to ketone bodies. The combined effects of insulin deficiency and the presence of glucagon suppress fat synthesis in liver. This reduces intrahepatic malonyl CoA, which together with carnitine stimulates the activity of hepatic acylcarnitine transferase I, facilitating the transfer of long chain fatty acids into mitochondria, where they are broken down via beta-oxidation and converted to ketone bodies. In addition, hypoinsulinemia, by decreasing ketone turnover, enhances the magnitude of the ketosis for any given level of ketone production. During diabetic ketoacidosis, ketone levels dramatically increase because of the concomitant release of counterregulatory hormones. The rise in glucagon accelerates hepatic ketogenesis, whereas elevations of catecholamines, GH, and cortisol act in concert to increase lipolysis and, in turn, the delivery of FFA to

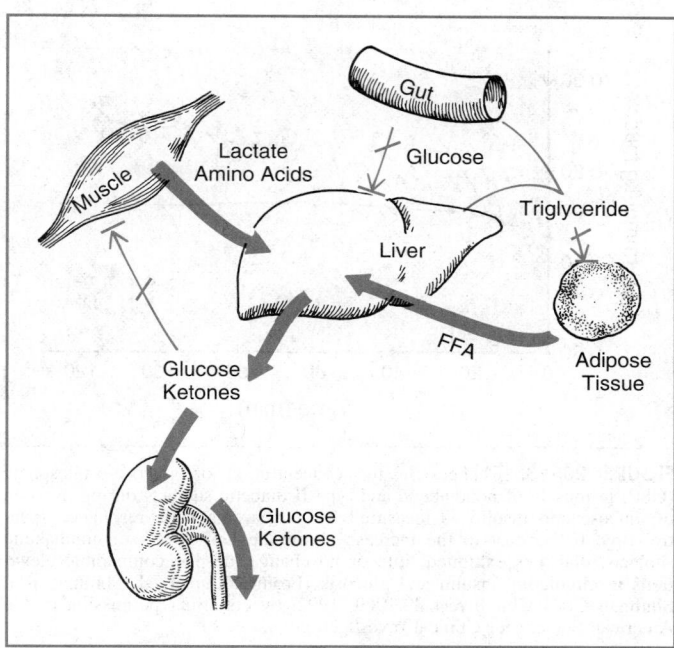

FIGURE 205–2. The effects of severe insulin deficiency on body fuel metabolism. Lack of insulin leads to mobilization of substrates for gluconeogenesis and ketogenesis from muscle and adipose tissue, accelerated production of glucose and ketones by the liver, and impaired removal of endogenously produced and exogenous fuels by insulin-responsive tissues. The net result is severe hyperglycemia and hyperketonemia that overwhelm renal removal mechanisms.

the liver (Fig. 205–2). The increase in substrate delivery may become so pronounced that it saturates the oxidative pathway, leading to a fatty liver and hypertriglyceridemia.

Diabetes is characterized by marked postprandial hyperglycemia after carbohydrate ingestion. In type II diabetes, the combined effects of delayed insulin secretion and hepatic insulin resistance impair the suppression of hepatic glucose production. Hyperglycemia ensues, even though insulin levels may rise to levels above those seen in nondiabetic individuals (insulin secretion remains deficient relative to the prevailing glucose level), because insulin resistance reduces the capacity of muscle to remove glucose and store it as glycogen. The normal increase in glucose-6-phosphate in muscle after insulin is markedly attenuated in diabetes, implying that the block in glycogen synthesis precedes glucose-6-phosphate formation and is mediated at either the level of glucose transport or its conversion to glucose-6-phosphate (by hexokinase) (Fig. 205–3). These defects are more pronounced in patients with severe hyperglycemia, in whom insulin secretion is further reduced. Type I patients show the most marked and prolonged elevations in blood glucose after ingestion of carbohydrate. These individuals have low portal vein insulin levels, which are not reversed by conventional subcutaneous insulin therapy. Consequently, the liver fails to reduce its glucose production or to appropriately take up glucose. In addition, glucose uptake by peripheral tissues is impaired by the lack of insulin and the development of insulin resistance secondary to chronic insulin deprivation. The net result is a gross defect in glucose disposal that is only partially compensated for by renal glycosuria. The insulin-deficient patient may exhibit defects in the disposal of ingested protein and fat as well. In the absence of a rise in insulin, meal ingestion may cause hyperaminoacidemia due to a failure to stimulate the net uptake of amino acids in muscle and hypertriglyceridemia due to reduced activity of lipoprotein lipase. Thus, type I diabetes may be viewed as a disorder of protein and fat tolerance as well as glucose tolerance.

PATHOGENESIS

Type I diabetes produces profound beta cell failure with secondary insulin resistance, whereas type II diabetes causes less severe insulin deficiency and a more severe impairment of insulin ac-

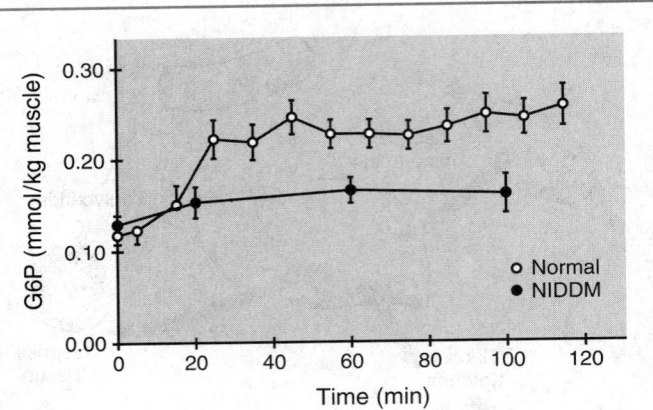

FIGURE 205-3. Changes in the concentration of glucose-6-phosphate (G6P) in muscle of nondiabetic and type II diabetic subjects during infusion of glucose and insulin as measured by nuclear magnetic resonance spectroscopy. In contrast to the increase in muscle G6P levels in nondiabetic subjects, diabetics exhibited little or no change, despite comparable elevations in circulating insulin and glucose. (From Rothman DI, Shulman RG, Shulman GI: J Clin Invest 89:1069, 1992, by copyright permission of the American Society for Clinical Investigation.)

tion. Given the similarity in the overall picture, it is not surprising that both forms of diabetes share many pathophysiologic features. However, despite the apparent phenotypic similarity, the underlying pathogenetic mechanisms leading to type I and type II diabetes are strikingly different.

TYPE I DIABETES. Type I diabetes results from an interplay of genetic, environmental, and autoimmune factors that selectively destroy insulin-producing beta cells. The role of genetic factors is underscored by data in identical twins showing concordance rates of 30 to 50%, rates much higher than those for nonidentical twins or siblings. It has been assumed that because concordance rates are not 100%, environmental factors must be important for disease expression. Even identical twins, however, do not have identical T cell receptor or immunoglobulin genes, and thus for autoimmune diseases, such as type I diabetes, total concordance would not be expected. Although all the genes linked to the disease have not been identified and are undoubtedly multiple, the HLA genes on the short arm of chromosome 6 play a dominant role. In nonaffected siblings, the risk of developing diabetes is 15 to 20% if they are HLA-identical, 5 to 10% if they share one HLA gene, and <1% if they are HLA nonidentical. Specific HLA haplotypes are linked to type I diabetes: 90 to 95% express DR3 and/or DR4 class II HLA molecules, compared with an incidence of 50 to 60% in the general population; 60% of patients express both alleles, a rate more than 10-fold that of the general population. Another class II allele, HLA-DR2, has a negative association with disease. Specific class II DQ haplotypes even more strongly correlate with disease susceptibility in Caucasians. Susceptibility is associated with polymorphisms of the allele encoding the beta chain of the DQ class II HLA molecule. The presence of aspartic acid at position 57 protects against disease, whereas substitution of a neutral amino acid at this position is associated with a much higher frequency. Other polymorphisms, such as a substitution of arginine at position 52 of the DQ alpha chain, may confer additional risk. It is likely, however, that no single class II gene accounts for HLA-associated susceptibility to disease and that significant genetic heterogeneity exists. The association of the disease with specific class II HLA genes implies the involvement of CD4 T cells in the autoimmunity process, because these molecules are critical for the presentation of antigenic peptides to CD4 T cells and for the selection of the T-cell repertoire.

Although environmental factors such as diet (e.g., milk protein in newborns) and toxins have been proposed as initiating factors, most attention has focused on viruses. Epidemics of mumps, coxsackievirus, and congenital rubella have been associated with an increased frequency of type I diabetes. In one instance, a coxsackievirus B4 was isolated from the pancreas of a child who died of diabetic ketoacidosis, and inoculation of the virus into mice caused

disease, fulfilling Koch's postulates. Viruses that produce acute, lytic infection, however, are probably responsible for only an occasional case. Instead, if viruses are involved, it is more likely that they trigger an autoimmune response. It has been postulated that if a virus contains an epitope that resembles a beta cell protein, infection with the virus could abrogate self-tolerance, triggering autoimmunity. Interestingly, sequence homology has been identified between coxsackievirus B and glutamic acid decarboxylase (GAD), an important autoantigen in type I diabetes.

About 80% of new-onset patients with type I diabetes have islet cell antibodies (ICA). A variety of antibodies with specificity against beta cell constituents have been identified, including insulin and GAD. The idea that type I diabetes is a chronic autoimmune disease with an acute presentation has come from evidence that ICA are present in approximately 3% of asymptomatic first-degree relatives of patients, and these individuals have a high risk of developing type 1 diabetes, often many years later. ICA-negative relatives rarely develop the disease. These antibodies, however, appear to be markers for rather than the cause of beta cell injury. Beta cell destruction is more likely mediated by a variety of cytokines released by T cells and macrophages that are toxic to beta cells or by the direct actions of cytolytic T cells. Patients dying soon after disease onset have a monocytic cellular infiltration restricted to islets, termed insulitis. The infiltrate is composed of CD8 and CD4 T cells, macrophages, and B cells. As the disease progresses, the islets become completely devoid of beta cells and inflammatory infiltrate, leaving intact alpha, delta, and pancreatic polypeptide cells, illustrating the exquisite specificity of the attack. At the time of clinical diagnosis, about 5 to 10% of the beta cell mass remains (see Fig. 205–1).

The damaged beta cells of newly diabetic patients overexpress antigen-presenting class I HLA molecules, which would promote increased susceptibility to attack by cytotoxic CD8 T cells. A role for CD8 T cells is supported by studies involving pancreatic transplantation in identical twins. Monozygotic twins with diabetes who received kidney and pancreas grafts from their nondiabetic, genetically identical sibling required little or no immunosuppression for graft acceptance. Nevertheless, the islets were soon selectively invaded with mononuclear cells, predominantly CD8 T cells, leading to the recurrence of diabetes. Thus, decades after the original onset of disease, the immune system still had the ability to selectively destroy beta cells. Evidence implicating T cells also derives from clinical trials using immunosuppressive drugs. Drugs such as cyclosporine slow or prevent progression of recent-onset diabetes, but immunosuppression must be administrated continuously to maintain the effect. Supporting data for a primary role for T cells derives from animal models that spontaneously develop diabetes. NOD mice develop insulitis and islet autoantibodies at about 4 weeks of age and ultimately progress to diabetes after 12 to 24 weeks. A variety of treatments designed to deplete T cells prevent diabetes. Most importantly, adoptive transfer of T cells isolated from acutely diabetic mice donors into irradiated NOD mice rapidly produces diabetes. Both CD4 and CD8 T cells are required for transfer of disease, suggesting that both are necessary for disease expression. The specific antigens recognized by these diabetogenic T cells remain uncertain. A potential role for GAD is suggested by data showing that if NOD mice are made tolerant to GAD early in life, they fail to develop insulitis and diabetes. The chronic smoldering nature of the disease suggests the presence of regulatory or protective influences. In keeping with this, T cells that protect the islet from immune attack have been isolated from the islets of NOD mice. Such findings suggest that the rate of appearance and clinical expression of disease may be modulated by the balance between diabetogenic and protective populations of T cells.

TYPE II DIABETES. Hyperglycemia in type II diabetes results from an undefined genetic defect(s) (concordance rates in identical twins are nearly 100%), the expression of which is modified by environmental factors. Inasmuch as hyperglycemia itself impairs insulin secretion and action, a phenomenon termed "glucose toxicity" (Fig. 205–4), by the time full-blown hyperglycemia has become manifest, virtually all patients exhibit both insulin resistance and defective insulin secretion. The sequence makes it impossible to determine which one started the vicious cycle leading to the disease.

Insulin Secretion. Fasting insulin levels in type II diabetes are generally normal or increased. Yet, they are relatively low if one takes into account the coexisting presence of hyperglycemia. As hyperglycemia becomes more severe, basal insulin fails to increase or

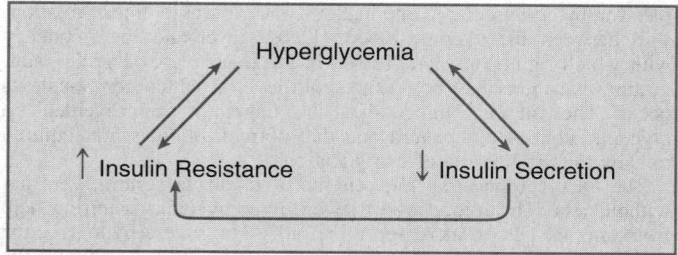

FIGURE 205-4. Elevations of circulating glucose initiate a vicious cycle in which hyperglycemia begets more severe hyperglycemia.

declines further. The insulin secretory defect usually correlates with the severity of fasting hyperglycemia and is more evident following carbohydrate ingestion. In its mildest form, the beta cell defect involves only the initial (or "first phase") secretory phase; the more delayed insulin response remains intact. When viewed in the context of simultaneous insulin resistance, however, a "normal" response is actually inadequate to maintain glucose tolerance. In these subjects, the beta cell defect is specific for glucose; i.e., it is spared from affecting other secretagogues (e.g., amino acids). Insulin deficiency is thus less pronounced during ingestion of mixed meals. Patients with more severe fasting hyperglycemia (>200 mg per deciliter), lose the capacity to respond to increases in circulating glucose. These observations suggest that a specific abnormality in recognition of glucose by the beta cell occurs in the earliest stages of type II diabetes and that this defect worsens as the disease progresses. Although the cause of beta cell failure is unknown, some French families with maturity-onset diabetes of the young (MODY) share a mutation in the gene encoding glucokinase, the key enzyme responsible for the phosphorylation of glucose within the beta cell and liver. A variety of glucokinase mutations have been identified in different families, each capable of interfering with transduction of the glucose signal to the beta cell. Because other families have no detectable glucokinase gene mutations, MODY appears to be a heterogeneous disorder much like more common type II diabetes, which is rarely associated with glucokinase gene mutations. Studies in rodents suggest that the loss of glucose-stimulated insulin secretion is associated with decreased expression of GLUT 2, the beta cell glucose transporter. This defect appears to be a secondary consequence of the diabetic state. Loss of GLUT 2 during the transition to the diabetic state could accelerate further loss in glucose-stimulated insulin secretion. Pathology studies of patients with longstanding type II diabetes have demonstrated amyloid-like deposits, within islets composed of islet amyloid polypeptide (IAPP) or "amylin," a peptide synthesized in the beta cell and cosecreted with insulin. Chronic hypersecretion of IAPP accompanying hyperinsulinemia may lead to precipitation of the peptide which, over time, might contribute to impaired beta cell function.

Insulin Resistance. With few exceptions (e.g., some African-American patients), type II diabetes is characterized by marked impairment in insulin action. The insulin dose-response curve for augmenting glucose uptake in peripheral tissues is shifted to the right (decreased sensitivity) and the maximal response is reduced, particularly with more severe hyperglycemia. Other insulin-stimulated processes, such as inhibition of hepatic glucose production and lipolysis, also show reduced sensitivity to insulin. The mechanisms responsible for insulin resistance remain poorly understood. Early studies focused on defects in insulin binding to its receptor. Mutations in insulin receptors result in the syndrome called Leprechaunism, characterized by severe growth retardation and insulin resistance. Two other rare syndromes of extreme insulin resistance have been identified, characterized by either a profound deficiency of insulin receptors (most often affecting young females with acanthosis nigricans, polycystic ovaries, and hirsutism) or the presence of anti-insulin receptor antibodies (associated with acanthosis nigricans and other autoimmune phenomena).

Although insulin receptors may be reduced in some type II diabetic patients, defects in more distal or "postreceptor" events appear to play the predominant role in insulin resistance. Abnormalities have been reported in β-subunit tyrosine kinase activity, protein tyrosine phosphatase, and the insulin-sensitive glucose transporter (GLUT 4) in adipose (but not muscle) tissue from patients with

type II diabetes. Whether the defects uncovered are primary or secondary to the disturbance in glucose metabolism is uncertain. Possibly, a variety of genetic abnormalities in the cellular transduction of the insulin signal may produce an identical clinical phenotype. No evidence suggests that the mechanisms of insulin resistance in nonobese patients differ from those of their obese diabetic counterparts, but the coexistence of obesity accentuates the severity of the resistant state. In particular, upper body or abdominal versus lower body or peripheral obesity is associated with insulin resistance and diabetes. It is now believed that intra-abdominal visceral fat (detected by CT or MRI) may be the real culprit. Abdominal fat cells have a higher lipolytic rate and are more resistant to insulin than fat derived from peripheral deposits. Cortisol hypersecretion and/or hereditary factors influence distribution of body fat, the latter contributing an additional genetic influence on expression of the disease.

What Is the Primary Defect? It remains uncertain whether insulin resistance or defective insulin secretion is the primary event leading to type II diabetes. Because it is difficult to resolve this issue once overt diabetes has developed, attention has focused on high-risk nondiabetic subjects. Studies in populations with high prevalence rates, such as Pima Indians and Mexican Americans, have found that insulin resistance is the initial predisposing defect. Similar results have been reported in nondiabetic first-degree relatives of type II diabetic patients and in healthy prediabetic offspring of two diabetic parents. Interestingly, hyperinsulinemia has been detected in prediabetic subjects one to two decades before the onset of diabetes, suggesting that the development of the diabetic syndrome is exceedingly slow. Although these studies support the view that insulin resistance generally antedates insulin deficiency, its presence was insufficient to produce overt diabetes. The finding implies that for diabetes to become manifest, the additional factor of impaired insulin secretion is required (Fig. 205-5). It is unclear whether the appearance of a secretory defect is a secondary phenomenon (e.g., due to beta cell exhaustion) or the result of a second independent defect that becomes evident only upon chronic beta cell stimulation (e.g., a subtle genetic defect in beta cell signal transduction). This sequence of events, although common, does not occur in all patients. The demonstration of functional glucokinase gene mutations in some MODY patients clearly indicates that primary beta cell defects are capable of producing an identical phenotype. Furthermore, a significant number of African-Americans with type II diabetes exhibit little or no insulin resistance, and diminished glucose-stimulated insulin secretion has been reported to be a feature of the subgroup of women with gestational diabetes who later develop type II diabetes. Thus, it is unlikely that a single pathogenetic mechanism is responsible for type II diabetes.

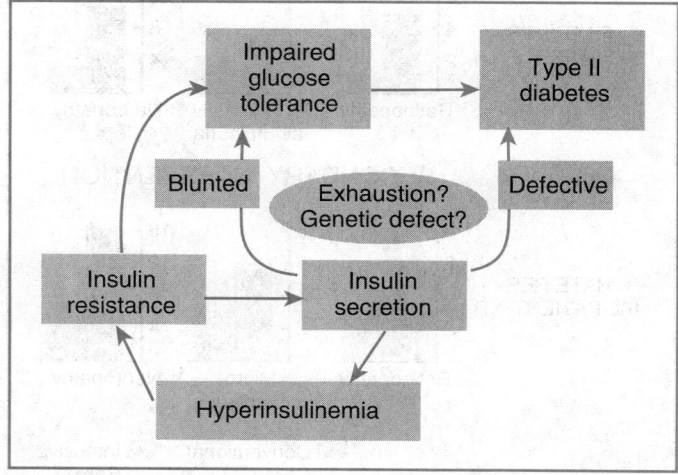

FIGURE 205-5. A proposed sequence of events leading to the development of type II diabetes: insulin resistance resulting from genetic influences, central obesity, inactivity, or a combination of these factors leads over time to a progressive loss of the beta cell's capacity to compensate for this defect.

RELATIONSHIP BETWEEN DIABETES CONTROL AND ITS COMPLICATIONS

Whether the vascular and neuropathic complications of diabetes can be prevented or delayed by improved glycemic control has been debated for more than a half century. To answer the question, the National Institutes of Health initiated the Diabetes Control and Complications Trial (DCCT) to determine if intensive insulin therapy can prevent diabetic complications and/or retard the progression of mild retinopathy. The 9-year trial involved 29 medical centers in North America and included 1441 type I patients aged 13 to 39 years who agreed to be assigned randomly to either intensive insulin therapy or conventional care. Intensive care consisted of three or more insulin injections per day or an insulin pump, self-monitoring of blood glucose at least four times per day, and frequent contact with a diabetes health care team. Conventional care consisted of one or more commonly two injections of insulin mixtures per day, less frequent monitoring, standard education, and less frequent visits. The target goals of therapy were markedly different. The intensive care group sought premeal blood levels of 70 to 120 mg per deciliter, postprandial blood levels of < 180 mg per deciliter, and a glycohemoglobin as close to normal as possible. In the conventional care group, the goal was clinical well-being. Patients were divided into two groups of comparable size: (1) a primary prevention group with diabetes for 1 to 5 years and no detectable complications, and (2) a secondary intervention group with diabetes for 1 to 15 years who had mild nonproliferative retinopathy. Remarkably, nearly 99% of the patients completed the trial.

The DCCT achieved a clear separation of glucose levels between the groups over the entire study period. Glycohemoglobin and mean glucose levels in the intensive care group were 1.5 to 2.0% and 60 to 80 mg per deciliter lower than those receiving conventional care. Although there was considerable variability among individual patients, most of the intensive care group failed to achieve normal glucose levels (glycohemoglobin averaged 1.1% above normal, or a glucose level of about 155 mg per deciliter). Despite this, intensive care reduced the development of retinopathy by 76% in the primary prevention group and the progression of retinopathy by 54% in the secondary intervention group (Fig. 205–6). The latter effect became apparent only after 4 years. In addition, intensive care reduced the risk of developing microalbuminuria by 39%, frank proteinuria by 54%, and clinical neuropathy by 60% compared with conventional care. The incidence of major cardiovascular events also tended to be lower, but the number of events was insufficient to provide statistical proof. At the least, intensive therapy did not seem to pose a risk for macrovascular complications. There was a linear relationship between the average blood glucose level and the frequency with which retinopathy progressed in the intensive care group, suggesting that there may be no threshold level at which complications occur. The findings imply that any degree of improvement in glycemic control has benefit and that normalization is not required to slow the progression of complications.

The DCCT found that the benefits of intensive control were not without risk. The frequency of severe hypoglycemia requiring help from another person increased threefold. Also, severe hypoglycemia often occurred without classic warning symptoms (often while the patient was asleep). This is in keeping with data showing suppression of adrenergic responses to hypoglycemia in subjects treated with intensive insulin regimens. Weight gain was more common. These changes indicate that in some patients the risks of intensive therapy may outweigh the benefits. Included are patients with recurrent severe hypoglycemia and hypoglycemic unawareness, patients in whom the dangers of hypoglycemia are greater because of other coexisting medical conditions or their occupation, patients with far-advanced complications, young children, the elderly, and patients who are unable or unwilling to participate in their management (e.g., self-monitoring of blood glucose). Such individuals are likely to benefit from less aggressive therapy designed to lower glucose levels without provoking hypoglycemia. It is noteworthy that despite a higher rate of hypoglycemia, intensive care did not have any detectable effect on cognitive functioning.

What conclusions can be drawn from the DCCT? The primary message is that "control matters." In type I diabetic patients who are willing and able to participate actively in their management, the goal should be the best level of glycemic control possible without placing them at undue risk. It is crucial that there be in place a health care team that is able to provide the resources, guidance, and support required to achieve treatment goals. Although the DCCT did not involve type II patients, it is likely that the results of the DCCT apply to them as well. However, a larger subgroup of type II patients are not ideal candidates for tight control when viewed in the context of its potential risks. This is particularly true in elderly patients with coexisting cardiovascular disease. The DCCT suggests there are benefits to be gained in nearly all patients from lowering glucose from levels > 200 to levels in the 150 mg per deciliter range; for most type II patients this is achievable with diet, oral agents, or less complicated insulin regimens than are required in type I patients. The greatest challenge to the DCCT results relates to how they can be effectively applied to clinical practice, a formidable task. The study group was highly motivated and more compliant than the average patient with diabetes. Management was supervised by an experienced health care team that was able to devote more time to patients than is possible in most practices. Also, the immediate costs of intensive treatment are greater, although the long-term cost savings of having healthier, more productive patients is obvious. An important lesson from the DCCT experience was that successful treatment was largely accomplished by the efforts of the patients themselves as well as nonphysicians, principally nurse educators and dietitians. Thus, it may be more practical to use physician-directed health care teams to translate the findings of the DCCT.

TREATMENT

Treatment of diabetes mellitus involves changes in lifestyle and pharmacological intervention with insulin or oral glucose-lowering drugs. In type I diabetes, the primary focus is to replace insulin secretion; lifestyle changes are required to facilitate insulin therapy and optimize health. For most patients with type II diabetes, changes in lifestyle are the cornerstone of treatment. Pharmacologic intervention represents a secondary treatment strategy for individuals unable to adopt lifestyle changes. Although therapeutic strategies for the two forms of diabetes differ, the short-term and long-term goals of treatment are identical (Table 205–3).

Type I Diabetes

INSULIN PREPARATIONS AND PHARMACOKINETICS. A variety of highly purified insulin preparations are commercially available that differ mainly in their time of onset and duration of action (Table 205–4). Nearly all contain 100 units per milliliter (U-100), although a more concentrated regular insulin with a more prolonged action (500 units per milliliter or U-500) can be obtained for

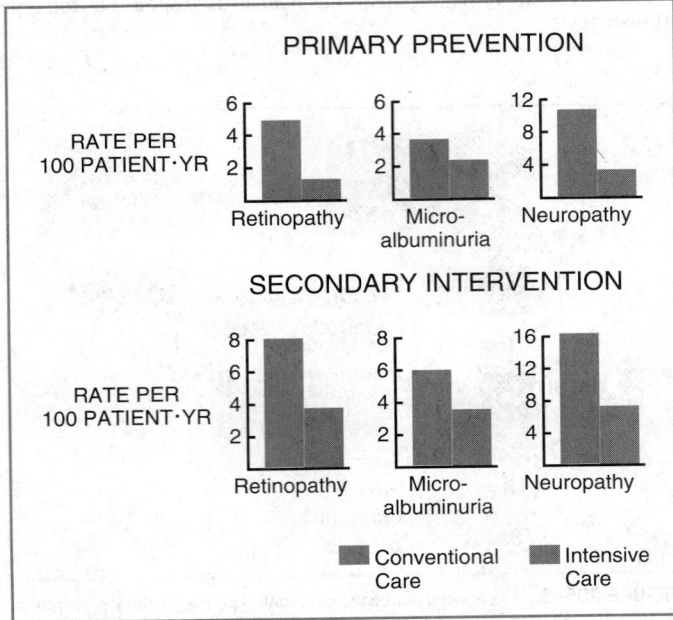

FIGURE 205–6. A summary of the results of the Diabetes Control and Complications Trial (DCCT).

TABLE 205-3. TREATMENT GOALS

I. *Short Term*
  A. Restore metabolic control to as close to normal as possible
  B. Improve sense of well-being
II. *Long Term:* Minimize risk of diabetic complications
  A. Accelerated atherosclerosis
  B. Microangiopathy (retinopathy, nephropathy)
  C. Neuropathy

resistant patients. Pure insulin preparations result in fewer problems related to insulin antigenicity, such as insulin allergy, insulin resistance, and lipoatrophy. Human insulin is the principal form of insulin sold in North America and other industrialized countries. Although animal (beef, pork, and beef/pork combination) insulins are still sold, they will be less available in the years to come. Human insulins are slightly less antigenic than porcine and much less antigenic than bovine insulin. Because they generate lower titers of insulin antibodies, human insulins act more rapidly after injection, and their effects tend to persist for a shorter time. This allows for better synchrony between insulin peaks and meal absorption after injection of rapid-acting insulin with meals but may produce earlier peaks of intermediate-acting insulin that cause hypoglycemia during sleep and/or fail to sustain effects for a full 24-hour period, thereby necessitating twice-daily injections. Human insulin is most useful in patients who are initiating insulin therapy and do not already have antibodies or who have the potential to require insulin intermittently (e.g., type II diabetics during an illness) because intermittent insulin use increases its antigenic potential. There is little clinical benefit in introducing human insulin to patients who are well controlled using animal preparations.

After subcutaneous injection regular insulin begins to act in about 30 minutes and therefore should be given 20 to 30 minutes before a meal. Because it acts quickly, it is most effective in blunting elevations in glucose following meals and in allowing for rapid adjustments in insulin dosage based on measurements of blood glucose by the patient. This is especially helpful in managing glucose elevations that occur during illness or with consumption of large meals. Because rapid-acting insulins afford much greater flexibility, they have assumed a greater role in intensive treatment regimens. Other insulin preparations are modified to delay their absorption from injection sites so as to prolong their action. Either protamine is added, yielding intermediate-acting NPH insulin, or the size of the zinc-insulin crystal is enlarged by adjusting the preparation process. The latter yields Lente (intermediate-acting) and Ultralente (long-acting) insulin. The intermediate-acting insulins (NPH and Lente) have a similar time course of action. They offer the compromise of some degree of coverage for meals coinciding with their peak actions and provision of basal levels of insulin when given twice per day. Longer-acting insulins (Ultralente), because they have less evident "peaks," offer some advantages for basal insulin replacement. Human Ultralente has a shorter duration of action and generally requires twice-daily dosing. Among individuals, the time course of a given preparation is highly variable, owing in part to differences in circulating insulin antibodies. Even in the same patient, a preparation may produce variable responses. This phenomenon is partially explained by the fact that insulin absorption depends on the site of injection. Absorption is faster when insulin is injected into the abdomen than into an extremity, and is faster in an upper than in a lower limb. Moreover, absorption is accelerated if it is injected into an extremity that is subsequently involved in exercise or if the injection site is massaged or warmed. The depth of injection is also a critical variable. Absorption is much faster if insulin is injected intramuscularly rather than subcutaneously, and intramuscular injection in thin individuals often may occur. These confounding factors lead to variations in blood glucose responses and frustration for the patient. Furthermore, insulin preparations are predominantly in hexameric form, which delays its absorption from subcutaneous injection sites because of the slow dissociation of hexamers into monomers. This factor has led to using recombinant DNA technology to construct monomeric insulin analogues that are more rapidly absorbed from subcutaneous tissues. Although the clinical utility of monomeric insulins is not established, the use of genetic engineering to design novel insulins is a promising development.

INSULIN REGIMENS. During the first few years of type I diabetes some degree of beta cell function typically persists, allowing many patients to achieve glycemic control with less intensive effort. Because intermediate-acting insulins generally are not sustained over a 24-hour period and because insulin requirements tend to increase early in the morning, most patients should be started on two daily injections of a mixture of intermediate-acting and rapid-acting human insulin before breakfast and dinner. Although Lente insulin has a theoretical advantage over NPH insulin because it does not contain a foreign protein (protamine), this appears to have negligible clinical significance. There is some advantage to using NPH when insulin mixtures are used. If regular insulin is mixed with NPH, it retains its pharmacokinetic characteristics, whereas if it is mixed with Lente, the excess zinc may cause regular insulin to precipitate out of solution, delaying its absorption. Initially, the doses of intermediate-acting insulin are adjusted to optimize predinner and fasting glucose levels. Once this is accomplished, the doses of rapid-acting insulin are varied so as to optimize prelunch and bedtime glucose values. Patients should inject in the same region but different locations at the same time each day, i.e., in the abdomen in the morning to optimize insulin delivery and in the leg or buttock at night to slow absorption. Some patients may experience a brief "honeymoon" period during which there is partial recovery of beta cell function and a need to reduce insulin doses. This should not be used as a signal to reduce efforts aimed at glycemic control; optimized insulin therapy may help preserve beta cell function.

Several years after the onset of type I diabetes, residual insulin secretion typically stops and twice-daily insulin injections no longer suffice. Optimal glycemic control requires that insulin delivery be directed toward more closely simulating the normal pattern of insulin secretion, namely continuous "basal" insulin secretion throughout the day and night and brief increases in insulin levels coinciding with ingestion of meals. The major problem with regimens relying on twice-daily injections is that the glucose-lowering effect of predinner intermediate-acting insulin is greatest at the time when requirements are lowest (i.e., 2:00 to 3:00 A.M.), whereas when requirements are increasing early in the morning (i.e. 5:00 to 8:00 A.M.) insulin levels decline. The result is a tendency to nocturnal hypoglycemia and/or fasting hyperglycemia.

It has become evident that successful management must begin with control of fasting glucose levels. Failure to do so leads to perpetuation of hyperglycemia for the remainder of the day or attempts at corrective measures with supplemental insulin that miss the mark. The therapeutic obstacle imposed by fasting hyperglycemia is best appreciated in the context of its pathogenesis, namely, glucose overproduction. Once hepatic gluconeogenesis has been activated in the morning, it is not readily suppressed by subcutaneous injections of insulin and hyperglycemia persists after breakfast. The key factors responsible for fasting hyperglycemia are inadequate overnight delivery of insulin and sleep-associated GH release. The "dawn phenomenon" is most pronounced in patients with type I diabetes because of their inability to compensate by raising endogenous insulin secretion. The magnitude of the dawn phenomenon can be attenuated by designing insulin regimens to ensure that the effects of exogenous insulin do not peak in the middle of the night and become dissipated by morning. Several approaches can deal with the problem (Fig. 205–7). The simplest is to use three injections, i.e., mixtures of intermediate- and short-acting insulin before breakfast, short-acting insulin before dinner, and intermediate-acting insulin at bedtime. The primary disadvantage of this approach is that meal schedules must be fixed rather rigidly. Alternative multidose regi-

TABLE 205-4. INSULIN PREPARATIONS: TIME-COURSE OF ACTION

Class	Preparation	Onset of Effect	Peak Effect	Duration of Action
Rapid-acting	Regular	30 min	2–4 hr	5–8 hr
Intermediate-acting	NPH or Lente	1–2 hr	6–10 hr	16–24 hr
Long-acting	Ultralente			
	Human	4–6 hr	8–20 hr	24–28 hr
	Bovine	4–6 hr	14–24 hr	28–36 hr

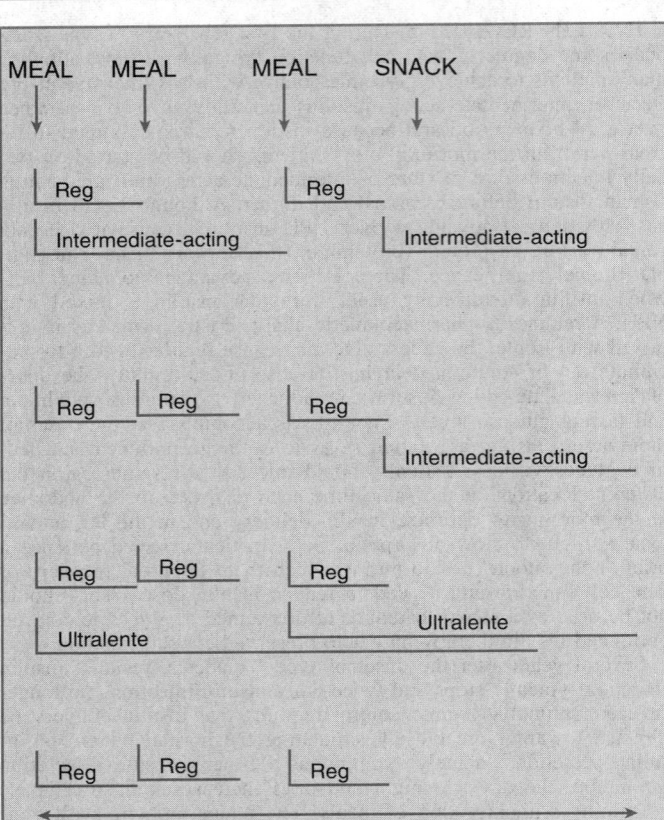

FIGURE 205–7. Several intensive insulin regimens commonly used in the treatment of diabetes. Each is designed to provide a continuous supply of insulin around the clock and to make extra insulin available at the time of meals, thereby simulating more closely the normal physiologic pattern of insulin secretion.

mens include (1) Ultralente (twice daily if human insulin is used) to replace basal insulin secretion and short-acting insulin before each meal, or (2) short-acting insulin before each meal and intermediate-acting insulin at bedtime. Pen injectors containing cartridges filled with insulin make multidose insulin regimens more convenient.

An alternative that provides greater flexibility in insulin dosing while minimizing variations in absorption is continuous subcutaneous insulin infusion (CSII). This method administers rapid-acting insulin around the clock using a battery-powered, externally worn, computer-controlled infusion pump. The pump delivers basal rates continuously and can be programmed to vary the flow rate automatically for set time periods, such as reducing the flow rate at 1:00 to 4:00 A.M. and then increasing it to compensate for increased insulin requirements early in the morning (i.e., 5:00 to 8:00 A.M.). Boluses determined by self-monitoring of blood glucose are given before meals by manually activating the pump. Most pumps contain a syringe filled with insulin attached to an infusion set consisting of a catheter and a 27-gauge needle which is inserted subcutaneously, preferably in the abdomen, to optimize absorption. Unfortunately, the approach has problems that limit its use. The most obvious disadvantage is wearing the pump itself. Because CSII uses short-acting insulin, any interruption in the flow (most commonly due to insulin precipitation within the catheter) leads to rapid deterioration in control. Local infections at the catheter site occasionally occur. Also, maintenance of the pump and appropriate infusion rates requires effort and sophistication. The intensive treatment regimens

described above are not for everyone. In patients appropriate for such care, however, intensive insulin therapy should be encouraged. An absolute indication for intensive therapy is pregnancy. In order to eliminate the excess neonatal morbidity and mortality which, in the past, were associated with diabetic pregnancy requires maintaining glycemic control. Ideally, intensive insulin therapy should be instituted prior to conception to minimize the higher risk of fetal anomalies. After conception, blood glucose targets are more stringently applied than at other times, with the aim to restore glucose levels to those found in nondiabetic pregnant individuals.

LIFESTYLE CHANGES. The management of diet and exercise contributes importantly to the care of patients with type I diabetes (Table 205–5). The patient must be advised of the need for a careful balance between calorie intake and energy expenditure (exercise), while taking into account the availability of injected insulin. The introduction of intensive insulin regimens has permitted more flexibility in meal planning by allowing more latitude in varying the size, content, and timing of meals. This offers the opportunity for a more normal lifestyle, minimizing compliance problems and optimizing patient acceptance. Meals should be nutritionally sound and provide sufficient calories to meet the energy needs of growing children, active young adults, or pregnancy. The 1800-kcal diet commonly used in type II patients is grossly insufficient in such active individuals. Furthermore, diets should be specifically aimed at minimizing long-term cardiovascular risk. Because type I patients depend on exogenous insulin, management is facilitated by using a meal plan designed to match the time course of the insulin dosage regimen selected. Patients should learn a system that allows for consistent nutrient (especially carbohydrate) intake each day (such as the Exchange System developed by the American Diabetes Association) to allow the appropriate substitution of foods within the meal plan and learn to compensate for departures from the meal plan by adjusting insulin doses or for periods of increased activity by consumption of extra food. Efforts should be made to avoid long delays between meals; frequent small snacks may be needed at times of peak insulin action to avoid hypoglycemia. Most patients, regardless of their regimen, require a bedtime snack to reduce the risk of nocturnal hypoglycemia. The potential for weight gain requires special emphasis on portion control and appropriate (but not excessive) food intake for treatment of hypoglycemia.

Regular exercise is important to promote well-being and reduce vascular complications. Little evidence suggests, however, that exercise substantially improves glycemic control in type I diabetes, even though it reduces overall insulin requirements by enhancing insulin sensitivity. Exercise may rapidly reduce blood glucose levels, particularly when it coincides with the time of the peak action of an insulin injection or if it accelerates insulin absorption from its injection site. Exercise also produces a marked increase in glucose uptake by muscle. Blood glucose levels nevertheless remain stable in normal subjects because insulin levels fall, promoting increases in hepatic glucose production that match the rate of glucose consumption. In the diabetic receiving insulin exogenously, this "finely

TABLE 205–5. LIFESTYLE MODIFICATIONS FOR THE PATIENT WITH DIABETES

I. Diet prescription
  1. Weight reduction (when appropriate)
  2. Carbohydrates: 45–60% (depending on severity of diabetes and triglyceride levels)
  3. Restriction of saturated fat (to < 10% of calories)
  4. Increased monounsaturated fat (depending on the need to limit carbohydrate)
  5. Decreased cholesterol intake to < 300 mg per day
  6. Sodium restriction in patients prone to hypertension
II. *Exercise prescription**
  1. *Type:* Aerobic strongly preferred. Avoid heavy lifting, straining, and Valsalva maneuvers that raise blood pressure.
  2. *Intensity:* Increase pulse rate to at least 120–140, depending on the age and cardiovascular state of the patient.
  3. *Frequency:* 3–4 days per week
  4. *Duration:* 20–30 minutes preceded and followed by stretching and flexibility exercises for 5–10 minutes.

* Limitations are imposed by pre-existing coronary or peripheral vascular disease, proliferative retinopathy, peripheral or autonomic neuropathy, and poor glycemic control.

tuned" homeostatic mechanism is disturbed. The continued presence of exogenous insulin further accelerates glucose uptake and, more importantly, blocks the compensatory increase in glucose production, so that circulating glucose falls. Because the magnitude of the fall is not easily titrated, hypoglycemia may be a complication. The tendency to overeat when hypoglycemic symptoms occur may lead to a rebound increase in blood glucose to hyperglycemic levels. Thus, if the patient is unable to adjust diet and insulin, intermittent exercise may intensify glucose fluctuations rather than improve glycemic control.

Type II Diabetes

In most type II diabetic patients, diet and exercise are the key or the only therapeutic intervention required to restore metabolic control (Table 205–5). They are especially effective in obese, sedentary persons who constitute the majority type II diabetic patients. For the obese patient, modest weight reduction (e.g., 5 kg), irrespective of starting weight, leads to a rapid decline in blood glucose levels. The dramatic impact of weight loss is mediated by changes in insulin-responsive tissues as well as the beta cell: Insulin resistance diminishes, glucose production declines, and the resulting fall in glucose leads to improved glucose-stimulated insulin secretion. The effect of weight loss is not restricted to glucose; lipoprotein profiles and blood pressure also improve. In general, *it matters little how weight loss is achieved* provided that adequate nutrition is maintained. In sedentary diabetic patients daily caloric requirements for weight maintenance are as low as 25 to 30 kcal per kg body weight per day. In such individuals the classic 1800-kcal diet commonly prescribed is generally ineffective. It is sensible to begin with a nutritionally sound, individually tailored restrictive diet aimed at producing a caloric deficit of about 500 kcal per day. Because a caloric deficit of 3500 kcal is required to lose 1 pound of body fat, weight loss can be expected to be approximately 1 pound per week. For some very obese patients with a history of failed weight loss attempts, very low calorie diets (600 to 800 kcal per day) can be useful when done under medical supervision. Regardless of the method used, most patients are unable to maintain a diet for an extended period of time, and if they are successful, most regain the lost weight. Although the reasons for the failure of most diet programs are unclear, confounding factors may make weight loss more difficult in type II diabetes. The normal decrease in basal metabolic rate during weight loss is accentuated in diabetic patients because the metabolic improvement produced by weight loss reverses the accelerated gluconeogenesis and futile cycling of substrates commonly seen in poorly controlled diabetes, both of which waste energy. Moreover, dieting reduces glycosuria, lessening urinary caloric loss. Success is best achieved by a combination of a supportive environment that emphasizes long-term goals (short-term weight changes mean little in the big picture), regular exercise to increase energy expenditure, behavior modification, and, most importantly, the patient's commitment.

Even when weight loss is not successful, the meal plan can remain a valuable tool to reduce the risk of cardiovascular disease in the patient with diabetes. This is best achieved by reducing saturated fat and in turn raising the carbohydrate content of the diet. Although it was originally thought that carbohydrate intake should be restricted, it is now appreciated that a diet high in carbohydrate (50 to 60%) can improve insulin action and glycemic control. This is particularly true in patients with mild hyperglycemia. In patients with more severe fasting hyperglycemia or with triglyceride elevations that may be aggravated by high-carbohydrate diets, a moderate carbohydrate intake (45 to 50% of total calories) may be preferable. It has been assumed that carbohydrate intake should be focused on complex carbohydrates (starches) and that simple sugars should be limited. Little evidence supports this assumption; simple sugars raise glucose levels to about the same extent as complex carbohydrates when they are consumed by diabetic patients. Thus, the total amount of carbohydrate in the diet rather than the source of carbohydrate should be the primary consideration. The optimal source of carbohydrate may be foods containing water-soluble fiber (e.g., oats, gums, legumes, fruit pectin). Such fiber blunts the meal-induced rise in blood glucose by delaying gastric emptying and, in turn, the rate of meal absorption. A mild lowering of triglycerides and LDL-cholesterol may occur as well. It is commonly believed that sucrose leads to excessive glycemic excursions and therefore must be omitted. This may not be the case, especially when modest

amounts of sucrose are eaten within the context of mixed meals. Glucose excursions are not significantly different when equivalent amounts of sucrose and complex carbohydrates are added to meals. This may be because other foods (e.g., protein and fat) act to delay the absorption and promote insulin secretion. Thus, it is unnecessary to forbid the use of foods containing sucrose, provided it is done in moderation. Such restrictions can lead to poor adherence to the meal plan.

A key component of the diabetic meal plan is to reduce or change the composition of dietary fat. The typical diet of Western countries, high in saturated or animal fat, appears to contribute to the development of atherosclerosis in patients with diabetes. Although substituting monounsaturated fatty acids (MUFA) rather than carbohydrates for saturated fat in the diet has been advocated to reduce LDL-cholesterol without raising triglycerides, the approach is difficult to achieve as the major sources of MUFA are olive, canola, and peanut oils.

Regular exercise is a useful adjunct in the therapy of diabetes (Table 205–5). It can improve insulin action and facilitate weight loss, but its major advantage is to lower cardiovascular risk. Experiments in monkeys fed atherogenic diets and retrospective population studies strongly suggest that regular exercise attenuates coronary artery disease. This is thought to apply to diabetic patients as well. In support of this view, regular exercise produces a fall in VLDL-triglyceride and a rise in HDL-cholesterol and fibrinolytic activity in type II diabetes. Limitations may be imposed by pre-existing coronary or peripheral vascular disease, proliferative retinopathy, peripheral or autonomic neuropathy, and poor control.

Pharmacologic Intervention

The temptation to use pharmacologic agents should be restrained in type II diabetes, particularly in obese patients. However, the clinician must also resist the temptation to stop at diet and exercise, if they are sufficient only to eliminate symptoms.

ORAL GLUCOSE-LOWERING AGENTS. Oral glucose-lowering agents are generally effective in patients in whom diet and exercise fail to achieve treatment goals. Oral agents tend to be favored as first-line therapy if hyperglycemia is mild, the patient is older, and obesity is pronounced. The response cannot be predicted with certainty based on clinical characteristics, and few circumstances contraindicate their use (e.g., severe insulin deficiency, allergy, pregnancy). Patients presenting with severe hyperglycemia generally require insulin to lower glucose levels in the initial phases of treatment. Once glucose levels have stabilized and the "toxic" effects of severe hyperglycemia on beta cell function and insulin action have been minimized, many such patients become responsive to oral agents.

Sulfonylurea drugs were the only class of oral agents available in the United States before 1995. Initially they enhance insulin secretion by virtue of their ability to bind to potassium channels on the surface of the beta cell, thereby facilitating cellular depolarization. The reduction in glucose that follows is accompanied by a decline in insulin levels toward baseline. Insulin resistance commonly diminishes, mainly due to partial reversal of postreceptor defects that are produced either by extrapancreatic effects of the drug or improved glycemic control *per se*. The clinical benefits of sulfonylureas are due to their combined effect on insulin secretion and action. The importance of the former is underscored by the fact that sulfonylureas are totally ineffective in type I diabetes. Although the sulfonylureas differ in relative potency, effective dosage, duration of action, metabolism, and side effects, from a clinical standpoint these differences have marginal practical significance (Table 205–6). Each drug has similar hypoglycemic effects when used in maximal doses. *Tolbutamide* has the shortest duration of action and is metabolized by the liver and therefore has advantages in elderly patients with impaired renal function who are more vulnerable to hypoglycemia. Because it usually must be taken two or three times a day, it tends to be less effective because of problems with compliance. *Chlorpropamide* is the longest-acting sulfonylurea and therefore requires only once per day dosing. It is partially metabolized in the liver, but it and its active metabolites are removed by the kidney. These properties enhance the risk of hypoglycemia in the patient who omits meals or has renal insufficiency. Chlorpropamide can cause significant hyponatremia by virtue of its capacity to pro-

TABLE 205–6. CHARACTERISTICS OF GLUCOSE-LOWERING AGENTS

Generic Name	Daily Dosage Range (mg)	Duration of Action (hr)
Tolbutamide	500–3000	6–12
Chlorpropamide	100–500	60
Tolazamide	100–1000	12–24
Glipizide	2.5–40	12–24
Glyburide	1.25–20	16–24
Micronized glyburide	0.75–12	12–24
Metformin	850–2550	8–12

mote the action of antidiuretic hormone. This effect is more common in elderly patients, especially when they are taking diuretics. Thus, chlorpropamide has the greatest potential for serious side effects. *Sulfonylureas* with an intermediate duration of action offer a reasonable compromise, although they still have a risk of producing severe hypoglycemia. These drugs may be given once per day, although twice-daily dosing may be required in patients with more severe hypoglycemia. After choosing an oral agent, treatment is initiated using low doses and then increasing dosage every 1 to 2 weeks until treatment goals or maximally effective doses are reached. Most patients (about 75%) initially respond with a lowering of glucose levels. It is not uncommon to see slippage after years of therapy owing to failure to sustain enthusiasm for diet and exercise, to progression of beta cell failure, to superimposition of other medical problems or drugs, or to drug tolerance. The deteriorating glycemic control begets even poorer control owing to the phenomenon of glucotoxicity (see Fig. 205–4). Secondary drug failure occurs at a rate of 5 to 10% per year. Early signs of secondary drug failure should provoke renewed attempts to enforce diet as well as an increase in drug dosage. Persistent hyperglycemia despite maximal drug doses signals the need to switch to insulin therapy or to add metformin; rarely is it helpful to switch to another oral agent.

Recently, the biguanide metformin became available in the United States as an alternative oral glucose-lowering agent. (The drug has been used for many years in Canada and Europe.) Unlike sulfonylureas, this drug acts mainly by reducing hepatic gluconeogenesis and diminishing intestinal glucose absoption. As a result, insulin levels fall, a potential advantage if the theory implicating hyperinsulinemia in the development of atherosclerosis proves correct. Because metformin tends to induce mild weight loss, it may be particularly suitable for obese patients either as monotherapy or as an additive drug when sulfonylureas are ineffective alone. The drug does not produce hypoglycemia when used as monotherapy; however, it can rarely produce lactic acidosis (approximately 0.03 cases per 1000 patient years) and should therefore not be given to patients with renal insufficiency, liver disease, or a history of hypoxemia or alcohol abuse. The major side effects are gastrointestinal, particularly anorexia and nausea, which may contribute to its effect on weight loss. Metformin has a relatively short half-life (it is eliminated exclusively by the kidney), generally necessitating administration as two or three divided doses given with meals.

INSULIN THERAPY. Insulin is most commonly used as first-line therapy for nonobese, younger, or severely hyperglycemic patients and is temporally required during severe stress (e.g., injury, infection, surgery) or in pregnancy. Insulin should not be used as first-line therapy in poorly compliant patients who are unwilling to self-monitor glucose levels or for patients possessing a high risk of hypoglycemia. In patients with severe obesity, profound insulin resistance often necessitates the use of large doses of insulin, which sometimes interferes with efforts to restrict caloric intake to achieve weight loss. In newly diagnosed patients or those with relatively mild fasting hyperglycemia who continue to maintain endogenous insulin secretory capacity, relatively small doses of insulin (e.g., 0.3 to 0.4 unit per kilogram of body weight per day) given once or twice a day may be sufficient to achieve target goals. Such patients retain some degree of meal-stimulated endogenous insulin secretion and therefore may require less rapid-acting insulin. Although it is common practice to administer a single dose of intermediate-acting insulin in the morning, frequently its glucose-lowering effect does not extend over a full 24-hour period. Because a key element of successful insulin treatment is to diminish accelerated rates of morning glucose production, it is generally more effective to split the dose, administering sufficient amounts of intermediate-acting insulin in the evening (before dinner or preferably at bedtime) to optimize control of the fasting glucose level. Alternatively, a single small dose of intermediate-acting insulin given at bedtime to control fasting hyperglycemia may be effective throughout the remainder of the day in patients who have retained the capacity to secrete insulin with meals. This approach has the advantage of greater simplicity and may be combined with oral glucose lowering agents during the day to facilitate endogenous insulin release with meals.

In practice, most insulin-treated patients are obese, have more severe hyperglycemia, and have already failed oral therapy. These patients are more insulin deficient and insulin resistant. As a result, they often require multiple-dose regimens involving insulin mixtures to control hyperglycemia. As in type I patients, it is best to distribute their insulin as evenly as possible throughout the day. The complexity of the regimen must be individualized based on the total clinical context of the patient's disease, the level of diabetes education and ability to perform self-care, and most importantly on the patient's motivation. Although some specialists have advocated combinations of insulin and oral hypoglycemic drugs in patients requiring large doses of insulin, combination therapy is no more effective than insulin alone in controlling blood glucose. However, less insulin may be required.

Monitoring

SELF-MONITORING OF BLOOD GLUCOSE (SMBG). SMBG has revolutionized diabetes management. It actively involves patients in the treatment process, allows more rapid treatment adjustments, and reinforces diet therapy. SMBG provides the patient with the tools necessary for crucial self-management. SMBG is especially useful in the care of patients receiving insulin or oral glucose-lowering agents during periods of stress and of patients susceptible to hypoglycemia. Urine glucose testing is unreliable and should be used only in patients who cannot or refuse to apply SMBG or in whom the treatment goal is only prevention of symptomatic hyperglycemia.

The newer glucose meters are small, portable, and accurate, give a digital readout, and have computerized memory to facilitate record keeping. These factors make them, for most patients, preferable to visual estimates from test strips. Blood sampling is facilitated and made less painful by automated spring-operated lancet devices. SMBG is of value only if the patient performs tests on a regular basis, can accurately measure glucose levels, and can make use of the results. The patient must become familiar with what a normal glucose value is, what the glucose targets are, and how they may vary with changes in diet, activity, and insulin absorption. Day-to-day adjustments in short-acting insulin, based on premeal values and a "sliding scale," can be readily accomplished by most patients. The patient also needs to examine the effects of longer-acting insulins and make small adjustments if glucose levels (e.g., prebreakfast and predinner values) are not within the target range. At a minimum, patients need to be able to adjust to repetitive patterns of hypoglycemia or hyperglycemia as well as to periods of illness ("sick days"). In the latter circumstance, urine testing for ketones should be done as well.

The success of insulin therapy depends on the frequency with which the patient monitors. Patients with type I diabetes should be encouraged to monitor before each meal and at bedtime. Periodic checks 90 to 120 minutes after meals help to control postprandial hyperglycemia, and patients may occasionally need to monitor blood levels in the middle of the night (e.g., 3 AM) to avoid nocturnal hypoglycemia. Type II patients who are treated with insulin should conduct SMBG daily, before breakfast and dinner and at bedtime. Here the aim is to reduce the risk of hypoglycemia. Those taking oral agents may benefit from less frequent testing (e.g., before breakfast or dinner, every 2 or 3 days), depending on their metabolic status. Type II patients on diet therapy should, at the very least, learn SMBG to prevent metabolic decompensation. They may benefit from monitoring glucose levels periodically so that they can better appreciate how individual foods or deviations from the meal plan adversely affect their glycemic control.

GLYCOHEMOGLOBIN. Glycohemoglobin (or glycated hemoglobin) assays have emerged as the "gold standard" by which glycemic control is measured. The test does not rely on the patient's ability to monitor or accurately record blood glucose levels, and it is not influenced by acute changes in blood glucose or by the interval since the last meal. Glycohemoglobin is formed when glucose reacts nonenzymatically with the hemoglobin A molecule and is composed of several fractions, the major one being hemoglobin A_{1c} (HbA_{1c}). Total glycohemoglobin (HbA_1) and HbA_{1c} (expressed as the percentage of total hemoglobin) vary in proportion to the average level of glucose over the lifespan of the red blood cell (RBC), thereby providing an index of glycemic control during the preceding 6 to 12 weeks. Several assay methods have been developed that vary in their precision, yield different ranges for nondiabetic values, and lack common standardization procedures. Clinicians must therefore become familiar with the assays used in their own laboratory and use that specific assay when evaluating changes in glycemic control in individual patients. Although the ambient glucose level is the dominant factor influencing glycohemoglobin, other factors may confound interpretation of the test. For example, any condition that increases RBC turnover (e.g., pregnancy or hemolytic anemia) spuriously lowers glycohemoglobin, regardless of the assay employed. Some assays yield spuriously low values in patients with hemoglobinopathies such as sickle cell disease or trait and hemoglobin C or D, or spuriously high values when hemoglobin F is increased (e.g., thalassemia, myeloproliferative disorders) or large doses of aspirin are consumed. Thus, for unexpected high or low values, factors that alter the specific test used should be excluded, including hemoglobin variants. In most cases, however, discrepancies between SMBG and glycohemoglobin results reflect problems with the former rather than the latter. Although glycohemoglobin provides the most accurate estimate of overall glycemic control, it is less valuable in determining what specific changes in therapy are indicated. Blood glucose measurements are essential to adjust the components of the insulin regimen appropriately.

MANAGEMENT PLAN/TREATMENT GOALS. A management plan should take into consideration the life patterns, age, work and school schedules, psychosocial needs, educational level, and motivation of the individual patient. The plan should include medications, recommendations for lifestyle changes, a meal plan, monitoring instructions (including "sick day" management), and hypoglycemia prevention and treatment strategies. Each component of the plan must be understood and agreed upon by the patient. Active patient participation in problem solving as well as ongoing, continued support from the health care team are critical for successful management. At each visit the management plan should be reviewed and an assessment made of the patient's progress in achieving target goals. If the goals are not met, the causes need to be identified and the plan modified accordingly. The history and physical examination should focus on early signs and symptoms of retinal, vascular, neurologic, and foot complications and reinforcement of the diet and exercise prescription. A complete ophthalmologic examination and a timed urine collection for albumin should be obtained annually in most patients.

The formulation of target glycemic goals must take into account the results of the DCCT, the patient's capacity to implement the treatment plan, the risk for hypoglycemia, and other factors that would alter the risk-benefit ratio. The risk-benefit ratio for intensive pharmacologic therapy may be less favorable for patients with type II than type I diabetes. However, in those patients considered appropriate for more intensive management, the glycemic targets should be much the same, regardless of the form of diabetes. Table 205–7 presents target glycemic guidelines for nonpregnant diabetic patients and targets for other factors that increase the potential for diabetic complications.

Pancreas/Islet Transplantation

Intensive insulin treatment rarely, if ever, restores glucose homeostasis to levels achieved in nondiabetic individuals. The search for more effective methods of treatment thus remains a long-term goal of diabetes research. Efforts have focused on transplantation of insulin-producing tissue, resulting in substantial improvement in the outcome of such pancreas transplant surgery in recent years. In major centers, most patients emerge from the perioperative period with a functioning graft, and, once insulin independence is established, the majority stabilize for many years. Unfortunately, because of the need for long-term immunosuppression, pancreas transplantation is, at present, an option for only a select group of patients, mainly for

TABLE 205–7. THERAPEUTIC TARGETS FOR NONPREGNANT DIABETIC PATIENTS

Parameters	Normal	Goal	Signals Possible Intervention*
Premeal glucose (mg/dl)	<115	80–120	<80 or >140
Bedtime glucose (mg/dl)	<115	100–140	<100 or >160
HbA_{1c}† (%)	<6	<7	>8
LDL-cholesterol (mg/dl)	<130	<130	>130
HDL-cholesterol (mg/dl)	>35	>35	<35
Fasting triglycerides (mg/dl)	<150	<150	>250–300
Blood pressure (mm Hg)	<140/90	<130/85	>130/85

* Targets may vary depending on assessment of risk-benefit ratio.
† Targets need to be adjusted for local laboratory differences in assay method and nondiabetic reference ranges.

type I diabetes requiring immunosuppression for renal allografts. In such individuals successful pancreas transplantation may be more effective in preventing nephropathy in the grafted kidney. The application of islet transplantation to humans with diabetes has proved exceedingly difficult, largely because of difficulty in obtaining sufficient numbers of viable human islets. Thus far, only a few patients have become insulin independent. Interestingly, islet transplantation has been much more successful in patients with chronic pancreatitis who have undergone total pancreatectomy followed by intraportal injections of their own islets. The implication is that the use of immunosuppressive drugs and/or chronic low-grade rejection of the foreign islet grafts accounts for the high incidence of failure reported with early attempts. If correct, the future of islet transplantation therapy may depend more on the manipulation of the islet or the immune system to prevent rejection than on technical surgical advances.

COMPLICATIONS

Acute Metabolic Complications

HYPERGLYCEMIC STATES. Metabolic decompensation in diabetes manifests as severe hyperglycemia with or without ketoacidosis. Although diabetic ketoacidosis (DKA) generally is seen in type I patients and nonketotic hyperosmolar syndrome generally is seen in type II patients, exceptions are common. In both conditions mortality increases with age and is usually due to an associated catastrophic illness (e.g., myocardial infarction, cerebrovascular accident, sepsis) or acute complications (e.g., aspiration, arrhythmias, or cerebral edema). Thus, treatment does not simply depend on insulin to reverse the metabolic abnormalities that dominate the picture; it also depends on detection and treatment of precipitating illnesses as well as prompt attention to fluid and electrolyte disturbances.

DIABETIC KETOACIDOSIS. DKA may herald the onset of type I diabetes, but it most often (>80%) occurs in established diabetic patients as a result of an intercurrent illness (e.g., infection), an inappropriate reduction in insulin dosage, or missed injections (especially in adolescents). A common scenario is the patient who fails to increase insulin therapy and consume extra fluids during illness. Prevention requires education in "sick day" management and assessment of urine ketones whenever blood glucose monitoring shows severe hyperglycemia or physical illness is noted.

The two cardinal biochemical features of DKA—hyperglycemia and hyperketonemia—are caused by the combined effects of severe insulin deficiency and excessive secretion of counterregulatory hormones that interact synergistically to magnify the effects of insulin lack. These changes mobilize the delivery of substrates from muscle (amino acids, lactate, pyruvate) and adipose tissue (FFA, glycerol) to the liver, where they are actively converted to glucose (via gluconeogenesis) or ketone bodies (beta-hydroxybutyrate, acetoacetate) and ultimately released into the circulation at rates that greatly exceed the capacity of tissues to utilize them. The net result is hyperglycemia (greater than 300 mg per deciliter), acidosis (pH < 7.35), and an osmotic diuresis leading to marked dehydration. Typically, the history indicates deterioration over days with symptoms of increasing hyperglycemia. Other features may include abdominal pain, anorexia, and nausea. The pain is normally periumbilical and constant in nature and can mimic that pain associated with surgical emergencies. Reduced motility of the gastrointestinal tract, or a paralytic ileus in severe cases, may further contribute to the diagnostic confusion. Vomiting is a threatening symptom, as it precludes oral replacement of the excessive fluid loss caused by the osmotic diuresis; severe volume depletion follows quickly. Physical findings are mainly secondary to dehydration and acidosis and include dry skin and mucous membranes, reduced jugular venous pressure, tachycardia, orthostatic hypotension, depressed mental function, and deep and rapid (termed Kussmaul) respirations. Ketosis is recognizable by a sweet, sickly smell on the patient's breath.

The diagnosis is usually straightforward and should be made promptly. The clinical picture and the presence of severe hyperglycemia should alert the clinician to test for serum ketones, and if possible, to measure arterial pH. The severity of hyperglycemia can vary from 250 to 300 mg per deciliter to > 1000 mg per deciliter, serum bicarbonate is depressed, and there is an increase in the anion gap (the difference between the serum sodium and the sum of the chloride and bicarbonate concentrations) that is generally proportional to the decrease in serum bicarbonate. There may be superimposed hyperchloremia if the patient maintains adequate glomerular filtration rate (GFR) and is able to exchange ketoacid anions for chloride in the kidney. The depression of arterial pH depends on the degree of respiratory compensation; in mild cases pH ranges from 7.20 to 7.35 and in severe cases it may be as low as 6.8 to 6.9. Usually the severity of the clinical presentation depends more on the magnitude of the acidosis than of the hyperglycemia. Occasionally a degree of superimposed metabolic alkalosis (e.g., caused by vomiting or diuretic use) may obscure the true severity of ketoacidosis. An increase in the anion gap out of proportion to the level of bicarbonate should suggest this possibility. Because quantitative measurements of beta-hydroxybutyrate and acetoacetate are not readily available, rapid diagnosis requires qualitative assessment of serum ketones using dilutions of serum and reagent strips (Ketostix) or tablets (acetest). These methods depend on a nitroprusside reaction with acetoacetate. Acetone, however, reacts weakly with nitroprusside and beta-hydroxybutyrate reacts not at all, making the test sometimes misleadingly low. Because of the presence of intracellular acidosis, beta-hydroxybutyrate levels are often much higher than acetoacetate, and the frequent present of concomitant lactic acidosis farther reduces acetoacetate. Conversely, once insulin therapy begins, the nitroprusside reaction often remains "positive" and gives the false impression of sustained ketosis for many hours or days because some beta-hydroxybutyrate is converted to acetoacetate, and nonacidic acetone is cleared slowly from the body. Other laboratory abnormalities in DKA include reduced serum sodium (due to hyperosmolarity and the shift of water from the intravascular to the extravascular space), prerenal azotemia, and hyperamylasemia, which is usually of nonpancreatic origin but can lead to the erroneous diagnosis of pancreatitis. Normal, elevated, or reduced concentrations of potassium, phosphate, and magnesium may exist at the time of presentation of DKA. Nevertheless, large deficits of these electrolytes invariably accompany the osmotic diuresis and become apparent during the course of treatment. Mortality rates for DKA vary between 5 and 10%. For the most part, death occurs in elderly patients (> 65 years) in whom DKA is initiated or complicated by a serious underlying illness. DKA also remains a major cause of death in children with type I diabetes, especially if complicated by the development of cerebral edema.

NONKETOTIC HYPEROSMOLAR SYNDROME. Nonketotic hyperosmolar syndrome is characterized by severe hyperosmolarity (greater than 320 mOsm per liter), hyperglycemia (greater than 600 mg per deciliter), and dehydration. The major reason such severe hyperglycemia occurs is that patients cannot drink enough fluid to keep pace with the osmotic diuresis caused by hyperglycemia. This results in impaired renal function that reduces glucose loss via the kidney, leading to remarkable elevations in blood glucose. The history is usually of an insidious onset with a deterioration over weeks. Patients are often elderly with either mild or undiagnosed type II diabetes. They may be on medications that contribute to the diuresis as well as the impairment in insulin secretion (e.g., thiazide diuretics), or they may be demented or institutionalized and unable to recognize thirst or have access to fluids. Unlike DKA, severe acidosis and ketosis are absent. However, some type II patients with depressed endogenous insulin secretion may be unable to suppress ketone production in the face of elevations in counterregulatory hormones produced by physical illness. Because they have higher portal vein insulin concentrations than type I diabetic patients, ketone production by the liver and in turn the severity of the acidosis are usually mild. The level of consciousness generally correlates with the severity and duration of hyperosmolarity. Only about 10% of patients present in coma, and an equal number show no signs of mental obtundation. A variety of often reversible neurologic abnormalities may exist, including grand mal or focal seizures (about 10% of cases), extensor plantar reflexes, aphasia, hemisensory or motor deficits, delirium, and exacerbation of a pre-existing organic mental syndrome. Clinical signs show profound dehydration; gastrointestinal symptoms are less frequent than in DKA. The laboratory picture is dominated by the effects of uncontrolled diabetes and dehydration; renal function is invariably impaired, hemoglobin is elevated, liver function tests may be abnormal owing to fatty liver, and hypertriglyceridemia may lead to a falsely low serum sodium ("pseudohyponatremia"). Although the severe hyperosmolarity would be expected to lower serum sodium as well, it is not uncommon to see "normal" or even elevated levels due to the severe dehydration. The severity of the hyperosmolar state can be measured directly or estimated according to a formula that excludes urea because it is freely diffusible throughout the body and therefore has little influence on the osmotic pressure gradient:

$$\text{Effective osmolarity (in mOsm/L)} = 2[Na^+ + K^+ (mEqL)] + \frac{\text{plasma glucose (mg/dl)}}{18}$$

A value greater than 320 mOsm per liter reflects hyperosmolarity and greater than 350 mOsm per liter indicates a severe hyperosmolar state. Recent data suggest that mortality is approximately 10 to 20%. Poor outcome is related to age as well as elevated BUN and sodium concentrations. The syndrome may be complicated by thromboembolic events, aspiration, and rhabdomyolysis. Surprisingly, acute renal failure and cerebral edema are relatively uncommon.

MANAGEMENT. The goals of therapy for both DKA and nonketotic hyperosmolar syndrome are to reverse the metabolic disturbance and replace fluid and electrolyte deficits. This requires the prompt delivery of water, electrolytes, and insulin, as well as attention to potential complications that might arise during therapy and treatment of underlying precipitating events.

In the initial stages of therapy, the primary consideration is to restore vascular volume and correct hypoperfusion. At this time a massive total body deficit of water (5 to 12 liters) and sodium (about 5 to 10 mEq per kilogram) requires prompt attention (deficits usually are more profound in nonketotic hyperosmolar syndrome). Although water loss is greater than sodium, it is usually preferable initially to replace fluid deficits with isotonic normal saline (0.9% NaCl solution) so as to restore intravascular volume as quickly as possible. Fluid replacement regimens vary, but it is common to administer 1 liter of normal saline in the first 30 to 60 minutes followed by another liter over the next hour. Therefore, the regimen (normal or half-normal saline) and the rate of infusion (commonly 0.5 liter per hour) should be adjusted over the next 6 hours (and thereafter) based on the response to fluid replacement and the clinical status of the patient (e.g., underlying cardiovascular disease or oliguria). In general, normal saline and hypotonic solutions are alternated for DKA. For nonketotic hyperosmolar syndrome or older patients with DKA, hypotonic solutions are more commonly used. In the latter circumstance, normal saline generally provides more sodium and chloride than the patient needs and may result in hypernatremia; in DKA hypotonic solutions may accelerate the shift of water into the intracellular space and in turn contribute to the development of cerebral edema that may be seen in young patients. During the course of treatment, once blood glucose falls to 250 to 300 mg per deciliter, glucose should be added to the solution to avoid eventual hypoglycemia and to minimize the risk of cerebral edema.

Although insulin resistance is present in both DKA and nonketotic hyperosmolar syndrome, large supraphysiologic doses of insulin are not necessary and are more likely to provoke hypokalemia, hypophosphatemia, and delayed hypoglycemia. A typical insulin replacement regimen is to give an intravenous bolus of 0.1 U per kilogram of rapid-acting (regular) insulin followed by 0.1 U per kilogram per hour thereafter. Intravenous administration is the most predictable way of delivering insulin to target tissues, particularly in the severely hypovolemic patient with reduced peripheral blood flow. If this is not possible, the intramuscular site is preferred to the subcutaneous site because the latter predisposes to unpredictable absorption. It is ideal if blood glucose falls at a steady and predictable rate (about 100 mg per deciliter per hour), so it is important to monitor blood glucose closely after starting insulin to check that the rate of fall is appropriate. Blood glucose should not fall too rapidly, especially in young children, as a rapid fall may be associated with cerebral edema. A steady fall in blood glucose also means that the time at which glucose is added to the regimen may be predicted in advance. When reviewing the progress of treatment, it is important to consider a failure in insulin delivery if blood glucose fails to drop. In some this is due to severe insulin resistance and necessitates an increase in the insulin dose. Because the primary mechanism for lowering plasma glucose in the early stages of treatment is disposal of glucose via the urine rather than by insulin-stimulated glucose consumption, the problem may reflect inadequate replacement of intravascular volume and restoration of GFR or the development of renal failure.

Potassium replacement needs close attention because both hyperkalemia and hypokalemia are associated with cardiac arrhythmia. At the time of presentation, patients have a severe total body deficit of potassium (about 5 mEq per kilogram), yet serum potassium levels may be low, normal, or high (especially if acidosis or renal failure exists). Once one starts intravenous fluid and insulin, serum potassium falls quickly because of an insulin-mediated shift of potassium into the intracellular space. In addition, fluid replacement causes extracellular dilution of potassium and increases potassium removal because of improved renal perfusion. This trend can be countered by potassium replacement based on serum levels. A low potassium requires prompt treatment with 30 to 40 mEq per hour, whereas a normal serum potassium signals the need to ensure an adequate urine output before starting therapy at approximately 20 mEq per hour. In patients who may have lost potassium for other reasons such as diuretic use or gastrointestinal loss, one should anticipate the need for greater potassium supplementation. Patients with circulatory collapse or compromised renal function may not be able to tolerate a potassium load. Electrocardiograms may provide a more direct assessment of intracellular potassium and are recommended. Flat or inverted T waves suggest a low and peaked T waves a high intracellular potassium. The intracellular potassium deficit in renal tubular cells further promotes potassium loss by the kidneys, and this abnormality does not correct immediately. As a result, excess potassium loss may continue for days or weeks.

In most patients with DKA, acidosis disappears with standard therapeutic measures. Artificial correction with alkali (bicarbonate) is unnecessary. Insulin suppresses lipolysis, reducing FFA flux to the liver and ketogenesis. The remaining ketoacids are oxidized, leading to the regeneration of bicarbonate. In severe acidosis, bicarbonate is indicated. The hyperventilatory drive of severe acidosis is uncomfortable, and severe acidosis has a negative inotropic effect and causes vasodilation. However, bicarbonate must be used with caution because it may provoke hypokalemia, which in the context of a falling serum potassium may precipitate a cardiac arrhythmia. In addition, by causing a sudden left shift of the dissociation curve for oxyhemoglobin, bicarbonate may impair oxygen delivery to tissues. At the time of presentation, the dissociation curve for oxyhemoglobin is approximately in the normal position, as the expected right shift caused by acidosis is offset by a left shift due to reduced red cell 2,3-diphosphoglycerate. Sudden correction of acidosis moves the curve to the left, as red cell 2,3-diphosphoglycerate levels recover only slowly during the course of therapy. If alkali is given, small amounts should be slowly administered (44 mEq every 1 to 2 hours) when there is evidence of severe acidosis (pH < 7.0 to 7.1). Therapy should be discontinued when pH rises to about 7.1. Although substantial phosphate depletion occurs with both DKA and nonketotic hyperosmolar syndrome, the prophylactic use of phosphate in DKA has failed to show any significant benefit. Hypocalcemic tetany may complicate phosphate therapy unless magnesium supplements are provided. Because the longer prodro-

mal period associated with nonketotic hyperosmolar syndrome may lead to more severe phosphate losses, they may need to be replaced as potassium phosphate together with magnesium.

The patient's fluid and cardiovascular status must be carefully monitored throughout treatment. When there is severe hypovolemia or renal dysfunction, central venous pressure monitoring is indicated. The presence of cardiac dysfunction or adult respiratory distress syndrome, both recognized complications in severe cases, calls for measuring pulmonary wedge pressure. Urinary catheterization is essential in unconscious or oliguric patients, and gastric decompression may be required to minimize the risk of aspiration. As in any intensive care situation, an accurate record of fluid input and output and key laboratory measurements (every 1 to 2 hours), such as plasma glucose, arterial pH, and electrolytes, allow an ongoing review of progress. Even more important is the need to search for a possible coexisting illness; serious medical illness may easily be overlooked for several hours during the early phases of therapy. In children, monitoring of mental status is crucial because of their risk of cerebral edema. Leukocytosis often accompanies DKA or nonketotic hyperosmolar syndrome and should not be taken as a rationale for antibiotic prophylaxis.

ALCOHOLIC KETOACIDOSIS. This syndrome may be confused with DKA, particularly when hyperglycemia is present. It typically is seen in people who have consumed large amounts of alcohol and then abstain from food or drink for an extended period. Commonly, the patient is anorectic and has nausea and vomiting, prolonging the period of starvation. The syndrome is characterized by severe ketoacidosis and dehydration. Hyperglycemia is inconsistent; it may exist in association with underlying diabetes (or pancreatitis) or be mildly present in nondiabetic subjects. The stress of the illness, volume depletion, activation of the sympathetic nervous system following alcohol withdrawal, prolonged starvation, or probably a combination of these factors results in a fall in insulin and a rise in glucagon levels. The combination markedly accelerates ketogenesis. Hyperglycemia is probably limited because hepatic metabolism of alcohol leads to an increase in the NADH/NAD ratio, which inhibits gluconeogenesis despite insulin deficiency. Alcoholic ketoacidosis is rapidly reversed by intravenous administration of fluids and glucose; insulin is rarely needed, except in diabetic persons.

HYPOGLYCEMIA. Severe hypoglycemia is the most frequent complication in type I diabetes. It symptomatically affects 10 to 25% of these patients at least once a year. The condition can vary widely, from requiring just the help of another person to being severe enough to require emergency medical assistance. The frequency of less disabling hypoglycemia is even higher. From a practical standpoint, data showing that near-normoglycemia prevents the long-term vascular complications of diabetes has resulted in a much greater frequency of severe hypoglycemia in insulin-treated patients and renewed interest in its physiology and prevention. The less common event of hypoglycemia induced by oral glucose-lowering agents should not be overlooked. This tends to occur in elderly diabetics with impaired renal function and is generally associated with the longer-acting sulfonylureas. The management is no different from the treatment of insulin-induced hypoglycemia, but because of the long-acting nature of oral agents hypoglycemia may recur for 24 to 48 hours after drug withdrawal. Prolonged and severe hypoglycemia can cause irreversible brain damage; it has been less clear what, if any, neurologic damage is caused by milder episodes of hypoglycemia. Some studies have shown that EEG abnormalities are more prevalent in young children who have a history of recurrent hypoglycemia. The DCCT, on the other hand, reported no evidence of neuropsychological impairment after an average of 7 years of intensified treatment, even in patients with recurrent severe hypoglycemic episodes. Nevertheless, hypoglycemia may provoke seizures, accidental injury, and a catecholamine response that can induce arrhythmias or cardiac ischemia in patients with underlying cardiac disease. Hypoglycemia is thought to account for 3 to 4% of deaths in insulin-treated diabetic patients. It also has far-reaching social implications. At a personal level, it can become the patient's greatest fear and lead the patient and clinician to aim deliberately for less than optimal glycemic control.

In normal persons, hypoglycemia provokes a response that returns blood glucose to normal. This involves three defense mechanisms: (1) insulin dissipation, (2) counterregulatory hormone secretion and action, and (3) a subjective awareness of hypoglycemia, resulting in ingestion of carbohydrate. The brain cannot synthesize or store more than a few minutes' supply of glucose and, in the short term, is wholly dependent on a constant supply of glucose. If glucose efflux from the circulation exceeds exogenous and endogenous influx, hypoglycemia results. Spontaneous recovery of blood glucose involves a complex response that includes activation of hepatic glucose production and, to a lesser extent, diminution of peripheral glucose uptake. These changes are triggered when plasma glucose begins to approach the hypoglycemic range (60 to 70 mg per deciliter). The rise in glucose production is initiated by the release of glucagon as well as epinephrine in conjunction with a fall in endogenous insulin release and, at the outset, probably reflects mainly the stimulation of hepatic glycogenolysis. When hypoglycemia is sustained, other hormones such as GH and cortisol help to ensure the continued glucose production via gluconeogenesis. Multiple factors contribute to the diminution in glucose uptake, including epinephrine's inhibitory effect on insulin-stimulated glucose uptake, insulin disappearance, elevations of free fatty acids and hypoglycemia *per se*.

Type I diabetic patients are much more prone to hypoglycemia for several reasons. Insulin enters the circulation from a nonphysiologic source (e.g., a subcutaneous depot) that is unaffected by regulatory responses to a falling blood glucose. In addition, these patients for unclear reasons have attenuated or absent glucagon secretion during hypoglycemia, although glucagon responses to other stimuli persist. Most patients develop defective glucagon responses after 2 to 5 years, about the time they become totally insulin-dependent. Consequently, they must rely heavily on their ability to release epinephrine. Unfortunately, nearly half of type I patients with disease for over 10 years also undergo a stimulus-specific diminution of their epinephrine response to hypoglycemia that increases its risk. The ability of type I patients to recognize hypoglycemia and take corrective action may be impaired as well, further adding to the risk. Symptoms result from changes in autonomic activity and brain function. Autonomic symptoms, including sweating, tremor, and palpitations, are often the earliest subjective warning of hypoglycemia. Symptoms and signs of glucose deficiency in the central nervous system, termed neuroglycopenia, may be nonspecific. (e.g., fatigue or weakness) or more clearly neurologic (e.g., double vision, oral paresthesias, slurring of speech, apraxia, and behavioral disturbances). The irritability and confusion that occur during hypoglycemia may prevent a patient's awareness of their cause. Some diabetic patients lose their normal autonomic warning symptoms of hypoglycemia and may recognize the condition only when somatic neurologic function becomes impaired. The loss of awareness of symptoms is more likely to be found in patients with long disease duration and is associated with an absent or impaired sympathoadrenal response. The duration of diabetes, however, is not the only factor responsible for impaired adrenergic and symptomatic responses to hypoglycemia. Similar phenomena may also occur when patients are switched to intensive insulin regimens, which at least partly may explain the increased frequency of severe hypoglycemia reported in the DCCT. Recent studies indicate that the introduction of intensified treatment regimens may lower the glucose level that triggers epinephrine release and adrenergic symptoms (Fig. 205–8). The major cause for this phenomenon is the increased appearance of iatrogenic hypoglycemia during intensified insulin therapy because brief periods of hypoglycemia suppress counterregulatory hormone responses and symptoms during subsequent hypoglycemia for several days. Defective glucose counterregulation induced by intensive insulin regimens appears to be reversible by scrupulous avoidance of hypoglycemia and a readjustment of treatment goals, underscoring the need to prevent hypoglycemia by improving self-management skills.

Pathogenesis of Chronic Diabetic Complications

The pathogenesis of the microvascular and neuropathic complications of diabetes remains poorly understood. Proteins are readily glycosylated *in vivo* in direct proportion to prevailing levels of glucose. The relative nonspecificity of the process is underscored by the fact that nonenzymatic glycosylation involves not only hemoglobin but also serum and membrane proteins, low density lipoproteins (LDL), peripheral nerve protein (tubulin), and structural pro-

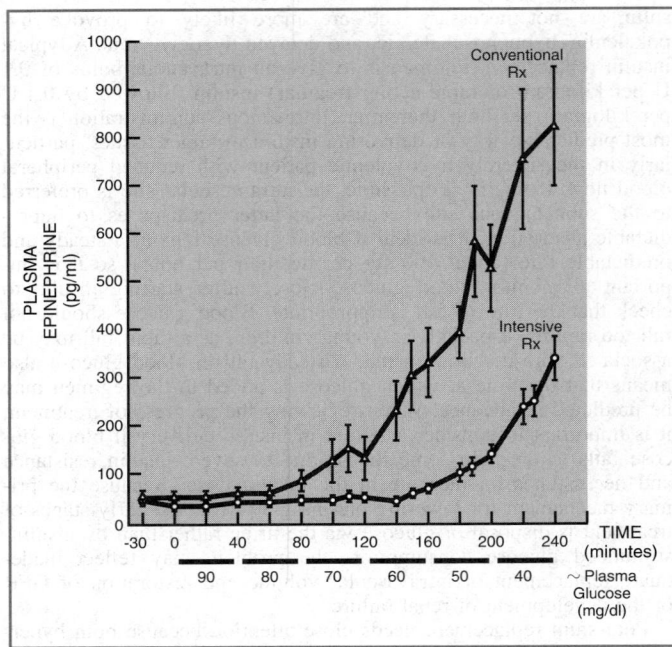

FIGURE 205–8. Plasma epinephrine levels during a stepwise reduction in plasma glucose levels from 90 to 40 mg per deciliter over 4 hours in patients with type I diabetes before *(triangles)* and after several months of intensive insulin treatment *(circles)*. (Adapted from Amiel SA, Sherwin RS, Simonson DC, Tamborlane WV: Diabetes 37:901, 1988.)

teins. This has led to the idea that hyperglycemia induces widespread modifications of cellular and structural proteins that contribute to long-term complications. Available data suggest that advanced glycosylation end products (AGE's) have adverse functional consequences. AGE's are generated by the nonenzymatic glycosylation of long-lived proteins (e.g., collagen, laminin) that are further modified by the Maillard reaction, resulting in accumulation of proteins with glucose-derived cross-links in a variety of tissues, including the kidneys and blood vessels. In experimental diabetic animals, inhibition of AGE formation not only reduces tissue deposition of AGE's but also inhibits the expansion of glomerular volume and urinary protein excretion in the absence of changes in circulating glucose levels. These observations suggest that at least some complications may be amenable to agents that do not depend on reversing hyperglycemia. Another potential biochemical mechanism through which hyperglycemia could impair cell function involves the polyol pathway through which nonphosphorylated glucose is reduced to sorbitol by aldose reductase and sorbitol is converted to fructose by sorbitol dehydrogenase. Polyol pathway activity is regulated by the intracellular concentration of free glucose and therefore varies according to glucose levels in insulin-independent tissues. It has been postulated that accumulated sorbitol might exert osmotic effects that could lead to cell injury or to depletion of myoinositol. Beneficial effects of aldose reductase inhibitors and myoinositol therapy, however, have not been convincingly shown in patients.

Hemodynamic changes in the microcirculation may also contribute to microangiopathy. In the kidney, GFR is increased out of proportion to plasma flow owing to an elevation in the transglomerular pressure gradient. It has been postulated that the raised glomerular pressures contribute to renal disease based on the observation that single-nephron hyperfiltration after partial renal ablation in the nondiabetic rat causes proteinuria and progressive glomerular damage in the remnant kidney. Similarly, the hemodynamic alterations of diabetes may cause transglomerular passage of proteins and AGE's; with time their accumulation in the mesangium could trigger proliferation of mesangial cells and matrix production, eventually leading to glomerulosclerosis. Less affected glomeruli would develop compensatory hyperfiltration but ultimately succumb, as does the remnant kidney. Clinical studies support this view. Unilateral renal artery stenosis diminishes diabetic pathologic lesions in the affected kidney, and angiotensin-converting enzyme inhibitors, which reduce intraglomerular pressure, slow progression of diabetic nephropathy. The diabetes-associated increase in microcirculatory hydrostatic pressure also may contribute to the generalized capillary leakage of macromolecules in diabetic patients.

The above theories would predict the benefits of optimal glycemic control reported by the DCCT in patients with few or no complications. Whether similar benefits can be expected once severe damage has occurred is less clear. Extensive glycosylation of proteins with slow turnover rates would not be readily affected by correction of hyperglycemia. Moreover, the hemodynamic theory for nephropathy predicts that once glomerular injury causes compensatory hyperfiltration, progressive injury would continue in the remaining glomeruli, regardless of the metabolic state.

Diabetic Retinopathy

Diabetes is the leading cause of blindness in persons aged 30 to 65 years. Blindness occurs 20 times more frequently in diabetic patients than others and is most often seen after the disease has been manifest for at least 15 years. Approximately 10 to 15% of type I diabetic patients become legally blind (visual acuity of 20/200 or worse in the better eye), whereas in type II diabetic patients the risk is less than half that value. The primary cause of visual loss is retinopathy.

The earliest retinopathic changes are classified as nonproliferative. The first sign is microaneurysms (small red dots 20 to 200 μm), which typically arise in areas of capillary occlusion. Microaneurysms develop after about 3 to 5 years of diabetes and are seen in most conventionally treated patients who have had diabetes for 10 years. Subsequently, retinal blot hemorrhages (round with blurred edges) and hard exudates (variable size, sharply defined and yellow) appear due, respectively, to extravasation of blood and lipoproteins. Infarctions of the nerve fiber layer, called "cotton wool spots" or "soft exudates," may be observed as white or gray rounded swellings. These lesions generally do not affect visual acuity. Advanced nonproliferative lesions occur if retinal ischemia becomes more severe, including intraretinal microvascular abnormalities (IRMA), dilated capillaries that are very permeable, and venous irregularities. They compose the "preproliferative phase" of retinopathy, which predicts a high risk for proliferative retinopathy within 1 to 2 years. Proliferative retinopathy is characterized by the growth of fine tufts of new blood vessels and fibrous tissue from the inner retinal surface or optic nerve head. The vessels and fibrous tissue begin on the retinal surface and later grow into the vitreous, leading to retinal detachments and hemorrhages, the most important contributors to blindness. Occasionally, new vessels may invade the anterior chamber angle, leading to intractable glaucoma, severe pain, and blindness. Some patients without proliferative changes may also develop severe visual loss due to vascular leakage (macular edema) and/or vascular occlusion in the area of the macula. Macular edema may be suggested by the presence of large deposits of hard exudates surrounding the macular area but is often undetectable by direct ophthalmoscopy. Maculopathy is more common in type II diabetes and represents an important cause of decreased visual acuity in this group. Visual loss in diabetes is further complicated by high prevalence rates of cataracts and open angle glaucoma. Diabetic patients commonly report changes in vision resulting from osmotic swelling of the lens due to hyperglycemia. These changes are reversed by improved glycemic control and must be distinguished from more serious ocular pathology.

The eye provides a unique window through which to follow the appearance and progression of retinopathy. Regardless of the type of diabetes, the severity of retinopathy increases with increasing duration of the disease. The one exception is early childhood diabetes; before puberty retinopathy (as well as other complications) is less common regardless of disease duration. Prevalence rates of both nonproliferative and proliferative retinopathy are higher in type I than in type II diabetes. In conventionally treated type I diabetes, patients rarely, if ever, exhibit retinopathy when first diagnosed. Thereafter, the frequency of retinopathy rises to 20 to 25% at 5 years, 50 to 70% at 10 years, and >95% after 15 years. Proliferative retinopathy is rare within the first 10 years of type I diabetes, but increases to 50% after 20 years. It is less common in type II diabetes, appearing in about 10 to 15% of patients after 20 years. Retinopathy affects about 15 to 20% of type II diabetic patients at the time of disease detection, implying that the disease had previously been undetected.

Although retinopathy may be triggered by hyperglycemia, eventually retinal vascular perfusion diminishes, and this is believed to accelerate the process. New vessels generally appear in areas of nonperfusion. Ischemia may provoke local production of insulin-like growth factor I, a stimulator of retinal angioneogenesis in animals and other growth factors. Epidemiologic studies show a higher prevalence of retinopathy and macular edema in patients with hypertension; nephropathy and pregnancy also appear to accelerate retinopathy. At present, medical therapy is restricted to optimization of glycemic control, which delays and slows progression of nonproliferative retinopathy. Little evidence suggests that improving glycemic control benefits the more advanced stages of retinopathy. In addition, it makes sense to treat hypertension aggressively. Surgical therapy using retinal photocoagulation is the treatment of choice when progressive retinopathy threatens vision. Its value was established by the prospective Diabetic Retinopathy Study involving patients with proliferative retinopathy. The risk of severe visual loss in treated eyes was less than half of that in untreated eyes. The study also defined the advantage of panretinal photocoagulation for proliferative lesions (e.g., involving the disc, associated with hemorrhage), which posed the highest risk for visual loss. The more recent Early Treatment Diabetic Retinopathy Study involved patients at an earlier stage and showed an even more striking reduction in the risk of visual loss after laser therapy. It established the benefit of photocoagulation for all patients with new vessels, regardless of severity, and for macular edema. The trial found that interventions at the nonproliferative stage had no detectable value. In more advanced proliferative retinopathy, vitrectomy may be required to remove vitreous hemorrhage or to cut extensive fibrous bands causing retinal detachments. In such cases, surgery may restore vision although vitrectomy has risks, including retinal detachment, cataract formation, and glaucoma.

The above considerations make it imperative for physicians to identify prospectively patients at risk. Nonspecialists, including house officers, internists, and diabetologists, have difficulty in diagnosing proliferative retinopathy; in one study they correctly diagnosed proliferative retinopathy in less than half the cases! Accordingly, diabetic patients should be advised to have annual ophthalmologic examinations. In type I diabetes ophthalmologic visits should begin within 5 years, whereas type II diabetic patients should be seen from disease onset.

Diabetic Nephropathy

End-stage renal disease (ESRD) from diabetic nephropathy is a major cause of death, particularly in type I diabetes, in which it affects 30 to 35% of patients. Although it is less frequent (about 15 to 20%) in the type II diabetic population, this more common form of the disease still constitutes the majority of diabetic patients seeking therapy for ESRD. Overall, diabetes is the leading cause and accounts for one third of the ESRD cases in the United States.

The natural history of diabetic nephropathy has been well characterized in type I diabetes (Fig. 205–9); much less data are available in type II. Soon after diagnosis, GFR is commonly increased, associated with renal hypertrophy and an increase in glomerular volume and capillary surface area. Hyperfiltration appears to depend on hyperglycemia because it is reversed by intensive treatment. After several years glomerulosclerosis appears, characterized by thickening of the glomerular capillary basement membrane and the expansion of collagen matrix material within the mesangial region, as well as arteriolosclerosis. In the early years of this histologic evolution, renal function is not impaired and on routine urinalysis test strips show no evidence of proteinuria. Although most patients continue to develop mesangial and capillary wall change as the duration of diabetes increases, only a minority develop sufficiently extensive glomerulosclerosis to cause ESRD. Renal biopsy specimens from these individuals generally show more pronounced expansion of mesangial volume and diffuse deposits of mesangial matrix that presumably encroach on glomerular filtering capacity. Accordingly, routine tests of renal function (e.g., serum creatinine and urinalysis) remain normal during a long "silent" period as glomerular compromise gradually progresses.

In patients destined to develop ESRD, gross proteinuria (greater than 0.3 gram of albumin per day) begins approximately 15 years after the diagnosis of diabetes. At this time, renal function remains

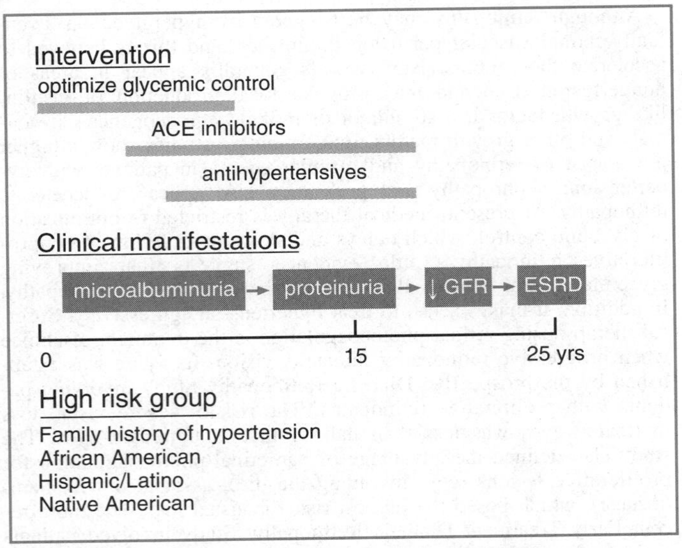

Intervention

optimize glycemic control

ACE inhibitors

antihypertensives

Clinical manifestations

microalbuminuria → proteinuria → ↓ GFR → ESRD

0   15   25 yrs

High risk group

Family history of hypertension
African American
Hispanic/Latino
Native American

FIGURE 205–9. The natural history of diabetic nephropathy and the time sequence of various medical interventions.

normal, but hypertension is often present. After a variable period of time, however, (about 3 years), GFR diminishes, as reflected by an increase in serum creatinine. The appearance of massive proteinuria and the nephrotic syndrome is common in this context and often heralds progression to renal insufficiency. Once serum creatinine rises (reflecting a 40 to 50% decline in GFR), most patients develop ESRD within 10 years. The course is highly variable, however, particularly in type II diabetes, in which moderate proteinuria may persist for many years without substantive deterioration in renal function. A simple but useful method of following progression of renal failure is to plot the reciprocal of the serum creatinine as a function of time. This allows better assessment of therapeutic interventions and the time when dialysis will be necessary.

Several potential complications accentuate renal dysfunction in diabetes. Azotemic patients are at higher risk to develop acute renal failure after injection of contrast for diagnostic studies. When such tests are necessary, special attention should be given to ensure adequate hydration before and immediately after the procedure. Other types of renal disease are also more prevalent in diabetes. Asymptomatic bacteruria and pyelonephritis are about twice as common, especially in women. This is due to multiple factors, including autonomic bladder dysfunction, impaired perfusion, and glycosuria, which enhances bacterial growth. Papillary necrosis is associated with diabetes in over half the cases, and renal artery stenosis is more common in patients with diabetes. Particularly in patients receiving ACE inhibitors, hyperkalemia may develop. A variety of other factors contribute to this, including insulin deficiency, metabolic acidosis, reduced GFR, tubulointerstitial disease, and the syndrome of hyporeninemic hypoaldosteronism commonly seen in older patients with impaired renal function.

A genetic predisposition to hypertension and persistent elevations of GFR predict an increased risk of nephropathy. Erythrocyte sodium-lithium countertransport, a marker of essential hypertension that is increased in some type I patients with nephropathy, may provide the link between a family history of hypertension and nephropathy. The risk of nephropathy is three- to six-fold higher in African-Americans, Latinos, and Native Americans with type II diabetes, a frequency similar to that seen in type I diabetes (Fig. 205–9). Although type I patients destined to develop nephropathy may have no signs on routine testing, they pass through a stage during which they excrete small amounts of albumin (or microalbuminuria) detectable only by sensitive assay techniques (40 to 300 mg per day). The appearance of hypertension increases the likelihood that microalbuminuria will progress to nephropathy. In patients with type II diabetes, progression of microalbuminuria to clinical proteinuria is slower and may reflect severe generalized vascular disease rather than nephropathy. The importance of detecting microalbuminuria is underscored by evidence that its progression to nephropathy can be prevented or delayed by optimized glycemic control, angiotensin-converting enzyme (ACE) inhibitors, and hypertension control. Albumin excretion rates should be confirmed at least once before intervening because transient microalbuminuria can be induced by nonspecific factors such as severe hyperglycemia or heavy exercise.

Treatment of nephropathy varies depending on the stage of disease (Fig. 205–9). Early in the course of diabetes (no microalbuminuria), primary efforts should focus on optimizing glycemic control, especially in higher-risk patients. Other measures should include aggressive treatment of coexisting hypertension as well as routine screening for asymptomatic urinary tract infections and bladder dysfunction. We recommend strict glycemic control for patients with microalbuminuria. ACE inhibitors appear to have special value, with benefits such as retarding proteinuria, that are independent of their blood pressure–lowering effects. Once clinical nephropathy becomes evident, aggressive efforts at glycemic control have marginal value; reducing hypertension and intraglomerular pressure remain the only proven means of slowing progression. In addition to ACE inhibitors alone or in combination with other antihypertensives, calcium channel blockers have potential value, although their long-term benefits have not been formally tested. Dietary protein restriction (i.e., 0.8 gram per kilogram of body weight) may add limited benefit once GFR becomes subnormal. As ESRD approaches, long-term treatment plans should proceed much as they would in nondiabetic uremic patients, but therapy should be instituted earlier. Diabetic patients tolerate uremia poorly: retinopathy and neuropathy deteriorate more rapidly, hypertension becomes more difficult to control, glycemic excursions increase, and protein wasting is aggravated. Generalized atherosclerosis accelerates, leading to significant morbidity during dialysis or following transplantation. The decision between transplantation and dialysis should be individualized. Renal transplantation represents the treatment of choice for most young patients, especially if one can find a matched living-related donor. Survival rates for recipients of cadaver grafts remain high and are only about 10% less than for nondiabetic graft recipients. Cardiovascular disease provides the major cause of morbidity and mortality following transplantation. Accordingly, transplant candidates should be evaluated prospectively and treated for vascular insufficiency. Most older type II patients are offered dialysis. The preference between continuous ambulatory peritoneal dialysis and hemodialysis varies among centers. However, many diabetic patients have problems caused by the rapid shifts in blood volume that accompany hemodialysis. Although survival rates are considerably worse for dialysis than transplantation, this difference largely reflects the fact that the patients are older and have more severe underlying disease. Mortality is substantially higher in diabetic than nondiabetic patients receiving dialysis owing to the more rapid development of vascular insufficiency.

Diabetic Neuropathy

Symptomatic, potentially disabling neuropathy affects nearly 50% of diabetic patients. It may be symmetrical or focal and often involves the autonomic nervous system as well. The prevalence of symmetrical neuropathy is similar in type I and II diabetes, whereas focal neuropathy is more common in older type II patients. Because it is a heterogeneous collection of clinical syndromes, multiple pathogenetic factors are likely involved. Hyperglycemia figures prominently; however, other factors may also be important, especially ischemia. The chronic, more insidious neuropathic disorders may be mediated by a "metabolic" process, whereas the more acute, often self-limiting neuropathies may have a vascular cause. Nerve growth factor is diminished in nerves of patients with neuropathy, perhaps limiting regenerative capacity. Autonomic nerve bundles and ganglia from type I diabetic patients with autonomic neuropathy show monocytic infiltration, and their sera may contain complement-fixing antibodies to sympathetic ganglia, suggesting that autoimmune mechanisms contribute to this complication. Because the mechanisms producing such a heterogeneous clinical picture are poorly understood, neuropathy is classified according to areas affected (Table 205–8). Currently, therapy is limited to improving glycemic control. This is effective mainly before clinical symptoms have developed. The usefulness of aldose reductase inhibitors has been difficult to establish, perhaps because more advanced cases were studied.

TABLE 205-8. CLASSIFICATION OF DIABETIC NEUROPATHY

Polyneuropathies	Mononeuropathies
Distal symmetrical	Isolated nerve lesions
Chronic sensorimotor	Peripheral
Acute sensory	Cranial
Proximal motor	Radiculopathy
Autonomic	

DISTAL SENSORIMOTOR NEUROPATHY. This syndrome, characterized by axonal loss, is the most common presentation of diabetic neuropathy. The process involves all somatic nerves but has a distinct predilection for distal sites, i.e., the distal sensorimotor nerves of the feet and hands. Patients complain of numbness and tingling in the extremities, especially the feet. Symptoms characteristically worsen at night, and function usually declines relentlessly with time. In early cases, the neuropathy can be asymptomatic and may be discovered only during a clinical examination. Sometimes, distal neuropathy first expresses its presence via complications, such as foot ulceration or spreading cellulitis from a traumatic cut (see below). Bedside clinical testing typically demonstrates a symmetrical loss of sensation distally, with variable loss of distal reflexes (e.g., ankle) and muscle wasting of the intrinsic muscles of the hands and feet. Damage usually affects sensory more than motor fibers and usually encompasses both small (pain and temperature) and large (position and touch) sensory fibers. In less obvious cases, subtler deficits may be detected by testing thermal discrimination, vibration sense thresholds, and nerve conduction. Because the clinical picture is not distinguishable from other forms of distal neuropathy (e.g., alcohol, heavy metals, uremia, amyloidosis), the diagnosis is one of exclusion.

ACUTE SENSORY NEUROPATHY. This less common form of neuropathy is symptomatically distressing but usually self limiting. It may develop after a period of altered metabolic control, such as an episode of DKA. It is characterized by severe pain, hyperesthesias, and a worsening of pain at night. The hyperesthesia can be so severe that even contact with bedclothes brings on distressing pain. Some cases are associated with weight loss and depression. Pathologic studies show a loss of small sensory fibers. Occasionally, small fiber injury is selective, leaving vibratory and position sense and motor function intact.

PROXIMAL MOTOR NEUROPATHY. This syndrome, also known as diabetic amyotrophy or femoral neuropathy, affects males more than females and tends to occur in elderly type II patients. It is characterized by wasting and weakness of the major proximal muscle groups of the pelvis and may be accompanied by sensory defects, often with a femoral nerve distribution. The anterolateral muscles of the calf are less often involved. Occasionally there is extension plantar response. There is some overlap with the clinical features of acute sensory neuropathy in that most such patients have suffered recent severe weight loss and many are depressed. Nerve biopsies show ischemic changes in keeping with a vascular cause. This form of neuropathy has a good prognosis; most cases resolve within 12 months.

MONONEUROPATHIES. The mononeuropathies are a collection of isolated lesions affecting cranial or peripheral nerves. They usually have a sudden onset and occur most often asymmetrically. The oculomotor, trochlear, and abducens nerves mark the most common sites for a cranial nerve lesion, with lesions of the oculomotor nerve characteristically sparing the pupillary reflex. The median, radial, and lateral popliteal nerves are the most common sites of peripheral nerve lesions. The cause of such lesions is unknown, but the sudden onset suggests a vascular component. Nerve entrapment may contribute to peripheral nerve lesions. Painful radiculopathies may also occur in the distribution of one or a number of spinal roots, presenting as an asymmetric lesion in a well-defined dermatome(s) that may be confused with herpetic neuralgia or occasionally with abdominal or cardiac disease. The mononeuropathies and radiculopathies are symptomatically distressing, but all tend to resolve with time.

AUTONOMIC NEUROPATHY. Symptomatic, autonomic diabetic neuropathy produces a wide range of problems and carries a poor prognosis. It usually accompanies other chronic complications of diabetes and through disturbed regulation of local blood flow may play a role in their pathogenesis. Neuropathic lesions may result in abnormalities of the cardiovascular system, skin, gastrointestinal tract, bladder, and sexual function. In recent years a battery of tests of cardiac autonomic function based on reduced changes in the RR interval of the ECG following a Valsava maneuver or standing have proved useful diagnostically. The most disabling cardiovascular effect is orthostatic hypotension, caused by an impaired sympathetic vasoconstrictor response and possibly impaired cardiac reflexes. Medications that cause volume depletion or vasodilation may worsen the hypotension. More commonly, cardiac denervation results in a rapid heart rate and an impaired rate response to stress. Patients with cardiovascular autonomic neuropathy are more likely to have silent myocardial ischaemia or infarction, an abnormal prolongation of the QT interval, and defective heart rate and blood pressure responses to exercise, each of which is potentially capable of precipitating an acute cardiac event. Autonomic sudomotor dysfunction is characterized by distal anhidrosis, compensatory truncal and facial sweating, heat intolerance, and on occasion, gustatory sweating. Heat stroke and hyperthermia are the most serious risk, especially when vascular disease is present. It may also facilitate foot infections by creating breaks in the skin. Altered gastrointestinal function is frequent. The most common symptom is constipation, but diarrhea is often the most distressing. Diarrhea may have a variety of causes, including hypermotility due to impaired sympathetic inhibition, hypomotility leading to bacterial overgrowth, pancreatic insufficiency, or a spruelike syndrome. The problem may be compounded by fecal incontinence due to the loss of sphincter control and intensification of diarrhea during sleep. Gastroparesis may lead to complaints such as bloating and early satiety after meals, or nausea and vomiting. This is a problem for patients on insulin, in whom unpredictable food absorption may adversely affect glycemic control and exacerbate hypoglycemia. Bladder dysfunction caused by neuropathy leads to infrequent urination, incomplete bladder emptying, dribbling, and overflow incontinence. Bladder residual volumes may exceed 150 ml, predisposing to urinary tract infection. Psychologically, the most disturbing complication of autonomic neuropathy is impaired sexual function consisting of male impotence and retrograde ejaculation. The prevalence may be as high as 50% in males and 25% in females at some point in the disease. One must exclude psychogenic or other organic causes of impotence due to medications, alcohol, or vascular insufficiently which may be correctable.

TREATMENT. In the absence of specific ways to reverse established neuropathy, pain control is the highest priority. Some patients respond to standard analgesic therapies, and tricyclic antidepressants have shown some efficacy in prospective randomized trials. Intravenous lidocaine or the analogue oral mexiletine may be of benefit when pain is severe. Occasionally, opiates are the only option. Autonomic neuropathy causes specific problems for which more therapeutic interventions are available. Stocking supports, 9α-fluorohydrocortisone, pindolol (a β blocker with partial agonist properties), and clonidine have all been used with mixed success for orthostatic hypotension. Metoclopramide and cisapride can stimulate gastric emptying in cases of gastroparesis. Erythromycin also stimulates gastric emptying and may be helpful. These patients should avoid high-fiber diets, which interfere with treatment. Diarrhea may respond to broad-spectrum antibiotics, clonidine, or agents such as diphenoxylate or Imodium, and bladder emptying may be enhanced by drugs such as bethanechol. The treatment of impotence in males includes vacuum erection aids, intracorporeal papaverine or phentolamine injections, and penile prosthetic implants.

Diabetic Foot

The "diabetic foot" results from a complex interplay of factors. The syndrome is characterized by plantar ulcers that heal slowly and follow apparently insignificant trauma. In severe cases gangrene may be a complication and amputation the outcome. Diabetes accounts for about one half of nontraumatic limb amputations. To varying degrees, the diabetic foot is characterized by chronic sensorimotor neuropathy, autonomic neuropathy, and poor peripheral circulation; visual loss may also contribute to the difficulties with self-care. Sensorimotor neuropathy results in a loss of normal sensation, preventing detection of traumatic events. Accordingly, sharp objects left in the sole of the shoe or ill-fitting shoes may erode the skin surface without signalling pain. Neuropathy also produces abnormal motor function of the intrinsic muscles of the foot and abnormal proprioception, thereby altering weight distribution on the sole. Unnatural weight bearing on the metatarsal heads and clawing of the metatarsophalangeal joints result. Also callous formation occurs at these sites which may erode the softer underlying tissues. In severe cases the abnormal distribution of weight endured by the foot can result in repeated painless fractures and displacement of normal joint surfaces producing the so-called Charcot joint. Impaired peripheral circulation often coexists. Atheromatous plaques in the descending aorta, major vessels of the leg, or distal sites compromise flow. Diminished cardiac output due to cardiovascular disease and/or disturbed autoregulatory mechanisms of the microcirculation may contribute to impaired peripheral blood flow. Characteristically the diabetic foot, in the absence of severe atheromatous disease, appears well perfused with a skin surface that is normally warm and dry. This is thought to be due to increased skin blood flow and reduced sweating, both features of impaired autonomic regulation. Treatment of the diabetic foot is aimed primarily at prevention. This involves education (Table 205–9) and regular checking of the state of the feet of patients at risk during routine visits and by foot care specialists. Proper preventive foot care can reduce the rate of amputations by 50%. In cases of deformed feet, orthotics to minimize abnormal weight bearing or orthopedically fitted shoes may be required. It is essential that ulcers be treated early with antibiotics, dead tissue debridement, and appropriate dressings. Cast immobilization made for the foot may be a useful adjunct to the treatment of foot ulcers by redistributing weight away from an ulcerated area. Surgical removal or débridement is required for nonviable tissues such as gangrenous toes or deep soft tissue infections with evidence of gas gangrene. In extensive cases, foot or even leg amputation may be necessary; a compromised peripheral circulation makes this outcome more likely. If poor circulation is a dominant feature, one must attempt to improve distal flow by surgery or angioplasty.

Atherosclerosis and Hypertension

Atherosclerosis involving the arteries of the heart, lower extremities, and brain is the major cause of death from diabetes. The atherosclerotic process is indistinguishable from that affecting the nondiabetic population but begins earlier and is more severe. The predilection to atherosclerosis is uniformly observed over the entire spectrum of diabetes—from difficult-to-control insulin-dependent patients to patients with mild hyperglycemia not requiring insulin. For unclear reasons, the disparity between diabetic and normal subjects is more pronounced in women.

Accelerated atherosclerosis in diabetes is an independent risk factor not solely attributable to an increased frequency of the other recognized factors, e.g., hypertension or dyslipidemia. Whereas microvascular and neuropathic complications develop more commonly in individuals showing the highest glucose levels, this is not true for atherosclerotic complications. Other abnormalities induced by diabetes could be responsible such as small dense atherogenic LDL, oxidized or glycated LDL, increased platelet aggregation, hyperviscosity, endothelial cell dysfunction, decreased fibrinolysis, and increased clotting factors and fibrinogen. Clinical studies indirectly support the concept that hyperinsulinemia *per se* may contribute to macrovascular disease in diabetes, perhaps because of its stimulatory effects on smooth muscle proliferation. Both type II and type I diabetic patients (because they receive insulin via the systemic route) commonly have elevated insulin levels in the systemic circulation, despite the presence of hyperglycemia.

Diabetes may be accompanied by other risk factors for atherosclerosis that markedly increase the incidence of macrovascular complications. The prevalence of hypertension is increased at least twofold in patients with type II diabetes, owing in part to the clustering of both disorders in patients with obesity and insulin resistance. Hypertension is not associated with type I diabetes in the absence of renal disease but develops in most patients with nephropathy. Although LDL-cholesterol levels are not higher in diabetes, dyslipidemia characterized by elevated triglycerides, decreased HDL cholesterol, and smaller, denser LDL cholesterol commonly develops in type II diabetic patients and in poorly controlled type I diabetes. The major cardiovascular risk factors—hypertension, hypercholesterolemia, and smoking—synergize with diabetes to promote atherosclerosis. As a result, the risk of myocardial infarction is two- to three-fold greater in diabetes, but increases to about eight-fold in the presence of hypertension, and to about 20-fold if hypercholesterolemia coexists. Smoking enhances the risk even further. The diagnosis of diabetes should prompt a careful search for other risk factors for atherosclerotic vascular disease and initiate aggressive preventive measures.

Because hypertension accelerates not only atherosclerosis but also nephropathy and probably retinopathy, it is important to treat even minimal elevations of blood pressure that in nondiabetics might be dismissed. The normal nocturnal fall in blood pressure may be lost in diabetic patients, leading to more sustained hypertension throughout the day. Initially, nonpharmacologic measures such as weight loss, exercise training, and sodium restriction should be tried. If blood pressure is not lowered *below* 130/85 mm Hg, drug therapy is indicated. Among the various therapeutic options, ACE inhibitors offer special advantages, especially when there is concomitant renal disease. Unlike thiazide diuretics and β-adrenergic blockers, they do not adversely effect glycemic and lipid control. Their use should, however, be restricted in patients with hyperkalemia. Calcium channel blockers, α-adrenergic blockers, and vasodilators have no adverse metabolic effects and therefore are good alternatives. The selection of drugs should be individualized, taking into consideration other coexisting medical problems. Diuretics may be helpful as adjuncts if there is a volume component to the hypertension. If thiazides are used, they should be given in small doses to minimize their adverse metabolic effects. β blockers should be avoided in patients who are at risk for hypoglycemia.

Elevations of LDL cholesterol must also be treated. Because women with diabetes have a cardiovascular risk similar to that of men, all diabetic patients should be viewed as "high risk," regardless of gender. The goals should be an LDL-cholesterol below 130 mg per deciliter, and lower if there is already evidence of vascular disease (e.g., below 100 mg per deciliter). The first step lies in reinforcement of diet and optimization of glycemic control. If this fails, bile acid sequestrants or HMG CoA reductase inhibitors are recommended. Nicotinic acid is less useful because it increases insulin resistance and hyperglycemia. More commonly, diabetes is associated with elevations of VLDL-triglyceride and reductions of HDL-cholesterol. These variables often respond to weight reduction, diet modification, regular exercise, and other measures aimed at improving glycemic control. Only if this fails should drug therapy (e.g., fibric acid derivatives) be considered. Unfortunately, drug treatment is more effective in lowering triglycerides than raising HDL-cholesterol. Low-dose aspirin therapy reduces cardiovascular events in diabetic patients similarly to its effect in nondiabetic individuals. Large vessel disease in diabetics is as well treated surgically as it is in nondiabetic illness. Similarly, neither the frequency of multiple coronary vessel disease nor the outcome of coronary vascular surgery differs between diabetic and nondiabetic persons.

The association of diabetes with premature atherosclerosis may only represent the "tip of the iceberg." Impaired insulin-stimulated glucose metabolism commonly affects seemingly healthy people living in industrialized western countries but is generally counterbalanced by increased insulin secretion. Although this state of chronic hyperinsulinemia may successfully defend against the de-

TABLE 205–9. FOOT CARE PRESCRIPTION FOR HIGH-RISK PATIENTS (E.G., NEUROPATHY AND/OR VASCULAR INSUFFICIENCY)

Never walk barefooted
Do not apply hot water or heating pads to feet
Inspect feet daily (use mirror for plantar surfaces)
Keep feet clean, dry between toes
Lubricate dry skin using a nongreasy lotion or cream to avoid cracking
Wear properly fitting soft shoes
Break in new shoes slowly
Use second pair of shoes at night (larger size for edema)
Cut toenails straight across
Visit foot care specialist regularly
Stop smoking

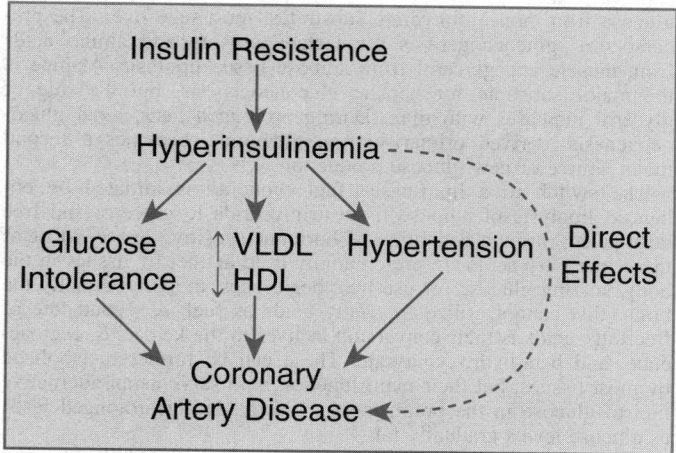

FIGURE 205–10. Syndrome X, a hypothesis based on the premise that insulin resistance accounts for the clustering of cardiovascular risk factors within a given individual.

velopment of diabetes, Reaven suggests that the price paid may be substantial (Fig. 205–10). According to his hypothesis, compensatory hyperinsulinemia has adverse effects on other systems affected by insulin such as sympathetic nervous system activity, renal sodium reabsorption, hepatic triglyceride synthesis, and arterial smooth muscle proliferation. Healthy, nonobese nondiabetic individuals with hyperinsulinemia have higher blood pressures, glucose, and triglyceride levels and lower HDL cholesterol concentrations than do subjects with normal insulin levels. The term syndrome X has been coined to describe this phenomenon, namely the clustering within the same persons of hyperinsulinemia, mild glucose intolerance, dyslipidemia, and hypertension, each of which is a risk factor for atherosclerosis. Several prospective population studies have found that the presence of hyperinsulinemia is closely related to the subsequent appearance of cardiovascular disease. Although statistical associations of this sort do not prove causality, they strongly suggest that insulin resistance has a potential role in the pathogenesis of atherosclerosis. If true, it further underscores the importance of lifestyle changes that improve insulin action in the treatment of type II diabetes and suggests that the same approach could benefit insulin-resistant patients with more subtle metabolic abnormalities (syndrome X). These data should not be a signal to lower therapeutic insulin doses, because the long-term adverse effects of hyperglycemia in diabetics are likely to be much greater than those caused by hyperinsulinemia. Instead, these observations suggest the

potential value of distributing smaller doses of insulin more evenly throughout the day to increase biologic effectiveness of the insulin regimen.

SUMMARY

The long-term goals of diabetes care consist of minimizing vascular and neurologic complications and maintaining a sense of well-being. These are best attained by early detection and treatment. Considering the wide array of potential problems and their multifactorial nature, diabetes care must be comprehensive in nature rather than limited to glycemic control. Attention should be devoted to risk factors that compound the adverse effect of diabetes on atherogenesis, the principal cause of mortality from the disease. Because the complications of diabetes develop slowly and are not readily reversible, it is crucial for the clinician to take a prospective approach, as is summarized in Figure 205–11.

American Diabetes Association: Position Statement: Standards of medical care for patients with diabetes mellitus. Diabetes Care 17:616, 1994. *An up-to-date summary of current standards of care for the management of diabetic patients, including the goals of treatment.*

Bouchard C, Despres J-P, Mauriege P: Genetic and nongenetic determinants of regional fat distribution. Endocrinol Rev 14:72, 1993. *This review summarizes the metabolic and clinical implications of variations in body fat distribution as well as the genetic and nongenetic factors influencing body fat topography.*

Brownlee M: Glycation products and the pathogenesis of diabetic complications. Diabetes Care 15:1835, 1992. *A short review of the process by which glucose modifies macromolecules and how these changes might lead to diabetic complications and be prevented.*

Castano L, Eisenbarth GS: Type I diabetes: A chronic autoimmune disease of man, mouse, and rat. Annu Rev Immunol 8:647, 1990. *A review of the evidence supporting the role of autoimmune mechanisms in the pathogenesis of type I diabetes.*

Consensus statement: Detection and management of lipid disorders in diabetes. Diabetes Care 16 (Suppl 2):106, 1993. *A summary of a consensus conference organized by the American Diabetes Association to develop strategies to better define and reduce the risk of vascular disease associated with diabetes.*

Cryer PE: Iatrogenic hypoglycemia as a cause of hypoglycemia-associated autonomic failure in IDDM. Diabetes 41:255, 1992. *A short review of the various clinical syndromes that lead to an increased risk of hypoglycemia in patients with type I diabetes.*

Davis MD: Diabetic retinopathy: A clinical overview. Diabetes Care 15:1844, 1992. *A review article that presents a description of the natural history of diabetic retinopathy and analyzes the results of clinical trials assessing treatment.*

Deckert T, Grenfell A: Epidemiology and natural history of diabetic nephropathy. *In* Pickup J, Williams G (eds.): Textbook of Diabetes. Oxford, Blackwell Scientific, 1992, p. 651. *A review of the natural history of diabetic renal disease and the factors influencing its development.*

DeFronzo RA, Bonadonna RC, Ferrannini E: Pathogenesis of NIDDM: A balanced overview. Diabetes Care 15:318, 1992. *A comprehensive review article dealing with the pathophysiology of type II diabetes and pathogenetic factors leading to its development.*

Diabetes Control and Complications Trial Research Group: The effect of intensive treatment of diabetes on the development and progression of long-term complications of insulin-dependent diabetes mellitus. N Engl J Med 329:927, 1993. *The report summarizes the results of the landmark multicenter prospective trial that evaluated the impact of intensive insulin therapy on its long-term complications.*

Fajans SS: Classification and diagnosis of diabetes. *In* Rifkin H, Porte D Jr (eds.): Diabetes Mellitus: Theory and Practice. New York, Elsevier, 1990, p 346. *Summarizes the classification of the various forms of diabetes and the diagnostic criteria used to detect disease.*

Greene DA, Sima AAF, Albert JW, Pfeifer MA: Diabetic neuropathy. *In* Rifkin H, Porte D Jr (eds.): Diabetes Mellitus: Theory and Practice. New York, Elsevier, 1990, p 710. *A general review of the pathogenesis and the management of diabetic neuropathy.*

Groop LC: Sulfonylureas in NIDDM. Diabetes Care 15:737, 1992. *A comprehensive review of the actions, pharmacokinetics, and clinical use of sulfonylurea drugs.*

Kreisberg RA: Diabetic ketoacidosis. *In* Rifkin H, Porte D Jr (eds.): Ellenberg and Rifkin's Diabetes Mellitus, 4th ed. New York, Elsevier, 1990, p 591. *A thorough and current review of the pathogenesis and treatment of this disorder.*

Lasker RD: The Diabetes Control and Complications Trial: Implications for policy and practice. N Engl J Med 329:1035, 1993. *This editorial discusses the health care implications of the DCCT results.*

Lewis EJ, Hunsicker LG, Bain RP, Rohde RD: The effect of angiotensin-converting enzyme inhibition on diabetic nephropathy. N Engl J Med 329:1456, 1993. *A report of a well-designed multicenter trial to examine the use of angiotensin-converting enzyme inhibitors in slowing the progression of diabetic nephropathy.*

Physician's Guide to Insulin Dependent (Type I) Diabetes: Diagnosis and Treatment, 2nd ed. Alexandria, VA, American Diabetes Association, 1994. *A monograph that provides a detailed review of the diagnosis and treatment of type I diabetes.*

Physician's Guide to Non–Insulin-Dependent (Type II) Diabetes: Diagnosis and Treatment, 3rd ed. Alexandria, VA, American Diabetes Association, 1994. *A monograph that reviews the diagnosis, pathogenesis, and treatment of type II diabetes.*

Reaven GM: Role of insulin resistance in human disease. Diabetes 37:1495, 1988. *A detailed review of the evidence linking insulin resistance with a variety of risk factors associated with atherosclerosis.*

Trucco M: To be or not to be Asp 57, that is the question. Diabetes Care 15:705, 1992. *A short review of the role of HLA genes in the pathogenesis of type I diabetes.*

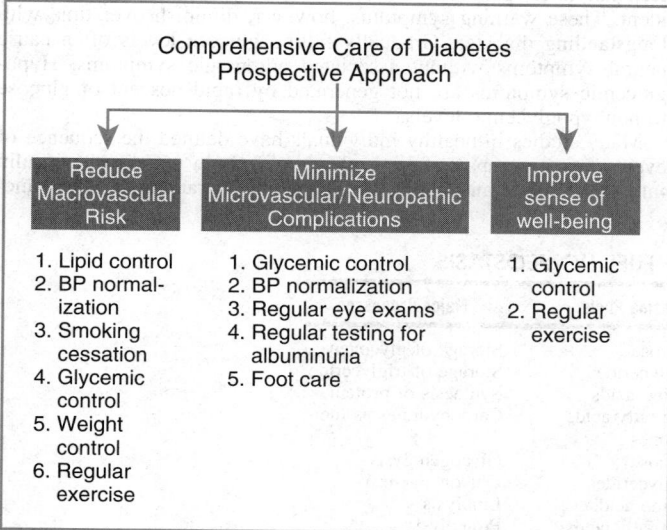

FIGURE 205–11. The key elements of a comprehensive management plan for patients with diabetes.

206 HYPOGLYCEMIA/PANCREATIC ISLET CELL DISORDERS

Jeffrey S. Flier

206.1 Hypoglycemia

In spite of food intake being intermittent and the unavoidability of periodic fasting, normal human plasma glucose concentrations remain within narrow limits. An abnormally low plasma glucose concentration, or hypoglycemia, may result from a variety of clinical disorders. Because glucose is the primary fuel of the brain, and the brain cannot synthesize glucose, transport it against a concentration gradient, or substitute alternative fuels in the short term, the consequences of hypoglycemia for brain function may be severe, including death. As a result, numerous and redundant adaptive mechanisms have evolved to prevent hypoglycemia. When these fail or become overwhelmed, the clinical syndrome of hypoglycemia results.

FUEL HOMEOSTASIS

Hypoglycemia is best viewed within the framework of disordered fuel homeostasis. Highly regulated changes in the rates of glucose production and use, coordinated with changes in the metabolism of muscle and fat, maintain glucose concentrations within narrow limits (usually between 70 and 150 mg per deciliter) despite intermittent and variable food intake. This is best seen as occurring in two contrasting physiologic conditions—the fed and fasted states (Table 206–1).

After food ingestion, circulating insulin levels rise, stimulated by increased plasma glucose and potentiated by meal-induced enteric hormones (incretins). Insulin is the dominant hormone of this anabolic postprandial period, and counterregulatory hormones are suppressed. Insulin shuts off hepatic glucose production, promotes the utilization of glucose as opposed to fat as an energy substrate, and directs storage of ingested nutrients such as glycogen, fat, and protein. In contrast, within 4 to 6 hours of food ingestion, metabolism switches to a fasted or catabolic phase characterized by falling insulin levels and rising levels of four counterregulatory hormones—glucagon, epinephrine, growth hormone, and cortisol. These hormonal changes result in critical changes in fuel metabolism: a switch from glucose use to production to maintain glucose levels sufficient for normal brain function and the change from a carbohydrate- to a lipid-based fuel economy for most other tissues of the body.

Hepatic glucose production derives initially from preformed glycogen, but the capacity of hepatic glycogen to sustain plasma glucose levels is limited to 8 to 12 hours, or even less after periods of exercise or illness. Thus, for more sustained fasting, including the normal overnight fast, gluconeogenesis, the generation of new glucose from noncarbohydrate substrates, must take over. The precursors of gluconeogenesis are lactate/pyruvate and amino acids from muscle and glycerol from adipose tissue lipolysis. Alanine is the major substrate for hepatic gluconeogenesis, but the role of glycerol increases with time. During prolonged fasts, renal gluconeogenesis, derived primarily from glutamine, becomes a second major source of new glucose production.

The switch to a lipid-based fuel economy is initiated by enhanced lipolysis of adipose tissue triglyceride to glycerol and free fatty acids, through activation of hormone-sensitive lipase. Most of these free fatty acids are preferentially used as fuel by tissues in the body, sparing glucose for use by other tissues, most importantly the brain, that cannot utilize free fatty acids as fuel. A second fate of free fatty acids is their conversion in liver to the ketoacids, acetoacetate, and beta-hydroxybutyrate. These can be further metabolized by most tissues, but their main function is to serve as an alternative fuel to glucose in the brain, most critically during prolonged fasts, as glucose levels gradually fall.

The defense against hypoglycemia requires both a fall in insulin levels and a rise in the four counterregulatory hormones. The fall in insulin levels is dominant, since if insulin fails to fall, hypoglycemia may result despite maximal counterregulatory response. A rising level of glucagon, by increasing hepatic glucose production, is the primary defender of the plasma glucose level under most circumstances. Epinephrine plays a secondary role, both by increasing glucose production and limiting its use, but may be critical under circumstances in which glucagon is deficient, as often occurs during the course of diabetes mellitus. Permissive levels of cortisol and growth hormone contribute to the defense against hypoglycemia by antagonizing insulin action. They also promote gluconeogenesis by enhancing provision of substrate and inducing the enzymes responsible for hepatic gluconeogenesis.

SIGNS AND SYMPTOMS OF HYPOGLYCEMIA

Hypoglycemia produces two distinct categories of symptoms (Table 206–2). The first results from secretion of the adrenal hormone, epinephrine; this provides a potential warning of hypoglycemia while simultaneously contributing to glucose counterregulation. Adrenergic symptoms include pallor, sweating, tachycardia, tremor, anxiety, and hunger. The second consists of central nervous system (CNS) symptoms of "neuroglycopenia," including headache, dizziness, altered mentation, visual disturbance, motor dysfunction, confusion, erratic behavior, convulsions, and loss of consciousness. Hypoglycemic patients often report a stereotyped subset of these symptoms with repeated episodes. No feature of these neuroglycopenic symptoms suggests their being caused by hypoglycemia as opposed to the many other structural or metabolic etiologic factors. This accounts for the common delay in considering hypoglycemia as a cause of altered mental status in other than insulin-treated diabetics. When glucose drops rapidly to hypoglycemic levels, as in response to exogenous insulin, adrenergic symptoms are usually evident. These warning symptoms, however, diminish over time with longstanding diabetes. Gradually falling glucose levels often cause neural symptoms without associated adrenergic symptoms. Hypoglycemic symptoms are not generated by rapid descent of glucose to nonhypoglycemic levels.

Many studies in healthy individuals have defined the sequence of events that accompany falling glucose levels in response to insulin infusions. Subtle and clinically inapparent alterations in CNS func-

TABLE 206–1. PHASES OF FUEL HOMEOSTASIS

Phase	Hormonal Determinants	Plasma Fuels	Major Processes
Fed (anabolic)	Rising insulin Falling glucagon	Glucose Triglycerides Amino acids Free fatty acids Ketones	Storage of glycogen Storage of triglyceride Synthesis of protein Carbohydrates as fuels
Fasted (catabolic)	Falling insulin Rising glucagon	Glucose Triglycerides Amino acids Free fatty acids Ketones	Glycogenolysis Gluconeogenesis Lipolysis Proteolysis Ketogenesis Lipid fuel economy

TABLE 206–2. SYMPTOMS OF HYPOGLYCEMIA

Adrenergic
  Sweating
  Tremor
  Anxiety
  Palpitations
  Weakness
  Hunger
Neuroglycopenic
  Headache
  Dizziness
  Altered mentation
  Visual disturbance
  Motor disturbance
  Convulsions
  Unconsciousness

tion may be detected in response to decrements in plasma glucose of only 15 mg per deciliter below that of an overnight fast. In one study, glucagon and epinephrine release appeared at 53 mg per deciliter, growth hormone at 52 mg per deciliter, and cortisol at 43 mg per deciliter. Neuroglycopenic symptoms generally develop when the plasma glucose level falls below 45 mg per deciliter, and major dysfunction is expected below 20 mg per deciliter. These figures are only guidelines, however, since considerable variability may be seen, some of which is predictable. Counterregulation typically occurs in diabetics with chronic hyperglycemia. These diabetics may have symptoms at higher glucose levels, and individuals with frequent hypoglycemia, including tightly controlled diabetics, have a lowered threshold for symptoms; they remain completely unaware of hypoglycemia prior to the onset of major CNS dysfunction. These adaptations may reflect changes in the system for transporting glucose into the CNS.

CAUSES OF HYPOGLYCEMIA

When the possible causes of hypoglycemia are being addressed (Table 206–3), the most important clinical distinction is to separate hypoglycemia induced by eating (reactive) and hypoglycemia occurring in the fasting state. The former is diagnosed excessively and rarely indicates a serious underlying disorder, while the latter demands a thorough search for a specific cause. Reactive hypoglycemia is not associated with hypoglycemia during a fast, but patients with true fasting hypoglycemia may experience the problem within 6 hours after ingesting food.

TYPES OF HYPOGLYCEMIA

POSTPRANDIAL HYPOGLYCEMIA. The most serious form of reactive hypoglycemia is alimentary hypoglycemia. Affected persons most often have had gastrectomy, but may also have had gastrojejunostomy, pyloroplasty, or vagotomy. Typically such patients develop adrenergic or neuroglycopenic symptoms of hypoglycemia from 30 to 120 minutes after a meal, and the blood sugar fall may be sufficient to produce seizures or coma. The pathogenesis is thought to involve rapid absorption of glucose, stimulating brisk insulin release, and, ultimately, inappropriately elevated insulin levels. The possible involvement of gut-derived incretins in causing the insulin hypersecretion has been suggested. Early diabetes is frequently cited as a condition that predisposes to reactive hypoglycemia, but the association appears to be exceedingly rare or nonexistent. Hypoglycemia may develop after ingestion of fructose or galactose in individuals with fructose intolerance or galactosemia.

Idiopathic reactive hypoglycemia includes two syndromes. The first is true idiopathic reactive hypoglycemia and is quite rare. Affected persons repeatedly exhibit symptoms of hypoglycemic-induced adrenergic excess following meals. Ingestion of carbohydrate relieves the symptoms as glucose levels rise. No specific mechanism for this disorder has been defined, and the hypoglycemia virtually never causes serious neuroglycopenia. A far more common situation involves patients with what has been called the idiopathic postprandial syndrome or pseudohypoglycemia. These individuals report symptoms suggesting either adrenergic discharge or mild neuroglycopenia in the 2 to 5 hours after meals but have normal accompanying glucose levels. Substantial confusion

has arisen from performance of oral glucose tolerance tests that were interpreted as demonstrating hypoglycemia, often defined as values below 60 mg per deciliter. Tests performed on control groups without symptoms demonstrate similar glucose values, suggesting that the "low" glucose levels are unrelated to the symptoms. It is no longer recommended that oral glucose tolerance tests be performed when evaluating postprandial "hypoglycemia." Instead, persistent symptoms in the postprandial state should be evaluated by measuring glucose levels during episodes as they occur during the course of a normal day. Patients with pseudohypoglycemia often remain convinced that they suffer from hypoglycemia even after such studies have proven normal. The popular press has proposed many remedies and unusual diets to deal with pseudohypoglycemia, but scientific explanations for the symptoms are lacking.

FASTING HYPOGLYCEMIA. Fasting hypoglycemia results from a mismatch between the rates of glucose production and glucose utilization. This can be due to impaired glucose production or to combinations of decreased production and increased utilization. Isolated increases in utilization with appropriate glucose production are not known to exist. The causes of isolated failure of hepatic glucose production can be divided into several categories based on pathogenetic mechanisms. These include defects in hormones that promote gluconeogenesis; defects in one or more of the enzymes critical to gluconeogenesis; severe generalized liver disease; deficiency of gluconeogenic substrates; and certain drugs. Overutilization of glucose may be caused by endogenous or exogenous insulin or insulin-like factors, by certain large metabolically active tumors, and by specific metabolic disorders that impair the availability of fat as a substrate for energy production. One clinical clue regarding the role of underproduction versus overutilization of glucose is the rate of glucose infusion needed to prevent hypoglycemia. Since the rate of glucose production during a fast approximates 2 mg per kilogram per minute, whereas the maximal rate of glucose utilization under the action of insulin is 12 mg per kilogram per minute,

TABLE 206–3. CLINICAL CLASSIFICATION OF HYPOGLYCEMIAS

I. Postabsorptive (fasting) hypoglycemia
  A. Drugs
    1. Insulin, sulfonylureas, ethanol
    2. Pentamidine, quinine, salicylates, propranolol
    3. Others
  B. Critical organ failure
    1. Liver disease
    2. Renal failure
    3. Cardiac failure
    4. Sepsis
    5. Inanition
  C. Hormone deficiencies
    1. Hypopituitarism
    2. Adrenal insufficiency
    3. Glucagon and epinephrine deficiency (esp. in diabetes)
  D. Non-beta cell tumors
  E. Endogenous hyperinsulinism
    1. Insulinoma
  F. Autoimmune
    1. Autoantibodies to insulin
    2. Autoantibodies to insulin receptor
  G. Factitious
    1. Insulin
    2. Sulfonylureas
  H. Hypoglycemia of infancy and childhood
    1. Ketotic hypoglycemia
    2. Enzyme deficiencies in pathways of glycogenolysis and gluconeogenesis
    3. Defects in amino acid, fatty acid, and ketoacid metabolism
II. Postprandial (reactive) hypoglycemias
  A. Alimentary hypoglycemia
  B. Idiopathic reactive hypoglycemia
  C. Deficiencies of enzymes of carbohydrate metabolism
    1. Galactosemia
    2. Hereditary fructose intolerance
  D. (Pseudohypoglycemia)

glucose requirements substantially above 10 grams per hour strongly suggest that overutilization must exist.

DRUG-INDUCED HYPOGLYCEMIA. When use of insulin and sulfonylureas in patients with diabetes is included, drugs are the most common cause of hypoglycemia. Drug-induced hypoglycemia is more likely to occur at the extremes of age, in the acutely or chronically undernourished, and in the presence of renal or hepatic dysfunction. Alcohol predictably inhibits hepatic gluconeogenesis. Ethanol oxidation generates reduced nicotinamide adenine dinucleotide (NADH) and increases the ratio of NADH to nicotinamide adenine dinucleotide (NAD). This inhibits gluconeogenesis at multiple steps, including the transformation of pyruvate to oxaloacetate, which is further transformed into phosphoenolpyruvate via the rate-limiting enzyme of gluconeogenesis, phosphoenolpyruvate carboxykinase. Even quite modest amounts of alcohol will induce hypoglycemia under conditions in which gluconeogenesis is driving hepatic glucose production, for example, when starvation has depleted hepatic glycogen. The CNS consequences of hypoglycemia may mimic intoxication, and alcoholic hypoglycemia can have serious consequences if not identified promptly. Salicylates may cause hypoglycemia, especially in children, by an uncertain mechanism. Propranolol may contribute to fasting hypoglycemia by reducing the glycogenolytic response to epinephrine and, in diabetics, by blunting the awareness of hypoglycemia due to epinephrine release. Pentamidine exerts a toxic effect on pancreatic beta cells to release insulin acutely and cause hypoglycemia; chronic effects can cause diabetes. Quinine treatment of malaria has been described as causing hypoglycemia secondary to drug-induced insulin release. Many other drugs have been associated with hypoglycemia as a rare event.

INSULINOMA. Insulinoma is a rare disorder that occurs in approximately one per 250,000 individuals. The median age of onset is about 50 years, except for those who develop it in the context of multiple endocrine neoplasia type I (MEN I), in which it occurs in the mid 20's. Such tumors are uncommon below the age of 20 years, and very uncommon below the age of 5 years. Most insulinomas are small, benign, and single. Tumors are multiple in 7% and malignant in about 5%. Eight percent of patients with insulinoma have MEN I, and these are much more likely to be multiple. These tumors will occasionally secrete other hormones, including gastrin, ACTH, glucagon, somatostatin, and 5-hydroxyindoles. Nesidioblastosis is a rare condition affecting neonates in which pancreatic duct epithelium gives rise to endocrine cells that are distinct from true islets. The condition is more common than insulinomas in producing hyperinsulinism and hypoglycemia in this age group; its occurrence in adults is very rare.

Clinical Picture. Patients with insulinoma have varying combinations of neuroglycopenic and autonomic symptoms that tend to occur five or more hours after a meal, as after an overnight fast. The symptoms and extent of hypoglycemia are affected by exercise, diet, ingestion of ethanol, or religious fasts. Rarely, symptoms may occur only in the 2 to 4 hours after a meal rather than during fasting. Common symptoms include diplopia, blurred vision, palpitations, weakness, and confusion or bizarre behavior. Some patients will have a refractory seizure disorder in the absence of other symptoms. In such instances, insulinoma may be overlooked for prolonged periods. As many as 20% of patients may be mistakenly viewed as suffering from neurologic or psychiatric disorders. Many patients remain unaware that eating prevents attacks.

Diagnosis. The diagnosis of insulinoma is based on the presence of *Whipple's triad* (appropriate symptoms in association with hypoglycemia and relief of symptoms after elevation of the blood glucose level) together with inappropriately elevated plasma insulin and C-peptide levels in the absence of sulfonylurea in the plasma. The diagnosis is most straightforward when insulin, C-peptide, and sulfonylurea determinations are obtained concurrently during an episode of hypoglycemia. It is often useful to retain a separate aliquot of plasma for subsequent measurement of proinsulin, cortisol, anti-insulin, or receptor antibodies in the event that the diagnosis is unclear after measurement of insulin and C-peptide.

If the history suggests hypoglycemia but neither symptoms nor hypoglycemia can be identified at the initial evaluation, supervised fasting is usually the next step. The goal is to determine whether

hypoglycemia develops and, if so, whether it is accompanied by endogenous hyperinsulinism. While extended overnight fasts may be useful in initial outpatient evaluation, the gold standard for safe and thorough evaluation is an inpatient fast of up to 72 hours. Plasma glucose, insulin, C-peptide, and cortisol should be measured every 6 hours, with the frequency of testing influenced by the patient's history and the obtained glucose values. The patient should be tested repeatedly for cognitive function. The diagnosis of hypoglycemia during a fast is complicated by the fact that normal individuals may have quite low levels of glucose during a 72-hour fast in the absence of symptoms. Although the mean minimal levels of glucose in one study were 62 mg per deciliter and 52 mg per deciliter in men and women, respectively, values as low as 22 mg per deciliter have been recorded in asymptomatic normal women. It is therefore essential to continue the fast to the point at which symptoms occur, or to 72 hours. In one large series, Whipple's triad was demonstrated within 12 hours of the last meal in 29% of patients, within 24 hours in 71%, within 36 hours in 79%, within 48 hours in 92%, and within 72 hours in 98%. At the time of symptoms, plasma glucose concentration was below 46 mg per deciliter in all patients. Rarely, exercise at the end of a fast will provoke hypoglycemia that is otherwise not demonstrable. Given the results in normal persons, the clinician should be wary of diagnosing hypoglycemia in the absence of symptoms that are relieved by food ingestion. Interpretation of insulin levels during a fast may also be a source of confusion and must be evaluated in the light of simultaneous glucose values. Insulin levels are of no value if simultaneous glucose values are normal or elevated; any measurable insulin level in the presence of hypoglycemia less than 45 mg per deciliter must be viewed as suspicious.

Some centers aim to avoid the use of the prolonged fast in diagnosing insulinoma. Several provocative tests rely on the tendency of insulinomas to release insulin excessively in response to specific secretagogues, including tolbutamide and glucagon, but these are not in wide use. The C-peptide suppression test is based on the fact that after exogenous insulin–induced hypoglycemia, patients with insulinoma have impaired suppression of endogenous insulin and C-peptide. These results are influenced by age and obesity. Proinsulin levels, both absolute and as a fraction of total immunoreactive insulin, are elevated in most patients with insulinoma.

Once insulinoma has been confirmed biochemically, the tumor should be localized before surgery. Preoperative and intraoperative ultrasonography has replaced celiac angiography and CT in many centers as the method of choice, with intraoperative sonograms approaching 90% sensitivity. If a tumor cannot be localized, a skilled surgeon may identify a tumor intraoperatively, and failing that, distal pancreatectomy may be successful, because tumors are evenly distributed through the pancreas, and ectopic insulinomas are exceedingly rare. Malignant insulinoma metastasizes to regional lymph nodes and liver but rarely produces distant metastases. Persistent hypoglycemia in patients with malignant insulinomas, in patients whose tumors could not be found at exploration, or in patients refusing surgery is best treated with diazoxide, which inhibits insulin release. Phenytoin, propranolol, and verapamil have been reported to be useful in some cases. A long-acting analogue of somatostatin, octreotide, reduces hyperinsulinemia and symptoms in many but not all patients with insulinoma. A chemotherapeutic regimen reported to have some benefit in malignant insulinoma consists of streptozotocin plus fluorouracil or chlorzotocin. Although the prognosis is generally poor, a few patients with metastatic insulinomas survive in relatively good health for long periods.

FACTITIOUS AND AUTOIMMUNE HYPOGLYCEMIA. Hypoglycemia induced by the surreptitious administration of insulin or sulfonylureas is probably more common than insulinoma. As a result, the coexistence of hypoglycemia and inappropriate insulin levels does not establish the diagnosis of insulinoma (Table 206–4). Most often, factitious hypoglycemia occurs in medical personnel or in family members of patients with diabetes. Insulin has been used for suicide, homicide, and child abuse. The best means to distinguish insulinoma from surreptitious insulin administration is to measure C-peptide along with insulin during hypoglycemia. C-peptide is released on an equimolar basis with endogenous insulin into the portal vein, and its level is elevated parallel to insulin in insulinoma. Exogenous insulin suppresses insulin secretion in normal

TABLE 206–4. DIFFERENTIAL DIAGNOSIS OF INSULINOMA AND FACTITIOUS HYPOGLYCEMIA

Test	Insulinoma	Exogenous Insulin	Sulfonylureas
Plasma glucose	Low	Low	Low
Plasma insulin	Inappropriately high	Inappropriately high (possibly very)	Inappropriately high
C-peptide	Increased	Not increased or low	Increased
Proinsulin	Increased	Not increased or low	Increased
Insulin antibodies	Absent	May be present	Absent
Sulfonylurea levels	Absent	Absent	Present

individuals, and C-peptide levels are similarly suppressed. Antibodies to insulin, if present in persons not known to have received insulin therapy, can also indicate surreptitious insulin use. Both insulin and C-peptide levels are increased as a consequence of sulfonylurea administration; this can be diagnosed only by identifying the drug in plasma or urine.

Hypoglycemia can be the result of autoimmune disease, due either to the occurrence of spontaneous autoantibodies against insulin or the insulin receptor. Both syndromes commonly occur in the context of other autoimmune features. The mechanism for hypoglycemia caused by anti-insulin autoantibodies has never been clearly defined, but is probably a consequence of erratic release of insulin bound to antibodies in the circulation. Hypoglycemia may be severe, may accompany either fasting or the postprandial state, and is typically self-limited. Autoantibodies to the insulin receptor most often cause insulin-resistant diabetes and the skin condition acanthosis nigricans. Such antibodies can act as insulin-like agonists after binding to the insulin receptor, thereby causing hypoglycemia. Patients with hypoglycemia due to anti-insulin receptor autoantibodies may have pure fasting hypoglycemia, they may develop fasting hypoglycemia after a previous phase of insulin-resistant diabetes, or they may have the otherwise very unusual combination of fasting hypoglycemia together with postprandial hyperglycemia. Such patients typically do not have acanthosis nigricans as a clue to diagnosis, and the diagnosis may be suggested by the presence of one or more findings suggestive of autoimmunity. During hypoglycemia caused by such insulin-mimetic antibodies, C-peptide levels are suppressed. Insulin levels may be suppressed, normal, or slightly elevated because of the ability of receptor autoantibodies to reduce clearance of the hormone. Glucocorticoids may be effective therapy, either by inducing cellular resistance to the agonist properties of the antireceptor antibodies or in some cases by lowering the antibody titer.

NON–BETA CELL TUMOR HYPOGLYCEMIA. Hypoglycemia may occur in a variety of extrapancreatic tumors of mesenchymal or epithelial origin, and some malignant hematologic diseases can result in systemic hypoglycemia. Sarcomas and fibromas are the most common, but renal, adrenal, and gastrointestinal cancers and hepatomas may have a similar effect, along with several other rare associations. The mesenchymal tumors are typically large tumors that arise in the retroperitoneum or thorax. Characteristic of these hypoglycemias is the suppression of plasma insulin levels. In some cases, very large tumors appear capable of inducing hypoglycemia through massive utilization of glucose that exceeds the capacity for hepatic compensation. In other cases, a humoral mediator apart from insulin has been sought; very high levels of insulin-like growth factor-II (IGF-II) mRNA have been identified in several such tumors. IGF-II bears homology to both insulin and IGF-I and may produce hypoglycemia through receptors for either or both of these ligands. IGF-II may also suppress growth hormone levels, and this additional consequence of IGF-II expression may contribute to hypoglycemia.

HYPOGLYCEMIA IN HEPATIC, RENAL, AND ENDOCRINE DISORDERS AND MISCELLANEOUS CONDITIONS. Although the liver has substantial reserve capacity, hypoglycemia may accompany fulminant hepatic failure and sometimes occurs for unclear reasons in association with less severe hepatic dysfunction due to viral hepatitis; cirrhosis; and hepatic congestion caused by severe right-sided heart failure. The hypoglycemia that sometimes accompanies renal failure is often multifactorial and may be due to reduced clearance of hypoglycemic drugs, reduced food

intake, and reduced gluconeogenesis, possibly secondary to deficient gluconeogenic substrates. Most patients with hypopituitarism and adrenal insufficiency do not develop hypoglycemia, although this can occur, especially during fasts. Hypoglycemia is a common development in children below 6 years of age with hypopituitarism. Isolated deficiencies of glucagon and epinephrine are not known to cause hypoglycemia.

Children are susceptible to hypoglycemia because of a number of inherited or acquired abnormalities affecting the enzymes that regulate fuel metabolism. These include defects that affect the rate of glycogen breakdown, such as glucose-6-phosphatase deficiency; glycogen synthesis as in the glycogen storage diseases; and gluconeogenesis, as with deficiency of fructose-1,6-diphosphatase. Ketotic hypoglycemia of childhood may be due to substrate limitation, and alanine turnover is reduced. Hypoglycemia may also result from defects in the ability to utilize fatty acids or ketones, in which case the tissues become dependent on glucose for fuel, and the liver cannot meet the demand. Defects in the pathway of fatty acid oxidation or ketone formation can cause this result, as can systemic deficiency of carnitine, a molecule necessary for the transport of fatty acids into mitochondria, the site of their oxidation.

Hypoglycemia accompanies starvation and may occur in anorexia nervosa as well as in persons following unusual faddist diets. It may also accompany any state of extreme inanition or cachexia, during sepsis, or after prolonged, severe exercise, especially in the physically untrained.

THE APPROACH TO THE PATIENT WITH HYPOGLYCEMIA (Fig. 206–1)

Hypoglycemia may be suspected on the basis of symptoms that are nonspecific or identified through a blood test in a patient otherwise not suspected of being hypoglycemic. In the latter situation, the possibility of artifactual hypoglycemia, due to utilization of glucose by erythrocytes or leukemic leukocytes in the test tube, must be considered, as must the possibility that the patient has adapted to longstanding or mild hypoglycemia by nutritional or other modifications.

In the initial phase of consideration of hypoglycemia, several major questions must be addressed. These include the distinction between fasting and reactive hypoglycemia and the relationship between hypoglycemia and any symptoms or signs. This requires a careful history from both patient and family members including detailed evaluation of medication use, and an effort to obtain specimens for assay during any spontaneous episodes if possible before administration of food or intravenous glucose, should that be necessary. If hypoglycemia is suspected, 10 to 20 ml of blood should be drawn beyond that needed for glucose determination. Additional analyses, including insulin, C-peptide, cortisol, sulfonylurea level, and others can be determined on the basis of clues generated from the history and physical examination. If hypoglycemia is noted in a patient who is ill or if history and physical examination point to specific syndromes known to be associated with hypoglycemia, the subsequent evaluation should be led by this information and may be quite limited. If hypoglycemia is documented without a clear indication of its relationship to fasting or symptoms and the patient is generally healthy, fasting hypoglycemia and its provocation of symptoms should be documented. Once fasting hypoglycemia is demonstrated, insulinoma should be distinguished from hypoglycemia due to ingestion/administration of insulin or sulfonylureas or, less commonly, from hormone deficiency or inapparent solid tumor.

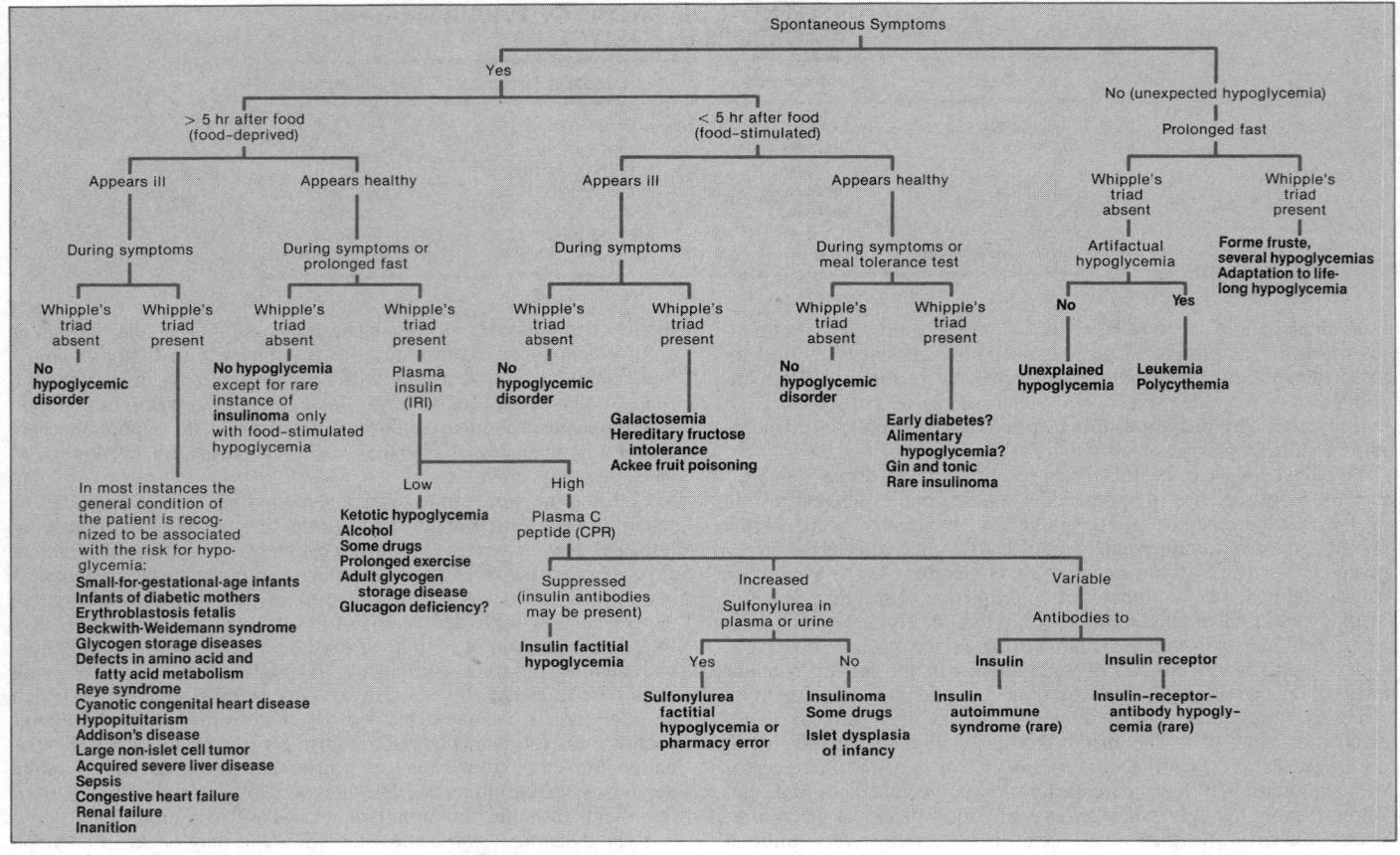

FIGURE 206-1. Evaluation of hypoglycemic disorders.

Cryer PE: Glucose counterregulation: Prevention and correction of hypoglycemia in humans. Am J Physiol 264:E149, 1993. *Review of the physiologic response to hypoglycemia.*

Davis SN, Cherrington AD: The hormonal and metabolic responses to prolonged hypoglycemia. J Lab Clin Med 121:21, 1993.

De Feo et al.: Modest decrements in plasma glucose concentration cause early impairment in cognitive function and later activation of glucose counterregulation in the absence of hypoglycemic symptoms in normal man. J Clin Invest 82:436, 1988. *Evidence for subtle defects in cognitive function when glucose levels fall modestly below the fasting level.*

Grunberger G, et al.: Factitious hypoglycemia due to surreptitious administration of insulin: Diagnosis, treatment and long-term follow-up. Ann Intern Med 108:252, 1988. *An approach to this vexing disorder.*

Lowe WL, Roberts CT, JR, Leroith D, et al.: Insulin-like growth factor-II in nonislet cell tumors associated with hypoglycemia: Increased levels of messenger ribonucleic acid. J Clin Endocrinol Metab 69:1153, 1989. *Nonislet cell tumors associated with hypoglycemia were found to produce large amounts of IGF-II mRNA.*

Moertel CG, et al.: Streptozocin-doxorubicin, streptozocin-fluorouracil, or chlorozotocin in the treatment of advanced islet-cell carcinoma. N Engl J Med 326:519, 1992. *Comparative regimens for treatment of islet cell carcinoma.*

Palardy J, Havrankova, Lepage R, et al.: Blood glucose measurements during symptomatic episodes in patients with suspected postprandial hypoglycemia. N Engl J Med 321:1421, 1989. *Importance of measuring glucose during occurrence of spontaneous symptoms of hypoglycemia clearly demonstrated by data in this paper. When self-collected capillary blood specimens on filter paper were analyzed for glucose, only 5% had values less than 2.8 mM/L (50 mg/dl).*

Pandit MK, et al.: Drug-induced disorders of glucose tolerance. Ann Intern Med 118:529, 1993.

Service FJ: Hypoglycemias. J Clin Endocrinol Metab 76:269, 1993. *Excellent clinical review.*

Zeiger MA, et al.: Use of intraoperative ultrasonography to localize islet cell tumors. World J Surg 17:448, 1993. *Efficacy of this technique in identifying small insulinomas.*

206.2 Islet Cell Tumors

The islets of Langerhans are nests of endocrine cells dispersed throughout the exocrine pancreas. Each islet may be viewed as a miniature organ in which four distinct cell types, each producing a single hormone, are organized in a specific manner. The insulin-producing B cells comprise 60% of islet cells and are located in the core of the islet. They are surrounded by a rim of glucagon-secreting A cells and pancreatic peptide-secreting PP cells. D cells containing somatostatin are found primarily between the A and B cells. Several other peptides, such as gastrin and vasoactive intestinal polypeptide (VIP), have less clear cells of origin and may be expressed only in perinatal islets under normal circumstances.

ISLET CELL TUMORS

Tumors can arise from any of the hormone-producing cells of the islets of Langerhans. Patients with islet cell tumors may seek medical attention as a result of distinct syndromes caused by hormone hypersecretion or because of the consequences of growth of either the primary tumor or its metastases. Nearly all benign islet cell tumors and more than 80% of carcinomas secrete clinically significant amounts of hormone; some secrete multiple hormones. Clinical presentation usually reflects the dominance of one hormone. The tumor is named after the hormone responsible for the clinical syndrome, or in asymptomatic patients, the hormone found in highest concentration in the circulation or in the tumor.

DIAGNOSIS. Islet cell tumors are generally slow growing and are compatible with prolonged survival. Nonfunctioning tumors are typically found during evaluation of symptoms or signs due to the pancreatic mass, and the diagnosis is made histologically. Alternatively, patients may have a characteristic clinical syndrome, which stimulates the measurement of circulating tumor products. Further evaluation often requires provocative or suppressive tests, evaluation to identify physiologic consequences of hormone oversecretion, and exclusion of alternative causes for elevated levels of the hormone.

Once biochemical criteria for a hormone-secreting tumor are satisfied, imaging studies are used to assess the site and extent of the tumor and the possibility of surgical cure. The combination of endoscopic and intraoperative ultrasonography plus computed tomography (CT) has proven the most sensitive approach, largely displacing angiography in most centers. Selective venous sampling has been applied with limited success. Preliminary indications suggest that external scanning after administration of a radiolabeled analogue of somatostatin can identify islet cell tumors based on their expression of somatostatin receptors.

PATHOLOGY. Benign and malignant islet tumors cannot be readily distinguished on the basis of histologic appearance. The diagnosis of carcinoma requires the identification of metastases.

ASSOCIATED SYNDROMES. Pancreatic islet cell tumors may occur as part of the multiple endocrine neoplasia (MEN) syndrome. The islet cell tumors most commonly present in MEN I are gastrinomas and insulinomas. Compared with sporadic tumors, pancreatic tumors in MEN I are more likely to be multiple and malignant. The diagnosis of the MEN I syndrome should be considered when hypercalcemia is present in a patient with an islet cell tumor, as more than 90% of patients in whom MEN I is diagnosed have hyperthyroidism.

THERAPY. The initial aim of treatment is curative resection of the tumor. If this proves impossible, tumor syndromes may be attenuated either by diminishing hormone secretion or by blocking their untoward physiologic effects. Residual tumors can be palliated with chemotherapy or surgical debulking. Octreotide, a long-acting 8-amino acid analogue of somatostatin, reduces hormone production and has proven to be a mainstay in the treatment of symptoms due to hormone-secreting islet cell tumors. Unfortunately, gradual loss of efficacy of this agent often develops, presumably in association with advancing tumor burden.

TYPES OF TUMORS

INSULINOMA. Insulinoma is the most common islet cell tumor. This subject is discussed in Ch. 206.1.

GASTRINOMA. The second most common islet cell tumor is the gastrinoma, associated with the Zollinger-Ellison syndrome, in which recurrent gastric ulcers are produced as a result of hypersecretion of gastric acid. This is discussed in Ch. 99.6.

VIPOMA. VIP is a 28-amino acid peptide that has considerable homology with members of the secretin family. It was purified as a vasodilating activity from normal intestine in 1970 and was shown to have widespread distribution in the central and peripheral nervous systems. Although purified from this source, it is apparently not expressed in the endocrine cells of the normal gastrointestinal tract, where it plays the role of a local neurotransmitter, modulating ion and water transport as well as vascular tone.

Several years earlier, Verner and Morrison described the association of severe watery diarrhea with a non–insulin-producing islet cell tumor. The disorder subsequently was identified with VIP-producing tumors and circulating VIP, and it was shown that VIP infusion would produce secretory diarrhea, hypokalemia, and metabolic acidosis. Accordingly, the term *VIPoma* has superseded other designations, including Verner-Morrison syndrome, watery diarrhea hypokalemia achlorhydria (WDHA), and pancreatic cholera. These tumors may produce other peptides that can contribute to the features of this disorder. These include peptide histidine methionine (PHM), which is derived from a common precursor with VIP and has similar actions on intestinal secretion, as well as neurotensin and somatostatin.

Clinical Features and Diagnosis. The diagnosis of VIPoma is suggested by watery diarrhea that exceeds 3 liters per day in 80% of patients and hypokalemic acidosis due to major losses of potassium and bicarbonate in the stool. The volume depletion and hypokalemia can cause profound weakness, flaccid paralysis, and hypokalemic nephropathy, and may be fatal. Diabetes or glucose intolerance is common, due either to a glucagon-like effect of VIP or to an effect of hypokalemia to inhibit insulin secretion. Half of the patients may develop hypercalcemia, which may be due to co-expression of parathyroid hormone-related peptide by the tumor, rather than parathyroid adenomas; VIPomas rarely associate with the MEN syndrome.

Diagnosis requires demonstration of elevated levels of VIP in plasma. The sample should be carefully prepared with protease inhibitors, as the VIP molecule is highly unstable and may be degraded if such precautions are not carried out. Mild elevations of VIP below the range seen in VIPomas sometimes occur in diarrheal states associated with short bowel syndrome and inflammatory bowel disease. Secretory diarrhea may be seen in three other endocrine tumors (gastrinoma, carcinoid, and somatostatinoma), but peak volume of diarrhea rarely exceeds 3 liters per day in these disorders. The diarrhea in gastrinoma is caused by hypersecretion of

gastric acid and is reversed by treatments that reverse acid hypersecretion, whereas VIPomas are associated with hypochlorhydria or achlorhydria.

Pathology. Among patients with the VIPoma syndrome, 80% have islet cell tumors, of which approximately half are malignant, with hepatic metastases at the time of presentation. Pancreatic VIPomas are often large, up to 7 cm in diameter, and may be identified by immunocytochemistry using antibodies to the prepro-VIP molecule. Association with MEN I syndrome is rare. VIPoma may also be associated with neuroblastoma, ganglioneuroma, pheochromocytoma, and small cell tumors of the lung.

Treatment. The optimal treatment is surgical extirpation of the primary tumor. Localization of the tumor and identification of any metastases can be carried out with CT. In the occasional case in which localization of a biochemically identified tumor is impossible, including efforts at intraoperative ultrasonography, a blind distal pancreatectomy can be performed. Surgery may also be indicated to treat local effects or to remove a large primary tumor in the presence of metastases, although this is controversial.

Medical treatment includes support with fluid and electrolyte repletion, as well as an effort to limit the secretory diarrhea. Glucocorticoids may reduce diarrhea without affecting levels of VIP, and transient responses to clonidine, indomethacin, and a variety of other agents have been described. A major advance in the medical treatment of VIPomas has been the introduction of octreotide, which both reduces tumor output of VIP and reduces intestinal chloride secretion in response to VIP. Symptoms are ameliorated in most patients, although gradually increasing doses may be required, sometimes ending in loss of clinical response. In patients with inoperable tumors, chemotherapy with regimens combining streptozotocin and fluorouracil or streptozotocin and doxorubicin has induced partial remissions with lowered levels of VIP and reduction of symptoms. Hepatic embolization has also been used to reduce VIP production by hepatic metastases.

GLUCAGONOMA. Glucagon, a 29-amino acid peptide produced in the A cells located in the periphery of the islets of Langerhans, plays a key role in the regulation of hepatic glucose production. The glucagon gene is also expressed in the small intestine, where processing of preproglucagon yields the glucagon precursor enteroglucagon, as well as the glucagon-like peptides 1 and 2. These may function as "incretins," enhancing glucose-induced insulin secretion. Patients with glucagonoma typically have large forms of glucagon and glucagon-like peptide in the circulation, in addition to native glucagon.

Clinical Features and Diagnosis. Patients with glucagonomas most commonly present between the ages of 40 and 70 years. The disorder is most often brought to attention by a characteristic necrolytic, erythematous rash, which affects more than 80% of the patients and is usually a major source of disability. Located most often on the face, intertriginous areas, and extremities, the rash is initially erythematous and scaly, tends to become raised and bullous and then crusty, and heals as a hyperpigmented and indurated lesion. The rash may become superinfected, and glossitis, stomatitis, angular cheilitis, nail dystrophy, and thinning of the hair may also be seen. The etiology of the rash is linked to hyperglucagonemia and associated amino acid deficiency, although a role for zinc deficiency has been suggested based on similarities to the rash seen in zinc deficiency (acrodermatitis enteropathica) and a claimed response of some patients to treatment with zinc.

Mild, asymptomatic diabetes mellitus accompanies glucagonomas. The condition is evident only as an abnormal glucose tolerance test; ketoacidosis does not occur, presumably because of adequate insulin to suppress lipolysis. Other common clinical features are weight loss, anemia, psychological depression, and thromboembolic disease, as well as nonspecific abdominal complaints.

The diagnosis of glucagonoma requires finding elevated levels of glucagon in the plasma, and exclusion of other conditions associated with elevated, although typically much lower, levels of glucagon, such as uncontrolled diabetes mellitus, chronic renal failure, cirrhosis, sepsis, stress, or fasting. Normal circulating glucagon levels lie between 50 and 150 pg per milliliter. Most patients with glucagonoma have levels above 1000 pg per milliliter, often much higher. Patients usually seek attention for evaluation of the skin rash or thromboembolic disease; routine consideration of the diagnosis of glucagonoma in the patient with new-onset diabetes is not warranted in their absence.

Pathology. Glucagonoma is most often caused by single, large (3 to 5 cm) pancreatic tumors located in the body and tail of the organ. Although these tumors are typically slow growing, by the time of diagnosis as many as three quarters will have metastasized, most often to regional lymph nodes and liver, occasionally to distant sites. The syndrome accompanies MEN I.

Treatment. After localization of the tumor and assessment of metastatic disease, most often with CT, surgical cure can be achieved in approximately one third of patients. Surgery may also be indicated to relieve local effects or in an effort to reduce the tumor burden. Octreotide usually reduces glucagon levels and improves symptoms. The rash often resolves after several days of octreotide treatment or after successful surgery. Zinc supplementation and amino acid infusions also have been reported to diminish the severity of the rash. Arterial embolization or chemotherapy with combinations of streptozotocin, fluorouracil, doxorubicin, and dacarbazine may reduce hormone production from the tumor and induce partial remission. Tumor burden may gradually increase over a period of 2 to 10 years despite these treatments, and the clinical course may be complicated by production of additional hormones, such as gastrin.

SOMATOSTATINOMA. Somatostatin, an inhibitor of growth hormone secretion, is widely distributed in the nervous system and the gut. It acts as a neurotransmitter in the nervous system, as a paracrine regulator within endocrine glands, and as a hormone in the hypophyseal-portal system. Somatostatin inhibits the secretion of many hormones, including insulin, glucagon, growth hormone, prolactin, gastrin, and secretin, and in addition inhibits gastric acid and enzymes as well as pancreatic exocrine secretion. Somatostatin is produced by the D cells of the islets, which account for approximately 10% of islet cells.

Clinical Features and Diagnosis. Somatostatinoma may occur with a complex of symptoms, including mild diabetes mellitus, cholelithiasis, and diarrhea with steatorrhea. These result from the action of somatostatin to inhibit insulin release, gallbladder motility, and pancreatic enzyme and bicarbonate secretion. Patients may also develop weight loss, hypochlorhydria, anemia, and flushing. The diagnosis can be difficult, as somatostatinoma is very rare, its symptoms are nonspecific and often mild, and its associations (such as diabetes and cholelithiasis) occur much more often in its absence. As a result, at the time of diagnosis two thirds of patients have hepatic metastases. Some patients with documented somatostatinoma may lack any features of the syndrome, and in these cases the disorder is found incidentally or during the evaluation of jaundice or weight loss. Somatostatinomas have been documented to produce other hormones, including insulin, glucagon, adrenocorticotropic hormone (ACTH), calcitonin, gastrin, VIP, and prostaglandins. Somatostatin-producing tumors may also arise in the duodenum, where they are more typically small, well circumscribed, and amenable to resection. Duodenal somatostatinomas may be associated with neurofibromatosis, but are not associated with high circulating levels of somatostatin or the associated syndrome.

Pathology. Most somatostatinomas arise in the pancreas, where they are typically single, large, and metastatic at the time of diagnosis. Most other cases arise in the duodenum or jejunum. Secretion of somatostatin by other tumors, including pheochromocytomas and medullary carcinoma of the thyroid, has been reported.

Treatment. The treatment of pancreatic somatostatinomas resembles the treatment of other islet cell tumors, including surgery if possible, and palliation with hepatic embolization or chemotherapy. There is little evidence for utility of octreotide.

OTHER HORMONES PRODUCED BY ISLET CELL TUMORS. Pancreatic islet cell tumors that produce ACTH account for nearly 10% of cases of Cushing's syndrome due to ectopic ACTH production. However, in patients with islet cell tumors in the context of MEN I, the Cushing phenotype is more often a consequence of a pituitary adenoma. Some islet cell tumors have also been shown to produce corticotropin-releasing hormone, but Cushing's syndrome in a patient with islet cell tumor has yet to result from this mechanism. Acromegaly has been reported in patients with islet cell tumors secreting growth hormone-releasing factor, as has hypercalcemia due to secretion of parathyroid hormone-related pep-

tide. Many endocrine tumors of the pancreas and gut produce pancreatic polypeptide (PP) as a second hormone, and PP therefore can serve as a useful marker for islet cell tumors. PP is a 36-amino acid peptide from a family that includes neuropeptide Y and peptide YY. PP comprises 10% of islet cells, and although it is evolutionarily conserved, is released in response to food, and has biologic effects when given to experimental animals or humans, its precise physiologic role has not been defined. Most patients with PP-secreting tumors are asymptomatic.

NONFUNCTIONING ISLET CELL TUMORS. Approximately 10% of islet cell tumors have no identified syndrome of hormone excess. Some of these express peptides such as PP, and others undoubtedly express genes encoding presently unknown peptides. These tumors frequently reach a large size at the time of diagnosis and present symptoms such as malaise, abdominal pain, and jaundice. A mass can often be palpated, and at least half have hepatic metastases at first evaluation. Surgery cures approximately 20%, and chemotherapy with streptozotocin with or without fluorouracil provides objective palliation in approximately half of the remaining. Although 5-year survival is approximately 40%, many patients with metastatic disease enjoy a substantially longer survival.

Gorden P, Comi RJ, Maton PN, Go VL: Somatostatin and somatostatin analogue (SMS 201-995) in treatment of hormone secreting tumors of the pituitary and gastrointestinal tract and non-neoplastic diseases of the gut. Ann Intern Med 110:35, 1989. *Thorough review of somatostatin analogue as therapy.*

Kvols LK, Brown ML, O'Connor MK, et al.: Evaluation of a radiolabeled somatostatin analog (I-123 octreotide) in the detection and localization of carcinoid and islet cell tumors. Radiology 187:129, 1993. *Technique evaluated in 28 patients. Previously undetected lesions were found in four.*

Moertel CG, Lepkopoulo M, Lipsitz S, et al.: Streptozotocin-doxorubicin, streptozotocin-fluorouracil or chlorozocin in the treatment of advanced islet cell carcinoma. N Engl J Med 326:519, 1992. *Comparison of chemotherapeutic regimens.*

Rosch T, Lightdale CJ, Botet JF, et al.: Localization of pancreatic islet cell tumors by endoscopic ultrasonography. N Engl J Med 326:1721, 1992. Describes advantages of the technique.

Vinik AI, Moattari AR: Treatment of endocrine tumors of the pancreas. Endocrin Metab Clin North Am 18:483, 1989. *Comprehensive review with 186 references.*

207 DISORDERS OF SEXUAL DIFFERENTIATION

Maria I. New and Nathalie Josso

Gonads, genital ducts, and external genitalia become sexually dimorphic during fetal life, depending upon the presence or absence of genetic and endocrine factors, all of which actively impose maleness. Female differentiation requires no specific stimulus, occurring constitutively in the absence of male-determining factors. The asymmetric mechanism of sex differentiation has an important bearing upon the pathogenesis of intersex disorders: Male pseudohermaphroditism, defined as incomplete virilization of a 46,XY male, results from defects in the synthesis, metabolism, or action of one or several masculinizing factors. In contrast, female pseudohermaphroditism results from inappropriate exposure of female anlagen to masculinizing agents.

ANATOMY OF NORMAL SEX DIFFERENTIATION

MALE SEX DIFFERENTIATION. Testicular Differentiation. The gonadal primordium is represented by the gonadal ridge, which is progressively colonized by extraembryonic primordial germ cells. The first recognizable event of testicular differentiation, at 7 weeks' gestation, is the development of primordial Sertoli cells, which aggregate to form seminiferous tubules and produce anti-müllerian hormone (AMH). Leydig cells differentiate at 8 weeks of gestation and increase until 12 to 14 weeks, when they begin to degenerate. At birth, very few remain in the interstitial tissue; the Leydig cell population reappears at puberty.

Somatic Sex Differentiation. After gonadal differentiation, the internal reproductive tract consists of two pairs of ducts: the wolffian ducts and the müllerian ducts. In males, müllerian duct regression begins at 8 weeks and is more or less complete at 10 to 12 weeks. The wolffian ducts develop into the vasa deferentia, epididymides, and seminal vesicles. Prostatic buds develop around the opening of the ducts at 10 to 11 weeks of age while fusion of outgrowths of the urogenital sinus forms the prostatic utricle, the male equivalent of the vagina (Fig. 207–1). At 10 weeks, the genital tubercle elongates and the urethral folds fuse over the urethral groove, leading to formation of the penile urethra, while the genital swellings move posteriorly and fuse, forming the scrotum. Male anatomic development is completed by 90 days of gestation, but penile growth occurs only between 20 weeks and term, at a time when, paradoxically, serum testosterone levels are declining.

FEMALE DIFFERENTIATION. *Ovarian Differentiation.*
Slower than the testis to differentiate initially, the fetal ovary eventually reaches a more advanced stage of maturation. At 12 to 13 weeks, some oogonia, located in the deepest layer of the cortex, have entered meiotic prophase. By 7 months' gestation, all germ cells have entered or completed meiotic prophase. Fetal granulosa cells produce estrogen at the same developmental stage at which fetal testes produce testosterone, but ovarian production of AMH can be demonstrated only after birth.

Somatic Sex Differentiation. Female fetal sex differentiation is characterized by degeneration of the wolffian ducts at 10 weeks, while the müllerian ducts develop into fallopian tubes, uterus, and upper vagina. The vagina differentiates at the level of the müllerian tubercle, between the openings of the wolffian ducts where the prostatic utricle forms in males. Whereas in males the prostatic utricle opens just beneath the neck of the bladder, in females, the lower end of the vagina slides down the posterior wall of the urethra to acquire a separate opening on the body surface (Fig. 207–1). Feminization of the external genitalia begins by the formation of the dorsal commissure, between the genital swellings, which in the fe-

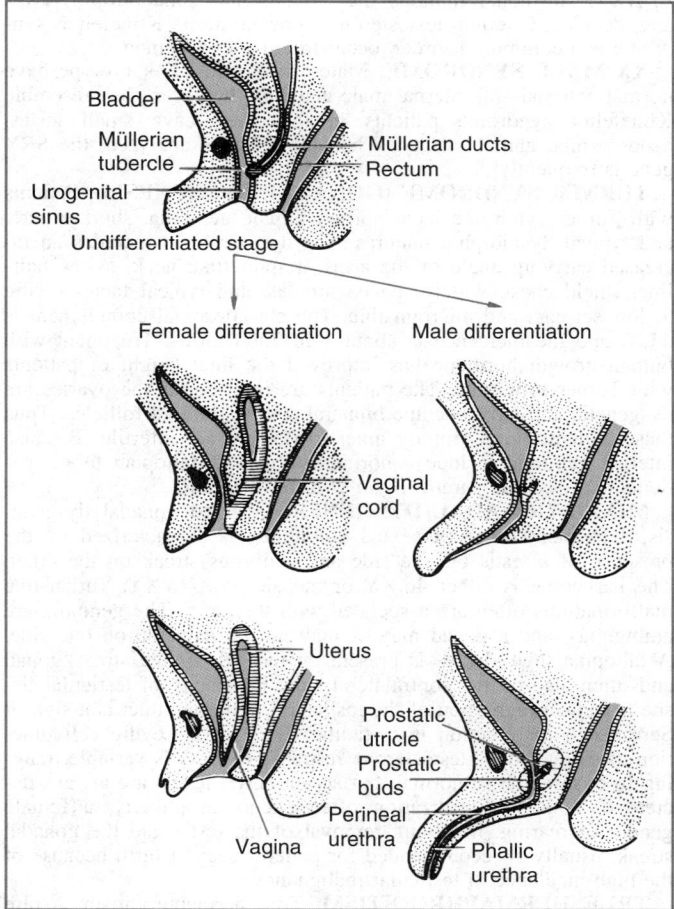

FIGURE 207–1. Differentiation of the urogenital sinus. (From Josso N: Physiology of sex differentiation: A guide to the understanding and management of the intersex child. *In* Josso N [ed.]: The Intersex Child. Basel, Karger, 1981, p 1.)

male do not migrate posteriorly or fuse, and give rise to the labia majora. Because the genital folds do not fuse, they become the labia minora, and the genital tubercle becomes the clitoris. In the female, all these steps are constitutive and occur in the absence of hormonal stimulation.

MECHANISMS OF GONADAL SEX DETERMINATION: THE SRY GENE. Sex determination in mammals is governed primarily by gene(s) lying on the Y chromosome; the number of accompanying X chromosomes is irrelevant. The X and Y chromosomes each contain pseudoautosomal regions of approximately 2.6×10^6 base pairs, which enter into homologous recombination between the sex chromosomes at meiosis, ensuring their correct segregation. Loci on the Y chromosome proximal to the pseudoautosomal boundary normally are not involved in an exchange with the X chromosome and exhibit patrilineal inheritance. It is essential to the chromosomal basis of sex determination that the testis-determining gene be located in the nonrecombining, Y-specific region. The testis-determining gene (SRY), which is located on the short arm of the human Y chromosome, is conserved and Y-specific among a wide range of mammals and encodes a testis-specific transcript. Mutations of the SRY gene have been reported in sex-reversed XY individuals. Conversely, translocation of SRY leads to maleness in XX subjects, but these are sterile because XX germ cells do not survive in a testicular environment.

Although fetal ovarian development is constitutive, female germ cells survive only in the presence of two X chromosomes; 45,X individuals experience early loss of germ cells, leading to fibrous degeneration of the ovaries usually associated with Turner syndrome. Recently, it has been found that male to female sex reversal occurs in individuals with duplications of the short arm of the X chromosome, suggesting that there also may be a gene for femaleness. This locus has been termed DSS for dosage-sensitive sex reversal and has been localized to a 1.6×10^5 base pair region of the short arm of the X chromosome.

MECHANISM OF SOMATIC SEX DIFFERENTIATION. Sex differentiation of the reproductive tract is mediated by two discrete hormones produced by the fetal testis: AMH and testosterone (Fig. 207–2). In the absence of both, female differentiation proceeds unimpeded.

AMH, which is synthesized by immature Sertoli cells and by postnatal granulosa cells, is responsible for müllerian regression. The gene, located on chromosome 19, is a member of the transforming growth factor-β (TGF-β) superfamily and acts via a serine threonine kinase receptor located on chromosome 12.

Androgens are responsible for maintenance of the wolffian ducts and virilization of the urogenital sinus and external genitalia. Testosterone production by the fetal testis is detectable at 9 weeks in the human fetus, increases to a peak at 15 to 18 weeks, then falls sharply, so that serum concentrations of testosterone overlap in males and females in late pregnancy. In adult Leydig cells, the capacity to respond to sustained gonadotropin stimulation by increased androgen production is curtailed by the development of a refractory state, due to receptor down-regulation, which does not occur in the fetus. When human chorionic gonadotropin (hCG) declines in the third trimester, the hypothalamic-pituitary axis gains control over testicular functional activity.

Testosterone is the major steroid released by fetal testes in the bloodstream, and it enters cells by passive diffusion or pinocytosis. A local source of androgen is important for wolffian duct development, which does not occur if testosterone is supplied only via the peripheral circulation, as in female pseudohermaphroditism due to adrenal hyperplasia. Testosterone is converted intracellularly to dihydrotestosterone (DHT) by the enzyme 5α-reductase (Fig. 207–3). Two distinct isoforms of 5α-reductase have been cloned: Type 1 is present in very low levels in the prostate and the sebaceous glands; type 2 is present in high levels in the prostate and in the area of the external genitalia. DHT binds to the androgen receptor with greater affinity and stability than does testosterone. Therefore, in tissues equipped with 5α-reductase at the time of sex differentiation, such as the prostate, urogenital sinus, and external genitalia, DHT is the active androgen. However, at high concentrations, testosterone interacts with the androgen receptor similarly to DHT. The gene coding for the androgen receptor is located on the X chromosome.

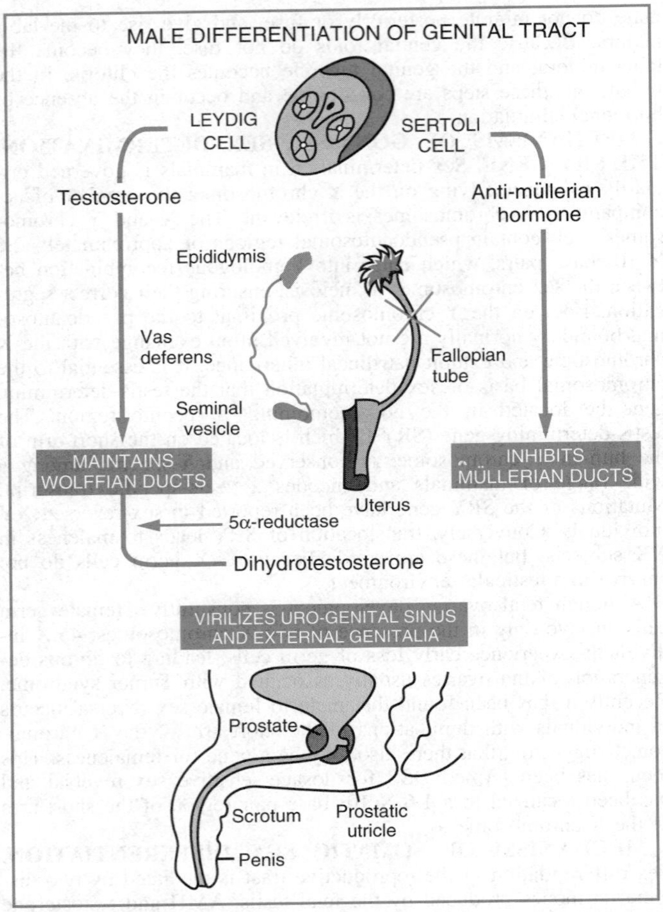

MALE DIFFERENTIATION OF GENITAL TRACT

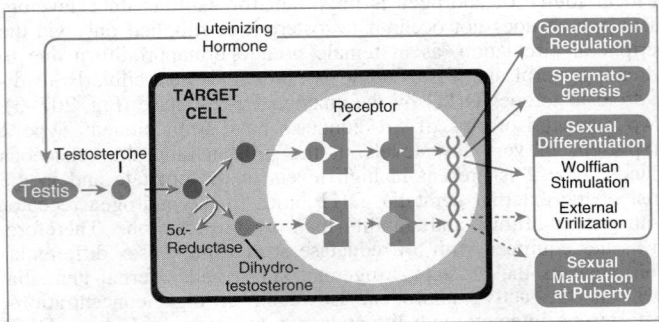

FIGURE 207-2. Hormones involved in male differentiation of the reproductive tract. Testosterone, synthesized by Leydig cells, maintains the wolffian ducts and virilizes the urogenital sinus and external genitalia after reduction to dihydrotestosterone. Antimüllerian hormone, produced by fetal Sertoli cells, inhibits the development of the müllerian ducts, which would otherwise develop into uterus and tubes. (From Josso N: Physiology of sex differentiation: A guide to the understanding and management of the intersex child. *In* Josso N [ed.]: The Intersex Child. Basel, Karger, 1981, p 1.)

CLASSIFICATION OF INTERSEX STATES

Normal sex differentiation occurs at various levels (Fig. 207-4): Genetic sex is established at fertilization by the nature of the sex chromosome donated by the spermatozoon. The presence or absence of the SRY gene primarily determines gonadal sex, and the presence or absence of fetal testes determines somatic sex through the secretion of testosterone. Gender identity is established early in life by the sex of rearing but can exceptionally be disrupted at puberty by hormonal factors.

FIGURE 207-3. General scheme of androgen action. (From Wilson JD: Syndromes of androgen resistance. Biol Reprod 46:168, 1992.)

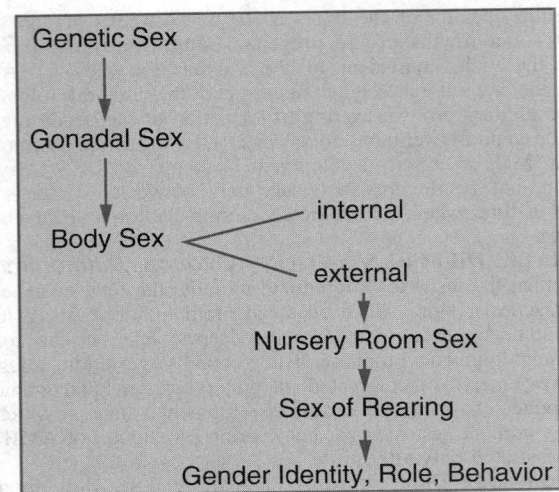

FIGURE 207-4. Stages of sex differentiation. Genetic sex specified at fertilization determines gonadal sex, which in turn determines somatic and legal sex. Gender identity usually is determined by the sex of rearing. (From New MI, Levine LS: Congenital adrenal hyperplasia. *In* Harris H, Hirschhorn K [eds.]: Advances in Human Genetics. New York, Plenum Press, 1973, p 251.)

DISORDERS OF CHROMOSOMAL SEX

KLINEFELTER SYNDROME. In this condition, males have normal development of the penis and scrotum, but the testes are small and firm. At adolescence, gynecomastia is frequent and infertility is common owing to azoospermia. The usual karyotype is 47,XXY. Hormonal findings include elevated gonadotropin levels and decreased serum testosterone concentration. Klinefelter syndrome is a common disorder, occurring in 1 in 500 men.

XX MALE SYNDROME. Males with a 46,XX karyotype have normal external and internal male genitalia; however, they resemble Klinefelter syndrome patients in that they have small testes, azoospermia, and infertility. When the DNA is analyzed, the SRY gene is frequently present.

TURNER SYNDROME (GONADAL DYSGENESIS). Patients with Turner syndrome have normal female genitalia, short stature, and typical dysmorphic features. The dysmorphism includes an increased carrying angle of the arms, a sphinxlike neck, a low hairline, shield chest, widely spaced nipples, and typical facies owing to low-set ears and micrognathia. The chromosomal complement is 45,X, and the incidence is about 1 in 2500 births. Treatment with human growth hormone has improved the final height of patients with Turner syndrome. The patients are infertile, as the ovaries are dysgenetic and have become bilateral streaks without follicles. Thus these patients have primary amenorrhea and are infertile. Because internal genitalia include a normal uterus and fallopian tubes, patients may become parents by *in vitro* fertilization.

MIXED GONADAL DYSGENESIS. Mixed gonadal dysgenesis, a frequent cause of sexual ambiguity, is characterized by the presence of a testis on one side and a fibrous streak on the other. The karyotype is either 46,XY or mosaic 45,X/46,XY; Turner-like malformations often are associated with the latter. The genitalia are ambiguous, and a gonad may or may not be palpable on one side. A fallopian tube always is present on the side of the streak gonad and often also on the contralateral side; incapacity of testicular tissue to induce regression of the ipsilateral müllerian duct is a sign of Sertoli cell malfunction in testicular dysgenesis. Leydig cell function as evaluated by testosterone response to hCG is variable, ranging from minimal to normal, but serum AMH levels are always decreased. Although virilization often occurs at puberty, a female gender of rearing, involving removal of the testis and the gonadal streak, usually is recommended for patients seen at birth because of the high incidence of testicular malignancy.

TRUE HERMAPHRODITISM. True hermaphroditism, a rare and usually sporadic disorder, is defined as coexistence of seminiferous tubules and ovarian follicles in the same subject. Most patients have an ovotestis with either an ovary or a testis on the opposite side; a testis is usually in the scrotum, an ovotestis more seldom. Histologically, ovarian tissue is more or less normal, whereas testicular tubules are markedly dysgenetic and may harbor gonadoblastomas or seminomas.

The genitalia are usually ambiguous; rare cases of completely masculine or feminine genitalia have been reported. The anatomy of the internal reproductive tract depends on the nature of the gonads. A uterus is present in approximately 90% of cases. Testosterone response to hCG is variable, and AMH levels are usually low. Most patients experience breast development, ovulation, and even menstruation at puberty; pregnancy and successful childbirth are possible if selective removal of testicular tissue is feasible. Unless gender has already been assigned, male orientation should be restricted to patients with no uterus and descended testicular tissue, because testicular tissue is usually dysgenetic and prone to malignant degeneration. The majority of true hermaphrodites have no Y chromosome: 68% have a 46,XX karyotype, 12% are 46,XY, and the remainder are mosaics. To resolve the discrepancy between the presence of testicular tissue and the lack of a Y chromosome, the DNA of 46,XX true hermaphrodites has been examined with probes for SRY. True hermaphrodites usually lack SRY, suggesting that the condition, at least in familial cases, is due to constitutive activation of a gene normally triggered by SRY.

DISORDERS OF GONADAL SEX

PURE GONADAL DYSGENESIS, TESTICULAR REGRESSION SYNDROME. Patients with pure gonadal dysgenesis have a normal female phenotype, including uterus and tubes, but have fibrous streaks instead of gonads; they are free of Turner-like malformations and develop to normal height. Familial cases have been described, with either a 46,XX or a 46,XY karyotype; in the latter, mutations of the SRY gene have been identified. Other 46,XY patients with absent gonads present with various degrees of sexual ambiguity and no müllerian derivatives. The implication that some testicular tissue was functional at least up to 10 weeks and subsequently regressed has led to the name "fetal testicular regression syndrome." Testicular regression may occur in late pregnancy or even postnatally; these fully virilized males present only with bilateral cryptorchidism. This condition also is known as *anorchia*.

TESTICULAR DYSGENESIS. Testicular dysgenesis is characterized by seminiferous tubule degeneration and invasion by connective tissue arranged in whorls as in a streak gonad. Germ cells are rare or absent; the gonad is often maldescended and prone to malignant degeneration. The clinical picture, as in true hermaphroditism, combines defects of AMH- and testosterone-dependent steps of sex differentiation, depending on the extent and timing of testicular degeneration. The incidence of gonadal tumors may reach 30%, making castration and subsequent hormonal replacement the safest therapeutic option.

DYSGENETIC MALE PSEUDOHERMAPHRODITISM. Patients with dysgenetic male pseudohermaphroditism have bilaterally differentiated dysgenetic testes. Their external genitalia are ambiguous and müllerian derivatives are always present. The clinical, endocrine, and cytogenetic picture is similar to that of mixed gonadal dysgenesis.

NONDYSGENETIC MALE PSEUDOHERMAPHRODITISM. Patients with bilateral nondysgenetic testes fail to masculinize because of biochemical alteration of the synthesis or action of a single testicular hormone. This is in contrast to subjects with true hermaphroditism or testicular dysgenesis, characterized by defects of testosterone- and AMH-dependent steps of sex differentiation. Defects of testosterone-mediated steps of sex differentiation are the most frequent and are characterized, in 46,XY subjects, by a variable degree of penile development and hypospadias. Usually, a single perineoscrotal opening leads into a urogenital sinus; the blind vaginal pouch opens into the posterior wall of the urethra, usually at the junction of the vertical and horizontal segments of the urethra. Extreme situations occur more rarely. Sometimes, the vagina and urethra have separate perineal orifices as in a normal female, or, in deeply virilized patients, the vaginal orifice opens beneath the bladder neck, differing only by size from the prostatic utricle of a normal male. Müllerian derivatives, the uterus and upper segment of the vagina, are always regressed. Serum levels of AMH are normal or elevated. Insufficient production of active androgens or androgen end-organ resistance may be involved. However, a large number of cases cannot be classified. "Idiopathic" male pseudohermaphroditism can be considered to be a malformation masquerad-

ing as a testosterone defect. Association of genital ambiguity with other developmental defects frequently is observed, sometimes as one of the several components of a recognized syndrome such as Smith-Lemli-Opitz; the WAGR syndrome, including Wilms tumor, aniridia, gonadal abnormalities, and mental retardation; or the hand-foot-genital syndrome.

DISORDERS OF PHENOTYPIC SEX

FEMALE PSEUDOHERMAPHRODITISM. Female pseudohermaphroditism, defined as the sexual ambiguity of a 46,XX fetus with two normal ovaries, is the most frequent type of intersex. Rarely, the female fetus is masculinized owing to transplacental transfer of androgens from an ovarian or adrenocortical tumor in the mother or from exogenous steroids. Most female pseudohermaphrodites have been exposed to endogenous androgens prenatally owing to congenital adrenal hyperplasia (CAH).

Virilization due to androgen excess is limited to the androgen-responsive external genitalia (the lower vagina, genital folds and swellings, and phallus). Masculinization ranges from minimal clitoromegaly and a mild degree of posterior labial fusion to formation of a urogenital sinus with the orifice located distally along the urethral groove, ending in extreme cases at the tip of the phallus. Because there is no testicular tissue, testosterone is not produced locally to support development of wolffian duct structures, nor is AMH produced; therefore the fallopian tubes, uterus, and upper vagina are normal. Thus, with proper medical treatment and vaginal reconstruction, there is capacity for normal childbearing.

CAH should be suspected in sexually ambiguous newborns with a uterus but no palpable gonadal tissue. Such patients should be karyotyped and have endocrine evaluation done immediately because of the life-threatening salt loss found in many cases of CAH.

CONGENITAL ADRENAL HYPERPLASIA. CAH is a family of monogenic autosomal recessive disorders of steroidogenesis in which enzymatic defects result in impaired synthesis of cortisol by the adrenal cortex (Table 207–1). Subsequent adrenocorticotropic hormone (ACTH) oversecretion via the negative feedback system stimulates the adrenal to become hyperplastic. As a result, both precursor steroids proximal to the enzyme block and hormonal products of unimpeded pathways are overproduced. In some forms, diversion of precursor steroids into androgen pathways results in excessive levels of potent androgens and virilization of the female fetus. In other forms, sex steroids are underproduced in both the adrenal and the testes, leading to ambiguous genitalia in genetic males. Abnormal secretion of mineralocorticoids in some cases results in disturbances in the regulation of electrolytes, plasma volume, and blood pressure.

STEROID 21-HYDROXYLASE DEFICIENCY. *Classic 21-Hydroxylase Deficiency.* Steroid 21-hydroxylase deficiency is the most common enzymatic defect causing CAH. Classic 21-hydroxylase deficiency occurs in about 1 in 14,000 live births, but the incidence may vary by population and geographic area (Fig. 207–5). The classic disorder has two forms: salt wasting and simple virilizing (non–salt wasting); both result in sexual ambiguity in the newborn genetic female. In the salt-wasting form, which occurs in about three fourths of cases, adrenal production of aldosterone and of cortisol is inadequate. Salt-wasting crises are associated with hyponatremia, hyperkalemia, and hypovolemia, with metabolic acidosis, loss of vascular tone, and, in some cases, shock and death. Crises usually arise between 7 days and 2 weeks of life, after discharge from the hospital. Thus, the affected first-born male who has normal genitalia is particularly at risk for a salt-wasting crisis at home. Ambiguous genitalia in the female usually prompt diagnostic procedures, placing females at lower risk. Salt wasting should be carefully ruled out even in newborns with mild genital ambiguity. Unlike salt wasters, simple virilizers can synthesize sufficient amounts of aldosterone for salt retention.

Nonclassic 21-Hydroxylase Deficiency. Nonclassic 21-hydroxylase deficiency, a genetic variant of the classic form, is associated with a milder enzyme defect and does not cause prenatal virilization in the genetic female. However, signs of androgen excess may appear postnatally in both sexes. Nonclassic 21-hydroxylase deficiency occurs in 1 in 100 births in the general population and with a higher frequency in specific ethnic groups, making this the most frequent autosomal recessive disease in humans.

TABLE 207–1. THE FORMS OF CONGENITAL ADRENAL HYPERPLASIA: CLINICAL AND HORMONAL ASPECTS

Deficiency	Genital Ambiguity	Postnatal Virilization	Salt Metabolism	Renin	Steroid Pattern	
					Increased	*Decreased*
21-hydroxylase				High		
A. Classic salt wasting	F	Yes	Salt wasting		17-OHP; Δ^4-A	aldo; cortisol
Simple virilizing	F	Yes	Normal		17-OHP; Δ^4-A	cortisol
B. Nonclassic (symptomatic and asymptomatic)	No	Yes	Normal		17-OHP; Δ^4-A	—
11β-hydroxylase				Low		
A. Classic	F	Yes	Salt retention		DOC; compound S	cortisol $\pm$ aldo
B. Nonclassic	No	Yes	Normal		Compound S $\pm$ DOC	
3β-hydroxysteroid dehydrogenase				High		
A. Classic	M/F	Yes	Salt wasting		17-OH-pregnenolone; DHEA	aldo; cortisol; T
B. Nonclassic	No	Yes	Normal		17-OH-pregnenolone; DHEA	—
17α-hydroxylase	M	No	Salt retention	Low	DOC; compound B	cortisol; T
17,20-lyase	M	No	Normal		None	DHEA; T; Δ^4-A
Cholesterol desmolase	M	No	Salt wasting	High	None	All

17-OHP = 17-hydroxyprogesterone; Δ^4-A = Δ^4-androstenedione; aldo = aldosterone; DOC = deoxycorticosterone; compound S = 11-deoxycortisol; DHEA = dehydroepiandrosterone; T = testosterone; B = corticosterone.

Clinical Presentation. In 21-hydroxylase deficiency, 17α-hydroxyprogesterone (17-OHP) and progesterone are overproduced and are converted to the androgens dehydroepiandrosterone (DHEA), Δ^4-androstenedione (AD), and testosterone, which cause virilization. Postnatally, in untreated classic and nonclassic children, growth accelerates in the early years but the epiphyses close prematurely, resulting in a tall child but a short adult. Even when treated, most patients do not reach the height potential indicated by family height. Pubertal development under hypothalamic-pituitary control may be suppressed by excess adrenal androgens, and fertility potential may not be achieved until proper treatment is instituted to suppress ACTH and adrenal androgen secretion. Without treatment, males may evidence pseudopuberty marked by phallic growth, small testes, and precocious growth of pubic, axillary, and body hair. Male internal and external genital development is normal. Untreated females may suffer from excessive androgenic symptoms such as cystic acne, secondary amenorrhea/oligomenorrhea, or polycystic ovarian syndrome (Fig. 207–6).

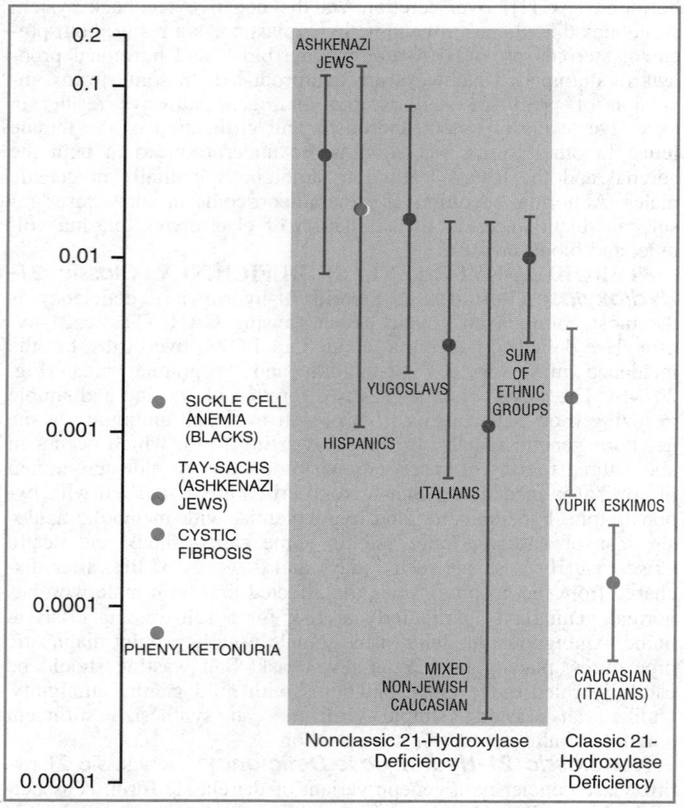

Molecular Genetics. The gene encoding 21-hydroxylase is located on the short arm of chromosome 6 within the human major histocompatibility complex. The gene locus for the 21-hydroxylase enzyme, termed CYP21, has a closely neighboring homologue, the pseudogene CYP21P, which is not expressed. Two forms of mutations observed are gene deletions, which result from chromosomal misalignment as well as unequal crossing over during meiosis, and gene conversions, which apparently involve the transfer of short sequences resident on the pseudogene to the active gene.

Diagnosis and Treatment. Screening of newborns for elevated serum 17-OHP identifies males and females with classic 21-

FIGURE 207–5. Disease frequencies of classic 21-hydroxylase deficiency (in two populations), nonclassic 21-hydroxylase deficiency (in five ethnic groups), and four other relatively common autosomal recessive disorders compared. (From Speiser PW, Dupont B, Rubinstein P, et al.: High frequency of nonclassical steroid 21-hydroxylase deficiency. Am J Hum Genet 37:650, 1985.)

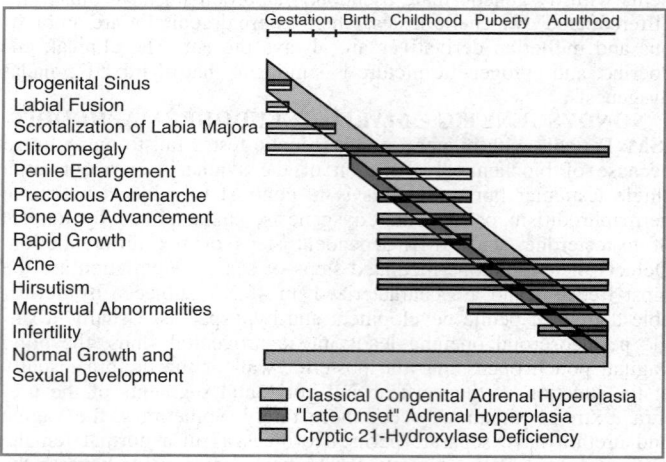

FIGURE 207–6. Clinical spectrum of HLA-linked steroid 21-hydroxylase deficiency. Clinical presentation in 21-hydroxylase deficiency ranges from prenatal virilization with labial fusion to precocious adrenarche, to pubertal or postpubertal virilization. During their lifetime, patients may change from symptomatic to asymptomatic with 21-hydroxylase deficiency. (From New MI, Dupont B, Grumbach K, et al.: The adrenal hyperplasias. In Stanbury JB, Wyngaarden JB, et al. [eds.]: The Metabolic Basis of Inherited Disease. 5th ed. New York, McGraw-Hill, 1983, p 973.)

hydroxylase deficiency irrespective of genital phenotype. In the United States, newborns currently are screened in 15 states. In suspected cases, the chromosomal or genetic sex should be determined by buccal smear for Barr bodies, karyotyping, fluorescent Y, or SRY analysis. Elevated 17-OHP, which may be several hundred times normal, confirms the enzyme defect. Routine screening does not detect the nonclassic form of 21-hydroxylase deficiency. In the nonclassic form, 17-OHP levels may be elevated in early morning readings but normal in midmorning and afternoon. Thus, the deficiency is best diagnosed with an ACTH stimulation test (an intravenous bolus injection of 0.25 mg synthetic ACTH and assay for serum 17-OHP at 0 and 60 minutes). The coordinates of the baseline and the ACTH-stimulated 17-OHP concentrations aggregate on a regression line into three diagnostic groups. Classic cases fall into the highest group on the regression line, nonclassic cases aggregate lower than classic cases, and an overlap of heterozygote carriers and unaffected cases appears in the lowest group (Fig. 207–7).

The female with classic 21-hydroxylase deficiency should almost always be assigned to the female gender, as she has the potential for normal sexual and reproductive function. In classically affected untreated females, surgical correction of genital ambiguity is required. Recent experience indicates that early one-stage vaginal and perineal reconstruction, which avoids a second-stage surgical procedure and decreases delayed vaginal stenosis, is effective in correcting the ambiguity.

Postnatal management involves lifelong hormonal replacement. It is necessary to monitor 17-OHP serum concentration (or daily urinary excretion of pregnanetriol) as well as plasma renin activity in the classic salt-wasting form. Hydrocortisone generally is given in infancy and childhood in a dose range of 10 to 25 mg per square

meter per day in order to maintain the serum 17-OHP concentration between 500 and 1000 ng per deciliter. Attempts to bring the 17-OHP concentration to normal results in cushingoid features and retarded growth. In adolescence and adulthood, hydrocortisone may be replaced with dexamethasone or prednisone. Mineralocorticoid (9α-fluorohydrocortisone) administration and added salt to the diet are necessary in patients with salt-wasting disease and may improve hormonal control in simple virilizers. Treatment of nonclassic 21-hydroxylase deficiency with dexamethasone in low doses (0.25 mg at bedtime) is usually effective in reversing symptoms of androgen excess, including reduced fertility.

Prenatal Management. Prenatal diagnosis is best performed with a direct molecular genetic approach but can also be achieved by assessment of 17-OHP or AD in amniotic fluid. Diagnosis by DNA testing requires sampling of chorion frondosum obtained by chorionic villus sampling or amniotic fluid cells obtained by amniocentesis. Chorionic villus sampling performed in the eighth to tenth week of gestation allows diagnosis earlier than amniocentesis performed in the second trimester. Direct examination of the CYP21 gene locus is carried out by Southern blotting for identification of gene deletions (10 to 35% of cases) and with allele-specific oligonucleotide probes for point mutations. Together, these two tests routinely identify about 90% of all mutations.

The recommended prenatal treatment of 21-hydroxylase deficiency is oral dexamethasone, 20 μg per kilogram per day (prepregnancy weight) divided in three equal doses and administered to the mother starting before the ninth week of gestation (Fig. 207–8). Therapy should continue to term if the fetus is found to be an af-

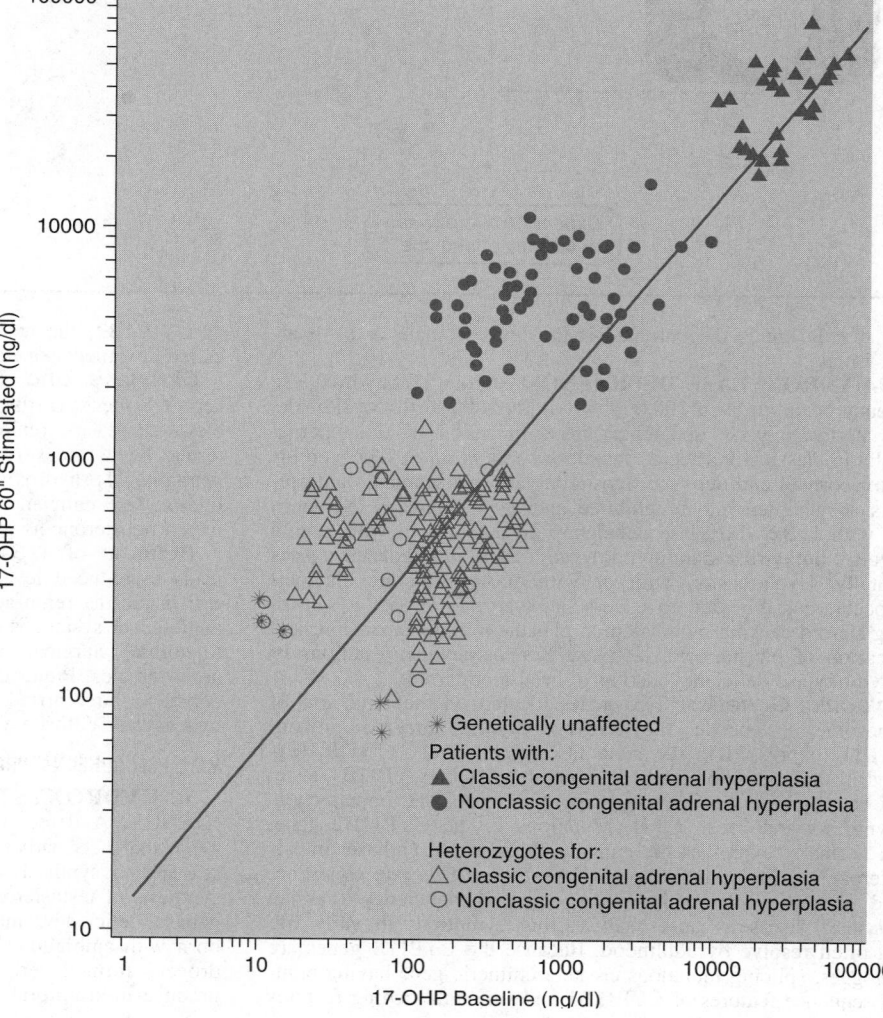

FIGURE 207–7. Nomogram relating baseline to ACTH-stimulated serum concentrations of 17-hydroxyprogesterone (17-OHP). The scales are logarithmic. A regression line for all data points is shown. The data for this nomogram were collected between 1982 and 1991 at the Department of Pediatrics, The New York Hospital–Cornell Medical Center, New York, New York.

17-OHP NOMOGRAM FOR THE DIAGNOSIS OF STEROID 21–HYDROXYLASE DEFICIENCY

60 MINUTE CORTROSYN STIMULATION TEST

Y-axis: 17-OHP 60" Stimulated (ng/dl)

X-axis: 17-OHP Baseline (ng/dl)

✳ Genetically unaffected

Patients with:
▲ Classic congenital adrenal hyperplasia
● Nonclassic congenital adrenal hyperplasia

Heterozygotes for:
△ Classic congenital adrenal hyperplasia
○ Nonclassic congenital adrenal hyperplasia

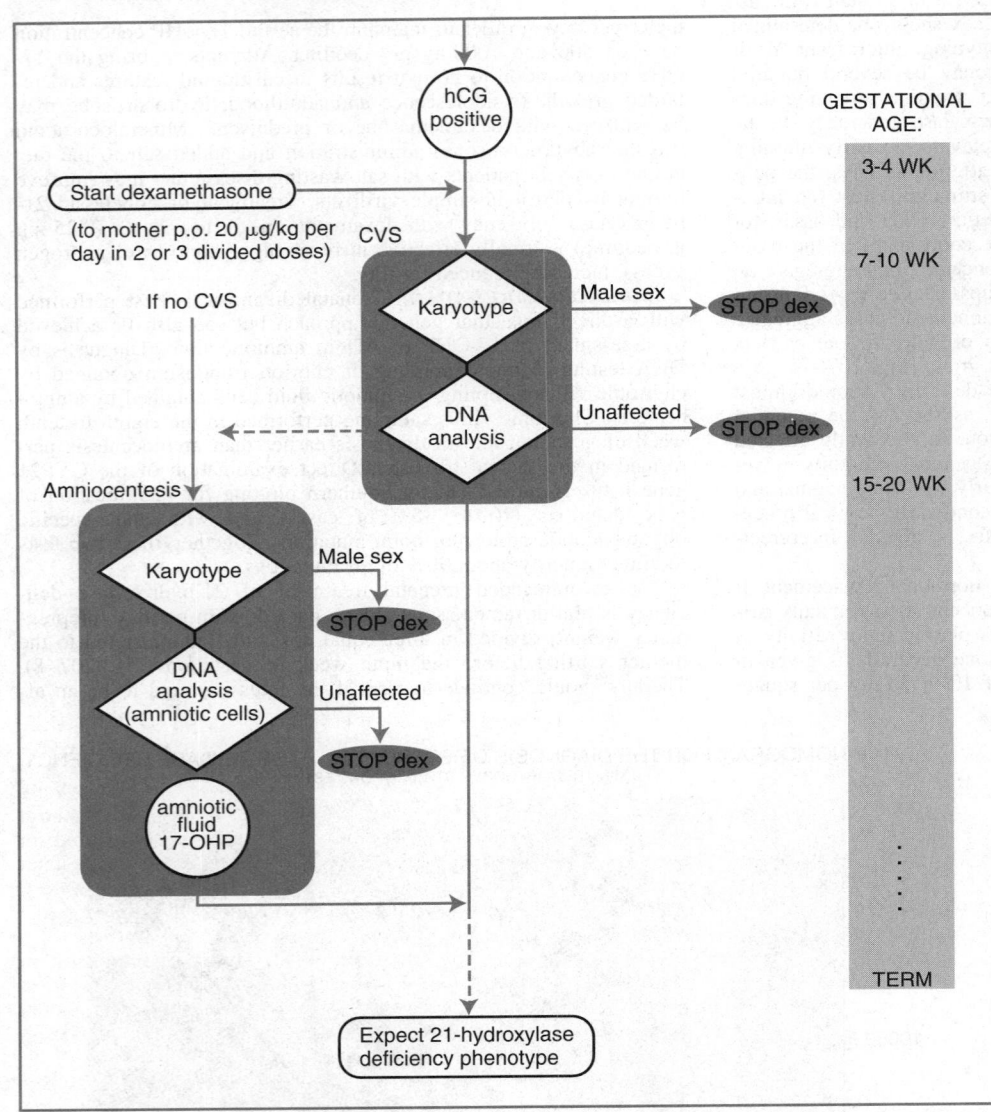

FIGURE 207-8. Algorithm depicting prenatal management of pregnancy in families at risk for a fetus affected with 21-hydroxylase deficiency. (From Speiser PW, Laforgia N, Kato K, et al.: First trimester prenatal treatment and molecular genetic diagnosis of congenital adrenal hyperplasia [21-hydroxylase deficiency]. J Clin Endocrinol Metab 70:838–848, 1990. © The Endocrine Society.)

fected female but is discontinued if the fetus is male or an unaffected female.

11β-HYDROXYLASE DEFICIENCY. Steroid 11β-hydroxylase deficiency occurs in 1 in 100,000 to 1 in 200,000 births worldwide. As in 21-hydroxylase deficiency, masculinization of the external genitalia in classically affected females occurs *in utero*. The steroids 11-deoxycortisol and deoxycorticosterone are oversecreted, and precursors are shunted into uninhibited androgen pathways. Newborn males with 11β-hydroxylase deficiency do not present with genital ambiguity, but virilization in untreated males and females ensues postnatally. Hypertension with or without hypokalemic alkalosis may occur, possibly due to excess deoxycorticosterone, a salt-retaining steroid causing hypokalemia; plasma volume expansion; and suppression of plasma renin activity. Nonclassic manifestations of 11β-hydroxylase deficiency also have been recognized.

Molecular Genetics. Two genes located on the long arm of chromosome 8 encode the 11β-hydroxylase enzyme protein: CYP11B1 (expressed in the zona fasciculata) and CYP11B2 (expressed in the zona glomerulosa). Mutations in the CYP11B1 gene, which has regulatory sequences responsive to ACTH, impair cortisol synthesis and cause CAH. Mutations in the CYP11B2 gene, which normally expresses the enzyme aldosterone synthase, impair aldosterone synthesis but not cortisol synthesis. This rare condition, termed corticosterone methyloxidase type II deficiency (Persian salt-wasting disease), causes salt-wasting symptoms in early life which often resolve by adulthood. Because the CYP11B genes are homologues, splicing mutations create a chimeric gene having regulatory sequence features of CYP11B1 and structural coding features

of CYP11B2; the result is a rare form of low-renin hypertension called dexamethasone-suppressible hyperaldosteronism.

Diagnosis and Treatment. In 11β-hydroxylase deficiency, serum 11-deoxycortisol (compound S) and deoxycorticosterone are elevated. Plasma renin activity is suppressed and/or plasma aldosterone levels are very low. In the genetic female with ambiguous genitalia, 11β-hydroxylase deficiency can be distinguished from 21-hydroxylase deficiency by elevated levels of compound S and deoxycorticosterone as well as suppressed plasma renin activity.

Treatment of 11β-hydroxylase deficiency with glucocorticoids leads to reduced levels of deoxycorticosterone with natriuresis, a rise in plasma renin activity, and normotension. Because the renin-angiotensin system is no longer suppressed, aldosterone levels rise to normal. Surgical correction may be necessary in untreated genetic females. Prenatal diagnosis and treatment of 11β-hydroxylase deficiency are carried out with the same protocol as in steroid 21-hydroxylase deficiency.

MALE PSEUDOHERMAPHRODITISM

3β-HYDROXYSTEROID DEHYDROGENASE DEFICIENCY. A defect in 3β-hydroxysteroid dehydrogenase, an enzyme that acts early in the pathway of cortisol synthesis, impairs sex steroid synthesis in both the adrenal and the gonads. As the synthesis of testosterone is impaired in 3β-hydroxysteroid dehydrogenase deficiency, males are incompletely masculinized and are born with ambiguous genitalia. In the genetic female fetus, Δ4 androgens formed peripherally from the excess secretion of DHEA produce mild clitoral enlargement. In the case of a severe enzyme block in either gender, salt wasting owing to aldosterone deficiency may develop.

A gene for the peripheral form of 3β-hydroxysteroid dehydrogenase (type I) and a gene for the adrenal-gonadal form of 3β-hydroxysteroid dehydrogenase (type II) have been identified and mapped to chromosome 1. Mutations in the type II gene have been described only in the classic form of the disorder.

Steroid 3β-hydroxysteroid dehydrogenase deficiency is diagnosed by a high ratio of Δ^5 to Δ^4 steroids. Elevated levels of pregnenolone, 17-hydroxypregnenolone, and DHEA are evident in serum; urinary Δ^5 metabolites pregnanetriol and 16-pregnanetriol are elevated. Steroid values in the newborn period may not be informative, as Δ^5 steroids are normally high during this time in unaffected persons. Glucocorticoid administration, with the addition of a mineralocorticoid to correct salt wasting, is effective.

Some women exhibiting clinically significant signs of androgen excess show a pattern of elevated Δ^5 to Δ^4 steroids; this may represent an underlying mild (nonclassic) 3β-hydroxysteroid dehydrogenase defect. No mutation has been identified to date in the nonclassic form. The nonclassic defect is diagnosed by 60-minute ACTH testing. Treatment consists of oral dexamethasone administration in small doses (0.25 mg at bedtime).

17α-HYDROXYLASE/17,20-LYASE DEFICIENCY.
Combined 17α-hydroxylase/17,20-lyase deficiency, a rare form of CAH, impairs the synthesis of cortisol and sex steroids. Males at birth may present with ambiguous genitalia or be mistakenly assigned to the female gender. Wolffian duct formation is incomplete owing to deficient androgen production, whereas normal AMH secretion by Sertoli cells inhibits formation of the uterus and fallopian tubes. Genetic females appear normal at birth and throughout childhood but may present with primary amenorrhea at puberty. Plasma gonadotropins are elevated in both sexes. Hypertension with hypokalemia due to excess deoxycorticosterone may develop and present clinically in childhood or may be found incidental to failure of puberty. The structural gene for P450c17 is located on chromosome 10.

The deficiency is diagnosed by high serum deoxycorticosterone and extremely high corticosterone (B) levels. Aldosterone levels are low owing to suppressed renin and hypokalemia from excess deoxycorticosterone. Before puberty, 17α-hydroxylase/17,20-lyase deficiency is treated with glucocorticoids. Sex steroids appropriate to the gender of rearing are given at pubertal age to induce the development of secondary sex characteristics. In genetic males raised as females, gonadectomy and vaginal reconstruction are required.

Isolated 17,20-lyase deficiency also can occur, in which the 17-hydroxylase function of the enzyme is intact and allows the synthesis of cortisol, but C_{19} steroid production is deficient.

CHOLESTEROL DESMOLASE DEFICIENCY.
Cholesterol desmolase deficiency (lipoid adrenal hyperplasia or Prader's syndrome), an extremely rare condition, involves a block in the conversion of cholesterol to pregnenolone. Affected males and females have a female external genital phenotype. Biochemical findings include profound deficiencies of all steroids, low plasma volume, hyperkalemia, and hyponatremia. Neonatal mortality is high from total adrenal insufficiency, but some patients maintained on hormonal replacement can survive to adulthood. The gene for the cholesterol desmolase enzyme has been cloned and mapped to chromosome 15.

LEYDIG CELL APLASIA.
Leydig cell aplasia or hypoplasia is a rare syndrome characterized by high basal luteinizing hormone (LH), normal follicle-stimulating hormone, and low testosterone, which does not respond to hCG stimulation. Adrenal steroidogenesis is normal, suggesting that the defect may reside at the level of the LH receptor.

5α-REDUCTASE DEFICIENCY.
Deficiency of 5α-reductase is a rare autosomal recessive disorder (Table 207–2). The membrane-bound enzyme 5α-reductase type 2 is responsible for the conversion of testosterone to DHT. A defect in 5α-reductase causes selective impairment of DHT-dependent steps of male sex differentiation. In patients with 5α-reductase deficiency, plasma testosterone levels are normal to elevated, whereas DHT levels are low. LH levels are normal or slightly elevated. Most patients have severe perineoscrotal hypospadias, and there may be a blind vaginal pouch opening into the urogenital sinus or the urethra. As the wolffian ducts are maintained by testosterone, patients have normal vasa deferentia, seminal vesicles, and epididymides. DHT-mediated virilization of the urogenital sinus and the external genitalia is impaired, and the prostate is small or absent. Patients have a female habitus without breast development but lack female internal genital structures. At puberty, testosterone-dependent masculinization occurs to a variable degree; affected males develop rugation and hyperpigmentation of the scrotum, growth of the phallus, an increase in muscle mass, and deepening of the voice. Some may have testicular descent (Fig. 207–9A). Gender change from female to male in untreated affected subjects has been documented.

Patients diagnosed with 5α-reductase deficiency in infancy and early childhood are best reared as males once hypospadias, ventral contraction and bowing of the penis (chordee), and cryptorchidism are surgically corrected. Because DHT is not available for general use, adults are usually treated by high doses of testosterone esters. In the absence of 5α-reduction, 19-nortestosterone is active and can be given by injection in an esterified form.

5α-Reductase isoform 2 is the major isoenzyme expressed in genital tissues, and a deletion in the type 2 gene has been found in affected subjects. Eighteen different mutations have been identified in 25 families, and approximately 40% of affected individuals are compound heterozygotes.

ABNORMALITIES OF THE TESTOSTERONE RECEPTOR: ANDROGEN INSENSITIVITY.
Masculinization of the reproductive tract depends upon androgen binding to the androgen receptor protein. Mutations of the X-linked gene coding for the androgen receptor in subjects hemizygous for the mutated gene therefore lead to androgen insensitivity, known in its complete form as testicular feminization syndrome (see Table 207–2). Androgen insensitivity is one of the most frequent forms of male pseudoher-

TABLE 207–2. DISORDERS OF SEXUAL DIFFERENTIATION IN MALES

| Disorder | Defective Protein | Gene Localization | Phenotype | | | | Endocrinology | |
			Müllerian Ducts	Wolffian Ducts	External Genitalia	Other	Testosterone	AMH
Defects in enzymes involved in testosterone synthesis or metabolism	Side chain cleavage	15q23–24	Absent	Present	Ambiguous		Low	Normal
	17α-hydroxylase	10	Absent	Present	Female	Hypertension	Low	Normal
	3β-HSD type 2	1p13	Absent	Present	Ambiguous	Salt loss	Low	High*
	17β-HSD type 3	9q22	Absent	Present	Female		Low	Normal
	5α-reductase type 2	2p23	Absent	Present	Ambiguous		High	Normal
Androgen insensitivity A. CAIS	Androgen receptor	Xq11–12	Absent	Absent	Female		Normal	High*
B. PAIS	Androgen receptor	Xq11–12	Absent	Present	Ambiguous		Normal	High*
Persistent müllerian duct syndrome	AMH	19p13	Present	Present	Male		Normal	Low
	AMH receptor	12q13	Present	Present	Male		Normal	Normal

* In the neonatal and pubertal period; normal at other times.

AMH = anti-müllerian hormone; 3β-HSD = 3β-hydroxysteroid dehydrogenase; 17β-HSD = 17β-hydroxysteroid dehydrogenase; CAIS = complete androgen insensitivity; PAIS = partial androgen insensitivity.

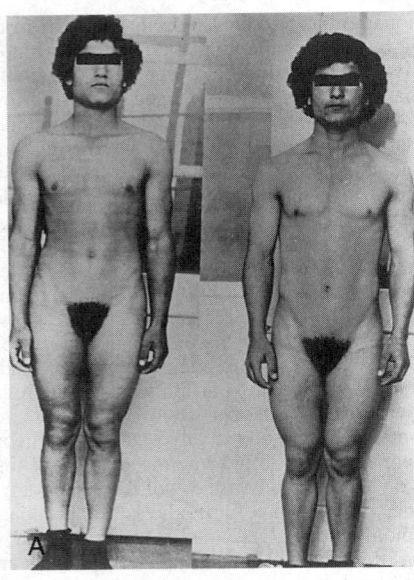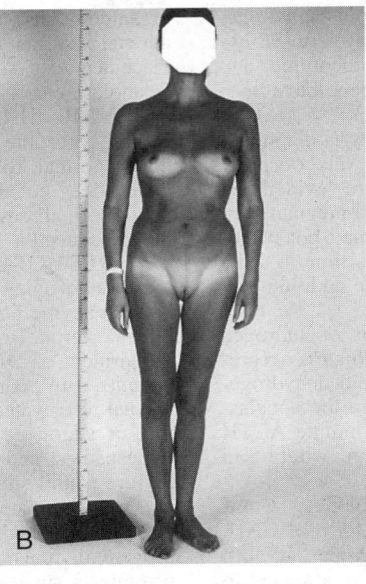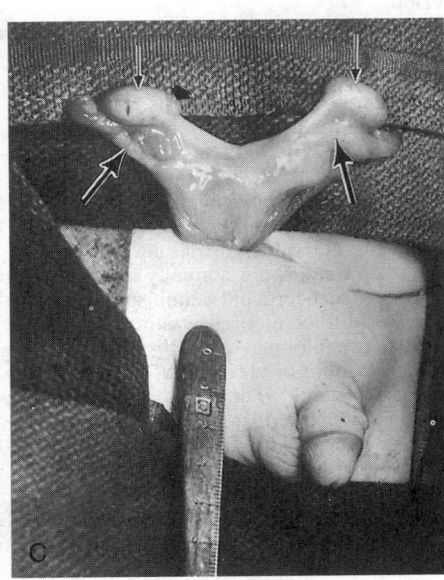

FIGURE 207-9. *A,* Pubertal virilization in brothers with 5α-reductase deficiency. (From Savage MO, Preece MA, Jeffcoate SL, et al.: Familial male pseudohermaphroditism due to deficiency of 5α-reductase. Clin Endocrinol 12:397, 1980.) *B,* Picture of patient with complete androgen insensitivity. *C,* A case of persistent müllerian duct syndrome; operative field. Above the normal, infantile, male genitalia are the contents of the right hernia sac. This consists of the testes *(small arrow)* and fallopian tubes *(large arrow)* which are separated by the uterus. A portion of an epididymis *(arrowhead)* caps the right testis. The vas deferens was palpable posteriorly on both sides. (From Harbison MD, Magid MLS, Josso N, et al.: Anti-Müllerian hormone in three intersex conditions. Ann Genet 34:226, 1991.)

maphroditism; estimates of incidence vary from 1 in 20,000 to 64,000 male births. It causes a spectrum of phenotypic abnormalities.

Clinical Features. Subjects affected by the complete form of androgen insensitivity have a normal female phenotype. They are rarely discovered before puberty unless masses are palpated in the groin or labia and discovered to be testes at surgical exploration. The vagina is usually shallow and ends blindly. Internal genital structures usually are absent, although some cases with residual müllerian derivatives have been described. The testes may be located in the abdomen or in the labia majora and do not undergo spermatogenesis. Testosterone and LH levels are elevated owing to a defective feedback regulation caused by androgen resistance at the level of the hypothalamus. Testicular estrogen production usually is increased; coupled with androgen insensitivity, this results in an unopposed estrogen effect and is the most likely explanation for breast development at puberty. Pubic and axillary hair is scant or absent (Fig. 207–9*B*).

Partial androgen insensitivity, also termed Reifenstein syndrome, presents with a variable degree of genital ambiguity, and both virilization and breast development occur at puberty (see Table 207–2). Partial androgen insensitivity also is consistent with a male phenotype with gynecomastia and infertility as the sole manifestations.

Molecular Genetics and Prenatal Diagnosis. The androgen receptor gene is located on the X chromosome, between Xq13 and Xp11, consistent with the sex-linked recessive mode of inheritance observed in affected families. *De novo* cases are not uncommon, contributing to the negative family history exhibited by approximately one third of complete androgen insensitivity sufferers.

At the cellular level, androgen insensitivity usually can be recognized by studying the affinity of cultured genital skin fibroblasts for DHT, but mutations can affect DNA binding and other aspects of receptor function. Prenatal diagnosis of androgen receptor defects is possible using chorionic villus tissue biopsy and DNA analysis.

Management. Management depends on the severity of the androgen receptor defect. Patients with complete androgen insensitivity should be raised as girls, and the testes should be removed to avoid malignant degeneration, which occurs in 1 to 2% of cases. The optimal time for castration is controversial. Some physicians prefer to delay it until after adolescence, to allow spontaneous feminization to occur. Estrogen treatment is then required to preserve breast development. Management of patients with partial androgen insensitivity is less straightforward because the diagnosis cannot always be confirmed by molecular studies in the neonatal period.

When the phallus is very small and other causes of male pseudohermaphroditism have been excluded, female gender assignment is the best option. Patients with partial androgen insensitivity who are raised as girls should have their testes removed early to avoid unwanted virilization.

PERSISTENT MÜLLERIAN DUCT SYNDROME. Male pseudohermaphroditism due to an isolated defect of AMH synthesis or action is a rare autosomal recessive disorder, characterized by the presence of uterus and tubes, tightly linked to the testes in otherwise normally virilized males. When these are held in the pelvis by the round ligament, they prevent the testes from descending and lead to bilateral cryptorchidism (Fig. 207–9*C*). In most cases, however, müllerian derivatives are mobile and are dragged into the inguinal canal and scrotum by the descending testis, resulting in an apparent inguinoscrotal hernia with contralateral cryptorchidism. The condition usually is discovered only at operation.

A dozen different mutations of the gene coding for AMH have been described in patients with low or undetectable serum concentrations of the hormone. End-organ insensitivities, perhaps due to mutations of the AMH receptor gene, are probably involved in subjects with normal serum levels of AMH. Treatment should aim at preserving fertility through early correction of cryptorchidism, paying great attention to the integrity of the vas deferens, which often is incorporated in the wall of the uterus and cervix.

CONCLUSIONS AND GENERAL MANAGEMENT

Sexual ambiguity, at least in the newborn, should be treated as a pediatric emergency. It may threaten the life of the patient if, as in most cases, the intersex condition is due to CAH and is associated with salt loss. Even if this is not the case, it is important to assign gender as early as possible. Gender identity is established very early in life, certainly by the time speech is established. Gender confusion owing to indeterminant or wrong assignment of gender may lead to severe emotional disorders later in life.

Three diagnostic clues are helpful: gonadal location, presence of a uterus, and karyotype. If no gonads are palpable in a 46,XX chromatin-positive baby, CAH should be suspected before the possibility of true hermaphroditism or idiopathic female pseudohermaphroditism is entertained. In patients with at least one palpable gonad, if a uterus can be visualized by ultrasonography, the most likely diagnosis is testicular dysgenesis in 46,XY subjects and true hermaphroditism or XX maleness in 46,XX subjects. If there are no müllerian derivatives, male pseudohermaphroditism due to testosterone defects or malformations should be considered. It is prudent to wait a few days to assign the gender until common causes of sexual ambiguity are investigated. However, once gender is assigned, the physician should proceed with certainty in counseling parents on the sex of rearing, thus avoiding confusion of gender.

Donahoe PK, Powell DM, Lee MM: Clinical management of intersex abnormalities. Curr Probl Surg 28:519, 1991. *A compendium of surgical approaches in the reconstruction of genital abnormalities.*

George FW, Wilson JD: Sex determination and differentiation. *In* Knobil E, Neill JD (eds.): The Physiology of Reproduction. 2nd ed. New York, Raven Press, 1994, p 3. *An up-to-date overview of the physiology of sex determination.*

Josso N, Cate RL, Picard JY, et al.: Anti-Müllerian hormone, the Jost factor. Rec Progr Hormone Res 48:1, 1993. *An update on AMH.*

McPhaul MJ, Marcelli M, Zoppi S, et al.: Genetic basis of endocrine disease: The spectrum of mutations in the androgen receptor gene that causes androgen resistance. J Clin Endocrinol Metab 76:17, 1993. *A study of the relationship between phenotype and genotype in androgen insensitivity.*

New MI: Congenital adrenal hyperplasia. *In* DeGroot L (ed.): Endocrinology. 3rd ed. Philadelphia, WB Saunders, 1994. *A comprehensive chapter on the various forms of congenital adrenal hyperplasia.*

New MI, White PC, Speiser PW, et al.: Congenital adrenal hyperplasia. *In* Emery AEH, Rimoin DL: Principles and Practice of Medical Genetics. 3rd ed. New York, Churchill Livingstone, 1995. *An overview of the molecular genetics of congenital adrenal hyperplasia.*

Polin RA, Fox WW (eds.): Fetal and Neonatal Physiology, vol 2. Philadelphia, WB Saunders, 1992. *Section XXVIII of this book comprises six chapters on the ovary and testis. Notable is the chapter "Germ Cells and the Indifferent Gonad" by Jirasek.*

Wachtel S (ed.): Molecular Genetics of Sex Determination. New York, Academic Press, 1994. *Articles on the basic biology of sex determination as well as human genetics of sex determination and clinical aspects of syndromes of abnormal sex differentiation.*

Wilson JD, Griffin JE, Russell DW: Steroid 5 alpha-reductase-2 deficiency. Endocr Rev 14:577, 1993. *A study of the molecular genetics of 5α-reductase deficiency.*

208 ENDOCRINOLOGIC DISEASES UNIQUE TO WOMEN

208.1 The Ovaries
Robert W. Rebar

The ovaries episodically release female gametes (oocytes or eggs) and secrete sex steroid hormones, principally androstenedione, estradiol, and progesterone. Oocytes are released only during the adult reproductive years, when sex steroid secretion is also greatest, but the ovaries are physiologically active throughout life.

Sex steroids affect the growth, differentiation, and function of a variety of tissues and organs throughout the body; therefore, abnormalities of the ovaries and of sex steroid secretion should be recognized by all physicians. A rational approach to the diagnosis and treatment of reproductive disorders in women requires an understanding of the functions of the ovaries and of their most important unit, the follicle, throughout life.

EMBRYOLOGY AND ANATOMY OF THE OVARIES

EMBRYOGENESIS AND DIFFERENTIATION (see also Ch. 207). Prior to 6 to 7 weeks of fetal age the gonads are paired, undifferentiated gonadal ridges overlying the mesonephros. By the sixth week of gestation, the primordial germ cells have migrated from their site of origin in the yolk sac to the gonadal ridges. Beginning during the sixth to eighth weeks the ovaries rapidly differentiate, and the number of germ cells, now called oogonia, increases by mitosis to 6 to 7 million. The germ cells next undergo meiosis such that all germ cells (now called oocytes) are arrested in meiotic prophase by the seventh month of gestation. From midgestation onward the number of germ cells progressively decreases until the menopause, by which time virtually no oocytes remain (Fig. 208–1). The germ cells are eliminated from ovaries by *ovulation* and by *atresia* (degeneration), which accounts for the elimination of 99.9% of all germ cells. The development of the ovaries is described in greater detail in Ch. 207.

THE ADULT OVARY. The adult ovary consists of two principal parts: a central medulla surrounded by the predominant outer cortex

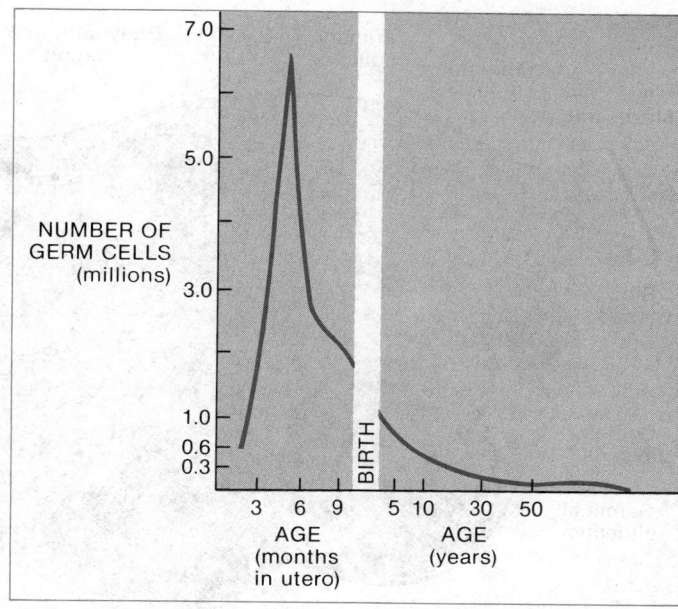

FIGURE 208–1. The number of oocytes present in both ovaries at different ages. (Adapted from Baker TG: *In* Austin CR, Short RJ [eds.]: Reproduction in Mammals. I. Germ Cells and Fertilization. London, Cambridge University Press, 1972, pp 14–45. Reproduced from Rebar RW: Semin Reproduct Endocrinol 1:169–176, 1983.)

(Fig. 208–2). The entire ovary is limited by a single cell layer termed the germinal epithelium. The medulla contains the blood vessels and nerves as well as nests of steroid-secreting hilus or ovarian Leydig cells. The cortex contains the *follicle complexes,* composed of the *oocyte, granulosa cells,* and *theca cells.* Characteristic changes occur in each component during follicle growth and differentiation. Interactions among the follicular components give rise to the gamete (ovum) and to sex steroid hormones necessary for establishing and maintaining early pregnancy following fertilization of the ovum.

Follicles can be divided into two major classes, nongrowing and growing. The nongrowing or *primordial* follicles comprise 90 to 95% of the ovarian follicles throughout the reproductive life of the female. The ability of a woman to menstruate and reproduce depends totally upon the pool of primordial follicles. Each primordial follicle contains a small oocyte arrested in meiotic prophase, surrounded by a layer of squamous cells from which granulosa cells originate. These cells are bounded by the basal lamina, which is selectively permeable to solutes in plasma. This complex is surrounded in turn by stroma, which consists of supporting connective tissue cells, contractile cells, and steroid-secreting thecal interstitial cells. Primordial follicles are recruited sequentially to become growing follicles, which then pass through primary, secondary, and tertiary (or graafian) phases. Atresia may occur in any phase.

Erickson GF, Schreiber JR: Morphology and physiology of the ovary. *In* Becker KL, (eds.): Principles and Practice of Endocrinology and Metabolism. Philadelphia, JB Lippincott, 1990, p 776. *A treatise on follicular growth and development.*

OVARIAN FUNCTION IN CHILDHOOD AND PUBERTY

PHYSICAL CHANGES AT PUBERTY. Puberty extends from the earliest signs of sexual maturation until the attainment of physical, mental, and emotional maturity. Pubertal changes in girls result directly or indirectly from maturation of the hypothalamic-pituitary-ovarian unit. Hormonally, human puberty is characterized by a resetting of the negative gonadal steroid feedback loop, the establishment of new circadian and ultradian (frequent) gonadotropin rhythms, and the acquisition in the female of a positive estrogen feedback loop controlling the menstrual cycle as interdependent expressions of the gonadotropins and ovarian steroids. In girls, pubertal development generally occurs between 8 and 14 years of age. The age of onset and the rate of progress through puberty are vari-

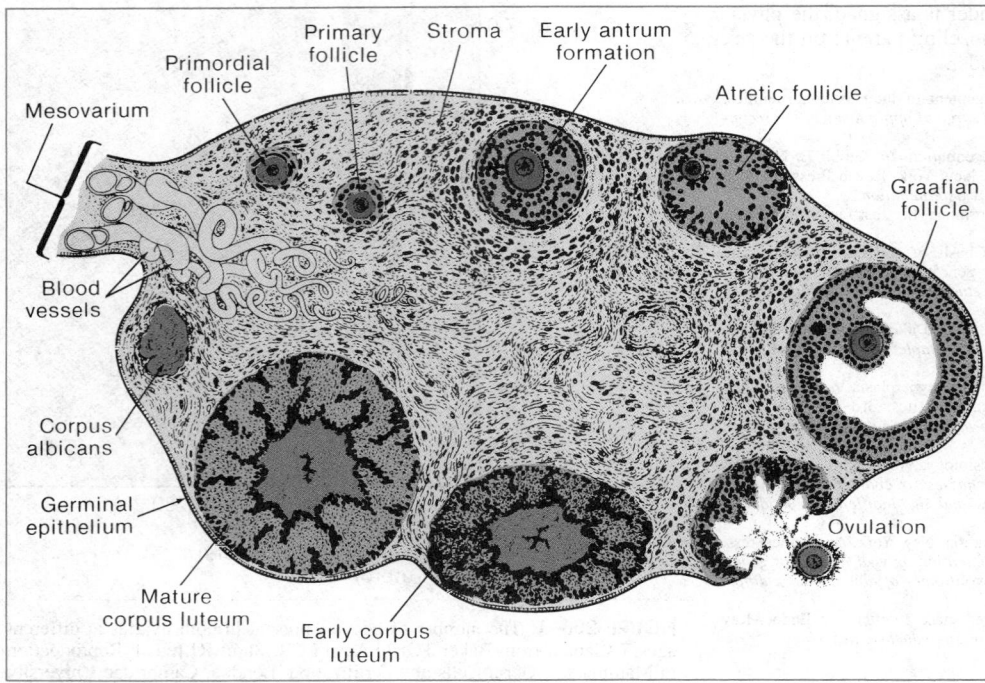

FIGURE 208–2. Diagrammatic illustration of the microscopic anatomy of the ovary. Changes in the components of the follicular complex occurring during atresia and ovulation are shown, progressing clockwise, from a primordial follicle (*upper left*) to a corpus albicans (*lower left*). (Adapted from Ross GT, Schreiber JR: *In* Yen SSC, Jaffe RB [eds.]: Reproductive Endocrinology—Physiology, Pathophysiology and Clinical Management, 2nd ed. Philadelphia, WB Saunders, 1986, p 115.)

able and depend upon genetic, socioeconomic, nutritional, physical, and psychological factors.

Physical changes occur in an orderly sequence over a definite time frame during puberty (Fig. 208–3). Breast budding in girls is usually the first pubertal change, followed shortly by the appearance of pubic hair, with menarche occurring late in pubertal development. The time from breast budding (median age of onset 9.8 years) to menarche approximates 2 years. Breast development results from increasing ovarian estrogen production and pubic and axillary hair from increasing ovarian androgen production. Estrogens are required for growth of pubic hair as well.

The ovarian sex steroids join with growth hormone and adrenal androgens to produce the adolescent growth spurt. Peak growth velocity is achieved relatively early with little growth observed following menarche. Lean body mass, skeletal mass, and body fat are equal in prepubertal boys and girls, but by maturity women have twice as much body fat and less lean body mass and skeletal mass as men, as a result of differences in sex steroid secretion beginning at puberty. Estrogens are necessary for normal formation, mineralization, and maturation of bones. Well-established standards exist for determining radiographically, typically by examining radiographs of the bones of the wrist, whether bone age is appropriate

for chronologic age. Estrogen deficiencies retard and excesses advance bone age in relation to chronologic age.

HORMONAL CHANGES. The ovaries function even in early childhood. The low levels of luteinizing hormone (LH) and follicle-stimulating hormone (FSH), which are normally present, increase if the ovaries are removed prior to puberty, just as they do later in life, indicating exquisite sensitivity of the hypothalamic-pituitary unit to extremely low circulating sex steroid levels. As puberty nears there is a progressive decrease in sensitivity of the hypothalamic-pituitary unit to sex steroids, leading to increased secretion of pituitary gonadotropins, stimulation of sex steroid output, and the

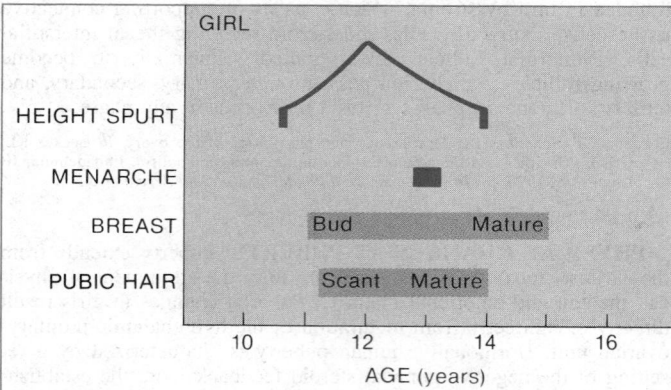

FIGURE 208–3. Temporal sequence of events for the "average" girl during puberty. (Reproduced from Rebar RW: *In* Yen SSC, Jaffe RB [eds.]: Reproductive Endocrinology—Physiology, Pathophysiology and Clinical Management, 3rd ed. Philadelphia, WB Saunders, 1991, p 830.)

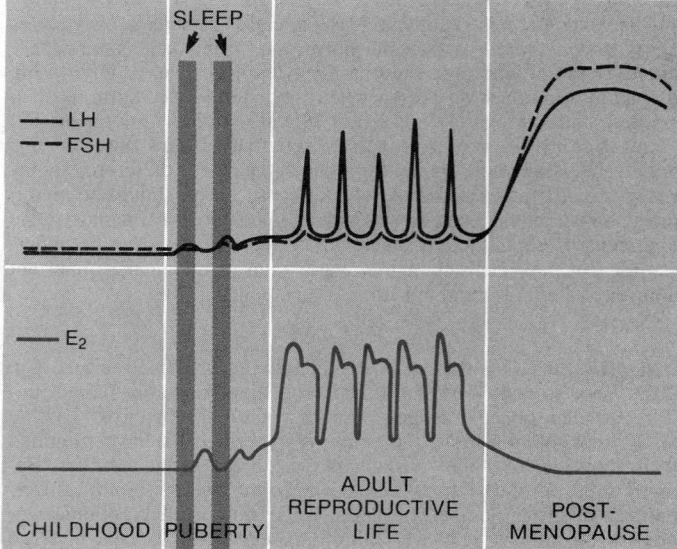

FIGURE 208–4. The changing patterns of LH, FSH, and estradiol (E_2) concentrations in peripheral blood throughout the life of a woman. The elevated levels of LH and FSH present in the first several weeks of life are not shown, nor is the fact that both LH and FSH are secreted in a pulsatile fashion. The pubertal period has been expanded to illustrate the sleep-associated increases in LH and FSH followed by morning increases in E_2 that are observed during puberty. (Reprinted with permission from *Endocrine and Metabolism Continuing Education Quality Control Program*, 1982. Copyright American Association for Clinical Chemistry, Inc.)

development of secondary sex characteristics. Increased secretion of both LH and FSH initially occurs at night with sleep and is associated with increased estradiol secretion the following morning (Fig. 208–4). As is true for most hormones, both LH and FSH are secreted in an episodic or pulsatile rather than a continuous fashion. It is possible that the sleep-entrained pulsatile secretion of gonadotropins commences in response to increased pulsatile secretion of gonadotropin-releasing hormone (GnRH). Later in puberty, secretion of LH and FSH is increased, relative to childhood, throughout the 24-hour period, except during the early follicular phase when nighttime increases still occur. Basal levels of estradiol, the major estrogen secreted by the ovaries, increase throughout puberty. A "critical body mass" may be required for positive estrogen feedback and ovulation. During the first 2 years after menarche, up to 90% of menstrual cycles may be anovulatory because of a delay in the synchronization of the hypothalamic-pituitary-ovarian axis.

ABERRATIONS IN PUBERTAL DEVELOPMENT

DEFINITION. Abnormalities of pubertal development can be divided into four major categories (Table 208–1):

1. *Precocious puberty* represents any pubertal changes before the age of 8 years. The precocious development is *isosexual* when the development is common to the phenotypic sex of the individual and *heterosexual* when the development is characteristic of the opposite sex. *True* or *central precocious puberty* is due to premature maturation of the hypothalamic-pituitary axis. In the absence of increased hypothalamic-pituitary activity, *precocious pseudopuberty* (also known as precocious puberty of peripheral origin) exists.

2. *Delayed (or interrupted) puberty* is defined as the absence of any secondary sex characteristics by the age of 13 years or of menarche by age 16 or by passage of 5 or more years from breast budding to menarche.

3. *Asynchronous pubertal development* occurs when there is deviation from the normal pattern of pubertal development.

4. *Heterosexual pubertal development* is development occurring at the appropriate time, but with some features characteristic of the opposite sex.

PRECOCIOUS PUBERTY. *Differential Diagnosis.* The temporal sequence in which the signs and symptoms of sex steroid hormone excess appear is most important. *Incomplete isosexual precocious puberty* indicates premature development of only a single pubertal feature. If breast budding occurs prior to the age of 8 years in the absence of any other development, the diagnosis may be *premature thelarche.* Premature thelarche is believed due to transient increases in estrogen secretion or increased breast sensitivity to the small quantities of circulating estrogens present prior to puberty. If pubic and/or axillary hair develops alone and persists, *premature pubarche* and *adrenarche* must be considered. These abnormalities are associated with slight increases in adrenal androgen secretion, but not with clitoromegaly or other signs of virilization. These syndromes require no treatment, and affected girls typically begin true puberty at the usual age.

When precocious development is isosexual, the purpose of evaluation is to determine if the cause is central (true precocious puberty) or not. Careful questioning of the patient and her parents may indicate inadvertent ingestion or absorption of sex steroids (ia-

TABLE 208–1. ABERRATIONS OF PUBERTAL DEVELOPMENT

I. **Precocious development (before age 8)**
  A. Isosexual precocity
    1. Incomplete sexual precocity
      a. Premature thelarche
      b. Premature pubarche
      c. Premature adrenarche
    2. True (central) precocious puberty
      a. Idiopathic (constitutional)
      b. Due to CNS lesions
      c. Primary hypothyroidism
      d. Silver-Russell syndrome
    3. Precocious pseudopuberty (of peripheral origin)
      a. Ovarian neoplasms
      b. Adrenal neoplasms
      c. Iatrogenic (estrogen-containing preparations)
      d. hCG-secreting neoplasms distinct from CNS and ovarian tumors
      e. McCune-Albright syndrome
  B. Heterosexual precocity
    1. Ovarian neoplasms
    2. Adrenal neoplasms
    3. Congenital adrenal hyperplasia
    4. Other rare disorders of sexual differentiation
II. **Delayed pubertal development**
  (no development by age 13; absence of menarche by age 16; passage of 5 years or more from breast budding without menarche)
  A. Anatomic abnormalities
    1. Müllerian agenesis or dysgenesis (Rokitansky-Küster-Hauser syndrome)
    2. Distal genital tract obstruction
      a. Transverse vaginal septum
      b. Imperforate hymen
      c. Vaginal agenesis
  B. Hypergonadotropic hypogonadism (FSH > 30–40 mIU per milliliter)
    1. Gonadal dysgenesis
      a. With stigmata of Turner's syndrome
      b. Pure (46,XX or 46,XY)
      c. Mixed
    2. Ovarian failure with normal ovarian development
      a. Autoimmune disorders
      b. Gonadotropin receptor and/or postreceptor defects (?resistant ovary or Savage syndrome)
      c. Enzymatic defects (17α-hydroxylase deficiency, galactosemia)
  d. Physical causes
    i. Irradiation
    ii. Chemotherapeutic agents
    iii. Viral agents
  e. Idiopathic
  C. Hypogonadotropic or normogonadotropic hypogonadism (LH and FSH < 10 mIU per milliliter or LH and FSH 6–25 mIU per milliliter with at least one being > 10 mIU per milliliter)
    1. Isolated gonadotropin deficiency
      a. In association with midline defects (Kallmann's syndrome)
      b. Independent of associated disorders
    2. Neoplasms of the hypothalamic-pituitary axis
      a. Craniopharyngiomas
      b. Pituitary tumors
      c. Others
    3. Infiltrative processes (Langerhans-type histiocytosis)
    4. Idiopathic hypopituitarism
    5. "Hypothalamic" forms of amenorrhea
      a. Psychogenic
      b. Exercise associated
      c. Associated with malnutrition
      d. Anorexia nervosa
    6. Miscellaneous disorders
      a. Prader-Labhardt-Willi syndrome
      b. Lawrence-Moon-Bardet-Biedl syndrome
      c. Primary hypothyroidism
    7. Constitutional delayed puberty
III. **Asynchronous pubertal development**
  A. Incomplete forms of androgen insensitivity
  B. Complete forms of androgen insensitivity
IV. **Heterosexual pubertal development**
  A. Polycystic ovary syndrome
  B. Congenital adrenal hyperplasia (female pseudohermaphroditism)
    1. 21-Hydroxylase deficiency
    2. 11β-Hydroxylase deficiency
    3. 3β-ol-Hydroxysteroid dehydrogenase deficiency
  C. Male pseudohermaphroditism due to 5α-reductase deficiency
  D. Male pseudohermaphroditism due to partial androgen insensitivity
  E. Mixed gonadal dysgenesis
  F. Androgen-producing neoplasms
    1. Ovarian
    2. Adrenal
  G. Cushing's syndrome

trogenic or factitious). About 10% of individuals with true precocious puberty have one of several organic brain diseases, including neoplasms, tuberous sclerosis, neurofibromatosis, encephalitis, meningitis, and hydrocephalus. The seriousness of intracranial lesions mandates that girls with precocious puberty have radiographic evaluation of the central nervous system, most effectively by magnetic resonance imaging (MRI). In almost 90% of girls with true precocious puberty, however, no cause is identified (idiopathic or constitutional).

The physical examination may also provide critical information about the cause of the precocious development. Cutaneous café-au-lait spots, facial asymmetry, polyostotic fibrous dysplasia and other skeletal abnormalities, cranial nerve deficits, and multiple ovarian follicular cysts suggest *McCune-Albright syndrome* in a girl with precocious puberty. It is now known that various clones of cells in the endocrine glands of girls with this disorder function autonomously with respect to cyclic AMP (cAMP) production as a consequence of a mutation within exon 8 of the G protein α subunit. This same mutation probably accounts for the bone lesions and café-au-lait hyperpigmentation. Precocious development associated with short stature, congenital bodily asymmetry, a triangular facies, and clinodactyly suggests the *Silver-Russell syndrome*. Characteristic signs and symptoms may suggest the coexistence of primary hypothyroidism and precocious puberty, especially if galactorrhea is also present. In these patients, thyroid hormone replacement therapy halts progression of pubertal development until the expected age of puberty. (Enigmatically, primary hypothyroidism may also lead to delayed pubertal development. Thyroid hormone replacement permits the onset of puberty.)

Abdominal and rectal examination may reveal a mass, suggesting an adrenal or ovarian tumor. Because palpable ovarian cysts may develop rarely prior to ovulation in true precocious puberty, the presence of a mass need not confirm the diagnosis of precocious pseudopuberty.

When vaginal bleeding is the only sign of development, the diagnosis of sexual precocity should be suspect. Common causes of bleeding in this age group include irritation from a vaginal infection or foreign body, sexual assault, prolapse of the urethral meatus, and ingestion of estrogen-containing medications (most commonly oral contraceptive preparations). A vaginal or cervical neoplasm is also a rare possibility. Thus, vaginal bleeding dictates the need for vaginal examination, often best performed under anesthesia, before further evaluation is undertaken.

Heterosexual precocity in an apparent prepubertal female is almost always due to congenital adrenal hyperplasia or to an androgen-secreting adrenal or ovarian neoplasm. Only very rarely must another disorder of sexual differentiation be considered (see Ch. 207). It is important to examine the external genitalia carefully because congenital adrenal hyperplasia is usually associated with some degree of sexual ambiguity.

Excessive androgens produced endogenously by abnormal fetal adrenal glands *in utero* or diffusing across the placenta to the fetus from the mother can virilize the external genitalia and result in female pseudohermaphroditism. The extent of virilization varies from an enlarged clitoris only to sexual ambiguity sufficient to make gender assignment difficult.

Excessive maternal androgen secretion, typically from an ovarian or adrenal neoplasm, can lead to virilization of a female fetus. This occurs very rarely, because of the great capacity of the placenta to aromatize naturally occurring androgens to estrogens. Virilization of a female fetus is much more likely to occur if a pregnant woman has ingested a synthetic steroid preparation with androgenic properties because available synthetic compounds generally cannot be aromatized.

Excessive androgen secretion beginning *in utero* is usually associated with defective cortisol synthesis. As a consequence, ACTH secretion is increased, resulting in congenital adrenal hyperplasia and excessive androgen secretion. The three different enzyme defects in the steroidogenic pathway that can lead to virilization of the female fetus are described in Ch. 207. 21-Hydroxylase deficiency is the most common form of congenital adrenal hyperplasia, accounting for the disorder in more than 90% of affected individuals. The defect may vary from partial to complete deficiency of the enzyme.

Diagnostic Tests. **Measurement of Peptide and Steroid Hormones.** Increased levels of immunoreactive human chorionic gonadotropin (hCG) may suggest an hCG-secreting neoplasm, most commonly an ovarian teratoma or dysgerminoma. In such cases, the hCG, which is antigenically and biologically similar to LH, stimulates ovarian steroid secretion and pseudopubertal development. Because even specific LH immunoassays show some cross-reactivity with hCG, values for serum LH may be elevated in individuals with hCG-secreting tumors. Immunoreactive hCG is always elevated in the presence of such tumors. Levels and ratios of FSH and LH typical of pubertal as opposed to prepubertal girls help in diagnosing true precocious puberty. Timed urine collections rather than blood samples can be used to measure gonadotropin secretion if necessary. The use of exogenous GnRH to stimulate endogenous LH and FSH secretion can be useful in differentiating gonadotropin-dependent from gonadotropin-independent precocious puberty. Excessively high circulating levels of estrogen suggest an estrogen-producing neoplasm. High levels of serum testosterone suggest an ovarian source of excess androgen in girls with heterosexual development, whereas increased levels of dehydroepiandrosterone (DHEA) or its sulfate (DHEA-S) (the principal precursors of 17-ketosteroids) suggest an adrenal source. High levels of serum 17-hydroxyprogesterone imply congenital adrenal hyperplasia (CAH) secondary to 21-hydroxylase deficiency, whereas high levels of serum 11-deoxycortisol imply an 11β-hydroxylase deficiency. In CAH these hormone levels should decrease promptly following oral administration of suppressive doses of dexamethasone. Suppression in response to exogenous corticoids occurs much less consistently in individuals with adrenal cortical adenomas and carcinomas and rarely in those with ovarian androgen-secreting neoplasms (see Ch. 204.1, 207).

Additional Studies. Ultrasonic scanning of the adrenals and ovaries and computed tomography (CT) of the adrenals may be indicated to confirm clinical suspicions. In girls with ovarian or adrenal neoplasms the tumor can almost always be localized radiographically. Catheterization of the ovarian and adrenal veins and measurements of the effluent steroids from each gland should be pursued only when CT, ultrasonography, or MRI fails to identify what is suspected to be a neoplasm. Although plain skull films are of use in screening for pituitary and parapituitary tumors, CT or MRI of the skull is indicated in the presence of definite neurologic deficits or if true precocious puberty is suspected. Radiographic estimation of bone age is indicated in all cases and serves as a useful tool to follow the results of treatment.

Treatment. Treatment for precocious puberty should be initiated promptly so that: (1) The patient's ultimate height is not compromised as a result of sex steroid–induced premature epiphyseal closure. (2) Emotional disturbances in the patient and her parents are prevented or attenuated.

GnRH analogues are now the preferred therapy for suppressing gonadotropin secretion and also may prevent early bone maturation. The analogues are not effective in children with McCune-Albright syndrome, and ketoconazole or testolactone has been only marginally successful. Medroxyprogesterone acetate (100 to 200 mg intramuscularly every 2 to 4 weeks) also may be used to suppress gonadotropin secretion. Medroxyprogesterone acetate, however, does not always prevent premature epiphyseal closure and the resultant short stature.

Individuals with CNS or steroid-secreting neoplasms must undergo therapy appropriate for the particular lesion. Girls with congenital adrenal hyperplasia are appropriately managed with glucocorticoids (plus mineralocorticoids when indicated) as outlined in Ch. 207.

DELAYED PUBERTY. Typically girls with delayed puberty present at the age of 16 years or later because of primary amenorrhea, but younger girls may present because of failure to initiate pubertal development. Because of the anxiety generated by delayed puberty, some evaluation is always indicated regardless of the age of the patient.

When pubertal development progresses normally but menstruation does not begin, an abnormality in the genital tract should be considered. Congenital malformations of the müllerian ducts are uncommon, occurring in 0.02% of all women. Most do not cause amenorrhea, and many do not impair reproduction. The anomalies associated with amenorrhea vary in severity from an imperforate hymen to complete aplasia of all müllerian duct derivatives with vaginal atresia. Although aplasia generally involves all of the müllerian duct derivatives, defects may involve only a single part of the distal genital tract.

A müllerian duct anomaly is suggested by (1) normal levels of serum gonadotropins and steroids, (2) an abnormal outflow tract, (3) a history of cyclic abdominal pain with or without a palpable mass, and (4) normal development of secondary sex characteristics. Normal ovarian function still induces endometrial growth and shedding after menarche if the uterus is normal. In the absence of a normal outflow tract, however, the menstrual effluent is retained and may or may not be able to escape into the abdominal cavity. Free in the abdominal cavity, the effluent may cause endometriosis. Constrained to the uterine cavity, the effluent causes hematometra and a large abdominal mass. In the absence of a mass or cyclic pain, a karyotype is indicated in girls with evidence of an abnormal genital tract to rule out any of several disorders of sexual differentiation (see Ch. 207). Such disorders, however, almost never occur together with completely normal pubertal development. In girls with a normal karyotype and a genital tract anomaly, examination under anesthesia and diagnostic laparoscopy should be undertaken to delineate the extent of the defect. When the abnormality consists of an imperforate hymen or transverse vaginal septum only, surgical restoration can be accomplished relatively simply. Attempts to provide an outflow tract for the uterus should not be undertaken if there is no cervix because of the high risk of recurrent pelvic infection. Even with a functional cervix, the creation of an outflow tract that will permit successful pregnancy is unlikely. A functional vagina can be created surgically or by the daily use of ever-larger dilators. To prevent shrinkage and scarring, surgery should be deferred until the patient is willing to use dilators postoperatively on a daily basis or she is about to become sexually active.

Other causes of delayed puberty and primary amenorrhea are the same as those that may cause amenorrhea in older women (see below). When no apparent cause for delayed development is found, constitutional delayed puberty must be entertained as a diagnosis of exclusion. A strong family history of delayed maturation adds support to this presumption. Small doses of estrogen may be administered to induce some pubertal development but may obscure a pathologic cause for the delay and may compromise linear growth and ultimate height.

ASYNCHRONOUS PUBERTAL DEVELOPMENT. Asynchronous pubertal development is characteristic of male pseudohermaphroditism due to androgen insensitivity, especially complete testicular feminization. This syndrome of androgen insensitivity is inherited either as an X-linked recessive or as a sex-limited autosomal dominant trait. Despite the presence of intra-abdominal or inguinal testes, there is complete failure of virilization. Affected individuals develop breasts (but only to Tanner stage 3) and a typical female habitus with unambiguous female external genitalia but with absence of internal female structures, generally having only a foreshortened blind-ending vagina. Little or no pubic and axillary hair develops. The karyotype is obviously 46,XY in these individuals. Circulating testosterone levels are equivalent to or higher than those found in normal men, and LH levels are elevated while FSH levels are normal compared to those in menstruating women. This syndrome is further discussed in Ch. 207.

HETEROSEXUAL PUBERTAL DEVELOPMENT. *Polycystic ovary (PCO) syndrome,* by far the most common cause of heterosexual pubertal development, is associated with the development of some secondary sex features characteristic of males at the normal age of puberty. Feminization occurs in affected girls, and they develop normal breasts and a typical female habitus, but masculinization also occurs. (In contrast, girls with congenital adrenal hyperplasia generally show little if any female development at puberty.) A heterogeneous syndrome, PCO syndrome most typically begins at or near puberty with hirsutism and irregular menses from the time of menarche. Menarche may be delayed as well, so that young women may present with primary amenorrhea. Basal LH levels tend to be somewhat elevated in perhaps 80% of cases, and circulating levels of all androgens are elevated moderately.

Congenital adrenal hyperplasia is generally diagnosed prior to puberty, and heterosexual precocious pseudopuberty is typical. However, if the defect is mild and changes to the external genitalia are minimal, masculinization may occur at the expected age of puberty. This attenuated or nonclassic form of 21-hydroxylase deficiency seems to occur in families with a strong family history of

hirsutism. Affected girls generally have some defeminization with flattening of the breasts, severe hirsutism, relatively short stature, and obesity.

Mixed gonadal dysgenesis designates asymmetric gonadal development, with a germ cell tumor or a testis on one side and an undifferentiated streak, rudimentary gonad, or no gonad on the other. The extent of genital virilization prior to puberty is variable in this rare disorder. The vast majority are reared as girls, in whom virilization occurs at puberty; some may note breast development as well. Affected individuals generally have a mosaic karyotype, with 45,X/46,XY being most common. Short stature and other stigmata associated with a 45,X karyotype in Turner's syndrome are less common in patients with tumors than in patients with testes. Gonadectomy is indicated in all individuals with a Y chromosome to eliminate the increased neoplastic potential of such dysgenetic gonads and in all patients in whom virilization occurs at puberty to remove the source of androgen. Estrogen replacement therapy is warranted following gonadectomy. Other causes of male pseudohermaphroditism associated with heterosexual pubertal development are described in Ch. 207.

An androgen-producing neoplasm or Cushing's syndrome may occur rarely during the pubertal years and lead to heterosexual development.

Marshall WA, Tanner JM: Variations in the pattern of pubertal changes in girls. Arch Dis Child 44:291, 1969. *A classic paper that is required reading for all serious students.*
Simpson JL, Rebar RW: Normal and abnormal sexual differentiation and development. *In* Becker KL, et al. (eds.): Principles and Practice of Endocrinology and Metabolism. Philadelphia, JB Lippincott, 1990, p 710. *A detailed discussion of the disorders of sexual differentiation organized similarly to the discussion in this chapter.*
Styne DM, Grumbach MM: Puberty in the male and female. Its physiology and disorders. *In* Yen SSC, Jaffe RB (eds.): Reproductive Endocrinology, 3rd ed. Philadelphia, WB Saunders, 1991, p 511. *A detailed and excellently referenced discussion of normal and abnormal pubertal development.*

THE NORMAL MENSTRUAL CYCLE

CHARACTERISTICS OF THE MENSTRUAL CYCLE. Between menarche at approximately age 12 years and the menopause at about age 51 years, the reproductive organs of normal women undergo a series of closely coordinated changes at approximately monthly intervals that together comprise the normal menstrual cycle. The menstrual cycle is the expression of the coordinated interactions of the hypothalamic-pituitary-ovarian axis, with associated changes in the target tissues (endometrium, cervix, vagina) of the reproductive tract.

A menstrual cycle begins with the first day of genital bleeding (day 1; menses) and ends just prior to the next menstrual period. The median menstrual cycle length is 28 days, but normal ovulatory menstrual cycles may range from about 21 to 40 days in length. Menstrual cycles vary most greatly in length in the years immediately following menarche and in the years immediately preceding menopause, largely because of an increased incidence of anovulatory cycles. Irregularities in menstrual cycle length also may be caused by abrupt changes in diet, exercise, or environment; serious emotional disturbances; and following parturition or abortion. The menstrual cycle can be divided into three distinct phases: *follicular, ovulatory,* and *luteal.*

The Follicular or Preovulatory Phase. Variable in length, the follicular phase begins with the first day of menstrual bleeding and extends to the day prior to the preovulatory LH surge. A rise in serum FSH begins in the late luteal phase of the previous menstrual cycle, continues into the early follicular phase, and initiates growth and development of a group of follicles (Fig. 208–5). The preovulatory follicle destined for ovulation is selected from this cohort in a manner that is not yet understood. Circulating LH levels rise slowly throughout the follicular phase, but FSH levels fall after the early follicular phase increase. Approximately 7 to 8 days before the preovulatory LH surge, estradiol (E_2) and estrone (E_1) begin to increase, generally reaching a maximum on the day before or the day of the LH surge. The divergence in LH and FSH levels may be related to the follicular secretion of *inhibin* (folliculostatin), a hormone that specifically inhibits the release of FSH. Several days before the LH surge, plasma androgens (androstenedione and testosterone) and some progestins (17α-hydroxyprogesterone and 20α-dihydroprogesterone) begin to increase. They peak on the day

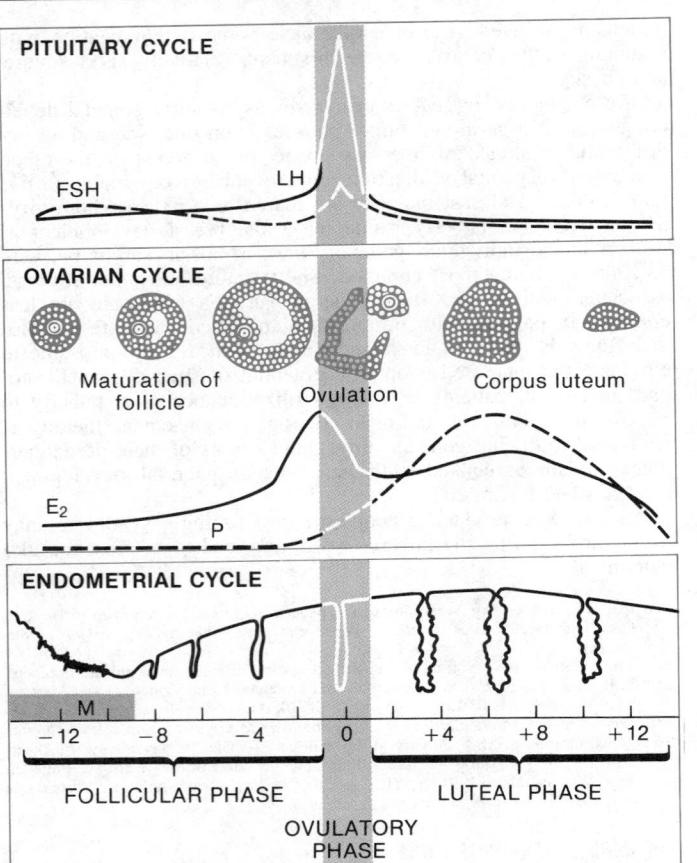

PITUITARY CYCLE

FSH   LH

OVARIAN CYCLE

Maturation of follicle   Ovulation   Corpus luteum

E₂   P

ENDOMETRIAL CYCLE

M

−12   −8   −4   0   +4   +8   +12

FOLLICULAR PHASE   LUTEAL PHASE

OVULATORY PHASE

FIGURE 208–5. The idealized cyclic changes observed in gonadotropins, estradiol (E_2), progesterone (P), and uterine endometrium during the normal menstrual cycle. The data are centered on the day of the LH surge (day 0). Days of menstrual bleeding are indicated by M. (Reprinted with permission from *Endocrine and Metabolism Continuing Education Quality Control Program*, 1982. Copyright American Association for Clinical Chemistry, Inc.)

of the LH surge. Progesterone itself does not increase until just prior to the onset of the LH surge.

The Ovulatory Phase. During this phase the ovum is released from the mature graafian follicle about 32 to 34 hours after the onset of the preovulatory surge of LH by the pituitary gland. The ovulatory phase extends from 1 day prior to the LH surge to 1 day following the LH surge. Some women experience brief (a few minutes to few hours in length), dull, unilateral pelvic pain near the time of ovulation, termed *mittelschmerz*. The association of this pain to ovulation is unknown, but it may be due to leakage of follicular fluid into the abdominal cavity at ovulation. *Mittelschmerz* may occur before or after actual ovulation or not at all in ovulatory women. During the ovulatory phase a rapid rise in plasma LH results in response to positive estrogen feedback, leading to final maturation of the follicle and to ovulation. As peak LH levels are reached, E_2 levels drop, but progesterone levels continue to increase.

The Luteal or Postovulatory Phase. The more constant half of the menstrual cycle, the luteal phase, is approximately 14 days in length and ends with the onset of menses. This phase represents the functional lifespan of the corpus luteum ("yellow body") of the ovary, which supports the released ovum by secreting progesterone. In the luteal phase, progesterone secretion increases to peak 6 to 8 days after the LH surge. Parallel but smaller increases in 17α-hydroxyprogesterone, E_2, and E_1 levels also occur. Progesterone levels decrease toward menses unless the ovum is fertilized and pregnancy results. The finding of serum progesterone levels greater than 10 ng per milliliter 1 week prior to menses is probably diagnostic of normal ovulation. Progestins increase basal morning body temperature so that a "thermogenic shift" of more than 0.3° C occurring after a nadir is a presumptive sign of ovulation and proges-

terone secretion. Unfortunately, taking basal temperatures on a daily basis is tedious, subject to error, and not very reliable.

CYCLIC CHANGES IN TARGET ORGANS. *Endometrium.* During the menstrual cycle the endometrium undergoes remarkable histologic and cytologic changes, which culminate with menstrual bleeding when the corpus luteum ceases to secrete progesterone. The *basal layer of the endometrium,* which is not lost during menses, then regenerates the *superficial layer* of compact epithelial cells lining the uterine cavity and an *intermediate layer of spongiosa,* both of which are shed at each menstruation. Endometrial glands in these layers proliferate under the influence of estrogen in the follicular phase so that the mucosa thickens. In the luteal phase, under the influence of progesterone, the glands become coiled and secretory, with increased vascularity and edema of the stroma. As both E_2 and progesterone decline in the late luteal phase, the stroma becomes increasingly edematous, endometrial and blood vessel necrosis occurs, and endometrial bleeding ensues. Local release of prostaglandins may initiate vasospasm and ischemic necrosis in the endometrium as well as the uterine contractions accompanying menstrual flow. Thus prostaglandin synthetase inhibitors can relieve dysmenorrhea (menstrual cramping). Fibrinolytic activity in the endometrium also peaks at the time of menstruation, accounting for the noncoagulability of menstrual blood. Because the histologic changes during the menstrual cycle are so characteristic, endometrial biopsies are used to date the stage of the cycle and to assess the tissue response to gonadal steroids.

Cervix and Cervical Mucus. During the follicular phase, cervical vascularity, congestion, and edema increase progressively under the influence of estrogen. The external cervical os opens to a diameter of 3 mm at ovulation and then decreases to 1 mm. Cervical mucus increases in quantity (10- to 30-fold) and in elasticity. "Palm leaf" arborization (ferning) becomes prominent just prior to ovulation (if cervical mucus is allowed to dry on a glass slide and is examined microscopically). Under the influence of progesterone during the luteal phase, cervical mucus thickens, becomes less watery, and loses its elasticity and ability to fern. The characteristics of cervical mucus are useful clinically to evaluate the stage of the cycle and the amount of estrogen present.

Vagina. When ovarian estrogen secretion is low, as in the early follicular phase, vaginal epithelium is pale and thin. In the follicular phase under the influence of estrogens the epithelium thickens, and the number of mature cornified epithelial cells increases. During the luteal phase, progesterone causes a decrease in the percentage of cornified cells and an increase in the number of precornified intermediate cells and polymorphonuclear leukocytes. There is also increased cellular debris and clumping of shed desquamated cells. Histologic changes in the vaginal epithelium and in the cervical mucus are the most sensitive indicators of estrogen status in the body. However, the reliability of vaginal smears depends upon the absence of infection or exogenously administered steroid hormones that have antiestrogenic effects. Steroid hormones also facilitate progression of spermatozoa toward the ovaries and of ova toward the uterine cavity through effects on the fallopian tubes.

Ovary. A small primordial follicle with a diameter of 50 μm transforms and grows into a mature graafian follicle 1 to 2 cm in diameter in two distinct phases: (1) The oocyte and follicle grow to form a *primary follicle,* apparently independent of gonadotropin control. The oocyte increases tenfold in diameter (from 15 to 150 μm) and becomes surrounded by a zona pellucida, a translucent "shell" of glycoproteins. In addition, the single layer of cells surrounding the oocyte becomes cuboidal and takes on the characteristics of granulosa cells. (2) In a second phase completely dependent upon gonadotropin and steroid hormones, the follicular unit develops into a *mature graafian follicle,* which is capable of being released in response to the midcycle surge of LH and FSH. Under the influence of FSH, granulosa cells acquire specific receptors for FSH, undergo mitosis, multiply to form secondary follicles consisting of several granulosa cell layers, and also acquire the ability to aromatize androgens to estrogens. Simultaneously, thecal interstitial cells begin to develop around the basement membrane surrounding the granulosa cells, develop specific cell membrane receptors for LH, and synthesize and secrete androgens, primarily Δ⁴-androstenedione and testosterone, in response to LH. The androgens can diffuse across the basement lamina where they are aromatized to estrogens. The rising E_2 in the follicular phase then feeds back on the hypothalamic-pituitary unit via the systemic circulation (Fig. 208–6).

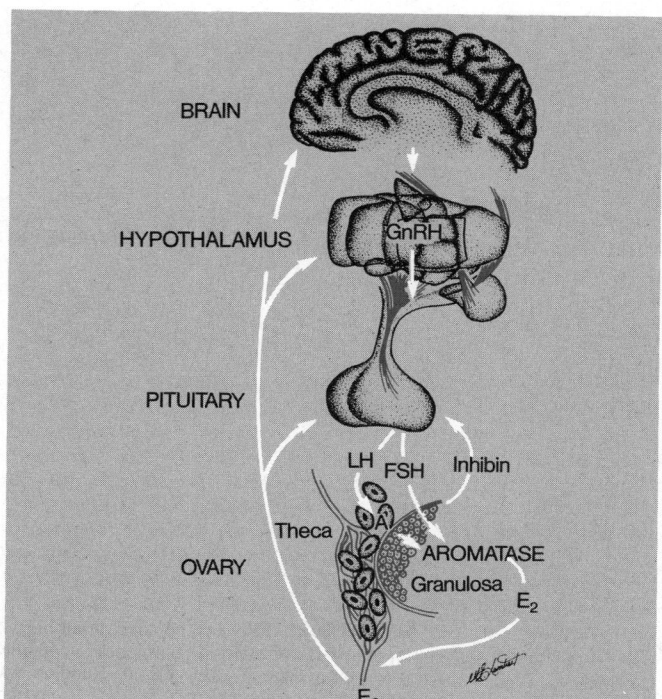

FIGURE 208-6. The hypothalamic-pituitary-ovarian axis in the regulation of follicular maturation and steroidogenesis. A = androgens; E_2 = estradiol. (Modified from *Endocrine and Metabolism Continuing Education Quality Control Program,* 1982. Copyright American Association for Clinical Chemistry, Inc.)

The so-called *two-cell theory* holds that both granulosa and theca cells are required for estrogen biosynthesis and maturation of the follicle.

A tertiary graafian follicle that contains an antrum or fluid-filled cavity increases from 200 μm to 1 to 2 cm in diameter, primarily because of accumulation of follicular fluid, again under the direct control of FSH. In tertiary follicles, FSH induces the appearance of specific LH receptors on granulosa cell membranes. These LH receptors are responsible for the stimulation of progesterone secretion prior to ovulation (luteinization) and for continued production of progesterone in the luteal phase.

Approximately 2 weeks are required for the presumptive preovulatory follicle to complete its growth and expel a mature oocyte. The oocyte is inhibited from resuming meiotic maturation by granulosa cell–oocyte interaction and an oocyte maturation inhibitor (OMI) until following the LH-FSH surge. Within 36 hours of the onset of the surge, the oocyte completes the first meiotic division (reduction to 22 + X chromosomes) and a first polar body is extruded. The second meiotic division is completed only if the oocyte is fertilized by a spermatozoon. During the LH-FSH surge the preovulatory follicle bulges above the surface of the ovary. A stigma or avascular area develops on the follicle surface. Under the influence of local prostaglandins, plasminogen activator, and other hormones, a cluster of granulosa cells surrounding the oocyte and the oocyte itself (together known as the cumulus oophorus) are extruded.

The corpus luteum is formed from the granulosa and theca cells of the former preovulatory follicle following ovulation and secretes progesterone and E_2 for approximately 14 days. It then degenerates unless fertilization occurs. The lifespan of the corpus luteum may depend in part upon prostaglandins and prolactin as well as upon progestin. If fertilization occurs, hCG, which is similar to LH, is secreted by the developing blastocyst and helps to support the corpus luteum until the fetoplacental unit can support itself. Pregnancy tests in common use have been developed utilizing antibodies to the specific β subunit of hCG and have little if any cross-reactivity with LH.

OVARIAN STEROIDOGENESIS. The ovaries and the developing follicles synthesize sex steroid hormones (estrogens, androgens, and progestins), which play important roles in feedback regulation of the menstrual cycle and in preparing the uterus to accept a fertilized ovum via two separate pathways: (1) the so-called Δ^5 pathway, in which 17α-hydroxypregnenolone and DHEA with double bonds between carbons 5 and 6 are intermediates, and (2) the Δ^4 pathway, in which pregnenolone is converted to progesterone and in which 17α-hydroxyprogesterone and androstenedione with double bonds between carbons 4 and 5 are the alternative intermediates (Fig. 208-7).

Although cholesterol as substrate for steroid synthesis is obtained normally from circulating low-density lipoproteins (LDL's), it can be synthesized *de novo* from two-carbon fragments (acetate). Different structures and cells within the ovary synthesize different steroids, in part because of stimulation by the gonadotropins. Gonadotropin binding to its receptor activates adenylate cyclase and stimulates cAMP production. The cAMP in turn activates protein kinases that catalyze phosphorylation of proteins to mediate the cellular effects of each gonadotropin (see Ch. 199). LH also increases phosphatidylinositides within the ovary. LH acts primarily to regulate the first step in steroid hormone biosynthesis, that is, the conversion of cholesterol to pregnenolone. FSH acts to aromatize androgens to estrogens. Thus, LH acts to enhance substrate flow and the synthesis of androgens and/or progesterone. In the absence of LH, FSH action is reduced because of diminished substrate for aromatization.

Androgens, primarily androstenedione and testosterone, are secreted by interstitial and theca cells and serve as the substrate for the granulosa cell aromatase enzyme for synthesis of estrogens. Androstenedione, the major ovarian androgen, can also be converted to testosterone and estrogens in peripheral tissues. When ovarian androgen synthesis is excessive, as in ovarian androgen-producing tumors, or when conversion of androgen to estrogen in the ovary is reduced, as in PCO syndrome, hirsutism and even virilism can result. Testosterone, the most biologically potent androgen, is bound tightly to sex hormone–binding globulin (SHBG; also known as testosterone-estradiol–binding globulin, TeBG) so that only about 1% of circulating testosterone is biologically free and active. Secretion rates and circulating concentrations in normal adult premenopausal women are given in Table 208-2.

Estrogens are produced predominantly in ovarian follicles by granulosa cell aromatization of the A ring of theca cell androgens. Naturally occurring estrogens are 18-carbon steroids, which by definition stimulate proliferation of the endometrium and bind to specific, saturable cytosolic receptors. The amount of estrogen secretion depends on the phase of the menstrual cycle (Table 208-2). In the early follicular phase the secretion rates of E_2 and E_1 are almost equal (60 to 170 μg per day). As the dominant follicle is selected, E_2 secretion increases to as much as 800 μg per day, with almost all the E_2 synthesized by the dominant follicle. The corpus luteum also produces significant quantities of E_2 (250 μg per day). In the late follicular and luteal phases, E_1 secretion is about one-fourth that of estradiol. The dominant follicle and corpus luteum synthesize about 95% of circulating E_2; E_1 is of little significance in the ovulating woman. In the postmenopausal years, however, E_1 becomes the predominant estrogen in the absence of functioning follicles. E_1 is synthesized by peripheral conversion of adrenal androgens, especially androstenedione. As much estrogen is synthesized during the 9 months of pregnancy as would be synthesized during 100 years of normal menstrual cycles.

Progesterone synthesis is low in the follicular phase, but increases to 10 to 40 mg per day during the luteal phase (Table 208-2). Should pregnancy occur, progesterone production increases to as much as 300 mg per day at term. Why the corpus luteum atrophies at about 14 days is not known, but it may be due to the effects of intraovarian estrogen and/or prostaglandins. However, LH stimulation is required for progesterone production by the corpus luteum. Progesterone induces secretory changes in the endometrium in preparation for implantation of the fertilized ovum.

INTRAOVARIAN CONTROL OF FOLLICULAR DEVELOPMENT. Although the secretion of E_2 by granulosa cells is critical for the occurrence of normal menstrual cycles, any role for E_2 within the ovary in regulating follicular development in women is now questioned. Nuclear estrogen and progesterone receptors do not appear in the granulosa cells of the dominant follicle in women until just prior to the LH surge, and androgen receptors cannot be

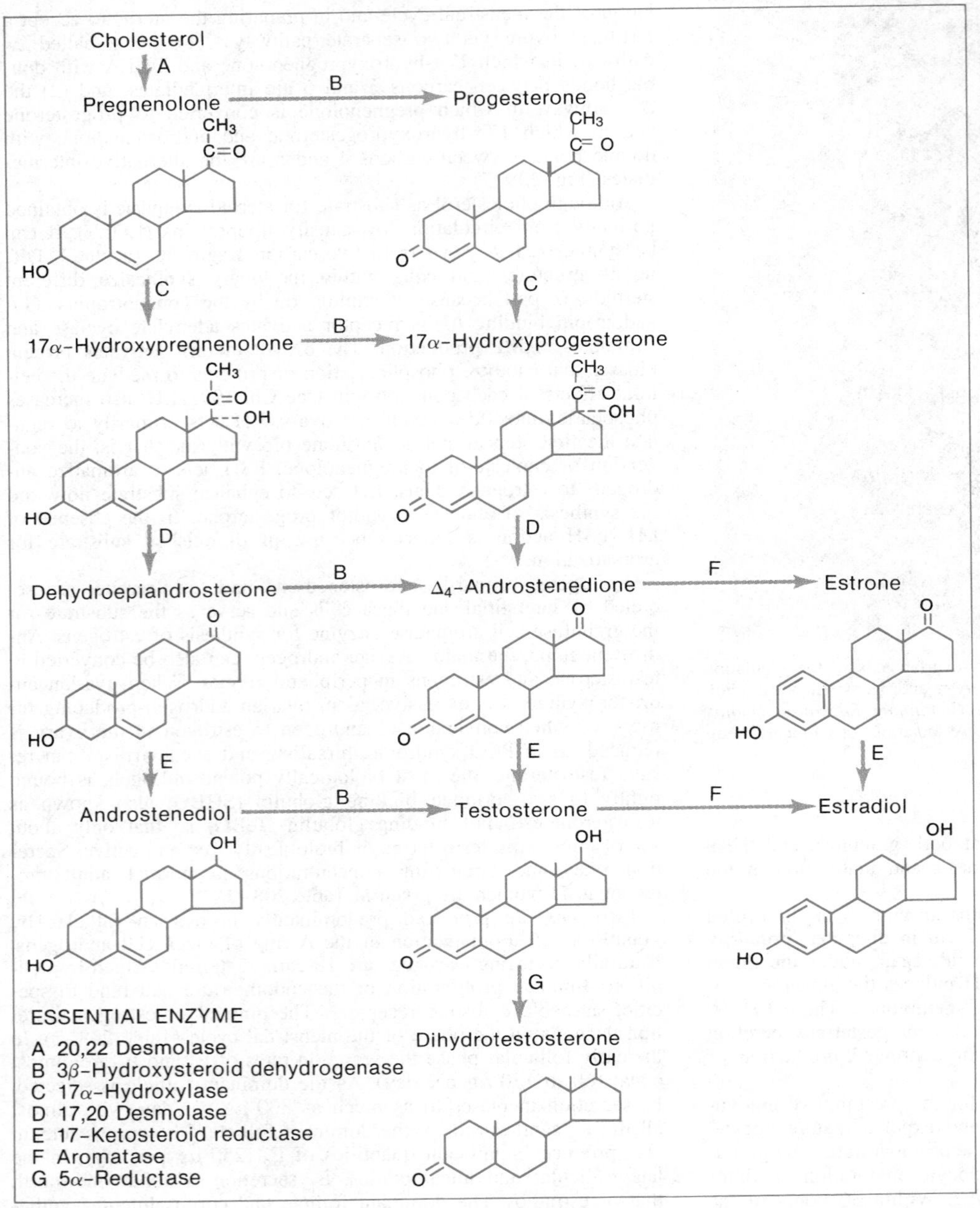

FIGURE 208–7. Steps in ovarian biosynthesis of steroid hormones. (Modified from data of Ross GT: *In* Rudolph AM [ed.]: Pediatrics 16:1726, 1977. Copyright American Academy of Pediatrics 1977.)

ESSENTIAL ENZYME

A 20,22 Desmolase
B 3β–Hydroxysteroid dehydrogenase
C 17α–Hydroxylase
D 17,20 Desmolase
E 17-Ketosteroid reductase
F Aromatase
G 5α-Reductase

identified in either granulosa or theca cells until the secondary stage of development. Because steroids act by binding to these receptors, it appears that steroids are not essential for follicular development. Consistent with this conclusion is the surprising observation that normal follicular growth and development and successful fertilization *in vitro* can be accomplished with use of exogenous gonadotropins in women with 17α-hydroxylase deficiency, who have no ability to synthesize androgens and estrogens (Fig. 208–7).

Several peptides secreted by granulosa cells appear to play critical roles in intraovarian regulation of follicular development, whereas steroids are important for neuroendocrine feedback regulation and preparation of the endometrium to receive the fertilized oocyte. Although the physiologic roles of these peptides remain to be defined precisely, inhibin, insulin-like growth factors (IGF) I and II and their binding proteins, and perhaps other growth factors as well appear to have modulatory effects on follicular development. At present this is an evolving area of knowledge with potential implications for developing new strategies to induce ovulation in anovulatory women.

NEUROENDOCRINE REGULATION OF THE OVARIES. Neurons containing various peptide hormones that can release or inhibit secretion of the gonadotropins are found in the hypothalamus

(see Ch. 201). Specifically, cells containing GnRH occur in the area including the arcuate nucleus and median eminence and the preoptic area. Axons from these neurons run in the tuberoinfundibular tract and terminate on capillaries within the median eminence; this allows for delivery of their products through the portal vascular system to the anterior pituitary gland. It appears that classic neurotransmitters, including norepinephrine, dopamine, and serotonin, as well as neuromodulators, such as endogenous opiates and prostaglandins, influence secretion of GnRH by the hypothalamus. In addition, estrogens and androgens bind to cells in the hypothalamus and the anterior pituitary, and progestins bind to cells in the hypothalamus to influence hypothalamic-pituitary regulation of ovarian function.

GnRH is secreted in a pulsatile fashion (perhaps because of an inherent oscillator within the arcuate nucleus) and is responsible for pulsatile release of gonadotropins. Pulsatile gonadotropin release in turn appears to account for the pulsatile secretion of sex steroids from the ovaries. The ovarian sex steroids then feed back on the hypothalamic-pituitary unit to modulate both the frequency and amplitude of the gonadotropin pulse (see Fig. 208–6). Thus, gonadotropin pulses vary throughout the menstrual cycle. Pulses occur at approximately 60- to 90-minute intervals in the

TABLE 208-2. CONCENTRATIONS, METABOLIC CLEARANCE RATES, PRODUCTION RATES, AND OVARIAN SECRETION RATES OF SEX STEROID HORMONES IN BLOOD

Steroid	Plasma MCR (liters/day)	Binding	Phase of Menstrual Cycle or Stage of Life	Plasma Concentration (ng/dl)	Plasma Production Rate (μg/day)	Ovarian Secretion Rate (μg/day)
Androstenedione	2000	Albumin	Premenopausal	40–240	3200	800–1600
			Postmenopausal	30–120	1600	
Testosterone	700	TeBG, albumin	Premenopausal	19–70	260	
			Postmenopausal	15–70	150	
Estradiol	1350	TeBG, albumin	Early follicular	2.5–6	70–200	60–170
			Late follicular	20–40	445–945	400–800
			Midluteal	15–25	270	250
			Postmenopausal	< 1.0–2.5		
Estrone	2200	Albumin	Early follicular	2–6	70–200	60–170
			Late follicular	10–20	300–600	250–500
			Midluteal	10–15	240	160
			Postmenopausal	1.5–5.0	55	
Progesterone	2200	CBG, albumin	Follicular	3–10	700–2500	1500
			Luteal	10–25	3000–30,000	24,000

CBG = Cortisol-binding globulin; MCR = metabolic clearance rate; TeBG = testosterone-estradiol–binding globulin.

follicular phase and at intervals of >180 minutes in the luteal phase.

Gonadal steroids can exert both negative and positive feedback effects on gonadotropin secretion. Among ovarian steroids, 17β-estradiol is the most potent inhibitor of gonadotropin secretion, acting on both the hypothalamus and the pituitary. For women to ovulate, E_2 must also elicit a positive feedback effect on gonadotropin release. The feedback effects are both time and dose dependent. In the normal menstrual cycle the positive feedback action of E_2 leading to the LH surge is preceded by a period when lower E_2 levels are present with their negative feedback effects.

It appears that the ovary is the "clock" for the timing of ovulation, with the hypothalamus stimulating pulsatile release of the gonadotropins. The follicle complex and corpus luteum develop in response to gonadotropin stimulation. For appropriate ovarian regulation of reproductive function in women, three biologic characteristics are necessary: (1) an appropriate balance and sequence of negative and positive feedback actions; (2) differential feedback effects on the release of LH and FSH; (3) local intraovarian controls on follicular growth and maturation, separate from but interrelated to the effects of gonadotropins on the ovaries.

Erickson GF, Schreiber JR: Morphology and physiology of the ovary. In Becker KL (eds.): Principles and Practice of Endocrinology and Metabolism. Philadelphia, JB Lippincott, 1990, p 776. A detailed discussion of ovarian function.
Richardson GS: Steroidogenesis. In Sciarra JJ (ed.): Gynecology and Obstetrics. Vol. 5. Philadelphia, Harper and Row, 1986 (rev. ed.), p 1. A detailed summary of the steroidogenic pathway.
Speroff L, Glass RH, Kase NG: Regulation of the menstrual cycle. In Clinical Gynecologic Endocrinology and Infertility, 5th ed. Baltimore, Williams & Wilkins, 1994, p 183. A detailed and up-to-date summary of what is currently known about the human menstrual cycle.

ABNORMALITIES OF THE REPRODUCTIVE YEARS

DYSMENORRHEA AND ENDOMETRIOSIS. Dysmenorrhea, perhaps the most common of all gynecologic disorders, affects about 50% of postpubertal women. Dysmenorrhea can be classified as primary or secondary.

Primary dysmenorrhea occurs only in ovulatory cycles. Prostaglandins that are released from the endometrium just prior to and during menstruation cause contraction of uterine smooth muscle and produce dysmenorrhea by initiating painful, exaggerated uterine contractions and myometrial ischemia. Associated systemic symptoms include nausea, diarrhea, headache, and emotional changes. Primary dysmenorrhea is much more common than is secondary dysmenorrhea.

In *secondary dysmenorrhea* there is a pathologic cause for the dysmenorrhea. Endometriosis, the ectopic occurrence of endometrial tissue generally within the abdominal cavity, is the most common cause in severe cases. Other possible causes include pelvic inflammatory disease, congenital abnormalities such as atresia of a portion of the distal genital tract and cystic duplication of the paramesonephric ducts, and cervical stenosis.

Prostaglandin synthetase inhibitors such as naproxen, ibuprofen, mefenamic acid, and indomethacin are the mainstays of treatment. If the dysmenorrhea is still severe, addition of an oral contraceptive preparation to inhibit ovulation and limit prostaglandin release is generally effective. In cases in which the pelvic pain still remains intractable, additional evaluation is warranted. If thorough evaluation of the gastrointestinal and urinary tracts fails to reveal a definitive cause, examination under anesthesia and diagnostic laparoscopy may be indicated.

If endometriosis is diagnosed at laparoscopy, treatment varies, depending on the severity of the disease and the goals of the patient regarding fertility. It may be possible to fulgurate implants or lyse adhesions through the laparoscope. In general, endometriosis should be treated medically, with additional surgery deferred until infertility (if present) becomes manifest. Medical therapy can consist of continuous suppression with GnRH analogues, progestins, oral contraceptive agents, or danazol for 3 to 6 months. GnRH analogues are rapidly becoming the most frequent form of medical suppressive therapy. After a course of therapy, use of oral contraceptive agents probably should be continued until fertility is desired. Conservative surgical resection of endometriotic tissue should almost always be deferred until it is established as the cause of infertility. Surgery may be required, however, for continuing severe pain, severe endometriosis, or large ovarian cysts containing endometriosis (endometriomas). If symptoms continue despite adequate treatment or if psychological overlay is suspected, psychiatric evaluation may be indicated. Medical causes of dysmenorrhea, however, should be eliminated first.

PREMENSTRUAL SYNDROME. Premenstrual syndrome (PMS), also known as premenstrual tension (PMT), is a complex of physical and/or emotional symptoms that occur repetitively in a cyclic fashion before menstruation and that diminish or disappear with menstruation. Typically these cyclic symptoms are sufficiently severe to interfere with some aspects of life. Women with established psychiatric disturbances probably should not be included among those with PMS. More than 150 different symptoms are now thought to vary with the menstrual cycle (Table 208–3). Estimates of the prevalence of PMS range from 25 to 100%. For most women the syndrome is merely annoying; it is likely that PMS causes serious difficulties for no more than 5 to 10%. The diagnosis is best established by requiring patients to keep prospective daily records of symptoms over a 2- to 3-month period. Fewer than 50% of women complaining of PMS are found to have the syndrome when such records are examined.

Most women seek help for PMS in their 30's after 10 or more years of symptoms. Many report that their symptoms began at menarche; approximately half state that symptoms followed childbirth. Severity and duration of symptoms are often reported to increase following each successive pregnancy, and to become more severe with advancing age. Women with severe longstanding PMS almost always describe associated psychological reactions, including social difficulties, such as marital discord, difficulty relating to their children, difficulty maintaining friendships, and withdrawal from social activities.

The cause of PMS is unknown and patients should be informed that no one therapy has been effective in all women. Women with mild premenstrual symptoms often benefit from simple changes in

TABLE 208–3. COMMON SYMPTOMS OF CYCLIC PREMENSTRUAL SYNDROME

Somatic Symptoms

Abdominal bloating	Constipation or diarrhea
Acne	Headache
Alcohol intolerance	Peripheral edema
Breast engorgement and tenderness	Weight gain
Clumsiness	

Emotional and Mental Symptoms

Anxiety	Insomnia
Change in libido	Irritability
Depression	Lethargy
Fatigue	Mood swings
Food cravings (especially salt and sugar)	Panic attacks
	Paranoia
Hostility	Violence toward self and others
Inability to concentrate	Withdrawal from others
Increased appetite	

lifestyle, including addition of mild aerobic exercise each day; reduction in intake of xanthine-containing beverages, salt, and refined sugar in the day, particularly in the luteal phase; stress reduction; and adequate rest. Women with more severe PMS may benefit from treating predominant complaints symptomatically. Thus bromocriptine* (generally 2.5 mg twice a day) or danazol (100 to 400 mg daily in two divided doses) may be given continuously for relief of mastalgia, with the understanding that both may have unpleasant side effects. Prostaglandin synthetase inhibitors may help reduce dysmenorrhea and may benefit headaches. Mild sedatives and tranquilizers may help reduce insomnia and anxiety. Low doses of fluoxetine (20 mg) either administered daily or for the last 2 weeks of each menstrual cycle have been reported to reduce the emotional symptoms associated with PMS. Mild diuretics (especially spironolactone at doses up to 100 mg each morning) may benefit cyclic edema if such can be confirmed.

Because PMS requires the occurrence of cyclic ovulation, oophorectomy is occasionally considered for patients with particularly intractable symptomatology. However, oophorectomy may create new problems related to estrogen deficiency for women with PMS treated in this permanent fashion. Several recent trials employing a GnRH agonist together with exogenous steroids (so-called add-back therapy) have been described as reducing PMS. Whether such therapy can be utilized long-term remains to be determined.

Natural progesterone, particularly in the form of vaginal suppositories given at doses of up to 800 mg per day, has been used but results of double-blind placebo-controlled trials have provided no evidence of efficacy. Likewise, the use of large quantities of multiple vitamins or of oil of evening primrose, containing the essential fatty acid γ-linolenic acid, a precursor of prostaglandins, is unsubstantiated.

Keye WR Jr (ed.): The Premenstrual Syndrome. Philadelphia, WB Saunders, 1988. *A simple multiauthored text detailing what is known about this disorder.*
Stillman R: Endometriosis. *In* Becker KL (ed.): Principles and Practice of Endocrinology and Metabolism. Philadelphia, JB Lippincott, 1990. *A succinct summary of this enigmatic disorder.*

ABNORMAL UTERINE BLEEDING. *Differential Diagnosis.*

The causes of abnormal uterine bleeding in the reproductive years include complications from the use of oral contraceptive preparations; complications of pregnancy (especially threatened, incomplete, or missed abortion and ectopic pregnancy); coagulation disorders (most commonly idiopathic thrombocytopenic purpura and von Willebrand's disease); and pelvic disease such as intrauterine polyps, leiomyomas, and tumors of the vagina and cervix. Clear-cell adenocarcinoma of the vagina or cervix may occur in women exposed to diethylstilbestrol (DES) during fetal life as a result of maternal ingestion. Affected women also may have congenital abnormalities of the upper vagina, cervix, and uterus. Because a history of DES exposure is not always obtained and because this malignant tumor may be fatal, clinical suspicion should remain high.

Women with a history of DES exposure should be reassured, however, that the incidence of malignancy is extremely low. Trauma (coital or otherwise), foreign bodies, systemic illnesses including various endocrinopathies (such as diabetes mellitus, hypothyroidism and hyperthyroidism, Cushing's syndrome, and Addison's disease), leukemia, and renal disease may also be associated with abnormal bleeding as the presenting manifestation.

Dysfunctional uterine bleeding (DUB), abnormal uterine bleeding with no demonstrable organic genital or extragenital cause (75% of cases), is most frequently associated with anovulation. Postmenarchal bleeding in adolescents secondary to immaturity of the hypothalamic-pituitary-ovarian axis accounts for about 20% of all cases, and premenopausal bleeding consequent to incipient ovarian failure constitutes more than half of the cases. Most anovulatory bleeding is due to either estrogen withdrawal or estrogen breakthrough bleeding. In anovulatory women, estrogen stimulates the endometrium unopposed by progesterone. As a consequence, the endometrium proliferates, becomes thicker, and may shed irregularly, especially if estrogen levels drop. Anovulatory bleeding tends to occur at less frequent intervals, while organic lesions tend to cause bleeding more frequently than cyclic menses.

Evaluation and Treatment. All cases of abnormal bleeding should be evaluated, including obtaining a thorough history with special emphasis on the amount and duration of blood loss. Prospective charting of the days on which bleeding occurs may be required to evaluate the bleeding pattern. Complications of pregnancy or a bleeding diathesis must always be ruled out.

The physical examination (including the Papanicolaou smear) is normal in dysfunctional bleeding except for signs of anemia in the more severe cases. Laboratory tests should include a complete blood count, platelet count, coagulation studies, thyroid function tests, and fasting blood glucose. DUB must be a diagnosis of exclusion. Management of DUB depends upon the age of the patient and the extent of the bleeding. A sample of the endometrium should be obtained by biopsy or by dilatation and curettage from all women over age 35 and from those at increased risk of developing endometrial carcinoma because of prolonged anovulatory bleeding.

Even profuse bleeding in anovulatory women can almost always be successfully treated by administering one combination oral contraceptive pill every 6 hours for 5 to 7 days. Bleeding should cease within 24 hours, but patients should be warned to expect heavy bleeding 2 to 4 days after stopping therapy. If anemia and signs of acute blood loss are profound, blood transfusion may be necessary. If the bleeding continues despite therapy, curettage can be carried out. Recurrence can be prevented by giving the patient combination oral contraceptive agents cyclically for 3 or more months. If spontaneous cyclic menses do not resume and pregnancy is not desired, the patient can be treated with cyclic progestin (medroxyprogesterone acetate 5 to 10 mg for 10 to 14 days each month) or oral contraceptive agents. If pregnancy is desired, ovulation can be induced, as discussed subsequently.

Acute episodes of anovulatory bleeding also can be treated with conjugated estrogens administered intravenously (25 mg every 4 hours for up to three doses) until bleeding ceases. Progestin therapy (medroxyprogesterone acetate 5 to 10 mg orally for 10 days) should be started simultaneously. Withdrawal bleeding will occur after cessation of therapy, and the patient can then be treated with oral contraceptive agents for at least three cycles.

For individuals with anovulatory bleeding without an episode of profuse bleeding, treatment with cyclic oral contraceptive agents or progestin can be provided unless pregnancy is desired, in which case ovulation must be induced.

Speroff L, Glass RH, Kase NG: Dysfunctional uterine bleeding. *In* Clinical Gynecologic Endocrinology and Infertility, 5th ed. Baltimore, Williams & Wilkins, 1994, p 531. *A detailed and logical approach to the treatment of abnormal uterine bleeding.*

AMENORRHEA. *Definition and Etiology.*

Amenorrhea is the absence of menstruation for 3 or more months in women with past menses *(secondary amenorrhea)* or the absence of menarche by the age of 16 years regardless of the absence or presence of secondary sex characteristics *(primary amenorrhea).* If an intact genital outflow tract exists and there is no primary disease of the uterus, amenorrhea is a sign of failure of the hypothalamic-pituitary-ovarian axis to produce cyclically the hormones necessary for menses. Amenorrhea is a sign of any of several disorders involving different organ systems. Amenorrhea is physiologic in the prepubertal girl,

---
* This use is not listed in the manufacturer's directive.

during pregnancy and early in lactation, and after the menopause. At any other time it is pathologic and demands evaluation. Use of the term *post-pill amenorrhea* to refer to failure to resume menses within 3 months of discontinuing oral contraceptives is inappropriate. Women so affected should be evaluated in the same manner as for any woman with amenorrhea. Similarly, individuals with menses occurring at infrequent intervals of greater than 40 days or having fewer than 9 menses per year, termed oligomenorrhea, should be evaluated identically to women with amenorrhea.

Clinical Evaluation. In patients with amenorrhea even subtle hormonal abnormalities may be manifested by obvious signs and symptoms. Breast development indicates exposure to estrogens, and the presence of pubic and axillary hair indicates androgenic stimulation.

Patients should be questioned especially closely for evidence of psychological disturbances, dietary and exercise habits, lifestyle, environmental stresses, a family history of genetic anomalies, and abnormal growth and development. Patients should also be asked about and examined for the presence of any signs of hyperandrogenism, including hirsutism, temporal balding, deepening of the voice, increased muscle mass, clitoromegaly, and increased libido, as well as for any signs of defeminization, including decreasing breast size and vaginal atrophy. Any history of galactorrhea, the nonpuerperal secretion of milk from the breasts, should be determined (see Ch. 208.4). A history of symptoms related to thyroid and adrenal dysfunction should also be sought.

The physical examination should focus on evaluating (1) body dimensions and habitus, (2) the extent and distribution of body hair, (3) breast development and secretions, and (4) the genitalia.

In normal adult women the arm span is similar to the height, whereas in hypogonadal women the span is generally more than 5 cm greater than the height. The general appearance of the patient should be evaluated to determine if the habitus is that of an adult female. The distribution and quantity of body hair should be considered in view of the family history. The extent of any hirsutism should be recorded, preferably by photographs. Other signs of virilization should be sought carefully. Breast development should be graded according to the method of Tanner (Table 208–4). Breast secretion should be sought by applying pressure to the breasts while the patient is seated. Any secretion should be examined microscopically for the presence of perfectly round fat globules of varying size, which are always present in milk and indicate galactorrhea. Finally, the female genitalia should be examined carefully because they are such sensitive indicators of hormonal milieu. The Tanner stage of pubic hair development should be noted (Table 208–4). Because the sensitivity of the genitalia to androgens decreases onward from early in fetal development, the extent of any virilization is important. Fusion of the labia and enlargement of the clitoris with or without formation of a penile urethra are observed in women exposed to androgens during the first 3 months of fetal development (see Ch. 207). Significant clitoromegaly in the absence of other signs of sexual ambiguity and in the presence of other signs of virilization requires marked androgenic stimulation and strongly implicates an androgen-secreting neoplasm in the absence of a history of ingestion of exogenous steroids. The development of the labia minora in postpubertal women indicates the influence of estrogens. Overt anomalies of the distal genital tract and especially any evidence of obstruction to the escape of menstrual blood should be sought in the remainder of the pelvic examination. The vaginal mucosa and the cervical mucus are exquisitely sensitive to estrogen. Under the influence of estrogen the vaginal mucosa changes during sexual maturation from a tissue with a shiny, bright red appearance with sparse, thin secretions to a dull, gray-pink rugated surface with copious, thick secretions.

The history and physical examination quickly differentiate among several causes of amenorrhea, regardless of the age of the patient (Table 208–5). The various disorders of sexual differentiation and the other peripheral causes are often apparent on inspection. Distal genital tract obstruction should be identified at the time of pelvic examination even if the specific abnormality is not obvious. The physical stigmata of Turner's syndrome, discussed subsequently, generally make the diagnosis simple. Any sexual ambiguity indicates the need for chromosomal analysis and the measurement of 17α-hydroxyprogesterone to rule out congenital adrenal hyperplasia. Pregnancy and gestational trophoblastic disease may be suspected and confirmed by measuring circulating concentrations of hCG. The possibility of intrauterine synechiae or adhesions (Asherman's syndrome) must be considered in individuals developing amenorrhea following curettage or endometritis. Tuberculous endometritis, especially in younger women, may also lead to this disorder. Without hormonal measurements it may be impossible to distinguish among individuals with chronic anovulation, in whom hypothalamic-pituitary-ovarian function is insufficiently coordinated to produce cyclic ovulation, and those with ovarian failure, in whom in most cases the ovaries are devoid of oocytes. Still, it is generally possible to form some strong clinical impressions about the cause of the amenorrhea. It can be noted if the patient has absence of, incomplete, or complete development of secondary sex characteristics. The presence of excess body hair or galactorrhea may provide clinical evidence of the pathogenesis of the amenorrhea. Signs and symptoms of adrenal or thyroid dysfunction may be important as well.

The administration of a progestin has been advocated to assess the level of endogenous estrogen. This test is of limited value, however, because almost half the young women with premature ovarian failure experience withdrawal bleeding in response to progestin.

To ascertain if the outflow tract is intact, an orally active estrogen, such as 2.5 mg conjugated estrogen daily for 21 days, with 5 to 10 mg of oral medroxyprogesterone acetate for the last 5 to 10 days, may be administered. Withdrawal bleeding should occur if the endometrium is normal. Still, hysterosalpingography and hysteroscopy may be required to diagnose Asherman's syndrome because some patients do continue to have some withdrawal bleeding.

Laboratory Evaluation. Basal levels of FSH, prolactin, and TSH should be measured in all amenorrheic and oligomenorrheic women to confirm the clinical impression (Fig. 208–8).

TABLE 208–4. CRITERIA FOR DISTINGUISHING TANNER STAGES 1 TO 5 DURING PUBERTAL MATURATION

Tanner Stage	Breast	Pubic Hair
1 (Prepubertal)	No palpable glandular tissue or pigmentation of areola; elevation of areola only	No pubic hair; short, fine vellous hair only
2	Glandular tissue palpable with elevation of breast and areola together as a small mound; areolar diameter increased	Sparse, long, pigmented terminal hair chiefly along the labia majora
3	Further enlargement without separation of breast and areola; although more darkly pigmented, areola still pale and immature; nipple generally at or above midplane of breast tissue when individual is seated upright	Dark, coarse, curly hair, extending sparsely over mons
4	Secondary mound of areola and papilla above breast	Adult-type hair, abundant but limited to mons and labia
5 (Adult)	Recession of areola to contour of breast; development of Montgomery's glands and ducts on areola; further pigmentation of areola; nipple generally below midplane of breast tissue when individual is seated upright; maturation independent of breast size	Adult-type hair in quantity and distribution; spread to inner aspects of the thighs in most racial groups

Data from Ross GT: Disorders of the ovary and female reproductive tract. *In* Wilson JD, Foster DW (eds.): Textbook of Endocrinology, 7th ed. Philadelphia, WB Saunders, 1985, p 206; Speroff L, Glass RH, Kase N: Clinical Gynecologic Endocrinology and Infertility, 3rd ed. Baltimore, Williams & Wilkins, 1983, p 377; and Kustin J, Rebar RW: Menstrual disorders in the adolescent age group. Primary Care 14:139, 1987.

TABLE 208-5. CAUSES OF AMENORRHEA

Disorders of sexual differentiation
  Distal genital tract obstruction (müllerian agenesis and dysgenesis)
  Gonadal dysgenesis
  Ambiguity of external genitalia (male and female pseudohermaphroditism)
Other peripheral causes
  Pregnancy
  Gestational trophoblastic disease
  Amenorrhea traumatica (Asherman's syndrome)
Chronic anovulation or ovarian failure
  Degree of sexual development
  Galactorrhea
  Evidence of androgen excess
  Evidence suggestive of adrenal or thyroid dysfunction

Increased TSH levels with or without increased levels of prolactin imply primary hypothyroidism, and further evaluation for this disorder is indicated (see Ch. 203). Although hypothyroidism commonly results in anovulation, amenorrhea occurs in only some hypothyroid women. Menorrhagia and oligomenorrhea may occur as well. The very sensitive immunoassays for TSH permit identification of women with hyperthyroidism as well because TSH levels are suppressed in those individuals.

If the prolactin concentration is increased (typically > 20 to 30 ng per milliliter) and the TSH level is normal (generally < 5 μU per milliliter), measurement of the prolactin concentration in the basal state should be repeated before more extensive evaluation is undertaken. This is the case because prolactin levels are increased by nonspecific stressful stimuli, sleep, and food ingestion. Prolactin levels may be elevated in as many as one third of women with amenorrhea. Evaluation of galactorrhea and hyperprolactinemia is detailed in Ch. 208.4.

Increased FSH levels (generally > 30 to 40 milli International Units [mIU] per milliliter) imply ovarian failure and require further evaluation. Chromosomal evaluation is indicated in all individuals with elevated FSH levels who are under the age of 30 years at the time the amenorrhea begins.

If prolactin and TSH concentrations are within normal ranges and FSH levels are low or normal, the measurement of total testosterone levels may be helpful whether or not there is any evidence of hirsutism or virilization. Hyperandrogenic women need not be hirsute because some have relative insensitivity of the hair follicles to androgens. Mildly increased levels of testosterone (and perhaps DHEA-S as well) suggest PCO syndrome. However, total circulating androgen levels are rarely not elevated because of the alter-

ations in metabolic clearance rate and SHBG that are present in PCO syndrome. Circulating levels of LH and FSH may aid in differentiating PCO syndrome from hypothalamic-pituitary dysfunction. LH levels are frequently elevated in PCO syndrome such that the ratio of LH to FSH is increased; however, LH levels may be identical to those observed in normal women in the follicular phase. In contrast, levels of LH and FSH are normal or slightly reduced in hypothalamic-pituitary dysfunction. There is some overlap between women with "PCO-like" disorders and those with hypothalamic-pituitary dysfunction. Radiographic assessment of the sella turcica is indicated in all amenorrheic women in whom both LH and FSH levels are very low (both < 10 mIU per milliliter) to exclude a pituitary or parapituitary neoplasm. Other pituitary functions should be evaluated in any individual with significantly impaired LH and FSH secretion, as detailed subsequently. Both total testosterone and DHEA-S levels should be measured in hirsute or virilized women. Testosterone levels of > 200 ng per deciliter should lead to investigation for an androgen-producing neoplasm, most likely of ovarian origin. DHEA-S levels > 7.0 μg per milliliter should lead to evaluation for an adrenal neoplasm, and DHEA-S levels between 5.0 and 7.0 μg per milliliter should lead to evaluation for "adult-onset" congenital adrenal hyperplasia (see Ch. 207).

Hypergonadotropic Amenorrhea (Presumptive Ovarian Failure, Primary Hypogonadism)

Differential Diagnosis. Gonadal failure may begin at any time during embryonic or postnatal development and may result from many causes (Table 208–6). Normally the ovaries fail at menopause when virtually no functioning follicles remain. However, premature loss of oocytes prior to age 40 may occur and lead to premature ovarian failure, possibly from abnormalities in the recruitment and selection of oocytes. Because FSH is the principal regulator of folliculogenesis, most causes of premature ovarian failure may somehow involve FSH secretion or action. Circulating gonadotropin levels increase whenever ovarian failure occurs because of decreased negative estrogen feedback to the hypothalamic-pituitary unit.

Genetic Abnormalities. Several pathologic conditions with dysgenetic gonads have elevated gonadotropin levels and amenorrhea. The term *gonadal dysgenesis* refers to individuals with undifferentiated streak gonads without any association with either extragonadal stigmata or sex chromosomal aberrations. Because individuals with gonadal dysgenesis have the normal complement of oocytes at 20 weeks of fetal age but virtually none by birth, this disorder is a form of premature ovarian failure.

Turner's syndrome describes patients with streak gonads composed of fibrous stroma and four cardinal features: (1) a female phenotype, (2) sexual infantilism, (3) short stature, and (4) several physical abnormalities, sometimes including a webbed neck, lowset ears, multiple pigmented nevi, double eyelashes, micrognathia, epicanthal folds, shieldlike chest with microthelia, short fourth

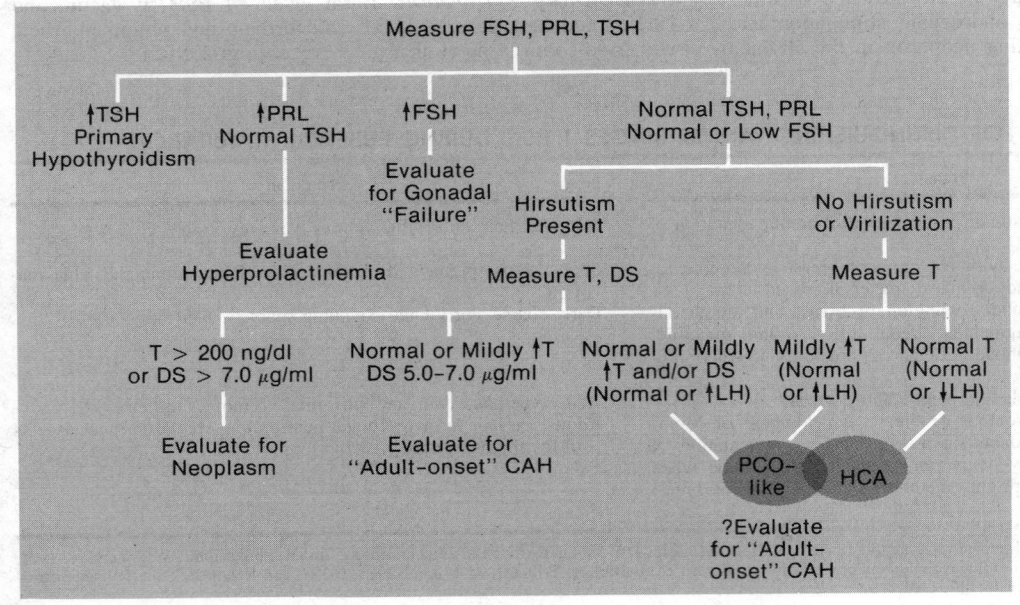

FIGURE 208–8. Biochemical evaluation of amenorrhea. This schema must be considered as an adjunct to the clinical evaluation of the patient. See text for details. **Abbreviations:** FSH = follicle-stimulating hormone; PRL = prolactin; TSH = thyroid-stimulating hormone; T = testosterone; DS = dehydroepiandrosterone sulfate; LH = luteinizing hormone; PCO-like = polycystic ovarian–like; HCA = hypothalamic chronic anovulation; CAH = congenital adrenal hyperplasia.

TABLE 208-6. CLASSIFICATION OF HYPERGONADOTROPIC AMENORRHEA (FSH > 40 mIU per milliliter)

I. Menopause
II. Genetic abnormalities
    A. Genetically reduced cell endowment
    B. Accelerated atresia
    C. Gonadal dysgenesis
       1. With stigmata of Turner's syndrome (45,X)
       2. Pure (46,XX or 46,XY)
       3. Mixed
    D. Trisomy X with or without chromosomal mosaicism
    E. In association with myotonia dystrophica
III. Physical causes
    A. Gonadal irradiation
    B. Chemotherapeutic (especially alkylating) agents
    C. Viral agents
    D. Surgical extirpation
IV. Autoimmune disorders
    A. Polyglandular, involving ovarian failure and any combination of thyroiditis, hypoadrenalism, hypoparathyroidism, diabetes mellitus, myasthenia gravis, vitiligo, mucocutaneous candidiasis, and pernicious anemia
    B. Isolated ovarian failure
V. Enzymatic defects
    A. 17α-Hydroxylase deficiency
    B. Galactosemia
VI. Defective gonadotropin secretion and/or action
    A. Resistant ovary or Savage syndrome
    B. Secretion of biologically inactive forms
    C. α or β subunit defects
VII. Congenital thymic aplasia
VIII. Circulating gonadotropin antibodies
IX. Idiopathic premature ovarian failure

metacarpals, an increased carrying angle of the arms, and certain renal and cardiovascular defects (most commonly coarctation of the aorta and aortic stenosis). The diagnosis can sometimes be made at birth because of unexplained lymphedema of the hands and feet. The syndrome is associated with an abnormality of sex chromosome number, morphology, or both. Most commonly the second sex chromosome is absent (45,X). This is the single most common chromosomal disorder in humans, but more than 95% of such fetuses are aborted so that the incidence in newborns is approximately 1 in 3000 to 5000. Chromosomal breakage and mosaicism occur frequently as well. In mosaic individuals with a normal 46,XX cell line, sufficient follicles may persist postnatally to initiate pubertal changes and to cause ovulation so that pregnancy is possible.

Pure gonadal dysgenesis is the term given to phenotypically female individuals with streak gonads who are of normal stature and have none of the physical stigmata associated with Turner's syndrome. Such individuals have either a 46,XX or 46,XY karyotype. The 46,XX defect may be inherited as an autosomal recessive, with 10% having associated nerve deafness. The 46,XY defect may be inherited as an X-linked recessive, with clitoromegaly occurring in 10 to 15% and gonadal tumors developing in 25% if the gonads are not removed.

Trisomy X (46,XXX karyotype) is also associated with premature menopause, while many such individuals actually have normal reproductive lives. Premature menopause can also occur in mosaic individuals with cell lines with excess X chromosomes. When gonadal abnormalities occur in women with excess X chromosomes, they seem to occur after ovarian differentiation so that some ovarian function is possible. Only later in life do such women develop secondary amenorrhea and premature ovarian failure.

Other Causes. *Physical, Chemical, and Infectious Causes.* Irradiation and chemotherapeutic agents, especially alkylating agents, utilized to treat various malignant diseases also may cause premature ovarian failure. Ovulation and cyclic menses return in some of these patients even after prolonged intervals of hypergonadotropic amenorrhea associated with signs and symptoms of profound hypoestrogenism. Rarely, mumps affects the ovaries and causes ovarian failure.

Autoimmune Disorders. Premature ovarian failure may occur in conjunction with a variety of autoimmune disorders. The most well-known syndrome involves hypoadrenalism, hypoparathyroidism,

and mucocutaneous candidiasis together with ovarian failure (see Ch. 210). Thyroiditis is the most commonly associated abnormality. Antibodies to the FSH receptor have been identified in a very few cases. These associations make it mandatory to rule out other potentially life-threatening endocrinopathies in young women with hypergonadotropic amenorrhea.

Enzymatic Defects. In girls with the rare syndrome of 17α-hydroxylase deficiency who survive until the expected age of puberty, sexual infantilism and primary amenorrhea occur together with elevated levels of gonadotropins. Increased synthesis of desoxycorticosterone leads to hypertension with hypokalemic alkalosis; serum progesterone levels are elevated as well. As with other causes of congenital adrenal hyperplasia, the hypertension is controlled by replacement therapy with glucocorticoids (see Ch. 207). Women with galactosemia also develop ovarian failure early in life, even when a galactose-restricted diet is introduced early in infancy (see Ch. 169).

Defective Gonadotropin Secretion and/or Action. The resistant ovary (Savage) syndrome occurs in young amenorrheic women who have (1) elevated peripheral gonadotropin concentrations, (2) normal (although immature) follicles present on ovarian biopsy, (3) a 46,XX karyotype with no evidence of mosaicism, (4) fully developed secondary sex characteristics, and (5) ovarian resistance to stimulation with human menopausal or pituitary gonadotropins. There seems to be some block to gonadotropin action within the ovary in this syndrome.

Therapeutic Considerations. Women with hypergonadotropic amenorrhea and ovarian failure should be treated identically whether or not they have signs of hypoestrogenism or desire pregnancy. Ovarian biopsy is not indicated to document the existence of follicles because only a small portion of each ovary can be sampled and because pregnancies have resulted in patients who had biopsies devoid of follicles. Estrogen replacement is warranted to prevent the accelerated bone loss known to occur in affected women (see Ch. 217). The estrogen should be given sequentially with a progestin to prevent endometrial hyperplasia. Young women with ovarian failure may require twice as much estrogen as postmenopausal women for relief of signs and symptoms of hypoestrogenism.

Women with hypergonadotropic amenorrhea are rarely able to become pregnant. Pregnancy is more likely to occur with estrogen replacement therapy than with any other therapy. It is not clear why pregnancy may rarely occur in such women. Even with estrogen replacement the pregnancy rate is less than 10%. The most successful treatment of young women with hypergonadotropic amenorrhea involves hormone replacement to mimic the normal menstrual cycle and embryo transfer utilizing donor oocytes. Pregnancy rates are higher than in other women undergoing *in vitro* fertilization and typically exceed 30% per cycle.

Differential Diagnosis and Treatment of Chronic Anovulation. Chronic anovulation, the most frequent form of amenorrhea encountered in women of reproductive age, implies that functional ovarian follicles remain and that cyclic ovulation can be induced or reinitiated with appropriate therapy (Table 208–7). Appropriate management requires that the cause of the anovulation be determined. The pathophysiologic bases for several forms of anovulation are unknown, but the anovulation can be interrupted transiently by nonspecific induction of ovulation in the majority of affected women. It is important to recognize that anovulation can result in either amenorrhea or irregular (generally less frequent) menses.

Hypothalamic Chronic Anovulation (HCA). HCA represents a heterogeneous group of disorders with similar manifestations. Emotional and physical stress, exercise, diet, weight loss, body composition, malnutrition, environment, and other unrecognized factors may contribute in varying proportions to the anovulation. Abrupt cessation of menses in women under 30 years of age who have no anatomic abnormalities of the hypothalamic-pituitary-ovarian axis and no other endocrine disturbances suggests a diagnosis of HCA. Affected individuals tend to be bright, educated, and engaged in intellectual occupations and may well give a history of psychosexual problems and socioenvironmental trauma. HCA is characterized by low to normal levels of gonadotropins and relative hypoestrogenism. Rarely, however, do affected women present with signs and symptoms of estrogen deficiency. Psychological counseling and/or a change in lifestyle, especially for those women engaged in strenu-

TABLE 208-7. CAUSES OF CHRONIC ANOVULATION

I. **Chronic anovulation of hypothalamic-pituitary origin**
  A. Hypothalamic chronic anovulation
    1. Psychogenic
    2. Exercise associated
    3. Associated with diet, weight loss, and/or malnutrition
    4. Anorexia nervosa and bulimia
    5. Pseudocyesis
  B. Forms of isolated gonadotropin deficiency (including Kallmann's syndrome)
  C. Due to hypothalamic-pituitary damage
    1. Pituitary and parapituitary tumors
    2. Empty-sella syndrome
    3. Following surgery
    4. Following irradiation
    5. Following trauma
    6. Following infection
    7. Following infarction
  D. Idiopathic hypopituitarism
  E. Hypothalamic-pituitary dysfunction or failure with hyperprolactinemia (multiple causes)
  F. Due to systemic diseases

II. **Chronic anovulation due to inappropriate feedback** (i.e., polycystic ovary syndrome)
  A. Excessive extraglandular estrogen production (i.e., obesity)
  B. Abnormal buffering involving sex hormone–binding globulin (including liver disease)
  C. Functional androgen excess (adrenal or ovarian)
  D. Neoplasms producing androgens or estrogens
  E. Neoplasms producing chorionic gonadotropin

III. **Chronic anovulation due to other endocrine and metabolic disorders**
  A. Adrenal hyperfunction
    1. Cushing's syndrome
    2. Congenital adrenal hyperplasia (female pseudohermaphroditism)
  B. Thyroid dysfunction
    1. Hyperthyroidism
    2. Hypothyroidism
  C. Prolactin and/or growth hormone excess
    1. Hypothalamic dysfunction
    2. Pituitary dysfunction (microadenomas and macroadenomas)
    3. Drug induced
  D. Malnutrition

Modified from Rebar RW: Chronic anovulation. *In* Serra GB (ed.): The Ovary. New York, Raven Press, 1983, p 217.

ous exercise programs, may be effective in inducing cyclic ovulation and menses. For women desiring pregnancy, ovulation can also be induced with clomiphene citrate (50 to 100 mg per day for 5 days beginning on the fifth day of withdrawal bleeding). Treatment with human menopausal gonadotropin and human chorionic gonadotropin (hMG-hCG) or with GnRH administered in a pulsatile fashion may be effective in women who do not ovulate in response to clomiphene. Most physicians advocate the use of exogenous steroids to prevent osteoporosis. A regimen can be used consisting of oral conjugated estrogens (0.625 to 1.25 mg); ethinyl estradiol (20 μg), or micronized estradiol-17β (1 to 2 mg) or transdermal estradiol-17β (0.05 to 0.10 mg) daily, with oral medroxyprogesterone acetate (5 to 10 mg) added for the first 12 to 14 days of each month. Sexually active women can be given oral contraceptive agents as an alternative. If steroid therapy is administered, patients must be informed that the amenorrhea probably will be present when therapy is discontinued. Other physicians believe only periodic observation is indicated, with barrier methods of contraception recommended for fertility control. Adequate ingestion of calcium should be ensured regardless of therapy. Contraception is needed for sexually active women with HCA, because the functional defect is mild in these disorders and may resolve spontaneously at any time, with ovulation occurring prior to any episode of menstruation.

Individuals with amenorrhea and significant weight loss should be examined for the possibility of *anorexia nervosa* (see Ch. 195). This disorder may be the most severe form of functional HCA, or it may be a distinct entity.

Kallmann's syndrome (isolated gonadotropin deficiency or familial hypogonadotropic hypogonadism) is a familial disorder consisting of gonadotropin deficiency, anosmia or hyposmia, and color blindness in men or, more rarely, in women. Other midline defects such as cleft lip and palate can occur in the affected individual or in family members. The trait is transmitted as an X-linked recessive or a male-limited autosomal dominant trait, but genetic heterogeneity may occur. Partial or complete agenesis of the olfactory bulb is present on autopsy, accounting for use of the term *olfactogenital dysplasia*. The disorder affects only gonadotropin secretion, and all other pituitary hormones are secreted normally. Isolated gonadotropin deficiency in the absence of anosmia occurs as well. Sexual infantilism with a eunuchoid habitus is the clinical hallmark of this disorder, but moderate breast development may occur. Circulating LH and FSH levels are quite low, but almost always detectable. Ovulation induction requires use of hMG-hCG or pulsatile GnRH. Estrogen replacement therapy is indicated in these women until such time as pregnancy is desired. It may not be possible to distinguish between partial isolated gonadotropin deficiency and functional HCA in all cases.

Hypopituitarism may be obvious upon cursory inspection or sufficiently subtle to require endocrine testing (see Ch. 202.1). The clinical presentation depends on the age of onset, the cause, and the nutritional status of the individual. Failure of development of secondary sex characteristics or for development to progress once puberty is initiated must always raise the question of hypopituitarism. Ovulation can be induced successfully with exogenous gonadotropins when pregnancy is desired and after the hypopituitarism is treated appropriately. Replacement therapy with estrogen is indicated to prevent signs and symptoms of estrogen deficiency.

Galactorrhea associated with hyperprolactinemia, whatever the cause, almost always occurs together with amenorrhea caused by hypothalamic-pituitary dysfunction or failure. Many conditions can cause excess prolactin secretion (see Ch. 208.4). It is unclear if all individuals with chronic anovulation associated with hyperprolactinemia and no other cause have pituitary microadenomas, even in the absence of identifiable radiographic changes of the sella turcica. Hirsutism may be observed occasionally in association with amenorrhea-galactorrhea and hyperprolactinemia. Elevated levels of the adrenal androgens DHEA and DHEA-S may be observed and may account for the PCO-type ovaries present in some hyperprolactinemic women.

The hypothalamic-pituitary unit also may fail to function normally in a number of stressful, debilitating, systemic illnesses that interfere with somatic growth and development. Chronic renal failure, liver disease, and diabetes mellitus are the most prominent examples.

Chronic Anovulation Due to Inappropriate Feedback. PCO syndrome, which causes anovulation because of inappropriate feedback signals to the hypothalamic-pituitary unit, is a heterogeneous disorder in which there is considerable clinical and biochemical variability among affected individuals. Although patients usually present with amenorrhea, hirsutism, and obesity, affected women may instead complain of irregular and profuse uterine bleeding, may not have hirsutism, and may be of normal weight. Excess androgen from any source or increased extraglandular conversion of androgens to estrogens can lead to the typical findings of PCO syndrome. Included are such diverse disorders as Cushing's syndrome, mild congenital adrenal hyperplasia, virilizing tumors of adrenal or ovarian origin, hyperthyroidism and hypothyroidism, obesity, and primary PCO syndrome with no other recognizable cause. In the primary syndrome the irregular menses, mild obesity, and hirsutism begin during puberty and typically become more severe with time. Obesity alone can lead to a PCO-like syndrome, with the degree of obesity required to cause anovulation varying widely from individual to individual. All such patients are well estrogenized regardless of whether they present with primary or secondary amenorrhea or dysfunctional bleeding. As noted, LH concentrations tend to be elevated, with relatively low and constant FSH levels, but both may be in the normal range compared with levels in women in the follicular phase of the menstrual cycle. Levels of most circulating androgens, especially testosterone, tend to be mildly elevated. The cause of PCO syndrome is unknown, but current evidence suggests that the hypothalamic-pituitary unit is intact and that a functional derangement, perhaps involving insulin-like growth factors such as insulin-like (IGF-I) within the ovary, results in abnormal gonadotropin secretion.

The aim of the diagnostic evaluation is to rule out any causes (such as neoplasms) that require definitive therapy. Hirsutism should be evaluated as detailed in Ch. 208.3. PCO syndrome itself is a benign disorder. Patients generally require therapy for hirsutism, for induction of ovulation if pregnancy is desired, and for prevention of estrogen-induced endometrial hyperplasia and cancer. No ideal therapy exists, but rather the therapeutic approach must be individualized to the needs of each patient.

In the anovulatory woman not desiring pregnancy who is not hirsute, therapy with intermittent progestin administration (such as medroxyprogesterone acetate 5 to 10 mg orally for 10 to 14 days each month) or oral contraceptives can be provided to reduce the increased risk of endometrial carcinoma that is present in such a woman with unopposed estrogen. All women utilizing intermittent progestin administration should be cautioned about the need for effective contraception if they are sexually active, because these agents do not inhibit ovulation when administered intermittently.

The approach to the hirsute anovulatory woman not desiring pregnancy is detailed in Ch. 208.3. Oral contraceptive agents are the first line of therapy for such women with mild hirsutism and offer protection from endometrial hyperplasia.

In women with PCO syndrome desiring pregnancy, clomiphene citrate is the first approach to inducing ovulation because of its simplicity and high success rate. Approximately 75 to 80% conceive with such therapy. Other possible methods of inducing ovulation include use of hMG-hCG, purified FSH, pulsatile GnRH, wedge resection of the ovaries at laparotomy, and laser or cautery destruction of follicles at laparoscopy. Surgical treatment is warranted only rarely and only in women in whom all other methods fail, in whom there is a question of an ovarian tumor because of ovarian size or circulating androgen levels, and in whom fertility is not an issue (because of the risk of pelvic adhesions from the surgery leading to infertility).

A particularly severely affected subset of women present with marked obesity, anovulation, mild glucose intolerance and high levels of circulating insulin with insulin resistance, acanthosis nigricans, hyperuricemia, and severe hirsutism with markedly elevated circulating androgen levels. These women have *hyperthecosis of the ovaries* in which the androgen-producing cells in the stromal, hilar, and thecal components of the ovaries are increased greatly in number. Although considered a separate entity by some clinicians, hyperthecosis probably should be viewed as a part of the spectrum of disorders constituting PCO syndrome.

Chronic Anovulation Due to Other Endocrine and Metabolic Disorders.
Adrenal hyperfunction appears to cause chronic anovulation by inducing a PCO-like syndrome secondary to increased adrenal androgen secretion, but other possible mechanisms also exist.

Both hyperthyroidism and hypothyroidism are associated with a variety of menstrual disturbances, including dysfunctional uterine bleeding and amenorrhea as a result of alterations in the metabolism of androgens and estrogens. These metabolic changes in turn result in inappropriate steroid feedback and chronic anovulation.

Rebar RW: Premature ovarian failure. *In* Lobo RA (ed.): Treatment of the Postmenopausal Woman. Basic and Clinical Aspects. New York, Raven Press, 1994, p 25. *A detailed discussion of the diagnosis and treatment of premature ovarian failure.*

Yen SSC, Jaffe RB (eds.): Reproductive Endocrinology, 3rd ed. Philadelphia, WB Saunders, 1991. *Detailed chapters describe practical evaluation of hormonal status and chronic anovulation caused by peripheral endocrine disorders as well as by CNS-hypothalamic-pituitary dysfunction.*

DISORDERS OF FOLLICULOGENESIS. Recognized disorders of folliculogenesis cannot be identified before ovulation begins. They are believed to reflect abnormalities in follicular development.

Luteinized Unruptured Follicle (LUF) Syndrome.
The LUF syndrome describes development of a dominant follicle without its subsequent disruption and release of the ovum. The abnormality can be diagnosed by ultrasonography or by the absence of evidence of ovulation when the ovary is viewed at laparoscopy. The disorder is believed to occur infrequently and sporadically and is probably not a significant cause of infertility. Menstrual cycles in which no ovum is released are characterized by presumptive evidence of ovulation, including biphasic basal body temperatures, secretory endometrium, a normal LH surge, and normal progesterone production in the luteal phase. In fact, although the syndrome is believed to occur, data to substantiate its existence are only circumstantial (although strongly suggestive) at present.

Luteal Phase Dysfunction.
Progesterone secretion in the luteal phase may be reduced in duration (termed luteal phase insufficiency) or in amount (termed luteal phase inadequacy). More rarely the endometrium may be unable to respond to secreted progesterone because of the absence of progesterone receptors. These disorders are believed to represent causes for infertility (because of inability of fertilized ova to implant) in approximately 5% of infertile couples. Abnormalities of the follicular phase, especially in the frequency of gonadotropin pulses, may account for most luteal phase defects. Luteal phase defects also may occur sporadically in normally ovulating women approximately once each year.

Luteal phase dysfunction may be associated with several clinical entities, including mild or intermittent hyperprolactinemia (of any cause), strenuous physical exercise, inadequately treated 21-hydroxylase deficiency, and habitual abortion. Luteal dysfunction occurs more commonly at the extremes of reproductive life and in the first menstrual cycles following full-term delivery, abortion, or discontinuation of oral contraceptives. It also may occur during ovulatory cycles induced with clomiphene citrate or hMG-hCG.

The diagnosis of luteal phase dysfunction can be made either by endometrial biopsy or by serial progesterone determinations. Endometrial biopsies obtained from the uterine fundus in the late luteal phases of two different cycles must be at least 2 days out of phase from the expected date of bleeding, as judged from the subsequent menstrual cycle, for the diagnosis to be made. The absolute concentration that progesterone must achieve and the length of time progesterone must be increased in the luteal phase to exclude luteal dysfunction are unclear. Luteal dysfunction is extremely rare in women with menstrual cycles greater than 25 days in length in whom a single random progesterone determination is greater than 15 ng per milliliter.

Treatment of luteal dysfunction is controversial. Any underlying defect should be treated. If subsequent luteal function depends on prior follicular development, modification of follicular development with either clomiphene citrate (25 to 100 mg daily by mouth for 5 days beginning on cycle day 3 to 5) or FSH (75 to 300 IU intramuscularly for 3 to 5 days beginning on cycle day 3 to 5) is reasonable. hCG (2500 to 5000 IU intramuscularly at 2- to 3-day intervals beginning with the shift in basal body temperature) or progesterone (12.5 mg intramuscularly in oil daily or 25 mg twice a day as rectal or vaginal suppositories) can be utilized as well. Bromocriptine may correct the abnormality in individuals with hyperprolactinemia. Synthetic progestational agents should not be used to treat luteal phase defects because of their possible (although unproven) association with congenital anomalies. Furthermore, the synthetic progestins produce an abnormal endometrium. None of these agents has been shown to increase the pregnancy rate.

Soules MR: Luteal phase deficiency: A subtle abnormality of ovulation. *In* Keye WR Jr, Chang RJ, Rebar RW, Soules MR (eds.): Infertility: Evaluation and Treatment. Philadelphia, WB Saunders, 1995. *A complete consideration of the etiology, diagnosis, and treatment of luteal phase abnormalities.*

INFERTILITY. *Infertility* may be defined as involuntary inability to conceive. *Sterility* is total inability to reproduce. In either case the situation may or may not be correctable, especially for each particular couple. Failure to reproduce thwarts a basic human instinct and causes anger, guilt, and depression. More than 10% of couples in the United States seek medical assistance for infertility.

The requirements for pregnancy to occur are several:

1. The male must produce adequate numbers of normal, motile spermatozoa.
2. The male must be capable of ejaculating the sperm through a patent ductal system.
3. The sperm must be able to traverse an unobstructed female reproductive tract.
4. The female must ovulate and release an ovum.
5. The sperm must be able to fertilize the ovum.
6. The fertilized ovum must be capable of developing and implanting in appropriately prepared endometrium.

Infertility is too frequently viewed primarily as a problem of the female. In fact, in approximately 40% of cases, infertility is caused by the male (Table 208–8). In perhaps one third of couples more than one cause contributes to the infertility.

TABLE 208-8. CAUSES OF INFERTILITY AND THEIR APPROXIMATE INCIDENCE (%)

I. **Male factors (40%)**
   A. Decreased production of spermatozoa
      1. Variocele
      2. Testicular failure
      3. Endocrine disorders
      4. Cryptorchidism
      5. Stress, smoking, caffeine, nicotine, recreational drugs
   B. Ductal obstruction
      1. Epididymal (postinfection)
      2. Congenital absence of vas deferens
      3. Ejaculatory duct (postinfection)
      4. Postvasectomy
   C. Inability to deliver sperm into vagina
      1. Ejaculatory disturbances
      2. Hypospadias
      3. Sexual problems (i.e., impotence), medical or psychological
   D. Abnormal semen
      1. Infection
      2. Abnormal volume
      3. Abnormal viscosity
   E. Immunologic factors
      1. Sperm-immobilizing antibodies
      2. Sperm-agglutinating antibodies

II. **Female factors**
   A. Fallopian tube pathology (20 to 30%)
      1. Pelvic inflammatory disease or puerperal infection
      2. Congenital anomalies
      3. Endometriosis
      4. Secondary to past peritonitis of nongenital origin
   B. Amenorrhea and anovulation (15%)
   C. Minor ovulatory disturbances (<5%?)
   D. Cervical and uterine factors (10%)
      1. Leiomyomas and polyps
      2. Uterine anomalies
      3. Intrauterine synechiae (Asherman's syndrome)
      4. Destroyed endocervical glands (postsurgery or postinfection)
   E. Vaginal factors (<5%)
      1. Congenital absence of vagina
      2. Imperforate hymen
      3. Vaginismus
      4. Vaginitis
   F. Immunologic factors (<5%)
      1. Sperm-immobilizing antibodies
      2. Sperm-agglutinating antibodies
   G. Nutritional and metabolic factors (5%)
      1. Thyroid disorders
      2. Diabetes mellitus
      3. Severe nutritional disturbances

III. **Idiopathic or unexplained (<10%)**

Peak age of fertility in the female is 25 years. For nulliparous women of this age the average time during which unprotected intercourse occurs until conception is 5.3 months. For parous women the average duration of intercourse until conception is 2.7 months. The reproductive performance of couples is influenced by the ages of the female and male partners, the frequency of intercourse, and the length of time the couple has been attempting to conceive. There is a decline in both female and male reproductive performance after age 25.

Couples who complain of infertility merit evaluation regardless of the length of infertility. If the couple believes there is a problem, it is the physician's responsibility to reassure them by appropriate evaluation and subsequent explanation of all findings and the prognosis.

The evaluation begins with a detailed history obtained from both partners and physical examinations of both individuals. The couple should be seen together for the first visit. Each couple should be questioned together and separately because separate interviews may uncover information that would not be imparted in the presence of the partner.

Initial evaluation for infertility generally includes (1) assessment of semen, (2) documentation of ovulation by basal body temperature, serum progesterone determination approximately 6 to 8 days before menses, or endometrial biopsy less than 3 days before onset of menses, and (3) evaluation of the female genital tract by hysterosalpingography. Basal serum levels of prolactin and thyroid hormones should be measured. Diagnostic laparoscopy with tubal dye instillation should be performed if results of all previous tests are normal because 30 to 50% of women are found to have endometriosis or tubal disease on surgical evaluation. Treatment must be predicated on the findings of the infertility evaluation.

Glass RH: Infertility. *In* Yen SSC, Jaffe RB (eds.): Reproductive Endocrinology, 3rd ed. Philadelphia, WB Saunders, 1991, p 689. *A summary of the approach to the infertile couple.*

SEXUAL FUNCTION AND DYSFUNCTION. Although sexual responses begin following puberty, they can continue for the duration of a woman's life. Sexual responses generally are divided into four phases: excitement, plateau, orgasm, and resolution.

With sexual arousal and excitement, vasocongestion and muscular tension increase progressively, primarily in the genitals, manifested by vaginal lubrication in the female. The lubrication is due to formation of a transudate in the vagina. Sexual excitement is initiated by any of a variety of psychogenic or somatogenic sexual stimuli and must be reinforced to result in orgasm. With continued stimulation, the excitement phase increases in intensity into a plateau phase during which a high state of sexual interest is maintained. The plateau phase may be short or long, and it is from this phase that an individual can shift to orgasm. The orgasmic phase tends to be brief and is characterized by rapid release from the developed vasocongestion and muscular tension. The orgasmic release is also known as the climax because peak psychological and physical intensity is achieved and there is an attendant feeling of satisfaction. Copious secretions and transudate may flow during orgasm in women. Although women may resolve toward sleep following orgasm, many remain responsive to sexual stimulation and may return to plateau and subsequent orgasm.

Characteristic genital and extragenital responses occur during these phases. Estrogens magnify the sexual responses, but responses may occur in estrogen-deficient women. For women these changes occur in the breasts and in the pudendal region and are variable from one response cycle to another. For some women, excitement proceeds quickly through plateau to orgasm, and orgasm is explosive and accompanied by vocalization and involuntary contractions of the pelvic skeletal muscles. For other women, the responses are slow in building, controlled in amplitude, and long lasting. For a few women orgasm never occurs; for many it is intermittently absent.

The somatic sensate focus enabling orgasmic release is variable and may include stimulation of the breast, vagina, or clitoris. The psychological aspect of coitus may involve concentration on the current partner or act or fantasies about other times and persons. Although orgasms may vary in physiologic intensity, what is important is psychological satisfaction. Satisfaction for both men and women may be had without orgasm.

Women may seek consultation because of disturbances in normal sexual arousal or orgasm. Such sexual dysfunction may be due to either organic or functional disturbances.

A variety of diseases affecting neurologic function, including diabetes mellitus and multiple sclerosis, may prevent sexual arousal. So, too, may local pelvic disorders, such as endometriosis and vaginitis, which cause dyspareunia and lead to sexual avoidance. Estrogen deficiency causing vaginal atrophy and dyspareunia is a relatively common cause of sexual dysfunction. Debilitating systemic diseases such as malignant disease may also affect sexual function indirectly.

In most cases the cause of sexual dysfunction is psychological. For instance, vaginismus involves involuntary contractions of the muscles surrounding the introitus and leads to dyspareunia. It is a conditioned response engendered by a previous imagined or real traumatic sexual experience. Feelings of guilt, caused by incest or rape as examples; of inadequacy, caused by hysterectomy or mastectomy; or of depression or anxiety may lead to failure to be aroused. Failure to achieve orgasm may be viewed as a dysfunction if the woman is frustrated or dissatisfied.

Treatment of sexual dysfunction is best accomplished by eliminating functional causes and providing the patient, often together with her partner, with appropriate psychological counseling. Behavioral modification is effective in treating many women with psychological sexual dysfunction.

Kaplan HS: The Evaluation of Sexual Disorders: Psychological and Medical Aspects. New York, Brunner-Mazel, 1983. *A good general text detailing sexual disorders.*

Kaplan HS: The Illustrated Manual of Sex Therapy, 2nd ed. New York, Brunner-Mazel, 1987. *A simple text graphically detailing the therapeutic techniques first introduced by Masters and Johnson.*

Kolodny RC, Masters WH, Johnson VE: Textbook of Sexual Medicine. Boston, Little, Brown and Company, 1979. *A widely used text detailing sexual problems and their therapy.*

Masters W, Johnson V: Human Sexual Response. Boston, Little, Brown and Company, 1966. *The classic work detailing human sexual response. Required reading for all individuals seriously interested in this field.*

Nadelson CC, Marcotte DB (eds.): Treatment Interventions in Human Sexuality. New York, Plenum Press, 1983. *A multiauthored text that considers sexual problems in detail.*

HORMONAL THERAPY DURING THE REPRODUCTIVE YEARS

INDUCTION OF OVULATION. Induction of ovulation should never be attempted until serious disorders precluding pregnancy are ruled out or treated. Furthermore, ovulation induction should be utilized only in women with chronic anovulation, because women with ovarian failure are unresponsive to any form of ovulation induction. In general, the use of pharmaceutical agents does not improve the quality of an ovum, and thus the chance of pregnancy is not improved in women who ovulate regularly.

Clomiphene citrate is the agent that usually induces ovulation most easily. Clomiphene should be utilized in individuals without hyperprolactinemia who have the ability to release LH and FSH. A typical course of clomiphene therapy is begun on the fifth day following either spontaneous or induced uterine bleeding. The initial dosage is 50 mg daily for 5 days. Clomiphene appears to act as an anti-estrogen and stimulates gonadotropin secretion by the pituitary gland to initiate follicular development. If ovulation is not achieved in the very first cycle of treatment, the daily dosage is increased to 100 mg. If ovulation is still not achieved, dosage is increased in a stepwise fashion by 50-mg increments to a maximum of 200 to 250 mg daily for 5 days. The highest dose should be continued for 3 to 6 months before the patient is regarded as a clomiphene failure. The quantity of drug and the length of time that it can be used, as suggested here, are greater than those recommended by the manufacturers, but conform with published series.

The ovulatory surge of LH may occur 5 to 12 days (average, 7 days) after the completion of the last day of clomiphene treatment in each course. Couples are advised to have intercourse every other day during this time interval. Ovulation can be documented by monitoring changes in basal body temperature or preferably by measuring serum progesterone approximately 14 days after the last clomiphene tablet is taken. In addition, menses should occur about 3 weeks after the last day of therapy. Withdrawal bleeding with progestin can be induced if the patient fails to bleed within 4 weeks of therapy and if a serum hCG level documents that the patient is not pregnant. Testing the urine for an LH surge with any of several commercially available tests may also be useful in timing ovulation.

Some clinicians give 5,000 to 10,000 IU of hCG intramuscularly 7 days after the last day of clomiphene therapy to trigger ovulation, but this approach has not been established to increase effectiveness. The administration of hCG, however, does serve to time ovulation and may be helpful in selected couples. Ovulation can be expected to occur approximately 36 hours after hCG administration.

Of appropriately selected patients, 75 to 80% will ovulate and 40 to 50% can be expected to become pregnant. About 15% of pregnancies can be expected with each ovulatory cycle. The multiple pregnancy rate is about 8%, with almost all being twins. The incidence of congenital anomalies is not increased.

Side effects of clomiphene are uncommon and rarely serious. The most serious ones include vasomotor flushes (10%), abdominal discomfort (5%), breast tenderness (2%), nausea and vomiting (2%), visual symptoms (1.5%), and headache (1%). Ovarian enlargement may occur but is rare (5%). Concern has recently been raised about the potential for clomiphene to increase the risk of epithelial ovarian cancer. The evidence is insufficient to change current practices but suggests that clomiphene be administered prudently and for only a limited number of cycles.

The addition of dexamethasone, 0.5 mg orally at bedtime to blunt the nighttime secretion of ACTH, may be useful in hyperandrogenic women with an adrenal component who fail to ovulate in response to clomiphene. Other individuals failing to respond to clomiphene typically require hMG-hCG or perhaps pulsatile GnRH to induce ovulation.

Bromocriptine, a dopamine agonist, is effective in inducing ovulation in hyperprolactinemic women (see Ch. 208.4). The drug should be stopped once pregnancy is confirmed. Ovulatory menses and pregnancy are achieved in about 80% of patients with galactorrhea and hyperprolactinemia. The majority of women with prolactin-secreting pituitary tumors remain asymptomatic during pregnancy. It is extremely rare for a patient with either a microadenoma or a macroadenoma to develop a problem related to the tumor that affects either the mother or the fetus during pregnancy. Monitoring during pregnancy need consist only of questioning the patient about the development of visual symptoms and headaches. Formal assessment of visual fields and CT or MRI should be carried out in any patient developing suspicious symptoms. Symptoms generally abate with institution of bromocriptine therapy. No adverse effects of bromocriptine on fetuses or pregnancies have been reported.

hMG, a purified preparation of gonadotropins extracted from the urine of postmenopausal women, must be administered intramuscularly. Each vial contains 75 units of FSH and 75 units of LH. Purified FSH has become available for use recently. Biochemically engineered preparations of both products will become available in the future. hMG is administered at doses of two to four vials for 5 to 12 days to achieve follicular development as monitored by ultrasonography and serum or urinary E_2 concentrations. hCG, 5,000 to 10,000 IU, is administered as a single intramuscular dose when follicular maturation is apparent. The hCG should be withheld if more than three follicles mature together. GnRH analogues are now being utilized to suppress endogenous follicular activity before initiating therapy with hMG and continued until hCG is given in older women and those with poor responses to hMG alone. Use of the analogues necessitates administration of larger quantities of hMG. Success rates, however, seem to be somewhat improved with this combined therapy.

Because of the expense and the complication rate, thorough evaluation should be carried out to exclude other causes of infertility before hMG-hCG is used. Ovulation can be induced in almost 100% of patients, but pregnancy occurs in only 50 to 70%. There is no increased risk of congenital anomalies with hMG-hCG. Concerns have been raised that hMG may increase the risk of ovarian epithelial cancer, but the data are too tenuous to require any change in current practice.

The rate of multiple pregnancies with hMG-hCG may approach 30%, with 5% being triplets or more. Ovarian hyperstimulation is the major side effect and may be life threatening. The ovaries enlarge remarkably in this treatment-induced syndrome, and multiple follicle cysts, stromal edema, and multiple corpora lutea are present. There is a shift of fluid from the intravascular space into the abdominal cavity with resultant hypovolemia and hemoconcentration. The cause of the ascites is unknown. Treatment is conservative, with monitoring of fluid and electrolyte status. Pelvic examinations should not be performed for fear of rupturing the ovaries. The hyperstimulation generally resolves slowly over about 7 days.

GnRH, administered intravenously or less effectively subcutaneously at doses of 5 to 20 μg every 60 to 120 minutes, also can be used to induce ovulation in women with an intact pituitary gland. It is most effective in individuals with hypothalamic chronic anovulation. hCG can be administered to support the corpus luteum after ovulation at a dose of 1500 IU intramuscularly every 3 days for three to four doses. The advantage of GnRH rests in the fact that hyperstimulation is extremely unlikely. However, reported pregnancy rates have been no greater than those achieved with hMG-hCG. Furthermore, some patients do not tolerate wearing the infusion pump that must be utilized.

Speroff L, Glass RH, Kase NG: Induction of ovulation. *In* Clinical Gynecologic Endocrinology and Infertility, 5th ed. Baltimore, Williams & Wilkins, 1994, p 897. *A detailed and practical survey of how to induce ovulation.*

STEROIDAL CONTRACEPTION. *Physiologic Actions and Metabolic Effects.* Oral contraceptive pills are the most widely used contraceptives worldwide, with more than 50 million users. Combination (estrogen-progestin) and progestin-only preparations are available. The estrogen may be either mestranol or ethinyl estradiol, while the progestin is usually one of eight derivatives of 19-nor-testosterone: norethindrone, norethindrone acetate, norethynodrel, ethynodiol diacetate, norgestrel, levonorgestrel, desogestrel, and norgestimate. Combination products containing one of the last two progestins were recently approved for use in the United States.

The low-dose combination pills currently in use (containing 30 to 35 μg of estrogen with reduced amounts of progestin) were developed to reduce the biochemical changes produced by contraceptive steroids, but the majority of studies were conducted with the older high-dose preparations. It is known that virtually all biochemical changes are dose related.

Combination oral contraceptives inhibit the midcycle gonadotropin surge by inhibiting GnRH release from the hypothalamus. Cervical mucus becomes thick, viscid, and scanty in amount, thus retarding sperm penetration. Fallopian tube motility and secretion are altered as well, and the endometrial glands produce less glycogen. Efficacy is substantiated by a failure rate of 0.1% during the first year of combination oral contraceptive use.

Oral contraceptives decrease maturation of the vaginal epithelium and somehow render the vagina more susceptible to candidiasis. The endometrium becomes atrophic with variable degrees of decidual change, leading to diminished menstrual flow. Follicular development is arrested with low estrogen and progesterone secretion. Both circulating LH and FSH levels are reduced and constant.

The general metabolic effects of oral contraceptives resemble those of pregnancy. Glucose tolerance is impaired, with an increase in plasma insulin levels. The "mini-pill" containing progestin only in low dosage may cause no changes in glucose metabolism. Levels of circulating triglycerides and of very low density lipoproteins (VLDL's) are often increased, almost entirely because of the estrogenic component (see Ch. 173). Only slight changes accompany the low-dose combination preparations. The new progestins desogestrel and norgestimate are less androgenic than the earlier agents and stimulate lipid formation less than did the earlier ones. Only very high estrogenic formulations will increase mean serum cholesterol levels. Because of a direct effect of estrogens on the endoplasmic reticulum in the liver, α_2 globulins, including angiotensinogen, and β globulins are increased, while serum albumin levels are decreased somewhat. A number of blood coagulation factors and carrier proteins (including thyroid-binding globulin, transferrin, ceruloplasmin, SHBG, and corticosteroid-binding globulin) are also increased.

Interactions with Other Drugs. Oral contraceptive steroids interact with several other drugs, leading to reduced effectiveness of the contraceptives or of the other drug. Such interactions occur because of altered drug absorption or metabolism. The majority of these interactions occur only with long-term use of the pharmacologic agent. By inducing hepatic microsomal enzymes, long-term administration of antibiotics may reduce the contraceptive efficacy of the steroids. The short-term use of antibiotics is probably of little concern. Anticonvulsants also sharply reduce the efficacy of contraceptive steroids, as do antacids, which may decrease the absorption of steroids. Conversely, contraceptive steroids oppose the therapeutic effects of anticoagulants, antidiabetic agents, and certain antihypertensive agents, such as guanethidine and α-methyldopa, because of their metabolic effects. Because of the impaired elimination of certain drugs, such as phenothiazines, oral contraceptive users may require lower doses.

Complications, Side Effects, and Benefits. Although the complications and side effects of combination oral contraceptives have been widely reported, the low-dose formulations currently available have minimized the side effects compared with the older, high-dose preparations without sacrificing contraceptive efficacy or reducing the substantial health benefits associated with oral contraceptive use.

The use of oral contraceptives increases the risk of *thromboembolism*, possibly as much as 4- to 13-fold with the doses of estrogens used in early preparations. The estrogen content of oral contraceptives appears to be correlated roughly with the risk of venous thromboembolic disease. Lower dosages of estrogen than were used initially in oral contraceptive preparations may not significantly increase the risk of any cardiovascular complications. Advanced maternal age and smoking seem to be the major risk factors for thromboembolic phenomena in users of oral contraceptives. In the absence of smoking and in women under the age of 45 years who do not suffer from obesity, hypertension, diabetes mellitus, or inherited lipoprotein abnormalities, there is little, if any, increased risk for cardiovascular disease, including myocardial infarction, with use

of low-dose combination oral contraceptives. Some clinicians believe that these preparations may be used safely in normal women until the menopause.

In the absence of smoking and hypertension, most recent epidemiologic studies indicate that the use of low-dose oral contraceptives approximately doubles the risk of fatal and nonfatal stroke in young women, compared with a fourfold risk associated with the earlier use of preparations containing larger amounts of estrogens. Some but not all women with migraine headaches may note increasingly frequent headaches with oral contraceptive use. Although anecdotes indicate otherwise, epidemiologic studies do not confirm that women with migraine headaches have a greater risk of stroke.

Women using oral contraceptives are more likely to become hypertensive, especially if over the age of 35 years. Smoking may contribute to the incidence of hypertension. Increases in blood pressure are generally reversible shortly after oral contraceptives are discontinued. Failure of the blood pressure to return to normal when oral contraceptives are discontinued suggests underlying disease.

Contraceptive steroids do not appear to be teratogenic. Derivatives of 19-nor-testosterone can virilize female fetuses when administered in large doses to women early in pregnancy, but the doses required are far in excess of those contained in oral contraceptives.

Use of oral contraceptives reduces the risk of benign breast neoplasia, including fibrocystic disease and fibroadenoma. Because benign breast disease is a significant risk factor for the subsequent development of breast cancer, oral contraceptives may afford protection against breast cancer in this manner. Indeed, the incidence of breast cancer does not seem to be increased by use of oral contraceptives. Furthermore, oral contraceptives reduce the risk of developing endometrial carcinoma by about half and of developing ovarian carcinoma by about 40%. In the cases of both endometrial and ovarian cancers, the protection is related to duration of use and persists for at least 10 years after stopping oral contraceptives.

Use of combined oral contraceptives may result in an increased risk for the development of *hepatocellular adenoma*, and this risk may increase with increased duration of contraceptive use. Rarely in patients with such adenomas the liver may rupture, and death may even occur because of hemorrhage. There is no evidence of any increased risk of developing liver cancer.

The relationships of oral contraceptive use to cervical carcinoma, pituitary tumors, and melanoma are unclear. Most studies show positive relationships between cervical dysplasia and oral contraceptive use. Cervical dysplasia is increased in women with first coitus at an early age and those who have multiple sexual partners. Current evidence suggests that the increased incidence of cervical dysplasia is not related to the oral contraceptive but to these behavioral characteristics. There is some evidence that the incidence of prolactinomas may be increasing in women, but the use of contraceptive steroids has not been shown to increase this risk.

So-called *post-pill amenorrhea* is sometimes regarded as a side effect of oral contraceptive use. The return to ovulation following discontinuation of contraceptive use is variable but occurs within 4 to 8 weeks in most patients. Approximately 1 in 500 patients have amenorrhea for 6 months or longer, with 15% of these having associated galactorrhea. This prolonged amenorrhea is probably caused by underlying disorders unrelated to oral contraceptive use. In normal women subsequent fertility is unimpaired.

Nausea and vomiting occur occasionally when use begins but generally abate with continued use. Mastalgia and increased breast size may occur but also tend to subside in several cycles. Chloasma (hyperpigmentation of the face) is a leading cause of pill discontinuation. Acne is usually improved, but occasionally may be exacerbated. Dizziness, headaches, visual disturbances, depression, and increased or decreased libido have been reported. Easy bruisability due to increased capillary fragility and edema also may occur.

Other therapeutic benefits exist with oral contraceptive use as well. The risk of pelvic inflammatory disease appears reduced by half. Decreased menstrual blood loss results in a lower incidence of iron deficiency anemia. Acne frequently improves and dysmenorrhea decreases in the majority of patients. Symptomatic relief of endometriosis occurs in some patients. The risk of functional ovarian cysts is decreased, as are the incidences of ectopic pregnancies and uterine fibroids. Women with PCO syndrome treated with oral contraceptives are afforded protection from endometrial carcinoma. Oral contraceptives have been linked to prevention of postmenopausal osteoporosis. Oral contraceptives may possibly afford protection against development of rheumatoid arthritis as well.

Absolute contraindications to the use of oral contraceptives include thrombophlebitis, thromboembolic disorders, cardiovascular disease, or a history of these conditions; markedly impaired liver function; known or suspected estrogen-dependent neoplasia; undiagnosed abnormal genital bleeding; known or suspected pregnancy; and congenital hyperlipidemia. Oral contraceptives generally should be administered with caution to smokers, women who are obese, and those with varicose veins. If headaches develop or become more frequent with pill use, oral contraceptives should be discontinued. Because of a possible increase in postsurgical thromboembolic complications in women using oral contraceptives, use of oral contraceptives should be discontinued 2 weeks prior to major surgery and begun again 2 weeks postoperatively.

Low-dose combination oral contraceptive pills offer superb protection for sexually active women not desiring pregnancy. For most such individuals the benefits of the low-dose preparations clearly outweigh the adverse effects, but possible side effects and complications must be considered in treating individual patients.

Two long-acting, implantable or injectable contraceptive steroid preparations are now approved for use in the United States. Levonorgestrel (Norplant) and depo-medroxyprogesterone (Depo-Provera) are extremely effective, contain no estrogen, and affect fertility by suppressing pituitary gonadotropin secretion. They also thicken cervical mucus and cause endometrial atrophy and irregular uterine bleeding.

Henzl MR: Contraceptive hormones and their clinical use. *In* Yen SSC, Jaffe RB (eds.): Reproductive Endocrinology, 3rd ed. Philadelphia, WB Saunders Company, 1991, p 807. *A detailed discussion of steroidal contraception.*

Speroff L, Darney P: A Clinical Guide for Contraception. Baltimore, Williams & Wilkins, 1992. *A monograph devoted to a consideration of contraceptive choices.*

THE MENOPAUSE AND POSTMENOPAUSAL YEARS

DEFINITIONS AND EPIDEMIOLOGY. The *menopause* is the final menstrual period denoting the cessation of cyclic ovarian function as manifested by cyclic menstruation. The *climacteric* is the physiologic period during which regression of ovarian function occurs. Its onset generally is signaled by alterations in the menstrual cycle or vasomotor symptomatology. Menopause occurs at a mean age of approximately 51 years. Today's average woman in the Western world can expect to live one third of her life in the postmenopausal phase.

SYMPTOMATOLOGY AND SIGNS. Most signs and symptoms associated with the postmenopausal years result from decreased circulating estrogen. Common symptoms include hot flushes, paresthesias, palpitations, cold hands and feet, headaches, vertigo, irritability, anxiety, nervousness, depression, fatigue, weight gain, insomnia, night sweats, forgetfulness, and inability to concentrate.

Vasomotor instability is perhaps the most common complaint. Over 75% of women experience hot flushes with decreasing estrogen levels, and these may persist for years. In a typical hot flush, the skin, especially of the head and neck, becomes red and warm for a few seconds to 2 minutes with cold chills thereafter. Accompanying physiologic changes include a rise in skin temperature, peripheral vasodilatation, increased heart rate, decreased skin resistance, and concomitant LH pulses. The mechanism for hot flushes is unknown but must involve thermoregulatory centers in the hypothalamus.

Any increase in bleeding or resumption of bleeding after 6 months of amenorrhea demands examination and sampling of the endometrium to exclude carcinoma. Women note relocation of fat deposits, with increased fat in the lower abdomen, hips, and breasts. The genital skin becomes thin and pale, with a decrease in the size of the labia minora, clitoris, uterus, and ovaries, and the women often complain of dyspareunia. Decreased elastic tissue of skin is noted, and osteoporosis may occur in about 25% of postmenopausal women (see Ch. 217).

Menopausal signs and symptoms may begin long before menses have ceased. Symptoms may be difficult to diagnose in women with previous hysterectomies. Following bilateral oophorectomy young women develop identical signs and symptoms.

ENDOCRINOLOGIC CHANGES. During the menopausal transition regular menstrual cycles may continue up to the menopause. The cycles may become shorter, due to shortened follicular phases, with increased FSH, normal LH, and decreased E_2 and progesterone levels compared with normal ovulatory cycles. Variable cycles also may occur prior to the menopause, with some being ovulatory and others being anovulatory. Waning ovarian follicular activity with decreasing E_2 production must be central to these changes, and yet some follicles have been found on occasion in ovaries of postmenopausal women.

In postmenopausal women, circulating FSH and LH concentrations are greatly increased. Estrogen levels are decreased markedly, but androgen levels are decreased only slightly. The postmenopausal ovaries continue to secrete substantial amounts of androgen (androstenedione and testosterone), which together with adrenal androgens are converted to estrogens by extraglandular conversion in the periphery. The peripheral conversion of androgens accounts for most circulating estrogen in postmenopausal women.

CLINICAL MANAGEMENT. Treatment of postmenopausal women must be individualized and based on a personal dialogue with each patient. Exogenous estrogen replacement stops or diminishes hot flushes, reverses atrophic genital changes, decreases osteoporotic fractures (see Ch. 217), and may decrease the incidence of atherosclerotic coronary artery disease.

Estrogen replacement therapy is absolutely contraindicated in postmenopausal women with estrogen-dependent tumors of the breast, uterus, or kidney; acute liver disease; cerebrovascular disease; active deep-vein thrombosis and embolism; malignant melanoma (?); and undiagnosed genital bleeding. Replacement therapy must be considered carefully and other therapy may require modification in women with estrogen-associated hypertension, diabetes mellitus, cholecystitis and cholelithiasis, pancreatitis, congestive heart failure, past endometriosis, and neuro-ophthalmologic vascular disease. Individual exceptions to even the absolute contraindications exist.

Many treatment regimens are currently being utilized. Estrogen should be administered together with a progestin in a cyclic fashion to women with a uterus to prevent an increased risk of endometrial hyperplasia and carcinoma. Oral estrone sulfate (0.625 to 1.25 mg), micronized estradiol-17β (1 mg), or transdermal estradiol (0.05 mg) may be given daily. To this should be added a progestin such as medroxyprogesterone acetate (5 to 10 mg orally for 12 to 14 days each month, beginning on the first day of the month). Menstrual bleeding occurs in more than half of the women. As a consequence, continuous daily administration of a combination of an estrogen and a progestin has been advocated. The ratios of estrogen to progestin utilized are empiric. Unfortunately, irregular breakthrough bleeding occurs frequently in the first several months of therapy, even though the majority of women eventually become amenorrheic. Although continuous combined therapy is an option, it cannot be advocated strongly until more data accumulate regarding its safety and efficacy. Similar dosages of estrogen alone may be administered continuously to women who have undergone hysterectomy, particularly because progestins may impact negatively on several beneficial metabolic effects of estrogen. Younger women may require twice as much estrogen as older women to alleviate symptoms.

Even the continuous combined replacement therapy differs from oral contraceptive preparations in that the doses of estrogen and progestin are lower. Moreover, the estrogens utilized in replacement therapy have fewer metabolic effects than do the synthetic estrogens used in oral contraceptives. There is no evidence that postmenopausal estrogen administration increases the risk of thromboembolic phenomena.

Before beginning estrogen replacement therapy, patients should have a complete history and physical examination. A pretreatment mammogram is indicated because estrogens stimulate glandular tissue and may make diagnosis of breast masses more difficult. Periodic Papanicolaou smears should be obtained, and patients should undergo endometrial biopsy for any breakthrough bleeding and perhaps at intervals of 1 to 2 years while receiving estrogen replacement therapy. Some clinicians believe endometrial biopsies are not needed so long as there is no abnormal bleeding and withdrawal bleeding does not begin until at least 11 days after beginning progestin.

Side effects of therapy are common and may require modifications of therapy. Breast tenderness occurs frequently if too much estrogen is given. The dose of progestin should be reduced in the woman who complains of depression and/or bloating.

Medroxyprogesterone acetate (20 to 40 mg) or megestrol acetate (40 to 80 mg) orally each day may be utilized to treat hot flushes in women who cannot or will not take estrogens. Clonidine skin patches programmed to deliver 0.1 mg per day may also reduce the intensity and frequency of hot flushes in individuals who cannot take estrogens. Postural hypotension, however, is a common side effect with this therapy. Vaginal lubricants may be used for symptomatic treatment of dyspareunia in such individuals.

EFFECTS OF ESTROGEN ON LIPIDS AND CARCINOMA.
Unlike with the use of oral contraceptives in younger women, estrogen replacement in postmenopausal women does not raise blood pressure. This may be true because some estrogens, particularly the synthetic ones used in oral contraceptives, increase hepatic synthesis of renin substrate (angiotensinogen). In standard doses, the naturally occurring estrogens E_2 and E_1 do not increase renin substrate.

Estrogen administration tends to lower total cholesterol levels, with the degree of reduction varying with the dose and potency of the estrogen. Furthermore, estrogen decreases the LDL-cholesterol and increases the HDL-cholesterol fraction. Thus the net effect of estrogen administration is to shift the HDL-LDL ratio to one associated with a decreased risk of cardiovascular disease. Overall, the risk of cardiovascular disease appears reduced by half in postmenopausal users of estrogen, but this reduced risk has not yet been confirmed by prospective studies. Estrogen administration to postmenopausal women may increase plasma triglycerides slightly, but these increases are generally of no significance except in some individuals with genetic disorders of triglyceride metabolism in whom marked elevations may occur.

Progestins, especially those derived from 19-nor-testosterone (such as norethindrone and norgestrel), oppose the effects of estrogens on plasma lipid and lipoprotein fractions. Even orally administered medroxyprogesterone, which is relatively neutral when given alone, appears to reduce the favorable changes induced by estrogens when given in combination with estrogen.

Estrogens exert their cardiovascular effects in many ways. They appear to retard the oxidation of LDL and thereby may decrease the atherogenicity of LDL. Estrogens also suppress the uptake of LDL by blood vessel walls, inhibiting the development of endothelial atheroma. Estrogens cause vasodilation of coronary vessels. These vasodilatory effects may be mediated by estrogen-induced alterations in prostaglandin metabolism and by increasing the levels of prostacyclin (a vasodilator) and decreasing the levels of thromboxane (a vasoconstrictor). Estrogen receptors exist in the endothelial cells of the vascular system, and binding to these receptors may stimulate the release of nitric oxide, a potent endogenous vasodilator. A positive inotropic effect of estrogen on cardiac function also has been observed.

Estrogen-containing oral contraceptive preparations have not been linked conclusively to increased risks of endometrial or breast cancer. However, as noted, estrogen given alone to postmenopausal women greatly increases the risk of endometrial cancer over that in women never given estrogen. The risk of endometrial carcinoma is reduced markedly, if not abolished, by the cyclic addition of a progestin. Whether estrogen therapy increases the risk of breast cancer is not clear. If so, the effect is approximately 25% with prolonged use of estrogen. Because the likelihood of death from cardiovascular disease is far greater than that from breast cancer, it appears that the benefits of estrogen replacement therapy outweigh the risks in most postmenopausal women.

Lobo R (ed.): Treatment of the Postmenopausal Woman. Basic and Clinical Aspects. New York, Raven Press, 1993. *A review by leading authorities on the physiologic changes and therapeutic approaches to the menopause.*

OVARIAN TUMORS

Ovarian tumors may cause ovarian dysfunction, either by secreting hormones or by stimulating adjacent non-neoplastic stromal cells. Only perhaps 5% of ovarian tumors, however, show functional activity. Most nonfunctional tumors are asymptomatic until late in their evolution; more than three fourths are diagnosed only in advanced stages. In contrast, women with functioning neoplasms commonly present with altered sexual development or reproductive abnormalities, and thus diagnosis is made much earlier. Ovarian tumors may occur in all age groups but are less common in younger women, especially before puberty.

Ovarian tumors generally are classified as (1) common epithelial tumors derived from coelomic epithelial cells; (2) sex cord stromal tumors composed of granulosa cells, theca cells, Sertoli-Leydig cells, or their progenitors; (3) lipid or lipoid cell tumors; (4) germ cell tumors, including teratomas, dysgerminomas, and choriocarcinomas; (5) gonadoblastomas; (6) soft tissue tumors not specific to the ovary; and (7) secondary metastatic tumors. Each of these major classes of tumors includes several different histologic types. Sex cord stromal tumors are most apt to be functioning.

Ovarian neoplasms must be distinguished from tumor-like conditions of the ovary, which include luteomas of pregnancy (nodular theca-lutein hyperplasia) that may result in virilization of the mother but regress spontaneously post partum; hyperplasia of ovarian stroma (hyperthecosis), frequently associated with severe hirsutism; functional follicle and corpus luteum cysts; germinal inclusion cysts lined by surface epithelium; simple cysts; paraovarian

TABLE 208–9. CLINICAL FEATURES OF HORMONE-PRODUCING OVARIAN TUMORS

Tumor	Hormones Produced*	Age in Years Peak	Age in Years Range	Malignancy	Bilaterality	Size Range in cm (per cent Palpable)	Miscellaneous
Androblastoma (arrhenoblastoma)	*Androgens,* estrogens	20–40	4–69	20%	Rare	<5->25 (85)	Most common virilizing ovarian neoplasm
Dysgerminoma	Androgens, *chorionic gonadotropin*	10–30	6–76	100%	15%	3–50 (60)	May be "mixed" with other tumors originating from germ cells
Gonadoblastoma	*Androgens,* estrogens	10–30	6–38	50%	40%	<1->30 (?)	Usually occur in genetic males with female external genitalia
Granulosa-theca cell	*Estrogens,* androgens, progestogens	30–70	<1–92	5–20%	10–15%	<1->30 (80–90)	Most common functioning ovarian neoplasm
Hilar cell	*Androgens,* estrogens	45–75	4–86	Rare	Rare	1–9 (50)	Hypertension in 50%, diabetes in 50%
Lipoid cell (adrenal-like)	*Androgens,* estrogens	20–50	6–78	20%	Rare	0.5–30	Diabetes associated with lesion in 50%
Teratomas, benign	Serotonin, thyroxine	10–40	<1–78	Rare	10%	2–45 (90)	Carcinoid syndrome only in patients with large carcinoid tumors
Teratomas, malignant	Chorionic gonadotropin	6–15	6–42	100%	Rare	>5 (100)	Not all secrete chorionic gonadotropin

Modified from data of Rose GI, Vande Wiele RL: *In* Williams RH (ed.): Textbook of Endocrinology, 5th ed. Philadelphia, WB Saunders, 1974, p 368.
* When more than one hormone is secreted, the major one is *italicized.*

cysts; inflammatory lesions; and endometrial cysts or endometriomas.

Ovarian neoplasms are diagnosed most commonly at the time of routine pelvic examination. Even most functioning neoplasms are palpable; those that are not may be identified by ultrasonography. As an ovarian tumor grows, it distends the abdomen, leading to pressure on the bladder or rectum and a sensation of pelvic fullness and discomfort. Ascites may develop if the neoplasm is malignant or sometimes when it is not (Meigs' syndrome). Abdominal and pelvic pain may occur with torsion, hemorrhage, or rupture of the tumor.

Functioning ovarian tumors can produce other clinical manifestations as well (Table 208–9). Some tumors are associated with clinical manifestations of decreased hormone production. Intervals of amenorrhea caused by steroid suppression of gonadotropins may alternate with excessive vaginal bleeding produced by steroid stimulation of the endometrium during the reproductive years. In some young girls, steroid-secreting ovarian tumors may cause pseudopubertal development. In postmenopausal women, increased estrogens, secreted by the tumor itself or from peripheral aromatization of androgens secreted by the tumor, may stimulate the endometrium and result in bleeding.

Any pelvic mass identified on examination must be investigated. What constitutes such a "mass" and what evaluation is indicated depend on the age of the individual. Adnexal masses < 5 cm in diameter may well be due to normal follicular development in women of reproductive age and may resolve with observation over 2 to 8 weeks. Even simple cystic masses > 5 cm in diameter, as documented by ultrasound examination, may resolve over a few weeks. Those that do not resolve require surgical removal. Any palpable, complex adnexal mass in a postmenopausal woman, in whom the ovaries normally atrophy and cannot be detected during examination, should be removed. Ultrasonography also may identify small simple cysts in postmenopausal women. Most regress spontaneously.

Yeh I-T, Zaloudek C, Kurman RJ: Functioning tumors and tumor-like conditions of the ovary. In Becker KL (ed.): Principles and Practice of Endocrinology and Metabolism. Philadelphia, JB Lippincott, 1990, p 848. An excellent discussion of the clinical manifestations of ovarian tumors for any physician who undertakes the medical care of women.

208.2 Ovarian Carcinoma
Howard W. Jones, III

Ovarian carcinoma is the most deadly of the gynecologic malignancies. The age-specific incidence gradually rises, reaching a peak at about age 70, at which time it is 55 per 100,000 among white women. The rate is somewhat lower among black women. The cause of ovarian cancer is unknown; except for some relatively rare familial groups, it has not been possible to identify any clinically useful high-risk groups for increased surveillance. The lifetime risk of ovarian cancer for women in the United States is about 1.4%, but women with one first-degree relative appear to have an increased risk of 3 to 5%. Rare familial groups with a high incidence of ovarian, breast, and colon cancer have been described. Multiple pregnancies and the use of oral contraceptives may be protective because of decreased ovulation and hormonal influences.

PATHOLOGY

Four types of ovarian tumors require separate consideration because of their clinical characteristics and prognoses: (1) The common epithelial tumors of the ovary include the serous, mucinous, endometrioid, clear cell, and otherwise unspecified adenocarcinomas. These tumors account for almost 90% of ovarian cancers and are most commonly found in postmenopausal women. (2) Germ cell tumors, which arise from the totipotent oocytes, are usually benign ("dermoid cysts"). They often occur in young women and are almost always unilateral. When malignant (e.g., dysgerminoma, teratoma), they are highly aggressive but respond very well to combination chemotherapy. (3) Stromal tumors are generally low grade, and because they arise from the granulosa, theca, and Sertoli-Leydig cells of the ovary, they may be hormonally functional. They are usually unilateral and may occur in any age group, but most typically in the fourth and fifth decades. Surgical excision alone may be all the therapy required, but combination chemotherapy is effective for metastatic or recurrent disease. (4) Malignancies of other sites that are metastatic to the ovary must always be considered in the evaluation of patients with a pelvic mass. In some cases a pelvic mass is the first indication of a primary gastrointestinal or endometrial carcinoma. Breast cancer also commonly metastasizes to the ovary.

DIAGNOSIS
Clinical Presentation

Early ovarian cancer is usually asymptomatic. Occasionally, ovarian enlargement is found on routine examination and cancer may be discovered incidentally at the time of abdominal or pelvic surgery for other indications. In most cases, however, widespread intra-abdominal metastases are present by the time the diagnosis is made. Symptoms of abdominal swelling, bloating, and pelvic fullness or pressure are common. It is not unusual for the patient to have had vague abdominal complaints or nonspecific gastrointestinal symptoms. Ascites or a palpable abdominopelvic mass may be found on examination. The presence of an irregular mass in the pelvis or cul-de-sac nodularity accompanied by ascites is often diagnostic. Some patients develop malignant pleural effusions and present with shortness of breath.

SCREENING TESTS. Screening tests for ovarian cancer are still controversial. Transvaginal ultrasonography, although quite effective for diagnosing ovarian cysts and tumors, is nonspecific and its use for screening results in surgical exploration of a large number of women with benign ovarian cysts. Even when a cancer is diagnosed by ultrasound screening in an asymptomatic patient, there is still no evidence that survival is improved. Serum levels of the tumor-associated antigen CA-125 above 35 U per milliliter are highly correlated with ovarian cancer in postmenopausal women. Unfortunately, many ovarian tumors do not cause elevated levels of CA-125, whereas endometriosis, pelvic inflammatory disease, and some benign ovarian tumors may do so. The relative rarity of ovarian cancer, combined with the nonspecific nature of currently available tests, makes ovarian cancer screening unsatisfactory.

DIFFERENTIAL DIAGNOSIS. A pelvic mass can be caused by either a benign or a malignant tumor of the ovary as well as by inflammatory conditions, physiologic cysts, and malignancies of other pelvic organs and structures. Initially, a careful history and physical examination are most helpful in suggesting possible primary sites. Pelvic ultrasonography may allow the dimensions and character of the mass to be determined. Smooth-walled, unilocular ovarian cysts are almost always benign, whereas malignancies are most commonly described as echogenically "complex," with both cystic and solid components. The possibility of ectopic pregnancy must always be considered, and a pregnancy test is therefore normally the first laboratory study done in women in the reproductive age group. A careful contraceptive history is important because functional ovarian cysts, including both follicle cysts and corpus luteum cysts, are common in ovulating women. Inflammatory masses and endometriosis can be confused with ovarian cancer and can cause an elevated CA-125 in addition to a complex adnexal mass. In the older age group, diverticular abscesses and carcinoma of the colon must be considered within the differential diagnosis.

Once a complete history and physical examination have been done and the size and character of the mass have been confirmed by ultrasonography, several additional studies may be helpful. A barium enema or colonoscopy is almost always indicated prior to surgery to rule out a primary lesion or secondary involvement of the colon. An abdominal and pelvic computerized tomography scan can identify evidence of upper abdominal metastases or ureteral obstruction.

Additional studies (e.g., brain scans, bone scans) should generally be reserved for patients whose symptoms or physical findings suggest involvement of the areas to be studied.

TREATMENT
Surgery

In almost all cases of suspected ovarian carcinoma, an exploratory laparotomy is the ultimate diagnostic procedure. If the diagnosis is sustained, tumor debulking, including total abdominal hysterectomy and bilateral salpingo-oophorectomy, if possible, should be done. At this point a definitive diagnosis can be made and the extent of the disease accurately staged (Table 208–10). Aggressive tumor debulking, even when all cancer cannot be removed, improves the length and quality of survival. If possible, this initial surgery should be done by a gynecologic oncologist whose special training and experience should provide the optimal surgical and postoperative management.

The goal of the initial operation for ovarian cancer is twofold. First, all tumor should be removed if possible to provide the greatest possibility of cure. In approximately two thirds of patients, however, widespread intra-abdominal metastases prevent complete surgical debulking. The second goal of surgery is accurate staging (Table 208–10). In addition to the stage of disease, the volume of residual tumor following initial surgery, the histologic type and grade of the tumor, and the age of the patient have important prognostic significance. Women with minimal residual disease and well-differentiated tumors have the most favorable outcome. Those under age 50 and those with tumors exhibiting mucinous and endometrioid histology also seem to do better.

Careful staging evaluation with peritoneal cytology and multiple biopsies of the upper abdomen (the omentum, diaphragm, and retroperitoneal nodes) is especially important in early-stage disease because microscopic metastases often escape clinical detection. Accurate staging guides the most appropriate postoperative management. Patients with Stage Ia well-differentiated epithelial ovarian cancers do not need additional therapy.

In patients with advanced disease, aggressive surgical debulking includes bowel resection or colostomy in as many as 25% of patients. Whether such extensive surgical resection actually improves 5- and 10-year survival rates is still controversial. It is agreed,

TABLE 208–10. DEFINITIONS OF THE STAGES IN PRIMARY CARCINOMA OF THE OVARY*

Stage I	Growth limited to the ovaries.
Stage Ia	Growth limited to one ovary; no ascites. No tumor on the external surface; capsule intact.
Stage Ib	Growth limited to both ovaries; no ascites. No tumor on the external surfaces; capsules intact.
Stage Ic	Tumor either Stage Ia or Ib, but with tumor on surface of one or both ovaries; or with capsule ruptured; or with ascites present containing malignant cells or with positive peritoneal washings.
Stage II	Growth involving one or both ovaries with pelvic extension.
Stage IIa	Extension and/or metastases to the uterus and/or tubes.
Stage IIb	Extension to other pelvic tissues.
Stage IIc	Tumor either Stage IIa or IIb, but with tumor on surface of one or both ovaries; or with capsule(s) ruptured; or with ascites present containing malignant cells or with positive peritoneal washings.
Stage III	Tumor involving one or both ovaries with peritoneal implants outside the pelvis and/or positive retroperitoneal or inguinal nodes. Superficial liver metastases equal Stage III. Tumor is limited to the true pelvis but with histologically proven malignant extension to small bowel or omentum.
Stage IIIa	Tumor grossly limited to the true pelvis with negative nodes but with histologically confirmed microscopic seeding of abdominal peritoneal surfaces.
Stage IIIb	Tumor involving one or both ovaries with histologically confirmed implants of abdominal peritoneal surfaces, none exceeding 2 cm in diameter. Nodes are negative.
Stage IIIc	Abdominal implants greater than 2 cm in diameter and/or positive retroperitoneal or inguinal nodes.
Stage IV	Growth involving one or both ovaries with distant metastases. If pleural effusion is present, there must be positive cytology to allot a case to Stage IV. Parenchymal liver metastases equals Stage IV.

* Nomenclature of the International Federation of Gynecology and Obstetrics (FIGO). Staging is based on findings at clinical examination and surgical exploration.

however, that optimal tumor debulking (< 1 cm residual) results in prolongation of good-quality survival. This is where the skills and experienced judgment of the gynecologic oncologist are most important.

Chemotherapy

Most patients with ovarian cancer require postoperative chemotherapy. Cisplatin or carboplatin, which has fewer renal and neurologic side effects, is the cornerstone of most regimens. They are usually given in combination with other agents, such as cyclophosphamide, doxorubicin, hexamethylmelamine, or etoposide. Taxol has also been shown to be effective and is being used as second line and sometimes as primary therapy. Most patients are treated with intermittent intravenous therapy at 4-week intervals for six monthly cycles, but some centers use intraperitoneal chemotherapy instead. Response rates of 60 to 80% are generally seen, but only about 30% of the treatment group experiences a complete response. Some debilitated patients are still treated with a single alkylating agent, such as oral melphalan, but this therapy is probably not as effective as cisplatin alone or in combination with other cytotoxic drugs. Carboplatin is almost as well tolerated as oral melphalan.

Radiation Therapy

Postoperative external radiation therapy to the whole abdomen is probably as effective as chemotherapy for patients with minimal residual tumor. The toxicity of such therapy, especially that of gastrointestinal obstruction, has usually been greater than that associated with chemotherapy.

Intraperitoneal radioactive colloidal chronic phosphate is also used to treat some women with Stage I or II disease with no gross residual tumor. Only patients with very early disease are good candidates for this therapy, which requires a complete and uniform intraperitoneal distribution of the radioactive suspension.

"Second-look" Surgery

A planned re-exploration in order to evaluate the extent of disease following a course of therapy and to resect any residual malignancy has been called "second-look" surgery. This approach allows an excellent research evaluation of the effect of the primary therapy, but it has not proven to be of significant clinical benefit to patients with ovarian cancer. Measurements of tumor-associated antigens, such as CA-125, used in conjunction with periodic physical examinations and selected radiographic studies, have been helpful in monitoring the disease status of treated patients. Until more effective salvage therapy is available, second-look surgery in the asymptomatic patient with a normal physical examination is probably not indicated.

Treatment of Recurrent, Metastatic Disease

The overall survival of patients treated for ovarian cancer is only 30 to 40%; many women develop progressive disease despite appropriate primary therapy. Salvage chemotherapy protocols for recurrent disease lead to only a 10% response rate, which is usually partial and short term. Widespread intra-abdominal metastases with bowel obstruction are frequent, but reoperation with resection, bypass, or enterostomy may provide significant palliation. Pleural effusion may require thoracentesis and pleural sclerosis. With the relative effectiveness of current primary chemotherapy, patients may survive to develop late metastases to the liver, brain, and meninges. Localized radiation has been helpful in some of these patients.

PROGNOSIS

The long-term survival rate of patients treated for epithelial ovarian cancer is still disappointing (Table 208–11). Almost 60% of patients have Stage III or IV disease at the time of diagnosis. Although the majority of women with advanced disease live 2 years with a reasonable quality of life, recurrent cancer eventually becomes symptomatic in most, and by 5 years only about 15% still survive. The results are much better for patients diagnosed at an earlier stage. Almost three fourths of women with Stage I ovarian cancer survive 5 years.

TABLE 208–11. CARCINOMA OF THE OVARY: DISTRIBUTION BY STAGE AND 3- AND 5-YEAR SURVIVAL IN THE DIFFERENT STAGES*

Stage	Patients Treated		3-Year Survival (%)	5-Year Survival (%)
	Number	(%)		
I	2230	26.1	79.8	72.8
II	1313	15.4	60.5	46.3
III	3339	39.1	27.1	18.6
IV	1391	16.3	10.1	4.8
Unstaged	268	3.1	31.7	21.6
TOTAL	8541	100.0	43.4	34.9

* Data from Carcinoma of the ovary. *In* Pettersson F (ed.): Annual Report on the Results of Treatment in Gynecological Cancer, Vol. 22. Stockholm, Panorama Press AB, 1994. The "Annual Report" is published at regular intervals by the International Federation for Gynecology and Obstetrics and contains vast quantities of statistics generated from institutions which submit their treatment results from throughout the world.

Baker VV: Molecular biology and genetics of epithelial ovarian cancer. Obstet Gynecol Clin North Am 21:25, 1994. *A good update on the rapidly expanding knowledge of the molecular genetics of ovarian cancer.*

Herbst AL: The epidemiology of ovarian carcinoma and the current status of tumor markers to detect disease. Am J Obstet Gynecol 170:1099, 1994. *An excellent review of epidemiology and screening for ovarian cancer. Part of a mini-symposium.*

Hoskins WJ: Surgical staging and cytoreductive surgery of epithelial ovarian cancer. Cancer 71:1534, 1993. *This paper discusses the importance and controversies related to staging and aggressive debulking of ovarian cancer.*

Ozols RF: Treatment of ovarian cancer: Current status. Semin Oncol 21:1, 1994. *A complete review on the therapy of ovarian cancer.*

Soper JT: Management of early-stage epithelial ovarian cancer. Clin Obstet Gynecol 37:423, 1994. *The indications for chemotherapy and radiation and the results that can be expected are reviewed.*

Thigpen JT, Bertelsen K, Eisenhauer EA, et al.: Long-term follow-up of patients with advanced ovarian carcinoma treated with chemotherapy. Ann Oncol 4(54):35, 1993. *The authors report 5- to 10-year follow-up in a series of patients treated with platin-based combination chemotherapy.*

208.3 Hirsutism
Roger S. Rittmaster

DEFINITION. Normal Hair Growth. Most body hair can be classified as vellus or terminal. Vellus hairs are fine and unpigmented, such as those that cover the face of children. Terminal hairs, pigmented and coarser, may be sex hormone–dependent (such as those over the chin and abdomen of men) or sex hormone–independent (such as eyebrows and eyelashes) (Fig. 208–9). Androgens convert vellus hair to terminal hair in sex hormone–dependent areas.

Hirsutism. Hirsutism is the presence of excess hair in women. This is usually an androgen-dependent process. Twenty-five to 35% of young women have terminal hair over the lower abdomen, around the nipples, or over the upper lip. Most women gradually develop more androgen-dependent body hair with age. Nevertheless, "normal" patterns of female hair growth are unacceptable to many women. At the other extreme, severe hirsutism may rarely be the earliest sign of masculinizing diseases. More often, however, severe hirsutism reflects only increased androgen production in women with no serious underlying disorder.

ETIOLOGY. Hirsutism may be divided into androgen-dependent and androgen-independent causes. Androgen-dependent hirsutism is restricted to areas where men typically become hirsute and often begins with adolescence. In women, androgens arise from the ovaries, the adrenal glands, or exogenous sources such as anabolic steroids (Table 208–12). Often, no definite abnormality exists; the hirsutism simply results from modestly increased androgen production and/or increased skin sensitivity to androgens.

Androgen-independent hirsutism is caused by drugs (cyclosporine, glucocorticoids, minoxidil, diazoxide, and possibly phenytoin) or starvation (anorexia nervosa); it may be associated with the skin lesions of porphyria; or it may be an inherited condition. Androgen-independent hirsutism is characterized by long, fine hairs occurring over much of the body, including such areas as the forehead and flanks. Androgens may exacerbate androgen-independent hirsutism, giving rise to a clinically confusing presentation. The pathophysiology of androgen-independent hirsutism is unknown.

PATHOPHYSIOLOGY OF ANDROGEN-DEPENDENT HIRSUTISM. To be active in skin, testosterone, the major circulating androgen, must first be converted to dihydrotestosterone by the enzyme 5α-reductase. Hirsute women have elevated skin 5α-reductase compared with nonhirsute women. Nevertheless, increased 5α-reductase alone is usually insufficient to induce hirsutism.

Hirsute women as a group also have increased androgen production from the adrenal glands, the ovaries, or both. Either testosterone itself is secreted, or androgen precursors such as androstenedione are secreted, which are then converted in the liver or skin to active androgens. Most hirsute women do not have an underlying disease, but simply fall at one end of the spectrum of androgen production and skin 5α-reductase activity.

The ovarian and adrenal causes of hirsutism listed in Table 208–12 lead to increased androgen production. Virilizing tumors secrete androgens directly. The pituitary adenomas in Cushing's disease release ACTH, which stimulates the adrenals to secrete both cortisol and androgens (see Ch. 204.1). The virilizing forms of congenital adrenal hyperplasia involve enzyme defects that impair cortisol synthesis, leading to increased ACTH secretion (see Ch. 204.1). The enzyme block causes shunting of cortisol precursors to androgens. The most common form, 21-hydroxylase deficiency, leads to an overproduction of 17-hydroxyprogesterone. Whereas severe forms of 21-hydroxylase deficiency cause ambiguous genitalia in female infants, milder forms may lead only to hirsutism and/or irregular menses. This "attenuated" form of 21-hydroxylase deficiency is present in about 1% of hirsute women.

In the polycystic ovarian syndrome, both the ovaries and adrenals secrete excess androgens, although the majority of the androgens are usually of ovarian origin (see Ch. 208.1).

CLINICAL MANIFESTATIONS. Androgen-induced hirsutism of benign origin usually begins in adolescence and becomes gradually worse with time. Family history is often positive. The hirsutism may vary from mild to severe. Usually hair growth begins over the lower abdomen, on the breasts, and over the upper lip. Widespread hirsutism over the upper back, upper abdomen, and upper chest implies severe hyperandrogenism. Some women may have only facial hair or other unusual patterns of hirsutism, probably due to local variation in skin 5α-reductase activity.

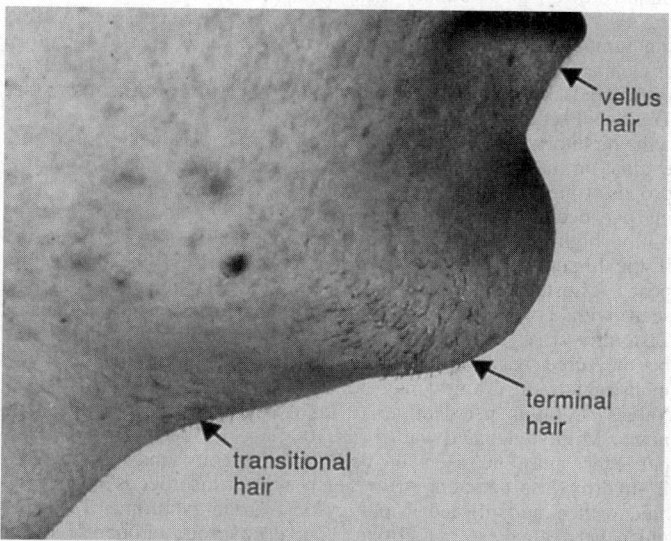

FIGURE 208–9. Facial hair growth in a hirsute woman. Vellus hair is fine, unpigmented hair. Terminal hair is coarse and pigmented. Transitional hair is intermediate between vellus and terminal. This woman also has mild acne, another androgen-dependent process. (Reprinted with permission from Rittmaster RS: Hirsutism. Med Clin North Am 14:2686, 1987.)

TABLE 208-12. CAUSES OF ANDROGEN-DEPENDENT HIRSUTISM

Ovarian causes
  Severe insulin resistance
  Virilizing ovarian tumors
Adrenal causes
  Congenital adrenal hyperplasia
    21-Hydroxylase deficiency
    3β-Hydroxysteroid dehydrogenase deficiency
    11-Hydroxylase deficiency
  Cushing's disease
  Ectopic ACTH-producing tumors
  Virilizing adrenal tumors
Combined ovarian and adrenal causes
  Polycystic ovary syndrome
  "Idiopathic" hirsutism
Exogenous androgens
  "Anabolic" steroids
  Danazol
  Postmenopausal hormone replacement formulations containing androgens

Severe, rapidly progressive hirsutism, beginning in childhood or beyond adolescence, suggests an androgen-secreting tumor. Such tumors can cause signs of virilization: deepening of the voice, excess muscle development, and marked clitoral enlargement. Signs of virilization, however, simply imply severe hyperandrogenism and can occasionally be seen with all causes of hirsutism. Androgen-secreting tumors are rare, and most severely hirsute women have either polycystic ovarian syndrome or hirsutism alone.

Attenuated congenital adrenal hyperplasia is clinically indistinguishable from simple hirsutism or polycystic ovarian syndrome, and the diagnosis must be made biochemically. Cushing's disease may be suspected when the patient presents with central obesity, hypertension, diabetes, and/or thinning of the skin (see Ch. 204.1).

DIAGNOSIS. The diagnostic evaluation of hirsutism is directed at ruling out a significant underlying cause. Important historical points include a drug history (including use of oral contraceptives), age of onset and rate of progression of hirsutism, presence of thinning of scalp hair or deepening of the voice, menstrual history, history of obesity, and family history of hirsutism. The physical examination should include an assessment of the quality and distribution of hair growth, signs of virilization or Cushing's syndrome, and presence of abdominal or pelvic masses.

Laboratory Evaluation. In women with androgen-dependent hirsutism, regular ovulatory menses, and no physical signs of Cushing's syndrome, hormonal evaluation is usually unnecessary. Virilizing tumors have not been reported in such patients, and hirsutism associated with attenuated congenital adrenal hyperplasia need not be treated differently from other benign forms of hirsutism (see Treatment section).

In hirsute women with irregular menses, a reasonable laboratory evaluation includes measurement of serum testosterone, 17-hydroxyprogesterone, prolactin, LH, and FSH. A testosterone level < 170 ng per deciliter (6 nmol per liter) makes an androgen-secreting tumor highly unlikely, although re-evaluation may be necessary if the hirsutism continues to progress or signs of virilization appear. Testosterone levels above 170 ng per deciliter may also be seen with polycystic ovarian syndrome. To rule out attenuated 21-hydroxylase deficiency, serum 17-hydroxyprogesterone should be measured between 7 and 9 A.M. during the first week of the menstrual cycle (values may be elevated during the luteal phase). Values < 200 ng per deciliter (6 nmol per liter) rule out this diagnosis. Mildly elevated values (< 1000 ng per deciliter) (30 nmol per liter) may be seen in both heterozygous and homozygous 21-hydroxylase deficiency (the heterozygous disorder is not associated with hirsutism) and in polycystic ovarian syndrome. To distinguish between these conditions, 17-hydroxyprogesterone should be measured 30 to 60 minutes after the intravenous administration of 250 μg synthetic ACTH. Levels are > 1500 ng per deciliter (45 nmol per liter) in homozygous 21-hydroxylase deficiency. Other forms of attenuated congenital adrenal hyperplasia are too rare to justify routine hormonal screening. Serum prolactin, LH, and FSH are used to evaluate the possibility that a prolactinoma, ovarian failure, or polycystic ovarian syndrome is contributing to the irregular menses. These tests are not directly relevant to the evaluation of hirsutism itself. Measurement of dehydroepiandrosterone sulfate (DHEAS) as an index of adrenal androgen production is generally unhelpful.

TREATMENT. Hirsutism is a cosmetic problem that may have severe psychosocial consequences. Because it is not a disease in itself, the benefits and risks of any therapy should be carefully weighed and the treatment individualized.

Mechanical Hair Removal. For mild hirsutism, bleaching and mechanical hair removal are adequate and safe. Shaving is the easiest method of temporarily removing visible hair. Although shaving does not increase hair growth rates, it may leave a stubble and is unacceptable to many women. Plucking and waxing may control mild hirsutism, but they also do not resolve the problem and may lead to scarring. Electrolysis can provide a safe, effective alternative for localized mild to moderate hirsutism and is a useful adjunct to medical therapy in more severe cases. Electrolysis is expensive, however, and long-term treatment may be necessary.

Drug Treatment. Successful medical therapy results in a gradual return of terminal hair to finer, less pigmented vellus hair. Younger women with mild hirsutism of brief duration respond best to medical therapy. More severe hair growth can be prevented, and resolution of the hirsutism is possible. Nevertheless, drug treatment is not a cure, and lifelong therapy may be necessary to prevent recurrence. Generally, 6 months is needed to judge the efficacy of a given therapy, although improvement may continue indefinitely. No drug is approved by the Food and Drug Administration for treatment of hirsutism.

Antiandrogens. Antiandrogens (spironolactone, cyproterone acetate, flutamide) block the androgen receptor and are the drug treatment of choice for hirsutism. They are effective in reducing hair growth in at least 70% of women, and hirsutism stabilizes in the remaining ones. Spironolactone is usually given in a starting dose of 50 mg twice daily. The most common side effect is increased frequency of menses, which can be controlled by combining spironolactone with an oral contraceptive. Spironolactone should not be given to women with renal insufficiency. Cyproterone acetate, a potent antiandrogen and progestin, is often given as 25 to 50 mg daily for the first 10 days of a birth control pill cycle. Although widely used in Europe and Canada, it is not available in the United States. Flutamide is given as 125 to 250 mg twice daily. Both flutamide and cyproterone acetate can cause a drug-induced hepatitis, and all antiandrogens should be avoided in pregnant women. Flutamide is more expensive than other antiandrogens.

5α-Reductase Inhibitors. This is a new class of drugs that blocks the formation of dihydrotestosterone. Finasteride, the only such inhibitor available at the time of publication, is approved for treatment of benign prostatic hyperplasia. Early studies suggest that it effectively treats hirsutism, but more experience is needed. It would be expected to cause ambiguous genitalia in the male offspring of women taking the drug during pregnancy.

Ovarian Suppression. Although oral contraceptives are often used to control menstrual cycles in women given antiandrogens, they are usually ineffective for treating hirsutism when used alone (although they may prevent the hirsutism from becoming worse). Birth control pills differ in the androgenicity of the progestational component, but this difference has never been shown to have clinical significance in the treatment of hirsutism. Gonadotropin-releasing hormone analogues suppress the ovary by suppressing LH and FSH secretion. They are effective in treating hirsutism associated with polycystic ovarian syndrome but are expensive and lead to menopausal symptoms unless estrogens are given concurrently.

Glucocorticoids. Glucocorticoids suppress adrenal cortisol and androgen secretion. They are frequently ineffective in low doses, and higher doses can cause Cushing's syndrome. They also can cause a drug-induced hirsutism in some women and cannot be recommended as a routine treatment. Although glucocorticoids have traditionally been used to treat congenital adrenal hyperplasia, antiandrogens are more effective in treating the hirsutism associated with this disorder.

PROGNOSIS. Untreated, hirsutism usually becomes gradually worse with time, and most therapies need to be continued indefinitely. However, worsening hirsutism is easily prevented with antiandrogen therapy, and most women experience a satisfactory improvement with the judicious use of mechanical and medical therapies.

Dunaif A, Givens J, Merriam G, Haseltine F (eds.): Polycystic Ovary Syndrome (Current Issues in Endocrinology and Metabolism). Cambridge, MA, Blackwell Scientific Publications, 1992. *A collection of excellent reviews on polycystic ovary syndrome.*

Jeffcoate W: The treatment of women with hirsutism. Clin Endocrinol 39:143, 1993. *A somewhat different approach (from mine) to the evaluation and treatment of hirsutism.*

Rittmaster RS: Hyperandrogenism. *In* Copeland LJ (ed.): Textbook of Gynecology. Philadelphia, WB Saunders, 1993, p 414. *A detailed review of the pathophysiology, evaluation, and treatment of hyperandrogenism.*

Rittmaster RS: Treating hirsutism. Endocrinologist 3:211, 1993. *An overview of recent advances in the evaluation and treatment of hirsutism.*

208.4 Nonmalignant Diseases of the Breast

Douglas J. Marchant

Approximately one in every four women in the United States requires medical attention for breast symptomatology. More than half of all women have some degree of fibrocystic changes during their lifetime, and most have histologic changes that could be described as "fibrocystic disease." It is recommended, however, that the term *fibrocystic disease* be abandoned and the term *fibrocystic change* or *condition* be substituted because it is more descriptive of the clinical entity.

The physician should be knowledgeable about these common benign conditions and provide treatment or referral when indicated. This chapter discusses growth and development of the breasts, puberty, pregnancy and lactation, and the common benign conditions for which consultation is requested. Diagnostic studies, including examination of the breast, aspiration, and indications for surgical biopsy and referral, are emphasized. Gynecomastia, the main nonmalignant abnormality of the male breast, is described in Ch. 209.1.

GROWTH AND DEVELOPMENT OF THE BREAST

The functional units of the breast are of ectodermal origin. The epithelial ridge that eventually forms the breast tissue, recognizable by the thirty-fifth day of embryonic life, undergoes a series of alterations to form the lactiferous ducts and alveolae. At 15 weeks, mesenchymal cells differentiate into the smooth muscle of the nipple and the areola. The breast unit is complete at birth, as demonstrated by the occasional appearance of "witch's milk" caused by high levels of maternal hormones. During the third trimester of pregnancy, placental hormones in the fetal circulation stimulate further development of the functional units. This colostral secretion declines within 3 to 4 weeks, the breast tissue involutes, and no additional differentiation occurs until puberty.

Development of the mature breast begins with the onset of puberty and continues for several years. Estrogen levels increase, and the areolae become enlarged and pigmented. Adipose tissue is deposited to form and shape the breast and to provide a steroidogenic milieu for the conversion of hormones directly in the breast. In addition to estrogen and progesterone, insulin, cortisol, thyroxin, growth hormone, and prolactin are required for complete functional development.

The mature breast consists of the functional units—the alveolae, lactiferous ducts, and their supporting tissues. The alveolae are inconspicuous in the nonpregnant, nonlactating breast. The much larger ducts lie embedded in a stromal network consisting of fibrous tissue, fat, blood vessels, and lymphatics.

ABNORMALITIES OF GROWTH AND DEVELOPMENT

A number of congenital anomalies may be referred to the clinician for evaluation and treatment. The most frequently observed is the accessory nipple, or polythelia. This tissue, which may be mistaken for a pigmented nevus, lies along the milk line extending from the axilla to the groin. Rarely, functioning breast tissue is found along this milk line. Most commonly this ectopic breast tissue is located in the axilla, where it may enlarge and become quite painful during pregnancy and lactation.

Patients may be referred for failure of breast development, premature development, and breast hypertrophy. Normal sexual development and puberty are discussed in Ch. 208.1. Complete absence of the breast is rare and usually is associated with defects in the chest wall and muscles. Premature development is usually associated with the appearance of a mass beneath the nipple-areola complex. Other manifestations of sexual maturation are absent and hormonal studies are normal. A vaginal smear reveals little or no estrogen effect, consistent with the prepubertal state. No treatment is required; in particular to be avoided is surgical removal of the mass in the mistaken belief that it represents a tumor. If this area is removed, breast tissue will not develop on the affected side. Asymmetric breast development is common and requires no further treatment. Breast hypertrophy, on the other hand, is often uncomfortable and disturbing both to the patient and to the parents. These patients require considerable counseling because if reduction mammoplasty is recommended too early, a repeat operation will be necessary. A reduction mammoplasty, if required, should be performed only after completion of breast development, which may take several years.

THE BREAST DURING PREGNANCY AND THE PUERPERIUM

With the completion of breast development during and following puberty, the breasts are quiescent until pregnancy. During pregnancy the breast grows and develops due to lobular alveolar growth, the formation of secretory cells, and changes in the supporting tissues. Insulin responsiveness also is acquired during pregnancy. Further growth requires estrogen, progesterone, prolactin, and human placental lactogen. During pregnancy, serum prolactin increases from a nonpregnant level of approximately 10 ng to 200 ng per milliliter or more at term. Human placental lactogen reaches serum concentrations of approximately 6000 ng per milliliter at term. Lactation is suppressed by estrogen and progesterone, which inhibit prolactin action at the receptor level. With the rapid drop in estrogen and progesterone levels following delivery, this inhibition is removed and milk production begins. A decrease in the prolactin-inhibiting factor (PIF) by suckling increases prolactin and further promotes lactation. In the final event oxytocin is released and acts on the myoepithelial cells to contract the duct system for the delivery of the milk. By the end of the third or fourth month, suckling is the only stimulus required for continued lactation. If breast-feeding does not occur, prolactin rapidly returns to nonpregnant levels.

Mastitis occasionally complicates lactation, usually following the first pregnancy. There is a localized area of inflammation and tenderness and slight elevation of temperature. Treatment includes continuation of breast-feeding and the use of appropriate antibiotics. Because the most common organism is *Staphylococcus aureus*, penicillin or one of its derivatives is the treatment of choice. If the patient does not respond and if the tenderness and fever persist, a breast abscess should be suspected, for which the treatment is adequate drainage under general anesthesia in an operating room setting. Antibiotics should be continued in full therapeutic doses for 7 to 10 days following adequate drainage. The breast rapidly returns to normal and the cosmetic result is excellent.

The discovery of a dominant mass during pregnancy or lactation requires careful consideration. Early in pregnancy, a dominant mass is easily distinguished from fibrocystic changes. Often the patient gives a history of a mass first discovered many years before and followed in the belief that it represented a benign fibroadenoma. With rare exception, the cause of all dominant masses discovered during pregnancy or the puerperium should be resolved. This requires an open biopsy using a local anesthesia. Biopsy can be safely performed during lactation. The patient is requested to empty the breast early on the day of the operation. The mass is removed with careful approximation of the breast tissues and a pressure dressing temporarily applied. This can be removed later in the day and often the patient can breast-feed on the operated side.

FIBROCYSTIC CHANGES

Fibrocystic changes, which represent an exaggerated physiologic response to a changing hormonal environment, include painful lumpy breasts (mastodynia, mastalgia), a dominant mass, and nipple discharge.

The peak incidence of fibrocystic changes occurs between the ages of 30 and 50. Breast tenderness often occurs premenstrually, which suggests that progesterone may play an important role in the development and symptomatology of these changes. In the resting breast there is minimal epithelial proliferation in the proliferative phase of the menstrual cycle and maximal proliferation in the secretory phase, a pattern quite different from that of the endometrium. Whether this dissimilarity between breast and endometrial epithelium reflects receptor content or some more indirect effect on proliferation is unclear. Estrogen is a mitogen for the endometrium but not for the breast, and the idea, derived largely from endometrial studies, that progestins are protective for the breast is difficult to sustain. The relative contributions of estrogen and progesterone to the origin of benign breast conditions require further investigation.

Most, if not all, women experience these fibrocystic changes, and to label this condition a "disease" is inappropriate. Physical examination usually reveals irregular thickening, particularly in the upper outer quadrants. The changes associated with this process and its symptomatology constitute one of the most difficult challenges in the office practice of the physician.

MASTODYNIA (MASTALGIA)

Breast pain is common; it may occur in as many as 50% of women. Usually the cause is unclear, and relief of symptoms often is proportional to the time that the physician spends with the patient. The discomfort generally is classified as (1) cyclic mastalgia or mastodynia occurring immediately prior to the menses; (2) fibrocystic changes, including duct ectasia and sclerosing adenosis; or (3) referred pain such as costochondritis.

Almost all women complain of occasional breast discomfort for the first few days preceding the onset of menses, and most do not seek medical attention. It is the discomfort occurring at other times during the menstrual cycle, or throughout the cycle, that brings the patient to the physician.

Perimenopausal patients not infrequently note breast discomfort. The cause is unknown. Postmenopausal patients should be carefully evaluated for referred pain. They often perceive the discomfort to be in the breast when in reality it is related to the pectoral muscles, the chest wall, or even the cardiovascular system. Trauma is not an infrequent cause of breast discomfort. The usual presentation is a tender erythematous or ecchymotic area. In some cases open biopsy must be performed to rule out carcinoma.

NIPPLE DISCHARGE

Nipple discharge may be physiologic or pathologic, provoked or spontaneous. In most cases the patient can be immediately reassured that cancer is unlikely because 10% or fewer of breast cancers present with nipple discharge. A careful and detailed history is essential. Is the discharge produced only at the time of breast self-examination when the nipple is squeezed? Does it occur only with sexual stimulation? What type of physical exercise does the patient do? Does she wear a sport brassiere? Does she take any medication? Has she ever been pregnant? What is the menstrual history? Most patients can describe the character of the discharge, although not necessarily in a reliable fashion. For example, many patients complain of bloody nipple discharge, but when the secretions are examined on a gauze or by cytology, the color is blackish green and no blood cells are found.

Three types of discharge deserve further comment: galactorrhea, serosanguinous or bloody discharge, and discharge from the postmenopausal breast.

GALACTORRHEA. Galactorrhea is the spontaneous secretion of a milky discharge not immediately associated with a pregnancy. Usually it is persistent and occasionally it is voluminous. Elevated prolactin levels may be associated with galactorrhea. Physiologic causes of hyperprolactinemia include breast stimulation, coitus, eating, exercise, pregnancy, sleep, and stress. Hyperprolactinemia may also be due to pathologic factors, including brain and pituitary disorders, encephalitis, and pituitary microadenomas or macroadenomas. In addition, a number of pharmacologic agents may produce hyperprolactinemia, as noted in Table 208–13.

Prolactin is secreted in a sleep-related circadian rhythm with maximal release between 3:00 A.M. and 5:00 A.M. Serum samples, therefore, should be obtained in a fasting state between 8:00 A.M. and 12:00 noon. Prolactin levels do not change during the menstrual cycle. A serum level of prolactin of >20 ng per milliliter

TABLE 208–13. CAUSES OF NONPUERPERAL GALACTORRHEA

I. **Central origin**
  A. Organic
    1. Suprahypophyseal lesions
      a. Hypothalamic disorders–infiltrative processes (histiocytosis, metastatic diseases); masses (craniopharyngioma, meningioma); infarction; embolism
      b. Pituitary stalk lesions–section; impingement by tumors (all types with suprasellar extension); vascular insult
    2. Hypophyseal tumors
      a. Prolactin secreting* (solitary; part of multiple endocrine adenomatosis syndrome mixed with GH, TSH, ACTH)
  B. Functional
    1. Drug related
      a. Psychotropic (butyrophenones, phenothiazines)*
      b. Antihypertensive (reserpine, α-methyldopa)
      c. Cannabinoids (morphine, heroin)
      d. Contraceptives
      e. Antigastroplegics (metoclopramide)*
    2. Unclassified (idiopathic, stress, empty sella syndrome)

II. **Peripheral origin**
  A. Due to pituitary prolactin
    1. Due to primary failure of target endocrine gland
      a. Hypothyroidism
      b. Addison's disease
    2. Due to excess estrogen formation from target endocrine glands
      a. Feminizing adrenal carcinoma
      b. Polycystic ovarian syndrome
    3. Due to decreased metabolic clearance of PRL
      a. Renal failure
      b. Liver failure
      c. Hypothyroidism
    4. Due to local breast conditions
      a. Mechanical stimulation or suckling
      b. Thoracic and/or breast trauma, burn
      c. Inflammation, i.e., mastitis, herpes zoster
  B. Due to ectopic prolactin production
    1. Renal neoplasia
    2. Bronchogenic neoplasia

* Most common causes of highest serum PRL levels.

may be abnormal and should be further evaluated. Other diagnostic studies include microscopic evaluation of the breast discharge, which may reveal refractile fat globules, confirming the diagnosis. A thorough history should be taken to rule out physiologic or pharmacologic causes, and the menstrual history should focus on amenorrhea, oligomenorrhea, infertility, or a short luteal phase.

Prolactinomas, or prolactin-secreting pituitary adenomas, are common causes for hyperprolactinemia in women. Prolactinomas may be microadenomas (<1 cm in diameter) or macroadenomas (>1 cm). The diagnosis usually is made by computed tomography (CT) scan using contrast media. Modern CT or magnetic resonance imaging has replaced older methods of diagnosing pituitary tumors, such as the cone view tomogram or plain skull film.

SEROUS OR BLOODY BREAST DISCHARGE. This type of nipple discharge must be investigated. Usually it is caused by a benign intraductal papilloma, but carcinoma occurs in 10 to 15% of these patients. Often it is difficult to demonstrate the exact quadrant of the breast from which the discharge appears at the nipple. A microscopic examination of the fluid may identify red blood cells, confirming the clinical impression and the need for open biopsy.

POSTMENOPAUSAL NIPPLE DISCHARGE. Any nipple discharge that occurs during the postmenopausal period must be viewed as suggestive of carcinoma of the breast. Careful examination of the breast may reveal a mass or other findings consistent with carcinoma, which must be followed up, as described in Ch. 208.5.

DETECTION AND DIAGNOSIS

HISTORY. The diagnostic evaluation begins with a careful history, noting the age of the patient, the date of the last menstrual period, family history of breast disease, use of medication, the date of birth of the first child, and any surgery related to previous breast disease. Inquiry should be made concerning the use of oral contraceptives, including the type of medication and for how long it has been taken. If the patient has received estrogen replacement therapy, the type of medication and the length of time that the medication has been used should be noted. Pelvic surgery, including oophorectomy and a history of pelvic malignancy, particularly ovarian carcinoma and endometrial carcinoma, should be recorded. Did the patient notice the symptom casually or by employing deliberate breast self-examination, or was it first noted by another health care provider? Does the patient wear a brassiere? What type of medication has the patient used to provide relief? Are there any emotional factors that should be considered? The history should be recorded with particular emphasis on the data of onset of the symptom, the exact location in the breast, and, finally, the disposition.

PHYSICAL EXAMINATION. For careful evaluation the breasts are first examined in the sitting or standing position. Contour, symmetry, and skin changes are noted. The vascular pattern is observed and the condition of the areola and nipple recorded. These changes may be exaggerated by asking the patient to elevate the arm or to place her hands on the hips, thus contracting the pectoralis major muscles and exaggerating any small change noted on routine observation. While the patient is in this position, the axilla is palpated, being careful to support the arm with the opposite hand. This relaxes the pectoralis muscle and permits careful evaluation of the axilla. While the patient is in the sitting or standing position, the supraclavicular area should be checked for a cervical rib or other unexpected finding. Examination of the neck may reveal thyroid enlargement.

Following these maneuvers, the patient is placed in the supine position. The breast is palpated in a systematic manner with the flat of the hand. The use of pHisoHex or talcum powder permits the identification of even minor alterations. Approximately 80% of American women discover their own lesions, often while taking a shower. The use of this so-called wet technique permits the identification of very subtle changes in breast texture. Following the careful evaluation of all quadrants, the areola and nipple should be carefully examined and the nipple gently squeezed. Any discharge is evaluated for location, consistency, and color.

The patient often presents with a chief complaint of a lump. This may or may not be confirmed by careful examination. The usual finding is a vague thickening, particularly in the upper outer quadrant.

The physician must carefully evaluate the chief complaint and then, on the basis of a thorough examination, decide whether the findings represent a dominant mass or an exaggeration of normal breast tissue associated with fibrocystic changes. In the obese patient with very large breasts, it is unlikely that any but the most obvious lesion will be discovered by routine examination. The large breast, therefore, is an indication for mammography to augment what in most cases is an inadequate physical examination.

Once a lesion has been characterized as a mass, a lump, or a dominant mass and has been measured or drawn, its cause must be established. There are no obviously benign lesions. The only exception is a mass in the teenager for whom elective treatment of an obvious fibroadenoma may be recommended.

CYST ASPIRATION

A mass may be cystic, solid, benign, or malignant. Attempts should be made to aspirate the mass with a fine (23 or 24) gauge needle. Local anesthesia is not required. The mass is immobilized with the fingers, the needle inserted, and the fluid withdrawn. If the fluid is clear or cloudy and no residual mass is palpated immediately following the aspiration, it is sufficient to arrange a follow-up examination in 1 month with reassurance and monthly self-examination of the breast. If the mass remains immediately following the aspiration, if the fluid is bloody, or if there is a residual mass on the first follow-up visit, open biopsy is mandatory. If the mass is solid, open biopsy is recommended except for a teenager, for whom excision biopsy can be performed on an elective basis.

Cytologic evaluation of nipple discharge or cyst fluid is seldom rewarding. On the other hand, it is probably advisable to examine spontaneous nipple discharge microscopically, particularly if it is unilateral and serosanguinous or bloody. A positive cytologic examination of cyst fluid in the absence of other indications for biopsy is exceedingly rare. Cytology is not, therefore, recommended as a routine examination.

FINE-NEEDLE ASPIRATION (FNA)

The accurate use of FNA requires an understanding of the techniques involved and a cytopathologist capable of interpreting the

smear. A standard disposable syringe can be used with a 23- to 25-gauge needle. Local anesthesia is helpful because several "passes" may be required to obtain an adequate sample of "tissue juice" for appropriate evaluation. The material should not enter the syringe and should be placed directly on the slide and fixed with an appropriate spray. The technique is most useful for the obvious dominant mass. FNA is useful only if positive; a negative finding is unreliable. Some radiologists prefer that a mammogram be performed prior to FNA because the procedure may distort the anatomy of the breast.

OTHER DIAGNOSTIC STUDIES

Ultrasonography is useful to confirm the presence or absence of macrocysts, particularly when these lesions are discovered by mammography and are nonpalpable. The procedure should not be performed on a routine basis because it is unsuitable for screening and is an extra expense to the patient. It is much simpler to immediately attempt aspiration with a fine-gauge needle. Thermography and diaphonography are experimental procedures and should not be employed, except with evaluative protocols.

Mammography may be used as a screening examination in the asymptomatic patient or to confirm the findings noted on physical examination. The accuracy of mammography depends upon a number of factors, including the size and density of the breast and the location of the lesion. False-negative results, which occur even in the best institutions, may reach 10% and in some centers approach 25%. The presence of a dominant mass and a negative mammogram clearly do not preclude the recommendation for referral and an open biopsy.

BREAST BIOPSY

Certain features of the breast biopsy are important when discussing such a recommendation with the patient. In the past, open biopsy was performed solely as a diagnostic procedure to determine the presence or absence of cancer. Currently, the biopsy often becomes part of conservative treatment, and therefore it must be executed by surgeons familiar with contemporary treatment for breast cancer (see Ch. 208.5). It is essential that the biopsy be performed in an operating room setting with trained personnel familiar with the biopsy technique and the use of local anesthesia.

MANAGEMENT OF BENIGN BREAST DISORDERS

The medical management of benign breast conditions often challenges even the most well-informed physician. For patients with mild fibrocystic changes and minimal symptomatology, reassurance only is indicated. Occasionally, a well-fitting brassiere, salt restriction, and a mild analgesic to control discomfort are all that is required.

For patients with greater discomfort, a detailed history is often the key to appropriate diagnosis and therapy. Mammography may be helpful in ruling out significant breast pathology and in reassuring the patient. Treatment strategy often depends upon the "complaint threshold of the patient and the safety threshold of the physician." In the absence of highly effective specific therapy, a number of treatment regimens have been proposed: the topical use of progestational agents, tamoxifen, bromocriptine, various vitamin formulations, and primrose oil. For most patients treatment is directed toward a reasonable and rational explanation rather than any specific medication.

Danazol is effective, but for most patients the cost and the side effects are prohibitive. Moderate doses of danazol decrease follicular maturation and increase anovulatory periods. Danazol has intrinsic androgenic activity and also decreases sex hormone–binding globulin, which increases free testosterone levels. Estradiol secretion is reduced because of the lack of follicular maturation. For some patients who have been incapacitated by breast discomfort and nodularity, a short course of danazol (400 to 600 mg daily for 6 months) may provide symptomatic relief and a marked change in the physical examination. The use of danazol should be restricted to those patients who have failed more conservative measures to control their symptomatology.

The treatment of patients with galactorrhea varies according to its cause and the patient's desires. For patients with a pituitary microadenoma, bromocriptine, 5 mg daily, is usually effective. Unfortunately, if bromocriptine is discontinued, hyperprolactinemia usually returns, leading to galactorrhea and amenorrhea. Therapy therefore must be continued indefinitely.

The objectives for therapy of prolactinomas are to normalize the prolactin levels and menstrual function, to preserve function of the anterior pituitary, and to reduce the tumor mass. Patients with macroadenomas or with extrasellar extension of the tumor should be treated first with bromocriptine, followed by surgery when maximal reduction of the tumor size has been obtained. Surgery should be performed without discontinuing bromocriptine because the adenoma may rapidly regrow.

Women with no evidence of pituitary adenoma but with unacceptable rates of galactorrhea may benefit from bromocriptine even if the serum prolactin level is normal. If galactorrhea is not symptomatic in such patients, however, treatment is not necessary. It is appropriate to refer most of these patients for further endocrine evaluation and to a reproductive endocrinologist if fertility is desired.

Occasional patients present with nonlactational mastitis, i.e., periodic drainage of purulent material from the nipple-areola complex in spite of previous attempts at drainage. In this condition, known as squamous metaplasia, it is not clear whether infection occurs initially followed by squamous metaplasia and intermittent discharge or whether squamous metaplasia occurs first followed by infection. The treatment, however, is complete excision of the involved duct system. Antibiotics are seldom helpful.

The most common benign neoplasm of the breast is the fibroadenoma, usually first presenting in the teenager but occasionally discovered on routine examination during the early reproductive years. Most of these lesions should be removed. In the occasional young patient with more than one mass, it is appropriate to use ultrasonography to document the actual number of lesions. Most surgeons prefer to remove the palpable lesion, usually as day surgery under local anesthesia, a procedure that is easy to do when the lesion is small. Patients who have discovered these lesions almost invariably request removal. The role of the primary care physician is to document the finding and then arrange for appropriate referral.

The diagnosis and treatment of nonmalignant diseases of the breast constitute one of the most difficult challenges facing the primary care physician. The symptomatology is extremely subjective, and conclusions based even upon the most careful examination are subject to error.

Even specific complaints, such as nipple discharge, require considerable judgment when recommending treatment or referral. No lesion is obviously benign. Because 80% of women with breast cancer have no identifiable risk factors, careful breast examination must be included as part of every physical examination.

Brookshaw JD: Danazol treatment of benign breast disease: A survey of U.S.A. multi center studies. Postgrad Med J 55:52, 1979. *Danazol has been approved by the FDA for the treatment of fibrocystic changes. It is costly, however, and there are a number of side effects. This article describes the results of a multicenter study in the United States.*

Feig SA: Decreased breast cancer mortality through mammographic screening: Results of clinical trials. State Art Radiol 167:659, 1988. *Although mammography screening can lead to a remarkable improvement in breast cancer survival, the degree to which any program achieves potential gain depends upon the technical quality of the study, the interpretive expertise of the radiologist, the screening facility, and the number of projections.*

Hindle WH: Fine needle aspiration. In Hindle WH (ed.): Breast Disease for Gynecologists, Norwalk, CT, Appleton and Lange, 1990, p 67. *This chapter covers the history and evolution of the fine-needle aspiration technique, including recommendations and contraindications for its use.*

Kleinberg DL, Noel GH, Frantz AG: Galactorrhea: A study of 235 cases including 48 with pituitary tumors. N Engl J Med 296:589, 1977. *This classic article is perhaps the most comprehensive report on the clinical entities associated with galactorrhea.*

Leis HP Jr: Management of nipple discharge. World J Surg 13:736, 1989. *This report of a series of over 8000 breast operations discusses the incidence of breast cancer in patients presenting with nipple discharge and the management of significant discharges.*

Love SM, Gelman SR, Silen W: Fibrocystic disease of the breast, a non disease. N Engl J Med 307:1010, 1983. *This article traces the history of fibrocystic "disease." Because most, if not all, women have these changes, the condition should not be called a disease. In most cases there is no relationship between fibrocystic changes and the later development of breast cancer.*

Yen SSC: Prolactin in human reproduction. In Yen SSC, Jaffe RB (eds.): Reproductive Endocrinology. Philadelphia, WB Saunders, 1986, p 237. *This chapter describes abnormalities in prolactin secretion and the treatment of the clinical sequelae.*

208.5 Breast Cancer

Brian J. Lewis and Robert M. Conry

EPIDEMIOLOGY AND PATHOGENESIS

In 1994, 182,000 new cases of female breast cancer and 1000 new cases of male breast cancer were projected for the United States. In terms of annual mortality, 46,000 women and 300 men die of breast cancer. These figures and the one in eight lifetime risk that a woman in the United States has for developing breast cancer make this disease a significant health problem.

The cause of breast cancer is unknown, but several factors correlate with its occurrence: age, family history, ethnic influences, and hormonal effects.

AGE. Only about 15% of cases of breast cancer occur before age 40. The age-adjusted incidence steadily increases thereafter, with two thirds of cases occurring in postmenopausal women.

FAMILY HISTORY. Daughters or sisters of breast cancer patients have a two- to threefold greater risk of developing breast cancer than do women without an affected first-degree relative. More specifically, this relative risk can range from 1.4 if only one first-degree relative is affected after age 60 to 4 to 6 if two first-degree relatives are affected. Unlike patients in the general population, women with the highest relative risk among those with a positive family history have a greater tendency to have their disease before age 40. Careful counseling, screening, and tracking of high-risk patients are essential. Increased monitoring should be performed on patients with prior definitive treatment for breast cancer because they have a 10 to 15% lifetime chance of developing a second primary breast cancer.

GENETICS. Five to 10% of breast cancer patients have inherited mutations leading to the disease. Two genes, BRCA1 and BRCA2, have recently been identified which together may account for most of these mutations (see Ch. 158.2). BRCA1, residing on the long arm of chromosome 17, is associated with female breast and ovarian carcinoma. BRCA2, residing on the long arm of chromosome 13, is associated with male and female breast cancer but not ovarian carcinoma. Mutations in either BRCA1 or BRCA2 are estimated to exist in 1% of all women and result in an extremely high risk of breast cancer, exceeding 50% before age 50 years and reaching 80% by age 65 years. Thus, as an inherited trait, breast cancer is among the most common genetic diseases in the world. BRCA1 and BRCA2 appear to be tumor suppressor genes, and their contribution to sporadic, nonhereditary forms of breast cancer remains uncertain. Diagnostic tests for mutations within these genes could be available within 2 years, raising numerous ethical, clinical, and psychological issues.

ETHNIC INFLUENCES. Ninety percent of breast cancer patients lack a positive family history. Although ethnic background has a role, it is necessary to control for the influences of allied cultural and nongenetic factors. Asian women have a much lower risk of breast cancer than women in Western countries, perhaps related to a later age of menarche. However, that these differences are not solely due to genetics has been suggested by studies of migrants. Japanese women immigrating to the United States were found to have an incidence of breast cancer almost equal to Caucasians in the same area.

HORMONAL EFFECTS. Estrogens have an impact on the development of breast cancer. Early menarche, late menopause, and late or no pregnancy correlate with a higher risk (relative risk of 1.3, 1.5 and 1.9, respectively). Conversely, premature loss of ovarian function, late menarche, early menopause, and early or more numerous pregnancies correlate with a decreased risk. The chance for developing breast cancer is increased in men with Klinefelter's syndrome or with other disturbances of estrogen metabolism.

Multiple trials examining the relationship between oral contraceptive use and the risk of developing breast cancer have yielded variable results. However, the data suggest that if oral contraceptives increase the overall risk of breast cancer, the magnitude of the increase is small and seen primarily among long-term users. Use of postmenopausal estrogen replacement therapy may be associated with a small increase in the relative risk of breast cancer in the range of 1.5 to 2.0 for moderate-dose conjugated estrogen therapy

TABLE 208-14. RISK FACTORS FOR BREAST CANCER IN WOMEN WITH PROLIFERATIVE BREAST DISEASE

Diagnosis	Relative Risk of Breast Cancer (95% Confidence Interval)
Nonproliferative lesions	1.0
Proliferative disease without atypical hyperplasia	1.9 (1.2 to 2.9)
Atypical hyperplasia	5.3 (3.1 to 8.8)
Atypical hyperplasia + family history of breast cancer	11.0 (5.5 to 24)

Data from DuPont WD, Page DL: Risk factors for breast cancer in women with proliferative breast disease. N Engl J Med 312:146, 1985.

over a 10- to 20-year period. Few data are available regarding the effects of long-term, low-dose therapy currently used for treatment and prevention of osteoporosis.

Historically, there has been a linkage between fibrocystic disease of the breast and an increased risk for breast cancer. A host of terms has been lumped under "fibrocystic disease" (i.e., macrocysts, microcysts, adenosis, apocrine change, fibrosis, fibroadenoma, and ductal hyperplasia). We now know that the majority of women (70%) who have a biopsy for benign disease are not at increased risk for cancer, but the presence of atypical hyperplasia and a family history of breast cancer greatly increase the probability of developing breast carcinoma (Table 208-14).

OTHER RISK FACTORS. Other risk factors include ionizing radiation and possibly diet. Surprisingly, consumption of even moderate amounts of alcohol is associated with an appreciable increase in risk. However, whether alcohol itself is responsible or whether it is associated with another responsible factor remains uncertain. Repeated chest fluoroscopy for tuberculosis, therapeutic radiation of mastitis, and exposure of Japanese women to the atomic bomb blast have been linked to increased rates of breast cancer. Animal models and geographic-ethnic differences in incidence suggest that dietary factors, in particular fat (increased in the Western diet), may contribute to the development of breast cancer.

DIAGNOSIS

Clinical Presentation

Breast cancer is usually noted as a painless lump and discovered incidentally by the patient, by routine physical examination, or by mammography. Pain and tenderness are nonspecific findings and herald cancer < 10% of the time. Physical findings suggestive of a malignancy include a hard, irregular mass and skin dimpling or nipple retraction. Nonbloody nipple discharges are rarely associated with cancer. Bloody discharges correlate with intraductal papillomas in about 30% of cases and with invasive cancer in about one third of cases.

Pertinent history includes a family history of breast cancer on the maternal side, especially in first-degree relatives, prior breast biopsies, whether the lump is new or old, and whether it fluctuates in size, consistency, and tenderness with the menstrual cycle. Such cycling is more suggestive of a benign process but by no means rules out cancer. Physical examination should include careful inspection and palpation of both breasts and assessment of the axillary, supraclavicular, and infraclavicular node areas.

Evaluating a Breast Mass

A suspicious breast mass requires systematic evaluation and follow-up. A negative mammogram or needle aspiration does not ensure that a mass is benign, and if it remains of concern, it must be excised. To avoid distortion of breast anatomy, a mammogram should precede any biopsy procedure. Breast imaging rules out contralateral lesions and multiple foci in the ipsilateral breast, and it is sometimes redone after biopsy to confirm that the area of interest was in fact removed.

Formerly, diagnosis and treatment were a one-step procedure. A woman with a suspicious lesion had an excision under general anesthesia with frozen section analysis of the tumor. If cancer was found, mastectomy immediately followed, and the woman awoke to confront both the diagnosis of cancer and the loss of her breast. A two-step procedure is now used. Fine-needle aspiration cytology or excisional biopsy under local anesthesia allows an outpatient diag-

nosis. If cancer is found, the patient and surgeon can then review treatment options.

Screening and Detection

Early detection of a tumor improves the chances for successful treatment. Efforts to screen for and detect early breast cancer have centered on self-examination, physician examination, and techniques for imaging the breast.

Self-examination is simple, without cost, and free of risk. It has been shown to result in earlier detection of tumors in several studies but has not been shown to reduce mortality. It is a reasonable practice to recommend for adult women, although its incremental benefit over that of mammography is uncertain. Any mass that is new and persists for more than a few weeks, is rapidly enlarging, or changes from a previously stable lump requires a physician's examination.

Examination by a physician as a screening tool is more costly and is applied less frequently than self-examination. Discovery of an unsuspected mass during a periodic examination by a physician leads to detection of tumors at an earlier stage than in patients who do not have periodic breast examinations. The American Cancer Society recommends that every woman over the age of 40 have a routine breast examination annually.

Breast imaging techniques include thermography, sonography, and radiographic mammography. Thermography has yet to prove sufficiently sensitive for widespread use. Sonography can help distinguish cystic from solid lesions initially found on radiography. Radiographic mammography is a well-studied and standardized methodology. Annual mammography lowers the mortality from breast cancer in screened populations by about 25% compared with unscreened control groups. It detects smaller lesions with fewer nodal metastases. Current technology allows a lower dose of radiation per examination. Table 208-15 shows guidelines for screening.

Breast cancer incidence rose gradually over the first half of the century and turned more sharply upward in the 1960's, concomitant with and possibly as a result of increased attention to education and screening. The mortality (deaths per 100,000), however, has remained constant. It may be that tumors are being found earlier and treated more readily, because more of the tumors found are smaller. Alternatively, a proportion of the early asymptomatic (subclinical) cancers being discovered may have a lower malignant potential than tumors that grow faster and more rapidly become clinically apparent. Thus, screening may appear more efficacious than it really is because some of the patients discovered to have an "early" cancer may represent a subpopulation with indolent disease who would not otherwise have had clinical expression of the tumor. Nonetheless, there has been a definite reduction in mortality from breast cancer in women who are screened with mammography.

TUMOR BIOLOGY

Breast cancer is more than just a local process; local control of tumor is necessary but not by itself sufficient to address the threat of distant metastases. Breast cancer is also a chronic illness with a potential for recurrence up to 40 years after removal of the primary tumor. Although one can extirpate apparent disease in the breast and in the axillary nodes in the majority of cases, at least 50 to 80% of women found to have tumor in the axillary nodes and 30% of those without axillary node metastases eventually have metastatic disease.

STAGING. The system for clinically staging breast cancer reflects the anatomic extent of tumor (Table 208-16). It allows consistent and comparable description and reporting of cases. The

TABLE 208-15. GUIDELINES FOR MAMMOGRAPHIC SCREENING OF ASYMPTOMATIC WOMEN

1. Mammography every 1 to 2 years for women aged 50 or older
2. Mammography annually for women at any age with a personal history of breast cancer
3. Mammography annually for women aged 40 and over who have a family history of breast cancer or who are otherwise at increased risk. The effectiveness of mammography in women aged 40 to 50 without increased risk is unproven.

TABLE 208-16. STAGING OF CARCINOMA OF THE BREAST

Stage I	Tumor ≤2 cm without skin or chest wall involvement and without regional lymph node metastases
Stage II	Tumor >2 cm without nodal metastases; tumor ≤5 cm with metastasis to moveable ipsilateral axillary nodes
Stage III	Tumor >5 cm with regional lymph node metastases; skin involvement or chest wall attachment; any size tumor with metastases to fixed ipsilateral axillary nodes or ipsilateral internal mammary nodes
Stage IV	Distant metastases

stages correlate with survival and are important in planning treatment, but they do not totally predict the clinical behavior of the tumor. A more complete classification scheme would ideally measure the balance between the inherent virulence of the cancer and the intrinsic antitumor defenses of the host. The combination of the presence and extent of metastases to the axillary nodes is the single most important prognostic factor for patients with breast cancer. Patients treated with radical mastectomy alone have 10-year survival rates of 70% with negative nodes, 50% with one to three positive axillary nodes, and only 20% with four or more positive axillary nodes. In addition to tumor size and nodal status, hormone receptor content and nuclear grade reproducibly correlate with prognosis. The infrequent histologic subtypes of papillary, colloid (mucinous), and tubular carcinoma are associated with a more favorable outcome. Other variables such as the percentage of cells in S-phase, oncogene expression, epidermal growth factor receptors, cathepsin-D, and stress response (heat shock) proteins may also predict who will have metastatic disease (Table 208–17), but the independent contribution of any of these factors remains to be established.

METHOD OF SPREAD. Breast cancer spreads directly to the bloodstream as well as to the draining lymphatics. Tumor emboli can traverse the lymph nodes and enter the venous system; and tumor cells can presumably reach lymph nodes by way of the bloodstream. In addition, upon discovery, a breast cancer mass usually contains 10^9 or more cells. Given what is known of doubling times, the cell number at diagnosis implies that the cancer may have been growing for a number of years. It seems logical that there will be shedding of the tumor cells into the venous and lymphatic circulation throughout the life of the tumor, especially early, when tumor growth rate is highest.

Accordingly, it is likely that many more patients with breast cancer have micrometastases than we see with clinical recurrence. Negative axillary nodes may not mean that the tumor was never present in the lymphatic system but rather that it had been there and was unable to flourish. Positive lymph nodes do correlate with subsequent metastases and poor survival. This could reflect simple anatomic spread of cancer past the last "line of defense" imposed by the lymph nodes (Halsted). More probably it implies that because the tumor persisted in the nodes, however it arrived there, it may also persist and grow in other organs.

CELL ORIGIN. Most breast tumors derive from mammary epithelium. Eighty percent of these are infiltrating ductal carcinomas. Less common are infiltrating lobular carcinoma, medullary carcinoma, comedocarcinoma, and tubular, papillary, and colloid carcinoma. Lobular and comedocarcinoma can be bilateral and require increased surveillance of the unaffected breast. Lobular carcinoma in situ poses a special problem. Although it is not an invasive lesion, it is associated with a 1% annual risk for the development of an invasive lesion in either breast. Some surgeons have therefore advocated prophylactic mastectomy. A more conservative approach is to do a "mirror image" biopsy of the contralateral breast to rule out invasive tumor and then to track the patient closely with periodic examinations and prompt biopsy of any suspicious lesions. Ductal carcinoma in situ carries a higher risk for evolving into invasive cancer and requires surgery. Inflammatory breast cancer represents a highly virulent pathologic variant. Clinically, the patient has a red, swollen, warm breast with a characteristic peau d'orange appearance. Microscopically, this is associated with involvement of dermal lymphatics by tumor. It has proven difficult to achieve long-term survival in patients with this diagnosis with local treatment, but the addition of systemic therapy has improved results somewhat.

HORMONE RECEPTOR PROTEINS. Estrogen and progesterone receptor proteins (ERP and PRP) are present in normal mammary epithelium and in a proportion of breast cancers. After binding to the steroid, the activated hormone-receptor complex interacts with specific sites on DNA, and this results in the initiation of steroid-specific protein synthesis. One product of estrogen stimulation is PRP, and the presence of PRP signifies functionally intact ERP. A tumor is considered ERP-positive when it contains more than 10 femtomoles of receptor per milligram of protein, as measured using a radioligand binding assay. Monoclonal antibodies against ERP are now available and permit microscopic visualization and enumeration of ERP-positive tumor cells.

ERP is found more frequently and in higher titer in tumors from postmenopausal patients (≥60% versus 30 to 40% positive in premenopausal women). ERP-positive tumors tend to be less virulent and are more likely to respond to hormonal therapy (see below). Tumors that contain both ERP and PRP have the greatest likelihood of regressing after an endocrine maneuver, and the probability of a response increases directly with the titer of the RP. Given the therapeutic and prognostic implications of hormone receptor levels, it is mandatory that all primary breast cancers be submitted for receptor analysis at the time of removal. There is an 80% concordance between the hormone receptor profile of a primary tumor and its metastases, in the absence of intervening hormone treatment. Breast cancers are heterogeneous in the sense that in RP-positive specimens, the majority but not necessarily all of the cells contain RP. When metastatic disease becomes refractory to hormonal therapy after initially responding, the progression reflects the outgrowth of hormone-independent cells that are usually RP-negative.

PRIMARY MANAGEMENT OF BREAST CANCER

Stage I and Stage II Disease

Since Halsted's time, almost three generations ago, the view of breast cancer as a local or regional process made radical mastectomy or one of its variants the standard approach to the management of resectable tumor confined to the breast and the axillary lymph nodes. Patients often received postoperative radiation therapy to the chest wall and the draining lymph node areas. These treatments have produced a local control rate of 95%, but variations in locoregional therapy have not differed significantly in their impact upon distant recurrence or overall survival. Furthermore, more extensive surgery or surgery followed by radiation increases the risk of arm edema.

These approaches entered general use without the testing of alternative approaches, but recently local tumor excision with breast irradiation has been gaining a wider acceptance. Older, largely uncontrolled studies seemed to indicate similar outcomes either with tumor excision and breast irradiation or with traditional mastectomy. Although one cannot refer to the decades of observation on local tumor control and side effects that exist for standard surgical approaches, multiple, controlled trials have recently shown that the techniques are equivalent in terms of tumor recurrence and overall survival.

Public interest in alternatives to mastectomy has increased, and patients are more informed and expect their physicians to provide a comprehensive overview of treatment possibilities, especially ones that would spare them the disfigurement and distress imposed by mastectomy. Likewise, the growing application of plastic surgery

TABLE 208-17. PROGNOSTIC FACTORS IN BREAST CANCER

Factor	Influence on Risk of Metastases
Tumor size	Risk increases with size
Nodal status	Risk increases with presence and number of nodal metastases
Hormone receptor status	Risk increased if receptors not present
Nuclear grade	Risk increased with high grade
Favorable histology	Risk decreases with favorable subtypes
Percent S-phase	Risk increases with percent S-phase
Oncogene expression	Risk appears to increase with increased oncogene expression
Cathepsin-D levels	Risk appears to increase with levels
Epidermal growth factor receptor levels	Risk appears to increase with levels
Stress response protein levels	Risk appears to increase with levels

for breast reconstruction after mastectomy has lessened the emotional trauma of the operation.

Breast conservation is appropriate therapy for Stage I or Stage II disease. Table 208–18 lists the requirements for its use. Mammography is essential to exclude patients with multifocal disease or with diffuse microcalcifications. (Even if the latter prove benign on biopsy, they will interfere with the subsequent mammographic follow-up used to screen for recurrent cancer.) An adequate surgical resection of the tumor with negative resection margins is essential and is facilitated by inking the margins of the specimen and orienting it for the pathologist. Axillary node dissection determines whether the patient requires adjuvant systemic treatment because of nodal metastasis. Extensive intraductal carcinoma *in situ* may be a contraindication to breast conservation because of a higher risk of recurrence in the treated breast.

The most common but not necessarily the preferred approach to the primary management of a Stage I or Stage II breast cancer is total mastectomy and axillary lymph node dissection. Postoperative radiation therapy is an individualized rather than "standard" therapy. It is employed when narrow resection margins, extensive nodal disease, the presence of residual tumor, or other high-risk factors for local recurrence are present. With the advent of adjuvant systemic therapy for Stage II disease (see below), there may be even fewer indications for adjuvant radiation therapy, because drug treatment alone decreases the local failure rate.

Clinically suspicious nodes are pathologically negative for tumor 25 to 30% of the time, and, conversely, clinically negative nodes are positive histologically with an equal frequency. With a proper axillary dissection, radiation to the axilla is not usually necessary (and increases the risk for arm edema). Although positive axillary nodes increase the likelihood of subclinical supraclavicular and internal mammary node metastases, no evidence indicates that adjuvant radiation to those areas improves survival.

Standard pretreatment evaluation for any of these techniques includes a complete blood count, a profile of serum chemistries with particular reference to studies suggestive of liver or bone involvement, and a chest radiograph. The yield of positive bone or liver scans is extremely low in the absence of symptoms or signs suggesting metastatic disease. On the other hand, with locally advanced tumor (Stage III), the yield of screening bone scans is sufficiently high (about 30%) to warrant their use. Likewise, with abnormal blood chemistries suggestive of liver involvement or with symptoms such as bone pain, scans would be required to avoid inappropriate use of a definitive local procedure in a patient with advanced, incurable disease.

Stage III Disease and Inflammatory Breast Cancer

If a patient's disease is Stage III solely on the basis of tumor size (tumor >5 cm), but the tumor appears to be as resectable as that of a Stage I or II patient, mastectomy has historically been the primary treatment. Recent studies have also shown satisfactory local control with the use of primary chemotherapy and breast conservation ther-

apy. For patients with locally advanced but unresectable disease (i.e., invasion of chest wall, fixation of axillary nodes, or positive supraclavicular nodes), control of persistent or recurrent regional disease as well as latent distant metastases is the dominant problem. Inflammatory breast cancer is aggressive locally as well as metastatically. It is properly considered a systemic disease from the outset, even though it appears to be confined to the breast. The treatment plan for the latter two presentations involves an individualized approach using chemotherapy to reduce the tumor volume, followed by radiation therapy and possibly resection of the breast and draining nodes. This strategy requires close consultation from the outset between surgeons, radiation oncologists, and medical oncologists. Prolonged remissions can be obtained in a fraction of patients.

Metastatic Breast Cancer

CLINICAL FEATURES. Breast cancer most frequently metastasizes to lymph nodes, skin, lung, pleura, bone, liver, brain, and pericardium. In autopsy series, the adrenals are involved in up to half the patients, but adrenal insufficiency is rarely seen. Likewise, the ovaries contain tumor in up to one quarter of patients at autopsy. Rarely metastatic breast cancer may be found incidentally at oophorectomy in a patient whose first sign of breast cancer is an involved ovary presenting as a pelvic mass. Breast cancer is the most common source of metastases to the eye in women.

PATIENT ASSESSMENT. Once a metastatic focus is found, routine studies to map tumor extent include a complete blood count (which can reflect myelophthisis secondary to marrow metastases) and the measurement of serum levels of liver enzymes, bilirubin, and calcium. The carcinoembryonic antigen titer and the CA 15-3 antigen titer can be useful markers for following response to therapy. A chest radiograph is indicated and can reveal lung nodules, mediastinal or hilar node involvement, or a pleural effusion. A bone scan is also mandatory, and positive areas, especially those that are symptomatic or in weight-bearing bones, require follow-up radiographs to distinguish metastatic involvement from coexisting benign bony disease and to determine whether radiation is needed to prevent collapse or pathologic fracture. If physical findings or laboratory studies suggest hepatic involvement, a radionuclide liver scan, a sonogram of the liver, or a liver CT scan confirms the presence of metastatic disease, gauges its extent, and allows comparison with follow-up studies during treatment. "Routine" liver imaging is widely employed, but its yield and cost-effectiveness in the absence of signs suggesting liver metastasis are open to question. The same statement applies to "routine" studies of the brain, although they are clearly indicated in the presence of neurologic symptoms or signs.

COMPLICATIONS. Certain complications occur with some frequency and require urgent attention in patients with metastatic breast cancer: hypercalcemia, metastases to weight-bearing bones, and metastases to the nervous system (the epidural space, the leptomeninges, or the brain).

Hypercalcemia requires standard methods of therapy, such as saline and furosemide, along with treatment of the breast cancer itself (see Ch. 214). Pamidronate and gallium nitrate are new effective agents for the treatment of hypercalcemia which function as potent inhibitors of bone resorption. A positive bone scan, especially in the femur or vertebral column, or bone pain in these areas requires radiographic analysis of the extent of structural damage. Femoral lesions may necessitate orthopedic stabilization and radiation therapy to prevent pathologic fractures. Vertebral body lesions may require radiation to diminish pain and avoid further collapse.

Patients with persistent back pain are at greater risk for *epidural metastases* and possibly cord compression. Motor or sensory changes in a segmental distribution greatly increase the possibility of an epidural lesion. However, in the presence of back pain, their absence does not exclude an epidural lesion. Magnetic resonance scanning is useful in establishing or excluding the presence of epidural lesions. Pain without a neurologic deficit means that there is still time to treat an epidural lesion with radiation before the cord becomes ischemic and permanently damaged.

Leptomeningeal metastases present with headache and focal sensory or motor changes suggestive of single or multiple nerve root involvement. The diagnosis depends upon the demonstration of breast cancer cells in the cerebrospinal fluid and may require multi-

TABLE 208–18. REQUIREMENTS FOR LIMITED SURGERY AND RADIATION THERAPY FOR EARLY BREAST CANCER

Patient Selection	Comments
Adequate resection of tumor without major cosmetic deformity	This requires a single discrete tumor, moderate sized breast, tumor diameter <4–5 cm.
Surgical Criteria	
Wide resection with specimen orientation	Grossly negative surgical margins are essential—re-resection may be required if margins are microscopically involved.
Hormone receptor analysis	
Separate axillary incision	
Radiation Therapy	
4500–5000 rad to entire breast ± boost to tumor bed	
Treatment of the Axilla	
Level I *and* Level II axillary dissection* (*not* an informal "sampling")	Permits adequate node sampling, controls local tumor, and obviates the need for axillary radiation. Does not impose a major risk for arm edema.

Sources: Harris et al., 1985; Danoff et al., 1985.
* Level I = Complete removal of nodes lateral to the pectoralis minor muscle.
Level II = Removal of nodes beneath the pectoralis minor.

ple spinal taps to yield a diagnosis (with appropriate studies beforehand, if indicated, to rule out a mass lesion in the brain). Intrathecal or intraventricular chemotherapy is usually necessary.

TREATMENT. The two major types of therapy for disseminated breast cancer are hormonal and cytotoxic. Hormonal therapy is less toxic but can require as long as 8 to 12 weeks to produce maximal benefit. The impact of chemotherapy is more rapid. Responses to all these treatments last a median of 6 to 18 months, and responders have a significantly prolonged survival compared with nonresponders. Whether the response itself is responsible or response to therapy identifies a more favorable subgroup of patients is uncertain.

The menopausal status of the patient and the hormone receptor profile of the tumor are the major determinants of whether to employ an endocrine maneuver and which particular therapy to use. Other important considerations are the tempo of the disease, the performance status of the patient, and the sites of metastases. A long interval between mastectomy and recurrence suggests indolent disease and would, along with a good performance status, permit the longer observation period needed to gauge response to an endocrine therapy. Bone, soft tissue, and limited pulmonary metastases may respond to hormonal therapy, whereas extensive lung or liver metastases greatly decrease the probability of a response and therefore require chemotherapy. Because treatment for metastatic disease is palliative, it may reasonably be delayed in the absence of symptoms or visceral metastases.

Premenopausal Patients. For premenopausal patients with ER-positive tumors, hormonal therapy is first-line treatment in the absence of the contraindications mentioned above. Oophorectomy is generally recommended as the first endocrine treatment. A good, probably equivalent, alternative is the antiestrogen tamoxifen. Most premenopausal women continue to menstruate while receiving tamoxifen, but its mechanisms of action are diverse. LHRH agonists are currently being examined as an alternative to oophorectomy. Oophorectomy produces tumor regression in 50 to 75% of patients with ER-positive tumors. Other surgical endocrine ablative procedures, such as adrenalectomy and hypophysectomy, are considered obsolete forms of therapy for metastatic breast cancer due to the availability of newer medical endocrine treatments. If a patient progresses after initial response to oophorectomy, then antiestrogens, progestins, or aminoglutethimide can be used in sequence until there is no longer a response. At that point, the patient should receive chemotherapy. The major source of estrogen following oophorectomy or in postmenopausal women is the adrenal gland, which produces androstenedione that is converted by an aromatase reaction in peripheral tissues to estrone and estradiol. Aminoglutethimide produces a medical adrenalectomy that is reversible once the drug is stopped. Patients receiving aminoglutethimide experience rash and somnolence 10 to 40% of the time, although these side effects wane after several weeks of treatment. The drug blocks all adrenal steroidogenesis by inhibiting conversion of cholesterol to pregnenolone. In peripheral tissue, it also blocks the conversion of androstenedione to estrone, a precursor of estradiol. Aminoglutethimide therapy at moderate to high dose requires replacement corticosteroid treatment with hydrocortisone, which also suppresses the increase in pituitary ACTH secretion produced by aminoglutethimide inhibition of cortisol production, an increase that could otherwise override the blockade. A periodic check of plasma dehydroepiandrosterone levels confirms the adequacy of adrenal suppression.

Premenopausal patients with RP-negative tumors, or those originally RP-positive who have become refractory to endocrine treatment, require chemotherapy. Drug classes active against breast cancer include alkylating agents (typically cyclophosphamide), antimetabolites (5-fluorouracil, methotrexate), antimicrotubule agents such as vinca alkaloids (vincristine, vinblastine) and paclitaxel, anthracyclines (doxorubicin), and mitomycin-C. In various combinations, these agents effect responses in 60 to 70% of patients, with 10 to 15% achieving a complete remission. However, these responses have a median duration of only 6 to 12 months. Studies are in progress using high-dose chemotherapy and autologous bone marrow rescue to see if selected patients can achieve permanent ablation of metastatic disease. Although this approach has produced high complete response rates (35 to 50%) among highly selected patients with Stage IV disease, the duration of response has not yet

TABLE 208–19. INDICATIONS FOR ADJUVANT SYSTEMIC THERAPY

Axillary lymph node metastases not present
1. Tumors ≤1 cm—no adjuvant therapy (risk of relapse <10%)
2. Tumors >1 cm and especially with adverse prognostic features (see Table 208–17)—consider adjuvant tamoxifen if receptor positive or chemotherapy if receptor negative
Axillary lymph node metastases present
1. Premenopausal, receptor positive or negative—combination chemotherapy
2. Postmenopausal, receptor positive—tamoxifen
3. Postmenopausal, receptor negative—consider chemotherapy

been convincingly shown to be prolonged over that with conventional treatments.

Postmenopausal Patients. For RP-positive tumors in postmenopausal patients who are candidates for endocrine therapy, the antiestrogen tamoxifen has replaced estrogen therapy (diethylstilbestrol, DES) as initial treatment. Tamoxifen has few side effects, in contrast to DES, which much more frequently produces nausea, anorexia, and salt retention. Both drugs have been associated with a tumor "flare" consisting of increased bone pain and hypercalcemia. This occurs in patients with skeletal metastases during the initial weeks of treatment, more commonly with DES. These reactions usually herald an antitumor effect and do not necessitate cessation of therapy as long as symptoms and calcium levels are controlled by standard supportive treatments. Withdrawal of DES, once the tumor progresses, produces further regression of tumor in 20 to 30% of patients (withdrawal effect is less common with tamoxifen). Once the disease progresses after this initial therapy, serial endocrine maneuvers are used, as discussed for premenopausal patients, until the tumor becomes refractory to hormonal therapy. Oophorectomy has no role in the treatment of postmenopausal patients. Again, for RP-negative tumors or for tumors resistant to endocrine treatment, chemotherapy becomes the treatment of choice.

Adjuvant Systemic Therapy

The goal of adjuvant systemic therapy after mastectomy is to control any micrometastases present and thus improve survival. Combination chemotherapy, tamoxifen, and ovarian ablation are all effective in subsets of patients. Table 208–19 summarizes the present indications for adjuvant systemic therapy. Ongoing clinical trials are likely to modify these guidelines in the near future. Currently available adjuvant therapy produces an overall reduction in the risk of death of at least 25% in the first 10 years following treatment. Thus, the absolute improvement in survival for a given patient depends on that patient's risk of death due to breast cancer. Consideration of the need for adjuvant systemic therapy should be a routine part of every patient's initial management. The decision should be based upon the individual risk of recurrence, the characteristics of the tumor, and the anticipated extent of improvement with the therapy selected.

The following points should be kept firmly in mind: (1) *Optimal* treatment for any subset of patients has yet to be defined, (2) physicians should continue to enroll their patients in controlled trials, and (3) the studies to date in axillary lymph node–negative patients show a statistically significant improvement in relapse-free survival and overall survival with adjuvant drug therapy. Because 70% of node-negative women survive 10 years or more following primary treatment, the challenge remains to identify and treat only the subset at high risk.

The best choice of drugs, dose, schedule, and duration for adjuvant treatment continues to evolve. The major delayed toxicity of adjuvant chemotherapy is irreversible amenorrhea. Severe long-term sequelae of chemotherapy are rare but include cardiomyopathy affecting <1% of patients receiving doxorubicin and acute leukemia in approximately 5 of 10,000 patients treated with cyclophosphamide-based regimens, especially higher dose or longer duration regimens.

NEW DRUGS AND TREATMENTS

TAXOL. Taxol, a mitotic spindle poison, is the most promising new drug for the treatment of breast cancer. Single-agent taxol has produced overall response rates of 55% as initial therapy for metastatic breast cancer and 26% among heavily pretreated patients with advanced disease, with median response durations ranging from 8 to 12 months. Taxol appears to merit broad investigation at the Phase III level both as a single agent and in combination.

AUTOLOGOUS BONE MARROW TRANSPLANTATION. Multiple Phase II studies in patients with Stage IV disease achieving a partial response to low-dose chemotherapy have demonstrated complete remission rates of 35 to 50% following high-dose chemotherapy with autologous bone marrow rescue. Approximately 20% of these patients remain disease-free without further therapy for several years. Despite the favorable impact on survival and quality of life achieved in this highly selected minority of patients, there is no evidence that broader application of this form of therapy will provide results superior to conventional drug treatments. Evaluation of high-dose chemotherapy with autologous bone marrow rescue in patients with advanced primary breast cancer (Stage III or Stage II with ≥10 positive axillary lymph nodes) is the subject of three national, randomized Phase III trials currently under way. Interim analysis of these trials is not planned until 1999.

SPECIAL CONSIDERATIONS

Male Breast Cancer

Carcinoma of the male breast occurs with 1% the frequency of female breast cancer. Its clinical presentation and primary therapy are similar to those in women. Abnormalities of estrogen metabolism are cited as a possible causative factor. The vast majority of tumors that have been examined are estrogen RP-positive. Orchiectomy and tamoxifen have similar efficacy for the initial management of metastatic disease. Responses to progestins, LHRH agonists, and aminoglutethimide have been reported. The approach to chemotherapy for these patients is similar to that used for women.

Breast Cancer and Pregnancy

Breast cancer complicates approximately one of every 3000 pregnancies. It has been held for some time that pregnancy adversely affects the outcome of breast cancer, with studies citing a high frequency of axillary lymph node metastases and shortened survival when the diagnosis is made during pregnancy. To some extent, these poor results may have related to a delay in diagnosis and in the initiation of treatment rather than inherently different biologic factors. The treatment considerations are the same as for the nonpregnant patients, and a standard surgical approach poses a ≤1% risk to the developing fetus. When patients present with disseminated disease in the first or second trimester, cytotoxic drug treatment may pose a significant risk to the fetus. If clinical considerations permit, treatment can be delayed to the third trimester to permit delivery of a viable fetus.

Patients who develop cancer during pregnancy tend to present with more advanced stages of disease than nonpregnant patients. However, when compared stage for stage, pregnant women have only a slightly less favorable prognosis than nonpregnant women. In a woman who has had successfully treated breast cancer, subsequent pregnancy is not associated with an excessive risk of recurrence. Patients with early stage breast cancer who bear children appear to have a survival equal to that of women who do not become pregnant. A 3-year interval between primary treatment of early breast cancer and a subsequent pregnancy has been advocated.

Beahrs O, Henson D, Hutter R, Myers M: Staging for cancer of the breast. In Beahrs O, Henson D, Hutter R, Myers M (eds.): Manual for Staging of Cancer, 3rd ed. Philadelphia, JB Lippincott, 1988, p. 145.
Bonadonna G: Evolving concepts in the systemic adjuvant treatment of breast cancer. Cancer Res 52:2127, 1992.
Dupont WD, Page DL: Menopausal replacement therapy and breast cancer. Arch Intern Med 151:56, 1991. *This important, authoritative review of a large number of studies concludes that menopausal therapy consisting of ≤ 0.625 mg or less of conjugated estrogens daily does not increase the risk of breast cancer.*
Early Breast Cancer Trialists' Collaborative Group: Systemic treatment of early breast cancer by hormonal, cytotoxic or immune therapy: 133 randomised trials involving 31,000 recurrences and 24,000 deaths among 75,000 women. Lancet 339:1, 1992. *This comprehensive meta-analysis of breast cancer trials worldwide provides the basis for current recommendations regarding adjuvant therapy of breast cancer.*
Fisher B, Costantino J, Redmond C, et al.: Lumpectomy compared with lumpectomy and radiation therapy for the treatment of intraductal breast cancer. N Engl J Med 328:1581, 1993. *This article, plus the reference by Veronesi, establishes the value of radiation therapy to reduce the risk of local recurrence following breast-preserving surgery.*
Friedman LS, Ostermeyer EA, Lynch ED, et al.: Special lecture. The search for BRCA1. Cancer Res 54:6374, 1994. *An overview of breast cancer susceptibility genes and their role in hereditary breast cancer.*
Harris JR, Morrow M, Bonadonna G: Cancer of the breast. In DeVita VT, Hellman S, Rosenberg SA (eds.): Cancer: Principles and Practice of Oncology. Philadelphia, JB Lippincott, 1993. *A comprehensive treatise detailing areas such as surgical technique, pathology, and chemotherapy.*
Miki Y, Swensen J, Shattuck-Eidens D, et al.: A strong candidate for the breast and ovarian cancer susceptibility gene BRCA1. Science 266:66, 1994. *A detailed description of the breast cancer susceptibility gene BRCA1 and its role in hereditary breast cancer.*
Seshadri R: Clinical significance of HER-2/neu oncogene amplification in primary breast cancer. J Clin Oncol 11:1936, 1993. *This report establishes HER-2/neu oncogene amplification as a significant prognostic factor in breast cancer.*
Spielmann M: Taxol in patients with metastatic breast carcinoma who have failed prior chemotherapy: Interim results of a multinational study. Oncology 51 (suppl) 1:25, 1994.
Veronesi U, Luini A, Del Vecchio M, et al.: Radiotherapy after breast-preserving surgery in women with localized cancer of the breast. N Engl J Med 328:1587, 1993.

209 ENDOCRINOLOGIC DISEASES UNIQUE TO MEN

209.1 The Testis
Alvin M. Matsumoto

The testis has three major physiologic functions: (1) During embryogenesis, testosterone and müllerian inhibiting substance produced by the fetal testis play vital roles in normal male sexual differentiation (see Ch. 207). (2) Beginning at the time of puberty and continuing into adulthood, testosterone produced by the testis is necessary for the development and maintenance of secondary sexual characteristics (virilization) and sexual functioning (libido and potency). (3) Production of spermatozoa by the testis is required for fertility.

Disorders of the testis are common and have profound effects on patients. Infertility due to disordered sperm production affects approximately 5 to 6% of all men wishing to father children. Klinefelter's syndrome, which results in permanent androgen deficiency and infertility, affects approximately one in 400 to 500 males. Testicular dysfunction occurs commonly as a result of systemic illness, malnutrition, and medications. Impotence and gynecomastia, which often result from testicular dysfunction, are very common complaints for which men seek medical attention. Finally, cancer of the testis remains one of the most common fatal neoplasms of young men.

Many disorders of the testis can be treated effectively. Testosterone replacement therapy in androgen-deficient men results in the development or restoration of secondary sexual characteristics and normal sexual functioning. Gonadotropin treatment of hypogonadotropic men often stimulates spermatogenesis and induces fertility in addition to restoring androgen secretion. Finally, seminomas are exquisitely responsive to radiation therapy, and the treatment of nonseminomatous testicular cancers with multidrug chemotherapy has markedly improved survival and cure rates.

TESTICULAR STRUCTURE AND PHYSIOLOGY
Functional Anatomy

The normal adult testis normally measures 3.5 to 5.5 cm in length and 2.0 to 3.0 cm in width and has a volume between 15 and 30 ml. About 90% of the volume of the testis is composed of seminiferous tubules, where spermatozoa are produced. Therefore, any significant reduction in testicular size is likely to be reflected in a decrease in total sperm production.

During fetal development, the testes descend from an intra-abdominal position into the scrotum. The scrotal location of the testes allows them to function at a temperature approximately 2°C lower than that of the abdomen. The pampiniform plexus of veins surrounds the testicular artery and cools the arterial blood supply to the testes. The lower testicular temperature is necessary for normal spermatogenesis in man. Failure of the testes to descend into the scrotum (cryptorchidism) or an abnormality in the venous cooling mechanism (varicocele) impairs sperm production.

The testis is composed of two structurally distinct compartments: the *interstitial* or *Leydig cell compartment* and the *seminiferous tubule compartment* (Fig. 209-1). These compartments are responsible for the two major products of the testis, testosterone and spermatozoa.

The interstitial compartment is composed of *Leydig cells* that produce sex steroid hormones, primarily testosterone. Leydig cells are in close proximity to seminiferous tubules, a location that facilitates delivery of high concentrations of testosterone to the seminiferous tubule compartment which is important in stimulating spermatogenesis.

The seminiferous tubule compartment is composed of developing *germ cells* and *Sertoli cells*. Spermatogenesis involves the differentiation and maturation of spermatogonia, the most primitive germ cell, into spermatozoa. In humans, spermatogenesis takes approximately 74 days. Sperm transport through the epididymis and vas deferens takes another 12 days. Therefore, processes that adversely affect early spermatogenesis may not be manifest by reduced sperm counts in the ejaculate until 2 to 3 months after the insult.

Sertoli cells play an important role in the development of germ cells and regulation of spermatogenesis. They maintain the structural integrity and compartmentalization of seminiferous tubules, deliver nutrients and produce proteins that support spermatogenesis, and regulate the movement and release of maturing sperm within the tubule. Sertoli cells also produce *müllerian inhibiting substance* (see Ch. 207), and *inhibin,* a glycoprotein that inhibits follicle-stimulating hormone secretion from the pituitary gland.

Central Nervous System Regulation of Gonadotropin Secretion

Normal testicular function depends on adequate stimulation by the gonadotropins, *luteinizing hormone (LH),* and *follicle-stimulating hormone (FSH),* that are secreted by the anterior pituitary gland (Fig. 209-1). Like thyroid-stimulating hormone and human chorionic gonadotropin (hCG), both LH and FSH are glycoprotein hormones composed of an α and a β subunit. The α subunits of all four glycoprotein hormones are identical and biologically inactive, whereas the β subunits are unique for each hormone and determine their biologic activity.

Measurements of serum gonadotropin levels are usually performed by immunoassays (e.g., immunofluorometric assays). In normal young men, LH and FSH levels range from 0.5 to 10 mIU per

milliliter depending on the specific assay used. Many gonadotropin assays cannot distinguish between low and low-normal gonadotropin levels. Therefore, a hormonal profile of low-normal gonadotropin levels and low testosterone levels is consistent with secondary hypogonadism (see below). Free α subunit is normally synthesized and secreted into the circulation by the pituitary. Gonadotropin-secreting pituitary adenomas and α subunit–secreting tumors, such as pancreatic islet cell tumors, secrete excessive amounts of free α subunit that can be measured using specific immunoassays.

Both LH and FSH are secreted into the peripheral circulation from the anterior pituitary in an episodic fashion (Fig. 209-2). Pulsatile gonadotropin secretion begins during sleep in early puberty, and by adulthood it is present throughout the day. The pulsatile secretion of gonadotropins is regulated primarily by the central nervous system through episodic stimulation of the pituitary by *LH-releasing hormone (LHRH)* (also known as *gonadotropin-releasing hormone [GnRH]*). LHRH, a decapeptide synthesized by hypothalamic neurons, stimulates release of both LH and FSH from the pituitary gland (see Fig. 209-1). Low-dose pulsatile LHRH administration is used to induce normal testicular function in patients with hypogonadotropic eunuchoidism, who lack endogenous LHRH. By contrast, administration of high-dose, continuous LHRH or potent LHRH agonists results in marked suppression of gonadotropin and testicular function. This paradoxic action of LHRH agonists has been used clinically to suppress endogenous testosterone production in the treatment of androgen-dependent tumors, such as prostate cancer.

The hypothalamic LHRH neuronal system plays an important integrative role in the regulation of testicular function (see Fig. 209-1). It receives input both from higher neural centers, such as the limbic system, through numerous stimulatory and inhibitory neurotransmitter and neuropeptide systems and from testicular feedback signals, primarily sex steroid hormones. The input from these sources alters LHRH output, which, in turn, regulates pituitary gonadotropin secretion and testicular function. Knowledge of how the central nervous system regulates LHRH secretion has clarified the mechanisms by which stress, malnutrition, and certain pharmacologic agents (such as opiate drugs) affect testicular function (see Ch. 201).

Gonadotropin Regulation of Testicular Function

LH REGULATION OF TESTOSTERONE PRODUCTION. LH binds to specific membrane receptors on Leydig cells of the testis and stimulates testicular steroidogenesis and secretion of *testosterone,* the major steroid product of the testis (see Fig. 209-1). Testosterone is secreted both locally within the testes and into the peripheral circulation. Healthy young men secrete approximately 5 to 7 mg of testosterone daily. Total plasma testosterone concentrations as determined by radioimmunoassay (RIA), range from 3 to 10 ng per milliliter. Like gonadotropins, testosterone is secreted in a pulsatile fashion (Fig. 209-2).

In early puberty, testosterone secretion increases from very low to near adult levels during sleep in response to sleep-associated rises in LH levels. In adults, testosterone secretion occurs throughout the entire day. In young healthy men testosterone levels exhibit a circadian variation of about 1.5 ng per milliliter, with maximal levels occurring at 8 A.M. and minimal levels occurring at 9 P.M.

Under LH stimulation, Leydig cells also convert testosterone to *estradiol.* However, secretion of estradiol by the testis accounts for only about 15% of the daily production of estradiol. The remainder of estradiol in blood is produced from testosterone and androstenedione (an adrenal androgen) by the enzyme aromatase in peripheral tissues.

TESTOSTERONE TRANSPORT. Like other steroid hormones, the majority of testosterone secreted into the circulation is bound to plasma proteins, primarily albumin and *sex hormone–binding globulin (SHBG).* Approximately 30 to 40% of total testosterone is bound to SHBG and is not biologically available. Only 1 to 2% is free (i.e., unbound to plasma proteins) and physiologically active. Albumin-bound testosterone is also available to act on many target organs. Therefore, measurement of non–SHBG-bound testosterone may provide the best estimate of biologically available testosterone. In certain clinical situations, alterations in SHBG levels result in total testosterone measurements that do not reflect bioavailable testosterone levels. SHBG (and total testosterone) levels are decreased with obesity, hypothyroidism, androgens, nephrotic syndrome, Cushing's disease, and acromegaly and increased with hepatic cir-

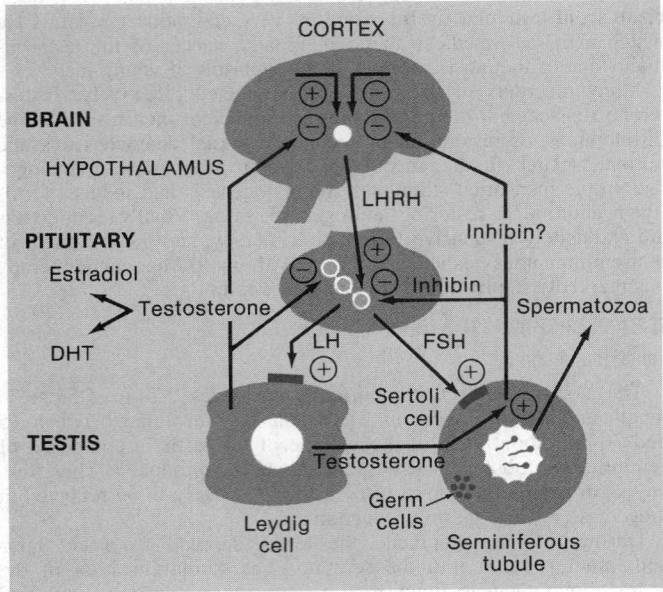

FIGURE 209-1. Diagram of the normal physiology of the hypothalamic-pituitary-testicular axis. (Adapted from Matsumoto AM, Bremner WJ: Endocrinology of the hypothalamic-pituitary-testicular axis with particular reference to the hormonal control of spermatogenesis. Bailliere's Clin Endocrinol Metab 1:71, 1987.)

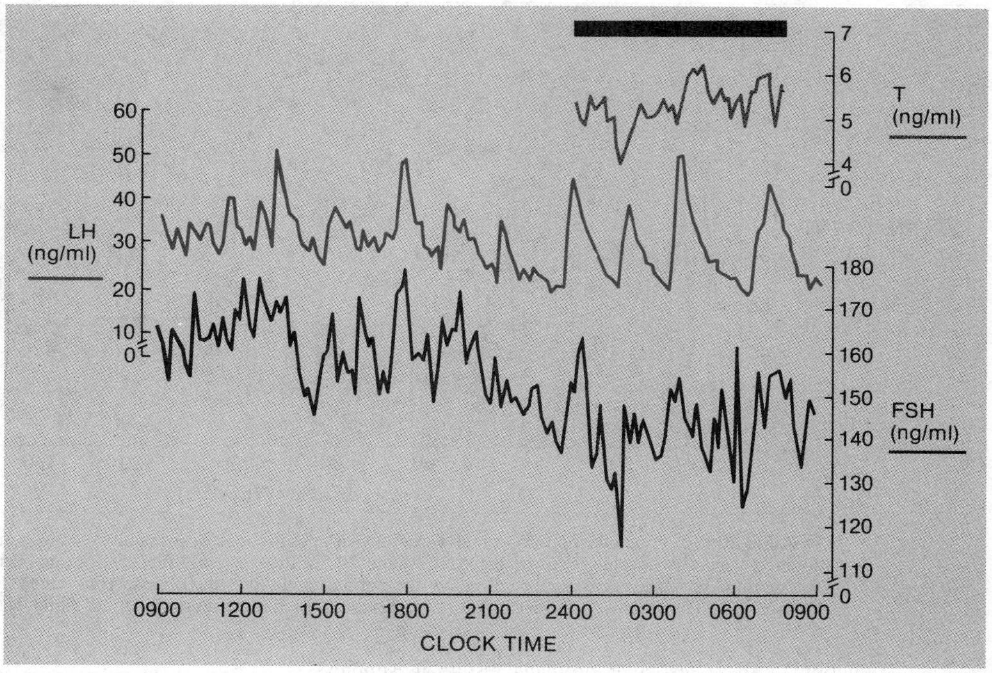

FIGURE 209-2. Example of pulsatile LH and FSH secretion throughout a 24-hour day and episodic testosterone secretion at night in a healthy young man. Blood samples were drawn at 10-minute intervals. Black bar denotes sleep, as documented by electroencephalogram.

rhosis, hyperthyroidism, and estrogens. In these situations, free or non-SHBG-bound testosterone levels should be obtained.

PERIPHERAL METABOLISM OF TESTOSTERONE. The metabolism of circulating testosterone plays a very important role in its biologic actions on target tissues. Testosterone may be converted in peripheral tissues to either *dihydrotestosterone (DHT)* or *estradiol,* which mediates many of the physiologic actions of testosterone (see Fig. 209-1).

In many androgen-dependent target tissues, testosterone is converted intracellularly to a more potent androgen, DHT, by the enzyme 5α-reductase. This conversion is required for normal male sexual differentiation (see Ch. 207). DHT mediates the androgenic effects of testosterone on skin and the prostate gland. In many peripheral tissues, especially in adipose tissue, testosterone is aromatized to estradiol, a potent estrogen. Obesity therefore results in increased peripheral estrogen formation. In men estrogens have diverse physiologic actions that may be agonistic or antagonistic to those of androgens. Therefore, the physiologic effects of testosterone result from the interactions of testosterone with its active metabolites, DHT and estradiol.

Circulating testosterone and its active metabolites are metabolized to inactive metabolites, mostly in the liver, and these metabolites are excreted primarily in the urine. In sexual tissue (including skin and prostate), DHT is efficiently metabolized to 3α-androstanediol and then to *3α-androstanediol glucuronide (3α-diol G).* Blood and urine measurements of 3α-diol G are useful markers of peripheral androgen action. In disorders in which DHT formation is reduced (such as 5α-reductase deficiency), 3α-diol G levels are reduced (see Ch. 207).

ANDROGEN ACTION AND FUNCTIONS. At the target cell, testosterone and DHT bind to intracellular androgen receptors, which interact with specific chromosomal sites to alter gene transcription and protein synthesis, resulting in expression of androgen action (see Ch. 199). Quantitative or qualitative abnormalities of the androgen receptor, resulting in impaired androgen action, cause varying degrees of male pseudohermaphroditism (see Ch. 207).

The major functions of androgens are the differentiation of male internal and external genitalia (primary sexual characteristics) during embryogenesis; the development and maintenance of secondary sexual characteristics, sexual functioning (libido and potency), certain behavioral characteristics (such as motivation), and feedback regulation of gonadotropins; and the initiation and maintenance of spermatogenesis.

FSH REGULATION OF SERTOLI CELL FUNCTION. FSH binds to specific membrane receptors on Sertoli cells of the seminiferous tubule compartment of the testis and stimulates the production of seminiferous tubule fluid and a variety of proteins thought to be important in regulating spermatogenesis (e.g., ABP, transferrin, plasminogen activator) and in feedback control of pituitary FSH secretion (inhibin and activin) (see Fig. 209-1). Testosterone produced by adjacent Leydig cells also regulates Sertoli cell functions through androgen receptors.

HORMONAL CONTROL OF SPERMATOGENESIS. Both FSH and LH stimulation are required for the initiation of spermatogenesis at the time of puberty. At this time, LH causes the differentiation of Leydig cells from interstitial connective tissue precursors and stimulates them to produce high intratesticular levels of testosterone, which are essential for sperm production. By stimulating Sertoli cell function, FSH also plays an important role in initiating spermatogenesis. In contrast to the hormonal requirements for sperm production at the time of puberty, normal levels of either FSH or LH do not appear to be absolute requirements for the maintenance of spermatogenesis in adult men.

Clinically, replacement of both FSH and LH activity is generally required to initiate sperm production in prepubertal hypogonadotropic hypogonadal patients. In contrast, initiation and maintenance of spermatogenesis in postpubertal men with acquired hypogonadotropic hypogonadism can usually be achieved with replacement of LH activity alone.

Seminal fluid analysis is used to evaluate the function of the seminiferous tubules. It is performed on seminal fluid samples obtained by masturbation after 48 hours of abstinence from ejaculation. Normal ejaculate volume ranges from 2 to 6 ml. Although the normal range of sperm concentration is generally considered to be 20 to 200 million per milliliter, sperm concentrations below 20 million per milliliter may be sufficient for fertility. In addition to determining sperm count, a careful microscopic examination of the seminal fluid is performed to assess sperm motility and morphology. Normally, >50% of sperm examined within 1 hour after ejaculation are motile, and >30% have a normal oval head morphology using stricter World Health Organization criteria.

The minimal levels of sperm concentration, motility, and oval forms compatible with fertility are not clearly defined. In any individual, sperm counts normally exhibit extreme variability (Fig. 209-3) and are often temporarily suppressed by illness. Therefore, estimates of sperm production require at least three seminal fluid analyses performed over approximately 2 months. Functional tests of sperm penetration into cervical mucus of various mammalian species or zona pellucida-free hamster ova may be helpful in assessing fertilizing capability of spermatozoa.

Testicular Feedback Regulation of Gonadotropin Secretion

Both steroid and nonsteroidal products of the testis are involved in negative feedback control of pituitary gonadotropin secretion. In-

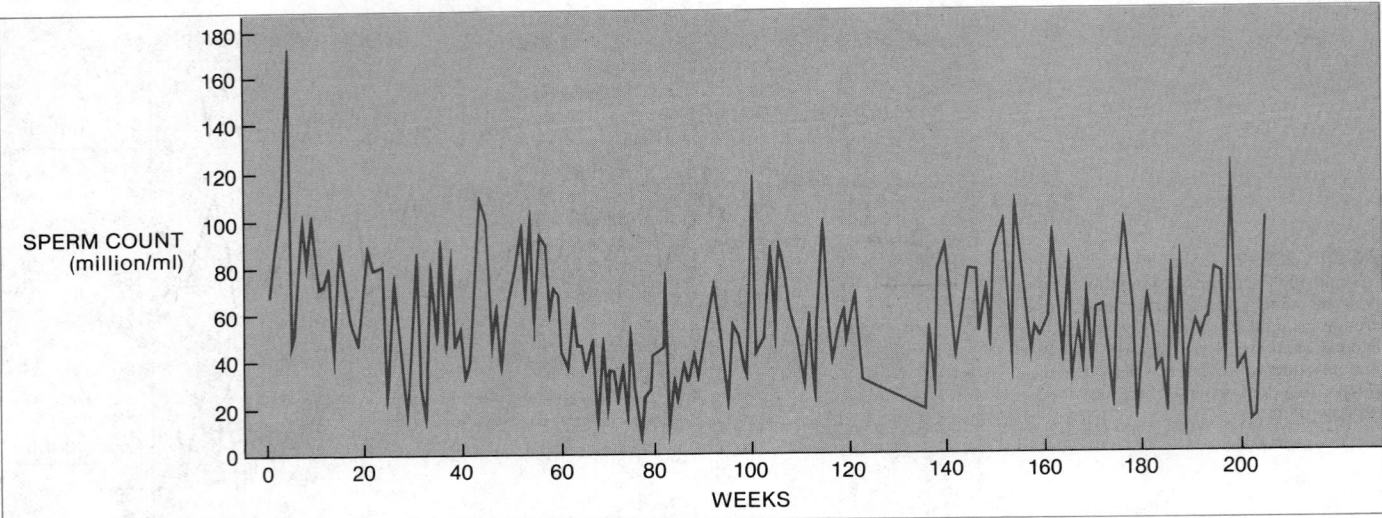

FIGURE 209-3. Example of the normal variations in sperm count in a healthy young man. Normal range of sperm count is generally considered to be between 20 and 200 million per milliliter. Despite good health and no medications, the sperm count may occasionally fall below the normal range, into the oligospermic range. (Adapted from Bardin CW, Paulsen CA: The testes. In Williams RH [ed.]: Textbook of Endocrinology, 6th ed. Philadelphia, WB Saunders, 1981.)

creased production of these testicular products results in suppression, whereas decreased production of these factors results in stimulation of gonadotropin secretion (see Fig. 209-1). Testosterone and its active metabolites, DHT and estradiol, exert profound inhibitory effects on both LH and FSH secretion, although the relative roles of these steroids are not clearly defined. Inhibin selectively inhibits FSH secretion. At present, the physiologic significance of inhibin is unclear. Knowledge of these negative feedback relationships is clinically useful in the diagnosis of hypogonadal states (see below).

Matsumoto AM, Bremner WJ: Endocrinology of the hypothalamic-pituitary-testicular axis with particular reference to the hormonal control of spermatogenesis. Bailliere's Clin Endocrinol Metab 1:71, 1987. *This paper reviews the normal physiologic regulation of testicular function, which forms the basis for understanding the pathophysiology and treatment of testicular disorders. An up-to-date discussion of the hormonal regulation of human spermatogenesis is also provided.*

Veldhuis J: The hypothalamic-pituitary-testicular axis. In Yen SCC, Jaffe RB (eds.): Reproductive Endocrinology: Physiology, Pathophysiology and Clinical Management, 3rd ed. Philadelphia, WB Saunders, 1991, p 409. *This chapter provides an excellent, detailed, and current discussion of the physiology and pathophysiology of the male reproductive axis.*

PHYSIOLOGY OF MALE SEXUAL FUNCTION

Normal male sexual function requires coordinated regulation of the following physiologic events: *libido* or sexual desire, sustained penile tumescence or *erection, ejaculation, orgasm,* and *detumescence.*

Libido

Libido is generated in the central nervous system (CNS) and stimulated by a variety of visual, tactile, imaginative, auditory, and gustatory stimuli. These stimuli are received in a number of cortical and subcortical regions of the brain, including the limbic system, and relayed via the preoptic–anterior hypothalamic area to spinal cord centers that control penile erection. Therefore, disturbances in libido are nearly always accompanied by disturbed erectile function or impotence.

Libido is regulated primarily by psychic factors and the sex steroid milieu, in particular serum testosterone concentrations. Thus, psychological disturbances of all degrees (from stress to major psychiatric illnesses), CNS lesions, drugs that alter brain function, and androgen deficiency may disturb normal libido and potency. Occasionally, castrated males maintain sexual desire and erectile function for long periods, suggesting that the requirement for androgens may be quite variable.

Erection

Erections are generated by two separate but synergistic mechanisms, one involving sensory stimulation of the genitalia, mediated through a spinal reflex arc (reflexogenic erections), and another involving psychogenic stimuli from higher brain centers (psychogenic erections). In reflexogenic erections, afferent sensory fibers from the penis travel in the pudendal nerve to the sacral spinal erection center (S2 to S4). Efferent parasympathetic fibers arising from this center travel in the nervi erigentes and innervate the blood vessels of the corpora cavernosa of the penis; efferent somatic fibers traveling in the pudendal nerve innervate the pelvic floor (ischiocavernosus and bulbocavernosus) muscles. Sympathetic fibers originating in the thoracolumbar spinal erection center (T12 to L1) innervate the muscles of the vas deferens, accessory sex glands, and internal sphincter of the bladder. In psychogenic erections, projections from higher brain centers descend in the lateral spinal columns and regulate both the thoracolumbar and sacral spinal erection centers.

Penile erectile tissue consists of paired corpora cavernosa on the dorsum of the penis and the corpus spongiosum that surrounds the urethra and forms the glans penis. The corpora are composed of spongelike, interconnected trabecular spaces lined by vascular epithelium and smooth muscle and are surrounded by a thick fibrous sheath, the tunica albuginea. Activation of the spinal erection centers results in relaxation of the penile smooth muscle and vasodilation of the cavernosal arteries (branches of the internal pudendal arteries). These actions are mediated by cholinergic and noncholinergic (e.g., vasoactive intestinal peptide) neurotransmitters, and endogenous vasodilators (e.g., nitric oxide). As a result, blood flow into the trabecular spaces of the corpora is increased, causing engorgement of the penis (tumescence). Expansion of the trabecular walls against the tunica albuginea compresses subtunical venules and impedes venous outflow, resulting in sustained tumescence, i.e., an erection.

Failure to achieve an adequate erection or impotence has many potential causes, including androgen deficiency, central and peripheral nervous system diseases, vascular disorders, and penile abnormalities. Impotence as it relates to the differential diagnosis of hypogonadism is discussed in a subsequent section of this chapter.

Ejaculation

Ejaculation is stimulated by sympathetic nervous system activation, which results in contractions of the vas deferens and accessory sex glands and emission of seminal fluid into the urethra. Emission is followed by reflex rhythmic contractions of the ischiocavernosus and bulbocavernosus muscles and expulsion of semen from the urethra, i.e., ejaculation. Like erection, the ejaculatory reflex is under considerable control by higher CNS centers. Sympathetic activation also stimulates closure of the internal urethral sphincter, thereby preventing retrograde ejaculation.

Premature ejaculation is usually due to performance anxiety or an emotional disorder and rarely has an organic cause. Retrograde ejaculation into the bladder usually occurs in patients with sympathetic neuropathy (e.g., with diabetes) or after bladder neck surgery. Reduced or absent ejaculation may occur with androgen deficiency, sympatholytic drugs, sympathectomy, or extensive retroperitoneal/pelvic surgery.

Orgasm

Orgasm, the pleasurable sensation that usually accompanies ejaculation, is primarily a CNS-mediated phenomenon that, under normal circumstances, is influenced by ascending pathways associated with ejaculation. However, orgasm can occur in the absence of erection or ejaculation (e.g., with temporal lobe lesions). Conversely, normal libido, erection, and ejaculation can occur without orgasm; this is nearly always due to a psychological disorder.

Detumescence

Detumescence results from contraction of the penile smooth muscle and α-adrenergic vasoconstriction of the cavernosal arteries, which reduce arterial blood flow into the penis. As a result, the trabecular spaces of the corpora collapse, subtunical venules are decompressed, venous outflow is increased, and the penis becomes flaccid. In many cases, premature detumescence may contribute to the pathophysiology of impotence (e.g., venous leak or incompetence). Failure of detumescence, priapism, is often painful and unrelated to sexual intercourse. It is commonly idiopathic but may be associated with spinal cord injury, sickle cell disease, chronic myelogenous leukemia, drugs (e.g., trazodone), and intracorporal injection of vasodilatory substances used in the treatment of impotence.

Korenman SG: Sexual dysfunction. *In* Wilson JD, Foster DW (eds.): Williams' Textbook of Endocrinology, 8th ed. Philadelphia, WB Saunders, 1992, p 1030. *This chapter contains a well-organized, clear, and comprehensive discussion of the physiologic and anatomic basis of male sexual function and dysfunction.*

HYPOGONADISM

Hypogonadism is the most common disorder of testicular function. The clinical manifestations of male hypogonadism differ depending on (1) whether there is *impairment of testosterone production,* which is nearly always accompanied by impairment of sperm production, or *isolated impairment of sperm production,* with normal testosterone production; (2) whether androgen deficiency occurs *during embryogenesis, before puberty,* or *after puberty;* and (3) whether testicular hypofunction is the result of a *primary* defect in the testis or is *secondary* to hypothalamic-pituitary dysfunction.

Androgen Deficiency

The clinical presentation of androgen deficiency depends on the stage of sexual development in which it occurs.

During early fetal development, testosterone and its active metabolite, DHT, mediate the differentiation of male internal and external genitalia. Androgen deficiency (e.g., due to a genetic androgen biosynthetic enzyme defect) or impaired androgen action (androgen resistance) occurring during this period of development results in varying degrees of ambiguous genital development, or *male pseudohermaphroditism* (see Ch. 207).

During puberty, testosterone is responsible for the development of male secondary sexual characteristics, such as (1) the growth of the penis and scrotum, (2) the development of accessory sexual organs (prostate and seminal vesicles) necessary to produce an ejaculate, (3) a male pattern of hair growth (face, external ear canals, chest, lower abdomen, pubis, perianal area, legs, and inner thighs) and frontal scalp regression, (4) the enlargement of the larynx and thickening of the vocal cords with consequent deepening of the voice, (5) the development of skeletal musculature and increase in strength (especially in the shoulder and pectoral muscles), (6) a redistribution of body fat, and (7) stimulation of erythropoiesis. Testosterone also stimulates the pubertal spurt of long bone growth and, eventually, the closure of long bone epiphyses, which results in cessation of bone growth. Finally androgens stimulate libido, potency, aggressive behavior, and motivation, and play an important role in initiation of spermatogenesis.

Patients who develop androgen deficiency before puberty usually present to physicians as adolescents or young adults with delayed puberty or poor male sexual development. Prepubertal testosterone deficiency results in *eunuchoidism* (Fig. 209–4), characterized by infantile genital development, failure to develop accessory sexual glands and an ejaculate (aspermia), lack of male hair pattern, high-pitched voice, poor muscular development and strength, lower abdominal–pelvic girdle fat distribution, and excessive long bone growth (due to lack of closure of long bone epiphyses). The testes are small, usually < 2 cm in length or 2 ml in volume. A eunuchoidal body habitus is characterized by excessively long arms and legs in proportion to height. Although there are racial differences in body proportions, eunuchoidal body measurements consist of an arm span that exceeds height, or a distance from the floor to symphysis pubis that exceeds that from the symphysis to the crown of the head by > 5 cm. Patients with prepubertal androgen deficiency fail to develop normal sexual functioning (libido and potency), are infertile, and may occasionally have gynecomastia (benign enlargement of breast tissue).

In the adult, testosterone is responsible for the maintenance of libido, potency, secondary sexual characteristics, and spermatogenesis. The major complaints of men with adult-onset androgen deficiency are poor sexual performance, as a result of diminished libido and/or impotence; infertility, as a result of impaired sperm production; and gynecomastia. Rapid development of severe androgen deficiency (e.g., with surgical castration) may also cause vasomotor instability or hot flushes, similar to those that many women develop at the time of menopause. Androgen deficiency may also result in behavioral changes, such as passivity, lack of motivation, and irritability.

Secondary sexual characteristics do not regress to the prepubertal state in men who develop testosterone deficiency as adults. However, with longstanding androgen deficiency, there may be significant loss of hair in androgen-dependent areas of the body, fine wrinkling of skin (most noticeable around the eyes and mouth), diminished muscle strength and mass, osteoporosis, and altered fat distribution. In hypogonadal men, pubic hair may assume a female type, inverted triangular pattern (female escutcheon), in contrast to the male type, diamond-shaped distribution, with hair extending to the umbilicus (male escutcheon). The testes are usually small in hypogonadal states. However, depending on the specific cause and severity of the disorder, testis size may be normal. For example, men with recent onset of gonadotropin deficiency from a destructive pituitary tumor may have normal size testes, despite severe testosterone deficiency.

Serum testosterone levels are low in states of androgen deficiency. Routinely available assays measure total testosterone and may give falsely low values in clinical states in which sex hormone–binding globulin is reduced (e.g., obesity). In these instances serum free or non–SHBG-bound testosterone levels should be measured.

Testosterone helps to maintain quantitatively normal spermatogenesis in man; androgen deficiency, therefore, almost always results in reduced sperm production. Impaired spermatogenesis is confirmed by a low sperm count on seminal fluid analysis. Because sperm counts are highly variable and often suppressed by illness, at least three sperm counts obtained over 2 months while patients are well should be performed before a diagnosis of oligospermia (low sperm counts) is made.

Isolated Deficiency in Sperm Production

In contrast to patients with androgen deficiency, men with an isolated deficiency of sperm production present postpubertally with infertility as their major complaint, without symptoms of testosterone deficiency. Testis size may be reduced or normal and an undescended testis or *varicocele* (varicose dilatation of the pampiniform venous plexus of the scrotum) may be found. The remainder of the physical examination is usually unremarkable. Sperm counts are usually low (< 20 million per milliliter) or zero (*azoospermia*), and there may be associated or isolated abnormalities of sperm motility and/or morphology on seminal fluid analysis. Serum testosterone levels are normal in disorders causing isolated impairment of sperm production.

Differential Diagnosis

The major manifestations of androgen deficiency in adults are impotence, infertility, and gynecomastia. Although hypogonadism resulting in testosterone deficiency is a major cause of these clinical manifestations, there are many other causes.

IMPOTENCE. Impotence is defined as a consistent inability to achieve or maintain penile erection that is adequate for completion of sexual intercourse. It is a commonly encountered complaint in

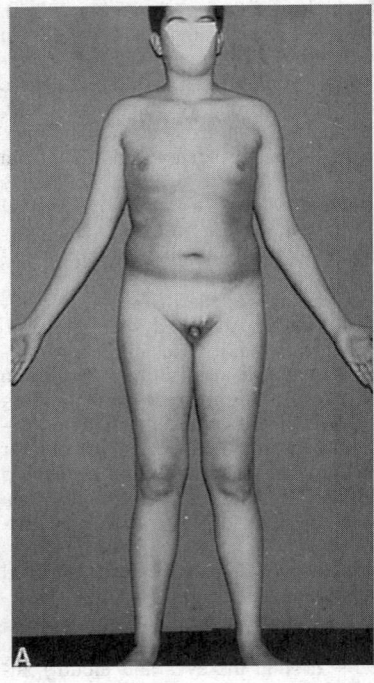
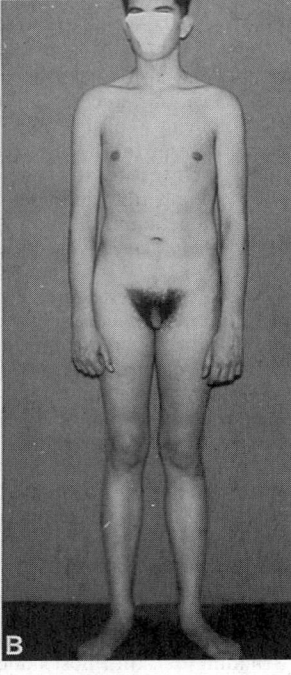
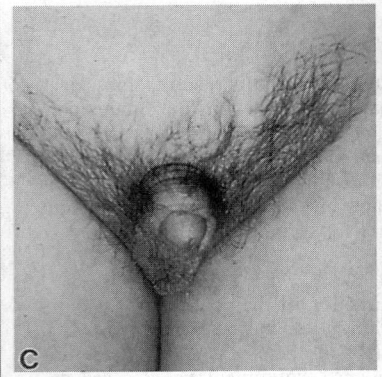
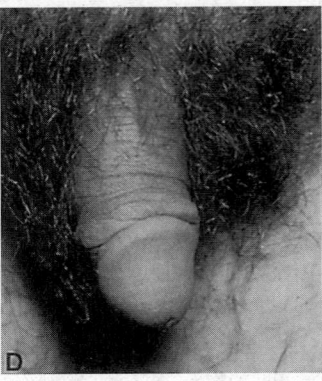

FIGURE 209–4. Example of eunuchoidism as a result of prepubertal androgen deficiency due to functional prepubertal castrate syndrome. *A* and *C,* Before androgen therapy, note the eunuchoidal features of infantile genital development, lack of male hair pattern, poor muscular development, pelvic girdle and lower abdominal fat distribution, and disproportionately long arms and legs. No testicular tissue was identified at the time of surgical exploration. *B* and *D,* After 18 months of testosterone treatment, scalp hair recession, penile development, and pubic hair growth have occurred. A masculine body habitus has developed, with an increase in pectoral and shoulder muscle development and loss of pelvic girdle and lower abdominal fat. (From Bardin CW, Paulsen CA: The testes. *In* Williams RH [ed.]: Textbook of Endocrinology, 6th ed. Philadelphia, WB Saunders, 1981.)

medical practice, occurring in 10 to 35% of adult men with medical problems and increasing in prevalence with advancing age. Impotence is often underdiagnosed because of reluctance of patients and physicians to discuss sexual dysfunction as a medical problem. Although psychogenic impotence is common, the majority of men with impotence who are followed in a general medical clinic have one or more organic causes of erectile dysfunction. Organic causes of impotence often result in performance anxiety and secondary psychogenic sexual dysfunction.

Penile erection sufficient to complete intercourse requires (1) normal *CNS* and thoracolumbar sympathetic and sacral parasympathetic *spinal cord* outputs to the penis; (2) an intact *arterial supply* and *venous drainage* of the penis; and (3) an *anatomically normal penis*. Dysfunction of any of these components interferes with normal initiation and maintenance of penile erection (Table 209–1).

Normal CNS function is necessary to produce adequate penile erections. *Libido* or sexual desire, mediated by the cerebral cortex and limbic system, has a profound influence on erectile function. In most CNS disorders that cause sexual dysfunction, reduced libido is usually associated with impotence. All degrees of *psychiatric disturbance,* from minor stress and performance anxiety to major psychiatric illness, such as depression and schizophrenia; *chronic debilitating illness,* such as cardiac, respiratory, renal, or liver disease or malignancy; and *drugs* that affect CNS function (sedatives, antipsychotics, antidepressants, centrally acting antihypertensive agents, and alcohol), are CNS causes of impotence that also generally reduce libido. *Androgen deficiency, hyperprolactinemia,* and *thyroid dysfunction* (hyperthyroidism and hypothyroidism) also impair libido and potency. Elevated prolactin levels may cause impotence by inducing secondary hypogonadism and androgen deficiency. In contrast to these disorders, *destructive or infiltrative diseases* of certain regions of the *brain* (such as tumor or infarction of the temporal lobe or limbic system) or *spinal cord diseases* (such as injury, tumor, multiple sclerosis, or syphilis) may cause impotence without associated loss of libido. Patients with high spinal cord le-sions (above T11) usually retain the ability to have reflexogenic erections.

In addition to intact CNS functioning, normal penile erection requires intact peripheral nervous system function, adequate blood flow to the penis, and normal erectile structures within the penis. *Disorders of peripheral autonomic nerve function* that cause impotence include extensive pelvic surgery, such as aortoiliac bypass, pelvic lymph node dissection, abdominoperineal resection of the rectum, lumbar sympathectomy, and prostatectomy; diabetes; and other conditions causing peripheral autonomic and sensory neuropathy. Atherosclerotic *peripheral vascular disease* involving the distal

aortoiliac arteries and *trauma* to these vessels are the most common causes of vascular impotence. These patients usually have diminished or absent femoral pulses and may present with *Leriche's syndrome,* although claudication may be absent in some cases. In addition, autonomic neuropathy and atherosclerotic macro- and microvascular disease are major factors contributing to erectile dysfunction in the 30 to 50% of diabetic men who develop impotence. Penile venous incompetence (venous leak) resulting in inadequate

TABLE 209–1. CAUSES OF IMPOTENCE

I. Disorders of Central Nervous System Control	II. Disorders of Peripheral Erectile Response
Psychiatric Illness	Drugs
Stress	Anticholinergic drugs
Performance anxiety	Antidepressants
Depression	Antihistamines
Major psychiatric illness	β-Adrenergic blockers
Chronic Illness	Sympathomimetic drugs
Cardiac disease	α-Adrenergic agonists
Respiratory disease	Antihypertensive agents
Renal disease	Autonomic Neuropathy
Liver disease	Pelvic surgery
Malignancy	Diabetes
Central Nervous System– Active Drugs	Other peripheral neuropathies
Sedatives	Vascular Disease
Antipsychotics	Distal aortoiliac atherosclerosis
Antidepressants	Diabetes
Central antihypertensives	Trauma
Alcohol	Venous incompetence
Endocrine Disorders	Penile Abnormalities
Hypogonadism (androgen deficiency)	Peyronie's disease
Hyperprolactinemia	Chordee
Thyroid disease	Priapism
Central Nervous System Disease	Trauma
Temporal lobe disorders	Microphallus or micropenis
Limbic system disorders	
Spinal Cord Disease	
Trauma	
Multiple sclerosis	
Syphilis	
Other spinal cord lesions	

veno-occlusion to sustain an erection is an uncommon cause of impotence. *Penile abnormalities,* such as Peyronie's disease, chordee, priapism, and microphallus, may also cause erectile dysfunction. *Drugs* may cause erectile dysfunction by inhibiting penile smooth muscle relaxation and arterial vasodilation (anticholinergic drugs, antidepressants, antihistamines, β-adrenergic blockers) or by inducing premature detumescence (sympathomimetic drugs, α-adrenergic agonists). The mechanism of impotence associated with certain antihypertensive agents (e.g., diuretics, vasodilators, sympatholytic agents) is unclear.

Normal testosterone levels are necessary for maintenance of libido and potency. Hypogonadism resulting in androgen deficiency is a cause of impotence in approximately 15 to 20% of men complaining of sexual dysfunction in a general medical clinic. Therefore, all impotent patients should have serum testosterone and gonadotropin levels measured as part of their diagnostic workup.

A thorough history and physical examination provide invaluable clues to the cause of impotence. Erectile dysfunction that occurs abruptly and is transient, intermittent, or temporally associated with stress is usually psychogenic in origin. Men with psychogenic impotence often have spontaneous nocturnal or morning erections and are able to achieve normal erections with some partners but not with others or with masturbation but not during sexual intercourse. Patients with impotence related to central or peripheral nervous system or vascular disease or penile abnormalities usually demonstrate clinical manifestations of the underlying disorder. A careful drug history may reveal offending medications that cause impotence.

Measurement of nocturnal penile tumescence (NPT) and buckling pressure may be used to differentiate psychogenic from organic impotence. NPT is usually present in psychogenic impotence but abnormal or absent if there is an organic cause of erectile dysfunction. Formal evaluation is done in a sleep laboratory with EEG monitoring to detect sleep disturbances that may disturb NPT. Resistance of the penis to buckling is also measured; this measurement correlates better than NPT alone with ability to have sexual intercourse. A simpler assessment of NPT can be made by wrapping the shaft of the penis with a snap gauge; NPT is detected by breaking of wires of different tensile strength.

Doppler determination of the ratio of supine penile systolic blood pressure to brachial systolic blood pressure (penile/brachial index) may be useful in diagnosing patients with penile arterial vascular insufficiency. An index >0.75 is normal; one between 0.75 and 0.60 is indeterminate; and one <0.6 is suggestive of arteriovascular impotence, which may be confirmed by arteriography. Recently, intracavernosal injection of vasodilatory agents with and without duplex ultrasonography or direct pressure monitoring has been used in the evaluation of impotence. Development of a sustained erectile response implies normal vascular status, whereas a short-lived, partial, or absent response suggests a hemodynamic abnormality. Corporal veno-occlusion is usually evaluated by cavernosometry and cavernosography following intracavernosal injection of a vasodilating drug. In the absence of neurogenic bladder dysfunction, electromyographic determination of the bulbocavernosus reflex latency and somatosensory evoked response of the dorsal nerve may be useful in detecting peripheral and sacral spinal abnormalities contributing to impotence.

Treatment of impotence is directed at the underlying causes of erectile dysfunction. Psychosexual education, counseling, and therapy are very successful in restoring sexual function in many men with psychogenic impotence. Testosterone therapy should be reserved for hypogonadal men with androgen deficiency in whom libido and potency are restored with adequate androgen replacement. Men with impotence and hypogonadism due to hyperprolactinemia may require agents to lower prolactin levels (e.g., bromocriptine) in addition to testosterone replacement to improve potency. Self-administration of intracavernosal injections of vasodilatory drugs (e.g., prostaglandin E, papaverine and/or phentolamine) induces penile erections sufficient for sexual intercourse in many patients with impotence. In general, it is very effective and well tolerated. Patients with severe arterial insufficiency or venous leaks are least likely to respond to this therapy. Select patients with vascular impotence are candidates for corrective surgical procedures.

In patients for whom effective therapy is not available, surgical implantation of a penile prosthesis offers rigidity sufficient for sexual intercourse without interfering with ejaculation or orgasm. Recently, vacuum-constriction devices have been introduced as a non-surgical alternative to penile prostheses for the treatment of impotence. A condom-like cylinder is placed over the flaccid penis; a vacuum is applied to generate negative pressure, drawing blood into the penis and resulting in an erection. A constrictive band is then placed around the base of the penis to prevent the drainage of blood from the penis, maintaining tumescence for the duration of intercourse.

INFERTILITY. Infertility is defined as the inability of a couple to achieve a pregnancy after 1 year of unprotected intercourse. An estimated 5 to 6% of men in the reproductive age group are infertile. Most causes of male infertility result in abnormal sperm count or semen quality, as reflected by an abnormal seminal fluid analysis. About 90% of male infertility is caused by hypogonadism resulting in impaired spermatogenesis; and 80 to 90% of these men have isolated deficiency of sperm production with normal androgen production of unclear origin, i.e., *idiopathic oligospermia or azoospermia* (see below). Other causes of male infertility include *coital disorders, ductal obstruction, ejaculatory dysfunction,* and *disorders of accessory sexual organs* (Table 209–2). Even if a cause of male infertility is diagnosed, the female partner should undergo diagnostic evaluation because a concomitant female factor causing infertility is found in 30% of infertile couples.

Although uncommon, *defects* in the *coital technique,* such as timing of intercourse during menses, rather than at the time of ovulation near mid-cycle, premature withdrawal of the penis, prior ejaculation, and infrequent intercourse are causes of male infertility. They are important to remember because they are potentially reversible with proper patient education. Basal body temperature measurements or rapid immunoassay kits measuring urinary LH levels are methods often used to estimate the timing of ovulation in the partner's menstrual cycle. *Erectile dysfunction* from any cause may result in unsuccessful intercourse and infertility.

Impediment of sperm transport from the testis to the urethra results in azoospermia and infertility. Causes of *ductal obstruction* include congenital absence of the vas deferens or seminal vesicles often associated with cystic fibrosis; congenital defects of the epididymis or vas, e.g., as a consequence of diethylstilbestrol exposure *in utero;* fibrosis as a complication of genitourinary infection, especially epididymitis; Young's syndrome, in which thickened, inspissated mucous secretions lead to blockage of the epididymis and vas deferens; and vasectomy.

Obstructive azoospermia must be differentiated from a severe defect in spermatogenesis. Measurement of a serum FSH level is often helpful because elevated levels generally indicate disordered seminiferous tubular function. Normal FSH levels may occur in either obstructive azoospermia or seminiferous tubule dysfunction. In obstructive azoospermia, radiologic examination, i.e., a vasogram, demonstrates the ductal obstruction, and a testicular biopsy reveals normal spermatogenesis. Evaluation of azoospermia is one of the few indications for performing a testicular biopsy. Vasectomy has been used widely and successfully to induce infertility in men who desire fertility control, without deleterious effects on the hypothalamic-pituitary-testicular axis or general health. Using microsurgical

TABLE 209–2. CAUSES OF MALE INFERTILITY

Coital Disorders
   Defects in Technique
      Poor timing with menses
      Premature withdrawal
      Infrequent intercourse
   Impotence
Hypogonadism (Deficiency of Sperm Production)
Ductal Obstruction
   Congenital Defects of Vas Deferens, Epididymides, or Seminal Vesicles
   Postinfectious Obstruction
   Cystic Fibrosis/Young's Syndrome
   Vasectomy
Ejaculatory Dysfunction
   Premature Ejaculation
   Retrograde Ejaculation
Disorders of Accessory Glands
   Epididymitis/Seminal Vesiculitis/Prostatitis
   Immunologic

techniques, vasovasostomy has been used successfully to restore fertility in vasectomized men. Despite return of sperm in the ejaculate in 80 to 90%, fertility is restored in only 30 to 50% of men after vasovasostomy.

Ejaculatory dysfunction, such as premature or retrograde ejaculation, can cause infertility by preventing the normal deposition of sperm into the female genital tract. Premature ejaculation is often successfully treated by sex therapy techniques. Retrograde ejaculation most commonly results from diabetic autonomic neuropathy, prostatic resection, pelvic surgery, or administration of sympatholytic drugs. It is suspected if orgasm produces little or no ejaculate and is confirmed by the presence of large numbers of sperm in a postejaculation urine sample. Sympathomimetic drugs, imipramine, and harvesting and concentrating of sperm from the urine for artificial insemination have been used to treat retrograde ejaculation.

Disorders of the *accessory sexual organs* result in infertility by a number of mechanisms. Infections of the epididymis, seminal vesicles, and/or prostate have been reported to cause infertility by affecting sperm maturation or function directly or by inducing antisperm antibodies that, in turn, affect sperm function. Offending organisms include *Neisseria gonorrhoea, Chlamydia trachomatis,* coliforms, *Ureaplasma urealyticum,* and *Mycobacterium tuberculosis.* Antisperm antibodies present in the semen may cause sperm agglutination and reduce sperm motility. Induction of these antibodies after vasectomy may be responsible for the discrepancy between the success rate for return of sperm in the ejaculate and restoration of fertility after vasectomy reversal. Glucocorticoid therapy can lower antisperm antibody titers and improve fertility in some patients.

GYNECOMASTIA. Gynecomastia, a benign glandular enlargement of the male breast, is usually asymptomatic, but its rapid development may cause pain and tenderness. It is often very difficult to distinguish between true gynecomastia and an increase in adipose tissue in obese boys or men. In order to adequately detect gynecomastia, fingers should be used to grasp the tissue surrounding the areola in a pinching action.

Although usually bilateral, gynecomastia may be markedly asymmetric or rarely unilateral. In these instances, gynecomastia must be distinguished from other benign chest wall tumors and male breast cancer. In contrast to benign lesions, breast carcinoma is usually eccentric in location, hard, and associated with skin or nipple retraction and bloody discharge; lymphadenopathy due to metastatic disease may also be found.

Gynecomastia usually occurs when the breast is exposed to a hormonal milieu of increased estrogen relative to testosterone concentration or action, i.e., an increased estrogen/testosterone ratio. An increased ratio may result from pathologic conditions or drugs that either increase estrogen or reduce testosterone levels or action of these hormones. Because both of these hormonal alterations commonly result in primary or secondary hypogonadism, hypogonadal states are major causes of gynecomastia. Unless hyperprolactinemia induces androgen deficiency by inhibiting gonadotropin secretion, elevated prolactin levels do not usually cause gynecomastia. The clinical causes of gynecomastia are summarized in Table 209–3.

Gynecomastia may sometimes be *physiologic* rather than pathologic. Transient gynecomastia is usually seen in neonatal boys, as a result of exposure *in utero* to high maternal estrogen concentrations. At the time of puberty, gynecomastia is observed in 60 to 70% of boys. Pubertal gynecomastia usually lasts for months to years and does not persist into adulthood. Finally, small amounts of palpable breast tissue (2 to 3 cm in diameter) can be detected by careful examination in 40% of healthy normal adult men, increasing in prevalence with advancing age.

In addition to *androgen deficiency* and *disorders of androgen action,* gynecomastia may be caused by a number of *drugs.* Gynecomastia may result from exposure to exogenous estrogen, e.g., from diethylstilbestrol treatment of metastatic prostate cancer, or accidental ingestion, use, contact, or occupational exposure. Excessive circulating estrogens inhibit endogenous gonadotropin secretion, resulting in secondary hypogonadism and reduced testosterone production that contributes to the development of gynecomastia. Administration of high doses of aromatizable androgens, especially to prepubertal boys or severely hypogonadal men, may induce gy-

TABLE 209–3. CAUSES OF GYNECOMASTIA

I. Physiologic Gynecomastia
  Neonatal
  Pubertal
  Adult
	V. Tumors
	  Estrogen-Secreting
	    Tumors
	    Adrenal carcinoma
	    Leydig cell or Sertoli
	      cell tumor of testis
	  Gonadotropin-Secreting
	    Tumors
	    Testicular carcinoma
	    Lung carcinoma
	    Liver carcinoma

II. Hypogonadism (Deficiency of Androgen Production)	
III. Androgen Resistance Syndromes	

IV. Drug-Induced Gynecomastia
  Hormones
    Estrogens
    Aromatizable androgens
    hCG
  Drugs Interacting with
    Estrogen Receptor
    Marijuana
    Digitalis
  Drugs Altering Androgen
    Production or Action
    Spironolactone
    Cimetidine
    Ketoconazole
    Cytotoxic agents
  Central Nervous System–
    Active Drugs
    Antihypertensive agents
    Tranquilizers
    Sedatives
    Antidepressants
    Amphetamines
	VI. Systemic Disorders
	  Hepatic Cirrhosis
	  Renal Failure
	  Thyrotoxicosis
	
	VII. Miscellaneous
	  Refeeding Gynecomastia
	  Familial
	  Increased Peripheral
	    Aromatization
	  Local Chest Trauma

necomastia analogous to that which occurs at puberty. hCG binds to LH receptors on Leydig cells, stimulates relatively greater testicular production of estradiol than testosterone, and may cause gynecomastia. Certain drugs result in breast enlargement by interacting with the estrogen receptor (marijuana, digitalis) or by interfering with androgen production or action (spironolactone, cimetidine, ketoconazole, certain cytotoxic agents). Finally, many CNS-active drugs, such as certain antihypertensives, sedatives, tranquilizers, antidepressants, and amphetamines, are associated with gynecomastia.

Although very uncommon, gynecomastia may be the initial manifestation of an *estrogen-secreting tumor* of the adrenal gland or testis. Feminizing adrenal tumors are usually malignant and present with a palpable abdominal mass. In contrast, estrogen-secreting tumors of the testis are often small and benign. *hCG-secreting tumors,* such as testicular, lung, and hepatic carcinoma, may cause gynecomastia by stimulating excessive estrogen relative to testosterone secretion by Leydig cells. A specific β-hCG assay should be used to confirm the diagnosis of an hCG-secreting tumor.

Certain *systemic disorders* are associated with gynecomastia. In hepatic cirrhosis, gynecomastia is associated with increased estrogen production, primarily as a result of accelerated peripheral conversion of adrenal androgens (androstenedione) to estrone. In addition, serum SHBG levels are elevated, and bioavailable serum testosterone levels are low, contributing to an increased estrogen/testosterone ratio. The gynecomastia observed in patients with renal failure is associated with androgen deficiency resulting from testicular failure, and estrogen production is not usually increased. High estradiol levels and relatively reduced bioavailable testosterone levels (as a result of increased SHBG levels) are commonly found in patients with thyrotoxicosis and contribute to the development of gynecomastia in this condition.

Gynecomastia is often associated with nutritional repletion and weight gain after a period of starvation and weight loss. This *refeeding gynecomastia* was originally described in former prisoners of war who developed tender gynecomastia following their liberation and resumption of a normal diet. A similar condition may occur upon recovery from any prolonged, severe illness associated with malnutrition and weight loss. Refeeding gynecomastia may contribute to the gynecomastia associated with hemodialysis in chronic renal failure patients. Malnutrition results in severe suppression of the hypothalamic-pituitary-testicular axis. Restoration of nutrition rapidly restores gonadal function ("second puberty") and may explain the gynecomastia associated with refeeding. *Familial* gynecomastia, chest wall trauma and pain, and idiopathic increase in peripheral aromatase activity are very rare causes of gynecomastia.

Treatment of gynecomastia should focus on the correction of the underlying disorder or withdrawal of the offending drug. Prophylactic low-dose irradiation of the breast prior to diethylstilbestrol treatment in men with prostatic carcinoma prevents gynecomastia. Testosterone treatment of androgen deficiency may occasionally result in resolution of gynecomastia. Experience with the estrogen antagonists (such as tamoxifen), nonaromatizable androgens (such as dihydrotestosterone), and aromatase inhibitors in treating gynecomastia has been limited and variably effective. Severe, longstanding gynecomastia of any cause is usually associated with increased fibrous tissue stroma and requires surgical reduction mammoplasty.

Braunstein GD: Gynecomastia. N Engl J Med 328:490, 1993. *A well-organized, clearly written, concise review of the causes, pathogenesis, evaluation, and treatment of gynecomastia.*

Dial LK (ed.): Geriatric sexuality. Clin Geriatr Med 7:1, 1991. *The entire issue is devoted to sexuality in older adults, with very good chapters on sexuality and impotence in aging men, urologic and endocrine considerations in geriatric sexual dysfunction, and the impact of medications and chronic diseases on sexual function in the elderly.*

Lipshultz LI (eds.): Male infertility. Urol Clin North Am 21:1, 1994. *An excellent, comprehensive discussion of the evaluation and treatment of male infertility by several authors.*

Morley JE, Kaiser FE: Impotence: The internist's approach to diagnosis and treatment. Adv Intern Med 38:151, 1993. *An excellent review of the etiology, diagnosis, and treatment of erectile dysfunction from an internist's perspective.*

NIH Consensus Development Panel on Impotence: Impotence. JAMA 270:83, 1993. *A consensus statement by an interdisciplinary panel of experts that reviews current knowledge regarding the epidemiology, etiology, risk factors, pathophysiology, diagnosis, management, and consequences of impotence.*

Skakkebaek NE, Giwercman A, deKretser D: Pathogenesis and management of male infertility. Lancet 343:1473, 1994. *An updated, concise review of the causes and treatment of male infertility.*

CAUSES OF MALE HYPOGONADISM

Once the diagnosis of male hypogonadism is suspected, the diagnosis is confirmed by measurement of serum testosterone level and sperm count.

The majority of hypogonadal men with *androgen deficiency* also have impairment in sperm production. Once androgen deficiency is diagnosed (low serum testosterone and sperm count), an effort should be made to distinguish between disorders that result from primary testicular disease (*primary hypogonadism*) and those that are secondary to inadequate gonadotropin stimulation of the testis (*secondary hypogonadism*), as a result of either pituitary or hypothalamic disease.

In addition to helping to determine the specific cause of androgen deficiency, the distinction between primary and secondary hypogonadism may have practical therapeutic implications. For example, regardless of the specific cause, primary hypogonadism is usually treated with androgen replacement. In the majority of cases, the infertility in primary hypogonadism is not treatable. However, secondary hypogonadism may result from destruction of pituitary gonadotropin-secreting cells, for example by a pituitary tumor. In this instance, in addition to androgen deficiency, the space-occupying effects of the tumor mass on brain function (such as visual fields and cerebroventricular flow) and alterations (both increase and decrease) in the secretion of other anterior pituitary hormones (such as ACTH, TSH, growth hormone, and prolactin) need to be considered in formulating a therapeutic plan (see Ch. 202.1). Furthermore, because the testes usually function normally in response to adequate gonadotropin stimulation in patients with secondary hypogonadism, gonadotropins (or LHRH for hypothalamic hypogonadism) may be administered in these patients to stimulate spermatogenesis and induce fertility.

The negative feedback relationship between gonadotropin secretion and circulating testosterone levels (see Fig. 209–1) provides the physiologic basis and rationale for the use of serum gonadotropin levels to distinguish between primary and secondary testicular disorders that result in androgen deficiency. Because the negative feedback effect of testosterone on gonadotropin secretion is reduced, men with *primary hypogonadism* have reduced serum testosterone and elevated serum LH and FSH levels; i.e., they have *hypergonadotropic hypogonadism*. Not uncommonly, serum FSH levels may be disproportionately elevated compared with LH levels, especially with severe seminiferous tubule dysfunction.

In contrast to primary testicular dysfunction, men with *secondary hypogonadism* are not able to increase gonadotropin secretion appropriately in the presence of reduced testosterone negative feedback and have inadequate gonadotropin stimulation of the testis. These men have a hormonal pattern of reduced serum testosterone and low to low normal serum LH and FSH levels; i.e., they have *hypogonadotropic hypogonadism*. Gonadotropin levels are often in the low normal range in men with secondary hypogonadism because most clinically available gonadotropin assays lack sufficient sensitivity to distinguish low from low normal values.

The majority of hypogonadal patients with *isolated impairment of sperm production* have primary testicular disease. These patients generally present with infertility and have no clinical manifestations of androgen deficiency. Serum testosterone and gonadotropin levels are usually normal. Infertile patients who present with no sperm in their ejaculate, i.e., azoospermia, may have either severe seminiferous tubule failure or obstruction of the genital tract. Measurement of serum FSH level may be helpful in evaluation of these patients. A selective elevation of serum FSH with normal LH levels in a patient with azoospermia implies severe germ cell dysfunction and poor prognosis for fertility. No further workup is usually necessary. A normal serum FSH level in an azoospermic patient leaves open the possibility of a surgically correctable ductal obstruction, and ultrasonography or vasography, and occasionally a testicular biopsy are performed. Selective elevation in serum FSH levels may also be observed in patients with gonadotropin-secreting pituitary adenomas. Uncommonly, isolated deficiency of sperm production results from inadequate gonadotropin stimulation of the testis. In these instances, serum gonadotropin levels are generally reduced, and very rarely selective FSH deficiency may occur.

The vast majority of adults with male hypogonadism have either primary or secondary testicular failure. Very rarely, *disorders of androgen action* may present in adults with a clinical picture of hypogonadism. Unlike the severe androgen resistance syndromes, which present at birth with male pseudohermaphroditism (see Ch. 207), these disorders are characterized by mild defects in androgen action, resulting in a nearly normal male phenotype (frequently with varying degrees of hypospadias). Both serum testosterone and gonadotropin levels are usually elevated.

In summary, clinical manifestations combined with measurements of serum testosterone, sperm count, and basal serum gonadotropin levels permit a physiologic classification of the causes of male hypogonadism into *primary* and *secondary hypogonadism* and subclassification into disorders that result in *deficiency of both sperm and androgen production,* and those with *isolated deficiency in sperm production* with normal androgen production (Table 209–4).

Primary Hypogonadism

DEFICIENCY OF SPERM AND ANDROGEN PRODUCTION. *Congenital or Developmental Disorders.* *Klinefelter's syndrome* is the most common cause of primary testicular failure resulting in impairment of both spermatogenesis and testosterone production. The syndrome is characterized by small, firm testes, azoospermia, gynecomastia, varying degrees of eunuchoidism and testosterone deficiency, and elevated gonadotropin levels. Klinefelter's syndrome is a very common disorder, affecting 1 in every 400 to 500 men. The incidence of Klinefelter's syndrome increases to 5% when maternal age is over 45 years. The fundamental defect in Klinefelter's syndrome and its variants is the presence of one or a number of extra X chromosomes.

Classically, the karyotype in Klinefelter's syndrome is 47 XXY, resulting from meiotic nondisjunction in either the maternal or paternal gamete. Variants of the syndrome demonstrate a variety of karyotypes, including XXYY, more than two X (poly X) plus Y, and mosaicism. In classic Klinefelter's syndrome (47 XXY), the presence of an extra X chromosome is responsible for the presence of a sex chromatin or Barr body in the nucleus of epithelial cells obtained on buccal smear, a normal finding in females, who carry two X chromosomes. The diagnosis of Klinefelter's syndrome is confirmed by karyotyping of lymphocytes or testicular tissue.

Clinical features of Klinefelter's syndrome are not evident prior to puberty. At the time of puberty, the testes fail to increase in size and become firmer in consistency. This is a result of fibrosis of the seminiferous tubules. The most remarkable clinical feature of Klinefelter's syndrome is the very small size of the testes, rarely exceeding 2 cm in length, in contrast to a lower limit of 3.5 cm in the nor-

TABLE 209-4. CAUSES OF MALE HYPOGONADISM

I. Primary Hypogonadism
Deficiency of Sperm and Androgen Production
    Congenital or Developmental Disorders
      Klinefelter's syndrome and variants
      Functional prepubertal castrate syndrome
      Noonan (Bonnevie-Ullrich) syndrome
      Myotonic dystrophy
      Polyglandular autoimmune disease
      Complex genetic disorders
      ? Normal aging
    Acquired Disorders
      Orchitis (mumps, leprosy, etc.)
      Surgical or traumatic castration
      Drugs (spironolactone, ketoconazole, H_2-receptor blockers, alcohol, marijuana, digitalis, cytotoxic drugs)
      Irradiation
    Systemic Disorders
      Chronic liver disease
      Chronic renal failure
      Malignancy (Hodgkin's, testicular)
      Sickle cell disease
      Paraplegia
      Vasculitis (periarteritis)
      Infiltrative disease (amyloidosis)
Isolated Deficiency of Sperm Production
    Congenital or Developmental Disorders
      Germinal cell aplasia (Sertoli cell–only syndrome)
      Cryptorchidism
      Varicocele
      Immotile cilia syndrome (Kartagener's syndrome)
      Myotonic dystrophy
    Acquired Disorders
      Orchitis (mumps, leprosy, etc.)
      Thermal trauma
      Irradiation
      Cytotoxic drugs
      Environmental toxins
    Systemic Disorders
      Acute febrile illness
      Paraplegia
    Idiopathic Oligospermia or Azoospermia

II. Secondary Hypogonadism
Deficiency of Sperm and Androgen Production
    Congenital or Developmental Disorders
      Hypogonadotropic eunuchoidism (Kallmann's syndrome)
      Hemochromatosis
      Complex genetic syndromes
      ? Normal aging
    Acquired Disorders
      Hypopituitarism
      Hyperprolactinemia
      Estrogen excess
      Progestins
      Androgenic anabolic steroids
      Opiate-like drugs
    Systemic Disorders
      Glucocorticoid excess (Cushing's syndrome)
      Acute stress or illness
      Nutritional deficiency (protein-calorie malnutrition, anorexia nervosa)
      Chronic illness
      Massive obesity
Isolated Deficiency of Sperm Production
    Androgen Excess
      Congenital adrenal hyperplasia (21- and 11β-hydroxylase deficiency)
      Androgenic anabolic steroids
      Androgen-secreting tumors
    Hyperprolactinemia
    Isolated FSH Deficiency

III. Androgen Resistance Syndromes
Reifenstein's Syndrome
Idiopathic Oligospermia or Azoospermia
? Celiac Disease

---

mal adult. Clinical androgen deficiency is usually present but variable in degree, resulting in varying degrees of eunuchoidism (Fig. 209–5). In contrast to other conditions that result in eunuchoidism, Klinefelter's syndrome often results in a disproportionate increase in lower compared with upper extremity long bone growth. Careful palpation usually reveals bilateral gynecomastia in 80 to 90% of patients. Although the incidence of mental retardation is greater, the majority of patients with Klinefelter's syndrome have normal intelligence. Most patients exhibit character and personality disorders that may be related, in part, to the psychosocial consequences of androgen deficiency. There is a slightly increased incidence of certain systemic diseases in Klinefelter's syndrome. These include diabetes, chronic obstructive pulmonary disease, autoimmune disorders (e.g., systemic lupus erythematosus, Hashimoto's thyroiditis), malignancy (breast cancer, lymphoma, germ cell neoplasms), and varicose veins.

The clinical manifestations of Klinefelter's syndrome variants differ from those of the classic 47 XXY syndrome. In general, the presence of more than two extra X chromosomes results in a much higher incidence of mental retardation and somatic abnormalities, such as hypospadias, cryptorchidism, and bony abnormalities of the radius and ulna. The majority of patients with mosaic Klinefelter's syndrome exhibit less severe clinical manifestations, particularly if a normal XY cell line is present. Indeed, fertility in patients with mosaic Klinefelter's syndrome (XXY/XY) has been documented. Patients with an additional Y chromosome tend to be tall and have extremely aggressive, antisocial behavioral abnormalities. Very rarely, a patient exhibits the classic features of Klinefelter's syndrome with a normal (46 XY) karyotype, a so-called mutant phenocopy. Finally, phenotypic males with a 46 XX karyotype may demonstrate the typical clinical manifestations of Klinefelter's syndrome, except for having shorter stature and a higher incidence of hypospadias. In some patients with this condition, Y chromosomal material is translocated onto the X chromosome (see Ch. 207).

Azoospermia is present in >95% of patients with classic Klinefelter's syndrome. Serum testosterone levels are usually low but may be in the low normal adult range. However, free testosterone levels are reduced in most patients with Klinefelter's syndrome. Serum estradiol levels are often elevated, resulting in elevated SHBG concentrations and contributing to the development of gynecomastia. Serum gonadotropin levels, especially serum FSH levels, are uniformly elevated.

Treatment of Klinefelter's syndrome is aimed primarily at correction of the androgen deficiency with testosterone replacement therapy. The infertility is irreversible. Gynecomastia may be a source of great social embarrassment, in which case reduction mammoplasty should be performed.

The *functional prepubertal castrate* or *vanishing testes syndrome (congenital anorchia)* is characterized by bilateral absence of functioning testes, occasionally associated with absent epididymides, in a genotypic man. The presence of otherwise normal male internal and external genitalia, without müllerian duct derivatives, and descent of the vas and testicular blood vessels into the scrotum imply that a normally functioning testis was present during fetal life. It is hypothesized that testicular damage during the fetal or prepubertal period results in atrophy of the testes. Patients with this syndrome usually present with delayed puberty, eunuchoidal features, absence of palpable testes, and short stature (see Fig. 209–4). Congenital anorchia must be distinguished from bilateral abdominal cryptorchidism, which also presents with absent scrotal testes. Because of the increased risk of malignancy, intra-abdominal testes require orchiectomy or orchiopexy. The absence of a testosterone response to exogenous hCG in patients with congenital anorchia may be helpful in distinguishing it from bilateral abdominal testes. However, laparoscopy or surgical exploration is often necessary to confirm the diagnosis. Treatment of this syndrome consists of androgen replacement therapy to induce full sexual maturation. Insertion of testicular prostheses may be of psychological value.

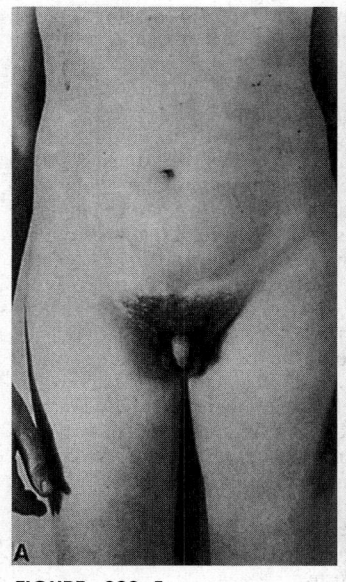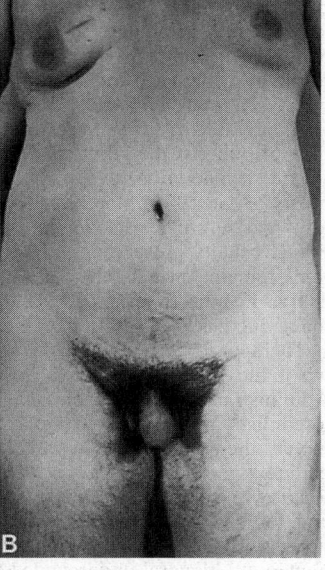

FIGURE 209–5. Two patients with untreated Klinefelter's syndrome, demonstrating the variability in degree of androgenization in this disorder. *A,* The small penis, diminished pubic hair with a female escutcheon, and sparse body hair indicate severe androgen deficiency. *B,* Normal penile development and adequate pubic and body hair indicate nearly normal androgen production by the testes. Gynecomastia is present in both patients, although only visible in the patient shown in *B.* The testes in both subjects were less than 2 cm in length. (From Bardin CW, Paulsen CA: The testes. *In* Williams RH [ed.]: Textbook of Endocrinology, 6th ed. Philadelphia, WB Saunders, 1981.)

Noonan (Bonnevie-Ullrich) syndrome, an autosomal recessive disorder, occurs in karyotypically normal males and females. It is characterized by a number of clinical features similar to those of females with Turner's syndrome. Characteristic findings include short stature, typical facies (hypertelorism, antimongoloid eye slant, ptosis, low-set ears, micrognathia, high-arched palate, and dental malocclusions), webbed neck, shield-like chest, pectus excavatum, cubitus valgus, mental retardation, cardiovascular anomalies (pulmonic stenosis and atrial septal defects), and lymphedema. Males with Noonan syndrome (also called male Turner's syndrome) exhibit primary testicular dysfunction with impairment of both sperm and androgen production and elevated serum gonadotropin levels. Cryptorchidism is frequently present. Treatment of this disorder consists of testosterone replacement to correct the androgen deficiency and orchiopexy for associated cryptorchidism, both for psychological reasons and to monitor the testes for malignancy.

Myotonic dystrophy (see also Ch. 454) is an autosomal dominant disorder characterized by progressive weakness and atrophy of muscles, especially those of the face, neck, and distal extremities. An important diagnostic feature in this disorder is the presence of myotonia, or prolonged contraction of muscles. Other characteristic findings include cataracts, cardiac arrhythmias, dysphagia, premature frontal balding, mild intellectual deterioration, and gonadal atrophy. Testicular atrophy that occurs in middle age is found in about 80% of men affected by myotonic dystrophy. The majority of these men have isolated impairment of spermatogenesis with normal androgen production. However, approximately 20% of men with myotonic dystrophy exhibit androgen deficiency. In addition to treating the androgen deficiency, testosterone replacement therapy may help to maintain or improve muscle function in these men.

Polyglandular autoimmune disease (see also Ch. 210.1) is a disorder in which there is concurrence of organ-specific autoimmune disease involving several endocrine and nonendocrine organs, associated with the presence of circulating autoantibodies to these organs. Specific conditions that occur in association with each other in this disorder are Addison's disease, Hashimoto's disease, insulin-dependent diabetes, pernicious anemia, ovarian failure, hypoparathyroidism, vitiligo, mucocutaneous candidiasis, Graves' disease, hypopituitarism, and alopecia. Although much less common than primary ovarian failure, primary testicular failure, associated

with antitesticular antibodies and resulting in androgen deficiency, may occur in males with polyglandular autoimmune disease.

Normal aging in healthy men is associated with significant reductions in testosterone and sperm production. Serum total and free testosterone levels in elderly men often fall below the normal range for younger men in association with slightly elevated or normal gonadotropin levels. Thus, a hormonal pattern suggesting either mild primary or secondary hypogonadism may be found in elderly men. The physiologic significance of reduced testosterone levels in aging men, however, is unknown. Normal aging in men is also accompanied by reductions in muscle mass and strength, bone mass, sexual interest and function, sleep, and vigor, and alterations in mood and cognition. Whether these changes in body function with aging are related to the reduction in testosterone levels remains to be determined.

Primary hypogonadism may present in a number of *complex genetic disorders,* such as *Alström ataxia-telangiectasia, POEMS, Sohval-Soffer, Weinstein,* and *Werner* syndromes. Rarely, patients with *Prader-Labhart-Willi* and *Laurence-Moon-Biedl* syndromes demonstrate primary, rather than the more commonly associated secondary, hypogonadism.

Acquired Disorders. In general, seminiferous tubule function and spermatogenesis are much more sensitive to external or environmental influences (such as irradiation, cytotoxic agents, or heat) than is Leydig cell production of testosterone. This greater sensitivity is due, in large part, to the fact that spermatogenesis involves active and coordinated cellular division and differentiation. As a result, most acquired primary testicular disorders causing hypogonadism result more commonly in isolated impairment of spermatogenesis (see below) than in androgen deficiency.

Viral orchitis, most frequently due to *mumps,* is a very common cause of acquired primary testicular failure. Approximately 15 to 25% of males with mumps develop acute orchitis. Acute mumps infection of the testes in prepubertal boys or adults usually results in permanent seminiferous tubule damage and, in severe cases, Leydig cell loss and androgen deficiency. Although clinical mumps orchitis is unilateral in the majority of cases, degenerative changes can occur in the clinically uninvolved testis. The use of mumps vaccine has significantly reduced the incidence of mumps orchitis. Orchitis may also complicate infections with viruses such as *echoviruses* and *arboviruses.* Uncommon causes of orchitis include *gonorrhea, leprosy, tuberculosis, brucellosis, glanders, syphilis,* and certain parasitic infections such as *filariasis* and *bilharziasis.* As in mumps, orchitis complicating these disorders results more commonly in isolated impairment of sperm production, although in severe cases androgen deficiency may develop.

Bilateral surgical or traumatic castration results in acute androgen deficiency. Castration after puberty often causes hot flushes and irritability, similar to women undergoing menopause.

Certain *drugs* may produce androgen deficiency by inhibiting testosterone biosynthesis and/or by blocking androgen action. *Spironolactone* inhibits testosterone synthesis and interferes with androgen action by competitively binding to the androgen receptor. *Ketoconazole* inhibits testosterone synthesis. H_2 *receptor blockers* (e.g., cimetidine) are weak androgen antagonists. *Alcohol* and *marijuana* (tetrahydrocannabinol) have direct toxic effects on both spermatogenesis and testicular steroidogenesis in addition to their CNS effects. *Digitalis* elevates serum estradiol, reduces testosterone levels, and interacts with both the estrogen and androgen receptors. A number of *cytotoxic drugs* used in cancer chemotherapy interfere with spermatogenesis and, rarely, with androgen production. In some *malignancies,* androgen deficiency occurs in the absence of exposure to chemotherapeutic agents (e.g., Hodgkin's disease or testicular cancer). Androgen deficiency may result from general debilitation and malnutrition associated with some malignancies. Exposure of the testes to very large doses of *irradiation* (over 600 to 800 rad) may compromise Leydig cell function.

Systemic Disorders. A number of systemic diseases cause deficiencies in sperm and androgen production, primarily by affecting testicular function directly, although gonadotropin secretion may also be affected in many of these conditions. In patients with *chronic liver disease* (cirrhosis), gynecomastia and testicular atrophy are commonly present (in 50 to 75%). Total serum testosterone levels are low or low normal. Because SHBG levels are elevated, free and non–SHBG-bound testosterone levels are low. Serum LH levels are usually elevated but may fall in the high normal range. Increased estrogen concentrations result from impaired hepatic clearance of adrenal androgens (androstenedione), leading to an increased substrate for peripheral aromatization to estrone and estradiol. The increased estrogen/testosterone ratio may contribute to the formation of gynecomastia. Treatment of androgen deficiency in patients with cirrhosis with an aromatizable androgen may result in worsening of gynecomastia.

Chronic renal failure usually causes reductions in both sperm and androgen production. LH and FSH levels are elevated, as a result of increased production as well as reduced renal clearance. The response of testosterone levels to hCG stimulation is impaired. Elevated serum prolactin levels and zinc deficiency may also contribute to testicular dysfunction in uremia. Hemodialysis does not significantly improve testosterone production. However, successful renal transplantation may result in some return of testicular function, which may be tempered by chronic immunosuppressive therapy to prevent graft rejection. In addition to treating androgen deficiency, testosterone replacement therapy may also improve the anemia of renal failure.

Sickle cell disease often results in primary testicular dysfunction with low serum testosterone and elevated serum gonadotropin levels. *Paraplegia* may result in a transient reduction in serum testosterone levels that return to normal in the chronic paraplegic state unless malnutrition is present. *Vasculitis* involving the testis (e.g., periarteritis nodosa) or *infiltrative diseases* (e.g., amyloidosis, leukemia) may also result in primary testicular failure.

ISOLATED DEFICIENCY OF SPERM PRODUCTION.
Congenital or Developmental Disorders. *Germinal cell aplasia, or Sertoli cell–only syndrome,* is an uncommon condition characterized on testicular biopsy by seminiferous tubules of moderately reduced size, lined with Sertoli cells but devoid of germ cells and having little or no tubular fibrosis. Patients with this syndrome are normally androgenized but infertile. They have slightly smaller than normal testes, azoospermia, and elevated serum FSH levels, indicative of severe seminiferous tubule dysfunction. Serum testosterone levels are normal, and LH levels are normal or slightly elevated. Congenital absence of germ cells is thought to be the basis for this syndrome. However, other gonadal disorders causing severe seminiferous tubule damage (such as mumps orchitis, cryptorchidism, irradiation, or cytotoxic drugs) may result in Sertoli cell–only syndrome. In these acquired causes, however, the tubules are usually extensively sclerosed and the testes are much smaller. Infertility in congenital germinal cell aplasia is irreversible.

In *cryptorchidism* the testes fail to descend normally into the scrotum and are usually located in the abdomen or inguinal canal. *Ectopic testes* are located outside the normal pathway of testicular descent and may be found in the perineal, femoral, or superficial inguinal areas. To avoid unnecessary treatment, cryptorchid testes must be distinguished from *retractile testes,* which are located in the scrotum but are withdrawn into the inguinal canal or abdomen with minimal stimulation.

The testes usually descend into the scrotum about the eighth month of fetal life. Undescended testes are found in approximately 3 to 4% of full-term newborn males, but the testes descend during the first year in all but 0.7 to 0.8%. The prevalence of cryptorchidism in adult males is about 0.3 to 0.4%. Inguinal hernia is associated with cryptorchidism in 50 to 80% of cases.

Bilateral cryptorchidism is associated with a number of disorders that cause androgen deficiency or resistance. When cryptorchidism is not associated with other hypogonadal disorders, it rarely affects Leydig cell function and usually causes isolated impairment of spermatogenesis. Even when cryptorchidism is unilateral, testicular dysfunction is very common, suggesting that both testes have altered function. In rare instances, normal testicular descent may be impeded by anatomic abnormalities along the pathway of descent, e.g., external inguinal hernias. In these instances, orchiopexy before puberty usually results in preservation of normal testicular function.

Careful physical examination of the scrotum should be performed to distinguish cryptorchidism from retractile testes, which is a more common condition. The diagnosis is particularly difficult in obese patients. Examination should be performed in the standing, squatting, and recumbent positions, and observation in warm water may

be helpful. The Valsalva maneuver and applied pressure to the lower abdomen are useful procedures to detect a mobile testis. In patients with retractile testes, elicitation of a cremasteric reflex may result in a localized puckering of the scrotal skin. Ultrasonography or CT scan may be helpful in localizing nonpalpable testes.

As a result of exposure to higher extrascrotal temperatures at the time of puberty, the germinal epithelium of cryptorchid testes shows severe degeneration, eventually resulting in seminiferous tubule fibrosis. Bilateral cryptorchidism causes infertility. Sperm counts are low, and serum FSH levels are usually elevated. Leydig cell function is usually preserved, and serum testosterone and LH concentrations remain normal. The risk of malignancy in undescended testes is five to nine times greater than in scrotal testes, and the risk remains increased even after orchiopexy.

Therapy for cryptorchidism should be instituted before puberty, when the degenerative changes of the germinal epithelium occur. Administration of hCG or LHRH to prepubertal boys with cryptorchidism may cause testicular descent in some patients. If hormonal therapy is unsuccessful in causing testicular descent, orchiopexy is performed in an attempt to preserve testicular function, to allow easier examination of the testis for malignant degeneration, and for cosmetic reasons. Despite orchiopexy, fertility rates in patients with cryptorchidism are usually reduced, particularly in patients with bilateral undescended testes.

A *varicocele* is an abnormal dilatation of the pampiniform plexus of veins surrounding the spermatic cord, caused by retrograde blood flow into the internal spermatic vein. Palpable varicocele occurs in about 10% of men and 30% of men with infertility. Although varicocele is clearly associated with infertility, approximately 50% of men with varicocele have normal seminal fluid analyses, and some men with varicocele and abnormal seminal fluid parameters are fertile. About 90% of varicoceles occur on the left side, as a result of valvular incompetence between the left internal spermatic vein and the renal vein. Occurrence of an isolated right-sided varicocele may be an early clue to venous obstruction by malignancy or to situs inversus. Varicoceles may affect testicular function by a variety of mechanisms, including increasing testicular temperature and blood flow. Seminal fluid analysis usually shows low sperm concentration with reduced motility and increased numbers of sperm with abnormal morphology. Testicular size and serum testosterone, LH, and FSH levels are usually normal. Surgical repair of varicoceles in infertile men has been reported to improve semen quality and fertility, although well-controlled clinical studies have not been performed.

Immotile cilia syndrome, or *Kartagener's syndrome,* is characterized by sinusitis, bronchiectasis, and situs inversus. Patients usually suffer from chronic respiratory infections because of impaired mucociliary clearance in the respiratory tract. In addition, these patients produce nonmotile spermatozoa. Cilia in the respiratory tract and the sperm tail are immotile in Kartagener's syndrome because of an abnormality in *dynein,* a protein that is important in microtubular filament movement. Other patients have a *deficiency of protein carboxyl methylase,* an enzyme that is important in sperm motility. Infertility in this syndrome is not treatable.

The majority of patients with *myotonic dystrophy* (see above) may have isolated impairment of spermatogenesis with normal androgen production.

Acquired Disorders. The majority of adults who develop mumps *orchitis* and orchitis due to other infectious agents sustain severe germ cell damage and isolated impairment of spermatogenesis with normal Leydig cell function (see above). Seminiferous tubule function is much more sensitive to damage from external or environmental agents than is Leydig cell function. Therefore, exposure of the testis to *thermal trauma, irradiation, cytotoxic drugs,* and *environmental toxins* often results in deficiency of sperm production without androgen deficiency. Even relatively minor thermal trauma, such as that induced by hot tubs, may result in suppression of sperm production.

The human testis is very sensitive to irradiation. Only 15 rad of x-irradiation may suppress spermatogenesis temporarily; >600 rad usually produces permanent infertility. Doses of radiation used in therapy of malignant lymphoma may result in permanent germ cell damage and infertility, despite shielding of the testis. Spermatogenesis is also very sensitive to damage by cytotoxic cancer chemotherapeutic agents, especially to alkylating agents. The likelihood of severe seminiferous tubule damage and permanent infertility is greater with combination chemotherapy regimens, such as

MOPP for Hodgkin's disease. Despite being very sensitive to radiation and cytotoxic drugs, the germinal epithelium has remarkable regenerative properties, and recovery of spermatogenesis may occur despite very severe germ cell loss. Both irradiation (> 800 rad) and cytotoxic agents occasionally produce androgen deficiency. Sperm banking offers some hope of fertility for patients who will develop permanent infertility as a result of irradiation or chemotherapy for malignant disease. Sulfasalazine has been reported to cause oligospermia, reduced sperm motility, and infertility.

Damage to the germinal epithelium has been reported in workers exposed to carbon disulfide, a solvent used in production of rayon, and to dibromochloropropane, an insecticide. A number of other chemical agents used in industry and laboratories have been implicated as direct testicular toxins (e.g., lead, deuterium oxide, cadmium, fluoroacetamide, nitrofurans, dinitropyrroles, diamines, α-chlorhydrin, other insecticides, and rodenticides).

Systemic Disorders. Minor *acute febrile illnesses* may result in temporary suppression of sperm production (e.g., minor viral infections). Over 50% of men with spinal cord lesions resulting in *paraplegia* exhibit diminished testicular function, the majority demonstrating impaired sperm production with normal androgen production. Reduced spermatogenesis may be a result of elevated testicular temperature, caused by loss of lumbar sympathetic innervation and the cremasteric reflex.

Idiopathic Oligospermia or Azoospermia. In most men who present with infertility and isolated impairment of spermatogenesis, no apparent cause can be found, leading to the diagnosis of *idiopathic oligospermia or azoospermia.* Because of the high prevalence of male infertility (5 to 6% of reproductive age men), idiopathic oligospermia or azoospermia is the most common cause of male hypogonadism. Because the pathogenesis of impaired sperm production is not known, therapy has been largely empiric and unsuccessful in improving fertility rates over those achieved by placebo or in untreated patients, who have a 20% fertility rate in 1 year. At present, infertility in these patients should be considered irreversible and couples should be offered artificial insemination using donor semen or adoption as alternatives. Recently, assisted reproductive technology using *in vitro* fertilization and intracytoplasmic sperm injection has been used successfully to achieve pregnancy in partners of men with idiopathic oligospermia and/or severely abnormal sperm function.

Secondary Hypogonadism

Secondary hypogonadism is testicular failure due to inadequate gonadotropin secretion as a result of either hypothalamic or pituitary dysfunction. In the majority of cases, both LH and FSH secretion are diminished, resulting in impairment of both sperm and androgen production. Rarely, there may be isolated deficiency of sperm production.

DEFICIENCY OF SPERM AND ANDROGEN PRODUCTION. Congenital or Developmental Disorders. *Hypogonadotropic eunuchoidism,* or *Kallmann's syndrome,* is a congenital and often familial disorder, characterized by isolated hypogonadotropic hypogonadism, eunuchoidism, and anosmia or hyposmia. Gonadotropin deficiency in this disorder is caused by a deficiency of LHRH, and chronic exogenous LHRH administration results in stimulation of normal testicular function. A developmental failure of the olfactory lobes is responsible for absent or reduced sense of smell. There is considerable genetic heterogeneity in Kallmann's syndrome, and inheritance may be autosomal dominant with male-predominant expression, autosomal recessive, or X-linked recessive.

Usually, patients with Kallmann's syndrome present with delayed puberty. They exhibit eunuchoidal features and prepubertal size testes. An early prepubertal manifestation of Kallmann's syndrome is micropenis. In addition to anosmia or hyposmia (present in approximately 80%), these patients may also exhibit other midline defects (e.g., cleft-lip or -palate, color blindness, renal agenesis, nerve deafness), cryptorchidism, and skeletal abnormalities (e.g., syndactyly, short fourth metacarpals, craniofacial asymmetry). Patients with Kallmann's syndrome are often aspermic (i.e., have no ejaculate). Serum testosterone, LH, and FSH levels are low, while other anterior pituitary functions are normal. The degree of gonadotropin deficiency, however, is highly variable.

The differentiation between Kallmann's syndrome and constitutional delayed puberty is very difficult in the absence of anosmia or hyposmia and cannot be reliably made in the prepubertal age range.

Usually, androgen therapy is initiated to induce sexual maturation in both of these conditions and is intermittently stopped to determine whether spontaneous onset of puberty occurs. Patients with Kallmann's syndrome continue to require androgen therapy to achieve and maintain sexual maturation, whereas patients with constitutional delayed puberty do not require treatment after spontaneous endogenous gonadotropin and testosterone secretion begin. When fertility is desired in men with Kallmann's syndrome, androgen treatment is stopped, and spermatogenesis may be induced with gonadotropin or LHRH therapy.

A variant of Kallmann's syndrome is *isolated LH deficiency,* also known as the *"fertile" eunuch syndrome.* In this syndrome, selective deficiency in LH secretion results in prepubertal androgen deficiency and eunuchoidism. Because FSH secretion is preserved, testis size is nearly normal and spermatogenesis is present. However, sperm production is not normal in these patients, and they are not fertile, as the name of the syndrome would imply. Treatment with hCG, which contains predominantly LH-like hormonal activity, stimulates Leydig cell production of testosterone, ameliorates androgen deficiency, and increases spermatogenesis.

Hemochromatosis is an autosomal recessive disorder in which there is parenchymal iron deposition in a variety of tissues, most prominently in the liver, skin, pancreas, and heart (see Ch. 189). Iron deposition in the pituitary gland selectively inhibits gonadotropin production without significantly affecting other anterior pituitary hormone secretion. The resulting hypogonadotropic hypogonadism and androgen deficiency are responsible for the common complaint of impotence in this disorder. Frequent phlebotomies or treatment with desferrioxamine to decrease iron overload may restore gonadotropin secretion in some patients. Even in the presence of significant iron overload, administration of gonadotropins can stimulate testicular function, including induction of spermatogenesis. Parenchymal iron deposition resulting in hypogonadotropic hypogonadism may also occur in patients with conditions that require frequent blood transfusions, such as thalassemia.

Secondary hypogonadism may be present in a number of *complex genetic syndromes,* such as *Prader-Labhart-Willi, Laurence-Moon-Biedl, Biemond, Carpenter, familial cerebellar ataxia, dyskeratosis congenita, familial ichthyosis, Börjeson, Kraus-Rupert, Lowe, steroid sulfatase deficiency, Rud, CHARGE, LEOPARD, Moebius, POEMS, Martsolf, Rothmund-Thomson,* and *Richards-Rundle* syndromes.

Acquired Disorders. *Hypopituitarism.* Any destructive or infiltrative lesion of the hypothalamus and/or pituitary may cause impairment of gonadotropin secretion, either selectively or in conjunction with deficiency of other anterior pituitary hormones (see Ch. 202.1). Specific pathologic conditions include functioning and nonfunctioning pituitary adenomas; suprasellar tumors, such as craniopharyngioma, meningioma, optic glioma, or astrocytoma; metastatic neoplasms; lymphoma; surgical ablation or irradiation of the pituitary; infarction; vasculitis; apoplexy; hypophysitis; aneurysm; abscess; trauma; granulomatous disease, such as tuberculosis, sarcoidosis, fungal disease, and histiocytosis X; and transfusional iron overload.

Usually, destructive processes involving the pituitary gland result in progressive loss of anterior pituitary function in the following order: Gonadotropin and growth hormone secretion are the first to be affected, followed by TSH production, and finally ACTH secretion. The combination of gonadotropin and growth hormone deficiency is important to recognize in prepubertal children with growth retardation. In adults, clinical secondary hypogonadism, in the absence of other anterior pituitary dysfunction, may be the initial manifestation of a hypothalamic or pituitary process. Because loss of TSH and ACTH secretion is associated with greater degrees of pituitary destruction, secondary hypothyroidism and hypoadrenalism usually do not occur without concurrent secondary hypogonadism.

Serum testosterone levels and sperm counts are low. Serum LH and FSH levels are low or in the low normal adult range. The gonadotropin response to single-dose LHRH administration does not reliably differentiate hypothalamic and pituitary causes of gonadotropin deficiency and is not a clinically useful test. Clinical evaluation of patients with secondary hypogonadism should include anatomic studies (such as CT scan and visual field examination) to determine the presence of hypothalamic or pituitary tumor and tumor mass effects, and investigation of other anterior pituitary hormone functions.

Treatment is aimed at the process causing hypopituitarism and correction of androgen deficiency with testosterone replacement therapy. If fertility is desired, androgens are discontinued and gonadotropin therapy is instituted.

Hyperprolactinemia, resulting from a pituitary adenoma, CNS-active drugs (such as phenothiazines and other antipsychotics, opiates, sedatives, antidepressants, stimulants), or adrenergic or dopaminergic antagonist drugs (antihypertensives, metoclopramide) may cause secondary testicular failure. Prolactin-secreting pituitary adenomas in men are usually large (macroadenomas), and gonadotropin deficiency results, in part, from destruction of pituitary gonadotrophs. Even in the absence of a tumor, prolactin has an inhibitory effect on gonadotropin secretion, resulting in secondary hypogonadism. Bromocriptine and other dopamine agonist drugs (such as pergolide) decrease pituitary prolactin secretion and are used to treat hyperprolactinemia. These agents may result in restoration of normal gonadotropin secretion and testicular function, and shrinkage of prolactinomas.

Estrogen excess in men causes inhibition of gonadotropin secretion and secondary hypogonadism. Estrogen excess may result from either exogenous administration of estrogens or estrogenic substances (e.g., diethylstilbestrol administration in men with prostate cancer) or endogenous secretion from an estrogen-producing neoplasm (e.g., feminizing adrenal carcinoma). Patients with estrogen excess usually manifest varying degrees of gynecomastia. *Progestins* (e.g., medroxyprogesterone or megestrol acetate), *androgenic anabolic steroids,* and *opiate-like drugs* (e.g., morphine, methadone, and heroin) also inhibit gonadotropin production and may cause secondary hypogonadism.

Systemic Disorders. *Glucocorticoid excess,* as a result of either Cushing's syndrome or high-dosage glucocorticoid administration, suppresses gonadotropin secretion, resulting in secondary testicular failure with loss of libido, impotence, and oligospermia. Activation of the hypothalamic-adrenal axis resulting in high circulating levels of endogenous glucocorticoids may contribute to the reduction in serum testosterone, LH, and FSH levels observed with *acute stress or illness,* such as emotional stress, trauma, myocardial infarction, surgery, burns, and sepsis. *Nutritional deficiency,* such as that associated with protein-calorie malnutrition or anorexia nervosa, inhibits gonadotropin production and may cause secondary hypogonadism. Concurrent primary testicular dysfunction may also be caused by inadequate nutrition. Malnutrition may contribute to the secondary testicular failure associated with a number of *chronic illnesses,* such as malignancy, AIDS, and chronic heart, respiratory, liver, and kidney disease. Moderate obesity results in reduction in SHBG and total testosterone levels, with normal free testosterone levels. Some men with *massive obesity* demonstrate clinical androgen deficiency with low free testosterone concentrations and reduced gonadotropin levels.

ISOLATED DEFICIENCY OF SPERM PRODUCTION. *Congenital adrenal hyperplasia* caused by either 21-hydroxylase or 11β-hydroxylase deficiency results in excessive production of adrenal androgens. Androgen excess suppresses gonadotropin secretion and sperm production. Excessive adrenal androgen production causes premature virilization and precocious pseudopuberty, rather than androgen deficiency. Secondary hypogonadism is therefore manifested by isolated impairment of spermatogenesis. Glucocorticoid treatment of some patients with congenital adrenal hyperplasia may result in true precocious puberty, with premature activation of the hypothalamic-pituitary-gonadal axis. Androgen excess caused by administration of *testosterone* or large doses of *androgenic anabolic steroids* or *androgen-secreting tumors* (e.g., Leydig cell tumors) also result in secondary hypogonadism presenting with isolated deficiency in sperm production. High doses of testosterone have been administered to normal men to suppress gonadotropin and sperm production in male contraceptive development trials.

Rarely, *hyperprolactinemia* impairs sperm production despite normal gonadotropin and testosterone levels. *Isolated FSH deficiency* is an extremely rare condition that causes impaired spermatogenesis.

Androgen Resistance Syndromes

Androgen resistance syndromes are caused by defects in androgen action (see Ch. 207). The severity of androgen insensitivity de-

termines the clinical presentation of these disorders. With severely defective androgen action, patients present at birth as either phenotypic females (testicular feminization) or with ambiguous genitalia (male pseudohermaphroditism). Men with mild, incomplete androgen insensitivity or *Reifenstein's syndrome* present as adults with mild androgen deficiency and a nearly normal male phenotype. Patients with Reifenstein's syndrome may have hypospadias, gynecomastia, varying degrees of virilization, a small prostate gland, impaired spermatogenesis, and cryptorchidism. They have elevated serum testosterone, LH, and FSH levels. Some men with very mild androgen resistance present with only oligospermia or azoospermia. Some men with celiac disease are infertile and have elevated serum testosterone and LH levels, suggesting androgen resistance.

Delayed Puberty

Puberty in boys usually begins between the ages of 9 and 14 years. With the maturation of the CNS mechanisms that regulate LHRH production, pulsatile gonadotropin and testosterone secretion begin, initially during sleep and then throughout the day. The first clinical indications of the onset of puberty are an increase in testicular size (>3 ml) and wrinkling and pigmentation of the scrotal skin. Subsequently, there are increases in penile length and appearance of pubic hair, followed by increasing long bone growth and development of other secondary sexual characteristics. The increase in testicular size precedes the appearance of pubic hair by about 2 years and the peak velocity in growth of height by 3 years. The onset and duration of puberty and the degree to which secondary sexual characteristics develop vary considerably and are largely attributable to the genetic background of an individual.

Delayed puberty is the lack of sexual maturation by 14 years of age. A number of the disorders that cause *hypogonadism* may result in delayed sexual maturation. *Severe systemic illnesses* (such as malabsorption, asthma, diabetes, malignancy) that also cause growth retardation and *thyroid hormone deficiency* may also cause delayed puberty. The majority of boys with delayed puberty, however, have physiologic or *constitutional delayed puberty.* This is a benign, frequently familial form of delayed adolescence that represents a normal variation in the onset of puberty. These boys eventually undergo a delayed but normal puberty and attain normal sexual maturation and height.

The diagnosis of constitutional delayed puberty can be strongly suspected in a healthy boy with retardation of growth and bone age, normal growth velocity in relation to bone age, a bone age between 12 and 13 years, a family history of delayed adolescence, and a testicular volume >2 ml. These clinical features are often not present and the diagnosis can be very difficult. Diagnostic evaluation should exclude organic causes of delayed puberty, i.e., hypogonadism, systemic illness, and hypothyroidism. In the absence of anosmia or other morphologic manifestations, constitutional delayed puberty cannot be distinguished from hypogonadotropic eunuchoidism.

Delayed sexual maturation often results in severe psychosocial distress to both the patient and his parents. Therefore, after systemic and endocrine disorders are excluded, boys with delayed puberty are usually treated with androgen replacement therapy to induce sexual maturation coincident with that of their contemporaries.

Handelsman DJ: Testicular dysfunction in systemic disease. Endocrinol Metab Clin North Am 23:839, 1994. *An excellent review of the effects of systemic illness on testicular function.*

Kletter GB, Kelch RP: Disorders of puberty in boys. Endocrinol Metab Clin North Am 22:455, 1993. *An excellent overview of delayed and precocious puberty in boys.*

Lee PA, St L O'dea L: Primary and secondary testicular insufficiency. Pediatr Clin North Am 37:1359, 1990. *A well-organized and well-written review of the diagnosis and treatment of primary and secondary testicular failure in the pediatric age group.*

Plymate SR: Hypogonadism. Endocrinol Metab Clin North Am 23:749, 1994. *An excellent, comprehensive discussion of disorders causing primary and secondary hypogonadism.*

Rosenfeld RL: Diagnosis and management of delayed puberty. J Clin Endocrinol Metab 70:559, 1990. *A concise review of the diagnosis and treatment of delayed sexual development.*

Wang C, Swerdloff RS: Evaluation of testicular function. Bailliere's Clin Endocrinol Metab 6:405, 1992. *A very complete review of the clinical and laboratory evaluation of testicular function.*

TREATMENT OF HYPOGONADISM

Androgen Therapy

Androgens are principally used to treat testosterone deficiency in hypogonadal men. In prepubertal androgen-deficient boys, the aim of androgen replacement is to stimulate and maintain male secondary sexual characteristics, somatic development, and sexual function without compromising adult height by premature closure of long bone epiphyses. In adult androgen deficiency, the objective of therapy is to restore and maintain libido, potency, and secondary sexual characteristics.

The long-acting 17β-hydroxyl esters of testosterone, *testosterone enanthate* and *cypionate,* are the most effective, safest, and most practical preparations currently available to treat androgen deficiency. In adults with androgen deficiency, replacement therapy is usually initiated with either testosterone enanthate or cypionate at a dose of 150 to 200 mg intramuscularly every 2 weeks. At these dosages, testosterone administration generally stimulates libido and potency, improves energy level, and social drive, restores male hair growth, and increases hemoglobin concentration.

In elderly androgen-deficient men, it is wise to begin testosterone therapy gradually at a reduced dosage. In elderly men who are not concerned about normal sexual functioning, low-dose androgen supplementation (e.g., testosterone enanthate or cypionate, 100 mg intramuscularly every 2 to 4 weeks) may suffice.

Recently, a transdermal delivery system consisting of a testosterone-containing scrotal skin patch was approved for androgen replacement therapy of hypogonadal men. Daily application of this patch maintains serum testosterone levels within the normal range; however, DHT levels are elevated (probably as a result of high 5α-reductase activity in scrotal skin). Except for minor skin irritation, the testosterone patch is tolerated well and offers an alternative to testosterone esters for replacement therapy of selected androgen-deficient men.

Androgen therapy is more complicated in boys with delayed puberty. Although testosterone is very effective in inducing secondary sexual characteristics and stimulating long bone growth, overly aggressive androgen therapy can result in premature closure of long bone epiphyses and compromise final adult height. Furthermore, it is often not possible to differentiate patients with constitutional delayed puberty, who require only temporary androgen replacement, from those with permanent hypogonadotropic hypogonadism. Therefore, in boys with delayed puberty whose height is far below the expected adult height, androgen therapy is begun with testosterone enanthate or cypionate, 50 to 100 mg intramuscularly every 2 to 4 weeks, and gradually increased to full adult replacement doses over several years. Androgen therapy is intermittently stopped for 3 to 4 months to determine whether spontaneous pubertal development will occur.

Androgen therapy is absolutely contraindicated in men with androgen-sensitive cancers, i.e., prostatic carcinoma and male breast carcinoma. Excessive stimulation of libido and erections by androgens is rare, usually occurring in prepubertal boys or in men with longstanding androgen deficiency given large doses of testosterone. These symptoms resolve with time or reduction in dosage. Acute urinary retention as a result of androgen replacement therapy is very uncommon in the absence of underlying prostatic carcinoma. Patients given testosterone to induce puberty may develop acne or gynecomastia, similar to that observed during normal puberty. Adult hypogonadal men develop acne less commonly and rarely develop gynecomastia, except when a predisposing condition such as hepatic cirrhosis exists. Androgens may cause mild weight gain as a result of sodium retention and protein anabolic effects, and patients with underlying edematous states may develop worsening edema during therapy. Erythropoiesis is stimulated by androgen administration. Occasionally, significant erythrocytosis occurs, requiring phlebotomy and reduction of testosterone dosage. Testosterone may also worsen or induce obstructive sleep apnea.

All oral androgens available in the United States are 17α-alkylated derivatives of testosterone. These oral preparations are weak androgens and have the potential for serious hepatotoxicity. They may cause hepatic cholestasis and occasionally clinical jaundice. Although rare, more serious and potentially life-threatening complications of oral androgens are the development of peliosis hepatis (blood-filled cysts in the liver), hepatic adenoma, hepatoma, or hepatic angiosarcoma. Hepatotoxicity does not result from replacement dosages of parenteral 17β-hydroxyl esters of testosterone. Because they carry greater risk, have reduced clinical efficacy, and are more expensive, oral androgen preparations should not be used for the treatment of androgen deficiency.

Androgens have also been used in the treatment of anemias related to renal and bone marrow failure, micropenis and microphallus, hereditary angioneurotic edema, female breast cancer, lichen

sclerosus, endometriosis, and osteoporosis. Androgen administration may induce virilization in women, manifested by acne, hirsutism, and menstrual dysfunction, and in severe cases frontal balding, voice changes, breast atrophy, and clitoral hypertrophy. The use of androgenic steroids has not been demonstrated to be of long-term value in promoting protein anabolism in catabolic states associated with a variety of acute and chronic illnesses.

Androgenic anabolic steroids are commonly used by competitive athletes with the hope of improving endurance, strength, and performance and increasingly by boys to improve their appearance. Androgens are of dubious value in increasing strength and performance, in the absence of intensive training and high-protein diets. Athletes often take multiple androgenic anabolic agents (including 17α-alkylated agents) in very high doses and in combination with other agents (e.g., growth hormone, hCG) with little regard for potentially serious side effects. Hepatotoxicity (including hepatoma) and impaired spermatogenesis resulting in infertility have been reported in athletes abusing androgenic steroids. Furthermore, the long-term sequelae of taking massive doses of 17β-hydroxyl ester preparations are unknown. The potential risks of high-dose anabolic steroid use far outweigh the potential benefits to athletic performance, and their use should be strongly discouraged.

Gonadotropin and LHRH Therapy

The aim of gonadotropin therapy is to stimulate spermatogenesis and establish or restore fertility in gonadotropin-deficient hypogonadal patients. The gonadotropin preparations usually used for this purpose are *hCG* that contains LH-like biologic activity almost exclusively; and *human menopausal gonadotropin (hMG,* Pergonal) that contains both FSH and LH activity. A more purified preparation of *human FSH (hFSH,* Metrodin) is also available for clinical use. Both hCG and hMG are expensive and require multiple injections per week. Therefore, testosterone, rather than gonadotropin therapy, is used to induce and maintain androgenization in patients with hypogonadotropic hypogonadism when fertility is not desired.

Initiation of spermatogenesis in prepubertal hypogonadotropic hypogonadism usually requires treatment with both hCG and hMG. Treatment is initiated with hCG alone, at a dosage of 1000 to 2000 IU subcutaneously or intramuscularly two to three times weekly for 6 to 12 months. Clinical evidence of sexual maturation and the increase in serum testosterone levels are monitored to determine the need for adjustments in dose. During hCG treatment, Sertoli cells mature and spermatogenesis is initiated to varying degrees of completeness. Occasionally, hCG alone stimulates spermatogenesis sufficiently for sperm to appear in the ejaculate. However, the majority of patients with prepubertal hypogonadotropic hypogonadism require FSH activity, in the form of hMG, in addition to hCG to complete spermatogenesis and induce fertility. Therefore, hMG, at a dosage of 75 to 150 IU subcutaneously or intramuscularly three times weekly, is administered together with hCG if there is no evidence of sperm in the ejaculate with hCG alone. Gonadotropin induction of sperm production may take as long as 2 to 3 years. Even with combined hCG and hMG treatment, sperm output in the ejaculate may not be normal. Despite very low sperm counts, fertility may be induced, however.

Once initiated, spermatogenesis may be maintained with hCG treatment alone in patients with prepubertal hypogonadotropic hypogonadism. In adults with acquired hypogonadotropic hypogonadism, sperm production may also be restored with hCG treatment alone. Previous androgen treatment does not alter testicular responsiveness to subsequent gonadotropin therapy. The presence of primary testicular disease, such as cryptorchidism, worsens the prognosis for induction of sperm production and fertility by gonadotropin treatment.

In patients with Kallmann's syndrome, pulsatile administration of low doses of LHRH may be used to stimulate endogenous gonadotropin secretion and spermatogenesis to induce fertility. Pulsatile administration more closely mimics the normal physiologic situation; however, a portable infusion pump must be used to deliver small doses of LHRH every few hours (5 to 20 μg subcutaneously every 2 hours) throughout the day, making LHRH therapy a much more complex management problem than gonadotropin therapy. The cost and effectiveness of LHRH and gonadotropin therapy to stimulate spermatogenesis in men with Kallmann's syndrome are comparable.

Matsumoto AM: Clinical use and abuse of androgens and antiandrogens. In Becker KL (ed.): Principles and Practice of Endocrinology and Metabolism. Philadelphia, JB Lippincott, 1990, p 991. This chapter reviews the pharmacology of androgen preparations, their clinical use in treatment of male hypogonadism and other conditions, the inappropriate use of androgens, and their potential side effects.

Matsumoto AM: Hormonal therapy of male hypogonadism. Endocrinol Metab Clin North Am 23:857, 1994. An up-to-date review of androgen, gonadotropin, and gonadotropin-releasing hormone treatment of male hypogonadal states.

PRECOCIOUS PUBERTY

Isosexual precocity is defined as the development of sexual maturation before the age of 9 years. In boys, premature development of secondary sexual characteristics results in virilization. This is accompanied by accelerated skeletal maturation and linear growth and premature closure of long bone epiphyses, resulting in short stature as an adult. True precocious puberty is caused by premature secretion of gonadotropins. Testicular androgen and sperm production are stimulated by gonadotropins, resulting in virilization and increased testis size. Precocious pseudopuberty results from secretion of androgens from the adrenal gland or testis. Androgen excess results in virilization, but normal sperm production is not stimulated and the testes remain small.

True Precocious Puberty

In the majority of cases of true precocious puberty no identifiable cause for premature activation of gonadotropin secretion is found. This condition is called idiopathic precocious puberty. It is often inherited as a male-limited autosomal dominant or X-linked recessive trait. Patients have an increased incidence of seizure disorders and abnormal electroencephalograms. The remaining cases of true precocious puberty are primarily caused by CNS lesions involving the posterior hypothalamus. Lesions include hypothalamic and pineal tumors, craniopharyngioma, hamartomas, hydrocephalus, postencephalitic lesions, congenital brain defects, neurofibromatosis, and tuberous sclerosis. CNS lesions may also result in disturbances of other hypothalamic functions, causing diabetes insipidus, eating disorders, somnolence, emotional lability, and altered temperature regulation, as well as mental and psychomotor retardation and seizures. Precocious puberty may precede the onset of a clinically detectable neurologic lesion. Therefore, a prolonged period of follow-up observation with repeated neurologic evaluation is necessary to exclude CNS lesions. Rarely, an hCG-secreting tumor (e.g., hepatoblastoma) or hCG administration for cryptorchidism (iatrogenic precocious puberty) causes true precocious puberty.

Precocious Pseudopuberty (see Ch. 207)

Adrenocortical hyperfunction, either from congenital adrenal hyperplasia (21-hydroxylase or 11β-hydroxylase deficiency) or a virilizing adrenocortical tumor, is the most common condition causing precocious pseudopuberty in boys. Patients with congenital adrenal hyperplasia caused by 21-hydroxylase deficiency usually have markedly elevated serum 17-hydroxyprogesterone and urinary pregnanetriol levels. Rarely, Leydig cell tumor of the testis, autonomous Leydig cell function (testotoxicosis), and administration of androgenic steroids may cause precocious pseudopuberty.

Treatment of these conditions is directed at the underlying cause. For idiopathic precocious puberty, drugs to inhibit pituitary gonadotropin secretion (medroxyprogesterone acetate, LHRH analogues), or androgen synthesis (spironolactone, ketoconazole), or to block androgen action (flutamide, cyproterone acetate) have been used with varying success to prevent further sexual maturation. With the exception of LHRH analogues, these treatments do not usually prevent premature closure of long bone epiphyses.

Kaplan SL, Grumbach MM: Pathophysiology and treatment of sexual precocity. J Clin Endocrinol Metab 71:785, 1990. A concise and up-to-date review of the pathophysiology and management of precocious pubertal development.

Wheeler MD, Styne DM: Diagnosis and management of precocious puberty. Pediatr Clin North Am 37:1255, 1990. This is an excellent, comprehensive review of the diagnosis and treatment of sexual precocity.

TUMORS OF THE TESTIS

Tumors of the testis are uncommon, representing about 1% of all cancers in men. They occur more commonly in white than in black males. The annual incidence of testicular tumors is 6 per 100,000 males. About 95% of testicular tumors are malignant and derive from the germ cells. The remaining 5% are non-germ cell or stromal tumors derived mostly from Leydig and Sertoli cells and are usually benign. Gonadoblastoma is a rare testicular neoplasm containing both germ cell and stromal elements, arising in dysgenetic testes containing a Y chromosome. The peak age of incidence of testicular cancer is 20 to 35 years. It is the most common malignancy in this age group. Advances in treatment have transformed testicular cancer from the most common cause of cancer death in this age group 20 years ago into one of the most curable of all cancers today.

The most significant risk factor for developing testicular cancer is cryptorchidism. In unilateral cryptorchidism, the contralateral, normally descended testis also carries an increased risk of malignant degeneration. Orchiopexy at an early age (2 to 3 years) permits easier palpation and detection of testicular cancer and may reduce the risk of neoplasm. Carcinoma in situ has been found in men with oligoazoospermia presenting with infertility and in the contralateral testes of patients with presumed unilateral testicular cancer, suggesting that these conditions may also carry an increased risk for testicular neoplasm.

Germ Cell Tumors

Germ cell cancers may be classified according to their pathologic characteristics into seminoma and nonseminoma. Nonseminomatous cancers include embryonal cell carcinomas, choriocarcinomas, and teratomas. Forty per cent of germ cell cancers contain a mixture of seminomatous and nonseminomatous elements. The presence of any nonseminomatous element in a tumor that is predominantly seminoma dictates its classification as a nonseminoma. The distinction between seminoma and nonseminoma is important for staging and subsequent therapy. Seminomas usually metastasize via regional lymph nodes to retroperitoneal, mediastinal, and supraclavicular lymph nodes and are very sensitive to radiation therapy. On the other hand, nonseminomas metastasize by both lymphatic and hematogenous routes (especially to liver and lungs) and are radioresistant.

Most patients with germ cell tumors present with a painless mass in the testis. A testicular mass in a patient over 50 years is more likely to be a lymphoma than a germ cell tumor. Rapid onset of a painful testicular mass is usually caused by bleeding into the neoplasm. Ultrasonography or MRI may be helpful in defining a mass in the testis. Back or abdominal pain (from retroperitoneal lymphadenopathy), shortness of breath (from diffuse pulmonary metastases), gynecomastia (from hCG secretion), supraclavicular lymphadenopathy, or ureteral obstruction may also be present.

Germ cell tumors, especially nonseminomatous cancers, often secrete biologic markers (see Ch. 158.2). Embryonal cell cancers may secrete α-fetoprotein. Pure seminomas never elaborate α-fetoprotein, and its presence in serum implies the presence of nonseminomatous elements in the tumor. hCG is secreted by nearly all choriocarcinomas, a third of embryonal cell carcinomas and teratocarcinomas and, rarely, by pure seminomas. This marker may be detected using a specific β-hCG assay. Both of these tumor markers may be used to monitor response to therapy. They may precede clinically detectable disease by weeks to months.

In seminoma, orchiectomy and radiation therapy to the periaortic and iliac lymph nodes or combination chemotherapy (for advanced disease) have resulted in cure rates of 80 to 95%. In nonseminomatous testicular cancer, the addition of cisplatin to aggressive, multiple-drug chemotherapeutic regimens following orchiectomy (and retroperitoneal lymph node dissection for more advanced disease) has resulted in response rates of >90% and long-term remission in 50 to 90% of patients.

Non–Germ Cell Tumors

Non–germ cell tumors are rare tumors that develop from the two major elements of testicular stroma, the Leydig and Sertoli cells. They are usually benign, but about 10% are malignant and metastasize via regional lymphatics. Both Leydig and Sertoli cell tumors may secrete a variety of steroid hormones, primarily androgens or estrogens, that may result in virilization or feminization, respectively. These tumors are usually small and difficult to diagnose; selective venous catheterization and sampling to determine the site of increased steroid production are often helpful. Gynecomastia is present in about 30% of patients with non-germ cell tumors. Children may present with either isosexual (virilizing) or heterosexual (feminizing) precocious pseudopuberty. Treatment consists primarily of orchiectomy.

Ozols RF, Williams SD: Testicular cancer. Curr Probl Cancer 13:285, 1989. *An excellent comprehensive review of the classification, epidemiology, staging, treatment, and prognosis of testicular cancer (98 references).*

Roth BJ, Nichols CR (eds.): Testicular cancer. Semin Oncol 19:1, 1992. *An up-to-date review of the treatment of testicular cancer, including therapeutic strategies, current controversies, and the direction of future research by several authors.*

209.2 DISEASES OF THE PROSTATE

Gary D. Steinberg and
Charles B. Brendler

This chapter discusses three common disorders of the prostate: prostatitis, benign prostatic hyperplasia, and adenocarcinoma of the prostate. A brief review of the normal anatomy, physiology, and biochemistry of the prostate is provided first.

THE NORMAL PROSTATE

ANATOMY. The normal adult prostate, a firm, elastic organ weighing about 20 grams, is located caudad to the base of the bladder and is traversed by the first portion of the urethra. It is bordered anteriorly by the symphysis pubis and posteriorly by the rectum. The paired seminal vesicles are attached to the prostate and are located posterior to the bladder (Fig. 209–6).

The human prostate has two concentric anatomic regions: an inner periurethral zone composed of short glands and an outer peripheral zone composed of longer, branched glands. These regions are separated by a thin layer of fibroelastic tissue, the so-called surgical capsule (Fig. 209–7). Benign prostatic hyperplasia (BPH) arises within the inner periurethral zone in a specific region near the verumontanum, called the transition zone. In contrast, prostatic carcinoma usually arises in the outer peripheral zone.

PHYSIOLOGY. The secretions of the prostate and other sex accessory organs presumably protect or enhance the functional properties of the spermatozoa. Of the total average human ejaculate volume of 3.5 ml, the prostate secretes 0.5 ml and the seminal vesicles secrete 2.0 to 2.5 ml.

The concentration of zinc is higher in the prostate than in any other organ in the body. Its function is uncertain, but it may protect the prostate against infection. Two other components of prostatic secretion, acid phosphatase and prostate-specific antigen (PSA), are important serum markers for prostate cancer. An elevated serum

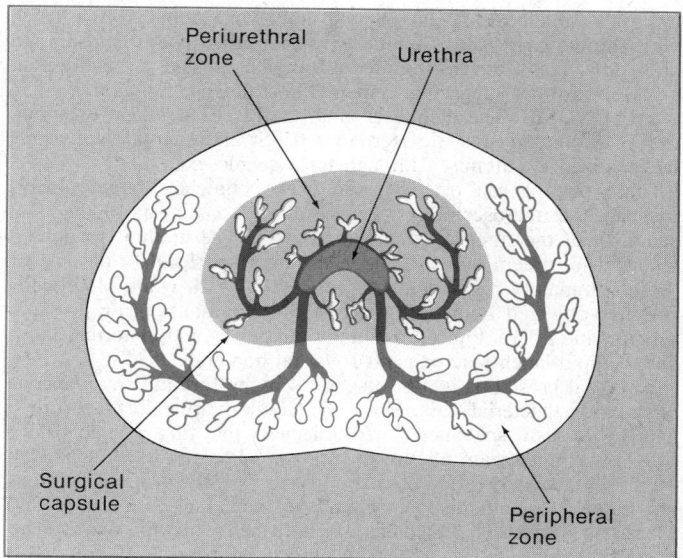

FIGURE 209–7. A coronal section through the prostate demonstrating the anatomic relationships among the urethra, periurethral tissue, surgical capsule, and peripheral tissue. (After Brendler H: *In* Glenn JF [ed.]: Urologic Surgery, 3rd ed. Philadelphia, J. B. Lippincott Company, 1983.)

prostatic acid phosphatase level, measured by enzymatic assay, is virtually diagnostic for metastatic prostate cancer. PSA is a serine protease that helps liquefy the ejaculate. The concentration of PSA is about 10-fold greater in prostate cancer than benign tissue. Since its discovery in 1979, PSA has emerged as the most important marker for prostate cancer. Serum PSA is useful in screening and staging prostate cancer, and it is the most sensitive indicator for monitoring response to treatment.

BIOCHEMISTRY. The growth and secretory function of the prostate depend on functioning testes; prostatic maturation does not occur in a male castrated before puberty. Testosterone, the major circulating androgen, is converted to dihydrotestosterone (DHT) by the enzyme 5α-reductase in prostatic epithelial cells. DHT, the major active androgenic metabolite within the prostate, binds to a cytoplasmic receptor, is transported to the nucleus, and there initiates RNA synthesis, protein synthesis, and cell replication.

Estrogens inhibit prostatic growth, largely by blocking the release of luteinizing hormone from the pituitary, thus inhibiting testicular synthesis of testosterone. If castrated animals are given both estrogens and androgens, normal prostate growth occurs, indicating that estrogens do not block androgen-induced growth in the prostate itself.

PROSTATITIS

INCIDENCE AND ETIOLOGY. About 50% of men experience symptoms of prostatic inflammation during adult life. Only about 5% of these cases are due to bacterial infection of the prostate. The etiology of these symptoms in the remaining 95% of patients is unclear.

Most bacterial infections of the prostate are caused by gram-negative organisms, most commonly *Escherichia coli.* Enterococci, staphylococci, and streptococci are rare causes of prostatic infection. *Chlamydia trachomatis* and *Ureaplasma urealyticum* probably cause prostatitis infrequently, but this topic remains controversial.

PATHOGENESIS. Most episodes of bacterial prostatic infection are due to a previous urethral infection with direct ascent of bacteria from the urethra through the prostatic ducts into the prostate. The organisms that cause bacterial prostatitis are the same as those that produce bacteriuria, and chlamydial and gonococcal infections of the urethra may involve the prostate.

Prostatic infection may also result from impairment of host defense mechanisms. The concentrations of prostatic antibacterial factor and magnesium, zinc, calcium, citric acid, spermine, cholesterol, and lysozyme are decreased in the prostatic fluid of men with chronic bacterial prostatitis. Whether these alterations contribute to

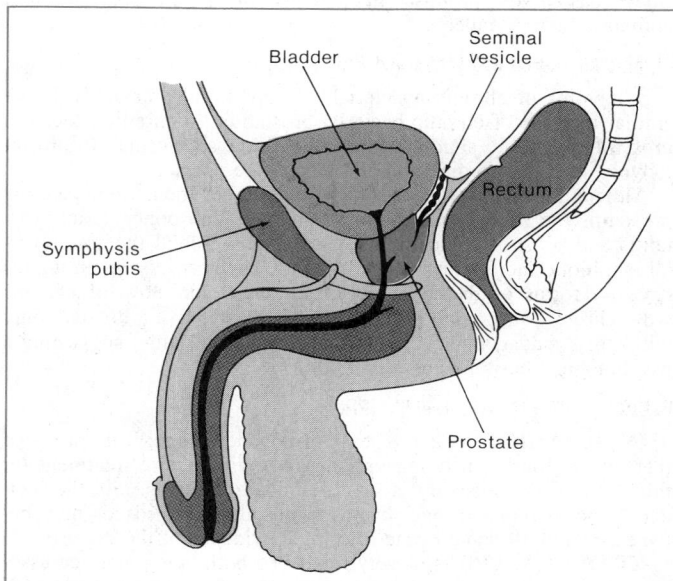

FIGURE 209–6. The anatomic relationship of the prostate to adjacent structures. (After Brendler H: *In* Glenn JF [ed.]: Urologic Surgery, 3rd ed. Philadelphia, J. B. Lippincott Company, 1983.)

or result from prostatic infection is unknown. About 10% of men with chronic bacterial prostatitis have more than one organism, and after cure, many develop reinfection of the prostate by a different organism, further suggesting impaired host defense function.

DIAGNOSIS. The diagnosis of prostatitis is based on examination of expressed prostatic secretions (EPS) and quantitative bacterial localization cultures. Although microscopic examination of EPS is important, it can be misleading. The clinician should always compare the microscopic appearance of EPS to smears of the spun sediment of the first voided 10 ml of urine (the urethral specimen) and the midstream urine (bladder specimen) to localize the site of the inflammatory response. The presence of >20 white blood cells per high-powered field (hPF) in EPS is abnormal. During prostatic inflammation, EPS typically contain leukocytes and abnormal numbers of lipid-laden macrophages (oval fat bodies).

Bacterial prostatitis is best diagnosed by performing simultaneous quantitative bacterial cultures of the urethral urine, bladder urine, and EPS. Four specimens are collected: the first voided 10 ml (VB1), the midstream aliquot (VB2), the EPS, and the first voided 10 ml immediately after prostatic massage (VB3). All specimens are cultured quantitatively by surface streaking onto blood and MacConkey agar. The diagnosis is confirmed when the quantitative bacterial colony counts of the prostatic specimens (EPS and VB3) significantly exceed those of the urethral (VB1) and bladder (VB2) specimens by at least 1 logarithm. Based on these diagnostic maneuvers, the inflammatory diseases of the prostate have been subdivided into four categories: (1) acute bacterial prostatitis, (2) chronic bacterial prostatitis, (3) nonbacterial prostatitis, and (4) prostatodynia.

DIFFERENTIAL DIAGNOSIS. A full urologic evaluation is required in all patients with lower urinary tract complaints. The differential diagnosis in patients with lower urinary tract irritative symptoms should include upper urinary tract infection with secondary colonization of the bladder, carcinoma of the bladder, neurogenic bladder, prostatic obstruction, and urethral stricture. Because the irritative urinary symptoms in men with prostatitis are identical to those in patients with carcinoma *in situ* of the bladder, urinary cytology and cystoscopy should be carried out in these patients to exclude the presence of bladder carcinoma.

Acute Bacterial Prostatitis

Acute bacterial prostatitis is a fulminant condition that occurs mainly between the ages of 20 and 40. There is acute onset of fever, chills, and malaise associated with marked urinary irritative and obstructive symptoms. Pain may be experienced in the suprapubic region, lumbar spine, and perineum.

On physical examination, patients frequently have a temperature as high as 39 to 40° C. Patients may have marked suprapubic tenderness if prostatic infection results in urinary retention. Rectal examination to rule out a prostatic abscess should be done very carefully, as it is extremely uncomfortable for the patient and may result in septicemia or secondary epididymitis if the prostate is massaged too vigorously. The prostate is variably enlarged, markedly tender, and hot to palpation. A prostatic abscess should be suspected if an abnormally fluctuant area is palpated within the prostate.

Patients with acute bacterial prostatitis almost always have associated bacteriuria, and therefore urinalysis and urine culture are helpful in establishing the diagnosis and identifying appropriate antibiotic therapy. With recurrent bacterial prostatitis, intravenous pyelography or abdominal ultrasonography should be done to rule out upper urinary tract pathology. Pelvic ultrasonography or computed tomography may be helpful in diagnosing a prostatic abscess.

Patients with acute bacterial prostatitis are frequently quite ill and need to be hospitalized for their initial treatment. Urinary retention may necessitate placement of a temporary suprapubic cystostomy or urethral catheter. Intravenous antibiotics are usually given; a combination of gentamicin to cover gram-negative organisms and ampicillin to cover enterococci should be used. Supportive measures include hydration, analgesics, and stool softeners. Following initial intravenous therapy, antibiotic therapy should be started with broad gram-negative coverage that diffuses readily into the prostatic fluid. Trimethoprim, trimethoprim-sulfamethoxazole, and the quinolone derivatives are the usual choices. Because bacterial infections may

be difficult to eradicate, oral antibiotics should be continued for 4 to 6 weeks after the acute episode. It is worthwhile to examine EPS and VB3 6 to 12 weeks after the start of therapy to be sure that the infection has resolved.

Granulomatous lesions of the prostate, observed in about 1% of tissue specimens obtained either by biopsy or by partial prostatectomy, usually result from previous bacterial infection or prior transurethral resection of the prostate. Systemic diseases commonly associated with granuloma formation, such as tuberculosis, account for only a small minority of cases. Granulomatous prostatitis may cause induration that mimics prostatic carcinoma, requiring a biopsy to distinguish the two conditions. Granulomatous prostatitis may result in irritative and obstructive urinary symptoms that usually resolve spontaneously. The value of antibiotics in this condition is controversial.

Chronic Bacterial Prostatitis

Chronic bacterial prostatitis is one of the most common causes of recurrent urinary tract infection in men. The symptoms, similar to but milder than those of acute bacterial prostatitis, include urinary frequency and dysuria along with vague lower abdominal, lumbar, and perineal pain. Fever and urethral discharge are uncommon. The diagnosis is made by examination of EPS and quantitative bacterial cultures. EPS should be considered abnormal if there are >10 leukocytes per hPF and more than one or two lipid-laden macrophages per hPF. Men with chronic bacterial prostatitis may have normal EPS while receiving antibiotic therapy, but may continue to have recurrent infections once antibiotics have been discontinued. Furthermore, 5% to 10% of men with no symptoms of prostatic inflammation have >10 leukocytes per hPF in their EPS.

An alternative approach to quantitative bacterial cultures, which are expensive and time consuming, is to obtain a quantitative culture of the bladder urine (VB2) and a nonquantitative culture of EPS on the first office visit. If these cultures are both negative, the prostate is probably not infected. Recovery of gram-negative bacteria from either of these specimens identifies patients who might have chronic bacterial prostatitis and provides a rationale for conventional bacterial localization cultures on the second office visit.

Chronic bacterial prostatitis is frequently difficult to treat. Antibiotic therapy alone eradicates only about 30 to 50% of the infections, but suppressive antimicrobial therapy usually results in complete symptomatic relief and reduces the risks of serious illness. The usual antibiotics used in this condition are trimethoprim-sulfamethoxazole, carbenicillin, or one of the quinolones, such as ciprofloxacin or norfloxacin, in a 4- to 12-week course of therapy. Suppressive antibiotic therapy with trimethoprim, trimethoprim-sulfamethoxazole, and nitrofurantoin is effective. Experimentally, direct injection of antibiotics, such as thiamphenicol and aminoglycosides, has given promise in patients in whom previous oral antibiotic therapy failed.

Chronic Abacterial Prostatitis and Prostatodynia

Symptoms of chronic abacterial prostatitis and prostatodynia are similar to those of chronic bacterial prostatitis. In chronic abacterial prostatitis, EPS are abnormal, but all cultures are normal. In prostatodynia, EPS are normal, and all cultures are normal.

Although cultures of prostatic biopsy specimens in abacterial prostatitis are rarely positive, some patients with nonbacterial prostatitis and prostatodynia improve with antimicrobial therapy. Overall, antibiotic therapy in these conditions has been disappointing, as have all forms of therapy to date. In one report 86% of patients with chronic abacterial prostatitis and prostatodynia treated only with stress management reported improvement or cure, suggesting a psychological basis for these conditions.

BENIGN PROSTATIC HYPERPLASIA (BPH)

INCIDENCE. BPH is a disease of advancing age; it is estimated that one in four men living until age 80 will require treatment for this disease. BPH usually is noted clinically after age 50, the incidence increasing with age, but as many as two thirds of men between 40 and 49 demonstrate histologic evidence of the disease.

ETIOLOGY. BPH is closely related to both aging and age-associated changes in circulating hormones. Circulating androgens clearly play a role; BPH does not develop in men who are castrated or who lose testicular function before puberty. Castration causes atrophy of prostatic epithelium.

With aging, serum testosterone levels decline while serum estrogen levels increase, resulting in an increase in the ratio of plasma estrogens to plasma testosterone. It is unclear, however, whether these shifts in circulating hormone levels are directly involved in the pathogenesis of BPH. Androgens and estrogens seem to act synergistically in the development of BPH in the dog, estrogens increasing prostatic androgen receptors by twofold. Levels of DHT are not actually elevated in BPH tissue, but enzymatic changes occur within the hyperplastic gland that would tend to favor the accumulation of DHT.

PATHOGENESIS. As the hyperplastic prostate enlarges, it compresses the urethra, producing symptoms of urethral obstruction that ultimately may progress to urinary retention. Urethral obstruction may cause incomplete emptying of the bladder, giving rise to urinary stasis, urinary tract infection, and bladder calculi. Furthermore, hypertrophy of the bladder muscle may cause hydronephrosis and bladder diverticula. The natural history of BPH is quite variable. In general, 1 to 2% per year of men with symptoms of BPH develop urinary retention.

SYMPTOMS. Symptoms due to BPH are either obstructive or irritative. *Obstructive symptoms* include hesitancy to initiate voiding, straining to void, decreased force and caliber of the urinary stream, prolonged dribbling after micturition, a sensation of incomplete bladder emptying, and urinary retention. These symptoms result directly from narrowing of the bladder neck and prostatic urethra by the hyperplastic prostate.

Irritative symptoms include urinary frequency, nocturia, dysuria, urgency, and urge incontinence. These symptoms may result from incomplete emptying of the bladder with voiding or may be due to urinary tract infection secondary to prostatic obstruction. More commonly, irritative symptoms result from reduced bladder compliance as a result of prostatic obstruction. It is important to recognize that irritative symptoms may be caused by other conditions such as bladder carcinoma, neurogenic bladder, and urinary tract infection unrelated to prostatic obstruction. All too frequently, patients with irritative urinary tract symptoms are presumed to have prostatic obstruction without an adequate diagnostic evaluation, resulting in delayed and sometimes inappropriate therapy.

PHYSICAL EXAMINATION. Other than a distended bladder, the usual physical findings in BPH are confined to the prostate. Examination of the prostate should be performed with the patient in either the knee-chest position or bent over the bed with his chest touching his elbows. The examining glove should be well lubricated, and the index finger should be inserted slowly into the rectum to allow the anal sphincter time to relax.

The normal prostate, the size of a walnut, has the consistency of a pencil eraser. The hyperplastic prostate is variably enlarged, usually no more than two or three times normal, but occasionally exceeding the size of a lemon. The consistency remains rubbery but is somewhat more fleshy, particularly in the larger glands. Rectal examination affords only a rough estimate of prostatic size and should never be relied upon to rule out prostatic obstruction. A much more accurate anatomic appraisal of the prostate can be obtained with transrectal ultrasonography and cystourethroscopy. The combination of a digital rectal examination (DRE) and serum PSA determination is the most effective means of screening for prostate cancer.

DIAGNOSTIC TESTS. The most valuable test for documenting urinary obstruction is measurement of the urinary flow rate. Inexpensive flowmeters allow accurate determination of the patient's voided volume and peak urinary flow rate, which can be plotted against the patient's age on a nomogram. A decreased flow rate *per se* is never an indication for prostatectomy, but, when used and interpreted correctly, uroflowmetry is an excellent physiologic test for prostatic obstruction.

An abdominal ultrasound examination is useful to rule out associated upper tract pathology, such as hydronephrosis, as well as to detect renal masses. Furthermore, ultrasound measurement of postvoid residual urine volumes and prostatic size is extremely accurate.

Cystourethroscopy, although often employed, may be misleading as a diagnostic test for prostatic obstruction. An anatomically small prostate may produce significant obstruction during voiding, while an anatomically large prostate may produce little or no obstruction. The place for cystourethroscopy is in making the decision whether the prostate is small enough to be resected transurethrally or sufficiently large to require open surgical removal. Before prostatec-

tomy, a careful inspection of the bladder is made to rule out bladder diverticula, stones, and most importantly tumors.

A retrograde urethrogram may be helpful in evaluating symptoms of BPH when a urethral stricture is suspected. Formal urodynamic pressure-flow studies may be indicated in patients with complex voiding symptomatology or suspected neurogenic bladder.

TREATMENT. Indications for treatment of BPH include (1) voiding symptoms that are troublesome to the patient; (2) urinary retention; (3) recurrent urinary tract infections caused by postvoid residual urine; (4) compromised renal function due to hydronephrosis from prostatic obstruction; (5) recurrent gross hematuria with no other explanation; and (6) urge incontinence due to prostatic obstruction.

Historically the most common treatment for BPH has been partial prostatectomy. The goal of partial prostatectomy is to re-establish a wide-open bladder neck and prostatic urethra by selectively removing all of the hyperplastic prostatic tissue down to the so-called surgical capsule, leaving the peripheral prostate intact (see Fig. 209–7). This is accomplished either by transurethral resection or by open surgical enucleation of the adenoma, depending usually on the size of the gland. Adenomas < 70 grams are usually approached transurethrally.

Transurethral prostatectomy (TURP) is generally regarded as a safe and effective procedure. Because of improvements in endoscopic instrumentation, antibiotics, anesthesia, and intraoperative management, most patients tolerate TURP well. The overall morbidity, however, is about 18% and mortality about 1%. Risk factors include age > 80 years, prostate size > 45 grams, surgical time > 90 minutes, and preoperative urinary retention. Although 80% of men report significant improvement in their symptoms following surgery, the morbidity of the procedure has stimulated interest in alternative treatments.

Alternative treatments for BPH include: (1) transurethral incision of the bladder neck, (2) α-adrenergic blockers, (3) 5α-reductase inhibitors, (4) aromatase inhibitors, and (5) laser or hyperthermic ablation of the prostate.

Transurethral incision is done by making one or two longitudinal incisions with an endoscope through the muscular fibers of the bladder neck and prostatic urethra to spring open the prostate and thus enlarge the caliber of the prostatic urethra. Transurethral incision can be performed as an outpatient procedure under local anesthesia, and operative time and blood loss are greatly reduced. Transurethral incision is probably as effective as transurethral resection in treating small prostates (< 20 grams) but appears less effective for larger, bulkier glands.

α-Adrenergic blockers relieve prostatic obstruction by decreasing α-adrenoreceptor-mediated smooth muscle tone of the prostatic capsule and bladder neck. Selective α_1-blockers, such as terazosin and doxazosin, have fewer side effects than nonselective α-blockers. Terazosin has the additional advantage of once-daily dosing. The response rate to these agents appears to be about 70%.

5α-Reductase inhibitors block the conversion of testosterone to DHT, the most active prostatic androgen, resulting in atrophy of the prostatic epithelium. Prostate size decreases an average of 30% after 3 to 6 months of therapy, but the prostate quickly regrows to its original size after cessation of therapy. Significant improvement in symptom score and urinary flow rate is achieved in about 30% of patients.

Multiple clinical trials have been performed in Europe using aromatase inhibitors to test the hypothesis that increased estrogen levels contribute to BPH in men. To date, no study has demonstrated efficacy of these agents in the treatment of BPH.

Transurethral laser ablation and transrectal hyperthermia are new treatments for BPH. The morbidity of these procedures appears to be markedly reduced from standard surgical intervention. Early results indicate, however, that laser ablation and hyperthermia may not be as effective as TURP. In addition, the instrumentation is expensive, and prostatic tissue is not obtained for pathologic examination to rule out unsuspected prostatic carcinoma.

For patients with urinary retention who are poor surgical candidates and in whom medical management is unlikely to be successful, options include either clean, intermittent urethral catheterization or long-term use of an indwelling urethral catheter. Alternatively these patients may benefit from placement of an intraurethral metal alloy prostatic stent. These stents serve to maintain an adequate channel in the prostatic urethra. They are initially associated with a high percentage of irritative voiding symptoms, but most patients ultimately tolerate them fairly well. At present, stents are available only at a limited number of investigational centers.

CARCINOMA OF THE PROSTATE

INCIDENCE. Carcinoma of the prostate is rare before age 50, but the incidence subsequently increases steadily with age. Overall, it is the most common malignant disease in United States men and the second most common cause of cancer deaths in men. Carcinoma of the prostate is more common among black American men (22 deaths per 100,000 men) than white American men (14 deaths per 100,000 men).

ETIOLOGY. The etiology of prostatic carcinoma is unknown. The disease does not occur in men castrated before puberty and partially regresses following castration or estrogen therapy, but a hormonal etiology has not been established. BPH does not appear to be causally related. Environmental factors may be involved, since men migrating from areas where prostatic cancer is uncommon to areas where it is more common develop the disease with increased frequency. The only known risk factor for prostate cancer is a positive family history. Men with a first-degree relative with prostate cancer have a twofold increased risk of developing the disease. The pattern of inheritance appears to be autosomal dominant, similar to hereditary breast cancer and nonpolyposis colon cancer.

PATHOGENESIS. Ninety-five per cent of prostatic cancers are adenocarcinomas, with the remainder being transitional cell carcinomas, squamous cell carcinomas, and sarcomas. Adenocarcinoma of the prostate usually arises in the posterior peripheral region of the prostate (Fig. 209–7), although it commonly invades the periurethral tissue where BPH originates, subsequently producing urethral obstruction. Prostate cancer may produce ureteral obstruction either by direct extension into the bladder or by spreading behind the bladder through the seminal vesicles. Distant spread occurs through lymphatic and hematogenous routes. Prostatic cancer most commonly metastasizes to the pelvic lymph nodes and skeleton, especially the pelvis and lumbar spine. Visceral metastases, which occur later and less commonly, most frequently involve the lungs, liver, and adrenals.

Prostate cancer has an extremely variable and largely unpredictable natural history. In some men the disease progresses very slowly, and they may do very well for 10 years without treatment. In others, the disease exhibits rapid metastatic spread, leading to early death.

SYMPTOMS. Early carcinoma of the prostate is asymptomatic. As the disease spreads into the urethra, it may cause symptoms of urinary obstruction indistinguishable from those produced by BPH. If the tumor has progressed to obstruct the ureters, the patient may have symptoms of uremia. Skeletal pain and pathologic fractures caused by metastatic disease may be the initial symptoms of advanced disease.

PHYSICAL EXAMINATION. The patient may have lymphadenopathy, signs of uremia, congestive heart failure, or urinary retention with a distended bladder. More commonly, the pathologic physical findings are confined to the prostate. On rectal examination the prostate feels harder than the normal or hyperplastic prostate, and the normal boundaries of the gland may be obscured. Approximately 50% of localized indurated areas within the prostate are malignant, with the remainder due to prostatic calculi, inflammation, prostatic infarction, or postsurgical change in a patient having previously undergone TURP or open prostatectomy for BPH. If induration is detected that is suggestive of carcinoma, the examiner should determine whether it is focal or diffuse in nature and whether it seems to extend beyond the border of the prostate.

DIAGNOSIS. As stated earlier, screening for prostate cancer is most effectively done by a combination of DRE and serum PSA determination. If the DRE is normal the chances of having prostate cancer are about 2%, 15%, and 35% for a serum PSA of <4, 4 to 10, or >10 ng per milliliter, respectively. If the DRE is abnormal the risks of having prostate cancer are about 10%, 35%, and 67% for a serum PSA of <4, 4 to 10, and >10, respectively. As a screening tool, transrectal ultrasound (TRUS), is relatively inaccurate, in that only 30% of the abnormal lesions detected on TRUS

are malignant. In men with an abnormal DRE and/or PSA, however, TRUS is much more accurate than digitally guided, "blind" biopsy in establishing the diagnosis of prostate cancer.

STAGING CLASSIFICATION. The treatment of prostatic carcinoma depends primarily on the stage of the disease, as illustrated in the TNM staging system (Fig. 209–8).

Stage T1 prostatic carcinoma refers to tumors that are discovered incidentally on histologic examination of prostatic tissue that has been removed for presumed BPH or by transrectal ultrasonography done because of an abnormal serum PSA. Stage T1 tumors are subdivided into stage T1a, which are well- or moderately-differentiated tumors involving <5% of the removed tissue; stage T1b lesions, which are either poorly differentiated or involve >5% of the removed tissue; and stage T1c lesions, which are detected because of an abnormal serum PSA. Stage T2 tumors are palpable on rectal examination and are confined within the boundaries of the prostate. Stage T2a and T2b include tumors involving less than one lobe of the prostate. Stage T2c includes tumors that involve one whole or both lobes. Stage T3 tumors have extended through the prostatic capsule and may involve the seminal vesicles. Stage T4 tumors have invaded other adjacent structures, such as the bladder neck or external urethral sphincter, or have extended laterally to involve the levator muscles and/or pelvic sidewall. Stage N+ and M+ tumors have metastasized—N+ to regional lymph nodes, and M+ distantly.

STAGING EVALUATION. The treatment of prostatic carcinoma is predicated largely on the stage of the tumor; accurate staging is therefore essential. The DRE is valuable in assessing the local extent of tumor, but transrectal ultrasonography and magnetic resonance imaging of the prostate may be useful when the findings on physical examination are not definitive.

Historically, enzymatic determination of serum prostatic acid phosphatase has been the basic screening test for metastatic prostate cancer, with an elevated value being about 70% sensitive and virtually 100% specific for metastatic disease. Because of its far greater specificity, however, serum PSA has replaced prostatic acid phosphatase in staging prostate cancer. Seventy per cent of prostate cancer patients who have a serum PSA < 10 ng per milliliter will have organ-confined disease, in contrast to only 35% of men with PSA levels between 10 and 20 ng per milliliter and only 20% with a

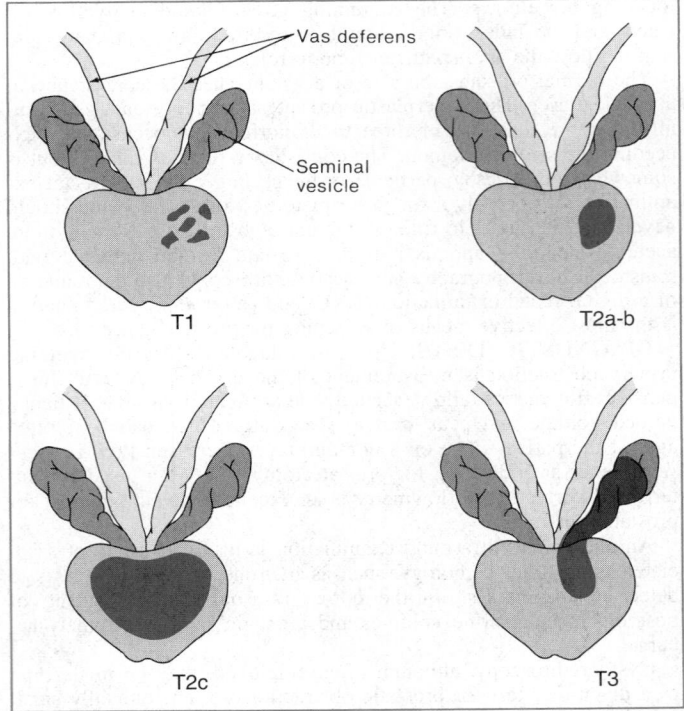

FIGURE 209–8. Whitmore staging classification of prostatic carcinoma. T1 = Microscopic disease in a clinically benign gland. T2a–b = Nodule involving less than one posterior lobe. T2c = Nodule involving one entire lobe or both posterior lobes. T3 = Extension beyond the peripheral capsule of the prostate.

PSA >20 ng per milliliter. In general, the higher the serum PSA level, the greater the likelihood of advanced disease.

Similarly, PSA is extremely useful in evaluating response to therapy, particularly radical prostatectomy. Since PSA is produced only in the prostate, serum PSA levels following successful radical prostatectomy should be undetectable. A measurable level of PSA postoperatively is thus essentially diagnostic of residual or recurrent disease and is almost always the first indicator of treatment failure.

The radionuclide bone scan is highly accurate and far more sensitive than conventional skeletal radiography in detecting osseous metastases. Pelvic lymph node metastases in prostatic carcinoma are more difficult to detect. Neither pedal lymphangiography nor pelvic computed tomography (CT) can reliably detect pelvic lymph node metastases. Neither technique is able to demonstrate microscopic nodal disease, and neither technique consistently demonstrates the obturator and hypogastric lymphatic chains, which are the primary sites of lymphatic drainage from the prostate. In patients with otherwise localized disease, a staging pelvic lymphadenectomy is usually done prior to performance of radical prostatectomy, either in conjunction with the operation, relying on a frozen-section evaluation of the lymph nodes, or several days earlier to allow a full histologic evaluation of the nodal tissue. Pelvic lymphadenectomy has a low morbidity rate and seems justified as a staging procedure to spare those patients with positive lymph nodes from a radical prostatectomy.

TREATMENT. *Watchful Waiting.* Since most prostate cancers are slow growing, watchful waiting with no immediate therapy may be appropriate. Watchful waiting is probably the best treatment for men with a life expectancy of less than 10 years who have well- or moderately-differentiated tumors. We believe, however, that watchful waiting is not appropriate for younger, healthier men or for those with more advanced or aggressive tumors. Patients with moderately differentiated tumors who are initially untreated have a 40 to 50% chance of developing metastatic disease within 10 years, compared with <10% of similar patients treated by radical prostatectomy.

Surgery. Radical prostatectomy is the most effective way of curing localized prostate cancer. In radical prostatectomy, the entire prostate and both seminal vesicles are removed through either a perineal or retropubic approach. The overall 10-year actuarial cure rate defined by an undetectable serum PSA is 70% following radical prostatectomy, and increases to more than 85% in men with clinical stages T1a–T2a disease. The major complications of radical prostatectomy are urinary incontinence and impotence. Recent advances in surgical technique, however, have reduced the risk of significant urinary incontinence to <5% and have allowed preservation of sexual function in the majority of men undergoing this procedure.

Radiation. Radiation therapy is administered either via external beam or via interstitial radioactive seeds that are implanted surgically into the prostate. Although the issue remains controversial, radiation therapy seems most appropriate in patients with localized disease who either are unwilling to undergo radical prostatectomy or are not surgical candidates for reasons of age and health. Radiation therapy also is the treatment of choice for patients with clinical stage T3 disease that has extended beyond the borders of the prostate and is therefore not curable surgically.

Endocrine. Hormonal therapy, the mainstay of treatment for patients with advanced disease, attempts to deprive prostatic tumors of circulating androgens and thereby produce regression of both primary and metastatic lesions. Hormonal ablation can be achieved either by medical or surgical castration. Historically, diethylstilbestrol (DES) was used to achieve medical castration, but has mostly been abandoned because of gynecomastia and cardiovascular complications. Medical castration is presently achieved with luteinizing hormone releasing hormone (LHRH) agonists that inhibit testosterone alone or in combination with antiandrogens that block androgen action in the prostate itself. These agents appear as effective as conventional hormone therapy with estrogens or orchiectomy, and the addition of an antiandrogen may provide an additional survival advantage of several months. Relapse following hormone therapy is due to continued growth of hormone-insensitive cells, and further attempts to lower serum testosterone levels provide little, if any, additional palliation.

Patient response to hormonal therapy varies considerably; 10% of patients live less than 6 months, 50% survive less than 3 years, and only 10% live longer than 10 years. The timing of endocrine therapy also appears to make little difference in the course of the disease. Initiation of treatment at the time of diagnosis may provide a longer symptom-free interval but little in the way of effective palliation once relapse has occurred. For this reason, it may be preferable to delay hormonal therapy until the patient has become symptomatic in the hope of providing increased long-term palliation.

Chemotherapy. Cytotoxic chemotherapy for carcinoma of the prostate has so far yielded discouraging results. A major goal for the future is to develop new forms of therapy that will be effective against the hormone-resistant cell population. The discovery of such agents will represent a major advance in the treatment of this disease.

Catalona WJ, Smith DS, Ratliff TL, et al.: Measurement of prostate-specific antigen in serum as a screening test for prostate cancer. N Engl J Med 324:1156, 1991. *This large study concluded that measurement of serum PSA levels is a useful addition to screening by rectal examination alone.*

Coffey DS: The molecular biology, endocrinology and physiology of the prostate and seminal vesicles. *In* Walsh PC, Retik AB, Stamey TA, et al. (eds.): Campbell's Urology, 6th ed. Philadelphia, WB Saunders, 1992, pp 221–266. *Excellent review of prostate biochemistry and physiology.*

Cooner WH, Mosley BR, Rutherford CL, Jr, et al.: Prostate cancer detection in a clinical urological practice by ultrasonography, digital rectal examination and prostate specific antigen. J Urol 143:1146, 1990. *Practical approach to detection of prostate adenocarcinoma.*

Fowler JE, Jr: Bacteriuria and associated infections of the reproductive system in men. *In* Urinary Tract Infection and Inflammation. Chicago, Year Book, 1989, pp 92–123. *Review of etiology, diagnosis, and treatment of male genital tract infections.*

Gittes RF: Medical progress: Carcinoma of the prostate. N Engl J Med 324:236, 1991. *Excellent review.*

McConnell JD, Barry MJ, Bruskewitz RC, et al.: Benign prostatic hyperplasia: Diagnosis and Treatment. Clinical Practice Guideline, Number 8, AHCPR publication No. 94-0582, Rockville, Md: Agency for Health Care Policy and Research, Public Health Service. U.S. Dept. of Health & Human Services, February, 1994. *Excellent recent review of diagnosis and treatment of benign prostatic hyperplasia.*

Osterling JE: Benign prostatic hyperplasia. Medical and minimally invasive treatment options. N. Engl J Med 332:99, 1995. *A comprehensive, highly readable review of the subject.*

Stamey TA, McNeal JE: Adenocarcinoma of the prostate. *In* Walsh PC, Retik AB, Stamey TA, et al. (eds.): Campbell's Urology, 6th ed. Philadelphia, WB Saunders, 1992, pp 1159–1221. *Provides a comprehensive review of all aspects of diagnosis and treatment of prostate carcinoma.*

210 MULTIPLE-ORGAN SYNDROMES

210.1 Polyglandular Disorders
Henry M. Kronenberg

Internists need to recognize diseases that involve independent abnormalities of more than one endocrine gland for a number of reasons: First, the known patterns of multiglandular disease can alert the clinician to look for a second disorder when one is diagnosed. Second, the treatment of many of the individual diseases in polyglandular disorders may differ from the treatment appropriate for the same diseases when they present in isolation. Third, because many of these diseases appear in characteristic familial patterns, the recognition of the syndromes can lead to useful family screening. Fourth, an understanding of the pathogenesis of these unusual disorders is likely to clarify the pathogenesis of more common single-gland disorders as well. This chapter discusses the best-characterized polyglandular disorders with these four considerations as the primary focus. Other chapters should be consulted for more detailed discussion of the diseases of individual glands.

POLYGLANDULAR NEOPLASIA

Three mechanistically distinct neoplastic syndromes involve more than one endocrine gland. Although given a variety of different names in the past, they are now most frequently called multiple endocrine neoplasia type 1, multiple endocrine neoplasia types 2a and 2b, and McCune-Albright syndrome.

MULTIPLE ENDOCRINE NEOPLASIA TYPE 1.

Multiple endocrine neoplasia type 1 (MEN 1) is an autosomal dominant disorder involving characteristically the parathyroid glands, the pancreatic islets, and the anterior pituitary. Less commonly, adrenal gland neoplasia, foregut carcinoids (primarily of thymus and lung), and lipomas occur. Because thyroid neoplasms are so common in the general population, their true association with MEN 1 is debated.

Parathyroid Disease. Hyperparathyroidism is the most common abnormality in MEN 1, found in more than 90% of patients. Elevation of blood calcium generally first appears between the ages of 20 and 40, considerably earlier than in sporadic primary hyperparathyroidism; this is not a disease of children, however. At first, the disease is asymptomatic but then can lead to all the expected consequences of primary hyperparathyroidism. Unlike sporadic hyperparathyroidism, the disease is relentlessly progressive and, with prolonged follow-up, always involves all four parathyroid glands. The involvement is characteristically asymmetric and asynchronous. This pattern can lead to inappropriately limited parathyroid surgery. If fewer than three parathyroid glands are removed, hypercalcemia always recurs, although not necessarily immediately. Surgical results in MEN 1 are generally less satisfactory than in sporadic four-gland parathyroid disease. At some centers all four glands are removed, and a portion of one gland is reimplanted in the easily accessible forearm in an attempt to avoid the hazards of too much or too little surgery. The difficulty in attaining long-term normocalcemia has led many clinicians to postpone surgery when the disease is asymptomatic. This strategy may need to be modified if the patient develops Zollinger-Ellison syndrome (see below), because hypercalcemia can dramatically increase the gastrin levels in such patients.

Pancreatic Islet Disease. As many as 80% of patients have pancreatic abnormalities at autopsy; a large number correspondingly have increased blood levels of gastrin, insulin, pancreatic polypeptide, somatostatin, vasoactive intestinal polypeptide, or glucagon during stimulation or suppression tests. The pancreas is often diffusely involved with microadenomas and macroadenomas and apparently hyperplastic lesions. Characteristically, more than one islet hormone is secreted from these multiple tumors. Despite this underlying pattern of multiple cellular involvement, patients characteristically present with symptoms of only one hormonal disorder. The most common disease is Zollinger-Ellison syndrome, peptic ulcer disease associated with gastrin-producing tumors. Identification of disease-causing tumors has proven difficult. The gastrinomas in MEN 1 are often multiple, very small, and found in the duodenal wall. Macroadenomas observed in the pancreas by computed tomography (CT) or intraoperative ultrasonography may well synthesize hormones other than gastrin. Although some centers continue to experiment with aggressive attempts at surgical cure, the high recurrence rate after surgery has limited the role for surgery in this disease. Medical therapy with H_2 receptor antagonists and H^+,K^+-ATPase inhibitors can usually adequately control the secretion of stomach acid. The tumors are slow-growing but frequently metastasize locally and to the liver. Chemotherapy is only partially effective and never cures the disease.

Insulinomas are the second most common clinically important islet tumor in MEN 1. These tumors are often small and multiple and are much less frequently malignant than the gastrinomas. Despite the frequently diffuse nature of the disease, dominant insulin-producing tumors can often be identified by selective portal venous sampling. Removal of the dominant tissue, or, if necessary, subtotal (80%) pancreatectomy is the primary therapeutic strategy.

Pituitary Disease. As in sporadic disease, pituitary disease can present with a hypersecretion syndrome or with symptoms due to a sellar mass or hypopituitarism. Pituitary tumors occur in more than half of MEN 1 patients. Prolactinomas are the most common tumors. Adrenocortical hyperfunction can result from a pituitary adenoma or from production of ACTH or corticotropin-releasing hormone by a foregut carcinoid. Although nonfunctioning adrenal neoplasms are common in MEN 1, primary adrenal neoplasms causing glucocorticoid excess are rare. Acromegaly can result from a pituitary neoplasm or as a consequence of production of growth hormone–releasing hormone by pancreatic islet tumors. After con-

sideration of ectopic hormone and releasing hormone production by nonpituitary tumors, the course and treatment of pituitary disease in MEN 1 resemble those of sporadic pituitary disease.

Pathogenesis. Family studies have mapped the gene responsible for MEN 1 to the long arm of chromosome 11, band 11q13. In addition to this genetic abnormality, inherited by all cells in the body, MEN 1 tumors harbor other tumor-specific genetic changes. In the majority of parathyroid and islet tumors studied, these additional genetic abnormalities consist of loss or mutation of DNA at loci that include 11q13. Strikingly, in every case, the loss of genetic information at 11q13 in tumors always involves the chromosome inherited from the normal parent rather than the chromosome carrying the inherited MEN 1 genetic mutation. This pattern strongly suggests that loss of function of both copies of the MEN 1 gene (one from the inherited mutation and one from the mutation found in the tumor) makes tumor formation likely. The tumors are thus clonal expansions that may result from loss of function of a so-called tumor suppressor gene. The gene involved in MEN 1 may be involved in the pathogenesis of sporadic parathyroid adenomas because 25% of such neoplasms also involve somatic (not inherited) abnormalities at 11q13. Still unclear are the direct consequences of the single inherited abnormality at 11q13 in MEN 1. A second, somatic mutation may be required for tumor formation in MEN 1. Alternatively, it is possible that the inherited abnormality alone can cause hyperplasia of the involved glands, which then evolves by clonal expansion. The two-hit, tumor suppressor model can explain many of the features of MEN 1. Clinical presentation of an inherited disorder in adulthood can be explained by the requirement for second mutations before clonal expansion. The asymmetric but relentless nature of the parathyroid disease may be explained by asynchronous but inevitable somatic mutations in each of the parathyroid glands. Multiple islet tumors might result from the same process. Definitive explanations of the pathogenesis of MEN 1 await the expected isolation of the MEN 1 gene.

Without identification of the gene, the identification of affected family members relies primarily on clinical screening. The most useful single test to complement a thorough history and physical examination is measurement of blood calcium, particularly ionized calcium, at intervals after age 15. Prolactin, gastrin, and fasting blood sugar measurements can also be useful. Research laboratories can identify affected family members by characterizing closely linked genetic markers in blood cells if specimens from more than one affected family member are available.

MULTIPLE ENDOCRINE NEOPLASIA TYPES 2A AND 2B.

Multiple endocrine neoplasia type 2a is an autosomal dominant disease that presents with medullary carcinoma of the thyroid (MCT), pheochromocytoma, and, less commonly, hyperparathyroidism. Multiple endocrine neoplasia type 2b is closely related to MEN 2a because it also presents with medullary carcinoma of the thyroid and pheochromocytoma and because both diseases map to the same genetic region—the pericentromeric region of chromosome 10. MEN 2b presents with a number of abnormalities not found in MEN 2a, however. These include mucosal neuromas of the tongue, lips, eyelids, and gastrointestinal tract and a marfanoid habitus. Hyperparathyroidism rarely occurs in MEN 2b. MEN 2b is less common than MEN 2a; both diseases are rarer than MEN 1.

In MEN 2a and 2b, the medullary cancers and the pheochromocytomas often present bilaterally. Careful prospective analysis of MEN 2a families has demonstrated that diffuse C cell hyperplasia precedes clinically obvious appearance of medullary cancer by decades. C cell hyperplasia can be detected by measurement of calcitonin after administration of gastrin. With current sensitive assays, the median age of presentation with C cell hyperplasia is 8 or 9. Virtually all MEN 2a patients eventually develop C cell disease. Complete thyroidectomy of patients with C cell hyperplasia has dramatically decreased the incidence of medullary cancer, which has been the major cause of death in MEN 2a.

Half the patients with MEN 2a develop pheochromocytomas. Family screening allows the detection of pheochromocytoma before the development of hypertension. The first laboratory abnormalities noted include an increase in urinary epinephrine and in the ratio of epinephrine to norepinephrine in the urine. Increases in urinary metanephrine and norepinephrine come later. The tumors are usually found in the adrenal glands and can be documented preoperatively by CT, magnetic resonance imaging, and [^{131}I]-metaiodobenzylguanidine scanning.

Most patients with MEN 2a have been found to harbor point mutations in the *RET* proto-oncogene. *RET* encodes a member of the tyrosine protein kinase family of cell surface receptors. The gene is expressed in spinal cord, in certain cultured blood cell lines, and in all tested medullary cancer and pheochromocytoma lines (both from MEN 2 patients and from sporadic tumors). The first characterized mutations have been found in four different cysteines located in the portion of the receptor predicted to form the extracellular, ligand-binding domain. In contrast to the pattern in MEN 1, no evidence for somatic mutations in the RET region of chromosome 10 have been found in MEN 2a tumors. It is likely that the mutant RET gene signals in a ligand-independent manner, thereby acting as an oncogene. The mutant RET genes can transform cultured cells, and the mutant ret protein can act as a ligand-independent protein kinase. The mutant RET genes are, therefore, likely to be inherited oncogenes.

The transition from diffuse hyperplasia of C cells or adrenal medullary cells to clonal neoplasms of the thyroid or adrenal probably requires subsequent somatic mutations. Such mutations include the loss of genetic markers on chromosomes 1p, 3p, 3q, and 22q that frequently occur in these tumors.

Patients with MEN 2b harbor a point mutation that changes methionine-918 to a threonine within the ret protein's intracellular kinase domain. Studies suggest that this mutation activates the kinase and may change its substrate specificity.

Carriers of the MEN 2 genes can best be identified by serial measurement of stimulated blood calcitonin levels, starting at an early age. Rapid progress in defining the *RET* lesions in MEN 2a (and perhaps 2b) now allows direct genetic testing, replacing calcitonin testing as a screening tool.

McCUNE-ALBRIGHT SYNDROME. The McCune-Albright syndrome is a noninherited disorder consisting of the triad of polyostotic fibrous dysplasia, light brown pigmented skin lesions (café-au-lait spots), and endocrinopathy, usually precocious puberty. Multiple endocrine abnormalities can occur. The precocious puberty, more often seen in girls than boys, is gonadotropin-independent. Hyperthyroidism is caused by autonomous thyroid nodules. Acromegaly is caused by pituitary adenomas that produce growth hormone and, usually, prolactin. Adrenocortical hyperfunction is caused by ACTH-independent adrenal adenomas. Hypophosphatemic rickets, with normal blood calcium, phosphate wasting, and low or inappropriately normal levels of $1,25(OH)_2D_3$, may result from release of a humoral factor from the dysplastic fibrous tissue.

This somewhat bewildering array of endocrine abnormalities has been rationalized by the observation that cells in the involved tissues harbor mutations in the α subunit of the G_S protein. The G_S protein links cell surface receptors to the activation of adenylate cyclase. The mutations in McCune-Albright syndrome are point mutations at arginine-201 in the G_S α subunit; these mutations lead to prolonged activity of G_S and inappropriate activation of adenylate cyclase. Increased levels of cyclic AMP lead to cellular proliferation and hormone secretion. McCune-Albright patients are genetic mosaics. Presumably, at an early stage in embryonic development, a point mutation occurs in the G_S α gene of a cell that then proliferates, differentiates, and variably populates normal bone, skin, and endocrine tissues. In cell types in which elevations in cyclic AMP lead to proliferation, abnormal cells become predominant and lead to disease. Because the disease is never inherited, the mutation is presumably lethal when present in all cells of the embryo. In contrast, the very same mutations at arginine-201 have been found in cases of isolated acromegaly and autonomous thyroid nodules. One can, therefore, speculate that McCune-Albright syndrome is the most dramatic example of a spectrum of disorders that vary in severity and presentation depending on the stage of development of the original mutant cell.

AUTOIMMUNE POLYGLANDULAR DYSFUNCTION

Organ-specific autoimmune disease, characterized by lymphocytic infiltration and organ-specific autoantibodies, commonly results in endocrine hypofunction or hyperfunction. Clinical manifestations of disease are usually limited to one gland. Not uncommonly, however, disorders of more than one endocrine gland appear in families or in individual patients. Characteristic patterns of disease presentation and genetic inheritance allow the definition of two syndromes with overlapping manifestations (Table 210–1).

TABLE 210–1. CLINICAL FEATURES OF AUTOIMMUNE POLYGLANDULAR SYNDROMES

	Type 1	Type 2
Mucocutaneous candidiasis	Very common	Not seen
Hypoparathyroidism	Common	Rare
Addison's disease	Common	Common
Primary hypogonadism	Common	Occurs
Autoimmune thyroid disease	Rare	Common
Autoimmune diabetes	Occurs	Common
Hypophysitis	Occurs	Occurs
Autoimmune hepatitis	Occurs	Not seen
Pernicious anemia	Occurs	Occurs
Vitiligo	Occurs	Occurs
Malabsorption syndrome	Occurs	Occurs in celiac disease
Alopecia	Common	Occurs
Myasthenia gravis	Not seen	Occurs
Keratopathy	Common	Not seen
Tympanic membrane calcification	Common	Not seen
Inheritance	Autosomal recessive	HLA association
Age of onset	Usually childhood	Usually adulthood

AUTOIMMUNE POLYGLANDULAR SYNDROME TYPE 1. This rare disease presents typically in early childhood. Mucocutaneous candidiasis occurs in virtually all patients and is usually the first manifestation of disease. Hypoparathyroidism and Addison's disease are the most common endocrine manifestations; each of these diseases occurs in 70 to 80% of patients. Hypoparathyroidism usually precedes Addison's disease; both diseases typically present before age 15. Premature ovarian failure (in 60% of affected women) usually presents as secondary amenorrhea; testicular failure occurs less frequently. Insulin-dependent diabetes mellitus occurs in 12% of patients, usually in adulthood; hypothyroidism is uncommon.

Nonendocrine components of this syndrome, in addition to the mucocutaneous candidiasis, include alopecia, vitiligo, corneal opacities, autoimmune hepatitis, enamel hypoplasia of teeth, tympanic membrane calcification, nail dystrophy that correlates only loosely with obvious candidiasis, parietal cell atrophy and vitamin B_{12} malabsorption, and more general intestinal malabsorption with steatorrhea. Asplenism, with Howell-Jolly bodies on peripheral blood smears, has been noted in several patients.

Each of the disease components should be sought when any patient presents with hypoparathyroidism, primary adrenal insufficiency, or mucocutaneous candidiasis. The hypoparathyroidism is treated like the sporadic disease with oral calcium and 1,25-dihydroxyvitamin D, although variable intestinal malabsorption can present a particular therapeutic challenge. The candidiasis can be satisfactorily controlled with ketoconazole.

Autoimmune polyglandular syndrome type 1 is an autosomal recessive disorder. The appearance of organ-specific autoantibodies precedes disease presentation and predicts the development of specific end-organ damage. The role of these antibodies and the precise pathogenesis of the syndrome are unknown, however.

AUTOIMMUNE POLYGLANDULAR SYNDROME TYPE 2. This syndrome is considerably more common than the type 1 syndrome and typically presents in adulthood. Insulin-dependent diabetes mellitus and thyroid dysfunction—either autoimmune hypothyroidism or Grave's disease—are the most frequent manifestations. Addison's disease is the third major endocrine component of this disorder. Although most patients who present with autoimmune diabetes or thyroid disease have clinical involvement of only one gland, a large fraction of patients with autoimmune Addison's disease develop clinically evident disease in other endocrine glands. Less common components of the type 2 polyglandular syndrome include primary hypogonadism and hypophysitis. Pernicious anemia, vitiligo, celiac disease, alopecia, and myasthenia gravis are also associated with this syndrome.

The treatment of each component of this syndrome is identical to the treatment of each disorder in isolation, although possible clustering of diseases must be kept in mind during the evaluation and follow-up of all patients with each individual component disorder. Thyroid hormone therapy can precipitate symptoms of adrenal insufficiency in patients with both disorders, for example. Consequently, careful history, including family history, physical examination, and a low threshold for specific laboratory testing for adrenal insufficiency should be part of the evaluation of every patient with autoimmune hypothyroidism. Further, combinations of hypothyroidism, adrenal insufficiency, and hypogonadism can mimic hypopituitarism, although specific hormonal testing can easily distinguish these disorders. Because multiple components of the syndrome can present asynchronously, periodic evaluation for early appearance of further disease components is indicated.

Autoimmune polyglandular syndrome type 2 is usually inherited in families with characteristic HLA associations. The HLA associations do not predict disease absolutely, even in identical twins, so environmental factors must contribute to disease presentation. Typically, several different autoimmune diseases occur in each family. Autoimmune vulnerability rather than specific organ disease is inherited. Diabetes, as part of the polyglandular syndrome, usually presents at an older age and develops more slowly than isolated autoimmune diabetes. The characteristic pattern of association with specific DQ loci does not differ between polyglandular and isolated diabetes, however. Presumably, genes not linked to the HLA complex modify the presentation of diabetes.

Organ-specific antibodies appear before clinical disease and predict subsequent disease. The role of these antibodies in organ hypofunction has not been established, however.

Ahonen P, Myllärniemi S, Sipilä I, et al.: Clinical variation of autoimmune polyendocrinopathy–candidiasis–ectodermal dystrophy (APECED) in a series of 68 patients. N Engl J Med 322:1829, 1990. *A large series with prolonged follow-up that presents a thorough summary of the clinical features of autoimmune polyglandular syndrome type 1.*

Eisenbarth GS, Jackson RA: The immunoendocrinopathy syndromes. *In* Wilson JD, Foster DW (eds.): William's Textbook of Endocrinology, 8th ed. Philadelphia, WB Saunders, 1992, p 1555. *An excellent general review stressing immune mechanisms.*

Gagel RF, Jackson CE (eds.): Proceedings of the fourth international workshop on multiple endocrine neoplasia. Henry Ford Hosp Med J 40:158, 1992. *A large collection of papers discussing both clinical and genetic aspects of MEN 1 and 2.*

Lips CJM, Landsvater RL, Höppener JWM, et al.: Clinical screening as compared with DNA analysis in families with multiple endocrine neoplasia type 2A. N Engl J Med 331:828, 1994. *The first "field" demonstration of the advantage of using DNA testing instead of calcitonin testing in MEN 2a families.*

Mignon M, Ruszniewski P, Podevin P, et al.: Current approach to the management of gastrinoma and insulinoma in adults with multiple endocrine neoplasia type I. World J Surg 17:489, 1993. *A useful survey of the varied surgical approaches to pancreatic islet disease in MEN 1.*

Santoro M, Carlomagno F, Romano A, et al.: Activation of RET as a dominant transforming gene by germline mutations of MEN 2A and MEN 2B. Science 267:381, 1995. *Elegant demonstration that mutant RET genes are the first inherited disease-causing oncogenes.*

Schwindinger WF, Levine MA. McCune-Albright syndrome. Trends Endocrinol Metab 4:238, 1993. *A succinct and thorough summary of the clinical and molecular aspects of the disease.*

210.2   Carcinoid Syndrome
John A. Oates

Carcinoid syndrome incorporates the constellation of signs and symptoms associated with malignant neoplasms of enterochromaffin cells. Cutaneous flushing, diarrhea, and cardiac valvular lesions are the most common endocrine consequences of these tumors.

THE NEOPLASMS

Tumors that cause the carcinoid syndrome have the characteristics of neuroendocrine cells of the enterochromaffin type. These tumors typically contain 5-hydroxytryptamine (serotonin) and tachykinins such as substance P. The metastatic tumors associated with carcinoid syndrome usually arise from primary tumors in the ileum. The syndrome also can be produced by neoplasms arising from the remainder of the small intestine, from organs derived from the embryonic foregut (e.g., bronchus, stomach, pancreas, and thyroid), and from ovarian or testicular teratomas. The usual carcinoid

tumor arising from the ileum has the histologic pattern of dense nests of cells with uniform size and nuclear appearance. Histochemically, they typically exhibit an argentaffin reaction in which the cells convert a silver salt to metallic silver. A positive argentaffin reaction is not required for the diagnosis, however, as carcinoid tumors arising from organs of the embryonic foregut may contain few if any argentaffin cells. Ultrastructural examination of carcinoid tumors reveals electron-dense secretion granules.

Carcinoid tumors have a proclivity to metastasize to the liver and may involve this organ extensively and predominantly. Extrahepatic metastases occur in bone, where they are often osteoblastic, and in the lung, pancreas, spleen, ovaries, adrenals, and other organs.

Primary carcinoid tumors of the appendix are common, but they rarely metastasize. Those from the large intestine may metastasize but almost never exhibit endocrine effects.

CLINICAL MANIFESTATIONS

Carcinoid tumors typically have a slow rate of growth, and many patients with carcinoid syndrome survive for a decade after the disease is recognized. For much of the duration of the illness, morbidity results largely from the endocrine functions of the tumor. Death usually is caused by cardiac or hepatic failure and by complications associated with tumor growth.

VASODILATOR PAROXYSMS. Cutaneous flushing is the most common clinical feature. The typical flush is erythematous and involves the head and neck (blush area). Some patients exhibit vivid color changes from red to violaceous to pallor. Prolonged flushing attacks may be associated with lacrimation and periorbital edema. The flush may be accompanied by tachycardia, and the blood pressure usually falls or does not change. A rise in blood pressure during flushing is rare, and carcinoid syndrome is not a cause of sustained hypertension. Flushing may be provoked by excitement, exertion, eating, and ethanol ingestion.

TELANGIECTASIA. In addition to paroxysms of cutaneous vasodilatation, some patients also develop telangiectasia, primarily on the face and neck and most marked in the malar area.

GASTROINTESTINAL SYMPTOMS. Intestinal hypermotility with borborygmi, cramping, and explosive diarrhea may accompany the episodic flushes. Chronic diarrhea is more common and may have a secretory component. When this is severe, malabsorption may occur.

CARDIAC MANIFESTATIONS. Plaquelike thickening of the endocardium of the valvular cusps and cardiac chambers occurs primarily on the right side of the heart but may involve the left side to a minimal degree. The endocardial thickening is composed of smooth muscle cells embedded in a stroma rich in mucopolysaccharides. The thickening and deformation of the valve cusps, chordae tendineae, and papillary muscles interfere with valvular function and may lead to regurgitation, stenosis, or combined functional lesions. There is a tendency for the fibrosing process to produce incompetence of the tricuspid valve and stenosis of the smaller pulmonary orifice, a deleterious hemodynamic combination. Cardiac dysfunction may be further compromised by impaired atrial and ventricular compliance and by the occasional occurrence of a high cardiac output that probably results from continuing release of a vasodilator.

PULMONARY. Bronchoconstriction, usually most pronounced during flushing attacks, is a less common feature of the syndrome, but it may be severe.

GENERAL. Intestinal obstruction may result from the primary tumor or from the desmoplastic reaction in the surrounding mesentery; infrequently, the primary tumors cause gastrointestinal bleeding. Necrosis of hepatic tumor masses may produce an acute syndrome of abdominal pain, tenderness, fever, and leukocytosis. Hepatomegaly from the metastatic disease is usually present, but extensive metastatic involvement of the liver by the slowly growing tumors may occur before liver function tests become abnormal. Generalized fatigue and debilitation are underappreciated features of carcinoid syndrome.

THE ENDOCRINE FUNCTION OF CARCINOID TUMORS

SEROTONIN. The most constant biochemical feature of carcinoid tumors is the presence of tryptophan hydroxylase, which catalyzes the formation of 5-hydroxytryptophan (5-HTP) from tryptophan (Fig. 210–1). The typical ileal carcinoid tumor also contains aromatic L-amino acid decarboxylase, which catalyzes the conver-

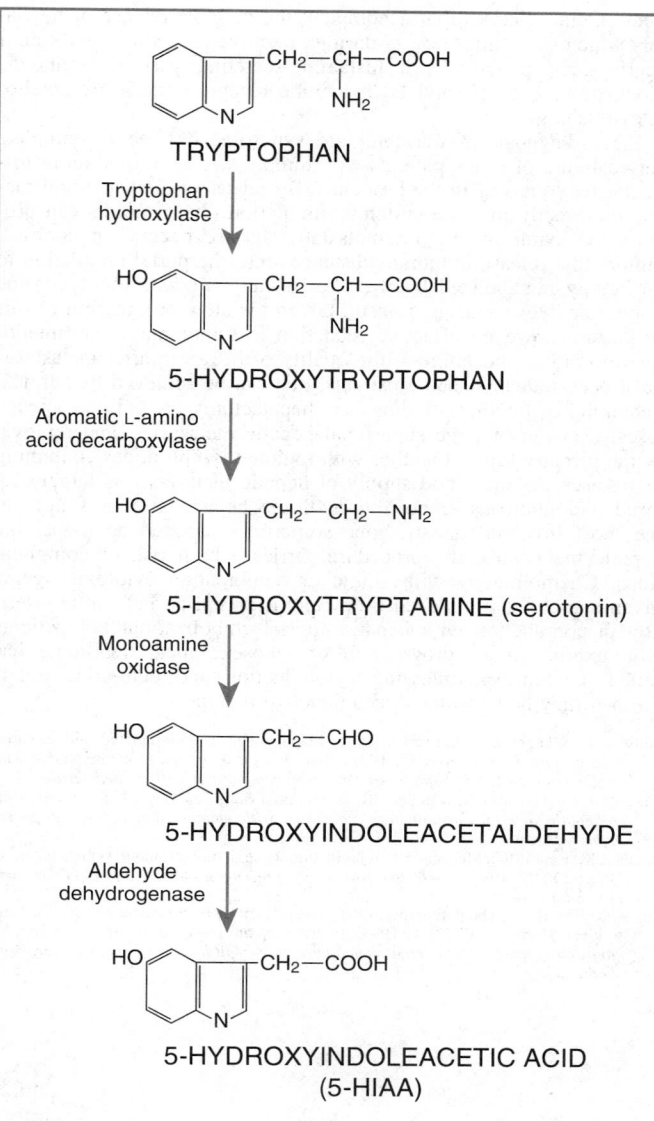

FIGURE 210–1. Synthesis and degradation of serotonin.

sion of 5-HTP to 5-hydroxytryptamine (serotonin). Gastric carcinoids, however, are frequently deficient in this decarboxylase and release 5-HTP from the tumor.

Following its release from the tumor, serotonin is inactivated primarily by monoamine oxidase; uptake in the platelets also contributes to removal of free serotonin from blood. Monoamine oxidase oxidizes serotonin to 5-hydroxyindoleacetaldehyde, which is rapidly converted to 5-hydroxyindoleacetic acid (5-HIAA) by aldehyde dehydrogenase (Fig. 210–1). This acid is rapidly excreted into the urine, and almost all circulating serotonin can be accounted for as urinary 5-HIAA.

TACHYKININS. Peptides of the tachykinin family are stored in carcinoid tumors and are released during flushing. Several tachykinins are derived from a common precursor β-preprotachykinin; of these, neuropeptide K, neurokinin A, and substance P have been identified in tumors and blood from patients with the carcinoid syndrome.

OTHER BIOLOGICALLY ACTIVE SUBSTANCES. Some carcinoid tumors, particularly those of gastric origin, release excessive amounts of histamine. This can be detected by an increased urinary excretion of histamine or its metabolite, *N*-methylhistamine.

Carcinoid tumors have been associated with a number of ectopic endocrine syndromes, including hyperadrenocorticism that results from ectopic production of adrenocorticotropic hormone and acromegaly due to secretion of growth hormone–releasing hormone by the tumor.

MECHANISM OF THE FLUSH. Flushing can be triggered by catecholamines, and this probably accounts for the association of flushing with exercise and emotional stimuli. For experimental induction of flushing, injection of isoproterenol in amounts of as little as 0.5 μg may be effective. Pentagastrin, in doses as small as 0.25 μg, also can trigger flushing, an action that may explain the provocation of flushes by eating in some patients. As the hemodynamic changes associated with such pharmacologically induced attacks can be severe, epinephrine and other β-adrenergic amines as well as pentagastrin should be administered with great caution. Flushing episodes can be blocked by somatostatin.

Most of the evidence points to the tachykinins as mediators of the carcinoid flush. Tachykinins, particularly neuropeptide K, can be identified in plasma during flushing. Tachykinin levels have been shown to be increased during pentagastrin-induced flushing, and when pentagastrin-induced flushing is inhibited by somatostatin, the rise in tachykinin levels also is blocked. Tachykinins are known vasodilators.

Serotonin does not cause flushing. In patients with gastric carcinoids that secrete histamine, the flushing attacks can be attributed to histamine.

PATHOPHYSIOLOGY OF SEROTONIN OVERPRODUCTION. Serotonin contributes to the intestinal hypermotility and diarrhea. A secondary effect of serotonin overproduction occurs when a large fraction of dietary tryptophan is shunted into the hydroxylation pathway, leaving less tryptophan available for the formation of nicotinic acid and protein. When urinary excretion of 5-HIAA exceeds 100 mg daily, low levels of plasma tryptophan and evidence of nicotinic acid deficiency are seen.

DIAGNOSIS

When all of its clinical features are present, carcinoid syndrome is easily recognized. The diagnosis also must be considered when any one of its clinical manifestations is present.

The diagnostic hallmark consists of overproduction of 5-hydroxyindoles accompanied by increased excretion of urinary 5-HIAA. Normally, excretion of 5-HIAA does not exceed 9 mg daily. Ingestion of foods containing serotonin may complicate the biochemical diagnosis of carcinoid syndrome; both bananas and walnuts contain enough serotonin to produce abnormally elevated urinary excretion of 5-HIAA after their ingestion. When dietary 5-hydroxyindoles are excluded, urinary excretion of 25 mg of 5-HIAA daily is diagnostic of carcinoid. Elevation in the range of 9 to 25 mg may be seen with carcinoid syndrome, nontropical sprue, or acute intestinal obstruction. Measurement of serotonin in blood or platelets is of interest but has less diagnostic value than assay of the major metabolite of serotonin in the urine.

DIFFERENTIAL DIAGNOSIS. Attacks of flushing in a patient with normal urinary excretion of 5-HIAA raises other diagnostic possibilities. Systemic mastocyte activation disorders, including systemic mastocytosis, produce flushing and diarrhea and should be considered when 5-HIAA excretion is not elevated. Flushing also occurs in genetically predisposed individuals following ethanol ingestion, in the postmenopausal state, and in conjunction with other neuroendocrine tumors such as VIPomas and medullary carcinoma of the thyroid.

VARIANTS OF THE CARCINOID SYNDROME. The origin of the tumor influences the biologically active substances produced and their storage and release. The typical carcinoid syndrome usually results from tumors of midgut origin, which almost invariably secrete serotonin. Tumor serotonin content is likely to be high, and the tumor usually contains dense nests of argentaffin-positive cells. In contrast, tumors arising from the embryonic foregut contain fewer argentaffin cells, have lower serotonin content, and may secrete 5-HTP. Ectopic hormone production (e.g., Cushing's syndrome and acromegaly) and multiple endocrine adenomas are more likely to be associated with tumors of embryonic foregut.

Patients with gastric carcinoids frequently exhibit unique flushing, which begins as a bright, patchy erythema with sharply delineated serpentine borders; these patches tend to coalesce as the blush heightens. Food ingestion is especially likely to produce flushes. The tumors are usually deficient in decarboxylase enzyme and secrete 5-HTP; histamine secretion is also common, as is a high incidence of peptic ulceration. In these patients, histamine is the principal factor causing flushing.

With carcinoid tumors arising from the bronchus, attacks of flushing tend to be prolonged and severe and may be associated with periorbital edema, excessive lacrimation and salivation, hypotension, tachycardia and tachyarrhythmias, anxiety, and tremulousness. Nausea, vomiting, explosive diarrhea, and bronchoconstriction may progress to a severe degree. This group is therapeutically unique in that severe flushes often can be prevented by corticosteroids.

TREATMENT

Treatment of the carcinoid syndrome is directed toward (1) pharmacologic therapy for humorally mediated symptoms and (2) the reduction of tumor mass.

The discovery that somatostatin can prevent the flushing and other endocrine manifestations of the carcinoid syndrome provided the basis for a major advance in the treatment of these patients. The development of analogues of somatostatin, with longer biologic half-lives than the native hormone, made subcutaneous administration a feasible route of therapy. One of the somatostatin analogues, octreotide, has been found to markedly improve the flushing and other endocrine manifestations of most patients with carcinoid syndrome. This is frequently associated with a reduction in urinary 5-HIAA excretion and in tachykinin levels in blood. With the improvement of these endocrine symptoms, including fatigue, a considerable improvement in quality of life may be achieved. Octreotide is administered subcutaneously at intervals of approximately 8 hours, usually beginning with 75 to 150 μg and titrating upward until maximum inhibition of flushing and other symptoms is achieved, which usually occurs at single doses of 750 μg or less. An uncommon but severe adverse effect of octreotide is hypoglycemia, probably as a result of the inhibition of glucagon and growth hormone secretion; the suppression of pancreatic exocrine function by octreotide can cause steatorrhea. In patients receiving octreotide, about 5% achieve tumor regression, and in the group as a whole there is less tumor progression and a longer median survival compared with historical controls. Octreotide can prevent or treat carcinoid crises that accompany the massive release of mediators which sometimes occurs during operative procedures and tumor necrosis. In patients with histamine-secreting gastric carcinoids, blockade of both H_1 and H_2 histamine receptors markedly ameliorates flushing.

Early diagnosis of the carcinoid syndrome has led to complete surgical cure of a few patients with tumors arising in ovarian or testicular teratomas or in the bronchus. By releasing their humoral mediators directly into the systemic circulation, these tumors can produce the syndrome before metastatic disease occurs. In contrast, tumors that release humoral substances into the portal circulation to be largely metabolized by the liver usually produce the syndrome only after liver metastases occur. Given the slow progression of this neoplasm, however, effective reduction in tumor mass can ameliorate morbidity and improve the quality of life even after metastases have occurred. In selected patients, this can be achieved by surgical debulking of tumor, including hemihepatectomy for unilobar metastases, excision of large superficial hepatic metastases, and removal of the primary tumor together with regional lymph nodes containing metastases. As the blood supply of hepatic metastases is largely arterial, percutaneous embolization of the hepatic arterial supply to the most involved hepatic lobe sometimes can reduce inoperable hepatic metastases; the procedure carries a high risk of complications. Chemotherapy with single or combination cytotoxic agents given acutely has produced little benefit except perhaps intra-arterially in conjunction with hepatic arterial embolization. For patients who exhibit tumor progression or whose clinical syndrome has failed to improve following cytoreduction and octreotide, interferon-α may be considered as adjunctive therapy.

Ahlman H, Wängberg B, Jansson S, et al.: Management of disseminated midgut carcinoid tumors. Digestion 49:78, 1991. *Describes an approach to cytoreduction with surgical resection and hepatic arterial embolectomy in a well-studied series.*

Hajarizadeh H, Ivancev K, Mueller CR, et al.: Am J Surg 163:479, 1992. *Describes intrahepatic arterial chemotherapy combined with embolization of the peripheral hepatic artery.*

Kvols LK, Reubi JC: Metastatic carcinoid tumors and the carcinoid syndrome. Acta Oncol 32:197, 1993. *A selective review that presents the results of octreotide therapy in 66 patients.*

Öberg K: The use of chemotherapy in the management of neuroendocrine tumors. Gastrointest Horm Med 22:941, 1993. *A review of the studies supporting the conclusion that acutely administered chemotherapy is of little or no benefit in carcinoid syndrome.*

PART XVIII

DISEASES OF BONE AND BONE MINERAL METABOLISM

211 MINERAL AND BONE HOMEOSTASIS

Stephen J. Marx

Calcium, phosphorus, and magnesium, three of the principal body elements, have diverse roles. The calcium ion is particularly versatile. In the crystalline phase, it contributes to the varied structural roles of bone. In a supersaturated solution in blood, it contributes to plasma membrane excitability, plasma enzyme activities, and accretion of all minerals in extracellular matrix of bone. In the cytoplasmic fluid, its extraordinarily low concentrations allow rapid rises of its local concentrations to transmit information among cell compartments via its interactions with high-affinity calcium-binding proteins, such as calmodulin or protein kinase C. Phosphate is the principal intracellular anion, with central roles in cytoplasm as a buffer, energy carrier (mainly via the high-energy phosphate bonds of adenosine triphosphate [ATP]), and molecular switch (through phosphorylation and dephosphorylation). Magnesium is the principal cation in cytoplasm, functioning as a cofactor in many chemical reactions (for example, as an Mg-ATP complex or as a cofactor in many steps of DNA or RNA metabolism).

MINERALS IN BLOOD

THE STATE OF CALCIUM, PHOSPHATE, AND MAGNESIUM IN BLOOD. Total calcium concentration is tightly regulated, so that typical diurnal fluctuations are not more than 5% from the mean value. Calcium in blood is divided among protein-bound, complexed, and ionized or free fractions (Table 211–1). Protein binding of calcium in blood is principally to albumin, and this binding is decreased by acid pH. The ionized calcium fraction is the focus for metabolic control by the parathyroid gland, and measurements of ionized calcium in blood give the most valid index of pathologic disruptions of calcium homeostasis.

Phosphate and magnesium in blood are principally unbound (Table 211–1), and the concentration of each is regulated over a broader relative variation from its mean than that for calcium. Neither phosphate nor magnesium has a unique endocrine system dedicated to its control. Rather, their blood concentrations are sustained indirectly by the hormones directed at calcium control and directly by poorly understood local processes in bone, kidney, and other organs.

STEADY-STATE FLOW OF MINERALS TO AND FROM BLOOD. Only 0.1% of the total body calcium is in blood and extracellular fluid (Table 211–2). This calcium pool is in a rapidly exchanging equilibrium with large calcium pools controlled by three organs (bone, intestine, and kidney), each of which is an important site for the regulation of mineral metabolism. The rate of these daily fluxes (Fig. 211–1) is sufficiently large that disturbance of mineral flux to or from any of these organs can result in abnormally high or low concentrations of one of these minerals in blood.

ORGANS EXCHANGING MUCH MINERAL WITH BLOOD

Bone

BONE FUNCTION AND ARCHITECTURE. Major functions of bone include support, locomotion, encasement of hematopoietic tissue, and reservoir for calcium, phosphate, and magnesium. The architecture of bone responds dynamically to changes in mechanical load. The mechanisms whereby the signals from altered load are transduced are poorly understood. Mature bone adopts one of two macroscopic organizations (Fig. 211–2). The cortices of all bones and the interior of certain bones have a continuous structure termed cortical or lamellar bone. Lamellar bone, which is predominant in the long bones, is characterized by little metabolic activity and few cells. It has a highly organized extracellular matrix of mineral and parallel bundles of type I collagen. During embryonic development or in states with pathologic increase of bone turnover, bone assumes a less organized "woven" architecture. Within the vertebral bodies and in portions of the interior of other bones, bone is organized as a series of thin, interdigitating plates; this is termed trabecular, cancellous, or spongy bone. Its ratio of surface to volume is higher than that found in cortical bone and is thus better suited to rapid turnover.

TABLE 211–1. CONCENTRATIONS AND STATES OF CALCIUM, MAGNESIUM, AND PHOSPHATE IN NORMAL HUMAN PLASMA OR SERUM*

State	Calcium (mM)	Magnesium (mM)	Phosphate (mM)
Protein bound	1.15 (47)	0.26 (31)	0.15 (13)
Filterable or free†			
Complexed	0.25 (10)	0.06 (7)	0.40 (35)
Ionized	1.06 (43)	0.52 (62)	0.60 (52)

* Number in parentheses indicates percentage of total for that mineral.
† Filterable or free = complexed + ionized.

TABLE 211–2. DISTRIBUTION OF CALCIUM, MAGNESIUM, AND PHOSPHATE IN THE BODY OF A 70-KG ADULT*

Compartment	Calcium (g)	Magnesium (g)	Phosphate (g)
Bones and teeth	1300 (99)	14.0 (54)	600.0 (86)
Extracellular fluid	1 (0.1)	0.3 (1)	0.2 (0.03)
Cells	7 (1.0)	12.0 (46)	100.0 (14)

* Most of calcium is in bone; almost half of magnesium is in cells. Phosphate, as the principal counterion to calcium and magnesium in their dominant pools, has an intermediate proportional distribution. Number in parentheses is the percentage of total for that mineral.

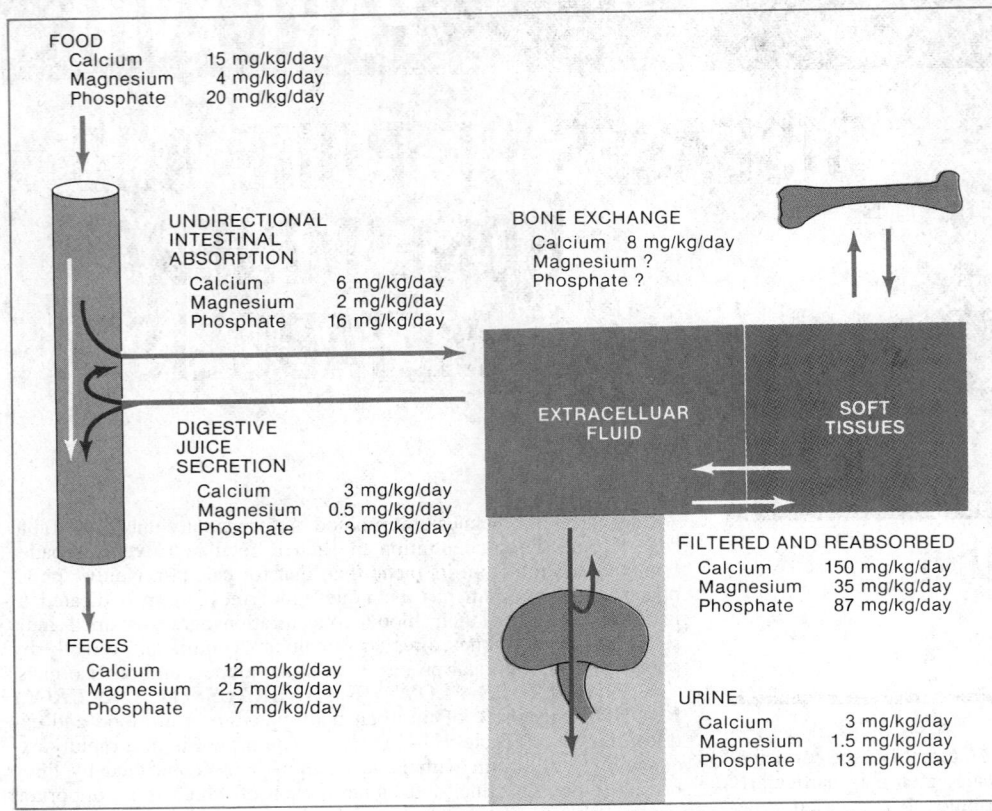

FIGURE 211–1. Typical mineral fluxes in adults. (Modified from Aurbach GD, Marx SJ, Spiegel AM: Parathyroid hormone, calcitonin, and the calciferols. *In* Wilson JD, Foster DW [eds.]: Williams Textbook of Endocrinology. 7th ed. Philadelphia, WB Saunders, 1985, p 1144.)

EXTRACELLULAR MATRIX. Newly deposited osteoid must undergo a poorly understood maturation process for 1 to 3 weeks until it is able to accumulate minerals. The mineral phase of bone extracellular matrix is a mixture of multiple amorphous and crystalline states, the latter principally as hydroxyapatite crystals $(Ca_5(OH)(PO_4)_3)$. Ninety to 95% of osteoid, the organic component of the extracellular matrix, is composed of bundles of type I collagen, a long triple helix of two alpha$_1$ (type I) chains and one alpha$_2$ (type I) chain. The principal collagen of cartilage matrix is type II as a homotrimer of three alpha$_1$ (type II) chains. Fibrils of collagen play a major role in the strength of bone (type I collagen), cartilage (type II collagen), and elastic tissues (type III collagen). Their disruption results in characteristic disturbances (osteogenesis imperfecta [type I collagen], chondrodysplasia [type II collagen], Ehlers-Danlos syndrome or arterial aneurysms [type III collagen], and even certain variants of familial osteoarthritis [type II collagen]). The second most prominent protein in bone matrix is osteocalcin (or bone gla-protein); it has a molar content of three residues of gamma-carboxyglutamic acid, an unusual amino acid that confers to the molecule high affinity for calcium on bone crystals. The roles of osteocalcin are unknown, but its concentration in blood is a potential index of osteoblast activity. Several other proteins, phosphoproteins, glycoproteins, and so on, in bone matrix have been identified in the search for molecules regulating bone mineral accumulation and bone growth.

BONE CELLS. Several cells are highly characteristic of bone. A flat bone-lining cell (perhaps derived from marrow stroma) with few organelles covers many bone surfaces thought not to be undergoing modification. This cell is perhaps one precursor of the osteoblast. The osteoblast is a cuboidal bone matrix-synthesizing cell. It lines any periosteal, endosteal, or trabecular surface at which bone formation takes place. Its plasma membrane is highly enriched with a bone-specific isoform of the alkaline phosphatase enzyme. This enzyme is believed to promote bone mineralization by catalyzing in supersaturated extracellular fluid of bone the hydrolysis of pyrophosphate and other inhibitors of calcium-phosphate crystallization. The osteocyte is the principal stable cell inside mature bone. It is probably derived from an osteoblast that has encased itself in bone. Osteocytes are interconnected with one another via long processes that traverse bone canaliculi. The role of the osteocyte is unknown, but it is appropriately located to modulate local mineral fluxes. The chondrocyte is the dominant cell of cartilage; it releases to the extracellular matrix type II collagen and vesicles that are rich in alkaline phosphatase and that may be a central organelle for accumulating calcium in preparation for mineralizing cartilage. The osteoclast is the main bone-resorbing cell. It is derived from precursors of the premonocyte lineage. It is a highly motile, multinucleated giant cell, with several specialized features for bone. These include organelles that mediate cell attachment to bone surface (podosomes), a strikingly redundant ruffled border at the bone face for ion transport, many enzymes that can function in bone resorption, and a high concentration of carbonic anhydrase II, which helps acidify the extracellular pocket between the osteoclast ruffled border and the skeletal resorption surface.

LOCAL REGULATORS OF BONE CELLS. Bone cells are under systemic and local regulation. Known systemic regulators include parathyroid hormone (PTH), calcitonin, and calcitriol, which are considered later in this chapter. There is also a highly complex network of local controls. The term "osteoclast-activating factors" was applied in the 1980's to components in incompletely characterized fluids that could activate bone resorption *in vitro*. Some of their active components have been identified. For example, interleukin-1 and lymphotoxin/tumor necrosis factor-beta are potential stimulators of bone resorption that seem to be released locally by some tumors in bone. They cannot act directly on mature osteoclasts but can act, rather, through nearby cells, such as osteoblasts or marrow stromal cells, that communicate with osteoclasts. Like the activators of bone resorption, the activators of bone formation are poorly understood, particularly because this process involves a complex interplay of osteoblast proliferation and differentiation. Some contributors to this process include type 1 insulin-like growth factor (IGF-1) and transforming growth factor-beta (TGF-β); the latter is present selectively and at high concentrations in osteoblasts and osteocytes. In addition, several newly identified proteins (osteogenesis-inducing factor, bone morphogenetic proteins [some of which are homologues of TGF-β], and so forth) can induce bone formation in soft tissue sites. Prostaglandins can stimulate bone formation or bone resorption, and they may be important mediators in inflammatory processes of the skeletal system.

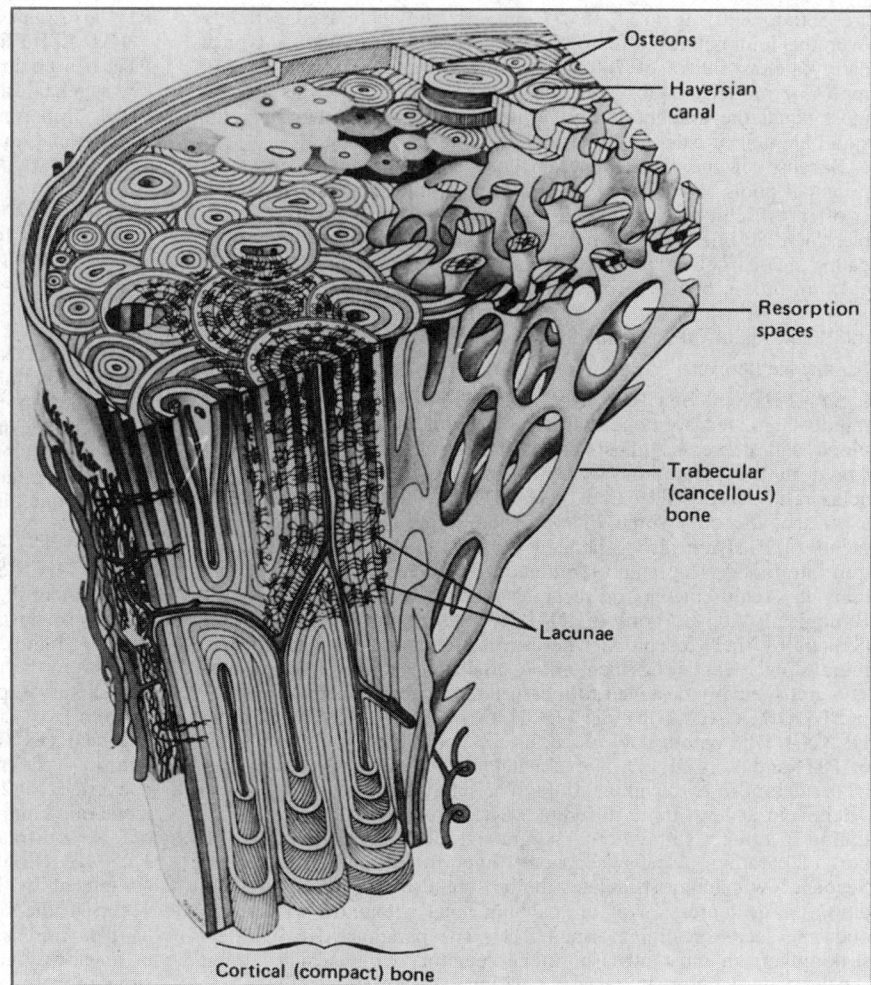

FIGURE 211–2. Bone organization. Microstructure of mature bone; areas of cortical (lamellar) and trabecular (cancellous) bone are shown. The central area in the transverse section shows differences in mineral density as degrees of shading. Note the organization of osteons, the distribution of osteocyte lacunae, and the organization of bone lamellae. (Adapted from Warwick R, Williams PL [eds.]: Gray's Anatomy. 35th ed. Edinburgh, Churchill Livingstone, 1973, p 217.)

BONE REMODELING. Bone growth or modeling occurs initially within a membrane or along the edge of cartilage (e.g., periosteum or epiphyseal growth plate). Although it contains few cells, cortical bone is constantly going through slow and orderly cycles of localized resorption and then rebuilding. This process is mediated by the local remodeling unit (alternately termed osteon or basic multicellular unit). Remodeling begins with osteoclasts excavating a cavity; as the resorption front advances, osteoclasts are replaced by other cells. Over an interval of several months, new bone is deposited in cylindrical lamellae around the rim of the cavity until it is refilled to complete this cycle. This cycle is an important example of the normal, coordinated relation between the bone resorption and bone formation processes. Most perturbations that modify one component of these two processes also modify the other in the same direction. The determinants of this coupling between bone resorption and formation are not known, but they probably include a host of growth factors present at high local concentrations in bone extracellular matrix and exposed or released by the skeletal resorption process.

Intestines

MINERAL ABSORPTION. The intestinal absorption of magnesium and phosphate is not subject to fine regulation and has not been studied intensively. By contrast, intestinal absorption of calcium is tightly regulated, and its quantitation has been analyzed in detail. Most calcium absorption is accomplished in the small bowel. Over a wide range of intakes, approximately 10% of dietary calcium is absorbed passively; the remainder of net intestinal absorption of calcium is regulated by active vitamin D metabolites, especially $1\alpha,25(OH)_2D$, in blood. With a normal diet, approximately 30% of calcium is absorbed. With low dietary calcium, the secon-

darily high blood $1\alpha,25(OH)_2D$ level can drive fractional calcium absorption to approach 90%.

Kidney

ION FILTRATION AND REABSORPTION. The non-protein-bound fractions of calcium, magnesium, and phosphate from plasma cross the glomerulus. The distal portions of the nephron have efficient and selective systems that can complete the reabsorption from tubular fluid of more than 99% of any one of these minerals. Tubular calcium reabsorption is stimulated principally by (PTH); thiazides or lithium can also increase tubular calcium reabsorption. Saline loading with or without loop diuretics can inhibit this. Tubular phosphate reabsorption is mainly under negative influence by PTH. The determinants of tubular reabsorption of magnesium are incompletely understood.

Integrated Fluxes: Mineral Balance and Nutrition

Skeletal growth is maximal throughout childhood, nearing completion during adolescence. Until this time, the rate of skeletal calcium accretion is typically 200 to 400 mg (5 to 10 mmole) per day. Fetal mineralization during the last trimester or milk secretion during lactation imposes similar daily increments on calcium efflux from maternal blood. The skeleton remains in a state of approximate zero mineral balance between ages 20 and 35, after which it slowly loses mass. This loss is greatest in the trabecular bone of the vertebrae, attaining peak rates about the menopause (3 to 10% per year during the first 1 to 4 years after surgically induced menopause).

Normal adults can sustain zero calcium balance with daily calcium intakes between 400 and 1500 mg (10 to 37.5 mmole), mainly as dairy products. Typical daily calcium intakes in the United States are 500 to 800 mg (12.5 to 20 mmole), and there is uncertainty over the minimal level for optimal skeletal health. With a typical daily calcium intake of 700 mg (17.5 mmole), one fourth, or 175 mg (43.7 mmole), is absorbed; during skeletal balance, this amount must equal the amount lost in urinary excretion (disregarding the small amount of calcium lost from skin).

Because of the large mineral fluxes between blood and three principal pools (bone, renal tubular lumen, and intestinal lumen), it is often difficult to assign mild disruptions to one pool. For example, there is uncertainty whether the slow bone losses with idiopathic age-associated osteoporosis reflect primary disturbances of calcium flux in bone, the intestine, or combinations of these.

HORMONAL REGULATORS OF MINERAL HOMEOSTASIS

Parathyroid Hormone

SYNTHESIS, SECRETION, AND METABOLISM. PTH is a rapidly regulated hormone that sustains calcium and $1,25(OH)_2D$ in blood and depresses phosphate in blood (Table 211–3). PTH is stored in the parathyroid cell mainly as a peptide of 84 amino acids. The parathyroid cell secretes PTH as the native molecule or as fragments, only some of which are biologically active. Fragments of PTH are also generated from its metabolism after secretion into blood. The amino terminus of PTH (residues 1 to 34) contains the requirements for receptor binding and biologic activity. Biologically active forms of PTH are cleared rapidly from blood, perhaps by their receptors, whereas inactive fragments are cleared more slowly, rendering them likely to be measured in immunoassays not specially designed to measure the intact molecule.

BLOOD CALCIUM EFFECT ON THE PARATHYROID GLAND. The parathyroid gland, as the coordinator of blood levels of PTH and $1,25(OH)_2D$, is exquisitely sensitive to changes of ionized calcium in extracellular fluid. The parathyroid cell responds to calcium in at least three different ways. First, low calcium concentration is a direct stimulus for the gradual increase in size and numbers of parathyroid cells (secondary hypertrophy and hyperplasia). Second, low calcium stimulates the biosynthesis of PTH over 1 to 2 days. Third, depression of the calcium level stimulates within seconds the secretion of preformed PTH. The parathyroid cell differs strikingly from most other hormone secretory cells, which exhibit accelerated secretion in response to increases of extracellular calcium.

PARATHYROID HORMONE MECHANISMS OF ACTION. PTH binds to a plasma membrane receptor; the PTH receptor then causes a rise of cyclic 3′,5′-adenosine monophosphate (cAMP) and other second messengers in the cytoplasm of its target cells. The consequence is rapid effects of PTH on the target cells in bone and kidney. A different peptide, termed "parathyroid hormone-related peptide," with homology to PTH at the amino terminus, is secreted by many cancers, causing hypercalcemia through its interactions with PTH receptors.

PARATHYROID HORMONE ACTION IN BONE. PTH in bone stimulates osteoblasts and osteoclasts. The effects on osteoclasts are indirect because these cells lack receptors for PTH. Very high PTH levels result in clear excess of bone resorption over bone formation. Controversy exists over whether mild PTH excess might have a net anabolic effect selectively in trabecular bone.

PARATHYROID HORMONE ACTION IN KIDNEY. PTH acts in the kidney to stimulate the synthesis of $1,25(OH)_2D$ by increasing the activity of $25OHD_3$ 1α-hydroxylase in the proximal tubules. PTH acts in the distal portions of the nephron to increase tubular reabsorption of calcium. In addition, PTH inhibits phosphate reabsorption in the distal, and perhaps also the proximal, tubules. PTH also inhibits bicarbonate reabsorption.

PARATHYROID HORMONE ACTION ON INTESTINE. PTH has no important direct action on the intestine. However, the direct renal effect of PTH to increase serum $1,25(OH)_2D$ causes highly important secondary effects in the intestine (see Intestinal Actions of Calcitriol, further on).

Calcitonin

CALCITONIN SYNTHESIS AND SECRETION. Calcitonin is a peptide of 32 amino acids that is normally synthesized and secreted by the parafollicular or C cells, which are neuroectodermal cells within the thyroid gland. Its secretion is stimulated by calcium and also by certain intestinal peptides (gastrin and glucagon) (see Ch. 215).

CALCITONIN ACTIONS. Calcitonin, at high concentrations, can directly inhibit osteoclast function. Calcitonin also can act in the kidney to cause mild natriuresis. These calcitonin actions have not been shown to be important in normal physiology. For the present, the principal interests in calcitonin are as a tumor marker, particularly for familial C cell neoplasia, or as a pharmacologic agent to treat bone disorders, such as Paget's disease.

Vitamin D and Its Metabolites

SYNTHESIS OF VITAMIN D. Vitamin D_3 is a seco-steroid (i.e., a steroid with one ring opened) synthesized from 7-dehydrocholesterol in the skin (Fig. 211–3), in a reaction catalyzed by ultraviolet light derived from the sun. Vitamin D_2, produced synthetically from the plant sterol ergosterol, is a vitamin D_3 analogue used as a dietary supplement or drug. The metabolism of vitamin D_3 and vitamin D_2 is similar in humans (see Ch. 212).

HYDROXYLATIONS OF VITAMIN D METABOLITES. Vitamin D ("D" refers to combinations of the D_3 and D_2 isoforms) is converted to 25OHD in hepatocytes. This reaction is not under metabolic control and is determined principally by the serum levels of its substrate, vitamin D. 25OHD is normally converted to $1,25(OH)_2D$ only in the renal proximal tubule by an enzyme system stimulated by PTH. A similar PTH-independent 1α-hydroxylation occurs in the normal placenta and abnormally in granuloma tissues, as in sarcoidosis. 25OHD and $1,25(OH)_2D$ can also be hydroxylated at other residues (C-23, C-24, C-26), but these and other conversions probably serve mainly to inactivate vitamin D metabolites.

ABSORPTION AND TRANSPORT OF VITAMIN D METABOLITES. Vitamin D metabolites enter the bloodstream like other sterols, and a small fraction of all vitamin D metabolites undergoes an enterohepatic recirculation. When cutaneous synthesis of vitamin D is marginal, any cause of intestinal malabsorption can result in vitamin D deficiency. Vitamin D metabolites are lipid soluble; they circulate in plasma bound to a specific 25OHD binding protein and, to a lesser degree, to other carriers.

MECHANISM OF ACTIONS OF VITAMIN D METABOLITES. Vitamin D is an inactive precursor; 25OHD and $1,25(OH)_2D$ are both active. Although the concentration of 25OHD is about 1000-fold higher than that of $1,25(OH)_2D$ in blood, the latter has far higher affinity for the vitamin D receptor and normally determines the degree of vitamin D receptor activation. Calcitriol binds to intracellular receptors in target cells and causes gradual changes in the nuclei of those cells. The vitamin D receptor is highly homologous to the receptors for other steroids and to those for thyroid hormone and retinoic acid. Although vitamin D receptors are present in many organs, only those in duodenal mucosa have been established as important in normal physiology.

TABLE 211–3. EFFECTS OF PRINCIPAL CALCIOTROPIC HORMONES

Hormone	Principal Target Tissues	Action
Parathyroid hormone	Renal proximal convoluted tubule	Increase serum $1,25(OH)_2D$
	Renal distal convoluted tubule	Increase calcium reabsorption
	Renal proximal and distal convoluted tubules	Decrease phosphate reabsorption
	Bone	Increase calcium and phosphate resorption
Calcitonin	Bone	Decrease calcium and phosphate resorption
$1,25(OH)_2D$	Small bowel	Increase calcium absorption
	Bone	Increase calcium and phosphate resorption
	Parathyroid gland	Decrease release of PTH

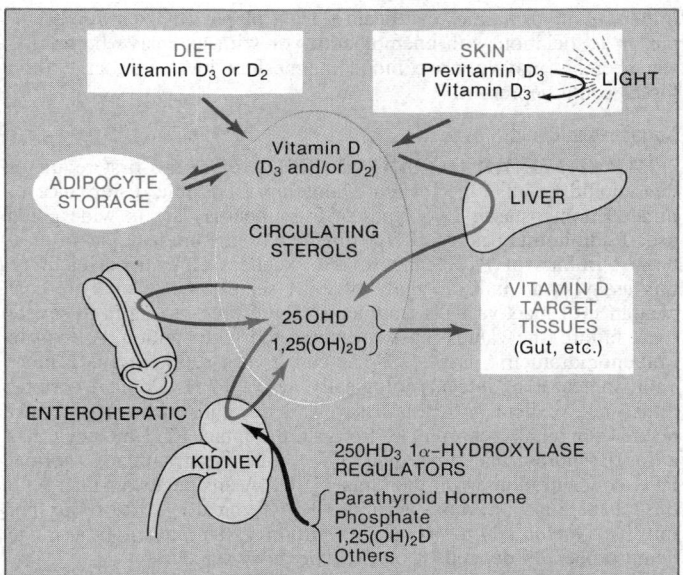

FIGURE 211–3. The vitamin D activation pathway. This involves steps in many different organs. Dysfunction at any step can have clinically important consequences.

INTESTINAL ACTIONS OF CALCITRIOL. Calcitriol (1,25(OH)$_2$D) increases the flux of calcium from the intestinal lumen to blood. Calcitriol, to a much lesser extent, increases the flux of phosphate and magnesium from intestinal lumen to blood. Calcium, magnesium, and phosphate ions have specific processes for their intestinal transport. Calcitriol induces in duodenal mucosa high concentrations of an intracellular calcium-binding protein, termed calbindin. Calbindin belongs to the calmodulin protein family, but its role, if any, in intestinal calcium transport is unknown.

SKELETAL EFFECTS OF CALCITRIOL. The principal effects of calcitriol on bone (antirachitic effects) are indirect results of its action to promote calcium influx from intestinal lumen to blood. The deficient mineralization in vitamin D deficiency states is the consequence of the combination of low calcium in blood and low phosphate in blood, the latter resulting from the renal phosphate-wasting effects from secondary hyperparathyroidism.

The supraphysiologic concentrations of vitamin D metabolites sometimes reached during pharmacotherapy can raise blood calcium in part by increasing osteoclast numbers and activity.

OTHER EFFECTS OF CALCITRIOL. Calcitriol can inhibit PTH biosynthesis and secretion; the direct negative effects of calcitriol might contribute a form of short-loop negative feedback to parathyroid function. Calcitriol exerts direct effects on the renal enzymes that hydroxylate 25OHD; calcitriol inhibits the 25OHD$_3$ 1α-hydroxylase and stimulates the other hydroxylases that catabolize 25OHD in the renal tubule and in other tissues. Possibly important effects of calcitriol in skin and hair are suggested by its protective effect on psoriatic skin at pharmacologic doses and by the striking association of total alopecia with the rare syndrome of severely defective vitamin D receptors. Vitamin D receptors are present in many additional organs, but no role for them has been identified in normal physiology.

Other Hormones

SEX STEROIDS. Sex steroids, particularly estrogens, have slow but extremely important anabolic effects on bone. The effects are exerted directly on the bone organ, perhaps through receptors in the osteoblast. Estrogen deficiency results in accelerated bone remodeling with disproportionate bone resorption, particularly in trabecular bone.

GLUCOCORTICOIDS. Glucocorticoids affect many of the cells that contribute to mineral metabolism. The most striking effect is bone thinning that results from high glucocorticoid concentrations. This thinning is probably a consequence mainly of inhibited osteoblasts. In addition, glucocorticoids antagonize the actions of vitamin D metabolites by unknown mechanisms.

THYROID HORMONE. Thyroid hormones also have direct effects on bone cells. Excess of thyroid hormones causes increased release of calcium from bone. The skeletal consequences of deficient thyroid hormone are most evident in the disordered growth of cartilaginous epiphyses associated with congenital hypothyroidism.

GROWTH HORMONE. Growth hormone stimulates the growth of bone and cartilage, in part by stimulating local production of IGF-1 by osteoblasts and chondrocytes.

ADAPTATIONS TO DISRUPTIONS OF MINERAL METABOLISM

Two principal calciotropic hormones, PTH and 1,25(OH)$_2$D, interact with each other and with multiple target tissues to control the metabolism of calcium, phosphate, and, to a lesser degree, magnesium (Fig. 211–4 and Table 211–3). These hormones allow for adaptations over time intervals that are short (minutes) or long (months).

Blood levels of ionized calcium are sustained at nearly invariant levels, with minimal diurnal changes reflecting mainly the sudden rises of calcium influx with meals. Serum levels of PTH and 1,25(OH)$_2$D also show only modest diurnal changes under normal conditions. Serum phosphate typically has broad diurnal fluctuations, with a nadir around 9:00 A.M. and peaks at around 6:00 P.M. and 4:00 A.M.

CALCIUM EXCESS STATES. States with long-term excess or deficiency of calcium are associated with deviations at multiple steps of the integrated mineral homeostasis system. The most common calcium excess state in adults is primary overfunction of the parathyroid gland. Of course, this has the potential to distort most of the normal calcium regulatory processes. Primary hyperparathyroidism results in high blood levels of PTH and often of 1,25(OH)$_2$D as well. The results are combinations of increased calcium influx to blood dependent upon the evoked dysfunctions in intestinal, skeletal, and renal pools of calcium. A very different integrated metabolic pattern results when calcium excess is caused by dysfunction outside the parathyroid—for example, with osteolytic metastases, skeletal immobilization, or dietary calcium overload (milk-alkali syndrome). In the latter disturbances, the parathyroid gland reacts appropriately and becomes suppressed by the increase of ionized calcium in blood; blood concentrations of PTH and 1,25(OH)$_2$D become low. The abnormally high filtered load of calcium without the anticalciuric effects of PTH results in severe hy-

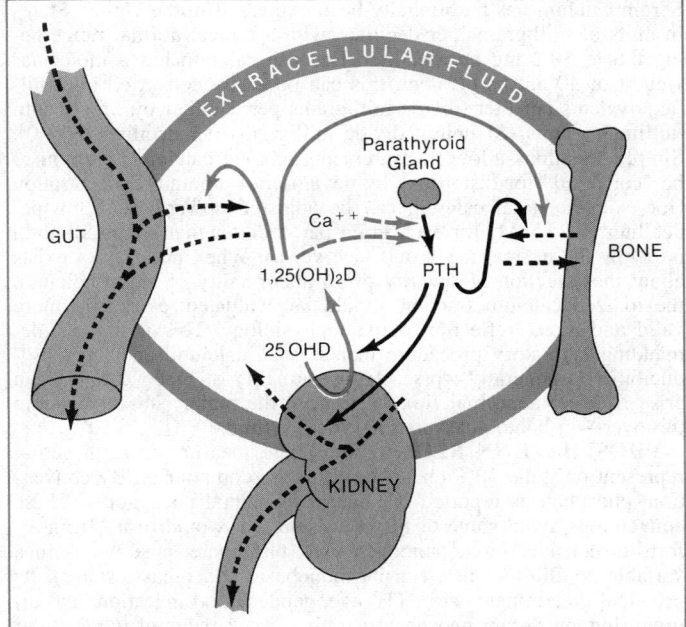

FIGURE 211–4. Integrated control of secretion and actions of parathyroid hormone (PTH) and calcitriol (1,25(OH)$_2$ vitamin D = 1,25(OH)$_2$D) with emphasis on calcium fluxes. Solid black lines show secretion of PTH and calcitriol. Interrupted black lines are calcium fluxes. Solid red lines show stimulatory effects; interrupted red lines show inhibitory effects.

percalciuria; irreversible renal damage can occur over a period of only a few weeks.

CALCIUM DEFICIENCY STATES. Calcium deficiency states generally result in the parathyroid gland's recognizing the signal of a low ionized calcium level in blood. Increased PTH secretion (within seconds), increased PTH biosynthesis (within days), and parathyroid cell hyperplasia (within weeks) activate the response pathways. The consequences of this secondary hyperparathyroidism are increased renal tubular secretion of $1,25(OH)_2D$ (if there is not underlying deficiency of 25OHD or 1α-hydroxylase) and increased net calcium flux into blood from the intestinal lumen, from bone, and from the renal tubular lumen. The relative contribution of each calcium pool to this integrated response depends in part on the chronic state of that pool and on the relative levels of PTH and calcitriol. Serum calcium typically begins to fall below normal only when the osteolytic response to PTH or $1,25(OH)_2D$ becomes weakened (from depletion of readily exchangeable calcium pools or other types of tachyphylaxis). Secondary hyperparathyroidism has important effects on phosphate homeostasis by directly affecting bone and kidney, increasing phosphate influx from bone and causing a similar increase in phosphate efflux into urine. With forms of hypoparathyroidism, some residual components of mineral homeostasis can be sustained despite a deficiency of PTH and secondarily of $1,25(OH)_2D$.

METABOLIC BONE DISEASES. Certain forms of metabolic bone disease are associated with dramatic imbalances in mineral flux to or from blood; these include increased calcium influx with aggressive osteolytic processes and decreased calcium influx with many forms of osteomalacia. Others, because they do not dramatically compromise the readily exchangeable pools of bone mineral, may have little or no long-term impact on the blood homeostatic system. For example, idiopathic osteoporosis has been categorized into two major forms (perimenopausal and aging associated), but no clear-cut changes in blood PTH or $1,25(OH)_2D$ as adaptations to altered serum calcium levels have been identified in either form.

USES OF LABORATORY TESTING
Electrolytes in Blood

CALCIUM IN BLOOD. To stabilize blood albumin concentration, total calcium should be measured in the fasting patient who is seated or recumbent. Most laboratories measure it inexpensively and with high precision. A high or low calcium value during multichannel screening is often the first indication of a treatable disorder. Serum calcium has traditionally been expressed in the United States in units of milligrams per deciliter, with a typical normal range being 8.8 to 10.2 mg per deciliter. Because calcium has a molecular weight of 40 and is divalent, this can be easily converted into milliequivalents per liter (divide milligrams per deciliter by 2.0) or into millimolar units (SI units); divide milligrams per deciliter by 4.0). Simple equations allow measurements of total calcium in serum to be "corrected" for distortions by deviation of albumin concentration (for example, total calcium can be adjusted upward by 1 mg per deciliter [0.25 mM] for each gram per deciliter that serum albumin is below the normal mean and vice versa). When uncertainty exists about the direction or severity of an abnormality of blood calcium, the ionized calcium fraction should be evaluated, as it is a more valid and direct reflection of pathophysiology. This is a more demanding laboratory procedure than is total calcium, and the reproducibility is generally worse. An abnormality of blood calcium can arise from an abnormal flux to or from the major sites of calcium turnover—in bone, gut, and renal tubular fluid.

PHOSPHATE IN BLOOD. Phosphate measurements in serum represent only the 30% that is in inorganic compounds. By convention, phosphate is reported in units of elemental phosphorus. These conventions avoid some of the confusion that would result from efforts to consider molar anion content (phosphate in serum is in a variable equilibrium between its monobasic and dibasic states). Its principal determinants are PTH, age, gender, food ingestion, and diurnal rhythm. Serum phosphate is only a weak index of intracellular phosphate stores. Its normal range is far wider than that for calcium.

MAGNESIUM IN BLOOD. Serum magnesium, like phosphate, is determined by its threshold for renal excretion and by total body pools. Primary disturbance of magnesium in blood is unusual, but important abnormalities can occur during major illnesses; for example, in association with chemotherapy or with extensive burns, tissue necrosis may increase blood magnesium levels, or large fluid losses could depress it.

Hormones in Blood

PARATHYROID HORMONE. PTH is often the first regulator that should be examined when evaluating a possible disturbance of mineral homeostasis. Two types of immunoassay are in widespread use. Radioimmunoassay (RIA) directed at the mid-region or carboxy terminus of PTH can provide excellent clinical correlations; this assay is an index equally of PTH secretion rate and of renal clearance of inactive PTH fragments. Therefore, with mild to severe renal failure, the values must be interpreted with caution. A two-site immunoradiometric assay (IRMA) can give a result that is a more valid indicator of intact, biologically active PTH. Clinical correlations are excellent with this assay, and no adjustment is generally needed for renal compromise. Because the intact PTH molecule has a much shorter half-time than do its inactive fragments, normal PTH concentrations with the "intact" IRMA are far lower than with the mid-region or carboxy terminus RIA (typically, 10 to 60 pg per milliliter versus 100 to 400 pg per milliliter, the latter normal range being especially dependent on the laboratory standard).

CALCITONIN. Calcitonin is measured by RIA. Clinical uses are limited. When the RIA is used in family screening for early stages of C cell neoplasia, it is particularly important that the laboratory provide normal ranges adjusted for the selected C cell challenge protocol and the patient's age.

25-HYDROXYVITAMIN D. Vitamin D itself is rarely measured in clinical settings. Two different vitamin D metabolites can be measured by most laboratories. It is essential to understand that these two metabolites, 25OHD and $1,25(OH)_2D$, are usually indicators of two entirely different types of process. Serum 25OHD is a useful index of vitamin D nutritional status. It is also a good index of sterol absorption. Low levels can arise from deficiency of sunlight, from deficiency of vitamin D nutritional supplementation, from fat malabsorption, and from accelerated hepatic catabolism of vitamin D metabolites. Because the body easily compensates for concentrations above normal, dangerously high levels occur only when consuming pharmacologic doses of vitamin D or of 25OHD.

1,25-DIHYDROXYVITAMIN D. $1,25(OH)_2D$ measurement in serum gives an index of the steroid hormone whose renal production is usually finely regulated by blood PTH. Even with vitamin D intoxication, the serum levels of $1,25(OH)_2D$ may be appropriately low because of this regulatory system. Serum $1,25(OH)_2D$ has only limited diagnostic use. However, certain states can be associated with otherwise unexplainable mineral disturbances that reflect high levels of $1,25(OH)_2D$ (sarcoidosis and other granulomas) or low levels (certain renal tubular disorders, such as X-linked hypophosphatemia).

Blood Indices of Bone Disturbance

Alkaline phosphatase enzyme in serum is an index of its sources in bone, liver, and placenta and of its excretion by the biliary tree. With increased osteoblastic activity, the amount of skeletal alkaline phosphatase enzyme in serum can rise dramatically. Skeletal alkaline phosphatase can be measured selectively through its physicochemical properties (it is the heat-labile component of total alkaline phosphatase) or otherwise (e.g., by RIA, a topic for research in several centers). High skeletal alkaline phosphatase levels can point to high bone turnover (hyperparathyroidism, Paget's disease). Specific portions of procollagen type I and other bone-specific proteins are also under investigation as possible specific indicators of skeletal processes. Osteocalcin (sometimes called bone gla-protein) is another osteoblast-specific protein that has been useful in some long-term studies of bone turnover, but its insensitivity to diffuse bone pathology has compromised its broad clinical use.

Measurements on the Skeleton

BONE RADIOGRAPHS AND SCANS. Standard radiography is often the starting point in evaluating bone disorders. Images can be specific for numerous conditions or can direct further diagnostic procedures (i.e., bone biopsy) to sites of focal disturbance. A bone scan with technetium-99m diphosphonate may identify a local disturbance that is not accompanied by radiographic change; the label adsorbs to bone mineral, and increased local blood flow without fracture is sufficient to give a positive signal.

BONE MASS INDICES. Bone mass can be measured noninvasively with a variety of techniques. These include dual-channel radiographs, single- and dual-channel photon absorptiometry, radiographs with computed tomography (CT), and other methods under development. The choice of one over another should depend largely on local expertise. For sequential studies in a patient, these methods are compromised, to varying degrees, by high cost and lack of precision.

BONE BIOPSY. Bone biopsy can be the final diagnostic tool in identifying local or generalized bone disturbances. It can be particularly useful in distinguishing osteomalacia from osteoporosis. Maximal information about the bone formation process can be obtained by prior administration of two pulses of tetracyclines 14 days apart (tetracyclines selectively adsorb to the mineralization front of osteoid and provide a fluorescent signal in the biopsy). When considering this test, the clinician should consult persons knowledgeable about its indications and the details of its processing.

Analyses of the Intestines in Mineral Metabolism

Specific tests of intestinal function are rarely used in current clinical practice. Metabolic balance studies are time consuming and expensive. Calcium absorption studies with radioactive or stable isotopes are not applied outside research settings. General indices of intestinal function are considered in other chapters.

Analyses of the Kidney and Urine

Renal biopsy should be done only for the standard indications related to intrinsic or systemic diseases in the kidney. Urinary excretion of hydroxyproline and other collagen metabolites is a useful index of bone resorption rates because 60% of urinary hydroxyproline is normally derived from collagen in bone. Pyridinum crosslinks, another collagen by-product in urine, may prove to be a more useful index of bone resorption.

Urinary excretion of calcium, magnesium, or phosphate is useful in screening for total body excess or deficiency of any of these minerals. Urinary excretion of calcium is central in the evaluation of urolithiasis. More detailed discussion of the workup of urolithiasis is presented elsewhere (see Ch. 88).

Aurbach GD, Marx SJ, Spiegel AM: Parathyroid hormone, calcitonin, and the calciferols. *In* Wilson JD, Foster DW (eds.): Williams Textbook of Endocrinology. 8th ed. Philadelphia, WB Saunders, 1991. *Detailed review of mineral metabolism with emphasis on calciotropic hormones. Other major textbooks of endocrinology have similar chapters.*

Avioli LV, Krane SM (eds.): Metabolic Bone Diseases and Clinically Related Disorders. 2nd ed. Philadelphia, WB Saunders, 1990. *A detailed review of the entire field from multiple authors.*

Favus MJ (ed.): Primer on Metabolic Bone Diseases and Disorders of Mineral Metabolism. Kelseyville, Calif., American Society for Bone and Mineral Research, 1990. *Concise chapters that quickly advance the reader to research on a topic.*

212 VITAMIN D
Bess Dawson-Hughes

Vitamin D, originally described as a fat-soluble vitamin that would prevent rickets, is a steroid hormone. Natural forms of the vitamin include cholecalciferol or vitamin D_3, produced in skin of humans and other vertebrates, and ergocalciferol or vitamin D_2, derived from plants and fungi. These forms are metabolized similarly in humans, and the term *vitamin D* in this chapter applies to both forms. To become biologically active, vitamin D is hydroxylated first in the liver to 25-hydroxyvitamin D (25(OH)D) and then in the kidney to form 1,25-dihydroxyvitamin D (1,25(OH)$_2$D).

SOURCES. Rich dietary sources of vitamin D include fish oil, cod liver oil, egg yokes, and fortified milk. Vitamin D from food and supplements is absorbed in the distal ileum by a process that requires bile salts. Gastrointestinal disorders of mixing and fat emulsification, decreased transit time, and fat malabsorption reduce vitamin D absorption. Aging also reduces vitamin D absorption effi-

ciency by about 40%, and about half of this loss may occur after age 65. Adults in the United States, Europe, and Japan typically consume 100 to 150 IU of vitamin D daily. Although the US recommended dietary allowance is 200 IU per day, 400 to 800 IU is increasingly recommended.

Vitamin D_3 is produced in the epidermal layer of the skin upon exposure to ultraviolet sunlight of wavelength 294 to 310 nm by photoconversion of the prohormone 7-dehydrocholesterol to previtamin D. The latter spontaneously isomerizes to vitamin D_3 over the 3 or 4 days following sun exposure and enters the circulation bound to vitamin D binding protein. Sun screens and the skin pigment melanin reduce cutaneous production of vitamin D_3 because they absorb solar ultraviolet light, leaving fewer photons available to initiate photosynthesis. Photoproduction declines with aging because of a twofold age-related reduction in epidermal 7-dehydrocholesterol concentration. Thinning of the skin and reduced sun exposure may also contribute to decreased vitamin D_3 production in the elderly.

In the heavily populated temperate zone, season and latitude regulate cutaneous vitamin D_3 production because they determine the intensity of ultraviolet rays reaching earth's surface. At 42 degrees North, the latitude of Boston, very little photosynthesis occurs between October and March and, in the winter, 25(OH)D levels typically decline by about 30% in ambulatory adults. This decline is accompanied by an increase in circulating levels of the bone-resorbing agent, parathyroid hormone (PTH).

METABOLISM. *Liver.* Vitamin D is hydroxylated by an hepatic microsomal cytochrome P-450 mixed-function oxidase to form 25(OH)D. This process is not tightly regulated and depends on the combined skin and dietary supplies of vitamin D. Several medications and diseases alter 25(OH)D metabolism. Anticonvulsants, rifampin, primidone, and other drugs that induce microsomal enzymes accelerate metabolism of 25(OH)D to inactive metabolites, thereby increasing the requirement for vitamin D. Cholestyramine increases the vitamin D requirement by binding 25(OH)D in the gut. Production of 25(OH)D is compromised by liver disease only when the disease is advanced.

Renal. In the final step of activation, 25(OH)D is 1α-hydroxylated in the proximal renal convoluted tubule to form 1,25(OH)$_2$D. Extrarenal production occurs in the normal placenta and sometimes in sarcoid and other granulomas. PTH and low blood levels of calcium and phosphorus promote renal 1,25(OH)$_2$D production. High blood levels of calcium and phosphorus and also 1,25(OH)$_2$D itself limit 1,25(OH)$_2$D production (Fig. 212–1). When 1α-hydroxylase is inhibited, 25(OH)D is metabolized by an alternate renal pathway to 24,25-dihydroxyvitamin D, a compound with no established function in humans. Advanced renal disease compromises 1α-hydroxylase, but the stage in renal failure at which 1,25(OH)$_2$D production starts to decline varies with calcium and phosphorus intake levels.

ACTIONS OF 1,25(OH)$_2$D. This hormone is part of the vitamin D/endocrine system that regulates blood calcium and bone mineralization by its actions on the intestine, bone, kidney, and other tissues (Fig. 212–2). 1,25(OH)$_2$D promotes absorption of intestinal calcium and phosphorus by acting on mucosal cell nuclear receptors to initiate the production of separate calcium- and phosphorus-binding proteins. These proteins ferry calcium and phosphorus across the intestinal mucosa. 1,25(OH)$_2$D is essential for both the formation and resorption components of bone remodeling. In concert with

TABLE 212–1. PHARMACOLOGIC PROPERTIES OF VITAMIN D METABOLITES

Metabolite	Time to Peak Serum Concentration	Onset of Hypercalcemic Action	Duration of Action
Ergocalciferol or cholecalciferol	—	12–14 hr*	6 mo or more
Calcifediol [25(OH)D]	4 hr	12–24 hr	15–20 days†
Calcitriol [1,25(OH)$_2$D]	2 hr	2–6 hr	1–2 days

* Therapeutic effect may take 10 to 14 days.
† Increased two to three times in renal failure.
From Dawson-Hughes B: Metabolic bone disease. *In* Bayliss TM (ed.): Current Therapy in Gastroenterology and Liver Disease. 3rd ed. Ontario, BC Decker, 1990.

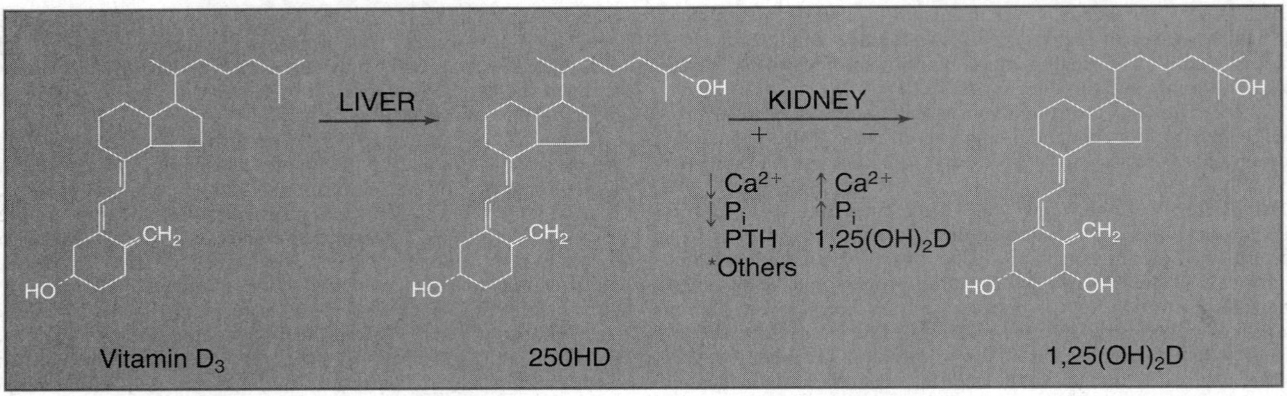

FIGURE 212-1. Activation of vitamin D. Estrogen, growth hormone, prolactin, placental lactogen, calcitonin, and insulin stimulate 1α-hydroxylase, but their role in the day-to-day regulation of $1,25(OH)_2D$ production is uncertain.

PTH, $1,25(OH)_2D$ stimulates bone resorption, perhaps by increasing the number of osteoclasts that are formed from macrophage stem cells. In addition to providing calcium for bone mineralization through increased intestinal absorption, $1,25(OH)_2D$ may also play a role in regulating osteoblast function. *In vitro*, $1,25(OH)_2D$ acts on osteoblast receptors to enhance production of alkaline phosphatase, osteocalcin, and several bone growth factors. In other actions, an elevated $1,25(OH)_2D$ level decreases PTH synthesis and release, and in concert with PTH, $1,25(OH)_2D$ reduces renal excretion of calcium.

PHARMACOLOGY. Selected properties of the major vitamin D metabolites are given in Table 212–1. Up to 99% of these three compounds circulates bound to vitamin D–binding protein, an α-globulin that protects them from rapid renal clearance. In nephrotic syndrome, the bound portion of each metabolite is reduced. Serum 25(OH)D reflects the solar and dietary contributions of vitamin D and is the best clinical measure of vitamin D status. Serum levels vary with sun exposure and intake, but typical values are vitamin D—1.5 ng per milliliter, 25(OH)D—35 ng per milliliter, and $1,25(OH)_2D$—30 pg per milliliter.

HYPOVITAMINOSIS D. Vitamin D insufficiency contributes to osteoporosis (see Ch. 217), and more severe deficiency results in osteomalacia (see Ch. 213).

HYPERVITAMINOSIS D. Vitamin D toxicity causes hypercalcemia and/or hypercalciuria because of increased calcium absorption. In animals vitamin D also enhances bone resorption, but this has not yet been confirmed in people. The clinical manifestations of vitamin D intoxication are associated with hypercalcemia (see Ch. 214). Hypervitaminosis D can result from excess intake or from altered metabolism of the vitamin.

Excess Intake. Long-term ingestion of 60,000 IU of vitamin D or more per day is required to produce hypercalcemia or hypercalciuria in healthy individuals. Toxicity may result from dietary excess but more often occurs when vitamin D is given therapeutically, as for hypoparathyroidism. A study of six patients with vitamin D intoxication from drinking overfortified milk revealed that the homeostatic regulation of 1α-hydroxylase is sometimes overridden by very high levels of the substrate 25(OH)D. Two of the six patients had elevated and four maintained normal serum levels of $1,25(OH)_2D$. The basis for hypercalcemia/hypercalciuria in the latter four is uncertain, although these findings demonstrate that at least one other vitamin D metabolite, perhaps 25(OH)D in very large amounts, influences calcium metabolism.

Altered Vitamin D Metabolism. Disordered calcium homeostasis sometimes occurs in granulomatous diseases, especially sarcoidosis, as a result of $1,25(OH)_2D$ production by macrophages in the granulomas. This hormone production is not regulated by factors that modulate renal synthesis of $1,25(OH)_2D$. Hypercalcemia occurs in about 10% of patients with sarcoidosis and can be the presenting feature. Sun exposure produces more substrate for $1,25(OH)_2D$ synthesis and can exacerbate the hypercalcemia.

Treatment. Hypervitaminosis D of any origin is treated by restricting calcium intake, rehydration, and administration of glucocorticoids. Up to 60 mg of prednisone per day may be needed to normalize serum calcium in vitamin D intoxication. If fat stores of vitamin D are large, toxicity can persist for well beyond 1 year. Intoxication from treatment with excess 25(OH)D or $1,25(OH)_2D$ resolves more rapidly. Glucocorticoids in low to moderate doses inhibit $1,25(OH)_2D$ production in granulomas and promptly reverse hypercalcemia in sarcoidosis and related diseases.

Jacobus CH, Holick MF, Shao Q, et al.: Hypervitaminosis D associated with drinking milk. N Engl J Med 326:1173, 1992. *A careful documentation of clinical and biochemical aspects of vitamin D intoxication.*
Reichel H, Koeffler HP, Norman AW: The role of the vitamin D endocrine system in health and disease. N Engl J Med 320:980, 1989. *An extensive review of the vitamin D endocrine system.*

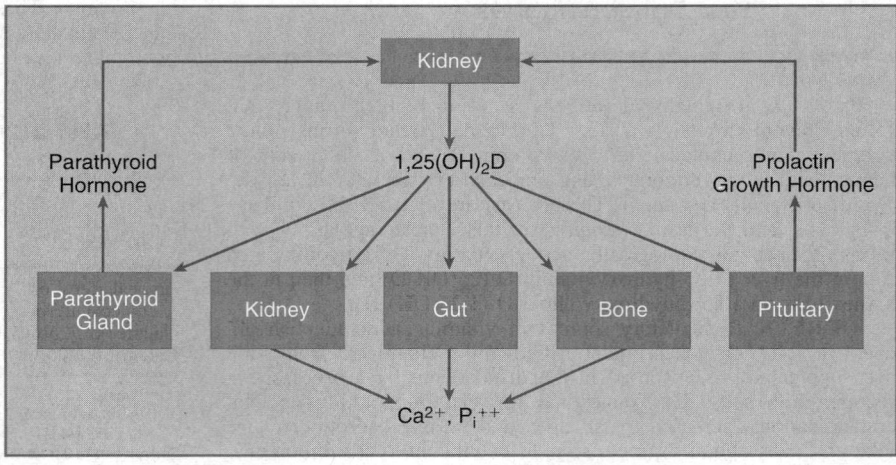

FIGURE 212-2. The vitamin D/endocrine system. The hormone $1,25(OH)_2D$ acts principally on the gut, bone, and kidney but also on other tissues to help regulate calcium (Ca^{2+}) and phosphorus (P_i) homeostasis. Parathyroid hormone regulates Ca^{++} and P_i homeostasis by direct actions on bone and kidney.

213 OSTEOMALACIA AND RICKETS

Marc K. Drezner

DEFINITION. Rickets and osteomalacia are diseases characterized by defective bone and cartilage mineralization in children and bone mineralization in adults. The abnormal calcification of cartilage occurs at epiphyseal growth plates, which also exhibit delayed maturation of the cartilage cellular sequence and disorganization of cell arrangement. The resultant profusion of disorganized, nonmineralized, degenerating cartilage causes widening of the epiphyseal plates with flaring or cupping and irregularity of the epiphyseal-metaphyseal junctions. The abnormal calcification of bone is restricted to the organic matrix at the bone-osteoid interfaces of remodeling tissue. The insufficient mineralization of newly formed matrix paradoxically results in enhanced bone volume and increased susceptibility to fractures or bone deformities. The various disorders associated with rickets and osteomalacia that have been identified and characterized to date are numerous (Table 213–1). Although the phenotypic expression of the defective bone and cartilage mineralization is similar in each of these, the associated biochemical abnormalities and the therapeutic approaches differ according to the pathogenetic defect. Therefore, when diagnosing rickets and/or osteomalacia, further systematic analysis is needed in order to determine cause and appropriate therapy for the disorder.

ETIOLOGY AND PATHOGENESIS. Mineralization of cartilage and bone is a complex process in which the calcium-phosphorus inorganic mineral phase is deposited in an organic matrix in a highly ordered fashion. Such mineralization depends on (1) the availability of sufficient calcium and phosphorus from the extracellular fluid; (2) adequate metabolic and transport function of chondrocytes and osteoblasts to regulate the concentration of calcium, phosphorus, and other ions at the mineralization sites; (3) the presence of collagen with unique type, number, and distribution of

---

TABLE 213–1. THE RICKETS AND OSTEOMALACIA SYNDROMES

I. Disorders of the vitamin D endocrine system
  A. Decreased bioavailability of vitamin D
    1. Deficient endogenous production
      a. Inadequate sunlight exposure
      b. Aging
    2. Nutritional deficiency
    3. Loss of vitamin D metabolites
      a. Nephrotic syndrome
      b. Peritoneal dialysis
  B. Vitamin D malabsorption
    1. Gastrointestinal disorders
      a. Partial/total gastrectomy
      b. Small bowel disease (e.g., celiac disease)
      c. Intestinal bypass
    2. Pancreatic insufficiency
    3. Hepatobiliary disease
      a. Biliary atresia
      b. Biliary obstruction
      c. Biliary fistula
      d. Cirrhosis
  C. Abnormal vitamin D metabolism
    1. Impaired hepatic 25-hydroxylation of vitamin D
      a. Liver disease
      b. Anticonvulsant therapy
    2. Impaired renal 1α-hydroxylation of 25-hydroxyvitamin D
      a. Hereditary vitamin D–dependent rickets type 1 (pseudo–vitamin D deficiency)
      b. Chronic renal failure
      c. Pseudohypoparathyroidism
  D. Target organ resistance to vitamin D and metabolites
    1. Hereditary vitamin D–dependent rickets type 2
      a. Hormone binding negative
      b. Defect in hormone-binding capacity
      c. Defect in hormone-binding affinity
      d. Deficient hormone-receptor nuclear localization
      e. Decreased affinity of the hormone-receptor complex
II. Disorders of phosphate homeostasis
  A. Dietary
    1. Low phosphate intake
    2. Ingestion of phosphate-binding antacids
  B. Impaired renal tubular phosphate reabsorption
    1. Hereditary
      a. X-linked hypophosphatemic rickets/osteomalacia
      b. Hereditary hypophosphatemic rickets/osteomalacia with hypercalciuria
      c. Autosomal dominant hypophosphatemic rickets
      d. Hypophosphatemic bone disease (nonrachitic hypophosphatemic osteomalacia)
      e. Adult-onset hypophosphatemic rickets
    2. Acquired
      a. Tumor-induced osteomalacia (oncogenous osteomalacia)
        (1) Mesenchymal, epidermal, and endodermal tumors
        (2) Fibrous dysplasia of bone
        (3) Neurofibromatosis
        (4) Linear nevus sebaceous syndrome
        (5) Light chain nephropathy
      b. Sporadic hypophosphatemic osteomalacia

  C. General renal tubular disorders
    1. Fanconi's syndrome type 1
      a. Hereditary
        (1) Familial idiopathic
        (2) Cystinosis (Lignac-Fanconi disease)
        (3) Hereditary fructose intolerance
        (4) Tyrosinemia
        (5) Galactosemia
        (6) Glycogen storage disease
        (7) Wilson's disease
        (8) Oculocerebral renal syndrome (Lowe's syndrome)
      b. Acquired
        (1) Renal transplantation
        (2) Multiple myeloma
      c. Intoxication
        (1) Cadmium
        (2) Lead
        (3) Tetracycline (outdated)
    2. Fanconi's syndrome type 2
III. Metabolic acidosis
  A. Distal renal tubular acidosis
    1. Primary
      a. Sporadic
      b. Familial
    2. Secondary
      a. Galactosemia (after galactose ingestion)
      b. Hereditary fructose intolerance with nephrocalcinosis (after chronic fructose ingestion)
      c. Hypergammaglobulinemic states
      d. Medullary sponge kidney
    3. Acquired
      a. Ureterosigmoidostomy
      b. Drug-induced
        (1) Acetozolamide
        (2) Ammonium chloride
IV. Disorders of calcium homeostasis
  A. Dietary calcium deficiency
V. Abnormal bone matrix
  A. Fibrogenesis imperfecta ossium
  B. Axial osteomalacia
VI. Primary mineralization defects
  A. Hereditary
    1. Hypophosphatasia
      a. Perinatal disease
      b. Infantile disease
      c. Childhood disease
      d. Adult-onset disease
      e. Pseudohypophosphatasia
VII. Mineralization inhibitors
  1. Etidronate
  2. Fluoride
  3. Aluminum

cross-links; remarkable patterns of hydroxylation and glycosylation; and abundant phosphate content which collectively permit and facilitate deposition of mineral at gaps, "hole zones," between the distal ends of two collagen molecules; (4) maintenance of an optimal pH (approximately 7.6) for deposition of calcium-phosphorus complexes; and (5) low concentration of calcification inhibitors (e.g., pyrophosphates, proteoglycans) in bone matrix.

Many of the disorders of mineralization occur secondary to known defects in these control steps. In this regard, most disorders resulting in rickets and/or osteomalacia result from disorders in the vitamin D endocrine system (see Ch. 212). Traditionally, a direct role has been assumed for vitamin D or more properly its active metabolite, 1,25-dihydroxyvitamin D, on production of normal collagen matrix and regulation of bone mineralization. However, more likely the abnormal mineralization in these disorders results from an associated calcium and phosphorus deficiency that diminishes the driving force for calcification. Primary disorders of phosphate homeostasis also underlie a large number of the rachitic/osteomalacic disorders. Diminished gastrointestinal absorption or renal wasting of phosphorus limits this essential mineral in such disorders. The isolated deficiency of phosphorus alone or in conjunction with a frequently occurring aberration in vitamin D metabolism underlies defective mineralization. In accord with the complex regulation of bone mineralization, however, decreases in calcium or phosphorus do not account for the rickets and osteomalacia in all forms of the disease. Indeed, certain forms of rickets and osteomalacia occur in spite of a normal or even elevated calcium-phosphate product. In such diseases, altered pH, abnormal collagen matrix, or excessive concentration of calcification inhibitors underlies the abnormal mineralization. In other forms of the disease, the precise mechanism causing the defective mineralization remains unknown.

Inadequate mineralization in rickets occurs in the matrix of cartilage in the growing epiphyseal plate. These characteristic changes are confined to the maturation zone of the cartilage, whereas the resting and proliferative zones of the epiphyses exhibit normal histologic features. In the maturation zone, the height of the cell columns is increased and the cells are closely packed and irregularly aligned. Moreover, calcification in the interstitial regions of this hypertrophic zone is defective.

In bone, the abnormal mineralization results in accumulation of excess osteoid, a *sine qua non* for the diagnosis of osteomalacia in most instances (Fig. 213–1). A supranormal amount of osteoid, however, may also occur in disease states associated with accelerated bone turnover, such as hyperparathyroidism. In addition, reduced mineralization activity may be observed without hyperosteoidosis in osteoporosis. Establishing the diagnosis of osteomalacia histopathologically, therefore, requires documenting abnormal mineralization with excess osteoid. These defects are manifest in bone by an increase in the forming surface covered by incompletely mineralized osteoid, an increase in osteoid volume and thickness, and a decrease in the mineralization front (the percentage of osteoid-covered bone-forming surface undergoing calcification) or the mineral apposition rate. The amount of osteoid in bone and the mineralization dynamics are determined in 3- to 5-μm-thick sections of undecalcified bone by special stains and the fluorescence of previously ingested tetracycline that is deposited at calcification fronts (Fig. 213–1).

CLINICAL MANIFESTATIONS. The clinical features of rickets, although variable to some degree according to the underlying disorder, are primarily related to skeletal pain and deformity, bone fractures, slipped epiphyses, and abnormalities of growth. In addition, hypocalcemia, when present, may be severe enough to produce tetany, laryngeal spasm, and seizures.

In infants and young children, symptoms include listlessness, irritability, and, in some forms of metabolic rickets, profound hypotonia and proximal muscle weakness. Indeed, as the disease progresses and muscle weakness is present, children often are unable to walk without support. Throughout early life, classic skeletal deformities appear. By age 6 months, frontal bossing with flattening at the back is evident. Later, a lateral collapse of both chest walls (Harrison's sulcus) and rachitic rosary may appear. If untreated, progressive bony deformities result in bowing—particularly in the tibia, femur, radius, and ulna—and fractures. In addition, dental eruption may be delayed and, in those forms of the disease with

hypocalcemia or hereditary hypophosphatemia, enamel defects and inadequate dentin calcification occur, respectively.

In contrast, clinical signs of osteomalacia are nondescript. Indeed, the disease-specific abnormalities may be overlooked and features of an underlying disorder (e.g., malabsorption) may predominate. Symptoms, when present, may include diffuse skeletal pain and muscular weakness. The pain, often described as dull and aching, is generally worsened by activity and prominent around the hips, resulting in an antalgic gait. The muscle weakness is primarily proximal and frequently associated with wasting, hypotonia, and a waddling gait. This myopathy is seen in almost all forms of rickets and osteomalacia, X-linked hypophosphatemic rickets/osteomalacia notably excepted. Clinical improvement in the myopathy usually results from specific therapy such as vitamin D repletion in nutritional osteomalacia, phosphate supplementation in disorders marked by renal phosphate wasting, or correction of acidosis. Fractures of the ribs, vertebral bodies, and long bones may occur and lead to progressive deformities, as well as point tenderness on palpation.

The radiographic abnormalities in both rickets and osteomalacia reflect the histopathologic changes. In rickets, alterations are most evident at the growth plate, which is wide and flared and displays an irregular hazy appearance at the diaphyseal line secondary to uneven invasion of the recently calcified cartilage by adjacent bone tissue. The trabecular pattern of the metaphyses is also abnormal, the cortices of the diaphyses are thinned, and the shafts frequently are bowed.

In osteomalacia, there is usually a moderate decrease in bone density associated with coarsening of trabeculae and blurring of their margins. When secondary hyperparathyroidism is present, subperiosteal resorption in the phalanges and metacarpals, erosion of the distal ends of the clavicles, and bone cysts may be observed. A more specific radiographic abnormality is the presence of Looser's zones, also called pseudofractures or milkman's fractures, in the shafts of long bones. These are ribbon-like zones of rarefaction, ranging from a few millimeters to several centimeters in length and usually oriented perpendicular to the bone surface. Often, they occur symmetrically and most commonly are present at the medial aspect of the femurs near the femoral heads, in the metatarsals, or in the pelvis. Long-standing osteomalacia may also result in additional characteristic radiographic abnormalities, including biconcave collapsed vertebrae and a trefoil (or triangular) pelvis.

In patients with renal tubular disorders (see Ch. 82), increased rather than decreased bone density may be present. In spite of the increased bone mass, histopathologic evaluation of biopsies reveals an abundance of unmineralized osteoid, and bones remain subject to fracture. Thus, the increased density likely reflects replacement of marrow air space with osteoid.

Biochemical abnormalities in patients with rickets and osteomalacia vary with the cause of the disorder. However, the rachitic and osteomalacic syndromes may be divided into calciopenic and phosphopenic forms, as well as those in which mineral availability is apparently normal. In general, patients with the calciopenic diseases exhibit a low or marginally normal serum calcium level, a decreased serum phosphorus concentration, and (secondary) hyperparathyroidism. If vitamin D deficiency prevails, the serum 25(OH)D levels are characteristically low, generally < 3 ng per milliliter. In contrast, the serum 1,25(OH)$_2$D concentration may not be overtly decreased secondary to the prevailing hyperparathyroidism. Alternatively, a defect in vitamin D metabolism often results in an isolated deficiency of 1,25(OH)$_2$D while end-organ resistance to this active vitamin D metabolite increases the circulating level of calcitriol.

A primary abnormality of transepithelial phosphate transport in the nephron, resulting in renal phosphate wasting, underlies the majority of the phosphopenic disorders. As a rule, patients with these disorders maintain a normal serum calcium concentration, whereas the serum phosphorus is characteristically low. In contrast to the calciopenic forms of disease, the serum 25(OH)D and parathyroid hormone levels are normal in patients with hypophosphatemic disease. Moreover, affected subjects commonly maintain a normal (or mildly decreased) serum 1,25(OH)$_2$D level in spite of the prevailing hypophosphatemia, which should increase production of this active vitamin D metabolite. However, an elevated serum 1,25(OH)$_2$D concentration was recently reported in two rare genetic phosphopenic disorders, hereditary hypophosphatemic rickets with hypercalciuria and Fanconi's syndrome, type 2. Whereas the elevated cal-

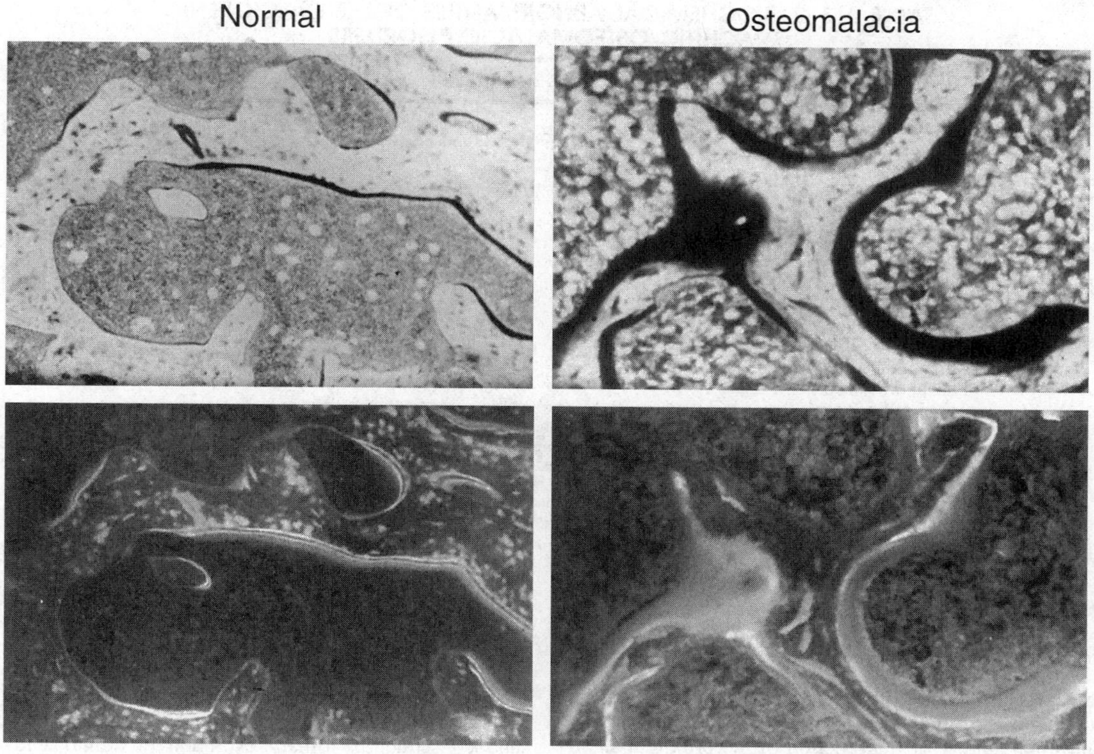

Normal

Osteomalacia

FIGURE 213–1. Microscopic appearance of bone biopsy sections from a normal and osteomalacic patient. In the upper panels the Villanueva-stained sections exhibit mineralized bone (white tones) covered by unmineralized osteoid seams (black tones). Normal bone has thin osteoid seams distributed over a limited portion of the bone surface. In contrast, osteomalacic bone is covered almost completely with thick osteoid seams. In the lower panels, the same bone sections are viewed under ultraviolet light in order to estimate mineralization activity by visualizing tetracycline labels. The normal bone reveals that the majority of the osteoid has crisp double tetracycline labels, indicative of normal mineralization activity. The osteomalacic bone, however, has evidence only of smeared tetracycline labels without the double label. Moreover, the tetracycline labels do not occupy the majority of the osteoid-bone interface. Such observations are representative of the abnormal mineralization that characterizes the osteomalacic bone disorder.

citriol level underlies increased gastrointestinal absorption of calcium and hypercalciuria in these diseases, the impact of abnormal vitamin D metabolism on the phenotypic expression of the phosphopenic disorders is less certain.

In those diseases with normal serum calcium and phosphorus concentrations, laboratory abnormalities are unique to each form of the disease. Nevertheless, alkaline phosphatase activity in plasma is generally elevated in all forms of rickets and osteomalacia. Even severe forms of disease, however, particularly those due to renal tubular disorders, may be associated with normal or only marginally elevated enzyme activity.

DIFFERENTIAL DIAGNOSIS AND THERAPY OF RACHITIC AND OSTEOMALACIC DISORDERS

Disorders of the Vitamin D Endocrine System

Rickets and osteomalacia due to disorders of the vitamin D endocrine system comprise a wide variety of calciopenic diseases. The variable biochemical abnormalities associated with these disparate disorders are summarized in Table 213–2. Although many of these diseases are no longer common causes of rickets and osteomalacia, others are often hidden causes of bone disease in a varying population of patients.

DECREASED BIOAVAILABILITY OF VITAMIN D. *Inadequate Sunlight and Nutritional Vitamin D Deficiency.* Adequate exposure to sunlight and fortification of dairy products with vitamin D have eliminated vitamin D deficiency secondary to inadequate endogenous production or nutrition in the majority of countries. However, in several populations, such as Asian immigrants in Britain, rickets and osteomalacia secondary to vitamin D deficiency occurs in neonates and infants, adolescents during pubertal growth, and less frequently among adults. Insufficient vitamin D intake secondary to using unfortified foods, racial pigmentation (which interferes with ultraviolet transmission through the skin), genetic factors, and social customs (such as avoiding sun exposure) contribute to

the development of disease in these subjects. Moreover, in the United States and other developed countries, a surprisingly frequent occurrence of vitamin D–deficiency osteomalacia has been recently recognized in alcoholics, institutionalized patients, and the elderly. Poor diet, in some cases including avoiding milk and milk products due to lactose intolerance, lack of sunlight exposure, and an age-related decline in the dermal synthesis of 7-dehydrocholesterol are among the factors predisposing to the vitamin D deficiency and consequent bone disease.

The clinical sequelae of decreased vitamin D bioavailability are generally preceded by a fall in circulating 25(OH)D levels. Measurement of this metabolite therefore serves to identify populations at risk for and facilitates early detection of vitamin D deficiency rickets and osteomalacia. Introducing vitamin D supplements (400 units per day) may, under these circumstances, prevent development of clinically significant disease.

Regardless, treating clinically evident vitamin D–deficient rickets and osteomalacia invariably results in healing of the bone disease. The disorder is best treated with vitamin D and restoration of normal dietary calcium and phosphorus intake. Ergocalciferol (vitamin D_2) is preferred because it provides the missing substrate that submits to physiologic regulation of vitamin D metabolite production.

Vitamin D Malabsorption. Gastrointestinal malabsorption associated with diseases of the small intestine, hepatobiliary tree, and pancreas may result in decreased absorption of vitamin D and/or depletion of endogenous 25(OH)D stores due to abnormal enterohepatic circulation. In general, malabsorption of vitamin D occurs as a consequence of steatorrhea, which disturbs fat emulsification and chylomicron facilitated absorption (see Ch. 103). Such abnormalities often are associated with rickets and/or osteomalacia. However, most affected patients are asymptomatic, and many exhibit only reduced bone volume rather than evidence of defective bone mineralization. Intestinal bypass surgery and adult celiac disease are common examples of disorders in which vitamin D malabsorption

TABLE 213–2. BIOCHEMICAL ABNORMALITIES OF THE CALCIOPENIC RACHITIC/OSTEOMALACIC DISORDERS

	VDDR	CRF	HVDDR 1	HVDDR 2	HP	PSH
Biochemistries						
Calcium	⇓	⇓	⇓	⇓	⇓	⇓
Phosphorus	N/⇓	⇑	N/⇓	N/⇓	⇑	⇑
Alkaline phosphatase	⇑	⇑	⇑	⇑	N/⇑	N/⇑
Parathyroid hormone	⇑	⇑	⇑	⇑	⇓	⇑
25(OH)D	⇓	N/⇓	N	N	N	N
1,25(OH)$_2$D	⇑	⇓	⇓	⇑	⇓	⇓
Renal function						
Urinary phosphorus	⇑	⇓	⇑	⇑	⇓	⇓
Urinary calcium	⇓	⇓	⇓	⇓	⇓	⇓
Gastrointestinal function						
Calcium absorption	⇓	⇓	⇓	⇓	⇓	⇓
Phosphorus absorption	⇓	⇓	⇓	⇓	⇓	⇓

VDDR = vitamin D–deficiency rickets (including sunlight or nutritional deficiency, vitamin D malabsorption, inhibition of 25-hydroxylation); CRF = chronic renal failure; HVDDR 1 = hereditary vitamin D–dependent rickets type 1; HVDDR-2 = hereditary vitamin D–dependent rickets type 2; HP = hypoparathyroidism; PSH = pseudohypoparathyroidism.
N = normal; ⇓ = decreased; ⇑ = increased; N/⇓ = normal or decreased; N/⇑ = normal or increased.

occurs and in which the suspicion for osteomalacia should remain high. In contrast, patients with cholestatic liver disease, extrahepatic biliary obstruction, and diseases of the distal portions of the small intestine, such as regional enteritis, may develop bone disease secondary not only to poor vitamin D absorption but to disruption of enterohepatic circulation as well.

Osteomalacia may also develop in patients who have had partial or total gastrectomy for peptic ulcer disease or other indications. Loss of gastrointestinal acidity or malfunction of the proximal small bowel underlies the vitamin D malabsorption in such circumstances. Absence of sufficient absorbing surface or failure of intestinal mucosal cells to respond to vitamin D or its metabolites may also cause vitamin D malabsorption and consequent bone disease.

The prevalence of osteomalacia in patients with gastrointestinal malabsorption varies widely from country to country. However, as many as 25 to 50% of British and European patients with partial gastrectomy, inflammatory bowel disease, and cholestatic liver disease have bone biopsy–proven osteomalacia.

Treatment of established disease generally requires pharmacologic amounts of vitamin D or its metabolites to overcome the defective absorption and the aberrant enterohepatic circulation or to offset end-organ resistance at the intestinal mucosa. Most patients respond well to calcium supplements, 1 to 1.5 grams per day, and ergocalciferol, 1250 to 5000 μg per day. If the severity of malabsorption makes oral vitamin D ineffective, parenteral ergocalciferol, 12,500 to 25,000 μg intramuscularly once a month is a practical alternative. Because magnesium deficiency often co-exists in malabsorptive diseases and may slow healing of the osteomalacia, adjunctive therapy with magnesium oxide may facilitate bone mineralization.

ABNORMAL VITAMIN D METABOLISM. *Liver Disease.* Because vitamin D is hydroxylated in the liver to form 25(OH)D, patients with severe parenchymal or obstructive hepatic disease (see Ch. 114) may have reduced production of this metabolite. These patients, however, rarely manifest biochemical or histologic evidence of osteomalacia. Indeed, an overt decrease of 25(OH)D generally requires concomitant nutritional deficiency or interruption of the enterohepatic circulation. Consequently, therapy for biopsy-proven osteomalacia, when present, is similar to that secondary to malabsorption of vitamin D.

Drug-Induced Disease. Decreased circulating levels of 25(OH)D may also occur in patients treated with drugs such as phenytoin or phenobarbital. This defect in vitamin D metabolism is due to induction of hepatic microsomal enzymes that metabolize 25(OH)D to inactive metabolites. Secondary to this abnormality and/or to the direct inhibitory effects of these drugs on intestinal calcium absorption and parathyroid hormone (PTH)–mediated calcium mobilization from bone, treated subjects often exhibit a decreased level of ionized calcium. These multiple influences commonly result in a bone disorder that may be mild osteomalacia or hyperparathyroid bone disease. Treatment of the bone disease and hypocalcemia generally requires modest vitamin D supplementation (150 to 400 μg per week).

Vitamin D–Dependent Rickets Type 1 (Pseudovitamin D Deficiency). Limited production of 1,25(OH)$_2$D due to hereditary or acquired diseases represents another abnormality of vitamin D metabolism that invariably results in rickets or osteomalacia. Vitamin D–dependent rickets type 1 is such a genetic disorder, transmitted as an autosomal recessive trait and characterized by hypocalcemia, hypophosphatemia, and elevated alkaline phosphatase activity. As a result of the hypocalcemia, PTH levels are elevated and consequently urinary excretion of amino acids and phosphate enhanced. In addition to these biochemical abnormalities, within the first year of life patients exhibit muscle weakness and hypotonia, motor retardation, and stunted growth. With progression patients develop the classic radiographic signs of vitamin D deficiency rickets and bone biopsy evidence of osteomalacia. Further, affected subjects have a decreased serum 1,25(OH)$_2$D concentration, likely due to an inherited deficiency of 25(OH)D-1α-hydroxylase activity, which limits production of this active vitamin D metabolite. This presumed abnormality has been substantiated by (1) experiments in humans that demonstrate serum calcitriol levels do not increase in response to classic stimuli of enzyme activity and (2) the absence of enzyme activity in renal cortical homogenates from the porcine homologue of this disease. Consistent with these observations, a physiologic dose of calcitriol (1 μg per day) generally promotes complete healing of the bone disease and resolution of the biochemical abnormalities, whereas a pharmacologic dose of vitamin D (20,000 to 100,000 U per day) or 25(OH)D (0.1 to 1.0 mg per day) is required to achieve similar effects. Regardless of the therapy used, in the majority of affected patients, therapy with vitamin D or its metabolites must be continued for life in order to prevent relapse. However, in a minority of subjects with a syndrome clinically identical to vitamin D–dependent rickets type 1, stopping treatment does not result in reappearance of biochemical or radiographic signs of the disease.

Chronic Renal Failure. Osteomalacia is common in patients with chronic renal failure and often tends to be the predominant type of renal osteodystrophy in younger patients (see Ch. 77). The defect in mineralization almost certainly results in part from a decreased conversion of 25(OH)D to 1,25(OH)$_2$D. Such abnormal vitamin D metabolism occurs secondary to either insufficient viable renal cortical tissue or the inhibitory effects of hyperphosphatemia on renal 25(OH)D-1α-hydroxylase activity. In addition, in some patients aluminum accumulated in bone underlies the abnormal mineralization. Indeed, the presence of aluminum may render the bone abnormality vitamin D resistant. Under such circumstances treatment with deferoxamine may be necessary to mobilize the aluminum from bone and other tissues and improve mineralization.

Hypoparathyroidism. Osteomalacia only rarely occurs in patients with hypoparathyroidism (see Ch. 214). Hypocalcemia and low or low-normal serum 1,25(OH)$_2$D are usually present and appear important in the pathogenesis of the bone disease. However, the underlying reason for the variable occurrence of bone pathology remains uncertain. The low serum 1,25(OH)$_2$D concentration results from the PTH deficiency. Bone pain suggests the diagnosis and generally the diagnosis depends on histomorphometric analysis of a bone biopsy. The majority of patients respond well to treatment with vitamin D and calcium supplements, but for unclear reasons some require therapy with 1,25(OH)$_2$D.

Pseudohypoparathyroidism. In pseudohypoparathyroidism apparent bone and kidney resistance to PTH results in hypocalcemia, retention of phosphate, and low serum 1,25(OH)$_2$D (see Ch. 214). Surprisingly, however, affected patients often manifest bone disease marked by increased resorptive activity and osteomalacia. Indeed, severe demineralization, including frank osteitis fibrosa cystica and occasionally rickets or osteomalacia has been observed in 24 patients with pseudohypoparathyroidism. More commonly, the bone disease is silent and diagnosis often depends on histomorphometric analysis of a bone biopsy. Undoubtedly, hypocalcemia, secondary hyperparathyroidism, and low serum 1,25(OH)$_2$D are important cofactors in the pathogenesis of the disease. Patients respond well to pharmacologic amounts of vitamin D or replacement doses of 1,25(OH)$_2$D.

TARGET ORGAN RESISTANCE TO CALCITRIOL. *Vitamin D–Dependent Rickets, Type 2.* Patients with clinical and biochemical abnormalities similar to those of subjects with vitamin D–dependent rickets type 1, but elevated 1,25(OH)$_2$D levels have recently been described. They have not only calciopenic rickets and/or osteomalacia but variably associated abnormalities, including alopecia, in 60% of patients, and in a minority of subjects additional ectodermal anomalies such as multiple milia, epidermal cysts, and oligodontia. The disease results from a group of genetic disorders that through heterogeneous mechanisms cause a decreased target organ responsiveness to 1,25(OH)$_2$D. The defects identified to date are (1) failure of 1,25(OH)$_2$D binding to available receptors; (2) a reduction in 1,25(OH)$_2$D receptor–binding sites; (3) abnormal binding affinity of 1,25(OH)$_2$D to receptor; (4) inadequate translocation of 1,25(OH)$_2$D-receptor complex to the nucleus; and (5) diminished affinity of the 1,25(OH)$_2$D-receptor complex for the DNA-binding domain secondary to changes in the structure of receptor zinc-binding fingers. Effective treatment of this disease likely depends on the nature of the underlying abnormality. Thus, patients with deficient affinity of 1,25(OH)$_2$D to receptor and inadequate nuclear translocation respond to high-dose vitamin D or 1,25(OH)$_2$D with complete clinical and biochemical remission. In contrast, patients with other forms of the disease generally remain refractory to treatment with vitamin D or its analogues. However, every patient should receive a 6-month trial of therapy with supplemental calcium (1 to 3 grams per day) and vitamin D (400,000 to 1,200,000 U per day), 25(OH)D (0.05 to 1.5 mg per day), or, in more severe cases, 1,25(OH)$_2$D (5 to 60 μg per day). If the abnormalities of the syndrome do not normalize in response to this treatment, clinical remission may be achieved by administering high-dose oral calcium or long-term intracaval infusion of calcium.

Disorders of Phosphate Homeostasis (see Ch. 190)

Rickets and osteomalacia occur in association with a variety of disorders in which phosphate depletion predominates. Most typically, these diseases have in common abnormal proximal renal tubular function, which results in an increased renal clearance of inorganic phosphorus and hypophosphatemia. However, the biochemical abnormalities characteristic of these disorders are quite variable (Table 213–3).

IMPAIRED RENAL TUBULAR PHOSPHATE REABSORPTION. *X-Linked Hypophosphatemic Rickets/Osteomalacia.* X-linked hypophosphatemic (XLH) rickets/ostemalacia represents the prototypic phosphate-wasting disorder, characterized in general by progressively severe skeletal abnormalities, growth retardation, and X-linked dominant inheritance. However, the clinical expression of the disease varies widely. The mildest abnormality is hypophosphatemia without clinically evident bone disease, and the most common clinically evident manifestation is short stature. Nevertheless, the majority of children with the disease exhibit enlargement of the wrists and/or knees secondary to rickets, as well as bowing of the lower extremities. Additional early signs of the disease may include late dentition, tooth abscesses secondary to poor mineralization of the interglobular dentine, and premature cranial synostosis. In spite of marked variability in the clinical presentation, bone biopsies in affected children and adults invariably reveal osteomalacia, the severity of which has no relationship to gender, the extent of the biochemical abnormalities, or the severity of the clinical disability. In untreated youths and adults, the serum 25(OH)D levels are normal and the concentration of 1,25(OH)$_2$D is in the low-normal range. The paradoxical occurrence of hypophosphatemia and normal serum calcitriol levels is due to aberrant regulation of renal 25(OH)D-1α-hydroxylase activity, most likely caused by the abnormal phosphate transport. Indeed, studies in *Hyp*-mice, the murine homologue of the human disease, have established that defective regulation is confined to enzyme localized in the proximal convoluted tubule, the site of the abnormal phosphate transport.

A primary inborn error that results in an expressed abnormality in the renal proximal tubule (and perhaps the intestine), which impairs phosphate reabsorption (and absorption), underlies the pathogenesis of XLH. Although controversy exists regarding the character of the inborn error, studies in *Hyp*-mice suggest that elaboration of a humoral factor underlies the observed inhibition of phosphate transport in affected patients.

Choice of therapy for this disease has been remarkably influenced by an increased understanding of the pathophysiologic factors that affect its phenotypic expression. Thus, current treatment strate-

TABLE 213–3. BIOCHEMICAL ABNORMALITIES OF THE PHOSPHOPENIC RACHITIC/OSTEOMALACIC DISORDERS

	XLH	HHRH	ADHR	AHR	FS I	FS II	TIO
Biochemistries							
Calcium	N	N	N	N	N	N	N
Phosphorus	⇓	⇓	⇓	⇓	⇓	⇓	⇓
Alkaline phosphatase	⇑	⇑	⇑	⇑	⇑	⇑	⇑
Parathyroid hormone	N	⇓	N	N	N	⇓	N
25(OH)D	N	N	?	N	N	N	N
1,25(OH)$_2$D	(⇓)	⇑	?	(⇓)	(⇓)	⇑	⇓
Renal function							
Urinary phosphorus	⇑	⇑	⇑	⇑	⇑	⇑	⇑
Urinary calcium	⇓	⇑	?	⇓	⇓	⇑	⇓
Gastrointestinal function							
Calcium absorption	⇓	⇑	?	⇓	⇓	⇑	⇓
Phosphorus absorption	⇓	⇑	?	⇓	⇓	⇑	⇓

XLH = X-linked hypophosphatemic rickets; HHRH = hereditary hypophosphatemic rickets with hypercalciuria; ADHR = autosomal dominant hypophosphatemic rickets; AHR = adult onset hypophosphatemic rickets/osteomalacia; FS I = Fanconi's syndrome type I; FS II = Fanconi's syndrome type II; TIO = tumor-induced osteomalacia (Oncogenous osteomalacia).
N = normal; ⇓ = decreased; ⇑ = increased; (⇓) = decreased relative to the serum phosphorus concentration.
Modified from Econs MJ, Drezner MK: Bone disease resulting from inherited disorders of renal tubule transport and vitamin D metabolism. *In* Coe FL, Favus MJ: Disorders of Bone and Mineral Metabolism. New York, Raven Press, 1992, p 937.

gies for children directly address the combined calcitriol and phosphorus deficiency characteristic of the disease. Generally, the regimen includes a period of titration to achieve a maximum dose of calcitriol, 40 to 60 ng per kilogram per day in two divided doses and phosphorus, 1 to 2 grams per day in four or five divided doses. Although youths occasionally prove refractory to such therapeutic intervention, combined therapy often improves growth velocity, normalizes lower extremity deformities, and induces healing of the attendant bone disease. Of course treatment involves a significant risk of toxicity that is generally expressed as abnormalities of calcium homeostasis and/or detrimental effects on renal function. Therapy in adults is reserved for episodes of intractable bone pain and refractory nonunion of bone fractures.

Hereditary Hypophosphatemic Rickets with Hypercalciuria (HHRH).

This rare genetic disease is marked by hypophosphatemic rickets with hypercalciuria. In contrast to other diseases in which renal phosphate transport is limited, patients with HHRH exhibit increased $1,25(OH)_2D$ production. The resultant elevated serum calcitriol levels enhance the gastrointestinal calcium absorption, which in turn increases the filtered renal calcium load and inhibits parathyroid secretion. The clinical expression of the disease is heterogeneous, although initial symptoms generally consist of bone pain and/or deformities of the lower extremities. Additional features of the disease include short stature, muscle weakness, and radiographic signs of rickets or osteopenia. These various symptoms and signs may exist separately or in combination and may be pres-ent in a mild or severe form. Relatives of patients with evident HHRH may exhibit an additional mode of disease expression. These subjects manifest hypercalciuria and hypophosphatemia, but the abnormalities are less marked and occur in the absence of discernible bone disease. The majority of evidence indicates that HHRH is inherited by autosomal recessive transmission.

Patients with HHRH have been treated successfully with high-dose phosphorus (1 to 2.5 grams per day in five divided doses) alone. In response to therapy, bone pain disappears and muscular strength improves substantially. Moreover, the majority of treated subjects exhibit accelerated linear growth, and radiologic signs of rickets are completely absent within 4 to 9 months. Despite this favorable response, limited studies indicate that such treatment does not heal the associated osteomalacia. Therefore, further studies are necessary to determine if phosphorus alone is truly sufficient for this disorder.

Autosomal Dominant Hypophosphatemic Rickets (ADHR).

Although many investigators assume that all familial renal phosphate wasting disorders are X-linked, several studies have documented an autosomal dominant inheritance of a hypophosphatemic disorder similar to XLH. The phenotypic manifestations of this disorder include the expected hypophosphatemia due to renal phosphate wasting, lower extremity deformities, and rickets/osteomalacia. However, long-term studies indicate that a few of the affected female patients demonstrate delayed penetrance of clinically apparent disease and an increased tendency for bone fracture, uncommon occurrences in XLH. Limited information is available regarding other aspects of the disease, and no data exist regarding localization of the genetic defect.

An apparent *forme fruste* of ADHR—(autosomal dominant) hypophosphatemic bone disease—has many of the characteristics of XLH and ADHR, but recent reports indicate that affected children display no evidence of rachitic disease. Because this syndrome is described in only a few small kindreds and radiographically evident rickets is not universal in children with familial hypophosphatemia, these families may have ADHR. Further observations are necessary to discriminate this possibility.

Adult-onset Hypophosphatemic Rickets.

In some patients older than 15, an acquired form of hypophosphatemic rickets and osteomalacia occurs. Presenting symptoms in affected patients include debilitating bone pain, a significant myopathy, and Looser's zones on bone radiographs. The pathogenesis of the disorder involves renal phosphate loss due to abnormal proximal tubule function. Usually the inheritance is sporadic, but a propositus occasionally passes the disease in an X-linked dominant mode, suggesting that spontaneous mutation may cause expression of the disease. Al-

ternatively, the disorder may represent tumor-induced osteomalacia in a patient with an undetected benign tumor or malignancy.

Tumor-induced Osteomalacia (Oncogenous Osteomalacia).

Since initial recognition of this disease, there have been reports of approximately 70 patients in whom rickets and/or osteomalacia have been associated with a coexisting tumor. The coexistent tumors have been of mesenchymal origin in the majority of patients. The cardinal feature of this disease is remission of the unexplained bone disease after tumor resection. In general, affected patients present with bone and muscle pain, muscle weakness, and occasionally recurrent fractures of long bones. Biochemical abnormalities include renal phosphate wasting marked by an abnormally low renal tubular maximum for the reabsorption of phosphate per liter of glomerular filtrate, decreased gastrointestinal absorption of phosphate, and consequent hypophosphatemia. In general, serum 25(OH)D levels are normal and serum calcitriol is profoundly decreased or inappropriately normal relative to the hypophosphatemia. Generalized osteopenia, pseudofractures, and coarsened trabeculae, as well as widened epiphyseal plates in children, comprise the common radiographic abnormalities of the syndrome.

Most investigators agree that tumor production of a humoral factor(s) that may affect multiple functions of the proximal renal tubule underlies the pathogenesis of this syndrome. This possibility is supported by (1) the presence of phosphaturic activity in tumor extracts from two of three patients with tumor-associated osteomalacia; (2) the coincidence of amino aciduria and glycosuria with renal phosphate wasting in some affected subjects, indicative of complex alterations in proximal renal tubular function; and (3) diminished renal 25(OH)D-1α-hydroxylase activity in heterotransplanted tumor-bearing athymic nude mice and in renal tubule cell cultures exposed to tumor extracts.

In contrast to these observations, patients with tumor-associated osteomalacia secondary to hematogenous malignancy exhibit abnormalities of the syndrome secondary to a distinctly different mechanism. In these subjects the nephropathy associated with light-chain proteinuria results in decreased renal phosphate reabsorption and consequent hypophosphatemia. At least 15 patients with this form of the disorder have been reported.

The primary treatment of this disorder is complete resection of the associated tumor. However, recurrence or metastases of tumors often preclude such definitive therapy. In such cases, calcitriol (1.5 to 3.0 μg per day) alone or combined with phosphorus supplementation (2 to 4 grams per day) completely heals the attendant bone disease or significantly improves the biochemical and histologic abnormalities. Careful serial assessment of parathyroid function, serum and urinary calcium, and renal function are essential to ensure safe therapy in affected subjects.

Fanconi's Syndrome (see Ch. 82).

Rickets and osteomalacia are frequently associated with Fanconi's syndrome, a disorder characterized by phosphaturia and consequent hypophosphatemia, amino aciduria, renal glycosuria, albuminuria, and proximal renal tubular acidosis. Although a wide diversity of congenital and acquired diseases are associated with this syndrome (see Table 213–1), damage to the proximal renal tubule represents the common underlying mechanism of disease (see Ch. 175). Resultant dysfunction results in renal wasting of those substances primarily reabsorbed at the proximal tubule. The associated bone disease in this disorder is likely secondary to hypophosphatemia and/or acidosis, abnormalities that occur in association with aberrantly (Fanconi's syndrome type 1) or normally regulated (Fanconi's syndrome type 2) vitamin D metabolism.

Metabolic Acidosis

Osteomalacia occurs secondary to renal tubular acidosis and the acidosis that follows ureterosigmoidoscopy. The bone disease results from the multifactorial influence of acidosis, which decreases the conversion of amorphous calcium phosphate to hydroxyapatite at the mineralization front, induces renal phosphate wasting, and possibly interferes with calcitriol production. Systemic acidosis also enhances dissolution of bone and results in hypercalciuria. Affected patients have a normal serum calcium, a low normal or decreased serum phosphorus, and an elevated alkaline phosphatase. Secondary to hypercalciuria, nephrocalcinosis and renal lithiasis often occur. Bicarbonate therapy alone effectively treats the osteomalacia associated with metabolic acidosis, although administering vitamin D and calcium when starting therapy facilitates healing of the bone disease.

Primary Disorders of Bone Matrix

Intrinsic disorders of bone in which apparently abnormal matrix is produced but not normally mineralized are extremely rare and poorly understood. These diseases may result from presumed abnormalities of collagen or other proteins in the matrix or aberrant enzyme activity essential for normal mineralization.

ABNORMAL BONE MATRIX. *Fibrogenesis Imperfecta Ossium.* Fibrogenesis imperfecta ossium is a rare, sporadically occurring disorder characterized by the gradual onset of intractable skeletal pain in middle-aged men and women. Pathologic fractures are a prominent clinical feature, and patients typically become bedridden. Although the serum calcium and phosphorus are normal, alkaline phosphatase is invariably elevated. The bones have a dense, amorphous, mottled appearance radiologically and a disorganized arrangement of collagen with decreased birefringence histologically. Most likely, the disorganized collagen matrix limits normal bone mineralization.

Axial Osteomalacia. Axial osteomalacia is another unusual sporadically occurring disorder that generally affects only middle-aged men. The majority of patients present with only vague, dull, chronic axial discomfort that typically affects the cervical region most severely. Abnormal radiographic findings are limited to the pelvis and spine, where the coarsened trabecular pattern is characteristic of osteomalacia. Although the alkaline phosphatase may be increased, histopathologic studies reveal a normal lamellar pattern of collagen. However, the osteoblasts appear flat and inactive, suggesting that an osteoblastic defect and perhaps attendant abnormal matrix inhibit normal mineralization.

ABNORMAL ENZYME ACTIVITY. *Hypophosphatasia.* Hypophosphatasia is an heritable disorder characterized by a deficiency of the tissue nonspecific (liver/bone/kidney) isoenzyme of alkaline phosphatase, increased urinary excretion of phosphorylethanolamine, and skeletal disease that includes osteomalacia and rickets. The severity of clinical expression is remarkably variable and spans intrauterine death from profound skeletal hypomineralization at one extreme to lifelong absence of symptoms at the other. As a consequence, six clinical disease types are distinguished (see Table 213–1). The age at which skeletal disease is initially noted delineates, in large part, the perinatal (lethal), infantile, childhood, and adult variants of the disorder. However, affected children and adults may manifest only the unique dental abnormalities of the syndrome and accordingly are classified as having odontohypophosphatasia. Finally, patients with the rare variant, pseudohypophosphatasia, have the clinical/radiologic/biochemical features of the classic disease without a decrease in the circulating levels of alkaline phosphatase. These individuals have defects in cellular localization and substrate specificity of the enzyme.

Affected infants exhibit hypercalcemia, hypercalciuria, enlarged sutures of the skull, craniostenosis, delayed dentition, enlarged epiphyses, and prominent costochondral junctions. Genu valgum or varum may develop subsequently. In older children disease may be limited to rickets. Surprisingly, the disorder in adults is mild despite the presence of osteopenia. Indeed, the disease may be limited to slowly healing metatarsal fractures or loss or fracture of teeth. Nevertheless, 50% of patients have an history of early exfoliation of deciduous teeth and/or rickets, and disease may reflect re-expression of the childhood disorder.

The perinatal and infantile forms of disease are inherited as autosomal recessive traits. The mode(s) of inheritance for odonto-, adult, and childhood hypophosphatasia remains unclear, although an autosomal dominant disease transmission has been described in some kindreds with mild disease. The physiologic basis for the bone disease likely relates to the role of alkaline phosphatase in cleaving pyrophosphate, an inhibitor of bone mineralization. Failure to hydrolyze this physiologic substrate results in inorganic pyrophosphate elevated to levels sufficiently high to inhibit the mineralization process.

Therapy of this disease has been generally unrewarding. Thus, supportive treatment is important and may include craniotomy in children (to manage craniosynostosis) and, in adults, insertion of load-sharing intramedullary rods to treat fractures. Expert dental care is also crucial to minimize tooth loss and prevent consequent malnutrition in youths.

Mineralization Inhibitors

DRUGS. *Etidronate.* Disturbances in mineralization may be seen in patients consuming etidronate daily at doses >5 mg per kilogram body weight. The etidronate is deposited at the bone surface and inhibits osteoblast function, as well as directly inhibits calcium-phosphate crystallization.

Fluoride. Although multiple studies document that fluoride stimulates new bone formation, administering the drug in high doses without adequate calcium supplementation results in poorly mineralized bone, consistent with osteomalacia. The mechanism(s) by which fluoride alters osteoblast function and/or directly inhibits mineralization remains unknown.

Aluminum. Excess aluminum accumulation in bone inhibits mineralization and is a potential mechanism for the osteomalacia observed in patients with chronic renal failure, as discussed above. In addition, accumulation of aluminum in bone likely underlies the osteomalacia observed in patients treated with total parenteral nutrition. In such cases aluminum contamination of casein hydrolysate, as well as albumin, phosphate, and calcium solutions, provides the major source of the mineral. Changing total parenteral nutrition solutions from those with casein hydrolysate to those with purified amino acids has markedly reduced the incidence of clinically evident bone disease.

Brenner RJ, Spring DB, Sebastian A, et al.: Incidence of radiographically evident bone disease, nephrocalcinosis, and nephrolithiasis in various types of renal tubular acidosis. N Engl J Med 307:217, 1982. *Discussion of the relationship between rickets and metabolic acidosis in youths.*

Cai Q, Hodgson SF, Kao PC, et al.: Inhibition of renal phosphate transport by a tumor product in a patient with oncogenic osteomalacia. N Engl J Med 330:1645, 1994. *Presentation of evidence that tumor-induced osteomalacia is caused by ectopic secretion of a heat-labile factor with a mass between 8000 and 25,000 which inhibits renal tubular reabsorption of phosphate.*

Econs MJ, Drezner MK: Bone disease resulting from inherited disorders of renal tubule transport and vitamin D metabolism. *In* Coe FL, Favus MJ: Disorders of bone and mineral metabolism. New York, Raven Press, 1992, p 935. *Extensive review of the classic vitamin D–resistant rachitic and osteomalacic disorders. The subjects discussed include clinical features, differential diagnosis, genetics, and therapy.*

Friedman NJ, Drezner MK: Osteomalacia, genetic. *In* Bardin CW: Current therapy in endocrinology and metabolism. 4th ed. Philadelphia, B.C. Decker, Inc. 1991, p 421. *Review of the concepts underlying and the specific details of treatment for hypophosphatemic rickets in all its varieties of clinical presentation.*

Tieder M, Arie R, Modai D, et al.: Elevated serum 1,25-dihydroxyvitamin D concentrations in siblings with primary Fanconi's syndrome. N Engl J Med 319:845, 1988. *First report and discussion of Fanconi's syndrome type 2.*

214 THE PARATHYROID GLANDS, HYPERCALCEMIA, AND HYPOCALCEMIA

Allen M. Spiegel

THE PARATHYROID GLANDS

EMBRYOLOGY AND ANATOMY. Normally, there are four parathyroids, averaging 120 mg in total weight, but as many as 5% of normal individuals may have more than four glands. The superior parathyroids are derived from the fourth (more caudal) branchial pouches and remain almost stationary during embryologic development. Their typical final location is near the upper poles of the thyroid. Aberrant locations include the tracheoesophageal groove and the retroesophageal space. The inferior parathyroids develop (in association with the thymus) from the third branchial pouches. During normal development, they migrate caudally, assuming a final position near the lower poles of the thyroid. The inferior parathyroids may fail to descend, remaining near the angle of the jaw or, at the other extreme, may descend into the anterior mediastinum in association with the thymus.

SYNTHESIS AND SECRETION OF PARATHYROID HORMONE. Parathyroid hormone (PTH), together with vitamin D (see Ch. 212), is the principal regulator of ionized calcium in extracellular fluid. PTH is synthesized in the parathyroid glands as "pre-proparathyroid hormone," a precursor composed of 115 amino acids. A hydrophobic "leader" peptide of 25 amino acids is first cleaved from the amino-terminus to yield the prohormone, followed by cleavage of a basic, amino-terminal hexapeptide to yield the mature 84-amino-acid hormone. The latter is the principal secreted form of the hormone. There is no evidence for secretion of either the preprohormone or the prohormone. The prohormone possesses <0.2% of the biologic activity of the native 84-amino-acid hormone. The full biologic activity of the intact hormone resides within the amino-terminal 1–34 fragment, whereas fragments from the midregion and carboxy-terminal regions lack biologic activity (Fig. 214–1).

Secretion of PTH is regulated primarily by the concentration of ionized calcium in the extracellular fluid. Normally, PTH secretion is regulated at a "setpoint" that maintains serum ionized calcium within a relatively narrow range. Deviations below the setpoint stimulate, and deviations above the setpoint inhibit, hormone secretion. Effects of calcium on hormone secretion occur acutely (within minutes); low calcium levels have a slower stimulatory action on hormone synthesis. At high calcium concentrations, there is evidence for intracellular degradation of synthesized hormone and possible release of biologically inactive fragments. High magnesium ion concentrations in extracellular fluid, like high calcium concentrations, inhibit PTH secretion, but hypomagnesemia, unlike hypocalcemia, may inhibit hormone secretion and action. The active metabolite of vitamin D, 1,25(OH)$_2$D (dihydroxycholecalciferol), suppresses both secretion and synthesis of PTH. Reduction in 1,25(OH)$_2$D is a major factor contributing to increased PTH secretion in renal failure.

FORMS OF PARATHYROID HORMONE IN PLASMA. PTH circulates in plasma as the intact hormone secreted from the gland and as fragments derived either from glandular secretion (particularly in hypercalcemic states) or from peripheral metabolism of the intact hormone. Most, if not all, of these fragments lack biologic activity but may, depending on antibody specificity, contribute to immunoreactivity in plasma (Fig. 214–1).

PARATHYROID HORMONE ACTION. PTH acts directly on kidney and bone, and indirectly on the gut, to maintain the normal concentration of serum ionized calcium (see Ch. 211 for a complete discussion of mineral homeostasis). In the kidney, PTH (1) enhances reabsorption of calcium, and also magnesium, from the glomerular filtrate; (2) increases excretion of phosphate and of bicarbonate; (3) activates the enzyme (1α-hydroxylase) that forms the active metabolite, 1,25(OH)$_2$D, of vitamin D. In bone, PTH causes the release of calcium and phosphate into the extracellular fluid. The hormone acts directly on osteoblasts, which secondarily affect osteoclast activity. The hypercalcemic action on bone and the anticalciuric action on kidney combine to raise the serum calcium level. The phosphatemic action on bone tends to blunt the hypercalcemic effect of the hormone owing to formation of calcium phosphate complexes, but the phosphaturic action counteracts the tendency to hyperphosphatemia. Stimulation of 1,25(OH)$_2$D formation promotes enhanced intestinal absorption of calcium, which also serves to maintain a normal serum calcium level (see Ch. 212). The clinical consequences of PTH excess (or in the opposite direction, hormone deficiency) follow directly from the actions of the hormone: (1) hypercalcemia, (2) a tendency to hypophosphatemia, (3) a tendency to reduced serum bicarbonate levels and hyperchloremia, (4) increased serum levels of 1,25(OH)$_2$D, and (5) relative reduction in urinary calcium excretion and increase in urinary phosphate excretion for a given filtered load.

MECHANISM OF PARATHYROID HORMONE ACTION. The first step in PTH action is binding to specific plasma membrane–bound receptors on target cells in bone and kidney. Such receptors are coupled to guanosine triphosphate (GTP)–binding proteins—in particular, the Gs protein that links receptors to stimulation of adenylyl cyclase (for a more general description of the mechanism of polypeptide hormone action, see Ch. 199). Adenylyl cyclase catalyzes the formation of the "second messenger," cyclic adenosine monophosphate (cAMP), which mediates hormone action by stimulating the phosphorylation of critical intracellular proteins. A diagnostically useful peculiarity of PTH action on proximal renal tubular cells is that not only are cAMP levels increased intracellularly but, because of overflow into the extracellular fluid, urinary cAMP excretion is also increased. "Second messengers" other than cAMP may also mediate certain actions of PTH.

ASSAY OF PARATHYROID HORMONE IN PLASMA. Normally, the concentration of biologically active PTH circulating in

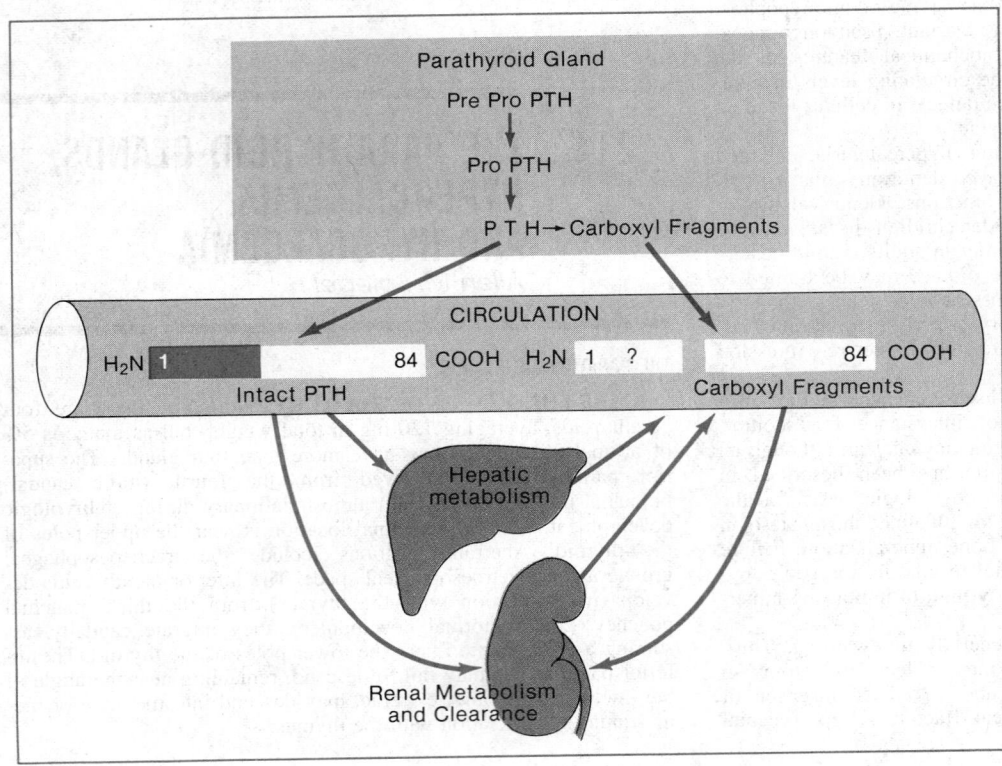

FIGURE 214–1. Secretion, metabolism, and clearance of PTH. *Top,* PTH is synthesized as a preprohormone and undergoes successive cleavages within the parathyroid to the mature (1–84), major secreted form of the hormone. Under certain conditions (e.g., hypercalcemia), some of the hormone is cleaved intracellularly into biologically inactive, carboxy-terminal fragments, which are also secreted. *Middle,* The major circulating forms of the hormone are the intact 1–84 species (the shaded region corresponds to the amino-terminal 1–34 portion possessing full biologic activity) and biologically inactive carboxy-terminal fragments. The presence of amino-terminal fragments in the circulation is unclear (indicated by "?"). *Bottom,* Peripheral metabolism of the hormone occurs in liver and kidney. The kidney also clears intact hormone and carboxy-terminal fragments from the circulation. (From Endres DE, Villanueva R, Sharp CF Jr, et al.: Measurement of parathyroid hormone. Endocrinol Metab Clin North Am 18:611, 1989.)

Parathyroid Gland

Pre Pro PTH

Pro PTH

P T H → Carboxyl Fragments

CIRCULATION

H$_2$N 1   84 COOH   H$_2$N 1 ?   84 COOH

Intact PTH   Carboxyl Fragments

Hepatic metabolism

Renal Metabolism and Clearance

plasma is quite low (<50 pg per milliliter). Bioassays sensitive enough to detect such low levels include a renal cytochemical assay and several assays based on stimulating cAMP formation in bone or kidney cells. Unfortunately, such assays are too cumbersome for routine clinical use. Total urinary cAMP excretion (normalized to creatinine clearance by simultaneously measuring serum and urinary creatinine) is an easily measured and sensitive index of circulating PTH bioactivity. It is elevated in primary hyperparathyroidism, is low in hypoparathyroidism, and falls within 1 hour of successful parathyroidectomy in patients with hyperparathyroidism. Increased urinary cAMP excretion, however, is not absolutely specific for PTH hypersecretion; parathyroid hormone-related peptide, secreted by many malignancies, similarly increases urinary cAMP excretion, and this must be taken into account when interpreting urinary cAMP measurements in subjects with hypercalcemia (see Hypercalcemia Associated with Malignancy, below).

Radioimmunoassays are sufficiently sensitive and practical for routinely measuring circulating PTH. Interpretation of assay results requires an understanding of what a particular antiserum is measuring. Immunoreactivity need not correlate with biologic activity. Indeed, the bulk of circulating PTH consists of biologically inactive mid-region and carboxy-terminal fragments. Because such fragments are cleared by the kidney, renal impairment causes them to accumulate at even higher concentrations (Fig. 214–1). Antisera with predominant specificity for mid-region and carboxy-terminal regions, therefore, measure predominantly biologically inactive hormone fragments. Such assays are reasonably useful for discriminating normal from hyperparathyroid subjects, but their utility is much more limited in subjects with renal failure. Even with normal renal function, such assays may show considerable overlap between patients with parathyroid-mediated hypercalcemia and those with non-parathyroid-mediated hypercalcemia. In part, this may reflect the parathyroid gland's release of inactive hormone fragments in non-PTH-mediated hypercalcemic states.

Most of these problems have been circumvented by the development of highly sensitive "two-site" immunoradiometric assays. Such assays employ two distinct antibodies, one against the amino-terminal region and one against the carboxy-terminal region. Effectively, only intact, biologically active hormone is measured. Such assays allow measurement of circulating hormone in most normal individuals, are scarcely affected by renal impairment, and allow excellent discrimination between PTH-mediated and non–PTH-mediated causes of hypercalcemia (Fig. 214–2).

Aurbach GD, Marx SJ, Spiegel AM: Parathyroid hormone, calcitonin, and the calciferols. *In* Wilson JD, Foster DW (eds.): Williams Textbook of Endocrinology. 8th ed. Philadelphia, WB Saunders, 1992, p 1406. *Detailed description of basic aspects of PTH synthesis, secretion, action, and assay.*

Endres DB, Villanueva R, Sharp CF Jr, et al.: Measurement of parathyroid hormone. Endocrinol Metab Clin North Am 18:611, 1989. *Complete discussion of methods for PTH assay, including comparison of two-site versus mid-region immunoassays.*

Juppner H, Abou-Samra A, Freeman M, et al.: A G protein–linked receptor for parathyroid hormone and parathyroid hormone–related peptide. Science 254:1024, 1991. *Describes cloning of receptor that helps define mechanism of action of parathyroid hormone.*

HYPERCALCEMIA

DEFINITION. Hypercalcemia is defined as an abnormal elevation in serum ionized calcium concentration.* Because total, rather than ionized, calcium is generally measured, one must be aware of factors that influence the fraction of total serum calcium that is ionized. Of these, serum albumin concentration is of greatest clinical relevance because albumin is the chief circulating calcium-binding protein. "Normal" total serum calcium concentration associated with a significant reduction in serum albumin (e.g., in patients with malignancy) may actually represent abnormally elevated levels of serum ionized calcium. Acid-base status also influences the proportion of total serum calcium that is protein bound (alkalosis decreases the ionized calcium concentration, and acidosis increases it).

ETIOLOGY. Many different diseases are potential causes of hypercalcemia. Of these, the most common are primary hyperparathyroidism (particularly in asymptomatic individuals whose hypercalcemia is detected by routine serum chemistry measurement) and malignancy (particularly in hospitalized individuals). These disorders, as well as some of the rarer causes of hypercalcemia, are considered in separate sections below.

PATHOGENESIS. Hypercalcemia results from excessive calcium influx into the extracellular fluid from bone and decreased efflux from the kidneys into the urine. Calcium mobilization from bone is mediated by activators of bone resorption. These activators include systemic factors (e.g., PTH, 1,25(OH)₂D) and locally acting factors, such as various lymphokines. Reduced renal calcium excretion may lead to hypercalcemia, particularly in states of increased

---

* See Ch. 211 and Part XXVIII for calcium and phosphorus reference range values in serum and urine.

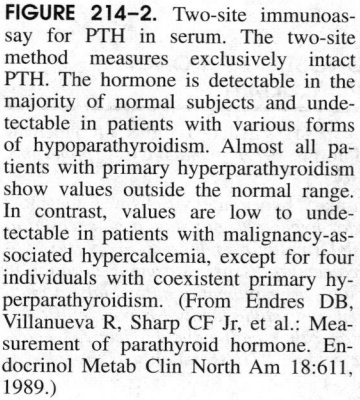

FIGURE 214–2. Two-site immunoassay for PTH in serum. The two-site method measures exclusively intact PTH. The hormone is detectable in the majority of normal subjects and undetectable in patients with various forms of hypoparathyroidism. Almost all patients with primary hyperparathyroidism show values outside the normal range. In contrast, values are low to undetectable in patients with malignancy-associated hypercalcemia, except for four individuals with coexistent primary hyperparathyroidism. (From Endres DB, Villanueva R, Sharp CF Jr, et al.: Measurement of parathyroid hormone. Endocrinol Metab Clin North Am 18:611, 1989.)

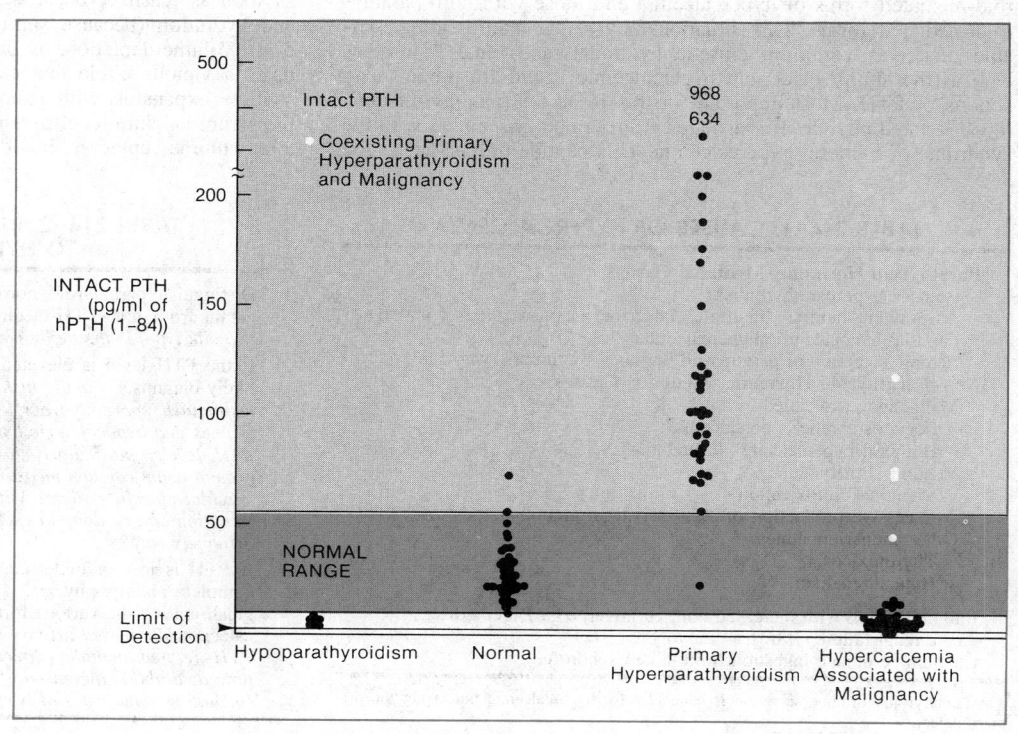

bone turnover. Renal impairment, volume depletion, and anticalciuretic agents, such as thiazide diuretics and PTH, are clinically relevant factors that can reduce renal calcium excretion and provoke hypercalcemia.

CLINICAL MANIFESTATIONS. Many manifestations are not specific to the underlying cause (specific disease manifestations are discussed under individual disease headings). Extreme hypercalcemia leads to coma and death. Neurologic manifestations in less severe cases may include confusion, lethargy, weakness, and hyporeflexia. Hypercalcemia may be detected by shortening of the QT interval on the electrocardiogram. Arrhythmias are rare, but bradycardia and first-degree heart block have been reported. Acute hypercalcemia may be associated with significant hypertension. Gastrointestinal manifestations include constipation and anorexia; in severe cases, there may be nausea and vomiting. Acute pancreatitis has been reported in association with hypercalcemia of various causes. Hypercalcemia interferes with antidiuretic hormone action, thereby leading to polyuria and polydipsia. Reversible reduction in renal function associated with significant hypercalcemia is followed by more permanent damage if hypercalcemia persists. Particularly if serum phosphorus is also increased, hypercalcemia can lead to nephrocalcinosis and interstitial nephritis. Hypercalciuria and nephrolithiasis may also occur. Deposition of calcium in other soft tissues, including skin and cornea, is most likely to occur in patients with associated hyperphosphatemia.

DIFFERENTIAL DIAGNOSIS. Potential causes of hypercalcemia are listed in Table 214–1. These may be divided into PTH-mediated (primary hyperparathyroidism) and non–PTH-mediated diseases (all others). Although ectopic secretion of PTH by tumors was long considered a potential cause of PTH-mediated hypercalcemia, there is now general agreement that ectopic secretion of authentic PTH (as opposed to PTH–related peptides; see below) by tumors is extremely rare. The first step in the differential diagnosis of hypercalcemia is to establish whether or not PTH hypersecretion is present because subsequent diagnostic maneuvers and definitive therapy critically depend on this distinction.

Readily measured blood and urine chemistries may offer some clues to diagnosis. In theory, PTH hypersecretion should be reflected by hypophosphatemia, hyperchloremia, hypobicarbonatemia, increased urinary phosphate excretion, and urinary calcium excretion that is relatively low for the filtered load. PTH secretion suppressed by hypercalcemia of non-parathyroid etiology should, in theory, reverse these parameters. In practice, there is considerable overlap in each of these parameters between patients with parathyroid-mediated forms of hypercalcemia and those with non–parathyroid-mediated forms. This situation may reflect confounding variables, such as vomiting, diuretic treatment, and renal failure, as well as the ability of certain hypercalcemic agents to mimic many actions of PTH. Most important in this respect is parathyroid hormone–related peptide, first isolated from tumors associated with the syndrome of humoral hypercalcemia. This peptide mimics all of the

known actions of PTH on kidney and bone, including increasing urinary cAMP excretion and stimulating renal formation of $1,25(OH)_2D$. Decreased urinary cAMP excretion (with normal renal function) strongly suggests non–PTH-mediated hypercalcemia, but increased urinary cAMP excretion is compatible with both primary hyperparathyroidism and tumor secretion of parathyroid hormone–related peptide. Serum $1,25(OH)_2D$ concentration also does not allow definitive diagnosis. It may be elevated in primary hyperparathyroidism and vitamin D–related causes of hypercalcemia and may be reduced in other non–parathyroid-mediated causes of hypercalcemia. For reasons that are not entirely clear, the serum $1,25(OH)_2D$ level is often low in patients with malignancies secreting parathyroid hormone–related peptide, despite the ability of the peptide to stimulate $1,25(OH)_2D$ formation.

Definitive distinction between parathyroid- and non–parathyroid-mediated causes of hypercalcemia relies primarily on PTH immunoassay. As discussed earlier, this distinction is best made with the two-site type of assays that measure intact PTH and are un-affected by renal function (Fig. 214–2). An elevated PTH level secures the diagnosis of primary hyperparathyroidism. In selected cases with coexistent malignancy, the unlikely possibility of ectopic PTH secretion may be excluded by selective venous sam-pling and assay of PTH, but generally this testing is unnecessary. Hormone levels in the normal range suggest the possibility of familial hypocalciuric hypercalcemia. This entity is discussed further in the section on hyperparathyroidism. Low to undetectable values for PTH place the patient in the non–parathyroid-mediated category. Additional testing is necessary to establish a specific diagnosis within this group. Immunoassays for parathyroid hormone–related peptide have been developed, and these may allow the diagnosis of hypercalcemia caused by a tumor secreting this agent. Complete clinical evaluation, including history (e.g., vitamin ingestion, chronicity of symptoms), physical examination (masses, lymphadenopathy), radiologic studies, and other blood tests (e.g., thyroid and adrenal function), may point to a diagnosis. The diagnostic approach to hypercalcemia is summarized in Table 214–2.

TREATMENT. The definitive treatment of hypercalcemia depends on the specific diagnosis and treatment of the underlying disease, e.g., parathyroidectomy for primary hyperparathyroidism, chemotherapy for a malignancy. The initial treatment of hypercalcemia can be instituted (and in acute hypercalcemic crisis, often *must* be instituted) without a specific diagnosis, but cumulative toxicity and loss of efficacy preclude long-term nonspecific treatment. Measures aimed at reducing the serum calcium level act by increasing urinary calcium excretion and by decreasing bone resorption. General measures applicable to every patient include mobilization as soon as feasible (because immobility increases bone resorption) and hydration (because significant hypercalcemia causes dehydration). Volume depletion, by limiting renal calcium excretion, perpetuates a vicious circle that can lead to acute hypercalcemic crisis. Volume expansion with isotonic saline often significantly reduces the serum calcium level by enhancing renal calcium excretion. Only after volume repletion should diuretics be used to enhance sodium

---

TABLE 214–1. CAUSES OF HYPERCALCEMIA

Parathyroid Hormone–Mediated Causes
  Primary hyperparathyroidism
    Sporadic, familial (multiple endocrine neoplasia types I and II)
  Familial hypocalciuric hypercalcemia*
  Ectopic secretion of parathyroid hormone by tumors (very rare)
Non–Parathyroid Hormone–Mediated Causes
  Malignancy associated
    Local osteolytic hypercalcemia
    Humoral hypercalcemia of malignancy
  Vitamin D mediated
    Vitamin D intoxication
    Excessive production of $1,25(OH)_2D$ in granulomatous disorders
  Other endocrinopathies
    Thyrotoxicosis
    Hypoadrenalism

  Immobilization with increased bone turnover, e.g., Paget's disease
  Acute renal failure with rhabdomyolysis
  Calcium carbonate ingestion (milk-alkali syndrome)

* Parathyroid hormone secretion is necessary for hypercalcemia but is not the primary defect.

TABLE 214–2. DIAGNOSTIC APPROACH TO HYPERCALCEMIA

1. Distinguish parathyroid hormone (PTH)–mediated forms of hypercalcemia from non–PTH-mediated forms: *PTH immunoassay (preferably two-site type) is the definitive test.*

2. If the PTH level is elevated, primary hyperparathyroidism is the most likely diagnosis: *Family history for hypercalcemia should be checked to distinguish sporadic from familial (multiple endocrine neoplasia syndromes and hypocalciuric hypercalcemia) disease. Marginal elevation in PTH levels, particularly in young, asymptomatic individuals, should prompt urine calcium measurement to exclude familial hypocalciuric hypercalcemia. In patients with coexisting malignancy, selective venous sampling can be done to exclude ectopic PTH secretion, but the latter is extremely rare.*

3. If PTH is low or undetectable, further laboratory tests (in addition to complete history, physical, and radiologic studies) are needed to distinguish among the various forms of non–PTH-mediated forms of hypercalcemia: *Increased urinary cAMP excretion suggests tumor secretion of PTH–related peptide (direct radioimmunoassays for this peptide are now available). Increased $1,25(OH)_2D$ suggests granulomatous disease (including some types of lymphoma).*

and thereby calcium excretion. With a vigorous saline diuresis, calcium excretion in the range of 1 to 2 grams per day can be achieved as a temporary measure to reduce the serum calcium level. In patients with renal failure, dialysis can be employed almost as effectively to remove calcium from extracellular fluid. Careful monitoring of cardiac function and serum electrolytes is necessary with both saline diuresis and dialysis treatment.

Measures aimed at reducing bone resorption by inhibiting osteoclast function are most effective in treating hypercalcemia, irrespective of the specific factor causing increased bone resorption. Available agents include calcitonin, bisphosphonates (diphosphonates), plicamycin (mithramycin), and gallium nitrate. Calcitonin has low toxicity and acts most rapidly, but even in doses up to 32 MRC units per kilogram per day by intravenous infusion, lowering of serum calcium is generally limited and transient. Bisphosphonates must be given parenterally, and their effect is both significant and often prolonged (days). Initially, only etidronate (7.5 mg per kilogram per day intravenously) was available, but this is being replaced by pamidronate (dose 30 to 90 mg intravenously over 24 hours), which is more potent and effective. Plicamycin (25 μg per kilogram intravenously) quite effectively lowers serum calcium, but it has cumulative toxicity in liver, kidney, and platelets and can no longer be justified as initial therapy. Gallium nitrate is an effective calcium-lowering agent and has recently been approved by the FDA, but it has potential nephrotoxicity and its place in treating hypercalcemia is not yet clear. Intravenous phosphate poses a serious danger of metastatic calcification in the hypercalcemic patient and should probably no longer be used, given availability of other safer and effective agents. Oral phosphate is safer and useful in patients with significant hypercalcemia who are awaiting definitive treatment and in whom hypercalcemic crisis should be prevented. Dosages in the range of 2 grams of elemental phosphorus (10 grams of phosphate salts) per day in divided doses can be given. Serum phosphate and renal function should be carefully monitored.

Glucocorticoids are highly effective in treating hypercalcemia caused by vitamin D–related mechanisms (vitamin D intoxication, overproduction of 1,25(OH)$_2$D in granulomatous disorders) and by certain malignancies (cytokine release associated with myeloma) but are ineffective in most other forms of hypercalcemia, including hyperparathyroidism and most malignancies. Forty to 100 mg per day of prednisone or the equivalent is the usual dose range.

PRIMARY HYPERPARATHYROIDISM

DEFINITION. Primary hyperparathyroidism is a disorder in which hypercalcemia is due to hypersecretion of PTH.

ETIOLOGY. In most cases (about 85%), hyperparathyroidism is caused by sporadic, solitary adenomas. Hyperplasia of all four glands occurs in about 10% of cases, and these are most often familial, in the context of three distinct autosomal dominant inherited diseases: multiple endocrine neoplasia (MEN) types I and II and familial hypocalciuric hypercalcemia. Carcinoma occurs rarely (<5% of cases). The gene for MEN type I has been linked to chromosome 11q13. Enlarged glands in this disease are monoclonal tumors, with a high percentage showing loss of alleles at 11q13. This suggests that the MEN type I gene may be a "tumor suppressor" whose loss leads to tumorigenesis. A significant percentage of sporadic parathyroid tumors also show allele loss at this locus, suggesting a similar pathogenesis. The gene for MEN type II has been identified as the *RET* proto-oncogene on chromosome 10q11. This facilitates genetic diagnosis and studies of pathogenesis. Very rarely, a rearrangement involving the PTH gene on the short arm of chromosome 11 and a cell cycle control gene termed cyclin D or PRAD 1 on the long arm of chromosome 11 appears to cause parathyroid adenoma formation. Epidemiologic evidence suggests that a history of neck irradiation predisposes to parathyroid tumor formation. Specific molecular defects have not been identified. Finally, longstanding secondary hyperparathyroidism (e.g., in response to renal failure) may evolve into autonomous hypersecretion, so-called tertiary hyperparathyroidism. Loss of tumor suppressor gene(s) on 11q13 may be involved in some of these cases.

INCIDENCE. The incidence of hyperparathyroidism has increased substantially, largely as a result of routine blood calcium measurement. Age-adjusted incidence rates are between 25 and 50 per 100,000, based on recent surveys. A prevalence between 0.1 and 0.5% has been estimated, with females affected about twice as commonly as males. The incidence rises sharply after age 40.

PATHOLOGY. Microscopic distinction between adenoma and hyperplasia is difficult, if not impossible. The distinction between single-gland and multigland disease relies on gross surgical identification of more than one enlarged gland. In MEN types I and II, there is always multigland involvement, although asymmetric gland enlargement is often present. The chief cell generally predominates in parathyroid tumors; oxyphil cell tumors are much rarer.

PATHOPHYSIOLOGY. The primary disturbance is inappropriate secretion of PTH for the level of serum calcium. Studies *in vitro* with isolated parathyroid cells show that most adenomas either fail to suppress secretion at high calcium levels or show an altered setpoint, i.e., a higher calcium level is required to suppress secretion than for normal cells. Cells from hyperplastic glands may show a normal calcium setpoint for secretion. Hypersecretion of PTH in such cases may be due to a primary defect causing cellular proliferation and to an inability to suppress hormone secretion completely because of increased cell mass.

Slight increases in PTH secretion act on bone to increase turnover and may reduce cortical rather than trabecular bone density. At very high levels, PTH causes radiographically detectable subperiosteal bone resorption and, eventually, marrow fibrosis and cystic, reparative bone lesions termed "brown tumors." This is the classic form of the disease called "osteitis fibrosa cystica." PTH increases renal calcium reabsorption, but nonetheless, at high filtered loads of calcium, hypercalciuria develops. Enhanced 1,25(OH)$_2$D formation by the kidneys is prominent in some patients and is associated with increased intestinal calcium absorption. Such patients may be at particular risk for renal stones.

CLINICAL MANIFESTATIONS. Most patients either are asymptomatic at presentation (discovered through incidental blood calcium measurement) or have vague, nonspecific symptoms, such as fatigue, weakness, and mental disturbance. Patients with significant hypercalcemia show many of the signs and symptoms of hypercalcemia discussed above. Nephrolithiasis, with or without renal colic, is not specifically associated with hyperparathyroidism but is most commonly seen in this setting. Subperiosteal bone resorption is rarely seen, and osteitis fibrosa cystica even less commonly. Neuromuscular abnormalities, particularly proximal muscle weakness affecting the lower limbs, may be prominent. Joint manifestations include chondrocalcinosis that may lead to pseudogout. It has been claimed that hypertension, peptic ulcer disease, and osteoporosis are manifestations of hyperparathyroidism, but these are all common, and there is no firm evidence for a causal relationship. No specific physical findings are present in hyperparathyroidism. A neck mass, if present, most commonly represents a coincidental thyroid nodule, less commonly a benign or malignant parathyroid tumor. "Band keratopathy," calcification at "3 and 9 o'clock" of the cornea, is best seen by slit-lamp examination and occurs most often when hypercalcemia is accompanied by hyperphosphatemia—thus less commonly in hyperparathyroidism than in other hypercalcemic disorders. Radiologic findings include subperiosteal resorption, which, when present, is best seen at the radial sides of the phalanges, distal phalangeal tufts, and distal clavicles. Lucent bone lesions, representing brown tumors, are seen in rare, severely affected patients. Soft tissue calcification may be evident in the joints, kidneys, and lungs. The calcification is best appreciated on bone scans.

DIAGNOSIS. The differential diagnosis of hypercalcemia is discussed above. PTH immunoassay, preferably one of the newer two-site assays, is the key to diagnosis. In distinguishing between hyperparathyroid and normal states (e.g., in patients presenting with nephrolithiasis), repeated careful serum calcium and PTH (including the mid-region type of assay) measurements are most useful. Hypercalcemic subjects taking lithium or thiazides should be retested for hyperparathyroidism after discontinuing the drug (this may not be feasible in some patients on lithium), because both drugs may alter serum calcium and PTH secretion. In relatively young, asymptomatic individuals, or if the serum PTH level is marginally elevated, hypercalcemia may be due to familial hypocalciuric hypercalcemia rather than hyperparathyroidism (see discussion below under Familial Hypocalciuric Hypercalcemia).

PROGNOSIS AND TREATMENT. Surgical parathyroidectomy is the only definitive treatment for hyperparathyroidism. Oral phosphate treatment can lower the serum calcium level, but the long-term safety and efficacy of this approach are unclear. In mildly affected, older women, estrogen treatment has been advocated, particularly to blunt bone resorption, but, again, long-term efficacy is unknown. Thus, the only alternative to surgery at present is conservative medical follow-up. Most experts recommend surgery for all patients with symptomatic disease and even for asymptomatic patients meeting other, somewhat arbitrary, criteria, such as age below 40 or a serum calcium level >11.5 mg per deciliter. The appropriate management of patients not fitting any of these criteria is controversial; some advocate surgery for all, and others conservative follow-up. The long-term course of untreated hyperparathyroidism is unknown. Controlled studies comparing surgery versus medical follow-up have not been performed. Small series of patients followed conservatively for several years suggest that mild biochemical disease rarely progresses to severe symptomatic disease, but it is difficult to exclude subtle abnormalities, such as reduced bone density. Because definitive treatment recommendations are not possible, therapy must be individualized. The author personally follows a policy of recommending surgery for all but older patients with only mild biochemical disease.

If the decision is to perform surgery, a highly experienced parathyroid surgeon must be found. A success rate as high as 95% can be expected for initial neck exploration by a skilled surgeon. The success rate is substantially lower with inexperienced surgeons. Preoperative localization is not needed by the skilled surgeon performing initial exploration. Neither localization studies nor neck exploration itself should serve as *diagnostic* maneuvers. Only after the diagnosis has been established biochemically (by PTH assay) should one recommend surgery. In patients undergoing repeat neck exploration for recurrent or persistent disease, localization studies are extremely helpful. Noninvasive studies include ultrasonography, technetium-99m-sestamibi scanning, computed tomography (CT), and magnetic resonance imaging. Invasive techniques include fine-needle aspiration of imaged lesions for PTH assay, selective arteriography, and selective venous catheterization for hormone assay. The latter techniques are best performed by radiologists with specialized experience.

After successful surgery, hypocalcemia is generally mild and transient and rarely requires treatment. In the rare case of subjects with extensive bone disease, severe, prolonged hypocalcemia secondary to "bone hunger" occurs. Persistent relative hypophosphatemia suggests that bone hunger, rather than hypoparathyroidism, is the cause of hypocalcemia in this setting. Acute treatment with calcium infusions and long-term treatment with vitamin D and oral calcium may be needed. Eventually, treatment can be discontinued if normal parathyroid tissue remains. In patients without residual normal parathyroid tissue, lifelong vitamin D therapy is necessary. Autotransplantation of parathyroid tissue in the forearm is an experimental alternative in such cases. Successful surgery generally halts formation of renal stones in patients with nephrolithiasis and allows skeletal remineralization in patients with bone disease. There is no definitive evidence that surgery corrects hypertension or other nonspecific manifestations of hyperparathyroidism.

FAMILIAL HYPOCALCIURIC HYPERCALCEMIA

DEFINITION. This is an autosomal dominant genetic disease with essentially complete penetrance that causes hypercalcemia and relatively low urinary calcium excretion for the filtered load.

ETIOLOGY. The disease is caused by mutations in a gene on the long arm of chromosome 3 encoding a calcium-sensing receptor. In some families, the disease may be caused by a gene localized to a different chromosome.

INCIDENCE. The disorder is relatively rare, but it is over-represented among patients presenting with unsuccessful neck exploration because of the difficulty in achieving normocalcemia by surgery.

PATHOPHYSIOLOGY. The primary disturbance appears to be in divalent cation transport and/or "sensing" in at least the kidneys and parathyroids. The kidneys show an exaggerated reabsorption of filtered calcium (and magnesium) that leads to hypercalcemia. The parathyroids, however, fail to suppress fully hormone secretion despite hypercalcemia. The process is PTH-dependent because totally parathyroidectomized subjects become hypocalcemic, but even small amounts of parathyroid tissue are sufficient to maintain hypercalcemia. Parathyroid gland mass is generally only mildly increased.

CLINICAL MANIFESTATIONS. The disease leads to few, if any, clinical manifestations—hence its other name, "familial benign hypercalcemia." Nephrolithiasis and bone disease are, in general, not seen. Pancreatitis has been reported, but the specificity of this association is unclear. Hypercalcemia is present at birth. In some neonates, a clinically severe form of the disease is present. This severe form may be due to inheritance of a double dose of the abnormal gene. Otherwise, the main morbidity is that resulting from unsuccessful neck exploration that has failed to distinguish this disorder from conventional hyperparathyroidism. There is no evidence of associated endocrinopathies, as in the MEN syndromes.

DIAGNOSIS. A high index of suspicion is needed to recognize this disease. Hypercalcemia associated with relatively young age, with only slight elevation in the serum PTH level, or with a family history of unsuccessful neck exploration should trigger further evaluation. Hypermagnesemia is suggestive; urinary calcium-creatinine ratios <0.01:1 strongly support the diagnosis. Screening first-degree relatives for hypercalcemia may also be helpful. For those families in which the disease gene is localized to chromosome 3q, specific genetic diagnosis is possible by screening for mutations in the calcium-sensing receptor gene. Distinct mutations in this gene have already been identified in several kindreds.

PROGNOSIS AND TREATMENT. Because the disease is compatible with normal life expectancy and is associated with little, if any, morbidity, neck exploration appears to be contraindicated. Successful surgical treatment, moreover, is quite difficult, with permanent hypoparathyroidism or, more commonly, recurrent hypercalcemia, the usual result.

HYPERCALCEMIA ASSOCIATED WITH MALIGNANCY

ETIOLOGY AND PATHOGENESIS. Malignancies can cause hypercalcemia through two non–mutually exclusive mechanisms. First, local osteolytic hypercalcemia is caused by tumor metastatic to bone. Tumor cells may release bone-resorbing factors or so-called osteoclast-activating factors, which indirectly lead to bone resorption. Cytokines such as lymphotoxin and interleukin-1 are potent osteoclast-activating factors. Second, humoral hypercalcemia of malignancy is caused by tumor-secreting factors into the circulation that act systemically to increase bone resorption. Such factors may show other PTH-like actions, including increasing urinary cAMP and phosphate excretion and decreasing renal calcium excretion. This condition leads to a syndrome with biochemical features closely resembling those of primary hyperparathyroidism. One such factor commonly associated with many tumors has recently been identified as a polypeptide roughly twice as large as PTH and homologous in amino acid sequence to the biologically active amino-terminus of PTH. This so-called parathyroid hormone–related peptide may also be secreted by tumors metastatic to bone, so that humoral and local osteolytic mechanisms may combine to cause hypercalcemia. Some tumors cause hypercalcemia through excessive synthesis of $1,25(OH)_2D$, in a manner analogous to that seen in sarcoidosis (see below). A role for additional, as yet unidentified, bone-resorbing agents secreted by tumors has not been excluded.

INCIDENCE. Malignancy-associated hypercalcemia occurs most commonly in patients with bone metastases. Breast carcinoma is one of the most frequent causes. Most subjects with bone metastases are not hypercalcemic because of adequate renal compensatory mechanisms. Slight renal impairment may then provoke hypercalcemia. Treatment of women with breast cancer metastatic to bone with tamoxifen has been associated with acute sharp increases in the serum calcium level. Certain hematogenous neoplasms, such as myeloma and human lymphotropic virus type I–associated leukemia/lymphoma, are frequently associated with hypercalcemia. Humoral hypercalcemia of malignancy is much rarer. It is seen most frequently with squamous carcinomas, but biochemical evidence indicates that almost any tumor type, including breast carcinoma, can produce PTH-related peptide.

CLINICAL MANIFESTATIONS. Malignancy-associated hypercalcemia often develops acutely, may be quite severe (hypercalcemic crisis), and is frequently a grave prognostic sign. In most cases, particularly of the local osteolytic hypercalcemia variety, the underlying neoplasm is clinically evident. An otherwise occult neoplasm may occasionally manifest with humoral hypercalcemia of malignancy. Accurate and rapid diagnosis is critical in such cases because successful tumor removal may be feasible.

DIAGNOSIS. As discussed earlier, PTH radioimmunoassay is the crucial test for excluding coexistent primary hyperparathyroidism. PTH-related peptide fails to cross-react in such assays. Recently, specific immunoassays for this peptide were developed, and these facilitate diagnosis of tumor secretion of the peptide. Increased urinary cAMP excretion (coupled with low or undetectable PTH measurement) also favors tumor secretion of PTH-related peptide. If both PTH and urinary cAMP levels are low, one is dealing with a vitamin D–mediated or local osteolytic hypercalcemia.

TREATMENT AND PROGNOSIS. Acute, nonspecific treatment of hypercalcemia is instituted if the diagnosis is unclear (see Ch. 163). Definitive treatment must be directed at the underlying neoplasm, if feasible. When tumor treatment is not possible, vigorous treatment of hypercalcemia may be irrelevant. In those cases mediated by vitamin D or lymphokine release, glucocorticoids are often uniquely effective in lowering the serum calcium level.

HYPERCALCEMIA DUE TO GRANULOMATOUS DISEASES

ETIOLOGY AND PATHOGENESIS. Hypercalcemia is caused by unregulated formation of $1,25(OH)_2D$ in granuloma-associated macrophages. Normally, 1-hydroxylation takes place in the kidney and is sensitive to feedback suppression by high serum calcium levels. Unregulated synthesis of $1,25(OH)_2D$ in patients with granulomatous diseases renders them hypersensitive to vitamin D (from the diet or through sun exposure).

INCIDENCE AND PREVALENCE. This form of hypercalcemia has been observed in almost any disease capable of causing granulomas. These diseases include sarcoidosis, tuberculosis and fungal infections, berylliosis, and some lymphomas, such as Hodgkin's disease. Overt hypercalcemia may be seen in only about 10% of patients with sarcoidosis, but hypercalciuria and intestinal hyperabsorption of calcium may occur in almost half of such individuals.

CLINICAL FEATURES. Manifestations are those of the underlying disease, as well as the superimposed effects of hypercalcemia. Because this form of hypercalcemia often coexists with relatively higher serum phosphorus levels than those seen in hyperparathyroidism, soft tissue calcification, nephrocalcinosis, and renal impairment are more common. Patients may present with hypercalcemia and relatively few other findings (e.g., subtle hilar adenopathy in sarcoidosis).

DIAGNOSIS. PTH and urinary cAMP are suppressed. The serum level of $1,25(OH)_2D$ is elevated (in cases of vitamin D intoxication, the serum $1,25(OH)_2D$ level may be normal and only serum $25(OH)D$ is increased).

TREATMENT AND PROGNOSIS. The prognosis depends on that of the underlying disease. Glucocorticoids are extremely effective in lowering the serum calcium level in such cases. Chloroquine has been used effectively in subjects who cannot tolerate glucocorticoid treatment.

Aurbach GD, Marx SJ, Spiegel AM: Parathyroid hormone, calcitonin, and the calciferols. *In* Wilson JD, Foster DW (eds.): Williams Textbook of Endocrinology. 8th ed. Philadelphia, WB Saunders, 1992, p 1429. *Detailed description of primary hyperparathyroidism and malignancy-associated and other forms of hypercalcemia, including differential diagnosis and treatment.*

Bilezikian JP: Management of hypercalcemia. J Clin Endocrinol Metab 77:1445, 1993. *Concise review focusing on treatment of mild, moderate, and severe hypercalcemia.*

Broadus AE, Mangin M, Ikeda K, et al.: Humoral hypercalcemia of cancer. N Engl J Med 319:556, 1988. *Review of pathogenesis of this syndrome and discovery of parathyroid hormone-related peptide.*

Deftos LJ, Parthemore JG, Stabile BE: Management of primary hyperparathyroidism. Annu Rev Med 44:19, 1993. *Brief review focusing on managing "asymptomatic" patients. Encompasses recommendations from 1991 Consensus Conference on hyperparathyroidism.*

Heath H III: Primary hyperparathyroidism: Recent advances in pathogenesis, diagnosis, and management. Adv Intern Med 37:275, 1991. *More detailed review on all aspects of the disease.*

Pollak MR, Brown EM, Chou YW, et al.: Mutations in the human Ca^{2+}-sensing receptor gene cause familial hypocalciuric hypercalcemia and neonatal severe hyperparathyroidism. Cell 75:1297, 1993. *Evidence that distinct mutations in this receptor gene cause familial hypocalciuric hypercalcemia in heterozygotes and that neonatal severe hyperparathyroidism can be caused by mutations in both alleles of the same gene.*

Singer FR, Adams JS: Abnormal calcium homeostasis in sarcoidosis. N Engl J Med 315:755, 1986. *Review of derangements in vitamin D metabolism causing hypercalcemia and hypercalciuria in granulomatous disorders.*

HYPOCALCEMIA

DEFINITION. Hypocalcemia is an abnormal reduction in serum ionized calcium concentration.* Reduction in total serum calcium, as may occur in patients with hypoalbuminemia, does not necessarily reflect a reduction in ionized calcium. Ionized, not total, serum calcium affects neuromuscular function and is therefore the clinically relevant parameter.

ETIOLOGY AND PATHOGENESIS. Normal serum ionized calcium concentration is maintained by the direct actions of PTH on kidney and bone and by the indirect actions (through $1,25(OH)_2D$) on the intestine (see Ch. 211). Hypocalcemic disorders can be divided according to pathogenesis into two broad categories: (1) primary hypoparathyroidism, in which hypocalcemia is due to deficient secretion and/or action of PTH (specific subtypes are discussed under individual headings below); and (2) hypocalcemia due to target organ malfunction (e.g., renal failure, intestinal malabsorption, vitamin D deficiency). Hypocalcemia occurs in this category despite normal or even increased PTH secretion (secondary hyperparathyroidism). In hypoparathyroidism, there is reduced mobilization of calcium from bone, reduced renal reabsorption of calcium, lowered phosphaturia, and reduced $1,25(OH)_2D$ formation with a resultant decrease in intestinal calcium absorption. The end results are hypocalcemia and hyperphosphatemia. Renal failure (see Ch. 216) and acute phosphate loads (as may occur with chemotherapy of certain tumors such as Burkitt's lymphoma) are other causes of hypocalcemia with hyperphosphatemia. With vitamin D deficiency or malabsorption, hypocalcemia occurs with normal or low serum phosphorus levels (the latter reflecting secondary hyperparathyroidism). Hypocalcemia with low or normal serum phosphorus levels is also seen in acute pancreatitis (attributed to calcium soap formation, but this is unproved) and in some patients with osteoblastic tumor metastases. Table 214–3 summarizes the causes of hypocalcemia.

CLINICAL MANIFESTATIONS. Hypocalcemia of any cause is associated with certain typical signs and symptoms. Most prominent among these is increased neuromuscular excitability. Paresthesias of the fingers, toes, and circumoral region are mild manifestations; in more extreme cases there may be muscle cramping, carpopedal spasm, laryngeal stridor, and convulsions. Symptoms reflect not only the degree of hypocalcemia but also the acuteness of the fall in serum calcium concentration. Patients with longstanding severe hypocalcemia may show surprisingly few symptoms. Factors that acutely alter the balance between ionized and protein-bound calcium may precipitate symptoms. For example, alkalosis lowers ionized calcium; thus hyperventilation may provoke symptoms of tetany. Signs of latent tetany include Chvostek's sign (twitching of the upper lip after tapping on the facial nerve below the zygomatic arch) and Trousseau's sign (carpal spasm after inflating a cuff on the upper arm above systolic blood pressure for 2 to 3 minutes).

Various mental disturbances, such as irritability, depression, and even psychosis, have been attributed to hypocalcemia. Papilledema and other signs of increased intracranial pressure have been reported. Intracranial calcifications, particularly of the basal ganglia, may be seen on plain radiographs and even more frequently on CT. Increased sensitivity to the dystonic effects of phenothiazines has been attributed to basal ganglia calcification. Longstanding hypocalcemia may lead to cataract formation. Cardiac effects of hypocalcemia include a prolonged QT interval and, rarely, congestive heart failure. Dental anomalies depend on age of onset; in children hypocalcemia can cause enamel hypoplasia and failure of the adult teeth to erupt.

DIFFERENTIAL DIAGNOSIS. Measuring serum calcium, phosphorus, and creatinine levels allows one to categorize the form of hypocalcemia. Hypocalcemia and hyperphosphatemia with normal renal function are pathognomonic of hypoparathyroidism. Low or undetectable PTH by immunoassay despite hypocalcemia confirms the diagnosis. (Rare forms of PTH-resistant hypoparathyroidism show elevated levels of PTH and are discussed further below.) Hypocalcemia and hyperphosphatemia caused by renal failure pose no diagnostic problem. Hypocalcemia with normal or low

---

* See Ch. 211 and Part XXVII for calcium and phosphorus reference range values.

TABLE 214–3. CAUSES OF HYPOCALCEMIA

Hypoparathyroidism
  Deficient parathyroid hormone secretion
    Idiopathic (autoimmune)
    Parathyroid hormone gene mutation
    Surgical
    Infiltrative (iron overload, Wilson's disease)
  Functional
    Hypomagnesemia
    Transient postoperative
  Deficient parathyroid hormone action (hormone resistance)
    Pseudohypoparathyroidism types Ia and Ib
Normal or Increased Parathyroid Hormone Function
  Renal failure
  Intestinal malabsorption
  Acute pancreatitis
  Osteoblastic metastases
  Vitamin D deficiency or resistance

serum phosphorus levels should prompt measurement of vitamin D metabolites and assessment of gastrointestinal function to check for vitamin D deficiency and malabsorption, respectively. Measurements of PTH should show increased values in such patients, as the normal parathyroids attempt to compensate for hypocalcemia.

TREATMENT. Acute, symptomatic hypocalcemia requires emergency treatment in the form of intravenous calcium infusion. Ten to 20 ml of 10% calcium gluconate solution (contains 10 mg of elemental calcium per milliliter) may be given over 10 to 20 minutes (this may be hazardous in patients taking cardiac glycosides). In less urgent settings, a slow intravenous infusion (over 4 to 8 hours) of 20 mg of elemental calcium per kilogram of body weight may be given. As with hypercalcemic disorders, definitive resolution of hypocalcemia requires treating the underlying disease. In patients with hypoparathyroidism, lifelong therapy with vitamin D (with or without oral calcium) is required. This is discussed further under treatment of hypoparathyroidism, below.

HYPOPARATHYROIDISM

DEFINITION. Hypoparathyroidism is defined as deficient PTH secretion and/or action. This condition may lead to overt hypocalcemia and hyperphosphatemia, as discussed above, or may only predispose to hypocalcemia (decreased parathyroid reserve) in times of increased calcium demand, such as pregnancy.

ETIOLOGY AND PATHOGENESIS. *Permanent Deficiency in Parathyroid Hormone Secretion.* This deficiency may result from surgical removal of the parathyroids, from glandular destruction by iron overload (e.g., transfusions in thalassemia) or copper overload (Wilson's disease), and from glandular destruction through a presumed autoimmune mechanism. The latter often has a genetic basis. The parathyroids may fail to develop as part of the DiGeorge syndrome. Some cases termed "idiopathic hypoparathyroidism" may be due to inherited mutations in the PTH gene that prevent synthesis and secretion of PTH.

Transient Deficiency in Parathyroid Hormone Secretion. Reversible hypoparathyroidism can be caused by hypomagnesemia. The latter may compromise both PTH secretion and action. Magnesium replacement corrects the defect. Transient hypoparathyroidism may also result from suppression of normal parathyroids by parathyroid adenomas or other causes of hypercalcemia. This condition rarely lasts more than 1 week. Surgical injury to the parathyroids is another postulated cause of transiently reduced hormone secretion.

Deficiency in Parathyroid Hormone Action. Secretion of a biologically inactive form of PTH is a theoretical, but unproven, cause of deficient PTH action. Target organ resistance to PTH appears to be the major cause of this form of hypoparathyroidism, which was termed "pseudohypoparathyroidism" by Albright, who described it as the first example of a hormone-resistance disorder. Subsequent studies indicated that the defect in this disease occurs before formation of cAMP (a second messenger of PTH action) because affected subjects lack the normal brisk increase in urinary cAMP excretion observed after infusing PTH in normal individuals. There are at least two forms of pseudohypoparathyroidism. In type Ia disease, a 50% deficiency has been found in the Gs protein that couples PTH (and many other) receptors to the enzyme that forms

cAMP, adenylyl cyclase. This deficiency may limit normal cAMP production in response to PTH as well as to other hormones, such as thyroid-stimulating hormone. As a result, patients with this form of the disease show many abnormalities (e.g., hypothyroidism, hypogonadism) in addition to hypoparathyroidism. In affected subjects from several families with type Ia disease, distinct mutations that prevent synthesis of normal Gs protein have been found in the gene encoding the Gs protein. Inheritance of the mutation is autosomal dominant. In subjects with type Ib disease, the Gs protein is normal, and resistance is limited to PTH. A defective PTH receptor is a likely, but unproven, basis for this disease. In some subjects, hypocalcemia and hyperphosphatemia are associated with radiographically evident osteitis fibrosa cystica. This finding suggests selective renal, as opposed to skeletal, resistance to PTH action. The pathogenesis is unclear.

INCIDENCE. All forms of hypoparathyroidism are relatively rare. The incidence of surgical hypoparathyroidism varies widely as a function of the skill of the surgeon.

CLINICAL MANIFESTATIONS. The manifestations generally associated with hypocalcemia have been discussed above. The clinical features unique to each form of hypoparathyroidism reflect the underlying disease. In autoimmune forms, there may be associated endocrine deficiency, most frequently Addison's disease, as well as a T cell defect predisposing to mucocutaneous candidiasis. Alopecia and vitiligo may also be seen. In pseudohypoparathyroidism type Ib, the appearance is normal, but in type Ia disease, affected individuals show a constellation of abnormal physical findings termed Albright's hereditary osteodystrophy (Fig. 214–3). These findings include obesity, short stature, round face and short neck, metacarpal and metatarsal shortening (most often fourth and fifth) as well as shortening and broadening of the distal phalanges, and subcutaneous calcifications. Such individuals often show slight mental retardation and associated endocrine abnormalities, most commonly

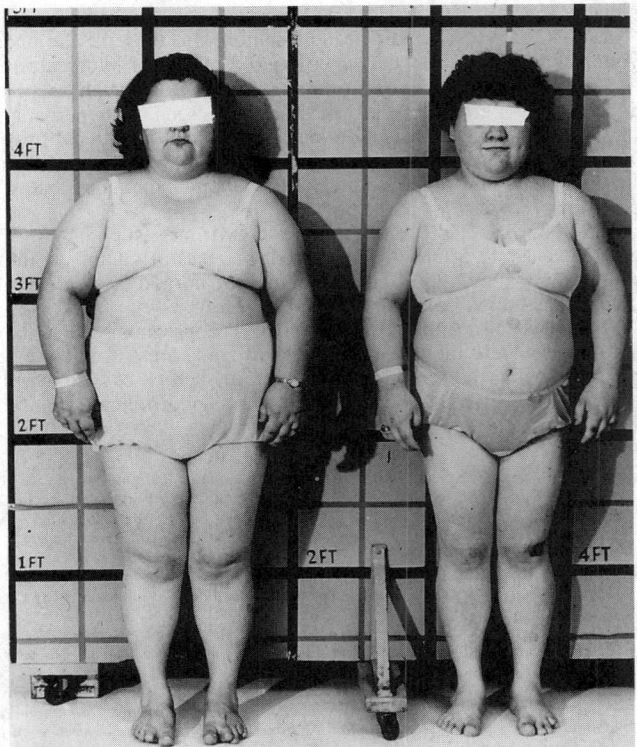

FIGURE 214–3. Phenotypic features of Albright's hereditary osteodystrophy. A mother *(left)* and daughter display many of the features of Albright's osteodystrophy, including obesity, short stature, round face, and short neck. Metacarpal and metatarsal shortening manifest as shortened fourth and fifth fingers (right hands of both subjects) and shortened fourth toes (left feet of both subjects), respectively. Both subjects show resistance to PTH and thyroid-stimulating hormone, as well as deficient Gs protein activity, characteristic of pseudohypoparathyroidism type Ia. (From Spiegel AM: Pseudohypoparathyroidism. *In* Scriver CR, Beaudet AL, Sly WS, Valle D [eds.]: The Metabolic Basis of Inherited Disease. 6th ed. New York, McGraw-Hill, 1989, p 2013; with permission.)

hypothyroidism (without goiter) and hypogonadism. First-degree relatives of patients with pseudohypoparathyroidism type Ia may show the physical features of Albright's osteodystrophy without evidence of hormone resistance. This condition has been termed pseudopseudohypoparathyroidism. Rarely, individuals with pseudohypoparathyroidism (more often of the Ib type) have radiographic evidence of osteitis fibrosa cystica and elevated serum levels of bone-derived alkaline phosphatase.

DIFFERENTIAL DIAGNOSIS. Low or undetectable serum PTH in the face of hypocalcemia, hyperphosphatemia, and normal renal function establishes the diagnosis of hormone-deficient hypoparathyroidism. Diagnosis of the underlying disease depends on history (e.g., neck surgery), physical findings (e.g., candidiasis, alopecia), and additional laboratory tests (e.g., evidence for hypoadrenalism). Antibodies to parathyroid antigens have been detected in the autoimmune form of the disease, but this test is not available for routine clinical use. An elevated level of serum PTH measured by immunoassay in a subject with hypocalcemia, hyperphosphatemia, and normal renal function suggests hormone-resistant hypoparathyroidism. PTH infusion (at present with commercially available synthetic 1–34 peptide) and measurement of urinary cAMP excretion can be performed to confirm PTH resistance. Physical appearance can help distinguish type Ia from type Ib pseudohypoparathyroidism, as can testing for other endocrinopathies, such as hypothyroidism. Measurement of Gs protein and detection of mutations in the corresponding gene are not routinely available tests.

TREATMENT. Transient forms of hypoparathyroidism may not require treatment. Reversible forms should be treated appropriately, i.e., magnesium replacement for hypomagnesemia. In permanent hormone-deficient hypoparathyroidism, hormone replacement therapy is not practical. Parathyroid autografting is effective in some patients with surgical hypoparathyroidism. When this is not feasible, and also in subjects with pseudohypoparathyroidism, lifelong treatment with oral vitamin D is required. Vitamin D_2, ergocalciferol (generally 50,000 units per day), is inexpensive by comparison with the active metabolite, $1,25(OH)_2D$ (generally 0.25 μg per day). The latter has the theoretical advantage of more rapid onset (and in case of toxicity, offset) of action, but with appropriate monitoring, vitamin D_2 can be used very effectively. Oral calcium salts (1 to 2 grams of elemental calcium per day in divided doses) may be added for individuals whose dietary calcium intake is highly variable or inadequate. The goal of treatment is the lowest serum calcium concentration compatible with avoidance of symptoms, because without PTH, urinary calcium excretion (and the possibility of nephrolithiasis) is increased at any filtered load of calcium. Both serum and urine calcium levels, as well as renal function, must be monitored. In forms of hypoparathyroidism that have associated endocrinopathies, appropriate hormone replacement therapy should be instituted.

Aurbach GD, Marx SJ, Spiegel AM: Parathyroid hormone, calcitonin, and the calciferols. *In* Wilson JD, Foster DW (eds.): Williams Textbook of Endocrinology, 8th ed. Philadelphia, WB Saunders, 1992, p 1456. *Detailed description of clinical and pathophysiologic features of hypocalcemic disorders and the multiple forms of hypoparathyroidism.*

Mallette L: Synthetic human parathyroid hormone 1–34 fragment for diagnostic testing. Ann Intern Med 109:800, 1988. *Description of use of this commercially available peptide in the differential diagnosis of hypoparathyroidism.*

Spiegel AM: Pseudohypoparathyroidism. *In* Scriver CR, Beaudet AL, Sly WS, et al. (eds.): The Metabolic Basis of Inherited Disease. 6th ed. New York, McGraw-Hill, 1989, p 2013. *Extensive discussion of clinical features and pathogenesis of hormone-resistant forms of hypoparathyroidism.*

215 CALCITONIN AND MEDULLARY THYROID CARCINOMA

Leonard J. Deftos

Calcitonin (CT) is a 32-residue peptide secreted primarily by the thyroidal C-cells in mammals and by the embryologically related ultimobranchial gland in submammals. The main biologic effect of CT is to decrease bone resorption by inhibiting the osteoclast. This effect decreases the concentration of blood calcium, with a nadir di-

rectly related to bone turnover; thus, the hypocalcemia may be slight in normal adults but considerable when bone resorption is increased pathologically in disease states or physiologically during bone growth. This property of CT makes it an effective drug for hyperresorptive diseases, such as Paget's disease, osteoporosis, and hypercalcemia. The physiologic significance of other reported effects of CT is not well established. The calciuric effect of CT is seen primarily with pharmacologic doses of the hormone. A stimulatory effect on bone formation may be attributed to a CT-related molecule rather than to CT itself. However, an analgesic effect of CT continues to receive considerable attention and may be related to neuroendocrine features of the hormone. In addition to its role in skeletal physiology and treatment, CT is a serum and tumor marker for medullary thyroid carcinoma (MTC), which is the signal tumor of multiple endocrine neoplasia (MEN) type II.

CALCITONIN

BIOCHEMISTRY. The 32-residue structure of CT, determined for nine species, reveals a common 1,7 amino-terminal disulfide bridge and carboxy-terminal proline. Seven of the nine amino-terminal residues are identical in all CT molecules. The interspecies structural differences in the rest of the molecule cause the submammalian (ultimobranchial) CT molecules to be more potent in mammals than the mammalian CT molecules. Thus, the potent salmon form of the hormone is widely used for treatment in humans. The greater chemical basicity of these submammalian CT species probably accounts for their increased potency. In contrast to the other major skeletal peptide hormone, parathyroid hormone (PTH), a biologically active fragment of CT has not been identified, and the entire molecule seems to be necessary for biologic activity.

SECRETION AND PRODUCTION. The most important secretory regulation of CT is mediated by ambient calcium. An acute increase in blood calcium concentration increases the secretion of CT, and an acute decrease in blood calcium level decreases the secretion of CT. The effects of chronic changes in blood calcium concentration on secretion have not been as well defined. Chronic hypercalcemia may stimulate CT production, but this compensatory response may be limited. Chronic hypocalcemia seems to increase CT storage in C-cells. Although a variety of other factors have been reported to stimulate CT secretion, only pentagastrin and its related peptides are consistent additional secretagogues. The high concentration of pentagastrin necessary to stimulate secretion does not support the presence of a normal entero–C-cell secretory pathway. Nevertheless, pentagastrin and calcium are clinically important agents for evaluating CT secretion by both normal and malignant C-cells.

The effect of gonadal steroids and age on CT production remains controversial. It is well established that blood concentrations of CT are higher in males than females and in children than adults. Some studies report a decline in CT secretion during adulthood and a stimulation of CT secretion by estrogens and testosterone. These observations have led to the hypothesis that age- and menopause-related declines in CT production contribute to the corresponding declines in bone mass seen in the elderly, especially postmenopausal women. These observations support the use of CT in treating osteoporosis, but more complex hormonal abnormalities underlie this skeletal disorder.

MEDULLARY THYROID CARCINOMA

Medullary thyroid carcinoma is a tumor of the CT-producing C-cells of the thyroid gland. These cells migrate from the neural crest to the thyroid gland and to other sites of the diffuse neuroendocrine system during embryogenesis in mammals. In submammals, these cells form their own distinct organ, the ultimobranchial gland. The neural crest origin of C-cells accounts for their production of a variety of biologically active substances. This embryologic origin may also explain the common association of MTC with other neuroendocrine tumors. Thus, MTC can occur as part of MEN type II or sporadically.

PATHOLOGY. A palpable tumor is the most common physical finding in the patient with MTC. The tumor is usually firm and located in the middle or upper lobes of the gland. Bilateral tumors are common in MEN. Calcification can be present in the tumor, and this may result in a radiographic pattern that is characteristic enough to help diagnose it clinically. Similarly, amyloid present in the tumor can assist in histologic diagnosis. However, cytologic diagnosis is made difficult by the fact that the cells of MTC can be arranged in a variety of patterns. Therefore, the diagnosis of MTC is conclusively made by demonstrating CT in the tumor by immunohistology. Hyperplasia of the C-cells antedates the frank malignancy of MTC, especially in the familial forms of the tumor. C-cell hyperplasia is often too subtle to be appreciated by light microscopy, and immunohistology for CT is necessary to make this diagnosis. The advent of genetic testing for MEN provides additional impetus for distinguishing MTC from other thyroid tumors.

TUMOR BEHAVIOR. The clinical behavior of MTC is usually intermediate between that of aggressive anaplastic thyroid cancer and that of indolent papillary and follicular thyroid cancer. Local lymph node spread is common, and metastases to lung and bone can occur. MTC in which all or most of the cells produce CT may have a better prognosis than a more heterogeneous tumor in which CT production is not uniform. Even in the most aggressive tumors, CT production is usually sufficient to serve as a specific marker for this thyroid cancer. However, there may be rare instances in which CT production has ceased. The 5-year survival of those with MTC approximates 50%. Survival can vary from several months to three decades after diagnosis. Patients under age 2 with metastatic disease and over age 50 with only localized disease have been reported. C-cell hyperplasia can occur in those as young as age 2 and as old as 45. Therefore, the tumor can be rapidly aggressive, leading to death within months after diagnosis, or it can be indolent and compatible with survival for decades.

PATHOGENESIS. MTC is preceded by C-cell hyperplasia, especially in the familial form of the disease. This progression from hyperplasia to cancer is best documented for MTC in the clinical setting of MEN type II. C-cell adenomas have also been observed. The progression of unregulated growth from hyperplasia to malignancy is similar to that seen in the progression of mucosal cells to a frankly malignant state in other tumors in which an oncogene cascade contributes to pathogenesis. It is thus interesting to speculate that an oncogene cascade is responsible for the progression of normal C-cells through hyperplasia to cancer in MTC. In the familial form of the tumor, an oncogene abnormality may be related to the chromosome 10 site, to which MEN type IIA and IIB have both been mapped. Abnormalities in expression of the RET oncogene have been observed in MTC, but the role in pathogenesis of this tyrosine kinase has not yet been elucidated. Abnormalities in this oncogene have recently been reported in familial MTC and Hirschsprung's disease. It is notable that this same progression of normal cells to hyperplastic and then neoplastic cells is also observed for the other two endocrine components of heritable MTC, pheochromocytoma and parathyroid neoplasia. Thus, the genetic abnormality on chromosome 10 may result in the overexpression (or undersuppression) of an endocrine cell growth factor.

DIAGNOSIS. Overexpression of the CT gene is the molecular hallmark of MTC. This overexpression results in the increased production of CT by the tumor and increased secretion of the hormone into blood. As a result, most patients with MTC have an increased circulating concentration of CT that can be detected by radioimmunoassay and increased tumor concentrations that can be demonstrated directly by immunohistology or through increased messenger RNA (mRNA) expression by in situ hybridization. Usually, the basal blood concentration of CT is sufficiently elevated to be diagnostic of the presence of the tumor. In the early stages of the diseases, however, the basal concentrations of CT cannot be readily distinguished from normal. In these circumstances, provocative testing of CT secretion can reveal the presence of the abnormal C-cells. Such testing is also clinically indicated for the relative of a patient with familial MTC when early diagnosis is sought. Screening is also recommended for apparently sporadic tumors because family history can be unreliable. The two most commonly used provocative agents for CT secretion are calcium and the synthetic gastrin analogue pentagastrin, alone or in combination. Most tumors respond to either agent with a diagnostic increase in CT secretion. CT blood measurements can also be used to evaluate therapy and monitor tumor recurrence. Interpretation must be made according to the specific parameters of the procedure used.

The primary genetic abnormality in MEN type IIA and IIB have been localized to chromosome 10. For MEN IIA, the genetic defect

has been localized to the RET oncogene, which encodes a tyrosine kinase. Molecular genetic techniques allow gene carrier status to be assigned in a patient at risk and with a well-documented pedigree. However, confounding factors such as mistaken diagnoses and non-paternity can complicate genetic analysis. The ethical considerations that surround all genetic screening should be considered in the light of the effective and curative treatment that is available for the components of MEN type IIA and IIB. Nevertheless, genetic diagnosis represents a substantial advance in management of the inherited forms of MTC.

CT GENE EXPRESSION. A variety of bioactive substances are overproduced by MTC. Some can be attributed to the neural crest origin of the C-cells and some to deregulated CT gene expression. This gene encodes peptides in addition to CT. The CT gene consists of six exons that generate—through differential mRNA splicing—two distinct mRNA's, one of them the CT precursor and the other a precursor for calcitonin gene–related peptide (CGRP). The CT precursor is processed into three peptides: CT; its amino-terminal flanking peptide, N-pro CT; and its carboxy-terminal flanking peptide, C-pro CT. The CGRP precursor is similarly processed. Thus, the CT gene encodes at least six peptides. The peptides derived from the CT precursor, including CT, act on the skeletal system, and the peptide derived from the CGRP precursor acts as a neurotransmitter. This remarkable genetic economy produces two CT precursor–derived peptides that have opposite skeletal effects, with CT inhibiting bone resorption and N-pro CT, its amino-terminal relative, promoting bone cell mitogenesis. Human CT gene expression and processing are summarized in Figure 215–1.

MULTIPLE ENDOCRINE NEOPLASIA (MEN)

MTC can occur in association with other endocrine tumors as part of a multiple endocrine neoplasia, designated MEN type II, to distinguish it from MEN type I, which consists of parathyroid, pancreatic, and pituitary tumors. MEN type II is an autosomal dominant syndrome that can be clinically classified into two subtypes, type IIA and IIB (Table 215–1).

PHEOCHROMOCYTOMA. Pheochromocytoma is a component of MEN type IIA and IIB. Bilateral and multifocal pheochromocytomas are very common in this clinical setting, with an incidence of >70%. This figure contrasts with a bilateral incidence of usually <10% for sporadic pheochromocytomas and only 20 to 50% for familial pheochromocytomas. Adrenal medullary hyperplasia is a precursor of the pheochromocytomas seen with MTC. The increase in adrenal medullary mass results from diffuse or multifocal proliferation of adrenal medullary cells, primarily those found within the head and body of the glands. The biochemical as well as clinical manifestations of this tumor may be subtle, so diagnostic tests for pheochromocytoma should be pursued vigorously in MEN type II.

HYPERPARATHYROIDISM. Hyperparathyroidism is much more common in MEN type IIA than in MEN type IIB (and it also occurs in MEN type I). The presence of hyperparathyroidism thus should always make one consider the possibility of MEN. Parathyroid hyperplasia is more common than adenoma, an important consideration for surgical treatment. Although a calcium-mediated functional relationship between hyperparathyroidism and MTC has been suggested, the two neoplasias are probably linked to the same gene.

MULTIPLE MUCOSAL NEUROMAS. The presence of neuromas with a centrofacial distribution is the most consistent component of MEN type IIB. The most common location of neuromas is the oral cavity. The oral lesions are almost invariably present by the first decade and in some cases even at birth. Mucosal neuromas can also be present in the eyelid, conjunctiva, and cornea. The most prominent microscopic feature of neuromas is an increase in the size and number of nerves. These hypertrophied nerve fibers are readily seen with a slit lamp and occasionally by direct ophthalmologic examination.

Gastrointestinal tract abnormalities are part of the multiple mucosal neuroma syndrome. The most common of these is gastrointestinal ganglioneuromatosis, which usually occurs in the small and large intestines but has also been noted in the esophagus and stomach. The lesions are sometimes associated with swallowing abnormalities, megacolon, diarrhea, and constipation. The diarrhea may also be due to excess production of bioactive substances by the MTC. In any case, diarrhea is the most common symptom of MTC.

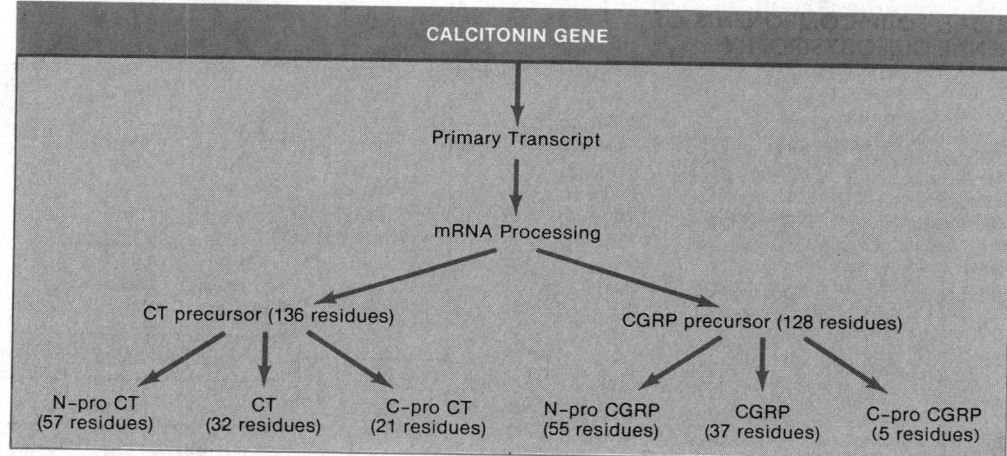

FIGURE 215–1. Summary of human calcitonin (CT) gene expression. The CT pathway occurs primarily in endocrine tissue (e.g., C-cells) and the calcitonin gene–related peptide (CGRP) pathway primarily in neural tissue. The gene has six exons whose primary RNA transcript is differentially spliced into an mRNA for the CT precursor and one for the CGRP precursor. A common 25-residue leader sequence is removed, and these two polypeptide precursors are each processed into their three respective peptide products. (Alternative designations for some of these peptides are as follows: for N-pro CT, PAS-57; for C-pro CT, PDN-21 and katacalcin; for N-pro CGRP, PAS-55). The functions of these other peptides are not firmly established.

MARFANOID HABITUS. Patients with this component have a tall, slender body with long arms and legs, an abnormal ratio of upper to lower body segments, and poor muscle development. Other features associated with the marfanoid habitus may include dorsal kyphosis, pectus excavatum or pectus carinatum, pes cavus, and high-arched palate. In contrast to patients with true Marfan's syndrome, these patients do not have aortic arch abnormalities, ectopia lentis, homocystinuria, or mucopolysaccharide abnormalities.

TREATMENT AND CLINICAL MANAGEMENT. Surgery is the treatment of choice for the three neoplasias in MEN type II. All are potentially lethal—especially MTC and pheochromocytoma—but all can be cured in their early stages by surgery. Aggressive therapy is thus warranted. Managing the individual components of MEN syndromes generally follows the accepted procedures for each of the neoplasias. However, the sequence of treatment is guided by the presence of multiple endocrine tumors. Pheochromocytomas, which are commonly bilateral, should be treated first because they can be life-threatening and pose risks for surgery of the other tumors. Thyroid and parathyroid surgery must be aggressive because all glandular tissue may be involved.

Evaluating family members is an essential feature of appropriate clinical management in MEN type II, because these tumors are transmitted in an autosomal dominant pattern. Family members must be re-evaluated periodically because of the varying penetrance of the component tumors. CT measurement remains the diagnostic procedure of choice. Genetic diagnostic techniques are being continually refined and are increasingly used to identify individuals at risk for the syndrome, especially now that the genetic abnormality has been identified for MEN IIA. Although such procedures may supplant CT measurement for diagnosis, measurement of the hormone will be useful for documenting the presence of neoplasia and monitoring therapy.

CALCITONIN AS A DRUG

CT's primary biologic effect of inhibiting osteoclastic bone resorption makes it useful for treating disorders characterized by increased bone resorption and certain forms of hypercalcemia. Thus, CT can be prescribed for treating Paget's disease, osteoporosis, and the hypercalcemia associated with malignancy. Both salmon CT and human CT are available, the former being more potent and the latter being less antigenic. Calcitonin is safer than most treatment alternatives, but its effects can be transient. The inconvenience of repeated parenteral administration may be avoided by transmucosally administering the peptide. In fact, a nasally administered preparation of CT has been recently approved by the FDA for treatment of osteoporosis.

Burns DM, Birnbaum RS, Roos BA: A neuroendocrine peptide derived from the amino terminal half of rat procalcitonin. Mol Endocrinol 3:140, 1989. *An exposition of the complexities of CT gene expression.*

Cance WG, Wells SA Jr: Multiple endocrine neoplasia. Curr Prob Surg 22:1, 1985. *A discussion of the surgical problems encountered in the treatment of multiple endocrine tumors.*

Deftos LJ: Radioimmunoassay for calcitonin in medullary thyroid carcinoma. JAMA 227:403, 1974. *Early study of the application of CT radioimmunoassay to the diagnosis of MTC.*

Deftos LJ, Roos BA: Medullary thyroid carcinoma and calcitonin gene expression. Bone Miner Res 6:267, 1989. *A detailed exposition of multiple endocrine neoplasia and the regulation of calcitonin-gene products.*

Gagel RF, Robinson MF, Donovan DT, et al.: Medullary thyroid carcinoma: Recent progress. J Clin Endocrinol Metab 76:809, 1993. *A recent review of the clinical features and molecular genetics of MTC.*

Mulligan LM, Kwok JBJ, Healey CS, et al.: Germ-line mutations of the *RET* proto-oncogene in multiple endocrine neoplasia type 2A. Nature 363:458, 1993. *Identification of the genetic abnormality in MEN IIA.*

Sobol H, Narod SA, Nakamura Y, et al.: Screening for MEN Type IIA with DNA-polymorphism analyses. N Engl J Med 321:996, 1989. *The application of RFLP to genetic analyses in MEN.*

van Heyningen V: One gene—four syndromes. Nature 367:319, 1994.

216 RENAL OSTEODYSTROPHY
Eduardo Slatopolsky

The main components of renal osteodystrophy are osteitis fibrosa and osteomalacia (Table 216–1). A lesser role is played by osteosclerosis and osteoporosis. Osteitis fibrosa, a consequence of an increased parathyroid hormone, is characterized by an increase in the number of osteoclasts and an increase in bone resorption and marrow fibrosis. Osteomalacia results from a decreased mineralization of osteoid tissue (shown histologically by an abnormal calcification front in bone). Osteosclerosis is due to localized areas of mineralized woven bone which appear as increased bone density on radiographic studies. Osteoporosis, defined as a decrease in the mass of normally mineralized bone, is an infrequent and minor component of renal osteodystrophy.

TABLE 215–1. COMPONENTS OF MULTIPLE ENDOCRINE NEOPLASIA TYPE II AND THEIR FREQUENCY BASED ON AVERAGE FIGURES FROM THE LITERATURE

Component	MEN Type IIA (%)	MEN Type IIB (%)
Medullary thyroid carcinoma	97	90
Pheochromocytoma	30	45
Hyperparathyroidism	50	Rare
Mucosal neuroma syndrome	—	100

TABLE 216-1. FOUR COMPONENTS OF RENAL OSTEODYSTROPHY

1. Osteitis fibrosa (high bone turnover)
   a. Phosphate retention
   b. Altered metabolism of vitamin D
   c. Skeletal resistance to PTH
   d. Decreased number of calcitriol receptors in parathyroid glands
   e. Unpaired degradation of PTH
   f. Altered feedback regulation of PTH by Ca^{2+}
2. Osteomalacia (low bone turnover)
   a. Altered metabolism of vitamin D
   b. Altered synthesis and maturation of collagen
   c. Acidosis
   d. Increased bone magnesium
   e. Increased pyrophosphate
   f. Retention of aluminum
   g. Retention of iron
3. Osteosclerosis ⎫
                  ⎬ of lesser quantitative importance
4. Osteoporosis ⎭

OSTEITIS FIBROSA (High-Turnover Bone Disease)

Chief cell hyperplasia of the parathyroid glands and high levels of immunoreactive parathyroid hormone (i-PTH) are among the earliest findings affecting mineral metabolism in most patients with chronic renal failure. Several factors contribute to the development of secondary hyperparathyroidism in renal insufficiency (Table 216–1 and Fig. 216–1).

THE ROLE OF PHOSPHATE RETENTION. Phosphorus retention plays an important role in the genesis of hyperparathyroidism. The mechanisms considered include (1) phosphorus-induced hypocalcemia, (2) phosphorus-induced decrease in the levels of calcitriol, and (3) other unknown factors. These mechanisms are closely interrelated and are not mutually exclusive.

PHOSPHORUS RETENTION AND HYPOCALCEMIA. A rise in serum phosphorus can evoke an increase in PTH secretion. An oral phosphorus load leads to an increase in serum phosphorus, a fall in ionized calcium, and increased levels of PTH in normal human subjects. Whether this sequence of events occurs in early renal failure has been questioned in that fasting or even postprandial levels of serum phosphorus are not consistently elevated. In fact, low levels of serum phosphorus are not uncommon. By contrast, in advanced renal failure, hyperphosphatemia plays a key role in the development of hypocalcemia, metastatic calcifications, peripheral vascular insufficiency, pruritus, and worsening of secondary hyperparathyroidism.

PHOSPHORUS RETENTION AND CALCITRIOL. Because phosphorus regulates the production rate of calcitriol by altering the activity of the enzyme 1α-hydroxylase, it is possible that the effects of phosphorus retention are mediated by a decrease in the synthesis of calcitriol. Conversely, the beneficial effects of phosphorus restriction in ameliorating hyperparathyroidism could be explained by increased levels of calcitriol. In patients with moderate renal insufficiency, dietary phosphorus restriction significantly increases plasma calcitriol levels with a concomitant normalization of plasma PTH. This occurs despite a lack of change in serum phosphorus levels.

OTHER MECHANISMS OF THE EFFECT OF PHOSPHORUS RETENTION. Although many investigators have focused their attention on the effects of phosphorus being mediated by changes in serum levels of calcium and/or calcitriol, there is evidence that phosphorus *per se* directly or indirectly may be involved. Several investigators have demonstrated that phosphorus restriction corrects secondary hyperparathyroidism in patients and dogs with advanced renal insufficiency. These studies suggest that a reduction in dietary phosphorus in advanced renal failure improves secondary hyperparathyroidism by a mechanism that is independent of the levels of calcitriol or serum ionized calcium.

In addition to the well-known effects of phosphorus in the regulation of calcitriol, a low-phosphorus diet may have an effect on the secretion of PTH. Although the mechanism of this effect is not yet known, phosphorus may potentially affect phospholipid composition of the parathyroid cell membrane, calcium fluxes in the parathyroid

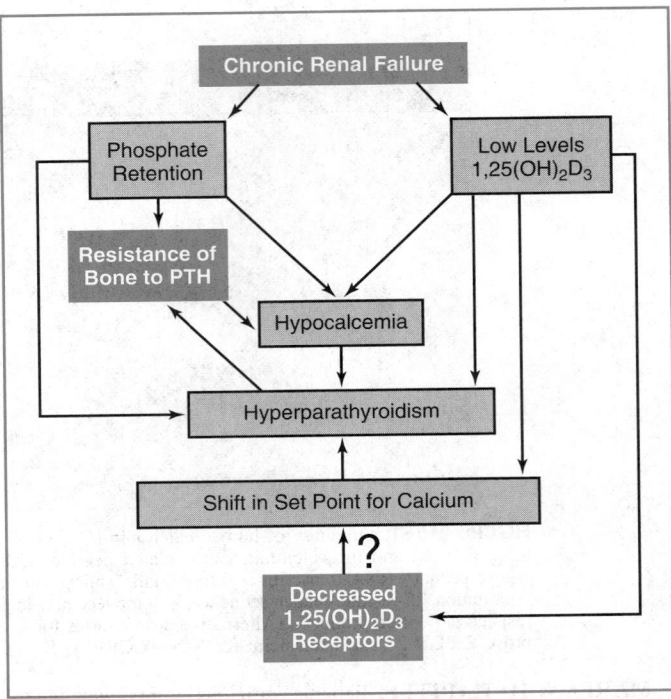

FIGURE 216–1. Diagrammatic representation of the factors involved in the pathogenesis of secondary hyperparathyroidism. (Modified from Slatopolsky E, Coburn J: Renal osteodystrophy. *In* Avioli L, Krane SM [eds.]: Metabolic Bone Disease, 2nd ed. Orlando, FL, Grune & Stratton, 1990.)

cells, and/or regulation of calcitriol receptors in the parathyroid cell (see Ch. 214).

ALTERATIONS IN VITAMIN D METABOLISM (see Ch. 212). Because the kidney is the major site of calcitriol production, it follows that a loss of renal mass, as renal disease progresses, may decrease the ability of the diseased kidneys to produce the active metabolite of vitamin D. PTH and low-phosphate or low-calcium diets stimulate the activity of the 1α-hydroxylase; lack of PTH, hyperphosphatemia, or hypercalcemia decreases the activity of the 1α-hydroxylase. Intestinal absorption of calcium is reduced in patients with far-advanced renal insufficiency, and low levels of calcitriol are found in serum as the probable cause.

SKELETAL RESISTANCE TO THE ACTION OF PARATHYROID HORMONE. Skeletal resistance to the calcemic action of PTH may also play a role in the development of hypocalcemia seen in patients with renal insufficiency. This supports the concept of desensitization/down-regulation of the PTH receptor-effective mechanisms and minimizes the direct role of calcitriol. Thus, higher circulating levels of PTH may be needed to maintain a normal serum calcium in patients with renal failure.

IMPAIRED DEGRADATION OF PTH SECONDARY TO REDUCED RENAL FUNCTION. PTH is metabolized by the liver and the kidney. The liver takes up the intact hormone exclusively; it does not remove either amino-terminal or carboxy-terminal PTH fragments from the circulation. In chronic renal insufficiency, therefore, the high levels of carboxy-terminal circulating i-PTH result both from increased PTH secretion due to chief cell hyperplasia and from a decreased catabolism of the hormone.

ALTERED FEEDBACK REGULATION BETWEEN IONIZED CALCIUM AND THE SECRETION OF PARATHYROID HORMONE (see Ch. 214). The control of PTH secretion by ionized calcium in extracellular fluid may be blunted in patients with chronic renal insufficiency (Fig. 216–1).

OSTEOMALACIA (Low-Turnover Bone Disease) (see Ch. 211 and 212)

Although the plasma levels of calcitriol are reduced in patients with far-advanced renal insufficiency, overt osteomalacia is found in only a small fraction of such patients and may be absent even in anephric patients. Thus, other factors could also participate in the pathogenesis of osteomalacia in uremic patients—the plasma level of phosphate, for example. Hypophosphatemia *per se* can produce severe osteomalacia even in patients with normal renal function. Additional factors include altered collagen synthesis and maturation, defective bone crystal maturation, increased bone magnesium, elevated levels of pyrophosphate, and diminished calcium carbonate. The combination of these factors may influence the maturation of bone and potentially contribute to osteomalacia. Acidosis also contributes to the skeletal disease. In chronic renal insufficiency the skeleton assists in buffering the retained acids. Administering bicarbonate and correcting the acidosis in azotemic patients can reduce fecal calcium excretion.

Another type of osteomalacia in renal insufficiency, and likely the most common one, that is resistant to vitamin D therapy results from excess aluminum. Patients with osteomalacia secondary to aluminum have pathologic fractures, severe bone pain, and characteristically have low levels of PTH. High aluminum content in the water and/or the ingestion of phosphate binders containing aluminum may be the causes. The aluminum is deposited in the interface between the osteoid tissue and the calcification front and is toxic to the osteoblast. Severe iron retention can induce a similar form of osteomalacia.

More recently, a form of low bone turnover called "adynamic" or aplastic bone disease has been described. Patients maintained on continuous ambulatory peritoneal dialysis (CAPD) suffer from this more commonly than those maintained on chronic dialysis. Aluminum accumulation has been implicated in approximately 50% of these patients. In the remainder, diabetes, aging, high calcium in the dialysate, and low levels of PTH have been implicated in the pathogenesis of this condition. Histologically, this lesion is characterized by a significant decrease in the amount of osteoid tissue and lack of osteoblasts. The clinical consequences of this lesion are as yet unclear.

CLINICAL MANIFESTATIONS

The symptoms related to renal osteodystrophy usually appear only when renal failure is advanced. On the other hand, certain biochemical alterations may appear much earlier. Detecting these alterations may direct the physician to early treatment and prevent severe complications in bone and mineral metabolism.

Bone pain can progress inexorably to a point where the patient becomes bedridden, without regard to whether the bone disease is predominantly osteitis fibrosa or osteomalacia. The bone pain is characteristically vague and commonly located in the lower back, hips, knees, and legs. Low back pain may result from the collapse of a vertebral body. Sharp chest pain may indicate spontaneous rib fracture. Physical findings are frequently lacking.

Muscular weakness, when present, is usually proximal, appears slowly, and progresses with time. Plasma levels of creatine phosphokinase and transaminases are usually normal, and the electron micrographic changes are nonspecific. The pathogenesis of this muscular weakness is uncertain. In patients with myopathy, the myofibrils are disorganized in a patchy fashion and the Z-band material may be dispersed. These changes revert to normal following treatment with $25(OH)D_3$. *Pruritus* due to calcium deposition in skin is a common symptom in uremic patients, particularly with severe secondary hyperparathyroidism.

Vascular calcification and peripheral ischemic necrosis may occur, producing lesions of the tips of the digits and violaceous discoloration of the skin. Ulcerations and scarring may occur, with clear demarcation of the lesions from the surrounding skin. Acute pain and swelling around one or more joints may also develop in uremic patients. The syndrome of *calcific periarthritis,* which may be caused by deposition of hydroxyapatite crystals, is accompanied by marked hyperphosphatemia.

Skeletal deformities are common in azotemic children who are growing. Bowing of the tibia and femur and deformities from slipped epiphyses are not uncommon. Children with renal rickets sometimes exhibit typical radiographic findings of vitamin D deficiency. In adults with renal failure, particularly those with osteomalacia, marked skeletal deformities with lumbar scoliosis, thoracic kyphosis, and deformity of the thoracic cage may be observed. Growth retardation is usually seen in young children before and during maintenance hemodialysis. See Ch. 213 for a further discussion of osteomalacia and rickets.

Many patients maintained on dialysis for ≥ 10 years may develop severe bone and joint pain secondary to amyloidosis. β_2-Microglobulins have been implicated in the pathogenesis of this condi-

tion. The presence of bone cysts in the hands, the head of the humerus, and other large joints is characteristic of this condition.

Another clinical manifestation of renal osteodystrophy may occur in some after renal transplant is aseptic necrosis of the femoral head. This condition is more frequently seen in patients with severe bone disease (osteitis fibrosa) before renal transplant and in those who receive large doses of glucocorticoids.

BIOCHEMICAL FEATURES

Circulating i-PTH is elevated early in the course of renal insufficiency (glomerular filtration rate [GFR] 60 to 80 ml per minute). As the disease progresses (GFR < 40 ml per minute), hypocalcemia and low levels of calcitriol appear. With advanced renal insufficiency, however, the serum calcium may remain close to normal and values < 7.5 mg per deciliter are infrequent. Usually hypocalcemia is more marked in severe osteomalacia or with profound metabolic acidosis. Occasionally, hypercalcemia may be observed in uremic patients, particularly in those undergoing long-term dialysis. This complication can arise from (1) severe hyperparathyroidism, (2) ingesting large amounts of calcium and vitamin D, (3) the presence of unrelated diseases such as sarcoidosis or malignancies, or (4) a "pure" mineralizing defect, as may occur in osteomalacia secondary to aluminum retention, and (5) adynamic bone lesion. Hyperphosphatemia is usually present in patients with GFR < 25 ml per minute. The degree of hyperphosphatemia depends on the amount of phosphate ingested, the fraction absorbed in the intestine, and the amount excreted in the urine. If the patient ingests phosphate binders, the serum phosphate may remain normal despite advanced renal insufficiency. Patients with severe hyperparathyroidism and advanced renal insufficiency usually have higher concentrations of serum phosphate in plasma.

Advanced renal insufficiency (GFR < 15 ml per minute) may be associated with hypermagnesemia and increased bone content of magnesium. This may adversely affect crystal formation.

Total serum alkaline phosphatase levels and osteocalcin (both markers of bone formation) are commonly higher in uremic patients with osteitis fibrosa than in those with osteomalacia. Coexistent liver disease should be excluded as a cause of an elevated alkaline phosphatase.

RADIOGRAPHIC FEATURES

Secondary hyperparathyroidism increases bone resorption, most commonly evident on the subperiosteal surfaces of bone. Erosions in conjunction with formation of new bone may appear as cysts or osteoclastomas (brown tumors). The presence of subperiosteal erosion correlates with serum i-PTH and with the histomorphometric features of osteitis fibrosa on bone biopsy. Subperiosteal resorption of the phalanges may be the most sensitive radiographic sign of secondary hyperparathyroidism (Fig. 216–2). The tuft of the terminal phalanx of the second or third digit commonly shows resorption. With severe tuft erosion the soft tissue may collapse and change of the contour of the tuft so that the finger appears to show clubbing. Bone erosions may also occur at the upper end of the tibia, the neck of the femur or the humerus, and the lower surface of the medial end of the clavicle. In the skull, resorption leads to the mottled and granular appearance commonly associated with altering areas of osteosclerosis.

Osteosclerosis is thought to be another feature of osteitis fibrosa arising from an increase in the thickness and number of trabecula in spongy bone. Osteosclerosis can lead to a typical "rugger jersey" appearance of the spine.

Osteomalacia is far less distinctive radiographically than is secondary hyperparathyroidism. The Looser zone or pseudofracture is the only pathognomonic radiographic finding of osteomalacia in the adult. Rickets, i.e., widening of the epiphyseal growth plate, cannot develop after epiphyseal closure and hence is limited to children. With mechanical stress following severe prolonged deficiency of vitamin D, a Looser zone may extend across the full width of the bone and produce a true fracture with displacement of fragments. In uremia, osteomalacia is commonly associated with secondary hyperparathyroidism with radiographic features of both. The diagnosis of osteomalacia rests on histologic examinations and can be established with certainty only by bone biopsy.

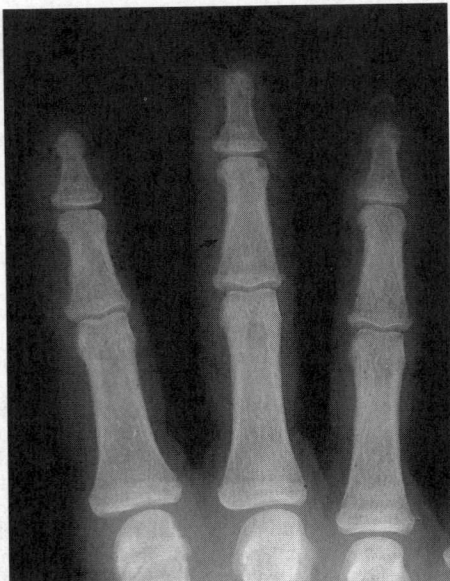

FIGURE 216–2. Radiographic manifestations of osteitis fibrosa. There are subperiosteal erosions of the phalanges and tuft of the terminal phalanx.

Soft-tissue calcification is presumed to be influenced by an increase in the calcium phosphate product in plasma, the degree of secondary hyperparathyroidism, the magnitude of alkalosis, and local tissue injury. Three major varieties include (1) calcification of the medium-size arteries, (2) articular or tumoral calcifications, and (3) visceral calcifications affecting the heart, lung, and kidney.

TREATMENT

The objectives of treating patients with renal osteodystrophy are (1) to return the blood levels of calcium and phosphate to normal, (2) to suppress secondary hyperparathyroidism, (3) to reverse the histologic abnormalities in the skeleton, and (4) to prevent and reverse extraskeletal deposits of calcium and phosphate. Guidelines for the management of renal osteodystrophy are summarized in Table 216–2.

CONTROL OF PHOSPHATE AND CALCIUM. To control phosphate, dietary phosphate intake should be reduced to 700 to 800 mg per day (determined as phosphorus) by restricting dairy products and by decreasing the amount of protein in the diet. In advanced renal failure, in addition to dietary control, phosphate binders are usually required to reduce its intestinal absorption. Phosphate binders should be ingested along with the meal in order to increase their efficiency. Aluminum-containing gels carry the potential of excessive aluminum absorption and accumulation. If the patient develops symptoms and signs suggesting aluminum-induced osteomalacia, this drug should be discontinued. Calcium carbonate (1 to 4 grams with each meal) helps bind phosphate and thereby reduces the amount of aluminum binders needed to treat hyperphosphatemia. During treatment with oral calcium carbonate, it is important to determine the amount of phosphate ingested in 24 hours and during each meal. In this way, the relative amount of calcium carbonate given can be adjusted to the phosphate-binding requirements of specific meals. Calcium carbonate also provides a calcium supplement that helps correct the negative calcium balance secondary to the calcium malabsorption of advanced renal insufficiency. The serum phosphorus should be maintained at normal or nearly normal levels, between 3.5 and 4.5 mg per deciliter, if the patient is not yet on dialysis. The serum calcium should be maintained in the upper limits of normal. Severe hyperphosphatemia should be corrected before administering calcium to reduce the risk of metastatic calcification. Supplemental calcium should be discontinued if the serum calcium increases above 11.0 mg per deciliter.

USE OF VITAMIN D AND ITS METABOLITES. Despite dietary control of phosphate using phosphate binders, adequate dietary calcium, and appropriate levels of calcium in the dialysate,

uremic patients may still develop skeletal disease. Thus, vitamin D and its metabolites are important agents for treating renal osteodystrophy. Calcitriol, the most active metabolite of vitamin D, is the drug of choice for treating hypocalcemia and secondary hyperparathyroidism (see Ch. 214). The usual dose is 0.5 to 1 μg per day. Recent evidence suggests that "oral pulse" (2 to 4 μg twice weekly) is more effective than the usual small dose (0.5 to 1.0 μg) given daily. Calcitriol, given intravenously during dialysis, at the dose of 1 to 3 μg three times per week, is the best approach to suppress secondary hyperparathyroidism. With the intravenous preparation of calcitriol, high concentrations of 1,25-$(OH)_2D_3$ can be obtained in serum. This is important because the low number of receptors in the parathyroid gland make the hyperplastic tissue more resistant to the action of calcitriol. Moreover, calcitriol can upregulate its own number of receptors.

PARATHYROIDECTOMY. The regimen outlined above can lead to improved homeostasis of calcium and phosphorus and reverse the symptoms of bone disease and suppression of PTH secretion. Such measures may not be entirely successful, however, and parathyroidectomy may be required. Indications for parathyroid surgery include severe secondary hyperparathyroidism (bone erosions and high levels of i-PTH) in the presence of any of the following: (1) persistent hypercalcemia, particularly when symptomatic; (2) intractable pruritus that does not respond to dialysis or other medical treatment; (3) progressive extraskeletal calcification in conjunction with a high calcium-phosphorus product that is consistently about 75 to 80 despite appropriate phosphate restriction; and (4) the appearance of ischemic lesions of soft tissues. Because of a lack of compliance, many patients are unable to control their serum phosphorus levels. In these cases, neither calcium supplements nor vitamin D or its metabolites can be recommended safely. Such patients are more likely to develop severe secondary hyperparathyroidism and require parathyroidectomy. Postoperative hypocalcemia may pose a problem if the remaining parathyroid tissue is inadequate and if severe osteitis fibrosa is present preoperatively. Preoperative treatment of such patients with calcitriol (1 to 2 μg per day) may obviate such problems. Serum levels of phosphorus and magnesium sometimes decrease after parathyroidectomy. Phosphate binders should be withheld if the serum phosphorus falls below 3.0 mg per deciliter. Rapid remineralization of the skeleton occurs during this period, but once the "hungry bones" have been

TABLE 216–2. GUIDELINES FOR MANAGING RENAL OSTEODYSTROPHY

Early treatment
  It is important to begin treatment early, i.e., when the GFR is 30–40 ml/min, especially for the control of serum phosphate.
Control of serum phosphate (P) (3.5–4.5 mg/dl)
  Restrict phosphorus intake in diet to 600–800 mg/day
  Phosphate-binding antacids; aluminum carbonate or hydroxide; individualize dosage: Basaljel, Dialume, Alucap, Amphogel, 1–4 capsules with each meal. *Minimize the use of aluminum binders. Preferentially use:*
    Calcium carbonate; 1–4 grams with each meal
    Calcium acetate 0.5–3 grams with each meal
    Hypophosphatemia should be avoided
    Predialysis phosphorus: 4.5–5.5 mg/dl
Adequate calcium intake
  Oral calcium supplements providing 1–2 grams/day when serum P is controlled: Os-Cal, Titralac, Tums
  Dialysate Ca, 5.0–5.5 mg/dl (2.5–2.75 mEq/liter)
Use of vitamin D sterols
  Vitamin D_2 or D_3, 50,000 to 250,000 IU (1.25–6.25 mg)/day
  25-Hydroxyvitamin D_3 (calcifediol), 20–100 μg/day (Calderol)
  1,25-Dihydroxyvitamin D_3 (calcitriol), 0.5–1.0 μg/day (Rocaltrol)
  1,25-Dihydroxyvitamin D_3 (calcitriol) ("oral pulse") 2.0–4.0 μg twice a week (Rocaltrol)
  1,25-Dihydroxyvitamin D_3 (calcitriol) IV, 1.0–3.0 μg three times a week (Calcijex)
Parathyroidectomy
  Severe secondary hyperparathyroidism (bone erosions and increased i-PTH) plus any of the following:
    Persistent hypercalcemia (serum Ca >11.5–12.0 mg/dl)
    Progressive or symptomatic extraskeletal calcification
    Persistently elevated serum calcium-phosphorus product
    Pruritus not responsive to medical treatment
    Calciphylaxis (ischemic ulcers and necrosis)
    Symptomatic hypercalcemia after renal transplantation

mineralized, serum calcium levels rise. A fall in a previously elevated serum alkaline phosphatase toward normal may indicate that rapid skeletal remineralization is nearly complete and that calcium supplements and vitamin D therapy may be reduced or discontinued. In the past, removing three and a half parathyroid glands was the procedure of choice. More recently, total parathyroidectomy followed by autotransplantation of some of the parathyroid tissue into the patient's forearm has been used. The transplanted tissue is more accessible if subsequent surgical removal is necessary. Total parathyroidectomy without autotransplantation has no place in managing renal osteodystrophy because it may predispose to the development of an isolated mineralization defect or osteomalacia in uremic patients. Cryopreservation of removed parathyroid tissue is a useful precaution so that hypoparathyroidism may be treated by reimplantation of parathyroid tissue.

Occasionally after a successful renal transplant, the patient may develop hypercalcemia. Usually this is due to persistent hyperparathyroidism and increased renal production of calcitriol. In the majority of cases, the hypercalcemia subsides several months after renal transplantation. In a few patients, however, severe hypercalcemia (calcium 12 to 13 mg per deciliter) may persist for several months and may affect renal function. In these patients, a subtotal parathyroidectomy is recommended.

TREATMENT OF ALUMINUM TOXICITY. If the patient has aluminum-induced osteomalacia, phosphate binders containing aluminum should be discontinued at once. Phosphate should be controlled by using a more restrictive phosphate diet, and serum phosphorus may be allowed to increase to 6 mg per deciliter. If the patient is not extremely symptomatic, discontinuing aluminum binders will greatly improve the skeletal abnormalities after a period of 6 to 18 months. Symptomatic patients bedridden with severe bone pain and pathologic fractures should receive desferoxamine, 0.5 to 1.0 grams once per week.

SECONDARY AMYLOIDOSIS. No specific treatment is available for this condition. Renal transplantation greatly improves symptoms.

Coburn JW, Slatopolsky E: Vitamin D, parathyroid hormone and renal osteodystrophy. *In* Brenner BM, Rector FC (eds.): The Kidney. 4th ed. Philadelphia, WB Saunders, 1990. *Comprehensive review of renal osteodystrophy.*

Delmez JA, Tindira C, Grooms P, et al.: Parathyroid hormone suppression by intravenous 1,25-dihydroxyvitamin D: A role for increased sensitivity to calcium. J Clin Invest 83:1349, 1989. *Demonstrates that administering IV calcitriol partially corrects the resistance of the parathyroid glands to calcium in uremic patients.*

Korkor AB: Reduced binding of [3H] 1,25-dihydroxyvitamin D_3 in patients with renal failure. N Engl J Med 316:1573, 1987. *Describes for the first time the decreased number of calcitriol receptors in the parathyroid glands of uremic patients.*

Slatopolsky E: Vitamin D. Semin Nephrol 14:99, 1994. *Comprehensive review (several papers) of vitamin D, vitamin D receptor, and analogues. Molecular interactions between vitamin D and PTH.*

Slatopolsky E, Weerts C, Lopez-Hilker S, et al.: Long-term effects of calcium carbonate and 2.5 mEq/liter calcium dialysate on mineral metabolism. Kidney Int 36:897, 1989. *Describes the effectiveness of calcium carbonate as a phosphate binder.*

Szabo A, Merke J, Beier E, et al.: 1,25(OH)$_2$ vitamin D_3 inhibits parathyroid cell proliferation in experimental uremia. Kidney Int 35:1049, 1989. *Demonstrates the antiproliferative effect of calcitriol on the parathyroid glands of uremic rats.*

217 OSTEOPOROSIS
Joel S. Finkelstein

Osteoporosis, the most common type of metabolic bone disease, is characterized by a parallel reduction in bone mineral and bone matrix so that bone is decreased in amount but is of normal composition. Osteoporosis affects 20 million Americans and leads to approximately 1.3 million fractures in the United States each year. During the course of their lifetime, women lose about 50% of trabecular bone and 30% of cortical bone, and 30% of all postmenopausal Caucasian women eventually sustain osteoporotic fractures. By extreme old age, one third of all women and one sixth of all men have a hip fracture. The annual cost of health care and lost productivity due to osteoporosis exceeds $10 billion in the United States.

ETIOLOGY AND PATHOGENESIS

At any point in time, bone density depends on both the peak bone density achieved during development and the subsequent adult bone loss (Fig. 217–1). Thus, osteopenia can result either from deficient pubertal bone accretion, accelerated adult bone loss, or both.

DETERMINANTS OF PEAK BONE DENSITY. Bone density increases dramatically during puberty in response to gonadal steroids and eventually reaches values in young adults that are nearly double those of children. Other factors that influence peak bone density are listed in Table 217–1. Of these, genetic factors account for up to 80% of the variance in peak bone mass. The impact of genetic factors on bone density has been demonstrated in several ways. For example, bone density is lower in the daughters of women with osteoporosis than in those without osteoporosis. Moreover, the concordance of bone density is much higher among monozygotic than dizygotic twins. Recent data suggest that most of the genetic differences in bone density can be accounted for by a gene closely linked to the vitamin D receptor gene, perhaps the receptor gene itself. A large cross-sectional analysis of Caucasian men and women revealed that allelic variations of the vitamin D receptor gene are associated with absolute differences in bone density of 10 to 12%, an effect as large as that caused by 10 years of estrogen deficiency. It is not known whether the differences in bone density associated with variations in vitamin D receptor genotypes reflect differences in bone accretion during development or in the rate of subsequent bone loss.

Men have higher bone density than women and blacks have higher bone density than Caucasians. These differences may account for a lower incidence of osteoporotic fractures in men and in blacks. Men with histories of constitutionally delayed puberty have decreased peak bone density, a finding that may be important in the pathogenesis of osteoporosis in some men. Similar findings have been reported in women with delayed menarche. Studies in identical twins suggest that moderate calcium supplementation can enhance prepubertal bone accretion. Associations between peak bone density and physical activity have also been reported.

PHYSIOLOGIC CAUSES OF ADULT BONE LOSS. After peak bone density is reached, bone density remains stable for years and then declines. Considerable evidence suggests that bone loss begins before menses cease in women and in the third to fifth decades in men. Once the menopause is established, the rate of bone loss is accelerated several-fold in women. During the first 5 to 10 years of the menopause, trabecular bone is lost faster than cortical bone with rates of approximately 2 to 4 and 1 to 2% per year, respectively. A woman can lose 10 to 15% of her cortical bone and 25 to 30% of her trabecular bone during this time, a loss that can be prevented by estrogen replacement therapy. Furthermore, rates of

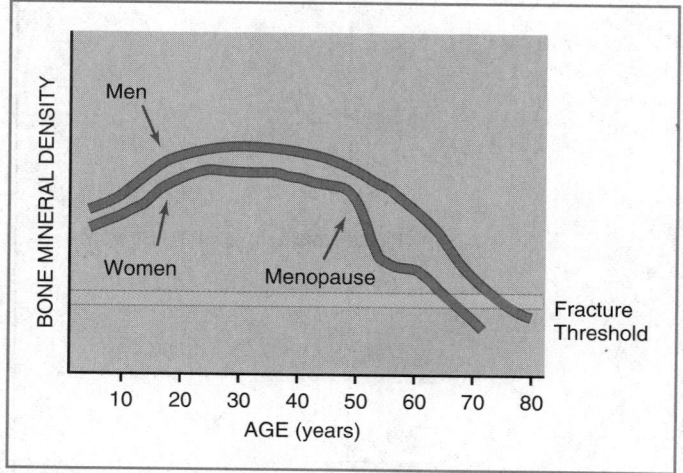

FIGURE 217–1. Cortical bone mineral density versus age in men and women. Women have lower peak cortical bone density than men and experience a period of rapid bone loss at menopause, thus reaching the fracture threshold (the level of bone density at which the risk of developing osteoporotic fractures begins to increase) earlier than men.

TABLE 217–1. FACTORS THAT MAY AFFECT PEAK BONE MASS

Gender
Race
Genetic factors
Gonadal steroids
Growth hormone
Timing of puberty
Calcium intake
Exercise

bone loss vary considerably among women. It is not clear why some postmenopausal women are "fast losers" of bone. A subset of women in whom osteopenia is more severe than expected for their age are said to have type I or "postmenopausal" osteoporosis (Fig. 217–2). Clinically, type I osteoporosis often presents with vertebral "crush" fractures or Colles' fractures. The mechanism whereby estrogen deficiency leads to bone loss is still not established. Recent evidence suggests that estrogen deficiency may increase local production of bone-resorbing cytokines such as interleukin-1 (IL-1), IL-6, and tumor necrosis factor. Bone resorption associated with estrogen deficiency can be attenuated by administering an IL-1 receptor antagonist or by knocking out the IL-6 gene, findings consistent with this hypothesis. Because estrogen also increases local production of growth factors that stimulate bone formation such as insulin-like growth factor-1 (IGF-1) and transforming growth factor-β (TGF-β), estrogen deficiency might diminish bone formation. Estrogen deficiency increases the skeleton's sensitivity to the resorptive effects of parathyroid hormone (PTH). Estrogen deficiency therefore leads to a small increase in serum calcium levels. According to one hypothesis, increased calcium levels suppress PTH secretion, thereby decreasing renal 1,25-(OH)$_2$ vitamin D formation, which then limits intestinal calcium absorption (Fig. 217–2). Finally, the discovery of estrogen receptors on osteoblasts suggests that estrogen deficiency may also alter bone formation directly.

Once the period of rapid postmenopausal bone loss ends, bone loss continues at a more gradual rate throughout life. The osteope-

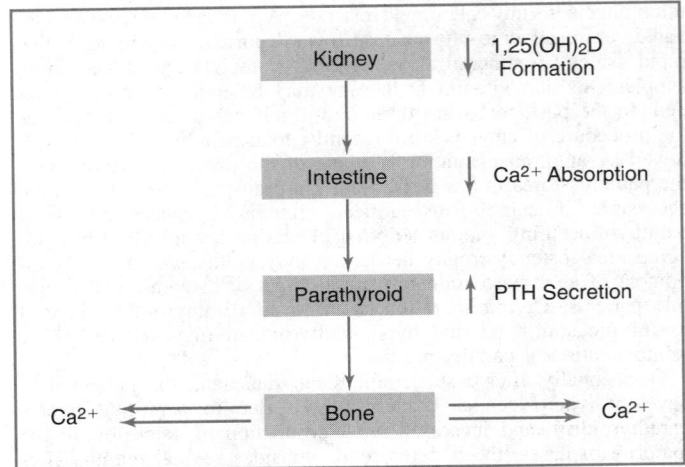

FIGURE 217–3. Physiologic alterations in women with type II ("senile") osteoporosis.

nia that results from normal aging, which occurs in both women and men, has been termed type II or "senile" osteoporosis (Fig. 217–3). Some data suggest that trabecular bone loss ceases after many years of estrogen deficiency but that slow cortical bone loss continues. Because type II osteoporosis is associated with a more balanced decrease in cortical and trabecular bone mass, fractures of the hip, pelvis, wrist, proximal humerus, proximal tibia, and vertebral bodies all occur commonly. Factors that may be important in the pathogenesis of type II osteoporosis include (1) a primary defect in the ability of the kidney to make 1,25-(OH)$_2$D and/or decreased intestinal sensitivity to 1,25-(OH)$_2$D, leading to diminished calcium absorption and mild secondary hyperparathyroidism; and (2) a decrease in osteoblastic bone formation with aging. Finally, the distinctions between type I and type II osteoporosis are often quite arbitrary, and there may be considerable overlap between these syndromes.

SECONDARY CAUSES OF ADULT BONE LOSS. Many disorders can lead to osteoporosis independent of the normal effects of the menopause in women and aging in both women and men (Table 217–2). For example, young women who develop estrogen deficiency due to hyperprolactinemia, anorexia nervosa, or hypothalamic amenorrhea frequently lose bone. Hypogonadism is also an important secondary cause of osteoporosis in men. Other endocrine disorders such as hyperthyroidism, hyperparathyroidism, hypercortisolism, and growth hormone deficiency can cause osteoporosis primarily due to increased bone resorption in the former two disorders and decreased bone formation and intestinal calcium absorption in the latter. Patients with gastrointestinal and hepatobiliary disorders most often have low-turnover osteoporosis, although some have osteomalacia or secondary hyperparathyroidism owing to calcium and/or vitamin D malabsorption. The osteoporosis in patients with marrow-related disorders may be due to local effects of cytokines on bone remodeling or to the release of systemic factors that activate bone resorption. Peak adult bone mass is compromised in certain connective tissue disorders such as osteogenesis imperfecta. Many drugs such as ethanol, heparin, glucocorticoids, suppressive doses of thyroxine, and anticonvulsants can cause osteoporosis. Ethanol is toxic to osteoblasts, whereas heparin increases osteoclastic bone resorption. In patients receiving anticonvulsant therapy, the combined effects of reduced 25(OH)D levels, secondary hyperparathyroidism, direct inhibition of intestinal calcium transport, and suppression of osteoblast function can lead to osteoporosis and/or osteomalacia. Bone resorption is accelerated in patients who are immobilized and in patients with rheumatoid arthritis. Finally, bone formation may be diminished in individuals with insulin-dependent diabetes mellitus.

CLINICAL MANIFESTATIONS

Osteoporosis is asymptomatic unless it results in a fracture—usually a vertebral compression fracture or a fracture of the wrist, hip, ribs, pelvis, or humerus. Vertebral compression fractures often occur with minimal stress, such as with sneezing, bending, or lift-

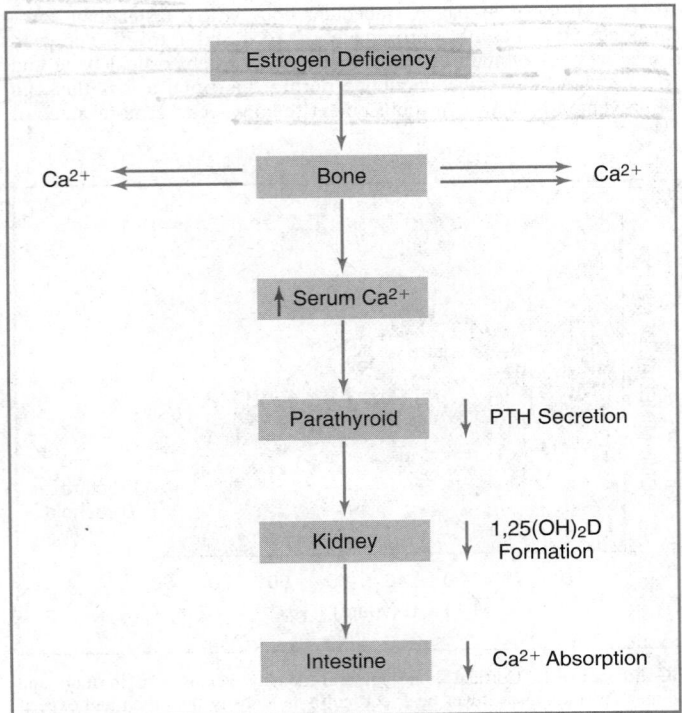

FIGURE 217–2. Physiologic alterations in women with type I ("postmenopausal") osteoporosis.

TABLE 217-2. SECONDARY CAUSES OF OSTEOPOROSIS

Endocrine diseases
  Female hypogonadism
    Hyperprolactinemia
    Hypothalamic amenorrhea
    Anorexia nervosa
    Premature and primary ovarian failure
  Male hypogonadism
    Primary gonadal failure (e.g., Klinefelter's syndrome)
    Secondary gonadal failure (e.g., idiopathic hypogonadotropic hypogonadism)
    Delayed puberty
  Hyperthyroidism
  Hyperparathyroidism
  Hypercortisolism
  Growth hormone deficiency
Gastrointestinal diseases
  Subtotal gastrectomy
  Malabsorption syndromes
  Chronic obstructive jaundice
  Primary biliary cirrhosis and other cirrhoses
  Alactasia
Bone marrow disorders
  Multiple myeloma
  Lymphoma
  Leukemia
  Hemolytic anemias
  Systemic mastocytosis
  Disseminated carcinoma
Connective tissue diseases
  Osteogenesis imperfecta
  Ehlers-Danlos syndrome
  Marfan's syndrome
  Homocystinuria
Drugs
  Alcohol
  Heparin
  Glucocorticoids
  Thyroxine
  Anticonvulsants
  GnRH agonists
  Cyclosporine
  Chemotherapy
Miscellaneous causes
  Immobilization
  Rheumatoid arthritis

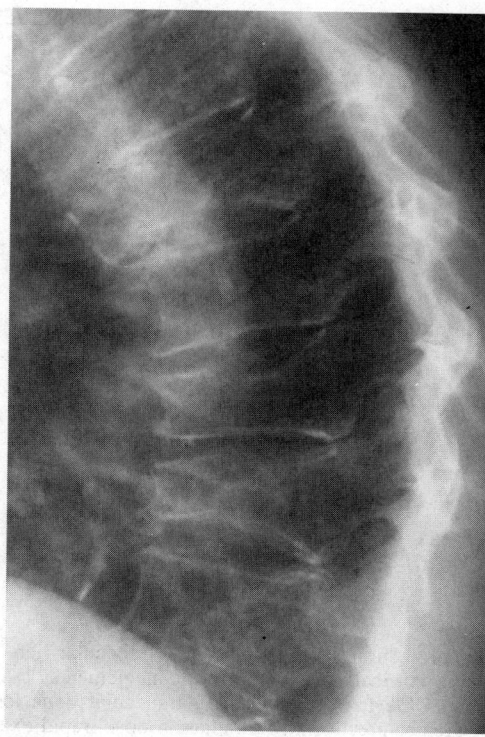

FIGURE 217-4. Radiograph showing radiolucency, compression fractures, and kyphosis in the spine of an osteoporosis patient.

terior and posterior height), anterior wedging (reduction in anterior height), or the so-called codfish deformity (due to weakening of the subchondral plates and expansion of the intervertebral discs). Protrusion of the intervertebral discs in the vertebral bodies produces "Schmorl's nodules." In the absence of fractures, radiographs are insensitive indicators of bone loss because a substantial reduction in bone mass is required before it is visible on radiographs.

DIAGNOSIS

The diagnosis of osteopenia can be made by either documenting a typical fragility fracture or measuring bone mineral density, in which case a bone density value below the lower limit of normal for sex-matched young adults establishes the diagnosis. Most individuals with osteopenia have osteoporosis, although only a histomorphometric analysis of bone can distinguish osteoporosis from osteomalacia with certainty. Several techniques are available for measuring bone mineral density in the axial and appendicular skeleton (Table 217-3). Large prospective studies have demonstrated that bone density measurements of the distal and proximal radius, os calcis, proximal femur, or spine can predict the development of the major types of osteoporotic fractures, including hip fractures. However, the techniques differ greatly in their sensitivity for detecting osteopenia, reproducibility, radiation exposure, examination time, and cost. Because it measures trabecular bone in the vertebral bodies, quantitative computed tomography (QCT) of the spine is the most sensitive method for diagnosing osteopenia. However, because the expense and radiation dose of QCT are high and its reproducibility is relatively poor, it is not an ideal technique when repeat measurements aimed at detecting small changes in bone density are needed. Single-photon absorptiometry of the proximal forearm has good precision and low radiation exposure but is relatively insensitive for detecting osteopenia because it measures cortical bone, which is lost more slowly than trabecular bone in the early menopause. Dual-photon absorptiometry (DPA), which measures bone density in the axial skeleton and proximal femur, is limited by poor reproducibility, long examination times, and artifacts caused by vascular calcifications and changes in the radioactive source. For most patients, dual energy x-ray absorptiometry (DXA) of the lumbar spine is currently the method of choice for measuring bone mineral density. Because DXA scans of the spine in the an-

ing a light object. The middle and lower thoracic and upper lumbar regions are most frequently involved. Back pain usually begins acutely and often radiates laterally to the flanks and anteriorly. The pain subsides gradually over a period of several weeks and recurs with the occurrence of new fractures. Patients with multiple fractures that result in spinal deformity may have a chronic backache that is made worse by standing. Such patients lose height and may develop the characteristic dorsal kyphosis and cervical lordosis known as the "dowager's hump." In some patients, vertebral collapse can occur slowly and without symptoms. Hip fractures are the most devastating complication of osteoporosis. They are of the femoral neck and intertrochanteric types, and the type is best predicted by the bone density of the trochanter. Hip fractures are associated with falls, occurring either as a result of modest trauma, or, in some instances, prior to the fall. The likelihood of suffering a hip fracture during a fall is also related to the direction of the fall so that fractures are more likely to occur in falls to the side, probably because less soft tissue is available to dissipate the impact. Secondary complications of hip fractures, such as pulmonary thromboembolism or nosocomial infections, carry a mortality rate of 15 to 20% in elderly patients and an additional 30% of hip fracture victims require long-term nursing home care.

RADIOGRAPHIC FINDINGS

A characteristic radiograph of osteoporosis of the spine is shown in Figure 217-4. With the loss of trabecular bone in the vertebral bodies, the vertebral end-plates appear to be accentuated. Loss of horizontal trabeculae causes the vertical trabeculae to be more prominent. The normal contrast between the radiodensity of the spinal column and the adjacent soft tissues also may be lost. Vertebral deformity may take the form of collapse (reduction in both an-

TABLE 217-3. TECHNIQUES FOR MEASURING BONE MINERAL DENSITY

Sites Measured	Precision (%)	Accuracy (%)	Scan Time (minutes)	Radiation Dose (mrem)
Quantitative computed tomography (QCT)	2–10	5–20	10–15	100–1000
Lumbar spine				
Proximal radius				
Distal radius				
Single-photon absorptiometry (SPA)	1–3	4–6	3–5	10–20
Proximal radius				
Distal radius				
Calcaneus				
Dual-photon absorptiometry (DPA)	2–6	4–10	20–40	10–15
Lumbar spine anteroposterior				
Lumbar spine lateral				
Proximal femur				
Total body				
Dual-energy x-ray absorptiometry (DXA)	1–2	3–5	2–8	1–3
Lumbar spine anteroposterior				
Lumbar spine lateral				
Proximal radius				
Distal radius				
Proximal femur				
Total body				

* For SPA, numbers refer to measurements of the proximal radius. For QCT, numbers refer to measurements of the lumbar spine. For DPA and DXA, numbers refer to AP measurements of the lumbar spine.

teroposterior projection include both the trabecular-rich vertebral bodies and the cortical-rich posterior spinal elements, DXA is not as sensitive as QCT for detecting early trabecular bone loss. However, its far greater precision, low radiation dose, rapid examination time, and lower cost make DXA preferable to QCT in most situations. Newer DXA scanners can measure spinal bone mineral density in both the anteroposterior and lateral projections. Lateral spine DXA is more sensitive than anterior-posterior spine DXA for detecting osteoporosis and has similar reproducibility.

Secondary causes of osteoporosis should be sought in patients with an established diagnosis of osteoporosis, particularly when the bone density is significantly lower than that of age- and sex-matched individuals. A history and physical examination that focus on the factors that may affect peak bone mass (see Table 217–1) and secondary causes of osteoporosis (see Table 217–2) and selected laboratory tests are sufficient in most patients. Levels of serum calcium, inorganic phosphate, and alkaline phosphatase are usually normal in patients with osteoporosis, although the latter may be transiently elevated after a fracture. A sustained elevation of the alkaline phosphatase level, in the absence of liver disease, may suggest osteomalacia, Paget's disease, or skeletal metastases. Other routine chemistries can help exclude renal or hepatic diseases, and a complete blood count may help uncover a hematologic or myeloproliferative disorder. Because multiple myeloma can mimic involutional osteoporosis, it should be considered when evaluating patients with osteoporosis, particularly those with severe disease. Measuring serum PTH and 25(OH)D levels is recommended to exclude hyperparathyroidism and vitamin D deficiency. A serum thyroid–stimulating hormone level should be checked when thyroid disease is suspected. In men with unexplained osteoporosis, a serum testosterone level should be measured. The clinical utility of measuring biochemical markers of bone formation (serum osteocalcin, bone-specific alkaline phosphatase, or type 1 procollagen carboxy-terminal propeptide) and bone resorption (urine hydroxyproline, urine pyridinium cross links, or urine cross linked N-telopeptides of type 1 collagen) has not been established. However, it is possible that these markers may help classify patients into high and low bone turnover states in the future and thereby provide a more rational basis for selecting therapies. Finally, in selected patients, iliac crest bone biopsy after double tetracycline labeling may be useful, particularly for distinguishing osteoporosis from osteomalacia.

TREATMENT

At present, it is not possible to reverse established osteoporosis. However, early intervention can prevent osteoporosis in most people, and later intervention can halt its progression once it has developed. The choice of treatment for osteoporosis depends on its cause and the stage of the illness. If a secondary cause of osteoporosis is present, specific treatment should be aimed at correcting it. During the acute phase of vertebral compression, attention is directed toward relieving pain with analgesics, muscle relaxants, heat, massage, and/or rest. Many patients with discomfort related to osteoporotic fractures or deformity benefit from a well-designed program of physical therapy. Some patients appear to benefit from a corset or an orthopedic back brace. Both weight-bearing and non–weight-bearing exercises appear to have beneficial effects on bone mass. For most patients, exercises to strengthen the abdominal and back muscles are appropriate and referral to a physical therapist with expertise in treating osteoporotic patients is often helpful. Precautions to prevent falls should be taken. Pharmacologic therapy is aimed at preventing further bone loss and decreasing the likelihood of future fracture.

CALCIUM. Both dietary calcium intake and fractional intestinal calcium absorption decrease with age. Most postmenopausal women consume <500 mg of calcium each day, far below the U.S. recommended dietary allowance (RDA) of 800 to 1000 mg. The effects of calcium supplementation on bone mass in early menopausal women have been examined in several prospective, randomized trials. The results are inconsistent. In general, it appears that calcium can retard, but not arrest, cortical bone loss from the forearm in women who are within the first several years of the menopause. However, calcium supplementation is clearly less effective than estrogen. Most studies have failed to demonstrate a protective effect of calcium on spinal bone loss in early menopausal women. Calcium therapy appears to be more effective in arresting bone loss in late menopausal women, although some studies indicate that administering calcium does not halt their bone loss completely. Overall, it appears that calcium therapy is somewhat beneficial in both early and late menopausal women. However, additional therapy clearly is needed if the goal of therapy is to prevent bone loss completely. Most experts recommend that postmenopausal women consume between 1000 and 1200 mg of calcium per day, either in their diet or from supplements. Because calcium may enhance peak bone mass, the RDA for adolescents and young adults in the United States is 1500 mg of calcium per day.

ESTROGEN. Estrogen replacement therapy inhibits osteoclastic bone resorption. It prevents both cortical and trabecular bone loss in estrogen-deficient women and is effective if administered orally or topically. Estrogen replacement therapy prevents bone loss in both early and late menopausal women, although its efficacy has not been tested adequately in women over age 75. Because bone loss is most rapid in the first years of the menopause, the benefits of estrogen therapy probably are greater if started before a substantial amount of bone loss has occurred. Case-control studies suggest that estrogen therapy significantly reduces the risk of forearm, vertebral, pelvic, and hip fractures in postmenopausal women. The minimally effective doses of estrogen to prevent bone loss are 0.625 mg per day of conjugated estrogens, 2 mg per day of estradiol, 25 μg per day of ethinyl estradiol, or 50 μg per day of transdermal estrogen, although some studies have shown that lower doses of conjugated estrogens (0.3 mg per day) prevent bone loss when combined with sufficient calcium intake. How long a women should remain on estrogen replacement therapy has not been established.

Although the beneficial effects of estrogen replacement therapy on bone mass are well established, <15% of postmenopausal women in the United States take estrogen replacement. The decision to treat with estrogen is influenced by several other factors and should be individualized. In some women, estrogen is prescribed to alleviate menopausal symptoms. In others, the prospect of adhering to a treatment program that will produce cyclic menstruation is unacceptable. The relationships between estrogen replacement therapy and endometrial cancer, breast cancer, and ischemic heart disease have been the subjects of numerous investigations. When given without concomitant progestin, estrogen replacement therapy increases the risk of endometrial carcinoma. Thus, in the woman whose uterus is intact, estrogen replacement therapy should be combined with a progestin, administered either cyclically (e.g., 5 to 10 mg medroxyprogesterone acetate for 10 to 14 days each month) or continuously (e.g., 2.5 mg medroxyprogesterone acetate per day). The latter regimen often eliminates menstrual bleeding after an initial period of 3 to 6 months during which irregular bleeding may occur. Progestins may also enhance the osteoprotective effect of estrogens. In the woman who has had a hysterectomy, unopposed estrogen should be given daily. Estrogen therapy is contraindicated in women with a history of endometrial cancer.

The relationships between estrogen replacement therapy and breast cancer or cardiovascular disease have been the subject of many case-control and cohort studies yet they remain unclear. Although authors of one meta-analysis concluded that long-term (>15 years) estrogen use is associated with an increase in the risk of breast cancer, other large cohort studies have failed to detect such a relationship. It has also been suggested that the risk of developing breast cancer is increased in women who take higher doses of estrogen (at least 1.25 mg of conjugated estrogen) and among women with a family history of breast cancer. Because the relationship between estrogen replacement therapy and breast cancer remains uncertain, estrogen replacement therapy is contraindicated in women with a history of breast cancer, and all postmenopausal women receiving estrogen therapy should have regular breast examinations and annual mammograms. Numerous case-control and cohort studies have reported that estrogen replacement therapy decreases the risk of major coronary disease by approximately 50%. However, the potential for bias due to patient selection or uneven diagnostic surveillance in these nonrandomized studies cannot be excluded completely. The potential beneficial effect of estrogen on coronary heart disease is often attributed to its ability to lower LDL cholesterol and raise HDL cholesterol. Still, because the reduction in cardiac events appears to be limited to current estrogen users and is independent of the duration of estrogen use, other mechanisms, including direct effects of estrogens on vascular wall function and coagulation factors, may be important.

CALCITONIN. Calcitonin inhibits osteoclastic bone resorption and is approved by the Food and Drug Administration (FDA) for treating postmenopausal osteoporosis. The effects of calcitonin therapy on bone loss in women who are within 5 years of the menopause have been inconsistent. Some groups have demonstrated that nasal calcitonin prevents spinal bone loss for up to 3 years while others have been unable to demonstrate such an effect. The reasons for these disparities are unclear. Calcitonin appears to prevent spinal bone loss in late menopausal women, although appendicular (i.e., cortical) bone loss continues. The effect of calcitonin therapy on the rate of osteoporotic fractures has not been well studied. At the present time, calcitonin is available only for parenteral use in the United States, although it is available as a nasal spray in some other countries. The recommended dose is 100 IU subcutaneously daily, given with adequate calcium and vitamin D, but it is possible that lower doses are equally effective. Side effects of parenteral calcitonin administration, including nausea, flushing, and local inflammatory reactions, occur in 10 to 15% of patients and can often be minimized by administering the medication at bedtime, starting at low doses (i.e., 25 IU) and increasing the dosage gradually over a period of several weeks. Calcitonin also appears to produce significant analgesic effects. Thus, it may be particularly useful in patients with osteoporosis who have chronic pain related to fractures or skeletal deformity.

BISPHOSPHONATES. Like calcitonin, bisphosphonates inhibit osteoclastic bone resorption. The only bisphosphonate that is currently available for oral administration in the United States is etidronate, although it has not yet been approved by the FDA for treating osteoporosis. Several other bisphosphonates are currently under investigation. Prospective studies have demonstrated that cyclic etidronate increases spinal bone mineral density slightly and decreases the incidence of vertebral fractures in late menopausal women when given for 2 to 3 years. However, further follow-up of these patients indicates that the previously reported beneficial effect of etidronate on fracture rate may be restricted to a subgroup of women at particularly high risk for fracture. Because the total number of fractures in these studies was small, it is difficult to draw firm conclusions regarding the effect of cyclic etidronate on osteoporotic fractures. The most commonly employed dose of etidronate is 400 mg per day for the first 2 weeks of every 3-month period. To ensure adequate absorption, it must be taken on an empty stomach.

The effects of bisphosphonates on bone loss in early menopausal women are less well studied. Short-term studies suggest that oral alendronate, tiludronate, and etidronate administration can prevent spinal bone loss in recently menopausal women.

VITAMIN D AND ITS METABOLITES. Calcium absorption decreases with age, especially after age 70. Because of low vitamin D intake, insufficient exposure to sunlight, and reduced ability to synthesize vitamin D in the skin, many elderly people are at risk for vitamin D deficiency. Furthermore, the ability to convert 25(OH)D to 1,25-(OH)$_2$D is impaired in many elderly people. Decreased vitamin D formation and calcium absorption in the elderly may lead to secondary hyperparathyroidism and accelerated bone loss.

Small doses of vitamin D (800 IU per day) plus calcium dramatically reduce the incidence of hip fractures and other nonspine fractures in elderly women. Because toxicity from such doses of vitamin D has not been reported, this therapy can be recommended to virtually all postmenopausal women. The role of 1,25-(OH)$_2$D therapy in postmenopausal osteoporosis is more controversial. At high doses (0.8 μg per day), 1,25-(OH)$_2$D plus calcium increases bone mass, but most patients develop hypercalciuria and/or hypercalcemia. At doses of 0.5 to 0.6 μg per day, 1,25-(OH)$_2$D plus calcium preserves spinal bone mass and decreases the rate of both vertebral and nonvertebral fractures with little toxicity. However, it is unclear whether 1,25-(OH)$_2$D therapy is superior to treatment with small doses of vitamin D. Because the therapeutic index of 1,25-(OH)$_2$D therapy is small, its use should probably be reserved for patients who are not candidates for other forms of pharmacologic therapy.

FUTURE THERAPIES. Several new types of therapeutic agents are currently in clinical trials. Antiestrogens such as tamoxifen can prevent spinal bone loss in postmenopausal women. Newer antiestrogens, which may have bone-sparing effects without causing endometrial hyperplasia, are being investigated. It is well known that sodium fluoride increases spinal bone density. However, the newly formed bone is qualitatively abnormal and cortical bone density sometimes decreases. A randomized controlled trial demonstrated that sodium fluoride therapy failed to reduce the risk of vertebral fractures and actually increased the incidence of fractures of the appendicular skeleton. However, lower doses of fluoride therapy and sustained-release preparations hold more promise and are under investigation. PTH, when given intermittently in low doses, is a potent stimulator of osteoblastic bone formation. In contrast to sodium fluoride, the bone formed in response to administered PTH is histologically normal and its strength is increased. Many animal studies have demonstrated that PTH can prevent or reverse estrogen-deficiency osteoporosis. Similar data have now been obtained in early human studies. Further investigation of the therapeutic potential of PTH is needed.

OSTEOPOROSIS IN MEN

Although osteoporosis is less common in men, men lose about 30% of trabecular bone and 20% of cortical bone during the course of their lifetime. By extreme old age, one in every six men has a hip fracture. Between 15 and 25% of men with hip or vertebral fractures are androgen deficient. Androgens have important effects on skeletal development. Peak bone mass is reduced in men who were androgen deficient during adolescence due to idiopathic hypogonadotropic hypogonadism or Klinefelter's syndrome and in men with histories of constitutionally delayed puberty (see Ch. 209). In adult men, castration or induction of androgen deficiency with long-acting GnRH analogues increases bone resorption and leads to rapid bone loss. Osteoporosis is also frequently observed in men with primary gonadal failure, hemochromatosis, hyperprolactinemic hypogonadism, or other disorders of the pituitary-hypothalamic axis.

Androgens may stimulate bone formation directly because osteoblastic cells possess androgen receptors. Androgens stimulate osteoblastic cell proliferation and differentiation, an effect that may be mediated by TGF-β or fibroblast growth factor. Like estrogens, androgens may inhibit bone resorption through mechanisms that involve alterations in the local production of bone-resorbing cytokines such as IL-1 and IL-6. In the majority of eugonadal osteoporotic men, bone formation and osteoblastic cell proliferation are decreased.

Other than androgen deficiency, secondary causes of osteoporosis in men are similar to those in women. Epidemiologic studies suggest that prior glucocorticoid use, gastric resection, and ethanol abuse are among the most common identifiable causes of osteoporosis in men.

In men with androgen-deficiency osteoporosis, androgen replacement is usually indicated, although beneficial effects on bone mass have been demonstrated only in men with hyperprolactinemic hypogonadism and idiopathic hypogonadotropic hypogonadism. A notable exception, however, is men with prostatic carcinoma in whom androgen replacement is contraindicated. In men with primary gonadal failure, testosterone replacement can be administered either parenterally or transdermally. In men with secondary hypogonadism, treatment with human chorionic gonadotropin or pulsatile GnRH may also be considered. The efficacy of antiresorptive agents such as calcitonin or bisphosphonates has not been investigated.

GLUCOCORTICOID-INDUCED BONE LOSS

Bone loss is a common complication of glucocorticoid excess, whether due to endogenous Cushing's syndrome or exogenous glucocorticoids. The most important adverse effects of glucocorticoids on bone metabolism appear to be suppressed osteoblast activity and a vitamin D–independent inhibition of intestinal calcium absorption. Enhanced osteoclastic activity may also be important. The ability of glucocorticoids to suppress bone formation appears to be mediated, at least in part, by suppression of local secretion of IGF-1 in bone.

The predominant effect of glucocorticoids on the skeleton is a loss of trabecular bone, although cortical bone mass also decreases. Bone loss is most rapid in the first 6 to 12 months of therapy, but accelerated bone loss appears to continue as long as therapy is continued.

Because the bone loss associated with glucocorticoids is largely irreversible, the decision to administer them should be made carefully. The dosage should be maintained as low as possible. If glucocorticoid therapy is expected to continue for several months or longer, treatment to prevent bone loss should be considered, particularly in estrogen-deficient women and when a high dosage of glucocorticoids is needed. Small studies have suggested that either calcitonin or bisphosphonates may prevent spinal bone loss in patients receiving long-term glucocorticoid therapy. Studies of the effects of vitamin D and its metabolites on glucocorticoid-induced bone loss have produced inconsistent results. Nonetheless, a recent controlled study demonstrated that 0.5 to 1.0 μg of calcitriol plus 1000 mg of calcium per day can prevent spinal bone loss for at least 1 year in patients who are starting treatment with glucocorticoids. However, because of the potential for hypercalciuria and/or hypercalcemia, patients receiving calcitriol therapy require careful monitoring. Calcitriol therapy seems most logical in patients with low urinary calcium excretion, suggesting poor intestinal absorption of calcium, and should be avoided in patients with hypercalciuria. Physiologic vitamin D replacement (400 IU per day) can be safely recommended in all patients receiving glucocorticoids. Calcium supplementation (1000 mg per day) should be added unless the urinary calcium excretion is excessive.

Christiansen CC (ed.): Consensus Development Conference on Osteoporosis. Am J Med 95(5A):1S, 1993. *Short, current reviews on such important issues in osteoporosis as the value of bone densitometry and use of biochemical markers of bone turnover in assessing osteoporosis, and reviews of major current therapies as well as potential future treatment strategies.*

Jackson JA, Kleerekoper M: Osteoporosis in men: Diagnosis, pathophysiology and prevention. Medicine 69:137, 1990. *The only comprehensive review of this topic.*

Lukert BP, Raisz LG: Glucocorticoid-induced osteoporosis: Pathogenesis and management. Ann Intern Med 112:352, 1990. *A thorough, well-balanced review of the pathogenesis and management of glucocorticoid-induced osteoporosis. Most important references are cited.*

Neer RM: Osteoporosis. In DeGroot LJ (ed.): Endocrinology. Philadelphia, WB Saunders, 1994, pp 1228–1258. *A thorough, scholarly review that carefully discusses the limitations of many prior studies. Virtually every significant reference is cited.*

Riggs BL, Melton LJ III: The prevention and treatment of osteoporosis. N Engl J Med 327:620, 1992. *A concise, up-to-date review of practical therapeutic options for women with postmenopausal osteoporosis.*

218 PAGET'S DISEASE OF BONE (Osteitis Deformans)
John A. Kanis

DEFINITION. Paget's disease of bone is a focal disorder of skeletal metabolism in which all the elements of skeletal remodeling (resorption, formation, and mineralization) are increased. Increased bone formation results in the disorganized assembly of collagen, giving rise to bony enlargement and deformity.

ETIOLOGY. The cause is unknown. A viral infection of osteoclasts is postulated on the basis of finding viral nucleocapsids of the paramyxoviridae in affected osteoclasts. Such findings are, however, not specific and are seen in some other rare disorders of bone turnover (pycnodysostosis and some cases of osteopetrosis [see Ch. 219]). Canine distemper is one of the paramyxoviridae, and an association between owning dogs and Paget's disease has been reported. A positive family history in approximately 10% of patients suggests a dominant pattern of susceptibility, with weak associations with the HLA Dqw1 antigens in the United States and with A9 and B15 in the United Kingdom (see Ch. 229).

PREVALENCE AND EPIDEMIOLOGY. Paget's disease is the second most common disorder of bone, outstripped only by osteoporosis. It is most commonly found in the United Kingdom, where the prevalence is 5% of the population over age 55 and is roughly equal between genders. The frequency of symptomatic disease rises with age. There is, however, little evidence for the occurrence of new lesions in symptomatic disease. This suggests a high modal incidence in early middle-age, which declines rapidly thereafter, but with a variable latency between the onset of the disorder and its radiographic or clinical expression.

Although most common in the United Kingdom, it is also common in countries such as Australia, New Zealand, South Africa, and the United States, where significant British immigration occurred in the past, but occurs with a lower frequency in native-born individuals than in immigrants. The disorder is extremely rare in the Nordic countries, the Arab Middle-East, China, and Japan and among Australian Aboriginals. Intermediate rates are found in France, Germany, Italy, and Spain. There is some evidence that the incidence of Paget's disease is falling in the United Kingdom and in the United States.

PATHOPHYSIOLOGY AND HISTOPATHOLOGY. The disease is characterized by increased metabolic activity of bone surfaces. Bone remodeling normally occupies 10 to 15% of bone surfaces, and at affected sites this may be increased 5- to 10-fold. Osteoclast numbers are increased, as is their size, and they may contain up to 100 nuclei. Osteoclast competence is decreased, but their plethora result in an increase in bone resorption with crenated resorption cavities subsequently in-filled by the activity of osteoblasts. The irregular cement lines give rise to a mosaic patchwork appearance at bone histology. New bone that is formed is often woven rather than lamellar and is structurally less competent and occupies more space. Mineralization rates are normal, but because abnormally large volumes of bone are undergoing mineralization, the surface covered with unmineralized osteoid is increased. Marrow fibrosis and hypervascularity are also features.

Remodeling throughout the cortex increases its porosity and blurs the distinction between cortical and cancellous bone. An imbalance between formation and resorption characteristically results in increased bone size and deformity.

CLINICAL AND LABORATORY MANIFESTATIONS. The extent of disease involvement is markedly heterogeneous. It may involve only one bone. More frequently, multiple sites are involved, typically in an asymmetric distribution. The most common sites are the pelvis, lumbar spine, and femur; one or more of these sites are affected in more than 75% of cases.

More than 95% of patients with Paget's disease are asymptomatic. The most common problems encountered are bone pain, skeletal deformity, and fracture (Table 218–1). Apart from fracture, the onset is insidious and 30% of patients have had symptoms at presentation for more than 10 years. It may be difficult to distinguish bone pain arising from Paget's disease from that due to arthritis, particularly of the hip and the spine. Deformity is a presenting complaint in one fifth of patients. Obvious bone enlargement is seen, particularly in the limbs and also in the skull and facial bones. Bone enlargement contributes significantly to the neurologic complications and more uncertainly to joint disease. The most frequent deformity of long bones is bowing, which is characteristically lateral in the case of the femur and anterior in the case of the tibia.

The incidence of fissure fractures is significantly greater in patients with bowing. Fissure fractures may be symptomatic and may herald complete fractures, but many patients have indolent pain, particularly on weight bearing associated with local tenderness. Complete fractures of the long bones occur most commonly in the femur, followed by the tibia and the forearm, which together account for up to 90% of pathologic fractures of long bones. They commonly follow trivial injury, and, unlike in osteoporosis, femoral fractures are less frequently cervical and more usually subtrochanteric or involve the shaft.

Neurologic complications are common and are among the more serious clinical problems. A variety of neurologic problems arise from platybasia. Cranial disease also results in deafness, vertigo, and tinintus. Spinal syndromes most frequently occur when Paget's disease affects the thoracic spine. They are usually associated with enlarged vertebrae and decreased diameter of the spinal canal with cord or root compression. Also, the highly vascular pagetic bone may divert the blood supply from neural tissue.

Cardiac output may be increased and give rise to high-output failure in patients with extensive disease when ≥30% of the skeleton is involved. Sarcoma arising in pagetic bone is rare but is a serious complication of the disorder, accounting for most cases of sarcoma in the population aged 50 or older. The pelvis and femora are common sites followed by the humerus, face, and skull. Benign and malignant giant cell tumors may also occur. New pain developing in a patient with long-standing Paget's disease not attributable to microfractures should arouse a high degree of suspicion. Other presentations include the development of a large mass or pathologic fracture.

Radiographic Features. The early phase of osteolytic activity is sometimes seen clearly in the skull as osteoporosis circumscripta or as a V-shaped advancing front in a long bone. A second mixed phase shows evidence of patchy osteolysis and sclerosis which is the most common radiographic finding. The third phase is that of predominant bone sclerosis (Fig. 218–1). Thickening of the cortices is characteristic with enlargement of the long bones (Fig. 218–2). Intracortical resorption results in a loss of the corticomedullary junction and accentuation of trabecular markings. The combination of all these features is virtually diagnostic, so that bone biopsy is rarely required. The average patient has six lesions affecting 14% of the skeleton. In approximately 10 to 20% of symptomatic patients, the disorder is mono-ostotic. As a general rule, scintigraphy is more sensitive than radiography, but 2 to 3% of radiographically overt lesions may not be associated with increased scintigraphic uptake (so-called burnt-out Paget's disease).

The pelvis is the most common site affected; evidence is found in approximately two thirds of patients. Narrowing of the joint space of the hip is common. Most patients show medial or concentric narrowing of the joint space; degenerative osteoarthrosis more frequently causes narrowing of the superior aspect. Computed tomography is also useful to assess the cause of pain at the spine and in the investigation for osteosarcoma.

Biochemical Manifestations. Extracellular calcium homeostasis is almost invariably normal, despite the massive increase in bone turnover. Hypercalciuria and more rarely hypercalcemia may occur with prolonged immobilization or fracture. Serum activity of alkaline phosphatase, in part derived from osteoblasts, is most often used to measure the extent of skeletal involvement. Increased bone resorption can be assessed by the urinary excretion of hydroxyproline, which in Paget's disease is derived largely from the collagen destruction of bone. The urinary excretion of pyridinoline cross-links is a more specific and sensitive marker. In untreated patients there is a close correlation between serum activity of alkaline phosphatase and urinary excretion of hydroxyproline, and both correlate

TABLE 218–1. CLINICAL FEATURES AND COMPLICATIONS OF PAGET'S DISEASE

Common
    Bone pain—pagetic, articular
    Fracture—long bones, vertebral bodies
    Neurologic—deafness
    Deformity and enlargement of bones
Uncommon
    Pain—fissure fracture
    Spinal neurologic syndromes
    Hypercalciuria of immobilization or fracture
    Vascular bleeding from bone during surgery
    Extraskeletal (aortic) calcification
    Osteosarcoma and other bone tumors
Rare
    Cardiovascular disease
    Cranial nerve lesions (except VIII)
    Brain stem and cerebellar lesions
    Hypercalcemia of immobilization
    Extramedullary hematopoiesis
    Epidural hematoma
Significance uncertain
    Gout
    Pseudogout
    Angioid streaks
    Hyperparathyroidism
    Urolithiasis

From Kanis JA: Pathophysiology and Treatment of Paget's Disease of Bone. London, Martin Dunitz, 1991.

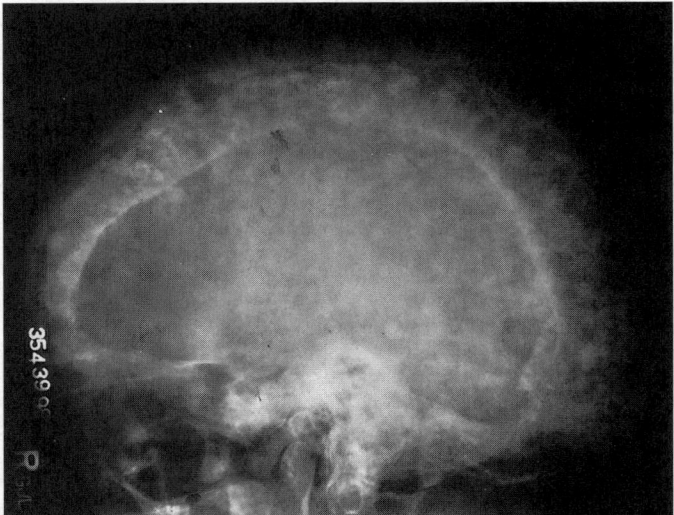

FIGURE 218–1. Advanced involvement of the skull with marked thickening of the entire vault, areas of osteolysis, and patchy new bone formation resulting in a "cotton-wool" appearance.

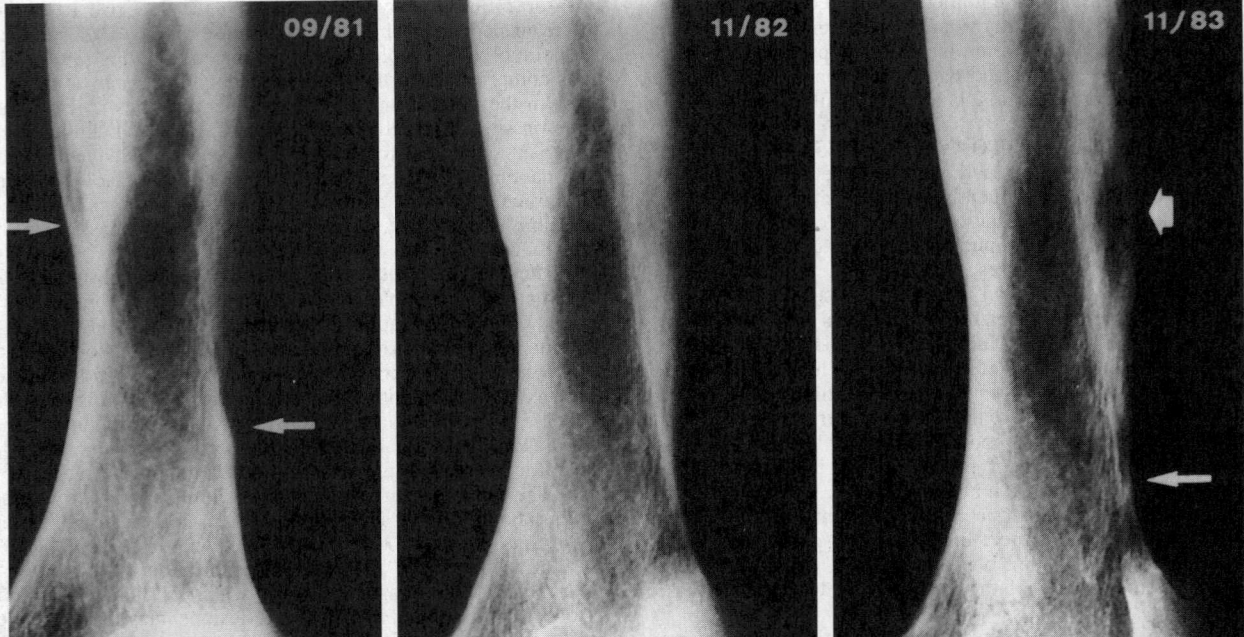

FIGURE 218–2. Sequential radiographs of the distal femur at the dates shown. *Left,* The distinction between Paget's and normal bone *(arrows),* the osteolytic front, and the expansion of bone diameter at the affected site. Treatment with a bisphosphonate–induced *(center)* infilling of the resorption front. Relapse after treatment *(right)* was associated with a new area of osteolysis *(thick arrow)* and progression of the resorption front. (From Kanis JA: Pathophysiology and Treatment of Paget's Disease of Bone. London, Martin Dunitz, 1991.)

with the extent of disease. Up to 10% of patients with symptomatic Paget's disease have values of alkaline phosphatase within the laboratory reference range, and this figure is even higher in the case of hydroxyproline.

TREATMENT. Data are insufficient to recommend medical treatment to asymptomatic patients, except in the presence of rapidly advancing osteolytic disease in the long bones of the lower limb where the risk of pathologic fracture is high. Medical treatment has centered on specific inhibitors of osteoclast-mediated bone resorption, including the bisphosphonates, calcitonins, mithramycin, and gallium nitrate.

Calcitonins. A variety of calcitonins have been used. The most common is synthetic salmon calcitonin (salcatonin), which may be given by subcutaneous injection, 50 to 100 units daily or on alternate days. In several European countries salcatonin is available as a nasal spray. Treatment results in an early decrease in bone resorption, which can be monitored by the fall in urinary excretion of hydroxyproline, and after several weeks a decrease in the serum activity of alkaline phosphatase. On average, these indices fall to 40 to 50% of pretreatment values. Treatment is associated with relief of bone pain, healing of osteolytic lesions, decreased cardiac output, and improvement of neurologic disease. Deafness is rarely reversed, but progression may be prevented.

Disease activity recurs once treatment is stopped, so if long-term control is required, calcitonin must be given indefinitely. In the case of bone pain, relief may occur for many months or years after treatment is stopped, so intermittent treatment is worthwhile. The escape phenomenon describes failure to maintain a biochemical response despite continued treatment or even increasing the dose. In some cases this acquired resistance appears to be associated with the development of salcatonin antibodies, in which case a biochemical response is elicited with an alternative calcitonin. No serious side effects of calcitonin are reported, but up to one third of patients develop transient nausea or flushing, and in 5 to 10% of patients long-term treatment cannot be tolerated.

Bisphosphonates. These pyrophosphate analogues are adsorbed onto hydroxyapatite, particularly at sites of resorption. As with calcitonin, an early effect of treatment is to decrease bone resorption, followed by a later decrease in bone formation, as marked by alkaline phosphatase. Etidronate is widely available and used at a dose of 5 mg per kilogram of body weight daily for up to 6 months. Disease activity is suppressed by approximately 50% from

initial values. Pain relief occurs, but radiographic improvement is unusual. Higher than recommended doses induce more complete responses but increase the risk of impairing mineralization of bone and should be avoided. Occasionally, bone pain may be associated with recommended doses, in which case treatment should be stopped. Intravenous treatment regimens with etidronate and other bisphosphonates are widely available in Europe. These include clodronate, alendronate, and pamidronate, but these drugs have not been approved by the FDA as of publication. They have, however, no adverse effect on the mineralization of bone, and their effects on disease activity, symptoms, and radiographic abnormalities (see Fig. 218–2) are more complete than in the case of the calcitonins or etidronate. Other nonapproved treatments include mithramycin, gallium nitrate, and the combination of calcium with thiazide diuretics.

Surgical Management. Elective surgery is often undertaken with effective medical treatment because this decreases bone vascularity and provides a more normal environment for prosthetic implants. Apart from fractures, the most common indication for surgery is joint disease at the hip. In the case of hip pain and some of the spinal neurologic syndromes, surgery can be avoided by medical treatment. Osteotomy has a role in managing deformities or the pain associated with fissure fractures in the presence of deformity.

PROGNOSIS. Pagetic bone pain almost invariably responds to medical treatment. In practice it may be difficult to distinguish pain due to Paget's disease from pain due to coexisting osteoarthropathy or joint pain arising from deformity. In patients in whom pain at the hip is not controlled by analgesics or specific treatment, replacement arthroplasty is the treatment of choice.

Long-term treatment results in the resumption of lamellar bone formation, and in the case of the calcitonins and newer bisphosphonates, more normal radiographic appearances. Overall, there appears to be a good correlation between the degree of biochemical control and attaining clinical improvement, so that biochemical monitoring of disease activity is of value. Decreased bone enlargement and deformity have been reported following long-term treatment with the bisphosphonates. Effective medical management improves spinal neurologic syndromes when these are slowly progressive. The long-term results are as good as those from surgery without the mortality of the latter. The rate of neurologic improvement seen with drug treatment is often more rapid than can be accounted for by remodeling of bone but is due to a decrease in soft tissue swelling and a redistribution of blood flow.

No good evidence indicates that medical treatment significantly alters the natural history of fissure fractures. These may be indolent, occasionally giving rise to pain and complete fracture. Limited experience suggests that in these patients pain decreases following osteotomy. Pathologic fractures of long bones generally heal well, but there is a higher than normal incidence of delayed union and nonunion. The occurrence of fracture provides an opportunity to correct deformity when managed either conservatively or with surgery. Long-term treatment may decrease the frequency of pathologic fracture, but this has not been assessed by long-term prospective studies.

The prognosis of patients with osteosarcoma is extremely poor, and no evidence indicates that medical treatment alters its natural history. Indeed, the role of radiation therapy, chemotherapy, or surgical intervention is not established except for symptomatic treatment.

Anderson DC: Paget's disease. *In* Mundy GR, Martin TJ (eds.): Physiology and Pharmacology of Bone. New York, Springer-Verlag, 1993, p 419. *A general account of Paget's disease.*

Kanis JA: Pathophysiology and Treatment of Paget's Disease of Bone. London, Martin Dunitz, 1991. *A comprehensive monograph of Paget's disease of bone.*

Singer FR, Wallach S (eds.): Paget's Disease of Bone: Clinical Assessment, Present and Future Therapy. New York, Elsevier, 1991. *A collection of review articles and recent abstracts of scientific contributions.*

219 OSTEONECROSIS, OSTEOSCLEROSIS, AND OTHER DISORDERS OF BONE
Michael P. Whyte

OSTEONECROSIS

Osteonecrosis (ischemic, aseptic, or avascular necrosis of bone) refers to skeletal *infarction*. Bone infarcts may be asymptomatic, cause self-limited discomfort, or engender painful collapse of subarticular bone and lead to joint destruction.

ETIOLOGY. Many conditions are associated with osteonecrosis (Table 219–1). In adults, the most common causes are long-term glucocorticoid therapy and ethanol abuse, which manifest dose-dependent effects.

PATHOGENESIS. Certain skeletal sites (often subarticular) are susceptible to osteonecrosis but differ for traumatic and nontraumatic processes and in children and adults. *Osteochondrosis* refers to necrosis of ossification centers; more than 50 eponymic types are recorded. The susceptibility of children to osteochondrosis and its pathogenesis are poorly understood. At all ages, the femoral head is especially prone to infarction. Nontraumatic osteonecrosis also commonly affects the femoral condyles, distal tibia, humeral head, and talus. Skeletal infarction may result from blood vessel destruction (e.g., joint dislocation, fracture), obstruction (e.g., thromboemboli, sickle cell disease, fat emboli, caisson disease), or, hypothetically, compression from local expansion of fatty tissue (e.g., ethanol abuse, glucocorticoid treatment, diabetes mellitus). However, symptoms may not occur unless, weeks later, resorption of dead bone during skeletal repair leads to pathologic fracture.

CLINICAL MANIFESTATIONS. Pain occurs acutely when there is skeletal collapse. Chronic arthralgia results from desquamated necrotic tissue and articular destruction.

DIAGNOSIS. Magnetic resonance imaging (MRI), demonstrating marrow edema, is especially sensitive for detecting early osteonecrosis. Bone scintigraphy discloses skeletal reconstitution with or without fracture. Relatively late in the process, radiographs first show patchy areas of osteopenia and osteosclerosis that reflect skeletal repair. A linear subchondral radiolucency (crescent sign) indicates bony collapse.

TREATMENT. Non–weight-bearing is advisable for an affected limb. Decompression by trephine insertion is used for some sites.

TABLE 219–1. CAUSES OF ISCHEMIC NECROSIS OF CARTILAGE AND BONE

Endocrine/Metabolic
  Ethanol abuse
  Glucocorticoid therapy
  Cushing's disease
  Diabetes mellitus
  Hyperuricemia
  Osteomalacia
  Hyperlipidemia
Storage diseases (e.g., Gaucher's disease)
Hemoglobinopathies (e.g., sickle cell disease)
Trauma (e.g., dislocation, fracture)
Dysbaric conditions (e.g., caisson disease)
Collagen vascular disorders
Irradiation
Pancreatitis
Organ transplantation
Hemodialysis
Idiopathic, familial
Burns
Intravascular coagulation

Arthrotomy to remove debris, transpositional osteotomy, arthroplasty, or joint replacement may be necessary.

OSTEOSCLEROSIS

Many conditions are associated with radiographic evidence of increased bone density, i.e., osteosclerosis. Skeletal dysplasias, metabolic disturbances, and a variety of other conditions can cause generalized or focal increases in bone mass (Table 219–2). Osteosclerosis is classified as affecting predominantly trabecular versus cortical bone or both. Osteosclerosis can occur with disturbances in bone growth, modeling (shaping), and/or remodeling (turnover).

Trabecular Osteosclerosis

Neoplastic, hematologic, and metabolic disorders may preferentially sclerose trabecular bone because it houses marrow and remodels more rapidly than cortical bone.

Cortical Osteosclerosis

PROGRESSIVE DIAPHYSEAL DYSPLASIA (CAMURATI-ENGELMANN DISEASE). This developmental disorder affects all races and is transmitted as an autosomal dominant trait with variable penetrance. New bone formation gradually involves both the periosteal and endosteal surface of long bone diaphyses. With severe disease, osteosclerosis also affects the axial skeleton.

Etiology and Pathogenesis. The gene defect has not been mapped. Osteoblast differentiation may be abnormal.

Clinical Presentation. During childhood there is limping or a broad-based and waddling gait. Muscular dystrophy can be diagnosed erroneously. Severely affected persons have a characteristic body habitus featuring an enlarged head with prominent forehead, proptosis, and thin limbs with little subcutaneous fat or muscle mass and tender thickened bones. Cranial nerve palsies and raised intracranial pressure can occur. Some patients have hepatosplenomegaly, Raynaud's phenomenon, and additional findings suggestive of vasculitis. Symptoms sometimes remit during or after puberty.

Diagnosis. Somewhat symmetric and irregular cortical hyperostosis of major long bone diaphyses slowly develops from periosteal and endosteal new bone formation. Femora and tibiae are most commonly affected. Metaphyses may become involved. Age of onset, rate of progression, and severity are variable. Clinical, radiologic, and bone scan findings are generally concordant. Routine biochemical parameters of bone and mineral metabolism are typically normal. Serum alkaline phosphatase activity, urinary hydroxyproline levels, and the erythrocyte sedimentation rate can be elevated. Histopathologic study reveals newly formed woven bone that matures and is incorporated into cortical bone. Electron microscopy of muscle may show myopathic changes and vascular abnormalities.

TABLE 219–2. DISORDERS THAT CAUSE OSTEOSCLEROSIS

Dysplasias
Craniodiaphyseal dysplasia
Craniometaphyseal dysplasia
Dysosteosclerosis
Endosteal hyperostosis
    van Buchem disease
    Sclerosteosis
Frontometaphyseal dysplasia
Infantile cortical hyperostosis (Caffey disease)
Melorheostosis
Metaphyseal dysplasia (Pyle disease)
Mixed sclerosing-bone dystrophy
Oculodento-osseous dysplasia
Osteodysplasia of Melnick and Needles
Osteoectasia with hyperphosphatasia (hyperostosis corticalis)
Osteopathia striata
Osteopetrosis
Osteopoikilosis
Progressive diaphyseal dysplasia (Engelmann disease)
Pyknodysostosis

Metabolic
Carbonic anhydrase II deficiency
Fluorosis
Heavy metal poisoning
Hypervitaminosis A, D
Hyperparathyroidism, hypoparathyroidism, and pseudohypoparathyroidism
Hypophosphatemic rickets or osteomalacia
Milk-alkali syndrome
Renal osteodystrophy

Other
Axial osteomalacia
Fibrogenesis imperfecta osseum
Intravenous drug abuse
Ionizing radiation
Lymphomas
Mastocytosis
Multiple myeloma
Myelofibrosis
Osteomyelitis
Osteonecrosis
Paget's disease
Sarcoidosis
Skeletal metastases
Tuberous sclerosis

From Whyte MP, Murphy WA: Osteopetrosis and other sclerosing bone disorders. *In* Avioli LV, Krane SM (eds.): Metabolic Bone Disease, 2nd ed. Philadelphia, WB Saunders, 1990.

Treatment. Glucocorticoid therapy (typically a low dose of prednisone on alternate days) can relieve bone pain and may normalize skeletal histology.

ENDOSTEAL HYPEROSTOSIS. Sclerosteosis and van Buchem disease, autosomal recessive disorders, are the principal types of endosteal hyperostosis.

Etiology and Pathogenesis. Sclerosteosis and van Buchem disease appear to reflect the same genetic defect in which differences are explained by the epistatic effects of modifying genes. The molecular basis is unknown. Enhanced osteoblast activity with failure of osteoclasts to compensate for the increased bone formation appears to explain the osteosclerosis.

Clinical Features. Sclerosteosis (cortical hyperostosis with syndactyly) occurs primarily in the Afrikaners of South Africa. Elsewhere, Dutch ancestry is also common. Gender distribution appears equal. Patients are tall and heavy beginning in childhood, and experience deafness and facial nerve palsy as a result of cranial nerve entrapment and have a prominent mandible of square configuration. Raised intracranial pressure and headache may reflect a small cranial cavity that shortens life expectancy. In van Buchem disease, progressive asymmetric enlargement of the jaw occurs during puberty, but there is no prognathism. Patients may be symptom free or suffer recurrent facial nerve palsy, deafness, and optic atrophy from narrowing of cranial foramina beginning as early as infancy. Long bones may hurt with applied pressure, but are not fragile.

Diagnosis. Radiologically in sclerosteosis, the skeleton is normal in early childhood except when syndactyly is present. Progressive bony thickening widens the skull and causes prognathism. Long bones have thickened cortices. Syndactyly, most often involving the index and third fingers, is common. Vertebral pedicles, ribs, pelvis, and other tubular bones may become dense. Computed tomography has shown fusion of ossicles and narrowing of the internal auditory canals and cochlear aqueducts. In van Buchem disease, endosteal thickening homogeneously widens diaphyseal cortices and narrows medullary canals. Bones are properly modeled. Osteosclerosis also affects the skull base, facial bones, vertebrae, pelvis, and ribs.

Serum alkaline phosphatase activity may be increased from enhanced skeletal production.

Treatment. Surgical decompression of narrowed foramina may alleviate cranial nerve palsies.

PACHYDERMOPERIOSTOSIS. Pachydermoperiostosis (hypertrophic osteoarthropathy, primary or idiopathic) is an autosomal dominant disorder that features clubbing of the digits, hyperhidrosis, and thickening of the skin (especially of the face), and periosteal new bone formation prominently in the distal limbs. Autosomal recessive transmission also seems to occur.

Etiology and Pathogenesis. No gene defect has been identified. A controversial hypothesis suggests that some circulating factor acts on the vasculature initially to cause hyperemia and thereby alters soft tissues, but later blood flow is reduced.

Clinical Presentation. Men appear to be more severely affected than women, and blacks more commonly than whites. Symptoms typically begin during adolescence, intensify during a decade, but then become quiescent. Arthralgias and fatigue are common. Stiffness and limited mobility affect both the appendicular and the axial skeleton. Progressive gradual enlargement of the hands and feet cause a pawlike appearance. Cutaneous changes include thickening, furrowing, pitting, and oiliness, especially of the scalp and face. Not all patients manifest all three principal features.

Radiologic Features. Periostitis thickens the distal portions of the tibia, fibula, radius, and ulna. Clubbing is obvious, and acro-osteolysis can occur. Ankylosis of joints, especially in the hands and feet, may affect older patients. Periosteal proliferation is exuberant and irregular and often involves epiphyses. Secondary hypertrophic osteoarthropathy (pulmonary or otherwise) typically causes a smooth, undulating periosteal reaction. Bone scanning in either condition reveals symmetric, diffuse, regular uptake along the cortical margins of long bones, especially in the legs. This feature results in a "double stripe" sign.

Treatment. Painful synovial effusions may respond to nonsteroidal anti-inflammatory drugs. Colchicine reportedly improved arthralgias, clubbing, folliculitis, and pachyderma in one patient. Contractures or neurovascular compression by osteosclerotic lesions may require surgical intervention.

Cortical and Trabecular Osteosclerosis

OSTEOPETROSIS. Osteopetrosis (marble bone disease) occurs in two major clinical forms—the autosomal recessive or "malignant" type that kills during infancy or early childhood if untreated, and the autosomal dominant or "benign" type that causes few or no symptoms. Other autosomal recessive types feature intermediate severity, neuronal storage disease, stillbirth, or renal tubular acidosis with cerebral calcification due to carbonic anhydrase II (CA II) isoenzyme deficiency.

Etiology and Pathogenesis. The defective gene loci are unknown except for CA II deficiency in which CA II gene mutations have been identified.

Histopathologic studies show that all true forms of osteopetrosis feature profound deficiency of osteoclast action. Primary spongiosa (calcified cartilage deposited during endochondral bone formation) occurs away from growth plates and constitutes the pathognomonic finding. Defective endosteal bone resorption precludes formation of marrow space. Quiescent skeletal remodeling leads to bone fragility from impaired interconnection of osteons and defective conversion of immature (woven) bone to mature (compact) bone. Hypothetically the various types of osteopetrosis could reflect abnormalities as distal as the microenvironment of osteoclast precursor cells in the marrow, or as proximal as bone tissue itself that is refractory to resorption. Viral-like inclusions in osteoclasts are of uncertain significance. Neuronal storage disease (ceroid lipofuscin) may reflect a lysosomal defect. Deficient superoxide production (necessary for bone resorption) can be a pathogenetic factor.

Clinical Manifestations.

Malignant osteopetrosis presents during infancy with nasal "stuffiness" from malformed mastoid and paranasal sinuses. Small cranial foramina compress optic, oculomotor, and facial nerves. Failure to thrive, delayed dentition, and fracture are characteristic. Hypersplenism and recurrent infection, bruising, and bleeding reflect myelophthisis. There are short stature, frontal bossing, large head, nystagmus, hepatosplenomegaly, and genu valgum. Untreated children usually die during the first decade of life from hemorrhage, pneumonia, severe anemia, or sepsis. Benign osteopetrosis occasionally causes fracture, and there may be facial palsy, deafness, mandibular osteomyelitis, impaired vision or hearing, psychomotor delay, carpal tunnel syndrome, and osteoarthritis. CA II deficiency has considerable clinical variability, including failure to thrive, fracture, developmental delay, mental subnormality, and short stature. Cerebral calcification develops during childhood, but defective skeletal modeling and osteosclerosis may correct spontaneously. Both proximal and distal renal tubular acidosis have been described.

Diagnosis.

Generalized symmetric osteosclerosis is the radiologic hallmark. In severe disease, modeling defects in long bones produce an "Erlenmeyer flask" deformity (Fig. 219–1). Alternating dense and lucent bands commonly occur in the pelvis and metaphyses. The cranium is usually thickened and dense, especially at the base, and the paranasal and mastoid sinuses are underpneumatized. Vertebrae may show, on lateral view, a "bone-in-bone" (endobone) configuration or end plate sclerosis causing a "rugger-jersey" appearance. Skeletal scintigraphy can disclose fractures and osteomyelitis. MRI helps to assess bone marrow transplantation, since successful engraftment normalizes marrow signals.

Serum levels of acid phosphatase and creatine kinase (brain isoenzyme), apparently from osteoclasts, are increased. In malignant osteopetrosis, hypocalcemia with secondary hyperparathyroidism and increased serum levels of calcitriol can accompany rachitic radiologic changes. In benign osteopetrosis, biochemical indices of mineral homeostasis are typically unremarkable, though serum parathyroid hormone levels may be increased.

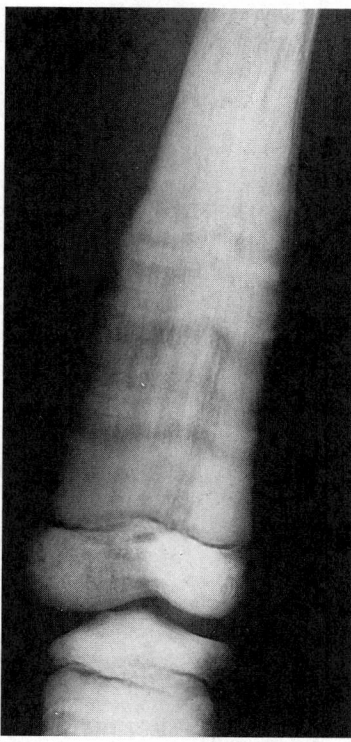

FIGURE 219–1. Osteopetrosis. Anteroposterior radiograph of the distal femur shows widened metadiaphyseal region with characteristic alternating dense and lucent bands. (From Whyte MP, Murphy WA: Osteopetrosis and other sclerosing bone disorders. *In* Avioli LV, Krane SM [eds.]: Metabolic Bone Disease, 2nd ed. Philadelphia, WB Saunders, 1990.)

Treatment.

Since the etiology, pathogenesis, and prognosis for osteopetroses differ, correct subclassification is crucial before treatment is attempted. It may be necessary to evaluate the family and disease progression. For the malignant form, HLA-identical bone marrow transplantation has remarkably benefited some children. Calcium-deficient diets have been helpful, but may be limited by hypocalcemia and rickets. Massive oral doses of calcitriol together with dietary calcium restriction (to prevent hypercalciuria/hypercalcemia), as well as human interferon-γ, that enhances superoxide production, stimulate osteoclast activity. Prednisone with a low-calcium/high-phosphate diet may be effective. High-dose glucocorticoid therapy stabilizes pancytopenia and hepatomegaly. Hyperbaric oxygenation helps treat osteomyelitis. Surgical decompression of optic and facial nerves can be beneficial. Early prenatal diagnosis by radiographs or ultrasound has not been successful.

PYKNODYSOSTOSIS.

Pyknodysostosis is believed to have affected the French impressionist painter Henri de Toulouse-Lautrec (1864–1901). Most descriptions have come from Europe and the United States, but the disorder appears to be especially common in Japan.

Etiology and Pathogenesis.

The molecular basis for this autosomal recessive condition is unknown. Diminished rates of bone resorption and skeletal turnover are reported. Degradation of collagen may be defective. In chondrocytes and osteoblasts, abnormal inclusions have been described.

Clinical Presentation.

During infancy or early childhood there are disproportionate short stature, fronto-occipital prominence, dental malocclusion with retention of primary teeth, proptosis, bluish sclerae, a beaked and pointed nose, as well as a relatively large cranium, obtuse mandibular angle, small facies and chin, and high-arched palate. Cranial sutures remain open. Fingers are short and clubbed from acro-osteolysis or aplasia of terminal phalanges, and the hands are small and square. Recurrent fractures cause genu valgum deformity. Mental retardation affects about 10% of patients. Adult height ranges from 4 feet 3 inches to 4 feet 11 inches. Recurrent respiratory infections and right-sided heart failure from chronic upper airway obstruction due to micrognathia may shorten life expectancy.

Laboratory Findings.

Osteosclerosis is uniform, first becoming apparent in childhood and increasing with age. Skeletal modeling defects do not occur, although long bones have thick cortices from narrow medullary canals. Clavicles are gracile and hypoplastic at their lateral segments. The calvarium and base of the skull are sclerotic, orbital ridges are dense, and wormian bones are present. Serum calcium and inorganic phosphate levels and alkaline phosphatase activity are typically normal. Anemia is not a problem.

Treatment.

There is no effective medical therapy. Fractures of the long bones usually mend satisfactorily. Internal fixation of long bones is formidable because of their hardness. Tooth extraction is difficult. Osteomyelitis of the mandible may require antibiotic, surgical, and/or hyperbaric therapy.

FIBROGENESIS IMPERFECTA OSSIUM.

This rare, sporadic disorder manifests generalized osteopenia, but features coarsening of remaining trabeculae. Thus it is included among osteosclerotic disorders.

Etiology and Pathogenesis.

The etiology is unknown. Subperiosteal bone formation and collagen synthesis in nonosseous tissue appear to be normal.

Clinical Presentation.

Typically, intractable skeletal pain begins gradually during middle age or later and rapidly progresses with a debilitating course and immobility. Spontaneous fractures are a prominent complication. Physical examination reveals marked bony tenderness.

Diagnosis.

Only the skull is spared. Initially, osteopenia and a slightly abnormal appearance of trabecular bone are noted. Subsequently the changes suggest osteomalacia. Corticomedullary junctions become indistinct as cortices are replaced by an abnormal trabecular bone pattern. The generalized osteopenia causes the remaining trabeculae to appear coarse and dense in a fish-net pattern. There is a mixed lytic and sclerotic appearance.

Alkaline phosphatase activity in serum is increased.

Histopathologic Findings.

The skeletal lesion is a form of osteomalacia that varies considerably in severity from area to area. In diseased regions, polarized light microscopy shows collagen fibrils that lack birefringence, and electron microscopy reveals thin and randomly organized collagen fibrils.

Focal Osteosclerosis

OSTEOPOIKILOSIS. Osteopoikilosis ("spotted bones") is a radiologic curiosity transmitted as a highly penetrant autosomal dominant trait. The bony lesions are asymptomatic. Incorrect diagnosis may lead to studies for other serious conditions, including metastatic disease. Some patients have connective tissue nevi called dermatofibrosis lenticularis disseminata, i.e., Buschke-Ollendorff syndrome.

Radiologic Features. Numerous small round or oval foci of bony sclerosis appear in cancellous bone in the tarsal, carpal, pelvic, and metaepiphyseal regions of tubular bones.

OSTEOPATHIA STRIATA. This autosomal dominant curiosity features linear striations in metaphyseal regions of long bones and in the ilium. Clinically important syndromes include osteopathia striata with cranial sclerosis or with focal dermal hypoplasia (Goltz's syndrome)—a serious X-linked recessive condition in which affected boys have widespread linear areas of dermal hypoplasia and various bony defects in the limbs.

MELORHEOSTOSIS. Melorheostosis causes changes likened to melted wax dripping down a candle. No mendelian basis for this disorder has been found. The anatomic distribution suggests a segmentary embryogenetic defect.

Clinical Presentation. Usually there is monomelic involvement; bilateral disease is generally asymmetric. Cutaneous changes over affected bones are not uncommon (e.g., linear scleroderma-like areas and hypertrichosis). Soft tissue abnormalities are often noted before the hyperostosis. Symptoms typically begin during childhood. Pain and stiffness are the major complaints. Joints may become contracted and deformed. Inequality of leg length results from soft tissue contractures and premature fusion of epiphyses. Skeletal changes appear to progress most rapidly during childhood. During adulthood, melorheostosis may or may not gradually extend. Pain is, however, more frequent.

Radiologic Features. Irregular, very dense, eccentric hyperostosis affects the cortex and medullary canal of a single bone or several adjacent bones. The lower limbs are most commonly involved. Endosteal thickening predominates during infancy and childhood and periosteal new bone formation during adulthood. Ectopic bone formation may occur, particularly near joints.

Treatment. It is difficult to surgically correct contractures; recurrent deformity is common.

MIXED SCLEROSING-BONE DYSTROPHY. This typically sporadic disorder features combinations of osteopoikilosis, osteopathia striata, melorheostosis, cranial sclerosis, or additional skeletal defects in one individual. Patients may experience the problems associated with the individual patterns of osteosclerosis, e.g., nerve palsy with cranial sclerosis, bone pain with melorheostosis.

OTHER DISORDERS OF BONE

FIBROUS DYSPLASIA. This sporadic, developmental, skeletal disorder features an expansile fibrous lesion(s) that can fracture, deform, or occasionally entrap nerves. Polyostotic disease typically presents before the age of 10 years; monostotic disease begins in adolescence or early adulthood. McCune-Albright syndrome refers to polyostotic fibrous dysplasia, café au lait spots (see Color Plate 10*D*), and endocrine hyperfunction (typically pseudoprecocious puberty in girls).

Etiology and Pathogenesis. Somatic mosaicism for activating mutations in the gene that codes for the alpha subunit of the receptor/adenylate cyclase–coupling G protein causes the McCune-Albright syndrome. Endocrinopathy generally results from end-organ hyperactivity. Imperfect bone forms because mesenchymal cells do not fully differentiate to osteoblasts.

Clinical Presentation. Monostotic fibrous dysplasia is more common than polyostotic disease. The skull and long bones are affected most often. Sarcomatous degeneration, affecting usually the facial bones or femur, occurs more frequently when there is polyostotic disease but is rare (incidence < 1%). Pregnancy may "reactivate" previously quiescent lesions. McCune-Albright syndrome usually is associated with pseudoprecocious puberty in girls. Less commonly there is thyrotoxicosis, Cushing's disease, acromegaly,

hyperprolactinemia, hyperparathyroidism, or pseudoprecocious puberty in boys. In some patients, renal phosphate wasting causes superimposed hypophosphatemic rickets or osteomalacia.

Radiologic Features. In the long bones, lesions are found in either the metaphysis or diaphysis. They are typically well defined with thin cortices and have a ground-glass appearance (Fig. 219–2). Occasionally they are lobulated with trabeculated areas of radiolucency.

Treatment. With mild disease, bone defects may not change. In severe cases, individual lesions can progress and new ones appear. Spontaneous healing does not occur. Pathologic fractures generally mend well. Stress fractures, however, can be difficult to detect and treat. When the skull is involved, nerve compression may require surgical intervention. In the McCune-Albright syndrome the aromatase inhibitor testolactone appears to help control the precocious puberty of affected girls.

HEREDITARY MULTIPLE EXOSTOSES. This relatively common, highly penetrant, autosomal dominant disorder features irregular bony excrescences that protrude from expanded metaphyses of long bones. There is evidence for a gene defect on chromosome 8 in some affected families. Osteocartilaginous exostoses arise from growth plates and expand until growth ceases. They may or may not become isolated from the parent bone. Their structure is relatively unremarkable with an outer cortex and an inner spongiosa. Disability results primarily from limb-length discrepancies; linear bone growth suffers at the expense of transverse growth. Compression of the nerve, spinal cord, and vascular system occasionally develops. Sarcomatous degeneration (0.5 to 2% of patients) must be suspected when a lesion enlarges rapidly, especially during adulthood.

ENCHONDROMATOSIS (DYSCHONDROPLASIA, OLLIER'S DISEASE). This sporadic condition features cartilaginous masses within the trabecular bone that arise from growth plates. The disorder occurs in childhood with swelling and interference with linear bone growth. At puberty, growth of cartilage masses ceases, and they can be replaced by mature bone. Enchondromas appear radiologically as radiolucent defects in metaphyses of tubular or flat bones, often with central calcific stippling. When enchondromatosis occurs with multiple hemangiomas (Maffucci's syndrome), the enchondromas or hemangiomas undergo malignant transformation in about 15% of cases.

ACHONDROPLASIA. Chondrodystrophies are disorders of cartilage growth that result in disproportionate short stature. Achon-

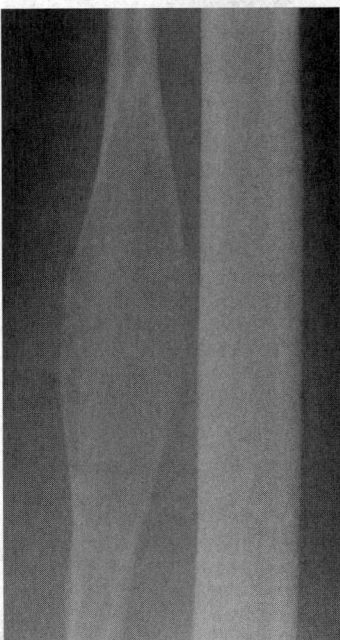

FIGURE 219–2. Fibrous dysplasia. A characteristic expansile lesion with ground-glass appearance has caused thinning of the cortex in the mid diaphysis of the fibula. (From Whyte MP: Fibrous dysplasia. *In* Favus MJ [ed.]: Primer on the Metabolic Bone Diseases and Disorders of Mineral Metabolism, 2nd ed. New York, Raven Press, 1993.)

droplasia is the most common. Mutations in the gene that encodes fibroblast growth factor receptor-3 cause achondroplasia. About 80% of cases are new mutations for this autosomal dominant trait. The mutation rate increases with paternal age. Short, tubular bones result from abnormal endochondral ossification in the limbs. A similar disturbance of the chondrocranium leaves membranous ossification undisturbed—thus the skull vault is normal. However, the cranial base and foramen magnum are small. Also, lumbar lordosis is greatly exaggerated, and the spinal canal narrows from the upper to lower lumbar spine, as revealed radiologically by decreasing interpeduncular distance. There is a notchlike sacroiliac groove. The head is large with frontal bossing and midface hypoplasia. The trunk is of relatively normal length, but the limbs have rhizomelic shortening and the hands have a trident configuration. The long bones appear massive, owing to their disproportionately normal width. Surprisingly, growth plates are not grossly disorganized, and chondrocytes appear normal. Complications can include brain stem compression, hydrocephalus, and spinal cord and root compression. Minimal impingement by a disc or osteophyte upon the small spinal canal can engender neurologic disturbances. Despite its problems, achondroplasia is compatible with good health and a normal lifespan.

Chang CC, Greenspan A, Gershwin ME: Osteonecrosis: Current perspectives on pathogenesis and treatment. Semin Arthritis Rheum 23:47, 1993. *Detailed overview of osteonecrosis.*
Horton WA, Hecht JT: The Chondrodysplasias. *In* Royce RM, Steinmann, B (eds.): Connective Tissue and Its Heritable Disorders, Somerset, NJ, Wiley-Liss, 1993. *Current, comprehensive description of connective tissue disorders including chondrodysplasias.*
McKusick VA: Mendelian Inheritance in Man: Catalogs of Autosomal Dominant, Autosomal Recessive and X-Linked Phenotypes, 11th ed. Baltimore, Johns Hopkins University Press, 1994. *Clinical features, patterns of inheritance, and molecular basis of heritable diseases in humans.*
Whyte MP: Genetic, Developmental, and Dysplastic Skeletal Disorders (Section VI) and Acquired Disorders of Cartilage and Bone (Section VII). *In* Favus NJ (ed.): Primer on the Metabolic Bone Diseases and Disorders of Mineral Metabolism, 2nd ed. New York, Raven Press, 1993. *General summary of metabolic bone diseases and disorders of mineral metabolism.*
Whyte MP, Murphy WA: Osteopetrosis and other sclerosing bone disorders. *In* Avioli LV, Krane SM (eds.): Metabolic Bone Disease, 2nd ed. Philadelphia, WB Saunders, 1990. *Detailed description of heritable disorders that increase bone mass.*

220 BONE TUMORS
Daniel I. Rosenthal

Tumors may involve bone as the result of (1) neoplastic transformation of bone or bone marrow cells, (2) metastatic dissemination of neoplasms arising in other organs, or (3) local invasion from contiguous tissues. Of these three mechanisms, metastatic involvement is by far the most frequent.

METASTATIC TUMOR

Several common cancers frequently involve the skeleton. In women, breast cancer is the most common primary tumor to result in skeletal metastases. Lung cancer is a distant second, although increasing in frequency. In men, prostate cancer is the most common primary tumor, followed by tumors arising in lung, kidney, gastrointestinal tract, and thyroid.

Whenever a destructive lesion of the skeleton is encountered, an effort should be made to determine whether it is primary or secondary. Metastatic bone lesions usually (but not always) produce an infiltrative pattern of bone destruction on radiography or other imaging studies. Compared with primary tumors, metastatic disease is usually accompanied by little or no soft tissue mass. Cancers arising in breast or prostate usually produce mixed lytic and blastic change within bone, whereas lung and renal cancers are purely lytic. A radioisotope bone scan is recommended to determine whether the lesion is solitary, as metastatic lesions are often multiple at presentation. Isotope bone scans are generally more sensitive than plain films for detecting metastasis; magnetic resonance imaging (MRI) is probably even more sensitive. Unfortunately, imaging of the entire skeleton by this modality is currently not practical. When more than one focus is present, the primary tumor is proba-

bly extraskeletal. Although bone sarcomas may metastasize to other parts of the skeleton, this phenomenon generally occurs late in the course of the disease, after lung metastases are present.

If multiple lesions are present and the primary tumor is not apparent, it may be desirable to consider biopsy for diagnosis rather than engage in an extended search for the primary. Needle biopsy can be done safely for most skeletal sites and is the most direct approach to diagnosis. Unfortunately, in a certain percentage of cases presenting as metastatic carcinoma, the primary tumor remains unknown despite all efforts.

Whether chemotherapy or hormonal therapy is useful in treating metastatic disease depends upon the primary tumor. Most metastatic lesions can be palliated with radiation. If there is important structural compromise of the skeleton and the patient's life expectancy justifies it, surgical stabilization should be considered to preserve function.

DIRECT INVASION

Direct invasion of bone by contiguous visceral or soft tissue tumors is uncommon. The most frequent cause of this complication is lung cancer invading the ribs or vertebrae (see Ch. 62). Paravertebral lymphadenopathy may sometimes invade the vertebrae. Deeply situated soft tissue sarcomas may also invade bone, but this is relatively rare considering the frequent proximity of these lesions to the skeleton. The radioisotope bone scan is useful to exclude bone involvement. However, a positive bone scan must be viewed with caution, as reactive changes at the margins of the tumor may cause the bone scan to be "hot." Confirmation of involvement by computed tomography (CT) scan or MRI is desirable.

PRIMARY BONE TUMORS

Primary bone tumors may arise from any of the cellular elements that are present. Tumors may be either malignant or benign. However, tumors of the mesenchymal tissues usually fall into a more or less continuous spectrum from benign to malignant. Not all lesions are clearly characterizable as either one or the other. For this reason, adequate diagnosis of most lesions requires not only the name of the tumor but its histologic grade. Further, individual tumors commonly exhibit a variety of cell types and grades. Features on imaging studies reflect the most abundant histologic elements, whereas clinical behavior is shaped by the most aggressive or malignant components. Generally speaking, the better differentiated the lesion (lower grade), the more it resembles the tissue from which it arose. Highly malignant lesions exhibit considerable similarity to each other on imaging studies.

Tumors may arise sporadically, as part of a generalized (and sometimes inherited) tendency to neoplasia, or as degenerations of precursor lesions. Almost any condition that causes a prolonged period of accelerated bone remodeling may lead to tumor formation, including Paget's disease, infections, radiation, bone infarctions, and benign bone lesions.

Adequate staging requires four pieces of information: tumor type, histologic grade, local extent, and presence of metastases. Tissue type and grade are learned from biopsy. Biopsy of these lesions requires considerable sophistication to avoid complicating future therapy. Biopsy should be performed in such a way as to obtain representative tissue, preserve structural integrity, and permit curative resection should that prove to be desirable. The latter usually requires that the biopsy track be excised along with the tumor.

Local extent can be determined by imaging studies. Plain radiographs are important in all cases. Either CT scan or MRI may be used to evaluate soft tissue and marrow extent. If the lesion is suspected of being malignant, a radioisotope bone scan is used to determine whether the lesion is solitary, and either chest radiography or CT is desirable to exclude pulmonary metastases.

Benign bone tumors are usually relatively small and often painless. Of these the most common (and least significant) is the *bone island*. These asymptomatic lesions arise during adult life, may slowly enlarge, and eventually regress. They are usually incidental findings on radiographs. Bone islands are not usually detected on isotope scans, although large lesions may show some uptake. Benign cartilage tumors, including osteochondroma and enchondroma, are next in order of frequency. These lesions are not generally painful unless complicated by pathologic fracture, adjacent soft tissue inflammation (bursitis), or malignant degeneration. Some painful benign tumors include osteoid osteoma, chondroblastoma, giant cell tumor, and chondromyxoid fibroma. Treatment by limited resection is adequate for these tumors. If the diagnosis is certain from imaging studies and resection is not required to relieve symptoms, observation may be adequate.

The most common malignant bone tumor is multiple myeloma, which is considered separately elsewhere (see Ch. 149). Osteosarcoma (or osteogenic sarcoma) is next in order of frequency and much more common than any of the others. Osteosarcoma exhibits two age incidence peaks—one in the second decade of life and another in the fifth and sixth decades, when it frequently represents a complication of a precursor lesion such as Paget's disease. It is most common in the distal femur and proximal tibia. Although low-grade osteosarcoma exists, most lesions are highly malignant. Ten per cent of patients have metastases at the time of presentation, and, if untreated, death ensues in less than 1 year. The alkaline phosphatase is usually elevated, and levels correlate with prognosis. In contemporary treatment a combination of chemotherapy, amputation, or if possible, limb-sparing surgery is used. With this approach survival rates of 85 to 90% are possible. Even for those patients presenting with pulmonary metastases, a combination of resection of the pulmonary lesion and chemotherapy may produce a 20% salvage rate.

Ewing's sarcoma is classified in a group of round cell lesions because of similar histologic and radiographic features. Lymphoma is another member of this group. Ewing's sarcoma tends to occur in children and young adults, whereas primary lymphoma of bone (usually non-Hodgkin's type) is seen in older individuals. The two entities may be difficult to differentiate. Ewing's sarcoma is of unknown pathogenesis and is highly malignant. It is remarkable for a tendency to produce both local and systemic symptoms that may simulate infection, including fever, malaise, and chills. Chemotherapy and surgery produce 60% cure rates.

Chondrosarcoma is usually a disease of people in the fourth, fifth, and sixth decades of life. Unlike osteosarcoma and Ewing's sarcoma, chondrosarcoma is of more variable grade, with most lesions of low or intermediate malignancy. Radiation and chemotherapy are relatively ineffective, but surgery may produce cure rates of 85%.

Goorin AM, Anderson JW: Experience with multi-agent chemotherapy for osteosarcoma. Clin Orthop Rel Res 270:22, 1991. *Current status of chemotherapy.*
O'Connor MI, Pritchard DJ: Ewing's sarcoma: Prognostic factors, disease control and the re-emerging role of surgical treatment. Clin Orthop Rel Res 262:78, 1991. *Improvements in survival related to local and systemic treatment.*
Schajowicz F: Tumors and Tumorlike Lesions of Bone and Joints. New York, Springer-Verlag, 1981. *A good general textbook providing incidence and age distribution for most lesions.*
Springfield DS (ed.): Limb salvage in the treatment of musculoskeletal tumors. Orthoped Clin North Am 22:1, 1991. *A comprehensive multiauthor review of the status of limb-sparing surgery.*

221 APPROACH TO THE PATIENT WITH IMMUNE DISEASE

J. Claude Bennett

The immune system consists of an integrated constellation of various cell types, each with a specifically designated functional role (Fig. 221–1). In addition, secreted molecules (cytokines) are responsible for interactions, modulations, and regulation of the system. These molecules and cells participate in specific interactions with immunogenic epitopes present on foreign materials, i.e., antigens introduced from the exterior world and foreign to the host. Recognition events are the beginning of the physiologic steps that make up the immune response; they initiate a series of processes causing a wide range of effects within the host. These include the pathways through which inflammation takes place, the killing of in-

vading microbial agents, and the disposal of foreign toxic compounds.

Events leading to specific molecular interactions depend upon the differentiation and expansion of the cell clones that are involved. These include production of specific cell-bound receptor molecules (TCR, T-cell receptors) and secreted or cell-bound immunoglobulins (antibodies). The cellular network (Fig. 221–1) results in an enormous array of specific molecular events. Abnormal regulation of the immune system may prevent the host from handling antigenic stimuli, resulting in a state of immune deficiency (see Ch. 223). At the other extreme it may allow the host to react to its own tissues, resulting in an autoimmune process (see Ch. 240).

In an immunocompetent individual, the immune response is initiated when introduced to an external agent that possesses an immunogenic structural epitope. The appropriate response depends upon the recognition by surface receptors of B and T lymphocytes of the foreignness of the introduced agent. These interactions lead to events that allow proliferation and differentiation of the antigen-stimulated cells. In order to appreciate the exquisite degree of specificity expressed by this remarkable system, one must understand the molecular interactions that result in antigen processing,

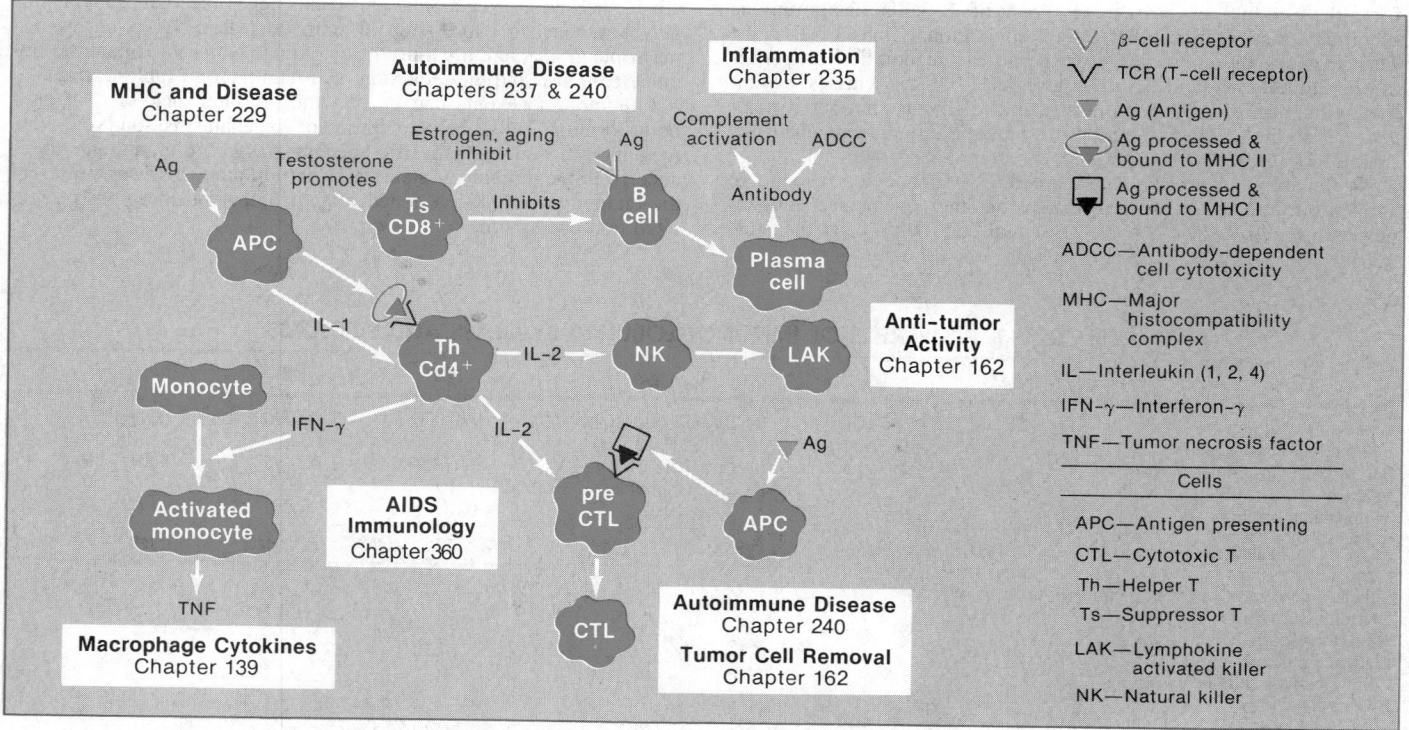

FIGURE 221–1. Schematic diagram of some of the major interactions among various cell types and secreted molecules of the immune system. Definitions of symbols are given on the right of the figure. The blocks at various stages in the pathways and their outcomes indicate their potential significance and refer to chapters elsewhere in this textbook for further reading and in-depth study.

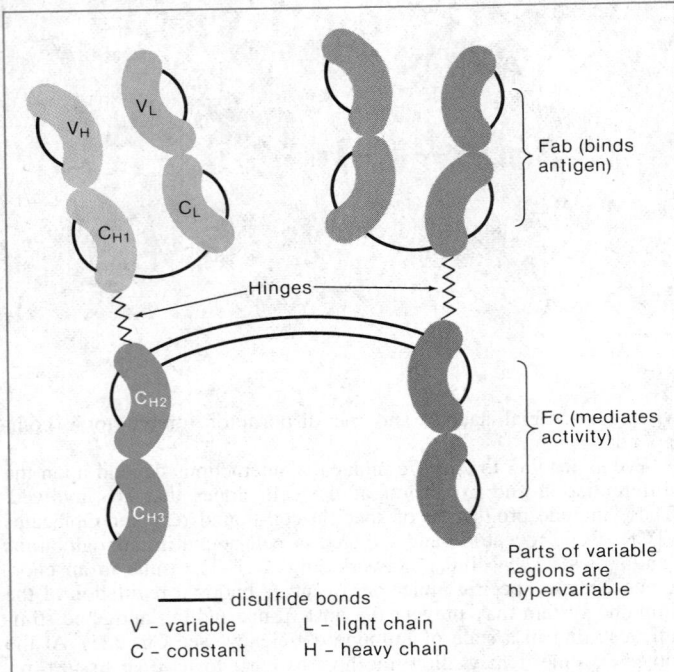

FIGURE 221-2. Diagram of the overall structure of immunoglobulin G, which is the basic structural pattern for all immunoglobulins (see text), drawn to highlight the various reactive areas and to emphasize the globular domain features of the immunoglobulin molecule.

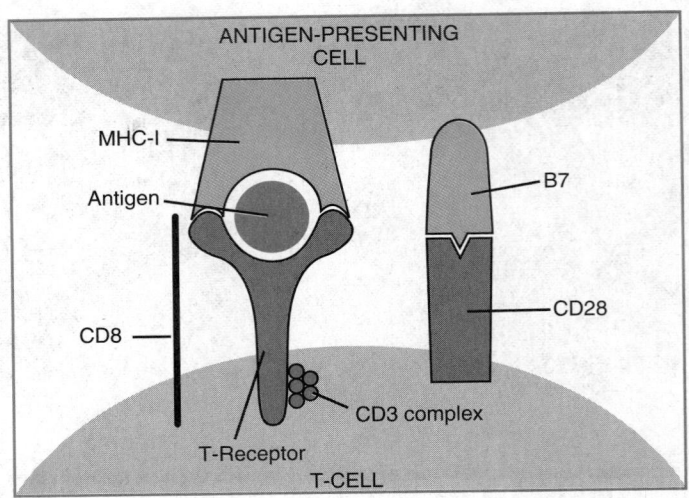

FIGURE 221-3. The molecular events involved in antigen presentation to the T cell. Shown are the interactions among the various molecules, including the major histocompatibility complex (MHC-I), the T-cell receptor, the CD8 or CD4 molecules, and the CD3 complex. Second signal events in the case of cytotoxin (CD8) T cells is shown by the interactions of B7 and CD28. See text for description of the polypeptide chain composition of the various molecules.

presentation, and cellular proliferation. B lymphocytes differentiate to produce specifically directed immunoglobulins (antibodies). All such immunoglobulins share an overall structure, but each contains its own antigen-binding area (Fab region) and within any class (e.g., IgG, IgM) a similar constant region (Fc) (Fig. 221-2). Therefore, the product of any given clone of B cells has a unique specificity distinct from that of all other clonal lines of B cells. This provides the enormous diversity in the recognition properties of the immune system. Furthermore, each of the classes of immunoglobulins is imbued with structural elements that set it apart and define its distinct function in biologic effector mechanisms (Table 221-1).

As the immune process is triggered, T lymphocytes respond to antigen on the surface of macrophages or other specialized antigen-presenting cells (APC) (Figs. 221-1 and 221-3). T cells then differentiate as they express various functions, such as cytotoxic potential, enhanced expression of immunity (helper T cells), or down-modulation of the immune response. Therefore, the T lymphocyte becomes pivotal in the development of both *humoral immunity* by way of its stimulation of B lymphocytes and the development of *cellular immunity* and regulation by virtue of its own intrinsic properties and its role in elaborating cytokines for cellular communication processes.

Reactions of the immune system may activate the complement cascade (see Ch. 222) and the production of arachidonic acid derivatives such as prostaglandins and leukotrienes (see Ch. 235), which play key roles in expressing inflammation. Both lymphocytes and macrophages secrete a variety of cytokines, which modulate the immune response and the induction of inflammation (Table 221-2).

Immunologic events can be regulated through networks of antibody-forming cells, helper/suppressor mechanisms, and cytokine mediation or through specific mechanisms of immunologic tolerance. Immunodeficiency states and autoimmune diseases represent the endpoints of either a genetically incompetent or a poorly regulated immune system.

TABLE 221-1. PROPERTIES OF IMMUNOGLOBULINS BY CLASS AND SUBCLASS

Class		IgG		IgA		IgM	IgD	IgE
Molecular weight		160,000		17,000 or polymer		900,000	80,000	90,000
Sedimentation constant		7S		7S (9, 11, 13)		19S	7S	8S
Serum concentration		1000–5000		250–300		100–150	0.3–30	0.0015–0.2
Valence		2		2 (monomer)		10	2	2
Molecular formula		$\gamma_2 L_2$		$(\alpha_2 L_2)_n$		$(\mu_2 L_2)_5$	$\delta_2 L_2$	$\epsilon_2 L_2$

Subclass	IgG1	IgG2	IgG3	IgG4	IgA1	IgA2	IgM	IgD	IgE
Subclass percent of class, in serum	65	20	10	5	90	10			
Complement fixation	++	+	++	−	−	−	++	−	−
Alternative complement fixation					+	+		±	±
Placental passage	+	+	+	+	−	−	−	−	+
Fixing to mast cells or basophils	−	−	−	−	−	−	−	−	+
Binding to									
Macrophages	+	±	+	±	−	−	−	−	−
Neutrophils	+	+	+	+	+	+	−	−	−
Platelets	+	+	+	+	−	−	−	−	−
Lymphocytes	+	+	+	+	−	−	+	−	−
Half-life (days)	23	23	8–9	23	6	6	5	3	2.5
Synthesis rate (mg/kg/day)	25	?	3.5	?	44	22	7	0.4	0.02

TABLE 221-2. CYTOKINES AND THEIR BIOLOGIC ACTIVITIES

Cytokines Interleukin	Cell Source			Major Activities
	T	**Macrophages**	**Other**	
Interleukin-1α and β (IL-1α and β)		+	+	Fever; bone resorption; prostaglandin release; stimulate cytokine production by macrophages and T cells.
IL-1α		+		
IL-1β				Some
IL-2	+		+	Activates cytotoxic T cells and NK cells.
				Stimulates proliferation of T cells and NK cells.
				Stimulates differentiation of T cells and LAK cells.
IL-3	+	+	+	Costimulates proliferation of B cells and antibody secretion.
				Supports proliferation of mast cells and pre-B cells.
IL-4	+		+	Supports differentiation of stem cells.
				Activates resting B cells and macrophages. Induces IgG and IgE secretion in LPS-activated B cells.
				Stimulates proliferation of T cells and mast cells.
IL-5	+			Suppresses TNF-α, IL-1, IL-6 in monocytes.
				Induces IgA production and IgM secretion from LPS-activated B cells.
				Proliferation of eosinophils; supports differentiation of cytotoxic T cells.
IL-6	+	+	+	Induces antibody secretion; differentiation of cytotoxic T cells; proliferation of megakaryocytes.
IL-7			Thymic strand cells	Promotes myeloma cell growth. Proliferation and differentiation of pre-B cells.
IL-8		+		Proliferation of thymocytes. Neutrophil and T-cell chemotaxis.
IL-9	+			Growth of T-helper cell clones.
IL-10	+	+	+	Inhibits production of (IFN-γ and TNF-α) and B-cell growth and differentiation.
IL-11			+	Proliferation and development of B cells, macrophages, and megakaryocytes.
IL-12			B cells	Proliferation of activated T cell induction of IFN-γ.
Tumor necrosis factor-α (TNF-α) (cachectin)	+	+		Fever; shock; activates macrophages; stimulates PMN chemotoxin; angiogenesis, bone resorption; cytotoxic to many cells.
Tumor necrosis factor-β (TNF-β) (lymphotoxin)	+			Activates endothelial cells, granulocytes, and B cells. Inhibits angiogenesis; cytotoxic to many cells.
Inteferon-γ (IFN-γ)			NK cells	Activated NK cells, cytotoxic T cells, endothelial cells, and macrophages. Has antitumor activity. Stimulates LAK activity; costimulates B-cell proliferation; inhibits T-cell proliferation.

B LYMPHOCYTE LINEAGE AND ANTIBODY PRODUCTION

Secreted antibodies are produced by plasma cells, which represent the terminal phase of differentiation of B lymphocytes. The latter are found in all peripheral lymphoid tissues and also in the circulating pool of lymphocytes. Within their surface membranes, B cells have receptors that allow them to recognize foreign antigenic determinants. These receptors are immunoglobulin molecules, and in the initial stages of differentiation are generally of the IgM and IgD classes. When stimulated by a specific antigen, in conjunction with appropriate cytokines, these B cells proliferate and secrete antibody (see Fig. 221-1).

In the earliest stages of differentiation (Fig. 221-4), B lymphocytes lack membrane immunoglobulin (mIg). However, these cells begin to express in their cytoplasm the μ chain, which is the heavy (H) chain of IgM. Later they produce the light (L) chain (either kappa [κ] or lambda [λ]) which allows IgM molecules to be expressed on the surface. The binding region on the mIg of each cell line is unique in its specificity and is identical to that of the antibody molecule that is to be secreted. This means that at a very early developmental stage, a given cell is locked into its own specificity. This process involves several gene rearrangements (see below).

B-cell activation, proliferation, and differentiation require a variety of cytokines. Perhaps the most important in humans is interleukin-2 (IL-2), which seems to play a central role in these events and thus facilitates the production of immunoglobulins of all isotopes. Although other cytokines (e.g., IL-4 and TGF-β) are identified as being able to amplify and modify antibody production, generally they cannot do this unless IL-2 is present (Table 221-2).

IMMUNOGLOBULIN FUNCTION AND STRUCTURE

The basic structure of all immunoglobulin molecules (see Fig. 221-2) is similar among the various classes. Essentially they consist of two types of polypeptide chains—the larger called the heavy

(H) chain, the smaller known as the light (L) chain. Each immunoglobulin subunit consists of two identical H and two identical L chains and would therefore have the molecular formula H_2L_2. The H and L chains are connected to each other by disulfide bonds, and similarly there are disulfide bridges between the two H chains (which vary in number for the different classes and subclasses). They are generally located in the center of the H chain region, known as the "hinge" region, which is unusually rich in cysteine and proline. The L chain has a molecular weight of about 25,000 daltons; the H chain varies between 50,000 and 65,000 daltons. H chain size is related to differences in the structure of the hinge region or to the presence of an extra globular domain, as in the case of the μ and ε H chains (in IgM and IgE, respectively). Globular domains, formed by intrachain disulfide bonds, each consist of about 110 amino acid residues; and there are four or five such domains in each H chain and two in each L chain. The domains are separated by extended regions known as interdomain stretches. These domain structures may have evolved to execute specialized biologic functions.

The amino terminal 110 to 120 residues of each immunoglobulin chain are known as the *variable* (V) region because the amino acid sequences of those molecules produced from a single clonal line differ from those of other lines. The remaining part of the immunoglobulin chain is identical for any given class and is referred to as the *constant* (C) region. Many direct lines of evidence indicate that the variable region contains the antibody-binding site into which antigen fits and that "hypervariable regions" are in the most intimate contact with the structural elements of the antigen. X-ray crystallography has confirmed these three-dimensional structures. The hypervariable regions are also largely responsible for the *idiotypic* determinants on an antibody molecule and tend to be similar on all antibodies that share specificities. The structures throughout the remainder of the V segments, which show less sequence variability, are referred to as the "framework" areas.

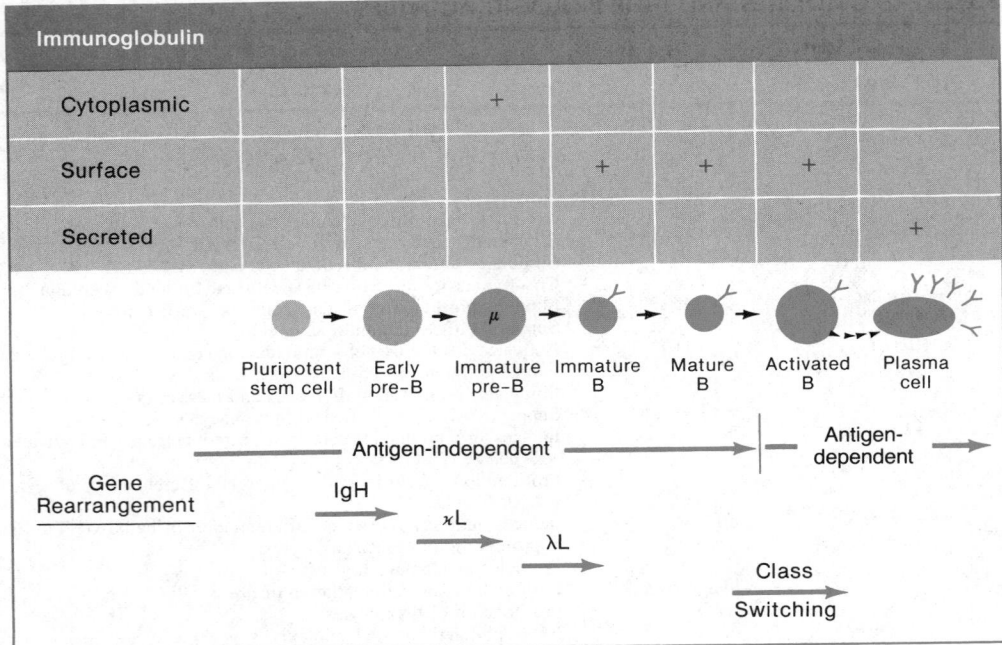

FIGURE 221–4. Presentation of B-cell pathway development in a sequential form showing when immunoglobulin appears in the cytoplasm or on the surface or is secreted. The gene rearrangements that take place at various stages of the differentiation pathway are indicated.

Although the amino acid sequences of the constant regions of the H chains show homologies among the Ig classes and subclasses, there are also very significant differences. The structural features appear to be important in giving the molecule its particular biologic function that distinguishes one class from another. Complement fixation, for example, seems to depend upon a structural determinant in the IgG CH2 domain, whereas features of the CH3 domain seem to be important for interacting with a variety of cells by way of the Fc receptors. More than one domain in the Fc region of the IgG H chain is required to react with the binding sites on rheumatoid factors (see Ch. 237).

Since Porter's original work on the structure of antibodies, much has been learned about their molecular structure by using proteolytic enzymes. For example, papain cleaves IgG into an Fc fragment and two Fab fragments, whereas pepsin degrades the Fc fragment and yields the two Fab fragments still joined by a disulfide bridge $(Fab)_2$ (see Fig. 221–2). Different enzymes cleave the various classes in different ways, and this approach has been important in defining structural corollaries to biologic properties.

Comparisons among the various classes of immunoglobulin are shown in Table 221–1. Certain immunoglobulins appear very different from IgG. For example, IgM is a large molecule but consists of five subunits of the same basic immunoglobulin pattern. It has 10 H and 10 L chains and, therefore, 10 antibody-binding sites per molecule. However, because of steric factors, when IgM reacts with large protein antigens, it tends to bind with a valence of five. This can best be seen in the case of IgM rheumatoid factor binding to IgG, which yields a 22 S complex with a formula $(\mu_2L_2)5$-(IgG)5.

TABLE 221–3. CHROMOSOMAL LOCATIONS OF THE HUMAN IMMUNOGLOBULIN AND T-CELL RECEPTOR GENES

Chain	Symbol	Locus
Immunoglobulin		
Heavy chain	H	14q32
Kappa light chain	κ	2p12
Lambda light chain	λ	22q11
T-cell receptor		
Alpha and delta chains	α, δ	14q11–12
Beta chain	β	7q32–35
Gamma chain	γ	7p15

IMMUNOGLOBULIN GENETICS AND GENE ORGANIZATION

Human immunoglobulin genes are contained on chromosomes 2, 14, and 22 (Table 221–3). Several sequences of events must take place for immunoglobulin genes to be expressed. This requires a random process of gene reorganization. As shown in Figure 221–5, each C region is coded by a single gene, but many gene segments are necessary to form the repertoire of V genes. The latter are formed by rearrangement of DNA to bring one V gene into proximity with a J (junction) gene in the case of the L chains; and in the case of the H chains, the V must be brought into proximity with a D (diversity) region and a J region. For any given H-chain gene, the total V region is formed from a single V region, a single D, and a single J (Fig. 221–5). Combination with a given constant region would determine the Ig class. Recombination activating genes (RAG) facilitate the V-D-J recombination, and this suggests that they may encode enzymes that have the properties of being V-D-J recombinases. The C region genes are located in tandem, so a switching process must occur in order to allow a given assembled V-D-J region to attach to any constant region. This process deletes

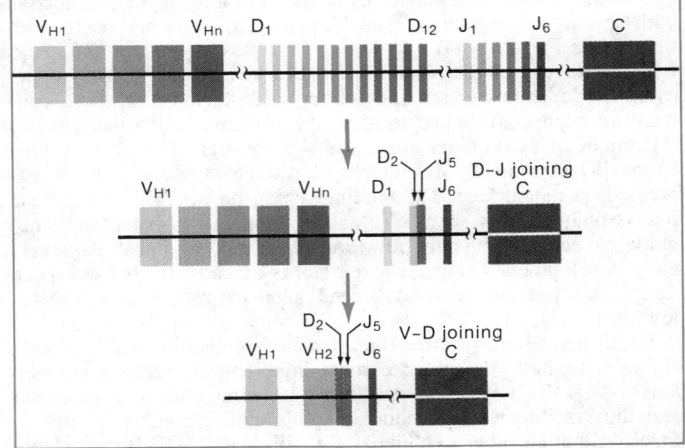

FIGURE 221–5. The mechanisms for DJ and VD joining to form the entire variable region of the heavy chain. Note that intervening gene sequences at each step of joining are deleted, giving rise to the final finished product of an entire V region with the constant region at some distance. This event would be followed by a messenger RNA developing and splicing to form the entire translatable message sequence (see text for details).

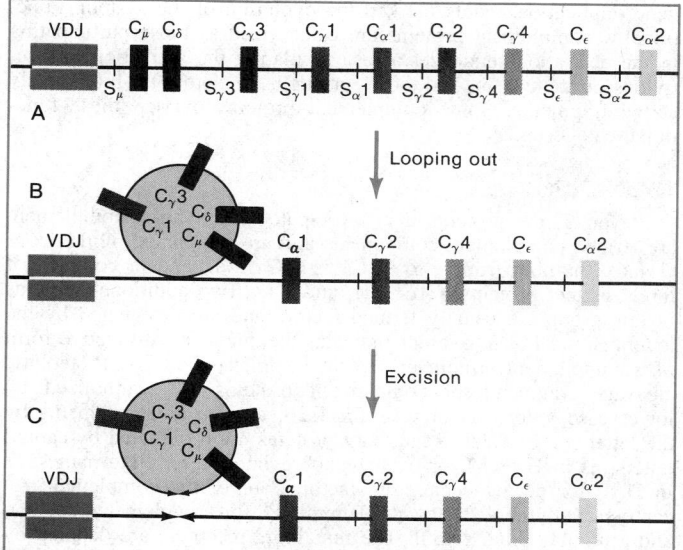

FIGURE 221-6. A diagrammatic representation of class switching to produce IgA$_1$. The switch sequence regions (S) identify places where looping can occur. This results ultimately in excision of the loop containing Cμ, Cδ, Cγ_1, and Cγ_3 and brings Cα_1 into close juxtaposition to the rearranged VDJ regions. (Adapted with permission from von Schwedler et al.: Nature 345:452–454, 1990. Copyright © 1990 Macmillan Magazines Limited.)

all intervening genes from that particular clone (Fig. 221–6). In some B lymphocytes both IgD and IgM are present on the cell membrane at the same time, and this occurs through alternative RNA splicing.

There are several mechanisms that generate antibody diversity which are inherent in the somatic process of forming Ig genes.

1. *Combinatorial diversity,* which results from the combination of various gene segments as described above
2. *Junctional diversity,* which results at the joining site because of some imprecision in codon formation
3. *Junctional insertion,* by which diversity may arise because of insertion of extra nucleotides
4. *Somatic mutational events*
5. *Exchange rearrangement* of the H segments
6. The *combination of associated H and L chains*

This process allows an essentially random extrapolation of combinations into the millions of possibilities; i.e., it *generates* antibody diversity.

T LYMPHOCYTES

T-Cell Receptors

The most common form of T-cell receptor consists of a disulfide-linked heterodimer of α and β chains. Both of these chains contain amino-terminal *variable* regions and carboxy-terminal *constant* regions, just as occur in immunoglobulins. These chains contain carbohydrate and are bound with the surface of the T cell with membrane-spanning regions. A subset of T cells possesses similar receptors made up of γ and δ chains that seem to be highly specialized and located in certain regions of the body, such as the gastrointestinal tract. A molecule called the T3 complex bears the CD3 determinant and is noncovalently linked to the T-cell receptor heterodimer (see Fig. 221–3). It is of special note that variable regions of the T-cell receptor genes are assembled from V-D-J segment joining just as the immunoglobulin V region genes are assembled. Much less if any somatic hypermutation occurs in the T-cell receptor V region genes. Thus, rearrangement occurs during the process of differentiation, and once it has occurred it produces a stable clone with a fixed specificity.

ANTIGEN PRESENTATION AND THE MAJOR HISTOCOMPATIBILITY COMPLEX

Certain cell types such as macrophages, dendritic cells, and epidermal Langerhans cells are able to take up antigens nonspecifically and, when they express major histocompatibility class I or II (MHC

I or II) molecules, present antigen to T cells (see Fig. 221–3). In some cases other cells, including activated B cells that may express class II MHC molecules, may also act as antigen-presenting cells. The antigen presented has often been processed so that only a relatively small peptide determinant is bound to the MHC for presentation. This event appears to involve the MHC molecule in conjunction with the processed antigen peptide on the surface of the antigen-presenting cell so that it can react with the T-cell receptor, and the CD4 molecule in the case of MHC-II, or with CD8 in the case of MHC-I, on the membrane of the T cell (see Ch. 229).

Similar membrane recognition events take place when cytotoxic T cells recognize and interact with cells bearing specific foreign antigens. In this case, the cytotoxic T cell may recognize the foreign antigen in conjunction with a class I MHC molecule, and it does so by virtue of its T-cell receptor in the presence of the CD8 molecule. Activation requires a second signal via B7 on the antigen-presenting cell and CD 28 on the T-cell surface. Such activated cytotoxic T cells can then destroy their target cells by a lytic process.

REGULATION AND MODULATION OF THE IMMUNE PROCESS

Complement

The complement cascade is important to modify the effector arm of the immune system. Activating complement allows important events such as removing infectious agents and expressing the inflammatory response to take place. These involve active fragments of the pathway that enhance chemotaxis of macrophages, alter blood vessel permeability, change blood vessel diameters, cause lysis to cells, alter blood clotting, and cause numerous other subtle points of modification. Complement is discussed in greater detail in Ch. 222.

IDIOTYPIC NETWORKS

As indicated previously, antibody molecules express unique antigenic determinants on their variable regions, thereby allowing secondary antibodies to be produced against them. Such determinants are designated *idiotopes.* Therefore, an idiotope of immunoglobulin is functionally equivalent to the *clonotypic* antigenic determinant of a clonal line of T cells. The idiotypic network concept (Fig. 221–7) holds that the immune system is in a dynamic regulatory equilibrium so that members of each clone within the system are recognized by members of other clones through these anti-idiotope interactions. Conceptually, this interrelated system provides mechanisms for regulation based on recognition of receptors without need for exogenous antigen. This method of regulation may allow certain idiotopes to become dominantly expressed and may be operative with unique *clonal markers,* such as those that are observed due to clonal expansion in malignant lymphoid diseases.

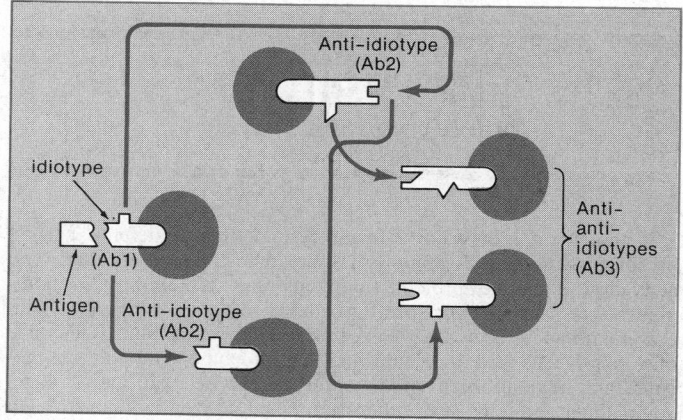

FIGURE 221-7. Diagrammatic representation of the idiotypic network showing the development of anti-idiotypes and anti-anti-idiotypes in sequential processes. This complementary fit mechanism provides the structural basis for the feedback network.

HELPER T-CELL SYSTEM

Helper T-cells may be divided into Th1 and Th2 populations. There is a feedback control mechanism for regulation of these subsets. Generally, Th1 cytokines promote Th1 activity and inhibit Th2 activity. The reverse is also true. Th1 cytokines are IL-1, IL-12, and IFN-γ and enhance the cellular immune response. Th2 cytokines are IL-4, IL-5, and IL-6 and enhance the humoral immune response.

SUPPRESSION

Regulating responses to antigenic stimulation and also controlling potential immune responses against self components are essential ingredients of a smoothly operating immune system. Suppressor T cells and the suppressor system represent a series of cell types that act in a highly complex fashion. Several distinct types of suppressor systems have been described, and their sequential action appears to have an amplification effect so that direct and graded regulation can take place. Suppressor effector cells can act on antibody-secreting cells and on T cells to downregulate their expression.

CYTOKINES

A growing array of molecules have been identified as products of cells that serve to regulate the immune system and to evoke responses in other cells, such as blood vessel endothelial cells and precursor cells in the bone marrow. Cytokines can regulate levels of response or induce differentiation and proliferation of cells. Table 221–2 summarizes the properties of some of these molecules which may be encountered in immune regulation (see also Ch. 235 and 264).

SUMMARY

The immune system is a highly orchestrated and coordinated system that allows a rapid response to foreign substances in a highly specific manner. The organization occurs at the level of the gene, the cell, and the mediator. Therefore, any qualitative or quantitative change in this system can produce profound effects. This is evident as one examines diseases of the immune system, such as those that occur as the result of altered immune regulation (see Ch. 237 and 240).

Inflammation, often immunologically mediated and often resulting in tissue damage, is a key feature of diseases of virtually any organ system. Therefore, a knowledge of basic immunology is critical to a clear understanding of the nature of these abnormalities. A student of medicine must be prepared to apply immunology to every branch of internal medicine and to recognize its importance in understanding disease and, hence, the care of the patient.

Engelhard VH: How cells process antigens. Sci Am 271:54, 1994. *Newest information on antigen breakdown and cell processing for presentation.*

Immunology Today 15:393–453, 1994 [entire issue]. *Ten papers bring together all the latest information on B-cell activation and regulation.*

Roitt IM: Essential Immunology. 8th ed. London, Blackwell Scientific, 1994. *An excellent introductory textbook of immunology; easy-to-read with good visual aids.*

222 COMPLEMENT

John E. Volanakis

Complement is a major effector system of host defense against invading pathogens. It comprises more than 30 proteins that upon activation elaborate protein fragments and protein-protein complexes that interact with specific cellular receptors or directly with cell membranes to mediate acute inflammatory reactions, clearance of foreign cells and molecules, killing of pathogenic microorganisms, and regulation of immune responses. In their native state, complement proteins are either serum soluble or associated with cell membranes (Table 222–1). Most of the serum-soluble proteins are synthesized in the liver. Complement proteins exhibit extensive structural homologies among themselves, remarkably conserving a small number of repeated structural motifs, indicating that multiple

gene duplication events marked the evolution of the system. Functionally, complement proteins are categorized as those participating in the activation sequences, those regulating the activation and activities of the system, and those serving as receptors for biologically active fragments. Some complement proteins overlap these functional categories.

NOMENCLATURE

Eleven of the proteins that participate in activating complement are termed complement components and are designated by the letter C and a number from 1 to 9. C1 is a Ca^{2+}-dependent complex of three distinct proteins, C1q, C1r, and C1s. Two additional proteins in this group are usually termed factors and are designated by the letters B and D. An overbar indicates the enzymatically active form of a complement protein or protein complex, as in $\overline{C1}$. Proteolytic cleavage fragments of complement proteins are symbolized by lower case letters, as in C2a and C2b, and inactive fragments by the letter i, e.g., C2ai. Regulatory proteins are designated by capital letters, as in H and I, or by their abbreviated descriptive names, as in DAF for decay-accelerating factor. Four of the complement receptors are symbolized by the letters CR, for complement receptor, and a number from 1 to 4. The remaining receptors are denoted by the symbol of the protein or protein fragment they bind followed by the letter R, as in C5aR.

COMPLEMENT ACTIVATION

The complement system must be activated to express biologic activity and is characterized by operational simplicity and economy of design. The most important host defense activities are derived from two proteins, C3 and C5, that are structurally homologous and probably represent gene duplication products. Expression of activity requires that C3 and C5 be cleaved by highly specific proteases, termed *convertases* (Fig. 222–1). There are two C3 and two C5 convertases. One of each is assembled during activation of the two pathways of complement, which are termed *classic* and *alternative*. The two activation pathways use different proteins to form these enzymes. In addition, the assembly of the convertases is initiated by different activators in the two pathways. However, the resulting enzymes have identical substrate and peptide bond specificity, giving rise to identical biologically active fragments. Characteristic of the simplicity and economy of design of complement activation is the fact that C5 convertases are derivatives of C3 convertases (Fig. 222–1). Furthermore, C3 and C5 are activated by their respective convertases in similar fashion: A single peptide bond near the NH_2 terminus of the α polypeptide chain of either C3 or C5 is cleaved to generate a small peptide, C3a or C5a, and a large two-polypeptide fragment, C3b or C5b. Each of these four fragments, as well as

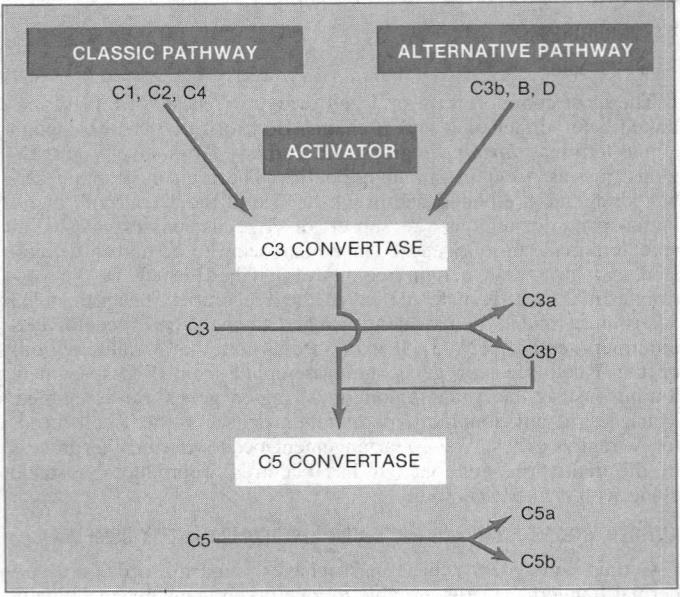

FIGURE 222–1. Activation of the complement system.

TABLE 222–1. PROTEINS OF THE COMPLEMENT SYSTEM*

Prevalent Form in Native State	Functional Group		
	Participating in Activation Sequences	*Regulatory*	*Receptors*
Serum soluble	Clq, Clr, Cls, D MBP, MASP C4, C3, C2, B C5, C6, C7, C8, C9	Cl INH C4bp, H, I, P C3a/C5a INA S protein	
Membrane associated		CR1 DAF, MCP HRF, CD59	ClqR, C3aR, C5aR CR1, CR2 CR3, CR4

* Established symbols have been used for most complement proteins. In addition, the following generally accepted abbreviations have been used: INH, inhibitor; C4bp, C4b-binding protein; INA, inactivator; R, receptor, e.g., CRI, complement receptor type 1; MBP = mannose-binding protein; MASP = MBP-associated serine protease; DAF = decay-accelerating factor; MCP = membrane cofactor protein; HRF = homologous restriction factor.

further cleavage fragments of C3b, expresses at least one activity important to host defense.

ASSEMBLY OF COMPLEMENT CONVERTASES

CLASSIC PATHWAY. In the classic pathway, assembly of the convertases is usually initiated by antibodies of the IgG or IgM class complexed with antigen. Several other substances, including CRP complexes, certain viruses, and gram-negative bacteria, can also activate this pathway. Activators are recognized by Clq, one of the three proteins in the C1 complex. Binding to an activator induces a change in the conformation of Clq that causes the autoactivation of Clr, which in turn activates proenzyme $\overline{C1s}$ to enzymatically active $\overline{C1s}$ (Fig. 222–2). In the next step, $\overline{C1s}$ cleaves C4, resulting in the covalent attachment of its major fragment, C4b, to the surface of the activator. C4b is attached through a transacylation reaction similar to that leading to covalent binding of C3b to activating surfaces (see below). C2 binds to C4b and is also cleaved by $\overline{C1}$ into two fragments, the larger of which, C2a, remains bound to C4b, completing the assembly of the $\overline{C4b2a}$ complex, which is the C3 convertase of the classic pathway. Cleavage of C3 by the C3 convertase results in the covalent binding of many C3b fragments to the surface of the activator and the eventual binding of one C3b to the C4b subunit of the C3 convertase. This leads to the formation of the $\overline{C3b4b2a}$ complex, which is the C5 convertase of the classic pathway. A novel C1-independent mechanism for activating the classic pathway was described recently. It uses mannose-binding protein (MBP), an acute-phase serum lectin with binding specificity for terminal mannose and *N*-acetylglycosamine. MBP binding to bacterial pathogens displaying these sugar residues results in activation of an associated protease, which in turn cleaves C4 and C2, leading to the assembly of a C3 convertase.

ALTERNATIVE PATHWAY. Alternative pathway activation is initiated by a variety of cellular surfaces, including those of certain bacteria, parasites, viruses, and fungi. Antibodies can also activate

this pathway, but they are not usually required. Assembly of the convertases is intimately related to certain structural features of the multifunctional protein C3. C3 is the most abundant complement protein in blood and is characterized by the presence on its α-chain of an unusual, for blood proteins, thioester bond. Under physiologic conditions, this bond is relatively stable, being hydrolyzed at very slow rates to give rise to C_{H_2O}, which can initiate the formation of the short-lived *initiation* C3 convertase. This is accomplished by the formation of a complex between $C3_{H_2O}$ and B and the subsequent cleavage of B by D to generate the $\overline{C3_{H_2O}Bb}$ complex, the initiation C3 convertase (Fig. 222–3). This series of reactions, starting with the hydrolysis of the thioester bond in native C3 and concluding with the cleavage of C3 into C3a and C3b by the initiation C3 convertase, is considered to occur in the blood continuously at slow rates. Thus, a constant supply of small amounts of freshly generated C3b is available at all times. The initiation C3 convertase is quickly inactivated by the control proteins H and I.

C3 cleaved by a C3 convertase induces a pronounced change in the conformation of C3b associated with an extremely labile (metastable) thioester bond that reacts either with water or with hydroxyl or amino groups on the surface of cells or proteins. Thus, C3b becomes covalently attached via an ester or amide bond to surfaces in the immediate vicinity of its generation. The fate of surface-bound C3b depends entirely on the chemical nature of the surface. C3b bound to a nonactivator of the alternative pathway, e.g., host's red cells, is quickly inactivated by the action of control proteins. In contrast, C3b bound to an activator, e.g., *Escherichia coli* cells, preferentially binds B, which is then cleaved by D, generating the $\overline{C3bBb}$ complex, which is the C3 convertase of the alternative pathway. This enzyme is stabilized by the binding of P and is termed the *amplification* C3 convertase because it generates many C3b fragments and thus additional molecules of C3 convertase. Binding of a single C3b molecule to the C3 convertase gives rise to

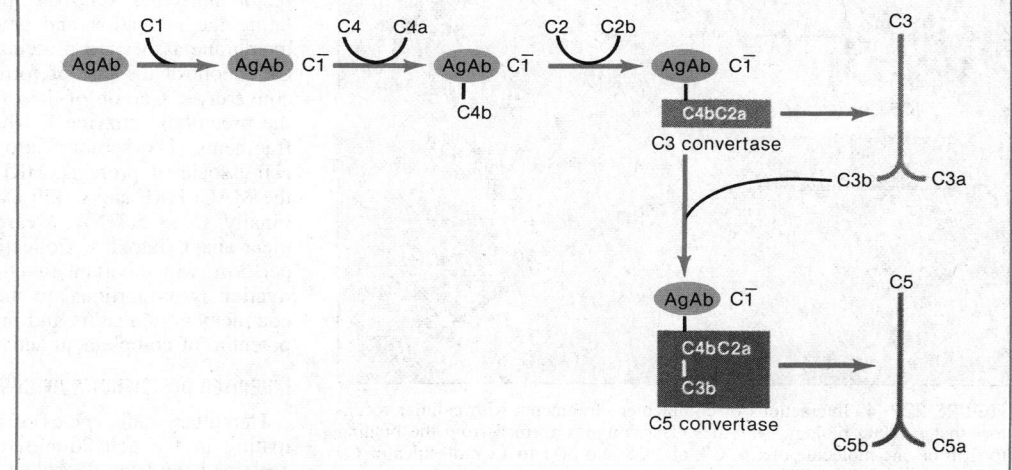

FIGURE 222–2. Formation of complement convertases in the classic pathway of activation.

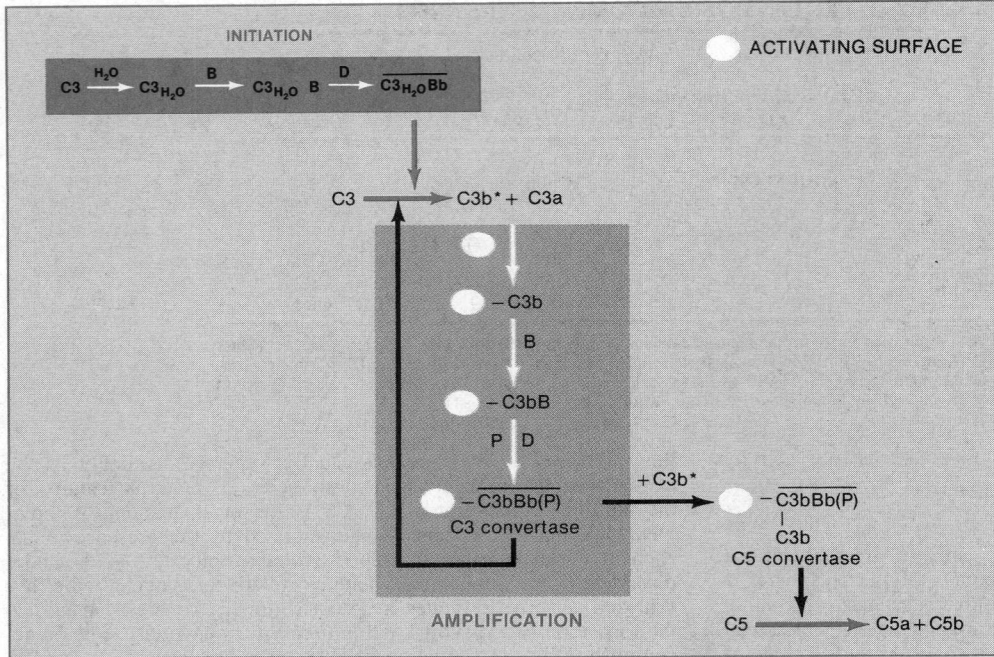

FIGURE 222-3. Formation of complement convertases in the alternative pathway of activation. Assembly of the *initiation* C3 convertase occurs at low levels continuously. When an activator is present, metastable C3b (C3b*) binds covalently to the activating surface and, because it is protected from the action of the regulatory proteins, initiates the assembly of the stable, *amplification* C3 convertase, which forms additional C3 convertase complexes and also the C5 convertase.

the $\overline{(C3b)_2Bb}$ complex, which is the C5 convertase of the alternative pathway (Fig. 222-3).

BIOLOGIC ACTIVITIES OF COMPLEMENT

With the exception of C5b, the fragments produced by the action of the convertases carry out their biologic functions by interacting with specific cellular receptors (Fig. 222-4). The complement *anaphylatoxins*, C3a and C5a, react with specific receptors to stimulate the release of histamine from mast cells and basophils mediating smooth muscle contraction and increased vascular permeability. In the presence of interleukin-3 (IL-3) or IL-5, C5a also causes release of leukotrienes from basophils. In addition, C5a evokes neutrophil and monocyte responses, including up-regulation of cellular receptors, adherence to vascular endothelia, chemotaxis, release of lysosomal enzymes, and generation of oxygen free radicals. Collectively, the anaphylatoxins allow for the recruitment of host defense molecules and cells to tissue sites invaded by pathogens. C3b and

its further cleavage fragments, C3bi and C3dg, react with multiple receptors distributed in a variety of cells (Table 222-2). C3b covalently attached to immune complexes binds to CR1 receptors on erythrocytes which transport the complexes to the liver where they are taken up by Kuppfer cells and cleared from the circulation. C3b and C3bi interact with CR1 and CR3, respectively, on phagocytic cells to promote ingestion of foreign cells and particles. Reaction of C3bi and C3dg with CR2 on B lymphocytes helps regulate immune responses. C5b initiates the assembly of a large protein-protein complex, termed membrane attack complex (MAC), by interacting sequentially with a single molecule of C6, C7, and C8 and with 1 to 12 molecules of C9. The MAC interacts directly with the lipid bilayer of biologic membranes through hydrophobic domains of the participating proteins and eventually forms a transmembrane channel that leads to killing of susceptible cells.

CONTROL OF COMPLEMENT ACTIVATION

The multiplicity and potency of the biologic activities generated when complement is activated and particularly the ability of complement to mediate acute inflammatory reactions and to produce lethal lesions in cell membranes present a threat not only to invading pathogens but also to the cells and tissues of the host. This self-damaging potential of complement activation is normally kept under effective control by a number of inhibitors and inactivators that act at points of enzymatic amplification and also at the level of effector molecules. C1 INH binds to and inhibits $C\overline{1r}$ and $C\overline{1s}$, regulating the activation and action of C1. A number of plasma and membrane-associated proteins, including C4bp, H, DAF, MCP, and CR1, control the rate of formation and the activity of complement convertases. Certain of these proteins act as obligatory cofactors for the proteolytic enzyme I, which cleaves C4b and C3b into smaller fragments. The serum S protein, also termed vitronectin, and two cell-associated proteins, HRF and CD59, inhibit the formation of the MAC. HRF and CD59 exhibit species specificity in their action. Finally, C3a/C5a INA, a carboxypeptidase, inactivates the complement anaphylatoxins. Collectively, the complement control proteins perform two important functions: They ensure that complement activation is proportional to the amount and duration of presence of complement activators and protect the host's cells from the harmful potential of complement activation products.

INHERITED DEFICIENCIES OF COMPLEMENT PROTEINS (Table 222-3)

Hereditary deficiencies of almost all complement proteins participating in the activation sequences and of several of the control proteins have been described. With two exceptions, complement deficiencies are inherited as autosomal recessive traits. C1 INH

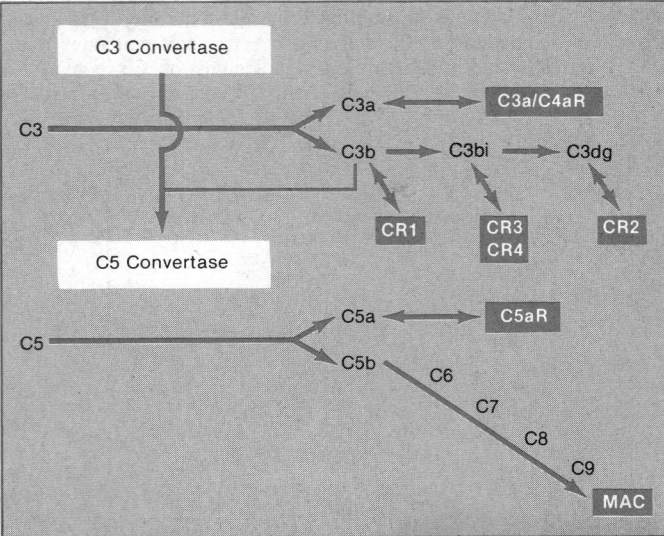

FIGURE 222-4. Interactions of complement fragments with cellular receptors that mediate biologic activities. The complex formed from the binding to C5b of one molecule of C6, C7, and C8 and of 1 to 12 molecules of C9 is termed MAC (membrane attack complex). It forms transmembrane pores by interacting directly with the lipid bilayer of biologic membranes.

TABLE 222-2. RECEPTORS FOR C3b AND ITS FRAGMENTS

Receptor	Ligands	Cellular Distribution	Functions
CR1	C3b, C4b, C3bi	Erythrocytes, neutrophils, eosinophils, monocytes, macrophages, B cells, T cell subsets, follicular dendritic cells, glomerular podocytes	Immune complex clearance, endocytosis, phagocytosis
CR2	C3dg, C3bi, Epstein-Barr virus	B cells, thymocytes, follicular dendritic cells, pharyngeal epithelial cells	Immunoregulation
CR3	C3bi	Neutrophils, monocytes, macrophages, large granular lymphocytes	Phagocytosis, leukocyte adhesion, enhanced cytotoxicity
CR4	C3bi	Neutrophils, monocytes, macrophages	Unknown

deficiency is inherited as an autosomal dominant and P deficiency as an X-linked trait. A rather limited number of clinical syndromes are associated with complement deficiencies. Deficiencies of C1q, C1r, C1s, C4, and C2 are associated with diseases of immune origin, including systemic lupus erythematosus (SLE), discoid lupus, glomerulonephritis, and nonspecific vasculitis. The underlying mechanisms are unclear, but impaired processing and clearance from the circulation of immune complexes and aberrant immunoregulation have been implicated in the pathogenesis of these syndromes. Clinically, SLE in complement-deficient individuals is characterized by early onset, extensive skin lesions, absent or mild renal involvement, and low levels of antinuclear and anti-DNA antibodies. Deficiencies of C3, H, I, or P predispose to severe recurrent infections with encapsulated pyogenic bacteria. Lack of or inefficient opsonization of the bacteria by C3b/C3bi apparently causes the susceptibility to infection. Individuals deficient in C5, C6, C7, or C8 are susceptible to disseminated neisserial infections. Direct lysis by complement is probably required for effective defense against gonococci and meningococci. Curiously, individuals with C9 deficiency are usually asymptomatic. Heterozygous deficiency of C1 INH results in hereditary angioedema (see Ch. 224), characterized by episodic attacks of circumscribed, nonpruritic edema of the skin or the mucosa of the respiratory or gastrointestinal tract.

Pathophysiology

In certain human diseases, uncontrolled or aberrant activation of complement plays an important pathogenetic role. The classic pathway activated at tissue sites by autoantibodies against tissue antigens or by immune complexes deposited at basement membranes results in accumulation of inflammatory cells and tissue damage. The former mechanism is exemplified by the renal lesions of Goodpasture's syndrome and the second by the vascular and renal lesions in SLE and other immune complex diseases. Hypocomplementemia is often present in patients with immune complex diseases, particularly SLE, but also in various other clinical syndromes. Measurement of serum complement levels thus provides a simple and widely used tool to diagnose and manage human diseases. The most commonly used assays in clinical practice are total hemolytic complement, C4, and C3. Total hemolytic complement, expressed in CH_{50} units, reflects the activity of all complement components. C4 and C3 are usually measured by immunochemical assays. Low complement levels by all three assays are often but not always seen in SLE, particularly in patients with renal involvement and during acute exacerbations of the disease. In patients with partial lipodystrophy with or without glomerulonephritis and in some patients with membranoproliferative glomerulonephritis, levels of total complement and C3 are very low, whereas C4 is usually normal. This is due to the presence of an IgG autoantibody, termed C3 nephritic factor, with specificity for the amplification C3 convertase. This au-

toantibody binds to C3bBb and creates a stable complex that is not regulated by control proteins and thus continuously cleaves C3. The alternative pathway is also activated during circulation of the blood through pump oxygenators or hemodialysis machines. The C5a generated during these procedures causes aggregation of neutrophils, leading to their sequestration in the pulmonary vasculature. In some patients this is manifested by symptoms of pulmonary dysfunction and hypoxemia. Complement activation may also play a role in the pathogenesis of myocardial reperfusion injury.

Ahearn JM, Fearon DT: Structure and function of the complement receptors CR1 (CD35) and CR2 (CD21). Adv Immunol 46:183, 1989. *Molecular biology, structure, and function of two important cellular receptors for C3 fragments.*

Campbell RD, Law SKA, Reid KBM, Sim RB: Structure, organization, and regulation of the complement genes. Annu Rev Immunol 6:161, 1988. *A review of the genetics and structure of complement proteins.*

Colten HR, Rosen FS: Complement deficiencies. Annu Rev Immunol 10:809, 1992. *An excellent review of genetic abnormalities of the complement system.*

Hebert LA, Cosio FG: The erythrocyte–immune complex–glomerulonephritis connection in man. Kidney Int 31:327, 1987. *Discusses immune complex processing, disposal, and tissue deposition.*

Volanakis JE, Fearon DT: The molecular biology of the complement system. *In* McCarty DJ, Koopman WJ (eds.): Arthritis and Allied Conditions. 12th ed. Philadelphia, Lea & Febiger, 1993 p 455. *A comprehensive description of the biochemistry and biology of the complement system.*

TABLE 222-3. DISEASES ASSOCIATED WITH INHERITED COMPLEMENT DEFICIENCIES

Deficient Protein	Diseases
C1q, C1r, C1s, C4, C2	SLE, SLE-like syndrome, discoid lupus, glomerulonephritis, vasculitis
C3, H, I, P	Recurrent pyogenic infections
C5, C6, C7, C8	Recurrent disseminated neisserial infections
C1 INH	Hereditary angioedema

223 PRIMARY IMMUNODEFICIENCY DISEASES
Rebecca H. Buckley

Since the first genetic defect in immunity was described in 1952, more than four dozen different primary immunodeficiency syndromes have been reported. Such diseases may involve any component of the immune system, including lymphocytes, phagocytic cells, and the complement proteins. This chapter focuses on abnormalities of lymphocytes. Deficiencies of the complement system (see Ch. 222) are mentioned briefly. A review of neutrophil dysfunction syndromes is presented in Ch. 139.1, and an overall review of the compromised host is given in Ch. 266. The acquired immunodeficiency syndrome (AIDS) is described in Part XXII.

Several of the primary immunodeficiency diseases have been mapped to specific chromosomal locations, and the fundamental biologic errors have been identified in a growing number of diseases (Table 223–1). Most are recessive traits, some of which are caused by mutations in genes on the X chromosome, others on autosomal chromosomes. Examples of the latter include an adhesion protein deficiency, now known to be due to mutations in the gene on chromosome 21q22.3 encoding the 95-Kd beta chain (CD18) common to three different leukocyte surface glycoprotein heterodimers, and combined immunodeficiencies due to abnormalities of purine salvage pathway enzymes, either adenosine deaminase (ADA, encoded by a gene on chromosome 20q13-ter) or purine nucleoside phosphorylase (PNP, encoded by a gene on chromosome 14q13.1) (see Ch. 181).

The faulty genes in many other immunodeficiencies are known to be on the X chromosome (Table 223–1). They have been localized

ITABLE 223–1. CHROMOSOMAL MAP LOCATIONS FOR FAULTY GENES IN PRIMARY IMMUNODEFICIENCY DISEASES

Chromosome	Disease
1q25	Chronic granulomatous disease (gp67^{phox})*
2p11	Kappa chain deficiency*
2g12	CD8 lymphocytopenia (ZAP70)*
6p21.3	(?)Common variable immunodeficiency and selective IgA deficiency
7q11.23	Chronic granulomatous disease (gp47^{phox})*
11	CD3 gamma chain deficiency*
11q22.3	Ataxia-telangiectasia
14q13.1	Purine nucleoside phosphorylase deficiency*
14q32.3	Immunoglobulin heavy chain deletion*
16q24	Chronic granulomatous disease (gp22^{phox})*
20q13-ter	Adenosine deaminase deficiency*
21q22.3	Leukocyte adhesion deficiency (CD18)*
22q11.2	DiGeorge syndrome
Xp21.1	Chronic granulomatous disease (gp91^{phox})*
Xp11.22–p11.23	Wiskott-Aldrich syndrome (proline-rich protein-WASP)*
Xq13	Severe combined immunodeficiency (gamma chain of IL-2R)*
Xq22	X-linked agammaglobulinemia (Bruton tyrosine kinase, BTK)*
Xq24–26	X-linked lymphoproliferative syndrome
Xq26	Immunodeficiency with hyper-IgM (CD40 ligand—gp39)*

* Gene cloned and sequenced, gene product known

to specific sites in the case of X-linked agammaglobulinemia, X-linked severe combined immunodeficiency, the Wiskott-Aldrich syndrome, X-linked lymphoproliferative disease, X-linked hyper-IgM, properdin deficiency, and X-linked chronic granulomatous disease (CGD). Until recently, there was little insight into the fundamental problems underlying most of these conditions. Recently, however, the molecular bases of four X-linked immunodeficiency disorders have been reported. These include X-linked immunodeficiency with hyper-IgM, X-linked agammaglobulinemia, X-linked severe combined immunodeficiency, and the Wiskott-Aldrich syndrome. Immune deficiency can also be associated with broad deficiencies of HLA class I and II antigens, and these have been shown to be due to different mutations in transactin factors governing the surface expression of these molecules. Table 223–2 lists the most prominent functional abnormalities and the presumed cellular level of the defect in 19 primary immunodeficiency syndromes.

In contrast to AIDS, which has a new case acquisition rate of more than 2500 per week, primary immunodeficiency diseases are rare. The incidence of agammaglobulinemia is estimated at 1 in 50,000. Selective absence of serum and secretory IgA, the most common, has a reported prevalence of 1 in 333 to 1 in 700.

APPROACHES TO THE PATIENT WITH SUSPECTED IMMUNODEFICIENCY

The number of patients suspected of having primary immunodeficiency will far exceed the incidences of these diseases. So it is important that the tests selected for immunologic assessment be broadly informative, reliable, and cost effective. Familiarity with certain clinical guidelines aids in the initial selection. Patients with antibody-, phagocytic-cell–, or complement deficiencies have recurrent infections with high-grade encapsulated bacteria. Therefore, those with only repeated viral respiratory infections are not likely to have any of these disorders. By contrast, patients with deficiencies in T-cell function usually manifest opportunistic infections. Most defects can be ruled out at little cost to the patient if the proper choice of screening tests is made. Among the most informative are the complete and differential blood counts and the sedimentation rate. Examining red cells for Howell-Jolly bodies helps exclude asplenia. A normal platelet count rules out Wiskott-Aldrich syndrome. If the sedimentation rate is normal, chronic bacterial infection is unlikely. If the absolute neutrophil count is normal, congenital and acquired neutropenia and severe chemotactic defects are eliminated. If the absolute lymphocyte count is normal, a severe T-cell defect is unlikely. Beyond this, it is good to keep in mind that tests of immune function are far more informative and cost effec-

tive than those measuring immunoglobulin concentrations or enumerating lymphocyte subpopulations.

In assessing B cell function, determinations of antibody titers to proteins (such as tetanus and diphtheria toxoids) and polysaccharides (such as pneumococcal antigens) following immunization are the most useful tests. As a rule, patients with B-cell defects for which there is an effective or indicated treatment do not produce antibodies normally. However, the presence of such antibodies does not exclude IgA deficiency, which would also be missed on a serum electrophoretic analysis. Immunoelectrophoresis is not quantitative and, for that reason, is not useful in evaluating immune competence. The quantification of serum IgA is particularly cost effective. If the IgA concentration is normal, this rules out not only IgA deficiency but all of the permanent types of agammaglobulinemia, because IgA is usually very low or absent in those conditions as well. A particularly uneconomical study is IgG-subclass measurement. It is far more helpful to know the results of antibody titer measurement because there are well-documented cases of antibody deficiency despite normal concentrations of all immunoglobulin classes and subclasses.

The most cost-effective test for assessing T-cell function is an intradermal skin test with 0.1 ml of a 1:1000 dilution of a known potent *Candida albicans* extract. If the test is positive, as defined by

TABLE 223–2. CHARACTERISTICS OF SOME PRIMARY IMMUNODEFICIENCY DISORDERS

Disorder	Functional Deficiencies	Molecular Defect
X-linked agammaglobulinemia	Antibody	Mutations in Bruton tyrosine kinase, BTK
Common variable immunodeficiency (CVID "acquired" hypogammaglobulinemia)	Antibody	Unknown, ? in MHC Class III region
Selective IgA deficiency	IgA antibody	Unknown, ? in MHC Class III region
Immunodeficiency with elevated IgM	IgG and IgA antibodies	Mutations in CD40 ligand on activated T cells
Transient hypogammaglobulinemia of infancy	None; immunoglobulins low, but antibodies present	Unknown
Antibody deficiency with near-normal immunoglobulins	Antibody	Unknown; ? related to CVID
X-linked lymphoproliferative disease	Anti-EBV nuclear antigen antibody	B cell; ? also T cell
DiGeorge syndrome	T cellular; some antibody	Microdeletions in chromosome 22q11
Nezelof syndrome (including PNP deficiency)	T cellular; some antibody	Unknown; PNP deficiency
Severe combined immunodeficiency syndromes (autosomal recessive; ADA deficiency; X-linked recessive; defective expression of HLA antigens; reticular dysgenesis)	Antibody and T cellular; phagocytic in reticular dysgenesis	ADA deficiency; mutations in gamma chain of the IL-2 receptor; other unknown defects
Wiskott-Aldrich syndrome	Antibody; T cellular	Mutations in a proline-rich protein, WASP
Ataxia-telangiectasia	Antibody; T cellular	Unknown
Cartilage-hair hypoplasia	T cellular	Unknown
Immunodeficiency with thymoma	Antibody; some T cellular	Unknown
Hyperimmunoglobulinemia E syndrome	Specific immune responses; excessive IgE	Unknown
Chronic mucocutaneous candidiasis	Variable cellular	Unknown
Leukocyte adhesion deficiency 1	Cytotoxic lymphocytes; phagocytic cell adhesion	Mutations in CD18
Leukocyte adhesion deficiency 2	Phagocytic cell adhesion	Unknown

erythema and induration of ≥ 10 mm at 48 hours, virtually all primary T-cell defects are excluded and the need for more expensive *in vitro* tests, such as lymphocyte phenotyping or assessments of responses to mitogens, is obviated. Killing defects of phagocytic cells, which should be suspected if the patient has problems with staphylococcal or gram-negative infections, can be screened for by tests measuring the neutrophil respiratory burst after phagocytosis or phorbol ester stimulation. Complement defects can be most effectively screened for in a CH50 assay, which measures the intactness of the entire complement pathway. If these tests are abnormal, or even if they are normal and clinical features of the patient still strongly suggest a host defect, the patient should be evaluated at a center where more definitive immunologic studies can be done before any type of immunologic treatment is begun.

ANTIBODY DEFICIENCY DISORDERS

Antibody deficiency may occur either as a congenital or an "acquired" abnormality, although in both situations it appears to be genetically determined. Most patients are recognized because they have recurrent infections, but some individuals with selective IgA deficiency or infants with transient hypogammaglobulinemia may have few or no infections.

X-LINKED AGAMMAGLOBULINEMIA (XLA). A majority of boys afflicted with this malady remain well during the first 6 to 9 months of life by virtue of maternally transmitted immunoglobulin. Thereafter, they repeatedly acquire infections with high-grade extracellular pyogenic organisms such as pneumococci, streptococci, and *Haemophilus* unless given prophylactic antibiotics or gammaglobulin therapy. The most common types of infections include sinusitis, pneumonia, otitis, septic arthritis, meningitis, and septicemia. Chronic fungal infections are usually not present, and *Pneumocystis carinii* pneumonia rarely occurs unless there is an associated neutropenia. Viral infections and live virus vaccines are also usually handled normally, with the notable exceptions of hepatitis and enterovirus infections. Several cases of paralysis after receiving polio vaccine have occurred, presumably because of muta-

tion of persistent vaccine virus to a more neurotropic form. In addition, a dermatomyositis-like syndrome accompanied by chronic, eventually fatal central nervous system disease caused by various echoviruses has occurred in more than 40 patients.

The diagnosis of XLA is suspected if serum concentrations of IgG, IgA, and IgM are below the 95% confidence limits for appropriate age- and race-matched controls (usually there is < 100 mg per deciliter total immunoglobulin). Demonstrated antibody deficiency in serum and in external secretions is of great importance in distinguishing this disorder from transient hypogammaglobulinemia of infancy. Tests for natural antibodies to blood group substances, for antibodies to antigens given during standard courses of immunization, and for antibodies to and ability to clear bacteriophage $\phi \times 174$ are markedly abnormal. Polymorphonuclear functions are usually normal, but some patients with this condition have had transient, persistent, or cyclic neutropenia.

Lymphopenia is uncommon, and the percentages of T cells and T cell subsets have been found to be normal or elevated in most instances. In contrast, blood lymphocytes bearing surface immunoglobulin, "Ia-like" antigens, or the EBV receptor, or reacting with a specific anti-B cell serum are absent or present in very low numbers. Hypoplasia of adenoids, tonsils, and peripheral lymph nodes is the rule; germinal centers are not present, and plasma cells are rarely found. Conversely, normal numbers of pre-B cells are found in the bone marrow. The abnormal gene in XLA was recently discovered by two groups, one using the technique of positional cloning and the other by seeking and finding a tyrosine kinase important in B-cell signaling that proved to be encoded by a gene on the X chromosome in the region where Bruton's disease had been mapped (see Tables 223–1 and 223–2 and Fig. 223–1). The tyrosine kinase has been named Bruton tyrosine kinase (or BTK) in honor of Dr. Bruton. BTK is a member of the Src-related nonreceptor cytoplasmic tyrosine kinase family, which includes Lck, Fyn, and Lyn, thought to be involved in signal transduction in many

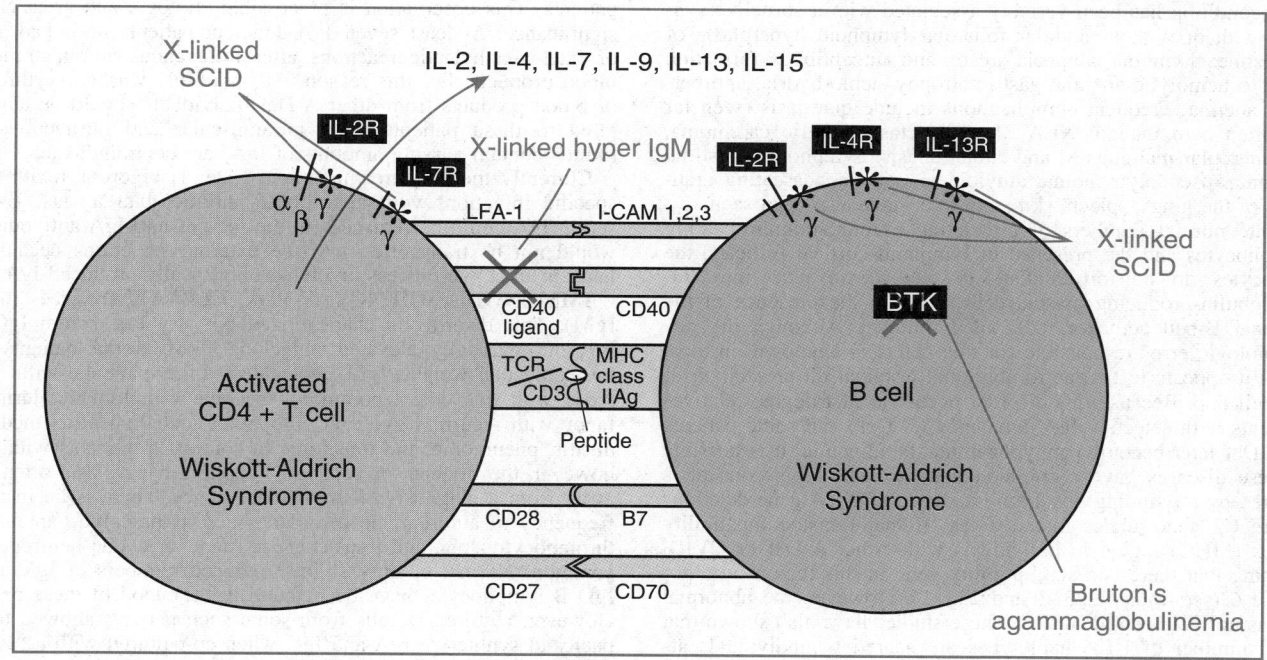

FIGURE 223–1. Schematic of molecules involved in T- and B-cell interaction and signal transduction, showing the location of newly defined molecular defects in four X-linked primary immunodeficiency diseases. Mutations in the gene encoding the cytoplasmic nonreceptor tyrosine kinase lead to Bruton's or X-linked agammaglobulinemia by preventing B-cell maturation beyond the pre–B cell stage. Mutations in the gene for the CD40 ligand, or gp39, prevent expression of this crucial molecule necessary for T cells to activate B cells by interacting with CD40 on their surface. These mutations are responsible for the defect in X-linked immunodeficiency with hyper-IgM that prevents the B cells from isotype-switching. Mutations in the interleukin-2 (IL-2) receptor gamma chain (IL-2Rγ) prevent the binding of not only IL-2 but of several other cytokines necessary for T- and B-cell development and function (IL-4, IL-7, IL-9, IL-13, and IL-15) because the IL-2Rγ chain is also a component of those cytokine receptors. IL-2Rγ mutations are thus responsible for the profound deficiencies in T, B, and natural killer (NK) cell function present in infants with X-linked severe combined immunodeficiency disease (XSCID). Finally, mutations in a novel gene encoding a 501–amino acid proline-rich protein (WASP) limited expression to lymphocytic and megakaryocytic cell lineages, resulted in the Wiskott-Aldrich syndrome.

hematopoietic cells. BTK is expressed at high levels in all B-lineage cells, including pre-B cells; it has not been detected in any cells of T lineage, but it has in cells of the myeloid series. Thus far, most males with known XLA (by family history) have had low to undetectable BTK mRNA and kinase activity due to point mutations in the catalytic (kinase) domain in BTK. Mixed lymphocyte responsiveness and lymphocyte responses to antigens and mitogens are normal. Cell-mediated immune responses can be detected *in vivo,* and the thymus has appeared normal in all autopsied cases.

Except in those unfortunate patients who develop polio, persistent echovirus infection, or lymphoreticular malignancy, the overall prognosis is reasonably good if humoral replacement therapy is instituted early. Systemic infection can be prevented by administering intravenous immune serum globulin (ISG, primarily IgG) at a dose of 400 mg per kilogram every 3 to 4 weeks. Such preparations are known to be free of the AIDS virus. Many patients go on to develop crippling sinopulmonary disease despite this therapy because no effective means exist for replacing secretory IgA at the mucosal surface. Chronic antibiotic therapy is also usually necessary for managing such patients.

COMMON VARIABLE IMMUNODEFICIENCY (CVID). Patients with this condition (formerly known as acquired hypogammaglobulinemia) may appear similar clinically in many respects to those with XLA. Although this disorder may occur in infants and young children, most patients present with a history of recurrent infection beginning several years after birth. CVID is distinguished from XLA by later age of onset, somewhat less severe susceptibility to infections, and almost equal gender distribution. In contrast to patients with the X-linked form, patients with CVID may have normal sized or enlarged tonsils and lymph nodes, and the latter may have cortical follicles. Additionally, such patients often have normal or nearly normal numbers of circulating immunoglobulin-bearing B lymphocytes. Nevertheless, the serum immunoglobulin and antibody deficiencies are usually just as profound, and the bacterial etiologic agents are the same as in the X-linked disorder. Echovirus meningoencephalitis is rare in patients with CVID.

This condition has been variably associated with a spruelike syndrome, with or without nodular follicular lymphoid hyperplasia of the intestine; thymoma; alopecia areata; and autoantibody formation leading to hemolytic anemia, gastric atrophy, achlorhydria, and pernicious anemia. Frequent complications include giardiasis (seen far more often here than in XLA), bronchiectasis, gastric carcinoma, lymphoreticular malignancy, and cholelithiasis. Lymphoid interstitial pneumonia, pseudolymphoma, amyloidosis, and noncaseating granulomas of the lungs, spleen, skin, and liver have also been seen.

Despite normal numbers of circulating immunoglobulin-bearing B lymphocytes and the presence of lymphoid cortical follicles, the lymphocytes do not differentiate *in vivo* or *in vitro* into immunoglobulin-producing plasma cells, even in the presence of the polyclonal B-cell activator, pokeweed mitogen. Although the primary biologic error responsible for this defect is unknown, in most patients it appears to be due to abnormal terminal differentiation of the B-cell line. Because this disorder occurs in first degree relatives of patients with selective IgA deficiency (A Def) and some patients with A Def later become panhypogammaglobulinemic, it is possible that these diseases have a common genetic basis. This concept is supported by the finding of a high incidence of C4-A gene deletions and rare C2 gene alleles in the Class III major histocompatibility complex (MHC) region in individuals with either A Def or CVID, suggesting that there is a susceptibility gene in this region on chromosome 6 (see Tables 223–1 and 223–2). However, the abnormal gene has not yet been identified. These studies have also shown that a small number of HLA haplotypes are shared by individuals affected with CVID and A Def, with at least one of two particular haplotypes being present in 77% of those affected. In one large family with 13 members, 2 had A Def and 3 had CVID. All of the immunodeficient patients in the family had at least one copy of an MHC haplotype shown to be abnormally frequent in A Def and CVID: HLA-DQB1 *0201, HLA-DR3, C4B-Sf, C4A-deleted, G11-15, Bf-0.4, C2a, HSP70-7.5, TNFα-5, HLA-B8, and HLA-A1. However, four immunologically normal members of the pedigree also possessed this haplotype, indicating that its presence alone is not sufficient for expression of the defects. Environmental factors, particularly drugs such as phenytoin, have been suspected to pro-

vide the triggers for disease expression in individuals with the permissive genetic background. The treatment of CVID is the same as that for the X-linked disorder.

SELECTIVE IGA DEFICIENCY (A Def). An isolated near-absence (i.e., < 10 mg per deciliter) of serum and secretory IgA is the most common primary immunodeficiency disorder, with a frequency of 1:333 being reported among some blood donors. Although A Def has been observed in apparently healthy individuals, it is commonly associated with ill health. The kinds of health problems experienced often reflect the type of clinic from which the patients are drawn. Among 75 from an allergy-immunology clinic, there were high frequencies of chronic or recurrent respiratory tract infection and atopic diseases. In contrast, 30 A Def patients drawn from a rheumatology clinic had a high frequency of autoimmune and/or collagen vascular disease.

IgA is the major immunoglobulin of external secretions. As would be expected, its deficiency is associated with infections occurring predominantly in the respiratory, gastrointestinal, and urogenital tracts. Bacterial agents responsible are essentially the same as in other types of antibody deficiency syndromes. There is no clear evidence that patients with this disorder have an undue susceptibility to viral agents. Serum concentrations of other immunoglobulins are usually normal in patients with A Def, although an IgG$_2$ subclass deficiency has been reported in some, and IgM (usually increased) may be of the low-molecular-weight variety. The defect may not always be permanent. Studies of T-cell function have been normal in most patients.

In addition to limiting the attachment of infectious agents to mucosal surfaces, secretory IgA antibodies probably act to prevent absorption of other foreign antigens, such as those in the diet. There is a high incidence of allergy and of IgG antibodies against cow's milk and ruminant serum proteins in patients with IgA deficiency. The antiruminant antibodies often falsely detect "IgA" in immunoassays that use goat (but not rabbit) antisera. Intestinal nodular hyperplasia has been seen in a few such patients. A spruelike syndrome may occur in adults with selective IgA deficiency and sometimes responds to a gluten-free diet.

Serum antibodies to IgA are found in as many as 44% of such patients. This observation is of possible etiologic and great clinical significance. At least seven IgA-deficient patients have had severe or fatal anaphylactic reactions after intravenous administration of blood products. For this reason, only multiply washed erythrocytes or blood products from other A Def individuals should be administered to these patients; both intramuscular and intravenous ISG (which contain varying amounts of IgA) are contraindicated.

Currently the only treatment for A Def is vigorous treatment of specific infections with appropriate antimicrobial agents. Even if serum IgA could be replaced (in the face of anti-IgA antibodies), it would not be transported into the external secretions because the latter is an active process involving only locally produced IgA.

IMMUNODEFICIENCY WITH ELEVATED IgM (hyper-IgM). This disorder is characterized by very low serum IgG and IgA but markedly elevated polyclonal IgM. Some patients have low-molecular-weight IgM molecules. Like patients with XLA, those with this defect commonly become symptomatic during infancy with recurrent pyogenic infections, including otitis media, sinusitis, pneumonia, and tonsillitis. In contrast to patients with XLA, however, the frequent presence of lymphoid hyperplasia often leads away from a diagnosis of immunodeficiency. There is an increased frequency of autoimmune disorders, such as hemolytic anemia and thrombocytopenia, and transient, persistent, or cyclic neutropenia is common. Normal or only slightly reduced numbers of IgM and/or IgD B lymphocytes have been found in the blood of these patients. However, cultured B cells from some such patients showed the capacity to synthesize IgA and IgG when co-cultured with a "switch" T cell line, suggesting that, in those patients, the defect lay in T lineage cells. A sex-linked mode of inheritance has been noted in many pedigrees. The abnormal gene in the X-linked type has been localized to Xq26 (see Table 223–1), and was recently isolated. The gene product is the gp39 ligand (CD40L, on activated T cells) (see Fig. 223–1) for CD40 on B cells (see Tables 223–1 and 223–2 and Fig. 223–1). Cross-linking of CD40 on either normal or hyper-IgM B cells by reacting them with a monoclonal antibody to CD40 or allowing CD40 to interact with normal T cell CD40L in the presence of certain cytokines (IL-2, IL-4, or IL-10) causes the B cells to undergo proliferation and isotype switching and to secrete various types of immunoglobulins. CD40L is a type II integral membrane glycoprotein with significant sequence homology to TNF; it is found only on activated T cells, primarily of the CD4 phenotype. Mutations in the CD40L on activated T cells from hyper-IgM patients result in failure of signaling of B cells to undergo isotype switching; thus, they produce only IgM. However, the facts that not all males with hyper-IgM have had a mutation in the CD40L, that B cells from such patients fail to isotype switch with monoclonal antibodies to CD40, and that there are several examples in females suggest that this condition has more than one genetic cause.

Because these patients are unable to make IgG antibodies, the treatment is the same as for agammaglobulinemia.

TRANSIENT HYPOGAMMAGLOBULINEMIA OF INFANCY. Unlike patients with XLA or CVID, those with this condition can synthesize antibodies to human type A and B erythrocytes and to diphtheria and tetanus toxoids normally, usually by age 6 to 11 months, well before immunoglobulin concentrations become normal. The finding of only 11 cases of transient hypogammaglobulinemia of infancy among > 10,000 sera tested by the author over a 12-year period suggests that this is not a common entity.

Gammaglobulin replacement therapy is not indicated in this condition. In addition to the known risks of inducing anti-IgG allotype antibodies, passively administered antibodies could block endogenous primary antibody formation in the same manner that RhoGAM suppresses anti-D antibodies in Rh-negative mothers delivering Rh-positive infants.

ANTIBODY DEFICIENCY WITH NEAR-NORMAL IMMUNOGLOBULINS. The author and her associates have studied the antibody-forming capacities of 12 patients with deficient antibody responses despite apparently normal T-cell function and normal or nearly normal immunoglobulin concentrations. This problem would not be detected unless functional tests of antibody-forming capacity are conducted. It may represent an early stage of "acquired" agammaglobulinemia (or CVID). Patients with this disorder are candidates for immunoglobulin replacement therapy.

X-LINKED LYMPHOPROLIFERATIVE DISEASE. This disorder, also referred to as *Duncan's disease* (after the original kindred in which it was described), is characterized by an impaired immune response to Epstein-Barr virus (EBV) (see Ch. 341). Affected persons are apparently healthy until they experience infectious mononucleosis. Two thirds of the more than 100 patients studied thus far died of overwhelming EBV-induced B-cell proliferation during mononucleosis. A majority of the survivors developed hypogammaglobulinemia or B-cell lymphomas or both. Such individuals have marked impairment in production of antibodies to the EBV nuclear antigen, whereas titers of antibodies to the viral capsid antigen have ranged from zero to markedly elevated. Antibody-dependent cell-mediated cytotoxicity against EBV-infected cells and natural killer function are depressed, and there is a deficiency in long-lived T-cell immunity to EBV. Despite normal numbers of B and T cells, there is an elevated percentage of lymphocytes of the suppressor (CD8$^+$) phenotype. In addition, lymphocyte immunoglobulin synthesis in response to polyclonal B-cell mitogen stimulation *in vitro* is markedly depressed. Thus, both EBV-specific and nonspecific immunologic abnormalities occur in these patients.

CELLULAR IMMUNODEFICIENCY DISORDERS

In general, patients with partial or absolute defects in T-cell function have infections or other clinical problems for which there is no effective treatment or which are often of a more severe nature than in those with antibody deficiency disorders. It is therefore rare that such individuals survive beyond infancy or childhood.

THYMIC HYPOPLASIA (DIGEORGE'S SYNDROME). This condition results from dysmorphogenesis of the third and fourth pharyngeal pouches, leading to hypoplasia or aplasia of the thymus and parathyroid glands. Other structures forming at the same age are also frequently affected, resulting in anomalies of the great vessels (right-sided aortic arch), esophageal atresia, bifid uvula, congenital heart disease (atrial and ventricular septal defects), a short philtrum of the upper lip, hypertelorism, an antimongoloid slant to the eyes, mandibular hypoplasia, and low-set (often notched) ears. The diagnosis is usually first suggested by the presence of hypocalcemic seizures during the neonatal period. DiGeorge's syndrome has occurred in both males and females, and consistent deletions and microdeletions of 22q11 have been found in a majority of cases (see Tables 223–1 and 223–2). Familial occurrence is rare but has been reported.

A variable degree of hypoplasia is more frequent than total aplasia of the thymus and parathyroid glands. Some children with the features of this syndrome have little trouble with infections and show evidence of some cell-mediated immunity. They are often referred to as having partial DiGeorge's syndrome. Those with marked thymic hypoplasia may resemble infants with severe combined immunodeficiency in their susceptibility to infection with low-grade or opportunistic pathogens (i.e., fungi, viruses, and *Pneumocystis carinii*) and to graft-versus-host (GVH) disease from nonirradiated blood transfusions.

Serum immunoglobulins are usually normal for age, but some fractions, particularly IgA, may be diminished and IgE may be elevated. T-cell numbers are decreased, and there is an increased number of B cells. Responses of peripheral blood lymphocytes following mitogen stimulation, like the intradermal delayed hypersensitivity response, have been absent, reduced, or normal. Careful postmortem studies have sometimes revealed tiny nests of thymic tissue containing Hassall's corpuscles and a normal density of thymocytes. Lymphoid follicles usually appear normal, but lymph node paracortical areas and thymus-dependent regions of the spleen show variable degrees of depletion, depending upon the degree of thymic hypoplasia. Because of variability in the severity of the immunodeficiency, it is difficult to evaluate claimed benefits of fetal thymus transplantation.

CELLULAR IMMUNODEFICIENCY WITH IMMUNOGLOBULINS (NEZELOF'S SYNDROME). This syndrome is characterized by lymphopenia, diminished lymphoid tissue, abnormal thymus architecture, and the presence of normal or increased immunoglobulins. Children with this condition may have recurrent or chronic pulmonary infections, failure to thrive, oral or cutaneous candidiasis, chronic diarrhea, recurrent skin infections, gram-negative sepsis, urinary tract infections, severe varicella, or combinations of these. An autosomal-recessive pattern of inheritance has been suggested in some cases, but an X-linked mode seemed more likely in others. Other findings include neutropenia and eosinophilia.

Studies of cellular immune function have shown delayed cutaneous anergy to ubiquitous antigens and low to absent *in vitro* lymphocyte responses to mitogens and allogeneic cells. Such patients have profound deficiencies of total T cells and T-cell subsets. Peripheral lymphoid tissues demonstrate paracortical lymphocyte depletion. The thymuses are very small and have a paucity of thymocytes and usually no Hassall's corpuscles; however, in contrast to AIDS, thymic epithelium is present. This is the primary immunodeficiency disorder most likely to be confused with AIDS. Fatal or serious infections have included varicella, vaccinia, *Pneumocystis carinii*, cytomegalovirus, rubeola, *Pseudomonas*, and *Mycobacterium kansasii*. Some patients have been reconstituted by bone marrow transplantation, but most other forms of therapy have been unsuccessful.

With Purine Nucleoside Phosphorylase Deficiency. More than 35 patients with Nezelof's syndrome have been found to have purine nucleoside phosphorylase (PNP) deficiency. In contrast to patients with adenosine deaminase (ADA) deficiency, serum and urinary uric acid are markedly deficient, and no characteristic physical or skeletal abnormalities have been noted. Some patients have suffered from a progressive neurologic disorder with spastic tetraplegia, some developed autoimmune hemolytic anemia, and others idiopathic thrombocytopenic purpura. Deaths have occurred from generalized vaccinia, varicella, lymphosarcoma, and GVH disease following blood transfusions. There is profound lymphopenia due to a marked deficiency of T cells and T-cell subsets, but there is usually an increased percentage of cells with natural killer (NK) phenotype and function. Attempts to correct the immunologic and enzymatic deficiencies of PNP-deficient patients by enzyme replacement or deoxycytidine therapy have not been successful. Some patients have been treated successfully with HLA-identical bone marrow transplants.

SEVERE COMBINED IMMUNODEFICIENCY (SCID) DISORDERS

The syndromes of SCID are characterized by their apparent congenital absence of all adaptive immune function and a great diversity of genetic, enzymatic, hematologic, and immunologic features. Unless immunologic reconstitution can be achieved through immunocompetent tissue transplants or enzyme replacement therapy or unless gnotobiotic isolation can be carried out, death usually occurs before the patient's first birthday. The major subcategories of this disorder are discussed below.

AUTOSOMAL RECESSIVE SEVERE COMBINED IMMUNODEFICIENCY DISEASE. Within the first few months of life, infants affected with this first-described SCID syndrome have frequent episodes of otitis, pneumonia, sepsis, diarrhea, and cutaneous infections. Growth may appear normal initially, but extreme wasting soon develops. Persistent infections with opportunistic organisms such as *Candida albicans, Pneumocystis carinii,* varicella, measles, parainfluenza 3, cytomegalovirus, and BCG frequently lead to death. These infants also lack the ability to reject foreign tissue and are therefore at risk for GVH disease. GVH reactions can result from maternal immunocompetent cells crossing the placenta or from the administration of blood products containing viable histoincompatible lymphocytes.

Immunologic evaluation reveals serum immunoglobulin concentrations to be diminished, and no antibody formation occurs following immunization. There is a lack of cellular immune function, with lymphopenia and absence of lymphocyte responses to mitogens or allogeneic cells, delayed cutaneous anergy, and inability to reject foreign tissues. Marked heterogeneity of lymphocyte subpopulations exists among SCID patients. Despite the uniformly profound lack of T- or B-cell function, some patients have had low numbers of both B and T lymphocytes, whereas others have had elevated numbers of B cells, and most of the lymphocytes of other infants with SCID are large granular lymphocytes with NK cell phenotype and function. Typically, these patients have very small thymuses (<1 gram), which usually fail to descend from the neck, contain few thymic lymphocytes, lack corticomedullary distinction, and lack Hassall's corpuscles. Despite the profound thymocyte depletion in SCID patients, thymic epithelium is present. Tonsils, adenoids, lymph nodes, and Peyer's patches are absent or extremely underdeveloped.

ISG fails to halt the progressively downhill course of SCID. Transplantation of bone marrow cells from HLA genotypically identical or D locus-compatible donors has resulted in apparent complete correction of the immunologic defect in >90 of these patients. For the past 12 years techniques to deplete all post-thymic T cells from donor marrow have also allowed the use of haploidentical (half-matched) bone marrow cells for correction of SCID. These employ either a combination of soy lectin agglutination and sheep erythrocyte rosetting (the most successful method) or incubation with monoclonal antibodies to human T cells and complement. Both methods leave the stem cells intact. To date, >200 infants with SCID who would have otherwise died because of lack of an HLA-identical donor have been treated successfully with T cell-depleted haploidentical bone marrow with few signs of GVH reaction.

With Adenosine Deaminase (ADA) Deficiency (See also Ch. 181). Absence of the enzyme ADA has been observed in approximately 40% of patients with the autosomal recessive form of SCID. Marked accumulations of adenosine, 2'-deoxyadenosine, and 2'-O-methyladenosine directly or indirectly lead to lymphocyte toxicity, which causes the immunodeficiency. Adenosine and deoxyadenosine are apparent suicide inactivators of the enzyme S-adenosylhomocysteine (SAH) hydrolase, resulting in the accumulation of SAH. SAH is a potent inhibitor of virtually all cellular methylation reactions. Although most such patients have had profound lymphopenia from the earliest age studied, a few have had early normal or fluctuating lymphocyte counts that declined by ages 6 weeks to 2 years. In contrast to "classic" SCID, ADA-deficient patients have been found to have rib cage abnormalities similar to a rachitic rosary and multiple skeletal abnormalities of chondroosseous dysplasia on radiographic examination.

Both matched sibling and haploidentical post-thymic T cell-depleted bone marrow transplants have resulted in lymphocyte chimerism and partial or complete correction of the immunologic defect in ADA-deficient SCID. Enzyme replacement therapy with irradiated packed normal erythrocytes or polyethylene-glycol–modi-

fied bovine ADA on a continuing basis has resulted in improvement in some patients. This condition was the first in which somatic cell gene therapy was attempted, but to date there has been only limited success.

X-LINKED RECESSIVE SEVERE COMBINED IMMUNODEFICIENCY DISEASE (XSCID). This is thought to be the most common form of SCID in the United States. Clinically, immunologically, and histopathologically, these patients appear similar to those with the autosomal recessive form except for uniformly low percentages of T and NK cells and an elevated percentage of B cells. The abnormal gene in XSCID was mapped by RFLP and linkage analysis to Xq13 (see Table 223–1). Recently, it was identified as the gene encoding the gamma chain of the IL-2 receptor (IL-2R). IL-2, formerly known as T-cell growth factor, plays a key role in intracellular signaling in T cells and, consequently, in the function and regulation of the immune system. Because genetically engineered IL-2–deficient mice and humans have T cells and a much less severe immunodeficiency, it was initially difficult to see how abnormalities in the IL-2R could lead to the devastating immunodeficiency of XSCID. However, the γ chain of the IL-2R has recently been shown to be a component of the receptors for several other cytokines that regulate the function and development of the immune system, IL-4, IL-7, and probably IL-9, IL-13, and IL-15 (see Fig. 223–1). One chain of each of the IL-2, IL-4, and IL-7 receptors is unique for each receptor, whereas the shared γ chain functions both to increase the affinity of the receptor for the respective cytokine and to enable the receptors to mediate intracellular signaling. IL-2, IL-4, and IL-7 are all facilitators of different stages of the growth and development of both T and B cells. Therefore, incapacitation of the receptors for all of these developmentally crucial cytokines by genetic mutations in their common γ chain provides an explanation for the severity of the immunodeficiency in XSCID. All XSCID infants reported thus far have been found to have point mutations in the IL-2R gamma chain. Carriers can be detected by demonstrating nonrandom X-chromosome inactivation in their T lymphocytes. Results of X-chromosome inactivation studies in obligate carrier mothers also suggest that the genetic defect affects their B and NK lineage cells, as well as their T cells. This is in keeping with the author's personal observations of very poor B- and NK-cell function in infants with X-linked SCID following nonablated bone marrow cell transplantation, despite excellent reconstitution of T-cell function by donor-derived T cells.

DEFECTIVE EXPRESSION OF MAJOR HISTOCOMPATIBILITY COMPLEX (MHC) ANTIGENS. There are two main forms: MHC class I antigen deficiency ("bare lymphocyte syndrome") and MHC class I antigen deficiency plus absence of MHC class II antigens. These autosomal recessive conditions are due to mutations in X-box binding proteins that result in failure of surface membrane expression of the HLA antigens. Sera from affected individuals contain normal quantities of MHC class I antigens and β_2 microglobulin. Patients (usually of North African descent) present with persistent diarrhea in early infancy and have oral candidiasis, bacterial pneumonia, pneumocystosis, septicemia, and undue susceptibility to enteroviruses, herpes, and other viral agents. Those with both class I and II antigen deficiencies also have malabsorption. There is variable hypogammaglobulinemia with decreased serum IgM and IgA and poor to absent antibody production. B-cell percentages are usually normal, but plasma cells are absent in tissues. Lymphopenia is only moderate; T-cell functions *in vivo* and *in vitro* are decreased but not absent. The thymus and other lymphoid organs are severely hypoplastic. A majority of affected infants die in the first 3 years of life. The associated defects of both B- and T-cell immunity and HLA expression reinforce the important biologic role for HLA determinants in effective immune cell cooperation.

SEVERE COMBINED IMMUNODEFICIENCY WITH LEUKOPENIA (RETICULAR DYSGENESIS). In 1959, identical twin male infants were described who exhibited a total lack of both lymphocytes and granulocytes in their peripheral blood and bone marrow. Seven of eight infants reported died between ages 3 and 119 days from overwhelming infections; the eighth underwent complete immunologic reconstitution from a bone marrow transplant. Autosomal inheritance seems likely from reports of familial occurrences.

IMMUNODEFICIENCY WITH THROMBOCYTOPENIA AND ECZEMA (WISKOTT-ALDRICH SYNDROME). This X-linked recessive syndrome is characterized clinically by the triad of eczema, thrombocytopenic purpura, and undue susceptibility to infection. Often there is prolonged oozing from the circumcision site or bloody diarrhea during infancy. Atopic dermatitis and recurrent infections usually develop during the first year of life. Infections are caused by pneumococci and other bacteria with polysaccharide capsules, resulting in episodes of otitis media, pneumonia, meningitis, and sepsis. Later, infections with *Pneumocystis carinii* and the herpesviruses become more frequent. Survival beyond the teens is rare; major causes of death are infections or bleeding, but a 12% incidence of fatal malignancy also occurs in this condition. A papovavirus has been recovered from a reticulum cell sarcoma of the brain and from the urine of patients with this syndrome.

The earliest evidence of immunodeficiency is an impaired humoral immune response to polysaccharide antigens. Absent or markedly diminished isohemagglutinin titers are uniformly found, and poor or no responses are seen following immunization with polysaccharide antigens. Antibody titers to protein antigens also fall with time, and anamnestic responses are often poor or absent. Studies of immunoglobulin metabolism have shown an accelerated rate of synthesis—as well as hypercatabolism—of albumin, IgG, IgA, and IgM, resulting in highly variable immunoglobulin concentrations. The predominant dysgammaglobulinemias are a low IgM, elevated IgA and IgE, and a normal or slightly low IgG concentration. Lymphocyte responses are moderately depressed, and cutaneous anergy is a frequent finding. Analyses of blood lymphocytes with monoclonal reagents have revealed moderately reduced percentages of cells reacting with antibodies to all T cells and to the helper (CD4+) and suppressor (CD8+) subsets. The molecular basis of this defect, which had been mapped to Xp11.22-p11.23, has been recently found to be mutations in a gene encoding a proline-rich protein restricted to cells of lymphocytic megakaryocyte lineages. This protein, named WASP, is likely to be a key regulator of lymphocyte and platelet function (see Fig. 223–1).

The thrombocytopenia is due to an intrinsic platelet abnormality because antiplatelet antibodies are not usually demonstrated, and survival times of allogeneic but not autologous ^{51}Cr-labeled platelets have been normal. Megakaryocytes are present in normal number in the bone marrow, but platelet size is small.

Treatment has been directed primarily toward controlling bleeding with platelet transfusions, splenectomy, or both and controlling infections by intravenously administering ISG. Several patients have had complete corrections of both the platelet and immunologic abnormalities by HLA-matched sibling bone marrow transplants after being conditioned with irradiation or busulfan and cyclophosphamide.

ATAXIA-TELANGIECTASIA. This is a complex syndrome with neurologic, immunologic, endocrinologic, hepatic, and cutaneous abnormalities. The most prominent clinical features are progressive cerebellar ataxia, oculocutaneous telangiectasias, chronic sinopulmonary disease, a high incidence of malignancy, and variable humoral and cellular immunodeficiency. Ataxia typically becomes evident soon after the child begins to walk. Telangiectasias usually develop by age 3 to 6. Recurrent, usually bacterial, sinopulmonary infections occur in roughly 80% of these patients; common viral exanthems have not usually resulted in untoward sequelae, but varicella was fatal in one of the author's patients.

The malignant tumors reported have usually been of the lymphoreticular type, but others have been seen. Cells from patients and heterozygous carriers have increased sensitivity to ionizing radiation, defective DNA repair, and frequent chromosomal abnormalities. The abnormal gene has been mapped to the long arm of chromosome 11 (11q22.3). An autosomal recessive mode of inheritance seems operative.

The most frequent immunologic abnormality is selective absence of IgA, found in 50 to 80% of these patients. IgG$_2$ or total IgG may also be decreased. IgE concentrations are usually low, and IgM may be of the low-molecular-weight variety. Specific antibody levels may be decreased or normal. *In vivo,* there is impaired but not absent cell-mediated immunity, as evidenced by delayed cutaneous anergy and prolonged allograft survival. Death from GVH disease has

not been reported. Enumeration of blood T cells and subsets reveals reduced percentages of total T cells and T cells of the helper (CD4) phenotype, with normal or increased percentages of cells of the suppressor (CD8) phenotype. An increase in T cells bearing the γ/δ T-cell receptor has been reported. *In vitro* studies of lymphocyte function have shown moderately depressed proliferative responses to mitogens, decreased T-helper cell function, and an intrinsic defect in B-cell IgA synthesis. The thymus is very hypoplastic and lacks Hassall's corpuscles. No satisfactory treatment has been found.

CARTILAGE HAIR HYPOPLASIA. An unusual form of short-limbed dwarfism with frequent and severe infections has been reported among the Amish. Features include short and pudgy hands; redundant skin; hyperextensible joints of hands and feet but an inability to completely extend the elbows; and fine, sparse light hair and eyebrows. Severe and often fatal varicella infections appear to be a particular hazard. Progressive vaccinia and vaccine-associated poliomyelitis have also been observed.

The severity of the immunodeficiency varies; in one series, 11 of 77 patients died before age 20, but two were still alive at age 76. Three patterns of immune dysfunction have emerged: defective antibody-mediated immunity, defective cellular immunity, and severe combined immunodeficiency. The most striking abnormality appears to be one of defective cell proliferation due to an intrinsic defect related to the G1 phase, resulting in a longer cell cycle for individual cells. The trait appears to be autosomal recessive with variable penetrance.

IMMUNODEFICIENCY WITH THYMOMA. These patients are adults who almost simultaneously develop hypogammaglobulinemia, deficits in cell-mediated immunity, and benign thymoma (see Ch. 232). The thymomas are predominantly of the spindle cell variety. Eosinophilia or eosinopenia, aregenerative or hemolytic anemia, thrombocytopenia, or pancytopenia may also occur. Antibody formation is poor, although percentages of immunoglobulin-bearing B lymphocytes are normal, and progressive lymphopenia develops.

HYPERIMMUNOGLOBULINEMIA E SYNDROME. The hyper-IgE syndrome is a primary immunodeficiency characterized by recurrent staphylococcal abscesses and markedly elevated serum IgE concentrations. The disorder was first reported by the author and her co-workers in two young boys in 1972. These patients all have lifelong histories of severe recurrent staphylococcal abscesses involving the skin, lungs, joints, and other sites. Persistent pneumatoceles develop as a result of their recurrent pneumonias. The pruritic dermatitis that occurs is not typical atopic eczema and does not always persist; respiratory allergic symptoms are usually absent. An autosomal-dominant form of inheritance with incomplete penetrance seems possible. Laboratory features include exceptionally high serum IgE concentrations but usually normal IgG, IgA, and IgM concentrations; pronounced blood and sputum eosinophilia; abnormally low anamnestic antibody responses; and poor antibody and cell-mediated responses to neoantigens. *In vitro* studies have shown normal percentages of CD2-, CD3-, CD4-, and CD8-positive lymphocytes, and there is no increase in the percentage of IgE-bearing B lymphocytes. Lymphocyte responses to mitogens are normal, but responses to antigens or to related allogeneic cells have been absent or very low. Histologic sections of lymph nodes, spleen, and lung cysts show striking eosinophilia.

Phagocytic cell ingestion, metabolism, and killing mechanisms and total hemolytic complement have been normal in all patients. Defects of mononuclear and/or polymorphonuclear chemotaxis are present in some but not most patients and thus are not the basic problem in this syndrome. Indeed, the fundamental biologic error remains to be identified in this condition.

The most effective therapy is chronic administration of therapeutic doses of a penicillinase-resistant penicillin, with adding other antibiotic or antifungal agents as required for specific infections.

CHRONIC MUCOCUTANEOUS CANDIDIASIS. This clinical syndrome, probably of multiple causes, is associated with chronic candidal infection of the skin and mucous membranes but only rarely life-threatening systemic infections of the types seen in patients with severe T-cell dysfunction. Some patients have endocrinopathies involving the parathyroid, thyroid, adrenal, and/or pancreatic glands (see Ch. 210.1); however, many have neither associated endocrinopathy nor any demonstrable immunologic abnormality. Ketoconazole (Nizoral) or fluconazole (Diflucan) have been found to be effective in controlling the fungal infection.

LEUKOCYTE ADHESION DEFICIENCY 1 (LAD 1 OR CD11/CD18 DEFICIENCY). This condition is due to an autosomal or recessively inherited mutation in the gene encoding the 95-Kd MW β subunit (CD18) shared by three adhesive heterodimers: LFA-1 on B, T, and NK lymphocytes; complement receptor type 3 (CR3) on neutrophils, monocytes, macrophages, eosinophils, and NK cells; and p150,95 (function unknown). Because these cells cannot adhere to vascular endothelium, there is a significant leukocytosis, even in the absence of infection. Patients have histories of delayed separation of the umbilical cord, omphalitis, gingivitis, recurrent skin infections, repeated otitis media, pneumonia, peritonitis, perianal abscesses, and impaired wound healing. Severe widespread and life-threatening bacterial and fungal infections account for the high mortality. All cytotoxic lymphocyte functions are markedly impaired due to a lack of the adhesion protein LFA-1; deficiency of LFA-1 also interferes with immune cell interaction and immune recognition. CR3 binds fixed iC3b fragments of C3 and β glucans; its absence causes abnormal phagocytic cell adherence and chemotaxis and a reduced respiratory burst with phagocytosis. Blood neutrophil counts are usually elevated. Deficiencies of these glycoproteins can be screened for by cytofluorography of blood leukocytes with appropriate monoclonal antibodies to CR3 (OKM1, MO1, MAC-1). The disease can be corrected by bone marrow transplantation.

LEUKOCYTE ADHESION DEFICIENCY 2 (LAD 2). Very recently, another adhesion molecule deficiency state has been described, designated LAD type 2, which is due to the absence of the neutrophil Sialyl-Lewis X ligand of E-selectin on vascular endothelium (see Table 223–2). This disorder was discovered in two unrelated Israeli boys, aged 3 and 5, each the offspring of consanguineous parents. Both have severe mental retardation, short stature, a distinctive facial appearance, and the Bombay (hh) blood phenotype, and both are secretor- and Lewis-negative. They both have had recurrent severe bacterial infections similar to those seen in patients with LAD type 1, including pneumonia, peridontitis, otitis media, and localized cellulitis. Similar to patients with LAD 1, their infections have been accompanied by marked leukocytosis (30,000 to 150,000 per cubic millimeter) but an absence of pus formation at sites of recurrent cellulitis. *In vitro* studies revealed a marked defect in neutrophil motility. Because the genes for the red cell H antigen and for the secretor status encode for distinct α1,2-fucosyl transferases and the synthesis of Sialyl-Lewis X requires an α1,3-fucosyl transferase, the authors have postulated a general defect in fucose metabolism as the basis for this disorder.

T-CELL ACTIVATION DEFECTS. These conditions are characterized by the presence of T cells that appear phenotypically normal by many criteria but fail to proliferate or produce cytokines in response to stimulation with mitogens, antigens, or other signals delivered to the T-cell antigen receptor (TCR). Recently a number of these have been characterized at the molecular level, including patients who had either (1) defective surface expression of the CD3/TCR complex, due to a selective deficiency of the CD3-γ subunit or to a mutation in the CD3 gene, leading to the synthesis of an abnormal and unstable CD3 subunit; (2) defective signal transduction from the TCR to intracellular metabolic pathways; (3) pretranslational defects in the synthesis of interleukin-2 (T-cell growth factor) and/or of multiple other cytokines due to a defective NFAT-1 transcriptional complex; and (4) CD8 lymphocytopenia due to mutations in a non–SRC-related protein tyrosine kinase, ZAP 70. These patients have clinical problems similar to those of other severely T cell-deficient individuals.

PRIMARY DEFICIENCIES OF THE COMPLEMENT SYSTEM

In addition to congenital or hereditary disorders of lymphoid cells, there are several well-defined primary immune defects involving the complement system. Genetically determined deficiencies have been described for all of the components of complement, and undue susceptibility to infection is a characteristic of deficiencies of C2, C3, C5, C6, and C7. The types of infections experienced in C2, C3, and in some with C5 deficiency are with gram-positive encap-

sulated organisms, whereas those in patients with deficiencies of the terminal components are usually meningococcal or gonococcal. A normal CH50 would exclude all heritable complement deficiencies. The complement system is discussed in detail in Chapter 222.

Anonymous: Primary immunodeficiency diseases—report of a WHO Scientific Group meeting. Immunodef Rev 3:195, 1992. *The most recent published report of the World Health Organization's classification and discussion of the diagnosis and treatment of primary immunodeficiency diseases.*

Arnaiz-Villena A, Timon M, Corell A, et al.: Brief report: Primary immunodeficiency caused by mutations in the gene encoding the CD3 subunit of the T lymphocyte receptor. N Engl J Med 327:529, 1992. *An excellent introduction to the concept of T-cell activation defects.*

Buckley RH: Breakthroughs in the understanding and therapy of primary immunodeficiency. Pediatr Clin North Am, 41:665, 1994. *A review of recent discoveries of the fundamental causes of four X-linked and seven autosomal recessively inherited immunodeficiency diseases and of advances in therapy.*

Buckley RH, Schiff RI: The use of intravenous immunoglobulin in immunodeficiency diseases. N Engl J Med 325:110, 1991. *A discussion of intravenous immunoglobulin preparations available in the United States, indications for their use, recommended doses, and adverse effects.*

Buckley RH, Schiff SE, Schiff RI, et al.: Haploidentical bone marrow stem cell transplantation in human severe combined immunodeficiency. Semin Hematol 30:92, 1993. *An update on the use of T-cell depletion techniques that allow non–HLA-identical bone marrow to immunologically reconstitute infants with severe combined immunodeficiency disease without lethal graft-versus-host disease.*

Derry MJ, Ochs HD, Francke U: Isolation of a novel gene mutated in Wiskott-Aldrich syndrome. Cell 78:635, 1994. *The latest discovery of the molecular basis for an x-linked immunodeficiency disorder.*

Elder ME, Lin D, Clever J, et al.: Human severe combined immunodeficiency due to a defect in ZAP-70, a T cell tyrosine kinase. Science 264:1596, 1994. *The latest discovery of the molecular basis for a T cell signaling defect.*

Puck JM: Molecular and genetic basis of X-linked immunodeficiency disorders. J Clin Immunol 14:81, 1994. *An excellent review of X-linked recessive immunodeficiency diseases and the molecular bases for their defects.*

224 URTICARIA AND ANGIOEDEMA
Michael M. Frank

DEFINITION

Urticaria (Table 224–1) is defined as the transient appearance of elevated, erythematous pruritic wheals (hives) or serpiginous exanthem, usually surrounded by an area of erythema. It commonly involves the trunk and extremities, sparing palms and soles, but may involve any epidermal or mucosal surface. The wheals are thought to result from local subcutaneous and intradermal leakage of plasma filtrate from postcapillary venules. In most cases there is associated increased blood flow to the localized area of swelling, resulting in a surrounding erythema. The lesions blanch on pressure, reflecting this pathogenetic process. The appearance of urticaria is thought to reflect an ongoing immediate hypersensitivity reaction.

Angioedema is formed by a similar extravasation of fluid, but in this case the leakage of fluid involves deeper structures, including dermal and subdermal sites. Because of its location in deeper cutaneous structures, it appears as brawny nonpitting edema, usually without well-defined margins. Although urticaria is almost always pruritic, indicating stimulation of nociceptive nerves supplying deeper cutaneous structures, angioedema may be unassociated with itching. Unlike other forms of edema, angioedema is not commonly distributed in dependent areas of the body. Angioedema often involves the lips, tongue, eyelids, genitalia, or dorsum of the hands or feet but also may involve any epidermal or mucosal surface. The transient nature of involvement is important in defining both urticaria and angioedema; these manifestations appear and peak in minutes to hours and disappear over hours to days.

INCIDENCE AND PREVALENCE

Acute episodes of urticaria/angioedema are arbitrarily defined as those lasting less than 6 weeks. More prolonged episodes are defined as chronic. Acute urticaria and angioedema are very common clinical problems occurring in as many as 10 to 20% of the population at one time or another. They may occur at any age and are the most common form seen in childhood. They occur in persons of all sexes, races, and occupations and at all seasons of the year. Chronic

TABLE 224–1. CLASSIFICATION OF URTICARIA/ANGIOEDEMA

I. Manifestation of hypersensitivity to a defined agent
   A. Drug reactions
   B. Foods and food additives
   C. Inhaled and contact allergens
II. Presumed immune complex–induced
   A. Collagen disease
   B. Endocrine disease (thyroid disorders)
   C. Serum sickness
   D. Transfusion-induced
   E. Malignancy (tumor antigen–induced)
   F. Infectious agents
   G. Urticarial vasculitis
III. Physical urticarias
   A. Dermatographism
   B. Familial and acquired cold urticaria
   C. Localized heat urticaria
   D. Cholinergic urticaria
   E. Exercise-induced anaphylaxis/urticaria
   F. Delayed pressure urticaria/angioedema
   G. Familial and acquired vibratory angioedema
   H. Solar urticaria
   I. Aquagenic urticaria
IV. Urticaria pigmentosa and systemic mastocytosis
V. Chronic urticaria and angioedema
VI. Defined complement-related disorders
   A. Hereditary angioedema
   B. Acquired Cl inhibitor deficiency
   C. Complement Factor I deficiency
VII. Angioedema induced by angiotensin-converting enzyme (ACE) inhibitors and IL-2

urticaria/angioedema also can occur in individuals of any age, but the peak incidence is noted in young adults. In general, symptoms of urticaria are more striking and are more easily recognized than those of angioedema, and these symptoms are often the presenting complaint. At presentation about 50% of patients are found to have both urticaria and angioedema, approximately 40% have urticaria alone, and about 10% only angioedema. Although the majority of patients clear their lesions spontaneously or respond rapidly to treatment with H_1 antihistamines, a minority of patients continue to have lesions over a period that may last years. It has been reported that of patients with chronic urticaria and angioedema, 75% have symptoms for longer than 1 year, 50% symptoms for longer than 5 years, and 20% symptoms for decades. At times these can be quite debilitating. This clinical syndrome represents a final common pathway of multiple initiating stimuli, and the natural course of disease undoubtedly reflects these multiple initiating factors.

PATHOGENESIS AND PATHOLOGY

Urticaria/angioedema appears to result from dilatation of small vessels with associated leakage of plasma from local postcapillary venules. Experimentally such leakage can be induced by multiple stimuli. Degranulation of cutaneous mast cells is thought to be the most frequent cause of disease. Mast cells are found in high frequency within the subcutaneous tissues and dermis. Their distribution is particularly rich around blood vessels. These cells stain poorly with the commonly used histopathologic stains and often must be visualized by specific staining techniques. Upon being activated by any of a number of stimuli, these cells degranulate, releasing preformed mediators present in the granules like histamine that induce capillary permeability and also synthesize various mediators in response to the activation signal that induce capillary permeability, including prostaglandins, HETES, leukotrienes C, D, and E, and platelet-activating factor (PAF). With appropriate stimuli, cellular regulatory factors like cytokines can be released without degranulating and releasing preformed mediators; these may control the function of other cells within the lesion. Under controlled conditions, triggering of cutaneous mast cells in normal volunteers induces a typical pruritic hive, lending support to the suggestion that these cells are crucial in urticarial reactions in humans.

Many stimuli induce mast cells to degranulate. Probably most important is the interaction of mast cell membrane–bound IgE antibody with specific antigen. Mast cells have on their surface a high-affinity receptor for IgE and in tissues are found coated with IgE antibody derived from plasma. Interaction of IgE antibody with its antigen cross-links IgE receptors, a required step in initiating the degranulation process by antigen-mediated cell activation. However, not only IgE meeting its antigen but also a series of peptides derived from various plasma mediator molecules can trigger degranulation. For example, peptides derived from activated complement proteins including C3a, C4a, and C5a and small fragments of C2 can induce mast cell degranulation. Similarly, peptides like bradykinin, derived from activation and cleavage of proteins of the kinin-generating system and neuropeptides like substance P can induce mast cell degranulation. Incompletely defined cellular products derived from circulating mononuclear cells and neutrophils can cause mast cell degranulation as well. Moreover, toxic products from neutrophils and monocytes, whose release is induced by many factors including mast cell products, can on injection induce a typical hive.

Inducing an immediate hypersensitivity response in an allergic individual by intradermally injecting a sensitizing antigen leads to rapid mast cell degranulation and the immediate appearance of a wheal and flare response that gradually fades. In many individuals 4 to 6 hours later a "late-phase" response is noted with an increase in local inflammation and swelling. Biopsy of such a late-phase reaction reveals that neutrophils and eosinophils are accumulated in the inflamed area and later they are gradually replaced by mononuclear cells. The factors that induce the late-phase reaction are not completely defined, but the recent demonstration that chemotactic cytokines are produced some hours after mast cell triggering suggests that these factors may contribute to late-phase inflammation.

An understanding of these experimental findings helps explain biopsy findings in patients with acute and chronic urticaria/angioedema. It should be emphasized that although the disease may be chronic, individual lesions may be quite evanescent, lasting hours to days. On biopsy, subcutaneous edema is prominent with flattened rete pegs, widened dermal papillae, and swollen collagen fibers. There is an increased number of cutaneous mast cells noted when compared with normal individuals. Even uninvolved skin from a patient with urticaria shows more mast cells than does the skin of normals. Some mast cell degranulation is seen on biopsy of lesions, and in chronic urticaria a modest mononuclear cell infiltrate around vessels containing lymphocytes (predominantly CD4+ helper T cells) and relatively few monocyte/macrophages are noted. An increase in eosinophils may be seen. Patients with the physical urticaria tend to have more neutrophils and eosinophils on biopsy than are observed in chronic urticaria/angioedema. In a minority of cases with typical urticarial lesions a typical leukocytoclastic vasculitis is observed. This latter finding, reported to be associated with the formation of IgG–anti-Clq autoantibody, indicates that the underlying diagnosis is vasculitis and places the patient in a different diagnostic and therapeutic group.

It must be emphasized that in most cases the cause of urticaria/angioedema is never found. In several large series ~70% of all cases remained in the idiopathic group after all other urticarial syndrome complexes were eliminated. These cutaneous manifestations appear, often are treated, and disappear with no cause ever defined. It is believed that most urticaria/angioedema cases represent hypersensitivity reactions to drugs, foods, or less commonly inhalants, because when a cause is defined it commonly involves one of these sensitizing agents. Penicillin is the drug still most commonly associated with acute urticaria, but aspirin and other nonsteroidal anti-inflammatory agents (NSAID's) may exacerbate urticaria, possibly by inhibiting prostaglandin synthesis, and diuretics, radiocontrast dyes, food additives, sulfonamides, and muscle relaxants all are associated with acute urticaria. Opioids can trigger direct mast cell release of histamine and cause urticarial lesions. Among foods, nuts, milk, eggs, chocolate, citrus fruits, tomatoes, fish, shellfish, and food dyes have all been associated with onset of urticaria in some individuals. Nevertheless, so many different antigens, including food additives, drugs, foods, and food contaminants, have been defined as causative in individual cases, and so little antigen may be required to precipitate attacks that it may be difficult or impossible to define the causative agent. In many patients in whom the disease becomes chronic, the patient is asked to keep a diary to determine whether a particular food or commercial product is involved with an attack. If it proves impossible to define the precipitating agent by this means, a severely restricted elimination diet, limiting foods to boiled rice and lamb, may be tried for several weeks to see if eliminating an offending ingested agent will terminate attacks. Too often these attempts are unsuccessful.

There are defined clinical situations in which urticaria and/or angioedema is a common presenting problem: Patients undergoing immune complex–mediated reactions, as occur in active systemic lupus erythematosus and serum sickness, may experience waves of urticarial lesions, in this case thought to be due to activation of mediator pathways by circulating immune complexes with generation of kinins and complement-derived anaphylatoxins.

Autoantibodies of various sorts interacting with antigen may induce urticarial reactions. IgG anti-IgE autoantibodies have been suggested as a major cause of chronic urticaria, and a recent study suggests that IgG-anti IgE receptor antibody is found in a subset of these patients. Thyroid autoantibodies have been singled out as a cause of urticaria; in one study 90 of 624 patients with chronic urticaria were found to have thyroid autoimmunity, being either hyperthyroid or hypothyroid. Similarly, blood transfusions and infusions of fresh frozen plasma are often associated with hives caused by antibodies in the infused materials encountering host antigen or circulating host antibodies binding antigens in the blood products. Similarly, some cancers, for example lymphomas, may be associated with urticarial lesions, thought to be due to an immunologic response to tumor antigens. A similar mechanism is clearly responsible for the hives that may be associated with many infectious agents, particularly viral agents. Here antigens on or released from the infectious agent are bound to antibodies induced in the patient and hives result. Hives are a frequent response to the antibodies formed in the early response to hepatitis A and B and Epstein-Barr virus infection. Rarely fungal antigens like those derived from *Candida albicans* may precipitate hives or angioedema. Given the rarity of this latter observation, it is inappropriate to treat patients with chronic urticaria/angioedema with nystatin unless a clear association with a hypersensitivity response to candidal antigens can be demonstrated. Although rare in the United States, many parasitic diseases can at times be associated with urticaria/angioedema with or without hypereosinophilia. Presumably the presence of the urticaria/angioedema reflects an ongoing immediate hypersensitivity reaction to parasite antigens.

The complex of urticaria, bone pain, and lymphadenopathy is termed Schnitzler's syndrome. Affected patients often have greatly increased IgM levels suggesting an ongoing immunologic reaction, but the cause of the syndrome is unknown.

PHYSICAL URTICARIAS AND ANGIOEDEMAS. It is important to consider the physical urticaria/angioedema complex when evaluating patients with chronic recurrent urticaria or angioedema because in one large series these represent 16% of all chronic urticaria/angioedema patients seen. In some patients a highly specific diagnosis can be made, a clear precipitating factor can be defined, and the patient can learn to avoid attacks. Moreover, specific therapy may be available. When one lists these causes of urticaria/angioedema, they appear to be so easily defined that it appears unlikely that they could be missed. However, in practice this is not the case; a detailed history is required to identify these factors. Indeed it is common for these patients to go years before a correct diagnosis is made. The physical urticarias have in common urticaria/angioedema precipitated by a known physical cause. This response may follow exposure to cold, heat, elevated body temperature, pressure, vibration, specific wave length ultraviolet rays, or rarely even water to the skin. In some cases these reactions are thought to be IgE mediated, as they can be passively transferred with serum of an affected donor to the skin of an unaffected recipient. In other cases the cause is unknown.

SYMPTOMATIC DERMATOGRAPHISM. As many as 2 to 5% of the general population may be dermatographic, with the appearance of blanching followed by a linear streak of edema and erythema within 2 to 5 minutes of stroking the skin. A small proportion of such individuals have sufficiently severe dermatographism that they become symptomatic. In some cases the symptoms can be transferred to a normal recipient by passive transfer of plasma, suggesting that in some way IgE antibody plays a

role. In general these individuals can be treated successfully with H_1 and H_2 antihistamines.

COLD URTICARIA. These patients experience urticaria/angioedema on exposure to cold and may become hypotensive on diving into a cold swimming pool. Careful studies have shown that mast cell degranulation with histamine release occurs in these patients on cold exposure. Degranulation may be even more extensive when the patient's tissues are warmed following cold exposure. Placing an ice cube on the skin for 5 minutes and then removing it reveals an area of blanching in the shape of the cube followed by edema formation in the same area surrounded by an erythematous flare caused by local hyperemia. Under appropriate conditions blood histamine is elevated. In some of these patients passive transfer to the skin of normals has been demonstrated. It has been suggested that upon cold exposure, certain dermal antigens undergo a conformational change that allows specific IgE autoantibody to bind and initiate mast cell degranulation. These patients are typically treated with cyproheptadine, sometimes with the addition of hydroxyzine. Cold urticaria has been described in a number of diseases associated with pathologic globulins, such as cryoglobulins, or cryofibrinogens. The symptom complex, however, is not associated with the presence of cold agglutinins. When cold urticaria is associated with underlying disease, treatment of those diseases is an essential part of therapy.

In some patients the disease is atypical in that the patient gives a history of typical urticarial symptoms but the ice cube test is negative. In occasional patients dermatographism is brought out by cold exposure; in others exercise-induced urticaria is noted only in the cold. There is a rare familial type of cold urticaria inherited as an autosomal dominant trait in which patients develop urticarial lesions 9 to 18 hours after cold exposure. This cannot be passively transferred with plasma and the cause is unknown.

Similarly, localized heat urticaria has been described with a wheal and flare response noted 2 to 5 minutes after applying localized heat to the skin.

CHOLINERGIC OR GENERALIZED HEAT URTICARIA. Typically these patients, representing about 4% of all patients with chronic urticaria, develop small (several millimeters), intensely pruritic wheals on an erythematous base on their upper trunk and arms following exercise with sweating or following hot showers. A rise in core body temperature is essential to develop lesions. It is generally believed that the parasympathetic nervous system supply to cutaneous vessels releases acetylcholine as well as a neuropeptide such as vasoactive intestinal peptide, causing mediator release. There is no evidence of an IgE-mediated reaction. In support of this hypothesis is the fact that some of these patients (30 to 50%) develop typical lesions as well as a series of local satellite lesions when intracutaneously injected with Mecholyl. Atropine may inhibit the skin test but does not successfully treat the disease. These patients are typically highly responsive to hydroxyzine therapy. There is a subset of patients who respond to heat exposure, developing large urticarial lesions rather than the typical lesions of cholinergic urticaria. These patients tend not to develop their hives with exercise and are less responsive to hydroxyzine therapy.

EXERCISE-INDUCED URTICARIA/ANAPHYLAXIS. These patients note urticarial lesions appearing 5 to 30 minutes after the onset of exercise. They last for 1 to 3 hours. In severe cases anaphylactic reactions may be noted. This is an illness generally of young adults. At times symptoms are difficult to distinguish from those of cholinergic urticaria; however, these patients do not develop urticaria on raising core body temperature as in a hot bath and tend to respond poorly to antihistamines.

PRESSURE-INDUCED URTICARIA. For unknown reasons, urticarial lesions are common at pressure points on the body, e.g., where clothing is tight. Some patients note that marked urticarial lesions develop 4 to 6 hours after pressure is applied to the body. For example, these individuals may note urticarial lesions on buttocks after sitting for a long time on a hard chair or angioedema or urticaria on their feet after prolonged standing in one place. The lesions may be provoked by placing over the shoulders for 20 minutes a 1-inch strap weighted at the ends with 15-pound weights. A systemic response with malaise and even fever is often noted. The response to antihistamines is often poor. The urticaria but not the systemic toxicity may respond to antihistamine therapy. The most severely affected of these patients may require every-other-day glucocorticoid administration for partial relief. They are reported to be unresponsive to NSAID's.

Similarly, some patients respond to local vibration by developing urticarial lesions. Typically symptoms are induced by placing a vibrator or vortex mixer on the arm for 5 minutes. Urticaria appears in 1 to 5 minutes.

SOLAR URTICARIA. In general these patients develop urticarial responses shortly after exposure to sunlight; the patients are divided into groups by the wavelength of light that provokes attacks. Patients whose attacks are provoked by light at 280 to 320 nm (type 1) and 400 to 500 nm (type 4) typically have disease that can be passively transferred with serum to nonaffected recipients. This observation suggests the presence of an IgE-dependent mechanism in these cases. Type 6, provoked by light at 400 nm, is present in some patients with erythropoietic protoporphyria. Glass absorbs light with wavelength below 320 nm, and patients with urticaria in response to light wavelengths below 320 nm can be protected easily. The erythema-causing band of the solar spectrum, UVB, is at wavelength 290 to 320 nm, and these patients can sometimes be helped considerably by PABA-containing sunscreens, which absorb light in this range. However, many are not protected by the PABA sunscreens. A sunscreen preparation, butyl methoxydibenzoyl methane, absorbs light in the UVA range and may be more useful for this patient group. There are many types of light sensitivity, and sorting these out may be confusing. They range from metabolic abnormalities (erythrogenic porphyria), in which products of metabolism absorb light energy and undergo chemical alteration, developing toxic products, to photoallergic reactions in which skin-sensitizing drugs induce allergic reactions when acted upon by sunlight, to phototoxic reactions in which drugs localized in cutaneous tissues directly cause tissue-damaging reactions when exposed to light of the proper wavelength. In many of these cases the light energy is absorbed by a complex ring structure in the drug, which subsequently releases photons and electrons that lead to local generation of toxic products such as singlet oxygen, hydrogen peroxide, and chloramines. Obviously in each case one attempts to identify the cause of the urticaria and eliminate the offending agent if it can be defined.

AQUAGENIC URTICARIA. These patients respond within 2 to 30 minutes with urticaria when water is applied to the skin. Typically this is noted in the course of baths or showers, even with water at tepid temperature. In many cases these individuals are probably exquisitely sensitive to additives in the water, e.g., chlorine, but it is reported that rare individuals develop urticaria in response to distilled water.

CHRONIC URTICARIA/ANGIOEDEMA. It should be clear from the material presented that chronic urticaria/angioedema can be caused by many agents, and identifying the agent may be difficult or impossible. Often after attempts at identifying the cause of the urticaria have failed, we are left with a patient who requires treatment. H_1 antihistamines are usually the agents of first choice. Some examples of therapeutic agents are listed earlier in the chapter; in patients with chronic disease, high-dose hydroxyzine and cyproheptadine are often effective. These agents make patients drowsy and may not be well tolerated initially, but drowsiness may pass if the drug is continued. Optimally the dose is increased until drowsiness persists and then the dosage is reduced slightly. It is common to find patients who, because the drugs have not been used properly, claim to have been unresponsive to these agents. Many more conveniently used and less sedating antihistamines have become available in the last few years and have been shown in controlled studies to be effective in chronic angioedema/urticaria. These include terfenadine, astemizol, loratidine, and cetirizine. H_2 inhibitory drugs are often added to H_1 inhibitors if the clinical response is not adequate. Other agents have also proven to be beneficial, including doxepin, a tricyclic antidepressant with anti-H_1 and anti-H_2 properties; nifedipine, a calcium channel blocker; and ketotifen, a drug shown to be efficacious in the physical urticarias. If these agents fail, a course of glucocorticoids may be required. In general one begins with 40 to 60 mg of prednisone per day in divided doses for 1 week. The dosage is then consolidated to a single dose a day, and then the drug is rapidly tapered on an every-other-day schedule until the patient is receiving glucocorticoids once every other day. The dose of glucocorticoids should be tapered to the lowest dose that will maintain the patient with minimal symptoms. Following a course of glucocorticoid therapy, patients often remain in remission for a prolonged time. The illness may recur at a later time or when glucocorticoids are tapered.

DIFFERENTIAL DIAGNOSIS

This set of diseases is multifactorial. Usually the diagnosis of urticaria/angioedema does not present a problem in the patient with clear episodes of pruritic wheals or localized brawny edema. Because many agents can cause these lesions, considerable detective work is required to define these diseases and to develop a suitable specific therapy. During the initial evaluation a number of points must be explored. A history of a fixed rather than evanescent eruption, burning, bruising, or vesiculating lesions must lead one to early biopsy. Similarly, fever or systemic signs and symptoms, including arthralgias, pulmonary symptoms, and abdominal pain, suggest that further exploration is needed. Patients with idiopathic chronic urticaria typically have a normal sedimentation rate, white cell count, and differential, and these should be examined. In appropriate cases, ANA, heterophile, STS, rheumatoid factor level, cryoglobulins and cryofibrinogen, cold hemolysin, C4, and C1 inhibitor levels should be studied for further clues to the underlying diagnosis. In the patient who responds poorly to therapy or who has atypical disease, a biopsy is clearly indicated. Patients with urticarial vasculitis are treated for the underlying vasculitis.

THERAPY

The use of antihistamines and glucocorticoids is discussed under the various entities and in the section on chronic urticaria/angioedema. Epinephrine is clinically useful in acute management of urticaria/angioedema. In this case the drug is administered as a series of injections (0.2 to 0.3 ml) of 1:1000 dilution subcutaneously, repeated at half-hour intervals two or three times until symptoms are controlled. Obviously the use of epinephrine is contraindicated in certain patient groups such as patients with severe cardiovascular disease. Longer-acting epinephrine preparations such as epinephrine in oil (Sus-Phrine) may be useful.

URTICARIA PIGMENTOSA AND SYSTEMIC MASTOCYTOSIS

Urticaria pigmentosa is characterized by the local accumulation of intradermal masses of infiltrating mast cells (see Ch. 231). The lesions may resemble freckles superficially but are raised, as might be expected of infiltrative lesions, and may be somewhat erythematous. They may urticate when stroked (Darier's sign). Systemic mastocytosis is associated with massive accumulation of mast cells in other organs, particularly the bone marrow and gastrointestinal tract. Although some affected patients may present with acute or chronic urticaria, that presentation is quite rare; systemic signs of histamine toxicity, gastrointestinal disorders, or disorders consequent to destruction of bone marrow or bone are more common.

HEREDITARY ANGIOEDEMA

Hereditary angioedema (HAE) presents clinically as episodic attacks of brawny nonpitting edema that usually involve the extremities but may affect any external body surface including the genitalia. Mucosal surfaces are affected as well and patients frequently have attacks of severe abdominal pain due to swelling of the submucosa of the gastrointestinal tract. On rare occasions attacks may affect the airway, where they can cause respiratory obstruction and asphyxiation. Although attacks are sporadic, about half of the patients note that trauma, particularly associated with local pressure, precipitates an attack, and half the patients note a marked increase in attack frequency at times of emotional stress. About one third of patients note an erythema marginatum–like rash at the onset of attacks which they often describe as nonraised, nonpruritic circles on the skin. In general, attacks become progressively more severe over about 1.5 days and then regress over a similar time period. Swelling of the gastrointestinal mucosa may be associated with exquisite abdominal pain.

Although relatively rare (incidence about 1:10,000), this disease has received a great deal of attention because of the high incidence of lethal complications, because its pathophysiologic basis is best understood of all of the angioedemas, and because adequate therapy is available for most patients. Presence of this disease is associated with either low levels or abnormal function of a plasma regulatory protein, the C1 inhibitor (see Ch. 222). This protein controls activation of the complement, kinin-generating, fibrinolytic, and intrinsic clotting pathways. Although the precise cause of the capillary leakage is unknown, it is believed that a peptide formed during activation of either the complement or the kinin-generating mediator pathway is the responsible factor. HAE has an autosomal dominant inheritance pattern, affecting 50% of the offspring of a patient and occurring with equal frequency in males and females. This autosomal dominant inheritance reflects the presence of one abnormal gene for C1 inhibitor on chromosome 11. This gene may yield no gene product (85% of patients; type 1) or may code for a nonfunctional protein (15% of patients; type 2).

HAE tends to be mild in childhood, becoming more severe at puberty. The factors that initiate attacks are unknown. There is no relationship between the level or activity of C1 inhibitor and the severity of disease. Patients are described who presumably had the defect from birth but whose attacks began at age 70. Diagnosis is established by finding low levels of C1 inhibitor antigen or function and low levels of the complement protein C4 and/or C2. C1 inhibitor inhibits the function of activated C1 of the classic complement pathway. C1 INH acts by binding to the substrate to be inhibited, and the product of one normal gene is insufficient to control mediator activation. When activated, C1 cleaves the next two proteins in the cascade, C4 and C2. Because the function of activated C1 is unregulated in the presence of a relative C1 inhibitor deficiency, C1 continues to cleave C4 and C2. Patients have low levels of circulating C4 and C2 during attacks and usually have low levels between attacks. Interestingly, because of the presence of other control proteins, the levels of C3, the most commonly measured complement protein, are almost always normal. Presumably because of the constant complement activation present in these patients, they have an immune dysregulation shown by the higher-than-normal incidence of autoimmune diseases. These include endocrinopathies, granulomatous bowel disorders, arthritides, and SLE.

Patients' angioedema attacks respond poorly to epinephrine, antihistamines, and glucocorticoids, the mainstays of treatment of urticaria and angioedema caused by immediate hypersensitivity reactions. Nevertheless, acute attacks are treated with epinephrine, both nebulized racemic epinephrine in the airway (1 : 1000 given by nebulization) and subcutaneous injections (0.2 to 0.3 ml 1 : 1000 SQ repeated q 20–30 min × 3). Epinephrine administered very early in an attack often produces some improvement. Patients also receive antihistamines for sedation. Patients often relate that intravenously administered FFP to supply the missing inhibitor proteins terminates attacks. Nevertheless, a rare patient becomes more edematous following FFP, presumably reflecting increased availability of mediator substrates, and FFP therefore is not recommended for treating life-threatening laryngeal edema. In this circumstance nasotracheal intubation in the operating room under conditions where tracheostomy can be performed is indicated. FFP can be given in nonemergency situations such as in preoperative patients to prevent attacks. The usual dose of FFP is 2 units, an arbitrary amount that has been used extensively and has proven to be effective. Evidence suggests that infusions of purified C1 inhibitor reliably terminate attacks; it is likely that this protein will be available for treatment of acute attacks within the next several years. Although short-term therapy and therapy of acute attacks of HAE have not been generally satisfactory, long-term therapy has been quite successful. Patients respond to all of the acetylated artificial androgens with increased C1 INH levels that in some cases approach normal values, a correction of serum C4 and C2, and a marked amelioration of symptoms. In the rare patient in whom the drug is ineffective or in whom drug toxicity is a problem, plasmin inhibitors such as ϵ-aminocaproic acid, have also been found to be effective. Their mechanism of action is unknown, and there is no change in the amount of C activation reflected in the persistent reduction in the serum level of C4 and C2. With all of these agents there is a high degree of patient-to-patient variation in dosage, and the lowest dose that controls symptoms is chosen. Women are often treated with danazol (200 to 400 mg per day), an impeded androgen that has

few masculinizing side effects. Men are often treated with the less expensive but more androgenic agent methyltestosterone (10 to 30 mg per day orally).

ACQUIRED C1 INHIBITOR DEFICIENCY

A number of syndromes have been recognized that are associated with a typical HAE symptom complex but are a reflection of acquired disease. A decade ago it was recognized that certain patients with malignancies, including lymphosarcoma, leukemia, lymphoma, and paraproteinemia, developed circulating or cellular factors that could activate C1 and deplete all the C1 inhibitor activity in serum. Later it was noted that rare patients with autoimmune disease also induced massive activation of the complement cascade with C1 inhibitor utilization and an HAE-like clinical picture. More recently, patients have been described with multiple myeloma and anti-idiotypic antibody causing the same symptom complex. Perhaps the most common of these rare individuals are recently described patients who form monoclonal or polyclonal autoantibodies to the C1 inhibitor, which destroy its activity. Clinically these patients cannot be distinguished from patients with HAE. However, their laboratory tests are unique. All of these patients have profound depressions in functional C1, C4, and C2. Patients with HAE commonly have normal C1 levels. Although their plasma C1 inhibitor antigen level may be normal, they have marked depression of C1 INH function. Their treatment focuses on the underlying disease where possible. Some of these patients respond to danazol or other anabolic steroids. Several of the patients with the anti–C1 INH autoantibody have responded to glucocorticoid therapy, and at least one of these patients has responded to cytotoxic therapy.

FACTOR I DEFICIENCY WITH CHRONIC URTICARIA

Factor I is one of the control proteins of the complement activation pathway. The rare individuals with an inherited deficiency of this protein continuously activate and cleave C3, generating the anaphylatoxins C3a and perhaps C5a. In vitro these cleavage peptides induce mast cell degranulation and cause chronic urticaria that disappears when the patient is infused with Factor I. In general, this form of urticaria is relatively mild and is treated symptomatically with antihistamines.

ANGIOEDEMA INDUCED BY ANGIOTENSIN-CONVERTING ENZYME (ACE) INHIBITORS AND INTERLEUKIN-2. Within hours to 1 week of therapy with ACE inhibitors, patients may note angioedema that becomes life-threatening. ACE plays an important role in the degradation of bradykinin and the neuropeptide substance P, and these mediators may be important in forming angioedema. Patients are treated with antihistamines and/or epinephrine as appropriate and the ACE inhibitor is discontinued. It has also been noted that systemic capillary leak or angioedema may follow the systemic infusion of IL-2 used to treat malignancy. It is reported that this cytokine activates both the complement- and kinin-generating pathways. It activates T cells, and it has been suggested that these activated cells directly damage the endothelium.

Casale TB, Sampson HA, Harrifin J, et al.: Guide to physical urticarias. J Allergy Clin Immunol 82:758, 1988. *Tables of information on the physical urticarias.*

Champion RH: Urticaria: Then and now. Br J Dermatol 119:427, 1988. *A report of the evaluation of 2300 cases and comments on the literature.*

Champion RH, Greaves MW, Kobza A, et al.: The Urticarias. Edinburgh, Churchill Livingstone, 1985. *The proceedings of a symposium on urticaria-angioedema.*

Frank MM: Hereditary angioedema. *In* Bayless TM, Brain MC, Cherniack RM (eds.): Current Therapy in Internal Medicine 2. Philadelphia, BC Decker, 1987, p 42. *Complete discussion of treatment.*

Frank MM, Gelfand JA, Atkinson JP: Hereditary angioedema: The clinical syndrome and its management. Ann Intern Med 84:580, 1976. *Although old, this represents the classic clinical review of this syndrome.*

Hide M, Francis DM, Grattan CE, et al.: Autoantibodies against the high-affinity IgE receptor as a cause of histamine release in chronic urticaria. N Engl J Med 328:1599, 1993. *First presentation of hypothesis that chronic urticaria is due to anti-IgE receptor autoimmunity.*

Leznoff A, Sussman GL: Syndrome of idiopathic chronic urticaria and angioedema with thyroid autoimmunity. A study of 90 patients. J Allergy Clin Immunol 84:66, 1989. *The best review of this patient group.*

Mehregan DR, Hall MJ, Gibson LE: Urticarial vasculitis, a histopathologic and clinical review of 72 cases. J Am Acad Dermatol 26:441, 1992. *Excellent clinical review.*

Monroe EN: Chronic urticaria. Review of nonsedating H₁ antihistamines in treatment. J Am Acad Dermatol 19:842, 1988. *Comparison of various H₁ agents and review of published studies.*

Wanderer AA: Cold urticaria syndromes. Historical background, diagnostic classification, clinical and laboratory characteristics, pathogenesis and management. J Allergy Clin Immunol 88:965, 1990. *A thorough review of this syndrome.*

225 ALLERGIC RHINITIS
Richard D. deShazo

DEFINITION

Allergic rhinitis is a symptom complex characterized by paroxysms of sneezing; itching of the eyes, nose, and palate; rhinorrhea; and nasal obstruction. It is often associated with postnasal drip, cough, irritability, and fatigue. Symptoms develop when persons inhale airborne antigens (allergens) to which they have been previously exposed and have made IgE antibodies. These IgE antibodies bind to IgE receptors on mast cells in the respiratory mucosa and to basophils in the peripheral blood. When IgE molecules on their surface are bridged by allergen, mast cells release pre-formed and granule-associated chemical mediators. They also generate other mediators and cytokines that lead to nasal inflammation and, with continued allergen exposure, chronic symptoms.

EPIDEMIOLOGY

Allergic rhinitis is common, accounting for at least 2.5% of all physician visits, 2 million lost school days per year, 6 million lost work days, and 28 million restricted work days per year. At least $1 billion is spent annually on prescription and over-the-counter medications for allergy. Between 10% and 20% of the United States population is affected, and the prevalence in urban areas is increasing. The prevalence is lowest in children under age 5, rises to a peak in early adulthood (as high as 24% in the U.S.), and declines thereafter. The 4-year remission rate is reported to be 10% in males and 5% in females.

PHYSICAL FINDINGS AND ASSOCIATIONS

The swollen nasal mucosa of patients with acute allergic rhinitis is pale and blue but becomes erythematous and indurated with chronic allergen exposure. Clear rhinorrhea may be visible anteriorly or, with nasal obstruction, dripping down a cobblestone-appearing posterior pharynx. Giemsa or Hansel's stains of these nasal secretions show cell populations to be predominantly eosinophils. A transverse nasal crease, a highly arched palate, mouth breathing, and dental malocclusion are common, especially in children. Venous dilation of the subcutaneous skin beneath the eyes may produce "allergic shiners."

Chronic allergic rhinitis may be associated with sleep disorders, sinusitis, secretory otitis media, and anosmia. Allergic rhinitis is also associated with other common allergic conditions, including allergic conjunctivitis, allergic asthma, and atopic dermatitis (eczema). Twenty-eight to 50% of patients with asthma and up to 30% with eczema have allergic rhinitis. These conditions have been termed "atopic diseases" and patients who have them are often called "atopic."

DIFFERENTIAL DIAGNOSIS

Syndromes of rhinitis may be divided into allergic, infectious, perennial nonallergic, and miscellaneous categories (Table 225–1). Allergic rhinitis should be differentiated from other forms of rhinitis, as the approach to management is different. Episodic exposure to inhaled allergens such as cat salivary proteins, horse dander, murine urinary proteins, pollen, or house dust mite feces may provoke acute allergic symptoms that are easily diagnosed as *acute allergic rhinitis*. If allergen exposure is seasonal—for instance, tree and grass pollen in the spring (rose fever) or ragweed pollen exposure in the fall (hay fever)—symptoms are predictable and reproducible and, thus, *seasonal allergic rhinitis* may be diagnosed by history (Fig. 225–1). When allergen exposure is chronic, *perennial allergic rhinitis* may result. This is common in subtropical regions with long pollinating seasons and ever-present mold and dust mite allergens and with occupational allergen exposure. This form of rhinitis may be difficult to distinguish from nonallergic forms of *perennial nonallergic rhinitis* and may require certain testing (discussed later) to diagnose accurately. Of all patients with rhinitis, 11% have seasonal symptoms, with 78% of these having an apparent allergic cause. Thirty-three percent of patients with rhinitis have perennial symptoms with a seasonal exacerbation, and 68% of these

TABLE 225–1. CLASSIFICATION OF RHINITIS

Allergic
  Seasonal
  Perennial
  Occupational
Infectious
  Acute: Viral, bacterial
  Chronic: Specific: Bacterial, fungal
      Nonspecific: Associated with immune deficiency (antibody deficiency, ciliary abnormalities)
Perennial nonallergic
  Idiopathic (vasomotor rhinitis)
  Nonallergic rhinitis with eosinophilia (NARES)
Miscellaneous forms
  Hormonal: pregnancy, hypothyroidism, etc.
  Drug-induced: Associated with aspirin and antihypertensives, rhinitis medicamentosa
  Food: gustatory, IgE-mediated, preservative-induced
  Atrophic rhinitis: (*Klebsiella ozenae*)
  Mechanical: hypertrophied turbinates, deviated nasal septum, foreign body, nasal polyps

patients have a probable allergic cause. Fifty-six percent of patients with rhinitis have perennial symptoms alone, and only about 50% of these have symptoms that can be attributed to allergens. Most patients with allergic rhinitis have allergic symptom triggers, eosinophil-rich nasal secretions, allergen-specific IgE to inhalant allergens, and a family history of allergic disease.

Nasal eosinophilia is not diagnostic for allergic rhinitis because nasal eosinophilia occurs in the *nonallergic rhinitis with nasal eosinophilia syndrome (NARES)*. This occurs in as many as 15% of patients with rhinitis and is characterized by perennial symptoms, an older average age than in patients with allergic rhinitis (39 versus 25 years), and milder symptoms of nasal itching and sneezing. The clear nasal secretions contain > 25% eosinophils, but the role of eosinophils in the disorder is unclear. Fifty percent of patients with NARES have sinusitis, 33% have nasal polyps, and 14% have asthma. IgE to inhalant allergens is usually absent. Another common form of perennial nonallergic rhinitis is commonly called *vasomotor rhinitis*. Patients with this disorder complain predominantly of chronic nasal congestion intensified by rapid changes in temperature and relative humidity, odors, or alcohol. Several lines of evidence suggest that they have nasal autonomic nervous system dysfunction. For instance, they have abnormal nasal responses to temperature stimuli applied to the skin and excess nasal sensitivity to topically applied acetylcholine congeners. They have little nasal itching or sneezing, but headaches, anosmia, and sinusitis are common. A family history of allergy or allergic symptom triggers is uncommon. Positive immediate hypersensitivity skin tests to inhalant allergens and nasal eosinophilia are unusual. *Atrophic rhinitis* is a syndrome of progressive atrophy of the nasal mucosa in elderly patients who report chronic nasal congestion and constantly perceive a bad odor. *Rhinitis medicamentosa* is a complication of chronically using vasoconstrictor nasal sprays. Patients develop chronic nasal obstruction and nasal inflammation manifest as beefy red nasal membranes on physical examination. *Rhinitis of pregnancy* and rhinitis associated with birth control pills or hypothyroidism reflect nasal obstruction that occurs on a hormonal basis. Nasal obstruction may also be a side effect of antihypertensive drugs. Unilateral rhinitis or nasal polyps are uncommon in uncomplicated allergic rhinitis. Unilateral rhinitis suggests the possibility of nasal obstruction by foreign body, tumor, or polyp, and the presence of nasal polyps suggests chronic sinusitis, aspirin hypersensitivity, or cystic fibrosis.

MECHANISMS OF ALLERGIC REACTIONS

The expression of allergic diseases reflects an autosomal dominant pattern of inheritance with incomplete penetrance. This is manifested as a propensity to respond to inhalant allergen exposure by producing high levels of allergen-specific IgE. The IgE response appears to be controlled by immune response genes located within the major histocompatibility complex (MHC) on chromosome 6 (see Ch. 229). The immunologic mechanisms for atopy have been studied in murine models and in humans and appear to center on the

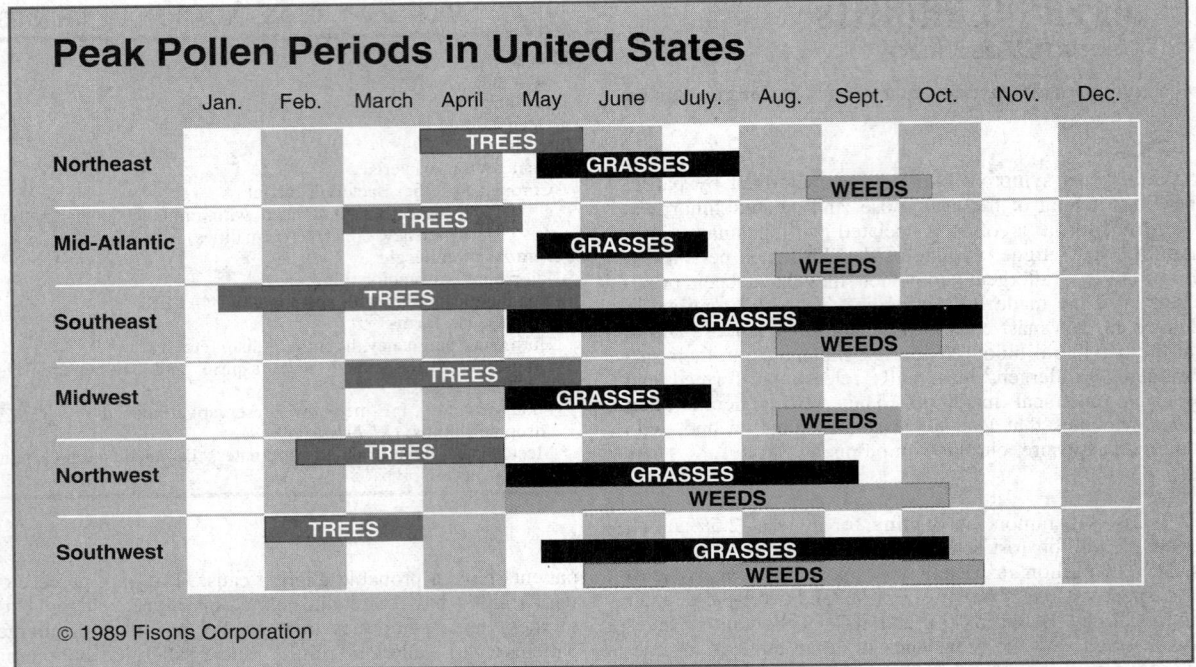

FIGURE 225-1. Peak pollen periods in the United States. (Reproduced with permission from Fisons Pharmaceuticals. © 1989, Fisons Corporation.)

expression of a repertoire of responses associated with the T_H2 type T-helper lymphocyte summarized below.

PRODUCTION OF IgE

Sensitization to allergen is necessary to elicit an IgE response (Fig. 225–2). After inhalation, the allergen must first be internalized by antigen-presenting cells, which include macrophages, dendritic cells, activated T lymphocytes, and B lymphocytes. After allergen processing, peptide fragments of the allergen are presented with class II (MHC) molecules of the host antigen-presenting cells to CD4+ T lymphocytes. These lymphocytes have receptors specific for the particular MHC-peptide complex. This interaction results in the release of cytokines by the CD4+ cell.

T-helper lymphocytes (CD4+) appear to be of two classes: T_H1 and T_H2. If the CD4+ cells that recognize the allergen are of the T_H2 class, a certain repertoire of mediators including granulo-cytemacrophage colony-stimulating factor (GM-CSF), interleukin (IL)-3, IL-4, IL-5, and IL-6, are released. IL-4, IL-5, and IL-6 are cytokines involved in B-cell proliferation and differentiation. Activated B lymphocytes, having bound allergen via their allergen-specific IgM-variable region binding sites, are stimulated by these cytokines to proliferate and secrete IgM. IL-4 from T_H2 cells promotes B-cell isotype switching to IgE antibody synthesis. Thus, atopy appears to be the result of a predisposition toward T_H2-type responses, which result in the formation of large quantities of allergen-specific IgE.

MAST CELLS AND EOSINOPHILS. After IgE antibodies specific for a certain allergen are synthesized and secreted, they bind to mast cells and basophils. When allergen is inhaled into the nose, the allergen or a hapten-allergen complex cross-links these allergen-specific cell-bound IgE antibodies on the mast cell surface, whereupon rapid degranulation and mediator release occur.

Mast cell mediators are either pre-formed, granule-associated, formed during degranulation, or generated after transcription (Fig. 225–3). The most important pre-formed mediator is histamine, which reproduces all of the symptoms of acute allergic rhinitis when sprayed nasally into normal volunteers. Histamine causes vasodilation that leads to nasal congestion, mucus secretion, and increased vascular permeability, which in turn leads to tissue edema and sneezing through stimulation of sensory nerve fibers. The cross-linking of IgE antibody on mast cells also initiates the release of arachidonic acid from cell membrane substrates. Mast cells then metabolize arachidonic acid—either via the cyclo-oxygenase pathway to form prostaglandin and thromboxane mediators or via the

lipoxygenase pathway to form leukotrienes. Prostaglandin D_2 (PGD_2), the sulfidopeptide leukotrienes LTC_4, LTD_4, and LTE_4 (SRS-A), platelet-activating factor (PAF), and bradykinin are formed during degranulation. PGD_2 is synthesized by mast cells but not basophils and appears more potent than histamine in causing nasal congestion. PAF is a potent chemotactic factor, and the sulfidopeptide leukotrienes and bradykinins are vasoactive. One leukotriene, LTB_4, is the most potent chemotactic factor in humans.

Mast cells are present in concentrations of 7000 per cubic millimeter in the normal nasal submucosa but only 50 per cubic millimeter in the nasal epithelium. The total number of nasal epithelial mast cells remains constant during the allergy season. However, the superficial nasal epithelium in allergic rhinitis patients has 50-fold more basophilic cells (mast cells and basophils) per specimen than the epithelium from nonallergic subjects. Increased concentrations of mast cells are found near postcapillary venules, where they increase vascular permeability; near sensory nerves, where they initiate the sneeze reflex; and near glands, where they facilitate secretion.

Once allergic reactions begin, mast cells amplify them by releasing not only vasoactive agents but also cytokines including GM-CSF, tumor necrosis factor-α (TNF-α), and IL-1 to -6. These cytokines further promote IgE production, mast cell growth, and eosinophil growth, chemotaxis and survival. For instance, IL-5, TNF-α, and IL-1 promote eosinophil movement by increasing the expression of adhesion receptors on endothelium. In turn, eosinophils secrete IL-1, which favors T_H2 cell proliferation, and the mast cell growth factor, IL-3. Eosinophils release oxygen radicals and proteins, including eosinophil major basic protein, which are toxic to the nasal epithelium.

MECHANISMS OF NASAL ALLERGIC REACTIONS

ANATOMY AND PHYSIOLOGY OF THE NOSE. Under normal conditions, the nose accounts for nearly 50% of the resistance to airflow in the airway. It is lined by pseudostratified epithelium resting on a basement membrane, separating it from deeper submucosal layers. The submucosa contains mucous, seromucous, and serous glands. The small arteries, arterioles, and arteriovenous anastomoses determine regional blood flow. Capacitance vessels, consisting of veins and cavernous sinusoids, determine nasal patency. The cavernous sinusoids lie beneath the capillaries and venules, are most dense in the inferior and middle turbinates, and contain smooth muscle cells controlled by the sympathetic nervous system. Withdrawal of sympathetic tone or, to a lesser degree, cholinergic

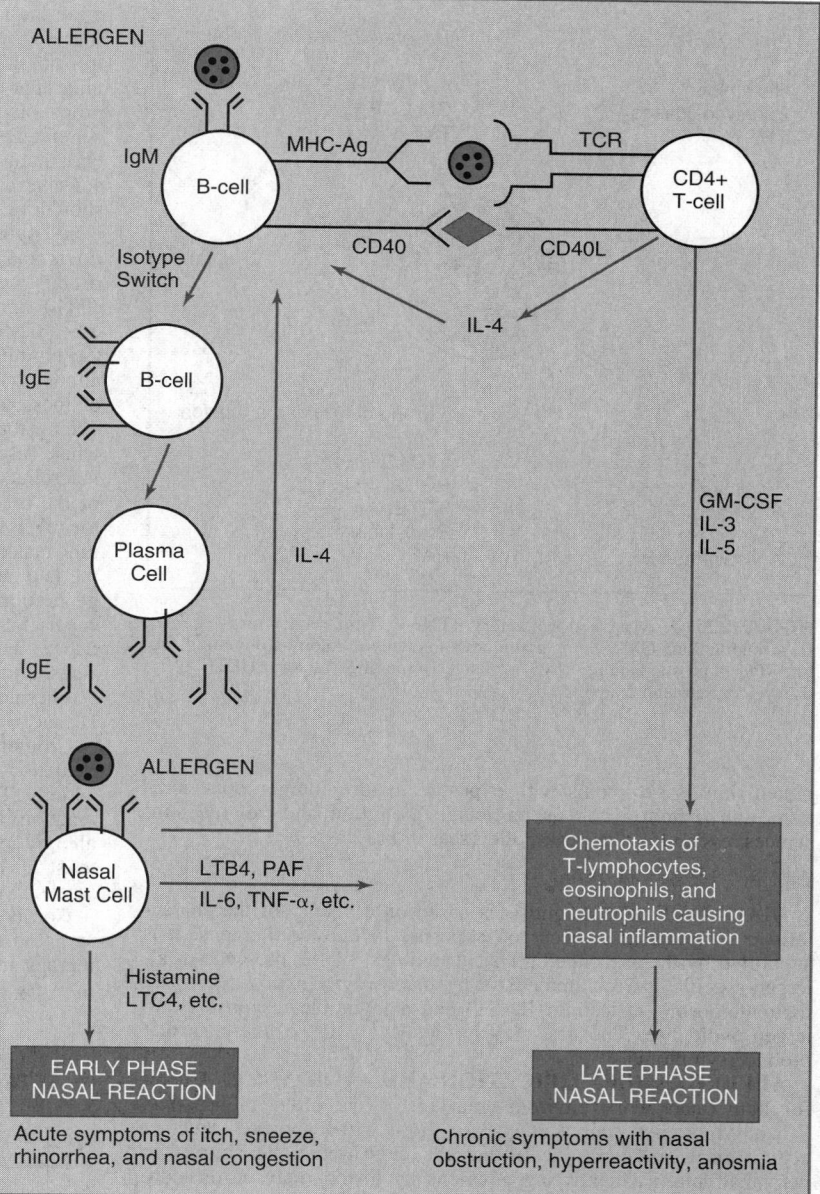

FIGURE 225–2. Pathophysiology of allergic rhinitis. Allergen is presented to T_H2 helper T lymphocytes by antigen-presenting cells (such as macrophages or B lymphocytes) in the context of major histocompatibility proteins. In atopic individuals, this leads to the production of cytokines including IL-4, GM-CSF, IL-3, and IL-5. The IL-4 from these T_H2 lymphocytes induces B-cell isotype switching to IgE. This isotype switch requires contact-dependent help from T cells via the interaction of the CD40 molecule on B cells and the CD40 ligand (CD40L) on T cells. B cells that produce allergen-specific IgE mature into plasma cells that produce IgE, which binds to mast cells in the nasal mucosa. When inhaled allergens bridge IgE molecules on mast cells, mast cell degranulation occurs, releasing pre-formed mediators. These mediators induce the *early phase nasal reaction,* characterized by rhinorrhea, sneezing, itching, and nasal obstruction. A second release of mast cell mediator may occur 2 to 6 hours later, leading to a recurrence of symptoms. This late-phase reaction is associated with an inflammatory response in the nose and the ongoing symptoms. Inflammation is promoted by the release of mast cell chemotactic factors such as LTB4 from mast cells and T_H2 lymphocytes. These cytokines promote eosinophil differentiation, activation, and survival. (GM-CSF = granulocyte-monocyte colony-stimulating factor; IL = interleukin; MHC = major histocompatibility complex; TNF = tumor necrosis factor; TCR = T-cell receptor.)

stimulation causes this sinusoidal erectile tissue to become engorged. Cholinergic stimulation causes arterial dilation and promotes the passive diffusion of plasma protein into glands and the active secretion by mucous glands in cells.

Novel neurotransmitters, including substance P, calcitonin gene-related peptide, and vasointestinal peptide, have been detected in nasal secretions after nasal allergen challenge of patients with allergic rhinitis. Because they can produce changes in regional blood flow and glandular secretion, their role in rhinitis may be important.

IMMEDIATE AND LATE NASAL REACTIONS. Exposing the nasal mucosa to ragweed in ragweed-sensitive subjects (nasal challenge) provokes the immediate onset of sneezing and nasal itching associated with significantly increased concentrations of inflammatory mediators. Histamine, PGD_2, the kininogen product tosylarginine-methylester (TAME-esterase), tryptase, kinins, and sulfidopeptide leukotrienes are present in nasal washes. After about half an hour, PGD_2 and histamine levels return to baseline, whereas TAME-esterase concentrations remain elevated. Sneezing correlates with the appearance of measurable histamine, TAME-esterase, and PGD_2 in nasal washes. Biopsy specimens of the nasal mucosa at this time show an increased number of degranulated mast cells.

Two to 6 hours after the initial allergen challenge, symptoms recur with a second release of mast cell mediators at the time of maximum mast cell cytokine production. This *late-phase nasal allergic reaction* occurs in approximately 50% of patients with seasonal rhinitis undergoing nasal challenge with allergen. This is associated with elevated levels of the same mediators noted in the immediate reaction except that PGD_2 is not detected. Thus, basophils appear partly responsible for such late-phase reactions because histamine is generated by both mast cells and basophils, whereas only mast cells can produce PGD_2. In support of this, a marked basophil influx into the nasal mucosa has been noted 3 to 11 hours after allergen challenge. Large numbers of neutrophils, mononuclear cells, and eosinophils also migrate into the nasal mucosa at this time. This inflammatory response is thought to cause the recurrence of symptoms and to induce chronic ones.

After allergen challenge, lymphocytes remain the predominant cells in the nasal mucosa. These cells actively transcribe messages for IL-3, IL-4, IL-5, and GM-CSF and have increased expression of the IL-2 receptor. Interleukins 1 through 5 and GM-CSF have been recovered from nasal washes after allergen challenge.

PRIMING AND NASAL HYPERREACTIVITY

When a patient is continually exposed to pollen, persistent nasal mucosal inflammation develops. In such patients, symptoms of rhinitis occur on exposure to lower doses of allergen (priming) and to nonspecific irritants (hyperreactivity). The clinical result is con-

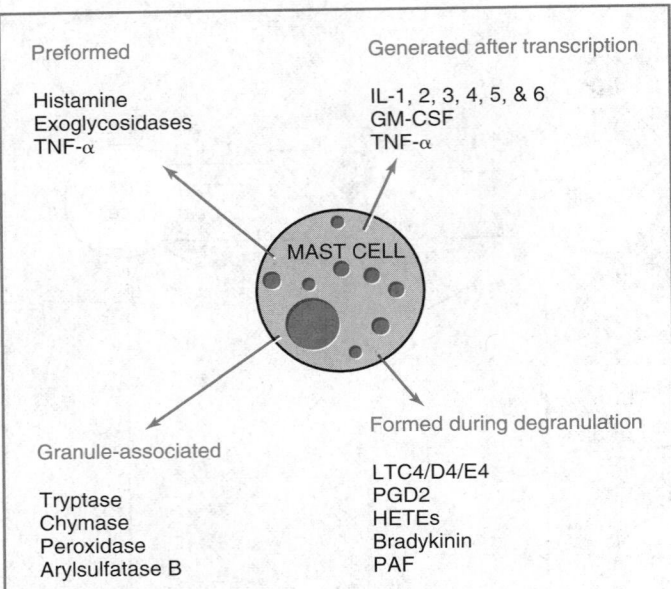

FIGURE 225–3. Mast cell mediators. (TNF-α = tumor necrosis factor-α; IL = interleukin; GM-CSF = granulocyte-monocyte colony-stimulating factor; PG = prostaglandin; PAF = platelet-activating factor; HETE = hydroxyeicosatetraenoic acid.)

tinued rhinitis symptoms with exposure to low allergen concentrations and irritants such as particulate pollution and volatile substances, even after the peak pollen season has passed.

MANAGING ALLERGIC RHINITIS

DIAGNOSIS. The diagnosis is based on a history of the characteristic symptoms that occur on exposure to known allergens. It is supported by the associated physical findings, by the presence of allergen-specific IgE on immediate hypersensitivity skin tests, or by radioallergosorbent testing (RAST) and a favorable response to allergen avoidance. The first step is identifying those allergens that produce symptoms.

ALLERGEN IDENTIFICATION AND AVOIDANCE. A careful home and work environmental history is often informative. When symptoms occur acutely, like those with exposure to cat or occupational allergens, identifying the culprit may be simple. In perennial rhinitis, identifying allergens by history may be difficult. In these circumstances, carefully performed immediate hypersensitivity skin testing (prick skin tests) is a quick, inexpensive, and safe way to identify the presence of allergen-specific IgE. In sensitive patients, testing with selected extracts of tree, grass, or weed pollen, mold, house dust mites and/or animal allergens results in a wheal and flare reaction at the skin test site within 20 minutes. A surrogate test, the RAST, although less sensitive and more expensive, gives similar information from a serum sample. Neither total serum IgE levels, elevated in only 30 to 40% of patients, nor peripheral blood eosinophil counts are sensitive enough to routinely diagnose allergic rhinitis. Stained nasal smears detect eosinophilia, helpful in narrowing the diagnosis to allergic rhinitis or NARES syndrome, and neutrophilia (>50%) associated with sinusitis.

Simple measures to avoid allergens include maintaining the relative humidity at 50% or less to limit house dust mite and mold growth and avoiding exposure to irritants such as cigarette smoke. Air conditioners decrease concentrations of pollens, molds, and dust mite allergens in indoor air. Avoiding exposure to the feces of the house dust mite—the most common cause of perennial allergic rhinitis—is facilitated by covering mattresses, box springs, and pillows with plastic and washing bedding in water hotter than 70°F once weekly. Synthetic pillows should also be used. Furry pets should be removed from the home unless testing shows they are not the source of symptoms.

PHARMACOLOGIC TREATMENT

If avoiding allergens does not result in improvement, antihistamine therapy is a reasonable next step. Antihistamines help control sneezing, rhinorrhea, and itching but may provide inadequate relief from nasal obstruction (Table 225–2). In this case, an oral antihistamine that contains a decongestant such as pseudoephedrine, phenylpropanolamine, or phenylephrine has been shown to be of added benefit. Because the latter agents may cause palpitations, insomnia or irritability, exacerbation of glaucoma, and urinary retention and are contraindicated in patients on monoamine oxidase therapy, they should be used cautiously. With use for more than 5 to 7 days, tachyphylaxis develops to nasal (decongestant) sprays of these drugs and rebound nasal congestion results. Continued use leads to rhinitis medicamentosa.

The first-generation H_1-receptor antagonists produce sedation and other CNS symptoms in 20% of patients and may cause drying of the mouth and urinary hesitancy. Newer second-generation antihistamines have sedative effects comparable to those of placebo. Two of these, terfenadine and astemizole, have been associated with inducing the complex ventricular tachyrhythmia, torsades de pointes, when used concomitantly with ketoconazole, itraconazole, or macrolide antibiotics that share hepatic metabolic pathways. Some of the second-generation H_1 antihistamines inhibit mast cell mediator release and inflammatory cell movement and function. This feature makes them effective in inhibiting not only the immediate but the late nasal reaction to allergen challenge. However, these second-generation agents have not yet been demonstrated to be clinically superior to other second-generation antihistamines. There is no evidence that pharmacologic tolerance develops to antihistamines. Thus, rotating from one antihistamine to another is not beneficial. Furthermore, clinical studies do not support using combinations of H_1 and H_2 antagonists to treat allergic rhinitis.

Cromolyn and nedocromil inhibit mast cell degranulation and mediator release from mast cells and have other anti-inflammatory actions. They thus inhibit both the immediate and late-phase nasal reaction. Both appear to be as effective as antihistamines in treating allergic rhinitis, with nedocromil the more effective. Both agents must be used frequently (three or more times a day), take 2 to 6 weeks to reach full efficacy, and have few side effects.

Corticosteroids given orally or parenterally usually abolish all symptoms of allergic rhinitis. The potential complications of such therapy make them unacceptable for treating allergic rhinitis except in very unusual circumstances. By contrast, topical intranasal

TABLE 225–2. REPRESENTATIVE ANTIHISTAMINES*

	Sedative Effects	Antihistamine Effects	Dosing Intervals (hr)
Ethanolamines			
Clemastine (Tavist)	2+	1–2+	12
Diphenhydramine (Benadryl)	3+	1–2+	6–8
Ethylenediamines			
Pyrilamine (Histadyl)	1+	1–2+	6–8
Alkylamines			
Chlorpheniramine (Chlor-Trimeton)	1+	2+	4–6
Phenothiazines			
Promethazine (Phenergan)	3+	3+	6–24
Piperidines			
Astemizole (Hismanal)	±	2–3+	24
Loratadine (Claritin)	±	2–3+	24
Terfenadine (Seldane)	±	2–3+	12–24
Azatadine (Optimine)	2+	2+	12
Cyproheptadine (Periactin)	3+	2+	8
Piperazines			
Hydroxyzine (Atarax)	3+	3+	12
Cetirizine (Reactine)	1+	2–3+	24
Miscellaneous			
Azelastine† (inves. drug)	±	2–3+	12
Levocabastine† (orphan drug)	±	2–3+	12

©1993 by Facts and Comparisons. Used with permission from Drug Facts and Comparisons. 1993 ed. St. Louis, Facts and Comparisons, a division of the JB Lippincott Company. Effects were graded 1–4+.

*Antihistamines in this listing have specific contraindications that require review prior to prescribing.

†Nasal spray.

TABLE 225–3. INTRANASAL STEROIDS AVAILABLE IN THE UNITED STATES

Name/Trade Name	Dose/Max. Dose	Approved for Children
Dexamethasone sodium phosphate (Decadron Turbinaire*)	2 sprays (168 μg) into each nostril 2–3/day; max = 1008 μg/day	>6
Flunisolide (Nasalide)	2 sprays (50 μg) into each nostril 2–3/day; max = 400 μg/day	>6
Beclomethasone dipropionate (Beconase, Vancenase, Beconase AQ, Vancenase AQ)	1 spray (42 μg) in each nostril 2–4/day; max = 336 μg/day	>6
Triamcinolone acetonide (Nasacort)	2 sprays (110 μg) in each nostril once a day; max = 440 μg/day	>6
Budesonide (Rhinocort)	2 sprays (64 μg) in each nostril twice a day; max = 256 μg/day	

©1993 by Facts and Comparisons. Used with permission from Drug Facts and Comparisons. 1993 ed. St. Louis, Facts and Comparisons, a division of the JB Lippincott Company.

*For short-term use only.

steroid therapy causes few side effects when used at recommended doses (Table 225–3). In experimental nasal allergen challenges, they decrease the amount of histamine release in the early nasal response to allergen by 75% and increase the threshold dose for a positive response to allergen. With regular use, they inhibit both the immediate and late-phase nasal reactions. Their maximal therapeutic effects are seen as quickly as 3 to 5 days. Corticosteroids have both vasoconstrictor and anti-inflammatory effects, including inhibiting mediator release and inflammatory cell chemotaxis. Topical nasal steroids are more effective than cromolyn and improve the symptoms of seasonal asthma in patients with both seasonal allergic rhinitis and seasonal allergic asthma. These preparations are available in both aqueous and Freon-propelled preparations. The aqueous preparations may be particularly useful in patients in whom Freon preparations cause mucosal drying, crusting, or epistaxis. Rarely, nasal steroids are associated with nasal septal perforation, probably secondary to nasal septal wall damage from inappropriately using the pressurized aerosol. Mucosal atrophy has not been noted even after years of usage. Treatment failures occur if mucus or other debris is not cleaned from the nose prior to their application. This cleaning can be facilitated by saline nasal sprays or washes.

Ipratropium bromide, a congener of atropine, has been found to reduce rhinorrhea when used intranasally. It does not block sneezing or nasal obstruction and thus is of greater use in nonallergic rhinitis with predominant rhinorrhea.

ALLERGEN IMMUNOTHERAPY

Allergen immunotherapy is the subcutaneous administration of increasing concentrations of allergen to which the patient has demonstrated sensitization and symptoms by skin test (or RAST) and history, respectively. Immunotherapy should be considered when pharmacotherapy and avoiding allergens fail to resolve symptoms or when pharmacotherapy produces unacceptable side effects or is not cost-effective. High-dose immunotherapy for allergic rhinitis has been shown to effectively relieve symptoms of allergic rhinitis in controlled studies. It should be strongly considered in patients with perennial symptoms, perennial rhinitis with seasonal exacerbations, constitutional symptoms (such as severe fatigue) or associated sinusitis, allergic conjunctivitis, or asthma. It is time-consuming and associated with a risk of anaphylaxis, especially when administered by health care professionals not properly trained in its use.

Allergen immunotherapy blocks both the immediate and the late-phase nasal reaction. The specific mechanism by which it relieves symptoms is unclear, although it increases allergen-specific IgG, reduces allergen-specific IgE, decreases allergen-induced mediator release, decreases eosinophil chemotaxis, and appears to favor a shift to cytokine profiles associated with T_H1 responses to allergen.

Badhwar AK, Druce HM: Allergic rhinitis. Med Clin North Am 76:789, 1992. *A practical and well-written review of the diagnostic approach and treatment of allergic rhinitis.*

Creticos P: Immunotherapy with allergens. JAMA 268:2834, 1992. *A well-written review of the rationale for allergen immunotherapy in allergic respiratory disease.*
Kaliner M, Lemanske R: Rhinitis and asthma. JAMA 268:2807, 1992. *An excellent review article with an extensive discussion of the pathophysiology of allergic disease.*
Mosimann BL, White MV, Hohman RJ: Substance P, calcitonin gene-related peptide, and vasoactive intestinal peptide increase in nasal secretions after allergen challenge in atopic patients. J Allergy Clin Immunol 92:95, 1993. *Provides evidence that neural reflexes and neurotransmitters play a role in allergic rhinitis.*
Naclerio RM: Allergic rhinitis. N Engl J Med 325:860, 1991. *An excellent review article covering all aspects of the topic.*
Naclerio RM, Proud D, Togias AG, et al.: Inflammatory mediators in late antigen-induced rhinitis. N Engl J Med 313:65, 1985. *A report on nasal allergen challenge studies that provided strong support that allergic rhinitis results from inflammatory processes.*
Pipkorn U, Proud D, Lichtenstein LM, et al.: Inhibition of mediator release in allergic rhinitis by pretreatment with topical glucocorticosteroids. N Engl J Med 316:1506, 1987. *Reports the results of corticosteroid administration on the production of the chemical mediators of allergic rhinitis.*
Sibbald B: Epidemiology of allergic rhinitis. In Burr ML (ed.): Monographs in Allergy. Basel, Karger, 1993, p 61. *A concise review of the epidemiology of allergic rhinitis.*

226 ANAPHYLAXIS
Allen P. Kaplan

The term *anaphylaxis* arose from the experiments of Richet and Portier in the early 1900's and meant the opposite of prophylaxis, i.e., a lack of protection rather than the expected immunity. Nevertheless, the reaction is indeed immune in nature and depends upon formation of IgE antibody, the immunoglobulin responsible for typical allergic reactions. The initial sensitization step induces formation of IgE specifically directed to the initiating substance. In anaphylaxis, the reaction is systemic in nature, occurs rapidly upon administration of minute concentrations of the offending material, and is potentially fatal. How the allergen is given can dictate the manifestations and magnitude of the ensuing allergic reaction; although all routes can lead to anaphylaxis, parenteral administration is more likely than inhaled or ingested allergens to cause elevated circulating levels of unaltered allergen and a systemic reaction. Thus, parenteral administration of medication and insect sting reactions (injected into cutaneous vessels) are among the most common causes of anaphylaxis. Anaphylactoid reactions are defined as systemic reactions that have the same symptoms as anaphylaxis but are not due to an IgE-dependent mechanism and are usually not immune. Examples include reactions to radiographic contrast agents and nonsteroidal anti-inflammatory drugs (e.g., acetylsalicylic acid, indomethacin, ibuprofen).

EPIDEMIOLOGY AND ETIOLOGY. The occurrence of anaphylaxis in the early 1900's was largely due to the use of serum from animals immunized with various toxins or bacteria to treat human illness. Most were due to diphtheria antitoxin injection. In the antibiotic era penicillin and sulfa drugs have become the leading causes of fatal anaphylaxis. In recent years, there have been between 100 and 500 deaths per year in the United States due to penicillin. The insect order Hymenoptera is responsible for about 40 deaths each year and is estimated to cause one significant reaction per 10,000 individuals per year, with a mortality of 0.2 per million in the United States. Estimates of penicillin-induced anaphylaxis are 10 to 40 per 100,000 injections. Most recently allergy to latex in surgical gloves is seen in health care workers or patients undergoing frequent procedures, e.g., children with meningomyelocele or spina bifida or congenital urogenital anomalies.

Although a history of atopy (allergic rhinitis, extrinsic asthma, atopic dermatitis) might be expected to be associated with an increased likelihood of anaphylactic reactions, atopic individuals appear to have, at worst, only a slightly greater risk than nonatopics. Thus, anyone can manifest an IgE response and clinical symptoms to the agents responsible for anaphylaxis. There is also no evidence that race, gender, age, occupation, or season intrinsically predisposes an individual to anaphylaxis.

TABLE 226-1. AGENTS CAUSING ANAPHYLAXIS

Type	Common	Rare
Proteins	Venoms (Hymenoptera)	Hormones (insulin, ACTH, vasopressin, parathormone)
	Pollens (ragweed, grass, etc.)	Enzymes (trypsin, penicillinase)
	Foods (eggs, seafood, nuts, grains, beans, cottonseed oil, chocolate)	Human proteins serum proteins, seminal fluid)
	Horse and rabbit serum (antilymphocyte globulin)	
	Latex	
Haptens and other low molecular weight substances	Antibiotics (penicillins, sulfonamides, cephalosporins, tetracyclines, amphotericin B, nitrofurantoin, aminoglycosides)	Vitamins (thiamine, folic acid)
	Local anesthetics (lidocaine, procaine, etc.)	
Polysaccharides		Dextrans, iron-dextran

Proteins, polysaccharides, and haptens are capable of eliciting systemic reactions in humans (Table 226-1). Proteins are the largest and most diverse group and include antiserum, hormones, seminal plasma, enzymes, Hymenoptera venom (e.g., phospholipase A_2), pollen allergens administered for immunotherapy ("allergy shots"), and foods. Polysaccharides such as dextrans are rarer causes. The most common etiologic agents are drugs, low molecular weight substances that are not antigenic themselves but act as haptens and become antigenic upon reaction with host proteins. These include antibiotics, local anesthetics, vitamins, and diagnostic reagents. Although the most common anaphylactic reactions are due to parenteral administration, food-induced anaphylaxis and anaphylactic reactions to an orally administered drug can occur in very sensitive individuals.

CLINICAL MANIFESTATIONS. IgE-mediated reactions can cause symptoms that include the cutaneous, respiratory, cardiovascular, gastrointestinal, and hematologic systems (Fig. 226-1). The onset and manifestations vary depending on route of administration, dose, release of and sensitivity to vasoactive substances, and differing sensitivities of the organs to these substances. These parameters can vary from person to person, and individuals tend to react in a characteristic pattern. The initial manifestations can begin in seconds or take as long as an hour to develop; in severe reactions the onset is usually within 5 to 10 minutes. Initial manifestations often include skin erythema, pruritus, a generalized feeling of warmth and/or impending doom, light-headedness, shortness of breath, nausea, vomiting, or a lump in the throat. Urticaria is the most common manifestation of anaphylaxis. The rash is generalized, intensely pruritic, and consists of well-circumscribed, erythematous, raised wheals with serpiginous borders and blanched centers. Angioedema may accompany urticaria and typically manifests as swelling of face, eyes, lips, tongue, pharynx, or extremities. The respiratory tract is commonly involved in fatal anaphylaxis. The early stages of upper airway edema consist of hoarseness, stridor, and/or dysphoria. Angioedema of the epiglottis and larynx can cause mechanical obstruction and death by suffocation. The swelling can extend to the hypopharynx and trachea. Between 25 and 50% of patients dying of anaphylaxis have pathologic changes consistent with severe asthma. There is pulmonary hyperinflation, peribronchial congestion, submucosal edema, edema-filled alveoli, and eosinophilic infiltration. The patient experiences shortness of breath, chest tightness, and wheezing. Severe hypoxemia and hypercarbia can manifest themselves rapidly.

Cardiovascular collapse is among the most severe clinical manifestations of anaphylaxis. The exact extent of fatal anaphylaxis is unknown, as anaphylaxis can be associated with myocardial ischemia and ventricular arrhythmias, each of which can cause or be caused by hypotension. Decreased blood pressure may be caused by diffuse peripheral vasodilatation due to release of vasodilatory mediators, decreased effective blood volume due to leakage of fluid into tissues, hypoxemia, or primary cardiac dysfunction.

Gastrointestinal manifestations can include nausea, vomiting, cramps, and diarrhea. Central nervous system abnormalities can include delirium and seizures, each of which may be due to hypoxemia and/or hypotension.

DIFFERENTIAL DIAGNOSIS. The diagnosis of systemic anaphylaxis may be obvious when there is a typical history of antecedent exposure to foreign antigenic material and a sequence of events consistent with the syndrome. Confirmation usually requires demonstration of IgE antibody to the substance by skin testing or by RAST (radioallergosorbent test). When the history is absent or when only a portion of the full syndrome is present, it may be difficult to exclude a vascular, cardiac, or neurologic disorder. Possibilities to be considered include acute myocardial infarction, pulmonary embolism, acute asthma, hereditary angioedema, cold urticaria, seizure disorder, anaphylactoid or idiosyncratic reaction, transfusion reaction, or vasovagal reaction. Vasovagal reactions may occur after an injection (e.g., penicillin, xylocaine) and include

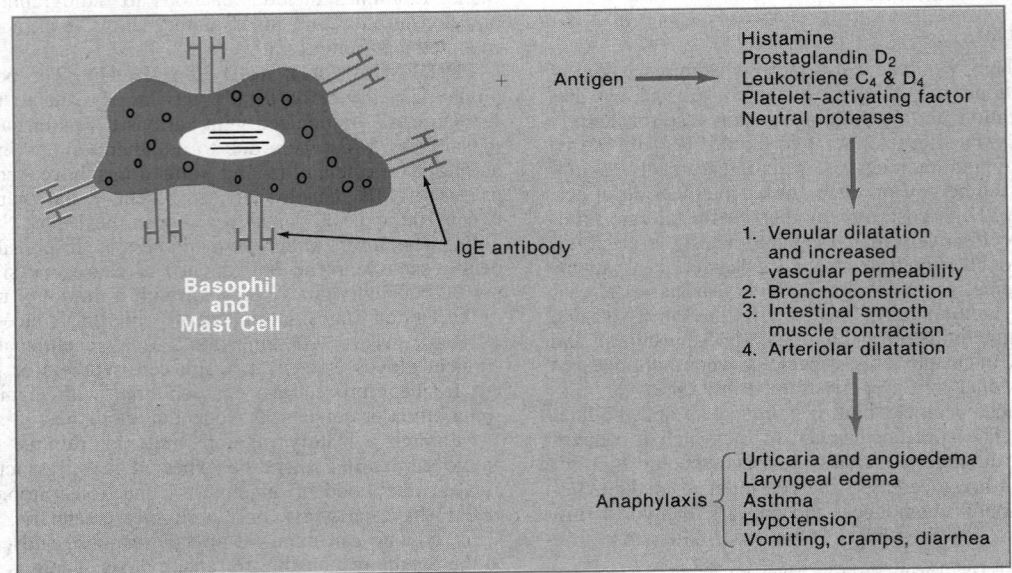

FIGURE 226-1. Acute anaphylaxis.

symptoms such as pallor, sweating, bradycardia, nausea, and hypotension, which can be confused with anaphylaxis. There is absence of any cutaneous manifestations or evidence of respiratory difficulty, and the diagnosis hinges on the cause of the hypotension. In such instances, skin testing is negative. Hereditary angioedema is due to absence or dysfunction of C1 inhibitor and is associated with laryngeal edema, peripheral angioedema, and acute abdominal pain. It is typically an autosomal dominant disorder with a family history or prior history of typical episodes. Trauma and infections may precipitate attacks of swelling. Patients with cold urticaria may have systemic symptoms due to water immersion such as while swimming; diffuse urticaria, angioedema, and hypotension may ensue. Anaphylactoid reactions can occur by substances causing direct nonimmune release of mast cell products (opiates, tubocurare, dextrans, sulfobromophthalein), which can cause urticaria, angioedema, chest tightness, wheezing, and hypotension. Aspirin and other nonsteroidal agents can cause upper and lower airway obstruction, urticaria, and/or angioedema with no IgE involvement. These agents all inhibit prostaglandin synthetase (cyclo-oxygenase). IgG–anti-IgA immune complexes may cause anaphylaxis-like symptoms when IgA-deficient patients receive blood. Complement activation appears to have a major role in such instances. Finally, radiocontrast media reactions occur in about 1% of studies that use them. The mechanism is unknown but may relate to their osmolarity. Newer agents seem to markedly diminish the incidence.

PATHOGENESIS. Antigenic induction of IgE formation requires antigenic processing (see Ch. 221) by dendrite cells or macrophages, T-cell help, and switching of B lymphocytes from IgG synthesis to IgE synthesis. Interleukin-4 may be critical for the latter switch and functions as a T-cell helper factor for IgE formation. Subsequent combination of antigen with IgE bound to high-affinity receptors on mast cells and basophils (see Fig. 225–2) causes secretion of a variety of vasoactive substances that may be responsible for the symptoms of anaphylaxis (Fig. 226–1). These include histamine, prostaglandin D_2, leukotrienes C_4 and D_4, and platelet-activating factor (PAF) (1-Ō-alkyl-2-sn-3 phosphoryl-choline). Histamine is the major secretory product of basophils and mast cells. It causes venular and arterial vasodilation, increases vascular permeability, and causes a decrease in diastolic blood pressure when systemic levels of approximately 2.5 ng per milliliter are reached. Histamine has direct inotropic and chronotropic action when injected directly into cardiac muscle, effects that are prevented by H_1 plus H_2 receptor antagonists. Prostaglandin D_2 is synthesized by mast cells but not by basophils. It is a peripheral vasodilator. Leukotrienes C_4 and D_4 are produced by basophils and mast cells and profoundly constrict peripheral arterial and coronary circulations and cause bronchoconstriction and decreased dynamic compliance. They also cause venular dilation and increase vascular permeability. PAF is synthesized by mast cells but not basophils and causes venular dilatation and an increase in cutaneous vascular permeability. When infused into rabbits, it causes profound hypotension, increased pulmonary resistance, pulmonary hypertension, cardiac arrhythmias, and decreased lung compliance, all manifestations of anaphylaxis.

Bradykinin is a nine–amino acid peptide that may also contribute to the symptoms of anaphylaxis and is generated by kininogen cleaved by enzymes known as *kallikreins*. Kinins are peripheral vasodilators, cause systemic hypotension, and constrict coronary vessels. Basophils and mast cells have a kallikrein-like enzyme; organs containing glands (lung, nasal mucosa) secrete a tissue kallikrein that digests low molecular weight kininogen to release bradykinin. Plasma kinin formation is associated with contact activation of Hageman factor, conversion of plasma prekallikrein to kallikrein, and digestion of high molecular weight (HMW)-kininogen.

Anaphylaxis is associated with depletion of clotting Factors V, VII, and fibrinogen, activation of complement, and depletion of HMW-kininogen consistent with acute intravascular coagulation. Clotting defects such as a prolonged partial thromboplastin time are commonly seen. Activation or depletion of these proteins is likely caused by enzymes released from cells that include not only mast cells and basophils but also monocyte/macrophages, eosinophils, and platelets. The latter group of cells possess low-affinity receptors for IgE (CD23) which may mediate cell secretion upon contact with antigen. The participation of these cells in allergic reactions is an area of current investigation.

PREVENTION AND TREATMENT. Patients who have previously experienced anaphylactic episodes should wear a Medic-Alert bracelet and be instructed regarding the importance of relating details of their specific drug reactions before taking medications. The medical history and medical record must include not only the allergic history but a description of the associated symptoms. The physician must be aware of drugs containing cross-reacting antigens. For example, patients with allergy to sulfa-containing antibiotics should avoid other sulfa-containing substances such as chlorthiazide diuretics, furosemide, sulfonylureas, and dapsone.

There is a 15% incidence of a reaction if a cephalosporin is substituted for penicillin because they share the presence of a β-lactone ring. Reactions with second- and third-generation cephalosporins may also occur, but aztreonam is an exception.

When the patient has a history of drug allergy or of taking a drug suspected of causing a reaction, it is appropriate to substitute another non–cross-reacting therapeutic agent whenever possible. Penicillin causes more anaphylactic reactions than any other drug, yet the history of "allergy" is unreliable because close to 80% of patients with such a history have negative skin tests to the major determinant (penicillin polylysine) or a minor determinant mixture (penicillin, penicilloic acid, penicillioylamine) and can tolerate the drug with impunity. Anaphylaxis is highly associated with IgE antibody directed to these minor determinants. Thus, a negative skin test to the commercially available major determinant is insufficient testing to administer the drug given a positive history. The addition of testing for minor determinants with negative results renders anaphylaxis or even any allergic reaction rare indeed. The number of alternative antibiotics that can be used in place of penicillin is ever increasing, and avoidance, in the sensitive patient, is the best approach. Nevertheless, there are circumstances in which use of penicillin or other agents by a known or suspected sensitive patient is necessary. In this circumstance, the patient can be desensitized by gradually administering increasing concentration of the drug—first intradermally, then subcutaneously, and finally parenterally. Such a procedure should be carried out by experienced personnel in an intensive care unit setting in which anaphylactic reactions can be effectively treated.

When an anaphylactic reaction is encountered, epinephrine given early quickly reverses most manifestations. Administered at a 1:1,000 dilution (0.01 ml per kilogram with a maximum dose of 0.5 ml subcutaneously repeated every 20 minutes as necessary), it is initial treatment once an adequate airway is in place. Further exposure to the inducing substance should be limited. When an anaphylactic reaction is initiated by an injection into the arm or leg, a tourniquet may be applied to limit antigen absorption. In the case of a honeybee sting, care should be taken to remove the stinger without compressing the venom sac. Upper airway obstruction must be differentiated from asthma because laryngeal and epiglottic edema may require endotracheal intubation or emergency tracheostomy to provide an airway. Asthma can be treated with epinephrine, administering an inhaled $β_2$ sympathomimetic, and/or intravenous aminophylline at a 6 mg per kilogram loading dose over 20 to 30 minutes, followed by 0.5 to 1 mg per kilogram per hour.

If any respiratory, vascular, or cardiac complications occur, an intravenous line should be placed promptly and a sample of arterial blood obtained for pH, Po_2, and Pco_2. Supplemental oxygen should be given to reduce hypoxemia. Pulse, blood pressure, and respiratory rate are monitored, and an electrocardiogram is obtained. Hypovolemic shock requires rapid intravenous fluid administration. Additionally, 5 ml of a 1:10,000 solution of epinephrine repeated every 5 to 10 minutes can be given intravenously in severe shock. A vasopressor such as dopamine (2 to 20 $μg$ per kilogram per minute) is indicated to manage hypotension unresponsive to volume expansion. This may increase cardiac output and improve blood flow to coronary, cerebral, renal, and mesenteric vascular beds. Higher doses of dopamine or norepinephrine yield significant $α$ receptor stimulation, which may increase blood pressure but constrict distal vascular beds. In case of significant cardiac dysfunction, an arterial line and a Swan-Ganz catheter should be placed.

Giving antihistamines at the onset of the acute episode may relieve pruritus, urticaria, and angioedema. Once an intravenous line is placed, 50 to 100 mg of diphenhydramine can be given slowly as a bolus. An H_2-receptor blocker may aid in the therapy of hypotension. Corticosteroids have no value during the acute episode, yet steroids are often also administered intravenously. It takes many hours before their first effect is seen. Thus, administration of steroids helps treat protracted asthma and late reactions that can ensue 1 to 2 days beyond the initial insult.

Bochner BS, Lichtenstein LM: Anaphylaxis—current concepts. N Engl J Med 324:1785, 1991. *An additional review including approaches to therapy.*

Dattwyler R, Kaplan AP, Austen KF: Human anaphylaxis. *In* Kaplan AP (ed.): Allergy. New York, Churchill Livingstone, 1985, p 559. *A textbook review of etiology, pathogenesis, and therapy.*

Gold M, Swartz JS, Braude BM, et al.: Intraoperative anaphylaxis: An association with latex sensitivity. J Allergy Clin Immunol 87:662, 1991. *A description of an increasingly recognized cause of anaphylactic reactions—namely, exposure to latex products.*

Sampson HA, Mendelson L, Rosen JP: Fatal and near fatal anaphylactic reactions to foods in children and adolescents. N Engl J Med 327:380, 1992. *Description of dangerous anaphylactic reactions to foods in children describing course and confirmation with assay of tryptase.*

227 INSECT STING ALLERGY
Lawrence M. Lichtenstein

The stings of insects of the order Hymenoptera have long been recognized as a potential cause of severe, often life-threatening reactions in susceptible individuals. These reactions are unrelated to the toxic chemicals in the venoms, being due to allergic sensitization. Insect sting allergy has recently become the most intensely studied model of anaphylaxis in humans, resulting in important advances that have had rapid clinical applications.

EPIDEMIOLOGY. The incidence of immediate hypersensitivity to insect stings based on history is 3%; more than 20% of the population, however, has positive skin test reactions to insect venoms. Other allergies do not seem to predispose to insect sting sensitivity. The frequency varies with exposure and is therefore greater in children and males as well as those inclined to outdoor activities. Systemic reactions to insect stings cause few fatalities, but the morbidity, fear, and change in life style caused by these reactions is significant. A large number of people suffer prolonged and unusually severe local inflammatory reactions to insect stings, which are allergic in nature. As with other allergies, there appears to be an inherited predisposition, since multiple family members are often affected.

ETIOLOGY. The only insects possessing true stingers are those of the order Hymenoptera. There are two families of importance, the bees (honeybees, bumblebees) and the vespids (yellow jackets, hornets, wasps). The bees have barbed stingers that remain in the skin after a sting. Yellow jackets are the most common culprits, but honeybees are more commonly implicated in the western United States. Wasps are more common in the south central United States (especially Texas). Sensitivity develops to antigens in the insect venom, most of which have enzymatic activity. A major allergen in both insect families is phospholipase A, but they do not cross-react with one another.

PATHOGENESIS. The injection of foreign proteins commonly causes the production of specific antibodies of the IgE and IgG classes. Individuals may develop venom-specific IgE antibodies after any sting, this response sometimes persisting for less than 3 months and in other instances persisting for more than 25 years. Tissue mast cells and circulating basophils bind IgE antibody, thereby becoming sensitized so that a repeat encounter with the offending allergen triggers release of the mediators of anaphylaxis (see Ch. 51). The initiation and persistence of this sensitization are related to inheritable and other unknown determinants. Sensitization may occur at any time in life, even after many uneventful stings. The sensitizing sting itself causes no unusual reaction and is often so remote as to evade recollection.

Generalized mediator release from sensitized basophils and mast cells (see Table 231–2) causes the many manifestations of anaphylaxis. Localization of symptoms to specific target tissues is not well understood. The pathology observed in fatal cases includes upper

airway edema and obstruction, the visceral consequences of hypotension, or occasionally no discernible abnormality (see Ch. 226 for a discussion of anaphylaxis).

Large local reactions are IgE dependent; their prolonged timecourse is characteristic of the so-called late phase response to antigen. These reactions involve a cascade of events beginning with mediator release from mast cells and culminating with local inflammation involving many cell types and numerous mechanisms. The potential roles of eosinophils, basophils, lymphocytes, and cytokines and chemokines are being elucidated.

The venom-specific IgG antibody response to a sting is usually short lived, lasting only a few months. Repeated stings (as in beekeepers) are associated with high titers of IgG antibodies, which protect against allergic reactions. Beekeepers who do not have anaphylactic reactions have high IgG titers, as do affected individuals immunized with venoms. Passive transfer of these IgG antibodies protects sensitive patients from a sting. These protective antibodies are thought to block the allergic reaction by competing with IgE for the allergenic venom proteins and have therefore been termed "blocking" antibodies.

CLINICAL MANIFESTATIONS. Allergic reactions to insect stings are either generalized (systemic) or large local reactions. *Systemic sting reactions* present the classic manifestations of anaphylaxis described in Ch. 226. The observed frequency of the most common symptoms in adult patients is presented in Table 227–1. The risk of a fatal outcome increases, as might be expected, with age and the use of certain drugs, especially antagonists of β-adrenergic receptors. Fatal anaphylaxis may occur without a history of sting allergy.

The onset of systemic symptoms is rapid, within 2 to 3 minutes, and rarely occurs more than 30 minutes after a sting. Symptoms presenting hours later (except large local reactions) are not usually associated with immediate hypersensitivity or IgE antibodies. Unusual reactions such as vasculitis, nephropathies, encephalitis, and other neurologic manifestations have been reported, but no causal relationship has been established. Allergic respiratory symptoms may occur in beekeepers and their families owing to sensitization to the dust in the hives that contain bee body proteins. This sensitivity is unrelated to sting reactions.

Large local reactions are slow in onset and occur with or without concomitant early systemic reaction. The area of induration increases in size progressively for the first 24 to 48 hours and then resolves gradually over several days. These reactions may be so large as to immobilize an entire limb and are a significant cause of morbidity in sensitive individuals. Red streaks resembling lymphangitis may be observed and are often treated with antibiotics despite a lack of evidence for true cellulitis.

NATURAL HISTORY. The natural history of insect sting allergy has been incompletely documented. The prevalence of venom sensitization in the general population was noted above. It is estimated that about 20% of those at risk by virtue of positive skin tests (but with no history of a systemic reaction) will react on sting. There is considerable variability in the reaction to a sting among those who are clearly allergic as demonstrated by positive skin tests and a history of a previous reaction. Recent studies indicate that 25 to 60% of adults had a systemic reaction when stung by the appropriate insect. In children, on the other hand, a repeat sting causes a reaction in only 8%. The incidence in adolescents and young adults must lie between these extremes. This variability confounds the prediction of risk associated with sensitization.

Although many patients and physicians believe that allergic sting reactions become progressively more severe with every sting, this is not true. Most of those affected maintain a similar pattern of symptoms with every sting. Factors favoring a systemic reaction include

TABLE 227–1. SYMPTOMS REPORTED BY 245 PATIENTS

Symptom	Percentage
Cutaneous only	14
Urticaria-angioedema	78
Dizziness-hypotension	61
Dyspnea-wheezing	53
Throat tightness-hoarseness	40
Loss of consciousness	33

multiple stings, or stings in close temporal proximity (only weeks apart).

Sensitization generally decreases or disappears in time. This is far more common in children than in adults. However, resensitization has been observed upon re-sting.

DIAGNOSIS. The acute presentation of anaphylaxis is easily diagnosed by the presence of classic symptoms and signs. The insect sting may be inapparent. Differential diagnosis is more difficult in localized reactions such as acute chest pain and dyspnea or syncope without urticaria.

The diagnosis of insect sting allergy currently rests on a convincing history and positive skin tests. Demonstration *in vitro* of venom-specific IgE by the radioallergosorbent test (RAST) is less sensitive than skin tests but is equally accurate when positive.

Skin tests are performed intradermally with venoms diluted to concentrations in the range of 1 to 1000 ng per milliliter. Five venoms are used: honeybee (HB), yellow jacket (YJ), yellow hornet (YH), white-faced hornet (WH), and *Polistes* wasp (POL). Positive intradermal skin tests, a wheal >5 mm in diameter with at least 20 mm of erythema, develops within 20 minutes. The degree of skin test sensitivity does not correlate with clinical sensitivity. Within a few months after a systemic sting reaction, skin tests are almost uniformly positive. Stings more remote in time are more commonly associated with an apparent loss of sensitivity (similar to the situation in penicillin-related anaphylaxis).

Honeybee venom sensitivity occurs independent of other venom allergies, but about 10% of patients are sensitive to both bee and vespid venoms. The vespid venoms are highly cross-reactive, so that almost all vespid-sensitive patients have positive YJ, YH, and WH skin tests even though most have been stung only by YJs. Half of these patients are also sensitive to POL venom. Very few individuals are allergic to only one or two of the vespid venoms. *In vitro* RAST inhibition techniques are useful to distinguish cross-reactivity from specific sensitivity. This is clinically relevant in patients with a positive skin test to *Polistes,* which is often due to cross-reactivity, and the patient may be spared considerable expense and unnecessary immunization by RAST inhibition analysis.

TREATMENT. The treatment of choice for anaphylactic reactions is subcutaneous epinephrine 1:1000, 0.5 ml initially and repeated twice at 10-minute intervals, if necessary, to reverse the progression of symptoms. Antihistamines and glucocorticoids do not contribute to the management of life-threatening symptoms but may reduce the duration and severity of cutaneous manifestations. Their use should not be considered until the acute episode has ended. Intravenous volume expansion or airway maintenance may be necessary. In a few individuals, the process is resistant to epinephrine; in such instances an α-adrenergic agent (i.e., norepinephrine) may be tried. Affected persons not yet protected by immunotherapy are advised to carry, and are instructed in the use of, a kit containing a syringe device preloaded with one or two recommended doses of epinephrine.

Venom immunotherapy is successful in virtually all patients. Less than 2% of those immunized have any systemic symptoms after a challenge sting, and these are uniformly less severe than their previous reactions. The indications for venom immunotherapy are now based on an improved understanding of the natural history of the disease. Those with a history of life-threatening reactions should be treated. The risk of progression from strictly cutaneous to life-threatening respiratory or vascular reactions is rare (<1%) in adults and children. Cutaneous reactors who are more likely to be stung in their daily activities or who for a variety of reasons (location, age, cardiovascular disease) can ill afford a reaction should be treated. The cost and inconvenience of treatment may deter other cutaneous reactors from undergoing immunotherapy. Children, much more commonly than adults, have cutaneous symptoms only. These children may be left untreated. Venom immunotherapy is usually contraindicated in the absence of positive venom skin tests or RAST. Although there are rare individuals who are sensitive without positive tests, treatment is currently recommended using all venoms that cause a positive skin test (for *Polistes,* see above). While other mechanisms may contribute, the induction of increased serum levels of venom-specific IgG antibodies is the most apparent mechanism of protection for venom immunotherapy; <3 μg per milliliter is associated with increased risk of sting anaphylaxis. In many European centers, the patient is re-stung in the hospital before therapy is begun.

Rapid immunization in six to eight weekly visits is recommended, since it is associated with a significantly greater and more rapid immune response and with fewer adverse reactions than a slower (>20 weeks) regimen. The maintenance dose of 100 μg of each venom is repeated monthly for at least 6 months, and is then continued at 6- to 8-week intervals for 5 years. If treatment is interrupted for more than 3 months, it is likely that protection will diminish to inadequate levels. Loss of venom sensitivity during maintenance immunotherapy occurs in some patients during the first 3 to 5 years of treatment. Skin tests should, therefore, be repeated every 2 years. After 5 years it appears that patients can stop therapy and suffer a sting without serious sequelae. Possible exceptions include patients with extremely severe reactions or those with complicating medical conditions. After stopping venom immunotherapy, venom sensitivity continues to decline and is not increased even after stings.

Adverse reactions to venom immunotherapy may be early or late. Immediate reactions include all the manifestations of anaphylaxis. During the initial course of treatment, 10 to 15% of patients report systemic complaints, only half of which require epinephrine. At maintenance doses, systemic reactions occur rarely. After a systemic reaction, the dose should be reduced by up to 50% on the subsequent visit and then increased gradually toward 100 μg again.

Large local reactions occur frequently—50% of treated patients experience at least one such reaction. These occur after 10 of every 100 injections in the induction phase, most commonly in the midrange of doses (10 to 50 μg) and much less often at maintenance doses. Large local reactions do not presage systemic reactions and require a reduction of dose only for the most severe reactions. Long-term side effects have not been observed with venom immunotherapy or in beekeepers stung frequently for over 30 years.

Golden DBK, Addison BI, Gadde J, et al.: Prospective observations on patients who discontinue Hymenoptera venom immunotherapy. J Allerg Clin Immunol 88:162, 1989. *Studies of when and how to discontinue venom immunotherapy.*

Golden DBK, Lawrence ID, Hamilton RH, et al.: Clinical correlation of the venom-specific IgG antibody level during maintenance venom immunotherapy. J Aller Clin Immunol 90:386, 1992. *The relevance of IgG "blocking" antibodies in venom immunotherapy.*

Golden DBK, Marsh DG, Kagey-Sobotka A, et al.: Epidemiology of insect sting allergy. JAMA 262:240, 1989. *A review of diagnostic and therapeutic problems in insect allergy.*

Hunt KJ, Valentine MD, Sobotka AK, et al.: A controlled trial of immunotherapy in insect hypersensitivity. N Engl J Med 299:157, 1978. *A comparison of venom immunotherapy with whole body extract and placebo. Demonstrates efficacy of venom therapy and the clinical consequences of challenge stings.*

Valentine MD, Schuberth KC, Kagey-Sobotka A, et al.: The value of immunotherapy with venom in children with allergy to insect stings. N Engl J Med 323:1601, 1990. *A prospective study of the epidemiology and immunotherapy of insect sting allergy in children, indicating that repeat reactions are rare and virtually never of increased severity.*

228 IMMUNE COMPLEX DISEASES
Richard D. deShazo

DEFINITION. Immune complex diseases are a group of conditions resulting from inflammation induced in tissues where immune complexes are formed or deposited. Clinical consequences may be local when immune complexes form in the tissues of a specific organ or systemic when complexes circulate and deposit widely. A variety of antigens have been associated with the induction of immune complex disease in humans (Table 228–1) (see Ch. 221).

PATHOPHYSIOLOGY. In their studies, von Pirquet and Schick observed that some children developed a "serumkrankheit" (serum sickness) 1 to 2 weeks after being injected subcutaneously with horse-derived diphtheria antiserum. The syndrome is characterized by fever, lymphadenopathy, arthralgias or arthritis, leukopenia, proteinuria, and cutaneous findings including urticaria. They postulated that the illness was caused by newly formed host antibody reacting to horse serum and resulting in the deposition of antigen-antibody

TABLE 228–1. REPRESENTATIVE ANTIGENS KNOWN TO CAUSE IMMUNE COMPLEX DISEASE IN HUMANS

Antigens	Syndrome
Therapeutic Agents	
Horse serum products: antilymphocyte globulin, snake venom antiserum, streptokinase, monoclonal antibody products	Serum sickness
Drugs: cephalosporins, penicillin, amoxicillin, trimethoprim-sulfamethoxazole, fluoxetine, iron-dextran, carbamazepine, and others	
Drugs: quinidine, chlorpromazine, sulfonamides	Hemolytic anemia (innocent bystander reaction)
Autologous (self) Antigens	
DNA	Vasculitis and glomerulonephritis of systemic lupus erythematosus
IgG, IgM	Vasculitis of rheumatoid arthritis and mixed cryoglobulinemia
Tumor antigens: Colon carcinoma (carcinoembryonic antigen)	Glomerulonephritis
Microbial Antigens	
Hepatitis B	Systemic vasculitis
Plasmodium malariae	
Schistosoma mansoni	Glomerulonephritis
β-Hemolytic streptococci	
Staphylococcus epidermidis	

complexes in tissue. Much later, Germuth and Dixon developed rabbit models of serum sickness that confirmed this hypothesis.

In the model of acute serum sickness, rabbits receive a single injection of radiolabeled foreign serum, e.g., bovine serum albumin. Initially, levels of antigen measured in the serum decrease rapidly as the antigen equilibrates in the animal's intravascular and extravascular fluid compartments over several days. Thereafter, serum antigen concentration falls at a steady rate associated with degradation. About 10 to 12 days after injection, there is a second rapid decrease in the concentration of free antigen in the serum. This coincides with the development of host antibody to the antigen and the formation and clearance of antigen-containing immune complexes by the reticuloendothelial system. At this time, serum complement levels drop, proteinuria develops, and histopathologic studies show inflammation in the rabbit's glomeruli, synovium, and arteries. Host immunoglobulin, complement, and antigen are deposited in a granular pattern along the glomerular basement membrane and near the internal elastic lamina of the coronary arteries. These findings occur when immune complexes of relatively high weight ($> 19S$) are present in serum and resolve rapidly after these complexes are no longer detectable. If additional doses of antigen are given, chronic symptoms develop.

The relative amounts of antigen and antibody detectable in this model of serum sickness form a "precipitin curve" (Fig. 228–1). The curve may be divided into zones of "free antigen" on the left, "equivalence" in the center, and "antibody excess" on the right. In antigen excess, the very small antigen complexes produced ($Ag_1 : Ab_{1-3}$) do not activate complement or induce inflammation. In antibody excess, the very large complexes present have difficulty diffusing across the endothelial barrier and are rapidly cleared by the reticuloendothelial system. Near the point of equivalence and in the area of slight antigen excess, little if any noncomplexed antigen or antibody is detectable and intermediate-size ($Ag_{2-3} : Ab_{2-6}$) ($> 19S$) soluble immune complexes circulate. At this point, a lattice of antigen and antibody molecules forms. This results from noncovalent bonding between antigen and antibody and between Fc portions of adjacent antibody molecules. The structure of this lattice depends on the valence of the antibody and the number of antigenic determinants on the antigen. In general, low-affinity antibodies form smaller immune complexes than do higher affinity antibodies.

BIOLOGIC PROPERTIES OF IMMUNE COMPLEXES. The biologic properties of antigen-antibody complexes depend on the nature of the antibodies and the degree of lattice formed and include (1) their ability to activate the complement system, (2) their ability to interact with cell receptors, and (3) their propensity to deposit in tissues.

Immune complexes may fix complement by either the classic or alternate complement pathway (see Ch. 222). Immune complexes that contain antibodies of the IgG (usually IgG_1 or IgG_3) or IgM class in an appropriate lattice structure activate the classic complement pathway by binding C1q, the first subunit of the first component of complement. Antibodies of the IgG_4 subclass are less efficient at activating complement than those of the other three subclasses. Immune complexes containing IgA may activate the alternate complement pathway but not the classic one.

Phagocytic cells and certain lymphocytes possess receptors for antibody molecules. Of these, the Fcγ receptors on these cells react with IgG molecules. The Kupffer cells of the liver possess a specific type of Fcγ receptor (Fcγ RIII), which helps remove IgG-containing immune complexes from the serum. Very large latticed immune complexes containing IgG may bind to this Fcγ receptor without activating complement. Once bound, they condense or rearrange to form even larger lattices that are phagocytosed.

Human erythrocytes have receptors for C3b, called *complement receptor type I* (CR1). The CR1 binds to immune complexes that contain molecules of C3b, iC3b, or C4b. When these erythrocytes circulate through the liver, the Kupffer cells effectively remove the

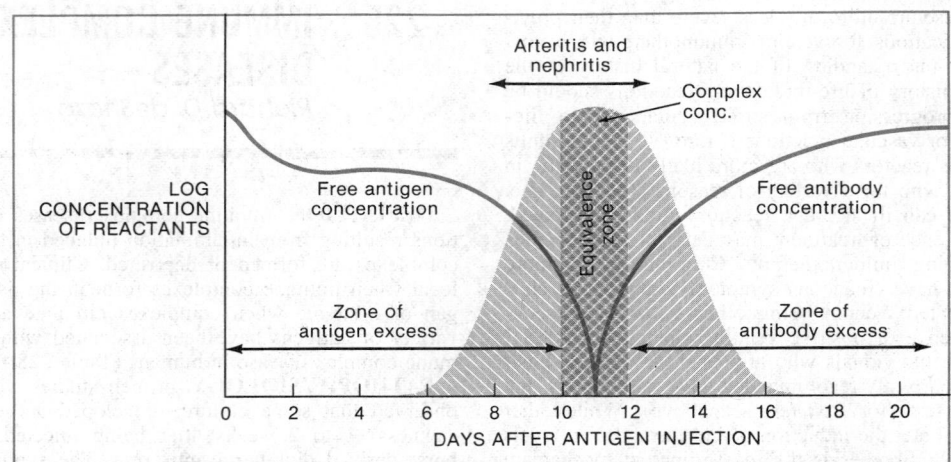

FIGURE 228–1. Natural history of acute serum sickness in rabbits following a single injection of radiolabeled bovine serum albumin (BSA) as antigen. The disease occurs when large quantities of soluble immune complexes are present in the circulation. (From Rich RR: Immune Complex Diseases. *In* Wyngaarden JB, Smith LH Jr, Bennett JC [eds.]: Cecil Textbook of Medicine. 19th ed. Philadelphia, WB Saunders, 1992, p 1468.)

large, complement-containing immune complexes without damaging the erythrocytes. This is accomplished by using their Fc receptors, which have a greater affinity for the complexes than does CR1 (Fig. 228–2).

The fate of immunocomplexes that contain IgA is less clear in humans. In experimental animals, immune complexes containing eight or more IgA antibodies are rapidly taken up by the liver.

FACTORS AFFECTING HOW IMMUNE COMPLEXES DEPOSIT. Experimental studies suggest that a number of factors determine the fate of immune complexes. These include the lattice structure, the presence of complement in the complex, the characteristics of antibodies and antigen in the complex, the numbers and functions of receptors on reticuloendothelial and other cells, and the charge of the immune complex. So far as *antibodies* are concerned, positive charges seem to facilitate deposition of immune complexes in the glomeruli. Moreover, certain nonglomerular cationic antigens like DNA appear to bind to glomeruli. They then serve as a nidus for immune complexes to form locally and deposit in the subepithelial area of the glomerular capillary membrane. IgA nephropathy (see Ch. 87) is a condition in which IgA-containing immune complexes deposit in the glomeruli, resulting in a focal glomerulonephritis. This form of glomerulonephritis, often subsequent to an infectious illness, may reflect the less efficient clearance of IgA-containing immune complexes that are unable to activate the classic complement pathway.

In respect to *complement*, patients with systemic lupus erythematosus (SLE) (see Ch. 240) have fewer CR1 receptors for C3b on their erythrocytes, a factor that may predispose them to immune complex disease. The presence of complement deficiency syndromes (C1q, C1r, C1s, C4, C2, and C3) is associated with lupus-like syndromes. This reflects, in part, the fact that complement components are not only proinflammatory in immune complex disease but also can inhibit immune complex deposition and resolubilize complexes from their sites of deposition. For instance, C1q fixation by immune complexes inhibits Fc-Fc interactions between IgG molecules and inhibits complex precipitation. Complex formation is inhibited, and deposited complexes are solubilized by the co-

valent attachment of C3b to antigen-antibody complexes. That Fc receptors can bind immune complexes to reticuloendothelial cells appears to influence their rate of clearance. In immune complex disease, Fc receptor function is often diminished. Finally, certain cells have receptors that facilitate interaction with immune complexes. Glomerular epithelium has receptors for C3; endothelial cells have receptors for C1q; renal interstitial cells, damaged endothelial cells, and platelets have Fc receptors.

INDUCTION OF INFLAMMATION BY IMMUNE COMPLEXES. Inflammation associated with immune complexes results when circulating phagocytic cells move into tissue sites where the complexes deposit. This movement is influenced by several processes. Tissue mast cells release vasoactive amines after antigen reacts with IgE or on contact with the anaphylatoxins C3a and C3b. These amines increase vascular permeability, which facilitates the movement of phagocytes responding to the chemotactic and adhesion-promoting factors, including C5a, that are released when immune complexes activate complement. This may explain why antihistamines may attenuate some of the cutaneous findings in experimental and human serum sickness. Subsequently, immune complexes binding to neutrophils and/or monocytes by their C3b and Fcγ receptors result in cell activation and the phagocytosis of the immune complexes. The activated phagocytes degranulate and release proteolytic enzymes and oxygen-derived free radicals. Cellular damage and loss of blood to local tissues result, and ischemic injury follows.

IMMUNE COMPLEX DISEASES IN HUMANS. Serum sickness occurs in humans, and the clinical and laboratory findings are much like those seen in the rabbit model. This most commonly occurs after using horse serum products, including Antivenin, used to treat rattlesnake bites, and antithymocyte globulin, used to treat aplastic anemia. The first sign of the syndrome in patients with serum sickness from antithymocyte globulin is a curious band of erythema located laterally on the hands, feet, fingers, and toes. Circulating immune complexes and decreases in serum C3, C4, and CH50 concentrations occur at the time of symptoms of serum sickness. Serum sickness also occurs with certain drugs, including β-lactam antibiotics, sulfonamides, thiouracil, hydantoin, thiazide diuretics, and para-aminosalicylic acid. Patients develop fever, malaise, arthralgia and arthritis, abdominal pain sometimes associated with melena, and urticaria and/or urticarial vasculitis. Similar symptoms may be noted in patients with mixed cryoglobulinemia, rheumatoid arthritis with high titers of rheumatoid factor, and SLE with high titers of antibody to double-stranded DNA.

Another immune complex disease in humans is the syndrome of leukocytoclastic (hypersensitivity) vasculitis. It is associated with the characteristic physical finding of recurrent episodes of palpable purpura. Findings are usually, but not always, limited to the skin and may occur as a reaction to drugs or in association with specific infections like hepatitis B, in certain connective tissue diseases like SLE, in cryoglobulinemia, or for no distinguishable cause. The histopathologic feature of a predominant polymorphonuclear cell infiltrate in postcapillary venules is associated with "nuclear dust" from leukocytoclasis, endothelial cell damage and proliferation, and distal infarction of tissues. Subendothelial electron-dense deposits in postcapillary venules appear in association with circulating immune complexes, which are detectable in a high percentage of patients.

TESTS TO DETECT CIRCULATING IMMUNE COMPLEXES. No available laboratory test detects all circulating immune complexes. *Complement assays,* including CH50, C3, and C4, are depressed only when large quantities of immune complexes that activate the complement system are present. *Physical methods,* such as precipitation, are laborious because they require separating immune complexes from other serum components. Each physical method has problems specific to it; e.g., cryoprecipitation is not a property of all immune complexes. *Biologic methods* depend on the interaction of immune complexes with complement components and receptors on cells. The binding and subsequent precipitation of radiolabeled C1q with immune complexes by polyethylene glycol is a widely used method that detects as little as 10 μg of aggregated IgG. Conglutinin assays detect only those immune complexes that contain C3bi. The most commonly used assay for immune complexes employs lymphoblastoid B cells, called *Raji cells.* These cells were derived from a patient with Burkitt's lymphoma. They

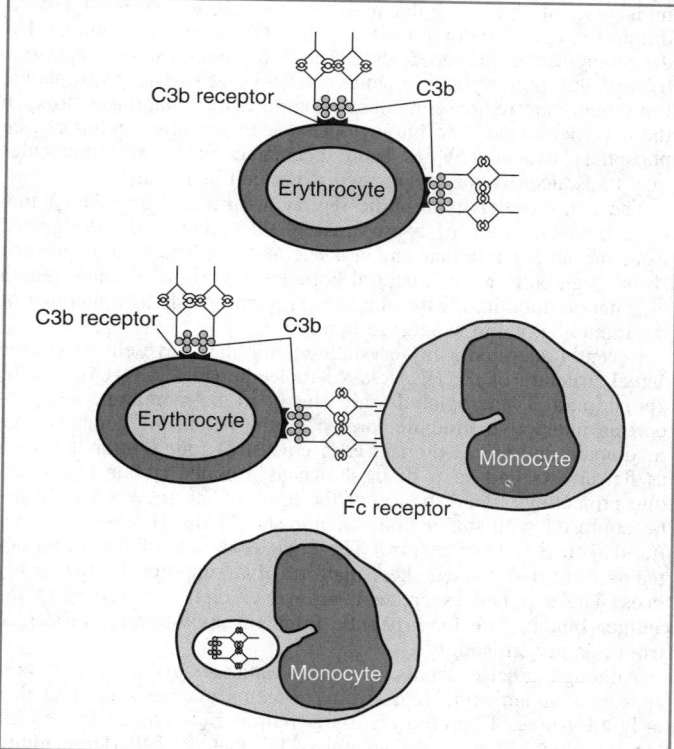

FIGURE 228–2. The role of hepatic mononuclear phagocytes (Kupffer cells) in removal of immune complexes from the circulation. Circulating complexes are bound to erythrocytes by the CR1 receptors for C3b. The complexes are removed from the erythrocytes by the Fc receptors of Kupffer cells, which have a greater affinity for the complexes. (From Virella G: Immunol Ser 58:379, 1993.)

lack surface immunoglobulins and have low-affinity receptors for IgG and high-affinity receptors for complement components.

Because immune complex assays are not antigen specific, they provide little insight into the cause of various immune complex diseases and do not provide a specific diagnosis. Some reports suggest that the presence of concentrations of immune complexes may correlate with the activity or prognosis of some diseases. Others suggest that they may be useful in the diagnosis of clinical diseases when immune complex deposition is a prominent component.

TREATMENT OF IMMUNE COMPLEX DISEASE. As with all diseases, the seriousness of the clinical syndrome determines the therapy. If the particular antigen that causes immune complex disease can be identified and avoided, for instance a drug, immune complex disease can be expected to resolve. When immune complex disease is a feature of an autoimmune disease such as SLE, controlling the disease with anti-inflammatory and/or immunosuppressive therapy usually resolves the related symptoms.

Serum sickness following drug therapy or therapeutic use of autologous serum proteins, such as rattlesnake horse antiserum, usually resolves spontaneously over 7 to 14 days. Symptoms usually respond to antihistamine therapy with or without corticosteroid treatment. Although controlled treatment studies are not available, moderate doses of prednisone (20 to 40 mg) given twice a day for 3 to 5 days followed by a tapering dose of corticosteroids over 10 to 14 days usually resolve symptoms in severe cases. The utility of plasmapheresis in immune complex disease is unproven.

Gauthier VJ, Abrass CK: Circulating immune complexes in renal injury. Semin Nephrol 12:379, 1992. *An extensive review of the mechanisms of immune complex–mediated renal disease.*

Hebert LA: The clearance of immune complexes from the circulation of man and other primates. Am J Kidney Dis 17:352, 1991. *A review of studies pertaining to the fate of immune complexes.*

Mannik M: Characteristics of immune complexes and principles of immune complex disease. *In* Arthritis and Allied Conditions: A Textbook of Rheumatology. 12th ed. Philadelphia, Lea & Febiger, 1993, p 495.

Virella G: Immune complex disease. Immunol Ser 58:379, 1993. *Two detailed reviews of the pathophysiology and clinical aspects of immune complex disease.*

229 THE MAJOR HISTOCOMPATIBILITY COMPLEX AND DISEASE SUSCEPTIBILITY

Benjamin D. Schwartz

The proper functioning of the immune system depends on its ability to distinguish "self" from "nonself." This crucial distinction is achieved via the molecules determined by the major histocompatibility complex (MHC), or HLA complex as it is known in humans. It is now clear that both foreign and self antigens are recognized by the T lymphocytes of the immune system only in conjunction with HLA molecules. During embryogenesis, a process of T-cell "education" takes place in the thymus whereby T cells recognizing self antigens (in the context of HLA molecules) are normally eliminated and T cells potentially capable of recognizing foreign antigens in the context of self HLA molecules are selected.

For a protein antigen to be recognized by the T lymphocytes of the immune system, it must undergo "processing." During processing, the protein is partially degraded into peptides, some of which are bound by HLA molecules. The peptide and HLA molecule form a complex that is the ligand recognized by the receptor on the T lymphocyte. There are two processing pathways used by the immune system. Intracellular antigens, such as viruses, are processed through the endogenous pathway and are presented by HLA class I molecules to CD8+ (generally cytotoxic) T lymphocytes. In contrast, extracellular antigens are processed through the exogenous pathway and are presented by HLA class II molecules to CD4+ (generally helper) T lymphocytes. Thus, HLA molecules are crucial in the recognition of antigen by the immune system.

HISTORY

The existence of a human MHC was first suggested in the mid 1950's when leukoagglutinating antibodies were discovered in the sera of multiparous women and multiply transfused leukopenic patients. Analysis of these sera indicated that these antisera were detecting alloantigens (i.e., antigens that were present on the cells of some individuals of a given species) which were the products of a polymorphic genetic locus. It was discovered shortly thereafter that these human leukocyte antigens (HLA) had a major role in determining the success of organ transplants, and this finding spurred the initial study of these antigens. In 1973, certain HLA antigens were found to be associated with specific diseases. In addition, at around the same time it was appreciated that the HLA complex regulates several aspects of the human immune response. These findings provided a second impetus for the study of the HLA complex. The application of molecular biology technology to the study of the HLA complex over the past 15 years has allowed additional HLA loci and alleles to be delineated and the sequence of many HLA genes to be determined. Most recently, x-ray crystallographic analysis of HLA molecules has allowed insight into their physiology. Together these findings have suggested how changes in the sequence of an HLA molecule may lead to predisposition to disease.

TISSUE DISTRIBUTION, FUNCTION, AND STRUCTURE

The HLA complex determines two distinct classes of cell surface glycoprotein molecules, designated class I and class II, with distinct structures, functions, and tissue distributions.

CLASS I MOLECULES. The HLA class I molecule consists of an HLA-encoded polymorphic glycoprotein of 44,000 molecular weight (MW) known as the heavy chain, in noncovalent association with a 12,000 MW nonpolymorphic protein known as β_2-microglobulin (Fig. 229–1A). The β_2-microglobulin is encoded by a gene on chromosome 15 and not by the HLA complex. The entire class I molecule is anchored in the cell membrane only by the heavy chain. This chain contains approximately 338 amino acids and can be divided into three regions. Starting from the amino terminal end of the molecule, these regions are an extracellular hydrophilic region (amino acids 1 to 281), a transmembrane hydrophobic region (amino acids 282 to 306), and an intracytoplasmic hydrophilic region (amino acids 307 to 338). The hydrophobic transmembrane region contains 24 amino acids, enabling it to span the cell membrane. The intracytoplasmic hydrophilic region can be phosphorylated, and it has been speculated that class I molecules may transduce external events across the cell membrane.

The extracellular hydrophilic region in turn can be divided into three domains, each of approximately 90 amino acids, designated from the amino terminal end α_1, α_2, and α_3. The α_3 domain and β_2-microglobulin have structural homology with the constant region of immunoglobulin, identifying the class I molecule as a member of the immunoglobulin supergene family.

Recently acquired x-ray crystallographic data have elucidated the actual structure of the HLA class I molecule (Fig. 229–1A). The α_3 domain and β_2-microglobulin are closest to the membrane and support an interactive structure formed by the α_1 and α_2 domains. The α_1 domain and the α_2 domain each consist of four β strands shown as flat arrows and an α helix shown as a coiled ribbon-like structure projecting toward the top of the figure. (The α helix should not be confused with the α domain, nor should the β strand be confused with β_2-microglobulin.) The eight β strands of these two domains form a β-pleated sheet platform that supports the two α helices. These α helices create a groove or cleft that serves as the antigen-binding site for a peptide fragment appropriately processed from a larger antigen.

Although precise details are not completely understood, it now appears that antigenic (e.g., viral) proteins synthesized intracellularly are subject to proteolysis by a multimeric complex termed the "proteasome." Two of the subunits, designated LMP (large multifunctional protease)-2 and LMP-7 proteins, are determined by genes within the HLA complex (see below). The resulting antigenic peptide fragments are then transported into the endoplasmic reticulum by a heterodimeric ATP-binding protein known as the transporter associated with antigen processing (TAP), whose subunits are determined by the TAP-1 and TAP-2 genes, also both within the HLA

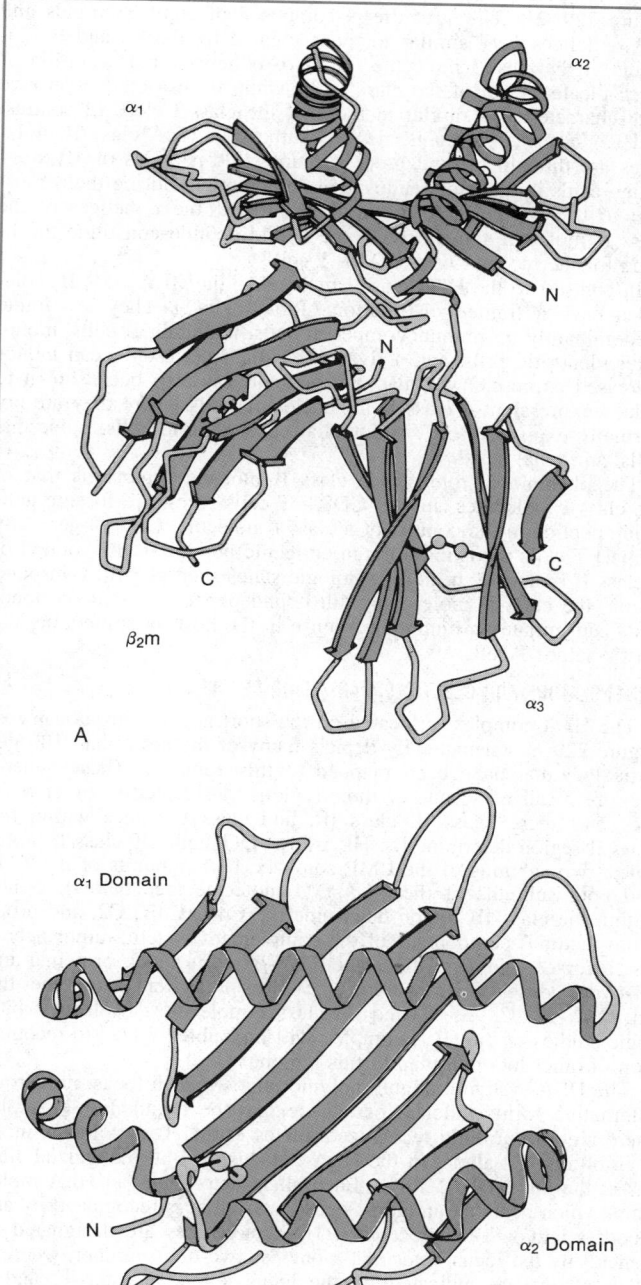

FIGURE 229–1. The HLA class I molecule crystal structure shown in both side view *(A)* and top view *(B).* The molecule consists of an α chain which anchors the molecule in the membrane, noncovalently associated with β₂-microglobulin (β₂m). The α_1, α_2, and α_3 domains and β₂m are labeled. β strands are depicted as thick arrows in the amino to carboxy direction, and α helices are represented as helical ribbons. Connecting loops are shown as thin lines. Disulfide bonds are two connected spheres. *A,* Side view. The molecule is shown with the α_3 domain and β₂-microglobulin at the bottom, and the α_1 and α_2 domains at the top. The α helices form the cleft into which peptide can fit. *B,* Top view. The α_1 and α_2 domains are seen from above. The β-pleated sheet platform and the cleft formed by the α helices are again visible. *(A and B* adapted by permission from Nature, Vol 329, p 506. Copyright © 1987 Macmillan Magazines Limited.)

complex (see below). In general, antigenic peptide fragments of 8 to 9 amino acids bind to the HLA class I molecule while all components are still in the endoplasmic reticulum, and the binding of peptide is necessary for the class I molecule to be transported to the cell surface. Once at the cell surface, the two α helices of the class

TABLE 229–1. COMPARISON OF HLA CLASS I AND CLASS II MOLECULES

	Class I	Class II
Molecules included	HLA-A, B, C	HLA-DR, DQ, DP
Structure	44,000 MW heavy chain	~34,000 MW α chain
	12,000 MW β₂-microglobulin	~29,000 MW β chain
Tissue distribution	On virtually every cell	Normal limited to immunocompetent cells, particularly B cells, macrophages, activated T cells
Function	Bind and present antigenic peptides to CD8+ T cells	Bind and present antigenic peptides to CD4+ T cells

I molecule together with the bound antigenic fragment comprise the ligand recognized by the T-cell receptor on a CD8+ T cell.

A top view of the class I molecule as it would appear to the T-cell receptor of a CD8+ T lymphocyte is shown in Figure 229–1*B.* The β strands of the α_1 and α_2 domains form the floor of the cleft, and the α helices of the same domains form the sides of the cleft. The majority of alloantigenic determinants recognized both by antibodies and by T cells have been shown to be located in the α_1 and α_2 domains.

The HLA class I molecules have been divided into the classic (class I-a) molecules and the nonclassic (class I-b) molecules. The majority of our knowledge pertains to the class I-a molecules, which are designated HLA-A, -B, and -C. The class I-a molecules are found on virtually every human cell (Table 229–1). This tissue distribution is well suited to the physiologic role of the class I molecules to present foreign antigenic peptides such as viral antigenic peptides to cytotoxic T lymphocytes (CTL's). Precursors of CTL's are specific for a particular viral antigenic peptide in the context of a particular class I molecule. When the precursors encounter this particular combination of the viral antigenic peptide and the class I molecule, they proliferate and differentiate to mature CTL's. The mature CTL's are restricted in their killing to those target cells that bear both the same viral peptide and the same class I molecule as were present on the sensitizing cells. That particular CTL does not kill a target cell with the same class I molecule infected with a different virus; neither does it kill a target cell with a different class I molecule infected with the same virus. Thus, CTL killing is both antigen-specific and class I restricted. In the nonphysiologic situation of a tissue or organ graft, the class I molecules, with bound peptide, on the graft are the principal antigens recognized by the host's CTL's during graft rejection.

The HLA class I-b molecules include HLA-E, -F, and -G. These molecules are associated with β₂-microglobulin and have a similar structure to class I-a molecules, but their tissue distribution and function appear to be different. HLA-G is found on trophoblast cells and may play a role in maternal-fetal interactions during pregnancy. The function of other class I-b molecules is not entirely defined, but recent data indicate that they play a role in host defenses against prokaryotes.

CLASS II MOLECULES

Each class II molecule consists of two glycoprotein chains, an α chain of approximately 34,000 MW, and a β chain of approximately 29,000 MW. Both of the chains span the membrane and therefore serve to anchor the molecule. Each chain can be divided into three regions. Beginning at the amino terminal end, there is an extracellular hydrophilic region, a transmembrane hydrophobic region, and an intracytoplasmic hydrophilic tail. Each extracellular region has been further divided into two domains of approximately 90 amino acids each. For the α chain these are designated α_1 and α_2, and for the β chain, β_1 and β_2. The α_2 and β_2 domains, like the α_3 domain of the class I molecule and β₂-microglobulin, show homology with the constant region domain of immunoglobulin, thus indicating that class II molecules are also members of the immunoglobulin supergene family. The crystallographic structure of an

HLA class II molecule has recently been delineated (Figure 229–2) and confirms that the class II α_2 and β_2 domains comprise the portion of the molecule proximal to the cell membrane which supports the distal interactive portion formed by the α_1 and β_1 domains. Somewhat surprisingly, the crystal structure demonstrated dimers of class II molecules, suggesting that a tetramer may be the natural state of class II molecules in the cell membrane. However, the existence of such a tetramer *in vivo* has not yet been proven or refuted.

A top view of the class II α_1 and β_1 domains, as they would appear to the T-cell receptor on a CD4+ T lymphocyte, is shown in

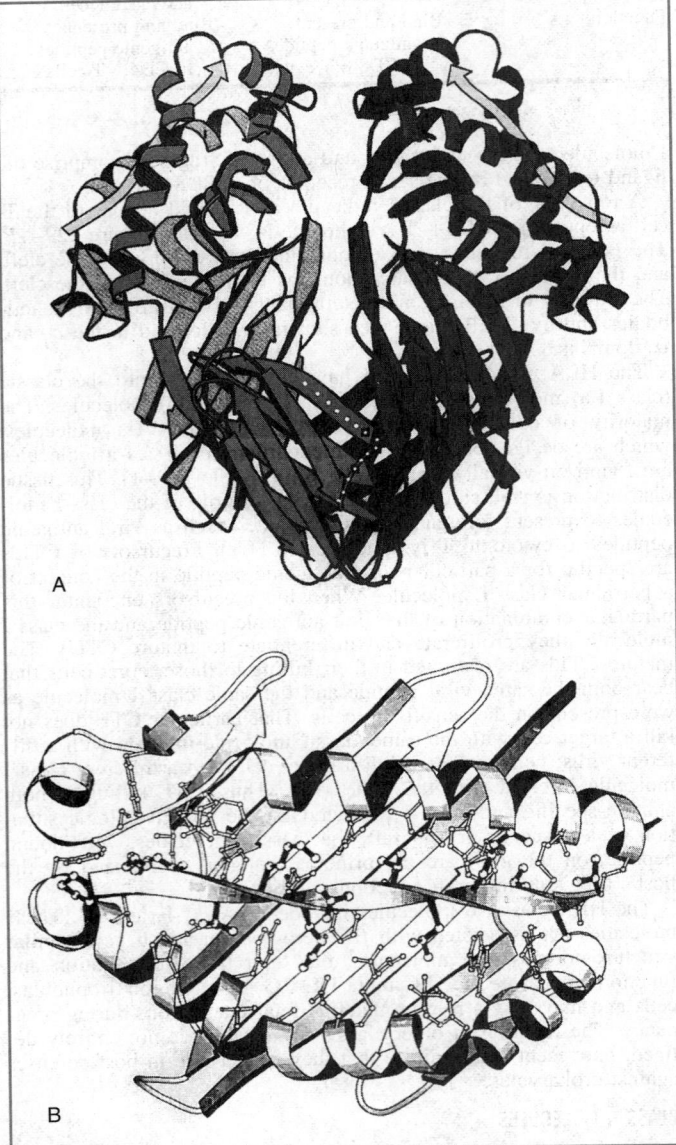

FIGURE 229–2. The HLA class II crystal structure shown in side *(A)* and top *(B)* views. The molecule consists of an α chain noncovalently associated with a β chain. Both chains anchor the molecule in the membrane. The α_1, α_2, β_1, and β_2 domains are indicated. The β strands are depicted as thick arrows in the amino to carboxy direction, and the α helices are represented as helical ribbons. *A,* The molecule is shown as a class II dimer (i.e., two class II molecules noncovalently associated), the form found in the crystal structure, although there is no evidence that this dimeric form does or does not exist *in vivo.* (In this view, the class II molecule is rotated approximately 90 degrees around the vertical axis from the side view shown of the class I molecule in Figure 229–1.) *B,* The cleft is very similar to that seen for the class I molecule. The α helices and a portion of the β-pleated sheet from the groove in which the peptide, shown as a twisted ribbon binds. (From Nature, Vol 364, p 33 Copyright © 1993, and Vol 368, p 215, Copyright © 1994, Macmillan Magazines Limited.)

Figure 229–2B. The structure is composed of eight β strands and two α helices very similar to those created by the α_1 and α_2 domains of the class I molecule. The two α helices and a portion of the β-pleated sheet of the class II molecule form a cleft or groove with characteristics similar to those of the class I cleft. In contrast to HLA class I molecules, newly synthesized HLA class II molecules are thought to bind processed antigenic peptides of 10 to 14 amino acids in an acidic endosomal compartment during their transport to the cell surface. On the cell surface, the α helices of the class II molecule together with the bound peptide constitute the ligand for the receptor on a CD4+ T cell.

In contrast to the HLA class I molecules, the HLA class II molecules have a limited distribution (Table 229–1). They are found predominantly on immunocompetent cells, including B cells, monocytes, dendritic cells, and activated T cells. Interferon-γ can induce increased expression on macrophages and has also been shown to induce expression of class II molecules on cells where they are not normally expressed, e.g., endothelial cells, thyroid cells, epidermal cells, and renal cells.

The physiologic role of the class II molecules parallels that of the class I molecules. Just as CD8+ T cells recognize foreign antigenic peptide in the context of a class I molecule, CD4+ (generally helper) T cells recognize foreign antigenic peptide in the context of a class II molecule. In nonphysiologic states such as graft transplantation, the class II molecules with bound peptide present on donor cells can initiate an immune response in the host by stimulating the host's helper T cells.

NOMENCLATURE AND GENETIC ORGANIZATION OF THE HLA COMPLEX

The HLA complex is located on the short arm of chromosome 6. Figure 229–3 schematically depicts many of the more than 100 genetic loci that have been mapped to this complex. These genetic loci are localized to one of three regions, designated in order from the centromere: class II, class III, and class I. Genes within the class II region determine the HLA-DR, -DQ, and -DP class II molecules, two subunits of the LMP complex, both subunits of the TAP, and both subunits of the HLA-DM molecule (see below). Genes within the class III region determine the C4A, C4B, C2, and properdin factor B components of the complement system, tumor necrosis factors α and β (TNF-α and TNF-β), heat shock proteins, and 21-hydroxylase. Genes within the class I region determine the HLA-A, -B, -C, -E, -F, and -G class I molecules. Molecular biologic studies of the HLA complex will undoubtedly lead to recognition of other loci that map to this region.

The HLA system is highly polymorphic. At each locus, numerous alternative forms (alleles) of a gene may be found. For example, there are 25 currently recognized alleles at the HLA-A locus, more than 60 distinct alleles at the HLA-B locus, and 60 recognized alleles at the HLA-DRB1 locus. Each allele determines an HLA molecule, which bears an antigenic determinant that is recognized by antibodies and/or T-cell receptors. HLA molecules are designated in general by the locus letter and a one- or two-digit number, whereas HLA alleles are indicated by the locus letter, an asterisk, and a four-digit number. The first two digits of this number correspond to the molecular designation. The last two digits allow discrimination among several distinct alleles that determine distinct molecules, all of which display a common antigenic determinant. Thus, for example, HLA-B27 refers to any of seven distinct HLA molecules, differing in 1 to 8 amino acids, all of which display the common antigenic determinant HLA-B27, but each of which is determined by a distinct allele, designated HLA-B*2701 through HLA-B*2707. A complete listing of the currently recognized HLA antigenic determinants is found in Table 229–2.

FIGURE 229–3. The current concept of the HLA complex, depicting the major HLA loci. The complex is divided into the class II, class III, and class I regions, in order, from the centromere, spanning approximately 4000 Kb. The designations of each region derive from the class of HLA genes that were first mapped to it. The types of loci are shown by different shadings. The insets indicate the different possible configurations of DRB genes and complement genes, respectively. (Adapted from Campbell RD, Trowsdale J: Map of the human major histocompatibility complex. Immunol Today 14:349, 1993.)

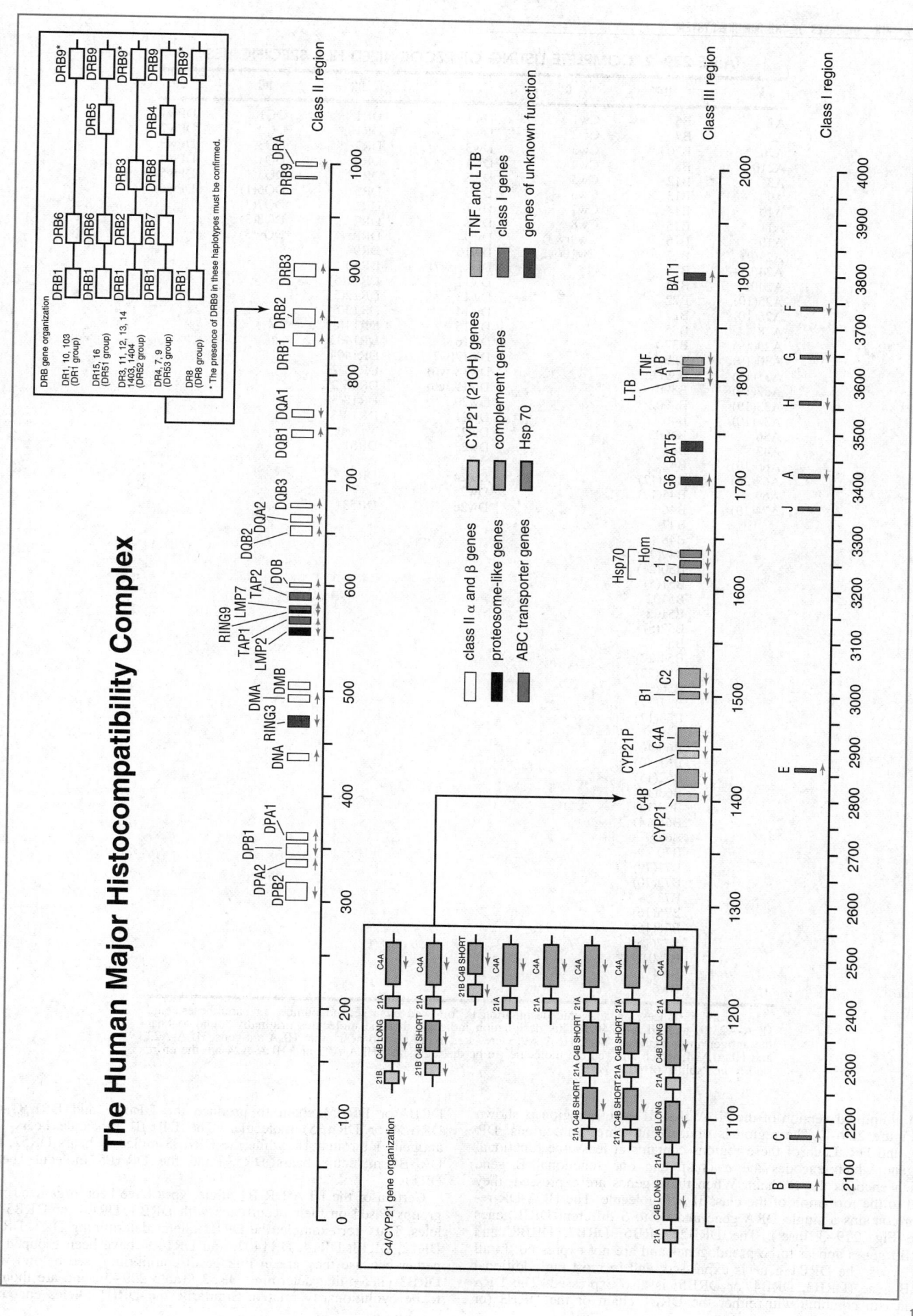

FIGURE 229-3 *See legend on opposite page*

TABLE 229-2. COMPLETE LISTING OF RECOGNIZED HLA SPECIFICITIES

A	B	C	D	DR	DQ	DP
A1	B5	Cw1	Dw1	DR1	DQ1	DPw1
A2	B7	Cw2	Dw2	DR103	DQ2	DPw2
A203	B703	Cw3	Dw3	DR2	DQ3	DPw3
A210	B8	Cw4	Dw4	DR3	DQ4	DPw4
A3	B12	Cw5	Dw5	DR4	DQ5(1)	DPw5
A9	B13	Cw6	Dw6	DR5	DQ6(1)	DPw6
A10	B14	Cw7	Dw7	DR6	DQ7(3)	
A11	B15	Cw8	Dw8	DR7	DQ8(3)	
A19	B16	Cw9(w3)	Dw9	DR8	DQ9(3)	
A23(9)	B17	Cw10(w3)	Dw10	DR9		
A24(9)	B18		Dw11(w7)	DR10		
A2403	B21		Dw12	DR11(5)		
A25(10)	B22		Dw13	DR12(5)		
A26(10)	B27		Dw14	DR13(6)		
A28	B35		Dw15	DR14(6)		
A29(19)	B37		Dw16	DR1403		
A30(19)	B38(16)		Dw17(w7)	DR1404		
A31(19)	B39(16)		Dw18(w6)	DR15(2)		
A32(19)	B3901		Dw19(w6)	DR16(2)		
A33(19)	B3902		Dw20	DR17(3)		
A34(10)	B40		Dw21	DR18(3)		
A36	B4005		Dw22			
A43	B41		Dw23	DR51		
A66(10)	B42					
A68(28)	B44(12)		Dw24	DR52		
A69	B45(12)		Dw25			
A74(19)	B46		Dw26	DR53		
	B47					
	B48					
	B49(21)					
	B50(21)					
	B51(5)					
	B5102					
	B5103					
	B52(5)					
	B53					
	B54(22)					
	B55(22)					
	B56(22)					
	B57(17)					
	B58(17)					
	B59					
	B60(40)					
	B61(40)					
	B62(15)					
	B63(15)					
	B64(14)					
	B65(14)					
	B67					
	B70					
	B71(70)					
	B72(70)					
	B73					
	B75(16)					
	B76(15)					
	B77(15)					
	B7801					
	Bw4					
	Bw6					

In certain instances, an antigenic designation is followed by a second number in parentheses, e.g., HLA-A23(9) and HLA-A24(9). This designation indicates that the molecules originally found to bear the antigen in parentheses, here, HLA-A9, were later found also to bear other HLA antigens, HLA-A23 and HLA-A24, which allowed the molecules to be distinguished. HLA-A23 and HLA-A24 are therefore said to be "splits" of HLA-A9.

A simplified version of the HLA class II genetic region is shown in Figure 229–4. The region is divided into three subregions: DP, DQ, and DR. Each of these regions contains at least one functional A gene which encodes the α chain and one functional B gene which encodes the β chain. When these genes are expressed, they lead to the formation of the class II $\alpha\beta$ molecule. The HLA-DR region contains a single DRA gene and up to 5 different DRB genes (see Fig. 229–3 inset). The DRB2, DRB6, DRB7, DRB8, and DRB9 genes appear to be pseudogenes and are not expressed. In all DR types, the DRB1 gene is expressed, and in most, an additional DRB gene (DRB3, DRB4, or DRB5) is also expressed. The DRα chain can combine with either the DRβ1 chain or the DRβ3 (or DRβ4 or DRβ5) chain to produce the DR$\alpha\beta$1 and DR$\alpha\beta$3 (or DR$\alpha\beta$4 or DR$\alpha\beta$5) molecules. The DR$\alpha\beta$1 molecule bears DR antigens 1 through 18, while the DR$\alpha\beta$3 molecule bears DR52, the DR$\alpha\beta$4 molecule bears DR53, and the DR$\alpha\beta$5 molecule bears DR51.

Certain of the HLA-DR B1 allele types have been organized into groups based on their occurrence with DRB3, DRB4, or DRB5 alleles. Thus, for example, the DRB1 alleles determining DR3, DR11, DR12, DR13, DR14, DR1403, and DR1404 have been grouped together because they are in linkage disequilibrium (see below) with DRB3 alleles that determine DR52 (Table 229–3), and are thought to be evolutionarily related. Similarly, the DRB1 alleles encoding

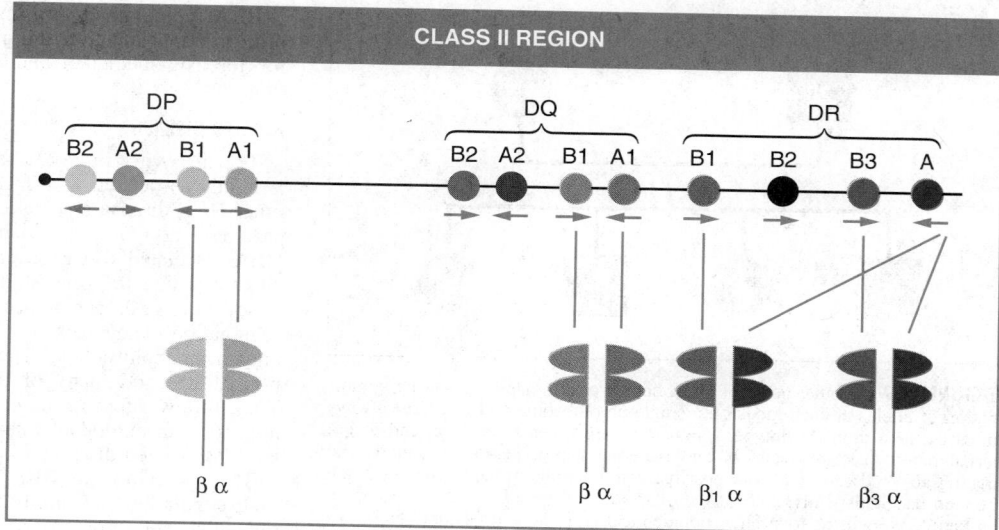

FIGURE 229–4. A simplified concept of the HLA-D region, showing the organization of the three subregions, DP, DQ, and DR. DPA2, DPB2, DQA2, DQB2, and DRB2 are pseudogenes and are not expressed. Pairs of expressed genes (DPA1 and DPB1; DQA1 and DQB1; DRA and DRB1; and DRA and DRB3) which encode class II molecules are indicated. (In other haplotypes, DRA and DRB4 or DRA and DRB5 would be the pair expressed in place of DRA and DRB3.) Arrows under genes give the direction of transcription (5′ to 3′).

DR4, DR7, and DR9 are grouped together because they are in linkage disequilibrium with DRB4 which encodes HLA-DR53, and are also evolutionarily related. Finally, the DRB1 alleles determining DR2 all are in linkage disequilibrium with DRB5. Linkage disequilibrium is also responsible for the association of particular DR antigens with particular DQ antigens (Table 229–4).

The DQ subregion contains two pairs of A and B genes. One pair, designated DQA2 and DQB2, are pseudogenes and are not expressed. The other pair, designated DQA1 and DQB1, are expressed and result in the formation of the DQ αβ molecule. Likewise, the DP subregion contains two pairs of A and B genes. One pair, designated DPA2 and DPB2, contain pseudogenes. The other pair, designated DPA1 and DPB1, encode the DPα and β chains that form the DPαβ molecule.

The polymorphism of the class II molecules (DR, DQ, and DP) varies somewhat for each set. For the DR molecules, the DRα chain is essentially nonpolymorphic between different DR types, whereas the DRβ chains are highly polymorphic. For the DQ molecules, both the DQα and DQβ chains demonstrate a high degree of polymorphism. For the DP molecules, the DPα chain shows relatively limited polymorphism, whereas the DPβ chains are again highly polymorphic.

Several additional genes have been mapped to the HLA class II region. These genes include the LMP (formerly low molecular weight polypeptide) genes, LMP-2 and LMP-7, which determine two subunits of the proteasome that digests protein antigens to peptides with the potential to bind to class I molecules; the TAP genes, TAP-1 and TAP-2, which encode proteins that transport proteasome-generated peptides from the cytoplasm to the endoplasmic reticulum; and the DMA and DMB genes, which are class II–like genes whose products have been implicated in processing antigen to peptides with the potential to bind to DR, DQ, and DP class II molecules.

It should be noted that there is no HLA-D locus or HLA-D molecule *per se.* The HLA-D antigens are defined and detected solely by a cellular reaction known as the mixed leukocyte reaction (MLR). Responder cells in the MLR appear to be detecting an array of antigenic determinants present on the HLA-DR, DQ, and/or DP molecules. In most cases, it is thought that antigenic determinants on HLA-DR molecules contribute most significantly to the MLR. As a result, HLA-D types tend to be most highly correlated with HLA-DR types.

HAPLOTYPE

Because of their close linkage, the alleles at each locus on a single chromosome are usually inherited in combination as a unit. This combination is referred to as the *haplotype.* Because each individual inherits one set of chromosomes from each parent, each individual has two HLA haplotypes. HLA genes are codominant; therefore, both alleles at a given HLA locus are expressed, and two complete sets of HLA antigens can be detected on cells. By simple mendelian genetics, there is a 25% chance that two siblings will share both haplotypes and be fully HLA compatible, a 50% chance that they will share one haplotype, and a 25% chance that they will share no haplotype and thus will be completely HLA incompatible (Fig. 229–5).

LINKAGE DISEQUILIBRIUM

Because of random matings, the frequency of finding a given allele at one HLA locus associated with a given allele at a second HLA locus should simply be the product of the frequencies of each allele in the population. However, certain combinations of alleles are found with a frequency greater than expected. This phenomenon is termed "linkage disequilibrium" and is quantitated as the difference (Δ) between the observed and expected frequencies. For example, the HLA-A*0101 allele, which determines HLA-A1, and the HLA-B*0801 allele, which determines HLA-B8, are found in the Caucasian population with frequencies of 0.161 and 0.104, respectively. Thus, the expected frequency with which the HLA-A*0101, B*0801 haplotype should be found is 0.161×0.104, or 0.0167. However, this haplotype is found with a frequency of approximately 0.0592, almost four times the expected frequency, for a $\Delta = 0.0592 - 0.0167 = 0.0425$. Table 229–5 lists some common exam-

TABLE 229–3. ASSOCIATIONS OF DRB1-ENCODED ANTIGENS WITH MOLECULES ENCODED BY DRB3, DRB4, OR DRB5 ALLELES

DRB3	DRB4	DRB5
DR3	DR4	DR15
DR5	DR7	DR16
DR6	DR9	
DR8		
DR11(5)		
DR12(5)		
DR13(6)		
DR14(6)		
DR17(3)		
DR18(3)		

TABLE 229–4. DQ ASSOCIATED HLA-DR ANTIGENS

HLA-DQ Antigens	Associated HLA-DR Antigens
DQ1	DR1, DR10, DR13(6), DR14(6), DR15(2), DR16(2)
DQ2	DR3, DR7
DQ3	DR4, DR7, DR9, DR11(5), DR12(5)
DQ4	DR8, DR15
DQ5	DR1, DR10, DR14(6), DR16(2)
DQ6	DR15(2), DR13(6)
DQ7	DR11(5), DR12(5), DR4
DQ8	DR4
DQ9	DR7, DR9

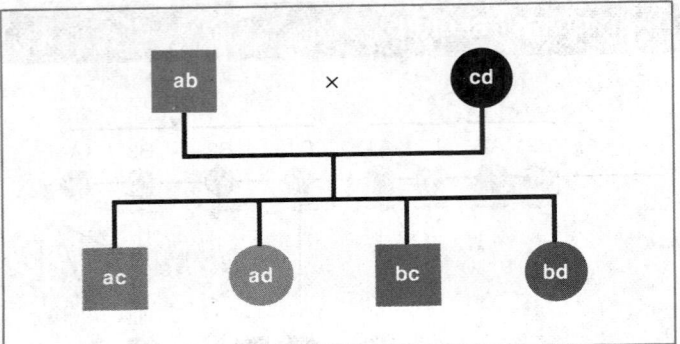

FIGURE 229–5. Inheritance of HLA haplotypes. A haplotype is the combination of alleles at each locus on a single chromosome and is almost always inherited as a unit. Haplotype designations are given by a, b, c, and d. Paternal haplotypes are a and b, and maternal haplotypes are c and d. The mating ab × cd can yield four possible combinations of haplotypes—ac, ad, bc, and bd. Statistically, 25% of the offspring will be HLA identical (e.g., ac and ac), 25% will be total HLA nonidentical (e.g., ac and bd), and 50% will be HLA-haploidentical (e.g., ac and ad).

ples of linkage disequilibrium. Several hypotheses have been put forth to explain linkage disequilibrium: (1) a selective advantage of a given haplotype, and (2) recent admixture of two inbred populations.

HLA TYPING

All HLA class I and class II antigens are present on the class I and class II molecules but are defined and detected by different methods. The HLA-A, -B, -C, -DR, and -DQ antigens are defined, detected, and typed serologically by the microlymphocytotoxicity assay. Although some monoclonal antibodies are available for particular HLA antigens, the majority of serologic typing is still done with sera obtained from multiparous women. Typing for the HLA class I antigens is done on purified populations of lymphocytes. Typing of the HLA-DR and -DQ class II antigens is performed on purified populations of B lymphocytes. Alternatively, a two-color dye procedure is used which allows B cells to be distinguished from T cells. HLA-DP antigens are defined and typed by a cellular reaction known as the primed lymphocyte test (PLT), but DP molecules can be detected by monoclonal antibodies. As noted above, HLA-D antigens are defined and typed by the mixed leukocyte reaction (MLR).

Molecular biologic techniques applied to HLA typing have made possible new and more precise methods. The most promising technique is the polymerase chain reaction (PCR) combined with oligonucleotide typing. The PCR is used to amplify the HLA gene(s) to be typed. Because each HLA allele has a unique nucleotide sequence that differentiates it from every other allele, it is possible to synthesize an oligonucleotide (or in some cases, a pair of oligonucleotides) which hybridize only to this unique sequence. A set of tagged oligonucleotides corresponding to various alleles can therefore be used for HLA typing at the DNA level. Oligonu-

TABLE 229–5. EXAMPLES OF LINKAGE DISEQUILIBRIUM IN CAUCASIANS

Haplotypes (listed as antigen phenotypes)	Δ (× 10⁻³)
HLA-A1, B8	53.2
HLA-A2, B44 (12)	14.8
HLA-A3, B7	32.4
HLA-B8, DR3	61.3
HLA-B7, DR2	36.8
HLA-DR2, DQ1	93.6
HLA-DR3, DQ2	37.4
HLA-DR7, DQ2	96.7
HLA-DR4, DQ3	87.5
HLA-A1, B8, DR3	28.0
HLA-A3, B7, DR2	11.5

cleotide typing is still in its infancy, and the vast majority of clinical HLA typing is currently done by conventional methodologies.

HLA typing is used primarily to determine HLA compatibility prior to transplantation and platelet transfusion, for paternity testing, for forensic medicine, and for establishing HLA disease associations.

HLA AND DISEASE

The discovery in 1973 that ankylosing spondylitis (see Ch. 238) is highly associated with HLA-B27 stimulated an intense search for other HLA-disease associations. Well over 100 diverse types of disease have now been associated with HLA. Despite this broad range, HLA-associated diseases for the most part share certain common characteristics. In general, these diseases have an hereditary tendency but weak penetrance and do not follow simple mendelian segregation. They lack a known causative agent and have an unknown pathophysiology. They are associated with immunologic abnormalities, and many of them are characterized as autoimmune. They follow subacute or chronic courses. Finally, they usually do not affect an individual's ability to bear offspring, thus allowing the HLA-associated diseases to persist.

The association of HLA and disease has been demonstrated by both population and family studies. These two types of studies provide different information. Population studies allow a statistically significant correlation between a particular HLA marker gene and a particular disease state. They do not constitute proof of genetic linkage between a disease susceptibility gene and the HLA marker gene because correlation does not necessarily imply genetic linkage. For example, if a disease susceptibility gene were not linked to HLA but required the presence of a particular HLA molecule for its expression, then an HLA-disease association would be demonstrated in population studies. In contrast, family studies provide an opportunity to determine linkage between a disease susceptibility gene and the HLA marker gene. Because population studies are easier to conduct, the majority of data on HLA and disease derives from this type of study.

It should be noted that no HLA-disease association is absolute. The majority of individuals with a given disease-associated HLA molecule do not contract the disease, and a given HLA-associated disease can occur in individuals who lack the usual disease-associated HLA molecule. It is now widely accepted that a combination of a particular HLA molecule, other genetic influences, and environmental agents is necessary for the disease to be manifest.

The strength of the association of a particular disease with a particular HLA molecule is quantitated by calculating the relative risk (Table 229–6). The relative risk (RR) is defined by the formula $RR = (P^+ \times C^-)/(P^- \times C^+)$, where P^+ is the number of patients possessing the disease-associated HLA molecule, C^- is the number of controls lacking that particular HLA molecule, P^- is the number of patients lacking that HLA molecule, and C^+ is the number of controls possessing that HLA molecule. The higher the relative risk above 1, the stronger the association between the HLA molecule and the disease. The relative risk can be stated as the chance of developing the HLA-associated disease for an individual with the disease-associated HLA molecule compared with an individual without that HLA molecule. Because there is usually a significant difference in the frequency of a given molecule among different racial groups, it is mandatory to compare a patient group with a control population of the same race. Thus, for example, HLA-B27 is found in 88% of American white patients with ankylosing spondylitis and approximately 8% of American white controls, yielding a relative risk of approximately 90. In contrast, HLA-B27 is found in 48% of American black patients with ankylosing spondylitis but in only 2% of American black controls, giving a relative risk of 37. Table 229–6 gives the relative risks for selected significant HLA-disease associations.

Because of the phenomenon of linkage disequilibrium and the order in which the HLA class I and class II molecules were defined, a particular disease may have appeared to be associated with a particular molecule determined by an allele at a given HLA locus when in actuality it is more highly associated with a particular molecule determined by an allele at a different HLA locus. Thus, for example, the alleles encoding HLA-DQ2, -DR3, and -B8 are known to be in linkage disequilibrium. Before any of the HLA class II molecules were well defined, celiac disease was associated with HLA-B8. The definition of the DR antigens allowed a stronger associa-

TABLE 229–6. SELECTED HLA AND DISEASE ASSOCIATIONS IN WHITE PATIENTS

Disease	Antigen	Approximate Relative Risk
Ankylosing spondylitis	B27	81.8
Reiter's syndrome	B27	40.4
Acute anterior uveitis	B27	7.98
Reactive arthritis (Yersinia)	B27	17.6
Rheumatoid arthritis	DR4	6.4
Juvenile rheumatoid arthritis		
Seropositive	DR4	7.2
	Dw4	25.8
	Dw14	47
	Dw4/Dw14	116
Pauciarticular	DR5	2.9
	DP2	3.9
Systemic lupus erythematosus	DR3	2.7
Behçet's disease	B5	3.3
Sjögren's syndrome	DR3	5.6
High-titer anti-SS-A antibody	DQ1/DQ2	
Graves' disease	DR3	3.8
Insulin-dependent diabetes mellitus	DR3	3.0
Celiac disease	DR3	13.3
Psoriasis vulgaris	B13	4.5
	B17	3.1
	Cw6	7.2
Pemphigus vulgaris	DR4	21.4
Dermatitis herpetiformis	DR3	18.2
Idiopathic hemochromatosis	A3	6.6
	B14	3.7
Goodpasture's syndrome	DR2	19.8
Multiple sclerosis	DR2	2.8
Myasthenia gravis (without thymoma)	B8	3.3
Narcolepsy	DR2	129

tion to be established between celiac disease and HLA-DR3. The subsequent definition of the HLA-DQ molecules suggested an even more significant association between celiac disease and HLA-DQ2. With molecular biology techniques applied to the study of HLA and disease associations, restriction endonuclease fragments have been identified in the HLA-DP region which yield even more significant associations. Thus, for example, it has recently been reported that 90% of patients with celiac disease have a genomic DNA fragment that can be detected using a DP β chain cDNA probe. Individuals with this fragment have a relative risk of 46 for contracting celiac disease.

In addition, because of linkage disequilibrium, a number of diseases have been associated with what has been termed extended haplotypes. Two such examples are the association of C2 deficiency with the haplotype A*2501, B*1801, C2*QO, BF*S, C4A*4, C4B*2, DRB1*1501, and systemic lupus with the haplotype A*0101, B*0801, BF*S, C2*C, C4A*QO, C4B*1, DRB1*0301.

Several hypotheses have been suggested to explain HLA-disease associations. Five of these apply to diseases associated with both class I and class II molecules. First, HLA molecules may act as receptors for causative agents. If only particular HLA molecules can act as receptors for agents that cause particular diseases, then the HLA-disease association would result. The second hypothesis suggests that the antigen-binding cleft of only a particular HLA molecule can accept the processed antigenic peptide fragment that is ultimately responsible for causing disease. The third hypothesis holds that the actual disease susceptibility genes are not the HLA genes themselves but rather T-cell receptor α and β chain genes. This hypothesis suggests that because a particular T-cell receptor α and β chain combination which predisposes to disease recognizes only a particular antigenic peptide fragment in the context of a particular HLA molecule, an *apparent* association with that HLA antigen is seen. The fourth hypothesis postulates that a TAP gene product, which normally transports antigenic peptides from the cytoplasm to the endoplasmic reticulum, is defective and that this defect predisposes to disease. Because fewer peptides are available for binding to class I molecules, there is an abnormally low surface density of HLA class I molecule–antigenic peptide complexes and a higher than normal density of empty class I molecules. Two alternatives are then possible. The low density of class I–peptide complexes may be insufficient to stimulate an immune response. If the pep-

tides are derived from a microorganism, the microorganism can produce disease by an unknown pathophysiologic mechanism. Alternatively, the empty surface class I molecules may bind peptides to which they would not normally be exposed intracellularly. These newly formed class I–peptide complexes could then induce an immune response that would produce disease. The fifth hypothesis, termed the molecular mimicry hypothesis, states that the disease-associated HLA molecule is immunologically similar to the causative agent for the disease and then postulates one of two alternatives. The first alternative suggests that because of the similarity of the causative agent and the HLA molecule, no immune response is mounted and therefore the agent can cause disease unabated. The second alternative suggests that a vigorous immune response is mounted against the agent, but because of the similarity of the agent and the HLA molecule, the immune response is turned against the HLA molecule and the resulting autoimmune response produces disease.

The majority of HLA-associated diseases have been associated with the class II molecules. The last hypothesis relates only to class II–associated diseases and suggests that class II molecules aberrantly expressed by cells which normally lack class II molecules may present self-antigenic peptide fragments to CD4+ T cells and thus induce an autoimmune response.

One recent noteworthy observation is that in certain diseases gene complementation between two different class II genes appears to play a role in disease predisposition. Thus, for example, the antibody response to the SS-A (Ro) antigen in patients with Sjögren's syndrome and SLE is highest in patients who are DQ1/DQ2 heterozygotes. A second example is that of insulin-dependent diabetes mellitus, which has been associated with both DR3 and DR4 but is most highly associated with DR3/DR4 heterozygosity, and, because of linkage disequilibrium, also with DQ2/DQ8 heterozygosity. Because both DQα and DQβ chains are polymorphic, DQ heterozygotes have the potential to form "hybrid" molecules, whereby the DQα chain encoded by one haplotype can pair with the DQβ chain encoded by the second haplotype. Thus, in such heterozygotes, it is possible to form DQ2α/DQ8β and DQ8α/DQ2β molecules. It is postulated that this "hybrid" molecule can present antigenic peptide fragments better than either "parental" molecule to the appropriate CD4+ T cell.

Recently, it has been found that individuals who are predisposed to insulin-dependent diabetes mellitus lack an aspartic acid residue at position 57 of the DQβ chain (e.g., the DQ8 β chain), whereas individuals who are protected from this disease possess an aspartic acid residue at this position (e.g., the DQ7 β chain). (It should be noted that DQ7 and DQ8 otherwise have very similar sequences.) Position 57 is found in the α helical portion of the class II peptide binding cleft. Thus, a single amino acid change in a crucial portion of a class II molecule can dramatically alter disease predisposition.

Finally, it has become apparent that certain regions of the class II molecule, rather than the entire class II molecule, may actually be the elements that confer disease predisposition. These regions have been termed *epitopes*. It has been found that in different populations, HLA-DR4 Dw4 subtype, HLA-DR4 Dw14 subtype, HLA-DR4 Dw15 subtype, HLA-DR1, HLA-DR10, and HLA-DR14 Dw16 subtype class II molecules all predispose an individual to rheumatoid arthritis (RA) (see Ch. 237). On further analysis, these predisposing DR molecules were found to share a common amino acid sequence in the α helix of the β chain, and it is thought that this amino acid sequence confers predisposition to RA. The fact that several different types of DR molecules share this common disease-predisposing epitope partially explains the lack of absolute HLA-disease associations. Of note, recent observations suggest that individuals who are homozygous for HLA-DR4 Dw4 subtype develop more severe RA.

Other mechanisms besides those noted above have also been suggested. It should be emphasized that different mechanisms may be operating to predispose to different diseases and that more than one mechanism may be operating concurrently to produce disease.

Dalton TA, Bennett JC: Autoimmune disease and the major histocompatibility complex: Therapeutic implications. Am J Med 92:183, 1992. *A discussion of the possible hypotheses for the association of HLA with disease.*
Germain RN: MHC-dependent antigen processing and peptide presentation: Providing ligands for T lymphocyte activation. Cell 76:287, 1994. *A complete and readable*

overview of the structure of the MHC class I and class II molecules, antigen processing, and antigen presentation to T cells.

Schwartz BD: Infectious diseases, immunity, and rheumatic diseases. Arthritis Rheum 33:457, 1990. *A clear discussion of the role of HLA molecules in antigen presentation and the models for HLA-disease associations.*

Tiwari JL, Terasaki PI (eds.): HLA and Disease Associations. New York, Springer-Verlag, 1985. *A comprehensive volume listing the majority of known HLA-disease associations.*

230 DRUG ALLERGY
James R. Bonner

The designation "drug allergy" should be reserved for adverse drug reactions caused by immunologic mechanisms. Although drug allergies are responsible for only a minority of adverse drug effects, the possibility of such reactions is a daily concern of most physicians. Drug allergy has a great variety of clinical manifestations and has been attributed to most categories of therapeutic agents. Because specific diagnostic tests are usually not available, physicians most often make decisions based on probabilities and the patient's need for treatment. This chapter provides an overview of drug allergy with emphasis on pathogenic mechanisms, diagnostic considerations, and preventive measures. Nonallergic reactions are discussed in Ch. 16.

EPIDEMIOLOGY/ETIOLOGY

Complications of drug therapy are the most common adverse events among hospitalized patients, and 10 to 14% of such drug reactions have an allergic basis. An estimated 5% of adult patients have at least one drug allergy, and many more patients incorrectly believe that they are allergic to medications. Drug allergy may be more common in women and may be expected to occur more frequently in patients given multiple courses of treatment. Atopic patients are not predisposed to drug allergy but may have more severe reactions. Drug allergy appears to be less common at the extremes of age, reflecting fewer sensitizing exposures in the very young and a decline in immune responsiveness in the very old. Risk factors for drug allergy are complex and include individual genetic differences in drug metabolism as well as immunologic reactivity.

Most drugs are capable of causing allergic reactions; the agents listed in Table 230-1 are among the most frequent offenders. Table 16-1 provides a more comprehensive listing of individual drugs by type of reaction.

Topical application of drugs has a higher risk of sensitization than oral or parenteral administration, although reactions occur most frequently when medications are given parenterally.

PATHOGENIC MECHANISMS

The process by which patients become immunologically sensitized to therapeutic agents is complex and for most drugs poorly understood. It is generally accepted that, to be an effective immunogen, a drug must have a molecular weight >4000 or, for polypeptides, have at least 7 amino acids. Some large molecular weight therapeutic agents such as antisera, vaccines, enzymes, and hormones are potentially immunogenic, but most drugs are much smaller and to elicit an immune response must form large hapten-carrier complexes by binding to tissue proteins. These carrier proteins may be free in plasma, intracellular, or incorporated into cell surface membranes. A high hapten density on the carrier proteins strengthens the immune response, which can be directed against the haptenated drug itself, a complex of hapten and protein, or a tissue protein conformationally changed by the binding of hapten. The binding of hapten to carrier proteins must be covalent rather than the reversible binding by which drugs are usually associated with plasma proteins. Indeed, allergy to β-lactam antibiotics may occur frequently because these drugs and the products of their spontaneous *in vivo* degradation can readily form covalent bonds with proteins. Most drugs do not bind well to proteins and must first be enzymatically metabolized to reactive forms by processes such as oxidation. Reactive forms can lose their ability to bind proteins by

undergoing further metabolism by processes such as acetylation and conjugation with glutathione. Therefore, risk factors for developing drug allergy in individual patients may include not only the ability to respond immunologically to hapten-carrier complexes but also the balance of genetically variable, drug-metabolizing enzymes.

All categories of immunologic hypersensitivity, as classified by Gell and Coombs, have been implicated in drug allergy (see Ch. 16); however, for many presumed allergic reactions the mechanism is unknown. Most hypersensitivity reactions require multivalent antigens to cross-link antibody such as IgE molecules bound to the high-affinity receptors on the surface of mast cells. Large molecular weight drugs may be inherently multivalent, and smaller drugs become effectively multivalent by binding to tissue proteins. To cause a generalized anaphylactic reaction, small drugs must bind *rapidly* to protein. Rapid protein binding is not as important in eliciting a primary immune response, and this might explain why some drugs that frequently evoke an antibody response are less commonly associated with clinical reactions. The specific organ location of some reactions may be due to hapten binding to particular tissue proteins or the production of reactive drug metabolites in specific locations such as the liver.

Some drug reactions that clinically resemble an allergic response have been shown not to involve specific immune recognition. Such *pseudoallergic* reactions can result from direct histamine release from mast cells and basophils, complement activation, generation of inflammatory mediators from arachidonic acid metabolism, or activation of the contact coagulation system. Examples of pseudoallergic reactions include aspirin-induced asthma, anaphylactoid reactions to radiographic contrast media, and angioedema attributed to angiotensin-converting enzyme (ACE) inhibitors (see below).

CLASSIFICATION

Allergic drug reactions can be classified as generalized or organ specific (Table 230-2). Descriptions of these reactions can be found elsewhere in this text. Urticaria, eosinophilia, cutaneous exanthems, contact dermatitis, and drug fever are the most common clinical manifestations of drug allergy.

TABLE 230-1. FREQUENTLY CAUSING ALLERGIC AND PSEUDOALLERGIC REACTIONS

Antimicrobials
  β-Lactams
  Sulfonamides
  Vancomycin
  Nitrofurantoin
  Antituberculous drugs
Anticonvulsants
  Phenytoin
  Carbamazepine
  Barbiturates
Cardiovascular agents
  Procainamide
  Hydralazine
  Quinidine
  Methyldopa
  ACE inhibitors
Macromolecules
  Heterologous antisera
  Enzymes
  Hormones
Anti-inflammatory agents
  Aspirin
  Other nonsteroidal anti-inflammatory drugs
  Gold salts
  Penicillamine
Antineoplastic agents
  Azathioprine
  Procarbazine
  Asparaginase
  Cis-platinum
Other
  Allopurinol
  Radiographic contrast media
  Opiates
  Sulfasalazine
  Neuromuscular blocking drugs
  Antithyroid drugs

TABLE 230–2. CLINICAL MANIFESTATIONS OF DRUG ALLERGY

Generalized
  Anaphylaxis
  Serum sickness
  Drug fever
  Vasculitis
  Drug-induced systemic lupus erythematosus
Organ specific
  Cutaneous
    Urticaria, angioedema, exanthems, hypersensitivity vasculitis, fixed eruptions, contact dermatitis, exfoliative dermatitis, erythema multiforme, toxic epidermal necrolysis, Stevens-Johnson syndrome
  Renal
    Acute interstitial nephritis, glomerulonephritis
  Pulmonary
    Asthma, acute infiltrates
  Hematologic
    Hemolytic anemia, granulocytopenia, thrombocytopenia, eosinophilia
  Hepatic
    Cholestatic hepatitis, hepatocellular damage

DIAGNOSIS

The following criteria should be considered when diagnosing drug allergy:

1. Enough time has elapsed for an immune response. For first use of most drugs, this requires a period of at least 7 to 10 days. Reactions with a more rapid onset are considered pseudoallergic or depend on prior sensitization during previous administration of the drug or a cross-reacting agent.
2. The character of the reaction does not suggest a pharmacologic or toxic effect of the drug.
3. The reaction does not appear to be dose-dependent and is not caused by drug interaction or abnormalities of absorption or elimination.
4. The reaction has characteristics that suggest a hypersensitivity response such as skin rash, fever, and eosinophilia.
5. Clinical improvement occurs promptly after the suspect drug is discontinued. For most reactions improvement is evident within 48 to 72 hours after stopping the drug.

Although it is not necessary that all these criteria be met, all should be considered when a patient is evaluated for possible drug allergy.

Patients suspected of having drug allergy are often receiving multiple drugs, and identifying the responsible agent can be difficult. It is sometimes helpful to make a flow chart listing the starting dates and times of all medications, including drugs that have been recently discontinued. The likely allergen may then be recognized by considering the above criteria and the drug categories most commonly implicated in allergic reactions (see Table 230–1). An allergic reaction to drugs that have been given continuously for long periods is much less likely than a reaction to recently introduced therapy. If the offending drug cannot be confidently identified, it may be necessary to discontinue all nonessential therapy and substitute treatment with chemically unrelated drugs.

Specific tests used to evaluate drug allergy include skin tests, measurement of serum antibody levels, and challenge administration of suspect drugs. Skin testing to detect specific IgE involves pricking the skin or intradermal injection with dilute solutions of the drug in question. If the test solution contains antigen able to cross-link IgE molecules on cutaneous mast cells, histamine and other mediators of inflammation will be released, producing a wheal and flare response. The significance of a skin response must be evaluated by comparison with control testing using both histamine and diluent solutions. This testing method can be used only to predict or confirm drug reactions of the immediate hy-persensitivity type, such as urticaria or systemic anaphylaxis. To get valid results, testing must be done with relevant antigens, which for most low molecular weight drugs are unknown metabolites. The lack of knowledge of the immunochemistry of most drugs severely limits the usefulness of skin testing. Negative tests are often uninterpretable, and false-positive reactions can result from nonspecific skin irritation. Skin testing has proved useful for evaluating peni-

cillin allergy when the relevant antigens are well known (see below) and for allergic reactions associated with anesthetic agents. Large molecular weight therapeutic agents such as heterologous antisera, peptide hormones (e.g., insulin), and vaccines are complete antigens that can appropriately be used for skin testing. Treatment with antihistamines must be discontinued before skin testing and, for safety, testing should always begin using the prick method. *In vitro* tests for drug-specific IgE, such as the radioallergosorbent test (RAST), are also limited by our incomplete knowledge of drug immunochemistry. Skin tests are generally more sensitive than measurement of specific IgE and have the advantage of immediately available results.

Challenge administration of a suspect drug offers the possibility of specific diagnosis or exclusion of drug allergy. However, challenges are inherently dangerous and should usually be avoided, especially if there is concern about possible anaphylaxis or other potentially life-threatening complications such as exfoliative dermatitis. When the drug in question is considered essential and the history is vague or suggests a mild reaction, challenge testing might be justified. Challenges should begin with a very low dose considered unlikely to cause a reaction.

MANAGEMENT

Discontinuing the responsible drug is often the only treatment necessary. Some reactions may require supportive measures directed at relieving symptoms and reducing inflammation. Antihistamines such as diphenhydramine, 25 to 50 mg every 4 to 6 hours, or hydroxyzine, 25 mg four times daily for adults, can relieve pruritus and may lessen the duration of some reactions. Corticosteroids should be reserved for the most severe or prolonged reactions. Treatment of anaphylaxis is discussed in Ch. 226.

In exceptional circumstances, it may be acceptable to continue drug treatment despite mild reactions such as delayed-onset urticaria, exanthems, and fever. Patients continued on the drug should receive supportive measures and should be followed closely; if the reaction increases in severity, the drug should be stopped.

Patients with a history of allergic reactions to multiple drugs, particularly antibiotics, present a difficult management problem. These reactions can sometimes be attributed to immunologic cross-reactivity, but often patients claim sensitivity to chemically dissimilar agents. In some cases a careful history reveals that allergy has been confused with other types of adverse drug reactions, such as side effects or drug toxicity. Some patients who have experienced severe allergic reactions become fearful of all drug use and experience reactions attributable to anxiety. However, the possibility of true allergy to multiple, chemically dissimilar drugs must also be considered. A prospective study demonstrated that patients with a history of allergic reactions to any antimicrobial agent were 10 times more likely to react to unrelated antimicrobial drugs than were history-negative controls. This suggests the existence of a group of patients predisposed to respond immunologically to drug haptens. Special care should be taken for patients with history of multiple drug allergy, including administering the first dose of any new drug in a physician's office or other supervised environment.

Another group of patients at risk for multiple drug sensitivities are individuals with HIV infection (see Part XXII). AIDS patients are reported to be at increased risk for reaction to multiple antimicrobial agents, including sulfonamides, amoxicillin, pentamidine, clindamycin, dapsone, quinolones, acyclovir, and antituberculosis drugs. Most drug reactions in HIV patients are characterized by a delayed-onset maculopapular rash and fever. Although these reactions do not usually resemble type I immediate hypersensitivity, they are probably caused by immunologic mechanisms related to the immune dysregulation caused by the HIV infection. The risk of drug reactions in HIV-infected patients can create difficult management problems. Successful rechallenge or desensitization of AIDS patients has been reported with trimethoprim-sulfamethoxazole, acyclovir, and dapsone. Although such procedures are inherently dangerous and have caused severe systemic reactions, the risk is sometimes justified for patients with opportunistic infections. Sensitivity to multiple antimicrobial agents has also been reported in patients with humoral immunodeficiency and patients with systemic lupus erythematosus.

PREVENTION

The most effective preventive measures are taking a careful history of previous drug reactions and avoiding unnecessary drug use. The history should be adequate to allow classification of the type of reaction experienced, and physicians should educate patients to distinguish allergy from other types of adverse reactions (see Ch. 16). Reactions attributable to drug toxicity or side effects do not necessarily preclude future use of the same or chemically similar agents.

Prior to prescribing any new drug, physicians should again inquire about past drug reactions. Skin tests can predict a type I hypersensitivity response to some drugs and should be done routinely prior before heterologous antisera is given. Patients should be kept under observation for 20 to 30 minutes after receiving parenteral medication.

When newly marketed drugs are used, physicians should be alert for unexpected complications, including allergic reactions. New drugs are not routinely evaluated for immunogenicity and animal studies may not predict human hypersensitivity. Premarketing clinical trials seldom include adequate numbers of patients to detect problems of low incidence such as drug allergy.

When treatment is considered essential despite well-documented allergic hypersensitivity, the drug can sometimes be administered by following a desensitization protocol. Successful desensitization regimens have been published for β-lactam antibiotics (see below), trimethoprim-sulfamethoxazole, vancomycin, allopurinol, tetanus toxoid, acyclovir, sulfasalazine, insulin, aspirin, and heterologous antisera. These regimens start with a very low drug dose, which is slowly increased as the patient is closely monitored. Reactions often occur during desensitization, and it is frequently necessary to drop back and repeat tolerated doses before proceeding. The mechanism of desensitization is uncertain but for some drugs may involve the gradual neutralization of IgE antibody with low drug doses. Desensitization is always a high-risk procedure that is undertaken only after obtaining informed consent from the patient or family and only by physicians who are prepared to treat severe reactions.

SPECIFIC DRUG ALLERGIES

β-LACTAM ANTIBIOTICS. β-lactam antibiotics—including penicillins, carbapenems, cephalosporins, and monobactams—are the most common cause of drug-induced immediate hypersensitivity reactions. The immunochemistry of penicillin is the best studied of any drug. Most protein-bound penicillin is in the form of penicilloyl, which is designated the major determinant. Other products of penicillin degradation, including penicilloate and penilloate, and penicillin itself are designated the minor determinants, indicating that these haptens are present in relatively small amounts. This terminology is somewhat confusing because the majority of patients who have had immediate reactions to penicillin are found to have IgE antibody to minor determinants rather than penicilloyl alone.

Most patients with a history of a penicillin allergy have no reaction if given the drug. This can be attributed both to inaccurate histories and the loss of sensitivity with time. The significance of a history of penicillin allergy can be clarified by skin testing. If skin testing is performed with both penicilloyl (available as Pre Pen) and minor determinants, the results are highly accurate in identifying patients at risk for immediate-type reactions, having a sensitivity of approximately 99%. Although minor determinants other than penicillin itself are not commercially available, skin testing with just penicilloyl and penicillin will identify about 93% of patients at risk. Details of penicillin skin testing are given in Table 230–3.

Whenever possible, alternative antimicrobial agents should be chosen for patients with a history of penicillin allergy of any type. If, however, the use of a penicillin or another β-lactam agent is considered essential for patient care, a decision to use a β-lactam can usually be made on the basis of the patient's history and skin test results. If the prior reaction is recalled as a delayed appearance of a morbilliform rash, the most common manifestation of penicillin sensitivity, then a β-lactam may be cautiously administered starting with a low dose. If the history is one of rapid-onset urticaria or anaphylaxis, skin testing can help determine the risk. Patients with a history of immediate-type hypersensitivity in the distant past and negative skin testing with penicillin and penicilloyl can be given a β-lactam agent starting with a low dose under

TABLE 230–3. PENICILLIN SKIN TESTING

Testing materials
    Penicilloyl polylysine (Pre Pen)
    Penicillin G, 10,000 U/ml
    Histamine, 1 mg/ml (positive control)
    Diluent (negative control)
Procedure
    Testing is usually done on the volar surface of the forearm or lateral surface of the upper arm. Begin with prick test using a 26-gauge needle to prick through a drop of test material. If the prick test is negative, proceed with intradermal testing, raising a bleb by intradermal injection of 0.02 ml of test material. Read test results at 15 minutes. For a patient with a history of a recent severe reaction to penicillin, begin testing with 100-fold dilution of test antigens.
Interpretation
    Skin tests can be interpreted only if the histamine control produces a wheal and flare response. A positive reaction includes a wheal of at least 4 mm accompanied by erythema. If the patient has dermatographia, manifested by a significant response to the diluent control, skin test results may not be interpretable. Questionable results should be repeated.

physician observation. For patients with positive skin tests or a recent history of anaphylaxis with penicillin, a formal desensitization protocol should be used. Examples of parenteral and oral desensitization regimens are given in Table 230–4. Oral desensitization may be safer and is preferred in most situations.

The reliability of skin testing with β-lactam antibiotics other than penicillin has not been established, and the degree of cross-reactivity among different classes of β-lactam varies. Published reports of patients with a history of penicillin allergy and positive penicillin skin tests who were given a cephalosporin antibiotic indicate a reaction risk of <10%, but most reported reactions have been anaphylaxis. The carbapenem antibiotic imipenem has considerable cross-reactivity with penicillin, but the monobactam antibiotic aztreonam has no significant cross-reactivity and can be safely used in patients with penicillin allergy. Aztreonam and the third-generation cephalosporin ceftazidime have the same side chain on the β-lactam ring and may have significant clinical cross-reactivity.

INSULIN. The incidence of significant allergic reactions to insulin has declined with the availability of recombinant human insulin. Most patients suspected of insulin allergy are found to have idiopathic urticaria or sensitivity to other medications. However, true immediate-type hypersensitivity reactions to human insulin do occur; such reactions are particularly likely in patients whose insulin therapy has been interrupted by attempts at management with diet and oral hypoglycemic agents. Sensitive patients usually have rapid-onset local reactions at insulin injection sites, and the presence of specific IgE antibody can be confirmed by skin testing. Effective desensitization regimens are available, and after desensitization patients should remain continuously on insulin treatment.

LOCAL ANESTHETICS. Immediate-type hypersensitivity to local anesthetics is rare. Most adverse reactions to these agents can be attributed to toxicity, anxiety, contact dermatitis, or coadministration of other drugs such as epinephrine. True allergy to local anesthetics is perhaps more common with benzoic acid esters such as procaine and benzocaine. When the history of past reactions is unclear or suggests immediate-type hypersensitivity, skin testing with dilute solutions of local anesthetics can be diagnostically useful. Skin testing is usually done with one of the amide local anesthetics such as lidocaine and mepivacaine. If skin tests are negative, incremental challenge doses of the anesthetic are usually well tolerated.

ANGIOTENSIN-CONVERTING ENZYME (ACE) INHIBITORS. Angioedema of the face and oropharyngeal structures is an important complication of ACE inhibitor therapy. Patients with such reactions appear to be sensitive to alternative ACE inhibitors that have the same pharmacologic action but different chemical structures. This suggests a pseudoallergic reaction not mediated by a specific immune response but possibly due to the drug's effect on kinin metabolism. The angioedema is characterized by nonpruritic swelling that is usually not accompanied by urticaria. Most reactions occur within the first week of therapy, but reactions have been reported as long as 7 years after the start of drug use. These reactions may be more common in women, blacks, and patients who have experienced idiopathic angioedema. Fatal episodes have been

✔ **TABLE 230–4. β-LACTAM DESENSITIZATION**

Penicillin Oral Desensitization Protocol*

Dose*	Penicillin V Elixir (U/ML)	Amount ML	Amount UNITS	Cumulative Dose (UNITS)
1	1000	0.1	100	100
2	1000	0.2	200	300
3	1000	0.4	400	700
4	1000	0.8	800	1500
5	1000	1.6	1600	3100
6	1000	3.2	3200	6300
7	1000	6.4	6400	12,700
8	10,000	1.2	12,000	24,700
9	10,000	2.4	24,000	48,700
10	10,000	4.8	48,000	96,700
11	80,000	1.0	80,000	176,700
12	80,000	2.0	160,000	336,700
13	80,000	4.0	320,000	656,700
14	80,000	8.0	640,000	1,296,700

Patients should be observed for 15 minutes between doses and for 30 minutes after the last dose prior to parenteral drug administration.

β-Lactam Intravenous Desensitization Protocol†

Dose No.	Concentration of Stock Solution (mg/ml)	Concentration of Infused Solution (mg/ml)	Amount of Antibiotic Administered (mg)
1	0.0005	0.00001	0.0005
2	0.005	0.0001	0.005
3	0.05	0.001	0.05
4	0.5	0.01	0.5
5	5	0.1	5
6	50	1	50
7	500	10	500

Stock solution is prepared by solubilizing the antibiotic with nonbacteriostatic saline to a final concentration of 500 mg/ml. Dilutions are prepared by adding 1 ml of each preceding dilution to 9 ml of diluent. One milliliter of stock solution is further diluted into 50 ml of saline and infused over 20 minutes.

* From Wendel GD Jr, Stark BJ, Jamison RB, et al.: Penicillin allergy and desensitization in serious infections during pregnancy. N Engl J Med 312:1229, 1985.

† From Borish L, Tamir R, Rosenwasser LJ: Intravenous desensitization to beta-lactam antibiotics. J Allergy Clin Immunol 80:314, 1987.

reported, and therapy with alternative ACE inhibitor drugs should not be attempted. The angioedema associated with these drugs is unrelated to ACE inhibitor–induced cough.

ASPIRIN AND OTHER NONSTEROIDAL ANTI-INFLAMMATORY DRUGS (NSAID's) (see Ch. 19). Two to 6% of asthma patients have a history of aspirin-induced symptoms, and challenge studies have demonstrated airflow obstruction in up to 20% of unselected asthmatics. Asthma patients with chronic rhinosinusitis and nasal polyps are at particularly high risk for aspirin sensitivity. Aspirin can also cause symptom exacerbation in patients with chronic urticaria. Aspirin-sensitive patients with asthma or chronic urticaria also react to most other NSAID's. This cross-reactivity between drugs with chemically different structures and similar pharmacologic action suggests that these reactions are not immunologically mediated. The reactions in asthmatics may be related to inhibition of cyclo-oxygenase with concomitant enhancement of leukotriene synthesis or to hyperresponsiveness to leukotrienes, which are potent bronchoconstrictors (see Ch. 19 for a description of the pharmacologic actions of NSAID's). Desensitization regimens have been effective for patients with aspirin-induced bronchospasm and produce cross-desensitization to other NSAID's. For most sensitive asthma patients, aspirin and NSAID's are easily avoided. Patients with both asthma and chronic rhinosinusitis/polyposis should probably avoid these drugs regardless of past history of aspirin sensitivity. NSAID's have been associated with other idiosyncratic inflammatory reactions including acute aseptic meningitis and hypersensitivity pneumonitis.

DeSwarte RD: Drug allergy. In Patterson R, Grammer LC, Greenberger PA, Zeiss CR (eds.): Allergic Diseases Diagnosis and Management. 4th ed. Philadelphia, JB Lippincott, 1993, p 395. A comprehensive review with 621 references.

Shepherd GM: Allergy to β-lactam antibiotics. Immunol Allergy Clin North Am 11:611, 1991. A good review and one of several useful articles on this monograph on drug allergy.

231 MASTOCYTOSIS
Dean D. Metcalfe

Mastocytosis is a rare disease characterized by an abnormal increase in mast cells in the bone marrow, liver, spleen, lymph nodes, gastrointestinal tract, and skin. Mastocytosis may present in any age group and demonstrates a slight male predominance (1.5:1.0). The prevalence of the disease is unknown. Familial occurrence is unusual.

The disease is divided into four categories on the basis of clinical presentation, pathologic findings, and prognosis (Table 231–1). Patients in the first category have a good prognosis, whereas patients in the other three groups do poorly. Indolent mastocytosis is divided into two subgroups: those with isolated skin involvement and those with systemic disease. In most cases such patients gradually accrue more mast cells with progression of symptoms but can be managed successfully for decades using medications that provide symptomatic relief. The second most common form of mastocytosis is that associated with a hematologic disorder, in which examination of the bone marrow and peripheral blood reveals the hematologic abnormality. The prognosis in these patients is determined by the associated hematologic disorder. The third category of mast cell disease is mast cell leukemia; it is the rarest form and has the most fulminant behavior. Mast cell leukemia is distinguished by its unique pathologic and clinical picture. The peripheral blood smear shows immature mast cells. The fourth category of patients has an aggressive form of mastocytosis; these individuals experience a rapid increase in mast cell numbers and have poor prognostic features but do not have a distinctive hematologic disorder or mast cell leukemia.

ETIOLOGY AND PATHOGENESIS. Mast cells originate from pluripotent bone marrow stem cells and migrate through the bloodstream and lymphatics to specific sites, where they mature into fully granulated cells. The targeting of mast cells to defined locations is determined by the sequential expression of cell surface adhesion molecules. Mast cells are often found along endothelial and epithelial basement membrane, along nerves, and around glandular structures. Tissues at interfaces between the external and internal environment, i.e., the skin and gastrointestinal tract, are particularly rich in mast cells.

Mast cell number and differentiation are regulated by factors produced both in the hematopoietic marrow and by cells in the tissues in which mast cells finally reside. Early mast cell differentiation depends on the colony-stimulating factor interleukin-3 (IL-3) and is inhibited by granulocyte-macrophage colony-stimulating factor (GM-CSF). Final maturation depends on the production of specific growth factors by fibroblasts and stromal cells such as c-kit ligand, or stem cell factor.

Regardless of the cause of the increased burden of mast cells, the pathogenesis of the disease is largely the result of the increased pro-

TABLE 231–1. CLASSIFICATION OF MASTOCYTOSIS

Indolent mastocytosis
  Skin only
    Urticaria pigmentosa
    Diffuse cutaneous mastocytosis
  Systemic
    Marrow
    Gastrointestinal
    ± Urticaria pigmentosa
Mastocytosis with an associated hematologic disorder (± urticaria pigmentosa)
  Dysmyelopoietic syndrome
  Myeloproliferative disorders
  Acute nonlymphocytic leukemia
  Malignant lymphoma
  Chronic neutropenia
Mast cell leukemia
Aggressive mastocytosis

duction of mast cell mediators, which have effects both at the site of their production and at remote sites. Mast cell mediators are three categories, all of which produce biologic effects typical of those observed in patients with mastocytosis (Table 231–2).

CLINICAL FEATURES. The categories of mastocytosis in general share similar clinical features, although some patterns of disease may predominate in a specific category. The skin, gastrointestinal tract, liver, spleen, lymph nodes, bone marrow, and skeletal system yield the most significant management problems. The respiratory tract and endocrine system are generally spared. Patients with mastocytosis do not suffer from recurrent infections.

The most common skin manifestation of mastocytosis is urticaria pigmentosa (Fig. 231–1). It is seen in >90% of patients with indolent mastocytosis and in <50% of patients with mastocytosis with an associated hematologic disorder or those with aggressive mastocytosis. The lesions of urticaria pigmentosa appear as scattered small reddish-brown macules or slightly raised papules. Scratching or rubbing the lesions usually causes urtication and erythema around the macules; this is known as Darier's sign. Urticaria pigmentosa is associated with pruritus, which may be exacerbated by changes in climatic temperature, skin friction, ingesting hot beverages or spicy foods, ethanol, and certain drugs. The diagnosis is confirmed by characteristic skin histopathology. Diffuse cutaneous mastocytosis consists of a diffuse mast cell infiltration of the skin. Solitary lesions called *mastocytomas* do occur but are quite rare. Young children with urticaria pigmentosa or diffuse cutaneous mastocytosis may have bullous eruptions.

Gastrointestinal disease often develops in patients with mastocytosis. The most common problem is gastric hypersecretion due to elevated plasma histamine with resultant gastritis and peptic ulcer disease. Diarrhea and abdominal pain are common and are followed by the onset of malabsorption in approximately one in three patients. Roentgenographic abnormalities fall into three major categories: peptic ulcers; abnormal mucosal patterns such as mucosal edema, multiple nodular lesions, coarsened mucosal folds, or multiple polyps; and motility disturbances. Histopathology of jejunal biopsies has shown moderate blunting of the villi; however, significant mast cell hyperplasia is uncommon.

Hepatic and splenic involvement in indolent systemic mastocytosis is relatively common, although liver function tests are usually normal. The most common chemical abnormality is an elevated alkaline phosphatase; this must be distinguished from bone-derived alkaline phosphatase, which may also be elevated. The most serious manifestation of hepatic and splenic involvement is portal hypertension and ascites associated with fibrosis of the liver and spleen. These conditions appear most commonly in patients who have mastocytosis with an associated hematologic disorder or in those with aggressive mastocytosis.

Bone marrow lesions consist of focal aggregates of spindle-shaped mast cells, often mixed with eosinophils, lymphocytes, and

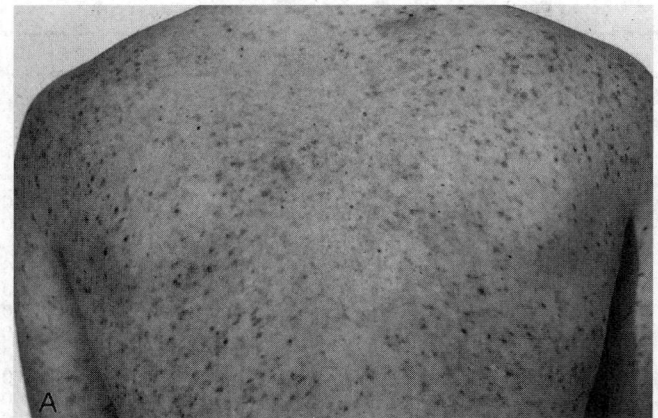
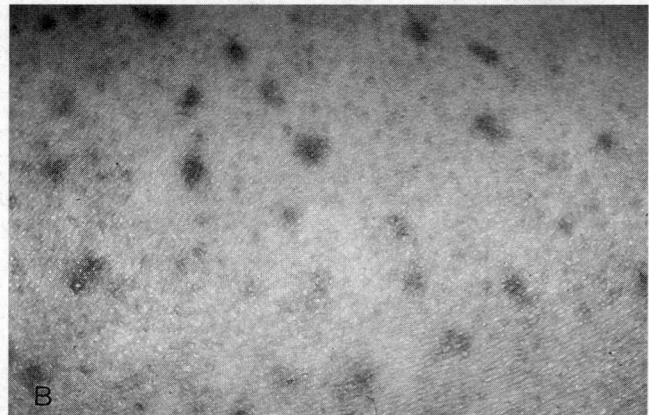

FIGURE 231–1. *A*, Urticaria pigmentosa in a patient with indolent systemic mastocytosis. *B*, Close-up view of urticaria pigmentosa.

occasional plasma cells, histiocytes, and fibroblasts (Fig. 231–2). Anemia, leukopenia, thrombocytopenia, and eosinophilia may occur in association with systemic disease. Bone marrow infiltration with mast cells may induce bone changes that cause radiographically detectable lesions in up to 70% of patients. The proximal long bones are most often affected, followed by the pelvis, ribs, and skull. Bone pain is the most common symptom and is present in 19 to 28% of patients. Skeletal scintigraphy (bone scans) is more sensitive than radiographic surveys in detecting and locating active lesions. In severe or advanced disease, pathologic fractures do occur.

Patients in every category of mastocytosis sometimes experience flushing or frank anaphylaxis. In occasional patients, anaphylaxis may be provoked by alcohol, aspirin, exercise, or infections.

Neuropsychiatric abnormalities have been reported. Problems include a decreased attention span, memory impairment, and irritability. Depression as a consequence of chronic disease or possibly mediated by mast cell products is a possibility.

DIAGNOSIS. The diagnosis of mastocytosis rests on histology, supported by clinical, biochemical, and radiographic data. Mast cells may be overlooked on histologic sections depending on the fixation and/or stain used. The most useful stains for mast cells include metachromatic stains, such as toluidine blue and Giemsa, and enzymatic stains, such as chloroacetate esterase and aminocaproate esterase. These procedures highlight the granules in the cytoplasm of the mast cell. In trephine core bone marrow biopsies, decalcification interferes with subsequent attempts to visualize mast cell granules.

The majority of patients with mastocytosis have urticaria pigmentosa. This diagnosis should be confirmed by skin biopsy. Blind skin biopsies are not recommended, as other skin conditions including eczema are associated with an increase in dermal mast cells.

In the absence of skin lesions, mastocytosis may be suspected in patients with one or several of the following: unexplained ulcer disease or malabsorption, radiographic or ^{99m}Tc bone scan abnormalities, hepatomegaly, splenomegaly, lymphadenopathy, peripheral blood abnormalities, and unexplained flushing or anaphylaxis. Ele-

TABLE 231–2. REPRESENTATIVE MAST CELL PRODUCTS AND THEIR BIOLOGIC EFFECTS

Granule-associated

Histamine	Pruritus, increased vasopermeability, gastric hypersecretion, bronchoconstriction
Heparin	Local anticoagulation
Tryptase, chymotryptic proteases	Degradation of local connective tissues

Lipid-derived

Sulfidopeptide leuko-trienes	Increased vasopermeability, bronchoconstriction, vasoconstriction (LTC_4); increased vasopermeability, bronchoconstriction, vasodilation (LTD_4 and LTE_4)
Prostaglandin D_2	Vasodilation, bronchoconstriction
Platelet-activating factor	Increased vasopermeability, vasodilation, bronchoconstriction

Cytokines

Proinflammatory factors	Fibrosis (TGF-β); activation of vascular endothelial cells, cachexia (TNF-α); IgE synthesis (IL-4)
Growth enhancing	Colony-stimulating factor (IL-3); eosinophilia (IL-5)

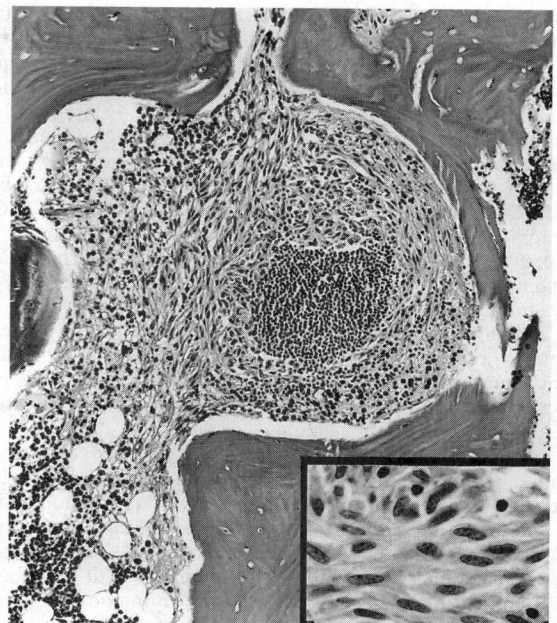

FIGURE 231–2. Bone marrow biopsy shows a characteristic lesion of systemic mastocytosis with nodular, paratrabecular infiltrate of mast cells surrounding a lymphoid aggregate. *Inset:* The mast cells are spindle-shaped, resembling fibroblasts or histiocytes. (Courtesy of W. D. Travis, Bethesda, MD.)

vated levels of plasma or urinary histamine or histamine metabolites, prostaglandin D_2 metabolites in the urine, or plasma mast cell tryptase are not diagnostic but do raise the index of suspicion of mastocytosis. Reliable tests for these substances, however, are not generally available except in research laboratories.

Patients suspected of having mastocytosis in the absence of skin lesions should have a bone marrow biopsy and aspirate for diagnosis. Patients with urticaria pigmentosa or diffuse cutaneous mastocytosis should also have this procedure if they have peripheral blood abnormalities, hepatomegaly, splenomegaly, or lymphadenopathy, to determine if they have an associated hematologic disorder. Other tissue specimens, such as lymph nodes, liver, and gastrointestinal mucosa, define the extent of mast cell involvement but are obtained only as necessary.

Patients suspected of having mastocytosis should have 24-hour urine 5-hydroxyindoleacetic acid (5-HIAA) measured to help eliminate the possibility of a carcinoid tumor. Patients with mastocytosis do not excrete increased amounts of 5-HIAA. Idiopathic anaphylaxis and flushing must also be considered. Patients with these disorders do not have histologic evidence of significant mast cell proliferation.

TREATMENT. In all categories of mastocytosis, a primary objective of treatment is to control mast cell mediator–induced signs and symptoms such as anaphylaxis, gastrointestinal cramping, and pruritus. H_1-receptor antagonists such as hydroxyzine and doxepin are helpful in reducing pruritus, flushing, and tachycardia. If insufficient relief occurs, adding an H_2 antagonist such as ranitidine or cimetidine may be beneficial. However, many patients continue to complain of bone pain, headaches, and flushing, resulting in part from the inability to block other mast cell mediators. Disodium cromoglycate (cromolyn sodium) inhibits degranulation of mast cells and may have some efficacy in the treatment of mastocytosis. Epinephrine is used to treat episodes of anaphylaxis. Patients should be prepared to self-administer this drug. If subcutaneous epinephrine is insufficient, intensive therapy for anaphylaxis should be instituted. Patients with recurrent episodes of anaphylaxis may be placed on H_1 and H_2 antihistamines to lessen the severity of attacks. Episodes of profound anaphylaxis may be spontaneous but have also been observed following stings from insects or administration of radiocontrast media.

Treatment of gastrointestinal disease is directed at controlling peptic symptoms, diarrhea, and malabsorption. Gastric acid hypersecretion leading to peptic symptoms and ulcerations is controlled

with H_2 antagonists. Diarrhea is difficult to manage, and H_2 antagonists are generally not effective. Anticholinergics may give partial relief. In patients with severe malabsorption, systemic steroids have been shown to be effective. Ascites is also difficult to manage. One patient with portal hypertension was successfully managed with a portacaval shunt. Another patient with exudative ascites was treated successfully with systemic steroid therapy.

Patients with mastocytosis and an associated hematologic disorder are treated as dictated by the specific hematologic abnormality. In mast cell leukemia, chemotherapy has not yet been shown to produce remissions. Chemotherapy has no place in the treatment of indolent mastocytosis. A recent study suggested that splenectomy may improve survival in patients with poor prognostic forms of mastocytosis.

PROGNOSIS. Prognosis must be addressed separately for each category of mastocytosis. One study found seven variables that were strongly associated with poor survival. These included constitutional symptoms, anemia, thrombocytopenia, abnormal liver function tests, lobated mast cell nucleus, a low percentage of fat cells in the bone marrow biopsy, and an associated hematologic disorder. Other poor prognostic variables include absence of urticaria pimentosa, male gender, absence of skin and bone symptoms, hepatomegaly, splenomegaly, and normal bone radiographic findings.

As a group, patients with indolent mastocytosis and skin involvement alone have the best prognosis. Among children with isolated urticaria pigmentosa, at least 50% improve by adulthood. Adults with urticaria pigmentosa usually progress gradually to systemic disease and rarely may convert to type II disease. Diffuse cutaneous mastocytosis is usually associated with indolent systemic disease. Patients with mastocytosis with an associated hematologic disorder have a variable course, depending on the prognosis of their hematologic disorder. With mast cell leukemia, mean survival is less than 6 months. Survival with lymphadenopathic mastocytosis with eosinophilia is 2 to 3 years without therapy. The prognosis appears to improve with aggressive symptomatic management.

Cherner JA, Jensen RT, Dubois A, et al.: Gastrointestinal dysfunction in systemic mastocytosis: A prospective study. Gastroenterology 95:657, 1988. *Describes patterns of gastrointestinal disease in mastocytosis and the implications for clinical management.*

Garriga MM, Friedman MM, Metcalfe DD: A survey of the number and distribution of mast cells in the skin of patients with mast cell disorders. J Allergy Clin Immunol 82:425, 1988. *A study of the value of determining mast cell numbers in skin biopsies.*

Horny H-P, Kaiserling E, Campbell M, et al.: Liver findings in generalized mastocytosis: A clinicopathologic study. Cancer 63:532, 1989. *A survey of liver histopathology in mastocytosis.*

Lawrence JB, Friedman BS, Travis WD, et al.: Hematologic manifestations of systemic mast cell disease. A prospective study of laboratory and morphologic features and their relation to prognosis. Am J Med 91:612, 1991. *An excellent review of the histopathologic and clinical features of mastocytosis.*

Mekori YA, Oh CK, Metcalfe DD: IL-3–dependent murine mast cells undergo apoptosis on removal of IL-3. J. Immunol 151:3775, 1993.

Schwartz LB, Metcalfe DD, Miller JS, et al.: Tryptase levels as an indicator of mast cell activation in systemic anaphylaxis and mastocytosis. N Engl J Med 316:1622, 1987. *Demonstration of mast cell tryptase in the serum of mastocytosis patients.*

232 DISEASES OF THE THYMUS
Max D. Cooper

NORMAL DEVELOPMENT AND FUNCTION. The essential role of the thymus is to generate clonally diverse T lymphocytes that can recognize a vast array of foreign proteins presented as peptides on host cells. An essential parallel thymic function is eliminating self-reactive T-cell clones that could damage normal tissues.

The embryonic thymus is formed initially from epithelial cells lining the third and fourth pharyngeal pouches. These specialized epithelial cells migrate through the neck region to form bilateral thymic lobes in the upper anterior mediastinum. The epithelial thymus begins to attract hemopoietic stem cells from the circulation around the eighth week of fetal life. Within the thymus these precursor cells are influenced to proliferate and differentiate along T-lymphocyte lines. This lifelong process begins in the outer cortex of the thymus, and the immature thymocytes migrate toward the medullary region as they proliferate and mature. Cortical regions of the lobules that collectively form the bilateral thymic lobes thus become filled with immature T lymphocytes, the extraordinary clonal diversity of which is manifested by differences in their T-cell receptor (TCR) specificities. Each developing T cell is selected for survival or death depending on the affinity of its receptor for self-peptides, which are presented initially on the surface of cortical epithelial cells. As maturing thymocytes approach the corticomedullary junction, they encounter macrophages or dendritic cell immigrants that can also present peptide fragments of antigenic proteins. Thymocytes that fail to receive any TCR-mediated signal are programmed to die. Immature thymocytes also receive a death signal if their TCR has relatively high affinity for a self-peptide, whereas moderate affinity for a self-peptide selects for survival. Only 1% or so of the thymic T cells survive this selection process to seed the peripheral lymphoid tissues.

Thymocytes also possess an array of non-TCR cell surface glycoproteins that they use to interact with their environment. Progression of thymocyte maturation can be conveniently monitored by the expression of the CD4 and CD8 molecules. The most immature thymocytes lack detectable CD4 and CD8. Intermediate-stage thymocytes express both CD4 and CD8; these double-positives predominate in the thymic cortex. Clonal selection occurs during this stage of differentiation, and the CD4 and CD8 molecules play key roles in the selection process. The peptide fragments of antigenic proteins are presented within the α-helical grooves of the major histocompatibility complex (MHC) class II and class I molecules. CD4 has an affinity for MHC class II molecules on specialized antigen-presenting cells, whereas the CD8 molecules can bind class I molecules present on all nucleated cells. The CD4 or CD8 molecules thus serve as co-receptors in the positive clonal selection, which leads to the development of either mature CD4+ cells with helper potential or CD8+ T cells with cytotoxic potential. Most of the positively selected helper or cytotoxic T cells exit the thymus via the small blood vessels in the corticomedullary region, and only a few settle within the thymic medulla. The cellular debris of dying thymocytes is apparently swept up by macrophages, perhaps aided by the epithelial cell whirls called *Hassall's bodies* that are located in the thymic medulla.

The lymphoid thymus reaches its maximal size of approximately 30 grams by around age 1, and it gradually decreases in size thereafter to ≤3 grams in most older individuals. Because the thymus-derived T-cell clones may have lifespans of several decades, normally there is little need for constant thymic replenishment. Nevertheless, thymocyte differentiation persists throughout life, albeit usually at low levels, which may vary according to an individual's hormonal balance and need for T-cell replenishment.

DEVELOPMENTAL DEFECTS OF THE THYMUS. *DiGeorge syndrome,* also called the third and fourth pharyngeal pouch syndrome, features hypoplastic thymus and parathyroid development in addition to facial and cardiac abnormalities, which may include a ventricular septal defect and aortic abnormalities. DiGeorge syndrome occurs in both males and females, a majority of whom may have submicroscopic deletions of chromosome 22q11. The initial clinical manifestations are neonatal seizures due to hypocalcemia, or cyanosis and other signs of cardiac insufficiency. Immunodeficiency is a later manifestation, the severity of which depends on the degree of thymic hypoplasia. Most affected individuals have a small ectopic but functionally normal thymus that can seed T cells to the periphery in numbers that may or may not be sufficient for immune defense. In rare instances, affected infants have no detectable thymus or peripheral T cells, and thymic transplantation must be considered in these cases. Thymic grafts and all blood products given to these patients need to be rigorously depleted of donor T cells by high-dose irradiation or other means because of the threat of lethal graft-versus-host disease.

Ataxia-telangiectasia is a hereditary disorder in which thymic hypoplasia and variable T-cell deficiency are seen in association with oculocutaneous telangiectasia and truncal ataxia (see Ch. 223).

ACQUIRED ABNORMALITIES OF THYMIC FUNCTION.
Infection. Human immunodeficiency virus (HIV) can drastically affect thymic development and function. First, massive thymocyte destruction occurs because most thymocytes express the CD4 mole-

cules that serve as HIV receptors. In addition, thymic epithelial components are damaged by the HIV-induced inflammation, which results in scarring and loss of thymopoietic activity. The capacity for thymic production of CD4+ T cells is thus severely compromised and may be lost entirely in AIDS patients. Consequently, severe immunodeficiency may occur relatively early in congenital HIV infections. In contrast, individuals infected with HIV later in life usually experience a latency period of 8 to 10 years before AIDS develops because of the gradual attrition of established CD4+ T-cell clones in the periphery.

Thymectomy. Removal of the thymus after the peripheral lymphoid compartments have been seeded with T-cell clones may have no discernible effects for many years, presumably because T-cell clones normally have very long lifespans. Thymectomy is rarely complete, moreover, in part because approximately 30% of individuals have extramediastinal thymic arrests. Nevertheless, the potential need for thymic function later in life dictates careful consideration before undertaking thymectomy.

Thymic Hyperplasia. Striking variability of thymic size can occur in apparently normal adults. The physiologic basis for thymic enlargement may include hormonal influences on thymopoietic activity. Pituitary hormones that can enhance thymic growth include growth hormone, luteinizing hormone, and follicle-stimulating hormone, whereas thyrotropin may inhibit thymic growth. Interleukin-7 (IL-7), a product of thymic stromal cells, is an important thymocyte growth factor. Other locally produced factors, including epithelial growth factor and transforming growth factor-α, may regulate thymic epithelial cell production of cytokines, such as IL-1 and -6, that can affect T-cell proliferation. Thymic enlargement can occur in adults without demonstrable pathology and rarely in patients with thyrotoxicosis, Addison's disease, or following orchidectomy.

Thymic Involution. This is a well-known consequence of stressful illnesses, including severe infections, burns, and other conditions that result in elevated levels of adrenal corticosteroids. The involution is due to the relative susceptibility of immature thymocytes to lysis by corticosteroids of endogenous or exogenous origin. Temporary thymic involution also occurs as a consequence of irradiation or treatment with cytotoxic drugs. Thymic involution is a physiologic consequence of pregnancy and elevated levels of estrogen.

Myasthenia Gravis and the Thymus. Myasthenia gravis is characterized by muscle weakness attributable to an autoimmune response against the acetylcholine receptors (see Ch. 459). Improvement in this disease is frequently observed after thymectomy, thus implying a causal link between the thymus and the autoreactive T- and B-cell clones. Germinal center formation is seen in the thymic cortex of most myasthenia gravis patients, and one hypothesis is that the autoimmune response is initiated by the acetylcholine receptors present on a minor population of thymic myeloid cells. Thymic tumors are diagnosed in approximately 10% of individuals with myasthenia gravis.

Thymoma. The term *thymoma* is usually reserved for thymic epithelial cell tumors which, although rare, are the most commonly diagnosed tumors of the anterior superior mediastinum. Thymomas are frequently associated with myasthenia gravis. They also occur in rare individuals with acquired hypogammaglobulinemia who stop producing B-lineage cells; bone marrow insufficiency in these individuals may also extend to the erythroid and myeloid lineages.

The diagnosis of thymoma is suggested when these associated conditions occur or when an anterior mediastinal mass is detected, which may be an incidental finding because approximately one third of affected individuals are asymptomatic. Others with thymoma may have chest pain, dysphagia, signs of tracheal impingement, or superior vena caval obstruction. The extent of the tumor mass can be estimated by imaging procedures, but accurate diagnosis depends on obtaining thymic tissues for histologic assessment. Even when an adequate sample is available, the diagnosis may be difficult, however. There are no reliable markers for neoplastic epithelial clones, and thymomas are rarely composed of obviously neoplastic epithelial cells. Instead they are usually formed by a mixture of apparently normal lymphoid thymocytes and epithelial cells that are either spindle-shaped or ovoid. Consequently, the most reliable prognostic indication is evidence for or against invasiveness by the epithelial tumor. For this reason, direct tumor visualization by thoracotomy is favored for both diagnosis and treatment. In the case of well-encapsulated thymomas, tumors rarely occur after surgical removal. When the thymoma has invaded the capsule or surrounding tissues, surgical removal and irradiation or intensive chemotherapy may prevent 5-year recurrences in more than half of the affected patients.

Other Tumors of the Thymus. **Lymphomas.** Thymic involvement may be a prominent feature in lymphoblastic neoplasms of T-cell origin. Hodgkin's disease, usually of the nodular sclerosing type, may primarily affect the thymus. Histiocytic lymphomas may also present as an anterior mediastinal mass in adults.

Carcinoid Tumors (see Ch. 210.2). These rarely arise in the thymus; those associated with elevated levels of ACTH-like hormones and Cushing's syndrome (approximately one third) are particularly invasive. Complete excision may be curative.

Germ Cell Tumors. These occur rarely in the thymus. These include seminoma, teratoma, embryonal cell carcinoma, and choriocarcinoma.

Day DL, Gedgudas E: The thymus. Radiol Clin North Am 22:519, 1984. *A review of thymic anatomy and function emphasizing evaluation with imaging techniques such as CT scans, sonography, and magnetic resonance imaging.*

Haynes BF: Human thymic epithelium and T cell development: Current issues and future directions. Thymus 16:143, 1990. *An analytic review of the different cellular elements that form the human thymus.*

Levine GD, Rosai J: Thymic hyperplasia and neoplasia: A review of current concepts. Hum Pathol 9:495, 1978. *A thoughtful consideration of normal thymic variation and neoplasias.*

Schnittman SM, Denning SM, Greenhouse JJ, et al.: Evidence for susceptibility of intrathymic T-cell precursors and their progeny carrying T-cell antigen receptor phenotypes TCR$\alpha\beta^+$ and TCR$\gamma\delta^+$ to human immunodeficiency virus infection: A mechanism for CD4+ (T4) lymphocyte depletion. Proc Natl Acad Sci 87:7727, 1990. *Infection of early stages of the T-cell lineage via the CD4 molecule may explain the inability of the T-cell pool to regenerate in HIV-infected individuals.*

PART XX

MUSCULOSKELETAL AND CONNECTIVE TISSUE DISEASES

233 APPROACH TO THE PATIENT WITH MUSCULOSKELETAL DISEASE

Duncan A. Gordon

Diseases of the musculoskeletal (MSK) system are common, disabling, and costly to the economy. This chapter provides a guide for approaching the patient with MSK symptoms by outlining the components necessary for identifying the patient's problems, formulating the diagnosis, and initiating treatment.

The pain, stiffness, and joint swelling of MSK disorders may be inflammatory, metabolic, degenerative, or combinations thereof. For the patient, however, it is the functional interference with daily activities that determines the impact of the condition. The value of a general medical approach to the patient with MSK complaints is paramount, keeping specialized assessment in perspective. At times, a limited workup may suffice, while in other instances, assessment by a number of laboratory, imaging, and other disciplines may be necessary. Before clinical approaches are considered, it is helpful to review the anatomy and pathophysiology of the structures affected.

ANATOMY. Knowledge of the anatomic structures will answer the question, "Where is the lesion?" In the case of MSK diseases, the joints are primarily affected. The structures that may be involved are shown in Figure 233–1 *(left),* the articular structures of the MSK system. Foremost is the joint cavity and lining membrane known as the synovium. Hyaline cartilage overlying the bony end-plates provides the lubricating surface for the joint. An intact bony end-plate is required to support the cartilage. The joint capsule and ligaments provide further support and blend with the periosteum.

The nonarticular anatomy of the MSK system is equally important (Fig. 233–1, *left*). This includes local structures such as tendons, bursae, or muscles associated with various joint regions or, more generally, the collagen, elastin, and ground substance known as the connective tissue system. These latter tissues are so widespread that any organ system of the body may be involved.

PATHOPHYSIOLOGIC PROCESS. After determining which anatomic structures of the MSK system are involved, one must answer the question, "What is the lesion?" The usual pathology is either inflammatory, metabolic, degenerative, or some combination thereof (Fig. 233–1, *right*). Joint neoplasms are exceptional. With inflammatory disorders such as rheumatoid arthritis (RA) or septic arthritis, the joint cavity and synovial membrane are primarily affected, whereas with degenerative conditions such as osteoarthritis (OA) the cartilage is primarily affected. Cartilage loss also may be secondary to synovial inflammation or trauma. Metabolic crystal deposition disorders such as gout or pseudogout also cause articular inflammation, whereas avascular necrosis of bone is associated with

cartilage damage after bony end-plate collapse. Moreover, the same pathologic processes noted above may affect extra-articular systems such as skin, muscle, and vasculature.

ROLE OF THE CLINICIAN. *History.* The interview should provide a detailed chronology of the illness: anatomic location of the pain, whether local or referred; its occurrence with activity, rest, or sleep; type of onset, whether sudden or insidious; the pattern of joint involvement, symmetric or not, and whether predominantly upper or lower limbs; influence of previous and current treatments; systemic symptoms such as fatigue, weight loss, or fever and duration of morning stiffness; an up-to-date account and systematic review of all the joints of the body; and a psychosocial history. A nonrestorative sleep pattern may be associated with morning stiffness and other diffuse aching. Symptoms should be interpreted in terms of the patient's functional ability to perform self-care and other daily activities. General weakness and fatigue may reflect that many MSK conditions affect the patient's body as whole and not just the joints.

Functional Disability Indices. A number of self-report questionnaires such as the Stanford Health Assessment Questionnaire (HAQ), Functional Disability Index (FDI), Arthritis Impact Measurement Scales (AIMS), or modifications of these have been developed for ongoing evaluation of patients with arthritis (Table 233–1). These instruments document the patient's functional status with results comparable with traditional measures of joint disease activity such as tender joint count, radiographic joint erosion score, and erythrocyte sedimentation rate.

Demography. An appreciation of the age, gender, marital status, and occupation of the patient is helpful. The age of the patient is relevant to developmental and heritable disorders of connective tissue. For example, arthritis is a major manifestation of hemophilia with onset during childhood. Juvenile RA refers to polyarthritis coming on before age 16. In young adults, seropositive, seronegative, and septic arthritic conditions may arise, whereas OA is exceptional. The onset for RA is the middle years, whereas the elderly are more prone to OA. RA and the collagen diseases are more common in women, whereas ankylosing spondylitis and the other B27 spondyloarthropathies are more common in men. Gouty arthritis is more common in men and rarely attacks women before the menopause. Arthritis in the elderly is often assumed to be degenerative, when in fact the patient may suffer from an inflammatory process such as polymyalgia rheumatica, RA, or systemic lupus erythematosus. Occupation is also important because of associated physical and psychological stresses. The clinician should find out exactly what the patient does to determine how demanding the job is. Occupational factors are important with repetitive joint trauma in individuals susceptible to OA. Symptoms may be associated with jogging or trauma from sports activities.

Physical Examination. Because many MSK/rheumatic disorders are systemic, physical examination may document the presence of extra-articular features. In RA these include subcutaneous nodules, digital vasculitis, and other systemic features described in Ch. 237. Any one of these may be mistaken for a nonrheumatic condi-

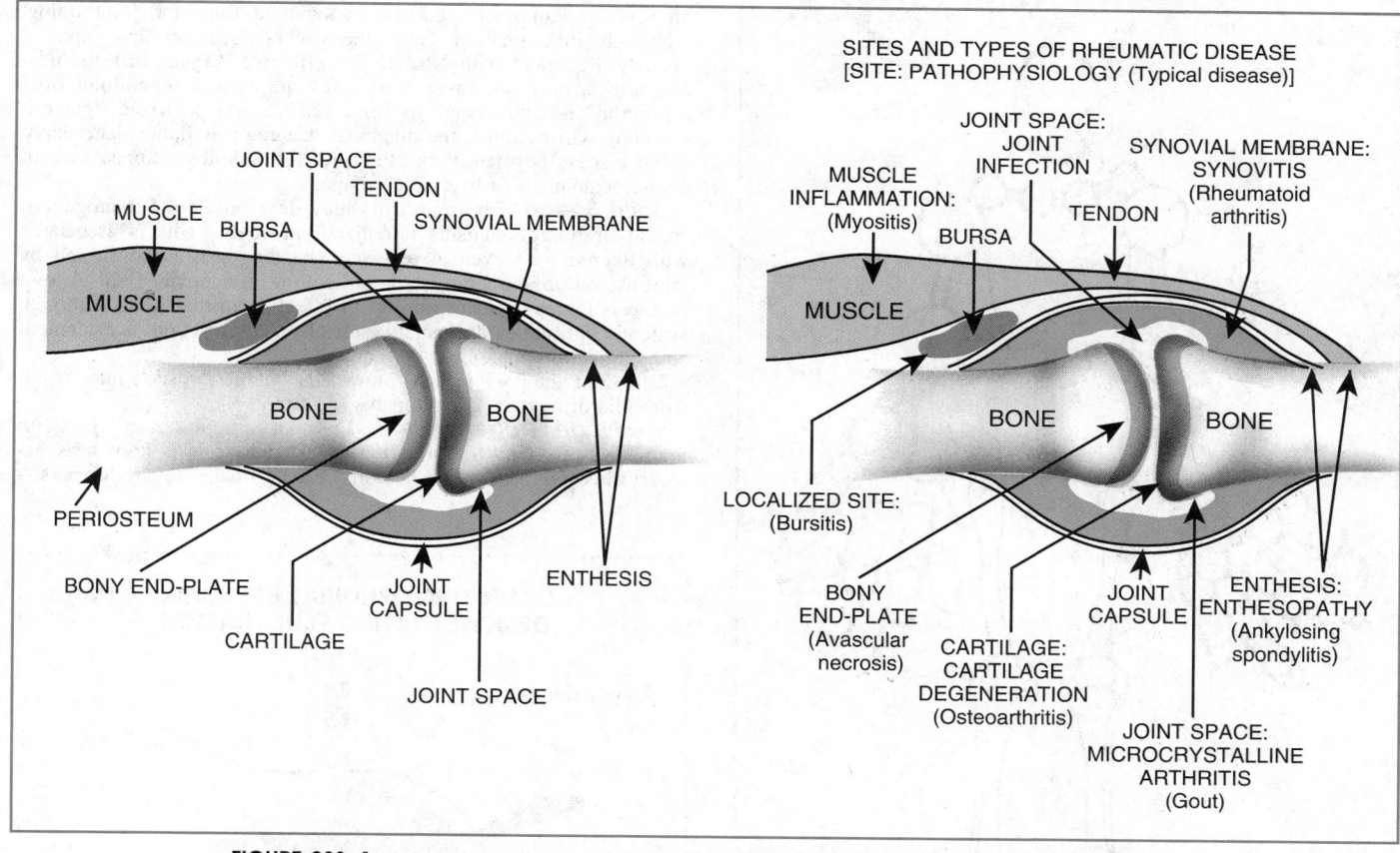

FIGURE 233–1. *Left,* Anatomic structures of the MSK system. *Right,* Location of MSK disease processes.

tion, and their presence may indicate more ominous disease. Any number of systemic features may be the result of an adverse drug reaction. The joints shown in Figure 233–2 should be examined systematically to determine if any are inflamed or damaged. The pattern of joint involvement, whether symmetrical, axial, or peripheral, should be recorded using the diagram.

Joint Inflammation. Key signs are tenderness and swelling. These may be associated with local heat, but erythema is not a feature of rheumatoid inflammation, whereas tenderness, heat, and erythema may be seen with septic or gouty arthritis. A joint is considered *active* if it is tender on pressure or passive movement with stress. Joint swelling may be periarticular or intra-articular. The latter is associated with a joint effusion detected by showing fluctua-

tion (see Fig. 233–3). It is important to note the difference between *tender joints* and deep referred *tender points* characteristic of a nonarticular syndrome known as "fibromyalgia" (see Ch. 258).

Joint Damage and Destruction. This may be assessed clinically or radiologically. Common observations include loss of range of movement, collateral instability, malalignment, subluxation, or cartilage loss causing bone-on-bone crepitus. Record a separate count of damaged joints, as with actively inflamed joints.

DIAGNOSTIC CONSIDERATIONS. Clinical evaluation enables us to establish which MSK structures are inflamed, which are damaged, and how function is impaired. Nine specific types of MSK involvement can be identified as a framework for various diagnostic possibilities or hypotheses to be considered (Fig. 233–1,

TABLE 233–1. SELF-REPORT QUESTIONNAIRE FOR ARTHRITIS

Please check (✓) the ONE best answer for your abilities.

At this moment, are you able to:	Without Any Difficulty	With Some Difficulty	With Much Difficulty	Unable to Do
a. Dress yourself, including tying shoelaces and doing buttons?				
b. Get in and out of bed?				
c. Lift a full cup or glass to your mouth?				
d. Walk outdoors on flat ground?				
e. Wash and dry your entire body?				
f. Bend down to pick up clothing from the floor?				
g. Turn regular faucets (taps) on and off?				
h. Get in and out of a car?				

From Pincus T, Callahan LF, Brooks RH, et al.: Self-report questionnaire scores in rheumatoid arthritis compared with traditional physical, radiographic, and laboratory measures. Ann Intern Med 100:259, 1989.

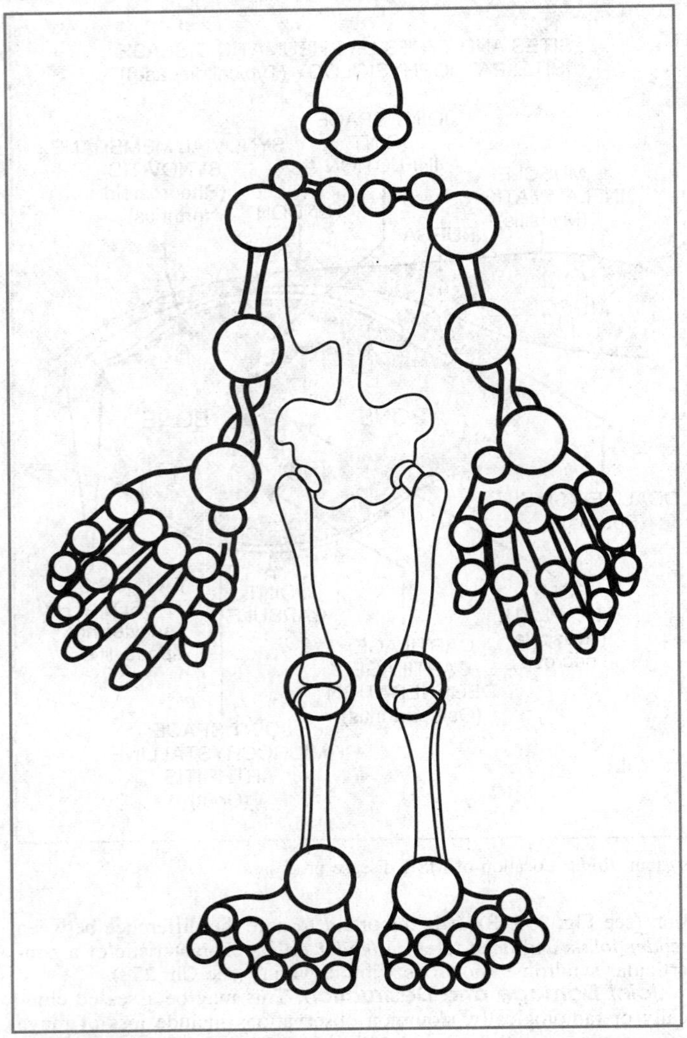

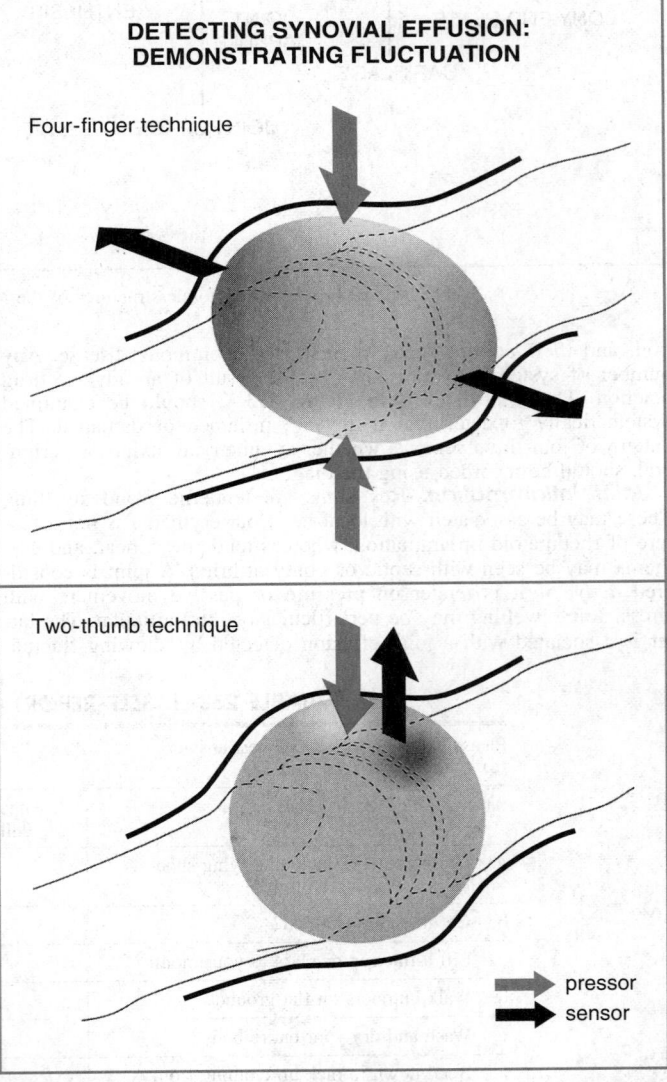

FIGURE 233–2. A pictorial method for indicating joint disease activity or destruction. The sketch may be used on a printed form or rubber stamp to chart which joints are active or deformed at the time of each assessment. (Courtesy Dr. Hugh A. Smythe, Toronto.)

right). The nine categories presented in the following paragraphs are listed in Table 233–2 along with typical diseases, examples of laboratory tests, and treatments. Table 233–2 and the descriptions below provide the basis for more detailed information contained in the following chapters of this section.

Synovitis. Inflammation of the synovial membrane lining of the joint is typical of inflammatory polyarthritis such as RA. If synovitis is persistent, irreversible joint damage results. The polyarthritis of RA is like that found in the diffuse connective tissue diseases associated with autoantibodies. These autoimmune collagen disorders include lupus, scleroderma, polymyositis, vasculitis, and Sjögren's syndrome. When these conditions are progressive or life-threatening, disease-modifying immunosuppressive drugs and/or corticosteroids are appropriate.

Enthesopathy. The enthesis is the anatomic transition zone where ligament attaches to bone. Inflammation in this region is the hallmark of a family of seronegative rheumatic diseases, of which ankylosing spondylitis is the prototype. Other members of this group include Reiter's syndrome, reactive arthritis, psoriatic arthritis, and the arthropathy associated with inflammatory bowel disease. All these conditions share in common the presence of the human leukocyte antigen HLA-B27. In ankylosing spondylitis, the sacroiliac joints and apophyseal joints of the spine show characteristic inflammation with a tendency to bony ankylosis. Nonsteroidal anti-inflammatory drugs (NSAID's) are usually effective, whereas prednisone is rarely needed.

Crystal-Induced Synovitis. Crystals of monosodium urate, calcium pyrophosphate, or hydroxyapatite are capable of inducing an acute inflammatory reaction in synovial fluid and joint lining. Although inflammation from these crystals may clear spontaneously, treatment with NSAID's is effective. Crystal arthritis usually affects only one or at most a few joints at a time. Joint fluid aspiration and synovianalysis for crystals using polarized light microscopy will establish the diagnosis. Calcium pyrophosphate deposition disease is often associated with the radiologic appearance of chondrocalcinosis of hyaline cartilage.

Joint Space. Septic arthritis may develop from hematogenous spread of microorganisms into the joint space. This is associated with intense pain even at rest, and the diagnosis is confirmed by joint aspiration and Gram stain and culture of synovial fluid. A joint prosthesis increases susceptibility to infection in that joint. Although systemic antibiotics are usually sufficient, arthroscopic debridement and surgical drainage may be required.

Blood in the joint space, known as "hemarthrosis," may result from microfractures, coagulopathy, or tumor.

Cartilage Degeneration. Loss of articular cartilage with bony repair leading to formation of osteophytosis is known as osteoarthritis (OA). It should be considered a final pathway for persis-

DETECTING SYNOVIAL EFFUSION: DEMONSTRATING FLUCTUATION

Four-finger technique

Two-thumb technique

⇨ pressor
➡ sensor

FIGURE 233–3. A demonstration of fluctuation for detecting a synovial effusion. An increase in fluid tension induced by finger pressure in one area is transmitted so that the sensor fingers can detect it elsewhere. In the two-thumb or four-finger technique, the pressure should be in a slightly different direction to the sensor finger to avoid false-positive results. (Reprinted courtesy Klippel JH, Dieppe PA: Rheumatology. London, Mosby–Year Book Europe, 1994, section 3, p 4.4.)

TABLE 233–2. CLASSIFICATION OF RHEUMATIC DISEASE

Category	Prototypes	Useful Tests	Treatments
Synovitis	Rheumatoid arthritis	Latex, erythrocyte sedimentation rate	Methotrexate
	Autoimmune collagen diseases	ANA test	Prednisone
Enthesopathy	Ankylosing spondylitis B27 spondyloarthropathies	Sacroiliac radiographs	Indomethacin
Crystal-induced synovitis	Gout	Joint fluid crystal examination	Indomethacin
	Pseudogout	Radiographic chondrocalcinosis Joint fluid crystal examination	Indomethacin
Joint space	Septic arthritis	Joint fluid culture	Antibiotics
Cartilage degeneration	Osteoarthritis	Radiographs of affected area	Physical therapy
			Analgesics
Osteoarticular	Avascular necrosis bone	Radiographs, magnetic resonance imaging	Prosthetic joint replacement
Polymyositis	Dermatomyositis Inclusion body myositis	Muscle enzymes, EMG, muscle biopsy	Corticosteroids
Local conditions	Tendinitis	None, radiographs of affected area	Local
General conditions	Fibromyalgia	Erythrocyte sedimentation rate	Fitness exercises

tent inflammatory conditions such as RA, ankylosing spondylitis, septic arthritis, and metabolic disorders with chondrocalcinosis. Joint hypermobility and previous trauma are other mechanical factors that may predispose to OA. Although hereditary OA may affect the distal interphalangeal (DIP) joints of the fingers, it usually only involves one or two larger joints such as a hip or knee. For this reason, OA disability can be more readily controlled by physical or orthopedic measures than RA. While NSAID's and analgesics may provide pain relief, they are largely palliative.

Osteoarticular Conditions. Avascular necrosis results after collapse of the bony end-plate from vascular insufficiency. The consequence is collapse and fragmentation of cartilage. Avascular necrosis may be associated with systemic conditions such as sickle cell disease or fatty liver after high-dose corticosteroids.

Inflammation of the periosteum, known as "periostitis," may be associated with hypertrophic pulmonary osteoarthropathy and clubbing. This syndrome may be a clue to underlying lung cancer.

Polymyositis. Inflammation and weakness of the proximal skeletal muscles are characteristic of polymyositis; with rash, it is called dermatomyositis. Elevated creatine kinase, electromyographic abnormalities, and histologic abnormalities of muscle biopsy are characteristic. Corticosteroids and immunosuppressives may control polymyositis, but older patients with dermatomyositis may have hidden malignancy and steroid resistance.

Local Conditions. Nonarticular disorders such as tendinitis, bursitis, and low-back strain are common medical problems. Local signs of inflammation are characteristic of these conditions that usually respond to physical therapy, protective splints, or injection of corticosteroids.

General Conditions. These nonarticular or extra-articular disorders are not usually associated with arthritis. This group includes polymyalgia rheumatica, sympathetic reflex dystrophy, and fibromyalgia. Polymyalgia rheumatica affects the elderly with persistent neck, shoulder, and hip pain; chronic fatigue; and high erythrocyte sedimentation rate. Sometimes it is associated with underlying giant cell and temporal arteritis. In the latter case, corticosteroids are mandatory because of the risk of blindness from ophthalmic arteritis.

"Fibromyalgia" refers to a common syndrome of widespread polyarthralgias associated with chronic fatigue and a nonrestorative sleep pattern. It is characterized by the presence of deep referred tender points described in Ch. 258.

TREATMENT CONSIDERATIONS. Treatment should be based on a correct diagnosis, which may not be initially obvious (see Table 233–2). Also important is whether the patient's problem is urgent, or whether treatment can be postponed until the diagnosis is established. For example, acute monarthritis due to sepsis or gout requires immediate attention, whereas widespread smouldering polyarthritis does not. However, a patient with polyarthritis who is systemically ill requires prompt investigation to exclude a diffuse connective tissue disease, underlying infection, or hidden malignancy.

Regardless of the diagnosis, educating the patient and family is crucial to successful management of any chronic MSK illness. The informed patient is more likely to comply with treatment and hold realistic expectations of outcome. For the patient with MSK disease, the goal of management is to maintain independence. For this reason, treatment should be individualized, based on early identification of problems, a firm diagnosis, and continued monitoring of response to treatment.

Gordon DA, Inman RD: Musculoskeletal disability and rheumatology. J Rheumatol 21:387, 1994. *This editorial draws attention to the frequency, types, risk factors, and economic impact of MSK disorders in the general population.*

Pincus T, Callahan LF, Brooks RH, et al.: Self-report questionnaire scores in rheumatoid arthritis compared with traditional physical, radiographic, and laboratory measures. Ann Intern Med 100:259, 1989. *Illustrates the value of self-report questionnaires in providing quantitative data that reflect traditional disease activity measures in arthritis patients.*

Schumacher HR (ed.): Primer on the Rheumatic Diseases. 10th ed. Atlanta, Arthritis Foundation, 1993. *Classic, authoritative, current descriptions of all rheumatic diseases and of all rheumatology, available as a public service at nominal cost.*

234 CONNECTIVE TISSUE STRUCTURE AND FUNCTION

Steffen Gay and Renate E. Gay

One of the fundamental characteristics of all connective tissues is the relatively large proportion of extracellular matrix in relation to cells. Until recently, the extracellular matrix was viewed as a passive framework serving mainly as an inert scaffolding for stabilization of the physical structure of tissues. In addition to maintaining this three-dimensional form during morphogenesis and tissue repair, it is now recognized as a dynamic milieu in which cells become organized, exchange signals, and differentiate. Study of these processes has led to discovery of a plethora of new matrix components, matrix receptors, and cell–matrix interactions. The extracellular matrix is composed of multidomain macromolecules that are linked together by covalent and noncovalent bonds to form a highly intricate composite. Two major types of matrices exist: the *interstitium,* which is synthesized by mesenchymal cells and forms the stroma of organs, and the *basement membranes,* which are produced by epithelial and endothelial cells. These matrices comprise four major classes of extracellular macromolecules: (1) the collagens, (2) elastin, (3) noncollagenous glycoproteins, and (4) glycosaminoglycans, which are usually covalently linked to proteins to form proteoglycans.

COLLAGENS. The collagens are the most abundant class of proteins in the human organism, constituting almost 30% of its total protein. The central feature of all collagen molecules is the stiff structure resulting from lengthy domains of triple-helical conformation. Three polypeptide chains, called α chains, are wound around one another to generate a ropelike fold. An absolute requirement for the formation of this triple helix, as well as the most distinctive feature of the α chains, is the presence of lengthy sequences of repeating Gly-X-Y triplets in which the X and Y positions are frequently occupied by prolyl and hydroxyprolyl residues.

Studies based on protein chemistry and complementary DNA (cDNA) sequencing have revealed a genetically determined heterogeneity with as many as 19 homopolymeric or heteropolymeric collagen types. As of this writing, 30 unique polypeptide chains have been identified. It is of interest that genes coding for the different chains are distributed among at least 12 chromosomes in the human genome (Table 234–1). Even simultaneously expressed genes, such as those coding for the two $\alpha_1(I)$ and one $\alpha_2(I)$ chains of the heteropolymeric type I molecule, are located on different chromosomes.

Functional diversity of the various collagen types is accomplished by formation of distinct extracellular aggregates. The most obvious are the interstitial linear polymers of fibrils, derived from collagen types I, II, and III. These fibrils with characteristic banding patterns can be visualized readily by electron microscopy. Type I collagen fibers are found in supporting elements of high tensile strength (e.g., tendon and cornea), whereas fibers formed from type II collagen molecules are restricted to cartilaginous structures. The fibrils derived from type III collagen are prevalent in more distensible tissues, such as blood vessels and parenchymal organs. In addition, collagen types V, VI, IX, and XII are also involved in fiber formation, but largely as adducts. This finding is illustrated by the association of collagen types IX, X, and XI with type II collagen in hyaline cartilage. Knockout experiments of the $\alpha_1(IX)$ gene in transgenic mice indicate that a lack of functional type IX collagen results in the development of a mild chondrodysplasia and osteoarthritis in these animals. Adaptation for a special function is shown by type VII collagen molecules, which aggregate as antiparallel overlapping dimers to form the anchoring fibrils required to stabilize the dermoepithelial junction of the skin. In contrast to the interstitial types of collagen, type IV molecules form large polygonal aggregates fulfilling the structural and support requirements of basement membranes.

ELASTIN. Elastic fibers are composed of two morphologically and structurally distinct components: elastin and the microfibrils. Elastin, whose gene has now been characterized, is an insoluble protein polymer. The biosynthetic precursor of elastin, tropoelastin, is a linear polypeptide composed of about 700 amino acids and is rich in nonpolar amino acids: glycine (>30%), valine, leucine, isoleucine, and alanine. Tropoelastin is synthesized by vascular smooth muscle cells and skin fibroblasts and subsequently incorporated into elastic fibers. Elastic fiber formation involves lysyloxidase-mediated formation of intermolecular crosslinks, called *desmosine* and *isodesmosine*. Since these crosslinks do not exist in other proteins and therefore are elastin-specific, determination of these two amino acid derivatives in tissue sample reflects the amount of elastin present. The microfibrillar components of interstitial elastic fibers are not fully characterized. However, disulfide-rich glycoproteins, such as *fibrillin* and *microfibril-associated glycoprotein* (MAGP) have been identified and may serve as a scaffold onto which tropoelastin is deposited.

STRUCTURAL GLYCOPROTEINS. The major noncollagenous glycoprotein present in the extracellular matrix is *fibronectin*. Fibronectins are dimeric cell adhesion glycoproteins composed of two disulfide-bonded subunits and found in rather large quantities in blood plasma (~0.3 mg per milliliter). The functions of fibronectin in cell adhesion are illustrated in Figure 234–1. Some of these functions can be mimicked by synthetic peptides that contain the sequence Arg-Gly-Asp (RGD sequence). Similar sequences are found in other cell adhesion proteins, such as vitronectin, laminin, and collagen type VI. Since fibronectin plays a major role in morphogenesis and tissue remodeling, the regulation of fibronectin biosynthesis by growth factors and cytokines has been

TABLE 234–1. POLYMORPHISM OF THE COLLAGEN TYPES

Type	Chain(s)	Major Molecular Species	Major Distribution
I	$\alpha_1(I)$ $\alpha_2(I)$	$[\alpha_1(I)]_2\alpha_2(I)$	Skin, tendon, bone, organ capsules
II	$\alpha_1(II)$	$[\alpha_1(II)]_3$	Hyaline cartilage
III	$\alpha_1(III)$	$[\alpha_1(III)]_3$	Blood vessels, parenchymal organs
IV	$\alpha_1(IV)$ $\alpha_2(IV)$ $\alpha_3(IV)$ $\alpha_4(IV)$ $\alpha_5(IV)$	$[\alpha_1(IV)]_2\alpha_2(IV)$	Basement membranes
V	$\alpha_1(V)$ $\alpha_2(V)$ $\alpha_3(V)$	$[\alpha_1(V)]_2\alpha_2(V)$	Smooth muscle
VI	$\alpha_1(VI)$ $\alpha_2(VI)$ $\alpha_3(VI)$	$[\alpha_1(VI),\alpha_2(VI),\alpha_3(VI)]$	Minor collagen of stroma matrices
VII	$\alpha_1(VII)$	$[\alpha_1(VII)]_3$	Anchoring fibrils of the dermoepidermal junction
VIII	$\alpha_1(VIII)$	$[\alpha_1(VIII)]_3$	Descemet's membrane, sclera, dura mater
IX	$\alpha_1(IX)$ $\alpha_2(IX)$ $\alpha_3(IX)$	$[\alpha_1(IX),\alpha_2(IX),\alpha_3(IX)]$	Hyaline cartilage
X	$\alpha_1(X)$	$[\alpha_1(X)]_3$	Hypertrophic cartilage
XI	$\alpha_1(XI)$ $\alpha_2(XI)$ $\alpha_1(II)$	$[\alpha_1(XI),\alpha_2(XI),\alpha_3(XI)]$	Hyaline cartilage
XII	$\alpha_1(XII)$		Tendons, ligaments, periosteum, skin, cartilage
XIII	$\alpha_1(XIII)$		Skin, gut
XIV	$\alpha_1(XIV)$		Skin, tendon, placenta, fetal cartilage
XV	$\alpha_1(XV)$		Fibroblasts
XVI	$\alpha_1(XVI)$		Placenta, fibroblasts
XVII	$\alpha_1(XVII)$		BP180 autoantigen in bullous pemphigoid
XVIII	$\alpha_1(XVIII)$		Liver, kidney, placenta

FIGURE 234-1. Multiple cell recognition sites in fibronectin. The fibronectin molecule contains a series of functional domains that bind the indicated ligands. The thick vertical bars indicate cell adhesive recognition sequences. SS = putative synergistic second site; RGD = Gly-Arg-Gly-Asp-Ser site; H = putative sites in the heparin-binding domain; CS1 = the CS1 site in the alternatively spliced IIICS region; REDV = the Arg-Glu-Asp-Val site. (Reprinted with permission from Yamada KM: Fibronectins: Structure, functions and receptors. Curr Opin Cell Biol 1:956–963, 1989. Copyright 1989 by Current Science.)

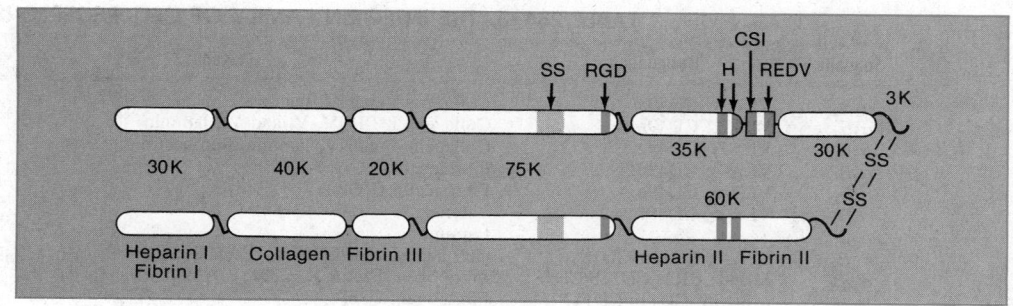

studied. For example, it is established that γ-interferon and transforming growth factor β (TGF-β) stimulate fibronectin synthesis, whereas tumor necrosis factor (TNF) and interleukin-1 (IL-1) inhibit synthesis.

Vitronectin is a 75-kD protein, which is considerably smaller than the 250-kD fibronectin polypeptide present in plasma and tissue. Vitronectin, also termed "serum spreading factor" and "complement S-protein," promotes cell attachment and spreading, inhibits cytolysis by the complement C5b–9 complex, and modulates antithrombin III–thrombin action in blood coagulation.

Tenascin is another large glycoprotein of the extracellular matrix. The previous other name *hexabrachion* refers to the disulfide-linked six-armed structure. Tenascin mediates cell attachment through an RGD-dependent receptor and is expressed in association with mesenchymal-epithelial interactions during morphogenesis and development of undifferentiated tumors. The same protein also has been referred to as myotendinous antigen, GP 250 protein, glial mesenchymal extracellular matrix protein, cytotactin, J1-protein, and brachionectin. As the names suggest, tenascin has been identified in tendons, development of smooth muscle, cartilage, and gut and in neuromuscular and neuronal-glial interactions. On the other hand, gene knockout experiments suggest that tenascin might be a superfluous nonfunctional protein and that other tenascin-like proteins, such as MHC-tenascin encoded in the human MHC class III regions, may compensate for the absence of tenascin.

Cartilage Glycoproteins. Several structural glycoproteins have been isolated from various cartilages. They include a 550-kD disulfide-bonded cartilage matrix glycoprotein (CMGP) composed of cartilage oligomeric protein (COMP) as well as two distinct 58-kD and 36-kD proteins. Fibromodulin, a 59-kD protein, and a 21-kD cell surface cartilage protein called "anchorin" are also localized in articular cartilage. In contrast, a 148-kD cartilage matrix protein (CMP) is prominent in adult tracheal cartilage but not present in articular cartilage.

PROTEOGLYCANS. Proteoglycans are proteins that carry one or more glycosaminoglycan side chains. Glycosaminoglycans are long, unbranched polysaccharide chains composed of repeating disaccharide units. One of the two sugar residues in the repeating disaccharide is always an amino sugar (N-acetylglucosamine or N-acetylgalactosamine). Glycosaminoglycans are highly negatively charged owing to the presence of sulfate and carboxyl groups on multiple sugar residues. In contrast, hyaluronic acid, also called *hyaluronan,* is a polymer of glucuronic acid and glucosamine that is not sulfated and not attached covalently to a protein core connected via a link protein. Proteoglycans of almost all sizes and shapes have been biochemically identified. Nevertheless, since cloning and sequence analysis have often identified the same core proteins, the number of distinct proteoglycans is limited (Table 234–2). With respect to their function, they have been referred to as a "multipurpose glue." Proteoglycans not only bind extracellular matrix components together and mediate cell binding to the matrix but also restrain soluble molecules such as growth factors in the matrix and at cell surfaces. Heparan sulfate proteoglycan, for example, binds basic fibroblast growth factor released from injured endothelial cells. The role of proteoglycans in cell

adhesion is best exhibited by a membrane-intercalated proteoglycan termed *syndecan.* This molecule binds to collagen and fibronectin through its heparan sulfate chains and mediates cell adhesion. Certain proteoglycans contain functional domains that are common for all the members of the aggrecan/versican family. These domains share further functional domains with other important proteins and include an immunoglobulin-like, epidermal growth factor–like, and complement regulatory protein–like sequence.

BASEMENT MEMBRANES. Basement membranes are thin, sheetlike structures deposited by endothelial and epithelial cells but also found surrounding nerve and muscle cells. They provide mechanical support for resident cells, function as a semipermeable filtration barrier for macromolecules in organs such as the kidney and the placenta, and act as regulators of cell attachment, migra-tion, and differentiation. The major constituents are collagen type IV, laminin, entactin (nidogen), and heparan sulfate proteoglycans. Collagen type IV molecules are $[\alpha_1(IV)]_2 \, \alpha_2(IV)$ heterotrimers comprising an N-terminal rod 30 μm long (7S), a linear triple helix containing over 20 noncollagenous sequences, and a C-terminal globular domain (NC1). These molecules can spontaneously aggregate into a network consisting of N-terminal tetramers (7S), lateral associations between the triple-helical rods, and C-terminal dimers (NC1). The network is eventually stabilized by disulfide- and lysyl oxidase–derived intramolecular and intermolecular crosslinks, which may provide the scaffold for basement membrane formation. Self-assembly also has been observed with *laminin,* a major basement membrane–associated glycoprotein. The typical features of the laminin molecule are a threadlike long arm terminating in a globular domain and three short arms, each con-sisting of two globular domains separated by short linear segments. Collagen type IV and laminin appear highly integrated in the basement membrane matrix and are closely associated with a 150-kD, sulfated glycoprotein called *entactin*

TABLE 234-2. STRUCTURAL FEATURES OF PROTEOGLYCANS

Location	Proteoglycan	GAG* (Number)
Extracellular matrix	Aggrecan	CS/KS (>100)
	Versican	CS/DS (20)
	Decorin	CS or DS (1)
	Biglycan	CS or DS (2)
	Fibromodulin	KS (4)
Cell surface	Syndecan	HS/CS (4)
	Betaglycan	HS/CS (2)
	CD44	HS or CS
	Glypican	HS
	Fibroglycan	HS
Intracellular	Serglycin	CS or Hep (8)
Basement membrane	Perlecan	HS (3)
Brain	Brevican	CS/DS (3)
	Neurocan	CS (7)
	Cerebroglycan	HS (5)

* Glycosaminoglycan (GAG) chains: HS = heparan sulfate; CS = chondroitin sulfate; Hep = heparin; KS = keratan sulfate; DS = dermatan sulfate.

TABLE 234-3. THE INTEGRIN FAMILY OF CELL RECEPTORS*

Subunits	Designation	Ligands	Distribution
$\alpha_1\beta_1$	VLA-1; CD49a	Collagens I and IV, laminin	F, BM, aT
$\alpha_2\beta_1$	VLA-2; CD49b	Collagens I, III, IV, V, and VI, laminin	F, En, Ep, aT, Pl
$\alpha_3\beta_1$	VLA-3; CD49c	Collagens I and IV, laminin, fibronectin	F, Ep
$\alpha_4\beta_1$	VLA-4; CD49d	Fibronectin, VCAM-1	F, Nc, T, B, M
$\alpha_5\beta_1$	VLA-5; CD49e	Fibronectin (RGD)	F, En, Ep, aT, Th
$\alpha_6\beta_1$	VLA-6; CD49f	Laminin	En
$\alpha_7\beta_1$		Laminin	En
$\alpha_L\beta_2$	LFA-1; CD11a/CD18	Cell adhesion molecules (ICAM-1, 2)	T, B, M, G
$\alpha_M\beta_2$	Mac-1; CR3; CD11b/CD18	Fibrinogen, Factor X, C3bi, ICAM-1	M, G
$\alpha_X\beta_2$	p150,95; CD11c/CD18	Fibrinogen, C3bi	M, G
$\alpha_{IIb}\beta_3$	gpIIb, IIIa; CD41/CD61	Fibronectin, fibrinogen, von Willebrand factor, thrombospondin	Pl
$\alpha_V\beta_3$	VNR; CD51/CD61	Fibrinogen, von Willebrand factor, vitronectin, thrombospondin	En
$\alpha_6\beta_4$	CD104	—	Ec
$\alpha_V\beta_5$	CD51/CD-	Vitronectin (RGD)	Ca

* Cloning of the α and β subunits has revealed cell surface proteins on other cells. These include the very late activation (VLA) antigens and the lymphocyte function–associated antigen 1 (LFA-1)/Mac-1/p 150.95 on leukocytes and the platelet IIb/IIIa glycoprotein.
F = fibroblasts; BM = basement membrane associated; aT = activated T lymphocytes only; En = endothelial cells; Ep = epithelial cells; Pl = platelets; Nc = neural crest melanocytes; T = T lymphocytes; B = B lymphocytes; M = monocytes; Th = thymocytes; G = granulocytes; Ca = UCLA-P3 lung adenocarcinoma cells.
Data from Springer TA: Adhesion receptors regulate antigen-specific interactions, localization, and differentiation in the immune system. Prog Immunol Springer 7:121–130, 1989; Hynes RO: Integrins: Versatility, modulation, and signaling in cell adhesion. Cell 69:11–25, 1992; and Schlossman SF, et al.: CD antigens 1993. J Immunol 52:1, 1994.

(nidogen) in a stable noncovalent complex. Amino acid sequence data of entactin have revealed epidermal growth factor (EGF)–like cysteine-rich motifs, segments showing homology to the EGF precursor, the low-density lipoprotein (LDL) receptor, and thyroglobulin. *Heparan sulfate proteoglycans* occur as an integral component in all basement membranes but play different roles in specific tissues. They control permeability of the glomeru-lar basement membranes and also have been implicated in the anchorage of acetylcholinesterase to the neuromuscular junction.

CONNECTIVE TISSUE MATRIX IN CELL REGULATION

It is well established that matrix components influence the maintenance of cellular phenotypes mediated through matrix receptors.
RECEPTORS FOR EXTRACELLULAR MATRIX COMPONENTS. Adhesive interactions between cells and their surrounding extracellular matrix are not only important in most developmental events but also essential for maintaining the fundamental life processes. Cell proliferation, polarization, migration, differentiation, and protein synthesis depend on interactions between cells and supporting matrix. Diverse families of structurally similar receptors for matrix components have been identified. They include the transmembrane integrin superfamily, peripheral membrane glycoproteins, glycosyltransferases, and proteoglycans. *Integrins* are a group of α/β heterodimers involved in cell binding, some of which involve recognition of an RGD sequence present in their ligands. The integrins consist of an α subunit with a molecular mass of 130 to 210 kD and noncovalently associated β subunits (95 to 130 kD). The cytoplasmic domain of the β subunit reveals homologies to the EGF, the insulin receptor, and the *neu* oncogene protein. Both subunits define the integrin subfamilies described in Table 234-3.

Since integrins localize in known junctional regions where actin bundles and myofibrils terminate at the cell surface, the major function of integrin receptors appears to be the linkage of extracellular matrix molecules with the intracellular cytoskeletal network. The connection is thereby mediated through the cytoplasmic domain of the subunits. That extracellular matrix components may influence gene expression by signal transduction is shown by the finding that fibronectin degradation products induce, via the fibronectin receptor, collagenase and stromelysin gene expression. The latter pathway may play a major role in inflammatory tissue destruction. The pivotal role of these receptors related to infectious diseases is further illustrated by the observation that bacteria use specific receptors to adhere to host connective tissue. For example, it has been shown that certain strains of *Es-*

cherichia coli express a fibronectin receptor that is involved in colonization.

The most provoking question remains: How do matrix receptors transmit information from the extracellular structure to affect gene expression? Figure 234–2 illustrates a model of "dynamic reciprocity," in which the extracellular matrix is postulated to influence gene expression at all levels, including transcription, messenger RNA (mRNA) processing, and translation, via transmembrane and cytoskeletal components. Elucidating the molecular mechanisms of this message system remains one of the key challenges in cell biology.

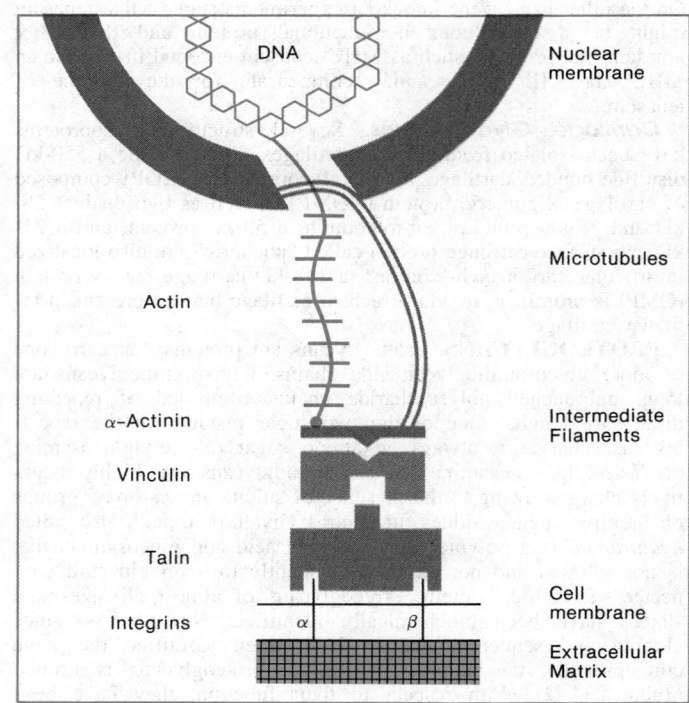

FIGURE 234-2. This refined model for the ultrastructural interaction of cells with extracellular matrix is based on a model of "dynamic reciprocity" whereby the extracellular matrix is postulated to exert an influence on gene expression via transmembrane proteins and cytoskeletal components, proposed originally by Bissell and Carcellos-Hoff (J Cell Sci Suppl 8:??7, 1987).

Some confusion remains about the role of collagen in a variety of diseases involving the connective tissues. Historically, the term "collagen disease"—describing a heterogeneous group of acute and chronic diseases, including rheumatoid arthritis, systemic lupus erythematosus, progressive systemic sclerosis, polymyositis, dermatomyositis, Sjögren's syndrome, arteritis, rheumatic fever, ankylosing spondylitis, and amyloidosis—was based on the erroneous notion that "collagen" was equivalent to "connective tissue." However, as outlined above, the different types of collagen and the macromolecular aggregates derived from them are now recognized as distinct structural and histologic entities that exist within a meticulously intercalated connective tissue matrix along with structural glycoproteins and proteoglycans. Consequently, no justification exists for using the anachronistic term "collagen disease" to encompass a group of such diseases initiated by vastly different pathomechanisms and affecting distinct connective tissue entities. The term "collagen diseases" now exclusively pertains to those inherited conditions in which the primary defect has been demonstrated to be at the gene level and to affect collagen biosynthesis, posttranslational modification, or extracellular processing directly. Recent technologies of gene cloning and gene analysis have led to the delineation of mutations in the fibrillar collagen genes. Collagen type I is the target of certain genetic mutations associated with classic clinical variants of dwarfing syndromes, osteogenesis imperfecta, and Ehlers-Danlos syndrome (types IV and VII) (see Ch. 182, 184, and 185). Moreover, polymerase chain reaction amplification of a series of overlapping segments encoding for the entire helical and telepeptide regions of the human α_1(I) collagen cDNA is expected to identify potentially all mutations and polymorphisms.

The acquired disorders of connective tissue involving collagen include conditions that result in repair from overt trauma; in diseases characterized by an excessive deposition of collagenous matrix, i.e., fibroproliferative disorders, or in pathologic loss of tissue matrix, including the breakdown of basement membranes in tumor invasion and rheumatoid joint destruction.

Although connective tissue repair after trauma largely depends on the type of injury and is, therefore, quite variable, the repair of various connective tissue lesions in wound healing follows a characteristic sequence of events. The initial events involve the synthesis of pericellular and basement membrane collagens in the proliferating epithelial and/or endothelial cells. Subsequently, a loose fibrillar network largely comprising fibronectin and collagen types III and V and single interspersed fibers derived from type I collagen are deposited. Finally, with the formation of scar tissue, the lesions become more fibrous and dense owing to a deposition of collagen fiber bundles derived largely from type I molecules. It is striking that the patterns of collagen deposition in fibroproliferative diseases show certain similarities. For example, liver damage is characterized by an initial accumulation of basement membrane collagens in the sinusoidal space of Disse, followed by a fine fibrillar material composed largely of type III collagen and, subsequently, in the case of the development of hepatic fibrosis (cirrhosis, Ch. 122), by an augmented deposition of type I collagen. A similar pattern appears in the development of fibrotic plaques in atherosclerosis (Ch. 40) or of cyclosporine-induced myocardial fibrosis in the transplanted human heart.

The major disease affecting almost exclusively the matrix of basement membranes is diabetes mellitus (Ch. 205). The histopathologic hallmark of diabetic microvascular disease is generalized basement membrane thickening. In the kidney, these changes include an increase in glomerular basement membrane permeability followed by decreased glomerular filtration. Evidence exists that accelerated nonenzymatic glycosylation (glycation) plays an important role in the development of diabetic microangiopathy.

The loss of a specialized connective tissue matrix plays a pivotal role in tumor progression and metastasis. With proliferation, malignant tumor cells acquire the capability to invade basement membranes actively and to migrate through the interstitial stroma. Despite the fact that tumor invasion requires a complex sequence of steps, such as the expression of receptors for basement membrane components by the malignant cells, invasion ultimately results in a loss of basement membrane integrity (Fig. 234–3). Severe recessive dystrophic epidermolysis bullosa features a loss of collagen type

VII anchoring filaments, which normally connect the epidermal basement membrane to the interstitial matrix of the dermis. In Goodpasture's syndrome, basement membranes are damaged by circulating autoantibodies against basement membrane collagen (Ch. 79). The Goodpasture antigen has been mapped to the C-terminal globular domain of type IV collagen, which explains the high cross-reactivity of the anti–glomerular basement membrane antibodies with alveolar basement membranes.

CONNECTIVE TISSUE MARKERS. The enormous progress in our knowledge of the structure and biology of the connective tissue matrix has caused considerable interest in the development of assays for diagnosis and monitoring therapy in diseases involving connective tissue. Historically, the determination of hydroxyproline as a measure of total collagen content or turnover has been a useful technique in connective tissue research. However, with the discovery of collagen polymorphism and a variety of molecules containing collagenous sequences, the measurement of hydroxyproline now appears to be of only limited value. This observation is based on the fact that there are varying levels of hydroxylation of the different collagens. For example, the type III collagen molecule contains about 30% more hydroxyproline than does type I, and other proteins such as C1q, acetylcholinesterase, and elastin also contain hydroxyproline. Specific immunohistologic and immunoserologic assays have been used to evaluate the complexity of collagenous proteins in normal and pathologic samples. As illustrated in Figure 234–3, using a monoclonal antibody specific for collagen type IV has been advantageous in studies assessing the integrity of basement membranes in neoplastic lesions. Several markers of collagen assembly and turnover have been employed to detect injury to a specific parenchymal organ or to diagnose organ fibrosis by noninvasive immunoserologic assays. The most widely applied test so far has been a radioimmunoassay to detect the N-terminal propeptide of type III procollagen in body fluids. The utility of this test was based on the notion that the propeptide is removed from type III procollagen molecules after synthesis to form new collagen fibrils. However, procollagen molecules may retain their propeptide as a part of the normal extracellular matrix. Thus the presence of the propeptide in serum may be related not only to neosynthesis but also to degradation from a preexisting matrix. Since both processes affect the results of this assay, increased levels of type III procollagen peptide have been reported in fibrotic diseases, i.e., liver cirrhosis, myelofibrosis, and lung fibrosis, and also have been correlated with destructive inflammation, such as that in acute viral hepatitis.

The development of molecular markers for joint diseases has focused on the immunochemical quantification of cartilage compo-

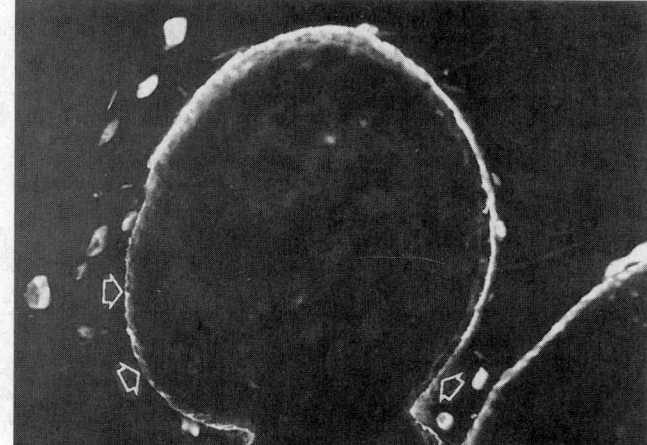

FIGURE 234–3. Frozen section of carcinoma *in situ* of the breast stained with monoclonal antibodies against human collagen type IV and fluorescence-labeled immunoglobulin antimouse G (IgG). In contrast to other atypical hyperplastic lesions, a thinning and focal loss of basement membrane integrity *(arrows)* is frequently observed in carcinoma *in situ* and suggests foci of preceding microinvasion.

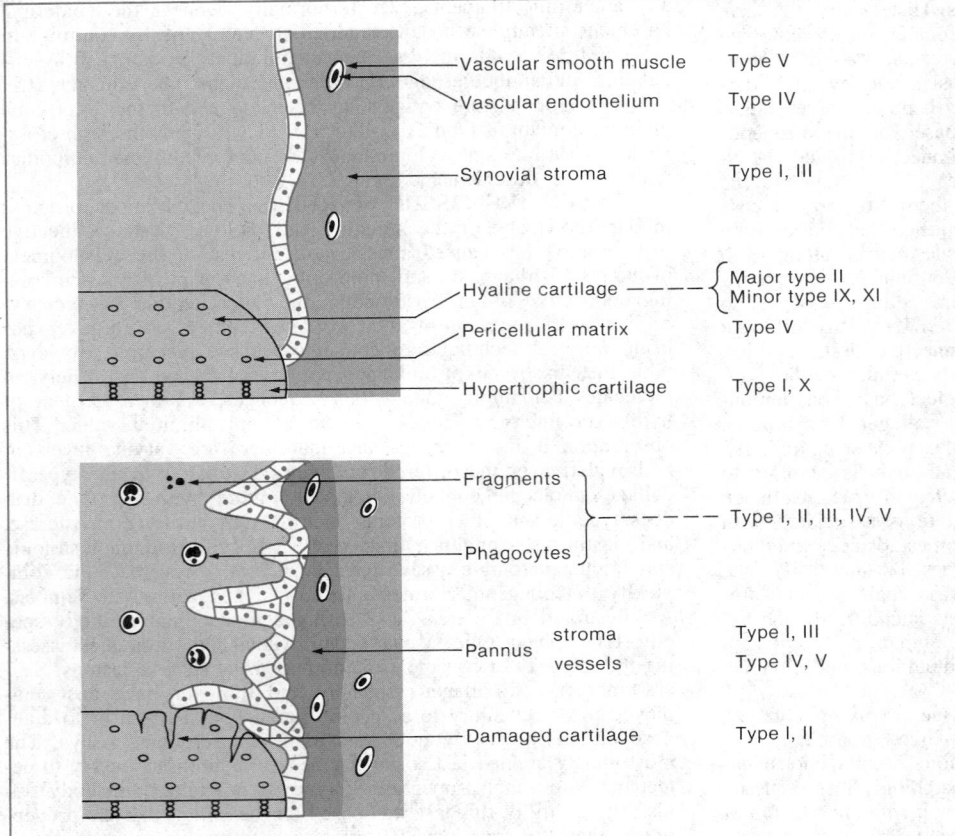

Vascular smooth muscle	Type V
Vascular endothelium	Type IV
Synovial stroma	Type I, III
Hyaline cartilage	{ Major type II / Minor type IX, XI }
Pericellular matrix	Type V
Hypertrophic cartilage	Type I, X
Fragments } Type I, II, III, IV, V	
Phagocytes	
Pannus stroma	Type I, III
Pannus vessels	Type IV, V
Damaged cartilage	Type I, II

FIGURE 234-4. Distribution of collagen types in a normal and rheumatoid joint. The normal synovial lining cell layer is supported by a loose fibrillar network composed of interstitial collagen types I and III, but lacking a continuous basement membrane. Basement membrane collagen type IV is restricted to the vascular endothelium. Vascular smooth muscle cells and pericytes are surrounded with fine, filamentous collagen type V, which is further associated with the interstitial fibers. The vast majority of the interstitial cartilaginous matrix is derived from type II collagen. Collagen types V, IX, and XI are distinctly associated with the hyaline articular interstitium. Synovial fluid normally does not contain collagen. Therefore, detection of collagen in synovial fluid and phagocytes indicates erosive and/or inflammatory joint disease. Detection of type IV collagen suggests endothelial damage and, if found concomitantly with type V collagen, implicates actual necrosis of the vessel walls, i.e., vasculitis. The detection of type I collagen indicates a high level of proteolytic breakdown of synovial stroma and/or bone matrix. Since type II collagen is restricted to the cartilage, the appearance of type II collagen epitopes in synovial fluid and serum represents a sensitive indicator of cartilage destruction and may serve as a tool for monitoring the effects and side effects of antirheumatoid drug therapy. (Reprinted with permission from Gay S, Gay RE: Cellular basis and oncogene expression of rheumatoid joint destruction. Rheumatol Int 9:105–113, 1989.)

nents using specific antibodies. In this regard, cartilage proteoglycan core protein and glycoproteins have been studied in serum and synovial fluid from patients with various arthritides. Keratan sulfate has been assayed as a marker of cartilage metabolism, and collagen type II as a marker of cartilage destruction (Fig. 234–4).

Bernfield M, Kokenyesi R, Kato M, et al.: Biology of the syndecans: A family of transmembrane heparan sulfate proteoglycans. Annu Rev Cell Biol 8:365, 1992. *This review article on a specialized novel structural proteoglycan supplements the review by Hardingham and Fosang.*

Christiano AM, Uitto J: Molecular pathology of the elastic fibers. J Invest Dermatol 103:55 (Suppl), 1994. *Provides the most updated information on structure and pathology of elastin.*

Hardingham TE, Fosang AJ: Proteoglycans: Many forms and many functions. FASEB J 6:861, 1992. *A concise survey of proteoglycans as modifiers of the organization of the extracellular matrices and modulators of the processes that occur there.*

Kivirikko KL: Collagens and their abnormalities in a wide spectrum of diseases. Ann Med 25:113, 1993. *Reviews mutations of the distinct collagen types and their putative role in connective tissue diseases.*

Lin CQ, Bissell MJ: Multifaceted regulation of cell differentiation by extracellular matrix. FASEB J 1993;7:737. *Summarizes the current data in which the extracellular matrix has been shown to be a crucial regulator of tissue-specific gene expression.*

Mayne R, Brewton RG: New members of the collagen superfamily. Curr Opin Cell Biol 5:883, 1993. *A concise review of previously described new collagen types XII–XIX.*

Miller EJ, Gay S: Collagen structure and function. *In* Wound Healing—Biochemical and Clinical Aspects. Philadelphia, WB Saunders, 1992, pp. 130–151. *An in-depth review on the biochemistry of collagens.*

Williams MJ, Hughes PE, O'Toole TE, Ginsberg MH: The inner world of cell adhesion: Integrin cytoplasmic domains. Trends Cell Biol 4:109, 1994. *A novel presentation of the integrin family of transmembrane receptors for transfer of signals across the cell membrane.*

Yamada H, Watanabe K, Shimonaka M, Yamaguchi Y: Molecular cloning of brevican, a novel brain proteoglycan of the aggrecan/versican family. J Biol Chem 269: 10119, 1994. *An example of the kind of experimental approaches currently applied to discover novel matrix components such as brevican and neurocan of the brain.*

235 TISSUE INJURY IN RHEUMATIC DISEASES

Gerald Weissmann

Acute inflammation and tissue injury in the rheumatic diseases are caused by host defense mechanisms that are designed to attack bacteria or viruses but become diverted instead into attacking the tissues of the host. The two major inflammatory diseases of rheumatology are rheumatoid arthritis (RA) and systemic lupus erythematosus (SLE), and we understand their pathophysiology thanks to three well-studied models of experimental pathology. Whereas some of their *acute* lesions resemble the Arthus and the Shwartzman reactions, in which neutrophils play the key role, the *chronic* features of RA mimic another model of experimental pathology, the tuberculin reaction and its late granuloma formation, in which cytokines, growth factors, and activated macrophages predominate. Joint injury and cartilage degradation result when synovial cells with activated proto-oncogenes form an invasive lesion called *pannus.*

THE ARTHUS LESION AS A MODEL FOR RHEUMATOID ARTHRITIS. Following the prescient observation of Magendie in 1839 that the second and third intravenous (IV) injections of foreign proteins into rabbits were followed by increasing distress, Richet coined the word "anaphylaxis" in 1902 to describe acute catastrophes mediated by repeated IV injections of antigens. Arthus, in 1903, then provoked "local anaphylaxis" in rabbits by repeated injections of antigen intradermally; inflammation and necrosis resulted. Opie, in 1924, confirmed that the lesions of Arthus were local antigen-antibody reactions in which inflammation was mediated by white cells and that proteolysis was crucial. Indeed, it was found that the Arthus lesions also could be provoked by planting antigen in the skin followed by specific antibody intravenously (the "passive Arthus reaction") or by injecting antibody in the skin followed by antigen intravenously (the "reversed passive Arthus reaction") (Fig. 235–1). In each case, one was dealing with the interactions at a surface of neutrophils that had been attracted by immune complexes localized beneath the endothelium of blood vessels. Comple-

ment, activated by immune complexes, releases anaphylatoxins (C5a and C3a), which liberate histamine. Histamine, in turn, causes reversible gaps to appear between endothelial cells, and once breached, the junctions permit egress of neutrophils. Stimulated by discrete receptors for C5a, C3a, and IgG's (FcγRII, FcγRIII), neutrophils release mediators of inflammation: reactive oxygen-derived products (O$_2^-$, H$_2$O$_2$), eicosanoids (see Ch. 19), and lysosomal enzymes. These products—especially superoxide (O$_2^-$), peroxide (H$_2$O$_2$), and proteases—cause irreversible tissue injury. Predictably, Arthus reactions can be abolished by rendering animals deficient in complement or in neutrophils. Antiproteases or antihistamines are somewhat less effective inhibitors of the Arthus lesion; antiplatelet agents or anticoagulants are useless. It is generally agreed that the local Arthus lesion is one model for immune complex vasculitis in humans, which is also due to interactions of neutrophils with immune complexes and complement. In generalized vasculitis of the Arthus type, the *homotypic* clumping of neutrophils to each other and their *heterotypic* sticking to endothelial cells are mediated by receptors for iC3b (CD11b/CD18), whereas the secretory responses of neutrophils are triggered by receptors for C5a and FcγRII.

The central role of neutrophils in this lesion is mirrored by their abundance in the synovial fluid of patients with RA. Their role in *periarteritis nodosa, leukocytoclastic vasculitis,* some of the *vasculitides of SLE,* and *allergic angiitis* is equally important. Although the *raison d'être* for the preponderance of neutrophils in rheumatoid synovial fluid is not yet clear, their sheer number is impressive. Neutrophils comprise over 90% of cells found in the synovial fluid of patients with RA, and it has been estimated that the daily turnover of neutrophils in 30 ml of a rheumatoid joint effusion is greater than a billion cells per joint. The cells take up self-associating complexes of IgG–IgG rheumatoid factor as well as the more common IgM/IgG complexes; complement is, predictably, activated. *Rheumatoid vasculitis* is another extra-articular problem mediated by neutrophils in seropositive *RA* patients.

THE SHWARTZMAN PHENOMENON AS ANOTHER MODEL OF VASCULITIS. Culture filtrates of gram-negative bacteria injected into the skin of rabbits prepare the site for hemorrhagic necrosis when similar filtrates are injected intravenously, a finding first made by Gregory Shwartzman in 1937. The two lesions require a latent, or "preparatory," period of 6 to 24 hours, and the second injection need not be of the same filtrate (Fig. 235–1). The systemic or generalized Shwartzman phenomenon provokes variable degrees of pulmonary or systemic vasculitis and bilateral renal cortical necrosis as its signature. Like the local lesion, it can be faithfully reproduced by purified endotoxins. Locally or systemically, the "preparatory" injection of endotoxin promotes modest adhesion of neutrophils to postcapillary venules with escape of some of the white cells from the vessels. The second, or "provocative," injection leads to microclumps of platelets and leukocytes within the circulation, and these tend to be sequestered in peripheral capillary beds or to attach to the sticky endothelium of venules of the prepared skin site.

The Shwartzman phenomenon can be elicited by second injections not only of endotoxin but also of various polyanions, glycogen, or antigen/antibody complexes, all of which share with endotoxin the capacity to activate complement via the alternative pathway. Moreover, local and systemic Shwartzman reactions can be prevented by rendering animals deficient in complement or neutrophils. In contrast to their inefficacy in the Arthus lesion, anticoagulants and antiplatelet drugs block the local and systemic Shwartzman phenomena. The final Shwartzman lesion is an intravascular insult with secondary damage to endothelial cells. It should be emphasized that the Shwartzman lesion is therefore an exception to the usual circumstances in which neutrophils fail to injure the endothelial cell layer from which they escape in response to chemoattractants.

Our modern interpretation of the Shwartzman phenomenon is based on recent studies with endotoxin tumor necrosis factor alpha (TNF-α) and cellular adhesive molecules displayed by activated endothelial cells and neutrophils. Both in the local and the systemic lesion, endotoxin elicits the formation of interleukin-1 (IL-1) by Langerhans cells, endothelial cells, or tissue histiocytes and of IL-1 and TNF-α from macrophages. These cytokines render venous en-

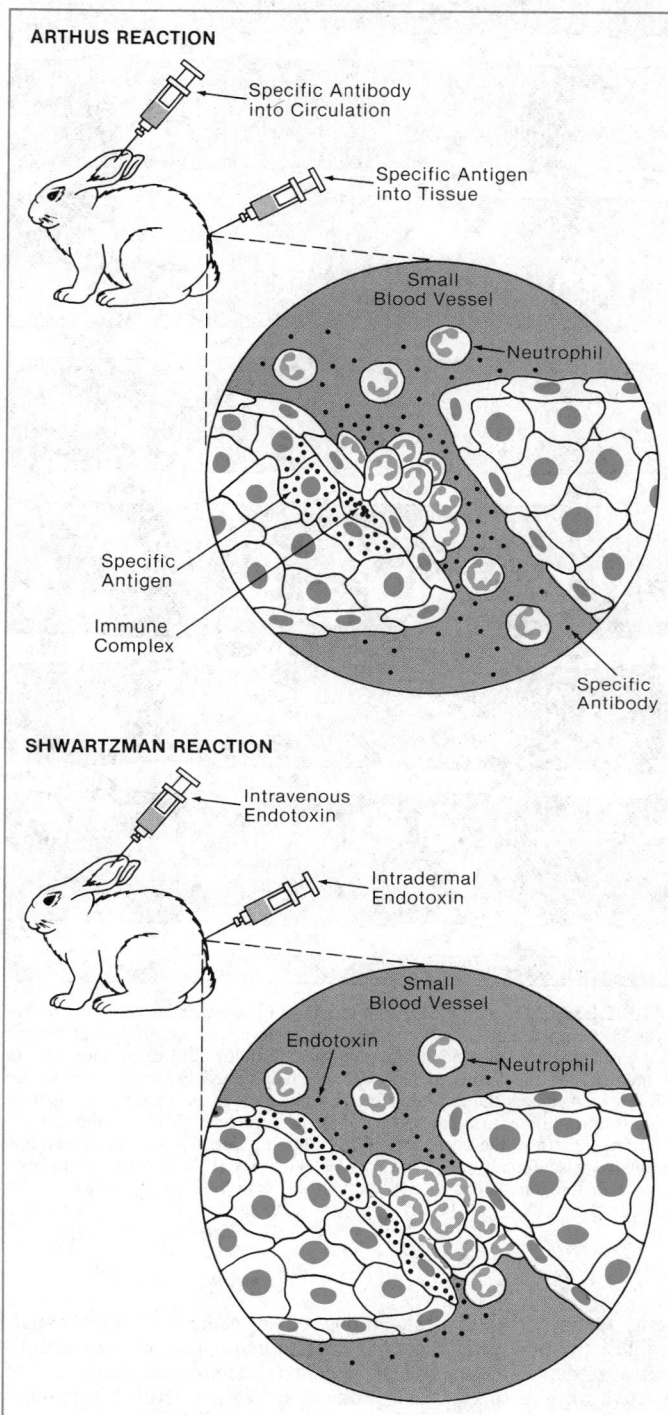

ARTHUS REACTION

Specific Antibody into Circulation

Specific Antigen into Tissue

Small Blood Vessel

Neutrophil

Specific Antigen

Immune Complex

Specific Antibody

SHWARTZMAN REACTION

Intravenous Endotoxin

Intradermal Endotoxin

Small Blood Vessel

Endotoxin

Neutrophil

FIGURE 235–1. In the Arthus model of vascular injury in SLE *(top)*, intradermal injection of an antigen following intravenous injection of specific antibody leads to immune complex (IC) deposition in vessel walls at the intradermal injection site, which triggers local complement activation, inflammation, neutrophil infiltration, and tissue destruction. In the Shwartzman model *(bottom)*, an intradermal injection of the antigen leads to intravascular alternate pathway complement activation. Antibody is not required, and no IC's are formed. Instead, neutrophils, primed by endotoxin and activated by complement, aggregate within small blood vessels at the intradermal injection site, plugging them and causing distal ischemia.

dothelium sticky—"prepared" in Shwartzman's terms—by inducing the display of adhesive, ligand-like molecules such as endothelial leukocyte adhesion molecule (ELAM-1) and by enhancing the procoagulant activity of endothelial surfaces (see below). The enhanced stickiness of endothelial cells induced by endotoxin, TNF, or IL-1 leads to *heterotypic* cell-cell adhesion of neutrophils by activating and upregulating the adhesive integrin CR3 (CD11b/CD18) on the neutrophil surface.

The second, provocative injection of endotoxin, glycogen, or immune complexes now causes massive *homotypic* neutrophil clumping. With C5a as the major culprit, neutrophils release inflammatory mediators such as hydroxl radical (OH^-), H_2O_2, eicosanoids, platelet activating factor (PAF), and lysosomal enzymes. As when complement is activated in experimental and clinical examples of the adult respiratory distress syndrome (ARDS) (Ch. 65 and 68), leukoaggregates become enmeshed in small capillaries, where the procoagulant effects of endotoxin (via platelets and Factor X) contribute to plugging of the vessels (Fig. 235–2). Tissue injury has been chiefly attributed to H_2O_2 and elastase. Neutrophils adhering to endothelial cells—as provoked by TNF, for example—are antagonized by another cytokine: transforming growth factor beta (TGF-β), which in turn is the most potent chemoattractant yet described.

It has now been appreciated that complement-mediated neutrophil aggregation may contribute not only to tissue injury in such diverse conditions as *ARDS, acute pancreatitis, Purtscher's retinopathy, acute thermal injury,* and the *extension of myocardial infarction* but also—especially in SLE—to florid vascular crises. Sera from patients with active SLE contain several factors (among them C5a) that cause normal neutrophils to aggregate. Neutrophil aggregating activity correlates with the activity of the disease and is most pronounced in patients with central nervous system (CNS) involvement. The availability of radioimmunoassays specific for complement split products permitted documentation of elevated levels of circulating C3a, C5a, and the C5b-9 membrane attack complex in patients with active SLE. Indeed, elevated C3a levels may predict flares of SLE, rising 2 months before disease becomes clinically apparent. Moreover, complement split products Ba and Bb (generated exclusively by the alternative pathway) are also elevated in active SLE; elevated levels of Ba and Bb are better predictors of clinical disease than conventional assays of total C3 and C4 or CH_{50}. In the course of SLE, microthrombosis without inflammation of the vessel wall (i.e., "vasculitis") has been described in lung, kidney, and brain, and histologic evidence has been found of intravascular leukoaggregation associated with elevated levels of circulating complement split products.

With C5a and C3a active in plasma, it is not surprising that cell receptors for complement become activated and upregulated: CR3 (CD11/CD18; see below) has been best studied. As expected, increases in CD11b/CD18 correlate with increased levels of circulating C5a and C3a. Increased expression of CD11b/CD18 on neutrophils has, again, been demonstrated in patients with active, but not inactive, SLE. The highest levels of neutrophil CD11b/CD18 are found in patients with the most severe disease, especially *cerebritis,* a group that had the highest levels of circulating C3a. CD11b/CD18 expression returns to control levels with improvement of clinical disease after these episodes of the "acute cerebral distress syndrome." In sum, whereas the normal emigration of neutrophils from endothelium does little injury to the vessel wall, the unique circumstances of the Shwartzman lesion—in which C3a and C5a are activated in the circulation—permit cytokine-activated endothelial cells to become susceptible to damage by complement-activated neutrophils.

RELEASE OF MEDIATORS OF INFLAMMATION FROM THE NEUTROPHIL. After engagement of its surface receptors by immune complexes (via FcγRII and FcγRIII receptors, CD32, and CD16, respectively) or chemottractants (receptors for C5a, and others), this motile, postmitotic cell becomes equipped to seek and destroy microbes by chemotaxis and phagocytosis. After neutrophils are engaged by membrane receptors, they (1) activate phospholipases and turnover of membrane phospholipids, (2) alter ion fluxes and membrane potential, (3) increase cytosolic calcium, (4) phosphorylate cellular proteins, and (5) assemble cytoskeletal compo-

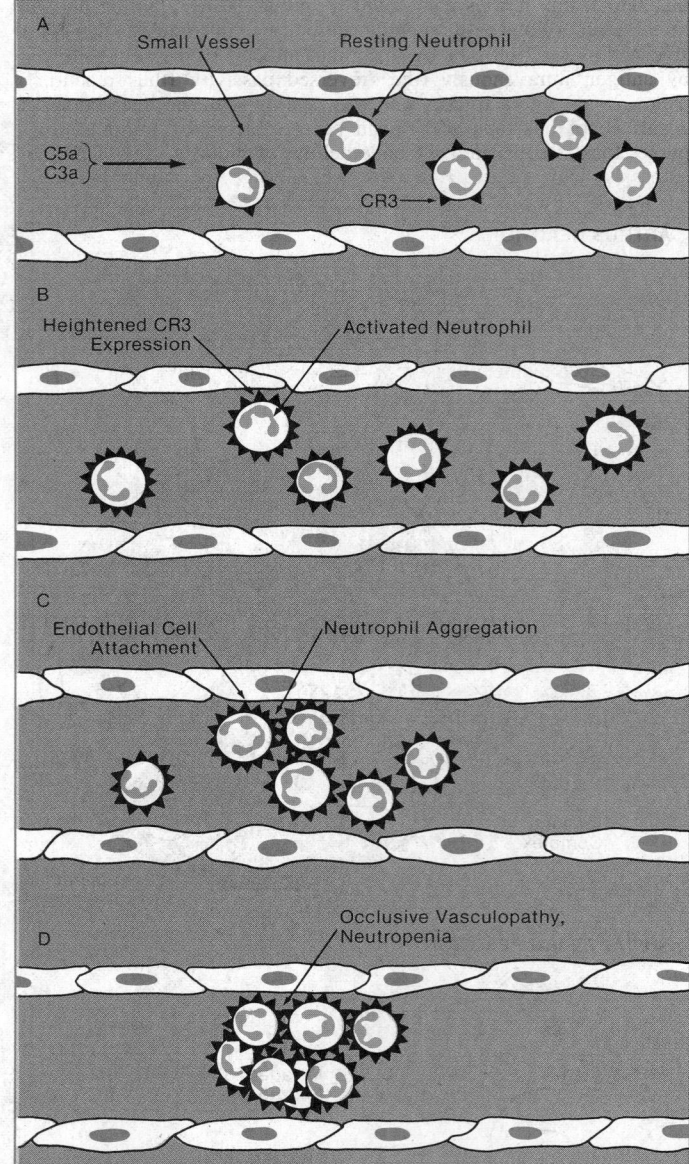

FIGURE 235–2. In active SLE, the process of intravascular complement activation, complement split product (CSP) release, and neutrophil activation may critically involve C5a stimulation of neutrophil CR3 expression *(A, B).* A hallmark of the activated neutrophil is heightened expression of surface CR3, which makes the cell stickier; this change can be induced *in vitro* by C5a. Neutrophils with increased numbers of surface CR3 would then aggregate and adhere to the vascular endothelium *(C),* leading to neutropenia and occlusive vasculopathy *(D).* The role of cytokines (IL-1 and tumor necrosis factor) in the interaction of neutrophils and endothelium in SLE is as yet unclear.

nents (actin, microtubules), among other responses. These events regulate the biological functions of *homotypic* and *heterotypic* cell-cell aggregation (see above), chemotaxis, degranulation, release of reactive oxygen species, and production of lipid-derived inflammatory substances such as platelet-activating factor (PAF), leukotriene B_4 (LTB_4), and lipoxin A.

Degranulation. During their maturation in the bone marrow, neutrophils acquire their characteristic populations of intracellular granules. These reservoirs, essentially lysosomes, serve as the main sources of enzymes responsible for destroying foreign substances and—by error, as it were—the tissue injury of inflammation. As they mature, neutrophils also acquire the enzymatic equipment with which to produce superoxide anion (O_2^-) and other mediators of tissue injury such as PAF or LTB$_4$. Primary (azurophil) granules, so named because of their early appearance in neutrophil maturation (or staining properties), contain myeloperoxidase, lysozyme, acid hydrolases, and several serine proteases, including elastase. Elastase is particularly important in connective tissue degradation because it is capable of breaking down not only elastin but also proteoglycans and collagen types III and IV. Secondary or specific granules are acquired later in maturation. These granules, like primary granules, also contain lysozyme, vitamin B$_{12}$–binding protein, lactoferrin, and the neutral proteinase collagenase. They also contain a reservoir of surface integrins (CD11b/CD18) and low-molecular-weight quanosine triphosphate (GTP)–binding proteins that bear homologies to the *ras* proteins of oncogenesis (see below). Collagenase has been detected in rheumatoid synovial fluid and degrades collagen types I, II, and III. Gelatinase, a third collagenolytic enzyme released by the neutrophil, has been localized to the C-particle compartment, an additional granule subclass. Gelatinase can degrade types IV, V, 1α2α3α, and denatured collagen. Thus neutrophil granules contain three enzymes—elastase, collagenase, and gelatinase—each with different substrate specificity and intracellular origin, which are capable of destroying collagen.

Neutrophils can discharge the contents of their intracellular granules either *overtly* or *covertly*. During uptake of particles, the neutrophil plasma membrane first invaginates to engulf particles such as immune complexes into a phagocytic vacuole. The vacuole then fuses with lysosomal granules to form a chamber called the "phagolysosome," and the granule contents are released into this chamber in the process called "covert degranulation." Sometimes, however, if the particle is too large, or if the opening of the chamber has not yet closed, lysosomal enzymes are freely discharged into the extracellular milieu, where they may attack host tissues. This "overt degranulation," a mechanism for extracellular secretion, has been termed "regurgitation during feeding," or when the material is too large to be ingested (e.g., immune complexes trapped in the matrix of cartilage), it has been given the picturesque name of "frustrated phagocytosis" (Fig. 235–3).

Antiproteases, such as α_2-macroglobulin and α_1-antitrypsin may prevent tissue damage caused by degradative proteases released inappropriately during overt degranulation. However, the effects of these antiproteases are readily overcome when they are exposed to hypochlorous acid, which inactivates them. Since hypochlorous acid (HClO$_3$) is formed in the neutrophil after interaction of myeloperoxidase, chloride anion, and H$_2$O$_2$ derived from O$_2^-$ via the NADPH oxidase of the cell, HClO$_3$ is an important mediator not only of bacterial killing (see Ch. 139) but also of tissue injury. The unfortu-

nate interaction of granule enzymes and oxygen metabolites released by neutrophils permits proteases to act unopposed and to elicit the inadvertent tissue injury that accompanies brisk phagocytosis.

Release of Toxic Oxygen Products and Lipid Mediators. The H$_2$O$_2$ used in the reaction just described is one of several oxygen metabolites, including O$_2^-$ and OH$^-$, released during neutrophil activation. The generation of these toxic compounds is governed by the membrane-associated NADPH oxidase system. In addition to contributing to the formation of hypochlorous acid, oxygen metabolites also can damage connective tissue directly. For example, OH$_2^-$ is capable of degrading bovine synovial fluid and depolymerizing purified hyaluronic acid.

Neutrophils respond to engagement of receptors for chemoattractants or immune complexes by mobilizing arachidonate from the sn-2 position of phospholipids. Arachidonate—a fatty acid abbreviated as 20:4 because of its 20 carbons and 4 unsaturated double bonds—is mobilized from membrane stores directly via a phospholipase A$_2$ (PLA$_2$) or indirectly via a phospholipase C (PLC) and followed by the action of a diacylglycerol lipase on diacylglycerol (DAG). PLA$_2$'s, which are associated both with neutrophil granules and the plasma membrane, have two pH optima (5.5 and 7.5). Purified preparations of PLA$_2$'s require high concentrations of calcium for activity. Neutrophils appear to contain at least two PLC's, one which acts specifically on phosphatidylinositol (PI) and a second which acts on phosphatidylcholine (PC) to yield DAG. Data on the remodeling of lipids show that not only PLA$_2$ activity but also the activity of PLC and PLD can explain these changes (see below). After treatment with calcium ionophore or zymosan particles opsonized by C3b, neutrophils release 20:4 from PI and PC to an almost equivalent extent.

Once released from neutrophil phospholipids, 20:4 is transformed to *eicosanoid* metabolites (*eicosa* = "twenty") such as 5-HPETE by 5-lipoxygenase; the peroxide of 5-HPETE spontaneously forms 5-hydroxyeicosatetraenoic acid (or 5-HETE) or reacts further with the 5-lipoxygenase to form LTA$_4$, which has an epoxide at the 5,6 position. The 5-lipoxygenase has been purified, sequenced, and cloned. It is a complex enzyme assembly that requires an activation step. LTA$_4$ is then acted on by LTA$_4$ hydrolase (LTB$_4$ synthetase) to form 5S, 12R, 6,14-*cis*, 8,10-*trans*-dihydroxyeicosatetraenoic acid, or LTB$_4$. Alternatively, LTA$_4$ made by the neutrophil can be processed by other cells as well; transcellular metabolism is a rule with eicosanoids (see Ch. 19). LTA$_4$ can break down nonenzymatically to 5S, 6S, or 5S, 6R-6,8,10-*trans* 14-*cis*-dihydroxyeicosatetraenoic acid. These nonenzymatic metabolites have, at best, one tenth the activity of LTB$_4$ in activating neutrophils. In the presence of exogenous arachidonic acid, neutrophils also show 15-lipoxygenase activity, which, in a parallel manner, produces 15-HPETE and 15-HETE. These products, in turn, are acted on by an LTA$_4$ synthetase-like enzyme to make a 14,15-dihydroxy product and finally, in concert with 5-lipoxygenase, to yield the trihydroxy compounds lipoxins A and B. Mononuclear cells, in contrast, produce stable prostaglandins (PGE$_2$) and the sulfidopeptide leukotrienes LTC$_4$, LTD$_4$, and LTE$_4$.

Two major candidates as inflammatory mediators made from neutrophils are LTB$_4$ and lipoxin A. LTB$_4$ is a potent chemoattractant that promotes adhesion of neutrophils to endothelial cells from a variety of arterial and venous sites of several species—an effect not shared with other eicosanoids. Prostacyclin from endothelial cells (PGI$_2$) does not inhibit LTB$_4$-stimulated adhesion. Finally, lipoxin A has potent vasodilating effects *in vivo* (but not *in vitro*) and does not mimic the action of EDRF (nitric oxide). Lipoxin A only has modest effects on neutrophil chemokinesis; since its major biological action appears to be inhibiting natural killer (NK) cell activity, lipoxin A may chiefly regulate IgG receptor (FcγRIII)—mediated signal transduction.

STIMULUS-RESPONSE COUPLING: THE BASIS OF CELL ACTIVATION IN INFLAMMATION. *Phospholipids and Intracellular Calcium.* When chemoattractants such as formyl-methionyl phenyl alanine (fMLP), C5a, C3a, or LTB$_4$ engage their receptors, neutrophils respond by generating inositol trisphosphate (IP$_3$) and DAG. Although signaling via Fc receptors and receptors for chemoattractants (Fig. 235–4) differs with respect

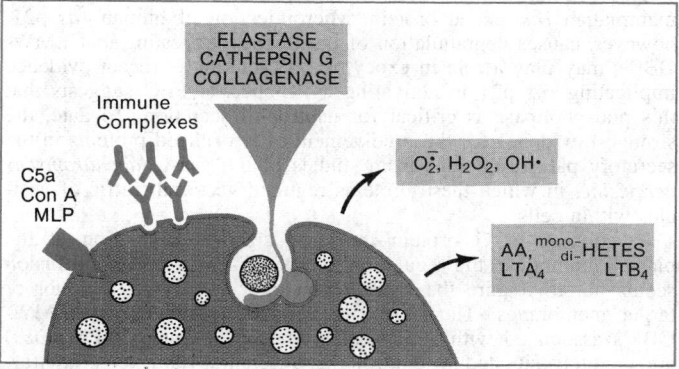

FIGURE 235–3. Release of mediators of inflammation by the human neutrophil. When neutrophils are engaged by chemoattractants of bacterial origin (fMLP, a bacterial peptide analogue), from the complement sequence (C5a), or by lectins (concanavalin A)—or by immune complexes—they release lysosomal enzymes from intracellular granules to the outside (overt degranulation), assemble and *activate* the NADPH oxidase that forms toxic oxygen species (O$_2^-$, H$_2$O$_2$, etc.), and turn over membrane phospholipids. These are the precursors for arachidonic acid (AA), which is transformed by an *activated* 5-lipoxygenase to the intermediate LTA$_4$, which can be used by neutrophils or other cells to form potent mediators: the leukotrienes (e.g., LTB$_4$).

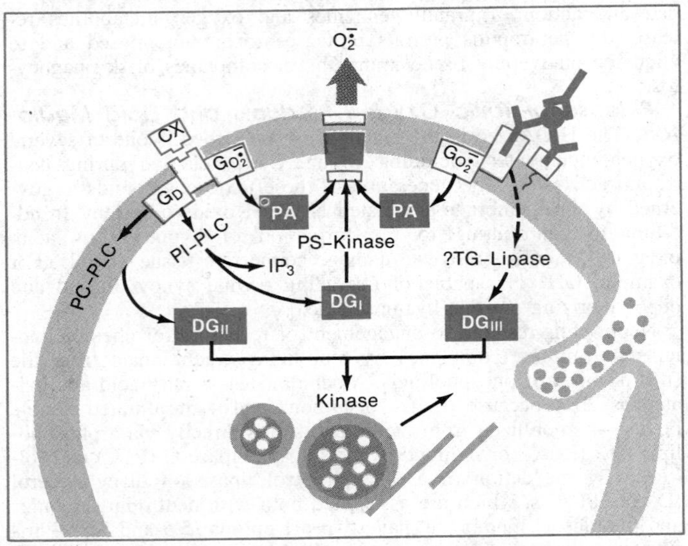

FIGURE 235–4. Stimulus-response coupling in the human neutrophil. Pathways for release of mediators of inflammation by chemoattractants (CX) on the left-hand side of the diagram differ from those launched by immune complexes (YY) on the right-hand side of the diagram. Three pools of diacylglycerol (DAG) are mobilized, only *one* of which (DAG III) is critical for secretion of lysosomal enzymes. Whereas CX-mediated generation of O_2^- is completely inhibited by pertussis toxin–sensitive G proteins, only some of the O_2^- assembly in response to immune complexes requires this intermediate. Phosphatidic acid (PA) seems to be the main intracellular messenger for assembly of the NADPH oxidase.

to some details, the *general* outline of stimulus-response coupling is similar, and neutrophils do not differ in these *general* pathways from other cells of inflammation.

Cellular IP_3 and DAG concentrations substantially increase within seconds after the fMLP receptor is engaged. By 5 seconds, IP_3 levels begin to decline. In contrast, both DAG and phosphatidic acid (PA) continue to increase over the course of the next 120 to 300 seconds. Although the exact sequence of enzyme reactions whereby the neutrophil generates these elevated levels of DAG and PA is not yet understood, it is likely that both PA and diglycerides play a crucial role in maintaining activation of the neutrophil. In order for neutrophils or macrophages to respond, over time and in space, two signals must be generated: a short "triggering" signal with an immediate increase in intracellular messengers (e.g., IP_3) and sustained "activation" signals (e.g., DAG or PA) required for the longer processes of chemotaxis and phagocytosis.

But lipid remodeling provides only *some* of the messengers needed for signal transduction. Calcium plays another key role. When treated with chemoattractants such as C5a or fMLP, neutrophils increase their levels of cytosolic calcium $[Ca]_i$, reaching a peak by 2 to 5 seconds. Over the next 2 minutes, $[Ca]_i$ slowly decreases and then returns *toward*—but not *to*—baseline. The peak levels (from 300 to 500 nM) are achieved primarily by IP_3-induced mobilization from intracellular stores, since similar levels are achieved in the absence of extracellular Ca. Influx of extracellular Ca begins approximately 5 seconds after Ca has been released from intracellular sites and while IP_3 levels are still dropping. Although IP_4 may in part regulate Ca channels, it is also possible that phosphatidic acid helps maintain Ca-dependent Ca influx.

Neutrophils break down PI to form DAG and PA within the first 5 seconds after chemoattractants or immune complexes engage receptors. Suggestions that one or another molecule in the PI-PA cycle mediate these changes in Ca permeability include the influx via PA-activated "Ca gates" or formation of IP_4 from inositol IP_3 by specific kinases. However, the turnover of IP_3/IP_4 as a consequence of specific phosphatases is extremely rapid (5 to 15 seconds), while DAG and PA continue to accumulate (30 to 120 seconds) after treating neutrophils with chemoattractants. In contrast, formation of DAG proceeds in a biphasic fashion. The first peak is at 2 to 5 sec-

onds, consistent with release of the "triggering" messengers IP_3 and DAG by the hydrolysis of polyphosphoinositides. Before this first wave is completed—by 15 to 30 seconds after treatment with fMLP—a second, more sustained wave of DAG formation commences. In contrast, PA rises throughout the time course of activation. Both PLC's and PLD's are involved in PA function. The concentration of DAG and PA remain elevated, compared with those of resting neutrophils, for more than 300 seconds in what has been called the "activation phase" of neutrophil responses. Although the evidence is by no means complete, it appears likely that the second wave of DAG is important in degranulation, whereas the increased levels of PA are important for assembly of the NAPH oxidase that is responsible for generating O_2^-.

GTP-Binding Proteins and Signal Transduction. The superfamily of GTP-binding proteins includes (1) the heterotrimeric proteins which transduce hormonal and sensory signals across the plasma membrane, (2) tubulin (each dimer binds 1 mole of GTP strongly and 1 mole loosely), (3) the elongation and initiation factors of protein synthesis, (4) products of the *ras* oncogene, and (5) putative GTP-binding proteins of cellular secretion. Whereas neutrophils clearly have GTP-binding proteins at their plasmalemma, the protein is neither a classic G_s or G_i protein and appears instead to be at least one novel G protein: G_n. In turn, at least one function of G_n is to couple receptors for chemoattractants to PLC. Composed of typical β/γ membrane components and an α subunit of the cytosol, 33 to 50% of the G_n protein is complexed to the β/γ dimer in the membrane, while the remainder is free in the cytosol. Pertussis toxin (PT) binds to the α subunit at sites distinct from the GTP site. Ribosylation by PT of the soluble α subunit is enhanced 12-fold by addition of β/γ subunits, whereas PT-ribosylation of membrane G_n is only modestly enhanced. G_n comprises between 1 and 3% of membrane proteins; no great excess of these molecules (10^6 per cell) is present over possible receptors (e.g., receptors for IgG and C5a). The neutrophil G protein (α subunit) is a substrate for ADP ribosylation both by pertussis and by cholera toxins (CT); both toxins inhibit high-affinity fMLP binding, and the protein is antigenically distinct not only from G_s and G_i proteins of other sources but also from the common G_o protein of brain. Predictably, for G protein–mediated functions, treatment of intact neutrophils with pertussis toxin inhibits ligand-mediated O_2^- generation, degranulation, chemotaxis, phospholipid turnover, high-affinity fMLP binding, release of eicosanoids, and Ca fluxes.

However, the G proteins of signal transduction are not the only G proteins of inflammatory cells; a rapidly growing family of "low-molecular-weight GTP-binding proteins" (LMW-GBP's) with molecular weights in the range of 20,000 to 30,000 are also present. These proteins are characterized by marked sequence homology to the *ras* oncogene product (*ras* p21). Unlike their high-molecular-weight counterparts, no clear function has been attributed to any mammalian *ras*-related protein. Microinjection of human *ras* p21, however, causes degranulation of mast cells, suggesting that LMW-GBP's may play a role in exocytosis. Furthermore, recent evidence implicating *ras* p21 in activating a PC-specific PLC suggests that this phospholipase is critical for neutrophil secretion. To date, the strongest evidence for the involvement of *ras*-related proteins in the secretory pathway comes from studies of the yeast *Saccharomyces cerevisiae*, in which these proteins regulate vectorial traffic of vesicles within cells.

In contrast to G protein–mediated signal transduction at the plasma membrane, the regulation of vesicular movement and fusion seems not to require the transduction of a signal across donor or target membranes. There is good reason to suspect that LMW-GBP's associated with neutrophil granule membrane GBP's (*rabs*) are uniquely situated to control the differential and vectorial trafficking of secretory granules in inflammatory cells. Indeed, these proteins can be considered as regulators of intracellular "docking" of secretory granules in the course of the inflammation.

SIGNALING VIA FC RECEPTORS: THE RESPONSE TO IMMUNE COMPLEXES. Three major classes of receptors have been described for the constant Fc region of human IgG's. FcγRI is *a high-affinity receptor* for monomeric IgG (K_a = approx. 10^{-8} M, 72 kDa) found mainly on mononuclear cells; recognized by monoclonal antibody 32, it is upregulated in response to interferon (IFN). Neutrophils also have *two low-affinity receptors* ($K_a = \sim 10^{-6}$ M) that bind aggregated IgG's or immune complexes much more avidly than monomeric IgG. FcγRII (or CD32) of approximately 40 kDa is present at 15,000 sites per cell (as recognized by monoclonal antibody IV-3) and is also present on B cells, macrophages, and platelets. FcγRII (1) is resistant to elastase, (2) is not linked to the plasmalemma via PI, (3) is present on neutrophils from patients with paroxysmal nocturnal hemoglobinuria (PNH), (4) appears to mediate O_2^- generation and degranulation, and (5) transduces all the signal for O_2^- generation and some of the signal for degranulation by means of a pertussis-sensitive G protein.

FcγRIII (or CD16) also prefers multimeric IgG and is expressed in heterogeneous fashion on neutrophils, macrophages, and NK cells. FcγRIII has a broad molecular weight range of 50,000 to 70,000, is present at approximately 120,000 sites per neutrophil, and is recognized by monoclonal antibody 3G8. The FcγRIII's on neutrophils and NK cells differ with respect to mass and are products of different but very homologous genes. FcγRIII's of the neutrophil are (1) elastase-sensitive, (2) linked to the external plasmalemma via PI, (3) reduced to 90% of controls at the plasmalemma—but not the Golgi region—of cells from patients with PNH, (4) an ineffective trigger of cells for O_2^- or enzyme release, and (5) polymorphic with respect to structure and antigenicity because there are two alleles (CNA1 and NA2). FcγRIII's are shed into the supernatant of neutrophils exposed to fMLP, whereas macrophages and NK cells—in which FcγRIII is a transmembrane structure—do not shed this receptor.

Since cells from patients with paroxysmal nocturnal hemoglobinuria respond as well as normal cells to IgG-opsonized particles by O_2^- generation and all O_2^- generating activity in response to IgG is PT-sensitive, we must conclude that the FcγRII is linked to GTP-binding proteins, whereas FcγRIII is not (see Fig. 235–4). Recent evidence shows that whereas stimulus-response coupling induced by immune complexes in the bulk phase is largely sensitive to PT, degranulation and O_2^- generation induced by immune complexes on a surface are relatively insensitive to PT. From these observations, it appears that FcγRIII may accumulate at the interface between neutrophils and the immune complexes trapped in the subendothelium. Moreover, signaling via Fc receptors *differs* from signaling via chemoattractant receptors in that the former is dependent on the integrity of cytoplasmic microtubules, whereas chemoattractant-induced signaling is independent of microtubules. *Colchicine therefore inhibits FcγR signaling.* FcγRIII receptors may serve to cluster Fc receptors in the service of "frustrated phagocytosis" when discharge of neutrophil contents is launched by an IgG-opsonized particle too large to digest. Therefore, of the two neutrophil Fc receptors for IgG, it appears that FcγRII triggers cells via classic G protein–mediated signal transduction as in synovial fluid. In contrast, FcγRIII receptors unlinked to G proteins mediate neutrophil discharge in vascular lesions where IgG's are trapped at subendothelial sites, as in vasculitis when release of mediators of inflammation is by "frustrated phagocytosis."

THE INTEGRINS AND INFLAMMATION. The adhesion of formed elements of the blood to endothelium and to each other is mediated by a superfamily of membrane proteins called "integrins." Three major families of mammalian integrins have been described: (1) receptors for extracellular matrix molecules such as fibronectin and T lymphocyte receptors known as "very late appearing antigens" (VLA's), (2) platelet surface glycoprotein IIb/IIIa and the vitronectin receptor, and (3) the LFA-1 family of leukocyte adhesion molecules. The most striking characteristic shared by these molecules is their noncovalently linked α/β heterodimer configuration in which the same β subunit is shared by all members of a family. In addition, many, but not all, integrins contain a domain that recognizes an Arg-Gly-Asp (RGD) sequence present in their respective ligands.

The LFA-1 family of leukocyte adhesion molecules includes three heterodimeric glycoproteins that share a common 95-kDa β chain (CD18): LFA-1, Mac-1 (also called Mo1, gp165/95, and CR3), and gp150/90, whose α chains have been designated CD11a, 11b, and 11c, respectively. The expression of these three molecules varies according to lineage and stage of maturation of various hematopoietic cells. In addition to mediating cell-cell adhesion, CD11b/CD18 functions as a receptor for iC3b (CR3) and thereby mediates phagocytosis of opsonized particles.

CD11b/CD18 is probably the major neutrophil adhesion molecule involved in *heterotypic* (neutrophil-endothelium) and *homotypic* (neutrophil-neutrophil) adhesion. A group of children genetically deficient in all three LFA-1 family adhesion molecules suffers from recurrent bacterial infections, impaired pus formation, delayed wound healing, and poor separation of the umbilical cord. Neutrophils from these patients are defective in functions related to adhesion such as aggregation, spreading on surfaces, directed migration, and attachment to endothelial monolayers. Normal human neutrophils treated *in vitro* with a subset of available anti-CD11b/CD18 monoclonal antibodies exhibit defects indistinguishable from those of neutrophils from patients with deficiency.

Although CD11b/CD18 is clearly implicated in the events of neutrophil adhesion, the molecular mechanisms are unclear. Under normal circumstances, neutrophil sticking must be suppressed to permit cells to circulate. Once they encounter ligands, cell activation is required to render neutrophils sticky. In heterotypic adhesion, the other agonist is the endothelial cell. The endothelial cell plays an active role in adhesion and displays to inflammatory cells an inducible endothelial surface glycoprotein designated ELAM-1 that partially mediates adhesion of leukocytes including neutrophils. Interleukin-1 (IL-1), tumor necrosis factor (TNF), lymphotoxin (LT), and endotoxin induce the expression of ELAM-1 on endothelial cells. Intercellular adhesion molecule 1 (ICAM-1), a similar but distinct antigen found on a variety of cells including endothelial cells, is the ligand for LFA-1 and is therefore one of several molecules that direct lymphocyte binding to high endothelial cells, especially those of the chronically inflamed rheumatoid joint. On the other hand, the endothelial side of the equation can be modified by transforming growth factor β (TGF-β). TGF-β inhibits the adherence of human neutrophils not only to normal endothelium but also to endothelial cells rendered sticky by ELAM-1, as induced by TNF-α.

In *homotypic* adhesion (neutrophil-neutrophil), the Cd11b/CD18 heterodimer receptor engages an as yet unknown ligand on an adherent neutrophil. The putative ligand is unlikely to be adsorbed iC3b, nor is the adhesive ligand likely to be CD11b/CD18 itself because normal neutrophils are capable of aggregating with neutrophils from CD11b/CD18-deficient patients.

CD11b/CD18 is constitutively expressed on the surface of resting neutrophils at a density of 10,000 to 20,000 molecules per cell. Upon activation by a number of stimuli, including especially chemoattractants, neutrophils upregulate their surface expression 5- to 10-fold. Since mature neutrophils synthesize few new proteins, it is not surprising that upregulation of CD11b/CD18 is due to translocation of preformed receptor to the plasma membrane from an intracellular source that co-sediments with specific granules.

Because each stimulus that enhances neutrophil adhesion also induces Mac-1 upregulation, it was widely believed that these two phenomena were causally related, but recent studies have dissociated neutrophil-neutrophil aggregation from upregulation of CD11b/CD18. Indeed, whereas the constitutive presence on the cell surface of CD11b/CD18 is *required* for neutrophil adhesion, regulation of cell-cell adhesion appears to involve a structural change in each receptor molecule rather than a quantitative change in the number of receptors.

RHEUMATOID ARTHRITIS AS A FORM OF THE TUBERCULIN REACTION. The histopathology of RA can be divided into two phases: (1) the acute inflammatory lesion—the Arthus-type lesion discussed earlier—and (2) the more chronic, mononuclear, cell-mediated, granulomatous disease proceeding in the deeper layers. This lesion—pannus—is marked by (1) focal collections of B lymphocytes and plasma cells that synthesize rheumatoid factors locally, (2) various subsets of T lymphocytes, (3) activated macrophages (Fig. 235–5), and (4) the proliferation of other mesenchymal cells of the synovium where genes for proto-oncogenes have been activated. The two types of activated cells, macrophages and synoviocytes, generate cytokines that cause chondrocytes to participate in their own destruction by releasing proteases and specific collagenase.

The lesions resemble those found in the tuberculin reaction, save for the clusters of B lymphocytes and plasma cells with rheumatoid factor. Indeed, for many years RA was thought to be a form of tu-

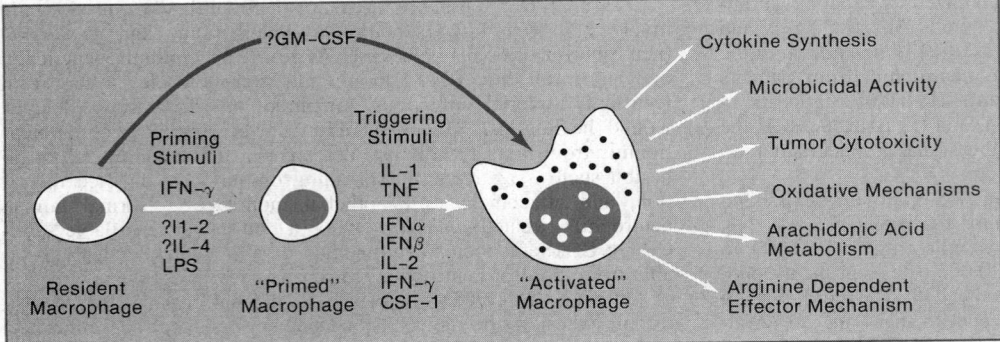

FIGURE 235–5. Schematic depiction of the role of cytokines in the two-stage hypothesis of macrophage activation. Unstimulated cells are primed by treatment with low-dose LPS, IFN-γ, and possibly IL-2. Primed macrophages can be triggered to an activated state by many other cytokines. Activation of the macrophages has classically been defined by demonstrating augmented effector functions as shown.

berculosis, and the gold salts that were used for treatment in the 1920's were first used for RA on this basis of this fuzzy correspondence. We may note that the earliest editions of this text classified RA as a form of "infectious arthritis."

Whereas the offending agent of RA is unknown, most modern speculation centers on the likelihood that one or another self-antigen looks very much like the product of a bacterium or virus. The major candidates have been (1) the Epstein-Barr virus (EBV), (2) type II collagen, (3) cartilage proteogylcan, and (4) heat shock (stress) proteins—especially a 65-kDa species against which many patients with RA mount a humoral and cellular immune response. Indeed, there is good evidence that stress proteins are present at the surface of antigen-presenting cells, and recently, it was found that a helper T-cell clone derived from a patient with tuberculous leprosy reacted with a synthetic peptide found in the third type variable region of the major histocompatability complex–DR2 β chain. The observation that cartilage proteoglycans share epitopes with acetone-extracted fractions of the tubercle bacillus suggests that when humans get RA, they respond to their own tissues as if these were products of the tubercle bacillus or EBV.

Whatever the offending antigen proves to be, the mediators released by T and B lymphocytes, by activated macrophages, and by activated synovial cells are the usual battery of cytokines found in chronic inflammation (Table 235–1). These cytokines in turn influence neutrophil function. Indeed, IL-1 (a pro-inflammatory cytokine produced chiefly by mononuclear cells but also by neutrophils) is capable of promoting thymocyte proliferation and synovial fibroblast activation and proliferation. Neutrophils display enhanced adherence to endothelial cells treated with IL-1. Among its many other properties, IL-1 also induces production of PGE$_2$ and type II collagenase by chondrocytes. These actions are regulated by an IL-1 inhibitor, which appears to be constitutively present in cartilage cells and in the neutrophil.

Treatment of neutrophils with the lymphokines, IFN-γ, or TNF-β augments neutrophil phagocytic capacity, especially when PMN's are at the surface of cartilage. TNF-β, the most potent chemoattractant, also promotes neutrophil adherence to endothelial cells and stimulates hydrogen peroxide release and degranulation. Granulocyte macrophage colony-stimulating factor (GM-CSF), produced largely by fibroblasts, facilitates phagocytosis by neutrophils, possibly by increasing Fc receptor expression. Although many cytokines have no effect on neutrophil chemotaxis, etc., IL-8, a macrophage-derived neutrophil chemotactic factor, is one of the most potent neutrophil activators yet found.

Abramson SB, Weissmann G: Complement split products and the pathogenesis of SLE. Hosp Pract 23:45, 1988. *How the Arthus phenomenon and the Shwartzman reaction apply to vasculitis in SLE.*

Bokoch GM: Signal transduction by GTP-binding proteins during leukocyte activation: Phagocytic cells. *In* Grinstein S, Rotstein OD (eds.): Mechanisms of Leukocyte Activation. New York, Academic Press, 1990, pp. 65–101. *A modern discussion of how the molecular biology of G proteins has permitted understanding of signal transduction control.*

Crofford LJ, Wilder RL, Ristimake AP, et al.: Cyclooxygenase-1 and -2 expression in rheumatoid synovial tissues: Effects of interleukin-1β, phorbol ester, and corticosteroids. J Clin Invest 93:1095, 1994. *How the two cyclo-oxygenases are influenced by interleukins and anti-inflammatory drugs in inflammation.*

Cronstein BN, Kimmel SC, Levin RI, et al.: A mechanism for the anti-inflammatory effects of corticosteroids: The glucocorticoid receptor regulates leukocyte adhesion to endothelial cells and expression of ELAM-1 and ICAM-1. Proc Nat'l Acad Sci USA 89:9991, 1992. *A modern view of how corticosteroids influence the display of adhesive molecules.*

Haines KA, Reibman J, Weissmann G: Triggering and activation of human neutrophils: two aspects of the response to transmembrane signals. *In* Poste G, Crooke ST (eds.): Cellular and Molecular Aspects of Inflammation. New York, Plenum Press, 1988, pp. 31–40. *A detailed analysis of the differences between immediate and prolonged responses to signals at the surface of inflammatory cells.*

Harris ED Jr: Pathogenesis of rheumatoid arthritis: A disorder associated with dysfunctional immunoregulation. *In* Gallin JI, Goldstein IM, Snyderman R (eds.): Inflammation. New York, Raven Press, 1985, pp. 751–774. *A review of rheumatoid inflammation with an emphasis on cell-cell interaction in chronic inflammation and cartilage destruction.*

Krane SM, Amento EP, Goldring SR, et al.: ML modulation of matrix synthesis and degradation in joint inflammation. *In* AM Glauert (ed.): The Control of Tissue Damage. Amsterdam, Elsevier, 1990, pp. 179–195. *How IL 1 appears to be crucial for the self-induced destruction in RA as mediated by prostaglandin E$_2$ and collagenase.*

Spaethe SM, Needleman P: Biosynthesis and release of lipid mediate of inflammation. *In* Poste G, Crooke ST (eds.): Cellular and Molecular Aspects of Inflammation. New York, Plenum Press, 1988, pp. 153–170. *A review of the cyclo-oxygenase and lipoxygenase pathways in inflammation, with a discussion of the role of essential fatty acid.*

Weissmann G: The role of neutrophils in vascular injury: Signal transduction mechanisms in cell/cell interactions. Springer Semin Immunopathol 11:235, 1989. *A review of the Arthus and Shwartzman models and how they relate to the vascular lesions of rheumatic diseases.*

West MA: Role of cytokines in leukocyte activation: Phagocytic cells. *In* Grinstein S, Rotstein OD (eds.): Mechanisms of Leukocyte Activation. New York, Academic Press, 1990, pp. 537–570. *A summary of the effects of cytokines—which are released in rheumatoid inflammation—on the activation of neutrophils and macrophages.*

Winfield JB: Stress proteins and autoimmunity. Arthritis Rheum 32:1497, 1989. *How heat shock proteins may be the link between autoantigens and microbial products in the perpetuating RA.*

TABLE 235–1. CELLULAR SOURCES AND TARGETS OF MAJOR CYTOKINES

Cytokine	Source	Target
IL-1α	Mφ, EC, fibroblasts	Lymphocytes, EC, HC, Mφ, fibroblasts, others
IL-1β	Mφ	Lymphocytes, EC, HC, Mφ, fibroblasts, others
IL-2	T cells	Lymphocytes, Mφ, others
IL-4	T cells	B cells, T cells, others
IL-8	Macrophages	PMN's
IFN-α	Lymphocytes	Multiple nucleated cells
IFN-β$_1$	Mφ	Multiple nucleated cells
IFN-β$_2$(IL-6)	Fibroblasts, Mφ	HC, lymphocytes, others
IFN-γ	T lymphocytes	Mφ, lymphocytes, others
M-CSF, CSF-1	Mφ	Bone marrow, Mφ, fibroblasts
GM-CSF	Fibroblasts	Mφ, PMN's
TNF-α	Mφ, fibroblasts	PMN's, Mφ others
TNF-β	Lymphocytes, Mφ	Multiple cells
TGF-β	T lymphocytes	PMN's, fibroblasts, Mφ
MDNCF	Mφ	PMN's

IFN = interferon; TNF = tumor necrosis factor; IL = interleukin; CSF = colony-stimulating factor; GM-CSF = granulocyte macrophage colony-stimulating factor; TGF-β = transforming growth factor β; Mφ = macrophage; PMN = polymorphonuclear neutrophil; EC = endothelial cell; HC = hepatocyte.

236 SPECIALIZED PROCEDURES IN THE MANAGEMENT OF PATIENTS WITH RHEUMATIC DISEASES

Robert W. Ike and William J. Arnold

Rheumatic diseases can account for an array of clinical presentations that range from signs and symptoms reflecting multiorgan involvement to pain and compromised function in a single anatomic area. Correct diagnosis of a suspected rheumatic process and optimal management of the patient with an established rheumatic disease rest on the physician's ability to identify the site(s) from which the patient's symptoms arise, ascertain the pathologic process affecting the identified site(s), determine why the process is occurring, and find measures to gauge the activity of the disease so that response to treatment can be followed. A directed history and physical examination provide the bedrock for this exercise, with suspicions regarding anatomy, process, and diagnosis supported or refuted by appropriate laboratory tests, imaging modalities, and invasive procedures. The number of specialized procedures applicable to rheumatic diseases continues to grow. Testing for relevant immunologic phenomena becomes ever more complex as newer tests, such as those for the antineutrophil cytoplasmic antibody (ANCA) system, join established tests that have become subdivided as the molecular bases for the measured phenomena become appreciated, as for the many specific target antigens in the antinuclear antibody (ANA) reaction. Certain anatomic abnormalities that had escaped detection previously can now be identified by newer imaging procedures—both direct (arthroscopy) and indirect (ultrasound, magnetic resonance imaging)—although these procedures present hurdles of cost, availability, and operator expertise. These new tests and the other procedures discussed below must always be interpreted in the context of a thorough, comprehensive, multifaceted evaluation.

ASPIRATION OF SYNOVIAL JOINTS AND BURSAE. In any patient with undiagnosed arthritis and an associated joint effusion, examination of the synovial fluid is mandatory. Gross appearance of the synovial fluid can provide an initial clue to the underlying process, and certain disorders such as crystalline arthropathies and bacterial infection are quickly confirmed by specialized microscopic examination. Successful joint or bursal aspiration depends on a thorough familiarity with certain principles.

Both the physician and the patient must be comfortable. The physician should have some experience and confidence concerning the particular joint to be tapped. Although most general internists can aspirate the knee or the olecranon bursa, other commonly inflamed structures, such as the shoulder, ankle, elbow, first metatarsophalangeal joint, and subdeltoid bursa, require special expertise for successful aspiration. The patient should be positioned to allow relaxation of muscles on both sides of the joint to be aspirated. For the knee, the patient should be supine with the knee in slight flexion, accomplished by resting it on a pillow. Palpation identifies landmarks for entry, discerns the region of the largest "bulge" in the joint capsule (crucial for small joints), and confirms relaxation of periarticular muscles. If the patella cannot be moved side to side, entry to the knee will be painful and difficult if not impossible.

After preparing the skin with iodine solution, the gloved aspirating hand determines point of entry. Most physicians find the knee easiest to enter from the medial aspect, just inferior to midpoint of the patella edge. Except for very large effusions that can be entered quickly with the aspirating needle, the skin and subcutaneous path to the joint capsule should be anesthetized with lidocaine, delivered while advancing slowly with the smallest-gauge needle available. This promotes patient comfort and marks the path to be taken into the joint. The joint space is entered with an 18-gauge needle to which a syringe of up to 20 ml is attached, depending on the size of the effusion. Failure to obtain fluid from a clinically swollen joint space can result from several processes, including presence of synovial fluid too thick to be withdrawn through the needle used, presence of intra-articular debris clogging the needle, a swollen space comprised mainly of tissue, or sequestration of fluid away from the needle point. When aspiration of fluid is critical, such as in suspected septic arthritis, ultrasound or arthrography can help guide the needle to the fluid-containing section of the joint. A 5-ml sample of synovial fluid is more than adequate for all routine studies, including cultures.

Synovial fluid analysis begins with a look at the fluid in the heparinized tube. Fluid that transmits light and can be read through (determined by holding the tube in front of a sample of printed text) will generally prove to have <2000 white blood cells (WBC's) per milliliter and is associated with "noninflammatory" disorders, most commonly osteoarthritis (OA) (Table 236–1). Translucent fluid that blurs print will have >2000 WBC's per milliliter but <100,000 WBC's per milliliter and is associated with a wide array of "inflammatory" conditions, such as rheumatoid arthritis (RA). Opaque fluid, usually quite thick, carries the usual concerns of pus obtained from any other body cavity and should place acute infection as the leading diagnosis until proven otherwise. Usually, such fluid will show 50,000 to 100,000 WBC's per milliliter, but other compounds in high concentrations (cholesterol, monosodium urate) can produce opaque synovial fluid that is relatively acellular. Bloody-appearing fluid carries a specific differential diagnosis but does not always connote true hemarthrosis, since it takes but a small amount of blood within the joint space to make

TABLE 236–1. SYNOVIAL FLUID ANALYSIS

	Noninflammatory (Group I)	Inflammatory (Group II)	Purulent (Group III)	Hemorrhagic (Group IV)
Color	Yellow	Yellow	Yellow-green	Red
Clarity	Transparent	Translucent	Opaque	Opaque
Leukocyte count (WBC/ml)	<2000	2000–50,000†	>50,000	†
% Polymorphonuclear leukocytes	<25%	>50%	>75%	†
Disease examples	Osteoarthritis	Rheumatoid arthritis	Bacterial infections	Trauma
	Trauma	Reiter's syndrome	Tuberculosis	Neuropathic joint
	Osteochondritis dessicans	Crystal synovitis, acute (gout, pseudogout)	RA (rare)	Coagulation disorders
	Osteonecrosis	Psoriatic arthritis	Reiter's (rare)	Hemophilia
	Amyloidosis	Viral arthritis	Pseudogout (rare)	von Willebrand's
	Scleroderma	Rheumatic fever		Heparin or warfarin
	Systemic lupus*	Behçet's syndrome		Sickle cell disease
	Polymyalgia rheumatica*	Lyme disease		Chondrocalcinosis
	Hypertrophic pulmonary osteoarthropathy	Some bacterial infections		Scurvy
				Tumor, especially pigmented villonodular synovitis, hemangioma

* Sometimes inflammatory.
† Wide range; WBC count should be interpreted in light of peripheral blood WBC and RBC counts.

synovial fluid appear bloody. Viscosity of the joint fluid is determined largely by molecular weight and concentration of hyaluronate, a proteoglycan polymer. Elaboration of enzymes that depolymerize hyaluronate can accompany synovial tissue inflammation in the absence of fluid phase inflammation. Hence "noninflammatory fluid" that appears "thin" and leaves a very short "string" when dripped from syringe into test tube can be due to synovitis that has not produced fluid phase inflammation and cloudy fluid. Bursal fluid cannot be classified by the same parameters as joint fluid. As a rule of thumb, the WBC count from bursal fluid is about one-tenth the WBC count that would be expected from a joint given the same phlogistic agent. For example, in gouty bursitis, an average bursal fluid leukocyte count is 2800 per milliliter compared with an average of 21,000 WBC's per milliliter in synovial fluid from an acute gouty joint. Thus bursal fluid with a leukocyte count of only a few hundred per milliliter should raise the same concerns—including the possibility of infection—as a joint fluid with several thousand WBC's per milliliter.

Examining synovial fluid under a polarized light microscope is essential for the diagnosis of crystal-associated arthropathies (see Color Plate 3C) and should be performed initially in all patients. Needle-shaped, negatively birefringent intracellular crystals of monosodium urate (MSU) confirm the diagnosis of gouty arthritis. Rhomboidal, positively birefringent intracellular crystals of calcium pyrophosphate dihydrate (CPPD) define the pseudogout syndrome. Intracellular CPPD and MSU crystals may be sparsely distributed on the microscope slide, and they are often identified only after a careful, thorough search guided by someone well versed in using the polarized microscope. Because other processes such as infection can "liberate" crystals into the joint fluid, identifying crystals in an acutely inflamed joint should not be taken as a complete explanation, particularly when CPPD is present. Other crystals and compounds identified by the polarized microscope include calcium oxalate (a positively birefringent tetrahedron found in some dialysis patients), corticosteroids from previous intra-articular injections (small and bright with variable birefringence characteristics), talc (positively birefringent clumps transferred from gloved hand to slide), lipid (round "maltese crosses" derived from bone marrow fat and indicative of fracture), and cholesterol (plate-like and brilliantly birefringent without a definite axis, associated with long-standing inflammatory effusions, especially when accompanied by bleeding as in hemophilia).

Bacterial infection should be considered in all patients with acute arthritis and in patients with established rheumatic disorders with exacerbation in one or several joints. Purulent, opaque synovial fluid is not present in all cases, and early-stage bacterial arthritis may not even produce "inflammatory" fluid. The most common pathogen is Staphylococcus aureus. Findings on Gram stain of synovial fluid can help guide initial therapy, but a negative study does not rule out infection. When clinical suspicion of septic arthritis is strong but not confirmed by initial studies of synovial fluid, empirical antibiotics should be given until culture results are available.

Arthritis due to other infectious agents may be more difficult to confirm. Neisseria gonorrheae is the most common gram-negative organism associated with infectious arthritis but is identified by Gram stain of synovial fluid in only a minority of cases. Chances for isolation of the gonococcus are improved if synovial fluid is plated directly onto chocolate agar and similar cultures are made from swabs of any skin lesions and of all potential portals of entry for the organism (urethra, cervix, anus, throat). Mycobacteria (tuberculosis and others) can cause an indolent monarthritis from which an inflammatory, mainly monocytic synovial fluid is obtained. Synovial fluid cultures are usually sterile, and signs of active extra-articular disease are minimal. A prompt, accurate diagnosis of tuberculous arthritis requires a high degree of suspicion and culture of synovial biopsy specimens. Extensive joint destruction is often present before a diagnosis of tuberculous arthritis is made.

Reduction in synovial fluid glucose to less than 50% of simultaneous serum measurement should raise suspicion for the diagnosis of infectious arthritis. In a patient with infectious arthritis, serial measurements of synovial fluid glucose levels can be one of the several parameters used to gauge the effectiveness of therapy.

ERYTHROCYTE SEDIMENTATION RATE AND ACUTE PHASE RESPONSE PROTEINS. The systemic response to tissue injury, regardless of cause, is characterized by a cytokine-mediated alteration in the hepatic synthesis of a number of different plasma proteins, known collectively as "acute phase reactants." These proteins, which include fibrinogen, haptoglobin, ceruloplasmin, α_1-antitrypsin, complement components C3 and C4, serum amyloid A protein, and C-reactive protein (CRP), rise in proportion to the severity of tissue injury, although the magnitude of rise in each component varies. Because some systemic rheumatic disorders cause chronic tissue inflammation and injury, assessment of the acute phase response is an important facet of rheumatic disease diagnosis and management (because the effectiveness of treatment is gauged by the extent to which the acute phase response is suppressed).

Measuring the erythrocyte sedimentation rate (ESR) has been a time-honored and simple method to approximate the acute phase response. "Extreme" elevation of the ESR (> 100 mm per hour) has come to have diagnostic significance, associated with polymyalgia rheumatica, giant cell arteritis, multiple myeloma, lymphoma, metastatic cancer, severe chronic infections such as subacute bacterial endocarditis and tuberculosis, and chronic renal failure. Reduction or normalization of the ESR is a goal of treatment for those treatable disorders associated with a rapid ESR. Sedimentation of erythrocytes is facilitated by certain plasma proteins that neutralize the negative charge on the erythrocyte surface, thus permitting the erythrocytes to aggregate and "fall" as a clump rather than as individual cells. Fibrinogen is among the plasma proteins capable of this action; thus the level of fibrinogen—which varies according to the intensity of the acute phase response—substantially affects the ESR. However, other proteins not associated with the acute phase response—notably immunoglobulin (particularly when present as a single paraprotein) and certain "middle molecules" in patients with chronic renal failure—also accelerate the ESR. Normal values for ESR span a wide range, slightly higher in women than in men and increasing with age in both sexes. Many individuals aged 70 and over may have ESR's in the range of 40 to 50 mm per hour without apparent inflammation or tissue injury. This confounds the utility of the ESR in supporting a suspected rheumatic disease diagnosis such as polymyalgia rheumatica in an elderly person. Finally, not all patients with clinically active rheumatic diseases have raised ESR's because of individual differences in hepatic function, alterations in erythrocytes, or abnormalities of other plasma proteins that counteract effects of acute phase reactants that speed the ESR.

Of the several acute phase reactants that can be measured directly, C-reactive protein (CRP), named for its binding of pneumococcal C-polysaccharide, is the most extensively studied and clinically useful. Most rheumatic diseases, including RA, juvenile chronic arthritis, ankylosing spondylitis, polymyalgia rheumatica, systemic vasculitis, Behçet's syndrome, Reiter's disease, and psoriatic arthritis, are associated with high levels of CRP (1 to 10 mg per deciliter) when they are active, with falling or undetectable levels when improving or inactive. For diseases in the spondyloarthropathy family (ankylosing spondylitis, Reiter's, psoriatic arthritis), the CRP is far more sensitive to fluctuations in disease activity than is the ESR. Systemic lupus erythematosus (SLE) disease activity, in the majority of patients, raises the CRP only slightly if at all (1 to 3 mg per deciliter); concurrent infection in SLE will raise the CRP, and extreme CRP elevation (> 10 mg per deciliter) in a lupus patient should provoke a hunt for infection.

AUTOANTIBODIES. Rheumatoid factors are immunoglobulins directed against the Fc portion of immunoglobulin G (IgG) (see Ch. 237). Measuring rheumatoid factor by tests that determine the highest dilution of serum capable of agglutinating IgG-coated latex particles is being replaced in many laboratories by automated methods such as nephelometry and enzyme-linked immunosorbent assay (ELISA). Thus the reporting of rheumatoid factor "titer" is often replaced by reporting an absolute concentration. Rheumatoid factor positivity with titers up to 1:320 may be found in otherwise normal people over age 70. While rheumatoid factor can be found in 70 to 80% of patients with RA, it is also present in other rheumatic diseases (Sjögren's syndrome, cryoglobulinemia, SLE) and non-rheumatic diseases, such as chronic infections (hepatitis, subacute bacterial endocarditis). In patients with RA, the presence of rheumatoid factor is associated with more severe disease, manifested by rheumatoid nodules, rheumatoid vasculitis, and bone erosions.

Testing serum for presence of *antinuclear antibodies (ANA's)* is useful primarily in the evaluation of suspected SLE (see Ch. 240). Many different antigen-antibody reactions underlie the various patterns detected by the ANA test, and identification of antibody to a specific antigen is diagnostically useful in several instances (Table 236–2). Antibodies to double-stranded DNA (particularly if raised one or more standard deviations above normal test range) and to the Smith (Sm) antigen are highly specific for lupus but not present in all cases. Antibodies to U1-nRNP, particularly if high titer, identify "mixed connective tissue disease" (MCTD), an overlap syndrome in which features of lupus, scleroderma, and myositis are likely to persist. An ANA pattern displaying fluorescence over centromeres in dividing cells associates with a range of scleroderma syndromes, usually with the milder CREST variant (Table 236–2) (but also with diffuse scleroderma), and sometimes identifies patients with isolated Raynaud's who will progress to a scleroderma syndrome. Tests for specific antibodies that associate with subsets of polymyositis (such as Jo-1) or scleroderma (ScL-70) should prove useful if diagnostic specificity holds as the tests become more widely available.

Most positive ANA's occur for reasons other than a rheumatic disease, since 1 to 2% of the normal population shows a positive, if low-titer, test. The frequency increases with age, with 20 to 25% of persons age 60 or older showing a positive test, and is higher in family members of patients with a rheumatic disease. Many drugs can produce a positive ANA test without inducing a lupus-like syndrome, although the list of responsible agents is similar for both. Chronic liver diseases, pulmonary disorders (pulmonary fibrosis, primary pulmonary hypertension), and endocrine syndromes (type I diabetes mellitus, autoimmune thyroid disease) show positive ANA's in a high proportion in patients, which in some instances can be taken as an overlap with a *forme fruste* rheumatic disorder (such as the patient with primary biliary cirrhosis and a positive ANA test). Certain leukemias, lymphomas, and solid tumors can be associated with ANA's. Because paraneoplastic phenomena can mimic rheumatic disease, the diagnosis of malignancy should be kept in mind when serologic tests suggest a rheumatic disorder in a perplexing multisystem illness that does not fit well with any

TABLE 236–2. ASSOCIATIONS BETWEEN SELECTED NUCLEAR AND CYTOPLASMIC AUTOANTIBODIES AND CERTAIN RHEUMATIC DISEASES

Substrate Immunofluorescence Pattern	Antibody	Antigen	Disease Association(s)	Comments
Human epithelial cells (Hep-2)				
Homogeneous ANA	Antihistone	Histones H1, H2A, H2B, H3, H4	Drug-induced lupus (>95%), infectious mononucleosis (5–10%), normals (1–2%)	Low titer (<1:320) in "normals"
Rim ANA	Anti-native DNA	Double-stranded DNA	SLE (50%)	Antibodies to *double-stranded DNA* highly specific for SLE; "Rim ANA" is rare pattern on Hep-2 cells
Speckled ANA	Anti-Sm	Nonhistone proteins DEFG complexed with small nuclear RNA's	SLE (30%)	Highly specific for SLE
	Anti-U1-nRNP	U1 small nuclear ribonucleoprotein	SLE (35%); MCTD (>95%)	High titer in MCTD
	Anti-Ro (SS-A)	Two proteins complexed with small RNA's Y1-Y5	SLE (35%); Sjögren's (70–80%)	Often missed on Hep-2 ANA; common in "ANA-negative" lupus
	Anti-La (SS-B)	Single protein + RNA polymerase III transcript	SLE (15%); Sjögren's (50–70%)	
	Anti-Ku	DNA binding protein	SLE (10%)	May identify SLE/PSS/myositis overlap
	Anti-Scl-70	DNA topoisomerase I	PSS (40–70%); CREST (10–20%)	
Nucleolar ANA	Anti-PM-Scl	Nucleolar protein complex	PSS (3%); PM (8%)	May identify "sclerodermatomyositis" overlap
	Anti-Mi-2	Nuclear protein complex	DM (15–20%)	Rare in PM
	Anti-RNA polymerase I	Subunits of RNA pol I	PSS (4%)	
Dividing cell-specific patterns	Anticentromere	Centromere/kinetochore protein	CREST (80%); PSS (30%)	In patients with isolated Raynaud's, may predict progression to CREST
	Anti-proliferating cell nuclear antigen	Auxiliary protein of DNA polymerase δ	SLE (3%)	
Cytoplasmic staining	Antisynthetases:			
	Anti-Jo-1	Histidyl tRNA synthetase	PM/DM (18–25%)	Often with ISLD
	Anti-PL-7	Threonyl tRNA synthetase	PM/DM (3%)	Often with ISLD
	Anti-PL-12	Alanyl tRNA synthetase	PM/DM (3%)	Often with ISLD
	Anti-SRP	Signal recognition particle	PM (4%)	No Raynaud's, rare ISLD, poor prognosis
	Antiribosomal P	Large ribosomal subunit	SLE (10%)	May associate with CNS manifestations
	Antimitochondrial	E2 component of pyruvate dehydrogenase complex at inner mitochondrial membrane	Primary biliary cirrhosis (PBC) 90–95%); normals (<1%)	PBC may show CREST, Sjögren's features
Alcohol-fixed human neutrophils				
Cytosol staining	C-ANCA	Neutrophil serine protease	Wegener's granulomatosis (90%)	
Perinuclear staining	P-ANCA	Myeloperoxidase	Microscopic polyarteritis (glomerulonephritis with or without extrarenal small vessel vasculitis); Churg-Strauss syndrome; miscellaneous vasculitides	

ANA = antinuclear antibody; SLE = systemic lupus erythematosus; MCTD = mixed connective tissue disease; PSS = progressive systemic sclerosis (diffuse scleroderma); CREST = calcinosis, Raynaud's phenomenon, esophageal dysmotility, sclerodactyly, and telangectasias; PM = polymyositis; DM = dermatomyositis; ISLD = interstitial lung disease.

rheumatic disease diagnosis. Finally, a number of infections raise ANA's, including malaria, schistosomiasis, trypanosomiasis, and liver flukes, along with tuberculosis, leprosy, and certain bacterial infections due to *Salmonella* and *Klebsiella*. In many patients, classic Epstein-Barr virus infection (infectious mononucleosis) shows ANA's that disappear with resolution of the illness. Some human immunodeficiency virus (HIV)–infected patients have ANA's, but the prevalence and significance of this phenomenon remain to be determined.

Use of human granulocytes as substrates for immunofluorescence testing has identified a group of antibodies directed against particles in the neutrophil cytoplasm (*anti-neutrophil cytoplasmic antibodies, or ANCA's*) that are of growing diagnostic significance. Antibodies against a serine protease contained in cytoplasmic granules (c-ANCA) can be found in 90% of patients with Wegener's granulomatosis (WG) (see Ch. 245) and in patients with chronic inflammation isolated to one or a few sites (e.g., sinuses, lung, or kidney) who do not have full-blown WG. While ANCA disappears in some WG patients with successful treatment and may reappear prior to a clinically evident flare, these fluctuations have not proved sufficiently reliable to guide treatment. Other ANCA patterns, mostly due to reaction with myeloperoxidase, are associated with a range of nephritic and vasculitic syndromes. However, these associations are not strong enough for ANCA's to be considered a "vasculitis test," and a positive ANCA test should not be substituted for biopsy confirmation of WG or vasculitis when cytotoxic therapy is being considered.

Antiphospholipid antibodies are encountered in many SLE patients and can be detected in patients without SLE but with sequelae of thrombosis in vessels of different sizes (e.g., livedo reticularis, gangrene, venous thrombosis, pulmonary emboli, strokes, transverse myelitis, recurrent spontaneous abortions). Results of several other tests in which phospholipids play an important role can be altered by antiphospholipid antibodies. The partial thromboplastin time (PTT) is prolonged by interference with the prothrombin activator complex (coagulation Factors V and Xa, platelet factor 3, and calcium), and this *in vitro* anticoagulation is not completely corrected by normal plasma (defining the "lupus anticoagulant"). Recognizing the phospholipid-rich cardiolipin–cholesterol–phosphatidyl choline target antigen in the venereal disease research laboratory (VDRL) turns this (and other tests for syphilis) falsely positive. Thrombocytopenia and a positive Coombs' test may be seen. A solid phase immunoassay for IgG and IgM antibodies to cardiolipin is the most widely used test for antiphospholipid antibodies.

IMAGING TECHNIQUES. *Plain radiographs* of the joints are relatively inexpensive and widely available. For many rheumatic diseases, information on plain radiographs—such as the presence, character, and distribution of bone erosions, soft tissue calcification, or swelling, alignment of bones, reaction of bone adjacent to joint surfaces, and space between joint surfaces indicating cartilage space—can define the problem and help in judging response to treatment of a chronic process. Plain radiographs may be normal or nonspecific at baseline yet become diagnostic as characteristic features evolve. However, the pathologic processes of many rheumatic disorders often occur in structures for which other means of imaging must be employed. *Arthrography* has mostly been replaced by less invasive techniques for investigating suspected loose bodies, meniscal derangements, or abnormalities of the rotator cuff; however, the technique still provides the standard for determining intraarticular volume and can help in entering a difficult-to-aspirate joint.

Computed tomography (CT) provides excellent spatial resolution of bone and soft tissue structures in an axial plane and is most useful in defining abnormalities of the spine, including herniated discs, sacroiliac joint abnormalities, narrowing of the spinal canal or neural foramina by bony outgrowths (spinal stenosis), and trauma. *Magnetic resonance imaging (MRI)* also provides superb spatial resolution of anatomic structures and characterizes tissue according to its morphologic appearance and physical properties. MRI has become the procedure of choice to delineate abnormalities of intraarticular and periarticular soft tissue structures in large joints, especially the shoulder (rotator cuff tears, glenoid labrum abnormalities) and knee (derangements of menisci and ligaments). For disorders of the spine, MRI can show structural abnormalities and their effect on

the adjacent spinal cord. Although most bony abnormalities are better shown by plain radiographs or CT, MRI can show features of *osteonecrosis* (dead marrow secondary to ischemia) and *osteomyelitis* (increased focal marrow signal indicating edema) before they can be seen on any other imaging study. Because of the high cost and limited availability of MRI, it should be used only when management will be significantly altered by possible findings.

Scintigraphy differs from other imaging techniques by providing information that pertains more to function than to structure. The distribution of tracer is a function of local blood flow, vascular permeability, and tissue uptake. ^{99}Tc-pyrophosphate is taken up by metabolically active bone and thus localizes where this is increased (fractures, blastic skeletal metastases, Paget's disease, periostitis, and "actively" degenerating joints). Because initial distribution of this radionucleide depends on blood flow, scintigraphy that measures activity at several time points ("triple-phase scan") will show uptake initially at sites of increased vascularity—such as synovitis, infection, or neoplasia—and then localize to bone later. While ^{99m}Tc-scanning is nonspecific, it can image the entire skeleton at modest cost and be used to screen for bone and joint abnormalities and metastatic disease. Gallium 67 binds to serum and cellular transferrin and lactoferrin and is preferentially taken up by neutrophils and some neoplastic tissues (e.g., lymphoma). Indium 111–labeled leukocyte scans permit more specific assessment of focal bone or joint infection. Site of tracer localization can be determined with some precision by subjecting the scanned image to single photon emission computed tomography (SPECT), which generates a virtual three-dimensional reconstruction of the image.

Ultrasonography (US) can discern boundaries between the various soft tissue structures comprising the musculoskeletal system and can evaluate pathology within these structures. Its ability to localize a fluid-containing structure can be useful in identifying a joint or bursa for aspiration that would have been difficult to enter using standard landmarks. Lesions of tendons, ligaments, and muscle can be identified and characterized. US is more operator-dependent than other imaging modalities but in experienced hands is the procedure of choice for defining the pathologic anatomy of a painful periarticular region when physical examination and plain radiography are not explanatory.

ARTHROSCOPY. Direct inspection of the joint interior for diagnostic and therapeutic purposes has grown in 25 years from a rarely utilized novelty to the major procedure most commonly performed on the musculoskeletal system (other than casting for fractures). Identifying and repairing traumatic injuries to specific intraarticular structures remain the major focus of arthroscopy. However, the use of arthroscopy in investigating and treating rheumatic disorders could increase as more rheumatologists take up the procedure by using smaller "needle" arthroscopes that can be employed in an office setting.

Arthroscopy has three generic capabilities: direct inspection of intra-articular anatomy, visually guided sampling (biopsy) of tissues, and modification/resection of pathologic tissue under direct visualization using specially designed instruments. During the procedure, the joint is distended and irrigated with a physiologic saline solution to clear away blood and debris. Conventional arthroscopy is usually done in a sterile operating room using a rigid glass lens magnifying scope coupled to a small camera that projects the intraarticular view to a videoscreen. Other instruments placed into the joint through additional punctures can be used to manipulate, cut, shave, and remove various tissues. Virtually all major joints can be arthroscoped, with the knee by far the most commonly entered, followed by the shoulder, ankle, elbow, wrist, and hip. "Needle" arthroscopy employs instruments about one-third the size of conventional arthroscopes (as small as a 16-gauge needle) and can be performed under only local and intra-articular anesthesia.

Some differential diagnostic possibilities that can be confirmed or ruled out by arthroscopy include processes that are treatable but lead to joint destruction if undetected, such as tuberculosis. Arthroscopy should be considered when these processes are even remotely possible. Closed synovial biopsy can be used if arthroscopy is not available but may miss areas of pathology sparsely distributed in the joint.

Arthroscopy can be used for patients with a diagnosed inflammatory arthropathy (such as RA) who have persistent knee symptoms not responding to conventional medical management. Patients with persistent synovitis can be treated by removing visibly inflamed or proliferative synovial tissue from all compartments of the knee under arthroscopic guidance (arthroscopic synovectomy). In other patients features do not suggest ongoing synovitis (pain with minimal swelling, "locking" or "giving way"), yet arthroscopy shows pathology—focal collections of proliferative synovium, areas of synovial scarring, or other consequences of prior inflammation such as softened and torn menisci or attenuated and eroded cruciate ligaments—for which arthroscopically guided resection often can be therapeutic.

In contrast to the "inflamed" knee, the painful knee with noninflammatory synovial fluid usually is diagnosed by defining a particular derangement of the intra-articular anatomy. The most common "derangement" is that of the articular cartilage surface, often suggested by grating, or *crepitus*, of the joint surfaces moving past one another and confirmed with some certainty by other features of OA found on plain radiographs (osteophytes, joint space narrowing, subchondral sclerosis). Other intra-articular abnormalities—torn or degenerated meniscal cartilage, loose bodies, focal synovial collections—can be identified and treated by arthroscopy. Some processes that disrupt joint surfaces through changes in underlying bone cannot be seen or modified at arthroscopy; these processes—osteonecrosis, stress fracture, malignancy—are often not apparent on plain radiographs and thus require more extensive imaging, such as MRI.

Adler RS, Martel W: Imaging techniques in the assessment of rheumatic diseases. *In* Schumacher HR (ed.): Primer on the Rheumatic Diseases, 10th ed. Atlanta, Arthritis Foundation, 1993, pp 74–81. *Concise, well-illustrated synopsis of capabilities and limitations of available imaging procedures.*

Kushner I: C-reactive protein in rheumatology. Arthritis Rheum 34:1065, 1991. *A succinct review of the CRP biology and clinical utility of its measurement, particularly in managing rheumatic diseases.*

O'Rourke KS, Ike RW: Diagnostic arthroscopy in the arthritis patient. Rheum Dis Clin North Am 20:321, 1994. *A review of the various situations in rheumatology when diagnostic arthroscopy—particularly with the "needle" arthroscope—can be useful, and why.*

Shmerling RH, Delbanco TL, Tosteson AN, et al.: Synovial fluid tests: What should be ordered? JAMA 264:1009, 1990. *Prospective analysis of 100 consecutive arthrocenteses judging contribution to diagnosis from several tests. Only WBC count and percent polys discriminated between "inflammatory" and "noninflammatory" diagnoses as determined independently.*

Tan EM: Molecular biology of nuclear autoantigens. Adv Nephrol 22:213, 1993. *Recent comprehensive review of identified autoantigens and corresponding autoantibodies, discussing clinical associations as well as known function of autoantigen.*

237 RHEUMATOID ARTHRITIS
Frank C. Arnett

Rheumatoid arthritis (RA) is a chronic systemic inflammatory disease predominantly affecting diarthrodial joints and frequently a variety of other organs. The American College of Rheumatology (ACR) revised classification criteria for RA to guarantee uniformity in investigative and epidemiologic studies (Table 237–1). Although these seven items include the most characteristic clinical features of RA, a variety of other disorders may mimic the disease (see Differential Diagnosis and Table 237–3).

RA occurs worldwide in all ethnic groups. Prevalence rates range from 0.3 to 1.5% in most populations, but frequencies of 3.5 to 5.3% have been found in several Native American tribes (Yakima, Chippewa, Inuit). The peak incidence of onset is between the fourth and sixth decades, but RA may begin at any time from childhood (see Juvenile Chronic Arthritis) to later life. Females are two to three times more likely to be affected than males.

ETIOLOGY. Despite intensive research over many decades, the cause of RA remains unknown. Three areas of interrelated research are currently most promising: (1) host genetic factors, (2) immunoregulatory abnormalities and autoimmunity, and (3) a triggering or persisting microbial infection.

Genetic susceptibility to RA has been clearly demonstrated. The disease clusters in families and is more concordant in monozygotic (30%) than in dizygotic (5%) twins. Certain major histocompatibility complex (MHC) class II alleles (and their encoded HLA, or human leukocyte antigens) occur with increased frequencies in affected individuals. Among Caucasians of western European origin,

TABLE 237–1. CLASSIFICATION CRITERIA FOR RHEUMATOID ARTHRITIS (RA)*

1. Morning stiffness (≥ 1 hr)
2. Swelling (soft tissue) of three or more joints
3. Swelling (soft tissue) of hand joints (PIP, MCP, or wrist)
4. Symmetric swelling (soft tissue)
5. Subcutaneous nodules
6. Serum rheumatoid factor
7. Erosions and/or periarticular osteopenia, in hand or wrist joints, seen on radiograph

* Criteria 1 to 4 must have been continuous for 6 weeks or longer and must be observed by a physician. A diagnosis of rheumatoid arthritis requires that four of the seven criteria be fulfilled.

PIP = proximal interphalangeal; MCP = metacarpophalangeal.

HLA-DR4 occurs in 60 to 70% of seropositive patients with RA compared with 25 to 30% of normal individuals. HLA-DR1 is found in the majority of HLA-DR4–negative patients and is most strongly associated with the disease in several other ethnic groups (Israelis, Asian Indians). Several subtypes of HLA-DR4 were defined initially by mixed lymphocyte culture (MLC) and more recently by DNA sequencing (Table 237–2). Only certain HLA-DR4 subtypes predispose to RA (Dw4 or DRB1*0401, Dw14 or DRB1* 0404, and Dw15 or DRB1*0405), while others do not (Dw10 or DRB1*0402 and Dw13 or DRB1*0403). HLA-DR4 subtypes result from only a few amino acid differences in the third hypervariable region of the HLA-DR beta chain. HLA-DR1 shares this same amino acid sequence as do several other HLA alleles that have more recently been associated with RA in some populations (see Table 237–2). Thus a "shared epitope" among several MHC class II molecules appears to predispose to RA. Moreover, homozygosity for the amino acid sequence, especially if carried on HLA-DR4 molecules, has been shown to correlate with disease severity, including more destructive joint disease, subcutaneous nodules, and the extra-articular manifestations, especially rheumatoid lung disease and Felty's syndrome. The crucial region for the shared epitope on HLA-DR molecules appears to be a combining site for the T-cell antigen receptor (TCR). Since MHC class II molecules present processed antigen to the TCR on helper (CD4+) T lymphocytes (see Ch. 221), it appears likely that an abnormal antigen-specific cellular and/or humoral immune response is inherent to the etiology of RA. The nature of the antigen, whether self or foreign, remains unknown, although candidates include type II collagen, proteoglycans, heat shock proteins, and immunoglobulins. Other genes also are probably necessary for RA, perhaps TCR and/or immunoglobulin loci.

RA appears to be an "autoimmune" disease, similar to other MHC class II–associated disorders (see Ch. 229). Autoantibodies to the Fc portion of immunoglobulin G (IgG) molecules, or RF's, are produced by B lymphocytes in the blood and synovial tissues of 80% of RA patients. Such cases are termed "seropositive." High titers of serum RF, typically of the IgM isotype when detected by the usual clinical methods, are associated with more severe joint disease and with extra-articular manifestations, especially subcutaneous nodules.

Despite the extremely strong association of RF's with RA, they clearly do not cause the disease. Production of RF occurs commonly in other disorders in which there is chronic antigenic stimulation, such as bacterial endocarditis, tuberculosis, syphilis, kala-azar, viral infections, intravenous drug abuse, and cirrhosis. Normal individuals occasionally produce RF, especially with increasing age.

An infectious origin for RA has been a continuing hypothesis. Streptococci, diphtheroids, mycoplasmas, and *Clostridium perfringens* have all been proposed and later discarded because of lack of definitive evidence. Viral infections such as rubella, Ross River virus, and more recently, parvovirus B19 have been shown to produce an acute polyarthritis, but no evidence exists that they initiate chronic RA. The Epstein-Barr virus (EBV) remains a viable but unproven candidate for a pathogenetic role. The EBV is a polyclonal B cell activator capable of stimulating autoantibody production, including RF. Increased numbers of EBV-infected B cells have been found in the blood but not the synovial tissue of RA patients. Anti-

TABLE 237–2. HLA ASSOCIATIONS WITH RA

	HLA Types (Alleles) and Methods of Detection			Third Hypervariable Region Amino Acid Sequences					Most Common Ethnic Groups
	Alloantisera (DR)	*MLC (Dw)*	*DNA (DRB1)*	70	71	72	73	74	
Associated with RA	DR4	Dw4	*0401	Q	K	R	A	A	Caucasians (West Europe)
	DR4	Dw14	*0404	•	R	•	•	•	Caucasians (West Europe)
	DR4	Dw15	*0405	•	R	•	•	•	Japanese, Chinese
	DR1	Dw1	*0101	•	R	•	•	•	Asian Indians, Israelis
	DR6 (14)	Dw16	*1402	•	R	•	•	•	Yakima Native Americans
	DR10	—	*1001	R	R	•	•	•	Spanish, Greeks, Israelis
Not associated with RA	DR4	Dw10	*0402	D	E	•	•	•	Caucasians (East Europe)
	DR4	Dw13	*0403	•	R	•	•	E	Polynesians
	DR2	Dw2	*1501	D	A	•	•	•	Caucasians
	DR3	Dw3	*0301	•	•	•	G	R	Caucasians

Abbreviations for amino acids: Q = glutamine, K = lysine, R = arginine, A = alanine, D = aspartic acid, E = glutamic acid.
• = the same amino acid in that position as DRB1*0401.

bodies against a nuclear antigen (EBNA) expressed in EBV-infected cells occur in the majority of RA patients, and a variety of other unusual immune responses to EBV are found in RA patients. More recently, an EBV protein has been shown to share the same five amino acids as the HLA-DR4 (Dw14) and HLA-DR1 molecules, which are implicated in susceptibility to RA, thus raising the possibility of "molecular mimicry" as a mechanism. A similar homology with an *E. coli* heat shock protein also has been found.

PATHOLOGY AND PATHOGENESIS. The pathologic hallmark of RA is synovial membrane proliferation and outgrowth associated with erosion of articular cartilage and subchondral bone. Often likened to a malignant tumor, proliferating inflammatory tissue (pannus) may lead subsequently to destruction of intra-articular and periarticular structures and may result in the joint deformities and dysfunction seen clinically.

The events initiating the process are unknown (Fig. 237–1). The earliest findings include microvascular injury and proliferation of synovial cells accompanied by interstitial edema and perivascular infiltration by mononuclear cells, predominantly T lymphocytes. Polymorphonuclear leukocytes and plasma cells are infrequent. As the process continues, there is further hyperplasia of lining cells, both DR-positive type A (macrophage-like) and DR-negative type B (fibroblast-like), and the normally acellular subsynovial stroma becomes engorged with mononuclear inflammatory cells, which may collect into aggregates or follicles, especially around postcapillary venules. The composition of cellular infiltrates varies, with some being predominantly T cells, usually CD4+ (helper/inducer), and others having a mixed population of lymphocytes (often CD8+ cytotoxic T cells), plasma cells, macrophages, and interdigitating (dendritic) cells. Mast cells are also commonly present. Occasionally, germinal centers rich in B lymphocytes can be seen. The proliferating synovium (pannus) becomes villous and is vascularized by arterioles, capillaries, and venules.

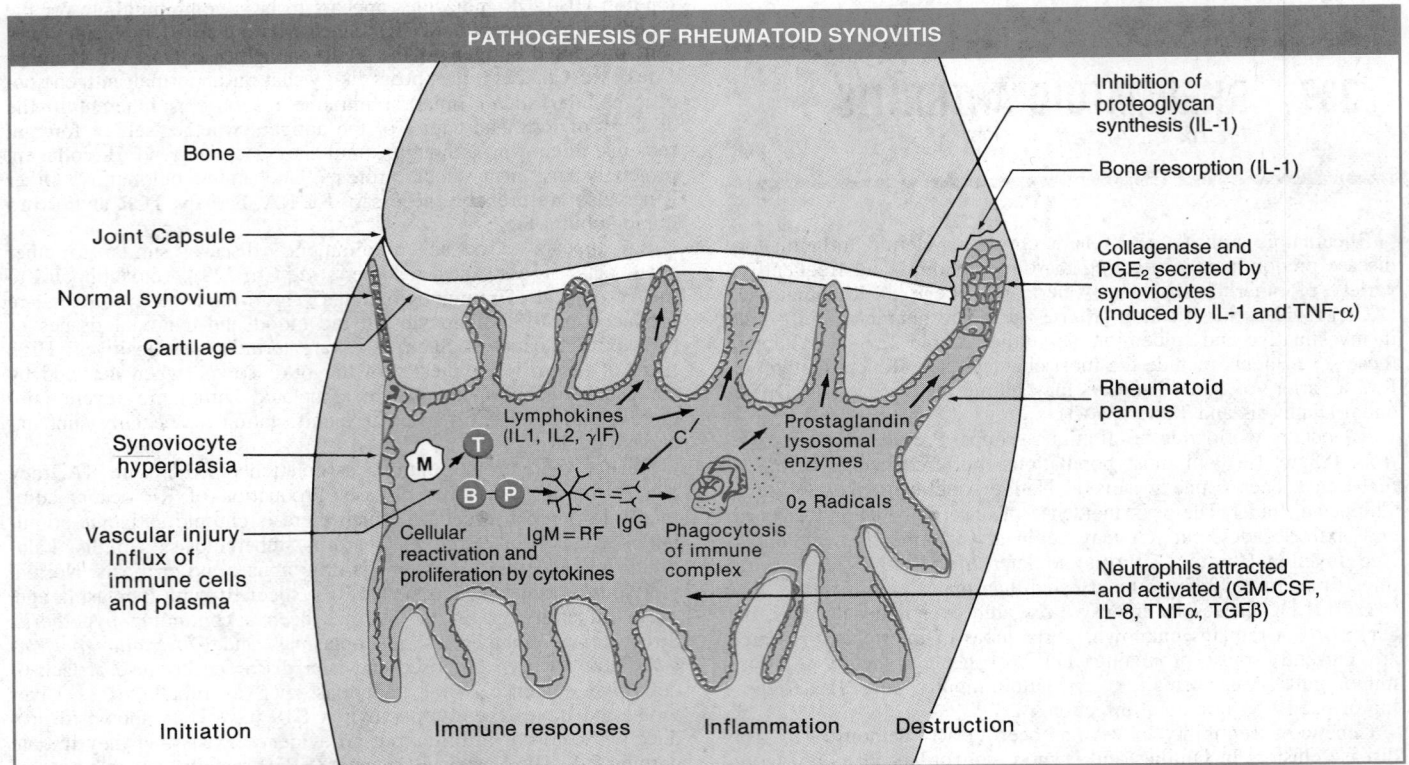

FIGURE 237–1. Events involved in the pathogenesis of rheumatoid synovitis progress from left to right. M = macrophage; T = T lymphocyte; B = B lymphocyte; P = plasma cell; Il = interleukin; TNFα = tumor necrosis factor alpha; TGFβ = transforming growth factor beta; GM-CSF = granulocyte-macrophage colony stimulating factor; γ If = gamma-interferon; RF = rheumatoid factor; PGE$_2$ = prostaglandin E$_2$; IgM = immunoglobulin M; IgG = immunoglobulin G; C = complement.

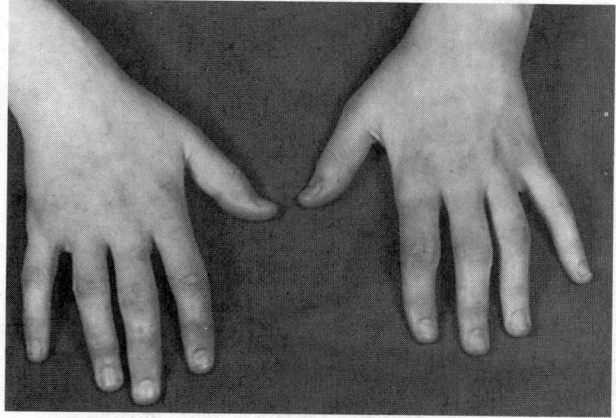

FIGURE 237–2. Early rheumatoid arthritis manifests as symmetric swelling and slight flexion deformities of proximal interphalangeal joints of the hands. Roentgenograms were normal except for evidence of soft tissue swelling.

Roles for both *cellular* and *humoral* immune mechanisms in the rheumatoid synovium are supported by molecular and immunopathologic findings. T lymphocytes appear to be activated, presumably by some unknown antigen(s) presented by DR-positive cells (type A synoviocytes, macrophages, dendritic cells, B lymphocytes). Studies of TCR gene expression suggest restricted Vβ usage and oligoclonality, but this area is controversial. Collectively, these interacting immune cells produce a variety of cytokines that promote further synovial proliferation and inflammation, as well as bone and cartilage destruction. Some of the cytokines that appear to play important and multiple roles include interleukins- (IL) 1, 2, 6, and 8, tumor necrosis factor α (TNFα), granulocyte-macrophage stimulating factor (GM-CSF), and transforming growth factor β (TGFβ). For example, IL-1 induces production of metalloproteinases (collagenase and stromelysin) and prostaglandin E$_2$ by synoviocytes. This cytokine also promotes degradation and inhibits synthesis of proteoglycan by chondrocytes, as well as enhances resorption of calcium from bone.

Humoral mechanisms are supported by the demonstration of local RF production within the synovium, the formation of IgM-activated B cells and IgG immune complexes, and activation and consumption of complement via the classic pathway. The sequelae of complement activation include increased vascular permeability and phagocytosis of the immune complexes by phagocytic cells. Aggregates of immune complexes within polymorphonuclear leukocytes are often seen in rheumatoid synovial fluid and have been termed "RA cells" or "ragocytes." Antigen-antibody complexes formed within the joint cavity can become trapped in hyaline cartilage and fibrocartilage, where they cause changes in matrix macromolecules. Within the synovial fluid, immune complexes activate the complement system, kinins, phagocytic cells, and the release of lysosomal enzymes and oxygen free radicals. Mediators produced in this process stimulate synovial cells to proliferate and to produce proteinases and prostaglandins. These products cause dissolution of the connective tissue macromolecules, as well as articular cartilage. They also may activate fibroblasts to produce a denser connective tissue matrix (fibrosis).

The ultimate destruction of cartilage, bone, tendons, and ligaments probably results from a variety of proteolytic enzymes, metalloproteinases, and soluble mediators. Collagenase, produced at the interface of pannus and cartilage, is probably largely responsible for the typical erosions.

CLINICAL FEATURES. The mode of onset of RA is highly variable. In the majority of cases, joint pain and/or stiffness develops insidiously over several weeks to months. One or more small joints of the hands, wrists, shoulders, or knees and/or the metatarsophalangeal (MTP) joints are frequently the first symptomatic areas. Malaise and fatigue, occasionally with low-grade fever, may accompany musculoskeletal discomfort. As the disease progresses, joint swelling, tenderness, and a red or bluish discoloration become apparent (Fig. 237–2). The pattern of joint involvement is typically polyarticular and symmetric, involving the proximal interphalangeal (PIP), metacarpophalangeal (MCP), wrist, elbow, shoulder, knee, ankle, and MTP joints. Distal interphalangeal (DIP) joints of the fingers are usually spared. Joint stiffness, especially if lasting more than 1 hour in the morning and after inactivity, is prominent. So characteristic is this symptom that the duration of morning stiffness is often used as a quantitative guide to the activity of the inflammatory process in both clinical practice and research studies. Over time the patient may experience increasing difficulty with pain and stiffness, as well as impaired joint function. The simple activities of daily living may be severely compromised, and the ability to continue a productive occupation is threatened. Sleep habits become disturbed, and the patient may experience depression and weight loss.

An "acute" onset occurring over 1 or several days is seen in about 20% of patients. Occasionally, an individual retires in the evening with no symptoms and awakens with acute, generalized RA. Such a rapid onset of pain involving joints, surrounding soft tissues, and muscle can mimic and must be differentiated from acute myositis, viral syndromes, or, if focal, even septic or crystal-induced arthritides. Rare patients experience recurrent (palindromic) episodes of acute monoarthritis, often so severe as to mimic gout, yet lasting only 24 to 48 hours. Such patients, especially if seropositive, eventually develop the typical chronic, symmetric polyarthritis of RA.

The course of RA, like its onset, varies widely. Fluctuating disease activity early in the disease process is usual. Ultimately, joint deformities and variable degrees of disability occur in most patients (Fig. 237–3). Some patients have a relentlessly progressive course leading to early disability or even death, but repeated periods of some degree of remission are the rule. The ACR has proposed criteria for clinical remission in RA. At least five of the following requirements must be fulfilled for at least 2 consecutive months: (1) duration of morning stiffness not exceeding 15 minutes, (2) no fatigue, (3) no joint pain (by history), (4) no joint tenderness or pain

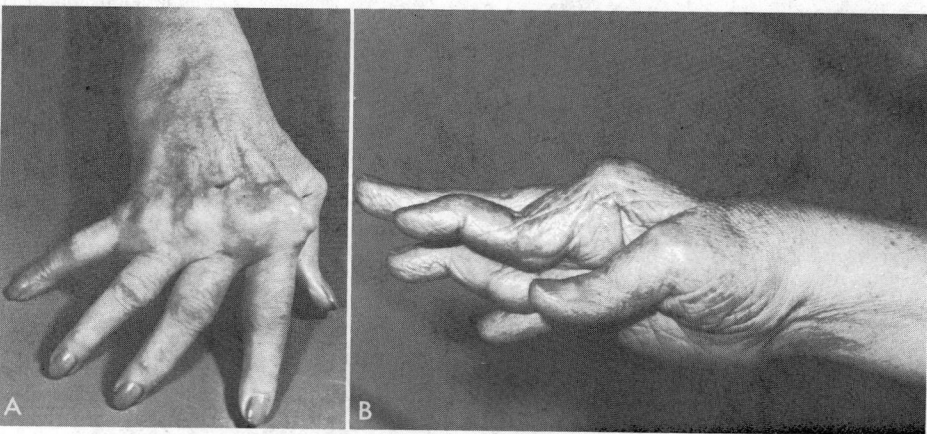

FIGURE 237–3. Hand deformities characteristic of chronic rheumatoid arthritis. *A,* Subluxation of metacarpophalangeal joints with ulnar deviation of digits. *B,* Hyperextension ("swan neck") deformities of proximal interphalangeal joints.

on motion, (5) no soft tissue swelling in joints or tendon sheaths, (6) an erythrocyte sedimentation rate (Westergren) <30 mm per hour for females or 20 mm per hour for males.

The assessment of functional capacity is frequently necessary in the RA patient. Although various schemes have been proposed, the simple classification that follows serves well in most situations:

Class I: No restriction of ability to perform normal activities.
Class II: Moderate restriction, but with an ability to perform most activities of daily living.
Class III: Marked restriction, with an inability to perform most activities of daily living and occupation.
Class IV: Incapacitation with confinement to bed or wheelchair.

DIFFERENTIAL DIAGNOSIS. Considerations in the differential diagnosis of RA are numerous (Table 237–3). Early RA, especially that of acute onset, is more difficult to diagnose than is the typical established case. The finding of subcutaneous nodules and the presence of RF are useful but are not absolutely specific differential features. Therefore, a complete medical evaluation, often including synovial fluid analysis, is indicated in all patients with significant joint manifestations.

ARTICULAR MANIFESTATIONS. RA can affect any diarthrodial joint. Those most commonly involved are the small joints of the hands, wrists, knees, and feet. With time, the disease also may affect the elbows, shoulders, sternoclavicular joints, hips, and ankles. The temporomandibular and cricoarytenoid joints are less frequently involved. Spinal involvement in RA is generally limited to the upper cervical articulations. In contrast to the spondyloarthropathies, RA does not cause sacroiliitis or clinically significant disease in the lumbar or thoracic spinal areas.

Hands. Swelling of the PIP joints, giving a fusiform or spindle-shaped appearance to the fingers, is one of the most common early signs. Bilateral and symmetric swelling of the MCP joints is also frequent (see Fig. 237–2). The DIP joints are usually spared, which is a useful sign in discriminating RA from osteoarthritis and psoriatic arthritis. Soft tissue laxity gives rise to ulnar deviation of the fingers at the MCP joints (Fig. 237–3A). Swan-neck deformities develop from hyperextension of the PIP joints in conjunction with flexion of the DIP joints (Fig. 237–3B). Boutonnière (buttonhole) deformities result from flexion contractures of the PIP joints associated with hyperextension of the DIP joints. These changes result in a loss of strength and dexterity in the hands, as well as the ability to maintain a good pinch. Synovial erosions of extensor tendons, usually at the dorsum of the wrist, may lead to sudden rupture and loss of the ability to extend one or more fingers.

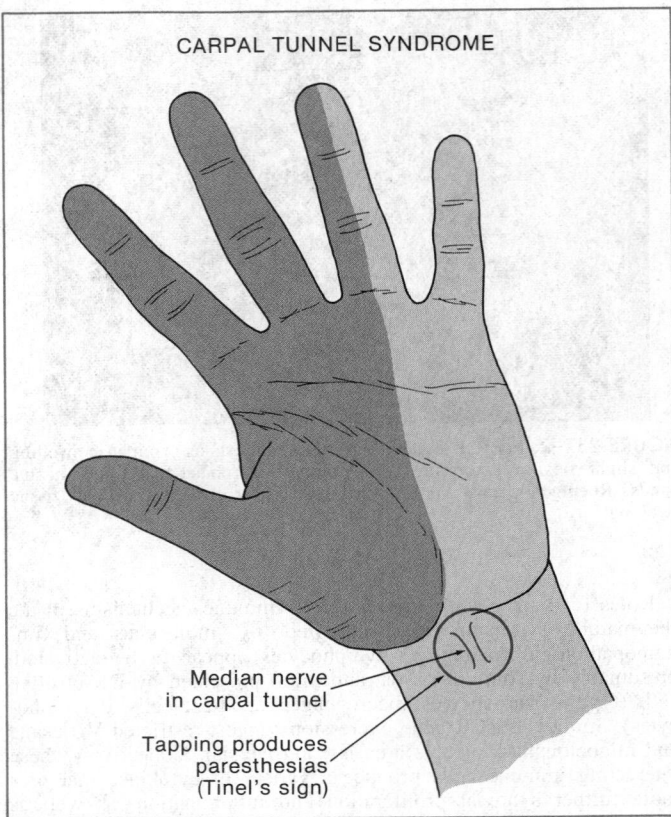

CARPAL TUNNEL SYNDROME

Median nerve
in carpal tunnel

Tapping produces
paresthesias
(Tinel's sign)

FIGURE 237–4. Distribution of pain and/or paresthesias *(shaded area)* when the median nerve is compressed by swelling in the wrist (carpal tunnel).

Wrists. The wrists are almost invariably involved in RA and frequently demonstrate easily palpable, boggy synovium, especially over the ulnar styloid. Loss of wrist motion, both flexion and extension, usually occurs to some degree. The median nerve on the volar side often becomes compressed by proliferating synovium, resulting in a carpal tunnel syndrome (Fig. 237–4). The patient notes paresthesias or pain in the thumb, second and third digits, and radial side of the fourth digit. Symptoms are typically worse at night or with other activities associated with sustained flexion of the wrist. *Tinel's* (Fig. 237–4) and *Phalen's* (Fig. 237–5) signs can usually be elicited, and thenar muscle wasting may be evident.

Knees. Synovial proliferation and effusion are common in these weight-bearing joints. Effusions may be detected by performing ballottement on the patella or by observing a "bulge sign" along the medial aspect of the patella when fluid is pushed into the suprapatellar pouch and then expressed back into the joint. Quadriceps atrophy may occur, and a flexion contracture of the knee may compromise walking. Eventually, destruction of soft tissue around the knee can produce marked joint instability. Popliteal (Baker's) cysts may form owing to effusion or synovial proliferation into the semimembranous bursa (Fig. 237–6). Such synovial cysts may dissect or rupture into the calf, producing symptoms and signs mimicking those of thrombophlebitis. Sonograms are useful to confirm the diagnosis. Venograms also may be necessary because venous occlusion by the cyst can occur.

Feet and Ankles. The MTP joints are the most commonly involved sites. Subluxation of the metatarsal heads into the soles, often with cock-up and valgus deformities of the toes, results in painful walking and difficulty with footwear.

Neck. Neck pain and stiffness are common. As in other joints, the rheumatoid process can lead to erosion of bone and ligaments in the cervical spine. Atlantoaxial subluxation (C1 on C2) can be seen radiographically in up to 30% of cases (Fig. 237–7). Spinal cord compression with neurologic manifestations occurs infrequently but is a neurosurgical emergency. Occipital and/or frontal headache is a common premonitory sign of weakness in the extremities, bladder or bowel incontinence, or frank quadriplegia. Vertebral arteries also may be compressed, resulting in vertebrobasilar insuffi-

TABLE 237–3. DIFFERENTIAL DIAGNOSIS OF RA

	Subcutaneous Nodules	Rheumatoid Factor (RF)
Acute viral arthritis (rubella, hepatitis B, parvovirus)	−	−
Bacterial endocarditis	+/−	+
Acute rheumatic fever	+	−
Serum sickness	−	−
Sarcoidosis	+	+
Reactive arthritis (Reiter's disease)	−	−
Psoriatic arthritis	−	−
Inflammatory bowel disease	−	−
Whipple's disease	−	−
Systemic lupus erythematosus	+	+
Sjögren's syndrome	−	+
Systemic sclerosis (scleroderma)	−	+/−
Polymyositis	−	+/−
Vasculitis syndromes	−	+
Polymyalgia rheumatica	−	−
Polyarticular gout	+ (tophi)	−
Calcium pyrophosphate disease	−	−
Amyloidosis	+/−	−
Paraneoplastic syndromes	−	−
Multicentric reticulohistiocytosis	+	−
Osteoarthritis (erosive)	−	−

− = not present; + = frequently present; +/− = occasionally present.

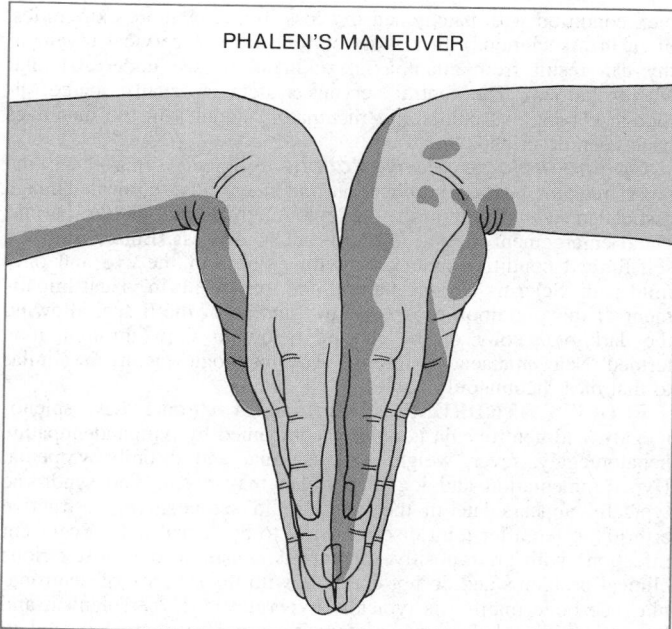

PHALEN'S MANEUVER

FIGURE 237–5. Pain and/or paresthesias are produced in the distribution of the median nerve (Fig. 237–4) when hands are held in forced flexion for 30 to 60 seconds (Phalen's maneuver).

ciency with vertigo or syncope, especially on downward gaze. Head tilt may occur from lateral mass collapse of the C1 and C2 vertebrae.

Elbows. Proliferative synovitis in the elbow often causes flexion contractures, even early in the disease. Supination of the hand may be impaired, especially if shoulder motion is concomitantly decreased. Rarely, ulnar or radial nerves may become entrapped.

Shoulders. Involvement of the glenohumeral, acromioclavicular,

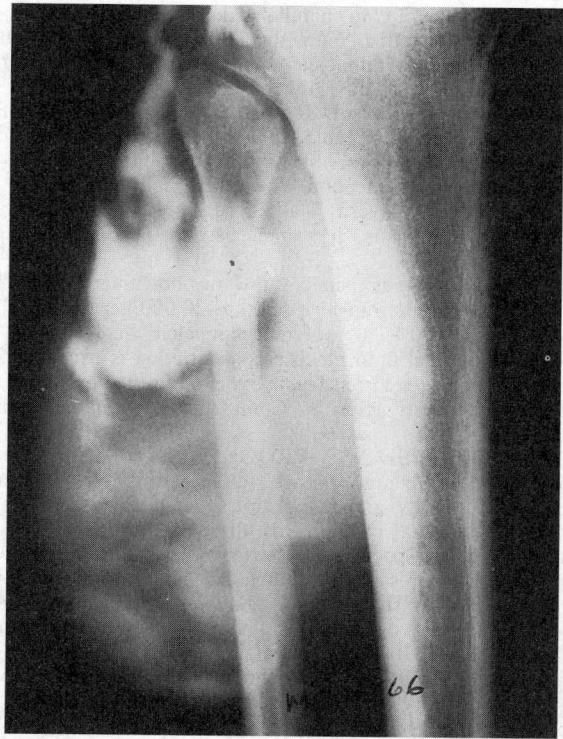

FIGURE 237–6. Arthrogram using a radiocontrast agent injected into the knee. The dye flows into the popliteal space and through a narrow channel into a large synovial cyst (Baker's cyst), which has dissected into the soft tissues of the calf.

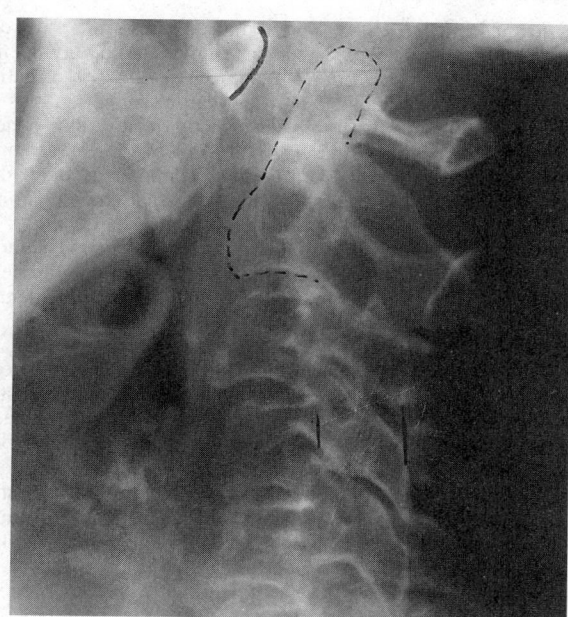

FIGURE 237–7. Lateral roentgenogram of the cervical spine in flexion. The body of C2 and its odontoid process are outlined by broken lines, and the posterior aspect of the anterior segment of C1 is indicated by a solid line. Normally, a space of only 2 to 3 mm separates C1 from C2. The space between C1 and the odontoid of C2 is markedly increased, indicating subluxation of C1 on C2. At a lower level, C3 is also displaced anteriorly owing to rheumatoid erosion of articular and ligamentous structures.

and thoracoscapular joints is common in advanced but not early RA. Limited motion and tenderness just below and lateral to the coracoid process are typical symptoms. Noticeable swelling is rare; however, large synovial cysts may occur (see Color Plate 3D). Joint destruction usually involves rupture of the joint capsule and subluxation of the humerus.

Hips. Pain in the groin, lateral buttock, or lower back may indicate hip involvement. Because the hip joint capsule has poor distensibility, severe pain can result if a large effusion occurs. Arthrocentesis should be done to relieve pain and to exclude infection in such cases. Rarely, extreme hip destruction results in protrusion of the femur into the pelvis.

Cricoarytenoid Joints. Synovitis of the cricoarytenoid joints may result in dysphagia, hoarseness, or anterior neck pain. The sudden onset of stridor and dyspnea in a patient with RA is an emergency. Prompt administration of intra-articular or parenteral corticosteroids and/or tracheostomy may be necessary.

EXTRA-ARTICULAR MANIFESTATIONS. Constitutional symptoms, including malaise, fatigue, weakness, low-grade fever, and mild lymphadenopathy, are common in RA. All the extra-articular complications occur almost exclusively in seropositive patients.

Skin. Subcutaneous nodules occur in 20 to 25% of RA patients and are almost always associated with serum RF and more severe articular disease. They occur most commonly in periarticular structures and areas subject to pressure, such as the elbows, extensor and flexor tendons of the hands and feet, Achilles tendons, and less commonly, occipital and sacral areas. They may occasionally become infected but are usually asymptomatic.

Palmar erythema and fragility of the skin, resulting in easy bruising, are common manifestations. Rheumatoid vasculitis occurs in two major forms. The first is manifested by small, splinter-shaped brown infarcts in the nail folds and digital pulp, often also present over subcutaneous nodules (see Color Plate 3E). Histologic examination may reveal leukocytoclastic vasculitis or a mild venulitis. This is a benign process in most patients and does not indicate serious systemic vasculitis. The second form is a severe necrotizing vasculitis of small and medium arteries indistinguishable from periarteritis nodosa. Digital infarcts, mononeuritis multiplex, fever, and other manifestations of systemic disease should prompt aggressive therapy.

Cardiac Manifestations. Pericardial disease is the most common cardiac feature of RA. Evidence of pericardial involvement with old fibrinous lesions is found in approximately 40% of patients at autopsy. A similar frequency of pericardial abnormalities can be detected by echocardiography in asymptomatic RA patients. Clinically evident pericarditis in RA, however, is infrequent. Large pericardial effusions with cardiac tamponade and death are rare. Constrictive pericarditis is somewhat more common and typically presents as dyspnea, right-sided heart failure, and peripheral edema. The pericardial fluid characteristics include a low glucose concentration, increased level of lactate dehydrogenase (LDH), elevated immunoglobulin levels, and low complement activity.

Rheumatoid nodules may develop occasionally in the myocardium or heart valves, and vasculitis may involve the coronary arteries. Conduction abnormalities, valvular incompetence or stenosis, and myocardial infarction are all rare clinical sequelae of rheumatoid heart disease.

Pulmonary Manifestations. Rheumatoid pleural disease, although frequently found at autopsy, is most commonly asymptomatic. Occasionally, a pleural effusion may cause respiratory limitation. Neoplasm and infection should be ruled out by a pleural tap. Typically, the pleural fluid is exudative, and white cell counts vary greatly but generally are <5000 per microliter. Glucose levels tend to be low, and the LDH enzyme level is high. Total hemolytic complement, C3, and C4 levels are low. Immune complexes and RF are frequently found in the pleural fluid.

Intrapulmonary nodules may also be seen (Fig. 237–8). Although they are usually asymptomatic, they may become infected and cavitate or rupture into the pleural space, producing a pneumothorax. Malignancy must be excluded in the RA patient, as in any other patient, with a solitary lung nodule. Similar but distinct nodular infiltrates also may be seen in rheumatoid lungs in association with pneumoconiosis (Caplan's syndrome).

Finally, a diffuse interstitial fibrosis with pneumonitis may progress to a honeycomb appearance on the roentgenogram, bronchiectasis, chronic cough, and progressive dyspnea. Pulmonary function tests show a diminished compliance and a restrictive ventilatory pattern. Large airways are not involved. An irreversible combination of respiratory insufficiency and resultant right-sided cardiac failure is possible. Rarely, small airway obstruction may develop into a necrotizing bronchiolitis. This complication also may result from therapies with gold and D-penicillamine.

Neurologic Manifestations. Peripheral neuropathies can be produced by proliferating synovium causing compression of nerves. Carpal tunnel syndrome (median neuropathy) (see under Articular Manifestations) is common, and a similar entrapment of the anterior tibial nerve (tarsal tunnel syndrome) can result in paresthesias with a foot drop. Rheumatoid vasculitis may cause a mononeuritis multi-

plex condition with patchy sensory loss in one or more extremities, often in association with a wrist or foot drop. A cervical myelopathy can result from atlantoaxial subluxation (see under Articular Manifestations). The central nervous system is usually spared, although cerebral vasculitis and rheumatoid nodules in the meninges have been described.

Ophthalmologic Manifestations. Sjögren's syndrome is the most frequent ocular complication and may cause corneal damage associated with dryness of the eyes. Xerostomia and/or parotid gland enlargement may accompany ocular dryness. Episcleritis is a self-limited condition associated with redness of the eye and only mild pain. Scleritis is more painful and may result in visual impairment. If this condition progresses to thinning of the tissue, allowing the dark blue color of the choroid below to show through, it is termed "scleromalacia perforans." The histologic picture is similar to that of a rheumatoid nodule.

FELTY'S SYNDROME. This triad of chronic RA, splenomegaly, and neutropenia is often accompanied by lymphadenopathy, hepatomegaly, fever, weight loss, anemia, and thrombocytopenia. Hyperpigmentation and leg ulcers also may occur. The syndrome typically appears late in the course of a seropositive, destructive arthritis, often after joint disease is felt to be "burnt out." Recurrent infections with gram-positive organisms constitute the most serious clinical problems and do not correlate with the severity of neutropenia. The bone marrow is typically hyperplastic. Hypersplenism and immune-mediated destruction of white blood cells are believed to cause the neutropenia. Splenectomy may correct the neutropenia and prevent further infections in some patients, but many do not improve. The "large granular lymphocyte syndrome," which is probably a premalignant disorder of T lymphocytes, may mimic Felty's syndrome in RA patients. Splenectomy should not be performed for this disorder because it may hasten the onset of malignancy.

LABORATORY FEATURES. A chronic normocytic, normochromic anemia with hematocrit values from 30 to 35% is usual. Typically, both serum iron levels and iron-binding capacity are low. The anemia does not respond to administration of iron, but erythropoietin may be effective when anemia is severe. The white blood cell count and differential are typically normal, but eosinophilia may occur in severe systemic disease. The platelet count may be moderately elevated owing to chronic inflammation. The erythrocyte sedimentation rate is elevated in most patients but only roughly parallels disease activity. The presence of RF is detected in more than 80% of cases and is useful in clinical diagnosis. Antinuclear antibodies detected by immunofluorescence, usually in low titer, can be found in 30 to 40% of cases. DNA typing of RA-associated HLA-DRB1 alleles (DR4, DR1, others; see Table 237–2) has no diagnostic utility because these genes occur in high frequencies in the normal population. However, detection of patients homozygous for these DRB1 "susceptibility/severity" alleles early in disease may predict the worst prognosis, in which early, aggressive therapy is indicated.

Synovial fluid analysis usually shows a poor mucin clot test and white cell counts in the range of 5000 to 20,000 per cubic millimeter, with 50 to 70% as polymorphonuclear leukocytes (Table 237–4). The synovial fluid glucose concentration is usually normal, but very low values occur occasionally, even in the absence of a superimposed infectious arthritis. Complement levels are typically low.

DISEASE COURSE AND PROGNOSIS. Although once considered a relatively benign disease, RA is now known to result in considerable disability and a higher than expected mortality rate. Approximately 20% of patients will improve spontaneously or even achieve remission, especially in the first year of disease; however, chronic disease progression and functional deterioration occur in the majority. Long-term studies have shown RA patients to have 6 times the probability of severe limitations of activities, 4 times as many restricted activity days, and 10 times the work disability rate as the general population, and approximately 50% are forced to stop working within 10 years of diagnosis. A higher mortality rate also correlates with the degree of disability and results from infections, systemic manifestations, and gastrointestinal bleeding or perforation. The economic impact on the health care system is also substantial.

THERAPEUTIC MANAGEMENT. Objectives of management include (1) relief of pain and stiffness, (2) reduction of inflamma-

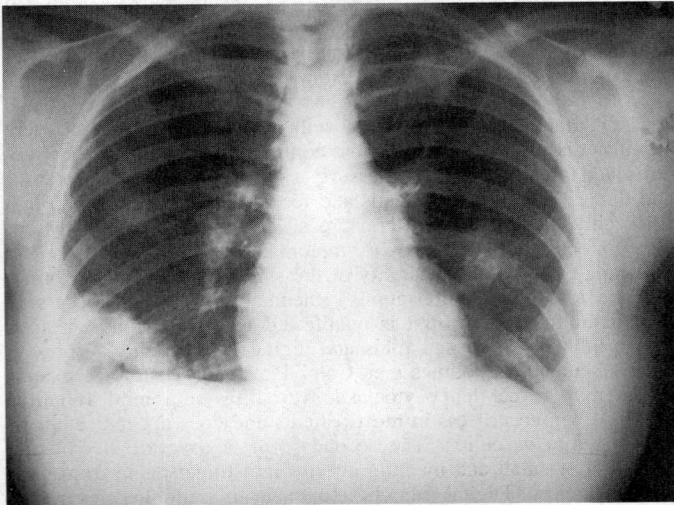

FIGURE 237–8. Chest roentgenogram demonstrating discrete rheumatoid nodules in both right and left lower lobes of the lungs. (Courtesy of Dr. Martin Lidsky, Houston, Texas.)

TABLE 237–4. SYNOVIAL FLUID FINDINGS IN RHEUMATOID ARTHRITIS AND OTHER FORMS OF ARTHRITIS

Synovial Characteristics	Rheumatoid Arthritis	Gout/Pseudogout	Reiter's/Psoriatic Arthritis	Septic Arthritis	Osteoarthritis, Traumatic Arthritis
Color	Yellow	Yellow-white	Yellow	White	Clear, pale yellow, or bloody
Clarity	Cloudy	Cloudy-opaque	Cloudy	Opaque	Transparent
Viscosity	Poor	Poor	Poor	Poor	Good
Mucin clot	Poor	Poor	Poor	Poor	Good
White blood cell count/mm^3	3000–50,000	3000–50,000 or higher	3000–50,000 or higher	50,000–300,000	< 3000
% polymorphonuclear leukocytes	>70	>70	>70	>90	<25
Glucose levels	10–25% less than serum*	10–25% less than serum	10–25% less than serum	70–90% less than serum	5–10 less than serum
Total protein	> 3.0 grams/dl	> 3.0 grams/dl	> 3.0 grams/dl	> 3.0 grams/dl	1.8–3.0 grams/dl
Complement	Low	Normal	High	High	Normal
Microscopic features	"RA cells"†	MSU and CPPD crystals	"Reiter's cells"†	Microbes (Gram stain)	Cartilage fibrils†
Culture	Negative	Negative	Negative	Positive	Negative

* Rarely, glucose levels are very low, as in rheumatoid pleural effusions.
† These are not disease specific or diagnostic.
MSU = monosodium urate; CPPD = calcium pyrophosphate dihydrate.

tion, (3) minimizing undesirable drug side effects, (4) preservation of muscle strength and joint function, and (5) maintenance of as normal a lifestyle as possible. The basic initial program that achieves these objectives for the great majority of patients consists of (1) adequate rest, (2) adequate anti-inflammatory therapy, and (3) physical measures to maintain joint function. An additional objective, (6) to attempt to modify disease course with early, aggressive drug therapies, recently has been advocated because of the prognosis studies and the findings that rheumatoid pannus invades and irreversibly damages articular cartilage within 1 to 2 years of disease onset. Identification of patients at highest risk for a poor outcome may be possible using high serum levels of RF and DNA typing of HLA-DRB1 alleles; however, this approach is currently unproven. Moreover, it is unclear that the current armamentarium of disease-modifying drugs can achieve this goal.

Any confusion arising from the complementary requirements of rest and exercise should be promptly dispelled. Bed rest tends to decrease the general systemic inflammatory response, and most patients soon learn that their midafternoon fatigue is significantly reduced by a period of rest. During acute attacks, longer rests and perhaps even remaining in bed for the duration of the attack may be required to treat the inflammation.

At the same time, the full range of joint motion should be maintained. This usually can be accomplished by the patient through graded exercise programs. However, during acute attacks, passive range-of-motion exercises by a physical therapist or instructed layperson may be indicated. Physical overexertion increases synovitis and inflammation in the joint affected by RA, but this does not contradict the usefulness of appropriate exercise. Exercise, as well as heat treatments such as showers, baths, warm pools, paraffin baths, or hot packs, should be used to loosen the joints and relieve stiffness. Exercise following the heat treatment maintains the motion of affected joints and prevents muscle atrophy.

NONSTEROIDAL ANTI-INFLAMMATORY DRUGS (NSAID's).
Anti-inflammatory therapy is crucial to the basic program. Salicylates are inexpensive, generally well tolerated, and demonstrably effective in controlling RA inflammation. The patient needs to understand that this requires a larger dose than would be used for analgesia alone. A constant blood level of 20 to 30 mg per deciliter is required. For most patients, this requires between 3 and 6 grams of aspirin per day. All patients should be monitored for toxic levels by blood tests and should be alerted to report deafness, ringing in the ears, or gastrointestinal intolerance. With the availability of buffered and coated aspirin, a suitable salicylate preparation can be found for almost any patient.

Many other NSAID's that are effective against pain, fever, and inflammation in RA are available. These include derivatives of propionic acid (ibuprofen, ketoprofen, flurbiprofen, oraprozin), naphthalene acetic acids (naproxen, nabumetone), pyrrolealkanoic acid (tolmetin), indoleacetic acid (indomethacin, sulindac), a halogenated anthranilic acid (meclofenamate sodium), piroxicam, diclofenac, di-

flunisal, and etodolac. Most of these drugs are beneficial in RA. They are generally no more effective than aspirin but may be tolerated in cases in which aspirin is not. Clinical experience suggests an occasional need to change from one to another of these drugs to minimize side effects and to give maximal benefit to the individual patient. Nonacetylated salicylates (sodium or choline) may be useful at times in patients intolerant of other NSAID's or those with aspirin hypersensitivity.

The NSAID's often cause silent gastrointestinal bleeding. Fortunately, this is usually minimal and tolerable. Overt gastrointestinal tract hemorrhage or ulceration is rare, but if this occurs or gastrointestinal bleeding is contributing to a constant anemia, the therapeutic regimen should be modified. NSAID's should be used cautiously or avoided in patients with impaired renal function.

DISEASE-MODIFYING THERAPIES.
The more slowly acting drugs include antimalarials, gold, penicillamine, sulfasalazine, and methotrexate. Antimalarials are usually given as hydroxychloroquine (Plaquenil), 200 mg once or twice daily. This, or chloroquine, may cause retinal lesions and loss of vision; therefore, the patient should be examined by an ophthalmologist at least twice a year.

Gold salts, especially weekly intramuscular injections, produce remission in many cases. An oral gold salt, auranofin, appears to be therapeutically effective and to have less toxicity than do intramuscular injections. A dose of 3 mg two to three times per day is recommended. A therapeutic effect should not be expected before 4 to 6 months. Many patients have been on oral or intramuscular gold therapy for a number of years. Common side effects include pruritic skin rashes and painful mouth ulcers. Severe manifestations include bone marrow suppression, usually leukopenia or thrombocytopenia, renal damage with proteinuria, and rarely a nephrotic syndrome. Therefore, frequent urinalysis and blood counts must be done, especially during early phases of treatment.

Penicillamine is also effective in inducing improvements and sometimes even remissions. Like gold, however, its effects are slow in coming, and it may affect both the bone marrow and the kidneys, so careful monitoring for toxicity is required. In addition, it may induce other autoimmune diseases, such as myasthenia gravis, Goodpasture's syndrome, or lupus erythematosus.

Sulfasalazine, given in a dose of 2 to 3 grams daily, may be effective in some patients. Headache and gastrointestinal upset are the most common side effects.

Immunosuppressive agents such as azathioprine, cyclophosphamide, chlorambucil, and methotrexate have been used to treat especially severe, unremitting RA. Currently, the most widely used and effective form of immunosuppressive therapy for RA appears to be methotrexate. An oral dosage of 7.5 to 15 mg one time per week is usually efficacious, and a therapeutic response can be anticipated in several weeks. Side effects include hepatotoxicity and possibly cirrhosis, bone marrow suppression, oral ulcers, and a potential life-threatening pneumonitis. Methotrexate also may cause a leukocytoclastic vasculitis and may promote the formation of rheumatoid nodules, including systemic nodulosis. Concomitant treatment with folic acid, 1 mg per day, reduces toxicity from metholrexate without impairing efficacy. Sulfonamides must be avoided because of potentiation of hematologic side effects.

Because of its side effects, long-term corticosteroid therapy should be reserved for patients with unresponsive and aggressive joint disease whose ability to function is threatened. When necessary, the smallest possible dose should be used, i.e., prednisone, 5 mg to 10 mg every other day or daily. Higher doses are necessary for patients with neuropathy, vasculitis, pleuritis, pericarditis, scleritis, and related conditions. Local steroid injections can sometimes be helpful for relieving persistent effusions and are the treatment of choice for a Baker's cyst of the knee.

Finally, reconstructive orthopedic surgery is of very great importance. Prosthetic devices for hip and knee joints have given excellent results, and devices for ankle, elbow, and shoulder replacement are improving.

JUVENILE CHRONIC ARTHRITIS. A chronic arthritis beginning in childhood and for which no underlying cause is apparent has been termed *juvenile rheumatoid arthritis*. Because the majority of these cases do not resemble adult RA, the term *juvenile chronic arthritis* (JCA) is a more appropriate designation. Several subgroups of JCA are recognized on the basis of modes of onset, other clinical features, and immunogenetic differences.

Arthritis of systemic onset, or Still's disease, accounts for about 20% of patients. It can begin at any age. Rheumatoid factor and antinuclear antibodies are generally not found. Clinical characteristics include high, spiking daily fevers; an evanescent, salmon-colored rash usually appearing with fever; lymphadenopathy; hepatosplenomegaly; polyserositis; leukocytosis; thrombocytosis; and anemia. Serum ferritin levels may be extremely high. Although the disease is rarely life threatening, it can be confused with leukemia or infection. It tends to run a self-limited course in the majority of patients but may recur. Chronic polyarthritis and joint deformities occur in only about 10% of patients.

Disease with a polyarticular onset occurs in approximately 40% of patients. There is a female predominance. The majority of patients are seronegative. Seropositive patients have the worst prognosis, and the disease usually follows a chronic course similar to that in adult RA. HLA-DR4 is strongly associated with seropositive disease, but HLA-DR8 and DP3 are significantly increased in the seronegative group.

Disease with a pauciarticular onset accounts for the remaining 40% of JCA patients. There are at least two subgroups within this group. One is characterized by early age of onset and female predominance. The serum is usually positive for antinuclear antibodies but not RF. Patients in this subgroup are at risk for chronic iridocyclitis, which may progress to blindness. Therefore, frequent ophthalmologic evaluations should be performed. The arthritis usually resolves without deformity. HLA-DR5, HLA-DR8, and HLA-DP2 are significantly increased in this subgroup. A second subgroup with pauciarticular onset has a strong male predominance and later age of onset. HLA-B27 occurs in the majority of these patients. The disease in these children follows a course consistent with spondyloarthropathy.

Treatment must be determined on the basis of disease severity. Aspirin is a basic standby, but tolmetin and naproxen can be used safely in children. Physical therapy and psychosocial support are also indicated.

ADULT-ONSET STILL'S DISEASE. Still's disease is one form of juvenile-onset chronic arthritis that may begin in adulthood. Cases have been recognized that span the entire adult age spectrum, including the elderly. The clinical features are the same as described above. Acute symptoms often respond to salicylates or other NSAID's, but prednisone may be necessary for short periods. The prognosis for complete recovery is good in the majority of patients.

Arnett FC, Edworthy SM, Block DA, et al.: The American Rheumatism Association 1987 revised criteria for the classification of rheumatoid arthritis. Arthritis Rheum 31:315, 1988. *An in-depth discussion of the development, recommended uses, and potential pitfalls of criteria for RA.*

Felson DT, Anderson JJ, Meenan RF: The comparative efficacy and toxicity of second-line drugs in rheumatoid arthritis. Arthritis Rheum 33:1449, 1990. *Large meta-analyses of clinical trials of most of the disease-modifying agents.*

Firestein GS: Mechanisms of tissue destruction and cellular activation in rheumatoid arthritis. Curr Opin Rheumatol 4:348, 1992. *An excellent review of molecular events in the rheumatoid synovium.*

Gregersen PK, Silver J, Winchester RJ: The shared epitope hypothesis: An approach to understanding the molecular genetics of susceptibility to rheumatoid arthritis. Arthritis Rheum 30:1205, 1987. *A well-written discussion of the molecular basis for different HLA associations with RA.*

Harris ED Jr: Rheumatoid arthritis: Pathophysiology and implications for therapy. N Engl J Med 322:1277, 1990. *An excellent review and extensive bibliography of current knowledge.*

Larsen EB: Adult Still's disease: Evolution of a clinical syndrome and diagnosis, treatment, and follow-up of 17 patients. Medicine 63:82, 1984. *An excellent clinical discussion.*

Pincus T: The paradox of effective therapies but poor long-term outcomes in rheumatoid arthritis. Semin Arthritis Rheum 21(Suppl 3):2, 1992. *An analysis of morbidity and mortality in RA patients.*

Weyand CM, Hicok KC, Conn DL, Goronzy JJ: The influence of HLA-DRB1 genes on disease severity in rheumatoid arthritis. Ann Intern Med 117:801, 1992. *A clinical-molecular study showing homozygosity for disease-associated HLA alleles correlates with RA severity.*

Wilske KR, Healey LA: Challenging the therapeutic pyramid: A new look at treatment strategies for rheumatoid arthritis. J Rheumatol 17(Suppl 25):4, 1990. *Advocacy for more aggressive treatment early in the course of RA.*

238 THE SPONDYLARTHROPATHIES

John J. Cush and Peter E. Lipsky

The spondylarthropathies are a heterogeneous group of disorders that share a number of clinical, radiographic, and genetic features. These disorders include ankylosing spondylitis, Reiter's syndrome, reactive arthritis, psoriatic arthritis, and the enteropathic arthropathies.

The spondylarthropathies share a constellation of characteristic clinical, radiographic, and immunogenetic manifestations that suggest a common or related etiopathogenesis (Table 238–1). Distinctive features include a propensity to axial arthritis (sacroiliitis and spondylitis), peripheral arthritis (often asymmetrical and oligoarticular), inflammation at tendinous, ligamentous, or fascial insertions (enthesitis), and a familial pattern of inheritance based on the presence of the class I major histocompatibility complex (MHC) antigen HLA-B27. These disorders can manifest extra-articular features that suggest a particular spondylarthropathy. Extra-articular manifestations may involve periarticular structures (enthesitis), eyes (uveitis), gastrointestinal tract (oral ulcerations, asymptomatic gut inflammation), genitourinary tract (urethritis), heart (aortitis, heart block), skin (keratoderma blennorrhagicum), or nails (onycholysis). Occasionally, patients with overlapping features of more than one condition or with HLA-B27(+) unclassifiable disease may be encountered. Thus approaching these conditions as a group of related disorders is important in understanding their pathologic consequences and in diagnosing them accurately.

New diagnostic criteria for the spondylarthropathies have been proposed (Table 238–2), because previous diagnostic criteria have been shown to exclude many spondylarthropathy patients. Broader definitions used in these criteria allow for earlier diagnosis and more liberal inclusion of many spondylarthropathy patients.

HLA-B27. The human leukocyte class I MHC antigen HLA-B27 was first linked with ankylosing spondyliitis in 1973. This genetic marker is found in nearly 8% of North American Caucasians. The actual risk of developing ankylosing spondylitis by an HLA-B27(+) person is estimated to be 1 to 2%. Only 20% of HLA-B27(+) individuals infected with arthritogenic bacteria (Table 238–3) will develop a reactive arthropathy. Moreover, only 20% of HLA-B27(+) first-degree relatives of HLA-B27(+) spondylitis patients will develop ankylosing spondylitis, suggesting that factors other than HLA-B27 must play a crucial role in determining disease susceptibility. The prevalence of HLA-B27 varies greatly among different ethnic groups. A higher prevalence is seen in the Haida and Pima Indians, and the lowest prevalence is seen among Africans and Asians. When North American Caucasians are compared with African-Americans, HLA-B27 is found in 90 versus 60% of ankylosing spondylitis and 75 versus 50% of Reiter's syndrome patients, respectively.

TABLE 238-1. COMPARISON OF THE SPONDYLARTHROPATHIES

	Ankylosing Spondylitis	Posturethral Reactive Arthritis	Postdysenteric Reactive Arthritis	Enteropathic Arthritis	Psoriatic Arthritis
Sacroiliitis	+++++	+++	++	+	++
Spondylitis	++++	+++	++	+	++
Peripheral arthritis	+	++++	++++	++	++++
Articular course	Chronic	Acute or chronic	Acute > chronic	Acute or chronic	Chronic
HLA-B27	95%	60%	30%	20%	20%
Enthesopathy	++	++++	+++	++	++
Common extra-articular manifestations	Eye Heart	Eye GU Oral/GI Heart	GU Eye	GI Eye	Skin Eye
Other names	von Bechterev's, Marie-Strümpell	Reiter's syndrome, SARA, NGU, chlamydial arthritis	Reiter's syndrome	Crohn's disease, ulcerative colitis	

Seven serologically defined subtypes of HLA-B27 have been defined, and five of these (B*2701, B*2702, B*2704, B*2705, and B*2707) are associated with ankylosing spondylitis. Other class I MHC antigens are termed the HLA-B27 cross-reactive antigens and include HLA-B7, -Bw22, -B40, -B42, and -B60, which are often present in HLA-B27(−) spondylarthropathy patients.

HLA-B27 has been shown to influence disease expression for most of the spondylarthropathies. HLA-B27(+) individuals are more likely to manifest an earlier disease onset, sacroiliitis, spondylitis, a severe clinical course, or acute anterior uveitis. By contrast, HLA-B27(−) patients are more likely to develop peripheral arthropathy, skin and nail disease, and inflammatory bowel disease or undifferentiated spondylarthropathy.

Strong evidence for the role of HLA-B27 in disease pathogenesis has been derived from experiments in which human HLA-B27 has been transfected into rats. These transgenic rats spontaneously develop typical features of spondylarthropathy, including gut inflammation, spondylitis, peripheral arthritis, psoriasiform skin and nail changes, uveitis, and orchitis. The role of environmental factors in disease pathogenesis is emphasized by the observation that many of these features do not develop when these animals are bred in a germ-free environment.

ANKYLOSING SPONDYLITIS. Ankylosing spondylitis is the most common inflammatory disorder of the axial skeleton. Epidemiologic studies have suggested that the prevalence of ankylosing spondylitis in a Caucasian population is 0.02 to 0.23%. Ankylosing spondylitis commonly affects young men more frequently than women, with an estimated male/female ratio ranging from 2.5 to 5:1. Ankylosing spondylitis in women is often underdiagnosed primarily because of milder axial disease and occult extra-articular manifestations. Women with ankylosing spondylitis tend to have a delayed disease onset, less hip involvement, less aggressive axial disease, more peripheral arthritis, severe osteitis pubis, and a higher incidence of isolated cervical spine disease.

Ankylosing spondylitis often begins in young adulthood. Up to 15% of children with juvenile chronic arthritis are classified with juvenile spondylitis. These children between ages 9 and 16 are often HLA-B27(+) and manifest low back pain or an asymmetrical oligoarthritis years before developing a fully expressed spondylarthropathy. In contrast, late-onset spondylarthropathy has been described in several HLA-B27(+) individuals over age 50 who developed sacroiliitis (without spondylitis), oligoarticular arthritis, an elevated erythrocyte sedimentation rate (ESR), and evidence of skeletal hyperostosis. This constellation of manifestations has been designated as the "RS3PE syndrome" ("remitting seronegative symmetrical synovitis with pitting edema").

The insidious onset of low back pain and/or stiffness is often the initial symptom of ankylosing spondylitis. The hallmark of ankylos-

TABLE 238-2. DIAGNOSTIC CRITERIA FOR THE SPONDYLARTHROPATHIES

Rome Criteria for Ankylosing Spondylitis (1961)	1981 ARA Criteria for Reiter's Syndrome
1. Low back pain and stiffness > 3 months, not relieved by rest	Peripheral arthritis > 1 month, in association with:
2. Pain and stiffness in the thoracic region	Urethritis and/or cervicitis
3. Limited motion of the lumbar spine	
4. Limited chest expansion	
5. History of iritis	
6. Radiographic evidence of bilateral sacroiliitis	

Diagnosis requires four of the first five criteria or sacroiliitis plus one of clinical criteria

ESSG Criteria for Spondylarthropathy (1992)	Criteria for Diagnosing Spondylarthropathies by Amor et al. (1993)	Score
Inflammatory spinal pain *or* peripheral synovitis (asymmetrical or lower limbs)	Lumbar pain at night or morning stiffness	1
	Asymmetrical oligoarthritis	2
Plus one or more of the following:	Buttock pain (or bilateral or alternating buttock pain)	1
Alternate buttock pain		
Sacroiliitis	Sausage-like toe or digit(s)	2
Enthesopathy	Heel pain or enthesitis	2
Positive family history	Iritis	2
Psoriasis	Nongonococcal urethritis/ cervicitis within 1 month of onset	1
Inflammatory bowel disease		
Urethritis, cervicitis, or acute diarrhea occurring within 1 month of the onset of arthritis	Psoriasis, balanitis, or inflammatory bowel disease	1
	Sacroiliitis (bilateral grade 2 or unilateral grade 3)	2
	HLA-B27(+) or (+) family history of a spondyloarthropathy	2
	Rapid (< 48 hours) response to NSAID's	2

Diagnosis requires score ≥ 6

Note: Older criteria *(top)* are being replaced by newer, more liberal criteria *(bottom)* for the spondylarthropathies.

TABLE 238-3. INFECTIOUS ORGANISMS ASSOCIATED WITH THE ONSET OF REITER'S SYNDROME

Enteric Pathogens	Urogenital Pathogens
Shigella flexneri (serotypes 2a, 1b)	*Chlamydia trachomatis*
Salmonella typhimurium	*Chlamydia psittaci*
Salmonella enteritidis	*Ureaplasma urealyticum*
Salmonella paratyphi	
Salmonella heidelberg	
Yersinia enterocolitica (serotypes 0:3, 0:8, 0:9)	
Yersinia pseudotuberculosis	
Campylobacter jejuni	
Campylobacter fetus	

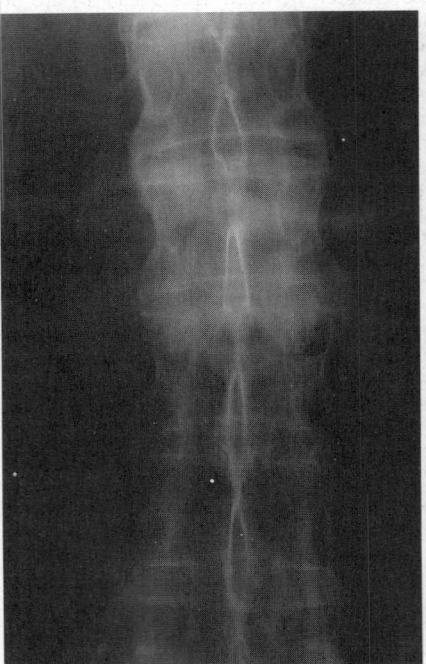

FIGURE 238-1. Bilaterally symmetrical sacroiliitis in ankylosing spondylitis.

ing spondylitis is symmetrical sacroiliitis that is often bilateral (Fig. 238–1). Sacroiliitis develops early but may take 7 to 10 years to become evident by conventional radiography. Pain is anatomically localized over the sacroiliac joints and less commonly radiates down the posterior thigh. Patients usually complain of prolonged morning stiffness that is relieved only by increased activity or anti-inflammatory therapy. Other constitutional features (e.g., fever, anorexia, weight loss) are not uncommon at the onset. With progressive axial involvement, pain and stiffness result in difficulty with ambulation and activities of daily living. The cervical spine is involved late in the disease.

A peripheral asymmetrical oligoarthropathy is seen in 30% of ankylosing spondylitis patients. Synovitis of the hip can be destructive and may lead to concentric loss of joint space, especially in men. Other involved joints include the ankles, wrists, shoulders, elbows, and small joints of the hands or feet.

Extra-articular disease in ankylosing spondylitis primarily affects the eye. Ocular involvement is seen in up to 40% of patients and is more frequently observed in HLA-B27(+) individuals. Uveitis presents as acute, unilateral orbital pain accompanied by photophobia and progressive loss of vision if untreated. Aortitis, aortic insufficiency, and conduction defects are uncommon. Other uncommon manifestations include mitral valve disease, myocardial dysfunction, pericarditis, pulmonary fibrosis, and amyloidosis.

Restricted spinal movement results from axial stiffness and paraspinal muscular spasm that accompanies inflammatory spondylitis, with or without intervertebral or zygapophyseal ankylosis. A loss of normal lumbar lordosis is a frequent observation in early disease. Fixed forward flexion, especially at the hip and neck, is seen after years of progressive disease. Chest expansion, as measured by the inspiratory minus expiratory chest circumference, is normally >5 cm. Ankylosing spondylitis patients demonstrate diminished expansion (<4 cm). Schober's test is performed to examine lumbar spine mobility. While the patient stands upright with heels together, a 10-cm span is marked from the fifth lumbar vertebrae cephalad. Upon maximal forward flexion, the distance between marks is remeasured. Normal spinal flexion expands the skin surface area over the flexed spine to >15 cm. Flexion in patients with spondylitis and limitation of spinal motion measures ≤14 cm.

Laboratory tests support the inflammatory nature of the disease with an elevated ESR or C-reactive protein, anemia of chronic disease, or mild elevations of the alkaline phosphatase. Elevated IgA may be present, but other autoantibodies are noticeably absent. HLA-B27 determination is seldom necessary to establish the diagnosis. However, in questionable cases without distinctive radiographic changes, the presence of HLA-B27 may be of diagnostic value.

Radiographs demonstrate normal mineralization before the onset of ankylosis. Once present, ankylosis results in marked immobility and subsequent generalized osteoporosis. Sacroiliitis is indicated by erosions (leading to "pseudowidening"), ileal sclerosis, or fusion of the inferior synovial-lined portion of the sacroiliac joint (see Fig. 238–1). These findings are easily observed on plain radiographs of the pelvis and seldom require computed tomography (CT) or magnetic resonance imaging (MRI) for diagnosis. In selected instances, MRI may accurately diagnose periarticular disease, such as plantar fasciitis. Axial radiographic findings also include marginal bridging syndesmophytes, interapophyseal joint fusion, and "squaring" of lumbar and thoracic vertebrae. Collectively, these findings may produce the classic appearance of a "bamboo spine" (Fig. 238–2).

The clinical course and disease severity are highly variable. Inflammatory back pain and stiffness are prominent early in the disease, whereas chronic, aggressive disease may produce pain and marked axial immobility or deformity. An earlier age of onset and

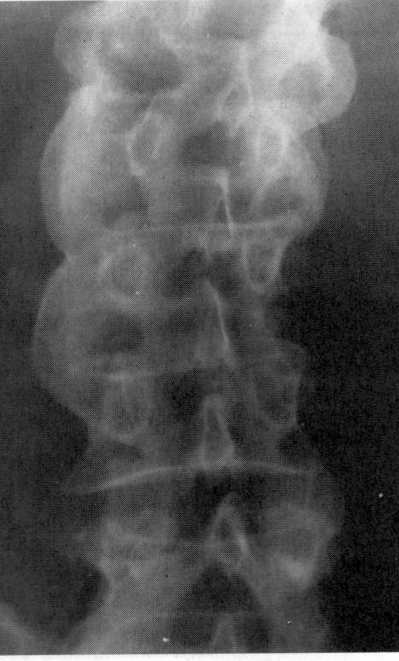

FIGURE 238-2. (Left) Lumbar spondylitis in ankylosing spondylitis with symmetrical, marginal bridging syndesmophytes and calcification of the spinal ligament. (Right) The bulky, nonmarginal, asymmetrical syndesmophytes of Reiter's syndrome with lumbar spondylitis.

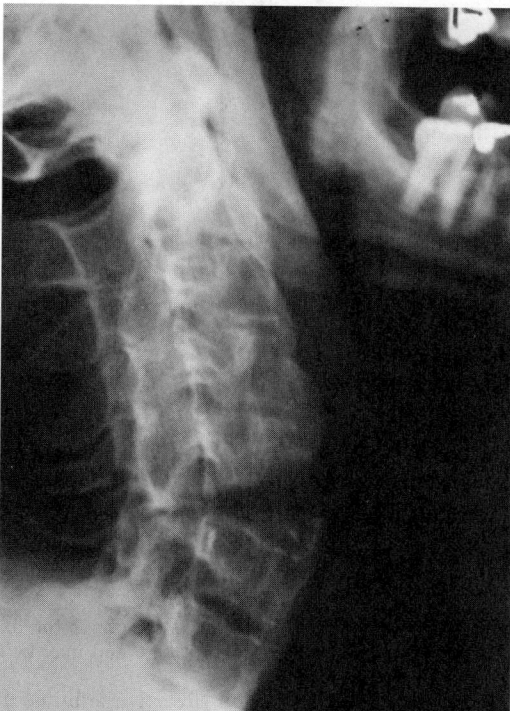

FIGURE 238–3. Posttraumatic fracture through the fifth cervical vertebrae in an ankylosing spondylitis patient with severe cervical ankylosis, interapophyseal ankylosis, and bridging syndesmophytes.

diagnosis portends a more severe outcome. Moreover, ankylosing spondylitis patients are at risk for complications, some of which may be life-threatening. These include restrictive lung disease, cauda equina syndrome, posttraumatic intervertebral fractures (Fig. 238–3), osteoporotic compression fractures, or spondylodiscitis.

Ankylosing spondylitis must be distinguished from other causes of mechanical or degenerative low back pain. The diagnosis of ankylosing spondylitis is suggested by (1) young age of onset, (2) strong family history of low back pain, (3) low back pain lasting more than 3 months, (4) prolonged morning stiffness, and (5) symptomatic improvement with activity or exercise. The differential diagnosis also includes other spondylarthropathies, osteitis condensans ilii, diffuse idiopathic skeletal hyperostosis (DISH), and other causes of hyperostosis (Table 238–4).

REITER'S SYNDROME. Reiter's syndrome is defined by the classic triad of arthritis, urethritis, and conjunctivitis. It most often affects young people, with a peak onset during the third decade of life. Like ankylosing spondylitis, however, it also has been reported in children and the elderly. Although men are most commonly affected, this predominance is often overestimated, because Reiter's syndrome in women may be associated with asymptomatic genitourinary disease and milder disease expression. Whereas postvenereal Reiter's syndrome is more common in males, postdysenteric Reiter's syndrome affects the sexes equally. Reiter's syndrome is

TABLE 238–4. CAUSES OF SKELETAL HYPEROSTOSIS

Spondyloarthropathies (ankylosing spondylitis, Reiter's syndrome, psoriatic arthritis, reactive arthritis)
Diffuse idiopathic skeletal hyperostosis (Forestier disease)
Vitamin A intoxication, retinoid therapy (i.e., etretinate)
Hypoparathyroidism
Familial hyperphosphatemia
SAPHO (synovitis, acne, pustulosis, hyperostosis, osteitis) syndrome
Pachydermoperiostitis
Hypertrophic osteoarthropathy
Plasma cell dyscrasia (POEMS syndrome)
Neurofibromatosis
Melorheostosis
Infantile cortical hyperostosis (Caffey's disease)
Fluorosis

one of the most common causes of acute inflammatory arthritis in young men. Case studies of epidemic dysentery suggest an estimated incidence of Reiter's syndrome of approximately 4 cases per 1000 dysenteric subjects per year. Analysis of epidemic dysentery secondary to arthritogenic bacteria suggests that Reiter's syndrome develops in 2 to 3% of infected individuals, whereas as many of 20% of the HLA-B27(+) infected individuals may develop arthritis. Similarly, 1 to 3% of patients with nongonococcal urethritis (NGU) secondary to *Chlamydia trachomatis* infection will develop a chronic arthritis. In Houston, the point prevalence of Reiter's syndrome was reported to be 33 per 100,000 men, and in Rochester, Minnesota, the age-adjusted incidence rate for males under age 50 was noted to be 3.5 cases per 100,000 per year.

The clinical triad of urethritis, conjunctivitis, and arthritis is observed in only 33% of patients with Reiter's syndrome. Thus many will not have evidence of prodromal enteric or urethral inflammation. Such patients are often designated as "incomplete Reiter's" or "sexually acquired reactive arthritis" (SARA). The remaining individuals can be diagnosed on the basis of an acute, additive lower extremity oligoarthritis that is accompanied by extra-articular features. The earliest features of Reiter's syndrome most frequently appear within 1 to 4 weeks of a putative microbial exposure. Disease onset is usually heralded by the development of one or more of the extra-articular features. Early genitourinary tract involvement may manifest as dysuria, urethral discharge, prostatitis in men, or cervicitis or vaginitis in women. Fever, malaise, fatigue, anorexia, weight loss, and ocular symptoms (e.g., conjunctivitis) are also common at the onset.

The arthritis is often the last feature to appear and manifests as an acute asymmetrical or ascending inflammatory oligoarthritis. Involvement of the lower extremity (first metatarsophalangeal joints, ankles, knees, and toes) is most common. Upper extremity involvement is rarely present at the onset. However, with chronicity, upper extremity involvement may occur. Involvement of the toes and fingers may result in dactylitis or the so-called sausage digit. Dactylitis is the net result of inflammatory changes affecting the joint capsule, entheses, periarticular structures, and/or periosteal bone.

Low back pain and other axial findings are present in up to 50% of individuals with Reiter's syndrome. However, radiographic evidence of sacroiliac or axial involvement is observed only with chronic and severe disease. About 20% of the most severely affected individuals demonstrate radiographic sacroiliitis.

Extra-articular Manifestations. Extra-articular manifestations are frequently seen in Reiter's syndrome. *Enthesitis* most commonly affects the insertion of the Achilles tendon and/or plantar fascia on the calcaneus with resultant heel pain. *Mucocutaneous features* may affect the genitourinary or gastrointestinal tract. Genitourinary involvement includes transient mucopurulent urethral discharge, urethritis, circinate balanitis, cervicitis, and/or vaginitis. Circinate balanitis appears as painless vesicles or large, shallow, serpiginous ulcerations or plaques on the glans or shaft of the penis. Painless lingual or palatal oral ulcerations may be seen in up to 50% of patients. Keratoderma blennorrhagicum is the most common of the cutaneous manifestations and presents as a painless papulosquamous eruption frequently found on the soles or palms and uncommonly on the penis, trunk, extremities, or scalp (Fig. 238–4). Patients with chronic disease may demonstrate nail changes of onycholysis or subungual hyperkeratosis. *Ocular manifestations* occur early in the disease and include conjunctivitis, uveitis, and rarely, keratitis. Conjunctivitis tends to be bilateral, painful, and recurrent and lasts days rather than weeks. Acute uveitis most often presents with unilateral ocular pain. *Other uncommon features* may include an asymptomatic conduction disturbance, prolonged PR interval, complete heart block, aortitis, aortic regurgitation, amyloidosis, central nervous system (CNS) involvement, serositis, or pulmonary infiltrates.

Radiographic abnormalities in Reiter's syndrome are commonly seen in the peripheral joints, primarily in an asymmetrical distribution affecting the feet, ankles, and knees. The sacroiliac and hip joints are less frequently involved. Soft tissue swelling, juxta-articular osteopenia, joint space narrowing, and/or ill-defined erosions are seen. Areas of periostitis or reactive new bone formation are common. Although bilaterally asymmetrical sacroiliitis is common (Fig. 238–5), unilaterally symmetrical inflammatory changes or ankylosis

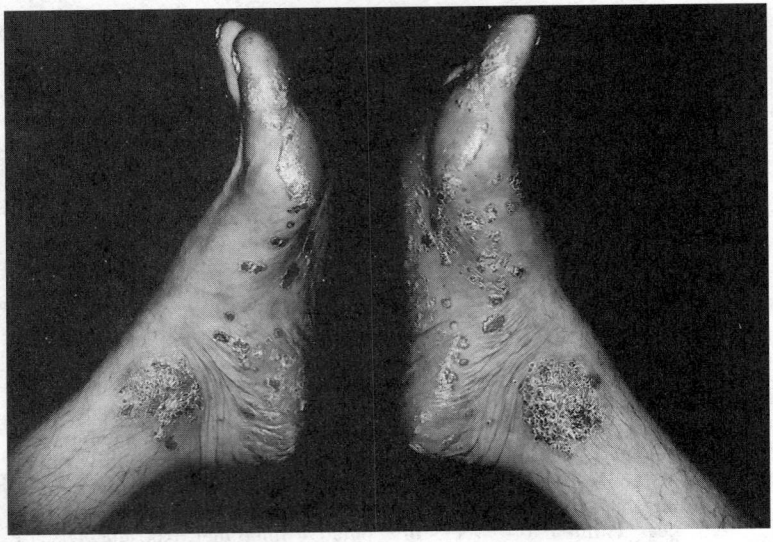

FIGURE 238–4. Keratoderma blennorrhagicum of the feet in Reiter's syndrome.

also has been observed. Involvement of the lumbar spine differs from ankylosing spondylitis with the presence of nonmarginal syndesmophytes or "bulky" osteophytes that are often unilateral or asymmetrical and tend to spare the anterior surface of the spine (see Fig. 238–2). Involvement of the cervical spine is uncommon in Reiter's syndrome.

Reiter's syndrome usually can be distinguished from rheumatoid arthritis (see Ch. 237) by the evolution, pattern of involvement, associated extra-articular features, clinical course, and absence of serum rheumatoid factor. Reiter's syndrome also should be distinguished from septic arthritis (especially gonococcal arthritis), crystal-induced arthritis, sarcoidosis, and erythema nodosum on clinical grounds and after appropriate laboratory and synovial fluid analyses. It is more difficult to distinguish Reiter's syndrome from the other spondylarthropathies and other reactive arthritides, such as that seen with *Yersinia, Chlamydia,* or AIDS-associated reactive arthritis. In such instances, a diagnosis of Reiter's syndrome is made after a careful history, identification of extra-articular features, and appropriate use of serologic testing and, most important, observation over time.

The prognosis and course of Reiter's syndrome are varied and unpredictable. The majority of patients demonstrate an initial episode usually lasting 2 to 3 months, but it may last up to a year. Recurrent attacks and prolonged disease-free intervals are common. A chronic peripheral arthropathy is observed in 20 to 50% of patients. These individuals have the greatest potential for axial progression and spondylitic changes. Death is rare and may be ascribed to cardiac complications or amyloidosis.

REACTIVE ARTHROPATHIES. "Reactive arthritis" refers to the occurrence of an acute, nonsuppurative, sterile inflammatory arthropathy arising after an infectious process but at a site remote from the primary infection. Reiter's syndrome is one of the most common examples of reactive arthritis. The microbial pathogens commonly associated with reactive arthritis are *Shigella, Salmonella, Yersinia, Campylobacter,* and *Chlamydia.* The reactive nature of these arthritides has been debated, since *Chlamydia, Yersinia,* and *Salmonella* microbial antigens have been identified at sites of tissue inflammation, suggesting that an ongoing immune response to disseminated material, rather than a reactive condition, may be the pathogenic mechanism. Many reactive arthritides occur after a known infection and therefore have been termed "postinfectious." Although the pathologic processes appear to be similar, this distinction may be important with regard to potential responsiveness to antibiotic therapy.

Reactive arthritis begins as an asymmetrical oligoarthritis, often preceded by an identifiable infectious event by one to four weeks. The temporal sequence suggests that these reactive disorders are triggered by an antecedent infectious process. Many patients without an identifiable infectious trigger have a similar constellation of signs and symptoms. The findings of sterile inflammatory synovial effusions, lymphocytes at sites of tissue inflammation, responsiveness to anti-inflammatory and immunosuppressive regimens, and the association with HLA-B27 suggest a common immunopathogenesis. A prominent feature of the reactive arthropathies is the inflammatory extra-articular process. Although frequently self-limiting, these disorders have the potential for chronicity and serious articular damage to the peripheral or axial joints.

Shigella. The occurrence of reactive arthritis following epidemics of *Shigella* dysentery has documented the arthritogenicity of this organism. Several reports suggest that 0.2 to 2% of infected individuals develop Reiter's syndrome following epidemic shigellosis. Infections with *S. flexneri* trigger Reiter's syndrome, whereas the more frequent *S. sonnei* does not. In most cases, the diarrheal illness resolves before the articular symptoms appear.

Salmonella. *S. typhimurium* is the most common *Salmonella* species inducing reactive arthritis. As many as 6 to 10% of infected individuals will develop a sterile arthropathy within 3 weeks of a *Salmonella* outbreak. Nearly 60% of patients will possess HLA-B27 or one of the cross-reactive antigens (HLA-B7 or HLA-B60). No clinical differences between *Shigella-* and *Salmonella*-induced reactive arthritis have been observed.

Yersinia. *Y. enterocolitica* is a common cause of reactive arthritis in endemic areas such as Scandinavia but is rarely encountered in England or the United States. *Yersinia* arthritis most commonly affects young adults as an acute, self-limiting gastrointestinal illness that may have associated joint complaints in 50% of cases.

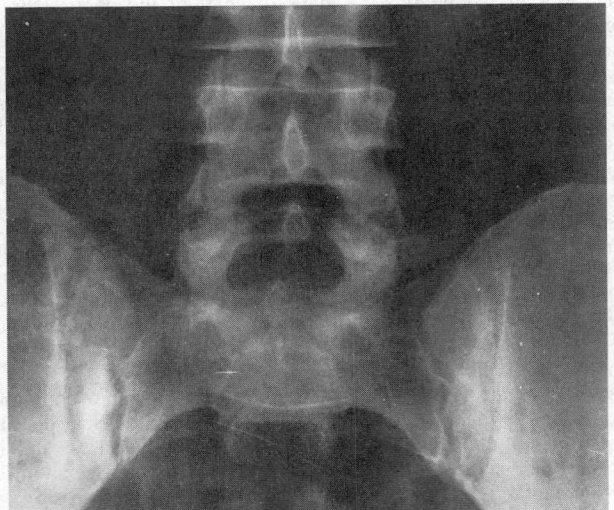

FIGURE 238–5. Bilaterally asymmetrical sacroiliitis in Reiter's syndrome. Erosions, pseudowidening, and ileal sclerosis are present.

Chronicity, severity, sacroiliitis, and ocular inflammation are more likely in HLA-B27(+) individuals. The arthritis is predominantly oligoarticular, affecting the lower extremities and hands, and may run a chronic or relapsing course. Chronic low back pain and sacroiliitis are seen in one third of patients, but severe spinal ankylosis is rare. Extra-articular features occur in 20 to 30% of individ-uals. Erythema nodosum and glomerulonephritis have been described in HLA-B27(−) individuals. Sustained elevations of IgA antibody titers correlate with persistent infection, chronic arthritis, and occult enteritis. Treatment is similar to that for other reactive arthropathies. However, appropriate antibiotic therapy should be used in patients with persistently positive stool cultures for *Yersinia.*

Chlamydia. *C. trachomatis* is thought to be responsible for as many as 10% of all cases of early inflammatory arthritis (see Ch. 323). As many as 1 to 3% of patients with chlamydial urethritis will develop arthritis. The incidence of *Chlamydia*-induced arthritis has been estimated to be 5 cases per 100,000 per year. Diagnosis is suggested by the presence of persistent arthritis in at least one joint, symptoms of genitourinary infection, detection of IgG or IgA anti-*Chlamydia* antibodies, or *Chlamydia* found in genitourinary swabs or urine culture. More than half of patients with Reiter's syndrome, NGU, or SARA will have antibodies to *C. trachomatis,* although positive cultures are seldom observed in patients with active disease.

The manifestations of *Chlamydia*-related reactive arthritis are similar to those described for classic Reiter's syndrome. However, only 20% of patients meet criteria for the diagnosis of Reiter's syndrome. Up to 15% of patients, especially women, have no urogenital manifestations at all. More than half develop a chronic arthropathy, with nearly one third having inflammatory low back pain, enthesitis, or radiographic sacroiliitis. Less than 50% of patients are HLA-B27(+). *Chlamydia*-induced arthritis apparently responds to antibiotic therapy, which is indicated in culture-positive or antibody (IgM or IgA)–positive patients. A prolonged course (i.e., 12 weeks) of doxycycline, minocycline, or lymecycline may improve symptoms.

ACQUIRED IMMUNODEFICIENCY SYNDROME (AIDS) AND REACTIVE ARTHRITIS (see Ch. 370). AIDS patients may develop an aggressive form of Reiter's syndrome. Early reports suggested that many of HIV(+) individuals developed Reiter's syndrome upon becoming profoundly immunosuppressed. Although it has been suggested that AIDS patients are at increased risk to develop reactive arthritis, a number of prospective analyses of HIV(+) populations failed to reveal an increased incidence or prevalence of Reiter's syndrome compared with that observed in an HIV(−) population matched for other risk factors. Each group, however, appeared to have a much higher prevalence of reactive arthritis than previously reported for young heterosexual males. Nevertheless, it seems clear that HIV infection alters the clinical expression of Reiter's syndrome. The vast majority of AIDS patients with Reiter's syndrome are HLA-B27(+) and present with incomplete symptoms and signs of Reiter's syndrome. The arthritis evolves in two main patterns: (1) an additive, asymmetrical polyarthritis or (2) an intermittent oligoarthritis that most commonly affects the lower extremities. Enthesitis, fasciitis, conjunctivitis, and urethritis are early and prominent symptoms. Although sacroiliitis does occur, HIV-associated reactive arthritis is rarely associated with axial disease or uveitis. HIV-associated disease also differs from classic Reiter's syndrome in the severity and chronicity of disease, prominent enthesitis, and a poor response to nonsteroidal anti-inflammatory drugs (NSAID's). Therapeutic options are somewhat limited in HIV(+) Reiter's patients, although some patients have responded to isotretinoin.

PSORIATIC ARTHRITIS. Psoriatic arthritis develops in roughly 5% of patients with cutaneous psoriasis. Although most cases arise in patients with established, active cutaneous disease, other patients (especially children) manifest articular disease that antedates the development of psoriasis. While the extent of psoriatic skin disease correlates poorly with the onset of arthritis, the risk of psoriatic arthritis increases with a family history of spondylarthropathy or extensive nail pitting. The age of onset is usually between 30 and 55 years, and psoriatic arthritis has been shown to affect men and women equally. Psoriatic spondylitis, however, has a male/female ratio of 2.3:1.

The genetic associations with psoriatic arthritis are heterogeneous. Cutaneous psoriasis is associated with HLA-B13, HLA-Bw17, and HLA-Cw6. By contrast, HLA-B39 and -B27 have been associated with sacroiliitis and axial involvement, and HLA-Cw6, HLA-Bw38, HLA-DR4, and HLA-DR7 have been associated with peripheral arthropathy. No etiologic agent or reactive process has been proven, although stress, trauma, the expression of heat shock proteins, and antecedent infection with *Streptococcus* or *Staphylococcus* have been suggested to play a role. Histopathology of psoriatic synovitis is similar to that seen in other inflammatory arthritides, with a notable lack of intrasynovial immunoglobulin and rheumatoid factor production and a greater propensity for fibrous ankylosis, osseous resorption, and heterotopic bone formation. Like HIV-associated Reiter's syndrome, disease severity in psoriatic arthritis is enhanced by coexistent HIV infection.

Psoriatic arthritis has an insidious onset and a progressive course. Five major variants of psoriatic arthritis have been described. These variants are not mutually exclusive, and patients may progress from one form to another. The first form is an asymmetrical oligoarthritis that is observed in 30 to 50% of patients and may involve both large and small joints. Dactylitis, or "sausage digits," may be seen in the fingers or toes. In this group, cutaneous features may be minimal and are often missed. The second variant involves the distal interphalangeal (DIP) joint and is seen in 10 to 15% of patients. It is strongly associated with nail changes of pitting, onycholysis, subungual hyperkeratosis, transverse ridging, and/or leukonychia (Fig. 238–6). Periungual erythema may reflect the extent of nail and joint disease. The third variant is a rheumatoid arthritis–like symmetrical polyarthritis that usually lacks serum rheumatoid factor or rheumatoid nodules. The fourth variant is psoriatic spondylitis, which is seen in approximately 20% of psoriatic arthritis patients, 50% of whom are HLA-B27(+). Finally, arthritis mutilans is seen in 5% of patients and presents as a destructive, erosive, polyarticular arthritis affecting the hands, feet, and spine. It often leads to progressive deformity and substantial disability.

Extra-articular features and laboratory findings are similar to those seen in Reiter's syndrome, although keratoconjunctivitis sicca, myopathy, and mitral valve prolapse are less common. Hyperuricemia may be found and often correlates with the severity of cutaneous psoriasis.

Radiographic changes in psoriatic arthritis are similar to those seen in Reiter's syndrome and include soft tissue swelling ("sausage digits"), erosions, periostitis, asymmetrical sacroiliitis, and spondylitis with asymmetrical nonmarginal bulky syndesmophytes (see Fig. 238–2). Patients with distal interphalangeal joint disease or arthritis mutilans may develop the typical "pencil and cup" deformity. Acro-osteolysis, paravertebral ossification, and pericapsular calcification also have been described.

The diagnosis of psoriatic arthritis depends on finding typical cutaneous or nail changes in association with one of the recognized articular variants. Cutaneous psoriasis should be distinguished from

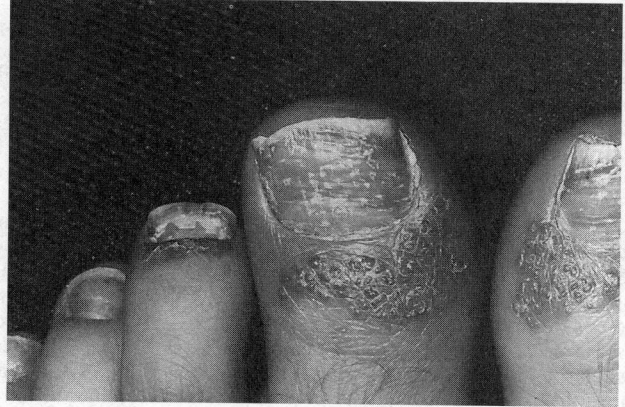

FIGURE 238–6. Nail pitting, onycholysis, and transverse ridging in psoriatic arthritis. Dactylitis of the second toe is present.

seborrheic dermatitis, fungal infection, exfoliative dermatitis, eczema, keratoderma blennorrhagicum, and palmoplantar pustulosis. The arthritis of psoriasis is often misinterpreted as erosive osteoarthritis, gout, rheumatoid arthritis, pauciarticular juvenile arthritis, ankylosing spondylitis, or Reiter's syndrome. A minority of psoriatic arthritis may exhibit clinical and radiographic features of Reiter's syndrome.

ENTEROPATHIC ARTHROPATHIES. "Enteropathic arthritis" refers to the arthropathies associated with Crohn's disease or ulcerative colitis (see Ch. 104). These disorders are unified by clinical and histologic gut inflammation, altered intestinal permeability, and the development of an inflammatory peripheral or axial arthritis. Peripheral arthritis is observed in nearly 20% and axial arthritis in 10 to 15% of patients, respectively. Peripheral arthropathy more frequently occurs in those with extraintestinal manifestations (i.e., erythema nodosum). Peripheral arthritis affects men and women equally. All age groups are affected, and while the onset of arthritis follows established intestinal inflammation in adults, the converse is true in children. Disease onset is sometimes heralded by low-grade fever, painful oral ulceration, ocular manifestations, cutaneous manifestations (i.e., erythema nodosum, pyoderma gangrenosum), or enthesitis. Rarely, a patient may have occult high fever, anemia, or weight loss. Peripheral arthritis manifests as an inflammatory, nonerosive, asymmetrical oligoarthritis or monarthritis affecting large joints (i.e., knees, ankles, elbows). Initially, the arthropathy may be migratory and may resolve in weeks or months. Peripheral articular activity often parallels gut inflammation. Thus measures to control colitis may prove beneficial for managing peripheral arthritis. With chronicity, peripheral arthritis may be misdiagnosed as seronegative rheumatoid arthritis, particularly when symmetrical joint disease or quiescent gut inflammation is present.

In contrast, with peripheral arthritis, axial disease may precede or coincide with the onset of colitis and is more common in men. Axial arthropathy is clinically and radiographically indistinguishable from ankylosing spondylitis. The course of sacroiliitis and spondylitis is independent of active bowel inflammation. Whereas no association between HLA-B27 and colitic peripheral arthritis has been noted, HLA-B27 is found in 50% of patients with spondylitic colitis. Therefore, inflammatory bowel disease should be considered in the setting of HLA-B27(−) ankylosing spondylitis.

The association between enteritis and arthritis is supported by the findings of ileocolonoscopic evidence of subclinical gut inflammation in a variety of spondylarthropathies. Histologic evidence of "acute" colitis (similar to bacterial enteritis) or "chronic" colitis (resembling chronic idiopathic inflammatory bowel disease) is commonly observed. Acute intestinal changes are commonly found in patients with postdysenteric reactive arthritis, whereas chronic lesions are more typical of ankylosing spondylitis and patients who will ultimately be diagnosed with enteropathic arthritis.

THERAPY OF THE SPONDYLARTHROPATHIES. Current therapies cannot cure the spondylarthropathies; therefore, treatment should be aimed at reducing pain and stiffness. An aggressive approach to patient education and joint protection will contribute to the maintenance of optimal function and the patient's sense of well-being and may slow progression to immobility, joint deformity, or axial malalignment. All patients should be counseled regarding a rational program of exercise, rest, physical therapy, diet, and vocational counseling. Patients with axial disease should engage in life-long physical therapy to maintain posture and prevent slow deformity. Once the diagnosis has been established, specific treatment can be initiated. Therapeutic options are largely the same for most of the spondylarthropathies and, as such, are considered together.

NSAID's. NSAID's have replaced the use of salicylates, since they have more convenient dosaging and are more efficacious. NSAID's effectively control the pain, stiffness, and/or joint swelling. While these agents modify symptoms, they are not thought to retard the underlying inflammatory disease or suppress disease progression. NSAID's are the mainstay of therapy in ankylosing spondylitis, Reiter's syndrome, reactive arthritis, and psoriatic arthritis. Their use in the enteropathic arthropathies is infrequently hampered by their potential to alter bowel permeability and/or induce exacerbations of colitis.

Although all NSAID's are potentially useful in the spondylarthropathies, only a few are of proven benefit and are FDA-approved for use in ankylosing spondylitis and/or Reiter's syndrome. These include indomethacin, diclofenac, naproxen, sulindac, and phenylbutazone. Of these, indomethacin, especially the sustained-release formula (1 to 2 mg per kilogram per day) is recommended because of its prolonged duration of effect and anti-inflammatory potency. Other NSAID's are used according to individual tolerability and efficacy. Phenylbutazone is a very effective agent but is reserved for intractable cases, primarily because of the risk of aplastic anemia.

Corticosteroids. Systemic corticosteroids are seldom used in the spondylarthropathies. They are most effective for controlling localized disease. They are used primarily as local therapy by intra-articular injection (i.e., mono- or oligoarthritis), topical management of ocular complications (conjunctivitis or uveitis), and on occasion intralesionally to control enthesitis. Systemic low-dose or high-dose "pulse" corticosteroids should be reserved for severe disease flares.

Slow-Acting Antirheumatic Drugs (SAARD's). When chronic, NSAID-unresponsive disease exists, adding certain SAARD's (e.g., sulfasalazine, methotrexate) should be considered. These agents have a delayed onset of action (2 to 6 months), and their efficacy in the spondylarthropathies is based on limited numbers of controlled trials and numerous anecdotal reports.

Placebo-controlled trials of sulfasalazine indicate that efficacy is greatest in patients with peripheral arthropathy and enthesopathy. Equivocal results have been observed in patients with longstanding disease and evidence of severe radiographic destruction or ankylosis. At a dose of 2 to 4 grams per day, it is most effective in patients with Reiter's syndrome, reactive arthritis, and enteropathic arthritis. The value of sulfasalazine in treating inflammatory axial disease has not been established but warrants consideration in poorly controlled spondylitis patients.

Methotrexate (7 to 15 mg per week) also may be effective in many spondylarthropathy patients. It is particularly effective for treating both cutaneous and articular disease in psoriasis, but higher doses and prolonged use may be associated with unacceptable hepatotoxicity. Azathioprine (1 to 2 mg per kilogram per day) should be reserved for those unresponsive to or intolerant of other SAARD's.

Additional therapeutic options exist for patients with psoriatic arthritis. Both methotrexate and sulfasalazine may be effective for managing articular and skin disease associated with psoriasis. Other patients may benefit from therapy with gold salts, antimalarials, etretinate, or cyclosporine. Although immunosuppressive regimens should be avoided in HIV-associated arthritis, agents such as sulfasalazine or etretinate may be considered.

Surgery. Surgery should be considered when pain and immobility markedly interfere with patient lifestyle. Total joint replacement is commonly performed in the hip or knee. The success of arthroplasty may be limited by postoperative heterotopic bone formation. Surgically correcting spinal deformities and/or fractures should be undertaken with extreme caution.

Arnett FC: Seronegative spondylarthropathies. Bull Rheum Dis 37:1, 1987. *An insightful overview of the clinical features of the spondylarthropathies and potential etiologic considerations.*

Bardin T, Enel C, Cornelis F, et al.: Antibiotic treatment of venereal disease and Reiter's syndrome in a Greenland population. Arthritis Rheum 35:190, 1992. *Suggested guidelines and treatment outcomes of Reiter's patients treated with antibiotics.*

Cush JJ, Lipsky PE: Reiter's syndrome and reactive arthritis. *In* McCarty DJ, Koopman WJ (eds.): Arthritis and Allied Conditions: A Textbook of Rheumatology. 12th ed. Philadelphia, Lea & Febiger, 1992, pp. 1061–1078. *A comprehensive overview of Reiter's and reactive arthropathies.*

Hammer RE, Malka SD, Richardson JA, et al.: Spontaneous inflammatory disease in transgenic rats expressing HLA-B27 and human β2m: An animal model of HLA-B27–associated human disorders. Cell 63:1099, 1990. *Describes the spectrum of clinicopathologic manifestations induced by introducing HLA-B27 into transgenic rats.*

Khan MA, van der Linden SM: A wider spectrum of spondylarthropathies. Semin Arthritis Rheum 20:107, 1990. *Clinical and pathologic similarities among the spondylarthropathies are described.*

Khan MA: Pathogenesis of ankylosing spondylitis: recent advances. J Rheumatol 20:1273, 1993. *Editorial review of the current understanding of the pathogenesis of HLA-B27–related disorders.*

Thomson GTD, DeRubeis DA, Hodge MA, et al.: Post-*Salmonella* reactive arthritis: Late clinical sequelae in a point source cohort. Am J Med 98:13, 1995. *Describes the incidence and long-term clinical consequences of reactive arthritis following epidemic dysentery caused by* Salmonella typhimurium.

239 INFECTIOUS ARTHRITIS
Luis R. Espinoza

Infectious or septic arthritis is a topic of increasing relevance in view of the continuous spread of the human immunodeficiency virus (HIV), Lyme disease, and gonorrhea and syphilis and the resurgence in recent years of more virulent strains of *Streptococcus* species and acute rheumatic fever.

In order of frequency, bacterial-nongonococcal and bacterial-gonococcal, viral, and fungal infections are the most common causes of inflammatory articular disease.

NONGONOCOCCAL BACTERIAL ARTHRITIS (Table 239–1). *Staphylococcus aureus* is the most common infectious agent in both adults and children over age 2. This is of extreme importance, since almost all strains of *Staphylococcus* are now resistant to penicillin and methicillin. Non-group A beta-hemolytic streptococci and *Streptococcus pneumoniae* are also common causative gram-positive microorganisms. Infections due to gram-negative microorganisms and anaerobes occur for the most part in patients with some degree of immunosuppression, prior joint damage (as in rheumatoid arthritis (RA), osteoarthritis, or a prosthetic joint), and underlying malignancy. *Hemophilus influenzae* is the most common infectious agent in bacterial arthritis occurring in children younger than age 2.

Most cases of bacterial arthritis result from hematogenous spread. Other routes of joint involvement include direct inoculation during diagnostic or therapeutic arthrocentesis or arthroscopies and by contiguous osteomyelitis, cellulitis, abscesses, tenosynovitis, and/or septic bursitis. Regardless of the route of infection, however, the histopathologic and biochemical changes are the same and include infiltration by polymorphonuclear (PMN) cells of the subsynovial space, neovascularization, synovial proliferation, granulation tissue, and if untreated, cartilage and bone destruction. Phagocytosis of microorganisms by PMN and/or synovial lining cells also may be found. As the inflammatory reaction progresses, increased amounts of synovial fluid, with inflammatory cells, predominantly polymorphonuclear, will be observed. The degree of synovial, cartilage, and bone destruction depends on multiple factors, including the direct toxic effect of the microorganisms or their products, the host response to the infection, and more important, the rapidity with which an accurate diagnosis and appropriate therapy are instituted.

Clinical Manifestations. The great majority of cases (80 to 90%) are monarticular, with the knee joint being affected most commonly. Polyarthritis may occur in patients with underlying connective tissue diseases or an immunosuppressed state and carries a worse prognosis, with a mortality rate of approximately 30%.

Most patients have constitutional complaints, including chills, fever, and general malaise. On physical examination, the affected joint(s) can be extremely painful, warm, and with fluid. These inflammatory signs, however, may be masked in debilitated, severely ill patients or in those receiving corticosteroids or immunosuppressive agents.

Diagnosis. The most important diagnostic test—to be performed as soon as possible—is arthrocentesis. This procedure is mandatory. Particular attention should be paid to performing the arthrocentesis through an area of uninvolved skin in patients with cellulitis or other skin involvement. In the presence of polyarticular involvement, all affected joints should be tapped. Joint aspiration should be followed immediately by Gram stain and culture of synovial fluid, leukocyte count with differential, and examination of a wet preparation for crystals. The findings of very high white blood cell count, usually over 100,000 per cubic millimeter, with a predominance of PMN's (>90 to 95%), low glucose levels, and high protein content are characteristic of bacterial arthritis. However, similar findings can be observed in other nonseptic inflammatory articular disorders, including "pseudoseptic" arthritis seen in patients with RA, Reiter's disease, and other arthritides.

Bacteriologic studies—cultures and Gram stains—of blood, skin lesions, cervical, urethral, and/or rectal swabs, urine, and any other sources of microorganisms should be part of the diagnostic workup of patients suspected of having bacterial arthritis. Imaging studies are helpful only in certain situations. Plain radiographs are seldom useful early on, although they may reveal joint abnormalities, i.e., loss of articular cartilage and bone erosions in untreated patients or in patients with aggressive disease. In patients suspected of deep-seated joint infections such as sacroiliac or facet joint involvement, scintigraphy with leukocytes labeled with technetium-99m diphosphonate or technetium-99m diphosphonate, computed tomography or magnetic resonance may be helpful.

Management. Treatment for nongonococcal arthritis includes appropriate antibiotics and joint drainage. Antibiotic therapy should be given to all patients suspected of septic arthritis until bacteriologic studies are completed. Otherwise normal individuals should be treated initially for infections due to gram-positive organisms, while treatment for both gram-positive and gram-negative microorganisms is indicated in debilitated, severely ill, immunocompromised individuals. Parenteral, not intra-articular antibiotics, often in high doses, should be given for two or four weeks or more. Methicillin or another penicillinase-resistant synthetic penicillin is the drug of choice. Vancomycin should be used to treat methicillin-resistant *S. aureus* infections. Gram-negative organisms should be treated with either a first- or third-generation cephalosporin or an aminoglycoside. Long-term administration of oral antibiotics is recommended in patients with chronic bone and joint infections (i.e., prosthetic joints). Closed-needle aspiration on a daily basis or as often as necessary is an important part of the medical management of bacterial arthritis. Most patients can be treated in this manner, although in certain situations—hip or shoulder involvement, joints anatomically altered by underlying pathology, joints not responding to appropriate antibiotic therapy, loculated synovial fluid, or contiguous osteomyelitis—surgical drainage is indicated. Arthroscopic surgery rather than open surgery is becoming the procedure of choice. Joint immobilization is not indicated, except in cases of incapacitating pain or following surgical drainage. Joint mobilization and functional splinting of the affected joint are recommended to prevent muscle atrophy and contracture and preserve joint function.

GONOCOCCAL ARTHRITIS. Disseminated gonococcal infection (DGI) (Table 239–2) is the most frequent type of septic arthritis among young adults of low socioeconomic status and accounts for up to two thirds of septic arthritis and tenosynovitis seen in the country. Women are affected two to three times as often as men.

DGI is always preceded by mucosal infection with *Neisseria gonorrhoeae*. This commonly involves the endocervix or urethra but may involve the pharynx and rectum and may or may not be symptomatic.

Clinical Manifestations. Mono-, oligo-, or polyarthralgia is the most common symptom of DGI, occurring in a diffuse, migratory, or additive pattern within a few days of the onset. Two thirds of patients develop tenosynovitis with or without arthritis, commonly affecting the wrists, fingers, ankles, or toes. Any joint may be involved, but the knees, wrists, hands, and ankles are usually affected. Fever and chills are common. Skin involvement occurs in approximately two thirds of patients with DGI. Rash is nonpainful, infrequent, and commonly found on the extremities. Rash presents

TABLE 239–1. MICROORGANISMS IN ACUTE NONGONOCOCCAL BACTERIAL ARTHRITIS

Microorganism	%
>**Age 2**	
Gram-positive	50–90
Staphylococcus aureus	40–60
Non-group A beta-hemolytic streptococci	15–30
Gram-negative	5–25
Escherichia coli	
Salmonella	
Pseudomonas spp.	
Anaerobes	1–2
Fusobacterium necrophorum	
Anaerobic cocci	
Bacteroides fragilis	
<**Age 2**	
Haemophilus influenzae	>90

TABLE 239–2. RISK FACTORS FOR DISSEMINATED GONOCOCCAL INFECTION (DGI)

Women during menses
Pregnancy
Immediate postpartum period
Homosexual men with asymptomatic pharyngeal or rectal infection
Inherited deficiency of complement (C5 to C8)
Human immunodeficiency virus infection(?)

as macules, papules, or pustules. They may progress to central necrosis and may develop up to 48 hours after starting antibiotics. Unusual clinical manifestations include pericarditis, meningitis, aortitis, endocarditis, myocarditis, and osteomyelitis.

Most patients with DGI have asymptomatic primary gonococcal infection of the genitourinary tract. The major differential diagnoses include Reiter's syndrome, bacterial arthritis, rheumatic fever, juvenile arthritis, bacterial endocarditis, hepatitis B infection, and meningococcemia.

Diagnosis. A definite diagnosis of DGI is established by identifying the rarely found *N. gonorrhoeae* in the synovial fluid, blood, or skin lesions. In most patients, the diagnosis is made indirectly by finding positive cultures from the genitourinary tract or, much less frequently, from the rectum or pharynx. If Gram stains and cultures are negative, a presumptive diagnosis is made by the typical clinical presentation associated with a rapid response to antibiotics.

Other laboratory findings may include leukocytosis, elevated sedimentation rate, and inflammatory synovial fluid, but they are nonspecific.

Management. Response to antibiotic therapy is excellent in most patients. Hospitalization may be indicated if endomyopericarditis and meningitis are present. Ceftriaxone, 1 gram intramuscularly or intravenously (IV) every 24 hours, or another β-lactamase–resistant cephalosporin is initially recommended because of the increasing number of penicillin (β-lactamase)–resistant strains. Penicillin G, 10 million units IV daily, or ampicillin 1 gram IV every six hours, can be administered when penicillin sensitivity is demonstrated. Parenteral therapy should be given until there is evidence of clinical improvement, 2 to 4 days, and then oral antibiotics may then be substituted; a penicillin derivative and cephalosporin should be given for another 7 to 10 days.

Joint effusions should be tapped on a daily basis with a large-bore needle. Open drainage is rarely indicated. Following completion of therapy, patients should be evaluated, repeat cultures obtained, and tests for syphilis and HIV infection considered.

MYCOPLASMA ARTHRITIS. *Mycoplasma*-induced mono- or oligoarthritis is not an uncommon occurrence, especially in agammaglobulinemic individuals. *Mycoplasma*-related superantigens also may induce arthritis in animal models.

VIRAL ARTHRITIS. The most important viral infections associated with a rheumatic syndrome are hepatitis viruses, rubella virus, parvovirus, and HIV. Hepatitis B virus (HBV) infection and to a lesser extent HCV and HAV may cause immune complex–mediated rheumatic syndromes. Acute and less commonly chronic arthritis and vasculitis, including that with essential mixed cryoglobulinemia, have all been described during the course of hepatitis infection. In HBV infection, acute arthritis is seen in the prodromal phase and is usually accompanied by fever and urticarial rash. As many as 40% of patients with HBV infection develop arthritis, and the joints most commonly affected are the small hand joints in a symmetrical fashion. Arthritis follows a migratory pattern and can be either additive or nonadditive, usually lasting an average of three weeks. In general, the inflammatory articular disease subsides as jaundice appears. Polyarteritis nodosa and mixed essential cryoglobulinemia are well-defined syndromes that may occur in patients with HBV and HCV infection and much less commonly HAV infection. Arthralgia and arthritis respond for the most part to conventional analgesic and/or anti-inflammatory therapy. Prednisone, cytotoxic therapy, and interferon-α with or without plasma exchanges have been shown to be beneficial for the most serious rheumatic syndromes.

Infection with HIV causes a wide clinical spectrum ranging from no symptoms to the acquired immunodeficiency syndrome (AIDS).

Rheumatic manifestations are an important part of the clinical findings of HIV infection (see Ch. 370). Arthralgia, usually of moderate intensity, intermittent and oligoarticular, is the most frequent rheumatic manifestation of HIV. It occurs in 35% of cases and predominantly affects knees, shoulders, and elbows. Other distinct rheumatic syndromes may be seen including Reiter's syndrome, psoriatic arthritis, vasculitis, myositis, Sjögren's syndrome, and fibrositis.

Any of these rheumatic disorders may occur in an otherwise completely asymptomatic HIV(+) individual but most often occur in late stages of the disease. HIV-induced "painful articular syndrome" and arthropathy also may occur. Septic complications in joint, bursa, bone, and muscle may occur rarely, usually in IV drug users. The pathogenic mechanisms underlying the rheumatic manifestations of HIV infection are not well understood. Their treatment includes conventional anti-inflammatory therapy. Antiretroviral therapy, particularly zidovudine (AZT), can effectively ameliorate some of the rheumatic manifestations, particularly psoriatic rash and myositis. It may induce a toxic mitochondrial myopathy, however, with the appearance of "ragged red fibers." Rapid improvement of the proximal muscle weakness seen in these patients follows AZT withdrawal. Methotrexate and other immunosuppressive drugs may be indicated in patients with refractory arthritis, myositis, and/or vasculitis. These agents always should be used in combination with antiretroviral therapy and antimicrobial prophylaxis to minimize the likelihood of serious complications, including the precipitation of AIDS and Kaposi's sarcoma. Rheumatic manifestations also have been recognized in association with human T-cell leukemia virus type I (HTLV-I) and HTLV-II infection.

Rubella-associated arthritis has a predilection for adolescent and adult women, but it can occur at all ages. Joint manifestations occur within days of the appearance of skin rash in natural rubella infection or 2 to 4 weeks after vaccination. The pattern of joint involvement is frequently that of a migratory polyarthralgia and less often polyarthritis. It may mimic RA, and wrists, small joints of the hands, and knees are affected most commonly. Synovial fluid, when obtained, is inflammatory in nature, and mononuclear cells are predominant. The acute episode usually lasts 3 to 21 days, but it may persist for several months. Rubella virus has been isolated from peripheral blood and synovial fluid in both the natural and the vaccine-induce syndrome. Its role as an etiologic agent in RA is questionable, however.

Human parvovirus B19 is a DNA virus that frequently causes widespread infection in the community. In adults, especially women, B19 infection causes adult erythema infectiosum, which may be associated with a rheumatoid-like syndrome of symmetrical polyarthralgia and polyarthritis. In most patients, joint symptoms subside in a few weeks without sequelae, but in a few, they may last for several months. In the latter situation, differential diagnosis with RA can be difficult, but B19 infection is seldom accompanied by a positive rheumatoid factor, subcutaneous nodules, or joint erosions. Elevated titer of specific IgM antibodies confirms the diagnosis, and treatment is symptomatic.

Other viruses less commonly causing arthralgia and polyarthritis include herpes zoster, cytomegalovirus, Epstein-Barr virus, echovirus, adenovirus, and coxsackieviruses. Chikungunya, O'nyong-nyong, and Ross viruses and Mayaro, Sindbis, and Barmah Forest viruses are all alphaviruses responsible for major epidemics of febrile polyarthritis in other parts of the world, especially Africa, Australia, Europe, and Latin America (see Ch. 346).

MISCELLANEOUS FORMS OF INFECTIOUS ARTHRITIS. *Lyme Disease* (see Ch. 321). Lyme disease is a systemic inflammatory tick-borne disorder caused by the spirochete *Borrelia burgdorferi*. Arthritis, usually monarticular or oligoarticular, with a tendency to involve large joints in a remitting fashion lasting for months or years, is the most common manifestation of late (persistent) infection, or stage 3. It may be seen in earlier stages but much less frequently. The knee joint is involved in almost all cases. Lyme arthritis seldom presents in a symmetrical or RA-like fashion, fails to respond to antibiotic therapy, and is associated with HLA-DR4. The diagnosis of Lyme disease is facilitated when patients in endemic areas exhibit the characteristic clinical picture. Laboratory diagnosis is based on serologic techniques, but interpretation of test results is often difficult. Treatment with appropriate antibiotics is effective in most patients with the correct diagnosis. However, some patients are refractory to conventional therapy, and in these, newer modalities (i.e., vaccination) may need to be tried.

Syphilis (see Ch. 318). Joint involvement may occur at any stage of congenital, secondary, and tertiary syphilis. It is extremely important to recognize the musculoskeletal manifestations of syphilis with its reported resurgence in recent years and because of its association with HIV infection. A variety of musculoskeletal manifestations may occur, including osteochondritis, periostitis, bilateral hydrarthrosis, usually involving knees and painless joints (Clutton's joints) in children with congenital syphilis, polyarthralgias, polyarthritis, tenosynovitis (not as common or as painful as in DGI), unilateral sacroiliitis, spondylitis, osteitis and periostitis in patients with secondary syphilis, and Charcot's joints, gummatous arthritis and osteitis, and chronic arthritis in patients with tertiary syphilis. Diagnosis can be difficult, especially in the setting of HIV infection, in which repeated serology testing is often necessary. Penicillin remains the agent of choice, and when appropriately given, results are excellent.

Tuberculous Arthritis (see Ch. 311). Tuberculosis is a rare cause of arthritis in industrialized countries. The recent increase in the incidence of pulmonary tuberculosis and its association (including the atypical forms) with HIV infection compel one to consider this etiology, especially in patients with chronic indolent mono- or oligoarthritis. Active pulmonary involvement is often not detected. The skin test is usually positive in most cases, but direct histologic evidence and cultures of synovial tissue are required for diagnosis. Joint involvement with atypical *Mycobacterium* infection should be considered in immunocompromised patients, after repeated intra-articular steroid injection, and in certain occupations, e.g., fishermen. Long-term therapy with isoniazid, ethambutol, and/or rifampin is indicated.

Fungal Arthritis (see Ch. 347 through 358). Musculoskeletal involvement secondary to fungal infection is rarely seen, although there is evidence of an increasing incidence of pathogenic and opportunistic fungal infections and emergence of new species of disease-causing fungi, particularly in immunosuppressed patients. Distribution is worldwide, clinical signs of infections can be mild, and chronic evolution as well as delayed diagnosis are common.

The most frequent species affecting the musculoskeletal system are *Coccidioides immitis, Histoplasma capsulatum, Blastomyces dermatitides,* and *Sporothrix schenckii* and in immunocompromised patients *Candida, Aspergillus, Cryptococcus,* and *Histoplasma.* For diagnosis, the organism must be identified in the synovial tissue or cultured from synovial fluid or tissue. Long-term therapy with amphotericin B and the newer antimycotic agents, with or without surgical debridement, is often effective.

Cuéllar ML, Silveira LH, Espinoza LR: Fungal arthritis. Ann Rheum Dis 51:690, 1992. *Comprehensively covers the rheumatic disorders caused by fungi.*
Espinoza LR, Cuéllar ML: AIDS and other immunodeficiency diseases. *In* Schumacher HR, Klippel JH, Koopman WJ (eds.): Primer on the Rheumatic Diseases. Atlanta, GA. Arthritis Foundation, 1993, pp. 258–261. *An overview of retrovirus-associated rheumatologic complications.*
Mikhail IS, Alarcón GS: Nongonococcal bacterial arthritis. Rheum Dis Clin North Am 19:311, 1993. *An excellent review of the clinical, diagnostic, and therapeutic aspects of nongonococcal bacterial arthritis.*
Scopelitis E, Martínez-Osuna P: Gonococcal arthritis. Rheum Dis Clin North Am 19:363, 1993. *Another good review of gonococcal arthritis, emphasizing pathogenesis and newer therapeutic modalities.*

240 SYSTEMIC LUPUS ERYTHEMATOSUS

Peter H. Schur

Systemic lupus erythematosus (SLE) is a disease of unknown cause that may produce variable combinations of fever, rashes, hair loss, arthritis, pleuritis, pericarditis, nephritis, anemia, leukopenia, thrombocytopenia, and central nervous system (CNS) disease. The clinical course is characterized by periods of remissions and acute or chronic relapses. Patients with SLE develop characteristic immune abnormalities, especially antibodies to a number of nuclear and other cellular antigens. The diagnosis is facilitated by determin-

ing whether the patient has 4 of the 11 clinical and/or laboratory criteria developed for the classification of SLE (Table 240–1).

EPIDEMIOLOGY. SLE can occur at any age but has its onset primarily between ages 16 and 55. It occurs more frequently in women. In children, the female:male ratio is 1.4 to 5.8:1; in adults, it ranges from 8:1 to 13:1; in older individuals, the ratio is 2:1. The prevalence of SLE is estimated to be between 4 and 250 cases

TABLE 240–1. CRITERIA FOR CLASSIFICATION OF SYSTEMIC LUPUS ERYTHEMATOSUS*

Criterion	Definition
1. Malar rash	Fixed erythema, flat or raised, over the malar eminences, tending to spare the nasolabial folds
2. Discoid rash	Erythematous raised patches with adherent keratotic scaling and follicular plugging; atrophic scarring may occur in older lesions
3. Photosensitivity	Skin rash as a result of unusual reaction to sunlight, by patient history or physician observation
4. Oral ulcers	Oral or nasopharyngeal ulceration, usually painless, observed by a physician
5. Arthritis	Nonerosive arthritis involving two or more peripheral joints, characterized by tenderness, swelling, or effusion
6. Serositis	a. Pleuritis—convincing history of pleuritic pain or rub heard by a physician or evidence of pleural effusion *OR* b. Pericarditis—documented by electrocardiogram or rub or evidence of pericardial effusion
7. Renal disorder	a. Persistent proteinuria >0.5 gram per day or >3+ if quantitation not performed *OR* b. Cellular casts—may be red cell, hemoglobin, granular, tubular, or mixed
8. Neurologic disorder	a. Seizures—in the absence of offending drugs or known metabolic derangements, e.g., uremia, ketoacidosis, or electrolyte imbalance *OR* b. Psychosis—in the absence of offending drugs or known metabolic derangements, e.g., uremia, ketoacidosis, or electrolyte imbalance
9. Hematologic disorder	a. Hemolytic anemia—with reticulocytosis *OR* b. Leukopenia—<4000/mm³ total on two or more occasions *OR* c. Lymphopenia—<1500/mm³ on two or more occasions *OR* d. Thrombocytopenia—<100,000/mm³ in the absence of offending drugs
10. Immunologic disorder	a. Positive LE cell preparation *OR* b. Anti-DNA: antibody to native DNA in abnormal titer *OR* c. Anti-Sm: presence of antibody to Sm nuclear antigen *OR* d. False-positive serologic test for syphilis known to be positive for at least 6 months and confirmed by *Treponema pallidum* immobilization or fluorescent treponemal antibody absorption test
11. Antinuclear antibody	An abnormal titer of antinuclear antibody by immunofluorescence or an equivalent assay at any point in time and in the absence of drugs known to be associated with "drug-induced lupus" syndrome

* The classification is based on 11 criteria. For the purpose of identifying patients in clinical studies, a person shall be said to have systemic lupus erythematosus if any 4 or more of the 11 criteria are present, serially or simultaneously, during any interval of observation.

per 100,000 population. In the United States, the highest incidence is among Asians in Hawaii, black Americans, and certain Native Americans (Sioux, Crow, Arapahoe). The risk to a black American female for developing SLE has been estimated to be 1:250. The prevalence is about the same worldwide; the disease appears to be common in China, Southeast Asia, and among blacks in the Caribbean but is seen infrequently in blacks in Africa. Limited observations suggest that the incidence of discoid lupus erythematosus is the same as that for SLE.

ETIOLOGY. The cause of SLE remains unknown, although many observations suggest a role for genetic, hormonal, immune, and environmental factors. The evidence for a genetic role is summarized in Table 240–2. Some of these genetic marker associations are found more frequently in SLE patients of different races and ethnicities. It has been calculated that at least four genes are involved in predisposing individuals to SLE. Each gene presumably affects some aspect of immune regulation, protein degradation, peptide transport across cell membranes, immune responses, complement, the reticuloendothelial system (including phagocytosis), immunoglobulins, apoptosis, and sex hormones. Thus combinations of dissimilar gene defects may result in distinct abnormal responses, producing separate pathologic processes and different clinical expression.

The evidence for hormonal abnormalities is based primarily on the observation that SLE is much more common among women in their childbearing years. In addition, SLE has been observed in some males with Klinefelter's syndrome, and some abnormalities of estrogen metabolism have been noted in both men and women with SLE. However, the clinical expression of SLE is the same in men and women. Furthermore, a lupus-like disease of New Zealand mice is more common, more severe, and has an earlier onset in females—and is ameliorated by oophorectomy or treatment with male hormones. However, in other strains of mice with a lupus-like disease, this gender difference is not noted.

Numerous immune abnormalities occur in patients with SLE, the etiology of which remains unclear; neither do we know which are primary and which are secondary. Some of these immune defects are episodic, and some correlate with disease activity. SLE is primarily a disease with abnormalities of immune regulation. These are thought to be secondary to a loss of "self" tolerance; that is, SLE patients (either before or during disease evolution) are no longer totally tolerant of all their "self" antigens and consequently develop an immune response to them. The number of suppressor T cells also decreases; these would normally be down-regulating (maintaining homeostasis) immune responses. Furthermore, mice with lupus and possibly humans with SLE have a (genetic) defect in apoptosis, resulting in abnormal programmed cell death. As a result of these defects, cells break down abnormally; certain (especially nuclear) antigens are processed by antigen-presenting cells (i.e., macrophages, B lymphocytes, dendritic cells) into peptides. The peptide–major histocompatibility complex (MHC) stimulates the expansion of helper (i.e., CD4) autoreactive T cells which, through release of cytokines (i.e., interleukin-6 [IL-6], IL-4), cause autoreactive B cells to become activated, proliferate, and differentiate into antibody-producing cells and make an excess of antibodies to many nuclear antigens (Fig. 240–1). Thus a characteristic immune profile develops in the SLE patient—the development of elevated levels of antinuclear antibodies (ANA's), especially to DNA,

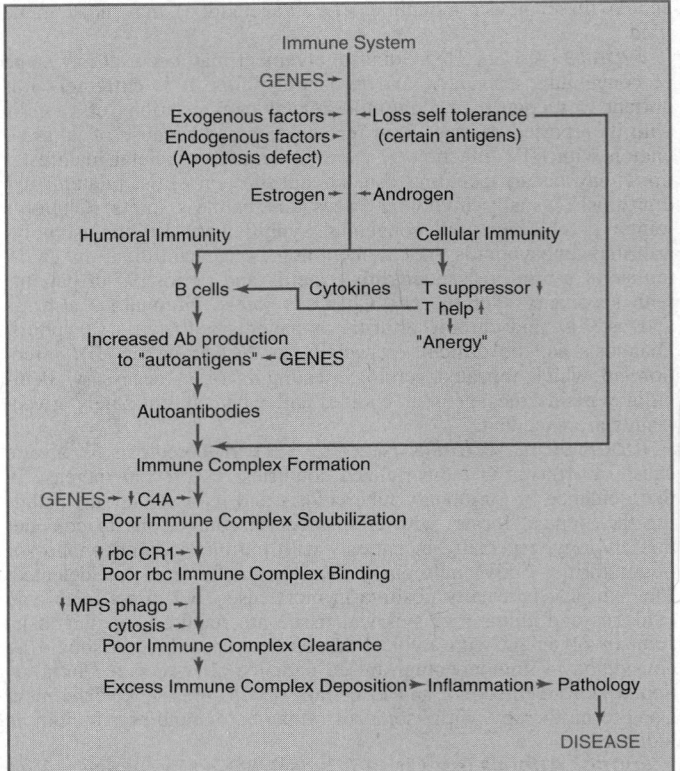

FIGURE 240–1. Pathogenetic events in SLE.

Sm, RNP, Ro, La, and others (see Ch. 236) (Table 240–3). ANA's are made to molecules involved in essential cellular functions (i.e., RNA splicing); antigens are active sites on these molecules. With continued pressure over time from "self" antigens, the immune response switches from low-affinity, highly cross-reactive IgM antibodies—via somatic (hyper)mutation—to high-affinity IgG antibodies and to more limited epitopes on "self" antigens. Unique idiotypes of antibodies may stimulate autoreactive T cells to expand, thereby helping unique clones of B cells to expand and thus making more specific ANA's with unique idiotypes. Female hormones promote B-cell hyperactivity, while androgens may have the opposite effect. Environmental factors such as microorganisms (i.e., viruses) may stimulate specific cells in this immune network. Furthermore, ultraviolet (UV) light—known to exacerbate lupus skin lesions—may stimulate keratinocytes to secrete more IL-1, which in turn stimulates B cells to make more antibody. Not all autoantibodies cause disease. In fact, all normal individuals make autoantibodies, albeit in low levels. The variability in clinical disease (different organs in specific patients) may thus reflect variability in the

TABLE 240–2. GENETIC RISK FACTORS FOR SLE

High concordance rate (14–57%) in monozygotic twins
Increased frequency (5–12%) of LE, autoantibodies, suppressor cell defects in first-degree relatives
Increased frequency: HLA-B8, DR2, DR3, DQA1, DQB1
                    C2, C4 (especially C4A), CR1 deficiency
                    Certain Gm markers
                    T-cell receptor (TCR) genes
Anti-DNA associated with DR2, DR3, DR7, DQB1
Anti-Sm associated with DR4, DR7, DQw6
Anti-RNP associated with DQw5, DQw8
Anti-Ro (SS-A) associated with DR2, DR3, DQA1/DQB1, C2D
Anti-La (SS-B) associated with DR3, DQw2.3
Antiphospholipid associated with DR4, DR7, DR53, DQw7

TABLE 240–3. AUTOANTIBODIES IN PATIENTS WITH SLE

Test	Sensitivity (%)	Specificity (%)	Predictive Value (%)
ANA	99	80	15–35
dsDNA	70	95	95
ssDNA	80	50	50
Histone	30–80	Moderate	Moderate
Nucleoprotein	58	Moderate	Moderate
Sm	25	99	97
RNP (U1-RNP)	50	87–94	46–85
Ro (SS-A)	25–35		
La (SS-B)	15		
PCNA	5	95	95

Cytoplasm: mitochondria, lysosomes, microsomes, ribosomes. RNA: dsRNA, ssRNA, rRNA. Cell membranes: red cells, white blood (T&B) cells, platelets, brain. Other: clotting factors (APL), thyroid, rheumatoid factors, BFP-STS. In SLE, anti-DNA and anti-Sm are associated with renal disease, anti-RNP with Raynaud's, and anti-Ro with photosensitivity. Anti-RNP is seen in SLE, RA, scleroderma, Sjögren's syndrome, and MCTD. Anti-Ro (SS-A) is seen in SLE, Sjögren's syndrome, primary photosensitivity, and primary biliary cirrhosis. Anti-La (SS-B) is seen in SLE and Sjögren's syndrome.

quality and quantity of the immune response. While these observations suggest possible triggering factors for disease, it remains unclear what causes exacerbations—although clinically they often follow infections and other stressful events—and what causes perpetuation of the immune abnormalities and waxing and waning of the disease.

PATHOGENESIS. Many manifestations are mediated by antibodies. The classic example is that of diffuse proliferative glomerulonephritis. Immune complexes (IC's), consisting of nuclear antigens (especially DNA) and high-affinity complement-fixing IgG (especially IgG1 and IgG3), ANA's (especially antibodies to DNA), form in the circulation and deposit in the glomerular basement membrane (GBM) or form *in situ;* histone may facilitate IC deposition. The complement system is then activated; chemotactic factors are generated, resulting in the attraction and infiltration of leukocytes, which then phagocytose IC's and release mediators (such as activators of the clotting system), which further perpetuate the glomerular inflammation. With continuing IC deposition, chronic inflammation may ensue, ultimately leading to fibrinoid necrosis and scarring (crescents) and loss of renal function. In lupus membranous glomerulonephritis, similar mechanisms occur, although IC-containing, poorly complement-fixing IgG2 and IgG4 form primarily *in situ* on the GBM; there is no cellular infiltrate. The mechanism for the GBM protein leakage, resulting in the nephrotic syndrome, is not clear. In lupus mesangial glomerulonephritis, mesangial cells (macrophage-like cells) have phagocytosed IC's, preventing them from depositing on the GBM. IC's also have been detected (by immunofluorescence and/or electron microscopy) at the dermal-epidermal junction in both skin lesions and normal skin, in the choroid plexus, in the pericardium, and in the pleural cavity. The pathogenic potential of IC's depends on the antibody (its specificity, affinity, charge, ability to activate complement or other mediators of inflammation), the nature of the antigen (size, charge), the ability of the IC to be solubilized by complement or bound to red blood cells (both systems may be defective in SLE), the clearance ability of the mononuclear phagocytosis system, as well as other factors.

SLE patients also make antibodies to cell surface antigens. Red blood cells (RBC's), white blood cells (WBC's), and platelets coated with such antibodies are cleared from the circulation either through (Fc) receptors on macrophages of the reticuloendothelial system, by complement-mediated cytotoxicity, or by antibody-dependent cellular cytotoxicity (ADCC)—resulting in (hemolytic) anemia, leukopenia, and thrombocytopenia. Antibodies to endothelial cells have been implicated in vasculitis, to neuronal cells in organic brain disease, and to renal glomerular and tubular antigens in lupus nephritis. Of recent particular interest are the antibodies to the phospholipid–β_2-glycoprotein I complex. These antibodies appear to interfere with the normal anticoagulant effect of β_2-glycoprotein I and are thus implicated in the arterial and venous thromboses (causing strokes and thrombophlebitis) and placental infarcts (causing miscarriages) complicating SLE.

Skin lesions are thought to be multifactorial in origin. UV light (1) damages DNA (the patient makes antibodies to DNA, IC's form, complement is activated, and a local inflammatory response ensues), (2) increases binding of anti-Ro, anti-La, and anti-RNP to UV-activated keratinocytes, (3) alters cellular membrane phospholipid metabolism, (4) increases IL-1 release from cutaneous keratinocytes and Langerhans cells, and (5) affects suppressor T cells.

PATHOLOGY. There are few unique pathologic features of SLE. In those patients with arthritis, the synovial histopathology tends to be nonspecific with superficial fibrin-like material and local or diffuse cell lining proliferation. Vascular changes include perivascular mononuclear cells, lumen obliteration, enlarged endothelial cells, and thrombi, but fibrinoid necrosis is uncommon. Biopsies of the malar erythema may reveal some minor basal layer abnormalities as well as IC deposits at the dermal-epidermal junction. Discoid skin lesions are characterized by hyperkeratosis, follicular plugging, and more basal cell layer changes, including IC's at the dermal-epidermal junction. Pleura and pericardium are infiltrated by mononuclear cells. Lupus pneumonitis is characterized by alveolar wall injury, hemorrhage, and edema, hyaline membrane formation, and IC deposits. Coronary arteries often demonstrate premature-onset atherosclerosis. Libman-Sacks endocarditis is characterized by the accumulation of IC's, mononuclear cells, hematoxylin bodies, and fibrin and platelet thrombi. Pathologic examina-

tion of the spleen often reveals an "onion skin" appearance of the splenic arteries, thought to represent healed arteritis.

Renal Disease. Minimal disease (type IIA mesangial disease) of glomeruli has IC deposits only in mesangial cells. Type IIB mesangial nephritis also has mesangial hypercellularity. Focal proliferative nephritis has segmental proliferation in glomerular tufts and in the mesangium and IC deposits in the mesangium and scattered granular deposits in the subendothelial, subepithelial, and intrabasement GBM. Active diffuse proliferative glomerulonephritis affects >50% of glomeruli with cellular proliferation, necrosis, "wire loops," subendothelial deposits, and hematoxylin bodies. When chronic, the process involves sclerosis, adhesions, crescents, and (tubular) atrophy. There are extensive "lumpy and bumpy" deposits of IC's. In membranous nephritis, diffuse, uniform thickening of the GBM is seen, with a fine granular deposition of IC's in the subendothelial region beneath fused foot processes. Tubular degenerative changes with interstitial mononuclear cells are not uncommon. Extensive crescent formation, representing scarring, indicates a poor prognosis.

The brain is notable for the paucity of pathologic changes. Some minor blood vessel abnormalities, an occasional microinfarct, and some perivascular infiltration have been noted.

CLINICAL MANIFESTATIONS. SLE is highly variable in onset as well as course. The initial symptoms may be nonspecific (Table 240–4) and include myalgia, nausea, vomiting, headaches, depression, easy bruising, or more specific symptoms or any combination thereof. These symptoms may be mild or severe, fleeting or persistent.

General Symptoms. Fatigue occurs in virtually all SLE patients. Fatigue may parallel the onset of SLE or its relapse but should be distinguished from the fatigue associated with other factors such as increased workload, sleep disturbance, depression, unhealthful habits, stress, deconditioning, anemia, the use of certain medications (including prednisone), and any intercurrent disease.

TABLE 240–4. CLINICAL FEATURES IN SLE

Manifestation	Approximate Frequency (%)	
	At Onset	*At Any Time*
Nonspecific:		
Fatigue	—	90
Fever	36	80
Weight loss	—	60
Arthralgia/myalgia	69	95
Specific:		
Arthritis	—	
Skin		
Butterfly rash	40	50
Discoid LE	6	20
Photosensitivity	29	58
Mucous ulcers	11	30
Alopecia	—	71
Raynaud's	18	30
Purpura	—	15
Urticaria	—	9
Renal	16	50
Nephrosis	—	18
Gastrointestinal	—	38
Pulmonary	3	50
Pleurisy	—	45
Effusions	—	24
Pnemonia	—	29
Cardiac	—	46
Pericarditis	—	48
Murmurs	—	23
ECG changes	—	34
Lymphadenopathy	7	50
Splenomegaly	—	20
Hepatomegaly	—	25
Central nervous system	12	75
Functional	—	Most
Psychosis	—	20
Seizures	—	20
Hematologic	—	90

Fever is seen in 80% of patients; it is usually episodic. Infections, which occur commonly in SLE patients, always must be considered.

Musculoskeletal Manifestations. Arthralgia and arthritis have been noted in 95% of SLE patients. Symptoms tend to be asymmetric and migratory, with complaints in a particular joint often gone in 1 to 3 days. Fingers, hands, wrists, knees, and less frequently, ankles, elbows, shoulders, and hips are affected. Morning stiffness is generally measured in minutes, in contrast to hours in rheumatoid arthritis (RA). Although joint deformities are considered to be more a feature of RA, damage to periarticular tissue can cause flexion deformities, ulnar deviation, soft tissue laxity, and swan neck deformities, particularly in those with longstanding disease receiving corticosteroids. Joint erosions are rare. Tenosynovitis is noted in 10 to 13% of patients. Synovial effusions are infrequent and usually small.

Avascular necrosis may occur, especially in the femoral head and less frequently in the humeral head, tibial plateau, and scaphoid naviculare. Involvement is often bilateral. High prednisone dosage, prolonged use, and pulse steroids are risk factors. The first symptom of hip involvement may be groin pain. Radiography may be negative or equivocal, but magnetic resonance imaging (MRI) is usually diagnostic. Osteoporosis is common, especially of the trabecular bones, which may not be worsened by corticosteroids. Muscle weakness may represent myositis (uncommon) or be due to medications (corticosteroids, antimalarials). Myalgia is very common.

Mucocutaneous Lesions. Photosensitivity, implying a rash after exposure to UVB light (e.g., sunlight, fluorescent light), occurs in >50% of patients. Some patients are also sensitive to UVA light—the clue, rash after exposure to sun filtered through glass. Fair-skinned individuals tend to be more susceptible. Photosensitivity may develop at any time or vary in intensity during the course of SLE. The classic butterfly rash, i.e., erythema over the cheeks and nose, develops after UV exposure in >50% of patients. The skin may feel warm and slightly edematous. Application of alcohol, found in many sunscreens, may cause vasodilation and thereby more erythema. The rash may last for hours or days and often recurs. A maculopapular eruption with fine scaling may ensue and last longer, although generally healing without residue.

Discoid lesions develop in 25% of patients with SLE but also may occur in the absence of any other feature of SLE. Discoid lesions are characterized by discrete round, annular, erythematous, slightly infiltrated plaques covered by a well-formed adherent scale that extends into dilated hair follicles. Follicular plugging is prominent. Lesions slowly expand with active inflammation at the periphery, leaving depressed scars, telangiectasia, and depigmentation; central scarring with atrophy is characteristic. Lesions tend to occur on the face, scalp, neck, ears, and around the shoulders. Some lesions may be hyperkeratotic and thus be confused with psoriasis. Patients with isolated discoid lupus have about a 10% chance of eventually developing SLE.

Subacute cutaneous lupus erythematosus (SCLE) occurs in about 10% of SLE patients. The lesions are small, erythematous, slightly scaly papules that evolve into annular or psoriasiform forms. Lesions appear typically on the forearms and upper torso; atrophy or scarring rarely develops, although telangiectasia does. There is a strong association with HLA-DR3 and anti-Ro antibodies.

Lupus profundus/panniculitis is a rare manifestation of SLE. Typically, painful nodules develop under a skin lesion on the scalp, face, arms, chest, back, thighs, and buttocks, resolving as a depression. Ulcerations are uncommon. The presence of IC deposits at the dermal-epidermal junction helps to distinguish lesions from those of the Weber-Christian syndrome. Bullous lesions are rare and can be distinguished from other bullous diseases by the difference in serum antibodies and dermal immune deposits.

Hair loss, on the scalp or elsewhere, occurs in 71% of SLE patients. The most common is premature hair loss (telogen effluvium), characterized by a diffuse thinning of the scalp. This may follow a flare of SLE, stress, pregnancy, or the use of steroids; hair generally grows back. Some patients have "lupus hair," hair that easily fractures and is thin and unruly. Discoid lesions of the scalp usually result in permanent hair loss.

Mucous membranes are frequently affected. Discoid lesions may appear on the lip. The soft or hard palate may be involved by discoid plaques, areas of erythema, and especially by painful ulcers. These lesions should be distinguished from lichen planus, candidiasis, aphthous stomatitis, bites, leukoplakia, and malignancy—by biopsy. Nasal ulcers have been noted in 20% of patients.

Vascular Lesions. Livedo reticularis, secondary to spasm of the dermal ascending arterioles, is often seen in the forearms, legs, and even the torso. Occlusion may result in ulcers. A strong association is seen with Raynaud's phenomenon and with antiphospholipid antibodies. Telangiectasias are found commonly on the face and elsewhere. They represent dilated blood vessels and *not* an active inflammatory lesion. Telangiectasias appear more prominent when the patient blushes, is in a hot environment (shower), or takes a vasodilator (e.g., alcohol, calcium channel blocker). Telangiectasias also may be associated with solar damage, aging, hypertension, diabetes, and other rheumatic diseases.

Raynaud's phenomenon occurs in 17 to 30% of patients. It is characterized by blanching of nail beds, fingers, toes, and occasionally ears, nose, and tongue. The vasospasm of small to medium-sized arteries may be induced by cold, cigarette smoke, caffeine, decongestants, stress, and other factors. Following ischemia, there may be bluing and graying followed by vasodilation with warming and reddening. Gangrene is rare.

Vasculitis of postcapillary venules with neutrophil or lymphocyte accumulation develops in 20% of patients, presenting as urticaria or purpura. When small arteries are affected, microinfarcts of fingertips, toes, nail cuticles, forearms, or about the ankle may develop; the lesions about the ankle may ulcerate. The blood vessels typically have fibrinoid necrosis, thrombosis, and a variable cellular infiltrate. Patients with vasculitis have low serum complement and high serum IC levels and may have antiphospholipid antibodies.

Other less common vascular lesions include Janeway's spots on the palms, Osler's nodes on fingertips, atrophie blanche lesions, and chilblain lupus (pernio) on fingers and toes.

Pulmonary Manifestations. Pulmonary involvement occurs in most patients, manifesting as pleurisy, coughing, dyspnea, abnormal pulmonary function tests, or chest radiography abnormalities. Pleurisy occurs in >50% of patients; the most common cause is chest wall pain on local pressure and/or movement. Pleuritis (inflammation of the pleura) also causes pleurisy. It is diagnosed by the presence of a pleural friction rub and/or the radiographic presence of a pleural effusion. Effusions typically have low complement and protein levels, few WBC's (the pleura has mononuclear cells), glucose levels approximating plasma levels (by contrast, they are low in RA), and LE cells. Cough usually represents an infection, but pulmonary edema secondary to cardiac or renal failure or fluid overload in a patient receiving corticosteroids should be considered.

Acute lupus pneumonitis occurs in 5 to 12%; it is characterized by fever, cough (even hemoptysis), pleurisy, and dyspnea. Radiography shows diffuse acinar infiltrates, especially in lower lobes. Subsequently, interstitial infiltrates and fibrosis may develop, with pulmonary function abnormalities. The prognosis is poor.

Pulmonary hypertension may complicate SLE but is more frequent with scleroderma or mixed connective tissue disease (MCTD). Raynaud's phenomenon is common. Late findings include dyspnea, hypoxemia, restricting lung disease, and reduced CO_2-diffusing capacity.

The shrinking or vanishing lung syndrome has been described in some patients. It is believed to result from weakening and elevation of the diaphragm (lung fields are radiographically clear).

Cardiovascular Manifestations. Pericardial effusion is observed by echocardiography in most patients, and clinical pericarditis, manifested as substernal chest pain, a pericardial rub, and electrocardiographic (ECG) changes, has been noted in up to 48% of patients. Tamponade and restrictive pericarditis are rare. The fluid has characteristics similar to SLE pleural fluids.

Myocarditis, characterized by resting tachycardia, arrhythmias, ECG nonspecific ST/T-wave abnormalities, and unexplained cardiomegaly with congestive heart failure (CHF), has been noted in 8 to 78% of large series.

Coronary artery disease is being recognized increasingly, particularly in patients with longstanding disease, especially those receiving chronic corticosteroids. As a result, more younger patients with angina, myocardial infarctions, and CHF are being seen. The cause of the premature atherosclerosis remains unclear, but steroid-induced lipid abnormalities, IC deposition along blood vessels, and hypertension may all play a role. Hypertension is common, especially with flares of nephritis, chronic renal disease, and steroid use.

Valvular disease has been noted in up to 25% of patients; most common is mitral valve prolapse. Murmurs are even more common and may represent valvular disease or be due to anemia, fever, and/or cardiomegaly. Echocardiography is very useful to detect Libman-Sacks verrucous endocarditis. Verrucae are typically near the edge of the valve. Bacterial endocarditis may develop on damaged valves.

Thrombophlebitis occurs in > 10% of SLE patients. It most commonly affects the lower leg and is often associated with antiphospholipid antibodies and oral contraceptives. The renal veins and inferior vena cava are rarely involved; their involvement may cause nephrotic syndrome—pulmonary embolisms are uncommon.

Hematologic Considerations.
Abnormalities of the formed elements of blood and the clotting and fibrinolytic systems are common. Anemia occurs in at least 50% of patients. The most common cause is chronic disease; red cells are normochromic and normocytic, the reticulocyte count is low, and iron stores are adequate. Anemia may reflect chronic gastrointestinal blood loss secondary to the use of nonsteroidal anti-inflammatory drugs (NSAID's) and/or steroids—or secondary to excessive menstrual bleeding. Hemolytic anemia frequently occurs, and the reticulocyte count is elevated, haptoglobin levels are low, and the Coombs' test is positive. A positive Coombs' test with both immunoglobulin and complement on RBC's is associated with hemolysis, while only a positive complement Coombs' test rarely features hemolysis. Antibodies are usually anti-Rh and are "warm." Medications, especially immunosuppressives, may induce anemia—here, reticulocyte counts will be low and haptoglobin levels normal.

Leukopenia, with a WBC count under 4500, has been noted in over 50% of patients, while counts under 4000 occur in only 17%. Granulocytes are affected more than lymphocytes. Leukopenia usually results from immune mechanisms (i.e., antineutrophil antibodies, IC's) or medications. Lymphocytopenia (which may be due to complement-fixing IgM or cold-reactive antibodies) may occur during active disease. Leukocytosis or an excess of neutrophils generally reflects infection or steroid use. There is an increase in activated T cells and a decrease in natural killer cells, especially during active disease.

Thrombocytopenia, with platelet counts under 150,000 per cubic millimeters, has been noted in >50% of patients, while counts under 50,000 have been noted in only 10%. Thrombocytopenia may reflect myeloproliferative diseases, ineffective thrombopoiesis (e.g., megaloblastic anemia), abnormal platelet distribution (e.g., splenomegaly), and abnormal immune mechanisms (antiplatelet antibodies, disseminated intravascular coagulation, and idiopathic thrombocytopenic purpuria, or ITP). ITP may be the first manifestation of SLE. Most patients with both hemolytic anemia and ITP (Evans' syndrome) have SLE. In SLE ITP, platelets are sensitized by IgG antibodies, which then bind to (splenic) macrophage Fc receptors with resulting phagocytosis—thrombocytopenia ensues when production fails to keep up with accelerated destruction. Platelet counts under 50,000 may rarely cause symptomatic bleeding, while counts under 20,000 per cubic millimeter may cause petechiae, purpura, nose bleeds, and gum bleeding.

Lymphadenopathy occurs in 50% of patients, especially during active disease. Nodes are typically small, soft, nontender, and discrete in the neck, axillary, and inguinal areas. Biopsies may reveal follicular hyperplasia. Infection and malignancy should always be considered. When in doubt, a biopsy should be done.

Splenomegaly occurs in 10 to 20% of patients, especially during active disease, and in association with lymphadenopathy. Splenomegaly does not necessarily cause hemolytic anemia but is usually associated with leukopenia. There is no apparent increase in lymphoproliferative malignancies in patients with SLE.

Antibodies to many clotting factors have been described in patients with SLE, including Factors VIII, IX, XI, XII, and XIII. These antibodies may induce bleeding. Antiphospholipid antibodies (APL's) are found in about 25% of SLE patients (see Ch. 236). They should be suspected when the patient has a prolonged partial thromboplastin time with arterial and venous thromboses, thrombocytopenia, false-positive tests for syphilis, and recurrent mid-trimester miscarriages. Weaker associations have been noted with livedo reticularis, renal disease, pulmonary hypertension, and cardiac valvular disease. Some individuals with APL's do not have

SLE. APL's can be detected as a lupus anticoagulant and as anticardiolipin antibodies. Clinical risks increase with higher titers.

False-positive tests for syphilis have been noted in 25% of SLE patients and in fact may precede SLE by years. The "false" nature is confirmed when a *Treponema pallidum* immobilization test (TPI) or fluorescent *Treponema* antibody absorption test (FTA-ABS) is negative. There is no rationale for performing tests for syphilis in patients with SLE unless syphilis is suspected.

The erythrocyte sedimentation rate is elevated in most patients with SLE and is thought by some observers to correlate with clinical activity (see Ch. 236).

Renal Manifestations.
Clinical lupus nephritis is observed in about 50% of SLE patients and is characterized by either urinary or functional (e.g., clearance) abnormalities. Also, many more patients have electron microscopic and/or immunofluorescence evidence of IC deposits in the glomeruli, even in the absence of light microscopic abnormalities. The presence of clinical lupus nephritis is of concern because of its potential for morbidity and mortality.

About 24% of patients develop minimal or mesangial nephritis (type II). Patients may have some urinary abnormalities, GFR is usually normal, complement levels may be somewhat depressed, and anti-DNA antibodies may be somewhat elevated. The prognosis is very good. Fifteen per cent of patients develop focal proliferative nephritis; the clinical picture is similar to that of mesangial (type IIB) disease but is somewhat more severe. Prognosis is good.

Diffuse proliferative glomerulonephritis occurs in about 43% of patients. There is an active urinary sediment, proteinuria may be marked, glomerular clearance is diminished, complement levels are significantly diminished, anti-DNA antibody and IC levels are elevated (especially during active nephritis), and patients are usually hypertensive. Initial creatinine levels > 1.2 mg per deciliter have a poor prognosis with regard to long-term renal function.

Membranous glomerulonephritis occurs in about 15% of patients. There is marked proteinuria; little urinary sediment; complement, anti-DNA antibody, and IC levels are normal; the glomerular filtration is normal; lipid levels are elevated; and hypertension is a late event. Mild proteinuria has a good prognosis, but nephrotic syndrome with persistent edema and high lipid levels has a poor prognosis.

Biopsies are useful in patients with clinical nephritis to determine the pathologic type of nephritis, whether there is active inflammation (which has the potential for reversal) versus fibrosis and sclerosis, and to distinguish lupus nephritis from other forms of renal disease.

Urinary tract infections are common. Azotemia (slight) may result from NSAID's.

Gastrointestinal Manifestations.
The gastrointestinal tract may be involved in 50% of patients. Up to 25% of patients have esophageal complaints, including difficulty swallowing. The lack of radiographic abnormalities suggests stress, while, if positive, scleroderma-overlap syndrome should be considered. Dysphagia also may result from hiatal hernia and gastric reflux. Dyspepsia is common, especially with stress and with NSAID and steroid use. Abdominal pain, nausea, and vomiting are also common. In the absence of peptic ulcers and adverse medication effect, a cause is rarely determined. On the other hand, one should always consider mesenteric vasculitis, characterized by intermittent lower abdominal pain eventually progressing to an acute abdomen. Diagnosis is usually confirmed by angiography. Pancreatitis (8% of patients) also should be considered in the presence of upper abdominal pain, nausea, and vomiting. Pancreatitis may reflect vasculitis and/or the use of steroids. Hepatomegaly is uncommon, but liver chemistry abnormalities (lactic dehydrogenase [LDH], serum glutamate pyruvate transferase [SGPT]) are common, especially in patients with active disease or those taking NSAID's. Persistent liver chemistry abnormalities may suggest cirrhosis; chronic, active, or persistent hepatitis; granulomatous hepatitis; cholestasis; infection (e.g., hepatitis); or drug toxicity—and may warrant a liver biopsy.

Neuropsychiatric Manifestations.
These symptoms occur in virtually all patients (Table 240–5). Many patients manifest anxiety and/or depression, often in response to their illness and the threat of loss of health, family, and job, disfigurement, disability, dependency, and death. Symptoms may include psychosomatic complaints, such as insomnia, anorexia, constipation, myalgia, arthral-

TABLE 240–5. NEUROPSYCHIATRIC MANIFESTATIONS—DIAGNOSTIC MANEUVERS

Functional Etiology	Functional or Organic	Organic Etiology
Depression	Psychosis	Seizures
Hypomania/mania	Cognitive defects	Neuropathy
Anxiety	Dysesthesia	Stroke
Conversion reaction	Headache	Movement disorder
Affective disorder		Organic brain syndrome
Mood swings		Coma
Adjustment disorder		Transverse myelitis
		Meningitis
Psych testing	EEG—evoked potentials	MRI
	CT	Angiography
	Brain scan	Antineuronal Ab
		Antiphospholipid Ab
		Lumbar puncture

gia, fatigue, palpitations, diarrhea, dizzy spells, hyperventilation, memory loss, emotional lability, confusion, decreased concentration, headaches, and cognitive defects. Frank psychosis may develop with compulsive-obsessive behavior, phobias, and even suicide. These symptoms also may precede a diagnosis of SLE for years, leading to frustration by the patient and physician regarding correct diagnoses. These psychological responses to illness should be differentiated from organic brain disease—which may cause the same symptoms. Most useful in discriminating functional from organic disease are tests of cognitive function and psychological tests (e.g., the Minnesota Multiphasic Personality Inventory [MMPI]); other tests such as MRI, electroencephalograph with evoked potentials, positron emission tomographic scans, SPECT scans, and antibrain and antiribosomal P-protein antibody determinations also may be useful. Cerebrospinal fluid (CSF) analysis is most useful to exclude infection, although some physicians note correlation of complement, anti-DNA, IC's, IL-6, elevated protein levels, and antineuronal antibodies with CNS activity.

Psychosis is said to occur in about 24% of patients. Psychosis also can be caused by renal failure (uremic encephalopathy), hypertension (with multiple cerebral infarcts), metabolic abnormalities, infection, or drugs (tranquilizers, antidepressants, narcotics, β blockers, NSAID's, cimetidine, antimalarials, alcohol, caffeine, benzodiazepine, and others). Steroids may cause or help clear a psychosis, suggesting that the psychosis had an organic etiology. Medications may cause other problems: aseptic meningitis from azathioprine, ibuprofen, and other NSAID's and, rarely, headaches, hallucinations, mental confusion, psychosis, seizures, and neuromyopathy from antimalarials.

Headaches are a frequent complaint and are usually due to stress and tension; migraine has been noted in 10 to 37% of patients. Other causes of headache include cold food, hangover, nitrites, monosodium glutamate, hunger, sinusitis, dental or eye disease, and malignancies.

Seizures are said to occur in 15 to 20% of patients, including grand mal, petit mal, temporal lobe, focal, and jacksonian. Seizures may reflect an old scar or an acute inflammatory episode or may be due to metabolic imbalances, uremia, hypertension, infections, tumors, head trauma, or vasculopathy. When associated with other aspects of a lupus exacerbation, a CNS etiology should be suspected. CNS vasculitis is rare.

Cranial or peripheral neuropathies develop in 10 to 15% of patients. They usually occur coincident with a lupus exacerbation. Cranial neuropathies include those affecting eye muscles, trigeminal neuralgia, facial weakness, and vertigo. Peripheral neuropathy is usually asymmetric and mild and affects more than one nerve (mononeuritis multiplex).

Stroke has been noted in up to 15% of patients secondary to hemorrhage or thrombosis, APL's, hypertension, ITP, and thrombocytopenia. Less common are movement disorders (e.g., ataxia, choreoathetosis, hemiballismus) and transverse myelitis. Meningitis is not uncommon and may be due to either microorganisms or medication.

The eye is frequently involved by rash involving the eyelid, conjunctivitis, or keratoconjunctivitis. A characteristic finding is retinal "cotton wool" exudates (cytoid bodies), usually near the disc. They reflect a microangiopathy of retinal capillaries and localized microinfarction of the superficial nerve fiber layers of the retina. While old textbooks cited a frequency of 10 to 25%, they are now only seen rarely.

Menses and Pregnancy. Some patients think that their SLE flares with menses. Some patients have heavy menses, which may reflect lupus anticoagulants, the use of NSAID's or steroids, or hormonal abnormalities. Lupus often becomes less active after menopause.

Approximately 25 to 30% of SLE pregnancies result in miscarriage; overall fetal loss approaches 50%, and patients are more likely to have a premature delivery. An increased fetal mortality is more likely (3×) to occur in the presence of major organ involvement, especially renal disease. APL's predispose to recurrent midtrimester fetal loss. Pre-eclampsia is a frequent complication and is difficult to distinguish from a lupus flare.

Neonatal lupus is a rare condition characterized by typical skin lesions shortly after exposure to UV light in a nursery. The rash generally clears within months; SLE rarely develops later in life. Sera from the infants (and their mothers) have antibodies to Ro and La. The risk of developing neonatal lupus is about 1 to 5% in those mothers with anti-Ro antibodies. If the mothers have other specific antibodies, hemolytic anemia or thrombocytopenia may ensue. Congenital heart block is very rare but is associated with anti-Ro, anti-La, and HLA-DR3 antibodies in the mother.

Drug-Induced Lupus. Some medications, such as sulfonamides, penicillin, and oral contraceptives, may exacerbate lupus. Hydralazine and procainamide can induce a lupus-like disease, especially in those who are slow acetylators and/or HLA-DR4+. Other medications may possibly induce lupus, or just ANA's, but the evidence is less convincing (Table 240–6). The symptoms and serology of drug-induced lupus are quite similar to those of SLE, with notable differences (Table 240–7). Furthermore, the disease tends to be mild, is not life-threatening, and is reversible. Between 50 and 100% of patients taking procainamide develop ANA's, while only 25% of those develop lupus. Therefore, the presence of a positive ANA test does not preclude continuing these medications. The mechanism for drug-induced lupus is unknown.

DIFFERENTIAL DIAGNOSIS. SLE usually begins with the nonspecific or specific symptoms and signs listed in Table 240–4, as well as easy bruising, splenomegaly, peripheral neuritis, myo- and endocarditis, interstitial pneumonitis, aseptic meningitis, or a positive Coombs' test. The presence of anemia (71%), leukopenia (56%), thrombocytopenia (11%), proteinuria, hematuria/pyuria,

TABLE 240–6. LUPUS-INDUCING DRUGS

Definite	Possible	Unlikely
Hydralazine	Phenytoin	Griseofulvin
Procainamide	Penicillamine	Phenylbutazone
	Isoniazid	Oral contraceptives
	Chlorpromazine	Gold salts
	Alpha-methyldopa	Penicillins
	Quinidine	Hydrazine
	Sulfonamides	L-Canavanine
	Propylthiouracil	Aminosalicylic acid
	Practolol	Streptomycin
	Acebutolol	Tetracyclines
	Lithium carbonate	Methylthiouracil
	P-Aminosalicylate	Oxyphenisatine
	Nitrofurantoin	Tolazamide
	Tartrazine	Methysergide
	Atenolol	Reserpine
	Metoprolol	Isoquinazepan
	Oxprenolol	
	Mephenytoin	
	Primidone	
	Trimethadione	
	Ethosuximide	
	Methimazole	
	Captopril	
	Chlorthalidone	
	Carbamazepine	
	Phenylethylacetylurea	

TABLE 240–7. CLINICAL AND LABORATORY FEATURES OF DRUG-INDUCED LUPUS

Clinical Features	Spontaneous SLE (%)	Drug-Induced Lupus (%)
Age	20–40	50
Sex (F:M)	9	1
Race	All	"No blacks"
Acetylation type	Slow-fast	Slow
Onset of symptoms	Gradual	Abrupt
Constitutional symptoms (fever, malaise, myalgia)	90	50
Arthritis/arthralgia	95	95
Pleuropericarditis	50	50
Skin rash	74	10–20
Renal disease	50	5
CNS disease	75	0
Hematologic disease	Common	Unusual
Immune abnormalities		
ANA	95	95
LE cells	90	90
Anti-dsDNA	80	Rare
Anti-ssDNA	80	Common
Anti-histone	25	90
Anti-Sm	20–30	Rare
Anti-RNP	40–50	Rare
Complement	Reduced	Normal
Immune complexes	Elevated	Normal

TABLE 240–9. CONDITIONS ASSOCIATED WITH ANA'S

Lupus erythematosus
Sjögren's syndrome
Rheumatoid arthritis
Juvenile arthritis
Leprosy
Infectious mononucleosis
Scleroderma
Liver disease
Primary pulmonary fibrosis
Vasculitis
Dermatomyositis/polymyositis
Mixed connective tissue disease
Mixed cryoglobulinemia
Aging
Medications

azotemia, hypergammaglobulinemia, IC's, cryoglobulins, APL's, and the Biologic False-Positive Serologic Test for Syphilis (BFP-STS) also should make one suspect SLE. On first examination, patients are often thought to have other connective tissue, rheumatic, or immune disorders (Table 240–8). Children tend to have more renal disease; older-onset patients have less rash, arthritis, and renal disease but more sicca; males tend to have more serositis and less arthritis.

Most physicians use the American Rheumatism Association (ARA) criteria for the classification of SLE (see Table 240–1) to help make a diagnosis—it should be noted that these criteria were developed for the *classification* of SLE, not for individual diagnoses. The sensitivity and specificity of these criteria are approximately 96% when compared with other rheumatic syndromes when patients have four of these criteria; however, their predictive value is less. Diagnosis in patients with three criteria should be "probable" SLE, and in those with two criteria, "possible" SLE.

The ANA test is a useful screening test. If the test is negative, the patient has a 0.14% probability of having SLE. A positive test has a 15 to 35% predictive value for SLE (see Table 240–3)—see Table 240–9 for a list of other diseases associated with a positive ANA test. Low titers (i.e., 1/40 to 1/80) have less predictive value. If the ANA test is positive, it is useful to test for antibodies to double-stranded DNA (dsDNA) and the Sm, RNP, Ro (SS-A), and La (SS-B) nuclear RNA proteins. Their sensitivity, specificity, and predictive value for SLE (as well as for some other specific ANA's) are detailed in Table 240–3.

Determining serum complement levels is also often helpful, both diagnostically and to assess lupus activity. Complement levels are rarely depressed in other rheumatic diseases. Levels of CH50 (total

hemolytic complement), C4, and C3 tend to parallel or even precede activity, especially renal disease.

THERAPY. Treatment must be individualized for each patient. Not all patients require steroids; steroids have the potential of doing more harm than good. The goals for each therapy and the potential of each for benefit and risk should be considered carefully. The goal is to maintain organ function and prevent permanent organ injury. The threat of a chronic disease can be very stressful, as can visiting a physician frequently and having many laboratory tests—and waiting for the results. Thus emotional support is essential, as well as counseling and the provision of written (and other) material. Patients should be assured that SLE is mild in most patients, that it is rarely life-threatening, and that serious organ involvement usually can be prevented. Support by family, friends, and organizations such as the Lupus Foundation of America and the Arthritis Foundation is often helpful.

It is important to determine whether symptoms and signs are due to SLE or something else (Table 240–10). For instance, fever is more likely to be due to an infection and fatigue due to lack of sleep. Low complement levels, high anti-DNA levels, and/or high IC levels suggest active SLE.

Preventive measures are useful. Patients should avoid using sulfonamides, penicillin, and (high-dosage) birth control pills, which may exacerbate lupus. Exercise has been demonstrated to ameliorate the fatigue of SLE. Patients should be questioned regarding their degree of photosensitivity; not all have this, and the degree may vary, including over time. Photosensitive patients should use sunscreens with an SPF of at least 15 daily—and for those who are very photosensitive, twice daily. Photosensitizing medications (e.g., tetracyclines, psoralens) should be avoided. In postmenopausal women, estrogen is recommended for its benefit regarding osteoporosis and coronary artery disease—SLE women are at excess risk for these—unless there are contraindications or the patient's SLE relapses. Immunization with flu and pneumococcal vaccines is advisable.

TABLE 240–8. DISORDERS RESEMBLING SLE

Common	Less Common
Drug-induced lupus	Polymyositis/dermatomyositis
Scleroderma	Rheumatic fever
Wegener's granulomatosis	Sarcoidosis
Cutaneous (discoid) lupus	Relapsing polychondritis
Rheumatoid arthritis	Weber-Christian disease
Chronic active hepatitis (lupoid hepatitis)	Mixed cryoglobulinemia
Vasculitis	Whipple's disease
Felty's syndrome	Familial Mediterranean fever
Juvenile (rheumatoid) arthritis	
Sjögren's syndrome	
Mixed connective tissue disease	
Fibromyalgia chronic fatigue syndrome	

TABLE 240–10. SIGNS AND SYMPTOMS SUGGESTING ACTIVE SLE

Malaise	Anemia
Poor appetite	Leukopenia
Weight loss	Thrombocytopenia
Fatigue	Hematuria
Pallor	Pyuria
Abnormal menses	Proteinuria
Fever	Azotemia
Arthritis	ESR elevation
Seizures	
Chest pain	
Edema	Decreased complement (C3, C4, CH50)
Hair loss	Immune complexes
Oliguria	Anti-dsDNA
Rashes	
Mouth sores	

TABLE 240–11. TREATMENT OF SPECIFIC PROBLEMS IN LUPUS

Fever: NSAID's → antimalarials → steroids
Arthralgia/myalgia: NSAID's → acetaminophen → amitriptyline
Arthritis: NSAID's → antimalarials → steroids (alternate day) or methotrexate
Rashes: Sunscreens → topical steroids → antimalarials → injection
Oral ulcers: Antimalarials
Raynaud's: No smoking, caffeine, decongestants → warm clothing → biofeedback → (long-acting) nifedipine → prazosin
Serositis: Indomethacin → steroids
Pulmonary: Steroids
Hypertension: Diuretics → ACE inhibitors → calcium channel blockers → β blockers → vasodilators
Thrombocytopenia/hemolytic anemia: Steroids → IV gamma globulin → immunosuppressives → splenectomy
Renal disease: Steroids → pulse steroids → immunosuppressives
CNS disease
  Organic: Steroids → antiseizure → immunosuppressives
  Functional: Antianxiety/depression

In treating SLE, one should consider which organ is involved and to what degree ("severity"). Table 240–11 provides an outline of therapy based on organ involvement; treatment starts conservatively and, if there is an inadequate response, becomes more aggressive.

Treatment of lupus nephritis (Table 240–12) should be based on whether the disease is considered active, the type of nephritis (see above), and the severity. The goal of treatment should be to improve, maintain, and prevent deterioration of renal function. For mesangial or focal glomerulonephritis, bed rest or a short course of prednisone (30 mg per day) will usually suffice to clear the urinary and serologic abnormalities. For diffuse proliferative glomerulonephritis, more vigorous treatment is usually given. Patients are generally treated with 1 mg per kilogram of prednisone. If there is azotemia (especially if the creatinine level is >1.2 mg per deciliter), an immunosuppressive should be added, either azathioprine in doses of 50 to 200 mg per day (a dose to achieve slight leukopenia) or cyclophosphamide. Pulse steroids may be useful acutely until the immunosuppressives start working (which may be 7 to 10 days). Cyclophosphamide given intravenously (in the morning) once monthly (×6) and then every 3 months (×8) appears to be as effective as and less toxic than the same drug given by mouth. The risks of this therapy (malignancy, infections, hair loss, infertility) should be discussed with patients. The initial dose is 0.85 gram per 1.7 square meters of body surface. The WBC count is determined 7 to 10 days later, and the next dose is adjusted (to a maximum of 2 grams per 1.7 square meter) so as to achieve a WBC count of about 4000. Acute membranous glomerulonephritis usually responds to high doses of prednisone or pulse steroids. If not, a trial of immunosuppressives should be instituted. Hypertension should be treated vigorously; angiotensin-converting enzyme (ACE) inhibitors appear to help proteinuria. Diuretics are useful to control edema and hypertension. There is no evidence that plasmapheresis benefits the management of lupus nephritis. For active renal disease, patients should be monitored once a week with urinalysis, serum creatinine determination, and immune function tests (complement, anti-DNA). When the disease becomes inactive, monitoring will be less frequent, depending on the degree of residual damage—patients with nephrotic-range proteinuria or those with azotemia need to be followed more closely.

Acute organic brain disease should be treated aggressively and quickly, in hopes of reversing the process. This usually means high doses of prednisone (1 to 2 mg per kilogram) as well as antipsychotics. Once the psychosis has cleared, the dosage of steroids should be tapered rapidly, because patients are at high risk for infection; adding immunosuppressives, particularly cyclophosphamide, may be beneficial. Steroids themselves may induce psychosis; therefore, it is important to serially monitor the patient with objective measures, including EEG, MRI, SPECT scans, and some antibrain antibodies, as well as CSF protein. However, often one must rely on clinical judgment. Seizure disorders are treated with anticonvulsants (e.g., phenytoin, phenobarbital, carbamazepine); no evidence exists that these medications exacerbate SLE. Multiple small strokes may be due to APL's.

Treatment of the APL syndrome remains controversial. Low levels of this antibody rarely cause symptoms. Patients with high levels without symptoms should be treated with low-dose aspirin; with symptoms, chronic Coumadin therapy is used.

Patients started on prednisone should be kept on high doses only until inflammation has subsided—thus the patient should be assessed frequently regarding specific organ function as well as the immune status (complement, anti-DNA antibodies). For acute, severe lupus, split doses are recommended, then a switch to a daily morning dose. For long-term management, the benefit:risk needs to be discussed. Prednisone dosage should then be tapered—the rate depending on the severity of organ inflammation and damage, the maximum dose, and side effects from prednisone (i.e., psychological changes, insomnia, weight gain, hypertension, diabetes, peptic ulcer, infections such as acne, cushingoid features, adrenal suppression, osteonecrosis, myopathy, impaired wound and fracture healing, skin atrophy, cataracts, atherosclerosis, growth retardation). Once a dose of about 10 to 20 mg per day is achieved and the disease is "quiet," the patient can be put onto every other day prednisone by decreasing the dosage progressively on alternate days. Patients on antimalarials should have an ophthalmologic examination every 6 months; those on NSAID's should be watched for gastrointestinal and renal toxicity.

PROGNOSIS. The prognosis for SLE patients in the United States has improved dramatically since the 1950's, when the life expectancy was approximately 50% at 5 years; in 1994, it was approximately 90% at 10 years. Prognosis is worse for those with CNS involvement, hypertension, azotemia, and early age of onset. The major cause of death is infection. While there is an impression of a greater awareness of the disease, the clinical expression has not changed in 20 years; neither is there evidence that it is being diagnosed earlier.

TABLE 240–12. TREATMENT OF RENAL LUPUS

Pathology	Symptoms	Urine	GFR	Complement	Treatment	Goal
Mesangial	0	RBC, WBC, protein	nl	± ↓	Monitor	Watch for progression
Membranous	Edema	Protein	nl	nl	Trial prednisone Immuno-suppressive Diuretic	Decrease proteinuria and edema
Focal — Active	0	RBC, WBC, protein	↓	↓	Prednisone	Improve renal function
— Chronic	BP ↑	Protein	↓	nl	Antihypertensive	
Proliferative						
Diffuse — Active	Edema BP	RBC, WBC, protein	↓ ↓	↓ ↓	Prednisone (pulse) Azathioprine, 200 mg Cyclophosphamide, 1 mg/m²	Improve renal function
— Chronic	Uremia	Protein	↓ ↓	nl	Antihypertensive	Prevent deterioration of renal function
Failure	Uremia	None	0	nl	Dialysis transplant	Decrease uremia

nl = normal.

Cervera R, Khamashta MA, Font J, et al.: Systemic lupus erythematosus: Clinical and immunologic patterns of disease expression in a cohort of 1000 patients. Medicine 72:113, 1993. *The largest cohort described in a cooperative European anthology—percentages of clinical and immunologic features.*

Hahn B, Wallace D (eds.): Dubois' Lupus Erythematosus. Malvern, PA, Lea & Febiger, 1993. *An excellent source.*

Lahita RG (ed.): Systemic Lupus Erythematosus. New York, Churchill Livingstone, 1992. *A comprehensive series of chapters on both mechanism and treatment divided up by organ systems.*

Schur PH (ed.): The Clinical Management of Systemic Lupus Erythematosus. New York, Grune & Stratton, 1983. *A book for internists and generalists on practical management of SLE patients.*

241 SYSTEMIC SCLEROSIS (SCLERODERMA)

E. Carwile LeRoy

Scleroderma (hard skin) is an uncommon disease marked by increases in connective tissue of skin and several visceral organs. It varies widely in extent and severity from isolated hardened skin patches of largely cosmetic importance to a life-threatening generalized condition that can restrict movement "by an ever-tightening case of steel" (Osler) and lead to insufficiency of the peripheral circulation, the lungs, the gut, the heart, and/or the kidneys. Fortunately, most persons with scleroderma are not at risk for the most severe of its consequences. Since the cause is unknown and no cure is available, the physician must distinguish as early as possible the attendant risks for each patient and manage these prospectively.

Distinctions between localized (skin only) and generalized scleroderma and the conditions that mimic each are shown in Table 241–1. Subsets of generalized scleroderma (systemic sclerosis, or SSc) are outlined in Table 241–2. SSc is a multisystem, multistage disorder in which each target organ progresses through stages of inflammation, induration (fibrosis), and atrophy, not always at the same pace.

DEFINITION. SSc is a generalized autoimmune disorder of small arteries, microvessels, and the diffuse connective tissue characterized by scarring (fibrosis) and vascular obliteration of the skin, gastrointestinal tract, lungs, heart, and kidneys, with hidebound skin as the clinical hallmark and organ compromise as the prognostic keystone.

PATHOGENESIS AND PATHOLOGY. *Fibrotic Events.* The mechanism(s) of fibrosis in SSc is (are) not understood. Mesenchymal cells (fibroblasts, smooth muscle cells, and endothelial cells) become activated by unknown stimuli, resulting in increased amounts of the usual components of connective tissue (types I, III, V, VI, and VII collagen, proteoglycans, fibronectin) being deposited in the interstitium and in the intima of small arteries. Endothelial cell changes, vasomotor and permeability changes, platelet activation, and perivascular mononuclear cell infiltrates are present in target tissues before fibrosis is prominent.

In SSc scar tissue, lesional fibroblasts can be shown to produce increased quantities of these connective tissue components (see above) on a per-cell basis even after being removed from the patient and propagated *in vitro*. One recognized profibrotic cytokine cascade playing at least a partial role in SSc is transforming growth factor beta (TGFβ) activation of fibroblasts with coordinate up-regulation of the platelet-derived growth factor AA (PDGF-AA) and its alpha receptor. The features of activation of the SSc lesional fibro-blast are outlined in Table 241–3. Understanding the regulatory defect of fibroblast growth may be the key to understanding the fibrosis in SSc and perhaps also in liver cirrhosis, atherosclerosis, and other examples of unregulated fibrosis.

Vascular Events. Prominent vascular and microvascular lesions dominate the early stages of both limited and diffuse cutaneous forms of SSc (see Table 241–2). The unusual cyclic vasoconstrictive-vasodilatory features of Raynaud's phenomenon are present in >90% of SSc patients. Edema is prominent, often occurring episodically, especially in the patient with diffuse involvement. Circulating evidence of endothelial cell perturbation (elevated levels of plasma Factor VIII–von Willebrand factor) and of platelet activation is present in many, but not all, patients. Histologically, vascular lesions are widespread.

TABLE 241–1. DIFFERENTIAL DIAGNOSIS OF SYSTEMIC SCLEROSIS

Vascular Changes

Peripheral vasospasm
Primary Raynaud's phenomenon
Occupational Raynaud's phenomenon
  Vibration and physical trauma (e.g., jackhammer operator)
  Chemical exposure
    Vinyl chloride (plastics industry)
    Mining exposure (coal, silicates, gold, heavy metals)
    Organic solvents (trichloroethylene, others)
Environmental and drug-associated Raynaud's phenomenon
  Toxic oil syndrome (ingestion of adulterated rapeseed oil, Madrid, 1982)
  Arsenic
  Bleomycin
  Cisplatin
  Ergotamine
  β blockers (high dose)
  5-Hydroxytryptophan and carbidopa → L-tryptophan and contaminants
Reflex sympathetic dystrophy (shoulder-hand, thoracic outlet)
Other diffuse connective tissue diseases (SLE, polyarteritis nodosa, DM/PM)
Intravascular causes (cryoglobulinemia, cold agglutinins, nondistensible RBC's, intravascular coagulation)
Telangiectasia
  Hereditary telangiectasia (Osler-Weber-Rendu syndrome)
  Hepatic and hormonal spiders (cirrhosis, contraceptives)

Skin Changes

Localized scleroderma
  Morphea (circumscribed, guttate)
  Generalized morphea
  Linear (with hemiatrophy)
  Other localized hamartomas (collagenoma, tuberous sclerosis, keloids, hypertrophic scars)
  En coup de sabre (with or without facial hemiatrophy)
Scleroderma-like skin changes
  Inflammatory-immunologic
    Undifferentiated connective tissue syndrome (mixed)
    Eosinophilic fasciitis (including diffuse fasciitis with eosinophilia and eosinophilia myalgia syndrome)
    Overlap syndromes (SSc with SLE, RA, DM/PM, Sjögren's syndrome [sicca complex and its overlaps])
    Chronic graft-vs-host disease (CGVHD)
  Occupational, enviromental, and drug-associated (see Vascular Changes above)
  Metabolic-genetic (pseudosclerodermas)
    Porphyrias
    Phenylketonuria
    Carcinoid syndrome
    Scleredema with or without paraproteinemia
    Scleromyxedema with or without paraproteinemia
    Lichen sclerosis et atrophicus
    Insulin-dependent diabetes mellitus (digital sclerosis)
    Acromegaly
    Amyloidosis
    Heritable premature aging syndromes (Werner's, progeria, Rothmund's)

Visceral Disease

Esophageal hypomotility (diabetes mellitus, aging)
Idiopathic pulmonary fibrosis
Sarcoidosis
Amyloidosis
Infiltrative cardiomyopathies
Intestinal hypomotility syndromes (pseudo-obstruction)
Malignant hypertension (hyper-reninemic, accelerated)
Occupational, environmental, and drug-associated interstitial pulmonary disease (see Vascular Changes above) (see also Ch. 54)

RBC's = red blood cells; SLE = systemic lupus erythematosus; RA = rheumatoid arthritis; DM = dermatomyositis; PM = polymyositis.

Immune Events. As in the other rheumatic or diffuse connective tissue disorders that show manifestations of autoimmunity, antinuclear antibodies (ANA's) are prominent in SSc (see Ch. 236) (Table 241–4).

Immunogenetic associations with SSc include loci of class II and III major histocompatibility regions (human leukocyte antigens [HLA's] in humans). DR associations include 1, 3, 5, 8, and 52; since these DR loci are in linkage disequilibrium with DQ loci,

TABLE 241-2. SUBSETS OF SYSTEMIC SCLEROSIS (SSc)

Diffuse Cutaneous SSc (dcSSc)

Onset of Raynaud's phenomenon within 1 year of onset of skin changes (puffy or hidebound)
Truncal and acral skin involvement
Presence of tendon friction rubs
Early and significant incidence of interstitial lung disease, oliguric renal failure, diffuse gastrointestinal disease, and myocardial involvement
Absence of anticentromere antibodies (ACA)

Limited Cutaneous SSc (lcSSc)*

Isolated Raynaud's phenomenon for years (occasionally decades)
Skin involvement limited to hands, face, feet (acral)
A significant late incidence of pulmonary hypertension, trigeminal neuralgia, skin calcifications, telangiectasia
A high incidence of anticentromere antibodies (ACA, 60%)
Dilated nailfold capillary loops without capillary dropout

Systemic Sclerosis *sine* Scleroderma (ssSSc)

Visceral disease without cutaneous involvement
Examples: (1) esophageal hypomotility, duodenal dilatation with malabsorption, wide-mouthed colonic sacculations; (2) Raynaud's phenomenon, dilated nailfold capillary loops, esophageal hypomotility, oliguric renal failure; (3) Raynaud's phenomenon, dilated nailfold capillary loops, esophageal hypomotility, pulmonary hypertension and/or interstitial lung disease

* Also termed CREST syndrome, i.e. *c*alcinosis, *R*aynaud's phenomenon, *e*sophageal hypomotility, *s*clerodactyly, and *t*elangiectasia.

TABLE 241-4. SSc AUTOANTIBODIES IN CAUCASIAN, AFRICAN-AMERICAN, AND JAPANESE PATIENTS

Present in 1 in 3 SSc patients (>33%)
  Anti-U1-RNP; Japanese, African-American
  Anti-U3-RNP (fibrillarin), African-American
Present in 1 in 5 SSc patients (<33, >20%)
  Anti-RNAP (RNA polymerase I, II, III), Caucasian*
  Antitopoisomerase I; Caucasian, Japanese*
Present in 1 in 10 SSc patients (<20, >10%)
  Anticentromere; Caucasian, Japanese†
  Antitopoisomerase, African-American*
  Anti-RNAP, African-American
  Anti-Ku, African-American
Present in <1 in 20 SSc patients (<5%)
  Anticentromere, African-American
  Anti-RNAP, Japanese
  Antifibrillarin; Japanese, Caucasian
  Anti-Ku; Japanese, Caucasian
  Anti-Th RNP in all
  Anti-PM-Scl in all
  Anti-Ro (SS-A)
  Anti-La (SS-B)
  Anti-Jo-1 (and other synthetases)

* Prevalence enriched in diffuse cutaneous SSc.
† Prevalence enriched in limited cutaneous SSc.
Adapted from Kuwana M, Okano Y, Kaburaki J, et al.: Racial differences in the distribution of systemic sclerosis–related serum antinuclear antibodies, Arthritis Rheum 37:902, 1994.

stronger associations with SSc and DQB1 alleles were suspected and have been observed. Strong associations between anticentromere serology and the presence of polar tyrosine or glycine at position 26 of a hypervariable region of the DQB1 chain, as well as a specific sequence at positions 67–71 of the same chain in association with antitopoisomerase serology, strengthen the case that an immunogenetic propensity to develop SSc exists and can be measured. The possibility of a gene dose effect (homozygosity) and preliminary evidence for a class III association with alleles of the fourth component of complement remain to be fully documented.

THE PATIENT. *Diffuse Cutaneous SSc.* The usual age of onset is the fourth decade but may range from the first to the eighth. There is no ethnic or geographic predilection; females outnumber males only slightly. The onset may be abrupt, with swollen hands, face, and feet associated with Raynaud's phenomenon (episodic pallor of the digits, nose, or ears following cold exposure or stress associated with cyanosis and followed by erythema, suffusion, tingling, and pain). Fatigue is common; overt weakness may be present. Skin examination reveals a nonpitting fullness, an inability to pinch skin folds, and the loss of skin lines and creases in involved areas. These changes may evolve over 12 to 18 months to include the fingers, hands, forearms, arms, face, thorax, and abdomen, as well as the toes, feet, legs, and thighs (Fig. 241–1). The fingers and toes may be dusky or overtly cyanotic and are usually cool to the touch. Blood pressure and pulse may be elevated, and evaluation of swallowing, breathing, urinary excretory, and cardiac function may reveal abnormalities. Patients with diffuse SSc should be followed closely for visceral involvement (see Table 241–2). The cumulative survival rate is reduced in diffuse SSc compared with limited SSc (Fig. 241–2).

Limited Cutaneous SSc. The typical patient with limited cutaneous SSc is a woman (or a man who has worked with vibrating machines, plastics, or in mining), aged 30 to 50, who presents with a 10- to 15-year history of numbness and a "dead" or "wooden"

TABLE 241-3. CHARACTERISTICS OF ACTIVATION OF SSc FIBROBLASTS

1. Increased expression of extracellular matrix genes [collagens $\alpha 1$ (I), $\alpha 2$ (I), $\alpha 1$ (III), $\alpha 3$ (VI), $\alpha 1$ (VII); proteoglycans; fibronectin]
2. Increased expression of cytokine receptors (interleukin-1α, PDGFRα and β, TGFβR)
3. Increased expression of cell adhesion proteins (ICAM-1, B_1 and B_2 integrins)

sensation associated with color changes (often pallor only) of at first the second and third fingers of the dominant hand. Full-fledged Raynaud's phenomenon usually develops symmetrically in both hands, fingers 2 to 5, with increasing frequency, especially in winter; there may be a history of hard crusting lesions on the fingertips, initially healing in warm weather. General stamina may be decreased, and there may be breathlessness with minimal exertion (see Table 241–2). Taut skin, often limited to the digits (sclerodactyly), may not be detectable until years after the onset of Raynaud's phenomenon.

DIAGNOSIS. The annual incidence of Raynaud's phenomenon is substantially greater than the incidence of all diffuse connective tissue syndromes combined (Table 241–5). When a careful history and physical examination reveal no features of connective tissue disease, including no signs of peripheral ischemia, the single best test to select those Raynaud's patients destined to develop scleroderma and related disorders is wide-field nailfold capillaroscopy, a noninvasive, reproducible, cost-effective, permanent identification of the connective tissue–prone patient that should be coupled with ANA testing.

The diagnosis of diffuse SSc is straightforward. A previously well person is now sick with the triad of Raynaud's phenomenon, nonpitting edema, and hidebound skin that may eventually cover virtually the entire body, sparing only the back and buttocks. There are very few alternative diagnoses that must be seriously entertained. Other causes of Raynaud's phenomenon are not usually accompanied by edema, and other causes of edema are not usually associated with Raynaud's phenomenon. The key questions in such patients are (1) Are features of other connective tissue diseases present? (2) Which internal organs are affected?

If symmetric, erosive polyarthritis is present, an overlap between SSc and rheumatoid arthritis (RA) should be considered; if fever and a characteristic malar rash are present, overlap with systemic lupus erythematosus (SLE) is likely. Most often these features are not present, and the second outcome becomes the primary focus. Each visceral target organ (esophagus, lungs, kidneys, heart) of SSc deserves screening.

Abnormal skin texture provides the definitive diagnostic criterion of SSc in >90% of patients. When distal to the metacarpophalangeal (MCP) joints only, it is called "sclerodactyly" and is *not* diagnostic of SSc. Firm, taut, hidebound skin proximal to the MCP joints represents the major diagnostic criterion. Skin biopsy is usually *not* more sensitive diagnostically than the experienced touch. Skin changes also distinguish the three prognostically different subsets. If truncal skin changes are present, the patient has diffuse cutaneous SSc, and systematic surveillance of visceral function is indicated. If skin changes are limited to the hands, fingers, and face,

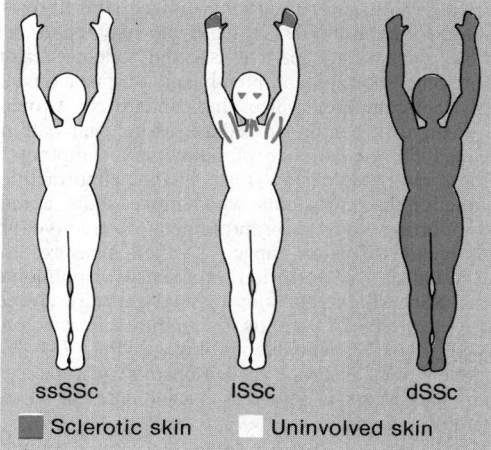

FIGURE 241–1. A pictorial representation of skin involvement in SSc. Note that the limited cutaneous SSc patient (see Table 241–2) may have subtle skin thickening of eyelid, neck fold, and armpit skin. ssSSc = systemic sclerosis *sine* scleroderma; lSSc = limited cutaneous systemic sclerosis; dSSc = diffuse cutaneous systemic sclerosis. (Adapted from Giordano M, Valentini G, Migliaresi S, et al.: Different antibody patterns and different prognoses in patients with scleroderma with various extent of skin sclerosis. J Rheumatol 13:911, 1986.)

limited cutaneous SSc is present, infrequent evaluation is adequate, and management should focus on the Raynaud's phenomenon. If the skin is of normal texture, two possibilities are suggested: The patient formerly had abnormal skin changes, either diffuse or limited in distribution, which have subsided (regressive systemic sclerosis), or the patient has visceral disease in the absence of skin changes, which occurs in approximately 5% of SSc patients (see Table 241–2, SSc *sine* scleroderma).

DIFFERENTIAL DIAGNOSIS. Connective tissue disorders are constellations of organ system involvement (skin, lungs, intestinal tract, serosal surfaces, joints, heart, central nervous system); each system involved can present immune-inflammatory, proliferative-erosive, or fibrotic-atrophic-insufficiency changes at different stages of the syndrome or disorder. Virtually none of the systems involved or the stages of involvement of those systems are entirely specific for the particular syndrome or disorder. It is not surprising, therefore, that the nomenclature is confusing. Terms such as "early," "mixed," or "undifferentiated connective tissue disease," as well as overlap syndromes, have emerged to describe the same patients.

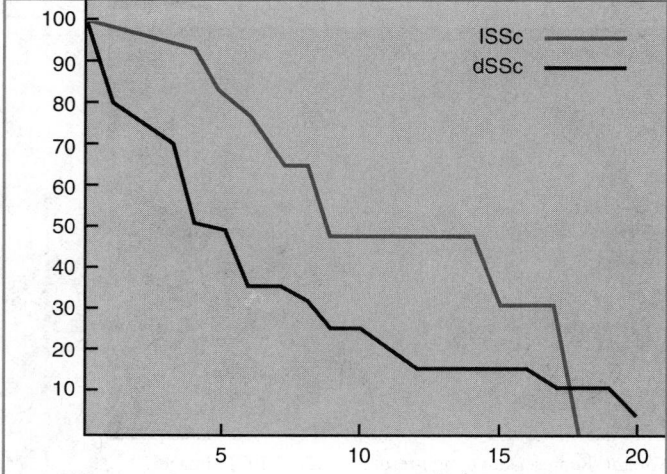

FIGURE 241–2. The cumulative survival rate (CSR, age-adjusted survival) in percent plotted against time in years for diffuse cutaneous SSc and limited cutaneous SSc patients showing the substantially reduced survival of diffuse cutaneous SSc patients (see Table 241–2). lSSc = limited cutaneous systemic sclerosis; dSSc = diffuse cutaneous systemic sclerosis. (Adapted from Giordano M, Valentini G, Migliaresi S, et al.: Different antibody patterns and different prognoses in patients with scleroderma with various extent of skin sclerosis. J Rheumatol 13:911, 1986.)

The time-honored term "overlap syndrome" remains the preferred term for established, stable connective tissue disorders with features of more than one traditional disorder (such as RA-lupus overlap). In the early-stage patient with inflammatory or edematous features that are insufficient for an established diagnosis, the term undifferentiated connective tissue disease (UCTD) is preferred.

Diffuse fasciitis with eosinophilia (also called eosinophilic fasciitis) is a syndrome which, when acute, is distinct from scleroderma and, when chronic, blends into the scleroderma spectrum of disorders. Occasionally after strenuous exertion, young, vigorous persons note the onset of swelling and tautness of the skin of the trunk and proximal extremities with a brawny texture that may be tender. Raynaud's phenomenon is consistently absent, the hands and feet are usually spared, and nailfold capillaroscopy is normal. Initially, visceral disease is absent. Deep skin and subcutaneous biopsies show inflammatory changes including the deep fascia, the subcutis, and the lower dermis. Eosinophilia is present, and eosinophils may or may not be present in the skin lesions. Symptoms subside with glucocorticoid therapy and also with no therapy over time. Eosinophilic fasciitis has been associated with aplastic anemia. In a substantial proportion of chronic patients, the visceral involvement of systemic sclerosis has been documented. In the tryptophan-associated epidemic variety of diffuse fasciitis, as well as the toxic oil syndrome, a fibrotic peripheral neuropathy may be present. Neuropathy is distinctly uncommon in SSc.

CLINICAL MANIFESTATIONS. *Peripheral Vascular System.* Pallor is the most definitive of the episodic triphasic responses of Raynaud's phenomenon (pallor, cyanosis, rubor). The circumstances that provoke pallor and the "dead" sensation of the fingers are usually reproducible in the individual patient (handling cold or frozen items, emotional disturbances). Persistent Raynaud's attacks may lead to a webbing phenomenon (as in the frenulum of the tongue), binding the fingernail to the fingertip skin of involved fingers. This is evidence of structural vascular and persistent ischemic disease, as are the more obvious fingertip calluses, digital ulcerations (of fingertips or over dorsal proximal interphalangeal joints), overt ischemic tissue, or calcification; the toes, the nose, and the ears may participate in Raynaud's attacks as well. The more widespread the areas involved, the more likely is systemic disease.

The Skin. The skin is the most distinctive diagnostic feature of SSc; the diagnosis can be made unequivocally by the texture and location of hidebound skin. In patients with diffuse SSc, skin tautness can limit movement at the wrists, elbows, shoulders, mouth, and thorax (less frequently the hips, knees, and ankles). When fully hidebound, the skin appears to become paper thin over points of bony protrusion, such as the proximal interphalangeal joints, the ulnar styloid process, the olecranon process, the bridge of the nose, and the cheek bones. Gentle pressure over these areas removes all blood from the capillaries; the refilling time can be used as a rough approximation of the degree of ischemia and the propensity to ulcerate.

Gastrointestinal System. If sensitive diagnostic techniques are used, esophageal hypomotility, by far the most common manifestation of gastrointestinal SSc, can be documented in over 90% of patients with both diffuse and limited cutaneous SSc. Many patients do not notice the subtle symptoms of esophageal SSc, which include a vertical substernal burning pain particularly at night, the occasional sense that a pill or large bit of meat "has not gone down," or "heartburn" on lying down soon after a full meal. The single best screening test for esophageal hypomotility is the radionuclide esophageal transit time; it is noninvasive, safe, and can be relied on when negative. Patients with slow transit times should be further studied with both barium swallow (using light barium and the re-

TABLE 241–5. POPULATION INCIDENCE OF MUSCULOSKELETAL DISEASE

Raynaud's phenomenon	1000*
Rheumatoid arthritis	750
Systemic lupus erythematosus	75
Systemic sclerosis	10
Dermatomyositis, polymyositis	10

* New cases per million adults per year.

From Kammer GM: Raynaud's phenomenon. *In* Andreoli TE (ed): Cecil Essentials of Medicine. Philadelphia, WB Saunders, 1990, p 657, with permission.

cumbent position) to detect structural abnormalities (hiatus hernia) and with esophageal motility studies, the definitive procedure for esophageal SSc. The earliest detectable abnormality is a reduction in resting lower esophageal sphincter (LES) pressure, which may be an isolated early finding or may be associated with reduced smooth muscle contraction (secondary and tertiary waves) of the distal two thirds of the esophagus. Upper third striated muscle dysfunction suggests an overlap syndrome with dermatomyositis. If peptic esophagitis with mucosal ulceration is well established, LES pressure may be increased, and the diagnosis of achalasia could be incorrectly entertained. The presence of other features of SSc and reduced LES pressure after treatment are helpful. Barrett's metaplasia and esophageal carcinoma are risks for all long-lived SSc patients.

Gastric hypomotility may be present but is not often of clinical significance. Small intestinal hypomotility, determined by upper gastrointestinal series with small bowel follow-through, occurs in 10 to 20% of patients, all of whom have esophageal hypomotility; this may occur in the absence of cutaneous scleroderma. It need not be searched for in the asymptomatic patient because it consistently declares its presence by postprandial bloating, abdominal distention with diffuse pain, intermittent diarrhea with or without steatorrhea, and weight loss from malabsorption (pseudo-obstruction). Abdominal attacks that mimic mechanical obstruction may lead to surgical intervention, from which some patients recover poorly and slowly, if at all.

Pulmonary System. Although renal failure was formerly the major threat to life in SSc, the combined impact of several pulmonary abnormalities now seems to be the number one cause of fatal involvement in this disease. Pleurisy and pleural effusions, pul-

monary hypertension, interstitial lung disease with fibrosis, and ultimately obstructive pulmonary disease all may be a part of pulmonary SSc. Because the patient is often sedentary from skin or joint restrictions, shortness of breath and dyspnea on exertion are surprisingly late complaints; also, the standard chest roentgenogram is not a sensitive screening procedure. More than half of SSc patients selected for the absence of pulmonary symptoms and for a normal chest radiograph show reproducible abnormalities on pulmonary function tests. Patients who smoke show a much higher positive proportion with more prominent obstructive phenomena. The single-breath diffusion capacity, which measures the balance between ventilation and perfusion, is a sensitive pulmonary screening tool for SSc. Mild reductions in vital capacity are common as well. The detection of alveolitis by high-resolution computed tomography (CT) or bronchoalveolar lavage (Fig. 241–3) identifies the SSc patient who is prone to demonstrate ventilatory deterioration over 4 to 6 years and who is a candidate for aggressive immunosuppressive therapy.

Pleural effusions are usually silent and noninflammatory. They take on clinical significance primarily in the patient with established restrictive lung disease (decreased vital capacity), in whom the aspiration of an effusion may improve ventilation. They are present in two thirds of patients at autopsy. In the immunosuppressed patient, infection may present with "silent" empyema.

Pulmonary hypertension, usually sudden in onset, constitutes a medical emergency. All patients with SSc should be followed closely for changes in the second heart sound over the pulmonic area and for the pulmonic valve closure component of that second sound, detected by the splitting of S_2 on deep inspiration. The appearance of tricuspid regurgitation or right ventricular enlargement is evidence of established pulmonary hypertension. The chest radi-

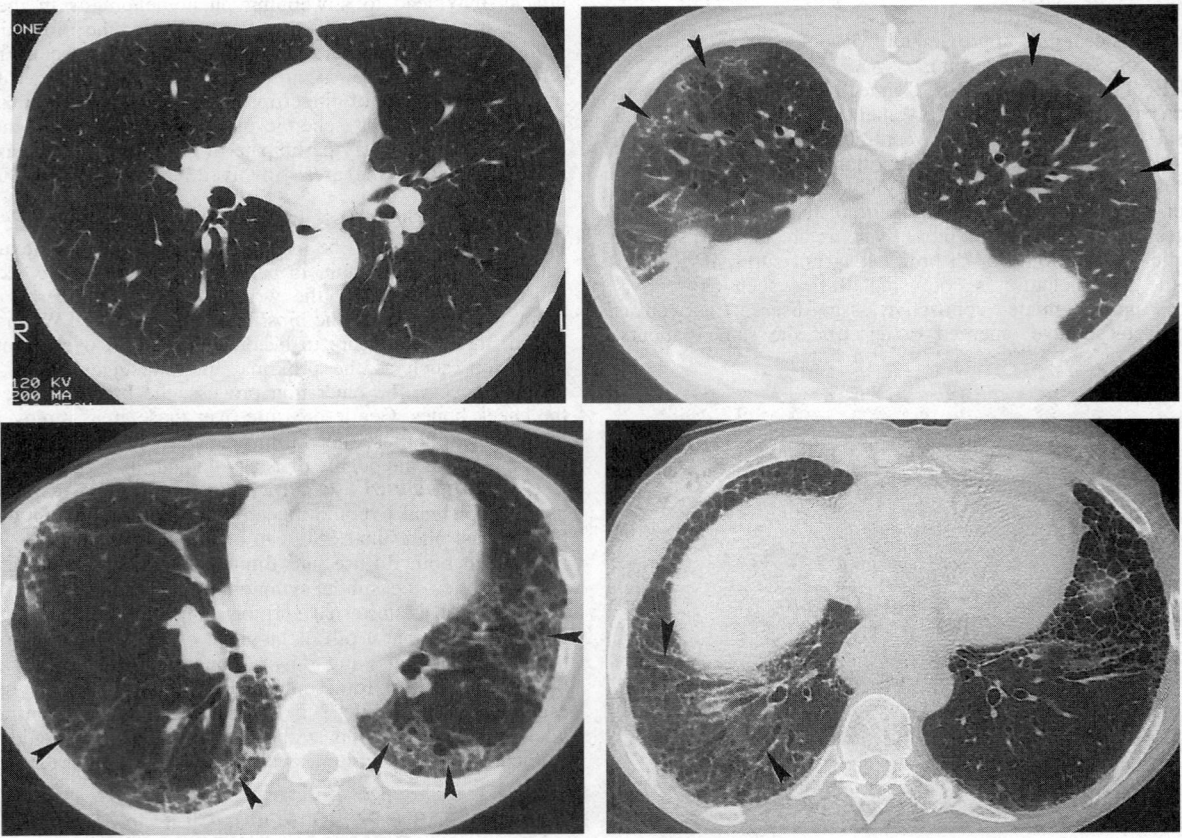

FIGURE 241–3. Computerized tomography of lung in SSc. *A, Normal.* Representative high-resolution CT (HRCT) image of normal lungs demonstrates branching pulmonary vessels tapering in diameter as they extend peripherally. With the available resolution, small vessels can only be visualized 3 to 4 mm deep to, but not extending out to, the pleural surface of the lung. *B, Alveolitis.* HRCT of a patient with early SSc shows subpleural "ground glass" opacities *(arrowheads)* in both lungs associated with and diagnostic of alveolitis. Unlike airspace opacities, these do not obscure the visibility of the small vessels. *C,* HRCT in SSc showing reticular opacities in the subpleural lung *(arrowheads)* caused by thickened intralobular and interlobular septa. Note that these are nontapering and extend all the way out to the pleural surface. Reticulonodular changes are associated with fibrosis. *D,* HRCT in advanced SSc showing honeycombing due to cystic distention of small airspaces of the lung, as well as traction bronchiectasis *(arrowheads)* caused by interstitial fibrosis. (Courtesy of M. Bhalla, M.D., Department of Radiology, Harvard University, Massachusetts General Hospital, Boston.)

ograph may provide evidence of enlarged pulmonary arteries but often does not; the echocardiogram has been useful in detecting pulmonary hypertension. Doppler techniques measuring tricuspid insufficiency (present in most patients with increased right ventricular pressures) in combination with echocardiography are promising for detecting pulmonary hypertension early. Aggressive attempts to lower pulmonary artery pressure should be instituted (see Ch. 38).

Renal System. At one time, the abrupt onset of accelerated hypertension and oliguria ("scleroderma renal crisis") accounted for the majority of deaths in SSc. Fortunately, with early identification and treatment with inhibitors of angiotensin-converting enzymes (ACE) (captopril, enalapril), the incidence of renal involvement and its consequences have been greatly reduced. All patients fulfilling the criteria for diffuse SSc should be suspected of having renal involvement and should be followed with 24-hour urine collections for protein excretion and creatinine clearance at least yearly. Excretions of >750 mg of protein per 24 hours or clearances of <60 ml per minute, or distinct changes in either proteinuria or glomerular filtration rate (GFR), should initiate measurements of resting renin level and, if elevated, treatment. The single most sensitive and cost-effective screening strategy is frequent blood pressure determinations at home, with patients asked to report a 20% increase in either systolic or diastolic level. Such increases in blood pressure and pulse rate, accelerated increases in edematous skin tightening (rapidly increasing skin score), or the appearance of microangiopathic hemolytic anemia or disseminated intravascular coagulation (see Ch. 153) also may herald the onset of renal involvement. The keys to managing renal SSc successfully are to identify the population at risk (those with diffuse SSc), to detect declining GFR early, and to treat expectantly. One remarkable feature of renal SSc is the ability of some patients to regain renal function after months to years (up to 4 years) of end-stage renal disease (ESRD) and hemodialysis. Very little is known about the mechanisms of this slow reparative process. Whatever the reason, it stays the hand that would undertake nephrectomy.

Cardiac System. More than 90% of patients with diffuse SSc (truncal skin involvement) have some form of cardiac involvement. Rarely, acute pericarditis with a friction rub is present; more frequently, a silent pericardial effusion appears slowly, with ankle edema and shortness of breath as presenting features. Echocardiography is the diagnostic procedure of choice. Pericardial effusions may predispose to renal failure by unknown mechanisms. By electrocardiographic monitoring and electrophysiologic studies, 80% of diffuse SSc patients *without* cardiovascular symptoms were found to have cardiac involvement; in more recent studies, 95% show reperfusion abnormalities of the intramyocardial circulation by thallium scanning. Most, but not all, of these patients have normal coronary arteries by coronary angiography.

Articular and Musculoskeletal Systems. Approximately 10% of SSc patients present with a symmetric small joint polyarticular synovitis initially indistinguishable from RA. Within a year, the pattern changes abruptly with subsidence of joint complaints and the appearance of Raynaud's phenomenon, edema, and diffuse cutaneous SSc. The presence of scleroderma-pattern nailfold capillary changes and a positive ANA pattern can identify these patients during their polyarticular phase, before cutaneous changes appear, as destined to develop SSc.

About one half of SSc patients develop stiffness and swelling of the fingers, wrists, knees, and ankles concomitant with cutaneous changes. Morning stiffness may be present. Signs of inflammation are usually mild. Polymorphonuclear leukocytes are usually present in synovial fluid. On biopsy, the synovium is mildly inflamed with a distinctive deposition of fibrin throughout the synovium. Obliterative microvascular disease and diffuse fibrotic changes occur at a later stage.

Indolent myopathy is common in SSc. It is difficult to distinguish from atrophy caused by taut skin. Most patients show diffuse atrophy of the extremities with slight elevations of muscle enzyme levels (creatine kinase and aldolase); these features are refractory to glucocorticoids or to immunosuppressive therapy. Mild SSc myositis is best left untreated. Less frequently, abrupt proximal muscle weakness develops and is associated with 10- to 50-fold increases in muscle enzymes, electromyographic features of acute myositis, and lymphoid cell infiltration with muscle fiber necrosis on biopsy. These patients generated the initial confusion regarding mixed, overlap, or undifferentiated connective tissue syndromes; they usually respond to glucocorticoid therapy. Rarely, their myositis is refractory, and methotrexate is warranted.

Other. In the second and third decades following the onset of Raynaud's phenomenon, a small but significant proportion of patients with limited cutaneous SSc develop unilateral or bilateral trigeminal neuralgia that can be disabling. Other entrapment peripheral neuropathies are less frequent and more subtle.

An increasing number of male SSc patients, especially those with diffuse disease, experience impotence, which is thought to be on an organic neurovascular basis because of diminished or absent nocturnal tumescence. It is refractory to treatment.

Dry eyes (keratoconjunctivitis sicca), dry mouth (xerostomia), or both occur in approximately one fourth of SSc patients. Salivary gland biopsies may show mononuclear cell infiltrates or replacement fibrosis. Supportive care with secretion substitution (artificial tears) and stimulation (lemon candy) provides some relief.

TREATMENT. No therapy has been shown to halt the progression of cutaneous or visceral SSc in a controlled, prospective study. A major source of confusion in assessing therapy is the dependence on softening skin as a key outcome measurement and the natural tendency for hidebound skin to soften after several years. Skin changes cannot be used as indications of the lessening of the critical vascular and microvascular disease.

The most distinctive change in the natural history of diffuse cutaneous SSc in the last decade is that fewer patients with SSc develop renal failure. This change has occurred with the advent of more powerful agents to control the accelerated hypertensive phase of renal failure, especially ACE inhibitors. Indications for immediate treatment are hypertension (an increase of 30 mm Hg systolic or 15 mm Hg diastolic blood pressure, no matter what the absolute level), a reduction in creatinine clearance of 30 ml per minute or to a clearance below 60 ml per minute, and microangiopathic anemia. If the serum creatinine value is < 4.0 mg per deciliter, ESRD can often, but not always, be averted. Continued intensive treatment is indicated even if hemodialysis is instituted, since some patients can regain function sufficient to discontinue dialysis after as long as 4 to 5 years.

D-Penicillamine has been advocated on the basis of retrospective studies that showed skin softening after 2 years. It probably functions as a mild immunosuppressant. The proportion of patients that develops significant side effects is 30 to 40%. Colchicine also has been proposed as capable of influencing cutaneous changes in SSc. Brief crossover studies were inconclusive, and longer open studies were promising but uncontrolled. It is better tolerated than D-penicillamine.

The management of Raynaud's phenomenon has improved in recent years (see Ch. 46); nonetheless, even the most successful management of vasoactive features does not affect the continuing appearance of new fibrotic or visceral manifestations. Sometimes a change in lifestyle is sufficient. Clothing should protect the trunk to encourage heat dissipation via peripheral vasodilatation. Extremes of cold, exhaustion, or stress should be avoided. Nitroglycerin ointment applied locally along the course of the digital arteries to only those fingers showing severe ischemia is helpful. Also, postganglionic alpha blockade with prazosin usually reduces symptoms but may be difficult to tolerate due to palpitation and orthostatic hypotension. Inhibitors of the slow calcium channels of cell membranes have been a significant advance for managing Raynaud's phenomenon. At present, nifidepine in gradually increasing doses is popular, and verapamil, diltiazem, and nicardipine have their proponents as well. When tissue necrosis is present (gangrene), prompt hospital admission for epidural sympathetic blockade is indicated.

Bronchoalveolar lavage and, more recently, high-resolution chest CT are useful to quantify the prefibrotic alveolitis in the interstitial lung disease of SSc; alveolitis is a consistent finding in SSc patients who gradually lose lung volume but not in pulmonary function–stable SSc patients. Furthermore, prednisone and cyclophosphamide, in open trials, seem to stabilize lung function in alveolitis-positive SSc patients. Defining alveolitis is key in selecting patients for aggressive immunosuppressive therapy (see Fig. 241–3).

Black C: The aetiopathogenesis of systemic sclerosis. J Intern Med 234:3, 1993. *A discussion of pathogenetic mechanisms in SSc with emphasis on immunogenetic association.*

Gay S, Trabandt A, Moreland LW, et al.: Growth factors, extracellular matrix, and oncogenesis in scleroderma. Arthritis Rheum 35:304, 1992. *A new hypothesis for the pathogenesis of SSc.*

LeRoy EC: A brief overview of the pathogenesis of scleroderma (systemic sclerosis). Ann Rheum Dis 51:286, 1992. *A concise discussion of our limited understanding of the pathogenesis of SSc with references for further study.*

LeRoy EC (ed.): Scleroderma. Rheum Dis Clin North Am 16:1, 1990. *A multiauthor and multifaceted group of reviews of many aspects of SSc.*

Rothfield NF: Autoantibodies in scleroderma in antinuclear antibodies. Rheum Dis Clin North Am 18:483, 1992. *An excellent summary of the immunology and clinical relevance of autoantibodies in SSc.*

242 SJÖGREN'S SYNDROME
Marc C. Hochberg

DEFINITION. Sjögren's syndrome (SS) is a chronic immune-mediated inflammatory disorder characterized by lymphocytic infiltration of the lacrimal and salivary glands associated with the clinical features of keratoconjunctivitis sicca and xerostomia. SS exists in both a primary and secondary form; the former comprises keratoconjunctivitis sicca and xerostomia with tissue confirmation of lymphocytic infiltration of the minor salivary glands, while the latter is either keratoconjunctivitis sicca or xerostomia occurring with a well-defined connective tissue disease, usually rheumatoid arthritis, systemic lupus erythematosus (SLE), systemic sclerosis, or polymyositis.

HISTORY. In 1933, Henrik Sjögren, a Swedish ophthalmologist, reported keratoconjunctivitis sicca with detailed histopathologic studies of the involved glands, the common occurrence of the disorder in postmenopausal women, the relationship with rheumatoid arthritis, and the ability to measure tear secretion with Schirmer's test.

EPIDEMIOLOGY. Classification. Numerous criteria were proposed for the classification of SS at the First International Conference on Sjögren's syndrome in 1986; however, none of these was universally accepted. In 1993, the European Community Study Group proposed preliminary criteria to classify SS (Table 242–1); the presence of four or more of six clinical and laboratory features classifies primary SS with a sensitivity of 93.5% and a specificity of 94%, while use of an algorithm has a sensitivity of 93.3% and specificity of 92.2% (Fig. 242–1). These preliminary criteria are currently undergoing validation.

Prevalence. The results of four small surveys suggest that between 2 and 5% of people aged 60 and above have primary SS. A large population-based study is currently in progress to estimate the prevalence of and investigate risk factors for the syndrome.

PATHOGENESIS AND PATHOLOGY. SS is an autoimmune disorder with a multifactorial etiology. Immunogenetic studies of patients with primary SS suggest a role for the HLA class II alleles DR3 and DQw2/DQw6 and a disease-associated haplotype DRB1*0301, DRB3*0101, DQA1*0501, DQB1*0201 in Caucasians, especially in those with antibodies to Ro(SS-A) and La(SS-B). Although different genes may be involved in patients of other racial/ethnic groups, they share a sequence homology in the first hypervariable region of the DQB1 gene from positions 58 to 69.

The role of viral infection as a trigger for the development of primary SS remains controversial; candidate viruses include Epstein-Barr virus and retroviruses, including a human intracisternal A-type particle and human T-cell lymphotropic virus type 1. Increased attention has been directed to this area because an SS-like illness, diffuse infiltrative lymphocytosis syndrome (DILS), was recognized in patients infected with human immunodeficiency virus (HIV). Patients with DILS differ from those with primary SS in that they are more likely to be male, have an absence of characteristic autoantibodies, have CD8+ rather than CD4+ T cells in biopsy specimens of lacrimal and minor salivary glands, and have an increased frequency of the HLA class II alleles DR5 and DRw6 and DRB1*1102 and *1301.

Studies of biopsies from lacrimal and minor salivary glands of patients with SS demonstrate infiltration by lymphocytes, predominantly the CD4+ subset of T cells bearing the CD45RO phenotype and expressing the $\alpha\beta$ T-cell antigen receptor, which is associated with destruction of acinar tissue and the resulting decrease in tear and saliva production, respectively. Based on the frequent discordance between the amount of acinar damage on biopsy and the physiologic decrease in fluid production, there appears to be a role for antisecre-

TABLE 242-1. PRELIMINARY CRITERIA FOR THE CLASSIFICATION OF SJÖGREN'S SYNDROME, EUROPEAN COMMUNITY STUDY GROUP

1. Ocular symptoms: A positive response to at least one of these questions:
   a. Have you had daily, persistent, troublesome dry eyes for more than 3 months?
   b. Do you have a recurrent sensation of sand or gravel in the eyes?
   c. Do you use tear substitutes more than three times a day?
2. Oral symptoms: A positive response to at least one of these questions:
   a. Have you had a daily feeling of dry mouth for more than three months?
   b. Have you had recurrent or persistently swollen salivary glands as an adult?
   c. Do you frequently drink liquids to aid in swallowing dry foods?
3. Ocular signs: Objective evidence of ocular involvement, determined on the basis of a positive result on at least one of the following tests:
   a. Schirmer 1 test (≤ 5 mm in 5 minutes).
   b. Rose Bengal score (≥ 4, according to the van Bijsterveld scoring system).
4. Histopathologic features: Focus score of 1 or more on minor salivary gland biopsy (focus defined as an agglomeration of at least 50 mononuclear cells; focus score defined as number of foci per 4 sq mm of glandular tissue).
5. Salivary gland involvement: Objective evidence of salivary gland involvement, determined on the basis of a positive result on at least one of the following tests:
   a. Salivary scintigraphy
   b. Parotid sialography
   c. Unstimulated salivary flow (≤ 1.5 ml in 15 minutes)
6. Autoantibodies: Presence of at least one of the following serum autoantibodies:
   a. Antibodies to Ro(SS-A) or La(SS-B) antigens
   b. Antinuclear antibodies
   c. Rheumatoid factor

Exclusion criteria: Pre-existing lymphoma, acquired immunodeficiency syndrome, sarcoidosis, or graft-versus-host disease.

Modified from Vitali C, Bombardieri S, Moutsopoulos HM, et al.: Preliminary criteria for the classification of Sjögren's syndrome: Results of a prospective concerted action supported by the European Community. Arthritis Rheum 36:340, 1992.

tory cytokines produced by these T cells. In addition, a neurogenic component is suggested by the presence of nerve fibers containing vasoactive intestinal peptide that innervate the acini and the therapeutic efficacy of pilocarpine, which augments neural stimulation.

CLINICAL MANIFESTATIONS. The typical patient with primary SS is a peri- or postmenopausal Caucasian woman; however, the disease affects both sexes and all ages and races.

Ophthalmologic. Patients usually complain of dry eye symptoms, including burning, itching, or a foreign body (gritty, sandy) sensation; this is worse at the end of the day rather than on awakening. Patients also may notice blurred vision, redness of the eye, ocular discomfort, photophobia, and a mucinous discharge.

Salivary. Oral dryness may range in severity; many patients describe difficulty in chewing and swallowing, oral soreness, changes in tasting or smelling, fissures of the tongue and lips (angular cheilitis), and an increase in dental caries. Often patients carry a bottle of water with them during the day and keep a glass of water or other liquid at their bedside at night. A helpful finding on history is a positive "cracker test," i.e., the patient reports difficulty chewing and swallowing a packet of Saltine crackers without fluids. Bilateral parotid and submandibular gland enlargement may be present.

Other. Dryness also may affect other mucous membranes, including the nose, pharynx, tracheobronchial tree, and larynx; skin; and vulva and vagina. Involvement of pancreatic exocrine glands may lead to a decrease in pancreatic secretions and intestinal malabsorption; acute pancreatitis is rare. Dysphagia and noncardiac chest pain from gastroesophageal reflux are presumably due to decreased salivary production and, possibly, altered esophageal motility. Joint involvement, particularly arthralgias and nondeforming arthritis, is common. Symmetric inflammatory polyarthritis with deformity and radiographic erosions implies the existence of rheumatoid arthritis with concomitant secondary SS rather than primary SS.

Extraglandular manifestations of SS are more common in patients with primary than secondary SS, especially those with antibodies to Ro(SS-A) and La(SS-B); the spectrum of extraglandular manifestations is summarized in Table 242–2. Skin features include nonthrombocytopenic palpable purpura of the lower extremities, some-

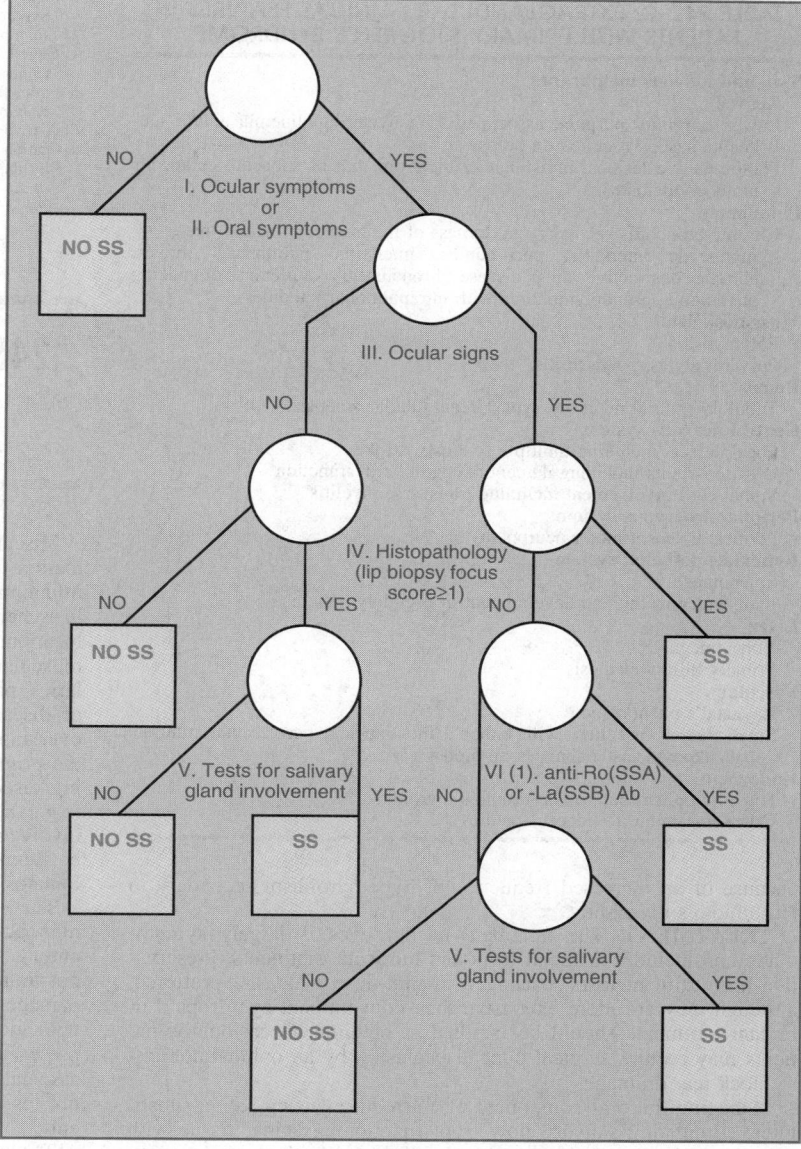

FIGURE 242–1. Algorithm for the classification of primary Sjögren's syndrome. The overall sensitivity was 93.3% in 149 patients with primary SS and the specificity was 92.2% compared with 90 control patients without connective tissue disease. See Table 242–1 for definitions of variables. (Modified with permission from Vitali C, Bombardieri S, Moutsopoulos HM, et al.: Preliminary criteria for the classification of Sjögren's syndrome: Results of a prospective concerted action supported by the European Community. Arthritis Rheum 36:340, 1993.)

times with leukocytoclastic vasculitis on biopsy, and photosensitive lesions indistinguishable from those of subacute cutaneous lupus erythematosus. Raynaud's phenomenon affects about one fifth of patients. Pulmonary features include lymphocytic pneumonitis, interstitial pulmonary fibrosis, and pseudolymphoma; pleurisy and pulmonary vasculitis are rare. Renal involvement, due to lymphocytes infiltrating the cortex, is manifest as type 1 distal renal tubular acidosis; the finding of glomerulonephritis should raise the question of coexistent SLE or cryoglobulinemia. Central nervous system involvement has been recognized only over the past decade, and its true frequency varies according to definition and referral patterns. Reported features include focal and diffuse defects, including multiple sclerosis, progressive dementia, and cognitive dysfunction, and spinal cord involvement similar to transverse myelitis. SS also has been associated with the liver secondary to primary biliary cirrhosis and, recently, hepatitis C infection.

DIAGNOSIS. *Ophthalmologic.* Keratoconjunctivitis sicca is demonstrated by decreased tear production with 5 mm or less wetting on Schirmer's test and the finding of devitalized cells and conjunctival and corneal defects with Rose Bengal staining observed during slit-lamp examination by an ophthalmologist. Other ocular tests, including measuring tear lysozyme and lactoferrin and impression cytology, have only a limited role in routine clinical diagnosis. The main differential diagnosis for the ocular findings is blepharitis; other conditions include reduced tear production after using antihistamines, diuretics, and antidepressant medications.

Oral. Salivary production can be evaluated by measuring unstimulated or stimulated flow rates; however, these tests lack specificity for SS because many conditions cause decreased production. Salivary gland scintigraphy, secretory sialography, ultrasound, and magnetic resonance imaging of the parotid glands, although useful for demonstrating glandular function and anatomy, have only a limited role in routine clinical practice. The major diagnostic tool is the labial salivary gland biopsy; the characteristic finding is focal lymphocytic infiltration. This is measured semiquantitatively by the number of foci, defined as 50 or more round cells, and a score of greater than one focus per 4 sq mm of tissue is diagnostic of SS. The biopsy is also useful in excluding other conditions that can cause xerostomia and bilateral glandular enlargement, including sarcoidosis, amyloidosis, hemochromatosis, and DILS.

Laboratory. Abnormalities in the complete blood count are common and include normochromic, normocytic anemia, leukopenia, and an elevated erythrocyte sedimentation rate; these are all nonspecific. Rheumatoid factor is present in one half to three quarters of patients, especially with secondary SS. Antinuclear antibodies are present in over three quarters of patients, and antibodies to Ro(SS-A) and La(SS-B) are found in about one-half to two thirds and one quarter to one third of patients with primary SS, respectively. Other immunologic abnormalities include a polyclonal hyperglobulinemia and positive tests for cryoglobulins; these cryoglobulins may contain monoclonal IgM_K proteins. Patients with myalgias and fatigue should have thyroid function tests performed

TABLE 242–2. EXTRAGLANDULAR CLINICAL FEATURES IN PATIENTS WITH PRIMARY SJÖGREN'S SYNDROME

Skin and mucous membranes
Xerosis
Lower extremity purpura, associated with hyperglobulinemia and/or leukocytoclastic vasculitis on biopsy
Photosensitive lesions, indistinguishable from that of subacute cutaneous lupus erythematosus
Pulmonary
Chronic bronchitis secondary to dryness of the tracheobronchial tree
Lymphocytic interstitial pneumonitis, interstitial pulmonary fibrosis, chronic obstructive lung disease, bronchiolitis obliterans organizing pneumonia, pseudolymphoma with intrapulmonary nodules
Musculoskeletal
Polymyositis
Polyarthralgias, polyarthritis
Renal
Tubulointerstitial nephritis, type 1 renal tubular acidosis
Central nervous system
Focal defects including multiple sclerosis, stroke
Diffuse deficits including dementia, cognitive dysfunction
Spinal cord involvement including transverse myelitis
Peripheral nervous system
Peripheral sensorimotor neuropathy
Reticuloendothelial system
Splenomegaly
Lymphadenopathy and development of pseudolymphoma
Liver
Hepatomegaly
Primary biliary cirrhosis
Vascular
Raynaud's phenomenon
Small vessel vasculitis, with either a mononuclear perivascular infiltrate or leukocytoclastic changes on biopsy
Endocrine
Hypothyroidism due to Hashimoto's thyroiditis
Other autoimmune endocrinopathies

because of an increased frequency of hypothyroidism secondary to Hashimoto's thyroiditis.

TREATMENT. The treatment of dry eyes is largely symptomatic and includes artificial tears and lubricant ointments. Preservative-free artificial tears, packaged in unit-dose vials, are preferred, although they are more expensive than conventional eye drops. Lubricant ointments should be instilled at bedtime. Occasionally, patients may require surgical punctal occlusion by an ophthalmologist to block tear drainage.

Managing the oral component of SS requires using saliva substitutes, stimulating salivary flow from functioning acinar tissue with pilocarpine hydrochloride at doses of 5 mg three times daily, treating oral candidiasis (a frequent complication of dry mouth) with nystatin or clotrimazole vaginal troches three times daily, and aggressively managing dental caries through both prevention and treatment.

Patients with extraglandular manifestations are usually treated with systemic corticosteroids, although no placebo-controlled studies have been conducted; hydroxychloroquine has been shown to be superior to placebo in these patients. Patients with secondary SS should receive appropriate therapy for their associated connective tissue disease. Patients with lymphoma should be treated in consultation with an oncologist.

PROGNOSIS. The ophthalmologic and oral manifestations of SS are generally nonprogressive. Patients with primary SS are at increased risk of developing lymphoproliferative disorders, including non-Hodgkin's lymphoma; in one study, the relative risk was estimated to be greater than 40. Patients with splenomegaly, bilateral parotid enlargement, and a history of radiation treatment to shrink these enlarged glands were at especially high risk. The lymphomas are B cell–derived, and the majority are IgM_K; recent studies have demonstrated a translocation of the bcl-2 t(14;18) proto-oncogene.

Young women with primary SS, especially those with antibodies to Ro(SS-A), should be counseled about the increased risk of delivering a child with neonatal SLE and congenital complete heart block; such women when pregnant should be followed closely by an obstetrician expert in high-risk pregnancies.

Fox RI (ed.): Sjögren's syndrome. Rheum Dis Clin North Am 18:507, 1992. Covers the history, pathology, immunopathogenesis, clinical features, and management of SS.
Homma M, Talal N (eds.): Proceedings IVth International Symposium on Sjögren's Syndrome. Amsterdam, Kluger Publications, 1994. Includes manuscripts of symposium papers of August 1993 in Tokyo.
St. Clair EW: Sjögren's syndrome and autoimmunity. In Cruse JM, Lewis RE (eds.): Clinical and Molecular Aspects of Autoimmune Disease. Concepts in Immunopathology. Basel, Karger, 1992, p 161. This chapter reviews SS immunopathogenesis.
Vitali C, Bombardieri S, Moutsopoulos HM, et al.: Preliminary criteria for the classification of Sjögren's syndrome: Results of a prospective concerted action supported by the European Community. Arthritis Rheum 36:340, 1993. Presents the results of the European Community Study Group's evaluation of criteria for the classification of both primary and secondary SS.

243 THE VASCULITIC SYNDROMES

Lanny J. Rosenwasser

Vasculitis is a clinicopathologic process characterized by inflammation and necrosis of the blood vessel wall. Associated with this inflammation may be compromise of the vessel lumen that results in ischemic changes in the tissues supplied by the vessel. Any size, location, and type of blood vessel may be involved, including large muscular arteries, medium-sized and small arteries, arterioles, capillaries, postcapillary venules, and veins. This heterogeneous category of diseases comprises unique syndromes as well as diseases with overlapping clinical and pathologic features. The vasculitis may be the primary process, or it may be a component of another underlying disease. Rarely, certain vasculitic disorders are life threatening (e.g., the hypersensitivity vasculitic syndromes in which cutaneous involvement usually predominates). Other vasculitic syndromes may be fulminant and, if untreated, rapidly fatal (e.g., Wegener's granulomatosis and polyarteritis nodosa).

The vasculitic syndromes are generally thought to result from immunopathogenic mechanisms; however, the evidence for this varies among the different syndromes. Among these mechanisms, the deposition of circulating immune complexes with subsequent vessel damage has emerged as a major immunopathologic event associated with most of the vasculitic syndromes (see Ch. 221 and 228). The presence of circulating immune complexes does not prove that the associated vasculitis is caused by them, and complexes per se need not result in vasculitis, even in diseases in which vasculitis is present.

The mechanism of tissue damage from immune complexes is thought to be similar to serum sickness. In this model, soluble immune complexes are formed in antigen excess and deposited in blood vessel walls in areas of increased vascular permeability. The increased permeability is attributed to release of vasoactive amines from platelets or mast cells under the influence of specific immunoglobulin E (IgE). Following deposition of complexes, various components of complement are activated, particularly C5a, which is strongly chemotactic for neutrophils. The neutrophils infiltrate the vessel wall at the site of immune complex deposition and release intracytoplasmic enzymes such as collagenase and elastase that directly damage the vessel wall. Compromise of the lumen occurs with resulting ischemic changes.

Certain of the vasculitides are characterized by granulomatous inflammation in and around the blood vessels. Although granulomatous responses are generally of the delayed hypersensitivity type, immune complexes themselves can trigger granuloma formation and thereby produce granulomatous vasculitis. Recently it has been found that the vessel wall itself, in addition to being a target for immune complex deposition, may actively participate in inflammation in the blood vessel by producing, locally, cytokines that are proinflammatory and that will attract other inflammatory cells, including cells that are involved in cell-mediated immunity. Hence, the mechanisms by which granulomatous inflammation may occur on the basis of immune complex initiation clearly will still involve the potential role of T cells, macrophages, and cytokines usually associated with delayed-type hypersensitivity.

The heterogeneity and the obvious overlap among the vasculitic syndromes have led to difficulties in classification of this group of diseases. The first report of a vasculitic syndrome was in 1866 by Kussmaul and Maier, who described the clinicopathologic features in a patient with what is now recognized as classic polyarteritis nodosa. It became evident that there were numerous vasculitic syndromes with diverse clinical and pathologic manifestations, but diagnostic criteria were controversial. More precise and accurate classification schemes now have emerged, based upon re-examination of clinical, pathologic, and immunologic features, as well as responses to certain therapeutic regimens. Table 243–1 is one such classification scheme.

The first group of vasculitides is the polyarteritis nodosa group. This syndrome is described in detail in Ch. 244. It is the prototype of the serious systemic necrotizing vasculitides and manifests features such as small and medium-sized muscular artery involvement, hypertension, visceral vessel involvement, and a noticeable lack of lung involvement. Eventually physicians recognized a systemic vasculitis that resembled classic polyarteritis nodosa except that lung involvement was a prominent feature and the patients generally manifested eosinophilia, granulomatous reactions, and a strong allergic diathesis, usually severe asthma. Most of these patients had what is now referred to as allergic angiitis and granulomatosis of the Churg-Strauss type. This disease is quite similar to classic polyarteritis nodosa except for the divergent features just mentioned. Many systemic necrotizing vasculitides manifest clinicopathologic characteristics that overlap these two syndromes as well as the hypersensitivity group of vasculitides (discussed below). This subgroup has been referred to as the overlap syndrome of systemic necrotizing vasculitis.

In addition to the polyarteritis nodosa group of systemic necrotizing vaculitides, certain other vasculitides are systemic and involve multiple organ systems. However, they are referred to by different names, since they possess characteristic clinical and/or pathologic features. This is true of diseases such as Wegener's granulomatosis (see Ch. 245), lymphomatoid granulomatosis, and the giant cell arteritides. In the last group, the two major subcategories—cranial or temporal arteritis (see Ch. 246) and Takayasu's arteritis—are systemic diseases involving large muscular arteries with mononuclear cell and often giant cell infiltration within the walls of the involved arteries. Despite the predisposition for certain vessels in these diseases (temporal artery in cranial arteritis and subclavian artery in Takayasu's arteritis), these are systemic diseases that involve multi-

ple arteries. Lymphomatoid granulomatosis is generally considered in the differential diagnosis of systemic necrotizing vasculitis with lung involvement such as Wegener's granulomatosis. However, it is not, strictly speaking, an inflammatory response in vessels, but an infiltration of blood vessel walls with atypical and often neoplastic-looking lymphoid cells. Lymphomatoid granulomatosis will often evolve into a lymphoma, and it has been suggested that these cases should be classified as angiocentric proliferative lesions.

Other vasculitic syndromes can be considered under the category of miscellaneous, for want of a better term. These include Kawasaki's disease and Behçet's disease, the major pathologic feature of which is a true vasculitis (see Ch. 249), and thromboangiitis obliterans, which is an inflammatory and occlusive disease of arteries and veins, although its true vasculitic character has been questioned. In addition to the granulomatous vasculitis of the central nervous system (CNS), which is seen in association with certain lymphoproliferative malignant neoplasms, there is also a rare syndrome of isolated vasculitis of the CNS that occurs in the apparent absence of systemic vasculitis or other systemic disease. Finally, erythema nodosum, erythema multiforme, and erythema elevatum diutinum are dermal vasculitides in this category.

HYPERSENSITIVITY VASCULITIS

Hypersensitivity vasculitis is a term applied to a heterogeneous group of disorders that are thought to represent a hypersensitivity reaction to an antigenic stimulus such as a drug or an infectious agent; hence the word hypersensitivity. Although the antigenic stimuli associated with this group are heterogeneous, these disorders generally involve the small vessels. They can be subdivided into two basic groups. The vast majority of patients manifest involvement of the postcapillary venules, and hence have a venulitis. A smaller group of patients falls into the second category, in which arterioles are predominantly involved (arteriolitis). Most important, there is predominant and often exclusive involvement of the vessels of the skin. Confusion in the literature generally resulted from grouping this category of vasculitis with the more serious systemic varieties, such as classic polyarteritis nodosa and related diseases. It is true that the hypersensitivity vasculitides may have variable degrees of organ system involvement other than of the skin. However, this is usually less severe than that of typical systemic vasculitis of polyarteritis nodosa and Wegener's granulomatosis. Most frequently the skin is exclusively involved, or if other organ systems are involved, the cutaneous disease still dominates the clinical picture.

ETIOLOGY. As indicated by the terminology, the cause is usually a recognizable antigenic stimulus, such as a drug, microbe, toxin, or foreign or endogenous protein. Etiologically the hypersensitivity vasculitides segregate into two distinct groups, depending on the source of the sensitizing antigen. In the classic original group, the antigen is foreign to the host. In the second group the antigen is endogenous.

INCIDENCE AND PREVALENCE. It is difficult to determine an accurate incidence for the hypersensitivity group of vasculitides owing to the marked heterogeneity among these diverse syndromes. However, the hypersensitivity group of vasculitides is much more common than the polyarteritis group and other syndromes such as Wegener's granulomatosis and Takayasu's arteritis. The disease can be seen at any age and in both genders; however, this varies considerably with the particular subgroup in question.

PATHOLOGY AND PATHOGENESIS. The histopathologic hallmark of the hypersensitivity vasculitides is leukocytoclastic venulitis. The term leukocytoclasis refers to nuclear debris derived from the neutrophils that have infiltrated in and around the involved vessels. In skin biopsies, this type of involvement is most common in the postcapillary venules just beneath the epidermis. When biopsies are obtained in the acute phase of active disease, the typical pattern of neutrophil infiltration is readily observed. In the subacute or chronic stages, biopsies often reveal mononuclear cell infiltration. In the second and smaller category of hypersensitivity vasculitis, arterioles and capillaries are predominantly involved. In the typical case of hypersensitivity vasculitis with a predominance of cutaneous involvement, the lesions are usually found in the lower extremities or in the dependent areas such as the sacrum in supine patients. This is most likely due to the increase in hydrostatic pressure within the postcapillary venules in these areas.

TABLE 243–1. THE CLINICAL SPECTRUM OF VASCULITIS

Polyarteritis Nodosa Group

Classic polyarteritis nodosa
Allergic angiitis and granulomatosis (Churg-Strauss disease)
Overlap syndrome

Hypersensitivity Vasculitis

Henoch-Schönlein purpura
Serum sickness and serum sickness–like reactions
Vasculitis associated with infectious diseases
Vasculitis associated with neoplasms
Vasculitis associated with connective tissue diseases
Vasculitis associated with other underlying diseases
Congenital deficiencies of the complement system

Granulomatous Vasculitides

Wegener's granulomatosis
Angiocentric immunoproliferative lesions (lymphomatoid granulomatosis)
Giant cell arteritides
    Cranial or temporal arteritis
    Takayasu's arteritis

Other Vasculitic Syndromes

Mucocutaneous lymph node syndrome (Kawasaki's disease)
Behçet's disease
Vasculitis isolated to the central nervous system
Thromboangiitis obliterans (Buerger's disease)
Erythema nodosa
Erythema multiforme
Erythema elevatum diutinum
Miscellaneous vasculitides

Although immune complex deposition is widely considered to be the pathogenic mechanism of this group of vasculitides, not every case of hypersensitivity vasculitis has had immune complexes demonstrated, even when carefully sought, as mentioned above.

CLINICAL MANIFESTATIONS. Just as the broad group is etiologically heterogeneous, so too are the clinical manifestations. However, the hallmark of the group is the predominance of cutaneous involvement. The skin lesions may appear as the classic palpable purpura, which results from the extravasation of erythrocytes into the tissue surrounding the involved venules. In addition, one may see macules, papules, vesicles, bullae, subcutaneous nodules, ulcers, and even recurrent or chronic urticaria.

Even though skin lesions generally dominate, various organ system involvement can be seen. Certain constellations of clinicopathologic findings define relatively distinct syndromes. For example, in Henoch-Schönlein purpura the typical syndrome consists of palpable purpura (usually over the buttocks), arthralgias, gastrointestinal symptoms, and glomerulonephritis. Henoch-Schönlein purpura is usually seen in children; however, adults of any age may be affected. The disease usually remits spontaneously after 1 week. However, the disease is remarkable for its tendency to recur a number of times over weeks to months before remission is complete. The characteristic skin lesions are present in virtually all patients, with most having arthralgias involving multiple joints, but frank arthritis is rare. The gastrointestinal involvement is usually manifested as colicky abdominal pain that may mimic an "acute surgical abdomen." Patients may experience nausea, vomiting, diarrhea, constipation, and occasionally the passage of blood and mucus per rectum. In the more severe and rare case, bowel intussusception may occur. Renal disease is a glomerulitis (see Ch. 79) that is usually expressed as microscopic hematuria without significant renal functional impairment. However, in rare cases, renal failure can occur. Most frequently, patients recover spontaneously and completely.

Other groups within the hypersensitivity category include serum sickness and serum sickness–like reactions. The classic manifestations are fever, urticaria, arthralgias, and lymphadenopathy occurring 7 to 10 days after primary exposure to the antigen in question, which for serum sickness is usually a heterologous serum protein and for serum sickness–like reactions is usually a drug such as penicillin. Very careful studies of serum complement levels demonstrate consumption of serum complement components C3 and C4 during the height of heterologous protein-related serum sickness. This depression of serum C3 and C4 is associated with increases in plasma level of C3a and other products that are indicative of complement activation. These alterations in serum complement correlate with the presence of immune complexes in the serum in these models of serum sickness. In addition, cases may occasionally progress to a typical systemic necrotizing vasculitis involving multiple organ systems.

A number of disorders have vasculitis as a manifestation of an underlying primary disease. Included in these diseases are systemic lupus erythematosus (SLE), rheumatoid arthritis, mixed cryoglobulinemia, and other connective tissue diseases. In these disorders the manifestations of the underlying disease usually predominate. When vasculitis is observed it is generally of the small vessel cutaneous type, which is virtually indistinguishable from the vasculitis seen in the hypersensitivity group with recognized exogenous antigens. However, patients with these disorders, particularly SLE and rheumatoid arthritis, may also develop a systemic necrotizing vasculitis that closely resembles the polyarteritis nodosa group in manifestations and severity. Nevertheless, in the typical case, the cutaneous vasculitis usually dominates the clinical picture with respect to the vasculitic process.

Other diseases that may fall into this category are the vasculitis associated with congenital deficiencies of various complement components, such as C1r, C1s, and C2, erythema elevatum diutinum; hypocomplementemic vasculitis; the vasculitis associated with certain neoplasms, particularly of the lymphoid type; and the vasculitis associated with other primary disorders such as ulcerative colitis, Crohn's disease, biliary cirrhosis, and retroperitoneal fibrosis.

DIAGNOSIS. The diagnosis of hypersensitivity vasculitis rests on demonstration of vasculitis on biopsy. Since the predominant organ involved is the skin, histopathologic material is usually readily available. Because cutaneous involvement is often present in severe systemic vasculitides, one should undertake a systematic workup of other organ systems in patients with apparently isolated cutaneous

vasculitis. Recently it has been suggested that the presence of antibodies against the cytoplasm of neutrophils (c-ANCA) is supportive evidence for a diagnosis of Wegener's granulomatosis (see Ch. 236 and 245).

TREATMENT AND PROGNOSIS. Therapy of the hypersensitivity group of vasculitides has in general been unsatisfactory. Since most cases resolve spontaneously, the lack of response to therapeutic regimens is of less importance. However, in those patients who develop persistent cutaneous disease or serious organ system involvement, several regimens have been tried with variable results. In cases in which a recognized antigenic stimulus is present, the sensitizing drugs or responsible organisms should be removed by appropriate antibiotic therapy when possible. In situations in which disease appears to be self-limited, no specific therapy is indicated. However, when disease persists or results in organ system dysfunction, a glucocorticoid is the drug of choice. Prednisone is usually administered in doses of 1 mg per kilogram per day with rapid tapering when possible, in some instances directly to discontinuation or initially to an alternate-day regimen followed by ultimate discontinuation. In cases that prove refractory to corticosteroid therapy, cytotoxic agents such as cyclophosphamide have been used. The efficacy of these regimens has not yet been fully evaluated in hypersensitivity vasculitis.

The prognosis of most of these diseases is generally excellent, with spontaneous and complete remissions in most patients. However, certain patients may develop persistent and debilitating cutaneous disease, and some cases may evolve into typical systemic vasculitis with a serious prognosis.

Calabrese LH, Michel BA, Bloch DA, et al.: The American College of Rheumatology 1990 criteria for the classification of hypersensitivity vasculitis. Arthritis Rheum 33:1108, 1990. *This paper is from an issue of Arthritis and Rheumatism that identified the American College of Rheumatology criteria for diagnosis of vasculitis using algorithms for patient symptoms and pathologic findings.*

Cupps TR, Fauci AS: The Vasculitides. Philadelphia, WB Saunders, 1981, pp. 1–21. *Comprehensive treatise on the entire spectrum of the vasculitis syndromes, discussing pathogenesis, clinicopathologic manifestations, and updated therapeutic approaches.*

Fries JF, Hunder GG, Bloch DA, et al.: The American College of Rheumatology 1990 criteria for the classification of vasculitis: Summary. Arthritis Rheum 33:1135, 1990.

Hiltz RE, Cupps TR: Cutaneous vasculitis. Curr Opinion Rheumatol 6:20, 1994. *Reviews in detail the various mechanisms and forms of cutaneous vasculitis and provides an interesting summary of cutaneous manifestations of hypersensitivity vasculitis.*

Lawley TJ, Bielory L, Gascon P, et al.: A prospective clinical and immunologic analysis of patients with serum sickness. N Engl J Med 311:1407, 1984. *Elegant description of changes in immune complexes and serum complement levels associated with horse antithymocyte globulin–induced serum sickness.*

Lipford EH Jr, Margolick JB, Longo DL, et al.: Angiocentric immunoproliferative lesions: A clinicopathologic spectrum of post-thymic T-cell proliferations. Blood 72:1674, 1988. *Detailed description of various stages of lymphomatoid granulomatosis.*

Michel BA: Classification of vasculitis. Current Opinion Rheumatol 4:3, 1992. *Provides algorithms and overviews necessary for differential diagnosis of a number of vasculitic syndromes and gives a very concise overview of all the vasculitic syndromes.*

244 POLYARTERITIS NODOSA GROUP

Lanny J. Rosenwasser

DEFINITION. In 1866 Kussmaul and Maier described a patient with polyarteritis nodosa and introduced the term *periarteritis nodosa* to describe segmental nodules of medium-sized muscular arteries. Because swelling of the arterial walls often leads to occlusion, many of the clinical manifestations are secondary to necrosis. Hence, polyarteritis nodosa is often classified as one of the systemic necrotizing vasculitides. Classic polyarteritis does not involve the lung, as do allergic angiitis and granulomatosis of Churg-Strauss (see Ch. 54). Polyarteritis associated with hepatitis B antigenemia was described in 1970 by Gocke and colleagues. The association of hepatitis B antigen-antibody complexes and polyarteritis provides strong support for the hypothesis that the vasculitides in general are secondary to the deposition of soluble immune complexes.

Some patients have manifestations of both classic polyarteritis nodosa and allergic angiitis and granulomatosis of Churg-Strauss. Such patients are classified in the group with the so-called overlap syndrome. Diagnosis, workup, and management are no different from those in other patients in the polyarteritis nodosa group. Polyarteritis nodosa occurs from infancy to old age, with a peak incidence in the fifth and sixth decades of life; the male-female ratio has been estimated to be 2 to 3 : 1.

PATHOLOGY. The lesions of polyarteritis affect arteries of medium and small caliber, especially at bifurcations and branchings. The segmental process involves the media, with edema, fibrinous exudation, fibrinoid necrosis, and infiltration of polymorphonuclear neutrophils, and extends to the adventitia and intima. Thrombosis and infarction or hemorrhage occur at this stage. Subsequently the regions of fibrinoid necrosis are replaced by granulation tissue, and the intima proliferates. Finally the involved segment is replaced by scar tissue with associated intimal thickening and periarterial fibrosis. These changes produce partial occlusion, thrombosis and infarction, and palpable or visible aneurysms with occasional rupture.

In allergic angiitis and granulomatosis the acute fibrinoid necrosis with cellular infiltration involves arterioles and venules as well as medium-sized muscular arteries. It is characteristic of the polyarteritis nodosa group for the vascular lesions to be in different stages of evolution, i.e., acute, subacute, and healed. In allergic angiitis and granulomatosis, the pulmonary granulomatous lesions in vascular and extravascular sites are accompanied by intense eosinophilic infiltration.

In patients with polyarteritis associated with hepatitis B antigenemia, the specific antigen has been recognized in immune complexes present in the circulation and deposited in affected vessels along with complement proteins. It is presumed that this pathogenetic mechanism prevails in the entire polyarteritis nodosa group, but the basis for arterial deposition is unknown. The deposition of immune complexes in venules and glomeruli is attributed to changes in permeability and to physical trapping.

CLINICAL MANIFESTATIONS AND DIAGNOSIS. The widespread distribution of the arterial lesions produces diverse clinical manifestations, which reflect the particular organ systems in which the arterial supply has been impaired. Among the early symptoms and signs of polyarteritis nodosa are fever, weight loss, and pain in viscera and/or the musculoskeletal system. Striking and specific presenting signs may relate to abdominal pain, acute glomerulitis, polyneuritis on occasion, or myocardial infarction. Pulmonary manifestations, especially intractable bronchial asthma, would indicate allergic angiitis and granulomatosis rather than classic polyarteritis nodosa.

Renal. Renal involvement in two forms, renal polyarteritis and glomerulitis, may occur separately or together. Approximately 70% of patients with polyarteritis nodosa and renal disease have renal vasculitis, whereas the other 30% have glomerulitis. Renal polyarteritis is the most common lesion seen at postmortem examination. Manifestations of the renal involvement include intermittent proteinuria and microscopic hematuria with occasional hyaline and granular casts. The glomerulitis is manifested by microscopic and even macroscopic hematuria, proteinuria, cellular casts, and progressive renal failure. Hypertension is common. Renal involvement is the cause of death in about two thirds of patients with classic polyarteritis nodosa and about one third with allergic angiitis and granulomatosis.

Gastrointestinal. Arterial lesions are commonly found in one or more abdominal viscera. The principal manifestation is pain; anorexia, nausea, and vomiting are less prominent. Impaired arterial blood supply to the bowel can produce mucosal ulcerations, perforation, or infarction with melena or bloody diarrhea. Involvement of appendix, gallbladder, or pancreas can simulate appendicitis, cholecystitis, or hemorrhagic pancreatitis. Liver involvement can range from hepatomegaly with or without jaundice to the signs of extensive hepatic necrosis. Splenomegaly is uncommon. No consistent relationship has been seen between the development of necrotizing vasculitis and the appearance of liver disease in patients with hepatitis B antigenemia. Some of the observed combinations include necrotizing vasculitis as the initial clinical finding, superimposed on chronic active hepatitis or appearing simultaneously with acute hepatitis.

Central and Peripheral Nervous System. Central nervous system (CNS) manifestations are generally late occurrences in the course of polyarteritis nodosa, and their particular presentation reflects the specific area of the brain that is compromised. Headache, seizures, and retinal hemorrhages and exudates occur with or without localizing signs referable to the cerebrum, cerebellum, or brain stem; meningeal irritation may occur as a result of subarachnoid hemorrhage. Multiple mononeuropathy, i.e., involvement of several or even many individual nerves at the same or different times, is common and is attributed to arteritis of the vasa nervorum. The peripheral neuropathy is usually asymmetric, with both sensory and motor distribution. The former can be extremely painful, but the latter has attendant muscular degeneration, which can be so severe as to dominate the clinical presentation.

Articular and Muscular. Arthralgias and myalgias are frequent in polyarteritis nodosa. Arthralgias are migratory, generally without swelling, and thought to be due to small, localized arterial lesions. Muscle pain or weakness reflects either direct involvement of the arterial supply or a peripheral neuropathy.

Cardiac. Polyarteritis of the coronary arteries and their branches has a frequency approaching that of renal polyarteritis, and heart failure is responsible for or contributes to death in one sixth to one half of the cases. Clinical manifestations are partial or complete arterial occlusion, as modified by the superimposition of renal hypertension and an appreciable incidence of acute pericarditis without effusion. Whereas the combination of infarction and hypertension commonly leads to left-sided failure, an occasional patient with allergic angiitis and granulomatosis has predominantly right-sided decompensation.

Genitourinary. Involvement of the ovaries, testes, and epididymis is frequent, though usually asymptomatic. Mucosal ulceration in the bladder can occasionally precipitate gross hematuria with dysuria.

Cutaneous. Cutaneous involvement of some form is believed to occur in >25% of those affected. The acute cutaneous manifestations include polymorphic exanthemas—purpuric, urticarial, and multiform in character—and severe subcutaneous hemorrhage, resulting from necrotizing arteritis, with secondary gangrene. Ulcerations and a persistent livedo reticularis are associated with the more chronic stage. A most characteristic but uncommon finding is cutaneous and subcutaneous nodules; these occur at any time in the disease course. The nodules tend to group, appear in crops, are usually movable, may regress in days or persist for months, range in size from a pea to a walnut, and may cause the overlying skin to become reddened or to ulcerate.

Pulmonary. Although the bronchial arteries can be involved in classic polyarteritis, only allergic angiitis and granulomatosis that involves the pulmonary arteries and parenchyma with granulomatous lesions give rise to clinical manifestations. Asthma, when present, is intractable and associated with marked peripheral eosinophilia. Pneumonic episodes are transient or progressive and may be accompanied by hemoptysis and/or pleuritic pain. Respiratory involvement accounts for about 50% of deaths, with the remainder being attributable to the arteritis in other organs.

COURSE UNTREATED. The course of polyarteritis nodosa is progressive with destruction of vital organs. Intermittent acute episodes resulting from thrombosis of vital or nonvital structures are prominent. Death is most frequently attributed to renal involvement in cases of classic polyarteritis nodosa and to pulmonary lesions in those cases classified as allergic angiitis with granulomatosis. Cardiac failure caused by a combination of infarction and renal hypertension is an additional frequent cause of death in both groups, and acute vascular accidents of the gastrointestinal tract or CNS account for much of the remaining mortality. In the retrospective postmortem study of Rose and Spencer, the 5-year survival rate was about 10% in classic polyarteritis nodosa and about 25% in allergic angiitis and granulomatosis if onset was dated from the start of respiratory symptoms. The report of the British Medical Research Council in 1960 placed the 54-month survival rate in polyarteritis nodosa at nearly 50%. Rare patients with polyarteritis limited to nonvital sites have been reported to experience an unusually long course or even a lasting remission.

LABORATORY FINDINGS. Leukocytosis, predominantly polymorphonuclear, is apparent in >75% of the cases of polyarteritis nodosa or allergic angiitis and granulomatosis, eosinophilia often being marked in the latter group. Hypocomplementemia, which has not been observed in classic polyarteritis nodosa, has been present in patients with hepatitis B antigenemia. The erythrocyte sedimentation rate is customarily elevated. Abnormalities in the urine sediment, especially hematuria and proteinuria, reflect renal involvement. Abnormalities of the electrocardiogram and electroencephalogram are those common to arterial occlusive disease or secondary to the metabolic disturbances of uremia. Lesions apparent on chest roentgenograms are the rule in patients with allergic angiitis and granulomatosis. The findings range from transient or progressive infiltration to consolidation, cavitation, or scarring; upper and lower lobes are involved with equal frequency. As none of these findings is specific, antemortem diagnosis of polyarteritis depends on biopsy. Since the arterial involvement is segmental and spotty in distribution, it is advisable to obtain tissue from a symptomatic site, and it is essential to section the entire specimen completely. A deep, open surgical biopsy, including subcutaneous tissue and underlying muscle, should be obtained whenever possible from a skeletal muscle exhibiting pain and tenderness. Involvement of the epididymis and testes is sufficiently common to make this a useful biopsy site if palpation reveals the typical nodularity of segmental vascular lesions. Needle and surgical biopsies of internal organs with clinical involvement, such as liver or kidney, are gaining in favor. As an alternative or additional procedure, angiography to detect aneurysms of medium-sized muscular arteries in renal, hepatic, or intestinal sites may be helpful.

DIFFERENTIAL DIAGNOSIS. This includes not only the constituent syndromes but also all those conditions associated with systemic necrotizing vasculitis. The key differences between classic polyarteritis nodosa and other causes of necrotizing vasculitis include the absence of extravascular granulomas, sparing of the pulmonary arteries, failure of venous involvement except by contiguous spread, and predilection for medium-sized arteries. For allergic angiitis and granulomatosis the striking granulomatous response excludes all but Wegener's granulomatosis. The prominence of bronchial asthma, peripheral eosinophilia, and the usual absence of necrotizing lesions in the upper respiratory tract permit tentative clinical distinction between allergic angiitis and granulomatosis and Wegener's granulomatosis. Underlying connective tissue diseases are still recognized by their clinical characteristics even when necrotizing arteritis becomes prominent. For example, patients with

rheumatoid arthritis with ulcerating cutaneous lesions and peripheral neuropathy often exhibit prominent rheumatoid nodules and a high titer of rheumatoid factor. The specificities of the immunoglobulins that accompany active systemic lupus erythematosus or mixed cryoglobulinemia are distinctive; in addition, in the presence of active renal disease both entities manifest a reduced serum complement level not generally observed in classic polyarteritis nodosa. The giant cell arteritides (i.e., temporal arteritis, Takayasu's arteritis) lack the glomerulitis, peripheral neuropathy, and cutaneous manifestations notable in polyarteritis nodosa. The combination of progressive nephritis and pulmonary hemorrhage seen in Goodpasture's syndrome is unlike polyarteritis nodosa. The drug-induced hypersensitivity vasculitis group may be difficult to separate on purely clinical grounds, although a history of antecedent drug administration, infrequency of gastrointestinal manifestations, and absence of nodules along arteries are useful points. The clinical presentation in Henoch-Schönlein purpura is distinctive.

TREATMENT. The commonly used nonsteroidal anti-inflammatory agents have no specific therapeutic role in polyarteritis nodosa; thus, corticosteroids have been employed most widely. Large doses, in the range of 40 to 60 mg of prednisone per day, afford symptomatic relief but probably have little effect on the 1-year survival statistics. In a series of 17 patients within the polyarteritis group, including 2 with allergic angiitis and granulomatosis and 6 with hepatitis B–associated polyarteritis, 14 experienced dramatic remission with 2 mg per kilogram per day of cyclophosphamide. It was subsequently possible to reduce the cyclophosphamide and to taper the steroid dose to every other day and yet maintain remission, and in some instances resolution of microaneurysms was noted on repeat celiac axis angiography (Fig. 244–1).

In patients who have polyarteritis nodosa associated with hepatitis B virus infection, recent reports from a European collaborative group have identified significant responses to treatment regimens that include the cytokine, interferon α2b, and plasma exchange. When these approaches are taken in conjunction with short-term steroid therapy and potential antiviral treatment with Vira-a, a sig-

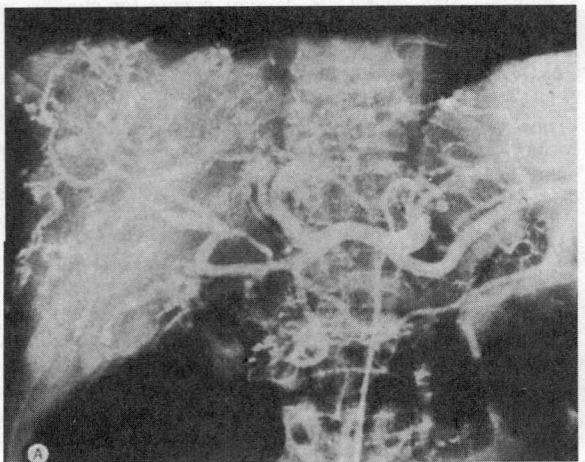
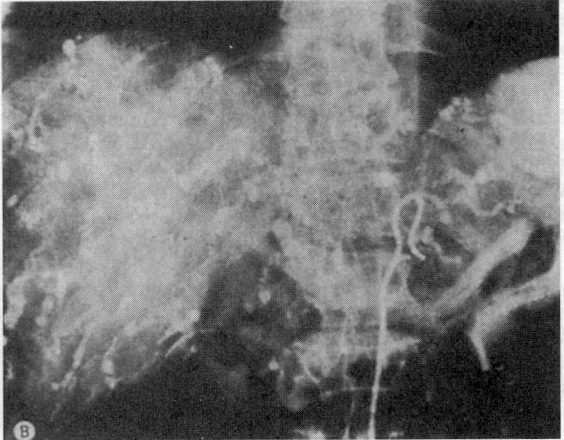
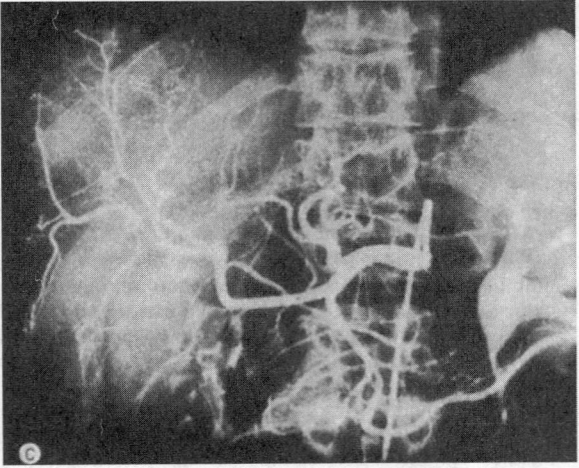

FIGURE 244–1. Selective celiac arteriogram demonstrates large hepatic arteries (*A*) and multiple aneurysms (*A* and *B*) throughout the liver. Resolution of aneurysms is seen after therapy (*C*). (From Fauci AS, Doppman JL, Wolff SM: Cyclophosphamide-induced remissions in advanced polyarteritis nodosa. Am J Med 64:891, 1978.)

nificant number of patients had long-term remission and seroconversion in terms of hepatitis. Obviously, initial interest in treating this subgroup of PAN patients, those who have documented hepatitis B virus infection, with alternative treatments to cytotoxic drugs and steroids, is promising.

Fauci AS, Katz P, Haynes BF, et al.: Cyclophosphamide therapy of severe systemic necrotizing vasculitis. N Engl J Med 301:235, 1979. *Most important contribution dealing with cyclophosphamide therapy effectiveness in management of a series of patients within the polyarteritis group and including such subgroups as allergic angiitis and granulomatosis and hepatitis B–associated polyangiitis.*

Guillevin L, Lhote F, Leon A, et al.: Treatment of polyarteritis nodosa related to hepatitis B virus with short term steroid therapy associated with antiviral agents and plasma exchanges. A prospective trial in 33 patients. J Rheumatol 20:289, 1993.

Guillevin L, Lhote F, Sauvaget F, et al.: Treatment of polyarteritis nodosa related to hepatitis B virus with interferon-alpha and plasma exchanges. Ann Rheum Dis 53:334, 1994. *This and the preceding report identify prospectively the response of patients with interferon-α2b and plasma exchange. The data suggest in these two trials that cytokine and antiviral therapy as well as plasmapheresis may have a role as a potential first-line treatment in proven virus-induced vasculitis and polyarteritis nodosa.*

245 WEGENER'S GRANULOMATOSIS
Nancy B. Allen

Wegener's granulomatosis (WG) falls within the spectrum of systemic vasculitides as a clinicopathologic syndrome involving upper and lower respiratory tract and kidneys and less commonly the eyes, joints, skin, and neurologic and cardiac tissues. Described in 1931 and 1936 by H. Klinger and F. Wegener, respectively, necrotizing granulomatous vasculitis is the hallmark disorder in the lower respiratory tract, and focal, segmental glomerulonephritis and small vessel or granulomatous vasculitis are found elsewhere. The disease is now known to be associated with the cytoplasmic pattern of antineutrophil cytoplasmic antibody (c-ANCA) and more specifically with antibodies against proteinase 3 (PR-3), a serine protease found in neutrophils.

ETIOLOGY. The cause of WG is not yet known, but much research is being done. Because of the almost universal upper and/or lower airway involvement, inhaled antigen(s) stimulating granuloma formation and altered immune reactivity with features of immune complex deposition and altered cellular immune responses are believed to play significant roles, along with host factors and/or genetic predisposition. As of this writing no single genetic marker, environmental agent, microorganism, or other factor can be identified as initiating this syndrome. Rare familial reports of WG in first-degree relatives exist.

INCIDENCE AND PREVALENCE. The demographics of WG may be changing with the presence of new laboratory markers (c-ANCA), enhanced education of physicians regarding this diagnosis, and expansion of the spectrum of clinical features and presentations. In the United States, the disease frequency is approximately 1 in 30,000. In recent studies, mean age of onset is approximately 40, equal in men and women, predominant in Caucasians, and occurring from childhood into older adulthood.

PATHOLOGY AND PATHOGENESIS. Classical histopathology in WG is necrotizing granulomatous vasculitis involving small arteries and veins, most reliably found on biopsies of the lung (Table 245–1). This typical pathology has been seen in many other tissues, including unusual clinical locations, such as muscle, prostate, and breast. Upper respiratory tract biopsies including nasal septum, sinus, and trachea most often show nonspecific acute and chronic inflammation with or without giant cells and generally without true vasculitis.

Renal biopsies typically show focal segmental glomerulonephritis, with crescent formation and necrosis in more severe forms. Generally, immunofluorescent staining yields pauci-immune deposits, but these findings are not specific to WG, as they can be seen in polyarteritis nodosa, other vasculitides, and some nonvasculitic conditions. Biopsy does help to exclude other conditions such as systemic lupus erythematosus (SLE), post-streptococcal disease, Goodpasture's syndrome, and cryoglobulinemia.

TABLE 245–1. PATHOLOGIC FINDINGS IN WEGENER'S GRANULOMATOSIS

Location	Pathology
Upper airways (sinus, nasal septum)	Acute and chronic inflammation, giant cells, necrotizing granulomas, rarely vasculitis
Lung	
Transbronchial	Acute and chronic inflammation, giant cells, granuloma, rarely vasculitis
Thorascopic or open	Necrotizing, granulomatous vasculitis* (negative special stains and cultures), eosinophils, hemosiderin-laden macrophages, capillaritis
Kidney	Focal segmental glomerulonephritis with or without crescent formation, pauci-immune deposits, rarely vasculitis ($<1\%$)
Orbital/ocular	Acute and chronic inflammation with or without granuloma and/or vasculitis
Skin	Leukocytoclastic vasculitis, occasionally granulomatous vasculitis with or without necrosis
Sural nerve/muscle	Acute axonopathy, denervation and/or renervation, occasionally vasculitis of vasa nervorum; myopathy, with or without inflammation
Liver/spleen	Granulomatous hepatitis, triaditis; granulomatous vasculitis in spleen
Cardiac	Pericardial inflammation; rarely true coronary arteritis or granulomatous inflammation in myocardium or conduction system

* "Diagnostic" pathologic triad in WG.

In the initial phase of WG, bronchoalveolar lavage shows neutrophilic alveolitis, phagocytosis of neutrophils by monocytes, and higher levels of c-ANCA in lavage fluid than in serum. A current theory about the pathogenesis of WG involves a stimulus (inhalant) of some type, activation of neutrophils, transfer of PR-3 to cell membrane, and increased levels of c-ANCA, rheumatoid factor, gammaglobulins, and circulating immune complexes. Both cellular and humoral immune factors then lead to vasculitis, tissue destruction, and granuloma formation, contributing to the clinical features of the disease.

CLINICAL MANIFESTATIONS. The spectrum of clinical presentations and organ system involvement in WG is broad (Table 245–2). As a multisystem disorder involving predominantly the upper and lower respiratory tracts and the kidneys, presentations vary from "classic," with sinusitis, serous otitis media, rhinitis with nasal ulcerations, cough, hemoptysis, and constitutional symptoms, to "fulminant," with rapidly progressive renal failure and respiratory failure requiring intensive care unit management, to "mild," with arthralgias, polymyalgia rheumatica–type symptoms, or inflammatory eye disease as examples. Astute clinicians must carry WG as a potential diagnosis in their differential diagnosis list for multisystem disease or unexplained illness, much as one keeps SLE or subacute bacterial endocarditis in mind. With greater understanding of systemic vasculitic syndromes and education of primary care providers, this diagnosis may be considered in more individuals than previously, leading to earlier diagnosis and selection of appropriate management.

Nearly three fourths of patients eventually diagnosed with WG initially seek help due to upper and/or lower respiratory complaints. These include seasonal allergic rhinitis symptoms, recurrent epistaxis, oral or nasal ulcerations, ear pain, cough, fever, or hearing abnormalities. Some patients experience months or years of these symptoms before diagnosis. Constitutional symptoms with fevers, weight loss, anorexia, fatigue, arthralgias, and myalgias, although nonspecific, are common in this condition.

Lung involvement may be symptomatic with cough, dyspnea, pleuritic chest pain, and hemoptysis or may be totally asymptomatic with abnormalities found only on chest radiographs. Fleeting or persistent pulmonary infiltrates are more commonly found in the upper lobes and may be due to pulmonary hemorrhage or granulomatous inflammation along with vasculitis (see Ch. 54). Solitary or multiple pulmonary nodules and, less commonly, bibasilar interstitial changes, may be seen. Some patients with lower respiratory symptoms but normal chest radiographs may have endobronchial lesions found only at bronchoscopy.

TABLE 245–2. CLINICAL MANIFESTATIONS OF WEGENER'S GRANULOMATOSIS

Region/Organ	Sign or Symptom
Upper airway (90–95%)	Sinusitis, serous otitis media, rhinitis, nasal ulcerations/septal perforation, epistaxis, oral ulcerations, saddle-nose deformity (later), headaches
Lower airway (90–95%)	Cough, dyspnea, hemoptysis; pulmonary infiltrates (may be fleeting or persistent), nodules, cavities, pleural effusions/pleuritis, subglottic stenosis, endobronchial lesions, interstitial lung disease
Kidneys (75%)	Urinary sediment abnormalities (microscopic hematuria, casts, proteinuria), with or without renal insufficiency, nephrotic syndrome, hypertension
Musculoskeletal (70–90%)	Polyarthralgias, myalgias, mono-, oligo-, or polyarthritis (may be in rheumatoid pattern), myositis, muscle weakness
Eye (50–65%)	Conjunctivitis, scleritis/episcleritis, uveitis, proptosis, nasolacrimal duct obstruction, orbital mass lesions, retinal vasculitis, corneoscleral ulceration
Skin (50%)	Palpable purpura, subcutaneous nodules, petechiae, vesicles, ulcers, Raynaud's phenomenon, digital ischemia, livedo reticularis, necrotic papules, pyoderma gangrenosum–type lesions (rare)
Neurologic (20–25%)	Mononeuritis multiplex, peripheral neuropathy, cranial neuropathy, central nervous system vasculitis (cerebral hemorrhage, cerebritis, syncope, diabetes insipidis)
Cardiac (20%)	Pericarditis, pancarditis, cardiomyopathy, arrhythmias, coronary arteritis
Gastrointestinal (15–30%)	Alkaline phosphatase and/or aminotransferase elevations, granulomatous hepatitis/triaditis, small bowel vasculitis, ascites, splenic granulomatous vasculitis
Miscellaneous (<1–5%)	Breast, prostate, testicle, pinnae, urethra, ureter, lymph nodes, parotid, pulmonary or temporal artery, vagina, other
Constitutional	Fatigue, weight loss, fever, malaise, anorexia

Renal involvement is certainly one of the most serious clinical aspects of WG. This may be asymptomatic, such that urinalysis and serum creatinine measurements are important and must be followed closely in patients suspected to have WG. Rapidly progressive renal insufficiency with or without hypertension, edema, and nephrotic syndrome requires prompt evaluation and management. Irreversible renal failure requiring dialysis may be part of the initial clinical presentation or may slowly develop during therapy or with recurrent disease.

Musculoskeletal manifestations occur in the majority of patients. Observations have included diffuse polyarthralgias, an arthritis ranging from monoarticular to oligoarticular, and a rheumatoid arthritis–like picture with polyarthritis involving wrists, metacarpophalangeal and proximal interphalangeal joints, knees, ankles, and other large or small joints. When rheumatoid factor occurs along with symmetric polyarthritis, the initial diagnosis may be rheumatoid arthritis; however, attention to extra-articular symptoms and/or signs and laboratory data may lead to a diagnosis of WG instead. Diffuse myalgias are often present, and in patients over age 50 a polymyalgia rheumatica–type onset of WG and/or overlap of WG and temporal arteritis has been described. True myositis, with creatine phosphokinase, aldolase, or aminotransferase elevations, proximal muscle weakness, and finding of granulomatous vasculitis or less specific myositis, has been observed in WG.

Ocular involvement occurs in one half to two thirds of patients with WG on the basis of either vasculitis or tracking granulomatous tissue through the lamina papyracea into the medial aspect of the orbit. Vasculitis is responsible for conjunctivitis, scleritis-episcleritis, uveitis, retinal vasculitis, and corneoscleral ulcerations. Granulomatous mass lesions contribute to proptosis, orbital masses, optic nerve compression, diplopia, and nasal lacrimal duct obstruction.

Cutaneous involvement is most typically seen as palpable purpura, predominantly in the lower extremities, but may occur in upper extremities and over bony prominences. Vesicles, verrucous/necrotic papular lesions, subcutaneous nodules, petechiae, and more severe pyoderma gangrenosum–type lesions have been described. Raynaud's phenomenon, digital ischemia/necrosis, and livedo reticularis are present in some patients with acute and fulminant disease, with small vessel vasculitis with or without vasospasm being the predominant cause. Biopsy of the skin most commonly shows leukocytoclastic vasculitis.

Neurologic involvement is most typical with mononeuritis multiplex, foot drop and/or wrist drop or both, with patchy sensory and/or motor abnormalities. A diffuse peripheral neuropathy and cranial neuropathy, particularly of cranial nerves I, VII, and VIII, have been described. Headaches, hypothalamic or pituitary disease with clinical diabetes insipidus, and cerebral or subarachnoid hemorrhage have been reported infrequently.

Cardiovascular manifestations include pericarditis, pericardial effusions, rarely coronary vasculitis, myocarditis, congestive heart failure (other than observed secondary to acute renal failure), valvular abnormalities, and arrhythmias. Miscellaneous clinical features are listed in Table 245–2.

DIAGNOSIS. The diagnosis is based on supportive clinical, pathologic, and laboratory confirmation. The diagnosis should be strongly suspected when a patient presents with multisystem illness

TABLE 245–3. LABORATORY ABNORMALITIES IN WEGENER'S GRANULOMATOSIS

	Typical	Occasional	Rare
Hematologic	Normochromic, normocytic anemia Leukocytosis Eosinophilia Elevated erythrocyte sedimentation rate	Thrombocytosis	Microangiopathic hemolytic anemia
Urine sediment	Microhematuria Proteinuria Cellular casts	Sterile pyuria	
Chemistries	Hypoalbuminemia Renal insufficiency (mild to severe)	Elevated alkaline phosphatase +/or aminotransferases; elevated creatine phosphokinase, aldolase	
Serologic	Positive c-ANCA Positive rheumatoid factor Hypergammaglobulinemia Elevated c-reactive protein	Positive ANA (any pattern) Positive p-ANCA Elevated circulating immune complexes	

involving upper and/or lower respiratory tract disease, glomeru-lonephritis, and vasculitis in any organ system. (See Table 245–3 for a listing of typical, occasional, and rare laboratory abnormalities in WG.) The gold standard for a diagnosis of WG has been patho-logic finding of necrotizing granulomatous vasculitis, particularly at open lung biopsy. However, active lung involve-ment is not always present initially. Localized disease may lead the clinician to enter-tain biopsy of other tissues, and thus knowledge of the array of pathologic findings in other organ systems is necessary.

Until relatively recently, laboratory features of WG were rela-tively nonspecific. A typical laboratory profile included normocytic normochromic anemia, elevated erythrocyte sedimentation rate, leukocytosis, and positive rheumatoid factor in 30 to 40% of pa-tients, with or without urine sediment abnormalities or elevated serum creatinine. In the past 10 years, c-ANCA and its relationship to WG has been studied. Clearly, this is a helpful test in WG, par-ticularly during active generalized disease, and may be confirma-tory. Because reports of false positives are increasing and because sensitivity varies from 30 to 90% in a clinician's diagnosis of WG, depending on extent of disease and disease activity level, the test cannot be used as a sole diagnostic criterion for WG. c-ANCA and more specific antibodies against PR-3 are somewhat analogous to a combination of antinuclear antibodies in SLE as a disease marker and anti-DNA in lupus as a disease activity marker. This topic con-tinues to attract much attention.

Radiologic imaging studies are helpful in diagnosing WG, includ-ing chest, sinus radiographs, and computed tomography. The differ-ential diagnosis is quite broad and depends on the patient's presen-tation. When the classic triad of involvement occurs, with confirmatory tissue biopsy and a positive c-ANCA, the diagnosis is easy. When the process is early and/or limited to upper airway or kidney, clinical challenge occurs. Destructive upper airway disease needs to be differentiated from infection such as fungal, mycobacte-rial, staphylococcal, syphilitic, substance abuse (particularly co-caine), malignancy (particularly T-cell lymphoma and squamous cell carcinoma), or rarely self-mutilating trauma. In the past, *idio-pathic midline granuloma* or idiopathic midline destructive disease was included in the differential diagnosis. Current investigators place this in the spectrum of *angiocentric immunoproliferative le-sions (AIL),* believed to be a prelude to lymphoma (see Part XIII).

Differential diagnosis of pulmonary involvement is broad but, particularly in combination with renal disease, should include Goodpasture's syndrome, SLE, lymphomatoid granulomatosis (also in the spectrum of AIL), infection (fungal, mycobacterial, bacterial), and malignancy.

TREATMENT AND PROGNOSIS. Optimal treatment for ac-tive WG, particularly with multisystem involvement including renal disease, includes cyclophosphamide and corticosteroids. Cyclophos-

TABLE 245–4. TREATMENT OF WEGENER'S GRANULOMATOSIS

	Indications	Initial dose	Monitoring	Duration
Cyclophosphamide	Moderate to severe	1–2 mg/kg/day (po)	CBC weekly; keep WBC >3000, PMN >1000 and monitor liver tests; urine cytology and/or cystoscopy if prolonged therapy	Approximately 1 year beyond clinical remission
	Fulminant	3–4 mg/kg/day IV for 2–3 day, then reduce to 2 mg/kg/day po or IV		
Corticosteroids	Moderate to severe	1 mg/kg/day prednisone equivalent (IV initially or po)	Glucose, lipids, bone density	Taper to low dose (5–10 mg/day) or alternate-day therapy over 2 months
Methotrexate	Mild to moderate; upper airway; or diffuse disease without significant renal involvement	Up to 15–25 mg once weekly	Monitor CBC and liver tests q 4–8 weeks	Taper to lowest dose controlling features; ? trial off 1 year past clinical remission; close follow-up
Antibiotics	Adjunctive, not primary, to treat secondary bacterial infections; consider chronic suppression in chronic upper airway disease (sulfa may be contraindicated with methotrexate)			Intermittent or chronic low-dose "prophylaxis"
Cyclosporine	Refractory disease; dialysis dependent; patients awaiting renal transplant	3–5 mg/kg/day	BP, chemistries (Cr, Mg)	1 year beyond clinical remission or until transplant

phamide is initiated in a dose of 1 to 2 mg per kilogram per day, with initially weekly monitoring of complete blood counts to keep total white count above 3.0 and neutrophil count above 1.0 to limit complications of infection due to neutropenia. The dose is adjusted based on blood counts, particularly as corticosteroids are tapered. The drug is generally continued for approximately 1 year beyond clinical remission, followed by discontinuation and close observation of the patient's clinical status, laboratory features, including blood counts, erythrocyte sedimentation rate, renal parameters, chest radiographs, and c-ANCA. This drug or alternative therapy is reinstituted in the case of recurrence or relapse. Complications include hemorrhagic cystitis (and thus patients should be instructed to drink at least 1.5 liters of liquids per day), bone marrow toxicity, infections, hair loss, nausea, infertility, and increased risk of malignancy (bladder carcinoma, leukemia, lymphoma).

Corticosteroids are used at the time of diagnosis for severe disease, initially at 1 mg per kilogram per day (may be used in divided dose, intravenous methylprednisolone for fulminant disease, followed by consolidation to daily or alternate-day therapy). Prednisone equivalent doses of 60 mg per day are then tapered to alternate-day therapy over 1 month and then to the lowest possible level to control upper airway and/or musculoskeletal symptoms, preferably discontinuing this drug by 3 to 6 months. The complications and side effects of corticosteroids are well known and provided elsewhere (see Ch. 18).

Whereas WG was once an invariably fatal disease, the combination of cyclophosphamide and prednisone has provided remission in 75% of all patients and improvement in 90%, as evidenced in the NIH series long-term follow-up studies. However, relapses occur in at least 50% of those achieving remission, at any time from several months to 15 to 20 years after stopping cytotoxic therapy. Thus, WG is a chronic disease and patients deserve close follow-up, patient and provider education, and sometimes creative therapeutic strategies.

Even though mortality due to WG and/or its therapy has improved significantly, disease-related morbidity occurs in the majority of patients, with chronic renal insufficiency, hearing loss, nasal deformity, tracheal stenosis, and ocular abnormalities leading the list. These also are reviewed thoroughly in the NIH series. More recently, alternative treatment strategies have been reported. Weekly low-dose (15 to 25 mg) oral or intramuscular methotrexate has provided hope and, owing to experience in the management of rheumatoid arthritis, may provide a less toxic alternative to cyclophosphamide in patients who relapse, particularly with significant upper airway disease. Azathioprine, pulse monthly cyclophosphamide, intravenous immunoglobulin, cyclosporine, and immune modulators have all been used in individual cases. Because of the relative infrequency of the disease, controlled, double-blind studies have not yet been performed.

An overview of treatment strategies is listed in Table 245–4. Antibiotic therapy has a role, but at present this is considered adjunctive, not primary therapy. Because of necrotic upper airway tissue, staphylococcal and other infections are quite common and could be part of the "chicken and egg" perpetuation of this condition. In WG patients taking immunosuppressives, fever, new pulmonary infiltrate, new headache, hematuria, and pyuria deserve careful evaluation for infection before symptoms are ascribed to disease flare.

Thus, WG is a multisystem, inflammatory, autoimmune disorder with a spectrum of clinical, laboratory, radiographic, and pathologic features, in which c-ANCA has been helpful diagnostically. Careful diagnosis, thoughtful management, and close follow-up are necessary for optimal outcome.

Gross WL (ed.): ANCA-Associated Vasculitides: Immunologic and Clinical Aspects. New York, Plenum Press, 1993. *Compilation of papers presented at the 2nd International Colloquium on Wegener's Granulomatosis and Vasculitic Disorders in Lubeck, Germany, in May 1992.*

Hoffman GS, Kerr GS, Leavitt RY, et al.: Wegener's granulomatosis: An analysis of 158 patients. Ann Intern Med 116:488, 1992. *Updated review of NIH series on WG, focusing on clinical manifestations, disease spectrum, chronicity, and morbidity/mortality issues.*

Hoffman GS, Leavitt RY, Kerr GS, et al.: The treatment of Wegener's granulomatosis with glucocorticoids and methotrexate. Arthritis Rheum 35:1322, 1992. *First article reviewing significant number of WG patients treated with MTX.*

Jennette JC, Falk RJ, Andrassy K, et al.: Nomenclature of systemic vasculitides. Arthritis Rheum 37:187, 1994. Lie JT: Nomenclature and classification of vasculitis:

Plus ca change, plus c'est la meme chose. Arthritis Rheum 37:181, 1994. *This pair of references provides point and counterpoint discussion of the classification of vasculitides. They are thought-provoking and interesting, providing perspective on Wegener's and other vasculitides in relation to diagnostic testing, particularly ANCA.*

Lieberman K, Churg A: Wegener's granulomatosis. In Churg A, Churg J (eds.): Systemic Vasculitides. New York, Igaku-Shoin, 1991, p 77. *A concise review of the topic with emphasis on pathologic findings. Beautiful color photomicrographs.*

246 POLYMYALGIA RHEUMATICA AND GIANT CELL ARTERITIS

Gene G. Hunder

Polymyalgia rheumatica and giant cell arteritis are common rheumatic diseases of middle-aged and older persons. Although the etiology of these conditions is unknown and their pathogenesis is poorly understood, it is clear that they are closely related. Some believe that a single agent causes both conditions and that host and other unknown factors determine whether a patient will develop one or both processes. A strong association with HLA-DR4 has been observed, indicating a hereditary link.

POLYMYALGIA RHEUMATICA

Polymyalgia rheumatica is characterized by aching and morning stiffness in the shoulder and hip girdles, the proximal extremities, the neck, and the torso. Usually, it is accompanied by evidence of an inflammatory reaction. The mean age at onset is about age 70, and it nearly always occurs after age 50, with women affected twice as commonly as men.

CLINICAL FINDINGS. Polymyalgia rheumatica may begin abruptly but usually develops gradually over a number of weeks. In mild or early cases, the symptoms may subside 1 to 2 hours after the patient arises in the morning, only to return later after a period of inactivity. Generally, the discomfort becomes severe enough to interfere with usual activities and may confine the patient to bed. Fatigue, loss of weight, and a low-grade fever may be present. Joint inflammation has been demonstrated in some cases, which supports the contention that polymyalgia rheumatica is a form of synovitis of the proximal joints and periarticular structures. Upon careful testing, muscle strength is found to be normal or nearly normal.

LABORATORY TESTS. A normochromic anemia is typical. Usually, the erythrocyte sedimentation rate is markedly elevated, averaging 70 to 80 mm in 1 hour (Westergren). Other acute-phase protein levels also are elevated. Some patients have mild hepatic dysfunction that reverts to normal with treatment. Other tests are normal.

INCIDENCE. Caucasians appear to be affected more frequently than other groups. The highest recorded incidence rates are from northern Europe and the northern United States. In one population study, the prevalence found was approximately 1 in 200 persons in the population aged 50 or older. Recent reports on incidence rates in Europe show similar findings.

DIAGNOSIS. Several criteria sets for diagnosing polymyalgia rheumatica have been suggested. Most are similar to those in Table 246–1. Morning stiffness should last at least one-half hour. The erythrocyte sedimentation rate is an indicator of systemic inflammation. An additional criterion of rapid response to 10 to 20 mg of prednisone per day is suggested by some. These criteria are only

TABLE 246–1. POLYMYALGIA RHEUMATICA: DIAGNOSTIC CRITERIA

>Age 50
Aching and morning stiffness in at least two of the following areas:
  Neck
  Shoulder girdle
  Pelvic girdle
Erythrocyte sedimentation rate (ESR) >40 mm in 1 hr
Duration of symptoms for 1 mo
No other disease present

TABLE 246–2. DIFFERENTIAL FEATURES IN POLYMYALGIA RHEUMATICA AND SIMILAR DISORDERS

	Polymyalgia Rheumatica	Giant Cell Arteritis	Rheumatoid Arthritis	Dermatomyositis	Fibromyalgia
Morning stiffness > 30 minutes	+	±	+*	±	Variable
Headache and/or scalp tenderness	0	+	0	0	Variable
Pain with active joint movement	+	0	+*	0	Inconstant
Tender joints	±	0	+*	0	Tender spots
Swollen joints	±	±	+	0	0
Muscle weakness	±†	0	+*	+	0
Normochromic anemia	+	+	+	0	0
Elevated ESR	+	+	+	±	0
Elevated serum creatine kinase	0	0	0	+	0
Serum rheumatoid factor	0	0	70%	0	0
Distinct electromyographic abnormality	0	0	0	+	0
Response to nonsteroidal anti-inflammatory drug (NSAID)	±	0	+	0	0

0 = absent, + = present, ± = present in minority of cases.
* = Associated with affected joints.
† = Pain inhibits movement. Disuse atrophy may occur.

guidelines, since patients occasionally have normal sedimentation rates at onset and may develop symptoms slightly before age 50.

DIFFERENTIAL DIAGNOSIS (Table 246–2). Some patients with early rheumatoid arthritis lack the more characteristic distal joint involvement and serum rheumatoid factor and have prominent proximal symptoms. In polymyositis, limitation is due to a lack of muscle strength; in polymyalgia rheumatica, limitation is due to pain. In polymyositis, muscle biopsy shows an inflammatory myopathy; in polymyalgia rheumatica, biopsy is normal or shows only atrophy.

Fibromyalgia usually affects younger individuals and tends to be associated with tender spots; laboratory tests are normal. When encouraged to do so, patients with fibromyalgia can move the joints through a full range of motion without great difficulty. Wakefulness in polymyalgia rheumatica is due to discomfort caused by movement in bed. In fibromyalgia, however, there is a more generalized, persistent discomfort that is less tangible.

Other conditions that occasionally need to be distinguished from polymyalgia rheumatica include chronic infections, such as subacute bacterial endocarditis or viral infections, malignancies, hypothyroidism, and other connective tissue diseases.

GIANT CELL ARTERITIS

Giant cell (temporal) arteritis affects large and medium-sized arteries, especially those branching from the proximal aorta that supply the neck and the extracranial structures of the head and arms. The lesions tend to be scattered irregularly along the involved vessels. A focal or diffuse granulomatous inflammatory infiltration is present with multinucleated histiocytic and foreign body giant cells, histiocytes, lymphocytes, and fibroblasts. Lymphocytes tend to be predominantly helper T cells.

CLINICAL FINDINGS. This disease affects the same population as polymyalgia rheumatica. The manifestations of giant cell arteritis are diverse, and many presentations have been described.

In most patients, symptoms or signs related to the vascular system develop at some time during the course of the disease (Table 246–3). Headache may be mild or severe. Scalp tenderness may be over the arteries of the head or at other sites.

Visual symptoms are present in about one third of patients; half are transient, and half are permanent. The former includes amaurosis fugax or diplopia. Permanent visual loss may be partial or complete and may occur without warning; about half are unilateral, and half are bilateral. The vision loss is due to narrowing or occlusion of the ophthalmic or posterior ciliary arteries.

Intermittent claudication occurs in about one half of patients, with the jaw muscles most frequently involved. During chewing of firm foods such as meat, fatigue or discomfort is noted. In a small percentage of patients, claudication of the tongue or throat develops with eating and repeated swallowing. Nervous system alterations are found in up to 30%; 14% have either mononeuritis or polyneuropathy, and 7% have transient ischemic attacks or strokes.

Polymyalgia rheumatica occurs in about 40% of patients with giant cell arteritis. It may precede other symptoms or become manifest only during the withdrawal of corticosteroid therapy given for the arteritis. Diffuse or asymmetric myalgias, arthralgias, or joint swelling may be present in other patients with giant cell arteritis.

PHYSICAL EXAMINATION. The temporal, occipital, or other scalp or cervical arteries may be enlarged, tender, and erythematous. Bruits or pulse deficits may be present over the carotid, subclavian, or brachial arteries. Large artery involvement may be present initially or later, as part of an exacerbation. Findings in the eyes of patients with recent visual loss include papilledema, hemorrhages, and exudates; later, optic atrophy develops.

LABORATORY TESTS. Blood tests are similar to those seen in polymyalgia rheumatica. The platelet count is generally increased. The erythrocyte sedimentation rate averages 80 to 100 mm in 1 hour (Westergren) but is occasionally normal.

INCIDENCE. Reported annual incidence rates have varied considerably and are highest (20 per 100,000) in persons age 50 and older in northern Europe and the United States. Although the reasons for the variable rates are unknown, ethnic and geographic factors have been suggested. Familial cases of giant cell arteritis and polymyalgia rheumatica have been reported. Giant cell arteritis appears to be one third as common as polymyalgia rheumatica.

DIAGNOSIS. Giant cell arteritis should be considered in any older person who has developed transient or sudden visual changes, unexplained fever, polymyalgia rheumatica or new headaches, and an elevated erythrocyte sedimentation rate. The arteries of the head, neck, and extremities should be examined carefully. Distinct tenderness, redness, and a palpable but nonpulsatile temporal artery are important clues to the presence of arteritis. In the absence of similar changes in the lower extremities, pulse changes or bruits over the

TABLE 246–3. GIANT CELL ARTERITIS: CLINICAL FINDINGS IN 94 PATIENTS*

Clinical Manifestation	Frequency (%)
Headache	77
Abnormal temporal artery	53
Jaw claudication	51
Scalp tenderness	47
Constitutional symptoms	48
Polymyalgia rheumatica	34
Fever	27
Respiratory symptoms	23
Facial pain	14
Diplopia/blurred vision	12
Transient vision loss	5
Blindness (partial or complete)	13
Hemoglobin < 11.0 gram/dl	24
Erythrocyte sedimentation rate > 40 mm/hr	97

* After Machado EBV, Michet CJ, Ballard DJ, et al.: Trends in incidence and clinical presentation of temporal arteritis in Olmsted County, Minnesota, 1950–1985. Arthritis Rheum 31:745–749, 1988.

axillary and brachial arteries are more likely to be caused by vasculitis than by arteriosclerosis.

A temporal artery biopsy is recommended for all patients suspected of having giant cell arteritis. A biopsy should be performed on the most clinically abnormal artery segment. When the arteries appear normal on examination, a segment several centimeters long should be removed from one temporal artery, and histologic sections should be examined at multiple levels in an effort to find an involved area. In the author's experience, if the first temporal artery biopsy is normal, the second side will yield approximately 10 to 15% additional positive cases.

Some patients with polymyalgia rheumatica may be followed carefully without a temporal artery biopsy. If polymyalgia rheumatica is of recent onset or has been present for a year or more in the absence of signs or symptoms of vasculitis, biopsy may be deferred and the patient should be followed closely.

DIFFERENTIAL DIAGNOSIS. Conditions that have been confused with giant cell arteritis include systemic infections, amyloidosis with prominent vascular involvement, neoplasms, arteriosclerotic vascular disease in patients with an elevated erythrocyte sedimentation rate that is due to some other cause, arteriovenous fistulas, and other forms of vasculitis.

Follow-up studies of patients who have had a negative temporal artery biopsy have shown that only approximately 10% develop findings of giant cell arteritis and require long-term corticosteroid therapy.

MANAGEMENT

Therapy for polymyalgia rheumatica is aimed at alleviating systemic symptoms and musculoskeletal discomfort. Corticosteroids are recommend for most patients with an initial daily dose of 10 to 20 mg of prednisone (or the equivalent dose of another corticosteroid). Prednisone acts rapidly, and the patient should notice significant improvement within 24 hours. The corticosteroid dose can be reduced as tolerated after one month or earlier. Nonsteroidal anti-inflammatory drugs may be added to control mild discomfort that may occur while corticosteroids are being withdrawn and discontinued.

In giant cell arteritis, the recommended dosage of prednisone is 40 to 60 mg per day. Vascular complications seldom occur after corticosteroids have been started. If the response to the initial dose of prednisone is incomplete, the dosage should be increased by 20 to 30 mg per day. Usually, if symptoms subside and laboratory values return to normal with a given dose, the disease process is adequately suppressed. Prednisone for both conditions may be administered as a single morning dose or in two to three divided doses per day.

The overall goal of therapy is to administer the lowest dose of corticosteroid that adequately controls the arteritis and prescribe it for the shortest necessary time. The dose needed to achieve control varies among patients and must be determined empirically. There is no evidence that corticosteroid therapy alters the natural course of the disease.

In a small proportion of cases, the corticosteroid dose cannot be reduced without an exacerbation of the disease. Cyclophosphamide, azathioprine, dapsone, and methotrexate have been reported as steroid-sparing drugs in some instances. However, no controlled studies of these drugs have been done. The average duration of both polymyalgia rheumatica and giant cell arteritis is about 2 years, during which time the intensity of the process may flare up at times but appears to resolve slowly. The course in individual patients, however, varies considerably, and some may continue with active symptoms for several years. Aortic aneurysm is a late complication of giant cell arteritis.

Aiello PD, Trautmann JC, McPhee TJ, et al.: Visual prognosis in giant cell arteritis. Ophthalmology 100:550, 1993. *A study of the ocular effects and outcome of vision in giant cell arteritis.*

Hunder GG, Lie JT, Goronzy JJ, Weyand CM: Pathogenesis of giant cell arteritis. Arthritis Rheum 36:757, 1993. *A critical review of factors involved in giant cell arteritis development.*

Weyand CM, Hicok KC, Hunder GG, Goronzy JJ: The HLA-DRB1 locus as a genetic component in giant cell arteritis. J Clin Invest 90:2355, 1992. *A disease-linked gene sequence is mapped to the binding site of the HLA-DR molecule.*

247 IDIOPATHIC INFLAMMATORY MYOPATHIES
Robert L. Wortmann

DEFINITION. The term "idiopathic inflammatory myopathy" represents a group of rare diseases of unknown cause that are characterized by symmetrical proximal muscle weakness and nonsuppurative inflammation of skeletal muscle. Specific diagnoses characterized by this term include polymyositis, dermatomyositis, cancer-associated myositis, myositis associated with another connective tissue disease (overlap syndromes), and inclusion-body myositis. Patients with any idiopathic inflammatory myopathy generally fulfill the criteria used to define polymyositis originally proposed in 1975 by Bohan and Peter (Table 247–1).

INCIDENCE. The idiopathic inflammatory myopathies are rare conditions, with an annual incidence ranging between 0.5 and 8.4 cases per 1 million population. The incidence is highest in blacks and lowest in Japanese. Women are generally more affected than men, with female predominance most pronounced between the ages of 15 and 44 and in persons having myositis associated with other connective tissue diseases. The gender ratio is equal in older age groups and in myositis associated with malignancy but is reversed in inclusion body myositis. Overall, the age of onset has a bimodal distribution with peaks in children between 10 and 14 and in adults between 45 and 54. The mean age of onset for the subset of myositides with other connective tissue diseases is similar to that for the associated condition. Individuals with myositis associated with malignancy or inclusion body myositis have a mean age over 60.

PATHOLOGY AND PATHOGENESIS. Abnormalities in skeletal muscle indicative of an idiopathic inflammatory myopathy include muscle fiber degeneration, regeneration, necrosis, phagocytosis, and mononuclear cell infiltration. In polymyositis, necrosis of single muscle fibers is common, and some non-necrotic fibers are invaded by T cells and macrophages. Collections of lymphocytes, plasma cells, and histiocytes are found primarily in the endomysium. Inflammatory aggregates contain high percentages of T cells but few B cells. Over time, fiber diameter variation increases, and interstitial fibrosis develops. Although abnormalities in muscle from patients with dermatomyositis may be similar to those in polymyositis, more commonly the inflammatory cells are grouped in the perimysium with a perivascular distribution and contain a higher percentage of B cells. In the childhood variety of dermatomyositis, vasculopathy, including endothelial hyperplasia, infarction, and perifascicular atrophy, is common, and deposition of IgG, IgM, and C3 occurs, particularly within the walls of intramuscular arteries and veins. In inclusion body myositis, light microscopy reveals inflammatory changes similar to those in polymyositis with the additional feature of characteristic intracellular vacuoles. The vacuoles are lined with basophilic granules on cryostat sections and eosinophilic material on paraffin sections. Intracytoplasmic or intranuclear

TABLE 247–1. CRITERIA USED TO DEFINE IDIOPATHIC INFLAMMATORY MYOPATHY*

1. Symmetrical weakness of limb girdle muscles and anterior neck flexors with or without dysphagia.
2. Elevation in serum of skeletal muscle enzymes, especially creative phosphokinase (CPK).
3. Electromyographic changes consistent with inflammatory myopathy: short, small polyphasic motor units; fibrillations; positive waves; and bizarre high-frequency repetitive discharges.
4. Muscle biopsy evidence of fiber necrosis, phagocytosis, and regeneration; variation in fiber size; and inflammatory exudate.

Note: Patients are classified as having definite disease with four, probable disease with three, and possible disease with two.

* These criteria were originally proposed in 1975 by Bohan and Peter to define polymyositis. At that time, the term "polymyositis" was used to represent a specific disease as well as a general term representing all the recognized forms of inflammatory myopathy.

tubulofilamentous inclusions are also seen with electron microscopy. These inclusions are straight, rigid, and have periodic striations resembling paramyxovirus. Using immunolocalization techniques, ubiquitin and β-amyloid protein (two proteins that have been identified in the plaques in brains from patients with Alzheimer's disease) have been observed in the vacuoles and tubulofilamentous inclusions.

The idiopathic inflammatory myopathies are believed to be immune-mediated processes that are triggered by environmental factors in genetically susceptible individuals. This is in part based on the prevalence of autoantibodies, inflammatory pathology, association with other autoimmune diseases, and response to corticosteroid therapy.

Many patients with idiopathic inflammatory myopathies have circulating autoantibodies (Table 247–2). Some are termed "myositis-specific autoantibodies" (MSA's) and are seen only in patients with polymyositis or dermatomyositis; others are those associated with other connective tissue diseases. Most MSA's are directed against cytoplasmic antigens and bind to evolutionary conserved epitopes. The percentage of patients with polymyositis and dermatomyositis who have circulating MSA's is uncertain, but estimates range between 10 and 50%. Eight different MSA's have been described. No more than one MSA has been found in an individual patient. The more common MSA's are directed against aminoacyl-tRNA (transfer RNA) synthetases and inhibit the activity of the respective antigenic enzyme protein *in vitro*. The most prevalent antisynthetase antibody is directed against histidyl-tRNA synthetase and is called "anti-Jo-1." Certain picornaviruses can substitute for tRNA and interact with aminoacyl-tRNA synthetase enzymes. Interestingly, there is some homology between amino acid sequences near the active site of histidyl-tRNA synthetase (Jo-1) and some capsid proteins in encephalomyocarditis virus, a picornavirus that induces a mouse model of polymyositis. Thus antibodies initially directed against virus or a virus-enzyme complex could cross-react with homologous areas of host proteins or the enzyme itself. This process is termed "molecular mimicry" and could explain the autoantibody production.

Several observations emphasize the importance of genetic factors in general and class II antigens in particular in the pathogenesis of inflammatory myopathy (see Ch. 229). Almost 50% of patients with polymyositis and dermatomyositis have the HLA-DR3 (HLA, human leukocyte antigen) phenotype. This is almost always linked with HLA-B8 and is most common in patients with anti-Jo-1 antibodies. HLA-DR52 is found in over 90% of patients who have myositis and anti-Jo-1 antibodies. The prevalence of the DR1 phenotype is increased compared with controls in inclusion body myositis.

Viruses, particularly picornaviruses, have been implicated as causes of myositis. Several viruses, especially coxsackie A9, have been associated with myositis in individual cases; elevated titers to coxsackievirus have been found in childhood dermatomyositis; mumps virus antigen has been demonstrated in inclusions in inclusion body myositis; and certain viral infections can induce inflammatory myopathy in mice, with inflammation persisting long after virus can be detected.

The pathologic changes in polymyositis and inclusion body myositis appear to result from cell-mediated, antigen-specific cytotoxicity. In these disorders, non-necrotic muscle fibers are found surrounded by and invaded by CD8+ mononuclear cells, with cytotoxic cells outnumbering suppresser cells by a ratio of 4:1. Studies of circulating mononuclear cells reveal decreased percentages of cells expressing CD8 and increases in those expressing the class II HLA antigen DR, as well as other T-cell activation antigens (interleukin-2 receptors; Ta-1, an activation marker also associated with anamnestic responses; and TLiSA-1, a late marker associated with cytotoxic T-cell differentiation). Different immune mechanisms are evident in dermatomyositis. Mononuclear cell invasion of non-necrotic fibers is rare, cellular infiltration is predominantly perivascular, B cells outnumber T cells, and the CD4/CD8 ratio is higher. In the circulation, DR+ cells and B cells (CD20+ cells) are increased, whereas T cells (CD3+ cells) are decreased. These findings indicate that humoral mechanisms play a significant role in the pathogenesis of dermatomyositis.

Loss of muscle fibers as a result of the immune response may contribute to muscle weakness in some patients with an idiopathic inflammatory myopathy. However, other factors also must be involved because weakness occurs in the presence of histology that has no inflammatory infiltrate or fiber necrosis. These observations suggest that abnormalities of the contractile process may underlie the muscle weakness. Energy (ATP) is required for normal muscle contraction and relaxation as well as the maintenance of membrane integrity. Altered muscle energy metabolism has been demonstrated *in vitro* using a coxsackievirus B1–induced mouse model of inflammatory myopathy. Muscles from these mice have increased glycolytic activity compared with controls as well as decreased activities of myophosphorylase and myoadenylate deaminase. A secondary deficiency of myoadenylate deaminase activity has been observed in muscle from some patients with polymyositis. *In vivo* ^{31}P magnetic resonance spectrographic studies of patients with polymyositis and dermatomyositis have shown lower levels of high-energy phosphate–containing compounds at rest, faster depletion of ATP with exercise, and slower recovery rates compared with normal individuals. These abnormalities reverse as patients improve with therapy, particularly in dermatomyositis. These studies support the hypothesis that metabolic changes contribute to the muscle weakness in the inflammatory myopathies.

CLINICAL MANIFESTATIONS. The onset of an idiopathic inflammatory myopathy is usually insidious, with no identified precipitating event. The cardinal feature of any inflammatory myopathy is symmetrical muscle weakness of shoulder and pelvic girdles, at times accompanied by mild pain and tenderness. Weakness of proximal leg and arm muscles, neck flexors, and pharyngeal muscles may follow. Early symptoms include difficulty getting up from a chair, climbing stairs, and using one's hands above shoulder level. Dysphagia, dysphonia, and dysarthria may develop when the disease affects the pharynx. Morning stiffness, fatigue, and other systemic symptoms are common. Arthralgias are noted with active disease, but frank synovitis is quite rare. With progression, weakness can become so severe that patients cannot lift their extremities against gravity, involved muscles become atrophic, and contractures develop. An explosive onset with rhabdomyolysis, myoglobinuria, and renal failure is rare. Typically, the neurologic examination is normal except for the motor component. Deep tendon reflexes are normal or appear slightly decreased because of muscle weakness. Cranial nerve function is normal. Dysphagia is primarily due to weakness of striated musculature in the posterior pharynx and is often associated with a poor prognosis. Patients may have difficulty swallowing liquids, are prone to aspiration, and may have nasal

TABLE 247–2. AUTOANTIBODIES FOUND IN PATIENTS WITH IDIOPATHIC INFLAMMATORY MYOPATHY

Autoantibody	Clinical Association
Myositis-specific autoantibodies	
Anti-tRNA synthetases	PM with interstitial
Anti-Jo-1	lung disease, arthritis,
Anti-PL-7	and fever; less
Anti-PL-12	common in DM
Anti-OJ	
Anti-EJ	
Anti-SRP	PM with poor prognosis
Anti-MAS	PM after alcoholic rhabdomyolysis
Anti-Mi-2	DM
Antinuclear antibodies associated with other connective tissue diseases	
Anti-SM	SLE
Anti-RNP	SLE, MCTD
Anti-SSA (anti-Ro)	SLE, Sjögren's syndrome
Anti-SSB (anti-La)	SLE, Sjögren's syndrome
Anti-centromere	CREST syndrome
Anti-SCL70	Scleroderma
Anti-PM-1	Scleroderma
Anti-Ku	Scleroderma

Anti-SRP = anti-signal recognition particle; PM = polymyositis; DM = dermatomyositis; SLE = systemic lupus erythematosus; MCTD = mixed (undifferentiated) connective tissue disease; CREST = *c*alcinosis, *R*aynaud's *e*sophageal dysmotility, *s*clerodactyly, *t*elangiectasia.

speech. These symptoms may be accentuated by spasm or fibrosis of cricopharyngeal muscles and may require surgical treatment. Esophageal dysfunction may occur but is not often clinically insignificant.

Pulmonary manifestations develop in some patients due to hypoventilation secondary to muscle weakness, swallowing abnormalities with aspiration, and infection. Approximately 5 to 10% develop interstitial lung disease (see Ch. 54). Some patients with interstitial pneumonitis have no respiratory symptoms, but others experience nonproductive cough and dyspnea, which may precede the onset of muscle weakness. The restrictive lung disease is associated with bibasilar fine crackles on chest auscultation and reduced diffusion capacity. Symptomatic cardiac problems are unusual, although conduction abnormalities and tachyarrhythmias may be seen on electrocardiograms. Congestive heart failure can result from hypoxemia, pulmonary hypertension, or cardiomyopathy. Raynaud's phenomenon is reported in a small percentage of patients (see Ch. 46).

Patients with polymyositis may develop periorbital edema. When other cutaneous manifestations are seen, the disease is termed "dermatomyositis." Typically, the rash is erythematous and appears on the face, neck, chest, and extensor surfaces of the extremities. The name "Gottron's patches" is given to raised, red to violet, scaly patches seen over the knuckles, elbows, and knees. A heliotrope rash on the upper eyelids is very characteristic. The term "mechanic's hands" is applied to the darkened or dirty-appearing horizontal lines that develop across the lateral and palmer aspects of the fingers (because of the similarity to changes seen in hands of people who do manual labor). Capillary nailfold changes are present in some individuals, especially those with Raynaud's phenomenon. These include dilated or distorted capillary loops sometimes alternating with avascular areas. Dermatomyositis in children is sometimes referred to by the specific term "childhood dermatomyositis." Childhood dermatomyositis is similar to dermatomyositis in adults, except that vascular involvement is more prominent. Fever, weight loss, and subcutaneous calcifications are more common, and gastrointestinal tract hemorrhage or perforation may occur.

When myositis occurs in association with another connective tissue or autoimmune disease, the associated conditions may dominate the clinical picture. The most frequently associated disease is systemic lupus erythematosus (SLE), but others include scleroderma, rheumatoid arthritis, polyarteritis nodosa, giant cell arteritis, autoimmune thyroid disease, insulin-dependent diabetes mellitus, dermatitis herpetiformis, myasthenia gravis, and primary biliary cirrhosis.

Approximately 20% of adults with polymyositis or dermatomyositis also have cancer. Although this may seem higher than expected for the general population, there appears to be no significant difference in the frequency of malignancy when compared with appropriate age-matched control populations. Most often the myositis and malignancy are diagnosed within a year of each other. In general, the type of the neoplasm is that expected for the patient's age. Overall, the most commonly associated tumors are of breast and lung. Ovarian and stomach cancers occur more frequently than in the general population; rectal and colon cancers are less frequent. Neoplastic disease is less common in patients with interstitial lung disease or in those with an associated connective tissue disease.

Inclusion body myositis occurs most commonly in older men and can differ from polymyositis by the additional features of distal muscle weakness, asymmetrical muscle involvement, and neuropathic findings or physical examination and electromyography.

CLINICAL COURSE AND PROGNOSIS. The overall 5-year survival rate is approximately 80%, with children having the best prognosis. About half of surviving patients with polymyositis or dermatomyositis essentially recover completely. Older patients, those with associated neoplasms, or those with significant pulmonary, cardiac, and gastrointestinal involvement have a poorer prognosis. Patients with antibodies to aminoacyl-tRNA synthetases (i.e., anti-Jo-1) have a very high prevalence of interstitial lung disease, arthritis, and fever and do not respond well to therapy. Those with circulating anti-SRP (SRP, signal recognition particle) antibodies have a high prevalence of Raynaud's and the worst prognosis of any subset. Although most patients with inclusion body myositis do not improve with therapy, their survival appears to be good. Typically, the weakness progresses very slowly and may become fixed in some cases.

LABORATORY DATA. Serum levels of muscle-derived enzymes are elevated at some time during the course of the disease in 99% of patients. Creatine phosphokinase (CPK) levels are the most sensitive, but levels of aldolase, aminotransferase (AST and ALT), and lactate dehydrogenase (LDH) are also useful. CPK levels can be used as an index of disease activity or therapeutic response in some but not all patients. When normal CPK values are encountered in the presence of active disease, possible explanations include circulating enzyme inhibitors, a possible associated malignancy, or longstanding disease with severe muscle atrophy. The MB isoenzyme of CPK may be increased in the absence of cardiac involvement due to the expression of that isoform in regenerating skeletal muscle fibers.

The erythrocyte sedimentation rate remains normal in over half the patients and when elevated does not correlate with the degree of weakness. Complete blood count, urinalysis, and other chemistries are usually normal unless there is an associated connective tissue disease or neoplasm.

Circulating autoantibodies are common in patients with idiopathic inflammatory myopathies (see Table 247–2). The most common MSA, anti-Jo-1, is found in polymyositis and less commonly in dermatomyositis. Certain antinuclear antibodies may herald an associated connective tissue disease: anti-SM and anti–double-stranded DNA for SLE; anti-SSA and anti-SSB for Sjögren's syndrome; anticentromere for CREST syndrome; and anti-PM-1, anti-Ku, and anti-SCL70 for scleroderma.

The electromyogram (EMG) is abnormal in 90% of patients. Classic changes include the triad of (1) small-amplitude, short-duration, polyphasic motor unit potentials; (2) fibrillation, positive waves, and increased insertional irritability; and (3) spontaneous bizarre high-frequency discharges. The complete triad may be found in only 40% of patients and in some patients changes are restricted to paraspinal muscles.

DIAGNOSIS AND DIFFERENTIAL DIAGNOSIS. Criteria are useful in establishing the diagnosis of an idiopathic inflammatory myopathy (see Table 247–1). These criteria can be used only after other causes are excluded, because no change or test is specific for the diagnosis. CPK elevation can occur in a wide number of conditions, as well as with blunt or sharp trauma, aerobic exercise, EMG studies, muscle biopsies, or drugs such as barbiturates or narcotics that retard the elimination of CPK from the serum. Normal blacks have higher levels of CPK than whites, frequently with values above the normals established for large populations. The EMG changes seen in polymyositis are not specific. Even in the classic case, the change can only be considered myopathic and consistent with inflammation. The EMG is useful in identifying areas of abnormality to be biopsied, but biopsy should not include the actual site of EMG needle insertion. Because of the symmetrical nature of this disease, it is best to limit the EMG to one side of the body and biopsy the other side. Magnetic resonance imaging (MRI) may provide an effective, noninvasive means for identifying the site for biopsy and for following the course of the disease, especially in dermatomyositis. Although the possibility of malignancy should be considered in each patient with myositis, extensive undirected testing is not advised. Clues to the coexistence of neoplastic disease are almost always apparent on history, physical examination, or routine laboratory tests. Routine screening should be that which is appropriate for the patient's age and sex.

A variety of other diseases may cause muscle weakness (Table 247–3), and patients with these may fulfill some or all four criteria for polymyositis (see Table 247–1); thus these diagnoses must be excluded before the diagnosis of an idiopathic inflammatory myopathy can be made. A careful history and physical examination coupled with the judicious use of laboratory tests allow one to sort through the extensive differential list efficiently. For example, a careful review of medication use may reveal an agent that induces muscle injury such as alcohol, chloroquine, corticosteroids, cimetidine, colchicine, lovastatin, penicillamine, or zidovudine (AZT). On physical examination, asymmetrical weakness and distal extremity involvement, as well as abnormal reflexes, altered sensation, or cranial nerve abnormalities, should suggest a neurologic disease. Patients with inclusion body myositis may prove the exception, because a subset may have distal or asymmetrical muscle involvement. Inclusion body myositis also may be difficult to separate from some cases of muscular dystrophy, but in the latter, family history is usually present, symptoms begin earlier in life, and the muscles involved differ.

TABLE 247-3. DIFFERENTIAL DIAGNOSIS OF MUSCLE WEAKNESS

Collagen-Vascular
Polymyositis
Dermatomyositis
Inclusion body myositis
Polymyalgia rheumatica
Temporal arteritis
Rheumatoid arthritis
Systemic lupus erythematosus
Polyarteritis nodosa
Scleroderma
Adult Still's disease
Eosinophilic fasciitis

Endocrine
Hypothyroidism
Hyperthyroidism
Hyperparathyroidism
Hypocalcemia
Cushing's disease
Addison's disease
Aldosteronism
Malabsorption
Diabetic amyotrophy

Infectious
Influenza, coxsackie, HIV, and other viruses
Infectious mononucleosis
Rickettsia
Toxoplasmosis
Trichinella
Schistosomiasis
Bacterial toxins
  Staphylococcal
  Streptococcal
  Clostridial

Toxic (Drug-Related)
Alcohol
Chloroquine/hydroxychloroquine
Clofibrate
Cocaine
Colchicine
Cromolyn
Cyclosporine
Emetine
Gemfibrozil
L-Tryptophan
Lovastatin
Penicillamine
Zidovudine (AZT)

Psychosomatic
Hysterical (?)

Miscellaneous
Hypereosinophilic syndromes
Rhabdomyolysis
Sarcoidosis
Fibromyalgia

Neurologic
Denervating disorders
  Amyotrophic lateral sclerosis
Neuromuscular junction disorders
  Myasthenia gravis
  Eaton-Lambert syndrome
Muscular dystrophies
  Limb-girdle
  Becker's syndrome
  Duchenne's syndrome
Neuropathies
  Guillain-Barré syndrome
  Diabetes mellitus
  Porphyria

Metabolic-Nutritional
Uremia
Hepatic failure
Hypercalcemia
Hypocalcemia
Hyperkalemia
Hypokalemia
Hypernatremia
Hyponatremia
Hypomagnesemia
Hypophosphatemia
Periodic paralysis
Vitamin D deficiency
Vitamin E deficiency

Carcinomatous
Neuropathy
Neuromyopathy
Myositis
Microembolization
Eaton-Lambert syndrome

Inherited Deficiency States
Glycogen storage diseases
  McArdle's syndrome (myophosphorylase)
  Phosphofructokinase
  Debrancher enzyme
  Brancher enzyme
  Phosphoglycerate kinase
  Phosphoglycerate mutase
  Lactate dehydrogenase
  Acid maltase
Lipid disorders
  Carnitine (primary and secondary)
  Carnitine palmitoyl-transferase
Purine disorders
  Myoadenylate deaminase
Mitochondrial myopathies

TABLE 247-4. PROTOCOL FOR FOREARM ISCHEMIC EXERCISE TESTING

Procedure

Venous blood samples are drawn for ammonia and lactate levels from non-dominant arm, preferably without a tourniquet.
A sphygmomanometer is inflated around the upper dominant arm to at least 20 mm HG above systolic pressure.
The subject then squeezes the dominant hand as vigorously as possible at a rate of one squeeze every 2 seconds for 2 minutes.
After 2 minutes of exercise, the cuff is deflated.
Two minutes after the cuff is deflated, venous samples are taken from the dominant arm for lactate and ammonia levels.

Interpretation

Normal individuals exercising with maximal effort increase lactate and ammonia levels at least threefold over baseline values. Individuals with a glycogen storage disease elevate ammonia levels normally but cannot raise lactate levels. Myoadenylate deaminase-deficient individuals raise lactate levels, but ammonia levels remain at baseline values. Falsely abnormal results may be obtained if the subject does not exercise with sufficient intensity. Abnormal results must be confirmed by a muscle biopsy to confirm the putative diagnosis.

TREATMENT. During the active stage of the disease, bed rest is essential, and physical therapy with passive range-of-motion exercises should be performed to maintain function and avoid contractures. Smoking is prohibited, and the head of the bed should be elevated in patients at risk for aspiration. Antacids or H$_2$ antagonists also may be useful to raise the pH of gastric fluids.

Treatment with corticosteroids is empiric but the standard. Initially, prednisone is used in single daily doses of 1 to 2 mg per kilogram. In responsive patients, muscle strength usually improves in 1 to 2 months, and the CPK normalizes in 3 months. Daily high-dose prednisone should be continued until strength has remained normal for 3 to 6 weeks. Once remission is attained, steroids are tapered very gradually, a process that may require up to 2 years. Alternate-day steroid use is recommended only when the disease is under excellent control.

Steroid failures may be attributed to inadequate initial dosage, tapering too quickly, inaccurate diagnosis, or an associated malignancy, refractory disease, or coincident steroid myopathy. An improvement in muscle strength when the steroid dose is raised indicates active disease; improved strength with a lower dose of steroid implicates steroid myopathy. Immunosuppressive agents are used in patients who do not respond adequately to corticosteroids. Daily oral azathioprine and weekly oral or parenteral methotrexate are the usual next choices. Cyclophosphamide, chlorambucil, cyclosporine, and intravenous immunoglobulin have been used in refractory cases. Only a small percentage of patients with inclusion body myositis achieve remission with steroid or other immunosuppressive therapy. Despite this poor prognosis, a therapeutic trial is indicated because remission occurs in some cases and progression may be delayed in others. However, if some benefit is not observed, drug therapy should be discontinued in order to avoid side effects and toxicity.

Love LA, Leff RL, Fraser DD, et al.: A new approach to the classification of idiopathic inflammatory myopathy: Myositis-specific autoantibodies define useful homogeneous patient groups. Medicine 70:360, 1991. *Review of 212 patients with idiopathic inflammatory myopathies, comparing them when classified by the traditional scheme versus when classified on the basis of myositis-specific antibodies.*
Plotz PH: Not myositis: A series of chance encounters. JAMA 268:2074, 1992. *Describes six cases that were confused with myositis, emphasizing the large number of conditions to be considered in the differential diagnosis of the idiopathic inflammatory myopathies.*
Sayers ME, Chou SM, Calabrese LH: Inclusion body myositis: Analysis of 32 cases. J Rheumatol 19:1385, 1992. *Review of clinical finding in larger series of this rare disease and discussion of expectations for therapy.*
Targoff IN: Autoantibodies in polymyositis. Rheum Dis Clin North Am 18:455, 1992. *Detailed review of the myositis-specific antibodies as well as autoantibodies associated with other connective tissue diseases.*
Wortmann RL: Inflammatory diseases of muscle. In Kelley WN, Harris ED Jr, Ruddy S, et al. (eds.), Textbook of Rheumatology. 4th ed. Philadelphia, WB Saunders, 1993, p 1159. *In-depth review of the inflammatory myopathies.*
Wortmann RL: Inflammatory muscle disease. In Weisman M, Weinblatt M (eds.), Drug Therapy for the Rheumatic Diseases. Philadelphia, WB Saunders, 1994. *Current status of treatments used.*

Serum electrolytes (sodium, potassium, calcium, phosphorous, and magnesium) should be measured. An abnormality of any electrolyte may interfere with the normal function of muscle fibers and result in weakness or myalgias. Uncovering an electrolyte abnormality usually reveals a reversible myopathy, especially if the cause of the electrolyte disturbance is identified. Some inherited metabolic myopathies can mimic inflammatory myopathy. Individuals with glycogen storage diseases such as myophosphorylase deficiency (McArdle's disease) or phosphofructokinase deficiency, as well as some with carnitine deficiency or myoadenylate deaminase deficiency, have proximal muscle weakness, elevated CPK levels, and myopathic EMG abnormalities. A forearm ischemic exercise test can be used to screen for the glycogen storage diseases and myoadenylate deaminase deficiency (Table 247-4).

248 THE AMYLOID DISEASES
Louis W. Heck

DEFINITION. Amyloidosis is not one clinical entity but a group of diverse structurally driven protein deposition diseases. They are similar in that protein deposition occurs extracellularly and these deposits stain eosinophilic using standard tissue histologic stains, bind Congo red dye, and emit an apple-green birefringence using polarized light microscopy; exhibit metachromasia with crystal violet; and have an array of 75- to 100-Å nonbranching fibrils by electron microscopy and a twisted β-pleated sheet antiparallel configuration by x-ray crystallography. They differ, however, in the biochemical nature of the proteinaceous deposits, the "etiology" of the associated diseases (neoplastic, inflammatory, degenerative, hereditary), the tropism of protein deposition, and the spectrum of disease manifestations. Thus amyloidosis is not a single disease but a variety of diseases ranging from the asymptomatic patient who has a focal deposit discovered as an incidental finding to generalized involvement with severe multiorgan failure.

Prior to the early 1970's, all amyloid deposits were thought to be chemically identical despite the clinical observations that systemic amyloidosis occurred in certain patients with either plasma cell myeloma or diverse chronic inflammatory states such as tuberculosis, osteomyelitis, rheumatoid arthritis (RA), ankylosing spondylitis, and Crohn's disease. The major breakthrough in the physicochemical characterization of amyloid proteins resulted from the discovery that many of the nonamyloid proteins in amyloid-laden tissue could be extracted using physiologic saline and the insoluble amyloid fibrils solubilized using dilute aqueous solutions and/or chemotropic agents such as urea and guanidine, isolated using column chromatography, and biochemically defined using amino acid sequence analysis. By studying amyloid-laden tissues and using the aforementioned techniques, many different amyloid proteins and precursor proteins associated with clinical syndromes or specific diseases have been identified (Table 248–1).

All the monomeric amyloidogenic proteins have a β-pleated sheet conformation in solution, and many have been demonstrated to form insoluble β-pleated sheet fibrils *in vitro*. The known properties of tissue amyloid deposits such as binding to Congo red, resistance to proteolysis, and insolubility in physiologic solutions are directly attributed to the periodic β-pleated sheet motif. The formation of β-pleated sheets *in vivo* is an extremely complex process involving crucial ion concentrations and hydrogen bonding between many similar monomeric polypeptide chains at high focal concentrations as well as molecular interactions with the myriad extracellular matrix components. Furthermore, most amyloid deposits contain P-component, an acute-phase circulating serum protein.

There is no satisfactory clinical classification of the amyloidoses. One method is to consider three major systemic forms—AA, AL, and ATTR; two major localized forms—Aβ₂ and Aβ; and several miscellaneous forms (Table 248–1). There are many clinical features of each form.

PATHOGENESIS AND CLINICAL MANIFESTATIONS. *Primary (AL) Amyloidosis.* This was the first amyloid protein defined biochemically and shown to be identical to the variable region of immunoglobulin light chain (Bence Jones protein). It is the most common of the systemic amyloidoses in the United States and is associated with plasma cell myeloma (20%) or plasma cell dyscrasias (80%) with involvement of skin and subcutaneous tissue, nerve, liver, spleen, heart, kidney, and lung. In a large retrospective series of AL patients, approximately 50% had presenting symptoms of fatigue and weight loss; less frequent symptoms included peripheral edema, dyspnea, paresthesias, lightheadedness, and hoarseness. Initial physical findings revealed a palpable liver and peripheral edema in one third to one half of the patients. Orthostatic hypotension, purpura, macroglossia, palpable spleen, skin papules, ecchymoses, and lymphadenopathy were found less commonly. The signs and symptoms result from amyloid infiltration of organs and tissues with subsequent dysfunction. Examples of syndromes include those related to nerve tissue such as carpal tunnel syndrome, peripheral neuropathy with paresthesias of the fingers and toes, and sympathetic dysfunction manifested by orthostatic hypotension, impotence, sweating abnormalities, and gastrointestinal disturbances due to autonomic nerve involvement and those related to congestive heart failure with either predominant right-sided failure with restrictive cardiomyopathy (see Ch. 43) with stiff, noncompliant ventricles and thick intraventricular septum (multiple discrete 3- to 5-mm highly refractile echoes with a "speckled" pattern on two-dimensional echocardiogram) or, rarely, a dilated cardiomyopathy with biventricular failure. Both forms may be associated with conduction disturbances. Renal involvement with albuminuria and the full expression of nephrotic syndrome (see Ch. 79), and slow progressive renal failure may be seen. Finally, ecchymoses and "pinch purpura" may result from minor skin trauma due to increased fragility from amyloid infiltration of the small blood vessels.

Secondary (AA) Amyloidosis. This was the second systemic type of amyloidosis shown to be due to protein deposition—in this case the precursor protein is a serum component (SAA) synthesized in the liver that may increase 100- to 200-fold following an inflam-

TABLE 248–1. NOMENCLATURE AND CLASSIFICATION OF THE AMYLOIDOSES, 1990

		Amyloid Protein	Clinical State(s)	Major Organ/Tissue Involvement*

Major systemic amyloidoses	1.	AA	1. Chronic inflammatory conditions
			  a. Infectious: tuberculosis, osteomyelitis, etc.
			  b. Noninfectious: juvenile rheumatoid arthritis, ankylosing spondylitis, Crohn's disease, etc.
			2. Familial Mediterranean fever
				K, L, S, GI, Sc
				H, unusual
				N, rare

	2.	AL	Plasma cell dyscrasia
			  10% multiple myeloma/macroglobulemia
			  90% idiopathic, "primary"
				H, L, S, T
				N, GI, Sc

	3.	ATTR	Various familial polyneuropathies and cardiomyopathies	N, H, K, E, GI, Sc
Major localized amyloidoses	4.	Aβ₂M	Chronic dialysis usually greater than 8 years	B, Sy, Ts
	5.	Aβ	1. Alzheimer's disease 2. Down syndrome 3. Hereditary cerebral hemorrhage, Dutch 4. Nontraumatic cerebral hemorrhage of elderly	C, CV
Miscellaneous amyloidoses	6.	A Apo AI	Familial polyneuropathy, Iowa	N, K
	7.	A Gel	Familial amyloidosis, Finnish	CN, E, Skin
	8.	A Cys	Hereditary cerebral hemorrhage, Icelandic	C, CV
	9.	A Scr	Creutzfeldt-Jakob disease	C
	10.	A Cal	Medullary carcinoma of thyroid	Th
	11.	AANF	Atrial amyloid	H
	12.	AIAPP	Diabetes mellitus, insulinomas	P

* B = bone; C = cerebrum; CN = cranial nerves; CV = cerebral vessels; E = eye; GI = gastrointestinal; H = heart; K = kidney; L = liver; N = nerve; P = pancreas; S = spleen; Sc = subcutaneous tissue; T = tongue; Th = thyroid; Ts = tenosynovium; Sy = synovium.

matory stimulus. Certain monocyte/macrophage cytokines such as interleukin-1 (IL-1), tumor necrosis factor, and IL-6 may up-regulate hepatic gene expression of this protein. Secondary amyloidosis usually involves the liver, spleen, and kidneys; heart involvement is less frequent than seen in primary amyloidosis; and nerve involvement is very infrequent. Some of the associated infectious diseases include osteomyelitis, tuberculosis, and bronchiectasis, and some of the noninfectious inflammatory states include RA, juvenile rheumatoid arthritis, ankylosing spondylitis, Crohn's disease, and familial Mediterranean fever. Curiously, the renal disease may be slow and indolent, with progressive proteinuria evolving into nephrotic syndrome and persisting for 5 to 10 years before end-stage renal disease. In Europe, renal amyloidosis has been reported as the major cause of death in juvenile rheumatoid arthritis patients, but this associated complication has not been seen in the United States. Another interesting observation is that AA may be resorbed *in vivo,* as manifested by reduction of an enlarged liver or spleen or reduction in proteinuria without defined treatment of the underlying disorder. Finally, the successful use of colchicine to reduce the attacks and development of amyloidosis in familial Mediterranean fever patients and decrease proteinuria and improve renal function in some cases mandates that AA be considered carefully and ruled out in all amyloid patients.

Familial (ATTR) Amyloidosis. This was the third systemic amyloidosis to be defined and shown to be associated with the presence of an abnormal plasma prealbumin protein, which normally functions to transport thyroxine and retinol-binding protein and subsequently was termed *transthyretin.* It was defined originally as an autosomal dominant inherited peripheral neuropathy (see Ch. 451) occurring in middle to late life that was progressive over the next several decades with additional autonomic neuropathy and variable organ involvement, primarily in Portuguese patients. Subsequently, many clinical manifestations defining different kindred in Europe and the United States have resulted from mutations in the gene for transthyretin with amino acid substitutions in this transport molecule, which have been associated with variable amyloid infiltration in heart, bowel, and kidney.

Dialysis-Related (β_2-Microglobulin) Amyloidosis (AB$_2$M). This localized amyloidosis occurs in most patients on maintenance hemodialysis or peritoneal dialysis for longer than 8 years and is due to the deposition of β_2-microglobulin amyloid in the periarticular, joint, bone, and carpal tunnel tissue. Some of the rheumatic complaints/findings include chronic shoulder pain with tenderness over the subacromial bursae, pain and swelling of the wrist and finger joints, proliferative tenosynovium over the wrist extensor tendons, and radiographic evidence of subchondral erosions of the carpal bones, femur, and humerus. Pathologic fractures of the humerus and femur have been described.

β_2-microglobulin is the noncovalently associated β chain of class I MHC molecules, which is present on virtually all human nucleated cells. The catabolism of this small protein depends on normal kidney filtration and excretion. In dialysis patients and those with end-stage renal disease, plasma levels of β_2-microglobulin are elevated. Efforts to effectively remove this protein using conventional dialysis membranes of cellulose acetate or cuprophane have not been successful owing to poor protein clearance. Furthermore, these membranes induce complement activation and generation of IL-1, which may result in β_2-microglobulin accumulation.

Beta Protein (Alzheimer's Disease) Amyloidosis (AD). Alzheimer's disease (AD) is the most common cause of dementia in elderly patients, afflicting 5 to 10% of the population over 65 (see Ch. 400). In neuropathologic studies of the brains of AD patients, neurofibrillary tangles and neuritic plaques are frequently found in the amygdala, hippocampus, and frontal, temporal, and parietal lobes. In addition, acellular thickening of the small and medium-sized arteries of the leptomeninges and cerebral cortex have been seen in AD and aged patients. By standard histologic techniques, the amorphous material in the walls of meningeal vessels and the central region of the neuritic plaques has the characteristic staining property for amyloid. The chemical nature of both amyloid deposits has been identified as a novel 40-amino-acid protein (β protein) that is generated by proteolysis of a much larger transmembrane glycoprotein termed "β amyloid precursor protein." In some forms of familial AD, point mutations have resulted in single amino acid substitutions in this precursor protein. Recent studies have reported that most patients with late-onset

sporadic AD have a strong association of ApoE$_4$ alleles and A$_\beta$ deposits within the cerebrum and cerebral vessels, which suggest the possibility that bimolecular complexes between ApoE$_4$ and A$_\beta$ may be important in the extracellular deposition and formation of cerebral amyloid.

There is evidence that the cerebrovascular deposition of β protein amyloid is an important etiology of nontraumatic/nonhypertensive brain hemorrhage in the elderly, usually presenting as cerebral lobe hemorrhage involving the cortex and subcortical white matter. In addition, a familial syndrome defined in a Dutch kindred in which certain family members died in their 40's or 50's from cerebral hemorrhages (hereditary cerebral hemorrhage with amyloidosis, Dutch type) has been shown to be due to an amino acid substitution in the β protein.

The suggestive signs and symptoms of the amyloidoses result directly from tissue/organ infiltration with subsequent dysfunction. As can be seen in Table 248–1, multiple organ involvement is common but variable in degree. This necessitates formulating a list of differential diagnoses to exclude other localized or systemic diseases. For example, carpal tunnel syndrome is a common clinical entity and is seen very frequently in patients on hemodialysis for longer than 8 to 10 years; it is due to Aβ_2M deposition in the tenosynovium of the carpal tunnel. This is also commonly found in the AL and ATTR forms and in nonamyloid diseases such as hypothyroidism, RA, and diabetes mellitus. Thus many disorders must be considered and subsequently excluded. The AA, AL, and ATTR forms may be associated with significant proteinuria or nephrotic syndrome, and many primary glomerular diseases must be excluded. AL and ATTR forms also may be the cause of vexing unexplained congestive heart failure with cardiomyopathy in patients who have had repeated heart catherization and coronary angiography without a clear answer. Clues to cardiac amyloidosis may be present on the standard 12-lead electrocardiogram, such as decreased QRS voltage, first-degree AV block with intraventricular conduction defects, and Q waves in precordial leads V_1 to V_3 (pseudoinfarction) or two-dimensional echocardiographic findings of a "speckled" pattern of intraventricular septum/myocardium. Peripheral neuropathies may be the initial and dominant expression primarily in the ATTR and other familial forms (see Table 248–1). Generally, the onset of symptoms occurs in early middle age (30 to 40 years old) in the lower extremity with progressive sensorimotor involvement including the proximal and truncal sensory nerves. Foot ulcers with secondary infections may occur. An autonomic neuropathy with orthostatic hypotension, impotence, and diminished peristalsis with pseudo-obstruction, diarrhea, or malabsorption may be present. Gastrointestinal bleeding and/or perforation may be associated with amyloid infiltration of the lamina propria and submucosal blood vessels. Often there are many interacting variables; for example, orthostatic hypotension in the amyloid patient may result from the combination of restrictive cardiomyopathy with diastolic dysfunction, diminished intravascular volume, and sympathetic dysfunction.

Two uncommon syndromes may be easily confused with amyloidosis. The POEMS syndrome (see Ch. 149) (*p*olyneuropathy, *o*rganomegaly, *e*ndocrinopathy, *m*onoclonal gammopathy, *s*kin findings) is a plasma cell dyscrasia with a constellation of diverse features similar to the systemic/localized amyloid syndrome, but no amyloid deposits have been described in these patients. Immunotactoid glomerulopathy (fibrillary renal deposits) is characterized by progressive proteinuria, microscopic hematuria, and hypertension. The renal biopsy tissue has variable glomerular deposits containing IgG, IgM, C_3, C_4, and λ and κ light chains (immunotactoid). On electron microscopy, fibrillary material is deposited within the mesangium and capillary walls and can be differentiated from the typical amyloid fibrils in that the fibrils are thicker and do not stain with Congo red.

DIAGNOSIS. *The diagnosis is made by detecting amyloid deposits in tissue preparations stained with Congo red and emitting an apple-green birefringence using polarized light microscopy.* If a patient is suspected of having one of the systemic amyloidoses (AL, AA, ATTR), aspiration and staining of abdominal subcutaneous fat tissue should be done, since this can be done rapidly and safely at the bedside. Fat tissue is obtained using a 16-gauge needle fixed to a 20- to 30-ml syringe—repeated movements of the needle with gentle pulling of the syringe barrel to produce a negative pressure is done to obtain fragments of the fatty tissue. The fatty fluid and fragments are placed on alcohol-cleaned glass slides, air-dried, and submitted for Congo red staining. Because variable false-negative results have been reported, a repeat biopsy of the subcutaneous tissue or of an alternative site such as the rectal mucosa is warranted. The redundant mucosal folds (valves of Houston) may be visualized directly and tissue (including the vascular submucosa) obtained by pincer forceps with bleeding controlled by cautery. Other biopsy sites include carpal tunnel tissue, kidney, sural nerve, heart (endomyocardial biopsy of right ventricle), bone, and synovium. Staining of amyloid deposits in synovial fluid of AL and $A\beta_2M$ patients has been described. In general, biopsy of the liver should be avoided due to the risk of bleeding. *Attempts to define the chemical amyloid type should be made.* For example, specific antisera to λ and κ light chains, SAA, β_2 microglobulin, and transthyretin are commercially available to stain the tissue using immunofluorescent or immunoperoxidase methods.

In patients with suspected AL with or without myeloma, agarose gel electrophoresis of serum and concentrated urine may be done easily. The monoclonal paraprotein is separated from other serum components by electrophoresis, interacted with separate antisera to λ and κ light chains, IgM, IgA, and IgG (immunofixation), and identified by protein staining. Bone marrow aspiration and biopsy are usually done to quantify the number of plasma wells and can be stained for amyloid. Scintigraphy using radiolabeled P-component, which binds to all amyloid types, remains experimental and cannot be justified as a screening or routine test.

TREATMENT. AL is treated with chemotherapy as a plasma cell neoplasm, even though only 10 to 20% of patients have plasma cell myeloma. The Mayo Clinic has used a treatment protocol of mephalan 0.15 mg per kilogram per day in two divided doses and prednisone 0.8 mg per kilogram per day in four divided doses. The duration of each treatment was 7 days with repeated cycles every 6 weeks. Diuretics may be necessary to treat fluid retention. Every patient with AL should be given a trial with this regimen, even though the response rate is disappointingly low at approximately 20%. However, dramatic resolution of multiorgan dysfunction/amyloid infiltration using cyclic prednisone and mephalan treatment has been reported.

The successful prevention and treatment of amyloidosis of familial Mediterranean fever with low-dose colchicine 0.6 mg once or twice daily has been a dramatic treatment development for AA. If the amyloidosis is related to an infectious process such as tuberculosis, it must be defined and treated aggressively. Likewise, any noninfectious inflammatory condition should be treated and patients given colchicine concomitantly.

Unfortunately, no standard treatment regimen for ATTR has been defined. The liver synthesizes the abnormal transthyretin protein in afflicted patients, and a small number of liver transplants have been performed but no results have been published. Furthermore, no guidelines for hepatic transplantation have been defined.

$A\beta_2M$ is a very common localized amyloidosis that is thought to result from poor clearance of β_2M by conventional dialysis membranes leading to high levels of this protein in serum and tissues enhancing fibril formation. A new group of synthetic high-flux, highly permeable dialysis membranes (polycarbonate, polymethyl methacrylate, polyacrylonitrile) is currently available but very expensive. Long-term studies are necessary to determine if these new synthetic membranes prevent dialysis-related $A\beta_2M$.

Finally, the loss of physical independence in older, frail patients with AD is devastating both emotionally and economically for these patients and their families. No preventative treatment is currently available. Much research is currently being performed to understand the mechanism(s) of $A\beta$ formation and the role of $ApoE_4$-$A\beta$ complexes in the formation of neuritic plaques.

Benson, MD: Amyloidosis: *In* Beaudet AL, Scriver CR, Sly WS: The Metabolic Basis of Inherited Disease. New York, McGraw-Hill, 1994. *A superb review of amyloidosis focusing primarily on the ATTR forms.*

Kyle RA, Griepp PR: Amyloidosis (AL): Clinical and laboratory features in 229 cases. Mayo Clin Proc 58:665, 1983. *Excellent reference for those interested in the various manifestations of AL.*

Natvig JB, Førre Ø, Husby G (eds.): Amyloid and Amyloidosis, 1990. New York, Kluwer Academic Publishers, 1991. Published proceedings of the VIth International Symposium on Amyloidosis, in Oslo, Norway. *Current status on nomenclature and scientific study of amyloidosis. Many references.*

Zemer D, Pras M, Sohar E, et al.: Colchicine in the prevention and treatment of the amyloidosis of familial Mediterranean fever. N Engl J Med 314:1001, 1986. *A review of 1070 patients on colchicine for 4 to 11 years with convincing evidence that long-term colchicine therapy prevents amyloidosis development and in some cases ameliorates already existing amyloid kidney involvement.*

249 BEHÇET'S DISEASE
Eugene V. Ball

Although there is no invariable feature of Behçet's disease (BD), certain features occur often enough to constitute a definable syndrome and serve as the basis for diagnostic criteria. One set in common use requires the presence of recurrent oral ulcers and any two of the following: genital ulcers, uveitis, cutaneous or large vessel vasculitis, arthritis, and meningoencephalitis. An "incomplete" form has been defined as recurrent aphthous ulcers and any one of the other features. Although oral ulcers are the linchpin of diagnostic criteria, a diagnosis of probable BD is tenable when several of these features occur together in the absence of aphthous ulcers, and other known causes can be excluded. Diagnosis has been possible in some patients only after as many as 20 years of minor symptoms.

CLINICAL MANIFESTATIONS. Table 249–1 lists manifestations of the disease in one group of 60 patients. Constitutional signs such as fever and weight loss were noted in 63%. Other significant manifestations include meningoencephalitis and abdominal pain. At least 24 patients from Mediterranean areas have had both BD and secondary (AA) amyloidosis.

Oral ulcers are painful, are round or oval, are usually multiple, and may be the only sign of BD; on the other hand, isolated genital ulcers are seldom indicative of BD. Ulcers occur elsewhere, as in the gut and on the skin, as do an assortment of nonulcerative skin lesions, such as erythema, erythema nodosum, photosensitivity, and spontaneous pustules. The pustular reaction of the skin to intradermal needle prick (sometimes referred to as "pathergy") denotes increased neutrophil chemotaxis and was once thought to be pathognomonic of BD, but this reaction occurs in no more than 70% of patients, usually in those with extensive disease. Furthermore, it is nonspecific, occurring in 7% of one group of healthy control subjects.

Ten to 15% of acquired blindness among Japanese is thought to be due to the uveoretinitis of BD. Decreased visual acuity results from inflammation, secondary glaucoma, cataracts, or vitreous hemorrhage; retinal vein thrombosis leading to sudden blindness is not rare.

Phlebitis or arteritis occurs in as many as a quarter of all patients and predisposes to thrombosis or aneurysms. For example, 10% of a group of 450 Tunisians had aneurysms, large artery occlusions, or both. Aneurysms are particularly common in pulmonary arteries and are most often single, but as many as 14 have occurred in one pa-

TABLE 249–1. MAJOR MANIFESTATIONS OF BEHÇET'S DISEASE

Manifestation	Prevalence (%)
Mouth ulcers	97
Genital ulcers	83
Cutaneous lesions	75
Uveitis	48
Joint pain	48
Phlebitis	17

tient in less than 1 year. Pulmonary vasculitis produces dyspnea, chest pain, cough, or hemoptysis and is a significant cause of death. Its radiographic signs include scattered infiltrates and pleural effusions.

The arthritis of BD is usually intermittent, self-limited, and localized to the knees and ankles; however, erosive changes have been observed in hip, heel, wrist, knee, ankle, and foot radiographs.

Aseptic meningitis occurs in almost all cases of neurologic BD; other manifestations include encephalopathy, seizures, corticospinal abnormalities, bulbar palsy, ataxia, transient ischemic attacks, strokes, and pseudotumor cerebri. These may be acute or gradual in onset, and they may resolve completely or cause death. Focal intracranial abnormalities are detected by imaging studies.

Small and large ulcers in the gut produce symptoms of inflammatory bowel disease and perforation and are more common in Japanese than in Turkish patients.

PREVALENCE. BD is rare in the Americas and Europe. It is more prevalent, as well as more virulent, in Turkey and the Middle and Far East. Evidence of BD was found in 19 of 1531 persons aged 10 or older in a field survey conducted in rural Turkey; on Hokkaido, Japan, its estimated prevalence was 1 in 1000 persons, but BD is less common in ethnic Japanese living in Hawaii. Its prevalence was estimated at 1 in 25,000 in Olmsted County, Minnesota.

GENETICS AND PATHOLOGY. Although not considered hereditary, BD was present in members of four HLA (human leukocyte antigen) B51–positive families. HLA-B51 has been detected in 51% of BD patients versus 16% of control subjects in Japan and in 62% with BD versus 29% of control subjects in Iraq. The HLA-B5101 allele of B51 was found in all 46 HLA-B51–positive Japanese BD patients. Histopathologic characteristics of BD are nonspecific. Despite its classification as vasculitis, fibrinoid necrosis of vessels is not usually found. Mononuclear cells, found in the epidermis and around small vessels in early lesions, are later replaced by neutrophils and plasma cells. Arteritis, which may be catastrophic, is due to inflammation of the vasa vasorum. Abnormalities of the immune system are inconstant, providing no clues to the cause and pathogenesis of BD, which remain unknown. The possible "cure" of retinitis by oral doses of retinal protein S supports the concept of autoimmunity to retinal-specific antigens in the pathogenesis of eye inflammation in BD.

TREATMENT. Numerous medications have been tried for symptomatic treatment as well as for prevention. Patients with thromboses of major vessels should receive anticoagulants. Corticosteroids are given in doses up to 1000 mg of prednisone or prednisolone per day for serious problems, such as central nervous system disease. Cyclosporine appears to be superior to colchicine in reducing the frequency and severity of ocular attacks. Other immunosuppressive drugs have been used with variable effectiveness and toxicity. Chlorambucil (0.1 mg per kilogram per day) moderates disease expression; however, long-term use is worrisome with respect to oncogenesis. Azathioprine (2.5 mg per kilogram per day) is superior to placebo in preserving visual acuity in patients with eye disease and in reducing the frequency of oral and genital ulcers and arthritis, and methotrexate may have a role in treatment of BD. Retinitis has been treated successfully with oral retinal protein S (personal communication).

Dilsen N, Konice M, Aral O, et al.: Behçet's disease associated with amyloidosis in Turkey and in the world. Ann Rheum Dis 47:157, 1988. *The features of 8 Turkish and 16 other patients with BD and amyloidosis are described.*

Hamza M: Large artery involvement in Behçet's disease. J Rheumatol 14:554, 1987. *Clinical descriptions of 10 of 450 patients evaluated over 20 years who had arterial aneurysms (7) and occlusion (3).*

Masuda K, Urayama A, Kogure M, et al.: Double-masked trial of cyclosporin versus colchicine and long-term open study of cyclosporin in Behçet's disease. Lancet 1:1093, 1989. *A randomized, 16-week, double-blind study comparing colchicine and cyclosporine in 49 and 47 patients, respectively. Thirty-six patients were enrolled in a long-term study of mean duration of 44 weeks.*

Mizuki N, Inoko H, Ando H, et al.: Behçet's disease associated with one of the HLA-B51 subantigens, HLA-B*5101. Am J Ophthalmol 116:406, 1993. *Of three HLA-B51 alleles, only B5101 was found in 46 HLA-B51–positive BD patients.*

Raz I, Okon E, Chajek-Shaul T: Pulmonary manifestations in Behçet's syndrome. Chest 95:585, 1989. *Seven of 72 patients had pulmonary vascular disease manifested as dyspnea, cough, chest pain, and hemoptysis. The clinical and radiographic data of these and 42 other patients were reviewed.*

250 PANNICULITIS AND DISORDERS OF THE SUBCUTANEOUS FAT

Gerald S. Lazarus

The subcutaneous tissue is a fibrofatty layer spread between skin and muscles. It functions not only as a thermal and mechanical insulator but also as an active metabolic organ. The characteristic "signet ring" lipocytes are organized into lobules by fibrous septa, which are continuous with the dermis and contain the blood and lymph vessels and reticuloendothelial cells.

The diagnosis of panniculitis frequently requires deep skin biopsy. The most important histologic characteristic is the location of the inflammatory process. Inflammation primarily in the septa is designated *septal panniculitis,* whereas inflammation primarily of the fat lobules is called *lobular panniculitis.* The presence or absence of vasculitis further differentiates panniculitis into four major groups.

LOBULAR PANNICULITIS WITHOUT VASCULITIS. Nodular Panniculitis—Weber-Christian Disease. Nodular panniculitis describes a group of syndromes or diseases characterized by subcutaneous nodules and inflammatory cells in the fat lobules. The term Weber-Christian disease is applied when cutaneous lesions are associated with systemic complaints; this eponym should be abandoned because lobular panniculitis includes a variety of distinctive disease entities.

The etiology of this group of diseases is unknown. In the early stages, the fat lobules are infiltrated with polymorphonuclear leukocytes. Later, macrophages appear and ingest fat, producing the characteristic lipophagic granuloma. The lesions heal with lobular fibrosis. Modest septal vasculitis may be observed.

Lobular panniculitis most commonly occurs in women between the ages of 30 and 60, although cases have been reported in all age groups. The lesions begin as red, slightly tender nodules deep in the skin. They appear more or less in symmetric crops on thighs and lower legs, but lesions also may occur on arms, trunk, and face. The number of lesions may vary enormously. The lesions become firmer, less red, and less tender over a period of weeks. They heal, leaving a depressed, hyperpigmented scar. *Liquefying panniculitis* is a variant in which the lesions become necrotic and drain an oily, yellow-brown fluid. Biopsy reveals polymorphonuclear leukocytes in the deep reticular dermis as well as in the fat. As many as 15% of patients with this clinical picture may have α_1 proteinase deficiency.

Systemic nodular panniculitis is a widespread process affecting cutaneous and visceral fat. Patients usually present with unequivocal cutaneous nodules and arthralgias, malaise, fatigue, weight loss, and abdominal pain. Involvement of the bone marrow may produce anemia, leukocytosis or leukopenia, and bone pain. Hepatomegaly, steatorrhea, and intestinal perforation also have been reported. Inflammation may occur in other internal organs, such as lungs, pleura, pericardium, spleen, kidney, and adrenal glands. Visceral involvement may be confined to the retroperitoneal space, producing abdominal pain, nausea, and vomiting. Mesenteric panniculitis resulting in abdominal pain, diarrhea, constipation, and occasional mass lesions may occur without cutaneous findings. Histiocytic cytophagic panniculitis is a disease characterized by panniculitis, fever, serositis, reticuloendotheliomegaly, hemorrhagic complications, and a poor prognosis; it is diagnosed by the presence of non-neoplastic T lymphocytes and histiocytosis with phagocytosis of erythrocytes, leukocytes, and platelets.

The prognosis of nodular panniculitis is good in patients with only cutaneous involvement. Remissions and exacerbations of the lesions are frequent. Some patients recover after a few months, and permanent remission is usual after several years. On rare occasions, visceral involvement may be fatal.

No specific therapy exists for this disease. Saturated potassium iodide, increasing by 1 drop per day from 5 drops three times per day to 30 drops three times per day, has been suggested. Hydroxychloroquine,* 200 mg two times per day, and cimetidine also have been advocated as treatment. High-dose prednisone, 40 to 60 mg for 1 to 2 weeks, with gradual tapering over 6 to 8 weeks, also has been reported to be of value in patients with severe disease; steroids should be used *only for acute* attacks and for limited periods. There are anecdotal reports that cyclosporine may be of value in patients with severe panniculitis.

Lobular Panniculitis Associated with Pancreatic Disease. The diagnosis is made by skin biopsy, which discloses acute fat necrosis with characteristic ghost cells. These patients often have associated arthritis, ascites, and eosinophilia. Acute pancreatitis, trauma to the pancreas, chronic pancreatitis, pancreatic cysts, and pancreatic carcinoma have been reported to be associated with this syndrome. Diagnosis depends on the histologic findings at skin biopsy and documentation of a specific pancreatic abnormality. Therapy is directed at the underlying pancreatic disease.

Poststeroid Lobular Panniculitis. Children who receive large doses of steroid for a short period, followed by abrupt discontinuance, may develop lobular panniculitis. Lesions may occur in the viscera, and a fatal case has been reported.

Physical Lobular Panniculitis. Physical trauma of any kind and cold injury, especially in children, can produce lobular panniculitis. A unique traumatic panniculitis occurs in the breasts of obese women in their 50's. Injection of silicone or other foreign materials into female breasts or buttocks and into the male genitalia may induce a granulomatous foreign body nodular panniculitis. Similar inflammatory lesions may be seen following injection of pentazocine (Talwin).

Lobular Panniculitis Associated with Systemic Disease. Lupus erythematosus, sarcoidosis, granuloma annulare, Sweet's disease, acute sudden weight loss from gastrointestinal surgery, and infections, including those caused by deep fungi, mycobacteria, and pyogens, may present as lobular panniculitis. Any patient with acquired immunodeficiency syndrome (AIDS) who has panniculitis must have a biopsy performed and the tissue sent for histologic study and culture to rule out infectious agents. Lymphoma or leukemia also may present as panniculitis; histologically, these lesions demonstrate malignant cells in the fat lobules. Lupus erythematosus confined primarily to the fat is known as "lupus profundus." The skin may be exclusively involved, or the panniculitis may be associated with systemic disease. Diagnosis is suggested by characteristic histology and the deposition of immunoglobulin at the dermal-epidermal interface.

Lobular Panniculitis with Vasculitis. This category of disease includes *nodular vasculitis* and *erythema induratum*. The eruption consists of recurring, tender, painful nodules on the calves, which often ulcerate and heal with scarring. It is much more common in females than in males. Increased erythrocyte sedimentation rate and hypertension have been associated with this syndrome. Bazin gave the name "erythema induratum" to this disease when histologic examination revealed caseation necrosis. These lesions may be associated with tuberculosis and especially a positive skin test.

Most patients experience remission of lesions with bed rest. Severe cases have been successfully treated with nonsteroidal anti-inflammatory drugs (NSAID's), dapsone, and prednisone. In cases of nodular vasculitis associated with a positive tuberculin skin test, appropriate antituberculous therapy is indicated.

SEPTAL PANNICULITIS WITHOUT VASCULITIS. This histologic picture in a patient with nodular, painful, tender lesions, especially on the anterior leg, is diagnostic of *erythema nodosum,* which is discussed in Ch. 475. A chronic disease similar to erythema nodosum clinically and histologically except that the lesions spread peripherally over months, forming rings, is called *subacute migratory panniculitis*. This disease responds to therapy with increasing doses of saturated potassium iodide as described for nodular panniculitis. Septal panniculitis without vasculitis also can be seen in scleroderma, dermatomyositis, and necrobiosis lipoidica diabeticorum. Eosinophilic fasciitis can mimic septal panniculitis. In-

---

* This use is not listed in the manufacturer's directive.

gestion of pharmacologic doses of tryptophan for pain or depression has produced a syndrome mimicking acute scleroderma or eosinophilic fasciitis. These diagnostic possibilities should be investigated in all patients.

SEPTAL PANNICULITIS WITH VASCULITIS. *Thrombophlebitis* may present with subcutaneous nodules. Histology reveals inflammation of veins with adjacent panniculitis (see Ch. 46).

Cutaneous polyarteritis is a chronic recurring painful nodular eruption, primarily of the legs. An associated mottled livedo vascular pattern is often present. Cutaneous polyarteritis is associated with myalgias, arthralgias, and increased erythrocyte sedimentation rate. Histologic examination demonstrates leukocytoclastic vasculitis of medium-sized arterioles. This disease is not usually associated with systemic involvement. It has a benign course, but lesions may recur for years.

Therapy includes NSAID's and short courses of corticosteroids. Cutaneous polyarteritis associated with granulomatous bowel disease has responded to short courses of cyclophosphamide (Cytoxan).

LIPOATROPHY. Subcutaneous tissue can be lost as a consequence of healing in almost any of the panniculitides described previously. The most common diagnosable cause of lipoatrophy is recurrent insulin injection. Insulin lipoatrophy is usually associated with repetitive injections of high doses of insulin in exactly the same location in females. Injections of pentazocine (Talwin) also may produce panniculitis and severe lipoatrophy.

Total lipoatrophy associated with diabetes may occur in children and adults. The clinical picture is dramatic, and there is almost complete loss of subcutaneous fat. Partial lipoatrophy usually begins in children or young adults. It is five times more common in females than in males. Patients often lose the fat in the face and the upper half of the body. In some cases, there is hypertrophy of the fat on the lower half of the body. Patients with partial lipodystrophy often develop progressive mesangiocapillary glomerulonephritis and hypocomplementemia. Diabetes develops in one third of these patients. Retinitis pigmentosa has also been reported with this disease. The prognosis depends upon the severity of the renal disease.

Ackerman AB: Panniculitis. *In* Ackerman AB (ed.): Histologic Diagnosis of Inflammatory Skin Diseases. Philadelphia, Lea & Febiger, 1978, pp 779–826. *An outstanding review of the classification and histology of panniculitis.*

Alegre VA, Winkelmann RK: Clinical and laboratory studies: Histiocytic cytophagic panniculitis. J Am Acad Dermatol 20:177, 1989.

Bondi EE, Lazarus GS: Panniculitis. *In* Fitzpatrick TB, Eisen AZ, Wolff K, et al. (eds.): Dermatology in General Medicine, 4th ed. New York, McGraw-Hill, 1993, pp 1329–1344. *A complete overview of panniculitis emphasizing clinical descriptions, mechanisms, and treatment.*

Peters MS, Su WP: Lupus erythematosus panniculitis. Med Clin North Am 73:1113, 1989. *An excellent review of this disease.*

Rademaker M, Lowe DG, Munro DD: Erythema induratum (Bazin's disease). J Am Acad Dermatol 21:740, 1989. *Correlation of erythema induratum with hypersensitivity to tuberculin.*

Smith KC, Su WP, Pittelkow MR, Winkelmann RK: Clinical and pathologic correlations in 96 patients with panniculitis, including 15 patients with deficient levels of alpha₁-antitrypsin. J Am Acad Dermatol 21:1192, 1989. *Clinical and pathologic correlations in 96 patients with panniculitis, including 15 with α_1-antitrypsin deficiency.*

---

251 GOUT AND URIC ACID METABOLISM
Michael S. Hershfield

Gout refers to the *inflammatory arthritis* induced by microscopic *crystals* of monosodium urate monohydrate (MSU) and to the pathognomonic deposition of aggregated MSU crystals *(tophi)* in various tissues and some organs. Chronic *hyperuricemia* is necessary for the development of gout, though not sufficient. *Urolithiasis* (renal stones composed of undissociated uric acid) may accompany gout or occur independently when renal urate excretion is excessive. Gout is chiefly a disease of adult men. It is mostly *idiopathic* and multifactorial in etiology. A few rare, inherited metabolic disorders markedly enhance urate production, causing urolithiasis and gout as primary manifestations. Other genetic and acquired disorders and some drugs cause secondary hyperuricemia and gout by impairing renal urate excretion or by indirectly increasing urate production (Table 251–1).

If untreated, gout can lead to painful, destructive arthropathy, and urolithiasis to renal failure. Correcting hyperuricemia and hyperuricosuria prevents these consequences and is achievable in most cases. However, because most hyperuricemic individuals will develop neither gout nor renal insufficiency and because therapy is not without risk and expense, *asymptomatic hyperuricemia per se* generally does not require therapy; observation and in some cases a search for a contributing, treatable disease are warranted.

PREVALENCE AND INCIDENCE. Surveys made in the 1960's estimated the prevalence of gout at about 0.5 to 0.7% for men and about 0.1% for women. Prevalence has been increasing over the past two decades. Gout is the most common inflammatory arthritis in men over 40 in the United States. A 1986 U.S. Health Interview Survey estimated 2.2 million cases of self-reported gout, about twice the physician-reported prevalence.

As Hippocrates observed, gout rarely occurs before puberty in males and seldom before menopause in females. Trends in serum urate values are consistent with this pattern. In normal children, serum urate averages 3.6 mg per deciliter in both genders. Levels rise at puberty, more so in males than in females. In the United States, the central 95% segment of the serum urate distribution ranges from 2.2 to 7.5 mg per deciliter in adult men and from 2.1 to 6.6 mg per deciliter in adult premenopausal women. Serum urate values increase with age; after menopause, mean values in women approach levels in men. Epidemiologic surveys have noted a trend toward increasing serum urate values in the United States in recent decades and significant variations among population groups, which reflect genetic and environmental factors. Obesity, alcohol consumption, and diuretic use are associated with hyperuricemia.

The incidence of gout increases with the degree and duration of hyperuricemia; age, obesity, hypertension, and alcohol intake show much weaker relationships when serum urate is factored out. Although lower levels are occasionally found during an attack, serum urate exceeds 7 mg per deciliter at some time in virtually all patients with gout. Nevertheless, the risk of gout is modest, even at higher serum urate levels. Among about 2000 initially healthy white males followed over a 15-year period, annual incidence rates for gout were 0.1% at < 7 mg per deciliter, 0.5% at 7.0 to 8.9 mg per deciliter, and 4.9% at ≥ 9 mg per deciliter. At levels over 9 mg per deciliter (the highest 1.8% of values observed), the cumulative incidence of gout after 5 years was 22%. Incidence rates were about threefold higher for hypertensive than for normotensive men in all age groups, reflecting the hyperuricemic effect of diuretics. Convincing studies have shown that hyperuricemia is not a risk factor for either renal failure or coronary artery disease.

PATHOGENESIS AND PATHOLOGY. Serum urate levels are very low, and gout is nonexistent, in nonhuman primates and other species that possess urate oxidase *(uricase),* a hepatic peroxisomal enzyme that converts urate to allantoin. The latter is 80- to 100-fold more soluble than urate and much more efficiently excreted by the kidneys. Mutational inactivation of the uricase gene occurred during evolution of *Homo sapiens* and a few other hominoid species. From this perspective, *uricemia per se* in humans is the abnormal result of an inborn error of urate catabolism. In terms of the pathogenesis of gout, which is caused by urate crystals rather than urate in solution, "hyperuricemia" is defined by the solubility of urate in body fluids, not by statistical distributions of urate levels. More urate produced than can be disposed of or maintained in solution leads over time to extracellular deposition of MSU crystals; urate solubility is much lower at the temperature of peripheral joints (about 32°C in the knee and 29°C in the ankle). Gout ensues when an inflammatory response is triggered.

Urate Production and Elimination. The total-body urate pool, with which sodium urate in plasma is miscible, is determined by rates of uric acid production and disposal and is expanded in patients with gout (Table 251–2A). Urate arises from the action of *xanthine oxidase* on its substrates, the purine bases hypoxanthine and xanthine (Fig. 251–1). Dietary purines are largely degraded to urate by catabolic enzymes, including xanthine oxidase, located in the intestinal epithelium. Purine restriction can modestly reduce serum urate by 0.6 to 1.8 mg per deciliter, but variation in absorption has not been implicated as a cause of hyperuricemia. The majority of urate is produced by hepatic xanthine oxidase acting on hypoxanthine and xanthine derived from the degradation of nucleic acids of senescent cells and from the metabolic turnover of cellular purine nucleotides. The latter arise from two biosynthetic pathways, termed *"de novo"* and "salvage" (or "reutilization") (see Fig. 251–1).

TABLE 251–1. CLASSIFICATION OF HYPERURICEMIA AND GOUT

Type	Disturbance in Uric Acid, Purine Metabolism	Inheritance
Primary		
I. Idiopathic (> 99% of primary gout)		
A. Normal urinary excretion (80–90% of primary gout)	Decreased renal clearance ± overproduction of urate	Polygenic
B. Increased urinary excretion (10–20% of primary gout)	Overproduction ± decreased renal clearance of urate	Polygenic
II. Due to specific inherited metabolic defects (< 1% of primary gout)		
A. PP-ribose-P synthetase over-activity	Increased *de novo* purine synthesis	X-linked
B. Hypoxanthine-guanine phosphoribosyltransferase deficiency	Impaired purine salvage + increased *de novo* purine synthesis	X-linked
Secondary		
I. Glucose-6-phosphatase deficiency (Gierke's glycogen storage disease)	Increased catabolism of adenine nucleotides + secondary increase in purine synthesis *de novo*	Autosomal recessive
II. Chronic hemolysis; erythroid, myeloid, and lymphoid proliferative disorders	Increased cell and nucleic acid turnover	
III. Renal mechanisms		
A. Familial progressive renal insufficiency	Reduced renal functional mass and various defects in renal tubular function	Variable
B. Acquired chronic renal insufficiency	Reduced renal functional mass	
C. Drugs (diuretics, cyclosporine, toxins, including lead)	Inhibit urate secretion or enhance reabsorption	
D. Endogenous metabolic products (lactate, ketoacids, β-hydroxybutyrate)	Inhibit urate secretion	

TABLE 251–2. URIC ACID PRODUCTION AND ELIMINATION

A. Urate Kinetics	Milligrams (mmol)
Total miscible pool	1200 (7.2)
Daily turnover	600–900 (3.6–5.4)
Daily production	750 (4.5)
Daily intestinal uricolysis	100–365 (0.6–2.2)
Daily urinary excretion	500–1000 (3–6) on normal diet
	420 ± 75 (2.5 ± 0.5)
	on purine restricted diet

B. Renal Clearance (Four-Component, Bidirectional Transport Model)	Relative Amount
1. *Glomerular filtration* • Complete • ↓ By diuretics, renal failure	100
2. *Tubular reabsorption* • Active, linked to Na⁺ reabsorption • Inhibited by *uricosuric drugs:* probenecid, sulfinpyrazone, benzbromarone, high-dose aspirin (>2 grams/d)	98–100
3. *Tubular secretion* • Active process • Inhibited by agents that cause *hyperuricemia:* pyrazinamide, low-dose aspirin, lactate, β-hydroxybutyrate, branched-chain ketoacids	50
4. *Postsecretory reabsorption*	40–44
Net clearance	**6–10**

Note: Gouty individuals have shown enlarged urate pools and in some cases increased urate turnover. Daily urinary excretion of uric acid is an index of urate production, provided renal function is normal. About 10% of patients with idiopathic gout are "urate overexcretors," defined as a daily urinary excretion exceeding the normal mean + 2 SD (i.e., >600 mg on a purine-restricted diet or >800 mg on an ordinary diet).

Most urate is eliminated by renal excretion (Table 251–2*B*). About one third is degraded by bacteria in the gut; this increases substantially in renal insufficiency. Uricosuric agents act by blocking urate reabsorption, while other drugs and weak organic acids raise serum urate by blocking renal urate secretion (see Table 251–2*B*). The latter mechanism contributes to the hyperuricemia associated with fasting, alcohol metabolism, and ketoacidosis.

Mechanisms of Hyperuricemia. About 10% of patients with gout show evidence of urate overproduction, as indicated by urinary excretion of uric acid exceeding the normal mean plus two standard deviations (>600 mg per 24 hours on a purine-restricted diet, >800 mg on an ordinary diet). The highest overproduction occurs in patients with either of two rare inherited defects in the regulation of purine nucleotide synthesis, deficiency of the salvage enzyme hypoxanthine-guanine phosphoribosyltransferase (HPRT) and overactivity of phosphoribosylpyrophosphate (PP-ribose-P) synthetase (see Fig. 251–1).

In the majority of patients with idiopathic gout, renal function is normal, but clearance of filtered urate is reduced, resulting in hyperuricemia. No specific renal abnormality has been identified to account for this.

Urate excretion diminishes with the onset of renal insufficiency, but in general, gout is uncommon in patients with chronic renal failure. However, several kindreds have been reported in which early-onset hyperuricemia, gout, and progressive renal failure (with or without hypertension), are associated (see Table 251–1). Other factors that have been implicated in causing hyperuricemia and gout through a renal mechanism include chronic lead nephropathy, alcohol abuse, and certain drugs (see Tables 251–1 and 251–2*B*). Hyperuricemia and idiopathic gout are associated with both obesity and hypertriglyceridemia. In some gouty patients, weight reduction and abstinence from alcohol reverse hypertriglyceridemia, hyperuricemia, and evidence of both overproduction and impaired renal clearance of urate.

Mechanism of the Acute Gouty Attack. A. B. Garrod noted correctly in 1859 that ". . . true gouty inflammation is always accompanied with a deposition of urate of soda in the inflamed part. . . . The deposited urate of soda may be looked upon as the cause, and not the effect, of gouty inflammation." The neutrophil is an essential mediator of acute inflammation in gout (Fig. 251–2). Ingestion of MSU crystals causes neutrophils to release leukotrienes, interleukin-1, and a glycoprotein "crystal chemotactic factor," which further amplify neutrophil infiltration into the involved joint. Activated neutrophils also produce superoxide and release lysosomal enzymes, owing to crystal-induced rupture of lysosomal membranes and to cell lysis. The resulting cleavage of complement peptides and kinins from precursors induces pain, vasodilation, and vascular permeability. Released lysosomal and cytoplasmic enzymes, as well as collagenase and prostaglandins produced by joint mesenchymal cells, contribute to chronic articular destruction and tissue necrosis.

Extracellular urate crystals are often found in asymptomatic joints of gouty individuals. Attacks may be initiated and terminated by plasma proteins that selectively adsorb to crystals and modify their interaction with neutrophils. Early in an attack, IgG antibody, possibly induced by MSU crystals acting as antigens, may serve as a nucleating agent that promotes MSU crystallization and increases their phagocytosis by neutrophils, enhancing release of lysosomal enzymes. Late in an attack, lipoproteins containing apoprotein B (Apo B) enter the inflamed joint from plasma and coat MSU crystals, inhibiting phagocytosis, neutrophil oxidative metabolism, superoxide production, and cytolysis. Qualitative and quantitative differences in protein modulators may account for the variable inflammatory response to urate crystals in gouty and nongouty individuals.

Tophi. A tophus is a deposit of fine, needle-shaped MSU crystals, surrounded by a chronic mononuclear cell reaction and a foreign body granuloma of epithelial and giant cells, which may be multinucleate (see Fig. 251–2). Tophi are commonly found in articular and other cartilage, synovia, tendon sheaths, bursae and other periarticular structures, epiphyseal bone, subcutaneous tissues, and the kidney interstitium.

Compared with the acute gouty attack, tophi evoke little inflammatory response and generally develop silently. In bone and articular cartilages they may be detected radiographically in gouty individuals who lack tophi in subcutaneous tissues and who rarely experience acute attacks of arthritis. In the joint, tophi gradually enlarge, causing degeneration of cartilage and subchondral bone, proliferation of synovium and marginal bone, and sometimes fibrous or bony ankylosis. The punched-out lesions of bone commonly seen on radiograph represent marrow tophi, which may communicate with the urate crust on the articular surface through defects in the cartilage. In vertebral bodies, urate deposits involve the marrow spaces adjacent to the intervertebral disks.

The Gouty Kidney. Interstitial deposits of MSU crystals in the medulla or pyramids, with surrounding mononuclear and giant cell reaction, are found commonly in gouty patients at autopsy and have been referred to as "urate nephropathy." Crystalline deposits of uric acid (not urate) within distal tubules and collecting ducts may occur and lead to dilatation and atrophy of the more proximal tubules. Renal disease is common in gout but generally mild and slowly progressive. Interstitial nephropathy may be due to urate deposits but also can be present in their absence. Other possible causes include nephrosclerosis due to hypertension, uric acid stone disease, infection, aging, and lead toxicity.

Uric Acid Nephrolithiasis. About 10 to 25% of gouty patients experience renal stones, over 200-fold higher than in the general population. The incidence of stones exceeds 20% when daily uric acid excretion >700 mg (see Table 251–2*A*) and is about 50% at 1100 mg. Prevalence of stones is also related to hyperuricemia and reaches 50% at serum urate levels >12 mg per deciliter. Over 80% of the stones are uric acid (not sodium urate); the remainder are mixtures of uric acid and calcium oxalate or calcium oxalate or phosphate alone.

For reasons that are unclear, both gouty and nongouty uric acid stone formers exhibit persistently low urinary pH, which favors uric

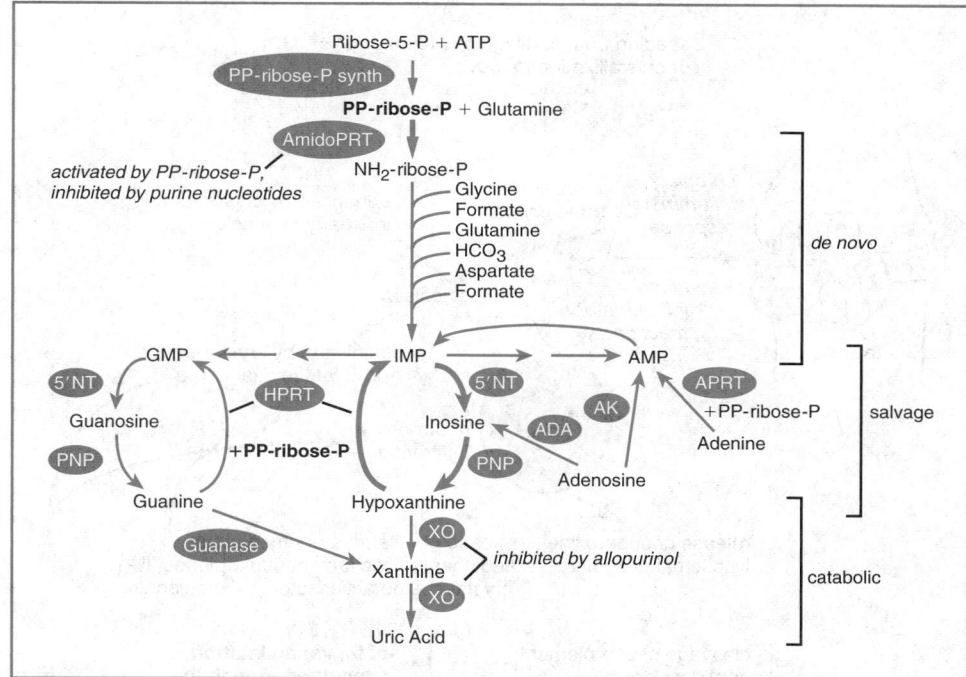

FIGURE 251–1. Intracellular purine metabolism and the basis for "metabolic" hyperuricemia. In the *"de novo"* pathway, the purine ring (hypoxanthine) of inosinic acid (IMP) is constructed from precursors on a ribose-5'-phosphate backbone derived from PP-ribose-P. At IMP the pathway branches, giving rise to AMP and GMP and their derivatives. In the "salvage" pathway, the preformed purine bases hypoxanthine, guanine, and adenine, derived from turnover of IMP, GMP, and AMP, are directly condensed with PP-ribose-P by HPRT and APRT to regenerate these ribonucleotides. Some of the hypoxanthine formed by nucleotide turnover is diverted to the liver and catabolized by XO to uric acid; the remainder is salvaged by HPRT.

Operation of the salvage pathway (the more economical in terms of energy required) reduces *de novo* activity because (1) HPRT and APRT have greater affinity for PP-ribose-P than amidoPRT (the first committed enzyme of the *de novo* pathway), (2) base salvage lowers the concentration of PP-ribose-P, which converts amidoPRT to an inactive form, and (3) the nucleotide endproducts of the HPRT and APRT reactions directly inhibit amidoPRT. Allopurinol, by blocking XO, enhances salvage of hypoxanthine, further inhibiting *de novo* activity; this reduces purine excretion more than is expected from inhibition of uric acid formation alone.

Deficiency of HPRT causes an obligatory loss of all hypoxanthine and guanine as urate. This also allows a compensatory increase in *de novo* pathway activity owing to reduced formation of inhibitory nucleotides and increased concentration and availability of PP-ribose-P for the amidoPRT reaction. In individuals with inherited "overactive" variants of PP-ribose-P synthetase, increased formation of PP-ribose-P stimulates amidoPRT, markedly enhancing *de novo* purine synthesis. The excess IMP formed is degraded to urate.

Increased nucleotide breakdown can cause hyperuricemia by increasing the production of XO substrates and by releasing inhibition of amidoPRT. This biphasic mechanism has been implicated in the hyperuricemia and gout associated with glucose-6-phosphatase deficiency (glycogen storage disease type I); glucose-6-phosphate accumulates at the expense of hepatic ATP, with degradation of AMP to urate. Hyperuricemia may occur acutely in various conditions that result in nucleotide catabolism: hypoxia, metabolism of some sugars, vigorous exercise in normal individuals, and moderate exercise in patients with metabolic myopathies. (PP-ribose-P synth = phosphoribosylpyrophosphate synthetase; AmidoPRT = amidophosphoribosyl transferase; 5'NT = 5'-nucleotidase; HPRT = hypoxanthine-guanine phosphoribosyltransferase; APRT = adenine phosphoribosyltransferase; PNP = purine nucleoside phosphorylase; ADA = adenosine deaminase; AK = adenosine kinase; XO = xanthine oxidase.)

acid stone formation. At pH 5 and 37°C, free uric acid has a solubility of only 15 mg per deciliter. Thus supersaturation is required to excrete an average uric acid load in a normal urine volume. The solubility increases more than 10-fold at pH 7 and more than 100-fold at pH 8.

CLINICAL MANIFESTATIONS. The peak age of onset of gout is about 45 in men, by which time the average gouty male has been exposed to 20 or 30 years of asymptomatic hyperuricemia and to varying degrees of tissue urate deposition. In predisposed women, gout usually occurs some years after menopause, when they become hyperuricemic.

Acute Gouty Arthritis. Gout usually presents as a fulminating arthritic attack affecting the lower extremity. Over 75% of first attacks are monarticular; at least half involve the metatarsophalangeal joint of the great toe (podagra). Next in order are the instep, ankle, heel, knee, wrist, finger, and elbow. Tenosynovitis, bursitis, or cellulitis also may occur. Minor episodes of "ankle sprain" or twinges of pain in the great toe may precede the first attack, sometimes by several years. More often the attack occurs explosively during apparent good health, often at night. Within minutes to hours the affected joint becomes hot, dusky red, and exquisitely tender and

painful. With very severe attacks, there may be fever, leukocytosis, and increased erythrocyte sedimentation rate, suggesting infection. The course of an untreated attack is variable, resolving in hours or a few days when mild and lasting many days to several weeks when severe. As the attack subsides, desquamation of inflamed skin over the affected joint may occur. Once the attack has broken, recovery is generally rapid and complete. The patient then re-enters an asymptomatic phase, often termed "intercritical" or "interval" gout.

The subsequent course is variable, but commonly a pattern of recurrences develops. Attacks often follow a precipitating event such as a long walk, trauma, surgery, alcohol or dietary overindulgence, starvation, infection, or the start of hypouricemic drug therapy. In the untreated patient, attacks often increase in frequency, and they may become more severe, last longer, and are more often polyarticular. Later attacks may involve the shoulder or hip or rarely the sacroiliac, sternoclavicular, or mandibular joints or even the spine. The more distal the site, the more typical is the attack. Eventually, attacks may be refractory to usually effective measures; they resolve incompletely, and disability may become permanent.

Chronic Tophaceous Gout. Progressive inability to dispose of urate results insidiously in tophaceous crystal depositing in and

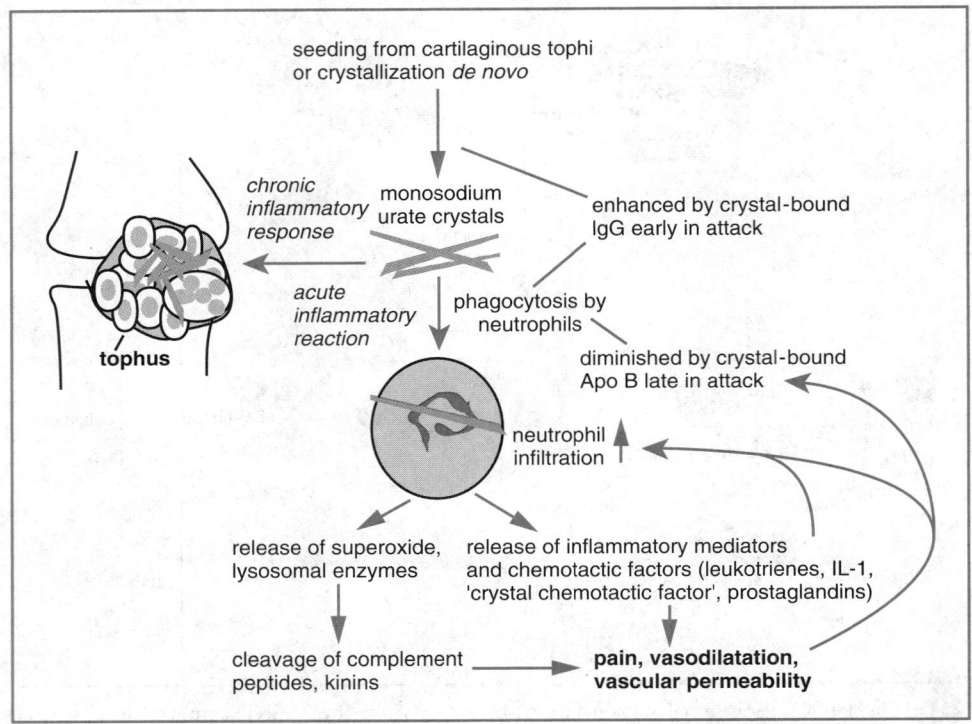

FIGURE 251-2. Inflammatory responses to monosodium urate crystals.

around joints. Tophi may first appear as superficial yellowish-white infiltrates on the fingertips, palms, and soles and later as irregular, asymmetric enlargement of joints, fusiform or nodular enlargements of the Achilles tendon, or saccular distensions of the olecranon bursa (Fig. 251–3). A classic, though relatively infrequent, site of tophi is the helix or anthelix of the external ear. Visible tophi develop in 10 to 25% of gouty patients and in >50% of those who are noncompliant; time of appearance after the initial attack is correlated with the degree and duration of hyperuricemia and with renal insufficiency. In rare patients, often those with gout secondary to a myeloproliferative disease, tophi are present at the time of the initial attack.

Although tophi themselves are relatively painless, they often result in stiffness and persistent aching that limit use of affected joints. Destruction of cartilage and bone by tophi leads to radiolucent "punched-out" lesions and to cortical erosions with characteristic "overhanging margins" (see Fig. 251–3). Eventually, extensive destruction of joints may be disabling, and large subcutaneous tophi may cause grotesque deformities. The stretched, thin skin over tophi may ulcerate and extrude white chalky or pasty "milk of urate" composed of myriads of fine, needle-like crystals. The olecranon bursa may be massively distended with this material, which may be mistaken for pus if not examined by polarized light microscopy. Rarely, tophi may involve the tongue, larynx, corpus cavernosum and prepuce of the penis, aortic or mitral valves, and cardiac conducting system, causing rhythm disturbances. They do not involve the liver, spleen, lungs, or central nervous system.

Gouty Nephropathy. Progressive renal failure due to urate nephropathy may occur in patients with inherited metabolic disorders that cause extreme urate overproduction and possibly in rare forms of inherited renal disease and chronic lead poisoning. Isosthenuria and mild intermittent proteinuria occur in about one third of patients with idiopathic gout. Decline in renal function is correlated with aging, hypertension, renal calculi, pyelonephritis, or independently occurring nephropathy. Hyperuricemia *per se* is not a risk factor for renal insufficiency.

Acute oliguric renal failure can result from bilateral tubular obstruction by uric acid crystals. This occurs in several clinical settings, including untreated leukemia and lymphoma, during chemotherapy for these disorders (tumor lysis syndrome), and in the presence of severe dehydration and acidosis. This condition is preventable by maintaining a high urine volume, with alkalinization, and by pretreating with allopurinol.

DIAGNOSIS. The sudden onset of severe inflammatory arthritis in a peripheral joint, especially of the lower extremity, suggests gout. A history of discrete attacks separated by completely asymptomatic periods is helpful for diagnosis. The diagnosis is established by demonstrating brilliant, negatively birefringent, needle-shaped MSU crystals by polarized light microscopy in the leukocytes of synovial fluid (see Ch. 236) (Fig. 251–4). The synovial fluid leukocyte count ranges from 5000 to over 50,000 per cubic millimeter, depending on the acuteness of inflammation. A Gram stain and culture of synovial fluid should always be obtained to evaluate infection, which may coexist.

Determining the 24-hour urinary excretion of uric acid can be informative, particularly in the young, markedly hyperuricemic patient in whom a metabolic etiology may be suspected. The sample should be collected after 3 days of moderate purine restriction, during an intercritical period. Values >600 mg per 1.72 square meters per day under these conditions suggest overproduction, and those >800 mg per day warrant additional studies for a specific subtype of primary gout, such as HPRT deficiency or PP-ribose-P synthetase overactivity, or of secondary gout, such as a myeloproliferative disorder. Elevated urinary uric acid excretion also predicts a higher risk for renal stones and is an indication for allopurinol rather than uricosuric drug therapy for gout.

DIFFERENTIAL DIAGNOSIS. Acute gout must be differentiated from pseudogout, acute rheumatic fever, rheumatoid arthritis, traumatic arthritis, osteoarthritis, pyogenic arthritis, sarcoid arthritis, cellulitis, bursitis, tendinitis, and thrombophlebitis. Gout can coexist with most of these conditions. Podagra, the most common initial presentation of gout, can be mimicked by trauma, degenerative arthritis, acute sarcoidosis, psoriatic arthritis, pseudogout, Reiter's syndrome, infection, and in the immediate postoperative period following parathyroidectomy can be caused by hydroxyapatite crystals. Pseudogout (see Ch. 252), which is manifested by acute attacks of arthritis of knees and other joints, is often accompanied by calcification of joint cartilage; the synovial fluid contains nonurate crystals of calcium pyrophosphate. When gout and pseudogout coexist, both types of crystals will be found in synovial leukocytes.

TREATMENT. Understanding the rationale for treatment by both the physician and patient is essential for long-term success. One aspect is aimed at terminating the acute inflammatory gouty attack, and the other is aimed at correcting the underlying metabolic problem (Table 251–3).

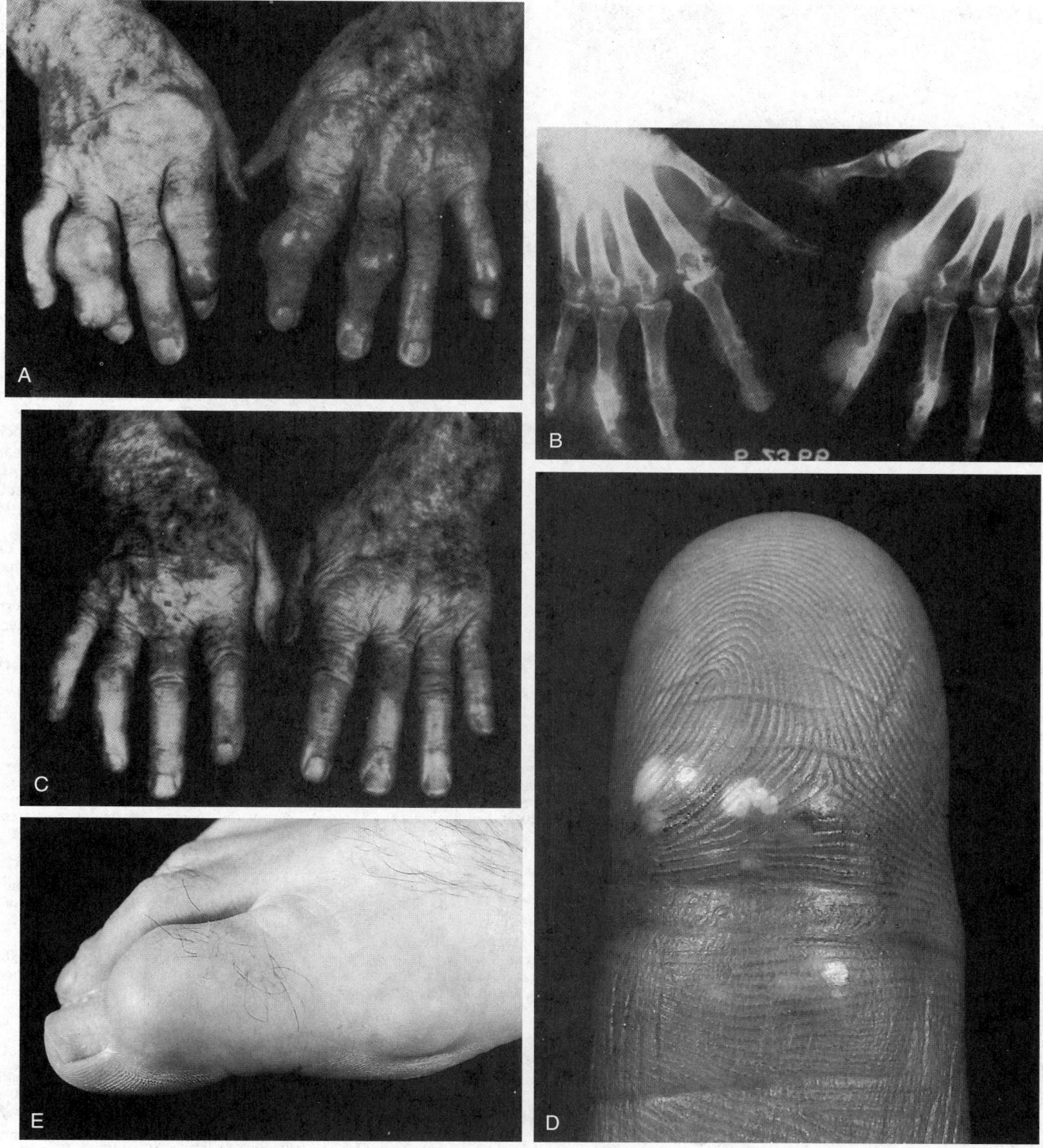

FIGURE 251–3. Tophaceous gout. *A–C,* Chronic gouty arthritis with tophaceous destruction of bone and joints *(A, B)* and improvement after 3 years of treatment with allopurinol, prophylactic colchicine, and a moderately low purine diet *(C). D,* Tophaceous deposits in digital pad of a 28-year-old man with systemic lupus erythematosus under treatment with diuretics. A single attack of gout had occurred 2 years earlier. *E,* Tophaceous enlargement of the great toe in a 44-year-old man with a 4-year history of recurrent gouty arthritis.

Acute Attack. The affected joint(s) should be kept at rest and therapy begun promptly with full doses of an oral nonsteroidal anti-inflammatory drug (NSAID). Salicylates should not be used because of their effects on urate excretion (see Table 251–2). The typical monarticular acute attack responds within 24 hours and resolves in 48 to 72 hours; established or polyarticular attacks may require longer treatment. Once the attack subsides, the NSAID is tapered over several days and discontinued. Hypouricemic therapy should not be initiated during an acute attack because it is ineffec-

tive in relieving inflammatory symptoms and may induce a recurrent attack by mobilizing urate from tissues.

Oral colchicine is effective therapy for acute gout but has a low therapeutic index; relief of pain often coincides with gastrointestinal toxicity. If an attack does not respond in 48 hours, alternative therapy should be used. If oral medication is precluded, intravenous colchicine may be used *with caution.* Colchicine is a microtubule poison; it is retained in cells (half-life about 30 hours) and is not dialyzable. Dose-related toxicity includes alopecia, bone marrow

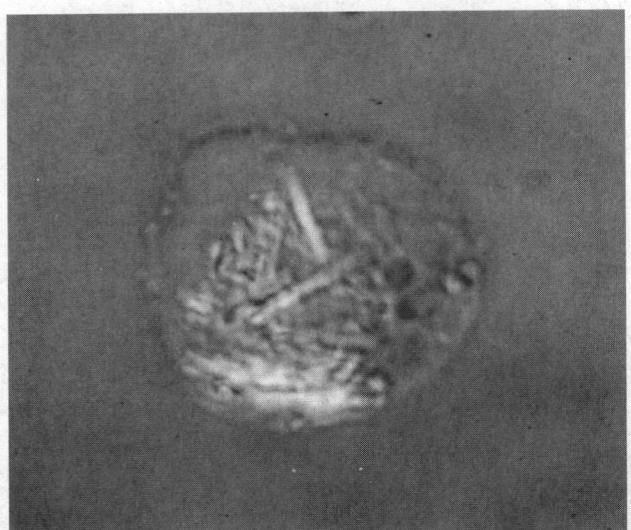

FIGURE 251-4. Sodium urate monohydrate crystals phagocytosed by leukocyte in synovial fluid from acute gouty arthritis, examined by polarized light.

suppression, and hepatocellular damage. Deaths from overdosage have been reported. Blood counts should be monitored during intravenous use of colchicine and periodically during long-term oral therapy. Dosage should be reduced in the presence of renal or hepatic disease, and it should not be used in patients with advanced disease. Reversible myopathy has occurred in elderly patients on daily colchicine prophylaxis who have been treated with larger doses for an acute attack.

Interval Phase. Patients should be warned that acute attacks

may still occur, particularly in the first 6 months or so after beginning hypouricemic therapy. Oral colchicine is effective prophylaxis to prevent recurrent attacks, but an NSAID should be taken at the first sign of prodromal symptom, if recognizable. Although hypouricemic therapy should not be initiated during an acute attack, once begun, it should *not* be interrupted during subsequent attacks. Hypertension should be treated vigorously; if hyperuricemia worsens, antihyperuricemic drug therapy can be initiated or appropriately increased.

Long-Term Management. Use of a drug to lower the serum uric acid level to ≤6 mg per deciliter is indicated in all patients with visible tophi or radiographic evidence of urate deposits or with a history of two or more major attacks of gouty arthritis. Allopurinol is preferred unless the patient is already well managed with a uricosuric agent. With either type of agent, the number of acute attacks may increase during the first few months unless prophylactic colchicine is given; after 12 to 18 months, the frequency of attacks should decline.

Allopurinol reduces urate production by inhibiting xanthine oxidase, with secondary reduction of *de novo* purine synthesis (see Fig. 251-1). Its major active metabolite, oxypurinol, has a long half-life (28 hours) and is primarily responsible for these effects during maintenance. In contrast with uricosuric agents, allopurinol reduces urinary uric acid excretion, is effective in renal failure and very useful in controlling urolithiasis, and its action is not blocked by salicylate. In the presence of renal insufficiency, the maintenance dose of allopurinol should be reduced, since the half-life of oxypurinol is prolonged. Allopurinol-induced xanthinuria has resulted in xanthine renal stones on rare occasions in patients with HPRT deficiency and during chemotherapy for leukemias.

Allopurinol is well tolerated but may cause gastric irritation, diarrhea, or skin rash in about 3% of patients. In about 0.4%, allopurinol causes a serious hypersensitivity syndrome, with worsening renal function, hepatitis, and severe dermatologic injury (epidermal necrolysis, exfoliative dermatitis, erythema multiforme, Stevens-Johnson syndrome), often with fever, leukocytosis, and eosinophilia. Patients with renal insufficiency are at higher risk, particularly if dosage has not been appropriately reduced. Allopuri-

TABLE 251-3. TREATMENT OF GOUT

Acute Gout	Interval Gout	Long Term
Therapeutic goal: Terminate acute inflammatory attack	**Therapeutic goal:** Prevent recurrent attacks	**Therapeutic goals:** Prevent attacks; resolve tophi; maintain serum urate at ≤6 mg/dl
NSAID's *(preferred):* Indomethacin 50 mg qid *or* ibuprofen 800 mg tid (or other NSAID's in full doses) *(lower dose in renal insufficiency; contraindicated with peptic ulcer disease).* OR	**Colchicine, oral:** 0.6–1.2 mg daily as prophylaxis against recurrent attacks.	**Colchicine, oral:** 0.6–1.2 mg daily for 1–2 weeks before initiating hypouricemic therapy and for several months afterwards to prevent recurrent attacks during initial period of hypouricemic therapy.
Colchicine, oral *(used infrequently:* 0.6–1.2 mg (1–2 tablets), then 0.6 mg (1 tablet) q1–2h until attack subsides, *or* until nausea, diarrhea, or GI cramping develops. Maximum total dose 4–6 mg. If ineffective in 48 hr, do not repeat *(see text for discussion of colchicine toxicity).*	Start hypouricemic agent if indicated by frequent attacks, severe hyperuricemia, presence of tophi, urolithiasis, or urate overexcretion.	**Allopurinol:** Dose variable; usually 300 mg once daily, but up to 900 mg may be needed in occasional patient; dose should be reduced to 100 mg daily or every other day in patients with renal insufficiency *(see text for discussion of allopurinol hypersensitivity).* OR
Colchicine, IV *(only if oral medication is precluded):* 1–2 mg in 20 ml 0.9% saline infused slowly *(extravasation causes tissue necrosis);* dose may be repeated once in 6 hr. Few GI symptoms with IV use. Maximum total dose 4 mg per attack. Monitor blood counts.	High fluid intake to promote uric acid excretion in a dilute urine. Diet—moderate protein, low fat; avoid excessive alcohol. Treat hypertension if present.	**Uricosuric agent** (reduced efficacy if creatinine clearance <80 ml; ineffective if <30 ml): Probenecid 0.5–1 gram bid or sulfinpyrazone 100 mg tid or qid; usually well tolerated but may cause headache, GI upset, rash.
Steroids *(only if oral medication is precluded and NSAID's or colchicine are contraindicated, e.g., postoperatively):* Prednisone, 20–40 mg daily, or ACTH 25 U by slow IV infusion. Intra-articular steroids may be used to treat a single inflamed joint: triamcinolone hexacetonide 5–20 mg or dexamethasone phosphate 1–6 mg.		High fluid intake, particularly at night, to promote uric acid excretion in a dilute urine. Acetazolamide 250 mg at bedtime may be used to keep urine pH >6. Diet—moderate protein, low fat; avoid excessive alcohol. Treat hypertension if present.
Hypouricemic agents of no benefit for inflammatory attack and may initiate recurrent attack. Should not be started until attack has resolved, but *ongoing use should not be interrupted during an attack.*		

nol interferes with the metabolism and increases the half-life of azathioprine and 6-mercaptopurine used to treat leukemia and to prevent allograft rejection, conditions in which significant hyperuricemia and gout may be associated with renal insufficiency.

If the serum urate level can be maintained below saturating levels, some tophi resolve, and bone erosions may be reduced. In selected patients, surgical treatment of chronically draining tophi or removal of large extra-articular urate deposits may be advisable. Effective treatment of severe gout is difficult in certain situations, particularly in patients with renal failure and allopurinol hypersensitivity and if allopurinol may interfere with drug therapy necessary for allograft rejection or malignancy. Desensitization to allopurinol has been used in some patients with mild allergic reactions but is considered dangerous in those who have had severe hypersensitivity reactions.

Asymptomatic Hyperuricemia.

Asymptomatic hyperuricemia is frequent in family members of patients with gout and in the general population. Less than a fifth of hyperuricemic individuals ever develop gout, and effective therapy can be begun when attacks do occur. In patients with a strong family history of tophaceous diseases or gout and renal problems, treatment with allopurinol should be begun before articular or renal complications develop.

Arellano F, Sacristan JA: Allopurinol hypersensitivity syndrome: A review. Ann Pharmacother 27:337, 1993. *Reviews over 100 reports of a serious potential complication of allopurinol therapy.*

Delaney V, Sumrani N, Daskalakis P, et al.: Hyperuricemia and gout in renal allograft recipients. Transplant Proc 24:1773, 1992. *Analyzes the risk of hyperuricemia and gout in over 200 renal transplant patients.*

Gaudry M, Roberge CJ, de Medicis R, et al.: Crystal-induced neutrophil activation: III. Inflammatory microcrystals induce a distinct pattern of tyrosine phosphorylation in human neutrophils. J Clin Invest 91:1649, 1993. *Signal transduction pathways involved in triggering the inflammatory response to urate crystals.*

Wallace SL, Singer JZ: Review: Systemic toxicity associated with the intravenous administration of colchicine—guidelines for use. J Rheumatol 15:495, 1988. *Provides guidelines for the cautious use of colchicine for treating gout.*

252   OTHER CRYSTAL DEPOSITION ARTHROPATHIES

H. Ralph Schumacher, Jr.

At least three different calcium-containing crystals are now known to deposit in joints and to be associated with a variety of patterns of arthritis in much the same way as urate crystals cause the various features of gouty arthritis. Calcium pyrophosphate and occasionally calcium oxalate produce linear or punctate calcifications in menisci and articular cartilage that can be readily seen on roentgenograms (Fig. 252–1). These calcifications are termed "chondrocalcinosis." Both these crystals and calcium apatite also can deposit diffusely in synovium and periarticular tissues, giving a soft tissue pattern on roentgenograms. Radiographs may not show obvious calcifications when crystals are relatively few. Definitive diagnosis is made only by aspiration of synovial fluid for identification of the crystal type. In addition to the crystals discussed below, others of various implications may be seen in joint fluids (Table 252–1).

Schumacher HR, Reginato AJ: Atlas of Synovial Fluid Analysis and Crystal Identification. Philadelphia, Lea & Febiger, 1991. *An extensively illustrated compendium of all joint fluid findings, including less common crystals and artifacts.*

CALCIUM PYROPHOSPHATE DIHYDRATE (CPPD) CRYSTAL DEPOSITION DISEASE (Pseudogout Syndrome)

CPPD crystals are rod- or rhomboid-shaped 2- to 20-μm-long, weakly birefringent crystals with positive elongation. CPPD crystals can be present without symptoms or can cause several patterns of arthritis. They are most frequent in the elderly. Up to 27% of nursing home patients in their 80's have radiographic evidence of chondrocalcinosis. Familial cases have been described in populations of various ethnic origins. Both genders are affected.

The cause of CPPD crystal deposition is not established, but local overproduction of pyrophosphate related to excessive activity of

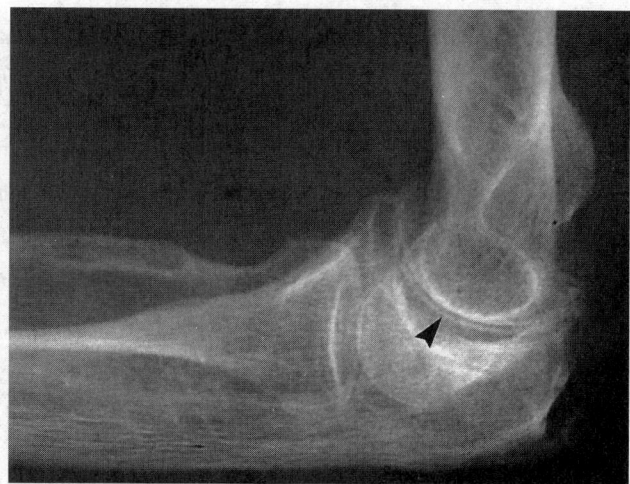

FIGURE 252–1. Chondrocalcinosis *(arrow)* at the elbow joint of a patient with CPPD deposition disease.

nucleoside triphosphate pyrophosphohydrolase, deficiency of phosphatases, and local changes in matrix proteoglycans and collagen are probably important. CPPD crystals deposit only in joints and adjacent tendons or bursae, where they produce hematoxyphilic clumps replacing the normal tissue. Virtually any joint can be involved, but knees, wrists, and second and third metacarpophalangeal joints are most common, so chronic cases can be confused with rheumatoid arthritis. Acute bouts of crystal-induced arthritis at one or more joints can mimic gout and lead to "pseudogout." Fever with bouts can mimic infection. CPPD crystal deposition often complicates osteoarthritis; this association is more prominent at knees than at hips. Whether crystals contribute to cartilage degeneration in osteoarthritis or are purely an epiphenomenon is not yet clear. Occasional severe arthritis mimics the destruction seen in neuropathic joints. Radiographic evidence of calcification can be present in some cases for years without inducing any symptoms. Others may have crystals in joint fluid with osteoarthritis-like radiographic changes but no visible chondrocalcinosis.

Synovial effusions may have leukocyte counts up to 100,000 per cubic millimeter and with 80 to 90% neutrophils during acute attacks. Between attacks or in osteoarthritis, crystals can be seen in clear, noninflammatory joint effusions.

CPPD crystal deposition can be an important clue to a number of associated diseases, many of which have specific treatments that can control systemic features if not the arthropathy. Some clearly associated diseases are shown in Table 252–2. CPPD crystal deposition is increased in knees after meniscectomy and may complicate advanced arthritides.

Treatment of inflammatory episodes with thorough aspiration and use of nonsteroidal anti-inflammatory drugs (NSAID's) is generally successful. Intra-articular steroid injections may provide relief in refractory involvement of individual joints. Intravenous colchicine may also be helpful. Chronic therapy with 0.6 to 1.2 mg of colchicine per day can decrease the frequency of acute attacks. Otherwise the prognosis is for slow progression. Joint replacement has been successful when needed.

Alvarellos A, Spilberg I: Colchicine prophylaxis in pseudogout. J Rheum 13:804, 1986. *Colchicine seems well worth trying to prevent acute exacerbations.*

Rachow JW, Ryan LM: Partial characterization of synovial fluid nucleotide pyrophosphohydrolase. Arthritis Rheum 28:1377, 1985. *Overproduction of pyrophosphate by this soluble extracellular enzyme is one possible factor in CPPD crystal deposition.*

Rahman MU, Shenberger KN, Schumacher HR: Initially unrecognized calcium pyrophosphate dihydrate deposition disease as a cause of fever. Am J Med 89:115, 1990. *Even mild crystal-induced joint findings can cause potentially confusing fever.*

APATITE CRYSTAL DEPOSITION DISEASE

Individual apatite crystals can be seen only by electron microscopy, but clumps of these crystals appear as 2- to 25-μm shiny (but not generally birefringent) globules that can suggest the diag-

TABLE 252-1. DIFFERENTIAL DIAGNOSTIC FEATURES FOR SOME OF THE CRYSTAL-ASSOCIATED ARTHROPATHIES

	Crystal Size (μm)	Crystal Shape	Crystal Birefringence and Elongation	Other Points	X-ray Findings
Calcium pyrophosphate	2–20	Rods, rhomboids	Weak positive	Elderly and consider associated metabolic diseases	Chondrocalcinosis, bony sclerosis
Apatite	2–25	Chunks or globules*	Nonbirefringent	Clumps stained with alizarin red S	Soft tissue calcification
Oxalate	2–15	Rods, bipyramids	Positive	Renal failure	Chondrocalcinosis or soft tissue calcification
Monosodium urate	2–20	Rods, needles	Bright negative	Middle-aged men and elderly women	Cysts and erosions; tophi may calcify
Liquid lipid crystals	2–12	Maltese crosses	Positive	Unexplained acute arthritis	
Cholesterol	10–80	Notched rectangles	Positive or negative	May complicate RA and OA	
Depot corticosteroids	4–15	Irregular or rods	Bright positive or negative	Can cause iatrogenic inflammation	
Immunoglobulins, other proteins	3–60	Rods or irregular	Positive or negative	Cryoglobulinemia	
Charcot-Leyden	10–25	Spindles	Positive or negative	Eosinophilic synovitis	

* Aggregates are seen by light microscopy. Individual needle-shaped crystals are seen only by electron microscopy.

nosis. Apatite crystal deposition and crystal-induced inflammation are common factors in bursitis and periarthritis. Apatites also occur in some otherwise unexplained acute arthritis, and in osteoarthritic joint effusions. Most joints or bursae can be involved, with more common sites including shoulders, hips, knees, and digits (including the first metatarsophalangeal joint). Joint or periarticular inflammation can be acute or chronic. An extremely destructive arthritis has been noted especially at shoulders ("Milwaukee shoulder"), hips, and knees in elderly patients. Radiographs can show soft tissue calcifications with or without bone erosions. Definitive diagnosis of the crystal type is only by electron microscopy with electron probe elemental analysis, x-ray diffraction, or infrared spectroscopy. Other calcium phosphates, such as octacalcium phosphate, can be seen along with the apatite; the significance of amounts of other associated calcium phosphates is not known. Synovial or bursal effusions can have many or few leukocytes. Serum studies are generally normal except that phosphate levels are often elevated in renal dialysis patients, who are at high risk of apatite deposition, and in tumoral calcinosis due to renal retention of phosphate.

Apatite deposition also can be associated with scleroderma and the other connective tissue diseases, repeated depot corticosteroid injections, central nervous system injury, and high-dose vitamin D therapy. In most instances, the cause of soft tissue apatite deposition is not known. Treatment for acute arthritis or periarthritis is with NSAID's or colchicine. Aspiration of crystals and local injection with depot corticosteroids also can be effective.

Doherty M, Holt M, MacMillan P, et al.: A reappraisal of "analgesic" hip. Ann Rheum Dis 45:272, 1986. *Destructive hip arthritis like the "Milwaukee shoulder" is felt to be related to apatite crystal deposition.*

Paul H, Reginato AJ, Schumacher HR: Alizarin red S staining as a screening test to detect calcium compounds in synovial fluid. Arthritis Rheum 26:191, 1983. *This describes a simple office screening test for apatite and other calcium-containing crystals.*

Pinals RS, Short CL: Calcific periarthritis involving multiple sites. Arthritis Rheum 9:566, 1966. *This recurrent calcific periarthritis is related to apatite crystals.*

OXALATE CRYSTAL DEPOSITION DISEASE

Calcium oxalate deposition can occur in joints along with other tissues of patients with renal failure who are on chronic hemodialysis or peritoneal dialysis, producing radiographic evidence of soft tissue calcification or chondrocalcinosis. Acute or chronic joint effusions with intracellular crystals can be seen. Masses of vertebral ox-

TABLE 252-2. SYSTEMIC CONDITIONS ASSOCIATED WITH CPPD DEPOSITION DISEASE

Hyperparathyroidism
Hemochromatosis
Hypophosphatasia
Hypomagnesemia
Myxedematous hypothyroidism
Ochronosis

alates can cause spinal cord compression. Diagnosis is made by identification of typical bipyramidal crystals in joint fluid or biopsy specimens. When less characteristic crystals are seen, other techniques as described under apatite deposition can be used. Vitamin C may potentiate oxalate deposition, so this might be avoided.

Hoffman EC, Schumacher HR, Paul H, et al.: Calcium oxalate microcrystalline-associated arthritis in end stage renal disease. Ann Intern Med 97:36, 1982. *Three cases with oxalosis and arthritis are described. Methods to identify oxalate crystals are included.*

Reginato AJ, Kurnik BRC: Calcium oxalate and other crystals associated with kidney disease and arthritis. Semin Arthritis Rheum 18:198, 1989. *Extensive oxalosis can involve skin, bursae, tendon sheaths, vessel walls, and joints, as well as kidneys and various viscera.*

GOUT

Monosodium urate (MSU) crystal deposition (see Color Plate 3C) in joints and other connective tissues accounts for the most frequent clinical manifestations of gout. The complex genetic, metabolic, and renal factors that interact to produce hyperuricemia and eventually gout are described in detail in Ch. 251. Gouty arthropathy and the gross tophaceous deposits in chronic gout are also described in Ch. 251 but are summarized here, as gout is the most common and prototypical of the crystal deposition diseases.

MSU crystals are rods or needles up to 15 to 20 μm in length and are brightly birefringent with negative elongation when viewed with compensated polarized light. Those from visible tophi or synovial microtophi tend to be more often needle-like, while some in acute arthritis can be very short. At least some crystals are intracellular during gouty arthritis. Leukocyte counts during attacks usually range from 10,000 to 50,000 per cubic millimeter, with 80 to 90% neutrophils. Gout is most common in middle-aged men but is increasingly seen in women after the menopause. It is very rare in premenopausal women but may occur with chronic renal failure. A variety of lower extremity joints are commonly involved, in addition to the classic first metatarsophalangeal joint, but any joint or bursa, including those in the upper extremities, can be affected by either acute or chronic arthritis. Chronic or recurrent acute gout can be polyarticular, can mimic rheumatoid arthritis, and may be misdiagnosed, especially if the typical dramatic early short-lived attacks are not appreciated and synovial fluid is not examined. Tophaceous gout can slowly destroy joints. Crystals are often present in joint fluids even between attacks and may contribute to low-grade inflammation and joint damage.

Radiographs show only soft tissue swelling early in gout but later can reveal cystic erosions with thin, overhanging edges of bone suggestive of gout. Soft tissue tophi are common around joints, in bursae, in Achilles tendons, and at the extensor surface of the forearm; ear tophi appear to be less common than in the past. Gout should be recognized as a syndrome resulting from the many possible causes noted in Ch. 251.

Treatment of acute gouty arthritis can be with NSAID's (although relatively high doses are needed), oral or intravenous colchicine, adrenocorticotropic hormone (ACTH), or prednisone. The latter two agents may be needed in complicated patients with renal failure, liver disease, or gastrointestinal disease. Colchicine is most effective early in attacks (see also Ch. 251). Joint aspiration with instillation of depot corticosteroids also may be used if a single joint is involved and infection is excluded. If recurrent attacks develop, chronic low doses of NSAID's or colchicine can suppress inflammation, but crystal accumulation will likely continue. Thus, with more frequent attacks or visible tophi, patients should be considered for long-term lowering of urate levels with a uricosuric agent such as probenecid (if renal function is good and the patient is not overexcreting uric acid) or, in other cases, allopurinol, a xanthine oxidase inhibitor.

Lawry GV, Fan PT, Bluestone R: Polyarticular versus monoarticular gout. A prospective, comparative analysis of clinical features. Medicine 67:335, 1988. *Polyarticular gout and other crystal-associated diseases continue to be misdiagnosed without synovial fluid analysis. Fever and other constitutional symptoms are common.*
Moreland LM, Ball GV: Colchicine and gout. Arthritis Rheum 34:782, 1991. *Some of the complex situations involved in colchicine use for acute and chronic gout are reviewed. There are risks both from disease progression and from drug toxicities. Colchicine, NSAID's, and allopurinol all require care in appropriate use.*

253 RELAPSING POLYCHONDRITIS
H. Ralph Schumacher, Jr.

This uncommon disease is characterized by recurrent inflammation and destruction of cartilaginous and other connective tissue structures. Frequently involved cartilages are the pinnae of the ears, nasal cartilages, and tracheal rings. Polychondritis occurs nearly equally in both genders and at any age, but with a peak of onset between the ages of 40 and 60.

The pathologic lesion seen by light microscopy consists of loss of matrix staining, predominantly superficial infiltration with polymorphonuclear neutrophils or lymphocytes, and eventual destruction of normal structures followed by fibrosis. Electron microscopy in addition shows alterations of superficial chondrocytes, matrix, and elastic fibers. The cause of polychondritis is unknown, but the location of lesions and frequency of associated systemic diseases suggest the importance of systemic factors. Antibodies to types II, IX, and X collagen and the presence of cell-mediated immunity to proteoglycan and type II collagen are evidence of immunologic aberrations. An association with HLA-DR4 has been noted.

Inflammation of the cartilaginous structures of the ears is the most common initial finding (see Color Plate 10C). There may be acute onset of pain and tenderness with erythema and swelling of one or both helices. The lobe is spared. Inner and middle ear involvement can occur, causing hearing loss or vertigo. Nasal cartilage involvement can produce a saddle nose. Laryngeal and tracheal disease can cause hoarseness or life-threatening upper respiratory obstruction. Ocular manifestations are common and include conjunctivitis, episcleritis, iridocyclitis, proptosis, and rarely other problems, such as optic neuritis. Antigens in the eye that are cross-reactive with cartilage proteoglycans and their link protein have been identified.

Cardiac involvement, especially of the aortic root with aortic insufficiency, is seen in up to one fourth of cases. There also may be aortic aneurysms. Arthritis is reported in about three fourths of cases. This is generally nondestructive. Fever, rashes, oral or genital ulcers, and neurologic and renal disease can occur. Renal involvement can include glomerulonephritis and immunoglobulin A (IgA) nephropathy.

There are no diagnostic laboratory tests, although the erythrocyte sedimentation rate is often elevated. Antineutrophil cytoplasmic antibodies (ANCA's) have been reported. There may be anemia and leukocytosis. Roentgenograms can detect advanced tracheal narrowing. Computed tomographic (CT) scans and pulmonary function tests can detect more subtle airway obstruction.

Relapsing polychondritis is associated with other diseases in one third or more of cases. These include rheumatoid arthritis, systemic lupus erythematosus, Sjögren's syndrome, thyroid disease, ulcerative colitis, psoriasis, spondylarthropathies, Behçet's disease, vasculitis of various types, cryoglobulinemia, diabetes mellitus, biliary cirrhosis, panniculitis, malignancies, myelodysplastic syndromes, sinusitis, and mastoiditis. Wegener's granulomatosis and infections can cause potentially confusing chondritis.

In mild cases, nonsteroidal anti-inflammatory agents can be used for symptomatic treatment, although adrenocorticosteroids in the range of 30 to 60 mg of prednisone per day are generally needed for acute inflammatory episodes and severe respiratory involvement. Immunosuppressives and cyclosporine have been used with apparent benefit. Dapsone has been used with variable results in several series. Tracheostomy or stents may be life-saving if tracheal collapse occurs.

The course is unpredictable, with about 55% of subjects surviving for 10 years. Infection and systemic vasculitis caused more deaths than did airway obstruction in a recent series. Remissions do occur. Aortic valve disease has required surgery.

Chang-Miller A, Okamura M, Torres VE, et al.: Renal involvement in relapsing polychondritis. Medicine 66:202, 1987. *Glomerulonephritis often responds to corticosteroids or cytotoxic agents.*
Lang B, Rothenfusser A, Lanchbury JS: Susceptibility to relapsing polychondritis is associated with HLA-DR4. Arthritis Rheum 36:660, 1993. *HLA-DR4 was seen in 56% of 41 cases, suggesting similarities to rheumatoid arthritis, which is also DR4-associated.*
Michet CJ, McKenna CH, Luthra HS, et al.: Relapsing polychondritis. Survival and predictive role of early disease manifestations. Ann Intern Med 104:74, 1986. *Anemia, saddle nose deformity, and vasculitis appear to be poor prognostic signs.*
Pazirandeh M, Ziran BH, Khandelwal BK: Relapsing polychondritis and spondylarthropathies. J Rheum 15:630, 1988. *In addition to the many associated autoimmune diseases, one must also consider a possible relationship to psoriasis and spondylarthropathy.*
Yang CL, Brinkmann J, Rui HF, et al.: Autoantibodies to cartilage collagens in relapsing polychondritis. Arch Dermatol Res 285:245, 1993. *Immune mechanisms appear to be important.*

254 OSTEOARTHRITIS (Degenerative Bone Disease)
Thomas J. Schnitzer

Osteoarthritis (OA) is a disorder of diarthrodial joints characterized clinically by pain and functional limitations, radiographically by osteophytes and joint space narrowing, and histopathologically by alterations in cartilage integrity. The most common of all joint diseases, its importance derives from its economic impact, in terms of both productivity (single greatest cause of days lost from work) and cost of treatment (chronic use of analgesics and anti-inflammatory drugs). Although the etiology of the disorder is still not clearly understood, OA has been shown to be a family of disorders with cartilage as a target organ in which biomechanical factors play a central role and with risk factors such as age, weight, and occupation also of major importance. Since there is currently no treatment to prevent or ameliorate the basic disease process, medical treatment is aimed primarily at relieving pain, with orthopedic intervention largely reserved for those situations which cannot be controlled with more conservative therapy.

EPIDEMIOLOGY. OA is by far the most common joint disorder, one of the most common chronic diseases in the elderly, and a leading cause of disability. Because OA can be defined both radiographically and clinically and because there is little correlation between the two, the prevalence of this condition has been variously estimated in epidemiologic studies. Using radiographic criteria, prevalence of the joint findings steadily increases from <2% in women under age 45 to 30% in those aged 45 to 64 and to 68% in those older than 65. Prevalence in men is slightly higher in the younger age groups (younger than 45), while women are affected more commonly at ages over 55, except for disease of the hip.

The pattern of joint involvement in OA is strikingly affected by age, gender, and previous occupational history. Prior to age 55, there is little difference in joint pattern between men and women. In older men, hip OA is more common, while older women tend to have more involvement of the proximal interphalangeal (PIP) joints and the base of the thumb. Joints subjected to repeated trauma or overuse demonstrate a higher prevalence of OA. Cotton and mill workers have increased OA of the hand and involved fingers, miners demonstrate increased knee and spine involvement, and pneumatic drill workers experience increased elbow and wrist disease.

Racial and genetic factors are also important in OA prevalence and pattern. Chinese, Jamaican blacks, South African blacks, and Asian Indians have been shown to have a lower incidence of OA of the hip than Caucasians, while Japanese have an increased incidence, apparently related to the more frequent occurrence of congenital hip dysplasia. African-American women have a higher prevalence of knee OA than Caucasian women but a lower prevalence of involvement of the distal interphalangeal (DIP) joints of the hand (Heberden's nodes). Involvement of the DIP joints of the hands is particularly common in women and is often found to have a familial pattern of inheritance, with the female relatives of the proband having similar joint findings with a two- to fivefold increased prevalence.

Additional modifiable risk factors for OA also have been identified in recent studies. Weight demonstrates by far the strongest association with OA; and importantly, weight reduction has been shown to correlate with a reduction in the risk of later OA. Certain types of repetitive activities have been correlated with increased OA in the stressed joint (see above), while, interestingly, others have not. In particular, there appears to be no increased prevalence of knee OA in marathon runners, but this may be due to a self-selection process, with those experiencing knee pain unable to continue the activity. Smoking and osteoporosis have both been shown to be negatively associated with OA, but the explanation for this association is unknown.

PATHOLOGY. The hallmarks of OA on gross or arthroscopic examination are focal ulcerated areas of cartilage exposing underlying eburnated (ivory-appearing) bone that occur at the load-bearing areas of the joint surface as well as the juxta-articular osteophytes that grow at the joint margins. It is important to understand that these states represent the end stage of a continuum and that OA is a pathologic *process*. At its earliest stage, it presents as softening of the cartilage surface, progressing to fibrillation of the surface layers, loss of cartilage thickness, the development of clefts into the depth of cartilage, and eventual loss of cartilage integrity with release of shards of cartilage. Bone participates in this process as well, with reactive changes (bony sclerosis) underlying the areas of cartilage loss, the development of subchondral bone cysts that may communicate with the joint space and expand into geodes, and marginal osteophytes (new cartilage and bone growth) at non–weight-bearing areas.

The earliest histologic changes reveal loss of extracellular cartilage matrix, loss of chondrocytes in the surface layers of articular cartilage, and reactive changes in the deeper chondrocytes manifested by cellular division and "cloning" in an apparent attempt at repair. Later, there is progressive loss of chondrocytes at all levels, with marked thinning of the cartilage matrix and, in some instances, the development of fibrocartilage in place of lost hyaline cartilage. The surrounding synovium is largely unaffected, although in later disease cartilage fragments may incite focal inflammatory lesions without the progressive and destructive pannus seen in typical inflammatory arthropathies.

PATHOGENESIS. Articular cartilage serves two major functions: (1) to permit nearly frictionless joint motion and (2) to act as a "shock absorber" and transmit loads across joint surfaces to the surrounding tissues. The requisite properties of elasticity and high tensile strength are imparted by proteoglycans and collagen of the extracellular matrix that comprise over 90% of the cartilage substance. The proteoglycan elements of the matrix are actively being metabolized and turned over with a half-life of weeks. The highly negatively charged sulfated glycosaminoglycan components of the proteoglycans impart the elastic properties to cartilage. The collagen component is characterized by a unique structure (type II collagen), provides the tensile strength, and tightly constrains the proteoglycan molecules in a three-dimensional framework. The collagen fibers are covalently linked by other matrix molecules believed to provide

the "glue" to hold the matrix intact. Collagen itself is extremely slowly metabolized (half-life of many years) in the normal state.

In OA, there is chondrocyte "exhaustion" with loss of matrix and cells, loss of cartilage integrity, and eventual ulceration. The reasons for failure of collagen repair are unknown but may relate to the role of mechanical factors preventing appropriate apposition of cartilage matrix or the inability to re-form the complex three-dimensional architecture in mature individuals.

The processes responsible for degrading collagen and proteoglycans in OA are driven by proteolytic enzymes being synthesized and released from the chondrocytes themselves. Although chondrocytes can respond to cytokines released from inflammatory cells in synovial fluid, in OA it appears that chondrocytic chondrolysis is initiated primarily by changes in mechanical properties of the surrounding matrix. The release of potent proteolytic enzymes and their subsequent activation in the matrix overwhelm the natural matrix defenses and ultimately result in collagen breakdown and proteoglycan cleavage. Fragments from these molecules are then released into the synovial fluid and enter the circulation, where they provide "markers" and can be used as a means to detect and measure the degradative process.

The factors responsible for activating chondrocytes to degrade matrix in OA are not known but in most instances may relate to changes in mechanical forces on the cartilage itself. Those conditions causing biomechanical alteration of cartilage are known to lead to OA: joint injury, abnormal joint loading due to neuropathic changes (Charcot joint) or ligamentous damage (ACL or meniscus injuries), altered joint surface congruity as in dysplasias, and muscle atrophy in the elderly. A number of metabolic conditions are known to predispose to the early onset of OA: ochronosis with the deposition of homogentisic acid and hemochromatosis with the deposition of iron. Gene defects affecting matrix structures would be expected to possibly lead to OA, but thus far genetic factors have played a role only in the development of dysplasias with secondary OA changes. The pathogenetic mechanisms and feedback loops associated with altered cartilage structure and biomechanics are demonstrated in Figure 254–1.

CLINICAL FEATURES. The initial stages of the OA process are clinically silent, which explains the high prevalence of radiographic and pathologic signs of OA in patients who exhibit no clinical symptoms of the disease. Even in later stages of OA, there is a poor correlation between clinical symptoms and alterations in cartilage and bone integrity, defined arthroscopically or by indirect imaging techniques (radiography, magnetic resonance imaging [MRI]). The factors or events that make the OA process clinically apparent are unknown but are likely to be heterogeneous in nature and invoke processes within the synovium, bone, and surrounding supporting structures (muscle, ligaments) that produce pain rather than involve cartilage itself, a completely aneural tissue.

Pain is the predominant symptom that prompts the diagnosis of OA, initially often involving only one joint, with others becoming painful subsequently. The pain is most often described as a deep ache, accompanied frequently by joint stiffness that follows periods of inactivity (upon arising in the morning, after sitting). Pain is aggravated by using the involved joints, may radiate or be referred to surrounding structures, and in the early stages of the disease is commonly relieved by rest. With more severe disease, pain may be persistent, interfering with normal function and preventing sleep, even with medical management. Such patients are candidates for surgery. Even in severe disease, systemic manifestations such as fever, weight loss, anemia, and elevated erythrocyte sedimentation rate (ESR) are not present.

The joints most commonly involved in OA are the metatarsophalangeal (MTP) joint of the great toe (hallux valgus or "bunion"), the proximal (PIP) and distal (DIP) interphalangeal joints, the carpometacarpal (CMC) joint of the thumb, hips, knees, and both lumbar and cervical spine. Interestingly, other joints, even major weight-bearing joints such as the ankle, are regularly spared unless involved in secondary forms of OA (Table 254–1). On physical examination, the joints may demonstrate tenderness, crepitus, and a limited range of motion. Joint swelling may be due to an accompanying synovial effusion or bony enlargement and osteophytes. Joint instability is seen only in severe disease or after internal derangement of the knee with disruption of one or more of the major supporting structures (e.g., anterior cruciate ligament, medial collateral ligament). Patients with far-advanced disease exhibit gross defor-

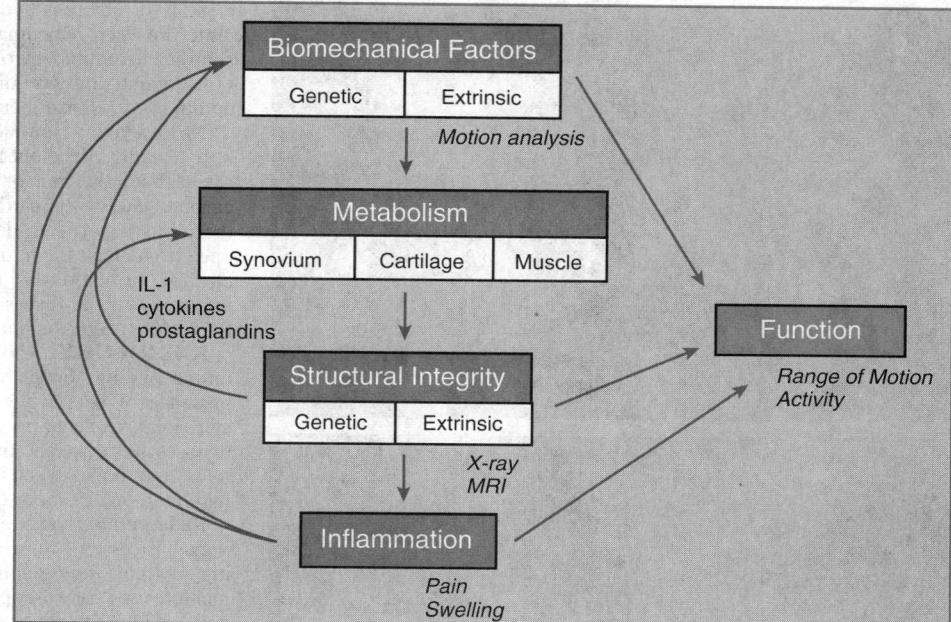

FIGURE 254–1. Pathogenetic pathways in osteoarthritis.

mity with subluxation of involved joints. Although OA is thought to be a uniformly progressive disease that invariably leads to joint replacement, this is not the case. The disease appears to stabilize in many patients with no worsening of signs or symptoms and actual improvement in some.

SPECIFIC JOINT INVOLVEMENT. *Hand.* Firm, slowly progressive bony enlargements of the DIP joints are called Heberden's nodes and represent marginal osteophytic spurs. Occasionally, the onset of symptoms is acute with sudden redness and tenderness in the involved joint. These changes can lead to deformity at these

TABLE 254–1. ETIOLOGIC CLASSIFICATION OF OSTEOARTHRITIS*

Idiopathic (primary)

Localized
  Hands: Heberden's nodes, erosive interphalangeal arthropathy
  Feet: hallux valgus, hammer toes; talonavicular osteoarthritis
  Knees: medial, lateral, patellofemoral compartments
  Hips: sites of cartilage loss—eccentric (superior), concentric (axial, medial), diffuse
  Spine: zygoapophyseal joints, osteophytes, intervertebral discs (spondylosis); ligaments, e.g., disseminated idiopathic skeletal hyperostosis
  Other single sites: shoulder, temporomandibular, carpometacarpal joints
Generalized—Includes three or more areas listed above
Mineral deposition diseases
  Calcium pyrophosphate deposition disease
  Hydroxyapatite arthropathy
  Destructive disease (e.g., Milwaukee shoulder)

Secondary

Post-traumatic
Congenital or developmental
  Legg-Calvé-Perthes hip dislocation
  Epiphyseal dysplasias
  Articular cartilage disorders associated with a gene deficiency (e.g., association with type II procollagen gene mutation)
Disturbed local tissue structure by primary disease, e.g., ischemic necrosis, tophaceous gout, hyperparathyroid cysts, Paget's disease, rheumatoid arthritis, osteopetrosis, osteochondritis
Miscellaneous additional diseases
  Endocrine: diabetes mellitus, acromegaly, hypothyroidism
  Metabolic: hemochromatosis, ochronosis, Gaucher's disease
  Neuropathic arthropathies
  Miscellaneous: frostbite, Kashin-Beck disease, caisson disease
  Mechanical: obesity, unequal lower extremity length; valgus/varus deformities, ligamentous laxity (including associations with type I procollagen gene mutations of Ehlers-Danlos syndrome).

*Compiled in part by Osteoarthritis Diagnostic Criteria Committee, American Rheumatism Association, 1983.

joints with lateral and flexor deviation. A related disorder, erosive OA, similarly produces repetitive episodes of acute symptoms and is differentiated by the additional finding of erosive changes on radiographs of the involved joints and a tendency to bony ankylosis. A genetic basis for Heberden's nodes appears to exist, the condition demonstrating a distinct female-dominant familial tendency (women are affected 10 times more commonly than men) (Fig. 254–2). Changes similar to those in the DIP joints occur in the PIP joints and are termed Bouchard's nodes. The only other joint to be commonly involved is the CMC joint of the thumb, often eliciting complaints of pain on use (wringing out clothes [washerwoman's hands] and grasping objects such as screwdrivers and doorknobs) and leading to a squared appearance of the base of the hand.

Knee. Idiopathic knee OA is a leading cause of painful ambulation and is directly related to weight; it is more common in women than in men. The medial compartment of the femorotibial joint space is most commonly affected, resulting in varus deformity (bow legs). Lateral compartment disease may lead to valgus (knock-knee) deformity. Patellofemoral disease has been shown recently to be common and may represent a substantial portion of knee pathology in patients presenting with knee pain. It is important to exclude other causes of knee pain such as internal derangements of the knee (which may lead to secondary knee OA), soft tissue sprains, bursal inflammation, and Baker's cysts (which may coexist with knee OA). In young women, the possibility of chondromalacia patellae should always be considered. Its cause is not known; it is almost always self-limited and is not thought to lead to OA. In idiopathic knee OA, physical examination of the involved joint often elicits crepitus, pain, and decreased range of motion. Effusions are not infrequently present but are often small and may be difficult to appreciate.

Hip. Although congenital (Legg-Calvé-Perthes disease) and developmental (slipped femoral capital epiphysis) abnormalities have long been implicated in secondary hip OA, the majority of primary hip OA is now believed to be the consequence of mild dysplasia of the femoral head and/or acetabulum resulting in incongruity of the articulating surfaces. With use of the joint, there is progressive cartilage degeneration and secondary bony productive changes typical of OA. Pain is typically referred to the groin, with anterior thigh and knee symptoms occasionally predominant. The majority of patients presenting with pain in their "hip" are suffering from OA of the lumbar spine. The earliest physical finding in hip OA is loss of internal rotation; with progressive disease, range of motion is limited further in all directions, and significant functional limitation occurs, often necessitating surgery.

Foot. The first MTP joint is the primary joint involved with associated bony swelling and deformity (bunion). Significantly more common in women than men, these changes have been attributed to

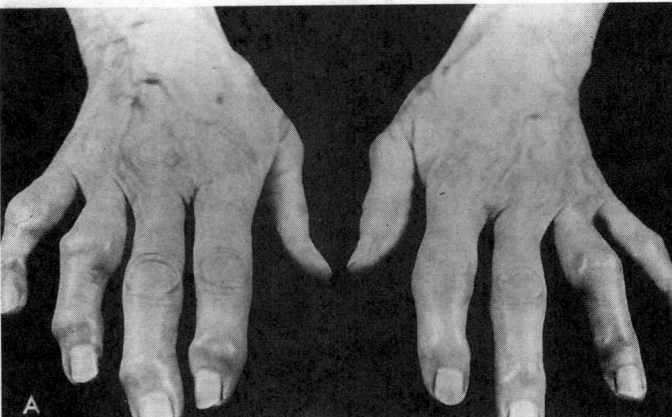

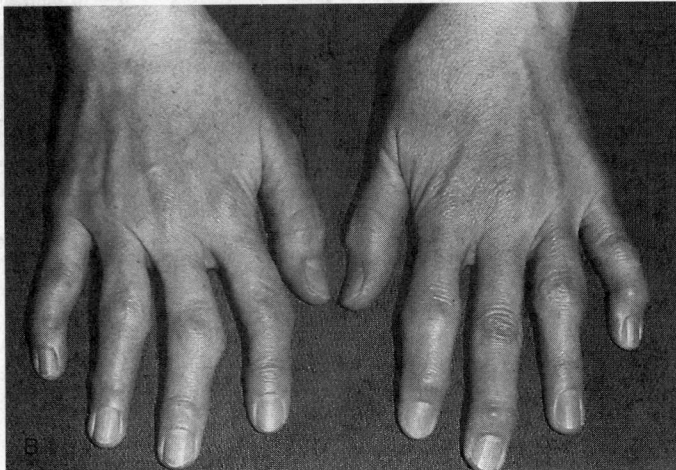

FIGURE 254-2. Typical hand deformities in osteoarthritis. *A,* Typical Heberden's and Bouchard's nodes comprise hypertrophic joint capsular and bony enlargement of the distal and proximal interphalangeal joints, respectively. *B,* Prominent Bouchard's nodes and minor subluxations may cause misdiagnosis of rheumatoid arthritis.

abnormal stresses imposed on the joint by footwear. In extreme cases, the joint space may be destroyed, leading to a condition known as "hallux rigidus," which may interfere with normal ambulation and necessitate surgical correction.

Spine. Technically, OA of the spine relates strictly to changes in synovial-lined joints (apophyseal and uncovertebral joints) that can lead to localized pain as well as irritation of adjacent nerve roots with referred pain in the form of radiculopathy. Nerve root compression resulting from apophyseal joint subluxation, prolapse of an intervertebral disc, or osteophytic spurring may occur and present with muscle weakness, hyporeflexia, and paresthesia or hypesthesia. In the cervical region, spinal involvement can lead to cord impingement with long tract signs or may affect the vertebral artery, producing posterior circulation insufficiency with associated symptoms. OA of the spine should be differentiated from diffuse skeletal hyperostosis (DISH), in which there is marked calcification of the paraspinous ligaments and sparing of the arthrodial spinal joints.

Primary Generalized OA. The pattern of involvement of three or more joints or joint groups with OA has been given this name and is seen most commonly in older women. Typically, the DIP and PIP joints of the hand, the knees, and the spine are involved. Whether this represents a distinct subset of OA is not known but has been suggested.

LABORATORY FINDINGS. OA involves a pathologic process that appears largely limited to cartilage and surrounding tissues with no evidence of systemic involvement. Typically, the ESR is normal, and there is no elevation of acute-phase reactants. The hemoglobin and leukocyte counts remain within normal limits. The synovial fluid itself demonstrates no evidence of an inflammatory

reaction with few leukocytes (typically <3000 per cubic millimeter) and good viscosity. Occasionally, fragments of cartilage and crystals of calcium hydroxyapatite or calcium pyrophosphate dihydrate are seen. Rheumatoid factor is absent in the majority, but a significant number of older individuals will exhibit low titer elevations which are not diagnostic of rheumatoid arthritis but are a common accompaniment of aging.

Various assays of biochemical markers of disease activity have been recently developed and hold great promise to more accurately assess both the rate of progression of the disease process and the current state of the cartilage. Cartilage matrix components unique to the joints have been identified, and sensitive tests have been developed to detect them in synovial fluid, serum, and urine. Further clinical correlations will need to be performed to determine their relationship to the disease process, activity, and state and their utility for earlier diagnosis and management of OA.

RADIOLOGY AND IMAGING TECHNIQUES. Pathognomonic findings on plain radiography of involved joints include the presence of osteophytes at the margins of involved joints, associated joint space narrowing representing areas of cartilage thinning or loss, and evidence of bony reaction marked by subchondral sclerosis and bone cysts in more progressive disease. Some patients may lack one or more of these findings.

Radiography has been shown to be very insensitive to the pathologic processes occurring in the cartilage, with many patients having normal radiographs but destructive cartilage changes documented by arthroscopy. Other techniques have therefore been developed with greater potential sensitivity to detect cartilage change. In particular, MRI has the advantage of demonstrating cartilage as a positive image and has been used widely to document major cartilage injury such as meniscal tears. Further refinement of this technology will enhance the resolution possible as well as increasing sensitivity to detect changes in hydration, which mark the earliest changes in OA. It is anticipated that such technology will be important in assessing disease progression in the future.

Other technologies being developed to evaluate the OA joint include scintigraphy and ultrasound.

TREATMENT. People with OA seek pain relief and improvement in their physical function. Because there is no known therapy in humans that affects the basic disease process (inhibits cartilage degradation or enhances synthesis), medical therapy has focused on providing symptomatic relief. Largely because of ease of administration and acceptance by patients, an unwarranted reliance has been placed on pharmacologic intervention, particularly nonsteroidal anti-inflammatory agents (NSAID's), as initial therapy at the expense of physical measures that have less morbidity and may provide longer-term benefit.

Pharmacologic Therapy. Symptomatic relief of pain in patients with OA is best achieved with simple analgesic agents such as acetaminophen. The effectiveness of NSAID's is due primarily to their analgesic rather than anti-inflammatory properties. Recent controlled studies have demonstrated that acetaminophen is as effective as NSAID's with considerably fewer serious side effects. Particularly in the elderly with decreased renal reserve and an increased incidence of upper gastrointestinal bleeding, acetaminophen and other simple analgesics should be the drugs of initial choice. If inflammation is present (erosive OA) or symptoms are not well controlled with simple analgesics, lower doses of NSAID's may prove to be effective. Intra-articular injection of various steroid preparations also can control joint symptoms. Controlled studies have demonstrated only short-term relief of symptoms, although some patients with OA may derive longer-term (months) benefit. Intra-articular injections should not be repeated more than three to four times per year in any given joint because of the possibility of the steroids potentiating cartilage breakdown. Systemic use of steroids has no place in the treatment of OA.

Other approaches to therapy are under investigation. Topical treatment with capsaicin, a substance-P inhibitor, has been shown to relieve pain in some patients with OA. The intra-articular injection of hyaluronan is undergoing clinical trials. The development of agents that can stimulate cartilage synthesis or prevent degradation is being actively pursued and should provide the next generation of agents used to treat this condition.

Physical Measures. Although often overlooked, physical therapy and exercise programs can provide important benefit to patients with OA. Muscle atrophy commonly accompanies OA. Because muscles serve to reduce load on cartilage, maintaining muscle function is crucial for cartilage integrity and can reduce pain. Both muscle strength and range of motion can be improved with appropriate physical therapy. Isometric exercises are preferred to isotonic because they place less stress on the involved joint.

Heat and cold are both used with varying effectiveness to provide symptomatic relief to patients and as an important adjunct to physical therapy regimens. Using transcutaneous nerve stimulation (TENS), particularly to relieve back pain, is effective in some patients and provides an attractive alternative to pharmacologic intervention.

Periods of rest throughout the day may be an important adjunct in the routine of patients with OA. Reduction in joint loading, either by resting or appropriately using a cane, often will permit increased periods of activity with reduced pain. Using cushioned shoes (commercial running or walking shoes) also may help lower extremity joint symptoms. Back pain may be reduced by muscle-strengthening exercises as well as a well-fitted brace.

Orthopedic Surgery.
Joint replacement surgery has been the single biggest advance in the treatment of OA in the past half century. Patients in whom optimal medical management has failed and who continue to have pain that interferes with sleep or activity or have significant limitations of joint function are candidates for an operation. Some individuals, those with altered limb alignment and early OA of a hip or knee, may benefit from osteotomy. Most patients have more advanced disease and require total joint replacement. Ideal candidates for total joint arthroplasty have well-maintained muscle strength and should be older than age 60. Younger patients are discouraged from undergoing joint replacement because of the small but real incidence of long-term failure of joint implants, mainly due to loosening. Revision arthroplasty is possible but has a higher failure rate and can be avoided by delaying initial arthroplasty as long as possible and putting less load on the replaced joint.

Arthroscopic surgery is useful for removing loose bodies and repairing intrinsic defects of the knee as well as shoulder (rotator cuff) and ankle pathology. Arthroscopic lavage (flushing of saline to remove cartilage debris) in patients with knee OA may provide pain relief. Abrasion arthroplasty (chondroplasty) has been widely used in patients with knee OA, but no data exist to demonstrate its efficacy, and it cannot be recommended currently.

Kuettner KE, Schleyerbach R, Peyron JG, et al.: Articular Cartilage and Osteoarthritis: Workshop Conference Hoechst Werk Kalle-Albert, Wiesbaden. New York, Raven Press, 1991. *Current understanding of cartilage biology and the pathogenesis of OA.*
McCarthy DJ: Arthritis and Allied Conditions. Philadelphia, Lea & Febiger, 1989. *Comprehensive overview of all aspects with illustrations.*
Moskowitz W, Howell DS, Goldberg VM, et al.: Osteoarthritis: Diagnosis and Medical/Surgical Management. Philadelphia, WB Saunders, 1992. *In-depth coverage of all aspects of OA.*
Silman AJ, Hochberg MC (eds.): Epidemiology of the Rheumatic Diseases. New York, Oxford Press, 1993. *A comprehensive review of definition, incidence, and prevalence of disease.*

255 THE PAINFUL SHOULDER
Dennis W. Boulware

Shoulder pain is a frequent complaint among adults and is likely to increase in prevalence as the population ages and active lifestyles remain popular. Pain can originate from many anatomic sites, including the glenohumeral joint, the periarticular soft tissue structures, or referred from the cervical spine, the thorax, the diaphragm, and the upper abdominal cavity. Although nonmusculoskeletal causes of shoulder pain are important, this chapter will focus on the musculoskeletal causes of isolated shoulder pain.

Most causes of shoulder pain are due to pathology involving the surrounding periarticular soft tissue structures: the *tendons* of the biceps and rotator cuff, the subacromial and subdeltoid *bursae*, and the *articular capsule* (Fig. 255–1). Infrequently, diseases of the *bone* and the *glenohumeral joint* can be responsible for shoulder pain. A basic knowledge of the anatomy of the shoulder joint and

the physical examination of these specific structures are essential for proper diagnosis and management.

TENDONS. In general, tendon lesions are painful only during active use. A bicipital tendinitis will hurt during active flexion of the elbow or forward flexion of the shoulder, and a rotator cuff lesion will cause pain on abduction of the shoulder. On examination, active testing of the myotendinous unit results in more tenderness than passive range of motion.

The Rotator Cuff.
All *lesions of the rotator cuff* will precipitate pain on active abduction of the shoulder, particularly the initial 90 degrees of motion. This pain is usually focused over the lateral aspect of the shoulder and frequently a problem at night. On examination of the shoulder, active abduction will elicit more tenderness than passive abduction done by the examiner. A "drop sign" is helpful in identifying the rotator cuff as the source of pain. With the patient's arm passively placed at full abduction, the patient will experience severe pain when the arm is slowly adducted from 120 to 60 degrees and the arm will reflexively "drop."

Rotator cuff tendinitis is the most common cause of shoulder pain and is usually due to overusing the arm in overhead activities. This abducted position impinges the cuff between the acromian and the humeral head. Chronic impingements also can occur from inferior osteophytes of the acromioclavicular joint encroaching into the acromiohumeral space. With time, chronic impingements can result in attenuation of the rotator cuff and an eventual tear.

Injury, overuse, or degenerative processes can lead to *rotator cuff tears* in the shoulder. The tear can exist as a complete rupture of the rotator cuff or as incomplete tears. The pain is worse with active abduction of the shoulder, particularly the initial 90 degrees. A complete tear of the cuff will make abduction of the initial 90 degrees impossible.

The diagnosis of *calcific tendinitis* is made in the clinical setting of a rotator cuff tendinitis coupled with the radiographic appearance of calcification of the rotator cuff, usually the supraspinatus tendon near its insertion on the humerus (Fig. 255–2).

Diagnostic plain radiography is helpful in chronic rotator cuff lesions. Chronic impingements with tendinitis will reveal sclerotic and cystic changes of the humeral greater tuberosity. Significant attrition or complete tears of the cuff will be demonstrated as narrowing or obliteration of the acromiohumeral space. *Magnetic resonance imaging* and *ultrasonography* are useful but expensive and difficult to interpret except by experienced musculoskeletal radiologists. *Arthrography* is the best study to document complete ruptures and often can detect incomplete tears (Fig. 255–3).

The *diagnosis of a rotator cuff lesion* often can be made by instilling an intralesional local anesthetic agent. When 2 to 4 ml of a local anesthetic is properly placed inferolaterally to the acromial process in the subacromial bursa, the patient should experience significant relief of pain and be capable of active, painless abduction. The exception will be the complete rupture of the rotator cuff, which will have pain relief but still be incapable of unassisted abduction.

The *treatment of lesions of the rotator cuff* is similar for all types of problems except a complete tear, which will require a surgical referral. Initial management with heat, physical therapy, and nonsteroidal anti-inflammatory drugs (NSAID's) is more effective when prescribed early. If ineffective, intralesional corticosteroid agents placed in the subacromial bursa may be required. Recalcitrant cases of impingement may eventually require surgery in the form of acromioplasty. Job modification for individuals with chronic impingement from occupational overuse will be essential.

Bicipital Tendon.
In *bicipital tendinitis,* the tendon of the long head of the biceps becomes inflamed as it traverses the bicipital groove of the humerus. Clinically, the patient experiences pain in the anterior aspect of the shoulder, especially upon actively using the biceps. Clinical examination can confirm the presence of bicipital tendinitis by one of several techniques. Directly palpating the tendon within the bicipital groove will result in tenderness, which can be accentuated by passively rotating the shoulder while maintaining pressure over the tendon. Alternatively, the patient can be placed in the initial position of maximal elbow flexion and wrist supination and asked to resist an attempt to suddenly extend the elbow and pronate the wrist. Tenderness in the anterior shoulder would be indicative of bicipital tendinitis (Yergason's sign).

Clavicle

Acromion

Subacromial bursa

Supraspinatus muscle

Coracoid process

Deltoid muscle

Glenohumeral fossa

Lesser tubercle

Greater tubercle

Intertubercular groove

Humerus

FIGURE 255–1. Anterior aspect of the shoulder joint showing palpable landmarks and their relationship to the subacromial bursa. (From Polley HF, Hunder GG [eds.]: Rheumatologic Interviewing and Physical Examination of the Joints, 2nd ed. Philadelphia, WB Saunders, 1978, p 63.)

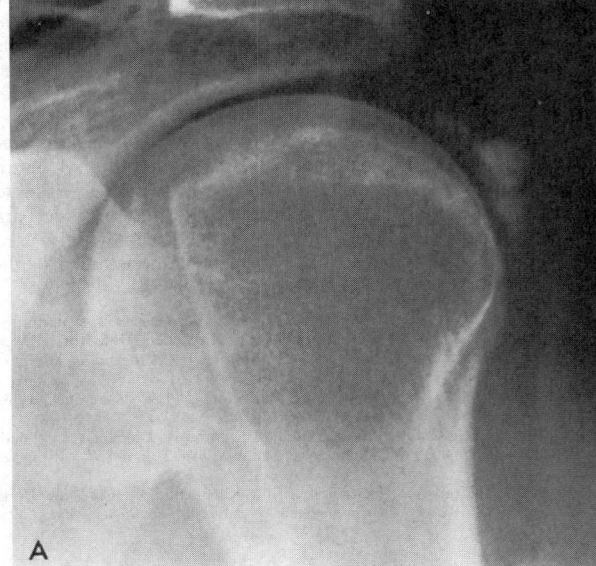

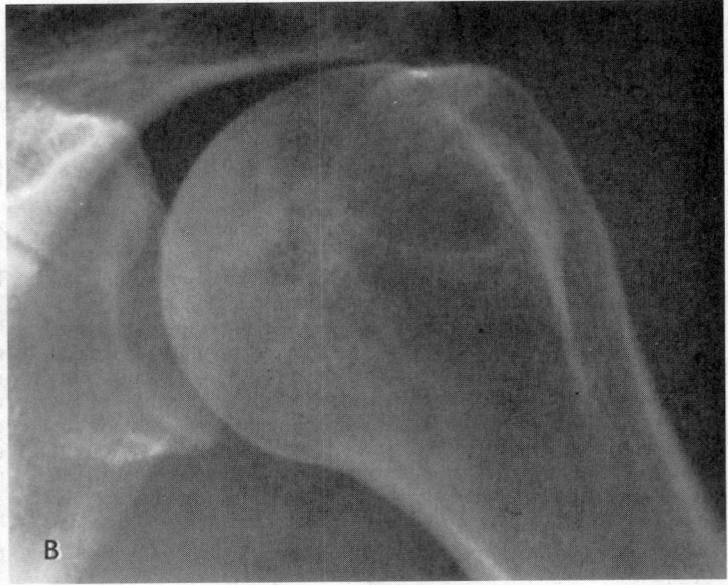

FIGURE 255–2. Calcific tendinitis. *A*, Two distinct deposits of calcium are present on the internal rotation view. *B*, External rotation projects the supraspinatus calcification above the greater tuberosity and superimposes the larger collection (within the infraspinatus tendon) over the humeral head. (From Forrester DM, Brown JC: The Radiology of Joint Disease, Vol 2. Philadelphia, WB Saunders, 1987, p 364.)

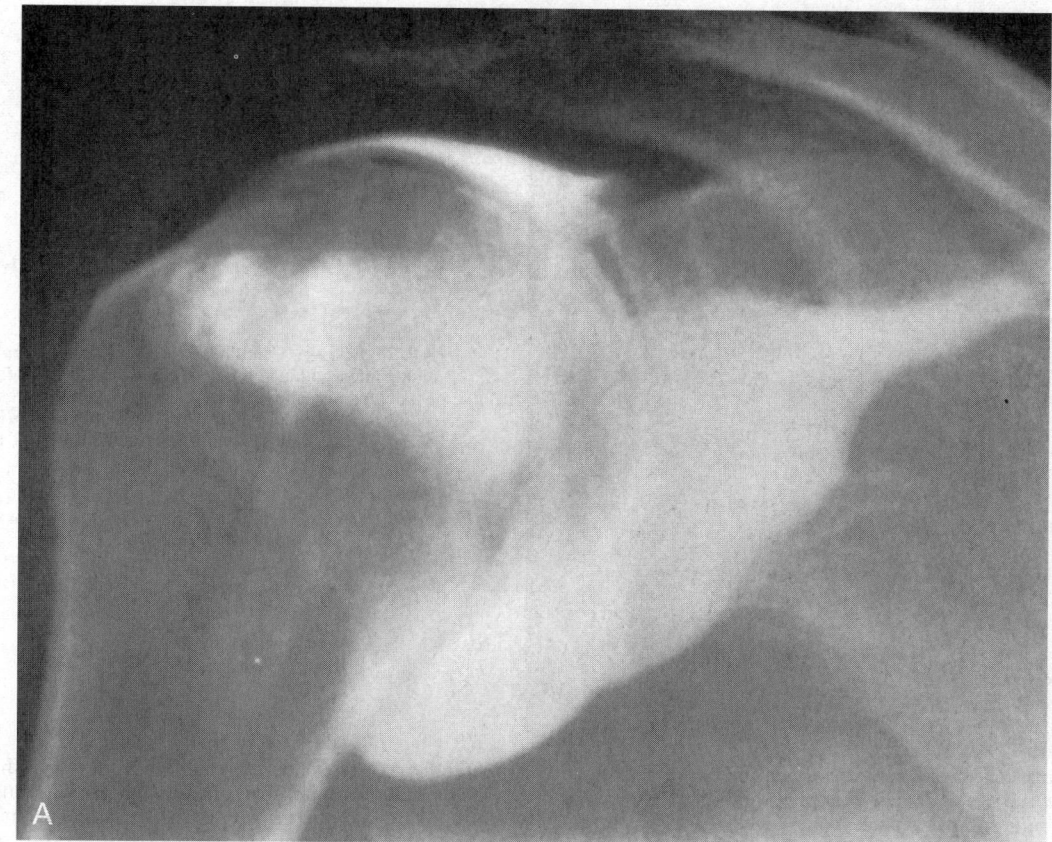

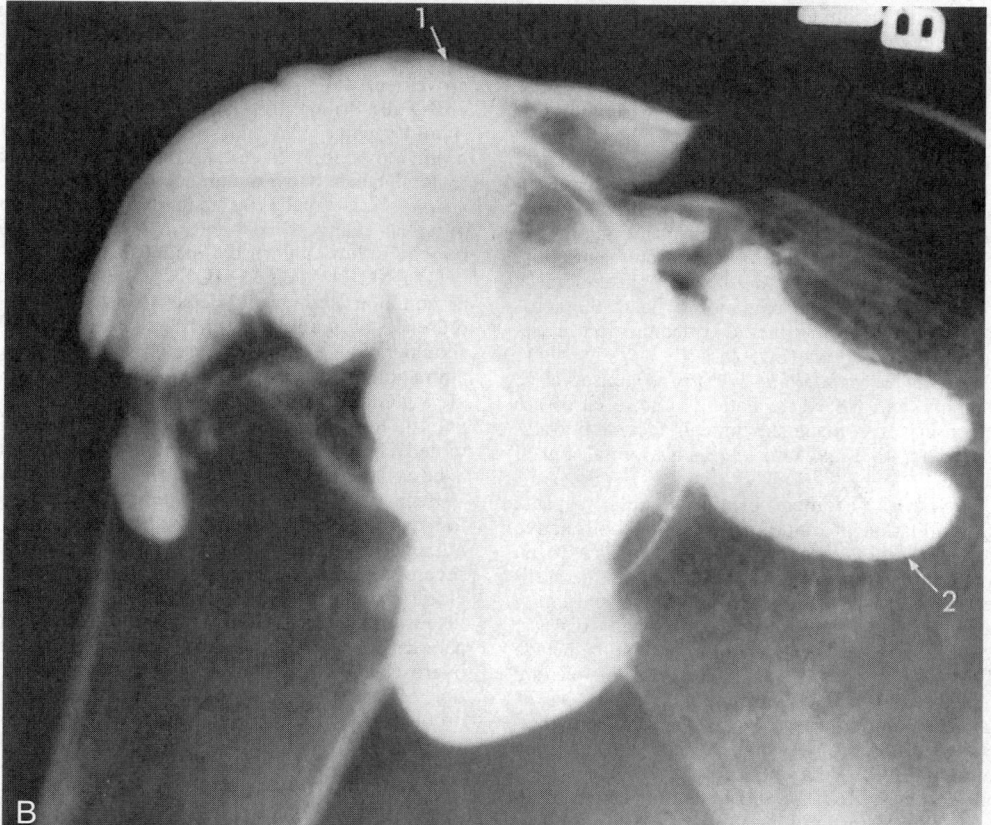

FIGURE 255–3. *A*, Arthrogram of normal shoulder. The extent of the joint capsule is delineated by contrast material. A prominent subscapular extension of the capsule is seen projecting toward the axilla. Filling of the subacromial bursa may occasionally occur normally. Extension of the capsule as a pouch around the long head of the biceps demarcates the intertubercular groove. *B*, Rotator cuff tear. Filling of (1) the subacromial bursa superiorly and (2) the subcoracoid bursa inferiorly indicates tear of the rotator cuff. The normal hyaline articular cartilage is seen as a radiolucent crescent over the head of the humerus. (From Forrester DM, Brown JC: The Radiology of Joint Disease, Vol 2. Philadelphia, WB Saunders, 1987, pp 362, 363.)

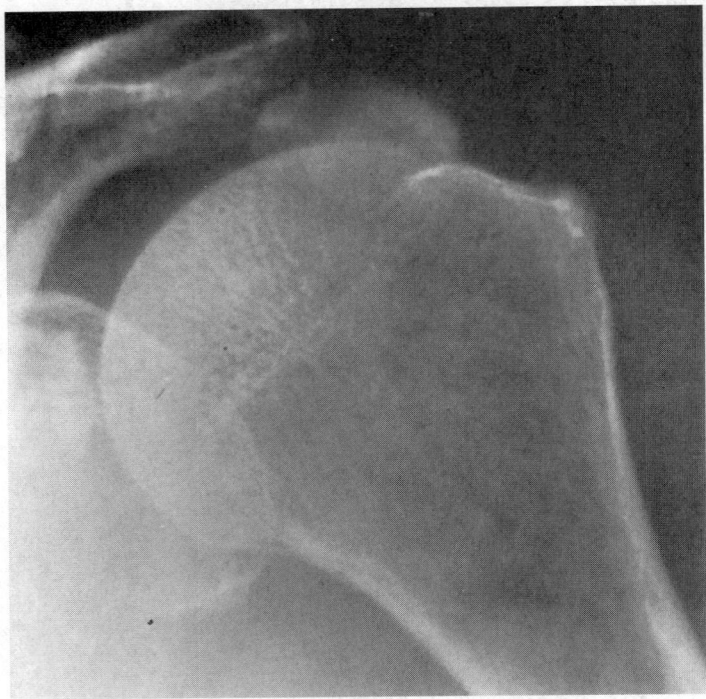

FIGURE 255–4. Calcific bursitis. A large amorphous collection of calcium lies within the subacromial bursa. In addition, a small fleck of calcium just above the greater tuberosity represents supraspinatus tendinitis. (From Forrester DM, Brown JC: The Radiology of Joint Disease, Vol 2. Philadelphia, WB Saunders, 1987, p 369.)

Chronic problems can cause attrition of the tendon and eventual rupture. Complete rupture will cause mild weakness of the biceps and a prominent bulge of the muscle belly. Integrity of the rotator cuff should be assessed in chronic bicipital tendinitis, because the two entities frequently occur concomitantly.

Treatment of bicipital tendinitis is initially conservative with rest and NSAID's. Physical therapy and intralesional corticosteroids are reserved for refractory cases. Successful treatment is more likely when initiated early. Surgery is essential for complete rupture and may be required for intractable cases of tendinitis.

BURSAE. The subacromial or subdeltoid bursa is the largest and most frequently inflamed bursa of the shoulder. Located beneath the acromian process between the rotator cuff and the deltoid muscle, *subacromial or subdeltoid bursitis* will cause pain in the lateral aspect of the shoulder similar to that caused by rotator cuff tendinitis. It differs from a rotator cuff tendinitis by the presence of tenderness upon passive abduction and upon direct palpation beneath the acromian process. *Plain radiography* sometimes can demonstrate calcification in chronic subacromial bursitis (Fig. 255–4).

Treatment of subacromial or subdeltoid bursitis is conservative with rest, physical therapy, and NSAID's. Patients whose cases are refractory to initial conservative management can receive intralesional corticosteroids given directly into the subacromial bursa, which are quite effective.

ARTICULAR CAPSULE. Disorders of the articular capsule will be evident by the limitation of range of motion by both active and passive abduction. *Adhesive capsulitis,* also known as "frozen shoulder," is a common entity that can occur in association with diabetes mellitus, tuberculosis, cervical spine disease, upper extremity injuries, coronary artery disease, and chronic pulmonary disease. Initially a painful condition, it will proceed through an adhesive phase characterized by the painless progressive loss of passive range of motion in all directions. Eventually, the shoulder "thaws" with the return of range of motion after several years. The diagnosis is best confirmed by arthrography, which reveals a contracture of the articular volume and loss of the axillary pouch. Pain is best managed by physical therapy, NSAID's, and judicious use of intra-articular corticosteroids. Early restoration of range of motion has been uniformly unsuccessful even when attempted by physical therapy, closed manipulation under general anesthesia, and hydraulic distention using large-volume intra-articular injections.

Reflex sympathetic dystrophy syndrome is similar to adhesive capsulitis except for more diffuse involvement with pain and vasomotor instability of the hand, wrist, and arm. More commonly seen after trauma of the upper extremity, it is seen in association with clinical situations similar to adhesive capsulitis. This condition can occur

bilaterally and responds more favorably to early therapy. Treatment should include aggressive physical therapy to maintain range of motion, non-narcotic analgesia for pain management, and a short, rapidly tapering course of corticosteroids. Best results have occurred when steroids are started at 40 to 60 mg of prednisone per day and tapered over a 3-week period. Stellate ganglion blocks and intra-articular corticosteroids are used but with less uniform improvement.

BONE. Primary diseases of the bone can manifest themselves as shoulder pain. *Avascular necrosis of bone* can affect the humeral head, although it is not as common as avascular necrosis of the femoral head. If avascular necrosis of bone is suspected, the *diagnosis* is best made by magnetic resonance imaging. Plain radiographic changes occur late in the disease process and should not be required to confirm the diagnosis.

GLENOHUMERAL JOINT. Arthritis of the glenohumeral joint is common and easily detected on physical examination by the presence of tenderness on passive rotation of the fully adducted shoulder. Soft tissue swelling is not to be perceived on routine examination, and tenderness on active rotation will not discriminate glenohumeral arthritis from lesions of the rotator cuff. Although painful for the patient, passive range of motion should be determined because it will be near normal in acute arthritis but not in adhesive capsulitis.

Because the glenohumeral joint is a common site of involvement for many forms of the polyarthritides, most episodes of glenohumeral arthritis are part of a polyarthritis. Alternatively, an isolated severe destructive degenerative glenohumeral arthritis seen in the elderly should make the clinician suspect *Milwaukee shoulder.* Predisposing factors for this condition include chronic renal failure, local calcium pyrophosphate dihydrate deposition, chronic joint overuse, and large tears of the rotator cuff. The long-term disruption of the rotator cuff seems to be the key factor in allowing this problem to occur.

Biundo JJ, Torres-Ramos FM: Common shoulder problems. Primary Care Rheumatol 4:1, 1991. *A practical approach to examination of the shoulder and diagnosing common problems.*

Boublik M, Hawkins RJ: Clinical examination of the shoulder complex. J Orthop Sports Phys Ther 18:379, 1993. *A comprehensive approach to the examination of the shoulder.*

Kozin F: Painful shoulder and the reflex sympathetic dystrophy syndrome. *In* McCarty DJ, Koopman WJ (eds.): Arthritis and Allied Conditions, 12th ed. Philadelphia, Lea & Febiger, 1993, pp 1643–1676. *A detailed and comprehensive resource of etiology, diagnosis, and treatment; 301 references.*

Thornhill TS: Shoulder pain. *In* Kelley WN, Harris ED, Ruddy S, et al. (eds.): Textbook of Rheumatology, 4th ed. Philadelphia, WB Saunders, 1993, pp 417–440. *A detailed and comprehensive resource of etiology, diagnosis, and treatment; 160 references.*

256 SYSTEMIC DISEASES IN WHICH ARTHRITIS IS A FEATURE

Eugene V. Ball

Eleven per cent of adult Americans interviewed in the National Health Survey claimed to have had one or more episodes of painful joints over a period of six weeks. Much of this pain was probably due to soft tissue rheumatism and common rheumatic diseases, such as osteoarthritis and rheumatoid arthritis (RA), that are defined by their own attributes and not by associated signs. The arthralgias of a fraction of these persons might have represented early symptoms of systemic diseases diagnosable only by the later appearance of other clinical signs or by laboratory testing. Table 256–1 illustrates the applicability of general medical laboratory tests to the evaluation of nonspecific joint symptoms. The tests afford significant diagnostic clues for certain systemic diseases in which arthralgias can be the earliest and only symptoms. Brief descriptions of musculoskeletal manifestations of a few systemic disorders follow.

PRIMARY BILIARY CIRRHOSIS (see Ch. 122). More than half of women with primary biliary cirrhosis (PBC) may have serologic abnormalities, such as rheumatoid factors and antinuclear antibodies, in addition to antimitochondrial antibodies. A large number, primarily in this group, have joint pains or outright rheumatic disease, mainly RA, Sjögren's syndrome, or limited scleroderma (CREST syndrome: *c*alcinosis, *R*aynaud's phenomenon, *e*sophageal dysfunction, *s*clerodactyly, and *t*elangiectasia). An asymmetric, nondeforming arthritis has been described in as many as 30% of patients. Other defined causes for bone or joint pains in PBC include osteomalacia and hypertrophic osteoarthropathy.

HEMOCHROMATOSIS (see Ch. 189). Arthritis is frequently the first sign of hemochromatosis and eventually develops in as many as half of all persons with the disease. Typically occurring between the ages of 40 and 50, the arthritis of hemochromatosis has been reported in persons younger than age 30 and is easily overlooked or confused with primary osteoarthritis, even though their distributions often differ. It also may be dismissed as idiopathic tendinitis or bursitis. Pain and stiffness frequently appear first in the metacarpophalangeal joints; other joints involved commonly include the wrists, hips, and knees. Signs of inflammation are negligible except during episodes of pseudogout. Chondrocalcinosis is common on radiographs, as are subchondral cysts, sclerosis, and joint space narrowing. The arthritis is not altered by phlebotomy; treatment is symptomatic and may necessitate arthroplasties, particularly in the hips.

SICKLE CELL DISEASE AND OTHER HEMOGLOBINOPATHIES (see Ch. 136). Almost all persons with sickle cell disease experience musculoskeletal symptoms. Large joint arthritis lasting a few days to a few weeks results from small vessel occlusion caused by local sickling. The aseptic bone infarcts of SC (or less often SS) disease resemble osteomyelitis, which is far more common in persons with sickle cell disease than in normal persons and is often caused by *Salmonella*. Osteonecrosis occurs in both SS and SC disease, often in the head of the femur; however, multiple areas may be infarcted. Hyperuricemia attributable to SS disease has culminated in gout in older patients. Pain due to microfractures in the lower leg, ankle, or foot, lasting up to 1 to 2 years, has been described in almost one half of a group of 50 patients with beta-thalassemia.

HYPOGAMMAGLOBULINEMIA (see Ch. 223 and 266). Arthritis as a complication of hypogammaglobulinemia is most typical of the X-linked variety (Bruton's disease) in children; however, it also occurs in other types of primary hypogammaglobulinemia. Septic arthritis is caused by common pathogens or by mycoplasmal organisms such as *Ureaplasma urealyticum.* Nonerosive arthritis, without evidence of infection or other demonstrable cause, often resolves following institution of immunoglobulin therapy. Its resolution with treatment does not necessarily constitute *a priori* evidence of an infectious etiology. Intravenous gamma globulin treatment might suppress arthritis through its complex modulating effect on the immune system (e.g., it has been shown to increase suppressor T-cell functional activity).

WHIPPLE'S DISEASE (see Ch. 103). The arthritis of Whipple's disease mimics that of rheumatic fever in some respects. It is painful; there is often warmth, redness, and swelling; it favors large joints; subcutaneous nodules have been noted in a few patients; recurrences are common; and it can be migratory. Less often, small joints of the hands and feet are inflamed, and the arthritis becomes chronic and resembles RA. The synovial fluid white cell count is sometimes elevated to 50,000 per cubic millimeter, and rod-shaped bacilli may be identified, usually by electron microscopy, in synovial biopsies. These organisms are also seen attached to circulating erythrocytes. Rheumatoid factors and antinuclear antibody are not features of Whipple's disease. The arthritis may antedate gastrointestinal symptoms by years, making diagnosis difficult.

HYPERLIPOPROTEINEMIA (see Ch. 173). An association exists between type II familial hypercholesterolemia (both homozygous and heterozygous forms) and musculoskeletal symptoms such as Achilles tendinitis, oligoarthritis, and polyarthritis. Transient pain in the Achilles tendon appears to be more common than frank inflammatory tendinitis, which can last a few days and recur two or three times yearly. A few patients have acute painful monoarthritis or pauciarthritis of the knees, ankles, or small joints that lasts a week or more and recurs frequently. Less common is an incapacitating polyarthritis resembling rheumatic fever, persisting a month or more. In one study, 40% of 73 heterozygous patients were symptomatic; articular manifestations appeared at times before the xanthomas that are the major diagnostic sign of familial hypercholesterolemia.

ENDOCRINE DISORDERS (see Ch. 202, 203, and 214). Aches and stiffness simulating fibromyalgia may appear early in hypothyroidism; untreated, this may progress to proximal myopathy with elevated creatine kinase levels, simulating polymyositis, or to a syndrome of synovial thickening and joint effusions, simulating RA. There also appears to be an association of hypothyroidism with calcium pyrophosphate deposition disease. Carpal tunnel syndrome is a more common manifestation of hypothyroidism. Hyperthyroidism may cause myopathy without elevations of the creatine kinase level but with muscle wasting, which may be severe. Thyroid acropachy, seen rarely in association with pretibial myxedema and Graves' disease, is characterized by diffuse swelling of the fingers and clubbing.

Hyperparathyroidism is another cause of diffuse, vague musculoskeletal pains resembling those of fibrositis. The other musculoskeletal complications of hyperparathyroidism include back pain due to vertebral body fractures, an erosive arthritis predominantly in the hands and wrists, and chondrocalcinosis (with pseudogout occurring most often after parathyroidectomy).

Carpal tunnel syndrome has been reported in almost one-half of persons with acromegaly. Raynaud's phenomenon is rare. The

TABLE 256–1. LABORATORY TESTS IN THE EVALUATION OF NONSPECIFIC JOINT SYMPTOMS

Test	Disease
Liver function tests	Primary biliary cirrhosis; chronic active hepatitis
Calcium and phosphorus	Hyperparathyroidism
Serum protein electrophoresis	Hypogammaglobulinemic arthritis; primary amyloidosis
Serum iron and total iron-binding capacity; ferritin	Hemochromatosis
Lipase or amylase	Pancreatic-arthritis syndrome
Thyroid-stimulating hormone (TSH); thyroxine	Thyroid myopathy or arthritis
Complete blood count	Leukemia; sickle cell disease
Lipid analysis	Hyperlipidemia-associated arthritis
Partial thromboplastin time; rapid plasma reagin (RPR) or VDRL	Vasculopathy; hemophilia Vasculopathy; syphilis
Anti-HIV (human immunodeficiency virus)	HIV arthritis
Antiparvovirus antibody	Parvovirus arthritis

arthritis of acromegaly is clinically indistinguishable from osteoarthritis.

SARCOIDOSIS (see Ch. 61). Joint or juxta-articular pains are experienced by as many as one third of patients with acute sarcoidosis and may be the only symptom of the disease; however, erythema nodosum often accompanies the arthritis and, together with hilar adenopathy, suggests the diagnosis (one should be aware that arthritis may accompany erythema nodosum of any cause). Arthritis often begins in the ankles and spreads symmetrically. The distal interphalangeal joints are typically spared, but any of the other peripheral joints, as well as the heels, may be painful out of proportion to signs of inflammation, which are meager. Episodes last a few days to a few months, and the arthritis usually resolves completely. The erythrocyte sedimentation rate is often elevated; antinuclear antibodies and rheumatoid factors may be present. Treatment with salicylates, nonsteroidal anti-inflammatory drugs (NSAID's), or prednisone is based on the severity of the arthritis. Progressive, deforming arthritis is a feature of chronic sarcoidosis, as are bone lesions, both lytic and sclerotic. Clinically significant sarcoid myopathy is rare.

FAMILIAL MEDITERRANEAN FEVER (see Ch. 139.2). Serositis, fever, and arthritis are the major signs of familial Mediterranean fever (FMF). Arthritis occurs in as many as one half of patients; it is usually monoarticular and confined to large joints in the lower extremities. Although it usually lasts < 1 week, arthritis has been reported to persist for several months. Synovial fluid contains large numbers of granulocytes, and there is intense infiltration of granulocytes and hyperemia in synovial tissue. Diagnosis is suggested by demographic and other clinical features of the disease. In the absence of these, FMF can be easily confused with juvenile RA. Colchicine most often prevents recurrent arthritis as well as amyloidosis.

257 MISCELLANEOUS FORMS OF ARTHRITIS
Eugene V. Ball

NEUROPATHIC JOINT DISEASE (CHARCOT'S JOINTS). Recognition of neuropathic joint disease and its association with syphilis preceded reports of its association with diabetes mellitus by 64 years, but syphilis has been superseded by the latter as the leading cause of this disorder. In syphilis, subacute combined degeneration of the spinal cord, paraplegia, and Charcot-Marie-Tooth disease, weakness, decreased pain sensation, and impaired position sense contribute to the massive destruction of the knee (or less often the hip or ankle) that typifies the disorder. In syringomyelia, upper limb involvement is typical. Neuropathic disease of the knee or ankle is suggested by effusions, crepitus, enlargement, and relatively little pain, although pain may become worrisome late in the disease. Neuropathic joint disease in diabetes mellitus (Fig. 257–1) is more likely to cause painless swelling of one or both feet in a patient with longstanding disease and sensory neuropathy. For mechanical reasons, the joints most frequently involved are the tarsometatarsals and the metatarsophalangeals. Destruction also occurs in the talus, the calcaneus, the ankle joints, and the distal tibia. Radiographs characteristically show loss of joint space, sclerosis, multiple irregular bodies representing chip fractures, and new bone formation; analogous changes are seen in osteomyelitis and malignancy. (Less severe, but similar, changes have been reported in calcium pyrophosphate deposition disease.) Attempts at stabilizing the involved joint with various orthotic devices are often unsatisfactory, and surgical fusion is difficult.

HEMARTHROSIS. Hemophilia (see Ch. 153) is the major medical cause of hemarthrosis, which (with muscle bleeding) accounts for >90% of all bleeding episodes in patients with hemophilia. The severity of hemarthrosis is related directly to the levels of clotting factors. For example, infants with severe factor deficiencies often experience hemarthrosis before the age of 1. By age 15, virtually all persons with severe, inadequately treated factor deficiencies have some form of chronic joint impairment.

Acute bleeding into a joint (most often the knees, elbows, or ankles) is frequently signified by stiffness or discomfort, followed by pain, swelling, and redness. The joint should be immobilized, and adequate factor replacement should be started as early as possible, preferably during the prodromal phase. The joint changes stimulated by repeated intra-articular bleeding resemble those of rheumatoid arthritis (RA). Hyperplastic synovium appears to be the source of proteases and other enzymes that destroy cartilage and bone, culminating in the absence of articular cartilage, joint disorganization, and fibrous contractures. Education of the patient and family, as well as home treatment, prevents or attenuates chronic, destructive arthritis. Joint replacements have been done successfully to relieve pain and restore function.

Bleeding into a muscle, which also should be treated with replacement factor, can lead to necrosis and fibrotic scarring. Pseudotumors are cystic bone swellings resulting from intraosseous bleeding and necrosis.

Von Willebrand's disease can produce hemarthrosis and joint destruction comparable to that of hemophilia.

Painful but nondestructive intra-articular bleeding is a common feature of scurvy, and intra-articular tumors such as pigmented villonodular synovitis frequently cause monoarticular bleeding.

MULTICENTRIC RETICULOHISTIOCYTOSIS. The chief manifestations of multicentric reticulohistiocytosis are arthritis and red to purple skin nodules varying in size from 1 to 10 mm. The nodules are found in any part of the skin but tend to concentrate on the face and hands and uncommonly coalesce. The arthritis is most often symmetric and polyarticular. Unlike adult RA, it does not spare the distal interphalangeal joints. It can be severely destructive and, in one third of cases, progresses to arthritis multilans. Systemic signs include fever and weight loss; less often, pericarditis and myositis are present, and it is frequently associated with a malignancy.

The disorder also has been termed "lipoid dermatoarthritis" because of the lipids contained within the histiocytes and granulomas that constitute the basic lesion. In the absence of a serum or lesional lipid abnormality, lipid deposition is now thought to be nonspecific. Improvement has been reported more consistently with alkylating agents than with prednisone. Methotrexate also has been used.

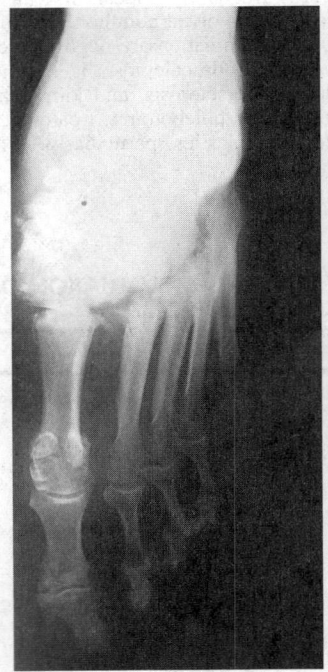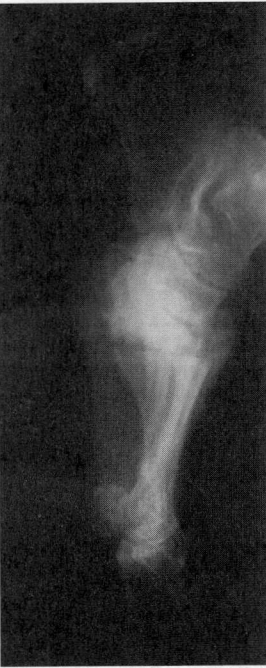

FIGURE 257–1. Diabetes mellitus and neuropathic arthritis. Note lateral displacement of metatarsals *(left)* and fragmentation and osseous debris *(right)*.

HYPERTROPHIC OSTEOARTHROPATHY AND CARCINOMATOUS POLYARTHRITIS.

Hypertrophic osteoarthropathy (HO) is a systemic disorder distinguished by periostitis of the distal ends of tubular bones. The lesions presumably begin with increased blood flow and periosteal edema, followed by new bone formation. Isotopic bone scans are positive at an early stage, often preceding radiographic evidence of periosteal new bone. Hypertrophic osteoarthropathy is often manifested as digital clubbing and frequently involves the tibiae, ulnae, radii, femora, metatarsals, and metacarpals. Painful articular swelling appears in approximately 30% of patients and may be debilitating; other variable features of the syndrome include gynecomastia and thickening and furrowing of the facial skin. Intrathoracic malignancies, especially squamous cell carcinoma, have supplanted pulmonary infections as the most common cause of HO. Pleural and diaphragmatic neoplasms and nasopharyngeal carcinomas are strongly associated with HO. Less common causes include chronic liver disease, inflammatory bowel disease, and cyanotic heart disease. There is also a hereditary form termed "pachydermoperiostosis," with strong male predominance and a curious bimodal distribution of disease onset during the first year of life or the midteens. No satisfactory unifying theory of pathogenesis exists. Successful treatment of the underlying disorder results in regression of HO. In fact, thoracotomy for cancer-causing pulmonary hypertrophic osteoarthropathy may result in a marked decrease in pain and swelling within 24 hours.

The "sudden" onset of polyarthritis resembling RA in an older adult should prompt suspicion of an associated malignancy. Carcinomatous polyarthritis may appear months before, or after, detection of malignancy of many types. Its incidence is unknown; in one small series it was almost as common as carcinomatous hypertrophic osteoarthropathy and more common than cancer-related dermatomyositis. Palmar fasciitis has been noted in association with ovarian cancer.

Ginsburg WW, O'Duffy JD, Morris JL, et al.: Multicentric reticulohistiocytosis: Response to alkylating in six patients. Ann Intern Med 111:384, 1989. *Five of six patients with multicentric reticulohistiocytosis manifesting as skin nodules and polyarthritis were treated with cyclophosphamide. The sixth was given chlorambucil. All had complete or near-complete remissions lasting as long as 32 months after cessation of treatment.*

Hoyer LW: Hemophilia A. N Engl J Med 330:38, 1994. *A review of the structure and function of Factor VIII, the molecular genetics of hemophilia A, its clinical manifestations, and treatment.*

Slowman-Kovacs SD, Braunstein EM, Brandt KD: Rapidly progressive Charcot arthropathy following minor joint trauma in patients with diabetic neuropathy. Arthritis Rheum 33:412, 1990. *This report of neuropathic arthropathy progressing rapidly after minor trauma in three patients is based on the authors' research in experimental arthritis.*

258 NONARTICULAR RHEUMATISM

Eugene V. Ball

FIBROMYALGIA (FIBROSITIS). Primary fibromyalgia (FM) has been defined as chronic, widespread musculoskeletal pain and tenderness at multiple sites, e.g., at 11 of 18 specific sites in the criteria of the American College of Rheumatology. Implicit in this definition is the absence of signs of connective tissue or other musculoskeletal disease. Because of its subjective nature and its frequent association with disturbed sleep, chronic fatigue, headaches, and irritable bowel syndrome, the validity of classifying FM as a disease rather than a "syndrome of being out of sorts" has been challenged. Patients often appear anxious and depressed, and studies have shown that they may feel dissatisfied with all aspects of their lives. Nevertheless, the specific characteristics of anxiety and depression have not been identified consistently on psychological testing, and it has been suggested that chronic pain and fatigue of any cause can engender anxiety and depression. Despite their subjectivity, symptoms of FM tend to be constant over many years; exceptionally, FM has been found to be premonitory of psychosis or hypothyroidism. There are no consistent biochemical, immunologic, or anatomic abnormalities in FM. Decreased threshold to pain on pressure over

certain sites and increased skin fold tenderness have led to numerous unsuccessful attempts to demonstrate localized peripheral abnormalities and to speculation that FM is a disorder of pain modulation.

Functional disability in FM may exceed that of rheumatoid arthritis, and in 1989, FM was the most frequent single reason for disability pensions among women in Norway, accounting for 7.2% of new pensions. Patients whose FM begins acutely after a specific traumatic event are more likely to be disabled than those in whom the disorder evolves insidiously. FM is significantly less common in men than in women and is either underreported or uncommon in developing countries. Treatment should emphasize its nondestructive nature, and the physician should be wary of overusing drugs to allay anxiety or induce sleep. Low-dose amitryptyline has been found to be valuable for decreasing pain and improving sleep in some patients.

BURSITIS. Bursae are small, synovial-lined, fluid-filled sacs located between tendons and bones which serve to reduce friction between opposing muscles or tendons. Most bursae are present from birth; however, others form in response to repeated pressure.

Of the approximately 80 bursae located on each side of the body, only a few are common sources of pain. The subdeltoid is the largest of the bursae around the shoulder; it is located between the deltoid muscle and the shoulder capsule and extends under the acromion. Acute inflammation of this or nearby bursae and tendons is apt to be exceedingly painful, resulting in restricted shoulder movement and tenderness over the rotator cuff. Intrabursal injection of lidocaine is diagnostic and often curative; however, recurrences are common. Bursal calcification predisposes to more frequent attacks. Infection is most common in the olecranon bursa.

Trochanteric bursitis is thought to occur as a result of chronic strain on weak quadricep muscles or overuse of hip and thigh muscles. Pain is often perceived to be in the lateral aspect of the thigh and the low back and is aggravated by abducting the affected leg and by lying on the affected side. Tenderness is present at the edge of the greater trochanter. Injections of lidocaine often abolish pain.

TENDINOUS LESIONS. Tendinous lesions include tenosynovitis, a lesion of the gliding surfaces of a tendon and its sheath; tendinitis, painful scarring within a tendon; and trigger lesions, which are localized enlargements of the tendon that engage a constricted part of the sheath (as in "trigger finger"). Tendinous lesions are common, occurring in many areas of the musculoskeletal system. An example is de Quervain's disease, which is stenosing tenosynovitis of the abductor pollicis longus and extensor pollicis brevis at the medial styloid. Pain can localize or radiate into the hand or back to the shoulder. This and carpal tunnel syndrome occur frequently during pregnancy.

CARPAL TUNNEL SYNDROME. The symptoms of carpal tunnel syndrome are paresthesias and pain in the palmar side of the first three fingers and at times the radial half of the fourth finger; the pain may radiate proximally to the shoulder, creating confusion with a cervical disc syndrome. Physical findings include sensory loss, weakness on abduction and opposition of the thumb, and atrophy of the thenar eminence. Carpal tunnel syndrome is caused by an array of conditions that result in pressure on the median nerve as it passes through the bony flexor compartment of the wrist. Some of these are listed in Table 258–1.

Diagnosis is confirmed by electrophysiologic nerve tests. (The clinical tests commonly used are of questionable value.) Magnetic resonance imaging may be useful in defining the cause and thus directing treatment, which might include splinting of the wrist, corticosteroid injections, and surgical release of the transverse carpal ligament. Oral pyridoxine is of questionable value.

TENNIS ELBOW. "Tennis elbow" refers to a lesion of the wrist extensor muscles causing pain at the outer elbow, along the back of the forearm, or less commonly, into the shoulder. The burning or aching pain is produced by resisted extension of the wrist, as in grasping and lifting, and rarely is felt as sudden, searing twinges of intensity sufficient to cause momentary grip paralysis. Tennis elbow usually results from repeated forceful extension of the wrist. A tear or area of degeneration most often occurs at the origin of the common extensor tendon from the lateral humoral epicondyle; much less frequently, the tear is in the muscle belly. Treatment includes

**TABLE 258-1. CONDITIONS CAUSING
CARPAL TUNNEL SYNDROME**

1. Trauma
2. Occupation
3. Infections: for example, Lyme disease and rubella
4. Rheumatoid arthritis and gout
5. Pregnancy
6. Hypothyroidism and acromegaly
7. Amyloidosis
8. Median artery aneurysm
9. Ganglion cyst, increased fat, hypertrophy of abductor pollicis muscle

injection of triamcinolone into the painful scar, manipulation, or partial tenotomy.

Like tennis elbow, "golfer's elbow" is a misnomer in that both conditions occur frequently in people who play neither sport. Golfer's elbow is less painful than tennis elbow; it represents a lesion of the common flexor tendon at the medial epicondyle. Pain is usually localized to the inner side of the elbow and is produced by resisted flexion of the wrist. Treatment includes triamcinolone injection or massage.

TIETZE'S SYNDROME. Tietze's syndrome is an uncommon cause of chest pain that can be mistaken for visceral pain. There is tender, most often unilateral, swelling at one or more costosternal junctions. Biopsy samples of involved areas have revealed chronic inflammatory fibrosis. The syndrome may result from prolonged coughing or hyperventilation, but it is often idiopathic. Injections into the painful area with triamcinolone are sometimes curative. Tietze's syndrome may be differentiated from the more common costochondritis, in which there are no signs of inflammation.

Bennett RM: Fibromyalgia and the facts: Sense or nonsense. Rheum Dis Clin North Am 19:45, 1993.
Block SR: Fibromyalgia and the rheumatisms: Common sense and sensibility. Rheum Dis Clin North Am 19:61, 1993. *These papers present opposing points of view concerning fibromyalgia as a distinctive syndrome with distinctive diagnostic criteria.*

259 ARTICULAR TUMORS
Eugene V. Ball

Articular tumors can be classified as those which arise within the synovium; those which arise from cartilage, bone, or contiguous structures; and neoplasms that are nonarticular in origin but which metastasize to joints or develop in multiple areas, including joints.

The most common of these are probably synovial chondromatosis and osteochondromatosis, which develop as cartilaginous synovial plaques that sometimes ossify. These cause episodic pain or swelling in a knee, hip, elbow, or shoulder. The joint may lock if the plaques become detached, forming loose bodies. Radiographs reveal multiple opacities if ossification has occurred; arthroscopy may be useful for both diagnosis and treatment.

Pigmented villonodular synovitis (PVNS) is a nonmalignant proliferative disorder of unknown cause that usually affects the entire synovium of a single joint. This condition occurs most often in early middle age and in the knee in 80% of cases. Uncommonly, two or more joints are involved; similar lesions occur in tendons and bursae. Pain and swelling are characteristic, as is serosanguineous synovial fluid. Radiographic signs include soft tissue swelling, subchondral cysts (particularly in the hip), and pressure erosions. Treatment is synovectomy. Hemangiomas, lipomas, and xanthomas may simulate PVNS.

Synoviomas (synovial sarcomas) are rare, aggressive tumors of young adults. They usually originate in the extremities adjacent to, but not within, a joint. Primary tumors histologically identical to synoviomas have been found in the head and neck, abdominal wall, retroperitoneum, heart, and mediastinum, supporting the view that the tumor originates from mesenchyme rather than synovium. Detection within tumor cells of both cytokeratin (an epithelial intermediate filament) and vimentin (a mesenchymal intermediate filament) has led to the suggestion that the synovioma is a carcinosarcoma. Synoviomas are usually discovered as deep swellings within a tendon sheath, a bursa, or a joint capsule. Pain and tenderness are variable, as are effusions. They metastasize early to lungs, bone, and lymph nodes. Tumor size > 4 cm, a high mitotic rate, and local recurrence after excision convey a poor prognosis.

Chondrosarcomas and fibrosarcomas are other malignancies arising within or near joints, and intrasynovial myeloma and lymphoma are rare causes of a swollen or painful joint.

Thorough investigation is required for unexplained pain or swelling within or adjacent to a single joint.

260 ERYTHROMELALGIA
Eugene V. Ball

Erythromelalgia (see Ch. 46) is a syndrome of episodic burning pain and redness in the extremities. Attacks may be confined to feet and, if severe and prolonged, may spread to the hands, or they may begin simultaneously in hands and feet. They are most often provoked by increasing environmental temperatures, although a few persons experience attacks only with febrile illnesses. The combination of increasing ambient temperatures and exercise often induces symptoms. Some persons maintain environmental temperatures at levels that are uncomfortably low for themselves, as well as others, to avoid attacks of erythromelalgia. Some sleep bundled up against the cold of an unheated room but with feet protruding uncovered from the blankets. Relief may require immersing the feet in ice water. The feet appear normal between attacks, except in those persons who habitually walk barefoot because attacks are provoked by wearing shoes.

Erythromelalgia is sometimes familial. In one remarkable kindred, the disorder is autosomal dominant, afflicting 29 members. Most often beginning between ages 2 and 8, it has been responsible for severe adjustment problems in youth, engendered in part by an inability to sit comfortably in a heated classroom or to participate in physical activities. In this kindred, the disorder has been frequently misdiagnosed as arthritis, reflex sympathetic dystrophy, or Raynaud's phenomenon; its pathogenesis is unknown, but it is not related to thrombocythemia.

By far the most common recognized cause of nonfamilial erythromelalgia is thrombocythemia, usually a feature of a myeloproliferative disorder. Erythromelalgia was the presenting symptom in 26 of 40 patients with platelet counts in excess of 500×10^9 per liter. Arteriolar inflammation and thrombotic occlusions were found on skin punch biopsy samples. Erythromelalgia disappeared for three or four days after a single dose of aspirin, which is the duration of its inhibition of platelet aggregation. In the absence of thrombocythemia, aspirins are likely to be ineffective for treating or preventing erythromelalgia.

Other reported associations with erythromelalgia include diabetes mellitus. In addition, nifedipine and bromocriptine can cause an erythromelalgia-like disorder.

Finley WH, Lindsey JR, Fine J-D, et al.: Autosomal dominant erythromelalgia. Am J Med Genet 42:310, 1992. *Clinical description of erythromelalgia in a large kindred.*
Michiels JJ, van Joost T, Vuzevski VD: Idiopathic erythromelalgia: A congenital disorder. J Am Acad Dermatol 21(S pt. 2):1128, 1989. *A brief report of idiopathic erythromelalgia in a female whose symptoms began at 2 years of age and increased in severity until age 14, by which time she was sleeping with her feet immersed in ice water.*
Millard FE, Hunter CS, Anderson M, et al.: Clinical manifestations of essential thrombocythemia in young adults. Am J Hematol 33:27, 1990. *Essential thrombocythemia was identified in 13 patients whose median age was 26. Erythromelalgia was the most common complication, occurring in 7 of the 13, of whom 7 were males.*

261 MULTIFOCAL FIBROSCLEROSIS

H. Ralph Schumacher, Jr.

In rare instances the delicate fibrous areolar tissue in a certain anatomic region becomes the site of a chronic low-grade inflammatory process, leading to deposition of dense sclerotic plaques, which may obstruct or limit the movement of adjacent viscera. When the process is in the active phase, there are characteristic findings of chronic or granulomatous inflammation, featured by mononuclear cell infiltration, plasma cells, some eosinophils, and occasional giant cells. Macrophage infiltration has recently been emphasized in retroperitoneal fibrosis. In the end stages, the pathologic lesion is simply that of scar tissue so that by the time this process causes clinical manifestations there may be little evidence of the initial inflammatory reaction. In at least some cases there is an accompanying vasculitis. As a general rule the process tends to originate in the midline, around the great vessels, and then to spread laterally. In most cases a clue to the inciting mechanism is lacking.

Syndromes that have been considered as manifestations of multifocal fibrosclerosis include retroperitoneal fibrosis, mediastinal fibrosis, sclerosing cholangitis (see Ch. 126), Riedel's thyroiditis (see Ch. 203), pseudotumor of the orbit, Peyronie's disease (a sclerotic induration of the corpora cavernosa of the penis), and sclerosing peritonitis. Other sites of a similar fibrosis, such as the testes, vagina, and suprasellar area, also have been reported. Pulmonary and myocardial fibrosis syndromes generally have not been seen as related to multifocal fibrosclerosis, although pleural fibrosis along with retroperitoneal fibrosis can be seen with ergotamine use.

Although most of these syndromes have been described as separate entities, several anatomic areas may become affected in one person. For example, retroperitoneal fibrosis and sclerosing mediastinitis may be present at the same time along with varying combinations of sclerosing cholangitis, Riedel's thyroiditis, and pseudotumor of the orbit. A possible genetic predisposition is suggested by familial cases and by an association between fibrosing syndromes and α_1-antitrypsin deficiency. Familial mediastinal or retroperitoneal fibrosis also may be associated with HLA (human leukocyte antigen)-B27 and seronegative spondylarthropathies.

Comings DE, Skubi KB, Van Eyes J, et al.: Familial multifocal sclerosis. Ann Intern Med 66:884, 1967. *Description of multiple sites of fibrosis in two brothers.*
Goldbach P, Mohsenifar Z, Salick AI: Familial mediastinal fibrosis associated with seronegative spondyloarthropathy. Arthritis Rheum 26:221, 1983. *Two siblings with both diseases.*

RETROPERITONEAL FIBROSIS. In retroperitoneal fibrosis, the process usually begins over the promontory of the sacrum and extends laterally across the ureters and as high as the second or third lumbar vertebra. Less commonly, the lesion develops in other extraperitoneal areas, e.g., contiguous with the kidneys, duodenum, descending colon, or urinary bladder. In some cases there has been an associated vasculitis in the skin and subcutaneous tissue, manifested by the formation of nodules, erythematous discolorations, and ulcerations. Similarly, inflammatory changes in small vessels at the sites of the sclerosis have been noted. Glomerulonephritis has been seen in a few patients.

The occurrence of retroperitoneal fibrosis in patients taking methysergide for migraine has been reported with greater frequency than could be due to chance. Occasional cases have been reported after use of other drugs such as ergotamine, various β-adrenergic blocking agents, hydralazine, and methyldopa. Associated diseases in patients with retroperitoneal fibrosis have included systemic lupus erythematosus; vasculitis; scleroderma; eosinophilic fasciitis; biliary cirrhosis; rubella-associated arthritis; renal, uterine, and other cancers; and carcinoid. Trauma, surgery, and occasionally ruptured echinococcal cysts have been reported as apparent causes. One patient with associated periarticular fibrosis had elevated plasma levels of a platelet-derived growth factor.

The disorder is about twice as common in males as in females, and the peak incidence is in the fifth and sixth decades. Cases have been reported in children. The manifestations are variable, depending on the anatomic location of the process. Pain is the most common symptom; it tends to be located in the low back and may be accompanied by symptoms referable to the gastrointestinal tract. The patient is likely to lose weight and have low-grade fever. There may be some anemia and an elevated erythrocyte sedimentation rate. Although the ureter is the structure most often affected, symptoms referable to the urinary tract are uncommon until obstructive uropathy has led to azotemia and other clinical manifestations of renal insufficiency. The fibrosing process may surround the inferior vena cava, but obstruction of that vessel is uncommon. Thromboembolism and hypertension can be complications. Arterial invasion has been described. Portal hypertension may occur. Retroperitoneal fibrosis occasionally develops in association with definable abdominal aortic aneurysm or aortitis and is considered in some cases to begin as a periaortitis. A possible element of reaction to atheromatous components has been described.

Diagnosis of retroperitoneal fibrosis has been most often suggested by the findings at intravenous pyelography: displacement of the ureters toward the midline and evidence of obstruction, usually at the level of the pelvic brim. One or both ureters may be affected. In rare instances a mass can be palpated in the pelvis or on the posterior abdominal wall. Ultrasonography, computed tomographic (CT) scanning, and magnetic resonance imaging (MRI) also can identify the fibrosing masses. Once a mass has been disclosed, the main problem in differential diagnosis lies in distinguishing retroperitoneal fibrosis from retroperitoneal tumor. Multiple deep biopsies should be made at the time of laparotomy.

Surgical treatment, if used before severe renal damage, is often highly successful. Inasmuch as the fibrosing process is seldom invasive, the constricted organ usually can be freed by blunt dissection so that normal movement or flow is restored. Relief of ureteral obstruction is usually achieved by bringing the ureter out on the anterior surface of the sclerotic mass. Occasionally, however, the obstruction recurs months or years after such treatment. Some surgeons wrap the ureters in omentum to decrease recurrent obstruction. Steroid therapy may be helpful in the rare case detected early or may be employed as an adjunct to surgical measures. Azathioprine has been used successfully in a few cases. Other drugs such as penicillamine, colchicine, and gamma-interferon, with theoretical ability to limit clinical fibrosis, have not been studied in this disease. Progesterone and tamoxifen have been reported to produce regression of fibrosis. When the inferior vena cava is obstructed, surgical relief is technically difficult and risky; here it may be preferable to temporize in the hope that development of collateral pathways may alleviate the circulatory block.

The long-term outlook is fairly good if the disease is recognized and if its obstructive consequences can be treated by surgical means. The disease often tends to run its course and subside. Most deaths have been caused by renal failure.

Benson JR, Baum M: Tamoxifen for retroperitoneal fibrosis. Lancet 341:836, 1993. *Regression of fibrosis also has been described with desmoid tumors.*
Cohle SD, Leil JT: Inflammatory aneurism of the aorta, aortic and coronary arteritis. Arch Pathol Lab Med 112:1121, 1988. *Inflammatory aneurisms of the aorta and other vasculitis may be associated with retroperitoneal fibrosis.*
Ewald EA, Gikas PW, Castor CW: Periarticular fibrosis associated with idiopathic retroperitoneal fibrosis. J Rheum 15:1443, 1988. *Elevated plasma platelet-derived growth factor is proposed as a possible pathogenetic mechanism.*

MEDIASTINAL FIBROSIS. Taut bundles of collagenous tissue form in the superior and anterior mediastinum, with impingement on the aorta, trachea, bronchi, esophagus, and pericardium. Patients may have thoracic pain, but the predominant manifestations are those caused by obstruction of the superior vena cava: puffy, suffused appearance of the face and conjunctivae; nonpitting edema of the face, neck, and upper extremities; and distended veins in the neck and upper extremities. Rarely, the principal vessels affected are the pulmonary arteries, causing pulmonary hypertension. More frequently, the pulmonary veins are involved, and here severe hemoptysis may be the most prominent manifestation. Pericardial fibrosis can lead to constrictive pericarditis. The main task in differential diagnosis is to distinguish this relatively benign condition from obstruction caused by tumor. Roentgenographic examination of the chest may reveal little or no abnormality or some pleural thickening. Angiographic studies show obstruction of the affected vessels. Thoracotomy may be required for histologic diagnosis.

Histoplasmosis and possibly tuberculosis may cause some mediastinal fibrosis. Mediastinal hemorrhage can lead to fibrosis, and cases have been associated with methysergide use. An interesting recent association has been with the SAPHO syndrome (synovitis, acne, pustulosis, hyperostosis, and osteomyelitis). Some patients with this syndrome have shown gradual improvement over months or years, presumably because of development of collateral circulation. Successful superior vena cava bypass surgery has been described. Corticosteroid therapy was ineffective in some reported cases.

Cunningham T, Farrell J, Veale D, et al.: Anterior mediastinal fibrosis with superior vena caval obstruction complicating the synovitis-acne-pustulosis-hyperostosis-osteomyelitis syndrome. Br J Rheumatol 32:408, 1993. *This idiopathic sterile inflammatory reaction most often involves the anterior chest wall.*

Mathiesen DJ, Grillo HC: Clinical manifestation of mediastinal fibrosis and histoplasmosis. Ann Thorac Surg 54:1053, 1992. Histoplasma *were still stainable in some resected specimens.*

Papandreou L, Panagou P, Bouros D: Mediastinal fibrosis and radiofrequency radiation exposure: Is there an association? Respiration 59:181, 1992. *Hemoptysis can be a presenting symptom. This and other reports raise the question of radiation as a cause.*

SCLEROSING PERITONITIS. A fibrotic syndrome has been observed in patients treated for prolonged periods with the now withdrawn β-adrenergic blocking drug practolol. Only a few cases have been reported with propranolol or other β blockers. Some cases have developed years after cessation of therapy. The peritonitis consists of a thick fibrous encasement of the small intestine, and the symptoms include abdominal fullness, back pain, ascites, weight loss, and signs of subacute obstruction. Surgery may be needed to peel away the fibrous tissue. Sclerosing peritonitis with many similarities also has been seen in idiopathic forms in association with systemic conditions, including drug abuse, sarcoidosis, and sicca syndrome, and now most importantly in patients treated with continuous ambulatory peritoneal dialysis (CAPD). A variety of factors used in dialysis have been suggested to contribute. Hemoperitoneum and peritoneal calcification have been reported in recent cases along with intestinal obstruction and ultrafiltration failure. Ultrasound findings can suggest the diagnosis.

Lo WK, Chan KT, Leung AC, et al.: Sclerosing peritonitis complicating prolonged use of chlorhexidine in alcohol in the connection procedure for continuous ambulatory peritoneal dialysis. Peritoneal Dialysis Int 11:166, 1991. *A mechanism is suggested and improvement noted with continued CAPD without the chlorhexidine.*

Pusateri R, Ross R, Marshall R, et al.: Sclerosing encapsulating peritonitis; report of a case with small bowel obstruction managed by long term hyperalimentation, and a review of the literature. Am J Kidney Dis 8:56, 1986. *This is a serious complication of peritoneal dialysis. Improvement in this patient occurred during parenteral nutrition.*

Introduction

262 INTRODUCTION TO MICROBIAL DISEASE
Gerald L. Mandell

Infectious diseases have profoundly influenced the course of human history. The black plague (caused by *Yersinia pestis*) changed the social structure of medieval Europe. The outcomes of military campaigns have been altered by outbreaks of diseases such as dysentery and typhus. Malaria influenced the geographic and racial pattern of distribution of hemgloblins and erythrocyte antigens. The development of *Plasmodium falciparum* is inhibited by the presence of hemoglobin S, and Duffy blood group–negative erythrocytes are resistant to infection with *Plasmodium vivax*. Thus populations with these erythrocyte factors are found in areas where malaria is common. Infections are the major cause of morbidity and mortality in the developing world. AIDS threatens to disrupt the social fabric in some countries of Africa and is severely stressing the health care system in the United States and other parts of the world.

Infection may be defined as multiplication of microbes (viruses, bacteria, fungi, protozoa, or multicellular parasites) in the tissues of the host. The host may or may not be symptomatic. For example, infection with the human immunodeficiency virus (HIV) may cause no overt signs or symptoms of illness or tissue damage for years. The definition of infection probably also should include instances of multiplication of microbes on the surface or in a lumen of the host, causing signs and symptoms of illness or disease. Certain strains of *Escherichia coli* may multiply in the gut and cause a diarrheal illness without invading tissues. This is also considered an infection. Microbes can cause diseases without actually infecting the host by virtue of toxin production. *Clostridium botulinum* may grow in certain improperly processed foods and produce a toxin that can be lethal upon ingestion. At no time does the microbe grow in or on the host. A relatively trivial infection such as that caused by *Clostridium tetani* in a small puncture wound can cause devastating illness because of a toxin released from the organism growing in the tissues.

We live in a virtual sea of microorganisms, and all our body surfaces have an indigenous bacterial flora. This normal flora actually protects us from infection. Reduction of gut colonization increases susceptibility to infection by pathogens such as *Salmonella typhimurium*. The normal florae are thought to exert their protective effect by several mechanisms: (1) utilizing nutrients and occupying an ecologic niche, thus competing with pathogens; (2) producing antibacterial substances that inhibit the growth of pathogens; and (3) inducing host immunity that is cross-reactive and effective against pathogens. In addition to the normal flora, transient colonization may be seen with known or potential pathogens. This may be a special problem in hospitalized patients (see Ch. 267).

Only a very small proportion of microbial species may be considered to be principal or professional pathogens, and even among these species only a relatively small number of clones have been shown to cause disease. This supports the concept that pathogenic organisms are highly adapted to the pathogenic state and have developed a set of characteristics which enables them to be transmitted, to attach to surfaces, to invade tissue, and to cause disease. In contrast, opportunistic pathogens cause disease principally in impaired hosts. Organisms that may be harmless members of the normal flora in healthy people may act as virulent invaders in patients with severe defects in host defense mechanisms. Pathogenic organisms may be acquired by several routes. Direct contact has been implicated in the acquisition of staphylococcal disease. Airborne spread, usually by droplet nuclei, is seen in respiratory diseases such as influenza. Contaminated water is the usual vehicle in *Giardia* infection and typhoid fever. Food-borne toxin illnesses may be caused by extracellular toxins produced by *Clostridium perfringens* and *Staphylococcus aureus*. Blood and blood products may be vectors for transmitting hepatitis B virus and HIV. Sexual transmission is also important for these latter two agents and for a variety of pathogens including *Treponema pallidum* (syphilis), *Neisseria gonorrhoeae* (gonorrhea), and *Chlamydia trachomatis* (nonspecific urethritis). The fetus may be infected *in utero,* and this may be devastating with rubella virus and cytomegalovirus. Insect vectors may be important, as illustrated by mosquitoes for malaria, ticks for Lyme disease, and lice for typhus.

Pathogens are able to cause disease because of a finely tuned array of adaptations. These include the ability to attach to appropriate cells, often mediated by specialized structures such as the pili on gram-negative rods. Microbes such as *Shigella* species have the ability to invade cells and cause damage in that way. Toxins may act at a distance or may intoxicate only infected cells. Pathogens have the ability to thwart host defenses by a variety of ingenious maneuvers. The antiphagocytic capsular coat of the pneumococcus is an example. Organisms may change their surface antigen display so as to outmaneuver the host immune system. This can be seen with influenza virus and trypanosomes. Certain pathogens have the ability to inhibit the respiratory burst of phagocytes (*Toxoplasma gondii*), and others can destroy phagocytic cells that have engulfed them (*Streptococcus pyogenes*). The environment plays an important role in infection, both in transmission and in the ability of the host to combat the invader. The humidity and temperature of air may affect the infectivity of airborne pathogens. The sanitary state of food and water is an important factor for the acquisition of enteric pathogens. The "bad air" of swamps associated with malaria turned out to be due to the mosquitoes, but the environmental association was appropriate. The nutritional status of the host clearly is a significant factor in certain infectious diseases. The establishment of infection is a complicated interplay of factors involving the microbe, the host, and the environment.

With rare exceptions, infections are treatable and often curable diseases. Thus it is important to make an accurate etiologic diagnosis and promptly institute appropriate therapy. In acute infections such as pneumonia, meningitis, or gram-negative sepsis, rapid institution of therapy may be life-saving, and thus a *presumptive* etiologic diagnosis should be established prior to a *definitive* diagnosis. This presumptive diagnosis can be based on the history, physical examination, epidemiology of illness in the community, and rapid techniques such as microscopic examination of appropriate gram-stained specimens. Antimicrobial therapy can then be instituted for the presumptive etiologic agents but must be re-evaluated as more definitive diagnostic information becomes available (see Ch. 270 and 327).

263 THE FEBRILE PATIENT
David C. Dale

Fever, or "pyrexia," is an elevation of body temperature to a level above normal, i.e., to >37.5°C (99.5° F), due to resettings of the thermoregulatory center in the medulla. To detect fever, oral, rectal, tympanic membrane, and pulmonary artery measurements are more reliable than axillary temperatures. Fever is a useful marker of inflammation; usually the height of the fever reflects the severity of the inflammatory process. Anorexia, malaise, myalgias, headache, and other constitutional symptoms often occur concomitantly. When the body temperature changes rapidly, chills and sweats are also observed. Fever with night sweats is a feature of many chronic inflammatory conditions. *Hyperthermia* is a term for fever due to a disturbance of thermal regulatory control: excessive heat production (e.g., with vigorous exercise or as a reaction to some anesthetics), decreased dissipation (e.g., with dehydration), or loss of regulation (e.g., due to injury to the hypothalmic regulatory center).

Most febrile patients have pain, tenderness, redness, and swelling at the site of inflammation, and the cause of the fever is readily identified. In a general medical practice, the most common causes of fever are upper respiratory illnesses, urinary tract infections, cellulitis, superficial abscesses, and pneumonia. In otherwise healthy individuals, fever alone is not a cause for hospitalization unless it is quite high (>39° C, or 102° F) or accompanied by shaking, chills, hypotension, a change in the sensorium, or other symptoms suggesting bacteremia. However, in immunosuppressed individuals, the elderly, and patients with recent surgery, greater caution is indicated.

FEVER OF UNKNOWN ORIGIN (FUO). An FUO is usually defined in adults as an illness lasting more than 3 weeks with temperatures >101° F (38.3° C) in which a diagnosis has not been made despite a good hospital or office evaluation. Ordinarily by this time the workup has included a history, physical examination, routine blood and urine tests and cultures, radiographs, and some specialized serologic tests. With careful further evaluation a diagnosis can be made in 70 to 90% of these cases.

Diagnoses for FUO's fall into six general categories: infections, noninfectious inflammatory conditions, neoplastic diseases, drug fevers, factitious illnesses, and a group of less common causes (Table 263–1). The pattern of fever is only occasionally helpful in pointing to a specific diagnosis, e.g., the alternate-day fever in established *Plasmodium vivax* infections, the sustained fever in untreated *Salmonella typhi* infections and other continuous bacteremias, and the relapsing (Pel-Ebstein) fever in Hodgkin's disease and other lymphomas.

Evaluation of the FUO Patient. In patients with persisting fevers, it is important first to carefully review the medical history and repeat the physical examination. New clues may be found in the social, occupational, travel, and medication history. On physical examination, special attention should be given to the skin, lymph nodes (including epitrochlear, postauricular, axillary), mucous membranes (including the conjunctivae), and abdominal region (masses, tenderness, and size of the liver and spleen). Usually the basic laboratory tests—CBC, differential, sedimentation rate, urinalysis, liver function tests, skin tests for delayed hypersensitivity (e.g., PPD, mumps), and stool for occult blood—should be repeated. Most patients with active inflammation are anemic, and the leukocyte dif-

ferential can provide valuable clues. Neutrophilia suggests an occult bacterial infection. Monocytosis suggests tuberculosis, brucellosis, inflammatory bowel disease, or other chronic inflammatory conditions. Severe lymphopenia suggests immunodeficiency or a malignancy. A very elevated sedimentation rate suggests giant cell/temporal arteritis, polymyalgia rheumatica, Still's disease, bacterial endocarditis, or other occult infections, and a normal test rarely occurs with any of these illnesses. If the alkaline phosphatase is elevated, obstructive or infiltrative disease of the liver is the most likely cause, although nonspecific elevation is not uncommon. Other tests, e.g., antinuclear antibodies, febrile agglutinins, complement assays, may be positive but are rarely helpful in the FUO evaluation.

A definitive diagnosis is usually made through a combination of imaging studies, microbiologic tests, and/or biopsies. Previous radiographs should be reviewed carefully for evidence of sinusitis, apical inflammation or small nodules in the lungs, hilar adenopathy, or an intra-abdominal mass. Abdominal ultrasonography, gallium and radioisotopically labeled leukocyte scans, computed tomography (CT), and magnetic resonance imaging (MRI) are very helpful to examine the liver, gallbladder, spleen, and pelvic areas for tumors and abscesses. These tests have reduced, but not completely eliminated, the need for exploratory laparotomies.

Cultures of blood (including for *Myobacterium avium* in HIV patients), urine (including mycobacterial cultures if tuberculosis is suspected), and other bodily fluids (e.g., cerebrospinal, peritoneal, pleural) should be obtained if at all suggested by the clinical examination. It is useful to do anaerobic cultures of materials from suspected abscess cavities and to examine blood cultures for fastidious bacteria, yeast, and fungi in difficult cases. A tissue diagnosis often can be made from a biopsy of abnormal skin or lymph nodes or the bone marrow. Biopsies or needle aspirations of liver, lung, bone, or other deep tissue sites are also valuable when abscesses or tumors are suspected.

THERAPY. Therapeutic trials with antibiotics, corticosteroids, or antipyretics before the diagnosis is clear can confuse the evaluation. In some instances, a trial may be justified but should be time limited, i.e., about 2 weeks. In patients with deep tissue abscesses,

TABLE 263–1. CAUSES OF FEVER OF UNKNOWN ORIGIN

Infections

Abscesses—hepatic, subhepatic, gallbladder, subphrenic, splenic, periappendiceal, perinephric, pelvic, and other sites
Granulomatous—extrapulmonary and miliary tuberculosis, atypical *Mycobacteria,* fungal infection
Intravascular—catheter-related endocarditis, meningococcemia, gonococcemia, *Listeria, Brucella,* rat-bite fever, relapsing fever
Viral, rickettsial, and chlamydial—infectious mononucleosis, cytomegalovirus (CMV), human immunodeficiency virus (HIV), hepatitis, Q fever, psittacosis
Parasitic—extraintestinal amebiasis, malaria, toxoplasmosis

Noninfectious Inflammatory Disorders

Collagen vascular diseases—rheumatic fever, systemic lupus erythematosus, rheumatoid arthritis (particularly Still's disease), vasculitis (all types)
Granulomatous—sarcoidosis, granulomatous hepatitis, Crohn's disease
Tissue injury—pulmonary emboli, sickle cell disease, hemolytic anemia

Neoplastic Diseases

Lymphoma/leukemia—Hodgkin's and non-Hodgkin's lymphoma, acute leukemias
Carcinoma—kidney, pancreas, liver, gastrointestinal tract, lung, especially when metastatic
Atrial myxomas

Drug Fevers

Sulfonamides, penicillins, thiouracils, barbiturates, quinidine, laxatives (especially with phenolphthalein)

Factitious Illnesses

Injections of toxic materials, manipulation or exchange of thermometers

Other Causes

Familial mediterranean fever, Fabry's disease, cyclic neutropenia fever usually persists despite antibiotics. In patients with noninfectious inflammatory diseases, e.g., sarcoidosis, Still's disease, or vasculitis, a good clinical diagnosis usually can be made before such therapies are begun. In patients with malignancies, rational therapy depends on a tissue diagnosis. Patients with factitious illness often have serious underlying psychiatric disorders. Care in confrontation is essential to prevent desperate acts including suicide.

Extensive workups of FUO's can be very expensive. In every patient the need for hospital care and testing should be continuously reassessed. When the patient is not severely ill, it is frequently worthwhile to use observation alone as a diagnostic tool. Sometimes even a short period of observation allows an obscure diagnosis to become obvious. In other cases, the fever disappears without the necessity for further diagnostic tests.

Bor DH, Makadon HJ, Friedland G, et al.: Fever in hospitalized medical patients: Characteristics and significance. J Gen Intern Med 3:119, 1988. *A careful review of the frequency and outcome of illnesses with fever in an acute care hospital.*

Kazanjian PH: Fever of unknown origin: Review of 86 patients treated in community hospitals. Clin Infect Dis 15:968, 1992. *FUO series from community hospitals, emphasizing the value of careful physical examination of the patient.*

Knockaert DC, Vanneste LJ, Bobbaers HJ: Recurrent or episodic fever of unknown origin: Review of 45 cases and survey of the literature. Medicine 72:184, 1993. *Episodic fever series, most cases with a long course before a diagnosis was made.*

Knockaert DC, Vanneste LJ, Vanneste SB, Bobbaers HJ: Fever of unknown origin in the 1980s: An update of the diagnostic spectrum. Arch Intern Med 152:51, 1992. *A series of 199 cases from the 1980's diagnosed using CT, ultrasound, and other newer modalities. Reference list includes many classic reports.*

Mackowiak PA, LeMaistre CF: Drug fever: A critical appraisal of conventional concepts: An analysis of 51 episodes in two Dallas hospitals and 97 episodes reported in the English literature. Ann Intern Med 106:728, 1987. *Illustrates the causes and courses of drug fevers in 51 cases, with a review of the literature.*

Rowland MD, Del Bene VE: Use of body computed tomography to evaluate fever of unknown origin. J Infect Dis 156:408, 1987. *Outlines the usefulness of CT for FUO patients.*

264 THE PATHOGENESIS OF FEVER

Bruce Beutler and Steven M. Beutler

DEFINITION. *Fever* (pyrexia) is defined as an elevation of core body temperature above the level normally maintained by the individual. Under normal circumstances, core body temperature (the temperature of blood in the right atrium) is tightly regulated, exhibiting circadian variations over a range that usually does not exceed 1°F (0.6° C), with a mean value of 98.6° F (37° C) (the normal "setpoint"). An array of thermoregulatory mechanisms, described in detail below, ensures that this temperature is maintained. During episodes of fever, the thermoregulatory setpoint is shifted such that the same thermoregulatory mechanisms are employed to maintain an abnormally elevated temperature.

It is important to realize that fever is not equivalent to an elevated core temperature but to an elevated setpoint. Under many circumstances, ranging from intense physical exertion to immersion in hot liquids, core temperature may be elevated yet fever does not exist, because the body is attempting to cope with the departure from homeostasis. Failure of thermoregulation also may be associated with elevated core temperature; this problem too (which occurs in malignant hyperthermia) is distinct from fever.

THERMOREGULATORY MECHANISMS. Core body temperature is determined by two opposing processes, each of which is regulated by the central nervous system (CNS). On the one hand, energy in the form of heat is generated by living tissues ("thermogenesis"). Energy may be passively absorbed from the environment as well. On the other hand, energy is inevitably lost to the environment, chiefly through the emission of infrared radiation and through transfer of energy to a surrounding medium. The temperature at which tissues are maintained is related to heat capacity (e.g., to the amount of energy required to elevate temperature by a defined increment) and to the quantity of energy lost or gained by the system.

Metabolic reactions proceed more rapidly at an elevated temperature. Therefore, the passive warming effect of a febrile state leads to accelerated energy production in the form of heat: for each temperature increment of 1° F (0.6° C), basal metabolic rate increases by approximately 10%. This may, at times, be quite significant from a nutritional point of view.

Muscle is a particularly flexible transducer of chemical energy. "Shivering thermogenesis" refers to the unconscious process whereby muscles are recruited to produce energy through the exercise of activity, leading to an enhanced metabolic demand. This is one mechanism responsible for the rise in body temperature in fever. Hence a sharp "chill" often heralds the onset of fever.

Conservation of energy is effected through piloerection in mammals other than humans. In humans, "gooseflesh" is the equivalent response. "Flushing" represents a redistribution of circulation to dermal vessels and facilitates heat loss; a blanched appearance of the skin indicates an attempt to conserve heat.

INITIATION OF FEVER. The neural pathways responsible for thermoregulation originate in the hypothalamus. A local sensing mechanism exists wherein the temperature of blood is coupled to the development of autonomic discharge. Elevation of body temperature depends primarily on sympathetic outflow, leading to shivering thermogenesis and dermal vasoconstriction, whereas cooling mechanisms (sweating and dermal vasodilation) involve a mixture of sympathetic and parasympathetic pathways.

Certain neurotropic drugs can disrupt the hypothalamic thermosensory mechanism, or blunt the hypothalamic response, and so may interfere with the development of fever. Among these, phenothiazines are the best known for their "poikilothermic" effect. These agents are not specifically active in febrile states; rather, they act to disable thermoregulatory mechanisms.

CLINICAL MANIFESTATIONS. Although fever patterns tend to be nonspecific, they may sometimes provide diagnostic clues (Table 264–1). Intermittent fevers are seen in many conditions and are therefore of little help in discriminating between various disorders. Intermittent fever also may be caused when a continuous fever is interrupted with antipyretics or cooling measures; such interventions must be taken into account in analysis of a temperature curve.

In addition to considering patterns of pyrexia, it is worthwhile to note the relationship between core temperature and other vital signs. For example, a dissociation between the temperature and pulse is sometimes seen in cases of typhoid fever, Legionnaire's disease, psittacosis, and brucellosis. Factitious fever is also accompanied by an inappropriately low pulse. In addition, the respiratory rate may remain unchanged and normal superimposed diurnal variations in temperature may be absent in factitious fever.

Drug fever may occur in association with nearly any medication (see Ch. 10). There is no characteristic fever pattern. Fevers due to drug allergy tend to be well tolerated and may be accompanied by other allergic phenomena such as rash, nephritis, or neutropenia in 20 to 60% of patients.

Extreme pyrexia (characterized by a core temperature > 106° F) often indicates failure of a distal mechanism of thermoregulation, occurring alone or in combination with infection. Examples of noninfectious causes of such extreme pyrexia include heat stroke (see Ch. 71), neuroleptic malignant syndrome (see Ch. 457), and malignant hyperthermia associated with succinylcholine.

CYTOKINES AND FEVER. Hypothalamic dysregulation and fever are triggered by proteins released from cells of the immune system (Fig. 264–1). This communication between the immune system and the nervous system is perhaps the most thoroughly studied "neuroimmunoendocrine" link. In response to invasive stimuli, including components of various microorganisms (e.g., lipoteichoic

TABLE 264–1. FEVER PATTERNS AS DIAGNOSTIC CLUES

Fever Pattern	Cause
Alternate-day fever	*Plasmodium vivax, P. ovale*
Fever every third day	*P. malariae*
Relapsing fever: daily for 3–6 days; fever-free interval for about 1 week supervenes	*Borrelia sp*, rat bite fever (*Streptobacillus moniliformis; Spirillum minus*)
Continuous "undulating fever"	Brucellosis; typhoid
Periodic pyrexia (Pel-Ebstein phenomenon) with variable cycles	Hodgkin's disease

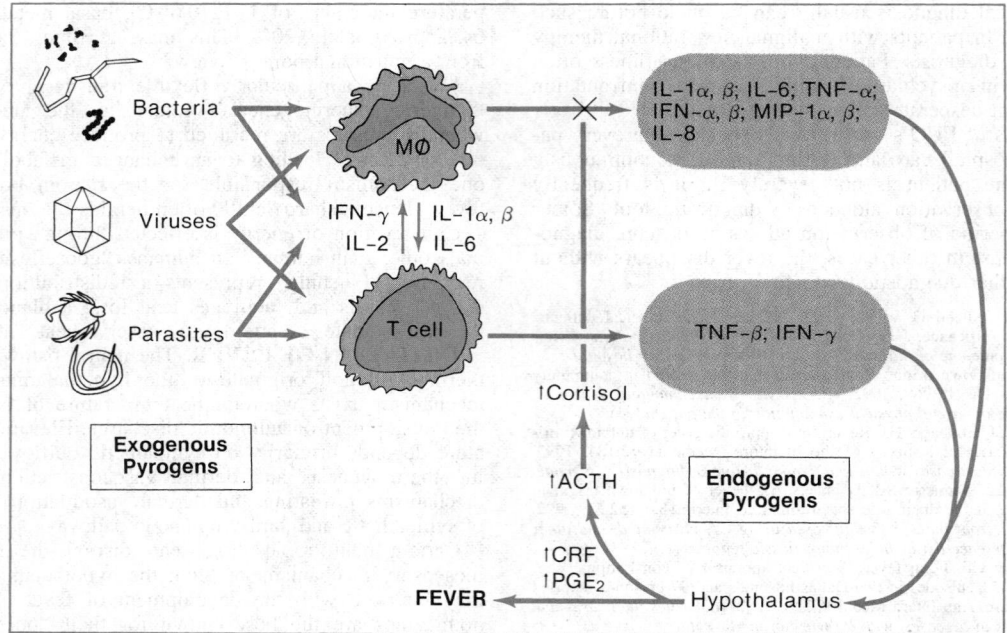

FIGURE 264–1. Production of endogenous pyrogens by macrophages and T lymphocytes. A variety of microbial pathogens produce molecules that function as exogenous pyrogens, triggering the release of endogenous pyrogens from mononuclear cells. ACTH = Adrenocorticotropic hormone; CRF = corticotropin-releasing factor; PGE_2 = prostaglandin E_2; other abbreviations are defined in the text and Table 264–2.

acid, lipopolysaccharides, and other collectively termed constituents ["exogenous pyrogen"]) or certain chemical agents (e.g., amphotericin and perhaps other drugs), cells of the immune system (principally macrophages and, to a lesser extent, lymphocytes) produce proteins that behave as "endogenous pyrogens." These proteins are designated as "monokines" and "lymphokines," respectively, and are often denoted under the more general heading of "cytokines." During the past decade, several of the cytokines active in the pathogenesis of fever have been isolated, and their structures have been determined by molecular cloning. As of this writing, 11 proteins with pyrogenic activity have been identified (Table 264–2); it is likely that many others exist. While mononuclear phagocytes comprise the principal source of pyrogenic cytokines, the same proteins may sometimes originate from nonimmune cells of neoplastic tissue, in which autonomous production and secretion may occur.

The pyrogenic cytokines are structurally diverse proteins with well-established effects in hematopoiesis, inflammation, and the regulation of cell metabolism. Individual agents are often markedly pleiotropic in their actions. In addition to their involvement in mediating fever, cytokines mediate the "acute phase response" (see Ch. 265), which is characterized by increased production of "acute phase reactants" in the liver (fibrinogen, C-reactive protein, complement proteins B, C3, C4, α_2 acid glycoprotein, serum amyloid A, and a variety of proteinase inhibitors among them), decreased production of albumin and transferrin, hypoferremia, hypertriglyceridemia, and other metabolic changes.

Pyrogenic cytokines are presumed to bind to receptors present on vascular endothelial cells that lie within the hypothalamus. They act to reset the hypothalamic thermoregulatory center, prompting an elevation of core body temperature. The resetting is believed to depend largely on endothelial cells producing prostaglandins (PGE_2 and perhaps $PGF_{2\alpha}$). Thromboxanes and lipoxygenase products also may affect the setpoint. Cytokines also may interact directly with neural tissues; there is evidence to suggest that the release of corticotropin-releasing factor (CRF) may trigger thermogenesis in response to at least one cytokine (interleukin-1β, or IL-1β).

Although no single cytokine is capable of provoking fever of a magnitude equivalent to that elicited by endotoxin, it is probable that combined production of several cytokines is sufficient to explain most fevers.

One monokine known as tumor necrosis factor-α (TNF-α) seems capable of reproducing many of the physiologic derangements ob-

served in septic shock and thus appears to mediate most of the deleterious effects of bacterial endotoxin, including fever. A lymphokine known as lymphotoxin (also referred to as tumor necrosis factor-β) is homologous to TNF-α, binds to the same receptor as TNF-α, and elicits many of the same effects. Two other cytokines (IL-1α and IL-1β), while incapable of causing shock by themselves, produce many effects similar to those of TNF-α, and in some instances, synergistic responses have been noted.

Many of the cytokines are mutually inducing, and the concept of a "cytokine cascade" has been offered to describe the production of several factors occurring in response to the elaboration of one member of the group. The temporal sequence of induction may be reflected in the course of fever *in vivo*. For example, injecting a bolus of TNF-α into a rabbit will immediately raise body temperature and cause a delayed rise, apparently related to secondary production of IL-1.

MECHANISMS OF ANTIPYRESIS. Nonsteroidal antipyretic agents inhibit fever by blocking the synthesis of prostaglandins (see Ch. 13) within the endothelium of the hypothalamic vasculature, which is accomplished through inhibition of cyclo-oxygenase. However, they do not diminish the elaboration of endogenous pyrogens and may actually increase the production of some of these proteins (notably TNF-α). Nonsteroidal antipyretics do not produce poikilothermic effects; they can reduce fever but cannot lower body temperature beneath its normal setpoint. It may reasonably be inferred from this observation that prostaglandins do not normally act to maintain core body temperature.

Glucocorticoid hormones directly impede the production of endogenous pyrogens by mononuclear phagocytic cells. Cytokine synthesis is inhibited at more than one level and has been studied most thoroughly in the case of TNF-α biosynthesis. Both transcription of the TNF-α gene and translation of the TNF-α mRNA are down-regulated by glucocorticoid agonists.

The cyclic (often circadian) course followed in many febrile illnesses has not been fully explained. In some instances (e.g., in malaria), a clear relationship to the life cycle of the pathogen has been demonstrated. Cyclicity may, in other cases, follow from the fact that cells comprising the chief source of endogenous pyrogens are rendered refractory by continued exposure to the stimulatory agent and must recover or be replaced.

TREATMENT. In the absence of specific knowledge concerning the benefits of fever, a conservative approach to the treatment of

TABLE 264-2. PROTEINS WITH PYROGENIC ACTIVITY

Endogenous Pyrogen	Other Names/ Abbreviations	Principal Source	Induced by	Principal Effects in Addition to Pyrogenesis	Physical Characteristics
Cachectin/tumor necrosis factor-α	TNF-α	Macrophages	LPS, other microbial products	Fever, shock, anorexia, wasting, tumor necrosis, bone resorption, ↓ adipocyte lipoprotein lipase, neutrophil activation, ↑ endothelial cell adhesiveness/procoagulant effect	Homotrimer; 17 kDa subunit size (nonglycosylated) $\updownarrow$ 26% identity
Lymphotoxin/tumor necrosis factor-β	TNF-β; LT	Lymphocytes (T & B)	Antigenic/mitogenic stimulation		Homotrimer; 20–25 KDa subunit size (glycosylated)
Interleukin-1α (IL-1α)	Leukocyte activity factor (LAF), leukocyte endogenous mediator (LEM), mononuclear cell factor (MCF), endogenous pyrogen (EP)	Macrophages and many other cell types	LPS, other microbial products, TNF	Fever, IL-2 production, bone resorption, pannus formation, neutrophil activation, ↑ endothelial cell adhesiveness/procoagulant effect	Monomer; 17 KDa (glycosylated) $\updownarrow$ 26% identity
Interleukin-1β (IL-1β)					Monomer; 17 KDa (glycosylated)
Interferon-α	IFN-α; leukocyte interferon	Leukocytes (esp. monocyte-macrophages)		Induction of antiviral state	22 KDa (glycosylated) $\updownarrow$ 23% identity
Interferon-β	IFN-β; fibroblast interferon	Fibroblasts	LPS, viral infection, double-stranded RNA		22 KDa (glycosylated)
Interferon-γ	IFN-γ; immune interferon; type 2 interferon	T lymphocytes		Macrophage activation Upregulation of Class I and Class II MHC molecules	20–25 KDa (glycosylated)
Interleukin-6 (IL-6)	Interferon-β₂, hepatocyte-stimulating factor (HSF), B-cell stimulating factor-2 (BSF-2), B-cell differentiation factor (BCDF)	Many cell types	LPS, TNF	↑ Synthesis of acute phase reactants Weak antiviral effect Terminal differentiation of B cells; T-cell activation	21–26 KDa (glycosylated)
Macrophage inflammatory protein 1α	MIP 1α		LPS		7.9 KDa (nonglycosylated) $\updownarrow$ 57% identity
Macrophage inflammatory protein 1β	MIP 1β	Macrophages		Neutrophil chemotaxis	7.8 KDa (nonglycosylated)
Interleukin-8 (IL-8)	Monocyte-derived neutrophil chemotactic factor (MDNCF)		LPS, TNF, IL-1		8.0 KDa (nonglycosylated)

fever is advisable. Core temperatures beneath 105° F are well tolerated by most individuals. Moreover, when its source has been defined, fever often serves as an important indicator of therapeutic effect.

Under certain circumstances, aggressive treatment of fever is warranted. Patients with myocardial ischemia, patients predisposed to seizures, and pregnant women may require treatment with antipyretics, since elevation of core temperature increases cardiac output and myocardial oxygen demand, increases the likelihood of seizures, and may exert a teratogenic effect. Acetaminophen or nonsteroidal anti-inflammatory agents prove adequate for this purpose in the majority of cases. Physical methods for increasing heat dissipation also may be employed.

Temperatures that exceed 106° F are life-threatening and must be lowered immediately. Antipyretics are often ineffective in such instances, since pyrexia of this degree does not result from an aberrant hypothalamic setpoint. It is advisable, in such cases, to lower temperature by any means possible; the most effective action to be taken is to immerse the patient in ice water while monitoring core temperature to be certain that a state of hypothermia is not induced.

Moltz H: Fever: causes and consequences. Neurosci Biobehav Rev 17:237, 1993. *An excellent review analyzing the neurochemistry and neuroanatomy of fever.*
Rothwell NJ: CNS regulation of thermogenesis. Crit Rev Neurobiol 8:1, 1994. *A current appraisal of the pyrogenicity of various cytokines.*

265 THE ACUTE PHASE RESPONSE

Charles A. Dinarello

ACUTE PHASE CHANGES. Infections, trauma, inflammatory processes, and some malignant diseases induce a constellation of host responses collectively referred to as the "acute phase response." The response is associated with characteristic metabolic changes in liver protein synthesis, but on closer examination, changes also occur in several other systems that include hematologic, endocrinologic, and immunologic dysfunctions. These changes are called "acute" because most are observed within hours or days following the onset of infection or injury, although some acute phase changes also indicate chronic disease. The full spectrum of the response includes dramatic increases in the synthesis of several unique hepatic proteins that are not produced in health. One of these, C-reactive protein, is a marker of the acute phase response and can be used to indicate disease. The increased plasma concentrations of acute phase hepatic proteins, glycoproteins, and globu-

1536 / XXI INFECTIOUS DISEASES

lins are responsible for elevated erythrocyte sedimentation rates. Although the liver is producing increasing amounts of a variety of proteins, hepatic albumin synthesis is decreased. Increases in gluconeogenesis, energy expenditure, and muscle proteolysis occur and contribute to weight loss. However, anorexia is often present and may account for most of the weight loss. Fever may be present, and increased sleep and lethargy are frequent clinical complaints. Leukocytosis with increased numbers of circulating immature neutrophils is common, and serum iron and zinc levels are depressed, while increased ceruloplasmin levels result in elevated serum copper. Thyroid dysfunction can be present, and there is often abnormal glucose tolerance and lipid metabolism. In addition, anemia develops despite adequate stores of iron, and hypergammaglobulinemia often occurs.

Although the most florid presentation of the acute phase response is observed in patients with bacterial infections, burns, or multiple injuries, clinicians also encounter acute phase changes in patients with occult infections or chronic illnesses such as rheumatoid arthritis, Crohn's disease, and several autoimmune diseases. The presence of acute phase changes also can serve as an indicator of silent disease and some cancers, particularly renal cell carcinoma and Hodgkin's disease. The acute phase response has the outstanding characteristic of being a generalized host reaction irrespective of the localized or systemic nature of the inciting disease. The various components of the response are remarkably consistent despite the considerable variety of pathologic processes that induce it. For example, plasma levels of several acute phase proteins are elevated following myocardial infarction, fracture of a bone, or bacterial pneumonia.

INDUCTION OF ACUTE PHASE CHANGES. How are infections, injuries, and immunologic and inflammatory reactions able to elicit acute phase changes in the host? The initiation of the acute phase response is linked to the production of hormone-like polypeptide mediators, now called cytokines. Several cytokines induce acute phase changes: interleukin 1 (IL-1), tumor necrosis factor, interferon-γ, interleukin 6 (IL-6), leukemia inhibitory factor, ciliary neurotropic factor, oncostatin M, and interleukin-11 (IL-11). These last five cytokines induce hepatic acute phase protein synthesis via the glycoprotein cell receptor 130. The ability of microbial and inflammatory substances to stimulate the production of these mediators in strategically located, specialized cells appears to be part of local pathologic changes in many diseases, as well as the systemic characteristics of the acute phase response.

Interferon-α is produced primarily during viral infections. Although it shares with IL-1 and tumor necrosis factor the ability to produce fever, sleep, and lethargy, interferon-α does not induce certain other acute phase changes, and hence elevated erythrocyte sedimentation rates and neutrophilia are not commonly observed during viral infections.

The patient with a localized bacterial infection represents an excellent example of the development of the acute phase response. At the onset of the infection, blood monocytes and tissue macrophages become activated either by phagocytosis of the invading microbe or by exposure to its products or toxins; the process results in the synthesis and release of various cytokines within 1 to 2 hours. These mediators enter the circulation and reach the brain where they initiate fever. Whereas fever is clearly one of the most obvious signs of the acute phase response, other components of the response can be present without apparent clinical manifestations. One of the most sensitive measures of the acute phase response is an increase in the number and immaturity of circulating neutrophils. In human subjects injected with small doses of IL-1 or related cytokines, neutrophilia can be measured in the absence of fever. Although not routinely measured, serum zinc and iron levels are depressed. Low serum iron associated with anemia in the face of adequate iron stores is characteristic of the acute phase response.

Within 8 to 12 hours after the onset of infection or trauma, the liver increases the synthetic rate of the so-called acute phase proteins. The response includes increases in proteins normally found in health as well as the appearance of new proteins that serve as markers of a pathologic event. Several normal plasma proteins increase several-fold during the acute phase response. These include haptoglobin, certain protease inhibitors, complement components, ceruloplasmin, and fibrinogen. However, true acute phase reactants increase several hundredfold. These include serum amyloid A protein, a precursor of the amyloid fibril in secondary amyloidosis, and C-reactive protein. C-reactive protein was named for its ability to interact with the C-polysaccharide of pneumococci and was the first acute phase protein described. Table 265–1 lists the characteristic pattern of increased plasma proteins observed during the acute phase response. Note one exception: The plasma concentration of albumin is decreased.

Of all the acute phase proteins, C-reactive protein is clinically the most important because its presence serves as an indicator of disease. C-reactive protein is particularly useful as a marker of the hepatic acute phase protein response and can be measured easily in most hospital clinical laboratories.

Despite the anabolic processes of the liver, the acute phase response is accompanied by a pronounced catabolism of muscle protein associated with loss of body weight and overall negative nitrogen balance. Fever increases oxygen and caloric demands (usually 7% per degree F), and most of the negative nitrogen balance results from oxidation of amino acids from skeletal muscle, which contributes to wasting. These amino acids are largely used for gluconeogenesis. Although the metabolic demands of elevated temperature contribute to the increased need for energy substrates, the host also requires a large supply of amino acids to synthesize new protein at a time when food intake may be impaired or appetite reduced. Amino acids are required for immunologic and reparative processes such as the clonal expansion of lymphocytes and the proliferation of fibroblasts. Also, they are needed for synthesis of hepatic acute phase proteins, immunoglobulins, and collagen. The mechanism of providing ample amino acids for these cellular functions seems to be well orchestrated during the acute phase response. The catabolism during infection and inflammation differs from that of starvation. Unlike starvation, in which large amounts of ketones are spilled into the urine, an individual with an infectious or inflammatory disease excretes protein with small amounts of ketones. IL-1, tumor necrosis factor, and IL-6 the primary mediators of acute phase changes, inhibit lipoprotein lipase and suppress appetite. In addition, these cytokines and interferons directly stimulate hepatic lipogenesis, contributing to the hypertriglyceridemia observed in patients with either acute or chronic disease.

MEASUREMENT OF ACUTE PHASE CHANGES IN CLINICAL MEDICINE. The acute phase response is nonspecific. However, the presence of certain acute phase changes in an otherwise healthy individual can alert the physician to hidden disease. Increased peripheral neutrophils and erythrocyte sedimentation rate are often used to detect an acute phase response. Measurement of C-reactive protein can help the physician determine the presence of disease in patients with vague, constitutional complaints. C-reactive protein levels are usually < 100 μg per liter but increase within hours 10- to 1000-fold. In severe bacterial infections, the serum level can rise from undetectable to over 100 mg per liter in 48 hours. The presence of elevated levels of C-reactive protein or serum amyloid A protein, even in the absence of fever or neutrophilia, may indicate occult infection or malignant change. Increases in C-reactive protein and serum amyloid A protein occur in

TABLE 265–1. PLASMA PROTEINS THAT INCREASE DURING THE ACUTE PHASE RESPONSE

C-reactive protein
Serum amyloid A protein
α_1-Glycoprotein
Ceruloplasmin
α-Macroglobulins
Complement components (C1–C4, factor B, C9, C11)
α_1-Antitrypsin
α_1-Antichymotrypsin
Fibrinogen
Prothrombin
Factor VIII
Plasminogen
Haptoglobin
Ferritin
Immunoglobulins
Lipoproteins

patients of any age and also in immunocompromised patients with opportunistic infections.

Not all inflammatory diseases are associated with elevated C-reactive protein. A refractory state can develop in certain diseases such as scleroderma, ulcerative colitis, and lupus erythematosus. Failure to develop hepatic protein changes and the neutrophilia of the acute phase response seems to be related to the presence of circulating inhibitors of cytokines, e.g., the IL-1 receptor antagonist.

TREATMENT OF ACUTE PHASE RESPONSES. Measurements of fever, acute phase plasma proteins, and peripheral leukocyte numbers are well-established procedures for monitoring many disease states. Although nonsteroidal anti-inflammatory agents are used to treat the fever and associated myalgias of acute phase responses, these drugs do not affect other acute phase changes in the liver, various endocrinologic parameters, or the bone marrow response. Antipyretic blood levels of aspirin and therapeutic concentrations of drugs such as indomethacin or ibuprofen do not reduce production of cytokines. On the other hand, corticosteroids are highly effective in reducing cytokine synthesis as well as the effect of these mediators on various tissue targets. Patients receiving therapeutic doses of corticosteroids have blunted acute phase responses with ongoing infections, inflammatory processes, or immunologic reactions.

The role of acute phase proteins in host defense and repair is not entirely clear. Studies suggest that the major role of C-reactive protein is to bind serum lipids or opsonize pneumococci, whereas serum amyloid A is thought to be immunosuppressive. Ceruloplasmin scavenges toxic free oxygen radicals that are injurious to many tissues. What is clear, however, is that the production and physical structure of these acute phase proteins have been conserved through 400 million years of evolution, and therefore they have presumably been useful to the host. The *Limulus* crab and fish make C-reactive protein that is nearly identical to human C-reactive protein. This argues that the acute phase response plays a role in survival.

Beisel WR: Magnitude of the host nutritional responses to infection. Am J Clin Nutr 30:1236, 1977. *Discussion of the metabolic imbalances seen in patients with infection and injury.*

Dinarello CA, Wolff SM: The role of interleukin-1 in disease. N Engl J Med 328:106, 1993. *Clinical role for IL-1 and IL-1 receptor antagonist in disease.*

Feingold KR, Soued M, Serio MK: Multiple cytokines stimulate hepatic lipid synthesis *in vivo.* Endocrinology 125:267, 1989. *Evidence that interleukin-1, tumor necrosis factor, and interferon may account for the hyperlipidemias observed in patients with acute or chronic inflammatory disease.*

Kushner I, Gewurz H, Benson MD: C-reactive protein and the acute-phase response. J Lab Clin Med 97:739, 1981. *A brief discussion of the usefulness of measuring C-reactive protein levels in clinical practice.*

Pepys MB, Baltz ML: Acute phase proteins with special reference to C-reactive protein and related proteins (pentaxins) and serum amyloid A protein. *In* Dixon FJ, Kunkel HG (eds.): Advances in Immunology, Vol 34. New York, Academic Press, 1983, pp 141-211. *A comprehensive discussion of the hepatic acute phase protein pattern observed during the acute phase response, with special attention to various autoimmune diseases.*

266 THE COMPROMISED HOST
Philip A. Pizzo

"Compromised host" is used to describe patients who have an increased risk for infectious complications as a consequence of a congenital or acquired qualitative or quantitative abnormality of one or more components of the host defense matrix (Table 266–1). Until the early 1980's, this term was largely restricted to patients with congenital immunodeficiencies (see Ch. 223) or to those who became immunocompromised as a consequence of cancer or its treatment, bone marrow failure, or treatment with immunosuppressive therapy. The advent of the acquired immunodeficiency syndrome (AIDS) has given the term "compromised host" a new meaning and relevance. The compromised host with AIDS is discussed in detail in Part XXII. In this chapter, the focus is on non-AIDS patients with altered immune defenses. However, many of the complications and approaches to diagnosis and management are generic.

PHYSICAL DEFENSE BARRIERS

The skin and mucosal surfaces represent the primary defense against both endogenous and exogenous sources of infection. Disruption of skin and mucosa may result from trauma, tumor invasion, the cytotoxic effects of chemotherapy or radiotherapy, the use of invasive diagnostic or therapeutic procedures (e.g., intravenous catheters), and effects of locally destructive infections such as oral herpes simplex. Such mucosal alterations provide a nidus for microbial colonization, a focus for localized infection, and a portal of entry for systemic invasion.

The skin and various mucosal surfaces are normally colonized by aerobic and anaerobic bacteria. However, in patients who have been hospitalized, who are neutropenic, or who have received prior broad-spectrum antibiotics, the normal gram-positive flora of the skin can be replaced by other gram-positive organisms such as CDC group JK *Corynebacterium* or *Bacillus* species or by gram-negative organisms (e.g., pseudomonads, enteric gram-negative rods), fungi (e.g., *Candida albicans* or *Aspergillus* species), and atypical *Mycobacterium* species such as *M. chelonei* or *M. fortuitum.*

Similarly, the gastrointestinal tract is normally colonized by an array of aerobic and anaerobic bacteria as well as some fungi, and disruption of its mucosa may lead to infections by a variety of pathogens including polymicrobial infections. A common cause for disruption of the gastrointestinal mucosal integrity is cytotoxic chemotherapy to patients with malignancy, particularly cytarabine (ara-C), the anthracyclines (daunorubicin and doxorubicin), methotrexate, 6-mercaptopurine, and 5-fluorouracil. Although stomatitis is usually the most clinically recognizable manifestation of gastrointestinal toxicity, diffuse gastrointestinal involvement is also likely. Frequently, the differentiation between chemotherapy-induced stomatotoxicity and localized infection (e.g., necrotizing gingivitis due to anaerobic bacteria or mucosal lesions due to herpes simplex virus) can be difficult, particularly in the neutropenic patient.

In addition to mucosal breakdown, mechanical obstruction of body passages also can increase the risk of serious localized infection due to stasis of local body fluids and resultant overgrowth of potentially pathogenic colonizing organisms. Common sites of secondary infection due to obstruction include the lung, urinary tract, biliary tract, and eustachian tube. One should consider an obstructive process when infection at any of these sites fails to respond to appropriate antibiotics.

Anatomic changes also can contribute to the risk of infection. For example, in patients with sickle cell disease, macrophage and splenic dysfunction predispose to the development of certain bacteremias, especially by *Streptococcus pneumoniae* and *Salmonella* species. Anatomic abnormalities of bones and joints as a result of vaso-occlusive crises caused by infarction of bone marrow, bony cortex, or synovium in patients with sickle cell disease also can predispose to development of infections such as osteomyelitis or arthritis caused by these organisms.

PHAGOCYTE DEFECTS

The polymorphonuclear leukocyte (PMN) and the monocyte are the two most important components of cellular host defense that protect against invasive bacteria and fungi. Both quantitative and qualitative defects affecting PMN's and monocytes may occur in compromised patients.

Quantitative Abnormalities of Phagocytes

Granulocytopenia is among the most important risk factors for serious infection in the compromised host. However, it is important to keep in mind that except for congenital neutropenias, there are often other alterations of the host defense matrix that occur in concert with granulocytopenia and can further alter the risk for infection as well as the types of infectious complications that occur. Granulocytopenia is most commonly associated with malignant disease and its treatment with cytotoxic therapy. This includes patients with hematologic malignancies and lymphomas as well as the increasing number of patients with solid tumors who receive cytotoxic chemotherapy. Patients with primary or secondary bone marrow failure also have neutropenia as their predominant risk for infection. In addition to the neutropenia *per se,* the patterns of infection are also influenced by the other disease- or treatment-related immune abnormalities. For example, despite equivalent degrees of granulocytopenia, the patient with acute myelogenous

TABLE 266-1. PREDOMINANT PATHOGENS IN COMPROMISED PATIENTS; ASSOCIATION WITH SELECTED DEFECTS IN HOST DEFENSE

Host Defense Impairment	Bacteria	Fungi	Viruses	Other

Neutropenia	Gram-negative
	  Enteric organisms
	    (*E. coli, K. pneumoniae, Enterobacter* spp., *Citrobacter* spp.)
	    Pseudomonas aeruginosa
	Gram-positive
	  Staphylococci
	    (coagulase-negative, coagulase-positive)
	  Streptococci, including viridans strep
	    (enterococci)
	  Anaerobes
	    (anaerobic streptococci, *Clostridia* spp., *Bacteroides* spp.)
		Candida species
		  (*C. albicans* > *C. tropicalis* > other species)
		Aspergillus species
		  (*A. fumigatus, A. flavus*)		

Abnormal cell-mediated immunity	*Legionella* *Nocardia asteroides* *Salmonella* spp. Mycobacteria (*M. tuberculosis* and atypical mycobacteria) Disseminated infection from live bacteria vaccine (BCG)	*Cryptococcus neoformans* *Histoplasma capsulatum* *Coccidioides immitis* *Candida*	Varicella-zoster virus Herpes simplex virus Cytomegalovirus Epstein-Barr virus Herpesvirus 6 Disseminated infection from live virus vaccines (vaccinia, measles, rubella, mumps, yellow fever, live polio)	*Pneumocystis carinii* *Toxoplasma gondii* *Cryptosporidium* *Strongyloides stercoralis*

Immunoglobulin abnormalities	Gram-positive
	  Streptococcus pneumoniae, S. aureus
	Gram-negative
	  Haemophilus influenzae
	  Neisseria spp., enteric organisms
			Enteroviruses
			Disseminated infection from live virus vaccines (vaccinia, measles, rubella, mumps, yellow fever, polio)
				Giardia lamblia

Complement abnormalities
  C3, C5
	Gram-positive
	  S. pneumoniae, staphylococci
	Gram-negative
	  H. influenzae, Neisseria spp., Enteric organisms			

C5–C9	*Neisseria* species (*N. gonorrheae, N. meningitides*)			

Anatomic disruption
  Oral cavity
	α-Hemolytic streptococci, oral anaerobes
	  (*Peptococcus, Peptostreptococcus*)
		Candida	Herpes simplex virus	

Esophagus	Staphylococci, other colonizing organisms	*Candida*	Herpes simplex virus Cytomegalovirus	

Lower gastrointestinal tract	Gram-positive
	  Enterococci
	Gram-negative
	  Enteric organisms
	Anaerobes (*B. fragilis, C. perfringens*)
		Candida		*Strongyloides stercoralis*

Skin (IV catheter)	Gram-positive
	  Staphylococci, streptococci
	  Corynebacteria, Bacillus spp.
	Gram-negative
	  P. aeruginosa, enteric organisms
	Mycobacteria
	  M. fortuitum, M chelonei
		Candida
		Aspergillus		

Urinary tract	Gram-positive
	  Enterococci
	Gram-negative
	  Enteric organisms
	  P. aeruginosa
		Candida		

Splenectomy	Gram-positive
	  S. pneumoniae
	Gram-negative
	  Capnocytophaga
	  H. influenzae
	  Salmonella (sickle cell disease)
				Babella

From Rubin M, Walsh TJ, Pizzo PA: Clinical approach to the compromised host. *In* Hoffman R, Benz EJ Jr, Shattil SJ, et al. (eds.): Hematology: Basic Principles and Practices, 2nd Ed. New York, Churchill Livingstone, 1994.

leukemia (AML) may have a different pattern of infection than the patient with aplastic anemia. The disruption of a mucosal defense barrier occurring in the patient with AML who is receiving cytotoxic therapy appears to increase the risk for infection with enteric gram-negative bacteria, α-streptococci, or anaerobes. In contrast, the patient with aplastic anemia who does not have impaired mucosal integrity may be able to sustain longer periods of granulocytopenia without developing a systemic bacterial infection. On the

other hand, if the patient with aplastic anemia is treated with steroids or cyclosporine, the risk for viral or fungal infection may be increased.

Regardless of these modifying factors, the relationship between granulocytopenia and serious infection has been established unequivocally by the classic study of Bodey and colleagues (Table 266–2). This study demonstrated that the risk of infection begins to increase significantly when granulocyte counts fall below 1000 per

TABLE 266–2. ASSOCIATION OF GRANULOCYTE LEVEL AND CHANCE OF DEVELOPING SIGNIFICANT INFECTION

Granulocyte Level (per cu mm)		Percentage of Serious Infections (Duration of Granulocytopenia in Weeks)							
Initial	Change	1	2	3	4	6	10	12	14
Any level	Any fall	12							
Any level	Fall to 2000	2							
Any level	Fall to 1500	5							
Any level	Fall to 1000	10	30	45	50	65	70	85	100
Any level	Fall to 500	19							
Any level	Fall to <100	28	50	72	85	100			

Adapted from Bodey GP, Buckley M, Sathe YS, Freireich EJ: Quantitative relationships between circulatory leukocytes and infection in patients with acute leukemia. Ann Intern Med 61:328, 1966.

microliter and is most marked when the counts are ≤ 100 per microliter. In addition to the absolute granulocyte count, the duration of granulocytopenia is also directly related to the direction of granulocytopenia as well as to whether the counts are rising or falling.

For practical purposes, granulocytopenia is usually defined as a count of ≤ 500 PMN's and band forms per microliter. However, a patient with an absolute granulocyte count of 500 to 1000 per microliter that is rapidly falling is probably at greater risk for infection than a patient with a count of 200 per microliter that is rising. Thus the absolute granulocyte count, the duration of granulocytopenia, and whether the neutrophil count is falling or rising must all be considered when assessing the risk to any individual patient. Some clinicians also include the monocyte count in this equation to generate an absolute phagocyte index.

Granulocytopenia primarily predisposes patients to bacterial and fungal infection and does not of itself appear to increase the incidence or severity of viral and parasitic infections. In the 1950's and 1960's, when cytotoxic therapy was first being developed, gram-positive bacteria (especially *Staphylococcus aureus*) predominated. In the early 1970's, with the availability of antibiotics to control gram-positive bacteria (e.g., methicillin), gram-negative organisms (e.g., *Escherichia coli, Klebsiella, Pseudomonas aeruginosa*) emerged as the predominant pathogens in neutropenic patients, perhaps because of the increasing use of more aggressive chemotherapy regimens and the use of broader-spectrum antibiotics. During the 1980's, gram-positive organisms re-emerged as common bacterial isolates, and at many centers they now represent the most frequently encountered organisms.

In addition to these changes in the pattern of infection, institutional variations in the causes of infection and the antibiotic sensitivity patterns of isolates cannot be overemphasized, making it imperative for physicians to have a working knowledge of the specific isolates encountered at their own clinical setting.

The gram-negative organisms encountered most commonly in granulocytopenic patients are *E. coli, K. pneumoniae,* and *P. aeruginosa.* Together, these have generally accounted for approximately 90% of the gram-negative isolates at most centers. A precise source for gram-negative bacteremia is identified in only a minority of cases, but the gastrointestinal tract, respiratory tract soft tissue, and urinary tract are the most probable sources for infection. Of these three organisms, *P. aeruginosa* is often the most virulent in neutropenic hosts, although in most developed countries the incidence of infection due to *Pseudomonas* declined in neutropenic patients during the 1980's. But as a general rule, virtually any organism can be pathogenic if the host defenses are severely impaired. *Enterobacter* species, *Citrobacter* species, and *Serratia marcescens* are less frequently encountered but are notable because they rapidly become resistant to β-lactam antibiotics through the induction of chromosomally mediated β-lactamases. Of concern, an increase in *Enterobacter* sepsis has been observed at a number of treatment centers. Other less common gram-negative isolates include *Acinetobacter* species, *Haemophilus* species (usually nontypable *H. influenzae*), and nonaeruginosa pseudomonads (often catheter-related and antibiotic-resistant).

The gram-positive organisms most frequently encountered are the coagulase-negative staphylococci (most commonly *S. epidermidis*), coagulase-positive staphylococci *(S. aureus),* enterococci, and α-hemolytic streptococci (e.g., *S. mutans* or viridans group strepto-

cocci). Both coagulase-positive and -negative staphylococci are most commonly isolated from the blood, often from patients with indwelling intravenous catheters, or from those with foreign bodies such as prosthetic heart valves or orthopedic implants. *S. aureus* tends to be significantly more virulent and its sensitivity to β-lactam antibiotics (e.g., methicillin, oxacillin, or nafcillin) can vary from center to center, making it imperative for physicians to be aware of the frequency of methicillin-resistant *S. aureus* (MRSA) at their institutions. In contrast, the coagulase-negative staphylococci tend to be relatively indolent. During the last decade, the coagulase-negative staphylococci have become increasingly resistant to β-lactam antibiotics, and the majority (50 to 80%) are methicillin-resistant and generally require treatment with vancomycin. Notable are the recent reports of α-hemolytic viridans streptococci that have been associated with septic shock and the adult respiratory distress syndrome (ARDS) in patients who are receiving high-dose cytosine arabinoside and who develop oral mucosal disruption. Other gram-positive bacteria that may be encountered in neutropenic patients include *Bacillus* species (often catheter-related), group CDC-JK *Corynebacterium* (often catheter-related and relatively antibiotic-resistant), *Enterococcus faecium* (may be resistant to vancomycin), and *Lactobacillus* (may also be resistant to vancomycin).

Infections due solely to anaerobic bacteria are less common and are usually associated with a concomitant abnormality in gastrointestinal mucosal integrity. While *B. fragilis* and *Clostridium perfringens* are the most common organisms, other *Bacteroides* species, as well as other *Clostridium* species (e.g., *C. tertium, C. septicum*), which are often clindamycin-resistant, can be clinically important. Anaerobes are frequent components of intra-abdominal infections, including peritonitis, intra-abdominal abscesses, and perirectal cellulitis or abscesses. *C. difficile* is a common cause of colitis in neutropenic patients treated with antibiotics or cytotoxic agents.

Although infections due to *Mycobacterium tuberculosis* have not been dominant in non-AIDS immunocompromised hosts, the rising incidence of tuberculosis (especially with multidrug-resistant strains) in homeless persons and people with AIDS increases the likelihood that these infections will occur in other immunocompromised hosts. Patients with hairy cell leukemia (HCL), who have profound monocytopenia in addition to neutropenia, appear to have an increased risk for developing atypical mycobacterial infection (e.g., *M. kansasii, M. fortuitum, M. chelonei,* and *M. avium-intracellulare* complex). Rapidly growing mycobacteria (*M. fortuitum* and *M. chelonei*) also may cause exit-site infections in patients with indwelling intravenous catheters, or wound infections following surgery.

In contrast to the bacterial infections, which are often associated with the onset of fever in neutropenic patients, fungal infections only rarely cause primary infection (i.e., initial infection in patients not yet receiving antibiotics). More commonly, fungal infections occur as a secondary process in patients receiving antibacterial agents. Although a variety of fungal infections may be encountered in the neutropenic host, *Candida* and *Aspergillus* species predominate.

The vast majority of infections due to *Candida* are caused by *C. albicans,* with other potential pathogens including *C. tropicalis, C. parapsilosis, C. krusei,* and *C. glabrata* (also known as *Torulopsis glabrata*). In neutropenic patients, *Candida* infections may include candidemia, catheter-related infections, invasive mucosal infections (e.g., oral, esophageal, or lower gastrointestinal), and disseminated disease, in which the most commonly affected organs are the liver and spleen (so-called hepatosplenic candidiasis), the eye (endophthalmitis), and the skin.

Aspergillosis is usually due to *A. fumigatus* and *A. flavus,* although *A. niger* and *A. terreus* also can result in infection. The upper airways (e.g., oral cavity, nasal cavity, or sinuses) and lung are the primary sites involved with *Aspergillus,* and spread is usually by direct invasion into contiguous areas, although widespread dissemination has been described in various sites including brain, liver and spleen, gastrointestinal tract, heart, and kidneys. However, positive blood cultures virtually never occur.

Other fungal pathogens that may occur in neutropenic patients include the Mucoraceae species (*Mucor, Rhizopus, Absidia,* and *Cunninghamella*—often clinically resembling *Aspergillus* infections), *Trichosporon beigelii* (which may cause disseminated visceral and cutaneous disease), *Fusarium, Drechslera, Pseudallescheria boydii,* and *Malassezia furfur.*

Qualitative Abnormalities of Phagocytes

The microbicidal activity of granulocytes and monocytes involves complex interactions between the cell and the organism or inflammatory site. Some of the major functions important for microbicidal activity include migration of the cell to the inflammatory site (or chemotaxis), cell activation, phagocytosis, and intra- and extracellular killing via both oxygen-dependent and -independent pathways. These qualitative abnormalities can be operationally divided into the following categories: (1) those associated with malignant or myeloproliferative disease itself, (2) those associated with diseases that do not primarily affect the leukocytes, (3) iatrogenic causes (such as administration of pharmacologic agents or radiation), and (4) primary disorders of phagocytes.

PATIENTS WITH MALIGNANT DISORDERS AND MYELODYSPLASIA. Significant functional defects in mature PMN's can occur in patients with AML and acute lymphoblastic leukemia prior to therapy. Although it has been largely assumed that granulocytes from patients with chronic myelogenous leukemia have normal microbicidal activity, some studies have documented significant impairment in neutrophil function of morphologically mature PMN's from patients with chronic myelogenous leukemia, including abnormalities in phagocytosis, random migration, chemotaxis, and bactericidal activity. Nevertheless, during the stable chronic phase of the disease, infectious complications are rarely seen in these patients.

In addition to immunoglobulin deficiencies that impair opsonization, patients with chronic lymphocytic leukemia and multiple myeloma also may have such abnormalities as defective granulocyte adherence, decreased granulocyte migration, a decrease in the number of granulocyte receptors for C3b and IgG, and decreased chemotaxis of monocytes.

Significant defects in granulocyte function also have been found in PMN's from patients with myelodysplastic syndromes and preleukemic states. The clinician should probably assume that neutrophils from patients with myelodysplastic syndromes or preleukemia are functionally defective, and thus patients with "borderline" granulocyte counts should be approached as if they had an absolute neutropenia.

NONMALIGNANT HEMATOLOGIC DISEASE. Although the predominant defect in host defense in most patients with aplastic anemia is neutropenia, followed by immune suppression as a result of therapy (e.g., steroids, antithymocyte globulin, or cyclosporine), deficient production of superoxide and a deficiency of myeloperoxidase can sometimes be observed. Patients with paroxysmal nocturnal hemoglobinuria (PNH) appear to have an increased susceptibility to bacterial infection. Impaired chemotaxis despite normal phagocytosis and bacterial killing has been described in PNH, and the Fc receptor type III (the major Fc receptor in blood and on neutrophils) also has been shown to be deficient in PNH.

In addition to splenic dysfunction, abnormal complement activation, and defective serum opsonizing capacity, defective phagocytic function has been described in patients with sickle cell anemia, although the significance of this is unclear. Neutrophils from infection-prone children with sickle cell disease have been shown to have defective bactericidal activity, perhaps secondary to zinc deficiency.

Some patients with severe G6PD deficiency appear to have an increased susceptibility to infections caused by catalase-positive bacteria. The clinical picture resembles that of chronic granulomatous disease of childhood, although only rarely are infections reported in the first decade of life. The granulocytes show normal phagocytosis and chemotaxis but defective bactericidal activity.

Although most studies address disseminated intravascular coagulation (DIC) secondary to overwhelming bacterial infection, the potential role of fibrinogen degradation products (FDP's) in modifying PMN function has been suggested by the finding that two FDP's (FDP D and FDP E) can cause substantial *in vitro* inhibition of PMN chemotaxis, oxidative metabolism, and killing of *E. coli.* DIC associated with infection, then, may represent a vicious circle in which the organism triggers the coagulation abnormalities, which in turn may result in neutropenia and defective PMN function, thus worsening the infection.

PHARMACOLOGIC AGENTS AND RADIOTHERAPY. Most cytotoxic drugs used for treatment of malignant and autoimmune diseases or transplantation have antiproliferative effects, resulting in neutropenia and monocytopenia. Among the antineoplastics, the most commonly implicated agents include methotrexate, 6-mercaptopurine, vincristine, vinblastine, anthracyclines, cyclophosphamide, carmustine, and platinum compounds.

Glucocorticoids are associated with increased susceptibility to infection. As a general rule, the signs and symptoms of even severe infections may be masked or greatly reduced in patients receiving steroids. Steroids impair neutrophil chemotaxis, and at high dosages, PMN phagocytosis, microbicidal activity, and antibody-dependent cytotoxicity also may be altered. In addition, steroids may cause monocytopenia as well as defects in monocyte chemotaxis, phagocytosis, and killing of bacteria and fungi. In addition to their action on granulocytes and monocytes, steroids may enhance susceptibility to infection by impairing wound healing, increasing skin fragility, and depressing lymphocyte function, the production of cytokines, and humoral immune responses.

Biologic agents (e.g., colony-stimulating factors [CSF's], interleukins, interferons) are being employed increasingly in clinical medicine. Studies to date suggest that granulocyte-macrophage (GM)-CSF or granulocyte (G)-CSF not only may increase cell number but also may enhance a number of neutrophil functions, including oxidative metabolism, phagocytosis, microbicidal activity, and antibody-dependent cytotoxicity. At the same time, in adults undergoing autologous bone marrow transplant, there appeared to be the unanticipated finding of a marked decrease in migration of PMN's toward a sterile, artificially created inflammatory site on the skin during periods of GM-CSF administration. Although the clinical significance of any of these effects has not yet been established, these data underscore the importance of carefully evaluating biologics as they are introduced into the therapeutic armamentarium. For example, although interleukin-2 (IL-2) appears promising in mediating tumor lysis (with either lymphokine-activated killer [LAK] cells, tumor infiltrating lymphocytes [TIL's], or interferon-α), impaired granulocyte function, decreased chemotaxis, and decreased Fc receptor γ-III expression have been noted in some patients receiving high doses of IL-2 and may be associated with an increased incidence of significant infections due to *S. aureus.* In contrast, other biologic agents such as interferon-γ may increase phagocyte function and decrease the risk for infection (e.g., in patients with chronic granulomatous disease).

PRIMARY DISORDERS OF PHAGOCYTE FUNCTION. Chronic granulomatous disease (CGD) has served as a prototype for diseases characterized by defective oxidative metabolism of phagocytes. Although CGD represents a heterogeneous group of disorders from a molecular and genetic perspective, the common denominator is that phagocytes lack essential components of oxidative metabolism and fail to generate the respiratory burst in response to various stimuli, including certain pathogenic organisms. The organisms that cause serious infections in patients with CGD are most often those which contain the enzyme catalase. In the absence of cellular production of H_2O_2, the peroxide generated by non–catalase-containing organisms is enough to ameliorate the neutrophil deficiency and allow microbicidal activity. However, if the organism also contains catalase, the H_2O_2 it produces is rapidly degraded and is not available for participation in oxidative-based killing. The majority of infections in patients with CGD are caused by *S. aureus,* although serious infections also can result from enteric gram-negative bacilli (e.g., *E. coli, K. pneumoniae,* or *Serratia* species), *P. cepacia, Nocardia asteroides,* and *Aspergillus* species.

Serious recurrent infections usually begin in the first year of life in children with CGD. The lung is the most common site of infection (pneumonias and abscesses), with other common infections including skin and soft tissue abscesses, visceral abscesses (particularly hepatic), osteomyelitis (especially of the small bones in the hands and feet), and suppurative lymphadenopathy. Uncommonly, CGD can present in adolescence or adulthood, although with careful history, infectious complications often date back to childhood.

Prophylactic antibiotics, with trimethoprim-sulfamethoxazole, have been advocated by many investigators. Interferon-γ also has been shown to reduce the incidence of serious infection and the number of hospital days for patients with CGD.

Myeloperoxidase (MPO) deficiency is perhaps the most common of all granulocyte disorders, with an estimated frequency ranging from 1 in 2000 to 1 in 4000. MPO is a lysosomal enzyme that catalyzes the formation of hypochlorous acid from H_2O_2 produced in the respiratory burst. Interestingly, most individuals identified with

MPO deficiency are healthy, and infectious complications are exceedingly rare. Systemic *Candida* infections have occurred in a small number of MPO-deficient patients who also had diabetes mellitus.

Chédiak-Higashi syndrome (CHS) is a rare disorder characterized by autosomal recessive inheritance, recurrent infections, partial oculocutaneous albinism, central and peripheral neuropathy, and increased bleeding time. Neutropenia also can be present. Infections result from combined effects of neutropenia and functional defects in phagocytes, which include impaired degranulation and defective chemotaxis. Infections frequently involve the skin, respiratory tract, and mucous membranes and are most commonly caused by *S. aureus* or gram-negative bacilli. Deficiency of the iC3b receptor (also known as CR3, Mo1, and MAC-1), which is important for adherence and phagocytosis, is a rare disorder. Accordingly, neutrophils demonstrate defects in aggregation, margination, chemotaxis, and phagocytosis. The most common infections are skin and subcutaneous tissue infections, otitis, mucositis, gingivitis, and periodontitis.

A number of disorders have been described that are characterized by defects in chemotaxis of granulocytes and/or monocytes. Infections in these patients tend to be cutaneous, and the most common pathogens are *S. aureus,* streptococci, *C. albicans, E. coli,* and *Trichophyton rubrum.* Depending on the specific syndrome, deep-seated infections also may occur. The "lazy leukocyte" syndrome also may be associated with neutropenia and is characterized by gingivitis, recurrent otitis media, rhinitis, and stomatitis. Hyperimmunoglobulin E syndrome (Job's syndrome) is usually associated with multiple cutaneous abscesses caused by staphylococci, but deep-seated infections and infections due to other organisms such as pseudomonads and *Candida* have also been reported. Wound healing does not appear to be a problem, as it is in CGD. Chemotaxis defects have been reported in patients with congenital ichthyosis and recurrent *T. rubrum* infections.

DEFECTS IN CELL-MEDIATED IMMUNITY (CMI)

Cellular immune dysfunction either may be primary, as in a number of congenital immunodeficiency states, or may occur secondary to other disorders or therapeutic interventions. Defective CMI may lead to infections caused by bacteria, fungi, viruses, and protozoa. The predominant pathogens are intracellular organisms (those microbes which survive inside of macrophages) and include mycobacteria (both *M. tuberculosis* and atypical mycobacteria), *Legionella, N. asteroides, Salmonella* species, *Cryptococcus neoformans, Histoplasma capsulatum, Coccidioides immitis,* varicella-zoster virus (VZV), herpes simplex virus (HSV), cytomegalovirus (CMV), Epstein-Barr virus (EBV), *Pneumocystis carinii, T. gondii, Cryptosporidium,* and *Strongyloides stercoralis.*

Patients with Malignant Disorders

Hodgkin's disease and the non-Hodgkin's lymphomas are associated with altered CMI not only when the malignancy is active but in some instances even when the malignancy is in remission.

CMI defects have been postulated to help explain the incidence of atypical mycobacterial infections in patients with hairy cell leukemia and also occur in relatively rare T-cell malignancies such as mycosis fungoides and T-cell chronic lymphocytic leukemia (CLL). CMI defects exist in children with ALL, as evidenced by their increased susceptibility to infections due to *P. carinii* or disseminated VZV, but it is likely that concurrent therapy plays a major role. Clinically significant impairment of CMI has not been well established for other malignancies.

Patients with Nonmalignant Hematologic Disorders

Impaired CMI is not a prominent feature of nonmalignant hematologic disorders unless associated with therapy or acquisition of HIV-1 infection. Abnormalities in CMI have been best described in patients with hemophilia who have received Factor VIII concentrates even in the absence of apparent HIV-1 infection. Patients with sickle cell anemia have been found to be anergic in association with zinc deficiency and decreased nucleoside phosphorylase activity.

A number of infections may produce impaired CMI either directly (e.g., by infecting key cellular components such as T lymphocytes or macrophages) or by affecting other immunoregulatory mechanisms. The most notable viral infection associated with impaired CMI is HIV-1. Other viral infections that also are associated

with CMI defects include CMV, EBV, RSV, hepatitis B, and influenza. Other nonviral infections that have been variably associated with impaired CMI by *in vitro* testing have included tuberculosis, leprosy, bacterial pneumonia, brucellosis, typhoid fever, coccidioidomycosis, syphilis, and a variety of parasitic diseases.

Noninfectious conditions that have been linked to abnormal CMI include chronic protein-calorie malnutrition, uremia, diabetes mellitus, surgery, anesthesia, sarcoidosis, and cystic fibrosis.

Pharmacologic Agents

Corticosteroids are the pharmacologic agents most often associated with CMI abnormalities, although they also may cause immune suppression due to effects on other host defense mechanisms. The degree of immunosuppression and the relative risk of infection depend on the dose and duration of corticosteroids as well as the underlying disease. Patients receiving pharmacologic doses of steroids (e.g., brain tumor patients, those with inflammatory bowel disease, and with autoimmune disorders) may have impaired CMI and should be considered at risk for mycobacterial, viral, and parasitic infections. Patients to be treated with corticosteroids with a known history of tuberculosis or a positive PPD skin test should be given prophylactic isoniazid (INH) to prevent reactivation and potential dissemination of disease.

A number of cytotoxic agents are also associated with impaired CMI, including methotrexate, cyclophosphamide, 6-mercaptopurine, and azathioprine. Cyclosporine is an immunosuppressant used to suppress transplant rejection and is associated with alterations in helper T cells, effector T cells, and natural killer (NK) cells. It has not been established, however, that cyclosporine *per se* is associated with an increased risk of infection.

Radiotherapy also may result in impaired CMI, especially when used in combination with other immunosuppressive agents or to treat patients with underlying diseases associated with intrinsic CMI defects (e.g., as a component of the preparatory regimen for bone marrow transplantation or for treatment of Hodgkin's disease).

Primary Disorders of Cell-mediated Immunity (see Ch. 223)

Defects in CMI are found as components of mixed primary B- and T-cell abnormalities, including severe combined immunodeficiency disease (SCID), Wiskott-Aldrich syndrome, ataxia-telangiectasia, and certain purine pathway enzyme deficiencies. Infections in patients with these disorders tend to begin early in life and may be caused not only by pathogens associated with CMI abnormalities but also by those seen with humoral defects such as the encapsulated bacteria.

SCID is associated with a marked decrease in both B- and T-cell numbers and extremely low levels of immunoglobulins. Patients fail to react to skin tests and have a negligible antibody response following immunizations. Failure to thrive and recurrent infections are seen within the first few months of life. Infections are due to *S. aureus, S. pneumoniae, H. influenzae, P. carinii, Candida,* and herpes group viruses. Affected infants usually die by 2 years of age. A variant of SCID has been described that is associated with chronic skin eruption, hepatosplenomegaly, eosinophilia, and histiocytic infiltration of the lymph nodes (Omenn's disease). *P. carinii* pneumonia may be a common presenting symptom in this disorder.

In patients with Wiskott-Aldrich syndrome, the major abnormality is an inability to respond to polysaccharide antigens. Infections are caused by polysaccharide-encapsulated bacterial pathogens such as *S. pneumoniae* and *H. influenzae.* However, patients also may lose T-cell functions and may have increased susceptibility to pathogens such as HSV and certain fungi and protozoa.

Ataxia-telangiectasia is associated with absent serum and secretory IgA. The thymus is hypoplastic, and thymus-dependent zones in lymph nodes are empty or unoccupied. Infection with encapsulated bacteria predominates, especially recurrent sinopulmonary infections. Many patients progressively lose T-cell function over time and may become susceptible to associated pathogens.

Purine pathway enzyme deficiencies (adenosine deaminase deficiency or nucleoside phosphorylase deficiency) may be associated with either combined B- and T-cell defects or isolated B- or T-cell abnormalities. The type of infection depends on the predominant immune defect. Infections may not appear until 6 to 12 months of age.

The primary cellular immunodeficiencies associated with T-cell abnormalities include thymic hypoplasia (DiGeorge's syndrome), combined immunodeficiency with predominant T-cell defect (Nezelof's syndrome), purine nucleoside phosphorylase deficiency, and chronic mucocutaneous candidiasis.

DiGeorge's syndrome develops when the third and part of the fourth pharyngeal pouches fail to develop during embryogenesis, resulting in absence of the thymus and parathyroid glands. Children with DiGeorge's syndrome lack T lymphocytes and have severe depression of CMI, making them susceptible to overwhelming infections due to a variety of organisms, including HSV, VZV, C. albicans, and P. carinii. Nezelof's syndrome can be differentiated from DiGeorge's syndrome by the absence of parathyroid and cardiac involvement.

Cartilage-hair hypoplasia is a form of short-limbed dwarfism associated with a virtual absence of T-cell function. Interestingly, susceptibility to infection is not as pronounced as in other T-cell deficiencies. Overwhelming viral infections due to vaccinia or varicella viruses may occur.

Chronic mucocutaneous candidiasis involves impairment in CMI, and infection is almost always limited to the skin and mucous membranes.

ABNORMALITIES OF HUMORAL DEFENSE MECHANISMS— IMMUNOGLOBULINS AND COMPLEMENT

Immunoglobulins and complement are among the most important components of the humoral immune system, and defects or deficiencies in either may be associated with serious infections. Other proteins that have been classified as part of the humoral defense system include lysozyme, lactoferrin, tuftsin, and fibronectin. Immunoglobulins may be opsonic (enhance phagocytosis), neutralizing (inhibit replication of viruses), or with complement mylyse microbes or cells. The humoral system functions predominantly against bacterial infections. Patients with either primary or secondary defects or deficiencies in these proteins are at highest risk for developing serious infections due to the encapsulated bacteria and to a lesser extent the enteroviruses and Giardia lamblia.

Patients with Malignant Disorders

The degree of humoral impairment in multiple myeloma appears to be related to the stage of the disease, primarily due to malignant plasma cell induction of a protein that is synthesized by macrophages and that selectively suppresses B-cell function. Myeloma patients are most susceptible to recurrent infections from encapsulated bacteria such as S. pneumoniae or H. influenzae early in the course of the disease. Infections due to enteric gram-negative rods and staphylococci are also encountered, especially in patients with refractory or advanced disease. Recurrent infection most often occurs in the upper respiratory tract, urinary tract, or skin.

Patients with B-cell CLL appear to have an unbalanced immunoglobulin chain synthesis and resultant hypogammaglobulinemia. The incidence of infection correlates with the duration and stage of the disease as well as the serum levels of immunoglobulins (particularly IgG). Encapsulated bacteria predominate, although infections due to staphylococci and enteric gram-negative bacilli also occur. Upper and lower respiratory tract infections are encountered most commonly, although other sites such as urinary tract and skin are frequently involved.

Nonmalignant states (e.g., nephrotic syndrome, burns, protein-losing enteropathy) can be associated with increased immunoglobulin catabolism or loss and may lead to decreased antibody levels and enhanced susceptibility to infection. Clinically significant acquired complement defects are unusual.

Primary Deficiencies

Isolated B-cell immunodeficiency states and their associated risks for infection in children include transient hypogammaglobulinemia of infancy, which is not usually associated with serious infections; sex-linked hypogammaglobulinemia, which is associated with recurrent pyogenic infections and septicemia due to S. pneumoniae, H. influenzae, S. aureus, N. meningitidis, and P. aeruginosa; hypogammaglobulinemia associated with hyperimmunoglobulin M, in which patients have recurrent respiratory, soft tissue, and gastrointestinal infections; selective IgM deficiency, in which patients have severe recurrent infections due to pyogenic bacteria; and selective IgA deficiency, in which certain patients may have increased numbers of upper respiratory tract infections, whereas others appear not to be at increased risk. Chronic diarrhea due to G. lamblia is also associated with IgA deficiency. Common variable hypogammaglobulinemia is associated with respiratory tract infections due to S. pneumoniae, H. influenzae, and S. aureus. Diarrhea due to G. lamblia also occurs.

Many patients with B-cell deficiencies, particularly those with congenital hypogammaglobulinemia, appear to be at risk for developing chronic central nervous system infections due to enteroviruses.

A number of primary defects in complement components also have been described. Although deficiencies of the early classic pathway components (C1, C2, C4) have been reported, associated infection is rare, probably because the alternative pathway remains functional and is able to compensate. Deficiencies of C3 or C5, on the other hand, often lead to severe infections due to encapsulated organisms, enteric gram-negative bacteria, and staphylococci. Absence of the later components (C5b, C6, C7, C8, C9) leads to an increase in infections, primarily due to Neisseria species, both N. gonorrhoeae and N. meningitidis. Although the defects in these later components may be present from birth, infectious episodes do not typically begin until the teenage years. Indeed, any patient with recurrent infections due to Neisseria species should be investigated for complement deficiency.

SPLENECTOMY AND SPLENIC DYSFUNCTION

Splenectomy may be performed either as a part of staging or as a therapeutic intervention in a number of disorders, including Hodgkin's disease, agnogenic myeloid metaplasia, paroxysmal nocturnal hemoglobinuria, hereditary spherocytosis, thalassemia, and a variety of autoimmune disorders.

The spleen probably plays an adjunctive role in host defense by removing organisms from the blood that have been ineffectively opsonized by complement. In addition, it participates in the primary immunoglobulin response and is involved in regulation of the alternative complement pathway, with low levels of immunoglobulins and properdin reported in patients following splenectomy. A decrease in the opsonic peptide tuftsin also has been reported following splenectomy, and alternative pathway defects may be important in patients with sickle cell disease and splenic dysfunction.

The risk of developing serious infection, as well as the types of infections, may vary depending on the reason for abnormal splenic function and the presence or absence of other immune abnormalities. Patients who undergo post-traumatic splenectomy appear to be at a lower risk for infection. An increased risk of Salmonella infections appears to be unique for the sickle cell population. Most asplenic patients or patients who have undergone splenectomy are at increased risk for serious bacterial infections, primarily due to S. pneumoniae and H. influenzae, as well as Neisseria species and Capnocytophaga. The initial presentation of even overwhelming infection may be deceptively subtle, with fever often being the only sign of infection. Asplenic patients with an underlying hematologic disease who present with fever should be managed initially as potentially septic.

EVALUATING AND MANAGING THE FEBRILE GRANULOCYTOPENIC PATIENT: A PARADIGM FOR THE COMPROMISED HOST

A classic tenet of infectious disease is that antibiotic therapy is based on isolating and identifying a specific organism or on reliably predicting a specific organism from a clinically involved site of infection. The overall management of neutropenic patients is based on use of empirical antibiotics directed against a wider array of potential pathogens. Indeed, it is well accepted that when a neutropenic patient develops a new fever (usually defined as one oral temperature $\geq 38.5°C$ or more than two successive readings of $\geq 38°$ C in a 12-hour period), an empirical broad-spectrum antibacterial regimen should be started expeditiously. The rationale for this approach evolved from the observation that bacteremias in neutropenic patients were rapidly lethal, especially those due to gram-negative organisms, if antibiotic therapy was delayed until an organism was isolated or a site of infection identified. Although the goal of the preantibiotic evaluation of a newly febrile neutropenic patient is to identify potential sources, the majority of patients will not have a source of infection identified to explain the fever.

The standard initial evaluation should include a careful physical examination with particular attention to areas that may "hide" an infection, notably the oral cavity and the perianal area. Examination of the perirectal area, including deep palpation, should be performed, and only if there are findings suggestive of a localized inflammatory site (e.g., pain or fluctuance) should a judicious digital examination be performed. At a minimum, two sets of blood samples for culture should be obtained. If the patient has an indwelling intravenous catheter, then at least one set should be drawn through the catheter and another from a peripheral vein. For patients with multilumen intravenous catheters, a culture should be obtained through *each* lumen and the specific lumen clearly identified on the culture bottle. This is important, because catheter infection may be limited to a single lumen. Because of the absence of granulocytes, microscopic examination of the urine may be normal even in the presence of a urinary tract infection. A chest radiograph can serve as a valuable baseline, although some investigators have questioned the use of this procedure in patients without pulmonary symptoms. In addition, accessible sites of potential infection should be aspirated or biopsied, with appropriate material sent for Gram stain, culture, and histologic examination.

Even with a comprehensive evaluation, an infectious cause for the fever is found in only 30 to 50% of patients. Nonetheless, even subtle indications of inflammation must be considered as sites of potential infection in the presence of granulocytopenia. For example, minimal perirectal erythema and tenderness may be harbingers of a perirectal cellulitis. Minimal erythema or serous discharge at the exit site of an indwelling intravenous catheter may herald a tunnel or exit-site infection.

Colonization with microorganisms often precedes development of significant infection. However, routine "surveillance" cultures are not of practical benefit in a neutropenic patient, since colonization of a single body site is not consistently predictive and multiple potential pathogens are usually isolated from any single site, making it difficult to predict the organism responsible for infection. Moreover, since empirical broad-spectrum antibiotics are administered under any circumstance, the expense of routine surveillance cannot be justified.

Tests such as nuclear scanning also have been used to define occult sites of infection. Although gallium citrate accumulates in inflammatory lesions because of its avid binding to lactoferrin, this test has not been shown to be useful in granulocytopenic patients. Autologous or allogeneic leukocytes labeled *in vitro* with indium-111 or indium-111 linked to IgG have been used with some success in the evaluation of febrile granulocytopenic patients.

Because of these diagnostic difficulties, even fevers that are temporally associated with the administration of blood products or with fever-producing antineoplastic agents should be considered potentially infectious and treated as such. In sum, virtually all new fevers in the neutropenic population warrant careful clinical and microbiologic evaluation, followed by prompt initiation of empirical antibiotic therapy. Conversely, any clinically evident site of potential infection mandates expeditious broad-spectrum therapy, even in the absence of fever.

Since the goal of empirical antibiotic therapy is to protect against the early morbidity and mortality that result from untreated bacterial infections, regimens have been formulated to maximize activity against commonly encountered organisms that are particularly virulent. However, empirical regimens cannot realistically be designed to cover every potential bacterial pathogen. Moreover, no regimen is capable of completely eliminating the risk of subsequent infections in persistently neutropenic patients.

Management of Indwelling Intravenous Catheters

Although gram-positive bacterial infections (especially staphylococcal) are the most frequent causes of catheter-related infections, other bacterial and nonbacterial species can be encountered, particularly in the neutropenic patient. These include resistant *Corynebacterium, Bacillus* species, gram-negative organisms, and fungi. In approaching the patient with a catheter-related infection, it is important to consider the specific type of infection, its location (i.e., bacteremia versus exit site versus tunnel), the type of access device (e.g., Hickman versus implantable subcutaneous reservoir), and the duration of symptoms.

In general, the vast majority of simple catheter-related bacteremias and exit-site infections can be cleared using appropriate antibiotics and do not require catheter removal. This applies to both neutropenic and non-neutropenic patients. If multilumen devices are used, the antibiotic infusion should be rotated among the ports, since infection may be limited to one lumen (failure to do so can be a cause of persistent infection despite antibiotics). If there is persistent bacteremia after 48 hours of appropriate therapy, the catheter should be removed. Failures of therapy are more common when the infections are due to certain organisms, such as *Bacillus* species or *C. albicans,* and when these are isolated, the catheter usually should be removed.

Infections extending to involve the tunnel of a Hickman catheter also mandate prompt removal of the device, because antibiotics alone rarely cure this "closed-space" infection, particularly in the granulocytopenic host. Likewise, infections around the reservoir of an implantable subcutaneous device may be difficult to eradicate without catheter removal. Patients with recurrent catheter infections (despite a history of appropriate therapy) are also candidates for prompt catheter removal.

It is unresolved whether a non-neutropenic patient with an indwelling catheter who becomes newly febrile should receive antibiotics empirically. The safest policy is to begin antibiotics (using a third-generation cephalosporin such as ceftriaxone or an aminoglycoside plus vancomycin) and continue them pending culture results and clinical response. This approach protects against rapid progression of undetected yet virulent infections (such as *S. aureus*) and may minimize the need for ultimate catheter removal. If by 72 hours the cultures are negative and the patient is stable, antibiotics can be discontinued.

Initial Management of the Neutropenic Patient Who Becomes Febrile

Although gram-negative bacteria still predominate at some institutions, there has been a trend in recent years toward more gram-positive infections, and these now comprise the majority of isolates at many centers. In general, the gram-negative infections tend to be more virulent, and early empirical regimens have been formulated to provide protection primarily against these organisms while maintaining a broad spectrum of activity against other potential pathogens. Indeed, adequate coverage of these gram-negative organisms is still an essential property of any empirical regimen.

Although there is no single best regimen or recipe, there are a number of appropriate options. The selection of a specific antibiotic regimen depends on many factors, including institutional sensitivity patterns, individual and institutional experience, and clinical parameters.

The standard approach to the empirical management of the febrile neutropenic patient has been to use combination antibiotic regimens. Until recently, this has been the only way to provide coverage broad enough to encompass the predominant gram-positive and gram-negative organisms. Moreover, some combinations have been considered to provide synergy and to have the potential for decreasing the emergence of resistant isolates. Aminoglycoside–β-lactam combinations were the first empirical regimens with acceptable efficacy in the setting of fever and neutropenia. Such combination regimens are still widely used and represent a standard against which newer regimens are tested. Many variations have been studied and include aminoglycosides combined with either an extended-spectrum penicillin or a cephalosporin, or as a component of a triple-drug regimen. If an aminoglycoside-containing combination regimen is to be employed, the choice of specific antibiotics should be based primarily on the institutional antibiotic sensitivity patterns and secondarily on toxicity and cost differences.

Non–aminoglycoside-containing combination regimens also have been studied. These have consisted of combinations of two β-lactam antibiotics, or so-called double β-lactam regimens, usually consisting of an expanded-spectrum carboxy- or ureidopenicillin plus a third-generation cephalosporin (e.g., piperacillin and ceftazidime).

New or Novel Antibiotics for Neutropenic Patients

The advent of β-lactam antibiotics with broad-spectrum activity which achieve high serum bactericidal levels has made monotherapy another option for the initial empirical therapy of the febrile neutropenic patient (Table 266–3). The third-generation cephalosporins and the carbapenems are the two classes that include potential candidates for empirical single-agent therapy. Ceftazidime

TABLE 266–3. MEDICATIONS IN PATIENTS WITH NEUTROPENIA AND FEVER

Agent	Comments
Antibiotic	
Third-generation cephalosporins	Only ceftazidime and cefoperazone are appropriate for coverage of *P. aeruginosa.*
Carbapenems	If *P. aeruginosa* is suspected or cultured, an aminoglycoside should be added.
Extended-spectrum penicillins	Because of the potential for resistance, piperacillin, azlocillin, or mezlocillin should be administered with either an aminoglycoside or a third-generation cephalosporin.
Monobactams	Aztreonam is an important alternative for patients allergic to β-lactam antibiotics, but it should be combined with vancomycin for empirical therapy.
Quinolones	Important for gram-negative infection and possibly for use in low-risk patients with neutropenia; to avoid resistance, do not use for prophylaxis.
Vancomycin	Pathogen-directed therapy generally suffices. Empirical use can be restricted to centers with a high incidence of methicillin-resistant *S. aureus.* Of concern, strains of vancomycin-resistant enterococci have been described.
Antifungal	
Amphotericin B	Still the best treatment. A dose of 0.6 mg per kilogram of body weight per day suffices for *C. albicans* and cryptococcus; 1 mg/kg/day is preferred for *C. tropicalis;* and 1.5 mg/kg/day is preferred for aspergillus.
Ketoconazole	Not an alternative to amphotericin B for empirical therapy. Useful for thrush or esophagitis.
Fluconazole	Very effective for thrush or esophagitis. Value for systemic mycoses, including hepatosplenic candidiasis, requires additional study.
Antiviral	
Acyclovir	Oral therapy is not advised for severely immunocompromised patients with varicella-zoster infections. For such patients parenteral therapy (1500 mg per square meter of body-surface area per day in 3 divided doses) is indicated. For patients with herpes simplex, oral or parenteral therapy (750 mg/m²/day in 3 divided doses) is satisfactory.
Ganciclovir	Of value for cytomegalovirus retinitis, prevention of pneumonitis, and combined with an intravenous immunoglobulin for pneumonitis.
Antiparasitic	
Trimethoprim-sulfamethoxazole	Best drug for *Pneumocystis carinii* prophylaxis. Not required in all cancer patients. Thrice-weekly schedule is satisfactory (150 mg of trimethoprim/m²/day in 2 divided doses).
Aerosolized pentamidine	Expensive and not as effective as trimethoprim-sulfamethoxazole in adults with HIV infection.

From Pizzo PA: Management of fever in patients with cancer and treatment-induced neutropenia. N Engl J Med 328:1323, 1993. Copyright by the Massachusetts Medical Society.

has been the most extensively studied of the third-generation cephalosporins as monotherapy because of its superior activity against *P. aeruginosa.*

A large, randomized study evaluating 550 consecutive episodes of fever and neutropenia was conducted at the National Cancer Institute (NCI). In this study, patients with fever and granulocytopenia underwent a standard initial evaluation and then were randomized to receive either a combination of antibiotics (cephalothin, gentamicin, and carbenicillin) or ceftazidime as a single agent. The overall results show that monotherapy compared favorably with a standard combination regimen. Approximately two thirds of the episodes in both groups were treated successfully for the entire duration of their granulocytopenia, without requiring *any* changes in their initial regimen. Another one third of the episodes required some change or modification (such as addition of an antibacterial,

antifungal, or antiviral drug) to ensure a successful outcome (see indications for modifications below), and an equally low number in both groups (about 5%) died of infection. None of the deaths was attributable to a specific deficiency in one regimen that was not present in the other.

Two subgroups of patients were identified who required more frequent modifications of the initial regimen in order to achieve a successful outcome: (1) those presenting with a documented source of infection to account for the initial fever and (2) those having relatively protracted periods of granulocytopenia (>1 week). The need for modification in these subgroups was identical for those episodes treated with monotherapy and those treated with combination therapy. In this study, these modifications did not represent a failure of either regimen *per se* but instead were reflective of the limitations of any regimen in treating patients who are at high risk for development of subsequent infections.

Results of an international cooperative study, which enrolled 876 episodes of fever and neutropenia (in 676 patients, 83% with acute leukemia) in a recently reported randomized trial comparing ceftazidime monotherapy with the combination of piperacillin and tobramycin, demonstrated comparable efficacy with both regimens but less toxicity with ceftazidime monotherapy.

Concerns regarding the use of ceftazidime as a single agent for fever and neutropenia include the lack of synergy against documented gram-negative infections, lack of activity against certain gram-positive isolates, poor antianaerobic activity, and the potential for developing resistance.

In addition to the third-generation cephalosporins, other antibiotics are also being evaluated in neutropenic patients. Imipenem, for example, is a member of the carbapenem class of antibiotics. It is formulated in fixed combination with cilastatin, which inhibits a renal enzyme that can degrade imipenem. Overall, it has the broadest spectrum of activity of any available antibiotic. Of note is its excellent *in vitro* activity against enterococci as well as many anaerobes.

Results of two randomized studies appear to corroborate its efficacy in this setting—one comparing it with an aminoglycoside-containing combination and another performed at the NCI comparing it with monotherapy with ceftazidime. Interestingly, neither of these studies appears to demonstrate superior efficacy for imipenem. Two potential drawbacks to its use include a relatively high incidence of the development of resistant *P. aeruginosa,* as well as its potential to decrease the seizure threshold in patients with central nervous system pathology. In addition, in the ongoing NCI trial, a higher than expected frequency of nausea has been found with imipenem.

Because of the increasing incidence of gram-positive infections in cancer patients during the 1980's and their increased resistance to β-lactam antibiotics, some authorities have recommended that vancomycin be added to empirical regimens. Conversely, it has been argued that since many of these organisms are of relatively low virulence, vancomycin may be safely withheld until the gram-positive isolate has been identified microbiologically.

At the present time, it seems reasonable not to routinely include vancomycin in all empirical antibiotic regimens. Its use, however, should be guided by institutional experience and sensitivity patterns. For example, in a center with a high incidence of methicillin-resistant *S. aureus,* routine use of vancomycin is clearly warranted, since this may be a particularly virulent organism if not treated. In addition, fluctuations in patterns of infecting microorganisms may occur over time. For example, penicillin-resistant α-hemolytic streptococci have recently been identified as particularly virulent pathogens in some centers (perhaps related to the use of high-dose cytosine arabinoside). Clearly, the emergence of new pathogens or pathogens with altered sensitivity profiles may force dramatic changes in how we use antibiotics in the future.

The appropriate role for the quinolones in the neutropenic patient has yet to be defined. Because of their relatively poor activity against certain gram-positive organisms, they should not be used for empirical therapy alone. They may, however, be useful to complete therapy in patients who initially respond to intravenous antibiotics and who have had either a fever of undetermined origin or a susceptible bacterial isolate.

A particularly useful feature of aztreonam is its apparent lack of cross-reactivity with the other β-lactams in patients who have penicillin or β-lactam allergies. In this group of patients, empirical therapy might begin with a combination of vancomycin, aztreonam, and an aminoglycoside.

Also recently introduced are combinations of β-lactams with β-lactamase inhibitors (i.e., clavulanic acid and sulbactam). Three preparations are now available, including amoxicillin + clavulanic acid (oral formulation only), ticarcillin + clavulanic acid, and ampicillin + sulbactam. A number of studies have documented the efficacy of ticarcillin + clavulanic acid combined with aminoglycoside for initial empirical therapy of fever in neutropenic patients. The expanded gram-positive coverage may obviate additional anti–gram-positive agents.

APPROACH TO THE PATIENT WITH PROLONGED GRANULOCYTOPENIA

How Long Should Antibiotics Be Continued?

A question of practical importance is how long empirical antibiotics should be continued in persistently neutropenic patients. Should they always be continued until the granulocyte count recovers, or can they be safely discontinued before that?

The question of duration of therapy can be approached by placing patients in two categories: those whose initial workup (at the time of presentation with fever and neutropenia) did not reveal a source of infection (i.e., a fever of undetermined origin, or FUO; see Ch. 263), and those whose initial workup revealed an infection to account for the fever (i.e., a positive culture, or clinically infected site, or both). Approximately 60% fall into the FUO category, although this varies with the institution, the therapy, and the patient population (Fig. 266–1).

FUO PATIENTS. There are only limited data that specifically address the issue of duration of empirical therapy in neutropenic patients presenting with an FUO. For patients with an expected short duration of granulocytopenia (e.g., < 1 week) and those with evidence of hematologic recovery, abbreviated courses of empirical therapy are safe and appropriate. However, the real dilemma arises in the population with more prolonged granulocytopenia.

In a study from the NCI, patients with FUO and persistent granulocytopenia were randomized either to discontinue antibiotics on day 7 of therapy or to continue them until the resolution of the neutropenia. Nearly 40% of afebrile patients in whom antibiotics were stopped developed recurrent fever, and 38% of febrile patients whose antibiotics were discontinued developed hypotensive episodes. It was concluded that day 7 was too early to discontinue antibiotics in this group.

A subsequent study randomized persistently neutropenic, afebrile patients to continue or discontinue antibiotics on day 14. Preliminary analysis showed no difference between the two groups: Approximately one third of patients became febrile again regardless of whether they stopped or continued antibiotics. However, those whose fevers recurred following discontinuation of antibiotics responded to a reinstitution of their initial regimens, whereas those remaining on antibiotics required addition of amphotericin B. On this basis, it seems reasonable to discontinue antibiotics and carefully observe FUO patients who are predicted to have a long duration of neutropenia and who have remained afebrile after 14 days of therapy.

PATIENTS PRESENTING WITH DOCUMENTED INFECTIONS. There are even fewer data that address the issue of duration of antibiotics in patients with defined sites of infection. For persistently neutropenic patients who have had clinical and microbiologic resolution of their infection and who are afebrile at day 14 (for a minimum of 7 days), antibiotics should be discontinued. The ultimate decision of whether to continue or discontinue rests on a number of clinical parameters, such as the degree of or potential for antibiotic toxicity, the predicted duration of neutropenia, the seriousness of the initial infection, and the presence or absence of a continued site of infection or other factors predisposing to subsequent infection. It should be emphasized that any neutropenic patient whose antibiotics are discontinued requires careful, meticulous follow-up in order to quickly detect new fevers or infection.

Modifications of Antibiotic Therapy During the Course of Granulocytopenia

Empirical antibiotics have their greatest impact early in the course of neutropenia. However, it is during a prolonged granulocytopenic episode when the patent is at highest risk for developing multiple types of secondary infections or superinfections. Many of these dictate specific modifications of the initial regimen (Table 266–4).

Bacterial isolates that are resistant to the initial empirical regimen are invariably encountered when managing neutropenic patients. For example, at most centers, the majority of coagulase-negative staphylococci are resistant to β-lactams, and breakthrough infec-

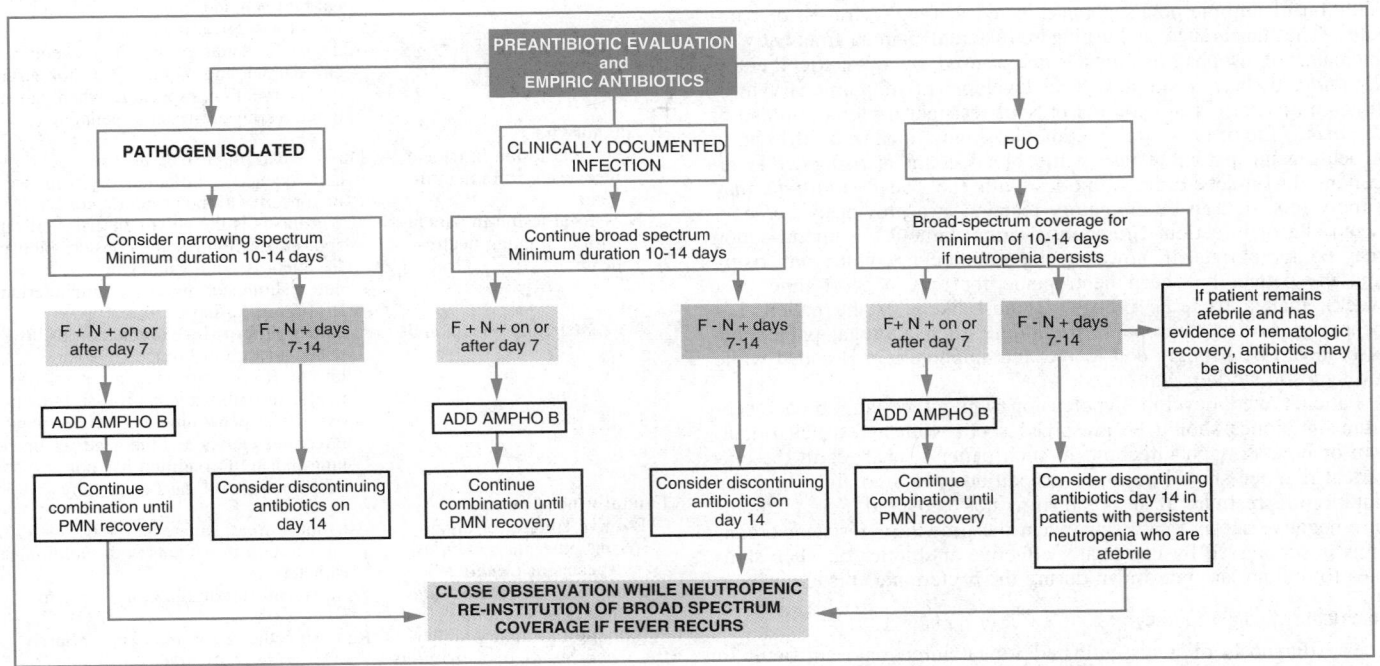

FIGURE 266–1. Management of fever and neutropenia. F + N + = Febrile, neutropenic. F − N + = Afebrile, neutropenic. FUO = No source for fever on preantibiotic evaluation. AMPHO B = Amphotericin B. (From Rubin M, Walsh TJ, Pizzo PA: Clinical approach to the compromised host. *In* Hoffman R, Benz EJ Jr, Shattil SS, et al. [eds.]: Hematology: Basic Principles and Practices, 2nd ed. New York, Churchill Livingstone, 1994.)

tions might be anticipated. Fortunately, coagulase-negative staphylococci are relatively indolent, and the risk for secondary infection can be balanced accordingly. Thus, for the patient who develops evidence of gram-positive infection while receiving β-lactam or who has evidence of a catheter site infection, vancomycin is an appropriate addition to the initial antibiotic regimen. Similarly, if the coverage of the initial regimen has limited antianaerobic activity, secondary infection with anaerobics might be anticipated.

The appearance of "secondary" resistance is seen more frequently with certain organisms. For example, *Enterobacter* species, *Citrobacter* species, and *Serratia* have inducible β-lactamases, and the appearance of a clinically significant clustering of resistant *Enterobacter* in a neutropenic population has been observed recently. Accordingly, when these organisms are isolated from a patient, careful observation for emergence of resistance is warranted, and for patients receiving monotherapy with a broad-spectrum β-lactam, an aminoglycoside should be added. *P. aeruginosa* may develop resistance to imipenem through a relatively novel mechanism involving a change in the porins. Hence patients receiving single-agent therapy for *P. aeruginosa* infection also should have an aminoglycoside added to their regimens. Secondary development of resistance by gram-positive organisms is somewhat rarer, although it has been increasingly described. Of note, recent studies have documented the emergence of vancomycin-resistant coagulase-negative staphylococci and enterococci in patients receiving vancomycin.

The appearance of a new site of infection (e.g., cellulitis or pneumonia) or the progression of a previously documented site of infection is an additional reason for changes or modifications of the antimicrobial regimen. For example, the development of marginal or necrotizing gingivitis is relatively common in patients who have received intensive cytotoxic therapy. Anaerobic organisms contribute to this process, and an antianaerobic agent such as clindamycin or metronidazole should be added to the empirical regimen if gingivitis is diagnosed.

The most common pathogens contributing to perianal cellulitis are the aerobic gram-negative bacilli, enterococci, and bowel anaerobes. Therefore, when it occurs in a patient already receiving broad-spectrum antibiotics, the addition of an antianaerobic agent as well as a change in the broad-spectrum coverage may be necessary. Similarly, any suspected intra-abdominal site of infection should prompt addition or inclusion of antibiotics active against aerobic gram-negative bacilli, enterococci, and bowel anaerobes.

The development of a new site of infection also may warrant the addition of antimicrobial agents directed at fungi, viruses, or parasites. The appearance of burning retrosternal pain is frequently an indicator of esophagitis, most often caused by cytotoxic therapy, *Candida,* or herpes simplex. The development of pulmonary infiltrates might raise suspicion not only of resistant bacteria but also of *P. carinii,* fungi, or a viral pneumonia. A new localized infiltrate in a neutropenic patient whose white blood count is rising while receiving broad-spectrum antibiotics with the "new" infiltrate may simply represent an inflammatory reaction at a previously unrecognized site of infection. Close observation without any modification may be appropriate. If, however, the granulocyte count is not rising and the patient has been neutropenic for only a short time (≤ 1 week), then a bacterial process is most likely. If the patient has been persistently neutropenic for longer, then a fungal pneumonia also should be strongly considered and amphotericin B added while a diagnostic workup is initiated.

Patients who develop hypotension while receiving broad-spectrum antibiotics should be presumed septic with a resistant organism or breakthrough infection. In such patients, changes in the empirical regimen should be made expeditiously and continued for the duration of treatment if an organism is not recovered. So-called culture-negative sepsis may occur when the growth of resistant organisms is suppressed by marginally effective antibiotics or when samples for culture are not drawn during the bacteremic episode.

Empirical Antifungal Therapy

The diagnosis of a disseminated fungal infection is difficult in an immunocompromised patient. Neutropenic patients who remain persistently febrile despite a 4- to 7-day trial of broad-spectrum antibacterial therapy are particularly likely to have a fungal infection. Empirical antifungal therapy might be expected to have a dual ef-

TABLE 266–4. COMMON MODIFICATIONS OR ADDITIONS TO INITIAL EMPIRICAL ANTIBIOTIC THERAPY IN PATIENTS WITH NEUTROPENIA AND FEVER

Status or Symptoms	Modifications of Primary Regimen
Fever	
Persistent for > 1 week	Add empirical antifungal therapy with amphotericin B.
Recurrence after 1 week or later in patient with persistent neutropenia	Add empirical antifungal therapy.
Persistent or recurrent fever at time of recovery from neutropenia	Evaluate liver and spleen by CT, ultrasonography, or MRI for hepatosplenic candidiasis, and evaluate need for antifungal therapy.
Bloodstream	
Cultures before antibiotic therapy	
Gram-positive organism	Add vancomycin pending further identification.
Gram-negative organism	Maintain regimen if patient is stable and isolate is sensitive. If *P. aeruginosa, Enterobacter,* or *Citrobacter* is isolated, add an aminoglycoside or an additional β-lactam antibiotic.
Organism isolated during antibiotic therapy	
Gram-positive organism	Add vancomycin
Gram-negative organism	Change to new combination regimen (e.g., imipenem plus gentamicin or vancomycin, or gentamicin plus piperacillin).
Head, eyes, ears, nose, throat	
Necrotizing or marginal gingivitis	Add specific antianaerobic agent (clindamycin or metronidazole) to empirical therapy.
Vesicular or ulcerative lesions	Suspect herpes simplex infection. Culture and begin acyclovir therapy.
Sinus tenderness or nasal ulcerative lesions	Suspect fungal infection with *Aspergillus* or *Mucor.*
Gastrointestinal tract	
Retrosternal burning pain	Suspect *Candida,* herpes simplex, or both. Add antifungal therapy and, if no response, acyclovir. Bacterial esophagitis also a possibility. For patients who do not respond within 48 hours, endoscopy should be considered.
Acute abdominal pain	Suspect typhlitis, as well as appendicitis, if pain in right lower quadrant. Add specific antianaerobic coverage to empirical regimen and monitor closely for need for surgical intervention.
Perianal tenderness	Add specific antianaerobic drug to empirical regimen and monitor need for surgical intervention, especially when patient is recovering from neutropenia.
Respiratory tract	
New focal lesion in patient recovering from neutropenia	Observe carefully, since this may be a consequence of inflammatory response in concert with neutrophil recovery.
New focal lesion in patient with continuing neutropenia	Aspergillosis is the chief concern. Perform appropriate cultures and consider biopsy. If patient is not a candidate for procedure, administer high-dose amphotericin B (1.5 mg/kg/day).
New interstitial pneumonitis	Attempt diagnosis by examination of induced sputum or bronchoalveolar lavage. If not feasible, begin empirical treatment with trimethoprim-sulfamethoxazole or pentamidine. Consider noninfectious causes and the need for open-lung biopsy if condition has not improved after 4 days of therapy.
Central venous catheters	
Positive culture for organisms other than *Bacillus* species or *Candida*	Attempt to treat. Rotate antibiotic administration in patients with multilumen catheters.
Positive culture for *Bacillus* species or *Candida*	Remove catheter and treat appropriately.
Exit-site infection with *Mycobacterium* or *Aspergillus*	Remove catheter and treat appropriately.
Tunnel infection	Remove catheter and treat appropriately.

From Pizzo PA: Management of fever in patients with cancer and treatment-induced neutropenia. N Engl J Med 328:1323, 1993. Copyright by the Massachusetts Medical Society.

fect: preventing a fungal overgrowth in patients with prolonged neutropenia and treating "subclinical" fungal disease early.

To date, the only proven agent for empirical therapy has been amphotericin B. Amphotericin B should be begun at 0.5 mg per kilogram per day and administered along with antibiotics until the resolution of neutropenia. If *Aspergillus* or *Mucor* is suspected, the dosage of amphotericin should be increased to 1 to 1.5 mg per kilogram per day. A number of new azole and triazole antifungal agents (fluconazole, itraconazole) offer less toxic alternatives to amphotericin B for certain patients.

Patients who remain febrile after the resolution of neutropenia should be evaluated for hepatosplenic candidiasis. The diagnosis is suggested by "bull's-eye" lesions on CT scan or ultrasonography of the liver and spleen. MRI scanning of the liver may be even more sensitive. Biopsy and histologic examination are essential. Patients with hepatosplenic candidiasis may require extended courses of antifungal therapy. The average amount of amphotericin B required to resolve these lesions is approximately 5 grams, often in conjunction with 5-flucytosine (100 mg per kilogram per day).

PREVENTION OF INFECTIONS

Because bacteria account for the majority of infections in compromised patients, prophylactic strategies have focused on these pathogens. The strategies that have been explored include mechanical techniques to prevent acquisition of new pathogens, absorbable or nonabsorbable oral antibiotic regimens to either prevent acquisition or decrease the number of potentially pathogenic colonizing organisms, and methods to improve the host defense matrix, including immunization and, more recently, biologic agents (e.g., the colony-stimulating factors) (Table 266–5).

Perhaps the most important infection prevention strategy of all, however, is handwashing. Although taken for granted, this simple procedure is frequently overlooked to the detriment of the patient.

Neutropenic Patients

MECHANICAL TECHNIQUES. Reverse isolation (i.e., single room with gowns, masks, and gloves) following the onset of neutropenia does not prevent infection. This is so because most of the infections arise from the patient's endogenous microbial flora. In addition, having patients wear a surgical mask outside of their room does little to protect against subsequent infection. Although some authorities have recommended that all foods be thoroughly cooked and that fresh fruits and vegetables be avoided to decrease the acquisition of gram-negative bacteria, the value of these measures in preventing infection remains unproven.

TABLE 266–5. METHODS STUDIED FOR PREVENTING INFECTION IN HIGH-RISK PATIENTS

Prevent Acquisition and/or Suppress or Eliminate Microbial Flora	Improve or Modify Host Defenses
Isolation	Immunization
Simple or reverse isolation	Active
Isolation with HEPA air filtration	*Pneumococcus*
Prophylactic antibiotics	VZV
Nonabsorbable antibiotics	Passive
Trimethoprim-sulfamethoxazole, erythromycin	J-5 core glycolipid
	Pooled immunoglobulins
Selective decontamination	Hyperimmune globulins
Quinolones	Monoclonal antibodies
Prophylactic antivirals	Cell-component replacement
Acyclovir	Leukocyte transfusions
Amantadine	Accelerate granulocyte recovery
Prophylactic antifungals	G-CSF
Nystatin	GM-CSF
Imidazoles	Immunomodulations
Triazoles	Interferons
Amphotericin B	Interleukins
Prophylactic antiparasitics	
Thiabendazole	
Trimethoprim-sulfamethoxazole	
Combination-comprehensive	
Total protective isolation	

Modified from Pizzo PA: Considerations for the prevention of infectious complications in patients with cancer. Rev Infect Dis 11:S1551, 1989.

The total protective environment (TPE) is a comprehensive regimen designed to reduce the patient's endogenous microbial burden as well as the acquisition of new organisms. The TPE includes a HEPA-filtered laminar airflow room together with an aggressive program of surface decontamination, including the sterilization of all objects that enter the room, and an intensive regimen to disinfect the microbial diet. A number of studies have documented that TPE can reduce infections in profoundly granulocytopenic individuals. However, TPE is expensive, and because of the improvement in treating established infections, it does not offer a current survival advantage to most patients. Thus TPE is not necessary for the routine care of the majority of granulocytopenic patients.

ORAL ANTIBIOTIC REGIMENS. Numerous studies have evaluated both nonabsorbable antibiotics (such as gentamicin, vancomycin, polymyxin, or colistin) and antibiotics that are absorbed from the gastrointestinal tract (e.g., trimethoprim-sulfamethoxazole, erythromycin, or quinolones). The goal of antibiotics has ranged from "total decontamination" of the alimentary tract with oral nonabsorbable antibiotics to "selective decontamination," in which the goal is to eliminate the potentially pathogenic aerobic flora (mostly the enteric gram-negative bacteria) while preserving the majority of anaerobic organisms and thus preserving "colonization resistance." Although the introduction of each new prophylactic regimen has been met with enthusiasm, over time these strategies have failed because of the emergence of resistant organisms.

The fluoroquinolones (mostly norfloxacin and ciprofloxacin) have been used in recent years for prophylaxis in neutropenic patients. These agents are well absorbed, and their use may really represent "early treatment" rather than prophylaxis. Although studies evaluating quinolones have demonstrated a reduction in gram-negative infections in the patients who receive them, caution about the widespread use of quinolones for prophylaxis should be underscored. Organisms resistant to the quinolones have been increasingly described, and the indiscriminate use of these agents only accelerates this process. Since the quinolones are useful for the treatment of both immunocompromised and immunocompetent individuals, the use of these antibiotics for prophylaxis should be discouraged.

PATIENTS WITH SICKLE CELL ANEMIA. Since patients with sickle cell anemia are prone to infections with encapsulated organisms (e.g., *S. pneumoniae, H. influenzae*), especially in young children, the pneumococcal vaccine and prophylactic penicillin have been used to prevent these infections. Unfortunately, the vaccination has not resulted in an effective antibody response. Prophylactic penicillin can, however, significantly reduce the incidence of infection, and it is recommended that penicillin prophylaxis be begun by 4 months of age in children with sickle cell anemia and that it be continued beyond the third birthday.

Prevention of Fungal Infections

Although the increasing incidence of fungal infection makes a preventive strategy desirable, to date no clear evidence of benefit has been demonstrated. It is hoped that newer azole and triazole antifungal agents may improve the ability to control these opportunistic pathogens.

Prevention of Viral Infections

HERPES SIMPLEX. Herpes simplex is a frequent cause of morbidity in compromised patients, particularly in association with bone marrow or renal transplantation or intensive chemotherapy regimens. Several studies have demonstrated that acyclovir administered either orally or intravenously at dosages of 250 mg per square meter every 8 hours can reduce the incidence of herpetic gingivostomatitis. Accordingly, it seems reasonable to administer prophylactic oral or intravenous acyclovir in patients who are HSV seropositive (titers ≥ 1:16) or who have a prior history of infection and are undergoing bone marrow transplantation or intensive therapy for acute leukemia.

VARICELLA-ZOSTER VIRUS. One of the most important ways to prevent VZV transmission is to prevent contact of immunosuppressed individuals with infected individuals. This includes patients with either primary VZV (chicken pox) or secondary VZV (zoster). If a seronegative individual has had contact with an infected individual, passive immunization with ZIG (zoster-immune globulin) has been shown to reduce the incidence of pneumonitis and encephalitis. Administration of ZIG (1 vial per 15 kg) must occur within 72 hours after exposure.

A varicella vaccine has been shown to reduce infection in children with leukemia. The live vaccine may be released soon for administration in normal healthy children and if effective should reduce the overall population of infected individuals.

CYTOMEGALOVIRUS. Successful strategies aimed at preventing CMV infection have included use of seronegative blood products in seronegative patients, passive immunization, and chemoprophylaxis with acyclovir or ganciclovir.

Prevention of Parasitic Infections

Pneumocystis carinii pneumonia can be largely prevented with trimethoprim-sulfamethoxazole. The decision to administer prophylaxis for *P. carinii* should be influenced by the patient's underlying disease, the intensity or immunosuppression of the therapy being delivered, and the center where treatment is being administered. Recent studies have demonstrated that trimethoprim-sulfamethoxazole can be effective and safe at a dosage of 75 mg per square meter twice a day given on 3 consecutive days each week. Alternatives include aerosolized pentamidine or atovaquone.

Improving Host Defense

Immunization against bacterial and viral pathogens has played an extremely important role in decreasing the incidence and/or severity of many infectious diseases. Unfortunately, active immunization is generally unsuccessful in immunocompromised hosts, since they are unable to mount or to sustain an antibody response to most vaccines.

Passive immunization, on the other hand, involves administration of preformed antibodies to high-risk patients. ZIG, for example, is effective in preventing infection and decreasing the incidence of morbidity and mortality associated with primary chicken pox in susceptible hosts. Another "hyperimmune" preparation that has been investigated in high-risk patients is the so-called J-5 antisera, collected from patients with high titers of antibody directed against the core glycolipid of Enterobacteriaceae. The results of early clinical trials with the J-5 antisera appeared encouraging, although confirmatory studies have not been consistent. Pooled immunoglobulin preparations do not appear to offer benefit for neutropenic hosts but are of benefit to patients who have either congenital or acquired (e.g., CLL, multiple myeloma) hypogammaglobulinemia. Monoclonal antibodies have been recently evaluated but were accompanied by unanticipated toxicity, impeding the use of current formulations.

Perhaps the most exciting new developments will be the therapeutic use of cytokines and lymphokines to enforce the host defense repertoire. Several studies have demonstrated that both GM- and G-CSF can shorten the duration of chemotherapy-induced neutropenia, abbreviate the durations of hospitalization, and decrease the need for antimicrobial therapy. The American Society of Clinical Oncology has recommended, on the basis of published data, that hematopoietic cytokines be used when the likelihood of a chemotherapy regimen resulting in fever and neutropenia >40%; when the interest is not in reducing the dose intensity of chemotherapy after a prior episode of fever and neutropenia; and when they are needed following autologous bone marrow transplantation. Conversely, these colony-stimulating factors are not indicated for patients with low-risk (i.e., short-duration) neutropenia. Clearly, as new factors become defined, the prospect for restoring function in the compromised host stands as the opportunity for the 1990's.

Ambrosino DM, Molrine DC: Critical appraisal of immunization strategies for prevention of infection in the compromised host. Hematol Oncol Clin North Am 7:1027, 1993.

Chanock SC: Evolving risk factors for infectious complications of cancer therapy. Hematol Oncol Clin North Am 7:771, 1993.

Freifeld AG, Hathorn JW, Pizzo PA: Infectious complications in the pediatric cancer patient. *In* Pizzo PA, Poplack DG (eds.): Principles and Practice of Pediatric Oncology, 2nd ed. Philadelphia, JB Lippincott, 1993, pp 987–1020.

Hathorn JW: Critical appraisal of antimicrobials for prevention of infections in immunocompromised hosts. Hematol Oncol Clin North Am 7:1051, 1993.

Heimenz JW, Greene JN: Special considerations for the patient undergoing allogeneic or autologous bone marrow transplantation. Hematol Oncol Clin North Am 7:961, 1993.

Pizzo PA: Management of fever in patients with cancer and treatment induced neutropenia. N Engl J Med 328:1323, 1993.

Roilides E, Pizzo PA: Biologicals and hematopoietic cytokines in prevention or treatment of infections in immunocompromised hosts. Hematol Oncol Clin North Am 7:841, 1993.

Rubin RH, Ferraro MJ: Understanding and diagnosing infectious complications in the immunocompromised host: Current issues and trends. Hematol Oncol Clin North Am 7:795, 1993.

Sloas M, Rubin M, Walsh TJ, et al.: Clinical approach to infections in the compromised host. *In* Hoffman R, Benz EJ Jr, Shattil SJ, et al. (eds.): Hematology. Basic Principles and Practices, 2nd ed. New York, Churchill-Livingston, 1994.

Walsh TJ: Management of immunocompromised patients with evidence of an invasive mycosis. Hematol Oncol Clin North Am 7:1003, 1993.

Weinberger M: Approach to the management of fever and infection in patients with primary bone marrow failure and hemoglobinopathies. Hematol Oncol Clin North Am 7:865, 1993.

267 PREVENTION AND CONTROL OF HOSPITAL-ACQUIRED INFECTIONS

William Schaffner

HISTORY. Hospitals are viewed today as institutions where scientific advances are used to provide the most up-to-date diagnostic and therapeutic services for patients. This optimistic view is tempered, however, by the realization that the hospital also can be a dangerous place for patients. The application of technology is not without hazards, and among these hospital-acquired infection has the longest history. When hospitals first were established in Europe during the Middle Ages, they were primarily places where the gravely ill were taken to die. Because facilities were primitive, infections that prompted the admission of some patients were readily spread to others. Hospital typhus and typhoid were commonplace, for example, and hospitals acquired the reputation of pest houses.

These circumstances remained basically unchanged until the mid-nineteenth century, when a Hungarian physician, Ignaz P. Semmelweis, was appointed to direct the obstetric service of the prestigious Allgemeines Krankenhaus (General Hospital) in Vienna. Semmelweis encountered a puzzling situation concerning the hospital's two obstetric wards. They were ostensibly similar and admitted patients on alternate days. Yet the mortality rates on the two wards were strikingly different. Semmelweis performed a seemingly elementary exercise but one that was unique in his time. He tabulated the monthly mortality rates on the two wards and documented that on Ward I the rates regularly were 8 to 10% or even higher, whereas on Ward II they rarely rose above 2%. The cause of this extraordinary mortality was puerperal sepsis (childbed fever), a rapidly fatal septic illness. Semmelweis worked before the formulation of the germ theory of disease, but we now know puerperal sepsis to be caused by the group A β-hemolytic streptococcus. He systematically examined a series of hypotheses attempting to explain the disparate mortality rates, but none proved valid. Among the more far-fetched notions was that the disease was psychosomatic and that intense anxiety was provoked when monks made their rounds, tolling hand-bells in mourning for those recently dead. Semmelweis persuaded the monks not to ring the bells and, of course, the occurrence of puerperal sepsis continued unaffected.

At that point a pathologist cut his finger while performing an autopsy of a woman who had died of puerperal sepsis. He soon developed a fatal illness with a clinical course that was entirely similar to puerperal sepsis. Because the pathologist had been inoculated with trace amounts of material during the autopsy, Semmelweis drew an insightful analogy: Perhaps the obstetric patients also were being inoculated with infectious material. It was then that a seemingly trivial difference between the two obstetric wards became important. The deliveries on the low-mortality ward were performed by midwives; on the high-risk ward they were performed by medical students and physicians. Furthermore, the autopsy room was directly adjacent to the ward, and Semmelweis deduced that the unwashed contaminated hands of students and physicians going from autopsies to the delivery room were the vehicles for transmitting infection to patients. Despite protestations from the medical staff, Semmelweis then insisted upon hand-washing after autopsies and before the examination of each patient. The mortality rate on Ward I promptly fell to levels even lower than those on the other ward.

Semmelweis is honored as the originator of hospital infection control efforts. His process of systematically gathering data, performing an analysis, and instituting control measures still is followed today. Furthermore, his emphasis on the hands of caregivers as the means for carrying pathogens from patient to patient remains valid. Unfortunately, as in the last century, contemporary physicians still require constant reminders to wash their hands during their patient care duties.

After the acceptance of the germ theory of disease, rapid advances in microbiology, disinfection, and aseptic technique around the turn of the century substantially enhanced the safety of patient care in hospitals. Starting in the 1930's, the introduction of antimicrobials made possible the development of progressively more elaborate surgery. However, predictions that hospital infections soon would become inconsequential have not come true. Rather, the types of hospital infection have changed in response to advancing medical science.

The 1950's and 1960's witnessed a global pandemic of hospital infections caused by *Staphylococcus aureus*. Previously very susceptible to penicillin, the new penicillin-resistant epidemic strain (phage type 80/81) became the scourge of hospitals worldwide. It stimulated research into all aspects of hospital-acquired infection and persuaded authorities that every hospital should have a formal infection-control program. For reasons still not clear, the staphylococcal pandemic waned in the 1970's and gram-negative bacilli, often antibiotic resistant, became the dominant nosocomial pathogens. In the 1980's there again was a shift; staphylococci returned (now methicillin resistant), enterococci rose in importance, and *Candida* and other yeast infections caused a larger proportion of nosocomial infections in seriously ill patients. During the 1990's, antibiotic-resistant organisms of all kinds assumed even greater importance in hospitals. Thus it seems that there will be no infection-free utopia; each era presents infection control challenges anew as yesterday's saprophyte becomes tomorrow's pathogen.

THE PROBLEM OF NOSOCOMIAL INFECTIONS. Infections that are acquired during hospitalization and are neither present nor incubating at the time of hospitalization are defined as *nosocomial** infections. The occurrence of a nosocomial infection does not *per se* indicate that the hospital or its personnel were at fault or committed an error in patient care. Current preventive measures still cannot prevent many nosocomial infections. Medicolegal liability regarding a nosocomial infection occurs when it can be demonstrated that physicians or hospital personnel have been negligent in not adhering to appropriate standards of care and that an infection resulted from the failure to perform consistent with the standard.

It is estimated that 5 to 8 nosocomial infections occur for every 100 admissions to acute-care hospitals in the United States, resulting in 2 to 4 million such infections annually. Some nosocomial infections are more serious than others, but taken together they are estimated to require over 6 million days of excess hospital stay a year and contribute to the deaths of many patients (Table 267–1).

Most studies of nosocomial infections have been performed in the high-technology hospitals of the developed countries. Although less attention has been given to delineating nosocomial infections in developing countries, it is clear that they are an important problem there as well. Hospital outbreaks of measles and shigellosis, as well as infections related to a lack of disinfectants and other supplies, occur regularly. Because developing countries have only modest resources, it is especially unfortunate that their efforts to provide medical care are so often thwarted by nosocomial infections. The World Health Organization has acknowledged that nosocomial infections are a substantial international public health issue.

PREDISPOSING FACTORS. All patients do not have an equal risk of developing a nosocomial infection. The inherent resistance of the patient to infection is probably the most important determinant of risk. The extremes of age, poor nutritional status, severity of underlying diseases, and breaks in the integrity of the skin and mucous membranes all increase a patient's risk of nosocomial infection.

The second strong influence on risk of nosocomial infection is the array of diagnostic and therapeutic manipulations undertaken for the patient's benefit. Every invasive procedure carries some risk of infection because it violates either a cutaneous or mucosal barrier to microbial invasion. The risk varies with the degree of invasiveness. For example, an intramuscular injection usually has virtually no risk of infection, whereas 15 to 20% of colorectal operations are complicated by wound infections despite meticulous surgical technique, preoperative bowel preparation, and appropriate antibiotic prophylaxis. Thus, physicians should weigh every invasive procedure's potential benefits against potential risks. Medical therapy also can make patients extremely susceptible to nosocomial infections. Cancer chemotherapy eliminates virtually all of a patient's circulating neutrophils, and the immunosuppressive regimens used in organ transplantation ablate the normal immune response to invading microorganisms (see Ch. 266). Infection control measures are designed to protect the patient until periods of such exquisite vulnerability have passed and the patient again has normal or nearly normal phagocytic and immune functions. In addition, the antibiotics used to combat infection can be considered a two-edged sword. Although their use does not generally confer an increased risk of complicating infection, when new infections occur in the face of antibiotic therapy, the pathogens often are resistant to the antibiotics being used (so-called suprainfections). Lastly, it follows that the longer a patient remains in the hospital, the more likely it is that a nosocomial infection will occur.

MODES OF TRANSMISSION. Nosocomial pathogens can be found in both the animate and inanimate environment of the hospital. It is not generally appreciated how clean the hospital's inanimate environment has become. The furniture, bedclothes, curtains, and other inanimate surfaces in the hospital only very rarely harbor microorganisms that cause infections in patients. Nevertheless, reservoirs of nosocomial pathogens still can be established in inanimate areas of the hospital occasionally, especially in specialty care areas. For example, if the countertop in the intensive care unit where urine specific gravity determinations are performed remains wet, it may harbor multiresistant gram-negative bacilli. Nurses' hands then become contaminated, and the organisms can be carried back to patients in the unit. Although similar infection hazards in the inanimate environment are detected periodically and need to be remedied, we cannot look to enhanced housekeeping of the general hospital environment to reduce nosocomial infection rates further.

Whereas the hospital's general inanimate environment has receded as a source of nosocomial infections, the role of contaminated medical devices has increased substantially; more than 100,000 device-related infections are estimated to occur each year. Medical devices are examples of imaginative medical technology that offer new benefits to patients. However, manufacturers often do not consider the potential infection risks of new devices fully, and physicians often employ devices in ways that were not initially anticipated. For example, when intravascular pressure transducers first

* Nosocomial is a new word constructed from Greek roots to define an event, such as an infection, originating in the hospital or other health care facility.

TABLE 267–1. IMPACT OF HOSPITAL-ACQUIRED INFECTIONS IN ACUTE-CARE HOSPITALS

Anatomic Site	Number of Infections per 100 Admissions	Proportion of All Hospital-Acquired Infections (%)	Estimated Direct Mortality (%)	Estimated Number of Excess Hospital Days per Infection	Proportion of All Excess Hospital Days (%)
Urinary tract	2.5	30–40	<1	2	19
Postoperative wound	1.5	20–25	1–2	7	33
Pulmonary	1	10–20	5–10	8	21
Bloodstream	0.5–1	5–15	25	14	16
Others	1	20–25	Varies with site	2	12

were introduced, their use was associated with outbreaks of bacteremia. Investigations revealed that instruments were being inadequately disinfected because the instruments were very fragile. When appropriate disinfection protocols were developed, this new infection risk associated with technologic innovation was virtually eliminated.

The animate hospital environment consists of the patients and their caregivers. These humans are the sources of most nosocomial pathogens, and the intimacies of patient care often result in their sharing their microbial flora.

A familiar scenario involves *Staphylococcus aureus,* a classic hospital pathogen. Hospital personnel have a higher rate of asymptomatic carriage of *S. aureus* (often >30%) than does the general population. Staphylococci may be transmitted from hospital workers to patients, in whom they later can produce, for example, postoperative wound infections. Such "hospital staph" pathogens often are more antibiotic resistant than community-acquired *S. aureus,* providing a distinctive marker that enables their movement to be readily traced. However, hospital personnel are not the only source of resistant microbial flora. Studies have demonstrated that when admitted to the hospital, some patients already may be colonized with small numbers of resistant bacterial strains. After antibiotic treatment, these resistant strains have a survival advantage and multiply to potentially cause nosocomial infection. Indeed, the endogenous flora is the major source of both the bacterial and viral pathogens that cause nosocomial infections in patients who receive organ transplants and are immunosuppressed for long periods.

More than 100 years have passed since Semmelweis implicated the hands of the students and physicians as the means of spreading pathogens to patients. Nevertheless, such direct contact continues to be the most common way patients are colonized with microorganisms of exogenous origin. At times the microorganisms may be from the caregiver's own flora. Usually, however, the hands of nurses or doctors are contaminated transiently while caring for one patient, and the pathogens then are carried over to the next patient (this process is aptly called cross-infection in Britain). Gram-positive skin flora (*S. aureus* and *S. epidermidis*), many gram-negative bacilli (*Enterobacter* and *Serratia*) and even viruses (respiratory syncytial virus, rotavirus) are spread by this means. Over a century ago Semmelweis introduced the most effective way to interrupt transmission by contaminated hands: hand-washing. To promote hand-washing after every patient contact, modern hospitals have located sinks conveniently and have provided disinfectant soap wherever patient examinations and manipulations take place, with special attention to intensive care areas, treatment rooms, and the like. However, persuading medical staff, especially physicians, to routinely wash their hands remains a challenge, especially in the hectic environment of the intensive care unit (ICU).

Airborne transmission once was thought to have an important role in the spread of pathogens in the hospital. Today this seems not to be the case, although occasional explosive outbreaks of tuberculosis and chickenpox strongly suggest airborne transmission from a source patient. *Aspergillus* infections have occurred in immunosuppressed patients whose rooms drew air from the vicinity of major construction sites in or adjacent to the hospital. Likewise *Legionella* infections have been produced by the contaminated water spray from an air conditioning cooling tower. Concern about the role of airborne infection in the operating room continues to influence the design and construction of these areas. Most studies indicate that the bacteria causing wound infections originate from the resident flora of either the patients themselves or the operating team. This suggests that transmission likely occurs by direct contact or droplet spread. Nevertheless, because only a few bacteria can incite infection in certain elaborate procedures that implant foreign bodies (such as total joint replacements), such procedures are performed in laminar airflow facilities where the airstream is designed to flow away from the operative field.

ANTIMICROBIAL RESISTANCE. Since the pandemic of the 1950's and 1960's caused by staphylococcal strains newly resistant to penicillin, it has become axiomatic that antibiotic resistance has been a major feature of nosocomial infections. Although antibiotic-resistant bacteria are not inherently more virulent than their susceptible counterparts, they reduce the physician's therapeutic options and often require the use of more expensive antibiotics.

Currently, both gram-positive and gram-negative hospital pathogens have developed patterns of antimicrobial resistance. *S. aureus* infections are resurgent, and many strains now have developed resistance to methicillin and other similar β-lactam antibiotics that have been mainstays of therapy until recently. Many physicians turned to the quinoline antibiotics as alternate therapy, but quinoline-resistant strains were recovered with extraordinary rapidity in hospitals where these drugs were used widely. *S. epidermidis* has become a notable nosocomial pathogen in some ICU's; these organisms have a very diverse pattern of antibiotic resistance. Likewise, gram-negative bacilli have developed distinctive resistance profiles in some hospitals; *Enterobacter cloacae, Pseudomonas aeruginosa,* and *Acinetobacter calcoaceticus* particularly have been involved. It has become clear that genes determining antibiotic resistance are often carried on extrachromosomal plasmids that can be transferred among bacterial species. Thus, some medical centers have had years-long outbreaks of resistant gram-negative bacillary infections. The distinctive antibiotic resistance pattern first was detected in one bacterial species (among *Serratia,* for example) and then over time also was found among other gram-negative nosocomial pathogens (among *Enterobacter* and *Klebsiella* sequentially). Investigations that combine studies of infections in hospital populations with molecular biologic studies of the pathogens have been called "molecular epidemiology."

During the early 1950's bacterial pathogens isolated from infections virtually anywhere in the United States had essentially identical antibiotic susceptibility patterns. Shortly after antimicrobial resistance was recognized, however, it became apparent that different hospitals began to develop antibiotic resistance patterns among their hospital pathogens that were distinctive and different from each other. Thus, one hospital might have a problem with multiresistant *Serratia,* whereas another directly across the street might encounter almost no such isolates. Although never precisely explained, these differences have been attributed to factors of patient populations, severity of illness, length of stay, and, most importantly, patterns and intensity of antibiotic use. Physicians needed to be aware of these differences, so clinical microbiology laboratories maintained surveillance of resistance patterns and reported them periodically to the medical staff. The more sophisticated surveillance systems were able to distinguish resistance patterns between community-acquired and hospital-acquired infections. More recently it has become clear that such hospital-wide surveillance is insufficient in large, complex medical centers. Rather than a uniform hospital-wide nosocomial flora, there are a number of independent subpatterns that are specific to each special care area. Thus, the burn unit, neonatal ICU, and surgical ICU each may have a distinctive nosocomial flora, each with its own localized resistance problem. Laboratories have started to adapt their computerized data management systems so that specialty unit–specific surveillance data can be provided to the physicians who practice in each unit.

COMMON NOSOCOMIAL INFECTIONS, BY ANATOMIC SITE (See Table 267–1)

URINARY TRACT INFECTIONS. Urinary tract infections (UTI's) continue to be the most common nosocomial infection, accounting for 30 to 40% of all hospital-acquired infections. They occur so frequently because almost all are linked to prior urinary tract instrumentation, most often with the seemingly innocuous bladder catheter. Even single in-and-out catheterization is associated with 2 to 3% bacteriuria in otherwise healthy persons. The urethral meatus is colonized with bacteria, and even after appropriate cleansing, some are inoculated into the bladder during the catheterization process. The healthy bladder almost always rids itself of small numbers of introduced bacteria. If the bladder and urethra are traumatized, however, an infection is more likely to be established. After complicated labor with its associated urethral and bladder trauma, 23% of postpartum women develop UTI after only a single catheterization.

Given these risks, the use of indwelling Foley catheters is preferred, and 10 to 20% of hospitalized patients are treated with these devices. Because of their frequent use, Foley catheters are the leading factor predisposing to nosocomial UTI's. The longer the catheter is in place, the more likely it is that an infection will occur; approximately 5% of patients with a catheter develop bacteriuria per day. The infecting strains colonize the urethral meatus. Through movement of the catheter as well as their own motility they gain entrance to the bladder. Contemporary urinary drainage systems are well designed so that ascending infection from the reservoir bag now is quite uncommon.

Most nosocomial UTI's are asymptomatic or mild, clear with little or no therapy after catheter removal, and do not prolong hospital stay very much (an average of 1 to 2 days only). They are important, however, for two reasons. They are occasionally severe, and 1 of every 200 nosocomial UTI's results in bacteremia. In addition, many nosocomial UTI's are caused by antibiotic-resistant bacterial strains. Thus, the infected catheter systems become reservoirs of resistant gram-negative bacilli, especially in ICU's where they can be spread easily to other very ill patients. The most common organisms producing nosocomial UTI's include *E. coli* (30%), enterococci (16%), *Pseudomonas* (12%), and *Klebsiella* (6%). Pseudomonads and other multiresistant gram-negative bacteria account for a gradually increasing proportion of these infections as the hospitalized population becomes older, is more severely ill, and receives more intensive antibiotic treatment.

The prevention of nosocomial UTI's has received sustained attention and considerable success. Of course, assuring that catheters are used only for patients who genuinely require continuous bladder drainage is the first guiding principle. It follows that catheters should be removed as soon as possible when patients no longer need them. Industry has been very responsive by producing reliable, sturdy, closed drainage systems. In the past, catheters were disconnected from drainage bags to empty the bags, obtain diagnostic urine specimens, and the like. Every such interruption was an opportunity to introduce bacteria into the catheter system. Contemporary designs maintain the system's integrity by allowing the catheter to be aspirated with a needle and syringe.

These systems work so well that catheters need not be changed routinely, nor is catheter irrigation required unless the catheter becomes obstructed. The use of triple-lumen catheters with a closed prophylactic antibiotic irrigation system has been proposed, but these systems offer no great advantage in preventing infection and are difficult to manage by ward nurses. They may be useful in some patients after urologic surgery to prevent obstruction by blood clots and proteinaceous debris. There is no need to culture the urine routinely when removing the catheter; the practice of cutting off the catheter tip and culturing it has no value.

Regular perineal hygiene and antibiotic-containing creams have not proven to reduce infection; neither have catheters impregnated with antibacterial materials. Use of prophylactic systemic antibiotics to "cover" an indwelling catheter has been decried for 30 years, yet some data suggest they may be efficacious for the first 4 days of catheterization. A serious prospective trial has not been undertaken, perhaps because of the fear of selecting antibiotic-resistant strains.

BACTEREMIA. If UTI's are the most frequent nosocomial infections, nosocomial bacteremias are the most serious. Bacteremias may be secondary to recognized infection at some site, or they may be primary and cannot be attributed to an obvious infection in another anatomic location. Identifying the source of secondary bacteremia permits one to treat it as well as the bacteremia and prevent recurrences.

The occurrence of primary bacteremia should always prompt a thorough review of all the patient's intravenous infusions as well as other intravascular devices, as they are frequent sources of bloodstream infections. More than 25% of hospitalized patients receive intravenous fluids. Other diagnostic and therapeutic procedures require access to the venous or arterial systems for either brief or prolonged periods. An intravenous pyelogram and cardiac catheterization are examples of abbreviated procedures, whereas intra-arterial pressure monitoring may continue for days. Although all these procedures create an access for bacteria to enter the bloodstream, they are remarkably safe. Nevertheless, the history of intravascular technology is punctuated with many studies of endemic and epidemic bloodstream infections. The procedures that offer assurance of reasonable safety today were hard won, and any lapse in appropriate care can result in a device-related bacteremia. As more patients have required admission to ICU's, the rate of nosocomial bacteremia gradually rose during the 1980's and 1990's.

Intrinsic contamination of intravenous fluid by the manufacturer is fortunately a rare event. Most episodes of infusion-related sepsis are caused by microorganisms that enter the system during its use (extrinsic contamination). The major locus of contamination is the cannulation site. The longer the catheter is left in place, the more

likely it is that infection will occur. The catheter site may be purulent, and phlebitis may be evident, but these overt clinical manifestations frequently are not present. Suppurative thrombophlebitis is an unusual event in which a substantial segment of vein becomes a linear abscess, the entire lumen being filled with pus. *S. aureus* and *S. epidermidis* are the most frequently isolated pathogens, but an array of gram-negative bacilli and *Candida* species also regularly are associated with catheter sepsis.

Any indwelling vascular access device can be associated with infection. Hickman-Broviac catheters that are tunneled under the skin of the anterior chest wall before they enter the subclavian vein were developed to provide long-term vascular access (as for cancer chemotherapy) and minimize the risk of infection. They have been largely successful. When infection does occur, it often is possible to treat the infection, leaving the catheter in place. Although such catheters have an enhanced risk for developing another infection, enough time is often gained to complete a course of chemotherapy.

The essentials of prevention begin with meticulous aseptic catheter insertion technique. Because the risk of infection increases with increasing duration of use, strict nursing protocols exist to ensure that use of all catheters is discontinued on a regular rotation and that new catheters are inserted at different sites. As a reminder, the dressings at the insertion site are dated; peripheral catheters should be left in place no longer than 72 hours unless there is no alternative. If a catheter must remain in place, a note providing the reasons should be written in the chart. Likewise, the infusions themselves also must be changed regularly; infusions should hang no longer than 24 hours. Because most infections originate at the insertion site, in-line filters have not reduced infection rates; they add expense without increasing safety. The catheter insertion site is protected by a single dressing for the duration of the catheter's routine use; daily dressings and antibiotic ointments are no longer considered useful.

NOSOCOMIAL PNEUMONIA. Hospital-acquired lower respiratory tract infections (including pneumonia and bronchitis) account for 10 to 15% of nosocomial infections. Almost 1% of patients admitted to the hospital develop pneumonia. Elderly patients with serious underlying illnesses are at risk, as are all patients receiving mechanical ventilation. These infections usually extend a patient's hospital stay for 7 days or more, produce substantial morbidity, and contribute to the deaths of already seriously ill patients.

In contrast to community-acquired pneumonia in younger patients, nosocomial pneumonia usually is a mixed infection involving more than one organism. Although a hospital's ICU may develop a dominant bacterial respiratory tract pathogen, the list of bacteria associated with nosocomial pneumonia is large. Aerobic gram-negative bacilli are associated with more than half the cases, including *P. aeruginosa, Enterobacter, Klebsiella, E. coli,* and *Acinetobacter,* among others. *Acinetobacter* particularly is associated with ventilated patients in busy ICU's. Among gram-positive organisms, *S. aureus* is isolated with regularity, but may not always have a major pathogenic role. Pneumococci contribute to about 3% of nosocomial pneumonias, usually in elderly patients with predisposing lung disease. Most clinical laboratory routines do not process respiratory tract specimens anaerobically, and even research methods have limitations in ascribing a role for anaerobes in lower respiratory tract infections. Although aerobic pathogens clearly are dominant, most authorities believe that anaerobes are involved in about one third of nosocomial pneumonias. *Legionella pneumophila* can be a vexing problem in some hospitals, where it can be isolated from the water supply. Viral respiratory infections are increasingly recognized as causes of nosocomial pneumonia and as infections predisposing to subsequent bacterial invasion. Respiratory syncytial virus, influenza, and cytomegalovirus are the viruses most commonly identified.

Endotracheal tubes and tracheostomies bypass the upper respiratory tract defense mechanisms and can traumatize mucous membranes. When managed improperly, these devices can provide direct access for hospital pathogens to be introduced on the hands of personnel or by contaminated suction tubing. Ventilator machines often produced contaminated aerosols in past years, but current maintenance protocols have made nosocomial pneumonia due to the machine itself an unusual event.

Aspiration of oropharyngeal secretions is the principal initiating event in nosocomial pneumonia. Patients who have an impaired gag reflex, are sedated, or have altered consciousness are more likely to aspirate. The volume and pH of the aspirate as well as its bacterial population contribute to the likelihood of lung injury. The bacterial population is determined by the organisms colonizing the oropharynx. The flora of the normal pharynx is largely gram-positive. Gram-negative bacillary colonization occurs in older persons with a variety of underlying diseases, after antibiotic therapy, and in patients who are leukopenic.

Gastric alkalinization can permit gram-negative bacteria to multiply in the stomach. These bacteria can then become the source of oropharyngeal colonization. Antacids and histamine type-2 (H_2) blockers are often given to patients in ICU's who are being ventilated to prevent stress ulcers. Because they raise gastric pH, these drugs promote the growth of bacteria in the stomach and increase the risk of nosocomial pneumonia. Because it does not neutralize gastric acidity, sucralfate is preferred for stress ulcer prophylaxis.

The prevention of nosocomial pneumonia is a daunting challenge. Positioning patients with their heads raised may reduce somewhat the occurrence of aspiration. Scrupulous hand-washing inhibits the transmission of nosocomial pathogens. Meticulous maintenance of ventilatory equipment and assiduous pulmonary toilet by nurses reduce risks. The role of selective decontamination of the gastrointestinal tract with combinations of oral and systemic antibiotics currently is being studied.

SURGICAL WOUND INFECTIONS. Postoperative wound infections account for 20% of nosocomial infections. These infections account for a substantial amount of morbidity, increase hospital stay considerably, and are costly. Some postoperative infections extend down from the skin incision to the depths of the surgical field where they can destroy vascular anastomoses or disrupt an implanted prosthetic device. Bacteremia may accompany such infections. The extent of the surgical procedure and its anatomic location, the severity of the patient's underlying illness, and the surgeon's skill are all important determinants of risk. When surgery involves tissues that normally are not subjected to a large microbial population during the procedure ("clean" operations), wound infection rates often are < 2%. Such operations include inguinal herniorrhaphy and vascular surgery in the neck, for example. When procedures transect mucosal surfaces, as in a colectomy ("contaminated" operations), up to 20% of patients have a postoperative wound infection. If patients are malnourished, at the extremes of age, or have serious underlying diseases, wound infections are more likely to occur. The longer the operation, the more likely that postoperative infection will occur. A surgeon's skill is critical. If tissues are traumatized, the vascular supply is unnecessarily interrupted, devitalized tissue or blood clots are left in the wound, or wound layers are not realigned properly, the risk of wound infection increases.

S. aureus and S. epidermidis are the most commonly isolated pathogens from wound infections, reflecting their common residence on human skin. A wide variety of other organisms contribute to these infections, including enterococci, E. coli, P. aeruginosa, and Bacteroides, largely determined by the organ undergoing surgery. The infecting bacteria most often originate in the patient's own endogenous microbial flora, whether on the skin or on a mucosal surface. A smaller contribution comes from the bacterial flora of the surgeon and other members of the operating team. Even clean wounds are not truly sterile; small numbers of bacteria can be recovered from virtually all wounds at the time of wound closure. Thus, for the most part, the infecting bacteria are in the wound when the patient leaves the operating room, unless there is a drain or packing in the incision. Occasionally bacteria originating from another infected site implant at the operative site; there have been a few well-described instances in which a wound was infected during postoperative care.

A whole array of techniques are used to minimize the occurrence of wound infection. The architecture, air handling, and housekeeping in the operating room have made the physical environment very clean. Special laminar flow rooms are used for some procedures, such as implantation of an artificial joint. An elaborate ritual of aseptic practice involves both the patient (shaving the surgical area, baths with disinfectant soap, skin preparation just before surgery, among others) and the surgeon (precise hand scrubbing, operating room gowns and masks, use of sterile gloves, and the like). The importance of the appropriate use of antibiotic prophylaxis cannot be

overemphasized. Indeed, some medical historians suggest that the most important consequence of the discovery of antibiotics was that their use permitted the development of the technologically adventurous procedures that characterize contemporary surgery. In recent years it has been amply confirmed that for antibiotics to be effective in preventing wound infection they need to be given only briefly, chosen to be effective against the most commonly expected pathogens at the surgical site, and given in amounts sufficient to provide killing concentrations in the tissues. The brevity of their use (often no longer than 24 hours) results in very little drug toxicity or development of bacterial resistance.

MISCELLANEOUS SITES. In addition to the most commonly occurring infections discussed above, nosocomial infections also occur in numerous other sites and circumstances. The extent of nosocomial infectious diarrhea is only now being recognized. Among children, the most common pathogen is rotavirus; among adults, Clostridium difficile colitis is a complication of antibiotic therapy. Epidemics of keratoconjunctivitis due to adenoviruses can be propagated by the contaminated hands of ophthalmologists as well as contaminated tonometers. Meningitis, usually caused by S. epidermidis, can follow the placement of shunts in the cerebral ventricles. Meningitis also can occur in immunocompromised organ transplant recipients. In renal transplant patients Cryptococcus and Listeria are the most frequent pathogens. Transfusions of blood and blood products have resulted in the transmission of hepatitis B virus and human immunodeficiency virus (HIV) as well as other viruses and bacteria.

INFECTION CONTROL PROGRAMS

Although many efforts were being made to prevent infections in hospitals, most institutions did not have a formal organized program until the 1960's. At that time it became apparent that the previous focus by hospitals on environmental hygiene was insufficient. Strongly influenced by the Centers for Disease Control, the American Hospital Association, and the Joint Commission on Accreditation of Health Care Organizations, every hospital now must have an active infection control program to secure accreditation. Central to the program is an Infection Control Committee whose members are broadly representative of hospital administration and the professional disciplines. A physician knowledgeable about infection control is designated the Hospital Epidemiologist. It is recommended that the hospital employ one infection control practitioner (usually a nurse with special infection control training) for every 250 beds. These practitioners organize a variety of infection control activities, but all who work in hospitals must realize that the practitioners alone cannot produce the safest milieu for patients. Rather, all who work in hospitals must assume responsibility: Infection control is everyone's business.

A critical element of the program is a system of surveillance for detecting nosocomial infections, analyzing the data, and reporting on distinctive events. Surveillance may involve reviewing microbiology laboratory reports, visiting wards, inspecting surgical wounds, and the like. It now has been well demonstrated that such surveillance provides more pertinent information than routinely culturing features of the environment, a practice that has largely ceased.

The infection control practitioners also orchestrate the institution's control measures, ranging from appropriate isolation systems to responses when an epidemic is detected. Each unit in the hospital contributes its own section of procedures to a hospital-wide infection control manual. Its procedures are reviewed on 1- to 2-year cycles and as needed when new developments occur.

Sophisticated support from the clinical microbiology laboratory is necessary for a successful infection control program. The laboratory provides its routine data for surveillance purposes, may be asked to process extra cultures when an outbreak is under investigation, and may undertake special studies with nosocomial pathogens.

Other hospital service units also provide critical support for the infection control program. Although the role of the inanimate environment has been de-emphasized, the housekeeping department must maintain a high level of cleanliness throughout the institution. They also are responsible for managing and disposing of the hospital's solid waste. Heavily contaminated wastes (as from the microbiology laboratory) must be incinerated. Solid waste disposal has become a major political issue over the last several years and has become very expensive, so this function has grown in importance.

The central supply operation cleans and either disinfects or sterilizes reusable materials that are used in the diagnosis and therapy of patients. The laundry collects and launders soiled linen. Linen need be sterilized only for use in operative procedures. The hospital kitchen or outside food service must adhere to strict hygiene standards in preparing the many and varied diets for patients. Fortunately, foodborne outbreaks in hospitals are not common.

The occupational health service has special responsibilities to protect hospital personnel from acquiring an infection from patients while performing their patient-care duties, and, in turn, also to prevent employees from transmitting their own infections to patients. In this regard, several diseases have assumed particular importance.

AIDS (see Part XXII). Although the risk of acquiring HIV infection from occupational exposure is very low, this disease has received great attention from hospital infection control programs over the past several years. AIDS has raised a number of scientific, ethical, social, and legal issues that have had an impact on the ability of the infection control team to devise solutions. Not every issue has as yet been adequately addressed, largely because certain essential data are lacking.

Because HIV is not transmitted through casual contact, routine interactions with patients are not hazardous. Exposures that are associated with a risk of acquiring HIV infection are injuries by "sharps" (needles and scalpels, primarily) contaminated with the body fluid (blood, most commonly) or tissue of an HIV-infected patient. A number of studies have indicated that approximately 1 of every 300 such exposures results in transmission of HIV infection to the health care worker. Transmission is more likely to occur when the exposures are multiple and deep and when a substantial volume of blood is inoculated during the injury. The prospective studies of exposures on skin or mucous membranes have not shown any seroconversions, but there have been anecdotal reports suggesting that such exposures rarely might result in transmission. Much remains to be learned in this regard.

Standard protocols have been developed to manage the hospital worker who sustains an occupational injury involving a patient's blood or other body fluid. These include testing the source patient for HIV infection (if the patient can be identified), counseling the hospital worker, and possibly offering zidovudine prophylaxis. Such injuries often are major anxiety-provoking events, and cooperation of the occupational health service and the infection control team in supportive counseling of the hospital worker is extremely important. See Ch. 363 for additional discussion of AIDS prevention and control.

TUBERCULOSIS (see Ch. 311). Health care workers have always been at greater risk than the general population for acquiring tuberculosis. The patient in whom tuberculosis is diagnosed is only a modest hazard. Respiratory isolation techniques and antituberculosis therapy quickly reduce the hazard of nosocomial transmission. Rather, the risk is from the cryptic case, the patient with as yet undiagnosed tuberculosis. After a steady decline for years, tuberculosis is again resurgent because of the recent wave of immigrants from Southeast Asia and Central America and the frequency with which tuberculosis complicates HIV infection.

All hospitals are obliged to have a tuberculosis control program. All personnel receive a tuberculin skin test on employment. Those who are skin test-negative are followed by periodic skin testing, usually at yearly intervals, although high-risk persons may be tested at shorter intervals. Those in whom the skin test converts to positive are evaluated for active disease and are candidates for isoniazid (INH) preventive therapy. There is no place for annual chest roentgenograms, a now discarded practice.

HEPATITIS B (see Ch. 117). Like HIV infection, hepatitis B is transmitted in the hospital by exposure to blood and other body fluids that contain the virus. Hospital personnel who are exposed to blood and use needles, scalpels, and other sharp objects are at increased risk of hepatitis B infection. Programs to prevent hepatitis B infection are two-pronged. First, strong attempts must be made to reduce injuries through education, designing safer devices, and providing for the secure disposal of sharps in impervious containers. These precautions help avert not only hepatitis B infections, but all other blood-borne pathogens, including retroviruses and other viral hepatitis agents. Secondly, hepatitis B vaccine must be offered to all workers at potential risk. Ideally, all students of the health care professions should be immunized early in their training. In addition, insistent attempts to immunize current health care workers, including physicians and nurses, must continue. After an injury, standard protocols are used by the occupational health service to evaluate the health worker and the source patient and to offer appropriate prophylaxis.

In addition to providing hepatitis B vaccine, hospitals should provide other vaccines for the protection of personnel. Measles, mumps, and rubella have produced outbreaks in hospitals resulting in a great deal of unnecessary illness, turbulence, and expense. In these outbreaks, hospital workers have both acquired these viral infections and transmitted them to patients. It now is recommended that hospital workers born since 1957 receive a second dose of measles vaccine. If this is provided as the combined measles-mumps-rubella (MMR) vaccine, protection is achieved against all three diseases.

Finally, as the United States population ages, as hospitals care for increasingly sicker patients, and as medical technology continues its aggressive advances in organ transplantation and other invasive therapy, the importance of nosocomial infections will likely continue to increase. Infection control programs must be alert to these changes and be prepared to respond to them with equally new and innovative preventive measures.

Centers for Disease Control and Prevention: Public health focus: Surveillance, prevention, and control of nosocomial infections. Morb Mortal Wkly Rep 41:783, 1992. *Examines knowledge about effectiveness of nosocomial infection surveillance, prevention, and control and their cost-benefits.*

Evans RS, Burke JP, Classen DC, et al.: Computerized identification of patients at high risk for hospital-acquired infection. Am J Infect Control 20:4, 1992. *Statistical method to predict risk—based on guidelines of the Study of Efficacy of Nosocomial Infection and the CDC—identified more nosocomial infections than did traditional methods. Computerized equations that can help identify patients at risk of having nosocomial infections can help focus prevention efforts.*

Goldrick B, Larson E: Assessment of infection control programs in Maryland skilled-nursing long-term care facilities. Am J Infect Control 22:83, 1994. *The CDC Infection Surveillance and Control Questionnaire is a reliable instrument to assess infection control programs in long-term care facilities. Nationwide study is planned to examine relationship between control activity and risk of nosocomial infection among US skilled-nursing long-term care facilities.*

Nathens AB, Chu PT, Marshall JC: Nosocomial infection in the surgical intensive care unit. Infect Dis Clin North Am 6:657, 1992. *ICU infections are commonly caused by endogenous organisms of low intrinsic pathogenicity, and contributions of these infections to the ICU outcome is controversial. Prevention is based on timely and definitive surgical therapy, judicious use of invasive devices and antibiotics, and early enteral feeding. Infection-control measures aimed at endogenous reservoirs show preliminary promise for certain subsets of patients but remain experimental; 85 references.*

Sepkowitz KA: AIDS, tuberculosis, and the health care worker. Clin Infect Dis 20:232, 1995. *HIV infection and tuberculosis, alone and together, pose increasing risks to health care workers. The hazards of occupationally acquired tuberculosis are described as well as methods used in hospitals to promote a safe working environment.*

268 ADVICE TO TRAVELERS

Richard D. Pearson

International travel has become increasingly common over the past three decades. Millions of North Americans and Europeans visit developing areas each year for business, vacation, study, or religious activities. Modern air transportation has brought even the most exotic locations within easy reach. In addition, hundreds of thousands of troops have been deployed at various times in Southeast Asia, the Middle East, Africa, and other areas.

The risks associated with international travel vary with the locations visited, the duration of the trip, and the traveler's health, age, and activities while abroad. In general, persons going to Australia, Canada, Europe, Japan, New Zealand, and the United States require no special prophylactic measures. In contrast, visitors to developing areas, especially in the tropics, may be exposed to serious and at times life-threatening infections, as well as significant noninfectious problems.

There is no typical traveler. The usual duration abroad is 1 to 3 weeks, but some stay longer and a few reside overseas for extended periods. Pretravel medical preparation should be tailored to the traveler's individual needs. The major issues to be addressed are immunizations, malaria prophylaxis, traveler's diarrhea, and other hazards that can be avoided or minimized. Travelers to developing areas should obtain advice on the ever-changing international health requirements and the epidemiology of diseases abroad. Detailed information about specific geographic areas can be obtained from the Centers for Disease Control and Prevention (CDC) through its publications (see bibliography) or by calling the CDC International Travelers Hotline [(404) 332-4559], through publications of the World Health Organization (WHO) and the American Society of Tropical Medicine and Hygiene, or through commercially available computer programs.

IMMUNIZATIONS (See Ch. 10)

GENERAL CONSIDERATIONS. Before travel, vaccines can be administered that are routinely recommended for residents of North America, that are needed to protect travelers against infectious diseases in developing or tropical areas, or that are legally required for entry into countries (Table 268–1). A number of countries require the yellow fever vaccine. Some apply these regulations to all entering travelers, even those arriving directly from the United States, while others require them only of travelers who have visited areas where yellow fever is endemic. They are listed in the CDC publications. A few local authorities require documentation of cholera immunization, although it is marginally effective. No immunizations are required for citizens returning to the United States. Required vaccines and other immunizations should be documented in the yellow booklet entitled, "International Certificate of Vaccination," as approved by the WHO.

Pregnant travelers and those immunocompromised by human immune deficiency virus (HIV), neoplasms, or chemotherapy present special challenges. Most live viral and bacterial vaccines are contraindicated in these persons, although there are exceptions. For example, the measles vaccine is safe in persons with HIV infection, while other live vaccines such as yellow fever, oral polio, and oral typhoid should be avoided. Inactivated vaccines can be used in immunocompromised travelers, but the immune responses they elicit may be impaired, leaving the traveler at increased risk.

With a few exceptions, vaccines can be given simultaneously without adversely affecting the immune responses they elicit. Exceptions include the cholera and yellow fever vaccines, which inhibit antibody responses to each other, and immune globulin, which can inactivate some live viral vaccines. Immune globulin should be

✔ TABLE 268–1. IMMUNIZATION OF INTERNATIONAL TRAVELERS

Routine Vaccines that Should Be Up-to-Date in All Travelers

Tetanus
Diphtheria
Pertussis (children <7 years)
Poliomyelitis
Measles
Mumps
Rubella
Haemophilus influenzae (children)
Hepatitis B

Routine Vaccines Indicated in Special Populations

Influenza
Pneumococcal

Vaccines Potentially Indicated for Travelers to Developing Areas*

Immune globulin (hepatitis A)
Typhoid
Yellow fever†
Meningococcal
Rabies
Japanese B encephalitis
Cholera†

* The choice of specific vaccines depends on the itinerary, activities, and duration of travel as well as cost, efficacy, and potential side effects of the vaccines.

† Required for entry by some countries. See Centers for Disease Control and Prevention: Health Information for International Travel and "Summary of Health Information for International Travel" for a listing of countries requiring vaccination for entry.

given at least 2 weeks after or 3 months before administering measles, mumps, and rubella vaccines. It has no apparent adverse effect on the oral polio vaccine or the yellow fever vaccine, but when possible, immune globulin should be given at a separate time. If live viral vaccines are not administered simultaneously, it is recommended that they be separated by at least 3 weeks. Immune globulin is given close to the time of departure because it has a limited duration of effectiveness.

Before vaccination, a thorough history should be obtained to identify allergies. A history of hypersensitivity reactions to egg proteins is important because many viral vaccines (e.g., yellow fever, mumps, measles, and influenza) are prepared in embryonated hen's eggs or chicken embryo cell culture. On rare occasions, there is hypersensitivity to thimerosal, neomycin, or other trace vaccine contaminants.

IMMUNIZATIONS TO PROTECT INTERNATIONAL TRAVELERS. *Cholera* (see Ch. 296). The currently available, nonviable, parenteral cholera vaccine provides approximately 50% protection for 3 to 6 months. Few experts recommend the vaccine, but travelers are strongly urged to follow food and water precautions (see below) and to institute rehydration and antibiotic treatment immediately if diarrhea develops. Cholera immunization is no longer required for entrance into any country, but documentation of immunization may be required by some local officials. In those circumstances, one dose of the vaccine properly recorded and given at least 6 days before travel is adequate.

Hepatitis A (see Ch. 117). Hepatitis A constitutes a major risk for travelers to areas where sanitation and hygiene are poor. The likelihood of acquiring hepatitis A has been estimated to be as high as 1 in 1000 travelers per 2- to 3-week trip in some areas. Hepatitis A infection can be prevented or rendered asymptomatic by immune globulin 2 ml given intramuscularly to adult travelers who will be in endemic areas less than 3 months and 5 ml to travelers going for 3 to 5 months. Transmission of HIV is not a concern with immune globulin preparations manufactured in North America.

It is worthwhile to determine the antibody status of travelers who may have been previously infected with hepatitis A. The presence of anti-hepatitis A IgG antibodies indicates that travelers do not need immune globulin. Several active hepatitis A vaccines are under development.

Japanese B Encephalitis (see Ch. 346). The Japanese B encephalitis vaccine is indicated for travelers who have intense and/or prolonged (>4 weeks) exposure in rural endemic areas in China, Korea, Southeast Asia, India, the lowlands of Nepal, Sri Lanka, and, to a limited degree, Japan. This mosquito-borne disease is most common in rural rice and pig farming areas. It occurs from June through September in temperate regions and throughout the year in tropical areas. Travelers to urban sites are usually at low risk of infection. Unfortunately, the vaccine is not without side effects. Allergic reactions, including rash, urticaria, anaphylaxis, and on rare occasions sudden death, occur in 0.1 to 10 per 100,000 vaccines. Persons with a history of hypersensitivity responses to other allergens seem to be at greatest risk. Vaccine recipients should be observed in the office for 30 minutes after immunization; however, reactions can occur days to weeks later, most within 10 days of immunization.

Meningococcal Disease (see Ch. 281). The quadrivalent meningococcal vaccine (A/C/Y/W-135) should be considered for travelers going to northern India, Nepal, Saudi Arabia during the Moslem Hajj, Kenya, Tanzania, Burundi, sub-Saharan Africa, or other sites where travel advisories have been issued.

Rabies (see Ch. 427). Rabies is endemic in many areas. Travelers should be warned about the disease and advised to avoid dogs and other animals. In general, long-term travelers (30 days or more) who live in areas where rabies is a threat should receive pre-exposure immunization with the human diploid cell rabies vaccine. Any short-term traveler who plans to have close contact with dogs, wild animals, or bat-infested caves also should be immunized. Simultaneous administration of chloroquine, and possibly mefloquine, can decrease the immunogenicity of intradermally administered rabies vaccine. If the drug cannot be stopped, the vaccine should be given intramuscularly. The high cost of the rabies vaccine has limited its use for pre-exposure prophylaxis.

All persons, whether or not they have received pre-exposure immunization, who are bitten by a potentially rabid animal should be advised to wash the site thoroughly with water and detergent and to seek medical care. Those who have received pre-exposure prophylaxis need additional doses of the human diploid cell vaccine; those who have not been previously immunized require full immunization plus human rabies immune globulin.

Typhoid (see Ch. 292). Typhoid is common in developing areas where sanitation is poor. The risk is relatively low among short-term travelers to urban areas who adhere to food and water precautions. The oral, live Ty21a typhoid vaccine has largely replaced the killed vaccine for adults and children older than 6. The oral vaccine has fewer side effects than the killed, parenteral vaccine, which can cause severe local pain, erythema, and constitutional symptoms. The oral typhoid vaccine should not be given to HIV-infected persons or those taking antibiotics or mefloquine, which can inactivate it. It is recommended that the oral series be repeated at 5-year intervals; the inactivated vaccine is boosted with a single dose at 3-year intervals.

Yellow Fever (see Ch. 345). Yellow fever is endemic in tropical areas of Africa and Latin America in a band ranging from approximately 15° north to 15° south of the equator. The yellow fever vaccine is a live, attenuated strain (17D). It is available only at licensed centers, which can be identified by calling local or state health offices. The vaccine is boosted at 10-year intervals. The yellow fever vaccine should not be given to HIV-infected travelers. They should be advised to avoid endemic areas. If they must travel, they should do all that they can to minimize mosquito bites and carry with them written evidence of medical exemption.

Other Vaccines (see Ch. 300). The plague vaccine is not available in the United States. It has been used for persons with intense field exposure in endemic areas, but it is seldom recommended for travelers. There are currently no vaccines to protect against a number of important viral diseases, including dengue, and parasitic diseases such as malaria.

TRAVELER'S DIARRHEA (See Ch. 298)

Traveler's diarrhea is the most common problem encountered by North Americans who visit developing areas. The incidence is as high as 40 to 60% in some areas of Latin America, Africa, and India if appropriate food and water precautions are not followed.

The risk of traveler's diarrhea can be reduced approximately fourfold by following the commandment, "Cook it, boil it, peel it, or forget it" and by eating only foods served piping hot. Even when these recommendations are followed, diarrhea may occur. The duration and severity can be reduced by early self-treatment. Travelers should be instructed in oral rehydration with solutions containing glucose and electrolytes. They also should have available and take an appropriate antibiotic; ciprofloxacin is widely used in adults. Use of an antimotility agent such as loperamide can further reduce the duration of secretory diarrhea, but it should not be taken by children or by adults with bloody diarrhea, high fever, or other evidence of inflammatory colitis.

PREVENTING MALARIA (See Ch. 374)

Malaria is a major health hazard for travelers to endemic tropical areas. The risk of exposure varies greatly throughout the tropics. The frequency of transmission is particularly high in sub-Saharan Africa. More than 80% of the cases of falciparum malaria diagnosed in the United States are acquired in East Africa. The mortality of falciparum malaria in returning travelers and immigrants to the United States is approximately 4%. Fortunately, malaria transmission is infrequent in most urban areas of Latin America and Asia.

Every effort should be made by travelers to minimize contact with *Anopheles* mosquitoes—the vector of malaria—which prefer to feed in the evening, at night, and in the early morning. Travelers outdoors at those times should wear long-sleeved clothing and apply insect repellents that contain *N,N*-diethylmethyltoluamide (DEET) at a concentration of 30 to 35% to exposed skin. DEET should be used cautiously in young children because of the potential for seizures and other neurologic side effects due to percutaneous absorption. Clothing and mosquito netting can be treated with permethrin, which confers further protection against mosquitoes for weeks.

Even with these measures, chemoprophylaxis is necessary (Table 268–2). For a full discussion of the efficacy and toxicity of these drugs, see Ch. 374.

✔ TABLE 268–2. CHEMOPROPHYLAXIS FOR MALARIA*

Travelers to areas with chloroquine-sensitive Plasmodium *species:*

Chloroquine phosphate, 300 mg base (500 mg salt) orally once a week[†]

Travelers to areas with chloroquine resistance:

Mefloquine, 250 mg orally once a week[†]
or
Doxycycline, 100 mg orally daily[†]

Alternative

Chloroquine phosphate as above[†]
plus
Presumptive treatment with pyrimethamine-sulfadoxine (Fansidar), 3 tablets self-administered for a febrile illness when medical care is not immediately available
or
Proguanil, 200 mg orally daily[†‡]
(in sub-Saharan Africa)

Prevention of late relapses with P. vivax *and* P. ovale[§]

Primaquine phosphate, 15 mg base (26.3 mg salt) orally each day for 14 days

---

* Based on recommendations of The Medical Letter on Drugs and Therapeutics (35:111, 1993). Insect repellents, insecticide-impregnated bed nets, and proper clothing are important adjuncts for preventing malaria. The potential toxicities and contraindications of antimalarial medications are discussed in Ch. 374 and should be reviewed before use. Chloroquine has been used extensively and safely in pregnancy, but other prophylactic medications are either contraindicated during pregnancy or their safety is uncertain. No prophylactic regimen guarantees protection, and travelers should be warned about the possibility of a relapse of malaria months to a year or more after returning.

† Adult dose; start 1 week prior to departure with chloroquine and mefloquine, 1–2 days with doxycycline, continue during travel, and for 4 weeks after return.

‡ Not available in the United States. Failures have been reported with chloroquine and proguanil in persons with chloroquine-resistant falciparum malaria in Kenya.

§ Some relapses have been reported with this regimen. Some experts prescribe primaquine during the last 2 weeks of malaria prophylaxis for travelers with presumed exposure to *P. vivax* or *P. ovale.* Others avoid primaquine and rely on early detection and treatment of *P. vivax* or *P. ovale* malaria if it occurs.

BEHAVIORAL MODIFICATIONS

INFECTIOUS DISEASES TO BE AVOIDED. *Sexually Transmitted Diseases (STD's)* (see Ch. 314–318, and Part XXII). A surprising number of U.S. and European travelers have sexual relations with local residents or casual contacts among other travelers while abroad, risking HIV infection and other STD's. These risks must be explicitly discussed with all travelers. Abstinence is the only fully effective way to avoid STD's. Travelers who choose to have sex abroad should use latex condoms. They should purchase them prior to departure because condoms manufactured abroad may not be protective. Some countries now require HIV testing before granting entrance visas.

Arthropod-Borne Diseases (see Ch. 345, 346, 374–377). A number of infectious diseases can be avoided by taking appropriate precautions. Every effort should be made to minimize exposure to arthropod vectors with clothing, insect repellents, and mosquito nets. Travelers to Latin America should not sleep in mud or adobe dwellings where reduviid bugs can transmit *Trypanosoma cruzi,* the cause of Chagas' disease.

Helminthic Infections (see Part XXIII). Travelers should not walk barefoot where hookworms and *Strongyloides stercoralis* are endemic. Persons visiting areas where *Schistosoma* species are found should avoid swimming or bathing in fresh or brackish water. People should not lie directly on beaches where dogs may have defecated leaving *Ancylostoma braziliensis,* the cause of cutaneous larva migrans.

OTHER IMPORTANT ISSUES. *Chronic Medical Problems.* Special attention should be directed to patients with chronic medical problems. They should wear medical alert identification. Travelers requiring medications should always keep these with them, since luggage may be unavailable, lost, or stolen. It is wise to keep a list of all medications. An extra set of glasses often comes in handy.

Jet Lag. When travelers cross multiple time zones, the following few days are frequently disrupted by jet lag. Dietary measures have not been rigorously evaluated, but it is thought that the symptoms may be minimized by avoiding excessive amounts of alcohol and food during flight. Short-acting benzodiazepines have been recommended by some to help with the adaptation to new time zones, but they can result in confusion.

Motion Sickness. Travelers with motion sickness may gain relief with short-term, over-the-counter preparations of diphenhydramine. For longer trips or cruises, sustained-release transdermal scopolamine may be preferred.

Altitude Sickness. Travelers to high elevations are at risk of acute mountain sickness, particularly if they ascend rapidly to heights greater than 9000 feet. Gradual ascent over a period of days is the best way to acclimatize. Acetazolamide, 250 mg two or three times a day, has been recommended for those who do not have time to acclimatize, but it is a diuretic, causes tingling and paresthesias that may interfere with climbing, and is contraindicated in persons with sulfonamide allergies. If mountain sickness develops, the safest course of action is to descend. Steroids and pressurizing bags are helpful. Anyone going to extreme elevations should seek advice from a mountaineering expert before the trip.

Venomous Snakes, Spiders, and Scorpions. In tropical areas it is advisable to hike on clear paths, to avoid thick grass or brush, and to check the inside of shoes, closets, and drawers before extending feet or hands into them. Hikers should always wear shoes or boots.

Accidents. Travelers frequently have a false sense of security. They should inquire about potential risks to their safety before exploring new areas or swimming, particularly in the ocean where tides may be dangerous. Information about civil unrest and political instability can be obtained from the Department of State [(202) 647-5225].

Centers for Disease Control and Prevention: CDC Health Information for International Travel 1994 [HHS Publication No. (CDC) 94-8280]. Atlanta, U.S. Department of Health and Human Services, Public Health Service, 1994. For sale by the US Government Printing Office, Superintendent of Documents, Washington, DC 20402-9328. *This is an excellent source of information on health risks in overseas locations as well as key information on vaccines and drugs. It is updated yearly.*

Centers for Disease Control and Prevention: Summary of Health Information for International Travel (HHS Publication No. 396). Atlanta, U.S. Department of Health and Human Services. *Published biweekly, listing countries or areas reporting yellow fever, cholera, and plague.*

Gardner P (ed.): Health issues of international travelers. Infect Dis Clin North Am 6:275, 1992. *This review summarizes preparations for international travel as well as the evaluation of returning travelers who are ill.*

Health Hints for the Tropics. 11th ed. Washington, American Society of Tropical Medicine and Hygiene, 1993. *A comprehensive review of health issues related to international travel.*

International Travel and Health. Vaccination Requirements and Health Advice. Geneva, World Health Organization, 1994. *Summarizes the WHO recommendations for vaccinations and malaria prophylaxis as well as other health advice for travelers.*

Bacterial Diseases

269 INTRODUCTION TO BACTERIAL DISEASE
Gerald L. Mandell

Bacteria are classified in the kingdom Procaryotae and contain DNA in a double-stranded loop not bounded by a membrane. The success of bacteria as life forms can be illustrated by the fact that fossils of bacteria 3.5 billion years old have been found. Bacteria are ubiquitous and can grow at temperatures as low as 0° C and as high as 110° C. All bacteria have a bilayered cytoplasmic membrane, and most bacteria (*Mycoplasma* are exceptions) have an outer cell wall containing muramic acid. Morphologic features are often used to categorize bacteria. Bacilli are rods or cylinders, with about half the species being motile, while cocci are spherical and nonmotile. It is useful to distinguish bacteria by their ability to retain a basic dye (crystal violet) after iodine fixation and alcohol decolorization (the Gram reaction). Gram-positive organisms retain the dye and contain techoic acids in their cell walls (Fig. 269–1), whereas gram-negative bacteria have an additional outer membrane containing lipopolysaccharide (endotoxin) (Fig. 269–2). Capsules may serve as major virulence factors by interfering with the ability of phagocytes to ingest the encapsulated organisms. The capsules of the pneumococcus and *Haemophilus influenzae* are important factors for the virulence of the organisms. Other virulence factors include exotoxins released from the microbe, such as tetanus toxin

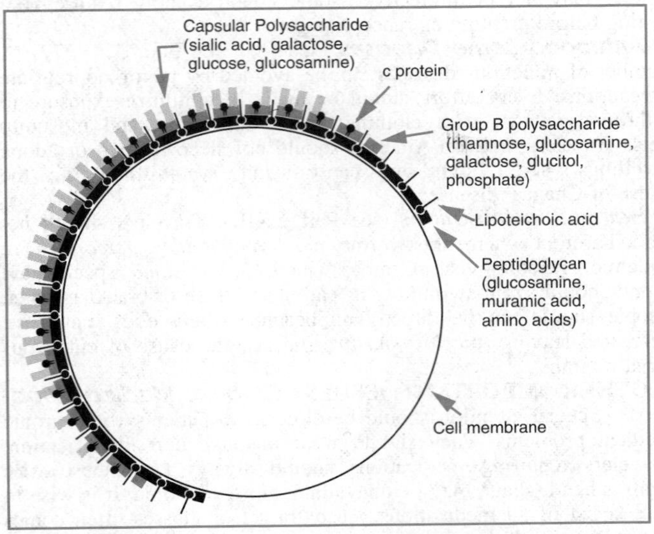

FIGURE 269–1. Schematic diagram of the cell wall of a gram-positive bacterium (group B streptococcus). (From Kasper S: Introduction to bacterial diseases. *In* Mandell GL, Douglas RG, Bennett JE [eds.]: Principles and Practice of Infectious Diseases, 3rd ed. New York, Churchill Livingstone, 1990, pp 1484–1489.)

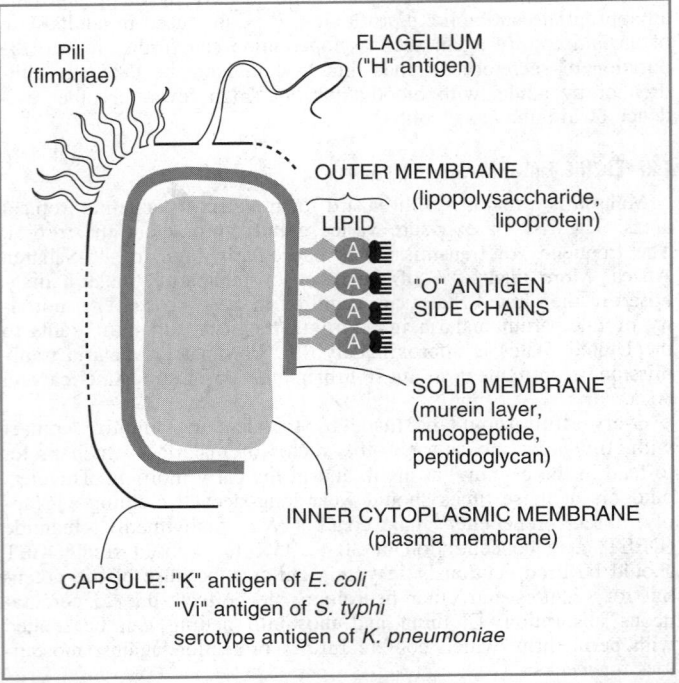

FIGURE 269–2. Schematic diagram of a gram-negative bacillus. (From Young L: Gram-negative sepsis. *In* Mandell GL, Douglas RG, Bennett JE [eds.]: Principles and Practice of Infectious Diseases, 3rd ed. New York, Churchill Livingstone, 1990, pp 611–636.)

and cholera toxin. Some bacteria, such as *Shigella flexneri,* can invade and damage host cells. Many gram-negative bacteria contain potent endotoxins that are important mediators of the sepsis syndrome. Pili or fimbriae are smaller hairlike structures that mediate bacterial attachment to various tissues and body surfaces. Only a very small proportion of species are pathogenic for humans, and new data suggest that even among those pathogenic species only certain clones are true pathogens.

Bacteria may be separated by their ability to reside and replicate intracellularly. Examples of intracellular bacteria include *Salmonella typhi, Legionella* species, mycobacteria, and chlamydiae. Extracellular pathogens include streptococci (including pneumococci), staphylococci, and most gram-negative enteric rods such as *Escherichia coli, Klebsiella* species, and *Pseudomonas* species. The main technique used for identification of bacteria in patient specimens is culture on artificial media. The ability to grow on the surface of such media in air defines aerobic organisms. Anaerobes cannot grow un-

der such conditions, and facultative organisms can grow either aerobically or anaerobically. Microscopy can be a very useful technique, especially when combined with appropriate staining procedures such as acid-fast stains for mycobacteria or Gram stain to differentiate gram-positive from gram-negative organisms. Newer techniques use direct immunofluorescence (e.g., for *Chlamydia trachomatis*), DNA probes (e.g., for *Legionella* species), and latex agglutination tests to detect antigen (e.g., for pneumococcal capsular antigen in spinal fluid). Assays using the polymerase chain reaction are now employed. Tests for antibodies are less useful but may be helpful in some diseases (e.g., Lyme disease).

Classification of bacteria has a historic basis and is based in large part on morphology and Gram-stain reaction. Genetic studies result in frequent changes in nomenclature. Table 269–1 is a much-abbreviated summary of potentially pathogenic microbes.

TABLE 269–1. CLASSIFICATION OF SELECTED BACTERIA THAT CAUSE DISEASE IN HUMANS

Aerobes
Gram-positive cocci
  Catalase-positive
    Staphylococcus aureus
    Staphylococcus epidermidis
    Other coagulase-negative staphylococci
  Catalase-negative
    Enterococcus faecalis
    Enterococcus faecium
    Leuconostoc sp.
    Streptococcus agalactiae
      (group B streptococcus)
    Streptococcus bovis
    Streptococcus pneumoniae
    Streptococcus pyogenes
      (group A streptococcus)
    Viridans group streptococci
      S. anginosus
      S. mutans
Gram-negative cocci
  Moraxella catarrhalis
  Neisseria gonorrhoeae
  Neisseria meningitidis
Gram-positive bacilli
  Bacillus anthracis
  Corynebacterium diphtheriae
  Corynebacterium jeikeium
  Erysipelothrix rhusiopathiae
  Gardnerella vaginalis
  Acid-fast organisms
    Mycobacterium avium-complex
    Mycobacterium kansasii
    Mycobacterium leprae
    Mycobacterium tuberculosis
    Nocardia sp.
Gram-negative rods
  Enterobacteriaceae
    Citrobacter sp.
    Enterobacter aerogenes
    Escherichia coli
    Klebsiella sp.
    Morganella morganii
    Proteus sp.
    Providencia rettgeri
    Salmonella sp.
    Salmonella typhi
    Serratia marcescens
    Shigella sp.
    Yersinia enterocolitica
    Yersinia pestis
  Fermentive non-enterobacteriaceae
    Aeromonas hydrophila
    Chromobacterium violaceum
    Plesiomonas shigelloides
    Pasteurella multocida
    Vibrio cholerae
    Vibrio vulnificus

  Nonfermentive non-enterobacteriaceae
    Acinetobacter calcoaceticus
    Alcaligenes xylosoxidans
    Eikenella corrodens
    Flavobacterium meningosepticum
    Pseudomonas aeruginosa
    Pseudomonas sp.
Gram-negative coccobacilli
  Actinobacillus actinomycetemcomitans
  Bartonella bacilliformis
  Brucella sp.
  Bordetella sp.
  Campylobacter sp.
  Haemophilus sp.
  Haemophilus influenzae
  Helicobacter pylori
  Legionella sp.
  Rochalimaea sp.
  Chlamydiae
    Chlamydia trachomatis
    Chlamydia pneumoniae
    Chlamydia psittaci
  Rickettsiae
    Rickettsia prowazekii
    Rickettsia rickettsii
  Myoplasmas
    Mycoplasma pneumoniae
  Treponemataceae (spiral organisms)
    Borrelia burgdorferi
    Leptospira sp.
    Treponema pallidum

Anaerobes
Gram-negative bacilli
  Bacteroides fragilis
  Bacteroides
  Fusobacterium sp.
  Prevotella sp.
Gram-negative cocci
  Veillonella sp.
Non–spore-forming gram-positive bacilli
  Actinomyces sp.
  Bifidobacterium sp.
  Eubacterium sp.
  Proprionibacterium sp.
Endospore-forming gram-positive bacilli
  Clostridium botulinum
  Clostridium perfringens
  Clostridium tetani
  Clostridium sp.
Gram-positive cocci
  Peptostreptococcus sp.
  Gemella morbillorum
  Peptococcus niger

Adapted from Bruckner DA, Colonna P: Nomenclature for aerobic and facultative bacteria. Clin Infect Dis 16:598, 1993, and Summanen P: Microbiology terminology update: Clinically significant anaerobic gram-positive and gram-negative bacteria (excluding spirochetes). Clin Infect Dis 16:606, 1993.

270 ANTIBACTERIAL THERAPY
Adolf W. Karchmer

The introduction of sulfonamides in the mid-1930's and of penicillin and streptomycin a decade later marked the beginning of the major developments in modern medicine. Subsequently there has been an expanded array of antimicrobics with increased potency and activity against the major bacterial pathogens. Not only has modern antibacterial therapy markedly reduced the morbidity and mortality of infections, but the judicious use of antimicrobics has also prevented disease and has contributed significantly to the development of modern surgery, trauma therapy, and organ transplantation. The broad application of antimicrobial agents in modern medicine has not, however, been problem free. These agents occasionally cause major adverse reactions among patients or untoward reactions when interacting with other classes of pharmacologic agents, and are a selective pressure for the increasingly widespread antimicrobial resistance among bacteria.

MECHANISMS AND TYPES OF ANTIBACTERIAL ACTIVITY

An effective antimicrobic should kill or inhibit the growth of a bacterium and not injure the human host. This selectivity results from targets that are either absent from mammalian cells or are more vulnerable to inhibition by the antimicrobic than are the analogous targets in mammalian cells. For example, the peptidoglycan rigid cell wall is unique to bacteria and thus a target for selective activity by β-lactam antibiotics. In contrast to humans who can use exogenous folic acid, bacteria cannot use exogenous tetrahydrofolic acid (folinic acid) in the synthesis of nucleic acids and must synthesize folinic acid from para-aminobenzoic acid. Inhibition of this pathway by sulfonamides or trimethoprim, independently or together, thus results in selective antibacterial activity. Antimicrobial agents that merely inhibit the growth of microorganisms are *bacteriostatic,* while those that kill bacteria at physiologically achievable concentrations are *bactericidal.* Growth inhibition and killing in general are the product of the drug's mechanism of action, but on occasion are concentration-dependent or unique to the interaction of a drug and a particular bacterial species. For example, chloramphenicol, which is generally bacteriostatic even at high concentrations, is bactericidal for *Haemophilus influenzae* at concentrations achieved in patients with standard doses. Conversely, penicillin G is generally bactericidal for susceptible organisms but is only bacteriostatic against *Enterococcus faecalis* and *E. faecium.* The site of action and antibacterial effect of major classes of antimicrobial agents are shown in Table 270–1. Combinations of antibiotics may produce an antibacterial effect greater than the sum of their independent activities; this is called *synergism.* The sequential inhibition of tetrahydrofolic acid by a sulfonamide and trimethoprim may cause synergism. Also, facilitated penetration of aminoglycosides into enterococci by penicillin, ampicillin, or vancomycin can result in bactericidal synergism.

MECHANISMS OF BACTERIAL RESISTANCE TO ANTIMICROBICS

In considering bacterial resistance to antimicrobial agents, it is useful to consider both the mechanisms of action of individual antibacterial compounds and the general properties of antibiotics that are necessary for efficacy. Antimicrobics must be able to (1) reach the molecular targets, which are primarily intracellular, in sufficient amounts; (2) interact with a target molecule in a manner that initiates an antibacterial effect; and (3) avoid inactivation by drug-modifying enzymes in the extracellular environment or within the bacterial cell. The molecular mechanism used by individual bacteria to resist specific antimicrobics can be viewed as a strategy to subvert one of these requirements for antimicrobial efficacy (Table 270–2). Frequently bacteria use more than one strategy; multiple mechanisms acting in concert may produce markedly enhanced antimicrobial resistance. Resistance to an antimicrobial agent may be an intrinsic property of a bacterial species or an acquired capability. To acquire resistance a bacterium must alter its DNA by mutating native DNA or by introducing foreign DNA. Resistance genes are often part of extrachromosomal plasmid DNA, which can transfer among organisms by conjugation, transduction, or transformation. Some resistance genes are part of DNA units called *transposons* that move between chromosomes and transmissible plasmids. Foreign DNA may be acquired through transformation, resulting in ex-

TABLE 270–1. MECHANISMS OF ACTION OF ANTIMICROBIAL AGENTS

Agent	Site of Action	Effect	Cidal	Static
Penicillins, cephalosporins, other β-lactams	Penicillin-binding proteins (peptidoglycan synthetic enzymes)	Inhibits cross-linking of peptidoglycan (transpeptidation), impairs cell wall synthesis	+	Occasionally
Vancomycin, teicoplanin	Terminal D-ala-D-ala of pentapeptide, peptidoglycan, precursor	Inhibits polymerization of disaccharide precursors to peptidoglycan (transglycosylation), impairs cell wall synthesis	+	Occasionally
Polymyxin B, colistin	Cytoplasmic membrane	Binds to phospholipid cytoplasmic membrane, disrupts membrane function	+	
Aminoglycosides	Ribosome, 30S subunit	Complex; inhibits peptide elongation, causes misreading of genetic code	+	
Tetracycline	Ribosome, 30S subunit	Inhibits binding of transfer RNA, inhibits protein synthesis		+
Chloramphenicol	Ribosome, 50S subunit	Blocks transfer of amino acids to peptide chains, inhibits protein synthesis	Occasionally	+
Erythromycin	Ribosome, 50S subunit	Inhibits translocation of ribosome on messenger RNA, inhibits protein synthesis	Occasionally	+
Clindamycin	Ribosome, 50S subunit	Blocks transfer of amino acids to peptide chain, inhibits protein synthesis	Occasionally	+
Rifampin	DNA-dependent RNA polymerase	Impairs RNA synthesis	+	
Metronidazole	Nucleic acids	Damages nucleic acid structure	+	
Quinolones	DNA topoisomerase (gyrase)	Impairs supercoiling in DNA synthesis	+	
Sulfonamides	Dihydropteroate synthetase	Competitive inhibition of synthesis of dihydrofolate from para-aminobenzoic acid		+
Trimethoprim	Dihydrofolate reductase	Inhibits reduction of dihydrofolate to tetrahydrofolic acid		+

TABLE 270–2. MECHANISMS OF ANTIBIOTIC RESISTANCE

Antimicrobic	Mechanism	Representative Organism
β-Lactam (penicillins, cephalosporins, carbapenems, carbacephems, monobactams)	Altered target (penicillin-binding protein)	*Enterococus faecium, Streptococcus pneumoniae,* methicillin-resistant *Staphylococcus aureus*
	Reduced permeability	*Enterobacter* species, *Pseudomonas aeruginosa*
	β-Lactamase	*S. aureus,* gram-negative bacilli, *Haemophilus influenzae, Neisseria gonorrhoeae, Enterococcus faecalis*
Aminoglycosides	Modifying enzymes (acetylation, adenylation, phosphorylation)	*S. aureus,* enterococci, *P. aeruginosa,* Enterobacteriaceae
	Reduced permeability or energy-dependent uptake	Enterobacteriaceae, *P. aeruginosa, S. aureus* (small cell variant), enterococci
	Decreased ribosomal binding	*S. aureus, E. faecalis* (streptomycin)
Chloramphenicol	Active efflux	*H. influenzae*
	Reduced permeability	Enterobacteriaceae
	Inactivating enzyme (acetylation)	*S. aureus,* enterococci, Enterobacteriaceae
Erythromycin, clindamycin	Decreased ribosomal binding (methylation of ribosomal RNA)	*S. aureus, S. pneumoniae,* streptococci, *Bacteroides fragilis*
	Reduced permeability	Enterobacteriaceae, *Staphylococcus epidermidis*
	Modifying enzymes	*E. coli, Klebsiella pneumoniae, S. aureus*
Quinolones	Target alteration (DNA gyrase)	Enterobacteriaceae, *S. aureus*
	Reduced permeability	Enterobacteriaceae, *P. aeruginosa*
	Active efflux	*Escherichia coli*
Tetracyclines	Altered target (ribosome)	*N. gonorrhoeae,* streptococci
	Active efflux	*E. coli*
	Permeability barriers	Enterobacteriaceae
	Drug detoxification	*B. fragilis*
Rifampin	Reduced RNA polymerase binding	*E. coli, S. aureus*
Sulfonamides, trimethoprim	Altered dihydropteroate synthetase or dihydrofolate reductase	Enterobacteriaceae, *Moraxella catarrhalis*
	Increased para-aminobenzoic acid	*S. aureus, N. gonorrhoeae*
	Reduced permeability	*P. aeruginosa,* Enterobacteriaceae
Vancomycin	Altered peptidoglycan precursor-binding site	*E. faecium*

changes of chromosomal DNA among species and subsequent interspecies recombination. Genetic mechanisms of resistance function constitutively (at a constant rate) or may be induced upon exposure to antimicrobial agents, which may confound detection of resistance by laboratory tests.

Exclusion of effective amounts of an antibiotic from intracellular compartments is a common mechanism of intrinsic resistance. Limited permeability is a property of the lipopolysaccharide outer cell membrane of gram-negative bacteria. The permeability of this membrane resides in special proteins, *porins,* which provide specific channels through which substances can pass to the periplasmic space and thereafter into the cell. Limited permeability accounts for the intrinsic resistance of gram-negative bacilli to penicillin, erythromycin, clindamycin, and vancomycin and that of *Pseudomonas aeruginosa* to trimethoprim. Similarly, the relative exclusion of aminoglycosides from the intracellular milieu of streptococci and enterococci accounts for intrinsic resistance of these organisms to this class of antimicrobics. Additionally, bacteria use this strategy in acquiring resistance. Thus, a mutational change in the specific porin of the outer cell membrane of *P. aeruginosa* through which imipenem usually diffuses can exclude the antibiotic from its target and render the *P. aeruginosa* resistant to imipenem. In general, however, mutations to decrease porin channels and reduce permeability are inefficient mechanisms for bacterial resistance and require a second mechanism, e.g., a coexisting β-lactamase, to generate higher-level resistance. The active pumping of antimicrobials from the intracellular milieu, i.e., active efflux, in effect excludes antibiotics from their targets and causes bacterial resistance. Plasmid-encoded resistance to tetracyclines among *Escherichia coli* results from active efflux.

Alteration of the target site at which an antimicrobic acts, such that an inhibitory or killing effect no longer occurs, constitutes a second major mechanism of resistance. Bacteria may acquire a gene that encodes a new antibiotic-resistant product that now substitutes for the original target. Thus, new forms of dihydropteroate synthetase and dihydrofolate reductase with lower affinity to sulfonamides and trimethoprim, respectively, mediate resistance to these drugs. Methicillin-resistant *Staphylococcus aureus* and coagulase-negative staphylococci have acquired the chromosomal gene *mecA* and produce a β-lactam–resistant penicillin-binding protein (PBP), called 2a or 2′, which is sufficient to maintain cell wall integrity during growth when other essential PBP's are inactivated by β-lac-

tam antibiotics. Alternatively, a newly acquired gene may act to modify a target, rendering it less vulnerable to an antimicrobic. Thus, a plasmid- or transposon-borne gene encodes an enzyme that methylates the 23S rRNA of the 50s ribosome and impairs the binding of erythromycins and clindamycin to their target. The resulting resistance to these antimicrobics, which has been noted in *S. aureus,* streptococci, pneumococci, clostridia, and *Bacteroides fragilis,* may be constitutive or inducible. Mutations in existing genes or homologous DNA acquired by transformation may result in antibiotic-resistant targets. Mutations leading to amino acid changes in RNA polymerase decrease the binding of rifampin to this enzyme and result in rifampin resistance. Similarly, mutations in the *gyrA* gene that alter amino acids in the A subunit of DNA gyrase have resulted in resistance to the fluoroquinolones among methicillin-resistant *S. aureus.* Perhaps the most striking alterations of native targets resulting in antibiotic resistance are those that occur among the various essential high molecular mass PBP's of gonococci, meningococci, *E. faecium,* and pneumococci and result in the decreased binding of penicillin to these targets. Alterations of PBP's in pneumococci have also resulted in the resistance of pneumococci to third-generation cephalosporins. In these naturally transformable bacteria, the acquisition of homologous DNA has resulted in mosaic genes, which in turn give rise to the penicillin-resistant hybrid PBP's. Pneumococci with relative and high-level resistance to penicillin due to PBP alterations are now widely distributed in the world and are an increasingly common cause of disease.

The third, and perhaps the most commonly used, mechanism by which bacteria are resistant to antibiotics entails the enzymatic alteration and inactivation of an antimicrobic. β-Lactamases hydrolyze the amide bond of the β-lactam ring, thus destroying the site at which β-lactam antibiotics bind to bacterial PBP's and through which they exert their antibacterial effect. Many different β-lactamases have been described. These enzymes are encoded chromosomally or extrachromosomally through plasmids or transposons and may be either produced constitutively or induced. The almost universal resistance of *S. aureus* to penicillin, ampicillin, the carboxypenicillins, and the ureidopenicillins is mediated by a plasmid-encoded, inducible β-lactamase. Staphylococcal β-lactamase, which is secreted into the surrounding environment, does not inactivate the penicillinase-resistant penicillins (oxacillin, nafcillin), the cephalosporins, or the carbapenems (imipenem, meropenem). Although occasionally hyperproduction of β-lactamase by *S. aureus* has engendered borderline resistance to oxacillin and nafcillin, these antibiotics retain antistaphylococcal activity in the presence of this β-lactamase. β-Lactams with minimal antibacterial activity that can bind irreversibly and inhibit β-lactamases have been developed. These compounds (clavulanic acid, sulbactam, tazobactam) have been combined with the penicillins to restore their activity despite the presence of staphylococcal β-lactamase. In gram-negative bacteria the role of β-lactamases in bacterial resistance is both complex and extensive. There are an abundance of structurally unique enzymes; many inactivate a broad range of β-lactam antibiotics; and the genes encoding these β-lactamases are subject to mutations that expand enzymatic activity and are both relatively easily transferred and widely distributed. In addition, in gram-negative bacteria β-lactamases are secreted into the limited confines of the periplasmic space where they act in concert with the permeability barrier of the outer cell wall to produce clinically significant antibiotic resistance. Among the more common of the plasmid-mediated β-lactamases are the TEM-1 and TEM-2 enzymes, the SHV-1 of *Klebsiella pneumoniae,* and the PSE-1 of *P. aeruginosa.* These confer resistance to penicillin, ampicillin, carbenicillin, ticarcillin, cephalothin, and cefamandole but not to the cephamycins (cefoxitin, cefotetan), third-generation cephalosporins, monobactams, or carbapenems. Plasmid-mediated, extended-spectrum β-lactamases (ESBL's) that inactivate third-generation cephalosporins and monobactams result from mutations in the TEM and SHV genes leading to amino acid substitutions in their products. Overproduction of TEM-1 β-lactamase by genes on multicopy plasmids have been encountered in *E. coli* that are resistant β-lactam/β-lactamase inhibitor combinations. Chromosomally mediated β-lactamases are produced at low levels by *P. aeruginosa, Enterobacter cloacae, Serratia marcescens,* and other gram-negative bacilli; when these organisms are exposed to β-lactam antibiotics, high levels of β-lactamase are induced, causing resistance to the broad-spectrum cephalosporins, cephamycins, and the β-lactam/clavulanic acid or sulbactam combinations. The third-generation cephalosporins are relatively resistant to hydrolysis by these enzymes. However, the limited entry of these cephalosporins into the periplasmic space allows even these β-lactamases to effectively mediate resistance. Some strains undergo a mutation resulting in fixed derepression of the chromosomal gene and constitutively produce these β-lactamases. Fortunately, β-lactam/β-lactamase inhibitor combinations and cephamycins remain active against organisms producing ESBL's, and imipenem remains active against organisms producing either ESBL's or chromosomal-type β-lactamases.

Resistance can result from constitutively produced modifying enzymes that acetylate amino groups and phosphorylate or adenylate hydroxyl groups on aminoglycosides. Permeability barriers to aminoglycosides may enhance this type of resistance. Several genes that encode different aminoglycoside-modifying enzymes may exist simultaneously in a bacterium. They are commonly on a plasmid, the chromosome, or a transposon. Modifying enzymes commonly cause aminoglycoside resistance in gram-negative bacilli. A bifunctional acetylating and phosphorylating enzyme that results in resistance to all clinically available aminoglycosides except streptomycin has been found increasingly in *Staphylococcus aureus* and coagulase-negative staphylococci, and enterococci. In enterococci this enzyme prevents the combination of penicillin, ampicillin, or vancomycin plus any aminoglycoside, except streptomycin, from exerting a bactericidal effect. The frequent coexistence in enterococci of this enzyme and streptomycin-adenylating enzyme renders strains resistant to all bactericidal combinations.

To effectively treat infection, physicians must be aware of resistance profiles for pathogens generally as well as in their immediate environment. For example, ceftriaxone has superseded penicillin as the drug of choice for gonorrhea because the frequency of penicillin-resistant strains in national surveillance data indicates unacceptable failure rates with continued penicillin therapy. In contrast, in any given hospital a physician must know the frequency with which wound infections are caused by methicillin-resistant *S. aureus* to choose between vancomycin and oxacillin as empiric therapy for the patient with apparent staphylococcal wound infection and bacteremia. Additionally, physicians must attempt to reduce the emergence of antimicrobial resistance among bacteria. Treatment with multiple antimicrobials, an effective strategy to decrease muta-

tional resistance among *Mycobacterium tuberculosis,* is less applicable to controlling antibiotic resistance among bacteria because bacteria become resistant to the multiple antimicrobials through acquiring a single plasmid or transposon rather than by multiple mutations. Antibiotics do not cause mutations and create resistant bacteria; nevertheless, their indiscriminate use provides enormous selective pressure to sustain and enrich resistant bacteria. Expanded antibiotic use is followed by increased frequency of resistant bacteria, which are then disseminated by poor sanitation and hygiene. Improved sanitation and hygiene and enhanced infection control in hospitals can reduce the dissemination of resistant organisms. While antimicrobic use cannot be eliminated, optimal antibiotic use not only requires judicious selection of an agent and duration of therapy but also avoidance of inappropriate use.

SELECTING ANTIMICROBIAL THERAPY

IDENTIFYING THE INFECTING AGENT. Effective therapy requires that the causative agent either be recovered and its antimicrobial susceptibility identified or reliably anticipated on the basis of the clinical presentation. Recovering the pathogen(s) by culture and subsequently determining antimicrobial susceptibility is highly desirable. Culture results, however, are usually not available when initial therapy is being selected, particularly for patients with more acute or severe infections. There are a few non–culture-based tests used to identify bacterial pathogens, e.g., group A streptococci in the pharynx, gonococci from genital secretions, pneumococci and *H. influenzae* in cerebrospinal fluid (CSF), and *Legionella pneumophila* antigen in urine. Examination of a Gram stain, or acid-fast stain, of material obtained from an infected site allows rapid assessment of bacterial content (semiquantitative) and the types of bacteria, and awareness of the local inflammatory response.

Physicians commonly initiate antimicrobial therapy empirically, and even when knowing the pathogen, must select antibacterial therapy without having specific antimicrobial susceptibility information. Various scenarios prompt empiric therapy: (1) The infection is immediately life threatening; (2) a less threatening infection is likely to worsen if therapy is delayed until culture results become available; (3) considering the predictability of the pathogens causing a syndrome, the inconvenience or hazards of acquiring a culture are unjustified; (4) the causative agent is predictable, therapy relatively simple, and the hazards of failed therapy are low. Meningitis with a polymorphonuclear CSF response (presumably bacterial) or clinical findings suggestive of septic shock mandate empiric therapy immediately after cultures are obtained. In contrast, pneumonia, even when not life threatening, is likely to progress if therapy is delayed. Hence, it is prudent to obtain blood and sputum cultures, examine a sputum Gram stain, and initiate empiric therapy. In contrast, the treatment of otitis media or acute bacterial sinusitis is initiated empirically based on the high probability that the bacterial infection is likely to be caused by pneumococci, *H. influenzae, Moraxella catarrhalis,* or less commonly, group A streptococci. Tympanocentesis or aspiration of the sinus for material to culture is reserved for patients in whom empiric therapy fails. Empiric treatment of recurrent uncomplicated cystitis in a young, otherwise healthy woman is an example of the fourth scenario. Although urine is easily cultured, the infection is probably due to *E. coli* or *Staphylococcus saprophyticus,* and successful empiric therapy with trimethoprim-sulfamethoxazole or a fluoroquinolone for 3 days will have been completed before culture results are available.

Culture results must be interpreted in the clinical context. Does the *E. coli* recovered from an abscess due to a ruptured appendix reflect the true microbiology or were the anticipated anaerobic bacteria not isolated because the specimen was mishandled? Furthermore, all isolates are not necessarily causing the infection; some may be contaminants or reflect colonizing flora. Thus, interpretation of the culture results is important, particularly if the specimen has been obtained across nonsterile surfaces. Some isolates from normally sterile material must be questioned. The coagulase-negative staphylococcus or *Corynebacterium* species recovered from a blood culture is possibly a contaminant, but in the patient with indwelling vascular catheters or leukopenia and fever after cancer chemotherapy, these isolates may be pathogens. Repetitive isolation or isolation of large numbers of organisms commonly considered contaminants, e.g., *S. epidermidis,* suggests that the bacteria are causing infection and warrants careful assessment.

Whether one is treating an infection empirically or on the basis of microbiologic data, the antimicrobial regimen should be as targeted as possible. The uncertainty inherent in empiric therapy necessitates broader-spectrum antimicrobial therapy. Nevertheless, judgment must be exercised to focus initial and subsequent (after culture data are available) antimicrobial therapy as much as the clinical syndrome allows. Using multiple antimicrobics or broad-spectrum therapy where more narrow spectrum therapy will suffice inevitably exposes the patient to increased risks of adverse effects and selects for increasingly resistant organisms.

EVALUATING ANTIMICROBIAL SUSCEPTIBILITY. Appropriate antimicrobial therapy is founded upon laboratory-documented inhibition of growth or actual killing of the organism by concentrations of antibiotics that can be achieved in a patient's serum using acceptable doses. Excretion by the kidney results in striking urine concentrations for some antibiotics; for an agent used only to treat urinary tract infection, e.g., nitrofurantoin, susceptibility is based on concentrations achieved in urine.

For most bacteria, antibiotic susceptibility cannot be adequately predicted and should be determined with *in vitro* tests. The predictable susceptibility of a few organisms obviates the need for their testing. Group A streptococci are universally susceptible to penicillin and cephalosporins, and *Neisseria meningitidis* is susceptible to penicillin, ampicillin, and chloramphenicol. These species do not require testing against those specific antibiotics. The susceptibility of these organisms to other antimicrobials is less predictable, and if other agents were used for therapy, testing would be required (e.g., erythromycin or tetracycline against group A streptococci or sulfonamides against meningococci). Resistance to penicillin has been noted among *Streptococcus pneumoniae* recovered worldwide. As a consequence, the antibiotic susceptibility of pneumococci isolated from blood or CSF must be evaluated as a guide for therapy.

PHARMACOLOGIC AND PHARMACODYNAMIC CONSIDERATIONS. Successful therapy requires that an antibiotic with *in vitro* activity be delivered to the site of infection in adequate concentration without inducing adverse reactions. Knowledge of the major pharmacologic and pharmacokinetic properties of the antimicrobic is necessary. The major pharmacologic properties of commonly used antibiotics are shown in Table 270–3. Penetration of antibiotics into some tissues and fluids is limited and drug specific. Lipid-soluble agents such as chloramphenicol, rifampin, sulfonamides, trimethoprim, ciprofloxacin, ofloxacin, metronidazole, and isoniazid penetrate into the CSF well, whereas penicillins, third-generation cephalosporins, and vancomycin penetrate adequately only when there is meningeal inflammation. Treatment of infection occurring in the CNS or other sites where antibiotic penetration is limited, e.g., the prostate or vitreous humor of the eye, requires special consideration and, on occasion, direct instillation. Most antibiotics are excreted primarily through the kidneys. Biliary excretion can be an advantage in treatment of biliary tract infection; however, excretion is markedly reduced if the biliary tract is obstructed. To achieve meaningful serum concentrations, aminoglycosides, carbapenems, and glycopeptides (vancomycin and teicoplanin) must be administered parenterally. Although parenterally administered antimicrobics are preferred for treatment of severe infections, the availability of well-absorbed potent penicillins, cephalosporins, quinolones, macrolides, and metronidazole allows early transition from parenteral to less costly oral therapy in many patients (exceptions include those with endocarditis, meningitis, or CNS infection).

Antibiotic penetration into cells, particularly polymorphonuclear leukocytes and macrophages, and intracellular antibacterial activity are necessary to effectively treat some infections (e.g., *M. tuberculosis, L. pneumophila, Listeria monocytogenes, Brucella* species, and *Salmonella typhi*).

The serum and tissue concentrations over time of an antimicrobic administered by a given route and the microbiologic activity of that antimicrobic when viewed together describe the pharmacodynamic properties of the agent. Bacterial killing by β-lactam antibiotics and vancomycin does not increase after antibiotic concentrations exceed an organism's minimum inhibitory concentration (MIC) by several multiples. Also, the postantibiotic effect (inhibition of an organism's growth resulting from immediately prior exposure to an antibiotic) of these antimicrobics is negligible. These interactions suggest that administration of β-lactam antibiotics and vancomycin to achieve sustained concentrations (four to five times the MIC) over longer periods is likely to result in more profound antibacterial action than

transient higher concentrations. Sustained concentrations may be achieved by more frequent dosing, by using higher doses, by using antibiotics with a long half-life, or by continuous infusion. Aminoglycosides and quinolones exhibit concentration-dependent killing wherein higher concentrations exert an increasingly bactericidal effect and cause a prolonged postantibiotic effect. These interactions suggest that larger doses administered less frequently provide greater antibacterial activity. Increasing numbers of controlled studies report that aminoglycoside therapy given as a single daily dose is as effective and less ototoxic and nephrotoxic than the same quantity of aminoglycoside divided in the standard multiple daily-dose regimen.

PATIENT-RELATED CONSIDERATIONS. Unique aspects of the patient and site of the specific infection are important in selecting an optimal antimicrobial agent, as well as the appropriate dose, route of administration, and duration of therapy. Recent treatment with an antibiotic, for example, increases the risk that the subsequent infection is caused by residual antibiotic-resistant bacteria. Residing in an environment that has an extensive antibiotic-resistant flora, e.g., an intensive care unit, a skilled nursing care facility, or a day care center, increases the risk for colonization and subsequent infection by antibiotic-resistant bacteria.

The patient's physiologic and metabolic status must be considered when therapy is selected. Premature infants and neonates have incompletely developed renal function, requiring adjustment of antibiotic doses. The hepatic glucuronyl transferase pathway through which chloramphenicol is metabolized is immature in newborns. As a result, chloramphenicol is likely to accumulate and cause circulatory collapse—the gray baby syndrome. Because tetracyclines deposit in growing bones and teeth and quinolones may damage cartilage, they are not used in children. Genetically determined drug metabolism also affects antibiotic selection. Antimicrobics, including sulfonamides, sulfones (dapsone), nitrofurantoin, chloramphenicol, and pyrimethamine, may cause hemolysis in patients with deficient glucose-6-phosphate dehydrogenase. Pridoxine is routinely given with isoniazid treatment or prophylaxis of tuberculosis to prevent the peripheral neuropathy that occurs among those who are "slow" acetylators of isoniazid.

Hypersensitivity to one member of an antibiotic class usually extends to all other compounds in that class, and if the reaction was severe, contraindicates their use. However, if the hypersensitivity reaction to penicillin, for example, was not an immediate or accelerated anaphylactic or urticarial reaction, cautious treatment with a cephalosporin is acceptable. From 3 to 7% of patients with a history of penicillin allergy experience an allergic reaction when treated with a cephalosporin, a rate 1.5 to 2 times that noted among patients who do not report a penicillin allergy.

Most antimicrobics cross the placenta and reach therapeutic concentrations in fetal tissues; thus, antibiotics, in general, should be administered during pregnancy only if absolutely required. The fetus should not be exposed to trimethoprim or rifampin, both of which are teratogens in animals; to metronidazole, which is mutagenic; or to clarithromycin, which has been associated with fetal toxicity in primates. Tetracyclines cause fetal bone changes, and in pregnant women are associated with increased risk for hepatotoxicity. If antimicrobial therapy is required during pregnancy, penicillins, β-lactam/β-lactamase inhibitor combinations, cephalosporins, and erythromycin are preferred. Data indicating safety during pregnancy are insufficient for clindamycin, vancomycin, azithromycin, and the aminoglycosides; hence these agents should be avoided, if possible. Many antibiotics appear in breast milk; antibiotics that pose a risk to the neonate or infant (chloramphenicol, sulfonamides, tetracyclines, and quinolones) must not be administered to nursing mothers. Generally, mothers are advised to temporarily discontinue nursing during periods of antimicrobial therapy.

The pharmacokinetics of antibiotics that are primarily excreted by the kidneys are significantly altered in patients with moderate to severe renal dysfunction. If antibiotic accumulation and potential toxicity are to be avoided, dosage adjustments, after an initial standard dose, are necessary when the antibiotics are administered to patients with renal dysfunction (Table 270–3).

Antibiotics that are metabolized in the liver or excreted in the bile should be used with caution when treating patients with severe liver failure (Table 270–3). The potential for antibiotics to interact

✓ **TABLE 270–3. DOSAGE, PHARMACOLOGIC FACTORS, AND ADJUSTMENT IN RENAL AND HEPATIC FAILURE**

Class/Agent	Dose* Systemic Infection	Oral Formulation	Peak Serum Concentration μg/ml	Protein Binding (%)	Normal Serum Half-Life (hr)	Dose Adjustment Hepatic Failure	Dose Adjustment Renal Failure	Serum Levels Affected by Dialysis‡
Aminoglycosides								
Amikacin	5–7 mg/kg/q8	—	35	0	2–3	No	Major	Yes (H, P)
Gentamicin	1.7 mg/kg/q8	—	7	0	2–3	No	Major	Yes (H, P)
Netilmicin	1.7 mg/kg/q8	—	7	0	2–3	No	Major	Yes (H, P)
Tobramycin	1.7 mg/kg/q8	—	7	0	2–3	No	Major	Yes (H, P)
Antituberculous Agents								
Ethambutol	15 mg/kg/d (PO)	Yes	2	10	1.5	No	Major	Yes (H, P)
Isoniazid	5 mg/kg/d (PO)	Yes	4.5	10	3	Yes	Minor	Yes (H, P)
Pyrazinamide	10 mg/kg/q8h (PO)	Yes	39	—	10	Yes	Yes	Yes (H)
Rifampin	10 mg/kg/d (PO)	Yes	7	70	3	Yes	Minor	No (H)
First-Generation Cephalosporins								
Cefadroxil	15 mg/kg/q12h (PO)	Yes	16	20	1.2	No	Yes	Yes (H)
Cefazolin	15 mg/kg/q8	—	80	80	2	No	Major	Yes (H) No (P)
Cephalexin	7 mg/kg/q6	Yes	18	15	1	No	Yes	Yes (H, P)
Cephalothin	30 mg/kg/q6	—	65	70	0.7	Minor	Yes	Yes (H, P)
Cephapirin	30 mg/kg/q6h	—	150	50	0.6	No	Yes	Yes (H, P)
Cephradine	30 mg/kg/q6h	Yes†	140	10	0.7	No	Yes	Yes (H, P)
Second-Generation Cephalosporins								
Cefaclor	7 mg/kg/q6 (PO)	Yes†	13	20	1	No	Yes	Yes (H) No (P)
Cefamandole	30 mg/kg/q6	—	150	70	1	No	Yes	Yes (H)
Cefmetazole	30 mg/kg/q12h	—	140	65	1.1	No	Yes	Yes (H)
Cefotetan	30 mg/kg/q12	—	230	85	3	No	Major	Yes (H)
Cefoxitin	30 mg/kg/q6	—	150	70	0.7	No	Yes	Yes (H) No (P)
Cefprozil	15 mg/kg/q12h (PO)	Yes	10	42	1.2	No	Yes	Yes (H)
Cefuroxime	15–20 mg/kg/q12h	—	100	50	1.5	No	Yes	Yes (H, P)
Cefuroxime axetil	7.5 mg/kg/q12h (PO)	Yes	9	50	1.2	No	Yes	Yes (H)
Third-Generation Cephalosporins								
Cefepime	30 mg/kg/q12h	—	193	20	2.1	No	Yes	Yes (H, P)
Cefixime	8 mg/kg/d (PO)	Yes	3.9	67	3.7	No	Yes	No (H, P)
Cefoperazone	30 mg/kg/q8–12	—	250	90	2	Some	No	Yes (H)
Cefotaxime	30 mg/kg/q6	—	130	50	1.2	Some	Minor	Yes (H) No (P)
Cefpodoxime proxetil	3–6 mg/kg/q12h (PO)	Yes	3.9	25	2.5	No	Yes	Yes (H)
Ceftazidime	30 mg/kg/q8	—	160	60	2	No	Major	Yes (H, P)
Ceftizoxime	30 mg/kg/q6–8	—	130	50	1.3	No	Minor	Yes (H) No (P)
Ceftriaxone	30 mg/kg/q12–24	—	250	90	8	No	No	No (H)
Penicillins								
Amoxicillin	7 mg/kg/q6 (PO)	Yes	6	20	1	No	Yes	Yes (H) No (P)
Ampicillin	30 mg/kg/q6	Yes†	100	20	1	No	Yes	Yes (H) No (P)
Azlocillin	50 mg/kg/q6	—	220	50	1	Minor	Major	Yes (H) No (P)
Carbenicillin	70 mg/kg/q4	—	300	50	1	Minor	Major	Yes (H, P)
Cloxacillin	7 mg/kg/q6 (PO)	Yes†	9	95	0.5	No	No	No (H, P)
Dicloxacillin	7 mg/kg/q6 (PO)	Yes†	18	97	0.5	No	Minor	No (H, P)
Methicillin	30 mg/kg/q4–6	—	100	30	0.5	No	Minor	Yes (H) No (P)
Mezlocillin	50 mg/kg/q6	—	260	50	1	Yes	Major	Yes (H) No (P)
Nafcillin	30 mg/kg/q4–6	—	160	90	0.5	Yes	No	No (H, P)
Oxacillin	30 mg/kg/q4–6	—	200	90	0.5	Yes	No	Yes (H, P)
Penicillin G	3–4 million U q4–6	Yes†	60	60	0.5	No	Yes	Yes (H) No (P)
Penicillin V	7 mg/kg/q6 (PO)	Yes	4	80	1	No	No	Yes (H) No (P)
Piperacillin	40 mg/kg/q6	—	240	50	1	Minor	Major	Yes (H)
Ticarcillin	40 mg/kg/q4–6	—	220	50	1	Minor	Major	Yes (H, P)
Quinolones								
Ciprofloxacin	7 mg/kg/q12 (PO)	Yes†	2–2.8	30	3	No	Yes	No (H, P)
Lomefloxacin	6 mg/kg/q24h	Yes	4	10	8		Yes	No (H, P)
Norfloxacin	6 mg/kg/q12 (PO)	Yes†	1.4–1.8	15	3	No	Yes	No (H, P)
Ofloxacin	6 mg/kg/q12h	Yes†	3–5	30	7		Yes	No (H, P)
Tetracyclines								
Doxycycline	1.5 mg/kg/q12–24	Yes	1.8–2.9	90	15–20	Avoid	No	No (H, P)
Minocycline	1.5 mg/kg/q12–24	Yes	2.2	90	15	No	Avoid	No (H, P)
Tetracycline	7 mg/kg/q6	Yes†	4	50	7	Avoid	Avoid	No (H, P)
Sulfonamides								
Sulfadiazine	15 mg/kg/q6	Yes	30	50	3	Avoid	Avoid	Unknown
Sulfamethoxazole	12 mg/kg/q8 (IV)	Yes	100	50	6	Avoid	Major	Yes (H) No (P)
Trimethoprim (used with sulfamethoxazole)	2.3 mg/kg/q8–12 (IV)	Yes	3–9	60	10	No	Avoid	Yes (H) No (P)
Sulfisoxazole	15 mg/kg/q6	Yes	60	50	6	Avoid	Major	Yes (H, P)
Macrolides-Lincosamides								
Azithromycin	4 mg/kg/q24h (PO)	Yes†	0.4	50	57 (tissue)	Unknown	Unknown	Unknown
Clarithromycin	7.5 mg/kg/q12h (PO)	Yes	2–3	70	7	No	Yes	Yes (H) No (P)
Clindamycin	7 mg/kg/q6	Yes	15	90	2.5	Some	No	No (H, P)
Erythromycin	7 mg/kg/q6 (PO)	Yes†	1.8	20	1.5	Some	No	No (H, P)
Other Agents								
Aztreonam	30 mg/kg/q8	—	250	60	2.0	No	Major	Yes (H, P)
Chloramphenicol	7–15 mg/kg/q6 (PO)	Yes	8–14	30	1.5	Some	No	Yes (H) No (P)
Imipenem	7.5 mg/kg/q6	—	40	15	1	No	Avoid	Yes (H)
Loracarbef	15 mg/kg/q12h (PO)	Yes†	18	25	1.2	No	Yes	Yes (H)
Meropenem	15 mg/kg/q8h	—	40		1.0	Unknown	Yes	Yes (H)
Metronidazole	7 mg/kg/q6	Yes	25	20	8	Yes	No	Yes (H) No (P)
Nitrofurantoin	1 mg/kg/q6 (PO)	Yes	nil	60	0.3	No	Avoid	Yes (H)
Spectinomycin	30 mg/kg/d	—	100	0	2	No	Avoid	Unknown
Vancomycin	15 mg/kg/q12h	Yes§	35	10	6	No	Major	No (H, P)

* mg/kg body weight at hour interval in patients with normal renal function; all doses are parenteral unless specified PO.
† Do not administer with food—absorption is decreased or delayed.
‡ H = hemodialysis; P = peritoneal dialysis.
§ Orally administered vancomycin is not absorbed; gastrointestinal tract lumen therapy only.

with other drugs that the patient is receiving is yet another important consideration that affects the selection of antimicrobial therapy (Table 270–4).

SPECIFIC ANTIMICROBIAL AGENTS

Although oversimplifying the process of selecting appropriate therapy, Table 270–5 lists the agents of choice and some of the alternative agents recommended for the treatment of infections caused by specific bacteria. Penicillin G remains the agent of choice for treatment of all stages of syphilis. Table 270–6 details the relative antibacterial activity of specific antimicrobics against organisms that

commonly cause infections. Because gram-negative bacilli commonly acquire resistance genes, antimicrobial susceptibility testing is required when treating serious infection caused by these organisms.

BROAD-SPECTRUM PENICILLINS AND RELATED COMPOUNDS. Selected side chains added to the β-lactam ring of the penicillin nucleus result in broad-spectrum penicillins that, while still inactivated by staphylococcal β-lactamase, possess enhanced activity against gram-negative bacilli. The aminopenicillins—ampi-

✔

TABLE 270–4. IMPORTANT ANTIBIOTIC-DRUG INTERACTIONS*

Antimicrobial Agent	Interacting Drug	Effect
Aminoglycosides	Amphotericin B, cyclosporin A, vancomycin	Increased nephrotoxicity
	Loop diuretics (bumetanide, furosemide, ethacrynic acid)	Increased ototoxicity (avoid)
	Carboxy/ureidopenicillins	Decreased aminoglycoside activity (renal failure only)
Cephalosporins		
MTT side chain	Warfarin, dicumarol	Increased anticoagulation, bleeding
MTT side chain	Alcohol	Disulfiram-like reaction
All	Loop diuretics	Nephrotoxicity
Chloramphenicol	Warfarin	Increased warfarin activity, increased anticoagulation
	Phenytoin	Increased serum phenytoin, phenytoin toxicity
	Sulfonylureas	Increased sulfonylurea, hypoglycemia
Clarithromycin,† erythromycin	Carbamazepine	Increased serum carbamazepine (avoid)
	Cyclosporin A	Increased serum cyclosporin A, nephrotoxicity
	Digoxin	Increased serum digoxin, toxicity
	Terfenadine, astemizole, loratadine	Increased antihistamine level, arrhythmia (avoid)
	Theophylline	Increased theophylline level, toxicity
Isoniazid	Warfarin	Increased warfarin activity, increased anticoagulation
	Alfentanil	Prolonged alfentanil activity
	Phenytoin	Increased serum phenytoin, phenytoin toxicity
	Disulfiram	Psychosis, behavioral change (avoid)
	Carbamazepine	Increased carbamazepine, toxicity (avoid)
	Rifampin	Additive hepatotoxicity
Metronidazole	Alcohol	Disulfiram-like reaction
	Disulfiram	Psychosis (avoid)
	Warfarin, dicumarol	Increased anticoagulation
	Phenobarbital	Decreased metronidazole
Penicillins		
Ampicillin/amoxicillin	Allopurinol	Increased rash
Ampicillin/carboxy-, ureidopenicillins	Oral contraceptives	Decreased contraceptive effect
	Probenecid	Increased serum penicillins
Fluoroquinolones		
All	Cimetidine	Increased antibiotic concentration
	Cyclosporin A	Increased serum cyclosporin A, nephrotoxicity
	Multivalent cations (Ca, Mg, Fe, Zn, Al orally)	Decreased absorption of quinolones
	Sucralfate	Decreased absorption of quinolones
	Warfarin	Increased anticoagulation
	Probenecid	Increased fluoroquinolone
Ciprofloxacin, enoxacin	Theophylline	Increased serum theophylline, toxicity
Norfloxacin, pefloxacin	Caffeine	Increased serum caffeine, insomnia, restlessness
Enoxacin	Fenbufen	Seizures
Rifampin‡	Corticosteroids	Decreased corticosteroid, supplement dose
	Cyclosporin A	Decreased cyclosporin A
	Methadone	Decreased serum methadone, withdrawal
	Phenytoin	Decreased serum phenytoin
	Warfarin, dicumarol	Decreased anticoagulation, need large doses
	Oral contraceptives	Decreased contraceptive effect
	Sulfonylureas	Decreased sulfonylurea, hyperglycemia
	Theophylline	Decreased serum theophylline
	Quinidine, β-blocker	Decreased quinidine, β-blocker
Rifabutin	Clarithromycin	Uveitis
Sulfonamides	Cyclosporin A	Decreased serum cyclosporin A
	Phenytoin	Increased serum phenytoin, toxicity
	Warfarin	Increased warfarin effect
	Sulfonylureas	Increased sulfonylurea, hypoglycemia
Trimethoprim	Azathioprine	Increased leukopenia
	Dapsone	Increased serum dapsone and trimethoprim, increased methemoglobinemia
Tetracycline	Multivalent cations (Ca, Al, Mg, Bi, Zn, Fe)	Decreased tetracycline absorption
	Barbiturates, carbamazepine	Decreased doxycycline
	Digoxin	Increased digoxin, toxicity
	Phenytoin	Decreased doxycycline
	Methoxyflurane (Penthrane)	Severe nephrotoxicity (avoid)

* Not all interactions have been listed.
† Interactions with azithromycin not adequately studied.
‡ Multiple other rifampin interactions mediated through cytochrome system.
MTT = methylthiotetrazole ring (cefamandole, cefotetan, cefmetazole, cefoperazone, moxalactam, cefmenoxime).

✔ TABLE 270–5. ANTIBACTERIAL DRUGS OF CHOICE FOR INFECTIONS CAUSED BY SELECTED BACTERIA

Infecting Organism	Agent of Choice*	Alternative Agent†
Gram-Positive Cocci		
S. aureus/coagulase-negative staphylococci		
Nonpenicillinase producing	Penicillin G or V	Cephalosporin§, vancomycin, clindamycin, erythromycin
Penicillinase producing	Nafcillin, oxacillin	Cephalosporin§, vancomycin, clindamycin, erythromycin, imipenem, β-lactam/β-lactamase inhibitor combinations
Methicillin resistant‡	Vancomycin	Trimethoprim-sulfamethoxazole, minocycline, teicoplanin (investigational)
β-hemolytic streptococci (groups A, B, C, G)	Penicillin G or V	Cephalosporin§, erythromycin, vancomycin, clindamycin
Viridans streptococci, *Streptococcus bovis*	Penicillin G	Cephalosporin§, vancomycin, erythromycin
Enterococci‡		
Uncomplicated urinary tract infection	Ampicillin, amoxicillin	Nitrofurantoin, quinolone¶
Moderately severe wound infection	Ampicillin	Penicillin G, vancomycin
Serious infection: Endocarditis or meningitis	Ampicillin plus gentamicin or streptomycin	Vancomycin plus gentamicin or streptomycin (test for high-level aminoglycoside resistance)
Streptococcus pneumoniae‡		
Pneumonia, upper respiratory tract infection	Penicillin G, amoxicillin	Cephalosporin, erythromycin, clindamycin, vancomycin
Meningitis	Ceftriaxone, cefotaxime	Ceftriaxone plus vancomycin ± rifampin, vancomycin + rifampin, penicillin G (if MIC < 0.1 µg/ml)
Gram-Negative Cocci		
N. gonorrhoeae	Ceftriaxone, cefixime	Second- or other third-generation cephalosporins**, quinolones¶, spectinomycin, trimethoprim-sulfamethoxazole, azithromycin (choices vary by sites of infection)
N. meningitidis	Penicillin G	Third-generation cephalosporin**, chloramphenicol, sulfonamide (if susceptible)
Moraxella catarrhalis	Trimethoprim-sulfamethoxazole	Amoxicillin/clavulanate, third-generation cephalosporin**, cefuroxime, clarithromycin
Gram-Positive Bacilli		
Bacillus anthracis (anthrax)	Penicillin G	Erythromycin, tetracycline
Corynebacterium diphtheriae	Erythromycin	Penicillin G
Corynebacterium species	Penicillin + gentamicin	Vancomycin
Listeria monocytogenes	Ampicillin or penicillin G ± gentamicin	Trimethoprim-sulfamethoxazole, vancomycin, tetracycline
Clostridium perfringens	Penicillin G	Metronidazole, chloramphenicol, imipenem, tetracycline
Clostridium difficile	Metronidazole	Vancomycin (oral only), bacitracin
Gram-Negative Bacilli‡		
Acinetobacter species	Imipenem ± gentamicin	Ureidopenicillin; aminoglycoside
Bordetella pertussis (pertussis)	Erythromycin	Trimethoprim-sulfamethoxazole, ampicillin
Brucella species (brucellosis)	Tetracycline + gentamicin or streptomycin	Tetracycline + rifampin, chloramphenicol ± streptomycin, trimethoprim-sulfamethoxazole
Campylobacter fetus spp. *jejuni*	Erythromycin, quinolone¶	Tetracycline
Enterobacter species	Imipenem, aminoglycoside††	Quinolone¶, third-generation cephalosporin**, cefepime, trimethoprim-sulfamethoxazole
Eikenella corrodens	Penicillin G, ampicillin	Trimethoprim-sulfamethoxazole, tetracycline, cefoxitin, third-generation cephalosporin**
E. coli		
Uncomplicated urinary tract infection	Trimethoprim-sulfamethoxazole	Ampicillin, cephalosporin§, trimethoprim, quinolone¶, tetracycline
Systemic infection	Third-generation cephalosporin**	Aminoglycoside††, β-lactam/β-lactamase inhibitor, aztreonam, trimethoprim-sulfamethoxazole

cillin and amoxicillin—have expanded the penicillin spectrum to include many of the gram-negative bacilli. However, subsequent acquisition of β-lactamase genes by many of these species, except *P. mirabilis,* has limited the use of aminopenicillins. Notably, 25% of *E. coli* and at least 15% of *H. influenzae* are resistant to these agents. Bacteria that are susceptible to penicillin G remain susceptible to ampicillin and amoxicillin. Although the *in vitro* antibacterial spectra of amoxicillin and ampicillin are equivalent, amoxicillin is more fully absorbed from the gastrointestinal tract than ampicillin. Amoxicillin is the recommended antimicrobic for prophylaxis against endocarditis at the time of dental procedures. Aminopenicillins are effective therapy for early Lyme disease (*Borrelia burgdorferi* infection) as are doxycycline, cefuroxime axetil, clarithromycin, and azithromycin.

The carboxypenicillins—carbenicillin and ticarcillin—and the ureidopenicillins—azlocillin, mezlocillin, and piperacillin—comprise the remaining broad-spectrum penicillins available in the United States. Carbenicillin and ticarcillin extended the antibacterial spectrum of penicillins to include indole-positive *Proteus* species, some *Enterobacter* species, *Acinetobacter,* and importantly *Pseudomonas aeruginosa.* The spectra of antibacterial activity of carbenicillin and ticarcillin are similar; however, the potency of ticarcillin against *P. aeruginosa* is twice that of carbenicillin. Mezlocillin and piperacillin are more active against the Enterobacteriaceae than are carbenicillin, ticarcillin, and azlocillin. While the

activity of mezlocillin against *P. aeruginosa* is similar to that of ticarcillin, piperacillin and azlocillin are more potent antipseudomonas agents than either ticarcillin or mezlocillin. The carboxypenicillins and ureidopenicillins are important agents for treating serious gram-negative infection; however, in this setting they are combined with an aminoglycoside because of their inactivation by various β-lactamases and the potential emergence of resistance.

To further expand their antimicrobial activity, agents from each group of broad-spectrum penicillins have been combined with a β-lactamase inhibitor. The β-lactamase inhibitors, which exert only weak antibacterial activity themselves, irreversibly bind and inhibit staphylococcal β-lactamase, many plasmid-mediated β-lactamases of gram-negative bacilli, the ESBL's, and the chromosomal β-lactamases of *Klebsiella* spp. and *Bacteroides* spp. Unfortunately, they do not inhibit the Bush class I chromosomal β-lactamases of *Enterobacter* spp., *Serratia,* and *P. aeruginosa.* Among the penicillin/β-lactamase inhibitor combinations, ampicillin-sulbactam, ticarcillin-clavulanate, and piperacillin-tazobactam are available for parenteral use, and amoxicillin-clavulanate is available for oral administration.

CEPHALOSPORINS. The cephalosporins contain a nucleus in which the β-lactam ring is fused to a six-membered dihydrothiazine ring (in contrast to the five-membered thiazolidine ring in the analogous position in penicillins). Substituent side chains are added to the β-lactam ring to alter antimicrobial activity and to the dihydrothiazine ring to alter metabolic and pharmacokinetic properties.

TABLE 270–5. ANTIBACTERIAL DRUGS OF CHOICE FOR INFECTIONS CAUSED BY SELECTED BACTERIA Continued

Infecting Organism	Agent of Choice*	Alternative Agent†
Helicobacter pylori	Tetracycline + metronidazole + bismuth subsalicylate	Amoxicillin + metronidazole + bismuth subsalicylate, tetracycline + clarithromycin + bismuth subsalicylate
Francisella tularensis (tularemia)	Streptomycin, gentamicin	Tetracycline, chloramphenicol
H. influenzae		
Meningitis, bacteremia	Ceftriaxone, cefotaxime	Trimethoprim-sulfamethoxazole, ampicillin (if β-lactamase negative)
Other infection	Ampicillin/clavulanate, amoxicillin/clavulanate	Trimethoprim-sulfamethoxazole, cefuroxime, quinolone,¶ third-generation cephalosporin**
Haemophilus ducreyi (chancroid)	Ceftriaxone	Azithromycin, erythromycin, amoxicillin/clavulanate, quinolone¶
Klebsiella pneumoniae/oxytoca	Aminoglycosides††, third-generation cephalosporin**	First- or second-generation cephalosporin, quinolone¶, ureidopenicillin, imipenem, aztreonam, β-lactam/β-lactamase inhibitor
Legionella pneumophila	Erythromycin ± rifampin	Quinolone¶ ± rifampin
Nocardia asteroides	Sulfonamides (high dose)	Trimethoprim-sulfamethoxazole, minocycline, amoxicillin/clavulanate
Pasteurella multocida	Penicillin G	Tetracycline, amoxicillin/clavulanate, third-generation cephalosporin**
Proteus mirabilis	Ampicillin	Cephalosporin†, trimethoprim-sulfamethoxazole, aminoglycoside††
Proteus (indole positive)	Third-generation cephalosporin	Imipenem, aminoglycoside††, trimethoprim-sulfamethoxazole, quinolone¶
Rochalimaea (Bartonella) henselae/quintana	Erythromycin	Tetracycline, clarithromycin
Salmonella spp.	Ceftriaxone, quinolone¶	Chloramphenicol, trimethoprim-sulfamethoxazole
Serratia marcescens	Aminoglycoside††, third-generation cephalosporin**	Imipenem, quinolone,¶ aztreonam
Shigella spp.	Quinolone¶, norfloxacin	Trimethoprim-sulfamethoxazole, ceftriaxone, chloramphenicol
Pseudomonas aeruginosa		
Urinary tract infection	Quinolone¶, ureidopenicillin	Aminoglycoside††, ceftazidime, imipenem, aztreonam
Pneumonia, bacteremia	Aminoglycoside†† + ureidopenicillin or ceftazidime	Imipenem + aminoglycoside††, aztreonam + aminoglycoside††
Vibrio vulnificus	Tetracycline + ceftazidime	Chloramphenicol
Xanthomonas multiphilia	Trimethoprim-sulfamethoxazole	Ticarcillin/clavulanate, quinolone¶
Yersinia pestis (plague)	Streptomycin, gentamicin	Tetracycline, chloramphenicol
Anaerobic Gram-Negative		
Bacteroides spp.		
Oropharyngeal isolates	Penicillin G	Metronidazole, clindamycin, cefoxitin, cefotetan, cefmetazole, chloramphenicol, β-lactam/β-lactamase inhibitor
Bacteroides fragilis group	Metronidazole	Cefoxitin, cefotetan, clindamycin, imipenem, β-lactam/β-lactamase inhibitor, chloramphenicol

* Dose and route of administration must be adjusted for severity of illness and host characteristics (organ dysfunction, allergy).
† List of alternative agents is not fully inclusive; confirm susceptibility *in vitro*.
‡ Must test susceptibility; resistant strains are increasingly frequent.
§ First-generation cephalosporin preferred (cephalothin, cephapirin, cephradine, cephalexin, cefazolin).
¶ Ciprofloxacin, lomefloxacin, ofloxacin (or for urinary tract infection, norfloxacin).
** Third-generation cephalosporins for this indication include ceftriaxone, cefotaxime, ceftizoxime.
†† Aminoglycosides for this indication include gentamicin, tobramycin, netilmicin, amikacin.

A widely accepted system classifies the cephalosporins into "three generations" on the basis of their spectrum of microbiologic activity. With each successive generation, cephalosporins have increasing antibacterial activity against gram-negative bacilli, and to a degree, decreasing antibacterial activity against gram-positive bacteria. For treatment of serious *S. aureus* infections in patients intolerant of antistaphylococcal penicillins, first-generation cephalosporins are preferred. The cephamycins (cefoxitin, cefotetan, and cefmetazole) are grouped with the second-generation cephalosporins and are active against many gram-negative anaerobic bacteria, including many *B. fragilis*. All cephalosporins are inactive against enterococci, methicillin-resistant staphylococci, and *L. monocytogenes*. Only ceftazidime and cefepime possess significant antipseudomonal activity, and only cefepime is active against *Enterobacter* spp. and related organisms that have been induced to produce Bush I chromosomal β-lactamases. ESBL production by *Klebsiella* spp. renders these organisms resistant to third-generation cephalosporins. Among the cephalosporins, only the third-generation agents retain clinically relevant activity against *S. pneumoniae* that are resistant to penicillin. Some strains of pneumococci have become resistant to third-generation cephalosporins. Cefazolin, the "workhorse" first-generation cephalosporin, is widely used for perioperative prophylaxis in surgical procedures involving foreign body implantation and for many clean and clean-contaminated operations, except those involving the colon. Cefotaxime, ceftriaxone, and ceftizoxime are the agents of choice for treatment of meningitis due to enteric gram-negative bacilli (except *Enterobacter* spp.) and are used widely in initial empiric therapy for meningitis in children (after the neonate period) and adults. Ceftazidime is the agent of choice for meningitis caused by *P. aeruginosa*. Ceftriaxone is the drug of choice for treatment of late stages of Lyme disease.

Adverse reactions caused by the cephalosporins are independent of their antibacterial spectra. Hypersensitivity cross-reactions between cephalosporins are not universal; nevertheless, they occur more frequently than penicillin-cephalosporin cross-reactions. There are no skin test reagents that predict cephalosporin hypersensitivity, and testing with the drug in question is not recommended. Whereas aztreonam can be administered to most patients with hypersensitivity to penicillins and cephalosporins, use of imipenem may result in cross-reactions. A methylthiotetrazole moiety on the dihydrothiazine ring (cefamandole, cefoperazone, cefotetan, moxalactam, cefmenoxime, and cefmetazole) is associated with unique reactions (Table 270–7).

COMBINATION ANTIMICROBIAL THERAPY

There are several rationales for administering antibiotics in combination: (1) A broader, more comprehensive antibacterial effect when treating a severe infection of unknown cause may be achieved; (2) the bacteria causing mixed infection may exceed the antibacterial range of a single agent; (3) combination therapy may

TABLE 270–6. ACTIVITY OF MAJOR ANTIBIOTICS AGAINST SELECTED ORGANISMS*

Antibiotic	Streptococci	Streptococcus pneumoniae†	Enterococci‡	Staphylococcus aureus (MS)	Staphylococcus aureus (MR)	Coagulase-negative staphylococci†	Listeria monocytogenes	Neisseria gonorrhoeae	Neisseria meningitidis	Moraxella catarrhalis	Haemophilus influenzae	Escherichia coli	Enterobacter spp.	Klebsiella spp.	Proteus mirabilis	Proteus vulgaris	Salmonella spp.	Serratia spp.	Shigella spp.	Acinetobacter spp.	Pseudomonas aeruginosa	Xanthomonas maltophilia	Pasteurella multocida	Vibrio vulnificus	Legionella spp.	Chlamydia spp.	Mycoplasma pneumoniae	Rickettsia spp.	Bacteroides fragilis group#	Clostridium spp. (not C. difficile)	Prevotella melaninogenicus	Actinomyces spp.
Penicillin G	+	±	+	0	0	0	+	±	+	0	0	0	0	0	±	0	0	0	0	0	0	0	+	±	0	0	0	0	0	+	+	+
Oxacillin[1]	+	±	0	+	0	±	0	0	0	0	0	0	0	0	0	0	0	0	0	0	0	0	0	0	0	0	0	0	0	0	0	0
Ampicillin[2]	+	+	+	0	0	0	+	±	+	0	±	±	0	0	+	0	+	0	±	0	0	0	+	+	0	0	0	0	0	+	+	+
Ampicillin-sulbactam[2]	+	+	+	+	±	±	+	+	+	+	+	+	±	+	+	0	+	0	±	±	0	0	+	+	0	0	0	0	+	+	+	+
Ticarcillin	+	±	+	0	0	0	+	+	+	0	+	+	±	0	+	+	+	0	+	0	+	±	+	+	0	0	0	0	0	+	+	+
Ticarcillin-clavulanate	+	+	+	+	±	±	+	+	+	+	+	+	±	+	+	+	+	±	+	±	+	±	+	+	0	0	0	0	+	+	+	+
Piperacillin	+	+	+	0	0	±	+	+	+	0	+	+	±	+	+	+	+	±	+	±	+	±	+	+	0	0	0	0	+	0	+	+
Piperacillin-tazobactam	+	+	+	+	0	±	+	+	+	+	+	+	±	+	+	+	+	±	+	±	+	±	+	ND	0	0	0	0	+	+	+	+
Aztreonam	0	0	0	0	0	0	0	±	+	+	+	+	±	+	+	+	+	+	+	0	+	0	0	ND	0	0	0	0	0	0	0	0
Imipenem	+	+	±	+	0	±	+	+	+	+	+	+	+	+	+	+	+	+	+	±	+	0	+	ND	ND	0	0	0	+	+	+	+
Cefazolin[3]	+	+	0	+	0	±	0	±	+	+	±	+	0	+	+	0	+	0	+	±	0	0	+	±	0	0	0	0	0	+	±	+
Cefotetan[4]	+	+	0	+	0	±	0	+	+	+	+	+	±	+	+	+	+	+	+	0	0	0	+	0	0	0	0	0	±	+	+	+
Cefoxitin	+	+	0	+	0	±	0	+	+	+	+	+	0	+	+	+	+	+	+	0	0	0	+	0	0	0	0	0	+	+	+	+
Cefuroxime	+	+	0	+	0	±	0	+	+	+	+	+	±	+	+	+	+	+	+	0	0	0	+	+	0	0	0	0	0	+	+	+
Cefotaxime	+	+	0	+	0	±	0	+	+	+	+	+	±	+	+	+	+	+	+	±	0	0	+	+	0	0	0	0	±	+	+	+
Ceftriaxone	+	+	0	+	0	±	0	+	+	+	+	+	±	+	+	+	+	+	+	±	0	0	+	+	0	0	0	0	0	+	+	+
Ceftazidime	+	+	0	+	0	±	0	+	+	+	+	+	±	+	+	+	+	+	+	±	+	±	+	+	0	0	0	0	±	+	+	+
Cefepime	+	+	0	+	0	±	0	+	+	+	+	+	+	+	+	+	+	+	+	±	+	0	+	ND	0	ND	0	0	0	ND	ND	ND
Cephalexin[3]	+	+	0	+	0	±	0	0	0	+	±	+	0	+	+	0	+	0	+	0	0	0	0	0	0	0	0	0	0	+	+	+
Cefuroxime axetil	+	+	0	+	0	±	0	+	+	+	+	+	0	+	+	0	+	0	+	0	0	±	+	0	0	0	0	0	0	+	+	+
Loracarbef	+	+	0	±	0	±	0	+	+	+	±	+	0	+	+	0	+	0	0	0	0	0	+	ND	0	ND	0	ND	0	ND	ND	ND
Cefixime	+	+	0	0	0	0	0	+	+	+	+	+	0	+	+	0	+	+	+	0	0	0	0	0	0	0	0	0	0	0	+	+
Cefpodoxime proxetil	+	+	0	+	0	0	0	0	+	+	+	+	0	+	+	0	0	+	0	0	0	0	+	+	0	ND	0	0	0	ND	ND	ND
Gentamicin[5]	C/S	ND	C/S	C/S	±	C/S	±	0	0	0	±	+	+	+	+	±	+	+	0	±	+	0	0	+	0	0	0	0	0	0	0	0
Clindamycin	+	+	0	+	±	±	ND	0	0	0	0	0	0	0	0	0	0	0	0	0	0	0	0	0	0	ND	0	0	+	+	+	+
Clarithromycin[6]	+	+	0	±	0	±	±	±	0	+	±	0	0	0	0	0	0	0	0	0	0	0	±	ND	+	+	+	ND	0	±	+	+
Erythromycin	+	+	0	±	0	±	±	0	+	+	±	0	0	0	0	0	0	0	0	0	0	0	0	ND	+	+	+	+	0	+	+	+
Doxycycline[7]	±	±	±	±	+	0	±	0	±	+	+	0	0	0	0	0	0	0	0	±	0	0	+	±	0	+	+	+	0	±	±	±
Vancomycin	+	+	+	+	+	+	+	0	0	0	0	0	0	0	0	0	0	0	0	0	0	0	0	0	0	0	0	0	0	+	+	+
Ciprofloxacin	±	±	±	±	0	±	±	0	+	+	+	+	+	+	+	+	+	+	+	±	+	0	+	0	+	+	+	+	0	0	0	ND
Ofloxacin	±	±	±	±	0	±	±	+	+	+	+	+	+	+	+	+	+	+	+	±	±	0	+	0	+	+	+	ND	0	±	0	ND

TABLE 270-6. ACTIVITY OF MAJOR ANTIBIOTICS AGAINST SELECTED ORGANISMS* *Continued*

	Streptococci	Streptococcus pneumoniae†	Enterococci‡	Staphylococcus aureus (MS)	Staphylococcus aureus (MR)	Coagulase-negative staphylococciø	Listeria monocytogenes	Neisseria gonorrhoeae	Neisseria meningitidis	Moraxella catarrhalis	Haemophilus influenzae	Escherichia coli	Enterobacter spp.	Klebsiella spp.	Proteus mirabilis	Proteus vulgaris	Salmonella spp.	Serratia spp.	Shigella spp.	Acinetobacter spp.	Pseudomonas aeruginosa	Xanthomonas maltophilia	Pasteurella multocida	Vibrio vulnificus	Legionella spp.	Chlamydia spp.	Mycoplasma pneumoniae	Rickettsia spp.	Bacteroides fragilis group#	Clostridium spp. (not C. difficile)	Prevotella melaninogenicus	Actinomyces spp.
Metronidazole	0	0	0	0	0	0	0	0	0	0	0	0	0	0	0	0	0	0	0	0	0	0	0	0	0	0	0	0	+	+	+	0
Trimethoprim-sulfamethoxazole	+	+	0	+	±	±	+	±	±	+	+	+	±	+	+	0	+	+	+	0	0	+	±	+	+	0	0	0	ND	ND	ND	ND
Chloramphenicol	+	+	0	±	0	0	±	+	+	+	+	+	0	±	+	±	+	0	0	0	0	+	+	+	C/S	+	+	+	+	+	+	+
Rifampin[8]	ND	C/S	ND	C/S	C/S	C/S	C/S	ND	+	ND	+	ND	0	±	ND	±	ND	0	ND	ND	0	ND	ND	ND	C/S	ND	ND	±	ND	ND	ND	ND

* Activity estimate is based on *in vitro* susceptibility and, where available, the results of treatment; activity against individual gram-negative facultative bacilli within a given species is difficult to predict. Discrepancies may exist between *in vitro* antimicrobial activity and clinical efficacy (especially for intracellular pathogens); review of disease-specific therapeutic recommendations is advised.

0 = uniformly or frequently resistant.
+ = usually susceptible.
± = variable susceptibility.
C/S = used in combination or for synergy.
ND = insufficient or no data.

1 Similar activity for methicillin, nafcillin, cloxacillin, dicloxacillin.
2 Similar activity for amoxicillin and amoxicillin/clavulanate, respectively.
3 Similar activity for other first-generation cephalosporins.
4 Similar activity for cefmetazole.
5 Similar activity against gram-negative bacilli for tobramycin, netilmicin; resistance of gram-negative rods to amikacin less frequent.
6 Similar activity for azithromycin.
7 Similar activity for other tetracyclines.
8 Broad spectrum of activity, but resistance emerges rapidly; limit use to combination therapy or eradication of meningococcal and *H. influenzae* pharyngeal carriage.

† Relative and full resistance to penicillin increasingly prevalent; resistant to first- and second-generation cephalosporins parallels that to penicillin.
‡ *E. faecium* intrinsically more resistant than *E. faecalis*; resistance to penicillin, ampicillin, vancomycin, and aminoglycosides (high level) increasingly frequent.
ø Many nosocomially acquired strains are methicillin resistant.
Some of the *Bacteroides fragilis* group (*B. thetaiotaomicron, B. distasonis, B. ovatus, B. vulgatus*) are more resistant than *B. fragilis*.

TABLE 270–7. UNTOWARD EFFECTS OF ANTIMICROBIAL AGENTS*

Agent	Target—Manifestation						
	General	Skin	GI Tract	Blood Cells	Kidney	Nervous System	Other
Sulfonamides	Hypersensitivity, anaphylaxis, serum sickness; fever	Rash, Stevens-Johnson syndrome, photosensitivity	Hepatitis	Hemolysis (G-6-PD deficiency), agranulocytosis, marrow suppression	Crystalluria	Neuropathy	Vasculitis
Trimethoprim with/without sulfamethoxazole†	Fever	Rash, erythema multiforme, Stevens-Johnson syndrome, TEN‡	Hepatitis, pancreatitis	Marrow suppression	Hyperkalemia, acute renal failure		
Penicillin	Hypersensitivity, anaphylaxis, Jarisch-Herxheimer reaction (syphilis), serum sickness	Rash, urticaria, erythema multiforme	Diarrhea (ampicillin, amoxicillin/clavulanate), hepatitis (oxacillin)	Coombs' test positive, impaired platelet function (carbenicillin, ticarcillin), leukopenia, thrombocytopenia	Nephritis (methicillin), hypokalemia, alkalosis (carboxy-, ureidopenicillins)	Seizures, twitching (high doses, renal failure)	Inactivate aminoglycosides when admixed, possible with concurrent therapy in renal failure
Cephalosporins	Serum sickness (cefaclor), hypersensitivity, anaphylaxis (rare)	Rash, urticaria	Diarrhea (cefoperazone), hepatic dysfunction, precipitates in bile (ceftriaxone), mild increase in LFT‡	Neutropenia, increased prothrombin time–bleeding (relates to MTT‡ side chain), impaired platelet function (moxalactam), Coombs' test positive	Enhance aminoglycoside toxicity, acute renal failure (rare), nephritis		Disulfiram-like reaction with concurrent alcohol use (MTT‡ side chain)
Carbapenems	Hypersensitivity	Rash, urticaria, erythema multiforme	Nausea, vomiting, abnormal LFT‡	Bone marrow suppression, Coombs' test positive	Renal dysfunction	Seizures, myoclonus	
Chloramphenicol	Fever			Marrow suppression (dose related), aplastic anemia		Optic neuritis, neuropathy	Circulatory collapse (gray baby syndrome–neonate)
Tetracyclines	Allergy	Photosensitization (doxycycline, demeclocycline)	Hepatotoxicity in azotemia or pregnancy, GI discomfort		Catabolic aggravation of azotemia (except doxycycline)	Vertigo (minocycline)	Deposition in bone (dysplasia) and teeth (staining)
Erythromycin	Fever	Rash	GI discomfort, nausea, cholestatic jaundice (erythromycin estolate)			Decreased hearing	Phlebitis if given through peripheral veins
Metronidazole	Headache, allergy		Nausea, metallic taste, pancreatitis	Leukopenia		Peripheral neuropathy, ataxia	Mutagenic, carcinogenic in rodents; disulfiram-like reaction with alcohol
Vancomycin	Allergy, fever	Rash		Leukopenia, thrombocytopenia	Nephrotoxic with aminoglycoside	Decreased hearing (serum > 50 µg/ml), neuropathy	Histamine release with flushing and hypotension (infusion <1 hr–antihistamines prevent)
Aminoglycosides	Fever	Rash			Renal failure	Irreversible vestibular toxicity (streptomycin, gentamicin, tobramycin), irreversible auditory damage (kanamycin, netilmicin, amikacin), neuromuscular blockade (with anesthetics and myasthenia–calcium reverses)	
Quinolones	Headache, allergy, anaphylaxis (rare)	Rash, photosensitization (pefloxacin, fleroxacin), urticaria	GI distress, LFT‡ abnormalities			Dizziness, insomnia, nervousness, tremors, visual changes, seizures, pseudotumor cerebri	Cartilage deposition and arthropathy (animal studies)

* Not all reactions are listed; check other sources for unusual reactions.
† Reactions to sulfonamides are not repeated.
‡ TEN = toxic epidermal necrolysis; MTT = methylthiotetrazole ring; LFT = liver function tests.

decrease the opportunity for the emergence of resistant bacteria; and (4) antibiotics administered concurrently may interact to exert an enhanced (synergistic) or additive antibacterial effect. An improvement in outcome of infection achieved by the enhanced antibacterial effect of combination therapy is seen in ampicillin-gentamicin therapy of enterococcal endocarditis, antipseudomonal penicillin-tobramycin therapy of *P. aeruginosa* endocarditis, and the synergistic β-lactam plus aminoglycoside therapy of bacterial infection in the neutropenic patient.

In spite of laudable goals, the end result of the combination therapy is not always favorable. Antibiotics administered as combination therapy may interact in antagonistic fashion (the net effect of the combination is less than that of the most effective of the agents acting individually). Antagonism was demonstrated clinically with penicillin and tetracycline treatment of pneumococcal meningitis. Antagonism is difficult to demonstrate clinically, but must remain a concern when antibiotics are used in combination. Additionally, administering multiple antibiotics may increase the risk for adverse events, especially unanticipated drug-drug interactions. Therapy with multiple antibiotics may increase selective pressure, leading to emergence of resistant bacteria or to colonization by fungi. For these reasons it is desirable to use targeted single-antibiotic therapy whenever possible.

DURATION OF THERAPY

There is no easy formula to determine optimal duration of therapy. One must weigh the site of infection, the patient as a host, the pathogen involved and its antimicrobial susceptibility, the response to treatment, the toxicity of the regimen, and the hazards of failure occasioned by terminating therapy prematurely. When the infecting organisms are vegetative, as in the vegetation of endocarditis, more prolonged therapy is required to eradicate the bacteria. Patients with impaired host defenses are treated with longer courses of therapy, assuming that host defenses will play less of a role in terminating infection. Superficial mucosal infection can be cured by single-dose therapy as noted with ceftriaxone, cefixime, or fluoroquinolone treatment of uncomplicated genitourinary gonorrhea. Single-dose therapy was also effective for bacterial cystitis, although 3-day short-course therapy is now preferred. Decisions regarding duration of therapy often are based on published trials and studies in which the goal was not to examine the impact of duration of therapy on outcome but rather to assess a predefined regimen. It is likely that antibiotic therapy is often excessive in length. This is not desirable in that it exacerbates cost of treatment, increases the risks of adverse events, and exerts unnecessary selective pressure on bacteria to become resistant.

ANTIBIOTIC TOXICITY AND UNTOWARD REACTIONS

Antibiotics commonly cause adverse drug reactions (Table 270–7). The majority of adverse events are mild, short lived, and resolve when the offending drug is withdrawn. Increasingly, untoward reactions are the manifestation of interactions between an antimicrobic and another medication that the patient is receiving (see Table 270–4).

FAILURE OF THERAPY

The persistence of fever and other signs of infection during antibiotic therapy calls for careful reassessment of the patient. The physician must reconsider the antimicrobials that have been administered in the light of available microbiologic data and seek new culture data that would explain the failure of therapy. Alternative explanations for fever must be considered; these range from a new superimposed infection, e.g., nosocomial intravenous catheter-related bacteremia, to a noninfectious complication, e.g., a pulmonary embolus, or a drug reaction. If the reassessment suggests that the diagnosis is correct, if the microbiology and clinical sequence of events support the antibiotic therapy given, and if no other explanations are noted, reasons for failure of appropriate therapy must be considered. These include (1) the presence of anatomic abnormalities or an obstructed drainage system; (2) an undrained abscess; (3) the presence of a foreign body or the equivalent (renal calculus, osteomyelitic sequestrum) at the site of infection; (4) infection in infarcted tissue; (5) emergence of resistance in the original pathogen or a resistant superinfecting organism; and (6) suboptimal effect of antibiotic therapy because of atypical disposition of the antibiotic, poor penetration to the site, or inactivation of the antibiotic. The physician must search diligently to explain and correct the antibiotic failure.

Bennett WM, Swan SK: Drug therapy in renal disease (chronic renal failure, appendix A). *In* Rubenstein E (ed.): Scientific American Medicine. New York, Scientific American, 1994, pp. A2–11. *Highly practical guide to dose reduction of antibiotics in renal failure. Updated annually.*

Davies J: Inactivation of antibiotics and the dissemination of resistance genes. Science 264:375, 1994. *Detailed discussion of the major mechanisms whereby bacteria inactivate antibiotics. The original sources of the genes conveying these abilities are considered.*

Mandell GL, Sande MA: Antimicrobial agents: Penicillins, cephalosporins, and other beta-lactam antibiotics. *In* Gilman AG, Rall TW, Nies AS, Taylor P (eds.): The Pharmacologic Basis of Therapeutics. Elmsford, NY, Pergamon Press, 1990, pp. 1065–1097. *Scholarly authoritative review of β-lactam antibiotics. This is best suited for reader seeking fundamental rather than clinical view of this core group of antibiotics.*

Neu HC: Pathophysiologic basis for use of third-generation cephalosporins. Am J Med 88:3S, 1990. *Detailed consideration of sophisticated clinical use of broad-spectrum cephalosporins.*

Neu HC: Quinolone antimicrobial agents. Ann Rev Med 43:465, 1992. *This well-referenced review of this important class of agents addresses chemistry, antibiotic activity, pharmacology, and appropriate clinical use.*

Neu HC: The crisis in antibiotic resistance. Science 257:1064, 1992. *Excellent review of mechanisms and epidemiology of antibiotic resistance, viewed from organism-by-organism perspective.*

Nightingale CH, Quintiliani R, Nicolau DP: Intelligent dosing of antimicrobials. *In* Remington JS, Swartz MN (eds.): Current Clinical Topics in Infectious Diseases. Boston, Blackwell Scientific Publications, 1994, vol. 14, pp. 252–265. *Clinically oriented, detailed discussion of pharmacodynamics and pharmacodynamic strategies for antibiotic dosing at one hospital. An important view of antibiotic dosing that may gain increasing support.*

Nikaido H: Prevention of drug access to bacterial targets: Permeability barriers and active efflux. Science 264:382, 1994. *Detailed consideration of permeability and active efflux mechanisms as used by bacteria in resisting antibiotics. Special attention is directed toward active efflux systems increasingly recognized as important in antibiotic resistance.*

Sande MA, Mandell GL: Antimicrobial agents: The aminoglycosides. *In* Gilman AG, Rall TW, Nies AS, et al. (eds.): The Pharmacologic Basis of Therapeutics. Elmsford, NY, Pergamon Press, 1990, pp. 1098–1116. *Provides a thorough consideration of this important class of antibiotics; other chapters on antibiotics are equally well written.*

Sanford JP, Gilbert DN, Gerberding JL, Sande MA: Guide to Antimicrobial Therapy 1994. Dallas, Antimicrobial Therapy, Inc., 1994. *Pocket guide to antibiotic use.*

Spratt BG: Resistance to antibiotics mediated by target alterations. Science 264:388, 1994. *Readable discussion of antibiotic resistance that results from changes in targets and resulting reductions in the affinity of antibiotics for their sites of action. Major focus is alterations in penicillin-binding proteins.*

271 PNEUMOCOCCAL PNEUMONIA
Richard J. Duma

DEFINITION. Pneumococcal pneumonia is an acute, suppurative infection of the lungs produced by an encapsulated bacterium, *Streptococcus pneumoniae* (pneumococcus). It is the most commonly occurring bacterial pneumonia in the world; in the United States, an estimated 150,000 to 570,000 cases occur annually.

MICROBIOLOGY. Virulent *S. pneumoniae* organisms are encapsulated, gram-positive cocci about 0.8 μm in diameter that occur in chains (streptococci) or pairs (diplococci) (see Color Plate 9E). When in pairs, cocci are characteristically lancet shaped; i.e., each coccus is pointed at the end like the tip of a lance, and the bases are in juxtaposition. The capsule, which is a complex polysaccharide and which varies in chemical composition and thickness, is not seen with Gram stain but may be recognized by negative staining (e.g., with India ink or methylene blue). In purulent clinical specimens, some pneumococci stain negatively rather than positively on the Gram stain, since aging, exposure of the cell wall to a variety of destructive host enzymes (e.g., lysozyme), and/or inhibition of cell wall synthesis by antibiotics (e.g., penicillin) result in incomplete or abnormal bacterial cell walls that no longer retain the iodine-fixed crystal violet stain.

Pneumococci are fastidious, facultative bacteria that grow best in the presence of blood or serum and in air supplemented with 10% carbon dioxide. Since they are fermentative and lactic acid is the usual end-product, concentrations of glucose in the culture media must be controlled and should not exceed 1%. In addition, since they produce hydrogen peroxide (H_2O_2) but not catalase, the addition of a catalase source (e.g., red blood cells) enhances growth. Viability is reduced by drying, a low pH (< 6.5), and prolonged incubation.

On blood agar after overnight incubation at 37°C, colonies generally appear mucoid, glistening, and dome shaped and are surrounded by an area of greening (α-hemolysis) within the blood agar. With continued incubation, as aged bacteria undergo autolysis, the colony domes of highly encapsulated strains collapse centrally and appear umbilicated. An important biologic feature that distinguishes *S. pneumoniae* from other streptococci is its bile solubility or susceptibility to surface-active agents, such as sodium deoxycholate and ethyl hydrocuprein chloride (optochin). The latter agent (optochin) is incorporated into a standardized 5-μg disc and is used worldwide to identify pneumococci rapidly. However, since optochin-resistant pneumococci occur, and since some nonpneumococcal, α-hemolytic streptococci are optochin sensitive, for purposes of species determination, the usefulness of this biologic property may be questioned.

Pneumococcal virulence is often studied in the mouse, since this animal is highly sensitive to encapsulated pneumococci (with the exception of type 14). Indeed, the sensitivity of mice to encapsulated pneumococci may be used for rapidly and selectively isolating virulent pneumococci from sputum specimens or from clinical materials containing other bacteria. If injected into the peritoneal cavity of the mouse, an exudate containing pneumococci may be harvested in 24 hours.

Unlike many other streptococci, particularly those belonging to Lancefield group A, and unlike other pyogenic bacteria that produce pneumonia, *S. pneumoniae* do not produce any major toxins, and particularly none that are tissue destructive. Some strains may elaborate hyaluronidase, and all contain pneumolysin, a hemolytic cytotoxic protein released when the organism undergoes autolysis, which disrupts the respiratory epithelium and slows ciliary movement.

The most important factor defining virulent *S. pneumoniae* is the presence of a high molecular weight complex polysaccharide capsule, which is a potent inhibitor of neutrophil phagocytosis. At least 84 different immunogenic types of capsules exist, and two different nomenclatures (Danish and American) are used to number them (which is often a source of confusion). Antigenically distinct capsules are easily identified with polyvalent antisera in an agglutination or precipitin test or by the Neufeld quellung reaction, a rapid test based on visualization of refractile swelling of the capsule after application of a polyvalent or monovalent type-specific antiserum to the bacterium in question. Nonencapsulated pneumococci, which are generally avirulent, do not react with antipolysaccharide antisera. Although the identification of pneumococcal capsular antigen in certain body fluids or secretions may suggest active pneumococcal infection (see below), immunologic tests to detect such antigens must be interpreted with caution, since antibodies against some pneumococcal capsular serotypes cross-react with polysaccharides of other streptococci (particularly group B), *Haemophilus influenzae* type B, *Escherichia coli, Klebsiella pneumoniae, Salmonella* species, and even human ABO blood group isoantigens.

Capsular polysaccharides consist of repeating di- or penta-oligosaccharides, some of which contain large proportions of acid constituents such as cellobiuronic, hexuronic, and pyruvic acid. Most are linear, although some are branched, and their antigenicities result principally from oligosaccharide epitopes of no more than six or seven sugar residues. The frequency of capsular types observed varies with time, geography, and the age of the patient; for example, types 6, 14, 18, 19, and 23 are common in infants and children, while types 1, 2, 3, 5, and 8 are common in adults.

The susceptibility of pneumococci to most chemotherapeutic antibacterials is generally excellent; however, this may be changing. Noteworthy among antipneumococcal drugs are the β-lactams, especially penicillins, cephalosporins, cephamycins, and carbapenems (but *not* monobactams). In addition, erythromycins, lincosines (e.g., clindamycin), vancomycin, chloramphenicol, and teicoplanins are usually effective. For penicillin G, the antibiotic against which all other antipneumococcal agents are compared, *susceptibility* is defined as inhibiting the growth of pneumococci at a concentration of <0.1 μg per milliliter (referred to as the *minimal inhibitory concentration,* or MIC). Indeed, the MIC of penicillin G worldwide for the majority of pneumococcal strains is predictably ≤0.1 μg per milliliter. However, since 1968, when penicillin-resistant strains were first identified in Australia, a significant but variable percent is now intermediately (i.e., the MIC is 0.1 to <2.0 μg per milliliter) or highly resistant (i.e., the MIC is ≥2.0 μg per milliliter). Isolates that are highly resistant are usually resistant to other antibacterials (Table 271–1), although such bacteria are uniformly susceptible to vancomycin and occasionally to third-generation cephalosporins or carbapenems. The resistance of pneumococci to β-lactams is *not*

due to bacterial production of a β-lactamase and is *not* plasmid mediated, but rather it results from chromosomal point mutations that dictate the production of aberrant target membrane penicillin-binding proteins (PBP's); it is the lack of affinity of these PBP's for penicillin G that distinguishes the penicillin-resistant strains from the penicillin-susceptible ones.

Pneumococci are relatively resistant to aminoglycosides; in fact, gentamicin may be incorporated into primary culture media for selective isolation of pneumococci from sputum, since it suppresses the growth of concurrent bacteria. Similarly, quinolones at low or clinically achievable concentrations are generally ineffective in inhibiting the growth of most pneumococci; further, in some studies, >50% of pneumococcal isolates are resistant to tetracyclines.

EPIDEMIOLOGY. Pneumococcal pneumonia is a sporadic disease that occurs most often during the coldest months of the year. The vast majority of cases occur after aspiration of "normal" oropharyngeal secretions that may contain encapsulated pneumococci, followed by an inability to clear such secretions; thus oropharyngeal carrier rates of pneumococci are important in the dynamics of acquiring pneumococcal pneumonia, its spread, and its frequency of occurrence within a population.

Since most data referable to oropharyngeal carrier rates were obtained prior to the use of pneumococcal vaccine, colonization rates with (or carriage of) certain serotypes and the relative importance of factors that impact on carriage must be interpreted with caution. Nevertheless, in longitudinal, prevaccine studies of pneumococcal oropharyngeal carriage by people living in temperate zones, serotypes with USA numbers of 23 or less are most frequently encountered, further suggesting that humans are infected by their own endogenous flora, since more than half the cases of pneumococcal pneumonia and bacteremia are caused by these strains. Clustering of one serotype within a family commonly occurs, and carriage rates do not appear to be affected by gender. Rates of carriage are higher in children, particularly those of a preschool age, than in adults; and among adults, rates are highest in those intimately exposed to preschool children. Oropharyngeal carriage appears to be highest during the coolest months of the year (fall, winter, and early spring), when respiratory infections are common, and spread may be enhanced during respiratory tract infections due to the pneumococcus or to certain respiratory viruses, such as the rhinovirus. Although the prevalence of oropharyngeal carriage in the surrounding community or within households affects the risk of individual acquisition, crowding does not appear to be important. The duration of oropharyngeal carriage of a particular serotype ranges from

TABLE 271–1. MIC$_{90}$ OF SOME COMMONLY USED BETA-LACTAM ANTIBIOTICS AGAINST PENICILLIN-RESISTANT PNEUMOCOCCI

Antibiotic	MIC$_{90}$ (μg/ml)* Intermediate Penicillin Resistance	High-Level Penicillin Resistance
Ampicillin	0.5	8
Oxacillin	4.0	31
Methicillin	—	64
Carbenicillin	32.0	64
Ticarcillin	64.0	128
Piperacillin	1.0	8–16
Mezlocillin	1.0–2.0	8–15
Azlocillin	1.0	16
Cephalothin	1.0	8–31
Cefaclor	4.0–16.0	16
Cefonicid	16.0	16
Cefoxitin	4.0–8.0	32–125
Cefamandole	0.5–2.0	8–31
Cefuroxime	0.25–0.44	—
Cefotaxime	0.125–1.0	1–4
Ceftriaxone	0.12–0.5	1
Ceftazidime	3.2–32.0	64
Cefoperazone	1.0–2.0	2–16
Moxalactam	2.0–4.0	128
Imipenem	0.06–1.0	1–2

* MIC$_{90}$ = Minimal inhibitory concentration at which 90% of strains are susceptible.
Adapted with permission from Klugman KP: Pneumococcal resistance to antibiotics. Clin Microbiol Rev 3:171, 1990.

TABLE 271–2. RISK FACTORS OR UNDERLYING CONDITIONS PREDISPOSING TO THE DEVELOPMENT OF PNEUMOCOCCAL PNEUMONIA OR SERIOUS PNEUMOCOCCAL INFECTIONS

Age (extremes)
Alcoholism
Bone marrow transplantation
Bronchiectasis
Cerebrovascular occlusions or severe neurologic impairment
Chronic bronchitis
Chronic lymphocytic leukemia
Chronic obstructive pulmonary disease (COPD)
Cirrhosis or chronic liver disease
Complement deficiency (particularly C'3)
Conditions associated with aspiration (e.g., seizures)
Congestive heart failure
Dementia
Diabetes mellitus
Immunologic deficiencies (acquired, hereditary, or iatrogenic)—humoral (IgG or IgA) or cellular (e.g., AIDS)
Institutionalization, homelessness, day care centers
Malignancy (particularly solid tumors of the lung)
Multiple myeloma
Nephrotic syndrome
Neutropenia
Smoking
Splenic dysfunction (e.g., in sickle cell disease) or asplenia
Viral diseases, especially influenza

2 weeks to years, the mean being 6 to 8 weeks. Reacquisition of the same serotype commonly occurs. In children, but usually not adults, initial acquisition within a family setting is frequently associated with rises in homotypic serum antibody and occasionally with illness.

Although epidemics of pneumococcal pneumonia may occur, they are *rare* and generally appear in special populations at high risk for pneumococcal disease, such as domiciliary populations of alcoholics, institutionalized elderly, Navajo Indians, New Guinea highlanders, Alaskan natives, and South African gold miners. In studies of ambulatory adult populations, a variety of risk factors appear to predispose to the development of pneumococcal infections (Table 271–2).

IMMUNOLOGY. In nonimmunized, untreated patients, specific anticapsular humoral antibody (immunoglobulin M [IgM] and immunoglobulin G [IgG]) can be detected in the blood 5 to 10 days after infection and correlates with the clearance of pneumococci and eventual recovery. Both classic and alternate pathway complement (C'3) and type-specific, opsonizing antibody, principally IgG (IgG1 in children and IgG2 and IgG4 subclasses in adults), enhance phagocytosis and intracellular killing of pneumococci by polymorphonuclear leukocytes and alveolar macrophages, the major host defense mechanism for eradicating pneumococci. Patients with deficiencies of biologically active IgM, IgG, and, to a lesser degree, IgA (particularly secretory) are more susceptible to developing pneumococcal pneumonia and other pneumococcal infections than are normal persons without such deficiencies. In normal persons, once specific anticapsular antibodies form, they generally persist for life.

If pneumococci escape this host defense mechanism, they may enter the bloodstream via lymph channels and the thoracic duct and produce bacteremia. Clearance from the blood also depends on opsonization via type-specific antibodies and activated complement; however, liver and spleen macrophages are principally responsible for removing pneumococci from the blood rather than polymorphonuclear leukocytes. Thus splenectomy or cirrhosis of the liver rather than neutropenia increases the risk for pneumococcal bacteremia, dissemination, and death.

PATHOGENESIS AND PATHOLOGY. Most cases of pneumococcal pneumonia result from the aspiration of oropharyngeal material containing indigenous, virulent pneumococci into terminal bronchioles and alveoli, followed by atelectasis and the inability to clear bacteria from these sites. Although microaspiration is a natural event that occurs commonly, pneumonia in normal individuals seldom results, because pulmonary bacterial clearance and/or local host defense mechanisms are adequate and intact and are not defec-

tive or suppressed. These important defense mechanisms, which serve as either a barrier against or a clearance for bacteria, are the epiglottic reflex, ciliary escalator and mucous blanket, secretory and humoral immunoglobulins, surfactant, alveolar macrophage and polymorphonuclear leukocyte activity, and lymphatic drainage. When these mechanisms are blunted or overwhelmed by aspirated noxious material, by large inocula of pneumococci, by a highly virulent strain, and/or by material containing additional pathogens, pneumonia may result. In addition, once infection occurs, further atelectasis from inspissated material may result.

After pneumococci establish themselves in the lung, the first visible evidence of an inflammatory response is localized capillary dilatation and hyperemia, the appearance of serous edema within alveoli, followed by margination, diapedesis, and chemotaxis of polymorphonuclear cells induced by immunoglobulins and/or activated complement. Fluid-filled alveoli enhance the passage of bacteria through the pores of Kohn and into terminal bronchioles, with spread to contiguous, uninfected alveoli, forming the advancing margins of the disease. If clearance and host immune mechanisms are adequate at this stage, the infection may resolve. However, if not, the disease may spread until the pleura and interlobar fissures are reached and consolidation with dense infiltrates of polymorphonuclear leukocytes and extravasated red blood cells occurs (see Color Plates 9A to 9C).

Pneumococcal pneumonia may involve an entire lobe (lobar pneumonia), multiple lobes (multilobar pneumonia), or just segments of a lobe, producing a patchy area (or areas) of pneumonia (pneumonitis). At times, infection spreads concentrically from bronchi (bronchopneumonia), a pattern occasionally seen in infants and in the elderly. In the central and oldest portions of infection, consolidation with massive numbers of polymorphonuclear leukocytes predominates, while peripheral to this are new areas of hemorrhage, infiltrating polymorphonuclear cells, and edema. Early pathologists referred to these areas in the lung as "gray hepatization" and "red hepatization," respectively, because of the gross resemblance of involved lung to liver tissue (see Color Plate 9A). In fully developed, untreated pneumococcal pneumonia, all stages of the cellular inflammatory process may be present.

In 5 to 10% of patients, infection may extend into the pleural space, resulting in an *empyema,* or in 15 to 25% of patients, bacteria may enter the bloodstream (*bacteremia*) via the lymphatics and thoracic duct. Invasion of the bloodstream by pneumococci may lead to serious metastatic disease at a number of extrapulmonary sites (Table 271–3), the most important and most frequent of which is the subarachnoid space (*meningitis*). Other infections that may occur from bacteremic spread are *septic arthritis, pericarditis, endocarditis* (infection of the heart valves), and, in patients with ascites, *peritonitis* (spontaneous bacterial peritonitis, or SBP). In addition, pneumococci may infect concurrently other tissues or organs, such as the sinopulmonary system, air sinuses (*sinusitis*), mastoids (*mastoiditis*), ears (*otitis media*), conjunctivae (pyogenic *conjunctivitis*), epiglottis (*epiglottitis,* particularly in infants), or rarely the soft tissues of the neck or retropharyngeal area (*Ludwig's angina*).

CLINICAL FINDINGS. The presentation of acute bacterial pneumonia due to *S. pneumoniae* may be highly variable, depend-

TABLE 271–3. CONCURRENT OR COMPLICATING PNEUMOCOCCAL INFECTIONS OCCURRING IN PNEUMOCOCCAL PNEUMONIA

Otitis media
Sinusitis/mastoiditis
Conjunctivitis (suppurative)
Epiglottitis
Tracheobronchitis
Pleuritis (empyema)
Soft tissue cellulitis (Ludwig's angina)
Pericarditis*
Endocarditis*
Meningitis*
Arthritis (septic)*
Peritonitis (in presence of ascites)*

* Usually blood borne.

ing on when the patient presents to the physician in the course of the disease, the patient's age, whether or not effective antibiotics were previously administered, the presence or absence of satisfactory host defenses, and the existence of risk factors for dissemination of pneumococci (e.g., asplenia, neutropenia, and agammaglobulinemia). The presentation may be mild or explosive and rapidly lethal. Classically, the onset of acute pneumococcal pneumonia is sudden and is characterized by an abrupt occurrence of cough, chills, high fever (up to 40°C), myalgias, tachypnea, shallow respirations, tachycardia, weakness, and often frank rigors. Initially, the cough may be productive of scant mucopurulent or blood-streaked sputum; later (after 24 to 48 hours), it may be thick, purulent, frankly bloody or rust-colored, and consistent with an alveolar, hemorrhagic, exudative process. If the infecting pneumococcus is highly encapsulated, a gelatinous, blood-tinged sputum may be seen. The presence of pleuritic pain is specific clinical evidence that the pneumonia is probably bacterial and, in the presence of most of the above findings, probably pneumococcal.

The patient with pneumococcal pneumonia is generally diaphoretic and, in addition, may be dehydrated and hypotensive. Anorexia, nausea, and vomiting are common. If allowed to continue untreated, single-lobe disease may progress to multilobe involvement, and the patient may become dusky, cyanotic, and confused. If bacteremia occurs, chills and rigors may persist, and rarely shock, a disseminated intravascular coagulopathy (DIC), and/or an adult respiratory distress syndrome (ARDS) may supervene and ultimately lead to the patient's death.

A history is frequently elicited of a recent upper respiratory or viral-like illness that has occurred prior to the appearance of clinical pneumonia, especially during the winter months, when influenza is common. Risk factors for aspiration, such as alcoholism, seizures, or vomiting, or for acquiring pneumococcal pneumonia may be present (see above).

On physical examination, the acutely ill patient is tachypneic and may be observed to use accessory muscles for respiration (intercostal, abdominal, and sternocleidomastoid) and even to exhibit nasal flaring. If pleuritic pain is severe, reflex splinting of the ipsilateral thorax is observed. Fever and tachycardia are present, and although hypotension may occur, frank shock is unusual, except in the later stages of infection or DIC.

Auscultation of the chest reveals bronchovesicular or tubular breath sounds and wet rales over the involved lung. As consolidation occurs, vocal and tactile fremitus is increased; however, if a concurrent pleural effusion is present, breath sounds and fremitus may be diminished or absent. A localized, grating pleural friction rub may occasionally be heard.

Examination of the upper respiratory passages may be helpful in suggesting a diagnosis of pneumococcal pneumonia. For example, in children, the absence of an exudative pharyngitis and the presence of otitis media might suggest pneumococcal involvement. In older children and adults, the air sinuses and/or mastoids may be acutely infected. (But these infections also can occur with streptococcal, staphylococcal, and H. influenzae pneumonia.)

Evidence of extrapulmonary infections may be present, particularly in untreated disease lasting more than 48 hours; for example, signs of meningeal irritation (stiff neck, Kernig's or Brudzinski's sign) with abnormalities in mentation may suggest meningitis; the appearance of pathologic heart murmurs, splenomegaly, and heart failure may be evidence of endocarditis; or the presence of pain, swelling, tenderness, heat, and possibly redness in one or more joints may point toward a septic arthritis of hematogenous origin.

Additional findings unrelated to pneumonia *per se* but related to sepsis and/or toxicity may be noted: a paralytic ileus with abdominal pain, distention, and loss of bowel sounds; mild jaundice due to a reactive hepatitis or to intrapulmonary hemorrhage; frank shock; purpuric lesions resulting from DIC; or symmetric gangrene and purpura of the fingers and/or toes (*purpura fulminans*) associated with bacteremia.

LABORATORY FINDINGS. The peripheral white blood cell (WBC) count is often two to three times the normal value; however, in alcoholics or immunosuppressed patients, it may be normal or low. Of more value is the WBC differential, which consists predominantly of bands and polymorphonuclear leukocytes (left shift). If DIC is suspected, thrombocytopenia, pleomorphism of red blood

cells (schistocytes and helmet cells), prolonged prothrombin and partial thromboplastin times, and hypofibrinogenemia and circulating fibrin-split products may be present.

In some patients, the total bilirubin and hepatic cellular enzyme levels may be slightly elevated. Since dehydration and hypovolemia commonly occur (owing to fever, diaphoresis, nausea, and vomiting), the hemoglobin, hematocrit, and serum sodium level may be elevated. When pneumonia is the dominant clinical event, arterial blood gas studies, which reflect pulmonary function and compensatory events, usually reveal hypoxemia (low Po_2), hypocarbia (low Pco_2), and alkalosis (blood pH > 7.4) resulting from hyperventilation and shunting. However, if frank shock intervenes, a metabolic acidosis may result (blood pH < 7.4); if it is not corrected, death may follow.

Good posteroanterior and lateral chest roentgenograms are important to obtain, first to confirm the presence and to ascertain the extent and radiographic character of the pneumonia and second to determine if underlying predisposing pulmonary diseases are present, such as bronchiectasis, bronchial obstruction, emphysema, tumor, or tuberculosis. In severely dehydrated or profoundly neutropenic or immunodeficient patients, early inflammatory infiltrates may not be seen radiographically or may be patchy and irregular in appearance, but after hydration or restoration of circulating levels of inflammatory cells, patterns of lobar consolidation may become apparent.

Characteristically, in immunocompetent patients with untreated, frank pneumococcal pneumonia, chest roentgenograms reveal a lobar distribution and an air space (or alveolar exudative) pattern of disease with an air bronchogram effect. However, if prior, partially effective antibiotic usage has occurred, the pattern may be atypical, and a lobar distribution may be the exception rather than the rule. Interlobar fissures may bulge, owing to considerable fluid content within the involved lung associated with large amounts of capsular material. In severe cases, more than one lobe may be involved (multilobar pneumonia). In 30% of cases, a pleural effusion may be present and may be readily detected by a lateral decubitus film. Such effusions may be sterile and represent parapneumonic collections of fluid, or occasionally they may be infected with pneumococci, in which case they are called *empyemas*.

If blunting of the costophrenic angle is noted radiographically, and the finding is believed to represent an effusion, then at least 300 to 500 ml of fluid is probably present, and a thoracentesis is indicated. Unless contraindicated, *every pleural effusion associated with an acute bacterial pneumonia in which the etiology of the pneumonia is unclear should be tapped and the fluid studied for microorganisms* (see Color Plate 9D). Ordinarily, fluid removed from the pleural space is sterile, so any bacteria seen on a Gram stain or cultured from the fluid represent pathogens until proved otherwise.

Other important laboratory studies *that must be obtained early in the patient's workup* are routine cultures of the blood, a microscopic examination of a Gram stain and a culture *of purulent material from the site of infection* (alveoli, bronchi, or lung), and an examination of any infected material that can be removed from a secondarily infected extrapulmonary focus. Results of blood cultures may not be available for 18 to 24 hours and thus cannot assist the physician in making a presumptive diagnosis or in selecting appropriate initial chemotherapy. Often, in asplenic patients, a high-grade bacteremia occurs, so examination of the peripheral WBC smear or of the buffy coat for pneumococci may be useful.

Microscopic examination and cultures of expectorated purulent sputum from a patient with acute bacterial pneumonia are essential if a correct presumptive etiologic diagnosis is to be made and an appropriate antibiotic is to be given. Ideally, these tests should be done before therapy is initiated; however, a significant delay in instituting therapy should not be permitted. Attention must be given to obtaining a diagnostically useful sputum sample; that is, material must be purulent to be presumed to be from the site of infection. Saliva or oropharyngeal contamination of the sample should be avoided.

In a patient with the clinical picture of acute bacterial pneumonia, the finding of gram-positive diplococci in expectorated sputum that contains many (≥ 50 bacterial cells per $100\times$ field) polymorphonuclear cells (purulent sputum) and few (< 10 squamous cells per $100\times$ field) or no squamous epithelial cells (which indicates little or no oropharyngeal contamination of the specimen) is strong presumptive evidence of pneumococcal pneumonia.

Cultures of expectorated sputum are also important but are not without problems; for example, since *S. pneumoniae* is fastidious, it may fail to grow in culture, but this does not exclude its presence. In addition, pneumococci may be overlooked, since they may be overgrown by other organisms or mixed with similar-appearing, nonpneumococcal, α-hemolytic streptococci, which are normally present in oropharyngeal secretions. On the other hand, since *S. pneumoniae* is often present normally in the oropharynx, its growth from sputum, especially from that which is expectorated, may not be indicative of pneumococcal disease. Perhaps the main value of securing a sputum culture is to confirm or question observations made from the Gram stain and, if pneumococci (and/or other bacteria) are ultimately isolated, to perform antibiotic susceptibility testing.

If the patient is unable to expectorate purulent sputum for microscopic examination and culture, and if other infected materials (e.g., pleural or joint fluid) are not available or are negative for pneumococci, various procedures for obtaining pus from the infected lung must be considered. Cough can be induced by having the patient inhale an aerosol of warm 3% NaCl; a plastic catheter can be inserted into the trachea via the nose or throat and suction applied; a direct transtracheal needle and catheter aspiration may be performed (a procedure not without complications); the patient may undergo endoscopy (provided the arterial Po_2 is ≥ 50 mm Hg), and alveolar washings or bronchial brushings may be obtained; or rarely, direct aspiration of the pneumonic infiltrate through the chest wall with a long, "skinny" needle (22 gauge) may be employed (a procedure also not without risks). Open-lung biopsies for pneumococcal pneumonia are not indicated, although they may be for certain complications, ill-defined superinfections, or underlying diseases. In any acute bacterial pneumonia, the guiding principles for deciding what procedure, if any, to use for obtaining purulent sputum from the involved lung are as follows: (1) If expectorated sputum is satisfactory (i.e., purulent and relatively free of contaminating oropharyngeal material), further efforts to obtain pus from the deeper recesses of the lung are probably not necessary; (2) if additional procedures are necessary, one should select first the procedure that is least traumatic and invasive and is risk free and then proceed, if necessary, in a stepwise fashion to the next least invasive, risk-free procedure until satisfactory material is obtained; (3) one should not delay more than several hours before beginning chemotherapy, and if the patient is extremely ill, one must rely on clinical judgment and not delay treatment at all; and (4) one must make every effort to identify the etiologic agent (or agents) responsible for the pneumonia early in the course of the illness, since once this goal is realized, the chances of managing the patient successfully are markedly enhanced.

A variety of other tests may be applied to sputum specimens to identify pneumococci in acute bacterial pneumonia; but in skilled hands, few, if any, are better, less costly, easier to do, and more informative than the Gram stain. All tests done on sputum possess a similar problem in interpretation, namely, determining whether or not bacteria present in the sample are responsible for the pneumonia observed. If blood or pleural fluid cultures are subsequently positive for *S. pneumoniae*, the etiologic agent is confirmed, although the presence of additional pathogenic bacteria within the lung may not be entirely excluded, as, rarely, blood or pleural fluid cultures may yield other bacteria (polymicrobial infection) in addition to pneumococci.

Detection of pneumococcal capsular antigen generally requires the presence of approximately 10^5 bacteria per milliliter, about the same concentration as required to observe an average of one bacterium per $1000\times$ field (or an oil-immersion field on a standard light microscope) on a Gram stain. Cross-reactions with other antigens of other bacteria are frequent, and with certain serotypes, false-negative results are common. Perhaps the greatest value of capsular antigen detection is to confirm the presence of pneumococci in those patients who have been partially treated and in whom sputum cultures may be negative and a Gram stain may reveal few, if any, intact bacteria.

Colony counts of bacteria from bronchoalveolar lavage (BAL) washings obtained during endoscopy are seldom available early in the course of illness. Specimens must be obtained with a special cuffed endoscope so that oropharyngeal contamination does not occur with insertion of the scope. Generally, counts of colony-forming units (CFU's) of bacteria higher than 10^3 to 10^5 per milliliter

of fluid removed are considered significant, but this is not invariably so.

DNA hybridization studies may be performed, but as with capsular antigen detection, adequate numbers of bacteria must be present for the test to be positive. Use of the polymerase chain reaction (PCR) may amplify pneumococcal DNA and improve the potential for detection; however, such enhanced sensitivity may lead to false-positive results caused by very small numbers of contaminating pneumococci.

Elastase or elastin fibers in sputum may suggest the presence of a gram-negative bacillary necrotizing pneumonia, particularly that due to *Pseudomonas,* but this test is of little value in the diagnosis of pneumococcal pneumonia (other than the test should be negative), since necrosis of tissue is not produced by pneumococci.

DIFFERENTIAL DIAGNOSIS (see also Ch. 55 and chapters dealing with specific organisms). The clinical picture and many of the routine laboratory and roentgenographic features associated with pneumococcal pneumonia are often indistinguishable from those of other acute bacterial pneumonias. Thus collecting appropriate microbiologic data is essential if the correct etiologic diagnosis is to be made.

In adults, the second most common community-acquired, acute bacterial pneumonia is that caused by *H. influenzae.* The Gram stain of purulent sputum from such patients often reveals myriads of tiny gram-negative coccobacilli, with the observation of an occasional filamentous form. Such an infection often occurs in a patient with chronic bronchitis or chronic obstructive pulmonary disease and usually is due to nonencapsulated *H. influenzae* (as opposed to highly encapsulated, serotype B strains commonly infecting young children).

Staphylococcus aureus is another bacterium occasionally producing acute pneumonia, but when this kind of pneumonia is community acquired, it usually occurs during or just after an epidemic of viral influenza. In the hospital setting, *S. aureus* may be seen year round, because it is a commonly occurring nosocomial infection. If a highly virulent, toxin-producing strain is responsible, the "toxic shock syndrome" may be observed. On a Gram stain of purulent sputum, clusters and characteristic tetrads of gram-positive cocci are seen. Late in the clinical course, abscess formation or destruction of the lung occurs.

Group A streptococci *(S. pyogenes)* also produce acute pneumonia, and in such instances, the patient may be more toxic-appearing than the extent of involvement of the lung might suggest. Classically, a small, peripherally located, wedge-shaped infiltrate is seen, and a thin, watery, serosanguineous, pleural effusion is present. A roentgenogram of the chest may suggest a pulmonary infarction. An upper respiratory tract infection, particularly an exudative or erythematous pharyngitis or tonsillitis (especially in children), may be present, and an erythematous rash produced by streptococcal erythrogenic toxin (scarlet fever) may be seen. A Gram stain of purulent sputum usually reveals numerous short chains of gram-positive cocci or diplococci. Thus the Gram stain may not differentiate group A streptococcal from pneumococcal pneumonia.

Branhamella catarrhalis may produce acute pneumonia, but usually this occurs in the elderly and particularly in those with chronic bronchitis or obstructive lung disease. It is a relatively benign infection, compared with those produced by other pyogenic bacteria, and is rarely, if ever, associated with bacteremia. A Gram stain of purulent sputum is again important, and the diagnosis should probably be made only when numerous gram-negative diplococci, in the absence of other potentially pathogenic bacteria, are seen. *N. meningitidis* (meningococci) are morphologically similar to *B. catarrhalis* and must be included in the differential diagnosis. However, in such instances, patients are generally young adults, and the infection is associated with significant toxicity.

Gram-negative bacilli, particularly those belonging to the family Enterobacteriaceae (e.g., *E. coli, Klebsiella, Enterobacter, Serratia,* and *Proteus*), also must be considered as causative agents in the differential diagnosis of pneumococcal pneumonia, particularly if the patient is debilitated and is residing in a nursing home or similar institution, and certainly if the patient is hospitalized. Aerobic gram-negative bacilli are often responsible for nosocomial but infrequently for community-acquired pneumonias. This is so because gram-negative bacilli rarely colonize the oropharynx of otherwise healthy people in the community, but they are common oropharyngeal residents in debilitated, hospitalized, or institutionalized patients. In addition, the patient in question may exhibit certain risk factors associated with invasion by gram-negative bacilli, such as the receipt of prior antibiotics, corticosteroids, inhalation therapy, or tracheostomy and the existence of profound neutropenia or severe debilitation. The pneumonic process is usually necrotizing, and gas formation may be detected on roentenograms. A Gram stain of purulent sputum usually reveals many large, bipolar-staining gram-negative rods. Elastin fibrils also may be seen on a KOH preparation of sputum from the site of infection.

Anaerobic bacteria also may produce acute suppurative pneumonia. Those most frequently involved are *Bacteroides* species (usually *B. melaninogenicus*), *Peptostreptococcus,* and *Fusobacterium.* Frequently, anaerobic infections are polymicrobial and may include bacteria other than strict anaerobes (e.g., *S. aureus*). The occurrence of anaerobic infection is usually preceded by gross aspiration and is enhanced if the individual has anaerobic oral infections or solid tumors of the oropharyngeal structures or tracheobronchial tree. The clinical presentation of anaerobic pleuropneumonic disease may be indolent rather than abrupt, and it may be accompanied by pus that has a fetid and nauseating odor. Necrosis of the lung with gas formation is often noted.

Mycoplasma pneumoniae, Chlamydia, and *Legionella* also may produce acute pneumonias, which are usually best described as atypical. With mycoplasmal pneumonia, patients are ordinarily young, and prolonged communicability, especially within households, may often be documented. The clinical, radiographic, and pathologic features are usually those of an interstitial pneumonia, rather than lobar consolidation and an alveolar exudative process. Serum cold agglutinin levels may be elevated, and the disease is rarely, if ever, fatal. Chlamydial pneumonia, especially that due to *C. psittaci,* is contracted from infected psittacine birds, while *C. pneumoniae* or the TWAR agent is acquired from other infected humans. *C. pneumoniae* is the most common species producing chlamydial pneumonia in humans, and the clinical picture is usually that of pharyngitis, often with laryngitis, and segmental pneumonia of a single lobe without pleural effusion. Seroepidemiologic studies reveal a higher prevalence of antibodies in males than females and in older adults than children. Legionnaires' disease, which may be produced by a variety of *Legionella* species but principally by *L. pneumophila,* is associated with considerable systemic toxicity (nausea, vomiting, and diarrhea) and may be very difficult to differentiate from pneumococcal pneumonia. However, in the temperate zones, community-acquired Legionnaires' disease usually occurs in the warmer months or summer; patients are typically male construction workers and smokers in their 50's whose clinical manifestations include fever, chills, myalgias, headache, dry cough, and nonspecific pulmonary infiltrates. Anti-*Legionella* fluorescein-labeled antibodies, which may be employed to examine sputum for *Legionella,* as well as antigen detection techniques applied to the urine, may be helpful in the early diagnosis of this disease.

Patients with the acquired immunodeficiency syndrome (AIDS) and acute pneumonia present considerable diagnostic problems. Although pneumococcal pneumonia and infections from encapsulated bacteria occur with greater frequency in patients with AIDS than in normal individuals, pneumocystosis and cytomegalovirus pneumonia occur frequently and thus must be excluded.

Finally, not only does pneumonia due to microbes other than the pneumococcus have to be considered in a differential diagnosis, but also a variety of noninfectious conditions may mimic the clinical picture of pneumococcal pneumonia. Pulmonary infarction, with emboli (e.g., in right-sided endocarditis) or without emboli (e.g., in sickle cell anemia), may present a considerable diagnostic challenge, even after differential lung scanning and pulmonary angiography. Chemical pneumonitis, localized or diffuse (Mendelson's syndrome), often caused by aspiration of gastric juice of low pH, also may be difficult to differentiate from pneumococcal or other bacterial pneumonias; however, in the absence of antibiotic therapy, a Gram stain of purulent sputum consistently reveals few or no bacteria.

TREATMENT. All patients with suspected pneumococcal pneumonia should be treated as promptly as possible with an effective antimicrobial agent. One should not wait for cultural confirmation of the diagnosis to initiate therapy. Although many patients may recover without antibacterial therapy, effective antimicrobial agents reduce morbidity, mortality, and complications.

At present, *penicillin G* is the therapy of choice, and it is the standard against which all other antipneumococcal agents are compared. Susceptible strains exhibit an MIC of < 0.1 µg per milliliter, levels that are easily achieved in a variety of tissues with therapeutic dosing of 1.2 to 2.4 million units per day. If complicating pneumococcal bacteremia occurs, only 10 to 15% of untreated patients may be expected to survive, while this figure increases to 85 to 90% with penicillin G treatment. A variety of other β-lactam antibiotics are also effective and may be used in special circumstances, such as when bacteria other than or in addition to pneumococci are considered in the differential diagnosis or when penicillin-resistant pneumococci are present. Ideally, initial therapy should be parenteral to ensure delivery and adequate serum and tissue levels. If the patient is in shock or has heart failure, the route of delivery should be intravenous. Later in the course of therapy, if the patient's progress is good, the route of administration may be changed to oral. Treatment with any effective agent should be for at least 5 to 7 days.

For patients who are believed to be allergic to penicillin, a variety of other antibacterial agents may be used. Usually, a first-generation cephalosporin is selected, since its molecular configuration is slightly different from that of penicillin G (a six-membered thiazole ring rather than a five-membered one) and since the frequency of serious reactions due to cross-allergenicity appears to be low. However, careful observation of the penicillin-allergic patient during the initial use of a cephalosporin must still be made. If the patient has a clear history of a type I (immediate) hypersensitivity reaction, all β-lactams should be avoided. For such patients, erythromycin is an excellent choice, even though an increasing frequency of resistance (MIC ≥ 1.0 µg per milliliter) to erythromycin is being observed worldwide. Tetracyclines should be avoided because the frequency of resistant strains is often widespread and high (up to 80% of isolates in some parts of the world). Similarly, quinolones also should not be used routinely because levels of susceptibility of most strains are often too high to predict a satisfactory outcome.

With the advent of penicillin-resistant pneumococci (see above), different strategies of therapy may have to be devised on the basis of susceptibility or resistance to other agents (Table 271–4). In the United States, such strains, although sporadic, localized to certain geographic areas, and generally of intermediate resistance (MIC between 0.1 and 2.0 µg per milliliter), appear to be increasing in frequency (up to > 30% in some locales). Nevertheless, each locale or hospital needs to monitor its own isolates, and therapeutic strategies should be based on these results. If strains are intermediate in resistance, simply increasing the dose of penicillin G to 6 million units per day will suffice (unless the complication of meningitis or endocarditis exists). However, if strains highly resistant to penicillin G (MIC ≥ 2.0 µg per milliliter) are repeatedly or frequently isolated, then penicillin G should not be routinely employed as initial therapy. In fact, such highly resistant isolates are generally resistant to most other β-lactam antibiotics (see Table 271–1), as well as to many other antimicrobials, so agents such as vancomycin, teicoplanin, clindamycin, fluoroquinolones, or rifampin may have to be used (with or without empirical penicillin) until the results

TABLE 271–4. CRITERIA FOR RESISTANCE OF *STREPTOCOCCUS PNEUMONIAE* TO SOME COMMONLY USED ANTIBIOTICS*

Antibacterial Agent	MIC (µg/ml)†
Penicillin G	
Intermediate	≥0.1 to <2.0
High level	≥2.0
Erythromycin	≥1.0
Trimethoprim-sulfamethoxazole	≥1.19
Rifampin	≥2.0
Chloramphenicol	≥8.0

* Based on criteria established by the National Committee for Clinical Laboratory Standards (NCCLS).
† MIC = minimal inhibitory concentration.

of susceptibility studies are available. Among currently available β-lactams, cefotaxime, ceftriaxone, cefepime, and the carbapenems are active against many highly resistant pneumococci (see Table 271–1).

If effective antibacterial therapy is employed, the patient's temperature usually falls to or below normal by crisis within 24 hours. However, in some instances, perhaps because of the nature of the pathology or complications that occur (e.g., pleural effusion), the patient's temperature may fall by lysis over 2 to 3 days. Resolution and recovery from pneumococcal pneumonia generally result in restoration of normal pulmonary architecture. Occasionally, healing may be via fibrosis, in which instance persistence of pulmonary infiltrates on roentgenograms may be evident for months after clinical recovery.

In addition to effective antibacterial therapy, a variety of supportive measures are generally used in the initial management of acute pneumococcal pneumonia; these include bed rest, monitoring vital signs and urine output, inserting a Swan-Ganz catheter to monitor cardiac output, administering an occasional analgesic to relieve pleuritic pain to permit effective breathing and coughing, replacing fluids if the patient is dehydrated, correcting electrolytes, oxygen therapy, and relieving an ileus with nasal gastric suctioning. In relieving pleuritic pain or in providing sedation in situations requiring it (e.g., in delirium tremens), care should be taken not to use excessively high doses of analgesics or sedatives that might depress the respiratory center. Intercostal nerve blocks, which do not interfere with respiratory drive, may be used. If possible, antipyretics also should be avoided, since these agents interfere with the evaluation of fever as a measurement of the patient's progress (or lack of).

COMPLICATIONS. Approximately 5% of patients with pneumococcal pneumonia develop an empyema, although a larger percentage (up to 30%) commonly develop sterile pleural effusions. Most effusions resolve with successful antibacterial therapy, although empyemas often require drainage. Empyemas usually consist of thick pus composed of fibrin, serous proteins, large numbers of leukocytes and/or their products, and pneumococci. Initially, such collections may be drained by needle aspiration; however, later, as loculations occur, drainage via chest tubes is usually necessary. Chest roentgenograms with lateral decubitus films are often useful in the early recognition of pleural effusions; however, at a later time and in the course of removal and follow-up, ultrasonography and/or computed tomography (CT) may be necessary. In any acute bacterial pneumonia, pleural fluid that is removed should be subject to a Gram stain, aerobic and anaerobic cultures, pH determination, cell count and differential, protein and sugar analysis, and a lactate dehydrogenase test to determine whether or not an empyema is present.

If pneumococcal bacteremia occurs, extrapulmonary complications, such as *meningitis, septic arthritis,* and *endocarditis,* must be excluded, since their therapy generally requires higher dosages of penicillin G and, in the case of septic arthritis, may require drainage. A spinal tap with examination of cerebrospinal fluid (CSF) should be done if meningitis is suspected, and multiple pretreatment blood cultures and echocardiography of the heart valves should be obtained if endocarditis is suspected. Other complications that might occur are *pyogenic pericarditis,* which may produce tamponade and require drainage, and *peritonitis* in those with ascites (e.g., cirrhosis or nephrotic syndrome).

PROGNOSIS. The case fatality rate for untreated pneumococcal pneumonia is about 25%, whereas in those treated promptly with penicillin G, it may be <5%. Fatality rates differ considerably among patient groups, depending on such factors as presence or absence of bacteremia, multilobe or single-lobe involvement, presence or absence of neutropenia or asplenism, underlying diseases (particularly of the heart and lung), age of the patient (the prognosis being poor at the extremes), complicating extrapulmonary pneumococcal infections (e.g., meningitis), the occurrence of shock, the serotype of pneumococcus responsible (type 3 being highly virulent), delayed therapy, penicillin susceptibility or resistance, and prior immunization with polyvalent pneumococcal vaccine. However, since the advent of penicillin G in the 1940's, the case fatality rate of pneumococcal pneumonia and bacteremia remains essentially unchanged.

PREVENTION. The most important preventive tool available is polyvalent pneumococcal vaccine. This type-specific vaccine contains 23 antigenic capsular polysaccharides, which in the United States account for up to 90% of bacteremic infections. In immunocompetent populations, it is estimated to be 79% protective, inducing antibodies of the IgG2 and IgG4 subclasses in adults, which enhance opsonization, phagocytosis, and killing of pneumococci by polymorphonuclear leukocytes and fixed macrophages. It is virtually free of life-threatening side effects and obviously cannot produce a pneumococcal infection, since it contains no viable, intact pneumococci. About 15 to 30% of patients who receive the vaccine may develop fever, localized swelling, and/or pain at the injection site. As with all polysaccharide vaccines, it is not immunogenic below ages 18 to 24 months and is poorly immunogenic in the very elderly and in those with a variety of conditions generally associated with decreased vaccine responsiveness. In normal individuals, if antibodies result from vaccination, colonization, or natural infection, they usually persist for several years, and then progressively decline. The vaccine is not associated with a booster effect, probably because it functions as a thymus-independent type 2 antigen. At present, highly immunogenic vaccines in which the capsular antigens are conjugated to proteins are under development. Revaccination of the elderly and other high-risk groups needs to be considered at 3- to 5-year intervals.

The U.S. Public Health Service specifically recommends the currently available pneumococcal vaccine for patients with underlying conditions that are associated with increased susceptibility to pneumococcal infections or increased risk of mortality from such infections, namely, healthy adults 65 years or older and those with chronic cardiac or pulmonary diseases, anatomic or functional asplenia, chronic liver disease, alcoholism, diabetes mellitus, and CSF leaks. Perhaps the greatest value of vaccination against pneumococci is to reduce bacteremia, dissemination, and mortality, especially in those with hepatic or splenic dysfunction. Type-specific antibody can be elicited with pneumococcal polysaccharides by subcutaneous vaccination even in splenectomized patients. In addition, recommendations for receiving the vaccine also are made for those with chronic renal failure or those on hemodialysis; for those with Hodgkin's disease, chronic lymphocytic leukemia, multiple myeloma, and AIDS; or for those receiving or about to receive chemotherapy for cancer, organ transplantation, or splenectomy.

Antibiotic prophylaxis with penicillin G or similar agents in otherwise healthy patients with viral upper respiratory infections is not routinely indicated, is not cost-effective, and may only lead to superinfections with antibiotic-resistant bacteria or to adverse side effects from the antibiotic itself. However, in individuals with seriously compromised pulmonary, cardiac, or immune function, a narrow-spectrum agent, such as penicillin G, may be given in low dosages during a viral syndrome for a limited time to reduce the risk of morbidity and mortality from potentially invasive pneumococci. Such prophylaxis may especially apply to those in households where pneumococcal infections recently occurred.

Finally, it should be appreciated that pneumococcal infections, including pneumonia, are generally not acquired by otherwise normal people from exposure to other patients with pneumococcal pneumonia; thus patients with pneumococcal pneumonia do not require isolation, and prophylaxis for medical staff exposed to such infections is not indicated.

Austrian R: Life with the Pneumococcus. Notes from the Bedside, Laboratory, and Library. Philadelphia, University of Pennsylvania Press, 1985. *An array of interesting observations, both clinical and laboratory, on pneumococcal infections by an outstanding authority and the father of the modern capsular polysaccharide pneumococcal vaccine.*

Austrian R, Gold J: Pneumococcal bacteremia with especial reference to bacteremic pneumococcal pneumonia. Ann Intern Med 60:759, 1964. *A landmark clinical study that clearly points out the major risk factors involved in pneumococcal pneumonia and bacteremia.*

Bruyn GAW, Zegers BJM, van Furth R: Mechanisms of host defense against infection with *Streptococcus pneumoniae.* Clin Infect Dis 14:251, 1992. *A thorough, up-to-date review of virulence factors of, and humoral and cellular mechanisms against, pneumococci.*

Friedland IR, McCracken GH Jr: Management of infections caused by antibiotic-resistant *Streptococcus pneumoniae.* N Engl J Med 331:337, 1994. *An excellent review of clinical responsiveness of infections due to penicillin-resistant pneumococci to various antibiotics with suggested therapeutic strategies.*

Hook EW III, Horton CA, Schaberg DR: Failure of intensive care unit support to influence mortality from pneumococcal bacteremia. JAMA 249:1055, 1983. *A clinical study that reveals that even intensive care and special units have not influenced the survival rate in pneumococcal pneumonia and bacteremia since the advent of penicillin, thus further emphasizing the need for prevention.*

Klugman KP: Pneumococcal resistance to antibiotics. Clin Microbiol Rev 3:171, 1990.

A complete, in-depth microbiologic, epidemiologic, and clinical review, evaluation, and update of the problem of penicillin resistance by an authority with considerable experience with such isolates.

Musher DM, Groover JE, Rowland JM, et al.: Antibody to capsular polysaccharides of *Streptococcus pneumoniae:* Prevalence, persistence and response to revaccination. Clin Infect Dis 17:66, 1993. *Presents new and reviews previously published data on the appearance, persistence, and fall of anticapsular antibodies against pneumococci after colonization, natural infections, and immunization.*

272 MYCOPLASMAL INFECTION
David Schlossberg

BACKGROUND. The mycoplasmas associated with humans include species from the genera *Mycoplasma, Ureaplasma,* and *Acholeplasma.* Since these genera all belong to the order Mycoplasmatales in the class Mollicutes, they are called collectively "mollicutes" or, more commonly, "mycoplasmas." There are over 150 species, and they are found in humans, animals, plants, and insects. Most of these organisms are commensals, but some of the human strains are pathogenic; rarely, some of the animal strains infect humans as well.

The mycoplasmas are the smallest free-living organisms. At 200 nm, they approximate the size of the larger viruses. Bound by a triple-layered cell membrane, they have no cell wall (thus the name "mollicute," Greek for "soft skin") and therefore are not seen on Gram stain and cannot be treated with cell wall–active antibiotics such as the β-lactams or vancomycin. Their small genome limits their genetic information, so mycoplasmas usually require media enriched with nucleic acid precursors and cholesterol.

Most mycoplasmas are facultative anaerobes. They grow down into agar and produce a dark center with a light periphery on the surface, the so-called fried-egg colonies. Mycoplasmas are distinguished from bacteria because they lack a cell wall and cannot produce cell wall precursors and from viruses, chlamydiae, and rickettsiae because the mycoplasmas can grow on cell-free media.

The mycoplasmas of humans are listed in Table 272–1. Some are established pathogens, some are commensals, and some infect immunocompromised patients.

IMMUNOLOGY. The mycoplasmas have a wide range of immunomodulatory effects. These include stimulating proliferation of T and B lymphocytes, inducing cytolytic activity of macrophages and cytotoxic T cells, stimulating cytokine production, inducing expression of major histocompatibility complex in macrophages and B cells, and producing chemotactic factors, Fc factors, Fc receptors, superantigens, and immunoglobulin proteases. This explosive and varied immunologic activity may contribute to disease expression. It is well known that rheumatoid factor, biologic false-positive tests for syphilis, antinuclear antibodies (ANA's), and other antibodies sometimes appear in the course of mycoplasmal infection.

MYCOPLASMA PNEUMONIAE. Mycoplasma pneumoniae accounts for 10 to 20% of all pneumonias and for at least half of all pneumonias in children and young adults. Although most cases occur in the first two decades of life, mycoplasmal infection is seen at all ages.

Infection with *M. pneumoniae* can occur in any season, with a 4-year periodicity for outbreaks. Since epidemics of pneumonia due to other agents usually peak in the winter, it is diagnostically help-

TABLE 272–1. HUMAN MYCOPLASMAS

Established Pathogens	Opportunists	Commensals
M. pneumoniae	M. salivarium	M. buccale
M. hominis	M. ovale	M. faucium
M. fermentans	M. genitalium	M. lipophilum
M. urealyticum	M. pirum	M. primatum
	M. penetrans	M. spermatophilum
	M. arginini	A. laidlawii
		A. oculi

ful when *Mycoplasma* pneumonia occurs in other seasons. College epidemics of *Mycoplasma,* for example, tend to peak in the fall.

The incubation period for *M. pneumoniae* averages $2\frac{1}{2}$ weeks but ranges from 4 days to over 3 weeks. This longer incubation period furnishes an important diagnostic clue, since incubation periods for most of the respiratory viruses are measured in days, not weeks. Because of the long incubation period and the lower efficiency of spread of *M. pneumoniae,* this infection spreads slowly through a population group or family. For example, several passages are needed to infect a large family, as opposed to the explosive swath through a household made by the influenza virus. Spread is person-to-person via droplet nuclei after close and prolonged contact. Patients shed the organism 2 to 8 days prior to the onset of clinical illness. They then transmit the disease during the acute phase of illness; patients with asymptomatic infection are not efficient transmitters of disease.

The attack rate of *M. pneumoniae* diminishes with age. Second infections can occur (especially if a patient is immunocompromised), but the second case is usually milder than the first. Extremely severe disease is seen in patients who have SS or SC hemoglobinopathy, Down syndrome, and hypogammaglobulinemia. Further, patients with humoral deficiency are more likely to become chronic carriers; normal patients shed the organism by 6 weeks, but immunodeficient patients may carry it for 4 months.

CLINICAL FINDINGS (Fig. 272–1). Most patients with *M. pneumoniae* infection are older children, adolescents, and young adults who develop a minor respiratory illness. In general, 75% of patients have a tracheobronchitis, 5% have an atypical pneumonia, and 20% are asymptomatic. Children under age 5 tend to have coryza and wheezing. Asthmatics may develop bronchospasm. In many patients, a sequence of symptoms occurs: The illness begins insidiously over days or a week with constitutional symptomatology (e.g., fever, myalgias, headache, and malaise); then upper respiratory signs and symptoms appear, with combinations of sore throat, cervical adenopathy, hoarseness, earache, coryza, and nonproductive cough; less commonly, croup or bronchiolitis may supervene, and in a small percentage, pneumonia ensues. At this point, the cough becomes productive.

Many patients report chilliness but not rigors. Protracted coughing results in tracheal tenderness and a sore chest, but actual pleuritic pain is rare. Signs include fever, an erythematous pharynx without exudate, and rarely, bullae on the tympanic membrane. The illness is usually self-limited and mild.

The insidious onset is usually followed by a gradual recovery. The upper respiratory symptoms may last for 2 to 3 weeks, and signs of pneumonia may persist for 4 to 6 weeks. Laboratory abnormalities are not specific; a slight leukocytosis ($<15,000$ per cubic millimeter) is seen in 25% of patients, with a normal differential count. Sputum Gram stain is very helpful in demonstrating inflammatory cells (polys or lymphs) but a paucity of bacteria.

Radiographic findings are manifold. Most patients have unilateral lower lobe segmental abnormalities on the right. The earliest signs are an interstitial accentuation of markings with subsequent patchy airspace consolidation and thickened bronchial shadows. Additional findings are platelike atelectasis, Kerley B lines, perihilar accentuations of markings, and nodular infiltrates. Hilar adenopathy is seen only occasionally in the adult but in 30% of children and may be unilateral or bilateral. A small effusion is seen in one-fourth of patients, but even in these patients pleuritic pain is rare. Complications seen on chest radiograph include pneumothorax, pneumatoceles, abscess, and in the rare case of fulminant disease, changes compatible with respiratory distress syndrome (see Ch. 65). In convalescence, an area of hyperlucent lung may persist on chest radiograph, but most of the changes resolve. Rarely, bronchiectasis, bronchiolitis obliterans, and progressive fibrosis are permanent sequelae.

Pathology of pulmonary involvement includes peribronchial and peribronchiolar mononuclear inflammatory infiltrates with intraluminal polymorphonuclear leukocytes. Occasionally seen are hyaline membrane formation and organizing pneumonia, with alveolar hemorrhage or proteinaceous material and, rarely, interstitial fibrosis.

Extrapulmonary complications are common and are usually superimposed on pulmonary disease so that a mycoplasmal etiology can be suspected. The most frequent extrapulmonary complication is neurologic.

Neurologic symptoms are seen as early as several days after the onset of respiratory symptoms or 2 weeks or more after the respira-

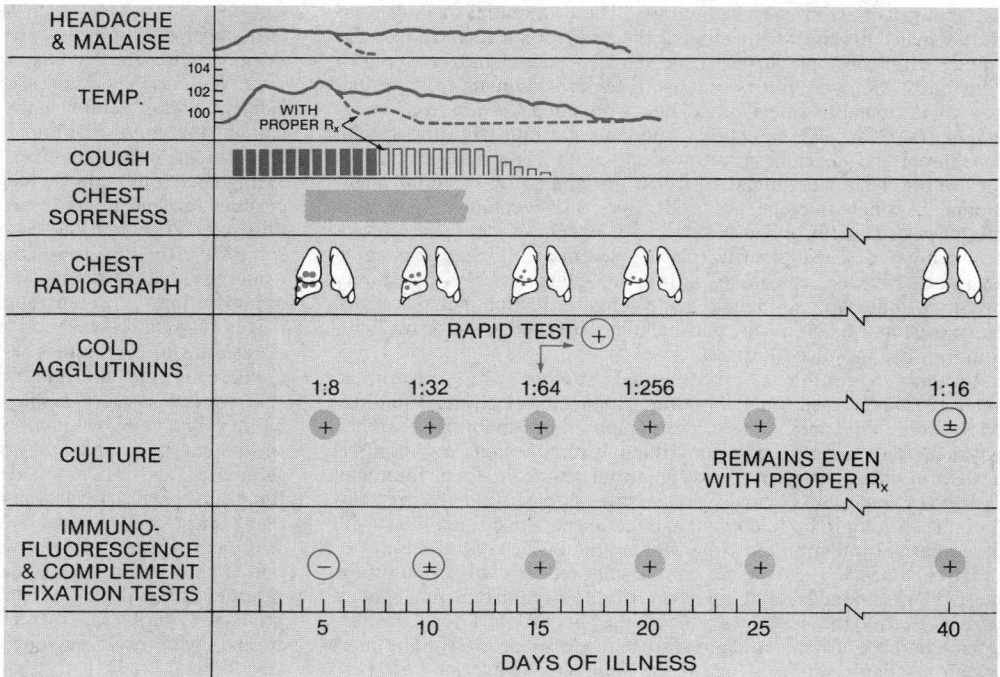

HEADACHE & MALAISE

TEMP.

COUGH

CHEST SORENESS

CHEST RADIOGRAPH

COLD AGGLUTININS

CULTURE

IMMUNO-FLUORESCENCE & COMPLEMENT FIXATION TESTS

FIGURE 272–1. Major clinical and laboratory manifestations of mycoplasmal pneumonia.

tory symptoms subside. Thus both infectious and postinfectious mechanisms seem to be involved. Respiratory disease may be absent in as many as 50% of patients at presentation. Most neurologic complications occur in children, and mycoplasmal infection accounts for 10 to 15% of childhood encephalitis. Cerebrospinal fluid typically displays a small number of lymphocytes (50 to 100) with normal or slightly elevated protein and occasionally lowered glucose.

Encephalitis may result in coma or psychosis or more focal phenomena such as stroke, ataxia, and choreoathetosis. A postinfectious leukoencephalitis has been described. Patients also may present with clinically characteristic meningitis. A number of types of myelitis are seen, including transverse myelitis and a polio-like syndrome. Finally, peripheral neuropathy may involve peripheral or cranial nerves; it is felt that *M. pneumoniae* accounts for 5% of cases of Guillain-Barré syndrome. Sequelae of neurologic involvement range from mental retardation to movement disorders and epilepsy. Corticosteroids and plasma exchange have been used as therapy, in addition to antibiotics, but there is no consensus on these additional modalities.

Rashes are seen in 10 to 20% of patients. Most are maculopapular, but they also may be vesicular, petechial, or urticarial, most commonly on the trunk and extremities. Less frequently, the face, buttocks, genitalia, hands, and feet are included. Rash usually begins during the acute illness but may precede or follow it. Most patients have obvious respiratory disease, and some have an associated conjunctivitis or an exanthem in the oropharynx. Other exanthemata associated with *M. pneumoniae* infection include pityriasis rosea, toxic epidermal necrolysis, erythema nodosum, and erythema multiforme or Stevens-Johnson syndrome. In fact, 15 to 20% of patients with erythema multiforme have been shown to have *M. pneumoniae* infection.

M. pneumoniae is the most common cause of rash and pneumonia, a combination also produced by viruses (herpes simplex, varicella-zoster, Epstein-Barr virus, enterovirus, adenovirus, and measles), *Chlamydia psittaci, Mycobacterium tuberculosis,* fungi (histoplasma, cryptococci, coccidioides), and meningococci.

Hematologic complications are well-known features of mycoplasmal infection. Anemia, hemolytic anemia, thrombocytopenia, disseminated intravascular coagulation, thromboembolism, thrombotic thrombocytopenic purpura, Pelger-Huët abnormality (polymorphonuclear leukocytes with monolobed or bilobed appearance), and hemophagocytic histiocytic syndrome are all described, but the most common hematologic complication is formation of cold agglutinins. These antibodies agglutinate red blood cells and are seen in

a variety of infections (influenza, mononucleosis, psittacosis, rubella, adenovirus, measles, and others) but usually occur at higher titer in mycoplasmal infection. If the titer is high enough, they may bind complement and cause hemolysis. These cold agglutinins are IgM antibodies directed against the I antigen of the red blood cell. They are seen in up to 70% of patients, especially those with severe disease. Appearing in the second week of illness, they peak at 4 weeks and disappear by 2 months. Thus, at the time the cold agglutinin titer is highest and hemolysis most likely to occur, the clinical disease is abating. A simple bedside test may be performed by adding 1 to 2 ml of the patient's blood to an anticoagulated tube. This tube is placed in a cup of ice water and tilted after 2 to 3 minutes to detect clumping, which represents agglutination of red blood cells. The tube is then warmed by holding it in the hands, and if the clumps redissolve, the test is positive and correlates with a titer of cold agglutinins of 1:64 or greater. Hemolysis is treated with corticosteroids as well as antibiotics; the role of plasmapheresis is uncertain, but patients (and any blood that is transfused) should be kept warm.

Cardiac complications include pericarditis with occasional hemopericardium and myocarditis, which can result in complete heart block or congestive heart failure. A migratory arthritis may be seen, involving medium-sized joints and occasionally resembling rheumatoid arthritis. Ophthalmologic complications include iritis and conjunctivitis, as well as optic neuritis with optic nerve atrophy. On occasion, retinal hemorrhages and exudates are seen. A number of other organ systems may be involved, with resultant bullous myringitis, glomerulonephritis, hepatitis, pancreatitis, splenomegaly, polymyositis, and Raynaud's phenomenon.

The differential diagnosis of *M. pneumoniae* infection includes most causes of the atypical pneumonia syndrome (Table 272–2). This syndrome refers to a generally benign febrile illness with prominent systemic complaints, nonproductive cough, and intersti-

TABLE 272–2. DIFFERENTIAL DIAGNOSIS OF *M. PNEUMONIAE* INFECTION

Common	Rare
Chlamydia pneumoniae pneumonia	Q fever
Legionnaires' disease	Psittacosis
Viral pneumonia	Acute fungal infection
Early bacterial pneumonia	Tularemia
	Tuberculosis

tial abnormalities on chest radiograph. The differential diagnosis includes many diseases with clinical or epidemiologic clues. For example, psittacosis should be suspected if a patient has had contact with birds, Q fever follows exposure to farm animals or cats, and *Legionella* tends to infect older men who smoke. *Chlamydia pneumoniae* (see Ch. 323) infection often causes a biphasic illness, with sore throat and hoarseness followed by cough. True viruses cause a more fulminant pneumonia. Early in the course of bacterial pneumonia, a cough may be nonproductive, but eventually sputum is produced with neutrophils and bacteria on Gram stain, in association with rigors and pleuritic pain. Tularemia follows exposure to an infected animal carcass or arthropod. Other illnesses that rarely mimic *M. pneumoniae* include acute fungal infection, such as histoplasmosis, and tuberculosis, particularly primary disease or reactivation in a compromised host.

Factors suggesting a mycoplasmal etiology are sore throat, headache, fever, rash, indolent course, a paucity of physical findings on examination, and a chest radiograph more abnormal than the physical examination predicted. Although rare, bullous myringitis is a helpful clue. *Against* a mycoplasmal etiology is a fulminant course, extreme leukocytosis, pre-existing disease, and recurrent infection. Although both coryza and hoarseness may be seen with mycoplasmal infection, they are more common in viral disease.

DIAGNOSIS. *Mycoplasma* can be cultured, but this capability is not widely available, and recovery of the organism from sputum does not prove the diagnosis, since it can persist for a long time after infection. Thus most diagnoses are made by serology. The most widely available serologic test is the complement fixation test (CF). Ninety percent of patients have either a fourfold rise in the CF titers (2 to 3 weeks apart) or a single titer of 1:32 or greater. There are problems with this test, however: First, the CF titer can remain elevated for a year after the infection. Second, the glycolipid antigen used in the test is not specific for *Mycoplasma* and is found in a variety of tissues, including human heart muscle, brain, and pancreas, as well as in some streptococci and leafy vegetables. Thus false-positive results may be seen, for example, in certain neurologic syndromes and pancreatitis. Third, there are false-negative reactions.

Other serologic tests include the ELISA, which can readily detect IgM as well as IgG antibody; this test is promising but is not as widely available as the CF. Other diagnostic tests that identify antibody in blood or nucleic acid in clinical samples (e.g., polymerase chain reaction [PCR]) are presently either under investigation or not widely available. Thus diagnosis is generally *proven* by a fourfold rise in CF titer or by a single IgM determination, and diagnosis is strongly *supported* by a single CF titer ≥ 1:32 or a titer of cold agglutinins ≥ 1:64.

THERAPY. From a practical standpoint, therapy for *M. pneumoniae* infection is empirical because culture takes time and may be misleading and serologic investigation is not diagnostic early in the course. Thus a compatible illness in a susceptible patient should be treated on the basis of clinical suspicion. There is a definite clinical response to tetracyclines and erythromycin, although treatment does not influence the carrier state, and the organism may persist in respiratory secretions despite appropriate antibiotic therapy.

Currently, erythromycin or tetracycline (either as 2 grams daily in divided doses) is standard therapy (Table 272–3). Doxycycline and the newer macrolides (azithromycin and clarithromycin) can probably substitute for tetracycline and erythromycin, respectively, and offer the advantage of greater patient convenience but at increased cost. Although most recommendations are for 10 to 14 days of therapy, longer courses of treatment (e.g., 2 to 3 weeks) may avoid the relapse that occurs in 5 to 10% of patients. Prophylaxis of contacts does not prevent infection but can prevent clinical disease. Tetracyclines should be avoided in children under the age of 8 and pregnant patients but are preferable if the differential diagnosis includes psittacosis, Q fever, or *M. fermentans* (see below). Correspondingly, erythromycin is preferred if the differential diagnosis includes legionellosis.

M. hominis is a commensal of the genitourinary tract, especially in women. It is seen in up to 50% of sexually active women and 30% of sexually active men. Occasionally, it is found in the pharynx. *M. hominis* may produce several different syndromes. It is a known pathogen of the female urogenital tract, causing Bartholin's gland abscess, pelvic inflammatory disease (PID), and pyelonephritis. It also causes postabortal and postpartum fever and wound infection following cesarean section. *M. hominis* can infect the fetus *in utero* or during birth, resulting in neonatal infection and stillbirth. Scalp wound infection may complicate fetal monitoring devices.

M. hominis also causes extragenital infection in the adult, typically following genitourinary manipulation in an immunosuppressed patient. Infection of surgical wounds should be suspected if a purulent exudate is negative on Gram stain and culture. Other sites of extragenital infection include brain, lung, prosthetic devices, skin, peritoneum, and joints (especially in patients with hypogammaglobulinemia). Although these organisms are not visible on Gram stain, some investigators have identified them in infected joint fluid by using the acridine orange stain and immunofluorescent staining. The organism may grow on routine media but is easily overlooked, and if it is suspected, the laboratory should be alerted. Since *M. hominis* is resistant to erythromycin, tetracycline is the drug of choice, with clindamycin and the quinolones as alternatives (see Table 272–3).

Ureaplasma urealyticum colonizes the genital tract of 75% of women and 45% of men who are sexually active (see Ch. 314). In the adult, it may cause nongonococcal urethritis as well as salpingitis and PID; outside the genitourinary tract, it can infect joints (especially in patients with hypogammaglobulinemia), transplant sites, and surgical wounds. In the neonate, it is associated with chorioamnionitis and with chronic lung disease of prematurity, but is not strongly associated with prematurity, and treatment to eradicate it during pregnancy does not reduce the incidence of premature birth or low birth rate. Tetracyclines are agents of choice, with erythromycin or possibly quinolones as alternatives (see Table 272–3).

Another definite pathogen has been recognized in *M. fermentans*. This organism has been recovered from the lower genital tract of men and women, the oropharynx, and the lower respiratory tract. Although associated with immunosuppression (leukemia, AIDS, and chemotherapy), it also has been described in normal patients who develop a febrile illness with fever, vomiting, and diarrhea and progress to fulminant disease with respiratory distress syndrome, multiple organ failure, and death. This organism is resistant to erythromycin and should be treated with doxycycline or a quinolone (see Table 272–3).

A variety of other mycoplasmas possibly cause disease, especially in immunosuppressed patients; *M. orale* has been isolated from the blood and marrow of children with leukemia; *M. pirum* has been recovered from lymphocytic cells from patients with AIDS; *M. genitalium* may cause urethritis or arthritis in hypogammaglobulinemic patients; *M. penetrans* is strongly associated with homosexual activity and has been isolated from the urine of patients with AIDS; *M. salivarium* causes periodontitis and septic arthritis in hypogammaglobulinemic patients; and *M. arginini*, an animal strain of *Mycoplasma*, has caused septicemia and pneumonia in an immunocompromised patient with lymphoma. Like *M. fermentans*, this strain of *Mycoplasma* is resistant to erythromycin and should be treated with tetracycline if suspected (see Table 272–3). Other human mycoplasmas, as noted in Table 272–1, are presently considered commensals.

Recent interest has focused on the relationship between mycoplasmas and human immunodeficiency virus (HIV) infection. It is possible that in patients with infection due to HIV-1, coincident infection with mycoplasmas may lead to accelerated disease via enhanced viral replication or cytopathic effects. This role of cofactor with HIV has been suggested for several strains of mycoplasmas, including *M. fermentans*, *M. pirum*, and *M. penetrans*, all of which

TABLE 272–3. ANTIBIOTIC SUSCEPTIBILITY*

	ERY	TCN	CLN	QUN
M. pneumoniae	sens	sens		
M. fermentans	res	sens	sens	sens
M. hominis	res	sens†	sens	
U. urealyticum	sens†	sens†	res	sens
M. arginini	res	sens		

* ERY = erythromycin; TCN = tetracycline; CLN = clindamycin; QUN = quinolones; sens = sensitive; res = resistant.
† Some resistance seen.

have been isolated from HIV-infected patients and are potent immunomodulators.

Couch RB: *Mycoplasma pneumoniae* (primary atypical pneumonia). *In* Mandell GL, Douglas RG Jr, Bennett JE (eds.): Principles and Practice of Infectious Diseases, 3rd ed. New York, Churchill-Livingstone, 1990. *A good general reference for all aspects of* Mycoplasma *infection.*

Koskiniemi M: CNS manifestations associated with *Mycoplasma pneumoniae* infections: Summary of cases at the University of Helsinki and review. Clin Infect Dis 17(suppl 1):S52, 1993. *An excellent and thorough review of neurologic complications.*

Lo S-C, Wear DJ, Green SL, et al.: Adult respiratory distress syndrome with or without systemic disease associated with infections due to *Mycoplasma fermentans.* Clin Infect Dis 17(suppl 1):S259, 1993. *Excellent clinical and laboratory description of this infection.*

McMahon DK, Dummer JS, Pasculle AW, et al.: Extragenital *Mycoplasma hominis* infections in adults. Am J Med 89:275, 1990. *Good concise review with helpful references.*

273 PNEUMONIA CAUSED BY AEROBIC GRAM-NEGATIVE BACILLI

Waldemar G. Johanson, Jr.

Over the past 30 years, the group of organisms known collectively as "aerobic gram-negative bacilli" (GNB) has assumed an increasing importance in clinical respiratory infections. There is no evidence that this phenomenon is due to increasing virulence of these organisms. Rather, it is due to changes in the human hosts they infect and, to some degree, to changes in the environment induced by antibiotics and other factors, especially in hospitals. Each of the GNB has its place (or places) in nature. Many are regular inhabitants of the human gastrointestinal tract, while others are found in water or other sites in the environment. None is especially virulent for the respiratory tract of healthy mammalian hosts; all are distinctly inferior to the pneumococcus, for example, in that regard. A careful review of the preantibiotic literature reveals that the presence of these organisms in the respiratory tracts of seriously ill patients is not a recent occurrence; rather, their presence was disregarded for many years, an approach that was not unjustified, considering the preeminence of the pneumococcus as a cause of fatal pneumonia before highly efficacious antibiotics were available. The emergence of GNB as respiratory pathogens in recent years is the result of more aggressive organisms being suppressed by effective therapy and the long-term survival of people who would have succumbed to other infections or other processes in an earlier era.

PATHOGENESIS. Pneumonias due to GNB are caused by one of three mechanisms: inhalation of contaminated aerosols, hematogenous infection of the lungs from another primary source of infection, or aspiration of oropharyngeal secretions that are colonized by these organisms.

Contamination of respiratory therapy equipment by GNB, usually *Pseudomonas aeruginosa,* was recognized as a major cause of nosocomial pneumonias in the 1960's. With the advent of disposable nebulizers and other control strategies, this problem has been largely eliminated.

Most instances of bacteremia from a nonpulmonary source, such as the gastrointestinal or urinary tract, associated with pulmonary infiltrates, fever, and hypoxemia, represent noncardiogenic pulmonary edema, or the "adult respiratory distress syndrome" (see Ch. 65 and 68), and not actual pneumonia. In fact, pneumonia due to this cause is sufficiently uncommon that the presence of gram-negative bacteremia in association with new pulmonary infiltrates should initiate a vigorous search for a primary site of infection outside the lungs before it is concluded that pneumonia is responsible.

Aspiration of oropharyngeal secretions that contain GNB is the usual event leading to pneumonia caused by these organisms. Colonization of the upper respiratory tract with GNB occurs in 10% or fewer of normal people but is markedly increased among patients with acute or chronic diseases. Colonization rates among populations with chronic disease, such as alcoholics and residents of

skilled nursing facilities, and previously healthy individuals with acute but severe illnesses or trauma approach 50%. Colonization of the oropharynx by GNB among healthy persons undergoing elective surgical procedures rises from essentially zero to 35 to 50% within 24 hours following surgery. The organisms responsible for colonization vary from one study to another, but only rarely can this sudden acquisition of GNB be attributed to demonstrable environmental sources. Instead, colonization appears to be caused by a translocation of the patient's fecal flora or the transfer of organisms from one patient to another on the hands of personnel. However, the root cause of this colonization is the great susceptibility of ill patients to acquire GNB from the immediate environment.

Once established in the oropharynx, GNB multiply, achieve high concentrations in secretions, and are aspirated in small liquid boluses into the lungs (see Ch. 55). Since lung defenses are often impaired by the same underlying conditions that promote changes in cell resistance to adherence and colonization, the ability of the lungs to handle this bacterial inoculum is insufficient, and pneumonia results. The specific lung defense mechanism that might be impaired in a given patient varies with the nature of underlying illness. For example, patients with chronic airway obstruction have impaired mucociliary transport and alveolar hypoxia that hinders the effectiveness of phagocytic cells. Some data suggest that the bronchial abnormalities in these patients allow persistent colonization of the distal airways by potentially pathogenic bacteria, a factor that affords the bacteria the advantage of access to the distal lung. Patients who are neutropenic are remarkably predisposed to develop pneumonias with GNB, a clinical observation that correlates nicely with the experimental finding that swift recruitment of circulating neutrophils into the lungs is a crucial aspect of host defense against *Pseudomonas* infection. Alcoholism seems to predispose to GNB pneumonias in several ways. Malnutrition promotes colonization of the upper tract by GNB, aspiration is facilitated by episodes of impaired consciousness, and acute alcohol intoxication hinders the ability of phagocytes to migrate to the site of inflammation.

Of the many species of gram-negative aerobic bacilli that colonize human hosts, only *Haemophilus influenzae* can be classified as a true respiratory pathogen, if the ability of the organism to produce infections in previously normal individuals is accepted as a reasonable criterion of pathogenicity. All the others together, including Enterobacteriaceae (*Escherichia coli, Klebsiella, Enterobacter, Serratia,* and *Proteus*), *Pseudomonas,* and *Acinetobacter,* account for 10 to 20% of community-acquired pneumonias, and these occur almost exclusively in patients with serious underlying disease. The genus *Klebsiella* contains four species, of which only *K. pneumoniae* and *K. oxytoca* cause pneumonia; infections due to *K. pneumoniae* are by far the most common.

Pneumonia caused by *Klebsiella* has been held separate from that caused by other gram-negative bacilli largely for historical reasons. It was the first such organism to be recognized as a pulmonary pathogen, and the pneumonia it caused was distinct from that caused by the pneumococcus, especially in its lack of response to early forms of treatment and its predilection to cause upper lobe pneumonias in alcoholic men. However, the classic features of *Klebsiella* pneumonia as described in the earlier literature, such as "currant jelly" sputum (a mixture of blood and mucus), the bulging fissure associated with upper lobe consolidation, and the syndrome of "chronic cavitary pneumonia," are rarely observed today. While *Klebsiella* remains an important pulmonary pathogen, the illness it causes cannot be clinically differentiated from that caused by other aerobic gram-negative bacilli, and its treatment is similar.

CLINICAL MANIFESTATIONS. Pneumonias caused by GNB may be community acquired or hospital acquired (nosocomial). Virtually all patients with community-acquired pneumonias caused by GNB have serious underlying chronic illnesses, especially chronic obstructive pulmonary disease (COPD), alcoholism, or malignancy. Nosocomial pneumonias resulting from GNB occur principally in patients with severe, acute illnesses whether or not they have underlying chronic disease as well. Thus these infections are most likely to be found in postoperative patients or patients who require intensive care for other reasons. The clinical manifestations of infection are influenced by the nature of the associated processes.

Community-acquired gram-negative bacillary pneumonias share the common features of all bacterial pneumonias—fever, cough productive of purulent sputum, chest pain, and shortness of breath. The illness tends to be abrupt and associated with prominent systemic signs and symptoms, such as mental confusion, vomiting, and hypotension. Physical examination reveals rales in most patients, but the classic findings of dense consolidation are uncommon. Pleural effusion is present in 15 to 20% of patients. Radiographic infiltrates may involve any lobe and are bilateral in about one third of patients. Although cavitation is most likely to occur in pneumonia caused by *Klebsiella,* it also occurs commonly with *Pseudomonas* infections and occasionally with other organisms. Laboratory features include leukocytosis or leukopenia, either of which is characteristically associated with a marked left shift. Leukopenia is a poor prognostic sign.

Nosocomial pneumonia produced by GNB can be an explosive illness similar to the community-acquired form but frequently proceeds with a more indolent but seemingly inexorable course. Often the patient is in respiratory failure, intubated, and receiving mechanical ventilation. GNB are initially found colonizing the oropharynx, and over the subsequent few days appear in tracheal secretions, followed by increasing numbers of neutrophils. Finally, the patient becomes febrile and develops new radiographic infiltrates and worsening hypoxemia. Another common presentation is fever on the second or third postoperative day. Postoperative pneumonias are most common after lateral thoracotomies (especially combined thoracoabdominal procedures) and upper abdominal incisions. When nosocomial GNB pneumonia complicates the course of an already seriously ill patient, it is frequently associated with evidence of multiple organ failures.

DIAGNOSIS. Confirmation that GNB are responsible for pneumonia is a difficult clinical problem created largely by colonization of proximal airways by these organisms. Thus GNB are often present in the secretions of ill patients whether they have pneumonia or not and whether or not the GNB are the cause of pneumonia. Blood cultures are positive in 20 to 30% of patients with community-acquired infections but in as few as 8% of those with nosocomial pneumonias. Nevertheless, because the information gained from a positive blood culture regarding the causative organism and its antimicrobial susceptibility is so important in patient management, blood cultures should always be obtained when GNB pneumonia is suspected. Similarly, while pleural effusion is usually not present, the yield of positive cultures from such fluid when it is present is about 30%, and a diagnostic thoracentesis should be performed if a sufficient volume of fluid is identified radiographically.

The usefulness of invasive sampling remains somewhat controversial. Transthoracic needle aspiration is rarely used in critically ill patients because of concern about complications, especially pneumothorax. Sampling via the fiberoptic bronchoscope using either bronchoalveolar lavage (BAL) or the protected specimen brush (PSB) technique offers a safe alternative. Both techniques have been studied extensively and accurately portray the lung's bacterial flora in the absence of antibiotic therapy. Using a cutoff of at least 10^3 bacteria by PSB to diagnose infection, over 50% of patients suspected of having nosocomial pneumonia on the basis of new-onset fever, leukocytosis, and radiographic infiltrates have been shown not to be infected. However, in patients who have received prior antimicrobial therapy, both techniques lose sensitivity and, in some studies, specificity. BAL has the added advantage of providing specimens for special staining and cytology and is especially useful in the diagnosis of infections in immunocompromised hosts. Despite the ready availability of bronchoscopy, the etiology of nosocomial pneumonias is often frustratingly difficult to establish with certainty.

TREATMENT. Recommendations for the antimicrobial treatment of pneumonia due to GNB are changing rapidly as new drugs aimed at this group of organisms are entering clinical practice. It must be remembered that GNB are relatively poor respiratory pathogens and that patients susceptible to infection by them are at even greater risk of pulmonary infection by more virulent organisms, such as the pneumococcus, *Haemophilus,* and *Staphylococcus aureus.* Thus, despite the presence of GNB in sputum, initial treatment of these pneumonias—particularly those acquired outside the hospital or in the absence of concomitant antibiotic therapy—should include coverage of the usual respiratory pathogens.

TABLE 273-1. EMPIRICAL ANTIBIOTIC THERAPY OF AEROBIC GRAM-NEGATIVE BACILLARY PNEUMONIA

Combination Therapy

Cefuroxime 1.5 grams every 8 hours + gentamicin 1.5 mg/kg every 8 hours*

Cefotaxime 2 grams every 8 hours + gentamicin 1.5 mg/kg every 8 hours*

Piperacillin 4 grams every 6 hours + gentamicin 1.5 mg/kg every 8 hours*

Monotherapy

Cefotaxime 2 grams every 8 hours

Ticarcillin/clavulanate 3.1 grams every 6 hours

Piperacillin/tazobactam 4.5 grams every 6 hours

Imipenem/cilastatin 500 mg every 6 hours

High Likelihood of *Pseudomonas aeruginosa*

Ceftazadime 2 grams every 8 hours + amikacin 7.5 mg/kg every 12 hours*

Ticarcillin 3 grams every 4 hours + amikacin 7.5 mg/kg every 12 hours*

Imipenem/cilastatin 500 mg every 6 hours + amikacin 7.5 mg/kg every 12 hours*

* Recommendations for adults with normal renal function; serum levels should be monitored.

Table 273-1 provides therapeutic options for the patient with a pneumonia suspected to be of GNB etiology. Agents must be given parenterally and in adequate dosage. Traditionally, therapy has consisted of broad-spectrum combination antibiotic therapy with an aminoglycoside in conjunction with a β-lactam agent. The rationale behind this approach has been (1) the identification and susceptibility of the infecting organism are unknown, and two agents allow better coverage, (2) emergence of resistance may be prevented by combining antibiotics, and (3) additive or synergistic effects may result from a two-drug combination. There is increasing evidence that monotherapy with a third-generation cephalosporin, imipenem/cilastatin, or a drug combining a β-lactam antibiotic with a β-lactamase inhibitor, such as ticarcillin/clavulanate or piperacillin/tazobactam, may be as efficacious as combination therapy.

Treatment of nosocomial infection is often made more difficult by previous antimicrobial therapy, and drug susceptibility studies are critically important. However, empirical therapy usually must be initiated before the results of such studies are available. Factors to consider when selecting appropriate therapy include knowledge of local resistance patterns, previous culture results, and prior treatment. For example, resistance of *P. aeruginosa* to gentamicin may approach 50% in some hospitals. If *P. aeruginosa* is strongly suspected on the basis of previous cultures or the clinical setting (respiratory failure, neutropenia), a β-lactam agent with antipseudomonal activity should be combined with an aminoglycoside (see Table 273-1). Amikacin is often used in this setting because of less frequent resistance to this agent. Because the pharmacokinetics of aminoglycosides vary widely, adjustments in dosing must be determined from peak and trough serum levels in the individual patient. Improved clinical outcomes in the treatment of pneumonia caused by GNB have been associated with peak plasma levels of 6 μg per milliliter for gentamicin or tobramycin and 24 μg per milliliter for amikacin.

When the pathogenic organisms have been identified and the susceptibility patterns are known, modifications can be made to optimize antibiotic therapy. Ideally, antibiotics with the narrowest spectrum of activity, the least toxicity, and the best lung penetration should be chosen. In neutropenic patients and in seriously ill patients with pneumonia caused by resistant organisms such as *P. aeruginosa, Serratia marcescens,* and *Acinetobacter,* continued combination therapy with an appropriate β-lactam agent and an aminoglycoside is recommended. Duration of therapy should be based on clinical response, but a minimum of 2 to 3 weeks is usually required.

PROGNOSIS. The mortality of GNB pneumonias remains high—in the range of 30 to 50%. It has been argued that this is the result of the underlying disease usually present in patients who develop these pneumonias. This notion could lead to therapeutic nihilism. Other data clearly indicate that GNB pneumonias increase hospital mortality among patients who have nonlethal disease processes, a finding that would support an aggressive diagnostic and treatment approach. It is probable that both conclusions could be correct, depending on the population of patients studied. There is little doubt that GNB pneumonias represent the terminal event for a number of patients with irreversible and lethal diseases and that such patients form a large fraction of all hospital patients. On the other hand, there is reason to expect recovery rates of 80% or more among patients who develop GNB pneumonias in the context of acute, severe, but nonlethal disease processes, and in these patients, aggressive diagnostic maneuvers and intensive therapy are clearly indicated.

COMPLICATIONS. Pneumonias caused by GNB are more likely than other pneumonias to be complicated by one or another adverse event. Important complications include empyema, lung necrosis, superinfections, and multiple organ failure; metastatic seeding of infection to other sites is an uncommon complication.

Empyema occurs in perhaps as many as 30% of patients with GNB pneumonias. Criteria for the diagnosis of empyema, besides the presence of gross pus, include the presence of bacteria on Gram stain, a pleural fluid pH ≤ 7.2, or a pleural fluid white cell count $> 30,000$ per deciliter. Each of these criteria indicates a condition that is unlikely to respond to antimicrobials alone, but that usually requires drainage of the pleural space as well. Thus the term "complicated effusion" has gained favor over "empyema" to identify pleural fluid collections for which drainage needs to be considered. The occurrence of a complicated effusion generally prevents the recovery of the patient until it is recognized and effectively treated. Signs and symptoms of continuing illness, such as fever, persistent leukocytosis, and the onset of multiple organ failure, in a patient undergoing treatment for a GNB pneumonia should raise suspicion of a complicated effusion. If pleural fluid is identified on upright posteroanterior and lateral chest radiographs, thoracentesis should be performed; useful studies of the fluid obtained include measurements of pH and glucose, white cell count, Gram stain, and cultures for aerobic and anaerobic organisms.

If the fluid qualifies as a complicated effusion, most authorities recommend prompt placement of a thoracostomy tube and drainage. Alternative approaches, principally repeated thoracentesis, are less successful owing to loculation of the pleural space. Surgical drainage of the pleural space, using localized resection of an overlying rib with creation of a larger drainage tract, is reserved for patients who do not respond to tube drainage. Decortication of the pleura may be necessary if the clinical signs of uncontrolled infection are not ameliorated by simple drainage plus antimicrobial therapy. In such patients, radiographic evidence of effusion persists, along with continued fever and leukocytosis. At surgery, the pleural space is found to contain numerous loculated pockets of pus. The timing of intervention with these techniques requires excellent clinical judgment, because the patients are usually seriously ill and poor candidates for surgical treatment of any kind; on the other hand, they will not recover unless the pleural space is adequately drained.

Extensive lung necrosis has been termed "lung gangrene" because of the rapid occurrence of pulmonary cavitation associated with marked systemic toxicity and the appearance of extensive devitalization of lung tissue at necropsy. Occasionally, an entire lung appears to dissolve within a few days, leaving multiple cavities with air-fluid levels. This complication occurs with all of the common GNB, although perhaps more commonly in infections produced by *K. pneumoniae* and *P. aeruginosa*. Lung necrosis may be caused by the extracellular products of these organisms. *P. aeruginosa* makes a number of "virulence factors," including exotoxin A, exoenzyme S, elastase, and a neutral protease. However, *K. pneumoniae* makes none of these, and the propensity of this organism to cause lung necrosis remains unexplained.

Extensive lung necrosis may be followed by massive hemoptysis, continued suppuration because of inadequate drainage of the massively disrupted lung parenchyma, or bronchopleural fistula caused by extension of the necrotizing process through the pleura. The last must be promptly treated by placing a chest tube because of the attendant pneumothorax. However, the definitive treatment of extensive lung necrosis is surgical resection of the involved lobe or lobes. As with management of complicated effusion, the timing of such an intervention must be carefully considered in light of the control of the underlying infection, the severity of complicating problems (hemoptysis, air leak, and so on), and the patient's general condition.

Assessment of the patient with multiple organ failure in the context of a serious illness complicated by a GNB pneumonia is always difficult. The major question is usually whether a new complication such as oliguria is due to the underlying disease, to the current treatment, or to the infection. Each of the common manifestations of multiple organ dysfunction—altered liver function, acute renal failure, hematopoietic abnormalities, upper gastrointestinal bleeding, and altered mental state—may be multifactorial in etiology, and the antimicrobial agents used to treat GNB pneumonia may cause most of them. The guiding principles are to treat the infection aggressively and to correct life-threatening complications as they occur.

Superinfections may develop during the treatment of GNB pneumonia, just as GNB pneumonia may occur as a superinfection of a previous pneumonia. Unfortunately, treatment of the patient's pneumonia does not prevent colonization of the oropharynx and tracheobronchial tree by additional GNB or fungi. Thus the clinician is often faced with evaluating a new set of microorganisms recovered from the patient's secretions. The guiding principle here is to treat patients, not culture results. If the patient is responding well and appears to be improving, the new cultures can be disregarded for the time being. On the other hand, if the new cultural data correspond to a worsening clinical course, the process of evaluation and revision of treatment must be begun again.

Dever LL, Johanson WG Jr: Nosocomial pneumonia. *In* Simmons DH, Tierney DE (eds.): Current Pulmonology, vol. 13, St. Louis, Mosby–Year Book, 1992, pp 1–28. *This review provides a current bibliography of 140 references with sections on pathogenesis, diagnosis, etiologic agents, therapy, and prevention.*
Dotson RG, Pingleton SK: The effect of antibiotic therapy on recovery of intracellular bacteria from bronchoalveolar lavage in suspected ventilator-associated nosocomial pneumonia. Chest 103:541, 1993. *This article highlights the difficulty encountered when patients have received antibiotic therapy.*
Fagon J, Chastre J, Hance AJ, et al.: Nosocomial pneumonia in ventilated patients: A cohort study evaluating attributable mortality and hospital stay. Am J Med 94:281, 1993. *Whether patients die of nosocomial pneumonia or with it has been controversial. This study found that nosocomial GNB pneumonias added significantly to patient mortality and length of hospital stay.*
Kollef MH: Ventilator-associated pneumonia. JAMA 270:1965, 1993. *Understanding risk factors for pneumonia might lead to effective forms of prevention. This study examines risk factors in a large group of patients who developed pneumonia in a university ICU setting.*

274 ASPIRATION PNEUMONIA
Waldemar G. Johanson, Jr.

Categorization of the various syndromes associated with aspiration of liquids into the tracheobronchial tree is not an area distinguished by precise terminology or even consistency in the use of terms. Most of the important syndromes are dealt with elsewhere in this volume: gastric acid aspiration (see Ch. 54.2), anaerobic pneumonias and lung abscess (see Ch. 56), lipoid pneumonia (Ch. 60), and hydrocarbon aspiration (see Ch. 54.2). In this chapter we concentrate on an infrequent but difficult problem: that of recurrent bacterial pneumonias associated with aspiration. Such pneumonias are defined as recurring clinical illnesses characterized by fever, purulent sputum, and new radiographic infiltrates in the lungs in a patient with known or suspected chronic aspiration of oropharyngeal contents.

ETIOLOGY. Most patients afflicted with this problem have serious problems with swallowing for one or another reason. Common predisposing conditions are carcinoma of the esophagus with obstruction, tracheobronchial fistula (usually following treatment for cancer), and neurologic diseases affecting deglutition. Strokes are certainly the most common cause of the latter, but amyotrophic lateral sclerosis (including bulbar palsy), multiple sclerosis, and the myopathies may be responsible. Recurrent nocturnal aspiration of gastric contents by patients with esophageal reflux represents the one situation in which the swallowing mechanism may be intact in this syndrome.

Impaired swallowing having neural or myopathic causes is most pronounced when the patient attempts to swallow liquids. By contrast, dysphagia caused by obstruction is always worst with solid foods. Thus it is not surprising that the patient with myoneural deficits of the pharyngeal musculature repeatedly aspirates oropharyngeal secretions. In patients with esophageal obstruction, secretions accumulate proximal to the obstruction, especially at night, and are aspirated. Gastric contents are normally sterile. However, as the patient with reflux aspirates gastric contents, a certain volume of oropharyngeal secretions is necessarily carried along.

Oropharyngeal secretions are massively contaminated, containing 10^6 to 10^8 aerobic bacteria per milliliter and about 10 times as many anaerobic organisms. Although the majority of organisms composing the normal flora of this region have little invasiveness for the normal host, highly pathogenic organisms, including *Streptococcus pneumoniae*, *Staphylococcus aureus*, and *Haemophilus influenzae*, may be present in the secretions of normal people. Since most of the patients susceptible to recurrent aspiration have serious underlying diseases, their upper respiratory tracts are likely to be colonized by enteric gram-negative bacilli and *Pseudomonas* as well.

Normal individuals aspirate small volumes of oropharyngeal secretions during sleep but do not develop recurrent pneumonias. The difference between normal people and those who do develop recurrent pneumonias is probably the volume of material aspirated and the underlying chronic illnesses of the latter patients; differences in the bacterial flora of secretions may play a role as well.

CLINICAL MANIFESTATIONS. Episodes of recurrent pneumonia associated with aspiration tend not to be acute, fulminant illnesses but rather are characterized by progressive fever, purulent sputum production, shortness of breath, and systemic symptoms (such as loss of appetite and malaise) over a period of days. The frequency of such episodes in an individual prone to recurrent aspiration varies widely. In patients with tracheobronchial fistulas, the episodes are essentially continuous until an effective preventive measure can be implemented or the patient dies. By contrast, patients with esophageal reflux may go years between episodes. The frequency of episodes is usually directly related to the frequency and volume of material aspirated and thus is increased in conditions in which aspiration is a daily event, especially if coupled with a decreased level of awareness, as occurs in some patients following strokes.

Physical findings include those related to the underlying illness and the presence of coarse rhonchi over dependent lung zones. Rales and signs of consolidation may or may not be present. Fever and leukocytosis are regularly present. Radiographs of the chest reveal infiltrates of varying intensity, with a preponderance of change in the dependent zones, i.e., posterior aspects of the lower lobes and posterior segments of the upper lobes. Pleural effusion is uncommon unless anaerobic infection is present.

DIAGNOSIS. Examination of expectorated sputum helps confirm the suspicion of aspiration pneumonia but is of little help in defining a specific bacterial etiology. Typically, the sputum of such patients is intensely purulent, with a wide spectrum of bacterial forms present on Gram stain. Culture of this material yields the same flora as in upper respiratory secretions, and the clinical problem consists of trying to discern which of several pathogenic organisms should be treated. Cultures should be obtained, however, since knowledge of the sensitivity of the organisms present may be needed to guide therapy. Blood cultures are rarely positive. The presence of food particles in tracheal secretions is clear evidence of aspiration. In patients receiving enteral feedings, the presence of glucose in secretions may be demonstrable by bedside tests. Since normal secretions contain an undetectable level of glucose, a positive result is highly specific for aspiration. Dietary lipids form large intracellular deposits when ingested by phagocytic cells, and examination of sputum with a lipid stain may confirm the clinical impression of chronic aspiration. The microscopic appearance of the large lipid deposits is important in differentiating this type of lipid inclusion from the foamy deposit that occurs in macrophages owing to the accumulation of endogenous lipid distal to an obstructing lesion in the airways.

When the diagnosis of recurrent aspiration is in doubt, cineradiographic studies of the patient swallowing a thin, water-soluble contrast material is usually definitive. Thick barium should be avoided because aspiration of this material compounds the

patient's problems and a thick solution is less likely to identify the swallowing difficulty. In questionable cases, the procedure may need to be repeated with the patient in the supine position. Follow-up films of the chest reveal the presence of contrast material in the airways.

Patients with infrequent episodes of recurrent pneumonia caused by esophageal reflux and nocturnal aspiration represent a somewhat different problem. The presence of a hiatus hernia or the demonstration of reflux during an upper gastrointestinal contrast study does not necessarily prove that pneumonia was caused by this mechanism, although that would be a reasonable presumption if other aspects of the patient's presentation were compatible with the diagnosis. One diagnostic test in uncertain circumstances is to monitor the pH in the upper esophagus during sleep. Reflux into the upper esophagus is marked by a sudden fall in pH, an event that is easily captured on a long-term strip chart recorder for review the next morning. Recent refinements in technique have improved the sensitivity of radioisotopic methods, which may become the diagnostic procedure of choice.

TREATMENT. Initial antibiotic therapy should provide coverage for gram-positive and gram-negative organisms as well as anaerobes. Pending the results of culture and susceptibility studies, empirical therapy with intravenous penicillin or clindamycin and an aminoglycoside is reasonable. Alternatively, monotherapy with a second- or third-generation cephalosporin, imipenem, or a drug combining a β-lactam antibiotic with a β-lactamase inhibitor such as ampicillin-sulbactam, ticarcillin-clavulanate, or piperacillin-tazobactam can be used. Supportive care, including aggressive tracheobronchial toilet, is required. Nutrition must not be overlooked despite the difficulties encountered in many of these patients. If swallowing is impossible and a small feeding tube cannot be placed in the intestinal tract via the nose or mouth, parenteral nutrition should be provided while a long-term solution to the patient's problem is sought. Failure to address the nutritional deficits of these patients is a common cause of protracted and often lethal complications.

Surgical intervention to prevent esophageal reflux is indicated for the patient in whom recurrent pneumonia can be reasonably attributed to this mechanism. Long-term solutions for the other patients with this syndrome often involve difficult choices. Bypassing the mouth to facilitate feeding can be accomplished with a feeding gastrostomy or enterostomy. The former can be performed noninvasively via fiberoptic gastroscopy, with the feeding tube being passed percutaneously into the stomach. In some patients, cessation of swallowing food diminishes the frequency and severity of aspiration and successfully ameliorates the clinical problem. However, in many it does not because patients must still handle their own secretions. Drug therapy aimed at reducing the volume of secretions in this situation is usually not successful. The only certain preventive measure is tracheostomy with all its complications. Even tracheostomy does not negate the possibility of aspiration around the tube unless the larynx is removed or the vocal cords are sewn together. The latter can be undone at a later date if the patient's condition improves. These procedures should not be contemplated in all patients with the syndrome of recurrent aspiration, since many patients have underlying conditions that will be lethal in a short time. However, if the patient has a reasonable chance of long-term survival in the absence of recurrent episodes of pneumonia, these steps should be considered.

Johnson ER, McKenzie SW, Sievers A: Aspiration pneumonia in stroke. Arch Phys Med Rehabil 74:973, 1993. *This study found that nearly 50% of stroke victims with dysphagia developed aspiration pneumonia within the first year. Pharyngeal transit time, as assessed by videofluoroscopy, was the best predictor of the subsequent development of pneumonia.*

Ruth M, Carlsson S, Mansson I, et al.: Scintigraphic detection of gastropulmonary aspiration in patients with respiratory disorders. Clin Physiol 13:19, 1993. *This carefully done study examined and corrected for artifacts produced by instilling radiolabeled materials into the stomach and demonstrated that aspiration could be detected in 20% of patients with a variety of pulmonary complaints, including asthma, chronic laryngitis, and recurrent infections. If properly controlled, this technique may be the method of choice for demonstrating aspiration because it is easily tolerated by patients.*

Torres A, Serra-Batlles J, Ros E, et al.: Pulmonary aspiration of gastric contents in patients receiving mechanical ventilation: The effect of body position. Ann Intern Med 116:540, 1992. *Aspiration occurs regularly in intubated patients receiving mechanical ventilation and is associated with the development of nosocomial pneumonia. Not surprisingly, nursing the patient supine, as contrasted with semirecumbent, promotes aspiration.*

275 LEGIONELLOSIS
Paul H. Edelstein

DEFINITION. "Legionellosis" is the term used to describe infections caused by bacteria of the genus *Legionella*. The most important of these diseases is pneumonia, called "legionnaires' disease." Either as part of legionnaires' disease or distinct from it, the legionellae may cause infections elsewhere in the body, usually in the form of abscesses. Pontiac fever, which is a self-limited mild febrile illness, is assumed to be caused by legionellae, although this is unproven.

HISTORY. Legionnaires' disease was first recognized when it caused epidemic pneumonia among members of the American Legion attending a convention in Philadelphia in 1976; this resulted in 29 deaths and in 182 cases of pneumonia. Charles McDade and William Shepard, of the United States Centers for Disease Control and Prevention, determined that this disease was caused by an ostensibly newly discovered bacterium, which was named *Legionella pneumophila*. Neither the disease nor the bacterium is new. The first documented epidemic of legionnaires' disease occurred in a meat packing plant in Minnesota in 1957, and the first recorded isolation of the bacterium was in 1943. In fact, three different *Legionella* species had been isolated from humans prior to 1976, although they were thought to be rickettsia-like agents. Several unsolved epidemics of pneumonia, including one in Philadelphia in 1974, were recognized to have been due to legionnaires' disease.

BACTERIOLOGY. Thirty-nine *Legionella* species have been recognized to date. About half of these have been isolated from patients with legionnaires' disease, and about half have been isolated only from the environment. The species that most commonly cause disease are *L. pneumophila, L. micdadei, L. bozemanii, L. dumoffii,* and *L. longbeachae*. Fifteen serogroups are recognized for *L. pneumophila,* while several other species contain up to two serogroups. *L. pneumophila* serogroup 1 causes up to 90% of cases of legionnaires' disease in nonimmunocompromised individuals. *L. micdadei* is probably the second most common cause of legionnaires' disease and commonly causes legionnaires' disease in immunocompromised patients.

The legionellae are small, gram-negative, obligately aerobic bacilli. *Legionella* requires complex growth media, having an absolute nutritional requirement for L-cysteine. Optimal growth occurs on a buffered charcoal yeast extract medium supplemented with iron, L-cysteine, and α-ketoglutarate (BCYEα). These bacteria do not grow on conventional bacteriologic media, such as tryptic soy blood agar, MacConkey's agar, or unsupplemented chocolate agar. Their usual habitat is natural and treated waters, such as lakes, ponds, and tap water. Legionellae are found in highest concentration in warm water, especially in water heaters, hot water plumbing fixtures, and cooling towers. They appear to be obligate or facultative parasites of freshwater amoebae, such as *Hartmannella* and *Acanthamoeba*. Humans are very likely accidental hosts of these bacteria.

Virulence factors have been examined for relatively few strains each of *L. pneumophila* and *L. micdadei* and are not well understood. The bacteria produce endotoxins and exotoxins, which may cause tissue damage independently or in concert with the host immune system.

PATHOGENESIS. Legionnaires' disease is acquired by inhaling aerosolized water containing *Legionella* organisms or possibly by pulmonary aspiration of contaminated water. The contaminated aerosols are derived from humidifiers, shower heads, respiratory therapy equipment, industrial cooling water, and cooling towers. Aerosols formed by contaminated water in plumbing systems and in cooling towers are the most common sources of infection. Inhaled organisms are phagocytosed by pulmonary alveolar macrophages, which are unable to kill the bacteria. The bacteria multiply within the phagosome. Eventually, the multiplying bacteria, which produce cytotoxins, kill the macrophage and are released extracellularly. The intracellular infection cycle is reinitiated in another macrophage. Continuing bacterial multiplication and consequent lung damage produce symptoms 2 to 14 days after initiation of infection.

Bacterial uptake and multiplication are curtailed by the action of cytokines (e.g., γ-interferon), which are produced by macrophages and lymphocytes. Natural killer and lymphokine-activated killer cells probably lyse infected macrophages, aborting the intracellular infection cycle. The role of polymorphonuclear phagocytes is unclear, although they probably have some part in eliminating bacteria, especially after activation by interleukin-2 and tumor necrosis factor. Antibody appears to have little function in host immunity or defense, whereas T lymphocytes play a major role in the immune process. The actual mechanism of pulmonary damage is not well understood and could be due to bacterial toxins, immune reactions to infection, or both. The bacteria may spread to extrapulmonary sites via the lymphatic system and bloodstream; they are likely transported in the blood by infected blood mononuclear cells. The mechanism whereby the pneumonia exerts systemic effects is unknown but could be the result of disseminated bacterial infection, the effect of toxin, or the production of host factors such as tumor necrosis factor.

The pathogenesis of Pontiac fever is a mystery. Inhalation of water contaminated with many different types of bacteria, including *Legionella* species, produces the disease. The incubation period of the disease, 12 to 36 hours, is too short to allow for bacterial infection and multiplication. It is possible that bacterial or fungal toxins present in the water produce this illness, as has been hypothesized for a closely related disease, "humidifier fever." Another possibility is an immune response to one or more of the multiple microorganisms found in the water. Antibody to *Legionella* species found in the contaminated water is present in most disease victims, but it is unclear what this means.

EPIDEMIOLOGY. Legionnaires' disease occurs worldwide but is primarily a disease found in technically advanced countries. Case reports from underdeveloped countries are rare, perhaps because of limited diagnostic facilities and also perhaps because of the infrequent use of air conditioning and complex plumbing systems. Normal children have this disease very rarely. Cigarette smokers, especially those 50 years of age or older, are at increased risk. The presence of chronic lung or heart disease may also increase risk. Glucocorticosteroid administration or its endogenous production is the major risk factor for legionnaires' disease. OKT3 administration also may predispose to this illness, but cyclosporine administration probably does not. Administration of cytotoxic agents is not a risk factor, nor are hematologic malignancies (except hairy cell leukemia) or neutropenia in the absence of glucocorticoid administration. Patients with the acquired immunodeficiency syndrome (AIDS) are at increased risk, although legionnaires' disease is an uncommon disease in such patients. Patients in the immediate postoperative period are at increased risk of acquiring legionnaires' disease, because of inhalation of contaminated water aerosols during anesthesia, transient paralysis of local lung defenses, or both. Males get legionnaires' disease about twice as often as females, although this does not hold true for several epidemics of legionnaires' disease. No good evidence exists for person-to-person spread of legionnaires' disease.

Legionnaires' disease may occur in epidemics originating in a single building or area. Outbreaks of the disease have occurred among hotel guests, hospital inpatients and outpatients, office building workers, and factory workers. There appears to be little, if any, increased risk of disease acquisition among people with occupational water exposure. The majority of Legionnaires' disease cases are nonepidemic in nature. Of these, perhaps 10% may be acquired in the home and the remainder through other exposures.

It is estimated that from 1 to 5% of all pneumonias in adults are due to legionnaires' disease. In some geographic regions, community-acquired legionnaires' disease is more common, with average prevalence rates of 10 to 20% of all pneumonias. When the disease occurs in endemic or epidemic nosocomial form, 1% to as many as 20% of hospitalized patients with pneumonia have this disease.

Pontiac fever has been recognized primarily as an epidemic illness, with attack rates in excess of 90%. It has been noted to occur in office and factory workers and in recreational bathers using spa or Jacuzzi-type baths. The disease very likely has a sporadic form, but the lack of specific diagnostic tests makes diagnosing this form very difficult.

TABLE 275–1. EXTRAPULMONARY INFECTIONS CAUSED BY *LEGIONELLA*

Dialysis shunt infection
Sinusitis
Pericarditis
Prosthetic valve endocarditis
Peritonitis
Abscesses
    Skin
    Brain
    Bowel
    Rectum
    Kidney
    Myocardium

PATHOLOGY. Specific pathologic changes are found only in the lung in the vast majority of fatal cases of legionnaires' disease. Intense inflammation is present in the alveolus, alveolar ducts, respiratory bronchioles, and alveolar septa. The inflammatory process consists of bacteria, polymorphonuclear leukocytes, and macrophages. On occasion, pleuritis, pleural empyema, pericarditis, and cavitary lung disease are found. Very rarely, abscess formation occurs outside the chest cavity.

CLINICAL PRESENTATION. Legionnaires' disease manifests as a febrile systemic illness with pneumonia. Several prospective and retrospective studies of patients with different types of pneumonia have shown that legionnaires' disease has few, if any, characteristic clinical features and that it cannot be distinguished clinically from pneumococcal pneumonia. However, clinical observations during epidemics of legionnaires' disease have often documented characteristic clinical findings. It is probable that the spectrum of clinical presentations is wide, ranging from a "typical" form of legionnaires' disease to one indistinguishable from other causes of pneumonia. This chapter describes the "typical" form of legionnaires' disease, which in reality may be present in the minority of patients. A prodromal illness consisting of malaise, low-grade fever, and anorexia may develop several days before the onset of more severe symptoms. Myalgia, extreme fatigue, and high fever then develop. Gastrointestinal complaints are common, such as generalized or localized abdominal pain, nausea, vomiting, and diarrhea; the diarrhea is generally watery and not dehydrating. Recurrent rigors and prostration may occur. Symptoms referable to the respiratory tract may not develop until later. It is this paucity of respiratory tract symptoms, despite evidence of a systemic febrile illness, that can either be a clue to diagnosis or mislead clinicians. When the patient is pressed for details regarding symptoms, a history of a nonproductive cough, or one productive of nonpurulent, sometimes bloody, secretions, is usually obtained. Production of large amounts of grossly purulent sputum is unusual. Pleuritic chest pain, sometimes in concert with hemoptysis, is present and may mislead the clinician into considering pulmonary infarction. Mental confusion is reported commonly in some series; obtundation, seizures, and focal neurologic findings may also occur less frequently.

Fever is almost uniformly present in cases of legionnaires' disease, although there are reports of short (days) afebrile periods in some immunosuppressed patients with *L. micdadei* pneumonia. Chest examination early in the disease may reveal only scattered rales or evidence of pleural effusion. However, later in the course, most patients have classic findings of consolidating pneumonia. Abdominal examination may reveal generalized or local tenderness and, in rare cases, evidence of peritonitis. Splenomegaly is uncommon. Findings of pericarditis, myocarditis, and focal abscesses are rare. No rash is associated with this disease, except that caused by other factors, such as drug therapy.

The fatality rate of untreated legionnaires' disease is about 3 to 30% in nonimmunosuppressed patients and up to 80% in immunocompromised ones. The majority of previously healthy people recover from untreated legionnaires' disease after 7 to 10 days of severe illness; those who do not recover die of progressive respiratory and multisystem failure.

Clinically significant extrapulmonary infection in patients with legionnaires' disease is quite rare (Table 275–1).

Pontiac fever is a nonfatal influenza-like disease, with symptoms of myalgia, fever, headache, and malaise occurring in 60 to 90% of patients. Arthralgia occurs with variable frequency, as do cough, anorexia, and abdominal pain. The illness is generally not severe enough nor long enough in duration to cause most patients to seek medical attention. Not much is known about physical findings early in the disease; findings after 3 to 5 days of illness are generally normal except for fever and possibly tachypnea. Pneumonia does not occur. The illness lasts about 3 to 5 days, although some patients may have persistent fatigue or nonfocal neurologic complaints for weeks to months afterward.

CHEST ROENTGENOGRAPHIC FINDINGS. Legionnaires' disease causes alveolar filling infiltrates that usually eventuate in consolidation. Interstitial infiltrates are rare, although they may occur early in the course of disease and then progress to consolidating infiltrates. The infiltrates may be unilateral or bilateral and can spread very quickly to involve the entire lung. Pleural effusion, usually small in volume, occurs commonly and may be the sole abnormal radiographic finding in early disease.

DIAGNOSIS. The results of multiple nonspecific laboratory tests may be abnormal in patients with legionnaires' disease. These abnormal findings include proteinuria, pyuria, hematuria, leukocytosis, leukopenia, and thrombocytopenia. Disseminated intravascular coagulation may be seen in patients with respiratory failure caused by legionnaires' disease. Hyponatremia, hypophosphatemia, hyperbilirubinemia, and elevated serum alanine transaminase (ALT), serum aspartate transaminase (AST), and alkaline phosphatase concentrations may also be found. Elevation of creatine kinase (MM

TABLE 275–2. SPECIFIC DIAGNOSTIC TESTS FOR *LEGIONELLA*

Type	Suitable Specimens	Sensitivity* (%)	Specificity (%)	Notes
Culture	Sputum, lung, pleural fluid, blood, abscess contents	—	100	Use of special and selective media required; 3 to 5 days required for growth
Immunofluorescent microscopy	Sputum, lung, pleural fluid, abscess contents	25–75	95–99.9	Species-specific monoclonal antibody available; not helpful for diagnosis of all species; highest specificity for *L. pneumophila;* relatively low specificity for other species; 2 to 3 hours required for testing
DNA probe	Sputum, lung	50–60	99.1–99.9	Genus specific; may have lower sensitivity for detection of some species and for detection of organism in pleural fluid and transtracheal aspirates; 2 to 3 hours required for testing
Urine radioimmunoassay (RIA)	Urine	90–95	99.9	Useful only for detection of *L. pneumophila* serogroup 1, the most common cause of legionnaires' disease; 2 to 3 hours required for testing
Antibody	Serum	60–70	90–99	Requires testing of paired specimens; seroconversion may not occur until 2 to 3 months after infection; most specific for *L. pneumophila* serogroup 1; cross-reactions e.g., with antibodies to many other bacteria.

* Sensitivity versus culture. Culture is the most sensitive diagnostic technique, but its absolute sensitivity is unknown; reasonable estimates are 80 to 90%.

TABLE 275–3. ANTIMICROBIAL DRUG THERAPY OF LEGIONNAIRES' DISEASE*

Drug	Route	Dosage	Duration (days)
First choice			
Erythromycin ± rifampin	Oral	500 mg four times daily	14–21
	IV	500 mg to 1 gram every 6 hours	
Second choices			
Azithromycin *or*	Oral	500 mg daily	3–5
Clarithromycin *or*	Oral	500 mg twice daily	10–14
Ciprofloxacin	Oral	500 mg twice daily	10–14
	IV	400 mg every 12 hours	
or			
Ofloxacin *or*	Oral or IV	500 mg twice daily	10–14
Doxycycline ± rifampin	Oral or IV	200 mg load, then 100 mg twice daily	14–21
or			
Cotrimoxazole ± rifampin	Oral or IV	5 mg per kilogram of trimethoprim three times daily	14–21
Rifampin†	Oral or IV	600 mg twice daily	3–5

* Only erythromycin is FDA-approved for the treatment of legionnaires' disease.
† Rifampin is administered only in combination with another antimicrobial agent.

isoenzyme) is common, and some patients develop myoglobinuria and renal failure. The cerebrospinal fluid is usually normal, although rare patients may have 25 to 100 white blood cells per microliter of cerebrospinal fluid.

Legionnaires' disease can be diagnosed using specific laboratory tests (Table 275–2). The most sensitive and specific test is culture of respiratory tract secretions, such as sputum. Sputum culture for *Legionella* should be performed on every patient suspected of having this disease. Serologic testing is more useful to epidemiologists than to clinicians, because of cross-reactions with antibodies to unrelated organisms. No laboratory test currently available is 100% accurate for the diagnosis of legionnaires' disease. Thus empirical therapy must be considered in appropriate clinical settings.

The diagnosis of Pontiac fever is based on demonstration of legionellae in water to which the patient was exposed, significant increases in antibody to the isolated *Legionella* species, and a clinical course compatible with this diagnosis. To be certain about the diagnosis of Pontiac fever, it is almost always necessary to perform extensive studies of unaffected people and their environments. This is so because recovery of legionellae from water and the elevation of antibodies to *Legionella* are relatively common events. Thus it is nearly impossible to diagnose nonepidemic cases of Pontiac fever specifically.

The differential diagnosis of legionnaires' disease is broad, since the disease usually presents as a nonspecific pneumonia. Mycoplasmal pneumonia is generally much less severe and causes significant respiratory system complaints. Pneumococcal pneumonia, in contrast to legionnaires' disease, is usually penicillin-responsive. Psittacosis and Q fever can have clinical presentations quite similar to that of legionnaires' disease.

THERAPY. Erythromycin (Table 275–3) is considered the drug of choice for this disease on the basis of retrospective studies, which show that the case-fatality rate is lowered about fivefold by prompt administration of erythromycin. Alternative drugs are listed in Table 275–3; there is not substantial clinical experience with any of these drugs. Intravenous drug therapy should be given until there is clinical improvement, which usually occurs in 2 to 4 days. After this, oral drug therapy is continued. Mild cases of legionnaires' disease can be treated with oral therapy exclusively. Quinolone antimicrobials (ciprofloxacin, ofloxacin) and the newer macrolide antimicrobials (azithromycin, clarithromycin) are more effective than are erythromycin, doxycycline, or cotrimoxazole (Septra or Bactrim) in experimental laboratory studies; with further clinical experience

they will likely become the drugs of choice. The quinolone drugs are preferred for organ transplant patients because of their lack of interference with cyclosporine levels. Because of its potent activity in experimental legionnaires' disease, many clinicians add rifampin for treatment of severe cases of legionnaires' disease. There are no clinical data indicating the superiority of such combination therapy. Penicillins, cephalosporins (first, second, and third generation), and aminoglycosides are ineffective for the therapy of legionnaires' disease. In fact, the failure of pneumonia to respond to these agents should prompt consideration of legionnaires' disease and perhaps initiation of erythromycin therapy. No effective therapy for Pontiac fever is known.

Most patients with legionnaires' disease respond within 1 to 4 days to specific antimicrobial therapy. The symptoms clearing most rapidly are rigors, mental confusion, myalgia, anorexia, fatigue, and abdominal complaints. Fever may persist for a week after initiation of therapy but starts a downward trend within a few days. Despite this clinical evidence of improvement, other findings may falsely imply disease progression, such as evidence of increased pulmonary consolidation on physical examination and on roentgenography. Weeks to months are required for the resolution of pulmonary infiltrates. Patients with respiratory failure have a relatively poor prognosis and tend to have a much slower response to therapy.

Barbaree JM, Breiman RF, Dufour AP (eds.): *Legionella:* Current Status and Emerging Perspectives. American Society for Microbiology, Washington, D.C. 1993. *Comprehensive reviews and experimental reports from a recent international meeting.*
Edelstein PH: Legionnaires' disease. Clin Infect Dis 16:741, 1993. *More extensive discussion of treatment and clinical diagnosis.*
Fang GD, Fine M, Orloff J, et al.: New and emerging etiologies for community-acquired pneumonia with implications for therapy: A prospective multicenter study of 359 cases. Medicine 69:307, 1990. *Excellent survey of community-acquired pneumonia, including legionnaires' disease.*

276 STREPTOCOCCAL INFECTIONS
Dennis L. Stevens

CLASSIFICATION AND IDENTIFICATION OF STREPTOCOCCI

Streptococci are gram-positive globular or coccoid bacteria that grow in chains. Streptococci colonize the mucous membranes of animals, produce catalase, and may be aerobic, anaerobic, or facultative. Streptococci require complex media containing blood products for optimal growth. On blood agar plates, streptococci may cause complete (β), incomplete (α) or no hemolysis (γ). The exhaustive work of Rebecca Lancefield has allowed hemolytic streptococci to be classified into types A through O based on acid-extractable antigens of cell wall material. Availability of rapid latex agglutination kits provides even small clinical laboratories with the means to identify streptococci according to Lancefield group. Bacitracin susceptibility, bile esculin hydrolysis, and the CAMP test (flame-type synergistic hemolysis on a *Staphylococcus aureus* blood agar streak) are useful presumptive tests for classifying groups A, D, or B streptococci, respectively. Modern schemes of classification of hemolytic and nonhemolytic streptococci use complex biochemical and genetic techniques.

GROUP A STREPTOCOCCAL INFECTIONS

EPIDEMIOLOGY. *Host Range.* The concept of group A streptococcus as a pure human pathogen is supported by the observations that (1) natural group A streptococcus infection in animals is rare; (2) laboratory animals are not useful models of streptococcal pharyngitis, scarlet fever, erysipelas, rheumatic fever, or poststreptococcal glomerulonephritis; (3) the inoculum needed to cause infection in laboratory animals is orders of magnitude greater than that estimated to cause infection in humans; and (4) streptococci have developed highly sophisticated defensive molecules which bind, inactivate, or destroy human immune response molecules (e.g., IgG antibody and complement [C5a]).

Age-Related Attack Rates. All group A streptococcal infections have the highest incidence in children younger than age 10. The asymptomatic prevalence is also higher (15 to 20%) in children compared with adults (< 5%). Age is not the only factor, because crowded conditions in temperate climates during the winter months are associated with epidemics of pharyngitis in school children as well as military recruits. Impetigo is most common in children from ages 2 to 5 and may occur year-round in tropical areas but largely in the summer in temperate climates. Similarly, 90% of cases of scarlet fever occur in children 2 to 8 years and, like pharyngitis, is most common in temperate regions during winter. An experiment of nature in the Faeroe Islands (Denmark) suggested that susceptibility to scarlet fever is not dependent on young age *per se*. Briefly, scarlet fever had disappeared from that isolated island group for several decades until it was reintroduced by a visitor with unsuspected scarlet fever. An epidemic of scarlet fever ensued, with significant attack rates in all age groups, suggesting that other factors, such as the lack of protective antibody against scarlatina toxin or the introduction of a new strain, rather than age predisposed those individuals to clinical illness.

In contrast to pharyngitis, impetigo, and scarlet fever, bacteremia has had the highest age-specific attack rate in the elderly and in neonates. Between 1986 and 1988, the prevalence of bacteremia increased 800 to 1000% in adolescents and adults in Western countries. Although some of this increase is attributable to intravenous drug abuse and puerperal sepsis, most of the increase is due to cases of streptococcal toxic shock syndrome (strepTSS).

Transmission of Group A Streptococcus. Human mucous membranes and skin serve as the natural reservoirs of *S. pyogenes*. Pharyngeal and cutaneous acquisition is by person-to-person spread via aerosolized microdroplets or direct contact, respectively. Epidemics of pharyngitis and scarlet fever also have occurred after consumption of contaminated nonpasteurized milk or food. Epidemics of impetigo have been reported, particularly in tropical areas, in day care centers, and among underprivileged children. Group A streptococcal infections in hospitalized patients occur during childbirth (puerperal sepsis), times of war (epidemic gangrene), surgical convalescence (surgical wound infection, surgical scarlet fever), or as a result of burns (burn wound sepsis). Thus, in most clinical streptococcal infections, the mode of transmission and portal of entry are easily ascertained. In contrast, among patients with strepTSS, the portal of entry is obvious in only 50% of cases.

PATHOGENESIS. Adherence of cocci to the mucosal epithelium is necessary but not sufficient to cause disease in all cases, since prolonged asymptomatic carriage is well documented. Complex interactions between host epithelium and streptococcal factors such as M-protein, lipoteichoic acid (LTA), and fimbriae are necessary for adherence. Fibronectin-binding protein (protein F) also contributes to adherence, because protein F–deficient mutants are incapable of binding to epithelial cells.

Within the tissues, streptococci may evade opsonophagocytosis by destroying or inactivating complement-derived chemoattractants and opsonins (C5a peptidase) and by binding immunoglobulins. Expression of M-protein, in the absence of type-specific antibody, also protects the organism from phagocytosis by polymorphonuclear leukocytes (PMN's) and monocytes. In tissues, streptolysin O (SLO) secreted in high concentration destroys approaching phagocytes. Distal to the focus of infection, lower concentrations of SLO stimulate PMN adhesion to endothelial cells, effectively preventing continued granulocyte migration and promoting vascular damage. In the nonimmune host, SLO, streptococcal pyrogenic exotoxin (SPE) type A, and other streptococcal components stimulate host cells to produce tumor necrosis factor (TNF) and interleukin-1 (IL-1), cytokines that mediate hypotension and stimulate leukostasis, resulting in shock, microvascular injury, multiorgan failure, and if excessive, death. A unique feature of the pyrogenic exotoxins and some M-protein fragments is their ability to interact with certain V_β regions of the T cell receptor in the absence of classic antigen processing by antigen-presenting cells (Fig. 276–1). This results in massive clonal proliferation of T lymphocytes. SPE type B is related to the proteinase precursor and may play a role in the pathogenesis of necrotizing fasciitis and myositis and may contribute to shock in

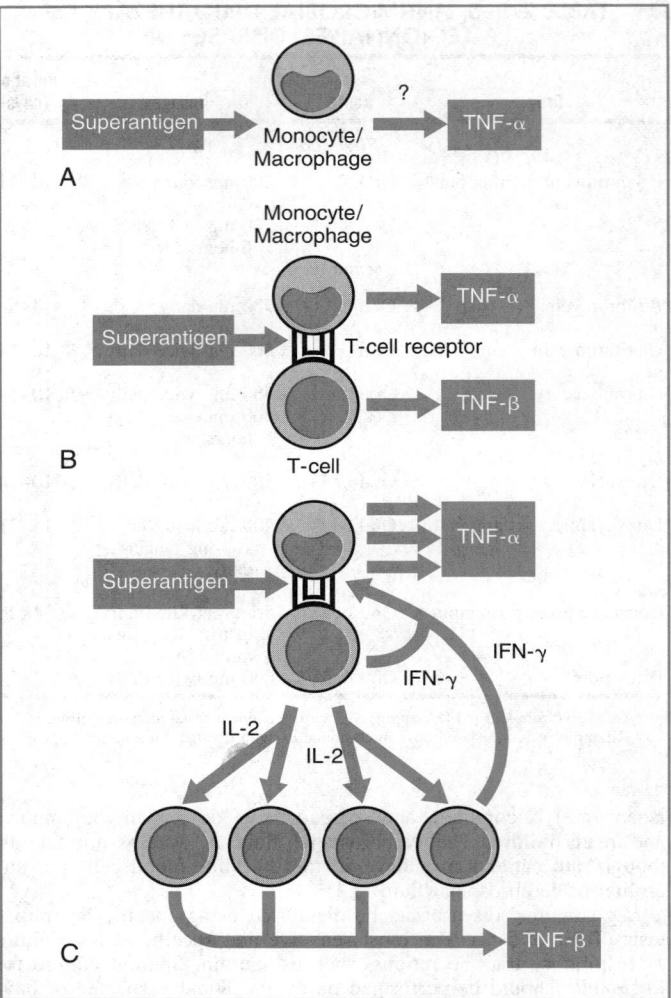

FIGURE 276–1. Superantigen-induced production of tumor necrosis factor-α (TNF-α) and lymphotoxin (TNF-β) by periperal blood mononuclear cells. *A,* Superantigens induce human monocytes to produce TNF-α; however, it is unclear whether such production results solely from direct stimulation of the monocyte by the superantigen. *B,* In mixed mononuclear cell populations, superantigens stimulate TNF-α synthesis in monocytes and, by binding to specific V_β regions of the T cell receptor, induce synthesis of lymphotoxin (TNF-β) from T cells. *C,* The T cell response to superantigen stimulation includes production of interleukin-2 (IL-2), resulting in clonal proliferation with concordant production of interferon-gamma (IFN-γ) and TNF-β. IFN-γ can then amplify monocyte synthesis of TNF-α, IL-1, and IL-6. (From Stevens DL, Bryant AE, Hackett SP: Sepsis syndromes and toxic shock syndromes: Concepts in pathogenesis and a perspective of future strategy. Current Opin Infectious Dis 6:374, 1993.)

strepTSS through its ability to cleave pre-IL-1β into active IL-1β. Thus, in strepTSS, lymphokines such as TNF-β, interferon-γ, and IL-2 may be crucial in the mediation of shock and microvascular injury.

BACTERIAL CELL STRUCTURE AND EXTRACELLULAR PRODUCTS. Capsule. Some strains of *S. pyogenes* possess luxuriant capsules of hyaluronic acid, resulting in large mucoid colonies on blood agar. Luxuriant production of M-protein also may impart a mucoid colony morphology, and this trait has been associated with M-18.

Cell Wall. The cell wall is composed of a peptidoglycan backbone with integral LTA components. The function of LTA is not well known, but both peptidoglycan and LTA have important interactions with the host.

M-Proteins. Over 80 different M-protein types of group A streptococci are currently described. The protein is a coiled coil consisting of four regions of repeating amino acids (A–D), a proline/glycine-rich region that serves to intercalate the protein into the bacterial cell wall, and a hydrophobic region that acts as a membrane anchor. Region A near the *N* terminus is highly variable, and antibodies to this region confer type-specific protection. Within the more conserved B–D regions lies an area that binds one of the complement regulatory proteins (factor H), stearically inhibiting antibody binding and complement-derived opsonin deposition and effectively camouflaging the organism against humoral immune surveillance. M-protein inhibits the phagocytosis of *S. pyogenes* by PMN's, though this property can be overcome by type-specific antisera. Observations by Lancefield suggest that the quantity of M-protein produced decreases with passage on artificial media and conversely increases rapidly with passage through mice. The quantity of M-protein produced by an infecting strain progressively decreases during convalescence and during prolonged carriage.

Streptolysin O. Streptolysin O (SLO) belongs to a family of oxygen-labile, thiol-activated cytolysins (TAC) and causes the broad zone of β hemolysis surrounding colonies of *S. pyogenes* on blood agar plates. TAC toxins bind to cholesterol on eukaryotic cell membranes, creating toxin-cholesterol aggregates that contribute to cell lysis via a colloid-osmotic mechanism. Cholesterol inhibits toxicity in isolated myocytes and hemolysis of red blood cells *in vitro*. In situations where serum cholesterol is high, i.e., nephrotic syndrome, falsely elevated ASO titers may occur because both cholesterol and anti-ASO antibody will "neutralize SLO." Striking amino acid homology exists between SLO and other TAC toxins.

Streptolysin S. Streptolysin S is a cell-associated hemolysin that does not diffuse into the agar media. Purification and characterization of this protein have been difficult, and its only role in pathogenesis may be in direct or contact cytotoxicity.

Deoxyribonucleases A, B, C, and D. Expression of deoxyribonucleases (DNases) *in vivo* elicits production of anti-DNase antibody following both pharyngeal and skin infection; this is most true for DNase B with group A streptococci.

Hyaluronidase. This extracellular enzyme hydrolyzes hyaluronic acid in deeper tissues, facilitating the spread of infection along fascial planes. Antihyaluronidase titers rise following *S. pyogenes* infections, especially those involving the skin.

Pyrogenic Exotoxins. SPE types A, B, and C, also called scarlatina toxin and erythrogenic toxins, induce lymphocyte blastogenesis, potentiate endotoxin-induced shock, induce fever, suppress antibody synthesis, and act as superantigens. The identification of these three different types of SPE's may in part explain why some individuals may have multiple attacks of scarlet fever. The gene for pyrogenic exotoxin A *(speA)* is transmitted by bacteriophages, and stable production depends on lysogenic conversion in a manner analogous to diphtheria toxin production by *Corynebacterium diphtheriae*. Control of SPE A production is not yet understood, though the quantity of SPE A produced varies dramatically from decade to decade. Historically, SPE A–producing strains have been associated with severe cases of scarlet fever and, more recently, with strepTSS.

Although all strains of group A streptococci are endowed with genes for SPE B *(speB)*, like SPE A, the quantity of toxin produced varies greatly.

Pyrogenic exotoxin type C (SPE C), like SPE A, is bacteriophage-mediated, and expression is likewise highly variable. Recently, mild cases of scarlet fever in England and the United States have been associated with SPE C–positive strains.

CLINICAL INFECTIONS. *Pharyngitis and the Asymptomatic Carrier.* Patients with streptococcal pharyngitis have abrupt onset of sore throat, submandibular adenopathy, fever, and chilliness but usually not frank rigors. Cough and hoarseness are rare, but pain on swallowing is characteristic. The uvula is edematous, tonsils are hypertrophied, and the pharynx is erythematous with exudates that may be punctate or confluent. Acute pharyngitis is sufficient to induce antibody against M-protein, SLO, DNase, hyaluronidase, and if present, pyrogenic exotoxins. Depending on the infecting strain, pharyngitis may progress to scarlet fever, bacteremia, suppurative head and neck infections, rheumatic fever, poststreptococcal glomerulonephritis, or strepTSS. Pharyngitis is usually self-limited, and pain, swelling, and fever resolve spontaneously in 3 to 4 days even without treatment.

Definitive diagnosis is difficult based only on clinical parameters, especially in infants, in whom rhinorrhea may be the dominant manifestation. Even in older children with all the preceding physical findings, the correct clinical diagnosis is made in only 75% of patients. Absence of any one of the classic signs greatly reduces the

specificity. Rapid antigen detection tests in the office setting have a sensitivity and specificity of 40 to 90%. A popular approach in clinical practice is to obtain two throat swab samples from the posterior pharynx or tonsillar surface. A rapid strep test is performed on the first, and if it is positive, the patient is treated with antibiotics and the second swab discarded. If the rapid strep test is negative, the second is sent for culture, and treatment is withheld pending a positive culture.

Scarlet Fever. During the last 30 to 40 years, outbreaks of scarlet fever in the Western world have been notably mild, and the illness has been referred to as "pharyngitis with a rash" or "benign scarlet fever" (see Color Plate No. XXI-0-1). In contrast, in the latter half of the nineteenth century, mortalities of 25 to 35% were common in the United States, western Europe, and Scandinavia. The fatal or malignant forms of scarlet fever have been described as either septic or toxic. "Septic scarlet fever" refers to patients who develop local invasion of the soft tissues of the neck and complications such as upper airway obstruction, otitis media with perforation, meningitis, mastoiditis, invasion of the jugular vein or carotid artery, and bronchopneumonia. "Toxic scarlet fever" is rare today, but historically patients initially developed severe sore throat, marked fever, delirium, skin rash, and painful cervical lymph nodes. In severe toxic cases, fevers of 107° F, pulses of 130 to 160 beats per minute, severe headache, delirium, convulsions, little if any skin rash, and death within 24 hours were common. These cases occurred before the advent of antibiotics, antipyretics, and anticonvulsants, and sudden deaths were the result of uncontrolled seizures and hyperpyrexia. In contrast, children with septic scarlet fever had prolonged courses and succumbed 2 to 3 weeks after the onset of pharyngitis. Complications of streptococcal pharyngitis and malignant forms of scarlet fever have been less common in the antibiotic era. Even before antibiotics became available, necrotizing fasciitis and myositis were not described in association with scarlet fever.

Erysipelas. Erysipelas is caused exclusively by *S. pyogenes* and is characterized by an abrupt onset of fiery red swelling of the face or extremities. Distinctive features are well-defined margins, particularly along the nasolabial fold, scarlet or salmon-red rash, rapid progression, and intense pain. Flaccid bullae may develop during the second to third day, yet extension to deeper soft tissues is rare. Surgical debridement is not necessary, and treatment with penicillin is effective. Swelling may progress despite treatment, although fever, pain, and the intense redness diminish. Desquamation of the involved skin occurs 5 to 10 days into the illness. Infants and elderly adults are most commonly afflicted, and historically erysipelas, like scarlet fever, was more severe before 1900.

Streptococcal Pyoderma (Impetigo Contagiosa). Impetigo is most common in patients with poor hygiene or malnutrition. Colonization of the unbroken skin occurs first, and then intradermal inoculation is usually initiated by minor abrasions or insect bites. Single or multiple thick crusted, golden-yellow lesions develop within 10 to 14 days. Penicillin orally or parenterally and bacitracin or mupuricin topically are effective treatments for impetigo and also reduce transmission of streptococci to susceptible individuals. None of these treatments, including penicillin, prevents poststreptococcal glomerulonephritis.

Cellulitis. Group A streptococcus is the most common cause of cellulitis; however, alternative diagnoses may be obvious when associated with a primary focus such as an abscess or boil (*Staphylococcus aureus*), dog bite (DF-2), cat bite (*Pasteurella multocida*), freshwater injury (*Aeromonas hydrophila*), seawater injury (*Vibrio vulnifica*), and so on (see Ch. 325 and 391). Clinical clues to diagnosis are important because aspiration of the leading edge or punch biopsy yields a causative organism in only 15 and 40% of cases, respectively. Patients with lymphedema of any cause such as lymphoma, filariasis, or after regional lymph node dissection (as in mastectomy or carcinoma of the prostate) are predisposed to developing streptococcal cellulitis, as are patients with chronic venous stasis. Recently, recurrent saphenous vein donor-site cellulitis has been attributed to group A, C, or G streptococci. Group A streptococci may invade the epidermis and subcutaneous tissues, resulting in local swelling, erythema, and pain. The skin becomes indurated and, unlike the brilliant redness of erysipelas, is pinkish. Streptococcal cellulitis responds quickly to penicillin, although when staphylococcus is of concern, nafcillin or oxacillin may be a better choice. If fever, pain, or swelling increases, if bluish or violet bullae or discoloration appears, or if signs of systemic toxicity develop, a deeper infection such as necrotizing fasciitis or myositis should be considered (see Necrotizing Fasciitis). When an elevated serum creatine phosphokinase level suggests deeper infection, prompt surgical inspection and debridement should be performed.

Lymphangitis. Cutaneous infection with bright red streaks ascending proximally is invariably due to group A streptococcus. Prompt parenteral antibiotic treatment is mandatory, because bacteremia and systemic toxicity develop rapidly once streptococci reach the bloodstream via the thoracic duct.

Necrotizing Fasciitis. Necrotizing fasciitis, originally called "streptococcal gangrene," is a deep-seated infection of the subcutaneous tissue that results in progressive destruction of fascia and fat but may spare the skin itself. Subsequently, "necrotizing fasciitis" has become the preferred term, since *Clostridium perfringens, C. septicum,* and *S. aureus* can produce a similar pathologic process. Infection may begin at the site of trivial or inapparent trauma. Within the first 24 hours, swelling, heat, erythema, and tenderness develop and rapidly spread proximally and distally from the original focus. During the next 24 to 48 hours, the erythema darkens, changing from red to purple and then to blue, and blisters and bullae form that contain clear yellow fluid. On the fourth or fifth day, the purple areas become frankly gangrenous. From the seventh to the tenth days, the line of demarcation becomes sharply defined, and the dead skin begins to reveal extensive necrosis of the subcutaneous tissue. Patients become increasingly prostrated, emaciated, and may become unresponsive, mentally cloudy, or even delirious. Aggressive fasciotomy and debridement ("bearclaw fasciotomy") and irrigations with Dakan's solution achieved mortality rates as low as 20%, even before antibiotics were available. The increased morbidity and mortality of necrotizing fasciitis could be due to increased virulence of streptococci (see section on Streptococcal Toxic Shock Syndrome).

Myositis. Historically, streptococcal myositis has been an extremely uncommon infection, only 21 cases being documented from 1900 to 1985. Recently, the prevalence of streptococcal myositis has increased in the United States, Norway, and Sweden. Translocation of streptococci from the pharynx to the deep site of trauma (muscle) must occur hematogenously. Symptomatic pharyngitis or penetrating trauma are uncommon. Severe pain may be the only presenting symptom, and swelling and erythema may be the only signs of infection. In most cases a single muscle group is involved; however, because patients are frequently bacteremic, multiple sites of myositis or abscess can occur. Distinguishing streptococcal myositis from spontaneous gas gangrene due to *C. perfringens* or *C. septicum* may be difficult, although the presence of crepitus or gas in the tissue would favor clostridial infection. Myositis is easily distinguished from necrotizing fasciitis anatomically by surgical exploration or incisional biopsy, although clinical features of both conditions overlap. In published reports, the case-fatality rate of necrotizing fasciitis is between 20 and 50%, whereas that of streptococcal myositis is between 80 and 100%. Aggressive surgical debridement is extremely important because of the poor efficacy of penicillin described in human cases, as well as in experimental models of streptococcal myositis (see section on antibiotic efficacy).

Pneumonia. Pneumonia caused by group A streptococcus is most common in women in the second and third decades of life and causes large pleural effusions and empyema. Chest tube drainage is mandatory even though management is complicated by multiple loculations and fibrinous effusions resulting in restrictive lung disease. Prolonged penicillin therapy, thoracoscopy, and decortication of the pleura may be necessary.

Streptococcal Toxic Shock Syndrome (strepTSS). Epidemiology. In the late 1980's, invasive group A streptococcal infections occurred in North America and Europe in previously healthy individuals ages 20 to 50. This illness is associated with bacteremia, deep soft tissue infection, shock, multiorgan failure, and death in 30% of cases. Although strepTSS occurs sporadically, minor epidemics have been reported. Most patients have either a viral-like prodrome, history of minor trauma, recent surgery, or varicella infection. The prodrome may be due to a viral illness predisposing to strepTSS, or these vague early symptoms may be related to the evolving infection. In cases associated with necrotizing fasciitis, the infection begins deep in the soft tissue at a site of minor trauma that frequently did not result in a break in the skin. Although surgical procedures and viral infections such as varicella and influenza may provide portals of entry, no portal can be ascertained in 45% of cases. Preceding symptomatic pharyngitis is rare.

Symptoms and Physical Findings. The abrupt onset of severe pain is a common initial symptom of strepTSS (Table 276–1). The pain most commonly involves an extremity but also may mimic peritonitis, pelvic inflammatory disease, acute myocardial infarction, or pericarditis. Treatment with nonsteroidal anti-inflammatory agents may mask the presenting symptoms or predispose to more severe complications such as shock.

Fever is the most common presenting sign, although some patients present with profound hypothermia secondary to shock (see Table 276–1). Confusion is present in over half the patients and may progress to coma or combativeness. On admission 80% of patients have tachycardia, and over half have systolic blood pressure < 110 mm Hg. Of those with normal blood pressure on admission, most become hypotensive within 4 hours. Soft tissue infection evolves to necrotizing fasciitis or myositis in 50 to 70% of patients, and these require emergent surgical debridement, fasciotomy, or amputation. An ominous sign is progression of soft tissue swelling to violaceous or bluish vesicles or bullae. Many other clinical presentations may be associated with strepTSS, including endophthalmitis, myositis, perihepatitis, peritonitis, myocarditis, meningitis, septic arthritis, and overwhelming sepsis. Patients with shock and multiorgan failure without signs or symptoms of local infections have a worse prognosis, because definitive diagnosis and surgical debridement may be delayed.

Laboratory Abnormalities. Hemoglobinuria is present and serum creatinine is elevated in most patients at the time of admission. Serum albumin concentrations are moderately low (3.3 grams per deciliter) on admission and drop progressively over 48 to 72 hours. Hypocalcemia, including ionized hypocalcemia, is detectable early in the hospital course. The serum creatinine kinase level is a

TABLE 276–1. CLINICAL AND LABORATORY FEATURES OF THE STREPTOCOCCAL TOXIC SHOCK SYNDROME

Symptoms
  Viral-like prodrome
  Severe pain
  Confusion
  Nausea
  Chills

Signs
  Fever
  Soft tissue swelling and tenderness
  Tachycardia
  Tachypnea
  Hypotension

Laboratory Findings
  Hematologic tests
    Marked left shift
    Red cell hemolysis
    Thrombocytopenia
  Chemistry tests
    Azotemia
    Hypocalcemia
    Hypoalbuminemia
    Creatine phosphokinase elevation
  Urinalysis
    Hematuria
  Blood gases
    Hypoxia
    Acidosis
  Radiographic
    ARDS
    Soft tissue swelling

Complications
  Profound hypotension
  ARDS
  Renal failure
  Liver failure
  Necrotizing soft tissue infections
  Bacteremia
  Death (30%)

TABLE 276–2. ANTIBIOTIC THERAPY OF GROUP A STREPTOCOCCAL INFECTIONS

Condition	Route	Dosages
I. Pharyngitis and impetigo		
Benzathine penicillin	IM	1.2 million units (>27 kg)
Penicillin G (or V)	PO	200,000 units q.i.d. for 10 days
Erythromycin	PO	40 mg/kg/day (up to 1 gram per day)
II. Recurrent streptococcal pharyngitis/tonsillitis		
Same as I above, *or*		
Ampicillin plus clavulinic acid	PO	20–40 mg/kg/day
Oral Cephalosporin		Check *PDR*
Clindamycin	PO	10 mg/kg/day
III. Cellulitis and erysipelas		
Penicilli G or V	PO	200,000 units q.i.d. for 10 days
Dicloxacillin*	PO	500 mg q.i.d. for 10 days (adults)
IV. Necrotizing fasciitis/ myositis/streptococcal toxic shock syndrome		
Clindamycin	IV	1800–2100 mg daily (adults)
Penicillin	IV	2 million units q4h (adults)
V. Prophylaxis for rheumatic fever (see Ch. 277)		

* Alternative to penicillin if *S. aureus* is of concern. Cephalosporins could be used; however, most (except ceftriaxone) have less activity than penicillin G against streptococci.

useful test to detect deeper soft tissue infections, such as necrotizing fasciitis or myositis.

The initial hematologic studies demonstrate only mild leukocytosis, but a dramatic left shift (43% of white blood cells may be band forms, metamyelocytes, and myelocytes). The mean platelet count is normal on admission but may drop rapidly by 48 hours, even in the absence of criteria for disseminated intravascular coagulopathy.

Clinical Course. Shock is apparent early in the course, and fluid management is complicated by profound capillary leak. Adult respiratory distress syndrome occurs frequently (55%), and renal dysfunction that precedes hypotension in many patients may progress in spite of treatment. In patients who survive, serum creatinine levels return to normal within 4 to 6 weeks; many require dialysis. Overall, 30% of patients die despite aggressive treatment including intravenous fluids, colloid, pressors, mechanical ventilation, and surgical interventions such as fasciotomy, debridement, exploratory laparotomy, intraocular aspiration, amputation, and hysterectomy.

Characteristics of Clinical Isolates. Group A streptococcus is isolated from blood in 60% of cases and from deep tissue specimens in 95% of cases. M types 1, 3, 12, and 28 are the most common strains isolated. Pyrogenic exotoxins A and/or B have been found in isolates from the majority of patients with severe infection. Infections in Norway, Sweden, and Great Britain have been primarily due to M type 1 strains that produce pyrogenic exotoxin B. Other novel pyrogenic exotoxins are being described that also may explain the recent enhanced virulence of group A streptococcus.

NONSUPPURATIVE COMPLICATIONS. The nonsuppurative complications of streptococcal disease are acute rheumatic fever and acute glomerulonephritis. These are discussed in Ch. 277 and 79, respectively.

TREATMENT OF GROUP A INFECTIONS. Prophylaxis. During epidemics, particularly when rheumatic fever or a poststreptococcal glomerulonephritis are prevalent, treatment of asymptomatic carriers may be necessary. Studies by the U.S. military have shown that monthly injections of benzathine penicillin greatly reduce the incidence of streptococcal pharyngitis and rheumatic fever in young soldiers living in crowded conditions.

Emergence of Resistance. Erythromycin resistance of *S. pyogenes* is currently 4% in Western countries; however, in Japan in 1974 the rate reached 72%. Sulfonamide resistance currently is reported in <1% of group A streptococcal isolates.

Therapeutic Failure of Penicillin. The recommended antibiotic therapies for group A streptococcal diseases are shown in Table 276–2. Resistance to penicillin has not been described, yet in some settings there is a lack of *in vivo* efficacy despite *in vitro* susceptibility to penicillin. Three mechanisms may explain this lack of efficacy.

1. *β-Lactamase production by co-infecting organisms.* Penicillin failure in pharyngitis, tonsillitis, or mixed infections may be due to inactivation of penicillin *in situ* by β-lactamases produced by cocolonizing organisms such as *Bacteroides fragilis, Haemophilus influenzae,* or *S. aureus.* For example, the failure rate of penicillin treatment of group A streptococcal pharyngitis may approach 25%, and if such patients are treated with a second course of penicillin, the failure rate may approach 80%, perhaps due to selection of β-lactamase–producing bacteria. In contrast, cures of 90% have been achieved when treatment consisted of amoxacillin plus clavulanate or clindamycin.

2. *Genotypic tolerance.* Genotypic tolerance to penicillin also may contribute to penicillin's lack of efficacy in tonsillitis or pharyngitis. In fact, penicillin-tolerant strains also have caused epidemics of pharyngitis. Tolerant strains demonstrate a slower rate of growth, a slower rate of bacterial killing by penicillin, and an absence of β-lactam–induced cell lysis. The role of tolerance in antibiotic treatment failure is not fully understood.

3. *Inoculum effect.* Studies in animals infected with group A streptococcus demonstrate that penicillin is effective only if given early or if small numbers of streptococci are used to initiate infection. It is likely that streptococci are not in a logarithmic phase of growth at the time the clinical diagnosis of necrotizing fasciitis or myositis is made. Penicillin is most effective against streptococci in log phase growth, a stage in their life cycle when five penicillin-binding proteins are expressed. Conversely, during stationary phase, the two penicillin-binding proteins with the greatest affinity for penicillin are absent. In contrast, clindamycin has much greater efficacy than penicillin even if treatment is delayed up to 16 hours. Clindamycin's greater efficacy could be due to its ability to suppress M-protein synthesis, its longer postantibiotic effect, an indifference to *in vivo* inoculum effect, or its effects on the host's immune system.

NON–GROUP A STREPTOCOCCAL INFECTIONS (Table 276–3)

Enterococcus faecalis. These gram-positive, facultatively anaerobic bacteria are usually nonhemolytic but may demonstrate α or β hemolysis. Enterococci were previously classified as group D streptococci because they hydrolyze bile esculin and possess the group D antigen. Based on nucleic acid hybridization studies, they

TABLE 276–3. NON-GROUP A STREPTOCOCCAL INFECTIONS

Organism	Lancefield Group	Type of Infection	Therapy
S. agalactiae	B	Neonatal sepsis Postpartum sepsis Septic arthritis Soft tissue infection Osteomyelitis	Ampicillin or penicillin
Enterococcus faecalis	D	Endocarditis Bacteremia UTI Abscesses, GI	Ampicillin + gentamicin
S. milleri	A, C, F, G, and nontypable	Abscesses Bacteremia	Penicillin
S. bovis	D	Bacteremia Abscesses	Penicillin
S. equi	C	Bacteremia Cellulitis Pharyngitis	Penicillin
S. canis	G	Bacteremia Cellulitis Pharyngitis	Penicillin
"Viridans" *S. salivarius*	Nontypable	Nonpathogen	
S. mutans		Endocarditis Caries	Penicillin
S. sanguis		Endocarditis	Penicillin
S. mitior		Endocarditis	Penicillin

are now designated *Enterococcus*. Enterococci are commonly isolated from stool, urine, and sites of intra-abdominal and lower extremity infection. Enterococci cause subacute bacterial endocarditis and have become an important cause of nosocomial infection, not because of increased virulence but because of antibiotic resistance. First, person-to-person transfer of multidrug-resistant enterococci is a major concern to hospital epidemiologists. Second, superinfections and spontaneous bacteremia from endogenous sites of enterococcal colonization are described in patients receiving quinolone or moxalactam antibiotics. Lastly, conjugational transfer of plasmids and transposons between enterococci in the face of intense antibiotic pressure within the hospital mileu have created multidrug-resistant strains, including those with vancomycin and teicoplanin resistance. Serious infections with enterococci such as endocarditis or bacteremia require a synergistic combination of antimicrobials such as ampicillin or vancomycin, together with an aminoglycoside. β-Lactamase–positive (Nitrocefin disc positive) strains can be treated with ampicillin and sulbactam.

Streptococcus bovis. *S. bovis* is also a cause of subacute bacterial endocarditis and bacteremia in patients with underlying gastrointestinal malignancy. Unlike entercoccus, it remains highly sensitive to penicillin.

Group C and G Streptococci. These organisms may be isolated from the throats of both humans and dogs, produce SLO, and resemble group A in colony morphology and spectrum of clinical disease. Before rapid identification tests were developed, many infections caused by groups C and G were mistakenly attributed to group A, such as pharyngitis, cellulitis, skin and wound infections, endocarditis, meningitis, osteomyelitis, and arthritis. Rheumatic fever following group C or G infection has not been described. These strains also cause recurrent cellulitis at the saphenous vein donor site in patients who have undergone coronary artery bypass surgery. Both organisms are susceptible to penicillin, erythromycin, vancomycin, and clindamycin.

Streptococcus milleri. *S. milleri* are usually β hemolytic and produce minute colonies on blood agar plates. They are found in the oropharynx, upper gastrointestinal tract, and appendix. Infections are most commonly related to contiguous abscess formation such as tooth abscess, periapendiceal abscess, and so on. Primary bacteremia with or without endocarditis and metastatic abscesses of the brain, lung, bone, joints, liver, and spleen are characteristic of *S. milleri*.

Streptococcus agalactiae. *S. agalactiae* (group B streptococci) colonize the vagina, gastrointestinal tract, and occasionally the upper respiratory tract of normal humans. They are recognized as gray-white colonies, slightly larger than group A streptococci, but with a narrower zone of hemolysis. They are resistant to bacitracin, do not hydrolyze bile esculin, demonstrate a positive CAMP test, and hydrolyze sodium hippurate. Definitive identification is made using group-specific antiserum or commercial kits that use agglutination endpoints. There are currently six different capsular polysaccharide types of group B designated Ia, Ib, II, III, IV, and V. Immunity results from the development of opsonic type-specific antibody.

Group B streptococci are the most common cause of neonatal pneumonia, sepsis, and meningitis in the United States and western Europe, with an incidence of 1.8 to 3.2 cases per 1000 live births. Preterm infants born to mothers colonized with group B streptococci and premature rupture of the membranes are at highest risk for early-onset pneumonia and sepsis. The mean time of onset is 20 hours, and symptoms are respiratory distress, apnea, fever, and hypothermia. Ascent of the streptococcus from the vagina to the amniotic cavity causes amnionitis. Infants may aspirate streptococci either from the birth canal during parturition or from amniotic fluid *in utero*. Radiographic evidence of pneumonia and/or hyaline membrane disease is present in 40% of neonates with infection, and meningitis occurs in 30 to 40% of cases. Type III group B streptococcus causes most cases of meningitis.

Late-onset neonatal sepsis occurs 7 to 90 days postpartum, with symptoms of fever, poor feeding, lethargy, and irritability. Bacteremia is common, and meningitis occurs in 80% of cases.

Adults with group B infections include postpartum women and patients with peripheral vascular disease, diabetes, or malignancy. Soft tissue infection, septic arthritis, and osteomyelitis are the most common presentations. Although penicillin is the treatment of choice, in practice many neonates are empirically treated with ampicillin (300 to 400 mg per kilogram per day) plus gentamicin. Once the diagnosis is established, penicillin at 200 to 500,000 units per kilogram per day should be given. Adults should receive 10 to 12 million units of penicillin per day for bacteremia, soft tissue infection, or osteomyelitis, but the dose should be increased to 18 to 24 millions units per day for meningitis. Vancomycin and a first-generation cephalosporin are alternatives for the penicillin-allergic patients. Intrapartum administration of ampicillin to women colonized with group B streptococcus who also had premature labor or prolonged rupture of the membranes prevents group B neonatal sepsis. Infants should continue to receive ampicillin for 36 hours postpartum. It is imperative that women during the third trimester be screened for risk factors for premature labor, and those at high risk should be cultured. Women presenting in labor without such definition could be screened with a rapid antigen detecting kit, even though the false-negative rate may be 10 to 30%. Passive immunization with IVIG or active immunization with multivalent polysaccharide vaccine shows promise and will likely be the best approach to prevent neonatal sepsis as well as postpartum infection of the mother.

Anthony B: Group B streptococcal infections. In Feign R, Cherry J (eds.): Textbook of Pediatric Infectious Diseases. 2d ed. Philadelphia, WB Saunders, 1987, p 1322. *A thorough review of the epidemiology, microbiology, and clinical aspects of group B neonatal infections, including medical management.*

Baker CJ, Edwards MS: Group B streptococcal infections. In Remington JS, Klein JO (eds.): Infectious Diseases of the Fetus and Newborn Infant. 3rd ed. Philadelphia, WB Saunders, 1991, p 820. *An excellent review of the clinical infections, virulence factors, and therapeutic approaches to group B streptococcal infections.*

Bisno AL: Group A streptococcal infections and acute rheumatic fever. N Engl J Med 325:783, 1991. *An excellent review article with emphasis on rheumatic fever; there are sections on virulence factors, epidemiology, and streptococcal infections in general.*

Cone LA, Woodard DR, Schlievert PM, et al.: Clinical and bacteriologic observations of a toxic shock–like syndrome due to Streptococcus pyogenes. N Engl J Med 317:146, 1987. *Case report of an early case of streptococcal toxic shock syndrome.*

Gossling R: Occurrence and pathogenicity of the Streptococcus milleri group. Rev Infect Dis 10:257, 1988. *An excellent review of the distribution of S. milleri in the human host. The types of human infection, the virulence factors of the organism, and its susceptibility to antimicrobial agents are discussed in detail.*

Herman DJ, Gerding DN: Screening and treatment of infections caused by resistant enterococci. Antimicrob Agents Chemother 35:215, 1991. *An excellent review of screening parameters and treatment regimens for infections caused by antibiotic-resistant enterococci.*

Martin PR, Hoiby EA: Streptococcal serogroup A epidemic in Norway 1987–1988. Scand J Infect Dis 22:421, 1990. *An excellent population-based study demonstrating a remarkable increase in bacteremia in age groups from 18 to 50.*

Murray BE: The life and times of the enterococcus. Clin Microbiol Rev 3:46, 1990. *Reviews recent changes in clinical findings, biochemical properties, and antibiotic resistance associated with the enterococcus.*

Schwartz B, Facklam RR, Breiman RF: Changing epidemiology of group A streptococcal infection in the USA. Lancet 336:1167, 1990. *A survey of group A streptococcal isolates sent to the CDC over the last decade. A clear indication that invasive infections are currently associated with M types 1 and 3.*

Stevens DL: Invasive group A streptococcus infections. Clin Infect Dis 14:2, 1992. *A review article describing the changing epidemiology of scarlet fever, necrotizing fasciitis, myositis, bacteremia, and the streptococcal toxic shock syndrome.*

Stevens DL, Bryant AE, Hackett SP: Sepsis syndromes and toxic shock syndromes: Concepts in pathogenesis and a perspective of future treatment strategies. Curr Opin Infect Dis 6:374, 1993. *Compares the cellular basis of cytokine- and lymphokine-mediated shock caused by gram-negative and gram-positive bacteria.*

Stevens DL, Tanner MH, Winship J, et al.: Severe group A streptococcal infections associated with a toxic shock-like syndrome and scarlet fever toxin A. N Engl J Med 321:1, 1989. *Reports clinical and laboratory features and complications of 20 patients with streptococcal toxic shock syndrome. An analysis of strains reveals that most were M types 1 and 3 and most strains produced pyrogenic exotoxin type A.*

277 RHEUMATIC FEVER
Alan L. Bisno

DEFINITION. Rheumatic fever is an inflammatory disease that occurs as a delayed, nonsuppurative sequel of upper respiratory infection with group A streptococci. The clinical manifestations include polyarthritis, carditis, subcutaneous nodules, erythema marginatum, and chorea in varying combinations. In its classic form, the disorder is acute, febrile, and largely self-limited. However, damage to heart valves may be chronic and progressive, causing cardiac disability or death many years after the initial episode.

ETIOLOGY. The development of acute rheumatic fever (ARF) requires antecedent infection with a specific organism, the group A *Streptococcus,* at a specific body site, the upper respiratory tract. Cutaneous streptococcal infection, a precursor of poststreptococcal acute glomerulonephritis, has never been shown to cause rheumatic fever.

Strains representing a number of the more than 80 M-protein serotypes of group A streptococci can cause ARF. There is a substantial body of evidence to indicate, however, that group A streptococci vary in their rheumatogenic potential. Strains causing clusters or epidemics usually belong to a limited number of serotypes (e.g., 3, 5, 18, 24, and others) and are often heavily encapsulated, as evidenced by their growth as mucoid colonies on blood agar plates. Streptococci epidemiologically associated with ARF outbreaks occurring during the 1980's in the United States exhibited these characteristics.

PATHOGENESIS. The mechanism by which group A streptococci elicit the connective tissue inflammatory response that constitutes ARF remains unknown. Various theories have been advanced, including (1) toxic effects of streptococcal products, particularly streptolysins S and O, both of which can initiate tissue injury; (2) inflammation mediated by antigen-antibody complexes, perhaps localized to sites of tissue injury; and (3) "autoimmune" phenomena induced by the similarity of certain streptococcal and human tissue antigens.

Efforts to discriminate among these potential pathogenetic mechanisms have been hampered by the lack of an animal model of rheumatic fever. Most authorities currently favor the theory that ARF is an "autoimmune" disorder in which tissue damage is mediated by the host's own immunologic responses to the antecedent streptococcal infection. This theory is rendered more credible by the relatively long latent period between the onset of pharyngitis and ARF and by the demonstration of numerous examples of antigenic similarity between somatic constituents of the group A *Streptococcus* and human tissues. The most intensively studied of these cross-reactions is that between streptococci and human heart. Many patients with ARF (as well as patients with uncomplicated streptococcal infections) have in their sera antistreptococcal antibodies that cross-react with heart tissue in a variety of test systems. Components of the streptococcal cell wall (including group A carbohydrate and M-protein) and of the cell membrane contain epitopes that share antigenic determinants with certain constituents of the human heart.

Antibodies to the cytoplasm of neurons located in the caudate and subthalamic nuclei of the brain have been identified in sera of patients with Sydenham's chorea, and such antibodies cross-react with group A streptococcal membranes. Streptococcal extracellular products appear to be present in immune complexes circulating in the blood of ARF patients. Taken together, these and other reported immunologic cross-reactions and toxic phenomena could theoretically account for most of the manifestations of ARF. As yet, however, there is no direct evidence that any of them is pathogenetically significant.

Patients with ARF have, on average, higher titers of antibodies to streptococcal extracellular and somatic antigens than do patients with uncomplicated streptococcal infections. Data relating to cellular immunity are more limited. ARF patients exhibit an exaggerated cellular reactivity to streptococcal cell membrane antigens, as demonstrated by inhibition *in vitro* of migration of peripheral blood lymphocytes.

Several observations suggest that development of rheumatic fever may be modulated, at least in part, by the specific genetic constitution of the host. These include (1) the tendency of rheumatic fever to affect more than one member of a given family, (2) the fact that only a small percentage of all individuals experiencing an immunologically significant streptococcal infection develop ARF, (3) the tendency of rheumatic individuals to experience recurrent attacks, (4) the propensity of rheumatic subjects to exhibit exaggerated immunologic responses to streptococcal antigens, and (5) the fact that certain class II histocompatibility antigens are encountered significantly more frequently in ARF patients than in controls. Recently, a unique antigen has been found to be strongly expressed on the B cells of virtually all ARF patients but in <20% of controls.

EPIDEMIOLOGY. The epidemiology of ARF mirrors that of streptococcal pharyngitis. The peak age of incidence is 5 to 15 years, but both primary and recurrent cases occur in adults. ARF is rare in children younger than age 4, a fact that has led some observers to speculate that repetitive streptococcal infections are necessary to "prime" the host for the disease. There is no clear-cut gender predilection, although females are more likely to develop certain manifestations such as Sydenham's chorea and mitral stenosis.

The frequency with which ARF develops following untreated group A streptococcal upper respiratory infection differs with the prevalence of highly rheumatogenic strains in the population and the epidemiologic circumstances. In the years following World War II, careful prospective studies were conducted among personnel in military camps suffering from exudative tonsillitis or pharyngitis caused by M-typable group A streptococci. Under such circumstances, in which cases of streptococcal pharyngitis tend to be clinically severe and to appear in epidemics, approximately 3% of untreated patients developed ARF. Studies of endemically occurring streptococcal infection among open populations of children are complicated by the difficulties of differentiating cases of streptococcal pharyngitis from viral pharyngitis occurring in streptococcal carriers; nevertheless, the ARF attack rate in such circumstances is clearly lower than in the military experience, with an overall attack rate of <1%.

Certain features of the antecedent streptococcal infection are associated with an increased risk of ARF. Among these are the magnitude of the antistreptolysin O (ASO) titer rise and the persistence of the infecting organism in the pharynx. Although ARF is more likely to occur following clinically severe exudative pharyngitis than following mild nonexudative illness, one third or more of cases occur after streptococcal infections that are asymptomatic or so mild as to have been forgotten by the patient.

Patients with a history of ARF are at greatly increased risk of recurrent disease following an immunologically significant streptococcal infection. In one long-term prospective study of rheumatic subjects at a rheumatic fever sanitarium, one of every five documented streptococcal infections gave rise to a recurrence of ARF. The risk of recurrence is greater in patients with pre-existing rheumatic heart disease and in those experiencing symptomatic throat infections; the risk declines with advancing age and with increasing interval since the most recent rheumatic attack. Nevertheless, rheumatic patients remain at increased risk well into adult life, perhaps indefinitely.

Rheumatic fever occurs in all parts of the world; there is no known racial predisposition. In temperate climates, ARF peaks in the cooler months of the year, in the winter and early spring or shortly after schools open in the fall. The major environmental factor favoring occurrence appears to be crowding, as in military barracks or similar closed institutions and large households. Crowding favors interpersonal spread of group A streptococci and perhaps enhances streptococcal virulence by frequent human passage.

ARF remains rampant in developing areas such as the Middle East, the Indian subcontinent, and many nations of Africa and South America. It has been estimated that rheumatic heart disease causes 25 to 40% of all cardiovascular disease in the Third World. In striking contrast, the incidence of ARF and the prevalence of rheumatic heart disease have declined both in North America and in western Europe during the course of the twentieth century. Rates of fewer than 2 per 100,000 school children have been reported from several areas of the United States. The disease has become extremely uncommon in the affluent suburbs of many U.S. cities, while persisting among lower socioeconomic groups, particularly in the densely populated core areas of major urban centers. The higher incidence rates reported for African-Americans than Caucasians thus appears to be due to socioeconomic rather than genetic factors.

The mid-1980's, however, witnessed some startling developments in the epidemiology of ARF in the United States. Outbreaks of the disease were reported in Salt Lake City, Utah, Columbus and Akron, Ohio, Pittsburgh, Pennsylvania, Nashville and Memphis, Tennessee, and a number of other communities. The largest outbreak was in Salt Lake City and its environs, where approximately 200 cases occurred between 1985 and 1989. Equally surprising was the fact that, in many of these outbreaks, the victims were predominantly white, middle-class children dwelling in the suburbs. Moreover, ARF epidemics occurred in military training bases in Missouri and California, a phenomenon that had not been observed for two decades. Group A streptococci recovered from ARF patients, their families, and community and training camp surveys were generally highly mucoid and belonged to well-established rheumatogenic serotypes (e.g., serotypes 3 and 18). There is as yet no evidence that these events presage a major national resurgence of ARF.

PATHOLOGY. ARF is characterized by exudative and proliferative inflammatory lesions in the connective tissues, especially those of heart, joints, and subcutaneous tissues. The early lesions consist of edema of the ground substance, fragmentation of collagen fibers, cellular infiltration, and fibrinoid degeneration. In the heart, diffuse degeneration and even necrosis of muscle cells may be observed. At a slightly later stage, focal perivascular inflammatory lesions develop. These so-called Aschoff nodules (Fig. 277-1), considered virtually pathognomonic of rheumatic fever, consist of a central area of fibrinoid surrounded by lymphocytes, plasma cells, and large basophilic cells, some of them multinucleate. Many of these cells have elongated nuclei with a distinctive chromatin pattern, sometimes called "caterpillar" or "owl-eye" nuclei, depending on their orientation in microscopic cross section. Cells containing these nuclei are called "Anitschkow myocytes," despite the fact that most authorities believe them to be of mesenchymal origin.

Cardiac findings may include pericarditis, myocarditis, and endocarditis. Foci of coronary arteritis also may be observed. A thickened and roughened area ("MacCallum's patch") is frequently present in the left atrium above the posterior leaflet of the mitral valve. Valvular lesions appear early as small verrucae along the line of closure. Later, as healing occurs, the valves may become thickened and deformed, the chordae shortened, and the commissures fused. These changes result in valvular stenosis or insufficiency. The mitral valve is involved most commonly, followed by the aortic, the tricuspid, and rarely, the pulmonic valves.

Pathologically, the arthritis of ARF is characterized by a fibrinous exudate and sterile effusion without erosion of the joint surfaces or pannus formation. Subcutaneous nodules have many histologic features in common with the Aschoff nodules. These consist of central zones of fibrinoid necrosis surrounded by histiocytes, fibroblasts, occasional lymphocytes, and rare polymorphonuclear cells. Inflammation of the smaller arteries and arterioles may occur throughout the body. Despite pathologic evidence of diffuse vasculitis, aneurysms and thrombosis are not typical features of ARF.

CLINICAL MANIFESTATIONS. Rheumatic fever may involve a number of different organ systems, most notably the heart, joints, skin, subcutaneous tissues, and central nervous system. The clinical picture of the disease may thus be quite variable (Table 277-1), depending on which systems are attacked, whether they are involved

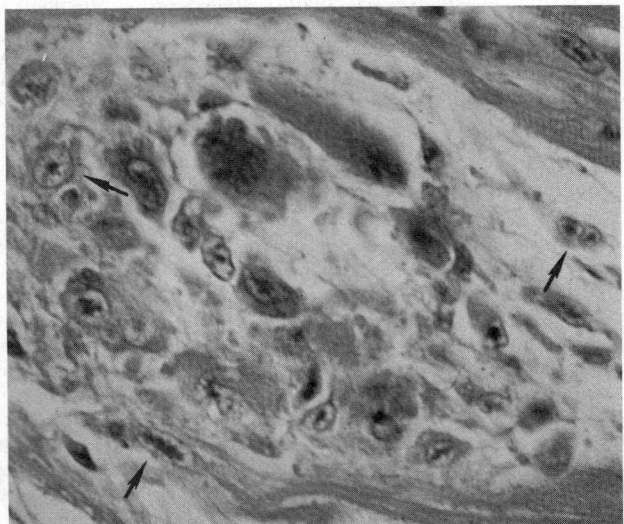

FIGURE 277-1. Myocardial Aschoff nodule demonstrates areas of fibrinoid degeneration and numerous large cells with polymorphous nuclei; several of the nuclei have "owl-eye" or "caterpillar" configurations *(arrows)*. X 630. (Courtesy of Robert Peace, M.D.)

TABLE 277-1. THE MANY FACES OF ACUTE RHEUMATIC FEVER: POSSIBLE PRESENTATIONS

High fever, prostration, crippling polyarthritis
Lassitude, tachycardia, new cardiac murmurs
Acute pericarditis
Fulminant heart failure
Sydenham's chorea, without fever or toxicity
Acute abdominal pain, mimicking appendicitis
Varying combinations of the above

singly or in combination, and the severity of the involvement. Five clinical features of the disease are so characteristic that they are recognized as "major manifestations" according to the revised Jones criteria (see below) for the diagnosis of ARF: carditis, polyarthritis, chorea, subcutaneous nodules, and erythema marginatum. Certain other findings, frequently present but nonspecific, have been designated "minor manifestations." These include arthralgia, fever, and certain laboratory findings (see below).

In cases in which it can be determined, the latent period between the antecedent streptococcal infection and the onset of symptoms of ARF ranges between 1 and 5 weeks. The average latent period is 19 days for both primary and recurrent attacks. When acute polyarthritis is the presenting complaint, the onset is often rather abrupt and may be marked by high fever and toxicity. If isolated carditis is the initial manifestation, the onset may be insidious or even subclinical. Between these two extremes, diverse gradations exist in the initial presentation of ARF (see Table 277-1). In most attacks, fever and joint involvement are the earliest clinical manifestations, although occasionally they may be preceded by abdominal pain localized to the periumbilical or infraumbilical areas. At times, the location and severity of the pain, as well as fleeting signs of peritoneal inflammation, may lead to a misdiagnosis of acute appendicitis. Carditis, if it is to appear, usually does so within the first 3 weeks of the illness. In contrast, chorea tends to occur later in the course of the disease, sometimes after all other manifestations have subsided. Fortunately, chorea and polyarthritis almost never occur simultaneously. Epistaxis may be a feature of ARF, occurring both at the onset and throughout the acute phase of the illness; it may be quite severe.

The incidence of major manifestations varies in reported series. Overall, however, arthritis occurs in approximately 75% of first attacks of ARF, carditis in 40 to 50%, chorea in 15%, and subcutaneous nodules and erythema marginatum in < 10%. The frequency of individual manifestations varies with age. Carditis is more frequent in the youngest age groups and is relatively uncommon in first attacks occurring in adults. Chorea occurs primarily in persons between age 5 and puberty. It is seen more frequently in females and virtually never occurs in adult males. Thus the majority of ARF attacks occurring in adults are manifested primarily by arthritis.

Arthritis. Joint involvement ranges from arthralgia alone to acute, disabling arthritis, characterized by swelling, warmth, erythema, severe limitation of motion, and exquisite tenderness to pressure. The larger joints of the extremities are usually involved—most frequently the knees and ankles but also the wrists and elbows. The hips and small joints of the hands and feet are affected occasionally. Involvement of shoulders and lumbosacral, cervical, sternoclavicular, and temporomandibular joints occurs in a relatively small percentage of cases. The synovial fluid contains thousands of white blood cells, with a marked preponderance of polymorphonuclear leukocytes; bacterial cultures are sterile. Characteristically, the articular involvement in ARF assumes a pattern of migratory polyarthritis. This does not mean that inflammation in one joint disappears before the next is attacked. Rather, a number of joints are affected in succession, and the periods of involvement overlap. Inflammation in one joint may subside while another is becoming symptomatic so that the process seems to migrate from joint to joint. In untreated cases, as many as 16 joints may be affected, and about half the patients develop arthritis in more than 6 joints. When effective anti-inflammatory therapy is administered early in the course of the disease, the involvement not infrequently remains monarticular or pauciarticular.

In most instances, inflammation in any one joint begins to subside spontaneously within a week, and the total duration of involvement is no more than 2 or 3 weeks. The entire bout of polyarthritis rarely lasts more than 4 weeks and resolves completely, leaving no residual joint damage. Some authors have described the rare occurrence of Jaccoud's arthritis, so-called chronic post-rheumatic fever arthropathy of the metacarpophalangeal joints, following repetitive bouts of rheumatic polyarthritis. This entity is not a true arthritis but a form of periarticular fibrosis; its relationship to rheumatic fever remains unresolved.

Carditis. Rheumatic fever may involve the endocardium, myocardium, and pericardium (Table 277–2), and thus the disease is capable of inducing a true pancarditis. Carditis is the most important manifestation of ARF because it is the only one that can cause significant permanent organ damage or death. Although the clinical picture may at times be fulminant, it is more frequently mild or even asymptomatic and may escape notice in the absence of more obvious associated findings, such as arthritis or chorea. The diagnosis of carditis requires the presence of one of the following four manifestations: (1) organic cardiac murmurs not previously present, (2) cardiomegaly, (3) pericarditis, or (4) congestive heart failure. In practice, the characteristic murmurs of ARF are almost always present in cases of rheumatic carditis, unless the ability to hear them is obscured (e.g., loud pericardial friction rub, large pericardial effusion, low cardiac output, severe tachycardia). The diagnosis of carditis should be made with caution in the absence of one of the following three murmurs: apical systolic, apical mid-diastolic, and basal diastolic. Such murmurs, if they are destined to develop, do so usually within the first week and almost always within the first 3 weeks of illness. (An exception to this rule may occur in the patient with "pure" chorea; see later discussion.) The apical systolic murmur of relative or actual mitral regurgitation encompasses most of systole. It is blowing, relatively high pitched, and heard best at the apex; it radiates to the axilla and at times to the base of the heart or the back. It must be distinguished carefully by quality, location, and radiation from a variety of functional precordial systolic murmurs heard in normal individuals, especially in children. The apical mid-diastolic (Carey-Coombs) murmur is a low-pitched sound replacing or immediately following the third heart sound and ending distinctly before the first heart sound. It may be heard in a variety of conditions associated with increased flow across the mitral valve and is thus not pathognomonic of ARF. It may be differentiated from the diastolic rumble of mitral stenosis by the absence of an opening snap, presystolic accentuation, or accentuated first sound at the mitral area. The high-pitched, decrescendo basal diastolic murmur of aortic regurgitation is best heard along the upper left sternal border or over the aortic area. It may be brief and faint, best heard after expiration with the patient leaning forward. The prognostic significance, if any, of echocardiographically recorded valvular regurgitation in the absence of audible murmurs remains to be determined.

Other prominent auscultatory findings in patients with active rheumatic carditis include tachycardia, which persists during sleep; protodiastolic, presystolic, or summation gallops; an indistinct or "mushy" quality to the first heart sound (resulting in some cases from first-degree heart block); pericardial friction rub; or muffling of heart tones caused by pericardial effusion. In the early stages of congestive heart failure, rapid distention of the hepatic capsule may lead to right upper quadrant aching and tenderness over the liver. All the usual clinical findings of pericarditis or congestive failure may be observed.

A number of different rhythm disturbances may occur during the course of ARF. By far the most common is first-degree atrioventricular block. Second- and third-degree heart block, nodal rhythm, and premature contractions also may be observed; atrial fibrillation, on the other hand, is usually a feature of chronic rather than acute rheumatic involvement. Conduction disturbances do not in themselves indicate acute carditis, and their presence or absence is unrelated to the subsequent development of rheumatic heart disease.

In cases of ARF with severe carditis, areas of patchy pneumonitis are sometimes seen. Many observers feel that these pulmonary infiltrates represent a specific rheumatic pneumonia. The case is difficult to prove, however, because of the confusion induced by such confounding clinical entities as pulmonary edema, pulmonary embolization, superimposed bacterial pneumonia, and the acute respiratory distress syndrome in these severely ill and toxic patients.

Sydenham's Chorea (Chorea Minor, "St. Vitus' Dance"). This neurologic syndrome occurs after a latent period that is variable but on average longer than that associated with the other manifestations of ARF. It frequently occurs in "pure" form, either unaccompanied by other major manifestations or, after a latent period of several months, at a time when all other evidence of acute rheumatic activity has subsided. Chorea is characterized by rapid, purposeless, involuntary movements, most noticeable in the extremities and face. The arms and legs flail about in erratic, jerky, uncoordinated movements that may sometimes be unilateral (hemichorea). Facial tics, grimaces, grins, and contortions are evident. The speech is usually slurred or jerky. The tongue, when protruded, retracts involuntarily, while asynchronous contractions of lingual muscles produce a "bag of worms" appearance. The involuntary motions disappear during sleep and may be partially suppressed by rest, sedation, or volition.

Patients with chorea display generalized muscle weakness and an inability to maintain a tetanic muscle contraction. Thus, when the patient is asked to squeeze the examiner's fingers, a squeezing and relaxing motion occurs that has been described as "milkmaid's grip." The knee jerk may have a pendular quality. There is no cranial nerve or pyramidal involvement, and sensory modalities are unaffected. The electroencephalogram may display abnormal slow wave activity.

Emotional lability is characteristic of Sydenham's chorea and often may precede other neurologic manifestations, leaving teachers and parents puzzled over apparently inexplicable personality changes.

Subcutaneous Nodules. These are firm, painless subcutaneous lesions that vary in size from a few millimeters to approximately 2 cm. The skin overlying them is freely movable and is not inflamed. The lesions tend to occur in crops over bony surfaces or prominences and over tendons. Sites of predilection include the extensor surfaces of the elbows, knees, and wrists, the occiput, and spinous processes of the thoracic and lumbar vertebrae (Fig. 277–2). Nodules are virtually never the sole major manifestation of ARF; they almost always appear in association with carditis, and the cardiac involvement in such cases tends to be clinically severe. Nodules ordinarily do not appear until at least 3 weeks after the onset of an attack, usually lasting 1 to 2 weeks. They may appear in repeated crops in patients with protracted carditis. Similar nodules may be seen in systemic lupus erythematosus (SLE) and in rheumatoid arthritis. Subcutaneous nodules in the latter disease are larger and more persistent than those in rheumatic fever.

Erythema Marginatum. The rash begins as an erythematous macule or papule which then extends outward while the skin in the center returns to normal. Adjacent lesions coalesce, forming circinate or serpiginous patterns. The lesions may be raised or flat, are neither pruritic nor indurated, and they blanch on pressure. They vary greatly in size and appear mostly on the trunk and proximal extremities, sparing the face. The lesions are evanescent, migrating from place to place, at times changing before the observer's eyes, and leaving no residual scarring. The erythema may be brought out by applying heat. Individual lesions may come and go in minutes to hours, but the process may go on intermittently for weeks to months uninfluenced by anti-inflammatory therapy; its persistence is not necessarily an adverse prognostic sign. In the great majority of cases, erythema marginatum is accompanied by carditis; it also tends to be associated with subcutaneous nodules.

LABORATORY FINDINGS. No specific laboratory test is diagnostic of ARF. Usually there is a leukocytosis with an increase in the proportion of polymorphonuclear leukocytes. A mild to moderate normocytic, normochromic anemia is the rule. In some patients,

---

TABLE 277–2. CLINICAL MANIFESTATIONS OF CARDITIS IN ACUTE RHEUMATIC FEVER

Murmurs*
    Apical systolic
    Apical mid-diastolic (Carey-Coombs murmur)
Basal diastolic
Pericarditis
Cardiomegaly
Congestive heart failure

* At least one of the characteristic murmurs is almost always present in acute rheumatic carditis (see text for details).

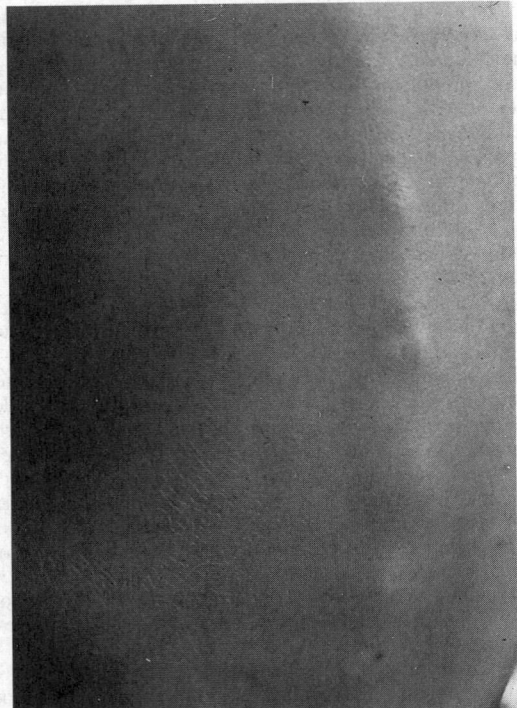

FIGURE 277–2. Subcutaneous nodules over spinous processes on the back of a patient with acute rheumatic carditis. (Courtesy of S. Levine, M.D.)

the serum aspartate aminotransferase (AST) level is elevated. Evidence of acute inflammation is prominent, including readily detectable quantities of C-reactive protein in the blood and elevation of the erythrocyte sedimentation rate. An exception is "pure" chorea, which may appear long after indices of inflammation have returned to normal.

The urine may contain protein, white cells, and red cells. Biopsy studies have revealed a variety of renal abnormalities, but the classic proliferative glomerular abnormalities that characterize poststreptococcal acute glomerulonephritis occur quite rarely in ARF. Electrocardiographic and radiographic studies may reveal evidence of rhythm disturbances, pericarditis, or congestive heart failure. Echocardiography may document myocardial and valvular dysfunction and pericardial effusion.

The major laboratory contribution to the diagnosis of ARF is the documentation of recent group A streptococcal infection. Throat culture should always be performed but is positive in only a minority of cases. The low rate of culture positivity remains unexplained, although it may be due in part to the time lapse of several weeks between the onset of the pharyngeal infection and the throat culture. The serum titer of ASO is elevated in 80% or more of ARF patients. If two streptococcal antibody tests, e.g., ASO plus either anti-DNase B or antihyaluronidase, are performed, an elevated titer of at least one will be found in 90% of ARF patients. A battery of three tests establishes the presence of recent, immunologically significant streptococcal infection in >95% of individuals experiencing an acute rheumatic attack. The definition of an "elevated" titer varies, depending on the test used, the patient's age, and geographic locale. ASO titers of at least 240 Todd units per milliliter in adults and 320 Todd units in children are generally considered elevated. At times, serial sampling may detect a rising titer of streptococcal antibodies in patients seen early in the course of a rheumatic attack.

COURSE AND PROGNOSIS. The average duration of an untreated attack of ARF is approximately 3 months. The duration tends to be longer, up to 6 months, in patients with severe carditis. Fewer than 5% of patients have continuing rheumatic activity for longer than 6 months. In a few of these the disease is limited to chorea and is otherwise benign. Other patients exhibit evidence of persistent inflammatory activity, including arthritis, carditis, and subcutaneous nodules. "Chronic rheumatic fever" occurs more fre-

quently in patients who have had one or more previous attacks; cardiac involvement in chronic rheumatic fever tends to be frequent and severe.

Death from intractable myocarditis during the acute phase of ARF is now very rare. Once the acute attack has subsided, the only long-term sequel is that of rheumatic heart disease, manifested primarily by scarring and/or calcification (Fig. 277–3) of the mitral and aortic valves (see Ch. 42) and leading to insufficiency and/or stenosis. The prognosis from a cardiac standpoint very much depends on the clinical findings when the patient is first seen. In one large study, for example, 347 patients were examined during an acute rheumatic attack and again 10 years later. Among patients who had been free of carditis during their acute attack, only 6% had residual heart disease on follow-up. Patients with no pre-existing heart disease and with mild carditis during their acute attack (i.e., apical systolic murmur without pericarditis or heart failure) had a relatively good prognosis in that only approximately 30% had heart murmurs 10 years later. About 40% of subjects with apical or basal diastolic murmurs and 70% of subjects with failure and/or pericarditis during their acute attacks had residual rheumatic heart disease. The prognosis was worse in patients with pre-existing heart disease and in those who had experienced recurrent attacks of ARF in the 10-year interval.

These data indicate that patients who do not develop carditis during an acute attack and are protected from ARF recurrences are most unlikely to suffer from rheumatic heart disease. The patient with "pure" chorea represents an exception to this rule. A significant proportion of such patients who have no evidence of carditis when first examined may develop rheumatic valvular disease on prolonged follow-up. Although the explanation for this phenomenon is unknown, it is conceivable that in view of the long latent period associated with chorea, signs of carditis might have been present earlier but subsided by the time the neurologic abnormality became evident.

DIAGNOSIS. Although ARF is readily recognized in the individual who presents with multiple major manifestations or in epidemic circumstances, at other times the disease may be extraordinarily difficult to diagnose with confidence. This is so because of the variability of its clinical presentation, the frequency with which only a single major manifestation is detected, and the fact that there is no definitive diagnostic laboratory test. Nevertheless, precise diagnosis is especially important in this disease because of the need to advise the patient regarding prolonged antimicrobial prophylaxis (see below).

The diagnostic criteria of T. Duckett Jones, initially proposed in 1944 and subsequently modified by committees of the American Heart Association, attempt to minimize overdiagnosis and underdiagnosis (Table 277–3). The most recent (1992) revision specifies that the guidelines are designed to assist in the diagnosis of the initial ARF attack. Although most patients with recurrent ARF fulfill the criteria, in some cases the diagnosis of a recurrence may be less apparent.

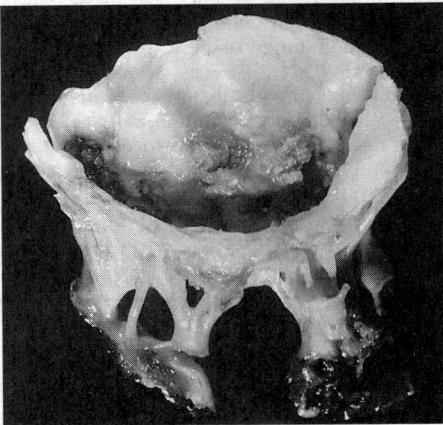

FIGURE 277–3. Calcified mitral valve from a patient with rheumatic heart disease. (Courtesy of A. Morales, M.D. From Bisno AL: Rheumatic fever. *In* Kelley WN, et al. [eds.]: Textbook of Rheumatology, 4th ed. Philadelphia, WB Saunders, 1993, p 1214.)

Two major manifestations, or one major and two minor manifestations, indicate a high probability of ARF, provided that there is supporting evidence of recent streptococcal infection. Although a positive throat culture or rapid antigen test for group A streptococci technically satisfies this requirement, streptococcal carriage rates of 15% are not uncommon among school-aged children during the fall and winter. Elevated titers of antibodies to streptococcal extracellular products, although not diagnostic of ARF, do indicate a recent, immunologically significant streptococcal infection. Conversely, if a battery of streptococcal antibody tests fails to reveal any evidence of recent infection, the diagnosis of ARF must be considered unlikely.

The modified Jones criteria are, of course, only guidelines. They are most difficult to apply confidently when polyarthritis is the single major manifestation. Under such circumstances, the diagnosis of ARF should be made only after excluding other causes of polyarthritis, such as rheumatoid arthritis, Still's disease, Lyme disease, viral arthritides (e.g., rubella, hepatitis B), the early prepurpuric phase of Henoch-Schönlein purpura, and septic arthritis, including gonococcal arthritis. The latter diagnosis cannot be excluded unequivocally by negative cultures of blood and synovial fluid. Therefore, if the clinical and epidemiologic picture is compatible with disseminated gonococcal infection, a trial of antigonococcal therapy should precede initiation of treatment with anti-inflammatory drugs.

Some patients have been described as manifesting polyarthritis that is atypical in time of onset and duration, does not respond dramatically to salicylate therapy, and is unassociated with other clinical features of ARF. Such individuals have on occasion been categorized as having "post-streptococcal reactive arthritis." The existence of this entity as a distinct syndrome, however, and its relationship to rheumatic fever remain uncertain. Pending further clarification, such individuals should be considered to have ARF if they fulfill the Jones criteria and alternative diagnoses have been excluded.

Serum sickness is frequently a serious consideration, particularly if the patient has received penicillin or other antibiotics for a preceding respiratory infection. SLE, sickle cell hemoglobinopathies, and infective endocarditis may involve the joints and the heart. Other differential diagnostic considerations include congenital heart lesions, viral and idiopathic forms of myocarditis and pericarditis, and functional heart murmurs. Nonfamilial forms of chorea have been described in SLE and rarely in association with the use of birth control pills. It remains uncertain how often episodes of chorea occurring during pregnancy ("chorea gravidarum") represent attacks of rheumatic fever. Other disorders that may at times be confused with ARF are gout, sarcoidosis, Hodgkin's disease, and acute leukemia.

There are certain circumstances in which ARF can be diagnosed even when the guidelines set forth in Table 277–3 have not been met. Patients whose only rheumatic manifestation is Sydenham's chorea may not fulfill the Jones criteria. Because of the long latent period between the antecedent streptococcal infection and the appearance of the neurologic abnormalities, evidence of inflammation encompassed in the minor manifestations may no longer be present, and previously elevated antibody titers may have declined to normal. A similar situation occasionally occurs in patients with indolent carditis, who may not come to medical attention until months after the onset of rheumatic fever. In patients with established rheumatic heart disease, it may be difficult to distinguish new from pre-existing cardiac involvement unless the patient has been under careful prospective follow-up, a previously undamaged valve is involved, or pericarditis is evident. Thus the diagnosis of recurrent ARF must be strongly entertained in the presence of suggestive clinical findings, provided there is evidence of recent group A streptococcal infection.

TREATMENT. Antibiotics neither modify the course of a rheumatic attack nor influence the subsequent development of carditis. Nevertheless, it is conventional to give a course of antibiotics designed to eradicate any rheumatogenic group A streptococci remaining in the tonsils and pharynx, in order to prevent spread of the organism to close contacts. The recommended regimens are those conventionally used for treatment of acute streptococcal pharyngitis (see Ch. 276). Benzathine penicillin G is preferred in non–penicillin-allergic patients. Following completion of this therapy, continuous antistreptococcal prophylaxis should commence (see below).

Treatment with anti-inflammatory agents is effective in suppressing many of the signs and symptoms of ARF. These agents do not "cure" the disease, nor do they prevent the subsequent evolution of rheumatic heart disease. They should be avoided in very mild or equivocal cases because, by suppressing the clinical manifestations, they may obscure the diagnosis. The two drugs most widely used are aspirin and corticosteroids. The former is used in patients with acute polyarthritis, provided that carditis is either absent or mild and there is no evidence of congestive heart failure. Aspirin is very effective in decreasing fever, toxicity, and joint inflammation. It should be given in a dosage of 90 to 100 mg per kilogram per day in children and 6 to 8 grams per day in adults. This is administered in equally divided doses, every 4 hours for the first 24 to 36 hours; thereafter it may be given in four doses during waking hours. A salicylate level of 25 mg per deciliter is usually satisfactory. The incidence of nausea and vomiting may be minimized by starting somewhat below the optimal dosage level and gradually increasing over a few days. The patient should be observed for evidence of significant gastrointestinal bleeding and for signs and symptoms of salicylism (see Ch. 19). After 2 weeks, the dosage is reduced to 60 to 70 mg per kilogram per day for an additional 6 weeks. These dosage schedules represent general guidelines only. The precise aspirin dose must be determined by the patient's clinical response, blood salicylate levels, and tolerance of the drug.

Corticosteroids are generally reserved for patients who have severe carditis manifested by congestive heart failure, who are unable to tolerate large doses of salicylates, or whose signs and symptoms are inadequately suppressed by aspirin. As with aspirin, the dosage must be individualized. Prednisone, 40 to 60 mg per day in divided doses, may be used initially. After 2 to 3 weeks it should be withdrawn slowly over an additional 3-week period. In cases of fulminating carditis with profound heart failure, intravenous corticosteroids may be used. As is the case for other patients receiving corticosteroids, the physician should be alert to problems such as

TABLE 277–3. GUIDELINES FOR THE DIAGNOSIS OF INITIAL ATTACK OF RHEUMATIC FEVER (JONES CRITERIA, UPDATED 1992)*

Major Manifestations	Minor Manifestations	Supporting Evidence of Antecedent Group A Streptococcal Infections
Carditis	Clinical findings	Positive throat culture or rapid streptococcal antigen test
Polyarthritis	Arthralgia	Elevated or rising streptococcal antibody titer
Chorea	Fever	
Erythema marginatum	Laboratory findings	
Subcutaneous nodules	Elevated acute-phase reactants	
	Erythrocyte sedimentation rate	
	C-reactive protein	
	Prolonged PR interval	

* If supported by evidence of preceding group A streptococcal infection, the presence of two major manifestations or of one major and two minor manifestations indicates a high probability of acute rheumatic fever.

Reprinted from Special Writing Group of the Committee on Rheumatic Fever, Endocarditis and Kawasaki Disease, American Heart Association. Guidelines for the diagnosis of rheumatic fever: Jones Criteria, 1992 update. JAMA 268 15:2069, 1992 with permission. Copyright, 1992, American Medical Association.

gastrointestinal bleeding, sodium and water retention, and impaired glucose tolerance. Suppression of the pituitary-adrenal axis or of the host immune system is a potential problem but not ordinarily a major one during this relatively short course of treatment. The role of nonsteroidal anti-inflammatory agents in managing ARF remains to be defined.

After cessation of anti-inflammatory therapy, clinical or laboratory evidence of ARF may reappear. Such therapeutic "rebounds" occur more frequently after corticosteroid therapy than after treatment with aspirin. They may be minimized by prolonging salicylate therapy for 9 to 12 weeks and, when corticosteroids have been required, by continuing aspirin for a month after corticosteroids have been discontinued. Congestive heart failure is managed by conventional measures. If digitalis is used, the potential risk of drug-induced arrhythmias in the patient with active myocarditis must be kept in mind. Patients with Sydenham's chorea require a quiet environment, and sedatives such as phenobarbital may be helpful.

Once the acute attack has subsided completely, the patient's subsequent level of physical activity depends on cardiac status. Patients without residual heart disease may resume full and unrestricted activity. It is important that patients not be subjected to unwarranted invalidism, because of either their own inaccurate perceptions of the nature of the rheumatic process or those of parents, teachers, or employers.

PREVENTION. "Primary prevention" of ARF consists of accurate diagnosis and appropriate treatment of streptococcal sore throat (see Ch. 276). Although straightforward in theory, primary prevention is often frustratingly difficult to achieve. In many of the densely populated indigent communities in which the risk of ARF is greatest, children with self-limited illnesses such as sore throats may never come to medical attention, and throat culture services are usually unavailable to aid in diagnosis. Moreover, in one third or more of cases, ARF may arise after a clinically inapparent streptococcal infection.

Perhaps the most effective strategy for avoiding the mortality and chronic cardiac disability associated with ARF is that of "secondary prevention." This strategy focuses on the group of persons who have already suffered a rheumatic attack and who are inordinately susceptible to a recurrence following an immunologically significant streptococcal upper respiratory infection. Recurrent attacks tend to be mimetic in nature, so patients who have suffered carditis with their previous attack are likely to have repetitive cardiac involvement and progressive cardiac damage. Because even patients who experienced only arthritis or chorea may develop carditis with recurrent attacks of ARF, all patients who have experienced a documented attack of ARF should receive continuous antimicrobial prophylaxis to prevent either symptomatic or asymptomatic streptococcal infections. The specific regimens to be used are indicated in Ch. 42 and 276. By far the most effective of these is intramuscular benzathine penicillin G every 4 weeks. Rheumatic recurrences are very unusual in patients faithfully adhering to this regimen. In areas of the world where the incidence of ARF and the risk of recurrence are extremely high, however, injections every 3 weeks may provide more complete protection.

The total duration of intramuscular or oral rheumatic fever prophylaxis remains unresolved. The risk of rheumatic recurrence is known to diminish with increasing age and increasing interval since the most recent rheumatic attack. Patients who escape carditis during their initial attack are less likely to experience rheumatic recurrences and less likely to develop carditis if a recurrence does ensue. These facts suggest that prophylaxis need not be perpetual for all rheumatic subjects. Continuous prophylaxis should be maintained indefinitely for those with clinically significant rheumatic heart disease. Other rheumatic subjects should be protected until reaching adulthood, for at least 5 years after their most recent attack, and if they are in an epidemiologic circumstance that places them at high risk of streptococcal acquisition (e.g., parents of small children, school teachers, military recruits, nurses, pediatricians, or residents of areas with a high incidence of ARF). The decision to remove a rheumatic subject from continuous prophylaxis should be an individualized one, based on the physician's assessment of the risk and likely consequences of recurrence, and taken with the patient's informed consent. Patients taken off prophylaxis must be instructed to

return immediately for medical follow-up whenever symptoms of pharyngitis occur.

Patients with rheumatic valvular heart disease must receive prophylaxis designed to avoid bacterial endocarditis whenever they undergo dental or surgical procedures likely to evoke bacteremia. This is not necessary in the rheumatic subject who is free of residual heart disease. The regimens to prevent endocarditis (see Ch. 278) are different from those prescribed for preventing ARF, and the fact that a patient is receiving rheumatic fever prophylaxis does not exempt him/her from endocarditis prophylaxis. This is a frequent point of confusion not only among patients but among physicians and dentists as well.

Berrios X, Del Campo E, Guzman B, Bisno AL: Discontinuance of rheumatic fever prophylaxis in selected adolescents and young adults. Ann Intern Med 118:401, 1993. *Presents new data, along with a review of previous studies, on the circumstances under which rheumatic fever prophylaxis might be discontinued.*

Bisno AL: Group A streptococcal infections and acute rheumatic fever. N Engl J Med 325:783, 1991. *Review of the biology of the group A streptococcus as it relates to civilian and military outbreaks of ARF in the 1980's and the more recent resurgence of life-threatening streptococcal infections.*

Stollerman GH: Rheumatic Fever and Streptococcal Infection. New York, Grune & Stratton, 1975. *A comprehensive, extremely readable summary of rheumatic fever. Detailed descriptions of clinical manifestations will be particularly valuable to physicians unfamiliar with the disease.*

Veasy LG, Tani LY, Hill HR: Persistence of acute rheumatic fever in the intermountain area of the United States. J Pediatr 124:9, 1994. *A summary of the demographic and clinical data on 274 cases of ARF hospitalized in Salt Lake City between 1985 and 1992.*

278 INFECTIVE ENDOCARDITIS
Matthew E. Levison

Endocarditis is characterized by the vegetation, a lesion that results from deposition of platelets and fibrin on the endothelial surface of the heart. Infection is the most common cause, the usual pathogen being one of a variety of bacterial species, microscopic colonies of which are buried beneath the surface of fibrin. However, other types of microorganisms, such as rickettsia, chlamydia, and fungi, may be involved, so that the more general term *infective,* rather than *bacterial,* endocarditis is preferred. Usually the heart valve is the site of the vegetation, but in certain instances vegetations may occur on other parts of the endocardium. Involvement of extracardiac intravascular sites, which can produce an illness clinically similar to endocarditis, is properly termed *endarteritis.*

PATHOGENESIS

Endocarditis is the result of the interaction among (1) host factors that predispose the endothelium to infection, (2) circumstances that lead to transient bacteremia, and (3) the tissue tropism and virulence of the circulating bacteria.

HOST. In population-based studies, the age- and gender-adjusted incidence of endocarditis is about 5 per 100,000 person-years. Advancing age and male gender are significant risk factors; the incidence rate ratio for those age 65 or older is almost 9 times that of those under 65 and for males 2.5 times that of females. The greater frequency in the aged is due in part to the increased prevalence of predisposing cardiac lesions (e.g., degenerative cardiac lesions and prosthetic cardiac valves) and circumstances that may lead to bacteremia (e.g., invasive urologic procedures, anorectal and colonic disease, and intravascular catheterization) in this age group, and in males, the increased prevalence of certain cardiac lesions, such as bicuspid aortic valves.

Local Host Factors. **Nonbacterial Thrombotic Endocarditis (NBTE).** The normal endothelium is nonthrombogenic, but when damaged or denuded the endothelium is a potent inducer of blood coagulation. Certain types of congenital or acquired heart disease can result in a high-velocity jet stream from a high to low pressure chamber (aortic or mitral insufficiency, ventricular septal defect, or patent ductus arteriosus), or create a pressure gradient across a narrowed orifice between two chambers (aortic stenosis or coarctation of the aorta). The high-velocity jet stream can lead to turbulent blood flow distal to the pressure gradient, which is thought to damage the valvular and endocardial endothelium in a predictable pattern distal to the pressure gradient (Fig. 278–1). Damage to the endothelium can be induced in an experimental animal by passing a catheter into the heart across the aortic or tricuspid valves, and intracardiac catheters can induce similar lesions in humans. Platelets are deposited on the surface of the damaged endothelium. The adherent platelets then degranulate and stimulate local deposition of fibrin. In the process, a sterile thrombus is formed on the endothelial surface, the so-called NBTE. For unknown reasons, NBTE are also found in some patients with chronic wasting illnesses (marantic endocarditis) and systemic lupus erythematosus (SLE) (Libman-Sacks endocarditis). NBTE can dislodge fibrin, embolize to block peripheral arteries, and produce sterile infarction of distal organs. The resultant clinical manifestations of NBTE in cachetic illnesses or SLE may simulate those of infective endocarditis (see below).

NBTE is the point of attachment and subsequent proliferation for certain microorganisms once they have gained access to the circulation. Following induced bacteremia in experimental animals without pre-existing NBTE, the endothelial surface is resistant to bacterial attachment and the subsequent development of infective endocarditis. The left side of the heart is apparently more susceptible to infection than the right side. For example, the left side is infected more readily with relatively avirulent microorganisms, such as α-hemolytic streptococci, whereas the right is infected only by virulent pathogens, such as *Staphylococcus aureus;* bacteria reach higher densities on the left side (e.g., 10^{10-11} colony-forming units [CFU] per gram) than on the right (e.g., 10^8 CFU per gram). Right-sided lesions tend to respond more readily to antimicrobial therapy than do left-sided lesions; right-sided lesions may even heal spontaneously, in contrast to persistence of infection on the left. Responsible factors may include differences between the left and right side of the heart in blood Po_2 and intracardiac pressures. Spontaneous resolution of right-sided endocarditis is probably also a consequence of bacterial clearance on the right side by polymorphonuclear leukocytes, a factor not operative to the same extent on the left for unknown reasons. Pre-existing cardiac lesions that are believed to promote the formation of NBTE are identified in about two thirds of patients with infective endocarditis. The cardiac defects most frequently found in patients with endocarditis are mitral valve prolapse (MVP), degenerative heart disease, congenital heart disease, rheumatic heart disease (RHD), and prosthetic cardiac valves. However, the degree of risk that each type of cardiac lesion poses for subsequent endocarditis cannot be inferred from their relative frequency because the prevalence of these cardiac defects in the general population varies widely. The absolute risk is indicated by incidence rate of endocarditis for each cardiac lesion (when the frequency of the cardiac defect in the general population is known) and the relative risk by the incidence rate ratio with reference to the incidence rate of endocarditis in the general population (Table 278–1).

TABLE 278–1. ABSOLUTE AND RELATIVE RISK FOR ENDOCARDITIS AMONG VARIOUS CARDIAC LESIONS (INCIDENCE RATE, CASES PER 100,000 PATIENT-YEARS)

Prosthetic valves	308–630	(63–129)*
Prior native valve endocarditis, non-IVDU	300–740	(61–151)
Rheumatic heart disease	380–440	(78–90)
Congenital heart disease	120	(25)
Coarctation of the aorta		
Tetralogy of Fallot		
Bicuspid aortic valve		
Transposition of the aorta		
Patent ductus arteriosus		
Ventricular septal defect		
Mitral valve prolapse with regurgitant murmur	52	(11)
Hypertrophic cardiomyopathy		
Other acquired valvular dysfunction (e.g., degenerative heart diseases)		
Marfan's syndrome		

*Incidence rate relative to rate of endocarditis in normal population, 4.9/100,000 patient years.

IVDU = Intravenous drug user.

Prosthetic cardiac valves are a major risk factor for endocarditis. Endocarditis occurs in 1 to 5% of patients with prosthetic valves over the lifetime of the valve, with an incidence rate of about 300 to 600 per 100,000 patient-years. Mechanical prosthetic cardiac valves probably have about the same risk as bioprostheses (e.g., porcine heterografts), and risk probably does not vary by site of prosthetic valve replacement but is greater when valves are placed in the presence of active endocarditis. Prior native valve endocarditis poses a significant risk factor for subsequent episodes as a consequence of both the continued presence of the risk factors that contributed to the initial episode (e.g., intravenous drug use or periodontitis) and the additional risk posed by the damage to the valve sustained in the initial episode. The decreasing relative frequency of RHD among patients with endocarditis in the United States reflects the decreasing prevalence of RHD in this country. Nevertheless, RHD is a major risk factor for endocarditis, with an incidence rate only slightly lower than that for prosthetic valves. RHD remains a frequent predisposing lesion for endocarditis in the developing world because of persistence of RHD in those populations. Congenital defects at increased risk for endocarditis are shown in Table 278–1. Although surgical correction of congenital defects such as ventricular septal defect lowers risk, it does not eliminate it. Nevertheless, the American Heart Association does not recommend preventive antibiotic therapy for patients 6 or more months after corrective surgery with prosthetic devices. As a general rule, cardiac lesions not associated with turbulent blood flow, such as cardiac lesions in a relatively low pressure system (e.g., on the right side of the heart) or abnormal flow through a wide orifice (e.g., secundum type of atrial septal defect) are less likely to be complicated by endocarditis. Because of its high prevalence in the population, MVP is the most frequent lesion predisposing to endocarditis. However, the absolute risk for endocarditis among patients with MVP and an audible murmur of mitral insufficiency is considerably lower than that of other cardiac abnormalities. Cardiac lesions that rarely predispose to endocarditis are shown in Table 278–2. Endocarditis can occur on structurally normal native valves in ≥25% of patients. In these patients, endocarditis is more likely to be nosocomial or

TABLE 278–2. CARDIAC LESIONS THAT RARELY PREDISPOSE TO ENDOCARDITIS

Isolated secundum type of atrial septal defect
Syphilitic aortitis
Previous coronary artery bypass graft
Mitral valve prolapse without murmur
Previous rheumatic heart disease without valvular dysfunction
Permanent cardiac pacemakers and implanted defibrillators
Surgical repair, without residua, of secundum atrial septal defect, ventricular septal defect, patent ductus arteriosus after 6 months

Adapted from Dajani AS, Bisno AL, Chung KJ, et al.: Prevention of bacterial endocarditis. Recommendations by the American Heart Association. JAMA 264:2919, 1990. Copyright, 1990, American Medical Association.

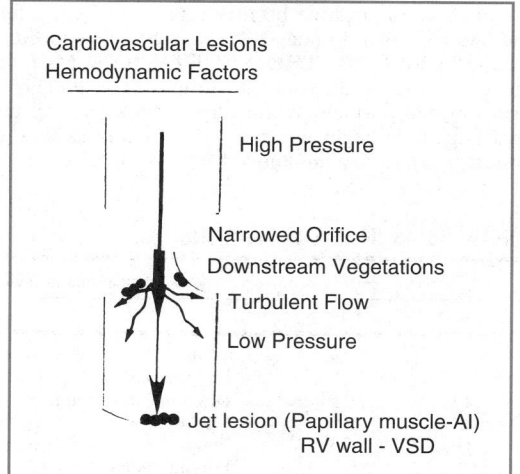

FIGURE 278–1. A schematic diagram of the hemodynamic factors favoring development of nonbacterial thrombotic endocarditis.

TABLE 278-3. CIRCUMSTANCES LIKELY TO LEAD TO TRANSIENT BACTEREMIA THAT CAN PRECEDE ENDOCARDITIS

Dental and periodontal procedure known to induce mucosal bleeding
Tonsillectomy and adenoidectomy
Bronchoscopy with rigid scope
Surgical procedure on the respiratory or intestinal mucosa
Gallbladder surgery
Esophageal dilatation and sclerotherapy for esophageal varices
Prostatic surgery
Vaginal hysterectomy
Cystoscopy or urethral dilatation
In the presence of infection, urethral catheterization or urologic surgery
In presence of infection, vaginal delivery, dilatation and curettage, therapeutic abortion, insertion and removal of intrauterine devices, sterilization procedures
Incision and drainage of infected tissue

Adapted from Dajani AS, Bisno AL, Chung KJ, et al.: Prevention of bacterial endocarditis. Recommendations by the American Heart Association. JAMA 264:2919, 1990. Copyright, 1990, American Medical Association.

caused by more virulent organisms, such as *S. aureus,* or the patient is more likely to be an intravenous drug user (IVDU).

Systemic Host Factors. Systemic host defenses (e.g., granulocytes, T lymphocytes, antibody, complement) most likely play a minor role in development or maintenance of endocarditis, except perhaps for granulocytes in right-sided endocarditis. Various immunodeficiency states, including HIV infection, do not seem to place the patient at increased risk for endocarditis.

CIRCUMSTANCES THAT LEAD TO TRANSIENT BACTEREMIA. Transient bacteremia is a common event and occurs as a consequence of trauma to skin or mucosal surfaces that are normally laden with an endogenous flora. The bacteremia is characterized by a low number of organisms per milliliter of blood (usually < 10 CFU per milliliter) and very short duration (15 to 30 minutes). The intensity of the bacteremia is related directly to the magnitude of the trauma, the density of the microbial flora, and the presence of inflammation or infection at the site of skin or mucosal injury. Mucosal sites that have a dense endogenous flora include the gingival crevice, oropharynx, terminal ileum and colon, distal urethra, and vagina. Minor trauma to the gingival crevice as routine as brushing teeth or chewing hard candy may account in part for the 75% of patients with viridans streptococcal endocarditis who fail to recall any unusual circumstance that could have resulted in an episode of transient bacteremia preceding the onset of endocarditis. Transient bacteremia likely to lead to endocarditis can also result from illicit intravenous drug use and nosocomial procedures. Circumstances known to predispose to transient bacteremia that can precede endocarditis are shown in Table 278-3.

A history of such procedures is obtained in only about 25% of patients with viridans streptococcal endocarditis, 40% of patients with enterococcal endocarditis, and 30 to 40% of patients with community-acquired staphylococcal endocarditis, but nevertheless this history is more frequent among patients with endocarditis than among matched controls without endocarditis. The source of bacteremia can be identified in >90% of cases of nosocomial endocarditis. However, some of these procedures may be associated with subsequent endocarditis only in the presence of high-risk underlying cardiac lesions, such as prosthetic valves or previous native valve

endocarditis. The prosthetic valve is usually infected at the time of surgical insertion of the valve or at any time following transient bacteremia in the postoperative period. Rarely the source is a prosthetic valve that was contaminated before insertion.

INFECTING MICROORGANISMS. Trauma to the skin or mucosal surfaces that harbor a prolific endogenous flora releases into the bloodstream many different microbial species. The array of microorganisms entering the circulation varies with the unique endogenous microflora at the particular traumatized site. Staphylococci and diphtheroids are characteristic for skin; oral anaerobes and streptococci for the oropharyngeal mucosa; and colonic anaerobes, enteric aerobic gram-negative bacilli, and enterococci for the genitourinary and lower intestinal mucosa. However, only a few of these species, e.g., most commonly oral streptococci, staphylococci, and enterococci, are likely to cause endocarditis. The frequency with which a particular organism causes endocarditis depends on the how frequently it can gain access to the circulation and its ability to survive in the bloodstream and adhere to components of NBTE, exposed subendothelial structures, or the endothelial surface itself.

A predictable array of microorganisms cause endocarditis for each of the specific conditions that predispose the patients to develop infective endocarditis (Table 278-4). For example, in community-acquired endocarditis in non-IVDU's, a variety of α-hemolytic streptococci (*S. mitis, S. sanguis, S. mutans,* and *S. intermedius*) and enterococci are the usual pathogens. *S. bovis,* a streptococcal species that contains group D polysaccharide capsular material, as does enterococci, causes endocarditis in patients who are likely to have an underlying gastrointestinal lesion. Isolating *S. bovis* from blood cultures should prompt a complete evaluation of the gastrointestinal tract, especially the colon, in that patient. Less frequent are fastidious gram-negative bacilli, the so-called HACEK microorganisms (*Haemophilus* species, *Actinobacillus, Cardiobacterium, Eikenella,* and *Kingella*). The *Haemophilus* species are usually *H. aphrophilus, H. paraphrophilus,* or *H. parainfluenzae,* and rarely *H. influenzae. S. aureus* causes >50% of cases of endocarditis occurring in IVDU's, and in many geographic locations the strains of *S. aureus* are resistant to all β-lactam antibiotics (i.e., usually designated as methicillin-resistant strains). Streptococci and enterococci are less frequent pathogens in IVDU. Gram-negative bacilli (usually *Pseudomonas aeruginosa, P. cepacia,* and *Serratia marcescens*) and fungi (usually non-albicans *Candida* species), unusual in non-IVDU native valve endocarditis, occur in about 8 and 5% of cases of IVDU endocarditis, respectively. Although uncommon in patients without prosthetic valves, coagulase-negative staphylococci, usually of the methicillin-resistant variety, are the predominant pathogen of prosthetic valve endocarditis (PVE) within 2 months after surgery, designated as early PVE. Indeed, the frequency of methicillin-resistant coagulase-negative staphylococci remains constant over the entire first 12 months, which suggests that a similar pathogenesis may extend over the first year after surgery, not just the first 2 months. After the first year, the array of organisms in PVE tends to resemble that of native valve endocarditis (NVE), i.e., streptococci. However, fungi, usually *C. albicans,* and aerobic enteric gram-negative bacilli occur more frequently in both early and late PVE than in non-IVDU native valve endocarditis.

DEVELOPMENT OF THE VEGETATION. Microorganisms adherent to the vegetation stimulate further deposition of platelets and fibrin on their surface. Within this secluded focus, the buried microorganisms then begin multiplying as rapidly as they would in broth cultures, apparently uninhibited by host defenses, e.g., phago-

TABLE 278-4. FREQUENCY OF INFECTING MICROORGANISMS IN ENDOCARDITIS (%)

Native Valve		PVE			Endocarditis in IVDU	
			Early	Late		
Streptococci	50	Coagulase-negative staphylococcus	33	29	*S. aureus*	57
Enterococci	10	*S. aureus*	15	11	Streptococci	13
Staphylococcus aureus	20	Gram-negative bacilli	17	11	Gram-negative bacilli	8
HACEK	5	Fungi	13	5	Enterococci	7
Other	10	Streptococci	9	36	Fungi	5
Culture-negative	5	Diphtheroids	9	3	Polymicrobial	5
		Other	4	5	Culture-negative	5

IVDU = Intravenous drug user.

cytes, antibody, and complement, to reach maximally dense populations of 10^{8-11} CFU per gram of vegetation. Over 90% of the microorganisms in these established vegetations are metabolically inactive and nongrowing, i.e., in a phase least susceptible to the bactericidal effects of β-lactam and aminoglycoside antibiotics.

Sustained bacteremia that is characteristic of endocarditis results from an equilibrium between the rate of release of microorganisms as the vegetation fragments and the rate of clearance of the circulating microorganisms by the reticuloendothelial system in the liver, spleen, and bone marrow. The vegetation enlarges as circulating bacteria are redeposited on the surface of the vegetation, which in turn stimulates further deposition of fibrin on the surface (Fig. 278–2). The resultant vegetation is composed of successive layers of fibrin and clusters of bacteria, with rare red cells and leukocytes, almost always covered by a layer of fibrin on the luminal surface. Enlargement of the vegetation tends to be counterbalanced by continued fragmentation. The ultimate size of the vegetation can vary from small sessile granular protuberances to a large pedunculated mass. The size of the vegetation itself and the fragments that break off depend to some extent on the type of infecting microorganism; e.g., *H. parainfluenzae* and *C. albicans,* tend to produce large friable vegetations and large emboli.

With effective antimicrobial therapy the vegetation becomes progressively organized as the edematous, vascular, and fibrogenic granulation tissue grows in from the base and is replaced by mature fibrous tissue with varying degrees of calcification. Healed vegetations are re-endothelialized, but the associated valve leaflet may become progressively more distorted as the healing proceeds. Thus, despite bacteriologic response, distortion of the healing valve may lead to hemodynamic decompensation and a highly susceptible site for development of repeated episodes of infective endocarditis in the future.

CLINICAL PRESENTATIONS (see Color Plates 11*A* through 11*D*)

Clinical manifestations include fever and cardiac and extracardiac findings that are the result of either (1) the valvular infection itself, (2) embolization of fragments of the vegetation, (3) suppurative complications on the basis of hematogenous spread of infection, or (4) immunologic response to the infection in the form of immune complex vasculitis.

NATIVE VALVE ENDOCARDITIS. Symptoms usually begin within 2 weeks of the inciting bacteremia. In the preantibiotic era, when endocarditis was uniformly fatal, a short duration of illness of <6 weeks prior to death was used to characterize acute endocarditis; in contrast, subacute and chronic endocarditis had a more indolent course until death of 6 weeks to 2 years. Chronicity is now used in reference to the duration of illness prior to presentation. Acute endocarditis is usually (50 to 70%) caused by *S. aureus,* especially when accompanied by marked signs of general infection and suppurative embolic phenomena and has a rapidly fatal course if treatment is delayed. Infection may develop on a previously normal valve. In the non-IVDU, the aortic valve is usually involved. Therefore, a diagnosis of acute endocarditis can serve as an effective guide to empiric antibiotic therapy, even before results of blood cultures are available. Subacute endocarditis, commonly caused by streptococci and enterococci, in contrast often develops on previously damaged endocardium, has less dramatic clinical manifesta-

tions of general infection, and is characterized by nonsuppurative peripheral vascular phenomena.

Systemic manifestations of endocarditis include fever most commonly and other symptoms that may accompany fever, such as drenching night sweats, arthralgias, myalgias (especially in the low back and thighs), and weight loss. Fever is usually low grade, the temperature peaks rarely exceeding 39.4° C. Fever may be absent in a few patients, e.g., those who are very elderly or severely debilitated, have significant renal or heart failure, or are taking antipyretics or antibiotics.

Cardiac manifestations include: (1) murmurs of valvular insufficiency due to a destroyed or distorted valve and its supporting structures, or valvular stenosis due to large vegetations. (2) Valve ring abscess due to local extension of the infection from the valve ring of the noncoronary cusp of the aortic valve. Valve ring abscesses can lead to persistent fever despite appropriate antimicrobial therapy, heart block as a result of destroyed conduction pathways in the area of the atrioventricular node and bundle of His in the upper interventricular septum, pericarditis or hemopericardium as a result of burrowing abscesses into the pericardium, or shunts between cardiac chambers or between the heart and aorta as a result of burrowing abscesses into other cardiac chambers or aorta. (3) Myocardial infarction from coronary artery embolization. (4) Myocardial abscess as a consequence of bacteremia. (5) Diffuse myocarditis possibly as a consequence of immune complex vasculitis. Murmurs are likely to be absent in tricuspid endocarditis or may be absent when a patient is first seen with acute endocarditis. Congestive heart failure (CHF) is the most common complication of endocarditis, developing in about 60% of patients as a consequence of valvular or myocardial involvement, or may precede the onset of endocarditis as a consequence of the underlying cardiac lesion. CHF is usually present on admission in patients with subacute or streptococcal endocarditis but may develop dramatically in patients with acute *S. aureus* endocarditis with an aortic diastolic murmur or sudden rupture of mitral valve chordae. CHF occurs more frequently with left-sided than right-sided endocarditis and with aortic more than mitral involvement.

Extracardiac manifestations include (1) embolic events that result in infarction of numerous organs, such as the lung in right-sided endocarditis or the brain, spleen, or kidneys in left-sided endocarditis; (2) suppurative complications that include abscesses, septic infarcts, and infected mycotic aneurysms; and (3) immunologic reactions to the valvular infection including glomerulonephritis, sterile meningitis, and polyarthritis, and a variety of vascular phenomena, such as mucocutaneous petechiae (Color Plates 11*A* and 11*C*), splinter hemorrhages, Roth spots (see Color Plate 11*B*), and Osler's nodes. Systemic embolization, often a devastating complication when it involves the cerebral circulation, occurs in about 20 to 40% of patients with left-sided endocarditis. Frank cerebral abscess is rare, except in *S. aureus* endocarditis, when it occurs in 1 to 5% of patients. Septic pulmonary emboli commonly occur in patients with right-sided endocarditis. On chest radiograms, these emboli appear as multiple round infiltrates that may undergo cavitation or be complicated by empyema. Emboli can occur at any time during the course of illness, even after an otherwise successful course of antibiotic therapy is completed, although the frequency of embolization decreases as the vegetation heals. Mycotic aneurysms are an unusual but important complication of endocarditis. Mycotic aneurysms (see Color Plate 11*D*) are commonly asymptomatic but can become clinically evident in 3 to 5% of patients, even months or years after completion of successful therapy. These aneurysms characteristically develop at arterial bifurcations, e.g., in the middle cerebral, splenic, superior mesenteric, pulmonary, coronary, and extremity arteries, the abdominal aorta, and the sinus of Valsalva. In a patient with endocarditis, unremitting headache, visual disturbance, or cranial nerve palsy suggests an impending rupture of a cerebral mycotic aneurysm. Signs of blood loss at any site in a patient with endocarditis should suggest rupture of a mycotic aneurysm once the aneurysm has enlarged beyond a critical size, probably about 1 cm in diameter. The development of clinically apparent splenomegaly and many of the various nonsuppurative peripheral vascular phenomena is related to the duration of illness prior to presentation. The frequency of these clinical manifestations (<50%) is currently less than in

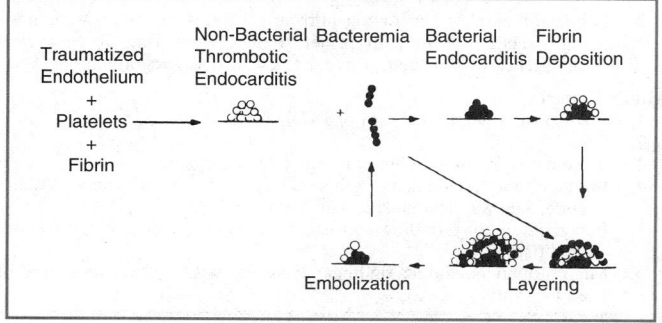

FIGURE 278–2. A schematic diagram of the pathogenetic events leading to development of infective endocarditis.

the past as a result of shorter durations of illness before antimicrobial therapy is given.

ENDOCARDITIS IN IVDU's. IVDU's with endocarditis tend to be younger than non-IVDU's with endocarditis, the disease is usually acute, and a previously normal tricuspid valve is usually involved. In tricuspid endocarditis, murmurs and heart failure are usually absent, but septic pulmonary complications occur in about 75% of these patients and *S. aureus* is the usual pathogen. Left-sided endocarditis in IVDU's resembles that in non-IVDU's, manifested by aortic or mitral murmurs, heart failure, neurologic damage, systemic embolization, peripheral mucocutaneous stigmata of endocarditis, or systemic metastatic infection such as osteomyelitis and septic arthritis. The pathogens isolated from IVDU's with left-sided endocarditis are similar those isolated from non-IVDU's, although *S. aureus* is probably disproportionately involved in IVDU's. Fever, the usual initial manifestation of endocarditis in the IVDU, also accompanies other major and minor illnesses in this population. Indeed only about 10% of febrile IVDU presenting to the emergency room have endocarditis. In most febrile IVDU's with a major infectious diseases such as cellulitis, endocarditis, pneumonia, or osteomyelitis, the cause of the patient's fever is obvious on presentation. However, in about one third of febrile IVDU's with endocarditis the cause of the patient's fever will be not apparent on presentation.

NOSOCOMIAL ENDOCARDITIS. Nosocomial endocarditis, which is defined as being due to a hospital-based procedure performed within 4 weeks preceding the onset of symptoms, accounts for 10 to 30% of cases of endocarditis, the frequency varying with the types of patients. Patients with nosocomial NVE tend to be elderly and have predisposing cardiac lesions, usually on the left-side of the heart. The major predisposing cardiac lesion for nosocomial endocarditis is a prosthetic cardiac valve (present in up to 50% of cases). The most important bacteremia-inducing event during hospitalization which results in endocarditis is use of an intravascular device, present in up to 50% of cases. Nosocomial *S. aureus* bacteremia is much more frequently complicated by endocarditis (5 to 10% of the time) than is enterococcal bacteremia (< 1%). The clinical presentation of nosocomial endocarditis is similar to that of community-acquired endocarditis. In patients with PVE, fever is usually present, although the classic clinical features of endocarditis, such as peripheral vascular phenomena, are frequently absent, especially in early infection. Although blood cultures are usually positive, the diagnosis is frequently delayed owing to failure to recognize the significance of the positive blood cultures.

ELECTROCARDIOGRAPHIC MANIFESTATIONS. A baseline electrocardiogram (ECG) should be obtained to assess the presence of conduction abnormalities that develop in about 10 to 20% of patients with endocarditis as a consequence of burrowing valve ring abscesses. A prolonged PR interval may be the initial indication of the sudden development of more severe conduction abnormalities, such as complete heart block. Other abnormalities that can be detected by ECG include myocardial infarction and pericarditis.

HEMATOLOGIC MANIFESTATIONS. Progressive anemia of chronic disease with normochromic, normocytic indices routinely develops in subacute endocarditis with relatively normal platelet, white blood cell, and differential counts. In acute endocarditis of short duration due to *S. aureus,* anemia may initially be absent, although the white blood cell count is usually elevated with a shift to the left and the platelet count is often low. PVE with an unstable prosthesis may cause acute hemolysis. The erythrocyte sedimentation rate is routinely elevated in endocarditis except when there is hypofibrinogenemia secondary to disseminated intravascular coagulation or congestive heart failure.

RENAL MANIFESTATIONS. Proteinuria and microscopic hematuria are common findings, occurring in up to 50% of patients. Renal emboli or focal glomerulonephritis can cause microscopic hematuria, but gross hematuria usually indicates renal infarction. Renal failure that develops in a patient with endocarditis is usually due to diffuse immune complex glomerulonephritis (see Color Plate 11E).

OTHER LABORATORY MANIFESTATIONS. Serologic evidence of circulating immune complexes (CIC) may by found in endocarditis, the frequency of which is related to the duration of illness. Occasional false-positive nontreponemal serologic tests for syphilis occur. The cerebrospinal fluid may show polymorphonuclear leukocytes and moderately elevated protein concentration in

up to 15% of patients. Frank bacterial meningitis, although unusual, occurs in *S. aureus* endocarditis.

DIAGNOSIS

Definitive diagnosis depends on microbiologic or pathologic proof of infection by histology or culture of vegetations obtained at surgery or autopsy or when an arterial embolus is surgically removed. In lieu of surgery or autopsy, definitive diagnosis can be established by demonstrating (1) a characteristic vegetation, valve ring abscess, or new prosthetic valve dehiscence with echocardiography and (2) intravascular infection with multiple blood cultures obtained over an extended period of time that are positive for a microorganism consistent with endocarditis. However, a blood culture or echocardiography is usually obtained only after the diagnosis is suspected based on history and physical findings. The diagnosis can be ranked in order of probability that endocarditis is present by distinction between major and minor criteria, which allows for weighting of clinical findings, echocardiographic findings, the type of microbial species isolated from blood, the frequency of positive blood cultures, and the absence of another source of infection (Table 278–5).

MICROBIOLOGIC INVESTIGATION. Isolating a pathogen from several blood cultures that are obtained over an extended period is important both to confirm the diagnosis of endocarditis and to enable determination of the antibiotic regimen that is optimal for therapy. Bacteremia in endocarditis is characterized by a constant number of organisms per milliliter of blood (usually 20 to 200 CFU per milliliter), unrelated to the height of the patient's temperature or the site of blood sampling (e.g., arterial versus venous blood), except for a slight fall in numbers across the hepatic or splenic circulation. Less than 5% of patients with endocarditis have sterile blood cultures if adequate blood culture methods are used. Three blood cultures should be obtained at least 1 hour apart to demonstrate that the bacteremia is continuous. If the cultures remain negative for 48 hours, two additional cultures should be obtained. However, in the absence of prior antibiotic therapy, the first three blood cultures are

TABLE 278–5. CRITERIA FOR THE DIAGNOSIS OF INFECTIVE ENDOCARDITIS (DUKE UNIVERSITY ENDOCARDITIS SERVICE)

1. Definitive diagnosis
   a. Pathology/microbiology of vegetations obtained at surgery or autopsy
   b. Two major criteria
   c. One major/three minor criteria
   d. Five minor criteria
2. Possible diagnosis: Findings consistent with but fall short of definitive diagnosis of endocarditis
3. No endocarditis: No pathology at surgery or autopsy or clinical resolution with 3 days of antimicrobial therapy; firm alternate diagnosis

Major Criteria
1. Blood culture
   a. 2 separate blood cultures positive for:
      i. Viridans streptococci, *S. bovis,* HACEK
      ii. Community-acquired *S. aureus* or enterococci, in absence of primary focus
   b. Positive blood cultures > 12 hours apart
   c. Positive blood cultures: 3 of 3, majority of ≥ 4 with 1st and last ≥ 1 hour apart
2. Echocardiography: Oscillating intracardiac mass on valve or supporting structure or in path of jet stream, valve ring abscess, new dehiscence of prosthetic valve, or new valvular regurgitation

Minor Criteria
1. Predisposing heart condition or IVDU
2. Fever ≥ 38°C
3. Systemic or pulmonary emboli, mycotic aneurysm
4. Immunologic phenomena: glomerulonephritis, Roth's spot, Osler's node, Janeway lesion, rheumatoid factor
5. Echocardiography finding consistent with but not definitive of endocarditis
6. Microbiologic/serologic findings consistent with but not definitive of endocarditis

Adapted from Durack DT, Lukes AS, Bright DK, et al.: New criteria for diagnosis of infective endocarditis: Utilization of specific echocardiographic findings. Am J Med 96:200, 1994.
IVDU = Intravenous drug user.

expected to be positive in >95% of patients with positive cultures. Prior antibiotic therapy, fastidious bacteria (such as the nutritionally deficient streptococci, the HACEK group of organisms, *Neisseria, Brucella,* and *Legionella*), fungi, chlamydia, and rickettsia can result in negative cultures. In acute endocarditis, when empiric antibiotic therapy should be initiated as soon as possible, two or three blood cultures should be drawn 1 hour apart before starting empiric therapy. In the face of a preceeding course of antibiotics, further antibiotic therapy should be held and blood cultures repeated until positive, if clinical conditions permit. The longer the time since the last dose of antibiotic or the shorter the preceding course of antibiotic, the more likely it is that the blood cultures will be positive. When fastidious bacteria and fungi are suspected, the clinical microbiology laboratory should be consulted for advice on the optimal methods to isolate these microorganisms, which may require more prolonged incubation (e.g., up to 3 weeks) or special media for isolation. Gram stain of the cultures may identify some pathogens not otherwise apparent in the blood cultures. Fungal endocarditis, which is likely to have negative blood cultures, tends to be complicated by large vegetations and embolization, in which case the organisms can be identified by Gram stain and culture of the surgically removed emboli. Serology techniques are needed to diagnose endocarditis due to *Chlamydia psittaci, C. trachomatis,* or *Coxiella burnetti* and may be helpful for *Brucella* endocarditis. Bacteriuria with either enterococci or *S. aureus* occurs in endocarditis due to the respective organism. Several *in vitro* tests must be done on the pathogen isolated from blood to assess susceptibility to potential bactericidal drugs (Table 278–6).

CARDIAC IMAGING PROCEDURES. Echocardiography has become second only to culture of blood for investigating patients who clinically are suspected to have endocarditis. Echocardiography can visualize valvular vegetations, satellite vegetations, flail valves, ruptured chordae, perivalvular abscesses, fistulas, valvular perforations, and mycotic aneurysms. Echocardiography can also identify predisposing cardiac lesions. Two-dimensional transthoracic echocardiography (TTE) and transesophageal echocardiography (TEE), the two currently performed types of echocardiography, are safe and portable to the bedside. TTE is rapid, noninvasive, and relatively inexpensive (see Ch. 33.3).

OTHER INVESTIGATIVE PROCEDURES. Although other studies may be suggestive, angiography is required for the definitive antemortem diagnosis of a mycotic aneurysm. Cardiac catheterization can provide important information and should not be avoided when indicated in selected patients with endocarditis for fear of dislodging emboli. Coronary angiography is used to assess the presence of significant coronary artery disease before elective placement of prosthetic cardiac valves in patients who are over age 40 and have additional atherogenic risk factors. Computed tomography is used to define the cause of focal neurologic findings and identify metastatic suppurative infection or embolic events that can impede clinical or bacteriologic therapeutic response.

DIAGNOSTIC STRATEGIES IN SPECIAL SITUATIONS. *IVDU* (see Ch. 12). Since outpatient follow-up in this population is rarely possible, admitting febrile IVDU's without a clinically apparent source for their fever is indicated for at least 1 week until results of blood culture are available. Blood cultures become positive within 1 week in most patients if fungi, fastidious gram-negative bacilli or streptococci, or anaerobes are involved or the patient has recently taken antibiotics. After obtaining blood cultures, empiric antimicrobial therapy should be initiated. Once the blood cultures are found to be positive, evidence of endocarditis should be sought initially by TTE, and if the TTE is negative, by TEE. If echocardiography reveals vegetations, valvular destruction or its hemodynamic effects, valve ring abscess or fistula, or predisposing valvular lesion and/or clinical evidence of left-sided or right-sided endocarditis (e.g., septic pleuropulmonary complications) exists, the diagnosis of endocarditis is made. Vegetations detected by TTE indicate a group of patients at greater risk of morbidity, i.e., prolonged fever or development of CHF. Evidence of CHF on echocardiogram defines a group of patients who may subsequently require valve replacement. Even if there is another potential source for the bacteremia and no echocardiographic or clinical evidence of endocarditis, but the organism isolated is likely to cause endocarditis, such as *S. aureus* or a streptococcus, the diagnosis of endocarditis should nevertheless be suspected. If there is no apparent source for the bacteremia, even if echocardiographic and clinical evidence is lacking, the patient should still be considered to possibly have endocarditis. With negative echocardiography, if the clinical course dictates and another diagnosis is still not apparent, the TEE should be repeated in about 1 week. If blood cultures remain negative after 1 week of incubation, the patient may be discharged from the hospital without echocardiography, unless there is clinical evidence of left-sided or right-sided endocarditis, in which case the diagnosis of endocarditis should nevertheless be suspected.

NOSOCOMIAL NATIVE VALVE ENDOCARDITIS. In patients with bacteremia related to intravascular devices, such as an arteriovenous fistula or graft for hemodialysis, indwelling central intravenous line, cardiac assist balloon pump, or pacemaker wire, the device should be removed, especially with *S. aureus* bacteremia or fungemia, or if an indwelling catheter is associated with a tunnel or exit site infection. In patients with clinical evidence of endocarditis, echocardiography should be done to confirm the diagnosis and to assess local complications. Catheter-associated coagulase-negative staphylococcal nosocomial bacteremia, which rarely eventuates in NVE, should not be investigated with echocardiography after antibiotics are begun unless a prosthetic cardiac valve is present. Indeed, catheter removal may not be necessary to cure coagulase-negative staphylococcal catheter-associated bacteremia. Catheter-associated nosocomial fungemia probably should be investigated with echocardiography after the catheter is removed and an-

TABLE 278–6. *IN VITRO* ASSAYS

Viridans streptococcus	Broth dilution test	Penicillin MIC
Enterococcus	Broth dilution test	Penicillin MIC
		Vancomycin MIC
	Growth in 500 μg/ml 1000 μg/ml	High-level resistance to: gentamicin streptomycin
	Nitrocephin	β-Lactamase production
Staphylococcus aureus, coagulase-negative staphylococcus	Nitrocephin	β-Lactamase production
	Oxacillin/methicillin sensitivity	MRSA/MRSE
	Broth dilution test	Vancomycin MIC Rifampin MIC TMP-SMX MIC
Other pathogens	Broth dilution tests	Antibiotic MIC/MBC
All pathogens	Serum bactericidal activity*	Bactericidal activity at peak
	Serum antibiotic level	Peak and trough gentamicin and vancomycin levels

*May be useful for nonstandard antimicrobial regimens or unusual pathogens.
MIC = Minimal inhibitory concentration; MBC = minimal bactericidal concentration; MRSA = methicillin-resistant *S. aureus;* MRSE = methicillin-resistant coagulase-negative staphylococci; TMP-SMX = trimethoprim-sulfamethoxazole.
From Levison ME: *In vitro* assays. In Kaye D (ed.): Infective Endocarditis. 2nd ed. New York, Raven Press, 1992, p 151.

tifungal chemotherapy begun, whether or not clinical evidence of endocarditis is present.

PROSTHETIC VALVE ENDOCARDITIS. The diagnosis of PVE is usually suspected because of fever and confirmed by the presence of multiple blood cultures positive for the same microorganism. In a recent study, 43% of patients with a prosthetic valve who developed fever and bacteremia had or developed PVE. Any organism in blood cultures in these patients must be taken seriously as potential causes of endocarditis. In those presenting with clinical evidence suggestive of PVE, empiric antibiotic therapy can be initiated after three or four sets of blood cultures are obtained. After antimicrobial therapy is started, blood cultures should be repeated to assess for clearance of bacteremia. In bacteremic patients with no evidence of endocarditis despite these studies, antimicrobial therapy has traditionally been recommended for 2 weeks, but new data suggest that even therapy continued beyond 2 weeks may not prevent PVE from occurring as a result of the initially transient bacteremia.

ANTIBIOTIC THERAPY

PRINCIPLES. Effective antimicrobial therapy of endocarditis optimally requires identification of the specific pathogen and assessment of its susceptibility to various antimicrobial agents. Therefore, every effort must be made to isolate the pathogen before initiating antimicrobial therapy, if clinically feasible. In those patients who are in immediate danger of death, empiric antibiotic therapy should be started as soon as possible after obtaining blood cultures. Empiric therapy should be targeted at the most likely pathogens in that particular clinical setting (see Table 278–4). The minimal requirements for an effective antimicrobial regimen include the following:

1. Bactericidal Activity. Bacteriostatic agents are not able to clear the pathogen from infected tissues unaided by host defenses, such as polymorphonuclear leukocytes, antibody, and complement. Because host defenses are thought not to operate within vegetations (except in tricuspid valve vegetations, in which polymorphonuclear leukocytes may aid the effect of an antimicrobial agent) clearing bacteria from these vegetations requires bactericidal action from the antibiotics. In fact, complete eradication of pathogens from the vegetation is thought to be essential to cure endocarditis. If any bacteria remain after completion of antibiotic therapy, the residual organisms regrow and result in relapse. If the pathogen cannot be eliminated completely by antimicrobial therapy, e.g., if relapse occurs or the patient has persistent bacteremia, the infected vegetation may need to be excised surgically for cure. Table 278–7 shows the various antimicrobial agents that have bactericidal activity. For microorganisms without predictable susceptibility, bactericidal activity of an antimicrobial agent for the particular patient's pathogen must be assessed by determination of the minimal inhibitory (MIC) and minimal bactericidal concentrations (MBC) of the antimicrobial agents *in vitro* (see Table 278–6).

The enterococcus illustrates the problems in selecting appropriate bactericidal therapy for endocarditis. Enterococci are relatively resistant to penicillin. In contrast to viridans streptococci, which are inhibited by 0.1 μg per milliliter of penicillin G, most *E. faecalis* require up to 6.3 μg per milliliter to be inhibited. Unlike viridans streptococci that are killed by relatively low concentrations of penicillin, penicillin G alone, even at concentrations of up to 1000 μg

TABLE 278–7. BACTERICIDAL AGENTS

β-lactams	Penams (e.g., penicillin, ampicillin, amoxicillin, nafcillin, ticarcillin)
	Penems (none as yet marketed)
	Carbapenem (imipenem)
	Cephems (cephalosporins, cefoxitin)
	Carbacephems (loracarbef)
	Monobactam (aztreonam)
Aminoglycosides	E.g., gentamicin, tobramycin, amikacin
Quinolones	E.g., ciprofloxacin, ofloxacin, norfloxacin, enoxacin
Glycopeptides	Vancomycin, teicoplanin
Other	Trimethoprim-sulfamethoxazole
	Metronidazole
	Rifampin

Adapted from Levison ME: *In vitro* assays. *In* Kaye D (ed.): Infective Endocarditis. 2nd ed. New York, Raven Press, 1992, p 151.

per milliliter, is only inhibitory or at best slightly bactericidal against enterococci. The aminoglycosides are also poorly effective at low concentrations ($<$ 500 to 1000 μg per milliliter) owing to inadequate permeability. Antibiotic synergism does occur, however, as the result of enhanced intracellular uptake of the aminoglycoside in the presence of a β-lactam (such as penicillin, ampicillin, or piperacillin) or a glycopeptide (such as vancomycin or teicoplanin), the so-called cell wall–active antibiotics. The definition of synergism requires that the reduction in bacterial count at 24 hours with the drug combination be at least 100-fold greater than that with the cell wall–active antibiotic alone. Synergism is predicted on routine screening of strains by inhibition of growth with 500 μg per milliliter of gentamicin or 1000 μg per milliliter of streptomycin (see Table 278–6). No bactericidal therapy exists for strains that exhibit high-level resistance to both gentamicin and streptomycin or strains that exhibit high-level resistance to both β-lactam and glycopeptide antibiotics.

2. High Concentrations of the Antimicrobial Agent in the Vegetation. Doses of the antimicrobial agent must achieve blood concentrations of the antimicrobial agent high enough to facilitate passive diffusion of the antimicrobial agent into the depths of the vegetation where the microcolonies of the pathogen are located. Dosing sufficiently large to attain bactericidal activity in a $\geq$ 1:8 dilution of the patient's serum against the patient's pathogen at the peak time after administrating the antimicrobial agent has traditionally guided therapy (although more recent data suggest that dilutions of $\geq$ 1:64 have more predictive accuracy for bacteriologic cure).

3. Prolonged Duration of Antimicrobial Therapy. Over 90% of the microbial population in the vegetation is nongrowing and metabolically inactive once the infection has become well established. Nongrowing organisms are more likely to be found in the central portions of the microcolonies in the deeper regions of the vegetation. As a result, microorganisms in vegetations for the most part are not susceptible to commonly used antibiotics that are effective only against actively growing bacteria, such as the β-lactams and aminoglycosides. Optimally the antimicrobial agent should be active against nongrowing microorganisms. However, when the drug is active only against growing microorganisms, each dose of the bactericidal drug is able to effect a reduction in the microbial count only in that minor portion ($<$ 10%) of the population that happens to be growing at the time of drug administration. The duration of drug therapy therefore must be prolonged in order to completely clear the pathogen from the vegetation.

Duration of therapy varies with the specific pathogen, the site of the infection, and the type of antibiotic. For example, bacterial clearance is more rapid for viridans streptococci than for staphylococci, in tricuspid than in aortic vegetations, with antistaphylococcal β-lactams than with vancomycin, or with combinations of cell wall–active agent plus aminoglycoside than with single drugs. More rapid clearance in these special circumstances may permit a shorter course of therapy to achieve cure.

4. Dosing Should Be Frequent Enough to Prevent Regrowth of Microorganisms Between Doses. The organisms that remain after a brief *in vitro* exposure to an aminoglycoside or a β-lactam antibiotic frequently exhibit a postexposure delay in further *in vitro* growth, the so-called postantibiotic effect. Unfortunately, no such effect occurs with some organisms, such as enterococci or *P. aeruginosa* in vegetations. Thus, even though a bactericidal effect can be achieved in the vegetation in the early portions of a dosing interval when levels of the drug are high, if antibiotic levels are not maintained in the vegetation at least above the MIC during the rest of the dosing interval, the residual organisms may regrow and efficacy may be compromised.

Standardized regimens have been recommended for the most common pathogens—viridans streptococci, enterococci, and staphylococci on native and prosthetic valves (Table 278–8). Standardized regimens are not available for more unusual pathogens, including strains of *E. faecalis* that both produce β-lactamase and are highly aminoglycoside-resistant; strains of enterococci that exhibit high-level resistance to vancomycin, ampicillin, and aminoglycosides; and gram-negative bacilli, anaerobes, and diphtheroids. *In vitro* susceptibility testing should be performed for these organisms and the patient treated with the regimen that demonstrates the best bactericidal activity. Bactericidal activity for anaerobic gram-negative bacilli can frequently be achieved with metronidazole, for HACEK organisms with ceftriaxone, for aerobic enteric gram-negative bacilli or *P. aeruginosa* with a cell wall–active agent–aminoglycoside combination or ciprofloxacin, for diphtheroids with a vancomycin-aminoglycoside combination, and for methicillin-resistant coagulase-negative staphylococci causing PVE with vancomycin-aminoglycoside-rifampin combination.

SURGICAL THERAPY (see Ch. 41.3)

Prosthetic valve surgery is indicated in the following situations: (1) Increasing or refractory CHF secondary to valvular dysfunction. In those patients who are hemodynamically unstable, emergency cardiac valve replacement should not be delayed to allow further antibiotic therapy. Although operative mortality and PVE are higher in this situation than when a prosthetic valve is placed in the absence of active infection, the overall outcome is better if the prosthesis is replaced promptly, the patient's clinical condition permitting, despite active infection. If the patient is hemodynamically stable, prosthetic valve replacement is best delayed until a course of antimicrobial therapy is completed or has been given for at least 7 days. (2) Multiple clinically significant emboli, despite antibiotic therapy for 2 weeks. (3) Infection due to certain pathogens such as fungi, which rarely respond to medical therapy, high level ampicillin/aminoglycoside/vancomycin-resistant enterococci, β-lactamase producing/high-level aminoglycoside–resistant *E. faecalis,* and β-lactam or quinolone resistant gram-negative bacilli. Surgical indications for valve ring abscess, which may heal with antimicrobials alone, include extension of infection, development of prosthetic valve dehiscence, heart block, or CHF, and persistence of infection despite medical therapy. Patients with valve ring abscess should be monitored for conduction abnormalities, which may require placing a transvenous pacemaker because of the risk of high-grade heart block.

✔ TABLE 278–8. ANTIBIOTIC THERAPY (ADULT DOSES) FOR INFECTIVE ENDOCARDITIS

Regimen	Dose and Duration
Highly penicillin-susceptible streptococci (MIC ≤ 0.1 µg/ml)	
1. Aqueous penicillin G, 10–20 million U daily IV for 4 weeks	
2. Aqueous penicillin G, 10–20 million U daily IV	
plus	
Streptomycin, 7.5 mg/kg (maximum 500 mg) q12h IM[a]	
or	
Gentamicin, 1 mg/kg (maximum 80 mg) q8h IV/IM[b] for 2 weeks	
3. Aqueous penicillin G, 10–20 million U daily IV for 4 weeks	
plus	
Streptomycin, 7.5 mg/kg (maximum 500 mg) q12h IM[a]	
or	
Gentamicin, 1 mg/kg (maximum 80 mg) q8h IV/IM[b] for the first 2 weeks	
4. Ceftriaxone, 2 grams q24h IV for 4 weeks	
Highly penicillin-susceptible streptococci in penicillin-allergic patients	
1. Cefazolin,[c] 1 gram q8h IV/IM	
or	
Ceftriaxone, 2 grams q24h IV for 4 weeks	
or	
2. Vancomycin,[d] 30 mg/kg daily (maximum 2 grams/day unless serum levels are monitored) divided q6h or q12h IV for 4 weeks	
Streptococci relatively resistant to penicillin (MIC > 0.1 and < 0.5 µg/ml)	
Aqueous penicillin G, 20 million U daily IV for 4 weeks	
plus	
Streptomycin, 7.5 mg/kg (maximum 500 mg) q12h IM[a]	
or	
Gentamicin, 1 mg/kg (maximum 80 mg) q8h IV/IM[b] for the first 2 weeks	
Enterococci or other streptococci (MIC ≥ 0.5 µg/ml)	
Aqueous penicillin G, 20–30 million U daily IV, or ampicillin, 12 grams daily IV	
plus	
Gentamicin, 1 mg/kg (maximum 80 mg) q8h IV/IM[be]	
or	
Streptomycin, 7.5 mg/kg (maximum 500 mg) q12h IM[ae] for 4 to 6 weeks	
Enterococci or other streptococci in penicillin-allergic patients (MIC ≥ 0.5 µg/ml[f])	
Vancomycin,[g] 30 mg/kg daily (maximum 2 grams/day unless levels are monitored) divided q6h or q12h IV	
plus	
Gentamicin, 1 mg/kg (maximum 80 mg) q8h IV/IM[be]	
or	
Streptomycin, 7.5 mg/kg (maximum 500 mg) q12h IM[ae] for 4 to 6 weeks	

278 INFECTIVE ENDOCARDITIS / 1603

✔ TABLE 278–8. ANTIBIOTIC THERAPY (ADULT DOSES) FOR INFECTIVE ENDOCARDITIS *Continued*

Regimen	Dose and Duration
Methicillin-susceptible staphylococci	
Nafcillin, 2 grams q4h IV	
or	
Oxacillin, 2 grams q4h IV for 4 to 6 weeks	
with or without	
Gentamicin,[h] 1 mg/kg (maximum 80 mg) q8h IV/IM for first 3 to 5 days only	
Methicillin-susceptible staphylococci in penicillin-allergic patients	
Cefazolin, 2 grams q8h IV	
with or without	
Gentamicin,[h] 1 mg/kg (maximum 80 mg) q8h IV/IM for first 3 to 5 days only	
or	
Vancomycin,[d] 30 mg/kg daily (maximum 2 grams/day unless serum levels are monitored) divided q6h or q12h IV for 4 to 6 weeks	
Methicillin-resistant staphylococci	
Vancomycin,[g] 30 mg/kg daily (maximum 2 grams/day unless serum levels are monitored) divided q6h or q12h IV for 4 to 6 weeks	
Methicillin-resistant staphylococci in the presence of a prosthetic device	
Vancomycin,[g] 30 mg/kg daily (maximum 2 grams/day unless serum levels are monitored) divided q6h or q12h IV	
plus	
Rifampin,[i] 300 mg q8h PO for 6 weeks or longer	
plus	
Gentamicin, 1 mg/kg (maximum 80 mg) q8h IV/IM[b] for first 2 weeks	
Methicillin-susceptible staphylococci in the presence of a prosthetic device	
Nafcillin,[j] 2 grams q4h IV	
or	
Oxacillin, 2 grams q4h IV for 6 weeks or longer	
plus	
Gentamicin, 1 mg/kg (maximum 80 mg) q8h IV/IM[b] for the first 2 weeks	
with or without	
Rifampin,[k] 300 mg q8h PO for 6 weeks or longer	

[a]Peak serum levels should be approximately 20 µg/ml.
[b]Peak serum levels should be approximately 3 µg/ml.
[c]Streptomycin or gentamicin may be added for the first 2 weeks as in Regimen 3.
[d]Vancomycin is preferred if immediate-type hypersensitivity is suspected. The dose should be infused over 1 hour, and peak levels at 1 hour after the end of infusion should be approximately 30 to 45 µg/ml when given every 6 hours or 20 to 35 µg/ml when given every 12 hours.
[e]Choice of an aminoglycoside should be based on *in vitro* susceptibility testing. Enterococci should be tested for high-level resistance.
[f]Penicillin desensitization should be considered. Cephalosporins are not acceptable alternatives.
[g]Vancomycin should be infused over 1 hour, and peak levels at 1 hour after the end of infusion should be approximately 30 to 45 µg/ml when given every 12 hours or 20 to 35 µg/ml when given every 6 hours.
[h]The benefit of additional aminoglycoside has not been established.
[i]Rifampin should be added in cases of coagulase-negative staphylococci; its use for coagulase-positive staphylococci is controversial.
[j]Cefazolin or vancomycin should be used in penicillin-allergic patients. Vancomycin is preferred if there is immediate-type hypersensitivity.
[k]The use of rifampin for methicillin-susceptible staphylococci is controversial.
Adapted from Bisno AL, Dismukes WE, Durack DT, et al.: Antimicrobial treatment of infective endocarditis due to viridans streptococci, enterococci and staphylococci. JAMA 261:1471, 1989.

The surgical indications for PVE are the same as those outlined for NVE and include relapse after a course of appropriate antibiotic therapy. To avoid the complications of prosthetic valve replacement (e.g., PVE, bleeding, thromboembolic events, and valve deterioration), new surgical options, which have been proposed as an alternative to a prosthetic valve, include valve debridement, valvuloplasty, and repair or replacement of the paravalvular structure with pulmonary root autograft. Prosthetic valve replacement in an IVDU is problematic, because the prosthetic valve places the patient at continued risk of PVE. Alternatively for tricuspid valve endocarditis, tricuspid valve resection without prosthetic replacement can be tolerated hemodynamically for extended periods of time in many of these patients.

Intrathoracic, intra-abdominal, or peripheral mycotic aneurysms usually require surgical excision. Cerebral aneurysms may heal on medical therapy alone. If symptomatic, cerebral aneurysms should be followed closely with serial angiography and may require surgery if enlarging or bleeding.

Myocardial revascularization should be performed at the time of elective valve surgery if significant coronary artery disease is present. However, patients who require emergency placement of the

TABLE 278-9. REASONS FOR INADEQUATE CLINICAL RESPONSE

1. Inadequate therapy: wrong drug, wrong dose
2. Infarcts secondary to emboli
3. Metastatic abscesses of the spleen, kidney, brain, etc., that may require surgical drainage
4. Suppurative thrombophlebitis at site of an IV catheter, with or without superinfecting endocarditis
5. Other superinfections: e.g., *Clostridium difficile* colitis, urinary tract infection
6. Febrile reaction to the antimicrobial agent or another drug
7. Another unrelated febrile illness

TABLE 278-10. CURE RATES (ANTIMICROBIAL THERAPY + SURGERY) (%)

Native valve endocarditis	
Non-IVDU	
Viridans streptococci*	> 90
Vancomycin, ampicillin, aminoglycoside–susceptible enterococci*	75–90
*Staphylococcus aureus**	60–75
Fungi	40–50†
IVDU	
S. aureus, left-sided	50
S. aureus, right-sided	95
Prosthetic valve endocarditis	
Early onset	12–44
Late onset	47–70

*Deaths due to complications, not failure of antibiotic therapy.
†Antimicrobial therapy plus surgery.
IVDU = Intravenous drug user.

✔ TABLE 278-11. PROPHYLACTIC REGIMENS FOR BACTERIAL ENDOCARDITIS

*Genitourinary/gastrointestinal procedures**
Standard regimen

Ampicillin, gentamicin, and amoxicillin	IV or IM administration of ampicillin, 2.0 g, plus gentamicin, 1.5 mg/kg (not to exceed 80 mg), 30 min before procedure; followed by amoxicillin, 1.5 g, orally 6 hr after initial dose; alternatively, the parenteral regimen may be repeated once 8 hr after initial dose.

Ampicillin/amoxicillin/penicillin–allergic patients

Vancomycin and gentamicin	IV administration of vancomycin. 1.0 g, over 1 hr, plus IV or IM administration of gentamicin, 1.5 mg/kg (not to exceed 80 mg), 1 hr before procedure; may be repeated once 8 hr after initial dose.

Alternate low-risk patients

Amoxicillin	3.0 g orally 1 hr before procedure; then 1.5 g 6 hr after initial dose.

*Dental, oral, or upper respiratory tract procedures in patients who are at risk**
Standard regimen

Amoxicillin	3.0 g orally 1 hr before procedure; then 1.5 g 6 hr after initial dose

Amoxicillin/penicillin–allergic patients

Erythromycin	Erythromycin ethylsuccinate, 800 mg, or erythromycin stearate, 1.0 g, orally 2 hr before procedure, then half the dose 6 hr after initial dose
or	
Clindamycin	300 mg orally 1 hr before procedure and 150 mg 6 hr after initial dose

Patients unable to take oral medications

Ampicillin	IV or IM administration of ampicillin, 2.0 g, 30 min before procedure; then IV or IM administration of ampicillin, 1.0 g or oral administration of amoxicillin, 1.5 g, 6 hr after initial dose

Ampicillin/amoxicillin/penicillin–allergic patients unable to take oral medications

Clindamycin	IV administration of 300 mg 30 min before procedure and IV or oral administration of 150 mg 6 hr after initial dose

Patients considered high risk and not candidates for standard regimen†

Ampicillin, gentamicin, and amoxicillin	IV or IM administration of ampicillin, 2.0 g, plus gentamicin, 1.5 mg/kg (not to exceed 80 mg), 30 min before procedure; followed by amoxicillin, 1.5 g, orally 6 hr after initial dose; alternatively, the parenteral regimen may be repeated 8 hr after initial dose

Ampicillin/amoxicillin/penicillin–allergic patients considered high risk†

Vancomycin	IV administration of 1.0 g over 1 hr, starting 1 hr before procedure; no repeat dose necessary

*Initial pediatric doses are as follows: ampicillin or amoxicillin, 50 mg/kg; erythromycin ethylsuccinate or erythromycin stearate, 20 mg/kg; clindamycin, 10 mg/kg; gentamicin, 2.0 mg/kg; and vancomycin, 20 mg/kg. Follow-up doses should be one half the initial dose. *Total pediatric dose should not exceed total adult dose.* The following weight ranges may also be used for the initial pediatric dose of amoxicillin: < 15 kg, 750 mg; 15 to 30 kg, 1500 mg; and > 30 kg, 3000 mg (full adult dose). Follow-up amoxicillin dose is 25 mg/kg.

†Includes those with prosthetic heart valves and other high-risk patients.

Adapted from Dajani AS, Bisno AL, Chung KJ, et al.: Prevention of bacterial endocarditis. Recommendations by the American Heart Association. JAMA 264:2919, 1990.

prosthetic valve for hemodynamic decompensation secondary to acute endocarditis usually cannot tolerate the dye load necessary for coronary angiography and the additional bypass surgery.

Anticoagulant therapy, although it may impede further enlargement of a vegetation, is relatively contraindicated in endocarditis due to conversion of a unsuspected cerebral infarct into an intracerebral bleed.

SHORTER INPATIENT THERAPY

Shorter courses of antibiotic therapy, oral regimens, and parenteral antibiotic therapy administered at home have been investigated in selected patients to shorten the course of hospitalization. Having a focal infection that would require more than 2 weeks of antimicrobial therapy, PVE, and significant renal or eighth nerve impairment precludes use of short-course β-lactam–aminoglycoside combination therapy. Absorption of orally administered agents may be unreliable, and oral therapy is generally not recommended. Patients can be selected for parenteral therapy at home by their being at low risk for complications of endocarditis, the most frequent of which are CHF and emboli. In streptococcal endocarditis, heart failure, if not present on admission, rarely first develops during therapy. Emboli most often occur before or within the first few days of antimicrobial therapy. Before considering outpatient therapy, most patients should first be evaluated and stabilized in the hospital, although some patients may be managed entirely as outpatients. The standard regimens used to treat penicillin-sensitive streptococci require either continuous infusion of penicillin or frequent intravenous administration. A single daily dose of ceftriaxone is an attractive alternate to penicillin for antibiotic therapy at home. Because of its long half-life and good potency against these streptococci, serum levels of ceftriaxone remain well above the MIC and MBC for over 24 hours.

RESPONSE TO THERAPY

Once on appropriate antimicrobial therapy, most patients note a sense of well-being, less fatigue, and improved appetite, and their temperature usually falls to normal levels within 2 to 5 days. However, the erythrocyte sedimentation rate, anemia, and renal function may take weeks to months to improve. CIC and related serologic findings that include hypocomplementemia, mixed cryoglobulinemia, and rheumatoid factor also tend to resolve with effective antibiotic therapy. Blood cultures for streptococci and enterococci should become sterile after 1 to 2 days of appropriate therapy and for *S. aureus,* after 3 to 5 days; however, with vancomycin therapy, blood cultures for *S. aureus* may take 10 to 14 days to become sterile. Blood cultures are obtained daily until sterile. If no organism is isolated from blood, but there is a good clinical response to an empiric antimicrobial regimen, empiric therapy should be continued. If no organism is isolated and there is no clinical response to empiric therapy after 1 to 2 weeks, endocarditis due to a fastidious pathogen, e.g., fungi or anaerobes, or a diagnosis other than endocarditis should be considered. If the pathogen is initially isolated from blood and appropriate antimicrobial therapy started but fever persists or recurs, blood cultures should be repeated to assess persistent or relapsing infection, among other possibilities, which include most commonly pulmonary or systemic embolization (Table 278–9). For nonstandard regimens or unusual pathogens, peak serum bactericidal activity may be assayed against the patient's pathogen early in the course of therapy, and if inadequate the dose of the antibiotic is increased (although not at the cost of toxicity) and the serum retested. Measuring vancomycin or aminoglycoside serum levels may be helpful to ensure adequate but nontoxic antibiotic levels. Blood cultures are repeated 2 and 4 weeks after therapy has been completed, relapse being most common within 1 month. The relapse organism should be evaluated for the development of antibiotic resistance.

OUTCOMES (Table 278–10)

Factors that affect mortality include the infecting organism (the mortality of endocarditis due to fungi and aerobic enteric gram-negative bacilli > staphylococci > enterococci > streptococci), the site of infection (aortic > mitral and left-sided > tricuspid infection), NVE versus PVE (early onset PVE > late onset PVE > NVE), age (higher in the elderly and very young), gender (men > women), and the presence of certain complications, such as heart or renal failure, rupture of a mycotic aneurysm, cardiac arrhythmias and conduction abnormalities, and cerebral emboli. Heart failure remains the leading cause of death. However, with increasing use of prosthetic valve replacement for heart failure, the leading cause of death may shift to neurologic complications due to embolic episodes or mycotic aneurysms or uncontrolled infection due to antibiotic-resistant microorganisms. Following cure of one episode of endocarditis, patients remain at increased risk for reinfection.

PREVENTION

The effect of endocarditis prophylaxis with antimicrobial agents has been estimated to be modest; i.e., < 10% of all cases are preventable by prophylaxis. For example, only about one half of cases have recognizable predisposing cardiac lesions, most cases do not follow an invasive procedure, and only about two thirds of cases are due to microorganisms (viridans streptococci and enterococci) against which prophylactic regimens are directed. However, in those patients who are known to have a risky cardiac lesion (see Table 278–1) and are to undergo a procedure that is likely to induce bacteremia (see Table 278–3), with organisms having predictable susceptibility to antibiotics with minimal inconvenience, toxicity, and cost, the American Heart Association has made the recommendations shown in Table 278–11. Additional preventive measures are minimizing invasive procedures, avoiding intravascular catheters (a major predisposing event for PVE), aggressively treating focal infections, and maintaining good dental hygiene in patients at increased risk for endocarditis.

Durack DT: Prevention of infective endocarditis, N Engl J Med 332:38, 1995. *Discusses prevention as a complex issue involving diverse aspects of medicine, microbiology, dentistry, surgery, epidemiology, and decision analysis.*

Durack DT, Lukes AS, Bright DK, et al.: New criteria for diagnosis of infective endocarditis: Utilization of specific echocardiographic findings. Am J Med 96:200, 1994.

Kaye D (ed.): Infective Endocarditis. 2nd ed. New York, Raven Press, 1992. *This multiauthored text is a thorough, up-to-date review of every aspect of infective endocarditis, written by experts.*

Wilson WR, Steckelberg JM (eds.): Infective endocarditis. Infect Dis Clin North Am 7:1, 1993. *This issue highlights important new developments in pathogenesis, diagnosis, and treatment.*

279 STAPHYLOCOCCAL INFECTIONS
Gordon L. Archer

Staphylococcus aureus has been recognized as one of the most important and lethal human bacterial pathogens since the beginning of this century. Until the antibiotic era, >80% of patients growing *S. aureus* from their blood died; most of those dying had been healthy with no underlying disease. Though infections caused by coagulase-positive *S. aureus* were generally known to be potentially lethal, coagulase-negative staphylococci had been dismissed as avirulent skin commensals incapable of causing human disease. However, over the past 20 years, coagulase-negative staphylococcal infections have emerged as one of the major complications of medical progress. They are currently the pathogens most commonly isolated from infections of indwelling foreign devices and are the leading cause of hospital-acquired bacteremias in United States hospitals. This ascendancy of staphylococci as pre-eminent nosocomial pathogens also has been associated with a major increase in the proportion of these isolates that are resistant to multiple antimicrobial agents. If the trend continues, we may be forced to revisit the serious staphylococcal infections of the preantibiotic era that textbooks had long since relegated to medical history.

BACTERIOLOGY. The name staphylococcus means "bunch of grapes" and describes the clusters and clumps of gram-positive cocci seen on Gram stain of both infected material and organisms recovered from culture bottles and agar plates. Staphylococci produce catalase, breaking down hydrogen peroxide to H_2O and O_2; streptococci do not. This is the definitive test for separating the two

TABLE 279-1. STAPHYLOCOCCAL SPECIES FOUND ON HUMAN SKIN AND MUCOUS MEMBRANES

Coagulase-positive	Coagulase-negative	
S. aureus	S. epidermidis	S. cohnii
	S. saprophyticus	S. xylosus
	S. haemolyticus	S. auricularis
	S. warneri	S. similans
	S. capitis	S. schleiferi
	S. hominis	S. lugdanensis
	S. saccharolyticus	

genera of gram-positive cocci. Staphylococci are nonmotile and are facultative anaerobes. The latter characteristic predicts that these organisms should grow equally well in both aerobic and anaerobic media. The coagulase test identifies the exoenzyme produced by *S. aureus* that interacts with a prothrombin-like plasma factor, converting fibrinogen to fibrin and causing plasma to clot. This is the test that traditionally separates the pathogenic species, *S. aureus,* from the numerous nonpathogenic staphylococci, collectively referred to as "coagulase-negative staphylococci." However, in current practice, many clinical microbiology laboratories use rapid tests for identifying *S. aureus* that rely on the clumping of latex beads coated with plasma factors that interact with *S. aureus* cell-surface components rather than coagulase.

S. aureus comprises a homogeneous species, as determined by biochemical testing and nucleic acid analysis, while coagulase-negative staphylococci are sufficiently varied to be assigned to numerous species. Coagulase-negative staphylococci are found as normal skin flora on all mammals, and currently, 30 different and distinct species are recognized. Of these, 14 species are found colonizing the cornified squamous epithelium and mucous membranes of humans. Each species has a unique niche on the body, but *S. epidermidis* is the predominant species in terms of numbers and different colonization sites. Since many laboratories report specific species of coagulase-negative staphylococci to clinicians, a list of the most prevalent human pathogenic species is shown in Table 279-1. Because only 60 to 70% of coagulase-negative species identified from specimens processed by the clinical laboratory are *S. epidermidis,* it is clearly improper to refer to coagulase-negative staphylococci as "*S. epidermidis.*" However, since no specific pathogenic potential has been recognized for one coagulase-negative staphylococcus versus another, routine species identification of these organisms is useful only for purposes of epidemiology.

EPIDEMIOLOGY. *S. aureus* is carried asymptomatically on the mucous membranes in the anterior nares, nasopharynx, vagina, and/or rectum in 20 to 40% of normal, healthy adults without underlying diseases. Carriage can be transient, lasting hours to days; intermittent, lasting weeks to months; and recurring or chronic, persisting for months to years despite attempts at eradication. Intact cornified squamous epithelium will not support intermittent or chronic carriage of *S. aureus* for reasons that are not clear but may involve bacteriostatic skin lipids, absence of *S. aureus*-specific receptors, or interference by colonizing coagulase-negative staphylococci. However, transient hand carriage clearly occurs and is an important means of exchange between patients and hospital personnel. Certain conditions have been described, however, that markedly increase skin carriage as well as nasal carriage of *S. aureus.* These include a variety of acute and chronic skin conditions, most prominently burn injuries, atopic dermatitis, eczema, psoriasis, and decubitus ulcers. In addition, needle use by insulin-dependent diabetics and intravenous drug abusers has been associated with increased *S. aureus* carriage; health care workers have been found to have a higher prevalence of nasal colonization that those individuals not involved with patients or hospitals; and patients on chronic hemodialysis have a higher-than-expected colonization rate.

S. aureus is extremely hardy and can survive drying, extremes of environmental temperature, wide ranges of pH, and high salt. It can therefore survive in the hospital on inanimate objects such as pillows, sheets, and blood pressure cuffs (called "fomites") for some time. However, the major reservoir of *S. aureus,* in both hospitals and nature, is humans (see Ch. 267).

In certain cases, *S. aureus* infections result when patients who are carriers infect themselves. This has been shown to be true for most hemodialysis shunt and peritoneal dialysis catheter infections, for infective endocarditis in intravenous drug abusers, and for both individuals and families who suffer from recurrent staphyloccal furunculosis. Eradicating nasal carriage in patients by using topical mupirocin ointment has been shown to reduce the incidence of shunt infections and recurrent furunculosis in hemodialysis patients.

Coagulase-negative staphylococci colonizing the skin and mucous membranes of hospitalized patients and some hospital personnel have been shown to be more resistant to antimicrobial agents than staphylococci found on the skin of outpatients or hospital personnel not working on inpatient units. The alteration in skin flora is associated with antimicrobial use that selects more resistant organisms on patient skin. This comprises a huge hospital reservoir for multiple-antibiotic-resistant coagulase-negative staphylococci that can be transferred among patients, can be acquired by hospital personnel, and may eventually be inoculated into wounds in association with implanted, indwelling foreign devices.

IMMUNITY AND PATHOGENESIS OF INFECTIONS. *S. aureus* causes disease syndromes by two different mechanisms. The organism can become locally or systemically invasive by producing molecules that thwart host defense mechanisms, or it can elaborate toxins that cause disease without the need for the organism itself to invade tissue (toxinoses).

Local Infection. The hallmark of the localized staphylococcal infection is an abscess—a walled-off lesion consisting of central necrosis and liquefaction and containing cellular debris and multiplying bacteria surrounded by a layer of fibrin and intact phagocytic cells. The abscess may be superficial, in skin (furuncle), or deep, in organs (renal carbuncle), as a result of bacteremic dissemination. The factors that result in initial *S. aureus* infections are not clear; normal individuals seem to be fairly resistant to local infection. Intact cornified squamous epithelium is normally a barrier both to colonization and infection by *S. aureus,* and even injecting virulent organisms into the skin will cause infection only if a foreign body (e.g., suture) is also present. Furthermore, most adult serum contains both heat-labile and heat-stable opsonins (complement and specific antibody) that are highly efficient at mediating the phagocytosis and killing *S. aureus* by neutrophils. Since humoral immunity and opsonophagocytosis are the body's major defense against pyogenic microorganisms such as *S. aureus,* most individuals are well equipped to resist infection. The role of neutrophils and opsonophagocytosis as the primary antistaphylococcal host defense is illustrated by patients with neutrophil defects (see Ch. 139.1 and 266) who have an increase in *S. aureus* infection. These include defects in intracellular killing (chronic granulomatous disease and Chédiak-Higashi syndrome) and impaired neutrophil chemotaxis and humoral immunity (Job's syndrome). Once the balance is tipped in favor of the organism, *S. aureus* possesses a number of factors that may produce an abscess and promote its survival inside the lesion. While no single factor has been shown to be the major abscess-forming virulence factor and mutants deficient in each of the factors have been recovered from full-blown infections, there is a general feeling that, since most of these factors differentiate the pathogenic *(S. aureus)* from nonpathogenic (coagulase-negative staphylococci) members of the genus, they probably play some coordinate role in initiating and maintaining of infection. Table 279-2 outlines *S. aureus* factors that may contribute to the establishment of local infections.

Disseminated Infection. A small percentage of local infections progress to dissemination, where *S. aureus* gains access to the blood. Dissemination is characterized by *bacteremia* and *metastatic infection.* The factors leading to dissemination and the type and appearance of local infections that are more likely to disseminate are not known.

S. aureus produces such enzymes as *staphylokinase* (a fibrinolysin), *hyaluronidase,* and various *proteases* that may enable it to escape the abscess, invade tissue, and eventually enter the blood. Once in the blood, the most lethal immediate consequence is *sepsis* or *septic shock* (see Ch. 70). This syndrome is mediated chiefly by *enterotoxins* and *toxic shock syndrome toxin* (TSST-1), all of which contain similar motifs (superantigens) that enable them to bind to T cells and macrophages, stimulating the production of such sepsis-associated cytokines such as interleukin-1, tumor necrosis factor, and interleukin-6. Approximately 60% of *S. aureus* isolates contain a gene for one of the five serotypes of enterotoxin (A to E) or TSST-1.

TABLE 279–2. S. AUREUS FACTORS THAT MAY PROMOTE LOCAL INFECTIONS BY THWARTING HOST DEFENSE

Factor	Proposed Mechanisms for Interfering with Host Defense
Coagulase	Prevents neutrophil access to infection site
Microcapsule	Inhibits phagocytosis
Protein A	Inhibits IgG-mediated opsonization (binds Fc fragment)
Clumping factor (fibrinogen receptor)	Inhibits opsonization (fibrin coating)
Catalase	Interferes with intracellular killing
Proteases, nuclease, lipase, and cytolysins (alpha, beta, and delta)	Liquefaction necrosis and phagocyte dysfunction
Leucocidin and gamma toxin	Neutrophil cytolysis
Fatty acid metabolizing enzyme	Inactivates bactericidal lipids

One of the target cells for bacteremic *S. aureus* is the endothelial cell. Organisms adhere to and are internalized by endothelial cells, where, by releasing cytolysins, the bacteria can disrupt the endothelial cell layer and invade underlying tissue. *S. aureus* also can exist inside intact endothelial cells. The ability for the organisms to survive inside phagocytes and endothelial cells may explain their propensity to cause recurrent and refractory bacteremia despite seemingly appropriate therapy.

Toxinoses. *S. aureus* produces three toxins, or classes of toxin, that produce specific syndromes without the need for the organism itself to invade and disseminate. *Staphylococcal food poisoning* occurs when a preformed, heat-stable *enterotoxin* is ingested and interacts with parasympathetic ganglia in the stomach, producing vomiting. Five closely related toxin serotypes (A to E) can all produce the characteristic symptoms. *Staphylococcal scalded skin syndrome* results from the production of *exfoliative toxin* by *S. aureus* isolates that colonize or infect the skin of newborns. The characteristic exfoliation of the superficial stratum granulosum layer of the epidermidis is due to the action of the toxin on desmosomes that hold the cells of this skin layer together. There are two exfoliating serotypes, A and B. The variety of *toxic shock syndrome* associated with tampon use in young women is due to TSST-1 entering into the blood through the vagina, produced by *S. aureus* that colonize the mucosa.

DIAGNOSIS. The diagnosis of staphylococcal infections requires that the organism be seen on Gram stain of an infected specimen and be grown on artificial media, preferably in pure culture. Since coagulase-negative staphylococci are the most common contaminants of any culture obtained by crossing skin, it is important that multiple cultures grow the same organism. This is a major reason for drawing blood cultures in pairs from two different sites. While various tests for serum antibody to *S. aureus* antigens (e.g., teichoic acid antibody) have been evaluated for their ability to differentiate serious, deep-seated infection from trivial infections or self-limited bacteremia, none has proved to have a sensitivity or specificity sufficient to warrant its use as a basis for making clinical decisions.

CLINICAL MANIFESTATIONS: *S. AUREUS* INFECTIONS. Skin and Soft Tissue Infections. The most common *S. aureus* infections are *folliculitis* and the *furuncle*, or boil (Table 279–3). These infections involve a single hair follicle or a localized area of the epidermidis and dermis. While most *S. aureus* furuncles are without systemic symptoms, those on the face should be treated aggressively because of their potential to migrate directly to the brain via the venous circulation. Furuncles can coalesce and spread through deeper skin layers or extend down to and along a fascial plane causing a much more extensive and serious infection called a "carbuncle." Carbuncles are most common over the upper back and back of the neck, where they can form multiple draining sinuses; bacteremia results in approximately one-quarter of patients. A boil or furuncle also may be called a skin abscess if it becomes large but remains circumscribed, confined to one area, and fluctuant. A nonlocalized *S. aureus* skin infection is called "cellulitis" and may resemble the skin infections caused by *Streptococcus pyogenes,* the most common cause of cellulitis (see Ch. 276). *S. aureus* cellulitis also can lead to bacteremia, proving the staphylococcal etiology of

some of these infections. *S. aureus* cellulitis is particularly common in individuals with pre-existing chronic skin disease such as stasis dermatitis and diabetic, trophic, or decubitus ulcers. Adults also can develop a form of impetigo, called "bullous impetigo." The lesions are characterized by erythema with a crusty surface and small or large bullous lesions. The bullae are thought to be the result of the elaboration of exfoliative toxin and are the localized, adult equivalent of the scalded skin syndrome (Ritter's disease) seen in infants.

The most common nosocomial *S. aureus* skin and soft tissue infection is the *wound infection,* where surgical or catheter exit-site wounds are contaminated with *S. aureus* and become erythematous, draining purulent or serosanguineous fluid. *S. aureus* is the most common and most serious cause of hospital-acquired wound infections, leading to local, deep-wound infections and systemic, metastatic infections due to bacteremia.

Recurrent furunculosis can occur in members of families, usually due to persistent nasal or perineal carriage in family members with autoinoculation of skin due to scratching. The infections are commonly superficial and without systemic symptoms but are painful and annoying. Interruption is not possible until the carrier state is eradicated in all family members. While most individuals with recurrent furunculosis have normal immune systems, a syndrome called Job's syndrome (see Ch. 139.1) is recognized in individuals with recurrent *S. aureus* furunculosis. In addition to recurrent furunculosis, patients have high levels of serum IgE, neutrophil chemotactic defects, and a generalized disorder of immunoregulation. Adults with this syndrome usually not only describe a long history of recurrent skin infections since childhood but often also have had recurrent sinopulmonary infections as well.

Pleuropulmonary Infections. *S. aureus* is an uncommon cause of pneumonia in otherwise healthy, unhospitalized adults, accounting for <10% of community-acquired pneumonia. However, following influenza A infections, the incidence of *S. aureus* pneumonia markedly increases. Chest radiographs of patients with community-acquired *S. aureus* pneumonia may show abscesses and thin-walled cysts, resembling the pneumatocoeles seen in infants.

In contrast to community-acquired pneumonia, *S. aureus* is a prominent cause of nosocomial pneumonia, particularly in intubated patients on mechanical ventilation. Cultures obtained from intubated patients by techniques designed to minimize contamination of specimens by organisms colonizing the upper airway have found *S. aureus* in up to a third of patients. Pneumonia in ventilator-dependent patients is a particularly lethal event, with one-quarter to one-half of the patients dying as a direct result of their pulmonary infection. There seems to be nothing that distinguishes the radiographic appearance of nosocomial *S. aureus* pneumonia from that of pneumonia due to other nosocomial pathogens. *S. aureus* bacteremia due solely to nosocomial pneumonia also is uncommon.

Septic pulmonary emboli in patients with right-sided *S. aureus*

TABLE 279–3. INFECTIONS CAUSED BY S. AUREUS

Common or Usual Etiologic Pathogen	Less Common Etiologic Pathogen	Uncommon or Rare Etiologic Pathogen
Furuncle or skin abscess	Cellulitis	Community-acquired pneumonia
Bullous impetigo	Hospital-acquired pneumonia	Ascending urinary tract infection
Surgical wound infection	Brain abscess	Meningitis
Hospital-acquired bacteremia	Empyema	Enterocolitis
Acute or right-sided bacterial endocarditis		
Hematogenous osteomyelitis		
Septic arthritis		
Pyomyositis		
Renal carbuncle		
Scalded skin syndrome		
Toxic shock syndrome		
Food-borne gastroenteritis (short incubation)		
Botryomycosis		
Paraspinous or epidural abscess		

endocarditis (see below) also can present like a primary pneumonia. However, these patients will all have *S. aureus* bacteremia and usually have discrete lesions in multiple lobes, often accompanied by hemoptysis and chest pain.

S. aureus is cultured from the pleural space in up to 15% of adults with empyema, but it is found in pure culture in fewer than 10%. The incidence of *S. aureus* as a cause of empyema seems to have decreased overall in the past 20 years but is still a prominent etiologic pathogen in patients with nosocomial empyema.

Endocarditis (see also Ch. 278). There are two different and distinct populations who develop endocarditis caused by *S. aureus;* these are compared in Table 279–4. One group consists of older patients with underlying diseases who develop primarily left-sided endocarditis and have a high mortality rate (20 to 30%). Approximately half will develop heart failure, half will have central nervous system (CNS) manifestations, and 40 to 50% will have had either a skin infection or an intravenous catheter as the presumed portal of entry. Although it is important to realize that patients with left-sided *S. aureus* endocarditis can present acutely, with symptoms compatible with the sepsis syndrome, and that *S. aureus* can infect previously normal valves, the majority of patients will have had more subacute symptoms of fever, malaise, and fatigue for 1 to 2 weeks, and three quarters will have evidence by history or echocardiography of previously damaged or abnormal valves. An increasing proportion of patients in this category infect cardiac valves as a result of a hospital-acquired bacteremia (see below). Patients with nosocomial *S. aureus* endocarditis may be infected with methicillin-resistant staphylococci.

The second population developing *S. aureus* endocarditis consists of those who inject illicit drugs intravenously. These individuals are younger, healthier, usually have no known valvular heart disease, and infect the tricuspid valve in 80 to 90% of cases. The patient is the source of the infecting organism. The major presenting symptoms in these patients are those of septic pulmonary emboli. The chest film typically shows multiple nodular infiltrates in various lobes that often cavitate and occasionally form pneumatocoeles. Most of these patients have pure right-sided endocarditis and only rarely will have any peripheral left-sided manifestations. However, a murmur of tricuspid insufficiency is heard in less than half the cases. The mortality rate is extremely low for these patients, usually only 2 to 5%, but recurrence is relatively common, given the individuals' proclivity for continued drug abuse.

Bacteremia. *S. aureus* is second only to coagulase-negative staphylococci as a cause of hospital-acquired bacteremia. The usual source of nosocomial bacteremia is intravenous catheters. The consequences of nosocomial bacteremia are usually only fever and malaise, but they can include endocarditis, osteomyelitis, metastatic abscesses in various organs, and death from overwhelming sepsis. Treatment, therefore, is prolonged in order to eradicate the organism from tissues and organs. Bacteremia caused by *S. aureus* is usually high-grade, with the organism grown from all blood cul-

tures drawn over a period of time even if there is no endocarditis or infected foreign body present. Furthermore, bacteremia may persist for several days even with appropriate therapy and removal of an infected catheter. This is felt to be due to the organism's ability to survive host phagocytic defense and to be sequestered inside cells.

In contrast to nosocomial *S. aureus* bacteremia, the source of community-acquired bacteremia is often obscure. It may originate from a skin infection, intravenous injection of illicit drugs, or an infected focus in the heart or at a peripheral site. In all patients with community-acquired *S. aureus* bacteremia, a diligent search should be made for an infected source. If none is found, patients should be treated as if they have endocarditis.

Osteomyelitis (see also Ch. 283). *S. aureus* is the most common cause of acute hematogenous osteomyelitis. While most cases occur in children, adults are also at risk, particularly those who have had documented *S. aureus* bacteremia. Children develop osteomyelitis almost exclusively in long bones, while in adults from a third to a half of the cases of hematogenous osteomyelitis are in the lumbar or thoracic vertebrae. Vertebral osteomyelitis results when *S. aureus* initially seeds the intervertebral disc space and then spreads from the disc space to involve contiguous veretebrae. A paraspinous or epidural abscess frequently occurs as an extension of the initial intervertebral focus. Patients present with fever and back pain and may have neurologic symptoms from cord compression. Radiographs typically show narrowing of one or more intervertebral disc spaces with collapse of adjacent vertebrae. A magnetic resonance imaging scan is particularly helpful in defining the extent of vertebral osteomyelitis. Long bones may be involved following hematogenous dissemination of *S. aureus,* but osteomyelitis in these locations is more typically the result of contiguous spread from an infected decubitus, trophic ulcer, or traumatic wound. One of the most common causes of *S. aureus* osteomyelitis of the foot bones is infection of ulcers in diabetics with vascular disease. Occasionally, hardware used to repair long bone fractures will become infected with *S. aureus.* These infections are particularly refractory to therapy without removal of the foreign body.

Septic Arthritis (see also Ch. 239). *S. aureus* is a common cause of acute septic arthritis, although spontaneous *S. aureus* septic arthritis in otherwise normal joints is usually seen in children rather than adults. In adults, *S. aureus* septic arthritis typically occurs in joints that previously have been damaged by a chronic inflammatory arthritis or osteoarthritis; that have been violated by needle aspiration, injection, or surgery; or that contain a prosthetic device. Occasionally, an otherwise normal joint will be seeded by the hematogenous route or the joint space will be invaded from a contiguous focus of osteomyelitis. These infections need to be differentiated from such other causes of acute monarticular arthritis in adults as gout and gonococcal infection. In all cases of septic arthritis, arthrocentesis should be performed before beginning therapy so that a specific cultural diagnosis can be made. *S. aureus* pyarthrosis can be present with relatively little systemic toxicity in patients with chronic inflammatory arthritis taking large doses of anti-inflammatory medication; this may be particularly difficult to diagnose. One unique form of *S. aureus* septic arthritis is infection of the sternoclavicular joint usually seen in intravenous drug users or in patients who have had subclavian intravenous catheters.

Genitourinary Tract Infections. The only important *S. aureus* infections of the genitourinary tract are those which result from hematogenous dissemination. These include microabscesses, renal carbuncles, and perinephric abscesses. The presence of *S. aureus* in the urine, therefore, is either the result of contamination in individuals asymptomatically colonized in the vagina and/or rectum or an indication that the kidney has been infected during an episode of *S. aureus* bacteremia. The absence of cells in the urine should suggest contamination. However, if *S. aureus* is repeatedly cultured from urine or present in the urine together with pyuria or hematuria, the patient should be evaluated for bacteremia, for a deep focus that might have caused disseminated infection, and for an intrarenal or perinephric abscess. The presence of *S. aureus* in the urine should *never* be assumed to be secondary to an ascending urinary tract infection.

Central Nervous System Infections. While brain abscess and meningitis can be caused by *S. aureus,* they are relatively rare. Fewer than 10% of cases of meningitis and 20 to 30% of cases of brain abscess are caused by *S. aureus.* They are usually due to metastatic seeding as a result of bacteremia from an identified focus, to direct inoculation following trauma or a neurosurgical proce-

TABLE 279–4. *S. AUREUS* ENDOCARDITIS IN DIFFERENT PATIENT POPULATIONS

Patient and Disease Characteristics	Intravenous Drug Abusers	Nonintravenous Drug Abusers
Mean age (yr)	30	50
Underlying disease	No	Yes
Portal of *S. aureus* entry	Skin (IV injection)	Skin (infection or IV catheter)
Valves involved	Tricuspid	Mitral, aortic
Pre-existing valve abnormality	No	Yes
Presentation	Chest pain, fever hemoptysis	Fever, fatigue, malaise; sepsis (less common)
Peripheral manifestations	Septic pulmonary emboli	Skin manifestations; central nervous system abnormalities; metastatic infection in bone, kidney, and spleen
Heart failure	Rare	Common
Mortality	<5%	20–30%
Treatment duration	2–3 weeks	4–6 weeks

TABLE 279-5. DIFFERENTIATION OF DESQUAMATING SYNDROMES

	Staphylococcal Scalded Skin Syndrome	Toxic Epidermal Necrolysis
Etiology	*S. aureus* exfoliative toxin	Drug hypersensitivity
Pathology	Intraepidermal cleavage plane; no inflammatory cells	Involvement of entire epidermis; infiltration with inflammatory cells
Clinical appearance	Involvement of epidermis only; positive Nikolsky's sign	Involvement of skin, mucous membranes, and multiple organs; negative Nikolsky's sign
Outcome	Low mortality; heals without scarring	High mortality; often heals with scarring

TABLE 279-7. CHARACTERISTICS OF COAGULASE-NEGATIVE STAPHYLOCOCCAL INFECTIONS

1. Hospital-acquired
2. Caused by species *S. epidermidis* (70–80%)
3. Resistant to multiple antimicrobial agents (>80% methicillin resistant)
4. Involve indwelling foreign devices (catheters, prosthetic heart valves and joints, vascular grafts)
5. Exhibit a long latent period between device contamination and clinical presentation

dure, or to infection of an indwelling foreign body, such as a ventricular shunt. The prognosis of patients infected as a result of metastatic seeding is particularly poor, with a mortality rate of 30 to 50%. The one infection associated with the CNS that is uniquely caused by *S. aureus* is a paraspinous or epidural abscess, usually secondary to vertebral osteomyelitis.

Pyomyositis. Infection of the large skeletal muscles is due to *S. aureus* in >80% of cases. It is prevalent in tropical countries, giving it the name "tropical pyomyositis," but it is being increasingly described in temperate climates. Patients in tropical countries usually are adults who have no underlying disease and present with fever, pain, and swelling in the involved muscle, but there is often little evidence of local inflammation. Diagnosis is made by needle aspiration of pus. Because eosinophilia is common in patients in tropical countries who have pyomyositis, parasites are felt to have a role in the pathogenesis of this disease. Pyomyositis in temperate climates presents in much the same manner but more often is seen in children or in adults with underlying diseases, is associated with muscle trauma in more than half of patients, and more frequently involves more than one noncontiguous muscle group.

Toxinoses. *Staphylococcal scalded skin syndrome,* also known as Ritter's or Lyell's syndrome, is usually a disease of neonates and is due to the action of the exfoliative toxins, A and B. This syndrome results from *S. aureus* colonization or local infection, usually of the umbilical stump, and results in generalized desquamation of the superficial granulosum cell layer of the epidermis. The adult equivalent is bullous impetigo, associated with localized skin involvement, but adult cases of more generalized desquamation have been described. However, it is important to differentiate staphylococcal scalded skin syndrome from toxic epidermal necrolysis (TEN). Table 279-5 contrasts the two syndromes.

The *toxic shock syndrome* was initially described in young, menstruating women and was associated with tampon use in women vaginally colonized with *S. aureus* that produced TSST-1. However, the number of tampon-associated cases has decreased markedly in recent years. The majority of cases are now secondary to *S. aureus* infections of skin or other sites, and the etiologic toxin is often one of the enterotoxins rather than TSST-1. The criteria for the diagnosis of staphylococcal toxic shock syndrome are shown in Table 279-6. Staphylococcal toxic shock syndrome has a relatively low mortality and is a true toxinosis; bacteremia is rare.

Gastroenteritis or *staphylococcal food poisoning* is due to ingesting preformed staphylococcal enterotoxin. Enterotoxin-producing *S. aureus* are inoculated into food by a colonized food handler. If the food sits at room temperature before being cooked, the organism will multiply and produce toxin. Subsequent cooking will not inactivate the heat-stable toxin, and ingestion will produce symptoms predominantly of vomiting after a short (2 to 8 hours) incubation period.

Miscellaneous Infections. The older literature describes "botryomycosis," a chronic *S. aureus* infection of skin, lung, or bone that produces granules resembling those seen in actinomycosis, and "enterocolitis," a necrotizing infection of bowel in surgical patients associated with sheets of organisms seen on Gram stain of stool. These infections are rarely seen today.

CLINICAL MANIFESTATIONS: COAGULASE-NEGATIVE STAPHYLOCOCCAL INFECTIONS. The major infections caused by coagulase-negative staphylococci are hospital-acquired and involve indwelling foreign devices. Table 279-7 outlines the characteristics of these infections. In general, coagulase-negative staphylococci are of low virulence, rarely causing metastatic infections, even though they are the most common cause of hospital-acquired bacteremia. Bacteremia is usually the result of intravascular catheter infection. However, coagulase-negative staphylococci can be lethal when they infect prosthetic cardiac valves. They are the most common cause of prosthetic valve endocarditis, presenting in the first year after surgery, presumably inoculated into the area of the sewing ring during valve implantation. Valve dysfunction results from dehiscence or obstruction of the valve orifice, and most patients require surgery for cure. The exception to infections described in Table 279-7 are those caused by *S. saprophyticus*. This organism is second only to *Escherichia coli* as a cause of ascending urinary tract infections in young, sexually active female outpatients, implicated in 15 to 20% of cases in this population. In addition, low colony counts of this staphylococcal species have been recovered from urine obtained by suprapubic aspiration in some women with the anterior urethral syndrome or symptomatic abacteriuria.

THERAPY. Antimicrobial agents effective for treating *S. aureus* infections are listed in Table 279-8. Treatment of hospital-acquired infections is limited by resistance to many of these agents. Methicillin-resistant isolates are *cross-resistant* to *all* β-lactams (penicillins, cephalosporins, and imipenem) and are usually also resistant to at least three additional classes of antimicrobial agents (multiresistant). However, while only 20 to 30% of nosocomial *S. aureus* isolates are methicillin-resistant, >70% of nosocomial coagulase-

TABLE 279-6. DIAGNOSTIC CRITERIA FOR STAPHYLOCOCCAL TOXIC SHOCK SYNDROME

1. Fever (usually ≥38.9°C, or 102°F)
2. Rash (diffuse macular erythroderma, sunburn or scarlet fever–like)
3. Desquamation, 1 to 2 weeks after onset of illness, particularly of palms and soles
4. Hypotension (systolic blood pressure <90 mm Hg or orthostatic syncope)
5. Involvement of three or more of the following organ systems: gastrointestinal (nausea and vomiting), muscular (myalgias), mucous membrane (hyperemia), renal, hepatic, hematologic (↓ platelets), central nervous system, or pulmonary (ARDS)
6. *S. aureus* infection or mucosal colonization

TABLE 279-8. ANTIMICROBIAL AGENTS EFFECTIVE FOR TREATING *S. AUREUS* INFECTIONS

Agents	Resistance* Hospital-Acquired	Resistance* Community-Acquired
Penicillin G	>90	>90
Antistaphylococcal penicillins and cephalosporins	30	S
Erythromycin	40	10
Clindamycin	40	10
Sulfamethoxasole-trimethoprim	20	S
Tetracycline	20	10
Minocycline	S	S
Rifampin	S	S
Gentamicin	30	S
Quinolones	30	S
Vancomycin	S	S

* Numbers are percentage of isolates from patients with hospital-acquired or community-acquired infections resistant to each agent; S = >95% susceptible

negative staphylococci are methicillin-resistant and multiresistant. Thus, while the treatment of hospital-acquired *S. aureus* infections should be guided by susceptibility testing, infections caused by nosocomial coagulase-negative staphylococci are usually treated with vancomycin.

Treating staphylococcal infections usually consists of administering antimicrobial agents, surgical or catheter drainage of abscesses, and removal of foreign bodies. The duration of therapy is usually 1 to 2 weeks for localized, drained infections not associated with bacteremia or a foreign body. In general, infections can rarely be cured if the foreign material is left in place. Infections requiring more specialized therapeutic decisions are detailed below.

Bacteremia and Endocarditis. For *S. aureus,* all patients with community-acquired bacteremia who have evidence of a metastatic infection or who have no obvious source for bacteremia should be treated as if they have endocarditis. For intravenous drug abusers with right-sided endocarditis: 2 to 3 weeks of an antistaphylococcal penicillin (nafcillin or oxacillin) or vancomycin, plus gentamicin for the entire treatment period; for left-sided endocarditis: 4 to 6 weeks of an antistaphylococcal penicillin or vancomycin, with gentamicin for the first week. However, in patients with hospital-acquired *S. aureus* bacteremia from a removable focus (usually an intravascular catheter), the decision becomes more difficult. Those patients whose fever and bacteremia resolve within 3 days after removing the infected focus, those who have no complications or evidence of metastatic infection, and those who have no abnormality of cardiac valves can receive 2 weeks of therapy. All other patients with nosocomial bacteremia who do not meet all the exclusions should be treated as if they have endocarditis (see Ch. 278).

Osteomyelitis. Patients with *S. aureus* osteomyelitis require a minimum of 6 weeks of therapy, with the initial 2 to 4 weeks being parenteral. Therapy of osteomyelitis of long bones often will be unsuccessful if sequestra are left in place.

PREVENTION. Preventing hospital-acquired infections is accomplished by paying attention to tenets of infection control. These include handwashing and regloving between patients and strict adherence to aseptic technique when creating or caring for any kind of wound. Patients undergoing procedures that may result in wound or implanted device infections also should receive prophylactic antibiotics before and during the procedure. Patients with recurrent *S. aureus* infections of skin, catheters, or dialysis shunts should have their nares cultured, and if they are *S. aureus* carriers, they should be treated with topical mupirocin ointment. Chronic carriers resistant to topical *S. aureus* eradication may be given oral rifampin plus sulfamethoxazole-trimethoprim, a fluoroquinolone (ofloxacin or ciprofloxacin), or minocycline.

Chambers HF: Methicillin-resistant staphylococci. Clin Microbiol Rev 1:173, 1988. *A good overview of antibiotic resistance among staphylococci.*
Novick RP: Staphylococci. *In* Davis BD, Dulbecco R, Eisen HN, et al. (eds.): Microbiology. 4th ed. Philadelphia, JB Lippincott, 1990, pp 539–550. *An excellent summary of basic staphylococcal biology and pathogenic factors produced by* S. aureus.
Raad LI, Sabbagh MF: Optimal duration of therapy for catheter-related *Staphylococcus aureus* bacteremia: A study of 55 cases a review. Clin Infect Dis 14:75, 1992. *An excellent study and review of a difficult problem.*
Rupp ME, Archer GL: Coagulase-negative staphylococci: Pathogens of medical progress. Clin Infect Dis 19:231, 1994. *The most recent review of infections caused by coagulase-negative staphylococci.*

Bacterial Meningitis

280 BACTERIAL MENINGITIS
Morton N. Swartz

Meningitis is an inflammation of the arachnoid, the pia mater, and the intervening cerebrospinal fluid (CSF). The inflammatory process extends throughout the subarachnoid space about the brain and spinal cord and regularly involves the ventricles. Pyogenic meningitis, considered in this chapter, is usually an acute infection with bacteria that evoke a polymorphonuclear response in the CSF. One of its major forms, that caused by meningococci, is considered in Ch. 281; less acute forms of bacterial meningitis, characterized by a mononuclear cell response in the CSF, are discussed in Ch. 311 and 406.

ETIOLOGY AND INCIDENCE. In the 1970's and 1980's, 20,000 to 25,000 cases of bacterial meningitis occurred annually in the United States. If all cases are included regardless of the age of patients, data from the Centers for Disease Control and Prevention indicate that *Haemophilus influenzae* type b was the most frequent bacterial cause (45%), followed by *Streptococcus pneumoniae* (18%) and *Neisseria meningitidis* (14%). About 70% of all cases occurred in children under age 5. The relative frequencies with which the different bacterial species cause meningitis are age related (Table 280–1). In the newborn, group B streptococci and gram-negative bacilli (most frequently *Escherichia coli,* but also other enteric bacilli and *Pseudomonas*) are the principal causes. Beyond the first month of life and extending through childhood, *H. influenzae* and *N. meningitidis* have been the most frequent causes of bacterial meningitis. The pre-eminent position of *H. influenzae* as a cause of meningitis in infants and young children (and as the leading cause of bacterial meningitis overall) has changed dramatically since immunization with the *H. influenzae* type b conjugate vaccines was introduced in the late 1980's. Whereas the rate of *H. influenzae* meningitis in the United States had been about 40 per 100,000 children under age 5 in the mid-1980's, it had fallen to about 2 per 100,000 in this age group by 1993. Consequently, the relative frequencies of *S. pneumoniae* and *N. meningitidis* have increased among children. In adults, *S. pneumoniae, N. meningitidis,* and *Listeria monocytogenes* are responsible for most cases of community-acquired bacterial meningitis. Meningococcal meningitis is the only type that occurs in outbreaks; its relative frequency among the meningitides depends on whether statistics have been gathered in a hyperendemic area or during an epidemic period. In about 10% of patients with pyogenic meningitis, the bacterial cause cannot be defined. Simultaneous mixed meningitis is rare, occurring in the setting of neurosurgical procedures, penetrating head injury, erosion of the skull or vertebrae by adjacent neoplasm, or intraventricular rupture of a cerebral abscess; the isolation of anaerobes should strongly suggest the latter two of these.

Important changes have occurred in the frequencies of several types of bacterial meningitis over the past 25 years. Gram-negative bacillary meningitis has doubled in frequency in adults, reflecting more frequent and extensive neurosurgical procedures as well as other nosocomial factors. *L. monocytogenes* has increased eight- to tenfold as a cause of bacterial meningitis in urban general hospitals, reflecting the enlarging immunosuppressed population at particular

TABLE 280–1. BACTERIAL CAUSES OF MENINGITIS*

	Neonates (≤ 1 month) (%)	Children (1 month– 15 years) (%)	Adults† (> 15 years) (%)
S. pneumoniae	0–5	10–20	40–50
N. meningitidis	0–1	25–40	15–30
H. influenzae	5	40–60¶	2–4
Streptococci	40–50‡	2–4	5–10
Staphylococci	5	1–2	5–10
Listeria	5–10	1–2	5–10
Gram-negative bacilli	30–45§	1–2	5

* In the United States in the 1980's.
† These represent cases of community-acquired meningitis.
‡ Almost all isolates from neonatal meningitis are group B streptococci.
§ Of all cases of neonatal meningitis, *E. coli* accounts for about 40% and *Klebsiella-Enterobacter* for about 8%.
¶ Markedly lower in the 1990's.

risk. *Listeria* infections appear to be foodborne (dairy products, uncooked vegetables) and involve particularly organ transplant recipients, patients in hemodialysis units, other patients receiving corticosteroids and cytotoxic drugs, patients with liver disease, pregnant women, and neonates. Meningitis due to coagulase-negative staphylococci, essentially unheard of 30 years ago, now represents about 3% of cases in large urban hospitals. It occurs as a complication of neurosurgical procedures and may present a particular therapeutic problem due to methicillin resistance of many of the involved strains.

In large urban tertiary-care general hospitals, the distribution of bacterial etiologies of adult meningitis differs from that in smaller community hospitals, where community-acquired disease predominates. For example, at the Massachusetts General Hospital about 40% of cases of bacterial meningitis in adults are of nosocomial origin. In this category, the leading etiologies are gram-negative bacilli (primarily *E. coli* and *Klebsiella*), accounting for about 40% of nosocomial episodes, and various streptococci, *Staphylococcus aureus,* and coagulase-negative staphylococci, each responsible for 10% of nosocomial cases.

CLINICAL SETTINGS. The clinical setting in which meningitis develops may provide a clue to the specific bacterial cause. Meningococcal disease, including meningitis, may occur sporadically and in cyclic outbreaks. In the past, military recruits were particularly susceptible, but now meningococcal vaccine (polysaccharides of groups A, C, Y, and W135) is employed for protection. Large urban outbreaks can occur.

Certain predisposing factors are frequently associated with the development of *pneumococcal meningitis. Acute otitis media* ($\pm$*mastoiditis*) occurs in about 20% of adult patients. *Pneumonia* is present in about 15% of patients with pneumococcal meningitis, a much higher frequency than in meningitis caused by *H. influenzae* or *N. meningitidis. Acute pneumococcal sinusitis* is occasionally the initial focus from which infection spreads to the meninges. A significant head injury (recent or remote) has occurred in about 10% of patients with pneumococcal meningitis. CSF rhinorrhea (usually caused by a defect or fracture in the cribriform plate) is present in about 5% of patients with pneumococcal meningitis. Meningitis occurring in young children with sickle cell anemia is most likely to be caused by *S. pneumoniae*. A variety of defects in host defenses (primary or acquired immunoglobulin deficiencies, the asplenic state) may predispose to severe pneumococcal disease, particularly bacteremia and meningitis. Alcoholism is an underlying problem in 10 to 25% of adults with pneumococcal meningitis in urban hospitals.

S. aureus meningitis is seen most commonly as a complication of a neurosurgical procedure, following penetrating skull trauma, or occasionally secondary to staphylococcal bacteremia and endocarditis. Meningitis caused by *gram-negative bacilli* takes one of three forms: neonatal meningitis, meningitis following trauma or neurosurgery, or spontaneous meningitis in adults (e.g., bacteremic *Klebsiella* meningitis in a patient with diabetes mellitus). The most common causes of gram-negative bacillary meningitis in the adult are *E. coli* (about 30%) and *Klebsiella-Enterobacter* (about 40%). The most frequent causes of bacterial meningitis in patients with neoplastic disease are gram-negative bacilli (particularly *Pseudomonas aeruginosa* and *E. coli), L. monocytogenes, S. pneumoniae,* and *S. aureus.* Meningitis caused by *group A streptococci* is uncommon but occasionally occurs following acute otitis media.

The age-related incidence (children under 5 years) of *H. influenzae* type b meningitis has been so striking that the occurrence of this disease in an adult should raise the question of the presence of an underlying anatomic or immunologic defect, circumventing the usual barrier interposed by serum bactericidal mechanisms.

Neonatal Meningitis. The incidence of meningitis is higher in the first month of life than in any other single month. In the newborn, the group B *Streptococcus* can produce either an "early-onset" (occurring within 8 days of delivery and characterized by a fulminant illness with septicemia, severe respiratory distress, and sometimes meningitis) or a "late-onset" (occurring 10 days to 2 months after delivery and presenting a more insidious, slowly progressive illness which usually includes meningitis) infection. The second leading cause, *E. coli* strains containing K1 capsular antigen, is usually acquired by the neonates from their mothers, who carry the organism in their stool.

The clinical signs in neonatal meningitis suggest sepsis but not necessarily central nervous system (CNS) involvement: fever (in only 60%), jaundice, diarrhea, lethargy, poor feeding or vomiting, respiratory distress (including apnea), seizures, irritability, bulging fontanel (in only 30%), and nuchal rigidity (15%). Frequently, only by examining the CSF can the presence of meningitis be ruled in or out.

PATHOLOGY. The purulent exudate is distributed widely in the subarachnoid space, most abundant in the basal cisterns and about the cerebellum initially, but also extending into the sulci over the cerebrum. There is no direct invasion of cerebral tissue by the infecting organism or the inflammatory exudate, but the subjacent brain becomes congested and edematous. The effectiveness of the pial barrier accounts for the fact that cerebral abscess does not complicate bacterial meningitis. Indeed, when these two processes coexist, the sequence usually has been that of an initial abscess subsequently leaking its contents into the ventricular system, producing meningitis. There are two possible exceptions to the aforementioned generalization: (1) neonatal meningitis due to *Citrobacter,* in which the organisms appear to invade the brain after producing a necrotizing vasculitis of small penetrating blood vessels, and (2) *Listeria* rhombencephalitis, a very rare process in which brain stem infection can occur simultaneously with *Listeria* meningitis (or alone). Structures adjacent to the meninges may show a variety of pathologic changes secondary to bacterial meningitis. *Cortical thrombophlebitis* results from venous stasis and adjacent meningeal inflammation. Infarction of cerebral tissue may follow. *Involvement of cortical and pial arteries* with peripheral aneurysm formation and vascular occlusion occurs occasionally in bacterial meningitis. Rarely, narrowing of the supraclinoid portion of the internal carotid artery at the base of the brain occurs as a result of arteritis and arterial spasm. In fulminating cases (particularly meningococcal meningitis), *cerebral edema* may be marked even though the pleocytosis is only moderate. Rarely such patients develop temporal lobe and cerebellar herniation, resulting in compression of the midbrain and medulla. *Damage to cranial nerves* occurs in areas where dense exudate accumulates; the third and sixth cranial nerves are also vulnerable to damage by increased intracranial pressure. *Ventriculitis* probably occurs in most cases of bacterial meningitis; rarely this progresses to the accumulation of pus, *ventricular empyema. Hydrocephalus* can develop during meningitis from obstruction to CSF flow within the ventricular system (obstructive hydrocephalus) or extraventricularly (communicating hydrocephalus). *Subdural effusions* are sterile transudates that develop over the cerebral cortex in about 15% of infants with bacterial meningitis. Rarely such effusions become infected, producing a subdural empyema. In the past the diagnosis was made almost exclusively in infants, in whom abnormal transillumination or increasing head size can be detected. Now, sterile or infected (showing peripheral contrast enhancement) subdural collections can be demonstrated readily by computed tomographic scan as low-density areas about the cerebrum.

PATHOGENESIS. Bacteria may reach the meninges by several routes: (1) systemic bacteremia, (2) direct ingress from the upper respiratory tract or skin through an anatomic defect (e.g., skull fracture, eroding sequestrum, meningocele), (3) passage intracranially via venules in the nasopharynx, or (4) spread from a contiguous focus of infection (infection of the paranasal sinuses, leakage of a brain abscess). Bacteremic spread to the meninges is probably the most frequent path of infection. However, not all bacteremic organisms have the same likelihood of causing meningitis. Bacteremia with *H. influenzae* and *N. meningitidis* is usually initiated by pharyngeal adhesion and colonization by an infecting strain. Adhesion of such strains, as well as of *S. pneumoniae,* to mucosal surfaces is abetted by their capacity to produce IgA proteases (cleaving this antibody in the hinge region) and thus inactivating this local antibody defense. *N. meningitidis* adhesion to nasopharyngeal cells is effected by fimbriae or pili. In an *in vitro* nasopharyngeal organ culture these organisms injure ciliated epithelial cells and induce ciliostasis, selectively adhering to nonciliated epithelial cells. Meningococci invade the nasopharyngeal mucosal cells via endocytosis and are transported to the abluminal side in membrane-bound vacuoles. *H. influenzae,* in contrast, invades intercellularly by causing separation of apical tight junctions between columnar epithelial cells. When these meningeal pathogens gain access to the bloodstream, their intravascular survival is aided by the presence of polysaccharide capsules that inhibit phagocytosis and confer resistance to complement-mediated bactericidal activity.

Following entry into the bloodstream, CNS invasion occurs, but the mechanisms by which and sites at which this occurs are unclear. A high-grade and sustained bacteremia appears necessary. An important role for specific bacterial adhesion to elements of the blood-brain barrier is likely, as indicated by the preferential binding of fimbriated strains of *E. coli* to the endothelial cell surface of cerebral capillaries and the epithelial cell surface of the choroid plexus and ventricles. Evidence from animal models suggests that CNS invasion sites following bacteremia may develop at foci of nonspecific sterile inflammation above the cribriform plate and through the choroid plexus.

Most bacterial species causing meningitis (*H. influenzae* type b, *N. meningitidis*, *S. pneumoniae*, *E. coli* K1, group B *Streptococcus*) are antiphagocytic. Whether the capsular polysaccharide confers some special meningeal tropism, possibly through surface receptors, is not known. Although the primary focus initiating the bacteremia is usually in the upper respiratory tract or lung (pneumonia), it may be in the heart (endocarditis) or the gastrointestinal or urinary tracts. Once established in any part of the meninges, infection quickly extends throughout the subarachnoid space. Bacterial replication proceeds relatively unhindered, since CSF levels of complement are low early in meningeal inflammation, resulting in minimal opsonic and bactericidal activity (or none), and since surface phagocytosis of unopsonized organisms is meager in such a fluid environment. A secondary bacteremia may follow meningeal infection and itself contribute to continuing further inoculation of the CSF.

PATHOPHYSIOLOGY. Current experimental evidence suggests that meningeal inflammation follows bacterial entry and growth in the CSF and that specific bacterial components (e.g., pneumococcal cell walls or lipoteichoic acid, *H. influenzae* lipopolysaccharide [LPS]) are major elicitors of this response by causing release into the subarachnoid space of various pro-inflammatory cytokines such as interleukin-1 (IL-1) and tumor necrosis factor (TNF) from endothelial and meningeal cells. These cytokines increase adherence and transendothelial movement of neutrophils, as has been shown in endothelial cell monolayers in culture. Cytokines appear to enhance this passage of leukocytes by inducing several families of adhesion molecules that interact with corresponding receptors on leukocytes. The three likely families mediating endothelial-leukocyte adhesion are the (1) immunoglobulin superfamily, e.g., intercellular adhesion molecules (ICAM) 1 and 2; (2) integrins, e.g., CD11/CD18 subfamily; and (3) selectins, e.g., endothelial-leukocyte adhesion molecule (ELAM-1). Cytokines also can act to increase the binding affinity of a leukocyte selectin, leukocyte-adhesion molecule (LAM-1), for its endothelial cell receptor, contributing further to neutrophil trafficking into the subarachnoid space.

Once within the subarachnoid space, neutrophils are further activated to release products such as prostaglandins and toxic oxygen metabolites that increase local vascular permeability and may cause direct neurotoxicity. Evidence of breaching of the blood-brain barrier is found in animal models of meningitis where endothelial intercellular tight junctions are disrupted, where increased pinocytotic vesicles appear in endothelial cells, and where albumin escapes across postcapillary venules into the subarachnoid space.

The foregoing inflammatory changes can contribute to development of increased intracranial pressure and alterations in cerebral blood flow. Cerebral edema is commonly due to increased permeability of the blood-brain barrier (vasogenic), may be due to cellular

swelling in the brain as a result of toxic molecules released by bacteria and neutrophils (cytotoxic), and sometimes increased CSF pressure may result primarily from obstruction to CSF outflow due to inflammation at the level of the arachnoidal villi (interstitial). Whereas cerebral blood flow appears to be increased in the early stages of meningitis, subsequently it decreases, mirroring the severity of the disease. Localized regions of marked hypoperfusion (attributable to focal vascular inflammation or thrombosis) can occur in patients with normal blood flow. Impairment of autoregulation of cerebral blood flow may be a factor in cerebral edema or ischemia in some patients due to altered cerebral perfusion pressure.

CLINICAL MANIFESTATIONS. *History.* An acute onset of fever, generalized headache, vomiting, and stiff neck are common to many types of meningitis. The majority of patients with pyogenic meningitis of the three common causes have had an antecedent or accompanying upper respiratory tract infection or nonspecific febrile illness, acute otitis (or mastoiditis), or pneumonia. Myalgias (particularly in meningococcal disease), backache, and generalized weakness are common symptoms. The illness usually progresses rapidly, with development of confusion, obtundation, and loss of consciousness. Occasionally the onset may be less acute, with meningeal signs present for several days to a week.

General Physical Findings. Evidences of meningeal irritation (drowsiness and decreased mentation, stiff neck, Kernig's and Brudzinski's signs) are usually present. In certain patients, the findings of meningitis may be easily overlooked; infants, obtunded patients, or elderly patients with congestive failure or pneumonia may develop meningitis without prominent meningeal signs. Their lethargy should be investigated carefully, and meningeal signs should be sought; if any doubt exists, examination of the CSF is indicated.

The presence of a petechial, purpuric, or ecchymotic rash in a patient with meningeal findings almost always indicates meningococcal infection and requires prompt treatment because of the rapidity with which this infection can progress (see Ch. 281). Rarely, extensive petechial and purpuric lesions occur in meningitis caused by *S. pneumoniae* or *H. influenzae*. Very rarely skin lesions almost indistinguishable from those of meningococcal bacteremia occur in patients with acute *S. aureus* endocarditis who also have meningeal signs and a pleocytosis (secondary either to staphylococcal meningitis or to embolic cerebral infarction). Usually one or two of the lesions in such a patient are those of purulent purpura; aspiration of material reveals staphylococci on Gram stain. In the summer months, viral aseptic meningitis may produce meningeal signs, macular and petechial skin lesions, and a pleocytosis of several hundred cells, sometimes with neutrophils predominating initially.

Neurologic Findings and Complications. *Cranial nerve abnormalities,* involving principally the third, fourth, sixth, or seventh nerves, occur in 5 to 10% of adults with community-acquired meningitis. These usually disappear shortly after recovery. Persistent sensorineural hearing loss occurs in 10% of children with bacterial meningitis. In another 16% a transient conductive hearing loss develops. The most likely sites of involvement in persistent sensorineural deafness appear to be the inner ear (infection or toxic products possibly spreading from the subarachnoid space along the cochlear aqueduct) and the acoustic nerve. In children, permanent hearing impairment is more common following meningitis due to *S. pneumoniae* than to *H. influenzae* or *N. meningitidis*.

Seizures (focal or generalized) occur in 20 to 30% of patients and may result from readily reversible causes (high fever in infants; penicillin neurotoxicity when large doses are administered intravenously in the presence of renal failure) or, more commonly, from focal cerebral injury. Seizures can occur during the first few days or

TABLE 280–2. CENTRAL NERVOUS SYSTEM FINDINGS IN COMMUNITY-ACQUIRED BACTERIAL MENINGITIS IN ADULTS*

Time of Onset of Findings	Percentage of Episodes of Meningitis					
	Hemiparesis	Aphasia	Visual-Field Defect	Gaze Preference	Seizures	Other
Early (≤ 24 h)	9	6	2	10	15	5
Late (> 24 h)	2	1	0.3	0	8	1
Total†	11	7	2.3	10	23	6

* Based on data of Durand et al.
† Total percent of 279 episodes in which individual finding occurred (some episodes involved more than one finding).

can appear with associated focal neurologic deficits caused by vascular inflammation some days after the onset of the meningitis (Table 280–2). In adults with seizures accompanying meningitis, *S. pneumoniae* is more commonly the cause, but alcoholism is a confounding factor.

Brain swelling and increased CSF pressure are associated with seizures, third nerve dysfunction, abnormal reflexes, coma, hypertension, and bradycardia. In approximately one-quarter of fatal cases of community-acquired meningitis in adults, cerebral edema accompanied by temporal lobe herniation is observed at autopsy.

Papilledema is rare (1%) in bacterial meningitis even with high CSF pressures, probably because the patient is seen early in the process before changes have occurred in the nerve head. Its presence should indicate the possibility of some other associated or independent suppurative intracranial process (subdural empyema, brain abscess). Marked central hyperpnea sometimes occurs in patients with severe bacterial meningitis; CSF acidosis (principally caused by increased lactic acid levels) provides much of the respiratory stimulus.

Focal cerebral signs (principally hemiparesis, dysphasia, visual field defects, and gaze preference) occur in about 25% of adults with community-acquired bacterial meningitis (Table 280–2). They may develop during early meningitis secondary to occlusive vascular processes or some days later. Also, cerebral blood flow velocity may be decreased in the presence of increased intracranial pressure and lead to temporary or lasting neurologic dysfunction. It is important to distinguish lateralizing findings resulting from postictal changes (Todd's paralysis), which usually persist for no more than several hours.

Prompt treatment of bacterial meningitis usually results in rapid recovery of neurologic function. Persistent or late-onset obtundation and coma without focal findings suggests development of brain swelling, subdural effusion (in the infant), hydrocephalus, loculated ventriculitis, cortical thrombophlebitis, or sagittal sinus thrombosis. The last three are commonly associated with fever and continuing pleocytosis.

Residual neurologic damage remains in 10 to 20% of patients who recover from bacterial meningitis. Developmental delay and speech defects are each observed in about 5% of children. In infants surviving neonatal meningitis, significant sequelae are much more frequent (15 to 50%).

LABORATORY DIAGNOSIS. *Cerebrospinal Fluid Examination.* Initial CSF pressure is usually moderately elevated (200 to 300 mm H$_2$O in the adult). Striking elevations (> 450 mm H$_2$O) occur in occasional patients with acute brain swelling complicating meningitis in the absence of an associated mass lesion.

Gram-Stained Smear. By the time of hospitalization, most patients with pyogenic meningitis have large numbers (at least 10^5 per milliliter) of bacteria in the CSF. Careful examination of the Gram-stained smear of the spun sediment of CSF reveals the etiologic agent in 60 to 80% of cases. In most instances when gram-positive diplococci (or short-chaining cocci) are observed on stained CSF smear, they are pneumococci. In certain clinical settings it is important to distinguish this organism from the relatively penicillin-resistant *Enterococcus,* which would require adding an aminoglycoside to penicillin in treatment. This can be done by identifying pneumococcal polysaccharide in the CSF by latex particle agglutination (or by employing the quellung reaction). Rarely, three species may morphologically mimic *Neisseria* in the CSF or suggest a mixed infection with short gram-negative rods and meningococci: *Acinetobacter calcoaceticus, Moraxella* spp., and *Pasteurella multocida.* Culture of the CSF reveals the etiologic agent in 80 to 90% of patients with bacterial meningitis.

Special Immunologic and Serologic Procedures. In patients in whom the etiologic agent is not identified on Gram-stained smear of the CSF, rapid diagnosis may often be made by detection of specific bacterial antigens by latex agglutination (LA). This technique has been employed most extensively in the rapid diagnosis of meningitis caused by *H. influenzae* type b but also has been used in diagnosing meningococcal (groups A, B, C, and Y) and pneumococcal meningitis and meningitis due to group B streptococcus. Since *E. coli* K1 and *N. meningitidis* serogroup B share a common antigenic determinant, immunologic cross-reactivity may cause a false-positive reaction with the group B meningococcal reagent. Since the bacterial cause can be found on Gram-stained smear in most cases

of bacterial meningitis, the role of LA appears to be as an adjunct in rapid diagnosis when no organisms are observed or in providing a specific rather than a morphologic (Gram stain) diagnosis.

The limulus gelation assay for endotoxin is positive in the CSF of patients with meningitis caused by gram-negative but not by gram-positive bacteria.

Cell Count. The cell count in untreated meningitis usually ranges between 100 and 10,000 per cubic millimeter, with polymorphonuclear leukocytes predominating initially (≥ 80%) and lymphocytes appearing subsequently. Extremely high cell counts (> 50,000 per cubic millimeter) may occur rarely in primary bacterial meningitis but also should raise the possibility of intraventricular rupture of a cerebral abscess. Cell counts as low as 10 to 20 may be observed early in bacterial meningitis (particularly that caused by *N. meningitidis* and *H. influenzae*). Occasionally, in granulocytopenic patients or in the elderly with overwhelming pneumococcal meningitis, the CSF may contain very few leukocytes and yet may appear grossly turbid because of the presence of myriads of organisms. Meningitis caused by several bacterial species (*Mycobacterium tuberculosis, Borrelia burgdorferi, Treponema pallidum*) characteristically produces a lymphocytic pleocytosis. *L. monocytogenes* meningitis in infants may produce a primarily lymphocytic response in the CSF; in the adult there is usually a polymorphonuclear response, but rarely lymphocytes predominate.

Glucose. The CSF glucose is reduced to values of 40 mg per deciliter or below (or < 50% of the simultaneous blood level) in 50% of patients with bacterial meningitis; this finding can be very valuable in distinguishing bacterial meningitis from most viral meningitides or parameningeal infections. A normal CSF glucose does not exclude the diagnosis of bacterial meningitis. The simultaneous blood glucose level should be determined, because patients with diabetes mellitus (or those who are receiving intravenous glucose infusions) have an elevated level of glucose in the CSF, and its significance can be appreciated only on comparison with the simultaneous blood level. However, it may take 90 to 120 minutes for equilibration to occur after major shifts in the level of glucose in the circulation. The hypoglycorrhachia characteristic of pyogenic meningitis appears to be due to interference with normal carrier-facilitated diffusion of glucose and to increased utilization of glucose by host cells.

Protein. The level of protein in the CSF is usually elevated above 100 mg per deciliter, and the higher values are more commonly observed in pneumococcal meningitis. Extreme elevations, 1000 mg per deciliter or more, indicate subarachnoid block secondary to the meningitis.

Other Abnormalities in the CSF. Elevated levels of lactic acid occur in pyogenic meningitis. Although lactic dehydrogenase levels are higher in patients with bacterial meningitis than in those with viral infections of the CNS, these alterations are not of help in determining the specific etiologic agent involved. C-reactive protein is increased in about 95% of patients with bacterial meningitis and is not increased in most patients with viral meningitis. However, it does not seem to provide more information than the CSF cell count, is not helpful in diagnosing bacterial meningitis in newborns, and does not provide clues to the bacterial species involved.

Other Laboratory Tests. **Blood and Respiratory Tract Cultures.** Bacteremia is demonstrable in about 80% of patients with *H. influenzae* meningitis, 50% of those with pneumococcal meningitis, and 30 to 40% of those with meningococcal meningitis. Cultures of the upper respiratory tract are not helpful in establishing an etiologic diagnosis. Determining serum creatinine and electrolytes is important in view of the gravity of the illness, the occurrence of specific abnormalities secondary to the meningitis (syndrome of inappropriate secretion of antidiuretic hormone), and problems in therapy in the presence of renal dysfunction (seizures and hyperkalemia with high-dose penicillin therapy). In patients with extensive petechial and purpuric skin lesions, evaluation for coagulopathy is indicated.

Radiologic Studies. In view of the frequency with which pyogenic meningitis is associated with primary foci of infection in the chest, nasal sinuses, or mastoid, roentgenograms of these areas should be taken at the appropriate time after antimicrobial therapy begins when clinically indicated. Computed tomographic (CT) scans are not indicated in most patients with bacterial meningitis. If a mass lesion (cerebral abscess, subdural empyema) is suspected by history, clinical setting, or physical findings (papilledema, focal cerebral signs), then CT scans should be performed. *Bacterial meningitis is a medical emergency requiring immediate diagnosis and rapid institution of antimicrobial therapy.* Delay in performing a diagnostic lumbar puncture in order to obtain a CT scan should be avoided except on the basis of findings indicative of a parameningeal collection or other intracranial mass lesions, and in that case it would be reasonable to initiate antimicrobial therapy aimed at meningitis of unknown etiology or brain abscess before performing the CT scan. Changes may be observed on CT scan during meningitis itself: cerebral edema and enlargement of the subarachnoid spaces, contrast enhancement of the leptomeninges and the ependyma, or patchy areas of diminished density owing to associated cerebritis and necrosis. Patients with meningitis rarely have significant CT abnormalities in the absence of focal neurologic findings. In the patient with meningitis whose clinical status deteriorates or fails to improve, the CT scan may help demonstrate suspected complications: sterile subdural collections or empyema, ventricular enlargement secondary to communicating or obstructive hydrocephalus, prominent persisting basilar meningitis, extensive areas of cerebral infarction resulting from occlusion of major cerebral arteries, veins, or venous sinuses, or marked ventricular wall enhancement, suggesting ventriculitis or ventricular empyema. In about 10% of adults with bacterial meningitis, cranial CT scan findings (mastoid or sinus wall defect, eroding retrobulbar mass, pneumocephalus) are indicative of disruption of the dural barrier.

DIAGNOSIS. Diagnosis of bacterial meningitis is not difficult in a febrile patient with meningeal symptoms and signs developing in the setting of a predisposing illness. The diagnosis may be less obvious in the elderly, obtunded patient with pneumonia or the confused alcoholic patient in impending delirium tremens. Examination of the CSF should be carried out promptly whenever there is any question of meningitis.

Headache, fever, vomiting, stiff neck, and pleocytosis are features of meningeal inflammation and are common to many types of meningitis (e.g., bacterial, fungal, viral) and also to some parameningeal processes. The CSF findings are most helpful in distinguishing among these processes (see Ch. 421). In the patient with meningitis whose CSF does not reveal the etiologic agent on Gram-stained smear, particularly when the CSF glucose is normal and the polymorphonuclear pleocytosis is atypical, certain treatable processes which can mimic bacterial meningitis should be considered in differential diagnosis: (1) *Parameningeal infections.* The presence of infections (chronic ear or nasal accessory sinus infections, lung abscess) predisposing to brain abscess, epidural (cerebral or spinal) abscess, subdural empyema, or pyogenic venous sinus phlebitis should be sought. Neurologic findings may appear in the course of primary bacterial meningitis, but their presence should alert the physician to the need for close scrutiny for the presence of a space-occupying infectious process in the CNS. Neurologic symptoms or findings antedating the onset of meningeal symptoms should suggest the possibility of a parameningeal infection. The isolation of an anaerobic organism should suggest the possibility of intraventricular leakage of a cerebral abscess. (2) *Bacterial endocarditis.* Bacterial meningitis may occur during bacterial endocarditis caused by pyogenic organisms such as *S. aureus* and enterococci. In subacute bacterial endocarditis, sterile embolic infarctions of the brain may occur and produce meningeal signs and a pleocytosis containing several hundred cells, including polymorphonuclear leukocytes. A history of dental manipulation, fever, and anorexia antedating the meningitis should be sought; careful examination for heart murmurs and peripheral stigmata of endocarditis is indicated. (3) *"Chemical" meningitis.* The clinical and CSF findings (polymorphonuclear pleocytosis and even reduced glucose level) of bacterial meningitis may be produced by chemically induced inflammation. Acute meningitis following a diagnostic lumbar puncture or spinal anesthesia may be due to bacterial or chemical contamination of equipment or anesthetic agent. Chemical meningitis, characterized by a polymorphonuclear pleocytosis, hypoglycorrhachia, and a latent period of 3 to 24 hours, may occur following 1% of metrizamide myelograms. Endogenous chemical meningitis resulting from material from an epidermoid tumor or a craniopharyngioma leaking into the subarachnoid space can produce a

polymorphonuclear pleocytosis and hypoglycorrhachia. Birefringent material may be seen on polarizing microscopy of the CSF sediment.

Rarely, a patient develops meningitis characterized by subacute onset and persistent neutrophilic CSF pleocytosis lasting weeks or months without ready bacteriologic diagnosis. The etiologic agent in such cases of *chronic neutrophilic meningitis* has usually been either a fungus (*Aspergillus*, *Candida*, *Blastomyces*) or a bacterium such as *Nocardia* or *Actinomyces* species.

NON-NEUROLOGIC COMPLICATIONS. *Shock.* When shock occurs in pyogenic meningitis, it is usually a manifestation of an accompanying intense bacteremia, as in fulminant meningococcemia, rather than of the meningitis itself. Management is guided by the principles of septic shock therapy with appropriate modifications for myocardial failure (see Ch. 281).

Coagulation Disorders. Coagulopathies are frequently associated with the intense bacteremias (usually meningococcal, occasionally pneumococcal) and hypotension which can accompany meningitis. The changes may be mild, such as thrombocytopenia (with or without prolongation of prothrombin and partial thromboplastin times), or more marked, with clinical evidences of disseminated intravascular coagulation (see Ch. 281).

***Septic Complications.* Endocarditis.** Previously, 5 to 10% of patients with pneumococcal meningitis, particularly those with bacteremia and pneumonia as well, developed acute endocarditis, most commonly on the aortic valve. The incidence is currently much lower, as a result of earlier treatment of the initiating infection. In such patients, febrile relapse and a new murmur may appear shortly after completion of antimicrobial therapy for meningitis.

Pyogenic Arthritis. Septic arthritis may result from the bacteremia associated with meningitis caused by *S. pneumoniae*, *N. meningitidis*, or *H. influenzae*.

Prolonged Fever. With appropriate antimicrobial treatment of meningitis of the three most common bacterial causes, patients become afebrile within 2 to 5 days. Sometimes fever persists beyond this or recurs after an afebrile period. In the patient with persisting headache, obtundation, and cerebral findings, inadequate drug therapy or neurologic sequelae (cortical venous thrombophlebitis, ventriculitis, subdural collections) are important considerations. Reevaluation of the CSF, particularly Gram-stained smear and culture, is essential under these circumstances. Drug fever may be responsible in the patient who continues to show clinical improvement in all other respects. Metastatic infection (septic arthritis, purulent pericarditis, thoracic empyema, endocarditis) may be the cause of continuing or recurrent fever.

A syndrome consisting of fever, arthritis, and pericarditis 3 to 6 days after initiation of effective antimicrobial therapy of meningococcal meningitis occurs in about 10% of patients (see Ch. 281).

RECURRENT MENINGITIS. Repeated episodes of bacterial meningitis generally indicate a host defect, either in local anatomy or in antibacterial and immunologic defenses (e.g., recurrent *N. meningitidis* infections in patients with congenital or acquired deficiencies of complement, particularly late-acting components). Eleven percent of adults with pneumococcal meningitis have had more than one episode, whereas 0.5% of patients with meningitis caused by other organisms have had recurrent attacks. *S. pneumoniae* is the cause of one third of episodes of community-acquired recurrent meningitis; various streptococci, *H. influenzae*, and *N. meningitidis* are the causes of another one third of episodes. In contrast, in nosocomial recurrent meningitis, gram-negative bacilli and *S. aureus* are the causes of about 60% of episodes. A history of head trauma is much more frequent in patients with recurrent meningitis. Organisms may enter the subarachnoid space directly, through a defect in the cribriform plate (the most common site), in association with the empty sella syndrome, via a basilar skull fracture, through an erosive sequestrum of the mastoid, through congenital dermal defects along the craniospinal axis (usually evident before adult life), or as a consequence of penetrating cranial trauma or neurosurgical procedures. The anatomic defect may produce a frank CSF leak (rhinorrhea or, less commonly, otorrhea) or may entrap a vascular cuff of meninges which might subsequently serve as a direct route for organisms to reach the meninges. CSF rhinorrhea may be intermittent, and meningitis may occur months or years after head injury.

Any patient with bacterial meningitis, particularly if meningitis is recurrent, should be evaluated carefully for any congenital or post-traumatic defects. The presence of CSF rhinorrhea should be sought at admission and subsequently (rhinorrhea may clear during active meningitis only to recur when inflammation has resolved). Clinical clues suggesting the presence of a CSF fistula through the cribriform plate, pericranial air sinuses, or temporal bone include (1) salty taste in the throat, (2) positionally dependent rhinorrhea (rhinorrhea only in the lateral recumbent or prone position suggests an otic or sphenoid origin), (3) anosmia (cribriform plate leak), (4) hearing loss or full feeling in the ear, often with a finding of fluid or bubbles behind the tympanic membrane (leakage into the middle ear). Demonstration of glucose in nasal secretions with glucose oxidase "sticks" (Dextrostix) suggests the presence of CSF. Quantitative determination of glucose and chloride content of nasal secretions and detection by protein electrophoresis of transferrin bands unique to CSF can definitively establish the presence of CSF rhinorrhea.

Recurrent pneumococcal meningitis may occur without apparent predisposing circumstances, and cryptic CSF leaks should be sought actively in such patients by CT scanning of the frontal and mastoid regions and by radioisotope techniques. (Radioiodine-labeled albumin is introduced intrathecally, and pledgets of cotton placed in the nares are subsequently examined for the radionuclide. Radioisotopic cisternography has been used successfully.) Intrathecal introduction of fluorescein as a visual tracer (under ultraviolet light) can be employed similarly to detect active leaks. Surgical closure of CSF fistulas should be carried out to prevent further episodes of meningitis. Newer extracranial approaches via the ethmoid sinuses to repair cribriform plate or sphenoid sinus dural defects are successful and avoid the higher morbidity associated with craniotomy.

In most patients with CSF otorrhea and rhinorrhea following an acute head injury, the leak ceases in 1 or 2 weeks. *Persistent rhinorrhea for more than 4 to 6 weeks is an indication for surgical repair.* Prolonged administration of penicillin does not prevent pneumococcal meningitis and may encourage infection with more drug-resistant species.

Rarely, recurrent meningitis of nonbacterial etiology may mimic bacterial meningitis. *Mollaret's meningitis* consists of repeated febrile episodes of mild meningeal symptomatology, usually without neurologic abnormalities. Initially, large "endothelial" cells may be seen in the CSF along with polymorphonuclear leukocytes, which subsequently are replaced by lymphocytes. *Behçet's syndrome,* characterized by relapsing oral and genital ulcers and ocular lesions (hypopyon), may exhibit a variety of neurologic abnormalities, including recurrent meningitis.

PROGNOSIS. The introduction of antimicrobial agents has converted bacterial meningitis from a disease that was almost always fatal to one that the majority of patients survive without significant neurologic residua. The mortality rate for community-acquired bacterial meningitis varies with the etiologic agent and the clinical circumstances. With current antimicrobial therapy the mortality rate for *H. influenzae* meningitis is below 5% and that for meningococcal meningitis is about 10%. The highest mortality is with pneumococcal meningitis, in which the rate is about 25%. The mortality rate for gram-negative bacillary meningitis, commonly nosocomial in origin, in adults has been 20 to 30%, but it appears to be decreasing in the past 5 to 10 years. The mortality rate for recurrent community-acquired meningitis in adults (about 5%) is strikingly lower than the 25% rate for nonrecurrent episodes. Poor prognostic factors include advanced age, presence of other foci of infection, underlying diseases (leukemia, alcoholism), obtundation, seizures within the first 24 hours, and delay in instituting appropriate therapy.

TREATMENT. *Antimicrobial Agents.* Antimicrobial therapy should be begun promptly in this life-threatening emergency. Treatment should be aimed at the most likely causes based on clinical clues (age of the patient, presence of a purpuric rash, a recent neurosurgical procedure, CSF rhinorrhea). If the infecting organism is observed on examination of the Gram-stained smear of the CSF sediment, specific therapy is initiated. If the etiologic agent is not seen on smear (or not detected by LA), treatment for bacterial meningitis of unknown etiology should be carried out (see below).

With the exception of chloramphenicol, the commonly used antimicrobial agents do not readily penetrate the normal blood-brain barrier, but the passage of penicillin and other antimicrobials is enhanced in the presence of meningeal inflammation. Antimicrobial drugs should be administered intravenously throughout the treat-

ment period; reducing dosage as the patient improves should be avoided, because normalization of the blood-brain barrier during recovery reduces the CSF levels of drug that are achievable. Bactericidal drugs (penicillin, ampicillin, third-generation cephalosporins) are preferred whenever possible in the treatment of meningitis caused by susceptible bacteria. In animal models of bacterial meningitis, CSF levels of antibiotics at least 10 to 20 times the minimal bactericidal concentration appear to be needed for optimal therapy. Several antimicrobial drugs (first- or second-generation cephalosporins, clindamycin) do not provide effective levels in the CSF and should not be used.

Meningitis of Specific Bacterial Cause. The treatment of choice for pneumococcal meningitis in the adult has been penicillin (Table 280–3). For patients allergic to penicillin, chloramphenicol has been a reasonable alternative (see below). However, problems have developed because of the emergence of penicillin resistance in some pneumococcal isolates. Such resistance has arisen as a result of successive stepwise chromosomal mutations in genes for penicillin-binding proteins and is not due to β-lactamase production. Penicillin-resistant isolates are either relatively resistant (minimum inhibitory concentration [MIC] of 0.1 to 1.0 μg per milliliter) or highly resistant (MIC > 1.0 μg per milliliter). Penicillin-resistant pneumococcal strains have been found worldwide: 44% of isolates in parts of Spain, 45% in regions of South Africa, and almost 60% of isolates in Hungary. In the United States, currently almost 7% (range 0 to 32%) of pneumococcal isolates are penicillin-resistant, with higher percentages being noted in certain geographic areas such as Nashville, Tennessee, and parts of Texas and Kentucky. Cases of pneumococcal meningitis due to moderately and highly penicillin-resistant strains (some multiple antibiotic resistant) have now emerged in this country. Thus antimicrobial susceptibilities should be determined for all pneumococcal isolates from CSF, blood, or sterile body fluids (Table 280–3). Worrisome has been the recent appearance of cefotaxime resistance in pneumococcal isolates from children in South Africa and Texas. Since commercial MIC panels may not detect resistance to third-generation cephalosporins, it is necessary to determine the MIC to these drugs by means other than using such a panel. If the MIC for cefotaxime or ceftriaxone (< 1.0 μg per milliliter) indicates a highly susceptible isolate, cefotaxime or ceftriaxone would be the drug of choice. If the isolate is highly penicillin-resistant or is resistant to 1.0 μg per milliliter of ceftriaxone or cefotaxime, alternative therapy (vancomycin with or without rifampin intravenously) is indicated. If the patient has pneumococcal meningitis and comes from an area where highly resistant strains are known to occur, then initial therapy (pending susceptibility testing) with cefotaxime (or ceftriaxone) plus vancomycin intravenously is reasonable.

Although resistance to chloramphenicol is unusual among pneumococcal isolates from the United States, chloramphenicol has shown poor bactericidal activity against penicillin-resistant isolates from children with meningitis in South Africa. The relative chloramphenicol resistance of such strains may not be discerned on usual laboratory testing but is revealed when the minimum bactericidal concentration is determined. In areas where highly penicillin-resistant or chloramphenicol-resistant pneumococci are found, vancomycin replaces chloramphenicol in initial treatment of pneumococcal meningitis in the highly penicillin-allergic patient.

Penicillin G or ampicillin intravenously, in the dosage used to treat meningitis due to penicillin-susceptible pneumococci, is used to treat *N. meningitidis* meningitis. Recently, meningococci resistant to penicillin have been isolated occasionally in Spain, South Africa, Canada, and rarely the United States. Most of these isolates have been relatively resistant to penicillin (MIC 0.1 to 1.0 μg per milliliter), although a rare strain has had high-level resistance due to β-lactamase production. The latter-type strains require the use of third-generation cephalosporins, but "meningitis dosages" of penicillin or ampicillin may provide CSF levels that are sufficient for infections due to some strains of relatively penicillin-resistant *N. meningitidis.*

At present, 30 to 35% of isolates of *H. influenzae* type b in the United States are β-lactamase producers and ampicillin resistant; cefotaxime is the initial therapy of choice (see Table 280–3). Chloramphenicol combined with ampicillin is an acceptable alternative. If the isolate proves susceptible to ampicillin, the chloramphenicol

TABLE 280-3. THERAPY FOR MENINGITIS WITH KNOWN BACTERIAL CAUSE*

Therapy of Choice†	Penicillin Susceptibility	Alternative Therapy†
Pneumococcal Meningitis		
Penicillin, 24 million units qd in divided doses q2–4h *or* Ampicillin, 12 grams qd in divided doses q2–4h	MIC < 0.1 μg/ml	If penicillin allergic: chloramphenicol, 4–6 grams qd; cefotaxime or ceftriaxone; vancomycin
Cefotaxime, 2 grams q4–6h *or* Ceftriaxone, 2 grams q12h	MIC 0.1–1.0 μg/ml	Vancomycin
Vancomycin, 2–3 grams‡ qd in divided doses q8–12h ± rifampin	MIC > 1.0 μg/ml	
Haemophilus influenzae Meningitis		
For child: Cefotaxime, 180 mg/kg qd in divided doses q4–6h *or* Ceftriaxone, loading dose of 100 mg/kg followed by 50 mg/kg q12h (not to exceed 4 grams/d) *For adult:* Cefotaxime, 2 grams q4h		Chloramphenicol, 100 mg/kg qd *plus* Ampicillin, 300–400 mg/kg until β-lactamase status known Chloramphenicol, 4–6 grams qd *plus* Ampicillin, 12 grams qd until β-lactamase status known
Staphylococcus aureus Meningitis		
Methicillin-susceptible Nafcillin, 10–12 grams qd in divided doses q4h; in difficult cases may add rifampin, 600 mg qd IV or PO *Methicillin-resistant* Vancomycin, 2–3 grams‡ qd in divided doses q8–12h; in difficult cases may add rifampin, 600 mg qd IV or PO		If penicillin allergic: vancomycin, 2–3 grams qd in divided doses q8–12h
Listeria monocytogenes Meningitis		
Penicillin§, 24 million units qd in divided doses q2–4h *or* Ampicillin, 12 grams qd in divided doses q2–4h		If penicillin allergic: trimethoprim-sulfamethoxazole (20 mg/kg of trimethoprim component qd in divided doses q6–12h)
Meningitis Due to Susceptible Enterobacteriaceae		
Cefotaxime, 12 grams qd in divided doses q4h *or* (if susceptibilities not known) Ceftazidime, 6 grams qd in divided doses q8h and an aminoglycoside (e.g., gentamicin, 5 mg/kg qd in divided doses q8h) (if no response to initial therapy, consider adding intrathecal gentamicin, 3–5 mg dose q24h for first few days)		Aztreonam; trimethoprim-sulfamethoxazole; ciprofloxacin
Pseudomonas aeruginosa Meningitis		
Ceftazidime, 6–8 grams qd in divided doses q6–8h and an aminoglycoside (tobramicin or gentamicin); (if no response to initial therapy, consider adding intrathecal gentamicin)		Antipseudomonal penicillin (piperacillin or azlocillin) plus tobramicin (or gentamicin); ciprofloxacin; aztreonam

* All doses are intravenous for adults unless otherwise indicated.
† Dosages are for patients with normal renal function.
‡ Higher of the suggested vancomycin doses considered when serum levels inadequate on lower dose.
§ Addition of gentamicin may be considered.

may be discontinued. Although in areas of Spain > 50% of isolates are chloramphenicol resistant, < 1% have been resistant in the United States. Cefuroxime, a second-generation cephalosporin, has been used extensively in the past 8 years, but the third-generation cephalosporins are preferable because of reports indicating slower sterilization of CSF and a higher incidence of sensorineural hearing loss with cefuroxime.

Treatment for adult meningitis caused by methicillin-sensitive *S. aureus* is listed in Table 280-3. For the penicillin-allergic, vancomycin is the alternative of choice. Since penetration of vancomycin into the CSF is limited, adjunctive intrathecal (or intraventricular) therapy with vancomycin* (without preservative) has occasionally been resorted to when CSF cultures have remained positive after 48 hours of intravenous therapy alone and where CSF levels can be monitored. For adult meningitis due to methicillin-resistant *S. aureus,* intravenous vancomycin (with adjunctive intrathecal vancomycin as needed) is the treatment of choice. In refractory cases, adding another drug for systemic therapy (rifampin or gentamicin) may be warranted.

Cefotaxime (see Table 280-3) is used to treat meningitis known

to be due to susceptible gram-negative bacilli (*E. coli, Klebsiella, Proteus,* and so forth). It should not be used to treat meningitis due to less susceptible species such as *Pseudomonas aeruginosa* and *Acinetobacter.* Initial treatment (on the basis only of findings on Gram-stained smear of CSF) of adults with gram-negative bacillary meningitis is listed in Table 280-3. After identifying the specific pathogen and determining its drug susceptibilities, alterations in antimicrobial therapy may be indicated. If the organism is *P. aeruginosa,* use a third-generation cephalosporin with antipseudomonal activity (see Table 280-3).

Bacterial Meningitis of Unknown Etiology. Initial treatment of meningitis when the etiologic agent cannot be identified on Gram-stained smear of CSF is based on available clinical clues. *In the neonate,* a wide range of gram-positive (group B streptococci, *Listeria*) and gram-negative organisms (*E. coli, Klebsiella, H. influenzae*) may be the cause, indicating the intravenous use of combined therapy with drugs such as ampicillin with gentamicin (or amikacin), or ampicillin with cefotaxime (the combination favored by most pediatric infectious disease specialists), until results of cultures become available. *In children,* therapy is directed at the three most frequent pathogens: *H. influenzae, S. pneumoniae,* and *N. meningitidis.* The appearance of ampicillin resistance among strains of *H. influenzae* two decades ago necessitated the shift from single-drug therapy (ampicillin) to a two-drug approach (ampicillin-chloramphenicol) in the treatment of meningitis of unknown cause in

___
* Intrathecal use is not mentioned in the manufacturer's package insert approved by the U.S. Food and Drug Administration. Therefore, its use in these circumstances must be considered investigational.

this age group, pending results of culture. Now, ceftriaxone (same dosage as for *H. influenzae* meningitis) or cefotaxime is most commonly used in pediatric centers. *In adults*, therapy with ampicillin in combination with a third-generation cephalosporin (cefotaxime or ceftriaxone) is employed in view of the role of *L. monocytogenes* (susceptible to ampicillin but not to third-generation cephalosporins) in meningitis of older adults and in previously noted high-risk groups, the emergence of infections due to relatively penicillin-resistant pneumococci, and the increased frequency of aerobic gram-negative bacilli in nosocomial meningitis and meningitis in immunocompromised patients. In the penicillin-allergic individual, trimethoprim-sulfamethoxazole is a suitable alternative in the treatment of *Listeria* meningitis. In special settings (nosocomial meningitis or presence of endemic highly penicillin-resistant pneumococci) where more resistant species (resistant gram-negative bacilli, *S. aureus*, coagulase-negative staphylococci, or highly penicillin-resistant *S. pneumoniae*) are likely to be involved, broader initial therapy (addition of vancomycin) may be indicated.

Duration of Therapy. The frequency of CSF examinations depends on the clinical course, but a repeat examination should be done in 24 to 48 hours if there has not been satisfactory improvement. Routine "end-of-treatment" CSF examination is unnecessary in most patients with the common types of community-acquired bacterial meningitis. Meningococci are rapidly eliminated from the circulation and CSF with appropriate antimicrobial therapy, which should be continued for 5 to 7 days after the patient becomes afebrile. If the patient has responded well, a follow-up lumbar puncture is not necessary. *H. influenzae* meningitis should be treated for 10 days (at least for 7 days after the patient becomes afebrile). Follow-up CSF examination may be omitted in those patients who have responded with rapid clinical resolution of the meningitis. In pneumococcal meningitis, antimicrobial treatment should be continued for 10 to 14 days, and follow-up examination of the CSF should be done. More prolonged therapy is indicated with concomitant parameningeal infection. Treatment of gram-negative bacillary meningitis with parenteral antimicrobials is prolonged, usually for a minimum of 3 weeks (particularly in patients with a recent neurosurgical procedure) in order to prevent relapse. Repeated examinations of the CSF are necessary both during and at the conclusion of treatment to determine whether bacteriologic cure has been achieved.

Other Aspects of Treatment. Occasional patients with acute bacterial meningitis develop marked brain swelling (CSF pressure > 450 mm H$_2$O), which may lead to temporal lobe or cerebellar herniation following lumbar puncture. To decrease the possibility of this complication of increased pressure, only a small amount of CSF should be removed for analysis (the amount present in the manometer) and a 20% solution of mannitol (0.25 to 0.5 gram per kilogram) infused intravenously over 20 to 30 minutes, monitoring (if possible) the decline of CSF pressure to a lower level before the spinal needle is removed. Continued control of increased intracranial pressure, if needed thereafter, may be effected with mannitol, dexamethasone (10 mg intravenously, followed by 4 mg every 6 hours), or both. Brain swelling is about the only current indication for the use of corticosteroids in treating pyogenic meningitis in adults; they should be employed only when the appropriate antimicrobial drugs are administered. In the stuporous patient or one with respiratory insufficiency and markedly increased intracranial pressure, use of a ventilator to reduce the arterial PCO_2 to between 25 and 32 mm Hg is reasonable. Intravenous lidocaine can be used to block increased intracranial pressure associated with intubation, and subsequent transient increases associated with hyperactive airway reflexes can be mitigated by intratracheal instillation of lidocaine prior to vigorous suctioning. With continued elevations of intracranial pressure, a continuous intracranial monitoring device may be warranted.

Initial hypotension, if present, should be treated with fluid resuscitation in keeping with shock management principles. Over the next 24 to 48 hours, fluid limitation (1200 to 1500 ml daily in adults) to prevent brain swelling from the effects of inappropriate antidiuretic hormone secretion, sometimes associated with meningitis (particularly in children), is advisable.

Four prospective, controlled trials in children of the routine use of dexamethasone to reduce the pathophysiologic CNS conse-

quences of the inflammatory response during bacterial meningitis have been performed. Dexamethasone was administered intravenously (either 0.15 mg per kilogram every 6 hours for 4 days or 0.4 mg per kilogram every 12 hours for 2 days) either at the time of or 10 to 20 minutes before initiating antimicrobial therapy (third-generation cephalosporin). Corticosteroid use had no effect on mortality but did reduce the incidence of neurologic sequelae (primarily bilateral sensorineural hearing loss). Complicating gastrointestinal bleeding (usually occult) has been observed rarely but merits caution. On the basis of these studies, most pediatric infectious disease programs surveyed in 1992 used dexamethasone in bacterial meningitis of children over 2 months of age. Most of the children in the studies had *H. influenzae* meningitis, the most common type at the time, and the results reflect primarily the effects of dexamethasone on this form. Currently, *H. influenzae* meningitis has been sharply reduced in incidence by the use of protein-conjugate vaccines, but whether dexamethasone will have a similar effect in reducing neurologic sequelae of meningitis due to *S. pneumoniae* and *N. meningitidis* in children has not yet been established. As of this writing, use of adjunctive dexamethasone in cases of severe *H. influenzae* meningitis seems indicated, but whether adjunctive corticosteroid use will have a similar salutory effect in reducing the incidence of sensorineural hearing loss or neurologic sequelae in adults is not known and awaits results of a multicenter trial.

Patients with acute bacterial meningitis should receive constant nursing attention to ensure prompt recognition of seizures and to prevent aspiration. If seizures occur, they should be treated acutely with diazepam (Valium) administered slowly intravenously in a dose of 5 to 10 mg in the adult. Maintenance anticonvulsant therapy can be continued thereafter with intravenous phenytoin (Dilantin) until the medication can be administered orally. Sedation should be avoided because of the danger of respiratory depression and aspiration.

Surgical treatment of an accompanying pyogenic focus such as mastoiditis should be carried out when complete recovery from the meningitis has occurred, but under continuing antibiotic administration. Rarely, the mastoid infection (e.g., Bezold abscess) is so hyperacute that early drainage may be required after 48 hours or so of antibiotic therapy when the acute meningeal process has subsided somewhat.

Durand ML, Calderwood SB, Weber DJ, et al.: Acute bacterial meningitis in adults: A review of 493 episodes. N Engl J Med 328:21, 1993. *A detailed review of an extensive experience in adults between 1962 and 1988 in a large urban general hospital. Community-acquired, nosocomial, and recurrent forms of bacterial meningitis are categorized; the bacteriologic, clinical, CSF, and neurologic findings are well described.*

Feigin RD, McCracken GH Jr, Klein JO: Diagnosis and management of meningitis. Pediatr Infect Dis J 11:785, 1992. *A comprehensive review of bacterial meningitis in children (from neonate to adolescent). Epidemiology, bacteriology, pathogenesis and pathophysiology, neurologic features, CNS complications, and current treatment are emphasized.*

Odio CM, Faingezicht I, Paris M, et al.: The beneficial effects of early dexamethasone administration in infants and children with bacterial meningitis. N Engl J Med 324:1525, 1991. *This study showed that adjuvant dexamethasone treatment resulted at 12 hours in lowered CSF pressures and improved cerebral perfusion pressures and at follow-up, after 15 months, in decreased sensorineural hearing loss or neurologic sequelae.*

Pfister H-W, Feiden W, Einhaupl K-M: Spectrum of complications during bacterial meningitis in adults. Arch Neurol 50:575, 1993. *In this thorough prospective evaluation of 86 adults with bacterial meningitis, neurologic complications (cerebrovascular injury, brain swelling, cerebral herniation, hydrocephalus) are described. This study describes features helpful for identification of these complications and, particularly, their temporal relationships.*

Quagliarello V, Scheld WM: Bacterial meningitis: Pathogenesis, pathophysiology, and progress. N Engl J Med 327:864, 1992. *In this insightful and comprehensive review, particular attention is given to the role of bacterial components, cytokines and other mediators, and endothelial and leukocyte adhesins in the generation of the inflammatory response in the subarachnoid space.*

Roos KL, Tunkel AR, Scheld WM: Acute bacterial meningitis in children and adults. In Scheld WM, Whitley RJ, Durack DT (eds): Infections of the Central Nervous System. New York, Raven Press, 1991. *A thorough, particularly well illustrated consideration of all aspects of bacterial meningitis, including pathology, pathogenesis, clinical features, epidemiology, and treatment. Includes a helpful section on neuroimaging changes.*

Swartz MN, Dodge PR: Bacterial meningitis—A review of selected aspects. N Engl J Med 272:725, 1965. *Detailed account of Massachusetts General Hospital experience. Particularly good on clinical aspects, neurologic complications, and differential diagnosis.*

281 MENINGOCOCCAL INFECTIONS

Michael A. Apicella

Meningococcal infections are a major cause of mortality and morbidity in developed and developing nations. *Neisseria meningitidis* is the causative agent in meningococcal infections. It has become the most common cause of bacterial meningitis in United States children since using the *Haemophilus influenzae* type b protein-capsular polysaccharide conjugate vaccine in infants has dramatically reduced their incidence of meningitis due to this organism. Considerable progress has been made in managing and preventing infections due to *N. meningitidis* since the organism was first described in 1887 (Table 281–1). Because the meningococcal vaccine has limited effectiveness in the group at greatest risk for infection, children younger than age 2, meningococcal infection is still a major worldwide problem. The devastating nature of systemic meningococcal infection makes it imperative that preventive measures be developed to fully control this disease. In addition, an effective vaccine against meningococcal serogroup B infection has not been developed. Until this goal is realized, it is crucial that the clinician recognize and be able to successfully treat the infection as early as possible in its course to ensure an outcome with minimal mortality and morbidity.

MICROBIOLOGY AND PATHOGENESIS. *N. meningitidis* is a gram-negative diplococcus. Meningococci are considered a fastidious species, and media containing appropriate supplementation must be used to ensure reliable growth from clinical samples. Selective media such as Thayer-Martin medium have allowed the organism to be isolated from sites that contain diverse background flora, such as the nasopharynx. The organism grows best between 35 to 37° C in an atmosphere of 5% carbon dioxide. The organism will not grow below 32° C or above 41° C. Laboratory confirmation of the presence of the organism depends on the metabolism of glucose and maltose with the production of acid. Gas is not produced during this metabolic process.

The meningococcus has a very narrow environmental niche. It is a strict human pathogen that has only been isolated from human mucosal surfaces or body fluids. A number of factors contribute to the organism's ability to colonize and cause infection. The meningococcus has a typical gram-negative cell wall containing lipopolysaccharide or endotoxin, which is the primary toxin of the meningococcus. Meningococci express pili (attachment organelles) which they need to adhere to nasopharyngeal epithelial cells. Meningococci can express polysaccharide capsules; this is probably the most important virulence factor associated with this species.

TABLE 281–1. ADVANCES IN THE DIAGNOSIS, MANAGEMENT, AND PREVENTION OF MENINGOCOCCAL INFECTION

Year	Advance
1805	Epidemic cerebrospinal fluid fever (meningococcal meningitis) described in Geneva.
1885	Causative organism identified.
1904	Distinct serotypes of *N. meningitidis* described.
1909	Asymptomatic nasopharyngeal carrier state recognized.
1911	Use of serotherapy for management of meningococcal infection.
1933	Use of sulfonamides to treat meningococcal meningitis.
1942	Sulfonamide prophylaxis used in military camps to prevent epidemics.
1950	High-dose penicillin used successfully to treat meningococcal meningitis.
1963	Sulfonamide-resistant meningococci identified at Fort Ord, CA.
1971	Meningococcal capsular C polysaccharide used to successfully prevent meningococcal disease to prevent disease in U.S. Army recruits.
1989	*N. meningitidis* resistant to penicillin C first reported.

Thirteen serologically distinct encapsulated forms have been implicated in infection. Immunochemical differences in these capsules are the basis for the principal system used to serogroup encapsulated meningococci. Over 98% of cases are caused by five serogroups: A, B, C, W-135, and Y. Meningococci that lack capsular polysaccharides can be cultured. Called "nonencapsulated strains," they are frequently identified in nasopharyngeal cultures during screening in endemic periods. They have not been isolated from body fluids of patients with systemic meningococcal disease. In addition to serogrouping based on capsular antigens, meningococci also can be serotyped based on antigenic differences in their outer membrane proteins and lipopolysaccharides. These serotypes have become important in studies of the epidemiology of infection and in the development of new vaccines.

The pathogenesis of meningococcal infection is now beginning to be understood. The factors involved in colonization and invasion of the nasopharyngeal surface are shown in Figure 281–1A. The meningococcus can adhere to and enter the nonciliated cells of the nasopharyngeal mucosa. Organisms are able to transmigrate through these cells to the submucosal space, where they have access to enter capillaries and arterioles. If the organism can invade the vascular system, the capsular polysaccharide (in the absence of specific antibody) provides an antiphagocytic barrier that protects the organism against normal host clearing mechanisms. Figure 281–1B outlines the process by which endotoxin (lipo-oligosaccharide, or LOS), through the release of cytokines, leads to shock and disseminated intravascular coagulation (DIC) in meningococcal sepsis. Endotoxin and cytokine levels in meningococcal sepsis have been measured and high tumor necrosis factor alpha (TNFα) and interferon-γ levels correlate with a poor prognosis.

The propensity of the meningococcus to invade the central nervous system (CNS) and cause meningitis is poorly understood. The organism probably gains entry through the arachnoid villi. The release of endotoxin and peptidoglycan in the cerebrospinal fluid (CSF) evokes inflammatory factors that are chemoattractive for polymorphonuclear leukocytes (PMN's). Enzymes released by PMN's intensify the meningeal inflammation, leading to increased cerebral vascular permeability and brain edema.

EPIDEMIOLOGY. *N. meningitidis* can cause endemic and epidemic infection. At present, meningococcal infection is endemic in the United States, with approximately 2500 cases per year reported to the Centers for Disease Control and Prevention. This gives a case rate of approximately 1 in 10^5 total population. The fatality rate is approximately 12%. Disease rates in children younger than age 2 are approximately 10 times higher than in the overall population. Seasonal variation occurs, with the highest attack rates in February and March and the lowest in September. The male-to-female patient ratio is approximately equal. The predominate serogroups causing infection in the United States currently are serogroups B and C.

Before World War II, periodic epidemics of meningococcal infection ravaged American cities. These were caused primarily by the serogroup A meningococcus. With increasing standards of living, these epidemics have abated in this country, and infection due to the serogroup A has virtually disappeared in the United States.

Large-scale epidemics still occur with a deadly frequency in Africa, parts of Asia, South America, and the countries of the former Soviet Union. These epidemics are most commonly caused by serogroup A meningococcus and occasionally by the serogroup C meningococcus. In an area appropriately named "the meningitis belt" because it crosses the waist of sub-Saharan Africa, epidemics of meningococcal infection occur every 7 to 10 years. The case rate during these epidemics can be as high as 1 in 1000 total population. Case rates in children younger than 2 can be 1 in 100. In the developed nations of western Europe, epidemics due to serogroup B meningococcus have occurred over the past decade. Norway suffered such an epidemic with case rates of 1 in 10,000; a high attack rate was seen among teenagers.

The reason for the epidemic spread of the meningococcus is not known. The organism is considered a respiratory pathogen, and spread is most likely by the aerosol route. It is clear that the high attack rates seen in developing countries is in part due to poverty and the consequences of crowding, poor sanitation, and malnutrition. Factors such as herd immunity and specific virulence factors associated with "epidemic strains" have been implicated in the rapid spread of infection in these situations. Predisposition to meningococcal infection has been associated with preceding respiratory tract infection, particularly influenza.

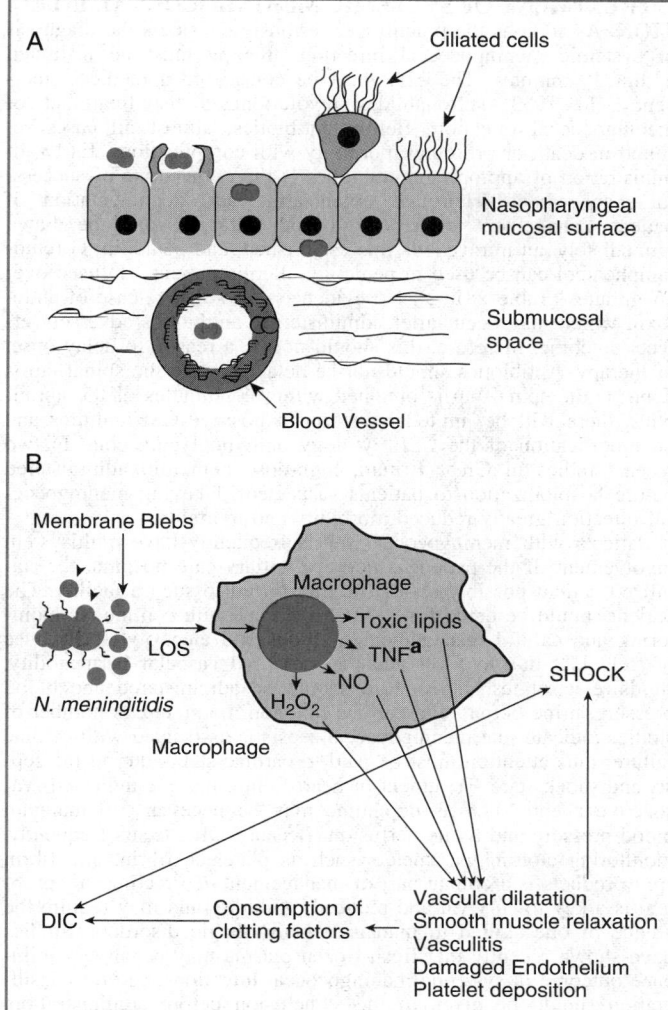

FIGURE 281–1. *A,* A schematic representation of nasopharyngeal invasion by the meningococcus. The process involves attachment to surface of nonciliated cells by meningococcal pili. Short-range attachment factors (meningococcal surface components) are probably involved in the endocytotic engulfment process as microvilli of the nasopharyngeal cell surround the organism. The nonciliated cells through which the organisms transmigrate do not appear to sustain damage. By contrast, the ciliated mucosal cells die and are extruded from the mucosal surface. Meningococcal lipo-oligosaccharide, peptidoglycan, and possibly other toxins are thought to be responsible for this cytolytic activity. Organisms in the submucosal space then have access to entry into capillaries and arterioles and can invade the vascular system. (Data from Stephens DS: Gonococcal and meningococcal pathogenesis as defined by human cell, cell culture, and organ culture assays. Clin Microbiol Rev 2:S104, 1989.) *B,* The rapid doubling time of the meningococcus and its ability to shed large amounts of endotoxin by a process called "blebbing" rapidly lead to a high-grade septic state with shock. Endotoxin (lipo-oligosaccharide, or LOS) interacts with macrophages to release cytokines, vasoactive lipids (prostaglandins), and free radicals such as H_2O_2, O^-, and NO. These substances damage vascular endothelium, resulting in platelet deposition and vasculitis. This leads to vascular disruption and the petechiae and ecchymoses that are frequently seen during meningococcal infection. Clotting factors are consumed, and DIC ensues, which is an ominous consequence of delayed treatment. Occasionally, the intravascular clotting can lead to occlusion of major arterial vessels in the extremities, requiring amputation. The most dire consequence of all these vascular effects is Waterhouse-Friderichsen syndrome, which is multiorgan failure due to shock and hemorrhagic diathesis. (Data from Brandtzaeg P, Ovstebo R, Kierulf P: Compartmentalization of lipopolysaccharide production correlates with clinical presentation in meningococcal disease. J Infect Dis 166:650, 1992.)

Epidemic infections in American military recruit camps were a major problem before vaccination was introduced. Throughout the nineteenth century, the unique susceptibility of military recruits can be attested to by the clinical descriptions of this infection that can be found in the records of the Crimean and American Civil Wars.

Since vaccinating recruits started in 1972 with a tetravalent vaccine containing serogroup A, C, Y, and W-135 polysaccharides, epidemics have not occurred.

Intimate contacts of cases, including family members, college roommates, and nursery school classmates are at 100- to 1000-fold increased risk of acquiring meningococcal infection. Such individuals should be told about the increased risk and monitored closely for emergence of co-primary cases (cases that arise within 48 hours of the primary case) and given chemoprophylaxis (see treatment section below) to prevent secondary cases of infection. Hospital personnel who care for patients with meningococcal disease are not at increased risk of acquiring infection. Exceptions would include individuals who suffer needle sticks contaminated with body fluids from untreated patients and health care personnel who give mouth-to-mouth resuscitation to infected individuals. It may be wise to manage such individuals with parenteral therapy rather than using chemoprophylaxis. Isolating patients in hospitals is a common practice—limited to respiratory isolation and terminated 24 hours after instituting appropriate antibiotic therapy.

CLINICAL SYNDROMES. *The Carrier State.* There are several different meningococcal infection syndromes. In the early twentieth century, the ability to isolate meningococci from the nasopharynx of otherwise healthy individuals led to the concept of asymptomatic carriage of bacterial pathogens. The observation that increased carriage rates coincided with onset of epidemics among military recruits during World War I first linked the relationship of the carrier state to disease. The nasopharyngeal carrier state is considered an active infection, because some individuals have symptomatic pharyngitis and develop rises in serologic titers to the infecting organism. It is considered that all cases of acute systemic meningococcal infection are preceded by recent nasopharyngeal colonization. Studies have shown that the carrier state can persist for long periods, with about 5% of the population carrying the meningococcus in their nasopharynx during endemic periods. The majority of these isolates are unencapsulated. During epidemics, the carrier rate can rise to over 30%, with the majority of individuals carrying the epidemic strains in their nasopharynx. Generally, most individuals who become carriers are asymptomatic. Evidence exists that the systemic immune system is primed during the period of nasopharyngeal carriage, since antibodies to the infecting strains can be shown to evolve concordant with colonization.

In a study of an epidemic among military recruits, it has been shown that nasopharyngeal colonization by the meningococcal strain responsible for the epidemic resulted in a 40% incidence of systemic infection if the person colonized also lacked bactericidal antibodies to the epidemic strain. This study confirmed the role of nasopharyngeal carriage as the source of systemic infection and the importance of the serum antibody in protecting against systemic meningococcal infection.

ized *Meningitis and Meningococcemia.* Acute systemic infection can be manifest clinically by three syndromes: meningitis, meningitis with meningococcemia, and meningococcemia without obvious signs of meningitis. Typically, an otherwise healthy patient develops sudden onset of fever, nausea, vomiting, headache, decreased ability to concentrate, and myalgia. The patient frequently tells the physician that this is the sickest he/she has ever felt. Many have an impending feeling of death. In children, the infection is rarely seen below age 6 months because they are protected by placentally transferred antibodies. Because children younger than age 2 cannot relate many symptoms, sudden onset of fever, leukocytosis, and lethargy become important findings. Initially, the physical examination may be unrevealing, with the exception of an acutely ill patient. The preceding symptoms of pharyngitis which may be associated with nasopharyngeal carriage can lead to a preliminary diagnosis of streptococcal infection. This frequently results in treatment with low-dose penicillin, which has little effect on the emerging meningococcal sepsis. Alternatively, the diagnosis of influenza is assigned to the patient because of complaints of fever, chills, and myalgia. In general, patients with meningococcal infection present considerably sicker than the majority of patients with streptococcal or viral infections. The vital signs will show a low blood pressure with an elevated pulse rate. Diaphoresis is common. In such patients, an intensive search for petechiae should be mounted (see Color Plate 10*A*). A complete examination of the skin with the patient completely undressed is essential. The physical examination should include provocative tests of meningeal irritability, the Kernig and Brudzinski signs. It must be remembered that patients with meningococcemia may not necessarily have meningeal signs but that from 50 to 80% will have petechiae upon presentation. An examination of the mucosal surfaces of the soft palate and ocular and palpabral conjunctivae for petechiae must be done.

The infection can progress rapidly. Depending on the patient's presentation, a critical situation can occur very quickly. Profound shock with DIC is the most ominous development in these patients. Coagulopathy, defined as a partial thromboplastin time of >50 seconds or a fibrinogen concentration of >150 μg per deciliter, is an excellent predictor of poor prognosis. A number of studies have demonstrated that myocardial dysfunction can occur in meningococcal sepsis. Signs of heart failure, including gallop rhythms and congestive heart failure with pulmonary edema, are not uncommon. In one large series, 15% of pediatric patients were admitted to intensive care units because of cardiovascular manifestations. Approximately 25% of patients who died of meningococcal sepsis had evidence of myocarditis. In France, a group of severely ill patients with meningococcal sepsis showed low stroke volume indices (29 ml per square meter) and tachycardia (>135 beats per minute), a profile suggesting a greater myocardial depression than usually observed in gram-negative sepsis. In infection due to meningococcal serogroup C, pericarditis with tamponade can seriously complicate the course of treatment unless recognized and managed. When DIC occurs, persistent bleeding at intravenous sites and sites of arterial punctures can complicate management of the tamponade.

Neurologic complications include signs of meningeal irritation, an encephalopathic state, and coma. Seizures can occur but are less common than in other forms of bacterial meningitis. In general, patients surviving meningococcal CNS infection have remarkably few sequelae (see Ch. 421), but cerebrovascular accidents secondary to intracranial bleeding can lead to paresis. Cases of posterior pituitary insufficiency have been reported in patients recovering from meningococcal infection.

Prognosis can vary depending on the presentation of the patient, the skill and completeness of the physician, and the nature of the facility. At tertiary care hospitals during endemic periods of infection, mortality rates as low as 8% have been reported. Patients who present with meningococcemia alone tend to have a higher mortality rate (up to 20%). During World War II, meningococcal mortality rates using sulfonamides were as low as 2%. Many of these patients were hospitalized and treated as soon as symptoms began. Recent studies in Norway and Africa have supported the concept that early onset of therapy significantly reduces mortality.

LABORATORY DIAGNOSIS. The laboratory diagnosis is based on isolating *N. meningitidis* from blood cultures or CSF. Blood cultures will be positive in 60 to 80% of untreated patients, while CSF cultures will be positive in 50 to 70%. Gram stain analysis of CSF requires a skilled patient observer but it can provide diagnostic results rapidly. Gram stain of the CSF can be useful as a rapid diagnostic tool, especially in patients with meningococcal meningitis. Approximately 50% of these patients will have a positive Gram stain. In cases of meningococcemia without overt meningitis, the CSF Gram stain will be positive in <25% of patients. Recent studies have suggested that Gram stain analysis of punch biopsy or needle aspiration of hemorrhagic skin lesions in meningococcal sepsis without clinical evidence of meningitis can lead to rapid diagnosis; approximately 70% of such skin lesions were positive. The tinctorial results for punch biopsy specimens were not affected by antibiotics, because Gram staining gave positive results up to 45 hours after antibiotic therapy was started. Cultures of these biopsies or aspirates also were useful diagnostically for as long as 13 hours after instituting antibiotic therapy. Detecting meningococcal capsular polysaccharide in CSF also can be used for rapid diagnosis; the test is most sensitive for the A and C polysaccharides and considerably less sensitive for serogroup B polysaccharide. In meningococcemia without clinically apparent meningitis, the antigen detection methods can be negative despite profound sepsis. Recently, polymerase chain reaction (PCR) has been demonstrated as a potentially rapid method for diagnosing CSF infection and serum. Further testing must be done to confirm the specificity and sensitivity of this technique.

TREATMENT OF SYSTEMIC MENINGOCOCCAL INFECTION. As soon as the practitioner seriously considers the diagnosis of systemic meningococcal infection, therapy must be instituted within 30 minutes. The case must be considered a medical emergency. In 1933, sulfonamides revolutionized the treatment of meningococcal infection. Before antibiotics, almost all cases resulted in death or profound morbidity with complications. Early administration of appropriate antibiotics is the cornerstone of successful management. Thorough organization and documentation of patient management are crucial. Blood cultures should be drawn immediately, an intravenous line established, and penicillin G (chloramphenicol can be used in penicillin-allergic patients) infused over 15 minutes (Table 281–2). No evidence exists that release of endotoxin which may occur after administering antibiotics adversely effects outcome; therefore, this should not be a reason to delay onset of therapy. Antibiotics should not be delayed while the spinal tap is done. If the spinal tap is obtained within 45 minutes of the antibiotics, there will be limited reduction in positive CSF cultures and no modification of the CSF cytology or hypoglycorachhia. In two recent studies in Great Britain, high-dose penicillin administered before hospitalization to patients suspected of having meningococcal infection greatly reduced morbidity and mortality.

Patients with meningococcal sepsis frequently have multisystem involvement. If the patient is not at a tertiary care hospital, the stabilized patient possibly should be transferred to such a facility. The patient should be cared for in intensive care with continuous monitoring and careful management of fluids and electrolytes. Because of fluid loss due to fever and the increased vascular permeability, fluids, electrolytes, and colloid should be administered and blood pressure, urine output, and cardiac function monitored. A number of studies indicate that meningococcal sepsis is associated with cardiac failure; thus attention must be paid to cardiac status during the sepsis and shock state. Treatment of heart failure may be indicated. Vasoactive agents such as dopamine may be necessary to maintain blood pressure and tissue perfusion. Because DIC occurs frequently, monitoring clotting parameters such as platelets, fibrin, and fibrin split products is a crucial part of management. Correcting this problem is a key to survival and reduced morbidity and may require the advice of one skilled in managing hemorrhagic disorders. Studies have shown recently that fresh-frozen plasma may negatively influence outcome in systemic meningococcal infections; careful consideration should be given to this conclusion before administration. Recent studies have suggested that exchange transfusion may improve the survival rate among patients with fulminant meningococcal sepsis. The beneficial effect is most likely not based on the elimination of endotoxin. One of the most serious causes of morbidity in fulminant meningococcal sepsis is skin necrosis and loss of distal digits and limbs. It has been suggested that epidural sympathetic blockade may preserve the lower extremities of such patients. Skin necrosis can be managed by debridement, grafting, and nutritional support after the patient has been stabilized.

Penicillin remains the cornerstone of therapy. The meningococcus is sensitive to a wide range of antibiotics, including third-generation cephalosporins and quinolones. Ampicillin is equivalent to penicillin G and can be used if there is uncertainty about the etiologic diagnosis at the time that therapy is instituted. Recent reports from southern Europe (primarily Spain and Greece) of the isolation of penicillin-resistant meningococci could have ominous consequences if epidemics occur due to these organisms. In Spain, the prevalence of *N. meningitidis* isolates that are moderately susceptible to penicillin and ampicillin has increased to almost 50%. These strains do not produce β-lactamase. In these strains, the basis of meningococcal resistance to penicillin is alteration in a group of inner membrane enzymes, the penicillin-binding proteins (PBP's), which are

TABLE 281–2. ANTIBIOTIC MANAGEMENT OF SYSTEMIC MENINGOCOCCAL INFECTION

Antibiotic	Dosage
Penicillin G	300,000 units/kg/d IV, up to 24 million units/day
Ampicillin	150–200 mg/kg/d IV, up to 12 grams/day
Ceftriaxone	2 grams/day IV
Chloramphenicol	For use in penicillin-allergic patients, 100 mg/kg/day IV, up to 4 grams/d

responsible for cell wall synthesis. Specifically, alterations in the PBP 2 result in decreased binding affinity of penicillin and ampicillin to these enzymes. Third-generation cephalosporins are usually effective against organisms that are resistant on this basis. However, careful antibiotic sensitivity testing should be performed to ensure that this is the case, since some third-generation cephalosporins also may not bind efficiently to these modified penicillin-binding proteins. Disk diffusion methods can still be used to analyze such strains, although plate dilution methods are preferred. Sulfonamide-resistant meningococci are still common in the United States; hence sulfonamides should not be used to treat acute infections.

Complement Deficiency and Meningococcal Sepsis.
Individuals with deficiencies in complement components appear to be uniquely susceptible to meningococcal infection. In properdin-deficient patients, fulminant meningococcal sepsis is a frequent cause of death. Families of such individuals should be investigated for a history of sudden septic death in relatives. Such families should be managed closely and undergo vaccination with the tetravalent meningococcal vaccine.

In patients with the late complement component deficiencies (LCCD), meningococcal infection occurs in older individuals (mean age 17) and tends to be milder (mortality ~ 2%) and caused by less common serogroups (serogroup Y and W-135) than occurs in the general population. LCCD patients respond normally to meningococcal capsular polysaccharide vaccine with the development of antibodies that are functional in both complement-dependent bactericidal assays and opsonophagocytic assays. These patients have a more rapid decline in capsular antibody than that seen in normal individuals, suggesting that LCCD patients are critically dependent on capsular antibody for protection against meningococcal disease. Vaccination, probably on a recurrent basis, is an important component in preventing meningococcal disease in LCCD patients.

OTHER CLINICAL SYNDROMES. Chronic Meningococcemia.
Chronic meningococcal sepsis, which is indistinguishable from the gonococcal dermatitis-arthritis syndrome, can occur. These patients have typical painful skin lesions usually on the extremities with migratory polyarthritis and tenosynovitis (see Ch. 239). This form of meningococcal sepsis can persist for weeks if untreated. This syndrome responds promptly to antibiotic therapy.

Respiratory Tract Infection.
Pneumonia due to *N. meningitidis* has been reported since the 1930's. In a recent study of community-acquired infections in Finland, *N. meningitidis* was implicated as the etiologic agent in 6%. Epidemic pneumonia due to serogroup Y strains has occurred at a military training center. Patients presented with chills, chest pain, and cough; rales and fever occurred in almost all patients, and infections were frequently multilobar (40%). The incidence of sepsis associated with these infections is quite low, and the diagnosis is usually made with transtracheal aspirations. There was no mortality, and all patients responded well to treatment with penicillin.

Meningococcal Pericarditis.
Pericarditis is usually associated with infections due to *N. meningitidis* serogroup C. It has been reported associated with meningococcemia and as an isolated syndrome. Patients can present with chest pain and signs of tamponade, but relatively asymptomatic disease can occur with detection made by sonography. Treatment with antibiotics and removal of the pericardial fluid usually results in a successful outcome. Pericarditis can occur in patients convalescing from meningococcal sepsis. It should be considered if fever and shortness of breath on minimal exertion occur when the patient is recovering from meningococcal sepsis. Echocardiogram will result in rapid diagnosis of this complication of infection. In convalescent patients, antibiotic therapy should be continued, and pericardiocentesis may be indicated. There is no evidence that steroids or anti-inflammatory agents have a role in management.

Meningococcal Urethritis.
Meningococci have been isolated from the urethra and can cause clinical urethritis. In a recent study of over 5000 urethral cultures from homosexual men, the isolation rate was 0.2%, compared with 4.7% for *N. gonorrhoeae* among the same population. Eight of these patients had symptomatic urethritis. In the same study, there were no isolates among almost 9000 urethral cultures from heterosexual males or almost 16,000 cervical cultures. This study strongly suggests that there is an association between orogenital sex and urethral acquisition of the meningococcus. Meningococcal urethritis has been managed successfully with penicillin and/or tetracycline.

CHEMOPROPHYLAXIS. The observation that sulfonamides could clear the nasopharynx carriage of meningococci for weeks after a single day of therapy led to the concept of chemoprophylaxis for preventing secondary infection in hyperepidemic situations. However, because of the profligate use of sulfonamides for chemoprophylaxis in the 1950's, the meningococcus developed resistance to these agents, and in 1963 epidemics were occurring on Vietnamese military bases. Military studies to find alternatives to sulfonamides resulted in an effective anticapsular vaccine in 1971 and use of minocycline and rifampin for chemoprophylaxis. Eradication of the carrier state in intimate contacts of index cases with chemoprophylaxis is an effective way to prevent secondary cases. The concept behind successful prophylaxis is the use of short-term antibiotic therapy (one to two doses) to achieve long-term (3- to 4-week) eradication of the meningococcus from the nasopharynx. Although physicians realize that prophylaxis is necessary, they fail to appreciate that specific antibiotics must be used for effective management. Penicillin, penicillin derivatives, and first- and second-generation cephalosporins are not effective for prophylaxis because they do not eradicate the meningococcus during the short courses of therapy. Rifampin and ceftriaxone have been shown to be effective agents for prophylaxis (Table 281–3). Recently, quinoline derivatives also have been shown to be effective for chemoprophylaxis.

PREVENTION. The immunologically different meningococcal serogroups were identified in the early 20th century, which led to the use of capsular-specific serotherapy to manage meningococcal infection before effective chemotherapy was developed. The ability of these polysaccharides to evoke a protective immune response is the basis for the meningococcal vaccines. An effective tetravalent capsular polysaccharide vaccine (containing A, C, Y, and W-135 polysaccharides) is available to prevent meningococcal infections in people older than age 2. Over 100 million doses of this vaccine have been given worldwide, with no serious side effects reported. Tetravalent vaccine should be administered to all intimate contacts of index cases at the start of chemoprophylaxis. This vaccine also has been used effectively in the U.S. military and in aborting epidemics caused by serogroup strains represented in the vaccine. A principal drawback of the vaccine is the lack of immunogenicity in children younger than age 2, limiting widespread application of the current vaccine in countries with recurrent epidemic infections. These children respond poorly to polysaccharides for reasons that are not clearly understood. Recent successes in vaccinating young children with *H. influenzae* polysaccharide conjugated to proteins suggest that a similar strategy might be useful for meningococcal polysaccharides. Such a vaccine is not currently available.

In addition, the lack of an antigen that can elicit protection against meningococcal serogroup B infection has limited the vaccine's use. The serogroup B polysaccharide is a poor immunogen, even in adults, perhaps because it resembles "self" antigens. Vaccine development in serogroup B strains has focused on other meningococcal subcapsular surface antigens (proteins and possibly lipopolysaccharide). These vaccines are based on serotypic protein antigens, and the vaccine must be tailored to the serotype of the specific meningococcal strain causing the epidemic. A recent noncapsular serogroup B vaccine has been tested in an epidemic in Brazil, and the results indicate that there was vaccine efficacy in children older than age 2.

TABLE 281–3. CHEMOPROPHYLAXIS FOR PREVENTING MENINGOCOCCAL INFECTION

Antibiotic	Dosage
Rifampin	Adults, 600 mg q12h for 2 days. Children, 10 mg/kg q12h for 2 days.
Ceftriaxone	Single 250-mg dose for adults, single 125-mg dose for children. Limited experience and at present should only be used if rifampin is contraindicated.
Ofloxacin	400 mg as a single dose. Limited experience and should be used only if rifampin is contraindicated. No experience in children.

Apicella MA: *Neisseria meningitidis. In* Mandell GL, Douglas RG, Bennett JE (eds.): Principles and Practices of Infectious Diseases, New York, Churchill Livingstone, 1990, pp 1600–1612. *Complete description of the biology and pathogenesis of* N. meningitidis *infection.*

Cartwright K, Reilly S, White D, et al.: Early treatment with parenteral penicillin in meningococcal disease. Br Med J 305:143, 1992. *Description of the improved outcome in meningococcal infection if therapy is instituted early.*

Densen P: Complement deficiencies and meningococcal disease. Clin Exp Immunol 86(suppl 1):57, 1991. *Review of the role of complement deficiencies and susceptibility to meningococcal infection.*

Durand ML, Calderwood SB, Weber DJ, et al.: Acute bacterial meningitis in adults. N Engl J Med 328:21, 1993. *Recent review of bacterial meningitis in an American hospital.*

Gilja HO, Halstensen A, Digranes A, et al.: Single-dose Ofloxacin to eradicate tonsillopharyngeal carriage of *Neisseria meningitidis.* Antimicrob Agents Chemother 37:2024, 1993. *This article demonstrates the usefulness of quinolones for meningococcal prophylaxis.*

McGee ZA, Baringer JR: Acute meningitis. *In* Mandell GL, Douglas RG, Bennett JE (eds.): Principles and Practices of Infectious Diseases. New York, Churchill Livingstone, 1990, pp 741–761. *Detailed discussion of the differential diagnosis and management of bacterial meningitis.*

Ni H, Knight AL, Cartwright K, et al.: Polymerase chain reaction for diagnosis of meningococcal meningitis. Lancet 340:1432, 1992. *Description of PCR to diagnosis meningococcal infection from clinical materials.*

Schwartz B: Chemoprophylaxis for bacterial infections: Principles of and application to meningococcal infection. Rev Infect Dis 13(suppl 2):S170, 1991. *Review of the concepts and strategies in chemoprophylaxis of meningococcal infection; studies validating using ceftriaxone.*

282 INFECTIONS CAUSED BY *HAEMOPHILUS* SPECIES

Michael S. Simberkoff

DEFINITION. The name *Haemophilus* is derived from the Greek nouns *haima,* meaning "blood," and *philos,* meaning "lover." *Haemophilus* species primarily infect the respiratory tract, skin, or mucous membranes of humans. From these sites, organisms can invade to cause bacteremia, meningitis, epiglottitis, endocarditis, septic arthritis, or cellulitis.

MICROBIOLOGY. The *Haemophilus* species are small, nonmotile, aerobic or facultative anaerobic, pleomorphic, gram-negative bacilli. The prototype of this genus, *H. influenzae,* was originally recovered from patients with influenza by Richard Pfeiffer in 1893, and it was considered the etiology of that disease for many years. The growth requirements of important *Haemophilus* species are summarized in Table 282–1. Primary isolation of *Haemophilus* species is best accomplished on chocolate agar medium in a CO_2-enriched atmosphere.

INFECTIONS CAUSED BY *H. INFLUENZAE*. General Considerations and Laboratory Characterization. *H. influenzae* is the most important pathogen in this genus. It can be recovered from sites where it colonizes, such as the nasopharynx and upper respiratory tract, and from sites where it causes disease, such as the blood, cerebrospinal fluid (CSF), sputum, pleura, middle ear, and joints (Table 282–2).

H. influenzae consists of encapsulated (typable) and nonencapsulated (nontypable) strains. The former are responsible for most of

TABLE 282–1. GROWTH REQUIREMENTS AND HEMOLYTIC PROPERTIES OF *HAEMOPHILUS* SPECIES

Species	X	V	CO_2	Hemolysis
H. influenzae	+	+	−	−
H. influenzae, b. aegyptius	+	+	−	−
H. parainfluenzae	−	+	−	−
H. aphrophilus	+*	−	+	−
H. paraphropilus	−	+	+	−
H. haemolyticus	+	+	−	+
H. parahaemolyticus	−	+	−	+
H. ducreyi	+	−	−	+†

* Hematin needed for primary isolation.
† Delayed hemolysis occurs in 11 to 89% of strains.

TABLE 282–2. SITES OF COLONIZATION AND INFECTIONS BY *H. INFLUENZAE*

Species	Normal Flora	Associated Disease(s)
H. influenzae	Nasopharynx Upper respiratory tract	Meningitis Epiglottitis Sinusitis Otitis Pneumonia Cellulitis Arthritis Osteomyelitis Obstetric infections Endocarditis
H. influenzae b. aegyptius	No	Purulent conjunctivitis Brazilian purpuric fever

the invasive infections in children, while the latter cause respiratory mucosal infections, including sinusitis and pneumonia, as well as invasive disease in adults. The capsules of *H. influenzae* consist of polysaccharide antigens. Six capsular serotypes (a through f) exist in the species.

Factors Affecting Virulence. The capsules of *H. influenzae* are important virulence factors that inhibit opsonization, clearance, and intracellular killing of the organisms. *H. influenzae* type b, the most common cause of meningitis in infancy and childhood worldwide, contains a pentose capsular polysaccharide consisting of polyribosyl-ribitol phosphate (PRP). Other serotypes contain hexose polysaccharides. It is believed that *H. influenzae* type b is more virulent than other serotypes because it is highly resistant to clearance once bacteremia has been initiated.

Fimbriae are important virulence factors that enhance the adherence of *H. influenzae* to mucosal surfaces. Both typable and nontypable *H. influenzae* isolates contain fimbriae. The lipo-oligosaccharides (LOS's) of *H. influenzae* also contribute to their virulence. LOS's appear to play a crucial role in facilitating the survival of *H. influenzae* on mucosal surfaces within the nasopharynx and in initiating invasive disease (bloodstream invasion) from these sites.

Outer membrane proteins (OMP's) also serve as virulence factors in *H. influenzae* disease. At least 15 different *H. influenzae* OMP's have been identified. One of these OMP's (P2, 39 to 40 kDa) functions as a porin, and others are associated with iron binding. Successful scavenging of iron within the human host is crucial for *H. influenzae* to multiply.

Host Defenses. Antibodies have been recognized for decades as an important part of the host defenses against *H. influenzae* diseases. The classic studies of Fothergill and Wright (1933) demonstrated that most cases of *H. influenzae* meningitis occurred in children during the ages between their losing passively acquired maternal antibodies and developing active humoral immunity to the organism. It is now recognized that these protective antibodies function primarily to opsonize and facilitate *H. influenzae* clearance rather than to directly kill virulent organisms.

Complement is also an essential component of the host defenses against some *H. influenzae* diseases. Children with congenital deficiencies of C2, C3, and Factor I have an increased incidence of *H. influenzae* infections. Patients who lack a functional spleen or who have undergone splenectomy also are at risk for developing overwhelming infection with *H. influenzae* type b.

Prevalence, Incidence, and Epidemiology. The precise prevalence and incidence of *H. influenzae* infections are unknown. This organism can be detected frequently in the nasopharynx of both children and adults. Between 3 and 5% of infants harbor *H. influenzae* type b in their nasopharynx. Nontypable *H. influenzae* can be detected in the nasopharyngeal culture of >70% of young children. Infections, however, occur in only a small fraction of colonized patients. The risk of infection in nonimmune household contacts of a patient with invasive *H. influenzae* disease is approximately 600-fold greater than the risk in the age-adjusted general population.

H. influenzae type b was the most common cause of meningitis in young children before effective vaccines were introduced in the 1980's. Vaccination dramatically reduced the incidence of this infection in young children. In a recent population-based study in Atlanta, Ga., over a 1-year period, invasive *H. influenzae* disease occurred in only 5.6 per 100,000 children and 1.7 per 100,000 adults. Forty of the 47 strains associated with invasive disease from adult patients in this study were serotyped. Twenty of these isolates (50%) were *H. influenzae* type b, 19 (47.5%) were nontypable, and 1 (2.5%) was a type f.

Patients with human immunodeficiency virus (HIV) infection are at increased risk for *H. influenzae* infection. Rates of invasive *H. influenzae* infection among men aged 20 to 49 with HIV infection and the acquired immunodeficiency syndrome (AIDS) were 14.6 and 79.2 per 100,000, respectively. The majority of these infections were caused by nontypable *H. influenzae* strains, although in a second study, 10 of 15 bacteremic *H. influenzae* type b infections observed in adults occurred in patients at risk for HIV infection, and AIDS was documented in 7 of these patients.

Other factors also increase the risk of *H. influenzae* infections. These include globulin deficiencies, sickle cell disease, splenectomy, malignancy, pregnancy, CSF leaks, head trauma, alcoholism, and race. Eskimo, Navajo, and Apache children have *H. influenzae* type b infection rates which are significantly greater than those in comparable non-native populations. In addition, day care attendance, crowding, presence of siblings, previous hospitalizations, and previous otitis media have been shown to increase the risk *H. influenzae* type b disease in young children, while breast-feeding decreases this risk.

Pathogenesis. *H. influenzae* is spread from person to person. Colonization of an individual depends on the virulence factors described above. When *H. influenzae* translocates across damaged epithelial cells, it invades the blood stream. Encapsulated organisms, particularly *H. influenzae* type b, are especially resistant to clearance.

The central nervous system (CNS) is primarily invaded via the choroid plexus. *H. influenzae* and its LOS's initiate an inflammatory process within the subarachnoid which is typical of pyogenic meningitis. This process can be transiently accelerated by using antibiotics that liberate LOS's from organisms if corticosteroids are not administered simultaneously.

Clinical Syndromes. **Meningitis.** *H. influenzae* meningitis commonly occurs in children under age 5 and in adults with histories of skull trauma or CSF leaks. *H. influenzae* type b strains cause the overwhelming majority of these. A review of 493 episodes of acute bacterial meningitis in adults over a 27-year period showed that 19 cases (4%) were due to *H. influenzae*.

H. influenzae meningitis is clinically indistinguishable from other forms of acute bacterial meningitis. Most patients with *H. influenzae* meningitis have CSF white blood counts > 1000 per cubic millimeter and hypoglycorrhachia. The CSF Gram stain shows pleomorphic gram-negative bacilli in 60 to 70% of untreated cases. In some patients, however, the bipolar staining may result in a mistaken diagnosis of pneumococcal meningitis. Thus Gram stain is neither sensitive nor specific for diagnosing *H. influenzae* meningitis.

A diagnosis of *H. influenzae* type b meningitis can be rapidly and reliably established by detecting PRP capsular antigens in CSF. The diagnosis can be established in most cases even when antibiotics have been given before CSF is obtained.

Epiglottitis. *H. influenzae* type b is the most common cause of acute epiglottitis in both children and adults. Epiglottitis is a life-threatening infection in children which usually occurs in patients younger than age 5. The symptoms are fever, drooling, dysphagia, and respiratory distress or stridor, which appear over the course of hours. In adults, fever, sore throat, dysphagia, and odynaphagia occur. Cervical tenderness and lymphadenopathy can be found at all ages. Laryngoscopy demonstrates a swollen, cherry-red epiglottis. However, this procedure should be avoided or undertaken only by experts, since it may precipitate an acute airway obstruction and thus make an emergency tracheotomy necessary. The diagnosis of acute epiglottitis is more safely confirmed by a lateral x-ray of the neck. The patient must be maintained in an upright position during this procedure, however, in order to avoid additional compromise of the airway. The etiology is usually established by blood culture. Cultures of the pharynx and other mucosal surfaces are less useful because *H. influenzae* may be part of the normal flora. A recent review suggests that while vaccination has effectively reduced the incidence of this disease in children, it is increasingly observed in adults.

Pneumonia. *H. influenzae* is a common cause of pneumonia in both children and adults. Nosocomial infections, including ventilator-associated pneumonia, also can be caused by these organisms. The clinical features of *H. influenzae* pneumonia include fever, cough, and signs and radiographic findings of lobar consolidation. Parapneumonic effusions or empyema occur commonly in patients with *H. influenzae* pneumonia. Gram-negative bacilli in sputum suggest the diagnosis, but isolation of *H. influenzae* from sputum culture alone is inadequate to prove an etiology because of the high frequency with which this organism colonizes the respiratory tract. A diagnosis can be established by isolating *H. influenzae* from either the blood or pleural fluid.

Tracheobronchitis. Tracheobronchitis is a condition characterized by fever, cough, and purulent sputum that occurs in the absence of radiographic infiltrates suggestive of pneumonia. It frequently occurs in patients with known chronic lung disease. Blood cultures are rarely positive. A combination of pleomorphic gram-negative bacilli predominating in purulent sputum, antibody titers to *H. influenzae* that rise following infection, and the response, at least transiently, to treatment for *H. influenzae* infection strongly suggest this diagnosis.

Sinusitis. *H. influenzae* and *Staplylococcus pneumoniae* are the most frequent bacterial isolates from antral punctures or surgical specimens of patients with acute purulent sinusitis. Most *H. influenzae* isolates are nontypable. While patients may respond initially to treatment directed against *H. influenzae*, the response is transient if sinus obstruction is not relieved. *H. influenzae* is not an important pathogen in patients with chronic sinusitis.

Otitis Media. *H. influenzae* is the most frequent cause of otitis media in young children. Approximately 90% of the *H. influenzae* isolates obtained by tympanocentesis are nontypable; *H. influenzae* type b causes most of the remaining 10% of infections. Patients with otitis media may present with ear pain or irritability. Drainage can be present. An inflamed, opaque, bulging or perforated tympanic membrane is usually demonstrated. The etiology can be proven by Gram stain and culture of purulent fluid obtained by tympanocentesis. Otitis caused by *H. influenzae* type b may occur in association with bacteremia and meningitis.

Cellulitis. *H. influenzae* type b is the cause of 5 to 15% of the cases of cellulitis in young children. Most of the infections occur on the face or neck. *H. influenzae* cellulitis is often described as causing a distinctive blue or violaceous discoloration of the skin. However, the fever, erythema, and tenderness observed may not be distinguishable from other causes. Diagnosis is established by culture of blood and/or tissue aspirates from the involved area.

Bacteremia Without a Primary Focus of Infection. *H. influenzae* causes primary bacteremia in both children and adults. In infants or children, occult meningitis or epiglottitis can be present. A rigorous clinical and laboratory evaluation is essential to avoid missing diagnoses of life-threatening focal infections in these patients. In adults, primary *H. influenzae* type b bacteremia often occurs in patients with underlying diseases such as lymphoma, leukemia, or alcoholism.

Obstetrical Infection. Pregnancy is associated with a significant risk for *H. influenzae* infection. In the Atlanta study, 7 of 47 adult *H. influenzae* invasive infections occurred in pregnant women.

Pericarditis. *H. influenzae* type b is an important cause of primary bacterial pericarditis in children. It rarely causes this infection in adults; however, pericarditis can occur in association with pneumonia, probably as a result of contiguous spread of the infection.

Endocarditis. *H. influenzae* is a very unusual cause of endocarditis, considering the frequency with which invasive disease occurs. Most infections occur in patients with pre-existing valvular heart disease. Because of its slow initial growth in blood culture media, the diagnosis of this infection may be delayed or missed. Patients with *H. influenzae* endocarditis are at high risk for arterial embolic phenomena.

Septic Arthritis. *H. influenzae* type b is a common cause of septic arthritis in young children; it is rare in adults. *H. influenzae* type b arthritis is clinically indistinguishable from other cause of pyogenic arthritis.

Treatment. Third-generation cephalosporins are currently considered to be the treatment of choice for serious *H. influenzae* infections, such as meningitis or epiglottitis. Treatment with ceftriaxone (adult dose: 1 gram IV every 12 hours) or cefotaxime (adult dose: 2 grams IV every 8 hours) should be started for patients with proven or suspected *H. influenzae* infection, and this should be continued at least until the full susceptibility data are available.

Ampicillin was considered to be the treatment of choice for all *H. influenzae* infections until the mid-1970's. Since the first reports of ampicillin-resistant *H. influenzae* isolates in 1972, however, this problem has been increasing. At present, 30% of *H. influenzae* type b isolates and 15% of nontypable *H. influenzae* isolates are resistant to ampicillin. The majority contain a plasmid-mediated, R-factor enzyme (TEM-1) β-lactamase, which can be detected rapidly in the laboratory. A small number of isolates, however, have altered penicillin-binding proteins. These proteins bind penicillin and other β-lactam antibiotics poorly. As a consequence, the isolates may be resistant to some cephalosporins such as cefaclor, cefamandole, and cefuroxime in addition to ampicillin. Therefore, patients with proven or suspected *H. influenzae* infections should not be treated with ampicillin or with second-generation cephalosporins until susceptibilities to these antibiotics are proven. Chloramphenicol resistance also occurs in *H. influenzae;* resistance is caused by an inactivating enzyme, chloramphenical acetyl transferase. A small number of *H. influenzae* isolates are resistant to both ampicillin and chloramphenicol.

Amoxicillin can be used for otitis media in children because of the lower prevalence of β-lactamases in nontypable *H. influenzae* isolates. Bactrim is also effective for most isolates. A combination of erythromycin and sulfisoxazole can be used in patients with documented penicillin allergy.

Prevention. The first *H. influenzae* type b vaccines were licensed for use in the United States in 1985. These contained purified PRP antigens. However, postlicensing studies of PRP vaccines in the United States showed variable efficacy. The PRP vaccines elicit a type 2, thymus-independent B-cell response, generate few (if any) memory B cells, and fail to stimulate a response in neonates and infants.

Protein-conjugated PRP vaccines were developed to overcome the problem of the lack of immune response in the most susceptible infants and some young children. Several are now licensed for use in infants. At present, protein-conjugated PRP vaccines are recommended for use in all infants over age 2 months, but not earlier than age 6 weeks. However, all patient populations are not equally protected. Additional studies are necessary to determine the optimal vaccine preparations and dosage schedules for the infants at greatest risk for *H. influenzae* type b disease.

Antibiotic prophylaxis should be used for unimmunized household or day care contacts of a patient with invasive *H. influenzae* type b disease. Rifampin is the treatment of choice. It should be given in a dose of 10 mg per kilogram once daily for 4 days to neonates younger than 1 month, 20 mg per kilogram (up to a maximum of 600 mg) once daily for 4 days to older children, and 600 mg daily for 4 days to adults.

INFECTIONS CAUSED BY *H. INFLUENZAE, BIOGROUP AEGYPTIUS* (PURULENT CONJUNCTIVITIS AND BRAZILIAN PURPURIC FEVER).

H. influenzae, biogroup *aegyptius* (Koch-Weeks bacillus) causes epidemic purulent conjunctivitis in children. This disease commonly occurs in hot climates or in the summer season. The infection causes conjunctival erythema, edema, mucopurulent exudate, and varying discomfort in the eyes. An unusually virulent clone of *H. influenzae,* biogroup *aegyptius,* causes an invasive infection called Brazilian purpuric fever (BPF). BPF is characterized by petechial or purpuric skin lesions and vascular collapse, which occur days to weeks after an initial episode of conjunctivitis in infants and children younger than 10 years. BPF is usually fatal.

INFECTIONS CAUSED BY OTHER *HAEMOPHILUS* SPECIES. H. parainfluenzae.

H. parainfluenzae can be found as part of the normal flora of the mouth and pharynx (Table 282–3). It is a rare cause of meningitis in children and an even rarer cause of meningitis in adults. It may cause dental infections or dental abscesses. Cases of brain abscess, epidural abscess, liver abscess, osteomyelitis, pneumonia, empyema, epiglottitis, peritonitis, septic arthritis, and septicemia caused by this organism have been reported. *H. parainfluenzae* also causes subacute endocarditis, often in young adults. *Haemophilus* species cause approximately 1% of cases of infective endocarditis in non–drug-abusing patients. *H. parainfluenzae* and *H. aphrophilus* (see below) are the species most frequently recovered from these patients. *H. parainfluenzae* forms

TABLE 282–3. SITES OF COLONIZATION AND INFECTIONS BY OTHER *HAEMOPHILUS* SPECIES

Species	Normal Flora	Associated Disease(s)
H. parainfluenzae	Mouth and pharynx	Endocarditis, brain abscess, liver abscess, pneumonia, epiglottitis, arthritis, osteomyelitis
H. aphrophilus	Mouth	Endocarditis, brain abscess, periodontal abscess, osteomyelitis
H. paraphropilus	Mouth and pharynx	Endocarditis, brain abscess, liver abscess
H. haemolyticus	Nasopharynx	?
H. parahaemolyticus	Mouth and pharynx	Endocarditis, empyema of gallbladder, ? pharyngitis
H. ducreyi	No	Chancroid

bulky vegetations on heart valves. Arterial embolization is common in patients with *H. parainfluenzae* endocarditis. Most isolates are sensitive to ampicillin, but some produce β-lactamases. Pending sensitivity reports, patients should be treated with a drug that combines a β-lactam antibiotic and a β-lactamase inhibitor (such as ampicillin/sulbactam; adult dose: 3 grams IV q6h) with ampicillin plus an aminoglycoside or with a third-generation cephalosporin.

H. aphrophilus. *H. aphrophilus* can be found as part of the normal oral flora (see Table 282–3). Like *H. parainfluenzae, H. aphrophilus* grows very slowly on primary isolation from blood cultures. It frequently causes bulky vegetations, and arterial emboli are common. *H. aphrophilus* is also a rare cause of brain abscess, periodontal abscess, meningitis, osteomyelitis, and suppurative pulmonary infections. Ampicillin or ampicillin plus an aminoglycoside should be used to treat infections.

H. paraphrophilus. *H. paraphrophilus* can be found as part of the normal flora of the mouth and pharynx (see Table 282–3). *H. paraphrophilus* is a rare cause of endocarditis, and arterial emboli have been observed in 50% of the cases *H. paraphrophilus* endocarditis. It is also a rare cause of brain abscess and liver abscess. Ampicillin is the treatment of choice for this infection.

H. parahaemolyticus. *H. parahaemolyticus* is an important pathogen in domestic animals, causing porcine pleuropneumonia. The organism can be found in the human mouth and pharynx. It is a rare cause of human subacute endocarditis and of empyema of the gallbladder (see Table 282–3). *H. parahaemolyticus* has been isolated from throat cultures of patients with pharyngitis. Animal isolates of *H. parahaemolyticus* are sensitive to tetracycline and sulfa drugs. There is insufficient information about human isolates to permit recommendations for therapy.

H. ducreyi. See Ch. 314.

Adams WG, Keaver KA, Cochi SL, et al.: Decline of childhood *Haemophilus Influenzae* type b (Hib) disease in the Hib vaccine era. JAMA 269:221, 1993. *Shows that, in children < age 5, there was a 71 to 82% reduction in H. influenzae type b meningitis in the year following licensing of the Hib conjugate vaccines in the U.S.*

Centers for Disease Control and Prevention. Recommendations for use of the *Haemophilus* b conjugate vaccines and a combined diphtheria, tetanus, pertussis, and *Haemophilus* b vaccine. Recommendations of the Advisory Committee on Immunization Practices (ACIP). MMWR 42 (No.RR-13):1, 1993. *Contains recommendations for use of Haemophilus b conjugate vaccines for infants beginning at age 2 months (but not earlier than age 6 weeks); also describes the safety, immunogenicity, efficacy, adverse reactions, contraindications, and precautions for vaccine use.*

Durand ML, Calderwood SB, Weber DJ, et al.: Acute bacterial meningitis in adults: A review of 493 episodes. N Engl J Med 328:21, 1993. *Summarizes data from a large series of adults with acute bacterial meningitis seen over 27 years. H. influenzae caused acute bacterial meningitis in 19 (4%) of the adults. Thirteen of these patients had community-acquired infections and six developed nosocomial H. influenzae meningitis after neurosurgery.*

Farley MM, Stephens DS, Brachman PS, et al.: Invasive *Haemophilus influenzae* disease in adults. Ann Intern Med 116:806, 1992. *A population-based study showing that 47 cases of invasive H. influenzae disease occurred in adults in metropolitan Atlanta from December 1988 through May 1990 (incidence 1.7 per 100,000 adults per year).*

Fothergill LD, Wright J: Influenzal meningitis: The relation of age incidence to the bactericidal power of blood against the causal organism. J Immunol 24:273, 1993. *The classic study showing that H. influenzae meningitis occurs in children during the ages between the loss of passively acquired maternal antibodies and the development of active immunity to this organism.*

Liu VC, Smith A: Molecular mechanisms of *Haemophilus influenzae* pathogenicity. Antibiot Chemother 45:30, 1992. *Reviews the virulence factors that have been associated with invasive* H. influenzae *infections, including the capsule, outer membrane proteins, fimbria, and lipo-oligosaccharides of the organism.*

Moxon ER: Pathogenesis of invasive *Haemophilus influenzae* disease. Molecular basis of invasive *Haemophilus influenzae* type b disease. J Infect Dis 165(Suppl 1): S77, 1992. *Studies of mutant strains of* H. influenzae *have clarified the mechanisms of colonization, mucosal damage, translocation, and multiplication of the*

organism within the vascular system to reach concentrations necessary for CNS invasion.

Steinhart R, Reingold AL, Taylor F, et al.: Invasive *Haemophilus influenzae* infection in men with HIV infection. JAMA 268:3350, 1992. *A population-based study shows that the rates of invasive* H. influenzae *among men aged 20 to 49 with HIV infection without AIDS and with AIDS were 14.6 and 79.2 in 100,000 respectively.*

Osteomyelitis

283 OSTEOMYELITIS

Barry D. Brause

DEFINITION. Osteomyelitis is an infection by microorganisms that invade bone. Three pathogenetic routes of infection define the major forms of osteomyelitis, with pathogens reaching osseous tissue by (1) hematogenous seeding, (2) contamination accompanying surgical and nonsurgical trauma (termed "introduced" infection), or (3) spread from infected contiguous tissue.

ETIOLOGY. Although virtually all microorganisms can infect bone, bacteria are the usual pathogens, and staphylococci are the most prominent etiologic agents. *Staphylococcus aureus* causes ap-

proximately 60% of hematogenous and introduced infections and is a principal agent when osseous sepsis spreads by contiguity. *S. epidermidis* has become a major pathogen in bone infections associated with indwelling prosthetic materials, such as joint implants and fracture fixation devices, responsible for 30% of these cases. Streptococci, gram-negative bacilli, anaerobes, mycobacteria, and fungi are etiologic agents in a variety of clinical settings (Table 283–1).

INCIDENCE, PREVALENCE, AND EPIDEMIOLOGY. The anatomic location of hematogenous osteomyelitis is age-dependent (Table 283–1). From birth to puberty the long bones of the extremities are the most frequently involved. In adults blood-borne osteomyelitis generally affects the spine, because vertebrae become more vascular than other skeletal tissue with maturation. Seventy percent of compound fractures are contaminated, but because of effective debridement and perioperative antibiotic therapy only 2 to 9% develop infection. Osteomyelitis develops by contiguous spread in 30 to 68% of diabetic patients with foot ulcers, and it is notable

TABLE 283–1. PREDISPOSITIONS, ANATOMIC SITES, AND PROMINENT PATHOGENS IN FORMS OF OSTEOMYELITIS

Form of Osteomyelitis	Predisposing Condition	Site	Prominent Pathogens
Hematogenous			
Childhood	None	Long bones	*S. aureus* Streptococci *Hemophilus*
	Sickle cell hemoglobinopathy	Multiple	*Salmonella*
Adult	Urinary tract infection or instrumentation	Vertebral	GNB Streptococci
	Skin infection	Vertebral	*S. aureus* Streptococci
	Respiratory infection	Vertebral	Streptococci
	IV drug abuse, or vascular catheters	Vertebral	GNB Staphylococci *Candida*
	AIDS	Multiple	Fungi Mycobacteria
Introduced type	Fractures	Fracture site	*S. aureus* *S. epidermidis* GNB
	Prosthetic joint	Prosthesis	*S. epidermidis* *S. aureus*
Contiguous spread	Skin ulcer	Foot, leg	Polymicrobial Staphylococci Streptococci GNB Anaerobes
	Sinusitis	Skull	Streptococci Anaerobes
	Dental abscess	Mandible Maxilla	Streptococci Anaerobes
	Human or animal bites	Hand	Streptococci Anaerobes *Pasturella*
	Felon	Finger	*S. aureus*
	Gardening	Hand	*Sporothrix*

GNB = gram-negative bacilli.

that more in-hospital days are spent treating foot infections than any other complication of diabetes.

PATHOGENESIS. In childhood hematogenous osteomyelitis the initial infective site is the long bone metaphysis due to its large blood flow. In adults bacteremias seed vertebral bodies preferentially at the more vascular anterior end-plates. Osteomyelitis commonly involves two adjacent vertebral bodies and the intervertebral disc space. Infection compromises the nutrient supply to the intervertebral disc, resulting in disc necrosis and disc space narrowing, which is often the earliest sign of vertebral osteomyelitis (Fig. 283–1). Table 283–1 lists examples of clinical conditions that predispose to the development of blood-borne bone infection.

With the introduced form of osteomyelitis, direct septic trauma breaches all protective tissue around the bone, allowing microorganisms into the osseous matrix. The risk of infection is increased further when metallic fixation devices or prosthetic joints are implanted. Indwelling foreign bodies decrease the quantity of bacteria necessary to establish infection in bone and permit pathogens to persist on the surface of the avascular material, sequestered from circulating immune factors and systemic antibiotics. Osteomyelitis is caused by contiguous extension from infected, adjacent soft tissue when the soft tissue process is sufficiently chronic or uncontrolled (see Table 283–1).

Once infection becomes established in bone, the microorganisms induce local metabolic changes and inflammatory reactions that increase necrosis. As the septic process spreads, local thrombophlebitis develops, further increasing ischemia, which results in necrosis of large areas of bone called "sequestra" (Fig. 283–2). When the osseous cortex is breached, subperiosteal abscesses can develop with periosteal inflammation that induces new bone formation in adjacent soft tissue.

CLINICAL MANIFESTATIONS. In the classic presentation of childhood hematogenous osteomyelitis, fever, chills, and malaise are present but are frequently absent in the other forms of bone infection. Localized pain is a characteristic feature of osteomyelitis, with overlying erythema, warmth, and swelling variably observed. Limb motion may be limited if infection is near an articulation, and joint effusions can occur but are usually sterile when the epiphyseal cartilage is intact.

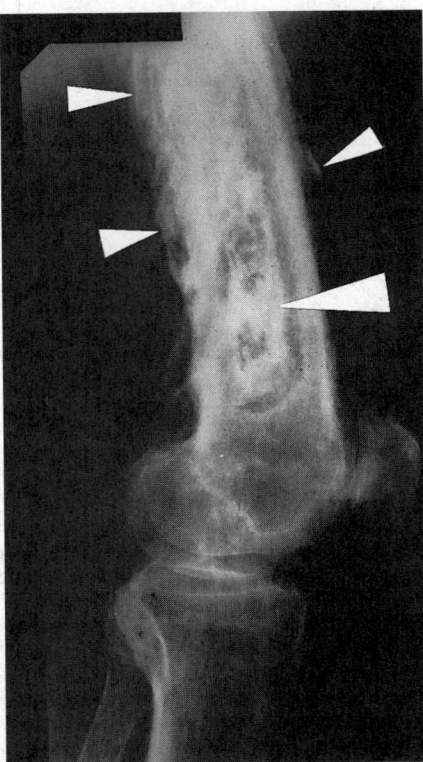

FIGURE 283–2. Femoral osteomyelitis. Hyperdense central zone is a sequestrum *(large arrowhead),* and peripheral linear densities are areas of periosteal elevation with periosteal new bone formation *(small arrowheads).*

Hematogenous vertebral osteomyelitis often presents with back pain, spine tenderness, and low-grade fever following urinary tract instrumentation or infection (30%), skin infection (13%), or respiratory infection (11%). The septic process extending beyond the vertebral column produces suppuration at the particular spinal level of infection such as retropharyngeal abscess, mediastinitis, empyema, subdiaphragmatic and iliopsoas abscesses, as well as meningitis. If paresis, sensory deficits, or bowel or bladder dysfunction develop, spinal epidural abscess—the most feared complication—should be suspected and evaluated immediately. *Mycobacterium tuberculosis* should be considered in relatively indolent infections of vertebrae (as well as at the hip and knee) (Table 283–1).

Osteomyelitis after trauma or bone surgery is usually associated with persistent or recurrent fevers, increasing pain at the operative site, and poor incisional healing, which is often accompanied by protracted wound drainage or dehiscence. Prosthetic joint infection presents with joint pain (95%), fever (43%), or cutaneous sinus drainage (32%).

Bone involvement by contiguous spread from an overlying chronic ischemic or neuropathic foot ulcer typically occurs in patients with longstanding insulin-dependent diabetes or other vascular disease and involves the metatarsals or the proximal phalanges. It is characterized by local cellulitis with inflammation and necrosis, but pain is only variably found due to the frequent presence of sensory neuropathy. Additional examples of osteomyelitis from contiguous spread of infection are listed in Table 283–1.

DIAGNOSIS. Diagnosis requires both confirming the osseous site of involvement and identifying the etiologic microbes. Bone infection must be differentiated from septic arthritis and bursitis, cellulitis and soft tissue abscesses, bone fractures, and neoplasms, as well as bone infarcts seen with sickle cell hemoglobinopathy and Gaucher's disease. Anatomic delineation of bone infection depends largely on radiologic techniques. In hematogenous infection, the earliest osseous changes by radiography are osteopenic or lytic lesions. They require 30 to 50% decalcification to be seen and take 2 to 4 weeks to develop. With further progression, periosteal elevation, thickening, and new bone formation are seen with sequestra and sclerotic changes occurring in chronic infection (see Fig. 283–2). Vertebral osteomyelitis appears initially as disc space nar-

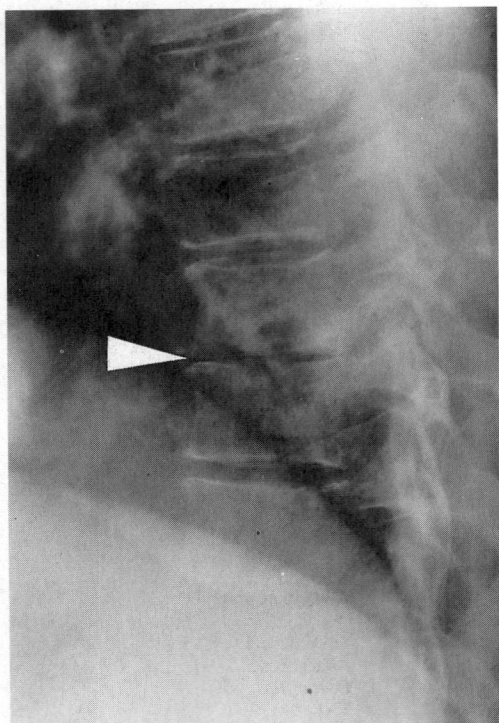

FIGURE 283–1. Vertebral osteomyelitis. Lateral view of spine illustrating disk space narrowing *(arrowhead)* and cortical destruction at the vertebral end-plates.

rowing followed by cortical destruction at the adjacent end-plates (see Fig. 283–1). Computed tomography (CT) is helpful to identify small osseous alterations and sequestra.

Technetium diphosphonate bone scans, gallium-citrate scans, and indium-labeled leukocyte scintigraphy are far more sensitive than radiography and usually reveal increased radionuclide uptake when symptoms begin. However, these techniques are plagued by inadequate specificity and spatial resolution, so they are not conclusively diagnostic. Inflammatory and degenerative processes in adjacent tissues, recent orthopedic surgery, bone fractures, and neoplasms produce abnormal scans in the absence of osteomyelitis. Magnetic resonance imaging (MRI) can detect osteomyelitis earlier than roentgenograms or CT scans with equivalent or greater sensitivity, specificity, and spatial resolution when compared with scintigraphic methods.

The exact microbial etiology of osteomyelitis should be determined, because it is never sufficiently predictable to permit routine presumptive therapy (see Table 283–1). Blood cultures are positive in 25 to 50% of acute childhood hematogenous osteomyelitis but are helpful in < 10% of the other forms of bone infection. When septic arthritis or soft tissue abscess accompanies the osseous process, arthrocentesis or abscess aspiration cultures can be diagnostic. However, superficial cultures of open wounds or skin ulcers and cultures of cutaneous sinus tracts do not delineate the true bone pathogen(s). In patients with deep chronic skin ulcers from which infection has spread to bone, curettage cultures from the base of the ulcer correlate with osseous tissue 75% of the time. Bone aspirate and biopsy cultures are positive in 70 to 93% of cases and should be sought (percutaneously or by operative debridement) when there is no overlying skin ulcer and the microbiologic diagnosis has not been otherwise established. Specimens for mycobacterial, fungal, and anaerobic cultivation should be considered when routine bacterial cultures are negative.

TREATMENT. Acute osteomyelitis is curable with adequate antimicrobial therapy and surgical debridement when necessary. Par-

enterally administered antibiotics are usually employed, but oral therapy is also effective when the pathogen is sufficiently susceptible and gastrointestinal absorption is ensured. The exact potency and duration of therapy required to eradicate bone infections are not known. Antibiotics that produce trough serum bactericidal activity at a 1:2 titer have been associated with high cure rates. Treatment should be given for 4 to 6 weeks. Surgery is indicated to drain abscesses, debride necrotic tissues, and remove foreign materials.

PROGNOSIS. Inadequate therapy of acute osteomyelitis results in relapsing infection and progression to chronic osteomyelitis; therefore, definitive treatment of acute infection is obligatory. Due to the presence of gross and microscopic foci of avascular bone, chronic osteomyelitis is not curable except by radical resection (occasionally amputation). Acute exacerbations of these chronic, recurrent infections can be suppressed successfully by debridement of identifiable sequestra followed by protracted courses of parenteral and oral antimicrobial agents.

Brause BD: Infected orthopedic prostheses. *In* Bisno AL, Waldvogel FA (eds.): Infections Associated with Indwelling Medical Devices. Washington, American Society for Microbiology, 1989, pp 111–127. *Detailed summary of the pathogenesis, microbiology, diagnosis, and treatment of osteomyelitis associated with prosthetic joints.*

Gold RH, Hawkins RA, Katz RD: Bacterial osteomyelitis: Findings on plain radiography, CT, MR, and scintigraphy. AJR 157:365, 1991. *Pictorial essay comparing all the different imaging techniques useful in diagnosing osteomyelitis.*

Norden CW (ed.): Osteomyelitis. Infect Dis Clin North Am 4:361, 1990. *A current and comprehensive evaluation of the epidemiology, clinical presentation, diagnosis, and therapy of osteomyelitis.*

Waldvogel FA, Medoff G, Swartz MN: Osteomyelitis: A review of clinical features, therapeutic considerations and unusual aspects, parts I, II, and III. N Engl J Med 282:198, 1970. *This detailed clinical description of the pathogenetic features of osteomyelitis remains best for in-depth understanding of the nature of these infections.*

Weinstein M, Stratton C, Hawley HB, et al.: Multicenter collaborative evaluation of a standardized serum bactericidal test as a predictor of therapeutic efficacy in acute and chronic osteomyelitis. Am J Med 83:218, 1987. *The best data collection for defining quantitatively effective antibiotic therapy for osteomyelitis.*

---

284 WHOOPING COUGH (Pertussis)

Richard B. Johnston, Jr.

DEFINITION. Whooping cough (synonym, pertussis) is a noninvasive, highly communicable bacterial respiratory illness. It occurs at all ages but is most common and most severe in infants and young children. The etiologic agent of the syndrome is usually *Bordetella pertussis*. The descriptive name derives from a distressing, prolonged inspiratory effort that follows paroxysmal coughing. Whooping cough is estimated to cause 500,000 deaths yearly, primarily in infants.

ETIOLOGY. When first isolated, *B. pertussis* is a small, nonmotile, weakly staining, gram-negative coccobacillus, 0.5 to 1.0 μ in length. Capsules can be demonstrated by special procedures, and bipolar metachromatic granules are present. The complex medium containing blood originally employed by Bordet and Gengou is still used (in modified form) for cultivation. *Primary isolates do not grow on conventional laboratory media.*

An estimated 5 to 10% of clinical whooping cough is caused by *B. parapertussis.* The animal pathogen *B. bronchiseptica* is responsible for a minor percentage of cases. These organisms can be differentiated from *B. pertussis* by growth requirements, enzyme production, and presence of species-specific antigens. It has been suggested that adenoviruses, alone or in concert with *B. pertussis,* and *Chlamydia trachomatis* may play an etiologic role in some cases of whooping cough.

EPIDEMIOLOGY. In nonimmune households the attack rate is 80 to 90%. Transmission is by droplet infection. Carriers of *B. per-*

Whooping Cough

tussis are found infrequently, but persons previously immunized have been shown during outbreaks of disease to excrete the organism in the absence of clinical symptoms or in the presence of mild or atypical illness.

The mortality rate from whooping cough has fallen since the beginning of the twentieth century owing to improved supportive therapy. The incidence of whooping cough, however, did not change until after the 1940's, when immunization of young children became standard practice. In the 1940's, approximately 200,000 cases of pertussis were reported annually in the United States, compared with about 5000 cases annually in recent years. Most deaths occur in children under 1 year of age. The case fatality rate in infants under 6 months of age is 1%.

Neither immunization against pertussis nor natural disease provides lifelong protection. In the case of immunization, an attack rate greater than 50% has been reported when the interval after immunization exceeds 12 years. Adolescents and adults represent a large reservoir of susceptibles who can transmit the disease to unimmunized infants, and pertussis is an important cause of persistent cough in adults.

PATHOGENESIS. *B. pertussis* adheres to ciliated epithelial cells of the respiratory tract and multiplies there without invading the tissues. Yet this colonization leads to profound changes in tissues which persist long after the responsible bacteria have been cleared. Such observations suggest that a toxin or toxins from the bacteria play an important part in the pathogenesis of the syndrome. A variety of biologic activities have been demonstrated by injecting *B. pertussis* products into experimental animals. An endotoxin and a heat-labile toxin that can cause tissue necrosis have been identified among these bacterial factors, but the exotoxin *pertussis toxin* (PT) is the best candidate at the moment for a major virulence factor. Immunization with chemically detoxified PT appears to prevent severe whooping cough with an efficacy similar to that achieved with the standard cellular vaccine. PT is believed to be responsible for the characteristic lymphocytosis of whooping cough.

PT is a protein composed of five noncovalently linked subunits (S1–S5). The subunits S2–S5 form a nontoxic unit that binds to the cell membrane; toxicity is mediated by the enzymatically active subunit, S1. Activity of S1 inhibits a subclass of guanosine triphosphate (GTP)–binding proteins (G proteins) that are essential for transmembrane signaling and, thus, certain types of receptor-mediated cell functions.

Adherence of *B. pertussis* to respiratory epithelium is required for the pathogenesis of whooping cough. Adherence appears to involve a bacterial outer membrane protein with a molecular weight of 69 kilodaltons, termed pertactin. An antigenically similar protein exists on *B. parapertussis* and *B. bronchiseptica*. Injection of this protein into mice or humans elicits agglutinating antibody to *B. pertussis* and protects the mice against lethal *B. pertussis* respiratory challenge. Synthesis of pertactin is controlled by a regulatory gene at the *vir* (virulence) locus, which modulates synthesis of PT and additional factors that may contribute to pathogenesis, including filamentous hemagglutinin.

PATHOLOGY. Lesions caused by *B. pertussis* are found principally in the bronchi and bronchioles, but changes are also seen in the nasopharynx, larynx, and trachea. Masses of bacteria and mucopurulent exudate are intertwined with the cilia of the columnar epithelium. There is necrosis of the midzonal and basilar epithelium with infiltration of polymorphonuclear leukocytes and macrophages. The most frequent findings in the lung are bronchopneumonia, interstitial pneumonitis, and numerous small areas of atelectasis. The brain can show edema and scattered petechiae at autopsy.

CLINICAL MANIFESTATIONS. The incubation period lasts 7 to 14 days (rarely over 2 weeks). It is customary to divide the clinical course into three stages.

Catarrhal Stage. Whooping cough begins with symptoms indistinguishable from those of a mild viral upper respiratory infection. Sneezing is frequent, conjunctivae are injected, and a nocturnal cough appears. The temperature may be slightly elevated. Infectivity is greatest at this stage.

Paroxysmal Stage. Seven to 14 days after onset, the cough becomes more frequent, then paroxysmal. In a typical paroxysm there is a series of 5 to 20 short coughs of increasing intensity and then a deep inspiration, making the "whoop." A tenacious mucus plug is usually expelled, and vomiting frequently follows. Paroxysms may occur as often as every half hour and are accompanied by signs of increased venous pressure, including deeply engorged conjunctivae, periorbital edema, petechial hemorrhages, particularly about the forehead, and epistaxis. During the attack, the infant may be cyanotic until the crowing whoop occurs. Between paroxysms, the child usually feels well, although justifiably apprehensive. This phase lasts 2 to 4 weeks.

Physical examination of the chest is often unremarkable except for scattered rhonchi. The chest roentgenogram sometimes reveals hilar and mediastinal nodal enlargement. The presence of fever should immediately suggest the development a secondary infectious process.

Convalescent Stage. Gradually the paroxysms become less frequent and less intense; vomiting ceases, and slow recovery ensues. Convalescence requires 4 to 12 weeks. For many months even a mild, unrelated respiratory infection can induce a return of paroxysmal cough and whoop.

In infants younger than 6 months old, the paroxysms and the whoop are often absent; choking spells and apneic episodes may be the major manifestations. Second attacks of whooping cough as well as disease occurring in previously immunized individuals often present simply as an upper respiratory illness or bronchitis.

Complications. Recurrent vomiting can lead to metabolic alkalosis or malnutrition. Central nervous system changes can result from cerebral anoxia or hemorrhages consequent to the elevated venous pressure. Rarely, cortical degeneration occurs, but the exact pathogenesis of the encephalopathy is unknown. A serous meningitis with lymphocytosis of the cerebrospinal fluid has been described. Pneumothorax and interstitial emphysema are infrequently seen. Secondary bacterial otitis media occurs frequently. The major cause of death in whooping cough is pneumonia, either primary or caused by other bacteria or viruses.

DIAGNOSIS. There is little difficulty in making the clinical diagnosis of whooping cough in a patient who, after a period of coryzal symptoms, develops paroxysmal coughing with a terminal inspiratory whoop. Lymphocytosis often occurs toward the end of the catarrhal stage or early in the spasmodic phase. Characteristically the leukocyte count ranges from 15,000 to 30,000 per microliter or higher, and 80% of the cells are small lymphocytes. Polymorphonuclear leukocytosis suggests a secondary bacterial complication.

Microbiologic identification of the organisms may be required to make the diagnosis in abortive or mild cases or in young infants. During the early stages, *B. pertussis* can be isolated from approximately 90% of patients. By the third or fourth week, the organism can be recovered in only 50% of cases, and in the convalescent stage it is unusual to obtain a positive culture.

Specimens for culture are best obtained by pernasal swab rather than by the cough plate method. A sterile cotton swab wrapped about a flexible copper wire is passed through the nares, and mucus is obtained from the posterior pharynx. *B. pertussis* is readily killed by desiccation, so the specimen should be quickly plated onto fresh medium, to which antibiotic has been added to prevent overgrowth of adventitious organisms.

A fluorescent antibody staining procedure can be applied directly to clinical specimens or organisms grown in culture, but false-positive and false-negative results are relatively common. Probes for *B. pertussis* DNA are available.

Serologic procedures are of little help in diagnosing whooping cough because a rise in titer of most antibodies does not occur until at least the third week of illness. Tests have not been well standardized.

TREATMENT. *Supportive Therapy.* Young infants, particularly those younger than 6 months of age, should be hospitalized. Supportive measures combined with careful nursing care are of paramount importance. Specific attention must be devoted to the maintenance of proper water and electrolyte balance, adequate nutrition, and sufficient oxygenation. Constant alertness for the presence of secondary infectious complications such as pneumonia is required. Mild cases require only supportive treatment.

Antimicrobials. Specific therapy of severe whooping cough has been disappointing despite the *in vitro* susceptibility of *B. pertussis* to various antimicrobial agents. Antimicrobials given in the catarrhal stage may ameliorate the disease. In the established paroxysmal stage, the organisms can be readily eliminated by antimicrobials, but the course of the illness is unaltered. Antibiotics may be justified in order to render the patient noninfectious. Erythromycin is the drug of choice. The daily dose is 50 mg per kilogram of body weight given in four divided doses. The organism is eliminated after a few days of therapy, but because bacteriologic relapse may occur, treatment should be continued for 14 days. Trimethoprim-sulfamethoxazole (8 mg per kilogram and 40 mg per kilogram per day in two doses) is a possible alternative for patients who do not tolerate erythromycin.

PREVENTION. Unfortunately, the diagnosis is usually not made until the end of the catarrhal stage, and by then, spread of the disease has already occurred. Exposed susceptibles should receive erythromycin prophylaxis for 14 days, and close (household, day care, classroom) contacts younger than 7 who have been previously immunized should receive a booster dose of vaccine in addition to erythromycin. Booster doses of vaccine or erythromycin chemoprophylaxis have been used to protect adults, such as hospital staff.

Active Immunization. Women of childbearing age generally do not have significant levels of protective antibody in their sera, and most newborns have received no passive protection. Consequently, active immunization is begun as early as is practicable. At present, it is recommended that the infant receive three injections of pertussis vaccine (inactive *B. pertussis* organisms) at 8-week intervals commencing at age 2 months. The pertussis suspension is mixed with alum-precipitated diphtheria and tetanus toxoids (DTP). A fourth injection is given 6 to 12 months after the third dose (15 to 18 months of age), and a booster is given before entering kindergarten. Administration of pertussis vaccine to those over age 6 is not generally recommended.

As previously noted, immunization does not confer lifelong protection. Approximately 80% of those vaccinated within 4 years of exposure are protected, whereas 80 to 90% of a matched unimmunized group with similar exposure contract pertussis. The prophylactic efficacy of pertussis vaccine was clearly demonstrated when epidemics occurred in the United Kingdom in 1977–79 and

1982 following a 3- to 5-year period during which vaccine acceptance had declined to very low levels. More than 170,000 cases of whooping cough were reported, including 42 deaths, principally among children under age 5. Similar outbreaks have followed diminished vaccine utilization in Japan and Sweden.

Reactions at the injection site as well as fever and hyperirritability occur commonly after injection of whole-cell pertussis vaccine. The incidence of postinjection acute encephalopathy is uncertain but apparently rare, and it is not clear whether administering DTP vaccine increases the overall risk in children of chronic nervous system dysfunction. It is clear that the risk of neurologic complications from pertussis immunization is far less than the hazards of whooping cough in the young child. Nevertheless, in infants with a personal history of convulsions or other neurologic disorders, pertussis immunization should be deferred until the condition has stabilized.

Acellular vaccines containing various combinations of pertussis toxin, pertactin, filamentous hemagglutinin, or other *B. pertussis* products are being studied for use in infants and adults, and one has been approved for the fourth and fifth injections. Acellular vaccines cause far fewer reactions than does the whole bacterial cell vaccine. If tests currently under way of their immunogenicity and prophylactic efficacy are convincing in field use, acellular vaccines should replace the killed whole-cell vaccine.

Edwards KM, Decker MD, Graham BS, et al.: Adult immunization with acellular pertussis vaccine. JAMA 269:53, 1993. *A report of the immunogenicity and safety of the new vaccine in adults.*
Gale JL, Thapa PB, Wassilak SGF, et al.: Risk of serious acute neurological illness after immunization with diphtheria-tetanus-pertussis vaccine. JAMA 271:37, 1994. *A careful (and unrevealing) population-based case-control study. Accompanying editorial on page 68.*
Howson CP, Howe CJ, Fineberg HV (eds.): Adverse Effects of Pertussis and Rubella Vaccines. Washington, National Academy Press, 1991. *A scientific, fully referenced review by the Institute of Medicine of DTP immunization and possible adverse events.*
Pittman M: The concept of pertussis as a toxin-mediated disease. Pediatr Infect Dis J 3:467, 1984. *A thorough, now classic review of pathogenesis, immunity, and immunization.*
Stratton KR, Howe CJ, Johnston RB Jr (eds.): DPT Vaccine and Chronic Nervous System Dysfunction: A new Analysis. Washington, National Academy Press, 1994. *A re-evaluation of this relationship by the Institute of Medicine.*

Diphtheria

285 DIPHTHERIA
Iain R. B. Hardy

Diphtheria is an acute communicable disease caused by *Corynebacterium diphtheriae*. The organism chiefly infects the respiratory tract, where it causes tonsillopharyngitis and/or laryngitis, classically with a pseudomembrane, and the skin, causing a variety of indolent lesions. If the infecting strain produces exotoxin, myocarditis and neuritis may ensue.

ETIOLOGY. *C. diphtheriae* is an aerobic, nonmotile, unencapsulated, nonsporulating, pleomorphic gram-positive bacillus. Its name comes from the Greek *korynee* ("club"), describing the shape of the organism on stained smears, and *diphtheria* ("leather hide"), for the characteristic adherent membrane. Both nontoxigenic and toxigenic strains exist. Toxigenicity is conferred when a nontoxigenic organism is infected by a β-phage carrying the gene for the toxin *(tox)*. *C. diphtheriae* has three biotypes, *gravis, mitis,* and *intermedius,* which are distinguished by colonial morphology and varying biochemical and hemolytic reactions. Strains may be distinguished for epidemiologic purposes by molecular techniques. There are a few reports of classic diphtheria, including toxic complications, due to infection with *C. ulcerans.*

EPIDEMIOLOGY. Humans are the only natural reservoir of *C. diphtheriae.* Spread occurs in close-contact settings via respiratory droplets or by direct contact with respiratory secretions or skin lesions. The organism survives for weeks on environmental surfaces and in dust, and fomite transmission may occur. Approximately one in seven individuals with nasopharyngeal infection develops clinical disease; asymptomatic carriers are important in transmission. Diphtheria immunization protects against disease but does not prevent carriage. In the prevaccine era, respiratory disease dominated in temperate climates, with a fall/winter peak in incidence, and most individuals developed natural immunity by adulthood. Cutaneous disease was primarily a problem in tropical countries, but over the last two decades, outbreaks of this form of diphtheria have occurred in the United States and Europe, typically among homeless and alcoholic inner-city adults.

Vaccination with diphtheria toxoid (formalin-treated toxin) was introduced in the 1920's and 1930's. Immunization of children in an era when the majority of older individuals had natural immunity resulted in a dramatic drop in diphtheria incidence and an even more rapid decline in the proportion of toxigenic strains isolated. This is believed to be because the selective advantage of the *tox* gene—promotion of greater replication and spread of the organism—is lost in the immune host. Currently in most Western countries, toxigenic *C. diphtheriae* has been virtually eliminated. In the United States, reported cases fell from 147,991 in 1920, to 15,536 in 1940, to a total of 40 cases from 1980–1993. Since 1988, all culture-confirmed cases have been caused by imported strains.

Vaccine-induced immunity to diphtheria wanes with time, and there is a growing cohort of individuals with no natural diphtheria immunity. Serosurveys indicate that 20 to 60% of adults in developed countries have antitoxin levels below 0.01 IU per milliliter, which is considered the lower limit of protection. As long as a high proportion of the population remains susceptible, the danger of reintroduction or re-emergence of toxigenic strains exists. Since 1990 there has been a major resurgence of diphtheria in several countries of the former Soviet Union. In Russia, the number of reported cases rose from 603 in 1989 to approximately 40,000 in 1994, with over two-thirds of cases among adults.

PATHOGENESIS. In classic diphtheria, *C. diphtheriae* colonizes the mucosal surface of the nasopharynx and multiplies locally without bloodstream invasion. Released toxin causes local tissue necrosis, and a tough, adherent pseudomembrane forms, composed of a mixture of fibrin, dead cells, and bacteria. The membrane usually begins on the tonsils or posterior pharynx. In more severe cases it spreads, extending progressively over the pharyngeal wall, fauces, soft palate, and into the larynx, which may result in respiratory obstruction. Toxin entering the bloodstream causes tissue damage at distant sites, particularly the heart (myocarditis), nerves (demyelination), and kidney (tubular necrosis). Nontoxigenic strains may cause mild local respiratory disease, sometimes including a membrane.

Diphtheria toxin is an extremely potent inhibitor of protein synthesis, with an estimated human lethal dose of 0.1 μg per kilogram of body weight. The extent of toxin absorption varies with site of infection, being much less from skin or nose than from the pharynx.

CLINICAL MANIFESTATIONS. *Respiratory Diphtheria.* Infection limited to the anterior nares manifests as a chronic serosanguineous or seropurulent discharge without fever or significant toxicity. A whitish membrane may be observed on the septum. The faucial (pharyngeal) form is most common. After an incubation period of from 1 to 7 days, the illness begins with a sore throat, malaise, and mild to moderate fever. There is initial mild pharyngeal erythema, usually followed by progressive formation of a whitish tonsilar exudate, which over 24 to 48 hours changes into a grayish membrane that is tightly adherent and bleeds on attempted removal. In more severe cases, the patient appears toxic, and the membrane is more extensive. Cervical adenopathy and soft-tissue edema may occur, resulting in the so-called bull neck and stridor. Laryngeal involvement, which may occur on its own or as a result of membrane extension from the nasopharynx, presents with hoarseness, stridor, and dyspnea.

The likelihood of toxic complications depends on the severity of disease at presentation and the interval between disease onset and administration of antitoxin. Myocarditis typically occurs between 1 and 2 weeks after the onset of respiratory symptoms and presents either suddenly or insidiously with signs of low cardiac output and congestive failure. Conduction disturbances, which may occur without other signs of myocarditis, include ST-T wave abnormalities, arrhythmias, and heart block. Neurologic impairment manifests as cranial nerve palsies and peripheral neuritis. Palatal and/or pharyngeal paralysis occurs during the acute phase; peripheral neuritis, symmetrical and predominantly motor, occurs from 2 to 12 weeks after disease onset. Motor deficit may range from minor proximal weakness to complete paralysis. Complete recovery is the rule. In fulminant, sometimes called "hypertoxic," diphtheria, toxic circulatory collapse with hemorrhagic features occurs.

In the United States, the diphtheria case-fatality rate has remained 5 to 10% over recent decades.

Cutaneous diphtheria lesions are classically indolent, deep, punched-out ulcers, which may have a grayish white membrane. However, the lesions may be indistinguishable from impetigo, or *C. diphtheriae* may infect chronic dermatoses, such as stasis dermatitis. There is frequently coinfection with *Streptococcus pyogenes* and/or *Staphylococcus aureus*. Toxic complications are rare.

Uncommonly, *C. diphtheriae,* both toxigenic and nontoxigenic, may cause *invasive disease,* including endocarditis, osteomyelitis, septic arthritis, and meningitis. Frequently, but not always, these patients have predisposing factors such as a prosthetic cardiac valve or underlying immunosuppression.

DIAGNOSIS. The decision to initiate therapy should be made on clinical grounds, since delayed treatment is associated with worse outcomes. A high index of suspicion is required. Cultures should be taken from beneath the membrane, from the nasopharynx, and from any suspicious skin lesions. Because special media are required, the laboratory should be alerted to the concern about diphtheria. *C. diphtheriae* is best isolated on selective media that inhibit the growth of other nasopharyngeal organisms; generally one containing potassium tellurite is used. Based on colonial morphology and Gram stain appearance, a presumptive diagnosis may be possible within 18 to 24 hours. Cultures may be negative if the patient received previous antibiotics. Toxigenicity testing should be performed on all *C. diphtheriae* isolates. Because both nontoxigenic and toxigenic strains may be isolated from the same patient, more than one colony should be tested. Traditional methods include guinea pig inoculation and the Elek test, where the isolate and appropriate controls are streaked on a culture plate in which a filter strip soaked with antitoxin has been embedded; toxin production is confirmed by an immunoprecipitation line in the agar. A recently developed polymerase chain reaction (PCR) test may allow both detection of the organism and determination of toxigenicity.

The differential diagnosis includes streptococcal and viral tonsillopharyngitis, infectious mononucleosis, Vincent's angina, candidiasis, and acute epiglottitis. A history of travel to a region with endemic diphtheria or of contact with a recent immigrant from such an area increases the possibility of diphtheria, as does a pre-antitoxin treatment serum antitoxin level of <0.01 IU per milliliter.

TREATMENT AND PREVENTION. Treatment goals are to neutralize toxin, eliminate the infecting organism, provide supportive care, and prevent further transmission. The mainstay of therapy is equine diphtheria antitoxin. Because only unbound toxin can be neutralized, treatment should commence as soon as the diagnosis is suspected. A single dose is given, ranging in quantity from 20,000 units for localized tonsillar diphtheria up to 100,000 units for extensive disease with severe toxicity. Antitoxin may be given intramuscularly or intravenously; particularly for more severe cases, the intravenous route is preferred. Tests for sensitivity to antitoxin should be performed before administering it and desensitization performed if necessary. Antibiotic therapy, by eliminating the organism, halts toxin production, limits local infection, and prevents transmission. Parenteral penicillin (4 to 6 million units per day) and erythromycin (40 mg per kilogram per day in 4 divided doses; maximum, 2 grams per day, usually orally if the patient can swallow) are the drugs of choice. General supportive care includes ensuring a secure airway, electrocardiographic monitoring for evidence of myocarditis, treating heart failure and arrhythmias, and preventing secondary complications of neurologic impairment such as aspiration pneumonia. The patient should be in strict isolation until follow-up cultures are negative. Convalescent patients should receive diphtheria toxoid.

The local health department must be notified. Close contacts should be cultured and commenced on prophylactic antibiotics. A positive culture in a contact may confirm the diagnosis if the patient is culture-negative. All contacts without full primary immunization and a booster within the preceding 5 years should receive diphtheria toxoid.

Immunization with diphtheria toxoid is the only effective means of prevention. The primary series is four doses of diphtheria toxoid (given with tetanus toxoid and pertussis vaccine) at 2, 4, 6, and 12 to 18 months; a booster is given at ages 4 to 6 years. Thereafter, Td (tetanus and diphtheria toxoid for adults) boosters should be given every 10 years, from the fifteenth birthday.

Dixon JMS, Noble WC, Smith GR: Diphtheria; other corynebacterial and coryneform infections. *In* Topley WWC, Parker MT, Collier L, et al. (eds.): Topley and Wilson's Principles of Bacteriology. 8th ed. Philadelphia, BC Becker, 1990, pp 56–75. *A useful review with especially comprehensive epidemiologic data.*
Farizo KM, Strebel PS, Chen RT, et al.: Fatal respiratory disease due to *Corynebacterium diphtheriae:* Case report and review of guidelines for management, investigation, and control. Clin Infect Dis 16:59, 1993. *Includes latest recommendations of the United States Centers for Disease Control and Prevention for case and contact management.*
Harnisch JP, Tronca E, Nolan CM, et al.: Diphtheria among alcoholic urban adults: A decade of experience in Seattle. Ann Intern Med 111:71, 1989. *Summary of last major outbreak of diphtheria in the United States.*
Pappenheimer AM: Diphtheria: Studies on the Biology of an Infectious Disease. The Harvey Lectures. New York, Academic Press, 1982, series 76, pp 45–73. *Detailed description of the cellular and molecular biology of diphtheria toxin.*

Clostridial Disease

286 CLOSTRIDIAL MYONECROSIS AND OTHER CLOSTRIDIAL DISEASES
Dennis L. Stevens

The genus *Clostridium* encompasses over 60 species of gram-positive anaerobic spore-forming rods that cause a variety of infections in humans and animals by virtue of a myriad of proteinaceous exotoxins (Table 286–1). *C. tetanii* and *C. botulinum* manifest specific clinical disease by elaborating single, but highly potent, toxins.

Though botulism is usually the result of ingestion of preformed toxin, tetanus requires the bacteria to proliferate at the site of penetrating injury (see Ch. 288 and 289). Frequently, signs of infection are not apparent even with lethal exotoxinemia. In contrast, other strains of clostridia, such as *C. perfringens* and *C. septicum,* cause aggressive necrotizing infections, attributable, in part, to bacterial proteases and cytotoxins.

CLOSTRIDIAL GAS GANGRENE

TYPES. Clostridial gas gangrene, or myonecrosis, occurs in three different settings. First, and most commonly, traumatic gas gangrene develops after deep, penetrating injury that compromises the blood supply (e.g., knife or gunshot wound, crush injury), creating an anaerobic environment ideal for clostridial proliferation. *C. perfringens* accounts for 80% of such infections. The remaining cases are caused by *C. septicum, C. novyii, C. histolyticum,*

TABLE 286–1. CLINICAL DISEASES CAUSED BY CLOSTRIDIA

Organism	Clinical Diagnosis	Clinical Features	Laboratory Features	Toxins
		Invasive Infections		
C. perfringens type a	Traumatic gas gangrene	Pain, necrotizing infection, renal impairment, shock	• Renal failure • ↑ CPK • Gas in tissues	α toxin θ toxin
C. septicum	Spontaneous gas gangrene	Pain, necrotizing infection, bowel portal	• Renal failure • ↑ CPK • Gas in tissues	α toxin
C. sordellii	Malignant edema	No pain, no fever, massive third spacing	• Leukomoid reaction • Hemoconcentration	?
C. tertium	Bacteremia in compromised hosts receiving antibiotics	Bacteremia, shock	• Positive blood cultures	?
		Gastrointestinal		
C. perfringens type a	Food poisoning	Nausea, vomiting, watery diarrhea	None	Enterotoxin
C. perfringens type c	Necrotizing enterocolitis	Bloody diarrhea, ruptured bowel	None	β toxin
C. septicum	Neutropenic enterocolitis, "typhlitis"	RLQ pain, abdominal distention	• Low white count	Unknown
C. difficile	Pseudomembranous colitis	Water, bloody diarrhea	• Stools positive for organism, toxin, blood and leukocytes	Toxin A Toxin B
		Neurologic		
C. tetanii	Tetanus	Spastic paralysis	None	Tetanospasmin
C. botulinum	Botulism	Flaccid paralysis	None	Botulinum toxin (A,B,E,F,G)

C. bifermentans, and *C. fallax.* Other conditions associated with traumatic gas gangrene are bowel and biliary tract surgery, criminal abortion, and retained placenta; prolonged rupture of the membranes; or intrauterine fetal demise or missed abortion in postpartum patients. Secondly, spontaneous or nontraumatic gas gangrene is most commonly caused by the more aerotolerant *C. septicum.* Lastly, recurrent gas gangrene caused by *C. perfringens* has been described in individuals with nonpenetrating injuries at sites of previous gas gangrene, where spores of *C. perfringens* remain quiescent in tissue for periods of 10 to 20 years and then germinate when minor trauma provides conditions suitable for growth.

TRAUMATIC GAS GANGRENE

CLINICAL MANIFESTATIONS. The first symptom is usually sudden and severe pain at the site of surgery or trauma. The mean incubation period is less than 24 hours but ranges from 6 to 8 hours to several days, probably depending on the degree of soil contamination or bowel spillage and degree of vascular compromise. The skin may appear pale initially but quickly changes to bronze and then purplish red and becomes tense and exquisitely tender. Bullae develop; they may be clear, red, blue, or purple. Gas present in tissue may be obvious by physical examination, soft tissue radiographs, or computed tomographic (CT) scan. Signs of systemic toxicity develop rapidly, including tachycardia, low-grade fever, and diaphoresis, followed by shock and multiorgan failure. Bacteremia occurs in 15% of patients and is usually associated with brisk hemolysis. Patients have been described with hematocrits of 0% for as long as 24 hours. Complications include jaundice, renal failure, hypotension, and liver necrosis. Renal failure is largely due to hemoglobinuria and myoglobinuria but complicated by acute tubular necrosis following hypotension. Renal tubular cells are likely directly affected by toxins, but this has not been proven.

DIAGNOSIS. Increasing pain at the site of prior injury or surgery, together with signs of systemic toxicity and gas in the tissue, supports the diagnosis. Definitive diagnosis rests on demonstrating large, gram-variable rods at the injury site. Note that although clostridia stain gram-positive when obtained from bacteriologic media, when visualized from infected tissues, they appear both gram-positive and gram-negative. Surgical exploration is essential and demonstrates muscle that does not bleed or contract when stimulated. Grossly, muscle tissue is edematous and may have a reddish blue to black coloration. Usually, necrotizing fasciitis and cutaneous necrosis are also present. Microscopic evaluation of biopsy material invariably demonstrates organisms among degener-

ating muscle bundles and, characteristically, an absence of acute inflammatory cells.

PATHOGENESIS. The initiating trauma introduces organisms (either vegetative forms or spores) into the deep tissues and produces an anaerobic niche with a sufficiently low redox potential and acid pH for optimal clostridial growth. Necrosis progresses within hours. At the junction of necrotic and normal tissues, no polymorphonuclear leukocytes (PMNL's) are present, yet pavementing of PMNL's is apparent within capillaries and in small arterioles and postcapillary venules, followed later in the course by leukostasis within larger vessels. Thus the histopathology of clostridial gas gangrene is completely opposite to that seen in soft tissue infections caused by organisms such as *Staphylococcus aureus,* in which an early luxuriant influx of PMNL's localizes the infection without adjacent tissue or vascular destruction.

Recent studies suggest that theta toxin, when elaborated in high concentrations at the site of infection, destroys host tissues and inflammatory cells. As the toxin diffuses into surrounding tissues or enters systemic circulation, it promotes dysregulated PMNL–endothelial cell adhesive interactions and primes leukocytes for increased respiratory burst activity. These actions lead to vascular leukostasis, endothelial cell injury, and regional tissue hypoxia. Such perfusion deficits expand the anaerobic environment and contribute to the rapidly advancing margins of tissue destruction that are characteristic of clostridial gangrene.

Shock associated with gas gangrene may be attributable, in part, to direct and indirect effects of toxins. Alpha toxin directly suppresses myocardial contractility *ex vivo* and may contribute to profound hypotension via a sudden reduction in cardiac output. Theta toxin contributes indirectly by inducing endogenous mediators that cause relaxation of blood vessel wall tension such as nitric oxide or the lipid autocoids, prostacyclin, or platelet-activating factor. Reduced vascular tone develops rapidly, and in order to maintain adequate tissue perfusion, a compensatory host response is required which either increases cardiac output or rapidly expands the intravascular blood volume. Patients with gram-negative sepsis markedly increase cardiac output; however, this may not be possible in *C. perfringens*–induced shock due to direct suppression of myocardial contractility by alpha toxin. The role of other endogenous mediators such as cytokines (e.g., tumor necrosis factor, interleukin-1, interleukin-6), as well as the potent endogenous vasodilator bradykinin, has not been elucidated.

TREATMENT. Penicillin, clindamycin, tetracycline, chloramphenicol, metronidazole, and a number of cephalosporins have excellent *in vitro* activity against *C. perfringens* and other clostridia.

No clinical trials have been conducted to compare the efficacy of these agents in humans. Experimental studies in mice suggest that clindamycin has the greatest efficacy and penicillin the least. Slightly greater survival was observed in animals receiving both clindamycin and penicillin; in contrast, antagonism was observed with penicillin plus metronidazole. Resistance of some strains to clindamycin suggests a combination of penicillin and clindamycin is warranted.

Aggressive surgical debridement is mandatory to improve survival and prevent complications. The use of hyperbaric oxygen (HBO) is controversial, though some nonrandomized studies have reported excellent results with HBO therapy when combined with antibiotics and surgical debridement. Experimental studies demonstrate slight benefit of HBO when combined with penicillin, though survivals were greater with clindamycin alone.

Therapeutic strategies directed against toxin expression *in vivo*, such as neutralization with specific antitoxin antibody or inhibiting toxin synthesis, may be valuable adjuncts to traditional antimicrobial regimens. Future strategies may target endogenous proadhesive molecules such that toxin-induced vascular leukostasis and resultant tissue injury are attenuated.

PROGNOSIS. Patients presenting with gas gangrene of an extremity have a better prognosis than those with truncal or intra-abdominal gas gangrene, largely because it is difficult to adequately debride such lesions. HBO could be useful in such patients, yet there are little data on this subject. In addition to truncal gangrene, patients with associated bacteremia and intravascular hemolysis have the greatest likelihood of progressing to shock and death.

PREVENTION. Aggressive debridement of devitalized tissue, as well as rapid repair of compromised vascular supply, greatly reduces the frequency of gas gangrene in contaminated deep wounds. Intramuscular epinephrine, prolonged application of tourniquets, and surgical closure of traumatic wounds should be avoided. Patients with contaminated wounds should receive prophylactic antibiotics.

SPONTANEOUS, NONTRAUMATIC GAS GANGRENE DUE TO *CLOSTRIDIUM SEPTICUM*

CLINICAL MANIFESTATIONS. The onset of disease is abrupt, often with excruciating pain, although the patient may sense only heaviness or numbness. The first symptom may be confusion or malaise. Extremely rapid progression of gangrene follows. Swelling advances, and blisters appear filled with clear, cloudy, hemorrhagic, or purplish fluid. The skin around such bullae also has a purple hue, perhaps reflecting vascular compromise resulting from bacterial toxins diffusing into surrounding tissues. Histopathology of muscle and connective tissues includes cell lysis and gas formation; inflammatory cells are remarkably absent.

Predisposing factors include colonic carcinoma, diverticulitis, gastrointestinal (GI) surgery, leukemia, lymphoproliferative disorders, and either chemotherapy or radiation therapy. Cyclic neutropenia is also associated with spontaneous gas gangrene due to *C. septicum*, and in such cases, necrotizing enterocolitis, cecitis, or distal ileitis are commonly found. These GI pathologies permit bacterial access to the bloodstream; consequently, the aerotolerant *C. septicum* can become established in normal tissues. Patients surviving bacteremia or spontaneous gangrene due to *C. septicum* should have appropriate diagnostic studies of the GI tract to rule out pathology in this area.

DIAGNOSIS. Unlike traumatic gas gangrene, bacteremia precedes cutaneous manifestations by several hours, causing delays in the appropriate diagnosis and, as a consequence, an increase in the mortality rate.

PATHOGENESIS. *C. septicum* produces four toxins—alpha toxin (α, lethal, hemolytic, necrotizing activity), beta toxin (β, DNase), gamma toxin (γ, hyaluronidase), and delta toxin (Δ, septicolysin, an oxygen-labile hemolysin)—as well as a protease and a neuraminidase. This alpha toxin does not possess phospholipase activity and is thus distinct from the alpha toxin of *C. perfringens*. Active immunization against alpha toxin significantly protects against challenge with viable *C. septicum*. The mechanism by which alpha toxin contributes to *C. septicum* pathogenesis is unknown; however, the recent cloning and sequencing of this toxin should facilitate studies in this area.

TREATMENT. Though no comparative human trials have evaluated the efficacy of antibiotics or HBO for treating clinical cases of spontaneous gas gangrene, *in vitro* data suggests that *C. septicum* is uniformly susceptible to penicillin, tetracycline, erythromycin, clindamycin, chloramphenicol, and metronidazole. The aerotolerance of *C. septicum* may reduce the efficacy of HBO therapy.

PROGNOSIS. The mortality of spontaneous clinical gangrene ranges from 67 to 100%, with the majority of deaths occurring within 24 hours of onset. Risk factors include underlying malignancy and compromised immune status.

OTHER CLOSTRIDIAL DISEASES

FOOD POISONING (ENTEROTOXEMIA) CAUSED BY *CLOSTRIDIUM PERFRINGENS* (see Ch. 109). *C. perfringens* accounts for nearly 20% of all reported cases of food poisoning. Ingesting large numbers of vegetative cells from inadequately prepared and stored food leads to multiplication and sporulation in the intestine. When mature spores are released, enterotoxin is liberated into the lumen of the GI tract. The alkaline environment of the proximal small intestine and the presence of trypsin (a pancreatic enzyme found in the gut lumen) cause a 2.5-fold increase in biologic activity of enterotoxin. Histologically, enterotoxin causes bleb formation and desquamation of the microvillus tips of the brush border. Physiologically, such cells are incapable of glucose and ion absorption. The net effect is loss of electrolytes and fluid across the brush border, with resultant diarrhea. Other symptoms that manifest 5 to 24 hours after ingesting contaminated food are nausea, vomiting, and abdominal cramping. The definitive diagnosis rests on demonstrating enterotoxin in stool samples. Reliable biologic tests, radioimmunoassays, and ELISA tests have been developed, though the ELISA is favored due its sensitivity, cost, and quick results.

NECROTIZING ENTERITIS. Neutropenic enterocolitis is a fulminant form of necrotizing enteritis that occurs in neutropenic patients. Neutropenia is often profound and may be related to cyclic neutropenia, leukemia, aplastic anemia, or chemotherapy. Symptoms include abdominal pain, chills, and malaise. Copious watery diarrhea, abdominal distention, and pain localizing to the right lower quadrant develop, followed rapidly by signs of toxicity, such as tachycardia, fever, and delirium. Radiographic examinations may reveal thickening of the wall of the colon or cecum and, in advanced cases, gas in the wall of the colon. Anecdotal reports suggest that CT scanning may be a superior means of diagnosing this condition. Complications include rupture of the bowel with peritonitis, bacteremia, and death in 100% of cases. Aggressive supportive measures, surgical intervention, and appropriate antibiotics (see section on Spontaneous Gas Gangrene) have reduced the mortality to 25%.

Postmortem examinations reveal that among children dying of leukemia, localized infection of the ileocecal region (typhilitis) is extremely common and may have contributed to death in nearly 40%. *C. septicum* is the most common organism isolated from the blood of such patients, and Gram stain and immunofluorescence studies demonstrate that these bacteria invade the bowel wall in most cases.

Other forms of necrotizing enteritis have occurred endemically in New Guinea (pigbel), in epidemic proportion in Germany following World War II (Darmbrand), and sporadically in Africa, Southeast Asia, and the United States. All cases are associated with ingesting meats contaminated with *C. perfringens* type c. Clinical courses vary between abdominal pain, fever, and diarrhea, which resolve spontaneously, to bloody diarrhea, ruptured bowel, and death. Beta toxin from *C. perfringens* type c has been implicated as causing these infections. Beta toxin paralyzes the intestinal villi and causes friability and necrosis of the bowel wall. Predisposing factors include malnutrition, specifically in those with diets low in protein and rich in trypsin inhibitors such as sweet potato or soy bean. In addition, *Ascaris lumbricoides* is found commonly in such patients, and it, too, secretes a trypsin inhibitor. These protease inhibitors protect beta toxin from intraluminal proteolysis.

Medical management should include aggressive fluid and electrolyte replacement, bowel decompression, and antibiotic treatment with penicillin or chloramphenicol. Surgical resection of necrotic bowel is necessary in 50% of patients, and mortality rates as high as 40% have been described. If peritonitis develops, broader antibiotic coverage may be necessary. Immunization of children in New Guinea with a beta toxoid vaccine has dramatically reduced the incidence of this disease.

C. SORDELLII INFECTION. Patients with *C. sordellii* infection present with unique clinical features including edema, absence of fever, leukemoid reaction, hemoconcentration, and later shock and multiorgan failure. Often *C. sordellii* infections develop after childbirth or after gynecologic procedures, though some cases involve sites of minor trauma such as lacerations. Unlike *C. perfringens* and *C. septicum* infections, pain may not be a prominent feature. The absence of fever and paucity of signs and symptoms of local infection make early diagnosis difficult. The mechanisms of diffuse capillary leak, massive edema, and hemoconcentration are not well established but clearly are related to elaboration of a potent toxin. Hematocrits of 75 to 80% have been described, and leukocytosis of 50 to 100,000 cells per cubic millimeter with a left shift is common.

C. TERTIUM INFECTIONS. *C. tertium* causes bacteremia in compromised hosts who have received long courses of antibiotics, thus explaining the organism's relative resistance to penicillin, cephalosporins, and clindamycin. *C. tertium* is, however, usually quite sensitive to chloramphenicol, vancomycin, and metronidazole. Because this organism can grow aerobically, it may be mistakenly disregarded as a contaminant such as a diphtheroid or bacillus species.

Farnell MB: Neutropenic enterocolitis: A surgical disease? Infect Surg 6(2):120, 1987. *Describes the clinical presentation of necrotizing lesions of the terminal ileum associated with neutropenic conditions; also describes the evidence that implicates Clostridium septicum as the cause of enterocolitis.*

Stevens DL, Bryant AE, Adams K, et al.: Evaluation of hyperbaric oxygen therapy for treatment of experimental *Clostridium perfringens* infection. Clin Infect Dis 17:231, 1993. *This study describes the efficacy of hyperbaric oxygen, alone and with various antibiotics, for treating experimental clostridial myonecrosis. In the same issue, editorials describe the pros and cons of hyperbaric oxygen treatment.*

Stevens DL, Laine BM, Mitten JE: Comparison of single and combination antimicrobial agents for prevention of experimental gas gangrene caused by *Clostridium perfringens.* Antimicrob Agents Chemother 31:312, 1987. *This study demonstrated superior efficacy of clindamycin alone and that neither synergy nor antagonism occurred when penicillin and clindamycin were both used to treat experimental clostridial myositis.*

Stevens DL, Musher DM, Watson DA, et al.: Spontaneous, nontraumatic gangrene due to *Clostridium septicum.* Rev Infect Dis 12(2):286, 1990. *A review article concerning clinical features of spontaneous gas gangrene (complete with color plates).*

Weinstein L, Barza M: Gas gangrene. N Engl J Med 289:1129, 1972. *A review of clinical features and management recommendations for gas gangrene.*

287 PSEUDOMEMBRANOUS COLITIS
Robert Fekety

DESCRIPTION. Pseudomembranous colitis (PMC) is a toxin-induced inflammatory process characterized by exudative plaques or pseudomembranes attached to the surface of the inflamed colonic mucosa. The disease is often referred to as "antibiotic-associated colitis" (AAC) because many patients who develop the disease after using antimicrobials have no grossly visible pseudomembranes but on biopsy have microscopically visible pseudomembranes.

ETIOLOGY. Although most patients with PMC develop it as a complication of antimicrobial therapy, the disease was recognized in the preantibiotic era. The etiologic agent in nearly all instances is *Clostridium difficile,* and the disease is caused by elaboration of two or more toxins during growth of *C. difficile.* Growth of the organism is promoted by poorly understood antibiotic-induced alterations in the normal intestinal flora. PMC is usually found in association with one or more underlying medical and surgical diseases, especially those involving the abdomen and requiring antibiotic therapy, although occasionally it occurs in healthy persons.

INCIDENCE AND EPIDEMIOLOGY. The disease occurs at all ages. The incidence of PMC depends on the frequency with which endoscopy and toxin tests on stools are performed to establish the diagnosis, on patterns of antimicrobial use, on antibiotic resistance patterns of the *C. difficile* isolates, and on epidemiologic factors favoring transmission of the organism. Nearly all antimicrobials have been implicated in PMC, but the most frequent are ampicillin, clindamycin, and the cephalosporins. Less frequent are

penicillins other than ampicillin, erythromycin, aminoglycosides, and sulfamethoxazole-trimethoprim. *C. difficile*–induced colitis occurs both sporadically in hospitals and communities and in clusters within institutions. Studies indicate that *C. difficile* may be detected in the colonic flora of 3 to 5% of healthy adults and that it is widely distributed in our environment, including soil and water. It is especially common in hospitals and nursing homes, where as many as 20 to 30% of patients who have received antibiotics may be asymptomatic carriers and where spread of the organism from patients who have colitis to others treated with antibiotics is likely to occur. Spread from patients who are healthy carriers or who have colitis seems most often the result of transmission via the hands of hospital personnel, although transmission by directly contacting contaminated surfaces or objects also can occur.

MECHANISM. *C. difficile*–induced colitis is a toxin-mediated disease in which there is attachment of one or more toxins to the colonic mucosa but rarely any invasion of it by the organism. Toxin A (an enterotoxin) appears to be responsible for most of the features of the disease, while toxin B, a cytotoxin detectable in cell cultures that does not attach to the intact mucosa, may cause additional damage in severe cases. About 75% of *C. difficile* isolates produce both toxins. Isolates that do not produce toxins do not cause colitis or diarrhea.

CLINICAL MANIFESTATIONS. The disease may begin as early as 1 day after antibiotic therapy is started or as late as 6 weeks after it is discontinued. The most frequent symptoms are profuse watery diarrhea and cramping abdominal pain. Most patients also have fever (while usually low grade, it may exceed 40° C). Leukoytosis as high as 50,000 per cubic millimeter is common. In some patients, fever and leukocytosis are the *only* early clues to the disease, and diarrhea may not begin until several days later. Other findings include marked lower abdominal tenderness, hypoalbuminemia, and edema. Mild colitis is much more common than severe colitis, and many patients simply have annoying watery diarrhea resembling that seen in benign antibiotic diarrheal states. Complications in severe cases include dehydration, anasarca, electrolyte disturbances, toxic megacolon, and colonic perforation. Unusual manifestations include reactive arthritis and the development of diarrhea and enterocolitis in very young children with Hirschsprung's disease. Colitis occasionally presents with fever, leukocytosis, and marked pain and tenderness *without* diarrhea, especially after use of opiates for postoperative pain. Symptoms may begin during the course of antimicrobial treatment, but in as many as 20% of patients, they may not begin until up to 6 weeks *after* therapy is discontinued. The differential diagnosis includes acute and chronic diarrhea caused by other enteric pathogens, an adverse reaction to medications other than antibiotics, idiopathic inflammatory bowel diseases, and intra-abdominal sepsis. Diarrhea beginning 3 or more days *after* admission to the hospital is not likely to be caused by enteropathogens other than *C. difficile.*

DIAGNOSIS. The role of various studies in the diagnosis of AAC is summarized in Table 287–1. The best and most rapid way to establish the diagnosis of PMC is by endoscopy.

The "gold standard" laboratory test for establishing the diagnosis and etiology of *C. difficile* colitis is still the demonstration in filtrates of diarrheal stools, a cytopathic effect (CPE) caused by toxin B that is neutralized by antitoxin. Computed tomography (CT) may be useful in detecting evidence of PMC, especially in patients presenting with an acute abdominal syndrome without diarrhea or in early detection of complications of PMC (Figs. 287–1 and 287–2).

TREATMENT. Discontinuing all antimicrobial agents is desirable, although not essential if specific antibiotic therapy for PMC is given. Discontinuing antibiotics and replacing fluid and electrolyte losses may resolve symptoms without further specific therapy, particularly if the patient has "simple" diarrhea without colitis. Patients with severe symptoms should have stool examinations performed to implicate *C. difficile* toxins and also should promptly receive specific therapy for colitis. Antiperistaltic drugs are best avoided because they may cause worsening of the illness, even though they usually do not.

Specific therapy with metronidazole or vancomycin is usually given for about 7 to 10 days, using antibiotics orally to prevent the organism from growing and producing toxins. Metronidazole given orally, 250 or 500 mg 4 times per day, is used for colitis of mild or

TABLE 287–1. DIAGNOSING *CLOSTRIDIUM DIFFICILE* COLITIS

Test	Comments
Laboratory Tests on Feces	
Test for fecal leukocytes	A simple screening test but sensitivity only 30 to 50%. *A positive test rules out benign or simple antibiotic diarrhea.*
Stool culture for *C. difficile*	Results delayed. *Not diagnostic,* since 10 to 25% of patients in hospitals may carry the organism, and only 75% of isolates produce toxins. May be used epidemiologically.
Tests for the presence of fecal toxins	
Cytopathic effect of toxin B in tissue cultures	*"Gold standard,"* but some cell lines are not as sensitive as others, so false-negatives may occur. Time consuming, expensive, and not widely available. Requires antitoxin neutralization for specificity.
Toxin A by ELISA	*Rapid, widely available, relatively inexpensive.* Sensitivity varies and may be only fair. If cut point is chosen to minimize false-negatives, false-positives become a problem.
Latex agglutination for *C. difficile*	Rapid and inexpensive. *Detects glutamic dehydrogenase* (neither a toxin nor specific for *C. difficile*). Many false-positives and false-negatives.
Counterelectrophoresis (antigen detection)	*Nonspecific.* Many false-positives and false-negatives.
Radiologic Studies	
Plain film of the abdomen	*Nonspecific* and useful only when colitis is far-advanced or complications such as toxic megacolon or perforation are present.
Barium enema	*Nonspecific* findings. May precipitate perforation or megacolon.
Computed tomography	Safe, but expensive, and not highly specific. *Can be useful,* especially when patients present with an acute abdomen without diarrhea. May demonstrate unsuspected PMC.
Radionuclide scans (indium) (labeled WBC)	May detect inflammation, but *doesn't diagnose etiology.*
Procedures	
Flexible sigmoidoscopy	*Most rapid way to make the diagnosis.* Expensive. Misses about 10% of cases (those with only minor or proximal colonic lesions). Biopsy of minor or nonspecific lesions increases yield.
Colonoscopy	Rapid and *most sensitive way to make the diagnosis.* Expensive and may be hazardous. Biopsy of minor or nonspecific lesions increases yield.

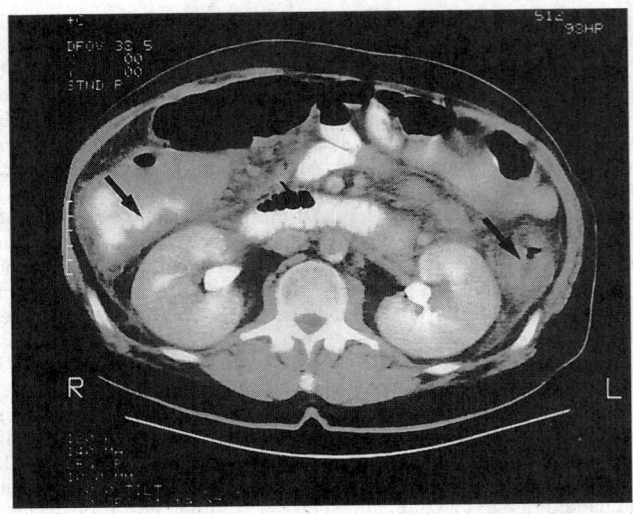

FIGURE 287–1. CT scan of abdomen of an elderly neurosurgical patient with fever and diarrhea postoperatively. Stools were positive for *C. difficile* cytotoxin. The arrow at left indicates irregularly thickened cecal mucosa; the arrow at right indicates lumenal narrowing, mucosal thickening, and edema of the descending colon. (From Fekety R: Infectious colitis. *In* Greenfield LJ et al [eds.]: Surgery: Scientific Principles and Practice. Philadelphia, JB Lippincott, 1992, p 1055.)

10 days) to bind the toxins of *C. difficile,* but they also bind vancomycin and teicoplanin. Oral bacitracin or teicoplanin has been an effective therapeutic alternate, but these drugs are not always readily available. Patients who cannot be treated orally or via a nasogastric tube should be given vancomycin in solution via a catheter passed to the cecum with a colonoscope, or via a long intestinal tube passed from above to the distal ileum, or via an ileostomy or colostomy, or if these are not possible, by colectomy. Therapy with intravenous metronidazole may be helpful in this setting, but is *not* reliable by itself.

Relapse or recurrence of colitis a few weeks or months after discontinuing antibiotic therapy occurs in 15 to 35% of successfully treated patients, whether the patient was treated with vancomycin or metronidazole. Attempts have been made recently to restore the normal fecal flora by giving live lactobacilli, mixtures of intestinal bacteria, or a live yeast *(Saccharomyces boulardii)* by mouth for a few weeks. *S. boulardii* reduced the frequency of relapses in a controlled study by about 50%, but it is not yet available in the United States.

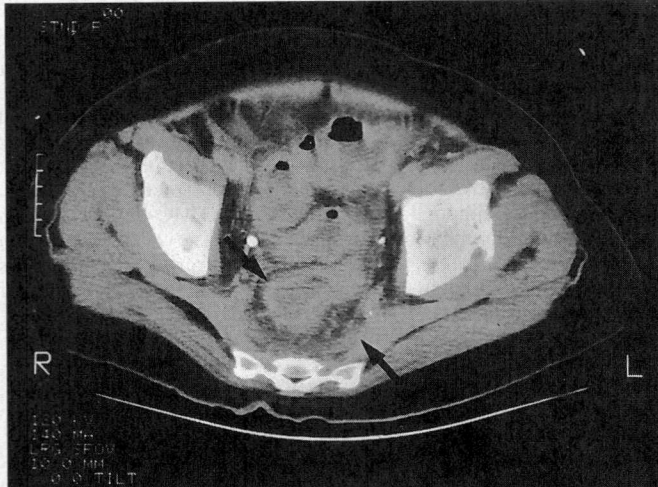

FIGURE 287–2. CT scan at another level of the patient with pseudomembranous colitis. The arrow at left points to thickening of the rectal mucosa; the arrow at right indicates edema and inflammation in the perirectal soft tissues. (From Fekety R: Infectious colitis. *In* Greenfield LJ et al [eds.]: Surgery: Scientific Principles and Practice. Philadelphia, JB Lippincott, 1992, p 1055.)

moderate severity but may produce side effects, and it should be noted that occasional isolates of *C. difficile* are resistant to metronidazole. The preferred treatment for seriously ill patients is vancomycin, 125 to 500 mg given orally 4 times per day for 7 to 14 days. Vancomycin is active against virtually all isolates of *C. difficile.* Major problems with vancomycin are its relatively high cost, bad taste, and unreliability when given intravenously to treat colitis. An alternative treatment uses anion exchange resins such as cholestyramine (4-gram packet given orally 3 times daily for 5 to

General	Outbreak Setting
Prudent use of antibiotics (narrow spectrum, short courses)	Education about the disease
Washing hands between patients	Emphasize handwashing before and after each patient
Enteric isolation of cases: stool precautions, use of gloves	Use of gloves for handling positive patients
Oral prophylaxis with *S. boulardii* (future)	Patient cohorting
Immunization with *C. difficile* toxoids (future)	Treatment of fecal carriers with oral metronidazole, bacitracin, or vancomycin to reduce fecal shedding of *C. difficile.*
Toxin adsorbents: Cholestryramine, sucralfate (still experimental)	Disinfection of unit and fomites to kill spores and vegetative forms with 2% alkaline glutaraldehyde or hypochorite solutions (1600 ppm)
	Closure of unit (as a last resort)

PREVENTION. The most important preventive measures are careful handwashing or use of gloves after contact with patients who have the disease or who may be carriers of the organism and judicious use of antimicrobial agents (Table 287–2).

Barbut F, Kajzer C, Planas N, et al.: Comparison of three enzyme immunoassays, a cytotoxicity assay, and toxigenic culture for diagnosis of *Clostridium difficile*–associated diarrhea. J Clin Microbiol 31:963, 1993. *A good review of diagnostic laboratory tests.*

deLalla F, Nicolin R, Rinaldi E, et al.: Prospective study of oral teicoplanin versus oral vancomycin for therapy of pseudomembranous colitis and *Clostridium difficile*–associated diarrhea. Antimicrob Agents Chemother 36:2192, 1992. *Comparison of this alternate to treatment with vancomycin or metronidazole, which is available in Europe but not yet in the United States.*

Fekety R, Shah AB: Diagnosis and treatment of *Clostridium difficile* colitis. JAMA 269:71, 1993. *Reviews the disease and presents an algorithim for diagnosing and managing the disease and its complications.*

Gumerlock PH, Tang YJ, Weiss JB, Silva J Jr.: Specific detection of toxigenic strains of *Clostridium difficile* in stool specimens. J Clin Microbiol 31:507, 1993. *Describes the use of PCR in diagnosis, which may eventually be the best diagnostic laboratory test.*

Kelly CP, Pothoulakis C, Lamont JT: *Clostridium difficile* colitis. N Engl J Med 330:257, 1994. *A good recent review.*

McFarland LV, Surawicz CM, Greenberg RN, et al.: A randomized, placebo-controlled trial of *Saccharomyces boulardii* in combination with standard antibiotics for *Clostridium difficile* disease. JAMA 271:1913, 1994. *Shows relapse rate was reduced by half with the use of this yeast as an adjunct to specific therapy.*

Waler KJ, Gilliland SS, Vance-Bryan K, et al.: *Clostridium difficile* colonization in residents of long-term facilities: Prevalence and risk factors. J Am Geriatr Soc 41:940, 1993. *Reviews important epidemiologic aspects of the disease in nursing homes.*

288 BOTULISM
John G. Bartlett

DEFINITION. Botulism is a severe neuroparalytic disease caused by botulinal toxin produced by clostridial species, usually *Clostridium botulinum*. There are four recognized disease categories: (1) foodborne botulism, (2) infant botulism, (3) wound botulism, and (4) unclassified cases.

ETIOLOGY. *C. botulinum* is a gram-positive, spore-forming obligate anaerobe that is widely distributed in nature and frequently found in soil, marine environments, and agricultural products. Adults regularly ingest *C. botulinum* spores from fresh agricultural products without deleterious consequences, and this organism is not recognized as a component of the normal fecal flora. Each strain produces one of eight antigenically distinct toxins of approximately 150,000 daltons, designated A through H. Human disease is caused by types A, B, E, and rarely by F and G. *C. barati* and *C. butyricum* have been implicated in infant botulism with production of type F and E toxins, respectively. Botulinal toxins are hematogenously disseminated to peripheral cholinergic synapses, where they bind irreversibly and block acetylcholine release. The result is hypotonia with a descending symmetric flaccid paralysis. Botulinal toxin is the most potent poison in humans; it has an estimated lethal dose in the bloodstream of 10^{-9} mg per kilogram. Type A

botulinum toxin is now available for injection as treatment for ocular muscle disorders, such as strabismus and blepharospasm, and dystonias, such as torticollis and hemifacial spasm.

FOOD POISONING. Foodborne botulism results from the ingestion of preformed toxin in inadequately prepared food, although *C. botulinum* in the intestine may be responsible or may serve as a continuing source of toxin. There are an average of 15 "outbreaks" annually in the United States, most of which involve a single case. The most frequently implicated vehicle in the United States is home-canned foods, which usually have a putrefactive odor. Meat and meat products are more commonly responsible in Europe, and preserved fish is most frequent in Japan, Scandinavia, and Russia. Type A and B organisms predominate in the United States, type A west of the Mississippi River and type B in eastern states. Type E organisms are usually, but not exclusively, associated with an aquatic source in northern latitudes, where they are found in coastal waters, lakes, and intestines of fish that inhabit these areas.

CLINICAL MANIFESTATIONS. The incubation period is usually 18 to 36 hours but may be as short as 2 hours or as long as 8 days. Persons with the shortest incubation period usually have the most severe disease. The bulbar musculature is affected first, with resultant diplopia, difficulty in focusing to a near point, dysphonia, dysarthria, and dysphagia. Involvement of the cholinergic autonomic nervous system may cause decreased salivation with a dry mouth and sore throat, ileus, or urinary retention. Common gastrointestinal symptoms include nausea, vomiting, and abdominal pain. Neurologic examination shows lateral rectus muscle weakness (cranial nerve VI), ptosis, dilated pupils with sluggish reaction, decreased gag reflex, or medial rectus paresis. This is followed by descending involvement of the motor neurons to peripheral muscles, including the muscles of respiration. Some patients have only mild illness, whereas others have severe paralysis that may require intensive supportive care for weeks. Mentation remains clear, there is no fever, and neurologic dysfunction is bilateral but not necessarily symmetric. The principal causes of death are respiratory or bulbar paralysis and infectious complications during the period of supportive care.

DIAGNOSIS. The usual laboratory test in suspected cases is analysis of serum, stool, gastric contents, and/or food for botulinum toxin and analysis of stool and/or food for *C. botulinum*. The classic toxin test is a mouse assay in which specimens are injected intraperitoneally to demonstrate a lethal toxin that is neutralized by type-specific antitoxin. Alternative antigen assays, such as the enzyme-linked immunoassay, have been developed but are not widely available. Among patients with clinical evidence of botulism, the toxin is detected in sera from one third, the toxin is found in the stool from one third, and the organism is recovered in stool from 60%.

Botulism should be suspected in patients with acute flaccid paralysis, especially when there is bilateral sixth cranial nerve dysfunction, associated gastrointestinal symptoms, prior ingestion of possibly contaminated food, and typical symptoms in other persons who shared this food. The differential diagnosis includes myasthenia gravis, Guillain-Barré syndrome, tick paralysis, cerebrovascular accident involving branches of the basilar artery, trichinosis, the Eaton-Lambert syndrome, hypocalcemia, hypermagnesemia, organophosphate poisoning, atropine poisoning, paralytic poisoning caused by shellfish or puffer fish, and psychiatric syndromes. Electromyography using repetitive stimulation at 40 Hz or greater is useful in differentiating botulism from other neurologic syndromes. This shows a diminished amplitude of muscle action potentials with a single supramaximal stimulus and facilitation of action potentials using paired or repetitive stimuli. These findings do not appear until the patient develops peripheral muscle weakness and are most likely to be positive in an affected limb.

TREATMENT. Sudden respiratory arrest is the most important serious complication, so patients must be carefully observed with monitoring of vital capacity and liberal use of ventilatory support. Elimination of the toxin from the gastrointestinal tract may be facilitated using gastric lavage, cathartics, and enemas early in the course. Antitoxin is usually given irrespective of the duration of illness, since the toxin may persist in the blood for extended periods. Treatment is initiated using two vials of the trivalent antitoxin, each containing 7500 IU type A, 5500 IU type B, and 8500 IU type E

1636 / XXI INFECTIOUS DISEASES

antitoxin; one vial is given intravenously, one is given intramuscularly. The antitoxin is horse serum and is associated with a 9% incidence of acute (5%) or delayed (4%) hypersensitivity reactions; 2% had anaphylaxis. Efficacy of the antitoxin is most clearly established with type B and type E botulism. Other therapeutic considerations include guanidine hydrochloride (15 to 50 mg per kilogram daily) to enhance acetylcholine release, but efficacy has not been established. Some advocate penicillin to help eradicate *C. botulinum* from the intestine, since this represents a potential source of additional toxin.

PROGNOSIS. The case fatality rate for foodborne botulism has decreased from > 60% to < 10% due largely to improved management methods, especially for ventilatory support. Patients who survive generally have complete recovery.

PREVENTION. Foodborne botulism is caused by germination of spores in food with toxin produced by vegetative forms, although the toxin also may be produced *in vivo* by simultaneously ingesting spores. The disease may be prevented by destroying spores in the original food source, inhibiting germination, or destroying preformed toxin. Specific measures are as follows:

1. Destroying spores with heat or irradiation. Spores of types A and B may survive boiling for several hours, especially at high altitudes (such as in Colorado), where the boiling point may be substantially lower. These spores may be destroyed if kept at 120°C for 30 minutes using pressure cookers. Spores of type E are most heat-labile and are killed with heating at 80°C for 30 minutes.

2. Germination may be inhibited by reducing pH, refrigerating, freezing, drying, or adding salt, sugar, or other inhibitory substances such as sodium nitrite.

3. Inactivation of preformed toxin is accomplished by terminal heating for 20 minutes at 80°C or 10 minutes at 90°C.

INFANT BOTULISM. Infant botulism results from botulinal neurotoxin produced *in vivo* following colonization of the gastrointestinal tract in children ages 1 to 9 months. This is the most common form of botulism in the United States, with 30 to 80 reported cases annually. Spores of *C. botulinum* (but not the toxin) have been found in about 10% of honey supplies, which previously accounted for one third of cases. The disease spectrum varies considerably, including "failure to thrive," "the floppy baby syndrome" (the most commonly recognized form), and sudden infant death syndrome or "crib death." Common symptoms in the floppy baby syndrome include lethargy, diminished suck, constipation, weakness, feeble cry, and diminished spontaneous activity with loss of head control, followed by extensive flaccid paralysis. The diagnosis is established by recovering *C. botulinum* or its toxin in stool. The toxin has rarely been detected in the serum. Fecal carriage of the organism and the toxin may persist for weeks to months following clinical improvement and hospital discharge. The major therapeutic need is supportive care with special attention to nutrition and maintenance of respiratory function. The role of antitoxin, guanidine, and antibiotics in this form of botulism has not been established, and generally their use is not advised. The mortality rate for hospitalized patients given supportive care is only 2%.

WOUND BOTULISM. This is a rare form of botulism in which a traumatic wound is infected by *C. botulinum* with toxin production *in vivo*. Types A and B have been implicated, reflecting their presence in soil. Clinical features are identical to those of foodborne botulism except that the incubation period from the time of injury is 4 to 14 days and there is a paucity of gastrointestinal symptoms. The diagnosis is established by recovering *C. botulinum* from the wound or by detection of the toxin in serum. Management includes wound debridement and other treatments described for foodborne botulism except for bowel cleansing.

UNCLASSIFIED BOTULISM. This category includes persons over the age of 12 months who have typical symptoms and signs of botulism with no identifiable vehicle. It is possible that some cases result from production of toxin *in vivo* by organisms colonizing the intestine in a fashion comparable with the mechanism described for infant botulism.

SPECIAL NOTE. Physicians may contact the Centers for Disease Control and Prevention (CDC) for advice on management of patients with botulism at (404) 639-2206; to obtain botulinal antitoxin, the 24-hour CDC contact number is (404) 639-2888.

Arnon SS: Infant botulism: Anticipating the second decade. J Infect Dis 154:201, 1986. *An authoritative review of infant botulism based on the 10-year experience following its original report in 1976.*

Black RE, Gunn RA: Hypersensitivity reactions associated with botulinal antitoxin. Am J Med 69:567, 1980. *The authors review the CDC experience with 268 patients who received botulinal antitoxin.*

Chia JK, Clark JB, Ryan CA, et al.: Botulism in an adult associated with food-borne intestinal infection with *Clostridium botulinum*. N Engl J Med 315:239, 1986. *This is a case report of an adult with the infant form of botulism and an accompanying editorial that places this observation in perspective.*

Dowell VR Jr, McCroskey LM, Hathaway CL, et al.: Coproexamination for botulinal toxin and *Clostridium botulinum*. JAMA 238:1829, 1977. *Reviews methods to establish the diagnosis in foodborne botulism.*

Woodruff BA, Griffin PM, McCroskey LM, et al.: Clinical and laboratory comparison of botulism from toxin types A, B and E in the U.S., 1975–1988. J Infect Dis 166:1281, 1992. *This is a review of clinical and laboratory observations in 309 cases of botulism. Patients with type A appeared to have a more serious illness.*

289 TETANUS

John G. Bartlett

DEFINITION. Tetanus is a neurologic syndrome caused by a neurotoxin elaborated at the site of injury by *Clostridium tetani*.

ETIOLOGY. *C. tetani* is an anaerobic, gram-positive, slender, motile bacillus. The sporulated form has a characteristic drumstick or tennis racket shape with a terminal spore. The vegetative form produces tetanospasmin, a protein neurotoxin with a molecular weight of approximately 150,000. Tetanospasmin ranks with botulism toxin as the most potent known microbial toxin; 1 mg is capable of killing 50 to 70 million mice. The vegetative forms of *C. tetani* are highly susceptible to heat, disinfectants, and other adverse environmental conditions, but the spores are highly resistant and can survive in soil for months to years. Killing of spores requires boiling for at least 4 hours or autoclaving for 12 minutes at 121°C.

EPIDEMIOLOGY. *C. tetani* can be found in 20 to 65% of soil samples and in stool from a variety of animals, house dust, operating rooms, and contaminated heroin. Approximately 10% of humans harbor *C. tetani* in the colon.

Tetanus is most common in warm climates and in highly cultivated rural areas. The greatest problem is in economically deprived countries, owing to poor immunization standards and unhygienic practices. An example is the practice of dressing the umbilical stump with animal dung or "dusting powder," a local dried clay sold for cosmetic purposes, after childbirth by unimmunized mothers. It is estimated that the annual toll from neonatal tetanus in developing countries is 1 million. In the United States, the incidence of tetanus declined dramatically when tetanus toxoid became available. The national tetanus surveillance system showed a decrease from 560 reported cases in 1947 to 36 in 1993. Nearly all cases currently reported occur in inadequately immunized persons due to failure to comply with guidelines for primary childhood vaccination, for a reinforcing dose at 10-year intervals, or for postexposure prophylaxis (most did not seek medical attention for the injury). Of 117 patients with tetanus reported in 1989–90, 86 (74%) had an acute injury (44 had a puncture injury), 14 (12%) had chronic wounds (skin ulcers, abscesses, or gangrene), 5 (4%) were injection drug users, and 10 (9%) had no defined pre-existing condition. Most patients (58%) were over age 60, and 6% were younger than 20. This predilection for the disease in the elderly appears to reflect waning immunity associated with aging.

PATHOGENESIS. Clinical tetanus requires a source of the organism, local tissue conditions that promote toxin production, and immunologic naiveté. The spores are ubiquitous in the environment, and most cases reflect contamination from exogenous sources. Important factors at the site of injury are necrotic tissue, suppuration, and the presence of a foreign body. These are responsible for a reduction in the local oxidation-reduction potential (Eh), thus promoting reversion of spores to the vegetative forms that produce tetanospasmin. Tetanospasmin is taken up by the peripheral nerve terminals and carried intra-axonally within membrane-bound vesicles to spinal neurons at a transport rate of approximately 250 mm per day. Upon reaching the perikarya of the motor neurons, the toxin passes to the presynaptic terminals, where it blocks release of neurotransmitters, including glycine, which is the neurotransmitter used by group 1A inhibitory afferent motor neurons. Loss of the inhibitory influence results in unrestrained firing with sustained muscular contraction. The result with spinal cord neurons is rigidity. In severe cases there is also involvement of the sympathetic chain causing autonomic dysfunction.

CLINICAL FEATURES. Forms of tetanus include generalized, localized, cephalic, and neonatal. In the United States, these account for 87, 9, 3, and 1% of reported cases, respectively.

"Generalized tetanus" is the most common. The extent of the associated trauma varies and may be trivial and forgotten or a severe crush injury. The usual incubation period is 4 to 14 days, depending largely on the distance of the site of injury from the central nervous system. Trismus is the presenting complaint in 75% of cases. Other early features include irritability, restlessness, diaphoresis, and dysphagia with hydrophobia and drooling. Sustained trismus may result in a characteristic sardonic smile, or "risus sardonicus," and persistent spasm of the back musculature may cause opisthotonos. These early manifestations reflect involvement of the bulbar muscles and paraspinous muscles, possibly because they are innervated by the shortest axons. Waves of opisthotonos are highly characteristic of the disease. With progression, the extremities become involved in episodes characterized by painful flexion and adduction of the arms, clenched fists, and extension of the legs. Noise or tactile stimuli may precipitate spasms and generalized convulsions, although they occur spontaneously as well. Involvement of the autonomic nervous system may result in severe arrhythmias, oscillation in the blood pressure, profound diaphoresis, hyperthermia, rhabdomyolysis, laryngeal spasm, and urinary retention. In most cases the patient remains lucid. Complications include fractures from sustained contractions and convulsions, pulmonary emboli, bacterial infections, and dehydration.

"Localized tetanus" refers to involvement of the extremity with a contaminated wound and shows considerable variation and severity. In the more severe cases, there are intense, painful spasms that usually progress to generalized tetanus. Cases that remain localized have a good prognosis.

"Cephalic tetanus" generally follows a head injury or occurs with C. tetani infection of the middle ear. The clinical symptoms consist of isolated or combined dysfunction of the cranial motor nerves, most frequently the seventh cranial nerve. This may remain localized or progress to generalized tetanus. The incubation period is only 1 or 2 days, and the prognosis for survival is extremely poor.

"Tetanus neonatorum" refers to generalized tetanus resulting from C. tetani infection in neonates. This occurs primarily in underdeveloped countries where various contaminated materials are used to sever or dress the umbilical cord in newborn infants of unimmunized mothers. The usual incubation period following birth is 3 to 10 days, and it is sometimes referred to as "the disease of the seventh day," reflecting the average incubation period. The child typically shows irritability, facial grimacing, and severe spasms with touch. The mortality rate > 70%.

DIAGNOSIS. The diagnosis of tetanus is usually made clinically. The following is the case definition used by the Centers for Disease Control and Prevention (CDC): "Acute onset of hypotonia and/or painful muscular contractions (usually the muscles of the jaw and neck) and generalized muscle spasms without other apparent medical cause." C. tetani is infrequently recovered with cultures of the wound. A confirmed history of immunization or a serum antitoxin level of ≥ 0.01 units per milliliter makes tetanus unlikely. Spinal fluid analysis is entirely normal, and the electroencephalogram generally shows a sleep pattern. The differential diagnosis depends on the dominant clinical features and includes oculogyric crisis secondary to phenothiazine toxicity, meningitis, dental abscess, seizure disorder, subarachnoid hemorrhage, hypocalcemic or alkalotic tetany, alcohol withdrawal, and strychnine poisoning. Strychnine poisoning produces very similar symptoms but differs from tetanus in that patients usually recover rapidly following supportive care.

TREATMENT. *Surgery.* Debridement of any associated wound. (This may pose a problem in "skin poppers," who often have multiple possibly infected sites.)

Antibiotics. Penicillin G should be given parenterally in doses of 1 to 10 million units daily for 10 days; tetracycline, erythromycin, and chloramphenicol are alternative agents for penicillin-allergic patients.

Antitoxin. Human tetanus immunoglobulin (TIG) should be given as soon as possible to neutralize toxin that has not entered neurons. The dose is arbitrary but averages 3000 IU. It may be administered intramuscularly as split doses and by infiltration into the wound. Some authorities advocate intrathecal administration of 250 IU of TIG. Equine tetanus immune globulin (10,000 to 100,000 IU intravenously or intramuscularly) is equally effective, but the rate of reactions is high owing to the equine source. Epinephrine 1:1000 should be readily available for severe reactions. This preparation is far less expensive and is consequently used most extensively in underdeveloped countries.

Active Immunization. Natural infection does not result in detectable levels of circulating antibody, so a full course of immunization with tetanus toxoid in three doses should be given.

Muscle Spasms. Chlorpromazine (50 to 150 mg every 4 to 8 hours in adults), meprobamate (400 mg every 3 to 4 hours in adults*), or diazepam (2 to 20 mg intravenously every 2 to 8 hours) is given to control spasms and convulsions, and short-acting barbiturates are useful for sedation. Overuse of these agents may lead to hypoventilation. When muscle spasms are severe or interfere with ventilation, therapeutic paralysis should be introduced using pancuronium bromide or metocurine combined with mechanical ventilation.

Supportive Care. Trismus, dysphagia, laryngeal spasm, respiratory muscle spasm, and sedatives all contribute to the high frequency of pulmonary complications. Maintaining a patent airway is imperative, often with intubation followed by a tracheostomy. The patient may then be maintained with mechanical ventilation in conjunction with diazepam in intravenous doses titrated to relieve rigidity without excessive sedation.

Patients with dysphagia should be fed via a nasogastric tube. Fluid balance needs to be followed assiduously, since large losses may occur and may be difficult to measure owing to profuse sweating. Autonomic nervous system involvement may result in tachycardia and hypertension with high cardiac output and cardiac arrhythmias. α- and β-adrenergic blocking agents were used formerly, but β blockade was sometimes complicated by cardiac arrest. Other considerations with autonomic instability include morphine, epidural blockade, or magnesium sulfate infusions. Additional concerns are pulmonary emboli requiring anticoagulation, gastrointestinal bleeding that may be prevented with sucralfate, rhabdomyolysis with myoglobinuria and renal failure that may require dialysis, superimposed infections requiring judicious use of antibiotics, hyperthermia requiring a cooling blanket, and hypotension requiring pressor agents.

Prognosis. The overall mortality rate for generalized tetanus has decreased in the U.S. from 91% in 1947 to 24% for 1989–90. Important prognostic features are the form of tetanus, as described above, the incubation period, the "onset period" (the period from first clinical symptoms of tetanus to the first generalized spasm), patient's age, and severity of symptoms. Patients with mild disease have only trismus with or without minor and brief muscle spasms. Moderate disease is characterized by trismus, dysphagia, rigidity, and intermittent muscle spasms. With severe tetanus there are generalized convulsions. Patients with moderate or severe generalized tetanus generally require 3 to 6 weeks for recovery. They may require intensive care during most of this time, but if they survive their recovery is usually complete. The highest mortality rates are at the extremes of age. The most frequent cause of death is pneumonia, but many patients have no obvious findings at autopsy, suggesting that death was directly due to the neurotoxin.

PREVENTION. Nearly all cases of tetanus occur in unimmunized or inadequately immunized individuals (see Ch. 10). The Immunization Practices Advisory Committee recommends active immunization of infants and children with DPT (diphtheria and tetanus toxoids and pertussis adsorbed) at 2 months, 4 months, 6 months, 15 months, and 4 to 6 years. Tetanus vaccination of school-age children is required in 47 states. Tetanus toxoid is a highly effective antigen, and protective levels of serum antitoxin in persons who complete the primary series persist for at least 10 years. Td (tetanus and diphtheria toxoids adsorbed for adult use) is

---

* May exceed manufacturer's recommended dosage.

TABLE 289-1. GUIDELINES FOR TETANUS PROPHYLAXIS IN WOUND MANAGEMENT

History of Adsorbed Tetanus Toxoid	Clean and Minor Wounds		Other Wounds*	
Number of Doses	Td†	TIG‡	Td†	TIG‡
Unknown or less than three	Yes§	No	Yes§	Yes
Three or more	Yes if over 10 years since last dose	No	Yes if over 5 years since last dose	No

* Included but not limited to wounds contaminated with dirt, feces, soil, saliva, puncture wounds; avulsions; and wounds resulting from missiles, crushing, burns, and frostbite.

† Td: Tetanus and diphtheria toxoids adsorbed. Children under 7 should receive DPT (diphtheria and tenanus toxoids are pertussis vaccine adsorbed). Too frequents booster doses of tenanus toxoid have been associated with hypersentivity reactions.

‡ TIG: Tetanus immune globulin in a dose of 250 to 500 IU intramuscularly. The usual dose is 250 IU. The usual prophylactic dose of equine tetanus immune globulin is 1500 t0 5000 IU intramuscularly. When tetanus toxoid is given concurrently there should be separate syringes and injection sites.

§ Unimmunized or incompletely immunized persons (1 or 2 doses of toxoid) should receive complete immunization with Td at times 0, 4–8 weeks later, amd 6–12 months later

recommended every 10 years at mid-decade ages (15 years, 25 years, 35 years). This is commonly neglected, as disclosed by surveys showing only 13% of persons older than 65 had received a dose of tetanus toxoid in the past 5 years and serosurveys showing 30 to 70% of older adults lack protective antibody levels. The recommended primary immunization series for unimmunized persons older than age 7 is Td at time 0, 4 to 8 weeks, 6 to 12 months after the second dose, and then every 10 years. About 90% of cases of tetanus in the U.S. involving patients with known vaccination status are in patients who failed to receive the primary immunization series. Immunized childbearing women confer protection on their infants through transplacental maternal antibody.

Preventing tetanus after injury requires managing wounds appropriately, assuring adequate immunity, and considering antibiotic prophylaxis. The aim of surgery is to eliminate necrotic tissue, purulent collections, and foreign bodies that promote the environmental conditions necessary for spore germination. Guidelines for immunoprophylaxis based on immunization status and wound characteristics are summarized in Table 289-1. Passive immunization is recommended only for "tetanus prone" wounds, preferably with TIG prepared from plasma of adults hyperimmunized with tetanus toxoid. The alternative is tetanus antitoxin equine prepared from hyperimmunized horses. The horse serum is associated with a high reaction rate, including pain at the injection site, serum sickness, and anaphylactic shock. Equine antitoxin also generates immune complexes that are rapidly excreted so that larger doses are required to produce sustained blood levels. The definition of "tetanus-prone" depends on the interval between injury and treatment, the degree of contamination, the extent of devitalized tissue or foreign bodies within the site of injury, and the depth of the injury. Antimicrobial agents such as penicillin, erythromycin, or metronidazole may be given to inhibit replication of the vegetative forms of *C. tetani,* but immunization and wound cleansing are considered more important so the use of antibiotics is generally dictated by other considerations.

Armitage P, Clifford R: Prognosis in tetanus: Use of data from therapeutic trials. J Infect Dis 138:1, 1978. *Data for 1385 patients with tetanus in India are reviewed to propose a prognostic classification.*

Bizzini B: Tetanus toxin. Microbiol Rev 43:224, 1979. *An extensive discussion of tetanus toxin.*

Centers for Disease Control and Prevention: Tetanus surveillance—United States, 1989-90. MMWR 41(55-8):1, 1991. *A review of the clinical experience with tetanus in the United States and the guidelines for tetanus prophylaxis.*

Dowell VR Jr: Botulism and tetanus: Selected epidemiologic and microbiologic aspects. Rev Infect Dis 6(suppl 1):202, 1984. *A review of the reported experience in the United States for these neurologic syndromes.*

Faust RA, Vickers OR, Cohn L Jr: Tetanus: 2,449 cases in 68 years at Charity Hospital. J Trauma 16:704, 1976. *The authors review a large clinical experience with tetanus in a United States hospital.*

Griffin JW: Local tetanus. Johns Hopkins Med J 149:84, 1981. *A good review of local tetanus and the pathophysiology of tetanospasmin.*

Olsen KM, Hiller FC: Management of tetanus. Clin Pharm 6:570, 1987. *A review of management guidelines with emphasis on the important role of benzodiazepines.*

Schofield F: Selective primary health care: Strategies for control of disease in the developing world XXII. Tetanus: A preventable problem. Rev Infect Dis 8:144, 1986. *The author reviews the tetanus problem in the developing world.*

Anaerobic Bacteria

290 DISEASES CAUSED BY NON–SPORE-FORMING ANAEROBIC BACTERIA

Ellie J. C. Goldstein

Anaerobic bacteria are the predominant indigenous, normal flora of the human body, including the skin and oral, gastrointestinal, and vaginal mucosa (Fig. 290–1; Table 290–1). Although these organisms perform beneficial functions, they are also consummate opportunistic pathogens and can cause serious and lethal infection, often in combination with aerobic bacteria. Their role in disease was first described 100 years ago and has been increasingly appreciated during recent decades. In almost all such infections, anaerobes are mixed with aerobes. Because the flora of these infections is often complex and culture results may be delayed, knowledge of the usual flora at the location of infection is an indispensable guide in selecting and instituting empirical antimicrobial therapy.

TAXONOMY

Anaerobic bacteria range from those that die with very brief exposure to oxygen and are usually isolated only in normal flora studies to those that can survive on the surface of a fresh agar plate even in the presence of atmospheric oxygen (e.g., *Bacteroides fragilis*). Most anaerobes require an environment with a low oxidation-reduction potential (eH gradient), which can be accomplished in association with low pH, tissue destruction, by-products from aerobic bacterial metabolism, or low oxygen content. Although not true anaerobes, some organisms such as microaerophilic streptococci and other capnophilic or hard-to-grow organisms are sometimes lumped together with anaerobes owing to their fastidious nature. Some genera such as *Lactobacillus* and *Actinomyces* contain both aerobic and anaerobic species.

Recent taxonomic advances have led to reclassification of many anaerobic species (Table 290–2). The term *"Bacteroides"* will ultimately be reserved for the 10 species of the *Bacteroides fragilis* group. What were previously considered "oral" *Bacteroides* and "pigmented" *Bacteroides* species have been reclassified as *Prevotella, Porphyromonas,* and other genera. Those that are capnophilic and not true anaerobes are often more related to *Campylobacter, Capnocytophaga,* and other genera. In addition, many new genera and several new species have been created to accommodate pathogens such as *Bilophila wadsworthia* and *Wolinella* species.

VIRULENCE FACTORS

Anaerobic bacteria possess a variety of virulence factors that differ among the species (Table 290–3).

DISEASES

BACTEREMIA. Transient anaerobic bacteremia occurs in approximately 85% of patients immediately after dental cleaning or

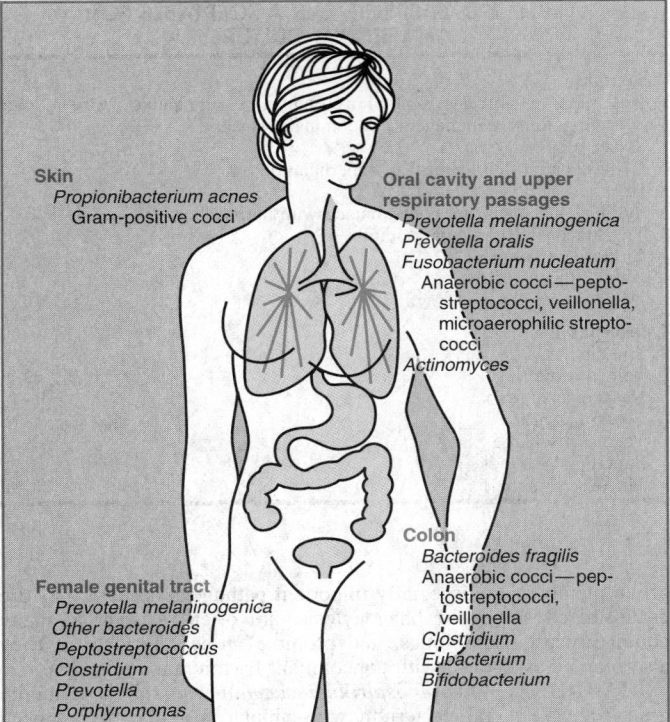

FIGURE 290–1. Anaerobes as predominant normal microflora of the human body by general anatomic location. (Adapted from Finegold SM, Sutter VL: Diagnosis and Management of Anaerobic Infections. Kalamazoo, MI, Upjohn, 1976. Copyright by Dr. Finegold.)

manipulation. More than 220 cases of endocarditis due to anaerobes have been reported and are usually associated with anatomic abnormalities or damaged valves. The majority of anaerobic bacteremias are intermittent and associated with serious intra-abdominal and female genital tract infections. Overall, it has been estimated that 10 to 20% of bacteremias are due to anaerobes, and in 80% of those anaerobes are the sole isolates.

HEAD AND NECK. Dental infections including periodontal disease, gingivitis, acute necrotizing ulcerative gingivitis, localized juvenile periodontitis, adult periodontitis, pericoronitis, endodontitis, dental abscess, and postextraction infection are associated with a variety of oral anaerobic bacteria.

Peritonsillar abscess is a deep-seated and potentially life-threatening complication of acute tonsillitis. It may extend into the various potential spaces of the neck or even the mediastinum and cause jugular vein thrombosis. Anaerobes may be isolated in >50% of such cases, usually in mixed culture with aerobes. Other regional infections include cervicofacial actinomycosis, Ludwig's angina, *Fusobacterium necrophorum* sepsis with metastatic infection (Lemiere's syndrome), and neck space infections. Whereas their

TABLE 290–1. LOCATION OF VARIOUS GROUPS OF NONSPORULATING ANAEROBES AS NORMAL MICROFLORA OF HUMANS

		Location		
Organism	Skin	Oral/ Respiratory	Gastrointestinal Tract	Genitourinary Tract
Actinomyces		+		
Bacteroides		+	+	
Eubacterium		+	+	
Fusobacterium		+	+	
Lactobacillus			+	+
Peptostreptococcus	+	+	+	+
Porphyromonas		+	+	
Prevotella		+	+	
Propionibacterium	+			
Veillonella		+	+	

TABLE 290–2. TAXONOMY OF ANAEROBIC BACTERIA

Current Name	Synonym/Comment
Bacteroides fragilis	⎫
Bacteroides caccae	
Bacteroides distasonis	
Bacteroides merdae	
Bacteroides eggerthii	B. fragilis group
Bacteroides stercoris	
Bacteroides ovatus	
Bacteroides thetaiotaomicron	
Bacteroides vulgatus	
Bacteroides uniformis	⎭
Bacteroides gracilis	Probably new species
Bacteroides ureolyticus	Probably new species
Prevotella bivia	*Bacteroides bivius*
Prevotella buccae	*Bacteroides buccae (ruminicola)*
Prevotella denticola	*Bacteroides denticola*
Prevotella disiens	*Bacteroides disiens*
Prevotella intermedia	*Bacteroides intermedius*
Prevotella melaninogenica	*Bacteroides melaninogenicus*
Prevotella oralis	*Bacteroides oralis*
Prevotella oris	*Bacteroides oris*
Porphyromonas asacharolytica	*Bacteroides asaccharolyticus*
Porphyromonas gingivalis	*Bacteroides gingivalis*
Porphyromonas salivosa	*Bacteroides salivosus*
Fusobacterium nucleatum subspecies: nucleatum, polymorphum, fusiforme	New subspecies
Fusobacterium necrophorum	
Fusobacterium ulcerans	New species
Anaerobiospirillum succiniproducens	New species
Bilophila wadsworthia	New species
Peptostreptococcus	Now includes almost all prior *Peptococcus* species of medical importance
Actinomyces	
Eubacterium nodatum	New species

acute counterparts are usually infections due to aerobes, chronic sinusitis and chronic otitis media often involve anaerobic bacteria of the normal oral flora.

PULMONARY. Because anaerobic bacteria are the predominant normal flora of the oral cavity and upper respiratory tract and most pneumonias are due to aspiration of indigenous oral flora, it is not

TABLE 290–3. POTENTIAL VIRULENCE FACTORS IN VARIOUS ANAEROBES

Factor	Species
Adhesion	
Capsule	*B. fragilis* group
Pili/fimbriae	*B. fragilis* group, *P. gingivalis*
Hemagglutinin	*P. gingivalis*
Lectin	*F. nucleatum*
Invasion/tissue damage	
Proteases	*F. necrophorum* *Bacteroides* species *Porphyromonas* species
Hemolysins	Many species
Fibrinolysin	*B. fragilis* group *Porphyromonas* species
Heparinase	*B. fragilis* group *Porphyromonas* species
Neuraminidase	*B. fragilis* group *Porphyromonas* species
Antiphagocytic	
Capsule	*B. fragilis* group *P. gingivalis*
Lipopolysaccharide	*B. fragilis* group *F. necrophorum, P. gingivalis*
Metabolic products	Most anaerobes

Adapted from Duerden BI: Virulence factors in anaerobes. Clin Infect Dis 18 (suppl 4): 253, 1994.

TABLE 290–4. OBSTETRIC-GYNECOLOGIC INFECTIONS THAT COMMONLY INVOLVE ANAEROBES

Abscesses
  Pelvic
  Vulvovaginal
  Vaginal cuff
  Tubo-ovarian
  Bartholin gland
  Skenes gland
Endometritis
Myometritis
Parametritis
Pelvic cellulitis
Pelvic thrombophlebitis
Bacterial vaginosis
Salpingitis
Chorioamnionitis
IUD-associated infection
Pelvic actinomycosis
Postabortal sepsis

TABLE 290–6. SPECIMENS ACCEPTABLE FOR ANAEROBIC CULTURE

Acceptable
Any aspirate: abscess, joint, lung, empyema, suprapubic (urine), brain, myringotomy, percutaneous abdominal, or pelvic
Tissue biopsy
Cellulitis after debridement of superficial debris
Bile
Surgical specimen (not contaminated with normal flora)
Transtracheal aspirate of sputum
Culdocentesis fluid
Antral sinus puncture
Deep gingival pocket

Unacceptable
Sputum
Voided urine
Nasal discharge
Feces/diarrhea
Vaginal discharge
Superficial wounds
Mucous membrane

surprising that anaerobes are important pulmonary pathogens. They are involved in aspiration pneumonia (both community-acquired and nosocomial), necrotizing pneumonia, empyema, and lung abscess. Aspiration of oral flora may be a result of altered consciousness, dysphagia, or mechanical devices such as intubation. Poor oral hygiene is associated with an increased anaerobic bacterial burden, and the presence of aerobes or tissue necrosis leads to a lowered eH, which in turn facilitates the growth of anaerobes. In community-acquired aspiration pneumonias, anaerobes are involved in 90% of cases, and in many cases may be the sole pathogens. Anaerobes can be isolated in 35% of nosocomial aspiration pneumonias. If one forgets to treat a routine aspiration pneumonia for its anaerobic component, then one must remember the propensity for anaerobes to cause abscess.

Management involves good pulmonary toilet and antimicrobial therapy. Because of the increasing resistance of the "oral *Bacteroides* species" (*Prevotella/Porphyromonas* species), penicillin alone is no longer recommended. Alternatives include penicillin plus metronidazole, β-lactamase inhibitor combinations, second-generation cephalosporins such as cefoxitin and cefotetan, carbapenems, and clindamycin plus penicillin. In choosing coverage, one must also consider the microaerophilic streptococci and the aerobic gram-positive and locally prevalent gram-negative components of the oral flora. Nosocomial aspiration frequently is a mixture of all these components.

INTRA-ABDOMINAL. Because anaerobes outnumber aerobes by 1000:1 in the large intestine, they play an important role in almost all intra-abdominal infections. Most visceral abscesses (e.g., hepatic), chronic cholecystitis, perforated and gangrenous appendicitis, postoperative wound infections and abscesses, diverticulitis, and any infection associated with fecal contamination of the abdominal cavity involve both aerobes and anaerobes. *B. fragilis*

group members are especially important pathogens because they are encapsulated and resist phagocytosis, are often resistant to many commonly used antibiotics, and promote abscess formation. They also may be associated with concomitant bacteremia and sepsis.

DIARRHEA. *Anaerobiospirillum succiniproducens* is a motile gram-negative spiral bacterium with bipolar flagellae. It has been isolated from the feces of asymptomatic dogs and cats and has been transmitted from them to humans. It may also be associated with bacteremia.

Although *B. fragilis* is part of the normal intestinal flora, evidence incriminating enterotoxin-producing strains as a cause of diarrhea in animals and humans has mounted.

OBSTETRIC-GYNECOLOGIC. Table 290–4 lists the various obstetric-gynecologic diseases that involve anaerobes. Bacterial vaginosis has been linked to a perturbation of the normal anaerobic vaginal flora and accounts for 45% of all cases of vaginitis. It is present in approximately 20% of college women, and up to 45% of women attending STD clinics. It can be diagnosed by the presence of a foul, gelatinous vaginal discharge, a vaginal pH >4.5, the presence of "clue cells," and a fishy amine odor after 10% KOH is added to vaginal secretions. Bacterial vaginosis has also been associated with premature rupture of membranes, chorioamnionitis, postpartum endometritis, vaginal cuff cellulitis, and postabortal pelvic inflammatory disease (PID). Culture of tubo-ovarian abscess, a complication of chronic PID, grows anaerobes in up to 85% of cases.

SKIN AND SOFT TISSUE. *Diabetes.* The infected fetid foot is the most frequent infectious cause for diabetics to be hospitalized. The role of anaerobes in >50% of these infections is well established. When present, anaerobes are often associated with the more severe cases, especially with vascular insufficiency and tissue necrosis and those that ultimately require amputation. In addition, the presence of fever, longstanding wounds, crepitus, foul odor, abscess, or prior antimicrobial therapy more often involves anaerobes.

TABLE 290–5. CLUES TO THE PRESENCE OF ANAEROBIC INFECTION

Infection in proximity to a mucous membrane
Foul odor to a discharge or wound
Gas or crepitus in a tissue
Infection associated with necrotic tissue or malignancy
Bacteremia with associated jaundice
Gram stain morphology consistent with anaerobes
"Sulfur" granules (actinomycosis)
Infection following human or animal bite
Dental infection
Infection following abdominal or pelvic surgery
No growth on routine bacterial culture (especially if Gram stain shows organisms)
Fistulous tracts
Any abscess
Typical clinical picture of gas gangrene or necrotizing fasciitis

Adapted from Finegold SM: Anaerobic Bacteria in Human Disease. New York, Academic Press, 1977, p 42.

TABLE 290–7. GENERAL PRINCIPLES OF THERAPY FOR ANAEROBIC INFECTIONS

Elimination of dead space
Debridement
Drainage
Irrigation
Provide adequate circulation when possible
Remove foreign body
Antimicrobials
  Activity against most likely pathogen(s): location-dependent, normal flora considered
  Absorption, appropriate route of administration
  Penetration into site of infection
  Dosage appropriate for local tissue levels, body mass of patient, renal and liver function
  Duration appropriate for condition
  Susceptibility testing of isolate to guide specific therapy

TABLE 290–8. ANTIMICROBIAL SUSCEPTIBILITY PATTERNS FOR ANAEROBIC BACTERIA*

Bacteria	Penicillin	β-Lactamase†	Cefoxitin	Cefotetan	Imipenem	Clindamycin	Metronidazole
B. fragilis	−	+	+	+	+	v	+
B. thetaiotaomicron	−	+	v	v	+	v	+
B. fragilis group, other	−	+	v	v	+	v	+
Prevotella species	v	+	+	+	+	+	+
Fusobacterium nucleatum	v	+	+	+	+	+	+
Fusobacterium necrophorum	+	+	+	+	+	+	+
Porphyromonas species	+	+	+	+	+	+	+
Peptostreptococci	+	+	+	+	+	+	v
Propionibacterium acnes	+	+	+	+	+	+	−
Veillonella	+	+	+	+	+	+	+
Actinomyces	+	+	+	+	+	+	−

* Based on a variety of *in vitro* susceptibility studies from different laboratories and utilizing different techniques.
† β-lactamase inhibitor—β-lactam combinations, e.g., ticarcillin clavulanate, ampicillin/sulbactam, pipericillin/tazobactam.
+ = Susceptible.
− = Resistant.
v = Variable.

Bites. Anaerobes are present in approximately 35% of animal bite wound infections (see Ch. 325), especially those that are more severe or are associated with tissue necrosis or abscess formation. These anaerobes are part of the oral flora of the biting animal. Consequently, the routine bacteriology laboratory may have difficulty in identifying them. Most are penicillin/ampicillin susceptible. Besides anaerobes, *Pasteurella multocida, Staphylococcus intermedius, Staphylococcus aureus,* and streptococci should be considered potential pathogens.

Human bites, both occlusional injuries and clenched fist injuries, tend to be more serious than animal bites. Anaerobes can be isolated from 55% of human bite wounds and are more frequently β-lactamase–producing and penicillin-resistant. There is also a higher frequency of septic arthritis and osteomyelitis associated with human bite wounds. One must consider anaerobes plus *Eikenella corrodens,* streptococci, *S. aureus,* and *Haemophilus* species as potential pathogens when choosing empirical antimicrobial therapy.

Gangrenes. Gangrene indicates necrosis, most often of skin and subcutaneous tissue, and is often rapidly progressive. Several types of "infectious gangrene" have been described and may sometimes be indistinguishable on a clinical basis. These include the following:

1. *Gas gangrene,* which can incidentally involve other anaerobes besides *C. perfringens* and other clostridia.
2. *Progressive bacterial synergistic gangrene* often involves microaerophilic streptococci and peptostreptococci as well as aerobic bacteria such as *S. aureus* and Enterobacteriaceae.
3. *Synergistic necrotizing cellulitis* involves a mixed aerobic and anaerobic bacteria including B. *fragilis* and peptostreptococci. Diabetic patients may be predisposed. The cellulitis is markedly painful, crepitus may be present, and the discharge has a foul odor.
4. *Fournier's gangrene* is a serious infection of the scrotum or perineum which starts with scrotal pain and erythema and rapidly progresses to necrosis and gangrene, which can lead to sloughing of tissue. It is more often seen in diabetics and can be associated with trauma.

PRINCIPLES OF DIAGNOSIS AND THERAPY

Clues as to when one should suspect anaerobic infection are listed in Table 290–5. Obtaining an appropriately collected and acceptable specimen (Table 290–6) must be an active process and specified in the orders.

General principles of therapy are listed in Table 290–7. In general, appropriate antimicrobial therapy coupled with prompt drainage and surgical debridement are essential for therapeutic success. Table 290–8 notes the susceptibility patterns of the various clinically important anaerobes.

Finegold SM, Goldstein EJC (eds.): Proceedings of the First North American Congress on Anaerobic Bacteria and Anaerobic Infections. Clin Infect Dis 16(suppl 4):159, 1993.

Finegold SM, Mulligan ME: Centennial Symposium on Anaerobes: A memorial to André Veillon, The Secret Pathogens. Clin Infect Dis 18(suppl 4):245, 1994.

Enteric Infections

291 INTRODUCTION TO ENTERIC INFECTIONS
Herbert L. DuPont

Enteric infections are second only to respiratory tract infections as common medical problems. In certain populations, enteric infections are hyperendemic: in poorly nourished children living in developing tropical countries where they are significant causes of pediatric mortality, in infants in day care centers, in residents of custodial institutions for the mentally retarded, in homosexual males, and in those who venture from industrialized to developing regions ("travelers' diarrhea").

In approaching a patient with an enteric infection, epidemiologic (Table 291–1) and clinical features (Table 291–2) are used to determine the proper approach to evaluation and management. One must work through the various considerations to be certain that the proper differential diagnosis and workup are developed. Recent travel to a mountainous region of North America should raise the possibility of infection by *Giardia lamblia.* Travel to Russia, particularly St. Petersburg, is associated with an increased risk of infection by *Cryptosporidium parvum* and *G. lamblia.* When diarrhea occurs during or after travel to a developing tropical region, a bacterial enteropathogen should be suspected.

A specific food or water vehicle cannot be suspected unless multiple cases of illness with a common exposure occur. In this situation, the incubation period will often help determine the etiologic diagnosis: <4 hours in the case of a *Staphylococcus aureus* or *Bacillus cereus* enterotoxin food poisoning or >8 hours in the case of intestinal infection. On evaluation of the clinical expression of the illness (see Table 291–2), a tentative diagnosis may be made. In the patient who is receiving an antimicrobial drug, or who has recently completed a course of therapy, and presents with an enteric infection manifested by diarrhea with or without fever and dysenteric disease, *Clostridium difficile* should be suspected. When a per-

TABLE 291-1. EPIDEMIOLOGIC FEATURES IMPORTANT IN DETERMINING POTENTIAL CAUSES OF ENTERIC INFECTION

Epidemiologic Feature	Etiologic Agent to Suspect
Travel to mountainous areas of North America	*Giardia lamblia*
Travel to Russia (especially St. Petersburg)	*Cryptosporidium, G. lamblia*
Travel to the developing tropical/semitropical world from an industrialized region	Enterotoxigenic *Escherichia coli, Shigella, Salmonella* (including *S. typhi*), other bacterial causes, *G. lamblia,* and *Cryptosporidium*
Presence of associated cases (an outbreak)	Use incubation period and clinical features (Table 291–2) to determine probable cause
Antibiotic use in the last 2 weeks	*Clostridium difficile*
Contact with day care centers	Any enteropathogen, often *G. lamblia, Cryptosporidium, Shigella,* or rotavirus
Homosexual male with diarrhea	Any organism spread by fecal-oral route, with proctitis suspect *Neisseria gonorrhoea, Chlamydia trachomatis,* herpes simplex, or *Treponema pallidium,* with AIDS any agent, especially *Cryptosporidium, Microsporidium, Cyclospora, Salmonella, C. jejuni, C. difficile, Mycobacterium avium-intracellulare,* cytomegalovirus

son has close contact with an infant or infants attending a day care center, a number of pathogens found in this setting should be suspected. Finally, the homosexual male with an enteric infection may have acquired it through fecal-oral contamination so common in this setting (and in this case multiple pathogens may be found in stool), through receptive anal intercourse, or when intestinal immu-

TABLE 291-2. CLINICAL FEATURES OF ENTERIC INFECTION

Clinical Syndrome	Etiologic Agents Suspected	Special Considerations
Enteric or typhoid fever	*Salmonella typhi, S. enteritidis, Campylobacter, Shigella, Yersinia enterocolitica*	Blood cultures; antibiotics generally needed
Acute watery diarrhea	Any agent may be responsible. Consider: *Vibrio cholerae,* enterotoxigenic *Escherichia coli, Shigella, Salmonella, C. jejuni*	Fluid and electrolyte therapy crucial for recovery in dehydration
Gastroenteritis	Viral agents (rotavirus or small round viruses) or enterotoxin mediated disease (*Staphylococcus aureus* or *Bacillus cereus*)	In case of an outbreak, incubation period suggests the etiology
Dysentery	*Shigella, C. jejuni, Salmonella,* enterohemorrhagic (0157:H7) or enteroinvasive *E. coli, Aeromonas hydrophilia, Vibrio parahemolyticus, Yersinia enterocolitica, Entamoeba histolytica,* or inflammatory bowel disease	Stool culture and occasionally parasite exam important to determining cause; hemolytic uremic syndrome may complicate diarrheal disease caused by *E. coli* 0157:H7 or *S. dysenteriae* 1
Persistent diarrhea	*Giardia lamblia,* small bowel bacterial overgrowth, bacterial diarrhea, lactase deficiency, Brainerd diarrhea	Stool culture and parasite exam indicated; empiric anti-*Giardia* therapy may be useful; milk should not be consumed; a history of raw milk or untreated (well or surface) water consumption suggests Brainerd diarrhea

nity has become depressed as a result of the acquired immune deficiency syndrome (AIDS).

Enteric infection syndromes may be divided into five groups based on the clinical presentation, including febrile systemic disease (enteric fever), acute watery diarrhea (small bowel secretory process), profuse vomiting (gastroenteritis), the passage of many small-volume stools containing blood and mucus (dysenteric disease), and diarrhea lasting longer than 2 weeks (persistent diarrheal disease). Table 291–2 lists the major syndromes along with the expected etiology. In the majority of cases of enteric infection, it is not possible to determine the cause of illness on clinical grounds. Laboratory tests are often useful, particularly in the more severe or intensely ill patients, to help establish cause and to develop the proper plan of treatment.

Treatment of diarrhea should be tailored to clinical syndrome. Oral rehydration with fluids and electrolytes is used in acute watery diarrhea and gastroenteritis and in all forms of enteric infection when any degree of dehydration occurs. For enteric fever and dysenteric disease, antimicrobial therapy is indicated. For patients with persistent diarrhea, workup for cause is indicated before a management plan is developed.

292 TYPHOID FEVER
Thomas Butler

DEFINITION. Typhoid fever is a bacterial disease caused by *Salmonella typhi.* It is characterized by prolonged fever, abdominal pain, diarrhea, delirium, rose spots, and splenomegaly and complicated sometimes by intestinal bleeding and perforation. Enteric fever is synonymous with typhoid fever, which is occasionally caused also by *S. enteritidis* bioserotype paratyphi A or B.

ETIOLOGY. The typhoid bacillus is a motile gram-negative rod in the family Enterobacteriaceae. It possesses a flagellar (H) antigen, a cell wall (O) lipopolysaccharide antigen, and a polysaccharide virulence (Vi) antigen located in the cell capsule. The polysaccharide side chain of the O antigen confers serologic specificity to the organism and is essential in virulence because salmonellae other than *S. typhi* and *S. enteritidis* bioserotype paratyphi A or B do not produce enteric fever in humans.

INCIDENCE AND PREVALENCE. Typhoid fever has been almost eliminated from developed countries because of sewage and water treatment facilities but remains a common disease in developing countries. In 1980, the number of cases occurring yearly was estimated as about 7 million in Asia, over 4 million in Africa, and 0.5 million in Latin America. About 500 cases are diagnosed each year in the United States, and over half of these are in recently arrived travelers who contracted their infections abroad.

EPIDEMIOLOGY. Adults and children of all ages and both genders appear equally susceptible to infection. In developing countries, most cases occur in school-age children and young adults. Although acquired immunity provides some protection, reinfections have been documented. Typhoid fever occurs during all seasons.

Transmission is by the fecal-oral route through contaminated water or food. The main human sources of infection in the community are asymptomatic fecal carriers and cases during either disease or convalescence. Females and older males are prone to become chronic fecal carriers because underlying cholecystitis enables them to harbor chronic infection in the gallbladder. *S. typhi* is resistant to drying and cooling, thus allowing bacteria to survive prolonged periods in dried sewage, water, food, and ice.

Vi-phage typing of *S. typhi* is a useful epidemiologic tool to trace cases of typhoid fever to a carrier or food source. Single-source outbreaks of typhoid fever are rare. In endemic situations, multiple phage types are present, and several phage types may be responsible for an epidemic.

PATHOGENESIS AND PATHOLOGY. After *S. typhi* is ingested, the part of the inoculum that survives stomach acid enters the small intestine, where bacteria penetrate the mucosa and enter mononuclear phagocytes of ileal Peyer's patches and mesenteric lymph nodes. Inocula of at least 10^5 bacteria are necessary to initiate disease, and inocula of 10^7 and more cause disease regularly. The incubation period ranges from 8 to 28 days, depending on inoculum size and immune status of the host. Bacteria proliferate in mononuclear phagocytes and spread by way of the blood to the spleen, liver, and bone marrow, where further proliferation in macrophages occurs. The earliest symptoms of fever and chills (Table 292–1) are associated with bacteremia. Inflammatory reactions occur in the spleen, liver, bone marrow, Peyer's patches mainly in the terminal ileum, and skin, consisting of mononuclear cell infiltration, hyperplasia, and focal necrosis. Focal collections of mononuclear leukocytes are called "typhoid nodules." Fever and other constitutional symptoms are probably caused by the release of cytokines, including tumor necrosis factor and interleukin-1, from infected mononuclear phagocytes. Endotoxemia does not occur in typhoid fever. Intestinal manifestations are caused by hyperplasia of Peyer's patches with ulcerations of overlying mucosa, resulting in pain, diarrhea, bleeding, or perforation.

CLINICAL MANIFESTATIONS. In the first days of illness, the nonspecific symptoms of fever, chills, and headache are mild and in the typical case build up in intensity during the first week, resulting in prostration. The evolution of disease syndromes occurs stepwise over 1 to 3 weeks (Table 292–1) but may be variable in the time of appearance. The early symptoms of fever, abdominal pain, and prostration tend to persist throughout the illness, which in untreated cases lasts a month or longer. Abdominal pain occurs in more than half of patients and is frequently diffuse or located in the right lower quadrant over the terminal ileum. Diarrhea occurs in about a third of patients and consists of either watery stools or semisolid stools. Melena occurs less commonly. Rose spots occur in more than half of light-skinned individuals but are often not visible in dark-skinned patients. The rash is seen most commonly on the shoulders, thorax, and abdomen and rarely affects the extremities. The lesions are erythematous macules or papules about 1 to 5 mm in diameter which typically blanch with pressure but may become hemorrhagic. Many patients display abnormal behavior or altered mental status that may be out of proportion to the severity of the systemic illness. Among the common presentations are "toxic" staring, delirium, aphonia, and coma. Seizures are common in children. Patients are rarely jaundiced.

In about 5% of patients, intestinal bleeding or intestinal perforation occurs, usually after the second week of illness. Bleeding occurs from ileal ulcers and may present as melena or bright red blood in stools. Brisk bleeding develops rarely but is an occasional cause of death. Intestinal perforation presents as the sudden onset of more severe abdominal pain, distention, and tenderness. Bowel sounds are diminished, and the abdominal radiograph usually reveals free air. Perforation most often occurs unexpectedly after a few days of treatment when a patient has started to improve. Other complications of typhoid fever include pneumonia, which develops as a superinfection due to other bacteria, myocarditis, acute cholecystitis, and acute meningitis.

Relapses occur in about 10 to 20% of patients treated with chloramphenicol. Patients with relapses experience the reappearance of typical symptoms about 7 to 14 days after the end of treatment. Relapses tend to be less severe than the initial episode.

DIAGNOSIS. The preferred method of diagnosis is isolation of *S. typhi* from a blood culture, which is positive in most patients during the first 2 weeks of illness. Urine and stool cultures are positive less frequently but should be taken to increase the diagnostic yield. The bone marrow culture is the most sensitive test, positive in nearly 90% of cases, and can be used when a bacteriologic diagnosis is crucially needed or in patients who have been pretreated with antibiotics. The duodenal string test to culture bile has also been used with success in typhoid fever.

The Widal test for agglutinating antibodies against the somatic (O) and flagellar (H) antigens of *S. typhi* is widely used for serodiagnosis. An O agglutinin titer of $\geq 1:80$ or a fourfold rise supports a diagnosis of typhoid fever, whereas the H agglutinins are more often nonspecifically elevated by immunization or previous infections with other bacteria. Serodiagnosis is of limited value because false-positive results are often obtained in endemic areas and false-negative results occur in some cases of bacteriologically proven typhoid fever.

Other laboratory findings are anemia of variable severity and a white blood cell count that is normal or decreased with an increased percentage of band forms. Platelets are often diminished, and signs of disseminated intravascular coagulation are present. Liver function tests frequently show elevated aminotransferases and bilirubin concentrations. Renal failure is an infrequent complication. In patients with diarrhea, the stool shows fecal leukocytes.

The differential diagnosis depends on infections that are endemic in the area where an individual contracted the infection. For returned travelers from developing countries, the common possibilities are malaria, hepatitis, typhus, amebic liver abscess, shigellosis, nontyphoid salmonellosis, and leptospirosis. In the United States one must consider septicemias originating from the urinary tract, gastrointestinal tract, or gallbladder as well as influenza, infectious mononucleosis, meningococcemia, miliary tuberculosis, and bacterial endocarditis.

TREATMENT. Chloramphenicol has remained the drug of choice since its introduction in 1948 because no other drug has been demonstrated to cause more rapid or consistent improvement of disease. Chloramphenicol is given orally in a dose of 50 to 60 mg per kilogram of body weight per day in four equal portions every 6 hours. After defervescence and clinical improvement the dosage can be reduced to 30 mg per kilogram per day to complete a 14-day course. In patients unable to take oral medication, the same dosage should be given intravenously until the patient can take capsules.

Alternative drugs should be considered when *S. typhi* resistant to chloramphenicol is isolated or strongly suspected. Several are nearly equal to chloramphenicol in efficacy. Trimethoprim-sulfamethoxazole is effective in a standard adult dose of 160 mg trimethoprim and 800 mg sulfamethoxazole given orally or intravenously twice a day for 14 days. Other drugs that are effective include ampicillin (intravenously), amoxicillin, cefoperazone, and ceftriaxone. In recent years, most isolates of *S. typhi* from cases in India and Pakistan have shown plasmid-mediated, multidrug resistance to chloramphenicol, ampicillin, and trimethoprim-sulfamethoxazole. These adults can be treated with ciprofloxacin, 750 mg twice daily for 7 to 14 days, or with other fluoroquinolones. Children with multidrug-resistant infections should receive ceftriaxone.

Patients who are dehydrated, anorectic, or suffering from diarrhea should receive intravenous saline with attention to electrolyte and acid-base disturbances. Patients with brisk intestinal bleeding require blood transfusion. Patients with suspected perforation should have an abdominal radiograph to look for free air and peritoneal

TABLE 292–1. EVOLUTION OF TYPICAL SYMPTOMS AND SIGNS OF TYPHOID FEVER

Disease Period	Symptoms	Signs	Pathology
First week	Fever, chills gradually increasing and persisting; headache	Abdominal tenderness	Bacteremia
Second week	Rash, abdominal pain, diarrhea or constipation, delirium, prostration	Rose spots, splenomegaly, hepatomegaly	Mononuclear cell vasculitis of skin, hyperplasia of ileal Peyer's patches, typhoid nodules in spleen and liver
Third week	Complications of intestinal bleeding and perforation, shock	Melena, ileus, rigid abdomen, coma	Ulcerations over Peyer's patches, perforation with peritonitis
Fourth week and later	Resolution of symptoms, relapse, weight loss	Reappearance of acute disease, cachexia	Cholecystitis, chronic fecal carriage of bacteria

fluid. Laparotomy should be undertaken as early as possible to suture the perforation.

In some high-risk patients with delirium, coma, or shock, high-dose dexamethasone in addition to antibiotics reduces mortality. The dose should be 3 mg per kilogram initially, followed by 1 mg per kilogram every 6 hours for 48 hours. One must be cautious with this therapy because signs and symptoms of perforation are masked by steroids. Antipyretic drugs such as aspirin should be administered with caution because they occasionally markedly reduce blood pressure.

Patients with relapses of typhoid fever should be treated the same as patients with a first attack. Chronic fecal carriers (asymptomatic excretion for a year or longer) should be given high doses of ampicillin or amoxicillin, 100 mg per kilogram per day, plus probenecid, 30 mg per kilogram per day for 4 to 6 weeks. Trimethoprim-sulfamethoxazole is also effective. Patients with multidrug-resistant infections can be treated with ciprofloxacin or other quinolones. Patients with gallstones or cholecystitis may require cholecystectomy to eradicate the carrier state. Chloramphenicol neither prevents nor effectively treats the chronic carrier state.

PROGNOSIS. Typhoid fever carried a case fatality rate of about 12% in the preantibiotic era which was reduced to about 4% after chloramphenicol became available. Case fatality rates >10% continue to be reported in developing countries despite availability of antibiotics, whereas developed countries show case fatality rates <1%. After treatment with chloramphenicol or other effective drug, most patients become afebrile in 4 to 7 days. In the preantibiotic era, about 10% of recovered patients had relapses, and chloramphenicol treatment has not reduced this rate. Intestinal bleeding or perforation occurs in about 5% of patients and may not be prevented by antibiotic treatment. Thus bleeding or perforation is occasionally detected after patients have defervesced during treatment. About 1 to 3% of patients become chronic fecal carriers after recovery.

PREVENTION. Travelers to developing countries should avoid consuming untreated water, drinks served with ice, peeled fruits, and other food that is not served hot. American international travelers face an overall risk of developing typhoid fever of <1 case in 10,000 trips, but travelers to high-risk countries like India and Pakistan have a probability of about 4 in 10,000 trips of getting typhoid fever. Travelers wishing immune protection should receive either live oral vaccine Ty21a (Berna Products [305-443-2900]) given as one capsule every other day for a total of four capsules or typhoid vaccine, U.S.P., administered as two subcutaneous injections of 0.5 ml each at intervals of 4 weeks, with booster doses given every 3 years if needed. These vaccines give only partial protection, and thus vaccinated persons should still exercise dietary precautions. The traditional method of controlling typhoid is to follow stool cultures of convalescent cases and report positive cultures to the health department. The health department investigates nonimported typhoid cases to identify possible food sources or contact with a chronic carrier.

Butler T, Ho M, Acharya G, et al.: Interleukin-6, gamma interferon, and tumor necrosis factor receptors in typhoid fever related to outcome of antimicrobial therapy. Antimicrob Agents Chemother 37:2418, 1993. *Plasma concentrations of cytokines were elevated but not to the same extent as in other causes of bacteremia.*

Butler T, Islam A, Kabir I, et al.: Patterns of morbidity and mortality in typhoid fever dependent on age and gender: Review of 552 hospitalized patients with diarrhea. Rev Infect Dis 13:85, 1991. *Severe and fatal disease in Bangladesh was more common in young children and adults and was correlated with high incidences of seizures, delirium or coma, intestinal perforation, and pneumonia.*

Islam A, Butler T, Nath SK, et al.: Randomized treatment of patients with typhoid fever by using ceftriaxone or chloramphenicol. J Infect Dis 158:742, 1988. *Study of treatment in Bangladesh showed that chloramphenicol remains the treatment of choice because of low cost and rapid defervescence, but newer cephalosporins are good alternatives.*

Levine MM, Ferreccio C, Black RE, et al.: Large-scale field trial of Ty21a live oral typhoid vaccine in enteric-coated capsule formulation. Lancet 1:1049, 1987. *In Chilean school children, three capsules given every other day conferred 67% protection during 3 years; oral vaccination is preferred to parenteral vaccine because of absence of toxic reactions.*

Trujillo IZ, Quiroz C, Gutierrez MA, et al.: Fluoroquinolones in the treatment of typhoid fever and the carrier state. Eur J Clin Microbiol Infect Dis 10:334, 1991. *Ciprofloxacin, norfloxacin, ofloxacin, and pefloxacin have been effective in limited trials against typhoid fever and chronic typhoid carriers.*

293 SALMONELLA INFECTIONS OTHER THAN TYPHOID FEVER

Donald Kaye

DEFINITION. *Salmonella*, a genus of the family Enterobacteriaceae, can cause an asymptomatic intestinal carrier state or clinical disease in both humans and animals. In humans, the most common clinical manifestation is enterocolitis, with diarrhea as the major symptom. Some patients develop bacteremia without gastrointestinal manifestations. Localization from bacteremia may result in osteomyelitis, a mycotic aneurysm, or other localized infection. *S. typhi*, a pathogen of humans only, causes enteric fever. Enteric fever produced by *S. typhi* is called "typhoid fever," whereas enteric fever caused by other salmonellae is named "paratyphoid fever."

An asymptomatic intestinal carrier state of variable duration may follow inapparent or symptomatic infection. Most carriers are transient carriers. A chronic carrier state, defined as lasting more than 1 year, is usually permanent and is most often related to persistent infection in the gallbladder. With the exception of *S. typhi*, in which a human carrier is always implicated, most *Salmonella* infections are acquired from food products derived from infected animals (e.g., eggs, poultry, meat, milk).

ETIOLOGY. Salmonellae are motile, gram-negative, non–spore-forming bacilli. They are differentiated from other Enterobacteriaceae by biochemical tests. They ferment glucose, maltose, and mannitol but not lactose or sucrose. Almost all salmonellae produce acid and gas with fermentation. Exceptions to the rules which are helpful in identification are the following: *S. typhi* does not produce gas, and *S. gallinarum-pullorum* is nonmotile. As another confounding exception, lactose-fermenting strains of salmonellae have been isolated.

Salmonellae can be differentiated into over 2000 serotypes by their somatic (O) antigens, which are composed of lipopolysaccharides and are part of the cell wall, and flagellar (H) antigens. Proper nomenclature has divided the salmonellae into three species: *S. typhi*, *S. choleraesuis*, and *S. enteritidis*. The first two consist of only one serotype each, whereas the third contains all the rest of the serotypes. These latter serotypes are recognized as *S. enteritidis* serotype _____ (e.g., *S. enteritidis* serotype typhimurium). However, in a less confusing and cumbersome system, each serotype is commonly referred to as a separate species and is so indicated in this chapter. In this system, using common O antigens, salmonellae have been divided into five major groups, A through E. Some of the important serotypes and their groups are *S. typhi* (group D), *S. choleraesuis* (Group C_1), *S. typhimurium* (group B), and *S. enteritidis* (group D).

S. typhimurium and *S. enteritidis* are the most common causes of human disease and represented 22 and 19% of *Salmonella* isolates from human sources reported in the United States in 1991. Other common isolates are *S. heidelberg*, *S. hadar*, *S. newport*, *S. agona*, *S. montevideo*, *S. poona*, *S. javiana*, and *S. thompson*. In 1991, these 10 serotypes accounted for 68% of the human isolates. In recent years, *S. enteritidis* outbreaks related to eggs have been increasing.

EPIDEMIOLOGY. *S. typhi*, *S. paratyphi A*, *S. schottmuelleri* (*S. paratyphi B*), *S. hirschfeldii* (*S. paratyphi C*), and *S. sendai* are either solely or almost always pathogens in humans only, and human-to-human transmission is important.

The remaining serotypes of salmonellae are widely spread in the animal kingdom, and salmonellae have been isolated from virtually all species, including birds, poultry, mammals, reptiles, amphibians, and insects. *Salmonella* infection in humans usually occurs from ingesting contaminated animal food products, most often eggs, poultry, and meat. Eggs usually become contaminated from feces on the surface of the egg, with small cracks allowing entry into the egg. However, infection of the ovary allows primary incorporation of salmonellae into the egg. Meat and poultry become widely contaminated at the slaughterhouse with salmonellae spread from carcass to carcass, usually on the surface. *S. choleraesuis* is associated with pig products and *S. dublin* with cattle and consumption of unpasteurized milk from cattle. Salmonellae may survive cooking at relatively low temperatures in the center of eggs or turkeys, or food may be contaminated after cooking from kitchen utensils or from the hands of food preparers who handle raw food.

Salmonella infections have been acquired following contamination of food or water with feces of pet turtles, chicks, birds, dogs, cats, and many other species. These pets become infected from their food.

Salmonella infection also can be acquired by eating food or less commonly drinking water contaminated by a human carrier who has not washed his/her hands adequately. Infection has been spread by the fecal-oral route in children, by contaminated enema and fiberoptic instruments, and by diagnostic and therapeutic preparations made from animal or insect products (e.g., pancreatic extract, carmine dye). Homosexual men are prone to fecal-oral infection.

Outbreaks of salmonellosis occur in institutionalized patients, who are probably more prone to develop *Salmonella* infections for three reasons. First, there are more underlying diseases which decrease host defense mechanisms against salmonellae such as disorders of gastric acidity and intestinal motility; second, use of antimicrobial agents reduces the normal, protective intestinal flora; and third, institutional food prepared in bulk is more likely to be contaminated than individually prepared meals. Outbreaks in nurseries and in the elderly in nursing homes have the highest mortality rates (i.e., >5%). Diabetes may be an additional risk factor for *Salmonella* infection.

Most cases of *Salmonella* infection occurring in the United States are sporadic rather than related to outbreaks. However, when an infection occurs in a family, other members of the household also tend to have positive stool cultures. About 40,000 cases of *Salmonella* infection have been reported to the CDC in recent years, a marked increase over the past 30 years. However, this undoubtedly represents only a fraction of actual cases. It has been estimated that over 1 million cases actually occur each year. A disproportionate number of infections occur in July through October, probably related to the warm weather. *Salmonella* infections are most common in infants and children under 5 years of age.

Salmonellae have become increasingly resistant to antibiotics, usually by acquiring resistance transfer factors. It is believed that much of the resistance has been related to widespread use of antimicrobial agents in farm animals.

PATHOGENESIS. Following ingestion of organisms, the determinants of whether or not infection results, as well as the severity of infection, are the dose and virulence of the *Salmonella* strain and the status of host defense mechanisms. Large inocula such as 10^7 bacteria are usually required to produce clinical infection in the normal host. Smaller inocula are more likely to result in no infection or to produce a transient intestinal carrier state. Gastric acid serves as a host defense mechanism by killing many of the ingested organisms, and intestinal motility is also probably a host defense mechanism. In the absence or decrease of gastric acidity (as in the elderly, following gastrectomy, vagotomy, or gastroenterostomy, with H_2-receptor antagonists, and with antacids) and with decreased intestinal motility (as with antimotility drugs), much smaller inocula can produce infection and the infection tends to be more severe.

Administration of antimicrobial agents prior to ingestion of salmonellae can markedly reduce the size of inoculum needed to produce infection, presumably by reducing the protective bowel flora.

While any *Salmonella* serotype can produce any of the *Salmonella* syndromes (transient asymptomatic carrier state, enterocolitis, bacteremia, enteric fever, and chronic carrier state), each serotype tends to produce certain syndromes much more often than others. For example, *S. anatum* usually causes asymptomatic intestinal infection, whereas *S. typhimurium* usually causes enterocolitis. *S. choleraesuis* is more likely to produce bacteremia (often with metastatic infection) than asymptomatic infection or enterocolitis, and some serotypes such as *S. typhi* are most likely to cause enteric fever as well as the chronic carrier state. Fortunately, most *Salmonella* serotypes are of relatively low pathogenicity for humans, and therefore, although food products are commonly contaminated, large outbreaks occur only when more virulent serotypes are involved.

In order to produce infection (even asymptomatic intestinal infection), enteric pathogens (including salmonellae) must first adhere to intestinal mucosal epithelial cells. Pili on the surface of salmonellae

adhere to specific receptor sites on the epithelial cells. Following adherence, invasion of the mucosal cell may result, or multiplication may occur without invasion, resulting in asymptomatic infection. When the organisms reach the lamina propria, polymorphonuclear leukocytes serve as a defense mechanism to prevent invasion of lymphatics. Certain serotypes seem more able than others to invade lymphatics and subsequently produce bacteremia. For example, *S. dublin*, which has been isolated from unpasteurized milk, commonly produces bacteremia following intestinal infection. Both the small intestine and colon are involved in the inflammatory process. The diarrhea in *Salmonella* enterocolitis results from the inflammation. In addition, watery stools may occur, apparently the result of secretion of water and electrolytes by small intestinal epithelial cells in response to an enterotoxin secreted by some of the *Salmonella* strains or in response to tissue mediators of inflammation.

Patients with diseases that impair host defense mechanisms seem to have an increased frequency of severe *Salmonella* infection. For many years, a striking association has been recognized between diseases producing hemolysis and *Salmonella* bacteremia. Specifically, *Salmonella* bacteremia is common in patients with sickle cell disorders, malaria, and bartonellosis. In fact, because of the frequency of *Salmonella* bacteremia in sickle cell diseases and the underlying bone disease in these patients to which salmonellae localize, these organisms are the most common cause of osteomyelitis in patients with sickle cell disorders. Prolonged *Salmonella* bacteremia occurs in patients with hepatosplenic schistosomiasis, probably related to localization on and in the intravascular schistosomes. Patients with lymphoma and leukemia also are more prone to develop *Salmonella* bacteremia. Recently, prolonged and recurrent refractory *Salmonella* bacteremia has been observed in patients with AIDS.

CLINICAL SYNDROMES. *Asymptomatic Intestinal Carrier State.* The asymptomatic intestinal carrier state may result from inapparent infection, which is the most common form of *Salmonella* infection, or may follow clinical disease (convalescent carrier). The carrier state is usually self-limited to several weeks to months, with the incidence of positive stool cultures rapidly decreasing. By 1 year, far less than 1% still have positive stools. The major exception is with *S. typhi:* About 3% of those infected excrete the organism for life. A patient who has had *Salmonella* in the stool for 1 year (chronic carrier) is likely to become a lifelong carrier. Patients with *Schistosoma haematobium* infections are predisposed to become chronic urinary carriers of *Salmonella.*

Enterocolitis. After an incubation period, which is usually 12 to 48 hours, the illness starts suddenly with crampy abdominal pain and diarrhea. A chill is common. Although occasional patients have nausea and vomit once or twice, vomiting is not persistent. The diarrhea may be watery and of large volume or small volume. The stools may contain mucus and occasionally blood. Polymorphonuclear leukocytes are present in the stool. Diarrhea may be mild or may be severe with up to 20 to 30 stools a day. Fever is present in most patients and may reach 40°C (104°F) or higher. The abdomen is tender to palpation. Transient bacteremia may occur and is most likely in infants, the elderly, and patients with impaired host defense mechanisms.

Symptoms usually improve over a period of days, with fever lasting no more than 2 to 3 days and diarrhea no more than 5 to 7 days. However, these symptoms may occasionally persist for up to 14 days. More severe disease is seen with malnutrition, inflammatory bowel disease, and AIDS. Reactive arthritis may follow enterocolitis in up to 7% of cases. It is especially frequent in those with the HLA-B27 phenotype.

Enteric Fever. Paratyphoid fever is an enteric fever syndrome identical to typhoid fever but produced by a serotype other than *S. typhi* (most often *S. paratyphi A, S. schottmuelleri,* or *S. hirschfeldii.* On occasion, it may immediately follow classic enterocolitis caused by the same organism. The syndrome, characterized by prolonged sustained fever, relative bradycardia, splenomegaly, rose spots, and leukopenia, is described in Ch. 292. Enteric fever produced by serotypes of *Salmonella* other than *S. typhi* is usually milder than typhoid fever, and the chronic carrier state follows less commonly than after typhoid fever.

Bacteremia. Patients with the syndrome of *Salmonella* bacteremia usually complain of fever and chills for a period of days to weeks. Gastrointestinal symptoms are unusual, but in some patients the syndrome of *Salmonella* bacteremia follows classic enterocolitis. Other symptoms are nonspecific such as malaise, anorexia, and weight loss. Metastatic infection of bones, joints, mycotic aneurysm (particularly of the abdominal aorta), meninges (mainly in infants), pericardium, pleural space, lungs, heart valves, cysts, uterine myomas, malignancies, and other sites is common, and symptoms may be related to the site of metastatic infection. Stool cultures are usually negative for *Salmonella*, but blood cultures are positive.

Although any *Salmonella* serotype can produce the syndrome of bacteremia, *S. choleraesuis* is most likely to cause this syndrome; over 50% of *S. choleraesuis* infections are bacteremic.

Salmonella bacteremia occurs with increased frequency in infants and the elderly and in patients with diseases associated with hemolysis (such as sickle cell diseases, malaria, and bartonellosis), with lymphoma, with leukemia, and perhaps with systemic lupus erythematosus. Localization to bone is common in patients with sickle cell diseases.

Prolonged *Salmonella* bacteremia lasting for months occurs in patients with hepatosplenic schistosomiasis. Patients with AIDS develop recurrent, relapsing *Salmonella* bacteremia that is difficult to cure with antibiotics.

DIAGNOSIS. The diagnosis of *Salmonella* infection is made by isolating the organism from the stool in enterocolitis, from the blood in bacteremia, from blood and stool in enteric fever, and from the local site in localized infection. Serologic studies are of little clinical value in salmonella infections other than typhoid fever, but they may be of use in epidemiologic studies. A stained smear of the stool usually demonstrates polymorphonuclear leukocytes in patients with *Salmonella* enterocolitis.

The differential diagnosis of *Salmonella* enterocolitis includes all causes of acute diarrhea, including invasive bacteria such as *Campylobacter jejuni*, *Shigella* species, invasive *E. coli*, *Yersinia enterocolitica*, and *Vibrio parahaemolyticus;* toxigenic bacteria such as *Vibrio cholerae*, enterotoxigenic *E. coli*, *S. aureus*, *B. cereus*, *C. perfringens*, and *C. difficile;* viruses; and protozoa such as *E. histolytica*, *G. lamblia*, and *Cryptosporidium* species. Invasive bacterial causes of diarrhea and *C. difficile* infection are also associated with polymorphonuclear leukocytes in the stool, whereas bacterial toxigenic causes (other than *C. difficile*), viruses, and protozoa generally are not. The bacterial toxigenic causes of diarrhea other than *C. difficile* do not produce fever.

Stool culture is definitive for the diagnosis of *Salmonella* enterocolitis, but by the time the results of the stool culture are available, most patients are recovering.

The differential diagnosis of *Salmonella* bacteremia includes all acute infectious and noninfectious causes of fever, including bacteremia caused by other organisms.

The differential diagnosis of enteric fever is the same as discussed in Ch. 292.

TREATMENT. *Enterocolitis.* The primary approach to treatment of *Salmonella* enterocolitis is fluid and electrolyte replacement. Drugs with antiperistaltic effects such as loperamide or diphenoxylate with atropine can relieve cramps but should be used sparingly because they can prolong the diarrhea.

Salmonella enterocolitis is self-limited, and the large majority of cases do not require antimicrobial therapy. However, infants, the elderly, and those with sickle cell disease, lymphoma, leukemia, or other serious underlying diseases who are severely ill and may have bacteremia may benefit from antimicrobial therapy. Amoxicillin, 1 gram every 6 hours orally, or trimethoprim-sulfamethoxazole, one double-strength tablet every 12 hours orally in adults, can be used in those who are able to take oral drugs. Ampicillin, 1 to 2 grams IV every 6 hours, and trimethoprim-sulfamethoxazole, 10 mg per kilogram per day IV of the trimethoprim component, have been used in those who are more severely ill. Antibiotic susceptibility studies should be performed on the isolates, as many strains are now resistant to ampicillin and trimethoprim-sulfamethoxazole. Therapy is continued for 5 days.

There has been a reluctance to treat *Salmonella* enterocolitis, since antibiotic therapy has been reported to have no effect on the clinical course and furthermore to prolong the period of time that salmonellae are excreted in the stool. In addition, most patients are improving by the time that salmonellae or other bacterial pathogens are isolated from the stool. Perhaps most important, effective, single-drug therapy active against *Salmonella, Shigella, Campylobacter,* and other bacterial causes of diarrhea was lacking until the availability of the fluoroquinolones (e.g., norfloxacin, ciprofloxacin, ofloxacin). These agents are active against virtually all bacterial pathogens that cause diarrhea except for *C. difficile,* and it is reasonable to use them empirically in the early therapy of severe diarrhea of presumed bacterial etiology. Furthermore, several studies indicate that these agents may decrease the duration of the clinical course of *Salmonella* enterocolitis, although prolonging the duration of fecal excretion while others have shown no differences from placebo. At present, routine use of these agents cannot be advocated for suspected *Salmonella* enterocolitis. Further caution is warranted concerning routine use of fluoroquinolones for acute diarrheal disease of unknown etiology because *Campylobacter* has been seen to develop resistance to these agents following treatment.

Bacteremia and Enteric Fever. The major therapeutic agents have been chloramphenicol, 50 mg per kilogram per day in four equally divided doses orally or IV, or ampicillin, 2 grams IV every 6 hours. With resistant organisms or when these agents cannot be used for other reasons, trimethoprim-sulfamethoxazole IV may be substituted at a dose of 10 mg per kilogram per day of the trimethoprim component. Ampicillin is preferred when localized infection (especially intravascular) is present. After response, oral amoxicillin or oral trimethoprim-sulfamethoxazole can be given in the doses described under enterocolitis. Although experience has not been extensive, third-generation cephalosporins such as cefotaxime, ceftizoxime, ceftriaxone, and ceftazidime and the fluoroquinolones appear to be as effective as the older agents, and resistance to these newer agents is less likely. Thus, with further experience, they may become the drugs of choice. Therapy is continued for 2 weeks for enteric fever and bacteremia without localization of organisms and for much longer periods of time with localization to bone, aneurysms, heart valves, and various other sites. Surgical drainage or removal of foreign bodies is often necessary to cure localized infection.

Curing schistosomiasis in patients with *Salmonella* bacteremia may cure the bacteremia. Patients with AIDS tend to relapse repeatedly after treatment courses for *Salmonella* bacteremia. Long-term suppressive therapy has been recommended by some.

Carriers. Chronic carriers (i.e., over 1 year) of salmonellae other than *S. typhi* are rare. Stools of convalescent carriers spontaneously become negative over a period of weeks to months, and no therapy should be given. The rare chronic carrier of non–*S. typhi* serotypes (usually infected with *S. paratyphi A*, *S. schottmuelleri*, or *S. hirschfeldii*) may be treated with 4 to 6 grams of ampicillin plus 2 grams of probenecid orally each day in four divided doses for 6 weeks. The fluoroquinolones are probably equally effective. Patients who relapse usually have gallbladder disease (most often calculi) and will not be cured with antimicrobial therapy. Cholecystectomy plus antimicrobial therapy may cure these patients, but it is doubtful that the carrier state *per se* is a sufficient indication for cholecystectomy.

PROGNOSIS. Mortality in *Salmonella* enterocolitis is rare; infants and the elderly are at greatest risk, with death occurring from dehydration and electrolyte imbalance. Mortality from *Salmonella* bacteremia or enteric fever is not uncommon and is most likely to occur in the very young and the very old. *S. choleraesuis* bacteremia has the highest mortality rate of any *Salmonella* serotype, as high as 20 to 30%.

PREVENTION. *Salmonella* infection is best prevented by properly managing the water supply and sewage disposal, cooking and refrigerating foods made from animal products, pasteurizing milk and milk products, and handwashing before preparing foods and after handling animals and uncooked animal products. Despite these precautions, because of the widespread presence of salmonellae in the animal kingdom, it is unlikely that the frequency of *Salmonella* infections will be significantly diminished.

There is no vaccine for any salmonellae other than *S. typhi.*

Centers for Disease Control and Prevention: *Salmonella* Surveillance: Annual Summary, 1991. Washington, U.S. Public Health Service, 1991. *A compilation of the serotypes of* Salmonella *isolated from human and nonhuman sources in the United States.*

Katz SG, Andros G, Kohl RD: *Salmonella* infections in the abdominal aorta. Surg Gynecol Obstet 175:102, 1992. *A review of* Salmonella *infections of the abdominal aorta demonstrating the importance of surgical therapy.*

Mäki-Ikola O, Granfors K: *Salmonella*-triggered reactive arthritis. Scand J Rheumatol 21:265, 1992. *A review of the clinical significance of reactive arthritis triggered by* Salmonella *infection.*

Sanchez C, Garcia-Restoy E, Garau J, et al.: Ciprofloxacin and trimethoprim-sulfamethoxazole versus placebo in acute uncomplicated *Salmonella* enteritis: A double-blind trial. J Infect Dis 168:1304, 1993. *A report of use of ciprofloxacin and trimethoprim-sulfamethoxazole in* Salmonella *enterocolitis with no differences from placebo in resolution of symptoms or clearance of salmonellae from the stool.*

Telzak EE, Zweig Greenberg MS, Budnick LD, et al.: Diabetes mellitus: A newly described risk factor for infection from *Salmonella* enteritidis. J Infect Dis 164:538, 1991. *A report of an outbreak of* S. enteritidis *infection in hospitalized patients demonstrating increased susceptibility of medication-dependent diabetes.*

Winstrom J, Jertborn M, Ekwall E, et al.: Empiric treatment of acute diarrheal disease with norfloxacin. Ann Intern Med 117:202, 1992. *A report of use of norfloxacin in acute diarrheal disease demonstrating clinical response in* Salmonella *enterocolitis. However, the duration of fecal excretion of* Salmonella *was prolonged by therapy, and emergence of resistance to norfloxacin occurred among* Camplyobacter *strains.*

294 SHIGELLOSIS
Thomas Butler

DEFINITION. Shigellosis is an acute bacterial infection caused by the genus *Shigella* resulting in colitis affecting predominantly the rectosigmoid colon. "Bacillary dysentery" is synonymous with shigellosis. The disease is characterized by diarrhea, dysentery, fever, abdominal pain, and tenesmus. Shigellosis is usually limited to a few days. Early treatment with antimicrobial drugs results in more rapid recovery.

ETIOLOGY. Shigellae are nonmotile gram-negative bacilli belonging to the family Enterobacteriaceae. Four species of shigellae are recognized on the basis of antigenic and biochemical properties: *S. dysenteriae* (group A), *S. flexneri* (group B), *S. boydii* (group C), and *S. sonnei* (group D). Among these species there are over 40 serotypes, each of which is designated by the species name followed by a specific Arabic number. *S. dysenteriae* 1 is called the "Shiga bacillus" and causes epidemics with higher mortality than other serotypes. With the exception of *S. flexneri* 6, they do not ferment lactose.

Serotypes are determined by the O polysaccharide side chain of the lipopolysaccharide (endotoxin) in the cell wall. Endotoxin is detectable in the blood of severely ill patients and may be responsible for the complication of the hemolytic-uremic syndrome. To be virulent, shigellae must be able to invade epithelial cells, as tested in the laboratory by keratoconjunctivitis in the guinea pig (Sereney test) or HeLa cell invasion. Bacterial invasion of cells is genetically governed by three chromosomal regions and a 140-megadalton plasmid. Shiga toxin is produced by *S. dysenteriae* 1 and in lesser amounts by other serotypes. It inhibits protein synthesis and has enterotoxic activity in animal models, but its role in human disease is uncertain.

INCIDENCE AND PREVALENCE. In the United States there were more than 23,000 reported cases of shigellosis annually in 1990–92. The predominant species in the 1980's was *S. sonnei* (64%), followed by *S. flexneri* (31%), *S. boydii* (3%), and *S. dysenteriae* (2%). Most cases were in young children, women of childbearing age, and low-income minority residents, and a large proportion occurred in population groups living in homes for the mentally ill or in nursing homes. A large outbreak in 1987 in Tennessee affected more than 1000 persons camping under unsanitary conditions at a mass gathering.

Worldwide, most cases of shigellosis occur in children of developing countries, where *S. flexneri* is the predominant species. During the past 20 years, major epidemics due to *S. dysenteriae* 1 have occurred in Central America, Central Africa, India, and Bangladesh.

EPIDEMIOLOGY. Shigellosis is transmitted by the fecal-oral route. Crowded living conditions, low standards of personal hygiene, poor water supply, and inadequate sewage facilities all contribute to an increased risk of infection. Transmission most often occurs by close person-to-person contact through contaminated hands. During clinical illness and for up to 6 weeks after recovery, organisms are excreted in the feces. Although the organisms are sensitive to desiccation, they may survive several months in food or water, which are occasional vehicles of transmission.

Children between 1 and 4 years old have the greatest risk of developing shigellosis. Inhabitants of custodial institutions, such as homes for retarded children, are at highest risk. Intrafamilial spread follows often when the initial case has occurred in a preschool child. In young adults, the incidence is higher in women than men, which probably reflects closer contact of women with children. The male homosexual population in the United States is at increased risk for shigellosis, which is one of the causes of the "gay bowel syndrome."

Humans and higher primates are the only known natural reservoirs of shigellosis. Transmission shows variable seasonal patterns in different regions. In the United States, the peak incidence is in late summer and early autumn.

PATHOGENESIS AND PATHOLOGY. Since the microorganisms are relatively resistant to acid, shigellae pass the gastric barrier more readily than other enteric pathogens. In volunteer studies, as few as 200 ingested bacilli regularly initiate disease in 25% of healthy adults. This contrasts strikingly with the much larger numbers of typhoid or cholera bacilli required to produce disease in normal individuals. During the incubation period, usually 12 to 72 hours, the organisms traverse the small bowel, penetrate colonic epithelial cells, and multiply intracellularly. An acute inflammatory response ensues in the colonic mucosa attended by prodromal symptoms (Table 294–1). Epithelial cells containing bacteria are lysed, resulting in superficial ulcerations and shedding of shigella organisms into stools. The mucosa is friable and covered with a layer of polymorphonuclear leukocytes. Advancing inflammation causes the formation of crypt abscesses. Initially, the inflammation is confined to the rectosigmoid colon but after about 4 days of illness may advance to involve the proximal colon also. In severe cases, there may be pancolitis with extension of inflammation into the terminal ileum; a pseudomembranous type of colitis may develop. Diarrhea results because of impaired absorption of water and electrolytes by the inflamed colon.

Although the colonic inflammation is superficial, bacteremia occurs occasionally, especially in *S. dysenteriae* 1 infections. Susceptibility of organisms to serum complement–mediated bacteriolysis may explain the infrequency of bacteremia and disseminated infec-

TABLE 294–1. EVOLUTION OF CLINICAL SYNDROMES IN SHIGELLOSIS

Stage	Time of Appearance After Onset of Illness	Symptoms and Signs	Pathology
Prodrome	Earliest	Fever, chills, myalgias, anorexia, nausea, vomiting	None or early colitis
Nonspecific diarrhea	0–3 days	Abdominal cramps, loose stools, watery diarrhea	Rectosigmoid colitis with superficial ulceration, fecal leukocytes
Dysentery	1–8 days	Frequent passage of blood and mucus, tenesmus, rectal prolapse, abdominal tenderness	Colitis extending sometimes to proximal colon, crypt abscesses, inflammation in lamina propria
Complications	3–10 days	Dehydration, seizures, septicemia, leukemoid reaction, hemolytic-uremic syndrome, ileus, peritonitis	Severe colitis, terminal ileitis, endotoxemia, intravascular coagulation, toxic megacolon, colonic perforation
Postdysenteric syndromes	1–3 weeks	Arthritis, Reiter's syndrome	Reactive inflammation in HLA-B27 haplotype

tion. Colonic perforation is a rare complication during toxic megacolon. Children with severe colitis due to *S. dysenteriae* 1 are prone to develop the hemolytic-uremic syndrome. In this complication fibrin thrombi are deposited in the renal glomeruli, causing cortical necrosis and fragmentation of red cells.

CLINICAL MANIFESTATIONS. Most patients with shigellosis begin their illness with a nonspecific prodrome (Table 294–1). The height of the temperature varies, and children may have febrile convulsions. The initial intestinal symptoms soon follow as cramps, loose stools, and watery diarrhea, which usually precede the onset of dysentery by 1 or more days. The average fecal output is about 600 grams a day for adults. The dysentery consists typically of flecks and small clots of bright red blood and mucus in stools that are small in volume. Frequency of passage is often as high as 20 to 40 times a day, with excruciating rectal pain and tenesmus during defecation. Some patients develop rectal prolapse during severe straining. The amount of blood in stools varies widely but usually is small because of the superficial colonic ulcerations. Abdominal tenderness is often most marked in the left lower quadrant over the sigmoid colon but also may be generalized. The fever is likely to abate after a few days of dysentery, making afebrile bloody diarrhea an occasional clinical presentation. After 1 to 2 weeks of untreated disease, spontaneous improvement occurs in most patients. Some patients with mild disease develop only watery diarrhea without dysentery.

Complications include dehydration, which can cause death, especially in children and the elderly. *Shigella* septicemia occurs mainly in malnourished children with *S. dysenteriae* 1 infections. The leukemoid reaction and hemolytic-uremic syndrome may develop in children late in the course after antimicrobial treatment when the dysentery has started to improve. Neurologic manifestations can be striking and include delirium, seizures, and nuchal rigidity.

The important postdysenteric syndromes are arthritis and Reiter's triad of arthritis, urethritis, and conjunctivitis (see Ch. 238). These are nonsuppurative phenomena that occur in the absence of viable *Shigella* organisms about 1 to 3 weeks after resolution of dysentery.

DIAGNOSIS. Shigellosis should be considered in any patient with acute onset of fever and diarrhea. Examination of the stool is essential. Blood and pus are grossly apparent in severe bacillary dysentery; even in milder forms of the disease, microscopic examination of the stool often reveals numerous leukocytes and erythrocytes. The fecal leukocyte examination should be performed with a portion of liquid stool, preferably containing mucus. A drop of stool is placed on a microscopic slide, mixed thoroughly with two drops of methylene blue, and overlaid with a coverslip. The presence of abundant polymorphonuclear leukocytes helps distinguish shigellosis from diarrheal syndromes caused by viruses and enterotoxigenic bacteria. The fecal leukocyte examination is not helpful in distinguishing shigellosis from diarrheal illnesses caused by other invasive enteric pathogens (nontyphoidal *Salmonella*, *Campylobacter*, and *Yersina*). Amebic dysentery is excluded by the absence of trophozoites on a microscopic examination of fresh stool under a coverslip. The peripheral white cell count is of little diagnostic value, since it may range from less than 3000 to more than 30,000. Sigmoidoscopic examination reveals diffuse erythema with a mucopurulent layer and friable areas of mucosa with shallow ulcers 3 to 7 mm in diameter.

Definitive diagnosis depends on isolating shigellae by selective media. A rectal swab, a swab of a colonic ulcer obtained by sigmoidoscopic examination, or a freshly passed stool specimen should be inoculated immediately on culture plates or into carrying media. Since isolation rates of shigellae from freshly passed stools of patients with shigellosis may be as low as 67%, culturing for 3 successive days is recommended. Stool cultures are generally positive within 24 hours after onset of symptoms and may remain positive for several weeks in the absence of antimicrobial therapy. Appropriate culture media include blood, desoxycholate, and *Salmonella-Shigella* (S-S) agars. Selected colonies should be diagnosed by agglutination with polyvalent *Shigella* antisera. S-S agar is inhibitory for *S. dysenteriae* 1.

Definitive bacteriologic diagnosis becomes critically important for distinguishing the more severe and prolonged cases of shigel-

losis from ulcerative colitis, with which it may be confused both clinically and on sigmoidoscopic examination. Patients with shigellosis have been subjected to colectomy because of a mistaken diagnosis of ulcerative colitis; a positive culture should prevent such a misadventure.

TREATMENT. Appropriate antimicrobial therapy instituted early may decrease the duration of symptoms by 50% and decrease the duration of excretion of shigellae (an important epidemiologic factor) by a far greater percentage. Because of the increasing frequency of plasmid-mediated antimicrobial resistance to *Shigella* infections, surveillance of drug susceptibility in an endemic area is important. In adults, ciprofloxacin given orally in a dose of 500 mg twice daily for 5 days or 1 gram as a single dose is the treatment of choice when the susceptibility of a strain is unknown. In children, treatment should be trimethoprim-sulfamethoxazole, ampicillin, or pivmecillinam, depending on susceptibilities of *Shigella* in a given location.

Fluid losses in shigellosis are qualitatively similar to those in other infectious diarrheal diseases, and the patient should be treated with appropriate intravenous or oral electrolyte repletion fluids in quantities adequate to correct clinical signs of saline depletion. The requirement for fluids is generally small, but fluid repletion is life-saving in exceptional cases.

Agents that decrease intestinal motility should not be used. Such preparations as diphenoxylate and paregoric may exacerbate symptoms, presumably by retarding intestinal clearance of the microorganisms. There is no convincing evidence that pectin- or bismuth-containing preparations are helpful.

PROGNOSIS. The mortality rate in untreated shigellosis depends on the infectious strain and ranges from 10 to 30% in certain outbreaks caused by *S. dysenteriae* 1 to < 1% in most *S. sonnei* infections. Even with infection caused by *S. dysenteriae* 1, mortality rates should approach zero if appropriate fluid replacement and antimicrobial therapy are initiated early.

About 2% of patients may develop arthritis or Reiter's syndrome weeks or months after recovery from shigellosis.

PREVENTION. Individuals excreting shigellae should be excluded from all phases of food handling until negative cultures have been obtained from three successive stool specimens collected after completion of antimicrobial therapy. In institutional outbreaks, strict and early isolation of infected individuals is mandatory. Targeted antimicrobial chemoprophylaxis has been disappointing. The most important control measure is rigorous handwashing with soap and water by all individuals involved in handling of food or changing diapers. Reporting of shigellosis cases to health authorities should be mandatory.

For the traveler to countries with major *Shigella* problems, no chemoprophylactic agent is an adequate substitute for good personal hygiene and avoiding contaminated food and water. A variety of vaccines has been developed and tested, but no vaccine is now commercially available.

Bennish ML, Harris JR, Wojtyniak BJ, et al.: Death in shigellosis: Incidence and risk factors in hospitalized patients. J Infect Dis 161:500, 1990. *Among more than 9000 infected inpatients, 9% died, with death more likely in infants, the malnourished, and patients with low serum protein concentrations and thrombocytopenia.*

Bennish ML, Salam MA, Khan WA, et al.: Treatment of shigellosis: III. Comparison of one- or two-dose ciprofloxacin with standard 5-day therapy. Ann Intern Med 117:727, 1992. *Ciprofloxacin given as a single dose of 1 gram cured patients with infections other than S. dysenteriae 1 as well as 500 mg given twice daily for 5 days. For* S. dysenteriae *1 infections, the 5-day treatment gave better results.*

Butler T, Islam MR, Azad MAK, et al.: Risk factors for development of hemolytic uremic syndrome during shigellosis. J Pediatr 110:894, 1987. *In children with S. dysenteriae 1 infection, hemolytic-uremic syndrome developed after antibiotic therapy, which was usually inappropriate for the susceptibilities of the isolated bacterial strains.*

Butler T, Speelman P, Kabir I, et al.: Colonic dysfunction during shigellosis. J Infect Dis 154:817, 1986. *Studies perfusing the human colon showed diminished colonic water absorption, increased potassium secretion, and normal ileocecal flow rates.*

Tauxe RV, Puhr ND, Wells JG, et al.: Antimicrobial resistance of *Shigella* isolates in the USA: The importance of international travelers. J Infect Dis 162:1107, 1990. *In the United States, resistance of Shigella isolates to trimethoprim-sulfamethoxazole occurred in 4% of domestically acquired cases and 20% of travel-related cases.*

Wharton M, Spiegel RA, Horan JM, et al.: A large outbreak of antibiotic-resistant shigellosis at a mass gathering. J Infect Dis 162:1324, 1990. *Poor sanitation at a camp site in Tennessee led to an attack rate of more than 50% in several thousand attendees; disease was caused by multiresistant* S. sonnei.

295 *CAMPYLOBACTER* ENTERITIS
Richard L. Guerrant

Enteric infection with a member of the genus *Campylobacter* usually results in an inflammatory, occasionally bloody diarrhea or dysentery syndrome, in industrialized, temperate areas. *Campylobacter jejuni* is often the most commonly recognized cause of community-acquired inflammatory enteritis. The diarrhea also may be watery, especially in developing, tropical areas. An enterocolitis or protocolitis syndrome similar to that seen with *C. jejuni* is also seen in homosexual males with several "*Campylobacter*-like organisms." The other major *Campylobacter* species that infects humans is *C. fetus,* a relatively uncommon cause of bacteremia and occasional intravascular infection in immunocompromised hosts. *Helicobacter pylori* (the cause of gastritis and peptic ulcers that was previously called *Campylobacter pylori*) is now classified separately.

ETIOLOGY. *Campylobacter* (meaning "curved rod") is a curved or spiral, motile, non–spore-forming, gram-negative rod measuring 1.5 by 3.5 μm which is distinguished from Enterobacteriaceae by its inability to ferment or oxidize carbohydrates. It was formerly called a "vibrio" but is now recognized as a separate genus on the basis of its distinctive DNA content. It is both oxidase- and catalase-positive and is a microaerophilic organism that requires reduced oxygen (5 to 10%) and increased carbon dioxide (3 to 10%). The organism does not grow at either aerobic or strictly anaerobic conditions. Perhaps reflecting its avian reservoir, *C. jejuni* also requires an increased temperature to 42°C for optimal growth. *C. jejuni* is distinguished from *C. fetus* by its higher growth temperatures, cephalothin resistance, and nalidixic acid sensitivity. As shown in Table 295–1, the additional *Campylobacter* species that infect humans include *C. laridis,* a thermophilic organism commonly found in healthy sea gulls that has been reported in children with mild recurrent diarrhea and in an elderly patient with sepsis and terminal multiple myeloma. The weak or non–catalase-producing *C. upsaliensis* may cause diarrhea or bacteremia, and *C. hyointestinalis,* like *C. fetus,* causes occasional bacteremia in compromised hosts. These organisms are also inhibited by cephalothin that is in some selective culture media. Up to three distinct species of "*Campylobacter*-like organisms" (including proposed species names *C. fennelliae* and *C. cinaedi*) are associated with protocolitis in homosexual males and occasionally with bacteremia or diarrhea in women and children. Like *C. fetus,* these *Campylobacter*-like organisms do not grow at 42°C or in the presence of cephalosporin antibiotics (present in some selective media for *C. jejuni*) and may require several days to a week or more to grow in culture. *C. jejuni* is further subdivided into over 90 serotypes on the basis of heat-stable O antigens or over 50 serotypes on the basis of heat-labile capsular and flagellar antigens, markers that are helpful in tracing the epidemiology of this common enteric pathogen.

EPIDEMIOLOGY. Although the frequency of other *Campylobacter* infections is either low or unclear, *C. jejuni* infections are extremely common throughout the world. In many studies, the frequency of *Campylobacter* enteritis exceeds that of *Salmonella* or *Shigella* infections, and it has been estimated that as many as 2 million *Campylobacter* enteritis cases occur annually in the United States. The reservoirs of *C. jejuni/coli* include a wide range of mammalian species. Between 30 and 100% of chickens, turkeys, and water fowl may be infected asymptomatically in their intestinal tracts, and commercially prepared poultry in supermarkets can often be shown to be culture-positive. In addition, swine, cattle, sheep, horses, and even household pets and rodents may carry *C. jejuni, C. coli,* or *C. fetus.* Enteric symptoms may be found, particularly in puppies, kittens, calves, or lambs, which may have diarrhea when infected. Furthermore, the organisms survive days to weeks in fresh or salt water and in milk and are killed most effectively by pasteurization, chlorination, drying, or freezing.

The transmission of *Campylobacter* infections is likely via the fecal-oral route. Fecal-oral spread may occur by contact among animals, homosexual males, and those in day care centers. Secondary transmission is relatively infrequent, and the infectious dose appears to vary from 500 to over 1 million organisms. The majority of infections are probably acquired by ingesting contaminated food, water, or milk vehicles. Many cases and outbreaks are associated with ingesting inadequately cooked poultry, unpasteurized milk, inadequately treated water, and even cake icing, salads, beef, and clams.

The majority of those infected in well-described outbreaks are symptomatic. Asymptomatic infection appears to be relatively infrequent in temperate climates and in adults. An exception is among young children in certain tropical developing areas such as Bangladesh, where as many as 39% of children under age 2 years may be infected asymptomatically (Table 295–2). These frequent asymptomatic infections in tropical areas raise important questions about possible strain differences in virulence, host susceptibility, and protective immunity against disease that might be acquired very early in developing areas.

Throughout the world, *Campylobacter* infections appear to predominate during the warmer or wet season. As with diarrheal illnesses in general, the highest age-specific attack rate is in young children. However, the greatest proportion of positive fecal cultures occurs in older children and young adults. The latter contributes a small peak in the age-specific attack rates during the "second weaning," when young adults leave home and lack experience with cooking poultry and other products. There is little, if any, sexual predominance of recognized *C. jejuni* infections.

PATHOGENESIS AND PATHOLOGY. *C. jejuni* and *C. coli* are reasonably susceptible to gastric acidity. However, the reported variation in infectious dose suggests considerable host or strain variability. After an incubation period of 1 to 7 (median 4) days, symptoms of the enteric infection begin. *C. jejuni* organisms are attracted toward mucus and fucose in bile, and the flagellae may be important in both chemotaxis and adherence to epithelial cells or mucus. Adherence also may involve lipopolysaccharide or other outer membrane components. Several laboratories around the world have documented the production by *C. jejuni* of a cholera-like, heat-labile enterotoxin that binds to ganglioside and is neutralized by anticholera toxin antiserum. However, the genetic code and role of this toxin in disease remain elusive to date. Studies from Mexico have shown that antitoxic immunity develops after infection, often with watery diarrhea, suggesting that this toxin is significant in those infections.

However, more characteristic in temperate areas is a diffuse, often bloody exudative enteritis involving the ileum and colon. These pathologic changes may include nonspecific crypt abscesses that on colonoscopy and histopathology may mimic the changes seen with inflammatory bowel disease. Such invasive pathology is also seen in rabbit, chick, mouse, dog, and monkey models of infection. Although *C. jejuni* is negative in the Sereny test for guinea pig con-

TABLE 295–1. HUMAN *CAMPYLOBACTER* INFECTIONS

Species	Growth Temperature	Reservoir	Clinical Manifestations
C. jejuni/coli	37–42°C	Poultry, mammals	Common cause of dysentery/diarrhea
C. fetus (sub sp. *fetus,* old sub sp. *intestinalis*)	25–37°C	Cattle, sheep	Uncommon, bacteremia; intravascular infections in debilitated hosts
C. laridis	30–42°C	Sea gulls	Uncommon, childhood diarrhea, one case of sepsis
C. upsaliensis	37–42°C	Dogs	Occasional diarrhea
C. hyointestinalis	37°C	Swine	Occasional bacteremia in compromised hosts
"*Campylobacter*-like organisms": (including *Helicobacter cinaedi,* *H. fennelliae*)	37°C	?	Proctocolitis, rarely sepsis, in homosexual males
H. pylori (formerly *C. pylori*)	37°C	?	Histologic gastritis ulcer or gastritis symptoms

**TABLE 295-2. CLINICAL PRESENTATIONS OF
CAMPYLOBACTER JEJUNI INFECTION**

	Industrialized Countries	Developing Countries
Percent of all diarrhea with *C. jejuni*	5–13	2–35
Percent of *C. jejuni* diarrhea with:		
Fecal PMN	78–93	22–46
Blood in stool	60–65	5–17
Asymptomatic infection rates (%)	<2	0–39*

* Depending on age—39% if less than 2 years old.

junctivitis, some have reported the production of cytotoxins by certain strains of *C. jejuni* that may be involved in the pathogenesis of the invasive colitis. The relative infrequency of bloodstream invasion by *C. jejuni*, compared with *C. fetus*, likely relates to the relative serum sensitivity of most *C. jejuni* strains and to the rapid development of bactericidal antibody with infection in normal individuals. Volunteer studies suggest that effective immunity develops to rechallenge with the homologous strain, and animal studies suggest that protective immunity may be transferred in immune milk to suckling offspring. Additional evidence of effective immunity comes with the decreasing illness/infection ratio among children in endemic areas as well as among regular consumers of raw milk.

Once patients are infected, they shed 10^7 to 10^9 organisms per gram of stool for a median duration of 2 to 3 weeks, if not treated with effective antibiotics. Although some may continue to excrete the organism for 2 to 3 months, chronic asymptomatic intestinal carriage is rare.

CLINICAL MANIFESTATIONS. As noted in Table 295–1, the major recognized disease with human *Campylobacter* infections is the characteristic diarrheal illness seen with *C. jejuni* or *C. coli* infections. Although asymptomatic infections and watery, noninflammatory diarrhea are seen with *C. jejuni* infections in tropical, developing areas as shown in Table 295–2, *C. jejuni* is characteristically associated with an inflammatory, febrile enteritis in industrialized countries throughout the world. After an incubation period of 1 to 7 days, a brief prodrome of fever, headache, and myalgias lasting for 12 to 24 hours is promptly followed in a case of *C. jejuni* enteritis in a child or young adult with the symptoms of acute enteritis. These characteristically include crampy abdominal pain, fever to 39 or 40°C, and diarrhea with up to 10 or more loose, often bloody bowel movements per day. Occasionally, the crampy abdominal pain may predominate as an appendicitis-like syndrome, with mesenteric adenitis or terminal ileitis being the predominant pathology. On physical examination, the abdomen is diffusely tender and may mimic appendicitis. Although the acute febrile enteritis is usually self-limited to 5 to 7 days, 10 to 20% of cases may last longer than 1 week and 5 to 20% of untreated cases may relapse with a similar illness.

Complications, particularly if antimotility agents are used, include toxic megacolon, pseudomembranous colitis, and colonic hemorrhage. In addition, hemolytic-uremic syndrome, postinfectious polyneuritis, or Guillain-Barré syndrome (GBS) may follow *C. jejuni* enteritis. Some suggest that *C. jejuni* (especially O type 19) may be a major recognized predisposing cause of GBS. As with many inflammatory colitis syndromes, reactive arthritis and full-blown Reiter's syndrome may follow weeks after *Campylobacter* enteritis. Bacteremia may occur relatively rarely (<1% of cases), particularly in the very young or the elderly, in whom meningitis, endocarditis, cholecystitis, urinary tract infections, and pancreatitis have been described. In patients with hypogammaglobulinemia or HIV infection, *C. jejuni* infections may be prolonged or severe despite appropriate antimicrobial therapy.

In striking contrast to *C. jejuni*, the slow-growing *C. fetus* is primarily an uncommon cause of bacteremia, often in immunocompromised hosts. Although *C. fetus* would be missed on most routine stool cultures for *C. jejuni*, studies with filtration methods suggest that it is a relatively infrequent cause of diarrhea. Instead, *C. fetus* tends to cause intravascular, meningeal, or localized infections such as arthritis, cellulitis, abscesses, cholecystitis, and urinary, placental,

or pleural infections, often in elderly or debilitated hosts. As it does in animals, *C. fetus* may cause stillbirth or septic abortions more often than generally recognized in humans. *C. fetus* infections are often recognized only by astute clinical microbiology technicians who methodically examine or subculture cultured specimens of blood or other body fluids after 1 week in the laboratory. The clinical course of *C. fetus* bacteremia is often related to its recognition and appropriate treatment as well as to the underlying disease.

DIAGNOSIS. The diagnosis of *Campylobacter* infections is related to a careful history for exposure or characteristic clinical syndromes, direct stool examination, and selective culture methods. *C. jejuni* enteritis should be suspected in anyone presenting with a febrile enteritis, especially if there is a history of recent ingestion of inadequately cooked poultry, unpasteurized milk, or untreated water. As suggested in Figure 295–1, such a history should prompt obtaining a fecal specimen in a cup if at all possible and direct microscopic examination using methylene blue or Gram stain for leukocytes as well as gross and/or occult blood. In many industrialized areas, the presence of blood or fecal leukocytes with fever strongly suggests the presence of a cultivable enteric pathogen such as *C. jejuni*, *Salmonella*, or *Shigella*, with *C. jejuni* being most common. Additional immediate clues to *C. jejuni* infection may be seen on dark-field or phase microscopy for characteristic darting motility or on a carbolfuchsin Gram stain of stool for characteristic curved rods or sea gull morphology. However, dark-field and Gram stains, while reasonably specific with trained observers, are each only 50 to 66% sensitive. Patients with febrile enteritis, particularly with blood and leukocytes in the stool, should be cultured for *C. jejuni*.

Additional differential diagnostic possibilities for febrile inflammatory enteritis include *Salmonella* and *Shigella* infections, for which one should seek a history of an outbreak or contact exposure (such as in day care centers or among homosexual males, respectively). If the patient has recently taken antibiotics, *C. difficile* colitis or *Salmonella* enteritis should be considered. Recent ingestion of raw seafood should prompt investigation for *Vibrio* infection that may present with either inflammatory or noninflammatory diarrhea. A history of sick pet exposure, persisting abdominal pain, or unexplained inflammatory diarrhea also should prompt consideration of *Yersinia enterocolitica* infections, and travel exposure to tropical areas or residence in an institution where careful hygiene is difficult should prompt an examination of stool and possibly rectal biopsy specimens for *E. histolytica* (which often destroys fecal leukocytes). Another frequent diagnosis that is considered, especially if *Campylobacter* enteritis has relapsed once or twice, is inflammatory bowel disease. However, it is imperative that anyone who is being considered for that diagnosis have treatable causes such as *Campylobacter* enteritis or amebiasis excluded by appropriate cultures or stains, as treatment with steroids may worsen *Campylobacter* or amebic enteritis with potentially devastating consequences. Additional noninfectious causes of bloody diarrhea with abdominal pain include intussusception and vascular insufficiency.

The diagnosis of *H. pylori* infections is best made by documenting the organism by culture and histology of gastric biopsies. Additional clues may be provided by ureases tests of biopsies, breath tests for urease degradation of ingested urea, or serologic tests for anti-*H. pylori* antibody (see Ch. 99.2).

THERAPY. The most important treatment for *Campylobacter* enteritis, as with all diarrheal illnesses, is adequate rehydration and maintenance fluid therapy, which can often be accomplished with oral glucose-electrolyte solutions. The effectiveness of specific antimicrobial therapy remains debated. Although most *C. jejuni* strains are sensitive to erythromycin as well as to tetracyclines, chloramphenicol, clindamycin, the quinolones, and aminoglycosides, they are characteristically resistant to penicillin, ampicillin, cephalosporins, and sulfamethoxazole-trimethroprim. Indications for antibiotic treatment remain controversial. Several studies have failed to show a significant reduction in the duration of illness with erythromycin treatment despite its prompt eradication of the organism from the stool. Some reserve antimicrobial treatment for those with particularly severe symptoms of high fever, bloody or severe diarrhea, young children in day care centers, or prolonged or relapsing illnesses. Antimotility agents should be avoided in *Campylobacter* enteritis, as with any inflammatory diarrhea.

It should be remembered that erythromycin orally may not be adequate for systemic *C. jejuni* or *C. fetus* endovascular infections,

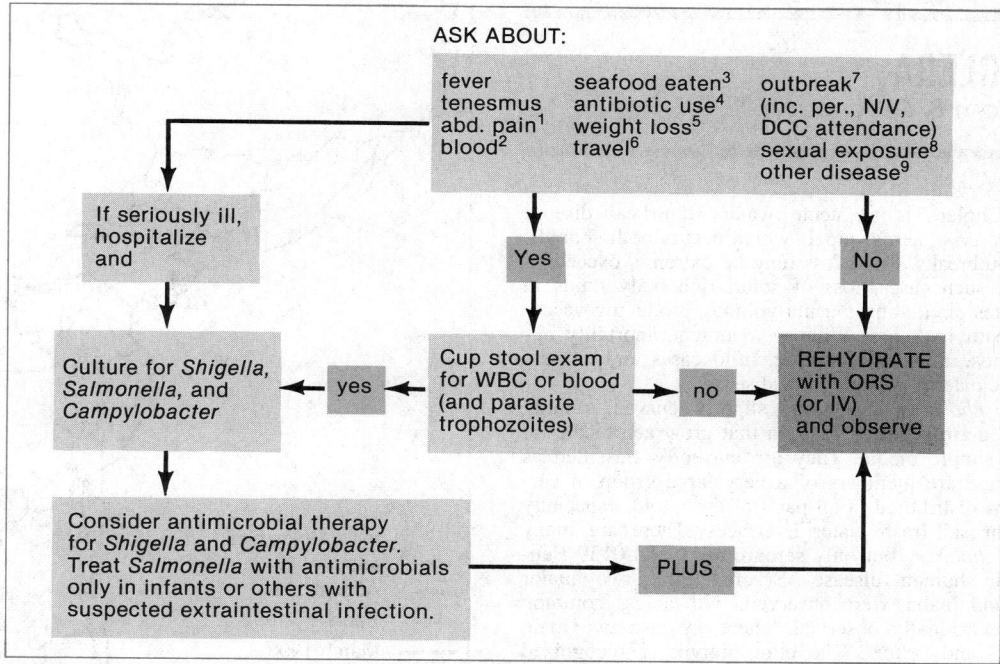

FIGURE 295–1. Approach to the diagnosis and management of acute infectious diarrhea.

1. If unexplained abdominal pain and fever persist or suggest an appendicitis-like syndrome, culture for *Yersinia enterocolitica*.
2. Bloody diarrhea, especially if without fecal leukocytes, suggests enterohemorrhagic (*Shiga* toxin–producing) *E. coli* O157 or amebiasis (where leukocytes are destroyed by the parasite).
3. Ingestion of inadequately cooked seafood should prompt consideration of *Vibrio* infections or Norwalk-like viruses.
4. Associated antibiotics should be stopped if possible and cytotoxigenic *C. difficile* considered.
5. Persistence (> 10 days) with weight loss should prompt consideration of giardiasis or cryptosporidiosis.
6. Travel to tropical areas increases the chance of enterotoxigenic *E. coli* as well as viral (ex. Norwalk-like or rotaviral), parasitic (ex. *Giardia, Entamoeba, Strongyloides, Cryptosporidium*), and, if fecal leukocytes are present, invasive bacterial pathogens as noted in the algorithm.
7. Outbreaks should prompt consideration of *S. aureus, B. cereus, Anisakis* (incubation period <6 hours), *C. perfringens*, ETEC, *Vibrio, Salmonella, Campylobacter, Shigella* or EIEC infection. If unexplained, consider saving *E. coli* for LT, ST, invasiveness, adherence testing, and serotyping, and save stool for rotavirus and stool + paired sera for Norwalk-like virus testing.
8. Sigmoidoscopy in symptomatic homosexual males should distinguish proctitis in the distal 15 cm only (caused by herpesvirus, gonococcal, chlamydial, or syphilitic infection) from colitis (*Campylobacter, Shigella, C. difficile*, or chlamydial [LGV serotypes] infections) or noninflammatory diarrhea (due to giardiasis).
9. Immunocompromised hosts should have a wide range of viral (ex. CMV, HSV, coxsackie, rotavirus), bacterial (ex. *Salmonella, Mycobacterium avium-intracellulare, Listeria*), fungal (ex. *Candida*), and parasitic (ex. *Cryptosporidium, Strongyloides, Entamoeba*, and *Giardia*) agents considered.

(Adapted from Guerrant RL, Shields DS, Thorson SM, et al.: Evaluation and diagnosis of acute infectious diarrhea. Am J Med 78:91, 1985; and Guerrant RL, Bobak DA: Bacterial and protozoal gastroenteritis. N Engl J Med 325:327, 1991.)

which probably warrant 2 to 4 weeks of parenteral bactericidal antimicrobial therapy.

H. pylori infections, although difficult to eradicate with a single agent, may be eradicated by combinations of agents such as bismuth compounds plus metronidazole, provided that the organism is susceptible (see Ch. 99.1).

PROGNOSIS. The prognosis of *C. jejuni* enteritis is generally quite good, and the disease is usually self-limited with or without specific therapy.

PREVENTION. Since most *Campylobacter* infections arise from fecal contamination, often from animal reservoirs, many if not most *Campylobacter* infections are potentially preventable by education. The most common recognized vehicles of spread are inadequately cooked food, unpasteurized milk, and inadequately treated water. Consequently, thoroughly cooking meat and poultry, careful hand-washing after preparing food, pasteurizing milk, and adequately chlorinating drinking water should greatly reduce the frequency of *Campylobacter* infections. Parents should be warned that sick pet kittens or puppies may harbor potential human pathogens such as *C. jejuni* and keep them away from small children and practice careful hygienic measures in their care.

Blaser MJ, Wells JG, Feldman RA, et al.: *Campylobacter* enteritis in the United States. Ann Intern Med 98:360, 1983. *Critical analysis of the presentation of* C. jejuni *and other enteritides in the United States.*

Butzler JP, Skirrow MB: *Campylobacter* enteritis. Clin Gastroenterol 8:737, 1979.

Good review of cultivation methods, epidemiology, clinical presentation, and models of C. jejuni *infections.*

Guerrant RL, Lahita RG, Winn WC, et al.: Campylobacteriosis in man: Pathogenic mechanisms and review of 91 bloodstream infections. Am J Med 65:584, 1978. *Review of both* C. fetus *and* C. jejuni *infections and their presentations as bacteremic illnesses.*

Guerrant RL, Bobak DA: Bacterial and protozoal gastroenteritis. N Engl J Med 325:327, 1991. *Update on epidemiology and pathogenesis as well as a practical clinical approach to diagnosis and management of bacterial and other causes of diarrhea.*

Mishu B, Blaser MJ: Role of infection due to *Campylobacter jejuni* in the initiation of Guillain-Barré syndrome. Clin Infect Dis 17:104, 1993. *Excellent update of data confirming a review of over 20 reports from 1984 showing that 20 to 40% of Guillain-Barré syndrome (GBS) cases may follow* C. jejuni *infections, especially those with LPS O type 19, which has been implicated in the pathogenesis of GBS.*

Nachamkin I, Blazer MJ, Tompkins LS: *Campylobacter jejuni:* Current Status and Future Trends. Washington, DC, ASM, 1992. *An excellent compendium of multiauthored chapters on epidemiology, microbiology, clinical manifestations, pathogenesis, immunity and therapy of* Campylobacter *infections.*

Perlman DM, Ampel NM, Schiffman RB, et al.: Persistent *Campylobacter-jejuni* infections in patients infected with the human immunodeficiency virus: Association with abnormal serological response to *C. jejuni* and emergence of erythromycin resistance during therapy. Ann Intern Med 108:540, 1988. *Report of persistent, severe* C. jejuni *enteritis and occasional bacteremia in patients with HIV infection who fail to mount a serum antibody response.*

Quinn TC, Corey L, Chaffee RG, et al.: The etiology of anorectal infections in homosexual men. Am J Med 71:395, 1981. *Review of the clinical manifestations and diagnostic approach to the wide range of enteric infections commonly seen in promiscuous homosexual males.*

Walker RI, Caldwell MB, Lee EC, et al.: Pathophysiology of *Campylobacter* enteritis. Microbiol Rev 50:81, 1986. *Excellent recent review of the virulence traits, pathogenic mechanisms, and animal models of* C. jejuni *infections.*

296 CHOLERA

William B. Greenough, III

DEFINITION. Cholera is an acute watery diarrheal disease caused by *Vibrio cholerae*, serogroup 1, which occurs both sporadically and as large outbreaks. Fluid loss may be extreme, exceeding 1 liter per hour. In such cases, loss of solute-rich body fluids in stools rapidly depletes circulating plasma volume, producing vascular collapse and death in hours. Without treatment, mortality approaches 60% of those affected; however, mild cases and carriers also occur and participate in the spread of disease.

ETIOLOGY. *V. cholerae* are short, slightly curved, rapidly motile, uniflagellate gram-negative bacteria that grow aerobically at 37°C on relatively simple media. They are currently classified as Enterobacteriaceae and are members of a very large group of surface water organisms distributed in all parts of the world, especially favoring brackish or salt-fresh water interfaces. There are many O serogroups of *V. cholerae*, but only serogroups 1 and 0139 Bengal cause epidemic human disease. Before 1992, two major serotypes, Ogawa and Inaba, were observed, with a less common Hikojima variant occasionally observed. There are also two main biotypes, "classical" and "eltor." The eltor biotype is recognized by its resistance to polymyxin B and by characteristic vibriophage susceptibility. These markers are of use epidemiologically. *V. cholerae* produces a potent exotoxin (choleragen) that binds to intestinal epithelium, producing a chloride ion–driven secretion and malabsorption of sodium ion and water. Other vibrios can produce exotoxins but do not have other biologic characteristics that lead to spreading epidemic disease. However, an entirely new serogroup (0139 Bengal) is currently responsible for major epidemics.

EPIDEMIOLOGY. Cholera is thought to be a disease of antiquity, with clear written descriptions dating before 500 B.C. The present global spread (seventh pandemic) has been due to an eltor biotype first recognized in 1911 at the El Tor quarantine station in the Persian Gulf. Epidemics due to this organism first appeared in the Celebes in the 1930's, spreading westward through Southeast Asia and reaching the Mediterranean and Africa in the 1970's. However, in the Ganges delta, epidemics of classic *V. cholerae* were replaced by eltor late in the 1960's. There have been small but regular outbreaks of cholera in the United States in the Mississippi delta regions since 1973. The eltor strains isolated have not been the same as the global epidemic strain. In 1991, *V. cholerae* 01 eltor caused explosive outbreaks of cholera in Peru and have subsequently spread throughout Latin America (Fig. 296–1). The newly arisen *V. cholerae* 0139 Bengal clearly has the potential for rapid global spread. *V. cholerae* serogroup 1 can be identified by gene amplification or immunofluorescent methods in many waters often associated with phytoplankton.

Mode of Spread. During epidemics, cholera is mainly waterborne. Large numbers of vibrios enter many water sources from the voluminous liquid stools that soak clothing and linens and contaminate the environment. The setting for epidemics is often extreme poverty with lack of safe water. However, an outbreak in Portugal affected the most careful travelers who used only bottled water, which unfortunately had been supplied from a spring contaminated with *V. cholerae*. Occasionally, contaminated foods spread disease. Most often raw or undercooked shellfish or fresh vegetables washed with contaminated water are responsible. These played an important role in the recent Latin American epidemics. There is a high risk of secondary spread in families or institutions in which water and food are shared. Contamination of household food and water sources is the rule. It is easy to understand how this occurs when an adult patient may produce 30 to 50 liters of stool in 2 to 3 days and is usually too weak to use a commode or toilet. Mild cases and convalescent carriers probably spread the disease between communities. True long-term carriers are rare enough to be reportable.

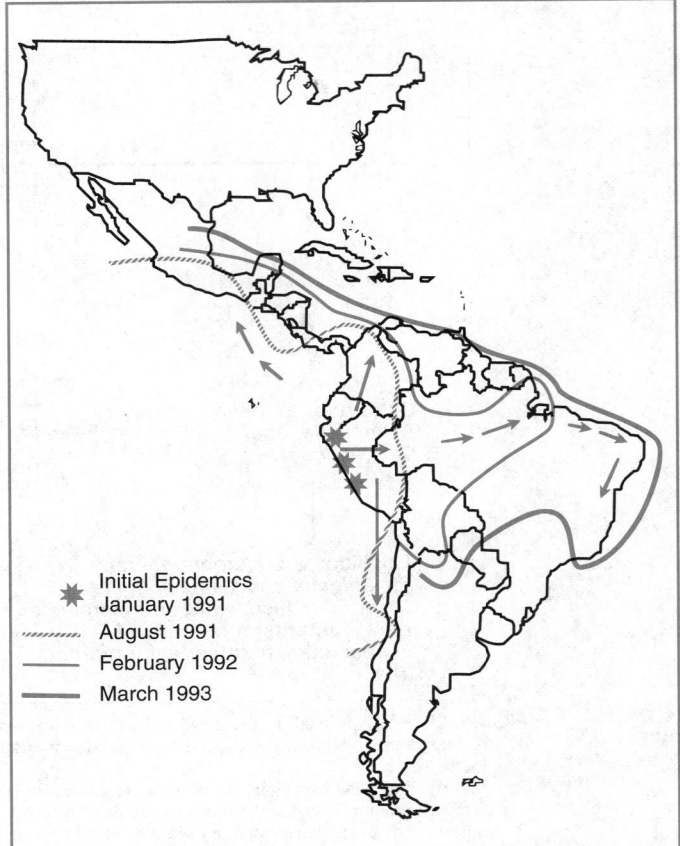

FIGURE 296–1. Geographic extent of the Latin American epidemic over time. Lines represent the advancing front of the epidemic at different times. By March 1993, all Latin American countries except Uruguay had reported cholera, and no cases had been reported from the Caribbean.

Legend:
- Initial Epidemics January 1991
- August 1991
- February 1992
- March 1993

Susceptibility to Cholera. In areas where cholera occurs each year, children younger than 5 are the main victims. Older children and adults in such endemic areas have acquired a lasting and strongly protective local intestinal immunity. Breast-fed infants in such circumstances do not get cholera and are solidly protected by antibodies from their mother's milk. When cholera attacks a population that has not experienced it for many years, as was true in recent spread to the Philippines and Africa, all ages are attacked equally, but morbidity and mortality are greatest among the very young and very old. Individuals with low gastric acid production, or those who are on acid-suppressing medications, or who have had gastrectomies are especially vulnerable, since *V. cholerae* is quite sensitive to acid. Cholera tends to attack persons of blood group O more frequently and with greater severity, whereas individuals with AB blood group have less severe disease. People with a safe, piped water supply and effective disinfected waste disposal are at least risk regardless of host susceptibility.

PATHOGENESIS. After *V. cholerae* is ingested, vomiting and diarrhea may begin as early as 12 hours or not appear for more than a week. Illness occurs when viable organisms reach the duodenum and jejunum where alkaline pH, nutrients, and bile salts favor rapid multiplication. Actively motile vibrios penetrate mucous layers and attach to the brush border of the intestinal epithelium, where they secrete a potent exotoxin. This toxin is a protein of 84,000 daltons consisting of five B subunits that bind irreversibly to a specific chemical receptor on the cell surfaces (GM1-ganglioside). The toxic moiety or A subunit is linked to the B aggregate and gains entry once binding has occurred. ADP ribosylates the α subunit of G protein, producing increased adenylate cyclase activity and consequent raised cyclic AMP levels in the enterocytes or any other affected cells. The most visible result in the small intestine is the profuse watery diarrhea resulting from abolition at the villous tips of the normal absorption of sodium ion and with it anions and water, and stimulation of crypt cells to secrete chloride, drawing with them cations and water from the blood stream into the gut lumen. The resulting solute-rich stream originating in the duodenum and jejunum is profuse, eliciting vomiting as it progresses cephalad and diarrhea as it flushes through the colon. The fluid lost in cholera is a slightly fishy-smelling nonfecal whitish mucous-flecked liquid ("rice water stool"). There is no cellular damage and no inflammation or loss of plasma proteins or formed elements of the blood. There is also increased secretion of hepatic and pancreatic fluids, prostaglandins, and other intestinal hormones. All signs and symptoms of cholera derive from the fluid losses, which approach in composition an ultrafiltrate of plasma enriched in potassium and bicarbonate (Table 296–1). There is no evidence for systemic effects by cholera toxin itself, since V. cholerae does not invade the body, nor is the toxin absorbed. It exerts all its effects topically by adhering to the intestinal lining and producing toxin that is bound at cell surfaces.

CLINICAL MANIFESTATIONS. Cholera can reduce a perfectly healthy, robust adult to shock and death in 4 to 6 hours. More usually, death ensues in 18 or more hours. In rare instances, "cholera sicca" shock and death occur before diarrhea appears, the voluminous secretions pooling in distended loops of bowel and not escaping as either diarrhea or vomiting. Despite the capacity of cholera to cause severe illness, many of the infected patients have only a mild diarrhea indistinguishable from that of ordinary gastroenteritis. In epidemics, about half those infected have either no symptoms or very mild illness.

Without fluid replacement, cholera patients demonstrate signs of severe volume depletion—sunken eyes, poor skin turgor, hoarse voice, extreme thirst, faint heart sounds, weak or absent peripheral pulses, and severe muscle cramps. Patients are oriented but appear apathetic except for thirst. If patients survive and have not received adequate hydration, fever secondary to sepsis and pneumonia are common, and pulmonary edema can ensue with even modest fluid replacement.

In children, unconsciousness and/or convulsions may signal hypoglycemia. In both children and adults, adequate early volume replacement with a correctly formulated oral hydration solution can prevent all signs and symptoms except diarrhea. Initial laboratory values from depleted cholera patients (Table 296–1) reflect the loss of isotonic fluid without larger molecules such as albumen. This results in increased concentrations of plasma proteins and blood cells. Loss of bicarbonate leads to acidosis with a low arterial pH and bicarbonate. Potassium depletion, which may be severe, is not reflected by low plasma values until acidosis has been corrected.

DIAGNOSIS. Cholera should be ruled out in any patient with acute watery diarrhea. Travel to or residence in a cholera-endemic area should raise the index of suspicion. In clusters of acute watery diarrhea, particularly where sanitation is poor, it is especially important to recognize cholera early to permit advance actions to prevent deaths of large numbers of people.

Treatment does not depend on an etiologic diagnosis. Fluid replacement should be started without delay as soon as diarrhea begins. After initiating treatment, stool should be examined directly for red and white blood cells. Except in mixed infections with invasive organisms, which do occur in cholera outbreaks, fecal red and white cells are not a feature of cholera. If phase or dark-field microscopy is available, the characteristic darting motility of vibrios

can be recognized in fresh wet preparations. To be certain that these motile bacteria are V. cholerae, serogroup 1 antisera can be applied to wet preparations, immobilizing the organisms in a rapid and specific diagnostic test. For greater sensitivity of this test, a stool sample or rectal swab can be incubated in an enrichment medium for vibrios, such as alkaline peptone water, for 12 to 18 hours. Stool culture is best done on a selective medium, since colonies of V. cholerae may be overgrown or are easily missed on standard enteric media. A simple method uses thiosulfate citrate–bile salt–sucrose (TCBS) agar, which is very stable and selective for vibrios. Opaque flat yellow colonies form on TCBS agar in 18 hours at 37°C. Confirmation of serogroup and serotype can be done by direct slide agglutination with specific antisera that are available commercially, including against the new 0139 Bengal strain. Biotyping requires more elaborate procedures, but resistance to polymyxin B is a quick way to recognize the eltor biotype.

Although the first line of immune defense is local at the intestinal epithelium, circulating antibodies occur to the specific O antigens. Testing for these is of use only as an epidemiologic tool to judge prevalence of disease in a specific population.

TREATMENT. Early and complete replacement of fluid losses averts death and all complications. Advanced oral hydration solutions based on rice or other starchy foods hydrate efficiently and reduce diarrhea and vomiting substantially (30 to 50%) as compared with intravenous treatment or glucose-based oral rehydration solutions. In all except the most severe cases, oral rehydration therapy is sufficient to treat cholera, especially if started as soon as diarrhea begins. All varieties of watery diarrhea lose fluid of similar composition, which varies with the rate of loss. Oral hydration therapy is the treatment of choice in all situations except when a patient is in shock or is comatose. Oral rehydration therapy should be used in hospitals, at home, or in the field, since it entails fewer risks, is much less costly, does not require trained medical personnel for administration, and is effective. The discovery that absorption of sodium by cotransport pathways in intestinal mucosa is spared during cholera and other diarrheal diseases opened the way for safe, inexpensive, and effective oral replacement solutions. Glucose, amino acids, and small peptides, when absorbed by separate cotransport pathways of the intestine, carry with them sodium ions. Water and anions follow down the osmotic and electrochemical gradients from the gut lumen to the bloodstream. Originally, oral rehydration solutions were based only on glucose. These remain very effective but do not diminish diarrheal fluid losses. The composition of available oral rehydration solutions is listed in Table 296–2, together with some standard intravenous solutions.

Intravenous fluid replacement should be reserved for neglected patients who have not received oral replacement and are in shock. In a cholera epidemic it is essential that all individuals at risk be thoroughly familiar with oral rehydration therapy and use it early to minimize deaths and the need for intravenous fluids. Thirst and urination are adequate guides to oral replacement therapy even in small children. This eliminates the need for accurate intake and output measurements and weighings, which even in excellent hospitals are difficult and are out of the question under epidemic conditions. Intravenous replacement for patients who are depleted and in shock should be given rapidly through a large-bore needle to ensure infusion rates of 50 to 100 ml per minute until a strong radial pulse has been achieved. Remaining fluid deficits may then be replaced less rapidly over 2 hours. The fluid deficit in a severely depleted patient is about 10% of body weight (for a 50-kg patient—5 liters). As soon as patients are strong enough to drink, oral rehydration therapy should begin, preferably with a rice- or other cereal-based solution of the proper solute composition. If this is done adequately, no further intravenous fluids are needed. In semicomatose patients who are unable to cooperate, nasogastric intubation permits adequate enteral replacement. For both intravenous and oral solutions the composition is crucial and should be within a range to properly replace losses of solutes and water (Table 296–2). It should be noted that many drinks ordinarily given to diarrhea patients are not adequate, although they may complement oral rehydration therapy. Vomiting is not a contraindication for oral rehydration therapy. However, fluids of high osmolarity should be avoided.

TABLE 296–1. TYPICAL CHEMICAL VALUES IN STOOL AND PLASMA FROM PATIENTS WITH SEVERE CHOLERA

	Stool	Plasma	
		Untreated	Treated†
Sodium*	138 (105)	141	142
Chloride*	102 (90)	107	106
Potassium*	18 (25)	4.5	3.6
Bicarbonate*	45 (30)	9	21
Arterial pH	–	7.21	7.43
Plasma specific gravity	–	1.040	1.026

*Milliequivalents per liter. Stool values in parentheses are for children less than 10 hours old.

†Four hours after water and electrolyte replacement.

TABLE 296-2. CHOLERA AND ACUTE DIARRHEA TREATMENT SOLUTIONS (ORAL AND INTRAVENOUS)

	Substrate (g/L)	Na$^+$	K$^+$ (millimoles/L)	Base*	Cl$^-$	Osmolality
Oral						
WHO/UNICEF	20 (glucose)	90	20	30	80	330
Pedialyte	25 (glucose)	45	20	30	65	300
Rice solution	80 (rice)	90	20	30	80	240
Infalyte	30 (rice digest)	50	25	34	45	200
Ceralyte‡	40 (rice digest)	90	20	30	65	235
Intravenous						
Dhaka solution	0	134	13	48 (bicarbonate)	99	294
Ringer's†	0	130	4	28 (lactate)	109	271

*Citrate is generally used but bicarbonate is equally effective, and lactate or acetate are used in intravenous solutions.
†Also contains calcium, 3.0 mEq per liter.
‡Available as dried powder in packets.

If a commercial preparation of oral rehydration salts is not available, a home solution can be prepared. The safest and most effective of these is a thick but drinkable suspension prepared from rice or other suitable ground starchy foods. If precooked products are available, these are very convenient but not essential. To a quart of water with cereal thickly suspended, a half level teaspoon (one three-finger pinch of salt) is added and the mixture cooked only long enough to soften the ground cereal powder. The mixture should be used within 6 hours and may be taken warm or cold. In cholera it may be necessary to drink a great deal of fluid every hour for the first day. The patient must be offered a small cup every few minutes to minimize overloading the stomach and consequent vomiting. This is labor intensive but does not require medical skills. Especially in epidemics, family members and friends are the backbone of a successful treatment program.

In treating either children or adults, fluid therapy should be guided by thirst, observations on the circulation, urine output, and presence of edema or rales at the lung bases. Feeding is important and should be initiated immediately. Breast feeding is especially useful in affected infants, although few breast-fed babies contract cholera except in nonendemic areas where maternal milk lacks protective antibodies. Feeding should be with appetizing complex carbohydrates and proteins culturally adapted to the taste of the patient.

Adjunctive antibiotic therapy may be indicated. This varies with the epidemic strain, but tetracycline and doxycycline have been effective when resistance is not present. As with other Enterobacteriaceae, resistance arises quickly and must be monitored to avoid wasting high-cost antimicrobics that are neither crucial nor lifesaving in cholera. Antibiotic prophylaxis has not been useful and encourages the emergence of resistant strains.

PREVENTION. Safe water supplies and appropriate disposal of human waste prevent spread of cholera but may not be achievable. Rapid loss of large volumes require the use of special beds (cholera cots) or fecal conduits that avoid widespread dissemination into surrounding areas. *V. cholerae* is a fragile organism and cannot withstand drying, mild oxidation, or acid conditions. Thus a variety of disinfectants are effective for soiled articles. Bleaching powder is frequently used. Handwashing with soap before food handling is important. Patients suspected to have cholera should be reported to state health authorities by telephone or fax because of epidemic risks.

The available injected cholera vaccine is not useful, but there are effective killed bacterial and toxoid oral vaccines as well as very promising genetically altered live vaccines. At present, none of these is available commercially.

Addressing emerging infectious disease threats: Preventive strategy for the U.S. MMWR 43:1, 1994. *Emphasizes risks of emerging infectious diseases, including V. cholerae 0139 Bengal.*

Barua D, Greenough WB III: Cholera. New York, Plenum Scientific Publishing Co., 1992. *A broad review of all aspects of cholera.*

Wachsmuth IK, Blake PA, Olsvik O: *Vibrio choloerae* and Cholera Molecular and Global Perspectives. Washington, ASM Press, 1994. *Comprehensive, current review on new epidemic strains, epidemiology, and microbiology of cholera.*

Weber JT, Levine WC, Hopkins DP, Tauxe RV: Cholera in the United States 1965–1991: Risks at home and abroad. Arch Intern Med 184:55, 1994. *Summary of risks of cholera in the United States.*

297 ENTERIC *ESCHERICHIA COLI* INFECTIONS

Richard L. Guerrant

Escherichia coli is the predominant aerobic, coliform species in the normal colon. However, *E. coli* also can be an enteric pathogen and cause intestinal disease, usually diarrhea. Diarrhea caused by *E. coli* may be watery, inflammatory, or bloody, depending on which genetic codes for virulence traits the organism happens to possess. Consequently, diarrheogenic *E. coli* must be defined more specifically according to its virulence traits. Specific virulence traits determine the type of disease the organism causes, such as enterotoxigenic, enteroinvasive, enterohemorrhagic, enteropathogenic, or enteroadherent *E. coli* diarrhea. Each of these categories is being further resolved by the type of enterotoxin (such as the cholera-like, heat-labile toxin, LT, or the heat-stable toxin, ST) or adherence (such as close, localized, epithelial cell effacing, or diffuse) it causes. Taken separately, organisms such as enterotoxigenic *E. coli* constitute major bacterial causes of diarrhea morbidity and mortality on a global scale, particularly among children in tropical, developing areas and in travelers. Taken together, the varied types of *E. coli* diarrhea not only constitute the major category of bacterial enteric pathogens but also illustrate the wide array of ways that enteric pathogens can cause disease.

As noted in Table 297–1, at least three different types of *E. coli* enterotoxins may cause intestinal secretion (ETEC), others are enteroinvasive (EIEC), still others cause foodborne hemorrhagic colitis (EHEC) and produce large amounts of Shiga-like toxin (EHEC), while the classically recognized enteropathogenic *E. coli* (EPEC) serotypes are neither enterotoxigenic nor invasive but attach and efface the epithelium. Further information is emerging on additional types of enteroadherent *E. coli* that exhibit aggregating (EAggEC) or diffuse adherence (DAEC) traits and may be associated with prolonged diarrhea among children in tropical, developing areas.

ETIOLOGY. *E. coli* is a small, catalase-positive, oxidase-negative, gram-negative bacillus in the family Enterobacteriaceae. It characteristically reduces nitrates, ferments glucose and usually lactose, and is either motile (with peritrichate flagella) or nonmotile. It gives a positive methyl red reaction and negative reactions with Voges-Proskauer, urease, phenylalanine deaminase, and citrate agents. *E. coli* constitutes the predominant facultative gram-negative bacillus in the intestinal tract of humans and other mammals. As with other gram-negative organisms, the lipopolysaccharide cell wall contains lipid A and 2-keto-3-deoxyoctanate (KDO), a core glycolipid that has been used to develop vaccines that provide cross-protection against systemic infections with other gram-negative organisms. Smooth (S) forms of *E. coli* have O-specific carbohydrate chains attached to this core glycolipid to provide 169 O serogroups as well as at least 60 heat-labile protein flagellar (H) antigens by which strains are currently serotyped. Historically, some 80 variably heat-labile capsular (K) antigens also have been described (L, B, and A), not to mention the more recently appreciated numerous adherence, enterotoxin, cytotoxin, and invasiveness factors that may be gained or lost by a particular serotype, since they are characteristically encoded on transmissible genetic elements such as plasmids or bacteriophages. Consequently, this common inhabitant of the normal human intestinal tract becomes a pathogen when it houses one or more specific traits contributing to its colonization and virulence in the intestinal tract. Other traits such as O and H serogroup also may be important for certain enteropathogenic and enteroinvasive organisms. For reasons that remain obscure, only a few O serogroups tend to predominate in the normal human colon (O groups 1, 2, 4, 6, 7, 8, 18, 25, 45, 75, and 81), while others noted in Table 297–1 tend (albeit not absolutely) to be associated with specific virulence traits and thus different types of pathogenesis in the intestine. The O antigens of invasive *E. coli* often cross-react with various *Shigella* species, suggesting further that, in addition to the 140-MDa plasmid, serotype also has a role in pathogenesis.

EPIDEMIOLOGY. Enteric *E. coli* infections are essentially acquired by the fecal-oral route, reflecting primarily a human reservoir for most recognized types of *E. coli* enteropathogens. Enterotoxigenic *E. coli* is also an important veterinary pathogen, especially in calves and piglets. However, the attachment traits of animal strains are different from those that infect humans and likely substantially influence their epidemiology.

The infectious doses of enterotoxigenic *E. coli* and enteroinvasive *E. coli* have been determined in volunteers to be 10^6 to 10^8, numbers that usually require multiplication in contaminated food or water vehicles for their transmission. Heavy contamination with enterotoxigenic *E. coli* has been documented in foods prepared in homes, restaurants, and at street vendors as well as in drinking water in many tropical areas, and contaminated water and foods likely represent the major sources of their acquisition, primarily in the warm or wet season. In the United States, major outbreaks of water- or food-borne *E. coli* diarrhea of different types have been documented in the last 10 to 15 years. A large waterborne outbreak of diarrhea at a popular national park was found to be caused by enterotoxigenic *E. coli* (ETEC), and a widespread outbreak of enteroinvasive *E. coli* (EIEC) enteritis was traced to consumption of French Camembert cheese. More recently, bloody, noninflammatory diarrhea has been increasingly associated with enterohemorrhagic *E.*

coli (EHEC) (O157) in rare hamburgers in several fast-food chains. EHEC infections are especially alarming because they are increasing in frequency and may cause hemolytic-uremic syndrome, which can be fatal despite antimicrobial therapy. Occasional nosocomial outbreaks of enterotoxigenic *E. coli* and enteropathogenic *E. coli* serotypes (EPEC) also have occurred in hospitalized infants in the United States and other industrialized countries.

As with most diarrheal illnesses, the highest age-specific attack rates of enterotoxigenic *E. coli* infections are in young children, especially at the time of weaning, when enterotoxigenic *E. coli* account for 15 to 50% of illnesses. Like immunologically inexperienced young children, the traveler visiting tropical areas has a 30 to 50% chance of acquiring travelers' diarrhea over a 2- to 3-week stay unless untreated water or ice and uncooked foods such as salads are strictly avoided. The most commonly recognized pathogen associated with travelers' diarrhea around the world is enterotoxigenic *E. coli* that produces either the STa, LT, or both enterotoxins (see Ch. 298).

Of potential immunologic significance is the continued occurrence of symptomatic infections with *E. coli* which produce the less immunogenic STa in adult residents of tropical or other areas endemic for enterotoxigenic *E. coli* infections. In contrast, adult residents in endemic areas often carry LT-producing *E. coli* asymptomatically, suggesting that they may be protected from symptoms, if not from colonization.

Limited data on invasive *E. coli* suggest that the infectious doses are relatively high. As with enterotoxigenic *E. coli* infections, such large numbers have been readily spread in food with high attack rates. Enteropathogenic *E. coli* have been recognized primarily in urban areas, especially among hospitalized infants in their first year of life, with apparent cross-infection in hospital nurseries. While sporadic cases still occur, nosocomial outbreaks of EPEC diarrhea during the summer appear to have become less common and less severe in industrialized countries in the last decade or two.

PATHOGENESIS AND PATHOLOGY. The pathogenesis of enteric *E. coli* infections begins with the ingestion of the organism in contaminated food or water, which then faces the normal gastric acid barrier. Both enterotoxigenic *E. coli* and enteroinvasive *E. coli* appear to be sensitive to gastric acid; neutralization by gastric acid

TABLE 297–1. DIFFERENT TYPES OF ENTERIC *E. COLI* INFECTIONS

Type	Mechanism	Predominant O Serogroups	Genetic Code	Detection	Clinical Syndromes
Enterotoxigenic E. coli (ETEC)					
1. Cholera-like, heat-labile toxin (LT)	Activates intestinal adenylate cyclase and adhesin fimbriae	6, 8, 11, 15, 20, 25, 27, 63, 80, 85, 139	Plasmid	ELISA, RIA, PIH, CHO, Y1 cells, 18 h loops, gene probe	Watery diarrhea, travelers' diarrhea
2. Heat-stable toxin (STa: STh or STp)	Activates intestinal guanylate cyclase and adhesin fimbriae	12, 78, 115, 148, 149, 153, 155, 166, 167	Plasmid (transposon)	ELISA, RIA, suckling mice, 6 h loops, gene probes	Watery diarrhea, travelers' diarrhea
3. Heat-stable toxin (STb)	?; Not cAMP or cGMP		Plasmid	Piglet loops, gene probe	?
Enteroinvasive E. coli (EIEC)					
4. Enteroinvasive *E. coli* (EIEC)	Cell invasion and spread	11, 28ac, 29, 124, 136, 144, 147, 152, 164, 167	Plasmid (140 MDa, pWR110)	Sereny test, gene probe, (lys⁻, NM, oft. lactose⁻)	Inflammatory dysentery
Enterohemorrhagic E. coli (EHEC)					
5. Enterohemorrhagic (EHEC)	Shiga-like toxin(s) and adhesin fimbriae	26, 39, 113, 121, 128, 139, 145, 157, occ 55, 111	Phage(s) & adhesin plasmid(s)	Serotype, HeLa, Vero cells, sorbitol, agar, SLT or eae gene probes	Bloody noninflammatory diarrhea; hemolytic-uremic syndrome
Enteropathogenic E. coli (EPEC)					
6. Focal attaching and effacing EPEC	Attach, then efface the mucosa	55, 111, 119, 125, 126, 127, 128, 142, 158,	Plasmid (60 MDa, pMAR2) + Chromosomal (eae and cfm)	Serotype, focal HEp2 adhesion, gene probes for EAF or eae	Infantile diarrhea
Enteroadherent E. coli					
7. Enteroaggregating *E. coli* (EAggEC)	Colonize (bundle-forming pili) ? toxins (EAST, EALT)	3, 15, 44, 51, 77, 78, 91	Plasmid	HEp2 cell adherence; AA probe	Persistent diarrhea
8. Diffusely adherent *E. coli* (DAEC)	Colonize (F 1845 fimbriate adhesin)	75 (F 1845), 15 (57-1), ? (189)	Chromosomal/ plasmid	HEp2 cell adherence; DA gene probe	Persistent diarrhea in children >18 mos. old

reduces the infectious dose by 100- to 1000-fold. This is followed by an incubation period of 2 to 7 days, during which colonization of the involved part of the intestinal tract and enterotoxin production or invasion take place. Best characterized is the colonization by enterotoxigenic *E. coli* in the upper small bowel, which involves one of at least five major colonization factor antigen groups (which are fimbriate or fibrillar protein structures on the surface of the organism). The colonization fimbriae bind the organism to cell surface receptors in the upper small bowel where the enterotoxin is delivered to reduce normal absorption and cause net electrolyte and water secretion. The heat-labile toxin (LT) with a molecular weight of about 86,000 has a binding and active subunit that, like choleratoxin, binds to a monosialoganglioside (Gm1) receptor. Also like choleratoxin, the active subunit ADP-ribosylates the regulatory subunit of adenylate cyclase to activate adenylate cyclase. The consequently increased chloride secretion and reduced sodium absorption combine to cause net isotonic electrolyte loss that must be replaced to prevent severe dehydration and hypotension and its potential consequences. Other strains produce the heat-stable toxin (STa), a much smaller molecule of 18 to 19 amino acids (molecular weight less than 2000), which activates intestinal particulate guanylate cyclase. Like cyclic AMP, the cyclic GMP thus formed also causes net secretion. A third type of *E. coli* enterotoxin (STb) causes secretion in porcine intestine without activating adenylate or guanylate cyclase; STb has no known role in human disease. Similarly, the roles of enterotoxins such as LTII, EAST, EIET, and others seen in ETEC, EAggEC, and EIEC, respectively, are unclear at present. Both the colonization traits and enterotoxin production are encoded on transmissible plasmids. Besides the complications of dehydration, the only significant pathologic change is depletion of mucus from intestinal goblet cells.

Other *E. coli,* often of certain serogroups noted in Table 297–1, have the capacity, analogous to *Shigella,* to invade and multiply in epithelial cells, cause conjunctivitis in guinea pigs (Sereny test), and cause inflammatory colitis and dysenteric or bloody diarrhea. As seen with shigellosis, a striking inflammatory response is seen, with sheets of polymorphonuclear leukocytes in the stool. The colon shows patchy, acute inflammation in the mucosa and submucosa with focal denuding of the surface epithelium but usually without deeper invasion or systemic spread. While epithelial cell invasiveness in both enteroinvasive *E. coli* and *Shigella* appears to be encoded on a large 120- to 140-MDa plasmid, several chromosomal determinants, including the O antigen, are crucial for full invasive virulence.

Classically recognized enteropathogenic *E. coli* serotypes often fail to produce known enterotoxins or to be invasive. Nevertheless, they are well-established causes of infantile diarrhea. The majority of classically recognized EPEC serotypes such as O55 and O111 exhibit both plasmid-encoded localized adherence to epithelial cells and chromosomally mediated attachment and effacement of the microvilli. There is also villus atrophy, mucosal thinning, inflammation in the lamina propria, and variable crypt cell hyperplasia. These morphologic changes are associated with a reduction in the mucosal brush border enzymes and may contribute to the impaired absorptive function and diarrhea.

Other *E. coli,* most notably serotype O157:H7 but also serogroups O26 and 39, are associated with foodborne outbreaks of bloody, noninflammatory diarrhea and with the hemolytic-uremic syndrome. These organisms produce Shiga-like toxins that may be responsible for the characteristic colonic mucosal inflammation, edema, and hemorrhage, as well as the complication of hemolytic-uremic syndrome. Sigmoidoscopy usually reveals only moderately hyperemic mucosa, and barium enema may reveal a thumbprint pattern of submucosal edema in the ascending and transverse colon. Some patients have superficial ulceration with mild neutrophil infiltration in the edematous submucosa. The mechanisms by which EAggEC (which adhere in an aggregative pattern to the mucosa and produce heat-stable and heat-labile "toxins"), DAEC, or colonization alone may cause diarrhea remain unclear at present.

CLINICAL MANIFESTATIONS. The most common clinical manifestation of enteric *E. coli* infections is the watery diarrhea that characterizes enterotoxigenic *E. coli* infections, particularly in young children and travelers to tropical or developing areas. This may range from mild to severe, cholera-like diarrhea that may be

life-threatening, especially in small children and elderly patients, who are particularly prone to suffer the most severe consequences of dehydration, undernutrition, and electrolyte imbalance (especially hypokalemia and acidosis).

The incubation period (2 to 7 days) varies with the size of the inoculum. Characteristic symptoms include malaise, abdominal cramping, anorexia, and watery diarrhea, occasionally associated with nausea, vomiting, or low-grade fever. The illness is usually self-limited to 1 to 5 days and rarely extends beyond 10 days or 2 weeks. Infections with *E. coli* which produce both ST and LT or ST alone may be more severe than those with only LT-producing *E. coli.* The persistence of impaired mucosal absorptive capacity for 1 to 3 weeks may further compound the cycle of malnutrition that complicates diarrheal illnesses in children in developing, tropical areas.

Infection with EIEC is characterized by inflammatory colitis, often with abdominal pain, high fever, tenesmus, and bloody or dysenteric diarrhea essentially like that seen with *Shigella,* to which this organism is closely related. The incubation period is usually 1 to 3 days with the duration usually self-limited to 7 to 10 days.

Outbreaks of EPEC infections in newborn nurseries have ranged from mild transient diarrhea to severe and rapidly fatal diarrheal illnesses, especially in premature or otherwise compromised infants. The more severe illnesses appear to have been more common in industrialized countries prior to 1950. However, more recent outbreaks and sporadic cases are well documented.

Hemorrhagic colitis associated with the Shiga-like toxin producing *E. coli* (EHEC) O157:H7 or O26:H11 is characterized by grossly bloody diarrhea with remarkably little fever or inflammatory exudate in the stool. Although the diarrheal illnesses have been self-limited, a significant number of children and adults have subsequently developed a potentially fatal hemolytic-uremic syndrome. Outbreaks of hemorrhagic colitis due to EHEC in nursing homes or other institutions may be quite severe and more common than previously appreciated. The incubation period in two outbreaks has been 3 to 4 days (range 1 to 7 days), and the illness is characteristically self-limited to 5 to 12 days (mean 7.8).

Enteroaggregative and diffusely adherent *E. coli* have been associated with persistent diarrhea in children in developing areas.

DIAGNOSIS. A definitive etiologic diagnosis of *E. coli* diarrhea requires the documentation of a specific virulence trait such as enterotoxin, invasiveness, enteroadherence, or serotype, which usually requires specialized immunologic, tissue culture, animal bioassay, or gene probes that are available only in research and reference laboratories. Such tests are rarely cost-effective or clinically indicated, except in outbreak or research situations. Fortunately, a likely diagnosis often can be suspected by the clinical and epidemiologic setting. For example, self-limited, noninflammatory diarrhea in tropical, developing areas is most likely due to enterotoxigenic *E. coli,* rotaviruses (young children), or Norwalk-like viruses (older children and adults). Noninflammatory diarrhea in winter months in temperate areas in older children or younger adults is more likely to be due to Norwalk-like viruses. Specific tests for the respective virulence traits of different types of *E. coli* are noted in Table 297–1. One should also consider *Vibrio* infections in areas endemic for cholera or in any coastal area where inadequately cooked seafood may be eaten. If noninflammatory diarrhea persists, especially with weight loss, one also should consider *Giardia lamblia* or *Cryptosporidium* infection. In outbreaks of food poisoning, *S. aureus,* *Clostridium perfringens,* and *Bacillus cereus* should be considered.

Inflammatory colitis with high fever, tenesmus, and leukocytes, mucus, and blood in the stool may well be due to enteroinvasive *E. coli* but should prompt a stool culture for more common invasive pathogens such as *Campylobacter jejuni, Shigella,* and *Salmonella* or even *Clostridium difficile, Yersina enterocolitica,* or noncholera *Vibrio* (see Ch. 295). On the other hand, bloody diarrhea without high fever and few, if any, fecal leukocytes should prompt consideration of the Shiga-like toxin producing enterohemorrhagic *E. coli* (EHEC) such as strain O157:H7. This organism is often suspected as a sorbitol-negative *E. coli,* which may require further study for serotype or Shiga-like toxin production.

THERAPY. As with all diarrheal illnesses, the primary treatment is replacement and maintenance of water and electrolytes. Losses of water and electrolytes may be particularly severe and even life-threatening with enterotoxigenic *E. coli* and can usually be replaced with a simple oral rehydration solution that uses the intact, sodium-coupled glucose, and/or amino acid absorption to replace fluid losses, as described in Ch. 296. This oral rehydration solution should be given *ad libitum* with free water and, in breast-fed infants, continued breast feeding and early refeeding to compensate for the nutritional losses.

Because most *E. coli* diarrhea is self-limited, the role of antimicrobial agents is debated and remains of secondary importance to rehydration. In areas where the enterotoxigenic *E. coli* remains sensitive, early initiation of sulfamethoxazole-trimethoprim, tetracycline, or new quinolone derivatives may reduce a 3- to 5-day illness to a 1- to 2-day illness if started with the first loose stool in travelers to endemic, tropical areas (see Ch. 298). The use of antimotility agents should be tempered by the potential added risk of worsening or prolonging inflammatory diarrheas and by their lack of effectiveness in reducing fluid loss even though abdominal cramping and overt diarrhea may be temporarily reduced. Because of the potential severity of the disease in infants, some pediatricians use neomycin, 100 mg per kilogram per day PO, divided into three daily doses for 5 days, for documented enteropathogenic *E. coli* infections in neonates. Bismuth subsalicylate may reduce symptoms in travelers' diarrhea but should be used with caution to avoid toxic doses of salicylate. A number of pharmacologic agents enhance absorption or reduce secretion with experimental diarrhea but remain inadequately studied or too toxic for recommended use to date.

The role of antimicrobial agents in treating EHEC infections or in preventing serious complications is controversial. The treatment of hemolytic-uremic syndrome may require plasma exchange as well.

PROGNOSIS. The overall prognosis in *E. coli* diarrheas of the various types noted, if fully and adequately treated, is generally excellent. However, the impact of *E. coli* and other common diarrheas on mortality and morbidity (particularly with repeated infections compounding malnutrition in young children) remains one of the major health problems on a global scale; this problem may actually be worsening in some transitional areas. The potentially serious complication of hemolytic-uremic syndrome may follow EHEC infection.

PREVENTION. The prevention of many *E. coli* enteric infections is ultimately related to basic economic development and adequate sanitary facilities and wide availability of sufficient quality and quantity of water. In the interim, especially in areas where adequate water supplies and sanitary facilities are not available, such measures as breast feeding for at least 6 to 12 months and hygienic measures like handwashing should reduce the likelihood of acquiring *E. coli* enteric infections. Travelers to developing or tropical areas should avoid drinking untreated or unboiled water or ice and eating uncooked fruits or vegetables that may have been "freshened" with highly contaminated water. Although a number of antimicrobial agents have been documented to be effective over short periods of time when taken prophylactically, their effectiveness is sharply limited by the rapidly emerging resistance to antimicrobial drugs as well as by the potential side effects of their indiscriminate, widespread use. For example, tetracycline resistance among enterotoxigenic *E. coli* is common, and combined sulfamethoxazole-trimethroprim resistance is rapidly emerging around the world. Finally, currently developing toxoid or colonization factor vaccines hold considerable promise for the prevention of enterotoxigenic *E. coli* diarrhea. EHEC infections can be largely prevented by adequately cooking beef, especially hamburgers, and by careful handwashing and other hygienic measures in day care centers and nursing homes.

Bhan MK, Raj P, Levine MM, et al.: Enteroaggregative *Escherichia coli* associated with persistent diarrhea in a cohort of rural children in India. J Infect Dis 159:1060, 1989. *A first report of a clinical role for new types of enteroadherent E. coli.*

Carter AO, Borczyk AA, Carlson AK, et al.: A severe outbreak of *E. coli* O157:H7 associated hemorrhagic colitis in a nursing home. N Engl J Med 317:1496, 1987. *A common source outbreak with secondary, probable person-to-person spread, of this cause of bloody diarrhea and hemolytic-uremic syndrome in the institutionalized elderly.*

Donnenberg MS, Kaper JB: Enteropathogenic *Escherichia coli*. Infect Immun 60:3953, 1992. *Excellent overview of recent advances regarding the pathogenesis of enteropathogenic E. coli infections.*

Griffin PM, Tauxe RV: The epidemiology of infections caused by *Escherichia coli* O157:H7 and other enterohemorrhagic *E. coli* and the associated hemolytic uremic syndrome. Epidemiol Rev 13:60, 1991. *Excellent review of the increasing problem of enterohemorrhagic E. coli infections and complications, often associated with rare hamburger and other foods and also seen in day care centers and institutions.*

Guerrant RL, Kirchhoff LV, Shields DS, et al.: Prospective study of diarrheal illnesses in northeastern Brazil: Patterns of disease, nutritional impact, etiologies and risk factors. J Infect Dis 148:986, 1983. *A detailed study of endemic diarrhea in a tropical area, including seasonality, risk after weaning, and nutritional impact, as well as relationship of enterotoxigenic E. coli to other pathogens.*

Guerrant RL, Hughes JM, Lima NL, Crane JK: Diarrhea in developed and developing countries: Magnitude, special settings and etiologies. Rev Infect Dis 12:S41, 1990. *Overview of community-based and hospital-based studies of diarrhea that reviews the relative importance of E. coli among other pathogens in developing and developed countries.*

Levine MM: *Escherichia coli* that cause diarrhea: Enterotoxigenic, Enteropathogenic, Enterohemorrhagic, and Enteroadherent. J Infect Dis 155:377, 1989. *A good overview of major pathogenic mechanisms of E. coli diarrhea.*

Microbial Toxins and Diarrheal Diseases. CIBA Foundation Symposium No. 112, 1985. *Thorough review of the mechanisms of enterotoxin action, relating the pharmacology of E. coli toxins (LT, STa, STb, Shiga) to those of such enteric pathogens as V. cholerae, Shigella, and C. difficile.*

NIH Consensus Development Conference on Traveler's Diarrhea. JAMA 253:2700, 1985. *A balanced critical appraisal of the epidemiology, etiologies, presentation, and treatment of travelers' diarrhea.*

Sansonetti PJ, Hale TL, Oaks EV: Genetics of virulence in enteroinvasive *Escherichia coli*. Microbiology, 1985, pp 67–82. *One of a series of three brief reviews that offer considerable new information on pathogenesis of the major types of E. coli enteric infection including ETEC, EIEC, EPEC, and EHEC.*

Thielman NM, Guerrant RL: *Eschericia coli*. In Emmerson AM, Hawkey PM, Gillespie SH (eds.); Principles and Practices of Clinical Bacteriology, New York, John Wiley & Sons, 1994. *Concise overview of 6 to 10 types of E. coli pathogenesis with update on new clinical and pathogenic studies of different types of E. coli pathogens.*

298 THE DIARRHEA OF TRAVELERS

R. Bradley Sack

Travelers from the developed world who visit the developing world are highly susceptible to an acute infectious diarrheal illness known as "travelers' diarrhea" or by more colorful names that fit the locale in which the travelers find themselves incapacitated. The etiologic agents of this syndrome are the same as those which cause endemic diarrheal illness, primarily in children, throughout the areas of the world in which sanitation is less than optimal. Travelers (see Ch. 268) from sanitized, developed countries are in a sense immunologically naive "children" who are suddenly transported to an endemic area of infection, where they are highly susceptible to the local pathogens. Other than during a common-source outbreak of diarrheal disease (such as a gross fecal contamination of a water supply), the attack rates among travelers are the highest known in any identifiable population. Approximately 25 to 50% of travelers will experience a diarrheal illness during their first 3 weeks of stay in a developing country; this will decrease markedly thereafter as immunity develops.

By way of contrast, travelers from developing countries who visit other developing countries usually have a considerably lower attack rate owing to their prior exposure and subsequent immunity to these organisms. As expected, these same visitors who visit the developed world do not develop the illness.

ETIOLOGY. Multiple studies have described the causes of this syndrome throughout the world, and it is clear that enterotoxigenic *Escherichia coli* is the most common pathogen. Other bacteria, viruses, and protozoa are also involved but with lesser frequency (Table 298–1). In certain localities and in certain seasons, the prevalence of *Campylobacter* or *Salmonella* may be particularly high. Even now, a considerable proportion of episodes (20 to 30%) cannot be diagnosed microbiologically, and new etiologic organisms continue to be discovered. Contrary to "popular" notions, relatively few cases of travelers' diarrhea are caused by *Entamoeba histolytica* or other protozoa.

PATHOGENESIS AND CLINICAL PICTURE. The clinical syndrome of travelers' diarrhea is typically that of a nonfebrile, secretory, watery diarrhea that is produced by the enterotoxins of bacteria, particularly *E. coli* (see Ch. 297). The watery diarrhea usually lasts 3 to 4 days and, when most severe, may result in 15 to 20 evacuations per day, with significant water and electrolyte loss, leading to clinical signs of dehydration. The vast majority of ill-

TABLE 298-1. ETIOLOGIC AGENTS OF TRAVELERS' DIARRHEA

Agent	Percentage
Enterotoxigenic *E. coli*	30–70
Shigella	5–10
*Salmonella**	<5
*Campylobacter**	<5
Enteroadherent *E. coli*	5–10
Rotavirus	<5
Giardia lamblia	<5
Entamoeba histolytica	<3
Cryptosporidium	<5
Cyclospora	<1
Unknown agents	20–30

* May be higher in certain geographic areas.

nesses are much milder, however, consisting of only 3 to 5 diarrheal stools per day, and are important primarily because they limit the activities of the traveler. Episodes due to invasive bacteria, such as *Shigella* or *Campylobacter,* may be dysentery-like in nature, with abdominal pain, fever, and blood in the stool (see Ch. 294).

Nearly all episodes are self-limited, but a few (<1%) may become persistent and require evaluation after the return home. Some of these prolonged episodes may be due to infection with *Cyclospora,* a newly recognized cyanobacterium-like organism.

TRANSMISSION. Transmission of the enteric pathogens occurs almost exclusively through fecally contaminated food and water. Of highest risk to the traveler are foods that are not cooked or peeled, foods obtained from roadside vendors, or foods kept unrefrigerated for long periods of time.

PREVENTION. Since the modes of transmission are known, prudent attention to the ingestion of uncontaminated food and water should entirely prevent the disease. This has been shown in the military or on board cruise ships, where all food is hygienically prepared and packaged. For the usual traveler, however, food must be obtained from local sources, and contamination cannot be entirely prevented. Even the "best" hotels in the developing world may have unsanitary kitchens, and "first class" travelers are therefore not exempt.

Many studies have now shown that a number of drugs can prevent 75 to 90% of diarrheal episodes when taken regularly during short-term travel (<3 weeks). Medication is begun on the day before reaching the locale and discontinued on the day after leaving. The antimicrobials that have been well studied are shown in Table 298–2. Doxycycline, which was the earliest antimicrobial shown to be effective, is no longer recommended because of marked increase in antibiotic resistance of enterotoxigenic *E. coli*. Because the antibacterial spectrum of the fluoroquinolones includes *Campylobacter,* these drugs provide the broadest spectrum of antibacterial coverage against the disease. A nonantimicrobial drug, bismuth sub-salicylate (BSS), taken four times a day also has given a significant but lesser degree (approximately 60%) of protection. Other antimicrobial drugs also have been used successfully (erythromycin, mecillinam, trimethoprim alone) but have not been tested as extensively.

Drugs that have been tested and found to be of little or no benefit include neomycin, streptotriad, hydroxyquinolines, and *Lactobacillus* preparations.

TABLE 298-2. PREVENTION AND TREATMENT OF TRAVELERS' DIARRHEA WITH ANTIMICROBIALS

Antimicrobial	Prevention* Daily Dose (mg)	Treatment† Dose (mg)	Duration‡ (days)
Trimethoprim-sulfamethoxazole	160/800	160–800 bid	3
Norfloxacin	400	400 bid	3
Ciprofloxacin	500	500 bid	3

* For periods up to 3 weeks.
† Loperamide given along with antimicrobials has given further improvement.
‡ Some studies have shown larger doses given as only a single dose to be effective.

THERAPY. Therapy is usually carried out by the patient, who must be able to recognize when to take the medication. Instructions for therapy should be given by the traveler's physician, who must be familiar with the disease. One aim of self-treatment is to avoid consultation by the traveler of local physicians (or diagnostic laboratories) for advice and medications. Therapy includes specific fluid replacement when indicated, specific antimicrobial therapy directed against the most likely causative agents, and, if necessary, symptomatic therapy directed at relieving the frequency of stooling and abdominal cramps.

Fluids may be replaced by increasing the amount of liquids ingested, such as soup and fruit juices, if the diarrhea is mild. For more severe diarrhea, an oral glucose electrolyte solution (ORS), which has been developed to treat all dehydrating diarrheas regardless of etiologic agent or age of the patient, should be taken. ORS is now available commercially in packets; the traveler can carry and use them as required by mixing the contents with appropriate volumes of potable water.

In many controlled studies, a short course (1 to 3 days) of appropriate antimicrobials has been shown to significantly shorten the disease to approximately 24 to 36 hours. The most widely used drugs (shown in Table 298–2) are also the ones that have been shown to be effective in prevention. In addition, some of the newer fluoroquinolones (oflaxacin, fleroxacin) and aztreonam have been shown to be equally effective.

Symptomatic therapy with antimotility agents, such as loperamide, may be useful for travelers who need to participate in certain vital events during which the need to evacuate frequently would be embarrassing and particularly inconvenient, such as during long bus rides or while giving lectures. The combination of loperamide with an effective antimicrobial has been shown to resolve the illness more quickly than would the antimicrobial alone.

BSS also has been shown to give significant but less striking symptomatic improvement, although the exact mechanism of action is unknown. Kaolin/pectin preparations are of no significant effect in treatment.

THE STRATEGY OF MANAGING TRAVELERS' DIARRHEA. Whether to give antimicrobials prophylactically or to rely on early patient-initiated treatment is the major question in management. The decisions should be based on the following considerations. It is known that all persons who travel to developing countries, regardless of whether they are taking antimicrobials, have an alteration in their microbial gut flora, which includes acquiring antibiotic-resistant bacteria. Antimicrobials are widely available without prescription in most developing countries and are used widely; therefore, the contribution of tourists taking antibiotics to the local microbial ecology is probably negligible. The real concern of giving antimicrobials prophylactically is side effects. Although adverse effects are known to be infrequent, some travelers will experience these when large numbers of persons are taking drugs. Contraindications include known allergies, pregnancy, and age. Therefore, the following suggestions are made when considering prophylaxis: Travelers should be on short-term visits (<3 weeks), they should request the use of antimicrobials, and they should be able to understand and accept the risk of side effects. Certain travelers with medical illnesses, for whom an episode of diarrhea would be particularly deleterious, also may be given special consideration for prophylaxis. The more widely recommended strategy is to have the traveler carry the medicines and self-administer them on recognition of the onset of illness.

The problem of travelers' diarrhea will continue until the general sanitation of the developing world approaches that of industrialized countries or until effective vaccines against the major diarrheal pathogens become available. Neither of these is expected soon; therefore, this common syndrome will need to be addressed for some time. Fortunately, this can now be done rationally and effectively based on our knowledge of causes and modes of transmission.

Black RE: Epidemiology of travelers' diarrhea and relative importance of various pathogens. Rev Infect Dis 12(suppl. 1):S73, 1990. *A summary of many studies worldwide on causes identified in persons with travelers' diarrhea.*

Consensus Conference: Travelers' diarrhea. JAMA 253:2700, 1985. *A summary of the NIH conference in which all aspects of the problem were reviewed; a complete publication of the conference is given in Rev Infect Dis 8(suppl. 2), 1986.*

DuPont HL, Ericsson CD: Prevention and treatment of travelers' diarrhea. N Engl J Med 328:1821, 1993. *A recent review of the problem with an extensive discussion of management options.*

299 EXTRAINTESTINAL INFECTIONS CAUSED BY ENTERIC BACTERIA

Elizabeth J. Ziegler

Bacteria constitute over half the dry weight of stool. *Bacteroides* species far outnumber other genera, at 10^{12} organisms per gram. Other anaerobes such as fusobacteria, clostridia, and peptostreptococci also are abundant. Among the facultative bacteria, members of the family Enterobacteriaceae predominate, at about 10^9 organisms per gram. Pseudomonads, enterococci, other nonhemolytic streptococci, and yeasts are present as well.

These bacteria that normally inhabit the human gastrointestinal tract perform important functions beneficial to the host. *Bacteroides fragilis,* clostridia, and enterococci deconjugate bile acids for participation in fat metabolism. Some intestinal bacteria synthesize menaquinone, or vitamin K, a cofactor for blood coagulation. Normal gut flora discourage colonization of the bowel with primary pathogens and overgrowth of bacteria usually present in small numbers. Colonization resistance is not understood completely, but it must involve bacteriocins, regulation of local oxidation-reduction potential, competition for receptors, and balance of nutrients as well as unknown factors. Breakdown of colonization resistance is illustrated by the increase in susceptibility of antibiotic-treated animals to *Salmonella* and by the emergence of fecal *Pseudomonas aeruginosa* and *Candida* in patients receiving antimicrobial agents.

PATHOGENESIS OF INFECTIONS

Enteric bacteria are not primary pathogens but cause disease when they escape from their usual gastrointestinal habitat. Direct penetration of the bowel wall by surgical, traumatic, or spontaneous rupture spills fecal contents into the peritoneal cavity and into open wounds. Gut bacteria on the perineal skin gain access to the urinary tract and proliferate there, especially when the flushing action of urine flow is disrupted by mechanical obstruction or neurologic dysfunction. When the biliary tract is obstructed by gallstones or tumor, the upper small bowel, which normally is sterile, becomes colonized with facultative bacteria (*Escherichia coli, Klebsiella,* enterococci) or, less often, with *Bacteroides* and *Clostridium,* which then infect the gallbladder and bile ducts. Intestinal flora can be introduced into the respiratory tract from contaminated skin or the environment; they proliferate there under the influence of antibiotics and loss of fibronectin and in the presence of underlying pulmonary disease and tracheal instrumentation. Penetrating foreign bodies, such as intravenous catheters and intraventricular cerebral pressure monitors, become colonized by gut flora on the skin and in respiratory secretions and then induce infection in adjacent tissues. In burns, destruction of the skin barrier, the rich culture medium of oozing tissue fluid, and a shift of surface flora by application of local and systemic antibacterial agents result in local necrotizing infection of the burn wound with gut flora and frequent secondary gram-negative bacteremia.

In the absence of mechanical and surface abnormalities such as those outlined above, systemic resistance to enteric bacteria is very strong. The mainstay of this resistance is the polymorphonuclear neutrophil, destruction or malfunction of which leads almost inevitably to bloodstream invasion by bowel bacteria. Serum complement must be protective against invasion of some organisms, since very few of the gram-negative bacilli isolated from blood are sensitive to complement-mediated bacteriolysis, whereas many enteric rods in feces are susceptible. Newborn infants, whose neutrophils and complement activity have not fully matured, are at high risk for disseminated infections with facultative enteric rods. Microbial factors are important, too. Although anaerobes predominate over facultative bacteria and aerobes in the gut, these anaerobes rarely cause bacteremia or metastatic infection even in neutropenia. The presence of certain bacterial polysaccharide capsules (e.g., *E. coli* K1) or production of large amounts of capsule (e.g., by *Klebsiella pneu-*

moniae in hyperglycemic or glycosuric diabetics) predisposes to systemic invasion by these organisms.

Infections with enteric bacteria have increased dramatically during the past four decades. The reasons should be apparent from the foregoing discussion. Advances in surgical and intensive care, trauma and burn management, blood transfusion, antimicrobial and cancer chemotherapy, transplantation, and immunosuppression all create opportunities for these infections. The average lifespan has lengthened, so that those receiving medical attention carry the added risks of advanced age. Many extraintestinal infections with enteric bacteria now arise in the hospital, and they exact a high toll in mortality and increased hospital costs. Furthermore, they jeopardize the success of the advanced treatments we have worked so hard to develop. Therefore, physicians should understand the pathogenesis of each infection so that they can effect a cure and prevent recurrence if possible.

SPECIFIC INFECTIONS WITH ENTERIC BACTERIA

The diagnosis and management of each of the following gram-negative infections are discussed in depth in the appropriate section elsewhere in the textbook. A few points are emphasized here.

PERITONITIS (see Ch. 111). It can be difficult to recover bacteria from patients with spontaneous bacterial peritonitis; large volumes of fluid should be submitted for culture. Patients undergoing chronic peritoneal dialysis frequently develop peritonitis. If the same organism is isolated from repeated episodes and especially if it is an enteric rod or *Pseudomonas,* infection of the subcutaneous catheter tunnel should be suspected. A radiolabeled white blood cell scan can be helpful in detecting such infections so that the infected catheter can be removed.

PYELONEPHRITIS (see Ch. 84). Urinary tract infections localized to the bladder or kidneys can have important implications for therapy. Symptoms may be misleading, selective ureteral catheterization carries considerable risk, and examination of urine for antibody-coated bacteria is not practical in most laboratories. A simple culture technique can differentiate between upper and lower urinary tract infections in difficult cases in which parenteral antibiotics would be required for kidney infection. In brief, the test employs a newly placed three-way bladder catheter through which a combination antibiotic and enzyme mixture (fibrinolysin and DNaase) is instilled to sterilize the bladder. Neomycin is used for most organisms; polymyxin can be used for *Pseudomonas* and amphotericin for yeast. Bladder instillation is followed by a large-volume sterile water wash. Then the catheter is clamped, and three 10-minute specimens are collected. Increasing bacterial counts after the wash point to pyelonephritis. If infection is limited to the bladder, this procedure can cure it. The test is unreliable in patients with low urinary output, and it should not be performed in those with neutropenia.

PROSTATITIS (see Ch. 209.2). Most antibiotics available for treating infections with enteric bacilli do not penetrate the prostate well. For this reason, chronic prostatitis rarely is cured. However, the role of chronic prostatitis as a nidus of recurrent acute urinary tract infection in males can be curbed by low levels of suppressive antibiotics in bladder urine, achieved by a single tablet of an oral antibiotic given daily.

MENINGITIS (see Ch. 280). Enteric rods, especially *E. coli* and *Klebsiella,* are a frequent cause of neonatal meningitis. In adults, meningitis with enteric bacilli is exceedingly rare except in cases of head trauma or neurosurgery. Bacteria may be infrequent and difficult to see on stained smears of spinal or ventricular fluid. Treatment with a third-generation cephalosporin that penetrates the blood-brain barrier at high dose may be sufficient, but infections with organisms resistant to such drugs may require chloramphenicol or a combination of intravenous and intrathecal aminoglycosides. Infected foreign bodies must be removed.

PNEUMONIA (see Ch. 19, 55, 274). Seeing gram-negative rods in respiratory secretions or growing them from the secretions does not necessarily imply infection. Susceptible patients often have severe chronic lung disease with abnormal chest radiographs. Many are on respirators with inflammation around endotracheal tubes and have abnormal gram-negative nasopharyngeal flora. Evidence of increasing infiltrates, fever, increasing leukocytosis, and/or worsening respiratory function should be sought before the diagnosis of gram-negative pneumonia is made in such cases.

INFECTIONS OF INTRAVENOUS CATHETERS. Critically ill patients may have limited numbers of sites for placing intravenous catheters. If catheter infection is suspected, it may be impractical or impossible to remove all the lines. Comparing simultaneous quantitative blood cultures drawn through each catheter and from one peripheral vein can identify the infected site and preserve the uninfected catheters in place.

INFECTIONS IN NEUTROPENIA (see Ch. 266). The most common bowel infection in neutropenia is perirectal abscess. Inflammation may be modest, but patients complain of severe pain. Examination can cause bacteremia. Surgical drainage may not be required unless neutropenia resolves and fluctuance develops. A less common but much more serious condition is typhlitis, an infection of the cecum associated with gas in the bowel wall, peritonitis, perforation, and bacteremia. This condition can be fatal within hours. Surgical resection has been helpful in a few cases, but surgical mortality is very high. Aggressive antibiotic therapy should be directed against *E. coli* and *P. aeruginosa,* the most common etiologic agents.

Necrotic skin lesions can accompany gram-negative bacteremia in neutropenic patients. These lesions are called ecthyma gangrenosum, and they are seen most frequently in *Pseudomonas* bacteremia. Cases have been reported with other gram-negative rods and with *Candida* and *Aspergillus* septicemia as well. The lesions can be scraped to search for the organism on smear. If nothing is seen, a punch biopsy for culture and histologic section can be done safely even in severe thrombocytopenia. In fungemia, the histologic section may be the only premortem specimen from which a diagnosis is obtained.

GRAM-NEGATIVE BACTEREMIA (see Ch. 70). Gram-negative bacteria gain access to the bloodstream from foci of tissue infection or, when host resistance is depressed, from sites of heavy colonization and minor trauma. Although bacteremia creates the opportunity for metastatic infections, a more immediate and serious consequence of gram-negative bacteremia is septic shock. The incidence of gram-negative bacteremia has risen steadily during the past three decades. It is estimated that at least 200,000 episodes occur in the United States each year, of which 20 to 60% are fatal. Mortality varies with the severity and nature of underlying disease, the source of bacteremia, and the incidence of serious sequelae. Rates of shock vary in different series from <20% to >50%. In comparable groups, shock is somewhat more frequent in gram-negative bacteremia than in gram-positive bacteremia or fungemia. However, gram-negative bacteremia is distinguished from the other septicemias by the fact that very small numbers of circulating bacteria are associated with hypotension. Figure 299–1 is a schematic representation of the complex relationship between sepsis, bacteremia, hypotension, and endotoxemia in gram-negative infection.

For therapeutic purposes, the diagnosis of gram-negative bacteremia cannot await the results of blood cultures but must be made on clinical grounds alone. The clinical setting is very helpful. A diagnosis of gram-negative bacteremia should be considered when sudden deterioration occurs in patients with focal infections usually caused by gram-negative bacteria (e.g., pyelonephritis, cholecystitis), in patients with significant focal infections from which gram-negative bacteria already have been isolated, and in patients with compromise in host defenses (e.g., neutropenia, burn injury), rendering them susceptible to their own bacterial flora. Neutropenic patients rarely have physical signs to localize the source of their bacteremia, but careful conversation often reveals a history of minor trauma, slight pain, or diarrhea. Gram-negative bacteremia and endotoxin infusion both cause transient neutropenia followed by neutrophilic leukocytosis. Large "toxic" vacuoles are seen. The first leukocyte count often is obtained after the leukopenic phase, but patients recovering from chemotherapy may have limited leukocyte reserves and thus exhibit only an apparent reversal of marrow recovery. Isolated thrombocytopenia or full-blown disseminated intravascular coagulopathy is not diagnostic of gram-negative bacteremia but, if present, is good supporting evidence. Arterial blood gas determinations may reveal unexplained hypoxemia without overt pulmonary disease, followed by metabolic acidosis.

TREATMENT. The correct choice of antibiotics is crucial to successful treatment of gram-negative bacteremia. When inappropriate drugs are used or the doses are too low, outcome is poor. It is never wise to give a single antibiotic to a patient at the onset of a bacteremic episode, even if the diagnosis and etiology seem certain. Many other infections can mimic gram-negative bacteremia, as discussed. Sometimes more than one bacterial species is involved. In neutropenia, the outcome of *Pseudomonas* bacteremia is much better if more than one effective antibiotic is used. The choice of empiric antibiotics should be made on the basis of the site of the focal infection (or infections) present, the known antimicrobial sensitivities of previous isolates from the patient and of agents of recent nosocomial infections in the hospital, and the patient's underlying diseases. In most patients the best regimen seems to be a combination of an aminoglycoside with a third-generation cephalosporin. An antistaphylococcal drug should be added if *S. aureus* infection is likely. If bowel perforation or infarction has occurred, *Bacteroides fragilis* must be covered. If *Clostridium perfringens* is suspected to be part of a mixed infection, concomitant high-dose penicillin should be used. (*C. perfringens* decolorizes easily in the Gram stain and may be distinguishable from gram-negative rods only by its boxlike rectangular shape.) A common mistake in use of aminoglycosides is to tailor the initial regimen to the first renal function tests. If azotemia is acute and attributable to poor perfusion, initial low doses will give inadequate levels as soon as hypotension is reversed. Renal toxicity from these drugs rarely occurs early; it is far more important to treat infection effectively in the first 24 hours than to avoid aminoglycoside toxicity.

Gram-negative bacteremia cannot be cured without eradicating the source of bacteremia. In cases of infection associated with ureteral or biliary obstruction, bacteremia and shock may persist in the face of adequate antibiotics until the obstruction is relieved. All likely sites of infection should be cultured, if possible, before antibiotics are given. However, antibiotic treatment should not be delayed for this reason. Wound cultures often remain positive after blood and urine have been sterilized. Physicians should not be content until they have found a satisfactory explanation for bacteremia. New fever or clinical deterioration can signal a new infection in a susceptible patient, the emergence of resistant bacteria, spread of the original focal infection, inadequate antibiotic levels, or a drug reaction. Such an episode requires complete re-evaluation with physical examination and repeat cultures.

Calandra T, Cometta A: Antibiotic therapy for gram-negative bacteremia. Infect Dis Clin North Am 5:817, 1991. *A good summary of recent studies.*

Kreger BE, Craven DE, Carling PC, et al.: Gram-negative bacteremia. III. Reassessment of etiology, epidemiology and ecology in 612 patients. Am J Med 68:332, 1980. *A recent classic clinical description of gram-negative bacteremia in an academic hospital setting with emphasis on the pathogenesis and the influence of the underlying condition on outcome.*

Uzun O, Akalin HE, Hayran M, Unal S: Factors influencing prognosis in bacteremia due to gram-negative organisms: Evaluation of 448 episodes in a Turkish university hospital. Clin Infect Dis 15:866, 1992. *A large recent series with good comments on prognostic factors.*

Van Deventer SJH, Buller HR, ten Cate JW, et al.: Endotoxemia: An early predictor of septicemia in febrile patients. Lancet 1:606, 1988.

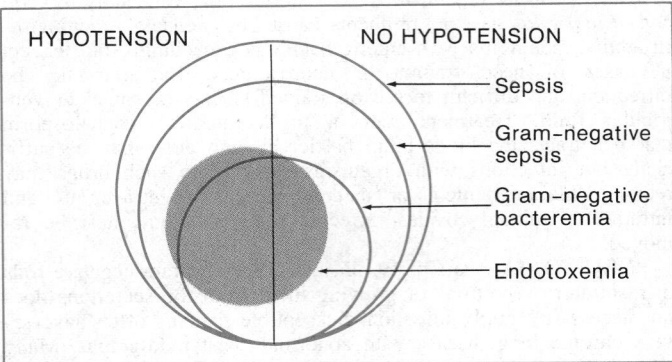

FIGURE 299–1. Schematic representation of etiologies of the sepsis syndrome. (Courtesy of Craig R. Smith.)

300 *YERSINIA* INFECTIONS

J. Glenn Morris, Jr.

The genus *Yersinia* contains at least nine species which have been isolated from humans. *Y. enterocolitica, Y. pseudotuberculosis,* and *Y. pestis* (the causative agent of plague) are well-recognized human pathogens; diseases associated with each of these three species are described in detail below. Within the past 15 years, DNA hybridization and other studies have resulted in the delineation of six additional *"Y. enterocolitica*–like" species: *Y. frederiksenii, Y. kristensenii, Y. intermedia, Y. aldovae, Y. mollaretii* (formerly biogroup 3A of *Y. enterocolitica*), and *Y. bercovieri* (formerly biogroup 3B of *Y. enterocolitica*). These latter species carry antigens that in some instances are identical to those of *Y. enterocolitica* strains (allowing strains to be serotyped with *Y. enterocolitica* typing sera), and may be identified as *Y. enterocolitica* in some laboratory identification systems. Although all have been isolated from humans, these species appear to have minimal pathogenic potential.

YERSINIA ENTEROCOLITICA

DEFINITION. *Y. enterocolitica* is an enteric pathogen that can cause gastroenteritis, mesenteric adenitis and ileitis ("pseudoappendicitis"), and sepsis. Infection may also trigger a variety of autoimmune phenomena, including erythema nodosum, reactive arthritis, and possibly thyroiditis.

Y. enterocolitica is a gram-negative bacillus within the family Enterobacteriaceae; when first identified, it was designated *Pasteurella* "X."

DISTRIBUTION AND EPIDEMIOLOGY. *Y. enterocolitica* is widely distributed in the environment (especially in cooler, temperate regions of the world) and frequently colonizes wild and domestic animals. The organism is a common pharyngeal commensal in swine, with potentially pathogenic strains isolated from 25 to 90% of pork tongues after slaughter. Fifty-eight per cent of *Y. enterocolitica* infections in Belgium (which has one of the highest rates of *Y. enterocolitica* disease in the world) have been attributed to eating raw pork. *Y. enterocolitica* outbreaks have also been linked with milk, in which the organism grows at refrigerator temperatures. *Y. enterocolitica* may also be introduced into a household by pets or by symptomatic or asymptomatic human carriers. Once the organism is present within a household, infants and young children appear to be at greatest risk for infection.

In parts of Canada and western Europe, *Y. enterocolitica* rivals *Salmonella* and surpasses *Shigella* as a cause of acute diarrheal disease. In the United States, isolation rates from diarrheal stool samples are somewhat lower, generally about one third of those for *Salmonella*. However, recent studies suggest that US rates are increasing. Isolation rates tend to be much lower in tropical areas. In one study in Bangladesh, *Y. enterocolitica* was isolated from only 0.06% of diarrheal stool samples from children under age 7; this very low rate may reflect both the decreased frequency of environmental isolation outside of cold areas and the dietary restrictions limiting pork consumption in Moslem countries.

PATHOGENESIS. *Y. enterocolitica* is an intracellular pathogen. It invades and survives within macrophages and may persist and grow within lymph nodes and other lymphoid tissue for extended periods. It can also produce one or more protein enterotoxins, which may be responsible for or contribute to the diarrheal disease caused by the organism. Autoimmune phenomena occurring after *Y. enterocolitica* infections appear to be due to cross-reactivity between host and bacterial antigens; several putative target antigens are under active investigation, including bacterial antigens that may cross-react with the HLA-B27 antigen (in reactive arthritis) (see Ch. 238), or with the human thyrotropin receptor (in Graves' disease) (see Ch. 203).

Human illness is most commonly associated with a group of *Y. enterocolitica* strains which share certain virulence characteristics, especially the ability to invade epithelial cells.

CLINICAL AND LABORATORY FEATURES. The most common clinical manifestation of *Y. enterocolitica* infection is diarrhea, frequently accompanied by abdominal pain and fever; vomiting occurs in 20 to 40% of cases. Diarrhea is mild to moderate in severity and may last 1 to 2 weeks. As many as 10 to 20% of patients are reported to have bloody diarrhea. The limited available data suggest that leukocytosis is common.

Abdominal pain may be quite severe, mimicking appendicitis, and may occur in the absence of diarrhea. This has resulted in several outbreaks of "pseudoappendicitis" associated with transmission of *Y. enterocolitica* in a common food item.

Y. enterocolitica can cause pharyngitis (8% of *Y. enterocolitica* cases identified in one large, multistate outbreak), hepatic and splenic abscesses, peritonitis, and septicemia. Sepsis has been closely linked with iron overload states (and the administration of deferoxamine, used in treating iron overload), and with the presence of underlying conditions such as cirrhosis, chronic renal failure, diabetes, and immunosuppression. Recent reports suggest that very young infants (<3 months) with intestinal *Y. enterocolitica* infections have an increased susceptibility to septicemia; these infants may or may not be febrile and may have protein-losing enteropathy and failure to thrive.

Infection with *Y. enterocolitica* can trigger myriad autoimmune processes, most notably erythema nodosum and a reactive polyarthritis. Arthritis generally occurs within 1 to 2 weeks of onset of gastrointestinal symptoms, usually in HLA-B27–positive patients. Viable organisms cannot be cultured from involved joints; however, *Yersinia* antigens have been identified in synovial fluid cells. *Y. enterocolitica* infections have also been implicated in the development of Reiter's syndrome, carditis, glomerulonephritis, Graves' disease, and Hashimoto's thyroiditis.

DIAGNOSIS. Diagnosis is based on isolation of the organism from stool, blood, or other clinical specimen.

Although not generally available in the United States, serologic diagnosis of *Y. enterocolitica* infections is widely used in Europe.

TREATMENT. Currently available data do not indicate that antimicrobial therapy is efficacious in cases of uncomplicated *Y. enterocolitica* enteritis, but it is indicated in systemic disease or focal extraintestinal infection. *Y. enterocolitica* strains are susceptible *in vitro* to aminoglycosides, chloramphenicol, tetracycline, trimethoprim-sulfamethoxazole, third-generation cephalosporins, and quinolones; isolates are resistant to penicillins and first-generation cephalosporins. Recent evidence suggests that fluoroquinolones may be the drug of choice for extraintestinal *Y. enterocolitica* infections, in combination with a third-generation cephalosporin or an aminoglycoside in severe cases.

PROGNOSIS. Most cases of *Y. enterocolitica* enteritis are self-limited, and recovery is complete. Mortality rates among persons with *Y. enterocolitica* sepsis were originally reported to exceed 50%. In more recent studies, with aggressive antimicrobial therapy and supportive care, mortality has been approximately 7.5%. Arthritis may persist for a period of months (mean of 3.2 months in one study), with mild residual symptoms occurring in 50% of patients; 1 to 2% develop chronic arthritis.

YERSINIA PSEUDOTUBERCULOSIS

Y. pseudotuberculosis is most commonly recognized as a cause of mesenteric adenitis. Cases of enteritis in children have been reported from Japan (Izumi fever), and septicemia is seen in patients who have underlying liver disease or immunosuppression. The organism is widely distributed in the environment and is carried by wild and domestic animals. Secondary immunologic complications, such as erythema nodosum, arthritis, and renal insufficiency, have also been observed.

YERSINIA PESTIS (PLAGUE)

DEFINITION. *Y. pestis* is the etiologic agent for plague. The most common clinical form is bubonic plague, or acute regional lymphadenitis; septicemic and pneumonic forms also occur. Although epidemics of plague have had a major impact on human history, cases today are confined largely to isolated endemic foci. Three biovars have been described: biovar orientatis is distributed worldwide; biovar antiqua is found in Central Asia and Central Africa, and biovar medievalis is found in Iran and in the former Soviet Union.

DISTRIBUTION AND EPIDEMIOLOGY. Among rodent populations, plague is spread by transmission from rodents to fleas and back to rodents (sylvatic plague). Soil can also be contaminated by infected dead fleas and rodents; rodents coming from noninfected areas can become infected when they dig burrows in previously infected areas. This cycle may be relatively stable (enzootic) or may result in periodic epidemics (epizootics) in susceptible rodent populations. Humans are an accidental host in this natural cycle, with cases occurring when infected fleas bite people, or, occasionally, after direct inoculation of the skin by body fluids of an infected animal (often rabbits or carnivores). Direct, person-to-person transmission is seen only in the setting of pneumonic plague.

In the United States, plague is found west of the 100th meridian, which runs from North Dakota to Texas. Animals most commonly involved have included ground squirrels, rock squirrels, and prairie dogs. Between 1983 and 1992, there were an average of 16 cases of plague per year in the United States, based on reports to the Centers for Disease Control and Prevention. Approximately one third of recent cases have occurred in Native Americans; this is presumably a function of lifestyle, which may involve herding animals, assisted by dogs, in enzootic areas. Two thirds of cases occur in persons under age 25.

CLINICAL AND LABORATORY FEATURES. Plague presents most commonly as an acute regional lymphadenitis, or bubonic plague. Symptoms generally occur after an incubation period of 2 to 6 days. Illness is marked by the sudden onset of fever, chills, weakness, and headache. Then or shortly thereafter, patients note an intensely painful swelling in one region of lymph nodes, usually the groin, axilla, or neck. This swelling, or bubo, is typically oval, varying from 1 to 10 cm in length; the overlying skin is elevated and warm and may appear stretched or erythematous. The bubo itself is firm, extremely tender to palpation, and nonfluctuant. Patients with bubonic plague usually do not have skin lesions. However, in studies in Vietnam, about one fourth of patients had pustules, vesicles, eschars, or papules near the bubo or in areas drained by the affected nodes; these were presumed to represent sites of flea bite inoculations.

In the absence of therapy, disease progresses rapidly to a septicemic phase, with marked toxicity, prostration, and shock. The white blood cell count is elevated, and evidence of disseminated intravascular coagulation may appear. Purpura may be seen, associated with vasculitis and thrombosis. Some patients do not develop a bubo and progress directly to septicemia (septicemic plague). Diagnosis in these cases may be particularly difficult, as initial symptoms are relatively nonspecific (fever, headache, sore throat, malaise, myalgia, nausea, diarrhea, vomiting).

One of the feared complications of plague is plague pneumonia. Secondary pneumonia results from hematogenous spread of *Y. pestis* to the lung. Patients develop cough, chest pain, and may have hemoptysis. Radiographically, there is patchy bronchopneumonia or confluent consolidation. Sputum is purulent and contains the etiologic organism. Plague pneumonia is highly contagious by airborne transmission; persons inhaling the organism, from either an infected person or an animal, are susceptible to infection (primary plague pneumonia). Plague meningitis is a rarer complication; it typically occurs more than a week after inadequately treated bubonic plague but may be seen as a primary manifestation, without associated lymphadenopathy.

DIAGNOSIS. Plague can be diagnosed by isolating *Y. pestis* from blood, from an aspirate of a bubo, or from sputum. A presumptive diagnosis can be made in the appropriate clinical setting by demonstrating (by Gram stain or fluorescent antibody) characteristic organisms in sputum or in an aspirate of the bubo. In the absence of culture results, infection can be diagnosed by serology.

TREATMENT AND PROGNOSIS. In the absence of therapy, plague has an estimated mortality of >50%; untreated primary septicemic or pneumonic plague is invariably fatal. Fatality rates of up to 22% continue to be reported in the United States, owing primar-

ily to delays in initiation of appropriate therapy. Because of this, therapy should be started immediately if the diagnosis of plague is suspected.

Streptomycin was the first drug to be shown to have activity against plague, and, in the absence of controlled trials with other agents, it remains the drug of choice. Chloramphenicol and tetracycline are thought to be acceptable alternative therapies. Other aminoglycosides, trimethoprim/sulfamethoxazole, and the fluoroquinolones may be effective, but data on which to base a recommendation for their use are limited. Penicillin and first-generation cephalosporins are not effective, are associated with a high mortality, and should not be used. Aggressive supportive care is essential for patients in shock or with disseminated intravascular coagulation.

PREVENTION. All suspected plague cases should be reported immediately to local health authorities. Patients with bubonic plague (with no cough and a normal chest radiograph) should be placed on drainage/secretion precautions; if any evidence of pneumonic involvement is present, patients should be placed in strict isolation with precautions against airborne spread of the organism. Isolation should be maintained for a minimum of 3 days after starting appropriate antimicrobial therapy. Clinical samples must be carefully handled to minimize the risk of skin contact or aerosolization of the organism. Close contacts of suspected or confirmed plague pneumonia cases (including medical personnel) should be provided with chemoprophylaxis with tetracycline or sulfonamides.

Persons living in endemic areas should be advised to protect themselves against rodents and fleas; this includes measures designed to reduce rodent populations near homes, and applying insecticides, as necessary, to control flea populations. A formalin-killed vaccine, plague vaccine, is commercially available. Its use is recommended for persons traveling to epidemic areas, for individuals who must live and work in close contact with wild rodents, and for laboratory workers who must handle *Y. pestis* cultures.

Crook LD, Tempest B: Plague: A clinical review of 27 cases. Arch Intern Med 152:1253, 1992. *A description of 27 plague cases seen at the Gallup, New Mexico, Indian Medical Center between 1965 and 1989; 19 patients had bubonic plague and 8 septicemic plague.*

Gayraud M, Scavizzi MR, Mollaret HH, et al.: Antibiotic treatment of *Yersinia enterocolitica* septicemia. Clin Infect Dis 17:405, 1993. *A comprehensive, albeit retrospective, review of the management of* Y. enterocolitica *sepsis.*

Tacket CO, Narain JP, Sattin R, et al.: A multistate outbreak of infections caused by *Yersinia enterocolitica* transmitted by pasteurized milk. JAMA 251:483, 1984. *A description of clinical and epidemiologic features of* Y. enterocolitica *infection in one of the largest outbreaks reported to date.*

301 TULAREMIA
Richard B. Hornick

DEFINITION. Tularemia is a rare infectious disease caused by a small gram-negative pleomorphic rod, *Francisella tularensis*. This organism is acquired from an animal reservoir, frequently cottontail rabbits, by direct contact with diseased animal tissues, the bite of an infected tick or deer fly, ingestion of contaminated food or water, and inhalation of aerosolized bacteria. Clinical manifestations usually include a cutaneous ulcer with enlargement of regional lymph nodes. Rarely, a pneumonitis results from inhalation of *F. tularensis* or secondary spread from the skin ulcer and lymph nodes. Confirmation of the diagnosis by cultural technique is not advocated because of the high contagion risk to personnel handling this organism. The therapeutic response to effective antibiotic therapy is rapid.

The typhoidal form of tularemia was first described in Japan in 1818. A clear description of the organism occurred in 1906 when McCoy uncovered a "plaguelike" disease among ground squirrels in Tulare County, California. In Japan, tularemia may be referred to as Ohara's disease or Yato-byo (wild hare disease).

F. tularensis is a small gram-negative pleomorphic rod-shaped bacterium. Organisms are not seen in smears of infected tissue unless special staining techniques are used. Fluorescent antibody conjugate staining and modified Dieterle staining are the best methods. All tularemia strains are serologically identical, but there are biochemical and virulence differences for mammals that have allowed differentiation of two strains. These are called Jellison A and B; the former, found only in North America, is lethal for domestic rabbits *(Oryctolagus)* and causes severe disease in humans. The unique biochemical capabilities of this strain—e.g., it ferments glycerol and contains citrulline ureidase—do not explain its increased virulence. Strain B lacks these biochemical features, is not lethal for cottontails, causes milder disease in humans, usually is isolated from rodents or from water, and is distributed over Europe, Asia, and North America. Reasons for the differences in virulence are unknown.

Culture Methods. The direct isolation of *F. tularensis* from blood (rarely), pus from ulcers or buboes, sputum, or pharyngeal or gastric aspirations in a patient with pneumonitis can be achieved by two methods. This is a class 4 organism requiring an effective hood or an adequate isolation laboratory to prevent human disease or epizootics. The two methods for isolation are intraperitoneal inoculation of guinea pigs and direct plating of a specimen onto glucose cysteine blood agar, cystine heart agar, or eugon agar. As few as one to five viable organisms will cause the death of guinea pigs in 5 to 10 days. Appropriate facilities are needed to prevent spread of the disease to other animals. The media used to isolate the organism usually contain drugs to suppress other flora and allow the tularemia colonies to be visible. Useful additions are 0.1 mg of cycloheximide and 20 units of penicillin per milliliter of media. The colonies are small on these media; they appear in 48 to 72 hours of incubation at 37° C.

Serologic Diagnosis. The measurement of serum agglutinating antibodies is a useful and safer method of diagnosing tularemia. Titers begin to rise in about 7 to 10 days and peak in 3 to 4 weeks. Paired serum specimens obtained 2 weeks apart and demonstrating a fourfold or greater rise are diagnostic of tularemia. However, a single specimen with a titer of 1:160 or greater in a patient thought to have tularemia on clinical grounds is diagnostic. Antibiotic therapy does not appear to dampen the antibody response. Titers remain elevated for 6 to 8 months and then decline in the subsequent 1 to 1.5 years to low or undetectable levels. There is a cross-reaction with brucella antigen during the early phase of the antibody response. The brucella titer falls off faster than and is never so high as the tularemia titer (see Ch. 308).

Skin Testing. A skin test antigen has proved to be reliable for diagnostic and epidemiologic purposes. A positive test result, similar in appearance to a tuberculin test response, is present during the first week of illness, frequently before the agglutinins are detectable, and remains positive for years. There is no known cross-reacting skin test antigen. The antigen is derived from *F. tularensis* by ether extraction; however, it is not commonly available. It can be obtained from the Centers for Disease Control and Prevention, Atlanta. In 10% of patients, the skin test antigen may boost pre-existing agglutinating antibody titers. Skin test reactivity can be shown to be associated with sensitized lymphocytes.

Epidemiology. Tularemia is a sporadic disease; humans acquire it when bitten by an infected tick or deer fly or when handling an infected animal. In the process of dressing a rabbit or skinning a muskrat, the hands may become contaminated with infected blood, subcutaneous abscesses, or liver and spleen that contain millions of organisms. The act of eviscerating the animal can create an aerosol that can be inhaled. Contaminated water or food is the least likely method of acquiring tularemia. Many carnivores such as dogs, cats, bull snakes, and others may feed on diseased rabbits, resulting in contamination of the teeth and saliva. These animals are relatively resistant to tularemia. Contact with the teeth of a pet dog or cat has resulted in ulceroglandular tularemia. Studies in volunteers have quantified the susceptibility of humans to infection and disease and the virulence of *F. tularensis* for humans. As few as 50 type A organisms injected subcutaneously cause ulceroglandular disease. Pneumonic tularemia can be induced by a similar inoculum size if the aerosolized and inhaled particles are small ($< 5 \mu m$). Type B organisms require an inoculum about 1000 times larger to induce ulceroglandular or respiratory disease in humans.

The incidence of tularemia is low, 150 to 300 cases a year having been reported in each of the past 20 years. The peak incidence was in 1939, when almost 2300 cases were reported. Laws passed at that time prohibited the sale of wild rabbits, especially cottontails, and this legislation plus increased public awareness of the danger of handling sick or dying wild animals has contributed to the decline. Most cases occur in the Midwest, but the disease is not restricted to any one geographic location in the United States. Cottontail rabbits in urban and suburban areas provide the reservoir from which tularemia can occur. Epizootics among these or other animals can cause epidemics in humans. Tularemia has been reported only north of the 30th parallel. The cottontail is not found in Europe; various rodents such as voles, muskrats, and hares carry *F. tularensis* (Jellison B type) in that part of the world. Diseased jackrabbits, found west of the Mississippi River, may be an important source of contamination of ticks and deer flies.

In the summer months, most cases of tularemia are caused by tick or deer fly bites. Ulceroglandular disease begins with an ulcer at the site of the bite, e.g., groin, axilla, or scalp. In the fall during hunting season, sporadic cases, usually ulceroglandular, occur among hunters and trappers. In Scandinavia, epidemics have occurred in winter when farmers handling stored hay contaminated by diseased voles inhaled *F. tularensis* and developed pneumonic tularemia.

MECHANISMS OF INFECTION AND PATHOLOGY. The most common form of tularemia results from *F. tularensis* penetrating the skin. This penetration may be through hair follicles or minute areas of trauma. Subsequent disease develops in 2 to 6 days, depending on the number of bacteria and their virulence. The organisms multiply in the dermis and induce a marked inflammatory process consisting primarily of mononuclear cells with a perivascular distribution. This process produces an erythematous tender papule. The inflamed area continues to swell until the induced ischemia causes the skin to ulcerate. The base of the ulcer becomes black and depressed and the edges sharply demarcated. At the time of penetration, some organisms may be phagocytized and transported in the lymph to regional nodes. There is no clinically apparent lymphangitis. The nodes enlarge and become painful when caseation occurs. Histologic sections reveal geographic necrosis and disruption of the capsule. Fluctuation of the node is a late and rare event. It may then rupture. The necrotic, purulent, painful lymph node is termed a bubo. Healing of a bubo takes months even with appropriate antibiotic treatment. Aspiration of an unruptured node may lead to an indolent draining sinus tract. *F. tularensis* may remain in the necrotic tissue and purulent drainage for many weeks. The ulcer heals slowly and usually leaves a depigmented, rounded area in the skin.

Oculoglandular tularemia may occur when the conjunctival sac is infected from an ulcer or contaminated finger. Small yellowish granulomatous lesions develop on the palpebral conjunctivae, accompanied by enlargement of the preauricular lymph nodes. In untreated patients the cornea may perforate.

Inhaled small particle aerosols ($< 5 \mu m$ in diameter) containing *F. tularensis* (usually type A) are ultimately deposited in the terminal bronchioles and alveoli, although infection of the trachea and large bronchi also occurs. A peribronchial inflammation develops, with infiltration by neutrophils and mononuclear cells. This produces necrosis of alveolar walls and results in localized pneumonitis. In humans, small areas of pneumonitis represent the most common findings on chest roentgenograms. Often these are ill defined and difficult to interpret. Lobar consolidation or lung abscesses, infrequent in humans, represent extensive spread and necrosis. Mediastinal and peritracheal lymph nodes enlarge and may be apparent on chest films. They may be partially responsible, along with the bronchitis, for the substernal burning common with tularemic pneumonia. The incubation period for this form of tularemia varies inversely with the size and virulence of the inhaled inoculum. Following an inoculum of 10 to 50 organisms, disease appears in about 4 to 7 days in volunteers.

Typhoidal tularemia follows systemic spread of *F. tularensis* from the oropharynx and probably the gastrointestinal tract when a huge inoculum is swallowed. Enlargement of cervical lymph nodes, and presumably nodes in the mesentery, occurs. This latter process causes abdominal pain and is associated with an ileus. This is the most unusual form of tularemia in this country.

CLINICAL MANIFESTATIONS. Disease initiated by a tick bite is manifested by an ulcer at the site or adjacent to it. The tick defecates after feeding, and the infected feces may be scratched into the epidermis. Usually the lesion is in the inguinal, axillary, or scalp skin. If contact with tularemia organisms results from handling an infected animal, an ulcerative lesion evolves in the skin of the hands, frequently around a fingernail. This lesion may be so trivial that it is ignored by the patient. The ulcer is depressed into the dermis, has sharply demarcated edges, and gradually develops a black base. Initially, the lesion produces a thick, yellowish exudate. Regional lymph nodes enlarge and are tender to palpation. Fever and chills are common. The temperature curve is usually remittent or continuous in character. Without antibiotic therapy, most patients remain febrile for several weeks, the ulcer heals slowly over weeks to months, and the enlarged lymph nodes persist for months. Untreated patients may occasionally develop a secondary necrotizing pneumonia as a consequence of bacteremia, causing acute illness.

Primary tularemia pneumonia involves the sudden development of substernal burning and a nonproductive paroxysmal cough associated with fever and chills. Headache, myalgia, photophobia, malaise, and prostration are common. The temperature elevates quickly to 39.4 to 40°C and remains at that level (continuous fever curve) until antibiotic treatment is given. Sixty to 70% of patients survive without specific therapy, and in these a slow defervescence occurs over several months. Radiographs of the lungs may reveal ill-defined, scattered oval areas of infiltration, with enlarged peritracheal lymph nodes. Pleural effusions, lobar consolidation, and lung abscess are other manifestations of this form of tularemia. Cervical lymph nodes are palpable and tender.

DIAGNOSIS AND DIFFERENTIAL DIAGNOSIS. The diagnosis of ulceroglandular tularemia is made on the basis of the clinical manifestations and serologic studies. Paired serum specimens collected over a 2- to 3-week period are required to demonstrate a fourfold rise in titer. A baseline agglutinin titer of 1:160 in a patient with a history of an indolent ulcer for 2 or more weeks is diagnostic of tularemia. Culture of an ulcer and blood should be performed only if the hospital laboratory has appropriate protective isolation hoods. Patients with sporotrichosis or *Mycobacterium marinum* infections may have ulcers suggestive of tularemia but are usually afebrile. Enlarged lymph nodes extending centripetally as a beaded chain are a characteristic finding in sporotrichosis. Lesions of the fingers infected with staphylococci or β streptococci usually produce more pus and may be associated with lymphangitis. *Bacillus anthracis* can produce an ulcer (anthrax) with black-based, sharply demarcated edges similar to that initiated by *F. tularensis*. A careful history and serologic data help in the differential diagnosis. In patients in whom any form of tularemia is suspected, the skin test antigen is helpful. The test result is usually positive before agglutinating antibodies develop.

Tularemia pneumonia must be differentiated from the more common bacterial, viral, and mycoplasmal pneumonias. The history and the presence of ulceroglandular disease are helpful. Skin testing and serologic studies are diagnostic. The chest radiographs may yield suggestive findings consisting of ill-defined, small, oval, multiple infiltrates but is not diagnostic.

Patients infected with *F. tularensis* usually have a normal leukocyte count with an elevated sedimentation rate. The white count is elevated when a bubo or a lung abscess is present.

COMPLICATIONS. Pericarditis and meningitis are rare events that usually occur in patients who have been misdiagnosed and have received inappropriate treatment. Pericarditis results from direct extension of the infection from the purulent, necroic mediastinal lymph nodes or the involved lung. Constrictive pericarditis has been reported. Meningitis develops rarely, represents a seeding of the meninges during bacteremia, and is characterized by a lymphocytic pleocytosis in the cerebrospinal fluid.

TREATMENT. Patients with all forms of tularemia respond to the antibiotics streptomycin, gentamicin, tetracycline, and chloramphenicol. The aminoglycoside antibiotics are recommended; they produce a prompt cure of patients with the most severe form of tularemia. Patients with pneumonitis are afebrile within 24 to 48 hours and do not relapse. Ulcers and tender lymph nodes heal in 7

to 10 days. Gentamicin, 5 mg per kilogram per day in divided doses, is given for 10 days. Streptomycin was the principal drug for treating tularemia before gentamicin; 1 gram is given every 12 hours for 10 days. Treatment with tetracycline or chloramphenicol may produce an equally rapid response, but relapses occur in 15 to 20% of the patients. These drugs are not recommended unless gentamicin and streptomycin are contraindicated. Doses of 3 to 4 grams of tetracycline or 3 grams of chloramphenicol daily for 10 days can be used. Naturally acquired resistance to any of these antibiotics has not been found. Ceftriaxone has excellent *in vitro* inhibitory activity but in one study failed to cure eight pediatric patients. *In vitro* studies also indicate the potential antibacterial effect of the quinolones. However, no systematic *in vivo* testing has been reported.

Patients with ulceroglandular tularemia respond well to these antibiotics. Fluctuant lymph nodes should not be aspirated until the patient has finished the course of the antibiotic treatment. Isolation of patients with any form of tularemia is not required; there is no evidence of person-to-person spread.

PROGNOSIS. The mortality for untreated ulceroglandular disease is about 5%. Patients infected with type B strains and untreated probably have a mortality <1%. Many cases probably go undiagnosed, as the disease is mild and self-limiting. Treatment with antibiotics prevents death and promotes healing in a week to 10 days.

The mortality for pneumonic tularemia in the preantibiotic period was 30 to 40%. Treatment with streptomycin or tetracycline has lowered this figure to <1%. Healing occurs without residual lung damage or deficits in pulmonary function.

PREVENTION. Patients who recover from tularemia have a high degree of resistance to reinfection. If *F. tularensis* is reintroduced into the skin, a positive skin test reaction ensues without ulceration. Resistance to pulmonary disease may be associated with sensitized lymphocytes and alveolar macrophages.

A live attenuated strain of *F. tularensis* has been prepared as a vaccine. This can be administered by the acupuncture route, and it produces excellent immunity. The vaccine can be obtained from the Commander, U.S. Army Medical Research Institute of Infectious Diseases, Frederick, Maryland 21701. Its use is limited to persons considered at high risk, such as selected laboratory workers, forest rangers, game wardens, and perhaps others known to be exposed during an outbreak. The vaccine works by stimulating cellular immune mechanisms. Circulating agglutinins are not associated with resistance to disease.

Capellan J, Fong IW: Tularemia from a cat bite: Case report and review of feline-associated tularemia. Clin Infect Dis 16:472, 1993. *Summarizes literature reports of patients acquiring tularemia from cats. Offers advice on management of cat bite wounds not healing with penicillin therapy.*
Enderlin G, Morales L, Jacobs RF, Cross JT: Streptomycin and alternative agents for the treatment of tularemia: Review of the literature. Clin Infect Dis 19:42, 1994. *Compares in vitro with in vivo results. A good guide to current therapy.*
Evans ME, Gregory DW, Schaffner W, et al.: Tularemia: A 30-year experience with 88 cases. Medicine 64:251, 1985. *An excellent summary of the clinical presentations of F. tularensis disease.*
Penn RL, Kinasewitz GT: Factors associated with a poor outcome in tularemia. Arch Intern Med 147:265, 1987. *A retrospective study of the factors leading to poor outcomes. One significant factor was delay in diagnosis and treatment.*
Scofield RH, Lopez EJ, McNabb SJ: Tularemia pneumonia in Oklahoma, 1982–1987. J Okla St Med Assoc 85:165, 1992. *Discusses factors influencing failure to diagnose pneumonic tularemia. This form is difficult to diagnose because of few distinguishing features.*

302 ANTHRAX
Jonas A. Shulman

DEFINITION. Anthrax is a zoonotic disease caused by *Bacillus anthracis,* a large gram-positive, spore-forming bacillus transmitted to humans by contact with infected animals or contaminated animal products. Other names for anthrax include woolsorter's disease, Siberian ulcer, malignant pustule, charbon, malignant edema, and ragsorter's disease. In 1877, Koch described *B. anthracis* as one of the first microbes identified as a cause of a specific disease, thereby making anthrax the prototype for Koch's postulates and the first disease to satisfy them. Anthrax has all but disappeared from North America, Western Europe, and Australia since being nearly eradicated in livestock following extensive veterinary programs, including vaccination. The disease is still prevalent in many developing countries, however, especially Asia, Africa, and Central America, where livestock are only marginally subjected to veterinary control and where environmental conditions are favorable for an animal-to-soil-to-animal cycle.

Anthrax occurs primarily in herbivorous animals, especially cattle, goats, and sheep, but many other animals, including pigs, buffalo, and elephants, have also been infected with the disease. Cattle are particularly susceptible to the systemic form of anthrax, which clinically progresses to death in 24 to 48 hours. The large numbers of organisms found in infected cattle may contaminate not only the animal but also its products and environs, thereby allowing infection to occur in animals more resistant to anthrax, such as humans.

The primary forms of anthrax in humans are cutaneous, inhalation, gastrointestinal, and oropharyngeal. Septicemia and meningitis may occur from any of these primary foci. By far the most common form of the disease in the United States is the cutaneous lesion, which accounts for >95% of clinical cases. Inhalation anthrax has occurred only rarely in the United States in the past 25 years, and gastrointestinal anthrax has never been reported in this country.

ETIOLOGY. *B. anthracis* is a large gram-positive, nonmotile, spore-forming bacillus (1 to 1.3 × 3 to 8 μm). Although spores of *B. anthracis* do not form in living tissue, they are induced by aerobic conditions in the external environment and may persist for years in the soil, in animal products, or in an appropriate industrial setting. The organism grows well aerobically on ordinary laboratory media at 35° to 37° C. The colonies produced are especially sticky (positive tenacity test, positive string of pearls test) and have a tendency to stand up in stalagmite fashion when lifted with a bacteriologic loop. The colonies are nonhemolytic, rough, and flat, with many comma-shaped outgrowths on blood agar. Microscopic examination of organisms growing on artificial media shows long, parallel chains of organisms frequently described as having a rather characteristic "boxcar" appearance. Spores are oval and occur either centrally or paracentrally but cause no swelling of the bacillus. Material from fresh lesions contains single or short chains of two or three bacilli, which may appear encapsulated, the ends of which are slightly rounded.

Anthrax organisms can be differentiated from the saprophytic *Bacillus* species by fluorescent antibody staining, lysis with a specific γ bacteriophage, and virulence for mice, guinea pigs, and rabbits. Parenteral inoculation into these species results in death in 1 to 3 days.

INCIDENCE AND PREVALENCE. *B. anthracis* is a soil organism that has worldwide distribution. Animal anthrax is endemic in some areas of Asia, Africa, and Latin America, especially in rural regions that have inadequate animal vaccination programs and poor animal husbandry. These areas are more likely to have a number of human cases as well. Certain areas within the United States and other parts of the world may provide a particularly favorable environment for large numbers of resistant spores to survive in the soil for many years. In fact, a number of epizootics related to focal regions of heavily contaminated soil have occurred.

Since no reliable reporting of anthrax exists, and in many instances the diagnosis may never be made, the actual worldwide incidence of anthrax is not known. Estimates in the past have ranged between 20,000 and 100,000 human cases per year, but these figures have more recently been estimated at 2000 to 20,000 cases per annum. In the United States, approximately one case of human anthrax per year was reported between 1970 and 1985, but only three cases have been documented since 1984. Reports of human anthrax have been especially frequent in Turkey, Pakistan, Iran, Haiti, and several Asian and African countries. There are probably many parts of the world with significant endemic problems but from which data are not available.

The potential for large outbreaks in animals and humans continues to exist, especially when economic or political upheaval is present. One of the largest epidemics of anthrax was reported in Zimbabwe between 1978 and 1980, when nearly 10,000 human cases of cutaneous anthrax and a few cases of gastrointestinal anthrax occurred, resulting in approximately 100 deaths. This outbreak was related to an extensive epizootic infection in cattle. Another major outbreak of anthrax occurred in Siberia in 1979. It was initially

thought by some to be related to inhalation, but more recently the route of infection has been identified as the ingestion and handling of infected "black market" meat. The source of anthrax in the cattle in this epidemic appeared to be a single 29-ton lot of bone meal used as animal feed that likely was made from the bones of animals that had died of anthrax the previous year.

Very rare cases of inhalation anthrax have developed in workers exposed to aerosolized anthrax spores generated during the processing of contaminated materials such as woolens, hides, or bone meal, and even more rarely in people who have simply been in the vicinity of a wool-processing mill or tannery but who were not directly involved in the processing of the product. Cases have even been reported in home weavers, such as those using contaminated goat yarn, or in individuals working with contaminated bone meal fertilizer.

In the United States, the average annual occurrence has diminished. From 1977 to 1988, the number of cases was only 0.8, as opposed to 127 cases reported to occur annually between 1916 and 1925. The case fatality rate of the 221 U.S. cases of cutaneous anthrax from 1955 to 1986 was approximately 5.0% (11 of 221), whereas the case fatality rate was 82% in the patients with inhalation anthrax (9 of 11). The overall mortality rate in these 232 American cases of anthrax was 8.6%.

EPIDEMIOLOGY. Cases of anthrax are classified generally as either agricultural or industrial. Most of the agricultural cases of human anthrax result from direct contact with contaminated discharges from infected animals. Occasional human cases have been transmitted by bites of flies that have fed on the carcasses of animals dead of anthrax. Others have been caused by ingestion of poorly cooked or raw infected meat. Industrial cases usually result from contact with anthrax spores contaminating animal products, such as goat hair, wool, hides, and skin, and animal bones, especially those imported from areas of high endemicity. Transmission usually occurs during the processing of these animal products, either by direct contact with the contaminated raw material or by indirect contact with a contaminated environment; rarely, transmission may occur via airborne particles produced during the manufacturing process. Because the *B. anthracis* spores can survive for long periods, a wide variety of unusual products have been associated with human infection, such as imported bongo drums made with goat skins, shaving brushes, various leather or woolen blankets, and ivory piano keys. Laboratory-acquired infections have been reported; however, human-to-human transmission of anthrax is not thought to occur.

Most cases of anthrax in the United States are sporadic, but occasional epidemics have been reported. In 1957, the largest and most serious of these occurred in New Hampshire, where nine employees of a textile mill acquired anthrax while processing a batch of contaminated goat hair imported from Asia. This outbreak included four cutaneous cases and five inhalation cases, with four fatalities reported in the latter group.

PATHOGENESIS. The virulence of *B. anthracis* is determined by both a plasmid-mediated group of exotoxins (plasmid pX01), and another plasmid-mediated antiphagocytic polydiglutamic acid capsule (plasmid pX02). Three toxic proteins (exotoxins) have been identified and cloned, including a protective antigen (PA), an edema factor (EF), and a lethal factor (LF). A combination of two of these proteins (PA and EF) has been demonstrated to decrease polymorphonuclear neutrophil function, suggesting that this is one of the ways that host susceptibility to infection with *B. anthracis* may be increased.

Furthermore, a combination of PA and EF causes local edema, whereas the combination of PA and LF may cause death in as little as 60 minutes. None of these three toxins, when administered alone, has any biologic effect in experimental animals. Protective antigen is able to bind to cell-surface receptors, in turn enabling them to be used by both EF and LF to reach the cytoplasm. Recently, EF has been found to be related to its ability to increase cyclic AMP. EF, in fact, is a calmodulin-dependent adenylate cyclase, and it is likely that the edema is produced through this mechanism.

As noted, virulent strains of *B. anthracis* contain two large plasmids, pX01 and pX02, both of which are necessary for virulence. Strains that contain only one of these plasmids are totally avirulent.

In cutaneous anthrax, the organism is introduced either through a wound or by means of infected animal fibers that disrupt the skin.

The organism is not known to penetrate intact skin. Once in the subcutaneous tissue, the anthrax spore is thought to germinate, multiply, and produce both its exotoxin and the antiphagocytic capsular material. The toxins are capable of provoking a marked edematous response and tissue necrosis with a paucity of neutrophil invasion. Phagocytosis of the organisms by local macrophages occurs, and these bacilli are then spread to regional lymph nodes, where further production of toxins produces a hemorrhagic, necrotic, and edematous lymphadenitis. Bacilli may enter the circulation, at times producing meningitis, pneumonia, and systemic toxicity.

Inhalation anthrax is fortunately a very uncommon clinical presentation of anthrax, as it is associated with close to 100% mortality. In the United States, inhalation anthrax is now essentially obsolete, with only two cases reported during the past 25 years; however, this is still a cause of significant disease in many parts of the world. Inhalation anthrax, commonly known as woolsorter's disease, occurs not as a result of direct contact with infected animals but rather by inhalation of an aerosol of spores in particle sizes < 5 μm. These aerosols usually occur during processing of contaminated material. In humans, spores are inhaled, reach the alveoli, and may then eventually be phagocytized by macrophages and carried by these cells to the mediastinal lymph nodes. Germination, growth, and toxin formation at this site can produce severe, massive hemorrhagic lymphadenitis and mediastinitis. B. anthracis may also directly affect the pulmonary capillary endothelium, causing thrombosis and respiratory failure. Pleural effusion is common. Anthrax is not thought to cause primary pneumonia, but secondary bacterial pneumonia may complicate inhalation anthrax. B. anthracis may also enter the bloodstream from this site, with the evolution of intense bacteremia. The number of organisms per milliliter of blood may be so great that in some instances the organism may be seen on smears of the peripheral blood. Hemorrhagic meningitis may ensue. Respiratory failure, shock, and pulmonary edema are frequent causes of death.

Ingestion of markedly contaminated, poorly cooked meat may result in either the oropharyngeal or the gastrointestinal form of infection. When oropharyngeal anthrax occurs, there is localized swelling of the pharynx, sometimes causing tracheal obstruction, and marked cervical adenopathy with overlying brawny edema. Similarly, the organism may reach the small and large intestines and cause a gastrointestinal syndrome. In this case, the spores that are deposited in the submucosa of the intestinal tract may germinate, multiply, and produce toxin, again resulting in marked edema, hemorrhage, and necrosis. Regional mesenteric lymphadenopathy is common, and findings associated with the syndrome include fever, vomiting, abdominal pain and distention, massive bloody diarrhea, mesenteric adenitis, hemorrhagic ascites, and septicemia. Gastrointestinal anthrax is a very severe form of the disease, has a high mortality rate (25 to 75%), and is rarely diagnosed during life except in the setting of an epidemic.

It is important to note that although antimicrobial agents may rapidly eradicate the organism, the persistence of the toxin that has been produced may result in continued development of the disease process until the toxin is metabolized. Thus, although the mortality rate may be diminished by appropriate antibiotic therapy, especially in the cutaneous form of the disease, the clinical process may continue to progress even after the institution of antimicrobial therapy. Antitoxins have been tried by some in the past, but such antitoxins are not currently available.

CLINICAL MANIFESTATIONS. Cutaneous anthrax is the most common form of the disease in humans, accounting for >95% of cases. After an incubation period of 1 to 5 days, the infection generally begins with a small, somewhat pruritic papule at the site of an abrasion, which over the next several days develops into a vesicle containing serosanguineous fluid teeming with organisms. The lesion generally occurs on the upper extremities, especially the arms and hands, or on the face, neck, or other areas that are likely to be exposed to the contaminated animal product or infected soil. As the lesion progresses, ulceration occurs, with formation of a necrotic ulcer base frequently surrounded by smaller vesicles. The characteristic black eschar evolves over several weeks to a size of several centimeters, gradually separating and leaving a scar. This black eschar accounts for the name anthrax, which comes

from the Greek word for coal. The edema is frequently nonpitting, gelatinous, and brawny and is very striking. It may be quite extensive, spreading over a wide area in severe cases. With involvement near the eye, periorbital swelling may be especially intense. The edema may be so dramatic that hypotension occurs in part because of the loss of intravascular volume as fluid enters the subcutaneous tissues. This edema, in combination with the vesicle progressing to the necrotic black eschar, forms the lesion that is highly characteristic of anthrax. Despite the dramatic appearance of the lesion, it is frequently painless.

In association with the localized cutaneous lesion, most patients have minimal constitutional findings, such as fever, malaise, myalgias, and headaches. In those with extensive edema, the systemic symptoms may be more severe. Localized lymphadenopathy may occur at times and may be complicated by bacteremia and even meningitis. Death is rare if appropriate antimicrobial therapy is instituted; in untreated cases of cutaneous anthrax, however, the mortality rate remains about 25%.

Bacterial adenitis due to staphylococci and streptococci, tularemia, plague, orf, cat scratch disease, localized herpes, and ecthyma gangrenosum are diagnostic considerations, and lesions seen in these diseases may be confused with those of anthrax. The diagnosis of cutaneous anthrax will rarely be missed if the disease is considered in any patient who has had exposure to an appropriate animal or animal product and who develops a painless ulcer surrounded by small vesicles, along with marked edema and eschar formation. Gram stains of the vesicular fluid and lesion usually readily demonstrate the characteristic gram-positive bacilli, as the organisms are present in large numbers in these lesions and are readily isolated by culture. Informing the bacteriology laboratory of the possibility of the diagnosis of anthrax is important to prevent the organism from being discarded as merely a probable contaminant of Bacillus species, which is frequently not fully characterized. At times, secondary bacterial infection may occur in these ulcers. Rarely, more than one lesion may be present, resulting from co-primary infections.

Inhalation anthrax is very rare, usually fatal, and extremely difficult to diagnose. The incubation period in this syndrome is generally 1 to 6 days, and the illness is generally biphasic. Initially, a brief, nonspecific "influenza-like" illness occurs, manifested by high fever, fatigue, myalgias, malaise, a nonproductive cough, and at times some chest discomfort. Few physical findings are noted at this time; however, within several days after a short period of clinical improvement, the patient becomes much more ill. This second phase is manifested by severe dyspnea, cyanosis, hypoxia, hemoptysis, stridor, chest pain, and diaphoresis. Physical examination may reveal some crepitant rales and evidence of pleural effusions. Some subcutaneous brawny edema of the chest wall and neck may be noted. The chest radiograph in these patients shows a rather distinctive clinical finding, namely, a widened mediastinum. Bacteremia, shock, and meningitis are frequently present, and death generally follows within 1 to 2 days of the onset of the respiratory distress. The mortality rate is 80 to 100%, even with appropriate therapy.

Inhalation anthrax should be considered in patients with appropriate exposure to an animal product, as in a weaver using imported goat hair or a textile mill worker. The most important clue is the presence of an appropriate epidemiologic history in a patient developing severe respiratory distress and a rapidly enlarging mediastinum.

Gastrointestinal anthrax is an extremely rare disease. It has an incubation period of 2 to 5 days, although there are some cases in which a more prolonged incubation period has been postulated. The diagnosis is rarely suspected before death except in areas where anthrax is highly endemic and in which multiple human cases are occurring. The symptoms include severe abdominal pain, hematemesis, melena, rapid onset of ascites, and at times, marked diarrhea. Paracentesis may reveal hemorrhagic ascites, and sometimes these cases may simulate "acute" or "surgical abdomen." The disease usually progresses to bacteremia, toxemia, shock, and eventually death in many patients. No cases of intestinal anthrax have been reported in the United States.

Oropharyngeal anthrax presents as severe sore throat with neck swelling, adenopathy, dysphagia, and at times tracheal compression and dyspnea. Cervical and submandibular lymphadenopathy is common. Again, bacteremia and its complications may ensue.

Meningitis may be a complication of any of the forms of anthrax and almost never is found without a primary focus of infection. It is frequently hemorrhagic and most often fatal.

DIAGNOSIS. The clinician who elicits a careful epidemiologic history and who has a high index of suspicion of anthrax will not have problems establishing the diagnosis in cutaneous anthrax and will even be alert to the rarer and more difficult to recognize cases of inhalation, gastrointestinal, or oropharyngeal anthrax.

Inhalation anthrax is rarely suspected before death and only if an epidemiologic history of aerosol exposure is obtained or if an epidemic is recognized. The major finding in the clinical evaluation, other than epidemiologic history, is the presence of a widened mediastinum or at times hemorrhagic pleural effusions or associated hemorrhagic meningitis. Ordinarily, Gram stains of sputum and cultures do not demonstrate *B. anthracis.* These patients frequently do develop bacteremia, however, and in these cases the organism can be readily isolated and sometimes seen on stains of the peripheral blood.

A number of serologic tests are available to diagnose anthrax retrospectively, but many of these very ill patients die so quickly that the initial serologic studies may not be especially helpful to the clinician. In some cases, however, serology has been a helpful diagnostic tool, especially when prior antibiotics have eradicated the bacteria before cultures or smears were obtained. Current serologic tests considered valuable include an enzyme-linked immunosorbent assay (ELISA), which detects antibodies to the capsular antigen, and an electrophoretic immunotransblot test, which detects antibodies to the PA exotoxin. Both of these serologic tests are quite sensitive and specific enough to be useful, but the test for antibody to the PA exotoxin may be more specific.

TREATMENT. Penicillin G is the drug of choice for treatment of anthrax. Only a few isolates of *B. anthracis* have been identified as resistant to penicillin G. In cutaneous anthrax, cultures of the infected blisters have become negative for the organism within 5 hours of the patient's receiving 2 million units of penicillin G. As previously mentioned, however, the presence of the toxin may persist, and the cutaneous lesion frequently goes through its various phases of evolution, even though the organism has been eradicated and the mortality rate reduced.

For cutaneous anthrax, intravenous penicillin G is given, 2 million units every 6 hours for several days, followed by a 7- to 10-day course of oral penicillin G. In patients with severe, overwhelming edema, corticosteroids have been thought by some to be helpful, although no controlled studies of their use have been performed. Severe neck swelling may require intubation or tracheostomy. In patients who are allergic to penicillin, effective alternatives include streptomycin, erythromycin, tetracycline, and chloramphenicol. No local surgery should be performed on these patients, because no pus requiring drainage is usually present and excision of the lesion has been reported to increase symptoms severity and organism spread. The lesion should be covered with a sterile dressing. No definite cases have been reported of spread of anthrax from human to human.

In inhalation, gastrointestinal, or oropharyngeal anthrax or in anthrax meningitis, high dosages of intravenous penicillin G, in the range of 24 million units per day, are recommended, along with excellent supportive care for the problems of hypotension and respiratory distress. Some physicians encourage parenteral streptomycin in a dosage of 1 to 2 grams per day to the penicillin G therapy in these cases. When the patient is hospitalized, good infection control practices are required. Soiled dressings must be incinerated or autoclaved.

PROGNOSIS. Inhalation anthrax is considered to be fatal in 80 to 100% of cases, and gastrointestinal anthrax has a case fatality rate of 25 to 75%. The case fatality rate for cutaneous anthrax is about 20 to 25% without treatment but generally is <1% with appropriate treatment.

PREVENTION. Control of anthrax in animals is essential to control of the disease in humans. All cases of anthrax—animal as well as human—should be reported to the state health department or the appropriate veterinary agency. Live avirulent animal vaccines are effective and may help control anthrax in endemic areas. Animals dead of anthrax should be cremated or buried, and care must be taken at autopsy to avoid additional environmental contamination by infected blood and tissues. Human anthrax can be partially prevented by proper disposal of the infected animals. In addition,

formaldehyde has been used successfully to decontaminate raw wool and hair. A cell-free filtrate vaccine has been shown to protect humans from anthrax and is available from the Michigan State Department of Health. This vaccine should be offered to workers likely to be exposed to contaminated animal products in high-risk industries. Newer vaccines are being evaluated, such as a PA toxoid vaccine and a PA-producing live vaccine. In the former Soviet Union, in addition to the chemical vaccine, a live anthrax spore vaccine has been widely used for prophylaxis against anthrax in both humans and animals.

Because none of the currently available vaccines is ideal, efforts at developing better agents are a major area of research. Among the newer approaches for anthrax vaccine development for human use are (1) combination of the PA with adjuvants derived from the BCG strain or killed cells of *Bordetella pertussis* and (2) PA cloned into a *Bacillus subtilis* as a recombinant vaccine that does not contain the *B. anthracis* genome.

Good personal hygiene, as well as the use of protective clothing and respirators when contaminated aerosols are likely to be encountered, may also prove to be helpful preventive measures. Gastrointestinal anthrax can be prevented by proper cooking of meat and by avoiding ingestion of potentially contaminated meat. Care must be taken by the laboratory personnel working with *B. anthracis,* since cases of anthrax have been acquired in this setting.

Farrar E: Anthrax: Virulence and vaccines. Ann Intern Med 121:379, 1994. *Excellent editorial outlining newer molecular biologic features of* B. anthracis *and the role of virulence factors in pathogenesis of the disease produced; also highlights new approaches to vaccine development.*
Harrison LH, Ezzell JW, Abshire TG, et al.: Evaluation of serologic tests for diagnosis of anthrax after an outbreak of cutaneous anthrax in Paraguay. J Infect Dis 160:706, 1989. *Serologic methods for diagnosis and detection of immunity.*
Ivins BE, Welkos SL: Recent advances in the development of an improved human anthrax vaccine. Eur J Epidemiol 4:12, 1988. *A approach to vaccines for anthrax.*
Ivins BE, Welkos SL, Little SF, et al.: Immunization against anthrax with *Bacillus anthracis* protective antigen combined with adjuvants. Infection Immunity 60:662, 1992. *Discusses the protective efficacy of immunization against anthrax with* B. anthracis *protective antigen combined with different adjuvants.*
Knudson GB: Treatment of anthrax in man: History and current concepts. Milit Med 151:71, 1986. *Reviews history of anthrax with emphasis on treatment.*
Shlyakov EN, Rubenstein E: Human live anthrax vaccine in the former USSR. Vaccine 12:727, 1994. *Describes the history of the development and use of the Soviet live spore human anthrax vaccine.*

303 DISEASES CAUSED BY PSEUDOMONADS
Stephen C. Schimpff

PSEUDOMONADS. Pseudomonads are gram-negative aerobic bacilli that prefer moist environments and are relatively noninvasive yet can cause serious and often fatal infection when the host defense mechanism is damaged or deficient. Each species is different in its pathogenic properties, each causes somewhat different types of infection, and each invades as a result of different host defense defects, but with each pseudomonad, the environmental source is usually water, moist soil, or a contaminated medical device, infusion, or injection.

Pseudomonads are divided into five major groups based on RNA homology (Table 303–1). Most human infections are caused by members of groups I, II, and V. For purposes of discussion, this chapter considers *Pseudomonas pseudomallei* (the cause of melioidosis), *Pseudomonas mallei* (the cause of glanders), *Pseudomonas aeruginosa* (which principally causes bacteremia, endocarditis, pneumonia, keratitis, and urinary tract infections), and *Pseudomonas cepacia, Pseudomonas pickettii,* and *Xanthomonas (Pseudomonas) maltophilia* (which cause bacteremia, pseudobacteremia, endocarditis, and urinary tract infections).

Pseudomonas pseudomallei. This organism causes melioidosis, often characterized as a glanders-like infectious disease. It was first described in Rangoon among debilitated morphine addicts. The term "melioidosis" means "a similarity to distemper of asses."

TABLE 303-1. CLASSIFICATION OF PSEUDOMONADS THAT HAVE BEEN ISOLATED FROM CLINICAL SPECIMENS

Group/Subgroup	Genus and Species
RNA group I	
Fluorescent group	P. aeruginosa
	P. fluorescens
	P. putida
Nonfluorescent group	P. stutzeri
	P. alcaligenes
	P. pseudoalcaligenes
RNA group II	P. mallei
	P. pseudomallei
	P. cepacia
	P. pickettii
RNA group III	P. acidovorans
	P. testosteroni
RNA group IV	P. diminuta
	P. vesicularis
RNA group V	Xanthomonas maltophilia

From Sanford JP: *Pseudomonas* species (including melioidosis and glanders). *In* Mandell GL, Douglas RG Jr, Bennett JE (eds.): Principles and Practice of Infectious Diseases, 3rd ed. New York, Churchill Livingstone, 1990, pp 1692–1696.

Despite the clinical resemblance to glanders, it has a totally different epidemiology. Melioidosis occurs in animals and humans in endemic areas of southeast Asia and northern Australia and has now been recognized to occur in epidemic-like form in specific areas, given the combination of the environment (an appropriate rainy season with water-covered rice paddies) and a susceptible host (abraded skin in barefoot farmers who have a high prevalence of diabetes mellitis, renal disease, or both).

P. pseudomallei is a gram-negative, motile, aerobic bacillus that is small and may grow in filamentous chains. Staining with methylene blue or Wright's stain shows a bipolar "safety pin" pattern. *P. pseudomallei* has a characteristic wrinkling appearance of the colonies on agar if held long enough. The organism, like most pseudomonads, can be isolated from soil and water and particularly streams, rice paddies, and ponds of the endemic areas and on plants, including commonly consumed vegetables. Most human infection probably occurs through skin abrasions. However, laboratory animals have been found to become infected by the respiratory route, so inhalation may be a possible human route of acquisition, which would explain the occurrence of primary pneumonia.

At the conclusion of United States involvement in the Vietnam war, 343 cases were reported, with 36 deaths; however, serologic surveys suggest that either mild or inapparent infection may be fairly common, with positive serologies found in 1 to 2% of healthy, nonwounded Army troops returning to the United States. This would suggest that as many as 225,000 military personnel may have had subclinical infection with *P. pseudomallei*. The importance of this observation is that recrudescence of disease has been observed many years after primary infection.

In addition to inapparent infection or asymptomatic pulmonary infection, the frequently observed forms of melioidosis are an acute, localized, suppurative soft tissue infection, an acute pulmonary infection, and an acute septicemic presentation. The localized infections are probably related to skin abrasion, with development of a nodule with secondary lymphangitis and regional lymphadenitis. An apparent primary pulmonary infection ranges from bronchitis to necrotizing pneumonia. The patient with pneumonia usually has high fever and signs and symptoms of consolidation, ordinarily in an upper lobe. It is an acute pyogenic process, frequently leading to early cavitation and giving a pulmonary appearance consistent with tuberculosis. Progression to bacteremia is rare.

Patients with the acute septic form characteristically present with a short history of fever and no clinical evidence of focal infection, although skin abrasion is the presumed site of origin. Most are profoundly ill, with signs of sepsis, such as tachypnea or Kussmaul's breathing, and occasional evidence of septic shock. Clinical and radiologic evidence frequently demonstrates progression to diffuse bilateral and patchy pulmonary infiltrate, which progresses to abscess

and cavity formation if the patient survives. Subcutaneous abscesses are relatively uncommon but can occur at multiple sites. Liver abscess, usually multiple, is not uncommon and is accompanied in more than 50% by multiple splenic abscesses, a combination unlikely for most other causes of liver abscess.

The diagnosis should be considered in any patient living in an endemic area who has a febrile illness and especially one occupationally at risk and, perhaps, at further risk of sepsis because of diabetes or renal disease. The diagnosis should be highly suspected in such an individual with a rapidly progressive, extensive pulmonary process if subcutaneous lesions are present or in one whose condition progresses to a cavitary form indistinguishable from tuberculosis. A Gram stain of pulmonary or abscess exudate shows small gram-negative bacilli, and methylene blue staining shows the characteristic bipolar "safety pin." The organism grows on standard media and is usually detected in blood cultures within 48 hours.

In northeast Thailand, a report from a hospital serving a population of nearly 2 million rural rice farming families determined that about 20% of all community-acquired bacteremias were caused by *P. pseudomallei* and that during the rainy season, when the paddy fields are under water (from June to September), *P. pseudomallei* was the single most common organism isolated from blood culture, representing nearly one half of all documented cases of community-acquired bacteremia in the month of August (Fig. 303–1). An interesting observation was the higher than expected frequency of both diabetes mellitus and renal calculi in patients with sepsis who are from this region, where both diabetes and calculi are common.

Treatment of pulmonary or suspected septic forms should probably begin with a combination of agents. The standard recommended treatment had been a combination of chloramphenicol, doxycycline, and trimethoprim-sulfamethoxazole. These agents, however, are bacteriostatic rather than bactericidal, do not represent a regimen one would wish to use for suspected community-acquired bacteremia, and are associated with a high mortality rate. The third-generation cephalosporin ceftazidime is now likely the drug of choice, with imipenem, piperacillin, or amoxicillin–clavulanic acid as reasonable alternatives. Adding an aminoglycoside during empirical therapy might be appropriate until culture results are known. Treatment apparently needs to be prolonged, including intravenous therapy (ceftazidime, imipenem, or piperacillin) for 2 to 4 weeks, followed by oral therapy (perhaps amoxicillin–clavulanic acid) for 6 months or longer to prevent recrudescence.

The prognosis for patients with localized disease should be excellent with appropriate therapy. However, those with the septicemic form are often gravely ill at the time of admission, and the mortal-

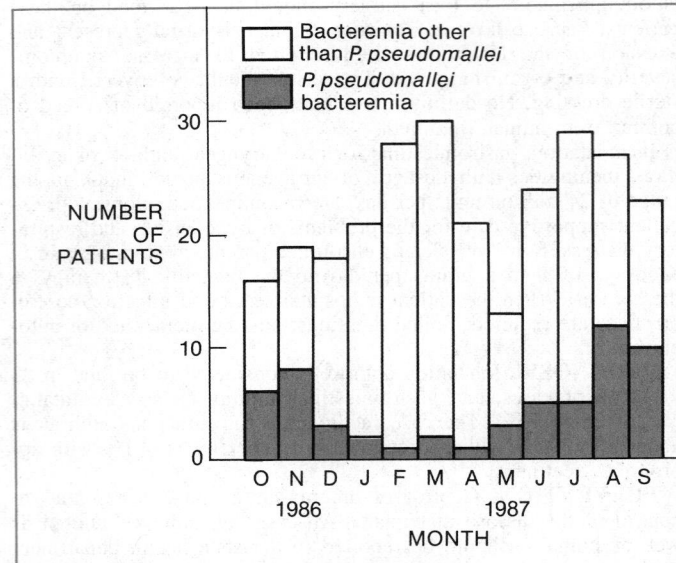

FIGURE 303-1. Number of persons with community-acquired bacteremia caused by *P. pseudomallei* and other organisms, in northeast Thailand from October 1986 to September 1987. (From Chaowagul W, White NJ, Dance DAB, et al.: Melioidosis: A major cause of community-acquired septicemia in northeastern Thailand. J Infect Dis 159:890, 1989; by permission of the University of Chicago Press, 1989.)

ity rate, even with current therapy, is about 40%. Patients with the highest mortality include those who are hypothermic, azotemic, or unable to produce a leukocytosis. Prompt early therapy with ceftazidime has now been found to reduce the mortality by 50% when historically compared with combination therapy with chloramphenicol, doxycycline, and cotrimoxazole as used before 1987. Relapses are common, perhaps 25% overall, with clinical severity and initial therapy the crucial risk factors (Fig. 303–2). Long-term oral treatment with amoxicillin–clavulanic acid appears logical to reduce relapses, since recurrence carries a high mortality rate.

Pseudomonas mallei.

P. mallei can cause an infection in horses, mules, and donkeys that occasionally has been transmitted to humans. The name "glanders" comes from the prominent pulmonary involvement, although the infection can, instead, be characterized by subcutaneous ulcerative lesions or lymphatic thickening with nodules (known as farcy).

Glanders was never a common human infection, and with the decline in the use of horses for day-to-day activities and with improved sanitation, glanders has become a very rare disease. Apparently, there have been no naturally acquired infections in the United States since 1938, although the occasional case occurs in other countries.

Like melioidosis, glanders tends to occur as an acute localized suppurative infection, an acute pulmonary infection, an acute septicemic infection, or a chronic suppurative infection. An abraded area of skin may lead to a local nodule with acute lymphangitis. Inoculation into an abraded mucous membrane can lead to extensive ulcerating granulomatous lesions. These forms of infection seem to have an incubation period of 1 to 5 days; in contrast, after inhalation, a primary pneumonia tends to develop 10 to 14 days later. Symptoms are relatively nonspecific and include fever, occasional rigors, malaise, fatigue, and headache. Examination findings depend on the form of infection. Leukocytosis is common. Chest radiographs of the acute pulmonary form usually show densities consistent with early lung abscess; however, lobar or bronchopneumonia-type infiltrates are common. Chronic suppurative disease involves multiple subcutaneous and intramuscular abscesses, especially on the extremities, with lymphatic involvement and, in many, a nasal discharge with or without ulceration.

The organism is usually difficult to find in exudates but, when seen with a Gram stain or methylene blue, appears similar to *P. pseudomallei*. The organism is reasonably easy to cultivate.

The treatment of glanders is uncertain because of its rarity—hence the inability to carry out clinical trials. A reasonable recommendation is to initiate therapy with regimens found effective for melioidosis, recognizing that the acute septicemic form has been uniformly fatal and suggesting that full dosage of intravenous combinations of agents be given initially.

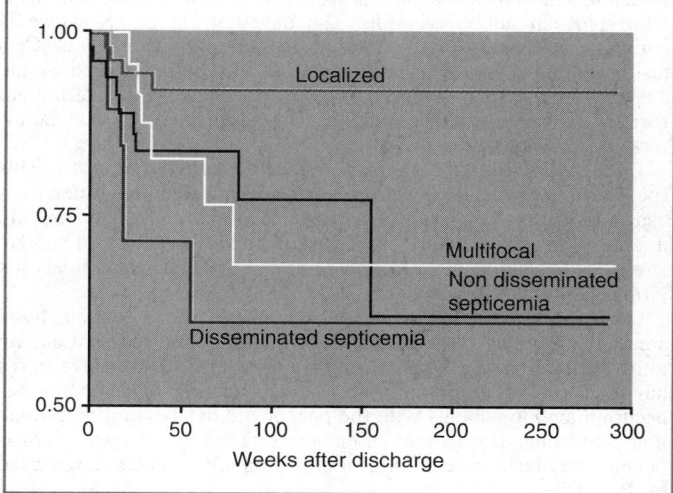

FIGURE 303–2. Relapse-free probability in survivors of acute melioidosis stratified by clinical severity on first admission. (From Chaowagul W, Suputtamongkol Y, Dance DAB, et al.: Relapse in melioidosis: Incidence and risk factors. J Infect Dis 168:1181, 1993.)

Pseudomonas aeruginosa.

The name "aeruginosa" comes from the fluorescent blue-green pigment pyocyanin, produced by many, but not all, strains. Other pigments produced by *P. aeruginosa* include pyoverdin (green) and, occasionally, pyorubin (deep red) and pyomelanin (black). Like other pseudomonads, *P. aeruginosa* grows well in multiple moist settings with limited nutrients. Found in soil, in water, and on plants, it also can be a normal commensal in animals and humans. Colonization in humans usually takes place in moist areas, such as perineum, auditory canal, axillae, and the lower alimentary canal. It is commonly found in faucet aerators, sink traps, ice machines, and kitchen settings in the hospital; it can become a particular problem when it contaminates medications or medical devices with a moist environment, such as ventilators, endoscopes, pressure monitors, and the like. It can withstand many disinfectants and is resistant to a broad variety of antimicrobial agents. In the nonhospital setting, infections have been related to growth in swimming pools, contact lens solutions, and hot tubs.

Infection with *P. aeruginosa* has become, to a large degree, a byproduct of medical advances in technology. In the 20 years prior to 1960 at the Johns Hopkins Hospital, only 91 cases of *P. aeruginosa* bacteremia occurred. In recent years, *P. aeruginosa* has been the fourth most common cause of primary nosocomial gram-negative bacteremia and the fourth most frequently isolated nosocomial pathogen, having caused about 10% of all hospital-acquired infections, 13% of all nosocomial pneumonias, 12% of urinary tract infections, and 7% of surgical wound infections.

The most common infections caused by *P. aeruginosa* include nosocomial bacteremia, nosocomial pneumonia, nosocomial urinary tract infection, surgical wound infection, endocarditis related to intravenous drug abuse or placement of artificial heart valves, respiratory infection associated with cystic fibrosis, external otitis, including "malignant" external otitis (see Ch. 421), corneal keratitis, and uncommon occurrences of spinal osteomyelitis in heroin addicts (see Ch. 283) and rare cases of meningitis or brain abscess. A common origin of bacteremia in the granulocytopenic patient is infection along the alimentary canal, especially perianal cellulitis, colonic lesions, and, occasionally, pharyngitis or esophagitis. Finally, extensive burns are commonly colonized by *P. aeruginosa*, with progression to sepsis and death.

P. aeruginosa almost never causes infection in the absence of (1) damage to a normal host defense mechanism (e.g., cancer chemotherapy–induced mucosal damage to the alimentary canal, granulocytopenia, or extensive third-degree burns), (2) deficiency or alteration in a defense mechanism (e.g., the progressive respiratory tract changes of cystic fibrosis), or (3) bypass of a normal defense mechanism (e.g., respiratory assist device directly inoculating organisms into the bronchial tree while concurrently limiting or damaging the mucociliary mechanism, or insertion of an indwelling urinary catheter, circumventing the normal bladder clearance mechanism). Thus infections with *P. aeruginosa* are seen most commonly in patients with a urinary catheter; those neutropenic from disease, chemotherapy, or both; those with cystic fibrosis; those with extensive thermal injuries; those in the intensive care unit who are subjected to any number of invasive procedures; those with head trauma, allowing entry either directly or via a pressure monitoring device; those with artificial heart valves or damaged endocardium from contaminants in illicit drugs; and those who have had extensive surgery, particularly when there is consequent need for open drainage. Pulmonary infection late in the course of AIDS may present as an acute infection or as an indolent, frequently recurrent infection mimicking that seen with cystic fibrosis.

Pollack has pointed out three distinct stages of *Pseudomonas* infection: stage I—bacterial attachment and colonization; stage II—local invasion; and stage III—bloodstream dissemination and systemic disease. Stage I is a prerequisite to stage II, which, in turn, is a prerequisite to stage III, although obviously not all colonized individuals have local invasion and not all those with local invasion progress to dissemination or systemic disease. The three stages relate to the fact that this organism is both invasive and toxigenic. Colonization in a normal person is relatively uncommon at most sites, although, over time, a fair proportion of the population will have transient colonization of the colon. However, hospitalized patients have a much higher frequency of colonization, related in part to changes in host defenses, as discussed above, and partly to the frequency of hospital reservoirs of this organism. In addition, broad-spectrum antimicrobial therapy suppresses other normal microbial flora, especially along the alimentary canal. This suppression reduces the body's normal mechanism of colonization resistance so that an organism such as *P. aeruginosa* or other species resistant to the antibiotics used can more readily colonize multiple locations in high concentration. Additional specific factors further predispose to colonization by *P. aeruginosa*. These include the presence of pili for attachment, flagella for motility, and exoproducts, especially proteinases. Also involved is the secretory protease-induced loss of fibronectin from epithelial cells during serious illness (among patients hospitalized or not), which in turn allows the pili or fimbriae to adhere to the oral, pharyngeal, and respiratory epithelium. Thus the illness determinants of protease production are major modulators of the oral flora. This colonization in turn can be accentuated by local damage caused by an endotracheal tube, by viral infection (such as influenza), by thermal injury, or by cancer chemotherapy and is exacerbated by antibiotics. *P. aeruginosa*, in some settings, can help protect itself from defense mechanisms by producing a glycocalyx, a carbohydrate produced by many bacteria, which, by surrounding the cell and anchoring it to epithelial cells or invasive devices such as an intravascular or urinary catheter, protects the bacterium from antibody, complement, and polymorphonuclear leukocytes or macrophages.

After colonization, *P. aeruginosa* can invade in the appropriate setting through the effect of extracellular enzymes (toxins). These include elastase, alkaline protease, and perhaps also cytotoxin and hemolysins. Elastase and protease have been demonstrated to cause necrotizing lesions in the skin, lung, and cornea, along with small vessel necrotizing lesions, which cause the characteristic skin finding known as "ecthyma gangrenosum." It is this combination of local necrosis and blood vessel destruction that is the essence of the initial invasive characteristic of *P. aeruginosa*.

The third stage of *Pseudomonas* infection, dissemination and systemic disease, is due, in the first case, to these same extracellular enzymes and, in the second case, to *Pseudomonas* liposaccharide (endotoxin) and exotoxin A. As with other septicemias caused by gram-negative bacilli, endotoxin is thought to be a critical factor in the activation of the clotting, fibrinolytic, kinin, and complement systems, along with the production of prostaglandins and leukotrienes, the release of β-endorphins, and the release of cytokines, including tumor necrosis factor. By some interaction of many or all of these factors come fever, shock, disseminated intravascular coagulation (which is relatively uncommon with *Pseudomonas* bacteremia), and the adult respiratory distress syndrome. The other factor, exotoxin A, is similar to diphtheria toxin in that it inhibits protein synthesis. It causes local necrosis and encourages bacterial dissemination to the systemic circulation and, in itself, has been shown to produce shock in animal models.

Pseudomonas bacteremia occurs most commonly in cancer patients who are receiving intensive chemotherapy that produces granulocytopenia in patients with extensive third-degree burns and, occasionally, in patients with immunoglobulin or hypocomplementemia states. It is also a common cause of bacteremia in the patient with urinary catheterization. It is the fourth most frequent cause of primary hospital-acquired gram-negative bacteremia. Sepsis in burn patients arises from the thermally damaged skin. Bacteremia in neutropenic patients arises principally from the lower intestinal tract and occasionally from primary pneumonia. Surveillance cultures have documented that granulocytopenic patients frequently become colonized, and nearly all colonized patients will develop bacteremia if profound (<100 per microliter) granulocytopenia persists for more than a few days. Ecthyma gangrenosum, usually a sign of fairly advanced systemic infection, is not pathognomonic but is most frequently associated with *P. aeruginosa* bacteremia. These skin lesions at first are small and indurated, and then rapidly enlarge, become necrotic, and may ulcerate. Bacteria, on histologic section, are seen to be invading small arteries and veins, with remarkably minimal evidence of inflammation. A histologically similar lesion can be found in the lungs as a secondary consequence of bacteremia. The mortality of *Pseudomonas* sepsis is high, with the underlying status of the patient's host defenses and the promptness of instituting empirical antibiotic therapy being the two

critical factors affecting survival. The presence of septic shock, the evidence of septic metastases, or both when antibiotics are started are usually considered adverse prognostic signs but, in reality, represent another measure of late institution of therapy.

The standard approach to suspected gram-negative sepsis, including that caused by *P. aeruginosa*, is a combination using an antipseudomonal β-lactam (penicillin or cephalosporin) with an aminoglycoside. Two newer drugs, imipenem and the antipseudomonal quinolones—again, in combination with an aminoglycoside—are also effective. Although in some cases, such as in the febrile neutropenic patient, monotherapy has been recommended with agents such as ceftazidime or imipenem, a two-drug regimen is advised for initial empirical therapy. Studies suggest that survival is improved when two antibiotics to which the organism is susceptible are given immediately and that survival is further improved if the two agents prove to be synergistic in activity. For example, in a study of 200 episodes of *P. aeruginosa* bacteremia, combination therapy yielded a mortality of 27%, whereas monotherapy mortality was 47%. A later study suggested that adding rifampin to the β-lactam–aminoglycoside would further improve response rates and reduce breakthrough or relapsing bacteremia, although survival was not affected. For the future, we must also look to immunologic approaches to bacteremia prevention and treatment, such as monoclonal antibodies to lipopolysaccharide.

Respiratory tract infections (see Ch. 273) can take the form of a primary pneumonia, a secondary pneumonia due to bacteremia, or a chronic infection with intermittent exacerbations. Primary pneumonia occurs almost exclusively in hospitalized patients whose oropharynx or tracheobronchial tree is colonized by *P. aeruginosa*, the latter as a result of intubation. Frequently, *Pseudomonas* pneumonia occurs in the setting of additional pulmonary damage, such as blunt trauma, substantial atelectasis, or hemothorax. Atelectasis appears to be a key contributing pathogenic factor. Early, aggressive physiotherapy for the chest sometimes clears what appears to be a pneumonia but in fact is atelectasis that has resulted in fever, purulent sputum production, and a positive chest radiograph. However, once actual pneumonia has begun, the prognosis is poor, and early empirical therapy is crucial.

The pneumonia that follows bacteremia is usually fulminant, with multiple areas of hemorrhage around small and medium-sized pulmonary arteries and lesions caused by necrosis of the small muscular arteries and veins in a fashion similar to ecthyma gangrenosum. Survival is limited even with prompt, aggressive therapy.

Chronic *Pseudomonas* respiratory infections are largely limited to patients with cystic fibrosis (see also Ch. 58), with the frequency of this infection increasing with age so that, ultimately, almost all patients will have significant *Pseudomonas* pulmonary infection. The age differential is probably related to the progressive development of airway obstruction, a crucial factor in development of *Pseudomonas* infection. This chronic infection is associated with chronic cough, nutritional losses, and progressive loss of pulmonary function. The standard treatment has been an antipseudomonal penicillin plus an aminoglycoside. The development of resistance is common, so therapy must be based on susceptibility patterns. Ceftazidime, imipenem, or a quinolone also may be considered. Acute exacerbations may be reduced or even prevented with intermittent therapy a number of times each year, irrespective of whether the infection is currently quiescent.

OTHER PSEUDOMONADS. *Pseudomonas cepacia*. This species of *Pseudomonas* can grow as well in distilled water as it can in trypticase soy broth; it is resistant to many of the commonly used hospital disinfectants; it can use penicillin as a carbon source; and it is resistant to many of the commonly used antimicrobials. Its virulence properties are not understood.

Community-acquired infections are rare. However, certain hosts are at substantially increased risk. Endocarditis has occurred among intravenous drug abusers; skin infections related to extensive burns have occurred; a necrotizing, occasionally recurrent pneumonia has occurred among patients with the phagocytic dysfunction of chronic granulomatous disease; and an emerging problem for cystic fibrosis patients has been a relentless, often fulminating pneumonia caused by *P. cepacia*.

Nosocomial infections and pseudoinfections are considered together because of a common origin and because it can be difficult to distinguish between the two. The source of hospital *P. cepacia* is usually a moist or water-based reservoir, which, given the technologic advances of medicine, suggests that *P. cepacia* has the potential to become a not infrequent cause of infection and pseudoinfection in the high-technology or intensive care setting. *P. cepacia* has been found to cause pneumonitis, endocarditis, wound infections, and urinary tract infections, along with primary bacteremia. The origins of iatrogenic bacteremia can be conveniently divided into those related to contaminated solutions, injectables, and medical devices. Among the contaminated solutions implicated in bacteremia or pseudobacteremia have been disinfectant solutions, heparinized flushing solutions, distilled water, topical anesthetics, and intravenous infusates, including human serum albumin and cryoprecipitate. Contaminated injectables have included saline, methylprednisolone, and fentanyl. The implicated devices all include a moist environment where the organism can multiply; pressure monitoring devices, respiratory assist devices, peritoneal dialysis machines, reusable hemodialysis coils, and blood gas analyzers have been documented as point sources.

Figure 303–3 shows an epidemic of *P. cepacia* bacteremia among patients at the Clinical Center of the National Institutes of Health. The figure indicates that *P. cepacia*–positive blood cultures were uncommon in the years preceding this outbreak and that the majority during the epidemic occurred within the medical intensive care unit. A blood gas analyzer in an adjoining laboratory was found to be contaminated, and this served as the point source for this series of bacteremias. Although some were apparently pseudobacteremias (i.e., the blood culture became positive owing to contamination by skin or other sources), others were true bacteremias with significant morbidity. Indeed, among those highly compromised patients, many with cancer and significant immune suppression, the mortality resulting from the *P. cepacia* infection itself was 38%. Respiratory colonization in an appropriately predisposed host can progress to pneumonia, as evidenced by 14 of 37 patients with colonization and hematologic malignancies who developed pneumonia during an 18-month outbreak. In another outbreak of 14 bacteremias among cancer patients, all had central venous lines flushed with a contaminated heparin solution.

P. cepacia is resistant to many of the commonly used broad-spectrum antibiotics but is usually susceptible to trimethoprim-sulfamethoxazole and ceftazidime.

Pseudomonas pickettii.
This is an uncommon cause of infection. In the past 30 years, 49 cases of bacteremia were reported. Thirty-eight of the 49 were caused by contaminated injected solutions; 7 more were related to contaminated ventilators or dialysis equipment. Four patients had bacteremia related to indwelling intravenous catheters; all were treated at one institution over a 2-year period. *P. pickettii* is usually resistant to aminoglycosides but susceptible to cephalosporins and antipseudomonal penicillins.

Xanthomonas maltophilia (Pseudomonas maltophilia).
X. maltophilia is atypical of the other pseudomonads in that the oxidase test is negative or equivocal. It is probably a fairly common commensal and a part of the transient flora, especially of hospitalized patients. In hospitals it is not infrequently found in moist or wet settings. The organism is resistant to most of the first- and second-generation cephalosporins, semisynthetic penicillins, and aminoglycosides, although it has variable susceptibility to the antipseudomonal penicillins. It is generally susceptible to many of the third-generation cephalosporins, trimethoprim-sulfamethoxazole, and rifampin. Synergy has been noted with trimethoprim-sulfamethoxazole plus carbenicillin and with the triple regimen of trimethoprim-sulfamethoxazole plus carbenicillin and rifampin.

X. maltophilia is an uncommon cause of a wide spectrum of diseases that, in general, are less severe than infections caused by other gram-negative bacilli in similar locations. *X. maltophilia* is susceptible to many, but not all, of the common broad-spectrum antibiotics. It is frequently resistant to cephalosporins, antipseudomonal penicillins, imipenem, and quinolones, and is usually susceptible to trimethoprim-sulfamethoxazole. The most common types of infection are pneumonia, endocarditis, urinary tract infection, and iatrogenic bacteremia or pseudobacteremia. Cholangitis and meningitis have been reported but are quite unusual, and wounds, although a common site for *X. maltophilia* isolation, are rarely infected by this organism. Pneumonias tend to occur in debilitated patients with prior antibiotic therapy in a nosocomial setting, but they are very uncommon, and the organism should be questioned as causative in the absence of a pure culture via bronchoscopy, thoracentesis, or blood. Endocarditis in the community occurs among intravenous drug abusers and in the hospital as a complication of open heart surgery, usually among those with abnormal valves. Traumatized victims, especially with contaminated wounds, develop serious infections in association with ventilatory assist and broad-spectrum antimicrobials. *X. maltophilia* is being increasingly recognized as a cause of serious infection (pneumonia, bacteremia, urinary tract and wound infection) among cancer patients who are granulocytopenic and have received broad-spectrum antibiotics, especially imipenem.

X. maltophilia bacteriuria is found occasionally in patients with indwelling long-term catheters; however, only rarely has the organism been shown to cause clinical infection. When infection has occurred, it has usually been in association with significant instrumentation, genitourinary surgery, or both. The morbidity has tended to be low, and therapy, especially with trimethoprim-sulfamethoxazole, has frequently been effective.

Iatrogenic bacteremia and pseudobacteremia caused by this organism have been reported often. In one epidemic of 25 patients with positive blood cultures, it was determined that these cases were pseudobacteremias due to contaminated blood collection tubes. In another setting, eight children were found to have bacteremia after open heart surgery, apparently as a result of contamination of the monitoring transducers in the intensive care unit. *X. maltophilia* has been found to contaminate the deionized water used for diluting disinfectants, and the organism can even survive in the diluted disinfectant. It is important to emphasize that not all of

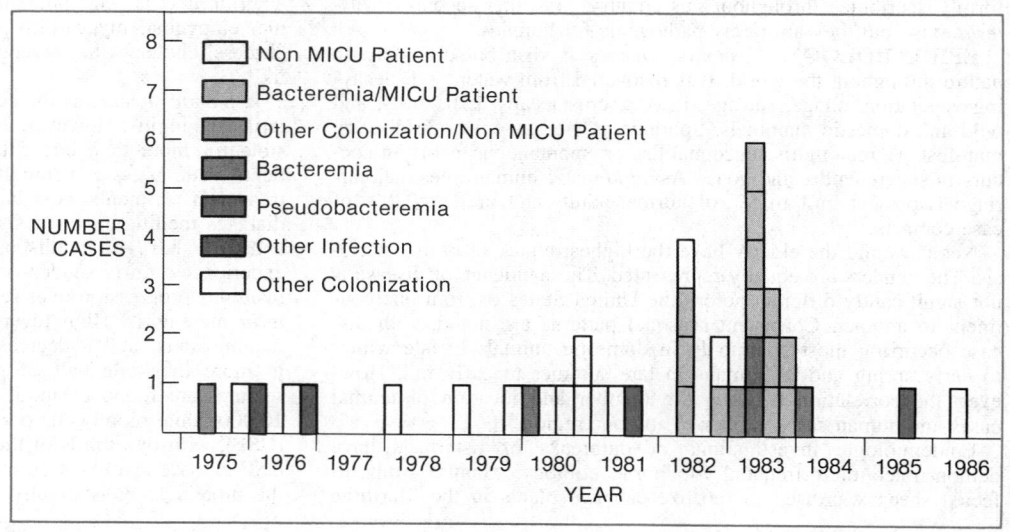

FIGURE 303–3. An epidemic of *Pseudomonas cepacia* bacteremia among patients at the Clinical Center of the National Institutes of Health. Note that the epidemic in 1982–1983 within the MICU was caused by a contaminated nearby blood gas analyzer. MICU = medical intensive care unit. (Reprinted with permission from Henderson DK, Baptiste R, Parillo J, et al.: Indolent epidemic of *Pseudomonas cepacia* bacteremia and pseudobacteremia in an intensive care unit traced to a contaminated blood gas analyzer. Am J Med 84:75, 1988.)

NUMBER CASES

□ Non MICU Patient
▨ Bacteremia/MICU Patient
▨ Other Colonization/Non MICU Patient
▨ Bacteremia
▨ Pseudobacteremia
▨ Other Infection
□ Other Colonization

YEAR

these bacteremias have been "pseudobacteremias"; for example, two fatal cases of endocarditis have been noted as a result of bacteremia caused by a contaminated device or solution. Permanent indwelling vascular catheters are a major source of bacteremias; imipenem therapy is an important predisposing factor.

Bodey GP, Jadeja L, Elting L: *Pseudomonas* bacteremia: Retrospective analysis of 410 episodes. Arch Intern Med 145:1621, 1985. *A review of P. aeruginosa bacteremia.*

Chaowagul W, Suputtamongkol Y, Dance DAB, et al.: Relapse in melioidosis: Incidence and risk factors. J Infect Dis 168:1181, 1993. *A 23% relapse rate was related to initial infection severity and therapy.*

Henderson DK, Baptiste R, Parillo J, et al.: Indolent epidemic of *Pseudomonas cepacia* bacteremia and pseudobacteremia in an intensive care unit traced to a contaminated blood gas analyzer. Am J Med 84:75, 1988. *A nice review of bacteremia and pseudobacteremia due to P. cepacia.*

Hilf M, Yu VL, Sharp J, et al.: Antibiotic therapy for *Pseudomonas aeruginosa* bacteremia: Outcome correlations in a prospective study of 200 patients. Am J Med 87:540, 1989. *A critical evaluation of antimicrobial therapy for P. aeruginosa bacteremia suggesting an advantage for combination therapy.*

Marshall WF, Keating MR, Anhalt JP, Steckelberg JM: *Xanthomonas maltophilia*: An emerging nosocomial pathogen. Mayo Clin Proc 64:1097, 1989. *A thorough review.*

Pollack M: *Pseudomonas aeruginosa. In* Mandell GL, Douglas RG Jr, Bennett JE (eds.): Principles and Practice of Infectious Diseases. 3rd ed. New York, Churchill Livingstone, 1990, pp 1673–1691. *A very thorough discussion of the microbiology, epidemiology, pathogenic factors, and clinical syndromes of P. aeruginosa.*

Raveh D, Simhon A, Gimmon Z, et al.: Infections caused by *Pseudomonas pickettii* in association with permanent indwelling intravenous devices: Four cases and a review. Clin Infect Dis 17:877, 1993. *A review of the few reported cases of bacteremia by this organism.*

Sanford JP: *Pseudomonas* species (including melioidosis and glanders). *In* Mandell GL, Douglas RG Jr, Bennett JE (eds.): Principles and Practice of Infectious Diseases. 3rd ed. New York, Churchill Livingstone, 1990, pp 1692–1696. *Broad discussion of melioidosis and glanders by an expert in infections of importance to the U.S. military.*

White NJ, Dance DAB, Chaowagul W, et al.: Halving of mortality of severe melioidosis by ceftazidime. Lancet 2:697, 1988. *New antibiotics have had a major impact on mortality.*

304 LISTERIOSIS
Alan M. Stamm

DEFINITION. Listeriosis is an infectious disease caused by the bacterium *Listeria monocytogenes*. The majority of afflicted patients are immunocompromised and present with meningoencephalitis.

ETIOLOGY. *L. monocytogenes* is a gram-positive bacillus but may stain unevenly and/or appear coccoid. It is facultatively anaerobic, non–spore-forming, and β-hemolytic on blood agar. It grows optimally at 35 to 37°C, grows less well at temperatures as low as 4°C, and exhibits tumbling motility at 20 to 25°C.

Although at least 16 serotypes of *L. monocytogenes* are identified, each of the types 1/2a, 1/2b, and 4b accounts for about 30% of human disease in the United States. These serotypes are uniformly distributed throughout this country. Six other species of *Listeria* exist, but they are rarely pathogenic for humans.

EPIDEMIOLOGY. *L. monocytogenes* is distributed widely in nature throughout the world. It is recovered from water, soil, decaying vegetation, silage, sewage, insects, crustaceans, fish, birds, and wild and domestic mammals. Sporadic as well as epizootic disease, manifest as meningitis, encephalitis, or spontaneous abortion, occurs in sheep, cattle, and goats. Asymptomatic human intestinal carriage is present in 1 to 5% of normal adults and in 10 to 20% of case contacts.

Neonates and the elderly have the highest attack rates of listeriosis. The genders are equally represented. The incidence of disease is not significantly different across the United States or from one continent to another. Consistent seasonal patterns are noted, with disease occurring most commonly in domestic animals in late winter to early spring and in humans in late summer to early fall. However, the correlation between the number and location of animal cases and human cases is poor in any one region.

Epidemiologic investigations of outbreaks of listeriosis have demonstrated their frequent foodborne etiology. Manure from infected sheep was used to fertilize cabbage plants in the Maritime Provinces of Canada; 41 cases of human disease in 1980–1981 were linked to the ingestion of cole slaw prepared from these cabbages. Milk from cows was pasteurized but nonetheless implicated in 49 cases of listeriosis in Massachusetts in 1983; whether the microorganism survived pasteurization or contaminated the product afterward remains controversial. The largest epidemic occurred in southern California in 1985; 142 cases were associated with the consumption of soft, Mexican-style cheese made with unpasteurized milk. Similarly, an outbreak of 122 cases in Switzerland during 1983–1987 was attributed to a soft cheese. During periods of increased disease activity, the organism causing an epidemic strain is differentiated from that causing sporadic disease by serotyping, electrophoretic enzyme typing, ribotyping, or DNA fingerprinting. All four of these outbreaks were due to *L. monocytogenes* serotype 4b.

Further evidence for foodborne acquisition of *L. monocytogenes* is provided by recent microbiologic investigations. The microorganism has been identified as a fairly common contaminant of raw and pasteurized milk; ice cream; soft cheese; raw beef, pork, and lamb; ready-to-eat meat products, including salami, sausages, paté, and hot dogs; retail poultry; cooked shrimp and crab; raw vegetables such as cabbage, cucumbers, potatoes, and radishes; and packaged salads. Although commercial food production methods may effectively kill the microorganism, products may become contaminated during subsequent processing and packaging before leaving the production facility.

PATHOGENESIS. Most adults with listeriosis have impaired cell-mediated immunity caused by cytotoxic chemotherapy for malignancy, immunosuppressive therapy for organ transplantation, or pregnancy. Both helper and suppressor T cells are centrally involved, whereas immunoglobulin and complement play lesser roles as opsonins. The gastrointestinal tract is the usual portal of entry. Bacteria are taken up from the lumen by endocytosis of epithelial cells covering intestinal villi. The inoculum required to cause disease may depend on the immunologic health and gastric acidity of the host as well as the virulence characteristics of the microorganism.

Dissemination occurs via simple bacteremia and/or circulation of infected monocytes. *L. monocytogenes* is a facultative intracellular parasite capable of multiplying within the nonimmune monocyte-macrophage. Listeriolysin O, a hemolysin structurally similar to streptolysin O, may be an important virulence factor in this process. Phagocytosis of the bacterium stimulates its production; it binds to cholesterol in cell membranes, leading to their disruption. This feature may allow the microorganism to escape from phagolysosomes but to persist and multiply within macrophages, ultimately leading to their destruction.

CLINICAL MANIFESTATIONS. The incubation period between acquiring the infection and disease onset varies from days to weeks. The clinical presentation of listeriosis is as meningitis in 50 to 60% of cases; bacteremia without evident localized disease in 25 to 30%; parenchymal disease of the central nervous system (CNS), with or without meningitis, in 10%; and endocarditis in 5%. Infrequent manifestations due to hematogenous dissemination include anterior uveitis, endophthalmitis, cervical lymphadenitis, pneumonia, empyema, myocarditis, pericarditis, peritonitis, hepatitis, liver abscess, cholecystitis, mycotic aneurysm, osteomyelitis, and arthritis.

L. monocytogenes is the cause in about 1% of cases of acute bacterial meningitis. However, among patients with cancer, it is responsible for more than one fifth of episodes. Conversely, among patients with *Listeria* meningitis, 25% have a malignancy; 25% are transplant recipients; 20% have another underlying disorder, such as diabetes mellitus or cirrhosis, or are receiving glucocorticosteroids; and 30% have no predisposing condition. Two thirds of patients experience a fairly sudden onset of symptoms, but one third note an insidious progression over several days. No features distinguish *Listeria* meningitis. High fever is almost always reported. Headache, meningismus, and a decreased level of consciousness are present in more than one half of patients. Focal neurologic deficits and seizures are found in about one fourth. Most patients have 100 to 10,000 white blood cells per cubic millimeter of cerebrospinal fluid (CSF), with two thirds of them being polymorphonuclear cells. The CSF glucose level is < 50 mg per deciliter in one half of cases, and the protein level is usually 50 to 300 mg per deciliter. The Gram stain of CSF is interpreted as revealing gram-positive bacilli in only 25% of cases. Cultures of blood are positive in 60%. The differential diagnosis includes disease due to *Streptococcus pneumoniae,* a gram-negative bacillus, or *Cryptococcus neoformans.*

Parenchymal disease of the CNS is associated with clinical and CSF findings of meningitis in only 50% of cases. Anatomically, the spectrum of disease includes diffuse and localized cerebritis, brain stem meningoencephalitis (rhombencephalitis), and macroscopic abscess formation in the brain or spine. All patients are febrile; other common symptoms and signs are decreased consciousness in two thirds of patients, headache and hemiparesis in one half, and seizures and cranial nerve palsies in one third. *Listeria* rhombencephalitis merits special mention. Eighty per cent of reported victims have been previously healthy. The illness has a biphasic course: A 3- to 10-day prodrome of fever, headache, and vomiting is terminated by the abrupt onset of asymmetric palsies of cranial nerves V, VI, VII, IX, and/or X, cerebellar signs, paresis, and hypesthesia. In patients without concurrent meningitis, the analysis of CSF is usually normal or reveals only a mild pleocytosis and increased protein; Gram stain and culture are positive in a minority. Blood cultures are positive in most patients with parenchymal CNS disease. The differential diagnosis includes tuberculosis, toxoplasmosis, nocardiosis, mycoses, and stroke.

Bacteremia without evident localized disease (primary bacteremia) occurs in patients with hematologic malignancies (33% of cases), organ transplant recipients (25%), pregnant women (13%), and individuals suffering from alcoholism or cirrhosis (11%). *Listeria* bacteremia has no distinguishing features. Up to one fourth have premonitory gastrointestinal symptoms: nausea, vomiting, abdominal pain, and/or diarrhea.

Endocarditis occurs not in immunocompromised hosts but usually in those with underlying valvular heart disease. The aortic valve is involved in two thirds of cases and the mitral valve in one third, and prosthetic valve disease is well described. The onset of illness is subacute, with a median duration of symptoms prior to hospitalization of 5 weeks. Fever is cited in 75% of reported cases, a new or changing murmur in 40%, splenomegaly in 35%, and hepatomegaly, CNS emboli, and pulmonary emboli each in 25%.

One third of all cases of listeriosis are associated with pregnancy. Most commonly, in the third trimester, the mother develops a "flu-like" illness with fever, sore throat, myalgias, crampy abdominal pain, and diarrhea. After 3 to 7 days, premature labor or abortion ensues. Transplacental transmission of disease becomes clinically evident in the newborn within hours of delivery; this severe septicemic illness is known as "granulomatosis infantisepticum." Babies also may acquire infection in the birth canal or nosocomially in the nursery; at a mean of 14 days of life, disease presents as anorexia, fever, or meningismus. *L. monocytogenes* is the third most common cause of neonatal sepsis and meningitis after *Escherichia coli* and group B streptococci.

The complete spectrum of listeriosis is seen among patients with acquired immunodeficiency syndrome (AIDS). Chemoprophylaxis of pneumocystosis with trimethoprim-sulfamethoxazole may prevent listeriosis.

DIAGNOSIS. The microbiologic diagnosis of listeriosis is established by culture of blood, CSF, or tissue. In cases of granulomatosis infantisepticum, meconium, amniotic fluid, and lochia are cultured. Initial growth in the laboratory may be slow and may require several days. Unwary technicians may misinterpret these gram-positive bacilli as diphtheroids and label them contaminants.

TREATMENT. Ampicillin is the antimicrobial agent of choice for listeriosis. Although no comparative trials have been conducted, it has an established record of efficacy and can be administered safely even during pregnancy and infancy. The standard dosage in patients with meningitis is 200 mg per kilogram per day in six divided doses given intravenously. The duration of therapy necessary for consistent cure is 3 weeks. Seriously ill and immunocompromised patients are treated with ampicillin plus gentamicin; the latter drug is administered intravenously in doses sufficient to yield peak serum concentrations of 5 to 8 μg per milliliter and predictable CSF concentrations of 1 to 2 μg per milliliter. Most *in vitro* studies and animal model trials suggest that these two drugs act synergistically against *L. monocytogenes.*

Trimethoprim-sulfamethoxazole has emerged as the preferred therapy for patients allergic to penicillins. The combination is bac-

tericidal at achievable serum and CSF concentrations. Many case reports have appeared in the literature, including those of immunocompromised patients with CNS disease, and all were cured. Experience to date suggests an initial dosage of 160 mg of trimethoprim plus 800 mg of sulfamethoxazole given intravenously every 6 to 12 hours in adults with normal renal function.

The inordinate number of treatment failures and relapses among patients treated with cephalosporins or chloramphenicol indicates that these agents are not to be used. Newer β-lactams, including imipenem, are not as active as ampicillin against *L. monocytogenes.* The quinolones do not appear to be sufficiently active at achievable concentrations to be useful clinically. There has been no significant change in the antimicrobial susceptibility profile of *L. monocytogenes* over the past two decades.

PROGNOSIS. The overall mortality rate of *Listeria* meningitis is 30%, being higher in patients with cancer, hypoglycorrhachia, or bacteremia and lower in previously healthy individuals. Parenchymal CNS disease and endocarditis are fatal in 50% of cases.

PREVENTION. Individuals at increased risk should avoid raw milk, wash raw vegetables carefully, and cook meats thoroughly. In the hospital, patients with listeriosis should be isolated from immunocompromised hosts.

Armstrong RW, Fung PC: Brainstem encephalitis (rhombencephalitis) due to *Listeria monocytogenes:* Case report and review. Clin Infect Dis 16:689, 1993. *A detailed analysis of the clinical aspects of this syndrome of immunocompetent adults.*

Farber JM, Peterkin PI: *Listeria monocytogenes,* a food-borne pathogen. Microbiol Rev 55:476, 1991. *An extensive review of the microbiology, epidemiology, and pathogenesis of foodborne disease.*

Jurado RL, Farley MM, Pereira E, et al.: Increased risk of meningitis and bacteremia due to *Listeria monocytogenes* in patients with human immunodeficiency virus infection. Clin Infect Dis 17:224, 1993. *Incidence, demographics, and clinical outcome were assessed in a prospective, population-based survey. The estimated incidence among patients with AIDS was 150 times higher than in the general population.*

Schuchat AM, Deaver KA, Wenger JD, et al.: Role of foods in sporadic listeriosis: I. Case-control study of dietary risk factors. JAMA 267:2041, 1992. *An interesting and enlightening description of the methods used to identify contaminated foods responsible for one third of sporadic disease. Provides detailed dietary recommendations for listeriosis prevention.*

305 ERYSIPELOID

Annette C. Reboli

DEFINITION. *Erysipelothrix rhusiopathiae,* the causative agent of swine erysipelas, causes three well-defined patterns of human infection: (1) a mild, localized cutaneous form (erysipeloid of Rosenbach); (2) a severe, diffuse cutaneous form without bacteremia; and (3) a bacteremic form, with or without cutaneous involvement, usually complicated by endocarditis. Sheep and swine erysipelas and diamond skin disease are animal diseases, whereas erysipeloid, whale finger, and seal finger involve localized cellulitis of the fingers and hands, which is the most common manifestation of infection with *E. rhusiopathiae* seen in humans. The term "erysipeloid" refers to cutaneous infection caused by *E. rhusiopathiae* and should not be confused with erysipelas, which is a superficial cellulitis due to streptococci or staphylococci.

ETIOLOGY. *E. rhusiopathiae* is a thin, pleomorphic, nonsporulating, microaerophilic, gram-positive rod. It may be confused with other gram-positive bacillary organisms, in particular *Listeria monocytogenes* and *Corynebacterium* species. It can be differentiated from *L. monocytogenes* by its lack of motility, lack of catalase and coagulase production, and resistance to neomycin. Most strains of *E. rhusiopathiae* produce hydrogen sulfide on triple sugar iron agar slants. This feature distinguishes *E. rhusiopathiae* from *L. monocytogenes* and from corynebacteria. Because α-hemolysis may be seen after 48 hours of incubation of *E. rhusiopathiae,* confusion with streptococci also may occur.

EPIDEMIOLOGY. *E. rhusiopathiae* is found worldwide as a commensal or a pathogen in a variety of animals, including swine, sheep, cattle, horses, dogs, and rodents; fowl, including chickens, ducks, turkeys, and parrots; and flies, ticks, mites, and lice. The greatest commercial impact of *E. rhusiopathiae* infection is due to disease in swine, but infection of sheep and poultry is also important economically. Although the organism colonizes the mucoid surface slime of fish, it does not appear to cause disease in these animals. Environmental surfaces in contact with infected animals or their products are potential sources of *E. rhusiopathiae*. It can persist for prolonged periods in contaminated soil. Although *E. rhusiopathiae* is resistant to smoking, salting, and pickling, it is killed within 15 minutes by heating to 55°C.

Infection in humans is usually the result of contact with infected animals or their products. Persons at greatest risk for infection include fishermen, fishmongers, butchers, slaughterhouse workers, and veterinarians. The organism gains entry via cuts and abrasions on the skin. The seasonal incidence of erysipeloid parallels that of swine erysipelas and is highest in the summer and early fall.

CLINICAL MANIFESTATIONS. Because of its mode of acquisition (contact with infected animals or their products, with organisms inoculating abrasions on the skin), lesions are usually confined to the fingers and hands. A well-defined, slightly elevated, violaceous lesion, accompanied by a very painful, throbbing, burning, or itching sensation, develops within 2 to 7 days of traumatic dermal inoculation. The infected area is swollen. Vesicles may be present, but suppuration is absent. The lesion spreads slowly to other fingers but rarely involves the fingertips or the skin above the wrist. As the lesion spreads peripherally, the central area clears. Systemic signs and symptoms are rare. There may be sterile arthritis of an adjacent joint. Regional lymphadenopathy or lymphadenitis occurs in about 20% of cases, and low-grade fevers occur in approximately 10%. Because *E. rhusiopathiae* is located only in deeper parts of the skin in cases of erysipeloid, biopsy of the entire thickness of the dermis from the edge of the lesion yields maximum recovery of the organism. *E. rhusiopathiae* grows on routine laboratory media. Lesions usually resolve within 3 weeks without treatment. Relapse occurs in 1% of cases.

The diffuse cutaneous form is rare. The cutaneous lesion progresses proximally from the site of inoculation or appears at remote areas. The patients often have fever and arthralgias, but blood cultures are negative.

Systemic *E. rhusiopathiae* infection is uncommon. Approximately 60 cases of bacteremia have been reported; 90% of the patients had endocarditis. All but two cases involved native valves. In 60% of cases, infection developed on apparently normal heart valves. One third of patients had an antecedent or concurrent skin lesion of erysipeloid. Clinical manifestations of endocarditis due to *E. rhusiopathiae* and other microorganisms are similar. *E. rhusiopathiae* endocarditis correlates highly with occupation, exhibits a tropism for the aortic valve, affects more males than females, and is associated with a high mortality.

TREATMENT. Most isolates of *E. rhusiopathiae* are susceptible to penicillins, cephalosporins, imipenem, clindamycin, and ciprofloxacin. Some resistance has been observed with erythromycin, tetracycline, and chloramphenicol. *E. rhusiopathiae* is resistant to vancomycin, aminoglycosides, trimethoprim-sulfamethoxazole, and sulfonamides. Penicillin G is the treatment of choice for infections caused by *E. rhusiopathiae*. Uncomplicated cutaneous lesions usually respond well to a 5- to 7-day course of oral penicillin. Treatment hastens healing, although relapse may still occur. Bacteremia should be treated with intravenous penicillin; cases of endocarditis should be treated with 12 to 20 million units of penicillin G daily for 4 to 6 weeks. Ciprofloxacin is an alternative therapy in the penicillin-allergic patient. Valve replacement may be necessary in patients with endocarditis.

Barnett JH, Estes SA, Wirman JA, et al.: Erysipeloid. J Am Acad Dermatol 9:116, 1983. *A complete review of the clinical and pathologic features of* Erysipelothrix *infections and their treatment.*

Reboli AC, Farrar WE: *Erysipelothrix rhusiopathiae:* An occupational pathogen. Clin Microbiol Rev 4:354, 1989. *Reviews epidemiology, clinical features, and bacteriology.*

Venditti M, Gelfusa V, Tarasi A, et al.: Antimicrobial susceptibilities of *Erysipelothrix rhusiopathiae*. Antimicrob Agents Chemother 34:2038, 1990. In vitro *susceptibility data on 10 isolates of* E. rhusiopathiae *to 16 antimicrobial agents.*

306 ACTINOMYCOSIS
Ward E. Bullock

DEFINITION. Actinomycosis is a chronic bacterial infection that induces both a suppurative and a granulomatous inflammatory response. It spreads contiguously through anatomic barriers and frequently forms external sinuses, from which may extrude "sulfur granules" that are characteristic but not pathognomonic. The most common clinical forms are cervicofacial, thoracic, abdominal, and, in females, genital.

ETIOLOGY. Members of the genus *Actinomyces* are prokaryotes with cell walls that contain both muramic acid and diaminopimelic acid. Unlike the cell walls of fungi, the cell walls of these organisms do not contain sterols and are insensitive to polyene antibiotics. *Actinomyces israelii* is the species most often recovered from human cases of actinomycosis. However, *A. naeslundii*, *A. odontolyticus*, *A. viscosus*, *A. meyeri*, and a related genus, *Arachnia propionica*, cause identical clinical infections and bear close resemblance in primary culture. *Actinomyces bovis* produces "lumpy jaw" in cattle but is not a human pathogen. These gram-positive bacteria are filamentous (0.5 to 1.0 μm in diameter) with branching and are non–acid fast, with a tendency to break up into coccobacilli. They require anaerobic to microaerophilic conditions for growth, which is quite slow; usually, 3 to 10 or more days are required before these organisms can be macroscopically detected in culture.

EPIDEMIOLOGY. Actinomycosis is observed throughout the world, and its prevalence is unrelated to climate, occupation, race, or age. The disease has been reported more commonly in men than in women (3:1). However, since the recognition of pelvic actinomycosis in association with the use of intrauterine contraceptive devices (IUCD's), the male prevalence ratio may be decreasing. The number of cases of actinomycosis reported annually to the Centers for Disease Control and Prevention is fewer than 100. These infections are not easily recognized by clinicians, and the organisms are fastidious; therefore, it is likely that the true incidence is substantially greater. Although many animal species are susceptible to actinomycosis, infection is neither transmissible from animal to human nor transmissible from person to person. *Actinomyces* species are part of the indigenous microbiota colonizing the teeth and oral cavity. They also may be found in the tonsillar crypts of asymptomatic individuals, in the fecal flora, and within the female reproductive tract.

PATHOGENESIS AND PATHOLOGY. The *Actinomyces* species maintain their niche within the microbial community of the mouth by adherence to oral surfaces, especially to dental plaque, a thin film of salivary proteins and glycoproteins that coats the enamel surface. Adherence is achieved by complex protein-protein stereochemical interactions and by lectin-carbohydrate interactions, the latter of which also mediate cellular coaggregation of oral *Actinomyces* with *Streptococcus milleri*, *Streptococcus sanguis*, and other mouth flora. This propensity for coaggregation may explain, in part, why actinomycotic infections often are polymicrobial, with "associate" mouth flora frequently isolated from cervicofacial, thoracic, and central nervous system (CNS) abscesses. The associate flora may play a synergistic role in infection by maintaining the low oxygen tension necessary for *Actinomyces* growth. To cause disease, these organisms must be introduced into tissue through a break in the mucous membrane resulting from dental infections and manipulations or from aspiration of infected dental debris. They may enter the abdominal cavity by perforation of the lower gastrointestinal tract or by ascending infection of the genital tract in women.

Actinomycotic infection evokes a combination of suppurative and granulomatous inflammatory responses accompanied by intense fibrosis. Plasma cells and multinucleated giant cells often are observed within lesions, as may be large macrophages with foamy cytoplasm around purulent centers. The infection spreads through fascial planes and ultimately may produce draining sinus tracts, especially in infections of the pelvis and abdomen. Sulfur granules within lesions and sinus drainage are a typical feature, not always present. These granules are gritty aggregates of organisms measuring 1 to 2 mm in diameter; the centers have a basophilic staining property, with eosinophilic rays terminating in pear-shaped "clubs" on the surface. They contain calcium phosphate, probably as a result of phosphatase activity of both the host and the organisms.

CLINICAL MANIFESTATIONS. Cervicofacial actinomycosis comprises 50 to 60% of reported cases. Infection is usually observed in a setting of poor oral hygiene with tooth decay, periodontal disease, or gingivitis, in which mucosal integrity is disrupted by dental manipulations or other injury. The infection generally evolves as a chronic or subacute soft tissue swelling or mass involving the submandibular or paramandibular region. The swelling may have a ligneous consistency caused by tissue fibrosis. More rapidly developing lesions often simulate pyogenic infections. Trismus may be present, and advanced lesions may discharge odorless pus containing "sulfur granules" through one or more sinuses. Fever, pain, and leukocytosis may be present. The infection can extend to the tongue, salivary glands, pharynx, and larynx. Bone (most commonly the mandible) may be invaded from the adjacent soft tissue. Cervical spine or cranial bone infection may lead to subdural empyema and invasion of the CNS. The differential diagnosis includes tuberculosis (scrofula), fungal infections, nocardiosis, suppurative infections by other organisms, and neoplasms.

Thoracic actinomycosis comprises 15 to 30% of the disease spectrum and usually results from aspiration of infective material from the oropharynx. Less commonly, thoracic infection may be introduced by esophageal perforation, by extension into the mediastinum from the neck, or by spread from an abdominal site; hematogenous spread to the lung is rare. Pulmonary actinomycosis commonly spreads from an early pneumonic focus across lung fissures to involve the pleura and the chest wall, with eventual fistula formation and drainage containing sulfur granules (Fig. 306–1). Granules rarely are present in the sputum. The incidence of this complication, as well as the destruction of thoracic vertebrae and adjacent ribs, has declined in the antibiotic era.

The complaints of patients with thoracic actinomycosis are nonspecific. The most common are a productive cough, dyspnea, weight loss, fever, and chest pain. Anemia, mild leukocytosis, and an elevated sedimentation rate are relatively common. There often is a history of underlying lung disease, and patients rarely present in an early stage of infection. The pulmonary lesions may resemble tuberculosis, especially when cavity formation occurs, and blastomycosis, which may destroy ribs posteriorly but rarely form sinuses. Nocardiosis, bronchogenic carcinoma, and lymphoma can also mimic thoracic actinomycosis.

ABDOMINAL-PELVIC ACTINOMYCOSIS. Actinomycosis of the abdomen and pelvis is a chronic, localized inflammatory process that often is preceded weeks or months by surgery for acute appendicitis with perforation or for perforated colonic diverticulitis or by emergency surgery on the lower intestinal tract after trauma. Occasionally, abdominal actinomycosis may manifest without identifiable predisposing factors. The ileocecal region is involved most frequently, with the formation of a mass lesion. The infection extends slowly to contiguous organs, especially the liver, and may involve retroperitoneal tissues, the spine, or the abdominal wall. Persistent draining sinuses may form, and those involving the perianal region can simulate Crohn's disease or tuberculosis. The extensive fibrosis of actinomycotic lesions, presenting to the examiner as a mass, often suggests tumor. Constitutional symptoms and signs are nonspecific; the most common are fever, weight loss, nausea, vomiting, and pain.

An association has been recognized between long-term use of IUCD's and actinomycosis of the genital tract. Manifestations of infection may range from a chronic vaginal discharge to pelvic inflammatory disease with tubo-ovarian abscesses or pseudomalignant masses. No association exists between actinomycotic infection and the type of IUCD used. Accurate data on the prevalence and incidence of infection among IUCD users are sparse, since cytologic criteria and fluorescent antibody staining techniques are the principal means of detecting *Actinomyces* in vaginal smears and other genital tract specimens. Anaerobic cultures of the female genital tract generally are unsuccessful.

Currently, it is generally agreed that *Actinomyces* species may be part of the indigenous genital tract flora of females and that demonstrating their presence by morphologic criteria and fluorescent anti-

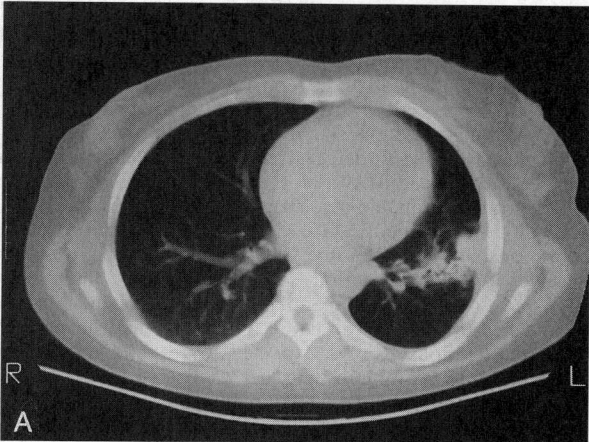

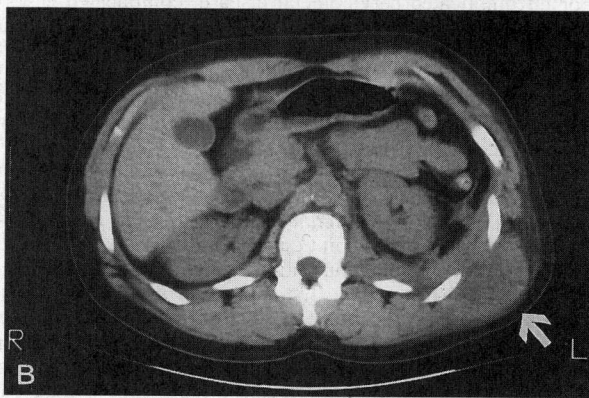

FIGURE 306–1. Thoracic computed tomographic scan of a 43-year-old woman with pulmonary actinomycosis. There is consolidation of the lung with pleural thickening adjacent to the parenchymal disease *(A)*. Abscess extended into the left breast and inferiorly to the costophrenic sulcus, to the retroperitoneum, and into the lateral abdominal wall *(B) (arrow)*.

body stains does not predict disease. However, colonization of the endometrium appears to require the presence of an IUCD. Although many cases of genital-pelvic actinomycosis associated with IUCD use have been reported, the actual incidence of disease appears to be low relative to the millions of those who use IUCD's.

CNS and disseminated actinomycosis are very uncommon. Most infections of the CNS manifest as encapsulated brain abscesses that are indistinguishable from those caused by other organisms. Most actinomycotic infections of the CNS are thought to be seeded hematogenously from a distant primary site; however, direct extension of cervicofacial disease is well recognized. Sinus formation is not a characteristic of CNS disease. The rare meningitis caused by *Actinomyces* is chronic and basilar in location, and the pleocytosis usually is lymphocytic. Thus, it may be misdiagnosed as tuberculous meningitis.

Unlike *Nocardia* species (see Ch. 307), *Actinomyces* species usually are not opportunistic in the immunocompromised host. To date, few systemic actinomycotic infections have been reported among patients with AIDS.

DIAGNOSIS. Crucial to the diagnosis is a high index of suspicion communicated to the microbiology diagnostic laboratory, along with material from draining sinuses, from deep needle aspiration, or from biopsy specimens. Anaerobic culture is required, and no selective media are available to restrict overgrowth of the slow-growing *Actinomyces* by associated microflora. The presence, in pus or tissue specimens of non–acid-fast, gram-positive organisms with filamentous branching is very suggestive of the diagnosis. The characteristic morphology of "sulfur granules" and the presence of gram-positive organisms within are helpful. However, the granules must be distinguished from similar structures that are sometimes produced in infections and that are caused by *Nocardia, Monospo-*

rium, *Cephalosporium*, *Staphylococcus* (botryomycosis), and others. *Actinomyces* and *Arachnia* generally can be differentiated from other gram-positive anaerobes by means of growth rate (slow), by catalase production (negative, except *A. viscosus*), and by gas-liquid chromatographic detection of acetic, lactic, and succinic acids produced in peptone-yeast-glucose broth. Direct fluorescent antibody conjugates can be used to detect *Actinomyces* in clinical material or culture but are not readily available to clinical microbiology laboratories. There are no reliable serologic tests or skin tests.

TREATMENT. Penicillin G is the drug of choice for treating an infection caused by any of the *Actinomyces*. It is given in high dosage over a prolonged period, since the infection has a tendency to recur, presumably because antibiotic penetration to areas of fibrosis and necrosis and into "sulfur granules" may be poor. Most deep-seated infections can be expected to respond to intravenous penicillin G, 10 to 20 million units per day given for 2 to 6 weeks, followed by an oral phenoxypenicillin in a dosage of 2 to 4 grams per day. A few additional weeks of oral penicillin therapy may suffice for uncomplicated cervicofacial disease; complicated cases and extensive pulmonary or abdominal disease may require treatment for 12 to 18 months. To date, little evidence exists of acquired resistance to penicillin G by *Actinomyces* during prolonged therapy. Radical excision of large sinus tracts should be considered in some cases. Alternative first-line antibiotics for treating *Actinomyces* infections include tetracycline, erythromycin, and clindamycin. First-generation cephalosporins and imipenem also are highly effective. Antifungal drugs are not active against these organisms. *In vitro* antibiotic sensitivity testing of *Actinomyces* is difficult, and the results may not be predictive of antibiotic activity *in vivo*.

The need to use combination antibiotic therapy to attack microorganisms that are isolated in association with *Actinomyces* has not been established. The generally good results obtained with penicillin G alone over nearly three decades indicate that monotherapy is effective in most cases. In complicated infections of the lower abdomen, where anaerobic gram-negative organisms, among others, may be the "associates," combination antibiotic therapy is appropriate.

The presence of organisms presumed to be *Actinomyces* on a Papanicolaou smear, obtained from an asymptomatic female with or without an IUCD in place, is not an indication for therapy. When patients experience well-defined IUCD-related symptoms and Papanicolaou smears demonstrate *Actinomyces* by specific fluorescent-labeled antibody, the device should be removed. Antibiotic administration for a 2-week period may be indicated. More serious infections require prolonged therapy as recommended above.

PROGNOSIS. The advent of antibiotics has greatly improved the prognosis for all forms of actinomycosis. At present, cure rates are high, and neither deformity nor death is common.

Bennhoff DF: Actinomycosis: Diagnostic and therapeutic considerations and a review of 32 cases. Laryngoscope 94:1198, 1984. *A general review.*

Bernardi RS: Abdominal actinomycosis. Surg Gynecol Obstet 149:257, 1979. *A thorough review of all aspects of actinomycosis, with emphasis on the abdominal form.*

Cisar JO, Sandberg AL, Clark WB: Molecular aspects of adherence of *Actinomyces viscosus* and *Actinomyces naeslundii* to oral surfaces. J Dent Res 68 (special issue) :1558, 1989. *A brief summary for those wishing to know more about adherence mechanisms.*

Evans DTP: *Actinomyces israelii* in the female genital tract: A review. Genitourin Med 69:54, 1993. *An up-to-date summary.*

Flynn MW, Felson B: The roentgen manifestations of thoracic actinomycosis. AJR 110:707, 1970. *An outstanding guide to roentgenographic diagnosis of pulmonary actinomycosis.*

Richtsmeier WJ, Johns ME: Actinomycosis of the head and neck. CRC Crit Rev Clin Lab Sci 11:175, 1979. *An excellent review, with an emphasis on infection of the head and neck.*

Smego RA Jr: Actinomycosis of the central nervous system. Rev Infect Dis 9:855, 1987. *A good review of 70 cases of CNS actinomycosis.*

307 NOCARDIOSIS
Ward E. Bullock

DEFINITION. Nocardiosis is a subacute or chronic bacterial infection that evokes a suppurative response. The most common sites of primary infection are, first, the lung and then the skin, from which bacteria may disseminate hematogenously to the central nervous system (CNS) and other tissues. The infection often pursues a more acute and aggressive course in immunosuppressed patients.

ETIOLOGY. The nocardiae are gram-positive, aerobic actinomycetes, many of which are weakly acid fast in tissue or on initial isolation. They reproduce by filamentous branching, with fragmentation into bacillary and coccoid forms. *Nocardia* species are distributed widely in nature and commonly are found in soil, grasses, and rotting vegetation. Of the species that cause most infections in humans, *N. asteroides* is by far the predominant pathogen. *N. caviae*, *N. farcinica*, *N. transvalensis,* and *N. brasiliensis* also produce pulmonary and disseminated infections, but much less frequently. *N. brasiliensis* is the most common cause of actinomycetoma in Latin and South America.

INCIDENCE AND PREVALENCE. A 1976 survey estimated the incidence of nocardiosis in the United States to be 500 to 1000 new cases per year. At present, the incidence undoubtedly is higher as a consequence of an expanding population of people who are immunosuppressed iatrogenically or by underlying diseases. Nocardiosis has been reported worldwide in all ages and races and is two to three times more common in men than in women. No occupational related risks have been found. Thus possible hormonal effects on bacterial growth or virulence have been postulated.

EPIDEMIOLOGY. The majority of infections caused by *N. asteroides* occur in patients with impaired cell-mediated immunity (CMI). However, the organism clearly is capable of infecting apparently normal persons. Nocardiosis presumably is acquired by inhaling airborne bacteria, since the primary site of infection is the lung in the majority of cases. Other mammals can be infected. However, no well-established evidence exists for animal-to-person transmission or for person-to-person transmission. Occasional clusters of nocardial infection have been reported among immunosuppressed hospital patients, suggesting possible nosocomial acquisition. *N. asteroides* has been recovered from the sputum, skin, and other body regions of patients who do not have apparent disease. Nevertheless, repeated isolation of *Nocardia* species from any immunocompromised person should be considered evidence of infection rather than colonization, and treatment should be initiated. Nocardiosis can manifest as a primary cutaneous infection (especially *N. brasiliensis*) after inoculation through local injury and may disseminate to other organs.

PATHOGENESIS AND PATHOLOGY. The typical nocardial lesion within the lung and other tissues is one of liquefactive necrosis with abscess formation. Polymorphonuclear leukocytes predominate in association with varying proportions of macrophages and lymphocytes. Granuloma formation is infrequent, and in contrast with actinomycotic lesions, fibrosis is rare. Confluent daughter abscesses are common. Sulfur granules are not present in visceral lesions, as they are in actinomycosis. However, they may be seen in nocardial lesions of the skin.

That CMI plays a major role in host defense against nocardiosis is suggested by the fact that immunocompromised patients are prone to this infection. The importance of antigen-specific T lymphocyte immune function is illustrated by the increased susceptibility of athymic nude mice to *Nocardia* infection and by the capacity of T lymphocytes from rabbits immunized with *N. asteroides* to augment phagocytosis and growth inhibition of these organisms by macrophages. Neutrophils exhibit poor nocardicidal activity *in vitro* but may inhibit growth of organisms during an early phase of infection prior to maturation of cellular immune responses.

N. asteroides may counter host defenses by inhibiting the phagolysosome fusion that enables phagocytic cells to kill ingested bacteria, by producing superoxide dismutase and catalase, and by blocking the acidification of parasitized phagolysosomes.

Nocardia species are not visible in tissue specimens stained by hematoxylin and eosin or by the periodic acid–Schiff procedure. They can be visualized by a tissue Gram stain or after slight overstaining by the Gomori methenamine silver method, which demonstrates the filamentous structure of the organisms. Many *Nocardia* are weakly acid fast and can be seen on a modified Ziehl-Neelsen stain.

CLINICAL MANIFESTATIONS. Pulmonary infection is the most frequent manifestation of nocardiosis (about 75% of the reported cases). The clinical manifestations are nonspecific and include fever, cough, weight loss, and dyspnea. The range of pulmonary involvement extends from transient or inapparent infection to confluent bronchopneumonia with complete consolidation. Radiographic examination of the chest may reveal one or more of the following: fluffy infiltrates, multiple abscess formation with cavitation in 10 to 20% of cases, bulging fissures, masses, nodules, and empyema. Hilar involvement and calcification are infrequent. *Nocardia* can disseminate to other organs from pulmonary lesions, especially in patients who are immunosuppressed following organ transplantation and in individuals with the acquired immunodeficiency syndrome (AIDS). Patients who have received extensive x-irradiation and chemotherapy for malignancies and those treated with high-dosage steroids also are prone to metastatic infection, and evidence thereof should be sought aggressively.

In 20 to 40% of patients with pulmonary nocardiosis, dissemination to the CNS occurs, and therefore, computed tomographic (CT) scanning of the head should be considered. Loculated brain abscesses, either singular or multiple, are common and are often accompanied by headache and focal neurologic findings; meningitis is infrequent. Other common sites of dissemination include the skin and subcutaneous tissues, kidneys, eyes, liver, and lymph nodes. In cases of apparently localized nocardial lesions of skin, it is important to distinguish between the possibilities of primary inoculation and hematogenous dissemination to the skin from another site.

DIAGNOSIS. The clinical and radiographic findings in pulmonary nocardiosis are nonspecific. Consequently, it may be confused with a variety of other bacterial infections of the lung, including actinomycosis and tuberculosis, as well as fungal infections and malignancies. Alertness to the possibility of nocardiosis can expedite the diagnostic workup, especially in immunosuppressed patients, in whom the disease may coexist with other opportunistic infections. Cultures and stains should be done on specimens of sputum, pleural fluid, bronchial lavage fluid, as well as on percutaneous lung aspirates or open lung biopsy specimens. Needle biopsy of cerebral mass lesions should be considered strongly in patients with AIDS who have pulmonary nocardiosis because of the multiplicity of infections and tumors that can manifest in a similar manner.

Skin lesions should be aspirated if fluctuant or biopsied, and specimens should be submitted for culture and the smear preparations or histologic sections examined for organisms. Nocardiosis often can be diagnosed with a high degree of confidence by direct examination of sputum or purulent material. The presence of gram-positive, filamentous branching rods that stain unevenly with crystal violet to give a beaded appearance is highly suggestive of either *Actinomyces* or *Nocardia*. If the organisms are acid fast on a modified Ziehl-Neelsen stain, the probability of *Nocardia* is high. However, lack of acid-fast staining does not exclude *Nocardia*.

Nocardia species are not fastidious and grow aerobically, though slowly, on routinely used media. Characteristic heaped, waxy colonies, often colored tan, orange, or even purple, may be seen after 2 to 7 days of culture. Longer times may be required. Thus the microbiology laboratory should be advised of possible nocardiosis to ensure that plates are held for 10 to 14 days and that steps are taken to limit overgrowth by microbial contaminants, particularly in sputum samples. The use of defined carbon-free medium to which paraffin is added may enhance the chances of isolating *N. asteroides* from sputum because it can use paraffin as a sole source of carbon, in contrast to most other organisms. Several simple tests can assist in the presumptive differentiation of *Nocardia* from other aerobic actinomycetes and from rapidly growing *Mycobacteria*, as, for example, the decomposition of casein, xanthine, and tyrosine. However, most clinical laboratories should rely on reference facilities for definitive taxonomic designations.

TREATMENT. The sulfonamides are equally efficacious and are first-line agents for treatment, as is the combination of trimethoprim-sulfamethoxazole (TMP-SMX). The dosage of sulfadiazine is 6 to 10 grams per day given in three to six divided doses, with adjustment as needed to achieve peak serum levels of 12 to 15 mg per deciliter. Dosing schedules of TMP-SMX range from 160 mg/800 mg to 320 mg/1600 mg every 6 or 8 hours. These antimicrobials penetrate the CNS and other body compartments well. A high percentage of *Nocardia* isolates are sensitive to sulfonamides and to TMP-SMX by *in vitro* testing. However, the techniques of *in vitro* sensitivity testing with *Nocardia* have not been standardized, in part because of technical difficulties created by slow growth in culture and problems in obtaining a homogeneous suspension of cells for standardization of the inoculum. Thus the results of *in vitro* tests frequently are poor predictors of *in vivo* efficacy and should be interpreted with caution.

Not all patients respond to sulfonamide or TMP-SMX therapy. Resistance developed to the sulfonamides during therapy has been documented, and metastatic lesions can appear during the course of apparently successful treatment. Hypersensitivity reactions, nephrotoxicity, or hemopoietic toxicity induced by these drugs may force discontinuation of treatment, especially in renal transplant recipients receiving cyclosporine and in patients with AIDS. The alternative antibiotics that have proved to be most efficacious, both *in vitro* and clinically, are minocycline, amikacin, and imipenem. Ceftriaxone, cefuroxime, and cefotaxime display *in vitro* activity against many, but by no means all, clinical isolates of the *Nocardia* species. However, it remains to be determined if the last-named three antibiotics will prove valuable for treating nocardiosis. Although some *in vitro* studies indicate that certain combinations of antibiotics may exert synergistic activity against *Nocardia*, no good clinical evidence exists that combination antibiotic regimens are superior to single-agent therapy.

Treatment should be prolonged, since relapse of nocardiosis is common. In patients with intact host defenses, treatment should be continued for at least 6 weeks after clinical recovery. In those who have AIDS or who are otherwise immunocompromised, treatment should be continued for a year or more. As a rule, it is necessary to perform surgical drainage of brain abscesses, empyema, and subcutaneous abscesses. Patients with cerebral nocardiosis or other deep abscesses should be monitored by serial CT scans. If patients are receiving immunosuppressive drugs, the dosage should be reduced if at all possible.

PROGNOSIS. The prognosis for clinical cure of nocardiosis is influenced by the location of the infection, by pre-existing impairment of cellular immunity from underlying disease or drug therapy, and by the aggressiveness of the patient's management. Mortality rates range from near 0% in patients with isolated skin lesions to more than 40% in cases of CNS involvement. The overall mortality rate in patients with pulmonary disease is in the range of 15 to 30%, including those who are immunocompromised.

Barnicoat MJ, Wierzbicki AS, Norman PM: Cerebral nocardiosis in immunosuppressed patients: Five cases. Q J Med 268:689, 1989. *Presentation of five cases with a good bibliography on the topic.*

Javaly K, Horowitz HW, Wormser GP: Nocardiosis in patients with human immunodeficiency virus infection: Report of 2 cases and review of the literature. Medicine 71:128, 1992. *A current discussion of nocardial infection in AIDS patients.*

Palmer DL, Harvey RL, Wheeler JK: Diagnostic and therapeutic considerations in *Nocardia asteroides* infection. Medicine 53:391, 1974. *A comprehensive literature review of 243 cases of nocardiosis (including 13 patients in the authors' own experience).*

Smego RA Jr, Moeller MB, Gallis HA: Trimethoprim-sulfamethoxazole therapy for *Nocardia* infections. Arch Intern Med 143:711, 1983. *This article provides an extensive literature review and discusses TMP-SMX in depth.*

Wallace RJ Jr, Steele LC, Sumter G, et al.: Antimicrobial susceptibility patterns of *Nocardia asteroides*. Antimicrob Agents Chemother 32:1776, 1988. *An examination of antibiotic sensitivity patterns among 78 clinical isolates of N. asteroides by a group experienced in the complexities of* in vitro *sensitivity testing with these organisms.*

Wilson JP, Turner HR, Kirchner KA, et al.: Nocardial infections in renal transplant recipients. Medicine 68:38, 1989. *A well-written review of nocardiosis, with emphasis on disease manifestations in renal transplant patients.*

308 BRUCELLOSIS
Robert A. Salata

DEFINITION. Bacteria of the genus *Brucella* cause disease with protean manifestations. Infection is transmitted to humans from animals as a consequence of occupational exposure or ingestion of contaminated milk products. Despite the attempt to institute effective control measures, brucellosis remains a significant health and economic burden in many countries.

ETIOLOGY. Brucellae are slow-growing, small, aerobic, non-motile, nonencapsulated, non–spore-forming, gram-negative coccobacilli. *B. abortus, B. suis, B. melitensis,* and *B. canis* are known to infect humans and are typed on the basis of biochemical, metabolic, and immunologic criteria. There are differences in virulence among these four species. *B. abortus,* with a reservoir in cattle, usually is associated with mild sporadic disease; suppurative or disabling complications are rare. *B. suis* infection, resulting from swine contact, is often associated with destructive, suppurative lesions and may have a prolonged course. *B. melitensis,* with a reservoir in sheep and goats, may cause severe, acute disease and disabling complications. *B. canis,* spread to humans from infected dogs, causes disease with an insidious onset, frequent relapse, and a chronic course that is indistinguishable from infection related to *B. abortus.*

EPIDEMIOLOGY. Over 500,000 cases of brucellosis are reported yearly to the World Health Organization from 100 countries. *B. melitensis* infection, distributed primarily in the Mediterranean region (particularly Spain and Greece), Latin America, and Asia (with increased occurrences in Iraq and Kuwait), accounts for the majority of cases. *B. abortus* infection occurs worldwide but has been effectively eradicated in several European countries, Japan, and Israel. *B. suis* occurs mainly in the midwestern United States, South America, and Southeast Asia, whereas *B. canis* infection is most common in North and South America, Japan, and Central Europe.

In association with effective control programs in animals, human brucellosis has decreased dramatically in the United States, from over 6000 cases in 1947 to fewer than 200 cases since 1980. States reporting the greatest number of cases include Texas, California, Virginia, and Florida. In North America, brucellosis occurs mainly in spring and summer and is most common in adult males, usually related to occupational exposure.

Brucella infection in the United States most frequently occurs in high-risk groups, including slaughterhouse workers, farmers and dairymen, veterinarians, travelers to endemic areas, and laboratory workers handling the organisms. More than one half of reported cases occur in the meat-processing industry, particularly in the kill areas, where infection is spread through abraded or lacerated skin and the conjunctiva, possibly by aerosolization, and rarely by ingestion of infected tissue. Many cases of *B. abortus* infection in veterinarians have accidentally occurred from the strain 19 vaccine used to immunize cattle. *B. melitensis* infection, transmitted through the ingestion of goat's milk cheese, has been seen in United States travelers to and immigrants from Mexico.

Brucellosis in children accounts for only 3 to 10% of all reported cases worldwide, is common in endemic areas (may account for 20 to 25% of cases), and is often a mild, self-limited process. Infection occurs most frequently in school-age children and in familial outbreaks; no convincing evidence exists to associate *Brucella* infection with abortion in humans.

PATHOGENESIS AND IMMUNITY. After penetrating the epithelial cells of human skin, conjunctiva, pharynx, or lung, *Brucella* organisms initially induce an exuberant polymorphonuclear neutrophil response in the submucosa. Following ingestion of organisms by neutrophils and tissue macrophages, spread to regional lymph nodes occurs. If host defenses within the lymph nodes are overwhelmed, bacteremia follows. The usual incubation period between infection and bacteremia is 1½ to 3 weeks. Bacteremia is accompanied by phagocytosis of free *Brucella* organisms by neu-

trophils and localization of bacteria primarily to the spleen, liver, and bone marrow, with the formation of granulomas.

If the inoculum is large and the patient is untreated, large granulomas may form, suppurate, and serve as a source of persistent bacteremia with the potential for multiorgan spread.

Both virulent and attenuated strains of *Brucella* are readily phagocytized by neutrophils after opsonization with normal human serum. Whole bacteria and extracts of *Brucella* species may inhibit neutrophil oxidative burst activity and degranulation. Intracellular killing of ingested bacteria has been demonstrated with *B. abortus* but not *B. melitensis;* this may explain differences in pathogenicity between these species.

Humoral factors may be important in the host defense against *Brucella.* Even in the absence of specific agglutinating antibody, normal human serum is bactericidal for *Brucella* organisms; *B. abortus* is more susceptible to serum lysis than is *B. melitensis.* The intracellular location of the organism may provide a means for the bacteria to escape the lethal effects of serum. Specific serum agglutinating antibody has opsonic activity but does not correlate with the development of protective immunity.

A role for mononuclear phagocytes and cell-mediated immunity in brucellosis has been demonstrated. Protection against *Brucella* infection in animals is associated with preceding infection with *Listeria monocytogenes* or *Mycobacterium tuberculosis,* both of which stimulate cell-mediated immune mechanisms. Skin testing with *Brucella* proteins elicits a typical delayed hypersensitivity response in infected individuals. Macrophages, activated with lymphokines, kill *Brucella in vitro.* In some cases of chronic brucellosis, depressed proliferative responses to classic T-cell mitogens or to *Brucella* antigen occur.

CLINICAL MANIFESTATIONS. Clinically, human brucellosis may be conveniently divided into subclinical illness, acute/subacute disease, localized disease and complications, relapsing infection, and chronic disease (Table 308–1).

Subclinical Illness. Detected only by serologic testing, asymptomatic or clinically unrecognized human brucellosis often occurs in high-risk groups, including slaughterhouse workers, farmers, and veterinarians. More than 50% of abattoir workers and up to 33% of veterinarians have high anti-*Brucella* antibody titers but no history of recognized clinical infection. Children in endemic areas frequently have subclinical illness.

Acute and Subacute Disease. After an incubation period of several weeks or months, acute brucellosis may occur as a mild, transient illness (with *B. abortus* or *B. canis*) or as an explosive, toxic illness with the potential for multiple complications (with *B. melitensis*). Approximately 50% of patients have an abrupt onset over days, while the remainder have an insidious onset over weeks. Symptoms in brucellosis are protean and nonspecific. More than 90% of patients experience malaise, chills, sweats, fatigue, and weakness. More than 50% of patients have myalgias, anorexia, and weight loss. Fewer patients complain of arthralgias, cough, testicular pain, dysuria, ocular pain, or visual blurring. Likewise, few localizing physical signs are apparent. Fever, often >39.4°C (103°F), occurs in 95%. An undulating or intermittent fever pattern is unusual. A relative pulse-temperature deficit may occur. Splenomegaly is present in 10 to 15%, lymphadenopathy occurs in up to 14% (axillary, cervical, and supraclavicular locations are most frequent, related to hand-wound or oropharyngeal routes of infection); hepatomegaly is less frequent. Other laboratory findings in acute or subacute disease may include mild anemia, lymphopenia or neutropenia (especially with bacteremia), lymphocytosis, thrombocytopenia, or (rarely) pancytopenia. The majority of infected individuals recover completely without sequelae if the diagnosis is appropriately made and prompt therapy is initiated.

Localized Disease and Complications. *Brucella* organisms may localize in almost any organ, most commonly in bone, joints, central nervous system (CNS), heart, lung, spleen, testes, liver, gallbladder, kidney, prostate, and skin. Localized disease may occur simultaneously at multiple sites. Localized complications most often appear in association with a more chronic course of illness, although complications may occur with acute disease due to *B. melitensis* or *B. suis.* In the United States, localized disease is most frequently related to *B. suis.*

Relapsing Infection. Up to 10% of patients with brucellosis relapse after antimicrobial therapy. This probably results from the intracellular location of the organisms, which protects the bacteria

TABLE 308–1. CLINICAL CLASSIFICATION OF HUMAN BRUCELLOSIS

	Duration of Symptoms Before Diagnosis	Major Symptoms and Signs	Diagnosis	Comments
Subclinical	—	Asymptomatic	Positive (low titer) serology, negative cultures	Occurs in abattoir workers, farmers, and veterinarians
Acute and subacute	Up to 2–3 mo and 3 mo to 1 yr	Malaise, chills, sweats, fatigue, headache, anorexia, arthralgias, fever, splenomegaly, lymphadenopathy, hepatomegaly	Positive serology, positive blood or bone marrow cultures	Presentation can be mild, self-limited (B. abortus), or fulminant with severe complications (B. melitensis)
Localized	Occurs with acute or chronic untreated disease	Related to involved organs	Positive serology, positive cultures in specific tissues	Bone/joint, genitourinary, hepatosplenic involvement most common
Relapsing	2–3 mo after initial episode	Same as acute illness but may have higher fever, more fatigue, weakness, chills, and sweats	Positive serology, positive cultures	May be extremely difficult to distinguish relapse from reinfection
Chronic	Longer than 1 yr	Nonspecific presentation but neuropsychiatric symptoms and low-grade fever most common	Low titer or negative serology, cultures negative	Most controversial classification; localized disease may be associated

from certain antibiotics and host defense mechanisms. Relapses occur most frequently within months after initial infection but may occur as long as 2 years after apparently successful treatment. Relapsing infection is difficult to distinguish from reinfection in high-risk groups with continued exposure.

Chronic Disease. Disease with a duration >1 year has been called chronic brucellosis. A majority of patients classified as having chronic brucellosis really have persistent disease caused by inadequate treatment of the initial episode, or they have focal disease in bone, liver, or spleen. About 20% of patients diagnosed as having chronic brucellosis complain of persistent fatigue, malaise, and depression; in many aspects this condition resembles the chronic fatigue syndrome. These symptoms frequently are not associated with clinical, microbiologic, or serologic evidence of active infection.

DIAGNOSIS. Many more common illnesses mimic the clinical presentation of brucellosis. The most conclusive means of establishing the diagnosis of brucellosis is by positive cultures from normally sterile body fluids or tissues. Isolation of the organism can be enhanced by use of special media. The culture of Brucella organisms is potentially hazardous to laboratory personnel. Therefore, most cases of brucellosis are diagnosed by serologic testing.

In acute brucellosis, positive blood cultures are obtained in 10 to 30% of cases (as high as 85% with B. melitensis). Blood culture positivity decreases with increasing duration of illness. With B. melitensis infection, bone marrow cultures are of higher yield than are blood cultures. Blood cultures processed in radiometric detection or isolator systems may yield positive cultures in <10 days. With localized brucellosis (e.g., lymph nodes, spleen, liver, or skeletal system), cultures of purulent material or tissues usually yield Brucella organisms. Culture of cerebrospinal fluid is positive in 45% of patients with meningitis. Antibody against Brucella may be demonstrated in cerebrospinal fluid by enzyme-linked immunosorbent assay (ELISA).

Most patients mount significant serologic responses to Brucella infections. The most frequently used test is the standard tube agglutination (STA) test, measuring antibody to B. abortus antigen. A fourfold or greater rise in titer to 1:160 or higher is considered significant. A presumptive case is one in which the agglutination titer is positive ($\geq$ 1:160) in single or serial specimens, with symptoms consistent with brucellosis. By 3 weeks of illness, >97% of patients demonstrate serologic evidence of infection. This test equally detects antibodies to B. abortus, B. suis, and B. melitensis, but not to B. canis. Serologic confirmation of B. canis infection requires B. canis or B. ovis antigen. Despite adequate antibiotic treatment, significant STA titers can persist for up to 2 years in 5 to 7% of cases. Because the STA titer may remain elevated, it is not useful in differentiating relapsing infection from other febrile illnesses in patients with past Brucella infections. Individuals with subclinical infection may demonstrate significant STA titers. In chronic localized brucellosis, STA titers may appear absent or low owing to a prozone phenomenon. This prozone effect appears to be related to the presence of immunoglobulin G (IgG) or immunoglobulin A (IgA) blocking antibodies; it can be eliminated if dilutions are carried out to at least 1:1280. False-positive STA titers due to immunologic cross-reactivity have been associated with Brucella skin testing, cholera vaccination, or infections due to Vibrio cholerae, Francisella tularensis, or Yersinia enterocolitica.

Immunoglobulin M (IgM) is the major agglutinating antibody formed in the first few weeks following infection with Brucella organisms. Thereafter, IgG levels also rise. The STA test measures both IgM and IgG. With prompt and adequate therapy, IgG antibody levels usually become undetectable after 6 to 12 months. If therapy is given, those patients who develop persistent Brucella infection usually maintain elevated IgG agglutinins. In the absence of rising STA titers, a single elevated 2-ME Brucella agglutination titer ($\geq$ 1:160) suggests either current or recent infection. Certain

TABLE 308–2. TREATMENT FOR BRUCELLOSIS

	Treatment	Comments
Acute With no endocarditis or CNS involvement	Doxycycline (200 mg/day) plus rifampin (600 to 900 mg/day) for 6 weeks	Treatment of choice by World Health Organization
	Tetracycline, streptomycin, chloramphenicol, rifampin, trimethoprim-sulfamethoxazole	Combination therapy indicated
	Fluoroquinolones, imipenem, and a variety of antimicrobial combinations	Being evaluated in trials
	Tetracycline (2 grams/day) for 6 weeks plus streptomycin (1 gram/day) for 3 weeks	Widely used; low rate of relapse; intramuscular administration of streptomycin may be difficult
In children	Trimethoprim-sulfamethoxazole	
CNS	Third-generation cephalosporin with rifampin	
Localized	Surgically drain abscesses plus antimicrobial therapy for 6 or more weeks	
Brucella endocarditis	Bactericidal drugs; early valve replacement may be necessary	Possible aortic valve destruction and/or major arterial emboli

newer antibody tests, including an ELISA and radioimmunoassay, are more sensitive than the STA; these methods have not been widely employed, and agglutination tests remain the standard for serologic diagnosis.

TREATMENT. Antibiotic treatment of *Brucella* infections is complicated by a number of complex issues, including the requirement for antibiotics that penetrate intracellularly, for prolonged therapy to prevent relapse, and for bactericidal antibiotics in treating CNS infection and endocarditis, as well as the lack of controlled, randomized, double-blind studies comparing different antimicrobial regimens. Debate is still considerable regarding which antibiotic regimens are clearly superior. Current recommendations are given in Table 308–2.

PROGNOSIS. Brucellosis appropriately treated within the first month of symptom onset is curable. Acute brucellosis often produces severe weakness and fatigue, and patients are frequently unable to work for up to 2 months. Immunity to reinfection follows initial *Brucella* infection in the majority of individuals. With early antimicrobial therapy, cases of chronic brucellosis or localized disease and complications are rare. Of patients who die of brucellosis, 84% have endocarditis involving a previously abnormal aortic valve, often associated with severe congestive heart failure.

PREVENTION. The control of human brucellosis relates directly to prevention programs in domestic animals and avoiding unpasteurized milk and milk products. In slaughterhouses, important means of prevention include careful wound dressing, protective glasses and clothing, prohibition of raw meat ingestion, and the use of previously infected (immune) individuals in high-risk areas.

Akova M, Uzun O, Akalin E, et al.: Quinolones in the treatment of human brucellosis: Comparative trial of ofloxacin-rifampin versus doxycycline-rifampin. Antimicrob Agents Chemother 37:1831, 1993. *The quinolone-rifampin combination was as effective as doxycycline plus rifampin regardless of the complications of the disease.*

Ariza J, Pujol M, Valverde J, et al.: Brucella sacroiliitis: Findings in 63 episodes and current relevance. Clin Infect Dis 16:761, 1993. *Epidemiologic, clinical, diagnostic, and treatment aspects of sacroiliitis reviewed over a 15-year period in Spain suggest that a mild disease exists with a good outcome similar to uncomplicated brucellosis.*

Buchanan TM, Faber LC, Feldman RA: Brucellosis in the United States, 1960–1972: An abattoir-associated disease. I. Clinical features and therapy. Buchanan TM, Sulzer CR, Frix MK, et al.: II. Diagnostic aspects. Buchanan TM, Hendricks SL, Patton CM, et al.: III. Epidemiology and evidence for acquired immunity. Medicine 53:403, 415, 427, 1974. *A very complete description of all aspects of brucellosis derived from a study of 160 patients in a large Iowa slaughterhouse.*

Gazapo E, Gonzalez Lahoz J, Subiza JL, et al.: Changes in IgM and IgG antibody concentrations in brucellosis over time: Importance for diagnosis and follow-up. J Infect Dis 159:219, 1989. *Patterns of antibody responses correlating with successful treatment, chronic disease, or drug relapses and failures were followed prospectively and proved clinically useful.*

Hall WH: Modern chemotherapy for brucellosis in humans. Rev Infect Dis 12:1060, 1990. *A comprehensive analysis of the world's literature related to therapy of brucellosis that stresses that prolonged combined chemotherapy in conjunction with surgery, where indicated, is the key to successful treatment.*

309 CAT SCRATCH DISEASE AND BACILLARY ANGIOMATOSIS

David A. Relman

Cat scratch disease and bacillary angiomatosis are manifestations of infection by members of the *Bartonella* genus (formerly the *Rochalimaea* genus). Cat scratch disease has been traditionally defined on the basis of a history of intimate cat exposure, the presence of an inoculation site lesion, local or regional (granulomatous) lymphadenitis, and a positive cat scratch antigen skin test. Bacillary angiomatosis involves skin and visceral sites with angioproliferative lesions whose gross appearance may be confused with that of Kaposi's sarcoma. Despite the two different histopathologic pictures, *Bartonella (Rochalimaea) henselae* causes both cat scratch disease and bacillary angiomatosis; *B. quintana* also can cause bacillary angiomatosis.

ETIOLOGY

In 1983, small pleomorphic weakly gram-negative but strongly argyrophilic bacilli were first described in cat scratch disease and bacillary angiomatosis tissues. An organism was subsequently cultivated from a small number of cat scratch disease lymph nodes on artificial media and on tissue culture cells, and was named *Afipia felis*. However, this organism and its DNA have not been detected often or consistently in patients with this disease; hence, the clinical significance of *A. felis* is in question. In 1990, a different bacillus was identified within tissues from patients with bacillary angiomatosis. Phylogenetic analysis revealed a novel *Rochalimaea* species: *R. henselae.* The close evolutionary relationships among the *Rochalimaea* and *Bartonella bacilliformis* (the cause of another human angioproliferative disease, verruga peruana; see Ch. 310), have led to a proposal to transfer all of the former *Rochalimaea* species to the *Bartonella* genus (Fig. 309–1). *B. henselae* and *B. quintana* (the etiologic agent of trench fever; see Ch. 324) have each been cultivated directly from and detected in tissues affected by bacillary angiomatosis. The relative importance of *B. henselae* and *B. quintana* in the causation of this disease is unclear.

A variety of data strongly incriminate *B. henselae* as an etiologic agent of cat scratch disease, as well as bacillary angiomatosis. Approximately 84 to 88% of patients who meet traditional diagnostic criteria for cat scratch disease demonstrate a significant elevation of serum IgG antibodies directed against *B. henselae;* approximately 20% of asymptomatic cat owners and 3 to 4% of the general population have elevated titers. In addition, *B. henselae* antigens and DNA can be detected in tissues from these patients with the polymerase chain reaction (PCR) and *in situ* immunohistochemistry. *B. henselae* DNA has been amplified from cat scratch antigen preparations. Finally, *B. henselae* has been cultivated from blood and tissues of patients with cat scratch disease. However, Koch's postulates have not been fulfilled for this organism, and a role for organisms other than *B. henselae* and *B. quintana* in either cat scratch disease or bacillary angiomatosis has not been ruled out.

B. henselae is a slightly curved, small (0.5×1 to 2 mm), self-aggregating, gram-negative bacillus that is capable of twitching motility. Optimal growth occurs on enriched media supplemented with 5% sheep or rabbit blood, at 35°C in a 5 to 10% CO_2 humified atmosphere. Colonies become visible after 9 to 15 days of primary culture (two different morphologies), and after 3 to 5 days on subsequent laboratory passage. *B. quintana* grows under similar conditions, especially after co-cultivation with endothelial cell monolayers. Species identification requires using specific antisera,

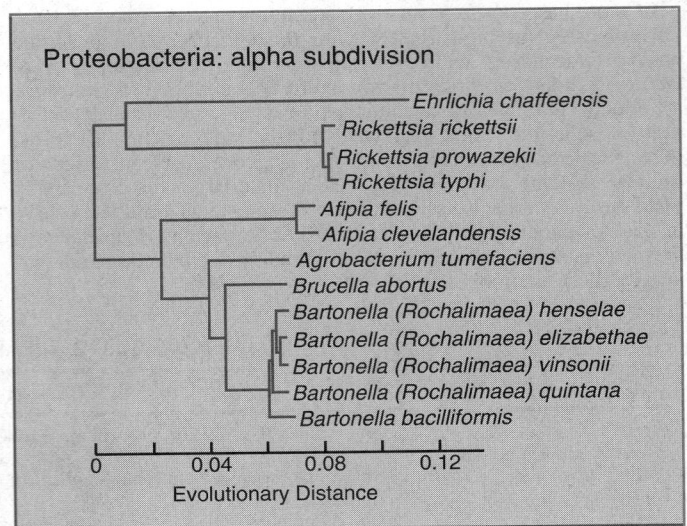

FIGURE 309–1. Phylogenetic relationships among the alpha-proteobacteria, based upon small subunit ribosomal RNA sequence analysis. Many of these organisms are endosymbiotic, and may have evolved in close association with insects or plants. Evolutionary distance is proportional to the length of horizontal line segments, and is expressed as the number of nucleotide substitutions per sequence position. (Modified from Mandell GL, Bennett JE, Dolin R [eds.]: Principles and Practice of Infectious Diseases. New York, Churchill Livingstone, 1995.)

cellular fatty acid profiles, or DNA polymorphism or sequence analysis.

EPIDEMIOLOGY

Cat scratch disease affects approximately 22,000 persons in the United States per year. The highest incidence of the disease occurs in the 5- through 14-year-old age group, and in the South. The incidence and prevalence of bacillary angiomatosis are unknown. Approximately 90% of individuals with this disease are co-infected with HIV or are otherwise immunocompromised.

Intimate or traumatic cat contacts are among the strongest risk factors for acquiring cat scratch disease and bacillary angiomatosis. In one study, 41% of cats had *B. henselae* bacteremia. Bacteremia is detected more often in younger cats, is asymptomatic, and may persist for the animal's lifetime. *B. quintana* has not been detected in cats, and cat exposure is uncommon among bacillary angiomatosis patients that are infected with this species. Unlike *B. quintana*-infected human body lice and the transmission of trench fever, it is uncertain whether arthropods play a role in either cat scratch disease or bacillary angiomatosis. Fewer than 5% of cases of cat scratch disease belong to a family cluster.

PATHOLOGY AND PATHOGENESIS

Histologic changes in lymph nodes evolve over a period of months in patients with cat scratch disease. Follicular hyperplasia and hypertrophy, and sinus histiocytosis and B cell proliferation are followed by granuloma formation and later by neutrophilic infiltration with central or stellate necrosis, and surrounding palisades of histiocytes. Microabscesses are common. Bacilli are best visualized with the Warthin-Starry silver impregnation stain early in the course of the disease.

The lesions of bacillary angiomatosis assume diverse macroscopic appearances, including an erythematous, polypoid or papular, cutaneous or mucosal pattern; deeply erythematous and indurated dermal plaques; and subcutaneous or visceral nodules. In all of these lesions, a distinctive lobular proliferation of capillaries is seen within a fibrous stroma. Hematoxylin and eosin reveal granular amphophilic material in the interstitium between vessels. This material corresponds to clumps of extracellular bacteria, as viewed with the Warthin-Starry silver stain or with electron microscopy. Bacillary peliosis is a histologic variant form of bacillary angiomatosis that is characterized by blood-filled cystic spaces, fibromyxoid stroma, and inflammatory cells; it is also associated with *B. henselae* and occurs most often within the liver and spleen.

CLINICAL MANIFESTATIONS

After an incubation period of 3 to 10 days, an erythematous papule develops at the inoculation site in more than half of those later diagnosed with cat scratch disease. These lesions may form a crust or become pustular; they resolve spontaneously in 1 to 3 weeks. Within a few weeks of inoculation, regional lymphadenopathy becomes apparent; usually a lymph node in the axillary or neck regions is found to be enlarged and tender (Table 309–1). Low-grade fever, malaise, anorexia, and nausea each occur in a minority of patients. Infrequently, inoculation of the eye results in a granulomatous lesion of the conjunctiva and in preauricular adenopathy, a condition known as the oculoglandular syndrome of Parinaud (4 to

6% of cat scratch disease patients). In a typical case of cat scratch disease, lymph nodes remain enlarged for at least 2 to 4 months.

Severe or systemic manifestations are reported in 2% of cat scratch disease patients, excluding those involving the central nervous system. These include persistent fever, weight loss, splenomegaly, diffuse papular rash, erythema nodosum, pleuritis, splenic abscess, central lymphadenopathy, osteolytic lesions, hepatitis, and thrombocytopenic purpura. An additional 2% of cat scratch disease patients experience neurologic complications. Encephalopathy or encephalitis are most common; other presentations include radiculitis, meningitis, cranial neuritis, neuroretinitis, and cerebral arteritis. Neurologic complications occur 2 to 3 weeks after onset of the initial illness.

Bacillary angiomatosis is most often manifested clinically by tender cutaneous or subcutaneous lesions. Mucosal lesions are also common. These lesions may be solitary or multiple, red, purple, or flesh-colored dome-shaped papules, nodules, polypoid tumors, or plaques. With age the lesions may ulcerate, form a crust, or develop a collarette of scale. Subcutaneous lesions sometimes erode underlying bone. In an undetermined percentage of cases, visceral bacillary angiomatosis occurs, sometimes in the absence of cutaneous disease. Visceral involvement may be asymptomatic or, as in disseminated cutaneous disease, may be associated with fever, chills, malaise, and anorexia. Liver, spleen, and internal lymph nodes appear to be the most frequent sites of extracutaneous disease. Biliary obstruction has resulted from external compression of periportal lymph nodes. Other sites affected by bacillary angiomatosis include bone marrow, lung, and brain.

A syndrome of *B. henselae* or *B. quintana* bacteremia has been reported sporadically in widespread regions of the United States. Signs of sepsis or localized (granulomatous or angioproliferative) disease are uncommon. Fever, headache, myalgias, and arthralgias may persist or recur over a period of weeks to months, despite therapy. Alcoholism and malnutrition characterize some urban clusters of *B. quintana* bacteremic disease. In addition, *B. henselae*, *B. quintana*, and *B. elizabethae* are reported agents of infective endocarditis. *B. henselae* is associated with lymphocytic meningitis.

DIAGNOSIS

The diagnosis of cat scratch disease and bacillary angiomatosis rests upon tissue examination and serologic tests in a compatible clinical setting. Typical histology in a hematoxylin and eosin-stained tissue is suggestive. Warthin-Starry stains will usually confirm a diagnosis of bacillary angiomatosis, and may confirm a diagnosis of cat scratch disease (i.e., reveal clumps of small, pleomorphic bacilli). Commercial laboratories, as well as the Centers for Disease Control and Prevention, offer an immunofluorescent or enzyme-linked immunosorbent assay for serum IgG antibodies directed against *B. henselae* and *B. quintana*. Most current assays do not distinguish between these species. Cultivation of *Bartonella (Rochalimaea)* and detection of specific genetic sequences by PCR or antigens by immunohistochemical methods are technically demanding and may currently exceed the capabilities of most clinical microbiology laboratories.

The differential diagnosis for localized cat scratch disease may include pyogenic lymphadenitis, mycobacterial infection, tularemia, brucellosis, lymphogranuloma venereum, syphilis, fungal disease, toxoplasmosis, and Epstein-Barr or Cytomegalovirus infection. Kaposi's sarcoma is the most important entity confused with bacillary angiomatosis. Visual detection of bacilli distinguishes the latter from the former. Lytic bone lesions in an HIV-infected individual should raise the possibility of bacillary angiomatosis because they are otherwise uncommon.

TREATMENT

Most patients with cat scratch disease do not require more than symptomatic support. A fluctuant or suppurative lymph node may benefit from needle aspiration. Antibiotic therapy should be reserved for immunocompromised individuals or those with evidence of severe or systemic disease. Because nearly all persons with bacillary angiomatosis fit into one of these latter categories, antibiotics should be routinely offered. *Bartonella (Rochalimaea)* bacteremia in the absence of localization also deserves antibiotic therapy.

TABLE 309–1. SELECTED CLINICAL FEATURES OF CLASSICAL CAT SCRATCH DISEASE

Feature	% of Cases
Site of lymphadenopathy	
Axilla	25–52
Neck	26–39
Groin	7–18
Elbow	2–13
Preauricular	5–7
Single node involvement	43–85
Lymphadenopathy only	48–51
Fever	31–48
Splenomegaly	11–12
Hospitalization	9–17

TABLE 309–2. TREATMENT SUGGESTIONS

Severe Cat Scratch Disease*

Trimethoprim-sulfamethoxasole	160–320 mg (TMP component) bid
Rifampin	300 mg bid
Ciprofloxacin	500 mg bid
Gentamicin sulfate	5 mg/kg qd

Bacillary Angiomatosis
B. henselae or B. quintana Bacteremia†

Erythromycin	250–500 mg qid
Doxycycline	100 mg bid
Azithromycin (anecdotal)	1 gram qd

* Treat for 7–14 days.
† Treat for at least 4 weeks; some patients may require more prolonged or lifelong treatment.

There are no data from prospective randomized studies to help a physician choose an antimicrobial regimen for cat scratch disease or bacillary angiomatosis. Nevertheless, in vitro susceptibility testing and retrospective or empiric clinical observations offer the basis for the suggested approaches in Table 309–2. Corticosteroids are not recommended for either disease.

Adal KA, Cockerell CJ, Petri WA: Cat scratch disease, bacillary angiomatosis, and other infections due to Rochalimaea. N Engl J Med 330:1509, 1994. Useful review of a rapidly evolving field. Emphasizes clinical features and microbiology. Contains helpful color photographs.

Koehler JE, Quinn FD, Berger TG, et al.: Isolation of rochalimaea species from cutaneous and osseous lesions of bacillary angiomatosis. N Engl J Med 327:1625, 1992. First isolation of R. henselae directly from lesions of bacillary angiomatosis, and first definitive association of R. quintana with this clinical syndrome. Excellent photographs.

Koehler JE, Glaser CA, Tappero JW: Rochalimaea henselae infection: A new zoonosis with the domestic cat as reservoir. JAMA 271:531, 1994. The first definitive demonstration that R. henselae bacteremia is common in asymptomatic domestic cats! Even though cat fleas were implicated, the mechanism(s) of R. henselae transmission from the cat reservoir to humans is presumed to be direct inoculation.

Margileth AM: Antibiotic therapy for cat scratch disease: Clinical study of therapeutic outcome in 268 patients and a review of the literature. Pediatr Infect Dis J 11:474, 1992. A large retrospective study of antibiotic efficacy in patients with classical (lymphadenopathic) cat scratch disease.

Relman DA, Loutit JS, Schmidt TM, et al.: The agent of bacillary angiomatosis: An approach to the identification of uncultured pathogens. N Engl J Med 323:1573, 1990. Describes the first clinical application of a molecular approach for identifying fastidious or uncultivated microbial pathogens directly from infected host tissue. The results of this study suggested a close relationship between the agent(s) of bacillary angiomatosis and R. quintana.

310 BARTONELLOSIS
C. Glenn Cobbs

DEFINITION. Bartonellosis (Carrión's disease) is an insect-borne bacterial disorder characterized by two well-defined clinical stages. It has a striking geographic restriction, occurring only on the western coast of South America at altitude. The first stage, Oroya fever, and the latter cutaneous stage, verruga peruana, were recognized in the nineteenth century. The common bacterial etiology of the two stages was established in 1885 when Daniel Carrión, a Peruvian medical student, died of acute hemolytic anemia 39 days after self-inoculation with material from a verruga lesion.

ETIOLOGY. In 1909, Barton described the causative microorganism, Bartonella bacilliformis, a small motile pleomorphic bacillus that requires enriched media for growth. It appears from recent genetic sequence analyses that B. bacilliformis is closely related to Rochalimaea quintana and Rochalimaea henselae, bacteria implicated in trench fever, bacillary angiomatosis, and cat scratch disease.

EPIDEMIOLOGY. Bartonellosis is generally restricted to the habitat of its main vector, the sandfly, Phlebotomus verrucarum,

which breeds and transmits the infection in river valleys of the Andes Mountains at an altitude between 2500 and 9000 feet. Humans provide the only known reservoir of the microorganism. Convalescent individuals may have low-grade bacteremia for months to years after infection, and B. bacilliformis may be recovered from 5 to 10% of apparently healthy persons in an endemic area. These carriers present the greatest transmission threat.

PATHOLOGY AND PATHOGENESIS. After inoculation by the vector, bacteria replicate, adhere to, and invade erythrocytes and endothelial cells. Red cell parasitization results in increased fragility and increased phagocytosis by the reticuloendothelial system. In severe cases, as many as 90% of the circulating erythrocytes may be parasitized. The ensuing hemolytic anemia causes fever, anemia, and weakness. Peripheral blood smears reveal a normochromic macrocytosis, striking polychromasia, Howell-Jolly bodies, Cabot rings, and nucleated erythrocytes, as well as the intracellular bacteria. The Coombs test and other assays for red cell agglutinins and hemolysins are usually negative. Reactive hyperplasia of lymphatic tissue is common.

Most untreated patients who survive the acute hemolytic episode go on to develop the chronic cutaneous lesions of verruga peruana. These hemangiomatous nodules consist of proliferating small vessels infiltrated by lymphocytes and macrophages and bear a distinct resemblance, clinically and histologically, to the lesions of bacillary angiomatosis (see Ch. 309). Verrugas also may occur in viscera, bone, and central nervous system.

CLINICAL MANIFESTATIONS. Within 2 to 6 weeks after the bite of an infected sandfly, the nonimmune host develops Oroya fever, characterized by the insidious onset of myalgias and low-grade fever, followed by high fever, headache, and painful muscles and joints. Tender lymphadenopathy is common, but splenomegaly is rare unless secondary infection is present. Anemia occurs rapidly, and the combination of anemia and jaundice results in a lemon color in light-skinned patients. In some, the disease is characterized by a febrile crisis, followed by rapid resolution of symptoms and signs, increased erythropoiesis, and gradual reduction in fever. Recurrence of fever after initial improvement suggests secondary infection. Salmonella disease is an especially important complication of bartonellosis, as it is of other hemolytic disorders.

After the febrile hemolytic anemia has resolved, immunity develops, and relapses of that syndrome are unusual. Following a latent period, which ranges in untreated patients from weeks to months, many patients manifest the second stage of bartonellosis, verruga peruana. This disorder is characterized by 1- to 2-cm reddish purple hemangiomatous nodules that typically evolve over 1 to 2 months in crops on exposed skin but also on mucous membranes and internal organs. The lesions are usually nontender and morphologically may vary, appearing as ulcers or secondarily infected pustules. The verrugas may persist for months to years in untreated patients.

DIAGNOSIS. The diagnosis is made by examining the peripheral blood film. There bacilli may be seen within red cells, either singly or in pairs or clusters. With a Giemsa stain, the bacilli appear as 0.3- to 1.5-μm red or reddish purple rods with some pleomorphism. The microorganism may be cultured from blood if appropriate media are used. It is difficult to identify the microorganisms in the verrucal lesion.

PROGNOSIS AND TREATMENT. Mortality in untreated Oroya fever approaches 50% and is a result of acute hemolytic anemia or secondary infectious disorders, e.g., Salmonella disease. Malaria, amebiasis, and tuberculosis also appear to be more common in these patients. Penicillin, chloramphenicol, and possibly tetracycline or streptomycin all appear to be effective. Because of the likelihood of associated Salmonella disease, chloramphenicol, at a dose of 2 to 4 grams daily for at least 7 days, is the therapy of choice. In patients so treated, fever generally disappears within 2 to 3 days, although blood smears may remain positive for some time longer. Verruga peruana may require more prolonged therapy.

PREVENTION. Insecticides are of use in eradicating the vector.

O'Connor SP, Dorsch M, Steigerwalt AG, et al.: 16S rRNA sequences of Bartonella bacilliformis and cat scratch disease bacillus reveal phylogenetic relationships with the alpha-2 subgroup of the class Proteobacteria. J Clin Microbiol 29:2144, 1991.

Schultz MG: A history of bartonellosis (Carrión's disease). Am J Trop Med Hyg 17:503, 1980. A fascinating summary of the initial historical accounts, medical descriptions, and investigations into the etiology and epidemiology of the disease.

311 TUBERCULOSIS
Michael D. Iseman

DEFINITION. Tuberculosis is an infectious disease caused by *Mycobacterium tuberculosis.* Characteristic features include a generally prolonged latency period between initial infection and overt disease, prominent pulmonary disease (although other organs can be involved), and a granulomatous response associated with intense tissue inflammation and damage.

ETIOLOGIC AGENT. Mycobacteria are small, rod-shaped, aerobic, non–spore-forming bacilli. In the genus *Mycobacterium,* there is a group of organisms so closely related that they are referred to as "the tuberculosis complex": *M. tuberculosis, M. bovis, M. africanum,* and *M. microti.* However, given the singular epidemiologic, clinical, public health, and therapeutic considerations associated with *M. tuberculosis,* the term "tuberculosis" should be reserved exclusively for infection or disease caused by this organism. Disease caused by other organisms of this genus should be referred to as "mycobacteriosis due to *M. x*" and not "atypical tuberculosis" or "tuberculosis due to . . ." (see also Ch. 312).

The mycobacteria are primarily soil or environmental organisms. However, *M. tuberculosis* has become so adapted to the human body that it has no natural reservoirs in nature other than infected/diseased persons; it is passed almost exclusively by aerosol transmission from the respiratory secretions of diseased patients to their contacts.

Mycobacterial cell walls contain high concentrations of lipids or waxes, making them resistant to standard staining techniques. They can be induced to take up a dye such as carbol fuchsin by alkalinity or by heating, and once so colored, they are resistant to the potent decolorizing agent acid-alcohol—hence the reference to "acid-fast" bacilli.

M. tuberculosis and most of the other mycobacteria grow quite slowly; their doubling time in most media is approximately 18 hours. Readily discernible colonies typically do not appear on solid media for 3 to 5 weeks; because of this, culture confirmation, speciation, and drug susceptibility testing have proven clinically problematic.

M. tuberculosis is an obligate aerobe and a facultative intracellular parasite. Tissues attacked are characterized by high regional oxygen tension. The ability to invade and spread throughout the human body has largely to do with the capacity of tubercle bacilli to survive and proliferate within mononuclear phagocytes.

TRANSMISSION. Infection is spread almost exclusively by aerosolization of contaminated respiratory secretions. Patients with *cavitary* lung disease are particularly infectious because their sputum usually contains 1 million to 100 million bacilli per milliliter, and they cough frequently.

However, the intact skin and respiratory mucous membranes of normal exposed individuals are quite resistant to invasion. For infection to occur, bacilli must be delivered to the distal air spaces of the lung, the alveoli, where they are not subject to bronchial mucociliary clearance. Once deposited in alveoli, bacilli are adapted to promote uptake by alveolar macrophages, which—depending on innate, genetically determined properties as well as immunologic experience—may be more or less permissive to bacillary proliferation (see below).

To reach the alveoli, which lie at the end of a ramifying system of progressively smaller airways, the bacilli must be suspended in very fine units that behave as the air itself and not as particles with significant mass. These units are the dehydrated residuals of the tinier particles generated by high-velocity exhalational maneuvers. These droplet nuclei are calculated to be approximately 1 to 5 μ in diameter, may remain suspended in room air for many hours, and when inhaled can traverse the airways to reach the alveoli.

Although patients with cavitary tuberculosis expectorate massive numbers of bacilli, the probability of generating *infectious* particles is relatively low. Household contacts of patients with extensive pulmonary disease who have had productive coughs for weeks or months before diagnosis have, on average, less than a 50% chance of being infected. Hence the usual case of pulmonary tuberculosis is of a low order of infectiousness compared with an airborne disease such as measles. However, infrequent cases demonstrate extremely high rates of transmission; specific factors in these instances have not been clearly elucidated.

The preponderance of transmission occurs as described above, but other mechanisms of transmission have been identified. Aerosols generated by debridement or by dressing changes of skin or soft tissue abscesses due to *M. tuberculosis* have been shown to be highly infectious. Also, tissue agitation associated with autopsies and direct inoculation into soft tissues via contaminated instruments or bone fragments also have been reported. Fomites do not play a significant role in transmission.

PATHOGENESIS AND IMMUNITY. The natural history and various clinical syndromes of tuberculosis are intimately related to the hosts' defenses. Tubercle bacilli do not elaborate classic endo- or exotoxins; rather, the inflammatory illness and tissue destruction are mediated by products elaborated by the host during the "immune" response to the infection (see Part XIX).

When an immunologically naive alveolar macrophage engulfs a tubercle bacillus, it initially provides a nurturing environment within its phagosome in which the bacilli survive and replicate. However, the infected macrophage releases a substance that attracts T lymphocytes; the macrophages then present antigens from the phagocytized bacilli to these lymphocytes, initiating a series of committed immune effector cells. The lymphocytes, in turn, elaborate cytokines which "activate" the macrophages, enhancing their antimicrobial capacity. Thus is set in motion an elaborate, delicately balanced struggle between the host and the parasite.

Among "normal" adult persons, the host initially prevails in over 95% of cases. However, this initial encounter typically extends over a few weeks to several months during which the bacillary population has proliferated massively and undergone variable degrees of dissemination. Tissues that are seeded during this bacillemia, such as the apices of the lungs, the kidneys, bones, meninges, or other extrapulmonary sites, are potential foci for subsequent "reactivation" tuberculosis. Through complex interactions involving mononuclear phagocytes and various T-cell subsets, host defenses are enhanced. This results in more competent macrophages capable of inhibiting the intracellular replication of mycobacteria. Also, disruption of permissive macrophages that support bacillary multiplication occurs in order that more competent macrophages may engulf and limit the growth of the mycobacteria. These phenomena are broadly referred to as "cell-mediated immunity" (CMI) and "delayed-type hypersensitivity" (DTH), respectively. DTH is associated clinically with the development of the tuberculin reaction, an indurated response 48 to 72 hours after the intradermal injection of tuberculosis protein antigens (such as purified protein derivative, or PPD). Skin test reactivity typically develops 4 to 6 weeks after infection, although intervals up to 20 weeks have been noted.

As these defenses gain momentum, involution of the numerous disseminated granulomatous foci in the lungs, lymph nodes, and scattered sites occurs. Typically, all that remains to overtly mark this encounter is the tuberculin skin test reactivity. In a minority of cases, a small single residual of the primary infection appears in the lung parenchyma (the Ghon focus); occasionally, this is accompanied by calcifications of the ipsilateral hilar nodes. Some patients also develop fibronodular shadowing in one or both lung apices ("Simon foci"); these presumably are the residua of subclinical disease at these sites.

The vast majority of cases occur due to late reactivation of the vestigial lesions of this primary infection, either in the lungs or in extrapulmonary sites. Rapid progression to overt disease occurs in a minority of newly infected persons who cannot mount sufficient immune responses. Groups at high risk include infants through age 4, the infirm elderly, and immunocompromised subjects, including those with human immunodeficiency virus (HIV) infection or acquired immunodeficiency syndrome (AIDS), organ transplant recipients, and those with other immunosuppressive illnesses or chemotherapy.

EPIDEMIOLOGY. Globally, tuberculosis is now the leading infectious cause of morbidity and mortality. However, in the more industrialized nations, the disease has retreated from the general populations, afflicting selected groups. Recognition of these high-risk groups is vital in terms of diagnosis, prevention, and control programs.

Global. The World Health Organization (WHO) estimated in 1990 that one third of the world's population, or 1.7 billion people, were latently infected with *M. tuberculosis.* From this pool, 8 to 10 million new active cases emerge per year, the majority of whom have communicable forms of pulmonary disease. Regions in the world where the infection and disease are most prevalent include the Pacific Rim nations (excluding Japan), Southeast Asia, Indo-Asia, sub-Saharan Africa, and Latin America. Due to delayed, inadequate, or unavailable therapy, 2 to 3 million persons die annually; indeed, WHO estimates that 26% of preventable deaths in the developing nations are attributable to tuberculosis.

United States. The United States has a considerably lower prevalence of infection, with only 4 to 6% of the population—10 to 15 million persons—harboring latent infections. From this pool, approximately 24,000 new active cases arose in 1992. These patients infected approximately 60,000 of their contacts, 3000 of whom went on to develop active disease in that same year—thus the cumulative morbidity of 27,000 cases in 1992.

Case numbers had declined steadily at 5 to 6% annually from 1953 to 1984; however, from 1985 to 1992 there has been a consistent increase in annual numbers of cases (Fig. 311–1). Indeed, from 1985 to 1992, there have been approximately 52,000 excess cases above those projected by the trend from 1953 to 1984; in 1992 alone, this "excess" constituted about 40% of the reported cases.

U.S. morbidity entails remarkable disparities according to race, age, and national origins. Among nonwhite Americans, it is largely a disease of young adults, with the peak incidence between ages 25 and 44 years; by contrast, the peak age among whites is 70 years and older, due presumably to latent early infections (Fig. 311–2). In 1992, 71% of U.S. tuberculosis cases occurred among minorities.

Immigration has contributed significantly to the upturn in morbidity. In 1992, roughly 27% of cases occurred among foreign-born persons (up 20% from 1985). Major sources of these cases include Mexico, the Philippines, Southeast Asia, the Caribbean, and Latin America, the bulk occurring within 5 years of arrival in the United States.

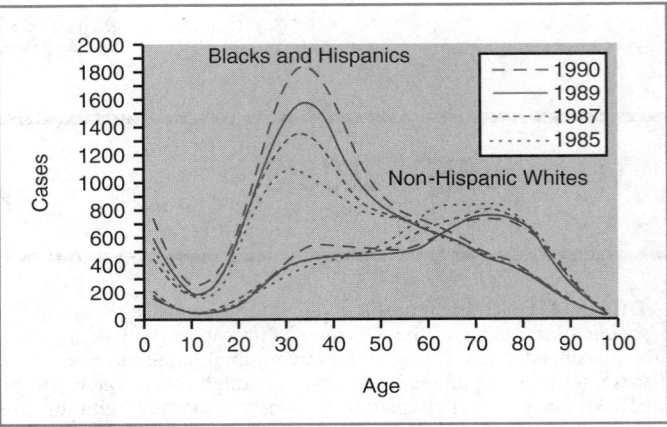

FIGURE 311–2. The majority of cases among non-Hispanic whites occurred between the ages of 60 to 90 years; the incidence declined over this interval. By contrast, the great bulk of cases among blacks and Hispanics occurred among 20- to 50-year-olds; the case numbers rose dramatically in this period. The incidence in 1992 per 100,000 population for non-Hispanic whites was 4 (*RR* = 1); for Hispanics it was 22.4 (*RR* = 5.6); for blacks it was 31.7 (*RR* = 7.9). (From Centers for Disease Control and Prevention, Division of Tuberculosis Elimination: Tuberculosis Statistics for the United States, Atlanta, 1990.)

HIV Infection/AIDS. HIV infection and AIDS have contributed to the rising case rates of tuberculosis through three broad pathways: (1) Individuals with latent tuberculosis infection who acquired HIV infection are at much greater risk of reactivation as their immune capacity diminishes; (2) persons with HIV infection or AIDS may well be at higher risk of acquiring new infections with tuberculosis, due probably to both biologic factors (they may be more prone to become infected on exposure due to impaired defenses) and situational factors (they are more likely to be exposed due to time spent in high-risk, congregate environments); and (3) young adults with HIV infection and active tuberculosis transmit it to people with whom they reside.

In the United States, the upsurge in tuberculosis from 1985 to the present has been clearly linked to the HIV epidemic, although full quantification of the association is not possible due to incomplete serologic testing. Conservatively, at least half the recent excess morbidity can be attributed to the effects of HIV. Direct evidence adduced in support of the relationship includes seroprevalence surveys in tuberculosis clinics located around the country; overall, 11% of U.S.-born tuberculosis patients were HIV-positive; these rates were higher in East Coast clinics and among persons ages 30 to 39. Inferential evidence includes temporal, geographic, and demographic associations between the two infections.

CLINICAL PRESENTATIONS. Since the primary pulmonary infection usually results in bacillemic dissemination, tuberculosis commonly entails disease in extrathoracic as well as pulmonary or pleural sites. As a generalization, hosts with more competent immunity tend to have disease limited to their lungs or other single sites, while those with less robust defenses experience multifocal or disseminated disease.

Normal Adults. Overall, excluding the influence of HIV infection, about 85% of adults present with pulmonary parenchymal disease, 15% with disease at extrapulmonary sites, and approximately 4% with simultaneously active disease at intra- and extrathoracic locations.

Two important comments should be made about clinical tuberculosis in normal adults: (1) The tuberculin skin test (TST) will be falsely negative in 20 to 25% at the time of diagnosis, and (2) although most complain of feeling "feverish," a substantial proportion do not have fever when measured. Thus a clinician should not be diverted from considering the diagnosis by nonreactive TST's or lack of fever in patients with other typical features of tuberculosis.

Pulmonary Disease. Classic symptoms include the following: Cough is nearly universal; typically, it is initially dry but then progresses with increasing volumes of purulent secretions and

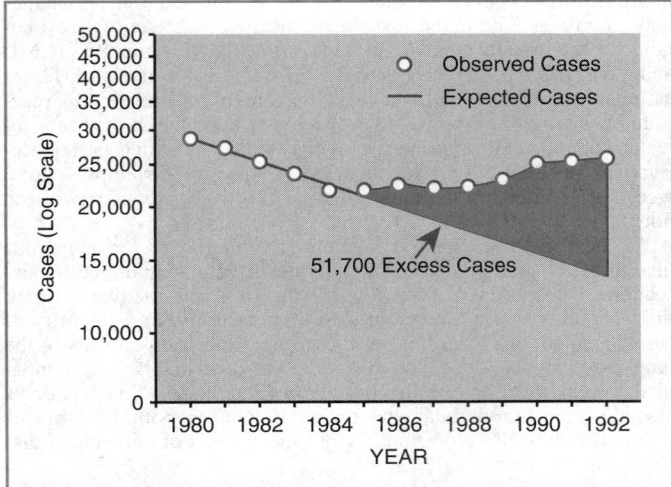

FIGURE 311–1. Excess cases, 1985–1992. CDC data indicate nearly 52,000 cases above the number anticipated based on constant decline of cases between 1953 and 1984. Major influences on this resurgence include HIV infection and immigration. (From Centers for Disease Control and Prevention: Tuberculosis morbidity, United States, 1992. MMWR 42:696, 1993.)

the variable appearance of blood streaking or gross hemoptysis. Feverishness is common as the disease advances; actual temperatures range from subnormal to extreme elevations. Sweating, including drenching night sweats, is quite typical. Other common complaints include malaise, fatigue, weight loss, nonpleuritic chest pain, and dyspnea.

Signs may be quite limited until the disease is in advanced stages. Fever with peaks as high as 40 to 41°C, typically occurring in the evening, is seen among patients with disease of various forms and extent. Localized rales are early findings; coarse rhonchi evolve as secretions become more voluminous and tenacious; signs of lung consolidation are rarely heard. Wheezing and/or regionally diminished breath sounds may be heard in cases with peri- or endobronchial airway compromise.

The chest radiograph is central to the diagnosis. Upper lung zone fibronodular shadowing involving one or both apices is seen in the majority of cases. As these lesions advance, they enlarge and become fluffy or softly marginated; coalescence occurs, and cavitation devolves as intense local inflammation produces necrosis and sloughing of lung tissue. The most common sites involved in reactivation adult tuberculosis are, in descending order, the posterior and apical segments of the right upper lobe, the apical-posterior segment of the left upper lobe, and the superior segments of the lower lobes. Lower zone disease is the presenting appearance in < 15% of HIV-negative adults; it is seen somewhat more commonly in diabetics and patients with prominent peribronchial and endobronchial involvement. Pleural effusions are uncommon in adults with reactivation-type pulmonary disease.

Sputum smears and cultures are the most specific components of diagnosis. Some contemporary laboratories still use the classic acid-fast stains (Ziehl-Neelsen or Kinyoun); however, most use a modified acid-fast method, the fluorochrome technique, which relies on the uptake and acid-fast retention of auramine-O, a dye that fluoresces when excited by ultraviolet light. With the fluorochrome technique, the tubercle bacillus is more easily discernible (bright yellow contrasted to an inky black background) than the older methods (red on a blue and white background); hence the fluorochrome system is visually more sensitive. Microscopic acid-fast bacilli (AFB) found in respiratory secretions associated with suitable clinical, epidemiologic, and radiographic findings highly suggests tuberculosis. However, microscopy is not specific, because other pathogenic or saprophytic mycobacteria may be found in sputum. The test is not very sensitive; the likelihood of positive smears depends heavily on the extent of pulmonary involvement. With readily visible cavities and no prior treatment, it would be rare to have negative sputum microscopy. However, with noncavitary fibronodular or miliary patterns on chest films, negative microscopy is common. Cultures are the gold standard for diagnosis; however, current methods typically entail 3 to 6 weeks to cultivate and identify species. More rapid cultivation and identification techniques that use liquid media with radiometric, molecular biologic, or chromatographic methods have reduced the required time substantially. The diagnosis is occasionally made on the basis of symptoms, radiographic findings, and response to empirical therapy *without* culture confirmation. Because of the rising prevalence of resistance to standard drugs, susceptibility testing on all initial M. tuberculosis isolates is recommended.

As noted earlier, the TST will be falsely negative in 20 to 25% of HIV-negative adults with pulmonary tuberculosis. Testing with other delayed-type hypersensitivity antigens may help identify persons who are broadly anergic; however, selective anergy to tuberculin occurs.

Extrapulmonary Tuberculosis (XPTB). XPTB occurs in roughly one sixth of HIV-negative adults in the United States with active disease. The most common sites and relevant features are displayed in Table 311–1 (see also Part XXII).

Clinically, it should be noted that the severe wasting seen with advanced pulmonary diseases—consumption—is rarely seen with

TABLE 311–1. COMMON FORMS OF EXTRAPULMONARY TUBERCULOSIS IN PATIENTS WITHOUT HIV INFECTION

Organ System	Relatively High Risk Groups	Common Clinical Manifestations	Diagnosis	Management
Lymphatic	Youngsters and young adults; F > M, Asian and Indian females high-risk	Unilateral, cervical; painless; sinus tracts late	Excisional biopsy with culture; PPD usually positive	May respond slowly to medication; rarely may require excision
Pleural	Young adults with primary infection; older adults with reactivation disease	May be acute or indolent; severe pleurisy or asymptomatic	Lymphatic exudate; AFB smear usually negative; biopsy with culture gives best yield	Usually responds well to medication; do not drain with tube thoracostomy
Genitourinary	Rare in young; more frequent among females, foreign born, and Native Americans	May involve kidneys, ureters, bladder, testes, epididymis, uterus, fallopian tubes	Culture urine; biopsy and culture masses and uterine scrapings	Usually responds well to medication; beware of early or late obstructive uropathy
Bone-joint	More common in elderly, although seen in all ages	Lumbar and low dorsal spine common in older; high dorsal in young; weight-bearing bones/joints	Needle biopsy and aspirate for spinal lesions; synovial biopsy and culture for joints	Debride and stabilize spine; try to avoid fusing joints
Disseminated	Most frequent in very young or old; blacks and Native Americans	Chest film abnormalities may lag; progressive fever and inanition; PPD negative in 50%	Smears and cultures of involved fluids, organs, and mesothelia; smear and culture urine	Early therapy vital; steroids of uncertain value
Meninges—CNS	Most common among infants/children with XPTB; higher risk for Hispanics, blacks, and Native Americans	Three stages: early fever, headache, and malaise; later confusion, obtundation, seizures, and coma	LP: ↑ protein and cells; ↓ glucose, ↑ pressure; smears rarely positive; special tests (see text)	Prognosis related to stage; steroids indicated in most cases; drugs must penetrate CNS
Peritoneal-GI	Increases with age; higher risk among minorities	Mainly mesothelial but ileal involvement may resemble Crohn's; abdominal swelling and vague pain common	Laparoscopic biopsy ideal; smear and culture ascites; stool cultures may be useful	Beware of adhesions and obstruction; steroids may be useful
Pericardial	Rare in children; more common in blacks	Acute pain rare; cough, dyspnea, and vague discomfort	Widened cardiac silhouette; left pleural effusion; ECG low voltage and chronic ST/TW changes; ↓ heart sounds, rubs rare	Steroids ↓ effusion, improve performance; may reduce late adhesive complications; pericardiectomy for tamponade

Note: Among persons without HIV infection, roughly 16% of tuberculosis presents as extrapulmonary involvement. Lymphatic and pleural disease are the most common forms.

XPTB. Feverishness occurs with more extensive disease, prominently including miliary, pleural, and genitourinary disease.

Diagnosis is problematic in most forms of XPTB due to the relative paucity of bacilli. Histopathology of involved tissues typically shows giant cell granulomas with caseating necrosis and few, if any, demonstrable AFB. Analysis of mesothelial effusions (pleural, peritoneal, or pericardial) characteristically reveals a lymphocyte-rich exudate with low concentrations of glucose; however, the *initial* inflammatory responses in these spaces may be polymorphonuclear (PMN) leukocyte predominant. Cerebrospinal fluid (CSF) in meningitis begins with a modest leukocytosis, shifting from PMN to lymphocyte dominance; leukocyte counts typically range from 50 to 300 cells per milliliter. The CSF protein concentration is typically moderately elevated. Glucose levels are progressively depressed in relation to the degree of leukocytosis. Because of the scarcity of AFB in the CSF, sophisticated markers, including the polymerase chain reaction, tuberculostearic acid levels, or antibody assays, appear to be useful in establishing the diagnosis, although they are not widely available.

Tuberculosis in Persons with HIV Infection/AIDS.
Early in the course of HIV infection, the clinical manifestations of tuberculosis are quite similar to those in normal hosts. However, with the progressive reduction in the T lymphocyte population, the following major changes ensue: (1) a steady reduction in the proportion who react significantly to tuberculin skin testing, reaching a nadir of 10 to 20% reactors among those with advanced AIDS; (2) substantially greater extrapulmonary involvement, reaching 60 to 80% prevalence of XPTB among those with CD4 counts < 50; and (3) changing patterns of disease on chest radiography, evolving from classic upper zone fibronodular, cavitary disease to lower zone, nondescript pneumonic patterns, infrequent cavity formation, interstitial or miliary shadowing, very prominent hilar or paratracheal adenopathy, and substantial pleural effusions.

TREATMENT. One unique aspect to the care of tuberculosis patients merits emphasis before discussing specific therapy: Because of the hazard of casual, airborne transmission of infection and of the potentially morbid or lethal consequences for the recipients, there is a singular public health mandate that *persons with communicable tuberculosis must either be treated or quarantined.* U.S. public health policy throughout the 20th century has empowered governmental representatives to quarantine patients with potentially lethal infectious diseases. In the case of tuberculosis, modern chemotherapy has, in effect, become "chemical quarantine"; thus nonadherence to treatment may be seen as breaching this quarantine. Because of the consequences of inadequate or incomplete treatment, directly observed therapy (DOT) to prevent noncompliance is being employed increasingly (see the section on nonadherence below).

Indications for Commencing Treatment.
Because it usually takes 3 to 8 weeks to culture and identify species, treatment for most patients is initiated before a "definitive" diagnosis is established, based rather on an amalgam of historical, epidemiologic, radiographic, tissue or fluid analysis, and microscopic findings. Beginning empirical therapy for patients with potentially rapid, life-threatening conditions such as central nervous system (CNS) or miliary disease usually entails a low threshold of suspicion; however, care should be taken to obtain optimal diagnostic specimens before commencing medication, lest the chemotherapy suppress growth from paucibacillary material.

The Principles of Multidrug Treatment.
Patients with active tuberculosis should receive multiple agents both to prevent the emergence of drug-resistant mutants as dominant strains and to accelerate the bacterial clearance. Of these, the former is more crucial, for the emergence of a substantial population of drug-resistant bacilli may significantly and permanently compromise the treatment outcome.

Biologically, tubercle bacilli have the well-documented capacity to undergo spontaneous mutations that confer resistance to the various antituberculosis medications. These mutations occur at predictable frequencies, usually in the range of 1 in 10^8 replications, and are unlinked, resulting in resistance to only one drug or drug category. In patients with cavitary tuberculosis, the population of bacilli is so numerous that small numbers of mycobacteria exist that are resistant to each of the standard medications. However, because the mutations are unlinked, there is an extremely low probability of spontaneous resistance to two or more drugs by a single microbe; e.g., the isoniazid-resistant mutants would be killed by rifampin (RIF) and the rifampin-resistant mutants killed by isoniazid (INH). Thus, early in treatment when the mycobacterial burden is greatest, it is vital that *at least* two effective agents be employed.

If patients are nonadherent, i.e., stop one of their medications unbeknownst to their clinician, the unopposed mutants are allowed to proliferate, resulting in treatment failures or relapses associated with acquired drug resistance. When this happens serially, multidrug resistance is created. Such organisms can be transmitted then to other persons, giving rise to initial drug-resistant tuberculosis.

In addition to combating drug resistance, multidrug regimens can shorten the required duration of treatment through unique contributions by the various agents. A regimen of INH and ethambutol (EMB) requires 18 months to cure the typical case of pulmonary tuberculosis; adding RIF to INH reduces the duration to 9 months; and when an initial 2-month phase of pyrazinamide (PZA) is added to INH and RIF, cure occurs in 6 months.

Choice of Regimen.
Due to concern over the rising prevalence of drug resistance, recent Centers for Disease Control and Prevention (CDC) recommendations advocate a four-drug regimen for most cases of known or suspected tuberculosis (Table 311–2). INH and RIF are the central agents of any regimen based on their

TABLE 311–2. RECOMMENDED REGIMEN OPTIONS FOR TUBERCULOSIS, UNITED STATES

Regimen	Medications	Total Duration	Comments
ATS/CDC (as modified by ACET)	INH and RIF daily for 6 mos. PZA and SM or EMB daily for 2 mos.	6 mos.	Add SM or EMB in areas/patients at risk for initial drug resistance. Stop PZA, EMB, or SM after 2 mos. if strain susceptible; continue or modify regimen if resistance present.
Denver	INH, RIF, PZA, and SM daily for 2 weeks; then twice weekly for 6 weeks. Follow with INH and RIF twice weekly for 18 weeks.	6 mos.	Stop PZA and SM at 8 weeks if strain is susceptible; continue through 6 mos. if there is initial INH resistance. May substitute EMB for SM. 24 weeks of twice-weekly therapy facilitates DOT.
Hong-Kong	INH, RIF, PZA, and SM or EMB thrice weekly for 6 mos. (may stop PZA, SM, or EMB after 2 mos.)	6 mos.	All-intermittent. If strain is susceptible, may stop PZA and SM or EMB after 2 mos. If there is INH resistance, stop INH and add the fourth drug (EMB or SM).
Arkansas	INH and RIF daily for 1 mo.; then INH and RIF twice weekly for 8 mos.	9 mos.	This regimen should only be employed in populations with a very low prevalence of drug resistance. Initial therapy probably should include a third drug until drug susceptibility is reported.

Note: Currently, the Advisory Council for the Elimination of Tuberculosis of the CDC advocates initial four-drug therapy for cases in communities with a background prevalence of initial drug resistance of 4% or greater. If susceptibility has been demonstrated or if resistance is deemed very unlikely, initial three-drug regimens may be used. INH = isoniazid; RIF = rifampin; PZA = pyrazinamide; SM = streptomycin; EMB = ethambutol.

TABLE 311–3. DOSAGE, TOXICITY, AND SPECIAL CONSIDERATIONS FOR STANDARD ANTITUBERCULOSIS MEDICATIONS

Drug	Daily	Usual Adult Dose Thrice ‖ Twice Weekly	Toxicity	Special Considerations	Comments
Isoniazid (INH)	300 mg PO	600 ‖ 900 mg	Hepatitis, neuritis, mood/cognition, lupus reaction	Pregnancy: safe Liver disease: caution Renal impairment: ↓ dose if severe	Monitor liver function tests monthly in most patients; clinically significant interactions with phenytoin and antifungals (azols)
Rifampin (RIF)	600 mg PO 450 mg in persons <50 kg body weight	600 ‖ (same)	Hepatitis, thrombopenia, nephritis, flu syndrome	Pregnancy: acceptable Liver disease: caution Renal impairment: safe	Key: multiple, profound drug interactions possible (see below); turns urine and fluids red
Pyrazinamide (PZA)	25–30 mg/kg PO	30–35 mg/kg ‖ (same)	Hepatitis, arthralgias and arthritis secondary to hyperuricemia, GI distress, rash	Pregnancy: unknown (avoid) Liver disease: caution Renal impairment: caution	Urate levels always rise; do not treat or stop PZA unless unmanageable gout develops
Ethambutol (EMB)	15–25 mg/kg PO	35 mg/kg ‖ 50 mg/kg	Optic neuritis	Pregnancy: safe Liver disease: safe Renal impairment: ↓ dose/frequency	Monitor visual acuity and color vision regularly
Streptomycin (SM)	12–15 mg/kg IM	15 mg/kg ‖ (same)	Vestibular and auditory, cation depletion	Pregnancy: high-risk (avoid) Liver disease: safe Renal impairment: ↓ dose/frequency	Reduce dose and/or frequency in case of renal impairment

Note: Rifampin drug interactions have been reported with oral contraceptives, anticoagulants, methadone, corticosteroids, estrogen replacement, calcium channel blockers, beta blockers, cyclosporine, antifungal azols, phenytoin, theophylline, sulfonylureas, haloperidol, and others (see *PDR*).

superior bactericidal activity and low toxicity. PZA has special utility in promoting rapid, early reduction in bacillary burden; in drug-susceptible cases, PZA need be given only for the initial 2 months to produce this effect. EMB is useful primarily to protect against the emergence of drug resistance in cases with unknown initial susceptibility patterns and large mycobacterial burdens; EMB may be terminated if susceptibility is reported or be continued throughout the duration of treatment if resistance is noted (see below). Streptomycin (SM), a parenteral agent, has found a diminishing role in modern therapy due to problems with regularly administering intramuscular injections; however, for patients with very extensive tuberculosis, SM may accelerate initial bactericidal activity. Dosage and toxicity for these agents are displayed in Table 311–3.

Does every patient need to receive such a four-drug regimen? In actual practice, clinicians should review every proven or suspected case and consider individual modifications or exemptions of this standard program. For example, (1) an elderly patient with known remote exposure to tuberculosis in the prechemotherapy era, with no recent contacts and no history of tuberculosis medical treatment, might reasonably be started on a three-drug (INH, RIF, EMB) or even two-drug (INH, RIF) regimen because of the very low likelihood of drug resistance; and (2) an injection drug–using 35-year-old HIV-positive man from the Bronx who has been hospitalized on multiple occasions over the prior 12 months might receive initial seven-drug treatment because of the substantial risk of disease due to one of the multidrug-resistant tuberculosis strains prevalent in the New York City area.

Common factors that might influence the initial choice of drugs are included in Table 311–4. Additional considerations in selecting therapy are noted below.

AIDS (see Part XXII). The most salient particular issue in patients with AIDS and tuberculosis is to ensure adequate absorption of the antituberculosis medications. Due to a variety of AIDS-associated enteropathies, there is a risk of grossly reduced serum drug concentrations, which can result in treatment failure and potentially promote acquired drug resistance. Direct determination of drug levels at some time early in treatment is the ideal means for addressing this issue. If this is not feasible, very close monitoring of responses to treatment and use of high-range drug dosing may be appropriate. Also, because of the polypharmacy typically used with AIDS, special attention should be given to the potential impact of RIF-induced hepatic catabolism of other medications (Table 311–4).

CNS Disease. Smaller un-ionized molecules such as INH and PZA cross the blood-brain barrier well, even in the absence of gross

inflammation. RIF crosses less well, although therapeutic effects are seen. EMB CSF levels are significantly lower than those in serum, and its use in meningitis is less well established. SM and the other aminoglycoside antibiotics are large, complex, and ionically charged molecules; they cross the barrier very poorly, even in the presence of inflammation.

Combating Nonadherence with Directly Observed Intermittent Chemotherapy. Treatment given intermittently, thrice or twice weekly, is generally comparable in efficacy with daily treatment. These intermittent schedules make it practical that patients either come to treatment centers or have visits by outreach workers at home or in shelters, schools, or work sites to observe ingestion or actually administer medications. Most reported regimens have begun with a daily phase of therapy and switched to an intermittent schedule after 1 or 2 months. However, effective treatment can either entail a brief (2-week) initial daily phase *or* be intermittent (thrice weekly) throughout. Not all patients need to receive directly observed therapy; many can be trusted to self-administer their drugs. However, it is extremely difficult to predict those who are likely to be compliant, and careful attention should be given to patient education and ongoing monitoring of medication-taking behavior for all patients. If nonadherence is demonstrated or reasonably anticipated (on the basis of risk factors such as homelessness, substance abuse, personality or thought disorders, language or cultural barriers), supervised treatment will benefit patients, their future contacts, and ultimately the community at large. Directly observed therapy may be the only feasible means of stemming the rising prevalence of tuberculosis in general and multidrug-resistant tuberculosis in particular in certain communities and populations.

Common Clinician Errors in Relation to Acquired Drug Resistance. Among the more common errors that contribute to the evolution of multidrug resistance are failure to recognize and cope with nonadherence in a timely manner, failure to identify an individual at high risk for pre-existing drug resistance resulting in use of an inadequate initial regimen, and adding a single drug to a failing regimen.

Monitoring for and Coping with Drug Toxicity. In the general population about a 5% incidence of significant reactions requiring transient or permanent discontinuation of one or more drugs is seen in a typical three- or four-drug regimen. Common drug toxicities are listed in Table 311–4. Vague gastrointestinal complaints are relatively common in association with all the first-line oral drugs. However, with coaching and encouragement, most patients can be induced to tolerate these drugs. Caution should be taken that pa-

TABLE 311-4. HIGH-RISK CANDIDATES FOR IPT

Candidates for preventive chemotherapy—persons at high risk for tuberculosis. Various persons with latent tuberculosis infection are at relatively great risk of developing active disease. The degree of tuberculin skin test reactivity to identify such persons varies based on epidemiologic and biologic factors. The recommended duration of therapy is 6 months for most candidates but 12 months for HIV-infected persons or patients with upper-zone fibronodular shadows on chest film.

High-Risk Groups

Certain groups within the infected population are at greater risk than others and should receive high priority for preventive therapy. *In the United States, persons with any of the following six risk factors should be considered candidates for preventive therapy, regardless of age, if they have not previously been treated:*

- Persons with human immunodeficiency virus (HIV) infection (≥ 5 mm) and persons with risk factors for HIV infection whose HIV infection status is unknown but who are suspected of having HIV infection.
- Close contacts of persons with newly diagnosed infectious tuberculosis (≥ 5 mm). In addition, tuberculin-negative (< 5 mm) children and adolescents who have been close contacts of infectious persons within the past 3 months are candidates for preventive therapy until a repeat tuberculin skin test is done 12 weeks after contact with the infectious source.
- Recent converters, as indicated by a tuberculin skin test (≥ 10 mm increase within a 2-year period for those < 35 years old; ≥ 15 mm increase for those ≥ 35 years of age).
- Persons with abnormal chest radiographs that show fibrotic lesions likely to represent old healed tuberculosis (≥ 5 mm).
- Intravenous drug users known to be HIV seronegative (≥ 10 mm).
- Persons with medical conditions that have been reported to increase the risk of tuberculosis (≥ 10 mm).

In addition, in the absence of any of the above risk factors, persons < 35 years of age in the following high-incidence groups are appropriate candidates for preventive therapy if their reaction to a tuberculin skin test is ≥ 10 mm:

- Foreign-born persons from high-prevalence countries.
- Medically underserved low-income populations, including high-risk racial or ethnic minority populations, especially blacks, Hispanics, and Native Americans.
- Residents of facilities for long-term care (e.g., correctional institutions, nursing homes, and mental institutions).

In addition to the groups listed above, public health officials should be alert for other high-risk populations in their communities. For example, through a review of cases reported in the community over several years, health officials may use geographic or sociodemographic factors to identify groups that should be targeted for intervention. Screening and preventive therapy programs should be initiated and promoted within these populations based on an analysis of cases and infection in the community. To the extent possible, members of high-risk groups and their health-care providers should be involved in the design, implementation, and evaluation of these programs. Staff of facilities in which an individual with disease would pose a risk to large numbers of susceptible persons (e.g., correctional institutions, nursing homes, mental institutions, other health-care facilities, schools, and child-care facilities) may also be considered for preventive therapy if their tuberculin reaction is ≥ 10 mm induration.

From Screening for Tuberculosis and Tuberculous Infection in High-Risk Populations and the Use of Preventive Therapy for Tuberculous Infection in the United States. Recommendation of the Advisory Committee for the Elimination of Tuberculosis. MMWR 39(No. RR-8):7, 1990.

tients, in an effort to diminish gastrointestinal intolerance, do not take their oral medications directly with meals, antacids, or H_2 blockers, any of which may substantially reduce absorption of certain of these agents. Regular monitoring of liver chemistries is indicated for all patients receiving multidrug therapy; monthly surveillance is common. In addition, patient education regarding the typical symptoms of hepatitis and regular reminders may be of major importance in preventing serious liver injury. When patients experience serious hepatitis, all potentially hepatotoxic drugs should be held until liver chemistries and symptoms normalize; then the drugs can be reintroduced one at a time at 3- to 4-day intervals, monitoring liver function tests and symptoms to identify the offending agent. Elderly patients receiving SM or other aminoglycosides should have baseline and periodic audiometry; in addition, surveillance of vestibular function is required. For younger patients who

are receiving only 2 months of SM, objective testing is generally not indicated.

Duration of Treatment and Posttreatment Surveillance. Currently, a 6-month regimen consisting of INH and RIF supplemented by an initial 2-month phase of PZA is regarded as sufficient and curative for the vast majority of cases caused by drug-susceptible strains. If these three agents cannot be used, the duration of treatment may be prolonged (see Table 311–3). Other situations in which therapy may be extended beyond 6 months include the following: *HIV infection/AIDS:* Although no well-controlled studies have demonstrated the superiority of longer therapy, some clinicians fear that impaired immunity will place these patients at higher risk of relapse. *Far-advanced, cavitary lung disease with delayed clinical response or sputum conversion:* About 95% of patients will become culture negative by 3 months of treatment; for those who remain positive longer than this, treatment for 3 months *after* conversion is recommended. *Irregular, interrupted therapy:* If patients fail to attend 10% or more of DOT encounters or are otherwise deemed to have been significantly nonadherent to their treatment, extended treatment is prudent. *Miliary or meningeal cases:* Due both to the concern that such patients may be less competent hosts and the implications of disease recurrence, therapy may be extended to 9 to 12 months.

A low and unavoidable risk of relapse exists following treatment; for the regimens described above in usual populations, the probability is $< 5\%$. The majority of such recurrences occur within 2 years and are usually associated with the same drug susceptibility profile as pretreatment. Current guidelines do not compel posttreatment surveillance. Rather, patients should be instructed to return after treatment when there are changes in their clinical status; suitable tests including sputa, chest radiographs, or other studies should be obtained if symptoms or signs appear.

Indications for Corticosteroid Therapy. Steroids may be used to reduce acute inflammation and limit delayed fibrotic complications. Acute reductions in inflammation with significant benefits in outcome have been demonstrated in meningitis and pericarditis cases treated with corticosteroids. Prednisone, at 1 mg per kilogram of body weight, is usual. Less well proven are the benefits of such therapy in pleural, peritoneal, miliary, or extensive pulmonary disease, although salutary effects may occur in individual cases. While high-dose corticosteroids may impair immune responses, there is no evidence that they adversely affect the outcome of treatment when given for 4 to 8 weeks to patients who are receiving adequate chemotherapy.

Adrenal insufficiency due to tuberculous destruction is uncommon in this era. However, among patients with marginal cortisol production, RIF may precipitate hypocortisolism by accelerating catabolism of endogenous steroids.

Drug-Resistant Tuberculosis. In a recent CDC survey, the national prevalence of resistance to one or more drugs was 14.2%. Resistance to INH was noted most commonly: 8.2% of new cases and 21.5% of recurrent cases. Resistance to INH and RIF was noted in 3.5% of strains studied; cases with resistance to INH and RIF, with or without resistance to other drugs, are referred to as "multidrug-resistant tuberculosis" (MDR-TB). This report indicated that the regional patterns of resistance varied widely, and it is incumbent on clinicians to consider this when choosing empirical therapy. For example, in New York City, resistance to INH and RIF was found in 12.9% of isolates. The particular importance of MDR-TB is that, in the absence of INH and RIF, the period required for treatment is doubled, the probability of cure drops substantially, and the ability to provide effective preventive therapy for infected contacts is sorely compromised.

Risk markers for the likelihood of drug resistance include prior treatment for tuberculosis, close contact to such persons, and time spent in communities/countries with known high prevalence. Cases proven or suspected to involve MDR-TB should be referred with alacrity to specialty facilities for expedited laboratory studies and individualized management.

CONTACT INVESTIGATION. It is vital that clinicians realize that their responsibilities are not complete when they have established the diagnosis and initiated chemotherapy for their patient. Tuberculosis is a reportable disease in all U.S. communities and states; clinicians are obligated to promptly notify public health authorities of all cases of proven or suspected tuberculosis. Contact investigation of the home, workplace, school, or other congregate facilities may well reveal other active cases or newly infected persons who are at substantial risk for tuberculosis. Priority must be given to investigations where infants or AIDS patients have been exposed due to their compressed incubation periods for potentially lethal forms of tuberculosis. Preventive chemotherapy of infected contacts is a highly efficient means of curtailing tuberculosis morbidity (see below).

PREVENTION OF TUBERCULOSIS. Multiple modalities are involved with the efforts to control tuberculosis. In the U.S. over the past 25 years, isoniazid preventive chemotherapy (IPT) has been relied upon. For the remainder of the world, vaccination with bacille Calmette-Guérin (BCG) has been the central element. The relative merits and limitations of these methods are discussed below.

Isoniazid Preventive Therapy: Principles and Efficacy. Because most U.S. tuberculosis cases arise from endogenous reactivation of latent infection acquired remotely in time, authorities reasoned that chemotherapy given to persons harboring such infections might be protective. In a series of randomized, placebo-controlled studies, IPT demonstrated 75% reduction of morbidity in the year of treatment and 54% protection in the posttreatment years; even higher rates of protection were shown in a large trial in Eastern Europe, ranging from approximately 70 to 90% with 6- and 12-month IPT, respectively.

Indications for IPT. The focus of IPT recommendations is on persons who are deemed to be at relatively higher risk for experiencing reactivation. Specific groups or conditions that are regarded at high risk and to be candidates for IPT are noted in Table 311–4.

In most instances, the TST is the central modality to identify latent infection. Interpretation of the TST, however, is influenced by circumstances. Thus, in some instances, IPT would be recommended despite nonreactivity, while in other cases ≥ 15 mm induration is required for significance.

Special Considerations in Preventive Therapy. HIV infection is probably the most potent risk factor for endogenous reactivation. Hence persons with positive HIV serology or strong epidemiologic or clinical markers for HIV risk should be assigned very high priority for IPT. In addition to protecting the individual patient from tuberculosis, IPT may extend survival by ameliorating the accelerated progression of HIV infection seen with active tuberculosis *and* could prevent transmission to other very vulnerable HIV-infected persons (e.g., in shared health care, social, or residential facilities).

Persons exposed to and presumed infected by resistant strains of *M. tuberculosis* pose problems for preventive therapy. If the strain from the source case is resistant only to INH, RIF likely would be a highly effective substitute. However, if the source-case strain is resistant to both INH and RIF, there are no really promising alternatives. For very high-risk persons (such as AIDS patients) exposed to an MDR-TB case, preventive therapy with ofloxacin and EMB or PZA may be indicated but should be undertaken only after expert consultation.

Monitoring for Compliance and Toxicity. Patients receiving preventive chemotherapy should be seen periodically to both provide adherence to the treatment and survey for signs or symptoms of drug toxicity. Intermittent, directly observed preventive therapy is not widely feasible; however, it may be applicable in selected circumstances such as prisoners, especially with HIV infection, or recently infected infants or children in chaotic households where reliable treatment is unlikely.

The major toxicity of INH is hepatitis, which may prove fatal if therapy is continued into the period of symptoms and gross chemical derangements. Therefore, it is important that initial education alert the patient and/or responsible family members to the early manifestations of liver injury (anorexia, nausea, malaise, loss of taste for cigarettes, dark urine) with instructions to stop the INH and report promptly for evaluation. Also, patients should have monthly communication with a health care worker, directly if possible but by telephone as an alternative, to inquire regarding their health and to reiterate the education. Biochemical monitoring of liver chemistries is indicated for persons 35 years of age or older, due to the age-related risk of hepatitis, and should be obtained at baseline and monthly intervals. Innocent increases in the transaminase levels three- to fourfold over baseline without symptoms are noted among up to 20% of persons on IPT; this is not an indication to discontinue the drug but to maintain close surveillance. However, liver chemistries elevated to higher levels or those associated with symptoms should result in discontinuation of the INH. The decision to rechallenge with this drug or to use an alternative agent should be made after expert consultation.

Vaccination with BCG. BCG is a live vaccine prepared from an attenuated strain of *M. bovis.* It has been used widely around the world, but its efficacy and utility are debated. The performance of various strains of BCG, given to different populations over time, has ranged from 80% protection to detrimental effects (more tuberculosis in those receiving the vaccine). A recent meta-analysis of published BCG studies indicated that vaccinations offered an overall 50% protective effect, with higher levels of protection against meningeal or disseminated tuberculosis. This study revealed that the efficacy of BCG diminished at sites near the equator. Although the calculated protection in this meta-analysis reached statistical significance, no explanation was offered for the failure to show efficacy in two large, recently conducted trials.

In addition, since BCG is presumed to work by conferring tuberculoimmunity to those *not* previously infected, it is not appropriate for widespread use in the United States, where most cases arise among those already infected with *M. tuberculosis.* Some have called for BCG vaccinations for health care workers at high risk for tuberculosis infection. However, given the disputable protection afforded by the vaccines and the loss of utility of the TST (due to reactivity induced by BCG) as a tool to mark recent infection and to qualify for preventive chemotherapy—which *has* proven efficacy—this seems to be a dubious proposition.

LIMITING NOSOCOMIAL TRANSMISSION. Substantial microepidemics of tuberculosis have been documented recently in various institutions, including hospitals, clinics, residential facilities, and prisons. To prevent institutional transmission, the CDC has advocated a three-tiered system: administrative measures, environmental programs, and personal respiratory protection. These measures are currently being employed by Occupational Safety and Health Administration (OSHA) as criteria to assess institutional tuberculosis control programs. *Administrative measures* include educational programs to alert staff on how to recognize and isolate possible active cases early. Also, staff tuberculin skin testing is required to assess the risks of intrainstitutional transmission. *Engineering or environmental programs* are intended to effectively isolate proven or suspected cases by placing them in negative-pressure rooms and diluting the air in the patients' environment through six or more air changes per hour, with the options of decontamination via the adjunctive use of HEPA filtration or ultraviolet germicidal irradiation. *Personal respiratory protection* entails respirators or masks that theoretically can filter out the infectious "droplet nuclei"; presently, HEPA filtration respirators most clearly meet federal guidelines. The optimal role for personal respirators is controversial. Perhaps the most suitable role would be to protect health care workers who have unavoidable exposure to smear-positive cases during cough-inducing procedures such as bronchoscopy or intubation. Use in other circumstances depends on source case and environmental factors. For considerations of both public health concerns and regulatory oversight, all institutions that might be involved with caring for tuberculosis patients should have an active program to limit the hazard of nosocomial transmission to health care workers and other patients or clients.

American Thoracic Society: Treatment of tuberculosis and tuberculosis infection in adults and children. Am J Respir Crit Care Med 149:1359, 1994. *Most recent guidelines for treatment and prevention in adults, children, and infants. Excellent overview of contemporary issues.*

Bloch AB, Cauthen GM, Onorato IM, et al.: Nationwide survey of drug-resistant tuberculosis in the United States. JAMA 271:665, 1994. *A careful delineation of the patterns, frequencies, and special risk-factors for drug resistance in the U.S. in the '90's. Helpful in selecting empirical drug regimens and preventive chemotherapy.*

Cantwell MF, Snider DE Jr, Cauthen GM, et al.: Epidemiology of tuberculosis in the United States, 1985–1992. JAMA 272:535, 1994. *Recent trends in demographics and special risk factors. Helps quantify the impacts of HIV infection and immigration upon case rates; also targets high-risk groups for screening, case detection, and prevention.*

Iseman MD: Treatment of multidrug-resistant tuberculosis. N Engl J Med 329:784, 1993. *Reviews recent epidemiology, management, and prevention of multidrug-resistant tuberculosis; discusses use of second-line medications and resectional surgery.*

312 OTHER MYCOBACTERIOSES

Laurel C. Preheim

MICROBIOLOGY. Among the mycobacteria, *M. tuberculosis,* *M. bovis,* and *M. leprae* have caused most human infections. In the 1950's, however, Timpe and Runyon established that other mycobacteria could cause disease in humans and classified these organisms based on pigment production, growth rate, and colonial characteristics. Photochromogens (group I) grow slowly on culture media (>7 days). Their colonies change from a buff shade to bright yellow or orange after exposure to light. Scotochromogens (group II) also grow slowly but demonstrate pigmented colonies when incubated in the dark or the light. Group III mycobacteria grow slowly and lack pigment in the dark or light. Rapid growers (group IV) also lack pigment, but they grow in culture within 3 to 5 days. Collectively, these four groups have been called the "atypical mycobacteria," "nontuberculous mycobacteria" (NTM), "mycobacteria other than tubercle bacilli" (MOTT), or "potentially pathogenic environmental mycobacteria" (PPEM).

EPIDEMIOLOGY. The rate of isolation of NTM is increasing and has surpassed that for *M. tuberculosis* in some areas. Ubiquitous in nature, many have been isolated from ground or tap water, soil, house dust, domestic and wild animals, and birds. Despite their wide distribution, some species are more common in certain geographic locations. Most infections, including those which are hospital-acquired, result from inhalation or direct inoculation from environmental sources. Ingestion may be the source of infection for children with NTM cervical adenopathy and for patients with AIDS whose disseminated infection may begin in the gastrointestinal tract. These infections are not considered contagious, since person-to-person transmission is extremely rare.

PATHOPHYSIOLOGY. The pathogenic potential for human disease varies among NTM. As a group, these organisms are less virulent for humans than *M. tuberculosis* and may colonize body surfaces or secretions without causing disease. Tissue invasion is most likely to occur in individuals with predisposing conditions associated with impaired local or systemic host defenses. In general, disease is slowly progressive, and histopathologic findings resemble those seen in tuberculosis.

DIAGNOSIS. The steps taken to diagnose tuberculosis generally apply to NTM infections. Standardized, specific skin test antigens for NTM, however, are unavailable. In addition, colonization of asymptomatic individuals and environmental contamination of specimens can yield positive cultures in the absence of clinical disease. NTM disease can be considered present in patients with a cavitary infiltrate on chest radiograph when (1) two or more sputums (or sputum and a bronchial washing) are smear-positive for acid-fast bacilli and/or yield moderate to heavy growth on culture, and (2) other reasonable causes for the disease process have been excluded, e.g., fungal disease, tuberculosis, malignancy. An additional criterion, (3) failure of the sputum cultures to convert to negative with either bronchial hygiene or 2 weeks of specific mycobacterial drug therapy, is applied in the presence of a noncavitary infiltrate not known to be due to another disease.

The diagnosis is also established if transbronchial, percutaneous, or open lung biopsy tissue reveals mycobacterial histopathologic changes and yields the organism. Extrapulmonary or disseminated disease is confirmed by isolating the organism from normally sterile body fluids, closed sites, or lesions, and environmental contamination of specimens is excluded. Radiometric culture systems, DNA probes, and polymerase chain reaction assays have increased the speed and accuracy of laboratory diagnosis of pulmonary and extrapulmonary infections.

CLINICAL DISEASE. NTM cause a broad spectrum of diseases (Table 312–1). The following discussion includes infections caused by selected species most likely to be encountered in clinical settings. It should be noted that therapeutic approaches continue to evolve and therefore remain controversial. Most conventional antituberculous agents have little or no activity against the majority of

TABLE 312–1. NONTUBERCULOUS MYCOBACTERIAL DISEASES AND ETIOLOGIC SPECIES

Clinical Disease	Etiologic Species (Runyan Group)*	
	Common	*Less Common*
Pulmonary	*M. avium* complex (III) *M. kansasii* (I) *M. abscessus* (IV) *M. xenopi* (II)	*M. simiae* (I) *M. szulgai* (II) *M. malmoense* (III) *M. fortuitum* (IV) *M. chelonae* (IV)
Lymphadenitis	*M. avium* complex (III) *M. scrofulaceum* (II)	*M. fortuitum* (IV) *M. chelonae* (IV) *M. abscessus* (IV) *M. kansasii* (I)
Cutaneous	*M. marinum* (I) *M. fortuitum* (IV) *M. chelonae* (IV) *M. abscessus* (IV) *M. ulcerans* (III)	*M. avium* complex (III) *M. kansasii* (I) *M. terrae* (III) *M. smegmatis* (IV) *M. haemophilum* (III)
Disseminated	*M. avium* complex (III) *M. kansasii* (I) *M. chelonae* (IV) *M. abscessus* (IV) *M. haemophilum* (III)	*M. fortuitum* (IV) *M. xenopi* (II)

* I = photochromogen; II = scotochromogen; III = nonpigmented; IV = rapid grower.

these organisms. Many treatment regimens contain new agents or older antimicrobials newly found to have activity against mycobacteria. In therapeutic decisions all potential drug toxicities and interactions must be weighed.

Mycobacterium avium-intracellulare. *M. avium* and *M. intracellulare* are closely related and commonly grouped as *M. avium-intracellulare* or *M. avium* complex (MAC). Distributed worldwide, they rank first among NTM isolates in the United States. MAC causes about 80% of NTM lymphadenitis cases. *M. scrofulaceum* is responsible for most of the rest. Excisional therapy without chemotherapy is curative in about 95% of cervical adenopathy cases. Pulmonary infection usually occurs in individuals with underlying lung disease and generally follows an indolent or slowly progressive course. Differentiation between colonization and true infection may be difficult initially. Extrapulmonary or disseminated disease, infrequently seen in immunocompetent patients, occurs in up to 40% of individuals with AIDS. It usually affects patients with advanced human immunodeficiency virus (HIV) disease. Therefore, prophylaxis with rifabutin (300 mg daily) is recommended for patients with CD4+ T lymphocyte counts <100 cells per microliter. Symptoms suggesting disseminated MAC include fever, weight loss, anorexia, abdominal pain, and diarrhea. Findings may include hepatosplenomegaly and generalized lymphadenopathy, including mediastinal adenopathy. Diagnosis of disseminated disease is commonly made by culturing the organism from blood, bone marrow, stool, or tissue biopsy.

Newer regimens for MAC infections are based on recent trials with patients with AIDS who received treatment for disseminated disease. These guidelines can be applied to patients with or without AIDS who have either pulmonary or disseminated infections. Treatment regimens should include at least two agents. Every regimen should contain either azithromycin (500 mg once daily) or clarithromycin (500 mg twice daily). Many experts prefer ethambutol (15 mg per kilogram once daily) as the second drug. One or more of the following may be added as second, third, or fourth agents: clofazimine (100 mg daily), rifabutin (300 to 600 mg daily), rifampin (600 mg daily), ciprofloxacin (750 mg twice daily), and in some situations amikacin (7.5 to 10 mg per kilogram daily). Isoniazid and pyrazinamide are not effective. No specific regimen has emerged as being superior for pulmonary or disseminated disease, and the optimal duration of therapy remains unknown. Immunocompetent patients probably should receive a minimum of 18 to 24 months of therapy. Therapy should continue for the lifetime of patients with AIDS if clinical and microbiologic improvement is observed.

Mycobacterium kansasii. *M. kansasii,* the most important photochromogen, often appears beaded or cross-barred on acid-fast stain. It ranks second among NTM in causing human infections. Most disease occurs in midwestern and southern United States. Pulmonary infection resembling tuberculosis is the usual clinical presentation. Although adult white men are most commonly affected, infection can occur in individuals of any age, gender, or race. Extrapulmonary disease can involve any organ system, and risks of dissemination are increased in immunocompromised patients.

Standard treatment of pulmonary disease is isoniazid (300 mg daily), rifampin (600 mg daily), and ethambutol (15 mg per kilogram daily) for 18 months. In patients who are unable to tolerate isoniazid, rifampin and ethambutol, with or without streptomycin for the first 3 months, is an alternative regimen. *M. kansasii* isolates are resistant to pyrazinamide. Patients with isolates resistant to rifampin can be treated with isoniazid (900 mg daily), pyridoxine (50 mg daily), ethambutol (25 mg per kilogram daily), and sulfamethoxazole (3.0 grams daily) for 18 to 24 months. This regimen can be combined with streptomycin or amikacin given daily or 5 times per week for 2 to 3 months, followed by intermittent streptomycin or amikacin for a total of at least 6 months. These treatment regimens apply to patients with pulmonary or extrapulmonary infection and have been used with some success in individuals with AIDS. The optimal agents and duration of therapy for disseminated disease in patients with AIDS are unknown.

Rapidly Growing Mycobacteria. Rapidly growing mycobacteria are acid-fast rods that resemble diphtheroids on Gram stain. Growth is rapid on subculture (1 to 3 days), but primary isolation from clinical specimens may require 2 to 30 days. Unlike other mycobacteria, they grow well on most routine laboratory media. Sporadic, community-acquired infections have been reported from most areas of the United States. The spectrum of diseases ranges from localized to disseminated, with cutaneous involvement being most common. Most infections are acquired by inoculation after accidental trauma, surgery, or injection. Nosocomial epidemics or clusters have been reported in numerous settings including augmentation mammaplasty, hemodialysis, plastic surgery, long-term venous catheter use, cardiac surgery, and jet injector use.

These NTM are highly resistant to conventional antituberculous drugs but may be sensitive to traditional antibiotics. Susceptibility testing of individual isolates is important, since resistance patterns vary by and within species subgroups. *M. fortuitum* is usually susceptible to amikacin, ciprofloxacin, sulfonamides, cefoxitin, and imipenem, and occasionally to doxycycline. *M. abscessus* is generally susceptible to amikacin and cefoxitin and occasionally erythromycin. In contrast, *M. chelonae* is most likely to be susceptible to tobramycin, amikacin, or erythromycin and occasionally to doxycycline.

Amikacin plus cefoxitin (12 grams daily) can be used for initial therapy of severe infections caused by all species except *M. chelonae*. The decision to change to oral therapy depends on clinical improvement and susceptibility testing results. Oral agents may include ciprofloxacin (500 mg twice daily), sulfamethoxazole (1 gram thrice daily), doxycycline (100 mg twice daily), and clarithromycin (500 mg twice daily). Because development of resistance has been reported during single-drug therapy with ciprofloxacin, the use of two agents should be considered. Treatment duration should be a minimum of 3 months for serious disease and 6 months for bone infections. Any regimen should include surgical débridement of infected wounds or excision of foreign bodies.

Other Nontuberculous Mycobacteria. *M. marinum* cutaneous infections commonly follow aquatic-related inoculation. Papules on an extremity, especially on the elbows, knees, and dorsum of feet and hands, may progress to shallow ulceration and scar formation. Therapeutic approaches have included simple observation for minor lesions, surgical excision, and antimicrobials. Acceptable regimens include doxycycline (100 mg twice daily), trimethoprim-sulfamethoxazole (160/800 mg twice daily), or rifampin (600 mg daily) plus ethambutol (15 mg per kilogram daily) for a minimum of 3 months. Recent studies indicate clarithromycin (500 mg twice daily) may be effective as a single agent. *M. xenopi, M. malmoense, M. szulgai, M. simiae, M. haemophilum,* and *M. terrae* are being reported with increasing frequency as causes of pulmonary or disseminated infections in Europe, England, Canada, and the United States. Patients with AIDS appear particularly prone to disseminated disease. Initial therapy for these infections should consist of isoniazid, rifampin, and ethambutol with or without streptomycin or amikacin. Optimal duration of therapy is unknown, but at least 18

to 24 months is recommended. *M. gordonae,* a scotochromogen also known as the "tap water bacillus," has been associated with nosocomial pseudo-outbreaks. It rarely, if ever, causes infection, and its isolation should suggest likely environmental contamination of a clinical specimen.

American Thoracic Society: Diagnosis and treatment of disease caused by nontuberculous mycobacteria. Am Rev Respir Dis 142:940, 1990. *Outstanding guidelines for the diagnosis and therapy of NTM.*

Centers for Disease Control and Prevention: Recommendations on prophylaxis and therapy for disseminated *Mycobacterium avium* complex for adults and adolescents infected with human immunodeficiency virus. MMWR 42(RR-9):13, 1993. *Authoritative, up-to-date therapeutic recommendations that can be applied to all types of MAC infections.*

Inderlied CB, Kemper CA, Bermudez LEM: The *Mycobacterium avium* complex. Clin Microbiol Rev 6:266, 1993. *An excellent review on the most common NTM.*

Straus WL, Ostroff SM, Jernigan DB, et al.: Clinical and epidemiologic characteristics of *Mycobacterium haemophilum,* an emerging pathogen in immunocompromised patients. Ann Intern Med 120:118, 1994. *A good description of a newly recognized NTM pathogen.*

Wayne LG, Sramek HA: Agents of newly recognized or infrequently encountered mycobacterial diseases. Clin Microbiol Rev 5:1, 1992. *An excellent, very comprehensive review; includes 244 references.*

313 LEPROSY *(Hansen's Disease)*
Gilla Kaplan and Zanvil A. Cohn*

DEFINITION. Leprosy is a bacterial disease of great chronicity and low infectivity that occurs worldwide. The primary host is the human, in whom the causative agent *Mycobacterium leprae* accumulates largely in the skin and peripheral nerves, leading to a variety of cutaneous lesions and loss of nerve conduction. Serious disfigurement and loss of digits may result and represent the stigmata of this biblical disease. The clinical manifestations are largely governed by the ability of the host to mount a cell-mediated immune (CMI) response to the organism and its antigens. Patients unable to generate an immune response develop widely distributed skin lesions of the "lepromatous" state and allow unrestricted growth of bacilli. In contrast, a moderate to vigorous immune response leads to the localized cutaneous lesions of the "tuberculoid" form. In addition to these polar states, there are intermediate forms that demonstrate gradations in reactivity. Spontaneous modulation of the disease toward more polar forms can occur and may lead to tissue damage via humoral (immune complex) and cellular (CMI) mechanisms. Multiple-drug therapy promptly reduces viable organisms and transmissibility but must be maintained for long periods for the disappearance of skin lesions and a reduction in bacterial load.

TRANSMISSION. Little detailed information is available about how the bacillus is transmitted from one individual to another. This deficit in our understanding is related to the long incubation period (> 3 years) and the absence of adequate techniques to identify the organism in the environment. Other than in humans, the disease has been discovered in feral armadillos studied in Louisiana and Texas. These animals contain large numbers of acid-fast bacilli in parenchymatous organs, which by DNA hybridization and restriction fragment length polymorphism analysis techniques are identical to bacilli obtained from humans. The sooty mangabey, a new world monkey, can become infected naturally in the wild or when injected with human bacilli. In both armadillos and monkeys it takes 18 to 24 months for the injected bacilli to reach high numbers. These infections are quite unlike the spectrum of human disease.

How the localized lesions of tuberculoid leprosy and the generalized cutaneous distribution of lepromatous disease evolved is unclear. Direct inoculation via trauma and puncture wounds might lead to an initial focus with environmental bacilli. Some suggest that the initial route may be through the respiratory or gastrointestinal tract. Biting insects have been considered, but no clear evidence

---

* Dr. Cohn is deceased.

exists on them as an intermediate vector. It seems reasonable, however, that at some point during the infection in lepromatous leprosy patients, hematogenous spread occurs with wide seeding of the body.

The extent of contact with environmental bacilli is correlated with transmission. The incidence of the disease within a household containing an infected tuberculoid or lepromatous index patient may be four to eight times that of the general population. In particular, lepromatous patients with lesions in the nasal mucosa discharge large numbers of organisms. Bacilli recovered from dry nasal discharges retain some viability for up to 7 to 10 days, with somewhat greater viability under conditions of higher humidity. Transmission of the disease from an untreated, infected mother to an infant is not uncommon and should always be considered. In general, clinical wisdom indicates that disease transmission takes place only after years of exposure. Little likelihood of transmission is present in a ward or hospital setting, and patients are now cared for on an ambulatory basis with a minimum of precautions.

SUSCEPTIBILITY. Leprosy occurs worldwide and in individuals of all ages. It appears more frequently in young adults, but this may be related to a parental index case and the long period of incubation. A large number of studies suggest, but do not prove, that the overall susceptibility to leprosy is not controlled by immune response genes and their expressed major histocompatibility class II antigens. Early analysis of the disease incidence and susceptibility in identical twins has not been conclusive. More recent studies suggest that the type of leprosy rather than overall disease susceptibility may be controlled by HLA determinants. No clear-cut conclusions on the genetic basis of susceptibility can therefore be accepted at this time. In this context, environmental factors such as nutrition and coincident microbial and parasitic infections must be considered as unproven alternatives.

The physiologic immunodeficiency of the newborn may lead to an early colonization with the bacillus. The AIDS pandemic has been associated with a rise in the incidence of other mycobacterial diseases, and this association, although not yet observed, may become more apparent in leprosy in the future.

EPIDEMIOLOGY. The worldwide number of leprosy cases has been estimated to be about 10 million in 1991. In many countries, valid statistics are not available, and the incidence in outlying, rural areas is poorly documented. The highest prevalence rates are in Asia and Africa, followed by Central and South America and Oceania. The highest rates do not usually exceed 55 per 1000 but may be as high as 200 per 1000 in selected villages. Many accept the fact that with effective chemotherapy the worldwide prevalence is dropping and will continue to do so with advanced diagnostic and public health methods. However, incidence does not appear to be changing.

The majority of leprosy cases are found in tropical areas. Socioeconomic condition, availability of health care, and body exposure to the environment may all contribute. The disease also occurs in the colder climates of Tibet, Nepal, Korea, and Siberia. In previous centuries, the disease occurred more commonly in Scandinavia and those countries bordering the North Sea. Small numbers (300 to 500 per year) of cases currently occur in the United States. The majority of these are in immigrant groups from Asia and South America, although occasional cases are seen in the southern states and those bordering Mexico.

The nature of the disease varies considerably with geographic distribution. African and Asian countries have a predominance of tuberculoid leprosy, and 20% or fewer of the cases are of the lepromatous type. In contrast, larger numbers of lepromatous cases are

reported in Brazil and Venezuela. Early infection and/or sensitization with cross-reacting antigens of other mycobacteria have been considered as an explanation for the variation in type of leprosy with which an individual presents.

ETIOLOGIC AGENT. M. leprae is the causative agent of human leprosy, and no evidence of strain variation has been noted by DNA-DNA hybridization or restriction fragment length polymorphism. The organism is acid-alcohol fast when stained by the Ziehl-Neelsen method. M. leprae is an obligate intracellular parasite and has never been cultivated extracellularly in laboratory media. It is a resident of the phagolysosomes of macrophages, Schwann cells, and endothelial cells. M. leprae is classified as a mycobacterium and contains mycolic acid, arabinogalactan, and phenolic glycolipid. The latter molecule is the only M. leprae–specific component. Most other carbohydrates, peptidoglycans, and proteins share antigenic determinants with other mycobacterial species, making serologic diagnosis especially difficult.

The absence of a culture system for M. leprae has complicated any investigations of the physiology and pathogenicity of the organism. Many advances in this field have resulted from the ability of the armadillo to support the growth of the mycobacteria. Eighteen to 24 months after inoculation, large numbers of bacilli (10^9 per gram) can be purified from liver and spleen and serve as a source for antigenic and chemical analysis. Many of the metabolic activities of M. leprae appear to be low compared with other mycobacteria. M. leprae lacks catalase activity, and de novo purine biosynthesis appears to be missing. M. leprae replicates very slowly within host cells and has a doubling time of approximately 13 days. It prefers ambient temperatures below 37°C and grows selectively in cooler portions of the body such as skin, testes, and nasal mucosa.

Determining bacillary viability and resistance to chemotherapeutic agents depends on its slow growth in the foot pads of mice—a bioassay taking about 12 months. Accelerated growth occurs in the athymic nude mouse but still requires 6 or more months. These properties impose severe restrictions on rapid diagnosis. Applying the polymerase chain reaction, in which selected DNA sequences are amplified a millionfold, may lead to the specific identification of as few as 10 bacilli within a few days.

IMMUNOLOGIC CONSIDERATION. A major immunologic defect occurs in patients with lepromatous leprosy. This is expressed as a selective unresponsiveness of T cells to M. leprae and is evident in skin test (Mitsuda) anergy and the in vitro lymphocyte transformation test for M. leprae antigens (Table 313–1). Patients with the tuberculoid form of the disease respond normally, and in neither form of the disease are there abnormalities in humoral immunity. The association between cell-mediated cutaneous responses, T-cell accumulation in lesions, T-cell–directed immunity, and the number of M. leprae in the tissues is shown in Table 313–1. These parameters are inversely related. In the absence of M. leprae–specific T-cell reactivity, lymphokine formation is depressed or absent and tissue macrophages fail to be activated into an antimicrobial state. Normally, macrophage activation occurs largely through the local release of interferon-gamma (IFN-γ), a lymphokine that enhances the production of toxic oxygen intermediates in these cells. Bacilli taken up by "resting" and "aged" macrophages of the skin are able to multiply intracellularly, leading in the case of lepromatous disease to multibacillary vacuoles. In tuberculoid forms, the bacilli are largely destroyed, and only small numbers survive to perpetuate the cell-mediated immune reactions.

Lepromatous patients, although unresponsive to M. leprae antigen, develop adequate reactions to other antigens to which they have been sensitized. These include skin test antigens such as PPD, mumps, Candida, trichophytin, and tetanus toxoid. The highly se-

TABLE 313–1. IMMUNOLOGIC FEATURES OF LEPROSY PATIENTS

	Tuberculoid	Borderline Tuberculoid	Mid Borderline	Borderline Lepromatous	Lepromatous
Acid-fast bacilli in skin lesion	−	−/+	+	+++	+++
Lepromin (Mitsuda) reaction	+++	++	−	−	−
Lymphocyte transformation test	95%	40%	10%	1–2%	1–2%
Anti-M. leprae antibodies	−/+	−/++	++	+++	+++
CD4+/CD8+ T-cell ratio in lesions	1.35	1.11	NT	0.48	0.20

lective anergy of leprosy may be related to the loss of *M. leprae*–specific T cells rather than suppressor cell phenomena.

CLINICAL DIAGNOSIS. Patients with leprosy are first seen and followed by dermatologists because the anesthetic cutaneous lesions are often the presenting complaint. The range in immunity to *M. leprae* is reflected clinically by a wide variation of skin lesions and peripheral nerve involvement. In this section we review the characteristics of the major polar and borderline forms.

Polar Tuberculoid Leprosy (TT). This form presents as one to a few asymmetric plaques or macules defined by a sharp, raised border. In dark-skinned patients, they are often centrally hypopigmented with a more erythematous border. The central area is scaly, lacks hair, and is anesthetic. Nerves leading to the area of the ear, elbow, and knee may be palpably enlarged. Almost any area of the skin may be affected except for the warmer regions of the scalp, axilla, and perineum. The disease is stable.

Borderline Tuberculoid and Borderline Lepromatous Leprosy (BT and BL). As the body burden of antigen increases, in association with a partial reduction in immunity, the number, distribution, and nature of the cutaneous lesions increase in complexity and the sequelae of peripheral nerve damage increase in severity. The skin exhibits a polymorphic array of macular, erythematous, hypopigmented lesions involving the trunk, extremities, and face. These vary randomly in number and distribution. Larger nerve trunks are infiltrated with a granulomatous reaction, leading to nerve damage resulting in foot drop, flexion contractions of the digits, and corneal abrasions. The anesthesia of hands and feet and the resulting damage from burns, trauma, and secondary infection leads to loss of digits, plantar ulcerations, and blindness. These widely dispersed lesions suggest hematogenous spread and a cell-mediated reaction that is not capable of fully controlling bacillary growth. Disease is unstable and may evolve toward the polar forms. Reactional states are common.

Lepromatous Leprosy (LL). Here there is little or no CMI, and tremendous numbers of organisms are dispersed throughout the skin. Again, the lesions are pleomorphic but often are less "angry" or erythematous than in borderline disease. Macules, papules, and nodules may cover wide areas of the trunk and extremities, and lesion distribution is often symmetric. Almost any area of affected or "normal" looking skin contains bacilli. Often there are no obvious lesions, but the skin looks shiny and "full," as the dermis is expanded with macrophages containing bacilli. This is particularly prominent on the ears, eyebrows, and face, giving rise to an appearance called "leonine facies." Eyebrow loss is frequent; a saddle nose deformity may result from cartilage destruction; gynecomastia from reduced testosterone levels secondary to testicular damage may be present; and blindness and iridocyclitis, laryngeal stenosis, loss of incisor teeth, and loss of digits may occur. Nerve damage in lepromatous leprosy is more slowly progressive but is eventually severe and diffuse and leads to a sensory polyneuropathy. Rigid, swollen nerves are palpable in many locations. Disease is stable. These results of long-term untreated lepromatous leprosy are the stigmata that ostracized the leper from his/her community and necessitated custodial care. This is almost never the case today, and patients undergoing chemotherapy remain members of their households.

REACTIONAL STATES. *Erythema Nodosum Leprosum (ENL).* Patients with BL and LL disease maintain high levels of circulating anti–*M. leprae* antibodies as well as high antigen levels in tissue depots. Following effective chemotherapy, a prompt and extensive kill of bacilli takes place, and large amounts of soluble antigens are liberated extracellularly. More than 30% of such patients develop ENL and present with painful subcutaneous erythematous nodules that arise diffusely and may eventually lead to necrosis and suppuration. These symptoms, accompanied by fever and malaise, can continue for months, are extremely debilitating, and are often accompanied by acute inflammation of the eyes, testes, nerves, lymph nodes, and joints. Some patients develop glomerulonephritis with the deposition of complement and immune complexes in the glomeruli. Enhanced production of tumor necrosis factor alpha (TNFα) has been associated with ENL. This serious complication requires prompt diagnosis and therapy.

Reversal Reactions. This reactional state also may occur after chemotherapy but differs from ENL in that acceleration or decrease of the local cell-mediated reaction is observed, accompanied by widespread erythema and induration of pre-existing lesions as well

as systemic symptoms, e.g., pyrexia. The onset of this state is slower, takes weeks to months, and may persist for many months if not properly treated. Rapid progression of pre-existing peripheral nerve damage may take place. These irreversible changes in nerve conduction should be considered a medical emergency and treated accordingly.

LABORATORY DIAGNOSIS. In addition to clinical manifestations, the primary method for diagnosing leprosy is identifying acid-fast bacilli in the skin. The slit smear technique is used throughout the world. Skin is incised with a scalpel, squeezing the area to maintain a bloodless field. The edges of the slit are scraped with the edge of the scalpel, smeared on a slide, fixed, and stained by the Ziehl-Neelsen method. A microscopic logarithmic score (1 + to 6 +; 5 + equals 100 to 1000 acid-fast bacilli per high-power field) is used to quantitate the bacterial load. Usually six sites on the earlobes, elbow, knee, and a lesion are prepared. This simple method, when skillfully applied, is as sensitive as any diagnostic procedure.

A more definitive estimate of bacillary numbers in the skin comes from biopsy material. A logarithmic score is made by counting the number of bacilli in high-power fields. This ranges from 1 + to 6 + and is a useful index in following the response of patients to therapy in terms of bacillary numbers and histopathologic classification. (Bacterial index: 0—no bacilli in 100 microscopic fields ($\times 100$); 1 + = 1 to 10 bacilli in 100 fields; 2 + = 1 to 10 bacilli in 10 fields; 3 + = 1 to 10 bacilli per field; 4 + = 10 to 100 bacilli per field; 5 + = 100 to 1000 bacilli per field; and 6 + = many 1000s per field.)

A skin test may be used which distinguishes the immunologically reactive (tuberculoid) and nonreactive (lepromatous) poles of the disease. A crude antigen consisting of heat-killed bacilli from lepromatous skin nodules is injected and induces local induration and the formation of granulomas in 3 to 4 weeks in most tuberculoid patients. Patients with lepromatous leprosy fail to react to the antigen and may remain unresponsive long after effective chemotherapy.

Serologic tests are useful in assaying the level of anti–*M. leprae* antibodies in multibacillary lepromatous but not in the paucibacillary tuberculoid forms. However, the many cross-reactive antigenic epitopes shared with other mycobacteria complicate interpretation and differential diagnosis. ELISA tests, which recognize antibodies against the carbohydrate moieties of the phenolic glycolipids, the only molecule that is *M. leprae*–specific, are positive in patients with lepromatous but not tuberculoid disease and decline after chemotherapy is initiated. Patients with lepromatous leprosy have a polyclonal hypergammaglobulinemia, acute phase reactants such as C-reactive protein, and immune complexes in the circulation. Ten percent give false-positive tests for syphilis and 30% have cryoglobulinemia.

HISTOPATHOLOGY AND IMMUNOPATHOLOGY. Microscopic analysis of tissue plays a primary role in diagnosing and classifying the various clinical forms of leprosy and uses the standardized classification described by Ridley and Jopling. Five groups have been defined spanning the spectrum from polar tuberculoid (TT) to polar lepromatous (LL) and include borderline (BB) as well as borderline tuberculoid (BT) and borderline lepromatous (BL). Our discussion focuses on the polar forms, and the details pertaining to the intermediate manifestations can be found in more specialized texts.

Lesions of the Skin. Tuberculoid Leprosy. Microscopic examination of H & E–stained sections of biopsies obtained from a TT macular plaque reveals heavy infiltration of the dermis by mononuclear leukocytes organized in well-developed granulomas. These contain large numbers of lymphocytes scattered between and surrounding other components of the granulomatous response, including macrophage-derived epithelioid cells and Langhans-type multinucleated giant cells (Fig. 313–1). Occasional plasma cells but no granulocytes are found. Langerhans cells are found within the dermal infiltrate in significant numbers. Staining with monoclonal antibodies shows that the majority of lymphocytes are T cells and that the CD4+ "helper type" phenotype predominates over CD8+ "suppressor/cytotoxic" cells.

The epidermis overlying the dermal infiltrate is thickened (two- to threefold), and individual keratinocytes are enlarged. The keratinocytes display large amounts of MHC class II determinants on

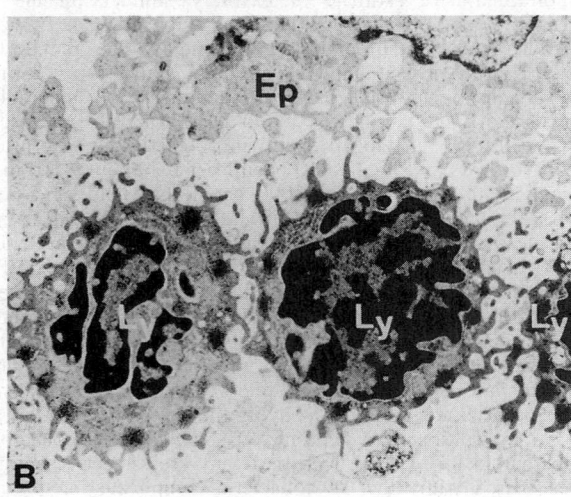

FIGURE 313-1. Transmission electron photomicrographs of cutaneous granulomas from a patient with tuberculoid leprosy. *A,* The granuloma contains large epithelioid cells (Ep) with multiple cytoplasmic organelles (×4500). *B,* Three T lymphocytes (Ly) and an epithelioid cell are observed (×9000).

their surface. This is a response to the local production of IFN-γ in the dermis and is accompanied by the expression of other IFN-γ–induced molecules by keratinocytes and other cell types.

Acid-fast staining of sections reveals an occasional bacillus or bacillary remnants within macrophages. BT lesions are similar except that acid-fast bacilli are more readily seen.

Lepromatous Leprosy. In contrast to TT lesions, the lepromatous lesion contains only small numbers of lymphocytes, predominantly of the CD8+ phenotype, scattered through a background of loosely organized dermal macrophages and collagen (Fig. 313–2). The macrophages often have a pale, foamy cytoplasm and may contain large clumps of *M. leprae* called "globi" (Fig. 313–3). By electron microscopy, these organisms are seen to reside within large cytoplasmic vacuoles, embedded in a lucent matrix that contains a phenolic glycolipid. Remnants of the osmiophilic bacilli are always present along with structurally intact organisms (Fig. 313–3B). A gram of skin may contain 10^9 bacilli. Langerhans cells are rarely seen in the dermis; the overlying epidermis is thin and atrophic and fails to show surface MHC class II antigens.

The loose bacilli-rich infiltrates of LL are present in almost every area of the skin, and individual infected macrophages may be observed surrounded by collagen bundles.

Lesions of Peripheral Nerve. **Tuberculoid Leprosy.** The paucibacillary granulomatous response is associated with significant destruction of peripheral nerve fascicles and late in the disease may lead to caseous necrosis of nerve trunks. Large numbers of T cells and mononuclear phagocytes breach the perineurium and lead to destruction of Schwann cells and axons alike. By the time the skin

lesion is apparent, nerve damage and sensory loss have occurred. The mechanism of the nerve damage in TT is unclear but is related to CMI and the granulomatous response.

Lepromatous Leprosy. Many bacilli are observed within Schwann cells and macrophages surrounding and within the perineural sheath in the majority of subcutaneously placed nerve trunks (Fig. 313–4). Nerve damage is relatively slow as compared with a TT but more extensive and insidious. Few, if any, lymphocytes are part of the lesion. Eventually, more enlargement and displacement by connective tissue result. Schwann cells are capable of taking up *M. leprae* and serve as permissive hosts for their replication (Fig. 313–4).

Other Organs. Granulomatous lesions can be seen in the lymph nodes, liver, spleen, bone marrow, endocrine organs, and eye. These contain bacilli but are not considered to be an important source of infection. Patients with untreated multibacillary disease can have a constant bacteremia of 10^5 AFB per milliliter, all of which are present within monocytes. The total body burden of *M. leprae* can reach 10^{12}.

Lesions of Reactional States. **Erythema Nodosum Leprosum (ENL).** Examination of the skin nodules of ENL shows extensive mixed leukocyte infiltration of neutrophils and mononuclear cells and tissue necrosis. Immune complexes are evident, and there is a panvasculitis of dermal arteries and veins. These are all hallmarks of an extensive acute inflammatory response resulting in tissue damage. TNFα and other monocyte cytokine–induced cell surface antigens can be demonstrated.

Reversal Reactions. Patients with BT, BB, or BL leprosy, who are partially responsive to *M. leprae* antigens, occasionally undergo an upgrading reaction after several months of therapy. This differs from ENL in the migration of a predominantly T-cell infiltrate into pre-existing inflammatory sites. Many of the T cells are of the helper phenotype and are secreting lymphokines into their environment. T-cell migration into skin lesions is associated with mononuclear phagocyte differentiation into organized granuloma and is often associated with the rapid progression of peripheral nerve damage. This enhancement of CMI leads to limited bacillary destruction. A downgrading or reduction in CMI also may occur. Such reactions may continue for weeks or months and are associated with severe morbidity leading to serious sequelae.

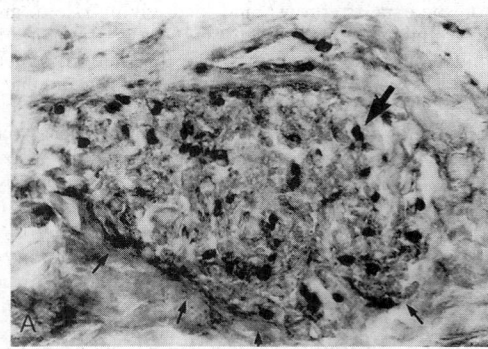
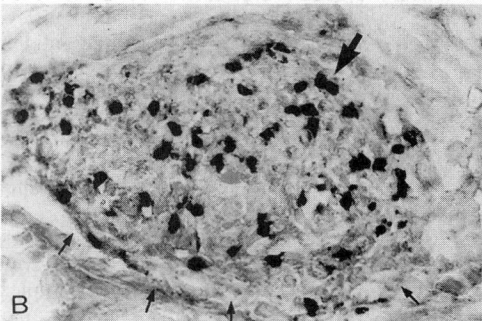

FIGURE 313-2. Lepromatous leprosy—cutaneous lesion. Frozen serial sections stained with Leu 3 (anti-CD4–helper T-cell subset) *(A)* and with Leu 2 (anti-CD8–suppressor/cytotoxic T-cell subset) *(B).* The inflammatory infiltrates *(small arrows)* contain few T cells. Cells of the CD4+ subset *(large arrow in A)* are less numerous than those of the CD8+ subset *(large arrows in B).* Immunoperoxidase, counterstained with hematoxylin (×200).

PATHOGENESIS. Recovery from infections with obligate intracellular parasites such as *M. leprae* requires the host to mount an effective CMI response. For this purpose, antigen-presenting cells must recognize and cluster with appropriate T cells, leading to T-cell stimulation, differentiation, and replication. T cells then follow two distinct pathways. In the first, helper cells synthesize and secrete a variety of hormone-like lymphokines which seem to enhance the microbicidal activity of monocytes and macrophages as well as stimulate other cells in the environment, e.g., keratinocytes, endothelial cells, and fibroblasts. A second pathway leads to the development of T cells which are of the CD4+ phenotype and are antigen specific and MHC class II restricted. Along with NK (natural killer) and LAK (lymphokine-activated killer) cells, they serve as potent specific and nonspecific cytotoxic effector cells.

In lepromatous leprosy, in the absence of local lymphokine production, bacilli multiply in macrophages that have the capacity neither to kill the organism nor to be activated by lymphokines. To modify this fertile intracellular culture environment, the host must destroy the heavily parasitized macrophage, liberating its contents into the extracellular milieu. Here, newly emigrated monocytes ingest, kill, and degrade *M. leprae* with the help of a lymphokine stimulus. This is the situation which applies in the tuberculoid form of the disease and is lacking in the lepromatous state.

RECOMMENDED TREATMENT SCHEDULES. The most commonly used drug in the therapy of leprosy is 4,4'-diaminodiphenylsulfone (dapsone, DDS). Because of the widespread emergence of dapsone-resistant strains of *M. leprae*, all patients now receive multidrug therapy. The components and schedules vary depending on the presence of dapsone-sensitive strains and the part

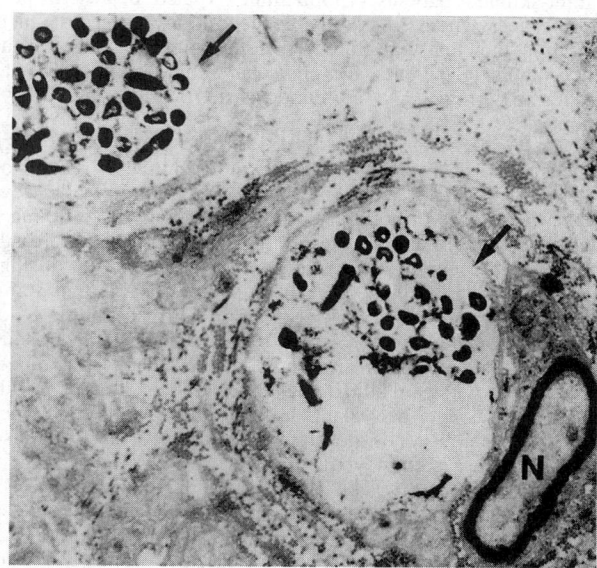

FIGURE 313–4. Transmission electron micrograph of an infiltrated peripheral nerve of a cutaneous lesion from a lepromatous leprosy patient. The myelinated neuron (N) and two *M. leprae*–infected Schwann cells *(arrows)* are observed (×9000).

of the world in which the patient resides. In the United States, the following recently modified regimens are employed:

1. *Paucibacillary disease of the TT and BT categories.*
   a. Dapsone-sensitive *M. leprae*—Dapsone is given in a daily dose of 100 mg and rifampin at a daily dose of 600 mg for 1 year.
   b. Dapsone-resistant *M. leprae*—Clofazimine at a daily dose of 50 to 100 mg is substituted for dapsone.
2. *Multibacillary disease of the BB, BL, and LL categories.*
   a. Dapsone-sensitive or dapsone-resistant *M. leprae*—Dapsone is given in a daily dose of 100 mg, rifampin is given in a dose of 600 mg per day, and clofazimine is given in a daily dose of 50 mg for 2 years.

To evaluate the dapsone sensitivity, the mouse foot pad assay must be used; this procedure is available only in specialized facilities.

A modified schedule for third world country control programs was issued in 1982 and is based on practical consideration by the World Health Organization (WHO), including the availability of slit smear facilities and financial constraints:

1. *Paucibacillary disease—a bacillary index of 0 at all six skin sites.* Dapsone is given daily at a dose of 100 mg, unsupervised. Rifampin is given at a dose of 600 mg once a month, supervised. Treatment is given for 6 months and is then discontinued.
2. *Multibacillary disease—a bacillary index of 1+ or more at any one of six skin sites.* Dapsone is given daily at 100 mg with clofazimine 50 mg daily, unsupervised. Rifampin 600 mg and clofazimine 300 mg are given once monthly, supervised. This therapy is continued for 2 years.

The WHO schedule for intermittent rifampin therapy is based in part on its expense and on clinical and laboratory trials. It should be noted, however, that many leprologists use rifampin at 450 to 600 mg daily for 2 to 3 years. Relapses under the WHO schedule are infrequent.

Rifampin is the most rapidly effective bactericidal agent and kills the majority of *M. leprae* within 2 to 3 weeks. This is evident by mouse foot pad assays. Resistance to rifampin is well known in the therapy of *M. tuberculosis* and is now becoming evident with *M. leprae*.

Therapy with clofazimine, a phenazine derivative, has certain unpleasant side effects based on its lipophilicity. The compound is a red-purple dye taken up and concentrated by macrophages of the

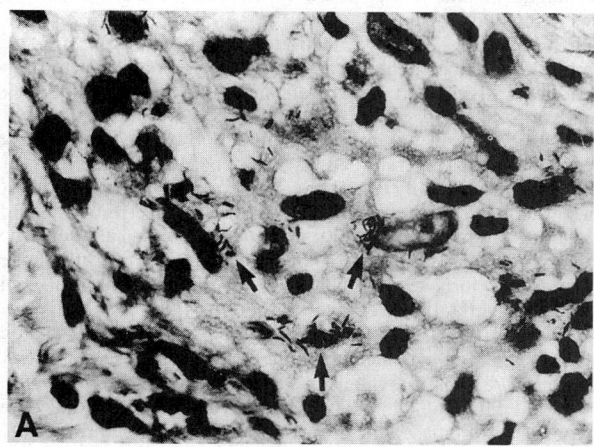

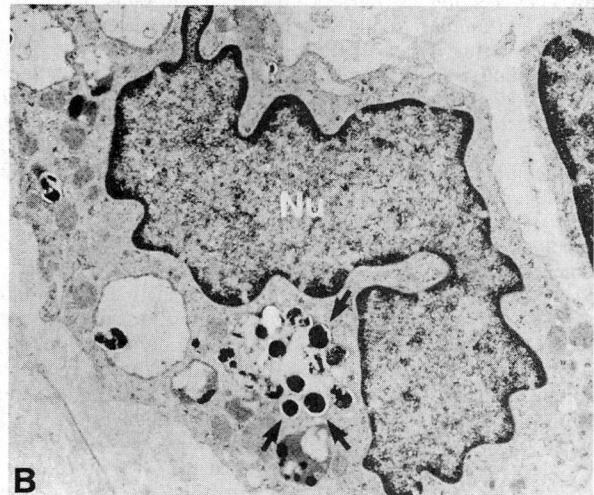

FIGURE 313–3. Lepromatous leprosy—cutaneous lesions. Acid-fast staining of histologic section *(A)* and transmission electron photomicrograph *(B)* of *M. leprae*–parasitized foamy macrophages *(arrows)*. The phagocytes have large nuclei and many light and electron lucent vacuoles containing darkly staining bacteria (*A*, ×500; *B*, ×9000).

skin, causing increased skin pigmentation. This is distressing to certain light-skinned patients. Clofazimine is also deposited in the small intestine, where it at high concentrations causes segmental thickening associated with crampy pain and diarrhea. If clofazimine is unacceptable to patients, the physician should consider substitution with 100 mg daily of minocycline or 400 mg daily of ofloxacin.

THERAPY OF REACTIONS. *Erythema Nodosum Leprosum.* The acute onset of ENL may be mild enough to require only salicylates or other cyclo-oxygenase inhibitors. With severe episodes, high doses of corticosteroids (prednisone 60 to 80 mg per day) are necessitated and should be tapered off as soon as feasible. However, exacerbations occur frequently, and repeated dosing is necessary. A particularly useful drug in severe ENL is thalidomide, a selective inhibitor of TNFα. It is given initially at 200 mg twice a day and then tapered to levels of 50 to 100 mg per day. Thalidomide is a potent teratogen and should be assiduously avoided if pregnancy is possible. Clofazimine also has been found useful in ENL but requires 4 to 6 weeks to achieve therapeutic effects. ENL in some patients responds poorly to thalidomide, and prednisone and/or clofazimine is employed.

Reversal Reactions. The chronicity and potential nerve damage of this cell-mediated reaction require high-dose steroids and careful evaluation of peripheral nerve condition. Thalidomide is not used in this condition, but clofazimine along with steroids allows the more rapid withdrawal of prednisone.

Other Complications. A number of surgical procedures are available at specialized leprosy hospitals to help correct foot drop, hand deformities, madarosis, and lagophthalmos. Plastic surgical procedures can replace nasal septa and help close large plantar ulcerations. On occasion, patients request the removal of glandular tissue for gynecomastia.

The presence of a cold abscess of a peripheral nerve with sudden increase in pain and functional loss requires immediate decompression by surgical drainage.

IMMUNOMODULATION. Recombinant lymphokines that can enhance the microbicidal properties of macrophages and stimulate the expression of CMI may find a place in the care of leprosy patients. Preliminary studies with the T-cell mitogen interleukin-2 (IL-2) have already been carried out in patients with lepromatous leprosy. The intradermal injection of IL-2 leads to a local cell-mediated reaction associated with induration, the destruction of parasitized macrophages, and a marked reduction in the bacillary load. Trials with more prolonged administration have demonstrated that a systemic response can be achieved.

PROGNOSIS. Tuberculoid leprosy is usually self-limited and responds well to chemotherapy. Nerve damage is, however, irreversible. In lepromatous disease, prolonged courses of multiple drugs arrest the progression of the illness when compliance is good. It is the ability of the public health infrastructure to monitor compliance that is central to effective therapy. Recurrences due to poor maintenance therapy are not infrequent.

PREVENTION AND PROPHYLAXIS. Education of the general public plays an important role in sensitizing individuals to the nature of leprosy lesions and the ability to cure the illness with medication. Once a case has been identified in a household, careful physical examination of all contacts with the biopsy of suspicious lesions should be carried out. The threat of contagion is much higher in children younger than age 16. In this adolescent category, the prophylactic use of dapsone should be considered.

A number of vaccine trials are currently underway, many sponsored by WHO. These are employing BCG vaccine with and without heat-killed *M. leprae* or other mycobacteria in highly endemic areas of Africa, Asia, and India. There is suggestive evidence that BCG alone may reduce the incidence of disease.

Cohn ZA, Kaplan G: Leprosy, cell-mediated immunity and recombinant lymphokines. J Infect Dis 163:1195, 1991. *Discussion of the regulation of CMI with cytokines.*

Guinto RS, Abalos RM, Cellona RV, Fajardo TT: An Atlas of Leprosy. Sasakawa Memorial Health Foundation, 1983. *Excellent pictorial of diagnostic signs.*

Hansen GA: Causes of leprosy. Norsk Laegevidensk 4:76, 1874. *The classic work on leprosy.*

Hastings RC, Franzblau SG: Chemotherapy of leprosy. Annu Rev Pharmacol Toxicol 28:231, 1988. *Current update of therapy and complications thereof.*

Job CK: Nerve damage in leprosy. XIII Leprosy Congress State of the Art Lectures. Int J Leprosy 57:532, 1989. *Good discussion of mechanisms of nerve damage.*

Kaplan G, Britton WJ, Hancock GE, et al.: The systemic influence of recombinant interleukin-2 on the manifestations of lepromatous leprosy. J Exp Med 173:993, 1991. *Systemic modulation of CMI with IL-2.*

Sexually Transmitted Diseases

314 INTRODUCTION TO SEXUALLY TRANSMITTED DISEASES AND COMMON SYNDROMES
P. Frederick Sparling

Sexually transmitted diseases (STD's) are a diverse group of infections, caused by biologically dissimilar microbial agents, that are grouped together because of certain common clinical and epidemiologic features. Advent of the acquired immunodeficiency syndrome (AIDS) has heightened public awareness of the importance of STD's and the dangers of unsafe sexual practices. New knowledge has accumulated rapidly about old diseases; for instance, it is now clear that cervical carcinoma is a complication of certain human papillomavirus (genital wart virus) infections. Some relatively less severe infections, such as chlamydial ones, are known to be alarmingly prevalent in young persons. This chapter discusses certain common features of some of these infections, as well as the differential diagnosis and management of several of the common syndromes of genital infections.

DEFINITIONS. Those infectious agents that are frequently transmitted by sexual contact, and for which sexual transmission is epidemiologically important, are considered STD's. In some cases, such as gonorrhea and genital herpes simplex virus infection, sexual transmission is the only important mode of transmission, at least between adults. In others, such as the hepatitis viruses, giardiasis, shigellosis, and amebiasis, there are also important nonsexual means of acquiring infection. Table 314–1 lists the important infectious agents commonly transmitted sexually, as well as their known or probable disease syndromes. "Sexual" includes the full range of heterosexual or homosexual behavior, including genital, oral-genital, oral-anal, and genital-anal contact.

EPIDEMIOLOGIC CONSIDERATIONS. Sexually transmitted infections are prevalent in many segments of society, but, for obvious reasons, are most prevalent in the groups with the most promiscuous sexual activity. It is not sexual activity *per se* but the number and type of different sexual partners that determine the risk of acquiring STD. The highest rates of gonorrhea are found in the young (15 to 30) and unmarried and in groups of low educational and socioeconomic status. Rates of gonococcal infection may be 50-fold higher in young, single inner-city persons than in married middle- to upper-middle-class persons. Decisions regarding the cost-effectiveness of screening for STD should be governed by these considerations; screening is most effective in high-risk groups.

Multiple infections are frequent in patients with sexually transmitted infection. In venereal disease clinics, about 20% of men with gonorrhea also have urethral chlamydial infection, and 30 to 50% of women with gonorrhea also have cervical chlamydial infection. In women with vaginitis, one study showed that 16% of cases were caused by mixed infection with various combinations of *Candida, Trichomonas,* and *Gardnerella vaginalis.* However, no convincing evidence exists that one sexually transmitted infection directly increases the risk of acquiring others. Rather, the frequent coexistence of multiple sexually acquired infections probably reflects the multiplicity of sexual partners among the subject patients.

Control of sexually transmitted infections is complicated by the frequent lack of significant symptoms. The majority of gonococcal and chlamydial infections in women probably are associated with few symptoms. From 10 to 50% of urethral gonococcal infections in men are oligo- or asymptomatic. Chlamydial infections are more common than gonococcal infections and frequently are asymptomatic. One of the crucial issues in management is proper diagnosis and treatment of the asymptomatically infected partner.

TABLE 314–1. SEXUALLY TRANSMITTED AGENTS AND THEIR SYNDROMES*

Microorganism	Syndromes
Bacteria	
Neisseria gonorrhoeae	Urethritis, cervicitis, bartholinitis, proctitis, pharyngitis, salpingitis, epididymitis, conjunctivitis, perihepatitis, arthritis, dermatitis, endocarditis, meningitis, amniotic infection syndrome
Mobiluncus species and Gardnerella vaginalis	"Nonspecific" vaginosis
Treponema pallidum	Syphilis (multiple clinical syndromes)
Haemophilus ducreyi	Chancroid
Calymmatobacterium granulomatis	Granuloma inguinale
Shigella species	Enteritis in homosexual men
Campylobacter species	Enteritis in homosexual men
Group B Streptococcus	Neonatal sepsis and meningitis
Chlamydiae	
Chlamydia trachomatis	Nongonococcal urethritis, purulent hypertrophic cervicitis, epididymitis, salpingitis, conjunctivitis, trachoma, pneumonia, perihepatitis, lymphogranuloma venereum, Reiter's syndrome
Mycoplasmas	
Ureaplasma urealyticum	Nongonococcal urethritis, ? premature rupture of membranes and abortion
Mycoplasma hominis	Postpartum fever, pelvic inflammatory disease
Viruses	
Herpes simplex virus (HSV)	Genital herpes, proctitis, meningitis, disseminated infection in neonates
Hepatitis A virus	Hepatitis in homosexual men
Hepatitis B virus	Hepatitis, ? periarteritis nodosa, hepatoma; especially prevalent in homosexual men
Cytomegalovirus	Congenital infection (birth defects, infant mortality, mental deficiency, hearing loss), mononucleosis syndrome
Human papillomavirus (HPV)	Condyloma acuminatum, cervical and perianal
Molluscum contagiosum virus	Molluscum contagiosum
Human immunodeficiency virus (HIV)	Acquired immunodeficiency syndrome (AIDS) and related illnesses
Protozoa	
Trichomonas vaginalis	Trichomonal vaginitis, occasional urethritis
Entamoeba histolytica	Enteritis in homosexual men
Giardia lamblia	Enteritis in homosexual men
Fungi	
Candida albicans	Vaginitis, balanitis
Ectoparasites	
Phthirus pubis	Pubic lice infestation
Sarcoptes scabiei	Scabies

* The relative importance of sexual transmission in the epidemiology of several of these agents remains to be defined; these include Group B streptococci, hepatitis A virus, cytomegalovirus, *Candida albicans*, and others.

INCIDENCE OF STD'S. The true incidence of STD's is not known in the United States because of serious problems of underreporting. Gonorrhea is the most common of the reported infectious diseases, with >500,000 infections reported annually. Although genital chlamydial infections generally are not reported, their prevalence certainly exceeds that of gonorrhea. Herpes simplex virus (HSV) and human papillomavirus (HPV) infections also are more prevalent than gonorrhea. The relative incidence of STD is quite variable in different areas of the world. For instance, chancroid is currently uncommon in the United States but is about as common as gonorrhea in certain areas of the Far East and Africa.

COMMON SYNDROMES *Urethritis in Males.* Urethritis in males is a very common syndrome. It is ordinarily classified as either gonococcal or nongonococcal urethritis (NGU), depending whether the presence of gonococci can be demonstrated by Gram stain or culture. In STD clinics, the prevalence of gonococcal and nongonococcal urethritis is similar, but NGU is considerably more common in private practice and in college infirmaries. Several studies of asymptomatic sexually active young persons found an incidence of up to 15% of genital chlamydial infection.

A large number of studies have established *Chlamydia trachomatis* as a cause of approximately 40% of cases of NGU. Case-control studies have provided evidence that suggests *Ureaplasma urealyticum* (formerly T-strain mycoplasma) is a significant factor in chlamydia-negative NGU. In addition, urethral inoculation of volunteers with pure cultures of *U. urealyticum* produced rather typical NGU. In practice, however, it is difficult to define the importance of *Ureaplasma* infection in patients with urethritis, because colonization of these organisms occurs in up to 70% of asymptomatic sexually active persons. A very small proportion of cases of NGU in men is due to *Trichomonas vaginalis* or HSV infection.

Diagnosis of urethritis requires demonstration of an inflammatory urethral exudate. A discharge may not be evident if the patient has recently voided, and patients preferably should be examined several hours after their last urination. The discharge may be present only in the morning, prior to urination. Demonstration of discharge often requires urethral "milking" and may require insertion of a small calcium alginate or similar swab into the anterior urethra, with examination of a direct gram-stained smear of the swab for leukocytes. Presence of an average of at least five polymorphonuclear leukocytes per high-power ($100 \times$) field suggests the diagnosis of urethritis.

The patient should be questioned for past history of urethritis and for symptoms suggestive of systemic diseases such as Reiter's syndrome or disseminated gonococcal infection. Examination should be made for signs of conjunctivitis, arthritis, dermatitis, and epididymitis. Prostatitis is rarely present unless there are symptoms of perineal, suprapubic, or rectal discomfort, and rectal examination is not routinely indicated. Rectal examination and urine culture are indicated in men with dysuria but without signs of anterior urethral discharge.

Laboratory studies are ordinarily limited to a Gram stain of urethral exudate. Demonstration of typical gram-negative diplococci, many of which are inside neutrophils, establishes the diagnosis of gonococcal urethritis. A Gram stain is positive in at least 90% of men with symptomatic culture-proven urethral gonorrhea. In occasional patients, especially those with an equivocal Gram stain, it may be necessary to culture the anterior urethra or freshly voided urine sediment for gonococci. This is particularly important in asymptomatic male contacts of patients with disseminated gonococcal infection or gonococcal salpingitis, since a Gram stain of urethral contents is positive in only about 60% of men with asymptomatic urethral gonorrhea.

Diagnosis of NGU usually is made by exclusion of gonorrhea. Immunoassays and a DNA hybridization test for chlamydia are widely available and have sensitivities of 70 to 80% and specificities of >90% for polymerase chain reaction (PCR) and culture. PCR is just now becoming widely available. Although culture is the "gold standard" for diagnosis of chlamydia, it is probably not as sensitive as PCR. There is no serologic test that is clinically useful. Tests for *Ureaplasma* are not readily available and rarely are indicated. Examination of a saline suspension of urethral exudate occasionally may reveal motile trichomonads in patients with recurrent urethritis who fail to respond to appropriate therapy. A serologic test for syphilis should be obtained, but the diagnostic yield is low.

Management is outlined in Figure 314–1 and is discussed further in Ch. 315. Sexual partners of men with gonococcal or nongonococcal urethritis should be treated to prevent both reinfection of the patient and development of complications in the partners.

The syndrome of *postgonococcal urethritis* (persistence or recrudescence of urethritis after administration of therapy that has eradicated gonococcal infection) is usually due to concomitant ure-

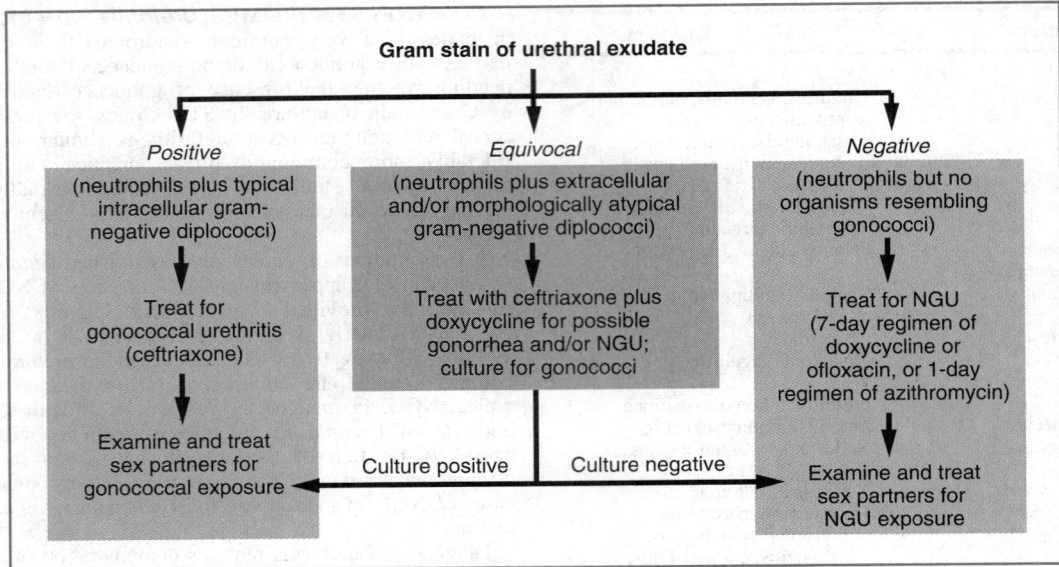

FIGURE 314–1. Management of male patients with urethritis.

thral chlamydial infection that was not eradicated by the original treatment. This syndrome is more common after therapy with a β-lactam antibiotic than after a regimen of tetracycline, undoubtedly because of the greater efficacy of tetracycline for treating chlamydial infections. Accordingly, there is considerable merit to use of oral tetracycline to follow up ceftriaxone therapy for genital gonorrhea.

Genital Ulcer Syndrome. Genital skin lesions may be either ulcerative or nonulcerative. In patients seen in a venereal disease clinic, the most common sexually transmitted nonulcerative genital lesions are due to scabies, genital warts, molluscum contagiosum, or *Candida* species, but differential diagnosis includes a long list of dermatologic conditions.

The most common cause of ulcerative genital lesions in patients in the United States is HSV, but differential diagnosis includes syphilis, chancroid, lymphogranuloma venereum (LGV), granuloma inguinale (GI), and trauma. Chancroid is becoming more common in certain cities in the United States; LGV and GI are rare. The most important distinction is among syphilis, genital herpes, and chancroid. Sometimes the appearance is virtually diagnostic: Grouped, painful, superficial vesicles are nearly diagnostic of herpes, whereas a single, clean-based, nonpainful ulcer with indurated margins suggests primary syphilis. In relatively recent studies, only about 60% of penile syphilitic chancres had this classic appearance. Painful ulcers suggest herpes or chancroid. Genital herpes may occur as a single ulcer, particularly in patients with recurrent herpes, and syphilis may occur with multiple ulcers. Secondarily infected lesions of primary syphilis may be painful.

It is a useful rule to obtain a serologic test for syphilis on all patients with genital ulcers, and, if the initial serologic findings are negative and if the diagnosis remains uncertain, to obtain a second serologic examination about 2 weeks later. A darkfield examination for syphilis should also be done, and it should be repeated twice on successive days if syphilis is seriously suspected and the initial examination is negative.

Infection by HSV may be efficiently diagnosed by viral culture or by immunofluorescent methods, but these are frequently unavailable in practice. Papanicolaou smear is suggestive of herpes in about two thirds of culture-positive cases. Giemsa's or Wright's stain of cells scraped from the base of a vesicle may reveal multinucleate giant cells (Tzanck's test), but this test is particularly insensitive in herpetic lesions that have become ulcerated. Serologic tests for herpesvirus are not helpful in management but may indicate persons with latent infection. Referral of patients to centers with capability of viral culture may be indicated in diagnostically difficult patients.

In addition to herpesvirus infection, chancroid should be sus-

pected in patients with painful genital ulcers. Chancroid is occurring in epidemics in certain United States cities, particularly among crack house clients. Attempts should be made to isolate the causative agent, *Haemophilus ducreyi;* selective culture media are an improvement over previously available methods. No serologic tests are available.

Therapy clearly depends on the correct diagnosis. Topical antibiotics are never indicated. Initial genital herpes (first infection) is best treated with topical or oral administration of acyclovir or intravenous administration for severe infections. Therapy of chancroid is with ciprofloxacin, azithromycin, erythromycin, or ceftriaxone. Occasional empiric trials of oral ciprofloxacin, azithromycin, or erythromycin are warranted in patients with persistent genital ulcers not readily attributable to herpesvirus or syphilis, but repeated attempts to isolate *H. ducreyi* should be made in such instances. It is not possible to arrive at an unequivocal diagnosis of the cause of genital ulcers in all patients.

Lower Genital Tract Infections in Women. Infections of the female genitourinary tract produce a variety of syndromes, often with overlapping symptoms (dysuria, vaginal discharge, vulvar irritation). These infections are very common, relatively poorly understood by most physicians, sometimes difficult to treat, and often frustrating for both doctor and patient. However, the various syndromes usually can be distinguished on relatively simple clinical and laboratory grounds, and a precise microbial cause often can be established.

It is most helpful first to determine the primary anatomic site of infection: urethra or bladder, endocervix, or vagina. This can sometimes be accomplished by history; women with urinary tract infection (UTI) usually experience "internal" dysuria, whereas women with dysuria associated with vaginitis usually experience "external" dysuria owing to passage of urine over inflamed labia. Cervicitis is diagnosed by physical examination; mucopurulent secretions emanate from the endocervical canal, and there is often a hypertrophic, mucoid, reddened "cobblestone" appearance to the cervical mucosa. The cervix may appear normal in women with culture-positive gonococcal or chlamydial infection of the cervix. Patients with cervicitis may also have urethritis or vaginitis. Vaginitis is associated with increased vaginal discharge of several types, as discussed below, and frequently there are associated signs and symptoms of vaginal, vulvar, and perineal irritation (dyspareunia, external dysuria, itching, pain). In patients with lower genitourinary infection, it is important to determine whether the upper genitourinary tract is involved (pyelonephritis, salpingitis).

The Urethral Syndrome. Bacterial cystitis with or without pyelonephritis is usually diagnosed in women with dysuria, urinary frequency, and pyuria if colony counts are at least 10^5 bacteria per milliliter of urine. If similar symptoms are present but routine cultures grow < 10⁴ bacteria per milliliter of voided urine, the "urethral syndrome" is likely.

In a study of young women with dysuria and urinary frequency, and who did not have vaginitis or active herpes simplex infection, 43% had the urethral syndrome (urethritis). Among women with urethritis, 25% had positive urethral cultures for *C. trachomatis*. Gonococci also were shown to cause this syndrome. Thus, women as well as men may have urethritis caused by gonococci and chlamydiae.

Patients with symptoms of UTI who do not have bacteriuria should have urethral and cervical cultures for *Neisseria gonorrhoeae*. If these cultures are also negative, a therapeutic trial may be made with a tetracycline, azithromycin, or ofloxacin.

Vaginitis. In a large study of women in a primary care clinic who had lower genitourinary complaints, vaginitis was more than five times as common as UTI's. In this and similar studies, there were three predominant types of vaginitis: yeast infection (*Candida albicans*), Trichomonas (*T. vaginalis*) infection, and bacterial vaginosis (BV) caused by organisms other than *Candida* and *T. vaginalis*. The incidence of these types of vaginitis varies in different patient populations, but in general *Candida* and BV are more common than *T. vaginalis* vaginitis.

Symptoms of vaginitis include increased volume of vaginal discharge, which is often abnormally yellow or green in appearance and may be malodorous. Vaginal and vulvar itching may be troublesome, especially in *Candida* infection. There may be vaginal tenderness and pain, dyspareunia, or dysuria.

The most common sign of vaginitis is an increased vaginal discharge. In *T. vaginalis* infections, there is often a profuse and frothy discharge. A curdlike, white discharge is common in *Candida* infections, and many patients with BV have an adherent, often gray, and frequently malodorous discharge. Microscopic examination shows many polymorphonuclear leukocytes in the discharge in all but BV. Speculum examination may show signs of endocervicitis as well, with purulent discharge issuing from the cervical os. In occasional patients, no objective signs of vaginal inflammation are found despite the presence of troublesome symptoms (Table 314–2).

Candida Vaginitis. Most vaginal yeast infections are due to *C. albicans*. Diagnosis is usually made by visualizing yeasts or pseudohyphae by microscopic examination of vaginal secretions suspended in normal saline or 10% potassium hydroxide (KOH). Microscopic examination is less sensitive than culture. However, many asymptomatic women have positive vaginal cultures for *C. albicans,* and therefore some authorities advocate using microscopy in preference to culture. The discharge in *Candida* vaginitis is not malodorous and has a pH of < 4.5 when a drop is applied to pH paper with a range of 4.0 to 5.5.

Therapy of *Candida* vaginitis is with one of the imidazole compounds (e.g., clotrimazole, miconazole, butoconazole, or terconazole) once each night for 3 to 7 days intravaginally, or an oral azole agent (ketoconazole, fluconazole, or itraconazole) for 1 to 5 days. The oral regimens are less well evaluated. No convincing evidence exists that attempts to eradicate yeast from the gastrointestinal tract significantly affect rates of cure or relapse of *Candida* vaginitis. There is no evidence to warrant therapy of sexual partners. Attempts should be made to correct ancillary conditions that increase susceptibility to vaginal candidiasis: antibiotic therapy, diabetes, or oral anovulatory steroids. Relapse is a significant problem in some patients. No therapy is indicated for asymptomatic vaginal carriers of *C. albicans*.

T. vaginalis Vaginitis. Diagnosis is made ordinarily by visualizing motile trichomonads in a normal saline suspension of vaginal secretions. The organisms are easily seen at high-dry (100 ×) magnification and may usually be seen under low-power magnification. The saline suspension should be examined promptly. Culture is more sensitive, but about 80 to 90% of culture-positive cases are detected by microscopy. Addition of a drop of 10% KOH to vaginal secretions usually results in liberation of a detectable fishlike odor, attributed to release of volatile amines. The pH of vaginal secretions is usually > 5.0. In these latter two respects, *T. vaginalis* vaginitis is similar to BV.

Therapy of trichomoniasis is with one of the nitroimidazoles, either metronidazole or newer compounds such as tinidazole. The latter is extensively used in Europe but is not approved in the United States. A single 2-gram oral dose of metronidazole is as effective as multiple-day regimens. Metronidazole is mutagenic, and there is evidence that it is a weak carcinogen in certain animal systems (but, so far, not in humans). Accordingly, it should be used with caution; it has been advocated for women with asymptomatic trichomoniasis, but others would reserve its use for women with symptomatic infections because of possible adverse effects. Metronidazole should not be used in the first trimester of pregnancy. Since more than one third of male sexual partners of women with trichomoniasis are asymptomatic urethral carriers of *T. vaginalis,* the male partners should also be treated with a single 2-gram dose of metronidazole.

Although *T. vaginalis* can be transmitted sexually, it probably is transmitted by other means as well. This conclusion is based on prevalence studies that show one peak in young, sexually active women and a second peak in older women who have no other evidence for sexually transmitted infection.

Bacterial Vaginosis (BV). This syndrome is probably due to infection by an organism formerly called either *Corynebacterium vaginale* or *Haemophilus vaginalis* but now termed *Gardnerella vaginalis,* in association with anaerobic bacteria, including the curved or comma-shaped rods now known as Mobiluncus species. *G. vaginalis* is a small, gram-variable coccobacillus that can be grown quite successfully on partially selective enriched media. Among women with abnormal vaginal discharge who do not have yeast infection or trichomoniasis, > 90% grow *G. vaginalis,* whereas < 10% of matched controls grow the same organism. There usually are increased numbers of anaerobic vaginal bacteria as well and decreased numbers of the normal vaginal lactobacilli. Development of full symptoms may require both *G. vaginalis* and vaginal anaerobes, although the precise pathophysiology of this syndrome is still under investigation.

Diagnosis of BV is by exclusion of trichomoniasis, candidiasis, and purulent cervicitis. Abnormal cells termed clue cells are often seen in a wet mount of vaginal secretions in normal saline; these are stippled, granular-appearing vaginal epithelial cells that contain large numbers of adherent *G. vaginalis*. Few polymorphonuclear leukocytes are present. Addition of a drop of 10% KOH usually results in production of an unpleasant fishy odor. The pH of the vaginal secretions is nearly always > 5.0.

Optimal therapy is being investigated. Metronidazole has only borderline activity *in vitro* against *G. vaginalis,* but in a dose of 500 mg by mouth twice daily for 7 days it was effective in eradicating both *G. vaginalis* and the symptoms of vaginitis from 80 of 81 patients in one trial; similar results have been obtained in other trials. This suggests that the principal cause of this syndrome is an anaerobe, since metronidazole is principally effective against anaerobes. Clindamycin (300 mg orally twice daily for 7 days) also is effective. More than 90% of male partners are urethral carriers of *G. vaginalis* and therefore probably should be treated with the same regimen as the patient, although data to support this are lacking at present.

Mixed Vaginitis. In 2 to 16% of patients, vaginitis may be due to polymicrobial infection with two or three organisms. Such mixed infection may account for some instances of treatment failure. Particular care should be given to identification of all causative organisms in patients who have recurrent or relapsing vaginitis.

Cervicitis. Two organisms are recognized as probable causes of mucopurulent endocervicitis: *N. gonorrhoeae* and *C. trachomatis*. Women who are sexual partners of men with chlamydia-positive NGU have a much higher rate of isolation of chlamydiae from the

TABLE 314–2. DIFFERENTIAL DIAGNOSIS OF VAGINITIS

Characteristics of Vaginal Discharge	Organism Causing Vaginitis		
	C. albicans	*T. vaginalis*	BV
pH	4.5	>5.0	>5.0
White curd	Usually	No	No
Odor with KOH	No	Yes	Yes
Clue cells	No	No	Usually
Motile trichomonads	No	Usually	No
Yeast cells	Yes	No	No

cervix than do women who are partners of men with chlamydia-negative NGU, and they also have significantly higher rates of mucopurulent cervicitis. HSV can also cause cervicitis, especially in primary infection. However, the clinical appearance in herpetic cervicitis is different, with cervical vesicles and ulcers rather than mucopurulent cervicitis.

True cervicitis should not be confused with cervical ectopy, which is merely the appearance of endocervical columnar epithelium on the exposed, visible exocervix. This results in a red-appearing cervix and may result in increased production of a mucoid vaginal discharge but does not require therapy.

Diagnosis of mucopurulent endocervicitis requires visualization of purulent discharge from the cervical os. There often is a roughened cobblestone appearance to the cervix. Gram stain is about 60% sensitive and > 90% specific for gonorrhea if typical intracellular gonococci are seen, but cultures for *N. gonorrhoeae* should be taken. Tissue culture for isolation of *C. trachomatis* may be employed if available. Cytologic methods are not sufficiently sensitive to warrant widespread use. Several nonculture diagnostic tests for *C. trachomatis* allow rapid, sensitive, specific diagnosis from patient secretions and undoubtedly should be more widely used to document cause and to initiate proper treatment for cervicitis due to chlamydiae.

Antibiotic therapy appears to result in clinical improvement in mucopurulent cervicitis. Patients with negative cultures for the gonococcus should be treated with doxycycline (100 mg twice daily for 7 days); alternatives are oral azithromycin in a single dose of 1 gram or oral ofloxacin in a dose of 300 mg twice daily for 7 days. No other form of cervicitis has been shown to respond to antimicrobial therapy.

Upper Genital Tract Disease in Women: Salpingitis.
Full coverage of this important topic is precluded by space considerations. This is a very important clinical problem, resulting in considerable morbidity in the estimated 250,000 to 500,000 women who are affected yearly in the United States.

Etiology. The gonococcus accounts for 20 to 50% of cases in the United States, particularly among women with relatively severe and first-episode salpingitis. About 15 to 20% of women with gonococcal cervicitis probably subsequently develop salpingitis. Strong evidence now implicates genital chlamydial infections as another significant cause of salpingitis. Salpingitis due to genital chlamydial infections may be mild, and patients may not seek medical care. Nevertheless, complications may follow, particularly tubal scarring and infertility. There is less convincing evidence that *Mycoplasma hominis* may occasionally cause a similar syndrome. Many cases of salpingitis are caused by mixed infection with microaerophilic streptococci and enteric bacilli, often including *Bacteroides* species. These polymicrobial infections appear to be more common in recurrent attacks of salpingitis.

Diagnosis. Clinical diagnosis of salpingitis is inexact. Perhaps only 20% of patients have the classic syndrome of lower abdominal pain and tenderness, cervical tenderness, fever, leukocytosis, and elevated sedimentation rate. The most common findings are lower abdominal tenderness, which is usually bilateral, and adnexal and cervical tenderness. Patients with gonococcal salpingitis are more likely to have fever and more commonly have onset near the menses, whereas patients with nongonococcal salpingitis more commonly have adnexal masses. Laparoscopy is commonly used to diagnose salpingitis in certain countries but is invasive and requires general anesthesia. In the United States, laparoscopy is usually used only in selected patients whose differential diagnosis includes ectopic pregnancy, appendicitis, ruptured abscess, or other potential emergencies.

Complications. Complications are primarily infertility and ectopic pregnancy. Rates of involuntary infertility are about 15% after one attack of salpingitis and about 75% after three or more attacks. Total hysterectomy may eventually be necessitated by symptoms of chronic salpingitis.

Therapy. Recommendations from the Centers for Disease Control and Prevention suggest initial therapy of outpatients with cefoxitin, 2 grams intramuscularly, along with probenecid, 1 gram orally, followed by doxycycline, 100 mg orally twice daily for 10 to 14 days. There are no controlled data on efficacy of various regimens used for hospitalized patients. Current recommendations call for doxycycline, 100 mg twice daily, plus cefoxitin, 2 grams intravenously four times daily; or clindamycin, 900 mg intravenously three times daily, plus gentamicin, 1.5 mg per kilogram three times daily. After discharge, doxycycline should be given in a dose of 100 mg twice daily to complete 10 to 14 days of therapy. Patients should usually be hospitalized if they are very ill, are pregnant, or have significant adnexal masses; if previous therapy failed; or if the differential diagnosis includes a surgical emergency such as appendicitis or ectopic pregnancy.

Prevention. Sexual partners of women with gonococcal salpingitis must be identified, examined, and treated to prevent subsequent reinfection of the patient. About one half of the infected male partners of women with gonococcal salpingitis are asymptomatic. Treatment of women with tetracycline (as compared with penicillin) to eradicate chlamydiae from the cervix reduces the incidence of posttherapy salpingitis, which suggests that increased emphasis on treatment of chlamydiae in the male and female genital tract will reduce the incidence of salpingitis.

Addiss DG, Vaughn ML, Ludka D, et al.: Decreased prevalence of *Chlamydia trachomatis* infection associated with a selective screening program in family planning clinics in Wisconsin. Sex Transm Dis 20:28, 1993. *Chlamydia can be controlled by screening and treatment.*

Brunham RC, Paavonen J, Stevens CE, et al.: Mucopurulent cervicitis—the ignored counterpart in women of urethritis in men. N Engl J Med 311:1, 1984. *Genital chlamydial infection causes mucopurulent cervicitis; proper diagnosis leads to effective treatment.*

Holmes KK, Mardh P-A, Sparling PF, et al. (eds.): Sexually Transmitted Diseases, 2nd ed. New York, McGraw-Hill, 1990. *The definitive textbook on STD's; heavily referenced.*

Nettleman MD, Jones RB, Roberts SD, et al.: Cost-effectiveness of culturing for *Chlamydia trachomatis*: A study in a clinic for sexually transmitted diseases. Ann Intern Med 105:189, 1986. *Cultures most cost-effective in low-risk women. Empiric therapy suggested in high-risk groups.*

Rees E: The treatment of pelvic inflammatory disease. Am J Obstet Gynecol 138:1042, 1980. *Treatment of chlamydial infection of cervix with tetracycline compared with penicillin reduced incidence of subsequent salpingitis.*

Stamm WE, Koutsky LA, Benedetti JK, et al.: *Chlamydia trachomatis* urethral infections in men: Prevalence, risk factors, and clinical manifestations. Ann Intern Med 100:47, 1984. *Asymptomatic male urethral carriers of chlamydiae are very common.*

Stamm WE, Wagner KF, Amsel R, et al.: Causes of the acute urethral syndrome in women. N Engl J Med 303:409, 1980. *Females may also develop a form of nongonococcal urethritis resulting from infection with Chlamydia trachomatis.*

Toye B, Laferriere C, Claman P, et al.: Association between antibody to the chlamydial heat-shock protein and tubal infertility. J Infect Dis 168:1236, 1993. *Evidence that Chlamydia causes tubal infertility.*

Wu C-H, Lee M-F, Yin S-C, et al.: Comparison of polymerase chain reaction, monoclonal antibody based enzyme immunoassay, and cell culture for detection of *Chlamydia trachomatis* in genital specimens. Sex Transm Dis 19:193, 1992. *One of many papers suggesting that PCR is the test of choice for Chlamydia.*

315 GONOCOCCAL INFECTIONS
P. Frederick Sparling

Neisseria gonorrhoeae is a common sexually transmitted organism that causes anterior urethritis in males and endocervicitis and urethritis in females. Other types of primary infection include pharyngitis, proctitis, conjunctivitis, and vulvovaginitis; the last-named occurs principally in prepubescent females. Complications may occur by direct extension of infection, including epididymitis, prostatitis, Bartholin gland abscess, salpingitis, and perihepatitis. Bacteremia may occur, with production of characteristic cutaneous lesions, arthritis, and tenosynovitis; rare complications include endocarditis and meningitis. Conjunctival infection formerly was a common cause of blindness in neonates.

Gonorrhea is the most common reportable infectious disease in the United States, with about 500,000 cases annually. The true incidence is probably at least 1 million cases annually. Incidence has declined dramatically in much of the industrialized West in recent years.

EPIDEMIOLOGY. The only natural hosts for *N. gonorrhoeae* are humans. The organism normally resides on the columnar epithelium of mucosal surfaces and is usually transmitted by intimate sexual contact. The incidence of gonorrhea varies greatly in different groups. As many as 5% of persons in high-risk populations may be infected at any time. Highest incidence is found in young (15 to 30) single persons of low socioeconomic and educational status, probably because these factors correlate positively with sexual promiscuity.

The risk of acquiring infection depends on the type of contact with an infected person. About 60 to 80% of females in contact with a male with urethral gonorrhea develop gonococcal cervicitis. By contrast, it is estimated that only 20 to 30% of males having sex with an infected female develop gonorrhea. This difference may be due to exposure of females to a larger inoculum of gonococci. A person having oral sex with a male with gonococcal urethritis has considerable risk of acquiring pharyngeal gonorrhea. Transmission of infection by oral contact with the genitals of an infected female is rare. Infection is apparently efficiently spread by penile-rectal contact.

Gonococci die rapidly upon drying, and transmission by fomites is rare. Epidemics were reported in prepubertal females living in proximity in orphanages, but such episodes are now very uncommon.

Control of gonorrhea is difficult because of the frequency of asymptomatic infection. Perhaps 50% of infections in females are asymptomatic or only minimally symptomatic, and at least 10% of infected males are asymptomatic.

In past years there was considerable emphasis on case finding by endocervical culture in young, sexually active females. The merit of this strategy depends on the prevalence of infection in the community and the lifestyle of the patient. A more cost-effective method for finding infected patients is to obtain a culture in patients about 6 weeks after treatment for gonorrhea; as many as 15 to 20% of such cases are culture positive, usually because of reinfection.

THE ORGANISM. *N. gonorrhoeae* is a gram-negative, aerobic diplococcus. Many strains require 3 to 10% CO_2 for optimal growth. They are highly autolytic and die rapidly when outside their normal human environment. They are sensitive to fatty acids and grow best on media with added starch to inhibit fatty acids present in agar. Several partially selective media are available; most employ antibiotics to inhibit growth of other microorganisms.

Presumptive identification *in vitro* is made by colonial morphology, Gram stain, and a positive oxidase test. Differentiation from the closely related meningococcus and the various nonpathogenic *Neisseria* is ordinarily by patterns of utilization of various simple carbohydrates; gonococci use glucose but not maltose or sucrose.

Gonococci are highly variable and occur in a number of different colonial forms. Small colonial types are piliated and more virulent in humans than the larger, nonpiliated variants. Variation is also found in certain outer membrane proteins. Gonococci undergo rapid variation in the antigenic type of pilus expressed, which probably contributes to prolonged infections without treatment and to the ability of persons to acquire repeat infections after treatment. The importance of surface components of the gonococcus in the pathogenesis of infection is under intense investigation.

Gonococci can be serotyped on the basis of antigenic differences in outer membrane proteins. These tests are not routinely available.

PATHOGENESIS. Surface pili undoubtedly help to attach the bacteria to the mucosal surface, and they also help prevent ingestion and killing by polymorphonuclear leukocytes. Typical urethral infections result in moderately severe inflammation, probably due to release of toxic lipopolysaccharide from gonococci and to production of chemotactic factors that attract neutrophilic leukocytes. Certain strains can cause asymptomatic urethral infection for reasons not completely understood. These strains are usually penicillin sensitive, resistant to the bactericidal effects of normal human serum, and particularly likely to cause bacteremia and septic arthritis.

In the preantibiotic era, symptoms usually persisted for 2 to 3 months before host defenses finally eradicated the infection. Host defenses include serum opsonic and bactericidal antibodies, as well as local (mucosal) antibodies of the IgG and IgA classes. All gonococci produce an enzyme, IgA protease, that cleaves the major class of secretory IgA, perhaps contributing to persistence of local gonococcal infections.

Serum bactericidal antibodies are undoubtedly important in preventing bacteremic infection. The best evidence for this has been provided by patients who suffer from homozygous deficiency of one of the complement components C6, C7, C8, or C9. This results in deficiency of serum bactericidal activity but no alteration of serum opsonic activity. Such individuals are particularly prone to recurrent bacteremic gonococcal infection or to recurrent meningococcal meningitis or meningococcemia.

CLINICAL PATTERNS OF DISEASE. *Gonorrhea in Males.* Gonococcal urethritis in males ("the clap" or "the strain") is characterized by a yellowish, purulent urethral discharge and dysuria. The usual incubation period is 2 to 6 days. The discharge in gonorrhea is slightly more copious and purulent than in nongonococcal urethritis (NGU). Symptoms are probably produced by 90% of infections, although asymptomatic infections do occur and may persist for many months. Males with asymptomatic infection do not seek treatment, whereas those with symptomatic infection are usually promptly treated and cured. This is the probable explanation for prevalence studies that show that up to 50% of infected males are asymptomatic. Asymptomatic infection in males and females is of great epidemiologic importance, since such carriers may continue to spread infection to new sexual partners for months if the infection is not properly diagnosed and treated.

Complications of gonococcal urethritis in males are now rare. Urethral stricture was formerly a common complication but was probably due in part to the use of caustic treatment regimens. Epididymitis and prostatitis, relatively common complications in the past, are seen only occasionally today. The principal complication is disseminated gonococcal infection, which is estimated to affect about 1% of persons with gonorrhea. This entity is discussed below. The differential diagnosis of gonococcal urethritis is discussed in Ch. 314.

Gonococcal infections of the pharynx and rectum are common problems in homosexual males. Most patients with pharyngeal infection are asymptomatic, but occasional patients have exudative pharyngitis with cervical adenopathy. Gonococcal infection of the rectum causes a wide spectrum of symptoms, ranging from no symptoms to severe proctitis with tenesmus and bloody, mucopurulent discharge. Although rectal cultures are also positive in approximately 40% of females with cervical gonorrhea, symptoms of proctitis in females are unusual. This has suggested that the trauma of rectal intercourse may contribute to the proctitis observed in males. Sigmoidoscopy may be indicated to exclude ulcerative colitis, Crohn's colitis, rectal lacerations, or other infections such as shigellosis, amebiasis, or syphilis, all of which are common in male homosexuals.

Gonococcal epididymitis is usually unilateral. Both *Chlamydia trachomatis* and the gonococcus are significant causes of epididymitis in men under 35, whereas coliform bacteria are the usual cause in older males. The differential diagnosis includes trauma, tumor, and torsion of the testicle, suggested by sudden onset and elevation of the testicle. If there is question of testicular torsion, consultation with a urologist is necessary. In epididymitis there is often a urethral exudate, which should be cultured for gonococci and other bacteria. Treatment of gonococcal epididymitis includes scrotal elevation and 7 to 10 days of appropriate antibiotics (Table 315–1).

Gonorrhea in Females. In incidence studies, approximately one half of women infected with the gonococcus are asymptomatic or have so few symptoms that they do not seek medical care. The most commonly involved site is the endocervix (80 to 90%), followed by the urethra (80%), rectum (40%), and pharynx (10 to 20%). Most pharyngeal, urethral, and rectal infections cause few or no symptoms. Cervical infection may result in vaginal discharge or abnormal menstrual bleeding. Neither of these symptoms is specific for gonococcal infection. Gonococcal urethritis may mimic cystitis caused by enteric bacilli, although standard urine cultures are negative because gonococci do not grow on culture media ordinarily used to diagnose urinary tract infection. Culture methods are discussed below under Laboratory Diagnosis. The differential diagnosis of cervicitis, vaginitis, and the urethral syndrome is discussed in Ch. 314.

The most important complication of gonorrhea is salpingitis. The less precise term "pelvic inflammatory disease" (PID) is often used synonymously. Although many other organisms can cause a similar syndrome, the gonococcus accounts for about half of the cases of PID in the United States. About 15% of women with gonococcal cervicitis develop PID, often in proximity to a menstrual period. Symptoms usually include abdominal pain, and often there is fever. Physical examination usually discloses cervical motion tenderness and bilateral adnexal tenderness; in a small proportion of cases the

1702 / XXI INFECTIOUS DISEASES

TABLE 315-1. ANTIBIOTIC REGIMENS RECOMMENDED FOR GONOCOCCAL INFECTION

Diagnosis	Treatment
Uncomplicated genital, rectal, or pharyngeal infection of men and women	Ceftriaxone, 125 mg IM once, plus doxycycline, 100 mg PO twice daily for 7 days *or* Cefixime, 400 mg PO once, plus doxycycline, 100 mg PO twice daily for 7 days *or* Ciprofloxacin, 500 mg PO once, plus doxycycline, 100 mg PO twice daily for 7 days *or* Ofloxacin, 400 mg PO once, plus doxycycline, 100 mg PO twice daily for 7 days
Gonorrhea in pregnancy	Ceftriaxone, 125 mg IM once, plus erythromycin base, 500 mg PO 4 times daily for 7 days *or* Spectinomycin, 2 grams IM, plus erythromycin (as in ceftriaxone regimen)
Salpingitis—outpatient	Cefoxitin, 2 grams IM, plus doxycycline, 100 mg PO twice daily for 10–14 days *or* Ofloxacin, 400 mg PO twice daily for 14 days, plus either clindamycin, 450 mg PO 4 times daily or metronidazole, 500 mg PO twice daily for 14 days
Salpingitis—inpatient	Doxycycline, 100 mg IV twice daily, plus cefoxitin, 2 grams IV 4 times daily until improved, followed by doxycycline, 100 mg PO twice daily to complete 14 days of therapy; alternative regimens include clindamycin plus an aminoglycoside
Disseminated gonococcal infection	Ceftriaxone, 1 gram IM every 24 hours *or* Spectinomycin, 2 grams IM every 12 hours (see text)

disease may be unilateral, causing confusion with appendicitis or ectopic pregnancy. There may be signs of generalized peritonitis. Laboratory studies often show elevation of the white blood cell count and sedimentation rate. The diagnosis of PID is inexact, as shown by laparoscopic examination; many cases of PID are missed if undue reliance is placed on presence of fever or elevation of white blood cell count or sedimentation rate.

Although PID is uncommon in pregnancy, it may be particularly severe, and pregnant patients with PID should probably be hospitalized. The incidence of gonococcal PID is increased about threefold in women using an intrauterine device (IUD) for contraception.

A single attack of gonococcal PID seems to increase twofold the risk of developing another with subsequent gonococcal cervicitis. About half of the male sexual partners of women with gonococcal PID are infected, and half of these infections are asymptomatic. Failure to diagnose cases and treat properly the male partners exposes the patient to the risk of further attacks of PID. After the patient has been effectively treated, it often is wise to refer her and her sexual partners to a public health clinic for follow-up.

The major complication of gonococcal PID is tubal scarring and infertility. The incidence of involuntary infertility is estimated as 15% after one attack of PID and about 50% after three attacks. The incidence of ectopic pregnancy is increased from seven- to tenfold in women with previous salpingitis, with resultant increased fetal and maternal mortality. Treatment is indicated in Table 315-1.

Gonococci may spread upward to the liver, causing perihepatitis (Fitz-Hugh–Curtis syndrome). Gonococcal perihepatitis causes tenderness and pain in the region of the liver, mimicking acute cholecystitis. However, it resolves promptly with appropriate antibiotic therapy. Peritoneoscopy may be indicated rarely for diagnostic purposes; "violin-string" adhesions between the liver capsule and the peritoneum are seen.

Gonorrhea in Children. Infants born to a mother with cervicovaginal gonorrhea may develop gonococcal conjunctivitis, although routine use of prophylactic 1% silver nitrate eye drops (or, in some hospitals, topical erythromycin or tetracycline) has

markedly reduced the incidence of this problem. Neonates may also acquire pharyngeal, respiratory, or rectal infection and may develop gonococcal sepsis. Older children up to 1 year of age usually acquire conjunctival or vaginal infection by accidental contamination from an adult, whereas from 1 year to puberty most childhood gonorrhea is the result of purposeful sexual abuse by an adult.

Gonococcal Bacteremia. Approximately 1% of adults with gonorrhea develop the syndrome of gonococcal bacteremia, dermatitis, and arthritis, or disseminated gonococcal infection (DGI). In most series, the majority of patients with DGI are women. The regional incidence of DGI probably varies because of geographic differences in prevalence of the usually antibiotic-sensitive, serumbactericidal-resistant strains of *N. gonorrhoeae* that cause this syndrome. The severity of the syndrome is variable, from a slowly evolving mild illness with little or no fever, mild arthralgias, and few skin lesions to a fulminant illness with high temperature and prostration. Most episodes of DGI are relatively mild in comparison with meningococcemia.

Many patients with DGI have no local symptoms of gonococcal infection. Initial manifestations are usually migratory asymmetric polyarthralgias and skin lesions that are often accompanied by fever. Many patients have tenosynovitis, typically involving the flexor tendon sheaths of the wrist or the Achilles tendon (colloquially known as "lover's heels"). Skin lesions are few in number (< 30 usually), are acral in distribution (fingers, toes, extremities), and may be painful before they are visible. The individual lesions may be papules, pustules, or bullae on an erythematous base; less commonly seen are petechiae or necrotic lesions. The rash is not pathognomonic but is sufficiently typical that it should strongly suggest DGI when seen in young patients with polyarthralgia. Blood cultures are often positive at this stage, and circulating immune complexes may be present. Gram stain of the skin lesions is positive in only about 5% of patients, but gonococcal antigens can be detected in these lesions in about two thirds of patients by use of immunofluorescent-labeled antigonococcal antibody.

The early stage of gonococcemia may subside spontaneously or may merge indistinctly after about 1 week into a second stage of septic arthritis. Skin lesions have usually disappeared by this time, and blood cultures are nearly always negative. Septic arthritis may occur without preceding skin lesions or polyarthralgia. One large joint (elbow, wrist, hip, knee, ankle) is usually involved, although some series report involvement of two joints in a significant minority of patients. On infrequent occasions symmetric involvement of the fingers may mimic acute rheumatoid arthritis. Physical examination typically discloses a swollen, warm joint with evident intra-articular fluid. Aspiration of the joint often reveals marked neutrophilic leukocytosis (50,000 to 100,000 leukocytes per cubic millimeter), although early in the development of the septic joint the synovial leukocyte count may be much lower. Cultures of joint fluid are often positive if the leukocyte count is ≥ 80,000, but are often negative when leukocyte counts are ≤ 20,000.

Other complications of gonococcal bacteremia include mild hepatitis, myocarditis, the Fitz-Hugh–Curtis syndrome, meningitis, and endocarditis. In the preantibiotic era, gonococcal infection accounted for up to 10% of all endocarditis, but it is now rare. Gonococcal endocarditis is often a rapidly progressive infection with severe valvular damage; it should be suspected in patients with a new murmur, severe prostrating illness, severe myocarditis, or evidence of renal failure, or in the presence of stigmas of peripheral embolization.

The differential diagnosis of the gonococcal bacteremia arthritis syndrome includes Reiter's syndrome, rheumatic fever, rheumatoid arthritis, systemic lupus erythematosus, other infectious or postinfectious arthritis, subacute bacterial endocarditis, meningococcemia, and viral hepatitis. In young males, Reiter's syndrome is the principal consideration. Conjunctivitis is rarely seen in gonococcemia but is common in Reiter's syndrome. In the absence of typical skin lesions, DGI may not be suspected until culture results are known.

Diagnosis of DGI is secure when gonococci are recovered from the blood, skin lesions, or synovial fluid. The diagnosis of DGI is probably correct in patients in whom the only positive cultures are from local mucosal surfaces but in whom there are both typical skin lesions and a prompt response to antigonococcal therapy.

LABORATORY DIAGNOSIS. Gram stain of urethral exudate in symptomatic males has a sensitivity of 90 to 98% and a specificity of 95 to 98%. Accordingly, urethral cultures are not ordinarily indicated in untreated symptomatic males. Since the sensitivity of the Gram stain is only about 60% in asymptomatic male urethral infection, cultures of the anterior urethra or fresh urine sediment are recommended when epidemiologic evidence suggests possible asymptomatic urethral infection. Gram stain of the endocervix is about 50 to 60% sensitive and about 82 to 97% specific in women with positive cervical cultures for *N. gonorrhoeae*. Care must be taken to avoid mistaking normal endocervical flora and neutrophils for gonorrhea; only smears showing several neutrophils with multiple, typical intracellular gram-negative diplococci should be read as presumptively positive for gonorrhea. Cultures for *N. gonorrhoeae* should be obtained in all women, even if the Gram stain appears positive.

Cultures should be plated immediately if possible onto chocolate agar or chocolate agar containing selective antibiotics (e.g., modified Thayer-Martin medium [MTM]). Holding media such as Amies' or Stuart's transport media may be used if necessary, but viability of gonococci drops after 12 to 24 hours in such media. In infected women, a single endocervical culture on MTM is about 80 to 90% sensitive, as judged by yields obtained with multiple cultures from multiple sites. In about 3 to 5% of women the only positive culture is at the pharyngeal, urethral, or rectal site. The yield from these sites is too low to warrant routine pharyngeal, urethral, or rectal cultures. Urethral cultures are indicated in women with the urethral syndrome. Both cervical and rectal cultures should be obtained as part of the test of cure in women after treatment, since inclusion of the rectal culture increases the diagnostic yield of treatment failures by as much as 50%. Pharyngeal cultures should be obtained from patients with symptomatic pharyngitis or from persons exposed by fellatio to infected males. Patients with possible DGI should have culture samples taken from all possible mucosal sites (pharynx, urethra, cervix, rectum), as well as blood and synovial fluid.

Cultures of the cervix should be taken under direct visualization during speculum examination, using a cotton-tipped swab. Lubricant jellies may be deleterious to gonococci and should be avoided. Cultures of the anterior urethra of males should be obtained with calcium alginate swabs or a sterile wire loop. Immediate culture of first-voided urine is also useful.

Positive cultures from the pharynx or rectum should be carefully evaluated by the microbiology laboratory to avoid confusion between gonococci and meningococci. Meningococci are more common than gonococci in throat cultures. No serologic test available is sufficiently sensitive and specific to merit use for screening or diagnostic purposes.

TREATMENT. Gonococci frequently have chromosomal mutations that result in relative resistance to penicillin, tetracycline, and other antibiotics. Strains with chromosomally mediated resistance (CMRNG strains) have become prevalent in certain areas of the United States and are more common in parts of Asia. These strains do not respond to penicillin but do respond to spectinomycin or ceftriaxone. As many as 5 to 10% of all gonococci in the United States now are CMRNG.

Gonococci that carry a β-lactamase (penicillinase) plasmid emerged in the Far East and elsewhere in 1975 and have spread to much of the world. Penicillinase-producing gonococci (PPNG) account for 30 to 50% of all gonorrhea in certain cities in Africa and the Far East but are less common in the United States. The incidence of PPNG is about 5% in the United States but varies in different locales. The gonococcal plasmids are similar to penicillinase plasmids found in *Haemophilus* species. PPNG are resistant to clinically attainable doses of penicillins but are sensitive to spectinomycin and to certain cephalosporins (cefuroxime, cefoxitin, ceftriaxone). PPNG are known to cause DGI and salpingitis.

Plasmid-encoded tetracycline resistance, Tc^r, is a newer problem. These strains do not respond to tetracycline but do respond to spectinomycin or ceftriaxone and may respond to penicillin. Incidence of Tc^r gonococci is increasing and approximates 5 to 15% in various U.S. cities.

The antibiotic regimens recommended for gonorrhea in the United States are summarized in Table 315–1. Ceftriaxone has replaced penicillin and ampicillin, because of the prevalence of CMRNG and Pc^r strains. Tetracyclines no longer are acceptable therapy for gonorrhea because of the prevalence of Tc^r strains. Because gonococcal infections commonly are associated with genital chlamydial infection, most authorities now recommend a 7-day

course of a tetracycline (usually doxycycline) for all patients with gonorrhea as follow-up to initial ceftriaxone therapy.

Each of the recommended regimens is highly effective for genital gonorrhea. In patients who do not respond, isolates can be tested for production of penicillinase, and spectinomycin should be used for retreatment. However, most apparent failures are really reinfections. Some studies show that 15% of patients are reinfected within 6 weeks of successful therapy. On this basis, many authorities recommend that recultures should be obtained 6 weeks after treatment.

In the absence of an effective vaccine, control of this disease depends on proper diagnosis and treatment of patients' sexual contacts. If patients are given simple instructions, many bring their contacts to the physician for examination. There are sound epidemiologic reasons for treating contacts immediately. Local health departments are not utilized sufficiently for help in examination and treatment of contacts.

Treatment of salpingitis (PID) has not been studied adequately (see Table 315–1). Most authorities recommend removal of IUD's in women with PID. It is crucial to examine and treat all sexual partners of women with gonococcal PID.

Therapy of gonococcal arthritis is ordinarily highly successful with each of the recommended regimens (see Table 315–1). Failure to improve in 3 days suggests that the patient does not have DGI. Septic joints should be aspirated, both to make the initial diagnosis and to remove inflammatory exudate. Open drainage is rarely indicated, except in infection of the hip in childhood. Repeat closed aspiration may be necessary if joint fluid rapidly reaccumulates, but most patients require only one or a few joint aspirations. Antibiotics should not be injected into the joint space. Most patients with DGI should be hospitalized initially, but outpatient therapy may be used to conclude a 7-day course of treatment. Oral therapy may be used initially in carefully selected, compliant patients with a definite diagnosis and only mild infection. Antibiotics for oral use in this situation include cefixime, 400 mg twice daily, or ciprofloxacin, 500 mg twice daily. Therapy should be continued for 7 days.

Gonococcal conjunctivitis should be treated by immediate saline irrigation and intravenous ceftriaxone.

PREVENTION. Although vaccines are currently under intense study, an effective gonococcal vaccine is still only a hope. Condoms prevent most infection. Certain contraceptive foams have antigonococcal activity but are of unproven efficacy clinically.

Centers for Disease Control and Prevention: Sexually transmitted diseases treatment guidelines. MMWR 42 (RR-14):1, 1993. *Current recommendations for treatment of gonorrhea and other STD's.*
Cohen MS, Sparling PF: Mucosal infection with *Neisseria gonorrhoeae*: Bacterial adaptation and mucosal defenses. J Clin Invest 89:1699, 1992. *A review of pathogenesis with emphasis on interactions with the host.*
Handsfield HH, Sparling PF: *Neisseria gonorrhoeae. In* Mandell GL, Bennett JE, Dolin R (eds.): Principles and Practice of Infectious Diseases, 4th ed. New York, Churchill Livingstone, 1995, pp 1909–1926. *Highly referenced overview of pathogenesis, epidemiology, clinical presentation, diagnosis, and treatment.*
Hook EW, Holmes KK: Gonococcal infections. Ann Intern Med 102:229, 1985. *Excellent, clinically relevant review.*
Luciano AA, Grubin L: Gonorrhea screening: Comparison of three techniques. JAMA 243:680, 1980. *Culture of the first-voided urine in asymptomatic males shown to be highly reliable method for diagnosis.*
Sparling PF, Cohen MS, Wyrick PB, Elkins C: Vaccines for bacterial sexually transmitted infections: A realistic goal? Proc Natl Acad Sci USA 91:2456, 1994. *Discussion of immunobiology of gonorrhea and prospects for a vaccine.*

316 GRANULOMA INGUINALE (Donovanosis)
*Edward W. Hook III**

Granuloma inguinale, also known as donovanosis, is a slowly progressive ulcerative disease involving principally the skin and subcutaneous tissues of the genital, inguinal, and anal regions. It is

* The author acknowledges the contribution of Dr. P. Frederick Sparling on this subject in the 19th edition of the *Cecil Textbook of Medicine.*

primarily transmitted sexually but probably can be transmitted by nonsexual contact as well. Multiple sexual contacts with an infected partner seem necessary for transmission of infection. The disease is uncommon in the United States, with < 100 recorded cases annually. It is quite common, however, in certain other areas of the world, especially Papua New Guinea.

ETIOLOGY. The causative organism is *Calymmatobacterium granulomatis*, a gram-negative bacterium immunologically related to certain *Klebsiella* strains. Current evidence suggests that *C. granulomatis* is not a member of the *Klebsiella-Enterobacter-Serratia* family; its exact taxonomic status is uncertain. The organism can be grown in yolk sacs, but only with great difficulty on artificial medium. It is apparently a facultative intracellular parasite because in infected lesions it is found primarily in histiocytes or other mononuclear cells.

CLINICAL MANIFESTATIONS. The initial lesion usually appears as a subcutaneous nodule that erodes through the surface and develops into a beefy, elevated granulomatous lesion. This usually is painless and unassociated with systemic symptoms. Secondary bacterial infection may cause a necrotic painful ulcerative lesion that may be rapidly destructive. A cicatricial form may also occur with a depigmented elevated area of keloid-like scar containing scattered islands of granulomatous tissue. Lesions in the genital area are commonly associated with pseudobuboes in the inguinal region; these swellings are usually not due to involvement of the inguinal lymph nodes but rather to granulomatous involvement of the subcutaneous tissues. Metastatic infection of bones or other viscera is occasionally seen. Clinical experience suggests that secondary carcinomas may be a complication of granuloma inguinale.

DIFFERENTIAL DIAGNOSIS. The differential diagnosis includes tumor, lymphogranuloma venereum, chancroid, syphilis, and other ulcerative granulomatous diseases. Chancroid is usually differentiated by its irregular undermined borders, which are not seen in the usual cases of granuloma inguinale. Darkfield examination and serologic tests should help to distinguish syphilis. Biopsies may be necessary to distinguish granuloma inguinale from certain tumors.

DIAGNOSIS. Diagnosis is made by demonstrating intracellular "Donovan bodies" in histiocytes or other mononuclear cells from lesion scrapings or biopsies. Wright's stain and Giemsa's stain of fresh impression smears or unfixed biopsies usually demonstrate the bacilli relatively easily, although multiple biopsies may be necessary in chronic cases. Culture is not practical at present. A serologic test has been devised but is not clinically available. Histologic examination of biopsies shows mononuclear cells with some infiltration by polymorphonuclear leukocytes but no giant cells.

TREATMENT. Treatment consists of tetracycline or sulfisoxazole in a dosage of 0.5 gram four times daily for at least 3 weeks. Other regimens that have proved effective include ampicillin, chloramphenicol, gentamicin, and co-trimoxazole. Limited experience suggests that lincomycin may be used successfully. Patients should be followed for at least several weeks after treatment is discontinued because of the possibility of relapse. Although the risk of communicability appears to be low, sexual contacts should also be examined; at present, treatment of contacts is not indicated in the absence of clinically evident disease.

PREVENTION. No effective prevention is known.

Breschi LC, Goldman G, Shapiro SR: Granuloma inguinale in Vietnam: Successful therapy with ampicillin and lincomycin. J Am Vener Dis Assoc 1:118, 1975. *Ampicillin was frequently effective in patients previously unresponsive to tetracycline.*
Garg BR, Lal S, Sivamani S: Efficacy of co-trimoxazole in donovanosis. A preliminary report. Br J Vener Dis 54:348, 1978. *Trimethoprim and sulfamethoxazole were effective.*
Kuberski T: Granuloma inguinale (donovanosis). Sex Trans Dis 7:29, 1980. *An excellent short review.*
Maddocks I, Anders EM, Dennis E: Donovanosis in Papua New Guinea. Br J Vener Dis 52:190, 1976. *A description of the epidemiology and clinical manifestations in an endemic area of granuloma inguinale.*
Rosen T, Tschen JA, Ramsdell W, et al.: Granuloma inguinale. J Am Acad Dermatol 11:433, 1984. *An American epidemic of this relatively rare disease is described.*

317 CHANCROID
Edward W. Hook III*

Chancroid is a sexually transmitted infection caused by the gram-negative bacillus *Haemophilus ducreyi.*

EPIDEMIOLOGY. Worldwide, chancroid is considerably more common than syphilis, and in parts of Africa and in Southeast Asia is nearly as great a problem as gonorrhea. In the United States it is an uncommon disease. In the mid-1980's, chancroid rates increased more than fivefold, peaking at 4986 cases in 1987. Since then rates have steadily declined. In North America there are strong epidemiologic links between chancroid and both prostitution and illegal drug use. Although all genital ulcer diseases are associated with increased risk for human immunodeficiency virus (HIV) acquisition, the association is particularly strong for chancroid. The majority of reported cases occur in males. An outbreak in Greenland was exceptional in that about 40% of cases were noted in women. It is quite likely that there has been significant underdiagnosis in women in the past.

CLINICAL MANIFESTATIONS. The usual incubation period is 2 to 5 days but may be up to 14 days. In the Greenland outbreak the incubation period averaged nearly 2 weeks in women. The clinical manifestations of chancroid are quite variable. Classically, the initial manifestation is an inflammatory macule that then becomes a vesicle-pustule and finally a sharply circumscribed, somewhat ragged, and undermined painful ulcer. The base is moist and may be covered with a grayish necrotic exudate. Removal of the exudate reveals purulent granulation tissue. There is usually surrounding cutaneous erythema. Lesions typically are single but may be multiple, possibly owing to autoinoculation of nearby tissues. There are rarely systemic symptoms. Inguinal adenopathy is noted in one half of patients, approximately two thirds of whom have unilateral adenopathy. Lesions are usually noted on the penile shaft or glans. In women lesions may occur on the cervix, vagina, vulva, or perianal area. Lesions may occasionally occur primarily on or spread to the abdomen, thigh, breast, fingers, or lips. Intraoral lesions are uncommon.

There are reports of a transient genital ulcer, followed by significant inguinal adenopathy. This may be difficult to distinguish from lymphogranuloma venereum. Other uncommon clinical variants include the *phagedenic type* of ulcer with secondary suprainfection and rapid tissue destruction; *giant chancroid,* which is characterized by a very large single ulcer; *serpiginous ulcer,* which is characterized by rapidly spreading, indolent, shallow ulcers on the groin or the thigh; and a *follicular* type with multiple small ulcers in a perifollicular distribution.

DIFFERENTIAL DIAGNOSIS. The differential diagnosis includes syphilis, herpes genitalis, lymphogranuloma venereum, traumatic ulcers, and granuloma inguinale. Of these the most commonly confused are syphilis and herpes genitalis. Multiple infections are relatively common. Outpatients with suspected chancroid should have a serologic test for syphilis and preferably a darkfield examination as well.

DIAGNOSIS. The diagnosis of chancroid is made on the basis of the clinical appearance of the lesions plus either morphologic demonstration of typical organisms in the lesions or recovery of *H. ducreyi* by culture. Culture is the preferred method, but selective culture media are often not available. Under optimal conditions, positive cultures can be obtained in > 80% of cases. Best culture results seem to be obtained with supplemented chocolate agar media containing 3 µg per milliliter of vancomycin and incubated at 33°C. Necrotic debris should be removed from the ulcer with physiologic saline. The base and edges of the ulcer should be swabbed with a cotton-tipped swab and inoculated directly onto the culture plate if possible; swabs may be put into Amies transport medium if culture plates are not immediately available. Smears obtained from the undermined edges should be gently rolled onto a slide. *H. ducreyi* is a small gram-negative bacillus with rounded ends, which

* The author acknowledges the contribution of Dr. P. Frederick Sparling on this subject in the 19th edition of the *Cecil Textbook of Medicine.*

typically forms chains or parallel aggregates in lesions. Typical organisms are seen in 50 to 80% of cases. Organisms may also be obtained by aspirating inguinal nodes. Nodes should be aspirated by placing the needle through normal skin to avoid formation of fistulous tracts. Nodes should not be incised. There is no commercially available serologic test for chancroid.

TREATMENT. The drug of choice is a single intramuscular dose of ceftriaxone, 250 mg. A single 1-gram dose of azithromycin, given orally, is highly effective. Erythromycin, 500 mg orally four times daily for 7 days, is also usually curative. Another effective agent is ciprofloxacin, 500 mg orally twice daily for 3 days. Ampicillin should not be used because some strains of *H. ducreyi* produce a typical TEM-type β-lactamase and are quite ampicillin resistant. Interestingly, the plasmids containing the gene for production of β-lactamase are very closely related to the penicillinase plasmids present in *H. influenzae* and *Neisseria gonorrhoeae.* Tetracycline resistance is common. Serologic testing for HIV is recommended for all patients treated for possible chancroid. All regular sexual partners should be examined and epidemiologically treated with a similar regimen.

PREVENTION. No vaccine is available. Use of a condom is presumably helpful. There are no data regarding efficacy of antibiotic prophylaxis.

Blackmore CA, Limpakarnjanarat K, Rigau-Perez JG, et al.: An outbreak of chancroid in Orange County, California: Descriptive epidemiology and disease-control measures. J Infect Dis 151:840, 1985. *A very large continental U.S. outbreak is described. Sulfa and tetracycline resistance was common, but erythromycin and cotrimoxazole were effective.*

Centers for Disease Control and Prevention: 1993 Sexually transmitted diseases treatment guidelines. MMWR 42(RR-14):20, 1993. *Current treatment and management recommendations for chancroid.*

Lykke-Olesen L, Larsen L, Pedersen TG, et al.: Epidemic of chancroid in Greenland 1977–78. Lancet 1:654, 1979. *A remarkable epidemic, affecting 3% of the adult population. Tropical climates are not necessary for disease transmission or expression.*

Schmid GP, Sanders LL, Blount JH, et al.: Chancroid in the United States: Reestablishment of an old disease. JAMA 258:3265, 1987. *A useful description of factors contributing to the chancroid resurgence in the mid-1980's.*

Taylor DN, Pitarangsi C, Echeverria P, et al.: Comparative study of ceftriaxone and trimethoprim-sulfamethoxazole for the treatment of chancroid in Thailand. J Infect Dis 152:1002, 1985. *Ceftriaxone appears to be effective for this infection as well, in a single intramuscularly administered dose of 250 mg.*

Telzak EE, Chaisson MA, Bevier PJ, et al.: HIV-1 seroconversion in patients with and without genital ulcer disease. Ann Intern Med 119:1181, 1993. *In this study of heterosexual men attending New York City STD clinics, a diagnosis of chancroid was associated with a more than threefold increased likelihood of HIV acquisition.*

318 SYPHILIS
Edward W. Hook III*

DEFINITION. Syphilis is a chronic infectious disease caused by the bacterium *Treponema pallidum.* It is usually acquired by sexual contact with another infected individual. Syphilis is remarkable among infectious diseases in its large variety of clinical presentations. It progresses, if untreated, through primary, secondary, and tertiary stages. The early stages (primary and secondary) are infectious. Spontaneous healing of early lesions occurs, followed by a long latent period. In about 30% of untreated patients, late disease of the heart, central nervous system (CNS), or other organs ultimately develops. At one time this disease was termed "the great imitator." Although the disease is less common now than previously, it remains a great challenge to the clinician because of its protean manifestations and is of great interest to biologists as well because of the long and tenuous balance between the host and the invading spirochete.

ETIOLOGY. The cause of syphilis was discovered in 1905 by Schaudinn and Hoffman when they visualized spirochetal organisms in early infectious lesions. The causative agent of syphilis, *T. pallidum,* is closely related to other pathogenic spirochetes, including those causing yaws *(T. pertenue)* and pinta *(T. carateum).*

T. pallidum is a thin, helical cell approximately 0.15 μ wide and

6 to 50 μ long. Ordinarily there are approximately 6 to 14 spirals. The organism is tapered on either end. It is too thin to be seen by ordinary Gram stain but can be visualized in wet mounts by darkfield microscopy (see below) or by silver stains or fluorescent antibody methods.

Recent studies have described several unusual characteristics of the *T. pallidum* outer membrane that may provide clues to syphilis pathogenesis. Unlike most bacteria having protein-rich outer membranes, the outer membrane of *T. pallidum* appears to be predominantly made up of phospholipids with few surface-exposed proteins. It has been hypothesized that because of this structure syphilis can progress despite a brisk antibody response (to non–surface-exposed, internal antigens). Between the outer membrane and the peptidoglycan cell wall are six axial fibrils. The axial fibrils are attached three at each end and overlap in the center of the organism. They are structurally and biochemically similar to flagella and may be in part responsible for the motility of the organism.

It is possible to culture *T. pallidum in vitro,* but sustained *in vitro* cultivation is not yet possible and yields are very low. Culture is of limited use in research but of no use in clinical practice. *T. pallidum* can be maintained by serial passage in rabbits without loss of virulence. Only a few strains have been isolated in rabbits and carefully studied, and little evidence is available regarding the genetic diversity of the organism. All studied isolates have been susceptible to penicillin and are similar antigenically. Immunity to the homologous strain develops after prolonged infection in rabbits. The only known natural hosts for *T. pallidum* are humans and certain monkeys and higher apes.

PATHOGENESIS AND HOST RESPONSE. *T. pallidum* may penetrate through normal mucosal membranes and also through minor abrasions of epithelial surfaces. In experimental rabbit syphilis, spirochetes can be found in the lymphatic system within 30 minutes of inoculation and are found in blood shortly thereafter. There have been occasional instances in humans of transfusion syphilis resulting from use of blood from a donor who was in the incubation stage of the disease. Therefore it seems clear that syphilis is a systemic disease from the onset in humans as well. However, the first lesions appear at the site of primary inoculation, presumably because of the large numbers of treponemes implanted at this site. In laboratory animals, there is an inverse relationship between numbers of treponemes inoculated and time required for development of the primary cutaneous lesion. The minimal number of treponemes required to establish infection is not known but may be as low as one treponeme. Multiplication of organisms is very slow, with a division time in rabbits of approximately 33 hours. Similarly slow growth of treponemes in humans probably accounts in part for the protracted nature of the illness and for the relatively long incubation period.

T. pallidum is not known to produce any toxins. Treponemes are capable of specific attachment to host cells, but it is not known whether attachment results in damage to host cells. Most treponemes are found in intercellular spaces, but occasional treponemes can be seen within phagocytic cells. However, there is no evidence for prolonged intracellular survival of treponemes.

The primary pathologic lesion of syphilis is a focal endarteritis. There is an increase in adventitial cells, endothelial proliferation, and presence of an inflammatory cuff around affected vessels. Lymphocytes, plasma cells, and monocytes predominate in the inflammatory lesion, and in some cases polymorphonuclear cells are seen as well. The vessel lumen is frequently obliterated. With healing there is considerable fibrosis. Treponemes may be seen in most early lesions of syphilis and in some of the late lesions such as the meningoencephalitis of general paresis.

Granulomatous reaction is also frequent in secondary syphilis and in late syphilis. The granuloma is histologically nonspecific, and cases of syphilis have been incorrectly diagnosed as sarcoidosis or other granulomatous diseases. Human inoculation studies suggest that the pathogenesis of the gumma, which is a granulomatous lesion, involves hypersensitivity to small numbers of virulent treponemes introduced into a previously sensitized host.

Intracutaneous inoculation of patients with syphilis in various stages with partially purified antigens of *T. pallidum* showed that delayed cellular hypersensitivity developed only in late secondary syphilis but was uniformly present in latent syphilis. There may be

* The author acknowledges the contribution of Dr. P. Frederick Sparling on this subject in the 19th edition of the *Cecil Textbook of Medicine.*

temporary hyporesponsiveness of lymphocytes from patients with primary and secondary syphilis to treponemal antigens. It is possible but not proved that the unusual waxing and waning of lesions in early syphilis depend on the balance between development of effective cellular immunity and suppression of thymus-derived lymphocyte function.

The host also responds to infection with production of numerous antibodies, and in some instances circulating immune complexes may be formed. The nephrotic syndrome has been recognized occasionally in secondary syphilis, and renal biopsies from such cases have shown membranous glomerulonephritis characterized by focal subepithelial basement membrane deposits. The deposits contain both IgG and C3, and treponemal antibody.

Antibodies useful in diagnosis are discussed under Serologic Tests, below.

EPIDEMIOLOGY. Syphilis, with the exception of congenital syphilis, is acquired almost exclusively by intimate contact with the infectious lesions of primary or secondary syphilis (chancre, mucous patches, condylomata lata). This is usually through sexual intercourse, including anogenital and orogenital intercourse. Health workers have sometimes been infected during unsuspecting examination of patients with infectious lesions. Infection by contact with fomites is extremely uncommon.

Syphilis is most common in large cities and in young, sexually active individuals. The highest rate in both men and women occurs at ages 20 to 24, followed by ages 25 to 29 and 15 to 19 years. Among predominantly rural areas in the United States the disease is most prevalent in the southeast.

Syphilis spares no class, race, or group but is more prevalent in the United States among the poorly educated and economically deprived than among more prosperous groups. In 1992, U.S. syphilis rates were more than 60-fold greater among African-Americans than among non-Hispanic whites (92.4 versus 1.5 per 100,000 population). Increased numbers of different sexual partners and perhaps indiscriminate choice of partner increase the risk of acquiring sexually transmitted disease. Patients with primary and secondary syphilis name on the average nearly three different sexual contacts within the previous 90 days. A traditional cornerstone of syphilis control has been epidemiologic investigation of sexual contacts of patients with primary or secondary lesions, and of patients with early latent disease. More recently, as syphilis has been associated with drug use and anonymous sex, epidemiologic investigations have become less efficacious.

In the 1970's and 1980's male homosexuals accounted for an increasing proportion of the total cases of infectious syphilis. The ratio of male:female cases of primary and secondary syphilis in the United States rose from 1.6:1.0 in 1965 to 2.5:1.0 in 1975 and about 3:1 in the mid 1980's. Similar trends were noted in other countries. From 1986 to 1990, U.S. syphilis rates nearly doubled to reach 50,578 cases in 1990. This epidemic disproportionately affected nonwhite heterosexual men and women and occurred contemporaneously with an epidemic of crack cocaine use. Many cases were related to the exchange of sex for drugs or money to buy drugs. After 1990, syphilis rates again declined and in 1993 there were 26,498 cases of primary and secondary syphilis reported, the lowest number since 1979. This epidemic is likely to have also contributed to the spread of HIV (see Syphilis/HIV Interactions, below) and to dramatic increases in congenital syphilis.

The annual incidence of syphilis has generally declined worldwide for approximately 100 years with the exception of periods of extensive war. With the introduction of penicillin there was a rapid decline in primary and secondary syphilis after World War II, to annual rates of approximately 4 cases per 100,000 in 1957. This resulted in declining federal expenditure for syphilis control, however, and there was a subsequent resurgence in infectious primary and secondary syphilis in the United States, reaching peaks of > 12 cases per 100,000 several times in the period 1965–1983. Because many cases of syphilis are not reported, the true incidence is much higher, perhaps 75,000 to 100,000 annually.

Reported deaths from syphilis declined from 2434 in 1965 to 200 in 1976. Infant deaths from syphilis fell by 98 to 99% by 1980, but rose sharply in 1988–1990. Patients with clinically manifest late syphilis, particularly those with gummas, are becoming less common, perhaps as a result of the effectiveness of penicillin therapy for early syphilis. However, surveys indicate that there still are sig-

nificant numbers of patients with untreated cardiovascular and neurologic syphilis, especially among older age groups. There is suggestive evidence that neurosyphilis may be presenting with atypical clinical manifestations and therefore may not be easily recognized.

NATURAL COURSE OF UNTREATED SYPHILIS. The incubation period from time of exposure to development of the primary lesion at the place of initial inoculation of treponemes averages approximately 21 days but ranges from 10 to 90 days. A painless papule develops and gradually breaks down to form a clean-based ulcer with raised, indurated margins. This persists for 2 to 6 weeks and then heals spontaneously. Several weeks later the patient characteristically develops a secondary stage characterized by low-grade fever, headache, malaise, generalized lymphadenopathy, and a mucocutaneous rash. There may be involvement of visceral organs. The secondary eruption may occur while the primary chancre is still healing or several months after the disappearance of the chancre. The secondary lesions heal spontaneously within 2 to 6 weeks, and the infection then enters latency. Some patients may later develop relapsing lesions similar to those of the secondary stage; rarely the relapse takes the form of recurrence of the primary chancre. About one third of untreated patients eventually develop late destructive tertiary lesions involving one or more of the eyes, CNS, heart, or other organs, including skin. These may occur at any time from a few years to as late as 25 years following infection.

The incidence of late complications of untreated syphilis is currently unknown but seems less than noted previously. Cases of gumma are at present so rare as to be reportable.

CLINICAL MANIFESTATIONS. *Primary Syphilis.* The typical lesion of primary syphilis is the chancre, a painless, clean-based, indurated ulcer. The chancre starts as a papule, but then superficial erosion occurs, resulting in the typical ulcer. The borders of the ulcer are raised, firm, and indurated. Occasionally, secondary infections change the appearance, resulting in a painful lesion. Most chancres are single, but multiple ulcers are sometimes seen, particularly when skin folds are opposed ("kissing chancres"). The untreated chancre heals in several weeks, leaving a faint scar. The chancre is usually associated with regional adenopathy, which may be either unilateral or bilateral. The regional nodes are movable, discrete, and rubbery. If the chancre occurs in the cervix or in the rectum, the affected regional iliac nodes are not palpable. See Figure 318–1.

Chancres may occur at any site of potential inoculation by direct contact. The majority of chancres occur at anogenital locations. Chancres may also be seen in the pharynx, on the tongue, around the lips, on the fingers, on the nipples, or in diverse other areas. The morphology depends in part on the area of the body in which they occur and also on the host immune response. Chancres in previously infected individuals may be small and may remain papular. Chancres of the finger may appear more erosive and may be quite painful.

The *differential diagnosis* of a genital ulcer should include genital herpes. Classically, herpetic ulcers are multiple, superficial, and, if seen early, vesicular. They are often painful. However, atypical presentations may be indistinguishable from a syphilitic chancre. Genital herpes is orders of magnitude more common than syphilis. Thus, genital herpes is now the most common cause of a "typical chancre" in North America. Herpetic ulcers, unlike syphilitic ulcers, may yield positive findings on Tzanck's test—multinucleated giant cells in the base of the ulcer. The ulcers of chancroid are usually painful, often multiple, and frequently exudative and nonindurated. Lymphogranuloma venereum may produce a small papular lesion associated with a regional adenopathy. Other conditions that must be distinguished include granuloma inguinale, drug eruptions, carcinoma, superficial fungal infections, traumatic lesions, and lichen planus. Final distinction in most cases is made on the basis of dark-field examination, which is positive only in syphilis.

Secondary Syphilis. Approximately 4 to 8 weeks after the appearance of the primary chancre, patients typically develop lesions of secondary syphilis. They may complain of *malaise, fever, headache, sore throat,* and other systemic symptoms. Most patients have generalized lymphadenopathy, including the epitrochlear nodes. Approximately 30% of patients have evidence of the healing chancre, although many patients, including male homosexuals and women, give no history of a primary lesion.

At least 80% of patients with secondary syphilis have cutaneous lesions or lesions of the mucocutaneous junctions at some point in

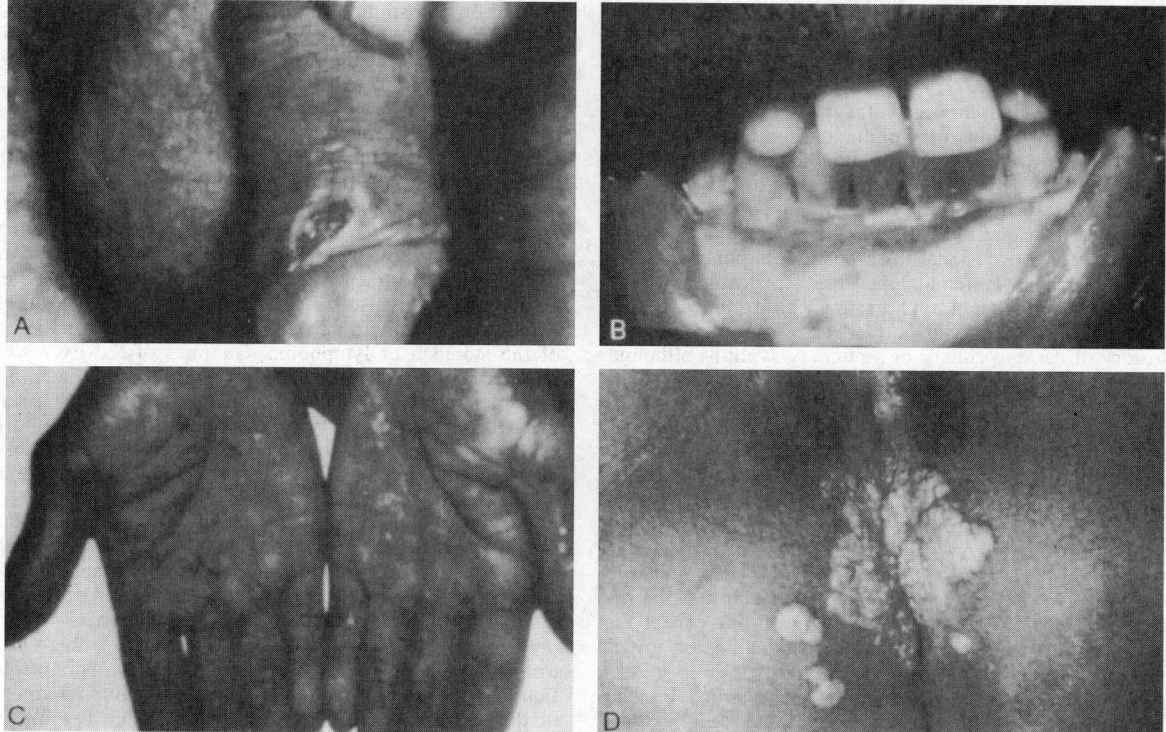

FIGURE 318–1. *A,* Primary syphilis, chancre. *B,* Secondary syphilis, mucous patch. *C,* Secondary syphilis, papulosquamous rash. *D,* Secondary syphilis, condylomata lata.

their illness. The diagnosis is usually first suspected on the basis of the cutaneous eruption. The rash is often minimally symptomatic, however, and many patients with late syphilis do not recall either primary or secondary lesions. The rashes are quite varied in their appearance but have certain characteristic features. The lesions are usually widespread and are symmetric in distribution. They often are pink, coppery, or dusky red, particularly the earliest macular lesions. They usually are nonpruritic, although occasional exceptions have been noted, and are almost never vesicular or bullous in adults. They are indurated except for the very earliest macular lesions and frequently have a superficial scale (papulosquamous lesions). They tend to be polymorphic and rounded, and on healing they may leave residual pigmentation or depigmentation. The lesions may be quite faint and difficult to visualize, particularly on dark-skinned individuals.

The earliest pink macular lesions are frequently seen on the margins of the ribs or the sides of the trunk with later spread to the rest of the body. The face is often spared except around the mouth. Subsequently a papular rash appears, which is usually generalized but is *quite marked on the palms and soles*. These rashes frequently are associated with a superficial scale and may be hyperpigmented. When the rash occurs on the face, it may be pustular, resembling acne vulgaris. On occasion the scale may be so great as to resemble psoriasis. Deep nodular lesions may cause confusion. Ulceration may occur, producing lesions resembling ecthyma. In malnourished or debilitated patients extensive destructive ulcerative lesions with a heaped-up crust may occur, the so-called rupial lesion. Lesions around the hair follicles may result in patchy alopecia of the beard or of the scalp.

Ringed or annular lesions may occur, especially around the face, particularly on black individuals. Lesions at the angle of the mouth or the corner of the nose may have a central linear erosion (the so-called split papule).

In warm, moist areas such as the perineum, large, pale, flat-topped papules may coalesce to form condylomata lata. These may also be seen in the axilla and rarely in a generalized form. They are extremely infectious. They are not to be confused with the common venereal warts (condylomata acuminata), which are small, often multiple, and more sharply raised than condylomata lata.

Other lesions of the mucous membranes are common. The palate

and pharynx may be inflamed. Approximately 30% of patients develop the so-called mucous patch. This is a slightly raised oval area covered by a grayish-white membrane, which when raised reveals a pink base that does not bleed. These may be seen on the genitalia, in the mouth, or on the tongue and, like condylomata lata, are highly infectious.

Other manifestations of secondary syphilis include hepatitis, which has been reported in up to 10% of patients in some series. Jaundice is rare, but an elevated alkaline phosphatase is common. Liver biopsy reveals small areas of focal necrosis and mononuclear infiltrate or periportal vasculitis. Spirochetes can often be visualized with silver stains. Periostitis with widespread lytic lesions of bone has been reported occasionally; bone scanning appears to be a sensitive test for early syphilitic osteitis. An immune complex type of nephropathy with transient nephrotic syndrome has been rarely documented. There may be iritis or an anterior uveitis. From 10 to 30% of patients have pleocytosis in the cerebrospinal fluid (CSF), but symptomatic meningitis is seen in <1% of patients. Symptomatic gastritis may be present.

Differential diagnosis of secondary syphilis includes a large number of diseases. The cutaneous eruptions may be mimicked by pityriasis rosea, which can be differentiated by the occurrence of lesions along lines of skin cleavage and frequently by the presence of a herald patch. Drug eruptions, acute febrile exanthems, psoriasis, lichen planus, scabies, and other diseases must also be considered in some cases. The mucous patch may superficially resemble oral candidiasis (thrush). Infectious mononucleosis may appear very similar to secondary syphilis, with sore throat, generalized adenopathy, hepatitis, and a generalized rash. Infectious hepatitis may also cause confusion. A high index of suspicion is required to make the diagnosis of syphilis in some cases. Unfortunately even classic cases with widespread, hyperpigmented, papulosquamous lesions involving the palms and the soles are not infrequently misdiagnosed today. Fortunately, if the serologic tests for syphilis are obtained, they are positive in 99% of patients. The condylomata lata and mucous patches contain large numbers of treponemes on darkfield examination. Aspiration of lymph nodes may occasionally reveal motile *T. pallidum.*

Relapsing Syphilis. Following resolution of primary or secondary syphilis skin lesions, approximately 30% of patients experience cutaneous recurrences. Recurrent lesions may be fewer or more firmly indurated than initial lesions and, like typical lesions of primary or secondary syphilis, are infectious for exposed sexual partners.

Latent Syphilis. By definition latent syphilis is that stage in which there are no clinical signs of syphilis and the CSF is normal. Latency begins with the passing of the first attack of secondary syphilis and may last for a lifetime thereafter. It is usually detected by reactive serologic tests for syphilis. The test must be shown to be reactive on more than one occasion to rule out technical errors. Diseases known to cause occasional false-positive treponemal reactions for syphilis, such as systemic lupus erythematosus, must be excluded. In addition, congenital syphilis must be excluded before the diagnosis of latent syphilis can be made. Patients may or may not have a history of earlier primary or secondary syphilis, although such history is obviously helpful in making a firm diagnosis of latent syphilis.

Latency has been divided into two stages: *early* and *late latency*. Evidence suggests that most infectious relapses occur in the first year, and epidemiologic evidence shows that the most infectious spread of syphilis occurs during the first year of infection. *Therefore early latency in the United States is defined as the first year after the resolution of primary or secondary lesions or as a newly reactive serologic test for syphilis in an otherwise asymptomatic individual who has had a negative serologic test within the preceding year.* Late latent syphilis is ordinarily not infectious except for the case of the pregnant woman, who may transmit infection to her fetus after many years.

Late Syphilis. Late, or tertiary, syphilis is the destructive stage of the disease and can be crippling. Late syphilitic complications are still important medical problems, but newly recognized cases of late syphilis have been declining steadily in the United States since World War II. Although the incidence of late syphilis is unknown, the prevalence of various types of late syphilis has been approximated (Table 318–1).

Late syphilis is usually very slowly progressive, although certain neurologic syndromes may have sudden onset owing to endarteritis and thrombosis in the CNS. Late syphilis is noninfectious. Any organ of the body may be involved, but three main types of disease may be distinguished: late benign (gummatous), cardiovascular, and neurosyphilis.

Late Benign Syphilis. Late benign syphilis, or gumma, was the most common complication of late syphilis in the Oslo Study of untreated patients (1891–1951). In the penicillin era gummas are rare. They typically develop from 1 to 10 years after the initial infection and may involve any part of the body. Although they may be very destructive, they respond rapidly to treatment and therefore are relatively benign. Histologically the gumma is a granuloma. The histologic findings are nonspecific and may be associated with central necrosis surrounded by epithelioid and fibroblastic cells and occasionally giant cells. There is sometimes vasculitis. *T. pallidum* is ordinarily not demonstrable by silver stains but can sometimes be recovered by inoculation of rabbits.

Gummas may be solitary or multiple. They are usually asymmetric and are often grouped. They may start as a superficial nodule or

TABLE 318–1. NEWLY DIAGNOSED TERTIARY SYPHILIS IN 105 PATIENTS IN DENMARK, 1961–1970

Type of Tertiary Syphilis	Number Observed*
Neurosyphilis	72
Asymptomatic	45
Tabes dorsalis	11
General paresis	13
Meningovascular	1
Optic atrophy	2
Cardiovascular syphilis	44
Aortic insufficiency	16
Aortic aneurysm	13
Uncomplicated aortitis†	15
Late benign syphilis (gumma)	4

*Some patients had more than one form of late syphilis.
†Autopsy diagnoses only.

as a deeper lesion that breaks down to form punched-out ulcers. They are ordinarily indolent and slowly progressive. They are indurated on palpation. There often is central healing with an atrophic scar surrounded by hyperpigmented borders. Cutaneous gummas may resemble other chronic granulomatous ulcerative lesions caused by tuberculosis, sarcoidosis, leprosy, and other deep fungal infections. Precise histologic diagnosis may not be possible. However, the syphilitic gumma is the only such lesion to heal dramatically with penicillin therapy. Another form of gumma is papulosquamous and may mimic psoriasis.

Gummas may also involve deep visceral organs, of which the most common are the respiratory tract, the gastrointestinal tract, and bones. In earlier centuries gummas of the nose and palate commonly resulted in septal perforations and disfiguring facial lesions. Gummas may also involve the larynx or the pulmonary parenchyma. Gumma of the stomach may masquerade as carcinoma of the stomach or lymphoma. Gummas of the liver were once the most common form of visceral syphilis, presenting often with hepatosplenomegaly and anemia, occasionally with fever and jaundice. Skeletal gummas typically produce lesions in the long bones, skull, and clavicle. A characteristic symptom is nocturnal pain. Radiologic abnormalities, when present, include periostitis and either lytic or sclerotic destructive osteitis.

Cardiovascular Syphilis. The primary cardiovascular complications of syphilis are aortic insufficiency and aortic aneurysm, usually of the ascending aorta. Less commonly other large arteries may be involved, and rarely involvement of the coronary ostia results in coronary insufficiency. These complications in all cases are due to obliterative endarteritis of the vasa vasorum with resultant damage to the intima and media of the great vessels. This results in dilatation of the ascending aorta and eventually in stretching of the ring of the aortic valve, producing aortic insufficiency. The valve cusps remain normal. Death may eventually result from congestive heart failure. There has been some success with placing prosthetic heart valves in patients with syphilitic aortic insufficiency. Aneurysms occasionally present as a pulsating mass bulging through the anterior chest wall. Syphilitic aortitis may involve the descending aorta, but this is almost always proximal to the renal arteries, unlike atherosclerotic aneurysms, which typically involve the descending aorta below the renal arteries.

The disease usually begins within 5 to 10 years after initial infection but may not become clinically manifest until 20 to 30 years after infection. Cardiovascular syphilis is thought to be more common in men than in women and possibly in blacks than in whites. Cardiovascular syphilis does not occur after congenital infection—a phenomenon that remains unexplained.

Asymptomatic aortitis is best diagnosed by visualizing linear calcifications in the wall of the ascending aorta by radiography. The signs of syphilitic aortic insufficiency are the same as for aortic insufficiency of other causes. In aortic insufficiency resulting from dilatation of the aortic ring, the decrescendo murmur is often loudest along the *right* sternal margin. Syphilitic aneurysms may be fusiform but are more typically saccular and do not lead to aortic dissection. Approximately 10 to 25% of patients with cardiovascular syphilis have coexistent neurosyphilis, and it is therefore mandatory to do a lumbar puncture in all patients with cardiovascular syphilis.

At present, syphilis is a relatively more common cause of aortic insufficiency among the elderly than among younger patients; this is due to the progressively decreasing incidence of new cases of late cardiovascular syphilis.

Neurosyphilis. Neurosyphilis may be divided into four groups: asymptomatic, meningovascular, tabes dorsalis, and general paresis. These are more fully described in Ch. 422. Division is not absolute, and overlap between syndromes is typical. Current cases of neurosyphilis are more likely than heretofore to be variants of the classic syndromes, possibly as a result of use of antimicrobials for other diseases.

Asymptomatic Neurosyphilis. Asymptomatic neurosyphilis is diagnosed when there are CSF abnormalities (pleocytosis, protein elevation, or a reactive VDRL*) in a syphilis patient in the absence of signs and symptoms of neurologic disease. Although numerous other processes may cause CSF pleocytosis or protein elevations, false-positive VDRL test results are very rare in CSF in the absence

---

* See Serologic Tests, p. 1710. Also refer to Table 318–2.

of a traumatic tap. The CSF usually shows an increased total protein and a lymphocytic pleocytosis. If the CSF is normal 2 or more years after the initial infection, the patient is not likely to develop a positive CSF later. Although up to 50% of patients with untreated secondary syphilis have an abnormal CSF, penicillin therapy apparently prevents progression to late symptomatic neurosyphilis. Because of this, routine lumbar punctures for examining CSF are not indicated in early syphilis unless the patient is known to have HIV infection. Unfortunately, it has become common practice to avoid lumbar punctures in later stages of syphilis as well. Instead, patients are treated with doses of penicillin thought to be effective for neurosyphilis, if present. As a result, there are few data on the present frequency and course of asymptomatic neurosyphilis.

Some laboratories perform an FTA-ABS* test on spinal fluid. Interest in tests such as this has been prompted by good evidence that patients with untreated neurosyphilis may have a nonreactive CSF-VDRL. Reports were published of positive FTA-ABS test results in the CSF of patients with otherwise normal spinal fluid, in whom there were clinical signs and symptoms compatible with neurosyphilis. However, the CSF FTA-ABS test has not been standardized, and some evidence exists that reactive CSF test results are caused by passive transfer of serum antibody into spinal fluid. At present, although a nonreactive CSF FTA-ABS may be useful to rule out the diagnosis, no diagnosis of asymptomatic (or symptomatic) neurosyphilis should be based solely on the CSF FTA-ABS* test.

Meningovascular Syphilis. An acute to subacute aseptic meningitis may occur at any time after the primary stage but usually within the first year of infection. It frequently involves the base of the brain and may result in unilateral or bilateral cranial nerve palsies. In about 10% of cases, the onset of meningitis coincides with the rash of secondary syphilis. The spinal fluid shows a lymphocytic pleocytosis with increased protein and usually normal glucose concentration. The CSF-VDRL is nearly always reactive. Rarely CSF glucose concentration is decreased. This syndrome can mimic tuberculous or fungal meningitis or nonpurulent meningitis of various causes.

In other patients, the meningeal involvement may be less prominent, but there is sufficient endarteritis and perivascular inflammation to result in cerebrovascular thrombosis and infarction. This usually occurs 5 to 10 years after the initial infection and is more common in males. There often is associated aseptic meningitis as well. Most cerebrovascular accidents are not due to syphilitic arteritis even in patients with a reactive serologic test for syphilis. However, syphilis should be considered as the cause in young patients with a history of syphilis and without other causes for cerebrovascular accidents.

Tabes Dorsalis. Tabes dorsalis is a slowly progressive degenerative disease involving the posterior columns and posterior roots of the spinal cord, resulting in progressive loss of peripheral reflexes, impairment of vibration and position sense, and progressive ataxia. There may be chronic destructive changes in the large joints of the affected limbs in far-advanced cases (Charcot's joints). Incontinence of the bladder and impotence are common. Sudden and severe painful crises of uncertain cause are a characteristic part of the syndrome. These most typically involve the lower extremities but may occur at any site. Not infrequently severe, sharp abdominal pains lead to exploratory surgery. These attacks may be triggered by exposure to cold or other stresses or may arise with no obvious precipitating cause.

Optic atrophy is seen in 20% of cases. The pupils are abnormal in 90% of cases, with bilaterally small pupils that fail to constrict further in response to light but that do constrict normally to accommodation (Argyll Robertson pupils).

The cause of tabes dorsalis is unclear. Spirochetes cannot be demonstrated in the posterior column or dorsal root.

Onset of the disease is usually delayed, often 20 to 30 years after initial infection. It is thought to be more common in whites and in men. Typical cases of patients presenting with lightning pains, ataxia, Argyll Robertson pupils, absent deep tendon reflexes, and loss of posterior column function are easy to diagnose. Atypical cases may be more troublesome, particularly because the VDRL test result in the serum is normal in as many as 30 to 40% of patients, and 10 to 20% of patients (even before the advent of penicillin)

have normal CSF-VDRL results as well. The FTA-ABS test in serum is nearly always reactive.

Treatment is unsatisfactory. Penicillin usually arrests progression but does not reverse the symptoms. Carbamazepine in doses of 400 to 800 mg per day has been reported to effectively treat the lightning pains.

Tabes dorsalis is now thought to be uncommon, although a survey of newly diagnosed late syphilis in Denmark in the decade 1961 to 1970 showed that in approximately 10% of all persons with late syphilis and 40% of all with clinical neurosyphilis there was evidence of tabes dorsalis.

General Paresis. This form of neurosyphilis is a chronic meningoencephalitis resulting in gradually progressive loss of cortical function. It typically occurs 10 to 20 years after the initial infection. Pathologically there is a perivascular and meningeal chronic inflammatory reaction with thickening of the meninges, a granular ependymitis, degeneration of the cortical parenchyma, and abundant spirochetes in the tissues.

The most devastating effect of general paresis is on the mind. With effective penicillin therapy this disease has become much less common; in the United States, first admissions to mental hospitals because of syphilitic psychosis declined from 7694 in 1940 to 154 in 1968, the last year for which definite figures are available.

In its early stages general paresis results in nonspecific symptoms such as irritability, fatigability, headaches, forgetfulness, and personality changes. Later there is impaired memory, defective judgment, lack of insight, confusion, and often depression or marked elation. The patients may be delusional, and seizures are sometimes seen. There may also be loss of other cortical functions, including paralysis or aphasia.

Physical signs are primarily those of the altered mental status. Cranial nerve palsies are uncommon. Optic atrophy is rare. The complete Argyll Robertson pupil is also uncommon, but irregular or otherwise abnormal pupils are not infrequent. Peripheral reflexes are often somewhat increased.

The CSF is nearly always abnormal, with lymphocytic pleocytosis and increased total protein. The VDRL is usually reactive in both spinal fluid and serum. The disease responds well to penicillin therapy if administered early, although as many as a third of treated patients may develop progressive neurologic decline in later years. Fever therapy induced with malaria was formerly an effective adjunct to treatment with arsenicals but has now been abandoned.

Even though classic general paresis is now infrequent, it remains reasonable to suspect syphilis as the cause of undiagnosed neurologic illness.

Syphilis/HIV Interactions. Syphilis and HIV infection interact on multiple levels. Thus, clinicians evaluating patients with newly diagnosed syphilis should consider whether coexistent HIV infection is present and how the two diseases might be interacting. Conversely, clinicians seeing patients with newly diagnosed HIV should be attuned to the possible existence of previously undiagnosed syphilis.

Syphilis, like other genital ulcer diseases, is associated with three- to fivefold increased risk for HIV acquisition. Presumably genital ulcers act as portals of entry through which HIV may more readily infect exposed individuals. In individuals with HIV infection who acquire syphilis, the natural history of the infection may be modified. HIV-infected syphilis patients are more likely to present with secondary syphilis than are non–HIV-infected patients. In addition, HIV-infected secondary syphilis patients are more likely to have coexistent chancres than are HIV-negative secondary syphilis patients, suggesting that either the healing of chancres is delayed or the appearance of secondary manifestations is accelerated in the presence of HIV coinfection.

Several reports have suggested that neurosyphilis may be more common in patients with HIV infection; however, no large or carefully controlled studies document this association. In HIV-infected syphilis patients in whom therapy fails, neurosyphilis may be a more common presenting feature than in patients without HIV infection.

Most experts agree that failure of treatment using currently recommended regimens for syphilis therapy is more common in patients with coexistent HIV infection. The magnitude of this increase, however, is probably small and as a result alternate

---

* See Serologic Tests, p. 1710. Also refer to Table 318–2.

treatment regimens are not currently recommended. Rather, closer follow-up is suggested to permit early detection of treatment failure and to help prevent disease progression or transmission of infection to others.

Congenital Syphilis. Congenital syphilis results from transplacental hematogenous spread of syphilis from the mother to the fetus. The incidence of congenital syphilis diagnoses in the United States fell below 1000 per year for the first time in 1975, and < 500 cases occurred per year until 1988, when the epidemic of syphilis in adults led to similar epidemic increases in congenital infections. From 1990 through 1993 > 3000 new cases of congenital syphilis have been reported each year. Each case of congenital syphilis represents a tragedy that could have been prevented by better case reporting and by proper prenatal care. A VDRL should be obtained in all expectant mothers at the beginning and near the end of pregnancy.

Spirochetes can be found in abortuses of as little as 9 to 10 weeks' gestation. The risk of fetal infection is greatest in the early stages of untreated maternal syphilis and declines slowly thereafter, but the mother may infect her fetus during at least the first 5 years of her infection. Adequate treatment of the mother prior to the sixteenth week usually prevents manifest clinical illness in the neonate. Later treatment may not prevent late sequelae of the disease in the child. Untreated maternal infection may result in stillbirth, neonatal death, prematurity, or syndromes of early or late congenital syphilis among surviving infants.

Manifestations of early congenital syphilis are often seen in the perinatal period but may not develop until the infant has been discharged from the hospital. The disease resembles secondary syphilis of the adult except that the rash may be vesicular or bullous, which is extremely rare in adults. There often is rhinitis, hepatosplenomegaly, hemolytic anemia, jaundice, and pseudoparalysis (immobility of one or more extremities) resulting from painful osteochondritis. There may be thrombocytopenia and leukocytosis. The early stages of congenital syphilis must be differentiated from rubella, cytomegalovirus infection, toxoplasmosis, bacterial sepsis, and other diseases.

Late congenital syphilis is defined as congenital syphilis of more than 2 years' duration. The disease may remain latent with no manifest late damage. Cardiovascular alterations have not been observed in congenital syphilis. Neurologic manifestations are common, and there may be eighth cranial nerve deafness and interstitial keratitis. The latter occurs in > 10% of patients but may not be apparent until the tenth year of life or later. Periostitis may result in prominent frontal bones, depression of the bridge of the nose ("saddle nose"), poor development of the maxilla, and anterior bowing of the tibias ("saber shins"). There may be late-onset arthritis of the knees (Clutton's joints). The permanent dentition may show characteristic abnormalities known as Hutchinson's teeth; the upper central incisors are widely spaced, centrally notched, and tapered in the manner of a screwdriver. The molars may show multiple poorly developed cusps (mulberry molars). Some of the late manifestations such as interstitial keratitis and Clutton's joints may be due to hypersensitivity responses and are benefited by corticosteroids in some cases.

DIAGNOSIS. Darkfield Examination. The most definitive means of making a diagnosis is finding spirochetes of typical morphology and motility in lesions of early acquired or congenital syphilis. The darkfield examination is often positive in primary syphilis and in the moist mucosal lesions of secondary and congenital syphilis. It may occasionally be positive in aspirates of lymph nodes in secondary syphilis. Problems arise, however, because of false-negative results in primary syphilis owing to application by the patient of soaps or other toxic compounds to the lesions. A single negative result is therefore insufficient to exclude syphilis. Optimally, patients with suspicious lesions but with an initially negative darkfield examination should be instructed to avoid washing the lesion and to return daily for two successive examinations. In practice, however, for high-risk individuals (drug users, homosexually active men), it may be more appropriate to treat patients with suspicious lesions presumptively after obtaining serologic tests. Confusion may also arise because of the presence of spirochetes that are morphologically indistinguishable from *T. pallidum* in the mouth, particularly around the gingival margins. For lesions in these areas

diagnosis often depends on clinical appearance, history, and serologic testing.

To perform the darkfield examination, the surface of the suspected ulcerative lesion should be cleaned with saline solution and gauze without producing bleeding. The presence of red cells in the specimen makes it difficult to visualize small numbers of *T. pallidum*. Squeezing of the lesion (with gloves on) may help produce serous fluid, which is picked up on a glass slide, covered with a coverslip, and examined with the darkfield microscope. Living *T. pallidum* organisms demonstrate gradual motion to and fro, rotational movement around the long axis, and rather sudden 90-degree bending near the center of the organism. Because most physicians do not have the proper equipment and are not familiar with the techniques of darkfield microscopy, the state public health authorities can be called for assistance.

T. pallidum may also be demonstrated in biopsies or pathologic specimens by fluorescent antibody stains or by silver stains.

Serologic Tests. Two basic types of serologic tests for humoral antibody are widely used to diagnose infection with *T. pallidum:* nontreponemal tests that detect antibodies reactive with diphosphatidylglycerol (cardiolipin), which is a normal component of many tissues; and specific treponemal antibodies. Nonspecific antibodies against cardiolipin were formerly designated "reagin," a term that should be discarded to avoid confusion with another "reagin," IgE. The kinds of tests used in syphilis are summarized in Table 318–2.

Nontreponemal Tests. Anticardiolipin antibodies were first discovered by Wassermann in 1907, using extracts of congenitally syphilitic livers as the antigen for a complement fixation test. Subsequently it was shown that normal livers contained the same antigen as do many other tissues; the antigen for this class of test is now extracted from beef heart. As yet there is no convincing explanation for why patients infected with *T. pallidum* develop increasing titers of antibody against a normal tissue component.

The Wassermann test has now been replaced by related tests. The standard test in use today to detect anticardiolipin antibody is the Venereal Disease Research Laboratories (VDRL) test, which is an easily quantified slide flocculation test. Many similar tests, including the rapid plasma reagin (RPR) test and the unheated serum reagin (USR) test, are frequently used for screening for syphilis.

The VDRL and related tests are simple, well standardized, cheap, and the screening tests of choice. The VDRL is readily quantified and, for that reason, is the test of choice for following the response of patients to treatment. Because the VDRL detects antibody against a normal tissue component, it may be falsely positive in a significant number of conditions. The relative proportion of patients with a false-positive VDRL depends on the prevalence of syphilis in the community; the lower the prevalence of syphilis, the higher the proportion of reactive VDRL tests that are due to nonsyphilitic causes.

The VDRL test begins to turn positive 1 to 2 weeks after the onset of the chancre. In large series of patients with primary syphilis, approximately two thirds have had a positive VDRL test result. Obviously, then, a nonreactive VDRL test does not exclude primary syphilis, particularly if the lesion is < 2 weeks old. The VDRL is positive in 99% of patients with secondary syphilis, the only exceptions being patients with such high titers of antibody that they are in antibody excess; dilution of the serum then paradoxically results

TABLE 318–2. SEROLOGIC TESTS FOR SYPHILIS

Type	Use
Nontreponemal (anticardiolipin) antibodies:	
VDRL (slide flocculation)	Screening, quantitation, following response to treatment
RPR (circle-card) (agglutination)	Screening
Specific treponemal antibodies:	
FTA-ABS (immunofluorescence with absorbed serum)	Confirmatory, diagnostic, not for routine screening
MHA-TP (microhemagglutination)	Similar to FTA-ABS but can be quantified and automated

VDRL = Venereal Disease Research Laboratories test.
RPR = Rapid plasma reagin test.
FTA-ABS = Fluorescent treponemal antibody absorption test.
MHA-TP = Microhemagglutination assay for *T. pallidum.*

in conversion of a negative test to positive. In patients with coexistent HIV infection, the serologic responses to syphilis may be modified. In large groups of syphilis patients nontreponemal test titers tend to be higher than for comparison groups of patients without HIV infection. In contrast, however, there are also case reports of patients with advanced HIV infection in whom development of a serologic response was delayed or absent and infection could be diagnosed only by biopsy. For most patients with HIV infection, however, serologic tests for syphilis remain useful for diagnosis and management. VDRL reactivity tends to diminish in later stages of the disease, and only about 70% of patients with cardiovascular or neurosyphilis have a positive VDRL test result.

The *quantitative titer* of the VDRL test is somewhat useful in diagnosis and quite useful in following therapeutic response. The titer is reported as the highest dilution that gives a positive response. Most patients with secondary syphilis have titers of at least 1:16. Most patients with false-positive VDRL tests have titers of < 1:8. No single titer is in itself diagnostic. Significant rises (fourfold or greater) in paired sera, however, are strongly indicative of acute syphilis.

Treponemal Tests. There are many varieties of specific treponemal antibody tests. The most widely used is the fluorescent treponemal antibody absorption (FTA-ABS) test. Patient serum is absorbed with extracts of nonpathogenic cultivable treponemes to remove cross-reacting group treponemal antibody. Agglutination of red cells to which *T. pallidum* antigens have been fixed is the basis of the microhemagglutination assay for *T. pallidum* (MHA-TP).

The precise nature of the antigens involved in these tests is not known. Characterization of the antigens of *T. pallidum* has been greatly hindered by inability to grow the organism in cell-free culture. Recent success in cloning *T. pallidum* antigens into *Escherichia coli* may circumvent this problem. Antibodies reactive in the various tests are found in all major immunoglobulin classes (IgG, IgM, IgA). A modification of the FTA-ABS test has been developed using fluorescein-labeled anti–human IgM (IgM FTA-ABS). The IgM FTA-ABS test is of some use in the diagnosis of early congenital syphilis but is of no use in distinguishing acute disease from old infections in adults.

The FTA-ABS test is best used as a confirmatory test. It is somewhat more difficult to perform than the VDRL test and cannot be easily quantified. It is sensitive and has a high degree of specificity, being reactive in only approximately 1% of normal individuals. It is reactive in 85% of patients with primary syphilis, 99% with secondary syphilis, and at least 95% with late syphilis. It may therefore be the only test positive in patients with cardiovascular or neurologic syphilis. In late syphilis the FTA-ABS test often remains reactive for life despite adequate therapy. It (as well as the MHA-TP) is positive in other treponemal diseases, such as pinta, yaws, and endemic syphilis (formerly bejel) (see Ch. 319).

The FTA-ABS test is reported in terms of relative brilliance of fluorescence, from borderline to 4+. Borderline reactivity has the same meaning as nonreactive for clinical purposes. Most laboratories report 1+ positive tests as reactive, but some studies have shown that such tests may be difficult to reproduce. Occasional laboratories therefore report as positive only tests with 2+ or greater reactivity. In patients lacking historical or clinical evidence of syphilis but with a reactive FTA-ABS test, one should repeat the FTA-ABS test. Use of another treponemal test such as the MHA-TP may be helpful in problem cases.

The MHA-TP test is less sensitive than either the VDRL or the FTA-ABS test in primary syphilis. Its sensitivity and specificity otherwise are nearly identical to those of the FTA-ABS test, being reactive in nearly all patients with secondary syphilis and in ≥95% of patients with late syphilis. The reactivity of serologic tests for syphilis in various stages of disease is shown in Table 318–3.

TABLE 318–3. FREQUENCY OF POSITIVE SEROLOGIC TESTS IN UNTREATED SYPHILIS

Stage	VDRL (%)	FTA-ABS (%)	MHA-TP (%)
Primary	70	85	50–60
Secondary	99	100	100
Latent or late	70	98	98

False-Positive Serologic Test Results for Syphilis. The VDRL or RPR test may be reactive in a variety of diseases other than syphilis. A false-positive result is defined as a reproducible positive test in a patient with no clinical or historical evidence of syphilis and whose serum FTA-ABS or MHA-TP test is negative.

"Acute" (<6 months) false-positive VDRL test results occur with low frequency in atypical pneumonia, malaria, and other bacterial or viral infections and may occur after smallpox or other vaccinations as well. *Chronic false-positive VDRL tests* (lasting >6 months) are relatively common in autoimmune disorders such as systemic lupus erythematosus (SLE), in narcotic addicts, in HIV infection, in leprosy, and in aged persons. From 8 to 20% of patients with SLE have been reported as having a false-positive VDRL test, and the false-positive result may develop many years prior to the onset of other manifestations of the disease. A chronic false-positive VDRL test in females aged 20 or younger carries a significant risk of future development of SLE, thyroiditis, or other autoimmune disorders, and such patients should be followed carefully for a considerable period of time. As many as one third of patients with narcotic addiction have a false-positive VDRL test. More than 1% of patients aged 70 and 10% of patients over age 80 have a low-titer false-positive VDRL test. Most false-positive VDRL tests have a titer of ≤1:8, although occasional patients with lymphoma and other diseases have been described with very high-titer false-positive VDRL tests.

A reactive FTA-ABS result is usually indicative of recent or past syphilis. However, there is an increased incidence of false-positive FTA-ABS results in SLE and in other chronic inflammatory diseases associated with hyperglobulinemia, including rheumatoid arthritis, biliary cirrhosis, and others.

Occasionally one encounters reproducible positive FTA-ABS results in patients with no clinical or historical evidence of syphilis and in whom there is no evidence of diseases associated with false-positive FTA-ABS results. It may be wise to obtain CSF for examination of total protein, cells, and VDRL reactivity in order to rule out neurosyphilis. If in doubt and if the patient is not allergic to penicillin, it is often wisest to treat such patients for possible syphilis.

IgM FTA-ABS Test for Congenital Syphilis. Mothers with a reactive VDRL or FTA-ABS deliver infants with a reactive VDRL and FTA-ABS because of passive transfer of the IgG antibodies reactive in these tests. Because many infants with congenital syphilis are clinically normal at birth but develop serious symptomatic disease some weeks later, it is important to determine whether a newborn with a reactive VDRL or FTA-ABS test has passively transferred maternal antibody or is actively infected. Because maternal IgM antibodies are not passively transferred to the fetus, an IgM FTA-ABS test has been developed to detect syphilis in the newborn. Unfortunately there is approximately a 35% incidence of false-negative IgM FTA-ABS test results in delayed-onset congenital syphilis. There also is a false-positive rate of approximately 10%. For these reasons the IgM FTA-ABS test is of limited use for diagnosing neonatal syphilis.

If the mother has been adequately treated for syphilis during pregnancy and the infant is clinically normal at birth, one may elect to follow the infant carefully by serial examination and VDRL titers. If the reactive VDRL in the infant is due to passively transferred maternal antibody, the titer of reactivity falls markedly in the first 2 months of life. A rising titer indicates active disease and the need for treatment. Many physicians are unwilling to risk failure of proper follow-up of VDRL-positive but clinically normal neonates and instead administer effective therapy immediately. The risk of penicillin allergy in neonates is very low.

TREATMENT. *T. pallidum* is highly susceptible to penicillin, being inhibited by <0.01 μg of penicillin G. Because treponemes divide slowly and because penicillin acts only on dividing cells, it is necessary to maintain serum levels of penicillin for many days. Studies in animals and in humans show that more therapy is required as the length of infection increases. Current recommendations for treatment of syphilis are summarized in Table 318–4.

Early (< 1 Year) Infectious Syphilis. Early syphilis may be treated with a single injection of 2.4 million units of *benzathine penicillin G,* which provides low but effective serum levels for >2 weeks. Extensive studies in the 1940's and 1950's with regimens

TABLE 318–4. PENICILLIN TREATMENT PRACTICE IN SYPHILIS AS RECOMMENDED BY UNITED STATES PUBLIC HEALTH SERVICE

Indications for Syphilis Therapy†	Dosage and Administration*	
	Benzathine Penicillin G	Aqueous Benzyl Penicillin G or Procaine Penicillin G
Primary, secondary, and early latent syphilis (< 1 year); epidemiologic treatment	Total of 2.4 million units; single IM dose of two injections of 1.2 million units in one session	Total of 4.8 million units IM in doses of 600,000 units daily for 8 consecutive days
Late latent (> 1 year) or when CSF was not examined in "latency"; cardiovascular syphilis, late benign (cutaneous, osseous, visceral gumma)	Total of 7.2 million units IM in doses of 2.4 million units at 7-day intervals, over 21 days	Total of 9 million units IM in doses of 600,000 units daily over 15 days
Symptomatic or asymptomatic neurosyphilis	2 to 4 million units of aqueous (crystalline) penicillin G IV every 4 hours for at least 10 days	2 to 4 million units procaine penicillin IM daily and probenecid, 500 mg orally 4 times daily for 10–14 days
Congenital Infants	CSF normal: Total of 50,000 units per kilogram IM in a single or divided dose at one session	CSF abnormal: Total of 50,000 units per kilogram IM per day for 10 consecutive days‡
Older children	CSF normal: Same as for early congenital syphilis, up to 2.4 million units	CSF abnormal: 200,000–300,000 units per kilogram per day IV aqueous crystalline penicillin for 10–14 days

*Individual doses can be divided for injection in each buttock to minimize discomfort.

†In *pregnancy*, treatment is dependent on the stage of syphilis.

‡For aqueous penicillin, give in two divided IV doses per day; for procaine penicillin, give as one daily dose IM.

that provided similar serum levels and duration of therapy showed that approximately 95% of patients were cured by such treatment. Many of the remaining 5% who had clinical or serologic evidence of relapse may actually have been reinfected. It is not necessary to examine the CSF at this stage because penicillin prevents development of later neurosyphilis. Motile treponemes disappear from primary lesions in 24 hours.

A single injection of 2.4 million units of *aqueous procaine penicillin,* which provides relatively high serum levels for a brief period, is ineffective in established early syphilis but is curative if the disease is still in the incubating stage. The ceftriaxone regimen currently useful for gonorrhea probably is curative for incubating syphilis, but data are few, and careful follow-up is indicated if there is reason to suspect exposure to syphilis in a patient treated for gonorrhea with ceftriaxone. The incidence of incubating syphilis in gonorrhea patients is ≥ 2% in several series.

For patients allergic to penicillin, doxycycline, 100 mg twice daily for 14 days, is recommended. Particularly careful follow-up is necessary in patients treated with drugs other than penicillin, because patients may not be fully compliant with these prolonged courses of oral therapy and these regimens have been less fully evaluated clinically. Ceftriaxone, 2 grams intramuscularly daily for 10 days, may be effective but has not been well studied. Chloramphenicol is of equivocal efficacy and for this reason, as well as because of the risk of toxicity, should not be used. Spectinomycin and quinolone antibiotics have essentially no effect on syphilis. Erythromycin is of questionable efficacy.

Syphilis of > 1 Year's Duration. Larger doses of penicillin are needed for *neurosyphilis* (see Ch. 422) than for syphilis of < 1

year's duration. In general, patients with general paresis respond better to treatment than do patients with tabes dorsalis, although patients with paresis should be expected to show residual effects of the infection. This is particularly true in advanced cases. Meningovascular syphilis usually responds well, except for residual damage resulting from ischemic infarcts. Published studies show that a total of 6.0 to 9.0 million units of penicillin G results in a satisfactory clinical response in approximately 90% of patients with neurosyphilis, in the absence of HIV infection.

Benzathine penicillin regimens have received relatively little study in neurosyphilis but were previously recommended. However, there are reports of patients who have failed standard benzathine penicillin therapy for neurosyphilis but who responded to intensive intravenous therapy that provided high serum levels of penicillin. Benzathine penicillin does not provide measurable levels of penicillin in the spinal fluid or aqueous humor of the eye. There are anecdotal reports of increased treatment failures in patients with concomitant HIV infection. *Therefore there is considerable rationale to treatment with intravenous penicillin G (20 million units per day for at least 10 days in hospital).* Therapy of neurosyphilis not infrequently results in increased CSF pleocytosis for 7 to 10 days after starting treatment and may transiently convert a normal CSF to abnormal.

Limited evidence suggests that treating *latent syphilis* with 7.2 million units total dose of benzathine penicillin is curative even if the patient has asymptomatic neurosyphilis. However, because of the possible lack of the efficacy of benzathine penicillin in some patients with CNS syphilis, it is preferable to examine CSF in all patients with latent syphilis to exclude asymptomatic neurosyphilis. This is particularly important in HIV-positive patients. Alternatively, a lumbar puncture may be performed at the conclusion of the follow-up period (2 years); if the CSF is normal, the patient can be reassured that neurosyphilis will not develop.

There is no evidence that therapy with antimicrobial drugs is clinically beneficial to patients with *cardiovascular syphilis.* Nevertheless, treatment of cardiovascular syphilis is recommended in order to prevent further progression of disease and because approximately 15% of patients with cardiovascular syphilis have associated neurosyphilis.

There is no evidence regarding the efficacy of other antimicrobials in the treatment of later syphilis. Therefore if patients are allergic to penicillin, it is mandatory that the CSF be examined before therapy is undertaken. Either tetracycline or doxycycline taken for 4 weeks is probably effective.

Syphilis in Pregnancy. All pregnant women should be examined with a VDRL or RPR test during pregnancy; if they are at high risk for syphilis, a second test should be obtained before delivery. Because of the risk to the fetus, evaluation and treatment of the VDRL-positive patient should be done as rapidly as possible, particularly for patients first seen in the later stages of pregnancy. If a confirmatory FTA-ABS is positive and the patient has not been treated, penicillin should be administered in doses appropriate for early or late syphilis as outlined above. Penicillin-allergic patients should not be treated with tetracycline or erythromycin because of toxicity (tetracycline) or lack of efficacy (erythromycin). Penicillin desensitization may be considered but also carries risks. For patients who are VDRL positive but FTA-ABS negative and who have no clinical signs of syphilis, treatment may be withheld. In such patients a quantitative VDRL test and another FTA-ABS test should be repeated in 4 weeks. If the VDRL titer has risen by fourfold or more, or if clinical signs of syphilis have developed, the patient should be treated. If after repeat examination the diagnosis remains equivocal, the patient should be treated to prevent possible disease in the neonate. After treatment a quantitative VDRL titer should be followed monthly; if it rises fourfold, the patient should be treated a second time.

Congenital Syphilis. Proper treatment of the mother usually prevents active congenital syphilis in the neonate. However, infected infants may be clinically normal at birth, and the infant may be seronegative if the mother's infection was acquired late in pregnancy. The infant should be treated at birth if the mother has received no or inadequate treatment, or has been treated with drugs other than penicillin, if the mother has not yet responded to possibly effective therapy, or if the infant cannot be carefully followed up for several months after birth. The CSF should be examined before the infant is treated. If the CSF is normal, treatment may be with a single injection of 50,000 units per kilogram of benzathine penicillin G. If the CSF is abnormal, treatment should be with aqueous penicillin G, 50,000 units per kilogram intramuscularly or intravenously daily, given in two divided doses, for a minimum of 10 days. Alternatively, a single daily intramuscular injection of procaine penicillin G, 50,000 units per kilogram, may be given for 10 days. These recommendations are based upon the failure of benzathine penicillin to provide adequate treponemicidal levels in spinal fluid and on evidence that aqueous or procaine penicillin does provide adequate CSF levels of penicillin. Many experts believe that all syphilis in infected infants should be treated with either procaine or aqueous penicillin to ensure adequate CSF levels. Tetracycline should not be used to treat children younger than age 8. Antimicrobial agents other than penicillin are not recommended for treating congenital syphilis.

Follow-up Examinations. All HIV-seronegative patients with early syphilis or congenital syphilis should return for quantitative VDRL titers and clinical examination 3, 6, and 12 months after treatment. Treatment failure is somewhat more common in patients with HIV infection and although more aggressive therapy is usually not required, more aggressive follow-up is suggested. Serologic tests should be repeated at 1, 2, 3, 6, 9, and 12 months. Patients with late latent syphilis should be examined also at 24 months after therapy; if CSF was not examined prior to therapy, a lumbar puncture should be done prior to discharge to rule out inadequately treated asymptomatic neurosyphilis.

In most patients with early (primary, secondary, or early latent) syphilis, quantitative VDRL titers become nonreactive in 12 to 24 months after therapy. Prolonged reactive VDRL test results are associated with higher initial VDRL titers, prolonged infection, more advanced stage (primary < secondary < early latent), or repeated infection. In a small percentage of patients with early syphilis, the VDRL remains reactive in low titer for long periods. Chronic low-titer VDRL reactivity after therapy is much more common in late syphilis and should not be viewed with alarm. The FTA-ABS test may remain positive for years, despite adequate therapy. A fourfold or greater rise of VDRL titer after therapy is sufficient evidence for retreatment. Patients with treated early syphilis are fully susceptible to reinfection, and many clinical and serologic relapses after therapy are probably reinfections. As such they represent failures of proper epidemiologic case finding and of preventive therapy of the patient's sexual contacts.

Patients with neurosyphilis should be followed with serologic tests for at least 3 years and with repeat examination of CSF at 6-month intervals. The CSF pleocytosis is the first abnormality to disappear, but cell counts may not be normal for 1 to 2 years. The elevated CSF protein level falls more slowly, followed by the positive CSF-VDRL test, which may take years to become negative. It is not known whether high-dose intravenous penicillin therapy accelerates the return of CSF to normal. Rising CSF cell counts, protein, and VDRL titer obtained at follow-up are an indication for retreatment.

Epidemiologic Investigation and Treatment. All patients with syphilis should be reported to public health authorities. In the absence of an effective vaccine, control of syphilis depends on finding and treating persons with infectious lesions of primary and secondary syphilis before they can further transmit the disease and on finding and treating persons with incubating syphilis before they develop infectious lesions. All patients with early syphilis (< 1 year) should be carefully interviewed by qualified persons to determine the nature of their recent sex contacts. Approximately 16% of the named recent contacts of patients with early syphilis are found to have active untreated syphilis on examination, and a similar proportion of individuals named as suspects or associates also have active syphilis.

Most authorities, particularly in the United States, recommend treating sexual contacts of patients with early syphilis even if the contacts are clinically and serologically normal on examination. This is justifiable, because 30% of clinically normal individuals named as contacts of persons with infectious lesions of syphilis within the previous 30 days go on to develop syphilis if untreated. In general, preventive treatment is given to all sexual contacts of the past 90 days, although nearly all cases of syphilis in contacts develop within 60 days of exposure.

Jarisch-Herxheimer Reactions. Up to 60% of patients with early syphilis, and a significant proportion of patients with later stages of syphilis, experience a transient febrile reaction after therapy for syphilis. This usually occurs in the first few hours after therapy, peaks at 6 to 8 hours, and disappears within 12 to 24 hours of therapy. Temperature elevation is usually low grade, and there is often associated myalgia, headache, and malaise. The skin lesions of secondary syphilis are often exacerbated during the Herxheimer reaction, and cutaneous lesions that were not visible may become visible. It is usually of no clinical significance and may be treated with salicylates in most cases. In patients with syphilis of the coronary ostia or of the optic nerve, there is a theoretical risk that local inflammation coincident with the Herxheimer reaction could precipitate serious damage. This is the subject of much discussion in the old literature, but there is little current evidence that "local Herxheimer reactions" constitute a significant risk to the patient. Corticosteroids have been used to prevent adverse effects of the Herxheimer reaction, but there is no evidence that they are clinically beneficial (other than reducing fever) or necessary. Institution of treatment with small doses of penicillin does not prevent the Herxheimer reaction.

The pathogenesis of the Herxheimer reaction is unclear. It may be due to liberation of antigens from the spirochetes. There is evidence that the complement cascade (see Ch. 222) is activated, including transient consumption of C3, C4, C6, and C7, and of transient decrease in treponemal antibodies coincident with the Herxheimer reaction. There is also evidence for endotoxemia, obtained by positive limulus amebocyte gelatin tests, at the time of the Herxheimer reaction, although *T. pallidum* does not contain biologically active endotoxin. These seemingly contradictory observations could be explained if the reaction resulted in release of endogenous endotoxin from the gut.

Persistence of Treponemes After Treatment. Studies in humans and in rabbits have shown that spiral forms may be visualized by silver stains in lymph nodes after effective treatment. Living virulent treponemes have occasionally been recovered by rabbit inoculation from lymph nodes, CSF, or ocular fluids after effective treatment has been given. These documented cases of treponemal persistence are very rare, however. At present there is little reason to worry about persistence of virulent treponemes after therapy with penicillin, with the possible exception of CNS syphilis, which needs further evaluation. No evidence exists for selection of penicillin-resistant mutants of *T. pallidum* to date.

PROSPECTS FOR PREVENTION. Solid immunity develops in rabbits following prolonged infection with virulent *T. pallidum*. It has not yet been possible to transfer immunity passively in laboratory animals by either immune serum or immune lymphocytes alone, suggesting that both cellular and humoral systems are necessary for immunity. Rabbits have been effectively immunized with multiple injections of treponemes that have been rendered avirulent by irradiation or by exposure to cold. However, a very large number of injections and a large mass of treponemes are necessary to effect immunity in the laboratory animal. For this reason and because *T. pallidum* cannot yet be grown in a virulent state in cell-free medium, there is no immediate prospect for a vaccine. However, significant immunity does develop in humans after prolonged infection. For the present, control depends entirely on clinical awareness on the part of physicians, adequate reporting to public health authorities, and vigorous application of epidemiologic investigation and preventive treatment of sexual contacts.

Cox DL, Chang P, McDowell A, Radolf JD: The outer membrane, not a coat of host proteins, limits the antigenicity of virulent *Treponema pallidum*. Infect Immun 60:1076, 1992. *New data regarding the causative agent of syphilis and the reasons humoral antibody does not control or prevent infection.*

Drusin LM, Singer C, Valenti AJ, et al.: Infectious syphilis mimicking neoplastic disease. Arch Intern Med 137:156, 1977. *A fascinating and frightening account of diagnostic problems caused by oral, rectal, or lymphatic syphilis, nearly leading to cancer surgery.*

Feher J, Somogyi T, Timmer M, et al.: Early syphilitic hepatitis. Lancet 2:896, 1975. *A description of the frequency and histology of early syphilitic hepatitis.*

Fischer A, Kristensen JK, Husfelt V: Tertiary syphilis in Denmark 1961–1970. A description of 105 cases not previously diagnosed or specifically treated. Acta Dermatovener 56:485, 1975. *One of few studies of the prevalence of newly diagnosed late syphilis in the antibiotic era.*

Gamble CN, Reardan JB: Immunopathogenesis of syphilitic glomerulonephritis: Elution of antitreponemal antibody from glomerular immune-complex deposits. N Engl J Med 292:449, 1975. *Clear evidence for an immune-complex cause of syphilitic nephrosis.*

Gjestland T: The Oslo study of untreated syphilis: An epidemiologic investigation of the natural course of the syphilitic infection based upon a re-study of the Boeck-

Bruusgaard material. Acta Derm Venereol 35:Suppl 34, 1955. *A medical classic, in which the long-term course of untreated syphilis is evaluated.*

Holmes KK, Märdh P-A, Sparling PF, et al.: Sexually Transmitted Diseases, 2nd ed. New York, McGraw-Hill, 1990. *The definitive text on sexually transmitted diseases.*

Hook EW III, Marra CM: Acquired syphilis in adults. N Engl J Med 326:1060, 1992. *A review of syphilis in the 1990's, including syphilis-HIV interactions.*

Lee TJ, Sparling PF: Syphilis. An algorithm. JAMA 242:1187, 1979. *An algorithm for management of patients who present with a positive VDRL or similar test.*

Lugar A, Schmidt B, Spendlingwimmer I, et al.: Recent observations on the serology of syphilis. Br J Vener Dis 56:12, 1980. *An evaluation of the merits of serologic tests for syphilis.*

Magnuson HJ, Thomas EW, Olansky S, et al.: Inoculation syphilis in human volunteers. Medicine 35:33, 1956. *A classic paper, in which prison volunteers were inoculated with virulent T. pallidum. Immunity to inoculation syphilis was observed only in individuals who had congenital or late syphilis.*

Raskind MA, Eisdorfer C: Screening for syphilis in an aged psychiatrically impaired population. West J Med 125:361, 1976. *Syphilitic disease of the CNS may be more prevalent than hospital surveys suggest.*

Tramont EC: Persistence of *Treponema pallidum* following penicillin G therapy: Report of two cases. JAMA 236:2206, 1976. *At least one of the cases of neurosyphilis probably was a true penicillin treatment failure.*

Wilner E, Brody JA: Prognosis of general paresis after treatment. Lancet 2:1370, 1968. *Neurosyphilis frequently shows clinical progression despite what is probably adequate therapy.*

Spirochetal Diseases Other Than Syphilis

319 NONSYPHILITIC TREPONEMATOSES

Edward W. Hook III*

DEFINITION. The nonsyphilitic treponematoses are the skin diseases called *yaws, endemic syphilis* (previously known as *bejel*), and *pinta*. They occur predominantly in tropical regions and are transmitted by skin contact with infected persons. Disfiguring ulcerations of the skin may be produced, and invasion of bone and other tissues has been described. Treatment with benzathine penicillin G is effective, and the World Health Organization (WHO) has carried out extensive treatment campaigns in endemic areas.

ETIOLOGY. Yaws is caused by *Treponema pallidum* subspecies *pertenue;* pinta is caused by *T. carateum;* and endemic syphilis is caused by *T. pallidum* subspecies *endemicum*. The *T. pallidum* subspecies causing nonsyphilitic treponematoses are closely related to *T. pallidum* subspecies *pallidum,* which causes venereal syphilis; there is a high degree of DNA homology, and they share unique, pathogen-restricted antigens. Like *T. pallidum,* these treponemes are spirochetal bacteria with helical structures and measure about 0.2 μ in diameter and 10 μ in length. They are visible by darkfield microscopy but cannot be cultivated for prolonged periods *in vitro*.

DISTRIBUTION AND EPIDEMIOLOGY. Yaws is prevalent in rural areas of tropical Africa, the Americas, Southeast Asia, and Oceania. The highest incidence is in children between ages 2 and 5 years. Endemic syphilis occurs in Africa, in Eastern Mediterranean countries, on the Arabian peninsula, in Central Asia, and in Australia. It is most prevalent in arid regions. Pinta occurs in rural areas of tropical Central and South America. Pinta affects mostly older children and adolescents. Humans are the only known carriers of the nonsyphilitic treponematoses. The spirochete enters the skin only after it is broken, as by a scratch or insect bite. Transmission is believed to occur by contacting the skin directly or indirectly by contaminated hands or fomites and is facilitated by conditions of poor personal hygiene and crowding.

CLINICAL FEATURES. *Yaws* produces a skin papule at the inoculation site after an incubation period of 3 to 4 weeks. The most common sites are the legs and buttocks. The papule enlarges, ulcerates, and develops a serous crust from which treponemes can be recovered. Regional lymphadenitis may accompany the papule, which will heal spontaneously within 6 months. A generalized secondary rash will occur before or after the initial lesion heals, and these rashes are also papular and often covered with brown crusts. Relapsing crops of lesions can occur. Papillomas may result, and the plantar surfaces of the feet are involved with hyperkeratotic lesions. Periostitis of long bones leads to tender bones, and fever may be present. Relapsing lesions may occur over several years, resulting in chronic ulcerations and destructive gummatous lesions affecting the skin and bones.

Endemic syphilis produces patches on the mucous membranes of the oral cavity and pharynx and can cause split papules at the mucocutaneous junction of the oral angles. Anal, genital, and other intertriginous skin areas can be affected by lesions that resemble secondary syphilis. Regional lymphadenitis is common, and generalized rashes are rare. Healing of these early lesions is followed by latency manifested by seropositivity or by late lesions that resemble tertiary syphilis. These include nodular ulcers of skin, deformities of bones, and gummatous lesions that can perforate the palate.

Pinta starts similarly as a cutaneous papule with regional lymphadenitis that is followed by a generalized maculopapular eruption. One to three years after healing of the initial lesion, large hyperpigmented macules that are brown or blue develop and subsequently lose their pigment and become white. The time required for lesions to pass through these stages varies, so that the same patient may have coexisting areas of increased pigment and loss of pigment.

DIAGNOSIS. By darkfield microscopy, the causative spirochetes from early skin lesions can be observed directly. Spirochetes have been demonstrated also in lymph node aspirates. There is no specific test for any of the nonsyphilitic treponematoses. Serologic tests for syphilis detect cross-reacting antibodies in these diseases. The VDRL test, the serologic test for syphilis, and the fluorescent treponemal antibody absorption test all give positive results if serum is obtained at least 2 weeks after the lesions initially appear.

TREATMENT AND PROGNOSIS. Long-acting benzathine penicillin G given as 1.2 million units intramuscularly is the preferred treatment for patients with early lesions. For patients with late manifestations, this therapy should be repeated twice at approximately 7-day intervals. The early lesions heal rapidly, and most seropositive cases convert to seronegative status. Late destructive lesions take longer to show improvement.

PREVENTION. The prevalence of these diseases has been reduced in several areas of the world by mass treatment campaigns using penicillin. The WHO has treated about 53 million cases of yaws and 350,000 cases of pinta in the field with good results. These campaigns, however, are not adequate to eradicate the disease, and in recent years the prevalence of yaws may have increased. It has been suggested that reduction in transmission requires improvements in the sanitation and economic standards of people living in endemic areas.

Engeikens HJ, Niemel PL, van der Sluis JJ, et al.: Endemic treponematoses. Part II. Pinta and endemic syphilis. Int J Dermatol 30:231, 1991.

Guthe T: Clinical serological and epidemiological features of framboesia tropica (yaws) and its control in rural communities. Acta Dermatovener 49:343, 1969.

Hackett CJ, Lowenthal LJA: Differential Diagnosis of Yaws. WHO Monograph Series No. 45. Geneva, WHO, 1960.

Kantor I, Wilentz JM, Berger BB: Yaws. Arch Dermatol 103:546, 1971.

Koff AB, Rosen T: Nonvenereal treponematoses: yaws, endemic syphilis, and pinta. J Am Acad Dermatol 29:519, 1993. *With worldwide travel there is a need to consider diagnosis of nonvenereal treponematoses in appropriate clinical and historical situations.*

Vorst FA: Clinical diagnosis and changing manifestations of treponemal infection. Rev Infect Dis 7(suppl 2):S327, 1985. *This paper shows that yaws in populations after mass treatment with penicillin assumes attenuated forms characterized by shorter duration of papillomas and lower antibody titers.*

---

* The author acknowledges the contribution of Dr. Thomas Butler on this subject in the 19th edition of the *Cecil Textbook of Medicine*.

320 RELAPSING FEVER
William A. Petri, Jr.

DEFINITION. Relapsing fever is a spirochetal infection with bacteria of the genus *Borrelia*. There are two modes of transmission: epidemic louse-borne and endemic tick-borne relapsing fever.

ETIOLOGY. *Borrelia* are spirochetes that measure 0.5 μ in diameter and 5 to 40 μ in length. They are aerophilic and require long-chain fatty acids for growth. Louse-borne relapsing fever is caused by *B. recurrentis*. Tick-borne relapsing fever organisms are named after their tick vector and include the closely related species *B. duttonii* (Old World) and *B. hermsii*, *B. turicatae*, and *B. parkeri* (North America).

EPIDEMIOLOGY. Louse-borne epidemic relapsing fever is carried from person to person by the human body louse. There is no animal reservoir. The spirochete lives in the hemolymph, and infection is transmitted to humans when the louse is crushed. Epidemics have occurred at wartime when breakdown in sanitation favors transmission of body lice. Louse-borne disease remains endemic in Ethiopia, Somalia, and the Sudan.

Tick-borne endemic relapsing fever is carried by *Ornithodoros* ticks, which become infected by feeding on wild rodents. In the United States, relapsing fever is limited to mountainous areas of the West at altitudes of 1500 to 8000 feet where the tick vector *O. hermsii* resides in forests of ponderosa pine and Douglas fir. A key diagnostic clue has been a history of sleeping in rodent-infested rustic cabins in western national parks.

PATHOLOGY AND PATHOGENESIS. *Borrelia* infection begins in the skin at the site of the louse or tick bite and is followed by rapid dissemination of the spirochetes via the bloodstream. Spirochetes are visible on Wright's stained peripheral blood smears during the initial febrile episode and during each relapse in most patients. Clearance of spirochetes from the blood is associated with the production of serotype-specific immune sera; anti-*Borrelia* antibodies have been shown in animal models to be the major mechanism of immune clearance of infection.

Relapses are associated with antigenic variation in the variable major proteins (VMP's), which are the abundant outer-membrane proteins of the spirochete that carry the serotype-specific epitopes. Antigenic variation is the consequence of recombination events occurring between VMP genes at silent and expression sites on linear plasmids.

CLINICAL FEATURES. An abrupt onset of fever to 38.5 to 40°C (>39°C in most patients), headache, myalgias, and shaking chills characterize the onset of illness. Cough, nausea and vomiting, and fatigue are less frequent complaints. Signs include fever, tachycardia, lethargy or confusion, conjunctival injection, and epistaxis. Hepatosplenomegaly, jaundice, and often a truncal petechial skin rash are common signs in louse-borne relapsing fever. Untreated louse-borne disease lasts 6 days, and relapses occur once after an afebrile period of 9 days. Tick-borne relapsing fever lasts about 4 days without antibiotic treatment and an average of two relapses occur after a 10-day afebrile period.

Relapsing fever in pregnancy results in miscarriage in one third of patients. Neonatal infection presents in both the tick- and louse-borne forms with jaundice, hepatosplenomegaly, and often sepsis and hemorrhage. Fever and hepatosplenomegaly are also common signs in children.

LABORATORY FEATURES. Spirochetes can be demonstrated in the Wright's stained peripheral blood smear of most patients. The white blood count is usually normal, but platelet counts <50,000 per cu mm occur in up to 90% of cases of louse-borne disease. Prothrombin and partial thromboplastin times are often prolonged. In louse-borne disease, elevations in hepatic enzymes and blood urea nitrogen are common. The degree of spirochetemia is often 10^5 organisms per cu mm.

DIAGNOSIS. Spirochetes can be demonstrated on peripheral blood smears taken during the febrile episodes in 70% of patients. With an average incubation period of one week, relapsing fever is often diagnosed in a nonendemic area after the individual has returned from a stay in the Rocky Mountains. Only a few patients will remember tick exposure, since *O. hermsii* is a night feeder and only remains attached for 15 minutes. Culture of the organism requires a special medium and is not practical in a clinical laboratory setting. Because the number of organisms in blood is extremely high, the diagnosis is most often made by direct visualization of the organism on a blood smear.

PROGNOSIS. Epidemics of louse-borne relapsing fever have been reported, with mortalities approaching 40%. With antibiotic treatment, mortality is <5% in all recent series, with complete recovery expected. Autopsies of patients with louse-borne disease have documented intracranial hemorrhage, brain edema, bronchopneumonia, hepatic necrosis, and splenic infarcts.

THERAPY AND PREVENTION. A single 500-mg dose of tetracycline may be as effective as longer treatments in clearing spirochetemia of louse-borne disease, although many physicians still treat with 500 mg tetracycline every 6 hours for 5 to 10 days. Erythromycin is also effective and should be used in children under age 7 (in whom tetracyclines can stain the permanent teeth). Penicillin treatment has been reported to clear the spirochetemia more slowly than tetracycline.

The Jarisch-Herxheimer reaction (typically characterized by a rise in body temperature of 1°C, rigors, a slight fall followed by a rise in blood pressure, and transient leukopenia) occurs 2 to 3 hours after treatment in many patients with louse-borne disease, less commonly in tick-borne disease, and should be anticipated and managed supportively. Deaths due to shock from the Jarisch-Herxheimer reaction occur rarely. The Jarisch-Herxheimer reaction has been associated with accelerated phagocytosis of spirochetes by neutrophils and transient elevations of tumor necrosis factor, interleukin-6, and interleukin-8.

Barbour AG: Antigenic variation of a relapsing fever *Borrelia* species. Annu Rev Microbiol 44:155, 1990. *Immunology and molecular biology of antigenic variation are reviewed.*

Common source outbreak of relapsing fever—California. MMWR 39:579, 1990. *Six individuals who had at different times spent the night in the same cabin at Big Bear Lake in California all developed relapsing fever with sudden onset of high fever, severe headache, prostration, nausea, and vomiting. Inhabited ground squirrel burrows were found under the cabin.*

Perine PL, Teklu B: Antibiotic treatment of louse-borne relapsing fever in Ethiopia: A report of 377 cases. Am J Trop Med Hyg 32:1096, 1983. *Tetracycline, doxycycline, erythromycin, and chloramphenicol were all effective as single-dose therapy but are associated with a Jarisch-Herxheimer reaction within 2 hours of drug administration.*

321 LYME DISEASE
Stephen E. Malawista

Lyme disease is a tick-borne inflammatory disorder caused by a newly recognized spirochete, *Borrelia burgdorferi*. Its clinical hallmark is an early expanding skin lesion, *erythema chronicum migrans* (ECM), which may be followed weeks to months later by neurologic, cardiac, or joint abnormalities. Symptoms may refer to any one of these four systems alone or in combination. All stages of Lyme disease may respond to antibiotics, but treatment of early disease is the most successful. Although cases of the illness are concentrated in certain endemic areas, foci of Lyme disease are widely distributed within the United States, Europe, and Asia.

"Lyme arthritis" was recognized in November 1975 because of unusual geographic clustering of children with inflammatory arthropathy in the region of Lyme, Connecticut. It soon became clear that this was a multisystem disorder (Lyme disease) occurring at any age, in both sexes, and often preceded by a characteristic expanding skin lesion, ECM. In Europe ECM had been associated with the bite of the sheep tick, *Ixodes ricinus*, and with tick-borne meningopolyneuritis. In the Lyme region, a closely related deer tick, *I. scapularis* (thought until recently to represent a new species, called *I. dammini*), was implicated as the principal disease vector on epidemiologic grounds. In 1982, Burgdorfer and associates isolated a spirochete, now called *B. burgdorferi*, from *I. scapularis* and linked it serologically to patients with Lyme disease. It was soon recovered from patient specimens.

DISTRIBUTION AND EPIDEMIOLOGY. Lyme disease is widespread. In the United States there are three distinct foci: the Northeast from Massachusetts to Maryland, the Midwest in Wisconsin and Minnesota, and the West in California, southern Oregon, and western Nevada. However, the illness has been reported in 46 states, as well as throughout Europe and Asia. The earliest known cases in the United States occurred on Cape Cod in 1962 and in Lyme, Connecticut, in 1965; annual cases now number in the thousands. Disease can occur at any age and in either gender. Onset of illness is generally between May 1 and November 30, with the peak in June and July.

The primary vectors of Lyme disease are tiny ixodid ticks. Major foci of disease correspond to the distribution of *I. scapularis* (Northeast, Midwest), *I. pacificus* (West), *I. ricinus* (Europe), and *I. persulcatus* (Eurasia, Asia), but other vectors, including the Lone Star tick, *Amblyomma americanum*, are likely in some areas. In one United States study, 31% of 314 patients recalled a tick bite at the skin site where ECM developed days to weeks later. The six ticks that were saved were invariably nymphal *I. scapularis*, whose peak questing period is May through July; the nymphal stage is primarily responsible for transmission of disease. Preferred hosts for *I. scapularis* nymphs are white-footed mice and, for adults, white-tailed deer, in whose fur they mate. A less successful transmission cycle involving the dusky footed woodrat has been described in California.

The rising incidence of Lyme disease in recent years in the United States may be explained by multiple factors, including an increase in the numbers of ixodid ticks, the outward migration of residential areas into previously rural woodlands (habitats favored by ixodid ticks and their hosts), an exploding deer population, and increased recognition.

In areas endemic for Lyme disease, the prevalence of *B. burgdorferi* in nymphal *I. scapularis* ranges from about 20 to >60% (cf. *I. pacificus*, 1 to 3%). The organism has been isolated, or specific antibody found, in blood and tissues of a wide variety of large and small animals, including domestic dogs and birds. Indiscriminate feeding on a variety of animals by immature *I. scapularis* may favor the spread of infection.

In high-risk areas, vaccines based on one of the outer surface proteins (OspA) of *B. burgdorferi*, which have been shown to protect animals against infection, are currently being tested in human volunteers.

PATHOGENESIS. Recovery of *B. burgdorferi* is straightforward from the tick but difficult from patients—except from ECM lesions, where the clinical diagnosis is usually obvious—in part because of a relative paucity of organisms in specimens of tissue and fluids from the latter. Nevertheless, rare positive cultures are reported at all stages of the illness—from blood (early), secondary annular lesions, meningitic cerebrospinal fluid (CSF), heart, joint fluid, ligament, and even a late skin lesion, *acrodermatitis chronica atrophicans*, that had been present for 10 years. Spirochetes have been identified by silver stain or by immunofluorescence in some histologic sections of ECM and rarely of secondary annular lesions, synovium, brain, eye, heart, striated muscle, ligament, liver, spleen, kidney, and bone marrow.

From these data, combined with clinical (see below) and epidemiologic features of Lyme disease, the following pathogenetic sequence is likely. *B. burgdorferi* is transmitted to the skin of the host via the tick vector. After an incubation period of 3 to 32 days, the organism migrates outward in the skin (ECM), spreads in lymph (regional adenopathy), or disseminates in blood to organs (e.g., central nervous system [CNS], joints, heart, and presumably liver and spleen) or other skin sites (secondary annular lesions; see below). Maternal-fetal transmission is distinctly uncommon. Although organisms are hard to find in later stages of Lyme disease, it is entirely possible that persistent live spirochetes are driving the illness throughout its course. Evidence for this interpretation includes the responsiveness of many patients to antibiotics, the rare sightings of spirochetes in affected tissues, the variable recovery from affected tissues and fluids of spirochetal DNA amplified by the polymerase chain reaction (PCR), and an expansion of the antibody response to additional spirochetal antigens over time. If live spirochetes are invariably present, it is not yet clear how they occasionally remain out of harm's way in the face of both antibiotic therapy and the body's usual phagocytic and other immune clearance mechanisms.

In the clinical laboratory, characteristic immune abnormalities are found. At disease onset (ECM), almost all patients have evidence of circulating immune complexes. At that time, the findings of elevated serum immunoglobulin M (IgM) levels and cryoglobulins containing IgM predict subsequent nervous system, heart, or joint involvement—i.e., early humoral findings have prognostic significance. Serial determinations of serum IgM are often the single most helpful laboratory indicator of disease activity. These abnormalities tend to persist during neurologic or cardiac involvement. Later in the illness, when arthritis is present, serum IgM levels are more often normal. By then, immune complexes are usually lacking in serum but are present uniformly in joint fluid, where their titers correlate positively with the local concentration of polymorphonuclear leukocytes. Mononuclear cells from peripheral blood increase their antigen-specific proliferative response as the disease progresses, but the greatest reactivity to antigen is seen in cells from inflamed joints. Adjacent to that joint fluid, on biopsy a proliferative synovium is seen, often replete with lymphocytes and plasma cells that are presumably capable of producing immunoglobulin locally. Thus an initially disseminated, immune-mediated inflammatory disorder becomes in some patients localized and propagated in joints.

Although *B. burgdorferi* seem not to destroy tissue directly, they nonspecifically activate monocytes, macrophages, synovial lining cells, B cells, and complement, resulting in the elaboration of a host of proinflammatory materials. These spirochetes adhere to extracellular matrix proteins, to endothelial cells (and penetrate endothelial monolayers), and to neural glycolipid. They can induce the production of cross-reactive antibodies and of specific immune B and T lymphocytes that may be associated histologically with endarteritic microvascular occlusive changes (e.g., in nervous tissue, hearts, joints), but it is not clear that these phenomena persist in the absence of live spirochetes.

In addition to factors related to the pathogenicity of specific isolates of *B. burgdorferi*, immunogenetic makeup may play a role in whether infected individuals can rid themselves of spirochetes, their antigens, or their effects. Patients with treatment-resistant chronic arthritis have been reported to have an increased frequency of the B-cell alloantigen HLA DR4.

CLINICAL CHARACTERISTICS. Lyme disease is conveniently divided into three clinical stages, but the stages may overlap, most patients do not exhibit all of them, and in fact seroconversion can occur in asymptomatic individuals. The illness usually begins with ECM and associated symptoms (stage 1), sometimes followed weeks to months later by neurologic or cardiac abnormalities (stage 2) and weeks to years later by arthritis (stage 3). Chronic neurologic and skin involvement also may occur years after onset.

Early Manifestations. ECM, the unique clinical marker for Lyme disease, begins as a red macule or papule at the site where the tick vector, usually long gone, had engorged. As the area of redness expands to 15 cm or so (range 3 to 68 cm), there is usually partial central clearing (see Color Plate 10*B*). The outer borders are red, generally flat, and without scaling. The centers are occasionally red and indurated, even vesicular or necrotic. Variations may occur—multiple rings, for example. The thigh, groin, and axilla are particularly common sites. The lesion is warm to touch, but not often sore, and is easily missed if out of sight. Routine histologic findings are nonspecific: a heavy dermal infiltrate of mononuclear cells, without epidermal change except at the site of the tick bite.

Within days of onset of ECM, one half of U.S. patients develop multiple annular secondary lesions (see Color Plate 10*B*; Table 321–1). They resemble ECM itself but are generally smaller, migrate less, and lack indurated centers; they are not associated with the sites of previous tick bites. Individual lesions may come and go, and their borders sometimes merge. Other occasional skin lesions are noted in Table 321–1. In addition, benign lymphocytoma cutis has been reported in Europe. ECM and secondary lesions fade in 3 to 4 weeks (range 1 day to 14 months). They may recur.

Skin involvement is often accompanied by musculoskeletal flu-like symptoms—malaise and fatigue, headache, fever and chills, myalgia, and arthralgia (Table 321–2). Even without ECM, this syndrome in summer, in an endemic area for Lyme disease, is grounds for treatment. Some patients have evidence of meningeal

TABLE 321–1. EARLY SIGNS OF LYME DISEASE

Signs	No. of Patients N = 314	(%)
Erythema chronicum migrans	314	(100)*
Multiple annular lesions	150	(48)
Lymphadenopathy		
Regional	128	(41)
Generalized	63	(20)
Pain on neck flexion	52	(17)
Malar rash	41	(13)
Erythematous throat	38	(12)
Conjunctivitis	35	(11)
Right upper quadrant tenderness	24	(8)
Splenomegaly	18	(6)
Hepatomegaly	16	(5)
Muscle tenderness	12	(4)
Periorbital edema	10	(3)
Evanescent skin lesions	8	(3)
Abdominal tenderness	6	(2)
Testicular swelling	2	(1)

Erythema chronicum migrans was required for inclusion in this study.
From Steere AC, Bartenhagen NH, Craft JE, et al.: The early clinical manifestations of Lyme disease. Ann Intern Med 99:76, 1983.

irritation or mild encephalopathy—for example, episodic attacks of excruciating headache and neck pain, stiffness, or pressure—but typically lasting only for hours at this stage of the illness and without CSF pleocytosis or objective neurologic deficit. Except for fatigue and lethargy, which are often constant, the early signs and symptoms are typically intermittent and changing. For example, a patient may have meningitic attacks for several days, a few days of improvement, and then the onset of migratory musculoskeletal pain. This last may involve joints (generally without swelling), tendons, bursa, muscle, and bone. The pain tends to affect only one or two sites at a time and to last a few hours to several days in a given location. The various associated symptoms may occur several days before ECM (or without it) and last for months (especially fatigue and lethargy) after the skin lesions have disappeared.

Later Manifestations. Neurologic Involvement. Within several weeks to months of the onset of illness, about 15% of patients develop frank neurologic abnormalities, including meningitis, encephalitis, chorea, cranial neuritis (including bilateral facial palsy), motor and sensory radiculoneuritis, or mononeuritis multiplex, in various combinations. The usual pattern is fluctuating meningoencephalitis with superimposed cranial nerve (particularly facial) palsy and peripheral radiculoneuropathy, but Bell's palsy may occur

TABLE 321–2. EARLY SYMPTOMS OF LYME DISEASE

Symptoms	No. of Patients N = 314	(%)
Malaise, fatigue, and lethargy	251	(80)
Headache	200	(64)
Fever and chills	185	(59)
Stiff neck	151	(48)
Arthralgias	150	(48)
Myalgias	135	(43)
Backache	81	(26)
Anorexia	73	(23)
Sore throat	53	(17)
Nausea	53	(17)
Dysesthesia	35	(11)
Vomiting	32	(10)
Abdominal pain	24	(8)
Photophobia	19	(6)
Hand stiffness	16	(5)
Dizziness	15	(5)
Cough	15	(5)
Chest pain	12	(4)
Ear pain	12	(4)
Diarrhea	6	(2)

From Steere AC, Bartenhagen NH, Craft JE, et al.: The early clinical manifestations of Lyme disease. Ann Intern Med 99:76, 1983.

alone. By now, patients with meningitic symptoms have a lymphocytic pleocytosis (about 100 cells per cubic millimeter) in CSF and sometimes diffuse slowing on electroencephalogram. However, the neck is rarely stiff except on extreme flexion; Kernig's and Brudzinski's signs are absent. Neurologic abnormalities typically last for months but usually resolve completely (late neurologic complications are noted below).

Cardiac Involvement. Also within weeks to months of onset, about 8% of patients develop cardiac involvement. The most common abnormality is fluctuating degrees of atrioventricular block (first-degree, Wenckebach, or complete heart block). Some patients have evidence of more diffuse cardiac involvement, including electrocardiographic changes compatible with acute myopericarditis, radionuclide evidence of mild left ventricular dysfunction, or, rarely, cardiomegaly. None has had heart murmurs. Cardiac involvement is usually brief (3 days to 6 weeks), but it may recur.

Arthritis. From weeks to as long as 2 years after the onset of illness, about 60% of patients develop frank arthritis, usually characterized by intermittent attacks of asymmetric joint swelling and pain primarily in large joints, especially the knee, one or two joints at a time. Affected knees are commonly more swollen than painful, often hot, and rarely red; Baker's cysts may form and rupture early. However, both large and small joints may be affected, and a few patients have had symmetric polyarthritis. Attacks of arthritis, which generally last from weeks to months, typically recur for several years, decreasing in frequency with time. Fatigue is common with active joint involvement, but fever or other systemic symptoms at this stage are unusual. Joint fluid white cell counts vary from 500 to 110,000 cells per cubic millimeter, with an average of about 25,000 cells per cubic millimeter, mostly polymorphonuclear leukocytes. Total protein ranges from 3 to 8 grams per deciliter. The C3 and C4 levels are generally greater than one-third, and glucose levels usually greater than two-thirds, that of serum. Rheumatoid factor and antinuclear antibody are absent.

In about 10% of patients with arthritis, involvement in large joints may become chronic, with pannus formation and erosion of cartilage and bone. Synovial biopsy findings may mimic those of rheumatoid arthritis: surface deposits of fibrin, villous hypertrophy, vascular proliferation, and a heavy infiltration of mononuclear cells. In addition, there may be an obliterative endarteritis and (rarely) demonstrable spirochetes. As noted above, B. burgdorferi stimulates mononuclear cells to produce cytokines (e.g., interleukin-1, TNFα, interleukin-6), and elevated concentrations of inflammatory cytokines have been found in synovial fluid. In one patient with chronic Lyme arthritis, synovium grown in tissue culture produced large amounts of collagenase and prostaglandin E_2. Thus in Lyme disease the joint fluid cell counts, the immune reactants (except for rheumatoid factor), the synovial histology, the amounts of synovial enzymes released, and the resulting destruction of cartilage and bone may be similar to those in rheumatoid arthritis.

Other late findings (years) associated with this infection include a chronic skin lesion—*acrodermatitis chronica atrophicans*—well known in Europe but still rare in the United States. One sees violaceous infiltrated plaques or nodules, especially on extensor surfaces, that eventually become atrophic. Uncommon late chronic neurologic disease includes transverse myelitis, diffuse sensory axonal neuropathy, and demyelinating lesions of the CNS. Mild memory impairment, subtle mood changes, and chronic fatigue states may also occur.

LABORATORY TEST RESULTS. The diagnosis of Lyme disease is based on recognizing clinical features of the illness in a patient with a history of possible exposure to the causative organism. Culture of *B. burgdorferi* from patients is definitive but has rarely been successful except from skin biopsy specimens. The organism can be isolated from blood in a significant minority of patients with systemic manifestations of early disease (it grows very slowly). Special tissue staining techniques generally have a low yield and are not readily available. Determination of specific antibody titers, usually performed by enzyme-linked immunosorbent assay (ELISA), is currently the most helpful additional diagnostic test for Lyme disease. In serum, specific IgM antibody titers against *B. burgdorferi* usually reach a peak between the third and sixth weeks after the onset of disease; specific immunoglobulin G (IgG) antibody titers rise more slowly and are generally highest months later when arthritis is present (Fig. 321–1). Individuals with Lyme disease of more than 6 weeks' duration can be expected to have elevated levels of specific antibodies. However, the tests employed are not yet standardized, and results from different commercial laboratories may vary, especially for borderline elevations. The vast majority of individuals with established Lyme arthritis have elevated specific IgG titers. This finding makes antibody titers against *B. burgdorferi* particularly useful in differentiating Lyme disease from other rheumatic syndromes, especially when ECM is missed, forgotten, or absent. This antibody cross-reacts with other spirochetes, including *Treponema pallidum,* but patients with Lyme disease do not have positive VDRL test results. Western blots can be helpful when false-positive ELISA's are suspected.

Another test of diagnostic interest uses the polymerase chain reaction (PCR) to detect spirochetal DNA in host material. Although this powerful tool is notorious for false-positive results when not performed under the most stringent conditions, it shows great promise, particularly in Lyme arthritis, in which synovial fluid from the large majority of untreated patients appears to be positive.

The most common nonspecific laboratory abnormalities, particularly early in the illness, are a high erythrocyte sedimentation rate, an elevated serum IgM level, or increased serum levels of aspartate transaminase (AST). The enzyme levels generally return to normal within several weeks. Patients may be mildly anemic early in the illness and occasionally have elevated white cell counts with shifts to the left in the differential count. A few patients have had microscopic hematuria, sometimes with mild proteinuria (dipstick); values for creatinine and blood urea nitrogen have been normal. Throughout the illness, serum C3 and C4 levels are generally normal or elevated. Rheumatoid factor and antinuclear antibodies are usually absent.

DIFFERENTIAL DIAGNOSIS. ECM is the unique herald lesion of Lyme disease (see Color Plate 10B). When present in its classic form, there is little else that might be confused with it. However, some patients are not aware of having had ECM, and in others, its appearance is not always characteristic. Secondary lesions might suggest *erythema multiforme,* but blistering, mucosal lesions, and involvement of the palms and soles are not features of Lyme disease. Malar rash may suggest systemic lupus erythematosus; an urticarial rash, hepatitis B infection or serum sickness. Evanescent blotches and circles may resemble *erythema marginatum,* but those of Lyme disease do not expand.

Early musculoskeletal flulike symptoms may be misleading, especially when ECM is absent or missed or is not the first manifestation. Severe headache and stiff neck may resemble aseptic meningitis, abdominal symptoms, hepatitis, and generalized tender lymphadenopathy and splenomegaly, infectious mononucleosis. As in the last infection, fatigue in Lyme disease may be a major and persistent complaint. However, initial presentations of an isolated chronic fatigue syndrome or of fibromyalgia-like complaints (diffuse aching, trigger points, sleep disturbance) are not characteristic of Lyme disease.

In later stages, Lyme disease may mimic other immune-mediated disorders. Like rheumatic fever, Lyme disease may be associated with sore throat followed by migratory polyarthritis and carditis, but without evidence of valvular involvement or of a preceding streptococcal infection. Migratory pain in tendons and joints may also suggest disseminated gonococcal disease. An isolated facial weakness may mimic Bell's palsy of other causes. Late neurologic involvement may suggest multiple sclerosis (transverse myelitis), Guillain-Barré syndrome (symmetric peripheral neuropathy), primary psychosis, or brain tumor. In adults with Lyme arthritis, the large knee effusions can resemble those in Reiter's syndrome, and the occasional symmetric polyarthritis, that of rheumatoid arthritis. In children, the attacks of arthritis, although generally shorter, may be identical to those seen in the oligoarticular form of juvenile rheumatoid arthritis, but without iridocyclitis.

TREATMENT. The major goal of therapy in Lyme disease is to eradicate the causative organism. Like other spirochetal diseases, Lyme disease is most responsive to antibiotics early in its course. Treatment regimens have evolved over time based on both controlled clinical data and on clinical experience. Because of the difficulty in proving that bacteria have been eradicated and the common persistence of some symptoms long after treatment, the endpoint of

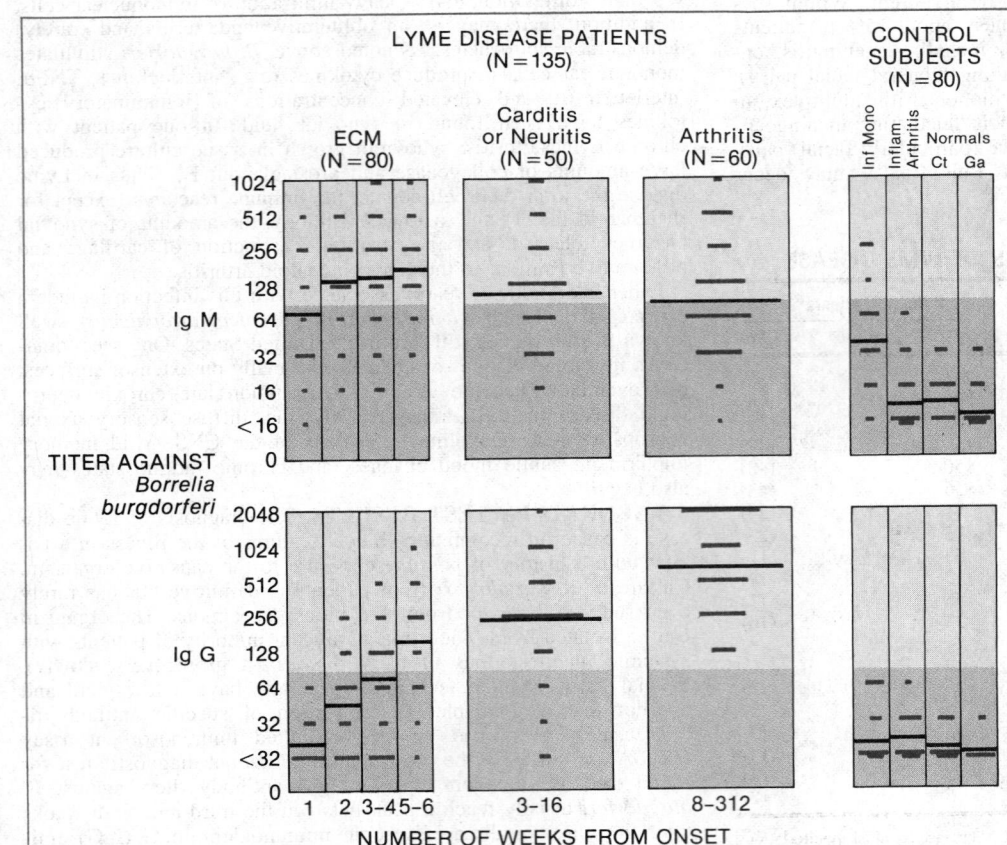

FIGURE 321–1. Antibody titers against *Borrelia burgdorferi* are shown in serum samples from 135 patients with different clinical manifestations of Lyme disease, and from 80 control subjects with infectious mononucleosis, inflammatory arthritis, or no disease (titers determined by indirect immunofluorescence). The black bar shows the geometric mean titer for each group; the pink shaded areas indicate the range of values generally observed in control subjects. Note that all patients with Lyme arthritis have elevated IgG antibody titers. (Adapted from Steere AC, Grodzicki RL, Kornblatt AN, et al: The spirochetal etiology of Lyme disease. N Engl J Med 308:733–740, 1983. Copyright 1983 Massachusetts Medical Society.)

antibiotic therapy is not always clear. The treatment regimens presented here represent guidelines that will no doubt be refined in time (Table 321–3).

Early Lyme Disease. If patients are treated early with oral antibiotics, ECM typically resolves promptly, and major later sequelae (myocarditis, meningoencephalitis, or recurrent arthritis) usually do not occur. Prompt treatment is therefore important, even though such patients may be susceptible to reinfection. For adults, antibiotic choices and doses are listed in Table 321–3; amoxicillin or doxycycline is favored. In children younger than 9, give divided doses of amoxicillin (30 mg per kilogram per day; not < 1 gram or > 2 grams per day) or, for the penicillin-allergic, erythromycin (30 mg per kilogram per day) for 10 to 20 days.

About 10% of patients with early Lyme disease experience a Jarisch–Herxheimer–like reaction (higher fever, redder rash, or greater pain) during the first 24 hours of antibiotic therapy. Whichever drug is given, 30 to 50% of patients have brief (hours to days) recurrent episodes of headache, musculoskeletal pain, and fatigue which may continue for extended periods. The etiology of these symptoms is unclear at present; they may result from undegraded spirochetal antigen(s) rather than persistence of live spirochetes. It is clear, however, that the risk of delayed resolution is greatest in individuals with disseminated manifestations of disease (multiple skin lesions, headache, fever, lymphadenopathy, or Bell's palsy) prior to the institution of antibiotics.

Later Lyme Disease. For Lyme meningitis, with or without other neurologic manifestations (cranial neuropathy or radiculoneu-

TABLE 321–3. RECOMMENDATIONS FOR ANTIBIOTIC TREATMENT OF LYME DISEASE[a]

Early Lyme Disease[b]
Amoxicillin, 500 mg three times daily for 21 days[c]
Doxycycline, 100 mg twice daily for 21 days
Cefuroxime axetil, 500 mg twice daily for 21 days
Azithromycin, 500 mg daily for 7 days[d]
  (less effective than other regimens)

Neurologic Manifestations
Bell's palsy (no other neurologic abnormalities)
  Oral regimens for early disease suffice
Meningitis (with or without radiculoneuropathy or encephalitis)[e]
  Ceftriaxone, 2 grams daily for 14–28 days
  Penicillin G, 20 million units daily for 14–28 days
  Doxycycline, 100 mg twice daily (oral or intravenous) for 14–28 days[f]
  Chloramphenicol, 1 gram four times daily for 14–28 days

Arthritis[g]
Amoxicillin and probenecid, 500 mg each, four times daily for 30 days[h]
Doxycycline, 100 mg twice daily for 30 days
Ceftriaxone, 2 grams daily for 14–28 days
Penicillin G, 20 million units daily for 14–28 days

Carditis
Ceftriaxone, 2 grams daily for 14 days
Penicillin G, 20 million units daily for 14 days
Doxycycline, 100 mg orally twice daily for 21 days[i]
Amoxicillin, 500 mg three times daily for 21 days[i]

Pregnancy
Localized early disease
  Amoxicillin, 500 mg three times daily for 21 days
Any manifestation of disseminated disease
  Penicillin G, 20 million units daily for 14–28 days
Asymptomatic seropositivity
  No treatment necessary

[a]These are guidelines, to be modified by new findings and to be applied always with close attention to the clinical context of individual patients.
[b]Without neurologic, cardiac, or joint involvement. For early Lyme disease limited to single ECM lesion, 10 days is sufficient.
[c]Some experts advise addition of probenecid 500 mg three times daily.
[d]Experience with this agent is limited; optimal duration of therapy is unclear.
[e]Optimal duration of therapy has not been established. There are no controlled trials of therapy longer than 4 weeks for any manifestation of Lyme disease.
[f]No published experience in the United States.
[g]An oral regimen should be selected only if there is no neurologic involvement.
[h]Amoxicillin is generally administered three times daily, but the only trial of this agent for Lyme arthritis employed a four times daily regimen.
[i]Oral regimens have been reserved for mild carditis limited to first degree heart block with PR ≤ .30 sec and normal ventricular function.
From Rahn DW, Malawista SE: Treatment of Lyme disease (special article). In Mandell GL, Bone RC, Cline MJ, et al. (eds.): 1994 Year Book of Medicine. St. Louis, Mosby–Year Book, 1994.

ropathy), intravenous penicillin G, 20 million units a day in six divided doses for 10 days, is effective therapy; in practice, courses are often extended to 3 weeks. Headache and stiff neck usually begin to subside by the second day of therapy and disappear by 7 to 10 days; motor deficits and radicular pain frequently require 7 to 8 weeks for complete recovery but do not require longer antibiotic courses. For Bell's palsy alone, oral regimens may suffice, but these patients may be at higher risk of later sequelae than are individuals with early disease without neurologic dissemination.

Although not studied systematically, carditis also responds rapidly (in days) to this regimen. Recovery from carditis was the rule even in the preantibiotic era, but untreated patients are at high risk for later manifestations of Lyme disease. Prednisone, 40 to 60 mg a day in divided doses, has, in the past, seemed to hasten resolution of high-grade heart block, but one should hesitate to institute glucocorticoids during antibiotic administration because they may impede eradication of infecting organisms. For patients with allergy to penicillin, doxycycline, 100 mg twice a day, is reasonable but unevaluated. If second- or third-degree heart block is present, patients should be admitted to hospital for cardiac monitoring; temporary pacing is occasionally required for complete heart block.

In clinical practice, ceftriaxone (2 grams daily for 14 to 21 days) has largely replaced penicillin for the therapy of disseminated Lyme disease. Arguments in favor of this practice are a once-daily administration schedule which is amenable to outpatient intravenous antibiotic programs and improved penetration of the CSF in comparison with penicillin. Penicillin and cefotaxime have been found equally effective for the treatment of acute neurologic Lyme disease (meningitis or radiculitis) in a group of patients studied in Germany. Ceftriaxone also appeared responsible for the complete recovery of 6 of 9 unusual Austrian patients with dilated cardiomyopathy attributed to Lyme disease.

Late Lyme Disease. Lyme arthritis has been successfully treated with both oral and parenteral antibiotics, but failures occur with any regimen chosen. Unless CNS involvement coexists, first-line treatment with a month-long course of doxycycline, 100 mg twice a day, or amoxicillin plus probenecid, 500 mg each four times a day, is recommended. The large majority of patients respond, although complete response can be delayed as long as 3 months or more after therapy is completed, and some patients may develop neurologic disease later. During treatment, the affected joint should be kept at rest and effusions drained by needle aspiration as for any infected joint. In patients who fail one or more courses of antibiotics, arthroscopic synovectomy can result in a long-term response and perhaps cure. Even without antibiotic or surgical treatment, persistent Lyme arthritis tends to resolve within several years.

Optimal therapy for the later neurologic complications of Lyme disease is also not yet clear, but 14 to 21 days of intravenous ceftriaxone or penicillin (see Table 321–3) are recommended. The frequency of subtle chronic encephalopathy and peripheral neuropathy is debated at present. These entities, when suspected, should be carefully documented through neurologic, neuropsychological, and electrophysiologic testing before aggressive or prolonged antibiotic therapy is instituted. Although some current thinking favors longer periods of the highest tolerated oral doses of amoxicillin (with probenecid), doxycycline, or even intravenous antibiotics in difficult cases, there is no controlled experience with courses of antibiotics longer than 1 month for any manifestation of Lyme disease. The infiltrative lesions of *acrodermatitis chronica atrophicans* are usually cured by 3 weeks of oral phenoxymethyl penicillin, 2 to 3 grams daily in divided doses.

Pregnancy. Because the spirochetes that cause relapsing fever and syphilis can cross the placenta, there has been concern regarding this possibility in Lyme disease. Maternal-fetal transmission of *B. burgdorferi* resulting in either neonatal death or stillbirth has been reported in rare instances in which symptomatic early Lyme disease occurred early in pregnancy and was either untreated or inadequately treated. In follow-up studies conducted by the Centers for Disease Control and Prevention, maternal Lyme disease was not directly implicated as a cause of fetal malformations. There have been no cases of fetal infection occurring when currently recommended antibiotic regimens for Lyme disease have been used during pregnancy. A lower threshold for initiating therapy for suspected Lyme disease in pregnancy is understandable, but women acquiring the illness during pregnancy should be reassured that the vast majority of infants born to women in these circumstances have been entirely well.

Tick Bites. A final treatment issue regards the advisability of administering antibiotics prophylactically to individuals sustaining ixodid tick bites in endemic areas. Studies completed to date have not supported this common practice. Because nymphal ixodid ticks must, in general, feed for a day or more before transmitting spirochetes (at least in mice), ticks removed prior to this time are unlikely to have transmitted *B. burgdorferi* even if infected. Tick bite sites should be observed for development of ECM and patients cautioned regarding the common associated symptoms of early Lyme disease. A watched tick bite allows for very early treatment of ECM in the small minority of patients in whom it will develop, and this is the stage of disease most amenable to therapy.

Barbour AG, Fish D: The biological and social phenomenon of Lyme disease. Science 260:1610, 1993. *The emergence of Lyme disease in the United States, unknown 2 decades ago, now its most common arthropod-borne illness.*

Bockenstedt LK, Malawista SE: Lyme Disease. *In* Rich RR (ed.): Clinical Immunology. St. Louis, Mosby–Year Book, 1995. *An expanded version of this chapter, with extensive recent references.*

Malawista SE, Steere AC, Hardin JA: Lyme disease: A unique human model for an infectious etiology of rheumatic disease. Yale J Biol Med 57:473, 1984. *The larger significance of Lyme disease, a disorder that is infectious in origin but inflammatory or "rheumatic" in expression.*

Rahn DW, Malawista SE: Treatment of Lyme disease (special article). *In* Mandell GL, Bone RC, Cline MJ, et al. (eds.): 1994 Year Book of Medicine. St. Louis, Mosby–Year Book, 1994. *Evolution of current recommendations for therapy, based on published studies, practical considerations, and clinical experience.*

Steere AC, Levin RE, Molloy PJ, et al.: Treatment of Lyme arthritis. Arthritis Rheum 37:878, 1994. *Oral antibiotics cured the large majority of patients with Lyme arthritis within 1 to 3 months, but a few developed neurologic disease later.*

Steere AC, Malawista SE, Snydman DR, et al.: Lyme arthritis: An epidemic of oligoarticular arthritis in children and adults in three Connecticut communities. Arthritis Rheum 20:7, 1977. *The first description of a new nosologic entity, recognized because it clusters geographically; rheumatoid arthritis does not.*

322 LEPTOSPIROSIS

William A. Petri, Jr.

DEFINITION. Leptospirosis is a spirochetal infection with bacteria of the genus *Leptospira*. The severe icteric form of infection is called Weil's disease, after the investigator who in 1886 described four men with an acute but self-limited infectious illness characterized by fever, jaundice, nephritis, and hepatomegaly and a biphasic course, with fever recurring 1 to 7 days into convalescence.

ETIOLOGY. There are two species of *Leptospira*, *L. interrogans*, which is pathogenic in humans and animals, and *L. biflexa*, which is free-living. *L. interrogans* is divided into >200 serovars grouped into 19 serogroups based on shared major agglutinins. Virulence does not in general correlate with serovars, although serovar classifications can be useful epidemiologically to identify common-source outbreaks. *Leptospira* are motile spirochetes 6 to 20 μ in length and 0.1 to 0.2 μ in diameter which are obligate aerobes with unique nutritional requirements for long-chain fatty acids.

EPIDEMIOLOGY. Leptospirosis is one of the most common, widespread, and underdiagnosed infections transmitted from animals to humans. *L. interrogans* can survive for months in the proximal convoluted tubules of the kidney in asymptomatically infected animals and upon excretion in urine survives in the environment for as long as 6 months. The optimal temperature for growth is 28 to 32°C, with slightly alkaline water ideal for growth and survival. Herbivores with alkaline urines, such as pigs, shed higher numbers of organisms than animals with acidic urine, such as dogs. The most common source of exposure in the United States is dogs, followed by livestock, rodents, and other wild animals. Humans become infected via recreational (e.g., windsurfing, kayaking, swimming) or occupational exposure to animal urine or urine-contaminated water and soil. Occupations with the greatest documented risks include New Zealand dairy farmers (incidence of 1.1 infections per 10 person-years), Glasgow sewer workers (3.7 infections per 10 person-years), and U.S. Army soldiers undergoing jungle

warfare training in Panama (4.1 infections per 10 person-years). Approximately 15% of veterinarians and abbatoir workers have serologic evidence of infection. Leptospirosis is up to 10 times more frequent in rural than in urban dwellers and three times more frequent in men, with a peak incidence in men at ages 30 to 39.

PATHOLOGY AND PATHOGENESIS. *Leptospira* penetrate intact mucous membranes and abraded skin and disseminate widely via the bloodstream. In the first week to 10 days of illness, spirochetes can be cultured with special media from blood and cerebrospinal fluid (CSF). Leptospirosis is an infectious vasculitis, with damage to capillary endothelial cells responsible for the major clinical manifestations of disease, including renal tubular and hepatic dysfunction, myocarditis, and pulmonary hemorrhage. Intra- to extravascular fluid shifts secondary to endothelial damage lead to hypovolemia, which complicates renal dysfunction and can lead to shock. Fatal cases are associated with widespread hemorrhage of mucosal, skin, and serosal surfaces. Examination of the kidneys from autopsies has revealed ischemic damage, including epithelial cell necrosis in the distal convoluted tubules and the ascending loop of Henle, and interstitial nephritis but only rarely glomerular damage. Liver pathology includes disorganization of liver cell plates, marked variation in the size and shape of parenchymal cells, mitotic figures, and evidence of cholestasis but not necrosis. Muscle biopsies have demonstrated focal necrotic changes with a mild mononuclear infiltrate. Only rarely is the spirochete visualized in the infected tissue. Hemorrhagic myocarditis has been observed frequently in autopsies. The secondary "immune" phase of leptospirosis is associated with the clearance of the organism from blood and CSF and the appearance of agglutinating anti-*Leptospira* antibodies.

CLINICAL FEATURES. Symptoms develop 7 to 12 days after exposure. Most patients have an abrupt onset of a self-limited 4- to 7-day anicteric illness characterized by the sudden onset of fever, mild to severe headache, myalgias, chills, cough, chest pain, neck stiffness, and/or prostration. An estimated 10% of patients will present with jaundice, hemorrhage, renal failure, and/or neurologic dysfunction (Weil's disease). Signs of leptospirosis include fever of 38 to 40°C (97 to 100% of patients), conjunctival suffusion (40 to 100%), hepatomegaly (80% of icteric cases), splenomegaly (15 to 25%), diffuse abdominal tenderness (5 to 30%), muscle tenderness (40 to 80%), meningeal signs (12 to 40%), disturbances in sensorium (50% of icteric cases), jaundice (10%), and a truncal rash that can be macular, urticarial, or purpuric (7 to 9%). Pretibial, raised, 1- to 5-cm erythematous lesions are seen characteristically in a form of leptospirosis called "Fort Bragg fever."

Classically, leptospirosis has been considered a biphasic illness, although many patients with mild disease will not have symptoms of the secondary "immune" phase of illness, and patients with very severe disease will have a relentless progression from onset of illness to jaundice, renal failure, hemorrhage, hypotension, and coma. Overall, about half the patients with leptospirosis will have a relapse. Typically 1 week after the initial fever resolves, fever, headache, and meningeal signs return. This immune phase of the illness can last several days to a month. A late complication is anterior uveitis, which may be seen in 10% of patients during and months to years after convalescence. Leptospirosis in pregnancy is associated with spontaneous abortion; children born with congenitally acquired leptospirosis have not been described to have congenital anomalies and have been treated successfully with antibiotics.

LABORATORY FEATURES. *Leptospira* can be cultured with special media from blood and CSF early in the illness, but incubation of the cultures for 5 to 6 weeks at 28 to 30°C is often required. Mild proteinuria is seen in most patients and may be accompanied by pyuria, casts, and microscopic hematuria. In patients with renal failure, the blood urea nitrogen level rarely exceeds 100 mg per deciliter, and the creatinine concentration is usually <8 mg per deciliter. Liver function tests are usually abnormal only in icteric patients, where two- to threefold elevations in aminotransferases and alkaline phosphatase are observed (lower than the elevations commonly seen in acute viral hepatitis), and a predominantly conjugated bilirubinemia is seen. Myositis with elevated serum creatine phosphokinase (MM band) occurs in about half of patients. Thrombocytopenia (usually ≥50,000 per microliter), anemia, and leukocytosis are commonly seen. Thrombocytopenia is seen most commonly in patients with renal failure. CSF examination shows a pleocytosis (<500 cells per cu mm) with an early neutrophilic and late mononuclear cell predominance, a normal glucose level, and mildly elevated protein level (50 to 110 mg per deciliter). Chest radiographs were abnormal in the majority of patients in one study, with small nodular densities showing a tendency to consolidate. First-degree atrioventricular block and changes consistent with acute pericarditis have been documented in one third of patients.

DIAGNOSIS. The presentation of the illness in anicteric cases is nonspecific. It is important to search for an exposure history to animal urine in a patient with a flu-like illness, respiratory illness, aseptic meningitis, acute hepatitis, acute renal failure, pericarditis, atrioventricular block, or anterior uveitis. In some developing countries, leptospirosis is more common than hepatitis A as a cause of acute hepatitis. Useful means to distinguish icteric leptospirosis from acute viral hepatitis include the prominent myalgias, conjunctival suffusion, elevated serum creatine phosphokinase, and the only two- to threefold elevations in aminotransferases seen in leptospirosis. The diagnosis is usually made retrospectively by a fourfold rise in agglutinating antibody titer. Agglutinins characteristically appear within the first 1 to 2 weeks of illness and peak at three to four weeks. It is possible to grow the organism from blood and CSF collected during the first week of illness, but it may take 4 to 6 weeks for the cultures to be positive because the organism is so slow growing.

PROGNOSIS. Case fatality rates for leptospirosis are <1% in studies where aggressive surveillance has been conducted (increasing the proportion of mild cases). The illness is usually self-limited. Liver and renal dysfunction are for the most part reversible, with return to normal function over 1 to 2 months. The mortality rate for icteric disease has been reported in different studies to be 2.4 to 11.3%, with deaths occurring secondary to renal failure, gastrointestinal and pulmonary hemorrhage, and the adult respiratory distress syndrome.

THERAPY AND PREVENTION. Antibiotic treatment is most beneficial when started within 4 days of illness; unfortunately, the diagnosis of leptospirosis is rarely made this rapidly. Doxycycline, 100 mg orally twice a day for 7 days, started within 48 hours of illness, decreased the duration of illness by 2 days in one study; penicillin at a dose of 2.4 to 3.6 million units per day also has been successful early treatment. A beneficial effect of antibiotic therapy later in disease course has not been uniformly seen. While a randomized, double-blinded trial of penicillin treatment (1.5 million units intravenously every 6 hours for 7 days) started on average nine days into illness showed a decrease in fever duration from 11.6 to 4.7 days and in elevated serum creatinine level from 8.3 to 2.7 days, a second randomized trial of penicillin in patients with icteric leptospirosis and a median duration of illness of 1 week demonstrated no beneficial effect. Jarish-Herxheimer reactions (fever, rigors, hypotension, and tachycardia) rarely occur upon initiation of antibiotic therapy. Supportive care and treatment of the hypotension, renal failure (including dialysis), and hemorrhage, which can complicate leptospirosis, are crucial for a good outcome.

Immunization of animals is not necessarily effective at preventing human disease, since leptospiruria can still occur in immunized animals. Because asymptomatically infected wild animals can chronically excrete large numbers of spirochetes in their urine, controlling environmental sources of leptospirosis is difficult if not impossible. Occupationally exposed individuals (abbatoir workers, veterinarians) should wear protective clothing to prevent exposure of skin and mucous membranes to potentially infected urine. Bodies of water associated with recreational exposures to leptospirosis may need to be placed off limits. Doxycycline, 200 mg orally once a week, has been 95% effective at preventing leptospirosis in U.S. troops undergoing training in the jungle warfare school in Panama and has a place in the short-term prevention of the disease in high-risk settings. No licensed vaccine is available in the United States for humans.

Lecour H, Miranda M, Magro C, et al.: Human leptospirosis—A review of 50 cases. Infection 17:8, 1989. *Epidemiologic and clinical aspects of 50 consecutive hospitalized patients with leptospirosis.*

Shaked Y, Shpilberg O, Samra D, Samra Y: Leptospirosis in pregnancy and its effect on the fetus: Case report and review. Clin Infect Dis 17:241, 1993. *Review of 16 cases of leptospirosis in pregnancy indicates that spontaneous abortion is a common consequence.*

Watt G, Padre LP, Tuazon ML, et al.: Placebo-controlled trial of intravenous penicillin for severe and late leptospirosis. Lancet 1:433, 1988. *Demonstration of the effectiveness of intravenous penicillin in severe leptospirosis.*

323 DISEASES CAUSED BY CHLAMYDIAE
Robert C. Brunham

Chlamydiae are obligate intracellular pathogens whose extreme biosynthetic defects in intermediate metabolism and energy generation cause them to be absolutely dependent on a host cell to grow and replicate. They are among the most common of all human infectious agents and produce much disability although little mortality.

CHLAMYDIAE AS ORGANISMS

Chlamydiae are a unique monophyletic bacterial family as defined by 16S rRNA sequences with an extremely ancient origin within the bacterial domain and are composed of four species (Table 323–1).

The chlamydial bacterial cell has a gram-negative cell wall structure consisting of an outer membrane and an inner cytoplasmic membrane. However, no peptidoglycan layer is found within the periplasmic space separating these two layers. The outer membrane is extremely protein-rich, composed of a single major outer membrane protein (MOMP 40 kDa) and two minor outer membrane proteins (60 and 12.5 kDa). All three proteins are extraordinarily rich in the amino acid cysteine, and inter- and intramolecular disulfide bonding produces a supramolecular protein complex that confers structural rigidity on the bacterial cell analogous to the role played by peptidoglycan in other bacteria. Within *Chlamydia trachomatis*, MOMP variation determines the serologic types that characterize the individual serovars. As with other gram-negative bacteria, the chlamydial outer membrane also contains lipopolysaccharide (LPS). Chlamydial LPS is a rough type without O-saccharides and is composed of a trisaccharide of 3-deoxy-D-manno-octulosonic acid (KDO). Although the core KDO sequences are shared by LPS from many other gram-negative bacteria, the chlamydial LPS is unique because two of the three KDO's are bonded through a unique 2.8 instead of a 2.4 linkage. Thus antibodies to chlamydial LPS are specific. Since all four species of chlamydiae share the same LPS structure, antibodies to chlamydial LPS are genus-specific.

Chlamydiae share a common and distinctive growth cycle. Figure 323–1 shows the distinctive developmental cycle typical for all chlamydiae. The size of the chlamydial genome is small at 1045 kilobases, containing enough information to code for approximately 600 different proteins. Most strains of chlamydiae also contain a 7-kilobase cryptic plasmid. Chlamydiae absolutely depend on host cells to obtain nutrients from the extracellular environment and convert them into forms they can use. Chlamydiae are obligate energy parasites of their host cells, and no net ATP-generating reactions have been observed in the organism. In comparison with other bacteria, chlamydiae are virtually unique in being able to transport phosphorylated compounds found in the host cell cytoplasm, and this undoubtedly represents their premiere adaptation to the intracellular environment. Despite sharing many characteristics in cell architecture and in the developmental cycle, chlamydiae are remarkably diverse at the DNA level. By DNA-DNA homology, the

TABLE 323–1. CLASSIFICATION OF BIOLOGIC VARIANTS (BIOVARS) AND SEROLOGIC VARIANTS (SEROVARS) OF THE GENUS *CHLAMYDIA*

	Biovar	Serovar
C. trachomatis	Trachoma	12
	Lymphogranuloma venereum	3
	Mouse pneumonitis	1
C. pneumoniae	TWAR	1
C. psittaci	Birds, mammals	Unknown, multiple
C. pecorum	Ruminants	Unknown, multiple

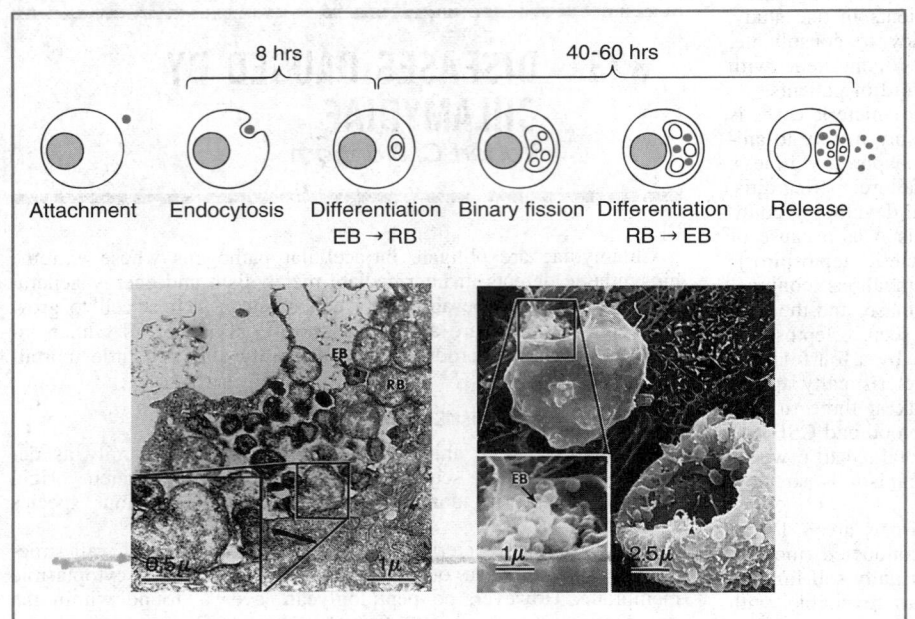

FIGURE 323–1. The top panel schematically shows the developmental cycle common to all chlamydiae. The red circles represent elementary bodies (EB's) and the open circles represent reticulate bodies (RB's). Chlamydiae infect eukaryotic cells through multiple attachment mechanisms, best understood for *C. trachomatis*. A trimolecular complex with a secreted heparan sulfate–like glycosaminogin synthesized by *C. trachomatis* acts as a bridge between ligands on the chlamydial EB and the eukaryotic cell surface. Different mechanisms exist among different chlamydial species and may explain their distinct trophism. After attachment, EB's enter the cell within a membrane-bound vacuole that remains unfused with lysosomes. EB's reorganize into RB's and asynchronously replicate 8 to 12 times with a doubling time of 2 to 3 hours. At the conclusion of the growth cycle, RB's differentiate back to EB's, and each inclusion yields 100 to 1000 new infectious EB's. The bottom left-hand panel is a transmission electron micrograph at 40 hours after infection showing the large RB's and the smaller EB's, which have a condensed nucleoid structure within their cytoplasm. The bottom right-hand panel is a scanning electron micrograph at 60 hours after infection showing a membrane-bound vacuole containing many EB's and apparently exiting from an infected HeLa cell.

chlamydial species share < 33% homology. Within each species, DNA-DNA homology varies between 14 and 95%.

CHLAMYDIAE AS PATHOGENS

Immune Responses

Chlamydiae produce intracellular infection, and, depending on the species of chlamydiae, macrophage or nonmacrophage host cells can support the organisms' replication. Macrophages appear to be the principal target cell for *C. psittaci* and *C. trachomatis* lymphogranuloma venereum (LGV) biovars. Columnar epithelial cells found in mucous membranes are the usual host cells for trachoma biovar and for *C. pneumoniae* replication. Host cell trophisms are correlated with the type of inflammation elicited by chlamydiae. LGV biovar and *C. psittaci,* which infect macrophages, produce granulomatous inflammation characteristic of delayed hypersensitivity reactions. Trachoma biovar, which infects epithelial cells, produces neutrophilic exudate during acute infection and submucosal mononuclear infiltration with lymphoid follicle formation during later stages of infection.

Chlamydiae elicit marked humoral and cellular immune responses. *C. trachomatis* elicits secretory IgA and circulatory IgM and IgG antibodies. Serum antibodies commonly recognize the chlamydial LPS as detected in the complement-fixation assay. *C. trachomatis* infection often elicits antibodies to serovar-specific epitopes on the MOMP. Women with reproductive sequelae such as tubal infertility or ectopic pregnancy due to prior *C. trachomatis* infection often have prominent antibody responses to a heat shock protein 60 antigen of chlamydiae.

Because chlamydiae produce intracellular infection, T cell–mediated immune responses are likely to be important. For chlamydiae that infect macrophages (LGV biovar and *C. psittaci*), granulomatous inflammation suggests the *in vivo* occurrence of T_h-1 activation. Interferon-gamma (IFN-γ), the principal cytokine of T_h-1 cells, has been detected in secretions from individuals infected with *C. trachomatis.* Cytotoxic T cells have not been detected during human chlamydial infection.

PATHOGENESIS AND MECHANISM OF HOST INJURY

Most animal model studies of chlamydial infection demonstrate an acute self-limited course. However, case reports of human LGV biovar and *C. psittaci* infections that last 10 to 20 years and observations from a longitudinal follow-up study of untreated cervical *C. trachomatis* infection showing that infection can last 15 months or more suggest that chlamydiae also can produce chronic persistent infection. Chronic persistent infection or repeated episodes of acute infection appear to elicit the immune mechanisms that cause host injury. Infection of a previously exposed host results in an accelerated and intensified inflammatory response, and tissue destruction appears to be directly correlated with the intensity of inflammation. This is best elucidated for *C. trachomatis* ocular infection. Inflammatory and scarring (cicatricial) trachoma are diseases of reinfection, and the more intense the initial inflammatory response, the more prominent is the late fibrotic response. Thus the mechanism for host injury with *C. trachomatis* infection is thought to be mediated by cellular immune responses.

CHLAMYDIAL DISEASES

Table 323–2 lists the most frequent chlamydial diseases.

Chlamydia trachomatis

The major diseases caused by *C. trachomatis* are trachoma produced by serovars A, B, Ba and C, sexually and perinatally transmitted diseases caused by serovars D through K, and sexually transmitted lymphogranuloma venereum caused by serovars L_1, L_2, and L_3. Trachoma and lymphogranuloma venereum are essentially restricted to developing areas of the world, whereas sexually and perinatally transmitted chlamydial infections are distributed globally. Trachoma and sexually/perinatally transmitted chlamydial infections are restricted to the mucosal surfaces of the body, and lymphogranuloma venereum causes systemic infection, principally of the lymphoid system.

TRACHOMA. *Epidemiology.* Trachoma is a distinctive ocular disease from infection by specific serovars of *C. trachomatis.* An estimated 500 million people worldwide are afflicted with trachoma, most of whom are young children. Trachoma is especially common in poor areas of sub-Saharan Africa. Trachoma is a major public health problem because 1 to 5% of infected individuals later develop scarring, which deforms the eyelid, causes inward turning of the eyelashes (entropion), and results in corneal abrasion (trichiasis). Corneal damage results in blindness. Trachoma is the most common preventable cause of blindness; an estimated 7 million people are blind as a result of trachoma. Most of these individuals are middle-aged and elderly adults. Active trachoma often occurs within the first 1 to 2 years of life but after the first month. Recurrences of active disease are common during childhood and spontaneously cease by age 10 to 15. Among children, the frequency of face washing, access to water, sharing a sleeping room with an affected individual, and intensity of eye-seeking fly exposure are important risk factors for trachoma. Active trachoma also can occur in adults, especially in mothers caring for young children with active disease. Trichiasis is related to repeated intense trachoma episodes in childhood, is more common in women than in men, and preferentially occurs in families.

The *C. trachomatis* serovars that produce trachoma are spread by direct contact with contaminated fomites such as washcloths or eye-seeking flies. Perinatal exposure to *C. trachomatis* from maternal genital tract infection is not important in transmitting trachoma.

Clinical Features. Trachoma is a chronic follicular conjunctivitis that causes macroscopically visible lymphoid follicles to form in the submucosa. These are especially apparent along the upper tarsal plate. The bulbar conjunctiva is minimally involved. Limited mucoid ocular discharge occurs; preauricular lymphadenopathy is rare and, if present, suggests other diagnoses such as adenovirus infection. The cornea may be involved with superficial vascularization and lymphocytic infiltration (pannus). Epidemic bacterial conjunctivitis due to *Haemophilus influenzae* can supervene on trachoma and cause a marked purulent conjunctivitis involving the bulbar conjunctiva. Bacterial conjunctivitis worsens the trachoma inflammatory damage. Tarsal conjunctival scarring deforms the eyelid structure and produces entropion and trichiasis in adulthood. Eventually, the corneal epithelium is eroded, and bacterial keratitis occurs. The cornea subsequently heals with opacification, resulting in blindness.

Diagnosis. Trachoma is most often a clinical diagnosis and is made if two of the following findings are observed:

1. Lymphoid follicles along the upper tarsal plate
2. Lymphoid follicles (or Herbert's pits) along the corneal limbus
3. Linear conjunctival scarring
4. Corneal pannus

Because most cases of trachoma occur in remote areas of the developing world without access to laboratory testing, most cases are diagnosed clinically. When laboratories are available, isolating *C. trachomatis* in cell culture provides definitive proof of the diagnosis. Culture is most often positive in young children with active disease and is rarely positive in adults with late scarring disease. Even in young children with active disease, culture is positive in only one-third to one-half of cases. Nonculture tests such as the direct immunofluorescent detection of elementary bodies (EB's) with monoclonal antibody or detecting chlamydial antigen by enzyme-linked immunosorbent assay (ELISA) are more frequently positive than are cultures. Detecting chlamydial DNA by the polymerase chain reaction (PCR) is the most sensitive diagnostic test, with about 70 to 80% of children with active trachoma testing positive. Few adults with late cicatricial disease are found to have positive tests for chlamydial EB's, antigen, or DNA.

Treatment and Prevention. Active trachoma in children can be treated with the topical ocular application of tetracycline or erythromycin ointment for 21 to 60 days. Because extraocular *C. tra-*

chomatis infection of the nasopharynx and gastrointestinal tract is relatively common during childhood trachoma, oral antibiotics such as erythromycin may be preferred. Single-dose oral azithromycin (20 mg/kg) seems as effective as 6 weeks of topical tetracycline. Trichiasis can be alleviated by depilation.

The prevalence of trachoma in a community responds dramatically to socioeconomic development. Mass chemotherapy for young school-aged children has a temporary impact on trachoma prevalence. No vaccine is available.

SEXUALLY AND PERINATALLY TRANSMITTED CHLAMYDIAL INFECTIONS. Epidemiology. Currently, *C. trachomatis* is the most prevalent sexually transmitted bacterial infection in the United States. More than 4 million chlamydial infections occur annually, and prevalence rates are highest (>10%) among sexually active adolescent females. Prevalence is higher in inner-city areas among lower socioeconomic status individuals and among minority ethnic groups such as African-Americans in the United States and Native Americans in Canada. Importantly, although prevalence rates are higher in these subgroups, with few exceptions, prevalences are ≥5% irrespective of geographic region, urban location, or ethnicity. In the United States, the direct and indirect costs of chlamydial disease exceed $2.4 billion annually. From a global perspective, sexually transmitted chlamydial infections are a major cause of total disease burden and healthy life years lost because of effects on the reproductive health of women.

Clinical Features. Urethritis. *C. trachomatis* causes 30 to 40% of cases of nongonococcal urethritis (NGU) in men, and an estimated 40 to 60% of urethral chlamydial infections are symptomatic with NGU. NGU is characterized by complaints of mild urethral discharge, urethral discomfort, and mild dysuria. On examination, a mild to moderate clear or cloudy urethral exudate can be detected. Often this is best observed in the morning prior to voiding. Sometimes, urethral discharge is apparent only on "milking" the urethra from the base of the penis to the glans. Gram stain of urethral exudate demonstrates ≥5 polymorphonuclear leukocytes per 1000× field and no gram-negative intracellular diplococci. Asymptomatic urethral infection is common with *C. trachomatis* infection and can be recognized by the urinary leukocyte esterase test on unspun first-void urine.

C. trachomatis urethral infection also occurs in women, in whom it produces the acute urethral syndrome. In such cases, the individual complains of dysuria, and pyuria (≥5 white blood cells per 1000× field) is found on urinalysis, but culture for uropathogens is negative. Urinary frequency and urgency are usually absent. Mild urethral exudate may be observed during pelvic examination when the urethra is compressed against the pubic ramus.

Epididymitis. In some men with urethral chlamydial infection (an estimated 1 to 3%), infection spreads from the urethra to the epididymis. This results in unilateral testicular pain, scrotal ery-

TABLE 323-2. MAJOR DISEASES CAUSED BY *CHLAMYDIA* AND CARDINAL EPIDEMIOLOGIC FEATURES

	Disease	Host Reservoir	Transmission Route	Epidemiologic Periodicity
C. trachomatis	Trachoma	Children	Fomites/flies	Endemic
	Urethritis/cervicitis	Sexually active teenagers and adults	Direct sexual contact	
	Epididymitis/salpingitis	Sexually active teenagers and adults	Direct sexual contact	
	Lymphogranuloma venereum	Sexually active teenagers and adults	Direct sexual contact	
	Inclusion conjunctivitis Infant pneumonia	Infected pregnant mothers	Direct perinatal contact	
C. psittaci	Atypical pneumonia Culture-negative endocarditis	Birds	Aerosol	Epidemic
C. pneumoniae	Bronchitis Atypical pneumonia	Humans	Respiratory droplet	Epidemic and endemic

thema and tenderness, or swelling over the epididymis. Epididymitis associated with urethritis is most commonly due to *C. trachomatis* or *Neisseria gonorrhoea* (see Ch. 315). Among men < 35 years of age, *C. trachomatis* is the principal cause of epididymitis. Among men > 35 years of age, complicated urinary tract infection with uropathogens is more commonly the cause of epididymitis.

Reiter's Syndrome. Reactive arthritis can complicate chlamydial infection (see Ch. 238). About 50% of men with nondiarrheal Reiter's syndrome have urethral *C. trachomatis* infection. It is estimated that approximately 1% of men with chlamydial urethritis develop Reiter's syndrome.

Mucopurulent Cervicitis. Mucopurulent cervicitis in women is the epidemiologic counterpart of NGU in men. As with NGU, *C. trachomatis* causes 40 to 50% of cases of mucopurulent cervicitis. Twenty to 50% of women with cervical chlamydial infection have mucopurulent cervicitis. Women with mucopurulent cervicitis may complain of mucoidy vaginal discharge. Unless concurrent infection with other pathogens is present, the vaginal discharge lacks odor, and vulvar pruritus does not occur. Mucopurulent cervicitis is best recognized during vaginal speculum examination with the cervix fully exposed and well illuminated. There is a yellow or cloudy mucoid discharge from the cervix, though the color may be better appreciated on the tip of a cotton swab than *in situ*. Gram stain of endocervical mucus shows > 10 polymorphonuclear leukocytes per 1000× field. Often, a red area of columnar epithelium is visible on the face of the cervix (ectopy). The area is erythematous, edematous, and bleeds easily when touched with a cotton-tipped swab.

Endometritis and Salpingitis. *C. trachomatis* infection can spread from the cervix to the endometrium to produce endometritis and to the fallopian tubes to produce salpingitis. Spread occurs in 10 to 40% of women with cervical chlamydial infection. If *C. trachomatis* spreads to the endometrium after therapeutic or postvaginal delivery, it can produce late onset postpartum or postabortal endometritis. More commonly, chlamydial infection spreads spontaneously to the upper reproductive tract. Although endometritis and salpingitis can occur subclinically, clinically patent disease includes the following features: subacute onset of low abdominal pain during menses or during the first 2 weeks of the menstrual cycle, pain on sexual intercourse (dyspareunia), and prolonged menses or intermenstrual vaginal bleeding. Fever is not a common feature of *C. trachomatis* endometritis or salpingitis.

Infant Inclusion Conjunctivitis and Pneumonia. Perinatally transmitted *C. trachomatis* infection is an important health problem for infants. Approximately, two of three infants perinatally exposed to *C. trachomatis* acquire infection. Clinically patent disease occurs in about 75% of infected infants, and 25% are subclinically infected. Inclusion conjunctivitis of the newborn develops in one in three exposed infants and a distinctive pneumonia syndrome in about one in six. Since 5 to 20% of pregnant women in the United States have *C. trachomatis* cervical infection, the morbidity due to perinatally transmitted chlamydial infection is substantial.

The distinctive pneumonia syndrome has a subacute onset in infants between ages 1 and 4 months. The natural history of illness is protracted, and importantly, fever is absent. The cardinal clinical characteristic is a distinctive staccato cough reminiscent of pertussis but without the whoop or posttussive vomiting. Hematologic examination consistently shows eosinophilia (≥ 400 eosinophils per cubic millimeter) and hypergammaglobulinemia (serum IgG ≥ 600 and IgM ≥ 110 mg per deciliter).

Lymphogranuloma Venereum. LGV is the result of sexually transmitted infection with *C. trachomatis* serovars L_1, L_2, or L_3. This is a systemic infection that involves lymphoid tissue. In the United States in 1992, 302 cases of LGV were reported to the Center for Disease Control and Prevention (CDC). In the developing world, especially sub-Saharan Africa, LGV is much more common, although accurate statistics are lacking.

The *C. trachomatis* serovars that produce LGV are much more invasive than are other *C. trachomatis* serovars. Similar to diseases due to other *C. trachomatis* serovars, LGV produces acute disease and late fibrotic complications. Among heterosexuals, primary LGV infection produces an evanescent and rarely observed genital ulcer

2 to 3 weeks after exposure. The ulcer spontaneously heals, and 2 to 4 weeks later painful bilateral inguinal lymphadenopathy develops, often associated with signs of systemic infection such as fever, headache, arthralgias, leukocytosis, and hypergammaglobulinemia. In the absence of treatment, LGV spontaneously heals, sometimes leaving lymphatic scarring. Late fibrotic complications of LGV include genital elephantiasis, strictures, and fistulas of the penis, urethra, and rectum.

In women and homosexual men, rectal infection with *C. trachomatis* L_1, L_2, or L_3 strains produces a severe febrile protocolitis illness. Patients complain of frequent painful defecation (tenesmus) with urgency and less commonly mucopurulent bloody discharge in stool. Biopsy of rectal mucosa shows submucosal granulomas, crypt abscesses, and diffuse mononuclear cell inflammation. The clinical, endoscopic, and histopathologic findings can mimic Crohn's disease of the rectum.

Laboratory Diagnosis. Empirical treatment for *C. trachomatis* infection should be initiated when a specific chlamydial syndrome is recognized. However, definitive diagnosis of *C. trachomatis* infection depends on laboratory identification of the organism. Laboratory diagnosis confirms the clinical diagnosis, assists in managing contacts of infected cases, and detects asymptomatic but infectious individuals.

The gold standard for diagnosing *C. trachomatis* infection is isolating the organism in cell culture. The development of culture-independent technologies to identify *C. trachomatis* infection was an important advancement. Culture-independent tests detect (1) *C. trachomatis* EB's in mucosal exudate by fluorescent labeled monoclonal antibody, (2) antigen (mainly lipopolysaccharide) in extracted mucosal exudate by ELISA, (3) plasmid DNA by direct probing, and (4) DNA by PCR amplification. The relative sensitivity of these tests is as follows: cell culture or PCR (capable of detecting a single EB) > LPS antigen detection by ELISA (lower limit of detection approximately 10^3 EB's) > chromosomal or plasmid DNA probe detection (lower limit of detection about 10^3 to 10^4 EB's). Because many chlamydial infections such as NGU, salpingitis, and trachoma are characterized by low numbers of organisms, amplification-based tests are preferred. At present, the higher costs of these tests will limit their widespread use, and antigen-based tests remain the most commonly used tests. Interpreting a positive ELISA test for chlamydia antigen can be difficult in situations where the prevalence of *C. trachomatis* is low (< 5%) because such tests typically have false-positive rates of 1 to 3%. For example, when an antigen-ELISA has a specificity of 98%, a sensitivity of 80%, and is used to screen 1000 individuals from a high-risk population with a *C. trachomatis* prevalence of 15%, the predictive value of a positive test is 88%. When the same test is used to screen 1000 individuals from a low-risk population with a *C. trachomatis* prevalence of 2%, the predictive value of positive tests falls to 44%. Clinicians should verify positive antigen-ELISA tests with a second *C. trachomatis* diagnostic test based on a different method if the risk of false-positive tests results in adverse medical, social, or psychological consequences.

Serology is infrequently used to diagnose *C. trachomatis* infection except in two circumstances: Specific *C. trachomatis* IgM antibody at a titer of 1:32 or more is useful to diagnose the infant pneumonia syndrome, and a complement-fixation antibody titer of 1:64 or more suggests LGV.

Treatment. *C. trachomatis* is uniformly susceptible to tetracyclines, macrolides, and sulfonamides. Recent data also suggest that selected quinolones (ofloxacin) are useful to treat *C. trachomatis* infection.

The recommended treatment for uncomplicated *C. trachomatis* urethritis and mucopurulent cervicitis is doxycycline (100 mg orally twice daily for 7 days) or azithromycin (1 gram orally in a single dose), although azithromycin is substantially more expensive than doxycycline. Alternate treatment regimens include erythromycin base (500 mg orally four times a day for 7 days), sulphisoxazole (500 mg orally four times a day for 10 days), or ofloxacin (300 mg orally twice daily for 7 days). *C. trachomatis* epididymitis and endometritis/salpingitis should be treated for 10 to 14 days. LGV should be treated for 3 weeks.

Sexual partners and parents of infants infected with *C. trachomatis* should be evaluated, tested, and empirically treated. Sexual contacts within the preceding 30 to 60 days should be seen.

Chlamydia pneumoniae

In 1986, a new chlamydial pathogen was recognized—*C. pneumoniae*—which causes respiratory illness. Although initially confused with *C. psittaci*, *C. pneumoniae* is a separate species with < 10% DNA homology with the other three chlamydial species. Pneumonia and bronchitis are the most frequently identified illnesses caused by *C. pneumoniae*.

EPIDEMIOLOGY. Much of what has been learned about *C. pneumoniae* epidemiology has resulted from serologic studies. More than 50% of adults in the United States and populations from other developed countries are seropositive. Most seroconversion occurs during childhood with rates of 6 to 9% per year for the age group 5 to 14. Many seroconversions occur subclinically. *C. pneumoniae* causes both endemic and epidemic atypical pneumonia syndromes. In Seattle, the average annual endemic incidence of *C. pneumoniae* pneumonia was 1.2 per 1000 population. Approximately 10% of pneumonia illnesses were attributed to *C. pneumoniae*. Periods of increased incidence were observed at 3- to 4-year cycles. The bacteria also has been documented to produce epidemics of atypical pneumonia in closed populations such as military recruits and university students. Case-to-case transmission appears to involve respiratory droplet spread with an average case-to-case interval of 1 month. Both diseased and asymptomatically infected individuals transmit infection.

CLINICAL FEATURES. Even though most acute infections occur in children, most *C. pneumoniae* disease occurs in adults, especially the elderly. It causes an afebrile, usually relative mild pneumonia. Extrapulmonary findings are not prominent. Nonproductive cough with sore throat and hoarseness are characteristic. The time from onset of illness to clinic presentation is long. On auscultation, localized crackles are often heard. Chest radiography shows a pneumonitis, most often evident as a single subsegmental lesion. Hematologic studies show a normal leukocyte count but a high erythrocyte sedimentation rate.

C. pneumoniae also causes bronchitis and sinusitis. Bronchitis is often subacute in onset, lasting several days or weeks. Some patients with the bronchitis illness unexpectedly have pneumonia on radiography. Sinusitis is often demonstrated by sinus percussion tenderness. Isolated pharyngitis is rarely attributable to *C. pneumoniae* infection, but when pharyngitis, sinusitis, and bronchitis are observed in association with pneumonia, *C. pneumoniae* is a likely cause.

LABORATORY DIAGNOSIS. Serology, isolation, and nonculture detection are the primary methods for laboratory disease of *C. pneumoniae* infection. A complement fixation titer of 1:8 or more has been considered a test for *C. psittaci* infection, but only 25% of hospitalized patients with *C. pneumoniae* pneumonia have a positive test result. The indirect microimmunofluorescent test for *C. pneumoniae* antibodies remains the best method for laboratory diagnosis but is restricted to the research laboratory. Isolating *C. pneumoniae* in cell culture (HL cell line) is successful in 50 to 75% cases of serologically confirmed infections but is technically demanding. PCR of *C. pneumoniae*–specific DNA is about 25% more sensitive than culture and likely will become the diagnostic test of choice. At present, no effective diagnostic method for *C. pneumoniae* is commercially available.

TREATMENT. *C. pneumoniae* is susceptible to tetracycline and macrolides but not sulfonamides. Antimicrobial therapy of *C. pneumoniae* infection can be difficult, and clinical response is not dramatic. Recommended treatment includes tetracycline or erythromycin base 500 mg orally four times a day for 10 to 14 days.

Chlamydia psittaci

EPIDEMIOLOGY. Strangely, *C. psittaci* is the least common but the only reportable chlamydial infection. This is so because it can produce common-source outbreaks of serious disease often related to infected imported birds. *C. psittaci* is a heterogeneous chlamydial species that naturally infects a variety of nonhuman mammals and birds. *C. psittaci* strains appear to be host-specific, and most human psittacosis infections are linked to bird and not mammal exposure. Approximately 100 to 200 cases of psittacosis are reported annually in the United States with no apparent periodicity. The annual incidence has been stable for the past 15 years. Psittacine birds (parrots, parakeets, budgerigars) are most commonly implicated as source contacts, although human cases have been traced to contact with pigeons, ducks, turkeys, chickens, and other birds. Among infected birds, *C. psittaci* is present in nasal secretions, guano, and feathers. Psittacosis in birds is a mild illness manifested by ruffled feathers and anorexia. Recovered and asymptomatically infected birds can shed the organism for months.

Transmission to humans is by the aerosol route to the respiratory tract. The infectious inoculum is likely very small, and brief contact with a contaminated environment can result in transmission. Person-to-person spread of *C. psittaci* rarely occurs.

CLINICAL FEATURES. Psittacosis is a systemic infection of the reticuloendothelial system and of the interstitium and alveoli of the lung by *C. psittaci*. Seven to 14 days following aerosol exposure, an abrupt febrile illness begins with shaking chills and a fever as high as 40°C. Headache, myalgias, and arthralgias can be disabling. Cough appears early in the illness but is usually nonproductive. Auscultation may be normal or show bilateral crackles. Chest radiograph shows single or multiple localized bronchopneumonic patches. Clinically, psittacosis can resemble legionnaires' disease. In distinction to *C. pneumoniae* pneumonia, psittacosis is more severe with high fever and absent or minimal upper respiratory complaints.

Extrapulmonary findings are usual with psittacosis, and myalgias can mislead the clinician to suspect meningitis or pyelonephritis. Fulminant psittacosis can produce meningoencephalitis, hepatitis, and a faint macular rash (Horder's spots) resembling the rose spots of typhoid fever. Like typhoid fever, psittacosis may cause abdominal pain, diarrhea, constipation, and splenomegaly. Occasional patients, especially with underlying valvular heart disease, develop endocarditis, and *C. psittaci* is a recognized, if rare, cause of culture-negative endocarditis. Untreated psittacosis can be fatal, but most patients recover slowly after an illness lasting 10 to 21 days.

LABORATORY DIAGNOSIS. The diagnosis can be established by isolating the organism in cell culture or by serology. Because laboratory-acquired *C. psittaci* infections are well documented, cell culture isolation is discouraged, and serology is the preferred test method. If culture is attempted, it is essential to contain the specimen in a biosafety cabinet for processing. Blood and respiratory secretions can be used to isolate the organism during acute disease. Psittacosis is most readily diagnosed by demonstrating a rising titer of complement-fixing antibody in the serum. Acute and 3- to 6-week convalescent sera should be tested.

TREATMENT. *C. psittaci* is susceptible to tetracyclines and macrolides but resistant to sulfonamides. Tetracycline has had the greatest clinical use. Psittacosis is the most gratifying of all chlamydial diseases to treat. Defervescence and marked symptomatic relief of systemic signs occur within 24 to 48 hours after starting tetracycline 500 mg four times a day. Treatment should be continued for 10 to 14 days.

PREVENTION. Epidemic psittacosis is a preventable disease by quarantining and giving all imported psittacine birds tetracycline. Preventing psittacosis acquired from nonpsittacine birds is more problematic and will remain a continuing source for human infection. No vaccine is commercially available.

Bailey RL, Arullendran P, Whittle HC, et al.: Randomised, controlled trial of single-dose azithromycin in treatment of trachoma. Lancet 342:453, 1993. *Single-dose treatment with azithromycin is remarkably effective in curing childhood trachoma.*

Centers for Disease Control and Prevention: Recommendations for the prevention and management of *Chlamydia trachomatis* infections, 1993. MMWR 42(RR-12):1, 1993. *Review of the major clinical syndromes due to sexually and perinatally transmitted* C. trachomatis *infection and a review of available diagnostic tests and how to screen for asymptomatic chlamydial infection.*

Grayston JT: Infections caused by *Chlamydia pneumoniae* strain TWAR. Clin Infect Dis 15:757, 1992. *A succinct review of the current status of* C. pneumoniae *as a human pathogen.*

Hedberg K, White KE, Forfang JC, et al.: An outbreak of psittacosis in Minnesota turkey industry workers: Implications for modes of transmission and control. Am J Epidemiol 130:569, 1989. *An interesting epidemiologic investigation of a large outbreak of psittacosis typifying many of the clinical and epidemiologic markers of this disease.*

Moulder JW: Interaction of chlamydiae and host cells in vitro. Microbiol Rev 55:143, 1991. *A masterful review of the cellular and molecular mechanisms of chlamydiae's interaction with host cells.*

Schachter J, Dawson CR: The epidemiology of trachoma predicts more blindness in the future. Scand J Infect Dis Suppl 69:55, 1990. *A good overview of the epidemiology of childhood trachoma and its relationship to blindness in adulthood.*

324 RICKETTSIAL DISEASES
Richard B. Hornick

Introduction

The rickettsiae are small obligate intracellular, gram-negative pathogens. They do not have a symbiotic relationship with human host cells and therefore cause metabolic derangements that result in cell death. Infections with the typhus and spotted fever groups of rickettsiae involve endothelial cells. This host-pathogen interaction results in a perivasculitis. Q fever induces granulomas in the liver plus interstitial pneumonia. Ehrlichiosis is a relatively new human disease, the cause of which continues to be investigated. It is caused by rickettsial organisms that are related to ones causing infections in dogs, horses, and so on. At least two species have been identified, *Ehrlichia chaffeensis* and an organism yet to be cultured which is related to the *E. phagocytophilia/E. equi* group. They are transmitted by ticks and cause illness in areas where Rocky Mountain spotted fever (RMSF) is endemic. Trench fever and cat scratch fever and three unusual infections occurring in immunocompromised hosts—bacillary angiomatosis, bacillary peliosis of the liver, and endocarditis—are caused by small gram-negative rods formerly classified as *Rochalimaea quintana, R. henselae,* and *R. elizabethae.* They are now included in the family Bartonellaceae and no longer part of the order Rickettsiales (see Ch. 310).

Each of the rickettsiae is transmitted to humans by ticks, mites, lice, fleas, or aerosols originating from animal products (placentas, Q fever) or from feces of the aforementioned insects. In the United States, there are relatively few cases of rickettsial infections. RMSF is the most prevalent, 600 to 700 cases having been reported annually since 1985. Fewer cases of Q fever and murine typhus are identified each year. Certain other rickettsial infections are major public health problems in developing countries but are not found in the United States, e.g., scrub typhus. The potential for tourists to return to the United States with an emerging rickettsial infec-tion is increasing. Because of the rarity of rickettsial infections in this country, diagnosis may be delayed. Delays in diagnosing these illnesses can adversely affect the potential for recovery.

In this chapter three tables (Tables 324–1 to 324–3) are included that summarize, first, the epidemiologic features of rickettsial infections; second, the host cells involved in the pathogenesis of the clinical manifestations of the disease; and third, those clinical features that will assist in differentiating the various forms of rickettsial infections. Additional details on the major rickettsial infections that occur in the United States or that represent potential threats to persons traveling abroad are found under separate sections in this chapter.

324.1 The Typhus Group

This group of conditions includes three established clinical and epidemiologic entities: epidemic louse-borne typhus fever, the oldest disease known to be caused by rickettsiae; Brill-Zinsser disease, a classic example of reactivation of a latent infection; and flea-borne murine typhus. The first two conditions are induced by *Rickettsia prowazekii,* a pathogen transferred from person to person by the bite of body lice. Persons who have recovered from epidemic typhus have persistent rickettsiae in various host cells, presumably in the reticuloendothelial cells; stresses that cause a defect in the suppressive lymphocytes will, years later, permit these rickettsiae to be reactivated, resulting in a mild typhus-like illness, called Brill-Zinsser disease. In 1975, *R. prowazekii* was isolated from flying squirrels in the southeastern United States. A number of persons acquired typhus fever from squirrels living in their attics and probably harboring infected fleas or lice or both.

Flea-borne murine typhus, caused by *R. typhi,* is a mild form of typhus fever occurring in the U.S. and elsewhere. It is transmitted by fleas from rodents. *R. canada* is a tick-borne (mouse-rabbit reservoirs), rickettsial organism, formerly classified with the typhus group. It is distinct from the typhus, as well as the spotted fever group. Whether it is a significant human pathogen requires more study. It has been implicated by serologic means as the cause of acute febrile cerebrovasculitis in one patient.

EPIDEMIC LOUSE-BORNE TYPHUS

INTRODUCTION. Synonyms include classic, historic, and European typhus; jail, war, camp, and ship fever; *Flichfieber* (German); *typhus exanthematique* (French); and *tifus exantematico* and *tabardillo* (Spanish). Many of these names indicate the location of the outbreaks—military and concentration camps, crowded ships with poor and starved immigrants, outbreaks in persons living in occupied countries during wartime, and so forth. Each implies crowded, unsanitary living conditions where bathing and laundry facilities are inadequate. These conditions allow for body lice to breed and propagate. The impact of typhus fever on military campaigns and immigration patterns is a fascinating and provocative story. The reader is referred to Woodward (1973) for an introduction to the effects of this disease on history.

DEFINITION. Classic typhus fever is manifested by the sudden onset of headache, fever, rash, and an altered mental state. (Typhus is derived from the Greek word meaning cloudy or misty. Applied to typhus, it describes the obtunded, lethargic state of mind.) *R. prowazekii* is transmitted by human body lice (*Pediculus humanus humanus*).

ETIOLOGY. *R. prowazekii* is a small obligate intracellular, gram-negative bacillus. In cells it stains red when exposed to Gimenez's stain. Viable rickettsiae stimulate the endothelial cell to act like a phagocyte to engulf the rickettsiae in a phagosome and internalize it. If rickettsiae do not break out of the phagosome promptly they begin to disintegrate, perhaps owing to enzymatic activities. The rickettsiae have an enzyme, phospholipase A, that enables them to lyse the phagosome wall and to multiply freely in the cytoplasm. *R. prowazekii* escape from the cell by destroying it. The necrotic cell stimulates an inflammatory response that leads to the vasculitis and subsequent clotting abnormalities.

TRANSMISSION AND EPIDEMIOLOGY. The unique feature of infection with *R. prowazekii* is that no animal reservoir has been implicated, at least until its isolation from the flying squirrel (*Glaucomys volans*). It is still uncertain how significant the flying squirrel will be in amplifying the incidence of this disease. Very few, if any, cases of classic typhus occur each year in the U.S. (Centers for Disease Control and Prevention [CDC] does not have an active surveillance for it). Fifteen cases were reported in 1980 and 1981, all in persons having contact with flying squirrels.

Classic typhus is a disease of humans. An individual with rickettsemia can infect body lice. The lice acquire the organisms in their blood meal. These ectoparasites may then find another person to whom they transmit the rickettsiae via infected feces. Body lice do not survive the ingestion of rickettsiae. The organisms multiply in the gut of the louse, destroy the epithelial cells, and the louse dies (usually in 1 to 3 weeks). However, during the period of infection, the louse passes feces heavily laden with rickettsiae. Either the human host scratches the site of the bite and thereby self-inoculates the rickettsiae, or the feces and rickettsiae contaminate minute apertures in the epidermis, allowing the organisms to find cells in which to multiply. Dried, contaminated feces can also become airborne, e.g., by shaking out clothing loaded with lice and feces and thereby creating an infectious aerosol. When inhaled, the rickettsiae can penetrate the mucosal cells and enter endothelial cells. Laboratory accidents frequently generate aerosols that induce infection in technicians. Nurses and other medical personnel are at risk for inhaling airborne particles when they remove the clothing from a patient.

When the body louse obtains a blood meal containing antibody-coated rickettsiae, the louse may modify the infectivity of the rickettsiae-antibody combination by partially digesting the antibody coating of the organism in its gut. This digestion destroys the Fc portion of the antibody that would have permitted attachment to macrophages. The rickettsia is then free of the inhibiting action of the antibody when it infects the next person.

TABLE 324-1. SUMMARY OF SOME EPIDEMIOLOGIC FEATURES OF SELECTED RICKETTSIAL DISEASES OF HUMANS

| Disease | Organism | Natural Cycle | | Usual Mode of Transmission to Humans | Common Occupational or Environmental Association | Geographic Distribution |
		Arthropod Vector	Reservoir/ Mammalian Host			
Typhus group						
Murine typhus	*Rickettsia mooseri* (*R. typhi*)	Flea	Rodents	Infected flea feces into broken skin or aerosol to mucous membranes	Rat-infected premises (shops, warehouses, grain elevators)	Scattered foci, worldwide
Epidemic typhus	*R. prowazekii*	Body louse	Humans*	Infected crushed louse or feces into broken skin or aerosol to mucous membranes	Lousy human population with louse transfer	Worldwide
Brill-Zinsser disease	*R. prowazekii*	Recrudescence months to years after primary attack of louse-borne typhus			Unknown; ?stress	Worldwide
Spotted fever group (selected examples)						
Rocky Mountain spotted fever	*R. rickettsii*	Ixodid ticks	Ticks/small mammals	Tick bite, mechanical transfer to mucous membranes, ?airborne	Tick-infested terrain, houses, dogs	Western hemisphere
Ehrlichiosis	*Ehrlichia chaffeensis*	Ticks	?Dogs	Tick bite	Tick-infested areas	At least 12 states in U.S., primarily southern states
	E. phagocytophilia/ E. equi group	Ticks	Ticks/Mammals	Tick bite	Tick-infested areas	Wisconsin-Minnesota
Boutonneuse fever	*R. conorii*	Ixodid ticks	Ticks/rodents, dogs	Tick bite	Tick-infested terrain, houses, dogs	Mediterranean littoral, Africa, ?Indian subcontinent
Rickettsialpox	*R. akrai*	Mouse mite	Mite/mice	Mouse mite bite	Unique mouse- and mite-infested premises (incinerators)	United States, former USSR, Korea, ?Central Africa
Scrub typhus Tsutsugamushi disease	*R. tsutsugamushi* (multiple serotypes)	Chigger	Chigger/?rodents	Chigger bite	Chigger-infested terrain; secondary scrub, grass airfields, golf courses	Asia, Australia, New Guinea, Pacific Islands
Q fever	*Coxiella burnetii*	?Ticks	Ticks/mammals	Inhalation of dried airborne infective material; ?tick bite	Domestic animals or products, dairies, lambing pens, slaughterhouses	Worldwide

* Recent isolations of putative *R. prowazekii* from flying squirrels in the eastern United States have not been evaluated as reservoirs for human infection. Previous claims of involvement of domestic animals are now largely discounted.

The louse does not transmit *R. prowazekii* transovarially to offspring and is not an amplifier for further propagation. Patients who recover from classic typhus have the opportunity to develop Brill-Zinsser disease and at that time have rickettsemia and are able again to infect body lice. However, this happens rarely, for few cases of Brill-Zinsser disease have been detected among the many hundreds of thousands of soldiers who acquired typhus in World War II; one estimate suggested a rate of 10 per 100,000 cases of primary typhus. More cases may be recognized as the geriatric population continues to increase. This group will have significant illness, surgical procedures, and chemotherapy that could cause reactivation of the latent rickettsiae.

Typhus fever remains a threat to persons living under unsanitary and deprived circumstances. As long as there are persons who are latent reservoirs for *R. prowazekii*, an epidemic can erupt. One country with persistent typhus is Ethiopia. There, prolonged drought, poverty, and malnutrition contribute to the perpetuation of the disease.

PATHOLOGY. The rickettsiae invade only endothelial cells, as described in the section on RMSF. This leads to vasculitis, with dif-

TABLE 324-2. RICKETTSIA TARGET CELL RELATIONSHIPS, PATHOLOGIC, LESIONS, AND CLINICAL MANIFESTATIONS OF HUMAN RICKETTSIOSES*

Disease	Target Cell	Host-Cell Association	Basic Lesion	Clinical Manifestations
Typhus-like fevers				
Typhus group	Endothelial	Free intracytoplasmic	Vasculitis	Acute self-limited fever
Scrub typhus	Endothelial	Free intracytoplasmic	Vasculitis	Acute self-limited fever
Spotted fever group	Endothelial, smooth muscle	Free intracytoplasmic and intranuclear	Vasculitis	Acute self-limited fever
Ehrlichiosis	Neutrophils/monocytes	Intracytoplasmic inclusion body (morulae)	Leukopenia, thrombocytopenia, liver cell damage	
Q fever	Reticuloendothelial	Intracytoplasmic vacuole	Granulomas	Acute self-limited fever, "atypical pneumonia," subacute hepatitis, subacute endocarditis

* Adapted from Stickland (ed.): Hunter's Tropical Medicine, Philadelphia, WB Saunders, 1984.

TABLE 324–3. SOME CLINICAL FEATURES OF SELECTED RICKETTSIAL DISEASES

Disease	Usual Incubation Period (Days)	Eschar	Rash Onset, Day of Disease	Rash Distribution	Rash Type	Usual Duration of Disease* (Days)	Usual Severity†	Fever After Chemotherapy (Hours)
Typhus group								
Murine typhus	12 (8–16)	None	5–7	Trunk → extremities	Macular, maculopapular	12 (8–16)	Moderate	48–72
Epidemic typhus	12 (10–14)	None	5–7	Trunk → extremities	Macular, maculopapular, petechial	14 (10–18)	Severe	48–72
Brill-Zinsser disease	—	None		Trunk → extremities	Macular	7–11	Relatively mild	48–72
Spotted fever group								
Rocky Mountain spotted fever	7 (3–12)	None	3–5	Extremities → trunk, face	Macular, maculopapular, petechial	16 (10–20)	Severe	72
Ehrlichiosis	7–21	None	?Rare	Unknown	Petechial	7 (3–19)	Mild	72
Boutonneuse fever	5–7	Other present	3–4	Trunk, extremities, face, palms, soles	Macular, maculopapular, petechial	10 (7–14) 7	Moderate	—
Rickettsialpox	?9–17	Often present	1–3	Trunk → face, extremities	Papulovesicular	7 (3–11)	Relatively mild	—
Scrub typhus (tsutsugamushi disease)	1–12 (9–18)	Often present	4–6	Trunk → extremities	Macular, maculopapular	14 (10–20)	Mild to severe	24–36
Q fever	10–19	None		None		(2–21)	Relatively mild‡	48 (occasionally slow)

* Untreated disease.
† Severity can vary greatly.
‡ Occasionally subacute infections occur (e.g., hepatitis, endocarditis).

fering pathologic changes in various organs. There is no eschar in this disease. The rash appears to have its origin in the leakage of blood and fluid from the damaged capillaries. The damage to the endothelial cells results in cell death, and at these sites platelet-fibrin thrombi form, platelet-active substances are released, and vasoconstriction and occlusion of small vessels occur. These changes can lead to infarcts in various organs, edema of tissue, leakage of inflammatory cells around small blood vessels ("typhus nodules" of the brain, for instance), stimulation of clotting mechanisms, and the development of shock. Almost all organs are involved in patients with untreated disease. The inflammatory exudate consists of mononuclear cells, plasma cells, histiocytes, and polymorphonuclear leukocytes. Gangrene of skin and limbs occurs in the presence of extensive thrombotic activity.

CLINICAL MANIFESTATIONS AND COURSE. The incubation period averages about 7 days but can range from 6 to 15 days. The onset is abrupt with intense headache, chills, fever, and myalgia. There is back or leg pain—presumably due to the muscle damage secondary to the vasculitis. Bites of lice may cause pruritus, and persons infested with lice may have numerous scratches in the skin. Sometimes the skin has a yellow-gold hue because of frequent lice bites. The headache is described as the "worst ever," and the pain is unremitting unless treated with narcotic analgesics. The temperature rises quickly during the first 2 days and persists for about 2 weeks, maintaining a continuous fever pattern if not altered by antibiotics or antipyretic medications. During the first week, there is a bradycardia relative to the temperature elevations of 39° to 41°C. Conjunctivae are injected, and photophobia is present. Deafness, tinnitus, and sometimes vertigo are prominent features. The patient appears to be in a toxic state, with a flushed face, obtundation, and profound weakness. There may be a cough, but no rales are apparent on auscultation of the lungs. The pharyngeal mucous lining is dry and inflamed.

The rash, characteristic of the typhus group, appears on the fourth to seventh day of disease. The lesions appear first on the trunk and axillary folds (areas of skin stress) and spread to the extremities but spare the palms and soles of the feet. The lesions are reddish-pink macules that fade on pressure. With treatment or in mild cases, the rash disappears within several days. In untreated patients, it can spread and coalesce, leading to gangrene of portions of

the skin, especially over regions of bony prominences. In 5 to 10% of patients, the rash may not be present.

These and other manifestations occur because of the initial unchecked multiplication and spread of the rickettsiae, involving ever-enlarging segments of the endothelial surface. The resulting damage to the organs evolves because of the compromised circulation and the associated acute inflammatory responses. Whether rickettsial toxin or endotoxin contributes to the pathologic changes is still debated. Whatever processes are involved, certain organs are regularly involved: the skin, heart, kidneys, and skeletal muscle. In patients with severe disease, hypotension and renal failure portend a fatal outcome.

The altered mental status that occurs as the disease progresses (in untreated patients) is striking. The patient may progress from stupor to coma. The stupor may be interrupted by brief periods of delirium. Patients may have to be restrained in order to protect them from trauma. At this stage, lymphocytic pleocytosis of the cerebrospinal fluid (CSF) may be present. Despite the seriousness of the patient's condition, complete recovery can ensue. Cranial nerve lesions are common. There are also temporary mental aberrations.

Patients who have acquired typhus fever in the U.S. from flying squirrels have had signs and symptoms of the classic disease. The rash was noted in 8 of 15, and it was evanescent. Significant central nervous system involvement was reported in five patients; two had coma and three had confusion or delirium.

Death in untreated patients occurs between the ninth and eighteenth days. Recovery from the disease begins with a rapid lysis of fever after about 2 weeks of disease. When the fever disappears, mental function returns quickly. Recovery of a sense of well-being is protracted owing to the need to counter the stresses of prolonged negative nitrogen balance, inanition, and loss of muscle mass.

Brill-Zinsser disease is manifested in a manner similar to classic typhus. All signs and symptoms are milder, presumably because the host has well-developed immune mechanisms that can regain control in a short time. Serologic studies in these patients demonstrate immunoglobulin G (IgG) rather than immunoglobulin M (IgM) antibodies. Occasionally, patients with unrecognized Brill-Zinsser disease die. An underlying disease or procedure may permit activation of the latent rickettsiae, and this combination can culminate in death. Reactivation has been noted following surgical procedures and the use of immunosuppressive drugs. In experimental animals that have recovered from the primary disease, isolation of rickettsiae at a future date is facilitated by steroid administration.

PROGNOSIS. The fatality rate in untreated groups of patients with classic typhus is 10 to 60%. Children usually have a mild illness with minimal risk of death. Patients over age 60 have the highest mortality rate. Recovery is the rule with appropriate antibiotic treatment.

TREATMENT. R. prowazekii responds well to tetracycline and chloramphenicol antibiotics. Doxycycline, 200 mg as a single oral dose, is the treatment of choice. Tetracycline, 25 mg per kilogram daily in four doses, or chloramphenicol, 50 mg per kilogram daily in four doses, is an effective alternative. Therapy should be continued for 2 to 3 days after the fever has defervesced. Most patients are afebrile within 48 to 72 hours and improve quickly from the debilitating headache or mental aberrations or both. Relapses occur in persons who are treated early, on day 1 or 2 of illness. Such patients do not develop the required immune mechanisms to contain the proliferation of the residual rickettsiae. Furthermore, both antibiotics are rickettsiostatic and do not eradicate all of these intracellular parasites even when specific immune mechanisms are introduced. Recovery from disease without antibiotics also allows rickettsiae to remain in cells, later to be activated and cause Brill-Zinsser disease. In the severely ill patient, fluid therapy and proper nutrition are mandatory. Fortunately, antibiotic therapy has simplified the need for supportive care.

PREVENTION AND CONTROL. To prevent and control the spread of classic typhus, the body lice (and feces) associated with patients and their clothes must be destroyed. The clothing should be carefully placed in plastic bags and sealed and carefully removed only in the area where they are to be treated. Clothes that can sustain boiling are boiled, and the rest should be subjected to steam and dry heat. It is also possible to kill the lice (also the eggs present in seams and elsewhere—these eggs will hatch in a week) with insecticides. Lice now are generally resistant to 10% DDT (chlorophenothane) and 1% lindane dust. Malathion (1%) and 2% temefos (Abate) are effective in most areas. These dusts are applied to the fully clothed individual. This approach controls the acute outbreaks of disease when applied to all persons in the community. Long-time use of insecticides is not effective because resistance develops, because long-term compliance is difficult, and because the insecticides may adversely affect the ecology of the region. Control requires improvement of sanitary conditions and standards of living as well as health education.

Health personnel treating patients with classic typhus are at risk for acquiring the disease from lice picked up from the patients or their clothing. There is no risk of direct human-to-human transfer of the rickettsiae other than by aerosolized, dried, contaminated feces. Once the patient has been deloused, no isolation barriers are required.

No vaccine is currently available for preventing classic typhus.

Travelers to endemic areas are rarely at risk unless, for example, they work in camps for displaced persons or carry out relief work that brings them in contact with persons with lice. Decontaminating the clothing overnight with insecticides or wearing insect repellent-treated clothes provides some protection. Prophylactic doxycycline has been effective when given weekly to prevent scrub typhus and would be expected to be effective in preventing R. prowazekii infections. This drug should be used only for short periods, 2 to 4 weeks. It is important under these circumstances to monitor the temperature for 2 weeks at least, as the drug may have masked the initial infection and delayed the onset of symptoms. Retreatment with doxycycline at the onset of the fever is curative.

MURINE TYPHUS

DEFINITION. Murine typhus, a milder form of classic typhus, is caused by *Rickettsia typhi* and is transmitted from rodents to humans by means of the rat flea (*Xenopsylla cheopis*). It is the only disease of the typhus group that occurs regularly in the United States, albeit in small numbers.

ETIOLOGY. R. typhi is a small gram-negative obligate intracellular pathogen. Like R. prowazekii, it can penetrate into endothelial cells by induced phagocytosis. Its disease potential resides in its ability to multiply in these cells, destroy them, and initiate a vasculitis. R. typhi is catalogued with the typhus group because it shares common antigens with R. prowazekii and R. canada. In addi-

tion, there is cross-immunity between R. prowazekii and R. typhi induced by infections. Despite these similarities, it is clear from DNA homology studies that the two are not closely related.

TRANSMISSION AND EPIDEMIOLOGY. R. typhi causes disease worldwide. Wherever there are large rodent populations, there is the potential for outbreaks. The rat and other small animals serve as reservoirs of this disease. *Rattus rattus* and *Rattus norvegicus* are two species of rats that can sustain the R. typhi, serve as a source of rickettsiae for the rat flea, and have no obvious illness from carrying this human pathogen. The rat flea disseminates the infection not through its bite but by placing contaminated feces on the skin. These may be rubbed or scratched into the skin; they can be carried to the conjunctival sac or mucous membranes on the fingers, where the rickettsiae can invade; or they can be aerosolized after drying and cause infection if inhaled. In the flea, the rickettsiae multiply in the enterocytes in the gut, do not kill the flea, and continue to be shed in the feces for the life of the flea. Transovarial transmission of R. typhi occurs in the oriental rat flea.

Murine typhus is a reportable disease. The CDC received 28 reports in 1992, 18 of which came from Texas. In the previous 10 years, the number ranged from 37 to 67 annually, with Texas and California having the highest numbers. Cases are probably underreported. A dramatic drop occurred in the number of reported cases after the mid 1940's. In 1944 there were over 5400 cases. By 1954 there were 163. This decline was due to intensive efforts at rodent control. Most of the cases occur in the warmer months, when rat fleas are plentiful.

PATHOLOGY. Descriptions of the pathologic lesions in this disease are few because of the rarity of fatal cases. Since the rickettsiae are known to invade endothelial cells, the pathologic consequences should mimic those seen in other rickettsial infections. The reasons for the differences in virulence of these rickettsiae and the varying severity of illnesses produced are unknown.

CLINICAL MANIFESTATIONS AND COURSE. Headache, fever, and myalgia are the principal symptoms and signs. These appear after an incubation period of about 1 to 2 weeks. A faint macular-papular pink-colored rash appears in about 80% of patients after 4 to 5 days of illness. It may be difficult to see in poor light. When present, it may be visible for 4 to 8 days before it gradually fades.

Rarely are there any significant complications of this infection, but as it is an infection of the endothelial cells, a vasculitis can cause widespread organ derangement. The patients, especially if older, are debilitated when not treated. They may remain febrile, with a temperature of 39° to 40°C for 2 weeks. This metabolic stress necessitates prolonged convalescence. Antibiotic therapy brings about a prompt recovery.

DIAGNOSIS. This disease has no distinguishing characteristics during the early days of symptoms. The rash appearing on the fourth or fifth day should alert the physician to the possibility of a rickettsial infection. The history of a possible exposure to areas where rats are known to exist, e.g., grain elevators, port facilities, and farm buildings, provides useful information. Flea bites, if seen early, are discrete and may have a central hemorrhagic punctum. The location and grouping of flea bites are important diagnostic features. They occur in covered parts of the body, in irregular groups of several to a dozen or more, in the region of the belt, shoulders, and hips, or on the legs.

Differentiating this disease from RMSF may be difficult. The rash of RMSF usually begins on the wrists and palms and on the soles of the feet and then extends to the skin of the thorax and abdomen. In murine typhus the lesions are on the skin of the chest and abdomen and rarely on the extremities. The history of a tick bite or exposure provides evidence for a clinical diagnosis of RMSF.

Serologic studies confirm the rickettsial infection. Weil-Felix OX-19 reaction is positive in most patients who have not received antibiotic treatment. This test, however, does not distinguish murine typhus from the spotted fever group of infections. The indirect immunofluorescent test can be used to identify R. typhi infections. However, because of the common antigens shared with R. prowazekii, the serum requires cross-absorption with special antigens from these two rickettsia strains. Isolating the organism is possible but should be done only in special laboratories where containment facilities are available.

PROGNOSIS AND TREATMENT. The mortality rate is <5% in untreated patients. Appropriate antibiotic treatment results in prompt cure, and the mortality rate is reduced almost to zero. Two deaths were reported between 1982 and 1991.

Tetracycline and chloramphenicol are effective for treating this rickettsial infection. A 5- to 7-day course of either is effective. The usual dosage of 25 mg per kilogram of tetracycline per day in four doses or chloramphenicol, 50 mg per kilogram per day in four doses, effects a prompt cure. The organisms are sensitive to these antibiotics. No resistant strains have been identified. Relapses do occur when antibiotics are administered early in the course of the illness. Retreatment with the antibiotic of choice provides prompt response.

PREVENTION AND CONTROL. There is no vaccine to prevent this disease. Control of rats has been shown to be very effective. When rat control programs are instituted, appropriate insecticides should be simultaneously used to prevent the fleas from seeking humans for feeding as the rat population is decreased.

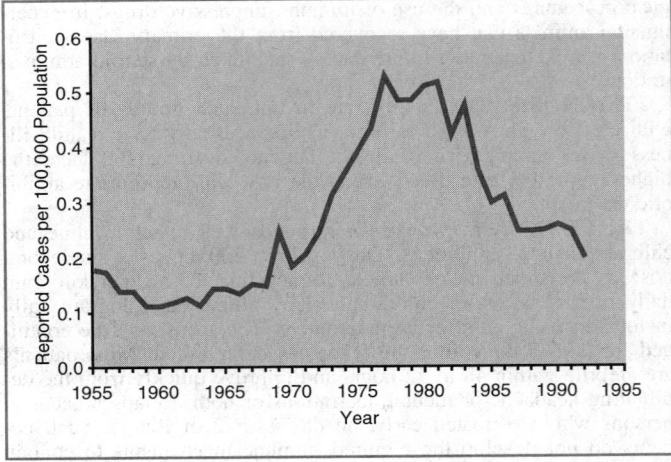

FIGURE 324–1. Rocky Mountain spotted fever in the United States, 1955 to 1992.

324.2 Rocky Mountain Spotted Fever

SYNONYMS AND DEFINITION. Rocky Mountain spotted fever (RMSF) is also known as typhus fever, tick-borne, by the CDC, *fiebre manchada* (Mexico), *fiebre petequial* (Colombia), and *febre maculosa* or Sao Paulo typhus (Brazil).

RMSF is a sometimes fatal systemic infection manifested by fever, severe headache, rash, and other organ disease caused by the vasculitis induced by *Rickettsia rickettsii*. The organism is usually transmitted to humans from animal reservoirs by a tick bite.

ETIOLOGY. *R. rickettsii* organisms are small gram-negative coccobacillary bacteria that can grow only inside eukaryotic host cells. They cannot be isolated on cell-free culture media. In human infections the rickettsiae invade and multiply within endothelial cells of arteries and veins. Different strains of *R. rickettsii* vary in virulence in human as well as animal hosts. Mortality rates appear to be higher in Montana than on the Eastern seaboard. Attempts to correlate virulence with structural components in the polysaccharide portion of the cell wall have been unsuccessful. However, two surface proteins, with molecular weights of 120,000 and 155,000, have been identified as possible virulence factors (protective antigens), and the latter has been produced from cloned genes in *Escherichia coli*. The antigenic material protects mice from lethal infection and will be studied as a potential vaccine.

DISTRIBUTION AND INCIDENCE. This disease was named for the geographic site of its original discovery; the causative agent was named for the discoverer, Howard T. Ricketts. By the 1940's the disease had become more common on the East Coast than in the West. The incidence rose sharply beginning in 1971 and peaked in 1981 at 5.2 per million population in the United States. In 1992, 502 cases were reported, for a low of 2.0 per million (Fig. 324–1). The decline occurred primarily in the southeast. Reasons for these fluctuations are unknown.

Serologic surveys in children and adults in North Carolina, the state with the highest number of reported cases, demonstrate that subclinical infections occur. Almost 20% of the children had OX-19 agglutination titers in the diagnostic range, and a smaller number had positive indirect fluorescent antibody titers, a more specific test. None of these children was previously diagnosed as having had RMSF.

TRANSMISSION AND EPIDEMIOLOGY. Ninety percent of reported cases occur between April 1 and September 30, with two thirds in May, June, and July. Children and young adults account for about 40% of cases. Ninety percent of patients give a history of a tick bite or attachment or of having been in a tick-infested area 14 days prior to onset of illness. Infected ticks are found in urban as well as rural areas. A park in New York City was the source of ticks that transmitted *R. rickettsii* to four children, one of whom died.

RMSF occurs in humans when an infected tick bites and injects *R. rickettsii* into the skin. Probably fewer than 10 organisms injected intradermally are sufficient to induce disease.

Several species of ticks are commonly involved in transmission of disease: *Dermacentor andersoni,* the wood tick, in the Rocky Mountain states; *D. variabilis,* the dog tick, in the East and Oklahoma; *Amblyomma americanum* in Texas and Oklahoma; and *Rhipicephalus sanguineus* in Texas and Mexico. These ticks feed on small mammals such as ground squirrels and rabbits as well as on larger animals such as bear and deer. Dogs serve as a reservoir to infect ticks and then other animals or humans. Figure 324–2 shows the distribution of cases of RMSF by state in the United States in 1992.

Laboratory-acquired infections have occurred in persons exposed to droplets from accidental generation of aerosols from solutions of the organism. However, even in circumstances conducive to airborne transmission, person-to-person transmission does not occur. RMSF can also be acquired by the transfusion of contaminated blood.

PATHOLOGY. The basis of the pathologic changes in this disease, as in other rickettsial infections, is the inflammatory response stimulated by the irreparable damage of the endothelial cells. In patients dying within 3 to 5 days of onset of disease, significant coagulation abnormalities are present. Causes may include damage to the endothelial cells with release of Factor VIII and stimulation of the release of platelet factors by damage to the endothelium or by activation of the kallikrein-kinin system by the Hageman factor. Microinfarcts result from occlusions of small vessels, and edema and hemorrhages occur secondary to increased permeability of the vasculature. Such lesions can be found in the heart, kidneys, adrenals, lungs, brain, skin, spleen, and subcutaneous tissues.

The rash is thought to result from the vasculitis and the associated permeability changes. Petechial lesions are caused by microhemorrhages secondary to the vasculitis and thrombocytopenia.

Patients with glucose-6-phosphate dehydrogenase (G6PD) deficiency appear to be prone to severe infections caused by *R. rickettsii* and other rickettsial agents. These patients have severe hemolytic reactions and significant thrombotic lesions in the glomeruli, resulting in oliguria.

CLINICAL MANIFESTATIONS. The incubation period of naturally acquired disease has a range of 2 to 14 days with an average of 7 days. The onset of disease in the typical case is sudden, with a severe headache, often retrobulbar in location, chills, fever, myalgia, malaise, nausea and vomiting, conjunctival injection, and photophobia. Tenderness may be present in large muscle groups. The duration of fever in untreated cases is about 2 weeks, but recovery from the debilitating effects of the disease requires several additional weeks.

Rash appears in 80 to 90% of patients—usually on the third or fourth day of fever, rarely after 5 or more days. It consists of pink macules, 2 to 5 mm, often noted first around the wrists and ankles. Lesions then spread to arms, chest, face, feet, and abdomen. Rarely does the rash involve the mucous membranes. Initially, these lesions blanch with pressure, but after 2 to 3 days they become fixed and turn dark red or purple and then slowly disappear during convalescence. The latter lesions represent microhemorrhages. Lesions

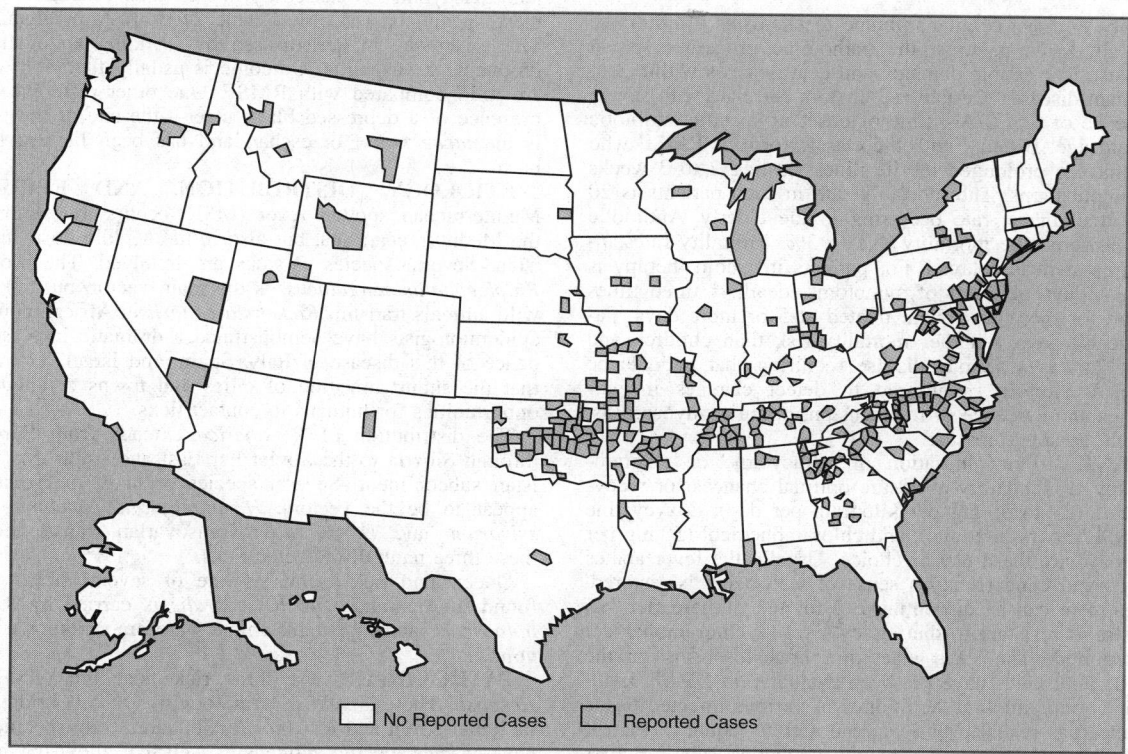

FIGURE 324-2. United States counties reporting cases of Rocky Mountain spotted fever, 1992.

on the palms and soles of the feet, in conjunction with the rash elsewhere, and petechial lesions in the skin folds of the axillae and around the ankles, constitute the classic distribution of the rash. Biopsy of the rash reveals perivascular round cell infiltration. Staining of the specimens of skin with fluorescent tagged antibodies to *R. rickettsii* shows the intracellular organisms.

In patients with unrecognized and inappropriately treated disease, the rash coalesces as the spread of the infectious process involves additional and larger vessels. This can result in large ischemic and gangrenous lesions. Especially susceptible is the skin of the tip of the nose, earlobes, digits, and scrotum. Involvement of the cooler portions of the body may reflect the optimal temperature for growth of *R. rickettsii* (32°C). Thrombosis of larger arteries can cause gangrene of a limb or hemiplegia. Patients with untreated disease may die of myocarditis and pulmonary edema.

The reported incidence of pulmonary abnormalities varies from 10 to 40% in large series of patients. Respiratory symptoms and signs as part of this illness have not been emphasized sufficiently. In fact, after the spleen, the heaviest concentrations of rickettsiae can be demonstrated by fluorescent antibody staining in the endothelial cells of the pulmonary vasculature.

Edema of the brain and ring hemorrhages may cause delirium and stupor and ultimately lead to death.

DIAGNOSIS. The diagnosis of RMSF is difficult in the patient presenting with nonspecific complaints such as sudden onset of fever, headache, myalgia, and malaise. A history of travel, camping, or outdoor recreational activities where tick exposure could occur and of recent tick bites is an especially important part of any workup of a febrile patient during the warmer months. The patient complains of a severe headache, photophobia, and pain when moving the eyes. There is no meningismus. Lumbar puncture usually reveals normal CSF. Patients with stupor or coma may demonstrate elevated CSF protein and a few mononuclear cells. The presence of a faint, pink-colored rash on wrists and ankles should raise a suspicion of RMSF. The information that the rash appeared after the fever helps make the diagnosis.

A search for an attached tick should concentrate on the scalp and groin. Hard body ticks such as *D. andersoni* tend to remain attached for long periods. The finding of an engorged tick should settle the clinical diagnosis. There usually is no ulceration or scar from the tick bite.

Most patients have thrombocytopenia but not significant clotting abnormalities. In severe cases, disseminated intravascular coagulopathy (DIC) occurs with hypofibrinogenemia and prolonged prothrombin and partial thromboplastin times. Other laboratory studies are not helpful in making a diagnosis. The white blood cell count is usually normal.

RMSF is confirmed by immunofluorescence staining of tissue specimens and by serologic analyses. The detection by immunofluorescence of rickettsiae in tissues, such as skin or rash biopsies, is the one test that can provide the most rapid (4 to 6 hours) and early (day 3 to 4) diagnosis. The state health department should be contacted about the availability of this test.

Serologic tests do not provide rapid diagnostic confirmation. The Weil-Felix reaction uses the polysaccharide antigens of three *Proteus* strains (OX-19, OX-2, and OX-K) to agglutinate antibodies produced by a rickettsial infection. Serum specimens from patients with RMSF agglutinate OX-19 and OX-2, but not OX-K. The peak titer occurs at about 2 to 3 weeks and then falls rapidly. Antibiotic treatment blunts the antibody response. The test is inexpensive, and with a fourfold or greater increase in titer of OX-19 or OX-2, or both, in paired specimens (drawn 2 weeks apart) confirmation is obtained. Indirect immunofluorescent antibody (IFA) testing is the most specific and sensitive serologic test available. It has replaced the complement fixation test and, in many laboratories, the Weil-Felix reaction. The IFA is now used in epidemiologic surveys because of the persistence of these antibodies compared with the short-lived antibodies demonstrated in the Weil-Felix reaction. A diagnostic rise (fourfold or greater) in titer also takes 2 to 3 weeks.

Differentiation of this disease from other infections is difficult without the history of a tick bite or the information about the fever preceding the rash. In children measles and atypical measles (in those who received killed vaccine) can mimic the early phase of RMSF illness. The location and type of lesions making up the rash, the presence of Koplik's spots, and a history of measles-like illness in close associates should permit a differentiation. Meningococcemia with meningitis usually produces petechiae or purpura, or both, in the patient earlier in the course of the disease than expected in all but rare patients with RMSF. Furthermore, the CSF indicates the septic nature of the meningitis caused by the meningococci.

PROGNOSIS. RMSF is a serious infectious disease that involves endothelial cells throughout the host. Prompt antibiotic therapy is necessary to assist cellular immune mechanisms to eliminate the pathogen. In some patients, the pathologic processes spread rapidly and cause irreversible damage, and death ensues within 3 to 5 days (fulminant disease). Certain risk factors correlate with severe diseases: presence of G6PD/A–, time of onset of specific antibiotic therapy, and old age. Patients with the classic form of RMSF who are untreated have a prolonged febrile illness lasting 2 to 3 weeks with many complications. The mortality rate in such patients is 20 to 30%, with the highest rate occurring in the elderly. Antibiotic treatment has lowered the mortality rate to 3%. Mortality rates increase when treatment is delayed. For patients in whom therapy is started within 4 days of onset of symptoms, death is three times less likely than for those who were treated at 5 or more days. Patients over age 40 have a higher mortality risk than children and young adults. This is a serious disease requiring that patients be hospitalized and carefully monitored to detect changes in pulmonary findings and evidence of hypotension, oliguria, myocarditis, or increasing intracranial pressure.

TREATMENT. Prompt initiation of tetracycline or chloramphenicol therapy is mandatory to ensure optimal chances for recovery. Tetracycline (25 to 50 mg per kilogram per day), doxycycline (100 mg every 12 hours in adults), and chloramphenicol (50 mg per kilogram per day) are the drugs of choice. Usually the fever abates in 2 to 3 days, and concurrently a sense of well-being is restored. Antibiotic treatment can be discontinued 2 to 3 days thereafter. No instances of strains resistant to the tetracyclines or chloramphenicol have been reported. The third-generation cephalosporins or the aminoglycoside antibiotics have not been evaluated in RMSF. Evaluation of four aminoquinolone antibiotics in various infected tissue culture cell lines has revealed antibacterial activity equal to that of tetracyclines. Clinical evaluations are not available. Relapses after tetracycline or chloramphenicol treatment are uncommon.

PREVENTION AND CONTROL. Immunity to reinfection after recovery from RMSF appears to be complete. No naturally acquired second cases have been reported. There is no effective vaccine.

The best method for preventing disease is to avoid contact with ticks. Ticks are brushed off grass onto clothes or skin. Ticks usually remain stationary until the host is quiet. They then seek warm, dark areas and migrate to the groin or the scalp, where they can grasp hair shafts while inserting their mouth parts into the skin. Small barbs on each side of the mouth make it difficult to withdraw the whole tick from the skin while it is feeding; the mouth parts may remain embedded. Ticks should be searched for at the end of each day spent in tick-infested country and removed with forceps or tweezers. A drop of acetone or a lighted match brought close to the tick may ensure that the tick withdraws its mouth parts. The tick should not be removed with exposed fingers because a tick crushed between the fingers may induce disease. Prophylactic antibiotics are not indicated for persons with known tick bites. They should be advised concerning the usual incubation period and urged to watch for development of fever or headache. Oral temperature should be recorded twice a day for 2 weeks. On elevation, medical attention should be obtained promptly. Therapy begun before the onset of fever could result in a prolongation of the incubation period.

Dalton MJ, Clarke MJ, Holman RC, et al.: National surveillance for Rocky Mountain spotted fever, 1981–1982; Epidemiologic summary and evaluation of risk factors for fatal outcome. Am J Trop Med & Hyg 52:405, 1995.
Donohue JF: Lower respiratory tract involvement in Rocky Mountain spotted fever. Arch Intern Med 140:223, 1980. *This retrospective review of pulmonary findings in patients with RMSF points out the delays that occurred in making the correct diagnosis because the respiratory symptoms were not considered to be a part of the clinical picture of RMSF.*

324.3 Other Tick-borne Rickettsioses

DEFINITIONS. *Mediterranean spotted fever,* also known as North African tick typhus, Kenya tick-bite fever, Indian tick typhus, and boutonneuse fever, is caused by *Rickettsia conorii*. A second disease, called North Asian tick-borne rickettsiosis, is induced by *R. siberica.* A third tick-borne rickettsial infection, called Queensland tick typhus, is caused by *R. australis.* The disease produced by these agents consists of headache, fever, rash, myalgia, and malaise. The rickettsiae induce disease by invading endothelial cells and producing a vasculitis. Outcome is usually favorable. The illnesses are mild compared with RMSF. One other difference is the usual presence of a depressed black ulcer—the site of the tick bite. This is the *tache noire,* or eschar, and has been likened to a cigarette burn.

ETIOLOGY, DISTRIBUTION, AND EPIDEMIOLOGY. Mediterranean spotted fever (MSF) occurs in countries bordering the Mediterranean Sea, but also in the Middle East, India, and Pakistan. Several species of ticks are involved. The brown dog tick, *Rhipicephalus sanguineus,* is the main vector, but ticks common to wild animals transmit *Rickettsia conorii* in African countries. Italian epidemiologists have demonstrated a dramatic increase in the incidence of this disease in Italy, Spain, and Israel. The assumption is that the suburbanization of cities and towns resulted in increased opportunities for humans to contact ticks.

The distribution of *R. siberica* extends from European Russia through Siberia to the Soviet Far East and south into the Indo-Pakistan subcontinent. Several species of hard, or ixodid, body ticks appear to be the vectors: *Haemaphysalis concinna, Dermacentor sylvarum,* and *D. nuttallii.* Transovarian transmission occurs in these three naturally infected ticks.

Queensland tick typhus is one of several rickettsial infections found in Australia. The *R. australis* is carried by the tick *Ixodes holocyclus,* and marsupial animals are among known animal reservoirs.

PATHOLOGY. These three rickettsiae are very similar to *R. rickettsii.* There is > 90% homology by DNA hybridization between the latter strain and *R. conorii.* All share group-specific antigens but have species-specific antigens as well that allow for their identification. These strains invade endothelial cells and cause cell death, resulting in a vasculitis (see above). Each of these three strains produces an eschar (*tache noire*) at the site of the tick bite.

SYMPTOMS, LABORATORY FINDINGS, AND DIAGNOSIS. The onset of disease caused by each of these three rickettsiae is sudden and characterized by fever, headache, malaise, myalgia, and conjunctival injection. These symptoms and signs appear about 5 to 7 days after the tick bite. The eschar is the distinguishing sign that confirms the diagnosis. It should be looked for in the scalp, axillae, and groin area, regions of the body favored by ticks. Because of the necrotic nature of the eschar, lymph nodes draining the region of the eschar are enlarged. The lesion has been appropriately likened to a cigarette burn, about 2 to 5 mm in diameter with a black center and a raised, erythematous rim. The lesion is only mildly tender.

As with RMSF, a generalized rash appears on the fourth to fifth day, including the palms and soles of the feet. The faint pink macular-papular lesions represent small hemorrhages in the skin. The duration of the disease is about 2 weeks. Death is unusual.

The Weil-Felix reaction demonstrates agglutinating antibodies to OX-19 antigen in most patients; these appear in the second to third week of disease. The microimmunofluorescence test for antibodies to *R. conorii* is the serologic test of choice, if available.

A skin biopsy stained with immunofluorescent antibody stain is the most rapid and earliest diagnostic procedure. This is indicated only when the diagnosis of spotted fever is suspected and a *tache noire* eschar is not present.

TREATMENT AND PROPHYLAXIS. Excellent outcomes are reported in patients receiving 200 mg of doxycycline every 12 hours for two doses. Tetracycline, chloramphenicol, and rifamycin can be used. Defervescence occurs over 2 days.

Tick bites should be avoided. Travelers into wild game country of Africa should check their clothes and skin carefully for ticks. Tourists traveling to southern European countries should search for ticks if they go hiking through suburban and rural areas during the spring and summer months.

Recovery from these rickettsial infections imparts solid immunity. In experimental animals *R. conorii* is relatively avirulent compared with most strains of *R. rickettsii.* However, animals recovered from infections with the former strain are protected against challenge with virulent *R. rickettsii.* This protection is mediated by T lymphocytes that recognize antigens on other species of rickettsial agents of the spotted fever group.

HUMAN EHRLICHIOSIS (SPOTLESS ROCKY MOUNTAIN SPOTTED FEVER). The first reported case of infection with a species of *Ehrlichia* in the United States occurred in 1986. A patient was found to have intracytoplasmic inclusions (morula) in monocytes and subsequently had an antibody rise to *E. canis*. This organism is known to cause severe pancytopenia in dogs. It is one of four species known to infect animals—*E. canis, E. equi, E. risticii,* and *E. phagocytophilia.* An additional species, *E. sennetsu,* was isolated from a patient in Japan in 1954, who had an infectious mononucleosis-like syndrome. This strain has not been identified outside of the Far East. In the United States since 1986, many investigators tried to isolate *E. canis* or a similar strain from patients with clinical and serologic evidence of ehrlichiosis. In 1990, the first isolation was made on a continuous cell line of canine macrophage cells using blood drawn from a patient with a 3-day history of fever, headache, pharyngitis, nausea, and vomiting. This isolate was named *E. chaffeensis* because the patient was an Army reservist stationed at Ft. Chaffee, Arkansas. This strain is different from but closely related to *E. canis* and is now used as the antigen for serologic studies. Patients suspected of having ehrlichiosis, but with no antibodies when tested with *E. canis,* do have antibodies to this human isolate. The organism can be stained in circulating monocytes. They are found in the cytoplasm as a clump of many organisms (0.2 to 1.5 μm) enclosed in a membrane; this mass is the morula (mulberry-like). These organisms have been found in *D. variabilis* ticks, one of the same tick species that transmits *R. rickettsii.* Most cases have been identified in Oklahoma, Missouri, and Arkansas—states in which RMSF is common.

In 1994 another *Ehrlichia* species was associated with human disease. Infection with this agent was confirmed in 12 patients in Wisconsin and Minnesota by serologic studies (IFA and/or polymerase chain reaction [PCR]). Two of these 12 died of infection. This strain has not been isolated as yet; it is different from *E. chaffeensis* as demonstrated by various serologic studies and is closely related to the *E. equi/E. phagocytophilia* group. None of the 12 patients was exposed to horses, sheep, deer, bison, and cattle, animals known to be infected with these strains. Eleven of the 12 had known tick exposure. *D. variabilis* and *I. scapularis* were identified in eight instances. The unique feature of infection with this strain was the location of the morulae. They were found in granulocytes in the circulation and in the bone marrow. Because of this, the current name for the disease is human granulocytic ehrlichiosis (HGE).

The clinical symptoms of both forms of ehrlichiosis are similar and can be difficult to distinguish from those found in patients with RMSF. Fever, chills, myalgias, headaches are common. Nausea, vomiting, and asthenia add to the patient's discomfort. The physical examination usually is nonrevealing. Rash has been reported in about 20% of patients infected with *E. chaffeensis,* but not in those infected with HGE. The rash has been described with a variety of lesions—macular or papular or both, petechial or erythematous. It is seen most frequently on the thorax, legs, and arms. The rash appears after the onset of symptoms; the median day of onset was 5 days in a series of 212 patients. Striking laboratory values are leukopenia, thrombocytopenia, and abnormal liver function tests. Liver abnormalities may be due to enlargement of cells of the reticuloendothelial system compressing adjacent parenchyma. The alanine aminotransferase (ALT) and aspartate aminotransferase (AST) values peak at the end of the first week of illness. The platelet count drops to its lowest level at about the same time. The leukocyte count falls quicker, within the first 3 to 5 days of disease. The presence of the morula in lymphocytes and monocytes *(E. chaffeensis)* and in granulocytes (HGE agent) is a significant laboratory diagnostic clue. This finding needs to be identified by skilled observers.

The severity of the clinical illnesses range from mild to fatal. Serologic evidence exists to indicate that more infections with *E. chaffeensis* are asymptomatic than those requiring medical attention. The PCR assay is now available at the CDC for precise diagnosis; when widely available it will provide a rapid diagnostic test.

Elderly patients are most prone to acquire the disease and to have the most severe illnesses. In the few patients who have died, the diagnosis was usually made late in the course of the disease. Therefore, there was a delay in onset of specific therapy, and frequently life-threatening complications were seen with severe infectious diseases, e.g., renal failure, meningitis, coma, DIC. The rapid appearance of pancytopenia in the sick patients has been postulated to be due to bone marrow hypoplasia, but more recent investigations point to sequestration or destruction of various blood elements (the hemophagocytic syndrome) as the most likely explanation.

The diagnosis of ehrlichiosis is based on epidemiologic information regarding possible tick exposure in areas where the tick-borne diseases are present, plus the aforementioned clinical and laboratory features. This febrile illness needs to be differentiated from Colorado tick fever and Lyme disease (see Ch. 321). The geographic location of the patient helps determine the possibility of Colorado tick fever. Differential features of Lyme disease include the classic erythema migrans lesion and the usual lack of leukopenia and thrombocytopenia. In the small percentage of patients with a rash more typical of RMSF, a mistaken diagnosis of RMSF is possible. Confusion with *R. rickettsii* disease is not a serious clinical management problem if the patient is treated with a tetracycline antibiotic or chloramphenicol. Failure to consider either disease and administer appropriate therapy can lead to serious consequences for the patient. Prompt antibiotic treatment needs repeated emphasis since delay is associated with the poorest prognosis.

Treatment of patients infected with either of the known strains of *Ehrlichia* requires doxycycline (100 mg every 12 hours for the first day and 100 mg once daily for at least 3 days after the fever abates). Tetracycline (500 mg once daily or chloramphenicol 500 mg once daily) can also be used. With early therapy the febrile course is short. Heparin therapy is not recommended because the pancytopenia disappears promptly as the disease is brought under control with antibiotics.

Bakken JS, Dumler JS, Chen S, et al.: Human granulocytic ehrlichiosis in the upper midwest United States. JAMA 272:212, 1994. *The first report on a new disease entity, caused by another species of* Ehrlichia.

Everett ED, Evans KA, Henry B, et al.: Human ehrlichiosis in adults after tick exposure. Ann Intern Med 120:730, 1994. *Presents data on 30 patients diagnosed and followed by this group.*

Fishbein DB, Dawson JE, Robinson LE: Human ehrlichiosis in the United States, 1985 to 1990. Ann Intern Med 120:736, 1994. *This report follows Everett et al. and is the usual excellent CDC review of 237 cases garnered by a laboratory surveillance.*

324.4   Rickettsialpox

DEFINITION. Rickettsialpox is a rare mite-borne infectious disease caused by *Rickettsia akari.* This mild, self-limited illness consists of headache, fever, an eschar at the site of the mite bite, and a papulovesicular rash.

ETIOLOGY. *R. akari* is classified with the spotted fever group of rickettsiae. It is a small, gram-negative, coccobacillus-shaped, obligate intracellular organism.

DISTRIBUTION AND INCIDENCE. Rickettsialpox was first described in 1946. In the subsequent few years, more than 500 cases were diagnosed, primarily in New York City. Since the early 1950's, only one outbreak has occurred, again in New York City. The disease is virtually unknown throughout the rest of the United States.

TRANSMISSION AND EPIDEMIOLOGY. The original description included *R. akari* isolated from persons with the disease, from mites *(Allodermanyssus sanguineus)* that feed on rodents, and from house mice *(Mus musculus).* Engorged mites were occasionally found on the mice; attachment was usually around the rump. The mites remain in the nest, where access to mice is readily available. Human intrusion into this animal-ectoparasite cycle can result in an infected mite's biting and inducing disease. The ecologic range of *A. sanguineus* covers most of the United States, and mice are ubiquitous animals. Thus the elements for potential epidemics exist. Isolated cases may develop from unusual exposure to mice, as in persons working in landfills or in homeless persons sleeping in abandoned buildings.

Rickettsialpox is fairly common in some urban areas of Ukraine, where rats appear to be the animal reservoir. In Korea small field mice are infected.

PATHOLOGY. The known pathologic changes are limited to the skin, since this is a nonfatal infection. Histologic examination of the eschar (site of mite bite) reveals intense inflammation with necrosis. Other findings are similar to those in RMSF: thrombosis and necrosis of capillaries, edema, and a monocytic perivascular infiltrate. The characteristic rash in this disease is papulovesicular. The lesions contain fluid that may yield *R. akari* on culture.

CLINICAL MANIFESTATIONS AND COURSE. The bite of the mite is not painful and goes unnoticed. This site undergoes a localized inflammatory reaction over the next week to 10 days. During this time the edema and cellular components of the reaction create a slowly enlarging, firm, erythematous papule, which may reach 1 to 1.5 cm in diameter. The involved skin separates gradually, creating a vesicle that finally breaks down to form an ulcer. The base of the ulcer is usually black and is surrounded by a rim of erythematous skin. This progression occurs over 3 to 7 days, at the end of which there is the sudden onset of fever, chills, sweats, headache, backache, and malaise. The lymph nodes draining the area of the eschar enlarge but are nontender. These symptoms and signs may be present for a week if no specific antibiotic treatment is administered.

As with other members of the spotted fever group, a rash appears after 2 to 3 days of illness. Initially the lesions are maculopapular, few in number, and distributed mostly on the trunk and abdomen, rarely involving the palms or soles. The lesions evolve quickly and uniformly into vesicular lesions; the vesicle appears to sit on top of an erythematous papule. These lesions persist for about a week; the fluid in the vesicle is slowly absorbed, and a scab forms, which leaves a brownish discoloration in the skin after it falls off. This gradually clears without leaving a scar. There is no significant internal organ involvement.

DIAGNOSIS. The diagnosis is made by clinical observation; the unique lesions of the rash, the presence of the eschar, and a history that suggests contact with rodents in the past 2 weeks provide sufficient evidence to make the diagnosis. Serologic studies confirm the diagnosis; complement-fixing antibody titers have been the standard, but indirect immunofluorescent antibodies are more specific, when available. Confusion exists regarding whether the Weil-Felix reaction can be used to diagnose rickettsialpox. In about 10% of patients in small series, significant titer rises to OX-19 and OX-2 have been observed. The test lacks sensitivity for confirming the diagnosis. The organism can be isolated from the vesicular fluid or from clotted blood specimens. These materials must be injected into animals or embryonated eggs. Laboratory tests are of no diagnostic help, although leukopenia is common.

The rash may be confused with the lesions of chickenpox, but no eschar is present in chickenpox (see Ch. 336). In addition, the lesions of chickenpox are usually in various stages of maturity, whereas the character of those in rickettsialpox is more uniform. Finally, the vesicle of rickettsialpox appears to sit on a papule, whereas those of chickenpox lack such a base.

PROGNOSIS AND TREATMENT. Rickettsialpox is a benign illness, and recovery occurs without therapy.

Treatment with tetracycline or doxycycline shortens the febrile period and hastens recovery. Antibiotic treatment need only be administered for 3 to 4 days to ensure a cure. No relapse will occur.

PREVENTION AND CONTROL. Rickettsialpox is a zoonosis involving a common house pest, the mouse. Control of this reservoir through elimination of mouse harborages and use of residual acaricides to walls adjacent to mice-infested areas should control mite populations. There is no available vaccine.

324.5 Scrub Typhus

DEFINITION. Scrub typhus is an acute febrile illness caused by *Rickettsia tsutsugamushi* (from the Japanese: *tsutsuga*, "dangerous"; *mushi*, "bug"). This rickettsia is inoculated into humans during the bite by a chigger. The site of the bite develops into an eschar.

ETIOLOGY. *Rickettsia tsutsugamushi (R. orientalis)* is a small gram-negative, obligate intracellular organism. Unlike other rickettsial infections, infection with *R. tsutsugamushi* does not induce solid protection against additional bouts of scrub typhus. This results from the variable antigenic compositions of the strains.

This is the only rickettsia whose polysaccharides bear an anti-

genic relationship to *Proteus* OX-K. This *Proteus* strain is used in serologic tests to confirm scrub typhus.

DISTRIBUTION. This disease occurs almost exclusively in the large triangular region extending from the northern islands of Japan southwest to Australia and southeast to the South Pacific Islands. This region contains the larval form of mites that are both vector and reservoir of rickettsiae.

TRANSMISSION AND EPIDEMIOLOGY. *R. tsutsugamushi* is transmitted to humans by the bite of the larva of trombiculid mites (chiggers). Chiggers are the only stage in the life cycle of these mites (*Leptotrombidium deliensis* and others) that can feed on humans. Chiggers are almost microscopic, often brilliantly colored (red bugs). The chiggers feed on rats and other small rodents. The word "scrub" was applied because of the type of vegetation—transitional between forests and clearings—that maintains the chigger-mammal relationship. But other regions (semiarid, sandy beaches, and so on) also support rodents and mites. Humans encounter scrub typhus when they enter such areas to build roads, to clear fields or forests, or on military expeditions. Circumscribed regions are highly endemic, a reflection of the lack of mobility of the chiggers and their rodent hosts. Mites transmit the rickettsiae to their offspring via the ova. Therefore they can serve as vector and reservoir of the etiologic agent.

This disease has been called river or flood fever because of the increased incidence during the rainy seasons. Chiggers and mites proliferate in warm, wet environments.

PATHOLOGY. *R. tsutsugamushi* invades endothelial cells to produce a vasculitis. The serious pathologic manifestations in untreated patients are predominantly myocarditis, meningoencephalitis, and pneumonitis. Coagulopathy develops but is less severe than in RMSF or typhus.

The site of the chigger bite develops into a papular lesion that ulcerates to form an eschar. This is associated with regional and later generalized lymphadenopathy.

CLINICAL MANIFESTATIONS AND COURSE. The incubation period for development of the primary papular lesion ranges from 6 to 18 days. This lesion can occur anywhere on the body. It enlarges, undergoes central necrosis, and crusts to form the eschar. As the eschar matures, the patient has the sudden onset of headache, fever, chills, and malaise. Over the next several days, these symptoms increase in severity with further elevation of the temperature. The patient, if untreated, may become stuporous as meningoencephalitis develops. Signs of cardiac dysfunction, including minor electrocardiographic abnormalities such as first-degree heart block and inverted T waves, can appear. The rash of scrub typhus appears at the end of the first week of disease. This is a faint, pink maculopapular rash appearing first on the trunk and spreading to the extremities.

Physical findings late in the first week of illness include generalized lymphadenopathy and palpable spleen and occasionally liver. Pulmonary findings are often absent despite radiographic evidence of interstitial pneumonia. In those patients with myocarditis, there may be a gallop rhythm, poor-quality heart sounds, and systolic murmurs.

Various cranial nerve deficits have been noted in untreated patients. Deafness, dysarthria, and dysphagia may occur but are usually transient, although deafness can last for several months.

All of 87 (nonimmune) soldiers in Vietnam who developed scrub typhus had fever and headache, 46% had an eschar, and 35% had a rash. Eighty-five percent had generalized lymph node enlargement. It is not surprising that many were misdiagnosed as having infectious mononucleosis.

Laboratory studies reveal leukopenia early in the disease with subsequent increase of white blood cell counts to normal levels. Coagulopathies can be demonstrated, but only rare patients develop the disseminated intravascular clotting syndrome. Liver enzyme values may be elevated, indicating hepatocellular damage. Proteinuria is common.

Patients with untreated disease remain febrile for about 2 weeks and have a long convalescence of 4 to 6 weeks thereafter.

DIAGNOSIS. The variable presentations in this disease make the clinical diagnosis difficult. The eschar and rash should suggest a rickettsial infection, but these may be found in fewer than one half of patients. Furthermore, the eschar and rash may suggest other rickettsial infections, such as tick-borne typhus. The endemic foci of scrub typhus and whether the patient has traveled or worked in such areas constitute important epidemiologic information. A therapeutic trial of tetracycline or chloramphenicol is indicated in patients in whom the diagnosis of scrub typhus is suspected. Defervescence should occur within 24 hours.

The specific serologic test is the detection of significant increases (greater than fourfold) of IFA's in paired serum specimens obtained 2 weeks apart. The *Proteus* OX-K antigen test is readily available and inexpensive, so that it is frequently employed in endemic areas. About 50% of patients have diagnostic titers. In Malaya, the sensitivity and specificity of both tests were found to be about the same, but their usefulness was enhanced when they were used concurrently.

R. tsutsugamushi can be isolated from a patient's blood by inoculating it, intraperitoneally, into white mice. The rickettsiae can be demonstrated in the tissues of the mice.

PROGNOSIS AND TREATMENT. Without treatment, the mortality rate ranges from 0 to 30% depending upon virulence and resistance factors; with treatment, survival is the expected outcome. Second or third attacks of scrub typhus, caused by different serotypes, usually result in a mild illness, usually with no eschar or rash.

Persistence of *R. tsutsugamushi* in lymph node tissues has been demonstrated 1 year after recovery. This finding raises the possibility of disease reactivating during immunosuppression.

Tetracycline, doxycycline, and chloramphenicol are all effective. The drug should be continued for at least 2 days after the patient has become afebrile.

PREVENTION AND CONTROL. Vaccines were developed and tested during and after World War II. Some were effective against homologous strains. However, no single antigen has been identified that induces protection against all of the antigenically diverse strains of *R. tsutsugamushi*. In military populations in endemic areas, weekly doses of doxycycline protect against scrub typhus.

Avoidance of chigger attachment can be accomplished by insect repellents applied to the skin and by use of protective clothing impregnated with benzyl benzoate. Diethyltoluamide preparations such as OFF and DEET are also effective if sprayed on clothing and exposed skin but are removed rapidly by water. Applying this chemical to socks is especially important in preventing chigger bites.

324.6 Q Fever

DEFINITION. Q fever is a systemic infection caused by inhaling small numbers of *Coxiella burnetii*. Domestic animals and pets are the usual sources of infection for humans. This highly infectious rickettsial agent induces mild febrile illness, occasionally associated with pneumonitis, but in a few patients causes chronic hepatitis and life-threatening endocarditis.

ETIOLOGY. *C. burnetii* is unique among the rickettsiae in the following ways: It is not transmitted to humans by arthropod vectors; rather, it is readily disseminated by aerosols. No rash ensues despite the similarity of the infection of endothelial cells (vasculitis) to that with *Rickettsia rickettsii*. The organism resides uniquely inside the phagolysosome in the cytoplasm of the infected cell. *C. burnetii* does not have cross-reacting antigens with *Proteus vulgaris,* and therefore antibodies developed during infection do not agglutinate in the Weil-Felix test. These rickettsiae are resistant to destruction by environmental stresses, e.g., sunlight, humidity.

Isolation of *C. burnetii* from pulmonary secretions, liver biopsies, and surgical cardiac valve specimens is possible but not recommended unless appropriate laboratory facilities are available. This is a highly infectious agent that can readily cause laboratory-acquired infections. These materials are injected into eggs and/or guinea pigs. In the latter, the production of agglutinating antibodies confirms the presence of the organism. *C. burnetii* can exist in two phases. Phase I organisms are usually associated with chronic, severe clinical illnesses, such as endocarditis. Phase II organisms evolve (through the loss of mono- and polysaccharide chains of the lipopolysaccharide surface antigens) following multiple transfers in eggs. Antibodies to Phase II organisms are predominant in most patients with Q fever. However, patients with endocarditis have higher titers of antibodies to Phase I organisms, specifically IgA and IgG; the latter two types of antibodies are diagnostic for this entity.

Virulence factors associated with *C. burnetii* include three plasmids. These appear to be specific for acute versus chronic disease; they control the production of proteins that may be involved in the infectious processes. The lipopolysaccharide antigen is another virulence factor. The antigen in strains causing chronic disease is different from that in strains involved in acute disease. The organism may resist destruction inside the phagolysosome by producing large quantities of acid phosphatase, which inhibits the superoxide production of the host cell, thereby avoiding lysis. In addition, its ability to survive in the acid milieu of the phagolysosome provides an environment that impairs the efficacy of most antibiotics. Raising the pH in tissue culture systems results in increased antibiotic efficacy. These virulence factors can enable *C. burnetii* to establish chronic infections.

EPIDEMIOLOGY. Human disease is acquired by inhaling aerosols containing *C. burnetii*. The organisms are disseminated from infected ruminants and pets (cats). The placentas from these animals contain huge concentrations of rickettsiae. During delivery of the placenta, aerosols are generated which may be wind borne to contaminate soil, clothing, and the wool or fur of other animals or may be transmitted hundreds of yards to susceptible persons. Trucks carrying sheep appear to disseminate organisms to persons passed on the streets. Sheep regularly transported to research laboratories through hallways in a medical center caused an epidemic that persisted for 6 months. Organisms are also found in amniotic fluid, feces, and the mammary glands and milk of sheep and cows. The ability of *C. burnetii* to form sporelike structures that resist environmental destruction allows these organisms to cause disease long after the initial contamination occurs and at sites distant from the original source.

The animals are infected by ticks. There are ticks that transmit the organisms among wild animals, such as the kangaroo in Australia. Spread to domestic animals occurs when the two populations of animals intermingle. Ticks have not been implicated in the transmission from animals to humans. Q fever is a mild and inapparent infection in animals. It may be responsible for placental deficiencies that lead to stillbirth of kittens and lambs. *C. burnetii* attach to the head of the sperm from infected mice. Males can infect female mice by sexual contact. Whether this occurs in humans is unknown.

Various volunteer studies, designed to evaluate vaccine effectiveness, have demonstrated that very few organisms, probably fewer than 10, are sufficient to induce disease. For this reason, as well as the ability to survive in most environments, *C. burnetii* is a hazardous organism with which to work. In one laboratory 21 of 50 cases diagnosed over a 15-year period occurred in persons working in laboratories (or offices) not directly involved in Q fever research. Presumably, these persons were infected by widely disseminated aerosols from laboratory accidents or from contaminated clothing of workers socializing outside their laboratory. Despite the infectious nature of the organism and its presence in sputum, human-to-human transmission does not occur and respiratory isolation for infected patients is not needed.

In the United States and Canada, *C. burnetii* (and antibodies) has been found in milk from numerous herds of cattle. Despite this evidence, documented cases of Q fever occurring after unpasteurized milk from such cows was ingested have not been identified. The ingestion of 10^5 organisms by mouth by volunteers failed to induce disease. If disease occurs, it could originate from aerosols created in the act of pouring the milk into a glass.

The incubation period varies indirectly with inoculum size. Large doses result in disease at about 7 days. Most persons develop symptoms at 13 to 18 days.

PATHOLOGY. Knowledge of the pathologic changes is greatest for the more severe form of this disease. For example, microscopic examinations of liver biopsies and autopsy material from patients dying of chronic hepatitis and from heart valves infected with *C. burnetii* are available. Patients with pneumonitis usually have a mild illness so tissue specimens are scarce. Animal studies have provided complementary pathohistologic data.

Hepatitis. Granulomas with fatty necrosis are typical microscopic findings. These granulomas are doughnut-shaped. While they are common in Q fever, they also are seen in patients with tuberculosis. Fatty metamorphosis is also seen. Patients with mild forms of Q fever may have elevated liver enzyme values indicative of minimal liver cell damage.

Subacute and Chronic Endocarditis. This is a life-threatening disease because it is difficult to eradicate the infection. These patients may have large vegetations on the aortic valve and less likely on the mitral valve. They have negative blood cultures and frequently have a history of a febrile illness with or without pneumonitis months previously. The vegetations have a histologic picture similar to that in other forms of endocarditis, an avascular collection of fibrin and platelets. These patients also have enlarged livers and spleens, plus signs of vasculitis associated with endocarditis, e.g., splinter hemorrhages, Roth spots, and petechiae.

Pneumonitis. In the few autopsies performed, consolidation similar to that of other bacterial pneumonias was the gross finding. The microscopic examination revealed an exudate loaded with histocytes and no polymorphonuclear leukocytes. This inflammatory response is compatible with a nonbacterial process. The histologic features have been described as those of a severe intra-alveolar, focally necrotizing, hemorrhagic pneumonia with associated necrotizing bronchitis and bronchiolitis.

The portal of entry of C. burnetii is the respiratory tract; small particles < 3 to 5μ in diameter can reach the terminal bronchioles. The pneumonia does not appear until the third or fourth day of fever. In a mouse model, the rickettsiae enter pneumatocytes, histocytes, and fibroblasts. The self-limiting nature of this infection is probably related to the destruction of the organisms in the macrophages. However, C. burnetii can persist for 2 months inside those cells. Some of the macrophages can be damaged by C. burnetii, leading to an inflammatory response. Cellular immune mechanisms attack these damaged cells. Numerous factors are involved in the pathogenesis of pneumonia—the number and virulence of the rickettsiae, particle size, and the functional status of the macrophages and parenchymal cells of the lung.

CLINICAL MANIFESTATIONS. The onset of Q fever is very abrupt; the manifestations are not specific. The patient develops a high fever that is associated with headache, chills, myalgia, and malaise. This flulike syndrome differs from influenza disease because of the height of the temperature, frequently 39.4° to 40°C. The fever also persists for 10 to 14 days. No rash occurs. Retro-orbital pain, common in other rickettsial infections, is reported by 10 to 15% of patients.

Patients may have a dry, nonproductive cough indicative of the bronchiolitis and the minimal pneumonitis produced by the invading C. burnetii. Physical findings of consolidated lung are lacking early in the course of the pneumonia. There may be decreased breath sounds, but rales are unlikely until the lesions start to resolve. The chest films reveal patchy infiltrates that frequently are multiple round, segmental opacities. These are discrete lesions. Larger areas of the lung may show consolidation, and linear atelectatic lesions occur in about half the patients with pneumonia. Resolution of the lesions is slow. The incidence of pneumonitis varies from 4 to 97% in series of cases reported from the United States (28%), Australia (4 to 75%), and Switzerland (97%). The reasons for these variations are unknown.

Most patients (85%) with Q fever have hepatic involvement as measured by abnormal liver cell enzymes. Hepatomegaly is noted in about 65% of patients, but few patients (10%) have liver tenderness. Jaundice is unlikely (about 5% of cases) unless chronic hepatitis ensues, a very rare manifestation. Liver biopsies have demonstrated, by direct immunofluorescent studies, rickettsia residing in hepatic cells. Q fever may account for a few cases of acute hepatitis. Patients with a strong exposure history should be evaluated for infection by C. burnetii.

The clinical manifestations of Q fever endocarditis are characteristic of those associated with the syndrome of endocarditis; e.g., splenomegaly, splinter hemorrhages, and heart murmurs. Few cases of C. burnetii–induced valvular infections are seen in the United States; small series are reported from countries in which Q fever is more common. Evidence of endocarditis in a patient occurs years after the acute infections. The lack of positive cultures contributes to a delay in diagnosis. The diagnosis is made by serologic means, demonstrating high ($> 1:800$ for IgG and $> 1:50$ for IgA) or rising titers of Phase I antibodies by indirect immunofluorescence. The

level of Phase I antibodies exceeding those for Phase II antibodies is indicative of chronic Q fever, whether it is endocarditis or a localized infection of bone, vascular prosthesis, aneurysm, liver, or joint. Phase II antibodies indicate a recent exposure or an acute infection.

PROGNOSIS. The key to diagnosing Q fever in a patient with a debilitating febrile illness is obtaining a history of contact with sheep, cattle, goats, or cats or the skins or wool from these animals. This history should be compelling enough to initiate antibiotic treatment and to obtain acute and convalescent serum for serologic studies. These latter studies are the practical and definitive diagnostic aids. Phase II antibodies (complement fixing [CF] or IFA) are present in two thirds of patients at the end of 2 weeks of illness and in 90% at 1 month. Phase I antibodies, if present, are found in titers lower than Phase II antibodies. IFA is more sensitive than CF in detecting early antibody formation (IgM) and also in demonstrating persistence of antibody at 1 year or longer. The presence of Phase I antibodies in excess of Phase II, and specifically Phase I IgA, is diagnostic of Q fever endocarditis.

The nonspecific clinical manifestations of early symptoms and signs of Q fever, e.g., headache, fever, myalgia, suggest numerous infectious diseases. Influenza infections are seasonal, the temperature is less than that of Q fever, and liver function tests are normal. The white blood cell count is not helpful, as it is normal in both infections. Other diseases such as typhoid fever and brucellosis can be diagnosed by bacterial cultures. Viral hepatitis can be mistaken for Q fever. Appropriate serologic studies and liver biopsy provide diagnostic evidence. In those patients with pneumonitis, the differential diagnosis includes viral or mycoplasmal etiologies, tularemia, psittacosis, and Legionella pneumophila. Serologic and culture results identify these organisms.

TREATMENT AND PROGNOSIS. C. burnetii is known to be susceptible to a number of antibiotics. Sensitivity studies have been conducted in eggs, guinea pigs, and in acute and chronically infected tissue culture cells. Tetracycline and doxycycline or chloramphenicol have been effective in vitro as well as in clinical studies. Early institution of tetracycline (within 3 days of onset) reduces the febrile course by half. Tetracycline, 500 mg four times a day, or doxycycline, 100 mg twice a day, should be continued for at least 1 week after the patient becomes afebrile (usually 2 to 3 days). The prognosis with such therapy is excellent, with no mortality expected. Those patients who receive no antibiotics also do well, with a recovery rate of $> 99\%$. If a febrile relapse occurs, retreatment with the same antibiotic is effective.

The recommended treatment of patients with Q fever endocarditis is not settled. Doxycycline and a quinolone have been somewhat effective, but cures have not been achieved even after 2 years of continuous therapy. The mortality rate remains high (24%). The location of the organism in an acid environment inside the phagolysosome interferes with the activity of antibiotics. Experimental studies designed to alkalize the fluid helped to eradicate the organisms in phagocytes. The combination of doxycycline and chloroquine in these studies was most effective and may be useful in patients with chronic Q fever. Surgical resection of infected valves is usually required because the large vegetations cause hemodynamic deficiencies in cardiac function.

PREVENTION. There is no commercially available vaccine for Q fever. Experimental vaccines using either Phase I or Phase II organisms have been effective in preventing disease in volunteers and in several field trials. For those persons at high risk, such as researchers working with sheep, veterinarians, or exposed laboratory workers, vaccine can be obtained under an investigational new drug (IND) application.

Focusing on controlling disease in the workplace is more effective than attempting to control the disease in animals. Three recommended measures include knowing the serologic status of the employees, not permitting pregnant women or persons with valvar heart disease to be in the high-risk jobs, and confining the research on sheep to a building dedicated solely to that purpose. Vaccination of employees should also be attempted.

Brouqui P, Dupont HT, Drancourt M, et al.: Chronic Q fever: Ninety-two cases from France, including 27 cases without endocarditis. Arch Intern Med 153:642, 1993. *An excellent review of chronic Q fever.*

Yeaman MR, Roman MJ, Baca OG: Antibiotic susceptibilities of two Coxiella burnetii isolates implicated in distinct clinical syndromes. Antimicrob Agents Chemother 33:2053, 1989. *A new method to evaluate sensitivities of Q fever isolates to antibiotics.*

325 ZOONOSES
Stuart Levin

"Zoonoses" are most simply defined as human infections derived from animals. There are approximately 200 different infectious agents that cause disease in humans and fulfill the definition of a zoonosis. Man's so-called best friend, the dog, has been targeted as facilitating the transmission of more than 50 different infectious agents and is credited with more than one million bite injuries each year in the United States. The risk of developing a zoonosis is increased by outdoor activities, with exposure to and inhalation of infectious air particles, direct animal contact, insect bites, contact with previously infected human blood products, and contact with and ingestion of infectious agents transmitted by animal-contaminated water and insufficiently cooked meat, eggs, dairy products, fish, and shellfish. Raw shellfish are the garbage filters of the ocean and can transmit at least 25 different infectious or toxic illnesses to humans. In addition, the farmer, pet owner, hunter, laboratory researcher, and cave explorer, among others, is at higher risk than the general population to develop a zoonosis. Infective agents transmitted by these routes from animal sources essentially include members of all microbial classes: viruses, bacteria, fungi, and parasites. Immunocompromised hosts such as splenectomized patients, trans-

TABLE 325-1. RESPIRATORY TRACT ZOONOSES

Disease	Microorganism	Clinical Syndrome and Diagnosis	Reservoir and/or Vector
Psittacosis	*Chlamydia psittaci*	Pneumonia, often severe; serology	Aerosols from parrots, ducks, turkeys
Q-fever	*Coxiella burnetii*	Pneumonia, hepatitis, or myocarditis; serology	Airborne from soil contaminated by sheep, goats, and cats, particularly if parturient
Tularemia	*Francisella tularensis*	Cutaneous ulcer and regional node; pneumonia and hilar node; pleural effusion, sepsis; serology	Rabbit contact (winter) and tick bites (summer)*
Plague	*Yersinia pestis*	Inguinal nodes, bubonic plague (10% will develop basilar pneumonia); hilar node enlargement; serology	Fleas from prairie dogs, rock squirrels, rats
Hantavirus adult respiratory distress syndrome	*Hantavirus muerto canyon*†	URI to LRI to ARDS; death; serology	Deer mouse fomites: urine, feces, saliva
Rhodococcus pneumonia	*Rhodococcus equi*	Pneumonia, often cavitate, in AIDS and other immunosuppressed patients; sputum culture	Horse manure, soil
Mycoplasma arginini pneumonia	*Mycoplasma arginini*	Pneumonia, sepsis, neutropenic hosts; special culture	Sheep, goats
Foot and mouth disease	Aphthovirus	Nonspecific URI, oral vesicles; serology	Cloven-footed mammals

Note: See Table of Contents and Index for more detailed discussion of each disease.
* Occurs in more than 1000 animal species.
† Proposed name.

TABLE 325-2. CENTRAL NERVOUS SYSTEM INFECTION: ZOONOSES

Disease	Organism	Clinical Syndrome and Diagnosis	Reservoir
Listeriosis	*Listeria monocytogenes*	Purulent meningitis during pregnancy and in neonate; immunosuppression; culture	Unpasteurized cheese and other dairy products; cattle, goats
Leptospirosis	*Leptospira interrogans*	Aseptic meningitis, hepatorenal syndrome; serology, culture	Asymptomatic dogs, cattle, water source common
Herpes B encephalitis	*Herpes simiae*	Diffuse, progressive encephalitis; culture	Bites or scratches of Macaques monkey
Lyme disease	*Borrelia burgdorferi*	Lymphocytic meningitis, motor-sensory neuropathy, facial palsy; serology	Tick bites, mouse hosts
Lymphocytic choriomeningitis	Lymphocytic choriomeningitis virus	Lymphocytic meningitis, occasionally with pneumonia; serology	Inhalation of mouse secretions, urine, feces, saliva
Mosquito-borne encephalitis, USA	Eastern, western equine encephalitis; St. Louis, California encephalitis	Diffuse encephalitis; least severe: California encephalitis; most severe: Eastern equine encephalitis; serology	Mosquito-borne from horses, birds
Rabies encephalitis	Rabies virus	Almost always fatal; encephalitis; serology	Bites from dogs, skunks, bats, raccoons, foxes
Toxoplasmosis	*Toxoplasma gondii*	CNS, multiple lesions, AIDS patient; CNS scan, serology, biopsy	Cat feces or ingestion of undercooked lamb, pork
Cerebral cysticercosis	*Taenia solium*	Epilepsy, CNS cysts, eosinophilic meningitis, hydrocephalus; scan, serology	Fecal-oral contamination of food; swine

Note: See Table of Contents and Index for more detailed discussion of each disease.

plant patients, and AIDS patients, as well as pregnant women and their fetuses, are at high risk of developing clinical disease when exposed to these various infectious agents.

Non–animal-associated environmental- or travel-related infectious diseases can be confused with zoonoses. The vast majority of clinical diseases caused by *Legionella pneumophila, Plasmodium falciparum, Entamoeba histolytica, Giardia lamblia, Pseudomonas pseudomallei, Chromobacterium violaceum, Aeromonas hydrophila, Francisella philomiragia,* and airborne fungi such as *Blastomyces dermatitidis, Coccidioides immitis,* and *Histoplasma capsulatum* are acquired through environmental exposure and are only rarely related to animal hosts.

Unfortunately, some descriptive disease titles can be misleading to clinicians and thus can interfere with the possible diagnoses that they consider. The transmission of tick-borne Rocky Mountain spotted fever actually occurs more commonly in the southeastern United States than in the Rocky Mountains and has even been acquired in the middle of the Bronx, New York. Vegetarians and other strict non–pork-eating persons have been seriously infected with the pig tapeworm, *Taenia solium,* as a result of fecal contamination of food from unsuspected infected human sources.

The influence of the animal host on human infection can be quite deceptive. Human influenza A is not typically considered a zoonosis; however, there is evidence that an initial incubation period within an animal host may facilitate the more dramatic antigenic change "shifts" that account for the devastating pandemics of the

TABLE 325-3. SKIN RASHES: ZOONOSES

Disease	Microorganism	Clinical Information and Diagnosis	Reservoir and/or Vector
Ehrlichiosis	Ehrlichia chaffeensis	Macular rash (one third of patients), central distribution; in south central U.S.; culture, serology	Tick bite
Leptospirosis	Leptospira interrogans	Central macular rash in 20%, with occasional enanthem; serology, culture	Urine-contaminated water, dogs, cattle
Lyme disease	Borrelia burgdorferi	Primary lesion is erythema chronicum migrans; 40% have multiple lesions; serology, culture	Mouse reservoir—tick bite
Rocky Mountain spotted fever	Rickettsia rickettsii	Acral or peripheral distribution of macular papular to hemorrhagic rash to gangrenous lesions; serology	Tick bite
Typhus (endemic)	Rickettsia prowazeckii	Central distribution, macular rash (can be hemorrhagic); serology	Flying squirrel fleas or fomites
Scabies	Mite Sarcoptes scabiei	Pruritic macules on trunk; skin burrow	Dogs—close contact. Up to one third of asymptomatic dogs have mite infection
Flea bite dermatitis	Pulex irritans	Pruritic papules, urticaria vesicles; fleas found on pets or in the environment	Fleas on dogs
Cat scratch disease	Rochalimaea henselae, Afipia felis	Large purplish skin nodules and papules in AIDS patients; bacillary angiomatosis, hepatic peliosis, cervical adenopathy, and local ulcer in normal hosts; culture, serology, silver stain biopsy	Cat scratch or bite

Note: See Table of Contents and Index for more detailed discussion of each disease.

TABLE 325-4. HIGHLY FATAL ZOONOSES

Disease	Fatality Rate (%)
Rabies	99
*Herpes simiae**	50–75
Ebola virus	70
Eastern equine encephalitis	50–70
Hantavirus pulmonary syndrome, U.S.†	60
Yellow fever‡	20–50
Lassa fever‡	15–25
Plague*	50–80
Rocky Mountain spotted fever*	20–60
East African sleeping sickness*	20–30
Anthrax*	20
Tularemia	10–15
Visceral leishmanias*	5–25
Louse-borne relapsing fever*	5–40

Note: See Table of Contents and Index for more detailed discussion of each disease.
* Fatality rate if untreated.
† If jaundiced.
‡ Case mortality of hospitalized patients.

TABLE 325-5. NEWLY CHARACTERIZED ZOONOSES

Disease	Clinical Information	Reservoir and/or Vector
Ehrlichia chaffeensis	Fever, myalgia, leukopenia	Tick bite
Cat scratch disease, Rochalimaea henselae, Afipia felis	Cervical lymphadenopathy in normal hosts and cutaneous and hepatic angiomatosis in AIDS patients	Cat scratch or bite
Enterohemorrhagic Escherichia coli 0157-H7	Rectal bleeding, dysentery, hemolytic uremia syndrome	Contaminated, undercooked meat
Hantavirus	Adult respiratory distress syndrome	Fomites of rodents
Cryptosporidium	Diarrhea	Contaminated water
Campylobacter jejuni	Dysentery, Reiter's syndrome, Guillian-Barré syndrome	Contaminated chicken
Capnocytophaga canimorsus	Sepsis, skin infection	Dog bites

Note: See Table of Contents and Index for more detailed discussion of each disease.

disease that appear every 10 to 30 years. Recent information suggests that avian (bird) influenza viruses common in domestic fowl (ducks) can intermix with human influenza A viruses in a third animal species, the domestic pig of China, leading to an antigen shift. Indeed, in areas of China the three species live together in very close quarters. This "new" influenza A virus is transmitted to the human host from the pig and then transferred rapidly from human to human around the world, with catastrophic health and economic consequences. Leprosy, a human-to-human–transmitted illness of biblical notoriety, is endemic in at least three animal species, including the armadillo, which occasionally has been implicated in the transmission of this disease to humans in the United States.

As clinicians evaluate an individual patient, they need consider only a limited number of historical details that generally will lead to an appropriate differential diagnosis. These include

1. Questions regarding direct contact with animals or animal products must be pursued. Details regarding animal bites, arthropod exposures, and food ingestion may offer clues to the correct etiology.

2. Consideration must be given to a patient's travel history, because a number of zoonoses are quite limited in their geographic distribution.

3. Details about occupational and recreational high-risk activities must be ascertained.

4. The patient's clinical presentation is used to focus simultaneously on the most likely cause and disease considerations. Tables 325–1 through 325–5 take advantage of this "syndrome" approach. Additional lists of zoonotic agents can be generated for the differential diagnoses of arthritis, jaundice, diarrhea, sepsis and shock, renal failure, fever of unknown origin, and endocarditis.

Cook GC: Canine-associated zoonoses: An unacceptable hazard to human health. Q J Med 70:5126, 1989.
Glaser CA, Angulo FJ, Rooney JA: Animal-associated opportunistic infections among persons infected with the human immunodeficiency virus. Clin Infect Dis 18:14, 1994.
Eastaugh J, Shepherd S: Infectious and toxic syndromes from fish and shellfish consumption. Arch Intern Med 149:1735, 1989.
Salgo MP, Telzak EE, Currie B, et al.: A focus of Rocky Mountain spotted fever within New York City. N Engl J Med 318:1345, 1988.
Schantz PM, Moore AC, Munoz JL, et al.: Neurocysticercosis in an orthodox Jewish community in New York City. N Engl J Med 327:692, 1992.

326 INTRODUCTION TO VIRAL DISEASES

R. Gordon Douglas, Jr.

Viruses are among the simplest and smallest of all forms of life. They are obligate intracellular parasites that require host cell structural and metabolic components for replication. They infect bacteria as well as plants and animals. More than 400 distinct viruses infect humans. They produce diseases ranging from subclinical infections and mild, self-limited, localized infections to common systemic infections and overwhelming, highly lethal infections such as meningoencephalitis or hemorrhagic fever with shock.

CHARACTERISTICS OF VIRUSES. Essentially, virus particles, or "virions," consist of nucleic acid enclosed in a protein coat. They lack metabolic activity and do not possess ribosomes or most enzymes necessary for replication. In addition, some possess a lipid envelope. Both the lipid and the protein coats protect the nucleic acid from enzymatic degradation. The nucleic acid may be either deoxyribonucleic acid (DNA) or ribonucleic acid (RNA). It may code for only a few or, in some cases, several hundred proteins. The protein coat, or "capsid," consists of repeating, identical subunits called "capsomeres." The capsid and nucleic acid together are called the "nucleocapsid." The smallest (parvoviruses) are only 18 nm in diameter; some poxviruses may be as large as 450 nm.

There are two major types of structures of virus particles. In the first type, capsomeres are arranged as a regular polyhedron with 20 triangular faces and 12 corners. Such a virus exhibits icosahedral symmetry. Many nonenveloped viruses are of this type. Other viruses exhibit helical symmetry in which a helix is formed of ribonucleoprotein and nucleic acid. Helical viruses are always enveloped, whereas icosahedral viruses may be enveloped or nonenveloped. The envelope is derived from host cell membranes and

modified by insertion of one or more spikelike glycoproteins. These and other proteins on the surface of enveloped or nonenveloped viruses are important for two reasons: They provide specific interaction with receptors on host cells, and they serve as the major antigens of the virus.

Figure 326–1 demonstrates schematically the marked variety in size, shape, and structure of human viruses. In addition, there is great diversity in the structure of the viral genome: Either RNA or DNA may be single stranded or double stranded. The genome may be linear or circular and may exist as single or multiple segments.

Viruses are classified by the International Committee on Taxonomy of Viruses according to the scheme presented in Table 326–1. The following order of virion characteristics is used: nucleic acid type, presence or absence of envelope, genome replication strategy, positive- or negative-sense genome, and genome segmentation.

Because virus structure varies and genomes are complex, mechanisms of replication are diverse. Following a random collision between a virus particle and a cell surface, attachment occurs by binding of a surface protein of a virus to a host cell virus receptor. The nature of the viral attachment protein has been identified for a number of viruses. Penetration of the plasma membrane of the cell occurs by endocytosis, a process similar to receptor-mediated endocytosis of nonviral ligands, or by nonendocytic pathways such as direct translocation across the plasma membrane. Following acidification of the endosome, the viral membrane fuses with that of the vesicle, releasing the nucleocapsid. After uncoating of the viral nucleic acid, macromolecular synthesis of nucleic acid and protein occurs. The strategy for genome replication depends on the type of nucleic acid. Assembly of virus components then occurs, with release of mature viruses by budding, in the case of enveloped viruses, or by lysis of the cell, in the case of some nonenveloped viruses. Such released virions are infectious for other cells.

Viruses cause cell injury by a number of mechanisms: directly by lysis resulting from viral replication, by lysis induced by antiviral antibody and complement, or by cell-mediated immune mechanisms recognizing infected host cells. As virus infection spreads and sufficient numbers of cells are injured, disease results. A role for viral toxins has never been established, and such enzymes as are virus

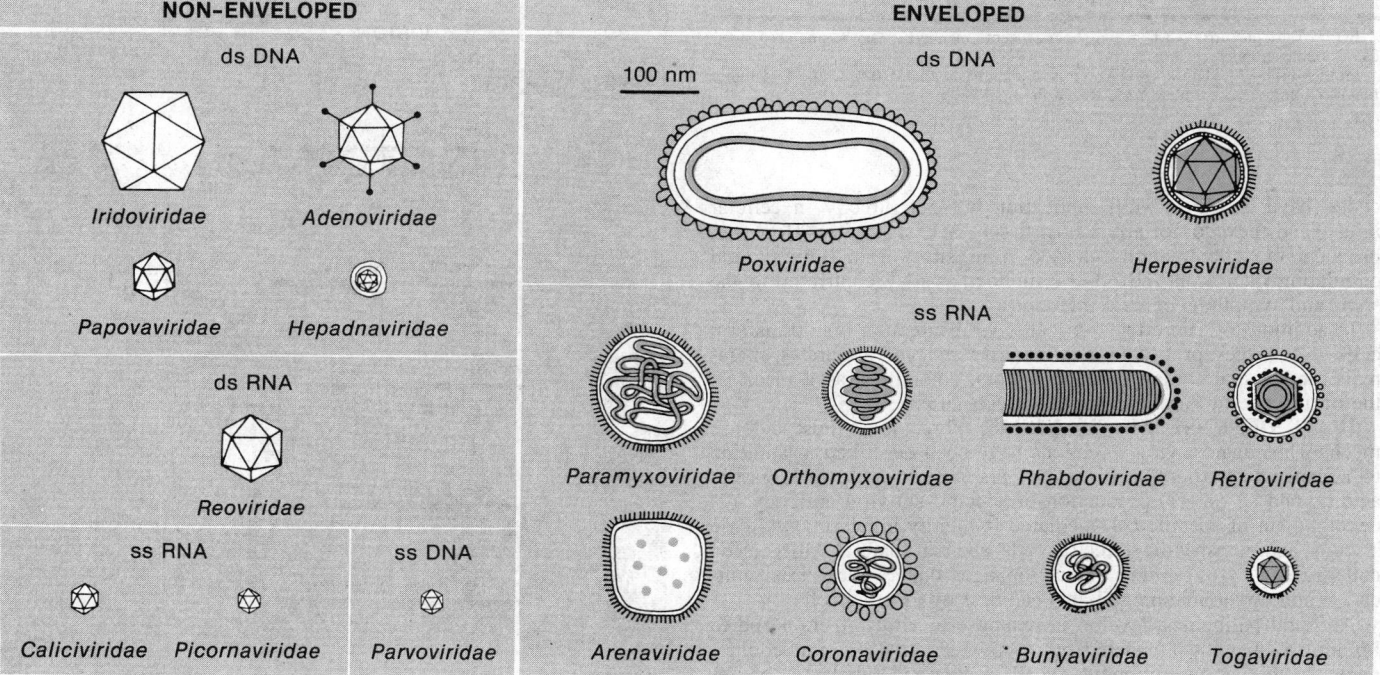

FIGURE 326–1. Structure and relative size of human virus families. (Modified from Matthews REF: Classification and nomenclature of viruses. Intervirology 12:158, 1979.)

TABLE 326-1. CLASSIFICATION OF HUMAN VIRUSES

Dividing Characteristics	Virus Families	Important Human Viruses
DNA Viruses		
dsDNA, enveloped	Poxviridae	Variola (smallpox) virus
		Vaccinia virus
	Herpesviridae	Herpes simplex virus types 1 and 2
		Varicella-zoster virus
		Human cytomegalovirus
		EB virus
		Human herpesvirus type G
dsDNA, nonenveloped	Adenoviridae	Human adenovirus
	Papovaviridae	Papillomavirus
	Hepadnaviridae	Hepatitis B virus
ssDNA, nonenveloped	Parvoviridae	Parvovirus B19
RNA Viruses		
dsRNA, nonenveloped	Reoviridae	Colorado tick fever virus
		Human rotaviruses
ssRNA, enveloped		
No DNA step in replication		
Positive-sense genome	Togaviridae	Alphavirus: Eastern equine encephalitis, Western equine encephalitis
		Rubivirus: Rubella virus
	Flaviviridae	Yellow fever virus
		Dengue viruses
		St. Louis encephalitis
	Coronaviridae	Human coronaviruses
Negative-sense genome		
Nonsegmented genome	Paramyxoviridae	Parainfluenza virus
		Measles virus
		Respiratory syncytial virus
	Rhabdoviridae	Rabies virus
	Filoviridae	Marburg and Ebola viruses
Segmented genome	Orthomyxoviridae	Influenza A and B viruses
	Bunyaviridae	California encephalitis virus
	Arenaviridae	LCM virus
		Lassa virus
DNA step in replication	Retroviridae	HTLV I, II
		HIV I, II
ssRNA, nonenveloped	Picornaviridae	Polioviruses, coxsackieviruses, echoviruses, rhinoviruses
	Caliciviridae	Norwalk virus

EB = Epstein-Barr; LCM = lymphocytic choriomeningitis; ss = single stranded; ds = double stranded.

From Murphy FA, Kinsbury DW: Virus taxonomy. *In* Fields BN, Knipe DM (eds.): Fields Virology. 2nd ed. New York, Raven Press, 1990.

coded have a role in viral replication but not directly in cellular injury, and they do not affect host tissues at distant sites. However, products of inflammation released from sites of cell injury and circulating interferon and other lymphokines may contribute to the signs and symptoms of viral infection.

In addition to lytic effects on cells, viral infection may transform cells so that they proliferate continuously and, in vertebrates, mammals, and humans, may produce tumors, sometimes as a result of the occurrence of viral oncogenes in such viruses.

HOST DEFENSE MECHANISMS. Three main host defense mechanisms against viral infections have been described in addition to nonspecific barriers such as skin, respiratory epithelium, gastric acidity, and so on: (1) production of specific antiviral antibody, (2) development of specific cell-mediated immunity involving cytotoxic T cells and nonspecific effector cells such as natural killer (NK) cells, and (3) proliferation of macrophages that restrict virus replication and dissemination and also can destroy infected cells.

Antiviral antibodies develop in response to viral infection and to immunization with attenuated or inactivated virus or viral components. In the serum, antibodies of all classes and subclasses of immunoglobulins are found; in addition, secretory antibodies consisting predominantly of immunoglobulin A (IgA) molecules develop on mucosal surfaces in response to infection of their surfaces. They

are of critical importance in diseases in which the primary site of inoculation is a mucosal surface.

The immune system may interact with extracellular (free) virus or cell-associated virus. Specific antibody inactivates (neutralizes) extracellular virus, and this activity may be enhanced by complement. Thus it can prevent initial infection or restrict cell-to-cell spread of virus through extracellular fluids. It cannot, however, penetrate into cells and neutralize intracellular virus. Thus virus may escape the effects of antibody by direct cell-to-cell transfer. Virus-infected cells possess viral antigens on their surface and may be lysed by specific antibody and complement, by specific cytotoxic T cells, or by nonspecific cells such as NK cells or macrophages. Virus released in the process may be neutralized by antiviral antibody.

Cytotoxic T cells (Tc), which are HLA class I antigen restricted, also develop in response to infection or immunization (see Ch. 221). They are important in limiting the growth of certain viruses in the infected host. This has been most clearly shown for influenza infections in mice, and Tc are undoubtedly important in a number of viral infections in humans.

NK cells are another important host defense mechanism against viral infections. During early stages of viral infection, the numbers of natural killer cells and their activity are greatly augmented by virus-induced interferon. Mice deficient in NK cells are more sensitive to cytomegalovirus infection, and NK activity has been demonstrated in a number of human infections.

Virus-induced interferons (α and β) have important roles in protection against virus infection through their ability to prevent viral replication in many cells throughout the body and by means of their regulatory function in the immune system. In experimental infections in animals in which interferon activity is neutralized by specific antibody, potentiation of viral infection occurs. In humans, in a number of infections, endogenous interferon developed in serum or secretions correlates with recovery: decreasing virus titers and amelioration of symptoms. Since administering interferon to humans produces a number of side effects, such as fever, leukopenia, and myalgias, interferon also may account, in part, for some of the systemic signs and symptoms that accompany viral infections.

Interferon-γ is induced as a result of immune stimulation. It also has antiviral effects and is a major immune regulatory protein that induces Tc, activates macrophages and NK cells, and regulates antibody production by B cells.

MECHANISMS OF PATHOGENESIS. Infection is initiated, often when one or a very few virus particles are deposited in the

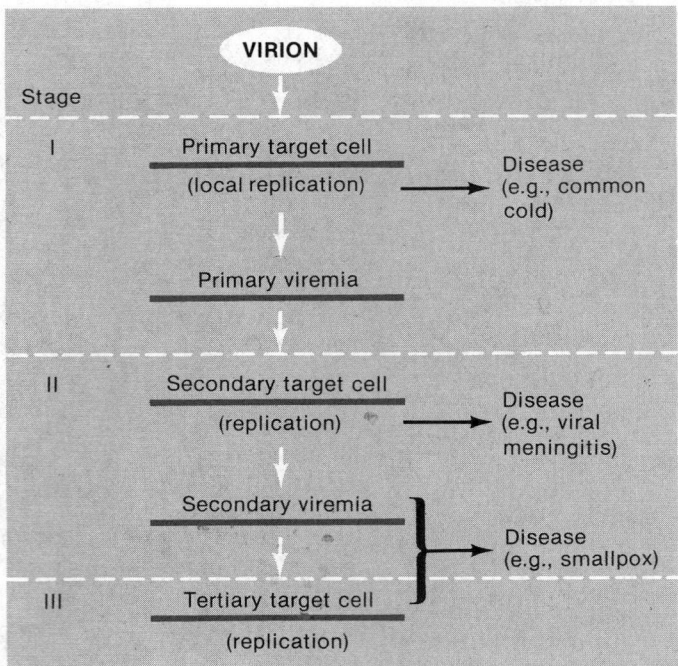

FIGURE 326-2. Stages of viral pathogenesis. Initial invasion may involve only primary target cells or may lead to secondary or tertiary target cell invasion, which results in the characteristic disease. (Courtesy of ED Kilbourne.)

TABLE 326–2. VIRUSES COMMONLY ASSOCIATED WITH DIFFERENT SYNDROMES

Disease Category	Common Associated Virus	Disease Category	Common Associated Virus
Respiratory Tract		*Gastrointestinal Tract*	
Upper respiratory infection (including common cold and pharyngitis)	Rhinoviruses Coronaviruses Parainfluenza 1–3 Influenza A, B Herpes simplex Adenoviruses Echoviruses Coxsackieviruses Epstein-Barr virus Respiratory syncytial	Gastroenteritis	Rotavirus Norwalk-like agents Adenovirus
		Hepatitis	Hepatitis A Hepatitis B Hepatitis C Hepatitis D Hepatitis E Epstein-Barr virus Cytomegalovirus
Croup	Parainfluenza 1–3 Influenza A, B Respiratory syncytial	*Skin*	
Bronchiolitis	Respiratory syncytial Parainfluenza 1–3	Maculopapular rash	Measles Rubella Parvovirus B19 Echoviruses Coxsackievirus A16 Enterovirus 71
Pneumonia (adults)	Influenza A	Hemorrhagic rash	Herpesvirus G Alphavirus Bunyavirus Flavivirus
Pneumonia (children)	Respiratory syncytial Parainfluenza 1–3 Influenza A	Localized lesions	Herpes simplex Human papillomavirus 1, 2, 4, 41 Molluscum contagiosum
Central Nervous System		*Neonatal*	
Aseptic meningitis	Mumps Coxsackievirus B1–5 Coxsackievirus A9 Echovirus 4, 6, 9, 11, 14, 18, 30, 31	Teratogenic effects	Rubella Cytomegalovirus
Paralysis	Polio 1–3	Disseminated disease	Coxsackievirus B1–5 Echoviruses Hepatitis B Parvovirus B19 Cytomegalovirus Herpes simplex
Encephalitis	Human immunodeficiency virus I Alphaviruses Flaviviruses Bunyaviruses Herpes simplex 1 Enterovirus 71 Mumps	Lower respiratory disease	Respiratory syncytial Influenza
Genitourinary Tract		Enteritis	Rotavirus
Vulvovaginitis, cervicitis	Herpes simplex 2	*Other*	
Penile and vulvar lesions	Herpes simplex 2 Molluscum contagiosum Human papillomavirus 6, 10, 11, 40–45, 51	Arthritis	Rubella Parvovirus B19 Hepatitis B
Acute hemorrhagic cystitis	Adenovirus 11	Myositis	Togaviruses Influenza B
Ocular		Carditis	Coxsackievirus B
Conjunctivitis	Adenovirus 3, 4, 7, 8, 19 Herpes simplex Varicella-zoster Measles	Parotitis, pancreatitis, and orchitis	Mumps
Acute hemorrhagic conjunctivitis	Enterovirus 70 Coxsackievirus A 24		
Immune System			
Acquired immunodeficiency syndrome	Human immunodeficiency virus I		

Modified from Manegus MA, Douglas RG Jr: Viruses, rickettsiae, chlamydiae, and mycoplasmas. *In* Mandell GL, Douglas RG, Jr, Bennett JE: Principles and Practice of Infectious Diseases, 3rd ed. New York, Churchill Livingstone, 1990.

respiratory, gastrointestinal, or genitourinary tract or are injected percutaneously or pass transplacentally. As shown in Figure 326–2, human viral infections may be classified according to mechanisms of pathogenesis. Many infections are limited to cells at the portal of entry, and dissemination does not occur. Conjunctivitis due to adenovirus type 8 and common colds due to rhinoviruses and to other respiratory viruses are excellent examples of this type of pathogenesis.

Other virus infections spread hematogenously to distal sites. Infection at the primary site may or may not result in symptoms, but viral replication in the distal site usually results in the characteristic illness associated with such a virus infection. Enteroviruses such as coxsackievirus and echovirus infect the gastrointestinal tract as their primary site, and this infection is usually clinically silent but produces a primary viremia, following which encephalitis, meningitis, or other central nervous system disease may occur as these tissues are infected. Other viruses reach target organs through nerves: rabies, varicella-zoster virus, and herpes simplex virus.

In other infections, viral replication in the secondary site pro-

duces a viremia that results in replication in still other sites. Such was the case with smallpox and may be the case with measles. Rash may be a manifestation of either primary or secondary viremia.

Many virus infections have clinical characteristics that permit diagnosis: measles, mumps, chickenpox, and poliomyelitis. However, many others do not, and many syndromes have multiple etiologies, as is shown in Table 326–2. In fact, as many as 200 serologically distinct viruses may cause the common cold and related disorders. In the case of some syndromes—for example, atypical pneumonia—the etiology may be shared with other infectious organisms: *Mycoplasma pneumoniae*, *Chlamydia pneumoniae*, and *Legionella pneumophila*. Others, however, are exclusively viral in etiology.

PREVENTION AND CONTROL. Recent advances in antiviral chemotherapy have produced a number of specific antivirals that are available and effective for prophylaxis or treatment, or both, of certain viral diseases. Drugs such as trifluridine, amantadine, ribavirin, acyclovir, vidarabine, zidovudine, ganciclovir, foscarnet, didanosine, zalcitabine, d4T, and interferon-α are available in the

United States. For many other viral infections, however, no specific therapy exists. Proper use of antivirals requires specific viral diagnosis. Fortunately, in the case of herpes zoster, the diagnosis can usually be made clinically, and in influenza, the diagnosis can often be made on clinical and epidemiologic grounds; however, for many infections, viral diagnosis is required. Viral diagnostic laboratories are more common than in the past, and rapid techniques are gaining acceptance.

Vaccines are available for a number of viral infections, and many have greatly affected morbidity and mortality due to specific infections. Antibodies induced by vaccination may block initiation of infection in a primary site, as in the case in influenza. Others, such as inactivated poliomyelitis vaccine, are designed to prevent primary viremia after initial infection has occurred. Live attenuated viruses induce cell-mediated as well as humoral immune response.

Fields BN, Knipe DM (eds.): Fields Virology, 2nd ed. New York, Raven Press, 1990. *Excellent definitive textbook of basic virology.*
Tyler UL, Fields BN: Introduction to viruses and viral diseases. *In* Mandell GL, Bennett JE, Dolin R (eds.): Principles and Practice of Infectious Diseases, 4th ed. New York, John Wiley & Sons, 1995. *Excellent detailed review of virus structure, virus-cell interactions, virus-host interactions, and virus transmission.*

327 ANTIVIRAL THERAPY (Non-AIDS)
Richard J. Whitley

Compared with the progress made in the treatment of bacterial infections over the past four decades, advances in the chemotherapy of viral diseases have come much more slowly. In the United States, only a few antiviral agents of proven clinical value are available and for a limited number of indications. The problems associated with the development of antiviral agents can be summarized as follows: (1) viruses are obligate intracellular parasites that use biochemical pathways of the infected host cell, so it is difficult to achieve clinically useful antiviral activity without also adversely affecting host cell metabolism; (2) early diagnosis of viral infection is crucial for effective antiviral therapy, yet by the time symptoms appear, several cycles of viral multiplication may have occurred and replication has begun to wane; (3) precise diagnosis is difficult for many viral infections because of the lack of specificity of symptoms; and (4) since many of the disease syndromes caused by viruses are common, relatively benign, and self-limiting, the therapeutic index (ratio of efficacy to toxicity) must be extremely high for therapy to be acceptable.

As with all infectious diseases, the effectiveness of therapy is related to host defenses. Not only is the incidence of reactivation of certain viral diseases high in the immunocompromised host, but these infections are often much more severe. These patients require high doses of antiviral agents for long periods of time and have a high morbidity and mortality with currently approved antiviral therapy.

ANTIVIRALS FOR HERPESVIRUS INFECTIONS
Acyclovir

MECHANISM OF ACTION. Acyclovir, 9-((2-hydroxyethoxy)methyl) guanine, is an acyclic analogue of guanosine. Virus-specified thymidine kinase phosphorylates acyclovir to its monophosphate derivative, an event that does not occur in uninfected cells to a significant extent. Acyclovir is then further phosphorylated by cellular enzymes to its triphosphate derivative. Acyclovir triphosphate binds viral DNA polymerase, acting as a DNA chain terminator. Because acyclovir is taken up selectively by virus-infected cells, the concentration of acyclovir triphosphate is 40 to 100 times higher in infected than in uninfected cells. Furthermore, viral DNA polymerase exhibits a 10- to 30-fold greater affinity for acyclovir triphosphate than does cellular DNA polymerases. The higher concentration in infected cells plus the affinity for viral poly-

merases results in the very low toxicity of acyclovir for normal host cells. Although Epstein-Barr virus (EBV) and cytomegalovirus (CMV) do not have virus-specific thymidine kinases, acyclovir does have minimal activity against these viruses.

LICENSED USES. Acyclovir is available in ointment, capsule, and intravenous formulations. In the topical form, acyclovir is licensed for managing primary herpes genitalis in both immunocompetent and immunocompromised hosts as well as in limited, non-life-threatening mucocutaneous herpes simplex virus (HSV) infections in immunocompromised hosts. It is less active topically than when delivered by other routes, and its use by this route should be discouraged.

Oral acyclovir is indicated in the management of most cases of primary or initial genital herpes in all patient populations and as suppressive therapy in normal hosts with frequently recurrent genital herpes (six or more recurrences a year). Oral acyclovir is also used as prophylaxis and treatment in immunocompromised patients with a history of HSV infections, e.g., herpes labialis or genital herpes. High-dose oral acyclovir (i.e., 800 mg five times per day) has recently been approved for use in immunocompetent patients with localized herpes zoster.

Intravenous acyclovir is indicated in severe initial herpes genitalis of immunocompetent patients and in the treatment of some initial and recurrent mucocutaneous infections in immunocompromised patients, as well as in the treatment of herpes simplex encephalitis (HSE). Intravenous acyclovir is approved for treatment of varicella-zoster virus (VZV) infections in immunocompromised hosts.

TOXICITY. Acyclovir has an excellent safety profile and is well tolerated. The major adverse effect of acyclovir is that it alters renal function. High-dose bolus injection of acyclovir can cause crystallization in renal tubules and subsequent acute tubular necrosis or simply a reversible elevation of serum creatinine. Dehydration, pre-existing renal insufficiency, and higher doses of acyclovir are risk factors for renal toxicity. Dosage alterations are required with renal impairment (Table 327–1). In addition, there have been a few brief reports suggesting central nervous system (CNS) toxicity after intravenous administration of acyclovir. Oral acyclovir has not been associated with renal toxicity, even when given in high doses (800 mg five times a day).

Because acyclovir is a nucleoside analogue that can be incorporated into both viral and host-cell DNA, it has been studied extensively for its potential as a carcinogen, teratogen, and mutagen. There is no significant evidence that acyclovir is a carcinogen in humans, and animal studies indicate that acyclovir is not a significant teratogen in clinically used doses. Acyclovir is not a significant mutagen *in vitro* but seems to be able to induce chromosomal events as does caffeine. Because of the many possible indications for acyclovir during pregnancy, as well as the likelihood of frequent first-trimester exposures to drug before pregnancy is established, it is extremely important to define its risk. An "Acyclovir in Pregnancy Registry" has been established to gather data on all reported prenatal exposures to oral acyclovir. Although no significant risk to the mother or fetus has been documented, the total number of monitored pregnancies remains too small to detect any risk that is not overwhelming. The safety of acyclovir in pregnancy, therefore, has not been unequivocally established. Since acyclovir crosses the placenta and can concentrate in amniotic fluid, there is valid concern about the potential for renal toxicity in the fetus.

RESISTANCE TO ACYCLOVIR. Resistance to acyclovir develops through mutations in one of two HSV genes, namely, those specifying viral thymidine kinase (TK) or DNA polymerase. Clinical isolates resistant to acyclovir are almost uniformly deficient in

TABLE 327–1. DOSAGE ADJUSTMENT FOR INTRAVENOUS ACYCLOVIR IN PATIENTS WITH IMPAIRED RENAL FUNCTION

Creatinine Clearance (ml/min/1.73 M²)	Percentage of Standard Dose	Dosing Interval (Hours)
>50	100	8
25–50	100	12
10–25	100	24
0–10*	50	24

* Administered after hemodialysis.

TK. Until recently, such resistance has been rare; all such mutants had reduced neurovirulence and did not readily establish latency. However, acyclovir-resistant HSV mutants are being reported more frequently in the immunocompromised patient population and in one normal host. These mutants are deficient in viral TK and sensitive to vidarabine and foscarnet, drugs that do not require viral TK for activation. Some isolates are fully neurovirulent and able to establish latency in a murine model. With the growing population of immunocompromised patients (due to both HIV infection and therapeutic immunosuppression) who suffer from frequent and severe herpesvirus infections, it is expected that acyclovir resistance will become more prevalent.

Ganciclovir

MECHANISM OF ACTION. Ganciclovir, also known as DHPG, is an acyclic nucleoside analogue of acyclovir that has increased *in vitro* activity against all herpesviruses as compared with acyclovir, including an 8 to 20 times greater antiviral activity against CMV. Like acyclovir, the activity of ganciclovir in HSV-infected cells depends on phosphorylation by virus-specific TK. Also like acyclovir, ganciclovir monophosphate is further converted to its di- and triphosphate derivatives by cellular kinases. In cells infected by HSV-1 or HSV-2, the triphosphate (DHPG-TP) competitively inhibits the incorporation of guanosine-TP into viral DNA and terminates chain synthesis. The mode of action of ganciclovir against CMV and EBV (which do not produce virus-specific TK) is not entirely known, but it has been suggested that these viruses may induce a cellular TK or viral kinase that efficiently promotes the obligatory initial phosphorylation of ganciclovir to its monophosphate.

LICENSED USES. Ganciclovir has been licensed by the United States Food and Drug Administration for treating CMV retinitis and life-threatening CMV diseases in AIDS and other immunocompromised patients.

TOXICITY. The most important side effects of ganciclovir are neutropenia and thrombocytopenia. Neutropenia occurs in approximately 35% of patients and is usually (but not always) reversible with dose adjustment or discontinuation. Thrombocytopenia occurs in about 20% of patients. Numerous other side effects possibly related to ganciclovir, such as nausea, vomiting, dizziness, and headache, are usually not of clinical significance. Agents with significant myelotoxicity, such as antimetabolites or alkylating agents, cannot be used concomitantly with ganciclovir. Zidovudine (azidothymidine, or AZT) may be used cautiously in low doses in patients receiving ganciclovir, but hematologic parameters must be monitored closely.

Ganciclovir also has significant gonadal toxicity in animal screening systems, most notably as a potent inhibitor of spermatogenesis. As an agent affecting DNA synthesis, ganciclovir has carcinogenic potential.

CLINICAL USE. Ganciclovir has been the most widely tested drug for the treatment of CMV infections. There is support for clinical benefit in immunocompromised patients with CMV retinitis and gastrointestinal infection. Benefit is suggested but has been less dramatic for CMV pneumonia in AIDS patients and organ transplant recipients. Ganciclovir has effectively suppressed the reactivation of CMV infections in organ transplant recipients.

Idoxuridine and Trifluorothymidine

Idoxuridine and trifluorothymidine are analogues of thymidine. When administered systemically, these nucleosides are phosphorylated by both viral and cellular TK to active triphosphorylate derivatives that inhibit both viral and cellular DNA synthesis. The result is antiviral activity but also sufficient host cytotoxicity to prevent the systemic use of these drugs. Toxicity of these compounds is not significant, however, when applied topically to the eye in the treatment of HSV keratitis. Both idoxuridine and trifluorothymidine, as well as vidarabine, ophthalmic ointments are effective and licensed for such treatment. Acyclovir as an ophthalmic preparation also appears to be effective but is not yet licensed. Trifluorothymidine appears to be the most efficacious of these compounds. Although these agents are not of proven value in the treatment of stromal keratitis and uveitis, trifluorothymidine is more likely to penetrate the cornea. Some forms of stromal keratitis and uveitis are thought to be caused by immune mechanisms and thus would not respond to antiviral drugs. The ophthalmic preparations of idoxuridine, vidara-

bine, and trifluorothymidine may cause local irritation, photophobia, edema of the eyelids and cornea, punctual occlusion, and superficial punctate keratopathy.

Vidarabine

Vidarabine has been shown to be effective when administered parenterally for HSE, neonatal herpes, and VZV infections in the immunocompromised host. Because of a lower therapeutic index than acyclovir, it is only available as an ophthalmic preparation for therapy of HSV keratitis.

Foscarnet

Foscarnet, a pyrophosphate analogue of phosphonoacetic acid, has potent *in vitro* and *in vivo* activity against herpesviruses. Foscarnet inhibits the DNA polymerase of all human herpesviruses by blocking the pyrophosphate binding site and preventing chain elongation. Unlike acyclovir, which requires activation by a virus-specific TK, foscarnet acts directly on the virus DNA polymerase. TK-deficient, acyclovir-resistant herpesviruses remain sensitive to foscarnet.

Foscarnet was recently approved for the treatment of CMV retinitis in HIV-infected patients. Data collected from the Soka clinical trial indicate the equal effectiveness of foscarnet and ganciclovir therapy of retinitis in this population. However, use of foscarnet in combination with zidovidine resulted in enhanced survival. These findings remain to be confirmed in a larger study population. Foscarnet has been used for induction therapy of retinitis as well as when ganciclovir is not tolerated. However, administration of foscarnet is not without toxicity. Renal toxicity has been documented as well as hypocalcemia and altered levels of serum magnesium. Foscarnet's lack of bone marrow toxicity offers an advantage over ganciclovir. Additionally, foscarnet also has been used to treat acyclovir-resistant herpes simplex genital disease.

ANTIVIRALS FOR RESPIRATORY VIRAL INFECTIONS

It is difficult to overestimate the impact of respiratory viral illnesses on human health. Almost 90% of the population experiences one of these illnesses each year, resulting in a staggering number of days lost from work and school, as well as significant potential for serious morbidity and even death. Nonetheless, since these conditions in most patient populations are self-limited and rarely fatal, the requirements for new drugs are stringent: an extreme degree of safety, moderate to high effectiveness, ease of administration, and low cost. Accordingly, only two such antivirals are approved for use in the United States, each with fairly limited indications. Because of the number of developmental programs identifying new antivirals for treatment of respiratory viruses, it seems likely that an expanded armamentarium will be forthcoming.

Amantadine and Rimantadine

MECHANISM OF ACTION. Amantadine and rimantadine have a narrow spectrum of activity and at concentrations achievable in humans are useful only against influenza A infections. Although amantadine was the first antiviral to be approved in the United States, its mechanism of action is not yet completely understood. Influenza A viruses differ in their susceptibility to amantadine, and the drug may have different actions depending on the concentration and virus strain. Early studies indicated that amantadine acted by preventing the penetration and/or uncoating the virus. More recently, low concentrations of the drug were shown to inhibit virus assembly by interacting with hemagglutinin; high concentrations appear to inhibit an early stage of the infection involving fusion between the virus envelope and the membrane of secondary lysosomes. Rimantidine has a similar mechanism of action.

LICENSED USES. As antiviral agents, amantadine and rimantidine are licensed for both the chemoprophylaxis and the treatment of influenza A infections. Both drugs can be used for any unimmunized member of the general population who wishes to avoid influenza A, but prophylaxis is especially recommended to control presumed influenza outbreaks in institutions housing high-risk persons. High-risk individuals include adults and children with chronic disorders of the cardiovascular or pulmonary systems requiring regular follow-up or hospitalization during the preceding year, as well as nursing homes and other chronic-care facilities residents. In these instances, drugs should be administered to all residents of the institution, whether or not they received influenza vaccination the previous fall. To reduce spread of virus and to minimize disruption of patient care, it is also recommended that amantadine prophylaxis be offered to unvaccinated staff who care for high-risk patients. Amantadine prophylaxis is also recommended in the following situations:

1. As an adjunct to late immunization of high-risk individuals. Amantadine does not interfere with antibody response to the vaccine.

2. For persons who have not been immunized and who care for high-risk persons in home settings, both to reduce spread of virus and to allow persons to maintain care for high-risk persons in the home setting.

3. For immunodeficient persons, who may be expected to have a poor antibody response to vaccine.

4. For persons for whom influenza vaccine is contraindicated, e.g., for persons hypersensitive to egg protein.

Both drugs are also indicated in the treatment of uncomplicated respiratory illness caused by influenza A. Studies have shown a beneficial effect on the signs and symptoms of acute influenza, as well as a significant reduction in quantity of virus in respiratory secretions. Because of the short duration of disease, amantadine must be administered within 48 hours of symptom onset to show benefit. The effect of amantadine on the prevention of complications in high-risk groups is under evaluation.

Rimantadine is a structural analogue of amantadine, with the same spectrum of activity, mechanism of action, and clinical indications. Rimantadine is somewhat more effective than amantadine against influenza type A viruses at equal concentrations. Absorption of rimantadine is delayed when compared with amantadine, and furthermore, equivalent doses of rimantadine produce lower plasma levels than does amantadine. The lower plasma levels may explain the lower incidence of side effects at similar doses. Rimantadine has similar CNS side effects even though, unlike amantadine, this drug does not affect CNS catecholamine release and is not effective in the treatment of Parkinson's disease. The efficacy of rimantadine in both the prophylaxis and treatment of influenza A infections is similar to that of amantadine. There has been a recent report of rimantadine-resistant strains of influenza isolated from patients treated for acute influenza A.

TOXICITY. Amantadine is reported to cause side effects in 5 to 10% of healthy young adults taking the standard adult dose of 200 mg per day. These side effects are usually mild, cease soon after amantadine is discontinued, and often disappear even with continued use of the drug. CNS side effects are most common and include difficulty in thinking, confusion, lightheadedness, hallucinations, anxiety, and insomnia. Activities requiring mental alertness (e.g., driving) should be avoided until it is reasonable to assume that these symptoms will not occur. More severe adverse effects, e.g., mental depression and psychosis, are usually associated with doses exceeding 200 mg daily. About 5% of patients complain of nausea, vomiting, or anorexia. Older individuals are more likely to experience side effects. Rimantidine appears to be somewhat better tolerated.

Patients with renal disease should receive doses based on their creatinine clearance (Table 327–2). Doses for older people and children are usually lower as well. Persons with an active seizure disorder may be at increased risk for seizures when amantadine is given at standard doses.

Ribavirin

MECHANISM OF ACTION. Ribavirin is a nucleoside analogue whose mechanisms of action are poorly understood and probably not the same for all viruses; however, its ability to alter nucleotide pools and the packaging of mRNA appears to be important. This process is not totally virus-specific, but there is a certain selectivity in that infected cells produce more mRNA than noninfected cells. The capacity of viral mRNA to support protein synthesis is markedly reduced by ribavirin. High concentrations also inhibit cellular protein synthesis.

LICENSED USES. The development of a mechanism to deliver ribavirin via a small-particle aerosol greatly enhanced the potential usefulness of this drug for respiratory viral infections. At this time ribavirin is licensed for the treatment, by aerosol administration, of carefully selected hospitalized infants and young children with severe lower respiratory tract infections caused by respiratory syncytial virus (RSV). The vast majority of infants and children with RSV infection have disease that is mild and self-limited and do not require ribavirin.

TOXICITY AND CLINICAL PROBLEMS. No adverse effect has been clearly attributable to aerosol therapy with ribavirin, although reports of adverse effects during or following therapy of infants with RSV have included bronchospasm, pulmonary function test changes, pneumothorax in ventilated patients, apnea, cardiac arrest, hypotension, and concomitant digitalis toxicity. Precipitation of drug within the ventilatory apparatus of patients on mechanical ventilation can be a serious problem. When proper precautions are taken, such as frequent changes in ventilator tubing, safe delivery of ribavirin to ventilated patients can be accomplished. Reticulocytosis, rash, and conjunctivitis have been associated with the use of ribavirin aerosol. Although there are no pertinent human data, ribavirin has been found to be teratogenic and mutagenic in nearly all species in which it has been tested. This drug is therefore contraindicated in women who are or may become pregnant. Some concern has been expressed about the risk to persons in the room with infants being treated with ribavirin aerosol, particularly females of childbearing age. Although this risk seems to be minimal with limited exposure, awareness and caution are warranted.

FUTURE ANTIVIRALS

Advances in molecular virology continue to define those sites of viral replication which may be vulnerable to attack without harm to the host cell. Further characterization of the viral DNA polymerase, required for replication but not used by the host cell, is a major research focus. In addition, classes of compounds, many of them nucleoside analogues, are being systematically evaluated in order to identify more efficacious and less toxic antivirals. A description of some of the most promising drugs follows.

Several compounds have activity against the herpesviruses, including 1-β-D-arabinofuranosyl-E-5-(2-bromovinyl) arabinosyluracil (BV-araU), fluoroidoarabinosyl cytosine (FIAC), valacyclovir, famciclovir, and (S)-1-((3-hydroxy-2-phosphonylmethoxy)propyl) cytosine (HPMPC).

Bromovinyl arabinosyl uracil, BV-araU, is a potent inhibitor of HSV-1 and EBV. More important, it is exquisitely active against VZV, being over 1000 times more potent than acyclovir. Like acyclovir, the mechanism of action of BV-araU is based on the phosphorylation of the parent compound by herpesvirus TK, which restricts its action to virus-infected cells. BV-araU appears to have a favorable toxicity profile and will soon begin clinical trials in the United States.

Valacyclovir is the prodrug of acyclovir. Plasma concentrations achieved with oral valacyclovir approximate that of 5 mg per kilogram of acyclovir administered intravenously. Controlled clinical studies indicate that valacyclovir is as good as acyclovir for both the treatment of herpes zoster in the normal host and recurrent genital HSV infections.

Famciclovir is the prodrug of penciclovir. Famciclovir has been administered orally to individuals with herpes zoster as well as genital HSV infection, both primary and recurrent etiology. For patients with shingles, famciclovir therapy is as good as, if not better than,

TABLE 327–2. DOSAGE ADJUSTMENT FOR ORAL AMANTADINE IN PATIENTS WITH IMPAIRED RENAL FUNCTION

Creatinine Clearance (ml/min/1.73 M²)	Suggested Oral Maintenance Regimen After 200 mg (100 mg bid) on the First Day
≥80	100 mg bid
60–80	100 mg bid alternating with 100 mg daily
40–60	100 mg daily
30–40	200 mg (100 mg bid) twice weekly
20–30	100 mg 3 times each week
10–20	200 mg (100 mg bid) alternating with 100 mg every 7 days
<10	100 mg every 7 days

acyclovir for managing infection. In the management of recurrent genital herpes, there appears to be accelerated healing of recurrent disease with episodic treatment. This drug was recently licensed for the treatment of shingles in the United Kingdom.

Fluoroiodoarabinosyl cytosine (FIAC) and fluoroiodoarabinosyl uracil (FIAU), its principal metabolite, are both potent selective inhibitors of herpesviruses. Like acyclovir and BV-araU, their activity depends on phosphorylation by herpesvirus TK. The parent compound is converted rapidly to the triphosphate in infected cells, selectively utilized by virus DNA polymerase, and incorporated into viral DNA, resulting in the formation of very short DNA chains. FIAU was proven to cause hepatic failure in patients with chronic hepatitis B infection.

HPMPC is a potent, broad-spectrum antiviral agent that is one of a new class of nucleotide analogues structurally characterized as phosphonylmethyl ethers of acyclic nucleoside derivatives. HPMPC has *in vitro* activity against HSV-1, HSV-2, CMV, VZV, EBV, adenovirus, and a retrovirus. The mechanism of action of HPMPC is thought to be similar to that of acyclovir, i.e., the triphosphate analogue inhibiting viral DNA polymerase. The difference, however, is that HPMPC is a monophosphate equivalent and does not require phosphorylation by a virus-specific TK, allowing HPMPC to have an expanded spectrum of activity. Of all of these compounds, HPMPC is emerging with the most clinical potential.

INTERFERONS

HISTORY AND INTRODUCTION. Interferons (IFN) are glycoprotein cytokines (intracellular messengers) with a complex array of immunomodulating, antineoplastic, and antiviral properties. The name *interferon* was derived from landmark experiments by Isaacs and Lindemann in 1957 demonstrating the existence of a biologic substance that "interfered" with viral replication in infected cells. Interferons are currently classified as α, β, or γ, with natural sources of these classes, in general, being leukocytes, fibroblasts, and lymphocytes, respectively. Each type of IFN can now be produced via recombinant DNA technology. The complexity of the response to IFN, including the variability of dose response, duration of therapy, and combination with other treatments, creates enormous challenges to determine appropriate clinical scenarios in which IFN might be a worthwhile therapeutic agent.

MECHANISM OF ACTION. Binding of IFN to the intact cell membrane is the first step in establishing an antiviral effect. Interferon binds to specific cell surface receptors; IFN-γ appears to have a different receptor from either IFN-α or β, which may explain the purported synergistic antiviral and antitumor effects sometimes observed when IFN-γ is given with either of the other two IFN species.

A prevalent view of IFN action is that following binding, there is synthesis of new cellular RNA's and proteins which mediate the antiviral effect. The antiviral state is not fully expressed until these primed cells are infected with virus. In addition to their antiviral effect, IFN's have a number of other biologic activities, including inhibition of cell proliferation and enhancement of the cytotoxic activities of lymphocytes, the expression of cell surface antigens, and the phagocytic and tumoricidal activities of macrophages. These properties may play an important role in the *in vivo* antiviral and antitumor effects of the IFN's.

LICENSED USES. Although promising for a number of viral infections and HIV-associated conditions, the only licensed use of IFN as an antiviral is its intralesional administration in the treatment of condyloma acuminatum, or genital warts, which are caused by human papillomaviruses, and therapy of chronic hepatitis B and C. Only IFN-α is licensed.

TOXICITY AND CLINICAL PROBLEMS. Side effects are frequent with IFN administration and are usually dose-limiting. Influenza-like symptoms, i.e., fever, chills, headache, and malaise, commonly occur, but these symptoms usually become less severe with repeated treatments. At doses used in the treatment of condyloma acuminatum, these side effects rarely cause termination of treatment and may be reduced in severity by pretreatment with acetaminophen. For local treatment (intralesional injection), pain at the injection site does not differ significantly from that in placebo-treated patients and is short-lived. Leukopenia is the most common hematologic abnormality, occurring in up to 26% of patients treated for condyloma. Leukopenia is usually modest, not clinically relevant, and reversible when therapy is discontinued. Increased alanine

aminotransferase levels also may occur, as well as nausea, vomiting, and diarrhea.

At higher doses of IFN, neurotoxicity is encountered, as manifested by personality changes, confusion, loss of attention, disorientation, and paranoid ideation. Early studies with IFN-γ show similar side effects as treatment with IFN-α and -β but with the additional side effects of dose-limiting hypotension and a marked increase in triglyceride levels.

CLINICAL TRIALS. IFN has potential use against virtually all viral infections. Its ultimate utility depends on a number of factors, including the acceptability of side effects, cost, and the availability of other antivirals. Of the many viral infections in which IFN has been tested, treatment of condyloma acuminatum, chronic hepatitis B, chronic hepatitis C, and recurrent respiratory papillomatosis and prophylaxis of rhinovirus and coronavirus upper respiratory infection have been promising.

Condyloma Acuminatum. Several large controlled trials have demonstrated the clinical benefit of IFN-α therapy of condyloma acuminatum. These studies have demonstrated clearance rates of treated lesions from 36 to 62%. Up to one-third of lesions treated with IFN recur. Much research remains to be done to examine the effects of different routes of administration, prolonged therapy, repeated courses of treatment, and combined treatment with other therapeutic modalities (i.e., cryotherapy podophyllin, and laser ablation).

Respiratory Papillomatosis. Recurrent respiratory papillomatosis is a disease in which squamous papillomata relentlessly recur within the larynx and trachea of both children and young adults. Standard management consists of careful microendoscopic excision, usually with a CO_2 laser. In recent years, there have been numerous case reports and uncontrolled studies supporting benefit from IFN as an adjunct to surgery. Results of placebo-controlled trials have suggested benefit.

Hepatitis. The inhibitory effect of human leukocyte IFN-α on hepatitis B virus (HBV) replication was first reported more than 10 years ago. Treatment with IFN-α in chronic hepatitis B subsequently has been investigated in several large, randomized, controlled trials. The earlier studies were encouraging, but the response rate was low at approximately 30%.

In an attempt to enhance the efficacy of antiviral therapy, combinations of IFN with other agents also have been studied. Vidarabine and acyclovir have been used in such studies with little success. It has been observed, however, that a short course of corticosteroids before treatment with IFN-α results in "immunologic rebound" after prednisone withdrawal. This phenomenon, which seems to be directed at virus-infected hepatocytes, is characterized by an acute hepatitis-like elevation of serum aminotransferases and a transient decline in levels of HBV DNA polymerase and HBV DNA. A large multicenter trial comparing patients randomly assigned to receive one of two doses of IFN-α versus prednisone followed by IFN-α or no treatment recently showed that a 4-month treatment regimen of subcutaneous IFN-α in a dose of 5 million units daily resulted in a complete response (loss of serum HBeAg and HBV DNA) in nearly 40% of patients and that reactivation of infection within 6 months after treatment was no greater than 2%. The beneficial effect of pretreatment with a tapering dose of prednisone was limited to patients with low baseline levels of alanine aminotransferase (<100 units per liter). The best predictor of response in this study was the HBV DNA level before treatment, with approximately half of the patients having levels <100 pg per milliliter experiencing a complete response. Long-term follow-up studies are required to determine the duration of antiviral effect and the impact on survival.

The efficacy IFN for treating chronic hepatitis C (non-A, non-B hepatitis) has been established. The first large, randomized, placebo-controlled study of IFN-α therapy in patients with chronic hepatitis C showed that the serum alanine aminotransferase levels declined to normal in 38% of patients treated with 3 million units of IFN-α for 6 months, compared with 4% of untreated patients. However, only 52% of the patients who initially responded to treatment remained in remission during 6 months of follow-up.

Respiratory Infections. The upper respiratory infection known as the "common cold" has a multitude of possible viral causes (see Ch. 328). It has been demonstrated that nasal spray or drops of IFN-α provide prophylaxis against the common cold caused by rhi-

TABLE 327-3. INDICATIONS FOR THE USE OF AVAILABLE ANTIVIRAL AGENTS

Indication	Antiviral Agent	Route	Dose	Comments
Respiratory syncytial virus infection (infants)	Ribavirin	Aerosol	Diluted in sterile water to a concentration of 20 mg/ml, then delivered via aerosol for 12–18 hrs/day for 3–7 days	Only for infants at high risk
Life- or sight-threatening CMV infections in immunocompromised hosts	Ganciclovir	IV	5.0 mg/kg q12h × 14 days	Maintenance therapy of 5.0 mg/kg/day recommended for AIDS patients. Leukopenia is a frequent complication; in bone marrow transplant patients with CMV pneumonia, CMV immune globulin may be a useful adjunct
	Foscarnet	IV		
Condyloma acuminatum	Interferon-α	Intralesional	1.0 million units injected into the base of each lesion, up to 3 times per week for 3 weeks	Flu-type symptoms may occur with administrations
Influenza A infection	Amantadine	Oral	Adults: 100–200 mg/day for 5–7 days Children ≤ 9 years: 4.4–8.8 mg/kg/day for 5–7 days not to exceed 150 mg/day	Normal person >65 years should receive 100 mg/day
Prophylaxis against influenza A virus infection	Amantadine	Oral	Adults: 100–200 mg/day Children ≤ 9 years: 4.4–8.8 mg/kg/day (not to exceed 150 mg/day)	Continued for the duration of the epidemic or for 2 weeks in conjunction with influenza vaccination (until vaccine-induced immunity develops); normal persons >65 years should receive 100 mg/day
	Rimantadine	Oral		
Herpes simplex virus (HSV) encephalitis	Acyclovir	IV	10 mg/kg (1 hour infusion) every 8 hours for 10–14 days	Morbidity and mortality are significantly lower in patients treated with acyclovir than with vidarabine
Neonatal herpes	Acyclovir	IV	10 mg/kg (1 hour infusion) every 8 hours for 10 days	Efficacy of vidarabine is established; vidarabine and acyclovir show equal efficacy
Mucocutaneous HSV in immunocompromised hosts	Acyclovir or	IV	250 mg/M² or 6.2 mg/kg (1 hour infusion) every 8 hours for 7 days	Choice of topical, oral, or intravenous preparation depends upon clinical severity and setting; topical acyclovir is appropriate only when it can be applied to all lesions; it does not affect untreated lesions or systemic symptoms
	Acyclovir or	Oral	400 mg 5 times/day for 10 days	
	Acyclovir	Topical	5% ointment; 4–6 applications/day for 7 days or until healed	Least desirable
Prophylaxis against mucocutaneous HSV during intense immunosuppression	Acyclovir or	Oral	200 mg 3–4 times/day	Oral therapy most convenient; lesions recur when therapy stops
	Acyclovir	IV	250 mg/M² every 8 hours or 5 mg/kg every 12 hours (1 hour infusion)	Lesions recur when therapy stops
Treatment of initial genital HSV infections	Acyclovir or	Oral	200 mg 5 times/day for 10 days	Drug of choice in most clinical settings; treatment has no effect on subsequent recurrence rates
	Acyclovir	IV	5 mg/kg (1 hour infusion) every 8 hours for 5–7 days	For patients requiring hospitalization or with neurologic or other visceral complications
Recurrent genital herpes	Acyclovir	Oral	200 mg 5 times/day for 5 days	No effect on subsequent recurrence rates; efficacy greater if used early in attack
Prophylaxis against frequently recurring genital herpes	Acyclovir	Oral	200 mg 3–5 times/day	Occasional "breaking through" attacks and/or asymptomatic virus shedding during treatment; re-evaluation every 6 months recommended
Treatment of HSV keratitis	Trifluorothymidine or	Topical	One drop of 0.1% ophthalmic solution every 2 hours while awake (up to 9 drops/day)	3% acyclovir ointment (ophthalmic) is equal or superior to idoxuridine, vidarabine, and trifluridine for treatment of HSV keratitis but is not available in the United States
	Vidarabine or	Topical	One-half-inch ribbon of 3% ophthalmic ointment 5 times/day	
	Idoxuridine	Topical	One-half-inch ribbon of 0.5% ophthalmic ointment 5 times/day	
Localized herpes zoster in immunocompetent hosts	Acyclovir	Oral	800 mg 5 times/day for 7–10 days	Shortens time to lesion healing, but not shown to decrease the incidence of postherpetic neuralgia
Chickenpox in immunocompromised hosts	Acyclovir or	IV	500 mg/M² (1 hour infusion) every 8 hours for 7 days	In the absence of comparative data, acyclovir is preferred because of its ease of administration and lower toxicity
	Vidarabine	IV	10 mg/kg/day (continuous infusion over 12 hours) for 5 days	
Treatment of severe localized or disseminated herpes zoster in immunocompromised hosts	Acyclovir or	IV	500 mg/M² or 12.4 mg/kg (1 hour infusion) every 8 hours for 5–7 days	Comparative trials in severe localized and disseminated herpes zoster are underway; pending results, acyclovir is preferred because of its ease of administration and lower toxicity
	Vidarabine	IV	10 mg/dg/day (continuous infusion over 12 hours) for 5–7 days	
Chronic hepatitis B	Interferon-α	SQ	10 × 10⁶ units tiw for 16 weeks or 5 × 10⁶ units daily for 16 weeks	Patients must have compensated liver disease
Chronic hepatitis C	Interferon-α	SQ	3 × 10⁶ units tiw for 24 weeks	Must have compensated liver disease

novirus or coronavirus infection. Although clinical benefit was demonstrated in these studies, administration of IFN-α for 2 to 3 weeks led to hemorrhage of nasal mucosa.

IMMUNOGLOBULIN THERAPY

Efficacy has been established for prophylactic immunoglobulin administration for several viral infections, but the use of immunoglobulin alone for therapy of established disease has not been proven unequivocally beneficial for any viral infection. Benefit has been shown for the administration of intravenous immunoglobulin or CMV hyperimmune globulin when combined with ganciclovir in the treatment of CMV pneumonia in bone marrow transplant recipients. Survival was increased to 52 to 79%, which is significantly better than that of historical controls treated with either agent alone.

Currently active areas of research include the efficacy of CMV hyperimmune globulin for prevention and treatment of disease in bone marrow, kidney, and heart transplant patients, and that of CMV monoclonal antibody in the treatment of established CMV disease in AIDS patients.

Although relatively few antiviral drugs are licensed for use at this time, there is significant interest in the development of antiviral compounds. Table 327–3 summarizes the use of currently available antivirals for indications other than therapy of HIV infections. Systematic approaches have revealed a number of promising new drugs and biologic agents in various stages of evaluation. A better understanding of the molecular biology of virus replication and pathogenesis should elucidate agents with enhanced virus-specific activity.

Buhles WC, Mastre BJ, Tinker AJ, et al.: Ganciclovir treatment of life- or sight-threatening cytomegalovirus infection: Experience in 314 immunocompromised patients. Rev Infect Dis 10:495, 1988. *Describes the clinical efficacy of ganciclovir when used to treat infections of the retina, gastrointestinal tract, and lungs.*
Couch R: Respiratory diseases. *In* Galasso G, Whitley R, Merigan T (eds.): Antiviral Agents and Viral Diseases of Man, 3rd ed. New York, Raven Press, 1990, pp 327–372. *This chapter contains a summary of the published work regarding the efficacy and toxicity of amantadine, rimantadine, and ribavirin for influenza and respiratory syncytial virus infections.*
Davis GL, Balart LA, Schiff ER, et al.: Treatment of chronic hepatitis C with recombinant interferon alfa. N Engl J Med 321:1501, 1989. *The first large, randomized, placebo-controlled trial of interferon therapy of chronic hepatitis C.*
Dorsky DI, Crumpacker CS: Drugs five years later: Acyclovir. Ann Intern Med 107:859, 1987. *A detailed analysis of the chemistry, antiviral activity, and clinical efficacy of acyclovir.*
Hayden FG, Belshe RB, Clover RD, et al.: Emergence and apparent transmission of rimantadine-resistant influenza A virus in families. N Engl J Med 321:1696, 1989. *Postexposure prophylaxis with rimantadine in families was not as effective as pre-exposure prophylaxis during community outbreaks.*
Hirsch MS, Kaplan JC: Antiviral Agents. *In* Fields BN, Knipe DM (eds.): Virology, 2nd ed. New York, Raven Press, 1990, pp 441–468. *A comprehensive text which includes a detailed analysis of antiviral therapy.*
Perillo RP, Schiff ER, Davis GL, et al.: A randomized, controlled trial of interferon alfa-2b alone and after prednisone withdrawal for the treatment of chronic hepatitis B. N Engl J Med 323:295, 1990. *A multicenter study of combination therapy for chronic hepatitis B.*
Reichman RC, Oakes D, Bonnez W, et al.: Treatment of condyloma acuminatum with three different interferons administered intralesionally. Ann Intern Med 108:675, 1988. *Intralesional injections of three different interferon preparations were found to be efficacious in the treatment of condyloma acuminatum.*
Reines ED, Gross PA: Antiviral agents. Med Clin North Am 72:691, 1988. *An excellent review of the principles and applications of antiviral chemotherapy.*

Viral Infections of the Respiratory Tract

328 THE COMMON COLD

J. Owen Hendley

DEFINITION. The common cold, also known as upper respiratory infection (URI) or acute coryza, is an acute, self-limited illness caused by a virus. Nasal symptoms including rhinorrhea and nasal obstruction are invariably present; sore/scratchy throat and/or cough may be present. Many myths surround the source of the virus causing colds. There are no normal viral flora of the respiratory tract in humans (two possible exceptions are human herpesvirus type 6 in saliva and adenovirus, which can be recovered from adenoid tissue of otherwise healthy children by co-cultivation with susceptible cells). In sharp contrast, luxuriant normal bacterial flora occur in the upper respiratory tract and mouth. Because viruses are not part of normal flora, the viruses that cause colds are not present in the host ready to be activated because "resistance" has been lowered by chilling, loss of sleep, or bad diet. Instead, the virus must be *passed* from another human in order to produce the cold.

ETIOLOGY. Colds are common because the viruses with few serotypes reinfect many times, and the viruses that infect an individual only once have multiple serotypes (Table 328–1). Rhinoviruses (*rhino* = "nose") cause 30 to 50% of colds in adults, and coronaviruses (*corona* = "crown") are responsible for 10 to 15%. Each of the other virus groups listed in Table 328–1 cause <5% of colds. Adults are susceptible to respiratory syncytial virus (RSV) and parainfluenza virus, but the illness in adults is usually a cold rather than the more severe involvement seen in infants. Some of the viruses that cause colds are characteristically associated with other syndromes. Influenza viruses cause febrile respiratory disease with lower tract involvement, adenoviruses cause pharyngoconjunctival fever or acute undifferentiated febrile illness, ECHO and other enteroviruses are an important cause of aseptic meningitis, and coxsackie A viruses cause herpangina.

EPIDEMIOLOGY AND TRANSMISSION. Colds are the most frequent disease of humans and the single most common cause of absenteeism from school and work. Frequency of colds varies with age. Even before widespread day care attendance, colds were particularly common in children younger than age 6. In the Cleveland family study in the 1950's, infants under age 1 had an average of 6.7 colds per year, 1- to 5-year-olds had 7.4 to 8.3 colds per year, and teenagers averaged about 4.5 colds per year. Mothers reported 4.5 colds and fathers 3.5 colds per year. The wider exposure to other preschoolers in day care has increased the frequency of colds in children under 6 even more. The number of colds in adults may

TABLE 328–1. IMMUNITY TO COMMON COLD VIRUSES

a. **Solid immunity not produced by infection (repeated infection with same serotype usual)**

Virus	No. of serotypes
Respiratory syncytial virus	1
Parainfluenza virus	4
Coronavirus	4

b. **Immunity produced by infection (reinfection with same serotype uncommon)**

Virus	No. of serotypes
Rhinovirus	>100
Adenovirus	≥33
Influenza	3 (type A subtypes change)
Echovirus	31
Coxsackie virus	
Group A	23
Group B	6

From Hendley JO: Immunology of viral colds. *In* Veldman JE, McCabe BF, Huizing EH, Mygind N (eds.): Immunobiology, Autoimmunity, Transplantation in Otorhinolaryngology. Amsterdam, Kugler Publications, 1985, pp 257–260.

increase for several years because of exposure to young children, which highlights the fact that children commonly introduce new viruses to their families. At least with rhinovirus, the home setting is the primary site for viral transmission. Co-workers in an insurance company office with simultaneous rhinovirus colds usually were infected with different serotypes of virus, but each worker's serotype was found in his/her family contacts.

In temperate climates, colds are epidemic in the winter months (Fig. 328–1). The epidemic starts with a sharp rise in frequency in September after children have returned to school; the incidence then remains at an almost constant level until spring. This epidemic curve is produced by successive waves of different viruses moving through the community. Although rhinovirus infections occur year-round, the epidemic is initiated by a sharp rise of rhinovirus infections in early fall. Parainfluenza viruses move through in October and November, followed by RSV and coronaviruses in winter months. Influenza viruses appear later in winter, then rhinovirus has a resurgence in spring. Summer colds are usually caused by rhinovirus or one of the enteroviruses. The wave of each virus moving through is not sharp, and many times two or three viruses may be overlapping. Adenovirus and parainfluenza virus type 3 contribute to the burden of illness throughout the epidemic.

Determinants of this yearly epidemic of colds are not established but certainly include human behavior, with more virus transmitted

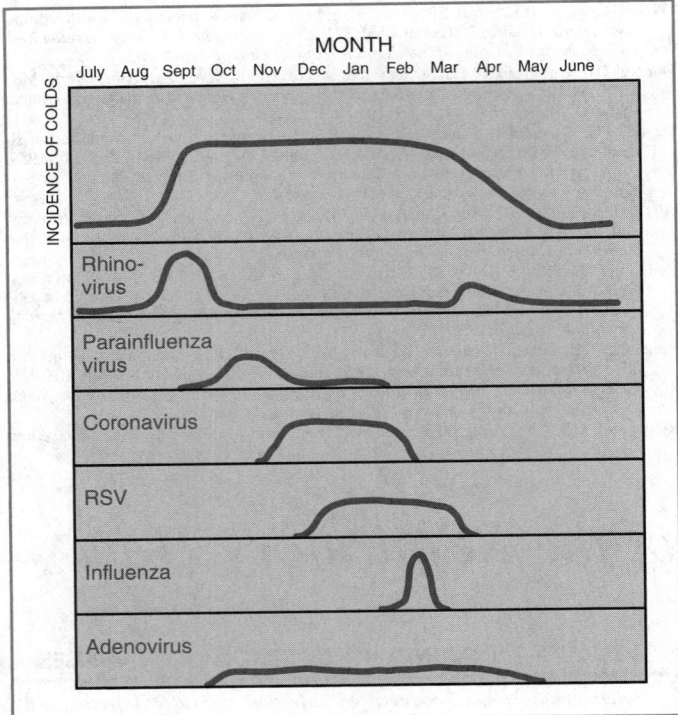

FIGURE 328-1. Schematic diagram of the incidence of colds and frequency of the causative viruses.

by higher indoor contact in colder months. Another determinant might be attributes of the viruses. Enveloped viruses, including RSV, parainfluenza virus, influenza virus, and coronavirus, may survive outside the host for longer periods in winter when the relative humidity of indoor (but not outdoor) air is very low.

Transmission of viruses causing colds could occur by one or more of three mechanisms: (1) small-particle ($<5\ \mu$ in diameter) aerosol in which virus may be suspended in air for an hour and infect by inhalation, (2) large-particle ($>10\ \mu$ in diameter) airborne droplets that travel <1 m and infect by landing on a mucosal surface such as conjunctiva or nasal mucosa, and (3) direct transfer of virus in secretions via hand contact from a person with a cold to a well person, who inoculates the virus onto his/her own conjunctival or nasal mucosa. Oral inoculation of rhinovirus or RSV does not result in infection, presumably because the stratified squamous epithelium of the mouth and oropharynx is not susceptible. The transmission route under natural conditions in the home has not been definitely established for any of the viruses. However, the importance of spread of colds in the home favors direct contact and/or large-droplet spread as being most likely. Influenza virus clearly can be transmitted by small-particle aerosol in some circumstances.

PATHOGENESIS. It had been assumed until recently that the symptoms of colds were produced by a viral cytopathic effect destroying the nasal mucosa. However, a recent study found that the histologic appearance of the nasal mucosa in biopsies taken during natural colds could not be distinguished from biopsies taken 2 weeks after illness except for an increased number of polymorphonuclear leukocytes (PMN's) during illness. The unexpected infiltration of PMN's in the nose in uncomplicated colds was confirmed in another study; the number of PMN's in nasal secretions increased coincidently when symptoms appeared in experimentally induced rhinovirus colds. Rhinovirus and coronavirus, in contrast to influenza virus and adenovirus, were not found to be destructive of nasal epithelium in organ cultures *in vitro*. Since mucosal damage by the virus during colds does not adequately explain the symptoms, the hypothesis that the viral infection of the nose triggers a cascade of inflammatory mediators that results in the symptoms is being explored. Support for this hypothesis was provided in volunteers with experimentally induced rhinovirus colds. Kinins (primarily bradykinin) and PMN's appeared in nasal secretions of infected volunteers at the time that they became ill, and their presence paralleled cold symptoms. Kinins sprayed into the noses of uninfected volunteers can reproduce many of the symptoms of a cold. Additional work on this hypothesis, with a focus on cytokines, is needed. How viral infection of the nose initiates the events leading to an influx of kinins, PMN's, and (possibly) cytokines into the nose and whether the sequence can be interrupted are of current research interest. However, the concept that it might be possible to ablate cold symptoms by blocking the mediators of the host response without having to kill the virus is exciting.

CLINICAL MANIFESTATIONS. The clinical manifestations of colds, which are familiar to all, are predominately subjective. In adults, rhinorrhea, nasal obstruction, and scratchy/sore throat are usually noted. The rhinorrhea is usually clear early in illness and may become white or yellow-green. Some malaise and nonproductive cough are common; sneezing is noted in some colds. Other common symptoms include sinus fullness and a "nasal" quality to the voice. Hoarseness is sometimes present. Objective findings in an adult with a cold are usually minimal. The nasal mucosa may be red but not to a degree that differs from normal. Mild erythema of the pharynx and redness around the external nares from nose blowing may be noted. Fever ($>38°C$) is uncommon in a cold in an adult; the presence of fever would suggest influenza or a bacterial complication of the cold. The symptoms of the cold usually abate in 5 to 7 days.

Colds in infants and children may be associated with more objective signs than in adults. In addition to rhinorrhea and nasal obstruction, moderate enlargement of the anterior cervical lymph nodes is frequent. Fever during the first 2 to 3 days of a cold in young children is not unusual, even when the child's parent or older sibling does not have an elevated temperature during the cold due to the same virus. In contrast to adults, the usual duration of cold symptoms in children is 10 to 14 days.

DIAGNOSIS. Self-diagnosis of a cold by the patient is usually accurate. Laboratory tests including white blood cell count and differential are not helpful. Sloughed ciliated cells may be present, and PMN's would be expected in nasal secretions during viral colds. The differential diagnosis of a cold includes an intranasal foreign body in a child and allergic or vasomotor rhinitis in adults and children. Examination of the nose should exclude a foreign body; the chronicity of symptoms with allergic or vasomotor rhinitis should differentiate these conditions from an acute cold.

Etiologic (virologic) diagnosis of a cold can be attempted by inoculation of a sample of nasal secretions into tissue cell cultures, but this is rarely needed or useful. Rhinoviruses can be grown in human embryonic lung fibroblast cultures; detection of rhinovirus using the polymerase chain reaction may soon be available. Coronaviruses cannot be detected accurately in cell cultures. Most coronavirus infections have been diagnosed by serologic titer rise in acute/convalescent paired sera. RSV in nasal secretions can be reliably detected by commercially available rapid tests. Influenza and parainfluenza viruses are usually grown in primary rhesus monkey kidney cell culture, and adenoviruses will grow in human embryonic kidney cells.

TREATMENT. Given the self-limited nature of colds, any treatment should be completely safe. Antibiotics have no place in therapy of uncomplicated colds, since they neither hasten nor delay recovery from the cold, nor do they reduce the frequency of bacterial complications.

Since the subjective symptoms of a cold disappear in 7 days without intervention, a variety of actually ineffective treatments have been reported to be effective due to inadequate blinding of placebo recipients. One example of this phenomenon was a study of large doses of vitamin C to prevent colds, in which many placebo recipients dropped out of the study because they could tell by tasting the medication that they were not receiving the vitamin C. Another example was the use of zinc gluconate lozenges as an antiviral treatment for colds. In the blinded trial, the only appropriate placebo that could be found to match the noxious taste of the zinc was denatonium benzoate, which is so bitter that it has been painted on the thumbs of children to discourage them from thumb-sucking.

No antivirals are currently available for treating colds. Individual symptoms may be treated. Malaise may be relieved by analgesics (e.g., aspirin, acetaminophen, ibuprofen). Nasal congestion may be relieved by decongestants by mouth (pseudoephedrine 60 mg, three times a day) or by topical application (oxymetazoline 0.05%, two sprays to each nostril twice daily). The benefit of oral antihistamines in colds remains controversial.

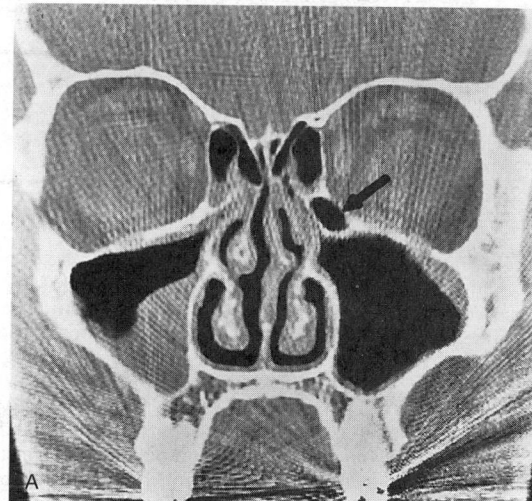 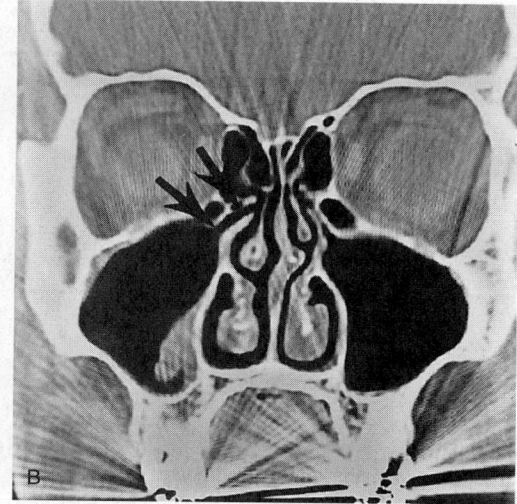

FIGURE 328–2. Sinus CT scan of adult during symptomatic cold *(left panel)* and 2 weeks later *(right panel)*. Arrow in the left panel denotes an infraorbital air cell (Haller cell). Bilateral abnormalities were observed in the ethmoid and maxillary sinuses during the cold, with an air-fluid interface in the right maxillary sinus. Two weeks later, all abnormalities had cleared except for a residual density in the right maxillary sinus. The infundibulum *(two arrows)* draining the maxillary antrum was now open. (Courtesy of Dr. Jack M. Gwaltney, Jr., Department of Internal Medicine, University of Virginia School of Medicine, Charlottesville, Virginia).

COMPLICATIONS. Secondary bacterial infection may complicate viral colds. The most common is bacterial suppurative otitis media, which occurs in some 5% of colds in preschool-aged children. Otitis media may be heralded by a secondary fever with associated ear pain. Bacterial sinusitis is estimated to occur in 0.5% of colds, primarily in adults. Sinusitis would be suggested by the presence of fever and/or facial pain (see Ch. 64). Bacterial pneumonia is thought to complicate colds, but it is very uncommon.

Clinical differentiation between primary viral and secondary bacterial infection of the respiratory tract is a challenge, since respiratory viruses may involve the middle ear or paranasal sinuses in the absence of bacterial infection. Tympanocentesis or maxillary sinus puncture provides definitive information on viral versus bacterial infection, but these are too invasive for routine use. Coronal computed tomographic (CT) scan is an accurate noninvasive method for imaging the paranasal sinuses. Recent work using CT scans has demonstrated that abnormalities in the sinuses may occur in colds not complicated by secondary bacterial infection. Coronal CT scans in 27 (87%) of 31 young adults during uncomplicated colds had abnormalities in one or more sinuses (Fig. 328–2). In 11 (79%) of the 14 subjects who had repeat scans 2 weeks later, the abnormalities had cleared or were markedly improved without antibiotic therapy.

An important complication of viral colds occurs in adults and children with underlying reactive airways disease or asthma. Wheezing occurs in 30 to 50% of episodes of viral colds in prospective studies of patients with asthma. Colds in these patients produce a large burden of illness, since up to 50% of asthma exacerbations in children and up to 20% of exacerbations in adults have been associated with an identified virus.

PREVENTION. Vaccine(s) to prevent common colds are unlikely to be useful given the multiplicity of immunotypes of some of the viruses and the lack of solid immunity to reinfection with the other viruses (see Table 328–1). Prophylaxis with topical interferon applied intranasally for 5 days after one family member appears with a cold has been shown to be moderately effective in preventing other family members from acquiring a cold, particularly colds due to rhinovirus. The practicality of this preventive approach may be argued, particularly in view of the fact that prolonged use of intranasal interferon is complicated by alteration or damage of the nasal mucosa.

Probably the only practical, albeit imperfect, means of preventing colds available is to prevent virus from reaching the nasal or conjunctival mucosa by way of one's own hands. If transmission occurs by inhalation of airborne small particles or by adherence of large droplets to a mucosal surface, infection is inevitable for those who enjoy contact with other humans. However, if transmission occurs by self-inoculation with virus on contaminated fingertips, the simple measure of ridding the fingers of viable virus before touching one's eye or nose might be helpful. The virus can be removed physically by rinsing the hands. Applying a virucide to the hands might be another approach.

Gwaltney JM Jr, Phillips CD, Miller RD, et al.: Computed tomographic study of the common cold. N Engl J Med 330:25, 1994. *Sinus CT scans during naturally acquired common colds demonstrated that one or more of the sinuses was abnormal in more than 80% of subjects. Most abnormalities had cleared on repeat scan after the cold was over.*

Hendley JO, Gwaltney JM Jr: Mechanism of transmission of rhinovirus infections. Epidemiol Rev 10:242, 1988. *Review of the various modes of transmission of rhinovirus common colds.*

Naclerio RM, Proud D, Lichtenstein LM, et al.: Kinins are generated during experimental rhinovirus colds. J Infect Dis 157:133, 1988. *Kinins, albumin, and PMN's appeared in nasal secretions of infected volunteers around the time they became ill but did not appear in secretions of subjects infected but not ill. Histamine in secretions did not correlate with illness.*

Pattemore PK, Johnston SL, Bardin PG: Viruses as precipitants of asthma symptoms: I. Epidemiology. Clin Exp Allergy 22:325, 1992. *Review of evidence incriminating viral respiratory infections as common precipitants of wheezing. Rhinovirus and RSV were most commonly associated with episodes of wheezing, but all respiratory viruses have been found.*

Winther B, Gwaltney JM, Hendley JO: Respiratory virus infection of monolayer cultures of human nasal epithelial cells. Am Rev Respir Dis 141:839, 1990. *Growth of rhinovirus and coronavirus in nasal epithelial cells produced no visible destruction of the epithelial layer, whereas influenza and adenovirus produced obvious disruption.*

329 VIRAL PHARYNGITIS, LARYNGITIS, CROUP, AND BRONCHITIS

Maurice A. Mufson

DEFINITION. Viral infections that localize to the upper and middle respiratory passages produce an acute inflammatory response and, depending on the anatomic site involved, evoke the clinical manifestations of pharyngitis, laryngitis, croup (laryngotracheobronchitis), and bronchitis. These infections do not ordinarily involve the pulmonary alveoli. Pharyngitis, laryngitis, and bronchi-

TABLE 329-1. VIRUSES THAT CAUSE PHARYNGITIS, LARYNGITIS, CROUP, AND BRONCHITIS

Virus	Serotype
Influenza	Types A, B
Parainfluenza	Types 1, 2, 3
Respiratory syncytial	Subgroups A, B1, B2
Adenovirus	Types 1, 2, 3, 4, 5, 6, 7 (also others)
Coronavirus	Types 229E, OC43 (also others)
Rhinovirus	Most or all of more than 100 serotypes
Enterovirus	At least some of more than 75 serotypes
Herpes simplex	Type 1

TABLE 329-3. EPIDEMIOLOGY OF VIRUSES THAT CAUSE PHARYNGITIS, LARYNGITIS, CROUP, AND BRONCHITIS

Epidemic	Endemic	Sporadic
Parainfluenza 1*	Parainfluenza 3	Parainfluenza 2
Influenza A†	Adenovirus	Herpes simplex
Influenza B	Coronavirus	
Respiratory syncytial‡	Rhinovirus	
	Enterovirus	

* Alternate years, usually.
† Epidemic and pandemic.
‡ Annual epidemics.

tis can occur in persons of any age. Croup occurs exclusively in children and mainly during the second year of life. Usually these illnesses begin abruptly with predominant upper respiratory tract signs and symptoms and limited systemic findings. The uncomplicated illness abates after 5 to 10 days.

ETIOLOGY. The major viral pathogens of the respiratory tract that can cause pharyngitis, laryngitis, croup, and bronchitis include members of the myxoviruses (influenza, parainfluenza, and respiratory syncytial viruses), adenoviruses, coronaviruses, picornaviruses (rhinoviruses and enteroviruses), and herpesviruses (Table 329-1). However, they differ in their propensity to cause these illnesses (Table 329-2). An etiologic diagnosis requires either isolation of virus or detection of viral antigen or demonstration of a rise in antibody during convalescence.

Pharyngitis also can occur as part of systemic viral illnesses associated with *Epstein-Barr virus* (see Ch. 341) or *cytomegalovirus* (see Ch. 340) infection, and laryngitis and bronchitis occur in *measles* virus infection (see Ch. 334). When coryza represents the main feature of an upper respiratory infection, the term "common cold" (see Ch. 328) prevails. When the infecting virus is an influenza virus, the designation *influenza* describes an acute respiratory tract infection with fever and prostration (see Ch. 332).

INCIDENCE AND PREVALENCE. Most children and adults experience three to five viral infections of the upper respiratory tract each year. In infants and children, croup is a serious illness that peaks in the second year of life, as high as 47 cases per 1000 children per year, and by age 4 to 5 it declines to under 15 cases per 1000 children per year.

EPIDEMIOLOGY. Viral pharyngitis, laryngitis, croup, and bronchitis occur during all months of the year, with peaks of occurrence paralleling epidemics of individual viruses. Respiratory syncytial virus, influenza A and B viruses, and parainfluenza virus type 1 occur in epidemics, mainly in the late fall, winter, and spring (see

TABLE 329-2. RELATIVE IMPORTANCE OF VIRUSES CAUSING PHARYNGITIS, LARYNGITIS, CROUP, AND BRONCHITIS

Virus	Pharyngitis	Laryngitis	Croup	Bronchitis
Influenza A	+ + + +	+ + + +	+	+ + + +
B	+ +	+ +		+ +
Parainfluenza 1	+ +	+ +	+ + + +	+ +
2	+	+	+ + +	+
3	+ +	+ +	+ + + +	+ +
Respiratory syncytial	+		+	+ + +
Adenovirus	+ + + +	+ +		+ +
Coronavirus	+	+		+ + +
Rhinovirus	+ + + +	+		+
Enterovirus	+			
Herpes simplex	+ +		±	+

* Graded from minimal (+) to major (+ + + +) importance; blank means unlikely occurrence; and ± means rare occurrence.

Table 329-3). The other viral pathogens occur endemically or sporadically. Virus infections of the respiratory tract spread by direct person-to-person contact, by infectious aerosols, or by fomites.

CLINICAL MANIFESTATIONS. *Viral Pharyngitis.* Acute viral pharyngitis is characterized by a scratchy and sore throat, but pain upon swallowing is not a prominent or constant feature. Dysphagia occurs infrequently in viral pharyngitis. Cough is not a feature of acute viral pharyngitis. Fever and malaise accompany influenza and adenovirus infections, but these findings are infrequent with the other respiratory viral pathogens. Pharyngeal erythema and edema and enlarged and tender lymph nodes may be the only physical findings. Adenovirus pharyngitis may be associated with conjunctivitis. Exudative tonsillitis occurs in adenovirus infections, infectious mononucleosis associated with Epstein-Barr virus infection, herpetic pharyngitis (with or without vesicles or small ulcers), as well as streptococcal pharyngitis. Exudative tonsillitis alone does not distinguish these infections. Bronchospasm occurs as a feature of herpes tracheobronchitis in elderly persons.

Viral Laryngitis. In acute viral laryngitis, hoarseness predominates, associated with difficulty in talking, pain on clearing respiratory secretions, and often fever, depending on the infecting virus. Cough and pharyngitis may be present. The larynx is erythematous and edematous, and the regional lymph nodes are slightly enlarged and tender. Wheezes may be audible upon auscultation.

Viral Croup. The clinical picture of croup characteristically includes inspiratory stridor, hoarseness, and a brassy cough. This distinctive triad of symptoms reflects the acute and intense edema and mucoid exudative secretions of the larynx and associated obstruction of the subglottic portion of the upper airway. These symptoms develop acutely, accompanied by fever, cough, tachypnea, and wheezing. Retractions of the chest wall occur. Hemoptysis does not occur. Rhonchi, rales, or wheezes, alone or in combination, may be audible upon auscultation of the lungs. Radiographic examination of the neck can demonstrate subglottic narrowing, and a chest roentgenogram may show hyperinflation of the lungs. In the uncomplicated case, the findings resolve in several days, but some children develop respiratory failure and pneumonia. Children who previously experienced multiple episodes of croup manifest hyperreactive airways several years later.

Viral Bronchitis. In acute viral bronchitis, cough, with or without sputum production, and fever are the main features. The sputum is slightly mucoid or watery and white. Other common symptoms include hoarseness, nonpleuritic substernal chest pain, and malaise. Rhonchi or rales may be heard upon auscultation of the chest. The chest roentgenogram may show increased intensity of the vascular pattern, but pulmonary infiltrates do not occur. Acute bronchitis associated with influenza or coronavirus infection occurs often as an exacerbation of chronic bronchitis.

TREATMENT AND PROGNOSIS. Viral pharyngitis, laryngitis, and bronchitis are self-limited illnesses and not severe, except for herpes tracheobronchitis infections. The symptoms of these illnesses should be treated with analgesics, fluids, and rest. Persistent cough can be treated with suppressant preparations. Antibiotics are not indicated, except when secondary bacterial infection occurs; it is likely to develop mainly with influenza virus infections. In pharyngitis, pharyngeal pain or dysphagia should be treated with analgesics and fluids.

The less serious cases of croup can be managed by having the child rest in bed at home. Vaporizers that produce a mist of moist air may be beneficial. Children with severe croup require hospitalization, supportive treatment, and constant monitoring for the devel-

TABLE 329–4. ANTIVIRAL DRUG THERAPY OF VIRUSES THAT CAUSE PHARYNGITIS, LARYNGITIS, CROUP, AND BRONCHITIS

Virus	Drug	Dose (Duration)	Route
Influenza A	Amantadine*	200 mg daily (7–10 days)	Oral
	Rimantidine*	200 mg daily‡ (7–10 days)	Oral
Respiratory syncytial	Ribavirin	20 mg/ml solution (12–18 hours)	Aerosol
Herpes simplex†	Acyclovir	8 mg/kg q8hr (7–10 days)	IV

* More commonly used for prophylaxis at same daily dose over longer periods of time until the virus leaves the community.

† Herpes simplex tracheobronchitis treated with IV acyclovir.

‡ In patients with hepatic dysfunction or renal failure and elderly nursing home residents, the dose for treatment and for prophylaxis is 100 mg daily.

opment of respiratory distress. If hypoxemia develops, oxygen therapy is essential; hypoxemia requiring oxygen can develop therapy even before cyanosis becomes evident. Subglottic edema may be reduced by the administration of racemic epinephrine. Administration of corticosteroids in the treatment of croup may have limited benefit. Antiviral drug therapy is available for influenza A, respiratory syncytial, and herpes simplex viruses (Table 329–4). Ribavirin lessens the severity of serious respiratory syncytial virus infection in the infant and child. Herpes tracheobronchitis responds to treatment with acyclovir. Influenza virus vaccine must be administered to persons in the high-risk group (unless contraindicated) to diminish the chance of infection (see Ch. 10).

Avila MM, Carballal G, Rovaletti H, et al.: Viral etiology in acute lower respiratory tract infections in children from a closed community. Am Rev Respir Dis 140:634, 1989. *One fifth of 94 children with bronchitis had virus infections; respiratory syncytial virus and adenoviruses were the most common.*

Houvinen P, Lahtonen R, Ziegler T, et al.: Pharyngitis in adults: The presence of coexistence of viruses and bacterial organisms. Ann Intern Med 110:612, 1989. *About one fourth of 106 adults with pharyngitis had virus infections; respiratory syncytial and influenza A viruses were most common.*

Inglis AF Jr: Herpes simplex virus infection: A rare case of prolonged croup. Arch Otolaryngol Head Neck Surg 49:551, 1993. *Croup due to herpes simplex type 1 in two children with 3- to 4-week illness; one child treated with acyclovir had a prompt response.*

Mufson MA, Åkerlind-Stopner B, Örvell C, et al.: A single season epidemic with respiratory syncytial virus subgroup B2 during 10 epidemic years, 1978 to 1988. J Clin Microbiol 29:162, 1991. *Annual winter-spring epidemics of respiratory syncytial virus. Subgroup A predominated. One third to one half of infections were limited to the upper respiratory tract.*

330 RESPIRATORY SYNCYTIAL VIRUS

Edward E. Walsh

DEFINITION. Respiratory syncytial virus (RSV), first identified in 1957, causes yearly outbreaks of respiratory illness during the fall, winter, and early spring. It is the single most important cause of bronchiolitis and pneumonia in young infants and is a common etiology of upper respiratory symptoms in older children and young adults. In addition, RSV is increasingly recognized as a cause of serious acute respiratory infection in the elderly. The name comes from the giant syncytial cells produced when it is grown in tissue culture.

ETIOLOGY. RSV is an enveloped virus of the family Paramyxoviridae, genus *Pneumovirus*. The single-stranded negative-polarity RNA encodes 10 proteins, of which 8 are found in purified virions. Two surface glycoproteins (G, attachment protein; F, fusion protein) protrude from a lipid bilayer encompassing three nucleocapsid proteins (N, P, polymerase) complexed with the genome. At least two additional proteins (M, 22K) are associated with the viral envelope. Neutralizing antibodies are directed at F and G glycoproteins, while F, N, and 22K are targets for cytotoxic T cells. Two major strains (A and B) are distinguishable, characterized by antigenically divergent G proteins and highly conserved F proteins. The closely related animal RSV strains (bovine, ovine, caprine) cause significant illness in farm animals but no human disease.

EPIDEMIOLOGY. Uniquely among respiratory viruses, worldwide RSV outbreaks occur annually. Epidemics generally begin in late fall, lasting until early spring. In the United States, RSV causes approximately 90,000 hospitalizations and accounts for 60% of bronchiolitis and 25% of pneumonia cases in infants. In the first year of life, over half of all infants become infected, with the remainder infected the following year. Family studies suggest that school children introduce RSV into the home with subsequent spread to parents and younger siblings, with infection rates of 43% and 62%, respectively. The virus readily infects infants and staff of day care centers, with attack rates approaching 100% for children below age 1. Like rhinovirus (see Ch. 328), RSV is transmitted principally by direct contact with large-particle fomites from respiratory secretions, in sharp contrast to the mode of spread of influenza virus, aerosolization. Direct inoculation of virus into the nose or eye by the hand appears to be the principal mode of spread. Since a virus survives for hours on hard surfaces and shorter times on clothing, inanimate objects also may play a role in transmission.

Approximately 0.5% of infected infants require hospitalization, but underlying prematurity, congenital cardiac abnormalities, bronchopulmonary dysplasia, and immunosuppression significantly increase the risk of serious disease. Lower socioeconomic status and being male also adversely influence severity. Hospitalization is most frequent between the ages of 1 to 6 months, with a median age of 2 months. Maternally derived antibody appears to protect in the first month of life when serious lower respiratory symptoms are infrequent, but this benefit is rather brief. Nosocomial spread of RSV on pediatric wards is a significant problem. Up to 32% of infants admitted to pediatric floors during the RSV season become infected while in the hospital. Infection among medical staff reaches 40%, and they probably serve as vectors for transmission to other infants. Careful attention to appropriate infection-control measures can reduce nosocomial transmission. Reinfection occurs frequently throughout life, although illness is less severe and hospitalization infrequent. However, older infants with serious underlying cardiac or pulmonary conditions, such as cystic fibrosis, may require inpatient care. Although primarily considered a pediatric disease, RSV infection in adults over age 65 may be serious and require hospitalization. Nursing home outbreaks are not uncommon. Both RSV strains usually co-circulate during outbreaks, although A strains usually dominate and may be associated with worse disease. Evidence suggests that strain variation alone does not solely account for reinfections. Partial immunity to RSV develops over time, as indicated by the resistance to both infection and illness. Clinical and experimental evidence indicates that neutralizing serum antibody diminishes the severity of illness, while mucosal IgA antibody reduces infection rates. Laboratory correlates of cell-mediated immunity can be identified; however, their role in illness and infection is unclear. The virus spreads from nasal epithelium to the lower respiratory tract, infecting the epithelium of small bronchioles; allergic mediators such as IgE, histamine, and leukotrienes also may contribute to the clinical symptoms.

CLINICAL MANIFESTATIONS. Following an incubation period of 3 days, the majority of previously uninfected infants develop signs and symptoms of upper respiratory infection. Asymptomatic primary RSV infection is considered rare. Conjunctival injection, copious mucopurulent nasal discharge, cough, and low-grade fever (38°C) are typical and indistinguishable from other respiratory infections. Otitis media occurs commonly, and RSV has been isolated from middle ear effusions, generally in association with bacteria. After several days, lower respiratory tract symptoms develop in 25 to 50% of infants. Cough, wheezing, increased respiratory rate, accessory muscle use, nasal flaring, intercostal retractions, and cyanosis are seen as the disease progresses. Expiratory wheezes, rhonchi, and fine rales are the most common findings on lung examination. With lower respiratory symptoms, arterial oxygen desaturation is universal, and hypercarbia and acidosis are ominous findings, suggesting impending respiratory failure. Ventilatory support is required in approximately 8% of hospitalized infants and is disproportionately high among infants with underlying cardiopulmonary disorders. Mortality for otherwise healthy children is about 1% but can reach 37% in infants with cardiac disorders.

Hyperinflation and diffuse interstitial pneumonitis are the most frequent radiographic findings. Infiltrates are usually diffuse, but consolidation is seen in up to one quarter. Although tachypnea is a universal respiratory pattern, sudden and irregular apneic spells can occur, especially in younger infants. RSV-induced apnea has been implicated in some cases of sudden infant death syndrome.

The usual hospital stay is 3 to 5 days, but the most severely ill infants may remain confined for several weeks. Virus is shed from respiratory secretions for 7 to 10 days, although immunocompromised infants (i.e., those with HIV infection) may excrete virus for considerably longer. Interestingly, clinical symptoms may not correlate with prolonged shedding. Co-infection with other viruses, such as influenza, adenovirus, parainfluenza, and enteroviruses, is not uncommon but is usually not clinically discernible. Bacterial superinfection may develop, with *Streptococcus pneumoniae* and *Haemophilus influenzae* being the most frequent organisms isolated. Treatment with antibiotics is indicated when bacterial superinfection develops. Clinical findings in primary RSV infection above age 1 are similar to those in younger infants but, in general, are milder. Long-term sequelae of lower respiratory tract infection include development of childhood asthma, although the precise contributions of RSV infection and allergic predisposition are unknown.

Longitudinal studies indicate that reinfection occurs in up to 75% of previously infected infants between the ages of 1 and 2 years. Reinfections are less severe than primary infection, and upper respiratory symptoms typically dominate, with the exception of infants with recurrent wheezing episodes. Adults are not spared reinfections and typically manifest nasal discharge, pharyngitis, and low-grade fever. Virus is shed for an average of 3 days. The very elderly with RSV infection may develop cough, dyspnea, fever, wheezing, and, in rare cases, respiratory failure. Analogous to the young infant, elderly patients with underlying chronic pulmonary and cardiac disease are most subject to severe disease and may require hospital care.

DIAGNOSIS. In the outpatient setting, a presumptive diagnosis is often suggested by typical symptoms occurring during the epidemic season, especially if RSV is known to be circulating in the community. However, since the clinical picture of RSV is often indistinguishable from illness caused by other infectious agents of respiratory disease, laboratory confirmation of RSV infection is required, especially if antiviral therapy is contemplated. Facilities for virus culture, immunofluorescence (IF) and enzyme immunoassay (EIA), are required for optimal speed and diagnostic accuracy. RSV is readily grown from respiratory secretions on HEp-2, human diploid fibroblast, and HELA cell lines. The sensitivity of viral culture varies with the method of collection and transport and the individual laboratory but is 100% specific when RSV is isolated. RSV is relatively labile, and samples should be kept at 4°C until placed on cell lines, preferably immediately. The characteristic giant cell cytopathic effect develops on average in 4 days but may require 10 days. Rapid diagnostic tests rely on detecting viral antigen in respiratory secretions. IF is the most widely used test and has a sensitivity of about 80%, while commercial EIA is less sensitive and less specific than IF. Serologic diagnosis can be made using a variety of highly sensitive methods but is not useful in immediate diagnosis.

THERAPY AND PREVENTION. Therapy for hospitalized infants includes hydration, oxygen, bronchodilators, and specific antiviral medication. Severely ill infants are commonly dehydrated and require intravenous fluid. Supplemental oxygen, administered as a humidified mist, should be given to all infants with hypoxia. The value of brochodilators for the treatment of wheezing is controversial, since most studies have not demonstrated clear benefit, but a trial of inhaled bronchodilators is probably indicated, especially in older infants. Specific antiviral therapy is currently limited to inhaled ribavirin (1-β-D-ribafuranosyl-1,2,4-triazole-3-carboxamide), a nucleoside analogue with activity against a number of RNA viruses. Ribavirin is administered via aerosol, typically for 4 hours three times a day for 3 to 5 days, although longer therapy has been used. Placebo-controlled clinical trials demonstrate more rapid resolution of respiratory symptoms and hypoxia and are associated with diminished virus shedding. Ribavirin treatment is indicated for infants at high risk of serious disease (congenital heart disease, bronchopulmonary dysplasia, prematurity, and immunodeficiency), those who

are severely ill, and infants who require mechanical ventilation. Although short- or long-term toxicity of ribavirin has not been recognized, hospital personnel and family members of patients should minimize exposure to the drug because of possible long-term side effects. It is recommended that pregnant health care workers avoid exposure altogether. Adhering to standard infection-control principles (e.g., gloves, gowns, and frequent handwashing) can substantially reduce nosocomial spread. RSV is inactivated by common detergents, soaps, and dilute bleach solutions. Thus far, efforts to control RSV infection by immunization with killed and live virus vaccines have been unsuccessful.

Collins PL: The molecular biology of human respiratory syncytial virus (RSV) of the genus pneumovirus. *In* Kingsbury D (ed.): The Paramyxoviruses. New York, Plenum Press, 1991, pp 103–162. *Provides a detailed overview of the molecular genetics and structure of RSV.*

Committee on Infectious Diseases: Use of ribavirin in the treatment on respiratory syncytial virus infection. Pediatrics 92:501, 1993. *Recommendations by clinical virology experts on appropriate use of aerosolized ribavirin.*

Falsey AR, Treanor JJ, Betts RF, Walsh EE: Viral respiratory infection in the institutionalized elderly: Clinical and epidemiologic findings. J Am Geriatr Soc 40:115, 1992. *This prospective study of respiratory illness in a long-term care facility describes clinical features of RSV infection in the elderly with comparison with other viral pathogens.*

331 PARAINFLUENZA VIRAL DISEASE
Edward E. Walsh

DEFINITION. Parainfluenza viruses are important causes of a wide spectrum of respiratory illness in infants and young children, producing syndromes ranging from the common cold and otitis media to severe croup, bronchiolitis, and pneumonia. In older children and adults, illness is usually limited to the upper respiratory tract, although immunocompromised individuals may develop fatal respiratory failure.

ETIOLOGY. The parainfluenza viruses are enveloped single-stranded nonsegmented RNA viruses and belong to the family Paramyxoviridae, which also includes measles, mumps, and respiratory syncytial viruses. The genome encodes for six structural proteins, of which the hemagglutinin-neuraminidase (HN) and fusion proteins (F) are exposed on the bilayered lipid envelope that surrounds a helical nucleocapsid-RNA complex. The two surface proteins, which mediate attachment and penetration of the virus into susceptible mammalian cells, have retained antigenic stability for over 30 years, unlike the influenza virus hemagglutinin protein.

There are four distinct serotypes of human parainfluenza viruses, types 1 through 4, with two subgroups (A and B) of type 1 and 4 viruses. In addition, numerous animal strains of parainfluenza viruses exist, including Sendai virus, which infects mice; SV5, which causes respiratory illness in dogs; and shipping fever virus of cattle and Newcastle disease virus of chickens, important causes of lost income for the livestock industry. These viruses do not cause human illness.

EPIDEMIOLOGY. The parainfluenza viruses are ubiquitous and have worldwide geographic distribution, as determined by both virus recovery and serologic studies. Spread principally by large-particle fomites and close person-to-person contact, each of the four serotypes displays somewhat different epidemiologic features, although none is so uniquely characteristic as to allow definitive diagnosis.

Over the years, parainfluenza type 1 activity has displayed both endemic and epidemic patterns (Table 331–1). Primary infection with parainfluenza viruses begins soon after birth, with each serotype favoring different age groups and causing distinct clinical syndromes. Significant overlap exists in this regard, thus precluding specific diagnosis based on clinical and epidemiologic grounds. Among the parainfluenza viruses, type 3 infects infants first, with over 50% showing serologic evidence of infection in the first year of life. Parainfluenza virus type 3 is second only to respiratory syncytial virus (RSV) as a cause of bronchiolitis and pneumonia in this youngest age group. Parainfluenza virus type 1 and type 2 infections occur later, with specific antibody developing slowly from

TABLE 331–1. PARAINFLUENZA PATTERNS

Type	Manifestation	Season	Comments
1	Epidemic croup	Fall of odd-number years	Since 1970
2	Epidemic croup	Fall or early winter	Less predictable than type 1; less widespread
3	Endemic epidemic bronchitis and pneumonia	Late winter, early spring	Recently epidemic, often following influenza season; low levels of virus year-round
4	Unknown	?	Mild illness; frequently unrecognized

ages 2 through 6. The peak incidence of infection, manifested principally as croup, occurs between ages 1 and 2. Virtually all adults have serologic evidence of infection with each of the serotypes. The lower infection rate with parainfluenza type 1 and 2 viruses in very young infants suggests that maternally derived antibody is protective, in contrast to parainfluenza virus type 3 infection, in which maternal antibody has only limited benefit. Following primary infection, a relatively brief period of immunity against homotypic reinfection develops, mediated principally by serum IgG and mucosal IgA. The fact that reinfections are common later in childhood highlights the lack of durable immunity. Although both genders are equally susceptible to infection with the parainfluenza virus, males manifest more severe illness.

CLINICAL MANIFESTATIONS. Illness associated with primary parainfluenza virus infection varies by age and the virus serotype, although substantial overlap occurs. Underlying medical conditions, such as cardiopulmonary or immune disorders, also will influence the severity of disease. In general, parainfluenza virus types 1 and 2 are associated with croup, while parainfluenza virus type 3 causes bronchiolitis and pneumonia. However, because of the greater frequency of parainfluenza virus type 3 infections, it is a more important cause of croup than is type 2 parainfluenza. Other causes of croup include influenza A and RSV.

Infection typically starts with upper respiratory signs and symptoms, notably coryza, rhinorrhea, pharyngitis without cervical adenopathy, and fever. If croup evolves, the child then develops a raspy, barking cough with notable inspiratory stridor, dyspnea, and respiratory distress. These latter symptoms, which may be spasmodic, are due to subglottic inflammation and edema. Typically, in mild to moderate illness symptoms last 3 to 5 days but may be quite unpredictable and result in sudden respiratory failure. In hospitalized infants, hypoxia is universal, and hypercarbia is present in half. Although imperfect as a guide, respiratory rate best correlates with the degree of hypoxemia. In severe stridor, differentiation from epiglottis due to *Haemophilus influenzae* type b (see Ch. 282) may be suggested by lateral neck radiography, which can show subglottic edema and narrowing, in contrast to epiglottic swelling.

Although also a cause of croup, parainfluenza virus type 3 more commonly causes disease indistinguishable from RSV: tracheobronchitis, bronchiolitis, and pneumonia. Cough, rales, and wheezing associated with hypoxia and air trapping on radiography are common. Although virus infection of the lower airway directly contributes to symptoms, parainfluenza virus–specific IgE is found frequently in respiratory secretions in infants who wheeze.

Reinfection with the parainfluenza viruses is less severe and typically causes cold symptoms, although nursing home outbreaks with a high incidence of pneumonia have been reported. More recently, reinfection with parainfluenza virus has been implicated in severe pneumonia in immunocompromised children and adults. In a large series of bone marrow transplant recipients, 27 parainfluenza virus infections caused 6 deaths due to respiratory failure.

DIAGNOSIS. Although the clinician may suspect parainfluenza virus based on clinical and epidemiologic grounds, specific diagnosis requires isolating the virus or detecting viral antigen in respiratory secretions. Monkey kidney or human embryonic kidney cell cultures are optimal for virus recovery. Although parainfluenza virus types 1 and 3 do not produce cytopathic effect in cell culture, in contrast to syncytial giant cells caused by type 2 virus, they can generally be detected by hemadsorption with guinea pig red blood cells by day 10 of culture. Parainfluenza virus type 4 grows more slowly, often requiring up to 3 weeks in culture. Specific serologic tests are also useful to diagnose both primary and reinfections.

THERAPY AND PREVENTION. Specific antiviral treatment

for parainfluenza virus is currently unavailable. Aerosolized ribavirin, approved for use in RSV infection, has *in vitro* activity against the parainfluenza viruses. Reports of ribavirin therapy of immunocompromised children and adults with severe parainfluenza virus pneumonia suggest possible benefit.

Treatment of croup, under usual circumstances, includes mist and supplemental oxygen. Aerosolized bronchodilators (racemic epinephrine) have definite but only transient benefit, while steroid use is controversial. Antibiotics are indicated only when bacterial superinfection is documented, an uncommon occurrence. Vaccination to prevent parainfluenza virus infection is under development.

Chanock RM, McIntosh K: Parainfluenza viruses. *In* Fields BN, Knipe DM (eds.): Fields Virology, 2nd ed. New York, Raven Press, 1990, pp 963–988. *Reviews the molecular biology, genetics, clinical diseases, and therapy for parainfluenza viruses.*
Denny FW, Murphy TF, Clyde WA, et al.: Croup: An 11-year study in a pediatric practice. Pediatrics 71:871, 1983. *Describes the viruses which account for 360 cases of croup in a single outpatient pediatric practice from 1964 to 1975.*
Welliver R, Wong DT, Choi T-S, Ogra PL: Natural history of parainfluenza virus infection in childhood. J Pediatr 101:180, 1982. *Describes immune response to parainfluenza virus infection in 130 infants, with correlation to protection from reinfection.*
Wendt CH, Weisdorf DJ, Jordan MC, et al.: Parainfluenza virus respiratory infection after bone marrow transplantation. N Engl J Med 326:921, 1992. *Clinical and therapeutic description of parainfluenza virus infection in bone marrow transplant recipients.*

332 INFLUENZA
Frederick G. Hayden

Influenza is an acute febrile respiratory illness that occurs in annual outbreaks of varying severity. The causative virus infects the respiratory tract, is highly contagious, and typically produces prominent systemic symptoms early in the illness. Influenza virus infection can produce various clinical syndromes in adults, including common colds, pharyngitis, tracheobronchitis, and pneumonia. Conversely, infections with other respiratory viruses, such as respiratory syncytial virus (RSV) or adenovirus, may produce influenzal illness. Influenza A viruses can cause worldwide epidemics (pandemics) and have done so four times this century (Table 332–1). The pandemic of 1918–1919 caused at least 500,000 deaths in the

TABLE 332–1. ANTIGENIC SUBTYPES OF INFLUENZA A VIRUS ASSOCIATED WITH PANDEMIC INFLUENZA

Year	Interval (Years)	Designation	Extent of Antigenic Change in Indicated Surface Protein*	Severity of Pandemic
1870	—	H2N8?	?	Moderate
1889	19	H3N8?	H+++N?	Severe
1918	29	H1N1†	H+++N+++	Very severe
1957	39	H2N2	H+++N+++	Severe
1968	11	H3N2	H+++N−	Moderate‡
1977	9	H1N1	H+++N+++	Mild§

* Compared with antecedent or co-circulating virus: + = minor change; ++ = moderate change; +++ = major change; − = no change.
† Formerly designated as H0N1 (swine virus prototype) or Hsw1N1.
‡ Population had some immunity to the N2 neuraminidase.
§ Most of population immune due to prior infection with earlier circulating identical virus.

TABLE 332-2. INFLUENZA VIRUS PROTEINS

Designation	Location (Approximate No. per Virion)	Function	Other
Hemagglutinin (HA)	Surface (500)	Cell attachment and penetration; fusion of virus and cell membranes	Subtype- and strain-specific antigens
Neuraminidase (NA)	Surface (100)	Virus release; enzymatic activity	Subtype- and strain-specific antigens
Membrane or M1 matrix	Internal (3000)	Major structural envelope protein; virus assembly	Type-specific antigen
M2 matrix	Surface (20–60)	Virus uncoating and assembly; ion channel	Site of action of amantadine/rimantadine
Nucleoprotein (NP)	Internal (1000)	Associated with RNA and polymerase proteins	Type-specific antigen
Polymerases (PB1, PB2, PA)	Internal (30–60)	RNA replication and transcription	Probable site of action of ribavirin
NS1, NS2	Nonstructural (infected cells)	Uncertain, regulation of virus replication	

Adapted from Murphy BR, Webster RG: Orthomyxoviruses. *In* Fields BN, Knipe DM (eds.): Fields Virology, 2nd ed. New York, Raven Press, 1990, p 1095.

United States and over 20 million worldwide. Influenza epidemics are associated with enormous morbidity, economic loss, and often substantial mortality. Excess deaths due to influenza average over 10,000 persons per epidemic in the United States.

ETIOLOGY. Influenza viruses belong to the family Orthomyxoviridae and are divided into three types (A, B, and C) distinguished by the antigenicity of their internal and external proteins (Table 332–2). The virion (Fig. 332–1) is a medium-sized enveloped pleomorphic particle covered with two types of surface glycoprotein spikes, the hemagglutinin (H or HA) and neuraminidase (N or NA). The envelope is composed of a lipid bilayer overlying the matrix

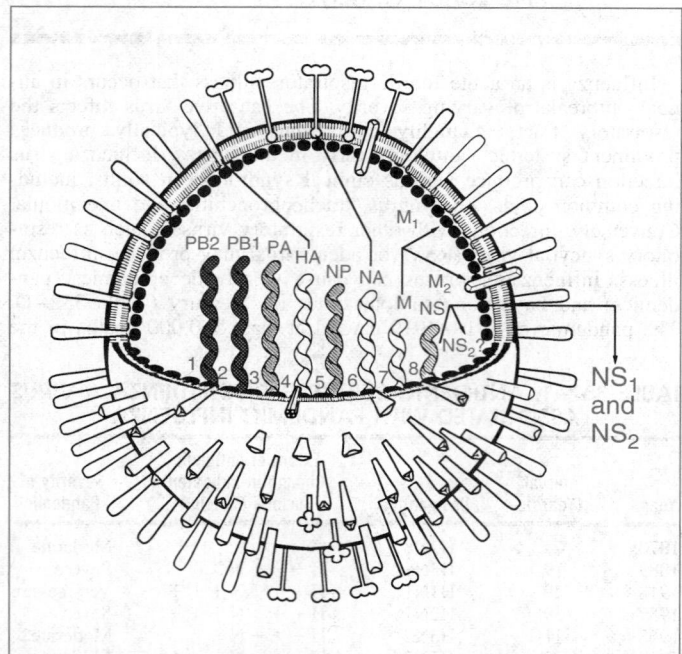

FIGURE 332–1. Diagram of influenza virus structure. Eight segments of viral RNA are contained within the envelope and matrix (M1) shell. Each codes for one or two proteins that form the virus or regulate its intracellular replication. The presumed functions of each are listed in Table 332–2. (Courtesy of Dr. Robert G. Webster.)

(M1) protein that surrounds the segmented viral genome. The genome comprises eight segments of single-stranded RNA. Influenza C viruses have seven segments and only a single surface glycoprotein. Whereas influenza B and C viruses are principally human pathogens, influenza A viruses infect diverse animal species, including birds, horses, swine, and marine mammals. Influenza A viruses are further classified into subtypes based on their HA and NA glycoproteins. As of this writing, three hemagglutinins (H1, H2, and H3) and two neuraminidases (N1 and N2) have been recognized in human influenza A viruses. Each strain within a subtype is identified by site, number, and year of isolation.

EPIDEMIOLOGY. *Antigenic Variation.* Influenza viruses are unique among the respiratory viruses with regard to their extent of antigenic variation, epidemic behavior, and association with excess mortality during community outbreaks. The changing antigenicity of the surface glycoproteins accounts in part for the continuing epidemics of influenza in humans. Antibody to the HA neutralizes viral infectivity and thus is the major determinant of immunity. Anti-NA antibody is not neutralizing but limits viral replication and therefore the severity of infection. Variation involves either relatively minor (antigenic drift) or major (antigenic shift) changes in antigenicity. Significant antigenic variation is much less frequent with influenza B than with influenza A and may not occur with influenza C.

Antigenic drift refers to small changes that occur frequently (every year or every few years) within an influenza A or B virus. For example, the original H3N2 variant, A/Aichi/68, has undergone successive drifts resulting in epidemic strains that include the recent circulation of A/Beijing/32/92(H3N2)-like viruses. Antigenic drift results from an accumulation of point mutations in the RNA segment coding for the HA that cause amino acid substitutions in at least one of five antigenic sites on the HA. Immunologic selection favors the new variant over the old for transmission because of the less frequent presence of antibody in the population to the new virus.

Antigenic shift results from the appearance of an influenza A virus with HA or NA (or both) glycoproteins new to humans or possible reappearance of virus after decades of absence. Because of the high level of immunity to the old strain and lack of immunity to the new strain within the human population, a virulent new strain can cause pandemic disease (see Table 332–1). Infection by one subtype does not provide cross-protection against another. The origin of new pandemic strains and the basis for their apparent recirculation remain incompletely defined. Reassortment of gene segments may occur when two influenza viruses simultaneously infect a single cell. The finding of 14 H and 9 N subtypes in animal influenza A viruses has lead to the hypothesis that viruses in nature, particularly those infecting birds, serve as the reservoir of new genes for human pandemic strains.

Epidemic or Interpandemic Influenza. An "epidemic" is an outbreak of influenza confined to one geographic location. In a given community, epidemics of influenza A virus infection have a characteristic pattern. They usually begin rather abruptly, reach a sharp peak in 2 or 3 weeks, and last 6 to 10 weeks. Increased numbers of school children with febrile respiratory illness is often the first indication of influenza in a community. This is soon followed by illnesses among adults and about a week later by increased hospital admissions of patients with influenza-related complications. Hospitalization rates in high-risk persons increase two- to fivefold during major epidemics (Table 332–3). School and employment absenteeism increases, as does mortality from pneumonia and influenza, especially in older persons (see Table 332–3). The latter finding is a highly specific indicator of influenza activity.

Epidemics occur almost exclusively during the winter months. In temperate areas, it is rare to recover influenza virus during nonepidemic periods. However, in the tropics, influenza activity may continue year-round. Regional differences in the time of occurrence of influenza outbreaks are common, and major outbreaks may occur in some communities or regions while others are experiencing no activity whatsoever. During epidemics, the overall attack rates typically average 10 to 20%. Attack rates of 40 to 50% are not uncommon in closed populations, including hospital and nursing homes, and in certain highly susceptible age groups. In recent years it has been recognized that two different strains within a single subtype, two different influenza A subtypes (H1N1 and H3N2), or both influenza A and B viruses may co-circulate. In addition, simultaneous outbreaks of influenza A and RSV have been found. Strains circu-

Age (years)	Physician Visits per 100	ARD Hospitalizations per 10,000	P + I Mortality per 100,000
<5	28	43	3
5–14	14	5	1
15–44	10	8	1
45–54	9	13	10
55–64	10	21	10
≥65	—	73	104

ARDS = acute respiratory disease; P + I = pneumonia and influenza; − = not stated.

Adapted from Glezen WP: Anatomy of an urban influenza epidemic. In Hannoun C, Kendal AP, Klenk HD, et al. (eds.): Options for the Control of Influenza II. Amsterdam, Elsevier Science, 1993, p 12.

lating at the end of one season's epidemic are likely to be responsible for the next season's outbreak (the so-called herald wave phenomenon). Furthermore, other than the association of influenza outbreaks with colder seasons, the factors are unknown that allow an epidemic to develop or those responsible for the tapering off of an epidemic, when only some susceptible persons have been infected.

Pneumonia and influenza (P + I) deaths predictably fluctuate annually, with peaks in the winter months. When such P + I deaths exceed the predicted number, this is due to influenza A or occasionally to influenza B virus or RSV activity. Although mortality is greatest during pandemics, substantial total mortality occurs with epidemics. Over 80% of P + I deaths occur among persons aged 65 and older (see Table 332–3). Other cardiopulmonary and chronic diseases also show increased mortality following influenza epidemics.

Pandemic Influenza. Pandemics of influenza A result from the emergence of a new virus to which the population contains no or limited immunity so that epidemics of influenza progress to involve all parts of the world (see Table 332–1). The pandemics of 1957, 1968, and 1977 all began in mainland China, and Southeast Asia has been postulated to be the epicenter for such strains. The interval between pandemics is variable and unpredictable. The most severe pandemics have resulted when there were major antigenic alterations in both the major surface antigens. Furthermore, it appears that intrinsic virulence is a virus-coded function that also varies among strains. The intrinsic virulence of recent H1N1 viruses appears to be milder than that of H3N2 viruses. After one or more waves of pandemic influenza, the level of immunity in the population increases. Such a chain of events provides a setting for emergence of a variant showing antigenic drift, since the level of immunity to it is less than that to the original strain. Repeated epidemics caused by strains showing antigenic drift within the subtype occur in subsequent years. After 10 to 40 years of circulation of variants within this given subtype, the population's immunity to all variants within the subtype is very high, and the conditions for the spread of a new virus are favorable.

PATHOGENESIS AND PATHOLOGY. Influenza virus infection is transmitted from person to person by virus-containing respiratory secretions. Small-particle aerosols appear most important, but transmission by other routes, including fomites, may be possible. Virtually all cells of the respiratory tract can support viral replication. Once the virus initiates infection of the respiratory tract epithelium, successive cycles of viral replication infect large numbers of cells and result in destruction of ciliated epithelium. The duration of the incubation period until onset of illness and virus shedding, which occur in close proximity, varies from 1 to 3 days. The quantity of virus in respiratory tract specimens correlates with severity of illness, which suggests that a major mechanism in producing illness is cell death resulting from viral replication. However, interferon is frequently detected in respiratory secretions and blood about a day after virus shedding and may contribute to systemic symptoms and fever. The roles of specific cytokines in producing and resolving illness are not defined. The duration of viral shedding depends on age and generally lasts for 3 to 5 days in adults and often into the second week in children. Viremia is rare.

Nasal and bronchial biopsy specimens from persons with uncomplicated influenza reveal desquamation of the ciliated columnar ep-

ithelium. Individual cells show shrinkage, pyknotic nuclei, and loss of cilia. In addition, the lungs in fatal influenza show extensive hemorrhage, hyaline membrane formation, and paucity of polymorphonuclear (PMN) cell infiltration. Secondary bacterial infections develop as a result of altered bacterial flora, damage to bronchial epithelium with depressed mucociliary clearance, decreased PMN and alveolar macrophage functions, and/or alveolar fluid.

Neutralizing, hemagglutination-inhibiting (HAI), antineuraminidase, complement-fixing, enzyme-linked immunosorbent assay (ELISA), and immunofluorescent antibodies begin to develop in the sera of persons with primary influenza virus infection during the second week after infection and reach a peak by 4 weeks. Secretory antibodies develop in the respiratory tract after influenza infection and consist predominantly of IgA antibodies that reach peak titers in 14 days. Cell-mediated immune responses also occur. Immunity to influenza appears to be subtype-specific and durable. Protection against infection is afforded by serum HAI titers of 1 : 40 or greater, serum-neutralizing antibody titers of 1 : 8 or greater, or nasal neutralizing antibody titers of 1 : 4 or greater.

CLINICAL FINDINGS. *Influenza Syndrome.* The abrupt onset of feverishness, chilliness, or frank rigors, headache, myalgia, and malaise is characteristic of influenza. Systemic symptoms predominate initially, and prostration occurs in more severe cases. Usually myalgia or headaches are the most troublesome early symptoms, and their severity is related to the level of fever. Arthralgia is common, and less often ocular symptoms, photophobia, tearing, burning, and pain on moving the eyes are helpful diagnostically. Respiratory symptoms, particularly dry cough and nasal discharge, are usually also present at the onset but are overshadowed by the systemic symptoms. Nasal obstruction, hoarseness, and sore throat also may be present. As systemic illness diminishes, respiratory complaints and findings become more apparent. Cough is the most frequent and troublesome and may be accompanied by substernal discomfort or burning. Nasal obstruction, discharge, pharyngeal pain, and injection are also common. Cough, lassitude, and malaise may persist for 2 more weeks before full recovery.

Fever is the most important initial physical finding. The temperature usually rises rapidly to a peak of 38 to 40° C and occasionally to 41° C within 12 hours of onset, concurrently with systemic symptoms. Fever is usually continuous but may be intermittent, especially if antipyretics are administered. As fever subsides, the systemic symptoms diminish. Typically, the duration of fever is 3 days, but it may last from 1 to 5 or more days. Uncommonly, a biphasic fever course occurs. Early in the course of illness, the patient appears toxic, the face is flushed, and the skin is hot and moist. The eyes are watery and reddened. Clear nasal discharge is common. The mucosa of the nose and throat are hyperemic, but exudate is not observed. Small, tender cervical lymph nodes are often present. Transient scattered rhonchi or localized areas of rales are found in < 20% of cases.

The pattern of illness just described occurs with any strain of influenza A or B virus. Illness is more frequent and severe in smokers, and attack rates are higher in children than in adults. Maximum temperatures are higher in children, cervical adenopathy may be more frequent, and gastrointestinal symptoms of nausea, emesis, or abdominal pain more common. Older adults (≥ 60 years) experience muscle aches, sore throat, and headache less often but have higher rates of pulmonary complications. Influenza C virus generally causes only sporadic upper respiratory tract illness.

Respiratory Complications. Three kinds of pneumonic syndromes have been described: primary influenza viral pneumonia, secondary bacterial pneumonia, and mixed viral and bacterial pneumonia. Influenza A and B virus infections may be associated with other respiratory tract complications, including exacerbations of chronic bronchitis, asthma, or cystic fibrosis; croup and bronchiolitis in young children; and otitis media, sinusitis, and rarely parotitis or bacterial tracheitis. Apparently uncomplicated influenza is often accompanied by abnormal tracheobronchial clearance, airway hyperactivity, and small airways dysfunction lasting weeks. A syndrome mimicking pulmonary embolism with transiently altered perfusion scans also has been described.

Primary influenza viral pneumonia occurs predominantly among persons with underlying pulmonary and cardiac disorders, pregnancy, or immunodeficiency states, although up to one-half of reported cases have no recognized underlying disease. Following a typical onset of influenza, there is rapid progression of fever, cough, dyspnea, and cyanosis. Physical examination and chest roentgenograms reveal bilateral findings consistent with the adult respiratory distress syndrome. Blood gas studies show marked hypoxia. Gram stain of the sputum may show abundant PMN's but scant bacterial flora. Viral cultures of sputum or tracheal aspirates yield high titers of influenza virus. Such patients do not respond to antibiotics, and mortality is high, exceeding 50%.

Bacterial superinfection is often clinically distinguishable from primary viral pneumonia. The patients are most often elderly or have chronic pulmonary, cardiac, metabolic, or other diseases. Following a typical influenza illness, a period of improvement lasting from 1 to 4 days may occur. Recrudescence of fever is associated with symptoms and signs of bacterial pneumonia, such as cough, sputum production, and a localized area of consolidation apparent on physical and chest roentgenogram examination. Gram stain and culture of sputum reveal predominance of a bacterial pathogen, most often *Streptococcus pneumoniae, Staphylococcus aureus,* or *Haemophilus influenzae* (see relevant chapters for specific bacterial diseases). Such patients usually respond to specific antibiotic therapy, although staphylococcal infections may be particularly virulent and cause destructive pulmonary lesions. Invasive aspergillosis occurs rarely following influenza.

In addition, during an outbreak of influenza, many less distinct cases are observed that do not clearly fit into either of these categories. These patients may have viral tracheobronchitis, milder forms of localized viral pneumonia, or mixed viral and bacterial infection. Many respond to antibiotics. Such cases are more likely to be confused with a pneumonia due to *Mycoplasma pneumoniae* than to that produced by other bacterial infection.

Nonpulmonic Complications. Reye's syndrome is a well-recognized hepatic and central nervous system (CNS) complication of influenza A and B virus infections, typically in children and rarely in adults (see Ch. 430). Toxic shock syndrome due to respiratory tract infection with toxin-bearing *S. aureus* has been reported. Outbreaks of meningococcal infections have been associated with both influenza A and B virus infections. Myositis with tender leg muscles and elevated serum creatine kinase (CPK) levels may develop uncommonly, more often in children. Disseminated intravascular coagulopathy (DIC) develops rarely, as does renal failure related to DIC or myoglobinuria. Myocarditis or pericarditis has been described rarely. Aseptic meningitis, myelitis, encephalopathy associated with acute illness, and postinfluenzal encephalitis also have been described. A possible relationship to Guillain-Barré syndrome remains to be substantiated.

DIAGNOSIS. In an individual case, influenza often cannot be distinguished from infection with a number of other viruses (and occasionally streptococcal pharyngitis) that produce headache, muscle aches, fever, and/or cough. In summer, enteroviruses produce a similar clinical picture, and the acute manifestations of many other infections, such as dengue, may mimic influenza. On the other hand, when public health authorities report an epidemic of influenza A and B virus infection in a given community and a patient is seen with typical illness, it is highly likely that these symptoms are caused by an influenza virus infection.

Definitive diagnosis depends on detecting infectious virus or viral antigen in secretions from patients or detecting a serum antibody response. Influenza virus is readily isolated from throat or nasal specimens, sputum, or tracheal secretion specimens in the first 2 or 3 days of illness. Usually infectivity is detected within 48 to 72 hours in cell cultures. Commercially available EIA tests can document influenza A virus infection rapidly and have sensitivities of 70% or better. Serologic methods are less useful clinically because they require a convalescent serum obtained 10 to 14 days after the onset of infection.

TREATMENT. Oral rimantadine or amantadine therapy shortens the duration of fever and of systemic and respiratory symptoms in uncomplicated influenza A by 1 to 2 days and speeds functional recovery. The possible effectiveness of these drugs in treating pulmonary complications of influenza is unknown. The usual dosage is 200 mg per day for 5 days. A daily dose of 100 mg should be used in older adults. Rimantadine has a lower risk of the CNS side effects that occur with amantadine. Amantadine is excreted un-

changed in the urine, so dose adjustments are needed for those with modest renal impairment. These agents are ineffective for influenza B infections. Treated persons sometimes transmit virus to close contacts.

Other symptomatic measures include antipyretics and cough suppressants. Many authorities recommend that aspirin not be used, especially for persons under age 16, because of its association with Reye's syndrome.

Influenza viral pneumonia in its severe form requires intensive respiratory monitoring and support. Oral amantadine, intravenous ribavirin, and aerosolized ribavirin have been used anecdotally. Secondary bacterial pneumonia should be treated with appropriate antibiotics. When studies of the sputum do not clearly indicate an infecting bacterium, use antibiotics that are effective against the likely pathogens, including *S. aureus.*

PREVENTION. The mainstay of prevention is using inactivated influenza virus vaccines. These vaccines provide about 60 to 90% protection against influenzal illness when vaccine matches the epidemic strain. Immunogenicity and hence protection rates are often lower in the elderly, particularly in infirm nursing home residents, and immunosuppressed patients, including those with advanced HIV infection or receiving chemotherapy. Among elderly nursing home residents vaccine is approximately 50 to 60% effective in preventing hospitalization and pneumonia. The antigenic composition is reviewed annually so that the vaccine contains the most recently circulating strains, usually one or more subtypes of influenza A and an influenza B virus. Between 1 and 2% of immunized adults have fever and less than 10% systemic symptoms peaking at 8 to 12 hours after vaccination, but 25% or more may have mild local reactions at the site of injection. Persons with malignant disease should receive vaccine between chemotherapy courses.

The priority groups for vaccine include those at highest risk for influenza complications and their immediate contacts (Table 332–4), although vaccine can be safely administered to anyone trying to avoid influenza. Vaccine should be given each year in the fall before the influenza season. The vaccine is contraindicated in persons with chicken egg anaphylactic hypersensitivity. Rarely reported and unproven complications of inactivated vaccine include Guillain-Barré syndrome, systemic vasculitis syndrome, and theophylline or warfarin toxicities. Intranasal attenuated vaccines and improved adjuvants are under study.

Rimantadine and amantadine are approximately 70 to 90% effective in preventing influenza A illness and can be used to supplement vaccine programs. Persons who are not vaccinated in the fall should be placed on prophylaxis when an outbreak occurs or throughout the influenza season for the highest-risk group. If vaccine is available, persons may be vaccinated simultaneously and drug therapy stopped after 14 days. Alternatively, if vaccine is not available, administration may be continued for duration of the outbreak. When given to patients and staff alike, these drugs may be helpful in

TABLE 332–4. TARGET GROUPS FOR INFLUENZA IMMUNIZATION

Groups at Increased Risk of Complications

Persons aged 65 and older
Residents of nursing homes and other chronic care facilities
Patients with chronic pulmonary (including asthma) or cardiac disorder
Patients with chronic metabolic disease (including diabetes), renal dysfunction, hemoglobinopathies, or immunosuppression
Children and teens receiving long-term aspirin

Groups in Contact with High-Risk Persons

Physicians, nurses, and other health care providers
Employees of nursing homes and chronic care facilities
Providers of home care to high-risk persons
Household members (including children) of high-risk persons

Other Groups

Providers of essential community services (e.g., police, fire)
International travelers
Students, dormitory residents
Anyone wishing to reduce risk of influenza

Adapted from Advisory Committee on Immunization Practices, Centers for Disease Control and Prevention. MMWR 43(No RR-9):1, 1994.

managing nosocomial outbreaks. Postexposure prophylaxis in households is also effective. Hospitalized patients should be placed in respiratory isolation.

Centers for Disease Control and Prevention. Prevention and control of influenza: 1. Vaccines. MMWR 43(no. RR-9):1, 1994. *Recommendations for influenza immunization that are updated on an annual basis.*

Hannoun C, Kendal AP, Klenk HD, et al. (eds.): Options for the Control of Influenza II. Amsterdam, Elsevier Science, 1993, pp 1–468. *Compilation of review articles and papers emphasizing virologic, immunologic, epidemiologic, and public health aspects of influenza.*

Hayden FG, Couch RB: Clinical and epidemiological importance of influenza A viruses resistant to amantadine and rimantadine. Rev Med Virol 2:89, 1992. *Review article summarizing data regarding this problem and suggesting management strategies.*

Kilbourne ED (ed.): Influenza. New York, Plenum Press, 1987, pp 1–359. *Single-authored, authoritative text covering all aspects of influenza virus infections.*

Leonardi GP, Leib H, Birkhead GS, et al.: Comparison of rapid detection methods for influenza A virus and their value in health-care management of institutionalized geriatric patients. J Clin Microbiol 32:70, 1994. *Examples of commercially available rapid diagnostic assays for detecting influenza.*

333 ADENOVIRUS DISEASES
John J. Treanor

VIROLOGY

The adenoviruses are found in a variety of animal species, including humans, simians, horses, pigs, goats, and dogs. These viruses have been the subject of intense investigation for many years because of their ability to undergo latency and to induce tumors in experimental animals; consequently, the molecular biology of the adenoviruses is among the most completely known of all viruses. However, despite much effort in this regard, there is no well-documented association between adenoviruses and any human tumor.

The virus is nonenveloped, with a double-stranded DNA genome (Fig. 333–1). The human adenoviruses are grouped into six subgenera (A–F) based on differences in genome content, pattern of hemagglutination, and ability to cause tumors in experimental animals. In addition, at least 47 distinct serotypes are defined based on neutralization tests. Specific disease syndromes or hosts are often associated with specific adenovirus serotypes (Table 333–1).

CLINICAL FEATURES

DISEASE IN NORMAL HOSTS. The adenoviruses can infect and cause disease in a variety of human epithelial tissues including those of the eye, respiratory tract, gastrointestinal tract, and urinary bladder. Most infections in immunologically competent individuals are subclinical. Virus may be shed for months following infection from either the gastrointestinal or respiratory tract.

Eye Disease. **Pharyngoconjunctival Fever** (see Ch. 329). The syndrome of pharyngoconjunctival fever (PCF) is characterized by bilateral conjunctivitis accompanied by mild pharyngitis without exudate. Fever, myalgias, and malaise also may be present. The eyes are itchy but not painful, with a boggy, hyperemic conjunctiva, and

TABLE 333–1. ADENOVIRUS SEROTYPES AND ASSOCIATED SYNDROMES

Host and Disease Category	Epidemiologic Features	Associated Adenovirus Serotypes
Immunocompetent Hosts		
Pharyngoconjunctival fever	Epidemics in schools, family and the military, associated with swimming pools.	3, 7
Epidemic keratoconjunctivitis	Sporadic epidemics in schools, families, and industrial sites; may cause nosocomial outbreaks. More common in fall and winter	8, 19
Endemic upper respiratory disease	Seen predominantly in children, in families and day care setting	1, 2, 5
Acute respiratory disease of military recruits		3, 4, 7, 14 21
Acute hemorrhagic cystitis	Male predominance	7, 11, 21, 35
Gastroenteritis	Predominant in children <2	40, 41
Immunocompromised Hosts		
Transplantation		7, 11, 31, 34, 35
Acquired immunodeficiency syndrome		Multiple, 35, 42–47

watery discharge. Occasionally, the syndrome may be complicated by punctate keratitis.

PCF is highly contagious (see Table 333–1) and can be spread by contact with the eyes and mouth for 8 to 10 days after the onset of symptoms. The incubation period is 5 to 8 days. The illness is self limited, with a duration of from a few days to as long as 3 weeks. There is no specific therapy.

Epidemic Keratoconjunctivitis. In contrast to PCF, epidemic keratoconjunctivitis (EKC) presents as unilateral disease in the majority of cases and is generally not accompanied by sore throat, fever, or systemic symptoms. The patient may complain of a mild foreign body sensation with watery tearing but is not in significant discomfort. Physical findings include a swollen eyelid, conjunctival hyperemia with edema and chemosis, and tender preauricular adenopathy. Keratitis eventually develops in about 80% of patients and is usually noted on about the eighth day of illness with the onset of pain, photophobia, lacrimation, and blepharospasm. Visual acuity also may be temporarily reduced during the height of illness. Subepithelial corneal infiltrates can be detected in about one third of patients and may take weeks or months to resolve.

Many EKC outbreaks (see Table 333–1) have been attributed to contamination of ophthamalogic equipment, such as tonometers, and stringent infection-control procedures often must be implemented to terminate nosocomial outbreaks.

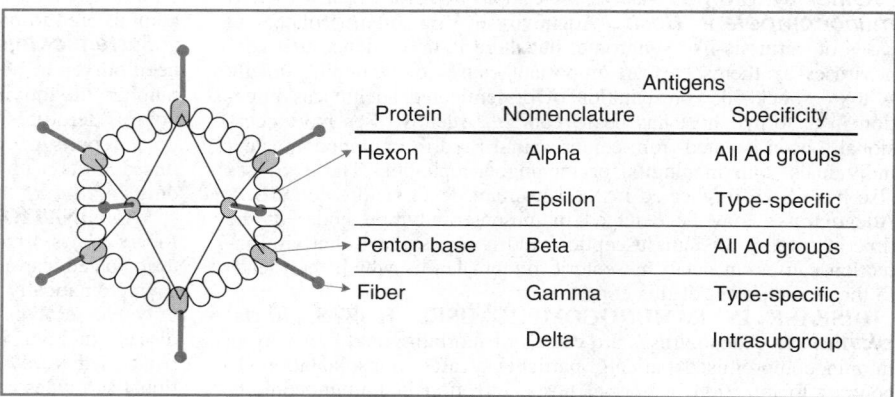

FIGURE 333–1. Structure of the capsid of adenovirus showing the major antigenic systems and capsid proteins. The viral capsid is an icosahedron composed of 252 capsomers arranged in 20 triangular faces and 12 vertices. The 12 vertex capsomers are called pentons because each is surrounded by five neighboring subunits. Each penton consists of a base and a fiber. The penton base is a toxic factor that causes cytopathology in cell culture. The nonvertex capsomers are called hexons, because each is surrounded by six neighboring subunits. (Adapted from Horwitz MS: Adenoviridae and their replication. *In* Fields BN, Knipe DM (eds.): Fields' Virology, 2d ed. New York, Raven Press, 1990, used with permission.)

Protein	Antigens	
	Nomenclature	Specificity
Hexon	Alpha	All Ad groups
	Epsilon	Type-specific
Penton base	Beta	All Ad groups
Fiber	Gamma	Type-specific
	Delta	Intrasubgroup

Respiratory Disease. **Upper Respiratory Tract Illness** (see Ch. 329). Acute pharyngitis is the most common respiratory syndrome attributed to the adenoviruses. Adenoviruses can cause an exudative tonsillitis similar to that caused by group A streptococci. In children, common associated syndromes include otitis media, coryza, and undifferentiated fever. Overall, adenoviruses are associated with about 7% of acute febrile illnesses in children, with a peak age of incidence between 6 months and 2 years. High secondary attack rates are seen in families or in the day care setting.

Lower Respiratory Tract Illness. Adenoviruses have been implicated as causing approximately 10% of childhood pneumonias. Clinical features are nondescript, and chest radiographs are similar to those in other forms of viral pneumonia, with the exception that hilar adenopathy is more common in children with adenoviral pneumonia than with other forms of viral pneumonia. Mixed bacterial/viral pneumonia is often present and may be suggested by elevations in band forms in peripheral blood.

Military recruits generally present with the atypical pneumonia syndrome (see Table 333–1), and illness clinically resembles that due to *Mycoplasma pneumoniae*. Although the illness is typically mild, more severe disseminated infections and deaths have been reported. Multiple radiographic patterns are noted; there may be large pleural effusions. Prodromal symptoms of upper respiratory infection are reported by most patients, and pharyngitis is often found on presentation. The disease is associated with the special conditions of fatigue and crowding found in military barracks and does not commonly occur in similarly crowded situations such as college dormitories. Bacterial superinfection, particularly with *Neisseria meningitidis,* may occur.

Adenoviruses rarely cause pneumonia in otherwise healthy adults, and adenovirus isolated from stool or respiratory secretions in normal adults with pulmonary infiltrates should be interpreted with caution.

Urinary Disease. **Hemorrhagic Cystitis.** Acute hemorrhagic cystitis (AHC) may be caused by adenoviruses (see Table 333–1). The patient complains of gross hematuria and dysuria. The presentation may be confused with glomerulonephritis, but laboratory tests of renal function remain normal, and fever and hypertension do not occur. AHC is generally self-limited.

Gastrointestinal Disease. **Gastroenteritis** (see Ch. 344). Although multiple adenovirus serotypes may be shed in the stool, only the so-called enteric adenoviruses, i.e., types 40 and 41, have been convincingly associated with acute gastroenteritis. These adenovirus types belong to the newly created group F and differ from other adenoviruses in being highly restricted in their ability to replicate in conventional cell culture. Development of alternative culture systems, such as use of the Ad 5–transformed HEK-293 cell line, allowed laboratory propagation of these viruses and clarification of their role in human disease.

Gastroenteritis due to enteric adenovirus is a disease predominantly of children under age 2. Clinical features include watery diarrhea and vomiting similar to those seen with infection with group A rotavirus. In contrast to gastroenteritis due to the rotaviruses and astroviruses, adenoviral gastroenteritis shows no significant seasonal variability. The frequency of illness is about 10% of that caused by rotavirus in the same age group. Adenoviruses are rarely causes of acute gastroenteritis in adults.

Other Syndromes Associated with Adenoviruses in Immunocompetent Hosts. Adenoviruses are often isolated in cases of pertussis-like syndrome, but there is no evidence that adenoviruses by themselves are important causes of whooping cough. A toxic shock–like presentation of disseminated adenovirus infection in a normal host has been reported. Adenoviruses have occasionally been isolated from cerebrospinal fluid in immunocompetent individuals with meningitis or meningoencephalitis. These viruses also have been implicated in sudden infant death syndrome (SIDS). Adenoviruses may be detected in mesenteric lymph nodes at the time of surgery for intussusception, and it is postulated that viral infection causes an acute mesenteric lymphadenitis which then leads to the development of this condition.

DISEASE IN IMMUNOCOMPROMISED HOSTS. Transplantation. Adenoviruses are causes of morbidity and mortality in immunocompromised patients, particularly after transplantation. In contrast to infection in normal hosts, infection in immunocompromised subjects tends to be disseminated, with virus isolated from multiple body sites, including lung, liver, and gastrointestinal tract, and in urine. In addition, the spectrum of serotypes includes both those found in immunocompetent individuals and a markedly increased frequency of higher-numbered serotypes found rarely in immunologically normal subjects (see Table 333–1). The source of infection may be reactivation of latent virus; nosocomial infection has also been documented.

Adenoviruses may cause hemorrhagic cystitis in bone marrow transplant recipients, which may be confused with that due to cyclophosphamide. Differentiation between these two possibilities is generally made by virus culture and by the timing of cystitis in relationship to drug administration. Individuals with cystitis may develop pneumonia, hepatic necrosis, gastroenteritis, and encephalitis. The case-fatality rate of disseminated infection can be as high as 60%. Disseminated disease after liver transplantation can be seen and frequently leads to loss of the transplanted liver. However, this does not appear to preclude successful transplant of a new liver if one is available. Adenovirus disease in renal transplant recipients is generally not as severe as that seen in other transplants. Hemorrhagic cystitis is the most commonly seen problem, with pneumonia seen more rarely.

AIDS. Adenoviruses also have been isolated frequently from the stool and urine of individuals with the acquired immunodeficiency syndrome (AIDS), particularly those with relatively low CD4 lymphocyte counts. The most remarkable aspect of this situation is the isolation of a wide variety of serotypes in these patients (see Table 333–1), including new, higher-numbered serotypes isolated for the first time in these subjects. In addition, antigenically intermediate types have been isolated which possibly reflect recombination events made possible by prolonged virus replication in these hosts.

Because adenoviruses are almost always isolated in these patients in conjunction with multiple other opportunistic pathogens, it is difficult to ascribe specific clinical syndromes to them. Described associations include pneumonia, meningoencephalitis, hepatitis, gastroenteritis, and colitis. Adenoviruses have been detected in the large bowel of such patients in association with chronic diarrhea, but generally these have not been the enteric adenoviruses most commonly associated with gastroenteritis in immunologically normal hosts.

DIAGNOSIS

Virus can be isolated efficiently from conjunctival swabs, respiratory secretions, urine, or stool in primary cells of human epithelial origin, such as human embryonic kidney cells. However, diagnosis is complicated by the prolonged time required for isolation. Other means of directly detecting viral antigen or nucleic acid in clinical specimens are therefore widely used, including enzyme immunoassays, immunofluoresecence tests, and nucleic acid hybridization techniques. In addition, the time required to detect virus in cell culture can be shortened to as little as 2 days by applying centrifugation culture systems coupled with detection of early virus replication in culture using immunofluorescent or other means.

TREATMENT AND PREVENTION

THERAPY. Conjunctivitis. Therapy is generally supportive. Steroids should be avoided in mild cases of conjunctivitis, since symptoms will usually recur when steroids are discontinued. In more severe cases of keratitis, mild topical steroids may be used with cycloplegics as needed for iritis. Topical antibiotics may be administered to prevent bacterial superinfection.

Systemic Infections. There is no antiviral therapy that has been proven to be effective in any systemic adenoviral syndrome. A number of antiviral compounds are active against common adenovirus serotypes *in vitro,* and there have been uncontrolled anecdotal reports of successful treatment of AHC in immunocompromised hosts with intravenous ribavirin, a broad-spectrum antiviral drug.

VACCINATION. Live adenovirus vaccines have been developed for serotypes 4 and 7. These vaccines are administered orally in enteric-coated capsules and bypass the respiratory tract to replicate asymptomatically in the intestine. They have been shown to provide effective serotype-specific protection against adenovirus respiratory disease in high-risk military recruits, but these vaccines have not been used in civilian populations because of the plethora of additional serotypes causing severe disease in this population.

Because relatively large portions of the adenovirus genome can be replaced without affecting viral viability, adenoviruses have received considerable attention in constructing recombinant vaccines for other infectious diseases, such as hepatitis B, and as a vector for the delivery of gene therapy.

Baum SG: Adenovirus. *In* Mandell G, Dolin R, Bennett J (eds.): Principles and Practice of Infectious Diseases. 4th ed New York, Churchill-Livingstone 1995, pp 70–75. *Readily accessible, detailed review of the clinical significance of the human adenoviruses.*

Hierholzer JD: Adenoviruses in the immunocompromised host. Clin Microbiol Rev 5:262, 1992. *A complete description of reported cases of adenovirus infection in individuals with primary and secondary immunodeficiencies, including AIDS.*

Horwitz MS: Adenoviridae and their replication. *In* Fields BN, Knipe DM (eds.): Fields Virology, 2d ed. New York, Raven Press, 1990, pp 1679–1722. *Detailed description of the molecular biology of adenovirus replication.*

Liu C: Adenoviruses. *In* Belshe RB (ed.): Textbook of Human Virology, 2d ed. St. Louis, Mosby–Year Book, 1991, pp 791–803. *An excellent overall review of the biology of the adenoviruses.*

Exanthems and Mumps

334 MEASLES
Philip A. Brunell

DEFINITION. Measles is an acute, highly contagious disease characterized by fever, coryza, cough, conjunctivitis, and both an enanthem and an exanthem.

ETIOLOGY. The virus is an enveloped, negative-stranded RNA paramyxovirus (genus *Morbillivirus*) measuring 120 to 250 mm in diameter, similar to other members of the Paramyxovirus family but lacking neuraminidase. Its single antigenic serotype has been remarkably stable throughout the world for many years. The virus contains six major polypeptides, which are responsible for a number of structural and functional properties, including hemagglutination (of primate erythrocytes), hemolysis, cell fusion, and others. Isolation of virus from clinical specimens is most successful with primary kidney cell cultures of human or simian origin. Selected laboratory strains grow well in other primary and continuous cell lines of mammalian and avian origin.

EPIDEMIOLOGY. With the introduction of routine immunization against measles in the United States in 1963, the incidence of measles fell by about 99%. Smaller outbreaks have occurred at increasing intervals in 1971, 1976, and 1986. A somewhat larger outbreak appeared in 1989. Prior to the advent of measles vaccine, almost every child got measles, most before entering school. The frequency increased every other year. This pattern still is seen in developing countries, where measles in the very young is common. It is estimated that there are from 1 to 2 million deaths annually worldwide. Many developed countries have a less stringent policy toward measles immunization than does the United States.

During the 1989–1990 epidemic in the United States, the highest attack rates were in infants, followed by preschool children. The largest number of measles deaths in over a decade, 89, was reported in 1990. About 30% occurred in those over 20 years of age, many in those who were immunocompromised. Almost all the remaining deaths occurred in those under 5 years of age, most of whom were unimmunized and otherwise normal. During the past few years, however, the reported cases of measles have been at an all-time low.

Communicability. Measles is one of the most highly contagious infections. Almost all unprotected household contacts are infected. Demonstration of virus in nasopharyngeal secretions during the prodromal, pre-eruptive phase and in the first days of rash is in accord with epidemiologic evidence of contagiousness. Close physical proximity or direct person-to-person respiratory droplet contact is the usual requisite for infection, although airborne transmission has been documented.

Immunity. An unmodified attack of measles is followed by lifelong immunity. Passively transferred maternal antibody protects the young infant during the early months of life.

PATHOLOGY AND PHYSIOLOGIC RESPONSES. Pathologic changes in fatal measles usually represent the compound effect of viral and secondary bacterial infection. Pneumonia is almost invariably present; it is most frequently interstitial. More representative are changes of the uncomplicated viral diseases within the tonsillar, nasopharyngeal, and appendiceal tissue removed during the prodrome. These changes consist of round cell infiltration and the presence of multinucleated giant cells. Giant cells also are observed in tissue cultures infected with measles virus. The skin and mucous membranes contain perivascular round cell infiltrates with congestion and edema. Koplik's spots are inflammatory lesions of the submucous glands with similar microscopic features.

Simultaneous with the onset of rash, measles-specific antibodies are detectable in serum. Leukopenia is observed on the first day of rash mainly due to a decrease in lymphocytes; subsequently, granulocytopenia ensues as well. Measles virus replicates in lymphoid tissues (spleen, thymus, lymph nodes), can be isolated from monocytes and other mononuclear cells during acute infection. The virus is propagable in suspension of leukocytes *in vitro.*

Immunosuppressive Effects of Measles. It has long been known that cell-mediated immunity is impaired during measles. There is transient suppression of the tuberculin reaction (observed also with measles vaccines); improvement in eczema and allergic asthma and the induction of remissions in nephrosis have been described. In severe disease, the magnitude of depression of the total lymphocytes has been positively correlated with a lessened chance of recovery.

CLINICAL MANIFESTATIONS. After an incubation period that averages 11 days, measles becomes clinically manifest with symptoms of fever, malaise, myalgia, and headache. Within hours, *ocular symptoms* of photophobia and conjunctival injection occur. The palpebral and, to a lesser extent, the bulbar conjunctivae are involved. There is usually no exudate. Sneezing, coughing, and nasal discharge occur almost simultaneously. Less commonly, hoarseness and aphonia may reflect laryngeal involvement. In this prodromal stage of 1 to 4 days' duration, tiny white spots on the buccal mucosa may herald the appearance of skin rash. The white lesions described by Koplik characteristically occur lateral to the molar teeth and typically are mounted on a bluish red areola of injected mucosa, superimposed on a diffuse red background. They generally appear a day or so prior to rash and disappear within 2 days after its appearance. They constitute a pathognomonic diagnostic sign. The enanthem may involve other mucous membranes such as the palpebral conjunctiva and vaginal lining.

The *rash* of measles follows the prodromal symptoms by 2 to 4 days, occasionally as late as 7 days. It first appears behind the ears or on the face and neck as a blotchy erythema, spreads downward to cover the trunk, and finally is manifest on the extremities. The hands and feet may escape involvement. Initially, the eruption consists of discrete red macules that blanch with pressure. Subsequently, these lesions become papular, tend to coalesce, and may develop a red, nonblanching component. In adults, the rash generally is more extensive, with a greater tendency to become confluent and slightly raised and redder than in children. This is particularly true on the face. The rash fades in the order of its appearance; its disappearance about 5 days after onset may be attended by a fine, powdery desquamation that spares the hands and feet. In adults, malaise may continue for 1 to 2 weeks.

The *fever* of measles may persist for about 6 days and frequently reaches 40 or 41°C. Throughout the febrile period, productive cough and auscultatory evidence of bronchitis may be evident. These manifestations may persist after defervescence, and cough is often the last symptom to disappear. Bronchopulmonary symptomatology is an integral part of the primary viral infection; roentgenographic evidence of pulmonary involvement is frequently seen in the uncomplicated disease in the absence of leukocytosis and obvious bacterial infection. Generalized lymphadenopathy accompanies the acute febrile illness and may persist for several weeks thereafter. Nausea and, less commonly, emesis appear to be more common in adults and are often accompanied by elevated serum aminotransferases.

COMPLICATIONS. The persistence or recurrence of fever and development of leukocytosis are presumptive evidence of the common bacterial sequela of otitis media or pneumonia. Transtrachial aspirates in patients with pneumonia have yielded a variety of organisms.

Laryngitis of sufficient severity to embarrass respiration has been observed. Keratoconjunctivitis is part of the acute phase. Electrocardiographic abnormalities may be found. Severe measles has been described in pregnant women with hepatitis and pneumonia, the latter sometimes ending fatally. Premature labor has resulted in prematurity and stillbirths.

Encephalomyelitis. A rare (0.1%) but serious consequence of measles is a demyelinating encephalomyelitis that may appear from 1 to 14 days after the onset of infection. This complication is associated with recurrence of fever and headache, vomiting, and stiff neck. Stupor and convulsions usually follow. Localizing neurologic symptoms may be present. Death ensues in about 10% of patients; more than half of survivors suffer permanent residuals of varying severity. Abnormal electroencephalograms were recorded in about half of children with measles without clinical signs of encephalitis.

Infection of brain cells results in an incomplete viral replicative cycle with production of defective virions lacking the matrix (M) measles virus protein. Studies of patients with acute measles encephalomyelitis and those with late-onset subacute sclerosing panencephalitis show high titers in serum and cerebrospinal fluid of antibodies to all the measles virus proteins except M.

Other late sequelae of measles are thrombocytopenic purpura and exacerbation or activation of pre-existing pulmonary tuberculosis. The late complication of subacute sclerosing panencephalitis is discussed in Ch. 428.4.

Giant-Cell Pneumonia. In patients who are immunocompromised, e.g., those with AIDS, measles virus may induce an interstitial pneumonia characterized by giant cells and intracellular inclusion bodies. The disease is often fatal.

Measles Modified by Administering Antibodies. Attenuation of the natural disease by antibody prophylaxis may result in an illness of lessened severity comparable with the milder infection as seen in infants with illness modified by maternally acquired antibody. Fever alone may be observed, but some degree of exanthem is usually apparent. Koplik's spots may not appear. In general, the course is truncated and relatively uncomplicated. Lasting immunity is uncertain. Later routine immunization of these individuals is probably indicated.

Atypical Measles. From 1963 to 1967, two types of measles vaccine, one live attenuated and the other inactivated or "killed," were available in the United States. The live attenuated vaccine has been the sole product licensed and used in this country since 1967. A severe illness was reported in killed vaccine recipients after exposure to natural measles. These patients had high fever, pneumonia with pleural effusion, obtundation, and an unusual rash. The exanthem was hemorrhagic and was most marked on the extremities. In some instances, vesicular, macular, or maculopapular phases have been observed. The rash is sometimes accompanied by edema of hands and feet. Concomitantly, these patients' sera revealed extraordinarily high titers of measles-specific antibodies.

Subsequent investigations showed that patients who had received inactivated measles vaccines failed to develop antibodies to the fusion (F) protein of the virus. Lack of antibodies to the cell fusion factor is believed to have permitted these patients to support measles infection. Thus the atypical measles syndrome is believed to be due to an anamnestic antibody response in the face of an abundance of measles antigens.

In addition to the rash and pulmonary findings, these patients may have elevated liver enzymes, disseminated intravascular coagulation, and marked myalgia. Nodular pulmonary changes have persisted in some patients. Some cases of pneumonia are reported to have occurred in the absence of rash. Initial diagnoses on presentation have included Rocky Mountain spotted fever and meningococcemia because of the similarities of rash and toxicity. Since inactivated vaccines were available only from 1963 through 1967, the past recipients are now young adults. This atypical measles syndrome is of increasing importance to the internist. Atypical measles has been reported in some patients who received live vaccine alone or after killed vaccine. Recipients of killed vaccine who later received live vaccine may have severe local and systemic reactions to reimmunization.

DIAGNOSIS. The diagnosis should be suspected during an epidemic or following history of exposure. Prior to the appearance of rash, the diagnosis may be difficult unless Koplik's spots are present. Finding an uncomfortable patient in a darkened room who has conjunctivitis, coryza, and cough should make one suspect measles. The rash in adults may be more violacious, confluent, slightly raised, and more extensive than in children. A history of having received measles vaccine does not preclude the diagnosis, because most individuals with measles of school age or older have had the vaccine.

Differential diagnosis (Table 334–1) includes consideration of rubella, scarlet fever, infectious mononucleosis, secondary syphilis, drug eruptions, toxic shock syndrome, and Kawasaki's disease. Of value in excluding these possibilities are the milder course, postauricular nodes, and pinker rash of rubella; the sore throat, eventual desquamation, strawberry tongue, and leukocytosis of scarlet fever; and serologic tests for infectious mononucleosis. Fever, enanthem, and catarrh are uncommon with the cutaneous manifestations of drug hypersensitivity. Erythema infectiosum is usually an afebrile illness with rash on the cheeks, arms, and legs. There is no prodrome or accompanying respiratory tract involvement. Kawasaki's disease is rare in adults.

Specific Diagnosis. Virus isolation is technically difficult. Increase in specific antibody may be detected as early as the first or second day of rash. Generally acute and convalescent sera are required. Demonstration of measles IgM is available in some laboratories.

Presumptive diagnosis may be made if giant cells are detected in stained smears of nasal exudate in the pre-eruptive period.

PROGNOSIS. Uncomplicated measles is rarely fatal, and complete recovery is the rule. Fatalities are almost always the result of pneumonia, occurring in adults or children younger than age 1. Congestive cardiac failure is a common cause of death in patients over 50 years old. The prognosis is particularly poor in patients with AIDS or other immunocompromised patients (see Ch. 360).

Antimicrobial drugs effective against the usual secondary in-

TABLE 334–1. A GUIDE TO THE DIFFERENTIAL DIAGNOSIS OF MEASLES

	Conjunctivitis	Rhinitis	Sore Throat	Enanthem	Leukocytosis	Specific Laboratory Tests Available
Measles	+ +	+ +	0	+	0	+
Rubella	0	±	±	0	0	+
Exanthem subitum	0	±	0	0	0	+
Enterovirus infection	0	±	±	0	0	+
Adenovirus infection	+	+	+	0	0	+
Scarlet fever	±	±	+ +	0	+	+
Infectious mononucleosis	0	0	+ +	±	±	+
Drug rash	0	0	0	0	0	0

0 Not usually present; no test available.
± Variable in occurrence.
+ Present: test available (virus or bacterial culture, serology).
+ + Present and severe.

vaders have reduced the case fatality rate of measles sharply. They have proved effective in therapy of bacterial complications, but not in prophylaxis.

Encephalitis occurs as frequently in mild as in severe measles (i.e., about one in 1000 cases); subacute sclerosing panencephalitis occurs about 7 years after measles and has essentially disappeared with widespread vaccine use.

TREATMENT. There is no specific antiviral therapy for measles with demonstrated efficacy, although ribavirin has been used in some cases.

Symptomatic Therapy. In the absence of complications, bed rest is the essence of treatment in this self-limited disease. Codeine sulfate may be useful to ameliorate headache and myalgia and is effective for cough. Analgesics and antipyretics may be useful. Fluids should be encouraged. Bright light is not an ocular hazard, but photophobia may require darkening the patient's room.

Antimicrobial Prophylaxis. The course of uncomplicated measles is not influenced by antimicrobial drugs, and their use during the acute illness has resulted in no decrease of secondary bacterial complications (otitis, sinusitis, pneumonia). Instead, the same rates of complications (about 10 to 15%) have been observed, but with organisms resistant to the antibiotics used during the viral illness. If careful observation of the patient is possible, rational therapy is based on promptly recognizing and defining the etiology of complications, followed by starting the appropriate antimicrobial drug in proper dosage.

PREVENTION. *Vaccination.* A highly effective vaccine available for preventing measles is derived from the Edmonston strain of virus isolated originally in the laboratory of Dr. John Enders. This live virus vaccine produces immunity by infection. A second dose now is recommended routinely. In children over age 1, seroconversion after vaccination in recent years is about 98 to 99%. Measles vaccine usually is given as a single preparation as measles, mumps, and rubella (MMR) vaccine. Failure of measles immunization was much more common prior to 1980. The reasons for this are unclear. It may be due to poor recall or faulty documentation of immunization, age of immunization, use of immune globulin with the vaccine, receipt of killed rather than live vaccine, or the type of live vaccine.

Vaccine recommendations vary depending on the measles experience in the community (see Ch. 10). The first dose is now recommended at age 12 months as MMR. During epidemics, it may be given as monovalent measles vaccine to infants as young as 6 months of age. In the latter case, it should be repeated in combination with mumps and rubella (MMR) after the first birthday. The second routine dose of MMR is given between ages 5 and 12. All entering college students and beginning health care workers born after 1956 should show evidence of measles immunity, e.g., positive serologic test, physician-documented measles, or receipt of two doses of measles vaccine or preferably MMR. The immune status of those contemplating foreign travel should be reviewed. A large number of military personnel have been reimmunized without significant side effects.

Contraindications to live virus vaccine include pregnancy, immunodeficiency, leukemia, and other systemic malignant diseases, active tuberculosis, and administration of resistance-depressing drugs such as corticosteroids and antimetabolites.

Annunziato D, Kaplan MH, Hall WW, et al.: Atypical measles syndrome: Pathologic and serologic findings. Pediatrics 70:203, 1982. *Excellent clinical description and explanation of a syndrome now seen in young adults.*

Atmar RL, Englund JA, Hammill H: Complications of measles during pregnancy. Clin Infect Dis 14:217, 1992. *A review of the complications and the treatment of measles in pregnancy.*

Centers for Disease Control and Prevention: Measles prevention: Recommendations of the Immunization Practices Advisory Committee (ACIP). MMWR 38:1, 1989. *Everything you want to know about the use of measles vaccine.*

Gilad M: Measles in adults: A prospective study of 291 consecutive cases. Br Med J 295:1313, 1987. *A brief summary of findings in a large number of adults.*

Gremillioin DH, Crawford GE: Measles pneumonia in young adults. Am J Med 71:539, 1981. *A large series of cases of measles pneumonia in young adults and other features of measles in this group.*

Gustafson TL, Brunell PA, Lievens AW, et al.: Measles outbreak in a "fully-immunized" secondary school population. N Engl J Med 316:771, 1987. *School outbreaks are described in a presumably well-immunized population.*

Katz SL, Gellin BG: Measles Control–Resetting the Agenda: A report of the children's vaccine initiative ad hoc committee on an investment strategy for measles control. J Infect Dis 170(suppl):S1, 1994. *An all-inclusive presentation of measles and its prevention throughout the world.*

Panum PL: Observations Made During the Epidemic of Measles on the Faroe Islands. New York, Delta Omega Society, 1940. *A classic clinical epidemiologic description of measles introduced into an isolated population with disease among all susceptibles born since the previous epidemic 65 years earlier.*

335 RUBELLA *(German Measles)*
Philip A. Brunell

DEFINITION. Rubella is an acute, usually benign infectious disease characterized by a 3-day rash, generalized lymphadenopathy, and minimal or no prodromal symptoms. Since 1941, it has been known to cause congenital malformations when infection occurs during the early months of pregnancy.

ETIOLOGY. Rubella is a small, spherical, enveloped virus containing single-stranded RNA of positive polarity. The structural proteins consist of membrane glycoproteins and a nucleocapsid protein. The virus is classified as a togavirus, genus *rubivirus*. It multiplies in a variety of primary cell culture systems and in some continuous cell lines in most systems without detectable cytopathic effects.

EPIDEMIOLOGY. Before rubella vaccines were available, the disease was worldwide in distribution, produced major epidemics at 6- to 9-year intervals, and was recognized mainly in school-age children; it also produced outbreaks in settings such as military recruit bases and college campuses where large numbers of susceptible young adults gathered in relatively crowded conditions. Since licensure in 1969 of the vaccine in the United States, there has been strikingly altered epidemiology. There has been no major epidemic since 1964–1965. In other nations, where rubella vaccine has not been widely used, the epidemiology has remained unchanged. Because the disease may be quite nonspecific clinically, with nearly one-third of adults undergoing infection without rash, epidemiologic reporting tends to underestimate its prevalence. Since 1966, congenital rubella has been a reportable disease. It is probable that rubella is spread by the respiratory route and by close and sustained personal contact. The incubation period in experimentally infected individuals was found to be 12 to 19 days, with most cases occurring 14 to 15 days following exposure. Although virus was isolated as early as 7 days prior to and as late as 21 days following onset of rash, infectivity probably is greatest throughout the period of prodromal symptoms and for as long as 7 days after the appearance of rash. Infants with congenitally acquired infection may excrete virus in respiratory secretions and in urine for months after birth and are contagious during this time. In hospital environments, especially in nurseries, the congenital rubella baby had been a source of nosocomial infection of personnel involved in his/her care.

Immunity is lifelong after initial infection. Authenticated second attacks are exceedingly rare and require serologic documentation because of the nonspecific nature of the clinical syndrome. Subclinical reinfection demonstrated by increase in IgG serum antibody has been documented. Such reinfections are not associated with viremia and thus pose little threat to pregnant women. IgM response has been used to distinguish primary infection from reinfection. Immunity that follows artificial immunization with live virus vaccine is apparently of equal duration even though the antibody titers induced may be somewhat lower.

PATHOLOGY. Death from postnatal rubella is usually due to encephalitis. Thus most autopsies describe only the brain findings. Since 1962, it has been possible to investigate the pathogenesis and to correlate clinical findings with virologic events. After initial invasion of the upper respiratory tract, virus spreads to local lymphoid tissue, where it multiplies and initiates a viremia of approximately 7 days' duration. Respiratory tract shedding of virus and the viremia rise to peak levels until the onset of rash, at which time the latter becomes undetectable, whereas respiratory secretions contain diminishing quantities of virus over the succeeding 5 to 15 days. Specific serum antibodies can be demonstrated with the onset of rash, and circulating immune complexes are detectable soon thereafter.

Congenital Rubella. Necropsies of fetal and neonatal victims of intrauterine infection have shown a variety of embryonal defects related to developmental arrest involving all three germ layers.

The virus establishes chronic persistent infection of many tissues, with resultant intrauterine growth retardation. Delayed and disordered organogenesis produces embryopathic structural defects of the eye, brain, heart, and large arteries; continued viral infection during the fetal and postnatal period causes organ and tissue damage, e.g., hepatitis, nephritis, myocarditis, pneumonia, osteitis, meningitis, cochlear degeneration, and pancreatitis with the development of diabetes.

CLINICAL MANIFESTATIONS. *Postnatally Acquired Rubella.* Twelve to 19 days after exposure, the onset of rubella is manifested by the appearance of a rash with mild accompanying constitutional symptoms of malaise and occasionally sore throat. Enlargement of the postauricular and suboccipital nodes generally appears about a week prior to rash. Moderate fever may accompany or precede the rash. Generalized peripheral lymphadenopathy and, more rarely, splenomegaly may occur.

The exanthem of rubella is usually apparent within 24 hours of the first symptoms as a faint macular erythema that first involves the face and neck. Characterized by its brevity and evanescence, it spreads rapidly to the trunk and extremities, sometimes leaving one site even as it appears at the next. The pink macules that constitute the rash blanch with pressure and rarely stain the skin. Rubella virus has been isolated from the skin lesions as well as from uninvolved sites. The truncal rash may coalesce, but the lesions on the extremities remain discrete. The eruption usually vanishes by the third day. Rubella may occur without rash. In the absence of an epidemic and of serologic or virologic confirmation, the clinical diagnosis of rubella is not reliable.

COMPLICATIONS. Recovery is almost always prompt and uneventful. In contrast to measles, secondary bacterial infections are not encountered in rubella. Transient polyarthralgia and polyarthritis are more common among adolescents and adults with rubella, particularly females. They appear 3 or more days after onset of rash and may last 5 to 10 days. The knees and joints of the hands and wrists are most often involved. Surveys during urban epidemics have revealed rates of 5 to 15% in males and 10 to 35% in females.

Thrombocytopenia, when sought by serial platelet counts, is common but rarely of clinical consequence. A meningoencephalitis of short duration may occur 1 to 6 days after the appearance of rash. Its incidence is estimated at 1 in 5000 cases, and it is fatal in approximately 20% of those afflicted. Rubella encephalopathy is not associated with demyelinization, in contrast to other postviral encephalitides. Survivors may have electroencephalographic abnormalities, but intellectual function seems to be preserved.

Congenital Rubella. Congenital transplacental infection of the fetus occurs as a consequence of maternal infection, usually in the first 4 months of pregnancy. Virus is demonstrable in placental and fetal tissues obtained by therapeutic abortion at that time. If pregnancy is not interrupted, fetal infection persists, and on delivery of the infant, virus is recoverable from the throat, urine, conjunctivae, bone marrow, and cerebrospinal fluid of the living infant and from most organs at autopsy. From 20 to 80% of infants born to mothers infected in the first trimester of pregnancy have stigmata of infection readily recognizable in the first year of life. These include cardiac lesions and eye defects, e.g., cataracts, glaucoma, retinitis, microphthalmia. Most infants in whom virus is detectable do not have evidence of disease at birth or may simply have intrauterine growth retardation. In others, more severe disease occurs. Most prominent of these manifestations is thrombocytopenic purpura, which disappears soon after birth. Hepatosplenomegaly with active hepatitis may persist for months. Other involvement includes interstitial pneumonia, meningoencephalitis, hearing loss of varying extent, and lesions of the long bones. Recently, a progressive panencephalitis simulating subacute sclerosing panencephalitis has been observed in the second decade following congenital infection. The long-term sequelae for infants with congenital rubella include psychomotor retardation, hearing loss, retinopathy, and diabetes.

A striking finding has been the persistence of virus in the pharynx, urine, and cerebrospinal fluid for as long as 1 year after birth in 7% of infants. Infective virus was found in a congenital cataract after 3 years. This evidence of continuing viral synthesis occurs coincidentally with circulating antibody. The character of the antibody changes during the first months from maternal IgG to IgM, indicating a primary response of the infant to the persisting viral antigen. Studies of older infants and children with stigmata of congenital rubella show them to be free of demonstrable virus and to possess the IgG immunoglobulins that characteristically persist after other viral infections.

DIAGNOSIS. Rubella may be diagnosed clinically with assurance only during an epidemic. Distinction from measles may be made on the basis of fainter, nonstaining rash, the milder course, and the minimal or absent systemic complaints. Sore throat is a more prominent complaint in scarlet fever; the course of infectious mononucleosis is often more protracted, and splenomegaly is more frequent than in rubella. Specific diagnosis of rubella is made by isolating the virus in any of several cell culture systems or by demonstrating a rise in hemagglutination-inhibiting (HI), ELISA, or complement-fixing antibody during infection.

PROGNOSIS. Complete recovery from postnatally acquired rubella is almost invariable. The rare deaths attributable to rubella follow the infrequent complication of meningoencephalitis. Infection in pregnancy constitutes a grave hazard to the fetus but not to the mother.

TREATMENT. There is no specific antiviral therapy. Few patients suffer discomfort severe enough to warrant symptomatic medication. Headache and myalgia or arthritis may be controlled by analgesics.

PREVENTION. *Passive Immunization.* Administration of gamma globulin to the pregnant woman may only mask her symptoms of infection and not protect the fetus from viral invasions. Thus its use may only obscure the picture and confound decision about the need to terminate the pregnancy.

Active Immunization. Rubella may be prevented in children and adults by parenteral attenuated live virus vaccines produced in cell cultures. Seroconversion rates after immunization are at least 98% with the current RA 27/3 vaccine. Joint symptoms are less common than with the older HPV 7-DE strain, occurring in about 2.5% of adults. Arthritis occurs 13 to 19 days following immunization and lasts 2 to 11 days. The fingers are most often affected, with the wrists and knees less commonly involved. Arthralgias generally begin 10 to 25 days following vaccination and last 1 to 9 days. Joint symptoms are less common in men than in women. In children, vaccination is attended by little or no reaction.

It was initially recommended in the United States that immunization be carried out principally in childhood. There now is a more aggressive attempt to immunize those remaining susceptible women and adolescent girls. Current policy recommends vaccinating all such persons who have no history of previous rubella immunizations. Postpartum immunization of those found to be seronegative during pregnancy is encouraged. Although occasionally vaccine virus has been transmitted to the newborn by breast milk, this has proven to be of little consequence. Only nonpregnant individuals should be immunized, and contraception, when appropriate, should be carried out for at least 3 months after vaccination. Inadvertent administration of vaccine to pregnant women has occasionally resulted in attenuated vaccine viruses infection of the fetus. In more than 500 such cases studied, no infant has been observed with congenital malformations as a result. The frequency of fetal infection with the RA 27/3 vaccine currently used is less than with the previous rubella vaccine. Use of vaccine in the United States prevented a large epidemic of rubella expected in the early 1970's and has reduced the reported annual occurrence from more than 50,000 cases annually, with epidemic peaks of 200,000 to 500,000, to an all-time low in 1988 of 221 cases. A slight increase in cases of rubella accompanied by cases of congenital rubella syndrome occurred in 1990.

Burke JP, Hinman AR, Krugman S (eds.): International symposium on prevention of congenital rubella infection. Rev Infect Dis 7(Suppl):1, 1985. *Fifteen years of vaccine use summarized by investigators from the developed nations.*

Centers for Disease Control and Prevention: Rubella and congenital rubella syndrome—United States. MMWR 38:173, 1989. *A summary report of progress in rubella "eradication" in the United States.*

Gregg NM: Congenital cataract following German measles in the mother. Trans Ophthal Soc Aust 3:35, 1941. *The original "classic" report associating rubella in pregnancy with congenital malformations.*

Proceedings of the International Conference on Rubella Immunization. Am J Dis Child 118, July 1969. *A compendium on rubella and congenital rubella.*

Sherman FE, Michaels RH, Kenny FM: Acute encephalopathy (encephalitis) complicating rubella. JAMA 192:675, 1965. *A clinical, pathologic, and epidemiologic study of rubella encephalitis.*

Townsend JJ, Stroop WG, Baringer JR, et al.: Neuropathology of progressive rubella panencephalitis after childhood rubella. Neurology 32:185, 1982. *A review of the clinical and neuropathologic findings.*

Weibel RE, Vilarejos VM, Klein EB, et al.: Clinical and laboratory studies of live attenuated RA 27/3 and HPV 77-DE rubella virus vaccines (40931). Proc Soc Exper Biol Med 165:44, 1980. *A description of the clinical and serologic response to rubella vaccine.*

336 VARICELLA (Chickenpox, Shingles)

Philip A. Brunell

DEFINITION. Varicella, or chickenpox, is an acute communicable disease characterized by a generalized vesicular rash. Because it is highly contagious, most individuals contract it in childhood. Herpes zoster, due to reactivation of varicella-zoster virus (VZV), is a dermatomal cutaneous eruption.

ETIOLOGY. Varicella is caused by VZV, a member of the α-herpes virinae subfamily. This enveloped herpesvirus contains a number of glycoproteins, some of which bear some homology to those of other members of the human herpesvirus group. The double-stranded DNA has a molecular weight of approximately 80 million. There is some diversity in the restriction enzyme patterns among wild isolates; there is only a single serotype. Although the human is the only known natural host, a closely related virus has been identified in a simian species.

EPIDEMIOLOGY. Varicella is a highly contagious disease. After continuing household exposure, as would occur in a family, almost all susceptibles are infected. The subclinical attack rate is believed to be no more than 4%. The results of nonhousehold exposure are less certain. Chickenpox may be most contagious the day prior to the onset of rash. Chickenpox is contagious for no more than 5 days after the appearance of the first lesion. Children may return to school at this time or earlier if the lesions are crusted. The incubation period is usually about 14 days. Ninety-nine percent of the cases occur 10 to 20 days following exposure. The disease is known to be spread by direct contact. Airborne spread also has been demonstrated, most notably in hospitals.

Nosocomial spread of varicella has been well documented. This has occurred room to room by airborne spread as well as by patient-to-patient or staff-to-patient contact. Adults with herpes zoster who are hospitalized are less likely to cause secondary cases of chickenpox among adult contacts than among children. The reason is that hospitalized children are more likely to be susceptible to chickenpox than hospitalized adults. Strict isolation is recommended for hospitalized patients with varicella and for children or immunocompromised adults with herpes zoster. Adults with localized herpes zoster require less stringent isolation procedures.

Most cases of chickenpox occur in childhood. Most children contract chickenpox either in day care situations or shortly after they enter school. Fewer than 2% of the cases occur following the second decade. Approximately 10% of hospital workers with a negative history are seronegative. Almost all individuals with a positive history are seropositive. A single attack of chickenpox usually confers lifetime immunity.

There appears to be more efficient transmission of disease in temperate than in tropical climates. The reason for this is uncertain but may be due to temperature rather than urbanization. Varicella occurs most commonly during the late winter and spring months, the peak being about in March. Sporadic cases occur into the early summer and start in late fall.

Varicella is more common than other childhood diseases during the early months of life. In this situation the disease is generally mild. Maternal antibody transferred across the placenta may not be as effective in protecting infants against this disease as are antibodies against other viruses. However, nursery outbreaks have been rare. Children who develop varicella during the early months of life or are exposed *in utero* have a greater risk of developing herpes zoster in childhood.

PATHOGENESIS. Replication of virus is believed to occur initially in the epithelial cells of the mucosa of the upper respiratory tract. Since VZV produces a disseminated rash, one can assume that bloodstream distribution must have occurred. Virus can be isolated from white blood cells from 5 days prior to 2 days following the appearance of rash. After clinical recovery, the virus infection continues in the absence of clinical symptoms in a latent phase. During this time, messenger RNA (mRNA) can be demonstrated in nonneuronal cells in dorsal root ganglia. The segmental distribution of herpes zoster (see Ch. 426.3), which usually occurs decades after the initial VZV infection, is consistent with a dorsal root ganglion site for the latent virus. In uncomplicated chickenpox, rises in serum aminotransferases levels have been demonstrated. This suggests that there is visceral involvement in the normal course of this disease.

The vesicular lesions of varicella contain a predominance of polymorphonuclear leukocytes even during the early phase of vesicle formation. Multinuclear giant cells are occasionally found in the base of the lesions, often containing eosinophilic intranuclear inclusions. Large amounts of virus can be demonstrated in vesicular fluid by electron microscopy.

Postmortem descriptions of patients with varicella have usually involved immunocompromised subjects. In these cases, inflammatory changes are usually found in multiple organs, including the lung, liver, spleen, and skin, together with anoxic changes in the brain. Similar involvement is found in the newborn. Focal areas of necrosis and intranuclear eosinophilic inclusions in mononuclear cells are common. Changes in otherwise normal individuals usually include myocardial and pulmonary lesions. On microscopic examination, the brain has demonstrated edema with some lymphocyte cuffing around the cerebral vessels.

CLINICAL MANIFESTATIONS. Varicella is characterized by a generalized eruption that is centripetal in distribution; erythematous macules, papules, vesicles, and scabbed lesions may be present at the same time. The vesicles are superficial, with varying amounts of erythema at their bases. Adults tend to have considerably more erythema than children. During the early phase of the eruption, lesions are found on the face, scalp, and trunk. By running the fingers through the hair, one often detects lesions that were not visible. Later, new lesions appear on the extremities. By this time, the earlier lesions have dried and crusted. Excoriations are common, attesting to the pruritic nature of the lesions. Mucous membranes of the conjunctiva and oropharynx are more frequently involved in adults than in children. New lesions continue to appear over a 3- or 4-day period, after which the rate of their appearance decelerates markedly.

There is a striking variation in the extent of systemic symptoms associated with varicella. Most children have a mild illness with few systemic complaints and an average maximal temperature of about 38.3°C. It is more common for adults to have considerable malaise, muscle ache, arthralgia, and headache. These may precede the first skin lesions by 24 to 48 hours.

In the immunocompromised subject, the disease often is very severe. Approximately 30% of children with leukemia or lymphoma who get varicella and receive no prophylaxis or treatment develop "progressive varicella." Vesicles continue to erupt into the second week of illness, accompanied by high fever. Lesions tend to be deep seated rather than superficial. Toward the end of the first week and the beginning of the second week, the lesions are more common on the extremities than on the trunk. Indeed, the distribution and lesions may resemble those with smallpox. Visceral involvement occurs in about 30% of these patients. The lung, liver, pancreas, and brain may be involved. Death occurs in about 9% of immunocompromised patients who develop varicella. The death usually is due to pulmonary involvement. Patients with HIV infections may have recurrent attacks of varicella in the absence of exposure or a persistent eruption that may continue for months.

Varicella in pregnant women is believed to be more serious than in nongravid females; fatalities have been reported. The rate of fetal wastage is not increased. About 1% of infants born to mothers who have had varicella early in pregnancy, however, have been found at birth to have "varicella embryopathy." The infants are born with cerebral damage and a variety of ocular findings, and characteristically they have a scarred, atrophic limb. The children are generally small for gestational age and may have other abnormalities as well. When mothers develop chickenpox within a few days of delivery, "varicella of the newborn" may occur. If the onset of varicella is between 5 and 10 days after birth, it is associated with a higher risk of serious disease and even death.

Bacterial infections of the skin are the most common complication of chickenpox in childhood. The rate of complications is much higher in adults than in children. Although fewer than 2% of the reported cases occur after the second decade, almost 35% of the deaths occur in this group. A disproportionate rate of hospitalization also is found in adults. The major complications of varicella in adults are encephalitis and pneumonia.

Approximately 1 in 400 adults with chickenpox are hospitalized for pneumonia. In a prospective study, however, it was found that only 6% of young adults with chickenpox had respiratory symptoms, whereas 16% had roentgenographic evidence of pulmonary involvement.

Infection produces a diffuse interstitial type of pneumonia with hypoxia resulting from poor diffusion of gases. Diffuse calcification of the lung parenchyma may be found years after recovery.

Encephalitis in childhood is most commonly manifested by a cerebellitis, which usually occurs at the end of the first week or during the second week following onset of rash. This complication is almost always self-limited. In contrast, an acute form of encephalitis usually occurring soon after the onset of rash often has a fulminating course; it is characterized by severe brain swelling. It has been estimated that as many as 20% of cases of Reye's syndrome may be preceded by chickenpox. A variety of other neurologic complications, including optic neuritis, transverse myelitis, and Guillain-Barré syndrome, may be associated with chickenpox. Hemorrhagic complications of chickenpox include thrombocytopenic purpura and purpura fulminans. Nephritis, myocarditis, and arthritis also have been described.

DIAGNOSIS. There is usually little difficulty in recognizing typical forms of chickenpox, particularly if there has been a history of exposure. The diagnosis may be more difficult in immunocompromised hosts, because they may have features of progressive varicella with visceral involvement. Modified cases of chickenpox may occur following passive or active immunization. These cases may require laboratory confirmation. The most common sources of confusion are insect bites, generalized herpes in the immunocompromised host, rickettsialpox, or "hand, foot, and mouth disease" caused by an enterovirus. The differentiation of disseminated herpes zoster from chickenpox may be difficult. The former usually has dermatomal involvement initially. Generalization usually does not occur until 3 to 5 days after onset of the zosteriform rash. In severely immunocompromised patients, e.g., bone marrow recipients, generalization may occur earlier and the clinical differentiation may be difficult.

The Tzanck smear is a frequently used laboratory aid for diagnosis. Multinucleated giant cells identify the lesions as being caused by one of the herpesviruses, but this is not specific for varicella. A properly stained smear also contains eosinophilic intranuclear inclusions. Virus can usually be isolated during the first 3 or 4 days after the onset of lesions. The virus is quite labile; it must be stored at $-70°C$ if cultures cannot be inoculated immediately. Our preference is to collect vesicular fluid in unheparinized capillary tubes and put the specimen directly into human embryonic lung fibroblasts at the bedside. Specimens from throat, urine, or stool are of little value for isolation of virus. Polymerase chain reaction (PCR) can be used to demonstrate the presence of virus in vesicular fluid and throat swabs.

Serologic confirmation of diagnosis can be made using a variety of techniques. The enzyme-linked immunosorbent assay (ELISA) and complement fixation are the most generally available. The laboratory director should be consulted regarding appropriate time of collection of specimens as well as interpretation of data. Because complement-fixing antibody generally does not persist, a single high titer often is confirmatory evidence of recent infection.

Determining the immune status of contacts can be done with the ELISA, latex agglutination test, or the fluorescent antibody test against membrane antigen (FAMA). The ELISA is a much simpler and technically less demanding test. Because complement-fixing antibody is lost rapidly after infection, it cannot be used for determining susceptibility. Fluorescence antibody test using fixed cells sometimes yields false-positive results. A number of laboratories have developed tests for VZV immunoglobulin M (IgM). It was hoped that these might differentiate varicella from herpes zoster in cases in which this was unclear. Unfortunately, these tests have not been very useful, as VZV IgM is present in the sera of many patients with acute herpes zoster.

TREATMENT. Major therapeutic objectives are the prevention of superinfection and relief of pruritus. The latter can be accomplished frequently by application of calamine lotion. Occasionally this does not suffice, and a systemic antipruritic agent such as trimeprazine may be necessary. It is advisable to trim and file nails to reduce the damage from scratching. Bacterial superinfection can best be prevented by encouraging daily bathing with an antibacterial soap. Following this with a colloidal starch bath also may be useful for relieving pruritus.

Relief of systemic symptoms may require additional medication such as acetaminophen, although this may increase pruritus. Salicylates are contraindicated, since there is an association between their use and development of Reye's syndrome in children. Special care should be taken to be certain that over-the-counter medications containing salicylates are avoided.

Some patients, particularly those who are immunocompromised, may require antiviral therapy. Intravenous acyclovir has been shown to be effective in immunocompromised children with varicella. A dose of 500 mg per square meter repeated every 8 hours has been used. VZV is generally less sensitive to acyclovir than herpes simplex. For this reason, larger doses are probably required. Studies on the use of oral antiviral drugs in the treatment of varicella have demonstrated some efficacy. Initial reports indicate that prophylaxis for 7 days starting 7 days following exposure is more effective. Patients who are sick enough to require antiviral therapy probably should be treated with parenteral rather than oral medication.

Patients on high doses of steroids or other immunosuppressive drugs who have been exposed to chickenpox are at high risk of developing progressive varicella. Steroids appear to be most deleterious when given during the incubation period. They have been used in the treatment of pneumonia after the eruption has occurred without any obvious deleterious effects.

PREVENTION. Immune serum globulin does not prevent varicella. Massive doses are required to produce measurable modification. If prevention or modification is indicated, varicella-zoster immune globulin (VZIG) should be given. Candidates are those who (1) are susceptible, (2) are at high risk of developing complicated varicella, and (3) have had an adequate exposure to the disease. Any individuals fulfilling the first two criteria who have had a household exposure should receive prophylaxis. It is often difficult to judge the degree of intimacy in other types of exposure. Reference to guidelines published by the Academy of Pediatrics or Centers for Disease Control and Prevention (CDC) may be helpful.

Patients considered at high risk are (1) those who are immunocompromised by virtue of either disease or immunosuppressive therapy, (2) infants born to mothers who have had varicella less than 5 days prior to or 2 days following delivery, (3) certain premature infants, (4) bone marrow transplantation recipients regardless of susceptibility, and (5) certain adults.

A history of varicella is usually reliable in both adults and children. Children who have a negative history are usually susceptible. Serologic testing of adults who have a negative history is useful if it does not delay administration of VZIG. VZIG should be given as soon as possible following exposure and has not been shown to be effective if delayed more than 96 hours.

Nosocomial infection following herpes zoster or varicella has been well documented. These outbreaks may result in significant morbidity and cause disruption of hospital routine. These situations are best managed by serologic screening of personnel and by permitting only those who are seropositive to care for patients with varicella or herpes zoster. Patients who are hospitalized with varicella should be isolated 7 days. Susceptible persons who are exposed to active cases should be isolated from the tenth to the twenty-first day after the last exposure if they cannot be discharged. Whenever possible, patients with chickenpox should be isolated in a room with negative pressure in order to prevent dissemination of infectious virus to other patients. Airborne spread in hospitals has been documented.

An attenuated live vaccine has been licensed for use abroad and is being considered for licensure in the United States. Susceptible adults who receive the vaccine have some local reactions and occasionally develop a varicelliform rash. Protection against infection is less complete than in children. Two doses 2 months apart are recommended for adults. In normal children, the vaccine is virtually benign and appears to offer very good protection. Initial data suggest that herpes zoster would be no more frequent and perhaps less common following immunization than following natural infection.

Advisory Committee on Immunization Practice: Varicella-zoster immune globulin for the prevention of chickenpox. MMWR 33:84, 95, 1984. *Guidelines for passive immunization against chickenpox.*

Brunell PA: Varicella in pregnancy, the fetus and the newborn: Problems in management. J Infect Dis 166:542, 1992. *A comprehensive review of varicella in pregnancy.*

Brunell PA: Varicella vaccine—where are we? Pediatrics 78:721, 1986. *A symposium on the epidemiology, cost burden, and complications of varicella and on varicella vaccine.*

Brunell PA: Varicella-zoster virus. *In* Rose NR, Friedman H, Fahey JL (eds.): Manual of Clinical Laboratory Immunity, 4th ed. Washington, DC, American Society for Microbiology, 1992, pp 560–562. *A review of serologic tests for varicella-zoster antibody.*

First International Conference on Varicella. J Infect Dis 166 (Suppl 1):S1, 1992. *A comprehensive review of basic and clinical information.*

Srugo I, Israele V, Wittek, AE, et al.: Clinical manifestations of varicella-zoster virus infections in human immunodeficiency virus–infected children. Am J Dis Child 147:742, 1993. *A description of the various manifestations of VZV infection in HIV-infected children.*

Varicella-zoster infections. Report of the Committee on Infectious Diseases, 22nd ed. Evanston, IL, American Academy of Pediatrics, 1994, pp 510–517. *A useful guide to management of patients exposed to varicella, including control of nosocomial infection.*

337 VARIOLA AND VACCINIA

Donald A. Henderson

The Thirty-third World Health Assembly "declares solemnly that the world and all its peoples have won freedom from smallpox" (Resolution 33.3, May 8, 1980, Geneva, Switzerland).

This announcement was made some 30 months after the last known endemic case, in Somalia, on October 26, 1977. In 1978, two additional cases of smallpox occurred in Birmingham, England, as a result of a laboratory infection, but except for these cases, no others have been found.

To confirm that eradication had been achieved, each country where smallpox had been endemic since 1967 and those at risk of importations conducted a search for cases for at least 2 years after the last known case. At the end of this period, World Health Organization (WHO)–appointed international commissions reviewed the records of work and conducted extensive field visits to confirm the results. Between 1973 and 1979, 21 different commissions visited and certified eradication in 49 countries.

Finally, a Global Commission for the Certification of Smallpox Eradication reviewed the findings and made special field visits. After satisfying itself that eradication had been achieved, the commission reported its findings to the World Health Assembly. The assembly members concurred and recommended that "smallpox vaccination be discontinued in every country except for investigators at special risk" and advised that "an international certificate of vaccination against smallpox should no longer be required of any traveller."

Thus concluded the first successful global program to eradicate a disease—one that had proved to be one of the most devastating known to humanity.

HISTORY (Fig. 337–1). Because of the need for variola virus to spread continually from person to person to survive, historians speculate that it emerged after the first agricultural settlements, about 10,000 B.C. In ancient times, only a few populated areas, probably in India, could have sustained its transmission. In the early Christian era, descriptions suggestive of smallpox appear in historical accounts of western Asia, and by the eighth century it had established itself in Europe. Central and southern Africa were probably infected sometime later.

Case-fatality rates of 20% and greater were characteristic, and where population densities permitted the disease to become endemic, virtually all persons eventually contracted smallpox. At the end of the eighteenth century, it was killing an estimated 400,000 Europeans each year and was responsible for one third of all cases of blindness.

VACCINATION. Edward Jenner discovered in 1796 that smallpox could be prevented by "vaccination" with material from a cowpox lesion. Before his discovery, the only defense against smallpox was deliberately to inoculate (variolate) scabs or pustular material from smallpox patients into the skin of susceptible persons. The resulting infection was usually less severe than infection acquired naturally by inhalation. Although case-fatality rates among those with in-

duced infection were sometimes as low as 1%, they readily transmitted infection to others.

During the nineteenth century, vaccination was increasingly widely practiced in temperate-climate countries, but the difficulties of sustaining the virus through arm-to-arm inoculation resulted in an uncertain supply.

In the industrialized countries, smallpox incidence declined steadily, and Europe and North America succeeded in interrupting smallpox transmission after World War II. In these areas, the impetus for vaccination had diminished early in the century when a less virulent strain, variola minor, with a case-fatality rate of about 1%, replaced variola major. In most of Africa, however, 5 to 15% died of smallpox, and in Asia the virulent variola major prevailed. Neither in Africa nor in Asia was vaccination widely practiced.

ERADICATION OF SMALLPOX. Smallpox was a problem to all countries. Even those without disease feared importations and conducted vaccination programs. Although the global control of smallpox was in everyone's best interests, progress was slow. Finally, in 1959, the World Health Assembly decided that a global eradication program should be undertaken. During the succeeding 7 years, a number of countries undertook campaigns, but few succeeded in interrupting smallpox transmission (see Fig. 337–1).

In 1967, when a definitive eradication program was decided, four geographic reservoirs of smallpox were identified: (1) Africa south of the Sahara, (2) a group of Southeast Asian countries extending from Bangladesh through India, Nepal, Pakistan, and Afghanistan, (3) Indonesia, and (4) Brazil. The estimated population of these countries was more than 1 billion persons.

WHO's strategy called for each country to undertake a program of vaccination with the objective of reaching at least 80% of the population during a 2- to 3-year period. During this time, a reliable reporting system was to be developed to identify foci of smallpox that would be eliminated by isolation of patients and vaccination of contacts. Extensive vaccination was believed necessary to increase population immunity and so reduce the number of cases to permit disease surveillance and containment activities to be effective.

Experience soon showed that the surveillance-containment strategy was more effective than had been thought, and this proved to be a key to success. In part, this was due to the unique characteristics of smallpox. An infected patient was able to transmit infection only from the time of first appearance of rash until the last scabs had separated. There were no chronic carriers or individuals with latent, transmissible infection and no animal reservoir. The rash was sufficiently characteristic to be diagnosed with a high degree of accuracy. The presence or absence of smallpox in an area could thus be reliably determined without laboratory studies. Moreover, approximately two thirds of recovered patients had characteristic residual facial scars. Thus it was possible to determine both the present status of smallpox and its past history in an area.

To persist, smallpox virus had to be transmitted from patient to susceptible contact. By isolation of the patient and by vaccination of contacts, a barrier to transmission was created. In small villages and in scattered populations, chains of transmission often terminated without intervention. Because smallpox did not spread rapidly, and then only to those in close contact, secondary cases usually were found among neighbors and relatives. A patient rarely infected more than two to three others. Because of these factors, early detection of outbreaks and their containment proved effective in stopping transmission.

Smallpox vaccine that conferred excellent and durable immunity was important to success. Studies revealed vaccine efficacy ratios of >90% after 20 years. Because the lyophilized vaccine retained its potency after incubation at 37°C for at least 1 month, the logistics of vaccine storage and distribution were comparatively simple. Vaccination was greatly facilitated by the inexpensive, newly developed bifurcated needle. The technique was learned quickly and produced a high proportion of successful vaccinations.

PROGRESS IN THE PROGRAM (see Fig. 337–1). By 1969, eradication programs were in progress in all the infected and immediately adjacent countries except for Ethiopia. Four years later, smallpox had been eliminated from most of Africa and in Asia, there remained only four smallpox-endemic countries: India, Pakistan, Nepal, and Bangladesh. However, the population of these four was over 700 million, and the techniques of surveillance and con-

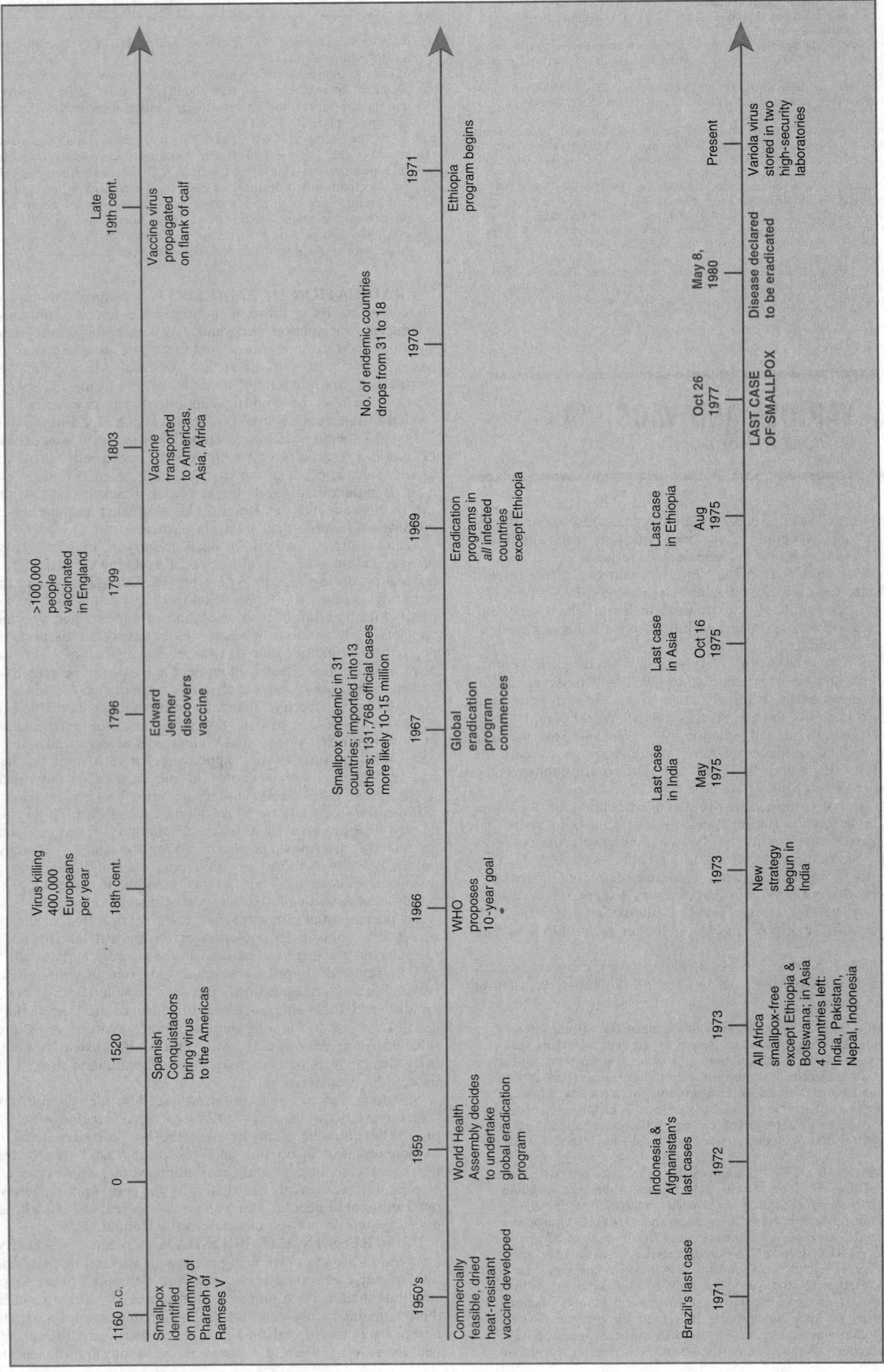

FIGURE 337–1. Smallpox timeline.

tainment that had been applied in other areas proved to be less successful.

A new strategy in India began in the autumn of 1973 (Basu and colleagues). Far more rapid case detection and more effective containment of outbreaks were required. Accordingly, for 1 week each month more than 100,000 health workers were mobilized to search house by house to detect cases. Hundreds of special teams contained the outbreaks that were found. Between searches, the teams asked questions at markets and in schools to uncover rumors of cases. By the summer of 1974, new cases began to decline, and a cash reward was offered to anyone who reported a case (see Fig. 337–1). In October 1975 the last case occurred in Asia and in October 1977 the world's last naturally occurring infection.

POSSIBLE SOURCES FOR A RETURN OF SMALLPOX. As of 1994, variola virus was known to exist in only two laboratories, where it was kept under high-security conditions.

Extensive studies had been conducted since 1967 to discover a possible animal or other natural reservoir of the virus. None was found. However, some 400 cases of a newly recognized disease that is clinically indistinguishable from smallpox but caused by the related monkeypox virus occurred in seven central and west African countries between 1970 and 1990. Genome maps of this and other animal poxviruses reveal many differences between them and variola.

The recurrence of smallpox resulting from a deliberate release of variola virus cannot be ruled out. However, the potential damage of such an act should not be exaggerated. Smallpox does not spread rapidly, and an outbreak caused in this manner should be able to be contained within 3 to 4 weeks.

Barring improbable circumstances, a human case of smallpox will never again be seen. However, the problem of mistaken diagnosis is a real one. For this reason, WHO medical officers with expertise in diagnosis remain on call to investigate rumors.

VARIOLA (Smallpox)

ETIOLOGY. Variola virus is one of a group of orthopoxviruses that includes vaccinia, monkeypox, rabbitpox, cowpox, camelpox, buffalopox, and ectromelia. The poxviruses are the largest viruses so recognized. The virions are brick-shaped structures with a diameter of about 200 μm. The genome consists of a single molecule of a double-stranded DNA.

INCIDENCE AND PREVALENCE. The disease was declared to be eradicated on May 8, 1980.

PATHOLOGY AND PATHOGENESIS. The site of entry of the smallpox virus was probably the respiratory tract. In the 12-day incubation period, the virus multiplied in the regional lymphoid tissues. Viremia occurred at the onset of fever and continued during the first 2 or 3 days of the pre-eruptive phase. During this time, the virus localized in mucous membranes, skin, and internal tissues. Virus multiplication in the epithelial cells of the skin and mucous membranes caused pustulation. Antibodies appeared as early as the fourth day of disease.

CLINICAL MANIFESTATIONS. The incubation period of smallpox was about 12 days with a range of 7 to 17 days. The illness began with severe malaise, prostration, head- and backache, and high fever lasting 2 to 5 days (Rao). Following the initial febrile period, a macular rash developed, which quickly became papular, and within 2 days the papules developed into vesicles and then pustules. On the eighth or ninth day of rash, crusting began. The scabs separated over the succeeding 2 to 3 weeks, leaving pigment-free skin. Subsequently, scarring or pitting developed. The eruption was characteristically more severe on the face and the distal parts of the arms and legs, and less severe over the trunk and abdomen. Lesions were often found on the palms of the hands and the soles of the feet.

VARIOLA MINOR AND INTERMEDIATE FORMS. In the early twentieth century, a milder clinical form of smallpox (variola minor, or alastrim) became prevalent in the Americas, Europe, and parts of southern and eastern Africa. Case-fatality rates were ≤1%. Variola major and minor were distinct, although at times coexisting. Each of the two types gave rise to illnesses with a wide spectrum of severity. There was cross-protection between each of these forms and vaccinia.

DIFFERENTIAL DIAGNOSIS. Most cases of smallpox could readily be identified by the typical deep-seated rash, the centrifugal distribution of lesions, and the fact that in any area on the body all

lesions were at the same stage of development. The infrequent severe hemorrhagic cases were frequently mistakenly diagnosed as meningococcemia, acute leukemia, or drug toxicity. Mild cases with few lesions were confused with varicella. Of help in diagnosis, however, was the fact that in any outbreak ≥80% of the cases were clinically typical.

LABORATORY TESTS. Diagnosis of a poxvirus infection can be rapidly established by electron microscopic identification of virus particles in vesicular or pustular fluid or scabs. Differentiation among poxviruses requires that the virus be isolated on chick chorioallantoic membrane and its properties characterized by specific biologic tests. WHO Reference Laboratories are prepared to undertake necessary diagnostic studies.

TREATMENT. No specific treatment is available.

IDENTIFICATION OF A SUSPECT CASE OF SMALLPOX. Because smallpox has been eradicated, the occurrence of a single case has profound international implications. Should a suspect case be identified, *immediate notification of local, state, and national health officials is essential.* Most suspected cases in recent years have been cases of varicella in adults. Should a case prove to be smallpox, the source of virus must be assumed to be inadvertent or deliberate release from a laboratory. A suspect patient should be placed under strict isolation. Additional measures will be dictated by epidemiologic circumstances.

VACCINIA (Vaccination)

No countries now require international certificates of vaccination, and none conducts civilian vaccination programs. Several countries, including the United States, continue to vaccinate military personnel. Vaccination is recommended only for investigators who are working with poxviruses in the laboratory.

THE VACCINE. Vaccinia virus is grown in tissue culture or on the scarified flank of a calf. After purification and the addition of stabilizing agents, the suspension is freeze dried. Inoculated intradermally, vaccinia virus induces a mild infection and confers protection against all orthopoxviruses known to infect humans—monkeypox, variola, and cowpox.

VACCINE PROTECTION. Following successful vaccination, protection against variola is virtually complete for 5 years, but effectiveness wanes over time. In poxvirus laboratories, vaccination at least every 3 years has been customary.

RISKS OF VACCINATION. Those who are candidates for vaccination are adults, a diminishing proportion of whom have received primary vaccinations as children. Although the risk of serious complications is very low, primary vaccination of adults once had been thought to be associated with a higher incidence of serious complications. However, a special study of vaccination complications among military recruits failed to document any cases of the most important, postvaccinal encephalitis, among an estimated 2 million primary vaccinees.

FIRST VACCINATION (PRIMARY TAKE). Three days after vaccination, a papule appears at the vaccination site; the papule changes to a vesicle and by the seventh day is a fully developed pustule. It is whitish, umbilicated, and multilocular and contains clear lymph. An erythematous areola expands to reach a maximal diameter about 9 days after vaccination. A crust forms and falls off about 3 weeks after vaccination, leaving a scar.

REVACCINATION. When persons are vaccinated a second time, a gradation of cutaneous responses is observed. Individuals who have not been vaccinated for several decades may develop what appears to be a primary take. In persons with an intermediate level of immunity, development of the lesion is more rapid, and the maximal diameter of erythema is reached in 3 to 7 days. In the highly immune person, virus multiplication may not occur. In such persons, a hypersensitivity response to vaccinial protein may occur. A papule and sometimes a vesicle with erythema may develop, reaching its peak in 48 hours.

To distinguish the hypersensitivity type of reaction, which may be caused by heat-inactivated vaccine, from one in which virus multiplication has taken place, the site of inoculation is examined between the sixth and eighth days. If there is evidence of induration or congestion, virus multiplication may be assumed.

CONTRAINDICATIONS. Four groups of persons are at special risk of complications: (1) persons with eczema or other forms of chronic dermatitis; (2) pregnant women; (3) patients with leukemia, lymphoma, other reticuloendothelial malignancies, and AIDS; and (4) those receiving immunosuppressive drugs, especially glucocorticosteroids. Vaccinees in close contact with persons with eczema may infect them, sometimes with serious consequences. If vaccination is required for persons at special risk, vaccinia immune globulin (0.3 ml per kilogram intramuscularly) should be administered simultaneously.

COMPLICATIONS. *Postvaccinal Encephalitis.* Encephalitis following vaccination is a rare event and occurs between the eighth and fifteenth days. Paralysis, when it occurs, is generally spastic in type. Residual paralysis and other central nervous system symptoms may persist. There is no treatment. Studies conducted in the United States in 1963 and 1968 (Neff and colleagues, Lane and associates) revealed 28 cases, 9 fatal, among 11.3 million primary vaccinees. No cases occurred among 16.3 million revaccinees.

Progressive Vaccinia (Vaccinia Gangrenosa). Progressive vaccinia is an exceedingly rare but often fatal complication among vaccinated persons who have deficient immune responses. The initial vaccinial lesion fails to heal and progresses to involve adjacent skin with necrosis of tissue. Dissemination may result in metastatic vaccinial lesions in other parts of the skin, bones, or viscera. Treatment with vaccinia immune globulin is beneficial.

Eczema Vaccinatum. Eczema vaccinatum is sometimes a serious complication, which may occur in vaccinated persons with active or healed eczema, or in subjects in contact with recent vaccinees. The disease tends to localize at sites where eczematous lesions are or have been present. Vaccinia immune globulin is of help in therapy.

Generalized Vaccinia. Generalized vaccinia represents a secondary eruption resulting from bloodborne dissemination of vaccinia virus. Almost all cases occur after primary vaccination. The lesions become evident between 6 and 9 days after vaccination. The number of lesions may range from a few to a generalized involvement of the skin. It is a self-limited illness, and complete recovery occurs without specific therapy.

Fetal Vaccinia. Fetal vaccinia results from a bloodborne dissemination of vaccinia virus in the pregnant woman given primary vaccination. It may occur during any trimester of pregnancy and frequently results in death of the fetus.

Miscellaneous Complications. A great variety of rashes have been reported to be caused by vaccination. Most common are erythema multiforme and variously distributed urticarial, maculopapular, blotchy erythematous eruptions.

Basu RN, Jerek Z, Ward NA: The Eradication of Smallpox from India. New Delhi, India, World Health Organization, 1979. *A well-written, detailed, profusely illustrated book describing the epidemiologic and operational aspects of the program in India.*

Fenner F, Henderson DA, Jerek Z, et al.: Smallpox and its Eradication. Geneva, Switzerland, World Health Organization, 1988. *This 1400-page, extensively illustrated and referenced book is the definitive text, providing an historical account of smallpox control and eradication as well as a summary of current knowledge regarding the epidemiology, virology, and pathogenesis of the disease.*

Hopkins DR: Princes and Peasants: Smallpox in History. Chicago, University of Chicago Press, 1983. *The only comprehensive history of smallpox prepared in this century, this interesting and readable book complements that by Fenner and associates.*

Lane JM, Ruben FL, Neff JM, et al.: Complications of smallpox vaccination, 1968. N Engl J Med 281:138, 1969. *With the paper by Neff and co-workers, one of the few detailed studies of the frequency of complications following smallpox vaccination.*

Neff J, Lane JM, Pert JH, et al.: Complications of smallpox vaccination. N Engl J Med 276:1, 1967. *With the paper by Lane and associates, one of the few detailed studies of the frequency of complications following smallpox vaccination.*

Rao AR: Smallpox. Bombay, India, Kothari Book Depot, 1972. *Written by a clinician who treated more than 3000 cases, this book is an excellent reference on the clinical aspects of variola major.*

338 MUMPS
John W. Gnann, Jr.

Mumps is an acute systemic viral infection that is usually self-limited, occurs most commonly in school-aged children, and is clinically characterized by nonsuppurative parotitis.

VIROLOGY. Mumps virus is classified as a member of the Paramyxovirus family. Mumps virions are pleomorphic, roughly spherical, enveloped particles with an average diameter of 200 nm. Glycoprotein spikes project from the surface of the envelope, which encloses a helical nucleocapsid composed of nucleoproteins and linear, nonsegmented, single-stranded, negative-sense RNA. Humans are the only natural hosts for mumps virus, although infection can be induced experimentally in a variety of mammalian species. *In vitro,* mumps virus can be cultured in many mammalian cell lines and in embryonated hens' eggs.

EPIDEMIOLOGY. In unvaccinated urban populations, mumps is a disease of school-aged children, and >90% will have mumps antibodies by age 15. Before the mumps vaccine was released in the United States in 1967, mumps was an endemic disease with a seasonal peak of activity occurring between January and May. Mumps epidemics occurred at 2- to 5-year intervals. The largest number of cases reported in the United States was in 1941, when the incidence of mumps was 250 cases per 100,000 population. In 1968, when the vaccine was first entering clinical use, the incidence of mumps was 76 cases per 100,000 population. In 1985, only 2982 cases of mumps were reported, an incidence of 1.1 per 100,000 population, representing a 98% decline from the number of cases reported in 1967. Between 1985 and 1987, the incidence of mumps in the United States increased fivefold to 5.2 cases per 100,000 population. More than one third of the cases reported between 1985 and 1989 occurred in adolescents and young adults, reflecting the slow acceptance of universal mumps vaccination during the 1970's when this cohort of children grew up. Renewed emphasis on vaccination has resulted in a further decline in the annual incidence of mumps. In 1993, the Centers for Disease Control and Prevention (CDC) reported only 1640 cases of mumps in the United States, the lowest annual total ever recorded. Epidemiologic studies during the 1980's of mumps epidemics in high schools, colleges, and military units demonstrated that outbreaks were due principally to failure to vaccinate. More recent studies have attributed smaller mumps outbreaks in the 1990's to primary vaccine failure and possibly to waning vaccine immunity.

PATHOGENESIS. Mumps is highly contagious and can be transmitted experimentally by inoculation of virus onto the nasal or buccal mucosa, suggesting that most natural infections result from droplet spread of upper respiratory secretions. The average incubation period for mumps is 18 days. Primary viral replication takes place in epithelial cells of the upper respiratory tract, followed by spread of virus to regional lymph nodes and subsequent viremia and systemic dissemination. Virus can be isolated from saliva for 5 to 7 days before and up to 9 days after the onset of clinical symptoms, meaning that an infected individual is potentially able to transmit mumps for a period of about 2 weeks. An estimated 30% of mumps infections in children are subclinical or associated only with nonspecific upper respiratory infection (URI) symptoms.

CLINICAL MANIFESTATIONS. *Parotitis.* Mumps usually begins with a short prodromal phase of low-grade fever, malaise, headache, and anorexia. Young children may complain initially of ear pain. The patient then develops the characteristic parotid tenderness and enlargement, which lifts the earlobe forward and obscures the angle of the mandible. The parotid glands are involved most commonly, although other salivary glands occasionally may be enlarged. Parotitis initially may be unilateral, with swelling of the contralateral parotid gland occurring 2 to 3 days later; bilateral parotitis eventually develops in 70% of patients with symptomatic salivary gland involvement. Painful parotid gland enlargement progresses over about 3 days, followed by defervescence and resolution of parotid pain and swelling within

Aseptic Meningitis. Symptomatic meningitis occurs in 15% of cases and is the second most common manifestation of mumps. About 50% of patients with mumps parotitis have cerebrospinal fluid (CSF) pleocytosis, although many have no signs or symptoms of meningitis. Symptoms of meningeal irritation (headache, neck stiffness, vomiting, and lethargy) plus high fever usually develop 4 to 5 days after the onset of parotitis, although the meningitis may occasionally precede the parotitis. Indeed, 40 to 50% of all cases of documented mumps meningitis occur in patients who never develop clinical parotitis. Symptomatic central nervous system (CNS) involvement with mumps is two to three times more common in males than in females. Examination of the CSF usually reveals a normal opening pressure and a mononuclear cell pleocytosis with an average cell count of 450 per cubic millimeter. A polymorphonuclear leukocyte predominance may be seen in some patients early during the course of mumps meningitis. The CSF protein is usually normal or mildly elevated (< 100 mg per deciliter). Hypoglycorrhachia, which is not usually seen in viral meningitis, may be present in 10 to 30% of patients with mumps meningitis. Mumps virus can be recovered from CSF. While the symptoms of mumps meningitis usually resolve within 7 to 10 days, the CSF abnormalities may persist for up to 5 weeks. Mumps meningitis is usually benign and significant neurologic complications are rare.

Encephalitis. The spectrum of mumps-induced CNS disease ranges from mild "aseptic" meningitis (which is common) to severe encephalitis (which is rare). Some cases of encephalitis develop concurrently with the parotitis and are thought to result from direct extension of viral infection from the choroid plexus ependyma into parenchymal neurons. Other cases of mumps encephalitis occur 1 to 2 weeks after the onset of parotitis and may represent a demyelinating postinfectious encephalitis. Clinical findings in mumps encephalitis include obtundation (and less commonly delirium), generalized seizures, and high fever. Other neurologic findings can include focal seizures, aphasia, paresis, and involuntary movements. Recovery from mumps encephalitis is usually complete, although complications such as aqueductal stenosis with hydrocephalus, seizure disorders, and psychomotor retardation have been reported. The overall mortality from mumps encephalitis is 0.5 to 2.3%.

Orchitis. Epididymo-orchitis is rare in boys with mumps but occurs in 15 to 35% of postpubertal men with mumps. Orchitis is most often unilateral (bilateral involvement occurs in 17 to 38% of cases) and results from replication of mumps virus in seminiferous tubules with resulting lymphocytic infiltration and edema. Orchitis typically develops within 1 week of the onset of parotitis, although orchitis (like mumps meningitis) can develop prior to or even in the absence of parotitis. Mumps orchitis is characterized by marked testicular swelling and severe pain, accompanied by fever, nausea, and headache. The pain and swelling resolve within five to seven days, although residual testicular tenderness can persist for weeks. Testicular atrophy may follow orchitis in about 35 to 50% of cases, but sterility is an uncommon complication even among men with bilateral orchitis (see Ch. 209.1).

Other Manifestations. Mumps can cause inflammation of other glandular tissues, including pancreatitis and thyroiditis. Oophoritis and mastitis have been reported in postpubertal women with mumps. Transient renal function abnormalities are common in mumps, and virus can be isolated readily from urine; significant renal damage is rare, however. Other infrequent manifestations of mumps include sensorineural deafness (either transient or permanent), arthritis, myocarditis, and thrombocytopenia. Maternal mumps infection during the first trimester of pregnancy results in an increased frequency of spontaneous abortions, but no clear association between congenital malformations and maternal mumps has been demonstrated.

IMMUNE RESPONSE. Transient IgM antibody responses are detected early in the course of mumps infection, followed by the appearance of IgG antibody and cytotoxic T lymphocytes. Mumps-specific IgG can be detected during the first week of acute infection, peaks at 3 to 4 weeks, and persists for decades. Lifelong immunity follows natural infection. Patients who report more than one episode of mumps probably had parotitis due to another etiology.

A variety of serologic tests have been designed to determine susceptibility to mumps. The neutralizing antibody (NA) assay has been considered the "gold standard" test but is technically demanding. The hemagglutination inhibition (HAI) assay is simple to perform but less specific due to cross-reactivity with other paramyxoviruses. Detection of complement-fixing (CF) antibodies against V (hemagglutinin-neuraminidase) and S (nucleocapsid) antigens previously has been the routine method for determining immune status but has been replaced by a sensitive and specific enzyme-linked immunosorbent assay. The mumps skin test is not a reliable indicator of immune status.

DIAGNOSIS. The diagnosis of mumps is usually made on the basis of clinical findings in a child who presents with parotitis, particularly if the individual is known to be susceptible and has been exposed to mumps during the preceding 2 to 3 weeks. However, an atypical clinical presentation (e.g., meningitis or orchitis without parotitis) may require laboratory confirmation. Culturing for mumps virus is definitive but frequently not available. Testing of acute and convalescent sera should demonstrate a diagnostic fourfold rise in mumps antibody titer. Alternatively, finding mumps IgM antibody provides good evidence of recent infection. About 30% of patients will have an elevated serum amylase level that may be due to parotitis or pancreatitis.

The differential diagnosis of parotitis includes infections caused by other viruses such as influenza A, parainfluenza virus, coxsackievirus, lymphocytic choriomeningitis virus, or bacteria such as *Staphylococcus aureus*. Parotid gland enlargement also can be associated with Sjögren's syndrome, sarcoidosis, thiazide ingestion, iodine sensitivity, tumor, or salivary duct obstruction. A careful examination should distinguish parotitis from lymphadenopathy.

THERAPY. Management of the patient with mumps consists of conservative measures to provide symptomatic relief and to ensure adequate hydration and nutrition. Therapy of orchitis includes bed rest, scrotal support, analgesics, and ice packs. Patients with significant CNS involvement will require hospitalization for observation and supportive care. There is currently no established role for antiviral drugs, corticosteroids, or passive immunotherapy.

PREVENTION. The cornerstone of mumps prevention is active immunization using the live attenuated mumps vaccine. In the United States, mumps vaccine is administered in combination with the measles and rubella (MMR) vaccines to children at age 15 months and produces protective antibody levels in $> 95\%$ of recipients. A second dose of MMR is recommended for children when they enter school. The mumps vaccine is also indicated for susceptible adults.

The "Jeryl-Lynn" strain of attenuated mumps virus used in the United States since 1967 is a very well-tolerated vaccine, although rare instances of fever, parotitis, and possibly aseptic meningitis have been reported following immunization. In 1988 and 1989, however, an apparent increased frequency of cases of vaccine-related mumps meningitis was recognized in Canada and Japan. These cases occurred after MMR vaccine was administered that contained the Urabe AM-9 mumps virus, and in several cases, the vaccine virus was isolated from CSF and positively identified by nucleotide sequencing. This problem has not been recognized in the United States, where the Jeryl-Lynn mumps vaccine continues to be used.

Questions regarding prevention often arise when an individual with no history of mumps (typically an adult male) is exposed to a patient with active mumps. The immune status of the exposed individual can be determined by serologic testing, although this may involve some delay. The vast majority of adults born in the United States before 1957 have been naturally infected and are therefore immune. Mumps vaccine can be safely administered to an individual of unknown immune status, although vaccine given to a susceptible individual after exposure to mumps may not provide protection.

Briss PA, Fehrs LJ, Parker RA, et al.: Sustained transmission of mumps in a highly vaccinated population: Assessment of primary vaccine induced immunity. J Infect Dis 169:77, 1994. *Investigation of a mumps outbreak attributed to vaccine failure.*
CDC: General recommendations on immunization: Recommendations of the Advisory Committee on Immunization Practices (ACIP). MMWR 43 (RR-1):1, 1994. *Current recommendations for mumps vaccination.*

The Herpes Group of Viruses

339 HERPES SIMPLEX VIRUS INFECTIONS

Richard J. Whitley

Herpes simplex virus (HSV), a member of the family Herpesviridae, has been implicated in human infections since descriptions of cutaneous spreading lesions in ancient Greek times. Scholars of Greek civilization define the word *herpes* to mean "to creep or crawl," in reference to the spreading nature of the observed skin lesions. More recently, infection has been defined by the spectrum of illnesses caused by HSV. In 1968, well-defined antigenic and biologic differences were demonstrated between herpes simplex virus type 1 (HSV-1) and herpes simplex virus type 2 (HSV-2). HSV-1 was more frequently associated with nongenital infection and HSV-2 with genital disease. Further study has revealed that, of all the herpesviruses, HSV-1 and HSV-2 are the most closely related, with approximately 60% genomic homology. These two viruses can be distinguished most reliably by DNA restriction enzyme analyses; however, differences in antigen expression and biologic properties also serve as methods for differentiation.

STRUCTURE. Membership in the family Herpesviridae is based on the structure of the virion (Fig. 339–1). HSV contains double-stranded DNA at the central core, has a molecular weight of approximately 100 million, and encodes at least 70 polypeptides. The DNA core is surrounded by a capsid that consists of 162 capsomers, arranged in icosapentahedral symmetry. The capsid is approximately 100 to 110 nm in diameter. Tightly adherent to the capsid is the tegument, consisting of amorphous material. Loosely surrounding the capsid and tegument is a lipid bilayer envelope derived from host cell membranes. The envelope consists of polyamines, lipids, and glycoproteins. These glycoproteins confer distinctive properties to the virus and provide unique antigens to which the host is capable of responding. Notably, glycoprotein G (gG) provides antigenic specificity to HSV and therefore results in an antibody response that allows for the distinction between HSV-1 (gG-1) and HSV-2 (gG-2).

A unique feature of HSV DNA is its genomic sequence arrangement. The genome consists of two components, L (long) and S (short), each of which contains unique sequences that can invert on themselves, leading to four isomers. Viral DNA extracted from virions of infected cells consists of four equimolar populations, differing only with respect to the relative orientation of the two unique components. Biologic relevance of this phenomenon is unknown.

REPLICATION. Replication of HSV is a multistep process (Fig. 339–2). Following the onset of infection, DNA is uncoated and transported to the nucleus of the host cell. This is followed by transcription of immediate-early genes, which encode for the regulatory proteins, and is followed by the expression of proteins encoded by early and then late genes. These proteins include enzymes necessary for viral replication and structural proteins.

Assembly of the viral core and capsid takes place within the nucleus. Envelopment at the nuclear membrane and transport out of the nucleus occur through the endoplasmic reticulum and the Golgi apparatus. Glycosylation of the viral membrane occurs in the Golgi. Mature virions are transported to the outer membrane of the host cell inside vesicles. Release of progeny virus is accompanied by cell death. Replication for all herpesviruses is considered inefficient, with a high ratio of noninfectious to infectious viral particles.

PATHOGENESIS AND LATENCY. A critical factor for transmission of HSV, regardless of virus type, is intimate contact between a person who is shedding virus and a susceptible host. With inoculation onto the skin or mucous membrane, HSV replicates in epithelial cells; the incubation period is 4 to 6 days (Fig. 339–3). As replication continues, cell lysis and local inflammation ensue, resulting in characteristic vesicles on an erythematous base. Regional lymphatics and lymph nodes become involved with the draining of infected secretions from the area of viral replication. Viremia and visceral dissemination may develop depending on the immunologic competence of the host. In all hosts, the virus generally ascends peripheral sensory nerves to reach the dorsal root ganglia. Replication of HSV within neural tissue is followed by spread of the virus to other mucosal and skin surfaces via the peripheral sensory nerves. Virus replicates further in epithelial cells, reproducing the lesions of the initial infection, until infection is contained through host immunity.

The histopathologic changes induced by HSV replication are similar for both primary and recurrent infection. Changes induced by

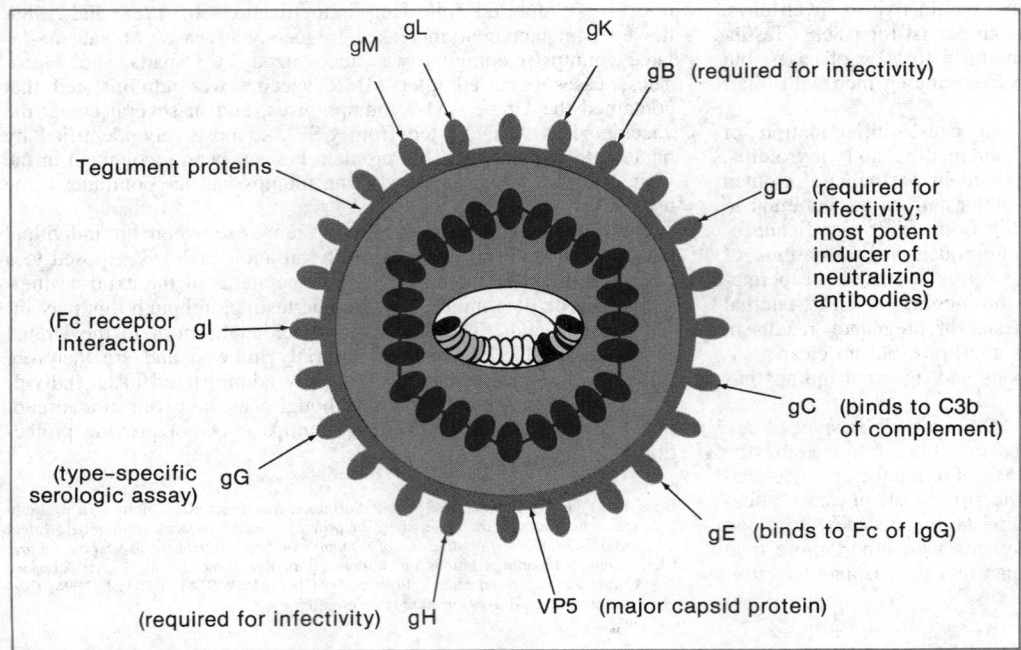

FIGURE 339–1. Schematic diagram of the HSV virion.

gM gL gK
gB (required for infectivity)
Tegument proteins
gD (required for infectivity; most potent inducer of neutralizing antibodies)
(Fc receptor interaction) gI
gC (binds to C3b of complement)
(type-specific serologic assay) gG
gE (binds to Fc of IgG)
(required for infectivity) gH VP5 (major capsid protein)

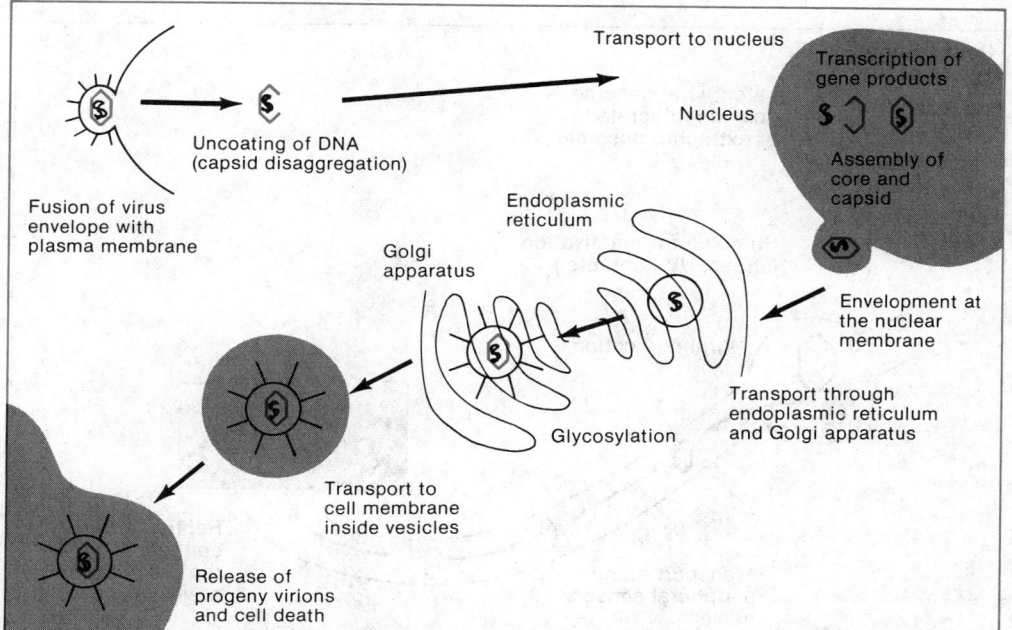

FIGURE 339–2. Schematic diagram of HSV replication.

viral infection include ballooning of infected cells and the appearance of condensed chromatin within the nuclei of cells, followed by subsequent degeneration of the cellular nuclei. Cells lose intact plasma membranes and form multinucleated giant cells. They also may demonstrate the intranuclear inclusion bodies known as Cowdry type A bodies, which are suggestive but not diagnostic of HSV infection. With cell lysis, a clear vesicular fluid containing large quantities of virus forms between the epidermis and dermal layer. The dermis reveals an intense inflammatory response, more so with primary infection than with recurrent disease. As healing progresses, the clear vesicular fluid becomes pustular with the recruitment of inflammatory cells. The pustule then forms a scab, with scarring being uncommon.

The vascular changes in the area of infection include perivascular cuffing and hemorrhagic necrosis. These changes are particularly prominent when organs other than skin are involved, as is the case with herpes simplex encephalitis or disseminated neonatal HSV in-

fection. Local lymphatics can show evidence of infection with intrusion of inflammatory cells due to the draining of infected secretions from the area of viral replication. As host defenses are mounted, an influx of mononuclear cells can be detected in infected tissue.

A unique characteristic of the herpesviruses is their ability to establish latent infection, persist in an apparently inactive state for varying amounts of time, and then be reactivated (Fig. 339–4). The latent viral genome may be either extrachromosomal or integrated into host-cell DNA.

Latency is established when HSV reaches the dorsal root ganglia after retrograde transmission via sensory nerve pathways. Latent virus may be reactivated and enter a replicative cycle at any point in time. The reactivation of latent virus is a well-recognized biologic phenomenon but not one that is understood from a molecular standpoint. Stimuli that have been observed to be associated with the reactivation of latent HSV have included stress, menstruation,

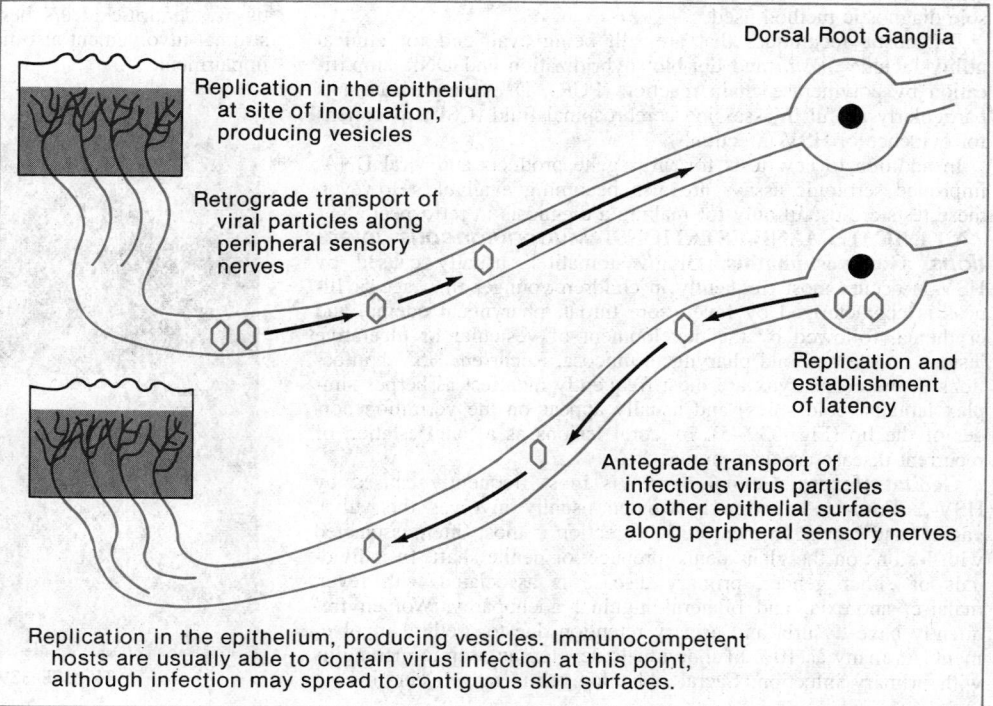

FIGURE 339–3. Schematic diagram of primary HSV infection.

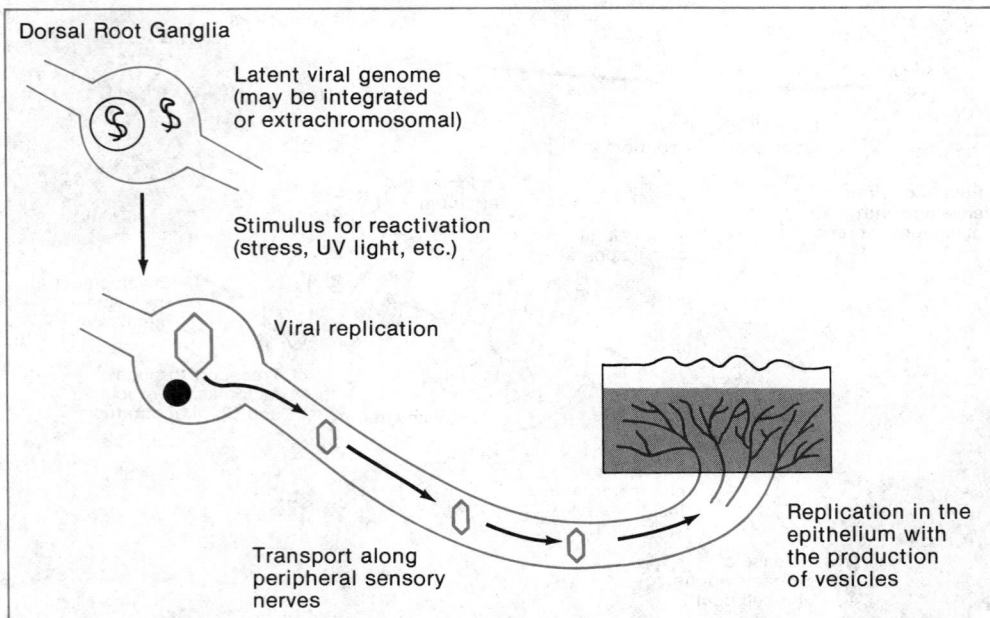

Dorsal Root Ganglia

Latent viral genome
(may be integrated
or extrachromosomal)

Stimulus for reactivation
(stress, UV light, etc.)

Viral replication

Transport along
peripheral sensory
nerves

Replication in the
epithelium with
the production
of vesicles

FIGURE 339–4. Schematic diagram of HSV latency and reactivation.

and exposure to ultraviolet light. Precisely how these factors interact at the level of the ganglia remains to be defined. Reactivation may be clinically asymptomatic, or it may produce life-threatening disease.

DIAGNOSIS. The definitive diagnosis of HSV infection requires isolation of virus. Swabs of clinical specimens or other body fluids can be inoculated into susceptible cell lines and observed for the development of characteristic cytopathic effects. This technique is very useful for the diagnosis of HSV-1 and HSV-2 infection because of the short replicative cycles.

In the absence of diagnostic virology facilities, cytologic examination of cells scraped from a clinical lesion may be useful in making a presumptive diagnosis of HSV infection. Material obtained from scraping the base of a lesion should be smeared on a glass slide and promptly fixed in cold ethanol. The slide can be stained according to the methods of Papanicolaou, Giemsa, or Wright. The presence of intranuclear inclusions and multinucleated giant cells is indicative, but not diagnostic, of HSV infection. This method has a sensitivity of only approximately 60 to 70% and should not be the sole diagnostic method used.

Diagnostic techniques that are still being evaluated for clinical utility include *in situ* and dot-blot hybridization and DNA amplification by polymerase chain reaction (PCR). DNA amplification is particularly useful in assessing cerebrospinal fluid (CSF) specimens for evidence of HSV infection.

In addition to new tests for virus gene products and viral DNA, improved serologic assays are also becoming available. However, these tests are useful only for making a diagnosis in retrospect.

CLINICAL MANIFESTATIONS. *Mucocutaneous Infections.* **Gingivostomatitis.** Gingivostomatitis (usually caused by HSV-1) occurs most frequently in children younger than age 5. Illness is characterized by fever, sore throat, pharyngeal edema, and erythema, followed by the development of vesicular or ulcerative lesions on the oral and pharyngeal mucosa. Recurrent HSV-1 infections of the oropharynx are most frequently manifest as herpes simplex labialis (cold sores) and usually appear on the vermilion border of the lip (Fig. 339–5). Intraoral lesions as a manifestation of recurrent disease are uncommon.

Genital Herpes. Genital herpes is most frequently caused by HSV-2. Primary infection in women usually involves the vulva, vagina, and cervix. In men, initial infection is most often associated with lesions on the glans penis, prepuce, or penile shaft. In individuals of either gender, primary disease is associated with fever, malaise, anorexia, and bilateral inguinal adenopathy. Women frequently have dysuria and urinary retention due to urethral involvement. As many as 10% of individuals develop an aseptic meningitis with primary infection. Sacral radiculomyelitis may occur in both

men and women, resulting in neuralgias, urinary retention, or obstipation. The complete healing of primary infection may take several weeks. It has been recognized that the first episode of genital infection is less severe in individuals who have had previous HSV-1 infections at other sites. Antibodies to HSV-1 appear to ameliorate the expression of HSV-2 clinical disease.

Recurrent genital infections in either men or women can be particularly distressing. The frequency of recurrence varies significantly from one individual to another. It has been estimated that one third have virtually no or few recurrences, one third have approximately three recurrences per year, and another third have more than three per year. Seroepidemiologic studies have found that between 25 and 65% of individuals in the United States in 1978 had antibodies to HSV-2 and that seroprevalence is correlated with the number of sexual partners.

Herpetic Keratitis. Herpes simplex keratitis is usually caused by HSV-1 and is accompanied by conjunctivitis in many cases. It is considered the most common infectious cause of blindness in the United States. The characteristic lesions of HSV keratoconjunctivitis are dendritic ulcers best detected by fluorescein staining. Deep stromal involvement also has been reported and may result in visual impairment.

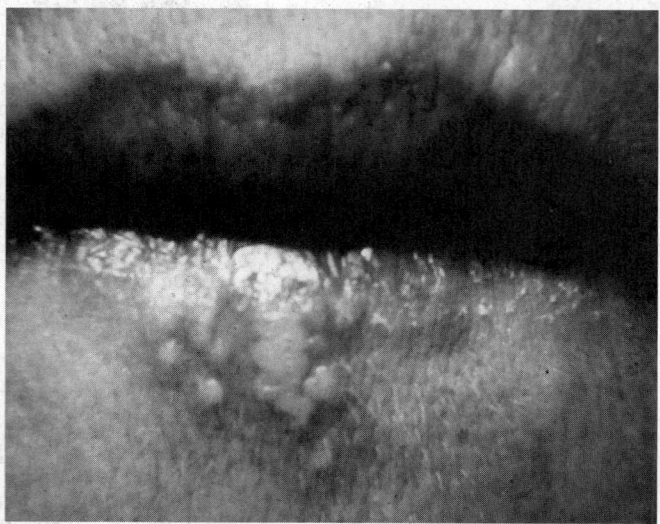

FIGURE 339–5. Herpes simplex labialis.

Other Cutaneous Manifestations. HSV infections can occur at any skin site. Common among health care workers are lesions on abraded skin of the fingers, known as herpetic whitlows. Similarly, wrestlers, because of physical contact, may develop disseminated cutaneous lesions known as herpes gladiatorum.

Neonatal Herpes Simplex Virus Infection. Neonatal HSV infection is estimated to occur in approximately 1 in 3500 deliveries in the United States each year. Approximately 70% of cases are caused by HSV-2 and usually result from contact of the fetus with infected maternal genital secretions at the time of delivery. Manifestations of neonatal HSV infection can be divided into three categories: (1) skin, eye, and mouth disease; (2) encephalitis; and (3) disseminated infection. As the name implies, skin, eye, and mouth disease consists of cutaneous lesions and does not involve other organ systems. Involvement of the central nervous system may occur with encephalitis or disseminated infection and generally results in a diffuse encephalitis. The CSF formula characteristically reveals an elevated protein and a mononuclear pleocytosis. Disseminated infection involves multiple organ systems and can produce disseminated intravascular coagulation, hemorrhagic pneumonitis, encephalitis, and cutaneous lesions. Diagnosis can be particularly difficult in the absence of skin lesions, which occurs in as many as 36% of cases. The mortality rate for each disease classification varies from zero for skin, eye, and mouth disease to 15% for encephalitis and 60% for neonates with disseminated infection, even with appropriate antiviral treatment. In addition to the high mortality associated with these infections, morbidity is significant in that children with encephalitis or disseminated disease develop normally in only 40% of cases, even with appropriate antiviral therapy.

Herpes Simplex Encephalitis. Herpes simplex encephalitis is characterized by hemorrhagic necrosis of the temporal lobe. Disease begins unilaterally, spreads to the contralateral temporal lobe, and is characterized by hemorrhagic necrosis (Fig. 339–6). It is the most common cause of focal, sporadic encephalitis in the United States today and occurs in approximately 1 in 150,000 individuals. Most cases are caused by HSV-1. The actual pathogenesis of herpes simplex encephalitis requires further clarification, although it has been speculated that primary or recurrent virus can reach the temporal lobe by ascending neural pathways, such as the trigeminal tracts or the olfactory nerves.

Clinical manifestations of herpes simplex encephalitis include headache, fever, altered consciousness, and abnormalities of speech and behavior, findings characteristic of temporal lobe involvement. Focal seizures also may occur. The CSF formula for these patients is variable but usually consists of a pleocytosis with both polymorphonuclear leukocytes and monocytes present. The protein concentration is characteristically elevated, and glucose is usually normal. Diagnosis can be achieved by PCR evaluation of CSF in experienced laboratories. The mortality and morbidity are high, even with appropriate antiviral therapy. At present, the mortality rate is ap-

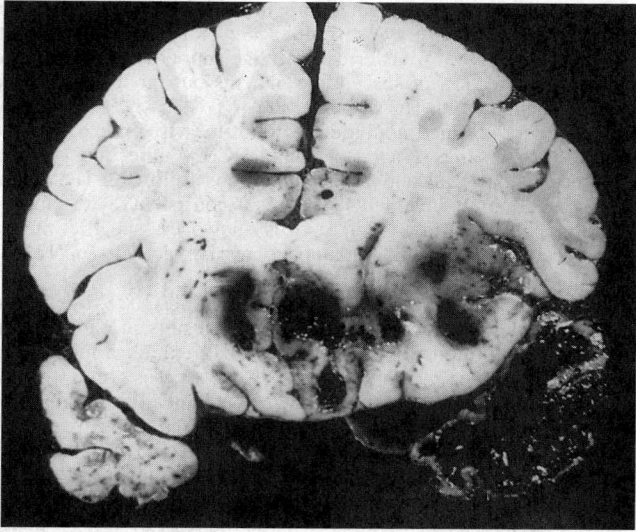

FIGURE 339–6. Hemorrhagic necrosis in herpes simplex encephalitis.

proximately 30% 1 year after treatment. In addition, approximately 50% of survivors have moderate or severe neurologic impairment.

Herpes Simplex Virus Infections in the Immunocompromised Host. HSV infections in the immunocompromised host are usually due to reactivation of latent infection and are clinically more severe, may be progressive, and require a longer time to heal. Manifestations of HSV infections in this patient population include pneumonitis, esophagitis, hepatitis, colitis, and disseminated cutaneous disease. Individuals suffering from human immunodeficiency virus (HIV) infection may have extensive perineal or orofacial ulcerations. HSV infections are also noted to be of increased severity in individuals with extensive burns.

EPIDEMIOLOGY. HSV infections are distributed worldwide and have been reported in both developed and underdeveloped countries. Animal vectors for human HSV infections have not been described, and there is no seasonal variation in the incidence of HSV infections. The virus is transmitted from infected to susceptible individuals during close personal contact, and virus must come in contact with mucosal surfaces or abraded skin for infection to be initiated. Since approximately one third of the world's population has recurrent HSV infections, and because infection is rarely fatal, a large reservoir of HSV exists in the community.

Although HSV-1 and HSV-2 are usually transmitted by different routes and involve different areas of the body, there is a great deal of overlap between the epidemiology and clinical manifestations of infections caused by these viruses. The mouth and lips are clearly the most common sites of HSV-1 infection. Primary HSV-1 infection in the young child is usually asymptomatic but may be manifest as gingivostomatitis. Primary infection in young adults has been associated with pharyngitis and sometimes a mononucleosis-like syndrome. Seroprevalence studies have demonstrated that acquisition of HSV-1 infection is related to socioeconomic factors. Antibodies, which indicate past infection, are found early in life among individuals of lower socioeconomic groups. This presumably is a consequence of crowded living conditions that provide a greater opportunity for direct contact with infected individuals. As many as 75 to 90% of individuals from lower socioeconomic populations develop antibodies by the end of the first decade of life. In contrast, only 30 to 40% of persons in middle and upper socioeconomic groups are seropositive by the middle of the second decade of life.

Because infections with HSV-2 are usually acquired through sexual contact, antibodies to this virus are rarely found until the onset of sexual activity. There is a progressive increase in infection rates with HSV-2 in all populations beginning in adolescence. As with HSV-1 infections, the rate of acquisition of HSV-2 infection appears related to socioeconomic factors. The number of sexual contacts is also an important risk factor for the acquisition of HSV-2. Importantly, genital herpes infection has been found to be a risk factor for another sexually transmitted virus, HIV.

Localized, recurrent HSV-2 infection is the most common form of HSV infection during gestation. Transmission of infection to the fetus is most frequently related to the shedding of virus at the time of delivery. Since HSV infection of the fetus is usually the consequence of contact with infected maternal genital secretions at the time of delivery, the determination of viral excretion at this time is of utmost importance. The incidence of cervical shedding in pregnant women with asymptomatic HSV infection is approximately 1%. Interestingly, most infants who develop neonatal disease are born to women who are completely asymptomatic for genital HSV infections at the time of delivery and who have neither a past history of genital herpes nor a sexual partner reporting a genital vesicular rash. These women account for 60 to 80% of all women whose children develop neonatal HSV infection.

PREVENTION. At present, there are no licensed vaccines directed against HSV. However, experimental vaccines for HSV-1 and HSV-2 are being evaluated. Acyclovir is currently being given to recipients of solid organ and bone marrow transplants in the immediate post-transplant period in an effort to prevent reactivation of latent disease.

TREATMENT. Infections caused by HSV-1 and HSV-2 are amenable to therapy with antiviral drugs (see Ch. 327). Both vidarabine and acyclovir have proved useful for managing specific infections caused by these viruses. At present, acyclovir is the treatment of choice for mucocutaneous HSV infections in the immuno-compromised host, herpes simplex encephalitis, and neonatal HSV infections. Intravenous administration is preferred for therapy of life-threatening disease. Intravenous acyclovir is also recommended for clinically severe initial genital herpes in the immunocompetent host. This includes patients with complications such as urinary retention or aseptic meningitis, and they should receive 5 mg per kilogram every 8 hours for 5 to 7 days. Caution must be exercised when acyclovir is used intravenously because it may crystallize in the renal tubules when given too rapidly or to dehydrated patients.

Immunocompromised individuals with mucocutaneous HSV infections that are not life threatening may be given oral acyclovir. Oral acyclovir is also useful in treating initial genital herpes. Recurrent episodes, however, are not as responsive to acyclovir. For individuals who experience severe or frequent recurrences of genital herpes, a "suppressive" regimen of acyclovir in doses of 600 to 800 mg per day may be useful. The efficacy of acyclovir for primary or recurrent oropharyngeal HSV in the immunocompetent host has not been well established.

Corey L, Spear P: Infections with herpes simplex viruses. N Engl J Med 314:686, 1986. *This two-article series is a concise review of herpes simplex virus infections.*
Goldsmith SM, Whitley RJ: Herpes simplex encephalitis. *In* Lambert HP (ed.): Infections of the Central Nervous System. Philadelphia, BC Decker, 1991, pp 283–299. *This chapter describes the clinical presentations, diagnostic evaluation, and treatment of herpes simplex virus encephalitis.*
Nahmias AJ, Lee FK, Bechman-Nahmias S: Sero-epidemiological and sociological patterns of herpes simplex virus infection in the world. Scand J Infect Dis 69:19, 1990. *A comprehensive analysis of herpes simplex virus seroepidemiology, utilizing new techniques for HSV-2-specific antibody.*
Roizman B: Herpesviridae: A brief introduction. *In* Fields BN, Knipe DM et al. (eds.): Fields Virology, 2nd ed. New York, Raven Press, 1990, p 1787. *This chapter provides an overview of the herpes family of viruses.*
Roizman B: New viral footprints in Kaposi's sarcoma (editorial). N Engl J Med 332:1227, 1995. *Discusses the discovery of human herpesvirus 8 by a novel technique and that the virus' footprints were found in cells affected by Kaposi's sarcoma.*
Straus SE: Clinical and biological differences between recurrent herpes simplex virus and varicella-zoster virus infections. JAMA 262:3455, 1989. *A concise article that emphasizes the distinctions between recurrent herpes simplex virus infections and recurrent varicella-zoster infections.*
Whitley RJ: Herpes simplex viruses. *In* Fields BN, Knipe DM, et al. (eds.): Fields' Virology. New York, Raven Press, 1990. *A comprehensive text that includes a detailed analysis of the molecular biology and clinical manifestations of herpes simplex virus.*

340 INFECTIONS ASSOCIATED WITH HUMAN CYTOMEGALOVIRUS

William J. Britt

Human cytomegalovirus (HCMV) is the largest and most structurally complex human herpesvirus. Its linear double-stranded DNA genome consists of 250,000 base pairs which can potentially encode over 200 different proteins. Two different types of infections have been defined, primary and recurrent. Recurrent infection may follow reactivation of previous infection or reinfection by a superinfecting viral strain. Host immunity is thought to be protective, because clinical evidence of infection rarely develops in the immunocompetent host. Abnormalities in immune responses caused by immunosuppressive drugs following allotransplantation, retroviral infections in patients with human immunodeficiency virus (HIV), or developmental immune dysfunction in the fetus predispose these unique populations to HCMV-induced disease.

EPIDEMIOLOGY. HCMV circulates within the population, and there is no evidence of epidemics or seasonal dependence. In most underdeveloped countries, HCMV is acquired early in childhood, likely as a result of either breast-feeding or secondary to crowded living conditions. Seropositivity reaches nearly 100% in these populations before childbearing age. In contrast, the seroprevalence in the United States is dependent on age and socioeconomic status. By

childbearing age, the seroprevalence often exceeds 90% in lower socioeconomic groups. In individuals of higher socioeconomic groups, approximately 50% are seropositive by early adulthood.

Several routes of virus transmission have been documented, including transmission following sexual contact. Previous studies have documented high levels of virus within semen and cervical secretions. Epidemiologic studies have demonstrated a correlation between a history of sexually transmitted disease with HCMV seropositivity. Transmission from young children represents another important source of HCMV infection. Careful epidemiologic studies within child care centers demonstrated virus transmission between young children, as well as transmission to adult caretakers and susceptible parents. The importance of children as a major source of virus can be appreciated if one considers that approximately 1% of all babies are born with HCMV infection (congenital) and that 30 to 70% of breast-fed babies of seropositive mothers will become infected. Because these infants often excrete large amounts of virus in their saliva and urine for months to years following infection, they provide an important reservoir of infectious HCMV.

Major sources of virus exposure among hospitalized patients include blood products and transplanted organs. Transfusion-acquired HCMV infection, prior to routine serologic screening of donor blood products, occurred at a consistent rate of approximately 2.5% per unit of whole blood. Numerous studies have demonstrated that leukocytes present within various blood products were responsible for the majority of transfusion-acquired HCMV infections. Measures that reduce leukocyte contamination within blood products or, alternatively, screening blood donors and matching HCMV serologic status of donor and recipient have reduced the incidence of transfusion-associated HCMV infection. Nosocomial transmission of HCMV to health workers is uncommon, even in personnel caring for patients excreting large amounts of HCMV, such as congenitally infected infants.

PATHOLOGY. Although HCMV can be consistently propagated *in vitro* only in human fibroblast cells, it can be isolated from a myriad of organs and cell types from infected humans. HCMV has been demonstrated in the endothelium of the vasculature, epithelium of almost every organ (including endocrine and exocrine organs), and neuronal cells of the central nervous system (CNS). Pathologic findings range from extensive tissue destruction to isolated cytomegalic cells. The typical cytomegalic cell consists of an enlarged cell with scant to reduced cytoplasm containing a large nucleus with prominent nucleoli and intranuclear inclusions.

PATHOGENESIS. Cellular-, antibody-, and cytokine-mediated immune responses have been proposed to limit HCMV infection, although direct evidence is lacking. A number of studies in bone marrow and solid organ allograft recipients have provided a strong correlation between the depression of HCMV-specific T lymphocyte responses and susceptibility to HCMV-associated infection and, more important, clinical disease. These responses have included both major histocompatability (MHC) class II–restricted CD4+ T lymphocytes and class I–restricted CD8+ cytotoxic T lymphocytes. Although the virus-encoded target antigens of these cellular responses are unknown, protein components of the virus itself are thought to induce protective responses. Several studies have documented that passively transferred antiviral antibodies failed to prevent HCMV infection in susceptible patients but modulated clinical disease associated with HCMV infection.

As yet poorly defined nonlytic effects of the virus may contribute to disease syndromes associated with HCMV infection. Clinical syndromes of bacterial and fungal infections following HCMV infection in allograft recipients are also consistent with an immunomodulatory activity of the virus; however, specific mechanisms accounting for this immunosuppressive activity of HCMV remain inadequately defined.

CLINICAL ASPECTS OF HCMV INFECTION. Although infection in the immunocompetent host rarely results in clinically apparent disease, infrequently, normal hosts will exhibit a mononucleosis-like syndrome. Approximately 8% of cases of infectious mononucleosis may be caused by HCMV. Clinically, this infection is indistinguishable from mononucleosis caused by Epstein-Barr virus, with the exception that it is heterophile-negative. Nonspecific constitutional symptoms predominate, including malaise, decreased appetite, and low-grade fever. Laboratory abnormalities include atypical lymphocytosis, chemical hepatitis and cholestasis, and less frequently, thrombocytopenia. Similar but often exaggerated findings have been associated with transfusion-acquired HCMV, including the previously described postperfusion syndrome that followed cardiopulmonary bypass.

Congenital HCMV infection (present at birth) is common, occurring in approximately 1% of all live births in the United States. Some 10% of these will suffer signs and symptoms of cytomegalic inclusion disease (CID), which include petechiae, hepatosplenomegaly, jaundice, and microcephaly. Thrombocytopenia, cholestasis, and evidence of hepatocellular damage are consistent laboratory findings. Although almost all end-organ disease is self-limited, CNS damage associated with congenital HCMV infection is permanent and often results in significant developmental delays, seizure activity, gross neurologic impairment, and most frequently, hearing loss. Subclinical congenital HCMV infection is less commonly associated with permanent CNS sequelae; however, up to 15% of infants with subclinical infection may exhibit evidence of CNS damage, such as sensorineural hearing loss. Both forms of congenital HCMV infection result in chronic virus excretion which may persist for years, thus providing an important source of HCMV exposure in the community.

HCMV infection following allograft transplantation is the most common infection in the post-transplant period. An estimated 60 to 100% of seropositive renal transplant recipients will excrete HCMV following transplantation. Although the vast majority of patients will not exhibit evidence of invasive HCMV infection, HCMV is a major cause of disease in heart, heart-lung, liver, and bone marrow transplant recipients. In the latter setting, HCMV pneumonia has been the leading infection-related cause of death, with mortality rates approaching 90%. Sources of HCMV infection in the allograft recipient include (1) reactivated infection of the HCMV-seropositive recipient, (2) exogenous blood products given in the post-transplant period, and (3) most commonly, from the transplanted organ obtained from an HCMV-seropositive donor. The highest risk for infection and disease is observed in the HCMV-seronegative recipient of an allograft from a HCMV-seropositive allograft donor (see Ch. 266). Other factors associated with clinically significant HCMV infections in solid organ allograft recipients include the use of cadaveric grafts, leukocyte-containing blood products, and immunosuppressive agents which deplete T lymphocytes such as antithymocyte globulin or anti-DC3 monoclonal antibodies. In bone marrow allograft recipients, the severity of HCMV infection often parallels the development of graft-versus-host disease (GVHD).

Clinical evidence of HCMV infection usually develops 4 to 6 weeks after transplantation and can present with a variety of end-organ diseases such as pneumonitis or hepatitis and more commonly as a syndrome similar to HCMV mononucleosis, which can include fever, leukopenia, thrombocytopenia, and hepatitis. Virus can be isolated from the urine in almost-infected patients and from the blood in a subset of patients. This latter finding may presage the development of invasive multiorgan disease. Potentially fatal invasive infections include pneumonitis, severe gastrointestinal ulcerative disease with perforation, and life-threatening hepatitis. HCMV pneumonitis most commonly presents insidiously as a diffuse interstitial pneumonia that progresses in the absence of specific therapy. Acute allograft loss may accompany HCMV disease either as a direct result of graft involvement, as seen in hepatic transplants, or secondary to the reduction in immunosuppression which may be necessary for treating invasive HCMV disease. Long-term allograft survival also appears to be reduced as a result of HCMV infection. In cardiac allografts this has been proposed to result from virus-associated acceleration of coronary artery atherosclerosis of the allograft, whereas in hepatic allografts it has been suggested that HCMV causes increased expression of MHC antigens resulting in enhanced immunologic recognition of the graft.

HCMV has become a major cause of morbidity and mortality in patients with acquired immunodeficiency syndrome (AIDS) (see Part XXII). Because of the importance of sexual transmission in the spread of HCMV in adult populations, it is not surprising that the rate of HCMV seropositivity approaches 100% in populations at high risk for HIV infection. Thus endogenous virus and frequent sexual exposure to reinfecting viral strains are likely sources of HCMV in these populations. The importance of HCMV coinfection to progression of AIDS has been proposed, and in vitro findings support a potential role of HCMV in HIV replication. Risk factors for the development of invasive HCMV disease in this population include a CD4+ lymphocyte count of <50 per cubic millimeter. In addition, it has been noted that the development of invasive HCMV disease is a grave prognostic sign, since overall survival is significantly shortened in patients with documented HCMV disease.

Invasive HCMV infections in patients with AIDS have included end-organ disease in almost all organ systems, with three systems being more frequently involved: the CNS, gastrointestinal (GI) system, and pulmonary system. HCMV infection of the CNS, although uncommon in allograft recipients, is not infrequent in HIV-infected patients. Encephalopathies, both diffuse and focal, as well as myelopathies and neuropathies, have been ascribed to HCMV. The most common and important disease associated with HCMV in this population is retinitis. It has been estimated that between 8 and 25% of long-lived patients with AIDS will develop this invasive HCMV infection. GI involvement includes both colitis and esophagitis and less frequently gastritis. Clinical and laboratory evidence of HCMV colitis is often found in association with other GI pathogens, thus raising questions about the importance of HCMV as a primary pathogen. Likewise, the significance of HCMV as a frequent cause of pneumonitis in AIDS patients has been challenged.

DIAGNOSIS. The diagnosis of HCMV has conventionally relied on isolating the virus from urine, saliva, blood, or biopsy specimens obtained from patients exhibiting symptoms compatible with HCMV infection. There is no convenient method to distinguish acute, invasive infection from peripheral shedding resulting from reactivation of a pre-existing infection. In the transplant and AIDS population, this has prompted diagnostic approaches for measuring viral burden, including HCMV blood cultures and cultures from biopsy specimens, both of which more closely correlate with invasive disease as compared with viruria. Adaptation of immunocytochemistry and centrifugation-enhanced culture techniques has shortened the time required to identify HCMV in clinical specimens to less than 24 hours.

Serologic determination of HCMV is valuable when both IgG and IgM virus-specific antibodies are measured and most frequently only in normal hosts. Measurement of IgG alone is of limited value because of the high seroprevalence of HCMV in the population and the persistence of antibody responses to the virus. Although HCMV-specific IgM antibodies persist for at least 2 to 3 months in normal individuals, their value in immunocompromised hosts is often limited.

Newer methods of diagnosis include the polymerase chain reaction (PCR) of several different body fluids as well as biopsy material. PCR has been used successfully to detect viremia and plasma HCMV DNA. Quantifying PCR results also should prove of prognostic value. A semiquantitative assay of viral burden that detects virus-encoded protein in polymorphonuclear leukocytes, the antigenemia assay, appears predictive of invasive disease in allograft recipients and patients with AIDS.

THERAPY. Until recently, effective antiviral therapy has not been available for HCMV infection. Two agents, ganciclovir and foscarnet, have been shown to be virostatic in vitro and in vivo. Clinical trials have documented efficacy of these agents in treating invasive HCMV disease in both transplant and AIDS patients. Both have significant toxicity, which often precludes their long-term administration. Ganciclovir causes dose-limiting hematopoietic toxicity, often resulting in clinically significant neutropenia. Foscarnet has significant nephrotoxicity, which limits its use in patients with azotemia. In addition, long-term therapy in immunocompromised patients has resulted in the development of viral resistance to both agents.

Perhaps the most beneficial use of these agents has been as prophylaxis in the immediate transplant period. Both foscarnet and ganciclovir have been used successfully to reduce the incidence of HCMV disease in the post-transplant period in both solid organ and bone marrow transplant recipients.

Immunoprophylaxis of HCMV infection has included passive transfer of antibody and limited clinical trials of a live-virus vaccine. The use of intravenous immunoglobulin containing anti-HCMV antibodies remains controversial, although a clinical trial in renal allograft recipients has provided evidence of its efficacy. Its use in bone marrow transplantation is contentious, but accumulating evidence suggests that any efficacy may result from poorly understood immunomodulatory properties that influence the severity of GVHD. Active immunization with a replicating HCMV virus as a means of inducing protective immunity has been attempted on a limited scale in renal transplant recipients. The results of this trial remain controversial, although there was some evidence suggesting that protective immunity was induced by the vaccine virus.

Alford CA, Britt WJ: Cytomegalovirus. In Roizman B, Whitley RJ, Lopez C (eds.): The Human Herpesviruses. New York, Raven Press, 1993, pp 227–255. Discussion of biology and clinical syndromes associated with HCMV.
Fowler KB, Stagno S, Pass RF, et al.: The outcome of congenital cytomegalovirus infection in relation to maternal antibody status. N Engl J Med 326:663, 1992. Recent information on the importance of maternal immunity and outcome of congenital HCMV.
Gallant JE, Moore RD, Richman DD, et al.: Incidence and natural history of cytomegalovirus disease in patients with advanced human immunodeficiency virus disease treated with zidovudine. J Infect Dis 166:1223, 1992. Prospective study of natural history of HCMV in HIV-infected patients.
Ho M: Cytomegalovirus Biology and Infection. New York, Plenum Press, 1991. Monograph on the biology of animal cytomegaloviruses including HCMV.
Mocarski ES: Cytomegalovirus biology and replication. In Roizman B, Whitley RJ, Lopez C (eds.): The Human Herpesviruses. New York, Raven Press, 1993, pp 173–226. Excellent overview of molecular biology of HCMV.
Pass RF, Britt WJ, Stagno S: Cytomegalovirus. In Lennette EH, Lennette DA, Lennette ET (eds.): Diagnostic Procedures for Viral, Rickettsial and Chlamydial Infections. 7th ed. Washington, APHA, 1994. Discussion of commonly used methodologies for diagnosing HCMV.
Schmidt GM, Horak DA, Niland JC, et al.: A randomized, controlled trial of prophylactic ganciclovir for cytomegalovirus pulmonary infection in recipients of allogeneic bone marrow transplants. N Engl J Med 324:1005, 1991. Early randomized trial of ganciclovir treatment of HCMV pneumonia in bone marrow allograft recipients.
Singh N, Yu VL, Mieles L, et al.: High-dose acyclovir compared with short-course preemptive ganciclovir therapy to prevent cytomegalovirus disease in liver transplant recipients. Ann Intern Med 120:375, 1994. Prophylaxis of HCMV following liver transplantation.
Winston DJ, Ho WG, Champlin RE: Cytomegalovirus infections after bone marrow transplantation. Rev Infect Dis 12:S776, 1990. Review of HCMV infections in bone marrow transplant recipients.

341 INFECTIOUS MONONUCLEOSIS: EPSTEIN-BARR VIRUS INFECTION

Elliott D. Kieff

DEFINITION. Infectious mononucleosis is a clinical syndrome characterized by malaise, headache, fever, pharyngitis, pharyngeal lymphatic hyperplasia, lymphadenopathy, atypical lymphocytosis, heterophile antibody, and mild transient hepatitis. The syndrome occurs most commonly in adolescents and young adults.

ETIOLOGY. Primary Epstein-Barr virus (EBV) infection is the cause of almost all typical infectious mononucleosis syndromes. EBV is a herpes virus. *In vitro*, it infects only human B lymphocytes. Virus infection of B lymphocytes *in vitro* results in lymphocyte proliferation and immunoglobulin secretion. EBV usually remains latent in the infected B lymphocytes and can be induced to replicate in these cells using a variety of chemicals.

EPIDEMIOLOGY. The usual mode of EBV infection is by direct contact of saliva from a previously infected person with the oropharyngeal epithelium of a nonimmune person. Infection in infancy commonly results from eating food premasticated by an infected mother, whereas infection in adolescence or as an adult is usually from salivary transfer during kissing. Virus survival in expectorated saliva is probably brief, since infection does not usually spread to susceptible roommates. Spread among young children sharing toys has not been studied.

Following oropharyngeal inoculation with infected saliva, the virus replicates in oropharyngeal epithelial cells. Although the amount of virus in saliva is highest during primary infection and for months thereafter, virus replication in the oropharynx occurs intermittently for many years, possibly for life. In the course of primary oropharyngeal infection, EBV infects tonsillar and peripheral blood B lymphocytes. Virus persists indefinitely in a small fraction of the peripheral blood B lymphocytes. Transfusion of whole blood, bone marrow, blood fractions, or tissue containing viable B lym-

phocytes to susceptible (nonimmune) persons can result in symptomatic primary infection. Following bone marrow transplantation, the donor's virus may predominate in the recipient and may emerge as the dominant virus in the oropharynx of the recipient, indicating that a bone marrow or blood cell such as B lymphocytes are a site of persistent latent infection and the source of virus for continuing infection of the epithelium. EBV has also been found in salivary gland secretions and in cervical secretions, indicating that latently infected B lymphocytes can transmit virus to other epithelial tissues.

Previously infected normal persons are immune to the development of infectious mononucleosis. In less industrialized societies or among lower socioeconomic groups in industrialized societies, most children experience primary infection in the first decade of life. Among middle and higher socioeconomic groups, primary infection usually occurs as a consequence of adolescent or postadolescent kissing. More than 90% of adults in all human populations have serologic evidence of previous primary EBV infection and are carriers of the virus. Although EBV infection is limited to humans, each Old World primate species is endemically infected with a related virus characteristic of that species. New World primates are free of EBV-related viruses and can be experimentally infected. Experimental infection of some species with a sufficient EBV inoculum results in acute fatal lymphoproliferation.

CLINICAL MANIFESTATIONS. The syndrome of infectious mononucleosis was a distinctive clinical entity for at least 40 years before the discovery of its etiologic agent. After a 2- to 5-week incubation period, most infected nonimmune adolescents and young adults develop malaise, headache, fever, pharyngitis, and lymphadenopathy lasting from 1 to several weeks. Temperatures may reach 40°C. Tonsillar or cervical lymph nodes may be quite enlarged, painful, and tender. Laboratory findings include relative or absolute lymphocytosis and a high titer of antibody to horse or ox red blood cells, referred to as a heterophile antibody. Up to 40% of the peripheral lymphocytes are atypical large cells with unusually abundant cytoplasm and a large pale pleomorphic nucleus. Other common manifestations are listed in Table 341–1. Malaise or weakness may recur over several months. Rashes are significantly more common in patients with primary EBV infection receiving penicillin or ampicillin treatment than in untreated patients or patients with other diseases who are treated with penicillin. Almost all normal people completely recover from acute infectious mononucleosis

TABLE 341–1. CLINICAL MANIFESTATIONS OF INFECTIOUS MONONUCLEOSIS

Common manifestations	(%)
Splenomegaly	50
Vomiting	20
Hepatitis	20–50
Jaundice	5
Palatal petechiae	
Skin rash	4
Albuminuria	10
Less frequent manifestations (0.5–1%)	
Cough	
Pneumonitis	
Neck stiffness	
Aseptic meningitis	
Cerebritis	
Cerebellar dysfunction	
Mononeuritis or polyneuritis	
Transverse myelitis	
Guillain-Barré syndrome	
Uveitis	
Subcapsular splenic hemorrhage or rupture	
Myocarditis	
Pericarditis	
Cardiac conduction abnormalities	
Nephrotic syndrome	
Renal dysfunction	
Diarrhea	
Hemolytic anemia with anti-i antibody	
Thrombocytopenia	
Agranulocytosis	
Pancytopenia	
Hemophagocytic syndrome	

within 3 to 4 months. Persistent systemic, hematologic, neurologic, or cardiac abnormalities are rare.

Outside of the adolescent and young adult populations, primary EBV infection frequently does not result in the full infectious mononucleosis syndrome. In younger children, fever and pharyngitis from primary EBV infection may be clinically indistinguishable from upper respiratory tract infections caused by other viruses, mycoplasma, or streptococci. At any age cerebritis, neuritis, pneumonitis, hepatitis, carditis, autoimmune hemolytic anemia, or thrombocytopenia may be the predominant clinical manifestation. Atypical lymphocytosis or heterophile antibody may be less prominent or absent.

Severe, progressive, and sometimes fatal primary EBV infections occur in children in X-linked lymphoproliferative disease (Duncan's syndrome). Non–X-linked, sporadic cases also occur. Although these children have no obvious pre-existing immune deficiency, primary EBV infection leads to massive lymphoproliferation, fever, anemia, hepatitis, or fulminant hepatic necrosis. The proliferating B lymphocytes are EBV-infected cells that express EBV-latent-infection–associated proteins. The early proliferation is polyclonal. Fulminant hepatic failure is a frequent cause of death. Recovery may be accompanied by persistent anemia, hypogammaglobulinemia, or pancytopenia. Oligoclonal or uniclonal EBV-infected B lymphomas may occur during the primary infection or after recovery. Similar illnesses with polyclonal lymphoproliferative disease occur in other immunosuppressed patients with primary EBV infection. Administration of high-dose cyclosporine as part of immunosuppressive regimens for heart, lung, liver, or bone marrow transplantation has been associated with severe EBV infection and polyclonal lymphoproliferative disease. The lymphoproliferative process may involve cervical, abdominal, or gastrointestinal lymphatics. Moreover, children with human immunodeficiency virus (HIV) infection are also at risk for severe EBV infection and lymphoproliferative disease (see Ch. 369), and EBV-infected lymphocytes are a frequent cause of the central nervous system lymphomas that occur in AIDS or organ transplant recipients. In AIDS patients, replicating EBV has also been found in hairy leukoplakia of the tongue, a proliferative epithelial lesion.

Very rare cases of chronic progressive primary EBV infection in otherwise normal young adults have been well documented. These few patients have had severe acute mononucleosis that persists with clinical manifestations that include lymphadenopathy or visceral organ involvement and abnormally high antibody titers to EBV replicative cycle antigens. These titers are characteristically 10- to 100-fold higher than those in normal persons after primary EBV infection. Some patients have lacked antibody to EBV nuclear antigens. Most patients eventually recover without specific treatment. In one patient, acyclovir treatment produced clinical remission.

Persistent active EBV infection has been proposed to be the cause of a more common chronic mononucleosis or *chronic fatigue syndrome*. This syndrome is characterized by recurrent episodes of malaise and weakness, sometimes accompanied by myalgias, arthralgias, pharyngitis, lymphadenitis, or mild fever. The persistent lack of significant objective clinical or laboratory abnormalities distinguishes most patients with this poorly defined syndrome from those with documentable infectious, autoimmune, oncologic, metabolic, or neurologic diseases that can also occur with chronic fatigue. EBV-specific antibody titers in most patients with the chronic fatigue syndrome do not differ significantly from those of normal infected adults (see below). Thus there is little to support the initial hypothesis that EBV is a frequent cause of this syndrome.

Latent EBV infection is also associated with B lymphomas in immunosuppressed patients, with Burkitt-type lymphoma in African children, with some of the sporadic Burkitt-type lymphomas that occur in developed societies, with about 50% of cases of Hodgkin's disease, with some T cell lymphomas in adolescents or young adults, and with anaplastic nasopharyngeal carcinoma. A substantial fraction of B lymphomas occurring in immunocompromised patients have EBV DNA in the tumor cells. In B lymphomas in which the virus is latent in all of the tumor cells, the virus probably provides an initial, and in some cases an ongoing, stimulus for cell proliferation. Malignant conversion in many late postinfection lymphomas requires at least one additional factor, since these cells frequently also have a chromosome translocation that enhances *c-myc* oncogene expression. In a prospective study of African children, a correlation was noted between children with higher EBV antibody

responses in the years after primary infection and tumor occurrence, suggesting that the extent of EBV replication is an important parameter in tumor induction.

In the last few years, considerable evidence has been amassed that EBV is an etiologic agent in Hodgkin's disease (see Ch. 146). EBV DNA is present in about 50% of Hodgkin's disease, with the highest incidence of EBV positivity being in younger patients, in Hispanic patients, and in patients with the mixed cellularity form of Hodgkin's disease. When present, EBV DNA is in all of the Hodgkin's disease "tumor" cells, and the cells are uniclonal with regard to EBV infection, indicating that infection did not occur after the onset of Hodgkin's disease.

EBV infection is also associated with anaplastic nasopharyngeal carcinomas. In retrospective and prospective clinical studies, high levels of IgA antibody to EBV antigens have been closely associated with anaplastic nasopharyngeal carcinoma. EBV has been uniformly found in each of the tumor cells of anaplastic nasopharyngeal carcinoma. The uniclonality of the virus genomes in these tumor cells indicates that the tumors arise in a single virus-infected cell. The virus is therefore likely to be necessary for this oncogenic conversion. Chinese and some North African and Canadian and U.S. Native American populations have a high incidence of nasopharyngeal carcinoma. Among peoples of Southern Chinese extraction, anaplastic nasopharyngeal carcinomas are the most common or second most common malignant growth. Genetic factors are therefore likely to be important determinants of tumor incidence. Other factors in the pathogenesis of nasopharyngeal carcinoma have not been defined.

PATHOLOGY AND PATHOGENESIS. EBV first infects pharyngeal epithelial cells and then spreads to subepithelial circulating B lymphocytes. The virus carries a gene similar to the human interleukin-10 gene, and the expression of this protein partially blocks the initial interferon, natural killer (NK), and T-cytotoxic responses. Infection may be confined to epithelial and B-lymphocyte tissues, since only these cells have EBV receptors. The EBV receptor is also the receptor for the C3d fragment of complement. Tonsils and regional and systemic lymph nodes enlarge because of follicular hyperplasia, due in part to virus-infected B lymphocytes and infiltration of sinuses and paracortex with reactive, atypical T lymphocytes. Loss of normal architecture and the presence of Reed-Sternberg–like cells may make EBV infection difficult to distinguish from Hodgkin's disease. Similar changes occur in the spleen. In patients with significant hepatitis, hepatic lobules or portal areas may be infiltrated with mononuclear cells. The bone marrow is usually unaffected. Early in the illness, up to 1 or 2% of the circulating leukocytes may be EBV-infected B lymphocytes. The predominant atypical lymphocytes in the peripheral blood, however, are reactive NK cells and T cells. EBV-infected B lymphocytes can be detected by their expression of EBV nuclear proteins (EBNA's) and latent infection membrane proteins or by their ability to proliferate continuously *in vitro* or in severe combined immunodeficiency (SCID) mice, a property that normal B lymphocytes lack. EBV infection of B lymphocytes stimulates both B-cell proliferation and Ig secretion, particularly IgM. The heterophile antibody may be the direct product of EBV-infected B lymphocytes, or it may be produced as a result of lymphokines produced by EBV-infected or reactive lymphocytes.

Lymphoproliferation following EBV infection of normal B lymphocytes *in vitro* is associated with the expression of six EBV nuclear proteins or EBNA's, two EBV integral membrane proteins or latent infection membrane proteins (LMP's), and two small RNA's. The same repertoire of genes is expressed in the peripheral B lymphocytes in acute infectious mononucleosis and in EBV-associated lymphoproliferative disease. The EBV-encoded nuclear proteins are transactivators of virus and cell gene expression. The virus LMP1 gene encodes the primary transforming protein of the virus. This protein is characteristically expressed in EBV-associated lymphoproliferative disease, in EBV-associated Hodgkin's disease, and in early nasopharyngeal carcinomas. The LMP2 gene encodes a protein that prevents reactivation of virus lytic infection in response to usual B-cell activators. In normal patients with primary EBV infection, the acute, non–B-lymphocyte response to EBV infection is multifunctional. Some T lymphocytes suppress both B-lymphocyte proliferation and Ig secretion. Other peripheral blood T lymphocytes and NK cells from patients with infectious mononucleosis are cytotoxic to autologous EBV-infected B cells. Most cytotoxic T lymphocytes are largely CD8+ and recognize EBNA or LMP epitopes in the context of class I histocompatibility molecules. Other T lymphocytes may augment the T- and B-lymphocyte immune responses. Two EBV types are endemic in humans. These two types differ in their EBNA proteins and in their ability to transform B lymphocytes *in vitro*. Some cytotoxic T-lymphocyte clones are specific for EBNA proteins. Some of these EBNA-specific cytotoxic T lymphocytes recognize only the EBNA protein of one virus type.

After the patient recovers from acute infectious mononucleosis, the proportion of circulating B lymphocytes infected with EBV is 1 in 10^5 to 10^6. Most of these lymphocytes express only the EBNA 1 protein, which is not usually recognized by immune cytotoxic T lymphocytes. These latently infected B lymphocytes are likely to be the site of virus persistence, since long-term suppression of virus replication in the oropharynx with antiviral chemotherapy does not decrease the number of circulating EBV-infected B lymphocytes; and after cessation of treatment, the virus rapidly returns to the oropharyngeal epithelium. Also after bone marrow transplantation, the donor's rather than the recipient's virus may persist in the oropharynx of the recipient. Long after primary EBV infection, T lymphocytes, which can suppress or kill HLA-related EBV-infected cells that express EBNA's or LMP's, continue to circulate in the peripheral blood. Cyclosporine administration for organ transplantation indirectly inhibits the EBV-specific T-lymphocyte immune response, thereby enabling EBV-infected B lymphocytes to overgrow in transplantation recipients receiving high doses of cyclosporine and other immunosuppressive drugs. In this patient group, EBV-associated lymphoproliferative diseases are a significant, albeit unusual, problem.

DIAGNOSIS. In normal adolescents the diagnosis of acute infectious mononucleosis can usually be made on clinical grounds and confirmed by the laboratory findings of atypical lymphocytosis and heterophile antibody to ox or horse erythrocytes. Bacterial throat culture should be obtained in patients with significant pharyngitis to exclude concomitant β-hemolytic streptococcal infection. The rapid heterophile tests are >95% sensitive and >95% specific in an adolescent or young adult population. Titers are substantially diminished by 3 months after primary infection and undetectable by 6 months. In patients with absence of or equivocal heterophile antibodies, EBV-specific serologic testing should be done. The differential diagnosis may include streptococcal or gonococcal pharyngitis; cytomegalovirus, hepatitis virus A or B, HIV, HHV6, adenovirus, or toxoplasma infection; leukemia, lymphoma, and Hodgkin's disease. Most heterophile-negative infectious mononucleosis with pharyngitis is also caused by EBV. In the absence of pharyngitis, however, cytomegalovirus, toxoplasma, hepatitis virus, or HIV infections are likely causes of heterophile-negative or low-titer heterophile-positive infectious mononucleosis. In some patient populations, acute HIV infection is a significant cause of typical or atypical infectious mononucleosis syndromes. HIV antigen or nucleotide sequence–specific detection may be necessary to diagnose HIV infection early in the illness. Later, seroconversion may establish the diagnosis.

Specific serologic testing for EBV infection involves determining antibody titers to latently infected (anti-EBNA), early replication cycle (anti-EA), or late replication cycle (anti-VCA) viral proteins (Fig. 341–1). This is usually done by indirect immunofluorescence microscopy or by enzyme-linked immunoassay. Infection titers are listed in Table 341–2. Those rare patients with chronically progressive EBV infection tend to have abnormally high titers of antibodies to some or many EBV antigens. On the other hand, serologic diagnosis may be misleading in immunosuppressed patients, including children with X-linked immunodeficiency. These infected children may have high or low antibody titers. EBV serologic studies are helpful in following patients with anaplastic nasopharyngeal carcinoma or in screening for early detection of this malignant disease in high-risk populations. Patients at risk for primary anaplastic nasopharyngeal carcinoma or for recurrences have high IgG or IgA EA antibody titers.

TREATMENT. No treatment is necessary for most EBV infections. Rest during the period of acute symptoms and slow return to normal activity are commonly advised, although the therapeutic efficacy of this regimen has not been firmly established. Patients with

splenomegaly should restrict their involvement in sports to avoid traumatic rupture. Acetaminophen or aspirin may be used to reduce temperature and pharyngeal pain in most patients who have normal or only slightly abnormal liver function. Very brief courses of glucocorticoid treatment (e.g., 60 mg prednisone per day for 4 days followed by rapidly decreasing doses) have been effective in shrinking obstructing tonsils, probably by ameliorating an overactive T cell response. Autoimmune hemolytic anemia, granulocytopenia, and thrombocytopenia usually respond to longer courses of glucocorticoid therapy. The use of glucocorticoids for other manifestations of EBV infection is less certain to be beneficial. Glucocorticoids have no antiviral activity and are contraindicated in most herpes virus infections. A few patients with severe hemorrhagic thrombocytopenia refractory to glucocorticoids have responded to intravenous immunoglobulin. Early plasmapheresis is indicated in patients with Guillain-Barré syndrome. Acyclovir and its derivatives have activity against EBV *in vitro* and *in vivo* but are not approved for use against EBV. These drugs should not be used in normal patients with EBV infections since they do not affect the length or severity of illness. Acyclovir can be used for AIDS patients with oral hairy leukoplakia or for pa-tients with well-documented chronically progressive EBV infection. Acyclovir has not affected the outcome of EBV-associated lym-phoproliferative syndromes in immunosuppressed patients. Partial restoration of immune function by lowering immune suppression has been beneficial. In one patient with X-linked lymphoproliferative disease, recombinant interferon-γ produced rapid clinical remission.

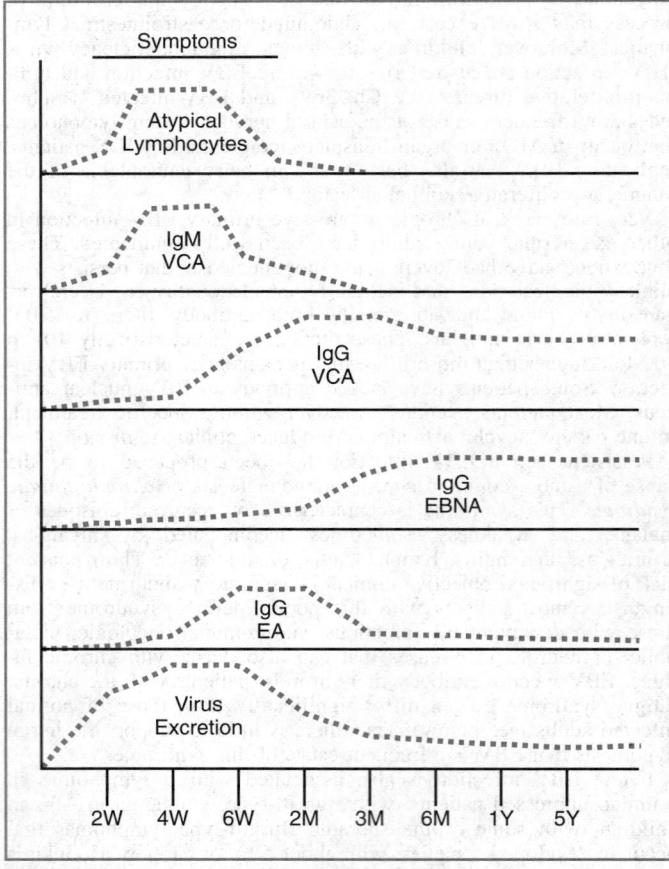

FIGURE 341–1. The usual incubation period after EBV infection is 10 days to 2 weeks. By the time headache, malaise, and fever develop there are usually a few atypical lymphocytes and the monospot or heterophile test may be slightly positive. By 4 weeks, symptoms, monospot test, atypical lymphocytosis, and IgM antibody against EBV viral capsid antigen (VCA) are usually at their maximum. They may persist for another 2 to 3 weeks. IgG anti-EBV early antigen (EA) and anti-VCA are frequently detectable at 4 weeks, but reach their maximum at 6 to 8 weeks. Anti-EBV nuclear protein (EBNA) IgG is usually not detectable until symptoms begin to resolve. Malaise may persist for 8 to 12 weeks. By 3 months, patients are usually fully recovered. IgG anti-VCA and EBNA titers persist at a high level for many years thereafter. EBV infection in normal humans is persistent but asymptomatic.

TABLE 341–2. ANTIBODY TESTS FOR EPSTEIN-BARR VIRUS

Acute primary infection	Titers
IgM EA and VCA	High
IgG VCA and EBNA	Low
Recovering from primary infection	
IgM EA or VCA	Lower
IgG VCA	Rising
EBNA	Low
After several months	
IgM EA and VCA	Low or normal
IgG VCA and EBNA	Persist at high for several years

Duncombe AS, Amos RJ, Metcalfe P, Pearson TC: Intravenous immunoglobulin therapy in thrombocytopenic infectious mononucleosis. Clin Lab Haematol 11:11, 1989. *Effect of Ig in two cases of refractory hemorrhagic thrombocytopenia.*

Ernberg I, Andersson J: Acyclovir efficiently inhibits oropharyngeal excretion of Epstein-Barr virus in patients with acute infectious mononucleosis. J Gen Virol 67:2267, 1986. *Effect of acycloguanosine on EBV infection.*

Kieff E: Epstein-Barr virus and its replication. *In* Fields B, Knipe D (eds.): Fields Virology, 3rd ed. New York, Raven Press, 1995. *Review of the biochemistry of Epstein-Barr virus and its effect on lymphocytes.*

Liebowitz D: Epstein-Barr virus—an old dog with new tricks (editorial). N Engl J Med 332:55, 1995.

Rickinson A, Kieff E: Epstein-Barr virus: Biology, pathogenesis and medical aspects. *In* Fields B, Knipe D (eds.): Virology, 3rd ed. New York, Raven Press, 1995. *Review of EBV-associated diseases.*

Schooley RT, Carey RW, Miller G, et al.: Chronic Epstein-Barr virus infection associated with fever and interstitial pneumonitis. Clinical and serologic features and response to antiviral chemotherapy. Ann Intern Med 104:636, 1986. *Illustrative case of chronic EBV.*

Retroviruses

342 RETROVIRUSES OTHER THAN HIV

William A. Blattner

The discovery in 1979 of human T-lymphotropic virus type I (HTLV-I) began a new age of medical virology. It resulted in discoveries that linked human retroviruses to diverse lymphoreticular and chronic degenerative conditions and to the discovery in 1983 of the human immunodeficiency virus (HIV), a lente-retrovirus, the cause of AIDS. These discoveries had scientific roots in the search for human cancer viruses in the early decades of this century; they were propelled by studies of mammalian cancer-causing retroviruses and the delineation of a replication cycle involving reverse transcriptase, which catalyzes the creation of a proviral DNA copy from a viral RNA template. This chapter focuses on the virologic, epidemiologic, and clinical correlates of the HTLV class of viruses; it reviews the distribution of HTLV-I and HTLV-II and presents the known and possible disease associations. Ch. 359 and 361 provide a comprehensive review of HIV and AIDS.

HTLV VIROLOGY

HTLV-I and -II are single-stranded RNA viruses containing a diploid genome that replicates through a DNA intermediary able to integrate into the host cell genome as a provirus. The integration process is essential to the ability of this class of virus to cause lifelong infection, evade immune clearance, and produce diseases of long latency such as leukemia and lymphoma. Morphologically, HTLV-I is approximately 100 nm in diameter with a thin electron-dense outer envelope and an electron-dense, roughly spherical core (Fig. 342–1). The genomic structure of HTLV-I is shown in Figure 342–2. The long terminal repeats (LTR) at the 5′ and 3′ ends of the genome contain regulatory elements that control virus expression and virion production. Retroviral genes generally code for large overlapping polyproteins that are later processed into functional peptide products by virally encoded protease and cellular proteases. The encoding genes of the virus are *gag* (group-specific antigen), *pol* (polymerase/integrase), *env* (envelope), and a series of accessory genes that regulate virus expression. The *gag* proteins function as structural proteins of the matrix, capsid, and nucleocapsid. The *pol* gene encodes for several enzymes—reverse transcriptase (involved in RNA to DNA transcription), endonuclease (ribonuclease-H), and integrase, which functions for viral integration. The *env* gene encodes the major components of the viral coat: the surface glycoprotein of 46,000 MW (gp46) and the transmembrane 21,000 MW (gp21). The regulatory region, pX, expresses *tax*, which is responsible for enhanced transcription of viral and cellular gene products; it has been postulated to play a crucial role in leukemogenesis. *Rex* (regulator of expression of virion proteins for HTLV) modulates, in a complex manner, the transport of virion components in the production of virus particles.

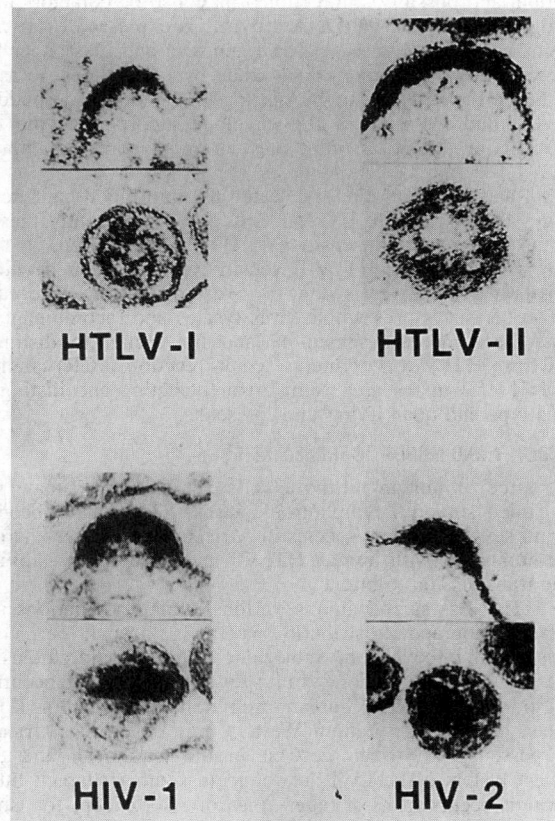

FIGURE 342–1. Morphology of human retroviruses. The budding particles are shown in the upper panel for each virus and the mature virion in the lower panel. The HTLV-I and -II viruses have a roughly spherical electron-dense core, in contrast to the more cylindrical core of human immunodeficiency virus, HIV. (From Blattner WA: Retroviruses. *In* Evans A [ed.]: Viral Infections of Humans, Epidemiology and Control, 3rd ed. New York, Plenum Publishing, 1989, p 545.)

The initial step in the life cycle of HTLV is attachment of the virus envelope glycoprotein to an unknown cell surface receptor, which results in preferential infection of CD4, T-helper cells, for HTLV-I, and CD8 cells for HTLV-II. Following uptake and uncoating, viral RNA is transcribed by *reverse transcriptase,* an RNA-dependent DNA polymerase complexed to the RNA in the core of the virus particle, into double-stranded DNA. This double-stranded viral DNA is integrated into the host cell nucleus by the virally encoded integrase, resulting in cell infection that may be lifelong.

The viral LTR elements are essential to integration: They form the sites for covalent attachment of the provirus to cellular DNA and important viral regulatory elements. The virus may remain "hidden" (unexpressed, not replicated) in cells for long periods.

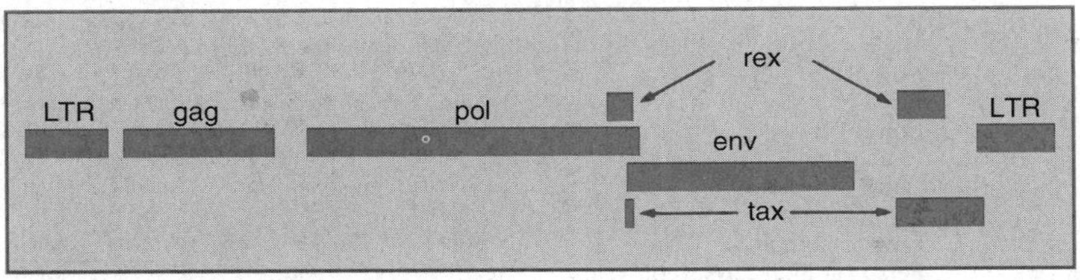

FIGURE 342-2. Genomic structure of human T-lymphotropic viruses. LTR = Long terminal repeat, which is organized into three regions: U5, R, and U3, which house the polyadenylation site; and the *rev* = response element—and the transactivating response element, which are involved in controlling virus expression. *gag* = group specific antigen, whose products form the skeleton of the virion (matrix, capsid, nucleocapsid, nucleic acid binding protein); *pol* = gene for reverse transcriptase, integrase, and protease; *env* = envelope gene; *tax* = transactivator gene; *rex* = viral regulatory gene involved in promoting genomic RNA production. (Courtesy of Dr. Robert C. Gallo.)

This may contribute to the long interval (sometimes many years to decades) between the time of infection and disease.

Factors that control viral replication (viral regulatory genes, cell stimulation, and possibly coinfections) may also be cofactors in disease progression. When the DNA provirus is expressed (transcribed by a cellular RNA polymerase), viral genomic and messenger RNA and subsequently viral proteins are made by the cell. These assemble at the cell membrane to be packaged and released (budding). During the budding process the envelope incorporates the cell's lipid bilayer, producing an infectious virion of about 100 nm (see Fig. 342-1).

HTLV-I and -II are routinely detected through blood bank screening assays that use whole HTLV-I virus lysates. Recently these assays were shown to be insensitive to HTLV-II detection, so newer test kits with enhanced HTLV-II sensitivity have been developed. Confirmation of positives is done by Western blotting. The current generation of assays uses whole virus lysates and recombinant viral antigens; these increase sensitivity and the ability to distinguish HTLV-I from HTLV-II. Polymerase chain reaction (PCR) is another technique useful in research settings for detecting and distinguishing virus type and quantifying viral presence.

EPIDEMIOLOGY AND MODES OF TRANSMISSION

The source of human retroviruses is not known. Primate retroviruses called simian T-lymphotropic virus (STLV) have been isolated from several primate species in Africa; these viruses share significant homology with human HTLV-I and raise the possibility of enzootic transmission to humans.

How HTLV has spread among various human populations is not known. The geographic distribution pattern is unusual; the inconsistent clusters of infection and molecular epidemiologic studies suggest that HTLV is an ancient virus showing patterns of occurrence similar to those of early human migrations. Clusters of HTLV-I have been detected throughout Western and Equatorial Africa and among persons of African descent in the Caribbean and South America. Clusters of HTLV-I are found in southern Japan; little or no infection occurs in most other areas of Asia except for isolated foci among Melanesian peoples in Papua New Guinea and northern Australia. The virus from Melanesia differs molecularly from the Japanese and African strains by 5 to 10%. This variability may be the result of the independent evolution of the virus in these populations of Africa and Asia, which have been separated for tens of thousands of years. A concentration of HTLV-I in northeastern Iran may have resulted from the cross-cultural migrations occurring along the trade routes from the Far East to the Middle East and Europe. HTLV-II has an equally intriguing worldwide distribution: Very limited clusters are found among Native American peoples throughout North, Central, and South America. An Asian focus was recently reported in remote areas of Mongolia, among people who share genetic links with Native American populations whose ancestors emigrated from this region during the Ice Age. HTLV-II has also been detected in Africa, originally among pygmies in Equatorial Africa but more recently in some areas of West Africa. Infections in Europe occur among injection drug users (IDU's) who may have acquired the virus via contact with US IDU's.

Table 342-1 summarizes the routes, cofactors, and viral characteristics associated with HTLV-I transmission; the basic modes of transmission for HTLV-I and HIV-1 are similar.

Sexual transmission of HTLV-I from male to female and female

to male as well as from male to male has been documented. HTLV-I transmission is cell-associated and appears to be at least an order of magnitude less infectious than HIV-1. Coincidental infection with other sexually transmitted diseases, particularly those associated with ulcerative genital lesions in males and inflammatory lesions in women, amplify the risk of transmission. For HTLV-I, elevated antibody titer, which appears to correlate with elevated virus load, is linked to heightened transmission. In viral endemic regions there is a characteristic age-dependent rise in HTLV-I seroprevalence. This increase first becomes evident in the adolescent years; it is steeper in women than in men and continues in women after age 40, whereas rates in men plateau around age 40. The most plausible explanation for this pattern is more efficient male-to-female transmission. For HTLV-II the pattern differs; here, the rates for both genders are equal. This finding suggests that there may be differences between the two viruses in the kinetics of transmission.

The second major route of transmission is from mother to child. For HTLV-I, breast-feeding is more efficient than *in utero* or perinatal transmission. For example, whereas 20% of breast-fed infants on average seroconvert to HTLV-I, only 1 to 2% of bottle-fed infants of HTLV-I–positive (HTLV+) mothers become infected. In this regard HTLV-I differs significantly from HIV-1; *in utero* and perinatal transmission accounts for virtually all HIV-1 transmission in the West, where breast-feeding is discouraged. The rate of breast milk–associated HIV-1 transmission is estimated to be approximately 15%. HTLV-II has been detected in breast milk, but mother to child transmission by this route has not been documented.

The third major route of transmission is parenteral, via either transfusion or injection drug use. Surveys of blood donors in the United States document that more than half of the HTLV infections are due to HTLV-II. Among IDU's the vast majority of infections are due to HTLV-II; it is projected that HTLV-II is more efficiently transmitted by this route than is HTLV-I.

Prospective studies of transfusion transmission indicate that both HTLV-I and -II are transmitted in association with cellular components. This is in sharp contrast to HIV-1, which is transmitted by

TABLE 342-1. TRANSMISSION OF HTLV-I/II

	Modes of Transmission	
	HTLV-I	*HTLV-II*
Mother to infant		
Transplacental	Yes	Not known
Breast milk	Yes	Probable
Sexual		
Male to female	Yes	Yes
Female to male	Yes	Yes
Male to male	Yes	Not known
Parenteral		
Blood transfusion	Yes	Yes
Intravenous drug use	Yes	Yes
	Co-factors	
Elevated virus load		
Mother to infant	Yes	Not known
Heterosexual	Yes	Not known
Ulcerative genital lesions	Yes	Not known
Cellular transfusion products	Yes	Yes
Sharing of "works"	Yes	Yes

cells, plasma, or plasma products. Approximately one half of the recipients of HTLV-I and -II+blood seroconvert; the percentage for HIV-1 is >95%.

The only documented illness linked to HTLV-I or -II transfusion transmission is the HTLV-associated demyelinating neurologic syndrome described below. Leukemia has not been associated with transfusion of HTLV+ blood. Among US blood donors who are confirmed HTLV+ (slightly less than half are HTLV-I and the others are HTLV-II), the major risk factors are intravenous drug use, birthplace in a viral endemic area, or sexual contact with a person with this profile.

Coinfection with HTLV-I and HIV-1 appears to increase the progression to AIDS through unexplained mechanisms, possibly related to the cell proliferative effects of HTLV-I on HIV-1–infected T cells. Such a relationship has not been shown for HTLV-II. Other modes of transmission involving "casual contact," mosquito transmission, and so on, do not seem to happen. Health care and laboratory workers who experience a needle stick, skin or mucous membrane exposure in the absence of protective barriers are at little or no risk for infection; a single case of such infection has been documented in a Japanese health care worker exposed to HTLV-I.

CLINICAL MANIFESTATIONS AND PATHOGENESIS

HTLV-I–associated diseases are listed in Table 342–2.

Adult T-Cell Leukemia/Lymphoma (ATL)

The most common malignancy caused by HTLV-I is ATL; this is more accurately classified as a form of peripheral T-cell lymphoma that may include peripheral blood involvement. The HTLV-associated lymphomas include several subtypes of ATL: acute, chronic, smoldering, and lymphoma-type. Their clinical features are summarized in Figure 342–3. These tumors represent high-grade lymphomas, usually of large, medium, and/or pleiotropic morphology and advanced clinical stage, and are associated with a poor prognosis.

The worldwide occurrence of these HTLV-I–associated malignancies is difficult to quantify because the incidence in any population depends on the prevalence of viral infection. In HTLV-I endemic areas such as southern Japan and the Caribbean Islands, the annual incidence of virus-associated leukemia is approximately 3 in 100,000 per year and may account for one half of adult lymphoid malignancies. The chance of an infected individual developing a malignancy over a lifetime is approximately 5%; early life exposure is associated with the greatest risk for subsequent disease.

The acute form of ATL (Fig. 342–3) is characterized by an aggressive mature T-cell lymphoma whose clinical course is often associated with high white count, hypercalcemia, and cutaneous involvement. Other cases resemble T-cell chronic lymphocytic leukemia and are termed chronic ATL. Smoldering ATL may clinically resemble mycosis fungoides/Sezary syndrome with cutaneous involvement presenting as erythema or as infiltrative plaques or tumors. Sometimes a long prodrome of symptoms is noted before transformation to an acute, rapidly fatal form of disease occurs. Sometimes ATL presents as a T-cell non-Hodgkin's lymphoma with no other clinical features of ATL except for monoclonal integration of HTLV-I in proviral DNA in the tumor cells. Most patients with acute and lymphoma-type ATL die within 6 months of diagnosis. The cause of death is usually an explosive growth of tumor cells, hypercalcemia, and various opportunistic infections including *Pneumocystis carinii* pneumonia and other infections observed in AIDS patients.

The age group ranges from adolescence to a peak in middle-aged adults. The diagnosis should be considered in an adult with mature T-cell lymphoma and hypercalcemia and/or cutaneous involvement, particularly if the individual is from a known risk group or endemic region. The diagnosis is established by testing serum for HTLV-I antibodies and finding leukemic T cells with the provirus in the blood or in biopsy specimens.

TABLE 342–2. HTLV-ASSOCIATED DISEASES

Diagnosis	Nature of Syndrome	Strength of Association
HTLV-I–associated diseases		
Adult T-cell leukemia/lymphoma	Aggressive lymphoproliferative malignancy of mature T lymphocytes	Strong
B-cell chronic lymphocytic leukemia	Tumor-associated immunoglobulin reacts to HTLV antigen	2 cases reported
Tropical spastic paraparesis (TSP)/ HTLV-associated myelopathy (HAM)	Chronic progressive demyelinating syndrome of long motor tracks of spinal cord	Strong
Polymyositis	Degenerative inflammatory syndrome of skeletal muscles	Probable
Infective dermatitis	Chronic generalized eczema of skin in children; potential for preleukemia and immunodeficiency	Strong
Uveitis	Inflammatory infiltration of the uvea of the eye	Strong
HTLV-associated arthritis	Large joint polyarthropathy; rheumatoid factor positive with HTLV-I positive cells infiltrating the synovia	Probable
Immune deficiency	Anecdotal reports of AIDS-like illness in HTLV-I positives; subclinical (e.g., decreased PPD response) or clinical (e.g., poor response to therapy for symptomatic strongyloidiasis)	Possible
Miscellaneous clinical conditions	Case reports or case series of Sjögren's syndrome, interstitial pneumonitis, small cell lung cancer with monoclonal HTLV-I integration, and invasive cervical cancer	Uncertain
HTLV-II–associated diseases		
T-hairy cell/ large granulocytic	Case reports of T-cell malignancy with either monoclonal or polyclonal integration	Possible
Leukemia	HTLV-II integration in T cells and either T-cell, NK-cell, or B-cell proliferation	
HTLV-associated myelopathy	Case reports of TSP/ HAM in association with HTLV-II. In some cases ataxic form of neurologic involvement reported	Probable
Miscellaneous clinical conditions	Case reports or case series of HTLV-II and mycosis fungoides, asthma, glomerular nephritis, pulmonary disease	Uncertain

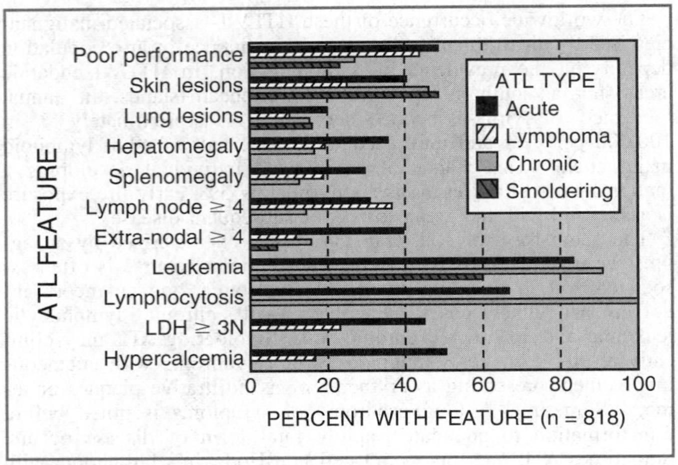

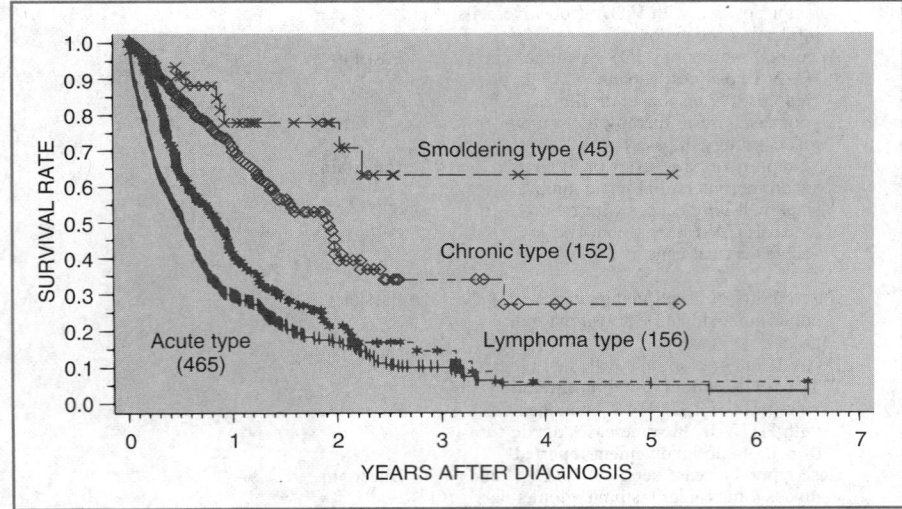

FIGURE 342–3. Features of adult T-cell lymphoma/leukemia in Japan. A combination of clinical and laboratory features is involved in defining the various subtypes of ATL (see text for details). (From Blattner W: Human T-cell lymphotropic viruses and cancer causation. *In* Devita VT, Hellman S, Rosenberg SA [eds.]: Cancer Prevention, Update. Philadelphia, JB Lippincott, 1993, p 1.)

ATL has proven refractory to most conventional and experimental chemotherapeutic regimens (Fig. 342–4). In general, smoldering ATL is the least aggressive form. The chronic type has a relatively poor prognosis with death occurring within a few years of diagnosis. Patients with chronic and smoldering ATL receive no therapy or they are treated with prednisone with or without cyclophosphamide. The more indolent forms of ATL have a high rate of complicating infections resulting from the immunosuppressive effects of aggressive therapy. Acute and lymphoma-type ATL's are aggressive high-grade lymphomas with a generally poor prognosis, although some cases do respond to multidrug regimens with prolonged remission.

Initial response rates, even for the poorest risk categories, are >50%, and complete remissions are achieved in 20% of the cases. Relapses often occur within weeks to months after treatment, although up to 15% of the patients have extended survival beyond 2 years (Fig. 342–4). Poor prognosis is associated with poor performance status at diagnosis: age over 40, extensive disease, hypercalcemia, and high serum LDH level. Relapses in long-term survivors often occur in the central nervous system (CNS) and prove refractory to subsequent therapy. Experimental approaches under investigation include using monoclonal antibodies to the interleukin-2 (IL-2) receptor linked with cell toxins selectively targeted to the leukemic cells and a combination of zidovudine and interferon.

A possible association was reported between HTLV-I and some cases of B-cell chronic lymphotropic leukemia. In these cases, chronic stimulation of B-cell proliferation by viral antigens, coupled with virus-induced impairment of CD4 cell function, resulted in malignant transformation in B cells with HTLV-I–specific cell surface antibodies.

Tropical Spastic Paraparesis/HTLV-1–Associated Myelopathy (TSP/HAM)

HTLV-I has been linked to a neurologic syndrome known as TSP/HAM. This disease is characterized by a chronic, slowly progressive development of spastic paraparesis resulting from the demyelination of the long motor neurons of the spinal cord. Symptoms often begin with a stiff gait, progressing (usually slowly) to increasing spasticity and weakness, with incontinence and impotence developing later in the course of the illness. Sometimes ataxia develops. In some cases, isolated lesions of the CNS are detected on a nuclear magnetic resonance scan. This syndrome differs from classic multiple sclerosis because of its generally slow, progressive course and the absence of a waxing and waning symptomatology. However, some cases are acutely progressive; such cases are sometimes associated with the transfusion of HTLV-I+ blood.

The incidence of disease is approximately half of the rate for ATL. The diagnosis is suspected in unexplained CNS disease with loss of pyramidal tract functions and is confirmed by testing sera for HTLV-I antibodies. Treatment with corticosteroids benefits some patients, particularly those with rapidly progressive disease; Danazol, an androgenic steroid, improves urinary and fecal incontinence but does not affect the underlying neurologic deficit.

TSP/HAM is the prototype for a series of immune-mediated syndromes characterized by high virus load, significant immune activation, and an indirect pathogenic mechanism produced by virally induced perturbations in immune function. Examples of these conditions include polymyositis of the skeletal muscle, uveitis of the eye, a large joint arthritis, and Sjögren's syndrome. Additional oncogenic effects are suggested by a Japanese case of small cell lung cancer with monoclonal HTLV integration and association with invasive cervical cancer. HTLV-I has also been linked to immunosuppression through clinical and laboratory observations of Japanese patients with AIDS-like illnesses associated with HTLV-I (in the absence of underlying malignancy), perturbations in skin test reactivity, and the finding that parasitic infestations (e.g., strongyloidiasis) are refractory to conventional treatments. The infective dermatitis syndrome first reported in Jamaica represents the first childhood HTLV-I syndrome; immunosuppression and preleukemia are possible features.

HTLV-II AND DISEASE

At this time HTLV-II continues to be an "orphan" virus with no true disease association. The virus was originally isolated from a patient with hairy T-cell leukemia, but surveys of hairy T-cell leukemia and related entities have identified only occasional HTLV-II positives. These include one case in which the virus was polyclonally infecting T cells while causing a B-cell malignancy. Large granulocytic cell leukemia (LGL), a malignancy with a natural killer (NK) cell phenotype, has also been linked to HTLV-II in

FIGURE 342–4. Survival by ATL subtype after polychemotherapy in Japan. Poorest survival is observed in patients with acute and lymphoma-type ATL. (From Tsukasaki K, Ikeda S, Murata K, et al.: Characteristics of chemotherapy-induced clinical remission in long survivors with aggressive adult T-cell leukemia/lymphoma. Leuk Res 17:157, 1993.)

some cases. In these instances, there is a pattern of polyclonal infection of T cells and malignant expansion of NK cells not infected with the virus. It has been hypothesized that in these cases HTLV-II is acting through an indirect mechanism.

Approximately a dozen TSP/HAM cases associated with HTLV-II have been reported. In some instances the clinical pattern had features of the ataxic form, but most had the more typical spastic paraparesis. Preliminary data suggest this syndrome is infrequent compared to its occurrence in HTLV-I carriers.

HTLV-I PATHOGENESIS

A great deal has been learned about the pathogenesis of HTLV-I–associated leukemia. Early in infection, HTLV-I infects only a small number of T cells and probably the monocyte/macrophage. The DNA provirus randomly integrates into the DNA of infected cells. Although HTLV-I may exist as a latent virus, the virus genes promote cell proliferation by direct and indirect mechanisms, including various lymphokine pathways. In the process they may promote the expression of additional activated target cells and thereby amplify virus spread. For example, when lymphocytes from HTLV-I–infected normal persons are placed in tissue culture, they undergo spontaneous (in the absence of exogenous antigens or mitogens) lymphocyte proliferation. Early in the infection phase, host immune responses to the virus are activated, producing viral antibodies and cytotoxic T cells targeted at viral antigens. In some cases persons with documented exposure (e.g., via blood transfusion) do not seroconvert and develop cell-mediated immune responses that presumably clear virus infection. Some healthy carriers develop T-cell polyclonal and oligoclonal proliferations that can later progress to malignancy or may disappear spontaneously. Morphologically distinct "flower cells," representing T cells with deeply lobulated nuclei resembling ATL leukemic cells, are seen on peripheral blood smears of healthy carriers but do not presage risk for subsequent disease. In ATL, the HTLV-I provirus is found integrated in the DNA of the leukemic cells in a clonal fashion with one (or occasionally two) copy of the provirus integrated in the same chromosomal location in each cell. This would indicate that ATL is tumor derived from a single transformed cell that sprouted from a virus infection before transformation and clonal expansion rather than afterwards as a passenger virus. Tumors from different patients have proviral integration in different locations. This indicates that cis-activation of a nearby cellular gene by the LTR of the virus, as occurs with some animal leukemia viruses, is not the mechanism for transformation in ATL.

The latent period for this process is years to several decades; it involves an interaction between viral expression and oncogenic mutations. For example, recent studies have identified abnormalities in the clearance of the p53 suppressor gene in HTLV-I infected cells; other studies demonstrate the binding of viral tax to a receptor on NF-kB. Immunosuppressive events may also play a role because the tumor necrosis factor-β (TNF-β) is turned on in ATL. Evidence is growing that at some stage, transformation involves the expression of the tax protein encoded by the px gene of HTLV-I. Because the tax protein induces expression of cellular genes critical for T-cell proliferation, including IL-2 and its receptor (IL-2R), an autocrine mechanism may be involved, particularly in the first steps of leukemogenesis, which involves polyclonal expansions of T cells. In order for malignancy to develop, additional genetic changes most probably take place (e.g., cytogenetic changes, oncogene alterations). Because tax gene expression is detectable in tumor samples,

even in some cases of antibody-negative ATL, this viral gene may be crucial in oncogenesis.

The pathogenesis of TSP/HAM is uncertain, but it appears to occur with a much shorter latency (sometimes acutely following transfusion-associated infection) than does ATL. Some researchers speculate a direct mechanism involving infection of nervous system cells; others conjecture an indirect mechanism involving immune- and autoimmune-mediated responses following from HTLV-I infection of regulatory T-cell populations.

PREVENTION

A major issue confronting practicing physicians is what to tell patients identified as HTLV+ based on blood bank screening. First and foremost, they must emphasize that disease complications related to HTLV-I are rare and that for HTLV-II no specific disease has been verified, and second, that the viruses are not easily transmitted. Third, the patient should be clearly counseled concerning the distinction between the HTLV and the HIV viruses because the greatest fear the patient may have is that he/she has the "AIDS virus." Recently, guidelines for prevention and counseling have been developed for HTLV-I and -II by a Centers for Disease Control and Prevention Working Group: (1) Blood for donation should be screened prior to transfusion and positive donors should be deterred from donating. (2) HTLV-I/II+ mothers should be discouraged from breast-feeding when practicable to prevent mother-to-infant transmission (except in particular settings, such as in the tropics, where diarrheal disease in non–breast-fed infants presents a high risk for morbidity and mortality). (3) Condoms should be used by discordant couples, but, given the relatively low frequency of sexual transmission per sexual encounter, couples who desire a pregnancy could time unprotected sexual intercourse to coincide with periods of maximal fertility. (Such decisions require careful discussion between physician and patient; there are no absolute guidelines in this area.)

Vaccines containing whole virus and recombinant HTLV-I envelope antigens have successfully prevented HTLV-I infection in monkeys and in a rabbit model; it is uncertain whether a vaccine for HTLV-I or -II will ever be implemented for humans. For example, in Japan epidemiologic data show that new infections are declining because of changing socioeconomic and lifestyle factors, whereas in developing countries rates as high as 1 to 1.5% per year are reported in sexually active populations. It is unclear whether the disease burden associated with these viruses warrants a vaccine.

Blattner WA (ed.): Human Retrovirology: HTLV. New York, Raven Press, 1990. *Comprehensive update of human T-cell leukemia virus including chapters on virology, immunology, epidemiology and clinical features, and management. In* Devita VT, Hellman S, Rosenberg SA (eds.).
Blattner W: Human T-cell lymphotrophic viruses and cancer causation. In Devita VT, Hellman S, Rosenberg SA (eds.): Cancer Prevention, Update. Philadelphia, JB Lippincott, 1993, p 1. *A clinically oriented review of HTLV-I and related diseases.*
Centers for Disease Control and Prevention: Guidelines for counseling persons infected with human T-lymphotropic virus type I (HTLV-I) and type II (HTLV-II). Ann Intern Med 118:448, 1993. *Presents important information to clinicians confronted with counseling persons referred with HTLV infection.*
Hall WW: Human T cell lymphotropic virus type I and cutaneous T cell leukemia/lymphoma. J Exp Med 180:1581, 1994. *A concise review of the pathogenic role of HTLV-I in the etiology of mature T-cell malignancies, including recent data exploring the role of this family of viruses in cutaneous T-cell malignancies in the United States and Europe.*
Takatsuki K (ed.): Adult T-cell Leukemia. Oxford, Oxford Press, 1994. *The most recent update of a monograph series on the subject of ATL and related diseases.*

Enteric Viral Infections

---

343 ENTEROVIRUSES
Michael N. Oxman

Enteroviruses, so named because they generally infect the alimentary tract and are shed in the feces, cause a variety of diseases in humans and lower animals. They comprise one of the five major subgroups, or genera, of the Picornavirus (*pico,* small; *rna,* ribonucleic acid) family. The other Picornavirus genera are: *Rhinoviruses,* which inhabit the upper respiratory tract and include the principal recognized etiologic agents of the common cold (see Ch. 328); *Cardioviruses,* recovered chiefly from rodents and only very rarely implicated in human disease; *Aphthoviruses,* named for the vesicular lesions that they produce in cloven-footed animals; and *Hepatovirus,* a newly designated genus with human hepatitis A virus as its only currently recognized member.

Enteroviruses are differentiated from *rhinoviruses* primarily by their resistance to acid; they are fully infectious at pH 3 or even lower. Consequently, enteroviruses that have undergone limited replication in the oropharynx survive passage through the stomach and implant in the lower intestinal tract, where they undergo more extensive multiplication. In contrast, rhinoviruses are acid labile; they begin to lose infectivity at pH 6 and are completely inactivated at pH 3. They are further distinguished from enteroviruses by their lower optimal temperature of replication (33°C versus 37°C for enteroviruses) and higher buoyant density in cesium chloride. Since rhinoviruses inhabit the nasopharynx, they have no obvious need for acid stability, and preferential replication at lower than body temperature probably reflects their adaptation to the cooler nasal passages.

Hepatitis A virus was originally classified as an enterovirus and designated enterovirus 72. However, it is more resistant to inactivation by heat than enteroviruses, and its genome has relatively little nucleotide sequence homology with members of the *Enterovirus* genus. Furthermore, in contrast to enteroviruses, hepatitis A virus does not cause a rapid shut-off of host cell protein synthesis, and the infected cells are not lysed. Because of these important differences, hepatitis A virus has been accorded its own genus, *Hepatovirus,* within the Picornavirus family. Hepatitis A virus is discussed in Ch. 117.

Within the *Enterovirus* genus, species are distinguished immunologically by the ability of specific antisera to neutralize only the homotypic virus. There are now 67 recognized human enterovirus species (*serotypes* or *immunotypes*), as well as numerous enteroviruses of lower animals. Humans appear to be the only natural host for the human enteroviruses, and, in general, the enteroviruses of lower animals are not natural pathogens for humans.

Historically, human enteroviruses have been subclassified into *polioviruses,* group A and group B *coxsackieviruses,* and *echoviruses* on the basis of antigenic relationships, differences in host range, and type of disease produced (Table 343–1). By 1969, 67 species (serotypes) of human enteroviruses had been identified and classified according to these criteria, although reclassification and redundancy have reduced this number to 63. The distinguishing characteristics of these enterovirus subgroups are outlined below.

POLIOVIRUSES. The first human enteroviruses to be recognized, *polioviruses* produce characteristic lesions when inoculated into the central nervous system (CNS) of primates. Clinical isolates replicate only in primates and in primate cell cultures (see Ch. 425). There are three poliovirus serotypes.

COXSACKIEVIRUSES. In contrast to polioviruses, *coxsackieviruses* produce paralysis and death when inoculated into suckling mice. This property was responsible for their detection and differentiation from polioviruses when they were first recovered in 1948 from the feces of two children in the village of Coxsackie, New York, who were suffering from a poliomyelitis-like paralytic illness. With the isolation of additional serotypes, it was recognized that when inoculated into suckling mice, some coxsackieviruses, designated *group A coxsackieviruses,* produced generalized myositis of skeletal muscles that resulted in flaccid paralysis, whereas others,

designated *group B coxsackieviruses,* produced only focal myositis but caused an encephalitis that resulted in spastic paralysis and a generalized infection that involved the myocardium, brown fat, pancreas, and other organs. Moreover, group B coxsackieviruses could be readily propagated in primate cell cultures, whereas group A coxsackieviruses grew poorly or not at all. Twenty-three group A and six group B coxsackievirus serotypes have been identified.

ECHOVIRUSES. The use of the cell culture techniques developed by Enders and colleagues led to the recovery, from the feces of healthy children, of additional enteroviruses that produced cytopathic effects in primate cell cultures but failed to produce disease in suckling mice or in the CNS of primates. These agents, initially considered "orphan" viruses because they were unrelated to any disease, were called *echoviruses* (enteric cytopathic human orphan). Echoviruses have now been associated with a variety of diseases, and 31 serotypes have identified. Most echoviruses are readily propagated in primate cell cultures.

SIMPLIFIED TAXONOMIC SCHEME. The detailed comparison of enterovirus genomes supports the validity of this classification scheme. Different serotypes within the same human enterovirus subgroup, e.g., group B coxsackieviruses, generally have 30 to 50% of their nucleotide sequences in common, whereas serotypes from different subgroups generally share < 20% of their nucleotide sequences. About 5% of the nucleotide sequences are conserved among all human enteroviruses.

Over the years, however, an increasing number of enterovirus isolates were identified that could not be subclassified unambiguously by these criteria (e.g., viruses serologically related to known echoviruses but with a host range characteristic of coxsackieviruses). Consequently it was agreed in 1970 that newly recognized human enteroviruses would be classified simply as *enteroviruses* and numbered sequentially, beginning with enterovirus 68. To avoid confusion with the older literature, the original classification (*poliovirus,* group A and group B *coxsackievirus,* and *echovirus*) has been retained for the first 63 serotypes. Since adoption of this simplified taxonomic scheme, four new human enteroviruses, enteroviruses 68–71, have been recognized.

ENTEROVIRUSES 68–71. Enterovirus 68 was initially isolated from the throat of an infant with bronchiolitis and pneumonia. Few isolates have since been reported, and the agent is little studied. Enterovirus 69 was recovered from the feces of an asymptomatic child, and this serotype has not yet been associated with disease. Enterovirus 70 is the principal cause of acute hemorrhagic conjunctivitis, a disease first recognized in 1969, which has subsequently affected tens of millions of persons throughout the world. Enterovirus 70 has an unusually broad host range; it causes meningoencephalitis in humans and in experimentally infected monkeys, and it infects both primate and nonprimate cell cultures. Genome analysis and serologic surveys raise the possibility that enterovirus 70 may be a zoonotic enterovirus that has recently extended its host range to include humans. Enterovirus 71, first recognized as the cause of an outbreak of aseptic meningitis and encephalitis in California between 1969 and 1972, is neurovirulent in monkeys and produces a myositis in suckling mice that is typical of that produced by group A coxsackieviruses. Enterovirus 71 has been recovered throughout the world in association with a variety of clinical

TABLE 343–1. CLASSIFICATION OF HUMAN ENTEROVIRUSES*

Enterovirus Group	Number of Serotypes	Numerical Designation	Growth in Primate Cell Culture	Pathogenicity for Suckling Mice	Pathogenicity for Monkeys
Poliovirus	3	1–3	+	−	+
Coxsackievirus, group A	23	A1–22, A24†	+/−‡	+	−α
Coxsackievirus, group B	6	B1–6	+	+	−
Echovirus	31	1–9, 11–27, 29–34¶	+	−	−
Enterovirus	4	68–71**	+	variable††	variable‡‡

* Many enterovirus strains have been isolated that do not conform to these criteria.
† Coxsackievirus A23 has been reclassified as echovirus 9.
‡ Except for a few serotypes (e.g., A7, A9, A16), primary isolates of group A coxsackieviruses grow poorly or not at all in cell culture; virus isolation requires inoculation of suckling mice.
α Coxsackievirus A7 is neurovirulent in monkeys.
¶ Echovirus 10 has been reclassified as reovirus type 1; echovirus 28 has been reclassified as rhinovirus 1A.
** Hepatitis A virus, formally classified as human enterovirus 72, is now classified as a member of the *Hepatovirus* genus.
†† Enteroviruses 70 and 71 are pathogenic for suckling mice.
‡‡ Enteroviruses 70 and 71 are neurovirulent in monkeys.

manifestations and many fatal infections. These have included respiratory infections, aseptic meningitis, hand-foot-and-mouth disease, maculopapular exanthems, and encephalitis. In addition, enterovirus 71 has been responsible for epidemics of acute paralytic disease indistinguishable from poliomyelitis.

The discovery of the enteroviruses, as well as the origins of modern virology, were closely associated with efforts to control poliomyelitis. Poliovirus type 1 is the prototype for the *Enterovirus* genus and for the Picornavirus family. It is one of the most extensively studied and thoroughly characterized agents of disease. While a number of nonpolio enteroviruses have also been well characterized and the genomes of several have been cloned and sequenced, much of our present understanding of enterovirus structure, replication, genetics, pathogenesis, and immunology is derived from studies carried out with wild type and vaccine strains of poliovirus.

The enteroviruses have many features in common, and they will be discussed as a group before considering the special features of individual members. Since polioviruses are the subject of Ch. 425, this discussion will be limited to the nonpolio enteroviruses.

PHYSICAL AND BIOCHEMICAL CHARACTERISTICS OF ENTEROVIRUSES

The enteroviruses share with all picornaviruses certain important physical and biochemical characteristics: They are small, spherical, nonenveloped viruses approximately 30 nm in diameter. Their genome consists of a linear, single-stranded, unsegmented molecule of RNA with a molecular weight of about 2.6×10^6 daltons (approximately 7500 nucleotides) which has the same polarity as messenger RNA, i.e., it is plus (+) stranded, and is thus infectious. In fact, purified enterovirus RNA can initiate the synthesis of complete infectious virions *in vitro* in cell-free extracts from susceptible cells. The viral genome is tightly packed within an icosahedral protein shell or *capsid* composed of 60 identical subunits or *protomers,* each of which has a molecular mass of 90,000 to 100,000 daltons and is itself composed of four nonidentical virus-encoded polypeptides (VP1, VP2, VP3, and VP4). VP1, VP2, and VP3 are exposed on the virion surface, whereas VP4 lies buried in association with the RNA core. Like all picornaviruses, enteroviruses exhibit a unique pattern of replication in which the viral genome is translated into a single giant *polyprotein,* which is then cleaved by endogenous viral proteinases into the individual viral structural and nonstructural proteins.

Enteroviruses are stable over a wide range of pH (pH 3 to 10) and retain infectivity for days at room temperature, weeks at refrigerator temperature, and indefinitely when frozen at $-20°C$ or lower. They are readily inactivated at temperatures above 50°C, but this inactivation is inhibited by molar magnesium chloride, which greatly enhances the stability of enteroviruses at all environmental temperatures. Thus, magnesium chloride is widely used as a stabilizer for oral poliovirus vaccines.

Enteroviruses are resistant to proteolytic enzymes and to inactivation by organic solvents, deoxycholate, and various detergents that destroy lipid-containing enveloped viruses such as herpesviruses, orthomyxoviruses, and paramyxoviruses. Enteroviruses are inactivated by formaldehyde, chlorination, and ultraviolet light but are protected from inactivation by dissolved organic matter, the formation of virus aggregates, and adsorption to particulate matter. Consequently, enteroviruses may survive secondary sewage treatment and chlorination as generally practiced, and are abundant in urban sewage and treated waste water. The agricultural use of treated sewage and recycled waste water may thus contaminate food and water supplies. Since sewage treatment that destroys fecal coliform bacteria does not eliminate enteroviruses, the use of fecal coliform counts to assess the sanitary quality of water is inadequate with respect to its potential for transmission of enteroviral diseases. Enteroviruses are often detectable in samples of recreational water judged acceptable on the basis of fecal coliform counts. Although person-to-person (fecal-oral) spread is the dominant mode of transmission, and water-borne outbreaks of enterovirus infection have rarely been documented, the hazard associated with the discharge of virus-laden sewage into coastal waters is demonstrated by the occurrence of shellfish-associated outbreaks of hepatitis A. Clams, mussels, and oysters are filter-feeders that concentrate virus and function as passive virus carriers. Most of the enteroviruses in sewage are associated with suspended solids, and virus adsorbed to sediment remains infectious for long periods in the marine environment. The reintroduction of specific en-

teroviruses into coastal populations when marine sediments are disturbed by storms, dredging, and so on, might explain the sudden occurrence of epidemics as well as the reappearance of certain enterovirus serotypes after years of absence from the human population.

EPIDEMIOLOGY

Human enteroviruses are worldwide in distributions, and humans are their only known reservoir. The prevalence of enterovirus infection varies markedly with season and climate, and with the age and socioeconomic status of the population studied. In tropical and semitropical regions, enterovirus infections are frequent throughout the year. In temperate climates, the incidence of infection is markedly increased in the summer and early fall; in Europe and North America 80 to 90% of enterovirus isolates are recovered from June through October, with peak recovery in August. Even within the United States, climatic and socioeconomic factors affect the prevalence of enterovirus infections. Enterovirus isolation rates from young children are twofold to threefold higher in southern than in northern cities, and threefold to sixfold higher in lower than in middle and upper socioeconomic districts. In developed countries, usually only one to three enterovirus serotypes are highly prevalent in a given community each year, with different serotypes prevalent in different years, and isolation rates in young children rarely exceed 10%. In developing countries with poor sanitation, a greater number of enterovirus serotypes circulate simultaneously, and isolation rates in children are regularly > 75%, with many fecal specimens yielding three or more enterovirus serotypes.

Some enteroviruses appear to be endemic, being isolated at low frequency in the same locality each year, whereas others produce local or regional epidemics and then disappear, only to return again years later. Occasionally an enterovirus will spread worldwide, infecting tens of millions of persons and producing pandemic disease. This pattern was observed with echovirus 9 in the late 1950's and with enterovirus 70, which caused a pandemic of acute hemorrhagic conjunctivitis beginning in 1969.

Enteroviruses exhibit a high rate of mutation during replication in the human gastrointestinal tract, and this can lead to the appearance of antigenic varients, as well as virus strains with altered tissue tropism and virulence. Such mutations are readily detected within days after administration of attenuated poliovirus vaccines to normal children. They have also been observed in a number of nonpolio enteroviruses. Recently isolated strains of several coxsackieviruses, echoviruses, and enterovirus 70 have been found to differ in many epitopes from the corresponding *prototype* strains isolated more than a decade earlier, a pattern of "antigenic drift" not unlike that seen with influenza viruses. In addition, recombination between the genomes of different enterovirus serotypes can be observed in multiply infected individuals, e.g., in young children in developing countries, and in recipients of trivalent oral poliovirus vaccines. Antigenic changes and alterations in cell tropism produced by mutation and recombination may help to account for the ability of individual enterovirus serotypes to persist in nature and to cause a variety of clinical syndromes.

Transmission of human enteroviruses is chiefly by the fecal-oral route directly from person to person or via fomites; spread by respiratory secretions plays a lesser role. After infection by most serotypes, virus can be recovered from the oropharynx and intestine of both symptomatic and asymptomatic individuals, but virus is shed in greater amounts and for a longer period (a month or more) in the feces.

Young children have the highest rates of infection, and enteroviruses are most efficiently disseminated by infected children younger than 2 years of age. Spread is from child to child, and then within family groups, and is facilitated by crowding and poor hygiene. Secondary attack rates of approximately 90% for polioviruses, 75% for coxsackieviruses, and 50% for echoviruses are observed in families. Middle-class parents with children in day care centers are at particular risk. Reared in circumstances that minimized their childhood exposure, they are likely to be susceptible to infection by many of the enteroviruses brought home from day care centers by their asymptomatically infected toddlers.

Although the epidemiology of most enteroviruses is similar, patterns of infection with some serotypes are distinctive. Enterovirus

70 and coxsackievirus A24, etiologic agents of acute hemorrhagic conjunctivitis, are transmitted by direct inoculation of the conjunctivae by fingers and fomites contaminated with infected tears. Replication of these viruses in the alimentary tract, if it occurs at all, is limited. Coxsackievirus A21 is shed primarily from the upper respiratory tract, where it produces a rhinovirus-like illness. It is transmitted by respiratory secretions.

The incubation period for illnesses caused by enteroviruses may vary from <1 day to >3 weeks, but it is generally 2 to 7 days. It is shortest when symptoms are the direct result of virus replication at the portal of entry (e.g., acute hemorrhagic conjunctivitis caused by enterovirus 70 or coxsackievirus 24) and longest when they reflect tissue injury that involves immunopathology in target organs infected following viremia (e.g., some forms of coxsackievirus myocarditis).

PATHOGENESIS OF ENTEROVIRUS INFECTIONS

The pathogenesis of enterovirus infections is understood best for polioviruses, which have been extensively studied in experimentally infected primates and in humans infected with attenuated vaccine strains. The pathogenesis of most nonpolio enterovirus infections appears to be similar, except for the principal target organs affected.

Following ingestion of fecally contaminated material, virus implants and replicates in susceptible tissues of the pharynx and distal small intestine. Within a day or two virus spreads to regional lymph nodes, and on about the third day small quantities escape into the bloodstream (the "minor viremia") and are disseminated throughout the reticuloendothelial system and to other receptor-bearing target tissues. In most cases, infection is contained at this stage by host defense mechanisms with no further progression, resulting in *asymptomatic infection*. In a minority of infected persons, replication continues in reticuloendothelial tissues producing, by about the fifth day, heavy sustained viremia (the "major viremia") that coincides with the "minor illness" of poliovirus infection (see Ch. 425) and with the "nonspecific febrile illness" caused by other human enteroviruses.

The major viremia disseminates large amounts of virus to target organs, such as the spinal cord, brain, meninges, heart, and skin, where further virus replication results in inflammatory lesions and cell necrosis. In most such patients, host defense mechanisms quickly terminate the major viremia and halt virus replication in target organs; only rarely is virus replication in target organs extensive enough to be clinically manifest. Although other host defense mechanisms (e.g., macrophages, interferon production) are doubtless involved, neutralizing antibodies play a major role in terminating viremia and limiting enterovirus multiplication in target tissues. Serotype-specific neutralizing antibodies may be detected in the serum within 4 or 5 days of the infection, and they generally persist for life. Evidence for the critical role of antibodies in terminating infection is provided by the occurrence of chronic persistent enterovirus infections in agammaglobulinemic children. Host defenses do not, however, terminate virus replication in the intestine, and fecal shedding continues for weeks after both symptomatic and asymptomatic enterovirus infections. Reinfection (i.e., virus excretion by a person with pre-existing homotypic antibodies) is relatively uncommon. When it occurs, infection is confined to the alimentary tract and is not associated with illness, and the duration of virus shedding is markedly reduced.

The clinical syndrome(s) caused by a given enterovirus reflect the particular target organs and tissues that it infects, i.e., its *cell tropism*. All of the determinants of cell tropism have not been elucidated, but a major factor is the presence on the cell surface of specific *receptor* molecules to which the virus attaches. Different groups of enteroviruses utilize different receptors, most or all of which are encoded by genes on human chromosome 19. A number of distinct receptors, each shared by multiple enterovirus serotypes, have been identified. The receptor used by all three polioviruses (PVR) and a receptor used by a subset of group A coxsackieviruses and by the majority of human rhinoviruses (ICAM-1) are both members of the immunoglobulin superfamily. A receptor used by a subset of the echoviruses (VLA-2) and another used by coxsackievirus A9 are members of the integrin family. Decay-accelerating factor (DAF), a surface glycoprotein that protects cells from complement-mediated lysis, is used as a receptor by another group of echoviruses. All six group B coxsackieviruses share the same receptor, a cell surface glycoprotein.

CLINICAL MANIFESTATIONS OF ENTEROVIRUS INFECTIONS

The majority of nonpolio enterovirus infections (50 to 80%) are asymptomatic. Most symptomatic infections consist of *undifferentiated febrile illnesses* ("summer grippe"), often accompanied by upper respiratory symptoms. These are generally mild and last only a few days. This syndrome is totally nonspecific; it can be caused by virtually any enterovirus serotype, as well as by members of a number of other virus families (e.g., adenoviruses, paramyxoviruses, orthomyxoviruses). The so-called characteristic enterovirus syndromes, such as aseptic meningitis, hand-foot-and-mouth disease, and pleurodynia, are in fact unusual manifestations of enterovirus infection. They represent the very small tip of a very large iceberg.

Some clinical syndromes are highly associated with certain enterovirus serotypes or subgroups (e.g., hand-foot-and-mouth disease with coxsackievirus A16, myopericarditis with group B coxsackieviruses), but even these associations are not specific. The same syndrome may also be caused by a number of other enterovirus serotypes. Conversely, a single enterovirus serotype may cause several different syndromes, even within the same outbreak (Table 343–2). The more important syndromes are discussed below.

CENTRAL NERVOUS SYSTEM SYNDROMES

ASEPTIC MENINGITIS. Aseptic meningitis is the most common significant illness caused by nonpolio enteroviruses, and these viruses are responsible for >80% of the cases of aseptic meningitis in which an etiologic agent is identified. Almost every enterovirus serotype has been implicated, but those most frequently associated include coxsackieviruses A2, A4, A7, A9, A10, and B1–5, echoviruses 3, 4, 6, 9, 11, 14, 16, 17, 18, 19, 25, 30, and 33, and enteroviruses 70 and 71, all of which have been responsible for outbreaks as well as sporadic cases. Although attack rates are generally highest in children, cases also occur in adults, especially during larger outbreaks. Initial symptoms, which are typical of the *undifferentiated febrile illness* (e.g., fever, headache, malaise, myalgias, and sore throat), are followed, usually within a day, by signs and symptoms of meningitis, including a more severe headache that is often retrobulbar, photophobia, meningismus, stiffness of the neck and back, and nausea and vomiting, especially in children. The illness is sometimes biphasic like poliomyelitis. The cerebrospinal fluid (CSF) is clear and under slightly increased pressure. The total cell count, which can vary from <10 per cubic millimeter to >3000 per cubic millimeter, averages 50 to 500 per cubic millimeter. Initially, neutrophils may predominate (although they rarely exceed 90%), but they are quickly replaced by mononuclear cells. The glucose concentration is usually normal, although levels <40 mg per deciliter are occasionally observed. The protein concentration is normal or slightly elevated, but rarely exceeds 100 mg per deciliter. Fever and signs of meningeal inflammation subside in 3 to 7 days, although pleocytosis may persist for an additional week or more. The great majority of children and adults recover fully without sequelae. However, enteroviral meningitis during the first year of life may, in up to 10% of affected infants, result in permanent neurologic damage as evidenced by reduced head circumference, spasticity, and impaired intellectual function.

In some cases, especially those caused by echoviruses and enterovirus 71, meningitis may be accompanied by a rash, which, if petechial, may raise the specter of meningococcemia. It is frequently necessary to distinguish enteroviral meningitis from partially treated bacterial meningitis. In bacterial meningitis, even when treated with appropriate antibiotics, the polymorphonuclear pleocytosis is usually more persistent, the protein concentration higher, and the glucose concentration lower. Aseptic meningitis may be caused by a number of other infectious and noninfectious agents, including mumps virus, arthropod-borne viruses, lymphocytic choriomeningitis virus (LCM), human immunodeficiency virus (HIV), herpes simplex virus, Lyme borreliosis, and leptospirosis. Differential diagnosis is aided by the distinct epidemiologic features and characteristic signs and symptoms of these other diseases.

PARALYTIC DISEASE. Paralytic disease may occur in the course of many nonpolio enterovirus infections. It is similar, but generally less severe, than that caused by polioviruses. Muscle weakness is far more common than frank paralysis, and recovery is nearly always complete, although occasional patients suffer cranial

TABLE 343–2. CLINICAL MANIFESTATIONS OF NONPOLIO ENTEROVIRUS INFECTIONS*

Clinical Syndrome	Group A Coxsackieviruses†	Group B Coxsackieviruses	Echoviruses	Enteroviruses
Asymptomatic infection	All serotypes	All serotypes	All serotypes	All serotypes
Undifferentiated febrile illness ("summer grippe") with or without respiratory symptoms	All serotypes	All serotypes	All serotypes	68, 70, 71
Aseptic meningitis	1, 2, 3, 4, 5, 6, 7, 8, 9, 10, 11, 14, 16, 17, 18, 22, 24	1, 2, 3, 4, 5, 6	1, 2, 3, 4, 5, 6, 7, 8, 9, 10, 11, 12, 14, 16, 17, 18, 19, 20, 21, 22, 23, 25, 30, 31, 33	70, 71
Encephalitis	2, 4, 5, 6, 7, 9, 10, 16	1, 2, 3, 4, 5	2, 3, 4, 6, 7, 9, 11, 14, 17, 18, 19, 22, 25, 30, 33	70, 71
Paralytic disease (poliomyelitis-like)	4, 5, 6, 7, 9, 10, 11, 14, 16, 21	1, 2, 3, 4, 5, 6	1, 2, 4, 6, 7, 9, 11, 14, 16, 17, 18, 19, 30	70, 71
Myopericarditis	1, 2, 4, 5, 7, 8, 9, 14, 16	1, 2, 3, 4, 5, 6	1, 2, 3, 4, 6, 7, 8, 9, 11, 14, 16, 17, 19, 22, 25, 30	
Pleurodynia	1, 2, 4, 6, 9, 10, 16	1, 2, 3, 4, 5, 6	1, 2, 3, 6, 7, 8, 9, 11, 12, 14, 16, 19, 23, 25, 30	
Herpangina	1, 2, 3, 4, 5, 6, 7, 8, 9, 10, 16, 22	1, 2, 3, 4, 5	6, 9, 11, 16, 17, 22, 25	
Hand-foot-and-mouth disease	4, 5, 7, 9, 10, 16	2, 5		71
Exanthems	2, 4, 5, 6, 7, 9, 10, 16	1, 2, 3, 4, 5	2, 4, 5, 6, 9, 11, 16, 18, 25	71
Common cold	2, 10, 21, 24	1, 2, 3, 4, 5	2, 4, 8, 9, 11, 20, 25	
Lower respiratory tract infections (broncheolitis, pneumonia)	7, 9, 16	1, 2, 3, 4, 5	4, 8, 9, 11, 12, 14, 19, 20, 21, 25, 30	68, 71
Acute hemorrhagic conjunctivitis‡	24			70
Generalized disease of the newborn	3, 9, 16	1, 2, 3, 4, 5	3, 4, 6, 7, 9, 11, 12, 14, 17, 18, 19, 20, 21, 22, 30	

* A great many enterovirus serotypes have been implicated in most of these syndromes, at least in sporadic cases. The serotypes listed are those that have been clearly and/or frequently implicated. Serotypes with the strongest association are underlined.

† Because isolation of many of the group A coxsackieviruses requires suckling mouse inoculation, they are likely to be underreported as causes of illness.

‡ Conjunctivitis without hemorrhage is frequently seen in association with other manifestations in patients infected with many group A and group B coxsackieviruses and echoviruses, especially coxsackieviruses A9, A16, and B1–5 and echoviruses 2, 7, 9, 11, 16, and 30.

nerve palsies or severe, sometimes fatal, bulbar involvement. Frequently implicated serotypes include coxsackieviruses A7, A9, and B2–5, echoviruses 2, 4, 6, 9, 11, and 30, and enteroviruses 70 and 71. In contrast to paralytic poliomyelitis, which in the prevaccine era occurred in epidemics, cases of paralysis associated with nonpolio enteroviruses are generally sporadic. However, several nonpolio enteroviruses produce paralytic disease with sufficient frequency to cause local outbreaks and epidemics. A variant of coxsackievirus A7 has caused outbreaks, as well as numerous sporadic cases of paralytic disease. In fact, coxsackievirus A7 was once thought to be a fourth serotype of poliovirus. Paralytic disease resembling poliomyelitis, with a significant incidence of residual paralysis and muscle atrophy, has been observed in patients with acute hemorrhagic conjunctivitis caused by enterovirus 70. Enterovirus 71 has caused outbreaks and epidemics of cutaneous and CNS disease in temperate regions around the world since its initial isolation in California in 1969. These have included epidemics of poliomyelitis-like paralytic disease with residual flaccid paralysis, encephalitis, and significant mortality.

ENCEPHALITIS. Encephalitis is a well-recognized but uncommon manifestation of enterovirus infection. Thus, despite their prevalence, enteroviruses account for only 10 to 20% of the cases of encephalitis in the United States of proven viral etiology. The most frequently implicated serotypes include coxsackieviruses A9, B2, and B5, echoviruses 4, 6, 9, 11, and 30, and enterovirus 71. In most cases, encephalitis complicates the course of aseptic meningitis; parenchymal involvement is indicated by the onset of confusion, coma, abnormalities of motor function, hemiparesis, vasomotor instability, cranial nerve palsies, cerebellar ataxia, and focal or generalized seizures, singly or in various combinations. Cerebral involvement is usually generalized, but focal encephalitis does occur and may occasionally be clinically indistinguishable from herpes simplex encephalitis. Recovery is usually complete, although neurologic sequelae and deaths do occur, especially in young infants and during enterovirus 71 epidemics.

OTHER REPORTED NEUROLOGIC COMPLICATIONS. Other neurologic complications, including Guillain-Barré syndrome, transverse myelitis, Reye's syndrome, and cerebellar ataxia, have been reported in patients with enterovirus infections. However, no clear epidemiologic or etiologic linkage to enteroviruses has been established. Given the high prevalence of asymptomatic enterovirus infections, these associations may be only coincidental.

EPIDEMIC PLEURODYNIA (BORNHOLM DISEASE)

Epidemic pleurodynia is an acute febrile viral illness characterized by the sudden onset of intense paroxysmal lower thoracic or abdominal pain. Synonyms include Bornholm disease, devil's grip, epidemic myalgia, epidemic benign dry pleurisy, and Sylvest's disease. The name, pleurodynia (*pleura,* side; *odyne,* pain) reflects the characteristic intercostal location of the pain and does not connote disease of the pleura. Pleurodynia is usually an epidemic disease, but sporadic cases do occur.

ETIOLOGY. The enteroviral etiology of epidemic pleurodynia was established in 1949. Group B coxsackieviruses, especially B3 and B5, are the principal cause. Other viruses associated with epidemic disease include echoviruses 1 and 6. Sporadic cases have also been associated with these viruses, as well as with many other enteroviruses, including coxsackieviruses A1, A2, A4, A6, A9, A10, and A16 and echoviruses 2, 3, 7, 8, 9, 11, 12, 14, 16, 19, 23, 25, and 30.

EPIDEMIOLOGY. Epidemics of pleurodynia have been recognized in Scandinavian countries for more than two centuries, but the disease was little known elsewhere until 1933, when the Danish physician Ejnar Sylvest described an epidemic on Bornholm, a Danish island in the Baltic Sea. Since then, epidemics and sporadic cases have been recognized in many parts of the world. As with other enteroviral infections, the majority of illnesses occur in summer and early fall. However, in contrast to the annual outbreaks of enteroviral aseptic meningitis, epidemics of pleurodynia are much less frequent, generally occurring at intervals of 10 to 20 years.

Transmission is primarily from person to person, and multiple family members may be attacked almost simultaneously or in rapid succession at intervals of 2 to 5 days. In epidemics, disease is observed in children and adults of both genders. Although the peak age of incidence is somewhat older than with other enterovirus syndromes, the majority of cases occur in persons under 30 years of age. The incubation period is generally 2 to 5 days.

PATHOGENESIS. Pleurodynia is a disease of skeletal muscle, not of the pleura or peritoneum. As in most enteroviral diseases, infection is initiated in the alimentary tract. Skeletal muscle is probably most often infected during the primary (minor) viremia, although it may be infected later, during the major viremia in the minority of patients in whom pleurodynia is preceded by a prodromal illness. Host immune responses terminate viremia and halt virus replication in the tissues, but they also contribute to the severity of local inflammation. Histopathologic data in humans are lacking because of the benign nature of the disease, but studies in murine models of coxsackievirus infection suggest that the myositis results from a combination of direct virus-induced cytolysis and immunopathology mediated by sensitized T lymphocytes.

CLINICAL MANIFESTATIONS. Pleurodynia is characterized by the abrupt onset of fever and sharp, paroxysmal pain over the lower ribs or upper abdomen. In about 25% of patients, this is preceded by a 1- or 2-day prodrome of headache, malaise, anorexia, sore throat, and diffuse myalgia. The pain varies in intensity, but is often severe. It is accentuated, sometimes elicited, by deep breathing, coughing, and movement. The pain of pleurodynia has been described as catching (a "stitch" in the side), stabbing, knife-like, lancinating, crushing, or vise-like. In adults, the pain is primarily in muscles of the thorax, especially the intercostals. In children, abdominal muscles are more often involved. Occasionally it may involve muscles in the neck or limbs. The pain is often unilateral, and is generally experienced in only one or two locations. Muscle tenderness and, occasionally, swelling can be detected at the site of pain, and characteristic paroxysms of pain can often be elicited by pressure on the affected muscles. Pleural friction rubs are uncommon, and peritonitis has generally not been observed in patients who have come to laparotomy. The level of creatine phosphokinase in the serum may be elevated, reflecting injury to striated muscle. Other laboratory values are usually normal, although there may be mild leukopenia in some patients.

During paroxysms of severe pain, the patient lies still in bed, sweating profusely and appearing acutely ill and apprehensive. Respiration, limited by pain, is shallow, rapid, and grunting, suggesting pneumonia or pleural inflammation. A temperature of 38°C to 40°C is present at the onset of pain, reaches its peak during the episode, and resolves between paroxysms. Multiple paroxysms of pain occur, each lasting from a few minutes to several hours. The initial paroxysm is usually the most severe, and patients frequently appear relatively well between paroxysms.

The acute illness generally lasts for 2 to 6 days, with a range of 12 hours to 3 weeks. The disease is often biphasic; the initial pain and fever resolve and the patient is asymptomatic for a day or more, and then the pain and fever recur, frequently at the same site. Rarely, patients will have several recurrences over a period of several weeks or will have a late recurrence after being symptom free for a month or more.

DIFFERENTIAL DIAGNOSIS. The most useful distinguishing feature of pleurodynia is the intermittent paroxysmal character of the pain. Epidemiologic information, such as the occurrence of similar illnesses in family members or in the community, may also suggest the diagnosis. Nevertheless, depending upon the location of the pain, pleurodynia may be confused with any of a number of more serious diseases. When the pain is thoracic, these include pneumonia, pulmonary infarction, rib fracture, costochondritis, and myocardial infarction. The absence of physical and roentgenographic evidence of fracture, costochondritis, or pulmonary parenchymal disease, lack of sputum production, absence of leukocytosis, and normal electrocardiogram help to exclude these diagnoses. When the pain is abdominal, it can be difficult to differentiate pleurodynia from serious causes of acute abdominal pain, such as peritonitis, cholecystitis, appendicitis, perforated peptic ulcer, and acute intestinal obstruction. Thus, during epidemics of pleurodynia, it is common to have as many children with the disease admitted to surgical wards as to medical wards, and in one epidemic 9 of 49 of these children underwent laparotomy with normal findings before the nature of their disease was recognized. The absence of signs of peritonitis and the normal white blood cell count are helpful in excluding these diagnoses, as are normal ultrasound and roentgenographic studies. Pleurodynia may also be confused with the pain of pre-eruptive herpes zoster, herniated intervertebral disc, and renal colic. However, the pain of pre-eruptive herpes zoster is usually more constant, and the localization of pain and tenderness to the affected muscle, normal roentgenographic and neurologic examinations (except perhaps for a local area of hyperesthesia over the affected muscle), and the absence of hematuria help to exclude the other two diagnoses.

TREATMENT AND PROGNOSIS. Treatment of pleurodynia is symptomatic. Episodes of pain can usually be controlled with salicylates or other mild analgesics, but opiate analgesics are recommended for severe pain once serious intraabdominal processes have been excluded. Heat applied to affected muscles may also be useful. Despite the tendency of the disease to relapse, patients with epidemic pleurodynia eventually recover completely. Occasionally, convalescence may be prolonged, with malaise or asthenia persisting for several months. Complications, which reflect dissemination of virus to other tissues, are relatively uncommon. When they do occur, they generally become apparent within several days after the onset of the disease. Aseptic meningitis is observed in approximately 5% of cases, and orchitis in a similar proportion of postpubertal males. Pericarditis and myocarditis are rare complications of epidemic pleurodynia.

MYOCARDITIS AND PERICARDITIS CAUSED BY ENTEROVIRUSES

Myocarditis and pericarditis have long been known to occur in association with epidemic viral diseases, including measles, mumps, rubella, varicella, influenza, poliomyelitis, and pleurodynia. Because many of these diseases have been controlled with vaccines, enteroviruses have emerged as the major recognized infectious cause of myocarditis and pericarditis in North America and Western Europe. The pathogenesis, clinical manifestations, and outcome of enteroviral infections of the heart vary markedly, depending on properties of the virus and characteristics of the host, especially age. Neonatal infections frequently result in severe myocarditis, widespread involvement of other organs, and high mortality, whereas in older children and adults, pericarditis often predominates, and the disease is generally benign and self-limited. In fact, it appears that the clinical manifestations are generally so subtle that cardiac involvement during enteroviral infections is often unrecognized. However, idiopathic dilated cardiomyopathy may, in many cases, be a late sequela of both recognized and unrecognized enteroviral myocarditis.

ETIOLOGY. The evidence linking specific enteroviruses with myocarditis or pericarditis varies markedly. Proof of causation requires isolation of virus from, or demonstration of viral proteins or nucleic acids in, the myocardium, pericardium, or pericardial fluid. Except in neonatal myopericarditis, virus is rarely isolated from cardiac tissue or pericardial fluid, and detection of viral proteins has been difficult, primarily because lack of specificity has led to false positive results. However, increasing use of endomyocardial biopsy and application of new techniques such as *in situ* hybridization and polymerase chain reaction (PCR) for detection and amplification of enteroviral nucleic acid has substantially improved our ability to establish the etiology in cases of myocarditis and pericarditis. While these techniques are not yet widely available, their limited application has already demonstrated the presence of enteroviral RNA in 20 to 30% of tissue specimens from patients with myocarditis and up to 15% of tissue specimens from patients with idiopathic dilated cardiomyopathy. In most instances, however, the association of a particular enterovirus with myocarditis or pericarditis is based only on isolation of virus from noncardiac sources (e.g., feces) and/or serologic evidence of recent or concurrent enterovirus infection. These associations may often be coincidental rather than causal.

Coxsackieviruses B1–6, A4, and A16 and echoviruses 9, 11, and 22 have been proven to cause myopericarditis in children and adults. Coxsackieviruses A1, A2, A5, A8, A9, and A14 and echoviruses 1, 2, 3, 4, 6, 7, 8, 14, 16, 19, 25, and 30 have also been implicated. The group B coxsackieviruses are the most common etiologic agents of myocarditis and pericarditis. They appear to account for approximately 50% of sporadic cases of acute myocarditis and for virtually all cases that have occurred in epidemics. Group B coxsackieviruses also appear to account for 30% or more of sporadic cases of acute nonbacterial pericarditis.

EPIDEMIOLOGY. Enteroviral myocarditis and pericarditis occur most frequently in the summer and early fall. Idiopathic myopericarditis also peaks during this period of maximum enteroviral prevalence; this is consistent with the notion that most cases of idiopathic myopericarditis are caused by enteroviruses.

The incidence of myopericarditis during enteroviral infections depends upon the virus and characteristics of the host, especially age. Myopericarditis has been the predominant manifestation of infection in only about 3% of group B coxsackievirus infections. However, 5 to 10% of infected adults and children older than 9 who sought medical care during coxsackievirus B5 epidemics were found to have evidence of acute myopericarditis. The incidence of myocarditis and disseminated disease during group B coxsackievirus infection is very high during the neonatal period. It drops to a minimum (e.g., ≤1% of symptomatic coxsackievirus B5 infections) in children 1 to 9 years of age and then increases again in older children and adults. Thus, despite the higher frequency of enterovirus infections in younger children, enteroviral myopericarditis is primarily a disease of adolescents and young adults. At least two thirds of the cases occur in males, and the risk of cardiac involvement also appears to be increased during pregnancy and immediately post partum. Enterovirus transmission associated with myocarditis and pericarditis is the same as that of enteroviruses in general: it is primarily fecal-oral.

PATHOGENESIS. When enteroviral infections involve the heart they almost always cause an inflammatory response in both the myocardium (myocarditis) and the pericardium (pericarditis). Although one or the other usually predominates, the term myopericarditis best describes the pathologic process. The hallmark of enteroviral myopericarditis is injury to myocytes with an adjacent inflammatory infiltrate. Cardiac myosites, which bear a receptor utilized by all 6 group B coxsackieviruses, are infected and lysed. The acute process may resolve completely or progress. Healing and progression are reflected by the development of interstitial fibrosis and loss of myocytes. Enteroviral pericarditis is almost always accompanied by focal subepicardial myocarditis, which has these same pathologic characteristics.

In neonatal enteroviral myopericarditis, the relatively short incubation period, the widely disseminated infection, and the presence of high titers of virus in the heart and other organs indicate that the primary pathogenic mechanism is direct cytolytic virus infection of the tissues involved. In myopericarditis in older children and adults, the longer incubation period, the presence of virus-specific antibodies and T lymphocytes at clinical presentation, the low frequency of virus isolation from the heart and pericardial fluid, and the later occurrence of relapses all suggest that immunopathologic mechanisms are involved. Patients with myocarditis have also been found to have cytotoxic T lymphocytes that react with normal cardiac myocytes, as well as high titers of antimyocyte antibodies.

Idiopathic dilated cardiomyopathy (see Ch. 43) may in many instances represent the end stage of an immunologically mediated chronic progressive enteroviral myocarditis. This notion is supported by the development of chronic cardiomyopathy in approximately 10% of patients observed long-term after group B coxsackievirus myocarditis, by demonstration of progressive fibrosis in such patients by serial endomyocardial biopsies, and by failure to isolate enterovirus from these biopsy specimens. The association of idiopathic dilated cardiomyopathy with group B coxsackievirus myocarditis has been further strengthened by the recent demonstration of group B coxsackievirus RNA in myocardial biopsies obtained from patients with the disease. These observations need to be confirmed and extended.

CLINICAL MANIFESTATIONS. Although the term myopericarditis best describes the pathologic process observed in enteroviral infections of the heart, myocarditis or pericarditis usually predominates, and the two syndromes are sufficiently distinct in clinical presentation and pathophysiology to warrant separate consideration. They are discussed in detail in Ch. 43 and 44.

Neonatal Myocarditis. Most severe neonatal enterovirus infections begin during the first week of life; the infant's mother has frequently been infected shortly before delivery and has transmitted

the virus transplacentally or by contact during or soon after delivery. However, the disease can be present at birth or may occur at any time during the first 3 months of life following a 2- to 8-day incubation period. It is usually a manifestation of generalized enteroviral disease of the newborn.

Myocarditis and Pericarditis in Older Children and Adults. In contrast to the neonate, enteroviral infections of the heart in older children and adults often present clinically as pericarditis rather than myocarditis, although the myocardium is almost always involved to some degree. Approximately 60% of older children and adults with symptomatic group B coxsackievirus-associated heart disease have a clinical diagnosis of pericarditis; approximately 40% have a clinical diagnosis of myocarditis. More than two thirds of the patients are male. See Ch. 43 and 44 for clinical features of myocarditis and pericarditis.

TREATMENT AND PROGNOSIS. Specific antiviral chemotherapy is not yet available for enterovirus infections, and treatment of neonatal myocarditis is supportive. Infants with neonatal myocarditis are unlikely to have received transplacental antibodies to the causative virus from their mothers. Thus it seems reasonable to administer human immune serum globulin, which contains high titers of neutralizing antibodies to a number of enterovirus serotypes, in an attempt to terminate viremia and limit further virus replication in infected tissues.

Treatment of enteroviral myopericarditis in older children and adults is primarily supportive. It should include control of pain with analgesics; careful monitoring for arrhythmias, heart failure, and hemodynamic compromise; and prompt treatment of these complications if they arise. Bed rest is an important component of therapy because of clear evidence in mice with coxsackievirus B3 myocarditis that exercise markedly increases the extent of myocardial necrosis and mortality during the acute phase of the disease. Adequate oxygenation should be assured and fluid overload avoided and promptly treated if it develops. In severe cases cardiac assist devices may be lifesaving.

Corticosteroids should not be administered to patients with suspected enteroviral myocarditis or pericarditis. Their use during the acute phase of viral myocarditis has been associated with rapid clinical deterioration.

The majority of children and adults with enteroviral myopericarditis recover without obvious sequelae. Acute mortality is low (0 to 5%), and deaths occur as a result of arrhythmias or congestive heart failure in patients with myocarditis; cardiac tamponade is extremely rare in enteroviral pericarditis.

Approximately 20% of patients experience one or more episodes of recurrent myopericarditis within 1 year of their initial illness and persistent electrocardiographic (ECG) abnormalities are observed in 10 to 20% of patients. Cardiomegaly persists in 5 to 10% of patients, and long-term follow-up suggests that ≥10% may develop chronic cardiomyopathy. Constrictive pericarditis rarely occurs following enteroviral pericarditis.

MUCOCUTANEOUS SYNDROMES CAUSED BY ENTEROVIRUSES

Enteroviruses are the leading cause of exanthematous disease in the United States and most other developed countries. Almost all enteroviruses can cause maculopapular eruptions, and most serotypes are occasionally responsible for petechial or papulovesicular exanthems and enanthems, as well. Moreover, a given enterovirus may cause more than one pattern of mucocutaneous disease, even within a single infected household. Consequently, except for hand-foot-and-mouth disease, which is usually caused by coxsackievirus A16 or enterovirus 71, there are no clinical or epidemiologic characteristics of any given enteroviral rash that point to a specific enterovirus as its cause.

EPIDEMIOLOGY. The epidemiology of enteroviral exanthems and enanthems is the epidemiology of enteroviral infections in general. The vast majority occur during the summer and early fall. The incidence of enanthems and exanthems in infected persons varies among different enteroviruses and even among different strains of the same enterovirus. For example, enanthems and exanthems are often seen in >50% of infected children during outbreaks of infection caused by echovirus 9 or coxsackievirus A16, but are rare during outbreaks caused by echovirus 6 or coxsackievirus A7. Host factors, especially age, are also important; infants and young children are more likely to develop mucocutaneous lesions, whereas other manifestations of enterovirus infection, such as aseptic meningitis, are more likely to develop in older children and adults. Thus during outbreaks of echovirus 9 infection, rash is often seen in the majority of infected children younger than 5 years of age, but in <5% of infected adults, and it is not uncommon when evaluating an adult with aseptic meningitis and no rash to find that a child in the same household is convalescing from an illness characterized by a maculopapular rash. Enteroviral exanthems and enanthems occur in outbreaks and as sporadic cases. Asymptomatic infections are common and are often the source of virus for symptomatic infections. Attack rates are highest in young children, who frequently introduce the virus into households where several members may become infected simultaneously or sequentially, with an incubation period of 3 to 10 days.

PATHOGENESIS. Enteroviral lesions in the oropharyngeal mucosa and skin are manifestations of a systemic virus infection. They result from the secondary infection of endothelial cells of small vessels in the underlying lamina propria and dermis, which occurs during the viremia that regularly follows enteroviral infection and replication in the alimentary tract. Their pathogenesis thus resembles that of the mucocutaneous lesions of measles, rubella, and varicella and contrasts with the pathogenesis of the lesions of acute herpetic gingivostomatitis, human papillomavirus infections (warts), and acute hemorrhagic conjunctivitis, which are the direct result of exogenous virus infection and replication in epithelial cells at the portal of entry.

The obligatory occurrence of alimentary tract replication and viremia before mucocutaneous lesions develop explains the 3- to 10-day incubation period and the frequent occurrence of prodromal signs and symptoms. Moreover, the simultaneous dissemination of virus to a number of target organs explains the concurrent appearance of other manifestations of enterovirus infection, such as aseptic meningitis and myopericarditis.

CLINICAL MANIFESTATIONS. *Enanthems.* The oropharyngeal mucosa is involved to some degree during most symptomatic enteroviral infections. This is usually manifest by mild pharyngitis and mucosal erythema, but it may also result in a variety of enanthems. These may consist of macules, papules, vesicles, petechiae, or ulcers, and they may occur alone or in association with exanthems and other manifestations of systemic enteroviral infection. They are often transient and frequently unrecognized, but they occasionally lead to diagnostic confusion, for example, when they resemble Koplik's spots and accompany a morbilliform exanthem in a child infected by echovirus 9. Two enanthems are sufficiently unique to warrant separate description.

Herpangina (*herpes,* vesicular eruption, *angina,* inflammation of the throat) is a syndrome characterized by sudden onset of fever, sore throat, pain on swallowing, and a vesicular enanthem of the posterior pharynx. It is seen primarily in children between ages 3 and 10. The disease begins abruptly, after a 3- to 10-day incubation period, with temperature ranging from 38° C to 41° C, sore throat, and pain on swallowing. Fever tends to be greater in younger children, who may suffer febrile convulsions; older children and adults frequently complain of headache and myalgia. On examination there is pharyngeal erythema but little or no tonsillar exudate. The characteristic lesions are discrete 1- to 2-mm vesicles and ulcers surrounded by 1- to 5-mm zones of erythema. Lesions are few, averaging 4 to 5 per patient, with a range of 1 or 2 to 20. They occur most frequently on the anterior tonsillar pillars, the posterior edge of the soft palate, and the uvula, and less frequently on the tonsils, the posterior pharyngeal wall, and the posterior buccal mucosa. They begin as small papules, progress to vesicles, and ulcerate within 24 hours. The shallow ulcers, which are moderately painful, may enlarge over the next day or two to a diameter of 3 to 4 mm. Symptoms generally disappear in 3 or 4 days, but the ulcers may persist for up to a week. Most cases are mild and resolve without complications, but herpangina is occasionally associated with exanthems, aseptic meningitis, or other serious manifestations of enterovirus infection.

Outbreaks of herpangina are common during the summer, and sporadic cases are also observed. Group A coxsackieviruses (A1–6, A8, A10, and A22) account for the majority of outbreaks, but outbreaks have also been caused by other enteroviruses, including coxsackievirus B1 and echoviruses 16 and 25. In addition, these viruses, as well as coxsackieviruses A7, A9, A16, and B2–5 and echoviruses 6, 9, 11, 17, and 22, have been isolated from sporadic cases.

A variant of herpangina has been described in children infected with coxsackievirus A10. The lesions have the same distribution as typical cases of herpangina, but instead of evolving into vesicles and ulcers, they remain papular and are infiltrated with lymphocytes to form 2- to 3-mm gray-white nodules surrounded by narrow zones of erythema. The disease, which has been called *acute lymphonodular pharyngitis,* is otherwise indistinguishable from herpangina.

Hand-foot-and-mouth disease (vesicular stomatitis with exanthem) is a mild enteroviral disease characterized by a vesicular eruption in the mouth and over the extremities. It occurs most frequently in children younger than age 5. After an incubation period of 3 to 6 days, the disease begins with mild fever ranging from 38° C to 39° C, anorexia, malaise, and, often, a sore mouth. Within a day or two, vesicular lesions appear in the oral cavity, most frequently on the anterior buccal mucosa and the tongue, but also on the labial mucosa, gingivae, and hard palate. In the majority of preschool children, but in only about 10% of infected adults, the oral lesions are accompanied by vesicular skin lesions, most often on the dorsal or lateral surfaces of the hands and feet and on the fingers and toes, but not infrequently on the palms and soles. Less often, lesions occur on the buttocks or more proximally on the extremities, and rarely on the genitalia. They are generally 3 to 7 mm in diameter and surrounded by a narrow zone of erythema. They range from 2 or 3 to 30 or more and consist of subepidermal vesicles containing a mixed inflammatory infiltrate of lymphocytes, monocytes and neutrophils, and accompanied by acantholysis and cellular degeneration in the overlying epidermis. Hand-foot-and-mouth disease is caused most frequently by coxsackievirus A16, less frequently by enterovirus 71 and coxsackieviruses A5, A9, and A10, and occasionally by coxsackieviruses A4, A7, B2, and B5. Outbreaks and sporadic cases occur primarily in the summer and early fall. It may be accompanied by more serious manifestations, especially when caused by enterovirus 71.

Exanthems. Enterovirus exanthems themselves are benign, but they are clinically important for at least three reasons: (1) They constitute direct evidence of enterovirus dissemination and thus provide a clue to the presence and the etiology of coexistent disease referable to other infected target organs, such as the heart and the CNS; (2) they represent the "tip of the iceberg" of enterovirus infection in the community; and (3) they are often confused with other infectious exanthems, some of which have more serious consequences, require specific control measures, or are amenable to specific anti-infective therapy. Since enteroviral rashes are not sufficiently distinctive to permit an etiologic diagnosis to be made on clinical grounds, laboratory diagnosis is required. However, the problem of confusing enteroviral rashes with other infectious exanthems can be approached by comparing the enterovirus rashes to the nonenterovirus rashes that they resemble.

The most common cutaneous manifestation of enterovirus infection is an erythematous maculopapular rash that appears together with fever and other manifestations of systemic infection. This is also a common manifestation of infection by a variety of other organisms, but it is more often caused by enteroviruses. Only certain enteroviruses (e.g., echovirus 9) cause this syndrome with high frequency, but almost all can produce it at least occasionally. The rash begins on the face and quickly spreads to the neck, trunk, and extremities. It consists of 1- to 3-mm erythematous macules and papules that may be discrete (*rubelliform,* resembling rubella) or confluent (*morbilliform,* resembling measles). It usually lasts for 2 to 5 days and does not itch or desquamate. Enteroviral exanthems are generally not accompanied by significant posterior cervical, suboccipital, or postauricular lymphadenopathy, but there are many exceptions. For example, posterior cervical and suboccipital lymphadenopathy similar to that seen in rubella has been observed in many children with exanthems caused by coxsackievirus A9.

Enteroviral rashes are sometimes petechial and occasionally purpuric. While this pattern is seen most frequently in echovirus 9 and coxsackievirus A9 infections, it is observed occasionally with many other enterovirus serotypes.

Vesicular exanthems are most often seen as a component of

hand-foot-and-mouth disease (see above), but several enteroviruses, including echovirus 11 and coxsackievirus A9, may cause vesicular exanthems without an associated enanthem. The lesions resemble those caused by varicella-zoster and herpes simplex viruses. In contrast to varicella, however, vesicular rashes caused by enteroviruses are usually peripheral in distribution and consist of relatively few lesions that heal without crusting. When they are not associated with hand-foot-and-mouth disease, vesicular lesions caused by enteroviruses are often confused with insect bites or poison ivy. Echovirus 11 and several coxsackievirus serotypes have been associated with skin lesions resembling papular urticaria, lesions that usually result from insect bites.

Enteroviral rashes are generally accompanied by fever; they develop at or within a day or two of its onset. In some cases, however, the rash does not develop until the fever subsides, a pattern resembling that of *roseola infantum* (exanthem subitem), a benign sporadic disease of infants 6 to 24 months old now known be caused by human herpesvirus 6. These roseola-like enterovirus infections are typified by the "Boston exanthem," caused by echovirus 16 and first described during an epidemic in Boston in 1951. It is characterized by fever (to 38° C to 39° C) lasting 2 to 4 days, followed by defervescence and then by the appearance of a salmon-pink maculopapular rash on the face and upper chest. The rash resolves in 1 to 5 days without sequelae. Frequently, multiple cases occur sequentially in households; the illness is mild in children and more severe in adults, who often develop high fever and aseptic meningitis without rash. In addition to echovirus 16, a number of other enterovirus serotypes have occasionally been associated with roseola-like illnesses.

DIFFERENTIAL DIAGNOSIS. Herpangina is most often confused with bacterial pharyngitis or tonsillitis, or with pharyngitis caused by other viruses. Other considerations include hand-foot-and-mouth disease, primary herpes simplex virus infections, particularly acute herpetic pharyngotonsillitis, and herpes zoster involving the palate.

The vesicular lesions of hand-foot-and-mouth disease resemble those caused by herpes simplex and varicella-zoster viruses. Patients with primary herpetic gingivostomatitis usually have more toxicity, cervical lymphadenopathy, and more prominent gingivitis. Their cutaneous lesions are usually perioral, but may occasionally involve a finger that has been in the mouth. Recurrent herpes simplex (herpes labialis) usually involves the vermilion border of the lip or the adjacent skin, is rarely accompanied by lesions on the hands or feet, often has a neuralgic prodome, and frequently has a history of recurrent episodes. The cutaneous lesions of varicella are generally more extensive and are centrally distributed, sparing the palms and soles. Oral lesions are far less prominent in varicella, and its prevalence in winter and spring further distinguish it from hand-foot-and-mouth disease. Aphthous stomatitis is distinguished from hand-foot-and-mouth disease by the absence of fever and other signs of systemic illness, the absence of cutaneous lesions, and often by a history of recurrence.

Maculopapular exanthems caused by enteroviruses are distinguished from measles and rubella by their summertime occurrence, the usual absence of posterior cervical, suboccipital, and postauricular lymphadenopathy, and their relatively short incubation period. The absence of significant coryza and conjunctivitis further distinguishes the typical enteroviral exanthems from measles. In addition, the probability of measles and rubella is markedly reduced in persons with a well-documented history of adequate immunization.

When enteroviral rashes are maculopapular they may be confused with drug reactions; when they are petechial they may be confused with bacterial or rickettsial rashes. When enteroviral rashes are petechial or purpuric it is impossible to rule out meningococcemia on clinical grounds alone, and when the rash is associated with aseptic meningitis (as is often the case in echovirus 9 and coxsackievirus A9 infections), it is clinically indistinguishable from meningococcal meningitis. Laboratory investigation is required, even during proven outbreaks of enteroviral disease, because concurrent enteroviral and meningococcal infections can occur.

TREATMENT AND PROGNOSIS. Enteroviral enanthems and exanthems are benign self-limited illnesses that require only symptomatic therapy for headache and sore throat. When illness mimics meningococcemia or meningococcal meningitis, antimicrobial chemotherapy should be initiated until bacterial infection is ruled out by appropriate cultures and antigen-detection assays.

RESPIRATORY TRACT DISEASE CAUSED BY ENTEROVIRUSES

A number of enteroviruses have been associated with mild upper respiratory tract illness in children and adults, especially coxsackieviruses A21, A24, and B1–5 and echoviruses 9 and 11, as well as 2, 4, 8, 20, and 25. Many of the enteroviruses, most notably coxsackievirus A21, produce illness that resembles the common cold, except for a higher incidence of fever. In contrast to most other enteroviruses, coxsackievirus A21 is shed primarily from the upper respiratory tract, rather than in feces. Enteroviruses have also been associated with lower respiratory tract illnesses in infants and children, though rarely in adults. These include tracheitis, bronchitis, croup, bronchiolitis, and pneumonia. Frequently implicated serotypes include coxsackieviruses A9, A16, and B1–5; echoviruses 4, 8, 9, 11, 12, 14, 19, 20, 21, 25, and 30; and enterovirus 68. In addition, respiratory tract symptoms frequently accompany the undifferentiated febrile illnesses (summer grippe) caused by most enteroviruses. Survillence data indicate that enteroviruses account for 2 to 10% of viral respiratory disease, and that 10 to 15% of symptomatic enterovirus infections are associated with respiratory symptoms. The respiratory illnesses caused by enteroviruses are clinically indistinguishable from similar illnesses caused by viruses more commonly considered to be respiratory tract pathogens, such as rhinoviruses, influenza viruses, parainfluenza viruses, respiratory syncytial virus, and adenoviruses. However, infections with these viruses occur most frequently during the winter, whereas enterovirus infections occur primarily in the summer and early fall. Viral respiratory tract infections are discussed in Ch. 328 through 333.

ACUTE HEMORRHAGIC CONJUNCTIVITIS

Acute hemorrhagic conjunctivitis (AHC) is an acute, highly contagious, self-limited disease of the eye characterized by sudden onset of pain, photophobia, conjunctivitis, swelling of the eyelids, and prominent subconjunctival hemorrhages. Since its first appearance in 1969, AHC has occurred in explosive epidemics throughout the world. The disease was initially nicknamed Apollo 11 disease because its appearance in Ghana coincided with the Apollo 11 moon landing.

ETIOLOGY. Enterovirus 70, a new enterovirus isolated from patients during the initial pandemic of AHC that began in Ghana in 1969, has been responsible for tens of millions of cases that have occurred in widespread epidemics during the past 25 years. A variant of coxsackievirus A24, which first appeared at about the same time as enterovirus 70, has been responsible for hundreds of thousands of cases of the disease that have occurred in a number of more circumscribed epidemics during the same period. Both viruses have been involved concurrently in some epidemics. To date, coxsackievirus A24 has been responsible for fewer cases of epidemic conjunctivitis than enterovirus 70, and it does not cause subconjunctival hemorrhages in as high a proportion of patients. Nucleic acid hybridization and serologic studies have shown that the two viruses are genetically and antigenically unrelated.

Enterovirus 70 is a most unusual enterovirus. In addition to being a naturally occurring temperature-sensitive virus that causes disease at its portal of entry and is not transmitted by the fecal-oral route, it has an exceptionally broad host range. Oligonucleotide mapping of a series of epidemic strains suggests that they all evolved from a hypothetical ancestor strain that did not exist before 1967. Serologic studies have reinforced the notion that enterovirus 70 has only recently emerged as a human pathogen; neutralizing antibodies to enterovirus 70 have generally not been found in human sera collected before 1969, even sera from elderly persons. Neutralizing antibodies to enterovirus 70 have been detected in animal sera from Japan and West Africa collected before 1969, indicating that enterovirus 70 or a very similar virus was circulating in animals before the first appearance of AHC in humans. These observations suggest that enterovirus 70 may represent a zoonotic picornavirus that extended its host range to humans, perhaps as a consequence of recombination with poliovirus type 3.

EPIDEMIOLOGY. Although mild conjunctivitis may occur as a minor manifestation of infection by many enteroviruses, especially in children, its occurrence as the major clinical manifestation of enterovirus infection was not observed until 1969, when explosive epidemics of AHC occurred in Ghana and almost simultaneously in Indonesia. Over the next 2 years the disease assumed pandemic proportions, with large epidemics occurring in many areas of Africa, Southeast Asia, the Far East, India, and Japan, and involving tens of millions of people. A number of smaller outbreaks also occurred in Europe. Scattered epidemics of AHC continued to occur in these same areas during the remainder of the decade, and the recurrence of epidemics in the same geographic areas suggests that immunity to AHC may be short-lived.

AHC is a highly contagious disease. In contrast to most enteroviral infections, it is transmitted by direct inoculation of the conjunctivae with virus-contaminated fingers or fomites (i.e., transmission is eye to finger or fomite to eye). Enterovirus 70 and the coxsackievirus A24 variant are both naturally occurring temperature-sensitive viruses that replicate optimally at 33°C to 35°C, the temperature of the conjunctivae. There appears to be little or no virus replication in the alimentary tract. Virus is abundant in the conjunctivae and in the ocular exudate, from which it can be readily isolated early in infection. During epidemics all age groups are affected; attack rates of clinical illness are highest in young adults, but infection rates are highest in children younger than 10 years, many of whom experience mild or inapparent infections. Infection rates are also substantially higher among the poor than in middle and upper socioeconomic groups. School-age children are most likely to introduce infection into households, where secondary attack rates are often > 50%.

PATHOGENESIS. In contrast to other enteroviral infections, AHC is transmitted by direct inoculation of the conjunctivae with virus on contaminated fingers or fomites (e.g., ophthalmologic instruments, shared towels). Disease results from local virus replication at the portal of entry; prior replication in the alimentary tract and viremia are not required to disseminate virus to ocular tissues. This explains the unusually short incubation period, generally lasting 24 hours or less (range, 12 to 72 hours).

The major complication of AHC is poliomyelitis-like flaccid paralysis, which occurs in a very small proportion of patients with AHC caused by enterovirus 70, but apparently not at all in patients with AHC caused by coxsackievirus A24. The pathogenesis of this AHC-associated paralytic disease is not clear, but infections and destruction of motor neurons appears to reflect axonal rather than viremic spread of enterovirus 70 to the CNS.

CLINICAL MANIFESTATIONS. AHC begins with the sudden onset of eye pain and foreign body sensation, lacrimation, photophobia, blurred vision, and bulbar conjunctivitis. Signs and symptoms rapidly increase in severity with the development of palpebral conjunctivitis, conjunctival edema, swelling of the eyelids, subconjunctival hemorrhages in the bulbar conjunctivae, and a serous or seromucoid ocular discharge containing large numbers of polymorphonuclear leukocytes. The subconjunctival hemorrhages, which are the hallmark of the disease, range from discrete petechiae to confluent hemorrhages that occupy virtually the entire bulbar conjunctiva. They are present, usually within 24 hours of onset, in 70 to 90% of patients with AHC caused by enterovirus 70, but are much less frequent in AHC caused by coxsackievirus A24. AHC often begins unilaterally, but it rapidly spreads to the other eye. Signs and symptoms peak within 24 to 36 hours of onset, by which time most patients have also developed hypertrophy of palpebral follicles and papillae, preauricular lymphadenopathy, and punctate epithelial keratitis with tiny corneal erosions that are often seen only by slit-lamp examination after fluorescein staining. Clinical improvement usually begins by the second or third day, and recovery is generally complete without sequelae within 7 to 10 days. Constitutional symptoms, including headache, low-grade fever, and malaise, occur in a minority of patients.

Poliomyelitis-like motor paralysis occurs as a rare complication of AHC caused by enterovirus 70, but not in AHC caused by coxsackievirus A24. It occurs predominantly in adult males. The neurologic disease generally does not begin until 2 to 5 weeks after AHC (range, 5 to 60 days or more), and thus its relationship to the conjunctivitis is often overlooked by physicians as well as by the patients themselves. Radicular pain and paresthesia, usually accompanied by headache, fever, and malaise, are followed in 1 to 3 days by acute asymmetric areflexic paresis or paralysis of one or more limbs. Proximal muscles are usually affected more than distal muscles and lower limbs more than upper limbs. Bulbar involvement, as evidenced by paralysis of one or more cranial nerves, is observed in one third or more of affected patients. The CSF is characterized by mononuclear pleocytosis and elevated protein concentration. Permanent paralysis and muscular atrophy occur in approximately 25% of affected patients. More than 200 cases have been reported to date, and the long interval between AHC and paralysis almost certainly accentuates underreporting. Nevertheless, in view of the many tens of millions of cases of AHC that have occurred since 1969, the incidence of this neurologic complication is probably less than 1 in 10,000 cases of AHC.

DIFFERENTIAL DIAGNOSIS. During major epidemics, AHC is unlikely to be confused with other eye infections. However, small outbreaks and sporadic cases may be mistaken for adenovirus infections, either acute follicular conjunctivitis or the more severe epidemic keratoconjunctivitis.

A variety of noninfectious conditions can produce the signs and symptoms of conjunctivitis (see also Part XXV).

TREATMENT AND PROGNOSIS. AHC almost always resolves spontaneously without sequelae, and treatment is symptomatic. Topical application of antihistamine/decongestant eye drops and cold compresses may be used to reduce discomfort. Corticosteroids, a component of many topical ophthalmic preparations, are contraindicated. Transmission of AHC can be prevented by careful hand-washing, avoidance of contaminated washcloths and towels, and sterilization of all ophthalmologic instruments. These practices should be routine in eye clinics.

CHRONIC MENINGOENCEPHALITIS IN AGAMMA-GLOBULINEMIC PATIENTS. Enteroviruses, primarily echoviruses, have been responsible for a syndrome of chronic meningoencephalitis in patients with inherited or acquired defects in B lymphocyte function, most often children with X-linked agammaglobulinemia. The majority of these patients also have a dermatomyositis-like syndrome, and many have chronic hepatitis. Surprisingly, despite the presence in their CSF of abundant virus, an increased number of lymphocytes, and elevated protein concentration, these patients generally exhibit few if any clinical signs of meningitis. Enteroviruses have been recovered from many sites in addition to the CSF, including cardiac and skeletal muscle. However, the pathogenesis remains to be elucidated.

DIAGNOSIS

The enteroviral etiology of a disease may be suspected on clinical and epidemiologic grounds, but the multiplicity of agents capable of causing most clinical syndromes makes it impossible to establish a specific etiologic diagnosis on the basis of such information alone. Virus isolation and/or serologic evidence are required, with serotype-specific IgM assays and direct detection of enterovirus RNA in tissues and CSF following PCR implification.

TREATMENT AND PREVENTION

Specific antiviral chemotherapy and chemoprophylaxis are not yet available for enterovirus infections. Treatment is symptomatic and, in severe disease, supportive. Corticosteroids, which have a deleterious effect on coxsackievirus-infected mice, should not be administered during acute enterovirus infections. Strenuous exercise and intramuscular injections, both of which may precipitate paralysis of the involved muscles during poliovirus and enterovirus 70 infections, should also be avoided during the acute, presumably viremic, phase of symptomatic enterovirus infections. Intravenous immunoglobulin (IVIG), which contains high titers of neutralizing antibodies to many enteroviruses, appears to have been useful in some agammaglobulinemic patients with chronic enteroviral meningoencephalitis. IVIG may also have a role in the treatment of enteroviral infections in other patients with severely compromised B lymphocyte function. Infants with generalized neonatal enterovirus infections are unlikely to have received transplacental antibodies to the causative virus from their mothers. Consequently it would seem reasonable to administer IVIG to such infants in an attempt to terminate their viremia and limit virus replication in infected tissues. Prophylactic IVIG should also be considered for patients with severely compromised B lymphocyte function, including bone marrow transplant recipients.

Live attenuated and inactivated poliovirus vaccines have been remarkably successful in preventing paralytic poliomyelitis (see Ch. 425). However, the large number of nonpolio enterovirus serotypes, and the benign nature of most nonpolio enterovirus infections, have precluded the development of vaccines for these agents. Pre-exposure administration of immune serum globulin reduces the risk of paralytic poliomyelitis. Since immune serum globulin also contains neutralizing antibodies to many nonpolio enteroviruses, it would probably prevent many nonpolio enteroviral diseases as well. This approach has proven effective for pre-exposure and postexposure prophylaxis of hepatitis A and probably reduces the frequency of severe enteroviral infections in agammaglobulinemic patients receiving replacement therapy. However, the benign nature of most enterovirus infections, the fact that exposures are rarely recognized (most result from contact with an asymptomatically infected person), and the relatively short half-life of exogenous immune serum globulin make this approach to prevention impractical in most situations. Nursery outbreaks of severe enteroviral disease provide an exception. The administration of IVIG to all infants in the nursery offers protection to those infants without transplancentally acquired neutralizing antibody who have not yet been infected.

McKinney RE, Katz SL, Wilfert CM: Chronic enteroviral meningoencephalitis in agammaglobulinemic patients. Rev Infect Dis 9:334, 1987. *Excellent review of this interesting syndrome with thoughtful discussion of pathogenesis and management.*

Melnick JL: Enteroviruses. *In* Fields BN, et al. (eds.): Fields Virology, 3rd ed. New York, Lippincot-Raven Publishers, 1996. *Authoritative review, with emphasis on epidemiology and extensive bibliography.*

Modlin JF: Coxsackieviruses, echoviruses, and newer enteroviruses. *In* Mandell GL, et al. (eds.): Principles and Practice of Infectious Diseases, 4th ed. New York, Churchill Livingstone, 1995, p 1620–1636. *Extensive review of epidemiology and clinical manifestations of nonpolio enterovirus infections with excellent bibliography.*

Rotbart HA: Enteroviruses. In Murray PR et al: Manual of Clinical Microbiology, 6th ed. Washington, DC, ASM Press, 1995. *A comprehensive treatment of laboratory diagnosis by the leader in PCR technology applied to enteroviral infections diagnosis.*

Rueckert RR: Picornaviridae and their replication. *In* Fields BN, et al. (eds.): Fields Virology, 3rd ed. New York, Lippincott-Raven Publishers, 1996. *Detailed summary of current knowledge of picornavirus structure, replication, and virus-cell interactions.*

Ryan MD, Jenkins O, Hughes PJ, et al.: The complete nucleotide sequence of enterovirus type 70: Relationships with other members of the Picornaviridae. J Gen Virol 71:2291, 1990. *Detailed comparison of genome of enterovirus 70 to genomes of other human and animal enteroviruses, with evidence for its unique nature and origin.*

Savoia MC, Oxman MN: Myocarditis and Pericarditis. *In* Mandell GL, et al. (eds): Principles and Practice of Infectious Diseases, 4th ed. New York, Churchill Livingstone, 1995. *Well-referenced review of etiology, pathogenesis, clinical manifestations, and diagnosis of myocarditis and pericarditis.*

344   VIRAL GASTROENTERITIS
Albert Z. Kapikian

DEFINITION

Viral gastroenteritis (acute infectious nonbacterial gastroenteritis, epidemic diarrhea, winter vomiting disease, sporadic infantile gastroenteritis) is a common acute infectious disease of all age groups, characterized by vomiting or watery diarrhea, or both, that may be accompanied by fever, nausea, anorexia, and malaise. It ranges from a mild, self-limited illness of short duration to life-threatening dehydration, especially in infants and young children.

The importance of this disease in a developed country was highlighted in the Cleveland Family Study, in which infectious gastroenteritis, presumably nonbacterial, was the second most common disease experience, accounting for 16% of approximately 25,000 illnesses in a period of almost 10 years. In developing countries the impact of diarrheal illnesses is staggering: In Asia, Africa, and Latin America, 3 to 5 billion cases of diarrhea and 5 to 10 million diarrhea-associated deaths occur annually, with the major impact in infants and young children. In addition, diarrheal illness was ranked first among infectious diseases in incidence and mortality in these developing areas.

In spite of major discoveries in bacteriology and parasitology in the past century, the etiology of most acute diarrheal illnesses remained elusive for many years. In the 1940's and 1950's, oral administration of bacteria-free stool filtrates from patients with acute diarrhea induced illness in volunteers, but the suspected viral etiologic agent could not be identified. In 1972, Kapikian and colleagues, employing immune electron microscopy (IEM), discovered the first virus-like particles that could be implicated as an important cause of acute gastroenteritis, in a stool suspension derived from a gastroenteritis outbreak in Norwalk, Ohio. In 1973, Bishop and associates, using electron microscopy (EM), discovered rotavirus particles in duodenal biopsies from infants and young children hospitalized with acute gastroenteritis. Rotaviruses have emerged as the major known cause of severe diarrhea of infants and young children worldwide.

ETIOLOGY

NORWALK VIRUS GROUP. The 27 nm Norwalk virus is the prototype strain of a group of fastidious, nonenveloped 27- to 40-nm particles usually named after the geographic location of the gastroenteritis outbreak from which they were first derived. They share these common characteristics: (1) are detected in feces of patients with gastroenteritis; (2) lack a distinctive morphologic appearance by EM; (3) have not been grown in cell culture; (4) possess an RNA genome; (5) have a buoyant density of 1:33 to 1:41 grams per cubic centimeter in cesium chloride; (6) possess a single primary virion-associated protein with a molecular weight of approximately 60,000. The Norwalk virus group includes at least four serotypes: Norwalk, Hawaii, Snow Mountain, and Taunton viruses. Related viruses include the Montgomery County (MC), Southampton, Desert Storm, Toronto (formerly minireovirus), Otofuke, and other small round-structured viruses (SRSV's). Although lacking the distinctive cup-like surface indentations of the "classical" caliciviruses (calix = cup in Latin), the Norwalk virus group is now classified definitively as a calicivirus in the family Caliciviridae. Recent molecular biologic studies established that the overall genomic organization of Norwalk and related strains was similar to that of feline calicivirus and rabbit hemorrhagic disease virus, another calicivirus. The Norwalk virus genome is composed of positive sense polyadenylated single-stranded RNA of 7642 nucleotides that encode three open reading frames. Previously, other noncultivatable human enteric viruses, which were associated with gastroenteritis in children or with outbreaks in the elderly, were considered to be "classical" caliciviruses morphologically. These viruses, which were recovered in the United Kingdom or Japan, were classified by IEM into five serotypes.

ROTAVIRUS. Rotaviruses are classified as a genus in the family Reoviridae and are etiologic agents of diarrhea in humans and in numerous animal and a few avian species. They are 70 nm in diameter, nonenveloped, and possess a distinctive double-layered capsid which surrounds the core that contains the genome consisting of 11 segments of double-stranded RNA, (Fig. 344–1). The name rotavirus (rota = wheel) was adopted because the sharply defined circular outline of the outer capsid was reminiscent of the rim of a wheel placed on short spokes radiating from a wide hub (the inner capsid). The virions have a density of 1.36 grams per cubic centimeter in cesium chloride and are antigenically distinct from the three reovirus serotypes. Rotaviruses possess three important antigenic specificities—group, subgroup, and serotype—which are mediated by different proteins: group specificity prominently by VP6 and subgroup by VP6 alone (encoded by RNA segment 6). Serotype specificity has been defined by VP7, a glycoprotein that is one of the two major neutralization antigens located on the outer capsid (encoded by RNA segment 7, 8, or 9). The other outer capsid protein VP4, which is encoded by RNA segment 4 and which protrudes from the smooth outer surface as a series of 60 short spikes of about 12 nm in length, also induces neutralizing antibodies. VP4 is the hemagglutinin in certain strains. Antibodies to both VP4 and VP7 are associated with protection against rotavirus illness. There are ten human rotavirus serotypes as defined by VP7 (also designated as "G" [for glycoprotein] serotypes), of which only four (nos. 1, 2, 3, or 4) are of epidemiologic importance. Many human and animal rotavirus strains share VP7 serotype specificity. Most animal and human rotaviruses share the common group antigen and are thus classified as group A rotaviruses, and these are further divided into subgroups. A serotyping scheme based on neutralization of VP4 (also designated "P" [for protease sensitive]) has been developed. The VP4 genotype of various strains has also been described, based on sequence analysis and/or nucleic acid hy-

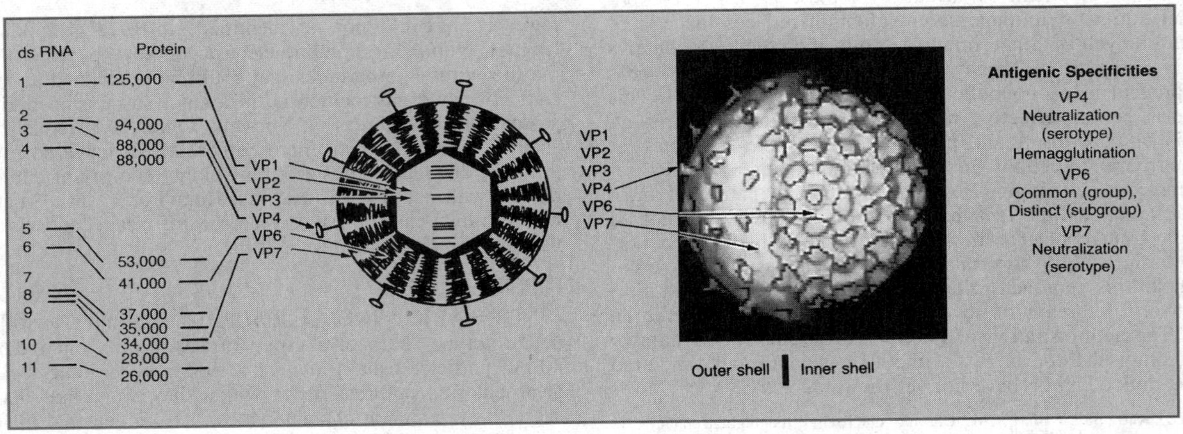

FIGURE 344–1. *Left,* Schematic representation of the rotavirus double-shelled particle. *Right,* Surface representations of the three-dimensional structures of a double-shelled particle (on the left half) and a particle (on the right half) in which most, if not all, of the outer shell and a small portion of the inner shell mass have been removed. (From Kapikian AZ, Chanock RM: Rotaviruses. *In* Fields BN, et al. (eds.): Fields Virology, 3rd ed. Philadelphia, Lippincott-Raven Publishers, 1996. Figure on right from Prasad BV, Wang GJ, Clerx JP, et al.: Three-dimensional structure of rotavirus. J Mol Biol 199:269, 1988.)

bridization of VP4. The human rotaviruses have only recently been grown efficiently in cell culture. Several human and animal rotavirus strains have been discovered that do not share the common group antigen and are classified as non-group A rotaviruses (groups B to G). In this chapter, when the term rotavirus is used, it is meant to describe only those rotaviruses belonging to group A, unless specified otherwise.

OTHER AGENTS. Other viral agents have been associated with gastroenteritis and include enteric adenoviruses belonging to types 40 and 41 (70 to 80 nm in diameter); astroviruses (28 to 30 nm); small, round viruses other than the Norwalk virus group (20 to 30 nm); putative coronavirus-like particles (100 to 150 nm); the pleomorphic, fringed, Breda or Berne virus-like particles (toroviruses) (100 to 140 nm); 35 nm "picobirnaviruses"; and a pestivirus antigen. The role of these viruses as etiologic agents of severe infantile diarrhea appears to be minor, with the exception of the enteric adenoviruses, which are associated with approximately 3 to 10% of the diarrheal illnesses of infants and young children requiring hospitalization. In addition, the role of these other agents in epidemic viral gastroenteritis appears to be minor. Additional studies are needed to assess the role of these other agents in gastroenteritis. It should be noted that about one third to one half of gastroenteritis episodes in developed countries have yet to be associated with an etiologic agent.

EPIDEMIOLOGY

NORWALK VIRUS GROUP. The Norwalk group of viruses comprises major etiologic agents of acute nonbacterial gastroenteritis, which typically occurs as a sharp outbreak affecting adults, school-age children, and family contacts. The location or source of contamination responsible for these outbreaks includes various settings such as schools, camps and recreational areas, nursing homes, swimming facilities, cruise ships, and restaurants. For example, the Norwalk virus was derived from an outbreak in an elementary school in Norwalk, Ohio, in which 50% of the students and teachers developed gastroenteritis within a 2-day period. Norwalk virus has been linked with 42% of 74 nonbacterial gastroenteritis outbreaks investigated from 1976 to 1980 and approximately 10% of all acute gastroenteritis outbreaks. In the United States, antibody to the Norwalk virus is acquired gradually in childhood and somewhat more rapidly in the adult years, so that by age 50 at least 50% of individuals have serum antibody. In developing countries, infants and young children acquire Norwalk antibody at an earlier age, and the virus is associated with mild gastroenteritis in this age group.

Norwalk virus is most likely transmitted via the fecal-oral route; however, it has also been detected in vomitus. Although sporadic cases attributed to person-to-person transmission may occur, the explosive nature of outbreaks associated with the Norwalk virus group often suggests a common source of infection, such as water or food. Common-source outbreaks have been attributed to contamination of community and noncommunity public water systems, stored water on cruise ships, or recreational swimming water and to inges-

tion of various foods, such as tainted oysters, lettuce, potato salad, cole slaw, or cake frosting. Secondary person-to-person transmission to contacts is relatively common. The incubation period ranges from 10 to 51 hours, with a mean of 24 hours, and symptoms usually last 24 to 60 hours. Norwalk virus outbreaks occur throughout the year without a peak season.

Norwalk virus infections have been detected in individuals with travelers' diarrhea. However, this agent is not considered to be an important cause of this disease.

The Norwalk virus or related agents have recently been shown to be important agents of acute gastroenteritis in military personnel deployed to different parts of the world. The "classical" caliciviruses have been associated primarily with pediatric gastroenteritis that characteristically is not severe enough to require hospitalization.

ROTAVIRUS. Rotaviruses are the major known etiologic agents of severe diarrhea in infants and young children in most areas of the world and are usually associated with sporadic infantile gastroenteritis, which differs from epidemic viral gastroenteritis associated with the Norwalk virus group in the following characteristics: (1) it usually does not occur in sharp outbreaks; (2) it can cause severe diarrheal illness in infants and young children; (3) it does not usually cause illness in adults; and (4) the attack rate among family contacts of index cases is low, although subclinical infections occur frequently in contacts. In addition, in contrast to Norwalk virus infections, about 90% of infants and young children in both developed and developing countries experience a rotavirus infection (as determined from antibody prevalence) by 3 years of age.

The most compelling evidence for the importance of rotaviruses in severe infantile gastroenteritis has emerged from numerous cross-sectional studies in developed and developing countries. In developed countries, including the United States, rotaviruses are associated with approximately 35 to 52% of acute diarrheal illness requiring hospitalization of infants and young children. The contribution of other enteric pathogens is consistently relatively minor. A similar pattern is also usually observed in developing countries, where rotaviruses are the most frequently detected pathogens in children younger than 2 who have severe gastroenteritis; however, bacterial agents also play an important role in such areas. It is estimated that in developing countries 873,000 infants and young children under age 5 die from rotavirus diarrhea each year. It should be noted that in developing countries during longitudinal studies in a community setting where all diarrheal episodes are monitored, the incidence of rotavirus diarrhea is lower than that of diarrhea caused by other pathogens, but dehydration is more often associated with rotavirus disease than with illness caused by other agents.

In temperate climates, rotavirus gastroenteritis has a characteristic seasonal occurrence during the cooler months of the year with peak prevalence in the winter months. In tropical countries it occurs throughout the year, with less pronounced peaks. Rotavirus diarrhea occurs most frequently in children between age 6 months and 24 months. Infants less than 6 months have the next highest frequency,

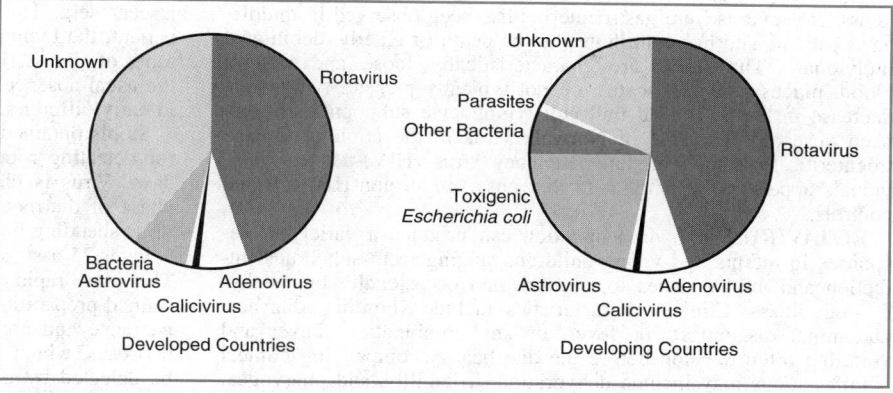

FIGURE 344–2. An estimate of the role of etiologic agents in severe diarrheal illnesses requiring hospitalization of infants and young children in developed countries *(left)* and in developing countries *(right)*. (From Kapikian AZ: Viral gastroenteritis. JAMA 269:627, 1993.)

although in certain studies the highest frequency is observed in this age group. The low frequency of clinical illness in neonates who undergo rotavirus infection is an unusual paradox that has not been explained. Rotavirus gastroenteritis occurs infrequently in adults, but subclinical infections are common.

Rotaviruses are likely transmitted by the fecal-oral route, although respiratory transmission remains a possibility, since there is such a rapid acquisition of serum antibody during the first 2 years of life regardless of hygienic conditions. Nosocomial rotavirus infections occur frequently. The incubation period of rotavirus illness is approximately 2 to 4 days. There are 10 recognized human rotavirus serotypes of which those numbered 1 to 4 appear to be clinically important. Group B rotavirus is responsible for widespread outbreaks of gastroenteritis in adults in China, and a relatively small number of group C rotaviruses have been recovered from individuals with gastroenteritis in various countries. With the exception of the group B rotaviruses in China, the role of the non–group A rotaviruses in other regions of the world appears to be relatively minor at this time.

Rotavirus infections have been observed in individuals with travelers' diarrhea. However, rotaviruses are not considered to be an important cause of this illness.

An estimate of the role of rotaviruses and other microbial agents in the etiology of severe diarrhea of infants and young children is shown in Figure 344–2. In addition, a summary of key findings regarding the epidemiology and importance of various viruses associated with acute gastroenteritis is shown in Table 344–1.

PATHOLOGY AND PATHOGENESIS

NORWALK VIRUS GROUP. Histopathologic lesions following Norwalk or Hawaii virus infection are characterized by a reversible involvement of the upper jejunum. The jejunal mucosa remains intact with marked broadening and blunting of the villi and shortening of the microvilli, along with mononuclear cell infiltration and cytoplasmic vacuolization. Functional alterations may include a transient malabsorption of fat, D-xylose, and lactose and a signifi-

cant decrease in levels of small intestinal brush border enzymes (alkaline phosphatase and trehalase). Adenylate cyclase activity in the jejunum is not elevated. Delay in gastric emptying may be responsible for the nausea and vomiting associated with these agents.

The nature of immunity to Norwalk virus is perplexing, because a high percentage (~ 50%) of adults are susceptible to both natural and experimental illness. In addition, although immunity has been observed in approximately 50% of adults, it appears to correlate inversely with the level of serum or local jejunal antibody.

ROTAVIRUS. The major histopathologic lesions are characterized by reversible involvement of the proximal small intestine. The mucosa remains intact, with shortening of the villi, mononuclear cell infiltration in the lamina propria, distended cisternae of the endoplasmic reticulum, mitochondrial swelling, and sparse, irregular microvilli. Functional alterations may include impaired D-xylose absorption and depressed levels of disaccharidases (maltase, sucrase, and lactase).

The mechanism of immunity to human rotaviruses is not clear. Although significant levels of serum antibodies correlate with resistance to illness, the role of local intestinal immunity has not been elucidated. Animal studies indicate that antibody in the small intestine is the major determinant of resistance to illness. A high rate of subclinical infection in neonates is well documented and may be related to passively acquired maternal antibody, host factors, or naturally attenuated rotaviruses that are able to persist in newborn nurseries.

CLINICAL MANIFESTATIONS

NORWALK VIRUS GROUP. Clinical characteristics of illness induced by the Norwalk group of viruses include nausea, vomiting, diarrhea, anorexia, or abdominal discomfort, or any combination. Accompanying clinical manifestations may also include myalgias, low-grade fever, headache, and chills. In children, vomiting occurs more often than diarrhea, whereas in adults the opposite is observed. The onset of illness may be abrupt, marked by vomiting, diarrhea, or both. The illness is usually mild and lasts about 24 to 60

TABLE 344–1. VIRUSES ASSOCIATED WITH ACUTE GASTROENTERITIS IN HUMANS

Virus	Size, nm	Epidemiology	Important as a Cause of Hospitalization
Rotavirus			
Group A	70	Single most important cause (viral or bacterial) of endemic severe diarrheal illness in infants and young children worldwide (in cooler months in temperate climates)	Yes
Group B	70	Outbreaks of diarrheal illness in adults and children in China	No
Group C	70	Sporadic cases and occasional outbreaks of diarrheal illness in children	No
Enteric adenovirus	70–80	Second most important viral agent of endemic diarrheal illness of infants and young children worldwide	Yes
Norwalk virus or Norwalk-like caliciviruses	27–32	Important cause of outbreaks of vomiting and diarrheal illness in older children and adults in families, communities, and institutions; frequently associated with ingestion of food	No
Caliciviruses ("classical")	28–40	Sporadic cases and occasional outbreaks of diarrheal illness in infants, young children, and the elderly	No
Astroviruses	28	Sporadic cases and occasional outbreaks of diarrheal illness in infants, young children, and the elderly	No

Adapted from Kapikian AZ: Viral gastroenteritis. JAMA 269:627, 1993.

hours. However, severe gastroenteritis has been observed in middle-aged patients and has contributed to the death of elderly, debilitated individuals. The stools are characteristically loose and watery; blood, mucus, and leukocytes are not typically present. A transient decrease in the T, B, and null cell lymphocyte subpopulations has been observed. The role of Norwalk virus in the etiology of gastroenteritis in human immunodeficiency virus (HIV)-positive individuals appears to be similar to that observed in non-HIV infected controls.

ROTAVIRUS. Rotavirus infection can produce a variety of responses in infants and young children, ranging from subclinical infection and mild diarrhea to a severe and occasionally fatal dehydrating illness. Clinical characteristics include vomiting, diarrhea, abdominal discomfort, or fever, or any combination. Fever and vomiting often develop before the diarrhea. Accompanying clinical manifestations may include dehydration, irritability, and pharyngeal or tympanic membrane erythema. In hospitalized patients, the mean duration of confinement is 4 days, with a range of 2 to 14 days. The stools are characteristically loose and watery and only infrequently contain blood or leukocytes.

Although rotaviruses can cause severe or fatal dehydrating illnesses in developing countries, deaths have also been documented in developed countries. In a study in Canada, rotavirus gastroenteritis was implicated in the deaths of 21 children 4 to 30 months old (mean 11 months) over a period of about 5 years. Twenty children were dead or moribund upon arrival at hospital, and one child was infected nosocomially. With the exception of the latter patient and one other, each child was considered healthy prior to the rotaviral illness. Death occurred within 1 to 3 days of onset of symptoms. Dehydration and electrolyte imbalance leading to cardiac arrest were believed to be the major cause of death in 16 patients; aspiration of vomitus was the cause of death in 3 patients; and seizures were a contributing factor in the remaining 2 patients.

Rotavirus can also induce chronic symptomatic diarrhea with prolonged fecal shedding of the virus and antigenemia in patients with primary immunodeficiency diseases. Infections with rotaviruses or other viral and bacterial enteric pathogens may be especially severe in individuals who are immunosuppressed for bone marrow transplantation. In one study, 8 of 78 such patients (average age of entire group, 20.5 years) shed rotavirus in stools and 5 of the 8 died. In addition, a non–group A rotavirus was associated with severe gastroenteritis in an 8-year-old bone marrow transplant patient. Rotavirus infections have also been persistent and severe in children with severe combined immunodeficiency. Rotavirus infections have also been associated with necrotizing enterocolitis and hemorrhagic gastroenteritis in neonates.

Outbreaks of rotavirus gastroenteritis have occurred in elderly individuals in nursing homes with several fatalities.

Rotaviruses do not appear to have an important role as etiologic agents of acute diarrhea in HIV-positive adults.

DIAGNOSIS

NORWALK VIRUS GROUP. Since a specific diagnosis of infection with this group cannot be made by clinical observation, the diagnosis must be made in the laboratory and relies on detection of virus in the stool or a serologic response to a viral-specific antigen. These tests include IEM (for the entire group), radioimmunoassay (Norwalk and Snow Mountain agents), and enzyme-linked immunosorbent assay (ELISA) (Norwalk, Snow Mountain, and Hawaii viruses). These are still research procedures, because reagents are not generally available. Virus shedding is maximal at or shortly after onset of illness and minimal at 72 hours following onset. The characteristic absence of fecal leukocytes in Norwalk infection may be helpful for differentiation from *Shigella* or *Salmonella* enteritis. Recent molecular biologic advances in the study of the Norwalk group of viruses should lead to a proliferation of diagnostic assays.

Although a specific clinical diagnosis of infection with Norwalk virus cannot be made in the individual patient, a tentative diagnosis of infection can be made during an outbreak if certain criteria are met: (1) bacterial or parasitic pathogens are not detected; (2) vomiting is present in at least 50% of cases; (3) incubation period is 24 to 48 hours; and (4) mean or median duration of illness is 12 to 60 hours.

ROTAVIRUS. The clinical manifestations of rotavirus gastroenteritis are not distinctive enough to enable diagnosis. Thus, diagnosis requires either detection of the virus or demonstration of a significant serologic response to rotavirus in paired acute and convalescent sera. The epidemiologic pattern relating to the age of the patient, the temporal occurrence of illness, and the signs and symptoms of illness, however, may suggest the diagnosis. In addition, the usual absence of fecal leukocytes in rotavirus diarrhea may help in early differentiation from *Shigella* or *Salmonella* enteritis.

Stools obtained from the first to fourth day of illness are optimal for detecting rotavirus, but virus shedding may continue up to 21 days. Virus is characteristically present in stools during the early phase of diarrhea, but diarrhea may continue for 2 to 3 days after virus shedding has ceased.

Over 25 assays have been developed to detect rotavirus in stools. The most rapid method is still direct EM because in negatively stained preparations these agents have a distinctive morphologic appearance and are present in large amounts. The non–group A rotaviruses, which do not share the common group antigen, can also be detected by EM. However, an electron microscope may not be readily available, and its use may be impractical when evaluating a large number of specimens. Thus, other rapid and highly effective methods for virus detection have been developed, including ELISA, counterimmunoelectroosmophoresis (CIEOP), radioimmunoassay (RIA), reverse passive hemagglutination assay (RPHA), latex agglutination (LA), RNA electrophoresis, dot hybridization, and recently by using the polymerase chain reaction. Commercial kits are now available for the ELISA, LA, and RPHA assays. A popular method is the confirmatory ELISA because it is simple to perform, is sensitive, does not require specialized equipment, and has a negative serum antibody control for detecting nonspecific reactions. An ELISA using monoclonal anti-VP7 antibody is also available. The non–group A rotaviruses cannot be detected by these assays, because they lack the common group antigen; however, an ELISA for group B rotaviruses has been developed. Diagnosis of group A rotavirus infection by growth in cell cultures is not practical.

There are many methods for measuring a serologic response to rotavirus infection, including IEM, complement fixation (CF), immunofluorescence, immune adherence hemagglutination assay, ELISA, neutralization, hemagglutination-inhibition (HI), inhibition of RPHA, and a competition solid-phase immunoassay that measures epitope specific immune responses to individual rotavirus serotypes. Complement fixation is an efficient assay for detecting a serologic response to rotavirus in patients age 6 to 24 months but is not as effective in adults or infants younger than 6 months.

Detection of rotavirus or demonstration of a serologic response does not necessarily establish an etiologic association with the patient's illness, especially in newborns and adults, who frequently undergo subclinical infection.

TREATMENT

NORWALK VIRUS GROUP. Since the Norwalk group of viruses characteristically causes a mild, self-limited gastroenteritis, replacement of fluid and electrolyte loss with orally administered isotonic fluids is usually sufficient. However, if severe vomiting or diarrhea occurs, parenteral fluid replacement may be necessary. Oral administration of bismuth subsalicylate significantly reduces the severity of abdominal cramps, with a decrease in the median duration of gastrointestinal symptoms from 20 hours to 14 hours. However, the number, weight, and water content of stools and the level of virus excretion are not affected significantly.

ROTAVIRUS. Because rotavirus gastroenteritis may lead to severe dehydration in infants and young children, the early replacement of fluids and electrolytes is essential. Intravenous fluids have been used effectively in treating dehydration. However, in many parts of the world where such treatment is not feasible, efforts have been made to evaluate the effectiveness of an oral rehydration salts (ORS) solution. In a double-blind study comparing ORS with intravenous fluids in children with rotavirus gastroenteritis, ORS solution containing either glucose (20 grams per liter) or sucrose (40 grams per liter) plus electrolytes was found to be as effective as intravenous therapy for rehydration. Glucose electrolyte solutions are recommended for optimal results. The recommended World Health Organization (WHO) ORS solution is made by adding the following to 1 liter of water: sodium chloride, 3.5 grams; trisodium citrate, dihydrate, 2.9 grams; potassium chloride, 1.5 grams; and glucose, anhydrous, 20 grams. Sodium bicarbonate, 2.5 grams, may be substituted for the trisodium citrate, dihydrate. The efficacy of oral glucose-electrolyte solutions that contained either 90 mmol of sodium per liter (as in the WHO formula above) or 50 mmol of sodium per liter, plus additional electrolytes, was examined in well-nourished ambulatory or hospitalized children with mild or moderate dehydrating diarrheal illnesses of varied etiology (including rotavirus but excluding cholera), and each was found to be safe and effective. After the initial calculated fluid deficit is corrected by the ORS, water or fluids without added electrolytes, such as breast milk or some other form of low-solute feeding, should be given orally in addition to the ORS solution, to replace both continued diarrheal fluid and electrolyte losses and to provide normal daily fluid requirements. If oral rehydration fails to correct the fluid and electrolyte loss or if the patient is severely dehydrated or in shock, or has depressed consciousness (see below), intravenous therapy must be given.

In recent studies, rice-based ORS solutions were also found to be effective in rehydrating infants and young children hospitalized with mild to moderate dehydration caused by diarrhea associated with various pathogens, including rotavirus. Both glucose-based or rice-based ORS solutions were effective in rehydration and maintenance therapy. Oral rehydration therapy should not be given to infants and younger children with depressed consciousness because of the possibility of fluid aspiration.

In a limited study, chronic rotavirus illness in immunodeficient children has been treated effectively by oral feeding of pooled human milk that contained rotavirus antibody. Oral administration of preparations containing rotavirus antibody has produced conflicting results regarding their efficacy for treatment of normal children during episodes of rotavirus gastroenteritis.

Orally administered bismuth subsalicylate (BSS) was evaluated in a placebo-controlled study as an adjunct to rehydration therapy in children age 4 to 28 months who were hospitalized with rotavirus diarrhea. The BSS group had a shorter course of diarrhea than the placebo group. Because of the reported association between the use of salicylates and Reye's syndrome, the authors reviewed the literature regarding the possibility of such an association with BSS and other non–acetyl-salicylic acid salicylates and were unable to find any such association.

PREVENTION

NORWALK VIRUS GROUP. There are no specific methods for preventing illness by the Norwalk virus group. However, because of the extremely infectious nature of these agents, careful handwashing and proper disposal of contaminated material should minimize transmission. In addition, hygienic preparation of food and measures to decrease contamination of drinking water or swimming facilities should limit the frequency of Norwalk virus outbreaks. Active immunization against this group of viruses is not yet feasible.

ROTAVIRUS. Epidemiologic studies indicate the global need for a rotavirus vaccine to prevent rotavirus diarrhea in the first 2 years of life, when illness is most severe. Current efforts are focused on developing a live, attenuated oral vaccine that is effective against all serotypes. A promising initial strategy involved the "Jennerian" approach, in which a related rotavirus from a nonhuman host (a bovine or rhesus rotavirus strain) was used as the immunizing agent. Efficacy trials of several such candidate rotavirus vaccines gave variable results and it soon became apparent that these vac-

cines did not induce satisfactory heterotypic immunity in infants not primed by previous rotavirus infection. The rhesus rotavirus vaccine (a VP7 serotype 3 strain) induced protection against rotavirus diarrhea in the 1- to 4-month age group in a study in which VP7 serotype 3 was predominant, but it failed in other studies to protect unprimed infants against illnesses caused by other than serotype 3 rotaviruses. Thus, the Jennerian approach has been modified with the goal being a quadrivalent vaccine composed of rhesus rotavirus (serotype 3) and three reassortant rotaviruses each containing 10 rhesus rotavirus genes and a single human rotavirus gene that encodes VP7 serotype 1, 2, or 4 specificity. Field trials of the quadrivalent vaccine in infants and young children have been encouraging, with approximately 80% efficacy against the development of severe rotavirus diarrhea observed in two separate trials in the United States.

Breast milk is generally considered to confer some degree of protection against clinically significant rotavirus diarrhea during infancy. The prophylactic oral administration of human serum globulin containing rotavirus antibody to low birth weight neonates provides significant protection against rotavirus diarrhea. In addition, passive oral immunization of infants and young children with bovine colostrum that contained antibodies to human rotavirus was effective in preventing rotavirus illness when compared with a control group.

Bernstein DI, Glass RI, Rodgers G, et al.: Evaluation of rhesus rotavirus monovalent and tetravalent reassortant vaccines in U.S. children. JAMA 273:1191, 1995. *A placebo-controlled vaccine trial in which the tetravalent vaccine induced > 80% protection against very severe rotavirus gastroenteritis.*

Guarino A, Canini RB, Russo S, et al.: Oral immunoglobulins for treatment of acute rotaviral gastroenteritis. Pediatrics 93:12, 1994. *A study reporting the benefit of oral human serum immunoglobulin in infants and young children hospitalized with acute viral gastroenteritis.*

Hoshino Y, Kapikian AZ: Rotavirus vaccine development for the prevention of severe diarrhea in infants and young children. Trends in Microbiol 2:242, 1994. *A concise review of rotavirus vaccine strategies and an up-to-date presentation of rotavirus serotypes.*

Jiang X, Graham DY, Wang K, Estes MK: Norwalk virus genome cloning and characterization. Science 250:1580, 1990. *A study describing the cloning of the fastidious Norwalk virus.*

Kapikian AZ (ed.): Virus Infections of the Gastrointestinal Tract. New York, Marcel Dekker, Inc., 1994. *An entire volume on viral infections of the gastrointestinal tract by numerous contributors. Includes relevant data on viral agents associated with gastroenteritis with extensive references.*

Kapikian AZ, Chanock RM: Norwalk group of viruses. In Fields BN, et al. (eds.): Virology, 3rd ed. New York, Raven Press, in press. *A detailed current review of the Norwalk group of viruses from a virologic, epidemiologic, and clinical point of view. 277 references.*

Kapikian AZ, Chanock RM: Rotaviruses. In Fields BN, et al. (eds.): Virology, 3rd ed. New York, Raven Press, in press. *A detailed current review of rotaviruses from a virologic, epidemiologic, and clinical point of view. 993 references.*

Molina S, Vettorazzi C, Pearson JM, et al.: Clinical trial of glucose-oral rehydration solution (ORS), rice dextrin-ORS, and rice flour-ORS for the management of children with acute diarrhea and mild or moderate dehydration. Pediatrics 95:191, 1995. *A study evaluating the efficacy of two rice-based rehydration solutions and a conventional glucose-based solution in hospitalized infants and young children with acute diarrhea associated with various pathogens, including rotavirus.*

Soriano-Brucher H, Avendano P, O'Ryan M, et al.: Bismuth subsalicylate in the treatment of acute diarrhea in children: A clinical study. Pediatrics 87:18, 1991. *A study evaluating oral BSS as an adjunct to rehydration in infants and young children hospitalized with acute diarrhea associated with various pathogens, including rotavirus.*

Hemorrhagic Fever Viruses

345 INTRODUCTION TO HEMORRHAGIC FEVER VIRUSES

Robert E. Shope

The viral hemorrhagic fevers encompass syndromes that vary from febrile hemorrhagic disease with capillary fragility to acute se-

vere shock leading rapidly to death. The causative agents include arthropod-borne and rodent-borne viruses. The rodent-borne viruses do not require an arthropod vector but are transmitted directly to vertebrates by aerosol spread or contact with infected excreta or body secretions of the rodent. The reservoir and natural mode of transmission for the African hemorrhagic fever viruses, Marburg and Ebola, are not known.

There are at least 18 viruses that cause human hemorrhagic fevers (see Table 345–1). They are in the families Flaviviridae, Bunyaviridae, Arenaviridae, and Filoviridae. All contain RNA, and all are zoonoses.

The hemorrhagic fevers form a special group of diseases charac-

TABLE 345-1. CLINICAL PARAMETERS OF VIRAL HEMORRHAGIC FEVERS

Disease	Viral Agent	Incubation Period (Days)	Clinical Syndromes				ARDS*	Case-Fatality Rate (%)
			Hemorrhage	Hepatitis	Encephalitis	Nephropathy		
Yellow fever	Yellow fever	3–6	major	major	absent	moderate	absent	2–20
Dengue hemmorrhagic fever	Dengue 1–4	5–8	moderate	moderate	absent	absent	absent	2–5
Rift Valley fever	Rift Valley fever	3–6	major	major	moderate	absent	absent	30–50
Crimean-Congo hemmorrhagic fever	Crimean-Congo hemmorrhagic fever	2–9	major	major	minor	absent	absent	30–50
Kyasanur Forest disease	Kyasanur Forest disease	3–8	minor	minor	moderate	absent	absent	5–10
Omsk hemmorrhagic fever	Omsk hemmorrhagic fever	3–8	minor	minor	moderate	absent	absent	0.4–2.5
Hemorrhagic fever with renal syndrome	Hantaan, Puumala, Dobrava, Seoul	2–42	moderate	rare	minor	major	absent	2–5
Hantavirus pulmonary syndrome	Sin Nombre Shelter Island I	12–16	minor	minor	absent	minor	major	40–50
Venezuelan hemorrhagic fever	Guanarito	7–14	moderate	rare	rare	minor	absent	60
Brazilian hemorrhagic fever	Sabiá	8–12	major	minor	minor	minor	absent	33
Argentine hemorrhagic fever	Junin	10–14	minor	rare	moderate	minor	absent	1–15
Bolivian hemorrhagic fever	Machupo	7–14	moderate	rare	moderate	minor	absent	15–30
Lassa fever	Lassa	3–16	minor	major	minor	minor	absent	10–25
African hemorrhagic fever	Marburg	3–9	major	major	minor	absent	absent	20–30
	Ebola	3–18	major	major	minor	absent	absent	60–90

* Adult respiratory distress syndrome.

terized by viral replication in lymphoid cells, followed by fever and myalgia and leading to hemorrhagic manifestations and hypovolemic shock. The basic physiologic defect in most is capillary leakage. In some, such as yellow fever, hepatocellular damage is prominent. In others, such as hemorrhagic fever with renal syndrome, renal lesions are striking. The mortality rates may be high, and the pathogenesis is poorly understood. Disseminated intravascular coagulopathy (DIC) is a feature in some cases, but probably not all. Antigen-antibody complexes may lead to release of mediators of shock in some cases, and direct effects of viral replication on capillary permeability in some have not been ruled out. It is important to understand the pathogenetic mechanism to manage the patient, but our knowledge is sparse at present.

Control can be achieved by interrupting the cycle, including peridomestic rodent control (Bolivian hemorrhagic fever), and, in those that are arboviruses, by vaccinating reservoir animals (Rift Valley fever), vector control, and education on methods to avoid the vector (dengue) or rodent reservoir (hantavirus pulmonary syndrome). Vaccines are available or under development for some of the agents such as Rift Valley fever, yellow fever, dengue, and Junin viruses. For others such as Lassa virus, we now have an antiviral drug, and for still another (Junin) pre-exposure and postexposure protection is afforded by human immune plasma.

345.1 Yellow Fever

DEFINITION. Yellow fever is an acute viral disease caused by infection with yellow fever virus. The disease is exemplary of the viral hemorrhagic fevers described in the following sections (Table 345–1). The infection is often subclinical but may lead to disease whose severity varies from mild and self-limited to a fulminant fatal outcome. Classic yellow fever is characterized by sudden onset, moderately high fever, nausea, bradycardia, prostration, vomiting of altered blood, jaundice, oliguria, and albuminuria. Natural cycles of the infection occur periodically in mosquitoes and primates of tropical South America as far north as Panama and in tropical west, central, and east Africa.

ETIOLOGY. Yellow fever virus is in the genus Flavivirus of the family Flaviviridae. Members of the family are single-stranded, negative-sense RNA viruses, spherical and approximately 40 nm in diameter. Particles form in the cytoplasm in close association with endoplasmic reticulum. They contain a lipid envelope and replicate in both arthropod and vertebrate cells. Other members of the Fla-

viviridae, including dengue, West Nile, and St. Louis encephalitis, cross-react with yellow fever virus in serologic tests and may confound the diagnosis. Minor antigenic differences exist between strains of yellow fever virus from Africa and South America, and among strains from different regions of Africa; however, the 17D yellow fever vaccine protects against all strains. The virus can be isolated in mosquitoes, arthropod and vertebrate tissue cultures, baby mice, and several monkey species. Rhesus monkeys regularly succumb following experimental inoculation and mimic severe human disease.

EPIDEMIOLOGY. Two epidemiologic types of yellow fever are distinguished: the urban and the sylvan (jungle) forms. Urban yellow fever is transmitted by Aedes aegypti mosquitoes from person to person, whereas sylvan yellow fever is maintained in a forest cycle of monkeys and forest-canopy mosquitoes; humans are infected when they enter the forest. The two types do not differ clinically.

A. aegypti is a peridomestic mosquito that breeds in abandoned tires, jars, cans, water storage containers, roof catchments, and drains in and around houses. Urban yellow fever was a major killer until the early 1900's, when mosquito control in Havana, Rio de Janeiro, Guayaquil, and the other large urban centers eliminated the disease. The last recorded urban case in the Americas was in Trinidad in 1954. A. aegypti continues to be prevalent in African cities, and A. aegypti-transmitted outbreaks still occur there. Major epidemics were recorded in Ethiopia, 1960–1962; Nigeria, 1969; Senegal, 1965 and 1979; Gambia, 1978; Ghana and Burkina Faso, 1983; and Kenya, 1993. In 1986, an epidemic involving at least 3000 persons occurred in Nigeria, in Benue and Cross River States, and extended into Oyo and Niger States in 1987. An estimated 39,000 cases, with 8400 deaths, were recorded.

Yellow fever virus in Africa is transmitted by A. aegypti not only in the cities but also in semirural areas. In addition, some African epidemics are maintained by other Aedes species, such as bromeliae and the tree hole-breeding africanus, leuteocephalus, and furcifertaylori, which transmit the virus in savannah and the transition forest-savannah zones of west Africa.

Sylvan yellow fever was recognized initially in Brazil in 1932. After urban yellow fever had been controlled in the Americas, sporadic cases continued to occur in persons exposed to mosquitoes in the jungles of South America and Africa. This sylvan form is maintained in tropical America by Haemagogus mosquitoes and forest primates, and sometimes by other sylvan animals. Evidence favors the hypothesis that the virus moves through the forest, cycling in one place until the monkeys are immune, then dying out and moving to areas where there are susceptible monkeys. People entering the forest are at risk. Sylvan yellow fever extends periodically outside the enzootic zone into forests such as those in Panama and Central America. The virus can be maintained over dry periods by transovarial transmission in mosquitoes, although it remains to be shown whether maintenance in mosquito eggs is more than a temporary mechanism.

The sylvan cycle in Africa is more complicated than in the Americas; in tropical Africa the virus cycles between *A. africanus* and monkeys. Another African mosquito, *A. bromeliae,* which feeds on both humans and monkeys, serves in some areas as a link between primates in the deep forest and people in the African villages.

A. aegypti was once carried on sailing ships between tropical ports and into temperate-zone cities. Modern ocean-going ships no longer harbor mosquito-breeding sites, but the mosquito continues to travel by small boats, airplanes, cars, and especially in the form of dried eggs transported by used tires. Cities such as Rio de Janeiro, which were once freed of the mosquito, are now reinfested. Dengue fever reappeared there in 1986. To control the mosquito again in this area will be difficult because of insecticide resistance and the high price of labor and materials. Jungle yellow fever continues to cycle, reappearing in the same locale every 5 to 40 years. The scene is thus set again for emergence of the virus from the jungle to reinitiate the urban cycle in the Americas.

A. aegypti is easily identified. It has white thoracic scales in the shape of a lyre and black legs with white bands. Mosquitoes that have fed on a viremic vertebrate become infective after an extrinsic incubation period of 9 to 30 days, the shorter periods correlating with higher ambient temperatures. This extrinsic incubation period in the mosquito accounts for the delay from the first human infection in an urban outbreak to subsequent clusters of infection.

Yellow fever is not found in Asia, although large areas harbor *A. aegypti* that are capable of transmitting the virus, should it be introduced. India and other Asian nations require vaccination of travelers from yellow fever-endemic regions.

All age groups and races are susceptible. However, sylvan yellow fever is found almost always in young males because they are the individuals who venture into the forest. Immunity following vaccination or infection is long-lasting. During an epidemic, the population at risk, therefore, may be limited to age groups not covered by prior immunization or those born since a prior outbreak. There is also some evidence that persons may be protected by antibody to heterologous flaviviruses.

During the 24-year period from 1965 to 1988, there were 3324 cases of yellow fever reported in the Americas, and 7701 in Africa. The numbers of cases are greatly underestimated, probably by a factor of at least 10. Case-fatality rates are usually about 20%, but are higher in some epidemics. Ratios of apparent to inapparent infection, estimated at 1:10, may vary greatly.

PATHOLOGY AND PATHOGENESIS. The lesions of yellow fever involve primarily the liver, heart, kidneys, and lymphoid tissues. Grossly, the skin is icteric, and there may be multiple hemorrhages or petechiae of the skin, mucous membranes, and multiple organs. The liver is normal in size, icteric, and fatty. The heart is soft and flabby, and the kidneys are swollen and a pink-gray color. Small peritoneal and pleural effusions are sometimes observed.

Histology is often characteristic in patients who die before the ninth day of illness, but the lesions are not always pathognomonic. The most striking lesion is the eosinophilic degeneration and coagulation of hepatocytes (Councilman's bodies). Hepatocyte destruction is most marked in the midzone of the lobule, with relative sparing of the central vein and portal areas. Intranuclear eosinophilic granular inclusions or enlarged nucleoli (Torre's bodies) are also described. Both microvacuolar and multivacuolar fatty changes are prominent, especially after the first week of illness. Inflammation is uncommon, and the reticulum framework is unaffected, probably accounting for the absence of postnecrotic fibrosis in convalescence and the regeneration of hepatocytes in recovered patients. The kidneys show cloudy swelling of tubular epithelium leading to acute tubular necrosis. The glomeruli are not obviously affected, but special stains indicate Schiff-positive alterations in the basal membranes, and proteinaceous material accumulates in the capsular spaces and lumina of the proximal tubules. The myocardium is characterized by granular or fatty infiltration of muscle fibers and of the atrioventricular (AV) conduction system and cloudy swelling and degeneration of myocytes without inflammation. Large monocytes replace lymphocytic cells in the splenic follicles and lymph nodes. Encephalitis is rare, although petechial hemorrhage in the brain stem and cerebral edema are observed.

Knowledge of the pathogenesis of yellow fever is sparse. Yellow fever cases occur in remote areas, and pathophysiologic studies of yellow fever patients are usually done with only rudimentary laboratory facilities. The virus replicates in the hepatocytes and myocytes, and it is presumed that lesions in these target cells are a direct effect of the virus. Jaundice and prolonged prothrombin time can be explained by hepatocellular damage; bradycardia and arrhythmias, by myocyte and AV node perturbation. The etiology of renal tubular necrosis is not clear, but it may be secondary to hepatic changes. Some, but not all, fatal cases are associated with thrombocytopenia; increased prothrombin, partial thromboplastin, and thrombin times; diminished Factor VIII and fibrinogen; and the presence of fibrin split products. The bleeding in these cases may be secondary to disseminated intravascular coagulopathy (DIC), but this is not generally accepted by all investigators. Hypoglycemia, metabolic acidosis, and hyperkalemia characterize the terminal stage and are probably the result of multiple organ system failure.

CLINICAL MANIFESTATIONS. Severe yellow fever is a fulminant febrile illness with ≥ 50% mortality. There is a great deal of variation, however; most cases are mild with a better prognosis, and only about 10 to 20% are in the severe category. The intrinsic incubation period is 3 to 6 days, exceptionally as long as 10 days.

The clinical syndrome is classified as very mild, mild, moderately severe, or malignant. Patients with very mild cases have fever and headache, and the patient recovers in 48 hours or less. Those with mild cases have sudden fever and headache with nausea, sometimes bleeding of the gums or epistaxis, bradycardia, or albuminuria. The patient recovers in 2 or 3 days. Those with moderately severe cases have more marked manifestations of bleeding, definite bradycardia in relation to the fever, nausea and vomiting, jaundice, and striking albuminuria. The illness may be aborted after 3 to 4 days or may develop serious hemorrhagic manifestations, such as black vomit, melena, and metrorrhagia. Moderately severe yellow fever may last 1 week or even longer.

Classic yellow fever is characterized as malignant and is divided into three periods. The period of infection involves sudden onset of fever and headache, with initial rapid pulse, but by day 2, the pulse slows in spite of continued fever (Faget's sign). Headache, back, and muscle pain may be severe, blood oozes from the gums, and other signs of bleeding become prominent. The face is flushed, the tongue is reddened (strawberry tongue), and the conjunctivae are injected; the patient is irritable, unable to sleep, and frequently constipated. The temperature is often 40° C or higher. On the third day of illness, there is nausea, vomiting of coffee-ground material, and notable albuminuria. The bleeding is usually gastric, not lower intestinal. In the period of remission, often on day 4, the patient feels better, the fever drops, and headache and nausea subside. Remission lasts a few hours to 2 days. It is followed by the period of intoxication in which the classic signs of fever, epigastric tenderness with vomiting of altered blood, nosebleeds, and albuminuria leading to oliguria or anuria occur. Dehydration may predispose to suppurative parotitis; the lungs are usually normal, but bacterial pneumonia may complicate the disease. Intoxication lasts from 3 days up to 2 weeks and may be accompanied by heart failure with drop in blood pressure, hiccup, coma, and death. Sometimes the patient is lucid until the end.

The clinical syndrome may be predominantly one of hepatic, renal, or cardiac failure. Meningoencephalitis has also been recorded. Death usually occurs between the seventh and the tenth day of illness. Patients who survive generally recover completely, although the convalescence may be prolonged, and late death from cardiac failure or arrhythmias is a rare complication.

CLINICAL LABORATORY FINDINGS. Early in the course there may be leukopenia with relative neutropenia (but sometimes with normal or elevated leukocyte count), decreased prothrombin time, and elevation of the serum bilirubin level. After the third day of illness, full-blown yellow fever is associated with abnormalities referable to the liver, kidneys, and heart. The total and conjugated bilirubin concentration values are elevated and rise together. The mean bilirubin value is 9 to 10 mg per deciliter but averages 15 to 20 mg per deciliter in severe cases and may be much higher. There are increased prothrombin and partial thromboplastin times and decreased platelets, blood glucose, and clotting Factors II, V, VII, IX, and X. Alkaline phosphatase levels are normal. Aminotransferase levels are of prognostic value; serum aspartate aminotransferase and alanine aminotransferase levels are consistently elevated in jaundiced patients.

Albuminuria usually appears on the fourth day, reaching levels of 3 to 5 mg per liter (in severe cases much higher). Blood urea averages 109 mg per deciliter, and creatinine averages 5.9 mg per deciliter in fatal cases; the averages are much lower in nonfatal yellow fever. The urine may contain bile and casts. Electrocardiogram abnormalities are sometimes present, including abnormal ST-T waves and prolonged PR and QT intervals. The cerebrospinal fluid (CSF) is under increased pressure and may contain increased protein with normal cell counts.

DIAGNOSIS. Diagnosis can be made by histopathologic examination of the liver, by isolation of yellow fever virus from blood during life and from liver and other tissues post mortem, by demonstration of specific nucleic acid, or by serologic tests. Yellow fever should be suspected in any febrile patient from endemic zones of Africa and the Americas and in areas of high *A. aegypti* prevalence where yellow fever may be introduced. Diagnosis post mortem by examination of liver taken by a viscerotome was successfully used in South America routinely for many years. Liver biopsy should not be attempted because of the danger of uncontrolled bleeding.

Yellow fever virus can be isolated from serum and blood during the first 4 days of fever by inoculation intracerebrally into baby mice or onto mammalian or mosquito cell cultures. Mice are observed for death; the virus causes cytopathic effect in Vero cells and is detected by immunofluorescence tests in mosquito cells 3 to 6 days after inoculation. The most rapid method of diagnosis is detection of antigen in acute phase blood by the antigen-capture enzyme-linked immunosorbent assay (ELISA). The test can be completed in a few hours, although detection of antigen by ELISA is less sensitive than virus isolation.

Serologic diagnosis is made by demonstrating immunoglobulin M (IgM) by the antibody-capture ELISA. Since IgM is relatively specific and is detectable for only a short time after infection, this technique is reliable using a single convalescent serum specimen. Alternatively, tests of sera collected during the acute and convalescent phases are diagnostic if they show a fourfold or greater rise (or fall) of yellow fever antibody. The neutralization test is highly specific, but the complement fixation, hemagglutination-inhibition, and ELISA methods are usually used because they are quicker and lend themselves to field laboratory use. The laboratory must also rule out cross-reacting antibody by related viruses such as dengue. A radio-labeled RNA probe detected yellow fever RNA in fixed human liver stored for more than 20 years.

DIFFERENTIAL DIAGNOSIS. The mild form of yellow fever is not clinically distinguishable from other tropical fevers. Severe yellow fever simulates viral hepatitis, including hepatitis D; other hemorrhagic fevers; leptospirosis; rickettsial fevers; malignant malaria; and drug- and toxin-related conditions.

PROGNOSIS. Two to 20% of patients with clinically evident yellow fever die, although as many as 50% of severely ill patients succumb. It is not clear whether these patients would survive if they received the most modern supportive treatment, because most cases are treated in primitive clinics in Africa and South America. Patients who enter the period of intoxication have a guarded prognosis, especially if they develop anuria, high levels of albuminuria and bilirubinemia, a prothrombin time prolonged beyond 25% of normal, a rapid, weak pulse, uncontrolled bleeding, persistent hiccup, delirium, hypotension, or coma.

TREATMENT. Treatment consists of complete bed rest, fluid and blood replacement, and supportive care, including monitoring of vital signs. Analgesics and antiemetics may be useful, but aspirin is contraindicated because it may exacerbate bleeding. Patients are placed under bed nets to prevent possible mosquito transmission to other patients and to hospital personnel. Malaria and bacterial complications should be treated if diagnosed. Electrolyte imbalance should be corrected. Dialysis has not been used in cases of renal tubular damage, but on theoretical grounds may benefit patients with renal failure. If DIC is evident by laboratory tests, heparin may be used cautiously, although there is insufficient experience to date to predict its efficacy. Interferon and other antiviral substances have not been tried in patients with yellow fever.

PREVENTION AND CONTROL. Yellow fever can be prevented by inoculation of 17D attenuated vaccine. This vaccine is safe and in >90% of vaccinees induces antibody that persists at least 10 years, and usually for life. The vaccine is produced in eggs and should not be given to persons with egg allergies. Travelers should be vaccinated at least 10 days before arrival in yellow fever–endemic areas. Since the presence of yellow fever often goes undetected and unreported in tropical Africa and South America, the vaccine should be given to travelers whether or not there is known active transmission. Human immunodeficiency virus (HIV) infection is not a contraindication to vaccination. Unless the risk of exposure to yellow fever is great, vaccine is not recommended during pregnancy; however, it is not known to have caused fetal damage. In an epidemic, mosquito control measures and use of bed nets and repellents are recommended until vaccine can be obtained.

345.2 Hemorrhagic Fever Caused by Dengue Viruses

DEFINITION. Dengue hemorrhagic fever (DHF) is an acute febrile illness characterized by decreased platelet counts and hemoconcentration in patients infected with any one of the four serotypes of dengue virus. The disease affects children mainly and sometimes adults. Capillary permeability and coagulation defects lead to hemorrhagic manifestations and, in the more severe cases, to hypovolemic shock (dengue shock syndrome), with death in 40 to 50% of untreated shock syndrome patients. The disease has been endoepidemic in Southeast Asia since 1953 and is increasing in prevalence. It was restricted to Asia and the Pacific until 1981, when epidemic DHF appeared in Cuba; it reappeared in Venezuela in 1990.

ETIOLOGY. DHF is caused by infection with dengue viruses, but it is not yet established why one patient develops hemorrhagic fever and another develops classic dengue fever. Initially, it was hypothesized that strains of dengue virus that caused DHF were more virulent than others; another current theory holds that infection is enhanced and the disease is more severe when the host has been sensitized by a prior dengue infection of different serotype.

EPIDEMIOLOGY. The epidemiology of DHF is that described for dengue fever with some added features. Epidemics of DHF are limited to Southeast Asia, the Pacific Islands, and, since 1981, the Caribbean and South America. It is estimated that <5% of individuals with dengue develop DHF. The attack rate in Thailand is highest in children, with a minor peak in infants, when maternal antibody is waning, and a major peak at ages 4 to 12 years, when second dengue infections are most common; adults as well as children develop DHF in some outbreaks, such as that in Cuba in 1981. Well-nourished children in Southeast Asia appeared to be at higher risk than the undernourished, and blacks in the Cuban epidemic had milder illness than whites; well-controlled studies are needed to substantiate these observations.

PATHOLOGY. Post mortem there are focal hemorrhages, vascular congestion, and edema in multiple organs. The spleen and lymphoid tissues show marked lymphocytolysis and phagocytosis of lymphocytes, primarily in the T cell-dependent zones. There is also proliferation of lymphoblasts and young plasma cells. Monocytic and lymphocytic non-necrotizing perivascular infiltration is found in skin lesions, resembling an antibody-dependent Arthus reaction.

PATHOGENESIS. Dengue virus infects the macrophages, lymphocytes, and endothelial cells. On rare occasions, DHF occurs in primary dengue, indicating that direct infection of these cells with the virus can lead to the syndrome; however, the vast majority of cases are secondary infections. In these cases there is a rapid anamnestic antibody response, with formation of antigen-antibody complexes. Experimentally, formation of complexes enhances infectivity of the virus for monocytes through attachment of complexes at the Fc receptor site and entry of virus into the cell. Between 0.05 and 0.1% of monocytes in the peripheral blood can be visualized carrying dengue antigen. The replication of dengue virus in the monocyte is postulated to be the effector pathway leading to vascular permeability. Monocyte infection is presumably responsible for the observed complement activation and consumption via the classic and perhaps the alternate pathway. This process may result in formation of C3a and C5a, which are anaphylatoxins, or some other as yet unknown mediator of vascular permeability may be activated. Another effector pathway leads to coagulation defects, including thrombocytopenia and abnormal clotting. The entire process is rapid. It may evolve in a few hours to shock and death or, if managed effectively, to complete recovery. Although the pathogenesis is not understood, the pathophysiologic events are known and can be treated rationally.

CLINICAL MANIFESTATIONS. DHF usually starts with sudden onset of high fever and the signs and symptoms of dengue fever, which include facial flush, anorexia, headache, nausea, and pains in the muscles and joints. Hepatic tenderness, epigastric or generalized abdominal pain, and sore throat are frequent. The liver is usually palpable, and the spleen is characteristically prominent on radiographs. The temperature continues high for 2 days to a week. A positive tourniquet test result, easy bruising, and fine petechiae on the face, soft palate, and extremities indicate a hemorrhagic disorder. Sometimes gum bleeding and epistaxis are noted. The majority of cases are moderately severe or mild, and the patients recover after lysis of fever. The lysis may be associated with sweating, coolness of extremities, and transient lowering of blood pressure.

More severe cases are associated with shock. The fall in blood pressure occurs suddenly on the third to the seventh day of illness and is accompanied by cool, blotchy skin, circumoral cyanosis, and tachycardia. The patient becomes restless and may complain of acute abdominal pain. The pulse pressure drops to ≤ 20 mm Hg, and in severe cases the blood pressure and pulse may not be detectable. Uncorrected shock may lead to metabolic acidosis and severe bleeding from the gastrointestinal tract and other sites. Death or recovery usually occurs in 12 to 24 hours. Surviving patients do not usually have sequelae. The white blood cell count is normal or slightly elevated, with lymphocytosis and atypical lymphocytes commonly seen. There is hemoconcentration and elevated serum aspartate aminotransferase and blood urea nitrogen levels.

DIAGNOSIS. The laboratory diagnosis is that of dengue fever, which is usually made retrospectively. DHF with shock syndrome is a medical emergency, and therefore early clinical diagnosis is essential. DHF presents with (1) acute onset of fever, which is high, continuous, and lasts 2 days or more; (2) positive tourniquet test result, with spontaneous petechiae or ecchymoses; bleeding from gums or nose; hematemesis or melena; (3) hepatomegaly, observed in >90% of Asian patients; (4) hypotension with cold, clammy skin, restlessness, and pulse pressure <20 mm Hg; (5) thrombocytopenia; (6) hematocrit increased 20% over the convalescent value; and (7) radiographic evidence of pleural effusion. Fever, hemorrhagic phenomena, thrombocytopenia, and hemoconcentration are the hallmarks of DHF, and, with hypotension or narrow pulse pressure, of dengue shock syndrome (DSS). Hepatoencephalopathy sometimes develops as a late manifestation. Bacterial endotoxic shock and meningococcemia can mimic DHF/DSS.

TREATMENT. There is no specific treatment. The object of therapy is to maintain hydration, to combat acidosis, and to correct coagulation abnormalities. Salicylates may contribute to bleeding and acidosis and are contraindicated. Paracetamol may be used. Steroids should not be used. Hematocrit should be determined frequently, at least daily, to measure the degree of plasma loss and the need for intravenous fluid. Fluid should be started at 20 ml per kilogram of body weight. One third to one half of fluid should be physiologic saline and the remainder, 5% glucose in water. If acidosis is present, one quarter of fluid should be 0.167 mol per liter of sodium bicarbonate. In shock cases, one should use Ringer's lactated solution, 5% glucose in physiologic saline, 5% glucose in one-half physiological saline, 5% glucose in one-half Ringer's, or 5% glucose in one-third physiologic saline (depending on degree of dehydration and age). One should monitor for signs of cardiac failure during rapid fluid administration.

In case of shock, one should administer fluid rapidly and under pressure if necessary. One should give plasma or another volume expander if shock persists and should follow the vital signs and hematocrit. The hematocrit should decline with fluid therapy, which is continued until the hematocrit is <40%, urine output is adequate, and the appetite returns. If electrolytes and blood gases indicate acidosis, sodium bicarbonate should be administered. Heparin for intravascular coagulopathy (prolonged prothrombin and partial thromboplastin times) is usually not needed but may be used cautiously in refractory cases. Chloral hydrate for sedation, oxygen for shock, and blood should be administered as needed.

PROGNOSIS. Case fatality from DHF is 2 to 10%; deaths occur in shock cases. Most patients will survive when treated early by experienced health care workers. Recovery is rapid and without sequelae.

PREVENTION. Prevention is as described for dengue fever.

345.3 Tick-Borne Flavivirus Diseases: Kyasanur Forest Disease and Omsk Hemorrhagic Fever

DEFINITION. Kyasanur Forest disease (KFD) of India and Omsk hemorrhagic fever (OHF) of western Siberia are tick-transmitted flavivirus fevers characterized by hemorrhage or encephalitis. Some patients manifest both syndromes.

ETIOLOGY. KFD and OHF viruses belong to the tick-borne complex of flaviviruses, which also encompasses the closely related viruses of central European tick-borne encephalitis, Russian spring-summer encephalitis, and Powassan encephalitis of North America and Asia.

EPIDEMIOLOGY. KFD was originally limited to the forests of Shimoga District of Karnataka State, India, but since its discovery in 1957 it has spread in an unpredictable fashion to three other neighboring forested districts. The largest outbreak occurred during 1982–1983 in a new focus in Nidle Forest. Many tick species are involved in transmission, especially nymphal *Haemaphysalis spinigera.* Small terrestrial mammals as well as birds and bats are infected in nature. When the forest is felled for plantations, the ecology is upset. Cattle brought in to graze at the forest fringe are not infected but serve as hosts that greatly increase the numbers of ticks. Infected ticks feed on black-faced langur monkeys and South Indian bonnet macaques, which become viremic, serve as amplifiers of infection, and often die. At the same time, epidemics occur in persons with forest occupations. People are infected incidentally and do not form part of the transmission cycle.

OHF occurs in the forest-steppe areas of the lake region of western Siberia. Epidemics of as many as 600 cases were recorded in the 1940's, but in recent years the disease has virtually disappeared. Numbers of cases peak in May and again in August and September. The virus is transmitted by *Dermacentor pictus* ticks and is maintained in small-mammal populations. Muskrats, which were introduced for hunting in the 1920's, are susceptible and apparently transmit OHF virus to other muskrats and to hunters by direct contact. Lake water contaminated by dead muskrats is said to be responsible for water-borne disease. Both KFD and OHF are transmitted transovarially and trans-stadially in ticks.

CLINICAL MANIFESTATIONS AND PATHOLOGY. The incubation period is 3 to 8 days. Onset is sudden, with temperature up to 40° C, headache, papulovesicular lesions of the soft palate, myalgia, and prostration lasting 1 to 2 weeks. In more severe cases, there may be nasal, enteric, uterine, or pulmonary hemorrhage. Leukopenia, thrombocytopenia, and albuminuria are found. Some patients have a diphasic course, with a more severe illness and meningoencephalitis after a 1- or 2-week afebrile period. The second phase is characterized by fever, severe headache, meningismus, mental disturbances, and tremors. Hemorrhagic manifestations or pneumonia may also be prominent in the second phase. The case fatality rate of KFD is 5 to 10%; that of OHF is 0.4 to 2.5%. There are no sequelae. Infections in laboratory workers are common but usually mild. Histopathology is minor in comparison to the gravity of the clinical disease. Findings include extravasation of red blood cells, edema, and thrombi in the small vessels.

DIAGNOSIS AND TREATMENT. Diagnosis is by isolation of virus from the blood during the first 10 days of illness and by demonstration of antibody rise or presence of specific immunoglobulin M (IgM) during convalescence. There is no specific treatment, but fluid and electrolyte balance should be maintained and blood transfused if needed. Analgesics other than aspirin may be indicated.

PREVENTION. Tick repellents, protective clothing, and spraying of forest tracts with acaricides are the only measures available for prevention.

345.4 Crimean-Congo Hemorrhagic Fever

DEFINITION. Crimean-Congo hemorrhagic fever (CCHF) is an acute febrile hemorrhagic tick-borne disease of Asia, Europe, and Africa. Mortality is high and hospital-based outbreaks are common.

ETIOLOGY. The disease is caused by CCHF virus of the *Nairovirus* genus, family Bunyaviridae. The virus kills baby mice and replicates in CER cells and several other cell culture systems.

EPIDEMIOLOGY. CCHF virus is transmitted in nature principally by hard ticks of the genus *Hyalomma*, but also by ticks in the genera *Rhipicephalus, Boophilus,* and *Amblyomma*. Virus is maintained by transovarial and trans-stadial passage in the tick and is amplified by hares and possibly hedgehogs, sheep, and cattle. Giraffe, rhinoceros, eland, buffalo, kudu, zebra, and dogs in southern Africa have antibody to CCHF virus.

The virus or its antibody is found in the distribution of *Hyalomma* ticks. Foci occur in the former Soviet Union, the Balkan nations, Iraq, Iran, Pakistan, Afghanistan, western China, the Middle East, and most of sub-Saharan Africa, including South Africa. Outbreaks occur among military personnel, campers, and in persons tending sheep and cattle. Medical workers are at high risk because of frequent spread in hospitals from infected human blood and tissues.

CLINICAL MANIFESTATIONS. The incubation period is usually between 2 and 9 days. Onset is sudden, with severe headache, fever, chills, myalgia, especially in the back and legs, sore throat, abdominal pain, nausea, vomiting, diarrhea, photophobia, and conjunctival injection. The fever is constant but may be remitting. The patient is often confused or aggressive with a marked mood change. Leukopenia and thrombocytopenia are usually observed. On days 3 to 6, hemorrhagic manifestations and a petechial rash on the trunk, limbs, and oral cavity appear. Epistaxis, hematemesis, melena, and uterine bleeding may be severe and require transfusion. The liver is sometimes enlarged and tender. In severe cases, hepatorenal failure or multiple organ system failure leads to death, usually on days 6 to 14 of illness. Death may also result from blood loss, cerebral hemorrhage, dehydration after diarrhea, or pulmonary edema. Patients recover gradually starting on day 10 when the rash fades. Asthenia may last for a month or more. Recovery is usually complete, although neuritis may persist for months. Liver function tests are abnormal, especially the aspartate aminotransferase, and serum bilirubin levels are often elevated late in the illness. Abnormal prothrombin, activated partial thromboplastin, and thrombin times, as well as increased fibrin degradation products, are indicative of disseminated intravascular coagulation (DIC).

DIAGNOSIS. Virus is easily isolated during the first 8 days of illness. Antibodies are detectable by the immunofluorescence and enzyme-linked immunosorbent assays (ELISA) in surviving patients. Specific immunoglobulin M (IgM) and immunoglobulin G (IgG) are present by days 7 to 9 of illness.

TREATMENT AND PROGNOSIS. Patients suspected of having CCHF should be housed in an isolation facility with needle and blood precautions. Health care personnel should use respirators and protective clothing. Treatment is supportive, including monitoring and correcting fluid and electrolyte imbalance and treating DIC. The vital signs and hematocrit should be tested frequently, and blood should be replaced by transfusion. Case-fatality rates range from 30 to 50%.

PREVENTION. Protection from tick bites and care in handling blood and tissues of sick sheep and cattle are the only preventive measures available in the case of exposure in natural foci.

345.5 Hemorrhagic Diseases Caused by Arenaviruses (Argentine, Bolivian, Venezuelan, and Brazilian Hemorrhagic Fevers and Lassa Fever)

DEFINITION. Argentine, Bolivian, Venezuelan, and Brazilian hemorrhagic fevers and Lassa fever are acute febrile diseases characterized by hemorrhagic diatheses, marked myalgia, and, in severe cases, shock. Case-fatality rates are between 5 and 30%.

ETIOLOGY. The diseases are caused by the viruses Junin (Argentina), Machupo (Bolivia), Guanarito (Venezuela), Sabiá (Brazil), and Lassa (West Africa) of the family Arenaviridae.

EPIDEMIOLOGY. The reservoirs are rodents that excrete virus in urine and possibly other body fluids. The rodents involved are Junin virus, *Calomys musculinus, Calomys laucha,* and *Akodon arenicola;* Machupo virus, *Calomys callosus;* Guanarito virus, *Sigmodon hispidus;* Sabiá virus, not known; and Lassa virus, *Mastomys natalensis*. People are believed to be infected by inhaling or eating contaminated excreta or by passage of virus through abraded skin or mucous membranes. In Argentina, exposure to Junin virus is primarily in workers harvesting corn in Cordoba and Buenos Aires provinces in the north. In Bolivia, domestic and peridomestic exposure to Machupo virus occurs in Beni province, and in Venezuela, similar exposure occurs to Guanarito virus in Portugesa and Barinas states. The site of exposure to Sabiá virus in São Paulo State, Brazil, is not known. Lassa virus is endemic in west and central Africa, especially in Liberia, Sierra Leone, and parts of Nigeria, where it is transmitted in and around homes that have an abundance of domestic rats.

Argentine hemorrhagic fever epidemics involving hundreds to thousands of farm workers are recorded annually. Bolivian hemorrhagic fever epidemics were common in the 1960's, but after institution of rodent control measures, the disease was not reported after 1974 until it reappeared in 1994. Lassa fever was recognized first in 1969 in a nosocomial outbreak in Nigeria. Several other nosocomial outbreaks were subsequently diagnosed, but studies in Sierra Leone established the basic endemic nature of the disease. In the eastern province, 8 to 52% of the population have antibody, and the annual seroconversion rate in susceptible subjects ranges between 5 and 22%. It is estimated that 5 to 14% of the fevers are Lassa virus infections and that Lassa fever accounts for 10 to 16% of the adult hospital admissions.

PATHOGENESIS AND PATHOLOGY. The diseases are characterized by multiple organ impairment, yet specific lesions are absent. The prominent findings are focal diapedesis and capillary hemorrhage, but inflammation is minimal. Focal areas of liver necrosis in Lassa fever are not sufficient to account for the profound shock and death. It is postulated that the virus infects cells of the reticuloendothelial system, including the B and T cells. It causes temporary inhibition of immune cell function, leading to prolonged and high-titered viremia. It is not known whether subsequent capillary damage and parenchymal edema are direct or indirect effects of the virus.

CLINICAL MANIFESTATIONS. The five diseases have many similarities. The incubation period of Lassa fever is 3 to 16 days; of Argentine hemorrhagic fever, 10 to 14 days; and of Bolivian hemorrhagic fever, 7 to 14 days. Onset is insidious, initially with fever, chills, malaise, asthenia, headache, retro-ocular pain, anorexia, nausea, vomiting, and muscle pain, (especially at the costovertebral angle in the South American forms and the legs in Lassa fever). Fever is nonremitting between 39 and 40.5° C. Sore throat is not prominent in the Argentine, Venezuelan, and Bolivian diseases, but purulent pharyngitis and aphthous ulcers are common in Lassa fever.

Signs include conjunctivitis, facial edema, exanthem with pharyngeal vesicles, exanthem of the face, neck, and upper thorax, tenderness of thighs, laterocervical and other polyadenopathy, and petechiae, especially in the axillae. There is no jaundice or hepatosplenomegaly. Leukopenia, thrombocytopenia, and albuminuria with casts are characteristic.

Late in the first week of illness, the signs and symptoms become more pronounced. Signs of dehydration, decreased blood pressure, and relative bradycardia are prominent. Hemorrhage from the gums, nose, stomach, intestines, uterus, and urinary tract indicates a severe hemorrhagic diathesis. Bleeding was observed commonly in the South American forms, but in only 17% of Lassa fever cases. Blood loss is not massive enough to account for the shock. The acute phase usually lasts 7 to 15 days. Death is the result of uremia or hypovolemic shock, usually in the second week of illness. Recovery is heralded by lysis of fever; there is usually a prolonged convalescence marked by periods of sweating, flush, and postural hypotension, but patients suffer no permanent non-neurologic sequelae.

Neurologic signs are prominent in Bolivian hemorrhagic fever; nearly 50% of patients have an intention tremor of the tongue and hands at about the fifth day of illness, and 25% of these progress to more serious encephalopathy with delirium and convulsions. The cerebrospinal fluid (CSF) is normal in these patients. A similar syndrome is occasionally seen in Lassa fever, and about 5% of patients develop unilateral or bilateral eighth cranial nerve damage, which may be permanent. Other transient complications are loss of hair and Beau's lines of the nails.

Most patients have leukopenia with depression of both lymphocytes and neutrophils; however, some Lassa fever patients have markedly elevated white counts. Thrombocytopenia is present during the first week of illness.

DIAGNOSIS. The diagnosis can be made definitively only with laboratory tests. Fever, muscle pain, and diminished white cell count in the endemic areas should alert the physician to the diagnosis. Virus can be isolated in Vero cells from blood, CSF, and throat washings during life and from most tissues at necropsy. Virus is recoverable even in the presence of antibody. Isolation of virus from Bolivian hemorrhagic fever cases is more difficult than from the Argentine or West African form. Virus isolation should be attempted only in laboratories with high biosecurity containment equipment because of the risk of infection of laboratory workers. Serologic diagnosis is made by the immunofluorescence test. Immunoglobulin G is present in 53% of Lassa fever patients on admission to hospital and immunoglobulin M (IgM), in 67%. The IgM test is useful for early and rapid diagnosis.

TREATMENT. Supportive therapy, including attention to electrolyte and fluid balance, is essential. Hematocrit and urine protein measurements aid in detection of hypovolemic shock. Plasma expanders are effective if used early, but may precipitate pulmonary edema late in the clinical course.

Specific Junin virus-immune human plasma given during the first 8 days of Argentine hemorrhagic fever reduced the case-fatality rate from 16 to 1%. A neurologic illness was observed about 3 weeks after the acute attack in some patients receiving this therapy. Most of these persons recovered completely.

Ribavirin given to Lassa fever patients early in the illness significantly reduced mortality. The drug was administered intravenously, 60 mg per kilogram per day for the first 4 days, and then orally, 30 mg per kilogram per day for 6 days more. Immune plasma was not effective in Lassa fever patients in controlled trials.

PROGNOSIS. In Lassa fever, bleeding manifestations, high levels of circulating virus in the blood, and elevated aspartate aminotransferase levels in serum are predictive of death. There are no such predictors for the South American arenavirus hemorrhagic fevers. Shock or abnormal neurologic findings indicate a poor prognosis.

PREVENTION AND CONTROL. Environmental sanitation, including rodent-proofing of homes, and proper storage of grains and other foods to diminish rodent populations are the only community control measures now available. A vaccine for Junin virus has proved efficacious in Argentina. Barrier nursing with use of gloves and gowns should be instituted in suspected cases of arenaviral

hemorrhagic fevers. Blood and other tissues are infective and should be decontaminated.

345.6 African Hemorrhagic Fever (Marburg-Ebola Disease)

DEFINITION. African hemorrhagic fever is an acute, often fatal, hemorrhagic disease. Fever, rash, hemorrhage, hepatic and pancreatic inflammation, and prostration are hallmarks of the illness.

ETIOLOGY. The disease is caused by Marburg and Ebola viruses of the family Filoviridae. The two viruses are distinct antigenically but of very similar morphology.

EPIDEMIOLOGY. Marburg disease was described in 1967 in Germany and Yugoslavia, where workers in vaccine manufacturing facilities sickened and died after they were exposed to infected tissues of African green monkeys from Uganda. Where the monkeys became infected is not known, although Marburg virus is indigenous to Africa. (Additional isolated cases in South Africa and Kenya are recorded.) Ebola virus epidemics in Sudan and Zaire in 1976 were traced to contact with infected patients and, in Zaire, spread by needle. The disease recurred in Sudan in 1979, and there was an isolated case in Kenya in 1980. The most recent outbreak was in Zaire in 1995, and a single case in Ivory Coast followed exposure of a Swiss ethologist during necropsy of a naturally infected chimpanzee in 1994. (The ethologist recovered.) The source of the outbreaks is unknown, and the natural history remains a mystery. A third filovirus, most closely related to Ebola virus, was isolated in 1989 from sick cynomolgus monkeys recently imported to the United States from the Philippines. Animal handlers in the United States seroconverted to the virus without associated illness.

PATHOLOGY. African hemorrhagic fever is a systemic disease with multiple organ involvement, most prominently the lymphatic system, testes, ovaries, and liver. Liver cell necrosis with eosinophilic inclusions, unlike that in yellow fever, is random and focal. Fibrin deposits are found in the renal glomeruli, consistent with disseminated intravascular coagulopathy (DIC). There is edema and diffuse inflammation in the brain.

CLINICAL MANIFESTATIONS. The incubation period is 3 to 9 days for Marburg virus infection and 3 to 18 days for Ebola. Onset is abrupt, with severe headache, backache, muscle pains, and sometimes abdominal pain. At this stage, the disease is not readily differentiated from malaria, typhoid fever, and other bacterial, rickettsial, or viral illnesses. On about the third day, nausea, vomiting, and profuse watery diarrhea with mucus and blood commence. Diarrhea may continue for several days. A maculopapular rash appears on the trunk and spreads to the rest of the body. On day 4 or 5, the patient's status becomes critical, with high, unremitting fever and an altered mental state, including confusion, aggression, or lethargy. There is spontaneous bleeding from injection sites, hematemesis, melena, hemoptysis, and, in pregnant patients, abortion, often with massive blood loss. Renal failure may be a terminal event. Death occurs from day 8 to 17, often on day 8 or 9. Recovery is marked by fatigue, anorexia, weight loss, hair loss, and, sometimes, psychological problems.

The pathophysiology is characterized by leukopenia, thrombocytopenia, increased prothrombin time, and other abnormalities in the liver function tests, increased serum amylase, proteinuria, and electrocardiographic changes indicative of myocardial disease. DIC has been documented in some cases.

DIAGNOSIS. Virus is isolated from acute phase blood, liver, and other organs by inoculation into guinea pigs or cell culture. The immunofluorescence and enzyme-linked immunosorbent assays (ELISA) become positive during the second week of illness.

TREATMENT AND PROGNOSIS. There is no specific treatment. Supportive therapy consists of maintenance of fluid and electrolyte balance and administration of blood, platelets, or fresh frozen plasma to control bleeding. Peritoneal dialysis for renal failure and heparin for DIC have been recommended, but their value in

African hemorrhagic fever is not established. The presence of bleeding indicates a poor prognosis. The case-fatality rate under relatively sophisticated hospital conditions in Marburg, Germany, was 22% in 1967, and under Third World rural conditions in Zaire during 1976, it was 90%. As of this writing, at least 30% of cases in the 1995 Zaire outbreak were fatal.

PREVENTION. Control activities are not carried out because the natural reservoir is unknown. Nosocomial spread can be minimized by barrier nursing and handling of blood and tissues in isolator laboratory units with proper decontamination.

345.7 Hemorrhagic Fever with Renal Syndrome

DEFINITION. Hemorrhagic fever with renal syndrome (HFRS) is a disease of Europe and Asia characterized by fevers, capillary dilatation, leakage of blood leading to hemorrhagic manifestations, and, in severe cases, shock and renal tubular disease.

ETIOLOGY. HFRS is caused by any one of several closely related viruses of the genus *Hantavirus,* family Bunyaviridae. The prototype is Hantaan virus, originally isolated from *Apodemus agrarius* field mice in the endemic region of Korea.

EPIDEMIOLOGY. The virus is transmitted from rodents. *A. agrarius* in Korea and other parts of Asia, *Clethrionomys glareolus* in Finland and west of the Ural Mountains, and *Rattus rattus* and *R. norvegicus* in cities of Japan, Korea, and Belgium serve as reservoirs. The rodent excretes virus in urine, saliva, and feces for weeks, and sometimes for months, after infection. Transmission is presumably by respiratory spread or direct contact with fomites contaminated by rodent excretions. Persons at risk include soldiers in field operations, campers, farmers, woodsmen, and, especially in the winter, family groups in houses harboring field rodents that seek shelter from the cold. Outbreaks have also occurred in laboratories housing field rodents or housing laboratory rats that carry the virus as an inapparent infection. Nosocomial infections are not reported. Viruses of the genus *Hantavirus* have been isolated from rodents in the Americas; the American viruses are associated with *Hantavirus* pulmonary syndrome (HPS).

PATHOLOGY. Patients who die of shock in the early stages demonstrate retroperitoneal gelatinous edema. There are macroscopic hemorrhages in the pituitary and right atrium. The renal medulla is congested and hyperemic, and patients who die later in the course of the disease have marked renal tubular necrosis. Petechial hemorrhages found in the skin and in multiple organs indicate widespread capillary fragility.

CLINICAL MANIFESTATIONS AND PATHOLOGIC PHYSIOLOGY. The incubation period ranges from 2 to 42 days but is usually about 2 weeks. Eighty percent of cases are mild (demonstrating only fever, facial flush, backache, and muscle aches) or moderate (fever plus proteinuria, and petechial hemorrhages). The remaining 20% are severe. They progress through five characteristic phases: febrile, hypotensive, oliguric, diuretic, and convalescent. The febrile phase lasts about 5 days, during which fever, facial flush, conjunctival injection, and backache precede the appearance of petechial hemorrhages and albuminuria. In the hypotensive phase, the temperature returns to baseline, and the patient manifests nausea, vomiting, abdominal pain, and about 3 days of capillary leakage with a rising hematocrit, heavy proteinuria, leukocytosis, thrombocytopenia, and decreased renal clearance. This is followed for about 4 days by the oliguric phase, when extravascular fluid is resorbed, leading to relative hypervolemia, hypertension, metabolic acidosis, and sometimes pulmonary edema and/or acute renal failure. The diuretic phase is accompanied by return of renal clearance to normal, but with marked electrolyte and fluid imbalance, which may lead to death if not adequately managed. The convalescent phase may last 1 to 3 months, with slowly recovering renal function. The clinical diagnosis may be reliable during an outbreak with classic severe cases but not with mild infections; serologic confirmation is obtained by the immunofluorescence, enzyme-linked im-

munosorbent assay (ELISA), and neutralization tests, which become positive at the end of the first week of illness. Antibody titers peak at 2 weeks and last for many years.

TREATMENT AND PROGNOSIS. Management includes careful monitoring of electrolytes and fluid intake and output with correction, especially during the oliguric and diuretic phases. Plasma expanders can be used for shock, and hemodialysis in cases of renal failure with hyperkalemia. Ribavirin improves survival if given within 5 days of onset. The case fatality rate in Korea is about 5% with hospital management; the disease in northern Europe is milder with a more favorable prognosis.

PREVENTION. Rodent control should be practiced where feasible, especially in urban settings.

345.8 Hantavirus Pulmonary Syndrome

DEFINITION. Hantavirus pulmonary syndrome (HPS) is a disease of North America first recognized in the Four Corners region of New Mexico and Arizona in 1993 and characterized by fever, muscle pain, and gastrointestinal symptoms, progressing to acute respiratory failure and shock. Case fatality approaches 50%.

ETIOLOGY. HPS is caused by any one of several closely related viruses of the genus *Hantavirus,* family Bunyaviridae. The prototype is Sin Nombre virus, originally characterized from human lung by reverse transcriptase-polymerase chain reaction (RT-PCR) analysis of its RNA.

EPIDEMIOLOGY. The viruses are transmitted from Cricetid rodent excreta, presumably by inhalation and percutaneous contamination. *Peromyscus maniculatus* in New Mexico and neighboring states, *Peromyscus leucopus* in New York and *Sigmodon hispidus* in Florida serve as reservoirs of different but related viruses. Transmission, seasonality, and risk factors are very similar to those of hantaviruses in Europe and Asia. No person-to-person transmission has been documented. Patients range in age from 12 to 69 years with a median of 35. The disease has not been recognized in young children. Fifty-four percent of patients are male and 62% white. Subclinical infections are rare.

PATHOLOGY. Pleural effusions and lung edema are found at autopsy. Microscopically, alveolar edema and pulmonary interstitial infiltrates of T cells and macrophages are evident in the absence of necrosis. There may be splenomegaly, but lymph nodes and other organs appear grossly normal. Infiltrates of atypical mononuclear cells are found in the spleen, liver, and lymph nodes. The hemorrhage, retroperitoneal effusions, and kidney lesions of hemorrhagic fever with renal syndrome (HFRS) are absent.

CLINICAL MANIFESTATIONS AND PATHOLOGIC PHYSIOLOGY. A prodrome of fever and myalgia, sometimes with abdominal pain, nausea, vomiting, and dizziness, lasts 3 to 6 days. A cardiopulmonary phase follows in which the patient has fever, cough, dyspnea, hypoxia, noncardiogenic pulmonary edema, and shock. Surviving patients recover completely, usually within a week after onset of respiratory signs, although there may be some continued fever. The partial thromboplastin and prothrombin times are prolonged, and thrombocytopenia and hemoconcentration are common, as are increased aspartate aminotransferase and serum lactate dehydrogenase levels. Leukocytosis, atypical lymphocytes, and immature granulocytes are noted in the peripheral blood. Severe cases develop metabolic acidosis. The only signs of renal involvement are proteinuria and mild elevation of creatinine levels. Viral antigen has been found in capillary endothelium of several organs. Diagnosis depends on demonstration of specific antibodies by immunofluorescence, enzyme-linked immunosorbent assay (ELISA), and Western blot. IgM detected with hantavirus antigens is usually present on admission to the hospital. RT-PCR and immunohistochemistry of lung or other tissues have also been used for diagnosis.

TREATMENT AND PROGNOSIS. Management includes adequate oxygenation and monitoring of hemodynamic status. Mechanical ventilation may be needed. Invasive monitoring is required in hypotensive patients and will guide therapy with pressors and/or inotropic agents. Crystalloids are recommended instead of colloids for volume replacement because of the increased pulmonary capillary permeability. Overhydration should be avoided. Ribavirin efficacy in HPS is not established; it is effective in treatment of HFRS if given early, and is available for intravenous administration to HPS patients under an investigational protocol.

Butler JC, Peters CJ: Hantaviruses and hantavirus pulmonary syndrome. Clin Infect Dis 19:387, 1994. *State-of-the-art clinical review of hantavirus pulmonary syndrome.*

Le Guenno B, Formentry P, Wyers M, et al.: Isolation and partial characterisation of a new strain of Ebola virus. Lancet 345:1271, 1995. *Description of the 1995 outbreak in Zaire.*

Preston R: The Hot Zone. New York, Random House, 1994. *Historical novel dealing with Marburg-Ebola Disease.*

Rev Infect Dis 11(suppl 4):5669–5896, 1989. *A comprehensive compilation of reviews of the viral hemorrhagic fevers, including DHF, Crimean-Congo hemorrhagic fever, arenaviral hemorrhagic fevers, African hemorrhagic fevers, and HFRS.*

Swanepoel R, Shepherd AJ, Leman PA, et al.: Epidemiologic and clinical features of Crimean Congo hemorrhagic fever in Southern Africa. Am J Trop Med Hyg 36:120, 1987. *Clinical description and review of CCHF literature.*

WHO Expert Committee Report: Viral Haemorrhagic Fevers. WHO Tech Rep Ser No 721, 1985. *Excellent review of hemorrhagic fevers by an international group of experts with detailed guide to management of patients, investigation of outbreaks, and vector control.*

WHO Scientific Group Report: Arthropod-borne and rodent-borne viral diseases. WHO Tech Rep Ser No. 719, 1985. *Authoritative discussion of epidemiologic principles, laboratory safety, vector control, and epidemic preparedness.*

WHO Technical Advisory Group Report: Dengue haemorrhagic fever: Diagnosis, treatment and control. Geneva, World Health Organization, 1986. *A most comprehensive manual for the physician faced with management of DHF patients.*

346 OTHER ARTHROPOD-BORNE VIRUSES

R. Gordon Douglas, Jr.

Arthropod-borne viruses (arboviruses) are transmitted by an arthropod to a vertebrate host, either a human or a lower animal. During an incubation period, the viruses replicate in the arthropod, which may be a mosquito, tick, phlebotomine sandfly, or culicoid midge. The viruses are transmitted by bite to the vertebrate, which becomes viremic and then can infect another biting arthropod. Some arboviruses also are transmitted vertically through the egg of the arthropod and may be maintained this way between seasons.

There are nearly 500 arthropod-borne viruses, and at least 100 of these infect humans. Most fit into five families—Togaviridae, Flaviviridae, Bunyaviridae, Rhabdoviridae, and Reoviridae. Within each family are one or more genera, each usually corresponding to an antigenic group. These groups are important, because the clinician must rely heavily on the laboratory for a serologic diagnosis or identification of an isolate.

Most infections are inapparent. The remainder are associated with one or more of five major syndromes: (1) undifferentiated fever, (2) fever with rash and/or arthritis, (3) pulmonary disease, (4) encephalitis, and (5) hemorrhagic fever (see Ch. 345).

This chapter describes several of the more important arboviruses known to infect people. Table 346–1 lists some that cause fever, rash, or polyarthritis in humans; those which cause encephalitis in humans are listed in Table 346–2.

The diseases described here are nearly all "zoonoses" (i.e., illnesses caused by viruses transmitted from animals to humans). They are more prevalent in the tropics and subtropics and are usually focal because of ecologic restrictions on their transmission. Diagnosis depends on a careful history encompassing exposure to vertebrate animals and arthropod vectors, age, season, and travel, including geographic site of exposure. The physician must have a high index of suspicion. Fevers are often diagnosed erroneously as malaria; indeed, in malaria-endemic regions, the patient frequently has malaria concomitantly with an arboviral infection.

Laboratory confirmation of infection is essential. Classically, the virus was isolated from acute phase serum or whole blood in laboratory animals or in tissue culture. Neutralization, complement-fixation, hemagglutination-inhibition, fluorescent antibody, and enzyme-linked immunosorbent assays (ELISA) tests of acute and 3-week convalescent sera also produced the correct diagnosis. Antigen detection and IgM-capture ELISA often permit diagnosis upon initial presentation and at least within a week of illness onset in most cases.

Treatment is symptomatic and may include bed rest, antipyretics, and analgesics. Ribavirin has shown some activity against certain viruses, but controlled clinical trials have not been done.

Control can be achieved by interrupting the cycle, including vaccination of reservoir animals, vector control, and education on vector avoidance. Vaccines are available or under development for some agents such as Rift Valley fever, Venezuelan encephalitis, yellow fever, Japanese encephalitis, and dengue.

FEVER AND RASH SYNDROMES

COLORADO TICK FEVER. Colorado tick fever (CTF) is an acute, benign tick-transmitted viral infection that occurs throughout the Rocky Mountain area. It is characterized by headache, myalgia, a biphasic febrile course lasting about 1 week, and leukopenia.

Etiology. CTF virus is an RNA virus in the coltivirus genus of the Reoviridae family; it is unrelated to other major arbovirus groups. The hard-shelled wood tick, *Dermacentor andersoni*, transmits the virus to humans by bite. Human cases are limited to the combined geographic distribution of the tick vector and the major mammalian rodent reservoirs, ground squirrels and chipmunks.

Epidemiology. Exposure usually occurs during the spring and summer in mountainous terrain and high plains between 4000 and 10,000 feet. Cases occur at lower altitudes during April and May and at higher altitudes during June and July, presumably because

TABLE 346–1. ARTHROPOD-BORNE VIRUSES THAT CAUSE FEVER, RASH, OR POLYARTHRITIS

Family (*Genus*) Virus	Human Disease	Distribution	Vector
Togaviridae (*Alphavirus*)			
Mayaro	Fever, arthritis, rash	South America	Mosquito
Ross River	Arthritis, rash, sometimes fever	Australia, South Pacific	Mosquito
Chikungunya	Fever, arthritis, hemorrhagic fever	Africa, Asia, Philippines	Mosquito
O'nyong-nyong	Fever, arthritis, rash	Africa	Mosquito
Sindbis	Arthritis, rash, sometimes fever	Africa, Europe, Australia	Mosquito
Flaviviridae (*Flavivirus*)			
Dengue (4 types)	Fever, rash, hemorrhagic fever	Worldwide (tropics)	Mosquito
Yellow fever	Fever, hemorrhagic fever	Tropical Americas, Africa	Mosquito
West Nile	Fever, rash, hepatitis, encephalitis	Asia, Europe, Africa	Mosquito
Bunyaviridae (*Bunyavirus*)			
Oxopouche	Fever	Brazil, Panama	Midge
Bunyaviridae (*Phlebovirus*)			
Sandfly fever viruses	Fever	Asia, Africa, tropical Americas	Sand fly, mosquito
Rift Valley fever	Fever, hemorrhagic fever, encephalitis, retinitis	Africa	Mosquito
Bunyaviridae (*Hantavirus*)			
Muerto Canyon	Pulmonary disease	Southwest U.S.	Rodent-borne
Reoviridae (*Coltivirus*)			
Colorado tick fever	Fever	Western U.S.	Tick

Note: Shown are the most important of over 100 arboviruses that infect humans.

TABLE 346–2. ARTHROPOD-BORNE VIRUSES THAT CAUSE ACUTE CENTRAL NERVOUS SYSTEM INFECTION AND ENCEPHALITIS

Virus by Group	Mode of Transmission	Geographic Distribution	Disease in Domestic Livestock
Viruses principally associated with the encephalitis syndrome; epidemic and endemic			
Togaviridae, alphavirus			
Eastern equine encephalitis	Mosquito	Eastern North America, Caribbean, South America	Equines, penned pheasants
Western equine encephalitis	Mosquito	Western North America, South America	Equines
Venezuelan equine encephalitis	Mosquito, possibly other	Florida, Central and South America	Equines
Flaviviridae, flavivirus			
St. Louis encephalitis	Mosquito	North America, Caribbean, Central and South America	None
Japanese encephalitis	Mosquito	East and Southeast Asia, India	Equines, swine
Rocio encephalitis	Mosquito	Brazil	None
Murray Valley encephalitis	Mosquito	Australia	(Equines)*
Tick-borne encephalitides	Tick, ingestion of milk	Europe, former U.S.S.R.	None
Russian spring-summer and Central European encephalitis			
Louping ill	Tick	British Isles	Sheep, equines, cows
Powassan	Tick	North America	None
Bunyaviridae, California subgroup			
California encephalitis, LaCrosse, Jamestown Canyon, snowshoe hare	Mosquito	North America, China, former U.S.S.R.	None
Viruses principally associated with other syndromes, but occasionally causing encephalitis; epidemic and endemic			
Togaviridae, alphavirus			
Sindbis (febrile illness with rash)	Mosquito	Africa, Europe	None
Semliki Forest (febrile illness)	Mosquito	Africa, Southeast Asia	(Equines)*
Flaviviridae, flavivirus			
West Nile (febrile illness with rash)	Mosquito	Africa, Middle East	(Equines)*
Kyasanur Forest disease†	Tick	India	None
Omsk hemorrhagic fever†	Tick	Central Asia	None
Bunyaviridae, phlebovirus			
Rift Valley fever (febrile illness, hemorrhagic fever, retinitis)	Mosquito, direct contact	Africa	Sheep, cows, goats
Crimean hemorrhagic fever†– Congo	Tick	Eastern Europe, former U.S.S.R., Africa	None
Reoviridae, orbivirus			
Colorado tick fever (febrile illness)	Tick	Western North America	None
Rare and sporadic infections associated with encephalitis			
Flaviviridae, flavivirus			
Ilheus‡	Mosquito	South America	None
Negishi	Tick	Japan, China	None
Langat†	Tick	Asia	None
Orthomyxovirus			
Thogoto	Tick	Africa	None

* Disease rare or suspected but not well documented.
† Tick-borne hemorrhagic fevers.
‡ Encephalitis recorded in laboratory infections or experimental infections of cancer patients only; significance in naturally acquired infections unknown.

ticks emerge later at higher altitudes. Most patients find attached ticks, but others may have seen ticks on their body or clothing. Postexposure travel during the incubation period or accidental transportation of infected adult ticks in clothing or bedding may result in cases outside the endemic area.

CTF virus has been recovered from up to 14% of *D. andersoni* collected in endemic areas. The virus overwinters in hibernating nymphal and adult ticks and in infected hibernating rodent hosts. Infected nymphal ticks feed on ground squirrels and chipmunks in the spring, and since viremia in the rodent reservoirs lasts for weeks or months, a cycle involving larval and nymphal ticks and their rodent hosts evolves. Humans are accidental hosts, resulting from the bite of an adult tick.

Incidence and Prevalence. The disease has been reported from most states in the Rocky Mountain area and from western Canadian provinces. The several hundred cases diagnosed annually in the endemic area probably represent only a fraction of the total. Mild or wholly subclinical infections probably occur.

The virus has been isolated from other species of ticks and from numerous species of small mammals, suggesting that the disease may occur over a wider geographic area than currently appreciated.

Pathogenesis. There is no unusual local reaction to the tick bite. The virus replicates in hematopoietic stem cells, and symptoms begin 3 to 6 days after tick exposure. Viremia can be demonstrated at onset of fever and in red blood cells long after the virus

has vanished from serum and neutralizing antibody has appeared. Transfusion-transmitted CTF has been documented.

Fatal cases are rare. Occasional patients have clinical evidence of central nervous system (CNS) or meningeal involvement, and CTF virus has been recovered from cerebrospinal fluid (CSF).

Clinical Manifestations. The disease begins abruptly, with chills, fever of 38 to 40°C, myalgias (especially in the back and legs), headache, retro-orbital pain, and photophobia. Malaise and nausea may occur, but vomiting is uncommon. Physical findings during the first 2 to 3 days of illness are nonspecific. The patient may be flushed with conjunctival and pharyngeal erythema. Mild splenomegaly is sometimes present. Up to 12% of patients suffer rashes, commonly macular or macropapular and distributed over the entire body, sometimes petechial and involving primarily the extremities. Tachycardia is in proportion to the temperature elevation.

In approximately one half of cases, a distinctly biphasic illness occurs, the so-called saddleback fever. Symptoms and fever abate after 2 to 3 days, and the patient feels relatively well for 1 or 2 days, after which there is an abrupt return of fever, headache, and back pain, often more intense than in the first phase. The second phase lasts 2 to 4 days and then subsides, leaving the patient with weakness and lassitude that disappear during the succeeding week or two. A prolonged convalescence of 3 weeks or more may ensue in patients over 30 years of age. Some patients do not exhibit the typical biphasic course, experiencing only one bout of fever, three phases of fever, or a single protracted febrile illness lasting 5 to 8 days.

Children are most susceptible to CNS involvement. Findings may include aseptic meningitis with nuchal rigidity and mononuclear pleocytosis or encephalitis with a depressed sensorium or stupor. Hemorrhagic manifestations have been described in a few children with encephalitis.

Laboratory findings very early in the illness are generally not helpful, but leukopenia usually is present by the third day and becomes even more pronounced during the second phase, reaching levels as low as 1000 per cubic millimeter. The most striking decrease is in the granulocyte series, with a relative lymphocytosis, and there is frequently an accompanying thrombocytopenia. Atypical, vacuolated lymphocytes are often observed. Bone marrow examination reveals a maturation arrest in the granulocyte series.

Diagnosis. CTF should be suspected in any person with a history of tick exposure in the endemic area 3 to 7 days before the onset of a febrile illness. Findings during the first phase, however, cannot be differentiated from many other acute febrile illnesses. A brief symptom-free interval followed by a second febrile illness should strongly suggest CTF.

Isolation of the virus from serum or whole blood, via inoculation of suckling mice, confirms the diagnosis. Direct immunofluorescent staining of virus in the patient's erythrocytes may provide more rapid identification. A diagnostic rise in antibody titers can be detected by indirect immunofluorescence or by neutralization test; an ELISA is also available.

The differential diagnosis can be troublesome, inasmuch as Rocky Mountain spotted fever (see Ch. 324.2) is transmitted in the tick fever endemic area by the same vector, *D. andersoni*. Paradoxically, Rocky Mountain spotted fever is abating in the state of Colorado; CTF now outnumbers it by at least 20-fold. Nevertheless, differential diagnosis may be impossible early in the course of disease, before the characteristic rash of Rocky Mountain spotted fever appears. A relatively symptom-free interval after 2 or 3 days would be most unusual in Rocky Mountain spotted fever and strongly favors the diagnosis of CTF.

Treatment and Prognosis. Therapy is entirely supportive. The disease is almost invariably benign, and the prognosis is excellent. Severe illness, complicated by CNS involvement, is seen infrequently and only in children.

Prevention. The most effective means of preventing CTF is for people outdoors in endemic areas during the spring and summer months to wear protective clothing or use tick repellents, together with frequent body inspection and prompt tick removal. Transfusion-associated disease can be prevented by excluding convalescent donors for a minimum of 6 months.

DENGUE. Dengue is an acute arbovirus infection that presents chiefly with fever, malaise, lymphadenopathy, and rash. Epidemics occur worldwide over large areas of the tropics and subtropics, including the Pacific Basin, Southeast Asia, and Africa. Outbreaks recurred in the Caribbean, including Puerto Rico and the U.S. Virgin Islands, in 1969. For the first time in 35 years, indigenous infections were recognized in the continental United States in 1980, but they have not recurred recently.

Dengue viruses are members of the Flaviviridae family. Single-stranded nonsegmented RNA viruses, they occur in four distinct serogroups, types 1 through 4.

Epidemiology. Dengue virus is transmitted from person to person primarily by *Aedes aegypti* mosquitoes, although other species of *Aedes* are involved in Asia and the Pacific. *A. aegypti* is peridomestic, biting humans readily or even preferentially. A single mosquito can infect a number of people. Small collections of water in backyard litter, especially tires, are favored breeding sites. *A. aegypti* has reappeared along the U.S. Gulf Coast; hence the threat of dengue reemerging in the United States is real.

Dengue viruses multiply in the midgut epithelium and salivary glands of mosquitoes without producing pathologic changes. Mosquitoes remain infectious for life.

Zoonotic cycles of dengue virus transmission involving monkeys and forest *Aedes* species occur in Malaysia and West Africa. The mechanism for maintaining the virus between epidemics has not been defined, but vertical transmission in *Aedes* has been documented experimentally.

Nonimmune individuals are uniformly susceptible, and susceptibility is not influenced by age. During outbreaks, attack rates in nonimmune individuals may be high; in Puerto Rico and the U.S. Virgin Islands, the overall rate of clinical disease was 20%, with infection rates as determined by serologic surveys as high as 79%. Immunity against homotypic reinfection is complete and probably lifelong, but cross-protection between different serotypes lasts < 3 months.

Clinical Features and Treatment. Dengue virus infection is often inapparent. When disease occurs, three overlapping clinical forms are recognized: classic dengue, a mild to moderate febrile illness; dengue hemorrhagic fever (DHF), a severe form; and the dengue shock syndrome (DSS). Classic dengue (breakbone fever) occurs primarily in nonimmune individuals, often nonindigenous children and adults. Disease begins abruptly after a 2- to 7-day incubation with severe splitting headache, retro-orbital pain, backache (especially in the lumbar area), leg pain, and arthralgia. Most patients complain of pain on moving their eyes. True rigors are common during the illness but usually do not herald the onset. Other common symptoms include insomnia, nausea, anorexia with taste aberrations, cutaneous hyperesthesia, and generalized weakness. Mild rhinopharyngitis occurs in one fourth of patients. Examination reveals a relative bradycardia, scleral injection (30 to 90%), tenderness on pressure on the ocular globes, and pharyngeal injection. A transient macular rash may appear on the first or second day. Within 2 to 3 days after onset, the temperature may decrease to nearly normal and other symptoms subside. Remission in this biphasic illness typically lasts 2 days. Fever then returns, as may other symptoms, although they are generally less severe. On the third to fifth day (with the second phase), a more definite maculopapular rash usually appears on the trunk and then spreads to the arms and legs while sparing the palms and soles. The rash is often characterized by 2- to 5-mm "islands of white in a sea of red." The rash is accompanied in some cases by complaints of burning in the palms and soles. On resolution, the rash may desquamate. Concurrently, generalized nontender lymphadenopathy, typically including posterior cervical, epitrochlear, and inguinal chains, develops. The biphasic febrile course is considered characteristic but often is not encountered. The entire illness lasts 5 to 7 days and terminates abruptly. Complaints of fatigue and depression for an additional several weeks are common.

In addition to the classic syndrome, a mild illness characterized by fever, anorexia, headache, myalgia, and evanescent rashes sometimes occurs and is usually not associated with lymphadenopathy. At onset in both classic and mild dengue, leukocyte counts may be normal or low; however, by the third to fifth day leukocyte counts are decreased (< 5000 per cubic millimeter with granulocytopenia). Thrombocytopenia (< 100,000 per cubic millimeter) also may be a feature. Urinalysis may show moderate albuminuria.

A history of travel to dengue-endemic areas and occurrence of other cases in a community are important reminders to include dengue in the differential diagnosis. Specific diagnosis depends on virus isolation or serologic tests. Viremia can be detected for the initial 3 to 5 days with dengue types 1, 2, and 3 by inoculation of mosquito tissue cell cultures. Viral titers in patients with dengue 4 are considerably lower than in patients with types 1, 2, and 3, making viral isolation less common. Of serologic tests, neutralization is most specific. IgM antibodies indicate recent dengue infection but do not provide a type-specific diagnosis and cross-react with other flavivirus antibodies, including those following immunization with yellow fever vaccine.

Treatment is entirely symptomatic. In the absence of DHF or DSS, mortality is nil. Preventing epidemics relies principally on reducing or eradicating *A. aegypti* by eliminating breeding sites and using larvacides. Ultra-low-volume aerial spraying of organophosphate insecticides (malathion) to reduce the population of adult female mosquitoes has been successful in emergency control of epidemics.

WEST NILE FEVER. Like dengue, West Nile fever is a mosquito-transmitted, acute, self-limited illness that presents chiefly with fever, malaise, lymphadenopathy, and rash. A flavivirus, West Nile fever viral strains from Africa, Europe, the former U.S.S.R., and the Middle East are antigenically distinct from strains isolated in India and the Far East.

Virus transmission involves mosquitoes and wild birds, with mammals, including humans, as incidental end-stage hosts. The mosquito vector species varies: *Culex univittatus, C. pipiens,* and *C. molestus* in the Middle East and Africa, *Mansonia metallicus* in Uganda, and *C. tritaeniorhynchus* in Asia. In endemic areas, human infections are extremely common, with over 60% of young adults having antibodies; this suggests a high prevalence of inapparent or undifferentiated febrile illness in children. There is no gender predominance.

Clinical Features. Following an incubation period of 1 to 6 days, the onset is usually abrupt without prodromal symptoms. The temperature rises quickly to 38.3 to 40°C, with rigors in one third of patients. Symptoms include drowsiness, severe frontal headache, ocular pain, myalgia, and pain in the abdomen and back. A small number of patients have dryness of the throat, anorexia, and nausea. Cough is common. Examination shows facial flushing, conjunctival injection, and coating of the tongue. The predominant finding is generalized lymphadenopathy. Nodes are of moderate size and nontender and usually include the occipital, axillary, and inguinal chains. The spleen and liver are occasionally slightly enlarged. The temperature curve may be biphasic. In one-half of patients, a pale roseolar maculopapular rash, predominantly on the trunk and upper arms, appears from the second to fifth day. It may be evanescent (several hours) or persist until defervescence and does not desquamate. Vesicular lesions may occur but are rare. The illness is self-limited and lasts 3 to 5 days in 80% of patients.

Infection also may result in aseptic meningitis or meningoencephalitis, especially in the elderly. CSF examinations may reveal a lymphocytic pleocytosis with some increase in protein concentration. Other rare complications include myocarditis, pancreatitis, and hepatitis. Convalescence is often prolonged, lasting several weeks with prominent symptoms of fatigue. Lymph node enlargement requires several months to regress. Laboratory findings include leukopenia (< 4000 per cubic millimeter in one third of patients).

Clinically, West Nile fever resembles dengue. West Nile virus can be isolated from the blood of three fourths of patients on the first day, with viremia persisting but decreasing over 5 days. Serologic diagnosis is possible using a number of tests; however, cross-reactions with other flaviviruses complicate interpretation.

Treatment is symptomatic. Ribavirin has activity against West Nile fever virus, but since the disease is self-limited and almost never fatal, its use does not seem indicated.

PHLEBOTOMUS FEVER. Phlebotomus (sandfly, pappataci, or 3-day) fever is an acute, relatively mild, self-limited infection transmitted by *Phlebotomus* flies.

The sandfly fever group of viruses are enveloped, single-stranded, trisegmented RNA viruses belonging to the phlebovirus genus of the Bunyaviridae family. There are at least five immunologically distinct phleboviruses (Naples, Sicilian, Punto Toro, Chagres, and Candiru). The principal vector of Phlebotomus fever viruses in the Mediterranean, Middle East, and northwest India is *Phlebotomus paptasii,* which breeds in dry sandy areas and feeds in early evening. In Central America, *Lutzomyia,* a forest-dwelling species is the primary culprit. Although undefined, sandfly fever viruses presumably are maintained in a vector-host wildlife cycle between epidemics. During epidemics, humans may act as the major host. Transovarial transmission probably serves as an alternative mechanism for virus perpetuation. Sandflies are small (2 to 3 mm), which enables them to penetrate screens and mosquito netting. There is no pain or itching after the bite; hence only about 1% of patients remember being bitten.

Clinical Features and Treatment. After an incubation period of 2 to 6 days, symptoms develop abruptly in >90% of patients. Temperatures rise to 37.8 to 40.1°C. Headache is nearly always present and often is accompanied by pain on ocular movement and retro-orbital pain. Myalgia is common and may be localized, for example, to the abdomen; if to the chest, it resembles pleurodynia. Other symptoms include vomiting, photophobia, alteration or loss of taste, and arthralgia. Conjunctival injection is seen in one third of patients. With severe illness, mild papilledema has been seen. Small vesicles occur on the palate. Malcular or urticarial rashes may erupt. The spleen is rarely palpable, and lymphadenopathy is absent. Pulse is proportional to the temperature on the first day, followed by relative bradycardia. Fever persists for 2 to 4 days in most patients and gradually decreases. Weakness and feelings of de-

pression are common during convalescence. Second attacks occur 2 to 12 weeks after the first in 15% of cases. Aseptic meningitis may develop. In one series, 12% of patients had lumbar punctures; findings included pleocytosis (average cell counts of 90 per cubic millimeter with either mononuclear or neutrophilic leukocytes). Laboratory findings include leukopenia (< 5000 per cubic millimeter) in 90% of patients. The leukopenia may not occur until the third day. Lymphopenia with an increase in band neutrophils early in the illness is followed by a relative lymphocytosis (40 to 65%). Urinalyses are usually normal.

Diagnosis is made on clinical and epidemiologic findings. Sandfly fever viruses replicate and produce plaques in Vero cell cultures. Serologic tests are not available.

Treatment is symptomatic. No fatalities have been reported.

RIFT VALLEY FEVER. Rift Valley fever (RVF) is an acute disease principally of livestock—sheep, goats, cattle, and camels—caused by the mosquito-transmitted RVF virus. The virus is an enveloped, single-stranded, trisegmented RNA virus belonging to the phlebovirus genus and the Bunyaviridae family. The virus multiplies readily in most common cell cultures, is cytopathic, and forms plaques.

RVF virus can be transmitted by a number of mosquito species; in Egypt, *Culex pipiens,* in South Africa, *C. theileri,* and in East Africa, *Aedes* species are the major vectors. Epizootics in large domestic animals have been associated with particularly wet rainy seasons and high mosquito density. In cattle and sheep, most pregnant ewes and cows abort, and mortality in newborn lambs is >90%. A wildlife-mosquito cycle during interepizootic periods has been postulated but not confirmed. Transovarial vertical transmission is an alternative. During an epizootic, disease occurs first in animals and then in humans. Direct transmission to humans by contact with blood or tissues of infected animals may be more frequent than mosquito transmission. Laboratory-acquired infections presumably due to aerosols are common. In addition to eastern and southern Africa, RVF virus has been isolated in western Africa. Zinga virus, a cause of sporadic human disease in central Africa, is a strain of RVF virus.

Clinical Features. After an incubation period of 3 to 6 days, illness begins with an abrupt onset, malaise, occasionally rigors, headache, myalgia, and backache. The temperature rises rapidly to 38.3 to 40°C. Later complaints include anorexia, loss of taste, photophobia, and epigastric pain. Findings may include facial flushing and conjunctival injection. Biphasic fever, with the initial elevation lasting 2 to 3 days, followed by remission and then a second febrile period, is common. Fever generally lasts a total of about 1 week. Convalescence is usually rapid. Normally a benign illness with almost no fatalities, rare cases with severe complications—meningoencephalitis, retinopathy, or hepatic or hemorrhagic manifestations—have resulted in death. Encephalitis with intense headache, confusion, and stupor may appear as the acute infection subsides. The CSF shows a lymphocytic pleocytosis with normal CSF glucose values. Ocular complications including visual loss occur 2 to 7 days after the onset. Findings on ophthalmoscopic examination include macular edema, cotton-wool exudates on the macula, hemorrhages, retinitis, and vascular occlusion. One half of such patients have some permanent loss of visual acuity. Hepatic and hemorrhagic manifestations may develop during the acute illness. Deaths from massive hepatic necrosis occur 7 to 10 days after onset. Hemorrhagic manifestations include epistaxis, hematemesis, melena, and intracranial hemorrhage. The fatality ratio in severely ill patients exceeds 50%. Laboratory findings include initial normal to increased total leukocyte counts initially, followed by leukopenia with granulocytopenia but an increase in band forms. Thrombocytopenia and clotting defects occur.

Diagnosis. Isolating virus from blood by inoculating mice confirms the diagnosis. Three fourths of patients are viremic at the onset of illness. Neutralizing antibodies appear as early as 4 days.

Treatment and Prevention. Treatment is symptomatic. In patients with hemorrhagic manifestations, transfusion of platelets and fresh frozen plasma may be beneficial. Ribavirin has been partially protective in experimentally infected animals. Thus one might consider administering ribavirin (2.0-gram loading dose IV, then 1.0 gram IV every 6 hours for 4 days, then 0.5 gram IV every 8 hours for 6 days) to patients with severe disease. Because the virus can be spread by contact with blood and tissues, and humans show high levels of viremia, blood and needle precautions are essential.

Fever, rash, and polyarthritis are caused by at least six viruses belonging to the alphavirus genus of the Togaviridae family. This group of single-stranded RNA viruses shares antigenic determinants and is transmitted by mosquitoes to vertebrate hosts.

CHIKUNGUNYA VIRUS. *Epidemiology.* Chikungunya virus (CK) is of major importance in Africa and Asia. CK virus is transmitted by *Aedes* mosquitoes in Africa; in the tropical forests of the continent, the mosquitoes belong to the subgenera *Stegomyia* and *Diceromyia*. Nonhuman primates—monkeys or baboons—serve as primary hosts, with transmission occurring mostly in the rainy season. Human involvement is largely secondary. *A. aegypti* also functions as a vector in villages and urban areas, where humans may serve as the vertebrate host. In sub-Saharan Africa, except in the dry areas and below 18 degrees latitude, antibody prevalence surveys range from 20% to > 90%. In Asia, transmission is primarily human to human via *A. aegypti*. CK virus is present in India, Southeast Asia, and the Philippines. Seroprevalence rates of 31% were observed in Bangkok. The potential exists for CK virus transmission outside the current distribution, i.e., Central and South America, as well as the southern United States.

Clinical Features. The incubation period is usually 2 to 3 days but may be as long as 12 days. The onset is usually abrupt, with temperatures rising to 38.3 to 40°C, often accompanied by rigors and incapacitating arthralgia. The arthralgias are polyarticular and migratory, involving predominantly the small joints of the hands, wrists, ankles, and toes. Pain is increased with motion and worse in the morning. Joint swelling is common, but effusions are not. The arthralgia is associated with generalized myalgia. Other symptoms include headache, photophobia, sore throat, anorexia, and vomiting. At onset there is flushing of the face and neck. Other signs include conjunctival injection and lymphadenopathy. A macropapular rash usually involving the trunk and limbs typically occurs on the second to fifth day. The rash lasts 1 to 5 days and may just fade or may desquamate. On the second or third day, the fever may remit for 1 to 2 days and then recur. However, the biphasic course is not as striking as that seen with dengue. Laboratory findings may include leukopenia with relative lymphocytosis, although leukocyte counts are usually normal. Mild thrombocytopenia may develop. The joint symptoms may persist for long periods, only one third of individuals being asymptomatic within a few weeks. About 5% of patients have persistent joint pain, stiffness, and recurrent effusions. Persistence may be more common in HLA-B27–positive patients. In African children, disease is milder, with arthralgia less prominent. In Asia, CK virus is responsible for a hemorrhagic fever syndrome closely resembling dengue hemorrhagic fever or the DSS. Other features may include encephalitis and myocarditis.

Diagnosis and Treatment. CK virus disease should be suspected clinically given the appropriate epidemiologic history and the triad of fever, acute arthralgia/arthritis, and rash. Most patients are viremic during the first 48 hours. Hemagglutination inhibition (HI) (III) antibodies appear by the fifth to seventh day. Treatment is symptomatic.

O'NYONG-NYONG VIRUS. The name *o'nyong-nyong* (in the language spoken in the Ugandan province of Acholi) means "weakening of the joints." Epidemics have occurred in Uganda and Kenya. *Anopheles funnestus* and *A. anogambiae* mosquitoes are o'nyong-nyong (ON) virus vectors.

Clinical features are similar to those of CK disease. The incubation period may be somewhat longer, at least 8 days. Fever is less prominent, exceeding 38.3°C only in one third of patients. Rash occurs in 60 to 70%. In contrast to CK virus disease, generalized lymphadenopathy is a common feature, and there appears to be less residual arthropathy. Diagnosis is based on virus isolation or seroconversion by HI assays, but cross-reactions with CK virus make interpretation difficult.

MAYARO VIRUS. Mayaro virus (MYV) has been associated with epidemics of acute polyarthritis in Brazil and Bolivia.

MYV exists in the forested areas of Central and South America with annual infection rates of 10 to 60% and a 2:1 male predominance. The vectors for MYV are *Haemagogus* mosquitoes. The virus causes high-level viremia in marmosets and other primates.

Clinical Features. After a 1-week incubation period, illness begins abruptly with fever, chills, severe frontal headache, myalgia, and dizziness. Arthralgia (which in some cases precedes the fever) is uniform, very prominent, and occasionally incapacitating, striking

small joints, wrists, fingers, ankles, and toes. Temperatures usually exceed 40°C. Other initial symptoms (less than one third of patients) include nausea, vomiting, and diarrhea. Initial clinical features include occasional conjunctival suffusion, inguinal lymphadenopathy (one half of patients), and joint swelling (one quarter of patients). About the fifth day, maculopapular rash develops over the chest, back, arms, and legs. Rash appears in 90% of children and one half of adults and lasts about 3 days. MYV's clinical course is usually 3 to 5 days except for the arthralgia, which may persist for several months. Laboratory findings include leukopenia (as low as 2500 per cubic millimeter). Urinalyses revealed albuminuria (2+) in one fourth of patients. Some patients showed increases in AST levels. Occasional fatalities have been reported.

Diagnosis. Diagnosis is confirmed by virus isolation. MYV-specific IgM responses have been observed.

ROSS RIVER VIRUS. Ross River (RR) virus outbreaks occur almost entirely between December and June. RR virus infection exists in Australia, New Guinea, and the Solomon Islands, Fiji, the Samoan, Cook, and some Melanesian islands. The natural vector-reservoir relationships have not been well established. *Culex annulirostris* is probably the major vector, although other species of mosquitoes may be involved. Several mammalian species, especially the New Holland mouse and wallabies, are important hosts in Australia. In the Pacific outbreak, *Aedes vigilax* also may have been an important vector, and human-mosquito-human transmission was likely. Infection rates are equal at all ages and in both genders, but clinical disease rates are 4% in patients under age 20 and 42% in those older than 20. The clinical attack rate of males to females is 1:1.7.

Clinical Features. In Australia, incubation is 7 to 9 days, while in the Pacific the incubation period is shorter. At onset, the illness is characterized by headache, myalgia, nausea, and vomiting, and occasionally tenderness of the palms and soles. Initially, fever may be absent or minimal (highest 38°C). About one half of patients experience arthritis involving mainly the small joints, wrists, and ankles. Knee involvement also is common. The joint swelling and paresthesias may precede a rash by 1 to 15 days. In the other half of patients, the rash precedes the arthralgia. The rash, which is usually maculopapular, appears on the cheeks and forehead, occasionally spreads to the trunk, or may be restricted to extremities. The rash may be pruritic. Vesicles occur rarely. Tender lymphadenopathy occurs in one fifth of patients. Recovery is slow, only one half being able to return to work by 1 month and 10% still having joint symptoms at 3 months. Laboratory findings are not striking; leukocyte counts are normal or minimally decreased. The erythrocyte sedimentation rate is increased acutely but normalizes over several weeks even with continued joint symptoms. Antinuclear antibodies and rheumatoid factor tests are negative. Synovial fluid changes are not striking: cell counts of 1000 to 60,000, predominantly mononuclear, normal viscosity. Urinalyses are normal, although recently RR virus has been associated with segmental sclerosing glomerulonephritis.

The diagnosis is usually based on clinical features. In Australia patients seldom have viremia on presentation, while in the Pacific outbreak viremia was readily detected. HI antibodies appear early. Treatment is symptomatic.

SINDBIS VIRUS (OKELBO DISEASE, POGOSTA DISEASE, KARELIAN FEVER). Sindbis virus has caused disease in Egypt, elsewhere in Africa, in Europe, and in Australia. In the former U.S.S.R. it is known as "Karelian fever," in Sweden as "Okelbo disease," and in Finland as "Pogosta disease." *C. univittatus* is the principal vector, and birds are the major hosts. Human infection is common where birds and *Culex* mosquitoes are in close proximity. Human antibody rates are commonly 20 to 30% in the Nile Valley of Egypt. Since Sindbis and West Nile fever virus share the same transmission cycles, Sindbis transmission often parallels West Nile fever virus. In northern Europe, symptomatic disease appears in late summer between 60 and 65 degrees of north latitude, usually affecting adults with forest occupations. The virus has been isolated from *Culiseta, Aedes,* and *Culex* mosquitoes. The host has not been identified.

Clinical Features and Treatment. The incubation period for Sindbis has not been defined. The illness more closely resembles Ross River virus disease than chikungunya or o'nyong-nyong disease. Clinically, fever is low grade and accompanied by malaise, myalgia, rash, and arthralgia in wrists, ankles, knees, and elbows. Periarticular involvement and tendinitis are common. The rash begins on the trunk as scattered macules and spreads to the extremities, palms, and soles. The rash may precede or follow the joint symptoms by 1 to 2 days. Unlike that caused by other alphaviruses, the rash frequently becomes vesicular, especially on the feet and hands. The rash fades within a week. In Europe, persistence of joint complaints is a common feature. In Sweden, >20% had joint symptoms longer than 1 month after onset.

Antibodies can be detected by HI tests within 7 to 10 days of onset. Treatment is symptomatic.

PULMONARY SYNDROMES

MUERTO CANYON VIRUS. Muerto Canyon virus is a recently discovered hantavirus responsible for an outbreak in 1993 of serious pulmonary disease (hantavirus pulmonary syndrome, or HPS) in the southwestern United States. The virus belongs to the hantavirus genus of the Bunyaviridae family, a group of large enveloped, negative-sense RNA viruses with tripartite genomes. Other hantaviruses cause hemorrhagic fever (see Ch. 345.8).

Muerto Canyon virus is a parasite of the deer mouse, *Peromyscus maniculatus*. Deer mice are found over most of the United States with the exception of the southeast and eastern seaboard states. The 1993 outbreak of approximately 50 cases involved predominantly the "four corners" region (New Mexico, Arizona, Colorado, and Utah), but at least 6 cases occurred in California, Nevada, Texas, and Oregon. Abundant deer mice populations were found in the southwestern United States in the summer of 1993. Transmission is thought to occur via aerosols contaminated with infectious rodent urine or feces.

Pathology. The lungs of patients dying from HPS show interstitial infiltration of T lymphocytes and alveolar pulmonary edema without marked necrosis or polymorphonuclear leukocyte infiltration. The major abnormality is thought to be an increase in vascular permeability via an immunopathologic mechanism.

Clinical Features. The disease begins abruptly with fever and myalgias, often accompanied by gastrointestinal symptoms and headache; it is indistinguishable from other nonspecific acute febrile illnesses such as influenza. Examination is unrevealing except for fever, tachycardia, and tachypnea. The respiratory symptoms begin after 4 to 5 days. The patient first notes cough and dyspnea, but acute pulmonary edema and hypotension develop rapidly in most patients. About three fourths of patients die.

Laboratory abnormalities include elevated hematocrit, marked leukocytosis (median count 26,000 per cubic millimeter) with shift to the left, abnormal lymphocytes on smear, thrombocytopenia, prolonged prothrombin and partial thromboplastin times, and mildly elevated alananine transaminase (ALT) and lactate dehydrogenase (LDH) levels. The severe renal abnormalities seen in hemorrhagic fever with renal syndrome (HFRS), characteristic of other hantavirus infections, are not seen, although mild elevations of serum creatinine and proteinuria have been observed. Blood gases reveal marked hypoxia of adult respiratory distress syndrome (ARDS).

Diagnosis. HPS should be considered when an otherwise healthy adult develops an ARDS-like picture without any of the known causes of ARDS. The diagnosis can be confirmed serologically: Virtually all patients will have specific IgM and IgG antibodies detectable by ELISA on admission to hospital. Virus recovery

from clinical specimens is difficult. Polymerase chain reaction and immunohistochemical staining can detect virus in tissue.

Treatment and Prevention. Intravenous ribavirin has been used to treat HPS in patients, but its efficacy has not been established. Nonspecific treatment of ARDS, shock, and other complications may be helpful.

Avoiding contact with rodent urine and feces and rodent control in the home form the basis of HPS prevention.

ARTHROPOD-BORNE VIRAL ENCEPHALITIDES

Arboviral encephalitis is a significant health problem in Europe, the former U.S.S.R., parts of Asia, and Central and South America but not Africa. The disease is of particular concern in the Americas not only because of its multiple etiologic agents and widespread occurrence but also because of its concurrent affliction of domestic animals and humans and its potential for epidemic spread.

The most important arthropod-borne viruses that cause encephalitis are shown in Table 346–2. Only a small fraction of persons infected with these viruses experience severe CNS manifestations, and human infection is most often subclinical (Table 346–3). The ratio of inapparent to clinically overt infections is a distinctive, age-dependent quality of each disease. The neurologic disease usually begins after a variable period of nonspecific, systemic symptoms and may take the form of aseptic meningitis, meningoencephalitis, or encephalitis. These syndromes are not distinguishable on clinical grounds alone from similar syndromes caused by other infectious agents.

Pathology and Pathogenesis. Two pathologic processes are common to the arboviral encephalitides: (1) neuronal and glial damage mediated by intracellular viral infection and (2) migration of immunologically active cells into the perivascular space and brain parenchyma. Endothelial cell swelling and proliferation, destruction of myelin sheaths in deep white matter areas, and vasculitis are present in some arboviral encephalitides.

After a bite by an infected arthropod, viral replication occurs in local tissues and in regional lymph nodes. Viremia, which seeds extraneural tissues, occurs and persists depending on the extent of replication in extraneural sites, the rate of viral clearance by the reticuloendothelial system, and the appearance of humoral antibodies. Sites of extraneural infection vary from virus to virus. Many alpha- and flaviviruses involve striated muscle and vascular endothelium, whereas Venezuelan encephalitis virus is associated with myeloid and lymphoid tissue invasion. During this viremia, the neural parenchyma may be invaded, but the mode of penetration of virus across the blood-brain barrier is not completely understood. Possible mechanisms include passive movement of virus across vascular membranes and virus replication in cerebral capillary endothelial cells. Factors that increase vascular permeability promote neuroinvasion. In experimental animals infected with some flaviviruses, virus enters the CNS via the olfactory neuroepithelium.

The immature brain is more susceptible to damage by western equine, Venezuelan equine, and California encephalitis viruses (see Table 346–3). St. Louis encephalitis principally affects the elderly, whereas Japanese encephalitis and eastern equine encephalitis have a bimodal incidence, striking both children and elderly persons. In endemic areas, immunity accumulated with increasing age may reduce the incidence of disease in older persons for some viruses; however, the reasons for increased severity of illness with other viruses remain unknown.

Differential Diagnosis. The most important consideration in diagnosis is to differentiate arthropod-borne viral encephalitis from

TABLE 346–3. DIFFERING FEATURES OF ARTHROPOD-BORNE ENCEPHALITIDES IMPORTANT IN THE UNITED STATES

	Western Equine Encephalitis	Eastern Equine Encephalitis	Venezuelan Equine Encephalitis	St. Louis Encephalitis	California Encephalitis
Incidence	0–200/year, mostly infants and children	15/year	Rare in U.S.; mostly children	0–2000/year, mostly adults	50–100/year, mostly children
Time of year	Early or midsummer	Late summer, early fall	Summer	Mid- to late summer	July–September
Case-fatality	3–5% in children	50–70%, highest in children <15 years and adults >55 years	35% in children; <10% in older persons	9% overall; 0% <20 years, 30% >65 years	<1%
Residual damage	33% in infants	30–50%, especially in children	Frequent in children	Frequent in elderly	Probably rare
Cerebrospinal fluid	<500 cells	500–2000 cells PMN's*	<500 cells	<500 cells	<500 cells

* Polymorphonuclear leukocytes.

acute CNS infection due to treatable organisms. The early prodromata resemble influenza, dengue, or other influenza-like illnesses. Bacterial meningitis (especially early or partially treated), infective bacterial endocarditis, brain abscess, subdural empyema, and cerebral thrombophlebitis may mimic viral encephalitis, and CSF changes are sometimes similar. Other infections that occasionally cause meningoencephalitis resembling arthropod-borne viral encephalitis include tuberculosis, cryptococcosis, histoplasmosis, coccidioidomycosis, Rocky Mountain spotted fever, leptospirosis, falciparum malaria, trichinosis, *Naegleria* meningitis, typhoid fever, Lyme disease, and *Mycoplasma* pneumonia.

Acute meningoencephalitis may result from infections with other viruses, including herpesviruses, human immunodeficiency virus (HIV), mumps virus, enteroviruses, lymphocytic choriomeningitis virus, rabies, influenza, and the exanthematous viral infections of childhood. Exposure history, presence of an outbreak of similar disease in the community, and summer-fall occurrence are principal clues to an arboviral etiology. Enteroviruses also cause summer-fall outbreaks, but the predominant syndrome is aseptic meningitis, and the occurrence of rash or pleurodynia is a helpful clue. Herpes simplex encephalitis presents an important diagnostic challenge, since chemotherapy is available. The presence of localizing neurologic signs, localizing findings on computed tomography (CT) or magnetic resonance imaging (MRI) scans, or brain biopsy may help distinguish herpes simplex encephalitis from that due to arthropod-borne viral encephalitides.

Noninfectious diseases of the CNS such as *cerebrovascular accident* may be confused with viral encephalitis. For example, St. Louis encephalitis, a disease of the elderly, has been misdiagnosed as a stroke. Subarachnoid hemorrhage produces meningismus, fever, headache, and neurologic signs that mimic an infectious etiology. *Metabolic encephalopathies* may present features suggesting infectious encephalitis. *Neoplastic* or *granulomatous diseases* involving the CNS and a variety of diseases of uncertain etiology (cat scratch disease, Behçet disease, Reye syndrome, acute multiple sclerosis, and systemic lupus erythematosus) must be considered in the differential diagnosis as well.

WESTERN EQUINE ENCEPHALITIS (WEE). *Etiologic Agent.* WEE virus is a member of the alphavirus genus of the Togaviridae family.

Epidemiology. **Incidence and Prevalence.** Since 1955, the number of cases of WEE reported annually in the United States has varied from 0 to 200. Most affected in recent years has been the area from the Mississippi River west to the Rocky Mountains. Mixed outbreaks of WEE and St. Louis encephalitis are common. Epidemics occur in early or midsummer and may follow heavy snow melt or flooding, conditions favorable for breeding of mosquitoes. Cases of encephalitis in equines often precede the appearance of human disease. The illness principally affects residents of rural communities, and the incidence is higher in males than in females. WEE is most severe in infants and young children. The case-fatality rate is between 3 and 5%. The ratio of inapparent to apparent infection is also age-dependent, ranging from about 1:1 in infants under age 1 year, to 58:1 in children aged 1 to 4 years, to over 1000:1 in persons over age 14 years.

WEE virus also occurs in South America. Equine epizootics in Argentina have been associated with human cases.

Transmission. WEE virus circulates between wild birds and *C. tarsalis* mosquitoes. *C. tarsalis* is responsible for infection of humans and equines, which develop low or undetectable viremias and do not perpetuate the chain of transmission. In temperate areas, transmission ceases during the winter months.

Clinical Features and Pathology. The disease usually begins with an influenza-like illness consisting of fever, headache, malaise, and myalgias lasting 1 to 4 days. Somnolence, lethargy, photophobia, vomiting, and neck stiffness may follow; neurologic involvement may rapidly progress to stupor, coma, and convulsions. Paresis, cranial nerve deficits, tremors, and abnormal reflexes may be present. In fatal cases, patients die 1 to 2 days after coma develops. Survivors generally experience a sudden and rapid recovery. However, about one third of surviving infants suffer retardation, cerebellar damage, choreoathetosis, and spastic paralysis. Children with protracted illnesses who develop convulsions during the acute stage are more likely to suffer long-term neurologic impairment. Adults may have a prolonged convalescent syndrome, but objective residua are rare. Congenital infections are documented and result in severe and progressive neurologic deterioration.

Leukocytosis and shift to the left are common. The CSF contains < 500 white cells (at first polymorphonuclear, then mononuclear) per cubic millimeter and elevated protein concentration (usually 90 to 110 mg per deciliter).

Pathologic examination of the brains of infants reveals massive neuroparenchymal destruction; children dying months or years after the acute insult often have large cystic lesions in many areas of the brain. In older children and adults, acute WEE is characterized by focal necrosis and perivascular cuffing, predominantly in the basal ganglia and thalamic nuclei but also in deep cerebral white matter.

Diagnosis. Viral isolation from blood or CSF is almost never successful. Diagnosis is achieved by demonstrating a rise in HI, fluorescent, complement-fixing (CF), ELISA, or neutralizing-antibody titers in appropriately timed (10 to 14 days apart) paired sera. IgM antibodies demonstrated in serum or CSF by ELISA provides a presumptive diagnosis.

Treatment. There is no specific therapy for WEE. Supportive care is essential and may reduce mortality. Control of high fever, cerebral edema, convulsions, fluid and electrolyte imbalances, and airways is critical.

Prevention and Control. An experimental formalin-inactivated vaccine grown in chick embryo cell cultures has been used to protect laboratory workers but is not indicated for others. In threatened or ongoing epidemics, residents should be advised to use protective clothing, insect repellents, and window screens and to restrict outdoor activity in the early morning, late afternoon, and evening (times of greatest mosquito activity). Public health measures include spraying insecticides aimed at the adult *C. tarsalis* vector.

EASTERN EQUINE ENCEPHALITIS (EEE). *Etiologic Agent.* EEE virus is a member of the Togaviridae family, alphavirus genus.

Epidemiology. **Incidence and Prevalence.** The disease in humans is relatively rare, with fewer than 15 cases occurring each year in the Gulf Coast and Atlantic states, usually associated with a predominantly equine epizootic involving 100 to 300 animals. Outbreaks usually occur during the late summer and early fall. The occurrence of equine cases or outbreaks of fatal encephalitis in penned exotic birds (pheasants, chukar partridges) precedes the appearance of human cases by several weeks or more. Epizootics of EEE have been reported in the Caribbean (Hispaniola) and South America.

Despite the small size of EEE epidemics, the severity is high. The case-fatality rate is 50 to 70%. Incidence and mortality are highest in children under age 15 and in persons over 55, with no gender predilection.

Transmission. In temperate areas, EEE virus circulates between wild birds and *C. melanura* mosquitoes in freshwater swamp habitat. Equine epizootics and associated human cases result from extension of the transmission cycle to involve *Aedes* and *Coquillettidia* mosquitoes, which feed on horses and humans.

Clinical Features and Pathology. The disease is more acute and rapidly progressive than the other arboviral encephalitides. Onset is abrupt, with high fever, vomiting, and somnolence. Stupor, coma, myoclonus, and generalized convulsions appear within 24 to 48 hours. Autonomic disturbances (sialorrhea) may be prominent, and respiratory difficulty and cyanosis are frequent. In children, facial, periorbital, or generalized edema may be present. Death usually occurs during the first week; in surviving patients, recovery begins during the second week and may progress rapidly. Good functional recovery is associated with a long prodromal course and absence of coma. Residual damage, found in 30 to 50% of the patients, is often severe, especially in children, and is characterized by retardation, spastic paralyses, and atrophy of brain substance.

A striking peripheral leukocytosis and shift to the left are frequent findings in patients with EEE. Examination of the CSF reveals 500 to 2000 white cells (predominantly polymorphonuclear) per cubic millimeter. As the total cell count falls, polymorphonuclear cells persist as a significant fraction. Red blood cells may be present, the protein is elevated, and glucose is normal.

In contrast to St. Louis encephalitis and WEE, the brain is grossly edematous and congested, and the inflammatory response is predominantly polymorphonuclear. The areas most affected are basal ganglia, thalamus, hippocampus, and frontal and occipital cortex. Focal vasculitis, endothelial cell swelling, intravenous and arteriolar thrombus formation, demyelination, necrosis, neuronolysis, and neuronophagia are prominent.

Specific Diagnosis. Isolating the virus from blood and CSF is rarely successful. Serologic diagnosis by demonstrating a rise in antibody titer using appropriately timed paired sera is the most practical and available test. Because of the rapid course of the clinical disease, sera should be obtained at 2- to 3-day intervals during the acute phase of illness.

Treatment, Prevention, and Control. Treatment is supportive (see previous discussion of WEE). An experimental formalin-inactivated chick embryo cell culture vaccine is used to protect laboratory and field workers. Reduction of mosquito populations by appropriate use of insecticides may be effective in threatened or established outbreaks.

VENEZUELAN EQUINE ENCEPHALITIS (VEE). Etiology. The causative agent of VEE is a member of the Togaviridae family and alphavirus genus. Six antigenic subtypes (I to VI) and multiple antigenic variants of subtypes I and III are recognized by serologic tests. Subtypes IAB and IC are responsible for epidemics involving humans and equines. In Florida, subtype II is enzootic and produces sporadic human disease.

Epidemiology. Incidence and Prevalence. Prior to 1973, large equine epizootics occurred at 5- to 10-year intervals in Venezuela, Colombia, Ecuador, and Peru, involving many thousands of animals and incurring mortality rates as high as 40%. Associated human morbidity also was great (up to 32,000 clinical cases). No outbreaks of equine or human disease have been recognized in over 12 years.

The predominant syndrome is a self-limited influenza-like illness; only about 4% of infected persons, principally children under age 15, develop encephalitis. Subclinical infections are rare. The case-fatality rate in children up to 5 years old with encephalitis is approximately 35%, but in older persons it is <10%. Laboratory infections are common in unvaccinated persons working with the virus or infected animals.

Transmission. A large variety of mosquito vectors, including species of the genera *Aedes, Psorophora,* and *Mansonia,* transmit subtypes IAB and IC during epizootic epidemics. Equines are the principal viremic hosts. Virus may be present in pharyngeal excretions of human patients; contact or aerosol person-to-person spread, although possible, is not epidemiologically important.

The other members of the VEE viral complex, including subtype II in Florida, have enzootic transmission cycles involving *Culex (Melanoconion)* species mosquitoes and small forest rodents and marsupials. Human disease is sporadic and relatively uncommon.

Clinical Features and Pathology. After an incubation period of 2 to 5 days, there is sudden onset of fever, chills, malaise, and headache, followed by myalgias, nausea, vomiting, and occasionally diarrhea. Physical examination reveals fever, tachycardia, conjunctival injection, and, in some cases, nonexudative pharyngitis. The acute illness generally subsides in 4 to 6 days, and convalescent symptoms may last up to 3 weeks. A biphasic course has sometimes been noted; acute symptoms reappear after a brief remission, within a week after the initial onset.

Some patients will exhibit evidence of mild CNS involvement (photophobia, somnolence, confusion) during the typical influenza-like illness. When it occurs, severe encephalitis is characterized by meningeal signs, convulsions, tremor, stupor, coma, spastic paralysis, abnormal reflexes, cranial nerve palsies, and central respiratory failure. Residual neurologic damage occurs in severe cases. Infections of pregnant women acquired during the first and second trimesters may result in fetal encephalitis and death.

The peripheral leukocyte count is often low, with decrease in both lymphocytes and neutrophils, or normal, with a relative lymphopenia. In patients with CNS signs, the CSF contains up to 500 cells, predominantly lymphocytes, per cubic millimeter. The serum LDH and glutamic-oxaloacetic transaminase levels may be elevated.

Pathologic changes in the CNS include edema, congestion, meningeal and perivascular inflammation, intracerebral hemorrhages, neuronal degeneration, and vasculitis. In addition, hepatocellular degeneration and necrosis, widespread lymphoid depletion and follicular necrosis, and interstitial pneumonitis are frequent findings. In the congenitally infected fetus, there are massive and widespread necrosis of brain tissue, hemorrhages, and resorption of brain material, resulting in hydranencephaly.

Diagnosis. In contrast to the other arthropod-borne encephalitides, VEE virus can be isolated from the blood or from throat swabs or washings during the first 3 or 4 days of illness. Serodiagnosis is usually more practical and is achieved by testing appropriately timed paired sera by HI, CF, ELISA, neutralization, or IgM immunoassay.

Treatment, Prevention, and Control. No specific therapy is available, and treatment of encephalitis cases is supportive. An experimental live, attenuated vaccine made from subtype IAB is used for adult laboratory personnel. It provides solid immunity to subtype IAB and its closest relative (IC) but incomplete protection against infection with other heterologous VEE viruses. Epidemics and epizootics can be prevented by effective vaccination of equines. Spraying insecticides to reduce adult (infective) mosquito populations is the only means of immediate control in the face of an ongoing epidemic. Individual protection against mosquitoes also is advised.

ST. LOUIS ENCEPHALITIS (SLEn). Etiology. St. Louis encephalitis virus, a member of the family Flaviviridae, shares close antigenic relationships with Japanese encephalitis, Murray Valley encephalitis, and West Nile viruses and is related to yellow fever and dengue viruses. Strains associated with *C. pipiens*–borne epidemics in the eastern United States are distinct from endemic strains transmitted by *C. tarsalis* in the western states.

Epidemiology. Incidence and Prevalence. The virus is present in all parts of the Western Hemisphere, but epidemics occur only in North America and some Caribbean islands. During epidemic years, the virus has been responsible for up to 80% of all reported cases of encephalitis of known etiology in the United States. In recent years, epidemics of up to 2000 cases have taken place, mainly in urban-suburban localities of the Ohio-Mississippi River basin, in eastern and central Texas, and in Florida. Small outbreaks also have occurred in the western United States. Epidemics usually transpire between July and September but may arise later in the year in warm areas such as Florida. Prior exposure and immunity to dengue may provide a degree of cross-protection against clinical SLEn.

The overall case-fatality rate is approximately 9%. Mortality is negligible in persons under age 20 but rises steeply after age 55 to approximately 30% in patients over age 65. The inapparent/apparent infection ratio is 800:1 in children up to age 9, 400:1 in persons aged 10 to 49, and 85:1 in persons older than 60.

Transmission. In most of the eastern United States, SLEn virus circulates between wild birds and *C. pipiens* mosquitoes, which breed in polluted water. In Florida and in parts of the Caribbean, *C. nigripalpus* is the principal vector. The cycle in the western United States also involves wild birds, but the vector is *C. tarsalis,* the vector of WEE. Because of the similar ecology of SLEn and WEE viruses in the west, mixed outbreaks occur, mostly in rural, agricultural areas.

Above-average summer temperatures and conditions such as deficient rainfall, which create stagnant pools suitable for *C. pipiens* breeding, are associated with epidemics in the eastern United States. SLEn in the western states is favored by warm spring temperatures, heavy snow melt, and flooding.

Clinical Features and Pathology. Three clinical syndromes are recognized: febrile headache, aseptic meningitis, and encephalitis. After an incubation period of 4 to 21 days, there is a variable period of nonspecific symptoms, including fever (38 to 41°C), headache, malaise, drowsiness, myalgias, and sore throat. This may be followed by the acute or subacute onset of meningeal or encephalitic signs or both. Nausea, vomiting, and photophobia are common. Neurologic abnormalities occur in up to 25% of patients. Extrapyramidal abnormalities (tremor of tongue, face, and limbs) and an altered state of consciousness are the most significant findings. Others include altered sensorium, meningismus, cranial nerve deficits (particularly N. VII), abnormal reflexes, tremors, myoclonic twitching, nystagmus, and ataxia. Motor abnormalities are infrequent and sensory changes extremely uncommon. Convulsions occur in 10% of patients and are a poor prognostic sign, as is a persistent high temperature of 40 to 41°C. Signs of markedly increased intracranial pressure are very unusual. Guillain-Barré syndrome has occasionally been associated with SLEn, both as an acute presentation and during the convalescent period. Approximately half the patients with fatal outcome succumb during the first week and 80% within 2 weeks after onset.

In uncomplicated cases of SLEn, there is a moderate peripheral neutrophilic leukocytosis and shift to the left. CSF pressure is elevated, protein mildly elevated, and sugar normal. Pleocytosis up to 500 cells per cubic millimeter is present. Polymorphonuclear cells predominate early, the change to lymphocytes occurring within several days. Serum creatinine phosphokinase, glutamic-oxaloacetic transaminase, and serum aldolase are frequently elevated. The electroencephalogram typically shows amorphous delta wave activity and diffuse generalized slowing most prominently in the frontal and temporal regions, but brain scans are normal. Inappropriate secretion of antidiuretic hormone is present in one third of patients.

Genitourinary tract symptoms (urgency, frequency, incontinence, and retention), microscopic hematuria, pyuria, and proteinuria, and elevated blood urea nitrogen are frequent. SLEn viral antigen in cells of the urinary sediment has been detected by fluorescent techniques and virus-like particles in urine by immunoelectronmicroscopy.

A convalescent syndrome characterized by weakness, fatigue, nervousness, tremulousness, sleeplessness, irritability, depression, difficulty in concentrating, and headaches occurs in 30 to 50% of older persons and clears in 80% of these within 3 years.

Pathologic changes in fatal cases are limited to microscopic findings. Leptomeningitis is characterized by lymphocytic inflammation. Parenchymal changes consist of lymphocytic perivascular cuffing, cellular nodule formation, and neuronal degeneration.

Diagnosis. SLEn virus is rarely isolated from blood or CSF obtained during the acute phase of illness. Serologic diagnosis is achieved by demonstrating changing antibody titers; the HI, fluorescent, ELISA, and neutralizing tests demonstrate antibody within the first week after onset, and titers rise during the ensuing 2 weeks. CF antibodies appear 10 to 20 days after onset. Rapid, early diagnosis is possible by detecting IgM antibodies by ELISA in serum and CSF. Serologic cross-reactions may occur in persons with prior exposures to dengue and other related flaviviruses.

Treatment, Prevention, and Control. Treatment is supportive. No vaccine is available for SLEn. Surveillance of viral activity in vectors and avian hosts is used to define the risk of human infection and initiate vector control efforts. In an established outbreak, avoiding mosquito bites and spraying to reduce infected adult mosquitoes are the only effective means of control.

CALIFORNIA ENCEPHALITIS. Etiology. At least four members of the California serogroup of the Bunyaviridae family (*Bunyavirus* genus)—LaCrosse, California encephalitis, Jamestown Canyon, and snowshoe hare virus—cause encephalitis. California encephalitis virus occurs in the western United States (California, New Mexico, Utah, Texas) and has been implicated in only three human cases. In contrast, LaCrosse virus, distributed more widely in the eastern half of the United States and southern Canada, is a major human pathogen. Recently, Jamestown Canyon and snowshoe hare viruses have been implicated in sporadic human encephalitis cases in the north central United States and Canada. California serogroup viruses have been implicated in human disease in the People's Republic of China and the former U.S.S.R.

Epidemiology. Incidence and Prevalence. California encephalitis occurs as an endemic rather than an epidemic disease, with individual or small clusters of cases scattered across the affected areas. An average of 80 cases are reported each year, generally occurring between July and September, with peak incidence in August. The virus primarily affects persons younger than 15 living in rural and suburban areas characterized by deciduous hardwood forests. It is most prevalent in the north central states, where it is responsible for as many as 20% of cases of acute CNS infection in children. Focal "hot spots" (communities, even backyards) of recurrent summertime viral activity are recognized. The case-fatality rate is less than 1%. The inapparent/apparent infection ratio has been estimated variably at between 26:1 and 157:1.

Transmission. The vector of LaCrosse virus is *A. triseriatus,* which breeds both in forest tree holes and in peridomestic artificial containers. The vector also serves as a reservoir of LaCrosse virus. Wild rodents (squirrels, chipmunks) contribute to a cycle of transmission as viremic hosts. Humans acquire the disease by being bitten by an infected mosquito.

A. communis, A. stimulans, A. triseriatus, and possibly anophe-line mosquitoes are involved in transmitting Jamestown Canyon virus, and deer are the principal vertebrate hosts.

Clinical Features. The clinical spectrum of California virus infection includes nonspecific febrile illness, aseptic meningitis, and meningoencephalitis. The disease begins with fever, headache, sore throat, and gastrointestinal symptoms, with appearance of the neurologic disorder within 1 to 3 days. In mild cases, CNS signs appear on the third day after onset and subside within 7 to 8 days. In the more severe form, neurologic signs appear within 24 to 48 hours of onset, usually in the form of generalized seizures and altered consciousness, and are more prolonged. Papilledema or abnormal optic disc margins have been noted. Encephalitis may be quite severe in the acute stage, but the disease is almost always self-limited, and death is extremely rare. The question of permanent sequelae is unsettled. Many researchers believe LaCrosse virus infection is responsible for residual psychological problems, emotional lability, hyperkinesis, infantilism, compulsive behavior, and auditory and visual perceptual problems. There are case reports of hemiparesis and persistent seizure disorders.

The peripheral white cell count is elevated, with a predominance of polymorphonuclear cells and a shift to the left. The CSF contains up to 500 lymphocytes per cubic millimeter, normal or mildly elevated protein, and normal glucose concentrations. The electroencephalogram reveals generalized slowing in the delta and theta range, indicating diffuse cortical dysfunction. Focal delta wave activity related to cortical destruction or focal seizures is also a common finding.

Histopathologic features in the CNS are qualitatively similar to those of other viral encephalitides; however, absence of inflammatory lesions in cerebellum, medulla, and spinal cord has been postulated to be a distinguishing feature of LaCrosse infection.

Diagnosis. The virus cannot be recovered from blood or CSF obtained during the acute phase. Diagnosis is best achieved by tests for antibody in paired acute and convalescent sera using counterimmunoelectrophoresis, HI, CF, fluorescent, ELISA, and neutralization tests. The most practical, sensitive, and reliable methods are the HI test using the LaCrosse viral antigen and IgM antibody capture ELISA.

Treatment, Prevention, and Control. Treatment is supportive. There is no vaccine for California encephalitis. Vector control methods are of uncertain usefulness in this disease. In defined "hot spots" of recurrent viral activity, efforts to eliminate breeding sites for *A. triseriatus* should be made. Parents should protect children by limiting exposure and using mosquito repellents.

JAPANESE ENCEPHALITIS (JE). Etiology and Epidemiology. Incidence and Prevalence. JE virus is a member of the Flaviviridae family. It causes epizootics of clinical encephalitis in equines. The disease occurs throughout Asia, including Japan, the Korean peninsula, Taiwan, the People's Republic of China, Okinawa, Vietnam, the Philippines, Burma, Malaysia, Bangladesh, east and south India, Sri Lanka, Thailand, and Indonesia. Over 30,000 cases occur annually. JE is a summertime disease in temperate areas but occurs sporadically year-round in the tropics. Epidemics have been most frequent at the northern fringe of the tropical zone. JE is predominantly a rural disease, and the incidence in males is often higher than in females. In hyperendemic areas, over 70% of adult populations surveyed have antibodies, and children under age 15 principally are affected by the disease. In areas without a high prevalence of background immunity (e.g., northern India), however, all age groups are affected. In Japan, where school children have been protected by vaccination campaigns targeted at this age group, occurrence of encephalitis in the elderly has become prominent. The inapparent/apparent infection ratio is over 500:1 in children and decreases with age; in Korea, the ratio among American servicemen was estimated at 25:1. The case-fatality rate probably is about 25%, but rates of 50% or more have been reported, which may reflect under-recognition of nonfatal cases.

Transmission. The natural cycle involves *Culex* mosquito vectors and wild birds and swine. Humans and equines are incidental hosts.

Clinical Features and Pathology. Manifestations of JE include febrile headache, aseptic meningitis, and meningoencephalitis. Onset is abrupt, with fever, headache, and gastrointestinal symptoms. Meningeal irritation develops within 24 hours and is followed on the second or third day by the appearance of irritability, impaired consciousness, convulsions (especially in children), muscular rigidity, masklike facies, ataxia, coarse tremor, involuntary movements, cranial nerve deficits, paresis, hyperactive deep tendon reflexes, and pathologic reflexes. Weight loss and dehydration are often striking findings. In mild cases, fever subsides after the first week and neurologic signs resolve by the end of the second week after onset. In severe cases, hyperpyrexia, progressive neurologic dysfunction, and coma result in death, usually between the seventh and tenth days. About 25% of patients undergo a prolonged recovery, often leaving permanent sequelae. Cardiorespiratory complications are frequent during the acute stage in these patients. A poor prognosis is associated with protracted high fever, frequent or prolonged seizures, high protein content in the CSF, Babinski signs, and early appearance of respiratory depression. Fetal death and abortion due to transplacental JE infection have been reported.

The occurrence of sequelae correlates with severity of the acute stage of illness. Young children are most susceptible, and sequelae such as mental impairment, emotional lability, choreoathetosis, tremor, parkinsonism, autonomic disturbances, motor paralysis, and pathopsychologic syndromes (including schizophrenia) have been reported in up to 75% of patients.

A moderate peripheral leukocytosis and neutrophilia occur early in the disease. Pleocytosis, protein elevation, and normal glucose in the CSF are usual findings.

Neuropathologic changes and distribution of lesions are similar to those described for St. Louis encephalitis (see earlier discussion of SLEn).

Diagnosis. Isolating JE virus from blood is uncommon; virus may be recovered from the CSF of about one third of patients who progress to a fatal outcome but rarely from patients who live. HI and neutralizing antibodies appear during the first and CF antibodies during the second week after onset. Cross-reactions with other flaviviruses make serodiagnosis difficult. Specific IgM antibodies in serum or CSF are detectable by immunoassays in over three fourths of patients at the time of hospital admission.

Treatment, Prevention, and Control. Treatment is supportive (see WEE). Uncontrolled trials of intrathecal interferon suggest a beneficial effect but require confirmation. Inactivated, partially purified mouse brain vaccines produced in Japan are safe and effective in preschool- and school-age children. Recently licensed for use in the United States, a vaccine produced in Japan is available to U.S. citizens traveling to high-risk areas. Information should be sought from state health departments or the Centers for Disease Control and Prevention. Since three doses of the inactivated vaccine are used and approximately 1 month is required to confer protection, vaccination is not a practical measure in the face of an ongoing epidemic. Reduction of vector mosquito populations by applying insecticides may help to abort outbreaks. Immunization of swine is an ancillary control strategy.

MURRAY VALLEY ENCEPHALITIS AND ROCIO ENCEPHALITIS. Murray Valley encephalitis and Rocio encephalitis are similar to JE in pathogenesis and clinical features and are caused by closely related flaviviruses. Murray Valley encephalitis has occurred in small epidemics in the Murray and Darling River valleys of Victoria and New South Wales, Australia. The virus is endemic in northern Australia and New Guinea, where it is maintained in a bird-mosquito cycle. Rocio encephalitis has caused epidemics of 1000 cases in São Paulo State, Brazil.

TICK-BORNE ENCEPHALITIS. Etiologic Agents. A complex of six antigenically related tick-borne flaviviruses cause encephalitis: Powassan, tick-borne encephalitis (TBE), louping ill, Kyasanur Forest disease (KFD), Omsk hemorrhagic fever (OHF), and Langat viruses. The predominant syndrome in KFD and OHF is hemorrhagic fever (see Ch. 345.3), but meningoencephalitis may be a component of the disease spectrum. Two subtypes of TBE virus (Central European encephalitis and Russian spring-summer encephalitis) are distinguished by special serologic tests, are ecologically distinct, and differ in virulence for humans. Powassan and louping ill viruses are rare causes of encephalitis in North America and the British Isles, respectively. These viruses are serologically easily distinguished from mosquito-borne flaviviruses but induce cross-reactions within the complex.

Tick-Borne Encephalitis (TBE). TBE occurs in Europe (including Eastern Europe and Ukraine), southern Scandinavia, and far

eastern Russia during summer months, corresponding to peak tick vector populations. Several hundred to 2000 cases are reported annually, with morbidity rates of up to 20 per 100,000 inhabitants. Inapparent infections are common. Adults over age 20 are mainly affected, and persons frequenting wooded areas that are heavily tick-infested are at highest risk. In Europe, the disease is relatively mild (case-fatality rate 1 to 2%), but in the Far East, it is severe (20 to 25%).

In Europe, the vector of TBE is *Ixodes ricinus,* and in the Far East, *I. persulcatus.* The tick vector also serves as a reservoir of the virus. Larval ticks parasitize small rodents, which serve as amplifying viremic hosts during the spring and summer. Large vertebrates (goats, sheep, cattle) are hosts for nymphal and adult ticks. Outbreaks have occurred in families or groups of individuals ingesting unpasteurized milk or cheese from goats or sheep.

TBE in Europe typically (but not invariably) has a biphasic course, beginning 7 to 14 days after exposure with an influenza-like illness lasting 1 week, followed by a period of clinical remission for several days and then abrupt onset of aseptic meningitis or meningoencephalitis. The latter is usually benign, although severe paralytic illness, myelitis, myeloradiculitis, and bulbar forms may occur. Convalescence is often prolonged, and residual paralysis may follow in severe cases. In the Far East, TBE begins suddenly with fever, headache, and gastrointestinal symptoms, followed rapidly by appearance of depressed sensorium, coma, convulsions, and paralysis. Bulbar paralysis and cervical myelitis are frequent findings. In fatal cases, death occurs in the first week after onset. Survivors have a high incidence of residual paralyses, especially lower motor neuron paralysis of upper extremities or shoulder girdle. Aseptic meningitis and milder forms of encephalitis also occur. Chronic forms of TBE have been described, with active clinical and pathologic abnormalities a year or more after onset.

In TBE, virus isolation from blood is also possible during the early phase of illness. Serologic diagnosis is achieved by the HI, CF, N, or ELISA techniques.

Treatment is supportive (see WEE).

In eastern Europe and the former U.S.S.R., TBE vaccines are used in high-risk groups (forestry and agricultural workers, military personnel). In Austria, immunization of the general population has resulted in a marked decline in incidence. Avoiding tick exposure by wearing protective clothing and using repellents may be recommended in areas of high TBE activity.

Louping Ill Encephalitis. Louping ill causes encephalitis in sheep (rarely in cattle, horses, and swine) in Scotland and in northern England and Ireland. Sporadic human cases have been recognized. Louping ill virus is maintained in nature by *I. ricinus* ticks and a variety of hosts, including small mammals, ground-dwelling birds (grouse), and probably sheep. The clinical features of louping ill resemble the European form of TBE.

Powassan Virus Encephalitis. Powassan virus encephalitis has been documented in a small number of cases in the northeastern United States and eastern Canada, with a case-fatality rate of 50%. The virus is not associated with animal disease. The transmission cycle of Powassan virus involves *I. cookei, I. marxi* (and possibly other tick species), and mammals, particularly rodents and carnivores. Powassan encephalitis is characterized by fever and nonspecific symptoms, followed by encephalitic signs, which are frequently severe. Residual paralysis may occur. Peripheral blood and CSF changes are similar to those described in other forms of flaviviral encephalitis.

Duchin JS, Koster FT, Peters CJ, et al.: *Hantavirus* pulmonary syndrome: A clinical description of 17 patients with a newly recognized disease. N Engl J Med 330:949, 1994. *Detailed clinical description of the first 17 patients with hantavirus pulmonary syndrome.*

Markoff L: Alphaviruses. *In* Mandell G, Bennett J, Dolin R (eds.): Principles and Practice of Infectious Diseases, 4th ed. New York, Churchill-Livingstone, 1995. *Clear description of alphaviruses and important syndromes including fever, polyarthritis, and encephalitis in a well-referenced, easily accessible source.*

Monath TP: Colorado tick fever. *In* Mandell G, Bennett J, Dolin R (eds.): Principles and Practice of Infectious Diseases, 4th ed. New York, Churchill-Livingstone, 1995. *A current, thoroughly researched review of Colorado tick fever.*

Peters CJ, Johnson KM: Bunyaviridae: California encephalitis viruses, *Hantavirus,* and other Bunyaviridae. *In* Mandell G, Bennett J, Dolin R (eds.): Principles and Practice of Infectious Diseases, 4th ed. New York, Churchill-Livingstone, 1995. *An up-to-date, well-referenced review of important Bunyaviruses and their infections in humans.*

Spach DH, Liles WC, Campbell GL, et al.: Tick-borne diseases in the United States. N Engl J Med 329:936, 1993. *Reviews recent advances in understanding these diseases, especially their microbiology, epidemiology, diagnosis, and treatment; 145 references.*

PLATE 9 INFECTIOUS AND PROTOZOAN DISEASES

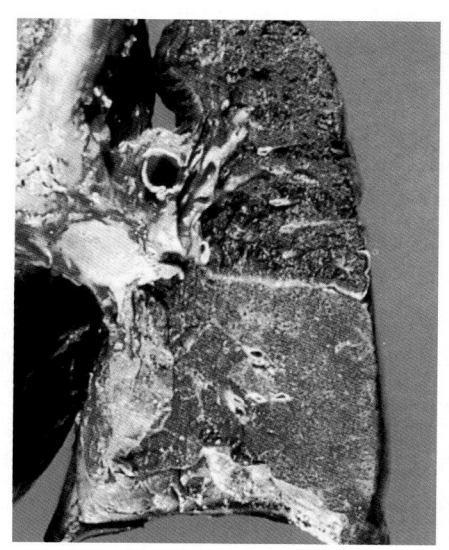

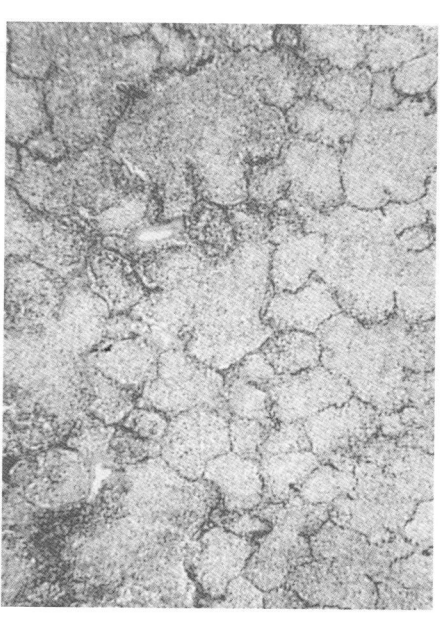

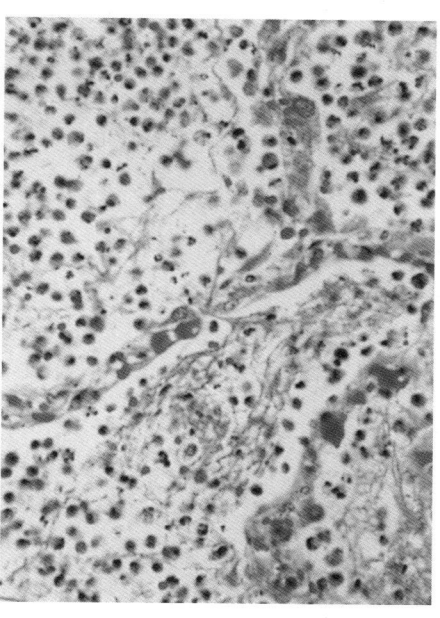

A, Autopsy specimen revealing lobar consolidation (gray and red hepatization) of the left lower lobe due to *Streptococcus pneumoniae.* Note the absence of abscess formation and the presence of dense consolidation extending from the hilum to the pleural surface.

B, Low-powered magnification (3 100) of hematoxylin and eosin (H & E) stain of tissue section from left lower lobar pneumonia pictured in *A.* Note intact alveolar walls and alveoli filled with edema and thick cellular exudate.

C, Higher magnification (3 500) H & E stain depicted in *B.* Note heavy infiltrate of polymorphonuclear cells and intact alveolar walls.

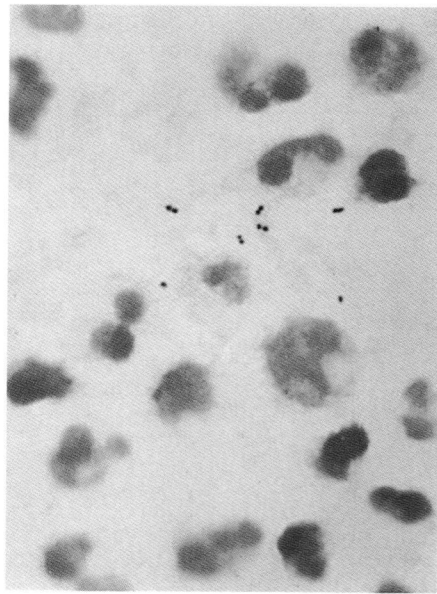

D, Fluid removed from the pleural space in a patient with early pneumococcal pneumonia and pleural effusion. The fluid may be serous, serosanguineous, green, or thick and white.

E, Gram stain of pleural fluid shown in *D,* revealing the presence of polymorphonuclear cells and typical gram-positive diplococci in pairs, consistent with pneumococci.

F, Cutaneous leishmaniasis due to *L. braziliensis.* (From Jeronimo SMB, Pearson RD: Subcell Biochem 18:1, 1992.)

G, Brazilian patient with mucosal leishmaniasis due to *L. braziliensis.* Note the destructive lesions involving the nose, nasal septum, and lips. (From Pearson RD, et al.: Rev Infect Dis 5:907, 1983.)

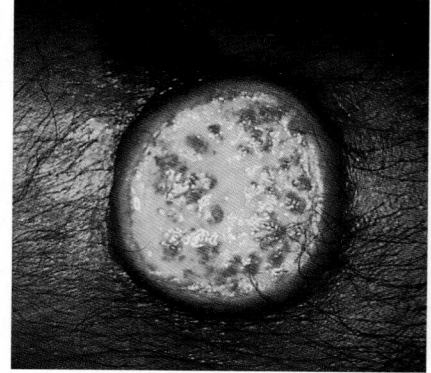

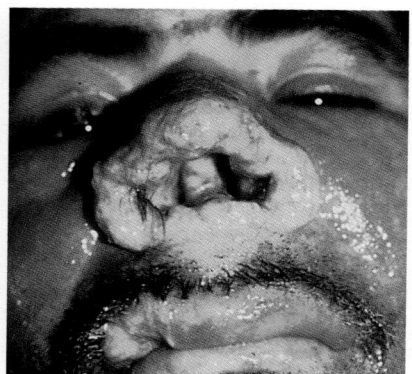

F

G

PLATE 10   INFECTIOUS, MUSCULOSKELETAL, AND PROTOZOAN DISEASES

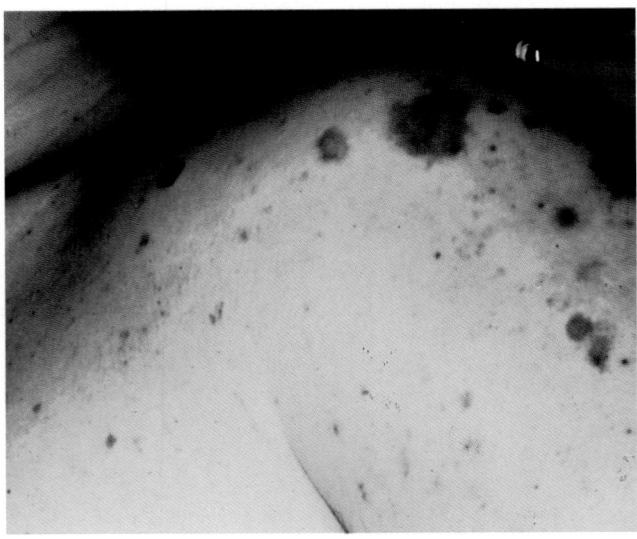

A, A patient with advanced meningococcemia who demonstrates multiple petechiae and ecchymoses on the shoulders, chest, and arm.

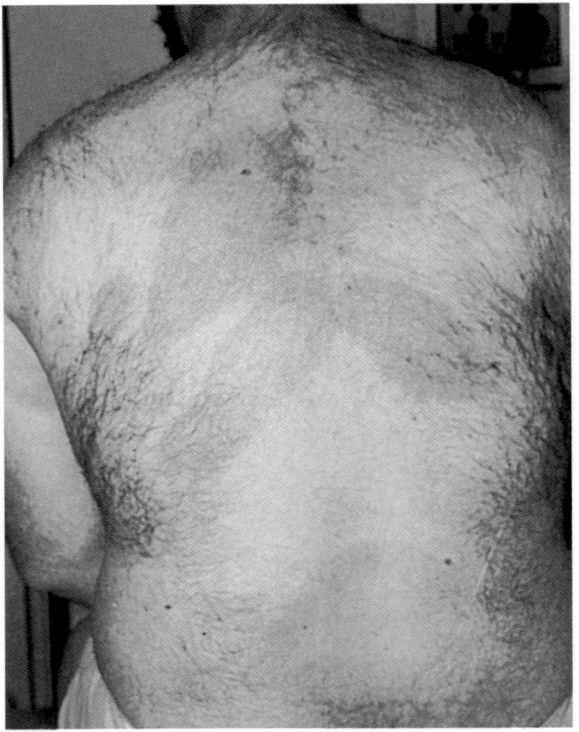

B, Erythema chronicum migrans (ECM), the major dermatologic manifestation of Lyme disease. Four days after onset of ECM, this patient has developed secondary annular lesions; some of their borders have merged. (From Steere AC, Bartenhagen NH, Craft JE, et al.: The early clinical manifestations of Lyme disease. Ann Intern Med 99:76–82, 1983; with permission.)

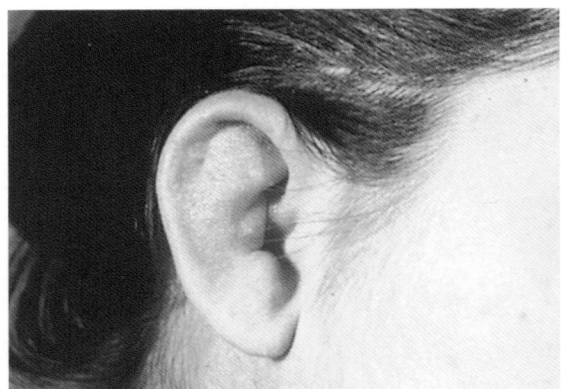

C, Polychondritis. Note nodularity of ear.

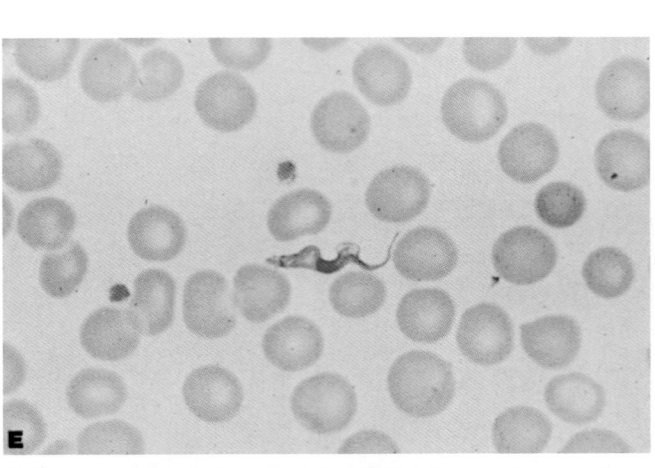

E, Trypanosoma rhodesiense in the peripheral blood. It has a nucleus, posterior kinetoplast, undulating membrane, and flagellum (× 1500).

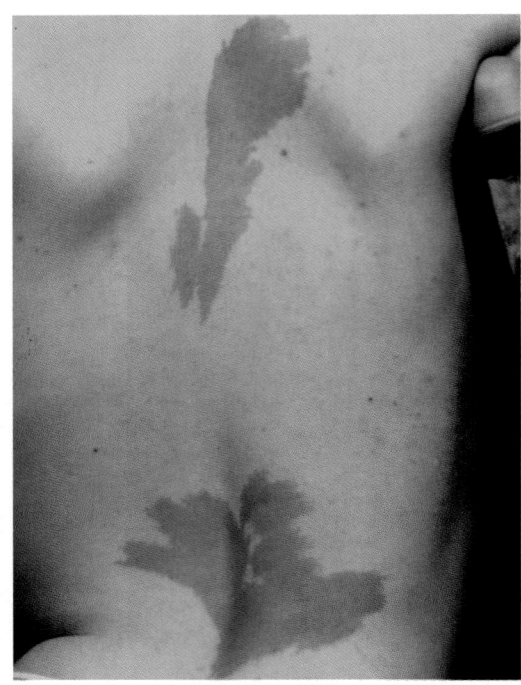

D, McCune-Albright Syndrome. Typical rough-border ("coast-of-Maine") pigmented café au lait spot (From Whyte MP: Metabolic and dysplastic disorders. *In* Coe FL, Favus MJ [eds]: Disorders of Bone and Mineral Metabolism, New York, Raven Press, 1992.)

PLATE 11   INFECTIOUS AND PROTOZOAN DISEASES AND HIV

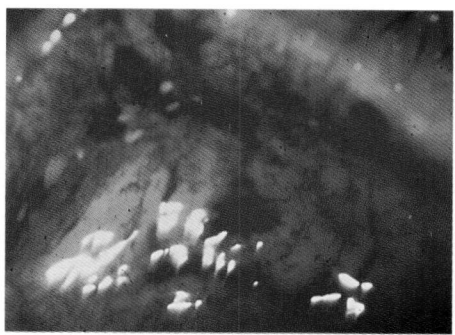

A, Conjunctival petechiae.

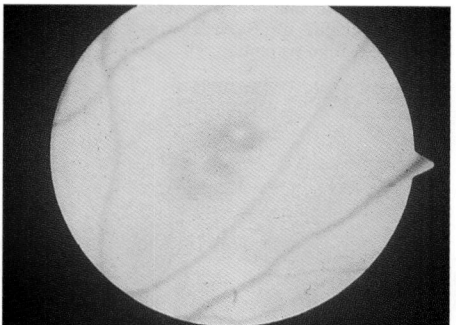

B, Roth's spots on retina.

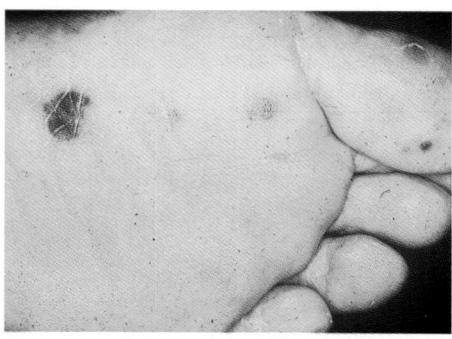

C, Janeway lesion: painless hemorrhagic macule on sole. (From Korzeniowski O, Kaye D: Infective endocarditis. *In* Braunwald E (ed.): Heart Disease, 4th ed. Philadelphia, WB Saunders, 1992.)

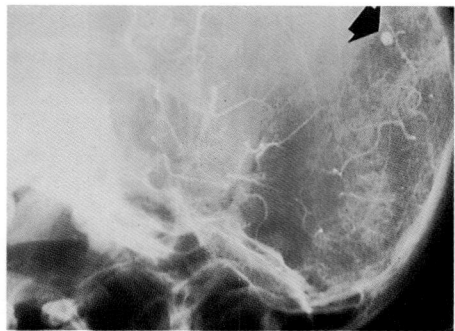

D, Cerebral angiogram illustrating a mycotic aneurysm *(arrow).* (From Kaye D [ed.]: Infective Endocarditis. Baltimore, University Park Press, 1976.)

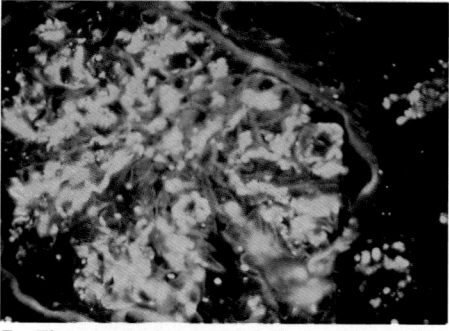

E, Fluorescent immunoglobulin staining of a glomerulus in a patient with glomerulonephritis. (From Kaye D [ed.]: Infective Endocarditis. Baltimore, University Park Press, 1976.)

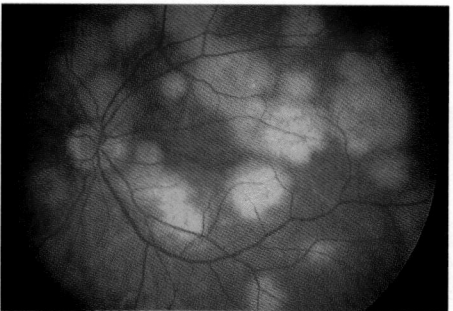

F, Photomicrograph of the indirect funduscopic examination of the left eye from a 35-year-old AIDS patient who was receiving aerosolized pentamidine for secondary prophylaxis of pneumocystis pneumonia. There is extensive choroidal exudation but, unlike CMV retinitis, there is sparing of the retina and minimal hemorrhage. (From Rao NA, Zimmermann PL, Boyer D, et al.: A clinical, histopathologic, and electron microscopic study of *Pneumocystis carinii* choroiditis. Am J Ophthalmol 107:218, 1989.)

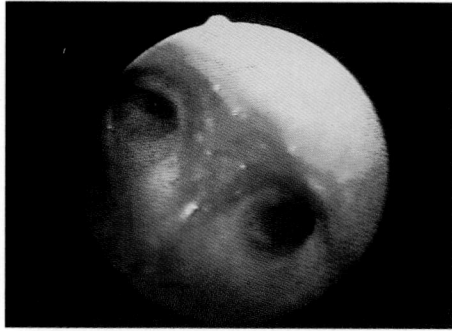

G, Bronchoscopic view of a typical endobronchial Kaposi's sarcoma lesion. The lesion is macular and bright red and straddles a carina. These lesions are sufficiently distinctive to be diagnostic of Kaposi's sarcoma.

H, Section of liver from a patient with zidovudine-induced steatosis. The hepatocytes are swollen with lipid vacuoles (mixed macrovesicular and microvesicular steatosis). A necrotic hepatocyte is seen at the center of the field (H & E, ×400). (Courtesy of Dr. D. Kleiner.)

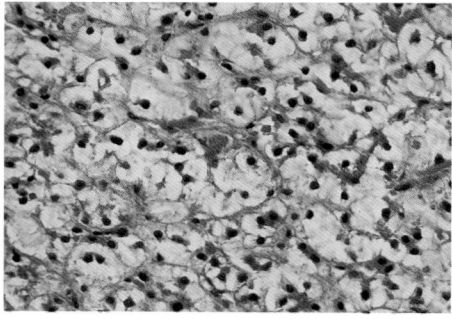

PLATE 12   HIV AND ASSOCIATED DISORDERS

A to *E* show dermatologic abnormalities in AIDS.

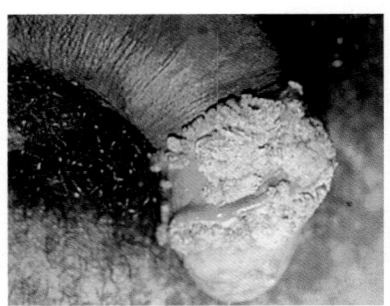

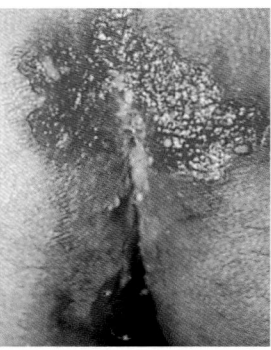

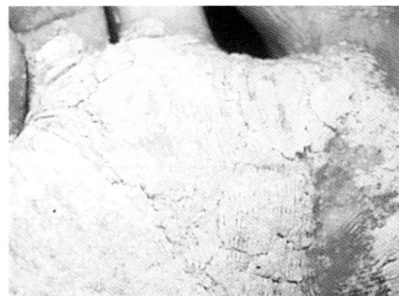

A, Prominent condyloma surrounding the corona and the shaft of the penis.

B, Chronic ulcerative herpetic infection is commonly seen in the intergluteal fold.

C, Marked hyperkeratosis characterizes keratoderma blennorrhagicum of Reiter's syndrome in HIV-seropositive patients.

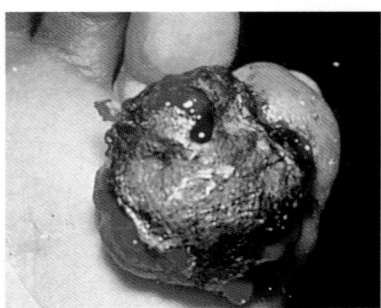

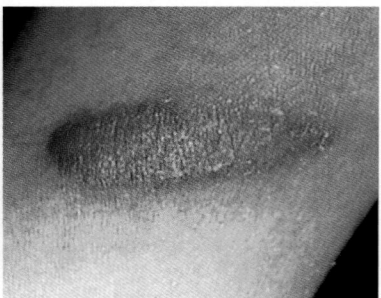

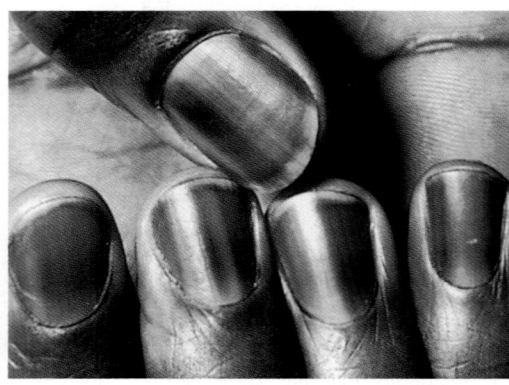

D, Left, An exophytic tumor of Kaposi's sarcoma on the sole. *Right,* Lesion demonstrating the linear configuration frequently noted in Kaposi's sarcoma of the skin in patients with AIDS.

E, Bluish discoloration of the nail plates developed during treatment with AZT.

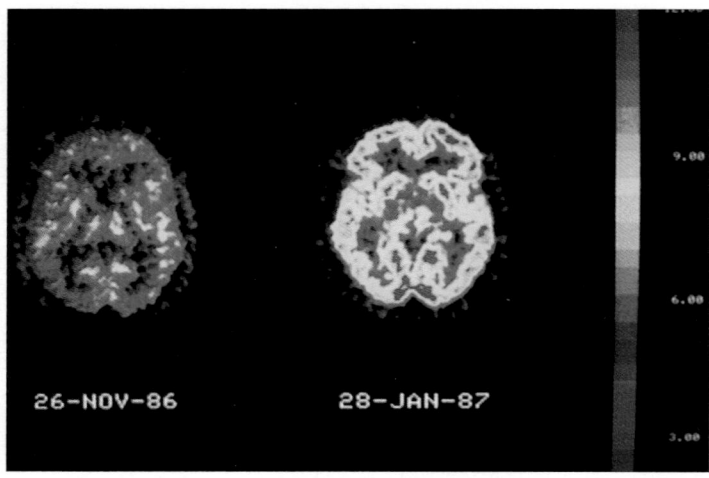

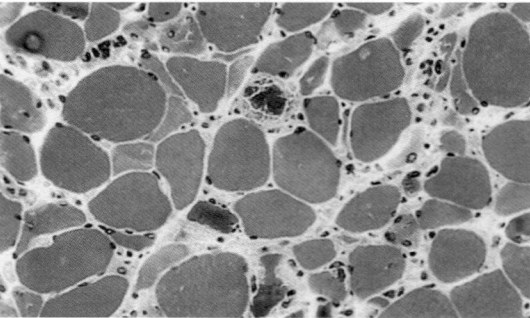

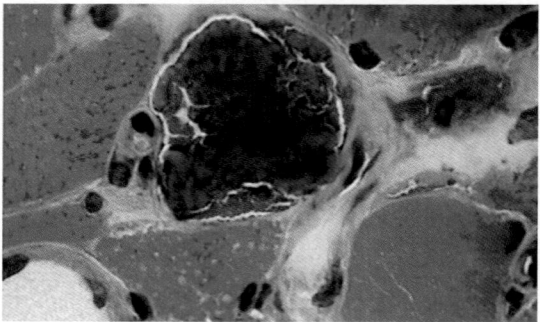

F, Positron emission tomography (PET) scan showing glucose metabolism in the brain of a patient with AIDS dementia before *(left)* and during *(right)* therapy with AZT. This patient had marked improvement in his cognitive function that was associated with a relative normalization of glucose metabolism in the brain. (Reproduced with permission from Brunetti A, Berg G, Di Chiro G, et al.: Reversal of brain metabolic abnormalities following treatment of AIDS dementia complex with 39-azido-29, 39-dideoxythymidine [AZT, zidovudine]: A PET-FDG study. J Nucl Med 30:581–590, 1989.)

G, Pathologic findings in a patient with AZT-induced myopathy. *Top,* Destructive changes with variation in fiber size and a "ragged-red" fiber. Inflammatory changes can be seen in both AZT-induced myopathy and the myopathy of HIV infection. However, ragged-red fibers are seen only in patients receiving AZT. Transverse section, stained with the modified Gomori trichrome stain (3 320). *Bottom,* Detail showing a ragged-red fiber (3 900). (Photographs courtesy of Dr. M. C. Dalakos.)

The Mycoses

347 INTRODUCTION TO THE MYCOSES

William E. Dismukes

Fungi are classified as eukaryotic microorganisms, in contrast to bacteria, which are considered prokaryotic. Eukaryotes, such as fungi, possess a discrete nuclear membrane and a nucleus that contains several chromosomes, whereas prokaryotes have no nucleus or nuclear membrane and possess only a single chromosome. Fungi also differ from bacteria in the ability of the former to reproduce sexually or asexually. Most fungi reproduce by asexual spore formation. When sexual mating of two closely related species, e.g., *Cryptococcus neoformans,* serotypes A and D, takes place, the "perfect state" (*Filobasidiella neoformans* var. *neoformans*) is produced. Fungi for which a perfect state has not been identified are referred to as fungi imperfecti (e.g., *Candida albicans* and *Coccidioides immitis*). The cell walls of fungi are rigid, usually composed of chitin, glucan, and mannoproteins, another feature that distinguishes fungi from bacteria. In addition, the cytoplasmic membrane of fungi contains sterols, principally ergosterol, which are the target sites of action for the major classes of antifungal drugs.

The terms "fungal diseases" and "mycoses" are used interchangeably. Fungal infections that involve only the skin and its appendages are referred to as cutaneous or superficial mycoses (e.g., ringworm of the scalp or groin and tinea versicolor). By contrast, fungal infections that are acquired primarily by inhalation and spread via lymphohematogenous dissemination to involve one or more organs, such as the lungs, skin, liver, spleen, and central nervous system, are referred to as systemic mycoses (Table 347–1). Candidiasis is a mycosis that may cause superficial disease (e.g., intertrigo, oral thrush, and vaginitis) or deep organ disease (e.g., candidemia and disseminated candidiasis).

Fungi causing systemic disease may also be classified by the morphologic or structural form of the organism. For example, *Aspergillus* species and zygomycotes (*Mucor* and *Rhizopus* species) are molds that grow as a hyphal structural form both in the laboratory (and nature) and in humans. By contrast, other fungi are dimorphic; i.e., they have the ability to transform morphologically into either a mold or a yeast form, depending on the environmental conditions. *Blastomyces dermatitidis, Coccidioides immitis, Histoplasma capsulatum, Paracoccidioides brasiliensis,* and *Sporothrix schenckii* exist as hyphal or filamentous forms in nature, but as yeasts (*B. dermatitidis, H. capsulatum, P. brasiliensis, S. schenckii*) or endosporulating spherules (*C. immitis*) in humans. *Cryptococcus neoformans* is a true yeast, growing as the same spherical form in both nature and humans.

Discussions of the epidemiologic features of the major systemic mycoses are provided in the individual chapters that follow. Soil and other environmental niches are the natural reservoirs for most of the causative organisms. Infections of humans primarily result from inhaling aerosolized spores (respiratory route of transmission). Exceptions include sporotrichosis, for which most cases are acquired via cutaneous inoculation, and candidiasis, which results either from an endogenous site of colonization such as the oropharynx, skin, or vagina, or from person-to-person contact. The other systemic mycoses are not transmitted routinely from human to human. The natural habitat of several fungal pathogens is limited to specific geographic areas. Consequently, persons living in these areas are at highest risk of acquiring infection. The diseases caused by such organisms are referred to as endemic mycoses and include blastomycosis, coccidioidomycosis, histoplasmosis, and paracoccidioidomycosis. These diseases typically are associated with asymptomatic or mild pulmonary infection that heals spontaneously. Progressive pulmonary infection or spread to extrapulmonary sites occurs less frequently.

Some fungal organisms are considered opportunistic pathogens and are especially prone to cause disease in the setting of altered host defense (Table 347–2). Common predisposing conditions or factors include interruptions in anatomic barriers (burns and endotracheal tubes) or indwelling foreign bodies (arterial or central venous catheters, urinary catheters, and prosthetic heart valves or joints); granulocyte dysfunction secondary to hematologic malignancies (leukemia) or cytotoxic chemotherapy; and depressed cell-mediated immunity associated with organ transplantation, AIDS, or immunosuppressive therapy, such as corticosteroids and azathioprine. Other conditions that may predispose to systemic mycoses include diabetic ketoacidosis (rhinocerebral mucormycosis) and intravenous drug abuse (*Candida* endocarditis and basal ganglia mucormycosis).

Culture for fungus and histopathologic studies using special stains of infected body fluids (sputum, blood, urine, and cerebrospinal fluid [CSF]) and tissues (skin, lung, liver, bone marrow, and lymph nodes) are the mainstays of diagnosis of the mycoses. If fungal disease is suspected, the microbiology laboratory should be alerted to use appropriate culture media. For example, the likelihood of recovering fungi in blood cultures is enhanced by using the lysis centrifugation method. Skin testing with fungal antigens has no place in the diagnosis of individual infections, although skin tests are useful as indicators of prior infection in epidemiologic studies of prevalence. Although most serologic tests for mycoses have limited value in diagnosis because of either low sensitivity and specificity or poor standardization of assay reagents and methods, there are exceptions. A positive latex agglutination test for cryptococcal antigen in CSF or blood is a highly reliable indicator of cryptococcal disease; similarly, a positive titer for complement-fixing antibody in serum or CSF is a reliable marker of coccidioidal disease. Widely available serologic tests that are both sensitive and specific would be very useful in the diagnosis of invasive aspergillosis and candidiasis.

Table 347–3 shows the currently available classes of antifungal drugs, with examples of each class and their mechanisms of action. Although amphotericin B remains the standard of therapy for many systemic fungal diseases, especially serious life-threatening infec-

TABLE 347–1. COMMON SYSTEM MYCOSES

Disease	Causative Fungus
Aspergillosis	*Aspergillus* species
Zygomycosis (mucormycosis)	*Mucor* and *Rhizopus* species
Candidiasis	*Candida* species
Cryptococcosis	*Cryptococcus neoformans*
Blastomycosis	*Blastomyces dermatitidis*
Coccidioidomycosis	*Coccidioides immitis*
Histoplasmosis	*Histoplasma capsulatum*
Paracoccidioidomycosis	*Paracoccidioides brasiliensis*
Sporotrichosis	*Sporothrix schenckii*

TABLE 347–2. ALTERED HOST DEFENSE AND OPPORTUNISTIC FUNGAL DISEASE

Alteration in Host Defense	Opportunistic Fungal Disease
Interruption of mechanical barriers or indwelling foreign bodies	Candidiasis (invasive)
Granulocyte dysfunction (quantitative or qualitative)	Aspergillosis Candidiasis Zygomycosis
Depressed cell-mediated immunity	Aspergillosis Candidiasis (mucosal) Coccidioidomycosis Cryptococcosis Histoplasmosis

TABLE 347–3. CURRENTLY AVAILABLE DRUGS FOR THERAPY OF SYSTEMIC MYCOSES BY CLASS AND MECHANISM OF ACTION

Class of Antifungal Drug with Examples	Mechanism of Action

Polyene
  Nystatin
  Amphotericin B
	Binds irreversibly to ergosterol, resulting in increased permeability of cell membrane with leakage of intracellular contents

Azole
  Clotrimazole
  Miconazole
  Ketoconazole
  Fluconazole
  Itraconazole
	Blocks synthesis of ergosterol via inhibition of cytochrome P-450 dependent enzyme, 14α-demethylase

Substituted pyrimidine Flucytosine	Inhibits both DNA and protein synthesis

tions in immunocompromised patients, this drug has two principal disadvantages—it must be administered intravenously and it is associated with a high toxicity profile, including azotemia, hypokalemia, and bone marrow suppression. Over the past two decades, much progress in antifungal therapy has been made, especially with regard to antifungal azoles. Miconazole, the first of this class of drugs and a parenteral preparation, is highly toxic and therefore of limited usefulness. The licensing of three orally administered azoles, ketoconazole (imidazole) in 1981, fluconazole (triazole) in 1990, and itraconazole (triazole) in 1992, represented a major breakthrough. Fluconazole possesses several pharmacologic advantages over ketoconazole and itraconazole, including availability as either an oral or parenteral formulation, significant urinary excretion of active drug, and excellent penetration into CSF (60 to 80% of plasma concentrations). In addition, the two triazoles, fluconazole and itraconazole, are better tolerated and less toxic than ketoconazole and are not associated with clinically significant suppression of endogenous steroid synthesis in humans, as is ketoconazole.

The only other antifungal drug currently approved for treating systemic mycoses is flucytosine, an oral preparation, which is often used in combination with amphotericin B to provide a synergistic effect against *C. neoformans* and *Candida* species and sometimes used alone as therapy for chromomycosis. Unfortunately, flucytosine is potentially toxic to the bone marrow and liver; in addition, its use, especially as a single agent, may be associated with rapid emergence of resistant organisms.

Several lipid formulations of amphotericin B, either encapsulated in liposomes or complexed with lipids, are currently in phase II and III clinical trials; these formulations include liposomal amphotericin B (Ambisome), colloidal dispersion of amphotericin B (Amphocil), amphotericin B lipid complex (ABLC), and amphotericin B intralipid. Preliminary evidence indicates that these investigational lipid preparations may offer advantages over currently available amphotericin B (Fungizone), including less toxicity, increased tropism for reticuloendothelial organs, and increased dosing of active drug.

Como JA, Dismukes WE: Oral azole drugs as systemic antifungal therapy. N Engl J Med 330:263, 1994. *An up-to-date review of the pharmacology, spectrum of activity and resistance, adverse effects, drug interactions, and clinical indications of the available oral azole drugs (118 references).*

Gallis HA, Drew RH, Pickard WW: Amphotericin B: 30 years of clinical experience. Rev Infect Dis 12:308, 1990. *A practical review of the pharmacology, clinical uses, and adverse effects of amphotericin B, the most important intravenous antifungal agent (190 references).*

Kwon-Chung KJ, Bennett JE (eds.): Medical Mycology. Philadelphia, Lea & Febiger, 1992. *An exhaustive, well-illustrated text that considers all fungal pathogens and their diseases, including the common and uncommon.*

348 HISTOPLASMOSIS
William E. Dismukes

DEFINITION. Histoplasmosis, the most common endemic systemic mycosis in the United States, is associated with a variety of clinical syndromes, the most frequent of which is an asymptomatic or self-limited influenza-like respiratory infection. Less frequently, histoplasmosis manifests as chronic cavitary pulmonary disease, progressive disseminated disease involving multiple organs, or immune-mediated disease of the mediastinum or eye.

HISTOPLASMOSIS	
Causative fungus	*Histoplasma capsulatum*
Primary geographic distribution	Worldwide; endemic in North and South Central United States
Primary route of acquisition	Respiratory (inhalation of spores)
Principal sites of disease	Lungs, lymph nodes, liver, spleen, bone marrow, adrenal glands, gastrointestinal tract
Opportunistic infection in compromised hosts	Frequent, especially in AIDS patients
Drug of choice for most patients	Itraconazole
Alternative therapy	Amphotericin B, ketoconazole, or fluconazole

ETIOLOGY. *Histoplasma capsulatum* is the imperfect state of a dimorphic fungus that grows as a mycelial form at temperatures below 35°C in the laboratory and in soil, its natural habitat, and as a yeast form at 37°C and in infected hosts. The perfect state is *Ajellomyces capsulatus.* The mycelial form bears two types of infectious spores, macroconidia and microconidia, both of which are readily airborne, but the smaller microconidia (2 to 6 μm versus 8 to 14 μm) more easily reach alveoli or small bronchioles upon inhalation. The oval yeast cells (2 to 3 $\times$ 3 to 4 μm) reproduce by single narrow-based buds, are unencapsulated, and are usually found within macrophages in viable tissue. A variant strain, *H. capsulatum* var. *duboisii,* which is found solely in Central Africa, is characterized by a larger yeast form (7 to 15 μm).

EPIDEMIOLOGY. Results of skin test surveys using histoplasmin antigen indicate that histoplasmosis is worldwide in distribution, with greatest prevalence in tropical and temperate zones. The disease is endemic in the South Central and North Central United States, especially along the Mississippi, Tennessee, Missouri, Ohio, and St. Lawrence River basins. A high prevalence has also been noted in selected areas of the eastern United States. In these endemic areas, over 80% of persons are infected by age 20. *H. capsulatum* can be readily recovered from soil, especially that enriched by bird and bat guano. Because of high body temperatures, birds are not infected, whereas bats are. Soil contaminated by chicken, pigeon, blackbird, or starling droppings and areas frequented by bats, such as caves, hollow trees, old buildings, and attics, are frequently identified sources of outbreaks. The disturbance of soil or sites by wind, bulldozing, demolition, or other construction-related activities may greatly increase the number of airborne spores and result in exposure of both nearby and distantly located persons. Although *H. capsulatum* is more prevalent in bird- or bat-related microenvironments, aerosolized microconidia are commonly present as "air pollutants" in endemic areas and may account for the majority of sporadic infections.

Pulmonary infection does not convey protective immunity; consequently, reinfection may occur. Person-to-person transmission of histoplasmosis is not known to occur. Although age, gender, and race do not significantly affect susceptibility to infection, middle-aged white men with pre-existing chronic obstructive pulmonary disease (COPD) appear to be at highest risk of developing chronic pulmonary histoplasmosis. Over recent years, *H. capsulatum* has emerged as an opportunistic fungal pathogen, especially in hosts with altered cellular immunity secondary to organ transplantation, corticosteroid or cytotoxic drugs, or infection with human immunodeficiency virus (HIV). In some endemic areas, disseminated histoplasmosis is the most common acquired immunodeficiency syndrome (AIDS)–defining opportunistic infection.

PATHOGENESIS AND PATHOLOGY. Aerosolized microconidia of *H. capsulatum,* after being inhaled into the lungs, undergo transformation into yeast forms at body temperature and are promptly phagocytized by macrophages. In nonimmune persons, macrophages are initially unable to kill the yeasts, which multiply intracellularly.

These infected macrophages migrate to the mediastinal lymph nodes and to other organs of the mononuclear phagocyte system (reticuloendothelial system) such as the spleen. Recent evidence indicates that L3T4+ cells are a critical determinant of an effective host response to *H. capsulatum.* In normal hosts, once antigen-specific cellular immunity becomes established, infection is usually contained by a sequence of events including a vasculitic response, granuloma formation with caseation necrosis, enlargement of regional lymph nodes followed by fibrosis, and ultimately, calcification. In contrast, in persons with impaired cell-mediated immunity, the mononuclear phagocyte system is unable to contain the infection and viable *H. capsulatum* organisms disseminate widely to macrophage-rich tissues, including liver, spleen, visceral lymph nodes, and bone marrow. In these individuals, because normal reaction of host tissue to parasitized macrophages is either minimal or absent, infection goes unchecked and progressive disseminated disease ensues. The pathogenesis of mediastinal fibrosis and ocular histoplasmosis, two uncommon but clinically significant complications of infection with *H. capsulatum,* is presumed to be immune mediated, at least in part. Mediastinal fibrosis appears to develop in hypersensitive persons with a large antigen load in caseous mediastinal nodes. Exuberant fibrous encapsulation of nodes and adjacent tissues may lead to bronchial or vascular occlusion or erosion.

In histopathologic specimens stained with periodic acid–Schiff (PAS), Giemsa, or Gomori methenamine silver (GMS), the characteristic ovoid yeast forms of *H. capsulatum,* surrounded by a clear space resembling a capsule but actually due to fixation artifact, are generally found in macrophages. Organisms are more difficult to visualize in tissue stained with hematoxylin-eosin. The likelihood of identifying organisms in tissue sections is directly related to the effectiveness of cellular immunity in a given host. In immune individuals with an intact host defense, fungi are rare, granuloma formation is well developed, and extent of disease is limited. By contrast, in compromised hosts with impaired cellular immunity, macrophages, including those in peripheral blood, are filled with intracellular yeasts, granulomas are poorly developed or absent, and disease is extensive.

CLINICAL MANIFESTATIONS. Pulmonary disease in histoplasmosis is conveniently classified into acute and chronic forms. Acute disease, which results from primary infection, most often resolves spontaneously but may be associated with early and late complications.

Acute Pulmonary Infection. The vast majority of primary infections with *H. capsulatum* are either asymptomatic or associated with a flulike illness, manifested by fever, chills, headache, nonproductive cough, pleuritic or substernal chest pain, malaise, and myalgias. The incubation period and severity of illness are directly related to the inoculum of inhaled spores and the prior immune status of the individual. In nonimmune persons with a heavy exposure, respiratory symptoms tend to be more severe and progressive and include severe dyspnea. A normal chest radiograph is most common, but abnormalities range from one or two patchy infiltrates, with or without mediastinal and hilar adenopathy, to diffuse miliary opacities, which frequently heal in a pattern of "buckshot" calcifications. Pleural effusion and cavitation are uncommon. Extrapulmonary symptoms and signs, including arthralgias, erythema nodosum, and erythema multiforme, may be present, especially in young women. Early and late complications of acute or primary pulmonary infection may result from vigorous host reactions causing enlarged mediastinal or hilar nodes and exuberant encapsulating fibrosis, which in turn lead to compression or erosion of adjacent mediastinal structures. These rare complications include acute pericarditis; tracheal, bronchial, or esophageal obstruction; esophageal diverticuli; bronchoesophageal fistula; broncholithiasis (secondary to erosion of a calcification into a bronchus); mediastinal granuloma; mediastinal fibrosis or fibrosing mediastinitis; and enlarging histoplasmoma (usually located in the peripheral lung parenchyma and recognized by concentric laminations of calcium). Mediastinal granuloma, which tends to develop more often in the right paratracheal area, is more circumscribed, smaller in size, and associated with fewer sequelae than is mediastinal fibrosis. Both entities are recognized causes of superior vena cava syndrome.

Chronic Pulmonary Infection. Chronic pulmonary histoplasmosis often resembles pulmonary tuberculosis in symptomatology and radiographic manifestations, although the course of this type of histoplasmosis tends to be milder and more indolent than that of tuberculosis. The pathogenesis and course of chronic pulmonary histoplasmosis are highly complex; pathologic studies indicate two basic lesions. An interstitial pneumonitis is characteristic of the early lesion, whereas the chronic lesion is manifested by organization of diseased tissue, with prominence of giant cells and progressive cavitation. In the thicker-walled cavities, infection is persistent, with continuing necrosis, leading to progressive cavity enlargement (marching cavity) at the expense of the surrounding lung parenchyma. In general, the symptoms and roentgenographic findings reflect the two types or stages of disease, namely, pneumonitis and progressive cavitation. Although symptoms overlap, they tend to be more abrupt in onset, with more severe constitutional symptoms, such as fever, night sweats, and malaise, in the pneumonitis stage; hemoptysis and progressive dyspnea are more typical of the cavitation stage. In 80% of cases, the pneumonitis stage tends to resolve spontaneously over 2 to 3 months, with a small fibrotic residuum, whereas the cavitation stage, especially that associated with thick-walled cavities, tends to be relentlessly progressive, leading to destruction and diminution of lung parenchyma, fibrosis, and, eventually, respiratory insufficiency.

Disseminated Histoplasmosis. This less common form of histoplasmosis develops primarily in persons with defective host immunity, including infants with immature immune systems; compromised hosts, such as corticosteroid-treated organ recipients and HIV-infected persons; and individuals with either no measurable defect or a highly selective defect, such as the failure of host lymphocytes to undergo *in vitro* blast transformation upon exposure to *H. capsulatum* antigen. The severity of the symptoms and signs of disseminated disease and the attendant histopathologic findings in a given patient mirror the level of immunocompetence of the individual. For example, in patients with the mildest and most chronic forms of disseminated disease, well-developed tuberculoid granulomas, typical of the response in normal hosts, can be found in reticuloendothelial tissues. In contrast, in patients with overwhelming multiorgan histoplasmosis superimposed on a severely immunocompromising condition, such as AIDS, the host response is suboptimal, with the pathologic findings consisting of large numbers of diffusely scattered macrophages filled with yeast forms and minimal or no granuloma formation.

Fever, chills, and other nonspecific constitutional symptoms, including malaise and weight loss, predominate. On initial presentation, many patients satisfy criteria for fever of unknown origin. Enlargement of liver and spleen is common; less frequently, peripheral lymphadenopathy is present. Mucous membrane ulceration, especially of the oropharynx, occurs in about 25 to 75% of patients with subacute disease and should alert the physician to the possibility of histoplasmosis. Laboratory clues may include anemia, leukopenia and thrombocytopenia as evidence of impaired bone marrow function or replacement of the marrow, elevated alkaline phosphatase levels, elevated erythrocyte sedimentation rate, and electrolyte abnormalities suggestive of adrenal insufficiency. In some patients, adrenal hypofunction may not be clinically manifest until years later. Chest radiographs may be normal or show findings suggestive of earlier primary infection or an interstitial pneumonitis consistent with hematogenous spread of infection. Unusual syndromes, including cardiac involvement with culture-negative endocarditis associated with large emboli, gastrointestinal involvement with bleeding secondary to mucosal ulceration, or central nervous system (CNS) involvement with chronic lymphocytic meningitis, occasionally dominate the clinical course. Cutaneous lesions, manifested by diffusely scattered papulonodules on an erythematous base, and CNS disease are more likely in HIV-positive persons. In some AIDS patients, disseminated histoplasmosis represents reactivation of dormant foci, as evidenced by the development of symptoms and signs during a period of residence in a nonendemic area, years after having lived in an endemic region.

Ocular Histoplasmosis. Vision loss associated with the triad of punched-out choroidal lesions or "spots," macular neovascular membranes, and peripapillary atrophy or scarring, in the absence of inflammatory changes in the vitreous or anterior chamber, has been labeled presumed ocular histoplasmosis syndrome (POHS). Although no direct relationship to active ongoing infection with *H. capsulatum* has been established, POHS is believed to represent a localized hypersensitivity response to *Histoplasma* antigen. In almost all instances, the syndrome occurs in young adults with no evidence of pulmonary or disseminated histoplasmosis. Antifungal therapy, either systemic or intraocular, is not indicated. Laser photocoagulation appears to be the most beneficial therapeutic modality to prevent or reduce vision impairment.

DIAGNOSIS. The diagnostic approach varies in part with the clinical syndrome under consideration. Special features or presentations that should raise suspicion of histoplasmosis include atypical pneumonia syndrome that occurs in a resident of an endemic area, right paratracheal adenopathy, superior vena cava syndrome secondary to adenopathy or a mediastinal mass, an oral ulcer resembling carcinoma, chronic progressive upper lobe cavitation associated with negative sputum smears and cultures for tuberculosis, adrenal insufficiency, "buckshot" calcifications in the lungs or spleen, and persistent unexplained fever in an HIV-infected person. In most instances, diagnosis should be based on demonstrated *H. capsulatum* by culture or by histopathologic study of involved organs. The histoplasmin skin test, although important in epidemiologic studies, is not recommended for diagnostic purposes, owing to the high positivity rate among persons residing in endemic areas. In addition, the skin test may falsely elevate titers of serum antibodies.

Among the serologic tests to detect serum antibody to *H. capsulatum,* complement fixation is the most widely used. Although a titer of 1:32 or more or a fourfold rise in titer provides presumptive evidence of active infection, a negative or lower titer does not exclude histoplasmosis. Similarly, titers do not parallel disease activity, correlate with response to therapy, or predict outcome. Testing of serum by immunodiffusion to detect precipitin bands to M and H antigens appears to be a more specific but less sensitive serologic method than complement fixation. All antibody tests are associated with frequent false-positive reactions to *Histoplasma* antigens among patients with tuberculosis and other fungal diseases, especially blastomycosis and coccidioidomycosis. On the other hand, use of radioimmunoassay to detect *H. capsulatum* polysaccharide antigen in body fluids such as serum and urine provides a relatively sensitive and specific marker of disseminated histoplasmosis. Antigen levels fall with treatment; consequently, this test is useful for both diagnosing and evaluating the response to therapy.

The diagnosis of primary pulmonary histoplasmosis should be suspected on the basis of clinical, radiographic, and epidemiologic clues, e.g., an acute febrile respiratory illness accompanied by scattered patchy infiltrates and hilar adenopathy in an individual with high risk of exposure to *Histoplasma* spores. An elevated complement fixation titer and/or precipitin bands in serum provide presumptive evidence. Whereas sputum cultures are rarely positive (only 10 to 20%) in primary pulmonary disease, the likelihood of positive sputum cultures is significantly higher in chronic pulmonary histoplasmosis. Among patients with chronic disease, about 60% with marching thick-walled cavities have positive cultures, and a significant percentage of these also have positive smears of stained sputum. Although serologic tests for antibody are only moderately helpful (positive results in only 50% of cases), an elevated complement fixation titer in a patient with characteristic radiographic findings provides strong supportive evidence. Definitive diagnosis of chronic pulmonary histoplasmosis must be based on a positive sputum culture or smear or on histopathologic studies and special stains of lung tissue obtained by bronchoscopy.

The diagnosis of disseminated histoplasmosis depends on either demonstrating intracellular yeast forms by histopathologic study or a positive culture of blood, bone marrow, lymph node, skin or mu-

cous membrane, liver, lung, or other involved site. A Wright-stained smear of peripheral blood is positive in >50% of acute or subacute cases. If possible, serum and urine should be examined for *H. capsulatum* antigen by radioimmunoassay. The cerebrospinal fluid of patients with chronic unexplained culture-negative lymphocytic meningitis should be tested for antigen and antibodies to *H. capsulatum.*

TREATMENT. For most patients with primary pulmonary histoplasmosis, no antifungal therapy is necessary. For those with severe or progressive primary infection, short-course intravenous amphotericin B (around 1000 mg total dose), oral ketoconazole, (400 mg daily for 3 to 6 months) or oral itraconazole, (200 to 400 mg daily for 3 to 6 months) is recommended, although none of these regimens has been prospectively evaluated in this setting. The treatment of chronic pulmonary histoplasmosis is even less standardized, in large part owing to the relative difficulty in clinically and radiologically distinguishing the pneumonitic and cavitary stages of disease. Although the early pneumonitic form of chronic pulmonary disease has been reported to resolve spontaneously in 80% of cases, rest and inactivity clearly promote healing. Traditionally, antifungal therapy has been advocated only for patients with progressive or marching cavitary disease, manifested by persistent or enlarging, thick-walled, >2 mm cavities. Amphotericin B (total dose 2.0 to 2.5 grams), ketoconazole (400 mg daily for at least 6 months), or itraconazole (200 to 400 mg daily for 6 to 9 months) is effective therapy. There may be merit in liberalizing criteria for treatment in patients with chronic pulmonary disease. Rather than reserving therapy only for patients with advanced cavitary disease, some authorities suggest that oral ketoconazole or itraconazole may be indicated for all patients with chronic pulmonary disease, regardless of the stage. Although itraconazole is better tolerated and less toxic, ketoconazole is less expensive.

In contrast to the somewhat controversial guidelines regarding therapy of pulmonary histoplasmosis, there is no question that all patients with disseminated histoplasmosis should be treated. For patients with severe life-threatening disease, immunocompromised hosts such as organ transplant recipients or corticosteroid-treated patients, and the rare patients with CNS or cardiac histoplasmosis, amphotericin B total dose (2.0 to 2.5 grams) is the drug of choice. Itraconazole, 200 to 400 mg daily for 6 to 12 months, is an effective alternative in immunocompetent patients with mild to moderate disease. Experience over the past decade with disseminated histoplasmosis in AIDS patients indicates that an aggressive approach to treatment is necessary in an attempt to prevent relapse. For AIDS patients with moderate to severe or life-threatening disease, intensive "induction" primary therapy with intravenous amphotericin B (total dose 1.0 to 2.0 grams) should be used to gain control of disease and reduce the organism load. For AIDS patients with milder disease, itraconazole (200 mg twice daily for 10 to 12 weeks) is highly effective primary therapy; fluconazole (400 to 800 mg daily) may be an effective alternative. Regardless of which primary therapy regimen is used, lifelong maintenance or suppressive therapy is required to prevent histoplasmosis relapse in patients with AIDS. At present, itraconazole (200 mg twice daily) is the drug of choice. In patients who cannot take itraconazole because of intolerance or drug interaction, fluconazole (200 to 400 mg daily) can be used. Ketoconazole is an inadequate primary or maintenance therapy in patients with AIDS. The approach of initiating therapy with intravenous amphotericin B and completing it with an oral agent may prove applicable to selected other patients with either chronic pulmonary or disseminated histoplasmosis.

The management of mediastinal fibrosis presumed secondary to *H. capsulatum* infection is largely unsatisfactory, as evidenced by progressive morbidity in many patients and a mortality rate of at least 30%. Antifungal chemotherapy is generally not recommended. In selected cases, surgical extirpation may be beneficial in alleviating entrapment or obstructive syndromes.

PROGNOSIS. Although primary pulmonary histoplasmosis may be associated with acute or chronic intrathoracic complications, this form of disease is usually self-limited. In contrast, chronic cavitary pulmonary histoplasmosis is usually progressive, resulting in respiratory insufficiency and death. Disseminated histoplasmosis is variable in its severity and course, depending on the immune status of the host. Although a single course of therapy may be curative in some patients, long-term maintenance therapy to prevent relapse is required in others, especially patients with AIDS.

Dismukes WE, Bradsher RW Jr, Cloud GC, et al.: Itraconazole therapy for blastomycosis and histoplasmosis. Am J Med 93:489, 1992. *In a prospective, nonrandomized open trial among 35 patients with non–life-threatening, nonmeningeal histoplasmosis treated for 2 or more months with itraconazole, the success rate was 86%.*

Wheat LJ: Diagnosis and management of histoplasmosis. Eur J Clin Microbiol Infect Dis 8:480, 1989. *A comprehensive review that includes an excellent perspective on the currently available serologic tests used to detect either antibody or antigen; includes 78 references.*

Wheat LJ, Connolly-Stringfield PA, Baker RL, et al.: Disseminated histoplasmosis in the acquired immune deficiency syndrome: Clinical findings, diagnosis and treatment, and review of the literature. Medicine (Baltimore) 69:361, 1990. *An informative review of disseminated histoplasmosis, a common opportunistic disease among AIDS patients living in or with history of exposure to the endemic area.*

Wheat LJ, Hafner R, Wulfsohn M, et al.: Prevention of relapse of histoplasmosis with itraconazole in patients with the acquired immunodeficiency syndrome. Ann Intern Med 118:610, 1993. *Results of this prospective, multicenter, open-label clinical trial indicate that itraconazole is safe and effective in preventing relapse of disseminated histoplasmosis in patients with AIDS.*

349 COCCIDIOIDOMYCOSIS

John N. Galgiani

DEFINITION. Coccidioidomycosis is a systemic infection due to the fungus, *Coccidioides immitis,* endemic to some deserts of the Western Hemisphere.

COCCIDIOIDOMYCOSIS

Causative fungus	*Coccidioides immitis*
Primary geographic distribution	Lower Sonoran deserts of the Western Hemisphere, including parts of Arizona, California, New Mexico, west Texas, and parts of Central and South America
Primary route of acquisition	Respiratory (inhalation of arthroconidia)
Principal site of disease	Lungs most common; spread to skin, bones, meninges, and other viscera uncommon but serious
Opportunistic infection in compromised hosts	Diffuse pneumonia and widespread infections common in patients with T lymphocyte defects or during high-dose corticosteroid therapy
Drug of choice for most patients	Usually no treatment required for primary pneumonia; usually fluconazole or itraconazole for extrapulmonary disease
Alternative therapy	Amphotericin B (especially with diffuse pneumonia); ketoconazole

ETIOLOGY. *C. immitis* is a dimorphic fungus that is classified as an ascomycete by ribosomal gene homology. In its vegetative state, mycelia with true septations mature to produce arthroconidia, single cells approximately 2 to 5 μm in size. After infection, an arthroconidium enlarges to as much as 75 μm in diameter as a spherule, undergoing internal septation to produce scores of endospores. When spherules rupture, packets of endospores are released, and these produce more spherules in infected tissue or revert to mycelia if removed from the body.

EPIDEMIOLOGY. *C. immitis* can be recovered from the soil of the low deserts of Arizona; the Central Valley of California; parts of other states, including New Mexico and Texas; and parts of Central and South America. Endemic regions follow the climatologic Sonoran life zone, which is characterized by modest rainfall, mild winters, and low humidity. *C. immitis* grows in a soil layer a few centimeters below the surface, and disruption of the dirt by windstorms or construction equipment increases the release of fungal particles into the air. The risk of exposure increases during dry months that follow rainy seasons. Primary infection outside the endemic regions occurs rarely from exposure to contaminated bales of cotton or other fomites. Person-to-person transmission of pulmonary infection has not been reported, and isolation precautions are unnecessary.

INCIDENCE AND PREVALENCE. Using dermal hypersensitivity to coccidioidal antigens as an indicator of prior infection, the annual conversion rate within strongly endemic areas is normally 3%, representing 50,000 to 100,000 new infections and producing an incidence of approximately 60% within the general population. However, in the years 1990 to 1994, the number of clinically diagnosed infections was manyfold larger than in past years; in situations where exposure is unusually intense, such as at archeology sites or during military maneuvers within endemic regions, infections can develop in the majority of persons exposed for only a matter of days.

PATHOGENESIS AND PATHOLOGY. Virtually all coccidioidal infections are the result of inhaling arthroconidia into the lung. Within the small airways, proliferation engenders both acute inflammation, including eosinophils, associated with spherule rupture, and granulomatous inflammation, associated with mature, intact spherules. Focal pneumonia is often associated with ipsilateral hilar adenopathy, and less frequently, infection enlarges peritracheal, supraclavicular, and cervical nodes. Lesions occurring elsewhere are the result of hematogenous dissemination and usually develop within months of the initial infection. Although progressive dissemination results from < 1% of infections, as many as 8% of persons with self-limited infection develop chorioretinal scars, suggesting that subclinical hematogenous spread may be frequent. Within weeks after infection, durable T-cell immunity normally arrests fungal proliferation, allowing inflammation to resolve and preventing reinfection in the future. However, control of the infection may not completely sterilize lesions, and reactivation of dormant infection or second infections is possible in patients whose cell-mediated immunity becomes deficient.

CLINICAL MANIFESTATIONS. At least two of every three infections are detected only by finding dermal hypersensitivity to coccidioidal antigens. Those who become ill usually experience a self-limited pulmonary syndrome. However, a minority of patients develop complications or progressive forms of infection that display a broad variety of manifestations and pose difficult problems for the clinician.

Primary Pulmonary Infections. Five to 21 days after exposure, symptoms develop; these may include fever, weight loss, fatigue, a dry cough, or pleuritic chest pain, and they are difficult to differentiate from those caused by other respiratory pathogens. Arthralgia without associated joint effusions is also frequent. Skin manifestations may also occur as a short-lived nonpuritic maculopapular rash, erythema multiforme, or erythema nodosum. The arthritic and dermatologic manifestations are thought to be mediated by circulating immune complexes or other immunologic phenomena and are referred to as "desert rheumatism." Radiographs of the chest may show no abnormalities or may demonstrate pulmonary infiltrates, either segmental or lobar. Hilar adenopathy is often a distinctive finding. Peripneumonic pleural effusions may occur and usually resolve without intervention, even though *C. immitis* is usually recoverable from the pleura. Eosinophilia is frequently a prominent finding in differential leukocyte counts of peripheral blood, and the erythrocyte sedimentation rate is usually elevated. Symptoms may persist for several weeks before improvement is clearly under way, and the illness, especially lassitude, may persist for months.

The primary pulmonary process produces a variety of sequelae. The most frequent is the development of a pulmonary nodule (Fig. 349–1), typically measuring 1 to 4 cm and lying within 5 cm of the hilus. Despite their harmless nature, coccidioidal nodules may engender concern because of their similarity to a malignant mass. For this reason, management usually requires percutaneous needle aspiration or resection. Another consequence of pulmonary coccidioidomycosis is cavitation of the infiltrate, which occurs in approximately 5% of pneumonias. Cavities are usually single, thin walled, in an upper lobe, and close to the pleura; they may cause pain, produce hemoptysis, or develop associated infiltrates. Infrequently a

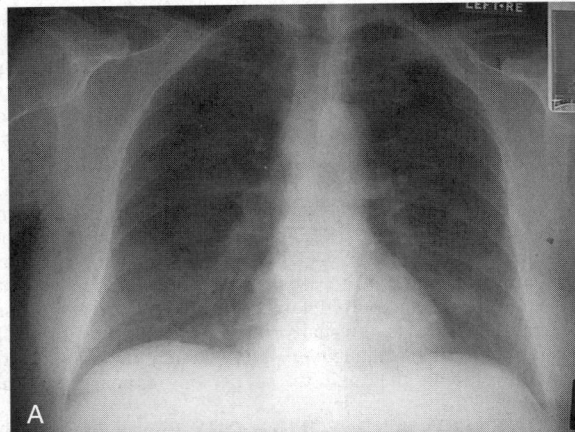

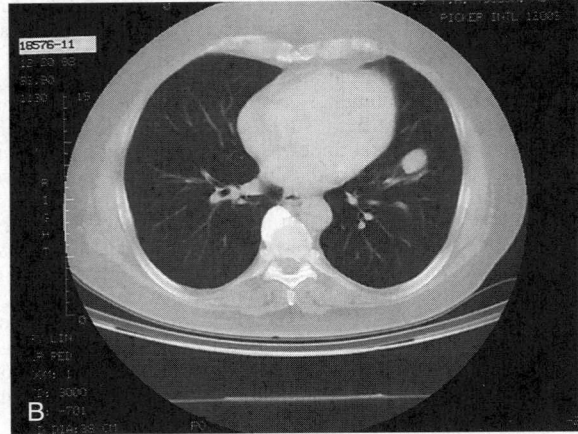

FIGURE 349–1. *A,* Benign nodule due to coccidioidomycosis. *B,* Computed tomographic image of the nodule in *A.*

cavity ruptures, forming a pyopneumothorax. This usually is the first symptom of coccidioidal infection and commonly occurs in otherwise healthy young males. An air-fluid level, detectable by roentgenography in the pleural space, often helps differentiate this problem from a spontaneous pneumothorax. Surgical resection of the cavity with closure of the bronchopleural fistula is the preferred treatment for this complication. The least common pulmonary complication is persistent fibrocavitary infection that progresses from involvement of lobes to involvement of both lungs.

Extrapulmonary Dissemination. Coccidioidomycosis usually results in dissemination beyond the lungs in immunosuppressed patients, such as organ recipients or those with AIDS or lymphoma. However, some patients have no underlying disease and do not manifest heightened susceptibility to other infections. The most common locations for disseminated lesions are skin (cutaneous papules or subcutaneous nodules); joints (especially the knee); bones, including vertebrae; and the basilar meninges. Such infections may produce one or many lesions and frequently are subacute or chronic in their presentation. When infections are more fulminant, they are usually in broadly immunosuppressed patients and produce fungemia detectable with blood cultures and diffuse reticulonodular embolic pulmonary infiltrates. Although the kidneys and the urinary bladder are rarely involved, *C. immitis* may be recovered from concentrated specimens of urine, because of either transient fungemia or focal dissemination to the prostate. In contrast to histoplasmosis, the gastrointestinal tract is rarely involved in coccidioidomycosis.

DIAGNOSIS. The diagnosis is firmly established by recovering *C. immitis* from clinical specimens. On direct examination of respi- ratory specimens or tissue, spherules can be seen as large structures with refractile walls and internal organization and also on hematoxylin-eosin, silver, or periodic acid–Schiff stains of histologic preparations. The Gram stain does not detect spherules. In culture, mycelial growth is often evident within the first week of incubation. Except in the case of coccidioidal meningitis, in which cerebrospinal fluid (CSF) cultures are usually negative, isolation of the fungus is nearly always possible in patients with infections sufficiently severe to warrant therapy. In contrast, recovery of *C. immitis* may be difficult in patients who have only scant respiratory secretions associated with the initial pneumonia.

A presumptive diagnosis of coccidioidal infection is often based on detecting specific antibodies in serum. Within the first weeks of initial infections, a precipitin-type antibody is detected, usually by immunodiffusion techniques. Later, complement fixing (CF)-type antibodies usually appear. When reported quantitatively, CF antibodies generally are found to be highest in the most extensive infections and to decrease in concentration in patients whose infections are controlled. An important means of diagnosing coccidioidal meningitis is by detection of CF antibodies in the CSF, along with other abnormalities, such as leukocytosis, elevated protein concentration, or low glucose concentration.

TREATMENT. Because the primary infection is usually self-limited, treatment has been limited to patients with progressive illness. This was typical when amphotericin B was the only effective therapy and still remains a rational approach despite the advent of other agents, since none has been shown to either hasten the resolution of initial symptoms or prevent subsequent complications. Amphotericin B has been used successfully in cumulative doses of 1.0 to 3.0 grams for treating all types of coccidioidomycosis. However, it has not been uniformly effective and frequently has produced treatment-limiting morbidity and toxicity. Binding amphotericin B in liposomes or lipid complexes is being explored as a means of improving the therapeutic to toxic profile. Treatment of coccidioidal meningitis has necessitated intrathecal administration, which imposes additional toxicity and risks.

Azole antifungals have expanded the alternatives for treating coccidioidomycosis. Ketoconazole is orally effective and less toxic therapy than amphotericin B, but absorption is variable, gastrointestinal intolerance is frequent, and signs of dose-dependent suppression of steroidogenesis occur in some patients. More recently, two triazoles, fluconazole and itraconazole, have demonstrated efficacy without hormonal suppression. Fluconazole is also efficacious in the treatment of meningitis. Unfortunately, cessation of therapy often is followed by recurrence of lesions and therefore protracted, and in some patients continuous courses of therapy are needed to maintain control.

PROGNOSIS. After resolution of the initial infection, most patients maintain lifelong immunity, and second infections are very infrequent. Similarly, late recurrence is unlikely in the absence of intercurrent profound immunosuppression. In those in whom the initial infection cannot be resolved, the disease frequently follows a protracted course. Although infection is more debilitating than fatal, fulminant respiratory failure can occur, and if untreated, coccidioidal meningitis is nearly always fatal within 2 years.

Ampel NM, Dols CL, Galgiani JN: Coccidioidomycosis during human immunodeficiency virus infection. Results of a prospective study in a coccidioidal endemic area. Am J Med 94:235, 1993. *Estimates that the risk of active infection within southern Arizona during a 41-month-period was between 8.2 and 41.1%. Risk factors for coccidioidal disease were low CD4 counts or other AIDS-defining illnesses but not a history of prior coccidioidomycosis or a positive skin test.*

Catanzaro A, Galgiani JN, Levine BE, et al.: Fluconazole in the treatment of chronic pulmonary and nonmeningeal disseminated Coccidioidomycosis. Am J Med 98:249, 1995. *Of 75 evaluable patients, 50 improved with 200 mg or 400 mg per day of fluconazole therapy. A comparison of fluconazole and itraconazole should be completed in 1996 by the Mycoses Study Group.*

Galgiani JN, Catanzaro A, Cloud GA, et al.: Fluconazole therapy for coccidioidal meningitis. Ann Intern Med 119:28, 1993. *In 50 patients treated with 400 mg per day of fluconazole as sole therapy for coccidioidal meningitis, overall response was 79%, which compares favorably with a response of 57% to intrathecal amphotericin B in earlier studies. However, even in patients who respond well to this therapy, the risk of relapse if fluconazole is stopped is probably greater than 60%.*

Pappagianis D, Zimmer BL: Serology of coccidioidomycosis. Clin Microbiol Rev 3:247, 1990. *Comprehensive review of diagnostic tests for coccidioidomycosis.*

350 BLASTOMYCOSIS

William E. Dismukes

DEFINITION. Blastomycosis (North American blastomycosis, Gilchrist's disease) is an endemic systemic mycosis that occurs primarily in noncompromised hosts. As with the other important endemic mycoses, such as coccidioidomycosis and histoplasmosis, infection follows inhalation of the aerosolized spore form of the fungus. Clinical disease most commonly involves the lungs, skin, skeletal system, and male genitourinary tract.

BLASTOMYCOSIS

Causative fungus	*Blastomyces dermatitidis*
Primary geographic distribution	Endemic in North and South Central United States
Primary route of acquisition	Respiratory (inhalation of spores)
Principal sites of disease	Lungs, skin, bone, joints, prostate gland
Opportunistic infection in compromised hosts	Infrequent
Drug of choice for most patients	Itraconazole
Alternative therapy	Amphotericin B, ketoconazole, or fluconazole

---

ETIOLOGY. *Blastomyces dermatitidis,* the imperfect or asexual state of *Ajellomyces dermatitidis,* is a dimorphic fungus, growing as a mycelial form in the environment and in the laboratory at room temperature and as a yeast form in mammalian tissue and in the laboratory at 37°C. The yeast cells, which are identical *in vitro* and *in vivo* in tissue and fluid specimens, vary from 8 to 15 μm in diameter, have a thick, highly refractile cell wall, and reproduce by single broad-based buds. In the laboratory, growth of *B. dermatitidis* is somewhat slow; mold colonies may not appear for 1 to 3 weeks.

EPIDEMIOLOGY. Because no sensitive and specific skin test exists, the epidemiology of blastomycosis is less well understood than that of coccidioidomycosis and histoplasmosis. The incidence of clinical disease as a manifestation of blastomycosis appears to be lower than the incidence of clinical disease associated with the two other endemic mycoses. The prevalence of subclinical blastomycosis is largely unknown. Isolated cases of blastomycosis have been reported worldwide, including Africa and Central and South America; however, the disease is concentrated or endemic in the South and North Central United States, especially in areas bordering the Mississippi and Ohio River basins, and the Great Lakes. In these endemic areas, small point-source outbreaks of blastomycosis have been associated with recreational or occupational activities in wooded areas along waterways. Current evidence indicates that *B. dermatitidis* exists in warm, moist soil enriched by organic debris, including decaying vegetation or wood. It is not surprising, therefore, that persons with occupational or avocational exposure to soil and the outdoors appear to be at highest risk of acquiring infection. Data from point-source outbreaks indicate that the median incubation period from exposure to infection is about 43 days. Animals, especially dogs and horses, are also susceptible to infection, which may progress to clinical disease. Among humans, clinical illness is most common among middle-aged men. Although *B. dermatitidis,* in contrast to the other dimorphic fungi, is a relatively uncommon opportunistic pathogen, studies over the past decade indicate that blastomycosis is being increasingly observed in immunocompromised hosts, e.g., corticosteroid- and cytotoxic drug-treated patients, organ transplant recipients, and AIDS patients. This observation suggests that reactivation blastomycosis may be more common than previously suspected.

PATHOGENESIS AND PATHOLOGY. Humans and animals, for the most part, acquire infection by inhaling aerosolized conidia that convert to the yeast form in the lungs at body temperature. Percutaneous inoculation of *B. dermatitidis* has been documented rarely, as a result of either a laboratory accident or a dog bite. The clinical manifestations of disease at body sites other than lung (and rarely skin) result from the hematogenous spread of organisms.

Cell-mediated immunity appears to be the most important arm of host defense against *B. dermatitidis.* Recent *in vivo* and *in vitro* studies indicate that macrophages, stimulated by lymphokines, are more effective in inhibiting or killing the organism than are granulocytes. A growth-inhibiting or protective role of humoral immunity in blastomycosis has not been established. The typical histopathologic picture of pulmonary blastomycosis and other nonmucocutaneous sites of disease consists of noncaseating granulomas as well as clusters of neutrophils. By contrast, cutaneous and mucous membrane lesions are characterized by pseudoepitheliomatous hyperplasia with microabscesses.

CLINICAL MANIFESTATIONS. In general, blastomycosis is a chronic indolent systemic fungal disease associated with a variety of pulmonary and extrapulmonary manifestations. Among the latter, cutaneous disease predominates, occurring in about 40 to 80% of cases. Multiple organ involvement occurs in approximately 50 to 60% of cases. Extrapulmonary disease may occur in the absence of clinical or radiologic evidence of lung disease.

Pulmonary. Although precise data are not available, most primary infections are believed to be either asymptomatic or unrecognized as being due to *B. dermatitidis* on the basis of nonspecific flulike symptoms. In patients with proven acute pulmonary blastomycosis, the radiologic findings usually consist of infiltrative or nodular air space opacities, most often in the lower lobes. Pulmonary blastomycosis usually manifests as a chronic pneumonia syndrome, characterized by productive cough, pleuritic chest pain, dyspnea, weight loss, and low-grade fever. Although there are no distinguishing radiologic characteristics, consolidation, one or more fibronodular infiltrates or mass lesions with or without cavitation, is common, often mimicking the findings in other granulomatous diseases or bronchogenic carcinoma. Although hilar adenopathy and pleural effusions occur, they are uncommon. Patients with overwhelming pulmonary blastomycosis may develop diffuse, bilateral, interstitial alveolar infiltrates on the chest radiograph and clinical evidence of acute respiratory distress syndrome.

Skin. The cutaneous lesions, which often prompt the patient with blastomycosis to seek medical evaluation initially, are of two general types, verrucous and ulcerative; both types tend to occur more commonly on exposed parts. The verrucous lesions, which begin as papulopustules, are more characteristic; these progress slowly over weeks to months to become crusted, heaped-up, and warty in appearance, often with a reddish-black or violaceous hue, an area of central healing and scarring, and a well-circumscribed outer border. Microabscesses, manifested by black dots on the surface, are typically located at the periphery of verrucous lesions; removing the crusted eschar often reveals purulent material in which the yeast form of the organism can be demonstrated by wet preparation. Ulcerative lesions overlying a bed of friable red granulation tissue are less common. Occasionally, mucosal ulcerations may be found in the mouth, nose, or larynx, mimicking the mucocutaneous lesions of histoplasmosis. Lymphadenopathy in the region corresponding to the skin lesion or lesions is distinctly uncommon in patients whose cutaneous disease is secondary to hematogenous spread of organisms from a primary pulmonary focus.

Other. After lung and skin disease, bone and joint involvement is next most common and is seen in 10 to 50% of cases. Osteolytic lesions, with or without sclerotic margins, are typically located in long bones and vertebrae. Often, patients with bone disease present as a result of overlying chronic draining sinuses or contiguous soft tissue lesions rather than bone pain. Septic arthritis, which is much less common than osteomyelitis, is frequently secondary to contiguous extension. Up to one third of men with blastomycosis have genitourinary tract disease, manifested most commonly by prostatic enlargement with obstructive symptoms and less frequently by epididymitis. Central nervous system (CNS) disease in the form of either granulomatous meningitis or a mass lesion (intracerebral blastomycoma) occurs in about 5% of cases. Clinically apparent blastomycotic involvement of other organs, e.g., gastrointestinal tract, liver, spleen, adrenals, and kidneys, is unusual, except in patients with fulminant disseminated disease.

DIAGNOSIS. As is true for all systemic mycotic diseases, the definitive diagnosis of blastomycosis requires a positive fungal culture from clinical specimens. A presumptive diagnosis may be based on the finding of characteristic yeast forms in a wet preparation of sputum, pus, or other body fluid or in a histopathologic section of tissue, e.g., skin, lung, bone, or prostate. *B. dermatitidis* in wet preparations of fluid specimens mixed with 10% KOH appears as a broad-based single budding yeast and in fixed-tissue specimens stained with hematoxylin-eosin or periodic acid–Schiff (PAS) reagents as single or budding yeast cells with a doubly refractile cell wall. Because a presumptive clinical diagnosis based on "characteristic" skin lesions or radiologic findings is associated with an unacceptably high error rate, obtaining fluids or tissue from involved sites for culture and histopathologic study is mandatory in the evaluation of all patients with suspected blastomycosis. Moreover, documented cutaneous and/or pulmonary disease should signal the possibility of bone or genitourinary disease and lead to appropriate diagnostic studies, such as bone scan and prostate examination and massage. As a diagnostic test, the blastomycin skin test lacks sensitivity and specificity and should not be used. Similarly, the complement fixation assay for serum antibody is highly cross-reactive and of no diagnostic value. Recent studies suggest that immunodiffusion, enzyme immunoassay, or radioimmunoassay tests for antibody to the A antigen of *B. dermatitidis* or antibody to other more purified antigens, e.g., 120 kD, are better serologic markers of disease.

TREATMENT. At present, three drugs, amphotericin B, ketoconazole, and itraconazole, are approved for the treatment of blastomycosis. Although intravenous amphotericin B has been traditionally considered the drug of choice for all forms of disease, studies and experience gained over recent years indicate that the oral azoles, ketoconazole and itraconazole, are highly effective, especially in patients with chronic indolent disease and noninvolvement of the CNS. Ketoconazole should be initiated at a dosage of 400 mg per day, advanced by 200-mg increments at monthly intervals, up to a maximum of 800 mg per day in patients with progressive disease, and continued for a minimum of 6 months. Itraconazole in a dose of 200 to 400 mg per day for 6 months or longer is even more effective than ketoconazole (90 to 95% success rate versus 80%) and associated with less toxicity. Accordingly, itraconazole is considered the drug of choice for most patients with blastomycosis. However, itraconazole is more expensive than ketoconazole. Fluconazole, at usual therapeutic doses of 200 to 400 mg per day, is not as effective as ketoconazole or itraconazole. Higher doses of fluconazole, which are associated with higher costs and increased potential for toxicity, appear necessary for cure. Amphotericin B, a total dose of 1.5 to 2.5 grams, should be reserved for patients with overwhelming life-threatening or CNS disease, those rare patients who are immunocompromised, and those in whom oral azole therapy has failed. In selected situations, some investigators advocate an induction course of amphotericin B (total dose of approximately 500 mg) for a rapid fungicidal effect to gain control of disease, followed by maintenance or "consolidation" therapy with ketoconazole or itraconazole for 3 to 6 months. Although controversy exists about whether or not to treat patients with acute pulmonary blastomycosis who are identified as part of point-source outbreaks, available data suggest that most such patients do not require therapy. However, careful long-term follow-up of untreated patients is important to monitor for evidence of disease activity.

PROGNOSIS. In contrast to the past, now most patients with blastomycosis are identified and treated before the development of overwhelming or fatal disease. Antifungal therapy with either amphotericin B or an oral azole drug is associated with cure rates of ≥80% and relapse rates of <10%.

Brown LR, Swensen SJ, Van Scoy RE, et al.: Roentgenologic features of pulmonary blastomycosis. Mayo Clin Proc 66:29, 1991. *A well-illustrated description of the varied radiographic findings in pulmonary blastomycosis. Consolidation and mass patterns are most common, whereas hilar adenopathy and pleural effusion are rare.*

Dismukes WE, Bradsher RW Jr, Cloud GC, et al.: Itraconazole therapy for blastomycosis and histoplasmosis. Am J Med 93:489, 1992. *In a prospective, nonrandomized open trial, the success rate for 40 patients with non–life-threatening, nonmeningeal blastomycosis treated with itraconazole for more than 2 months was 95%.*

Klein BS, Vergeront JM, Davis JP: Epidemiologic aspects of blastomycosis, the enigmatic systemic mycosis. Semin Respir Infect 1:29, 1986. *A valuable review that focuses on seven point-source epidemics and the ecologic niche of the organism.*

Meyer KC, McManus EJ, Maki DG: Overwhelming pulmonary blastomycosis associated with the adult respiratory distress syndrome. N Engl J Med 329:1231, 1993. *Overwhelming infection with B. dermatitidis can cause diffuse pneumonitis and the adult respiratory distress syndrome, even in immunocompetent hosts.*

Pappas PG, Threlkeld MG, Bedsole GD, et al.: Blastomycosis in immunocompromised patients. Medicine (Baltimore) 72:311, 1993. *This review documents the increasing occurrence of blastomycosis in compromised hosts, including corticosteroid-treated and oncologic patients, organ transplant recipients, pregnant patients, or those with AIDS, and describes the clinical manifestations and treatment approaches in these high-risk groups.*

351 PARACOCCIDIOIDOMYCOSIS
William E. Dismukes

DEFINITION. Paracoccidioidomycosis is a chronic granulomatous disease typically involving the lungs, skin, mucous membranes, and lymph nodes and limited to an endemic area extending from Mexico south to Argentina.

PARACOCCIDIOIDOMYCOSIS

Causative fungus	*Paracoccidioides brasiliensis*
Primary geographic distribution	Endemic in Central America and parts of South America
Primary route of acquisition	Respiratory (inhalation of spores)
Principal sites of disease	Lungs, mucous membranes, skin, lymph nodes, liver, and spleen
Opportunistic infection in compromised hosts	Infrequent
Drug of choice for most patients	Itraconazole
Alternative therapy	Sulfonamide, amphotericin B, or ketoconazole

ETIOLOGY. The causative agent, *Paracoccidioides brasiliensis,* is a dimorphic fungus that grows as a mycelial form in nature and as an oval or round yeast form in tissues or at 37°C. Identifying characteristic multiple budding or "pilot wheel," thick-walled yeast cells, 10 to 40 μm in diameter, in tissue provides presumptive evidence of disease. Because the organism grows slowly on primary isolation, fungal cultures should be held for at least 4 weeks before discarding.

EPIDEMIOLOGY. Most cases occur in persons living in or with a history of prior exposure to southern Mexico, Central America, or South America; in selected countries such as Brazil, paracoccidioidomycosis is the most common systemic mycosis. Owing to the long period of latency, overt disease may develop in persons many years after they have left the endemic region. Infection is acquired by inhaling spores. Neither human-to-human transmission nor common-source outbreaks have been documented. The majority of cases occur in adult males, especially those who labor in the outdoors. The preponderance of cases in men may also be related to the observation that estrogens inhibit the mycelium-to-yeast transformation of the organism. Although cases have been reported in compromised hosts, in general, paracoccidioidomycosis is not considered an opportunistic fungal disease.

PATHOGENESIS AND PATHOLOGY. After inhaling spores, infection may remain confined to the lungs or may spread by lymphohematogenous dissemination to multiple organs. The host pathologic response caused by *P. brasiliensis* is similar to that caused by tissue invasion with *Blastomyces dermatitidis* and *Coccidioides immitis,* i.e., both granulomas and suppuration may develop. The type of tissue pathology and the spectrum of clinical disease are in large part dictated by the integrity of the cell-mediated defenses of the host.

CLINICAL MANIFESTATIONS. Pulmonary paracocciioidomy-
cosis may be asymptomatic or result in symptomatic acute or
chronic disease. Whereas the acute form of pulmonary paracoccidioidomycosis is usually nonspecific and indistinguishable from
other influenza-like illnesses, the clinical and radiographic features
of the chronic form often resemble those of chronic pulmonary coccidioidomycosis. Any or all lobes may be infected, but the upper
lobes tend to be less frequently involved. In addition, cavities, if
present, are usually small (so-called microcavities). Extrapulmonary
disease, especially in persons younger than 30, may be acute in onset, is often manifested by lymphadenopathy and hepatosplenomegaly, and carries a poor prognosis. More typically, extrapulmonary disease in older adults is an indolent illness,
manifested by oropharyngeal and laryngeal mucous membrane ulcers; verrucous, ulcerative, or nodular skin lesions, often on the
face or mucocutaneous borders; and enlarged or necrotic, draining
lymph nodes, especially in the cervical region. Other sites of less
frequent involvement are the gastrointestinal tract, adrenal glands,
testes, epididymis, and skeletal system. Central nervous system and
eye disease secondary to *P. brasiliensis* are rare. A few cases of
paracoccidioidomycosis have been observed in human immunodeficiency virus (HIV)–infected persons.

DIAGNOSIS. Demonstration of the characteristic "pilot wheel,"
multiple-budding *P. brasiliensis* yeast cells by wet mounts or KOH
preparations of sputum, pus, or other body fluids or by special fungal stains of biopsy or cell-block specimens provides presumptive
evidence of paracoccidioidomycosis. A positive culture of body
fluid or tissue specimens is diagnostic. Two different serologic tests
(agar gel immunodiffusion and complement fixation) are available
through the Centers for Disease Control and Prevention in Atlanta.
Precipitin bands appear early in the course of active infection and
may persist for years, even after successful therapy. Complement-
fixing antibodies appear later and are more useful in evaluating response to treatment. Both tests have high specificity. Alternative
serologic tests, including enzyme-linked immunosorbent assay
(ELISA) and counterimmunoelectrophoresis (CIE) as well as newer
ones for detecting a 43-kD glycoprotein antigen and for antibodies
to this antigen, are under investigation. Skin tests have no role in
diagnosis.

TREATMENT. In the past, oral sulfonamides were the mainstay
of therapy; however, these have two major drawbacks, namely, a
high rate of relapse even after prolonged suppression therapy and a
high frequency of adverse reactions, especially skin rashes. Intravenous amphotericin B is effective therapy and is usually used for
more severe forms of paracoccidioidomycosis, such as pulmonary
or disseminated multiorgan disease, and for more refractory cases.
Follow-up chronic suppression therapy with sulfonamides is recommended. Oral antifungal azole drugs represent a significant advance
in the treatment of this disease. Ketoconazole, an imidazole, is
highly effective in both *in vivo* animal models and humans. Cure is
usually achieved with dosages of 200 to 400 mg per day, given for
at least 1 year. Itraconazole, a triazole, in a dose of 100 mg per day
for 6 to 12 months, is as effective as ketoconazole, is better tolerated, and is associated with a lower relapse rate. As a result, many
authorities now consider itraconazole the drug of choice for paracoccidioidomycosis. To date, experience in this disease with fluconazole, the other available oral triazole, has been limited. Because of the tropism of *P. brasiliensis* for the adrenal glands and
the possibility of adrenal insufficiency during active disease or even
after therapy is discontinued, periodic tests of adrenal function are
recommended.

PROGNOSIS. Untreated disseminated paracoccidioidomycosis is
generally fatal. As a rule, the more common indolent forms of adult
disease, usually associated with reactivation, are amenable to prolonged therapy, given over months to years. Unfortunately, clinically significant fibrotic sequelae often persist despite therapy.

Brummer E, Castaneda E, Restrepo A: Paracoccidioidomycosis: An update. Clin Microbiol Rev 6:89, 1993. *A comprehensive review of the disease, focusing on the
causative agent, epidemiology, pathogenesis, diagnosis, and therapy, with 329 references.*

Naranjo MS, Trujillo M, Munera MI, et al.: Treatment of paracoccidioidomycosis with
itraconazole. J Med Vet Mycol 28:67, 1990. *Forty-five of 47 patients had the
chronic form of disease. Itraconazole, 100 mg per day, given for a mean duration
of 6 months, was highly effective, as measured by radiographic and cultural responses, falling serologic titers, and improvement in clinical severity scores.*

352 CRYPTOCOCCOSIS
William E. Dismukes

DEFINITION. Cryptococcosis is a systemic mycosis that most
often involves the lungs and central nervous system (CNS) and, less
frequently, the skin, skeletal system, and prostate gland. *Cryptococcus neoformans,* the causative organism, is the most common agent
of fungal meningitis, and since the onset of the AIDS epidemic in
the early 1980's, it has been increasingly recognized as an opportunistic fungal pathogen.

CRYPTOCOCCOSIS	
Causative fungus	*Cryptococcus neoformans*
Primary geographic distribution	Worldwide
Primary route of acquisition	Respiratory (inhalation of spores)
Principal sites of disease	Lungs, CNS, blood, skin, bone, joints, prostate gland
Opportunistic infection in compromised hosts	Frequent, especially in corti-costeroid-treated and AIDS patients
Drug of choice in most patients	Amphotericin B (with or without flucytosine) or fluconazole
Alternative therapy	Itraconazole

ETIOLOGY. *C. neoformans* is a yeastlike round or oval fungus,
4 to 6 μm in diameter, which is surrounded by a polysaccharide
capsule and which reproduces by budding. Characteristics used to
distinguish genus *Cryptococcus* from other yeasts include a lack of
pseudohyphae, carbohydrate, and nitrate assimilation and production
of phenyloxidase, melanin, and urease. There are two varieties of *C.
neoformans:* var. *neoformans* and var. *gattii,* and four different
serotypes, A, B, C, and D (based on the antigenic specificity of the
capsule). In the laboratory, *C. neoformans* var. *neoformans*
(serotypes A and D) grows at 37°C on niger seed agar as smooth
brown colonies within a few days after inoculation. By contrast, *C.
neoformans* var. *gattii* (serotypes B and C) grows more slowly, and
nonpathogenic *Cryptococcus* species grow poorly or not at all at
37°C. Color reactions on canavanine-glycine-bromthymol blue
(CGB) agar are also used to determine varietal status. Nomenclature
of the perfect or sexual states is based on mating properties. For example, strains of serotypes A and D, which include the majority of
clinical isolates, can be mated to produce the perfect state (*Filobasidiella neoformans* var. *neoformans*).

EPIDEMIOLOGY. Cryptococcosis is worldwide in distribution.
C. neoformans var. *neoformans* is found in soil and other environmental areas, especially those contaminated by pigeon droppings;
pigeons themselves are not infected. Although less is known about
the ecologic niche of *C. neoformans* var. *gattii,* this organism has
been isolated recently from bark, wood, and leaves of river red gum
(*Eucalyptus calmaldulensis*) trees in tropical and subtropical regions, the areas of the world in which this variety of *C. neoformans*
is endemic. Although humans and animals acquire infection after
inhaling aerosolized spores, clusters of cases or mini-outbreaks of
cryptococcosis rarely occur. Only two unusual cases of presumed
person-to-person transmission of cryptococcosis have been observed. There is no obvious age, gender, or occupational predilection. Immunosuppression related to altered T-cell function is the
most common predisposing factor: Examples include corticosteroid
therapy, lymphoreticular malignancies (especially Hodgkin's disease), sarcoidosis (even in the absence of corticosteroid therapy),
HIV infection, organ transplantation, and perhaps diabetes mellitus.
The association of cryptococcosis and organ transplantation probably relates in large part to immunosuppression with corticosteroids.

Cyclosporine, at least in a murine model, inhibits growth of *C. neoformans*. Among patients with AIDS in the United States, the incidence of cryptococcosis ranges from 5 to 10%; by contrast, in Africa and other developing areas, the incidence of cryptococcosis in AIDS patients is much higher. Although cryptococcosis occurs most frequently in immunosuppressed hosts, about 20 to 30% of patients with the disease have no apparent underlying condition or predisposing factor (except for unexplained CD4 cytopenia in some).

PATHOGENESIS AND PATHOLOGY. After aerosolized spores are inhaled, most infections begin with an asymptomatic pulmonary focus. In individuals with normal host defense, cryptococci remain localized in the lungs and are eventually eliminated. By contrast, in immunocompromised individuals, there is hematogenous spread to extrapulmonary organs. Neutrophils and later monocytes clear cryptococci from inflammatory sites. Phagocytosis by neutrophils and macrophages appears to be mediated in part by complement and several cytokines including interferon-γ, tissue necrosis factor, and GM-CSF. Cryptococcal polysaccharide is a major virulence factor and may be immunosuppressive, inhibit phagocytosis, and impair migration of leukocytes. Paradoxically, cryptococcal polysaccharide has also been shown to activate the alternative complement pathway. In general, immunity depends on functioning, sensitized T cells and an intact cell-mediated arm of host defense. Consequently, patients with defective or altered T-cell immunity, such as those with HIV infection, are highly susceptible to infection with *C. neoformans* and progressive disease. The incidence of cryptococcosis in AIDS patients is highly associated with CD4 counts < 100 cells per cubic millimeter. The preferential involvement of *C. neoformans* for the CNS is explained by the absence of complement and soluble anticryptococcal factors (present in normal serum) in normal cerebrospinal fluid (CSF), as well as a decreased to absent inflammatory response to cryptococci in brain tissue. As a result, well-formed granulomas are generally absent in histopathologic sections of infected tissue. The characteristic lesion in cryptococcal meningoencephalitis consists of cystic clusters of fungi; the basal ganglia and the cortical gray matter are the sites of heaviest involvement. In other organs such as the lung, the inflammatory response varies in intensity from minimal to heavy and consists of an array of cells, including organism-containing macrophages, giant cells, plasma cells, and lymphocytes. No necrosis is present, and tissue is usually displaced by multiplying organisms. Yeastlike cryptococci with characteristic narrow-based buds stain poorly with hematoxylin-eosin but are easily visualized with Gomori methenamine silver (GMS) or periodic acid–Schiff (PAS) stains. Mucicarmine stain further aids identification by giving a rose color to the polysaccharide capsule.

CLINICAL MANIFESTATIONS. *Pulmonary Cryptococcosis.* The pattern of pulmonary cryptococcal infection is highly variable, ranging from the extremes of saprophytic airway colonization without clinical or radiographic evidence of disease to full-blown acute respiratory distress syndrome in compromised hosts, such as AIDS patients. More typically, radiographic findings include either patchy pneumonitis or solitary or multiple small nodules in asymptomatic persons or those with mild to moderate symptoms, e.g., fever, malaise, cough, scant sputum, pleuritic pain, or rarely hemoptysis. Although tumor-like masses mimicking carcinoma are not uncommon, cavitation and pleural effusions are less likely. The course of pulmonary cryptococcosis is also variable. In patients with normal host defenses, spontaneous regression of both clinical and radiographic manifestations is the rule, although chronic stable infection is known to occur. In contrast, pulmonary cryptococcosis in immunocompromised patients is more likely to progress and therefore requires antifungal therapy. Pulmonary disease may occur in the absence of extrapulmonary cryptococcosis, and conversely, extrapulmonary disease, such as meningitis, may develop in the absence of apparent lung involvement.

Central Nervous System Cryptococcosis. Meningitis, usually subacute or chronic in nature, is the most common manifestation of CNS cryptococcosis. Complications include hydrocephalus, encephalitis, involvement of the optic pathways, brain stem vasculitis, and mass lesions (cryptococcomas) of the brain parenchyma or spinal cord. The clinical presentation and course of cryptococcal meningitis vary greatly, related in part to the underlying condition and immune status of the host. In "normal" hosts, the onset is often insidious, whereas in compromised hosts, such as HIV-infected or corticosteroid-treated patients, the onset tends to be more acute and the course more rapidly progressive. The most common symptoms are headache and alteration in mental status, e.g., confusion, lethargy, obtundation or coma, and personality change. Nausea and vomiting are frequent; fever and stiff neck are less common. Ocular symptoms, such as blurred vision, photophobia, vision loss, and diplopia, secondary to perineuritic adhesive arachnoiditis, papilledema, optic nerve neuritis, chorioretinitis, or retinovitreal abscess, are present in about 25% of patients. Other findings include hearing deficits, seizures, ataxia, aphasia, and choreoathetoid movements. Dementia is important to recognize as a potential sequela because it may be curable. Cryptococcomas, which accompany cryptococcal meningitis in 5 to 20% of cases, are less common in patients with AIDS. Rarely, CNS cryptococcomas can be seen in the absence of meningeal disease. The mortality rate varies from 15 to 25%; most deaths occur in the first few weeks of illness.

Miscellaneous. After the lungs and CNS, the next most commonly involved organs in patients with disseminated cryptococcosis are the skin and skeletal system. Cutaneous manifestations occur in 10 to 15% of cases and usually take the form of papules, pustules, nodules, ulcers, or draining sinuses. Typically, cellulitis with prominent erythema and induration is seen in corticosteroid-treated transplant recipients, and umbilicated papules resembling molluscum contagiosum are observed in AIDS patients. Oral mucosal chancres have been reported rarely. Osteomyelitis is more common than septic arthritis. Less commonly involved sites of cryptococcal disease include pericardium, myocardium, muscle, liver, peritoneum, adrenal glands, kidneys, and prostate gland. Infections of these organs are being increasingly identified in AIDS patients. For example, the prostate has been reported to be a sanctuary of residual infection in this population group.

DIAGNOSIS. As with other systemic mycoses, the definitive diagnosis of cryptococcosis depends on demonstrating the characteristic yeastlike organism with its surrounding capsule in tissue or fluid obtained from involved sites, together with cultural confirmation. In addition, in patients with suspected cryptococcosis, the latex agglutination test to detect cryptococcal polysaccharide antigen in serum and CSF is an extremely important adjunct to diagnosis, unlike the situation for most other fungal disease, in which serologic tests lack specificity and sensitivity. Cryptococcal antigen is found in CSF in >90% and in serum in about 75% of patients with meningitis, especially if serial specimens are examined over time. Titers are particularly high in patients with AIDS. In patients with extraneural cryptococcal disease, antigen is detected in only 25 to 50% of cases. Proper controls are necessary to eliminate rheumatoid factor, which may give rise to a false-positive result. Serum of patients with disseminated infection caused by *Trichosporon beigelii* may also test positive for cryptococcal antigen. False-negative tests for cryptococcal antigen may be due to low numbers of cryptococcal organisms invading tissue or in CSF, unencapsulated or poorly encapsulated strains, or a prozone phenomenon. Tests for cryptococcal antibody are not useful for diagnosis.

Pulmonary cryptococcosis is difficult to diagnose in most cases without obtaining lung tissue via bronchoscopy, open lung biopsy, or thoracoscopy. Wet preparations of sputum are only occasionally helpful, and sputum cultures are positive for *C. neoformans* in only 20% of cases. In patients with pleural effusions, fluid tested for cryptococcal antigen may be positive, thereby obviating a more invasive procedure. In every patient with established pulmonary cryptococcosis, a lumbar puncture should be performed, whether or not CNS disease is apparent. Blood cultures and tissue for culture and histopathologic study of any other suspected sites of involvement, e.g., skin or bone, should also be obtained.

The diagnosis of cryptococcal meningitis is easier to establish than the diagnosis of cryptococcal pulmonary disease. Once the diagnosis of meningitis is considered, a lumbar puncture should be performed. Most patients, except for those with AIDS, have significant CSF abnormalities, including elevated opening pressure, depressed glucose levels (hypoglycorrhachia) in half the cases, elevated protein levels, and a lymphocytic pleocytosis. The India ink preparation of centrifuged CSF to detect budding yeast cells and surrounding capsule is positive in 50 to 75% of cases; because the incidence of false-positive smears is high, confirmation of findings by culture is imperative. Culturing of centrifuged sediment of large volumes (5 to 10 ml) of CSF obtained by repeated lumbar punctures is associated with a positive culture rate of 90 to 95%. In AIDS patients, the CSF formula is often normal or only minimally abnormal, owing to a diminished or absent inflammatory response. Yet in most cases, cultures are positive, cryptococcal antigen titers are high, and India ink preparations reveal organisms. The chest roentgenogram may or may not be abnormal. Blood should be cultured and tested for antigen in all patients; these tests are positive more commonly in AIDS patients than in patients without AIDS. In addition, computed tomographic scans (CT) or magnetic resonance imaging (MRI) of the head is indicated in most patients, especially those with coma, suspected hydrocephalus, focal neurologic findings, seizures, or clinical deterioration after initial improvement.

TREATMENT. Approaches to therapy of cryptococcosis vary according to site(s) of involvement and underlying host status. Whereas all patients with CNS cryptococcosis or other forms of extrapulmonary disease require treatment, the majority of cases of pulmonary cryptococcosis alone, especially in the "normal" host, resolve without antifungal therapy. By contrast, other patients with pulmonary cryptococcosis, including patients with AIDS and other immunocompromising conditions, those with accompanying extrapulmonary disease, and those with progressive disease, require antifungal therapy. Although specific guidelines are poorly defined, the two commonly used drugs are amphotericin B (total dose 1.0 to 2.0 grams) and fluconazole (200 to 400 mg daily for 3 to 6 months). Fluconazole should be reserved for patients with mild to moderate forms of cryptococcal lung disease. As a rule, therapy should be continued until clinical, radiographic, and mycologic resolution of disease is evident. Surgical resection may be an important adjunct to drug therapy in patients with extensive lobar consolidation and large mass lesions.

The therapy of cryptococcal meningitis has been more extensively studied than the therapy of any other systemic fungal disease. Data indicate that (1) all patients require treatment; (2) several treatment regimens, including oral azole drugs, may be used; (3) a combination of amphotericin B and flucytosine is the regimen of choice, especially for patients with moderate to severe disease including complications such as obtundation, coma, blindness, cranial nerve palsies, and hydrocephalus; (4) regardless of regimen, 15 to 25% of patients die of this disease; and (5) treatment considerations are somewhat different for AIDS patients with cryptococcal meningitis (see below). Although the standard regimen is combination amphotericin B (0.5 to 1.0 mg per kilogram per day) and flucytosine (100 mg per kilogram per day) for 4 to 6 weeks, both the daily dose and total dose should be individualized, balancing the risks of toxicities of the drugs and the potential benefits of synergy and increased efficacy. Both renal function and serum flucytosine levels should be closely monitored, and flucytosine doses should be regulated to maintain serum concentrations in the range of 50 to 100 μg per milliliter. Potential toxic effects of flucytosine include bone marrow suppression, hepatitis, diarrhea, and rash. Although experience with fluconazole in non-AIDS cryptococcal meningitis is limited, this drug may be an effective alternative therapy. Intrathecal therapy with amphotericin B is usually reserved for patients who relapse or whose disease is refractory to prolonged courses of high-dose intravenous amphotericin B.

Because cryptococcal meningitis in AIDS patients may be highly refractory and associated with a relapse rate of 50% if therapy is stopped, both aggressive primary therapy and long-term maintenance therapy are required. For primary therapy, several alternative treatment regimens may be used. First, combination amphotericin and flucytosine may be given for the entire period of primary therapy. However, some AIDS patients may not tolerate flucytosine because of a high incidence of drug-induced cytopenias, often superimposed upon pre-existing bone-marrow suppression secondary to zidovudine, cytotoxic chemotherapy, and opportunistic infectious diseases. In addition, flucytosine should not be used unless serum levels can be monitored. In such situations, amphotericin B may be used alone. Second, azole therapy alone is effective in selected patients, e.g., those with mild disease and normal mental status at time of diagnosis. Fluconazole is favored over itraconazole, another triazole, in cryptococcal meningitis because of fluconazole's water solubility, minimal protein binding, and good to excellent penetration into CSF (60 to 80% of serum concentration). In addition, an intravenous formulation of fluconazole is available. A major disadvantage of fluconazole and itraconazole is their less rapid sterilization of CSF than with amphotericin B. As a result, amphotericin B with or without flucytosine should be preferentially used as primary therapy in more seriously ill AIDS patients such as those who are obtunded or comatose or who have widespread disseminated cryptococcosis. Third, therapy with amphotericin B and flucytosine or amphotericin B alone may be given for an initial 2 weeks as induction primary therapy, followed by an oral azole for 8 additional weeks as consolidation therapy. This unique approach, currently being evaluated, represents an attempt to sterilize the CSF more rapidly, reduce the number of early deaths, and avoid the potential for prolonged toxicity of the drugs used in initial treatment. Fourth, the combination of two oral drugs, flucytosine and fluconazole, has been studied in both animal models and to a lesser extent in patients with AIDS-associated cryptococcal meningitis. Until more data are available about the efficacy of this novel regimen, it cannot be recommended routinely over more established treatments. Finally, recent data indicate that passive antibody in the form of murine or humanized monoclonal antibodies has the potential to enhance cellular immunity; trials are ongoing.

Chemotherapy alone is not adequate treatment for all patients. Ventricular shunting of CSF should be performed in obtunded or comatose patients with hydrocephalus demonstrated by imaging studies. Among patients with no overt hydrocephalus but abnormal mental status and elevated intracranial pressure, treatment approaches include frequent lumbar punctures to cautiously lower CSF pressure, high-dose dexamethasone therapy, and temporary ventricular drainage.

Once primary therapy has sterilized the CSF, i.e., converted the fungal culture from positive to negative, maintenance therapy in AIDS patients should be initiated. Fluconazole (200 mg daily) is more effective in preventing relapse than amphotericin (1 mg per kilogram weekly) and much better tolerated, resulting in better patient compliance. Fluconazole is also more effective than itraconazole. Chronic suppressive therapy must be continued for life.

PROGNOSIS. The outcome of cryptococcosis is significantly worse in AIDS patients than in the non-AIDS population, as evidenced by higher mortality and relapse rates. Pretreatment prognostic factors, in addition to HIV infection, which adversely affect outcome in patients with cryptococcal meningitis, include an underlying condition predisposing to T-cell dysfunction; absence of headache as a presenting symptom; altered mental status as evidenced by obtundation, stupor, or coma; positive extraneural cultures for *C. neoformans*, CSF white cell count ≤ 20 per cubic millimeter; and high cryptococcal serum and CSF antigen titers. Among these factors, HIV infection and abnormal mental status appear to be most important. A rise in CSF antigen during suppressive therapy is associated with relapse; by contrast, other abnormalities of CSF such as hypoglycorrhachia, elevated protein, or positive India ink preparation may persist for months after therapy has been discontinued and do not appear to correlate with relapse.

PREVENTION. Because an environmental source of infection cannot be determined in the vast majority of patients who develop cryptococcal disease, attempts at eliminating *C. neoformans* from soil or other habitats are not feasible or practical. With the availability of effective, safe, oral antifungal drugs such as fluconazole and itraconazole, use of these as prophylactic agents in high-risk groups such as HIV-infected persons has been evaluated. Preliminary data indicate that oral fluconazole, 200 mg daily, in patients with CD4 counts < 200 cells per cubic millimeter, is more effective than clotrimazole troches in reducing the frequency of systemic fungal disease, especially cryptococcosis, but not in prolonging survival.

Levitz SM: The ecology of *Cryptococcus neoformans* and the epidemiology of cryptococcosis. Rev Infect Dis 13:1163, 1991. *Reviews of the two varieties of* C. neoformans (var. neoformans *and var.* gattii) *with emphasis on their distribution in nature and epidemiologic characteristics of patients infected.*

Powderly WG: Cryptococcal meningitis and AIDS. Clin Infect Dis 17:837, 1993. *Focuses on clinical and laboratory features as well as different treatment options, including primary therapy for acute disease and maintenance therapy to prevent relapse.*

Powderly WG, Saag MS, Cloud GA, et al.: A controlled trial of fluconazole or amphotericin B to prevent relapse of cryptococcal meningitis in patients with the acquired immunodeficiency syndrome. N Engl J Med 326:793, 1992. *The definitive trial showing that daily fluconazole is superior to weekly intravenous amphotericin B as maintenance preventive therapy in AIDS-associated cryptococcosis.*

Rex JH, Larsen RA, Dismukes WE, et al.: Catastrophic visual loss due to *Cryptococ-*

cus neoformans meningitis. Medicine (Baltimore) 72:207, 1993. *A thorough review of 49 cases with emphasis on pathogenesis, natural history, and management of this devastating complication of cryptococcal meningitis.*
Saag MS, Powderly WG, Cloud GA, et al.: Comparison of amphotericin B with fluconazole in the treatment of acute AIDS-associated cryptococcal meningitis. N Engl J Med 326:83, 1992. *A large clinical trial indicating that fluconazole is an effective alternative to amphotericin B as primary treatment of cryptococcal meningitis in AIDS.*

353 SPOROTRICHOSIS
William E. Dismukes

DEFINITION. Sporotrichosis is a chronic mycotic disease that typically involves skin, subcutaneous tissue, and regional lymphatics as a result of cutaneous inoculation of *Sporothrix schenckii*. Extracutaneous disease secondary to either lymphohematogenous dissemination or inhalation of organisms is rare.

SPOROTRICHOSIS

Causative fungus	*Sporothrix schenckii*
Primary geographic distribution	Worldwide, mainly in temperate and tropical areas
Primary route of acquisition	Cutaneous inoculation
Principal sites of disease	Skin, lymphatics; less commonly, lungs and joints
Opportunistic infection in compromised hosts	Infrequent
Drug of choice for most patients	Itraconazole
Alternative therapy	Cutaneous disease: saturated solution potassium iodide, fluconazole, or surgery Excutaneous disease: amphotericin B

ETIOLOGY. *S. schenckii* is a dimorphic fungus that grows in nature and in the laboratory on Sabouraud's agar as a white mold, which, with time, becomes brownish black. In tissue and at 37°C, the organism exists as yeastlike cells, which appear as round, spherical, or cigar-shaped budding forms, 2 to 6 μm in size.

EPIDEMIOLOGY. Sporotrichosis is worldwide in distribution. *S. schenckii* appears to be ubiquitous in soil and in both living and decaying vegetation. Although the organism does not appear to infect plants, it may infect animals, especially cats and dogs, as well as humans, especially those who frequently handle or come in contact with mulch, sphagnum moss, hay, timber, and thorny bushes. Consequently, sporotrichosis is considered an occupational disease of certain groups, including farmers, nursery or forestry workers, gardeners, florists, landscapers, and carpenters. In 1988, the largest known epidemic of sporotrichosis in the United States occurred among 84 forestry workers exposed to sphagnum moss obtained from a single source. Transmission almost always results from the percutaneous introduction of organisms. In the majority of patients with extracutaneous disease, the route of acquisition is unclear. Rarely, pulmonary sporotrichosis may result from inhalation of aerosolized conidia. Although person-to-person transmission is not known to occur, transmission from animals, especially cats, to humans has been documented. The number of cases of cutaneous disease in males and females is similar; gender and age appear to play less of a role than does environmental exposure. By contrast, extracutaneous sporotrichosis is more common in males. *S. schenckii* is not considered an opportunistic fungal pathogen, although sporotrichosis in compromised hosts is being increasingly recognized. For example, cases have been observed in HIV-infected persons.

PATHOGENESIS AND PATHOLOGY. Cutaneous inoculation may follow either inapparent or obvious penetrating trauma. In the majority of patients, clinical disease does not extend beyond the site of inoculation or the draining lymphatics. Localized disease may persist for years, and cell-mediated immunity appears to be responsible for preventing or limiting the spread to extracutaneous sites. Conversely, multiorgan disease involving skin and distant sites, such as lungs, bones, and joints, is more common in immunosuppressed hosts.

The basic histopathologic pattern in cutaneous sporotrichosis is a combination of suppuration and granulomas, often accompanied by pseudoepitheliomatous hyperplasia. This pattern is not diagnostic, as it may also be seen in malignancy as well as other fungal diseases, such as blastomycosis, coccidioidomycosis, and chromomycosis. Because the yeastlike cells, typical of *S. schenckii*, are uncommonly identified in tissue sections, cultural confirmation is usually necessary for diagnosis. The finding of large asteroid bodies (radiate eosinophilic material surrounding fungal yeast cells) provides presumptive evidence of sporotrichosis.

CLINICAL MANIFESTATIONS. Two distinctive clinical forms of cutaneous and extracutaneous disease, which differ in management and prognosis, are seen.

Cutaneous. This form of sporotrichosis can be further divided into two types: plaque (or fixed) and lymphocutaneous. Plaque sporotrichosis, which is less common, consists of a single ulcerative or nodular lesion at the site of primary inoculation, usually on an exposed extremity or the face. The lesion begins as a small painless red papule, which gradually enlarges and finally ulcerates (sporotrichotic chancre). A violaceous hue and intermittent serosanguineous drainage are characteristic. Lymphocutaneous sporotrichosis, which is the more typical type and is found in about 75% of cases, represents an extension of the primary lesion. Subcutaneous nontender nodular lesions appear proximally along thickened lymphatics over days to weeks and occasionally ulcerate. Lymph nodes are rarely enlarged. Similarly, constitutional symptoms, such as fever and chills, are usually absent. This type of sporotrichosis, which usually remains confined to the primary site and its regional lymphatics, may wax and wane over years if untreated. Lymphohematogenous spread to distant organs is uncommon.

Extracutaneous. The pathogenesis of the majority of cases of extracutaneous sporotrichosis is uncertain because most cases are not accompanied by clinically apparent cutaneous disease. The skeletal system is the most commonly involved extracutaneous organ. Although indolent monarticular arthritis of the knees, ankles, wrists, and elbows is most frequent, osteomyelitis (especially of the tibia), tenosynovitis, and carpal tunnel syndrome have been reported. Multiarticular arthritis is more likely in compromised hosts with widespread hematogenous spread to multiple organs. Pulmonary sporotrichosis is far less common than osteoarticular disease. Fewer than 100 cases of pulmonary disease have been reported. This form of insidious infection occurs primarily in older male alcoholics and mimics reactivation tuberculosis. Thin-walled cavitary lesions in a single upper lobe are characteristic; bilateral fibrocavitary disease may be seen occasionally. Extrapulmonary spread of disease is uncommon. Ocular sporotrichosis results from traumatic inoculation of the conjunctiva or cornea; endophthalmitis is unusual. Chronic lymphocytic meningitis may be a complication of sporotrichosis, even in the absence of obvious extraneural disease. In any patient with chronic meningitis of unknown origin, cerebrospinal fluid (CSF) should be tested for antibody to *S. schenckii*.

DIAGNOSIS. As a rule, the diagnosis of sporotrichosis must be based on cultural demonstration of the organism in tissue or fluid obtained from involved sites, e.g., skin, subcutaneous nodule, joint, or lung. Histopathologic findings are usually nonspecific, and the characteristic yeastlike cells are often not identified by special stains such as Gomori methenamine silver or periodic acid–Schiff. Direct immunofluorescence, if available, may be helpful. Although testing of serum or CSF by latex agglutination or enzyme immunoassay for antibody to *S. schenckii* may be useful, especially in patients suspected of having extracutaneous disease, positive low-level antibody titers may be observed in normal persons. No skin test is commercially available.

TREATMENT. Conventional therapy for cutaneous sporotrichosis is saturated solution of potassium iodide, which is begun at a dosage of 5 drops three times a day and increased dropwise (3 to 5 drops per day) up to a maximum of 120 drops per day or until the development of iodine toxicity (manifested by rash, lacrimation, parotid swelling, or nonspecific gastrointestinal symptoms). Iodide therapy should be continued for at least 1 month after clinical resolution of the disease. Itraconazole in a dosage of 100 to 400 mg per day is an attractive alternative to iodide therapy for cutaneous sporotrichosis. Itraconazole is more effective than the other two oral azoles, ketoconazole and fluconazole, and better tolerated than potassium iodide. In addition, itraconazole (200 to 400 mg per day) is moderately effective in treating extracutaneous sporotrichosis. Amphotericin B should be reserved for patients with cutaneous or extracutaneous disease in whom iodide or azole therapy fails, and as therapy for immunocompromised patients with severe, life-threatening, widely disseminated sporotrichosis. In the latter group of patients, consideration may be given to switching to itraconazole after a successful induction course of amphotericin B. Cure rates may be improved in selected patients with bone and joint disease or single-cavity pulmonary disease by surgical resection of synovial tissue, bone, or lung, as an adjunct to antifungal therapy. Intra-articular amphotericin B may also be useful.

PROGNOSIS. Although untreated cutaneous sporotrichosis may remit and relapse for years, and rarely disseminate, the likelihood of cure with iodide or itraconazole therapy is high. In contrast, extracutaneous disease is more refractory, even to therapy including itraconazole, amphotericin B, and surgery; significant morbidity and mortality are frequent sequelae.

Calhoun DL, Waskin H, White MP, et al.: Treatment of systemic sporotrichosis with ketoconazole. Rev Infect Dis 13:47, 1991. *Oral ketoconazole was moderately effective in 11 patients with deep-seated sporotrichosis; durable responses were associated with prolonged treatment.*

Dixon DM, Salkin IF, Duncan RA, et al.: Isolation and characterization of *Sporothrix schenckii* from clinical and environmental sources associated with the largest U.S. epidemic of sporotrichosis. J Clin Microbiol 29:6, 1991. *A detailed microbiologic analysis of 21 clinical and 69 environmental isolates of* S. schenckii *associated with this sporotrichosis outbreak (84 cases).*

Sharkey-Mathis PK, Kauffman CA, Graybill JR, et al.: Treatment of sporotrichosis with itraconazole. Am J Med 95:279, 1993. *Results of this multicenter study in 27 patients show that itraconazole is effective and well-tolerated for lymphocutaneous and extracutaneous sporotrichosis.*

354 CANDIDIASIS
William E. Dismukes

DEFINITION. *Candida* species can cause a variety of clinical syndromes that are generically termed candidiasis and are usually categorized by site of involvement. Broadly speaking, the two most common syndromes are mucocutaneous candidiasis (e.g., stomatitis or thrush, esophagitis, and vaginitis) and invasive or deep organ candidiasis (e.g., fungemia, endocarditis, and endophthalmitis). In most patients, candidiasis is an opportunistic disease.

CANDIDIASIS	
Causative fungus	*Candida* species (*C. albicans* most common)
Primary geographic distribution	Worldwide; part of normal flora of humans and in environment
Primary route of acquisition	Endogenous; person-to-person
Principal sites of disease	Mucous membranes (oropharynx, vagina), skin, esophagus, blood, liver, spleen, kidneys, eyes, heart
Opportunistic infection in compromised hosts	Frequent; e.g., mucosal disease in AIDS patients and deep organ disease in granulocytopenic patients
Drug(s) of choice for most patients	Mucosal disease: topical or oral azole drug (clotrimazole or fluconazole)
	Deep organ disease: amphotericin B or fluconazole
Alternative therapy for deep organ disease	Amphotericin B plus flucytosine

ETIOLOGY. Among more than 150 recognized species of *Candida*, *C. albicans* is the most commonly identified pathogen in humans. Other clinically important species include *C. tropicalis*, *C. parapsilosis*, *C. krusei*, *C. pseudotropicalis*, and *C. guilliermondi*. *Candida* organisms share two morphologic features: small, spherical yeast forms (4 to 6 μm), which reproduce by budding; and pseudohyphae (pseudomycelia), which are chains of elongated yeasts separated by constrictions. In body fluids or tissue, both budding cells and fragments of pseudohyphae may be visualized. Identification and speciation in the microbiology laboratory are based on both morphologic characteristics and results of metabolic tests. The ability of *C. albicans* to produce germ tubes in serum allows presumptive identification. *Torulopsis glabrata,* the most commonly encountered pathogenic species in the genus *Torulopsis,* resembles the yeast forms of other *Candida* species; because it does not produce a pseudomycelial form, *T. glabrata* is generally not considered a member of the genus *Candida*.

EPIDEMIOLOGY. Candidiasis occurs worldwide. *C. albicans* is part of the normal human flora of the mouth, gastrointestinal tract, and vagina; normally lives in balance with other microorganisms in the body; and, in most individuals, exists as a saprophytic colonizer or commensal. When various drugs or conditions, such as broad-spectrum antibiotics, corticosteroids, diabetes mellitus, or human immunodeficiency virus (HIV) infection, upset this balance, endogenous *C. albicans* may become a pathogen and cause either mucocutaneous or deep disease. *C. albicans* may also be recovered from soil, hospital environments, food, and other substrates. In contrast to *C. albicans,* the other *Candida* species that are pathogenic for humans less frequently colonize the skin, gastrointestinal tract, or vagina of normal individuals. These species more often reside in the environment and on inanimate objects and thus reach the body from exogenous sources; consequently, they are generally regarded as opportunistic fungal pathogens. Unlike other fungi, *Candida* species may be transmitted from person to person, e.g., between sexual partners, by hands of medical personnel, and during birth from colonized vagina to neonatal oropharynx.

Candidiasis, both mucocutaneous and deep forms, has emerged as the most common opportunistic fungal disease, owing to the progressively increasing use of antibiotics (both prophylactic and therapeutic); immunosuppressive and cytotoxic drugs; indwelling foreign bodies, including prosthetic heart valves, prosthetic joints, and intravascular monitoring devices; venous, arterial, urinary, and peritoneal catheters; and organ transplantation. In addition, the AIDS epidemic has been highly contributory.

PATHOGENESIS AND PATHOLOGY. Several components of the host defense system are important in protecting against infection with *Candida* species. An intact integumentary barrier, including skin and mucous membranes, prevents invasion of normally colonizing organisms, which possess adherence properties as yet not fully understood. *C. albicans* and *C. tropicalis* appear to be more adherent than other species, accounting in part for the frequency of these organisms as pathogens. Disruption or loss of normal barriers as a consequence of percutaneous catheters, endotracheal tubes, severe burns, or abdominal surgery is a common predisposing factor, especially to deep invasive or disseminated disease. Polymorphonuclear leukocytes and monocytes are the major cellular defenses against *Candida* species; intracellular killing largely depends on the myeloperoxidase, hydrogen peroxide, and superoxide anion systems. Although the role of tissue macrophages is unclear, lymphocytes and cell-mediated immunity appear to play a role. Abnormalities of host defense include T-cell dysfunction, which predisposes to mucocutaneous disease (oropharyngeal or esophageal candidiasis in HIV-infected persons as well as chronic mucocutaneous candidiasis), and granulocytopenia secondary to underlying disease or therapy, which predisposes to deep disease (candidemia or invasive candidiasis). In cutaneous candidiasis, histopathologic evidence of chronic dermatitis with yeasts confined to the stratum corneum is characteristic. By contrast, microabscesses interspersed in normal tissue are the characteristic pathologic finding in visceral candidiasis. Neutrophils appear initially, followed by histiocytes and giant cells and, in some cases, a readily apparent granulomatous response. In severely immunocompromised patients, the inflammatory response may be minimal or absent. Both yeasts and pseudohyphae can usually be visualized by special stains, such as periodic acid–Schiff or Gomori-methenamine-silver.

CLINICAL MANIFESTATIONS. *Mucocutaneous Infections.* Thrush or oropharyngeal candidiasis is manifested by creamy white curdlike exudative patches on the tongue, buccal mucosa, palate, or other oral mucosal surfaces. These patches are actually pseudomembranes, which, upon removal, may leave a raw, bleeding, painful surface. Poorly fitting dentures may be a predisposing factor, and areas of erythema may be the only marker of disease. Cheilosis, an inflammatory reaction at the corners of the mouth, and atrophic changes, either acute or chronic, are less common presentations of oropharyngeal disease. Esophagitis, which may occur as an extension of thrush or may occur in the absence of thrush in up to one third of patients, is manifested typically by odynophagia, dysphagia, or substernal chest pain and uncommonly by bleeding. Thrush or esophagitis, occurring in the absence of any known predisposing condition, should raise the suspicion of HIV infection. Gastrointestinal candidiasis involving the mucosa of the stomach and small and large bowel is most common in patients with cancer and is an important source of disseminated infection.

Intertrigo, a cutaneous *Candida* infection involving warm, moist surfaces, such as the axillae, gluteal and inframammary folds, and groin, may be variable in appearance but is usually manifested as well-marginated, erythematous, exudative patches surrounded by satellite vesicles or pustules. Paronychia, a painful, tense, reddened swelling at the base of the nail or along the sides, is commonly caused by *Candida* species, especially in diabetics and persons whose hands are chronically immersed in water. Although *Candida* species may cause onychomycosis, this chronic deforming infection of the nails is most frequently due to one of the genera of superficial dermatophytes, such as *Trichophyton* or *Epidermophyton*. Vulvovaginitis, probably the most common *Candida* mucocutaneous infection in women, especially in association with pregnancy, oral contraceptives, antibiotic therapy, diabetes, and HIV infection, is characterized by thick, creamy vaginal discharge, erythematous labia, and intense pruritus. Balanitis in males, often acquired through sexual intercourse, is manifested by superficial vesicles and exudative patches, usually on the glans penis. *Candida* cystitis, which at cystoscopy resembles oral thrush, is most often a complication of an indwelling bladder catheter. Chronic mucocutaneous candidiasis, a rare condition manifested by a heterogeneous group of persistent, often disfiguring *Candida* infections involving skin, mucous membranes, hair, and nails, occurs primarily in persons with altered T-cell function or an endocrinopathy such as hypoparathyroidism or hypoadrenalism.

Deep Organ Candidiasis. Numerous diagnostic categories or labels for serious or deep *Candida* infection exist, including candidemia, disseminated candidiasis, systemic candidiasis, invasive candidiasis, visceral candidiasis, and terms indicating involvement of specific organs, such as hepatosplenic candidiasis and ocular candidiasis. Here, discussion focuses on two major categories: candidemia, which may or may not be associated with visceral organ involvement; and disseminated candidiasis, which implies systemic multiorgan disease and encompasses other subgroups, such as visceral, invasive, and hepatosplenic disease.

Candidemia. Candidemia, which is usually defined as one or more positive blood cultures for *Candida* species, may occur in the presence or absence of clinical manifestations, e.g., fever or skin lesions. The incidence of candidemia has risen dramatically over recent years in association with the increased number of compromised hosts (e.g., those with AIDS, cancer, or burns, those in the postsurgical intensive care unit, and organ transplant recipients) managed by aggressive interventions, including empiric antibiotics, cytotoxic chemotherapy, hemodialysis, intravenous and intra-arterial catheters, other intravascular devices, and parenteral alimentation. In many hospitals, *Candida* has become one of the three to five most common microorganisms isolated from blood cultures. Previously, "transient candidemia" was used to imply short duration (< 24 hours) of fungemia and indicate either clearing of the candidemia upon removal of an infected intravascular catheter or a benign condition not requiring antifungal therapy. Recent data argue against this concept and suggest that catheter removal alone is in-

sufficient, even in the noncompromised patient, to prevent metastatic hematogenous dissemination to visceral organs. Accordingly, most investigators now believe that all patients with candidemia, regardless of duration or circumstances, deserve some form of antifungal treatment. Controversy at present centers on which drug, at what dose, and for how long (see Treatment below).

C. albicans is the most common species identified in blood. Studies from multiple medical centers indicate that *C. tropicalis* is a likely pathogen in the leukemic population, while *C. parapsilosis* fungemia occurs frequently in patients with solid tumor or nononcologic diseases, especially in association with cannula-related sepsis and hyperalimentation. *T. glabrata* resembles *C. parapsilosis* in its predilection for patients with solid tumors or nononcologic disorders.

Cannulas of various types are the most important portals of entry, accounting for more than one half of the episodes of candidemia. In almost all cases, removing cannulas, either peripheral or central, is necessary to eradicate candidemia. Other common sites of infection are the gastrointestinal tract, especially in granulocytopenic patients, and surgical wounds. The urinary and respiratory tracts, although frequently colonized by *Candida* species, are less common sources of bloodstream infection. The mortality rate of candidemia caused by all species is high, ranging from 40 to 80%. Mortality is significantly associated with a high APACHE II score, a rapidly fatal underlying disease, and sustained candidemia. The mortality rate in cannula-associated candidemia is lower than in candidemia related to other sources.

The frequency with which candidemia results in localized single-organ disease (e.g., ocular candidiasis) or widespread disseminated multiorgan disease is 20 to 40%. Premortem diagnosis of invasive or disseminated candidiasis must be based on histopathologic demonstration of *Candida* organisms invading tissue. Because blood cultures are negative in at least 50% of patients with disseminated candidiasis and there are no other reliable markers, such as serologic tests, disseminated *Candida* disease may not be suspected and appropriate invasive diagnostic procedures may not be performed. Autopsy series indicate that disseminated disease involving kidneys, liver, spleen, brain, myocardium, and eyes is most likely in patients with some rapidly fatal underlying disease, such as leukemia complicated by neutropenia, and is least likely in patients with candidemia in the setting of nononcologic disease, especially cannula-related sepsis. In addition, patients whose candidemia is treated are less likely to develop disseminated disease.

Cutaneous Lesions of Disseminated Candidiasis. Papulopustules or macronodules on an erythematous base, usually widely distributed over the trunk and extremities, are the hallmark lesions associated with persistent candidemia. Hemorrhagic bullae have also been reported.

Ocular Candidiasis. This form of localized candidiasis may result from either hematogenous spread or direct inoculation, e.g., after cataract extraction or intraocular lens implantation. Any eye structure may be infected; endophthalmitis is the most fulminant manifestation and may result in blindness. Single or multiple fluffy white cotton ball–like chorioretinal lesions, often extending into the vitreous, are characteristic. These lesions can be easily recognized on funduscopic examination and should be serially looked for in all patients with known candidemia.

Renal Candidiasis. Infection of the kidneys may be secondary to ascending extension from the bladder (*Candida* cystitis), resulting in papillary necrosis, caliceal invasion, or formation of a fungus ball in the ureter or renal pelvis. More commonly, renal candidiasis is secondary to hematogenous spread, in patients with either documented or undocumented candidemia, resulting in pyelonephritis with diffuse cortical and medullary abscesses. The triad of candidemia, candiduria, and *Candida* organisms within casts in urinary sediment provides presumptive evidence of upper urinary tract involvement.

Hepatosplenic Candidiasis. This visceral form of deep infection occurs most commonly in patients with hematologic malignancies, especially leukemia, who are in remission after prolonged chemotherapy-induced neutropenia. Gastrointestinal candidiasis complicated by portal fungemia is the source in most patients; documented candidemia or evidence of disease in other organs is usually absent. Persistent unexplained fever, right upper quadrant tenderness and pain, elevated alkaline phosphatase levels and multiple, scattered "bull's eye" lesions in the liver and spleen, demonstrated by abdominal ultrasonographic examination or computed tomography (CT), are features. Diagnosis is established by characteristic histopathology on liver biopsy.

Pulmonary Candidiasis. Whereas colonization by yeasts of the tracheobronchial tree is common in seriously ill, debilitated intensive care unit patients on ventilators, *bona fide* pneumonia caused by *Candida* species is rare. Diagnosis should be based on histopathologic evidence of yeast invasion.

Cardiac Candidiasis. Disseminated candidiasis is complicated frequently by *Candida* myocarditis (>50% of cases) and occasionally by *Candida* pericarditis. *Candida* is the most common cause of fungal endocarditis and should be suspected in the setting of indwelling cardiac prostheses, intravenous drug abuse, and prolonged use of central intravenous catheters for chemotherapy, hyperalimentation, or hemodynamic monitoring. Because fungal valvular vegetations are large and friable, major embolic events involving the central nervous system (CNS), coronary arteries, and large peripheral arteries are common.

Central Nervous System Candidiasis. Meningitis and intracerebral microabscesses as well as macroabscesses frequently complicate disseminated candidiasis. Cerebrospinal fluid pleocytosis, most often lymphocytic, hypoglycorrhachia, and elevated protein levels are typical; yeast organisms can be identified by wet preparation, Gram stain, or culture, in fewer than one half of cases. *Candida* meningitis may be a complication of ventricular shunt infection.

Musculoskeletal Candidiasis. Manifestations include myositis (abscess) in neutropenic patients and costochondritis, arthritis, and osteomyelitis (special predilection for vertebrae and intervertebral discs) in intravenous drug users. All of these complications may develop in any patient with disseminated candidiasis, whatever the setting or source.

DIAGNOSIS. Mucocutaneous lesions are diagnosed on the basis of clinical appearance and by examination of potassium hydroxide wet mounts or Gram-stained smears of lesion material obtained by scraping or swabbing. Masses of spherical budding yeast forms and pseudohyphae are characteristic. Patients suspected of having *Candida* esophagitis should undergo not only endoscopy and brushing but also biopsy in an attempt to histopathologically demonstrate mucosal invasion of *Candida* organisms. Esophagitis caused by either herpes simplex virus or cytomegalovirus may mimic the symptoms and appearance of *Candida* esophagitis; infection in a single patient caused by more than one microorganism is not unusual. Fungal blood cultures in patients with suspected candidemia or disseminated candidiasis should be performed using the highly sensitive lysis centrifugation method; this technique also allows more rapid detection of growth. Multiple serial cultures should be obtained. Data gathered over the past decade indicate that a single positive blood culture for *Candida* species should be assumed to represent clinically significant candidemia that merits antifungal therapy. The finding of heavy growth of *Candida* species in cultures of sputum, tracheal aspirate, wounds, or urine may increase the likelihood of bloodstream invasion but does not prove that dissemination has occurred. Because blood cultures may be negative in as many as 50% of patients with disseminated candidiasis, diagnosis must often depend on the results of histopathologic study and fungal cultures of tissue obtained by biopsy. Diagnostic procedures that should be considered include CT of the head, thorax, and abdomen; echocardiography; thoracentesis; arthrocentesis; lumbar puncture; and biopsy of skin, liver, kidney, myocardium, bone, muscle, or lung. Although quantitative or semiquantitative cultures of selected tissue specimens have been advocated as useful predictors of disseminated disease, no correlative data support this concept. Skin testing with *Candida* antigen may be useful in assessing for anergy but has no role in diagnosing candidiasis. Although much effort has been devoted to the development of reliable, simple, sensitive, and specific serologic assays for detecting serum antibodies to *Candida,* circulating *Candida* antigen (e.g., cell wall mannan or cytoplasmic enolase), or a metabolite, controversy persists about the value of these serodiagnostic procedures. Because false-positive and false-negative results are common, the decision to initiate treatment cannot be based on results of serologic tests alone. Over the past decade, numerous strain-typing methods have been developed to assist in the epidemiologic investigation and control of *Candida* species as nosocomial pathogens. Examples of older phenotypic methods include biochemical markers, isoenzyme patterns, sensitivity toward killer yeasts, and serotyping; newer genotypic methods include electrophoretic karyotyping, DNA probes, restriction endonuclease analysis of genomic DNA, restriction fragment length polymorphism, and random amplified polymorphic DNA. At present, the genotypic typing methods appear to be the most practical and sensitive means of discriminating strains of *Candida* species.

TREATMENT. In most patients with mucocutaneous infections, any one of several topical preparations, including nystatin, clotrimazole, miconazole, econazole, and ketoconazole, provides effective therapy. Nystatin suspension and clotrimazole troches appear to be equal in efficacy as therapy for oral thrush, but clotrimazole is better tolerated. Although the clinical manifestations of *Candida* vulvovaginitis are usually eliminated by local topical therapy with nystatin, clotrimazole, butoconazole, terconazole, or miconazole administered for 3 to 7 days, the disease tends to recur frequently in some patients. Newer approaches to acute vulvovaginitis use single-dose therapy, e.g., clotrimazole, 500-mg vaginal pessary; miconazole, 1200-mg ovule; or fluconazole, 150-mg oral tablet. In refractory cases, prolonged therapy with a topical agent or an orally absorbed azole, such as ketoconazole or fluconazole, provided that pregnancy has been excluded, may be beneficial. Oral ketoconazole, 200 to 400 mg daily, is the treatment of choice for chronic mucocutaneous candidiasis and must be continued indefinitely to avoid relapse. HIV-infected patients with mucocutaneous forms of candidiasis respond less rapidly than other patient groups and often with incomplete clearance of exudative patches. Nystatin suspension appears to be less effective than either clotrimazole troches or an oral drug, e.g., ketoconazole or fluconazole, in AIDS patients with oropharyngeal or esophageal candidiasis. Fluconazole appears to be more effective than ketoconazole. However, recent clinical microbiologic and epidemiologic data indicate an emerging problem of resistance to fluconazole among AIDS patients with oral thrush who are exposed either to repeated short courses of low-dose fluconazole therapy (50 to 100 mg daily) or prolonged prophylactic therapy. Although cross-resistance may develop to itraconazole, this triazole has been an effective therapeutic alternative in many patients with fluconazole-resistant disease. In refractory cases associated with severe disease and/or fluconazole-resistance, low-dose amphotericin B can be used.

Recent studies have established important guidelines regarding therapy of serious *Candida* disease, e.g., candidemia or disseminated candidiasis. First, in most patients with catheter-related candidemia, the catheter, if still present, should be removed. Second, in patients with suppurative peripheral thrombophlebitis, surgical segmental venous resection is necessary. Third, because of the high risk of metastatic complications of candidemia, such as endophthalmitis, osteomyelitis, arthritis, nephritis, myocarditis, and endocarditis, all patients with candidemia, even non-neutropenic hosts, deserve a course of antifungal chemotherapy. For patients with candidemia, both amphotericin B and fluconazole are effective in selected populations. Fluconazole, 400 mg daily for 14 days (initial intravenous therapy followed by oral therapy), should be reserved primarily for non-neutropenic patients with catheter-associated candidemia. Amphotericin B, 0.5 to 0.8 mg per kilogram per day for 7 to 14 days, should usually be given to compromised hosts, especially those who are granulocytopenic, patients with persistent candidemia (whatever the cause), and patients with septic shock syndrome due to *Candida* species. Until additional guidelines are forthcoming from ongoing prospective studies, the decisions regarding which drug to use and at what dosage must be based on the host defense status of the patient, underlying conditions, predisposing factors, and results of serial blood cultures and physical examinations for complications of candidemia.

Patients with documented disseminated disease, manifested as either localized deep disease (e.g., hepatosplenic candidiasis, CNS candidiasis, renal candidiasis, or *Candida* endocarditis) or multiorgan disease, should be treated with amphotericin B (total dose 2.0 to 3.0 grams), often in combination with flucytosine (75 to 125 mg per kilogram per day). Fluconazole may have a role in the therapy of hepatosplenic candidiasis, either as primary therapy or consolidation therapy after an initial course of amphotericin B, with or without flucytosine. Valve replacement is a necessary adjunct to chemotherapy in patients with *Candida* endocarditis.

Candida cystitis, in contrast to renal candidiasis, can be cured by removing the bladder catheter in the majority of cases. Therapeutic options available for managing candiduria that is persistent after catheter removal or in diabetic patients include oral flucytosine, 75 to 100 mg per kilogram per day for 7 to 10 days, or oral fluconazole, 100 to 200 mg per day for 7 to 10 days. Although both of these antifungal agents are excreted by the kidneys, fluconazole is preferred because it is less toxic. Eradicating candiduria in patients whose condition justifies a persistent indwelling catheter can be attempted with amphotericin B (50 μg per milliliter) or miconazole (50 μg per milliliter) bladder rinses.

Therapy for *Candida* peritonitis, which most often is a complication of continuous ambulatory peritoneal dialysis, is less straightforward. Ideally, the peritoneal catheter should be discontinued, and either intravenous amphotericin B or oral fluconazole should be administered until clinical symptoms and signs resolve and cultures become negative. For patients in whom the catheter must be maintained, instilling either amphotericin B or fluconazole in the dialysate fluid, has been successful.

Managing ocular candidiasis requires close cooperation with an ophthalmologist experienced in eye infections. For most cases of endophthalmitis, systemic amphotericin B with or without flucytosine plus vitrectomy to remove vitreous abscesses is required. Findings at vitrectomy may also be used to confirm the diagnosis. Data, largely from animal models, provide conflicting results about the efficacy of azole drugs as therapy of *Candida* endophthalmitis.

PREVENTION. Given the increasing incidence of nosocomial candidemia and its potential severity, awareness of the problem and measures aimed at prevention assume increasing importance. The frequency and duration of use of intravascular catheters and monitoring devices should be reduced, and subclavian central catheters should be changed at least weekly. Special attention should be paid to long-term access devices for chemotherapy such as Hickman or Broviac catheters. Similarly, the frequency, breadth, and duration of courses of antibiotics should be reduced. Antifungal drugs are commonly used in seriously ill hospitalized patients, especially those with granulocytopenia, to prevent *Candida* infection. Although fluconazole, the drug most commonly used, appears to be more beneficial in bone marrow transplant recipients than in patients with acute leukemia (see references), several concerns persist. Widespread injudicious use of oral azoles in prophylaxis does not offer protection against natively resistant pathogenic fungi (*Aspergillus* species, *Mucorales*, *Fusarium* species, *C. krusei*, and *T. glabrata*), and it may increase the likelihood of emergence of resistant organisms and may not be cost-effective.

Edwards JE Jr, Filler SG: Current strategies for treating invasive candidiasis: Emphasis on infections in nonneutropenic patients. Clin Infect Dis 14(suppl 1):S106, 1992. *A thoughtful perspective on the various approaches to serious* Candida *disease, including data to support each approach.*

Fraser VJ, Jones M, Dunkel J, et al.: Candidemia in a tertiary care hospital: Epidemiology, risk factors, and predictors of mortality. Clin Infect Dis 15:414, 1992. *Detailed univariate and multivariate analyses of the risk factors and predictors of mortality among 106 patients with candidemia over a one-year period. Of 30 patients who did not receive antifungal therapy, 19 (63%) died.*

Goodman JL, Winston DJ, Greenfield RA, et al.: A controlled trial of fluconazole to prevent fungal infections in patients undergoing bone marrow transplantation. N Engl J Med 326:845, 1992; Winston DJ, Chandrasekar PH, Lazarus HM, et al.: Fluconazole prophylaxis of fungal infection in patients with acute leukemia: Results of a randomized placebo-controlled, double-blind, multicenter trial. Ann Intern Med 118:495, 1993. *The first trial in bone marrow transplant recipients showed that fluconazole (400 mg per day) was more effective than placebo in preventing both superficial and systemic fungal infections, but overall mortality between the two treatment groups was not significantly different. By contrast, in the second trial in patients with acute leukemia, the same dose of fluconazole did not decrease the frequency of invasive fungal disease, reduce the empirical use of amphotericin B, or decrease the mortality rate.*

Lecciones JA, Lee JW, Navarro EE, et al.: Vascular catheter-associated fungemia in patients with cancer: Analysis of 155 episodes. Clin Infect Dis 14:875, 1992. *A retrospective review of central venous catheter-associated fungemia, primarily candidemia, over a 10-year period; results argue strongly for catheter removal.*

Sobel JD: Candidal vulvovaginitis. Clin Obstet Gynecol 36:153, 1993. *A practical overview of the pathogenesis, clinical manifestations, and treatment of this common mucosal infection in women.*

355 ASPERGILLOSIS

David A. Stevens

DEFINITION. Aspergillosis refers to infection with any of the species of the genus *Aspergillus*. These are in mold form in the environment, on artificial media, and when invading tissues.

ASPERGILLOSIS	
Causative fungus	*Aspergillus* species: *A. fumigatus, A. flavus, A. niger, A. terreus*
Primary geographic distribution	Ubiquitous: human habitat, soil, water, air
Primary route of acquisition	Inhaling spores
Principal site of disease	Lung
Opportunistic infection in compromised hosts	Invasive form, pulmonary
Drug of choice for most patients	Amphotericin, itraconazole
Alternative therapy	None

ETIOLOGY AND EPIDEMIOLOGY. Aspergilli are ubiquitous in the environment and have been isolated with ease from soil and air, and even swimming pools and saunas. They are associated with decaying matter and may grow in temperatures of 40 to 50°C, e.g., self-heating organic compost. The ease with which they are isolated from composting materials, silos, and the cooling canals of nuclear power plants has been an environmental and industrial concern. They are easily isolated from houses, particularly from basements, crawl spaces, bedding, humidifiers, ventilation ducts, potted plants, wicker or straw material, and house dust; in surveys they have been found in, for example, condiments, pasta, and marijuana samples. This pervasiveness should not make it surprising that they are sometimes found in normal expectorated sputa. They are important pathogens of insects (of economic importance to beekeepers) and birds, both domesticated and wild, and cause abortion in cattle. As they grow, they produce toxins, such as aflatoxin—one of the most potent carcinogens known—which contaminates the food chain, posing a risk to animals and humans. Their threat to hospitalized patients has been revealed in outbreaks of infection, particularly pulmonary infection in compromised hosts, associated with renovation and new construction. The suspected vector has been unfiltered air, as from inlets contaminated with bird excreta and fireproofing materials.

The most common species infecting humans are *A. fumigatus, A. flavus, A. niger,* and *A. terreus.* Some are speciated by the clinical laboratory only with difficulty, and they may be reported only as "*Aspergillus* species." In tissues they may be seen as septate hyphae, dichotomously branched (resembling the divergence of fingers from one another), and they may produce their characteristic conidia in tissues or artificial media, which is one way to differentiate them. If the septation can be seen, they can be differentiated from the zygomycetes; they may be confused with *Pseudallescheria boydii*, however, unless the characteristic terminal spores of the latter are seen.

Aspergillosis generally results from airborne conidia and is not contagious.

SYNDROMES. The main forms of clinical aspergillosis are shown in Table 355–1.

The *invasive* form of the disease is generally a problem of im-

TABLE 355–1. ASPERGILLOSIS SYNDROMES

Invasive disease	Asthma
Aspergilloma (fungus ball)	Invasive airways disease
Superficial bronchial disease	Bronchocentric granulomatosis
Extrinsic allergic alveolitis	Pleural disease
Mixed forms	Local disease
Allergic bronchopulmonary disease	Endocarditis

munocompromised hosts (see Ch. 266), and more aggressive immunosuppression and anticancer therapy are the most important factors contributing to the rise of *Aspergillus* infections. Series have reported an incidence as high as 41% in those with acute leukemia at autopsy, and in 89% of these cases it played a significant role in the death of the patient. In 97%, pulmonary involvement was present, and in 25%, the infection was disseminated widely to various organs. Similarly, in a group of heart transplant patients, the incidence of infection was 28%. This is also a problem in diabetics and patients with the neutrophil defect of chronic granulomatous disease. Diagnosis is difficult because aspergilli are frequently contaminants in sputum and even in other cultures when handled in the laboratory. In patients with leukemia, there is particularly an association with relapses of the malignancy, and usually three or four of the following factors are present: leukopenia, glucocorticoid therapy, cytotoxic chemotherapy, and broad-spectrum antibacterials. The classic picture is that of fever and pulmonary infiltrates or nodules, especially progressing to a cavity (usually when granulocytopenia is reversed), or wedge-shaped densities resembling infarcts. The pulmonary pathology in all these entities is that of hemorrhagic infarction and pneumonia. Pulmonary emboli are common because of the organism's tendency to invade blood vessel walls. These processes often combine to produce a "target lesion" pathologically, consisting of a necrotic center surrounded by a ring of hemorrhage. The sputum culture is positive in only 8 to 34% of cases, and obtaining tissue is necessary to make the diagnosis. Prospective culturing of the nose of granulocytopenic patients has been of some value, because a positive nasal culture (and particularly the presence of nasal *Aspergillus* lesions) has led to the early diagnosis of concurrent pulmonary or sinus disease. However, negative nasal cultures are common in pulmonary aspergillosis.

Targets of *disseminated disease* include the central nervous system, where abscesses are characteristic. The cerebrospinal fluid (CSF) glucose level is normal, and cultures of the CSF are negative. Mycelia invading blood vessels may produce a microangiopathic hemolytic anemia. Dissemination can result in Budd-Chiari syndrome, myocardial infarction, gastrointestinal disease, or skin lesions. Esophageal ulcers may produce gastrointestinal bleeding. Abscesses are common in the kidney, liver, and myocardium.

Endocarditis is associated with cardiac surgery, particularly prostheses, or intravenous drug abuse. Major arterial emboli occur in 83% of patients, and neurologic presentations are common. Only 8% have positive blood cultures, and this positivity is usually delayed 14 to 20 days, contributing to the poor record of diagnosis ante mortem, which is usually made on histologic examination of an embolus. Overall survival is about 5%, and these individuals have had valve replacement. The disease should be suspected in any post-cardiac surgery patient who presents with endocarditis or emboli and negative blood cultures.

The typical picture of an aspergilloma is a fungus ball (matted hyphae and debris) in a cavity in an upper lobe (Fig. 355–1). This has been reported as a complication in as many as 11% of old tuberculous cavities. The patients present with cough (87%), hemoptysis (81%), dyspnea (61%), weight loss (61%), fatigue (61%), chest pain (31%), or fever (25%). The sputum culture is positive in most. Total immunoglobulin G (IgG) and immunoglobulin A (IgA) levels are elevated. Invasion of the parenchyma is rare.

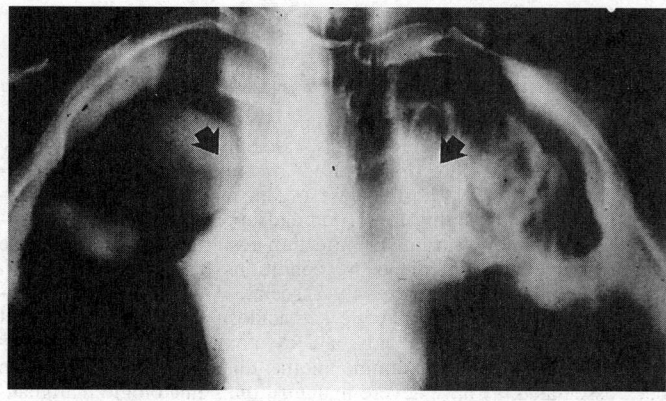

FIGURE 355–1. Tomogram of pulmonary aspergillomas.

Pleural disease is associated with tuberculosis and bronchopleural fistulas. It may occur after surgery or spontaneously.

Allergic bronchopulmonary aspergillosis is usually seen superimposed on a background of chronic asthma (see Ch. 51) or cystic fibrosis. It is characterized by episodic airway obstruction, fever, eosinophilia, mucous plugs, positive sputum cultures, and the presence of grossly visible brown flecks in the sputum (hyphae), transient infiltrates and parallel "tram-line" or ring markings on chest radiographs, proximal bronchiectasis, upper lobe contraction, and elevated levels of total IgA and immunoglobulin E (IgE) especially when the patient is symptomatic. It is more common in agricultural areas and in the winter, presumably representing an association with stored agricultural products (especially moldy hay) and spore production. The eosinophilia is present in blood, sputum, and the lung on biopsy. The mucous plugs contain mycelia, and the plugs may be the cause of the infiltrates, with collapse and inflammation occurring peripherally, or inflammatory edema may be responsible. The parallel or ring markings are caused by thickened ectatic bronchi, and the upper lobe changes are a result of progressive apical fibrosis. The infiltrates may be nonsegmental and transient, with a clinical presentation of "eosinophilic pneumonia" and asthma, with eosinophils in blood and sputum; alternatively, they may be segmental, associated with the blocking of bronchi by plugs, and asthma and eosinophilia may be absent. A biphasic skin test response may assist in the diagnosis. A scratch test with *Aspergillus* antigens produces an immediate type I wheal and flare reaction, mediated by IgE and blocked by antihistamines, but not by corticosteroids. An intracutaneous test with the antigens produces a later (6 to 8 hours) Arthus-type reaction, mediated by IgG antibody and complement and blocked by steroids. Similarly, bronchial challenge with the antigens can produce a biphasic response. Immediate, short-lived wheezing may result, reproducing the asthmatic symptoms and associated with increased airways resistance; this can be blocked by β-blockers, antihistamines, and cromolyn, but not by steroids. There may be a later (2 to 6 hours) reaction, of two types. One is increased airways resistance, as described. The other is a restrictive defect occurring peripherally, which may be associated with influenza-like symptoms, fever, leukocytosis, and infiltrates. These reactions are associated with IgG precipitins and are believed to account for some transient infiltrates.

Extrinsic allergic alveolitis is an unusual form of *Aspergillus* lung disease and has been most associated with A. *clavatus* in malt workers. The patients develop a hypersensitivity pneumonitis with dyspnea and fever 4 hours after exposure. Diffuse micronodular infiltrates may be present at the time of symptoms. The patients have IgG precipitins and cell-mediated immune reactions against *Aspergillus* antigens, and granulomas are present on biopsy. Eosinophilia is not a feature. The scratch test is negative, although an intradermal test produces a reaction in 4 hours, with immunoglobulins and complement present on biopsy. Bronchial challenge produces a reaction in 4 hours, with systemic symptoms and a restrictive defect but without airways resistance. The entity can progress to irreversible fibrosis. The same pathophysiology may be involved in episodes following massive inhalation of spores, usually in farm environments. Symptoms are present within 24 hours, and granulomas are found on biopsy.

Superficial bronchial disease, an acute or chronic bronchitis with brown-flecked sputum, *extrinsic asthma* due to airborne conidia, and *bronchocentric granulomatosis,* a peribronchial destructive disease with wheezing or fever and weight loss, are other important pulmonary diseases. The aspergilloma, allergic, alveolitis, and superficial forms rarely progress to invasive disease. However, more *invasive airways disease* with ulcerative, pseudomembranous, or plaquelike tracheobronchitis has been recently described, particularly in immunocompromised hosts, and may presage parenchymal invasion. *Chronic necrotizing pulmonary aspergillosis* is a poorly defined entity that usually occurs in patients with underlying lung disease, often with features of invasive disease and aspergilloma.

Examples of *locally invasive disease* abound and are usually severe. These include invasion of burn wounds, keratitis, external otitis (particularly in the tropics), focal rhinitis (particularly in immunosuppressed and/or granulocytopenic hosts), sinusitis (in these hosts or following dental procedures) and osteomyelitis or endophthalmitis (after fungemia, trauma, or surgery). Cutaneous ulcers have been associated with the use of adhesive tape. Bloodborne disease in addicts can produce foci of dissemination that are similar to those associated with the invasive pulmonary form of the disease. A noninvasive form of sinus disease has a predominantly allergic component and eosinophilia. It is responsive to drainage and corticosteroids.

DIAGNOSIS. Some of the modalities of diagnosis have been mentioned in connection with specific syndromes. Antibody to *Aspergillus* has been detected by a variety of techniques and with a variety of antigen preparations. Data from the more commonly reported techniques suggest a high degree of sensitivity in allergic disease or aspergillomas, but generally a low sensitivity in invasive disease. As the frequency of false-positive reactions, even in the presence of other mycoses, is low, a positive test in invasive disease may be useful. IgE and IgG antibody specific to *Aspergillus* antigens is another serodiagnostic adjunct in allergic disease. Detection of antigenemia and of antigen in bronchoalveolar lavage fluid is also promising in diagnosis of invasive disease. The problem with all serodiagnostic modalities is the lack of a generally available, standardized technique. The physician should know the background data for the laboratory to which the specimens may be sent, i.e., the sensitivity and specificity of the assay in the various syndromes. Serial antibody testing in groups of patients predisposed to aspergillomas (i.e., those with lung cavities), to endocarditis (cardiac surgery patients), or to invasive disease may increase the utility of otherwise problematic serodiagnostic methods.

In severe disease, an aggressive, invasive approach, as well as making a tissue diagnosis early in the illness, appears to be a key to survival. In the appropriate clinical setting, such as an immunocompromised host with fever and a pulmonary infiltrate, repeated isolation of the same species in culture, and particularly a bronchial lavage or other endobronchial culture, correlates with invasive disease; sometimes even a single sputum culture (especially with heavy growth) may have to be the stimulus for therapy if invasive procedures cannot be done. Negative cultures do not rule out invasive disease.

THERAPY AND PREVENTION. In invasive disease, prompt, aggressive chemotherapy has produced superior survival statistics at some institutions, although recovery from neutropenia is a necessary accompaniment of recovery in almost every success. The role of granulocyte transfusions or colony-stimulating factors is unclear. In endocarditis, in addition to prompt, aggressive chemotherapy, valve replacement appears necessary. Locally invasive disease in other sites also requires systemic or local chemotherapy, particularly intravitreal therapy or nephrostomy irrigation in renal disease. Surgical excision has an important role in the invasion of bone, burn wounds, epidural abscesses, vitreal disease, sinus disease of noncompromised hosts, and removal of catheters for peritonitis and of silk sutures in bronchial stump (postpneumonectomy) aspergillosis. It may have a function in invasive pulmonary disease for which chemotherapy has failed.

In cases involving aspergilloma, there is evidence that patients with fever, cough, weight loss, malaise, and hemoptysis have an element of allergy, which can be demonstrated by bronchial challenge or the presence of specific IgG and IgE. These patients symptomatically improve if given glucocorticoids. Intravenous amphotericin B therapy of patients with aspergilloma produces results no better than those with routine pulmonary toilet. Intracavitary amphotericin, instilled through a catheter, is a heroic form of therapy that has been attempted in some patients. The role of surgery in this entity is controversial. Seven to 15% of mycetomas undergo spontaneous lysis. The overall operative mortality aggregated from several series is 7% but may be as high as 14% in some large series. The frequency of various operative complications is 22%, aggregated from several series, with a range of 7 to 60%. Furthermore, new aspergillomas have later developed after surgical successes. On the other hand, in various series, 18 to 26% of patients with adequate follow-up treated without surgery died of disease complications, usually hemoptysis, whereas 50% have shown significant improvement symptomatically and radiographically. If any consensus exists, it is that surgical resection has a role in recurrent, significant hemoptysis. An alternative therapy, particularly for the nonsurgical patient, is selective bronchial arterial embolization to the bleeding vessel.

In pleural disease, locally instilling nystatin, amphotericin, or miconazole has succeeded. In allergic disease, measures that have *not*

worked include hyposensitization, avoidance of sites in the environment, and aerosolized corticosteroids. Cromolyn is inadequate in most patients. Aerosolized antifungals have produced remissions but do not prevent recurrences. Treating the clinical disease is more complicated than the effects of drug blockade demonstrable in challenge tests. The continuous use of systemic glucocorticoids can prevent the infiltrates and some accompanying symptoms. Intermittent use of glucocorticoids or raising the dose in patients on chronic therapy can produce rapid resolution of marked symptomatic episodes. The long-term beneficial effects of glucocorticoids are less clear; they are not so useful in arresting dyspnea or wheezing in the long term, and they do not prevent the development of the accompanying bronchiectasis. The proper approach to extrinsic alveolitis is to avoid the stimulus.

For those entities in which systemic chemotherapy is indicated, most clinical experience has been with amphotericin B. Its track record is generally poor in invasive or disseminated disease in compromised hosts (especially so in those with cerebral or hepatic disease or in bone marrow transplant patients). In the compromised host, it should be used aggressively, with prompt progression to a full therapeutic dose, which should be ≥ 1 mg per kilogram per day, if tolerated. Prophylactic therapy may have a role in patients who have survived invasive disease and will become neutropenic again. Rifampin almost always potentiates the activity of amphotericin *in vitro* against aspergilli, whereas results with flucytosine are unpredictable. Moreover, animal models have shown an enhanced effect of combinations of these drugs over that with amphotericin alone. Clinical data to support combination therapy are limited, but given the poor record of amphotericin alone in invasive disease, combination therapy appears a logical avenue to explore, particularly if synergy can be demonstrated. A few cures have been reported in invasive disease with flucytosine (which may have a role in cerebral or renal disease) or miconazole alone. Of the new azole drugs, itraconazole is clearly the most promising and as sole therapy has produced responses in invasive disease. Lipid-complexed amphotericin B and other drugs have demonstrated anti-*Aspergillus* activity *in vitro*, in models, and in some patients and may represent future avenues of exploration. Comparative clinical trials are needed to assess all alternative forms of systemic therapy.

In some centers, prophylaxis of susceptible patients, such as immunocompromised hosts, using intranasal, inhaled, or systemic antifungals, or allergic patients, using inhaled or systemic antifungals, has appeared to be a promising way to avoid disease and the need for therapy. Reducing airborne spores, such as by filtering hospital air and restricting contaminated materials (e.g., potted plants), is believed to be a worthwhile effort for patients who will be transiently immunosuppressed or neutropenic.

Denning DW, Stevens DA: The treatment of invasive aspergillosis. Rev Infect Dis 12:1147, 1990. *Reviews and tabulates data from more than 2000 published cases in 497 articles to give a current picture of therapeutic results.*
Vanden Bossche H, MacKenzie DWR, Cauwenbergh G (eds.): Aspergillus and Aspergillosis. New York, Plenum Press, 1988. *Contains 26 papers by experts on various clinical and microbiologic aspects of aspergillosis.*

356 MUCORMYCOSIS
Sandy F. S. Chun and David A. Stevens

DEFINITION. Mucormycosis is generally an acute and rapidly developing fungal infection caused by fungi of the class Zygomycetes. In healthy hosts, these organisms seldom cause infection. However, in debilitated or immunosuppressed hosts, they produce a fulminant opportunistic infection resulting in marked tissue destruction. Several predisposing conditions have been identified. The infection is most commonly associated with the acidotic patient, especially those in diabetic ketoacidosis. Prolonged treatment with antibiotics, corticosteroids, and cytotoxic drugs and, most recently, the use of deferoxamine in the dialysis patient have also been associated, as have severe malnutrition, hematologic malignancies, and extensive burns.

MUCORMYCOSIS

Causative fungus	The order Mucorales; *Rhizopus, Mucor* species most common
Primary geographic distribution	Ubiquitous: air, bread, fruit, vegetables, soil, manure
Primary route of acquisition	Inhaling spores
Principal sites of disease	Rhinocerebral, pulmonary, cutaneous, gastrointestinal, disseminated, central nervous system (CNS)
Opportunistic infection in compromised hosts	Pulmonary, rhinocerebral
Drug of choice for most patients	Amphotericin B
Alternative therapy	Amphotericin combined with rifampin, azoles, flucytosine

TABLE 356–1. CLINICAL MANIFESTATIONS OF MUCORMYCOSIS

Rhinocerebral	Gastrointestinal
Pulmonary	Widely disseminated
Cutaneous	Central nervous system

THE PATHOGENS. The pathogenic zygomycetes are largely in the order Mucorales, which is related to the term for this infection, mucormycosis. Zygomycosis has also been used to refer to the disease caused by organisms of the class, but that term would include diseases due to fungi of the order Entomophthorales. The latter diseases are different from those caused by the Mucorales (largely superficial infections) and are rare in North America. Phycomycosis is another older term in the literature describing the same infections. The Mucorales are morphologically distinct. Their hyphae are nonseptated, broad, and variable in size and shape. Furthermore, the branching of the hyphae is usually irregular and at right angles. Species of the genera *Rhizopus* and *Mucor* are the common pathogens of this group. Other genera, including *Absidia, Cunninghamella, Rhizomucor, Mortierella, Saksenaea, Syncephalastrum,* and *Apophysomyces,* have also been reported to cause disease. These fungi cannot be differentiated histopathologically. Further speciation requires culturing the pathogen and characterizing the isolates by their morphologic and physiologic features.

EPIDEMIOLOGY. The Mucorales are ubiquitous saprophytic fungi and are abundant in nature. They have been recovered from bread, fruits, vegetables, soil, and manure. These fungi have been isolated from the nose, stool, and sputum of healthy individuals. Despite their widespread distribution, they cause disease infrequently. Fortunately, even in the severely immunocompromised hosts, mucormycosis remains a rare opportunistic infection. The disease is not contagious.

PATHOGENESIS AND PATHOLOGY. Currently, there is no unifying concept of the pathogenesis of mucormycosis. In diseases of the airways (sinus, lung), the infection is presumed to originate from inhaled spores, although the lung may also be involved secondary to bloodstream invasion. Diabetic patients appear to be more frequently colonized. Whereas normal human serum can inhibit their growth, serum obtained from patients with diabetic ketoacidosis is not inhibitory and may even promote fungal growth. Undefined defects of macrophages and neutrophils contribute to the loss of immunity against this infection in the susceptible host. Corticosteroids weaken normal inhibitors of spore germination in tissue. Unlike most pathogenic fungi, these can grow in the absence of oxygen.

Invasion, thrombosis, and necrosis are the characteristic findings in this disease. Once the fungal spores have germinated at the site of infection, the hyphal elements are very aggressive and tend to invade blood vessels, nerves, lymphatics, and tissues. The infarction leads to further tissue hypoxia and acidosis, resulting in a vicious circle enhancing rapid growth and infection. The paucity of a granulomatous reaction is quite characteristic. The fungal hyphae sometimes have little or no inflammation around them.

CLINICAL MANIFESTATIONS. Mucormycosis can be manifested as at least six distinct clinical entities, dependent on the types of predisposing factors of the patient and the portal of entry of the organism (Table 356–1).

Rhinocerebral mucormycosis is the most frequent form of presentation, accounting for more than 75% of the cases in the literature. It commonly affects the poorly controlled diabetic patient who is also in ketoacidosis. It has also been reported in patients with hematologic malignancies who have been neutropenic for an extended period and who have received broad-spectrum antibacterial drugs or immunosuppressive therapy, in other acidotic patients, and in those with azotemia. This is one of the most rapidly fatal fungal diseases if left undiagnosed. Hyphae invade the paranasal sinuses and palate from the oronasal cavity. From the sinuses, especially the ethmoid sinus, the infection spreads to involve the retro-orbital region or the CNS. Epistaxis, severe unilateral headache, alteration in mental status, and eye symptoms such as lacrimation, irritation, or periorbital anesthesia are common symptoms. Examination of the nose may reveal the classic black necrotic turbinates (too often mistaken for dried blood) or even nasal septum perforation. However, at the early stage of infection, the nasal mucosa may appear only inflamed and friable. Facial cellulitis and palatal necrosis may be seen. The early eye findings include mild proptosis, periorbital edema, decreased visual acuity, or lid swelling. In more advanced orbital involvement, exophthalmos, complete ophthalmoplegia, conjunctival hemorrhage, blindness, fixed and dilated pupil, and corneal anesthesia may be found. These conditions result from fungal invasion of the roof of the orbit, affecting the nerves (third, fourth, and sixth cranial nerves and the ophthalmic branch of the fifth cranial nerve), muscles, and orbital vessels, a condition also known as the "orbital apex syndrome." The infection can spread through the superior orbital fissure or the cribriform plate to involve the brain. Cavernous sinus thrombosis is a frequent complication usually resulting from hematogenous spread from the ophthalmic veins.

This spread leads to additional cranial nerve involvement outside the orbital apex, specifically the trigeminal nerve ganglion and the root of the facial nerve, leading to ipsilateral paresthesia of the face or peripheral facial palsy. Internal carotid artery thrombosis, from retrograde spread from the ophthalmic artery or invasion from the cavernous sinus, is another late complication, leading to cerebral infarction. The middle ear may be involved via the blood, cerebrospinal fluid (CSF), or eustachian tube.

The radiographic manifestations are nonspecific. Plain roentgenograms of the sinuses and orbits may reveal nodular thickening of the mucosa of multiple sinuses, usually without air-fluid levels, or spotty destruction of the bone through the walls of the sinuses or into the orbit. Computed tomography or magnetic resonance imaging is useful in better defining the bone destruction and soft tissue involvement, which could be important in guiding subsequent surgical intervention. The CSF findings are usually nonspecific and often normal even in the presence of CNS involvement. The common findings are pleocytosis, with about 50% polymorphonuclear cells and slight protein elevation; hypoglycorrhachia is rare. Smear and culture of CSF are usually negative for fungus even in cases with documented meningeal involvement. Several infectious diseases can present a similar picture. Black necrotic lesions may also be seen with invasive aspergillosis and with infections by *Pseudomonas aeruginosa* or *Pseudallescheria boydii*. The only definitive method of differentiating between these possibilities is by examination of tissue. Cavernous sinus thrombosis due to *Staphylococcus aureus,* as well as rhinoscleroma, aggressive orbital tumor, midline granuloma, and other fungal infections, can mimic the disease as well.

Pulmonary mucormycosis occurs most frequently in patients with hematologic malignancies being treated with antibacterial drugs or immunosuppressive therapy. The presentation is usually acute, and the patients are often profoundly ill, with variable complaints of cough, fever, and sputum production. There is no specific lobar predilection. Pulmonary vascular thrombosis and infarction are universal findings. No pathognomonic clinical or radiographic findings exist. Sputum culture is usually negative. In fact, ante mortem diagnosis is seldom made because of the acuteness of the illness, the lack of consideration of the diagnosis, and the need for tissue to establish the diagnosis.

Invasive pulmonary aspergillosis or other mycoses, or nocardiosis, other bacterial infections, such as *Pseudomonas* infection, malignant invasion, hemorrhage, or pulmonary embolism and infarction may mimic the presentation of pulmonary mucormycosis.

Cutaneous mucormycosis is rare and is primarily a nosocomial infection in burn and blunt trauma victims. Local infection has also resulted from using contaminated elastic bandages. The involved area is erythematous and painful, with varying degrees of central necrosis that can progress to gangrenous cellulitis. This form of infection can also occur as a result of dissemination from another site of involvement. Skin and subcutaneous infection in diabetics can occur.

Gastrointestinal mucormycosis is the rarest form of infection. It is seen primarily in patients suffering from intrinsic abnormalities of the gastrointestinal tract or severe malnutrition. The infection is thought to arise from fungi entering the body with food. Any part of the gastrointestinal tract is susceptible to infection, with the stomach, terminal ileum, and colon being the most common sites. Wall invasion, ischemic infarction, and ulceration are characteristic. The diagnosis is frequently made at autopsy.

Disseminated mucormycosis is defined as infection occurring in two or more noncontiguous organ systems. The distant sites are infected by bloodstream invasion from a local site. Although any organ can be affected, the lungs and CNS are the two common sites. The outcome of this infection is almost invariably fatal.

Isolated CNS mucormycosis results from hematogenous spread and is seen primarily in intravenous drug addicts.

DIAGNOSIS. The diagnosis of any form of mucormycosis is dependent on direct and histologic examinations of scrapings and biopsies of necrotic material. In contrast to most fungi, these organisms are readily seen in hematoxylin and eosin-stained tissue. The Gomori methenamine silver stain is usually adequate, but some special fungus stains, such as periodic acid–Schiff, do not demonstrate the organism well. However, a more rapid but preliminary diagnosis can sometimes be made by demonstrating hyphal elements after potassium hydroxide digestion of fresh tissue scraping. The alkali digests some of the tissue debris, but not the fungus, and makes identifying the fungi easier. Swabs of discharge or abnormal tissue are not adequate and can give erroneous information. Fungal cultures are occasionally positive, but a negative culture result does not exclude the diagnosis nor make it less likely. The media used for culturing these fungi should not contain cycloheximide. At present, no skin tests or serologic methods are adequate for diagnosing mucormycosis. Blood cultures are not helpful.

THERAPY. The hallmarks of successful outcome in this aggressive infection rely on early diagnosis by invasive procedures, immediate correction of the underlying predisposing condition, aggressive surgical debridement, and early systemic amphotericin therapy. Amphotericin B is the only drug with proven clinical efficacy, and a high therapeutic dosage (such as 1.0 to 1.5 mg per kilogram per day, if tolerated) should be achieved as soon as possible. This may be reduced to alternate-day dosing once the patient is stabilized. Typically, a cumulative dose of 2 to 5 grams may be needed to achieve cure. Although local irrigation of infected sites with amphotericin is an unproven adjunct, given the difficulties in perfusion of infected areas because of the tendency to thrombosis, this measure seems logical. Similarly, potentiation of amphotericin with other drugs (such as rifampin, azoles, flucytosine) is of unproven benefit, but given the poor results with conventional therapy, this should be considered if susceptibility testing can be done *in vitro* with the patient's isolate to show synergy and exclude antagonism. The newer orally administered azole derivates have no proven activity alone against these fungi. Improvement of survival may necessitate repeated major surgical debridement of necrotic tissue, resulting in significant disfiguring. If the patient survives, major reconstructive surgery may be needed.

PROGNOSIS. Mucormycosis remains a disease with guarded prognosis. It is difficult to ascertain accurately the effectiveness of any therapeutic approach because the disease is relatively rare and there is a general bias toward reporting cases only if therapy is effective. With the introduction of amphotericin B in 1961, it is generally accepted that the survival rate significantly improved. Rhinocerebral mucormycosis is the most common form of infection and is thought to have an overall mortality rate of about 50%. Patients who develop hemiplegia, facial necrosis, or nasal deformity have a higher mortality. Pulmonary or disseminated mucormycosis frequently escapes ante mortem diagnosis, and only a handful of patients have been reported to recover from these. Superficial infections, particularly in immunocompetent patients, can be successfully treated with debridement and antifungal therapy. Deeper cutaneous infections of the extremities usually require amputation, and when the head or trunk is involved, the condition is commonly fatal.

At this time, the most aggressive approach we can take toward this lethal disease is rapid diagnosis and immediate institution of surgical debridement plus systemic and local chemotherapy.

Bigby TD, Serota ML, Tierney LM, et al.: Clinical spectrum of pulmonary mucormycosis. Chest 89:435, 1986. *This review emphasizes the pulmonary form and includes discussion of the microbiology, pathology, predisposing factors, clinical presentation, diagnosis, and treatment.*
Ingram CN, Sennesh J, Cooper JN, et al.: Disseminated zygomycosis: Report of four cases and review. Rev Infect Dis 11:741, 1989. *A presentation of four cases of disseminated disease and a comprehensive review of 181 cases reported in the English language literature. Hematologic malignancy is the major predisposing factor for dissemination. More than 90% of disseminated infections were diagnosed at autopsy.*
Sugar AM: Mucormycosis. Clin Infect Dis 14(Suppl. 1):S126, 1992. *A review of all forms of the disease.*

357 MYCETOMA
Michael S. Saag

DEFINITION. Mycetoma is a chronic, localized, subcutaneous infection characterized by draining sinus tracts that frequently discharge purulent material containing granules. The disease most often affects the lower extremities, with the majority of cases involving the foot. Originally described in the mid-1800's, the disease was initially referred to as "Madura foot," named after the region in India where it was first identified. Although still referred to as maduromycosis, the preferred name and the term used most often to describe the disorder is mycetoma.

EUMYCETOMA	
Primary geographic distribution	*P. boydii* (U.S.; N. America)
	L. senegalensis (W. Africa)
	M. grisea (S. America)
	M. mycetomatis (Worldwide; Saudi Arabia)
Primary sites of disease	Lower extremities; hands (direct inoculation)
Drug of choice	Itraconazole (as an adjunct to surgical debridement)
Alternative therapy	Ketoconazole Amphotericin B (resistant cases)

ACTINOMYCETOMA	
Primary geographic distribution	*A. madurae* (U.S.)
	S. somaliensis (Africa)
	A. pelletieri (S. America)
	N. brasiliensis (Mexico)
Primary sites of disease	Lower extremities; hands (direct inoculation)
Drug of choice	Trimethoprim/ sulfamethoxazole (as adjunct to surgery)
Alternative therapy	Dapsone Streptomycin

ETIOLOGY. More than 20 species of fungi and bacteria have been implicated as etiologic agents of mycetoma. Approximately 40% of cases are due to true fungi (eumycetoma), and 60% are caused by aerobic actinomycetes (actinomycetoma). The organisms are distributed throughout the world, and the predominant organisms responsible for disease are subject to regional variation. Etiologic agents of eumycetoma and actinomycetoma may be presumptively identified based on the characteristic pigment of their granules. A listing of the predominant causative organisms is given in Table 357–1.

EPIDEMIOLOGY. Mycetomas have been reported from all over the world but are endemic in tropical regions of Africa, India, Central and South America, and the Far East. The geographic distribution of the disease is more related to rainfall than any other climatic factor. Most of the etiologic agents have been cultured from the soil in endemic areas, and occasionally organisms have been identified on plant thorns, which may be responsible for intradermal inoculation. *Pseudallescheria boydii* is the most common cause of mycetoma in the United States and is readily isolated from the soil in the United States and Canada. *Nocardia brasiliensis* and *Actinomadura madurae* are the most frequently isolated organisms in Central America, South America, and the Caribbean.

The majority of cases occur in males, many of whom are field laborers or herdsmen who have long-term trauma to their feet while in wet or swampy soil. Although the disease afflicts people of all ages, most cases are reported in young adults. Person-to-person transmission is not believed to occur, and the disease is unrelated to animal contact.

PATHOGENESIS AND PATHOLOGY. In contrast to systemic mycoses, which are usually established via the respiratory route, mycetomas are initiated through direct inoculation of the organism into the skin or mucosal surface, frequently as a consequence of trauma. Although the foot is the most common site of infection, direct inoculation of organisms into the hand, back, neck, and back of the head can occur in individuals who carry loads contaminated with soil.

The precise mechanism of pathogenesis remains unknown. Once inoculated, the organism induces a subacute to chronic suppurative inflammatory response that is primarily neutrophilic in nature but that may be associated with a granulomatous reaction. Over time, localized necrosis, fibrosis, abscess formation, and, frequently, bone and joint disease ensue. Deep sinuses with fistulas commonly develop and present as draining sinus tracts on the skin surface. The purulent drainage from those tracts often contains grains or granules, which consist of the causative organism embedded in a host-derived, proteinaceous matrix. The size, character, and color of the granules suggest the underlying etiologic agent (see Table 357–1).

The inflammatory process usually extends along fascial planes and may result in substantial regional destruction of deep tissues and bone. Distal spread of disease via the lymphatics or the bloodstream may occur but is distinctly uncommon.

CLINICAL MANIFESTATIONS. Most cases of mycetoma present late in the course of a longstanding, chronic inflammatory disease. The initial lesion appears as a small, painless nodule several weeks to months after primary inoculation. The patient generally cannot recall a precipitating event or specific traumatic incident. The lesions slowly extend into deep tissues, and the resultant lymphatic obstruction, fibrosis, and tissue thickening give the foot a shortened, raised appearance. Skin nodules may break down, yielding granulomatous tissue with serosanguineous to purulent discharge. Later in the course of disease, sinus tracts begin to appear through which the characteristic fungal granules are expelled onto the skin surface. The sinus tracts spontaneously heal, only to be replaced by new tracts at nearby sites. Eumycetomas tend to be more circumscribed, remain localized, and progress more slowly than actinomycetomas, which have less well defined margins, merge with surrounding tissue, and progress more rapidly. The lesions tend to remain painless until deep bone involvement occurs, although many patients may complain of a deep itching sensation during active disease progression. Systemic involvement is rare, and patients feel remarkably well even in the presence of advanced localized disease.

DIAGNOSIS. The definitive diagnosis of mycetoma depends on culture of the causative organism from tissue specimens. The disease is suspected in the appropriate clinical setting, especially when grains are identified in the purulent discharge. Examination of the grains can establish a differential diagnosis of eumycetoma or actinomycetoma based on the presence of characteristic broad (fungal) or narrow (actinomycete) filaments. The characteristics of the granules, when combined with geographic and epidemiologic information, can yield a presumptive identification of the specific organism. However, cultural data are required for confirmation. Serologic tests are not routinely available.

TREATMENT. The response to therapy is dependent on the underlying etiologic agent. Eumycetomas are unresponsive to antimicrobial therapy, although partial responses to amphotericin B, liposomal amphotericin B, miconazole, ketoconazole, itraconazole, and thiabendazole have been reported. Fortunately, eumycetomas tend to be well circumscribed, yielding ready access to surgical approaches. If the lesion is not removed in its entirety and residual disease is present, relapse is inevitable.

Actinomycetomas are more responsive to antimicrobial therapy. Regimens consisting of high-dose penicillin (10 to 12 million units per day), sulfadiazine (3 to 10 grams per day), or minocycline (150 mg twice daily) have been reported to have some effect. The most successful regimens consist of trimethoprim-sulfamethoxazole (160 mg of trimethoprim and 800 mg of sulfamethoxazole given twice daily), combined with either streptomycin (1 to 3 grams per day for 3 weeks) or rifampin (600 mg per day for 3 to 4 months); or dapsone (100 mg twice daily) combined with streptomycin (1 gram per day for 1 month, given intramuscularly). The dapsone regimen is often preferred owing to its low cost. Amoxicillin-clavulanic acid therapy has been successful in some cases which were unresponsive to conventional therapy. The duration of therapy with either the trimethoprim-sulfamethoxazole or the dapsone regimen is usually 9 months, depending on response.

PROGNOSIS. If the disease is diagnosed early, the prognosis for mycetoma is good. Unfortunately, many cases are not identified until late in the course of disease, when response to therapy is limited, and amputation may be required. When disease is located on the back, neck, trunk, or abdomen, very little therapeutic intervention can be offered. The prognosis for survival is quite good; however, the quality of life may be dramatically lessened.

Fincher RM, Fisher JF, Lovell RD, et al.: Infection due to the fungus acremonium (cephalosporium). Medicine 70:398, 1991. *Case report and review of the literature of this saprophytic organism that may cause disease in humans, especially immunocompromised hosts.*

Hay RJ, Mahgoub ES, Leon G, et al.: Mycetoma. J Med Vet Mycology 30(suppl. 1):41, 1992. *Overview of the epidemiology, immunodiagnosis, and treatment of eumycetoma and actinomycetoma.*

Magana M: Mycetoma. Int J Dermatol 23:221, 1984. *A thorough review of clinical aspects of mycetoma and therapeutic approaches.*

Mahgoub ES: Medical management of mycetoma. Bull WHO 54:303, 1976. *Summarizes general principles of diagnosis and management.*

Smego RA Jr, Gallis HA: The clinical spectrum of *Nocardia brasiliensis* infection in the United States. Rev Infect Dis 6:164, 1984. *An important review of the pathogenesis, diagnosis, and therapy of the most common cause of mycetoma worldwide.*

TABLE 357–1. CAUSATIVE ORGANISMS OF MYCETOMA AND THE CHARACTERISTIC PIGMENT OF THEIR ASSOCIATED GRANULES

Eumycetoma	Actinomycetoma
White to yellow grains	
Pseudallescheria boydii	*Nocardia brasiliensis*
Acremonium species	*Nocardia asteroides*
Trichophyton species	*Nocardia cavae* (tiny grains)
Microsporum species	*Actinomadura madurae* (large
Fusarium species	grains)
Aspergillus nidulans	
Yellow to brown grains	
Neotestudina (Zophia) rosatii	*Streptomyces somaliensis*
Black grains	
Madurella mycetomatis	*Streptomyces paraguayensis*
Madurella grisea	
Exophiala jeanselmei	
Leptosphaeria senegalensis	
Leptosphaeria thompkinsii	
Red to pink grains	
	Actinomadura pelletieri

358 DEMATIACEOUS FUNGAL INFECTIONS

Michael S. Saag

DEFINITION. The term "dematiaceous" is applied to fungi that produce an intrinsic characteristic pigment. Diseases caused by dematiaceous fungi are divided into two groups: chromomycosis (chromoblastomycosis) and phaeohyphomycosis.

ETIOLOGY. Chromomycosis is caused by several species of related fungi, most notably *Fonsecaea*, *Phialophora*, *Cladosporium*, and *Acrotheca* species. These agents are brown-pigmented saprophytes commonly found in soil and wood. The microscopic appearance, which is virtually identical for all of the causative agents, consists of thick-walled, dark brown bodies ("sclerotic cells" or "copper pennies"), single or clustered. Sclerotic cells represent an intermediate form between yeasts and hyphae and multiply by horizontal and vertical separation, not by budding.

Phaeohyphomycosis may be caused by several organisms, frequently referred to as "black" fungi. They differ from the agents of chromomycosis in their clinical appearance and the absence of sclerotic cells. The black fungi usually exist in tissues as yeast-like cells (solitary or in small chains), as septated hyphae (branched or unbranched), or as a combination of yeast and hyphae. The hyphal forms are frequently confused with *Aspergillus* species but may be distinguished by using the Fontana-Masson staining procedure (a melanin-specific stain) or via *in vitro* culture. The most common agents of phaeohyphomycosis identified in humans include species in the following genera: *Curvularia*, *Bipolaris*, *Exserohilum*, *Alternaria*, *Mycocentrospora*, *Pyrenochaeta*, *Trichomaris*, *Wangiella*, *Xylohypha*, and *Exophiala*.

EPIDEMIOLOGY AND PATHOGENESIS. The organisms causing chromomycosis and phaeohyphomycosis are worldwide in distribution. Chromomycosis occurs predominantly in young males and is usually inoculated into the skin via thorns, splinters, and other penetrating wounds. The disease is more prevalent in rural populations, especially among those with suboptimal nutritional status and personal hygiene. Chromomycosis appears to be endemic in certain areas, such as Madagascar and Costa Rica.

Phaeohyphomycosis is becoming an important disease among immunocompromised hosts. Despite the ubiquity of black fungi in the environment, disease due to these organisms had in the past been sporadic. More recently, however, clusters of cases have been reported from major medical centers as opportunistic infections in transplant recipients, especially bone marrow transplant patients.

CLINICAL MANIFESTATIONS. Chromomycosis initially manifests as a wart-like papule that slowly enlarges into a verruciform plaque. The lesions may progress to ulceration with or without an exudate. Over time, the lesions become dry and crusted with a raised border, which may be serpiginous. Large plaques frequently develop central scarring. Occasionally, the lesions become pedunculated and acquire a cauliflower-like appearance. Systemic spread to distal sites is distinctly uncommon, although spread through autoinoculation or via lymphatic drainage may occur. Rarely, widespread disseminated disease to the pancreas, liver, bowel, lymph nodes, meninges, and brain is noted.

Phaeohyphomycosis may occur as a wide spectrum of clinical disease. Superficial phaeohyphomycosis is the most benign and is found in the stratum corneum or around the hair shaft. Tinea nigra and black piedra are examples of this disorder. More invasive skin disease involving nonliving layers of keratinized epithelium include the dermatomycoses and onychomycoses. Mycotic keratitis may result in extensive corneal damage and subsequent blindness. Subcutaneous disease usually results from direct inoculation of fungi through intact skin. Cystic lesions with well-defined walls and central abscess formation, occasionally surrounding a foreign body such as a splinter, are characteristic.

Invasive phaeohyphomycosis is a potentially life-threatening disease that occurs predominantly in immunocompromised hosts. Localized invasive disease frequently occurs in the paranasal sinuses, lower respiratory tract, and bone. Disease due to *Cladosporium*, *Curvularia*, *Bipolaris*, *Xylohypha*, and *Exserohilum* species is especially prone to invade the central nervous system.

DIAGNOSIS. The diagnosis of chromomycosis and phaeohyphomycosis is made by histopathologic examination of tissue biopsy specimens or KOH (10%) preparations. The brown sclerotic cells of chromomycosis are readily identified, and special stains are not usually required. Phaeohyphomycosis is best diagnosed using the Fontana-Masson technique, which distinguishes organisms producing melanin from *Aspergillus* species. Cultures are required to identify the specific genera causing chromomycosis and phaeohyphomycosis. All cultures should be held for at least 8 weeks, since some of the organisms grow slowly. No serologic or skin tests are available.

TREATMENT. Surgical excision, when feasible, is the most effective mode of therapy for subcutaneous or deeply invasive disease. Unfortunately, unless lesions are diagnosed and treated early, the rate of relapse is high. Systemic antifungal therapy with amphotericin B is often used; however, the results are generally disappointing. Flucytosine (5-FC; 150 mg per kilogram per day) has been used on an investigational basis in patients with chromomycosis, with some success (16 of 23 patients cured); however, resistance developed in several treated patients. The response to therapy of phaeohyphomycosis is highly dependent on the causative organism. Many black fungi are resistant to 5-FC, and amphotericin B therapy yields variable results. Newer triazole antifungal agents, such as fluconazole and itraconazole, show some promise as effective agents.

Adam RD, Paquin ML, Petersen EA, et al.: Phaeohyphomycosis caused by the fungal genera *Bipolaris* and *Exserohilum*. Medicine 65:203, 1986. *These fungi have been previously misclassified as* Helminthosporium *or* Drechslera *species, but the latter fungi appear not to produce human disease. This paper serves as an excellent review.*

Bennett JE, Bonner H, Jennings AE, et al.: Chronic meningitis caused by *Cladosporium trichoides*. Am J Clin Pathol 59:398, 1973. *Comprehensive review of cerebral infection with dematiaceous fungi.*

McGinnis MR: Chromoblastomycosis and phaeohyphomycosis: New concepts, diagnosis and mycology. J Am Acad Dermatol 8:1, 1983. *Clear-cut exposition of clinical and mycologic criteria for these diagnoses. A very important review.*

Sudduth EJ, Crumbley AJ III, Farrar WE: Phaeohyphomycosis due to *Exophiala* species: Clinical spectrum of disease in humans. Clin Inf Dis 15:639, 1992. *An in-depth review of infections due to* Exophiala. *Case report and review of the literature.*

PART XXII

HIV AND THE ACQUIRED IMMUNODEFICIENCY SYNDROME

359 INTRODUCTION TO HIV AND ASSOCIATED DISORDERS

Gerald L. Mandell

Disease, including the acquired immunodeficiency syndrome (AIDS), caused by the diabolically unique human immunodeficiency virus (HIV-1), has profoundly changed contemporary society and medical practice. The chapters in this part enable the physician to understand the virus and its effects on humans. In addition, there is an extensive discussion of involvement of various organ systems, both by the virus itself and by opportunistic infections. The management of patients with HIV infection is presented in detail.

In 1981, the first cluster of cases that we now call AIDS was recognized and reported. Nearly all of the early identified cases were in young homosexual men, but it was quickly learned that HIV infection could be transmitted by heterosexual contact and by blood transfer from infected to noninfected individuals.

After an initial flurry of fearful reactions by health care workers who believed that they were at a very significant risk for acquiring HIV infection, the facts are somewhat reassuring and protective procedures have been established. It is clear that the greatest risk to health care workers is needle stick (or other sharp) transmittal of blood from infected patients to health care workers, with an infection rate of about 3 per 1000. Universal precautions were established and appear to be a sensible and practical means for reducing nosocomial transmission of the virus. The premise is that blood and body fluids from all patients should be considered potentially infectious and appropriate precautions should be emphasized. Medical students and house officers training in many of our large medical centers are now just as likely to see patients with *Pneumocystis carinii* pneumonia as patients with pneumococcal pneumonia. The possibility of HIV infection must be considered in patients with a broad array of presenting symptoms because of the protean manifestations of this disease and its accompanying opportunistic infections and malignancies.

In the United States and other countries, governmental agencies are now reacting to the HIV infection pandemic. New civil rights and public health legislation has been passed. The potential penalty for acquiring a sexually transmitted disease has now escalated to death. Despite this, countries around the world have been relatively slow to realize that the rules of the game for sexual contact have changed. We can't wait for a magic vaccine to wipe out HIV infection. Educational efforts to reduce the spread of this disease have been supported by nearly all medical and public health groups but opposed by others on religious or moral grounds. The process for drug testing, development, and approval has been altered. Activist groups have caused re-examination of some of the processes and regulations regarding approval of new therapies. This has resulted in "fast tracks" for certain agents. The concept of "surrogate mark-

ers" for disease progression has emerged. In a disease where time from infection to death is close to 10 years, the use of survival measurements to determine efficacy of therapy would be impossibly slow. Therefore, surrogate markers such as CD4+ counts and number and severity of opportunistic infections are widely considered appropriate.

It is difficult to end this introduction on an optimistic note because, despite more than a decade of progress related to understanding the molecular biology of the virus and details of pathogenesis of the disease, neither a cure nor an effective vaccine is in sight. Despite intriguing observations and small gains, the big breakthrough has eluded us.

All practicing physicians must know the basics of AIDS pathogenesis, clinical disease presentation, and principles of management in order to effectively care for patients in the 1990's. A study of the following chapters will help to accomplish that.

360 IMMUNOLOGY RELATED TO AIDS

Bruce D. Walker

The clinical consequences of human immunodeficiency virus (HIV) infection are due to the ability of this virus to disarm the host immune system, a process that occurs by virtue of the fact that the primary target for the virus is the helper-inducer subset of lymphocytes. This lymphocyte subset, defined by its surface expression of the CD4 molecule, acts as the pivotal orchestrator of a myriad of immune functions. HIV infection can therefore be considered a disease of the immune system, characterized by the progressive loss of CD4-positive (CD4+) lymphocytes, (Table 360–1) with ultimately fatal consequences for the infected host.

Despite this immunosuppression induced by HIV, a number of specific immunologic defenses against the virus are generated in infected individuals and may contribute to the long asymptomatic phase following infection by keeping the virus at least partially contained. The potential significance of such responses is also underscored by the recent demonstration in animal AIDS models that

TABLE 360–1. POTENTIAL CAUSES OF CD4+ CELL DEPLETION

1. Direct toxic consequences of infection
2. Syncytia formation
3. Innocent bystander destruction of cells with adsorbed gp120
4. Impaired regeneration of the peripheral T cell compartment
5. Autoimmune destruction
6. Superantigens
7. Apoptosis

a state of vaccine-induced protective immunity can be achieved against retroviruses related to HIV. An understanding of the immunology related to HIV provides insight not only into the clinical sequelae of infection, but also into the prospects for development of an effective vaccine against HIV.

HIV-INDUCED IMMUNOSUPPRESSION

An understanding of HIV life cycle (see Ch. 361 and Fig. 360–1) is necessary to appreciate the induction of immunosupression.

The hallmark of HIV infection is progressive depletion of the CD4 helper-inducer subset of lymphocytes. Because of the central role of these cells in immunologic functioning, the clinical disease manifestations of immunosuppression and susceptibility to opportunistic infections and neoplasms are not surprising. The immunologic deficits associated with HIV infection are widespread and involve numerous interdependent effector arms of the immune system, including both cellular and humoral elements.

DIRECT IMMUNOSUPPRESSIVE PROPERTIES OF VIRAL PRODUCTS. Protein products of a number of retroviruses have been shown to have direct immunosuppressive properties independent of viral infection. A synthetic peptide corresponding to a highly conserved region in the HIV-1 gp41 transmembrane (TM) protein has been demonstrated *in vitro* to inhibit lymphocyte proliferative responses to mitogenic or antigenic stimuli. This region is analogous to a highly conserved immunosuppressive protein of human T-lymphotrophic virus I HTLV-I, and similar inhibitory TM proteins have been identified in other animal retroviral infections such as feline leukemia virus (FeLV). Whether such a phenomenon contributes to the global immunosuppression seen in HIV-infected individuals has not been determined, but the possibility that HIV proteins may be immunosuppressive has raised concerns about inclusion of such sequences in potential HIV vaccine candidates.

T LYMPHOCYTE ABNORMALITIES. Lymphocyte abnormalities associated with HIV infection can be classified as both quantitative and qualitative. Qualitative deficiencies become apparent soon after infection and before CD4 depletion is evident, and are largely related to intrinsic functional defects in the helper-inducer subset of lymphocytes. Studies using purified subpopulations of lymphocytes from AIDS patients have demonstrated a selective defect in soluble antigen (e.g., tetanus toxoid) recognition, although these cells are still able to undergo a normal degree of blast transformation and lymphokine production after exposure to mitogen (e.g., phytohemagglutinin). In other words, the weapon is loaded, but only mitogens and not antigens cause the trigger to be pulled. These studies also indicate that the central defect is lack of helper cell function rather than overabundance of suppressor cell activity. Other lymphocyte abnormalities observed with HIV infection include decreased lymphokine production, decreased expression of interleukin-2 (IL-2) receptors, decreased alloreactivity, and decreased ability to provide help to B cells. The functional T lymphocyte abnormalities also likely contribute to the loss of delayed type hypersensitivity reactions that become more prevalent as disease progresses.

The quantitative abnormality of T lymphocytes is the result of progressive depletion of the CD4+ helper T lymphocyte population (Table 360–1), which begins soon after primary infection. This downhill trend continues until the normal levels of 800 to 1200 CD4 cells per cubic millimeter drop below 50 cells per cubic millimeter and sometimes < 10 cells per cubic millimeter in the later stages of disease. CD4 cell depletion cannot be attributed solely to direct cytotoxic effects of virus infection, as only a minority of helper cells are actually infected, even in later stages of illness. Other factors potentially contributing CD4 depletion include (1) syncytia formation, in which a single infected cell fuses via its surface gp120 with the CD4 molecule on uninfected cells, forming multinucleated giant cells; (2) "innocent bystander" destruction of uninfected CD4 cells that have bound free gp120 to the CD4 molecule, rendering them susceptible to immune attack; (3) HIV infection of stem cells or HIV-induced thymic depletion, resulting in decreased helper cell production; (4) autoimmune mechanisms, whereby cross-reactive antibodies or cellular immune responses to the virus result in killing of uninfected CD4 cells; (5) superantigen effect, in which a viral protein would be hypothesized to lead to stimulation and ultimately depletion of CD4 lymphocytes bearing a specific T cell receptor; and (6) apoptosis, whereby virus or viral products would induce programmed cell death (PCD). Whatever the mechanisms of the CD4 cell depletion, the resultant consequence to immune function is so profound that total CD4 number is currently the best prognosticator of disease progression. The risk of certain opportunistic infections increases significantly when the total CD4 cell number is < 200 per cubic millimeter, which is why routine prophylaxis against *Pneumocystis carinii* pneumonic (PCP) is instituted at this stage. At levels below 50 to 100 cells per cubic millimeter the risk for other complications, such as disseminated mycobacterium avium or cytomegalovirus (CMV) infections, increases dramatically.

B LYMPHOCYTE ABNORMALITIES. As with T lymphocyte abnormalities in HIV infection, the B lymphocyte abnormalities are both quantitative and qualitative. Most characteristic, particularly in the early stages of infection, is intense polyclonal activation of B cells, evidenced clinically by elevated levels of immunoglobulins G and A, the presence of circulating immune complexes, and an increased number of peripheral blood B lymphocytes that secrete immunoglobulin spontaneously. These B cell abnormalities are unlikely to be a direct consequence of HIV infection of B cells. Whereas B cells can express low levels of CD4 and have been infected *in vitro,* there are no conclusive data indicating these cells became infected *in vivo.* Rather, the virus itself or viral proteins appear to directly interact with and stimulate uninfected cells. Other potential contributors to this polyclonal activation include concurrent viral infections. For example, CMV and Epstein-Barr virus (EBV) infection occur with greatly increased frequency in HIV-infected individuals and can lead to B cell hyperactivity.

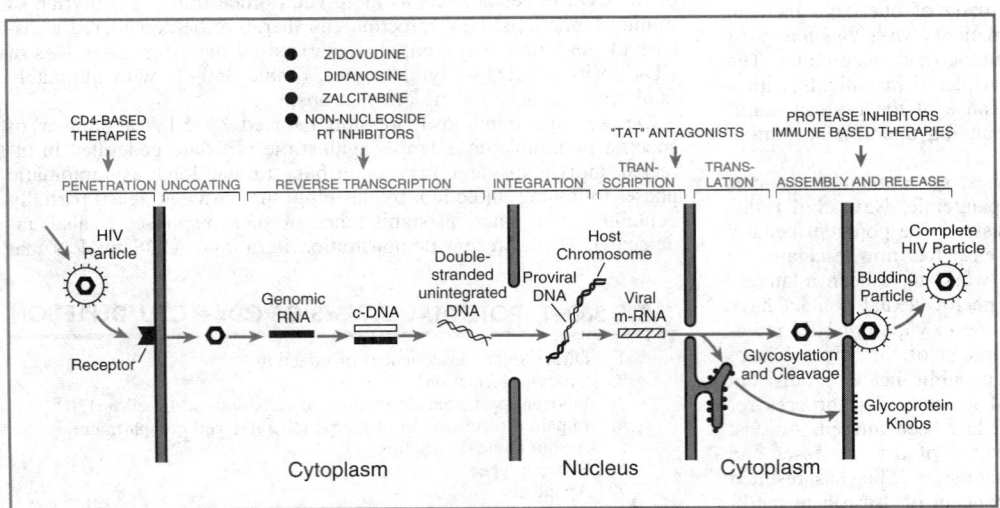

FIGURE 360–1. The life cycle of HIV. The target sites for antiretroviral agents are shown. (Reprinted with permission from Johnson VA, Hirsch MS: *In* AIDS Clinical Review. New York, Marcel Dekker, 1990, p 238.)

Functional abnormalities of B cells consist particularly of impaired antibody responses to antigenic stimuli, and impaired T cell helper function may also contribute to this problem. These impaired antibody responses may account for the increase in pyogenic infections seen in advanced HIV infection. In addition, decreased antibody responsiveness to vaccination against viruses such as influenza A and hepatitis B is also characteristic of late-stage HIV infection.

MONOCYTE/MACROPHAGE ABNORMALITIES. It has been clearly demonstrated that HIV also infects cells of the monocyte/macrophage lineage, probably by attaching to surface CD4 molecules on these cells. Infection and high-level replication of HIV have also been demonstrated in monocyte/macrophage progenitor cells of normal bone marrow and may contribute to the pancytopenia seen with HIV infection. Unlike CD4 lymphocytes, however, macrophages appear to be relatively resistant to the cytopathic effects of HIV infection and may therefore constitute a reservoir of infection. Macrophages may also play an important role in viral dissemination within the infected individual, in particular carrying virus across the blood-brain barrier to the central nervous system (CNS).

At least in part as a consequence of HIV infection, a number of monocyte/macrophage abnormalities have been detected in HIV-seropositive persons. The ability of monocyte/macrophages to act as antigen-presenting cells is impaired, particularly in later stages of illness. Some defects in these cells in AIDS patients may be a consequence of chronic *in vivo* activation, such as increased IL-2 receptor expression, IL-1 secretion, and increased chemotactic ligand receptor expression. The reasons for this chronic activation are likely multifactorial and may relate to exposure to viral proteins or lymphokines or to direct effects of HIV infection. These abnormalities may have immunopathogenic consequences, since defects in the ability to present antigens could ultimately impair the ability to sustain an immune response against HIV or other pathogens.

In the brain, cells of the macrophage lineage appear to be the major cell type infected with HIV and directly or indirectly may contribute to the CNS dysfunction observed in this disease. In the lung, infected alveolar macrophages may stimulate HIV-specific immune responses, the byproducts of which have been postulated to contribute to the observed alveolitis. Deficient T4 helper cell function may also indirectly contribute to the observed defects in monocyte/macrophages, since a minority of monocyte/macrophages appear to be actually productively infected *in vivo*.

NATURAL KILLER CELL ABNORMALITIES. Natural killer (NK) cells are thought to be an important component of immunosurveillance against virus-infected cells, allogeneic cells, and tumor cells. NK cells are typically large granular lymphocytes that recognize foreign antigens on cells, resulting in activation of lytic machinery. NK cells are phenotypically and numerically normal in AIDS patients, but they are functionally defective. This may relate in part to an observed defect in the trigger mechanism necessary to deliver the lethal blow to a target cell. In addition, defective lymphokine production in HIV-infected persons may also contribute to NK cell dysfunction. However, adding IL-2 to these cells *in vitro* only partially restores NK function.

AUTOIMMUNE ABNORMALITIES. Autoimmune phenomena are also part of the immunologic derangement in HIV infection and may also contribute to the disease manifestations seen clinically. When sensitive assays are used, circulating immune complexes can be detected in the majority of HIV-infected individuals. These may help to explain the occurrence of HIV-related arthralgias, myalgias, renal disease, and vasculitis.

Autoimmune mechanisms may also directly contribute to the immune suppression seen in AIDS. Sequence similarities exist between the HIV envelope transmembrane protein and human leukocyte antigen (HLA) class II proteins, and antibodies that cross-react with these two proteins have been detected in HIV-infected persons. Such autoantibodies could impair functioning of cells bearing class II antigens, either by directly eliminating these cells through antibody-dependent cellular cytotoxicity or by inhibiting their ability to interact with other cells.

VIRUS-SPECIFIC HOST IMMUNE RESPONSES (Table 360–2)

The initial phase of HIV infection is characterized by high-level viremia, associated with the ability to detect the viral core protein p24 in the serum. However, soon after infection the level of viremia and p24 antigenemia rapidly decreases (see Fig. 361–6). A long pe-

TABLE 360–2. HIV-SPECIFIC IMMUNE RESPONSES

1. Neutralizing antibodies
2. Antibody-dependent cellular cytotoxicity
3. Natural killer cells
4. Cytotoxic T cells
5. Cellular proliferative responses

riod of relatively asymptomatic infection ensues, suggesting that virus-specific immune responses may play a role in limiting viral replication and thereby disease progression. With the AIDS epidemic now entering its second decade, identification of the precise protective components of anti-HIV immunity remains an elusive goal, although significant progress continues to be made in characterizing HIV-specific humoral and cellular immune responses.

NEUTRALIZING ANTIBODIES. HIV infection induces B lymphocytes to produce antibodies directed against viral proteins, and some of these antibodies are capable of neutralizing the virus. Antibody responses are typically observed 1 to 3 months after primary infection, although longer periods before antibody responses develop have been documented in rare instances. Neutralizing antibodies directly neutralize free virus at a stage before the virus has entered the cell and become uncoated. In a number of viral infections, neutralizing antibody induced by immunization correlates with protection from subsequent viral infection. HIV-1 infection results in the production of HIV-specific antibodies directed at a number of viral proteins, and some of these antibodies demonstrate neutralizing activity. The primary target of neutralizing antibodies is the envelope glycoprotein, in particular a loop structure within a relatively hypervariable region of the gp120 glycoprotein termed the principal neutralizing domain or V3 loop, as well as epitopes in the region involved in CD4 binding that recognize conformationally determined regions that are composed of discontinuous segments brought together in the tertiary structure of the envelope protein.

Neutralizing antibodies have been demonstrated to be present at all stages of HIV infection, and although titers are generally lower in later stages of illness, attempts to correlate neutralizing antibody titers with disease progression have yielded conflicting results. Detailed studies in primary HIV-1 infection have demonstrated that antibodies capable of neutralizing the infecting strain of virus first appear after the clearance of the primary viremia, suggesting that other immune mechanisms may be important in the early control of viremia. In addition, it has been demonstrated that antibodies from infected persons at a given point in time tend to be poorly able to neutralize the infecting strain of virus, but much better at neutralizing isolates from other individuals or laboratory strains of virus. Although a number of animal studies have shown that neutralizing antibodies can confer protection against viral challenge, this protection has been largely in highly idealized situations in which maximal titers were induced just prior to challenge and a low inoculum of virus was given intravenously. Concern persists whether neutralizing antibodies alone would be able to confer protection against naturally acquired infection.

The ability of HIV-specific neutralizing antibodies to confer protection may be impaired in part by the high degree of antigenic variation exhibited by HIV. This antigenic variation is particularly pronounced in the envelope region of the virus, and virus variants may emerge within an infected individual that are neutralization resistant. This antigenic variation also has significant implications for vaccine design, since neutralizing antibodies generated in response to a single immunizing strain of virus are likely to neutralize only very closely related viruses, a phenomenon known as type specificity.

Antibodies also constitute the first line of defense at mucosal surfaces, in the form of secretory IgA. Such secretory antibodies have been found in blood, saliva, and other body fluids of persons infected with HIV, but their potential role as a protective immune response in HIV infection remains undetermined.

In sharp contrast to proposed protective attributes, HIV-specific antibodies have also been shown to promote HIV infection under certain experimental situations. Antibody binds to virions, and this complex appears to be taken up by some cells by binding of antibody through the cellular Fc receptor. This *in vitro* evidence for antibody-dependent enhancement is orders of magnitude less than that observed, for example, in dengue virus infection, and the clinical significance of this phenomenon is not known.

ANTIBODY-DEPENDENT CELLULAR CYTOTOXICITY (ADCC). Another mechanism the immune system can use to limit the spread of infection is ADCC, which involves both cellular and humoral components. ADCC is a process whereby virus-specific antibodies bind directly to viral proteins expressed on the surface of infected cells, thereby sensitizing these cells for lysis by cells that bind to the exposed Fc portion of the antibody. The cells mediating this response are typically NK cells, which express the CD16 Fc receptor for IgG. Antibodies that can mediate ADCC have been identified in the majority of HIV-infected individuals; these are present soon after seroconversion and are maintained throughout the disease course. The major ADCC target antigens are the envelope glycoproteins gp120 and gp41; *gag* proteins may also be involved. It has been postulated that ADCC may limit cell-cell spread of virus by providing an early cytotoxic host defense. ADCC may correlate with better clinical stage in children born to infected mothers, and ADCC titers have been shown to be higher in early stages of infection in some studies. However, the contribution of this immune response to protection from disease protection remains unclear.

NATURAL KILLER CELLS. *In vitro* evidence suggests that NK-type cells are not only important in ADCC, but also may bind free HIV-specific antibodies through their Fc receptors, arming them for attack against HIV-infected cells.

CYTOTOXIC T LYMPHOCYTES (CTL). Cytotoxic T lymphocytes have been demonstrated to be one of the protective host defenses generated in response to a number of viral infections. CTL can kill virus-infected cells by recognizing viral protein fragments on the infected cell surface, where these proteins form a binary complex with a surface HLA molecule. CTL recognition of this complex leads to lysis and elimination of the infected cell.

Although the hallmark of HIV infection is the development of profound immunosuppression, extremely vigorous HIV-specific CTL responses have been detected in the peripheral blood of infected individuals. These responses are directed not only against the major viral structural proteins, but also against the reverse transcriptase protein and regulatory proteins such as *vif* and *nef*. These responses appear to be mediated predominantly by CD8+ lymphocytes, which recognize processed HIV proteins on the surface of infected cells in conjunction with HLA class I (A,B,C) molecules. In addition to this so-called HLA-restricted CTL population, other cells appear to exist that can recognize HIV envelope protein on infected cells in an HLA-unrestricted fashion. These cells may be T cells or cells of the NK phenotype. Some studies have also suggested the existence of HIV-specific, CD4+ CTL restricted by HLA class II molecules.

Although a protective role for CTL has been demonstrated in numerous experimental models of viral infection, the question remains unresolved as to the possible protective role of CTL in HIV infection. Recent data demonstrate high levels of HIV-1–specific CTL in primary infection, and their appearance correlates with initial control of viremia. There is at least indirect evidence to suggest that the CTL response might indeed retard disease progression. For example, CD8+ lymphocytes from HIV-infected individuals can inhibit HIV replication in autologous CD4 lymphocytes *in vitro*. Similar inhibitory CD8 cells have also been identified in the SIV-infected macaque monkeys, and since cell contact is necessary for this inhibition to occur, it suggests that the cell mediating this response may be a classic CTL. Other indirect evidence that CTL may be important in retarding disease progression stems from studies quantifying HIV-specific CTL in infected persons. As clinical disease progresses, CTL numbers decline, which could help to explain the observed increase in viremia observed in later stages of illness.

Conversely, HIV-specific CTL have also been postulated to be deleterious to the host. These cells have been recovered from the lungs of subjects with lymphocytic alveolitis, suggesting that they may be inducing the alveolitis by attacking HIV-infected alveolar macrophages. In addition, CTL have been detected in the cerebrospinal fluid of HIV-infected individuals with neurologic disorders, prompting the hypothesis that CTL-mediated inflammatory reactions may contribute to the observed neurologic dysfunction. A possible mechanism may relate to the release of inflammatory cytokines by activated HIV-1–specific CTL. CTL could also contribute to the progressive decline in CD4 cells by eliminating those cells that become HIV infected.

CELLULAR PROLIFERATIVE RESPONSES. T cell immunity to viral pathogens consists not only of cytotoxic T lymphocytes, but also helper T cell proliferation and cytokine production in specific response to viral antigens. This CD4+ proliferative response is generally triggered by recognition of viral antigen in association with class II (HLA-D) molecules on the surface of antigen-presenting cells or B cells to be helped. Although HIV-specific proliferative responses are characteristically depressed in HIV-infected individuals, a number of epitopes eliciting these responses have been identified, particularly in the envelope glycoprotein gp120. Unfortunately, as with other HIV-specific immune responses, the precise contribution as a protective mechanism remains unclear. Recently it has been hypothesized that progression of HIV infection is associated with specific defects in T helper (Th) cell function. A switch from a predominantly Th1-type cytokine response, associated with the production of IL-2 and IFN-g following antigen or mitogen stimulation of peripheral blood mononuclear cells, to a predominantly Th2-type cytokine response, associated with the production of IL-4, IL-5, IL-6 and IL-10, has been observed by some investigators. Although this hypothesis remains quite controversial, it is perhaps intriguing that Th1-type responses to the HIV envelope protein have been detected in some exposed uninfected individuals.

IMMUNOTHERAPY FOR HIV INFECTION (Table 360–3)

Because the immune response elicited by HIV infection is ultimately incapable of protecting the host from disease progression, and because infection is associated with progressive deterioration of immune function, a number of approaches for immune-based therapy are being investigated. Passive immunotherapy with immunoglobulins as well as HIV-1–specific gamma globulins and monoclonal antibodies may have direct antiviral effects. Thymic hormones may influence the development of T cells, but clinical efficacy data are lacking. Cytokines may serve to regulate immune responses as well as HIV expression. Trials of intermittent IL-2 infusion are under way, with trials of IL-12 therapy planned. Preliminary *in vitro* studies have shown that IL-12 can restore some HIV-1–specific cell-mediated immune responses. Adoptive cellular therapy with autologous cloned HIV-1–specific CTL as well as polyclonal populations of CD8 cells are under way, and although efficacy has not yet been determined, the early data indicate that this approach seems to be safe. Trials of adoptive therapy with autologous uninfected CD4 cells to correct the CD4 cell deficit are being planned.

PROSPECTS FOR VACCINE DEVELOPMENT (Table 360–4)

Ultimate global control of the HIV epidemic will likely require a vaccine that can elicit protective immunity. Although efforts to define the components of protective immunity in infected persons have been unsuccessful thus far, recent data from animal models of retrovirus infection indicate that a state of protective immunity may be an attainable goal. When immunized with an attenuated, *nef*-deleted SIV, rhesus macaques were found to be protected when subsequently challenged with wild-type pathogenic SIV. Not only were the animals protected from low-dose challenge, but they were also protected from high-dose challenge. Although the precise mechanism whereby these animals were protected has not been deter-

TABLE 360–3. IMMUNE-BASED INTERVENTIONS FOR HIV INFECTION

Passive immunity
  Immunoglobulins
  Monoclonal antibodies
Thymic hormones
Cytokine treatment
  Interleukin-2
  Tumor necrosis factor
  Interferons
  Interleukin-12
Adoptive cellular therapy
Therapeutic vaccination

TABLE 360–4. POTENTIAL HIV-1 VACCINES IN CLINICAL TRIALS

1. Soluble protein/peptides
   gp160
   p24
   p17
   gp120
   V3 loop peptides
2. Recombinant live vaccines
   Vaccinia-HIV-1 gp160
   Canarypox gp160
3. Retroviral vectors
4. Pseudovirion vaccines
5. Whole inactivated HIV

mined, these results indicate that protective immunity may be an achievable goal for HIV infection.

Despite these promising results in the SIV model of HIV infection, a number of potential obstacles exist to the development of an effective AIDS vaccine (Table 360–5). Foremost among these is the genomic diversity of the viral genome. Most of this diversity occurs in the envelope gene, with as much as 20% divergence in nucleotide sequence among field isolates. Even within a single individual, multiple divergent strains of virus have been identified, reflecting an extremely high intrinsic mutation rate for the virus. The implications of such diversity for vaccine development are profound, since the virus acts as a moving target for any immune response that is generated. Another obstacle to be overcome is the type specificity of immune responses generated to candidate vaccines, since immune responses generated by an immunogen representing a single field isolate are unlikely to cross-react with all field isolates. In addition, although some of the protein-based HIV vaccine candidates have induced reasonably strong neutralizing antibodies when tested against laboratory strains of virus, these antibodies have been much less effective in neutralizing field isolates of HIV-1. The issue of antibody-dependent enhancement of HIV infection remains controversial and needs to be resolved so that high-risk individuals are not immunized and thereby potentially rendered more susceptible to infection. Once candidate immunogens are identified, animal testing for efficacy would be ideal, but may not be possible for a number of reasons. Unfortunately there is no good animal model of HIV infection. Although chimpanzees become infected with HIV, they do not develop disease. Rhesus macaques develop an immunodeficiency disease similar to AIDS when infected with SIV, but cannot be infected with HIV, are expensive to maintain, and are in limited supply. The potential utility of immunodeficient mice reconstituted with human fetal tissues, providing them with a "human" immune system, remains to be demonstrated. Perhaps the biggest obstacle will be demonstration of efficacy, which will require large field trials in populations showing a high enough incidence of new infection that statistically significant data can be generated in a reasonable period. Demonstration of efficacy in one population may not translate to other populations. For example, protection of persons infected by sexual exposure will not necessarily imply that such a vaccine would protect intravenous drug abusers as well, who may be exposed to a higher initial inoculum of virus. As with HIV-infected persons, the potential for discrimination against vaccines due to positive serology will have to be addressed.

Although these obstacles exist, a number of clinical trials are already under way with a variety of vaccine candidates. These include soluble *gag* or envelope proteins; recombinant vaccinia virus containing the HIV-1 envelope gene; pseudovirion vaccines that re-

TABLE 360–5. POTENTIAL OBSTACLES TO HIV VACCINE DEVELOPMENT

1. Genomic diversity of the viral genome
2. Type specificity of immune responses
3. Potential generation of enhancing antibodies
4. Lack of animal models of HIV infection and AIDS
5. Field trials to demonstrate efficacy
6. Indemnification of vaccinees from discrimination

semble whole HIV particles but are modified to exclude the viral genome or render it harmless; retroviral vectors; and whole killed virus vaccines. A number of these approaches are also being evaluated as potential therapeutic vaccines in an attempt to improve the host immune response to the virus. Combinations of some of these approaches are also under investigation. In subjects immunized with vaccinia-HIV-1 gp160, dramatic increases in HIV-1 envelope antibodies were observed when vaccinees were boosted with recombinant gp160 protein. Other approaches in various stages of preclinical development include use of recombinant BCG-HIV vectors as well as attenuated salmonella-HIV recombinants, which may be more effective at inducing mucosal immunity.

Cao Y, Qin L, Zhang L, et al.: Virologic and immunologic characterization of long-term survivors of human immunodeficiency virus type 1 infection. N Engl J Med 332:201, 1995. *Studies in seropositive subjects who have remained asymptomatic with normal and stable CD4 counts after 12 to 15 years of infection indicate low levels of plasma viremia, vigorous virus inhibitory CD8 lymphocyte responses, and strong neutralizing antibodies responses, as well as some degree of attenuation of the virus in a minority of subjects.*

Graham BS, Wright PF: AIDS vaccines. N Engl J Med 1995; submitted for publication. *Updated review on vaccines in Phase 1 and 2 trials.*

Koup RA, Safrit JT, Cao Y, et al.: Temporal association of cellular immune responses with the initial control of viremia in primary human immunodeficiency virus type 1 syndrome. J Virology 68:4650, 1994. *Characterization of the immune responses during primary infection.*

Levy JA: Pathogenesis of human immunodeficiency virus infection. Microbiol Revs 57:183, 1993. *Extensive review of HIV pathogenesis.*

Pantaleo G, Graziosi C, Fauci AS: The immunopathogenesis of human immunodeficiency virus infection. N Engl J Med 328:327, 1993. *A detailed review of the immunopathogenic mechanisms involved in HIV infection.*

Wei X, Ghosh SK, Taylor ME, et al.: Viral dynamics in human immunodeficiency type 1 infection. Nature, 373:117, 1995. *This study demonstrates that the life span of plasma virus and virus producing cells comprises a half-life of approximately 2 days, indicating that viremia is sustained by constant and rapid turnover of both free virus and infected cells.*

361 BIOLOGY OF HUMAN IMMUNODEFICIENCY VIRUSES
George M. Shaw

DISCOVERY OF HUMAN IMMUNODEFICIENCY VIRUSES

The identification of HIV-1 as the causative agent of acquired immunodeficiency syndrome (AIDS) just 3 years after the clinical syndrome was initially described represents a remarkable scientific achievement that had its roots in earlier discoveries of animal and human retroviruses (see Ch. 342). The selective loss of CD4+ helper T lymphocytes in patients with the disease implicated an agent with T-lymphocyte cell tropism. As expected for an etiologic agent, HIV-1 was shown to be uniformly present in subjects with AIDS and to reproduce the hallmark of disease, destruction of T lymphocytes, in tissue culture.

GENERAL BIOLOGIC PROPERTIES OF HIV-1

Soon after its discovery, HIV-1 was shown to be biologically, structurally, and genetically distinct from human T-lymphotrophic virus I (HTLV-I) and HTLV-II and more like members of the lentivirus subfamily of retroviruses (see Ch. 342). Unlike the leukemia viruses, which lead to immortalization of lymphocytes *in vitro* and *in vivo*, HIV-1 exhibits pronounced cytopathic properties for lymphocytes, causing syncytia formation and cell death. Morphologically, HIV-1 differs from HTLV-I and other type C oncogenic retroviruses in exhibiting a dense, cylindrical core surrounded by a lipid envelope typical of lentiviruses (Fig. 361–1).

The structural organization of HIV-1 is shown diagrammatically in Figure 361–2. Like all retroviruses, HIV-1 is a single-stranded plus-sense RNA virus. The RNA-dependent DNA polymerase, or reverse transcriptase, is packaged within the virion core and is responsible for replicating the single-stranded RNA genome through a double-stranded DNA intermediate, which in turn serves as the

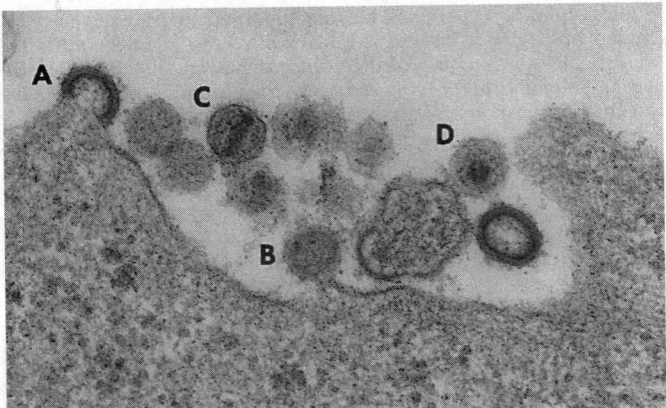

FIGURE 361-1. Transmission electron micrograph of HIV-1. Virions are shown at all stages of morphogenesis: early (A) and late (B) budding forms and cell-free mature virions (C and D) with condensed central cores. The diameter of virions is approximately 110 nm.

precursor molecule for proviral integration within the host cell genome. The major structural core proteins of HIV-1 are the p24 capsid protein and the p18 matrix protein, as shown. Surrounding the viral core protein structures is a bilayered lipid envelope that is derived from the outer limiting membrane of the host cell as the virus buds from the cell surface during replication. Studding this outer viral membrane are the envelope glycoproteins, gp120 and gp41, which are encoded by viral-specific genes and are responsible for cell attachment and entry.

The life cycle of HIV-1 is shown diagrammatically in Figure 361-3. Features of this life cycle distinguish retroviruses from all other viruses. The cell-free virion first attaches to the target cell through a specific interaction between the viral envelope and the host cell membrane. The specificity of this interaction between virus and cell has been shown to be due to a high-affinity specific interaction between the viral gp120 envelope glycoprotein and the target cell-associated CD4 molecule. Following virus adsorption, the viral and cellular membranes fuse, resulting in internalization of

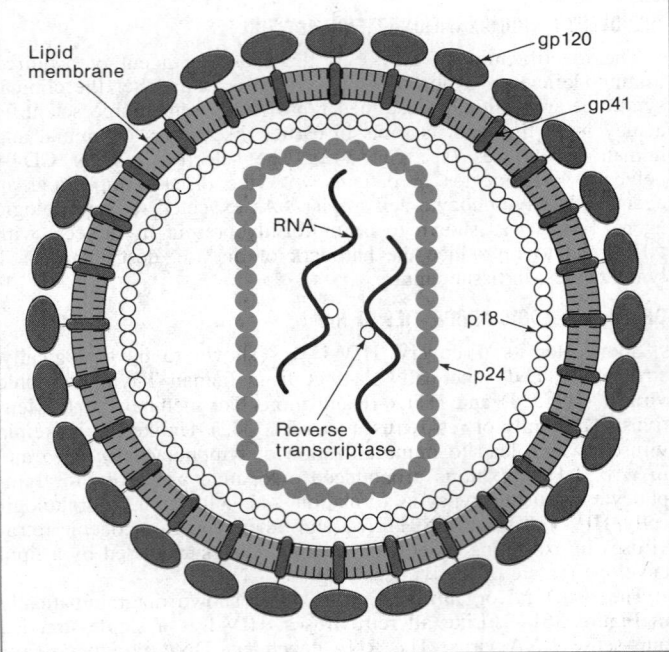

FIGURE 361-2. Structure of HIV-1. (Adapted from RC Gallo. Copyright © 1987 by Scientific American, Inc., and George V. Kelvin. All rights reserved.)

the nucleoprotein viral complex. Reverse transcription catalyzed by the viral reverse transcriptase generates a double-stranded DNA copy of the viral RNA within the nucleoprotein complex, and this migrates to the nucleus where covalent integration of viral DNA into the host chromosomes leads to formation of the provirus. Subsequent expression of viral DNA is controlled by a combination of viral and host cellular proteins that interact with viral DNA and RNA regulatory elements. Transcribed viral mRNA is translated into viral proteins, and new virions are assembled at the cell surface where genomic-length viral RNA, reverse transcriptase, structural and regulatory proteins, and envelope glycoproteins are assembled. Because the HIV-1 provirus is covalently integrated within the host cell chromosome, it represents a stable component of the host genome and is replicated and transmitted to daughter cells in synchrony with cellular DNA. Relevant to subsequent discussions of viral pathogenesis, the integrated provirus is thus permanently incorporated into the host cell genome and may remain transcriptionally latent or may exhibit high levels of gene expression with explosive production of progeny virus.

MOLECULAR STRUCTURE AND FUNCTION OF HIV-1

The genomic organization of HIV-1 is shown diagrammatically in Figure 361-4. The HIV-1 genome, like other retroviral genomes, is diploid, consisting of two identical viral RNA molecules assembled in a hydrogen-bonded 70S complex. These genomic subunits are plus strands of viral RNA in that they have the same chemical polarity as the mRNA from which viral products are translated. Like eukaryotic mRNA's, the genomic viral RNA contains a 5′ methylated-G nucleotide, a poly(A) tract of 100 to 200 nucleotides at its 3′ end, and a number of methylated(A) residues. Host cell–derived tRNA incorporated within the virion is base paired over a stretch of 18 nucleotides to the primer binding site of the genomic viral RNA near its 5′ terminus and serves to prime the synthesis of minus-strand DNA during the initial stages of viral replication following infection.

The HIV-1 genome is bounded by long terminal repeat (LTR) elements and contains genes encoding structural and enzymatic proteins (gag, pol, and env) found in all other replication-competent retroviruses. In addition to these, however, HIV-1 contains genes encoding other viral functions unique to this family of viruses that are responsible for their biologic behavior. The LTR sequences of HIV-1 direct and regulate expression of the viral genome (Fig. 361-5).

The gag gene encodes a precursor protein of 55 kilodaltons (p 55) which is cleaved into four smaller products with the linear order NH₂-p18-p24-p9-p7-COOH. These proteins constitute the core protein structure of the virus and also subserve nucleic acid and lipid membrane binding functions. The gag proteins of HIV-1, like those of other retroviruses, are synthesized as a polyprotein precursor that is subsequently cleaved during the viral maturation process. This facilitates the assembly of the different components of the virus core structure into a three-dimensional configuration that, when cleaved by a specific virus-derived protease, acquires the specialized functions characteristic of the mature virion. The polymerase gene products are translated from the same genomic RNA message as the gag proteins but in a different, overlapping reading frame as a result of ribosomal frame shifting. The pol gene encodes three proteins that are cleaved from a larger precursor polypeptide. These genes include NH₂-protease(p13)-reverse transcriptase (p66/p51)-integrase(p31)-COOH. The HIV-1 protease plays a critical role in virus biology, acting specifically to cleave gag and pol precursor polypeptides into functionally active proteins. The reverse transcriptase of HIV-1 is a magnesium-requiring RNA-dependent DNA polymerase responsible for replicating the RNA viral genome. The integrase protein is required for proviral integration into the host cell genome. The envelope gene (env) encodes a glycosolated polypeptide precursor (gp160) that is processed to form the exterior envelope glycoprotein (gp120) and the transmembrane glycoprotein (gp41), which anchors the envelope complex to the virus surface. It is the viral envelope that is responsible for CD4 binding, fusion, and virus entry.

Within the HIV-1 genome, there are additional genes that serve important viral functions and that distinguish HIV-1 from oncogenic retroviruses. These include the vif, vpr, and vpu genes located between pol and env; the nef gene located 3′ to the env and extending into the U3 region of the viral LTR; and the tat and rev genes, both

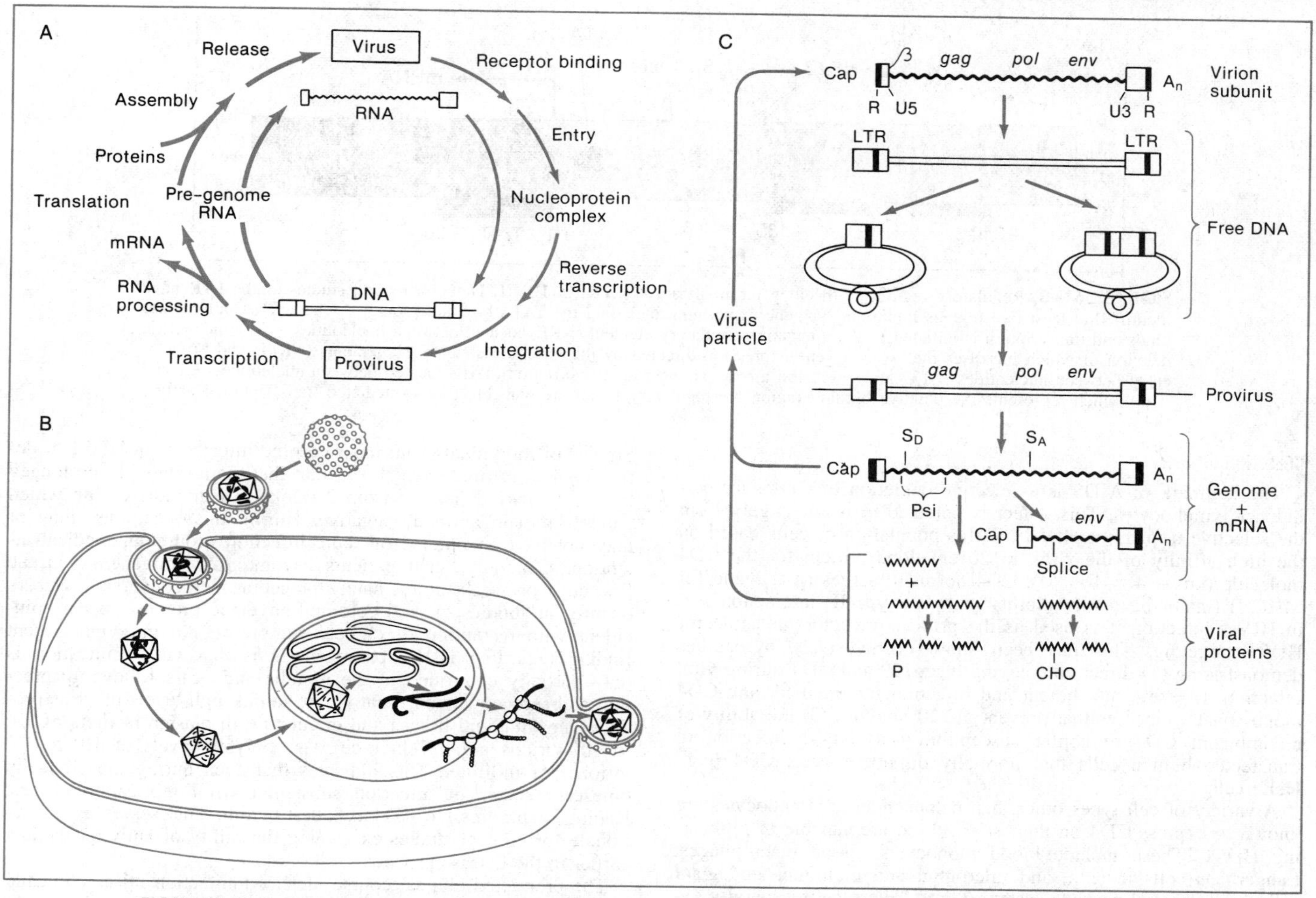

FIGURE 361-3. Different representations of the HIV-1 life cycle. *A,* An outline of the virus life cycle is shown, with thick arrows denoting amplification of viral products that may occur in the latter half of the replication cycle as a result of stimulation of virus expression. *B,* A pictorial overview of the virus life cycle outlined in *A,* beginning at the upper left and ending at the lower right. *C,* A detailed illustration of the major transformations of retroviral genetic information during the life cycle of HIV-1. Cap denotes the 5′ methyl-G-nucleotide, A_n the poly (A) tract, and S_D and S_A the splice donor and acceptor sites. Psi denotes the viral packaging signal sequence, P a phosphorylation site, and CHO a glycosylation site. (See text for discussion.) (Reprinted with permission from Varmus H, Brown P: Retroviruses. *In* Berg DE, Howe MM [eds.]: Mobile DNA. Washington, DC, American Society for Microbiology, 1989, p 53.)

of which exist as bipartite coding exons in the central and 3′ end of the virus. The *tat* gene encodes a 14-kDa protein that is essential for HIV-1 replication, upregulating HIV-1 expression at both transcriptional and post-transcriptional levels. The target sequence for *tat*-mediated upregulation of HIV-1 expression is the *trans*-acting responsive region (TAR) of the LTR, which apparently interacts with cellular factors induced by *tat* because the *tat* protein itself has not been shown to bind and activate TAR directly. The *rev* gene is also absolutely required for HIV-1 replication, facilitating transport of unspliced viral mRNA from the nucleus to cytoplasm. In the absence of *rev* genes, *gag* and *env* mRNA, transcripts are multiply spliced such that *gag* and *env* proteins are not made. The *vif* gene encodes a protein product of 23 kDa, which is required for the production of virions that are

fully infectious. The mechanisms of *vif* action are currently unknown. The *vpr* gene encodes a protein of 15 kDa which is involved in transport of the viral preintegration complex (see Fig. 361-3) to the nucleus. The *vpu* gene encodes a 16-kDa protein that is involved in virus assembly and release. The *nef* gene encodes a 27-kDa protein that decreases CD4 expression in virally infected cells, and by this or other means, accentuates viral pathogenesis *in vivo.*

In summary, HIV-1 encodes the usual structural and enzymatic proteins typical of other replication-competent retroviruses, including *gag, pol,* and *env,* but in addition it encodes a group of at least six regulatory or auxiliary proteins (*vif, vpr, vpu, tat, rev,* and *nef*) whose activities are critically important in regulating the life cycle and pathogenesis of the virus.

FIGURE 361-4. Genomic organization of HIV-1.

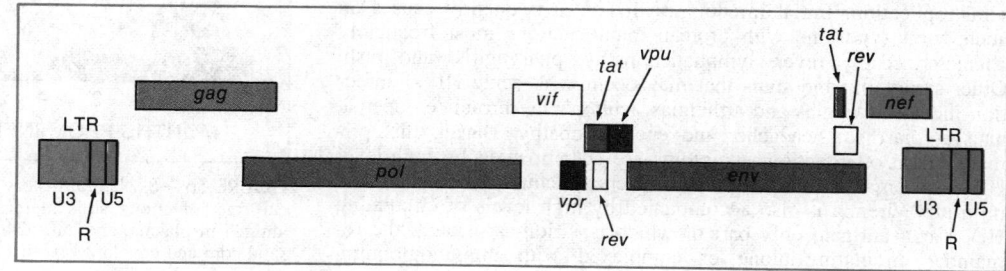

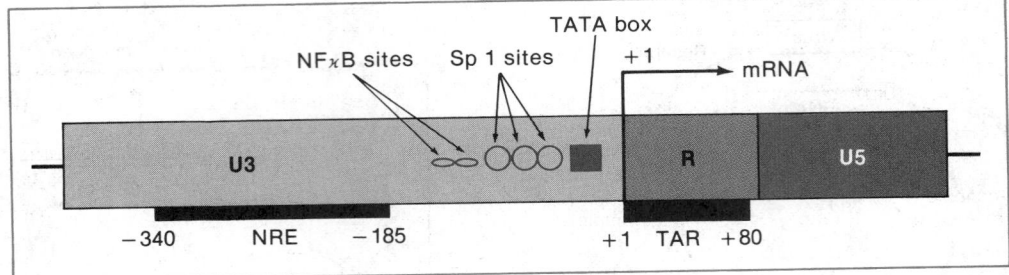

FIGURE 361–5. Regulatory regions in the long terminal repeat (LTR) of HIV-1. Deletion mutant studies of the LTR have identified at least five regions important for gene expression, including the TATA box and promotor where RNA polymerase binds and transcription is initiated (+1); a negative regulatory element (NRE) located between nucleotides −340 and −185, deletion of which increases the level of gene expression directed by the viral LTR; enhancer elements (NRκB and Sp1) located between nucleotides −137 and −17; and a *trans*-acting responsive region (TAR) located between nucleotides +1 and +80 which represents the putative binding region for regulatory factors responsible for *tat*-mediated transcriptional activation.

CELL TROPISM

The hallmark of AIDS is a selective depletion of CD4+ helper-inducer lymphocytes. This defect is believed to result largely from the selective tropism of HIV-1 for this population of cells based on the high affinity of the viral gp120 envelope protein for the CD4 molecule (km = 4×10^{-9}M). CD4 normally serves as a ligand for MHC II (major histocompatibility complex type II) interaction, but in HIV-1 infection it is used as the primary receptor molecule for HIV-1 targeting. This has been shown conclusively by studies demonstrating (1) direct complexing of gp120 and CD4 during viral infection; (2) viral attachment and infection inhibited by anti-CD4 monoclonal antibodies that prevent gp120 binding; (3) the ability of recombinant CD4 to confer susceptibility to HIV-1 infection to transfected human cells that normally do not express CD4 (e.g., HeLa cells).

A variety of cell types other than helper-inducer lymphocytes are known to express CD4 on their surface and are capable of replicating HIV-1. These include blood monocytes, tissue macrophages, Langerhans cells in skin, and microglial and multinucleated giant cells in the central nervous system (CNS). These cells generally express smaller amounts of CD4 on their cell surface but nonetheless have been shown to represent important reservoirs for HIV-1 *in vivo*. Infection of such cells, in fact, may play an important role in the pathogenesis of AIDS by sequestering the virus as described for other lentiviruses such as visna. Other cell types, including neurons, glial cells, B lymphocytes, colorectal epithelial cells, and myeloid precursors, which may or may not express small amounts of CD4 or CD4-related mRNA, have occasionally been shown to support HIV-1 replication, but the pathophysiologic significance of such findings in regard to viral pathogenesis *in vivo* is uncertain.

VIRAL PATHOGENESIS

Retroviral diseases are typically characterized by restricted viral gene expression, latency, and lifelong persistence of virus in the face of substantial host immune responses. From cohort studies of individuals infected with HIV-1 at known points in time, it is estimated that between 26 and 36% of infected individuals develop AIDS within 7 years of infection and that an additional 40% develop lesser signs of immune dysfunction. This protracted clinical course suggests that expression of the HIV-1 genome *in vivo* is downregulated as compared to *in vitro* infection of lymphocytes by HIV-1, which is characterized by explosive lytic viral infection.

Figure 361–6 depicts the natural history of HIV-1 infection of humans in relationship to clinical symptoms, immune function, and viral replication. Initial infection with HIV-1 frequently causes an acute viral syndrome with protean manifestations most frequently characterized by fever, lymphadenopathy, pharyngitis, and rash. Other symptoms and signs that may occur with acute HIV-1 infection include myalgias and arthralgias, leukopenia, thrombocytopenia, nausea, diarrhea, headache, and encephalopathy. During this primary phase of infection, symptoms are accompanied by high-level HIV-1 plasma viremia, with peak titers reaching 10^7 virions per milliliter. Viremia is also accompanied by high levels of circulating HIV-1 p24 antigen, only part of which is virion-associated, the remainder circulating alone or complexed with immunoglobulin.

Studies of individuals who have become infected with HIV-1 at defined points in time have shown that there is a relatively prolonged "window" period ranging from 2 weeks to 6 months during which patients remain antibody-negative. During this time, they may or may not have symptoms of acute infection prompting medical attention. Generally, such patients become p24 antigenemic in the few days or weeks immediately preceding seroconversion. Subsequently, antibodies to viral core and envelope proteins appear coincident with resolution of clinical symptoms. An important recent finding regarding HIV-1 pathogenesis is that viral replication is only partially controlled in the months and years following infection and seroconversion. That is, the initial high levels of virus produced in lymphoid tissues and circulating in plasma in titers of 10^6 to 10^7 virions per milliliter decrease only to levels of 10^3 to 10^5 virions per milliliter. This indicates that even during the clinically quiescent stages of infection substantial viral replication ensues, leading to progressive CD4 cell destruction. This serves as the rationale for clinical studies examining the utility of antiviral therapy earlier in the disease process.

The protracted clinical course of HIV-1 infection raises clinically relevant questions regarding viral pathogenesis: What are the mechanisms responsible for CD4+ cell loss *in vivo?* What are the viral and host interactions that underlie the chronicity of HIV-1 infection? The precise biologic mechanisms responsible for the cytopathic effects of HIV-1 *in vivo* are not known. Molecularly cloned HIV-1 proviral DNA, transfected into human cells, has been shown in cell culture experiments to contain all necessary information to generate infectious and cytopathic virus. Thus, there is no question that HIV-1 alone has the potential for direct cytopathic activity against CD4+ lymphocytes *in vitro* and *in vivo*. Expression of only the HIV-1 envelope on lymphocytes is sufficient for inducing fusion

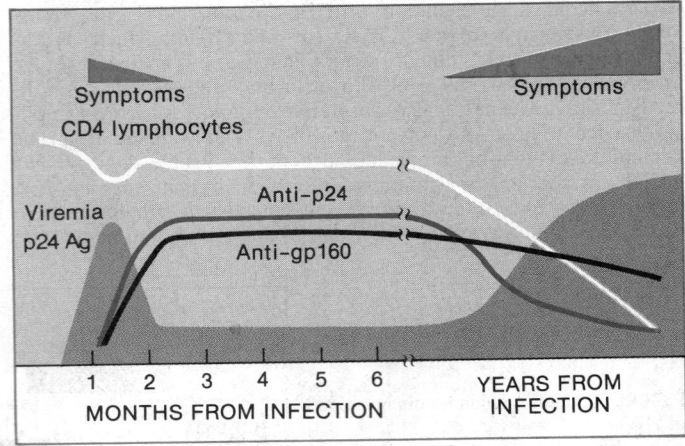

FIGURE 361–6. Natural history model for HIV-1 infection. Viremia denotes cell-free infectious virus in plasma, p24 Ag denotes circulating viral p24 antigen in plasma, and anti-p24 and anti-gp160 correspond to antibodies to viral core and envelope proteins.

of cells with normal uninfected CD4+ bystander cells, suggesting that syncytium formation mediated by gp120-CD4 interaction may also contribute to cell loss *in vivo*. However, other mechanisms of CD4 cell loss may also be operative. Cell-free HIV-1 gp120 envelope protein has been shown to adsorb to CD4+ cells and could serve as an effective antigen for mediating antibody-dependent cell-mediated cytotoxicity, and when processed by antigen-presenting cells, to constitute a target for direct T-cell cytotoxicity. The relative importance of these processes to CD4 cell loss *in vivo* remains to be determined. Similarly, in the CNS of infected individuals, wherein the predominant cell types infected with HIV-1 are cells of the monocyte/macrophage lineage, additional mechanisms of cytopathology are likely involved. Possibilities include the elaboration of cytotoxic factors from infected cells and interference with neurotropic factors, both leading to the clinically recognized AIDS dementia complex.

Viral and host factors responsible for the partial downregulation of HIV-1 replication following initial infection are also largely unknown. A strong humoral and cellular immune response to HIV-1 has been documented on the basis of ELISA, immunoblot, and radioimmunoprecipitation assays of patient sera and cell-mediated cytotoxicity to target cells displaying viral antigens. Neutralizing antibodies, antibody-dependent cell-mediated cytotoxicity, antibody-dependent complement-mediated cytotoxicity, MHC-restricted virus-specific cytotoxic T-lymphocyte-mediated cytotoxicity, and NK cell–mediated cytotoxicity have all been found to have activity against HIV-1 *in vitro* and may play an important role in the down-modulation of viral replication. However, the relative efficacy of the various immune effector arms and the changes that occur with time which eventually allow uncontrolled viral replication are unknown.

An additional component of the viral-host interaction of potentially great clinical importance is the regeneration capacity of the immune system. Recent studies of the clinical effects of novel, potent inhibitors of HIV-1 reverse transcriptase and protease genes indicate that patients with even severely depressed CD4 lymphocyte counts can experience substantial increases in such cells. Such responses have been of limited duration, however, owing to the development of viral resistance to these drugs. Yet they illustrate the potential benefits that may accrue if more effective antivirals are developed.

Genetic variability is a hallmark of HIV-1. The variability of the HIV-1 genome is characteristic of retroviruses in general because reverse transcription of viral RNA into proviral DNA and transcription of proviral DNA into genomic viral RNA are not subject to cellular proofreading mechanisms. The rate of nucleotide misincorporation by the viral reverse transcriptase is of the order of 10^{-4} per nucleotide per replication cycle. Because the HIV-1 genome is 10^4 nucleotides in length, this high rate of nucleotide misincorporation means that virtually no two viruses are identical and that HIV-1 isolates must, by definition, be described in terms of a "quasispecies" composed of populations of highly related but distinct viral genomes. Direct nucleotide sequence analysis of uncultured, virally infected human tissues using polymerase chain reaction amplification has confirmed these findings. The clinical importance of HIV-1 variability is still not fully understood. However, it is clear that viral resistance to reverse transcription inhibitors and protease inhibitors commonly develops and limits the effectiveness of these agents. Antigenic properties of the virus may also vary, thereby limiting the effectiveness of the immune response. Moreover, genetic variability leads to biologic changes in the virus over time, frequently resulting in the accumulation of virus strains with pronounced syncytium-inducing (SI) phenotypes in late stages of infection. Such a switch from non-SI to SI virus strains *in vivo* carries a worsened clinical prognosis.

HUMAN IMMUNODEFICIENCY VIRUS TYPE 2

Following the discovery of HIV-1 as the cause of epidemic AIDS in the United States, Europe, and Asia, patients in West Africa with AIDS-like symptoms were identified whose sera reacted more strongly with an immunodeficiency virus (SIV$_{MAC}$) isolated from captive rhesus macaques in US primate centers than with HIV-1. The identification of patients with serologic reactivity for SIV$_{MAC}$ raised the possibility that certain African human and simian populations could be infected with immunodeficiency viruses related to but distinct from HIV-1. An extensive survey of African primate species for such viruses led to the identification of distinct

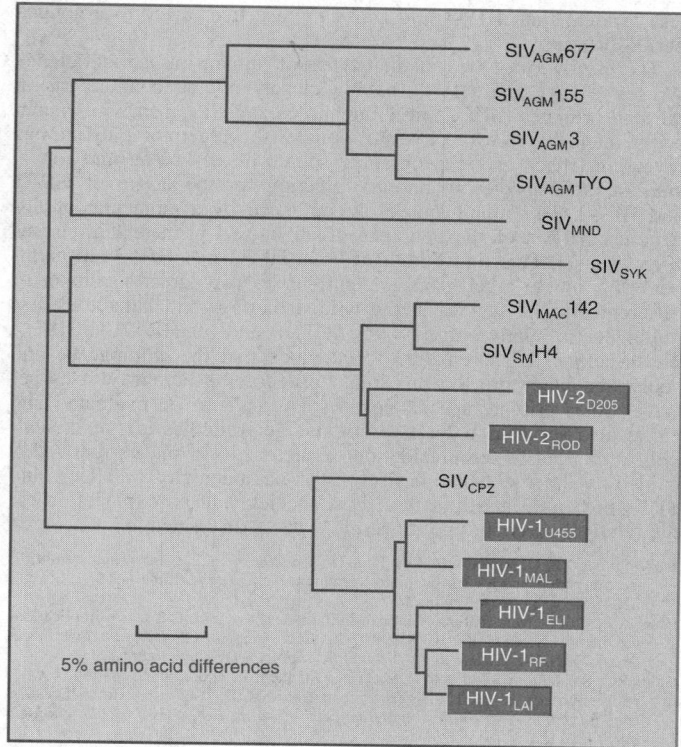

5% amino acid differences

FIGURE 361–7. Phylogenetic relationships among primate lentiviruses, inferred from *pol* protein sequences. Independent isolates of SIV obtained from African green monkeys (AGM), mandrill (MND), Sykes' (SYK), rhesus macaque (MAC), sooty mangabey (SM), and chimpanzee (CPZ) are depicted along with representative isolates of HIV-1 and HIV-2 (boxed). The horizontal branch lengths are drawn to scale and can be used to determine the percentage difference in *pol* protein sequences between the different virus strains. The figure shows five major and roughly equidistant phylogenetic lineages of viruses (SIV$_{AGM}$; SIV$_{MND}$; SIV$_{SYK}$; SIV$_{MAC}$/SIV$_{SM}$/HIV-2; and SIV$_{CPZ}$/HIV-1). HIV-1 and HIV-2 appear as members of larger viral lineages composed of both simian and human derived viruses. Such relationships are indicative of cross-species transmission. (Adapted with permission from Hahn BH: Viral genes and their products. *In* Broder S, Merigan TC, Bolognesi D (eds.): Textbook of AIDS Medicine. Baltimore, Williams & Wilkins, 1994, p 21.)

SIV viruses present in African green monkeys (SIV$_{AGM}$), mandrills (SIV$_{MND}$), sooty mangabeys (SIV$_{SM}$), and chimpanzees (SIV$_{CPZ}$) (Fig. 361–7). West African patients with AIDS-like symptoms and healthy individuals at risk for AIDS were identified who were infected with a virus closely related to SIV$_{SM}$. This virus was isolated, molecularly cloned and characterized, and shown to represent a second major class of human immunodeficiency viruses termed HIV-2. Although originally limited geographically to West Africa, HIV-2 has now been identified in patients in Europe, the United States, South America, and India. HIV-2 is approximately 40 to 50% similar to HIV-1 in overall nucleotide sequence homology. There are two major differences in the genomic organization of HIV-1 and HIV-2. The *vpu* gene of HIV-1 is not present in HIV-2, and HIV-2 contains an additional gene, *vpx*, in its central region that is not present in HIV-1. Although the function of *vpx* is not entirely clear, it is packaged in the viral particle, like *vpr*, and it may have a similar function related to nuclear transport or processing of the viral preintegration complex. Antigenically, HIV-2 and HIV-1 are distinct, with greatest cross-reactivity in structural proteins and least in envelope proteins. Currently licensed ELISA tests to detect HIV-1 infection generally include HIV-2 antigens. However, confirmation requires specific testing by Western immunoblot using HIV-2–specific proteins as antigen. Like HIV-1, HIV-2 selectively infects CD4+ cells. Although HIV-2 can cause profound immunodeficiency and an AIDS syndrome indistinguishable from that caused by HIV-1, evidence suggests that HIV-2 may in general be less virulent than HIV-1 and cause disease over a more prolonged period of time.

The discovery of two distinct types of human immunodeficiency viruses (HIV-1 and HIV-2) having closely related counterparts in African primates (SIV$_{CPZ}$ in chimpanzees and SIV$_{SM}$ in wild-caught sooty mangabeys, respectively), along with epidemiologic findings revealing Africa as the geographic source of all human and SIV's, suggest cross-species (zoonotic) infection for the origin of HIV-1 and HIV-2. This conclusion is strengthened by a molecular phylogenetic analysis of the genomes of all known primate lentiviruses (Fig. 361-7). This figure indicates that HIV-1 and HIV-2 are members of a much larger group of lentiviruses that infect a number of different primate species in the wild. It is apparent that the closest phylogenetic relative of HIV-1 is SIV$_{CPZ}$, and for HIV-2, is SIV$_{SM}$. Nevertheless, it is premature to conclude that the chimpanzee and sooty mangabey are the proximal hosts for the human viruses because other primate species in Africa remain to be evaluated and could also serve as natural reservoirs. Such studies are fundamentally important to the elucidation of the origin of the current AIDS epidemic, the molecular basis for the pathogenicity of HIV's and SIV's in natural and unnatural host species, and an explanation for the relatively recent appearance of AIDS as an epidemic.

Barre-Sinoussi F, Chermann JC, Rey F, et al.: Isolation of a T-lymphotropic retrovirus from a patient at risk for acquired immune deficiency syndrome (AIDS). Science 220:868, 1983. *Discovery of HIV-1.*

Fauci AS: Multifactorial nature of human immunodeficiency virus disease: Implications for therapy. Science 262:1011, 1993. *Excellent review of immunopathologic mechanisms in HIV-1 disease and the scientific rationale for early treatment.*

Gallo RC, Salahuddin SZ, Popovic M, et al.: Frequent detection and isolation of cytopathic retroviruses (HTLV-III) from patients with AIDS and at risk for AIDS. Science 224:500, 1984. *Initial report conclusively identifying HIV-1 as the etiologic agent responsible for AIDS.*

Hahn BH: Viral genes and their products. In Broder S, Merigan TC, Bolognesi D (eds.): Textbook of AIDS Medicine. Baltimore, Williams & Wilkins, 1994, p 21. *Comprehensive up-to-date review of the molecular biology of HIV-1.*

Piatak M Jr, Saag MS, Yang LC, et al.: High levels of HIV-1 in plasma during all stages of infection determined by competitive PCR. Science 259:1749, 1993. *First study to accurately and systematically quantify HIV-1 in plasma throughout the entire course of infection, demonstrating the persistent nature of viral replication in vivo.*

Sharp PM, Robertson DL, Gao F, et al.: Origins and diversity of human immunodeficiency viruses. AIDS93/94: A Year in Review, in press. *Excellent review of the phylogenetic origins and evolutionary relationships among all known human and simian immunodeficiency viruses.*

Shaw GM, Hahn BH, Arya SK, et al.: Molecular characterization of human T-cell leukemia (lymphotropic) virus type III in the acquired immunodeficiency syndrome. Science 226:1165, 1984. *First description of the molecular cloning and analysis of the HIV-1 provirus.*

Weiss R, Teich N, Varmus H, Coffin J (eds.): RNA Tumor Viruses. Cold Spring Harbor, NY, Cold Spring Harbor Laboratory, 1982; Weiss R, Teich N, Varmus H, et al. (eds.): RNA Tumor Viruses 2/Supplements and Appendixes. Cold Spring Harbor, NY, Cold Spring Harbor Laboratory, 1985. *Textbooks on current knowledge of all retroviruses, including the three major groups of onco-, lenti- and spumaviruses.*

Xiping W, Sajal KG, Taylor ME, et al.: Viral dynamics in human immunodeficiency virus type 1 infection. Nature 373:117, 1995. *First description of viral and cellular kinetics underlying HIV-1 pathogenesis.*

362 EPIDEMIOLOGY OF HIV INFECTION AND AIDS

James W. Curran

The first cases of what has become known as the acquired immunodeficiency syndrome (AIDS) were reported in mid-1981 from Los Angeles, California. One month following these five reports of *Pneumocystis carinii* pneumonia (PCP) in young homosexual men, 26 cases of Kaposi's sarcoma (KS) in homosexual men in New York and California and additional cases of PCP and other opportunistic infections were reported. Reports of cases in the United States continued to rise, and soon the occurrence of PCP, KS, or other serious opportunistic infections in a person with unexplained immune dysfunction became known as AIDS. In retrospect, sporadic cases may have occurred in the United States, Europe, or Africa as much as three decades earlier, but the worldwide epidemic was not apparent until the 1980's.

TABLE 362–1. 1993 REVISED CLASSIFICATION SYSTEM FOR HIV INFECTION AND EXPANDED AIDS SURVEILLANCE CASE DEFINITION FOR ADOLESCENTS AND ADULTS*

	Clinical Categories		
CD4+ T-cell categories	(A) Asymptomatic, acute (primary) HIV or PGL†	(B) Symptomatic, not (A) or (C) conditions	(C) AIDS-indicator conditions
(1) ≥ 500/μL	A1	B1	C1
(2) 200–449/μL	A2	B2	C2
(3) < 200/μL AIDS-indicator T-cell count	A3	B3	C3

* Shaded areas indicate conditions included in the 1993 AIDS surveillance case definition for adolescents and adults. Clinical conditions in C are listed in Table 362–2.
† PGL = persistent generalized lymphadenopathy.

The initial occurrence of AIDS in homosexual men and injecting drug users (IDU's) suggested by 1982 that a transmissible agent was the likely cause. The transmissible agent hypothesis gained credence by early 1983 with the documented occurrence of AIDS in persons with hemophilia and in recipients of blood transfusions. Within a year, the retrovirus, now termed human immunodeficiency virus (HIV), was isolated and shown to be the cause of AIDS.

HIV INFECTION AND AIDS IN THE UNITED STATES

Since 1981, more than 985,000 cases of AIDS have been reported from 190 countries. More than 40% of these were reported from the United States, reflecting the relatively high incidence of the syndrome here and a well-established national active surveillance system. All 50 states require that AIDS be reported to state health departments and subsequently without names to the Centers for Disease Control and Prevention (CDC). The surveillance case definition for AIDS was initially developed before its cause was known but was revised following the development of diagnostic tests for HIV infection and the widespread use of CD4 lymphocyte monitoring in clinical management of persons with HIV disease. The current definition provides a consistent method to monitor trends of serious HIV-associated morbidity and mortality (Tables 362–1 and 362–2). Patients infected with HIV exhibit a spectrum

TABLE 362–2. CONDITIONS INCLUDED IN THE 1993 AIDS SURVEILLANCE CASE DEFINITION

Bacterial infections, multiple or recurrent*
Candidiasis of bronchi, trachea, or lungs
Candidiasis, esophageal
Cervical cancer, invasive†
Coccidioidomycosis, disseminated or extrapulmonary
Cryptococcosis, extrapulmonary
Cryptosporidiosis, chronic intestinal (> 1 month's duration)
Cytomegalovirus disease (other than liver, spleen, or nodes)
Cytomegalovirus retinitis (with loss of vision)
Encephalopathy, HIV-related
Herpes simplex, chronic ulcer(s) (> 1 month's duration); or bronchitis, pneumonitis, or esophagitis
Histoplasmosis, disseminated or extrapulmonary
Isosporiasis, chronic intestinal (> 1 month's duration)
Kaposi's sarcoma
Lymphoid interstitial pneumonia and/or pulmonary lymphoid hyperplasia*
Lymphoma, Burkitt's (or equivalent term)
Lymphoma, immunoblastic (or equivalent term)
Lymphoma, primary, of brain
Mycobacterium avium complex or *M. kansasii,* disseminated or extrapulmonary
Mycobacterium tuberculosis, any site (pulmonary† or extrapulmonary)
Mycobacterium, other species or unidentified species, disseminated or extrapulmonary
Pneumocystis carinii pneumonia
Pneumonia, recurrent†
Progressive multifocal leukoencephalopathy
Salmonella septicemia, recurrent
Toxoplasmosis of brain
Wasting syndrome due to HIV

* Children < 13 years old.
† Added in the 1993 expansion of the AIDS surveillance case definition for adolescents and adults.

of manifestations ranging from no symptoms to AIDS. Systems have been developed to classify these manifestations in children and adults. In states that require reporting of all HIV infections, a standard classification system is used.

INCIDENCE AND TRENDS OF AIDS IN THE UNITED STATES

By December 1993, 361,164 cases of AIDS in adults and children had been reported to the CDC; >220,000 were reported to have died, including >80% of those diagnosed before 1990. Among cases reported in 1993, 47% of cases in adults were homosexual or bisexual men without a history of intravenous drug use, and 6% were homosexual or bisexual IDU's. More than 60% of the reported cases in heterosexual men and women had a history of IDU, including half of the cases in women. One per cent of adults with AIDS had hemophilia or other coagulation disorders; 2% of cases were associated with transfusions, the vast majority of which had been received before 1985, when HIV antibody screening of all blood and plasma donations was instituted. In 1993, 9% of all cases of AIDS, including 37% of cases in women, were attributed to heterosexual contact with a person with documented HIV infection or in one of the other main transmission categories.

By December 1993, 5228 cases of AIDS had been reported in children younger than age 13, with >54% reported to have died. In 1993, >93% of pediatric AIDS cases resulted from perinatal transmission of HIV infection, 3% were attributed to transfusions, and 2% occurred in children with hemophilia. In 1993, rates of reported AIDS varied substantially by age, gender, race-ethnicity, and geographic area, emphasizing that overall HIV/AIDS occurrence in the United States was a product of "hundreds of epidemics" of varying intensity. Figure 362–1 depicts 1993 case rates by gender throughout the United States, highlighting these substantial geographic disparities.

AIDS has disproportionately affected black and Hispanic minority populations in the United States. In 1993, 55% of reported cases were in these minority populations; 36% of adult and 55% of pediatric cases were black and 18% of adult and 27% of pediatric cases were Hispanic. In contrast, blacks and Hispanics are estimated to account for 11.6% and 6.5% of the US population, respectively.

In 1993, AIDS rates were approximately 15 and 6 times higher for black and Hispanic women than for white women. The rates for black and Hispanic men were five and three times higher than for white men. Racial disparities in pediatric AIDS rates reflect those in women (Table 362–3). During the 1980's and early 1990's, AIDS cases increased more rapidly in those racial and ethnic minority

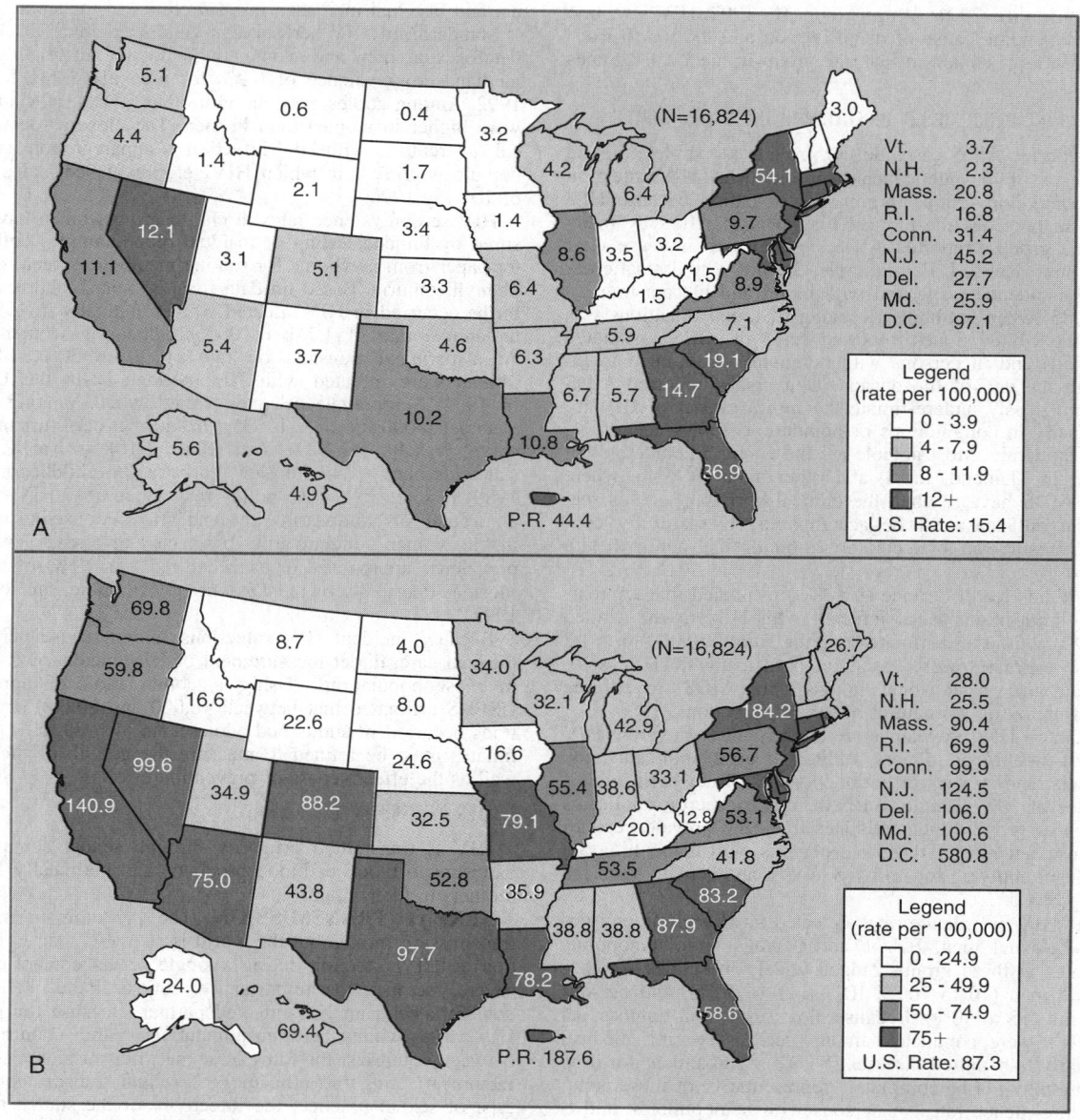

FIGURE 362–1. Adult/adolescent AIDS annual rates per 100,000 population, for cases reported in 1993 in the United States for *(A)* females and *(B)* males. (Source: Centers for Disease Control and Prevention: *HIV/AIDS Surveillance Report,* 5 (No.4):1, 1994.)

TABLE 362–3. NUMBER, PERCENTAGE, AND RATES* OF AIDS CASES, BY RACE/ETHNICITY—UNITED STATES, REPORTED IN 1993

| | Adult/Adolescent† | | | | | | | | | Children‡ | | |
| | Male | | | Female | | | Total | | | | | |
Race/Ethnicity	No.	%	Rate	No.	%	Rate	No.	%	Rate	No.	%	Rate
White, non-Hispanic	43,987	49	57	4,103	24	5	48,090	45	30	150	16	0.4
Black, non-Hispanic	28,792	32	266	9,220	55	73	38,012	36	162	532	55	7.2
Hispanic	15,301	17	146	3,324	20	32	18,625	18	90	263	27	3.6
Asian/Pacific Islander	665	1	21	97	1	3	762	1	12	5	1	0.3
American Indian/ Alaskan Native	281	<1	41	55	<1	8	336	<1	24	3	<1	0.6
Total minorities	45,039	51	179	12,696	75	47	57,735	54	111	803	84	4.8
Total¶	89,165	100	88	16,824	100	15	105,990	100	50	959	100	1.9

* Per 100,000 population. Population counts for 1993 were estimated from 1990 U.S. census data.
† Age ≥ 13 years.
‡ Age < 13 years.
¶ Includes 171 persons for whom race/ethnicity was unknown and one person for whom sex was unknown.

populations, particularly cases associated with injecting drug use or heterosexual HIV transmission.

HIV infection has a large impact on mortality in young adults in the United States, with three quarters of the nearly 37,000 deaths reported in 1992 in the 25 to 44 age group. By 1992, HIV infection had become the leading cause of death in men and the fourth leading cause of death in women in that age group in the United States (Fig. 362–2).

PREVALENCE AND INCIDENCE OF HIV INFECTION IN THE UNITED STATES

Trends in reported AIDS cases do not provide a complete picture of the prevalence of the public health problem that HIV infection poses for a population group, community, or nation because HIV infection *per se* precedes the clinical diagnosis of AIDS by many years. In some groups, reported AIDS continues to increase after HIV infection has declined. For example, despite very dramatic declines in HIV incidence associated with blood and plasma transfusions after 1985, when antibody screening of blood donations was instituted in the United States, reported cases of AIDS associated with transfusions and in persons with hemophilia continued to increase through the end of the decade. Conversely, reported AIDS case rates may grossly underestimate the future impact of HIV infection, especially in communities or populations more recently affected by the epidemic. Most notable are the emerging epidemics of HIV infection in Thailand, India, and other areas of Asia, where few cases of AIDS have reached the clinical horizon. For this reason, AIDS surveillance must be accompanied by carefully conducted HIV serosurveys to accurately monitor the public health problem.

The U.S. Public Health Service (USPHS) estimated that approximately 1 million persons were infected with HIV in the United States by 1990, with other estimates ranging from 750,000 to >1.2 million. These estimates were based on both available HIV seroprevalence data and on statistical models using AIDS surveillance data and information on the natural history of infection.

National data on HIV prevalence are directly measured from HIV testing of first-time blood donors, military recruit applicants, job corps applicants, and surveys of antibody status of newborn infants. The prevalence of HIV infection in both military recruit applicants and blood donors grossly underestimates true HIV prevalence rates because homosexual men, IDU's, and persons with hemophilia are discouraged from applying for military service and actively deferred from donating blood.

The highest HIV prevalence rates detected have been among homosexual or bisexual men, IDU's, and persons with hemophilia. Prevalence rates in these groups ranged widely in studies—homosexual/bisexual men (10 to 70%), IDU's, (1 to 50%), and persons with hemophilia (15 to 90%). Because most surveys in homosexual men and IDU's were conducted among persons seeking medical care for sexually transmitted diseases (STD's) or treatment for drug abuse, the data may not be completely representative of these populations. HIV prevalence rates in persons with hemophilia A and B were directly related to the amount of clotting factor received prior to 1985. HIV seroprevalence rates among female prostitutes varied

widely from 0 to >50%, with the differences largely attributed to the extent of injecting drug use in the population surveyed and the HIV prevalence among IDU's in the community at that time. HIV prevalence rates among male prostitutes parallel rates in homosexual and bisexual men seen in STD clinics in the same communities.

Standardized HIV serosurveys conducted in STD clinics among heterosexual men and women who do not inject drugs showed a median seroprevalence of 0.9% for men and 0.6% for women in 1992. Among adolescents, as with other STD's, HIV infection rates were higher in women than in men. The close association of clinical tuberculosis with HIV infection is apparent from surveys in tuberculosis clinics, in which HIV seroprevalence had a median rate of 10% by 1990.

HIV seroprevalence rates in childbearing women have been measured by blinded testing of residual blood samples collected on filter paper from newborns for routine metabolic screening such as for phenylketonuria. Based on data from 35 states, approximately 7000 births occurred in HIV-infected women annually in 1991–1992, for an annual rate of 1.7 per 1000 childbearing women nationwide. At a perinatal transmission rate of 20 to 30%, 1400 to 2100 infants were infected with HIV perinatally in the United States in 1992. Seroprevalence rates varied widely among states, from <1 per 1000 to >1 to 3% in northeastern urban areas. The survey results in New York State (HIV prevalence of 0.67% statewide and >1.4% in New York City in childbearing women in 1989) resulted in a state policy that encourages HIV counseling of all women of childbearing age and offers counseling and HIV testing to women contemplating pregnancy or already pregnant. Seroprevalence approached or exceeded 0.5% in New Jersey, Maryland, Florida, Puerto Rico, the District of Columbia, and New York by 1992.

Because incident HIV infections seldom cause persons to seek medical care, direct measurement of HIV incidence is very difficult in most populations. Using a combination of approaches, the USPHS estimated that between 40,000 and 80,000 new HIV infections occurred in adults and adolescents in 1989. HIV incidence estimates must be refined to measure the growth of the epidemic as well as the effectiveness of prevention efforts.

MODES OF TRANSMISSION OF HIV

HIV is transmitted primarily through sexual contact, parenteral exposure to blood or blood products, and perinatally from infected mothers to their infants.

SEXUAL TRANSMISSION. The predominant mode of HIV transmission throughout the world is sexual contact. The risk of acquiring HIV infection during a single sexual contact depends upon several factors. Most important, of course, is the likelihood that the contact is with an HIV-infected partner. Because the prevalence of HIV varies widely between populations within countries as well as between countries, the rates of sexual transmission also vary. Other factors affecting the efficiency of sexual transmission include the type of sexual practice; the infectivity of the source partner; coexisting genital infections in either partner, particularly those causing genital ulceration; and consistency of condom use. HIV transmis-

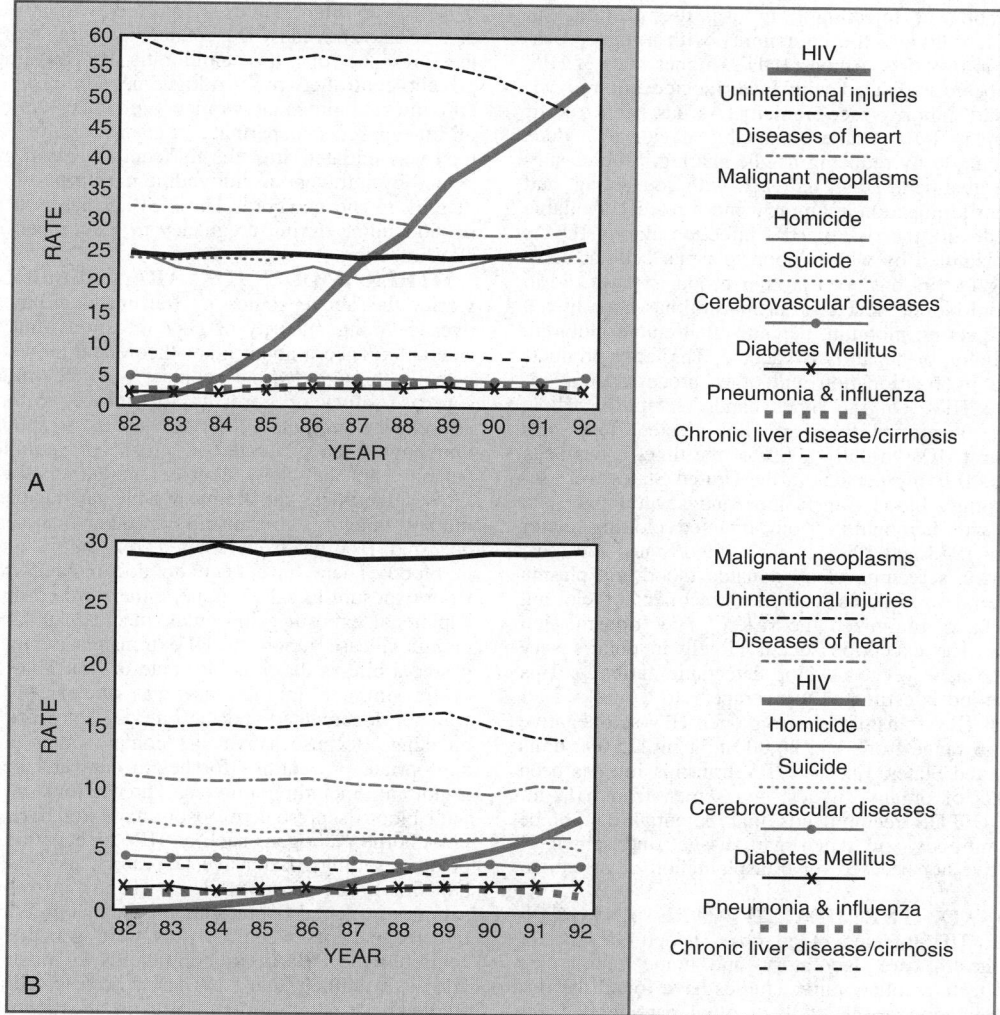

FIGURE 362–2. Death rates for leading causes of death among men *(A)* and women *(B)* aged 25 to 44, by year per 100,000 population in the United States, 1982–1992. (National vital statistics based on underlying cause of death, using final data for 1982 to 1991 and provisional data for 1992. Data for liver disease in 1992 were unavailable.)

sion has been attributed to vaginal, anal, and, less frequently, oral intercourse.

In epidemiologic studies among homosexual men, the risk of HIV acquisition increases with the number of sexual partners and the frequency of receptive anal intercourse, and practices associated with rectal trauma such as receptive "fisting" and anal douching. No sexual activity potentially involving the exchange of semen or blood, however, should be considered without risk. The relative efficiency of HIV transmission through various sexual practices was difficult to estimate precisely because most HIV-infected homosexual men in epidemiologic studies had engaged in multiple practices. Although the frequency of female-to-female transmission would seem to be quite low, such HIV infections associated with traumatic sexual practices have been reported. Most cases of HIV infection reported among bisexual women and lesbians are attributed to injecting drug use or heterosexual contact.

Most heterosexual transmission of HIV occurs during vaginal intercourse, although some studies suggest that receptive anal intercourse increases the risk of HIV transmission from an infected man to a woman. Some infected persons may be more efficient transmitters than others, perhaps owing to differences in viral strains or other factors. Transmission efficiency is inversely related to the immunologic status of the infected partner. In studies conducted among spouses and other steady sexual partners of HIV-infected persons, male-to-female, female-to-male, and male-to-male sexual transmission of HIV increased as the index partner's T-helper lymphocyte numbers declined. These findings are not surprising be-

cause the quantity of HIV in blood and semen increases as the disease progresses and the immune system weakens. Several studies have documented that infections such as *Haemophilus ducreyi, Treponema pallidum,* herpes simplex virus, and other pathogens causing genital or anal ulcers facilitate acquisition or transmission of HIV through sexual contact, most likely by disrupting the genital or anal skin and mucous membranes. Undoubtedly, the higher rates of untreated genital ulcer disease contribute to the high rates of sexual transmission of HIV observed in some areas of the developing world. Several investigators have reported increased risks of HIV acquisition for women with cervical infections with *Neisseria gonorrhoeae* or *Chlamydia trachomatis* or with cervical ectopy. To the extent that coexisting sexually transmitted infections increase the rate of HIV transmission, populations throughout the world with higher rates of these infections are at higher risk of HIV infection. Conversely, preventing and treating other sexually transmitted infections should have a beneficial effect on preventing HIV transmission. Cohort studies of couples discordant for HIV infection clearly indicate that consistent condom use reduces heterosexual as well as homosexual HIV transmission by ≥ 90% compared with inconsistent use or nonuse of condoms. Finally, preliminary studies suggest that antiretrovirals may reduce but not eliminate the risk of HIV transmission through sexual contact.

TRANSMISSION THROUGH PARENTERAL EXPOSURE TO BLOOD OR BLOOD PRODUCTS. HIV is transmitted to IDU's by parenteral exposure to contaminated injection equipment, including needles. Risk factors for infection include frequency of needle sharing, duration of injecting drug use, use of drugs in "shooting galleries," and living in a community with a high prevalence of HIV infection in IDU's. Among IDU's, higher rates of HIV infection have also been associated with lower socioeconomic status, homelessness, and minority race/ethnicity. As has been true of homosexual men, many IDU's have changed behavior to reduce their HIV risk, particularly by reducing needle sharing. Studies suggest that drug abuse treatment, street outreach with counseling, and measures to make sterile injection equipment more readily available all have a role in reducing the risk of HIV infection among IDU's.

HIV has been transmitted by whole blood, plasma, cellular components, and clotting factors but not by other products produced in the United States from blood. No HIV transmission has been linked to receipt of immune serum globulin, hepatitis B immune globulin, $Rh_o(O)$ immune globulin, or hepatitis B vaccine. The latter products have been produced by fractionation and other processes that remove and inactivate HIV. On the other hand, receipt of whole blood, packed cells, or plasma from an HIV-infected donor has been shown to transmit HIV virtually 100% of the time. It has been estimated that $>12,000$ living persons in the United States were infected with HIV through blood transfusions and several thousand additional persons with hemophilia from infected clotting factor concentrates between 1978 and 1985. In the United States and most industrialized countries, screening of all donated blood and plasma for HIV, donor deferral procedures, and heat treatment of clotting factor concentrates have minimized the risk of HIV transmission through transfusions. The exceptions occur largely in donors very recently infected who have yet to develop detectable antibody. This so-called window period is estimated to average 6 to 8 weeks after infection. The rate of HIV transmission from such HIV-seronegative donors is estimated to range from 1 in 36,000 to 1 in 225,000 units transfused in the United States. Because HIV transmission has been reported in recipients of organs, tissues, and semen from HIV-infected donors, the USPHS recommends that potential donors be screened for HIV antibody and that organ, tissue, and semen of those who test positive not be used for transplantation or insemination.

TRANSMISSION IN THE HEALTH CARE ENVIRONMENT. Exposure to HIV-infected blood poses a definite risk for HIV infection for health care, laboratory, and home health care workers. Large prospective collaborative studies have found the risk of seroconversion following needle stick or other parenteral exposures to the blood of HIV-infected persons to be approximately 0.3%. In addition, there are a few well-documented published reports of infections in health care workers following mucous membrane or extensive skin exposures. Such transmission can occur, but the risk is much lower than following parenteral exposures.

Transmission of HIV infection from an infected dentist to six patients remains the only documented transmission of HIV to patients from a health care worker. These patients had no other confirmed exposure to HIV and each was infected with an HIV strain nearly identical genetically to that of the dentist and dissimilar to that of other HIV-infected persons in the area. Rarely, HIV infection transmission has been reported through inadvertent intravenous injection of blood from HIV-infected patients in home health care or hospital settings. Major nosocomial HIV outbreaks resulted from improper sterilization or reuse of contaminated injection equipment in Romania and in the former Soviet Union.

The risk of transmission of HIV, hepatitis B and C viruses, and other bloodborne pathogens to and from health care workers and patients can be minimized by close adherence to recommendations, which include universal precautions when caring for all patients.

PERINATAL TRANSMISSION. HIV is transmitted from an infected woman to her fetus or newborn during pregnancy or delivery or through breast-feeding. HIV detected in fetal tissues and HIV isolated in cord blood provide suggestive evidence that transmission can occur *in utero*, but recent studies suggest much if not most transmission occurs during the intrapartum period. HIV can be detected at birth by culture or polymerase chain reaction in only 30 to 50% of infants ultimately found to be infected. There are several reports of mothers who were infected through postpartum transfusions and subsequently transmitted HIV to their infants through breast-feeding. For that reason, the USPHS strongly recommends that HIV-positive mothers avoid breast-feeding in the United States,

where nutritionally adequate and safe substitutes are available. The rate of perinatal transmission in published studies varies from 13 to $>40\%$ with higher rates associated with advanced maternal HIV disease and reduced CD4 count, higher rates of breast-feeding, and the presence of chorioamnionitis. In an important randomized placebo-controlled trial, zidovudine administered to asymptomatic HIV-infected pregnant women with CD4 counts >200 per cubic millimeter reduced perinatal transmission by two thirds. The regimen was initiated after the thirteenth week of gestation and accompanied by intravenous zidovudine during parturition and 6 weeks of therapy to the newborn. The USPHS has issued guidelines on use of zidovudine during pregnancy to reduce perinatal transmission of HIV infection.

OTHER MODES OF TRANSMISSION. Throughout the world, the above routes of transmission have accounted for the overwhelming majority of HIV infections, but there has been considerable concern about other theoretical modes of transmission, especially through "casual" contact with HIV-infected persons, exposure to saliva or aerosols, or insect vectors. More than 700 nonsexual household contacts of adults or children with HIV infection have been evaluated in prospective studies. In thousands of person-years of close contact, including sharing bathroom and kitchen facilities, and frequent personal interactions including kissing and hugging, no transmission other than sexual or perinatal has occurred. HIV has been isolated from saliva but less frequently than in blood. There have been no documented transmissions of HIV from exposure to saliva alone, either through kissing or through occupational exposures in dental, medical, or laboratory settings. Although a case report of HIV transmission between siblings suggested a bite as the possible route of transmission, the precise mode of transmission in this case was unclear because seroconversion was not documented and the bite did not break the skin or result in bleeding. Because saliva can contain other pathogenic organisms, appropriate precautions for health care and dental workers remain important, including universal precautions if gross contamination with blood is present. Aerosols have not been reported to transmit bloodborne pathogens such as HIV or hepatitis B in the health care or other settings. Extensive laboratory and epidemiologic studies of hepatitis B have failed to detect HBsAg in respirable particles in air samples in dental operatories or dialysis units during procedures on infected patients when aerosols were generated. Because the concentration of HBsAg in body fluids is much higher than that of HIV, it is unlikely that HIV would be detected. Extensive laboratory studies have failed to demonstrate replication of HIV in insects that were fed high concentrations of HIV or injected with HIV-contaminated blood. Epidemiologic studies in the United States, Haiti, and Central Africa show no evidence of insect-borne HIV transmission.

The possibility of previously unrecognized modes of HIV transmission cannot be entirely excluded, but they are likely to be rare, if found.

AIDS AND HIV INFECTION OUTSIDE THE UNITED STATES

Within 3 years after the syndrome was recognized in the United States, cases of AIDS were reported from every continent. By June 1994, nearly 1 million cases had been reported from 190 countries to the World Health Organization (WHO) (Table 362–4). WHO estimated that >40 million people would be infected with HIV by the end of the century. AIDS case reporting from developing countries is much less complete than in industrialized countries. Extensive HIV serosurveys in Africa, South and Central America, and parts of Asia provide evidence that AIDS case reports greatly un-

TABLE 362–4. CASES OF AIDS REPORTED TO WHO AS OF JUNE 30, 1994

Continent	Number of Cases	Number of Countries Reporting Cases
Africa	331,376	54
Americas	523,777	45
Asia	8,968	39
Europe	115,668	38
Oceania	5,330	14
Total	**985,119**	**190**

derestimate the magnitude of the HIV problem in many countries in these regions.

Modes of transmission of HIV are similar throughout the world, but the relative frequency varies considerably between countries and regions. In North America, Europe, Australia, New Zealand, and some areas of South America, the majority of HIV infections first occurred in homosexual men and IDU's; heterosexual and perinatal transmission initially resulted mostly from transmission from IDU's and their partners. In most countries in Africa and some in the Caribbean and South America, most HIV infections have occurred through heterosexual transmission. HIV seroprevalence rates are highest in urban prostitutes and sexually active young adults. High rates of infection in young women translate into a substantial amount of perinatal transmission. In some areas of Africa, pediatric HIV infection has significantly increased already high infant mortality rates. In many developing countries, transfusion of HIV-infected blood remains a substantial problem owing to inadequate blood banking and serologic testing capacity. Reuse of nonsterile needles and syringes and other medical practices have caused major HIV outbreaks in the former Soviet Union and Romania. In Asian countries such as Thailand and India, emergence of HIV infection as a major public health problem began in IDU's and prostitutes but rapidly spread more widely through heterosexual transmission to other young adult populations. In yet other countries, primarily in Eastern Europe, the Middle East, Asia, and the Pacific region, HIV has not yet been recognized as an important public health problem. The future course of HIV in these countries may depend upon their ability to anticipate and respond to the problem; it can be approximately predicted by the extent and pattern of sexually transmitted and transfusion-associated infections and the extent of injecting drug use which currently exists in each country.

A second human immunodeficiency virus, HIV type 2 (HIV-2), was first described in asymptomatic West Africans with AIDS in 1986. HIV-2 infection remains most prevalent in West Africa, although well-documented cases have been reported from Western Europe, Canada, Brazil, the United States, and Central Africa. HIV-2 is generally less virulent than HIV-1. The average viral titer is usually lower, perhaps explaining the lower rates of sexual and perinatal transmission and the slower rate of disease progression in persons infected with HIV-2 than HIV-1. HIV-1 and HIV-2 are closely related; tests for antibody for one virus often cross-react with those for the other. For example, licensed enzyme immunoassays for detecting HIV-1 find HIV-2 antibody in 60 to 90% of infected patients. In the United States combined HIV-1/HIV-2 assays are used to test donated blood. As of 1994, HIV-2 infection remained rare in the United States, with nearly all cases detected in persons from West Africa.

Recently additional HIV variants, classified together as subtype O, were reported from Cameroon. Although certain HIV antibody tests fail to detect these infections, these infections had not been detected in the United States by 1994 and were uncommon even in Cameroon. This situation reinforces the need for strong international collaboration in maintaining surveillance for variants of HIV and other emerging infections.

AIDS and human immunodeficiency virus infection in the United States: 1988 update. MMWR 38(S-4):1, 1989. HIV infection in the United States: A review of current knowledge. MMWR 36(S-6):1, 1987. The sentinel HIV seroprevalence surveys—special section. Pub Health Rep 105:113, 1990. National serosurveillance summary, Volume 3—Centers for Disease Control and Prevention, HIV/NCID/11-913/036; Gwinn M, Pappaioanou M, George JR, et al.: Prevalence of HIV infection in childbearing women in the United States. JAMA 265:1704, 1991. St. Louis ME, Connaugh A, Hayman CR, et al.: HIV infection in disadvantaged adolescents. JAMA 266:2387, 1991. *These articles summarize recent methods and data on HIV seroprevalence in the United States.*

1993 Revised classification system for HIV infection and expanded surveillance, case definition for AIDS among adolescents and adults. MMWR 41 (RR-17):1, 1992. Redfield RR, Wright DC, Tramont EA: The Walter Reed staging classification for HTLV-III/LAV infection. N Engl J Med 314:131, 1986. *These are the most widely used classification systems in the United States.*

Goedert JJ, Eyster EE, Biggar RJ, et al.: Heterosexual transmission of HIV: Association with severe depletion of T-helper lymphocytes in men with hemophilia. AIDS Res Hum Retroviruses 3:355, 1988. Holmberg SD, Horsburgh CR, Ward JW, et al.: Biologic factors in the sexual transmission of human immunodeficiency virus. J Infect Dis 160:116, 1989. Ellerbrock TV, Lieb S, Harrington PE, et al.: Heterosexual transmitted human immunodeficiency virus infection among pregnant women in a rural Florida community. N Engl J Med 327:1704, 1992. De Vincenzi I, et al.: A longitudinal study of human immunodeficiency virus transmission by heterosexual partners. N Engl J Med 331:341, 1994. Connor EM, Sperling RS, Gelber R, et al.: Reduction of maternal-infant transmission of human immunodeficiency virus type 1 with zidovudine treatment. N Engl J Med 331:1173, 1994. Recommendations of the U.S. Public Health Service Task Force on the use of zidovudine to reduce perinatal transmission of human immunodeficiency virus. MMWR 43(RR-1):1, 1994. *These summarize available information on factors related to heterosexual transmission of HIV and prevention of perinatal transmission.*

Mann JM, Tarantola DJM, Netter TW (eds.): AIDS in the World: A Global Report. Cambridge, Harvard University Press, 1992. *This volume summarizes what is known about HIV infection and prevention activities throughout the world.*

Update: Universal precautions for prevention of transmission of HIV, hepatitis B virus, and other bloodborne pathogens in health care setting. MMWR 37:337, 1988. Public Health Service statement on management of occupational exposure to HIV including considerations regarding zidovudine postexposure use. MMWR 39(RR-1):1, 1990. Recommendations for preventing transmission of human immunodeficiency virus and hepatitis B virus to patients during exposure-prone invasive procedures. MMWR 40(RR-8):1, 1991. *These documents summarize data on transmission of HIV in the health care setting and list recommended precautions.*

363 PREVENTION OF HIV INFECTION

Michael S. Saag

Prevention of HIV infection requires a thorough understanding of the modes of viral transmission, the populations at risk, and the established guidelines to avoid high-risk exposures. HIV has been identified in virtually every body fluid and tissue, including blood, semen, vaginal secretions, saliva, tears, breast milk, cerebrospinal fluid, amniotic fluid, urine, and fluid obtained from bronchoalveolar lavage. In most instances, the virus resides in lymphocytes present within body fluids; therefore, any fluid that contains lymphocytes could be implicated theoretically in the spread of the virus. Nonetheless, no cases of HIV transmission have been documented through any body fluids except blood and fluids grossly contaminated with blood, semen, vaginal secretions, and, rarely, breast milk. HIV has been transmitted through transplanted organs, including kidney, liver, heart, pancreas, and bone.

MODES OF HIV TRANSMISSION AND PREVENTION

SEXUAL TRANSMISSION. HIV infection is a sexually transmitted disease (STD). Like other STD's, HIV spreads bidirectionally and appears to be transmitted from male to female and female to male, with approximately equal efficiency. Although the majority of sexually transmitted cases reported in the United States occur via male homosexual activity, heterosexual transmission is one of the fastest growing modes of transmission reported in the United States and is the primary mode of disease acquisition in many African countries, where male-to-female prevalence ratios are approximately 1.1:1.

Certain cofactors are associated with an increased risk of acquiring HIV infection. Among homosexual men, receptive anal intercourse and contact with a large number of different sexual partners are the most important risk factors. Activities that may lead to damage of the rectal mucosa, such as rectal douching, manual penetration of the rectum ("fisting"), and concomitant ulcerative STD's, increase the likelihood of disease acquisition. Insertive rectal intercourse, fellatio, and ingestion of semen are associated with HIV transmission to a lesser degree. The likelihood of heterosexual acquired disease increases with a higher number of sexual partners, contact with intravenous drug users (IVDU's), prostitution, sexual practices that damage vaginal or rectal mucosa, and a previous history of other STD's. Female-to-female transmission has been reported via orogenital contact.

Prevention. Abstinence is the only absolute way of preventing sexual acquisition of HIV infection. Persons who have been engaged in a mutually monogamous relationship since the mid-1970's are at extremely low risk of acquiring disease; however, the assurance that both partners have remained "faithful" is sometimes difficult to confirm. For the majority of sexually active individuals it should be assumed that their partner is seropositive until demonstrated otherwise. Verbal claims of seronegativity should be viewed with skepticism. When a couple, heterosexual or homosexual, is establishing a long-term relationship, it may be recommended that they undergo serologic testing to determine their HIV status. However, the decision to be tested should be of mutual consent and viewed in the context that exposures outside the relationship may lead to seropositivity in the future.

In situations in which a decision to engage in sexual activity has been made and the HIV status of the partner is unknown or in doubt, safe sexual practices ("safe sex") should be implemented (Table 363–1). Mutual masturbation is considered "safe," assuming it is nontraumatic and not followed by ingestion of body fluids such as semen or vaginal secretions. Transmission of HIV has never been documented to occur through saliva; however, no group of patients has ever been studied who engage in deep "French" kissing as their sole means of sexual activity. Because HIV exists in saliva, albeit in very low titers, deep French kissing cannot be considered absolutely safe even though the likelihood of HIV transmission is extremely low. Condom use is the most effective means of preventing HIV infection among individuals who engage in vaginal or anal intercourse. To be effective, however, the condom should be made of latex and must be used properly. Natural skin condoms have been shown to leak in laboratory studies, whereas latex condoms maintain their integrity and are more durable. Nonoxynol-9, a spermicide with some antiviral activity, enhances the protective effects of condoms and should be used in conjunction with condoms either as a spermicidal jelly or impregnated into the latex condom itself. Petroleum-based lubricants enhance the likelihood of latex condom rupture and should be avoided. If needed, water-based lubricants such as K-Y Jelly should be used.

Both partners should be knowledgeable about the correct use of condoms. Discussions regarding condom use should occur before the need arises, and ideally, condom placement should be practiced in advance. A new condom should be used for each act of intercourse and each condom should be used only one time. Even under the best of circumstances, a 5 to 15% failure rate has been noted among couples using condoms as their sole means of contraception, and HIV transmission has been reported in discordant couples using condoms. Condom ineffectiveness is most often due to improper placement, falling off during intercourse, and rupture. Therefore, although condom use during intercourse is considered "safer" sex, it is not absolutely safe.

HIV TRANSMISSION IN INTRAVENOUS DRUG USERS. The primary mode of HIV transmission in IVDU's is sharing of contaminated needles and syringes. Sharing of injection paraphernalia ("works") is commonplace among IVDU's and is reinforced by the cultural, economic, and legal environment in the IVDU community. The risk of HIV transmission is highest among IVDU's who share needles and use drugs that are injected more often, such as cocaine. HIV is frequently transmitted from IVDU's to their sexual partners through both heterosexual and homosexual activity, and ultimately, the virus may be transmitted to their children via perinatal exposure. Many cases of heterosexual transmission, including transmission from prostitutes, are associated with intravenous drug use.

Prevention. The primary mode of preventing HIV transmission in IVDU's is to prevent the use of intravenous drugs in the first place. Education programs that are culturally sensitive and geared to young audiences have the best chance of preventing drug use. Access to treatment centers is the best approach for those individuals already using IV drugs. For those IVDU's who do not wish to seek treatment or who are unable to gain access to treatment, the

most effective way to prevent HIV infection is to avoid sharing needles and works. Where works are in short supply, needles and syringes should be cleaned after each use, preferably with readily accessible virucidal cleansers such as chlorine bleach (diluted 1:100). Some communities have adopted programs that provide free needles and syringes for IVDU's. Voluntary HIV testing and outreach programs that rigorously maintain confidentiality can be effective in reducing transmission to sexual partners of IVDU's. In order to be effective, antibody testing should be combined with intensive pretest and post-test counseling.

The efficacy of many community programs is limited, however, by cultural barriers, including lack of trust, fear of prosecution, misconceptions regarding the prevalence of HIV infection within the local drug-using population, and the use of ineffective language in delivering anti-HIV messages by program staff. When combined with the relative paucity of IV drug treatment resources, HIV education among IVDU's which ultimately results in behavioral changes represents the most challenging HIV prevention goal.

TRANSMISSION OF HIV THROUGH BLOOD PRODUCTS. HIV has been transmitted via transfusion of single-donor blood and blood products, including whole blood, fresh frozen plasma, packed red blood cells, cryoprecipitate, clotting factors, and platelets. Prior to May 1985, when the Red Cross began testing the blood supply for evidence of HIV antibodies, an estimated 10,000 to 12,000 individuals received blood products from HIV-infected donors. Most recipients develop infection after transfusion with HIV-tainted blood products, and recent data suggest that the time to development of advanced disease is shorter among transfusion recipients than among those who acquired their disease via sexual contact.

Since 1985, the rate of HIV transmission through transfusion has dropped precipitously. The current estimated rate of transmission is 1 in 40,000 to 1 in 200,000 units of blood, depending on the prevalence of HIV infection in the community where the blood was collected. Pooled plasma components often require 2000 to 30,000 donors per lot and represent a higher potential risk of transmission than single-donor blood products if the pooled product is not treated to eliminate infectious virus.

Prevention. Aggressive efforts by the American Red Cross have greatly reduced the risk of HIV transmission via transfusion in the United States. Voluntary self-deferral of donors at risk for HIV acquisition in the community was initiated in 1983. The effectiveness of self-deferral is limited, however, by social pressures. Some high-risk individuals view blood donation as a means of being tested for HIV and provide erroneous screening information in order to receive free, confidential evaluation of their HIV status. Other at-risk individuals may be coerced to participate in blood donation drives at work. Potentially infected donors may feel uncomfortable excusing themselves from donation and provide false information on screening in order to avoid possible disclosure of a high-risk lifestyle to their co-workers. Self-deferral programs are most effective when free, voluntary testing centers are readily available elsewhere in the community and when blood drives encourage potential donors to come to donation centers by themselves and not in groups.

The institution of HIV antibody testing of donated blood and blood products in 1985 has had the most dramatic effect on lowering the incidence of transfusion-related transmission. When combined with voluntary self-deferral, the blood supply has become relatively free of HIV. Heat inactivation processes for cryoprecipitate and clotting factor concentrates have virtually eliminated transmission of HIV through use of these products. Other products, such as immune globulin preparations and hepatitis B vaccines, are produced via methods that inactivate HIV and have never been associated with transmission of HIV.

TRANSMISSION OF HIV TO HEALTH CARE WORKERS. Transmission of HIV in the health care delivery setting has been the subject of intense investigation throughout the course of the epidemic. The percentage of health care workers with AIDS who have "no identified risk" for HIV infection has remained low (<10%) and has not increased over time, despite the dramatic increase in the number of AIDS cases and concomitant exposure of health care workers to patients with HIV disease. More importantly, detailed studies examining the risk of specific exposures, such as needle stick injuries and mucous membrane exposures, have demonstrated very low risk of disease acquisition in the workplace. More than

TABLE 363–1. SAFE AND UNSAFE SEXUAL PRACTICES IN ORDER OF "SURENESS" OF SAFETY

Safe
    Abstinence
    Monogamous relationship with confirmed seronegative partner
    Manual sex (mutual masturbation)
    Kissing
    Intercourse with latex condom (used in combination with nonoxynol-9)
Unsafe
    Intercourse with "natural skin" condom
    Intercourse with latex condom lubricated with petroleum-based lubricants
    Unprotected orogenital sex
    Unprotected vaginal intercourse
    Unprotected anal intercourse

3628 health care workers have been examined prospectively in carefully designed surveillance studies at 10 high-incidence medical centers. The overall risk of seroconversion after a percutaneous needle stick from a known HIV-positive source is 0.25% per exposure. Although mucous membrane exposures to HIV-positive blood have resulted in seroconversion in at least three health care workers, prospective studies of over 900 splash exposures have failed to identify any seroconverters, implying that the risk of infection is even lower after mucous membrane exposure than through percutaneous needle stick. To date, no transmission has occurred after exposure to body fluids other than blood or fluids heavily contaminated with blood. Therefore, although the potential for HIV transmission to health care providers clearly exists, the risk of infection is inherently low and can be further minimized by following routine precautions to prevent transmission.

Prevention. In August 1987, the Centers for Disease Control and Prevention (CDC) published guidelines designed to minimize health care worker exposure to blood and body fluids which may be infected with blood-borne pathogens, such as HIV. These so-called universal precautions are based on the premise that any patient may be infected with bloodborne infectious agents and it may be difficult, if not impossible, to differentiate those with infection from their uninfected counterparts. Thus, all specimens containing blood or blood-tinged fluids obtained from *any* patient should be considered hazardous and handled as such (Table 363–2).

Handwashing is the cornerstone of universal precautions, as it is with all infection-control practices. Gloves should be worn when spillage of blood or body fluids is likely. Gloves should *never* be washed and should be changed after soiling or after gross contamination, with handwashing immediately after the gloves are removed. Gowns, protective eyewear, and masks are usually not needed except in circumstances in which splattering or splashing of blood-containing fluids is likely to occur. Masks should always be worn in situations in which eyewear is required. Reusable equipment should be cleansed of visible organic material, placed in an impervious bag, and returned to central supply for decontamination. Although heat is the single best decontamination method, chemical agents that possess mycobactericidal activity are effective against both hepatitis B and HIV and are acceptable alternatives when heat inactivation is impractical. Blood spills should be cleaned with appropriate caution. After placing gloves and other appropriate barrier precautions, excess blood should be removed with absorbent materials (e.g., paper towels), the area then cleaned with soap and water, and the area disinfected with a 1:10 solution of sodium hypochlorite (household bleach) and water. Health care workers with denuded skin, open lesions, or active dermatitis should avoid direct patient contact and should not process contaminated equipment or materials. Private rooms are generally not required for patients known to be HIV infected unless a concomitant opportunistic disease is present which requires respiratory, enteric, or contact isolation. Food service should be provided as usual on reusable dishware.

Because *all* blood and body fluids should be handled as potentially hazardous and *all* patients presumed to be infected, it makes little sense to identify infected patients or their specimens with "blood and body fluid" labels. The use of such labels on *known* infected patients implies that unlabeled specimens or specimens from patients of unknown status are less hazardous and may be handled with less care. Indeed, studies have shown that more than half of the specimens containing antibodies to either HbsAg or HIV went to the laboratory unlabeled. The handling of sharp instruments ("sharps") represents the greatest risk of HIV transmission to health care workers. Although sharp injuries cannot be entirely eliminated, the number of exposures can be reduced substantially by adhering to guidelines put forth in universal precautions. Before a sharp instrument is used, thought should be given regarding where the instrument will be disposed after use. Impervious containers should be readily available in all patient care areas and identified by the health care worker *prior to* "sharp" utilization. The containers should be checked frequently and should not be allowed to overfill. Used needles should never be manipulated, bent, broken, or recapped. Recapping of needles is the single most common activity that results in needle stick injuries.

Despite their logical basis and relative ease of implementation, universal precautions have not been accepted by many medical centers and health care providers. Recent studies have shown that >50% of health care workers engage in inadequate infection control practices, even in high-impact AIDS centers, and up to 40% of the needle stick exposures were judged to be preventable. Although lack of adequate education may partly explain these findings, implementation of infection control practices has been generally poor historically. Between 200 and 400 health care workers die each year as a result of hepatitis B infection acquired on the job. The use of universal precautions helps minimize the transmission of many transmissible diseases in addition to HIV.

Even in the best of circumstances, accidental mucous membrane and percutaneous exposures to blood from HIV-infected patients do occur. Each institution and health care facility should adopt procedures for managing these exposures based on guidelines published by the CDC. The essential elements of management following needle stick or mucous membrane exposure include defining the type of exposure, appropriately evaluating the donor (patient) and recipient (health care worker) at the time of exposure, and follow-up of the health care worker for at least 1 year after exposure.

Proposed definitions of the types of exposure are summarized in Table 363–3. Health care workers with any kind of parenteral exposure should be counseled and evaluated for possible acquisition of HIV and receive routine prophylaxis against hepatitis B. The source patient (donor) should be evaluated for HIV infection; if the donor's HIV status is unknown, the donor should be informed about the incident and encouraged to allow voluntary, confidential screening of his/her blood for HIV and hepatitis B antibody. If the patient refuses or cannot give consent, he/she should be considered to be infected. In cases where exposure to HIV is documented or presumed to have occurred, the health care worker should be evaluated serologically for the presence of HIV as soon as possible after the exposure (baseline) and again at 6 weeks, 12 weeks, 24 weeks, and 1 year after the exposure to determine whether HIV transmission has occurred. The health care worker should report any acute illnesses that occur during the follow-up period, especially during the first 6 to 12 weeks after exposure. Exposed workers should follow the recommended guidelines for preventing HIV transmission, including using safe sexual practices, refraining from blood, semen, and organ donation, and avoiding breast feeding. If the source patient is seronegative for HIV and has no clinical manifestations of HIV disease, no further follow-up of the exposed health care workers is necessary, although some workers prefer follow-up for their own peace of mind. Serologic testing should be made available to all health care workers who are concerned about potential on-the-job exposure.

The use of zidovudine (AZT) prophylaxis following parenteral exposure to HIV remains controversial. Many clinicians favor using

TABLE 363–2. SUMMARY OF UNIVERSAL PRECAUTIONS

Specimens, including blood, blood products, and body fluids, obtained from *all* patients should be considered hazardous and potentially infected with transmissible agents.

Handwashing should be performed before and after patient contact; after removing gloves; and immediately if hands are grossly contaminated with blood.

Gloves should be worn when hands are *likely* to come in contact with blood or body fluids.

Gowns, protective eyewear, and masks should be worn when splashing, splattering, or aerosolization of blood or body fluids is *likely* to occur.

Sharp objects ("sharps") should be handled with great care and disposed of in impervious receptacles.

Needles should never be manipulated, bent, broken, or recapped.

Blood spills should be handled via initial absorption of spill with disposable towels, cleaning area with soap and water, followed by disinfecting area with 1:10 solution of household bleach.

Contaminated reusable equipment should be decontaminated using heat sterilization, or when heat is impractical, using a mycobactericidal cleanser.

Pocket masks or mechanical ventilation devices should be available in areas where cardiopulmonary resuscitation procedures are likely.

Health care workers with open lesions or weeping dermatitis should avoid direct patient contact and should not handle contaminated equipment.

Private rooms are not required for routine care; select circumstances, however, such as the presence of concomitant transmissible opportunistic diseases, may warrant respiratory, enteric, or contact isolation.

TABLE 363–3. DEFINITIONS OF EXPOSURES TO BLOOD AND BODY FLUIDS FROM HIV-INFECTED PATIENTS

	Zidovudine Prophylaxis*
Massive parenteral exposure	Recommended
Transfusion of blood	
High-inoculum injection of blood (>1 ml) or laboratory materials containing high viral titers	
Definite parenteral exposure	Encouraged
Deep intramuscular injury with a needle contaminated with blood or a body fluid	
Small volume injection of blood or body fluid (<1 ml)	
Laceration caused by instrument contaminated with blood or body fluids	
Laceration inoculated with blood, body fluids, or virus samples (research materials)	
Possible parenteral exposure	Available
Subcutaneous or superficial injury with an instrument or needle contaminated with blood or body fluids	
Injury with a contaminated instrument or needle which does not cause visible bleeding	
Previous wound or skin lesion contaminated with blood or body fluids	
Mucous membrane exposure to blood or body fluids	
Doubtful parenteral exposure	Discouraged
Subcutaneous injury by instrument or needle contaminated with noninfectious fluids†	
Contamination of a wound, previous skin lesion, or mucous membrane with noninfectious fluids	
Intact skin visibly contaminated with blood	

* Zidovudine 200 mg orally every 4 hours for 6 weeks; see text.
† Body fluids considered to be potentially infectious include blood, blood products, cerebrospinal fluid, amniotic fluid, menstrual discharge, inflammatory exudates, pleural fluid, peritoneal fluid, pericardial fluid, and any fluid visibly contaminated with blood. All other fluids are considered noninfectious.

prophylactic AZT after massive or definite exposures based on the proven antiviral effect of AZT, the relatively infrequent and apparently reversible nature of serious drug effects, and the demonstration in some animal models of retroviral infection that AZT, when given early after inoculation, modifies the course of disease. Others believe that AZT should not be administered based on the absence of postexposure prophylaxis data, the lack of information regarding toxicity in uninfected individuals, and the unknown long-term carcinogenic potential of AZT use. Although it is unlikely that any clinical trials will be able to resolve the issue owing to the large number of participants required (based on low rates of seroconversion) and the difficulty of enrolling exposed health care workers into placebo-controlled studies, very recent reports from the CDC indicate a 30% reduction in anticipated transmission rates of HIV to parenterally exposed health care workers who had received AZT prophylaxis. In many medical centers AZT prophylaxis has become a standard of practice. In those centers the option of AZT prophylaxis is offered to all health care workers with massive or definite exposures and discussed with those encountering possible parenteral exposures. Health care workers with doubtful parenteral or nonparenteral exposures generally should not take AZT prophylaxis. Those workers with massive or definite exposures who elect to take AZT prophylaxis should sign an informed consent that outlines the risks and benefits of AZT prophylaxis prior to starting therapy. The optimal timing and dosage of AZT prophylaxis are unknown; however, animal studies suggest that higher doses given as soon as possible after exposure have the best chance of being effective. Therefore, most centers that offer AZT prophylaxis to their employees have established mechanisms whereby the health care worker can be evaluated and the drug administered within 2 to 4 hours after the exposure. Dosing regimens vary from center to center but usually consist of 200 mg of AZT every 4 hours, with or without a 4 A.M. dose, for 4 to 6 weeks.

TRANSMISSION FROM INFECTED HEALTH CARE WORKERS TO THEIR PATIENTS. In July 1990, the first case of possible transmission of HIV from an infected health care worker (dentist) to his patients was reported. Six patients are believed to have acquired infection from the dentist based on the absence of other risk factors among the patients and the high degree of homology between the viruses isolated from the dentist and those isolated from the patients. Although each patient underwent an invasive procedure in the dental office, the precise mode of transmission remains unknown.

Based on the known transmission of other blood-borne pathogens from health care providers to their patients (e.g., hepatitis B), it was anticipated that HIV may also be transmitted in this fashion. Remarkably, despite the prolonged duration of the epidemic, the dentist described above remains the only documented case of transmission to patients in the health care setting. Several "look-back" studies of over 4000 patients who underwent invasive surgical procedures performed by HIV-infected physicians have failed to identify any additional cases of nosocomial transmission. Therefore, the risk of transmission from infected health care workers to patients is thought to be very low (between 1 in 42,000 and 1 in 420,000). Routine use of universal precautions should minimize the risk of transmission from HIV-infected patients to health care providers and vice versa.

VACCINE DEVELOPMENT

Education is the only means of HIV prevention currently available. Over the past few years significant efforts have been directed toward the development of an effective vaccine against HIV. Although substantial progress has been achieved, several obstacles still remain. Despite enormous advances in understanding the immunopathogenesis of HIV infection, the precise mechanism of protective immunity remains unknown. Without such knowledge, it is difficult to develop vaccines that are assured of targeting the appropriate arm of the immune system that confers long-term protective immunity. Another obstacle is the lack of correlation of data from animal models to the potential protective effects of vaccines in humans. Therefore, even if an effective vaccine were available, it would take years of human testing to demonstrate its effectiveness. Moreover, once a candidate vaccine is in human trials, the relatively low rate of HIV transmission and, in some cases, the difficulty in determining whether HIV infection has actually occurred will complicate the evaluation process. Despite the enormous progress made in vaccine development over the last few years, it will take several more years before protective efficacy can be established. Even if an effective vaccine is established, education will remain the primary mode of HIV prevention, owing to the difficulty in knowing how long the protective immune effect will last. Never before has so much been known about an epidemic during the time it was occurring. The challenge is to disseminate the knowledge to populations at risk in language they can understand and, ultimately, to modify activities so that the risk of transmission is minimized.

Centers for Disease Control: Recommendations for prevention of HIV transmission in health-care settings. MMWR 36(Suppl 2):1S, 1987. *Original description of universal precautions. Critical reading for all health care providers.*

Centers for Disease Control: Update: Investigations of persons treated by HIV-infected health-care workers—United States. MMWR 42:329, 1993. *Summary of look-back studies that examine the status of patients who received care from HIV-infected health care workers.*

Gerberding JL: Is antiretroviral treatment after percutaneous HIV exposure justified? Ann Intern Med 118:979, 1993. *Succinct overview of current thinking on postexposure prophylaxis. Cites key references.*

Lo B, Steinbrook R: Health care workers infected with the human immunodeficiency virus: The next steps. JAMA 267:1100, 1992. *Thoughtful review of the medical, epidemiologic, and ethical issues surrounding the practice of HIV-infected health care providers.*

364 NEUROLOGIC COMPLICATIONS OF HIV-1 INFECTION

Richard W. Price

The neurologic complications of HIV-1 infection are both common and varied. Indeed, only rarely do the central and peripheral nervous systems of HIV-infected patients remain unaffected through the course of their disease. Because each of the individual neurologic disorders is discussed in more detail elsewhere in this volume, the major purpose of this chapter is to provide an overview and a general guide to diagnosis and management. It is important to emphasize that differential diagnosis in these patients is far from an "academic exercise," because many of these conditions can be reversed, stabilized, or even cured with specific therapy.

Although the major susceptibility to neurologic complications occurs in the late phase of HIV-1 infection, at the time when immunosuppression leads to a marked increase in vulnerability to a host of conditions, patients may also manifest certain neurologic afflictions early in infection. Because the neurologic complications of early and late HIV-1 infection differ, they are considered separately. Indeed, because of these stage-related differences in susceptibility, when approaching diagnosis in HIV-infected patients it is important to characterize their "background" systemic HIV-1 infection, either clinically with respect to the presence or absence of previous opportunistic infections indicating compromised immunity or by assessment of surrogate markers, particularly the blood CD4+ lymphocyte count.

EARLY HIV-1 INFECTION

Although less common than in the late stages of HIV-1 infection, the nervous system may also be afflicted earlier, indeed as early as the stage of primary infection and seroconversion. Thus, individual reports have described examples of focal or diffuse encephalopathy, ataxia, myelopathy, and meningitis presenting either within the context of the mononucleosis-like HIV-1 seroconversion reaction or with minimal associated systemic symptoms. These conditions appear to evolve acutely or subacutely, to pursue a monophasic course, and to be followed by good, although not always complete, recovery. Peripheral nervous system disorders, including mononeuropathy involving cranial or segmental nerves, brachial plexopathy, and polyneuropathy, have also been reported during this phase. At times these peripheral and central nervous system (CNS) disorders occur together.

Subsequently, during the "clinically latent" phase of infection, several neurologic conditions have been reported. Among these is the Guillain-Barré syndrome and its more protracted counterpart, chronic idiopathic demyelinating polyneuropathy (CIDP), both of which are clinically indistinguishable from demyelinating polyneuropathies affecting non-HIV-1-infected individuals, except for higher cerebrospinal fluid (CSF) cell counts and perhaps a poorer prognosis. Response to treatment with corticosteroids, plasma exchange, and intravenous immunoglobulin has been noted, supporting presumption of an autoimmune pathogenesis. Because of the potential hazards of corticosteroids, plasma exchange and immunoglobulin are the preferred therapies. Isolated cases of a multi-

ple sclerosis–like demyelinating CNS disease have also been reported in this stage of HIV-1 infection, but this appears to be rare.

An additional important aspect of HIV-1 infection, with both diagnostic and pathogenetic implications, is the early development of CSF abnormalities, which presumably relate to early *asymptomatic HIV-1 infection of the CNS* soon after initial systemic infection. Prospective studies have reported that the majority of asymptomatic HIV-1-infected individuals exhibit mild CSF changes, including elevations in the cell count and protein and immunoglobulin levels as well as evidence of local "intra-blood-brain barrier" synthesis of anti-HIV-1 antibody. Additionally, in a substantial number of asymptomatic patients HIV-1 can be isolated from the CSF using culture techniques. These findings have not been shown to have an adverse prognostic significance for the subject; indeed, it is clear that patients with such abnormalities can continue to function without symptoms or signs of neurologic impairment. These "background" abnormalities may confound CSF analysis.

LATE HIV-1 INFECTION

The evolving, and eventually severe, impairment of immune defenses caused by HIV-1 renders the nervous system highly vulnerable to a broad spectrum of disorders. The following overview emphasizes general principles of pathogenesis and approach to diagnosis.

Pathophysiology

A number of pathophysiologic processes may lead to neurologic dysfunction in the late phase of HIV-1 infection (Table 364–1). These include conditions that distinguish the AIDS patient from other groups, such as *opportunistic infections, opportunistic neoplasms,* and several conditions that appear to relate to more *direct effects of HIV-1* itself. AIDS patients are also susceptible to the neurologic conditions that affect other acute and chronically ill populations, including metabolic brain disease resulting from systemic organ dysfunction, stroke related to nonbacterial thrombotic endocarditis or coagulopathies, toxic effects of medications, and primary psychiatric disturbances. Here we focus on those disorders that particularly distinguish AIDS patients.

OPPORTUNISTIC NERVOUS SYSTEM INFECTIONS. As with other organ systems, the spectrum of opportunistic infections of the nervous system results from the intrinsic vulnerabilities of the tissue (fertile soil) and the pattern of immunosuppression, in this case circumscribed impairment of T-cell/macrophage defenses. The patient's long-term history of exposure to particular organisms is also important because most of the opportunistic infections result from reactivation of latent infections rather than from new encoun-

TABLE 364–1. PATHOPHYSIOLOGIC CLASSIFICATION OF THE NEUROLOGIC COMPLICATIONS OF LATE HIV-1 INFECTION

Underlying Process	Examples
Opportunistic infections	Cerebral toxoplasmosis
	Cryptococcal meningitis
	Progressive multifocal leukoencephalopathy
	Cytomegalovirus encephalitis, polyradiculitis
Opportunistic neoplasms	Primary central nervous system lymphoma
	Metastatic lymphoma
Conditions possibly related to HIV-1 itself	AIDS dementia complex
	Aseptic meningitis
	Predominantly sensory polyneuropathy
Metabolic and vascular complications of systemic disease	Hypoxic, sepsis-related encephalopathies
	Stroke (nonbacterial thrombotic endocarditis, coagulopathies)
Toxic reactions	Dideoxyinosine, dideoxycytidine neuropathies
	AZT myopathy
Functional (psychiatric) disorders	Anxiety disorders
	Psychotic depression

ters with pathogens. An important implication of the pre-eminence of reactivated infection relates to serologic testing. Serology is most useful for assessing prior exposure to an organism and hence susceptibility to clinically important reactivation, but not for defining active infection. For example, patients with cerebral toxoplasmosis nearly always exhibit antecedent positive *Toxoplasma gondii* blood serology, and therefore a negative serum IgG antibody titer militates against this diagnosis. On the other hand, these serum antibody titers most often do not rise before or during the course of disease, and therefore a fourfold increase cannot be relied upon to establish disease activity. Moreover, as long as immunosuppression persists and therapy still cannot eliminate latent infection, suppressive antibiotic therapy must be maintained for the remainder of the patient's life.

The reason for the intrinsic vulnerability of the nervous system to certain infections (e.g., *T. gondii*) and not others (e.g., *Pneumocystis carinii*) in many cases remains uncertain. However, in some instances susceptibility relates to the capacity of local cells to support intracellular replication. Thus, the virus causing progressive multifocal leukoencephalopathy (PML), JC virus, causes a productive and lytic infection of oligodendrocytes and hence leads to spreading infection and demyelination as the processes of these myelin-producing cells disappear. In the case of HIV-1, productive infection appears to involve monocyte-derived macrophages and local microglial cells.

The circumscribed nature of the immunologic defect in AIDS determines the range of opportunistic infections, which therefore differs somewhat from that of other immunosuppressed states. For example, AIDS patients are particularly susceptible to cerebral toxoplasmosis but, unlike patients with organ transplants, are very unlikely to develop cerebral *Candida* or *Aspergillus* infections. For this reason, AIDS patients present a unique set of disease probabilities.

OPPORTUNISTIC NEOPLASMS. The major consideration in this category is primary brain lymphoma. These B-cell lymphomas arise in the CNS, usually are multicentric (at least microscopically), and only rarely metastasize systemically. Characteristically, they develop late in HIV-1 infection when blood CD4+ lymphocytes are low, i.e., in the same setting as major opportunistic infections. Indeed, the tumor cells are nearly always positive for Epstein-Barr virus (EBV), which likely plays an important role in their genesis. Radiation therapy usually results in tumor regression, but overall prognosis is poor, principally because other complications develop; the role of chemotherapy is uncertain, but aggressive treatment is often not possible because of reduced bone marrow reserves. Systemic lymphoma can also spread to the CNS, although usually to the leptomeninges rather than brain parenchyma. Although Kaposi's sarcoma has been reported to metastasize to brain, this is exceedingly rare.

EFFECTS OF HIV-1 ON THE NERVOUS SYSTEM. Several disorders have been suggested to relate in a more direct or fundamental way to HIV-1 infection. These include the AIDS dementia complex, aseptic meningitis, and perhaps predominantly sensory neuropathy. Although considerable uncertainty still exists regarding their cause and pathogenesis, the seeming uniqueness of these conditions in HIV-1-infected compared with other immunosuppressed patients, as well as more direct evidence of virus infection in some patients with the AIDS dementia complex, lends support to this contention.

Diagnosis: Neuroanatomic Approach

As with other neurologic disease, diagnosis in AIDS patients begins with localization of symptoms and signs and hence involves neuroanatomic classification (Table 364–2).

MENINGITIS AND HEADACHE. Several disorders may involve the leptomeninges in patients with advanced HIV-1 disease. The most important of these is infection by *Cryptococcus neoformans* (see Ch. 352). This condition usually presents subacutely with headache, nausea, vomiting, and confusion, just as in non-AIDS patients. However, importantly, in some patients initial symptoms can be remarkably benign, with only mild headache or fever. Likewise, the CSF findings may be bland, with few or no cells and little or no perturbation in either glucose or protein levels. For this reason the clinician should have a low threshold for lumbar puncture and

should routinely examine CSF for *Cryptococcus* (India ink stain, cryptococcal antigen determination, culture). Initial treatment is usually gratifying, although sterilizing the CSF is difficult and continued chronic therapy is required.

The syndrome of aseptic meningitis, presumably relating to direct HIV-1 infection of the leptomeninges, may complicate advanced HIV-1 infection but most often develops in the period of transition to AIDS. Both acute and chronic forms are accompanied by headache and meningeal symptoms, whereas signs of meningeal irritation are more characteristic of the acute group. Cranial nerve palsies affecting the seventh and, less often, the fifth and eighth nerves may complicate the course. The CSF shows a modest mononuclear pleocytosis, usually with normal glucose and mildly elevated protein. The presumption that this condition is due to direct HIV-1 infection of the meninges derives from the fact that the virus can be readily isolated from the CSF and no other cause has been identified. The syndrome itself is characteristically benign but may imply a poor prognosis in relation to impending progression to AIDS. The efficacy of antiretroviral or other therapies in this disorder has not been studied.

Other, less common meningeal disorders (including meningeal lymphoma, tuberculous meningitis, meningovascular syphilis) resemble their counterparts in the non-AIDS patient. A number of other conditions may present with symptoms resembling meningitis;

TABLE 364–2. NEUROANATOMIC CLASSIFICATION OF THE LATE COMPLICATIONS OF HIV-1 INFECTION

Meningitis and headache
  Cryptococcal meningitis
  Aseptic meningitis (HIV-1)
  Idiopathic, "HIV-1–related" headache
  Tuberculous meningitis *(Mycobacterium tuberculosis)*
  Syphilitic meningitis
  Lymphomatous meningitis (metastatic)
Diffuse brain diseases
  With preservation of consciousness
    AIDS dementia complex
  With concomitant depression of arousal
    Metabolic encephalopathies (alone or as an exacerbating influence)
    Toxoplasmosis ("encephalitic" form)
    Cytomegalovirus encephalitis
    Herpes encephalitis
Focal brain diseases
  Subacute
    Cerebral toxoplasmosis
    Primary CNS lymphoma
    Progressive multifocal leukoencephalopathy
    Tuberculous brain abscess *(M. tuberculosis)*
    Cryptococcoma
    Varicella-zoster virus encephalitis
    Herpes encephalitis
  Acute
    Vascular disorders
Myelopathies
  Subacute/chronic, progressive
    Vacuolar myelopathy
    HTLV-I–associated myelopathy
  Acute/subacute
    Transverse myelitis
      Varicella-zoster virus (herpes zoster)
      Spinal epidural or intradural lymphoma
    With polyradiculopathy
      Cytomegalovirus
Peripheral neuropathies
  Predominantly sensory polyneuropathy
  Toxic neuropathies (dideoxycytidine, dideoxyinosine)
  Autonomic neuropathy
  Cytomegalovirus polyradiculopathy
  Mononeuritis multiplex
  Herpes zoster
  Mononeuropathies associated with aseptic meningitis
  Mononeuropathies secondary to lymphomatous meningitis
Myopathies
  Polymyositis
  Noninflammatory myopathy
  AZT myopathy

for example, parenchymal brain diseases such as toxoplasmosis and primary CNS lymphoma may initially manifest with headache as an important symptom. More common, however, is the development of headache of uncertain cause. Although not well understood, this headache is not rare in late HIV-1 infection and at times can be a severe, debilitating problem. Whereas in some patients this headache may relate to systemic infection such as *P. carinii* pneumonia, in others the explanation is elusive and for this reason has been referred to as *HIV headache*.

PREDOMINANTLY FOCAL BRAIN DISORDERS. In approaching diagnosis of parenchymal brain disease, it is useful to separate the conditions that cause predominantly focal symptoms and signs from those producing more generalized brain dysfunction. Patients in the former group present with hemiparesis, aphasia, apraxia, hemisensory abnormalities, visual field loss, and the like, as a result of focal macroscopic lesions in cortical or subcortical brain regions. The most important of these are cerebral toxoplasmosis, which complicates the course of AIDS in 7 to 15% of patients, primary cerebral lymphoma developing in up to 5%, and PML, which occurs in perhaps 3%. Less common are a miscellany of other infections and cerebrovascular disorders.

Although the three major focal disorders all characteristically have a subacute onset and may be clinically indistinguishable, they tend to have somewhat different temporal profiles (Table 364–3). Thus, cerebral toxoplasmosis typically progresses most rapidly (over a few days) and PML evolves most slowly (over a few weeks), with primary CNS lymphoma somewhere in between. Each may cause similar neurologic deficits, but there are often differences in the associated findings. Thus, toxoplasmosis commonly presents with a combination of focal deficit and generalized encephalopathy with confusion or clouding of consciousness; fever and headache may also be present. This contrasts with PML, at least at onset, in which focal neurologic deficits are unaccompanied by either diffuse brain dysfunction or evidence of a systemic toxic state. CNS lymphoma, when accompanied by significant mass effect or when deep in the frontal or periventricular region, may cause more global mental dysfunction, but, again, these patients are usually afebrile without constitutional symptoms or signs.

Once the focal nature of the patient's symptoms and signs is recognized, use of neuroimaging techniques, including computed tomography (CT) or preferably magnetic resonance imaging (MRI), is critical both to confirm the presence of macroscopic focal disease and to determine the nature of the abnormalities (Table 364–3). Multiple lesions involving the cortex or deep brain nuclei (thalamus, basal ganglia) surrounded by edema strongly favor cerebral toxoplasmosis. In most cases *Toxoplasma* abscesses exhibit ringlike contrast enhancement on CT scan. Cerebral lymphoma may produce a similar neuroimaging appearance, although the lesions of lymphoma are usually less numerous (one or two definable lesions), commonly exhibit more diffuse or less clear-cut contrast enhancement, and are more often located in the white matter adjacent to the ventricles. PML characteristically involves the white matter, most often adjacent to the cortex, and is without mass effect or contrast enhancement.

After neuroimaging, the next step in diagnosing focal mass lesions often involves a trial of anti-*Toxoplasma* therapy. Pyrimethamine and sulfa therapy characteristically results in clinical improvement within a few days and distinct reduction of lesions on neuroimaging by 1 or 2 weeks. This rapid and consistent improvement allows treatment response to serve as a basis for diagnosis

and thereby obviates the need for brain biopsy in virtually all patients with toxoplasmosis. Biopsy is then reserved for cases with atypical clinical or laboratory features (including atypical neuroimaging appearance or negative *Toxoplasma* blood serology) along with those who fail to improve with treatment. It is important in the context of such therapeutic trial that, if possible, corticosteroids be avoided. Because the signs and symptoms, and even the neuroimaging abnormalities, of cerebral lymphoma may improve with corticosteroids, such treatment can confuse interpretation of the anti-*Toxoplasma* therapeutic trial. However, if cerebral edema threatens brain herniation, judicious short-term corticosteroids may be instituted along with appropriate specific therapy and subsequently tapered rapidly once the patient improves.

Other focal CNS disorders are uncommon but include some treatable lesions. This includes cryptococcoma, nearly always developing in the setting of meningitis. Varicella-zoster virus (VZV) can cause a demyelinating focal disease resembling PML, and cytomegalovirus (CMV) may rarely cause macroscopic lesions, sometimes with mineralization and contrast enhancement on neuroimaging, accompanied by focal clinical deficit. Herpes simplex viruses have also been reported to cause focal deficits. All of these evolve subacutely, as do the more common opportunistic problems. Acutely evolving neurologic deficits may follow seizures (Todd's palsy) or relate to poorly understood transient vascular syndromes resembling migraine clinically and pathogenetically. MRI and other studies are usually warranted in these patients to rule out other underlying disorders.

PREDOMINANTLY NONFOCAL BRAIN DISORDERS. The disorders presenting with more general or diffuse brain dysfunction and without focal features can be further divided into those in which consciousness remains fully preserved and those accompanied by a concomitant decrease in alertness. Most important among the former is the *AIDS dementia complex*, a clinical syndrome characterized by cognitive, motor, and, at times, behavioral dysfunction.

Both the incidence and severity of the AIDS dementia complex increase with advancing immunosuppression. The clinical syndrome is somewhat variable, and its pathologic substrate is heterogeneous. It appears to relate to effects of HIV-1 infection on the CNS rather than involving secondary opportunistic infection. Its early, mild form is usually characterized by impaired concentration and attention along with reduced mental agility, resulting in complaints of forgetfulness and slowness in performing complex mental tasks. In those who progress to more severe involvement, cognitive dysfunction worsens and involves other domains, and motor dysfunction becomes clinically manifest with gait unsteadiness and difficulty with rapid, fine movements of the hands. Personality change with apathy, lack of initiative, or, at times, hyperactivity and agitation may be part of the syndrome. In its most severe form, global dementia, paraplegia, and virtual mutism may evolve with resultant incapacity. Although it is in part a diagnosis of exclusion, the symptoms and signs of the AIDS dementia complex are sufficiently distinct to allow bedside diagnosis in most patients on the basis of their stereotypy. Neuroimaging characteristically reveals cerebral atrophy, and MRI may additionally demonstrate increased signal in white matter or basal ganglia. Several studies now suggest that zidovudine (AZT) can prevent and partially reverse the symptoms and signs of the AIDS dementia complex. Whether newer antiretro-

TABLE 364–3. COMPARATIVE CLINICAL AND RADIOLOGIC FEATURES OF CEREBRAL TOXOPLASMOSIS, PRIMARY CNS LYMPHOMA, AND PROGRESSIVE MULTIFOCAL LEUKOENCEPHALOPATHY

	Clinical Onset				Neuroradiologic Features	
	Temporal Profile	*Level of Alertness*	*Fever*	*Number of Lesions*	*Type of Lesions*	*Location of Lesions*
Cerebral toxoplasmosis	Days	Reduced	Common	Multiple	Spherical, ring-enhancing	Basal ganglia, cortex
Primary CNS lymphoma	Days to weeks	Variable	Absent	One or few	Irregular, weakly enhancing	Periventricular
Progressive multifocal leukoencephalopathy	Weeks	Preserved	Absent	Multiple	Nonenhancing	White matter

viral drugs have a similar therapeutic effect remains to be evaluated.

In the AIDS dementia complex there is relative preservation of alertness in relation to cognitive loss. This contrasts with most metabolic encephalopathies developing as sequelae of the systemic diseases suffered by AIDS patients; for example, hypoxia and sepsis are characteristically accompanied by a degree of lethargy and confusion which parallels the decline in cognition. Likewise, CNS-active drugs often cloud mentation and alertness together. Although such metabolic and toxic disorders may present alone, they may also have an exacerbating or unmasking influence on the AIDS dementia complex, resulting in a mixture of the two conditions. HIV-1-infected patients may also be more sensitive to neuroleptics and thereby manifest parkinsonian or other movement disorders as side effects at seemingly low doses.

Brain infections may also produce diffuse brain dysfunction. Although CNS toxoplasmosis characteristically causes focal neurologic symptoms and signs, in some patients generalized encephalopathy predominates. Similarly, CNS lymphoma may infiltrate deep structures and impair cognition and motor function without prominent focal symptoms or signs. The clinical importance of CNS CMV infection in this regard remains imprecisely defined. Scattered CMV infection of the brain is common at autopsy, but the clinical correlate of this finding is not clear, and likely it is often silent or mild. On the other hand, in a small number of patients CMV encephalitis may be severe with subacute clouding of consciousness and, at times, seizures. Herpes simplex virus types 1 and 2 may also cause subacute nonfocal encephalitis.

MYELOPATHIES. The most common spinal cord affliction in AIDS patients is the pathologically defined vacuolar myelopathy, which has been included within the broader clinical designation of the AIDS dementia complex because it is usually accompanied by evidence of concomitant brain dysfunction. The disorder is generally of subacute or gradual onset and progression with painless gait disturbance characterized by ataxia and spasticity. Bladder and bowel difficulty usually follow deterioration of gait, and sensory symptoms and signs are less prominent than gait dysfunction unless there is concomitant neuropathy. Patients do not manifest a distinct sensory or motor "level" as in transverse myelopathies but rather distal loss of large-fiber modalities accompanied by increased deep tendon reflexes (again, in the absence of neuropathy) and Babinski signs. The efficacy of AZT or other antiretrovirals in this subgroup of AIDS dementia complex patients is uncertain.

An additional, emerging cause of clinically similar myelopathy in HIV-1-infected patients relates to coinfection with a second retrovirus, human T-lymphotropic virus I (HTLV-I). Double infection results from the convergent epidemiologies of these infections related to intravenous drug abuse. Although pathologically distinct, clinical differentiation of vacuolar myelopathy and HTLV-I-associated myelopathy (HAM) may be very difficult. Diagnosis begins with suspicion based on risk and is supported by serologic documentation of HTLV-I infection, but the relative clinical contributions of the two viruses is problematic antemortem. In AIDS patients with myelopathy, laboratory diagnostic studies are principally directed at ruling out spinal cord disease other than vacuolar myelopathy because neither myelography nor spinal MRI usually detects vacuolar myelopathy or HAM.

PERIPHERAL NEUROPATHIES. The most common neuropathy in the late stages of HIV-1 infection is a distal, predominantly sensory, axonal neuropathy. Characteristically, sensory symptoms exceed both sensory and motor dysfunction. Although its prevalence has not been well defined, likely a mild form of this type of neuropathy is very common. In some patients these sensory symptoms become severe, and painful paresthesias and "burning feet" are disabling. Although suspected to relate to direct HIV-1 infection of nerve or dorsal root ganglia, this has not been directly confirmed, and the pathogenesis of this neuropathy is uncertain. Anecdotal experience suggests that it does not generally respond to AZT, and treatment therefore relies on symptom management with tricyclics and analgesics. Autonomic neuropathy has also been reported in AIDS patients, with presentation ranging from postural hypotension to cardiovascular collapse in the setting of surgery.

Of increasing importance in patient management are the toxic neuropathies caused by some of the newer antiretroviral nucleoside drugs, including dideoxyinosine, dideoxycytidine, and d4T. These drugs cause dose-dependent axonal neuropathies with clinical features very similar to the AIDS-related sensory polyneuropathy discussed above, often heralded by distal extremity pain.

CMV causes an uncommon but therapeutically important infection of nerve roots. This polyradiculopathy is usually of subacute but fulminant onset, with pain and sacral sensory loss followed by ascending progression to flaccid paralysis. The CSF reveals a characteristic pleocytosis with polymorphonuclear cell predominance. Early diagnosis and prompt institution of ganciclovir or foscarnet treatment can lead to arrest and clinical improvement.

Less common than these polyneuropathies are two forms of mononeuritis multiplex. A relatively benign form may be seen earlier in infection during "clinical latency" and is self-limiting. A later, severe form may be caused by CMV and can be fatal if not treated.

MYOPATHIES. Several types of myopathy may complicate HIV-1 infection. Although classification and characterization of these conditions remain imprecise, both inflammatory and noninflammatory myopathies have been described, ranging in severity from asymptomatic creatine kinase elevation to severe proximal weakness. Patients with inflammatory, polymyositis-like illnesses have improved with steroid therapy.

AZT can also cause proximal weakness and loss of muscle mass. This toxic myopathy appears to develop only after prolonged use of the antiretroviral and perhaps relates to the drug's effect on mitochondria; muscle biopsy may reveal excessive or abnormal mitochondria. Discontinuing the drug usually results in clinical improvement.

Baumbartner JE, Rachlin JR, Beckstead JH, et al.: Primary central nervous system lymphomas: Natural history and response to radiation therapy in 55 patients with acquired immunodeficiency syndrome. J Neurosurg 73:206, 1990. *Describes an extensive experience with primary CNS lymphoma in AIDS.*

Berger JR, Kaszovitz B, Post JD, et al.: Progressive multifocal leukoencephalopathy associated with human immunodeficiency virus infection. Ann Intern Med 107:78, 1987. *A review of experience with PML in AIDS.*

Navia BA, Cho ES, Petito CK, et al.: Cerebral toxoplasmosis complicating the acquired immune deficiency syndrome: Clinical and neuropathological findings in 27 patients. Ann Neurol 19:224, 1986. *Describes clinical features of cerebral toxoplasmosis in AIDS.*

Navia BA, Jordon BD, Price RW: The AIDS dementia complex. I. Clinical features. Ann Neurol 19517, 1986. *Report characterizing the clinical features of the AIDS dementia complex.*

Porter SB, Sande M: Toxoplasmosis of the central nervous system in the acquired immunodeficiency syndrome. N Engl J Med 327:1643, 1992. *A review of experience with cerebral toxoplasmosis in AIDS.*

Price RWP, Perry SW (eds.): HIV, AIDS, and the Brain. New York, Raven Press, 1994. *A volume devoted to the effects of HIV-1 on the CNS, particularly the AIDS dementia complex.*

Price RW, Worley JM: Management of the neurologic complications of HIV-1 infection and AIDS. *In* Sande MA, Volberding PA (eds.): The Medical Management of AIDS. 4th ed. Philadelphia, WB Saunders, 1994, p 261. *A general review with updated full bibliography.*

Simpson DM, Wolfe DE: Neuromuscular complications of HIV infection and its treatment. AIDS 5:917, 1991. *A general review of the neuropathies and myopathies complicating HIV-1 infection.*

Zuger A, Louie E, Holzman RS, et al.: Cryptococcal disease in patients with the acquired immunodeficiency syndrome: Diagnostic features and outcome of treatment. Ann Intern Med 104:234, 1986. *Describes the clinical features of cryptococcal meningitis in AIDS.*

365 PULMONARY MANIFESTATIONS OF HIV INFECTION

Philip C. Hopewell

Lung disease, specifically *Pneumocystis carinii* pneumonia (PCP), was the first recognized mode of expression of infection with the human immunodeficiency virus (HIV). Since the original clusters of cases of PCP were reported in 1981, the respiratory system has continued to be a common site of involvement in persons infected with HIV. Although pulmonary disorders are more frequent among persons who have advanced immunosuppression, meeting the current surveillance definitions for the acquired immunodeficiency syndrome (AIDS), lung diseases also occur with an increased frequency in individuals with HIV infection who have lesser degrees of immunosuppression. This chapter describes the relative frequency and spectrum of lung diseases that occur among persons infected with HIV and focuses on the approach to evaluating symptoms that originate from the respiratory tract in this unique group of patients.

EFFECTS OF HIV ON RESPIRATORY TRACT DEFENSES

The hallmark of the effect of HIV infection on host immune response is a progressive reduction in the number of circulating CD4+ lymphocytes or "T-helper" cells (see Ch. 360 and 361). The CD4+ lymphocyte plays a central role in orchestrating both cellular and humoral immune responses. Consequently, as HIV disease becomes progressively more severe, the ability of the host to ward off or contain infecting organisms becomes more and more limited. Many of the immune defects that have been described in HIV-infected persons can be attributed simply to a reduction in numbers of CD4+ lymphocytes. However, HIV infection also induces functional defects in these cells: Circulating CD4+ lymphocytes fail to proliferate in response to antigens that have been encountered previously. This loss of memory may account for failure to continue to contain infections, such as with *Mycobacterium tuberculosis* or *P. carinii*, and for the inability to prevent reinfection, as may occur with *M. tuberculosis*. Reductions in production of interleukin-2 (IL-2) and interferon-γ by CD4+ lymphocytes from HIV-infected persons have also been demonstrated. These cytokines are responsible for stimulating clonal proliferation of specifically activated alveolar macrophages and lymphocytes. Defects in production of IL-2 and interferon-γ are detectable early in the course of HIV infection and account for a functional decrease in immune response out of proportion to reduced numbers of circulating CD4+ lymphocytes (see Ch. 360).

Alveolar macrophages from persons with HIV infection have reduced chemotactic ability, but the ability to phagocytose and kill ingested organisms is thought to be normal. Alveolar macrophages express CD4 surface antigens and thus can be infected with HIV, yet they remain viable. It has been postulated that these cells can serve as reservoirs in which HIV may be sequestered. The protected virions may then infect other cells. It has also been demonstrated that cytokines, especially tumor necrosis factor-α and IL-3, stimulated by opportunistic infections such as tuberculosis, result in up-regulation of HIV production within macrophages. Given these findings, the alveolar macrophage may play roles in protecting both the host and the virus and may contribute to accelerated HIV disease in the presence of opportunistic infections.

CORRELATION OF RESPIRATORY TRACT DISORDERS WITH STAGE OF HIV DISEASE

The conceptual relationship between the frequency and spectrum of lung diseases and CD4+ lymphocyte count is shown in Figure 365-1. The data that support this concept have been derived from a large, national, multicenter investigation, The Pulmonary Complications of HIV Infection Study (PCHIS). The cohort that formed the basis for this study generally mirrored the characteristics of the known HIV-infected persons in the United States (that is, reported AIDS cases), had a broad range of severity of immune compromise (47% of the cohort had CD4+ lymphocyte counts >400 cells per microliter at the time of enrollment), and were followed for a median of 53 months.

Table 365-1 shows the diseases and their rates per 100 person-years of observation in the PCHIS. Because an HIV-negative control group made up of subjects from the two largest HIV transmission categories (homosexual/bisexual men and injecting drug users [IDU's]) was included, it was demonstrated that acute bronchitis, a disorder not usually regarded as opportunistic, is significantly more common among HIV-infected persons. It should be noted that because there were no study centers in areas in which histoplasmosis and coccidioidomycosis are endemic, there were few instances of these relatively common fungal infections of the lung noted in the cohort. This observation raises an important point: the spectrum of HIV-associated lung diseases varies with geographic location as well as with severity of immune compromise and the demographic (including transmission category) make-up of the HIV-infected population in any given medical center or geographic area.

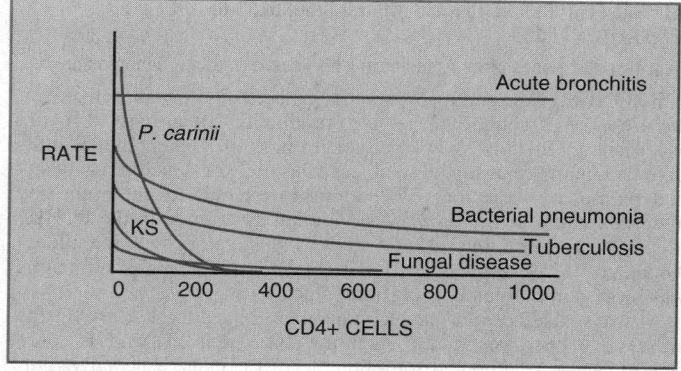

FIGURE 365-1. The relative frequency and spectrum of lung diseases change as the CD4+ lymphocyte count declines. This graph presents a conceptual depiction of these changes. The x-axis could also be equated with time following acquisition of HIV infection.

RELATIONSHIP OF RESPIRATORY TRACT DISEASES TO CD4+ LYMPHOCYTE COUNT, DEMOGRAPHIC CHARACTERISTICS, AND TRANSMISSION CATEGORY

PCP is the most common lung disease in persons with CD4+ counts <200 cells per microliter. However, in the PCHIS, 11 (6%) cases of PCP occurred in persons with CD4+ lymphocyte counts >200 cells per microliter. The patients with higher counts were marked by having other HIV-associated symptoms or findings such as fever, unintentional weight loss, oral thrush, and lymphadenopathy. Other lung diseases that usually occur only in persons with advanced HIV infection include fungal infections, pulmonary Kaposi's sarcoma (KS), lymphoma, and nontuberculous mycobacterial infections. In the case of *Mycobacterium avium* complex, it is difficult to determine if the organism is actually causing lung disease or is simply colonizing the airways. Thus, the frequency of *M. avium* complex lung disease is difficult to establish. The same difficulty applies to determining the frequency of cytomegalovirus (CMV) pulmonary disease.

Both demographic characteristics and HIV transmission category bear some relationship to the frequency of various lung diseases. Bacterial pneumonia tends to be more common among IDU's (with or without HIV infection) than in the other HIV transmission categories. Presumably, this relates, at least in part, to the effects of opiates on ventilation, cough, and ability to protect the airway. Tuberculosis is also more common in IDU's. Injection drug use had been shown to be a risk factor for tuberculosis prior to the HIV epidemic, so the finding of an increased amount of tuberculosis among drug users with HIV infection is not surprising.

Data from the PCHIS have shown that whites have a higher rate of PCP than blacks. Although the basis for this is unknown, the finding is consistent with the observation that PCP is rare in Africa. It has generally been assumed that the rarity of *P. carinii* in Africa is related to the organism being less common in the environment. However, the finding of a racial difference in risk suggests that genetic factors may play a role in predisposing whites to or protecting blacks from the disease.

TABLE 365-1. CUMULATIVE FREQUENCY OF DISEASES WITH RESPIRATORY TRACT INVOLVEMENT IN A COHORT OF PERSONS WITH HIV INFECTION (INCLUDES MULTIPLE EPISODES PER PERSON)

Diagnosis	Episodes per 100 Person-Years
Acute bronchitis	9.72
Pneumocystis carinii pneumonia	5.65
Bacterial pneumonia	5.63
Nontuberculous mycobacterial diseases	0.74
Interstitial lung disease	0.60
Pulmonary tuberculosis	0.58
Cytomegalovirus	0.42
Kaposi's sarcoma	0.33
Lymphoma	0.19
Cryptococcosis	0.16

CLINICAL FEATURES OF HIV-ASSOCIATED DISORDERS OF THE RESPIRATORY TRACT

Disorders Not Necessarily Associated with Severe Immune Suppression

BRONCHITIS. Acute bronchitis in the PCHIS was defined by the presence of cough with sputum production for at least 48 hours and a chest film that showed either no or stable parenchymal infiltrations occurring in a study subject who did not develop an identified pulmonary infection. Evaluations to attempt to determine the microbial cause of the bronchitis were not performed in the PCHIS. It was the general impression of the investigators that the illness tended to be self-limited but recurrent. Not surprisingly, bronchitis was more common among cigarette smokers.

Airways disease may be recognized on plain chest films by the presence of peribronchial thickening (Fig. 365–2A) and is more clearly seen on computed tomographic (CT) scans, especially thin-section scans (Fig. 365–2B). In addition, bronchiectasis may also occur without a recognized antecedent lung infection (Fig. 365–3). Bronchiectasis may also be a sequela of bacterial lung infection or, occasionally, PCP.

Although in the PCHIS cohort the episodes of acute bronchitis were neither associated with nor portended any other significant pulmonary diseases, the disorder may be problematic in that the symptoms may be mistaken as an indication for further, often invasive, evaluations. In general, however, bronchitis is recognizable by the absence of parenchymal infiltrations on chest films and, thus,

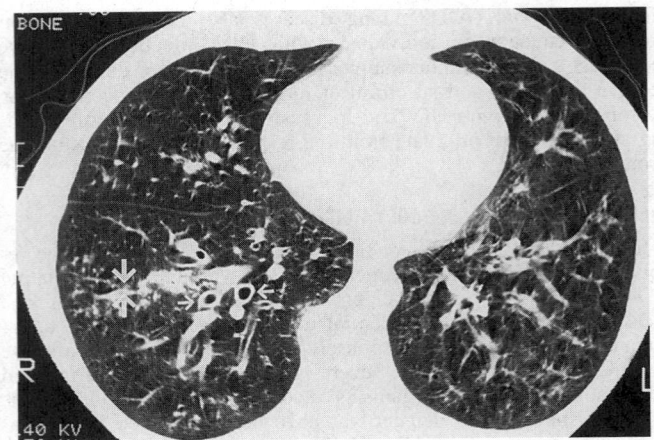

FIGURE 365–3. High-resolution CT scan of the chest of the patient whose films are shown in Figure 365–2. The scan is at a lower level and shows dilated airways with thickened walls indicative of bronchiectasis (*horizontal arrows*) and areas of mucus plugging and infiltration (*vertical arrows*). (Courtesy of Dr. James Gruden, Department of Radiology, San Francisco General Hospital.)

when the constellation of symptoms and findings described previously is noted, one should, generally, simply observe the patient, with or without antimicrobial therapy, and not undertake further evaluations.

BACTERIAL PNEUMONIA (see related chapter for each infection in Part XXI). As shown in Table 365–1, bacterial pneumonia occurred at a rate of 5.63 episodes per 100 person-years of observation in the PCHIS cohort. Bacterial pneumonia was defined as the presence of cough that was productive of purulent sputum, an area of parenchymal infiltration on chest film, and a response to antimicrobial therapy. A specific causative agent was identified in 35% of cases, a proportion that is consistent with the results of studies of the etiology of community-acquired pneumonia in persons without HIV infection.

Of the episodes for which the cause was established, *Streptococcus pneumoniae* accounted for 67% and *Haemophilus influenzae* 15%. These two agents have been generally ranked first and second in most reports of bacterial pneumonia in persons with HIV infection. In most reports, *Staphylococcus aureus* has been the third most common agent and seems to be especially common among persons with pulmonary KS. A long list of other bacterial pathogens has also been described as causing pneumonia in the setting of HIV infection (Table 365–2).

Bacterial pneumonia, especially pneumococcal pneumonia, commonly tends to be associated with bacteremia and, occasionally, sepsis syndrome. Other than the high frequency of bacteremia, the mode of clinical presentation of bacterial pneumonia does not differ in persons with and without HIV infection. Pneumonias caused by *S. pneumoniae* and *H. influenzae* tend to present as an acute illness of short duration characterized by fever, chills, and productive cough. Lobar consolidation is the most common finding on chest radiographs, and pleural fluid may be present.

The diagnostic evaluation should include sputum Gram stain and culture, Gram stain and culture of pleural fluid if present, and blood

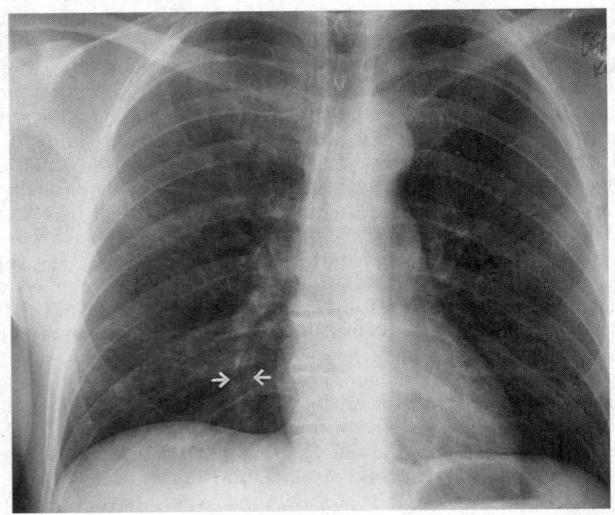

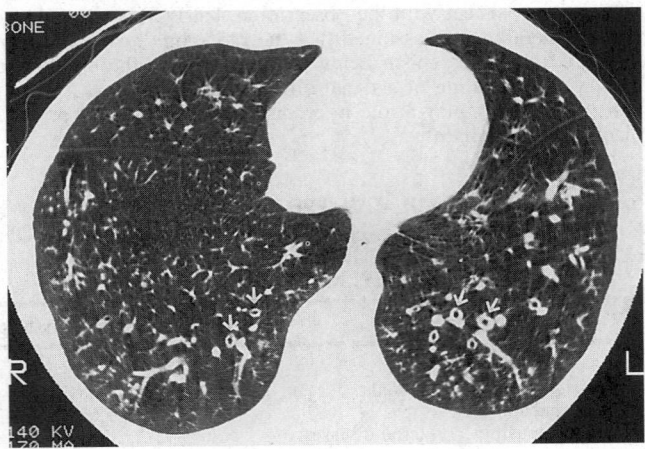

FIGURE 365–2. Bronchitis in HIV infection. *A,* A frontal view chest radiograph showing peribronchial thickening, right lower lung zone (*arrows*) consistent with bronchitis. *B,* A high-resolution CT scan of the chest showing bilateral peribronchial thickening (*arrows*) consistent with bronchitis. (Courtesy of Dr. James Gruden, Department of Radiology, San Francisco General Hospital.)

TABLE 365–2. REPORTED CAUSES OF BACTERIAL PNEUMONIA IN PERSONS WITH HIV INFECTION

Streptococcus pneumoniae
Haemophilus influenzae
Staphylococcus aureus
Nonpneumococcal streptococci
Pseudomonas aeruginosa
Moraxella catarrhalis
Rhodococcus equi
Neisseria meningitidis
Legionella species
Nocardia species
Actinomyces species

TABLE 365-3. FEATURES OF TUBERCULOSIS IN PATIENTS WITH HIV INFECTION

	Early in HIV Disease	Late in HIV Disease
Clinical course	More indolent Fewer systemic symptoms/signs	More acute Systemic symptoms/signs may predominate
Sites of disease	Predominantly pulmonary	Predominantly extrapulmonary and disseminated
Chest film	Upper lobe cavitary lesions	Diffuse or lower lobe infiltration Adenopathy Occasionally normal when lungs involved
Tuberculin test	Usually positive	Usually negative
Sputum smear/culture	Usually positive	Usually positive in patients with pulmonary disease
Infectiousness	Infectious when lungs are involved	Infectious when lungs are involved
Response to therapy	Excellent	Excellent

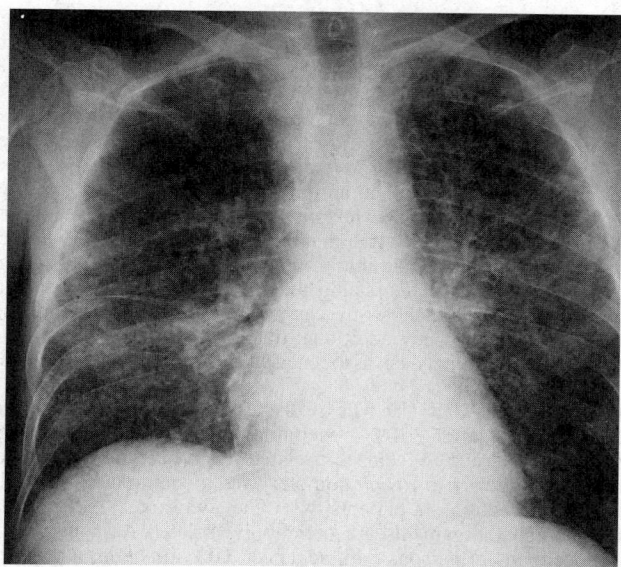

FIGURE 365-4. Frontal view chest radiograph showing diffuse pulmonary parenchymal infiltration and bilateral hilar and right paratracheal adenopathy. The patient had acid-fast bacilli seen on microscopic examination of his sputum, and *Mycobacterium tuberculosis* was isolated from sputum and blood. (Courtesy of Dr. James Gruden, Department of Radiology, San Francisco Hospital.)

cultures. Antimicrobial therapy should be guided by the usual principles for treating infectious disorders. The response to therapy should be prompt and comparable to the response of nonimmunocompromised patients. Clinicians should have a low threshold for initiating further diagnostic evaluations if the response is not prompt or is incomplete or there is worsening after an initial response. In a retrospective review of pneumococcal pneumonia in patients with HIV infection, all patients who failed to respond to usual antimicrobial therapy had superimposed PCP.

Another feature of HIV-associated bacterial pneumonia is the tendency for recurrence. This may be related to the failure to generate protective antibodies to the infecting organism or to bronchiectasis.

TUBERCULOSIS. Because *M. tuberculosis* is a very pathogenic organism, little or no immune compromise is needed for tuberculosis to develop. For this reason, tuberculosis tends to occur earlier in the course of HIV disease than diseases caused by less pathogenic organisms. The degree of immunosuppression present in a given patient has an important influence on the clinical features of tuberculosis in the presence of HIV infection, as described in Table 365-3. Persons with HIV infection and relatively well-preserved immune function tend to have "typical" features of tuberculosis, whereas tuberculosis that occurs among persons with advanced HIV disease commonly involves extrapulmonary sites and has diffuse lung infiltration with no cavitation and hilar and mediastinal adenopathy (Fig. 365-4). In terms of symptoms, tuberculosis may present as an acute illness or as a more indolent progressive process. When the lungs are involved, sputum smears and cultures are as likely to be positive in persons with HIV infection as in non–HIV-infected patients. However, because extrapulmonary sites are involved commonly, other diagnostic specimens are often necessary (Table 365-4).

Several studies have shown that persons with HIV infection and tuberculosis respond well to antituberculous therapy. In a series of patients, those who failed to respond to standard antituberculous therapy or who responded and then worsened had another superimposed disease, often PCP.

NONSPECIFIC AND LYMPHOID INTERSTITIAL PNEUMONITIS. In the PCHIS cohort, undiagnosed "interstitial disease" occurred at a rate of 0.33 cases per 100 person-years. It is not known, however, if these cases met the diagnostic criteria for either nonspecific interstitial pneumonitis (NIP) or lymphoid interstitial pneumonitis (LIP). LIP, although common in children with HIV infection, is thought to be rare in adults; thus, most of the cases in the PCHIS cohort were probably NIP. The cause of these conditions is not known, but it is speculated that they represent a response to the HIV itself. NIP tends to be self-limited in most instances and to resolve without therapy. LIP is more persistent and/or progressive but in some instances has seemed to respond to corticosteroids.

The diagnosis of both NIP and LIP can be made only by biopsy. Although transbronchial biopsy tissue is usually not sufficient to provide a definitive diagnosis, findings that are consistent with NIP in the absence of any other identified diagnosis is sufficient to infer a diagnosis of NIP. Because of the apparent benign course of the disease and the lack of any therapeutic modalities, invasive tests to establish a diagnosis of NIP are not warranted.

Disorders Associated with Severe Immune Suppression

***PNEUMOCYSTIS CARINII* PNEUMONIA** (see Ch. 383). PCP is the most common lung disease in persons with advanced HIV infection. The presentation tends to be indolent, characterized by slowly progressive shortness of breath and nonproductive cough, usually accompanied by fever. In the PCHIS cohort, it was noted that virtually all episodes of PCP were marked by cough or shortness of breath, or both. If at least one of these symptoms was not present, PCP was not found. This study also examined the utility of screening for *P. carinii* by performing chest radiographs, pulmonary function tests, and examination of induced sputum on asymptomatic subjects. No cases of PCP were found. Based on these data, an evaluation for *P. carinii* should not be undertaken unless an HIV-infected person complains of cough and/or shortness of breath.

The radiographic findings of PCP are extremely varied. Most frequently there is diffuse "interstitial" infiltration, but there may be

TABLE 365-4. RESULTS OF MICROSCOPIC EXAMINATION AND MYCOBACTERIAL CULTURES IN PATIENTS WITH ADVANCED HIV INFECTION AND TUBERCULOSIS

Specimen	No. Positive/No. Tested (%)	
	Acid-fast Smear	Culture
Sputum	43/69 (62)	64/69 (93)
Bronchoalveolar lavage	9/44 (20)	39/44 (89)
Transbronchial lung biopsy	1/10 (10)	7/10 (70)
Blood	—	15/46 (33)
Lymph node	21/44 (48)	39/43 (91)
Bone marrow	4/22 (18)	13/21 (62)
Cerebrospinal fluid	—	4/21 (19)
Urine	—	12/17 (71)
Other*	5/31 (16)	24/32 (75)

* Includes pleural fluid/biopsy, pericardial fluid/biopsy, stool, liver biopsy, abscess drainage, peritoneal fluid, bone biopsy.

Data from Small PM, Schecter GF, Goodman PC, et al.: Treatment of tuberculosis in patients with advanced human immunodeficiency virus infection. N Engl J Med 324:289, 1991.

any manner of focal infiltrations, nodules or cavitary lesions, pneumatoceles, or miliary infiltration (Fig. 365–5). Focal upper lobe involvement that mimics tuberculosis is more common in persons who have been given aerosol pentamidine as prophylaxis against PCP. Pneumatoceles and spontaneous pneumothorax may occur with first episodes of PCP but are more common with subsequent episodes.

Commonly, the response to antipneumocystis therapy is slow, and radiographic abnormalities and gas exchange may worsen during the first 4 to 6 days of treatment. Co-administration of corticosteroids may minimize this initial worsening. Generally, particularly if the diagnosis has been established by bronchoscopy, most clinicians who repeat bronchoscopy early in the course of therapy find that it does not yield any additional diagnoses. However, worsening later in the course may be associated with a second, superimposed disease.

NONTUBERCULOUS MYCOBACTERIAL DISEASES (see Ch. 312). Soon after AIDS was initially described, it was recognized that a group of closely related mycobacteria collectively named *Mycobacterium avium* complex was a common cause of disseminated infection in patients with the syndrome. Although *M. avium* complex organisms are commonly isolated from respiratory tract specimens in persons with advanced HIV infection, actual lung disease is unusual. Occasionally, however, the organism may cause focal lung disease. Endobronchial lesions may be seen on bronchoscopy, and on biopsy these lesions may contain granulomas, a histologic feature that is unusual in other organs involved in disseminated *M. avium* disease. Colonization of the lungs may precede

and be a marker for subsequent disseminated *M. avium* infection. Disseminated *M. avium* complex disease occurs late in the course of HIV disease, usually when the CD4+ lymphocyte count is < 50 cells per microliter. Fever, weight loss, diarrhea, and abdominal pain are common symptoms. Pulmonary involvement is usually indicated by cough. Because it is difficult to distinguish between colonization and infection, the radiographic features of *M. avium* pulmonary disease are not well-defined. As noted above, focal infiltration may occur. Rarely, there may be diffuse lung involvement with an interstitial pattern on chest films. However, in the presence of a diffusely abnormal chest film, *M. avium* complex should not be accepted as the cause until other diseases have been excluded.

Among the nontuberculous mycobacteria, *M. kansasii* is a distant second to *M. avium* complex as a cause of disease in HIV-infected persons. As with *M. avium* complex, *M. kansasii* infections tend to be disseminated in persons with HIV infection. However, when *M. kansasii* is isolated from a respiratory tract specimen, it is more likely to be a cause of lung disease than is *M. avium* complex. As with most lung infections, *M. kansasii* usually presents with fever, cough, and, subsequently, shortness of breath. *M. kansasii* is probably more likely to cause diffuse infiltration on chest film than *M. avium* complex (see Ch. 312).

FUNGAL INFECTIONS (see Ch. 347 to 358). Both histoplasmosis and coccidioidomycosis are common HIV-associated infections in the areas in which the causative organisms are endemic and are seen sporadically outside of the endemic regions. The presenting clinical features of both histoplasmosis and coccidioidomycosis are nonspecific and variable. Histoplasmosis is commonly a protracted, febrile, wasting illness. Both infections are usually dissemi-

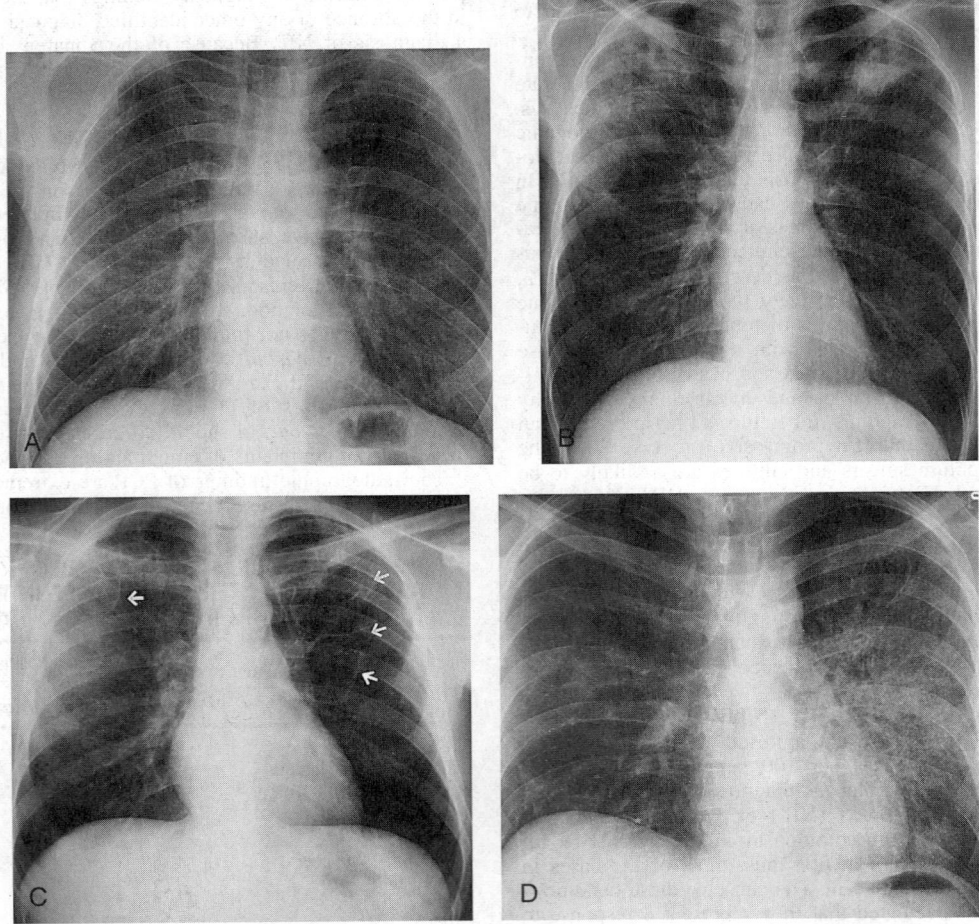

FIGURE 365–5. Radiographic findings of *Pneumocystis carinii* pneumonia (PCP). *A,* A frontal view chest radiograph showing diffuse hazy infiltration caused by early PCP. *B,* A frontal view chest radiograph with bilateral upper lobe infiltrations. *C,* A frontal view chest radiograph showing multiple bilateral thin-walled pneumatoceles *(arrows). D,* A frontal view chest radiograph with unilateral left-sided infiltration. (Courtesy of Dr. James Gruden, Department of Radiology, San Francisco General Hospital.)

nated, with respiratory symptoms and abnormal chest films reported in varying proportions. Both histoplasmosis and coccidioidomycosis can present with an acute sepsis syndrome including acute respiratory failure.

Chest radiographs are abnormal in the majority of patients, especially those who have respiratory symptoms. With histoplasmosis, the most common pattern is diffuse infiltration that is either reticulonodular or "alveolar." Coccidioidomycosis is associated with either localized or scattered nodular lesions or diffuse infiltration. For histoplasmosis, the diagnosis is commonly established by stain and culture of bone marrow, buffy coat, or blood. With coccidioidomycosis involving the lungs, specimens from the respiratory tract usually serve to establish the diagnosis.

Cryptococcosis is not limited to an endemic area. The presenting complaints are nonspecific and include fever, weight loss, fatigue, and headache, often present for a long period prior to diagnosis. Most often pulmonary involvement is silent, although in one large retrospective review, 31% of patients had respiratory complaints at the time of presentation. The findings on chest radiographs have been varied. Focal and diffuse infiltration, localized or scattered nodules, some of which may be cavitary, pleural effusions, and hilar adenopathy all have been described.

Aspergillosis has been diagnosed in a small number of patients with HIV infection. There are two patterns of *Aspergillus* pulmonary disease, one characterized by tissue invasion and the second largely an airway disease, obstructive bronchial aspergillosis. Reported risks in the setting of HIV infection have been neutropenia, use of corticosteroids, marijuana smoking, and use of broad-spectrum antimicrobial agents. Fever and cough that is sometimes productive of bronchial casts are the usual presenting complaints. The radiographic findings include focal infiltration, cavitary lesions, and pleura-based densities (Fig. 365–6). Atelectasis and airway filling patterns may be seen with obstructive bronchial aspergillosis.

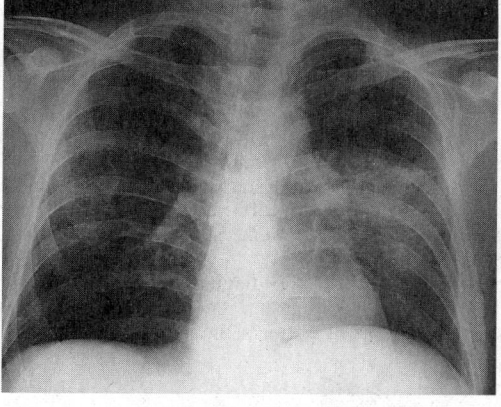

A

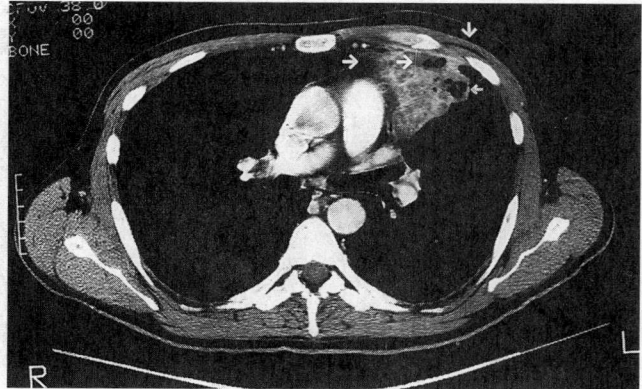

B

FIGURE 365–6. Invasive aspergillosis in an HIV-infected man. *A*, A frontal view chest radiograph showing infiltration in the right mid-lung zone. *B*, A CT scan of the chest at the level of the infiltration. The scan shows areas of necrosis *(horizontal arrows)* and probable chest wall invasion *(vertical arrow)*. (Courtesy of Dr. James Gruden, Department of Radiology, San Francisco General Hospital.)

CYTOMEGALOVIRUS. CMV is commonly isolated from respiratory tract specimens in HIV-infected patients. However, it is unusual for lung disease to be attributable to this agent even when specific cytomegalic cells are seen on biopsy specimens. Thus, the diagnosis of CMV pneumonia can be made only when the virus is isolated in culture, specific histopathologic changes are seen on biopsy, and no other diagnosis is established. Because it is difficult to determine if CMV is the cause of lung disease in a given patient, the radiographic features of CMV pneumonia are not well-defined. In general, however, it is thought to cause diffuse infiltration that is not distinguishable from the pattern caused by many other organisms and by nonspecific interstitial pneumonitis.

NEOPLASTIC DISEASES. In the PCHIS cohort, KS involving the lungs occurred at a rate of 0.33 cases per 100 person-years of observation (14 [13%] pulmonary cases of 105 total cases), and pulmonary involvement with lymphoma occurred at a rate of 0.19 cases per 100 person-years. However, among persons with advanced HIV disease, pulmonary KS has been diagnosed in 8 to 14% of patients being evaluated for respiratory symptoms, in 21 to 49% of patients with respiratory symptoms and mucocutaneous lesions, and in 47 to 75% of patients with known KS undergoing autopsy. It is likely that the reported frequency of KS is less than actually occurs because the lung involvement may be clinically silent.

The diagnosis of pulmonary KS is nearly always established by the appearance of lesions on bronchoscopy. Typically, endobronchial KS is seen as flat, red or purple submucosal lesions that are similar in appearance to submucosal hemorrhages induced by bronchoscope trauma (see Color Plate 11G). The lesions may be found in any location, from vocal cords to peripheral airways, and tend to favor airway bifurcations. Because of their submucosal location, the lesions are difficult to biopsy; however, the findings are sufficiently characteristic in appearance to enable a high degree of diagnostic certainty. In a few instances, pulmonary parenchymal KS has been diagnosed by transbronchial or open biopsy in persons with no endobronchial lesions seen.

The chest radiographs of patients who had pulmonary KS without coexisting infection showed lesions that were predominantly central and consisted mainly of bronchial wall thickening and nodules (Fig. 365–7). Kerley B lines and pleural effusions were noted in 71 and 52%, respectively. Hilar or mediastinal adenopathy was present in 15%.

Non-Hodgkin's lymphoma is the second most frequent malignancy involving the lungs in patients with HIV infection. The frequency of pulmonary involvement in reported series is 0 to 25%. The presentation, even in patients who have pulmonary involvement, is generally dominated by systemic symptoms. The most common chest radiographic findings are patchy parenchymal infiltrates, nodules, and solitary masses. Intrathoracic adenopathy has been reported in a minority of cases. The diagnosis can be established by transbronchial biopsy, needle aspiration biopsy, or thoracoscopic or open biopsy.

AN INTEGRATED APPROACH TO DIAGNOSIS

Although the differential diagnosis of lung disease in a person with HIV infection is quite broad, the probabilities of the various diagnoses can be reduced in a given patient by knowing the patient's symptoms, HIV transmission category, and CD4+ lymphocyte count and further refined by the findings on the chest film. A general approach to the diagnostic evaluation in patients with a CD4+ lymphocyte count of ≤ 300 cells per microliter is shown in Figure 365–8.

First define the patient's symptoms, especially whether or not the patient has cough and/or shortness of breath. If cough is present, it is important to ascertain if it is productive of purulent sputum. It is very uncommon for patients with PCP to have purulent sputum. Moreover, depending on the stain used, the presence of purulent debris in respiratory tract specimens makes it difficult to detect *P. carinii* in smears of sputum or bronchoalveolar lavage (BAL) fluid. As noted previously, acute bronchitis and bacterial pneumonia are relatively more frequent among persons with higher CD4+ lymphocyte cell counts. Additionally, IDU's have higher rates of bacterial pneumonia and tuberculosis than persons in other HIV transmission categories. Also as noted, the differential diagnosis varies somewhat with the geographic area, with histoplasmosis and

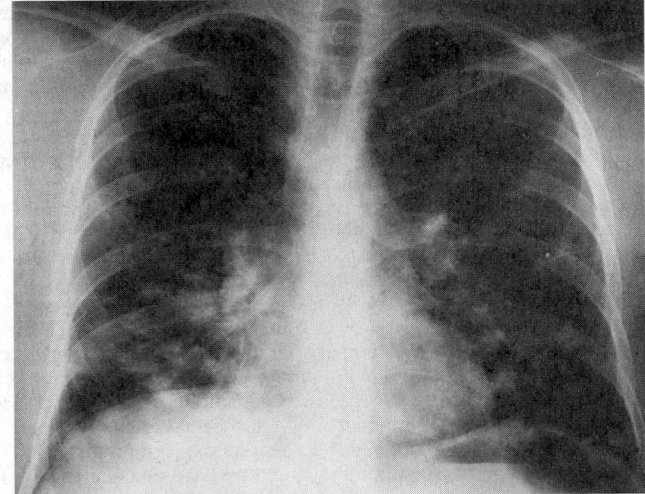

A

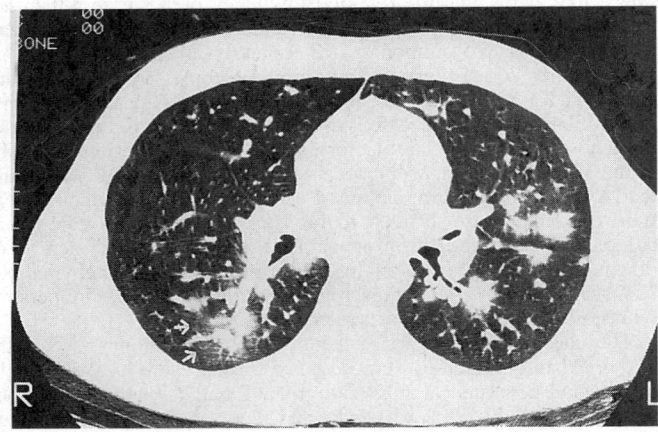

B

FIGURE 365-7. Kaposi's sarcoma (KS). *A*, A frontal view chest radiograph with typical findings of pulmonary KS. *B*, A high-resolution CT scan of the lower chest. Masslike peribronchovascular lesions typical of KS are seen. The lesions on the right side are surrounded by areas of fainter infiltration *(arrows)*, a so-called halo sign that is highly suggestive of KS. (Courtesy of Dr. James Gruden, Department of Radiology, San Francisco General Hospital.)

coccidioidomycosis being common in their respective endemic areas.

As in all patients with significant respiratory symptoms, radiographic examination of the chest is usually the first test. If the chest film shows no abnormalities in a patient with purulent sputum, the likely diagnosis is bronchitis. Patients with a diagnosis of bronchitis should be followed to be certain that the symptoms resolve and, if there is no resolution or worsening, further evaluation should be undertaken. It must be kept in mind that both tuberculosis and PCP may present with normal chest films.

Patients who have normal chest films and a nonproductive cough may also have bronchitis, but if the CD4+ lymphocyte count is <300 cells per microliter, *P. carinii* should be considered. In this circumstance, pulmonary function testing with measurement of the diffusing capacity for carbon monoxide (DLco) should be performed. If the DLco is <75% of the predicted normal value, further evaluation directed toward detecting *P. carinii* should be undertaken. A promising alternative approach that has not yet been fully evaluated is to replace measurement of the DLco with thin-section CT scanning using a limited number of images to reduce cost. This approach has the potential advantage of being able to distinguish among PCP, emphysema, and vascular obliteration caused by foreign particle embolization from intravenous drug use (Fig. 365-9).

If the chest film is abnormal, the next step depends on the type of abnormality. Focal infiltration, especially consolidation, in a pa-

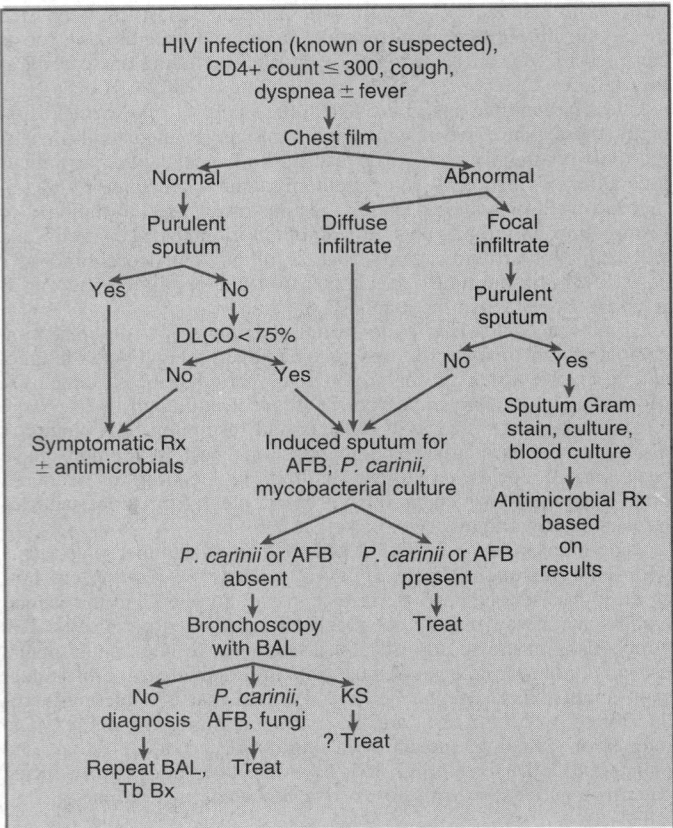

FIGURE 365-8. Algorithm of the diagnostic approach to patients who are known or suspected of having HIV infection resulting in significant immunocompromise, <300 CD4+ lymphocytes per microliter. DLco = Pulmonary diffusing capacity for carbon monoxide; AFB = acid-fast bacilli; BAL = bronchoalveolar lavage; Tb Bx = transbronchial lung biopsy.

tient with purulent sputum is most consistent with a diagnosis of bacterial pneumonia or tuberculosis (see Fig. 365-8). Sputum should be obtained for Gram stain, acid-fast stain, and cultures for pyogenic organisms and mycobacteria. If there is a poor response or worsening, further evaluation, especially for *P. carinii*, should be performed.

To this point much of the diagnostic approach is applicable for evaluating respiratory symptoms regardless of the HIV status of the patient. In the group of patients thought likely to have an HIV-re-

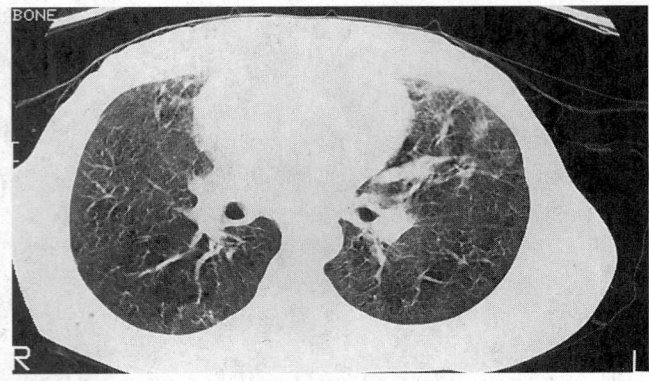

FIGURE 365-9. High-resolution CT scan of the chest of a patient who complained of shortness of breath but whose plain chest film was normal. The scan shows patchy "ground-glass" infiltration in the anterior portions of both lungs. The patient was found to have *P. carinii* in an induced sputum sample. The findings noted in the scan are typical of early *P. carinii* pneumonia. (Courtesy of Dr. James Gruden, Department of Radiology, San Francisco General Hospital.)

TABLE 365-5. EXAMINATION OF RESPIRATORY TRACT SPECIMENS

Specimen	Test
Spontaneous sputum	Gram stain, AFB stain, cultures for mycobacteria and pyogenic bacteria
Induced sputum	*P. carinii* stain, AFB stain, mycobacterial culture
Bronchoalveolar lavage fluid	*P. carinii* stain, AFB stain, mycobacterial and fungal cultures
Transbronchial biopsy tissue	Touch preparations and tissue stains for *P. carinii,* AFB stain, hematoxylin and eosin tissue stain, culture for mycobacteria and fungi
Needle aspiration biopsy tissue	*P. carinii* stain, AFB stain, cytologic examination, cultures for mycobacteria and fungi

AFB = Acid-fast bacilli.

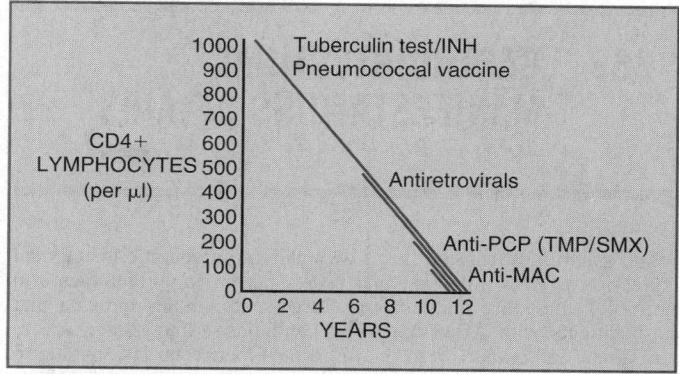

FIGURE 365-10. Schematic representation of the use of preventive interventions in persons with HIV infection. The timing of the interventions is based on the CD4+ lymphocyte count and the risk of the common HIV-associated lung infections. INH = Isoniazid; PCP = *P. carinii* pneumonia; TMP-SMX = trimethoprim-sulfamethoxazole; MAC = *Mycobacterium avium* complex.

lated opportunistic infection, however, there is considerable variation both in philosophy and in specific diagnostic tests used. Cogent arguments have been made for empiric treatment with antipneumocystis agents for patients thought highly likely to have PCP, with specific tests for the organism being reserved for patients who fail to respond. With or without an empiric therapeutic trial, when it is decided to seek a specific diagnosis, the approach used varies. In some institutions, as described subsequently, the first step is to examine induced sputum, with bronchoscopy being performed only in those patients with negative sputum examinations. In other institutions, bronchoscopy is the first procedure used to obtain respiratory tract specimens. Also, based on experience and preference, there are variations in the bronchoscopic procedure. Usually, BAL is performed with all procedures. Many clinicians also routinely perform a transbronchial biopsy at the time of initial bronchoscopy, whereas others perform biopsies on a case-by-case basis, and others do so only if the BAL does not provide a diagnosis (and perhaps not even then).

If there is diffuse or focal infiltration in a person with a nonproductive cough, generally the evaluation should be directed toward opportunistic organisms. In many institutions the next diagnostic step is to induce sputum by having the patient inhale a hypertonic (3%) saline mist generated by an ultrasonic nebulizer. Careful attention to the details of selecting patients and inducing, processing, and examining the sputum specimens is essential to obtain good results.

Diagnosis of mycobacterial disease and fungal infections can also be established by examining induced sputum. However, in HIV-infected patients, because of the high frequency of oral candidiasis, fungal cultures are frequently overgrown with *Candida* species.

Because the negative predictive value of a negative examination of induced sputum is in the range of 60%, patients having a negative sputum examination generally should undergo bronchoscopy with BAL unless another diagnosis has been established or the procedure is contraindicated. At San Francisco General Hospital, *P. carinii* infection, either alone or with another diagnosis, was found in 32% of bronchoscopic examinations in patients who had a negative sputum examination. KS was found in 15%, nontuberculous mycobacteria in 25%, *M. tuberculosis* in 5%, and fungal pathogens in 4%. In addition, nearly all of the pathogens were found by BAL, and only rarely did transbronchial biopsy provide additional information.

In patients whose chest films show focal or isolated nodular or mass lesions, needle aspiration biopsy, if the lesion is accessible, is an efficient diagnostic approach, and in some instances fluoroscopically guided transbronchial biopsy should be attempted. Enlarged intrathoracic lymph nodes may also be approached via needle aspiration biopsy, either through the bronchoscope (Wang needle) or via a transthoracic approach. The tests that should be performed on the various sorts of specimens described above are listed in Table 365-5.

PREVENTING LUNG DISEASES IN PERSONS WITH HIV INFECTION

Much of the improved survival for patients with HIV infection in recent years owes to the prevention of PCP. Hence, the use of antipneumocystis agents such as trimethoprim-sulfamethoxazole, dap-

sone, and pentamidine aerosol for persons with HIV infection and CD4+ lymphocyte counts < 200 cells per microliter is a high-priority intervention. This is described in more detail in Ch. 383.

Preventive interventions for tuberculosis also should be accorded a high priority. All HIV-infected persons should receive a tuberculin skin test, and, if the test is positive (≥ 5 mm induration), isoniazid preventive therapy should be given regardless of the CD4+ lymphocyte count. Isoniazid should also be given to all HIV-infected persons who have been exposed to a person with infectious tuberculosis regardless of the tuberculin test result. The use of isoniazid preventive therapy for nonexposed persons who are defined as anergic is not of proven benefit.

It is not established whether pneumococcal vaccine reduces the rate of pneumococcal disease in persons with HIV infection. However, because of the low likelihood of adverse reactions to the vaccine, any benefit would not be offset by risk. Data from the PCHIS cohort suggest that trimethoprim-sulfamethoxazole as antipneumocystis prophylaxis decreases the frequency of pneumococcal disease, thus providing an additional benefit for this preventive intervention.

Finally, it has been shown that prophylactic rifabutin reduces the frequency of *M. avium* complex disease by approximately 50%. Current recommendations are that rifabutin prophylaxis be given to persons with HIV infection and CD4+ counts of < 100 cells per microliter. Persons who are candidates for rifabutin should be carefully evaluated for tuberculosis. Rifabutin administered to a person who has undiagnosed tuberculosis would quickly result in resistance of *M. tuberculosis* to rifabutin *and* rifampin, a major antituberculosis drug. The relationship of preventive interventions to CD4+ lymphocyte count is summarized in Figure 365-10.

Chin DP: *Mycobacterium avium* complex and other nontuberculous mycobacteria in patients with HIV. Semin Respir Infect 8:124, 1993. *Describes the epidemiology, clinical presentation, diagnosis, and management of the nontuberculous mycobacterial diseases with a focus on* M. avium *complex.*
Hopewell PC: Tuberculosis and infection with the human immunodeficiency virus. *In* Reichman LB, Hershfield ES (eds.): Tuberculosis: A Comprehensive International Approach. New York, Marcell Dekker, 1993, p 369. *Describes the overall impact of HIV infection on all aspects of tuberculosis.*
Hopewell PC, Mazur H: *Pneumocystis carinii* pneumonia: Current concepts. *In* Sande MA, Volberding PA (eds.): The Medical Management of AIDS, 4th ed. Philadelphia, WB Saunders, 1994, p 367. *A comprehensive review of the epidemiology, pathogenesis, clinical features, diagnosis, and treatment of PCP.*
Irwin DH, Kaplan LD: Pulmonary manifestations of acquired immunodeficiency syndrome malignancies. Semin Respir Infect 8:139, 1993. *Describes the clinical features and management of pulmonary Kaposi's sarcoma and non-Hodgkin's lymphoma.*
Stansell JD: Pulmonary fungal infections in HIV infected persons. Semin Respir Infect 8:116, 1993. *Reviews the epidemiology, clinical features, diagnosis, and management of the fungal infections that involve the lungs in patients with HIV infection.*
Wallace JM, Rao V, Glassroth J, et al.: Respiratory illnesses in persons with human immunodeficiency virus infection. Am Rev Respir Dis 148:1523, 1993. *Describes the frequency and spectrum of lung diseases after 18 months of follow-up in a cohort of HIV-infected persons from the major transmission categories. Included are subjects who have little apparent immunosuppression.*

366 GASTROINTESTINAL MANIFESTATIONS OF AIDS

John G. Bartlett

The gastrointestinal tract is an especially common site for clinical expression of HIV infection and represents an important factor in morbidity, including malnutrition. Large-scale studies indicate that most patients with AIDS have oral candidiasis, many have severe periodontal infections, up to one third have perirectal lesions due to herpes simplex, 30 to 60% complain of chronic or intermittent diarrhea, and the average weight loss following an AIDS-defining diagnosis is 12 to 15 kg. Most of these complications represent opportunistic infections that occur only with advanced stages of immunosuppression when the T4 lymphocyte count is < 200 per cubic millimeter.

ORAL LESIONS. Oral candidiasis ("thrush") is encountered at some time in 80 to 90% of all patients with advanced stages of HIV infection. The usual finding is white patches that show yeast forms and pseudohyphae on KOH preparation. The diagnosis is usually made by visual appearance. The lesions usually respond to nystatin, clotrimazole troches, ketoconazole, or fluconazole, but relapse rates are high so that continuous therapy is often necessary. Oral hairy leukoplakia (OHL) is a newly recognized condition found exclusively in persons with HIV infection. *In situ* hybridization implicates Epstein-Barr virus. Typical lesions are patches of white fibrillar projections that are usually located on the tongue and often confused with thrush. OHL is usually asymptomatic, but occasional patients complain of pain or voice changes and respond to treatment with acyclovir. Herpes simplex virus (HSV) often causes painful oral lesions that have the typical appearance of vesicles on an erythematous base and break down to form ulcers. Herpetic lesions tend to be more severe and prolonged in patients with HIV infection. The usual treatment is acyclovir given orally or parenterally. The major source of confusion is aphthous ulcers of unknown origin that seem to respond best to topical or systemic corticosteroids. In patients with Kaposi's sarcoma, the oral cavity is often involved, most frequently with typical erythematous purplish raised lesions on the palate, although any site in the oral cavity may be involved. Most are asymptomatic; symptomatic lesions generally respond to radiation treatment. Periodontal disease is relatively common with either gingivitis or periodontitis. Treatment consists of topical chlorhexidine (Peridex) or systemically administered metronidazole.

ESOPHAGITIS. Odynophagia generally indicates an esophageal lesion. The most common cause is candidiasis, and most patients also have thrush. Alternative causes include HSV, cytomegalovirus (CMV), or aphthous ulcers. The diagnosis is optimally made with endoscopy showing grayish white plaques and smears or biopsy to demonstrate the causative agent. A presumptive diagnosis of *Candida* esophagitis is made in patients with thrush combined with odynophagia. Preferred drugs for *C. albicans* esophagitis are ketoconazole or fluconazole by mouth, or a brief course of amphotericin B by vein. HSV may be treated with acyclovir, CMV often responds to ganciclovir, and aphthous ulcers are optimally treated with systemic corticosteroids.

GASTRIC LESIONS. Patients with AIDS often have gastric achlorhydria; less common gastric lesions are Kaposi's sarcoma and opportunistic infections.

SMALL BOWEL AND COLON LESIONS. Acute and/or chronic diarrhea is a frequent complication, usually in the relatively late stages of HIV infection. In many instances, diarrhea is accompanied by severe weight loss, a combination referred to as "diarrhea-wasting syndrome" that is now included as an AIDS-defining diagnosis according to World Health Organization and Centers for Disease Control and Prevention definitions. The frequency of chronic diarrhea is usually reported at 30 to 60% for patients with AIDS, many have intermittent symptoms, and the small bowel is the most common site of pathologic changes. The most common opportunistic pathogens responsible for chronic diarrhea (intermittent or continuous loose or watery stools for > 1 month) are *Cryptosporidium,* Microsporida, *Mycobacterium avium,* and CMV; each of these account for 15 to 40% of cases in large series.

Cryptosporidia tend to cause intermittent diarrhea that persists for months and may be responsible for severe fluid losses, dehydration, and electrolyte abnormalities. Small bowel biopsies show villous atrophy, crypt hyperplasia, and intraepithelial lymphocytes with typical schizonts that appear adherent to the brush border, but are actually just inside the basement membrane of the enterocyte. Functional tests show D-xylose malabsorption, and stools show no fecal leukocytes. The usual diagnostic test is a stool examination for oocysts that appear like yeast but are easily detected using modified acid-fast stains. Complications include papillary stenosis and obstruction of the common bile duct. No antimicrobial therapy has proven effective.

Microsporida are a group of extremely small unicellular parasites, with the most frequent species in AIDS patients being *Enterocytozoon bieneusi.* The organism cannot be easily detected in stool, so small intestinal biopsy with electron microscopy is often required. Histopathologic changes are similar to those noted with cryptosporidiosis except for the unique morphologic features and location of the organism within the cytoplasm of the enterocyte. No antimicrobial therapy has proven effective.

M. avium may cause pathologic changes in the small bowel which appear identical to those of Whipple's disease, but with large numbers of acid-fast bacilli. Most patients have *M. avium* bacteremia. The usual treatment is a combination of clarithromycin with ethambutol, clarithromycin with clofazimine, or all three drugs (see Ch. 312).

CMV commonly causes disseminated infection in the late stages of HIV infection at any level of the gastrointestinal tract including the mouth, esophagus, stomach, small bowel, colon, and perirectal region. The most common is a diffuse colitis with superficial ulcerations seen with computed tomographic (CT) scan or endoscopy. Symptoms ascribed to this infection include diarrhea, abdominal pain, and bloody stools. Less common are a solitary ulcer, toxic megacolon, or intestinal perforation. The diagnosis is generally established by demonstrating typical viral inclusions in intestinal biopsies. Ganciclovir and foscarnet are sometimes effective, although many patients do not respond.

Isospora belli is a protozoan parasite that accounts for about 1 to 3% of cases of chronic diarrhea in patients with advanced HIV infection. Large acid-fast oocysts (20 to 30 × 10 to 20 μm) are seen in the stool and trimethoprim-sulfamethoxazole (TMP-SMX) is effective therapy. *Entamoeba histolytica* and *Giardia lamblia* are occasionally encountered, but their frequency is no greater than in immunocompetent persons. *Blastocystis hominis* is found in stools of 10 to 15% of healthy heterosexual persons and 35 to 50% of asymptomatic homosexual men; its role as an enteric pathogen is unclear. Nonpathogenic ameba (*E. hartmani, E. coli, E. nana,* and *Iodamoeba butchii*) play no established role in diarrhea in persons with or without HIV infection.

Among bacterial pathogens, *Salmonella,* especially *S. typhimurium,* is found at least 20-fold more frequently in patients with AIDS than in the general population. Unusual features include the lack of an identifiable source of infection in most, a high rate of bacteremia (enteric fever), and the propensity of the infection to recur when treatment is discontinued. The favored drugs include ampicillin or amoxicillin, TMP-SMX, third-generation cephalosporins, and quinolones. Antibiotic-associated diarrhea or colitis due to *Clostridium difficile* is also relatively common in patients with HIV infection owing to their high rate of antibiotic consumption. Additional microbial pathogens to consider in acute diarrhea are *Shigella, Campylobacter jejuni,* and enteric viruses.

Tumors of the gastrointestinal tract associated with HIV infection include Kaposi's sarcoma, non-Hodgkin's lymphoma, cloacogenic carcinoma of the rectum, and squamous cell carcinoma of the rectum and anus. The most common of these is Kaposi's sarcoma, which has been found in gut tissue at autopsy in 40 to 50% of persons with typical cutaneous lesions. Endoscopy typically shows raised red nodules, but histologic confirmation is difficult owing to the depth of pathologic changes. The great majority are asymptomatic; less common presentations include diarrhea, subacute intestinal obstruction, protein-losing enteropathy, and rectal ulcer. The lymphomas associated with HIV infection are usually high-grade B-cell lymphomas that are extranodal in origin. The gastrointestinal tract is affected in up to 20%, and there may be involvement of any site from the oral cavity to the rectum.

AIDS ENTEROPATHY. Endoscopy in patients with advanced AIDS often shows morphologic changes in the small bowel in the absence of evidence for a superimposed opportunistic infection. Characteristic features are villous blunting, a reduced villus-crypt ratio, and an inappropriately low number of mitotic figures. In the absence of an enteric pathogen the findings are sometimes referred to as "AIDS enteropathy." Studies of gastrointestinal function in the presence of AIDS enteropathy usually show malabsorption with abnormal D-xylose and ^{14}C-glycerol-tripalmitin absorption tests. The cause of these changes is not known, but the major considerations include direct invasion by HIV, an opportunistic infection that has not been detected, small bowel overgrowth, autonomic nervous dysfunction, or immune dysfunction (reflecting the fact that 25% of lymphatic tissue is in the gut).

MANAGEMENT GUIDELINES FOR PATIENTS WITH DIARRHEA. Recommended tests should be tailored to the specific clinical findings and likely etiologic agents. For most patients with HIV infection and diarrhea that is severe or prolonged, the initial evaluation should include cultures for bacterial pathogens (*Salmonella, Shigella,* and *Campylobacter jejuni*), direct examination for ova and parasites, and a *Clostridium difficile* toxin assay. Previous studies indicate that a likely etiologic agent will be detected in 30 to 50% of patients, the most common in chronic diarrhea being *Cryptosporidium*. Those with persistent and unexplained diarrhea or disabling abdominal pain may undergo additional testing, including radiography with contrast, abdominal CT, and/or endoscopy. Extensive use of upper or lower endoscopy in this setting is controversial because the conditions often cannot be readily treated, giving a poor cost-benefit ratio. These conditions include AIDS enteropathy and infections with Cryptosporidia and Microsporida. The treatment of diarrhea in the patient with advanced infection should include appropriate antimicrobial agents directed against identified pathogens (Table 366–1). Nonspecific agents such as imodium or loperamide, indomethacin, somatostatin, or bismuth salts are sometimes useful. Nutritional consequences of chronic diarrhea need to be addressed as described below.

NUTRITIONAL SUPPORT. The average patient with AIDS loses 15 to 20% of his/her baseline weight during the course of the infection. Protein-calorie malnutrition is a common and serious sequela to late disease that may accelerate progressive immunosuppression. Contributing factors to malnutrition include a hypermetabolic state associated with chronic infection (especially with fever), oral lesions causing pain, esophageal lesions resulting in odynophagia, reduced taste sensation, depression, HIV-associated subcortical dementia, gastrointestinal side effects of medications, AIDS en-

TABLE 366–1. TREATMENT OF ENTERIC PATHOGENS IN AIDS

Pathogen	Treatment
Candida albicans	
Thrush	Nystatin, clotrimazole, ketoconazole, or fluconazole
Esophagitis	Ketoconazole, fluconazole, or amphotericin B
Herpes simplex	Acyclovir
Cytomegalovirus	
Esophagitis	Ganciclovir
Enteritis/colitis	Ganciclovir (?) or foscarnet (?)*
Oral hairy leukoplakia	Acyclovir (symptomatic only)
Mycobacterium avium	Clarithromycin, clofazimine, ethambutol ± rifampin, ciprofloxacin or amikacin
Salmonella species	Ampicillin/amoxicillin, quinolone, trimethoprim-sulfamethoxazole, or third-generation cephalosporin
Clostridium difficile	Metronidazole or vancomycin
Campylobacter species	Erythromycin or quinolone
Entamoeba histolytica	Metronidazole + diloxanide
Giardia lamblia	Quinacrine or metronidazole
Isospora	Trimethoprim-sulfamethoxazole
Cryptosporidium	Paromomycin (?)*
Microsporidia	Albendazole (?)*

* (?) indicates that efficacy is not established.

TABLE 366–2. GASTROINTESTINAL LESIONS IN HOMOSEXUAL MEN AND PATIENTS WITH HIV INFECTION

Site	Immunocompetent Homosexual Men	Immune Deficiency with HIV Infection
Oral cavity	*Neisseria gonorrhoeae* Herpes simplex	*Candida albicans* Oral hairy leukoplakia Herpes simplex Aphthous ulcers Necrotizing gingivitis Kaposi's sarcoma
Esophagus		*Candida albicans* Cytomegalovirus Herpes simplex Aphthous ulcers
Small bowel	*Giardia*	*Cryptosporidium* *Isospora* Microsporidia *Mycobacterium avium* Cytomegalovirus *Salmonella typhimurium* "AIDS enteropathy" Lymphoma, B cell
Colon	*Chlamydia trachomatis* LGV serovars *Campylobacter* species *Shigella* *Etamoeba histolytica*	Cytomegalovirus
Anus, rectum	*Neisseria gonorrhoeae* *Treponema pallidum* Condyloma accuminatum Herpes simplex	Herpes simplex Cytomegalovirus

teropathy, and opportunistic infections causing malabsorption. Therapeutic approaches are optimally based on the cause. Patients with chronic diarrhea should receive small, frequent meals that are low in fiber, residue, lactose, fat, and caffeine. These patients often require additional nutritional support, preferably using the oral route. Supplementary enteral nutritional feedings may include polymeric formulas or, for patients with severe enteropathy, elemental formulas.

"GAY BOWEL SYNDROME." This term is used in reference to the enteric and perirectal infections that are commonly encountered in homosexual men. Relevant in the context of HIV infection is the fact that the homosexual lifestyle is a risk category for both. However, the pathogens observed with gastrointestinal lesions in immunocompetent homosexual men and immunosuppressed patients with HIV infection are very different (Table 366–2). The former includes a number of sexually transmitted diseases combined with several conventional enteric pathogens. By contrast, the listing for patients with HIV infection is largely restricted to opportunistic infections and opportunistic tumors, reflecting immunosuppression. The single pathogen encountered in both lists is HSV, although this infection is distinctive in the two groups; HSV infections in patients with AIDS are usually more extensive, more severe, more prolonged, and more likely to involve acyclovir-resistant strains.

HEPATOBILIARY DISEASE. Prevalence rates of hepatitis B and hepatitis C viruses are high in AIDS patients, reflecting their prevalence among homosexual men, intravenous drug abusers, and hemophiliacs. Other causes of hepatocellular injury are CMV, HSV, and drugs (e.g., nucleoside analogues, TMP-SMX, isoniazid, rifampin). Cholestatic changes in liver function tests suggest *M. avium*, tuberculosis, histoplasmosis, and lymphoma. Cholangiopathy with biliary obstruction is usually caused by cryptosporidia or CMV; less common causes are microsporidiosis, lymphoma, and Kaposi's sarcoma.

ABDOMINAL SURGERY. The most common clinical syndromes in persons with HIV infection that require abdominal surgery are peritonitis associated with perforation due to CMV infection; lymphoma of the gut (most frequently with involvement of the terminal ileum with obstruction or bleeding); Kaposi's sarcoma; and *M. avium* infection involving retroperitoneal lymph nodes or spleen. Patients with cholangiopathy due to CMV or cryptosporidiosis often respond to endoscopic retrograde cholangiopancreatography, but recurrence rates are high. The experience to date indicates that patients with HIV infection tolerate surgical procedures well and do not have an unusually high incidence of postoperative complications.

Bartlett JG, Belitsos P, Sears C: AIDS enteropathy. Clin Infect Dis 16:726, 1992. *This is a review of AIDS enteropathy with a literature review, suggested diagnostic evaluation, and possible causes of "idiopathic AIDS enteropathy."*

Kotler DP, Clayton F, Scholes JV, Orenstein JM: Small intestinal injury and parasitic diseases in AIDS. Ann Intern Med 113:444, 1990. *The authors review histopathologic findings including electron microscopy in AIDS patients with cryptosporidiosis and microsporidiosis.*

Laughon BE, Druckman DA, Vernon A, et al.: Prevalence of enteric pathogens in homosexual men with and without acquired immunodeficiency syndrome. Gastroenterology 94:984, 1988. *This is an exhaustive study of stool to detect bacterial, viral, fungal, and parasitic pathogens in homosexual men without AIDS, with AIDS, and with proctitis or diarrhea.*

Nelson MR, Shanson DC, Hawkins DA, et al.: *Salmonella, Campylobacter* and *Shigella* in HIV-seropositive patients. AIDS 6:1495, 1992. *Analysis of stool cultures from 654 AIDS patients with diarrhea.*

Smith PD, Quinn TC, Strober W, et al.: Gastrointestinal manifestations in AIDS. Ann Intern Med 116:63, 1992. *Reviews the spectrum of enteric pathogens by organism; also addresses issues of immunopathogenesis, diagnosis, and therapy.*

367 CUTANEOUS SIGNS OF AIDS
Neal S. Penneys

Cutaneous signs and symptoms associated with AIDS increase in frequency and severity as the disease advances. However, infection by human immunodeficiency virus (HIV) may produce a transient macular roseola–like eruption. As HIV infection progresses, infectious processes and neoplastic disease are most often seen. Patients also may have symptoms such as pruritus without visible skin lesions.

Cutaneous infections are a common feature of AIDS. Superficial infections such as dermatophytosis, candidiasis, and scabies may be extensive and have altered appearances. Superficial fungal infections may coexist with other pathogens such as herpesvirus or cytomegalovirus to produce unusual complex cutaneous infections.

Cutaneous viral infections also may have unpredictable presentations. Molluscum contagiosum occurs commonly, is persistent, and lesions may become quite large. Human papillomavirus–induced lesions may occur, ranging from persistent verrucae to severe anogenital condyloma (see Color Plate 12A). Molluscum contagiosum and human papillomavirus lesions frequently occur in cosmetically sensitive areas. Locally destructive treatments such as curettage and cryotherapy are effective, but lesions almost always recur or new lesions develop, particularly as CD4 counts decrease.

Herpes zoster may be a reliable sign of the presence or progression of HIV infection in an otherwise asymptomatic person. With the diminishing immune response, the usually self-limited herpetic infections become chronic and fail to heal (see Color Plate 12B). Chronic herpetic lesions may not have the characteristic morphology of acute lesions in immunocompetent individuals. Both herpes simplex and herpes zoster viruses may produce disseminated skin lesions in HIV-infected individuals. The diagnosis of herpetic infections can be made by morphology of the clinical lesion, examination of a Tzanck preparation (Wright stain of a scraping taken from the base of a lesion), skin biopsy, viral culture, and/or molecular diagnostic methods. For chronic or recurrent herpetic infection and for long-term suppression, oral acyclovir therapy is helpful.

Unusual primary and disseminated infections occur in the skin in the context of HIV infection. Mucosal and cutaneous lesions of histoplasmosis, cryptococcosis, and other systemic fungal disorders can be signs of disseminated infection in AIDS patients. Mycobacterial infections produced by *M. tuberculosis, M. avium–intracellulare, M. haemophilum,* and others affect the skin in patients with AIDS. A long list of unusual or unique infections has been observed, including disseminated amebiasis, *Trichosporon beigelei,* sporotrichosis, *Strongyloides* infection, alternariosis, and superficial pheohyphomycosis. A new entity, bacillary angiomatosis caused by

Rochalimaea henselae/quintana, produces vascular proliferations in the skin as well as in other sites. Reiter's syndrome, with typical cutaneous findings, is found with increased frequency in patients with AIDS (see Color Plate 12C). It is safe to predict that unusual presentations of disseminated infectious diseases will continue to be described in the skin of AIDS patients.

Mucous membranes are commonly affected by infectious processes in patients with HIV infection. Oral candidiasis may be present and is one harbinger of the progression of HIV infection. Human papillomavirus and herpesvirus can produce lesions in the oral cavity. Oral hairy leukoplakia, a mixed infectious process, produces a characteristic "hairy" appearance to the sides of the tongue. Severe necrotizing gingivitis and recurrent oral ulcers are common. Lastly, disseminated infectious disease and malignant lymphoma can affect the mucous membranes.

The most common neoplasm in the context of AIDS is Kaposi's sarcoma (see Color Plate 12D). In AIDS, however, Kaposi's lesions may be solitary or disseminated, vary in color from light tan to deep purple, vary in appearance from macules to tumor nodules, arranged in a follicular, zosteriform, or linear pattern, and are generally atypical when compared with the lesions of Kaposi's sarcoma occurring in non–HIV-infected individuals. Kaposi's sarcoma found in AIDS patients frequently affects the mucosae. Other malignant tumors have an increased incidence in the setting of HIV infection, including squamous cell carcinoma and a variety of lymphomas, and all may have cutaneous involvement.

A number of poorly classified eruptions occur in AIDS patients. Best known is seborrheic dermatitis, which occurs in the usual locations but can be persistent and difficult to treat. Patients with AIDS also may have persistent pruritic eruptions, annular eruptions that resemble granuloma annulare, folliculitis, vasculitis, alopecia areata, vitiligo, porphyria cutanea tarda, eosinophilic folliculitis, and others. Certain well-characterized dermatoses such as psoriasis and atopic dermatitis appear to be worsened by the presence of HIV infection. Many AIDS patients receive a panoply of therapeutic agents that in turn produce a spectrum of cutaneous reactions including certain recognizable reactions, such as discolored nails from azidothymidine therapy (see Color Plate 12E).

Koehler JE, Quinn FD, Berger TG, et al.: Isolation of *Rochalimaea* species from cutaneous and osseous lesions of bacillary angiomatosis. N Engl J Med 327:1625, 1992. *Describes the entity bacillary angiomatosis and the organisms associated with its development in HIV-infected individuals.*

Penneys NS: Skin Manifestations of AIDS, 2nd ed. London, Martin Dunitz, 1995. *This reference is the easiest way to see the most common skin changes associated with HIV infection; has primary references.*

368 OPHTHALMOLOGIC MANIFESTATIONS OF AIDS
Mark A. Jacobson

Infectious or noninfectious ocular disorders, some of which may lead to severe visual impairment, have been reported in 40 to 90% of patients with AIDS referred for formal ophthalmoscopy. The true incidence of ophthalmic complications of AIDS can best be estimated from prospective observational cohort studies in which the incidence of cytomegalovirus (CMV) retinitis (the most common ophthalmologic complication of AIDS) has been reported. In several such studies, a range of 20 to 40% of AIDS patients have been diagnosed with CMV retinitis.

The differential diagnosis of HIV-associated ocular disease is best considered by its anatomic location.

DISEASES OF THE CHOROID, RETINA, AND VITREOUS

RETINAL MICROVASCULAR DISEASE (Table 368–1). The most common ophthalmologic complication observed in patients with HIV infection is retinal microvascular disease, which usually manifests as asymptomatic cotton-wool spots or small retinal hemorrhages. Cotton-wool spots have been reported in at least half of patients with AIDS and in up to 40% of patients with symptomatic HIV disease. Histopathologically, these lesions represent areas of

TABLE 368-1. DIAGNOSTIC FEATURES OF IMPORTANT CAUSES OF HIV-ASSOCIATED RETINITIS*

Feature	Cytomegalovirus	Retinal Necrosis (VZV, HSV)	Toxoplasmosis	Syphilis
Ocular symptoms	Floaters, visual field defect, or decreased visual acuity; painless	Floaters, visual field defect, or decreased visual acuity; pain common	Floaters, visual field defect, or decreased visual acuity; ± photophobia	Floaters, visual field defect, or decreased visual acuity; ± photophobia
Associated clinical findings	AIDS	Orolabial herpes, trigeminal herpes zoster	AIDS, encephalitis	Rash, hearing loss
Typical retinal lesion	Cottage-cheese exudate with hemorrhage	Confluent, gray or pale retina	White or yellow exudate	Variable
Typical retinal location	Adjacent to major vessel	Peripheral	Multifocal	Focal or posterior retina
Risk of retinal detachment	+++	++++	++	+
Serology, culture	Not helpful	Viral culture of skin lesion	*Toxoplasma gondii* IgG titer	VDRL, FTA-ABS

* Modified from Culbertson WW: Infection of the retina in AIDS. Int Ophthalmol Clin 29:108, 1989.

retinal ischemia. Both immune complex deposition and direct HIV retinal infection have been implicated in the pathogenesis of cotton-wool lesions. On funduscopic examination, they typically appear as white spots with feathered edges on the surface of the retina. A common location is near major posterior retinal vessels, and these lesions can have small associated retinal hemorrhages. It may be difficult to differentiate between cotton-wool spots and early lesions of CMV retinitis, which can have a very similar appearance. Sometimes the distinction can be made only by serial ophthalmoscopic examination. Cotton-wool spots remain stationary or resolve, whereas the lesion of CMV retinitis increases in size. Because cotton-wool spots virtually never cause symptomatic loss of vision and often spontaneously resolve, no treatment is indicated.

Small retinal hemorrhages and other microvascular abnormalities have been reported in up to 40% of patients with AIDS. These lesions also are asymptomatic, except in the rare case in which perifoveal involvement may result in visual blurring.

CYTOMEGALOVIRUS RETINITIS. CMV retinitis is the most common sight-threatening ocular opportunistic infection in patients with AIDS. It usually occurs only in patients with < 50 CD4+ (T helper) lymphocytes per microliter. The typical appearance is a white, cottage cheese–like retinal exudate often associated with hemorrhage and frequently located adjacent to major retinal vessels. In tissue sections, full-thickness retinal necrosis and swollen retinal cells containing intranuclear and intracytoplasmic inclusions are observed.

Patients with CMV retinitis typically present with complaints of painless visual impairment—either blurred vision, decreased visual acuity, or visual field defects—almost always affecting one eye more than the other. Several studies of untreated CMV retinitis have demonstrated a natural history of progressive retinal destruction caused by new retinal lesions or increasing size of previous lesions, which is usually evident within 1 month of initial diagnosis.

CMV retinitis is diagnosed primarily by its typical clinical appearance. The differential diagnosis includes cotton-wool spots, retinal hemorrhages, choroidal granulomas, acute and progressive outer retinal necrosis syndromes, and toxoplasmic and syphilitic retinitis. Differentiating between these entities may be difficult and the therapy of CMV retinitis is expensive, time-consuming, and toxic; therefore, the diagnosis retinitis must be confirmed by an experienced ophthalmologist. Because CMV can be isolated from approximately one quarter of patients with advanced AIDS but not more than three quarters of those AIDS patients who have CMV retinitis, viral cultures are neither sensitive nor specific diagnostic tests and are of value only as research tools.

The current standard therapy for CMV retinitis involves chronic intravenous treatment with either ganciclovir or foscarnet (Table 368-2). Ganciclovir is a nucleoside analogue prodrug that is preferentially phosphorylated within CMV-infected cells to an active drug, ganciclovir triphosphate, which inhibits CMV replication. Foscarnet is a pyrophosphate analogue that does not require phosphorylation for its anti-CMV activity. Although ganciclovir and foscarnet equally halt retinitis progression in 90% of cases, most AIDS patients have progressive retinal necrosis occur within 1 month after discontinuing therapy. Hence, therapy must be given indefinitely to minimize further, irreversible visual impairment. Both ganciclovir- and foscarnet-resistant strains of CMV have emerged and have been associated with therapeutic failure. In such cases, higher doses of these agents or using these agents in combination may be effective in controlling retinitis progression. Of note, foscarnet therapy has been associated with increased survival compared with ganciclovir therapy.

Because atrophy occurs in areas of active CMV retinitis, patients are susceptible to rhegmatogenous retinal detachment (resulting from a scar in a thinned portion of the retina). This complication often occurs during the healing stage, even in patients whose active retinitis has been controlled with antiviral therapy. For such patients, surgical reattachment by removing the vitreous and injecting silicone oil can be effective in restoring functional vision.

TOXOPLASMIC CHORIORETINITIS. Toxoplasmic chorioretinitis is rare compared to CMV retinitis but may complicate up to 20% of cases of AIDS-associated toxoplasmic encephalitis. Unlike toxoplasmic retinitis in immunocompetent individuals, which typically results from reactivation of congenitally acquired cysts latent in the retina, the AIDS-associated version does not appear to originate in pre-existing retinochoroidal scars but from organisms disseminating from nonocular sites of disease. Necrotizing retinal lesions are often bilateral and multifocal, and (as in CMV retinitis) may result in rhegmatogenous retinal detachment. Vitreous inflammation and anterior uveitis are more common and associated hemorrhage less common than in CMV retinitis. Because nearly all cases of toxoplasmic chorioretinitis are associated with toxoplasmic encephalitis, a computed tomographic or magnetic resonance scan of the brain should be done whenever this diagnosis is considered. Specific antiparasitic therapy (pyrimethamine and sulfadiazine, or pyrimethamine and clindamycin, in the same doses used to treat toxoplasmic encephalitis) is usually effective in preventing further retinal necrosis, but chronic maintenance therapy must be continued indefinitely to prevent relapse.

ACUTE RETINAL NECROSIS SYNDROME. Widespread, often bilateral, necrotizing retinitis caused by herpes simplex (HSV) or varicella-zoster virus (VZV) is now a well-characterized, although rare, AIDS-associated condition. Unlike CMV retinitis, this disease is often associated with ocular pain and concomitant keratitis or iritis. Many individuals have had recent or concurrent trigemi-

TABLE 368-2. THERAPY FOR CYTOMEGALOVIRUS RETINITIS

Standard dosing regimen for CMV retinitis
Ganciclovir
    Induction therapy: 5 mg/kg IV q12h × 14 days
    Chronic maintenance therapy: 5–6 mg/kg qd or 5 days/wk
Foscarnet
    Induction therapy: 90 mg/kg IV q12h × 14 days
    Chronic maintenance therapy: 90–120 mg/kg qd
Adverse effects
Ganciclovir
    Granulocytopenia
    Thrombocytopenia
    Azoospermia
Foscarnet
    Nephrotoxicity
    Ionized hypocalcemia (seizure or arrhythmia with overdose)
    Hypomagnesemia, hypophosphatemia, hypocalcemia, hypokalemia
    Genital ulcers
    Nephrogenic diabetes insipidus

nal zoster or orolabial HSV infection, and evidence of concurrent viral meningoencephalitis may be present. On funduscopic examination, widespread, pale or gray, peripheral retinal lesions are noted. Although intravenous acyclovir is effective in preventing further retinal necrosis, subsequent retinal detachment is a frequent, sight-threatening complication.

PROGRESSIVE OUTER RETINAL NECROSIS SYNDROME. Progressive outer retinal necrosis is a recently described clinical variant of VZV retinitis occurring in patients with CD4+ lymphocyte counts < 100 cells per microliter and characterized by multifocal, deep retinal lesions that rapidly progress to confluence. Less inflammatory cell response is observed in this condition than in acute retinal necrosis. The clinical response to available antiviral therapies is poor.

OTHER CAUSES OF CHORIORETINITIS AND VITRITIS. Cases of syphilitic retinitis have been reported in individuals with AIDS, symptomatic HIV disease, and asymptomatic HIV infection. There is no characteristic ophthalmologic appearance, but nearly all reported cases have had markedly positive serologic tests for active syphilis and dermatologic or central nervous system manifestations of secondary syphilis. Generally, response to intravenous penicillin therapy has been good. Disseminated pneumocystosis, *Mycobacterium tuberculosis,* and *Mycobacterium avium* complex infection with choroidal infiltrates have been described, but these lesions generally have not been sight-threatening. *Pneumocystis* choroiditis has been associated with use of inhaled pentamidine prophylaxis against *Pneumocystis carinii* pneumonia. Several cases of indolently progressive retinitis have been attributed to endogenous bacterial infection on the basis of retinal histopathology and response to broad-spectrum antibiotics. Also, vitritis (i.e., endophthalmitis) due to disseminated candidiasis may occur in parenteral drug users who are HIV infected or AIDS patients with indwelling central venous catheters.

OPTIC NEUROPATHY

Opportunistic infectious diseases affecting the optic nerve of patients with symptomatic HIV disease or AIDS may result in visual impairment or blindness. The most common cause of optic neuropathy is CMV infection. When CMV retinitis involves the optic disc, swelling of the optic nerve head (papillitis) leads to decreased visual acuity. This may occur in the presence or absence of other areas of retinitis and alternatively may affect the intraorbital optic nerve (optic neuritis) or retrobulbar nerve (retrobulbar neuritis). The retinal necrosis syndrome caused by herpes simplex or VZV infection may cause papillitis, and syphilis may cause papillitis, optic neuritis, or retrobulbar neuritis in patients at any stage of HIV disease. The most serious ocular complication of crytococcal meningitis is an arachnoiditis compressing the retrobulbar optic nerve and occasionally causing blindness. The cause of optic neuropathy can usually be established by seeking the other characteristic features of the specific infection. However, specific antimicrobial therapy for the cause of optic neuropathy often fails to improve vision once significant visual loss has occurred.

ANTERIOR UVEITIS

Severe anterior uveitis is uncommon in patients with HIV disease, but when such cases occur, syphilis or VZV infection is the most common cause. Mild, asymptomatic anterior uveitis commonly is observed in patients with CMV retinitis, but inflammation severe enough to cause symptoms is extremely rare. Occasional cases of toxoplasmic anterior uveitis have also been reported.

KERATITIS

Inflammatory disease of the cornea (keratitis) is most frequently caused by VZV or HSV, and the clinical features usually make diagnosis relatively simple. Patients with advanced HIV disease who develop this complication may require intravenous acyclovir therapy in addition to topical trifluridine. Microsporida infection has also been reported to cause keratitis in HIV-infected patients.

DISEASES OF THE CONJUNCTIVA AND ADNEXA

Kaposi's sarcoma has a predilection to involve ocular structures. Twenty of 100 patients with Kaposi's sarcoma examined at UCLA had ophthalmic lesions, 16 involving the eyelid and 7 the conjunc-

tiva. In four of these patients, the ophthalmic lesion was the first and only clinically identified manifestation of Kaposi's sarcoma. Conjunctival Kaposi's lesions appear as bright red subepithelial nodules, and small lesions may be mistaken for subconjunctival hemorrhages. Periorbital edema may be caused by lymphangitic Kaposi's sarcoma, even in the absence of apparent ocular or cutaneous lesions. Most ocular lesions respond to local irradiation.

Nonspecific, nonpurulent conjunctivitis that often is self-limited has been reported in up to 10% of AIDS patients. Topical steroid and sulfa therapy may be beneficial for this condition. Other rare causes of conjunctivitis include syphilis, CMV, and molluscum contagiosum infection. Orbital Kaposi's sarcoma or Burkitt's lymphoma may present with ptosis and diplopia.

de Smet MD, Nussenblatt RB: Ocular manifestations of AIDS. JAMA 266:3019, 1991. *A practical clinical review that organizes ophthalmic complications of AIDS by anatomic structures.*

Gallant JE, Moore RD, Richman DD, et al.: Incidence and natural history of cytomegalovirus disease in patients with advanced human immunodeficiency virus disease treated with zidovudine. J Infect Dis 166:1223, 1992. *The largest prospective cohort study to evaluate the incidence of CMV retinitis in patients with HIV disease.*

Jacobson MA: Foscarnet therapy for AIDS-related opportunistic herpesvirus infections. *In* Volberding PA, Jacobson MA (eds.): AIDS Clinical Review 1992. New York, Marcel Dekker, 1992, p 173. *Reviews clinical pharmacology and rational therapeutic use of foscarnet.*

Studies of Ocular Complications of AIDS Research Group: Mortality in patients with the acquired immunodeficiency syndrome treated with either foscarnet or ganciclovir for cytomegalovirus retinitis. N Engl J Med 326:213, 1992. *The largest randomized trial to compare ganciclovir and foscarnet therapy for CMV retinitis.*

Winward KE, Hamed LM, Glaser JS: The spectrum of optic nerve disease in human immunodeficiency virus infection. Am J Ophthalmol 107:373, 1989. *A series of four patients with HIV-associated optic neuropathies (syphilitic, CMV, varicella-zoster virus, and cryptococcal).*

369 HEMATOLOGY/ONCOLOGY IN AIDS

David T. Scadden and
Jerome E. Groopman

HEMATOLOGIC ASPECTS OF HIV INFECTION

Hematologic abnormalities are frequent in HIV infection, and their pathogenesis is often multifactorial. Cytopenias are often the limiting factors in anti-infective and antineoplastic therapy for patients with HIV disease. Recombinant hematopoietic growth factors have been used to ameliorate anemia and neutropenia and can be important in treating such patients.

CYTOPENIA. HIV infection is associated most prominently with a decline in the number of CD4 lymphocytes over time. However, other cytopenias are also frequent, with anemia reported in 60%, thrombocytopenia in 40%, and neutropenia in 50% of patients with AIDS. These cytopenias occur in conjunction with progressive deterioration of immune function and are less common in the earlier stages of HIV infection. Thrombocytopenia is the exception and may constitute a manifestation of HIV infection during the asymptomatic phases. Many causes are frequently operative in the cytopenia in advanced HIV infection. Direct and indirect effects of HIV, opportunistic infections, neoplasms, and toxic antiretroviral, antimicrobial, or antitumor chemotherapy are the major factors to be considered. The differential diagnosis of cytopenia in HIV infection should primarily consider these causes. Evaluation of patients with low blood counts should focus on infectious processes and attendant myelotoxic effects of therapy. In addition to the usual laboratory approaches to cytopenia diagnosis based on impaired production, excess consumption, and/or sequestration, blood and marrow cultures and stains for fungi and mycobacteria should be performed. *Mycobacterium avium-intracellulare* (MAI), *Mycobacterium tuberculosis, Cryptococcus neoformans,* and *Histoplasma capsulatum* are often found within the marrow and lead to hematologic abnormalities. Cytomegalovirus (CMV) does not generally cause specific histopathologic changes of the bone marrow but may suppress hematopoiesis and is best cultured from the circulating buffy coat. Parvovirus infection may result in cytopenia (particularly anemia) and is often accompanied by characteristic giant pronormoblasts in the bone marrow. Neoplastic involvement of the marrow by B-cell lymphoma is frequent in AIDS patients with this malignancy, whereas Kaposi's sarcoma has only rarely been found in the bone marrow.

Bone marrow aspirate and biopsy in an HIV-infected patient with low blood counts is recommended, particularly in cases of fever of otherwise unknown cause and in staging of patients with non-Hodgkin's lymphoma.

Morphologic abnormalities of myeloid and erythroid lineages are often present in the bone marrow of patients with HIV disease in the absence of infection or neoplasm. These changes are nonspecific and include hypercellularity, dysplasia with frequent megaloblastosis, lymphoid aggregates, and increased eosinophils, plasma cells, and reticulin. The pathogenetic mechanisms for these morphologic abnormalities and the associated impaired hematopoiesis are not well defined. Laboratory studies of hematopoiesis in HIV infection have yielded variable and differing results. The bulk of evidence suggests that HIV does not directly infect early progenitors but may alter the proliferative capacity of progenitors by two possible mechanisms: (1) induction of inhibitory factors in the marrow microenvironment, or (2) interaction with the progenitor cell surface and induction of cell death (apoptosis) without infecting the cells.

THROMBOCYTOPENIA (see Ch. 152). Thrombocytopenia may be a presenting laboratory finding in an otherwise asymptomatic HIV-infected person. HIV infection should be considered in the differential diagnosis of thrombocytopenia, and the history should include questions regarding risk factors for this retrovirus. Clinically asymptomatic but thrombocytopenic HIV-infected patients have a similar rate of progression to AIDS as asymptomatic HIV-seropositive persons without thrombocytopenia. Thrombocytopenia is not a criterion for more advanced HIV disease according to the staging system developed by the Centers for Disease Control and Prevention (CDC). Multiple causes need to be considered in evaluating thrombocytopenia in HIV infection. Immune-mediated destruction and ineffective hematopoiesis are generally both operative. In addition, cases of AIDS with apparent hemolytic-uremic syndrome or thrombotic thrombocytopenic purpura have been described but are rare. Isolated thrombocytopenia is most often clinically similar to classic autoimmune thrombocytopenic purpura (ITP). Bone marrow examination reveals an increased number of megakaryocytes, and there are elevated levels of bound immunoglobulin on the platelet surface. However, the immunoglobulin is generally immune complexes often involving anti-HIV antibodies. Detection of antibody on platelet surfaces does not correlate with thrombocytopenia, possibly because reticuloendothelial cell dysfunction often occurs in AIDS and may reduce clearance of platelets. In addition to peripheral destruction of platelets, reduced production appears to be common in HIV disease. Even in patients with an ITP-like presentation, production is reduced. This mechanism predominates in patients with thrombocytopenia in the setting of AIDS.

The thrombocytopenia in HIV-infected patients has similar sequelae to classic immune thrombocytopenia, yet special attention to the issue of thrombocytopenia should be given in HIV-infected hemophiliacs. Complications from thrombocytopenia may be more severe in hemophiliacs, so therapy should be considered at a higher platelet count than in HIV-infected patients without other coagulation defects. An important observation has been the improvement in platelet count due to treatment with zidovudine (AZT) in HIV-infected patients with significant thrombocytopenia, regardless of risk group. Nearly two thirds of such patients may respond to AZT therapy and increase their platelet counts (mean of threefold increase) within 12 weeks of initiating treatment. If there is no response to AZT, then several treatment modalities may be considered, including interferon-α, splenectomy, corticosteroids, danazol, intravenous gamma globulin, anti-RhD preparations, or vincristine. Many of these have been successful in classic immune thrombocytopenia, particularly corticosteroids. Theoretical risk of steroid use exists in an HIV-infected individual including exacerbation of fungal infection, Kaposi's sarcoma, and activity of HIV itself. Nonetheless, most patients have tolerated corticosteroids for short intervals. Their long-term use in HIV-associated thrombocytopenia cannot be recommended.

ANEMIA. Anemia increases in incidence in HIV-infected patients as their degree of immune dysfunction worsens. The anemia is usually characterized as normochromic and normocytic, and iron studies are either normal or indicative of chronic disease. Occasionally the vitamin B_{12} level is decreased, but true vitamin B_{12} deficiency is uncommon; rather, transcobalamin transport may be altered and therapy with the vitamin does not lead to improved erythropoiesis. Should a low vitamin B_{12} level be found, then a true deficiency needs to be ruled out by a Schilling test and other studies (see Ch. 129).

The Coombs' test (antiglobulin) may be positive in the majority of patients with AIDS and in about a third of asymptomatic HIV-infected individuals. Although anti-i or other specific antibodies may occur, nonspecific binding of antiphospholipid antibodies or immune complexes to erythrocytes is more common. True hemolysis is unusual in HIV-infected patients as a cause of anemia.

Impaired erythropoiesis accounts for anemia in most HIV-infected individuals. Serum erythropoietin levels are often low for the degree of anemia in the patient without renal abnormalities and is of unclear origin. Parvovirus infection has been reported in HIV-infected patients and may result in red cell aplasia. Gamma globulin therapy has been reported to reverse this unusual cause of severe anemia.

The impairment in erythropoiesis due to HIV infection *per se* may be due to release of inhibitors and/or impaired production of trophic cytokines, as discussed above. Drug-induced anemia is frequent in HIV-infected patients. AZT is associated with both dose-related and idiosyncratic suppression of erythropoiesis. In the AZT Collaborative Working Group Study, anemia occurred in one third of AIDS patients following 6 weeks of treatment. This occurred at relatively high doses, and patients with severe immunosuppression were least tolerant of the drug. In other studies of AZT at doses of 300 to 600 mg per day, the decline in hemoglobin levels was less severe and the need for transfusion less frequent. The reductions in the recommended dosing have reduced the frequency and severity of anemia, but this toxicity remains a significant cause of anemia in AIDS patients. Of note, other antiretroviral drugs, dideoxyinosine (ddI) and dideoxycytidine (ddC), are not associated with anemia.

Macrocytic changes occur in the erythrocytes with AZT therapy. The mechanism of impaired erythropoiesis due to the drug appears to be impairment of DNA synthesis in developing progenitors. Recombinant erythropoietin therapy may decrease the transfusion requirement and increase the hemoglobin in anemic AIDS patients on AZT. The response to recombinant erythropoietin treatment is most clearly seen in patients with pretreatment serum erythropoietin levels below 500 mU per milliliter. Some anemic AIDS patients receiving AZT have developed red cell aplasia that does not improve with recombinant erythropoietin therapy.

NEUTROPENIA. Neutropenia occurs in the HIV-infected patient in concert with decreases in other cell counts with progressive deterioration of the immune system. As with the other cytopenias, neutropenia may be caused by impaired production and/or increased destruction of leukocytes. Antibody bound to granulocyte membrane structures has been observed in nearly one third of HIV-infected individuals. The presence of neutrophil-associated antibodies has not predicted the development of neutropenia. Impaired hematopoiesis is presumed to be the major cause of neutropenia due to HIV. In addition to neutropenia, neutrophil dysfunction has been reported in AIDS. The extent to which neutrophil defects, particularly in microbial killing, contribute to host immune impairment is unknown.

Neutropenia is most commonly caused by myelosuppressive therapy in AIDS patients. AZT treatment is at times limited by neutropenia, although neither ddI nor ddC seems to cause this problem. Other important therapies including trimethoprim-sulfamethoxazole for *Pneumocystis carinii* pneumonia, pyrimethamine-sulfadiazine for central nervous system (CNS) toxoplasmosis, acyclovir for disseminated herpes simplex or herpes zoster, and most prominently ganciclovir for CMV retinitis may be myelotoxic and result in neutropenia.

HEMATOPOIETIC GROWTH FACTORS. Suppression of leukocyte, as well as erythrocyte, production is a major issue in treating both HIV infection and its complicating infectious or neoplastic diseases. This problem may become less limiting as new antiretroviral therapies are developed and hematopoietic growth factors are used to over-ride myelotoxicity. The activity and safety of hematopoietic growth factors used to increase blood cell number in cytopenic HIV-infected individuals have been studied. The results have been quite encouraging with respect to the erythroid growth factor, erythropoietin, and the myeloid growth factors, granulocyte colony stimulating factor (G-CSF) and granulocyte macrophage colony stimulating factor (GM-CSF). It is clear that in most patients with anemia due to HIV infection and/or concomitant AZT therapy, with baseline serum erythropoietin concentrations <500 mU per milliliter, recombinant erythropoietin increases the hemoglobin and reduces the transfusion requirement. Use of the myeloid growth factors, G-CSF or GM-CSF, to ameliorate leukopenia due to HIV infection and/or therapy with AZT, interferon-α, or ganciclovir, has also been relatively successful. The myelotoxicity of these agents can be overcome using relatively low doses of G-CSF or GM-CSF. It is clear that with the myeloid growth factors as well as with erythropoietin, there is no sustained increase in blood cell production, so that therapy with the growth factor must be continued so long as the myelotoxic agent is administered.

The side effects of growth factor therapy seen in patients with HIV disease have been similar to those in other patients treated with these recombinant proteins. The major issue in the safety profile of the myeloid growth factors relates to their potential effects on replication of HIV. The preponderance of data indicate that HIV replication is stimulated *in vitro* by GM-CSF but not G-CSF. This is most clearly seen when isolates of HIV that are tropic for monocytes are studied. The data conflict as to whether this phenomenon occurs *in vivo*. There is also laboratory evidence that the antiretroviral effects of AZT in monocytes can be significantly augmented by the presence of GM-CSF. It appears that the growth factor increases the uptake and phosphorylation of AZT, resulting in higher intracellular concentrations of active drug. It is believed that GM-CSF should be considered for therapy only in combination with AZT based on these *in vitro* studies. G-CSF and erythropoietin do not appear to alter HIV expression and have been successfully combined with AZT, as stated above. Further clinical trials are required to demonstrate that adding the erythroid or myeloid growth factor not only allows for concomitant therapy with myelotoxic agents but significantly alters the natural history of patients with HIV disease.

ONCOLOGIC MANIFESTATIONS OF AIDS

Neoplasms, particularly Kaposi's sarcoma and B-cell lymphoma, are frequent in HIV-infected persons. Their development demonstrates the relationship of immune function to suppression of certain oncogenic events and provides a model to study the pathogenesis of these tumors. Clinical management of AIDS-associated neoplasia is complex because therapy should optimally address HIV and concurrent opportunistic infections as well as the tumors.

KAPOSI'S SARCOMA (see Ch. 110, 152, 367, and 475). Kaposi's sarcoma is the most frequent neoplastic manifestation of HIV infection. Indeed, it forms one of the CDC criteria that define an HIV-infected individual as having AIDS. Kaposi's sarcoma has been recognized in a number of other clinical and epidemiologic settings. The "classic" form of the neoplasm was described over a century ago in predominantly elderly men of Mediterranean and Jewish extraction. It generally involves lower extremities and is an indolent neoplasm. This form of Kaposi's sarcoma was also recognized in association with other malignancies, particularly lymphoma. This latter observation led to the hypothesis that immune surveillance was important in restricting the development of Kaposi's sarcoma. Another form of Kaposi's sarcoma was recognized in areas of Central Africa and has been termed the "endemic" form of the neoplasm. This occurrence in Africa was not related to infection with HIV. Again, the neoplasm was more frequently seen in men than in women but was generally more aggressive and involved lymph nodes and viscera.

Patients receiving immunosuppressive therapy, particularly for renal and hepatic transplants, were recognized to have a markedly increased incidence of Kaposi's sarcoma. This further supported the hypothesis that immunocompetence is important with respect to pathogenesis of this neoplasm. Of particular note has been well-documented resolution of Kaposi's sarcoma upon discontinuation of immunosuppressive therapy in these patients. Other disorders of the immune system, including systemic lupus erythematosus and pemphigus vulgaris, have also been associated with Kaposi's sarcoma.

The incidence of Kaposi's sarcoma has been estimated to be 20,000 times greater among HIV-infected individuals than in the general population. Although the neoplasm was originally diagnosed in 40% of AIDS patients when first reported in 1981, the incidence may be declining and is believed to now constitute approximately 15% of all AIDS patients in the United States. AIDS-associated Kaposi's sarcoma is more frequently seen among homosexual or bisexual men with HIV than in other risk groups with the virus. This suggests that HIV infection itself is not sufficient to account for the increased incidence of the disease; other factors may be important in the pathogenesis of the neoplasm. Early in the AIDS epidemic, it was suggested that CMV infection or the use of volatile nitrites could potentiate Kaposi's sarcoma. However, careful studies have not verified the importance of such candidate cofactors in the development of the neoplasm. Another hypothesis is that other cofactors of an infectious nature may be transmitted in tandem with HIV during intercourse and possibly during use of intravenous drugs. Molecular studies have recently identified a novel herpes virus genome in Kaposi's sarcoma lesions. A model of a neoplasm that distantly resembles Kaposi's sarcoma has been established in transgenic mice using the *tat* gene of HIV, but the significance of this to clinical Kaposi's sarcoma in AIDS is still unclear. It has been speculated that certain cytokines, such as interleukin-6, may be elaborated by the Kaposi's sarcoma cells and lead to autocrine proliferation. Reports of Kaposi's sarcoma in homosexual men not infected with HIV have provided further support to the hypothesis of an independent sexually transmitted infectious agent as an important cofactor in this neoplasm.

Histopathologically, these lesions are a mixture of different cell types. Endothelial cells are quite prominent within the Kaposi's sarcoma lesions, as is a prominent spindle cell proliferation surrounded by extravasated erythrocytes and macrophages. The cell of origin of the neoplasm is still debated, but permanent cell lines derived from the lesions suggest that the spindle cell is the primary neoplastic cell and is of mesenchymal origin.

Kaposi's sarcoma often is a cutaneous nonblanching red macule. As lesions increase in size, they often have surrounding ecchymoses and become more of a violet hue than red. At times, the lesions may become nodular and with advanced disease, the lesions may become confluent with large plaques developing, particularly on the legs. There is no orderly pattern of tumor progression, and presentation may be with lesions at multiple sites. The subsequent appearance of lesions is not affected if the primary lesion is excised. The rate of growth of the primary lesions, as well as the appearance of new lesions, can be quite variable. The lesions may occur on any cutaneous site and on mucous membranes. Lymphatic involvement is not unusual, and Kaposi's sarcoma may present as lymphadenopathy. Visceral involvement, particularly of trachea, lungs, and gastrointestinal tract, occurs commonly and may be seen in the absence of cutaneous disease. The most striking morbidity associated with Kaposi's sarcoma is that of lymph node involvement and consequent lymphedema involving the lower extremities, groin, and head and neck. Extensive parenchymal or pleural involvement of the lung may result in life-threatening respiratory compromise.

The diagnosis of Kaposi's sarcoma is relatively straightforward in HIV-infected individuals presenting with an erythematous or violaceous cutaneous or mucosal lesion. However, bacillary angiomatosis caused by *Rochalimaea* species may involve similar lesions. This process, which is treatable with antibiotics, should be excluded by Warthin-Starry staining of biopsy material. Following diagnosis, an assessment should be made of the rate of growth and distribution of the lesions. The presence of visceral disease does not necessarily correlate with poor response of lesions to therapy, so that an extensive evaluation for gastrointestinal or lymphadenopathic Kaposi's sarcoma is not indicated unless there are specific symptoms referable to such involvement. It should be pointed out that AIDS patients in general do not die of Kaposi's sarcoma, except for pulmonary Kaposi's sarcoma, but usually succumb to infectious complications. Thus, staging systems of the neoplasm have emphasized immunologic status and systemic symptoms in addition to the extent of the neoplasm. Recently, a classification system has been proposed which appears particularly useful for evaluating such patients. This system proposes a tumor (T), immunologic status (I), and systemic symptoms (S) staging (Table 369–1).

TABLE 369–1. KAPOSI'S SARCOMA (KS): RECOMMENDED STAGING CLASSIFICATION

	Good Risk (0) (All of the Following)	Poor Risk (1) (Any of the Following)
Tumor (T)	Confined to skin and/or lymph nodes and/or minimal oral disease*	Tumor-associated edema or ulceration Extensive oral KS Gastrointestinal KS KS in other non-nodal viscera
Immune system (I)	CD4 cells $\geq 200/\mu l$	CD4 cells $< 200/\mu l$
Systemic illness (S)	No history of OI† or thrush No "B" symptoms‡ Performance status ≥ 70 (Karnofsky)	History of OI and/or thrush "B" symptoms present Performance status < 70 Other HIV-related illness (e.g., neurologic disease, lymphoma)

* Minimal oral disease is non-nodular KS confined to the palate.
† OI = Opportunistic infection.
‡ "B" symptoms are unexplained fever, night sweats, > 10% involuntary weight loss, or diarrhea persisting more than 2 weeks.
Modified from Krown SE, Metroka C, Wernz J: Kaposi's sarcoma in the acquired immune deficiency syndrome: A proposal for uniform evaluation, response, and staging criteria. J Clin Oncol 7:1201–1207, 1989.

The clinician should pursue therapy of Kaposi's sarcoma in patients with symptomatic visceral disease, lesions associated with edema, or rapidly evolving extensive cutaneous disease. Such patients usually require chemotherapy. The most active chemotherapeutic drugs appear to be doxorubicin, etoposide, vinblastine, bleomycin, and vincristine. Combinations of these agents, particularly doxorubicin, bleomycin, and vincristine, have been associated with a response rate of $\geq 50\%$. The combination of bleomycin and vincristine has been recommended for patients with borderline marrow function because the drugs are minimally myelotoxic and may be given in conjunction with AZT. Recent experience with liposomal formulations of anthracycline agents suggests that these may be particularly active in Kaposi's sarcoma. Response to chemotherapy usually occurs within the first few weeks of treatment. Unfortunately, the lesions regrow when the chemotherapy is stopped so that treatment needs to be chronic.

Patients with Kaposi's sarcoma who do not have rapidly progressive disease and therefore do not require immediate intervention may be treated with several other approaches. These include observation, single-agent interferon-α, local radiation, intralesional chemotherapy, local cryotherapy, or combinations of these. Antiretroviral therapy alone is not effective as an antineoplastic therapy for Kaposi's sarcoma. Selecting the optimal therapeutic approach involves determining the clinical status of the patient, particularly utilizing the staging classification (Table 369–1), as well as lifestyle issues. Patients who are categorized as "good risk" by the TIS staging system are also good candidates for response to interferon-α. Interferon-α may have not only antineoplastic but also anti-HIV effects. Therapy of Kaposi's sarcoma with single-agent interferon-α requires relatively high doses of the agent (18 to 36 million units daily). Recently, it has been recognized that similar benefit may be obtained using lower doses of interferon-α in combination with AZT, although with limiting hematologic toxicity. Such hematologic side effects may be overcome by using myeloid and erythroid growth factors. Interferon-α is associated with flulike side effects, and many patients were not able to tolerate prolonged therapy. It is unclear whether the antiviral as well as the antitumor properties of interferon-α make it a superior agent in the therapy of AIDS-associated Kaposi's sarcoma compared with chemotherapy alone or AZT in combination with chemotherapy (Table 369–2).

"Poor risk" patients by TIS staging should be given antiretroviral therapy because their major life-threatening complication of AIDS is related to immune suppression and opportunistic infection. Local treatment of disfiguring Kaposi's sarcoma lesions may be achieved using radiation therapy, chemotherapy, or cryotherapy in these patients. Radiation therapy is often avoided for mucosal Kaposi's sarcoma lesions because severe mucositis may result.

NON-HODGKIN'S LYMPHOMA. B-cell lymphoma frequently occurs in immunosuppressed individuals. Genetic disorders of the immune system such as Wiskott-Aldrich syndrome, as well as immunosuppressive therapy used in organ transplantation, are associated with malignant transformation of B cells and an oligoclonal or monoclonal lymphoma. Non-Hodgkin's B-cell lymphoma is emerging as a frequent manifestation of HIV infection as individuals with the retrovirus live longer as a result of better control of opportunistic infections. The initial relative risk of lymphoma in HIV-infected individuals compared with matched uninfected controls was 60 times; it is likely that this is an underestimate of the current risk. Thus, we expect to see an increasing incidence of B-cell lymphoma in this population.

Causative factors operative in the development of lymphoma in AIDS are likely to be multiple (see Ch. 145). HIV itself appears not be play a direct role but rather provides a permissive environment in which lymphoma develops. Lymphoma in this setting may be regarded as an opportunistic neoplasm and is considered an AIDS-defining illness. Proliferative signals to B cells, whether from dysfunctional T cells, aberrant cytokine production, or infections (such as Epstein-Barr virus), may induce polyclonal expansion of the B-cell population (see Ch. 341). This expanded population may provide targets for genetic abnormalities that lead to malignant transformation and emergence of several dominant clones. The oligoclonal populations of malignant B cells seen in some HIV-infected individuals with lymphoma support such a model. Ultimately, a single malignant clone may emerge, leading to a monoclonal neoplasm. The chromosomal abnormalities frequently seen in B-cell lymphoma involve translocation of loci encoding the immunoglobulin genes with the c-myc oncogene. Genetic evidence of Epstein-Barr virus is found in about one half of B-cell lymphomas in AIDS patients and virtually all primary CNS lymphomas in AIDS. A number of interacting factors are likely to be important in the pathogenesis of lymphoma in those patients with HIV infection united by the disorganization of immune function induced by HIV.

Clinically, B-cell lymphoma in AIDS patients tends to be of high-grade histologic pattern and follows an aggressive clinical course. Small, noncleaved or immunoblastic histologies are most frequent and account for nearly three fourths of all lymphomas in this setting. The remaining are usually a diffuse, large-cell type. The lower-grade lymphomas reported among HIV-infected individuals may represent background rather than neoplasm directly associ-

TABLE 369–2. TREATMENT OF KAPOSI'S SARCOMA

Interferon-α
Single agent	Alpha-2a (Roche)	18–36 mU SC daily for 8 weeks, then three times weekly
	Alpha-2b (Schering)	30 mU SC three times weekly
Combined therapy	Zidovudine	Zidovudine 100 mg PO every 4 hours while awake, interferon-α 5–10 mU SC three times weekly

Chemotherapy
Single agent	Doxorubicin	20–40 mg/m² IV every 3 weeks
	VP-16	100 mg/m² IV every 3 weeks or 50 mg PO daily as tolerated
	Vinblastine	4–8 mg IV weekly
Combined therapy	Vincristine/vinblastine	2 mg IV vincristine every 2 weeks 4–8 mg IV vinblastine on alternate weeks
	Doxorubicin/bleomycin/ vincristine	Doxorubicin 20 mg/m² IV every 3 weeks Bleomycin 15 U/m² IV every 3 weeks Vincristine 2 mg IV every 3 weeks
	Bleomycin/vincristine	Bleomycin 15 U IV every 2–3 weeks Vincristine 2 mg IV every 2–3 weeks

ated with immunosuppression. Rarely, B-cell acute lymphoblastic leukemia or T-cell neoplasms have been reported.

Most patients have extranodular disease involving the gastrointestinal tract, CNS, liver, soft tissues, or bone marrow. In one large series, nearly 80% of all patients diagnosed with B-cell lymphoma in AIDS had non-nodular involvement. Lymphoma strictly confined to lymph nodes is uncommon. Gastrointestinal lymphoma may occur anywhere from the esophagus to the anus. Primary CNS lymphoma is usually immunoblastic in histologic type (see Ch. 364). Such patients generally have solitary mass lesions in the parenchyma of the brain, whereas CNS involvement in conjunction with systemic lymphoma is more often meningeal in location. All AIDS patients diagnosed with systemic non-Hodgkin's lymphoma should undergo careful CNS assessment with computed tomographic (CT) scan or magnetic resonance imaging (MRI) scan as well as lumbar puncture with cytology.

Most AIDS patients with B-cell lymphoma are classified as having stage III (involving both sides of the diaphragm without visceral involvement) or stage IV (visceral involvement). Systemic "B" symptoms are frequent, but fever should not be immediately ascribed to lymphoma in AIDS patients and secondary infectious causes need to be ruled out. Staging of patients should follow the approach used in other settings of non-Hodgkin's lymphoma, with particular attention to the gastrointestinal tract, bone marrow, and CNS. It is not clear that prognosis of lymphoma in AIDS is affected by stage, however.

The major differential diagnosis to be considered with primary CNS lymphoma is *Toxoplasma gondii* infection or progressive multifocal leukoencephalopathy (PML) (see Ch. 364). PML can usually be distinguished from CNS lymphoma by its lack of enhancement with gadolinium on MRI. CNS lesions due to lymphoma may be isodense or hypodense and contrast-enhancing on CT scan, and enhance on MRI, thereby resembling toxoplasmosis. Nonetheless, toxoplasmosis usually presents with multiple lesions throughout the neuraxis, whereas primary CNS lymphoma tends to be a single lesion located in a paraventricular site. Accessible lesions should be biopsied to distinguish between lymphoma and toxoplasmosis; lesions difficult to approach surgically may be empirically treated with antitoxoplasmal therapy for a limited time, generally 1 to 2 weeks. If no response is seen, lymphoma becomes more likely.

The treatment of AIDS-related B-cell lymphoma is controversial owing to the poor prognosis of the neoplasm and the limited tolerance of aggressive chemotherapy in this patient population. Both opportunistic infection and bone marrow suppression often limit the delivery of adequate dosage of chemotherapy on schedule. Patients with prior AIDS-defining illness, particularly a history of opportunistic infection, have a poor prognosis compared with patients who present with lymphoma as their initial manifestation of AIDS. Similarly, more severely immunocompromised patients with low CD4 cell numbers have a poor outcome and are less tolerant of chemotherapy than are those patients with more intact immune function.

Among "good prognosis" patients with relatively intact immune function and/or those presenting with lymphoma as their AIDS manifestation, aggressive therapy with combination regimens is indicated. For those patients who do not have CNS involvement at the time of presentation, prophylactic therapy to the CNS is often given to prevent CNS relapse. The response rate in these good-prognosis patients is similar to that of non-Hodgkin's lymphoma patients of stage IIIB or IVB without HIV (see Ch. 371), but the long-term survival rate is still poor owing to frequent relapse and intervening infections. Nonetheless, some patients have survived 12 months or longer disease-free following complete remission.

Patients with poor prognosis based on severe immune suppression and/or complicating opportunistic infections pose a particularly complex treatment dilemma. Some patients have opted for palliative therapy with corticosteroids because intensive chemotherapy may lead to further immune compromise and infection. Yet lymphoma is generally rapidly growing and fatal in patients who are not aggressively treated. Thus, the clinician needs to pursue therapy in such patients only with an informed discussion of the risks and benefits of treatment, honestly emphasizing the poor prognosis with or without chemotherapy.

Addition of antiretroviral therapy to chemotherapeutic regimens

is now possible with nonmyelosuppressive anti-HIV drugs. However, the benefit of such therapy remains unknown.

The outlook is generally poor for patients with lymphoma, and the majority die within 9 months. No chemotherapeutic regimen has been identified as superior to others for AIDS patients with this neoplasm. The survival is even poorer for those with primary CNS lymphoma, on the order of 2 to 4 months. Although radiation therapy may result in a tumor response in the majority of these patients, the advanced stage of immunosuppression in which primary CNS lymphoma tends to occur generally limits the prognosis.

OTHER MALIGNANCIES. There is active clinical surveillance to determine whether neoplasms other than Kaposi's sarcoma and B-cell lymphoma may ultimately arise at an increased incidence in immunocompromised patients with HIV infection. It now appears that the incidence of Hodgkin's disease may be increased among HIV-infected individuals. In addition, there may be important differences in the course of Hodgkin's lymphoma in such patients, including a higher incidence of advanced disease, mixed cellularity histology, and extranodular disease. Furthermore, HIV-infected individuals with Hodgkin's disease appear to tolerate chemotherapy less well and have a higher incidence of tumor relapse than do those without HIV infection. This is likely due to their impaired hematopoiesis and the potential for opportunistic infections in such patients. In general, patients with HIV infection and Hodgkin's disease have a survival of <12 months. Further work is needed to better understand the altered pattern of Hodgkin's disease in the setting of HIV infection.

Hodgkin's disease therapy among HIV-infected patients should be according to guidelines for non–HIV-positive individuals (see Ch. 146). The major difference is to incorporate prophylaxis against opportunistic infections, particularly *P. carinii* pneumonia, and to be particularly alert to infectious complications during therapy.

Anal cancer and cervical cancer, neoplasms associated with papillomavirus infection, may occur with higher incidence in HIV-infected patients. This is due to the high prevalence of papillomavirus infection in groups at risk for HIV (see Ch. 314) and the high frequency of the premalignant condition, intraepithelial neoplasia in HIV-infected women. Frequent careful cervical examinations including colposcopy are indicated in HIV-infected women to detect early malignant change. Ongoing surveillance programs of HIV-infected individuals using Papanicolaou smears on cells from the transitional zone of the anus and cervix should provide important data as to the increased incidence and optimal surveillance programs for these cancers in this population. Invasive cancer of the uterine cervix has recently been added as an AIDS-defining illness in women infected with HIV.

Although anecdotal reports abound of other malignancies in HIV-infected individuals, it is unclear whether these occur above that of the background prevalence in the general population. Nonetheless, consideration should be given to the significance of the HIV infection in clinical management. These patients have a propensity to develop opportunistic infections when starting chemotherapy or radiation therapy and, in general, have fared poorly because of these infectious complications.

Ballem PJ, Belzberg A, Devine DV, et al.: Kinetic studies of the mechanism of thrombocytopenia in patients with human immunodeficiency virus infection. N Engl J Med 327:1779, 1992. *A study on thrombocytopenia in HIV disease.*

Henry DH, Beall GN, Benson CA, et al.: Recombinant human erythropoietin in the treatment of anemia associated with human immunodeficiency virus (HIV) infection and zidovudine therapy. Overview of four clinical trials. Ann Intern Med 117:739, 1992. *A summary of controlled trials using recombinant erythropoietin in HIV infection.*

Koehler JE, Quinn FD, Berger TG, et al.: Isolation of *Rochalimaea* species from cutaneous and osseous lesions of bacillary angiomatosis. N Engl J Med 327:1625, 1992. *Report of bacillary angiomatosis that may be confused with Kaposi's sarcoma.*

Levine AM: Acquired immunodeficiency syndrome–related lymphoma. Blood 80:8, 1992. *A review of AIDS-related lymphoma with an excellent bibliography.*

Lilenbaum RC, Ratner L: Systemic treatment of Kaposi's sarcoma: Current status and future directions. AIDS 8:141, 1994.

Luft BJ, Hafner R, Korzun AH, et al.: Toxoplasmic encephalitis in patients with the acquired immunodeficiency syndrome. N Engl J Med 329:995, 1993. *A discussion of outcomes from anti-toxoplasmosis treatment of CNS lesions in patients with AIDS.*

Palefsky JM: Anal human papilloma virus infection and anal cancer in HIV-positive individuals: An emerging problem. AIDS 8:283, 1994.

Pluda JM, Mitsuya H, Yarchoan R: Hematologic effects of AIDS therapies. Hematol Oncol Clin North Am 5:229, 1991. *A review of myelosuppression caused by drugs used in AIDS care.*

Roizman B: New viral footprints in Kaposi's sarcoma (editorial). N Engl J Med 332:1227, 1995. *Discusses the discovery of herpesvirus 8 by a novel technique and that the virus' footprints were found in cells affected by Kaposi's sarcoma.*

Tirelli A, Serraino D, Carbone A: Hodgkin disease and AIDS. Ann Int Med 118:313, 1993.

Zauli G, Vitale M, Carla Re M, et al.: *In vitro* exposure to human immunodeficiency virus type 1 induces apoptotic cell death of the factor-dependent TF-1 hematopoietic cell line. Blood 83:167, 1994. *A report of a possible mechanism of myelosuppression by HIV.*

370 RENAL, CARDIAC, ENDOCRINE, AND RHEUMATOLOGIC MANIFESTATIONS OF HIV INFECTION

Michael S. Saag

Infection with the human immunodeficiency virus type I (HIV) is a multisystem disease. Manifestations of pulmonary, gastrointestinal, neurologic, hematologic, and oncologic disease are well described in the literature, owing mainly to their high prevalence and often dramatic modes of presentation. In contrast, HIV-related renal, cardiac, endocrine, and rheumatologic diseases are more insidious in presentation. As overall survival of HIV-infected individuals continues to improve and therapeutic regimens become more sophisticated, clinicians will undoubtedly encounter disorders of the latter organ systems with increasing frequency.

RENAL DISEASE

Renal disease associated with HIV infection may present as fluid-electrolyte and acid-base abnormalities, acute renal failure, coincidental renal disorders, or a glomerulopathy directly related to underlying HIV infection, the so-called HIV-associated nephropathy (HIVAN). Originally observed in patients with AIDS and referred to as AIDS-associated nephropathy, recent studies have described the characteristic renal changes of HIVAN in both asymptomatic HIV-infected individuals and those with early symptomatic HIV disease, thereby broadening the definition to include all HIV-infected patients.

FLUID, ELECTROLYTE, AND ACID-BASE DISORDERS. Fluid-electrolyte disorders are common in patients with advanced HIV infection. Hyponatremia is noted in up to 40% of hospitalized AIDS patients and occurs in the setting of both hypovolemia and euvolemia. Hypovolemia, most often due to gastrointestinal fluid losses, is the most common cause of hyponatremia among this group of patients. The syndrome of inappropriate antidiuretic hormone release (SIADH) is responsible for the majority of cases of euvolemic hyponatremia and is most often due to underlying *Pneumocystis carinii* infection, malignancy, or central nervous system (CNS) disease. The presence of hyponatremia is associated with increased morbidity and mortality, especially in conjunction with certain opportunistic infections, such as cryptococcosis.

Adrenal insufficiency is a less frequent cause of hyponatremia. Although abnormalities of the adrenal glands are frequently reported at autopsy, overt adrenal insufficiency occurs in <5% of patients. The typical findings of hyponatremia, hyperkalemia, non–anion gap metabolic acidosis, hypovolemia, renal salt wasting, and mild renal insufficiency are usually present in some combination.

Drugs are an important cause of fluid and electrolyte disorders in HIV-infected patients and can mimic the abnormalities associated with adrenal dysfunction. Hyperkalemia and non–anion gap metabolic acidosis have been noted in patients receiving parenteral pentamidine. Amphotericin B is associated with hypokalemia, hypomagnesia, renal tubular acidosis, and renal insufficiency. Foscarnet therapy is associated with decreased levels of ionized calcium and, on occasion, renal insufficiency. Chemotherapeutic agents used to treat AIDS-associated malignancies may lead to fluid and electrolyte disturbances through direct nephrotoxicity or gastrointestinal losses associated with prolonged vomiting or diarrhea.

ACUTE RENAL FAILURE. As with most chronic illnesses, acute renal dysfunction may develop as a complication in the management of HIV-infected patients. Prerenal azotemia often results from hypovolemia secondary to poor fluid intake, increased gastrointestinal losses, or both. Acute tubular necrosis can be ischemic in origin, usually secondary to hypotension or sepsis, or due to nephrotoxic agents. Acute interstitial nephritis is another complication associated with drugs used to treat HIV-related diseases. A listing of agents with nephrotoxic potential commonly used in HIV-infected patients is presented in Table 370–1.

Opportunistic infections, invasion of renal parenchyma with lymphoma or Kaposi's sarcoma, and amyloidosis, which occurs as a complication of subcutaneous narcotic abuse, all may result in interstitial nephritis. Other renal lesions, such as hepatitis B–induced membranous glomerulonephritis, IgA nephropathy, acute glomerulonephritis secondary to bacterial infection, direct infection of the renal parenchyma with cytomegalovirus (CMV), fungi, or mycobacteria, and the hemolytic-uremic syndrome have all been associated with renal dysfunction in HIV-infected individuals. The diagnosis and management of acute renal failure are no different in HIV-infected patients than in their uninfected counterparts.

HIV-ASSOCIATED NEPHROPATHY. *Definition.* HIVAN was first established as a unique clinical entity in 1984. Originally called AIDS-associated nephropathy (AAN), many investigators questioned whether AAN was indeed a unique manifestation of AIDS or simply represented heroin-associated nephropathy (HAN) occurring in intravenous drug users (IVDU's) who also happened to be infected with HIV. Although the lesions and clinical manifestations of HAN are similar to those of AAN, further studies have established clear distinctions between the two entities. Of note, AAN occurs in individuals, including children, who have never used intravenous drugs. Indeed, nearly half of the cases presenting with the manifestations of AAN have early (asymptomatic or minimally symptomatic) HIV disease. Therefore, HIVAN has replaced AAN as the most appropriate name for this entity.

Epidemiology. The first cases of HIVAN were described in major urban centers, such as New York and Miami, which also had many IVDU's among their HIV patient population. In contrast, centers whose HIV population consisted primarily of Caucasian homosexual and bisexual men, such as San Francisco and the National Institutes of Health, were not observing the renal changes of HIVAN in their patients, thereby implying that HIVAN was a manifestation of HAN. More recent epidemiologic data indicate that 50% of patients with HIVAN are IVDU's, with the remaining cases occurring in homosexual and bisexual men, immigrants from Haiti, women who have acquired HIV from heterosexual contacts, and children born to infected mothers, many of whom did not use intravenous drugs.

Over 90% of patients with HIVAN are black. No explanation regarding the high prevalence of cases among blacks has been established, although many investigators have speculated that cofactors such as superimposed infection(s) or specific immune response genes may be responsible.

Pathology and Pathogenesis. Focal and segmental glomerulosclerosis (FSGS) is the characteristic renal lesion identified in patients with HIVAN, occurring in 80 to 90% of patients. On gross inspection, the kidneys are usually enlarged and the cortical surface

TABLE 370–1. DRUGS WITH NEPHROTOXIC POTENTIAL COMMONLY USED IN THE TREATMENT OF HIV-RELATED DISEASE

Acyclovir	Nonsteroidal anti-inflammatory agents
Aminoglycosides	Penicillins
Amphotericin B	Pentamidine
Aspirin	Phenytoin
Cephalosporins	Rifabutin
Cimetidine	Rifampin
Cis-platinum	Spiramycin
Dapsone	Sulfonamides
Ethambutol	Tetracyclines
Foscarnet	Thiazides
Ganciclovir	Trimethoprim

is smooth, even in advanced uremia. Microscopic examination of early lesions reveals diffuse mesangial hyperplasia with minimal glomerular sclerosis over time. A variable number of glomeruli develop segmental sclerosis characterized by hyperplastic visceral epithelial cells with coarse cytoplasmic vacuoles, collapsed capillary walls or capillaries obliterated by protein deposits (hyalinosis), and foam cells (lipid-filled monocytes) in the lumina (Fig. 370–1). Bowman spaces are usually dilated and tubular damage is universal. Microcystic dilation of tubules is a unique feature of HIVAN not reported in the FSGS of HAN (Fig. 370–2). Interstitial changes consisting of mild edema with scattered mononuclear cells are usually evident in HIVAN kidneys but not nearly to the degree noted in HAN. Similarly, although interstitial fibrosis may be present in advanced HIVAN disease, it is not nearly as prominent as the marked interstitial fibrosis noted in HAN disease.

The etiology of HIVAN remains unknown; however, many investigators suspect that an infectious agent is responsible. Ultrastructural studies have demonstrated tubuloreticular structures in vascular endothelium as well as in circulating and tissue lymphocytes. Other findings, such as a large number of nuclear bodies existing as budding forms in renal and lymphoid tissues, have been interpreted by some investigators to suggest a viral etiology. *In situ* hybridization studies have demonstrated proviral HIV DNA in renal tubular and glomerular epithelial cells, implicating HIV as the causative agent. However, the predominance of HIVAN in blacks and the relative paucity of cases among Caucasian homosexual men suggest that other factors not yet identified must play a role in the pathogenesis of HIVAN.

Clinical Manifestations. HIVAN is characterized by the development of proteinuria, nephrotic syndrome, and rapidly progressive irreversible azotemia. The proteinuria is typically heavy and presents as an early manifestation. The time to the development of end-stage renal disease (ESRD) from the initial diagnosis of proteinuria is 4 to 16 weeks in patients with HIVAN, compared to 20 to 40 months among patients with HAN. Another clinical distinction between HIVAN and HAN is the relative absence of significant hypertension among patients with HIVAN. Accelerated hypertension is a hallmark of HAN. Peripheral edema and anasarca are conspicuously absent in a large number of HIVAN patients with high-grade proteinuria and hypoalbuminemia.

Nephropathy has been documented in patients months to years before the onset of clinical symptoms of early symptomatic HIV disease or AIDS. HIVAN is being reported with increasing frequency among HIV-infected children and appears to be independent of the risk factors for HIV infection in their mothers. It is anticipated that the incidence of HIVAN will continue to grow and should be considered as a diagnostic possibility in any HIV-infected patient who presents with unexplained proteinuria regardless of the stage of disease.

Diagnosis. Quantitative measurement of the amount of protein

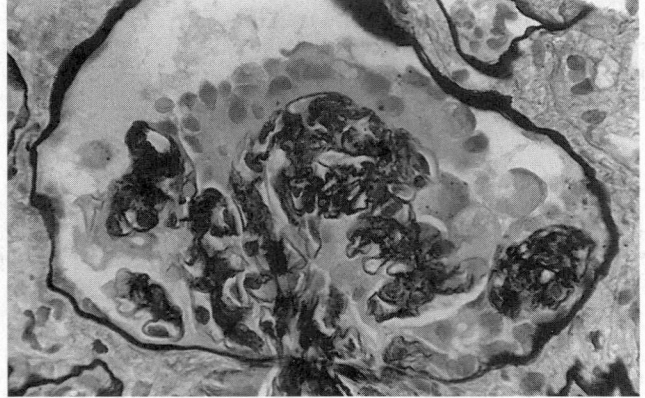

FIGURE 370–1. Glomerulus from a patient with HIV-associated nephropathy demonstrating global collapse of the glomerular capillaries, increased mesangial sclerosis, and a proliferative "cap" of visceral epithelial cells. (Silver methenamine; magnification ×400. Courtesy of Dr. William L. Clapp.)

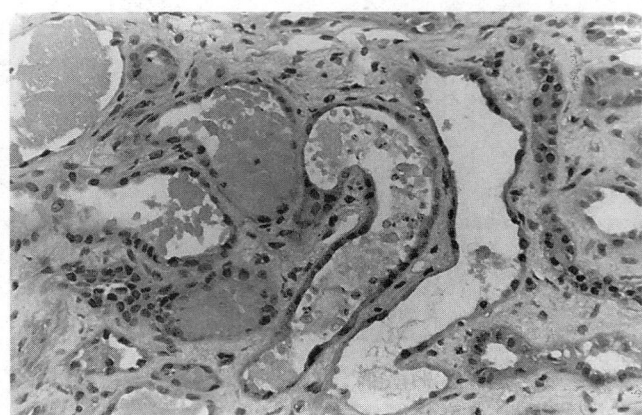

FIGURE 370–2. Dilated degenerated tubules demonstrating flattened epithelium and loss of nuclei and containing proteinaceous casts from a patient with HIV-associated nephropathy. (Hematoxylin-eosin; magnification ×200. Courtesy of Dr. William L. Clapp.)

excreted in the urine along with estimation of the creatinine clearance via a 24-hour urine collection should be performed early in the course of evaluation. Other reversible causes of renal insufficiency such as bacterial infection, crystalluria, and obstructive uropathy should be ruled out using urine culture, urinalysis, and ultrasonography. The kidneys are enlarged early in HIVAN and remain enlarged throughout the course of disease. The decision to perform renal biopsy should be made on a case-by-case basis depending on the clinical presentation, the likelihood of other diagnoses, and the therapeutic options available. Since a variety of other renal lesions, such as membranous nephropathy related to hepatitis B, membranoproliferative disease, and immune complex–related glomerular damage, may also present as nephrotic syndrome in HIV-infected patients, renal biopsy should be encouraged. The presence of the typical features of FSGS with tubular involvement as described above establishes the diagnosis of HIVAN when renal tissue is obtained.

Treatment. The lesions of HIVAN respond poorly if at all to currently available treatment regimens. In a few small studies, zidovudine has been shown to slow the progression of azotemia. Corticosteroids (60 mg prednisone daily over 2 to 6 weeks) recently have been shown to partially reverse the progressive azotemia and prevent the need for dialysis in a subgroup of patients. Until the use of corticosteroids is confirmed in larger studies, the treatment of HIVAN remains largely supportive. Nutritional support in the form of high-protein, high-calorie diets along with appropriate dosage adjustments of nephrotoxic drugs is crucial. Hemodialysis is of marginal benefit in prolonging survival of patients with advanced HIV disease once they have reached end-stage renal disease. Among patients with AIDS, hemodialysis provides short-term prolongation of life for 3 to 11 months. Patients who are asymptomatic or have early symptomatic HIV disease survive longer, with some patients living >4 years on chronic hemodialysis. Peritoneal dialysis should be considered in patients who are suitable candidates. Chronic ambulatory peritoneal dialysis (CAPD) may offer several advantages over hemodialysis, including avoiding leukopenia caused by the hemodialysis membranes, fewer problems with anemia, and theoretical advantages of less stimulation of HIV-infected T lymphocytes via membrane-induced cytokine release. A potential disadvantage of CAPD is the higher incidence of peritonitis. Renal transplantation is not considered a viable option in HIV-infected patients owing to the intensive immunosuppressive regimens required to prevent rejection. In some patients with advanced HIV infection or AIDS who develop HIVAN it may be appropriate to withhold dialysis support because of the generally poor prognosis. As always, such decisions should be individualized, taking into account the wishes of the patient, the family, and significant others.

CARDIAC DISEASE

A wide variety of cardiac abnormalities have been reported in HIV-infected patients, including ventricular dysfunction, myocarditis, pericarditis, endocarditis, and arrhythmias. Most often, cardiac involvement is clinically silent and is noted as an incidental finding at autopsy. When clinical symptoms are present, however, disease manifestations can be debilitating, and, in many cases, life threatening. Unlike HIV-associated renal disease, no specific cardiac syndrome or disease state has been described.

EPIDEMIOLOGY. Cardiac abnormalities have been observed in 25 to 75% of HIV-infected patients studied at autopsy. Myocardial disease is noted most frequently, occurring in >90% of subjects with cardiac findings. Pericardial disease, often with adjacent myocardial involvement, is observed in >20% of cases with cardiac abnormalities. Endocarditis is evident histologically in 3 to 5% of cases reported in autopsy series. No characteristic epidemiologic factor, such as age, gender, race, or means of acquiring HIV infection, has been identified which predisposes patients to cardiac disease. Although cardiac abnormalities are observed more frequently in AIDS patients, up to 30% of patients with early symptomatic HIV disease are noted to have abnormal findings on echocardiograms and electrocardiograms.

PATHOLOGY AND PATHOGENESIS. HIV-related heart disease may result from metastatic extension of a concomitant opportunistic infection or malignancy but most often is seen as lymphocytic infiltration of the myocardium or as an unspecified myocarditis. The mechanism responsible for the myocarditis remains unknown, although many investigators believe that HIV itself may be directly responsible. Other viruses, such as CMV, may be responsible for the development of myocarditis, although the typical "owl's eye" inclusion bodies are rarely seen in patients with HIV-associated cardiomyopathy. Additional mechanisms, such as postviral myocarditis or catecholamine-induced myocarditis, have been postulated, but little evidence exists to support their role.

A broad range of opportunistic infections and malignant diseases has been described in cardiac tissue examined at autopsy. Among the infectious disorders, fungal and viral pathogens are identified most often, followed by bacterial and protozoal infections (Table 370–2). Although the invading pathogen is frequently diagnosed at another primary site antemortem, cardiac involvement is rarely (<2%) identified before autopsy. This is largely due to the clinically silent nature of cardiac disease in HIV infection and a low index of suspicion by clinicians. Kaposi's sarcoma and metastatic lymphoma are the most common neoplastic diseases reported that invade the heart. Primary cardiac lymphoma has been reported rarely.

Pericardial disease is almost invariably associated with adjacent myocardial involvement. Pericarditis is usually nonspecific in origin, but when an etiologic process is identified, Kaposi's sarcoma or a pathogen such as *Mycobacterium tuberculosis* or *Cryptococcus neoformans* is responsible most often. Drugs used to treat HIV-associated disorders, such as doxorubicin for Kaposi's sarcoma, may cause myocardial damage. Other toxins, vitamin deficiencies, or metabolic abnormalities (e.g., hypothyroidism) may also result in myocardial dysfunction or pericardial disease.

Endocardial disease has been described in up to 3% of cases studied at autopsy and usually presents as either nonbacterial thrombotic (marantic) endocarditis or healed bacterial endocarditis.

TABLE 370–2. INFECTIOUS CAUSES OF CARDIAC DISEASE IN HIV-INFECTED PATIENTS

Bacteria
  Bacteria (endocarditis)
  Mycobacterium tuberculosis
  Mycobacterium avium-intracellulare
  Nocardia asteroides
  Actinomyces
Fungi
  Cryptococcus neoformans
  Histoplasma capsulatum
  Coccidioides immitis
  Candida species
  Aspergillus species
Viruses
  Cytomegalovirus
  Herpes simplex virus
  Human immunodeficiency virus
Protozoa
  Toxoplasma gondii
  Pneumocystis carinii

The precise etiology of marantic endocarditis is unknown, but it has been reported in other long-term wasting illnesses and malignant diseases. Vegetations are usually located on the mitral valve, although lesions on the tricuspid valve have been noted in up to 29% of AIDS patients with this disorder. Significant embolization to the spleen and brain was noted in >50% of patients with marantic endocarditis studied at autopsy. Bacterial endocarditis is reported rarely in AIDS patients. Healed lesions from previous bouts of bacterial endocarditis have been reported in autopsy series but are of little clinical significance.

CLINICAL FINDINGS. Most cardiac disease in HIV-infected patients is clinically silent. When symptoms are present they usually consist of the ordinary findings noted in non–HIV-infected patients with myocarditis or pericarditis, such as fever, dyspnea, chest pain, fatigue, cough, and orthopnea. Hepatomegaly and jugular venous distention are the most common signs noted on physical examination, followed by rales, systolic murmurs, and the presence of an S3 gallop. Signs of advanced pericardial disease with impending tamponade are among the most common clinical manifestations observed in patients who present with clinical symptoms of cardiac disease.

DIAGNOSIS. Demonstrated cardiomegaly on a chest roentgenogram is an important marker of underlying cardiac disease in HIV-infected patients. Right ventricular enlargement is usually the result of pulmonary artery hypertension, which in AIDS patients is often due to severe or recurrent opportunistic pneumonia. Left ventricular or biventricular enlargement is a characteristic finding of congestive cardiomyopathy due to any cause. Echocardiography is a more sensitive and specific noninvasive test that is used to assess the degree of ventricular dysfunction and to characterize the extent of pericardial effusion, if present. Several series have demonstrated echocardiographic abnormalities in up to 50% of HIV-infected patients who had no cardiac symptoms at the time of study. Ventricular enlargement, pericardial effusion, and ventricular hypokinesis were the abnormalities noted most frequently. In view of the overall silent nature of cardiac disease, the high likelihood that infiltrative processes will be evident and diagnosed at another site, and the often limited therapeutic options available for treating cardiac disease in HIV-infected patients, routine echocardiography should be discouraged in those without cardiac symptoms. The experience with endomyocardial biopsies in HIV-infected patients is quite limited; however, in those individuals who show signs of cardiac disease and have not had a specific diagnosis established, endomyocardial biopsy is a viable option for a definitive diagnosis.

Treatment. Supportive treatment consisting of diuretic therapy, reducing preload and afterload when appropriate, and correcting cardiac arrhythmias is the obvious initial approach to treating myocardial disease. Pericardial disease requires careful volume management with avoidance of aggressive diuresis or preload reduction. In the case of pericardial tamponade, surgical intervention is warranted. When the underlying etiology of the cardiac disease is known, appropriate therapy directed at the specific infectious agent or malignancy is indicated.

ENDOCRINE DISORDERS

Endocrine dysfunction has not been prominent in HIV infection. Nonetheless, all glands of the endocrine system may be infiltrated with opportunistic infections or malignancies or may be affected by drugs used to treat HIV-related disorders. The subtle presentations of endocrine diseases create difficult diagnostic challenges.

ADRENAL GLAND DYSFUNCTION. The adrenal gland is the endocrine gland most commonly affected in AIDS patients examined at autopsy, although clinical evidence of adrenal insufficiency is observed in <8% of AIDS patients. Widespread lipid depletion and varying degrees of adrenal necrosis are the most prevalent pathologic findings in postmortem examinations. Adrenal invasion by CMV is noted in up to 50% of patients with adrenal pathology. *Mycobacterium avium* complex, Kaposi's sarcoma, *C. neoformans,* and *Histoplasma capsulatum* involve the adrenal glands in 5 to 12% of cases. Drug therapy, with agents such as ketoconazole (adrenal dysfunction) or rifampin (increased clearance of cortisol) may also result in adrenal insufficiency. Fatigue, anorexia, nausea, vomiting, orthostatic hypotension, and hyponatremia are symptoms frequently noted in many HIV-infected patients; however, only a few with these symptoms are actually adrenal insufficient when evaluated using standard laboratory criteria.

Basal 8 A.M. plasma cortisol levels are usually higher in patients with advanced HIV disease than in asymptomatic patients and uninfected healthy controls. However, other ACTH-dependent steroids, such as desoxycorticosterone (DOC), compound B, and 18-hydroxy-DOC, are not elevated and show a blunted response to corticotropin (ACTH) stimulation, implying subnormal adrenal reserves. Patients who fail to achieve plasma cortisol levels > 20 μg per deciliter 60 minutes after ACTH stimulation should be considered to have, or be at high risk of developing, adrenal insufficiency. Plasma ACTH levels are frequently normal or subnormal even when plasma cortisol levels are depressed, suggesting that adrenal insufficiency in some HIV-infected patients is due to a primary pituitary or CNS disorder. Treatment of adrenal insufficiency in HIV-infected patients is the same as in other individuals with abnormal adrenal function.

HYPOGONADISM. The most common abnormality of endocrine function noted clinically is hypogonadism. Decreased libido occurs in over one half of male patients with AIDS, and impotence, usually associated with low serum testosterone levels, is reported in up to 30% of AIDS patients. Serum gonadotropin levels may be below normal or inappropriately within normal limits in hypogonadal men with AIDS. When pituitary responsiveness to gonadotropin-releasing hormone is assessed in these hypogonadotropic males, normal release of luteinizing hormone (LH) and follicle-stimulating hormone (FSH) has been observed, suggesting a hypothalamic basis for the central hypogonadotropism. Other studies have demonstrated appropriately elevated levels of LH and FSH in hypogonadal men, implying primary testicular dysfunction. Drugs, such as ketoconazole, ganciclovir, and acyclovir have been associated with low testosterone levels or decreased spermatogenesis. Studies of gonadal function in women are limited, although menstrual irregularities are common in women with advanced HIV disease.

THYROID DISEASE. Thyroid function remains remarkably normal throughout the course of HIV disease. Low levels of thyroxine (T_4), triiodothyronine (T_3), and free-thyroxine index (FTI) in the setting of low concentrations of thyrotropin (TSH), the so-called euthyroid sick syndrome, is remarkably uncommon among ambulatory HIV-infected patients. Decreased levels of T_3 resin uptake and elevated levels of T_4-binding globulin are frequently noted in ambulatory patients with advanced disease; however, concentration of T_3 and T_4 are most often within normal limits. Invasive disease due to CMV, *P. carinii, C. neoformans,* Kaposi's sarcoma, and lymphoma have all been described in the thyroid. Remarkably, even patients with infiltrating opportunistic diseases of the thyroid gland usually remain euthyroid throughout the course of their disease. Nonetheless, despite the relative infrequency of clinical disease, hypothyroidism represents a potentially reversible cause of fatigue, malaise, altered mental status, and "failure to thrive" in HIV-infected individuals and should be routinely evaluated.

Less common causes of hypothyroidism in HIV-infected patients include adverse effects of medications. Ketoconazole has been associated with primary hypothyroidism on rare occasions. In addition, drugs that are strong inducers of hepatic microsomal enzymes, such as rifampin, may lead to increased clearance of T_4.

METABOLIC ABNORMALITIES. Hyponatremia is the most common electrolyte disturbance noted in HIV-infected individuals (see discussion in renal section). Disorders of carbohydrate metabolism have been reported in association with direct pancreatic invasion by opportunistic processes and with drug therapy. Pancreatic lesions caused by CMV, toxoplasmosis, Kaposi's sarcoma, and lymphoma are noted in up to 35% of cases at autopsy. Yet the development of type I diabetes mellitus has been reported in only a few instances. Hypoglycemia is the most common alteration in glucose metabolism. Direct toxic effects of drugs may induce premature release of insulin by β cells, resulting in hypoglycemic episodes that may be severe and prolonged. Pentamidine isothionate is the most common cause of hypoglycemia, occurring in 4 to 33% of treated patients. Renal insufficiency is a predisposing factor in the development of pentamidine-induced hypoglycemia. Although most hypoglycemic episodes result from parenteral administration of pentamidine, several cases have been reported in patients receiving aerosolized drug.

Disorders of calcium metabolism are relatively uncommon but do occur. Hypercalcemia is associated with HIV-related leukemia and lymphoma. Hypocalcemia usually is the result of drug therapy with agents, such as amphotericin B and foscarnet, which induce magnesium wasting and decrease levels of ionized calcium, respectively. CMV has been observed in parathyroid tissue; however, CMV-induced hypoparathyroidism is extremely rare.

Hyperlipidemia is noted commonly in HIV-infected patients. Isolated elevation of triglycerides is reported in up to 50% of patients with either asymptomatic HIV disease or AIDS. Although hypertriglyceridemia is routinely noted among patients with HIV wasting syndrome, no relationship has been noted between the serum triglyceride level and the degree of wasting. Elevation of cachectin (tumor necrosis factor), inhibition of lipoprotein lipase, and decreased clearance of circulating lipoproteins have all been proposed as potential mechanisms of hypertriglyceridemia, but no clear association of any of these factors has been established.

RHEUMATOLOGIC DISEASE

Rheumatologic manifestations of HIV disease are being recognized with increased frequency. Musculoskeletal complaints are reported in 33 to 75% of HIV-infected patients and may present as a variety of rheumatologic disorders (Table 370–3). The severity of disease ranges from intermittent arthralgias to debilitating arthritis and vasculitis. An array of autoimmune antibodies, including antinuclear, antiplatelet, antilymphocyte, antigranulocyte, and antiphospholipid (anticardiolipin and lupus anticoagulant) antibodies are associated with HIV infection along with circulating immune complexes, rheumatoid factor, and cryoglobulins. Despite the presence of these antibodies in some patients, the precise mechanisms by which the rheumatologic abnormalities develop have not been elucidated and most likely are different for each particular disorder.

TABLE 370–3. RHEUMATOLOGIC DISEASES ASSOCIATED WITH HIV INFECTION

Autoimmune phenomena
  Anticardiolipin antibodies
  Antigranulocyte antibodies
  Antilymphocyte antibodies
  Antinuclear antibodies
  Antiplatelet antibodies
  Circulating immune complexes
  Cryoglobulins
  Rheumatoid factor
Dermatologic
  Dermatomyositis
  Malar flush
  Psoriasis
Joint disease
  Arthralgias
  Arthritis
  Enthesopathies
  HIV-associated arthritis
  "Painful articular syndrome"
  Psoriatic arthritis
  Reactive arthropathy
  Reiter's disease
  Septic arthritis
  Systemic lupus erythematosus (lupus-like syndrome)
Myopathies
  Infectious (septic) myositis
  Myalgias
    Idiopathic
    Zidovudine-associated
  Necrotizing, noninflammatory myopathy
  Nemaline rod polymyositis
  Polymyositis
  Pyomyositis
Sjögren's syndrome
  Sicca complex
Vasculitis
  Central nervous system angiitis
  Eosinophilic vasculitis
  Henoch-Schönlein purpura
  Hypersensitivity (drug-induced)
  Leukocytoclastic vasculitis
  Polyarteritis nodosa
  Unspecified vasculitis

ARTHRALGIAS. Arthralgia is a common manifestation of acute HIV seroconversion, in addition to fever, myalgia, headache, sore throat, abdominal cramps, and lymphadenopathy. Generalized arthralgias are reported in up to one third of HIV-infected patients with minimally symptomatic disease. Some patients develop arthralgias and myalgias when zidovudine therapy is initiated; however, these symptoms are usually self-limited and abate within 4 to 6 weeks after starting treatment. The "painful articular syndrome" is characterized by severe articular pain of 2 to 24 hours' duration. Although uncommon, this disorder is quite incapacitating and usually unresponsive to oral nonsteroidal anti-inflammatory agents (NSAID's) or narcotic analgesics. Its etiology remains unknown. With the exception of the painful articular syndrome, most of the arthralgias associated with HIV disease are treated with nonsteroidal agents.

MYOPATHIES. Polymyositis-like illnesses, characterized by myalgias, proximal muscle weakness, and wasting, have been reported in several HIV-infected patients and have been the initial HIV-defining presentation in a few. The findings of creatinine phosphokinase (CPK) elevation (> 5 times normal) and abnormal electromyography are indistinguishable from idiopathic polymyositis. Muscle biopsies reveal necrosis, fibrosis, and inflammation, but usually to a lesser extent than is noted in non–HIV-infected individuals. The presence of nemaline rods, often noted in muscle biopsies of older adults with myositis, suggests the likelihood of underlying HIV infection when noted in biopsy specimens obtained from younger adults, especially in the absence of inflammation.

Although virus-like particles have been demonstrated rarely in synovial tissue and HIV p24 antigen has been noted in the cytoplasm of degenerating muscle cells, no specific viral etiology has been determined. All attempts to culture HIV-1 from muscle tissue of patients with myositis have been unsuccessful.

Patients receiving long-term zidovudine therapy may develop myositis characterized by muscle weakness, elevated CPK levels, myalgias, and evidence of myopathy with a paucity of inflammatory cells on biopsy. Zidovudine-associated myositis usually responds to drug discontinuation and may recur on rechallenge. No definitive therapy exists for HIV-associated polymyositis, although corticosteroid therapy has been successful in reversing symptoms in some patients. If corticosteroid therapy is contemplated, the potential risks of superimposing immunosuppressive therapy on an immunocompromised host must be considered.

REITER'S SYNDROME. Reiter's syndrome is noted in up to 10% of HIV-infected patients who develop arthritis, and an additional 10 to 20% of patients are classified as having "reactive arthritis" because they lack the nonarticular features of Reiter's. Severe, persistent oligoarticular arthritis associated with urethritis, conjunctivitis, painless oral ulcerations, keratoderma blennorrhagicum, or circinate balanitis are the hallmarks of Reiter's disease in both HIV-infected and noninfected individuals. Clinical manifestations of Reiter's syndrome may precede or occur at the time of the initial diagnosis of HIV infection but most often follow the onset of immunodeficiency. HLA-B27 positivity is noted in 65 to 75% of HIV-infected patients with Reiter's syndrome. However, studies of African HIV patients with Reiter's disease or reactive arthritis revealed no increased incidence of HLA-B27, suggesting involvement of other gene markers in this group. *Shigella, Campylobacter, Ureaplasma,* and other bacterial species associated with the development of reactive arthropathies are rarely described in HIV patients with Reiter's syndrome. However, underlying concomitant sexually transmitted disease(s) may prove to be an important etiologic factor.

Treatment options for HIV patients with Reiter's disease are quite limited. Responses to NSAID's are minimal, and more potent immunosuppressive agents, such as methotrexate and azathioprine, frequently lead to opportunistic diseases and Kaposi's sarcoma shortly after initiation of therapy.

SJÖGREN'S SYNDROME. Xerophthalmia and xerostomia, the characteristic symptoms of Sjögren's syndrome (SS), have been reported with increasing frequency in AIDS patients. Features that closely resemble idiopathic SS, including sicca symptoms, a positive Schirmer test, abnormal salivary gland emptying, and abnormal salivary gland biopsies, have been reported in HIV-infected patients. As a result, it has been suggested that AIDS be an exclusionary disease for the diagnosis of idiopathic SS. The predominance of male patients, the absence of anti-Ro/SS-A and anti-La/SS-B antibodies, the absence of a well-defined connective tissue disease, the presence of HLA-DR52 and DR5 alleles instead of the characteristic A1, B8, DR3, DR2, and DQ1/DQ2 antigens, and a predominance of CD8 + lymphocytes instead of CD4 + cells infiltrating salivary tissue are the characteristic features of AIDS-associated SS, which differs from classic idiopathic SS. Treatment is primarily symptomatic.

SEPTIC ARTHRITIS. Joint space infection is remarkably uncommon in HIV-infected patients. Sporadic case reports have been published of septic arthritis due to fungal pathogens, such as *C. neoformans, H. capsulatum,* and *S. schenkii,* mycobacteria, and routine pyogenic organisms. The approach to diagnosis and treatment of septic arthritis is the same for HIV-infected patients as non–HIV-infected individuals.

HIV-ASSOCIATED ARTHROPATHY. A relatively uncommon arthritis has been described in patients with moderately advanced HIV disease who demonstrate no other signs of any recognizable rheumatologic disease. The so-called HIV-associated arthropathy (HIVAA) presents as a mono- or pauciarticular arthritis. The arthritis is usually severe, affects primarily the knees and ankles, and lasts from 1 week to 6 months. No extra-articular manifestations have been noted. The synovial fluid is noninflammatory in nature, although a mild synovitis consisting of a chronic mononuclear cell infiltrate is noted on biopsy. Rheumatoid factor, antinuclear antibodies, anti-DNA antibodies, and antibodies against RNP, Sm, Ro/SS-A, and La/SS-B are negative. No predominant HLA pattern has been described. NSAID's are of some benefit, but some patients require intra-articular steroid injections.

VASCULITIS. Several varieties of vasculitis have been reported in association with HIV infection. Necrotizing vasculitis of the polyarteritis nodosa type is reported most commonly and presents as a peripheral sensory or sensorimotor neuropathy. The vasculitis involves the medium-sized vessels of the nerves, skin, and muscle. None of the reported patients with HIV-related PAN were hepatitis B surface antigen positive. Primary angiitis of the CNS has been noted in two patients, one of whom had persistent varicella-zoster virus infection. Lymphomatoid granulomatosis has also been reported in HIV-infected patients. Henoch-Schönlein purpura has been reported rarely; however, no distinct etiology has been elucidated. Drug-induced hypersensitivity vasculitis, usually presenting as cutaneous disease, has been reported associated with penicillin, trimethoprim-sulfamethoxazole, amitriptyline, and griseofulvin. Recently, several cases of uveitis have been reported with rifabutin therapy, especially when this drug is administered with fluconazole and clarithromycin.

It is unclear whether HIV-associated vasculitis is the result of direct HIV invasion of the vessels, an immunologic reaction to an underlying viral infection, or a response to an opportunistic viral pathogen that invades vascular tissue. As with other serious rheumatologic manifestations of HIV disease, treatment options are limited by the underlying immunodeficiency of the host.

Buskila D, Gladman D: Musculoskeletal manifestations of infection with human immunodeficiency virus. Rev Infect Dis 12:223, 1990. *Extensively referenced review of the musculoskeletal complaints associated with HIV disease.*

Etzel JV, Brocavich JM, Torre M: Endocrine complications associated with human immunodeficiency virus infection. Clin Pharm 11:159, 1992. *A practical, easy-to-read overview of the endocrine abnormality seen in HIV-infected patients.*

Fernández SM, Cardenal A, Balsa A: Rheumatic manifestations in 556 patients with human immunodeficiency virus infection. Semin Arthritis Rheum 21:30, 1991. *One of the largest published reports on the rheumatological manifestations of HIV infection. Numerous tables, charts, and figures.*

Gherardi R, Belec L, Mhiri C, et al.: The spectrum of vasculitis in human immunodeficiency virus-infected patients. Arthritis Rheum 36:1164, 1993. *An up-to-date review of an uncommon yet diverse complication of HIV disease.*

Herskowitz A, Vlahov D, Willoughby S, et al.: Prevalence and incidence of left ventricular dysfunction in patients with human immunodeficiency virus infection. Am J Cardiol 71:955, 1993. *A study of 98 patients followed at Johns Hopkins Hospital Clinics who were evaluated for left ventricular dysfunction. Includes patients referred to the cardiology service as well as asymptomatic "controls."*

Kaul S, Fishbein MC, Siegel RJ: Cardiac manifestations of acquired immune deficiency syndrome: A 1991 update. Am Heart J 122:535, 1991. *Overview of the cardiac manifestations of HIV disease. Special focus on cardiomyopathy.*

Marks JB: Endocrine manifestations of human immunodeficiency virus (HIV) infection. Am J Med Sci 302:110, 1991. *A review of the pathologic and clinical reports in the literature regarding endocrinopathies in AIDS patients.*

Rao TKS: Human immunodeficiency virus (HIV) associated nephropathy. Annu Rev Med 42:391, 1991. *Succinct review of the renal complications of HIV disease, with special focus on the HIV-associated nephropathy.*

Smith MC, Pawar R, Carey JT, et al.: Effect of corticosteroid therapy on human immunodeficiency virus-associated nephropathy. Am J Med 97:145, 1994. *A recent study of a few patients successfully treated with corticosteroids for HIV-associated nephropathy.*

371 TREATMENT OF HIV INFECTION AND AIDS
Robert Yarchoan and Samuel Broder

Since the identification of AIDS as a new entity in 1981, dramatic changes have occurred in therapy for this disease and its related disorders. In 1984, therapy was either entirely supportive or directed at a bewildering array of infectious and oncologic complications. Identification of human immunodeficiency virus (HIV) as the causative agent of AIDS and elucidation of its life cycle have enabled the development of specific antiretroviral therapy. Such therapy is now recognized to be important in the treatment of AIDS. The available drugs, however, are not curative, and intense efforts to evaluate new therapeutic approaches to HIV infection and its associated conditions continue. In this chapter, we review some of the current approaches for treating AIDS patients. In addition, we discuss certain experimental approaches now being developed. In AIDS, as perhaps in no other disease, the line between approved and experimental therapy is difficult to draw.

The immunodeficiency in AIDS results, either directly or indirectly, from the progressive destruction of the immune system by HIV. In addition, HIV infection affects other organ systems (such as the central nervous system). T lymphocytes bearing CD4 antigen on their surface (CD4 cells or T4 cells), monocyte/macrophages, and monocyte-derived cells such as microglial cells are now recognized as the principal cellular targets for HIV. Although other cells are also susceptible to infection in certain settings, the clinical significance of this phenomenon is unclear. In infected individuals, the development and progression of disease require at least some level of ongoing infection of new cells by HIV. Thus, one could reason that interfering with HIV replication in vivo could halt (or even reverse) the progression of disease to AIDS. Indeed, the successful development of antiretroviral therapy has provided proof for this concept.

AZIDOTHYMIDINE (ZIDOVUDINE) AND OTHER DIDEOXYNUCLEOSIDES

The first three antiretroviral drugs to be developed and approved for the therapy of HIV infection are members of the class of compounds called dideoxynucleosides, special analogues of nucleosides that have a sugar and a purine or pyrimidine base. 3'-Azido-2',3'-dideoxythymidine, also called azidothymidine, zidovudine, or AZT (Fig. 371–1), was the first to enter clinical testing. Although this drug was initially synthesized as an anticancer agent, it was found to inhibit HIV replication in human T cells in vitro and was later found to have anti-HIV activity in monocytes and macrophages. In dideoxynucleosides, the 3'-hydroxy (—OH) group in the sugar is replaced by another group that does not form phosphodiester linkages. A number of dideoxynucleosides have been found to be potent inhibitors of HIV replication in vitro, and several, including AZT, have been shown to have clinical activity in patients with HIV infection.

Upon entering human cells, AZT and other dideoxynucleosides are activated (phosphorylated) to form a 5'-triphosphate moiety. This activation process, called anabolic phosphorylation, uses a series of enzymes (kinases) that usually serve to phosphorylate deoxynucleosides (Fig. 371–2). For many purposes, each drug in this broad family is unique. Even a one-atom shift in the sugar or the base of the parent compound can radically change activity and toxicity. There are substantial differences in the rates at which human cells phosphorylate these compounds and in their enzymatic pathways, and these differences may be important in their antiretroviral activity and differing toxicity profiles. For example, thymidine kinase, the enzyme responsible for the initial step in the phosphorylation of thymidine analogues such as AZT and 2',3'-didehydro-2',3'-dideoxythymidine (stavudine, d4T), is a cell cycle–dependent enzyme. As a result, the activity of this type of drug is relatively greater in replicating lymphocytes or cytokine-stimulated monocytes than in resting cells of the same lineage. By contrast, the activity of 2',3'-dideoxyinosine (ddI, didanosine) and 2',3'-dideoxycytidine

(ddC, zalcitabine) is not substantially affected by the state of activation of the cells. Therefore, these two classes of drugs may target different cell populations, and, as described below, this insight may be useful in guiding the development of combination regimens.

As triphosphates, dideoxynucleosides act as inhibitors at the level of HIV DNA polymerase (reverse transcriptase) (see Ch. 361). This unique viral enzyme catalyzes the conversion of HIV genetic information from RNA to DNA and subsequently catalyzes the formation of a second viral DNA strand, i.e., a copy complementary to the first. As 5'-triphosphates, dideoxynucleosides are believed to inhibit reverse transcriptase in two ways; as DNA chain terminators and as competitive inhibitors for binding deoxynucleoside 5'-triphosphates to relevant sites within reverse transcriptase. Reverse transcriptase, but not mammalian DNA polymerase alpha, preferentially uses dideoxynucleoside-5'-triphosphates in place of the respective physiologic 5'-triphosphates, and this is most likely one basis for their selective antiretroviral activity. Human mitochondrial DNA polymerase (gamma) is also relatively sensitive to inhibition by certain of these drugs, and, as discussed below, this may be a basis for clinical toxicities, including cases of hepatic steatosis and myopathy observed in patients receiving dideoxynucleoside therapy.

CLINICAL ACTIVITY OF ZIDOVUDINE. Phase I and II clinical trials of AZT conducted during 1985 and 1986 convincingly showed that the drug was effective at reducing morbidity and mortality in patients with advanced HIV infection (Fig. 371–3). The patients receiving AZT had increased numbers of CD4 cells, improved immunologic function, and a decreased viral load (as assessed by HIV p24 antigenemia). In addition, they had increased appetite, weight gain, and often reported feeling better, at least temporarily. In a 6-month multicenter double-blind randomized trial in which AZT was compared with placebo, patients who had severe early symptomatic HIV disease or who had had Pneumocystis carinii pneumonia were found to have a markedly reduced mortality and incidence of opportunistic infections upon receiving AZT compared with patients on placebo. Based on these studies, AZT was initially approved for patients with severe HIV infection at a recommended dose of 200 mg every 4 hours (1200 mg per day) around the clock. Since that time, it has been found that a maintenance regimen of 100 mg every 4 hours (600 mg per day), initiated after a month's therapy with 200 mg every 4 hours, is as effective as the initially recommended regimen and is less toxic. This is now the currently recommended dose schedule for patients with AIDS or advanced HIV infection. Many physicians do not use the higher dose during the first month of therapy and suggest that their patients omit the night-time dose, for a total of 500 mg per day. Also, many physicians believe that a regimen of 200 mg every 8 hours has equivalent activity and leads to increased patient compliance. Physicians should be alert for possible future modifications of the recommended dose of this drug. Of the dideoxynucleosides now available, AZT is generally recommended as the first-line drug for people with advanced HIV infection.

The pharmacokinetic profile of AZT is one of the factors that guide its usage. AZT is well absorbed by mouth; the average oral bioavailability is 63%. The circulating half-life is approximately 1.1 hours. Because of this relatively short half-life, a dosing schedule of every 4 hours was initially recommended. However, the active 5'-triphosphate moiety has an intracellular half-life of 1 to 3 hours, and as noted above, many physicians now use a regimen of 200 mg every 8 hours. Fifteen to 20% of an administered dose of zidovudine is excreted unchanged in the urine, whereas approximately 75% undergoes glucuronidation to an inactive form in the liver. AZT glucuronidation can be inhibited by certain other drugs, such as probenecid, which share this pathway, and these drugs can prolong the half-life of zidovudine. However, other drugs that undergo hepatic glucuronidation (e.g., acetaminophen) have no such effect. Studies are under way to evaluate the interactions of other drugs with AZT. Finally, AZT penetrates relatively well into the cerebrospinal fluid (CSF).

At the beginning of the epidemic, the expected survival of patients with fulminant AIDS was approximately 10 months. The expected survival of such patients has nearly doubled since that time. It is likely that a number of advances in diagnosis, prevention, and treatment of AIDS complications (particularly chemoprophylaxis for opportunistic infections such as P. carinii pneumonia) have contributed to this. However, when this specific factor has been looked at, the effect of AZT on survival has been observed over and above any contribution from chemoprophylaxis.

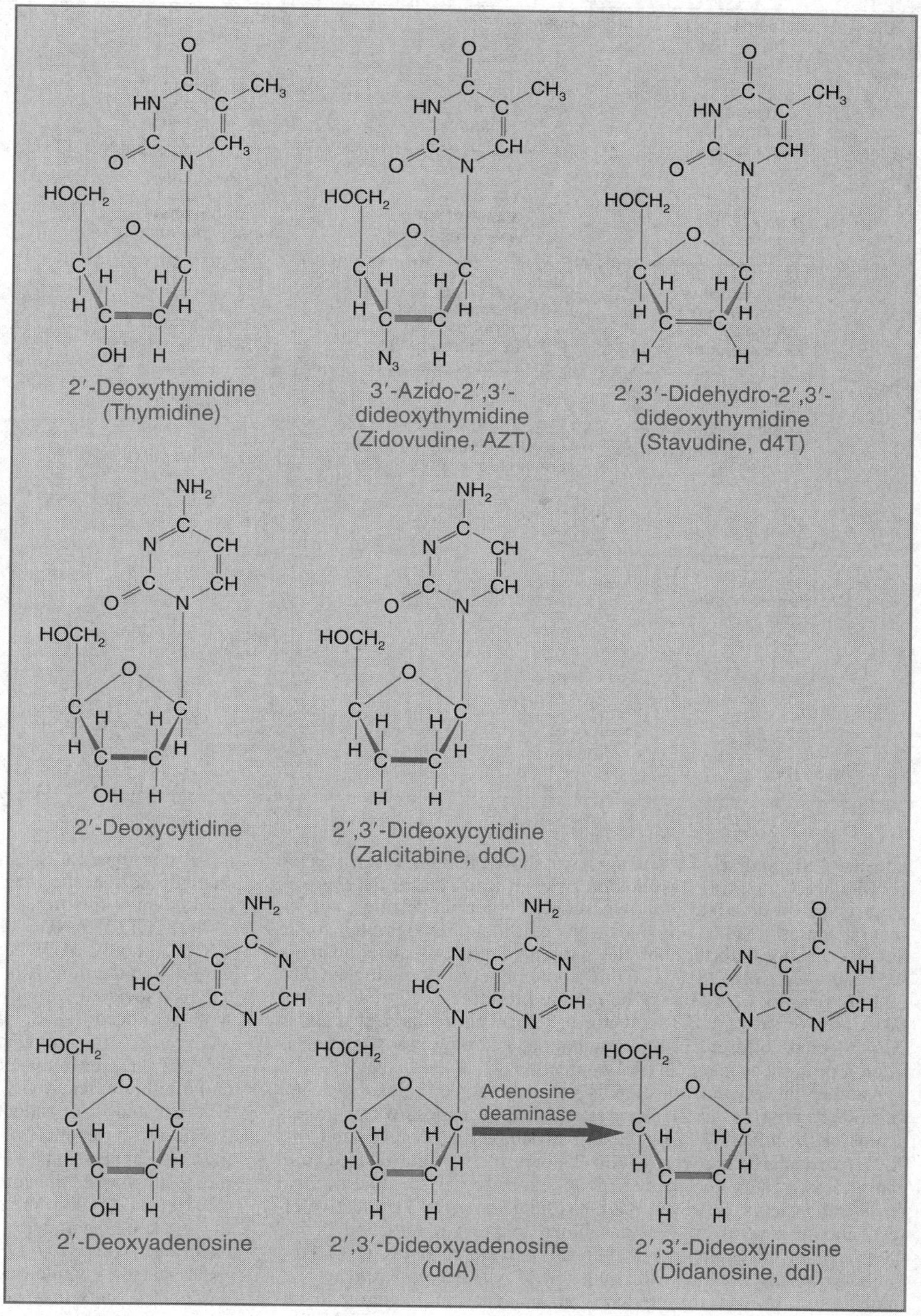

FIGURE 371–1. Structures of zidovudine (AZT), stavudine (d4T), zalcitabine (ddC), dideoxyadenosine (ddA), and didanosine (ddI), and their related physiologic deoxynucleosides. In each row, the physiologic deoxynucleoside is shown on the left and the related antiretroviral drug or drugs are shown to their right. In each case, a replacement of the 3′ hydroxy (—OH) group of the physiologic deoxynucleoside by an azido (—N₃) group or a hydrogen atom (—H) results in the formation of a potent antiretroviral drug. ddA is rapidly converted to ddI by the ubiquitous enzyme adenosine deaminase, and these can be considered alternate forms of the same drug for many purposes.

An unresolved issue is the optimal time to initiate AZT therapy. Five major double-blinded randomized trials of early AZT therapy have now been completed. Overall, these studies showed that AZT given to either asymptomatic or symptomatic patients with 200 to 500 CD4 cells per cubic millimeter resulted in a somewhat reduced progression of disease over 1 to 2 years. As a result of these observations, AZT was approved for HIV-infected patients with 500 CD4 cells per cubic millimeter or less. However, one study showed that the reduction in quality of life from the side effects of AZT was about equal to the increase associated with the effect on disease progression. Moreover, two of the studies specifically looked for an effect on survival, and in each case, no overall survival advantage was seen in patients given AZT early as opposed to those in whom the drug was withheld until symptoms developed. The consensus from these trials is that in regard to overall survival as an endpoint, administering AZT early is not proven to be better than later admin-

istration. It should be stressed that these results in no way refute the earlier findings that AZT initiated at the time of advanced HIV infection improves survival. Also, it should be remembered that these trials all involved AZT as a single agent, and the results do not necessarily apply to combination regimens.

Based on an informed discussion, some physicians and patients may elect to use AZT early whereas others may not. In either case, the physician should explain the results from the available clinical trials to the patient. Physicians should keep informed of changes in these recommendations as new trials are completed and analyzed.

In considering initiating therapy with AZT, physicians may weigh two factors: the presence of HIV-related thrombocytopenia and HIV-related dementia. HIV-infected patients sometimes develop thrombocytopenia, which can be rather severe. Several studies have now shown that AZT can reverse this process and is better tolerated in this population than are corticosteroids. Also, AZT can penetrate

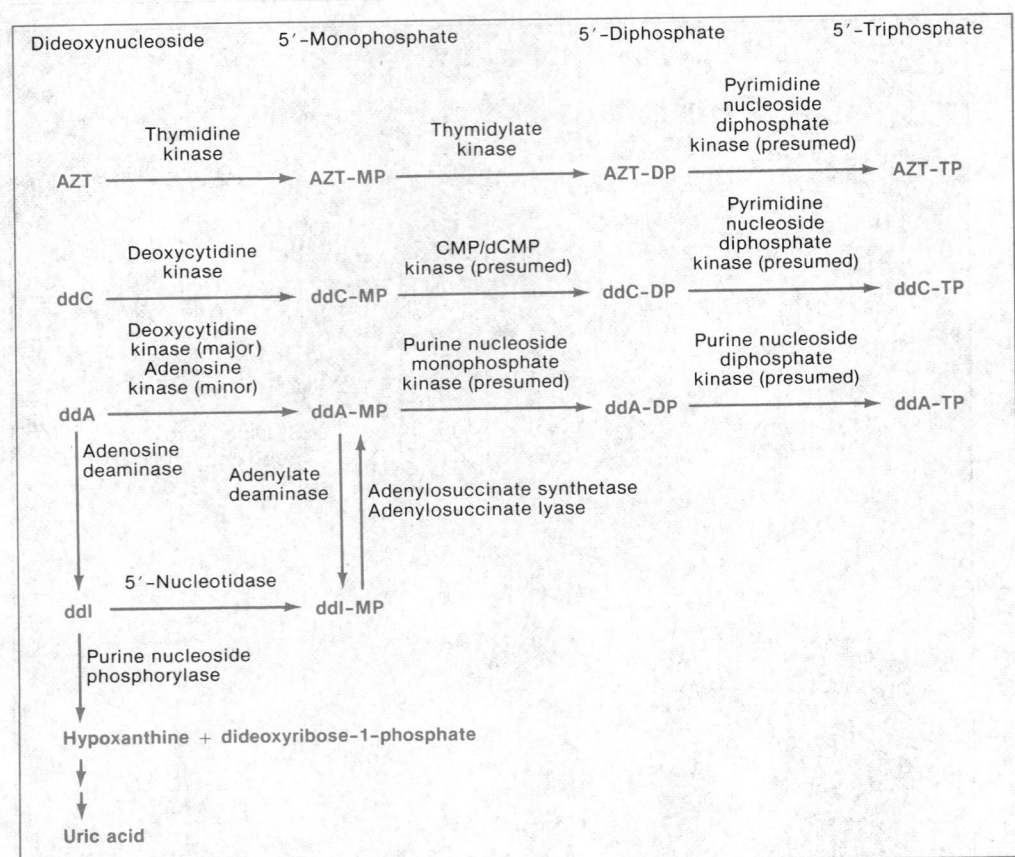

FIGURE 371–2. Activation pathways for zidovudine (AZT), zalcitabine (ddC), dideoxyadenosine (ddA), and didanosine (ddI) to the active triphosphate moieties in human cells. MP = 5′-monophosphate; DP = 5′-diphosphate; TP = 5′-triphosphate.

into the CSF, and several studies have shown that AZT can reverse HIV-induced cognitive dysfunction or even frank dementia. Patients have been observed to improve on psychometric testing, and, in several cases studied by positron emission tomography, there has been a normalization of the pattern of glucose metabolism in the brain (see Color Plate 12*F*). In some patients, doses higher than 500 mg per day of AZT may be required to effectively treat dementia. The reversal of HIV dementia has been particularly striking in HIV-infected children. In this population, neurologic dysfunction is often a prominent feature of HIV infection.

Another unresolved question is under what conditions AZT (or any other anti-HIV drug) given at the time of exposure can protect against HIV infection. Several animal studies have suggested that AZT (particularly if given within 2 hours of the time of infection) can at least reduce the degree of infection. In certain other animal retroviral systems, however, AZT has failed to yield a protective effect, and in several cases it has failed to prevent infection in humans even when given soon after the parenteral exposure to HIV. No data, however, address the question of whether postexposure administration of AZT may reduce the incidence of infection in humans. Many hospitals now offer a 4- to 6-week course of AZT to employees who have a substantial exposure to HIV, e.g., a needle stick with HIV-infected blood or a laboratory accident. In considering such therapy, physicians should weigh the risk of HIV infection occurring (about 1 in 200 for a needle stick), the short-term side-effects of AZT, and the unknown long-term sequelae of this drug.

Recent evidence from a recently conducted placebo-controlled trial, ACTG 076, indicates that AZT can reduce the transmission of HIV from the infected mother to her infant. In this study, the treatment consisted of a regimen of AZT administered to the mother during pregnancy (100 mg five times daily by mouth starting between weeks 14 and 34) and during labor and delivery (by the intravenous route), as well as to the infant during the first 6 weeks of life. Transmission of HIV infection was found to be reduced from 25.5% in the placebo control group to 8.3% in the treated group. The mothers in this study all had > 200 CD4 cells per cubic millimeter and had never received anti-HIV therapy. No increase in congenital defects was seen in the AZT-treated infants. It should be noted that the results cannot be extrapolated beyond the population studied and that the long-term effects of AZT exposure *in utero* are not known at this time.

TOXICITY AND OTHER LIMITATIONS OF AZT THERAPY. Although AZT has clearly been shown to benefit patients with HIV infection, it is by no means a perfect drug. Its long-term use is associated with a number of toxicities, particularly in patients with advanced AIDS, and on occasion the side effects may be lethal. Also, the immunologic and virologic improvement induced by AZT may be only temporary, especially in patients with AIDS, and a reduced sensitivity to the drug has been observed in strains of HIV isolated from patients on long-term therapy.

The most frequent toxicity associated with AZT therapy is bone marrow suppression (Table 371–1). The earliest sign is often anemia with marked macrocytic changes; a mean corpuscular volume of 110 to 120 cubic microns is not uncommon. AZT is now a leading cause of macrocytosis in several medical centers. Some patients have been observed to develop hypocellular or (rarely) aplastic bone marrows while receiving AZT. Later in the course of AZT therapy, patients may become neutropenic or thrombocytopenic. In some patients, the platelet count remains stable or paradoxically increases for some time, perhaps reflecting an effect against underlying HIV-induced thrombocytopenia. AZT-induced bone marrow suppression is most common in patients with advanced AIDS, low CD4 cell counts, pretherapy anemia, and pretherapy neutropenia. It is less problematic with the recently recommended dosage of 600 mg per day; however, even with this dosing schedule, it can occur in 30% or so of patients with advanced disease during the first year of therapy. HIV-infected patients often have vitamin deficiencies, particularly of vitamin B_{12}, and megaloblastic anemia from folic acid or vitamin B_{12} deficiency bears a certain similarity to AZT toxicity. It may thus be prudent to measure serum levels of folic acid and vitamin B_{12} and give replacement therapy if they are low; however, this intervention has not been shown to prevent or reverse AZT toxicity. It has been shown that genetically engineered erythropoietin (epoetin alfa) can partially ameliorate AZT-induced anemia, particularly in patients who do not have markedly elevated erythropoietin levels (see Ch. 369). For patients who develop severe

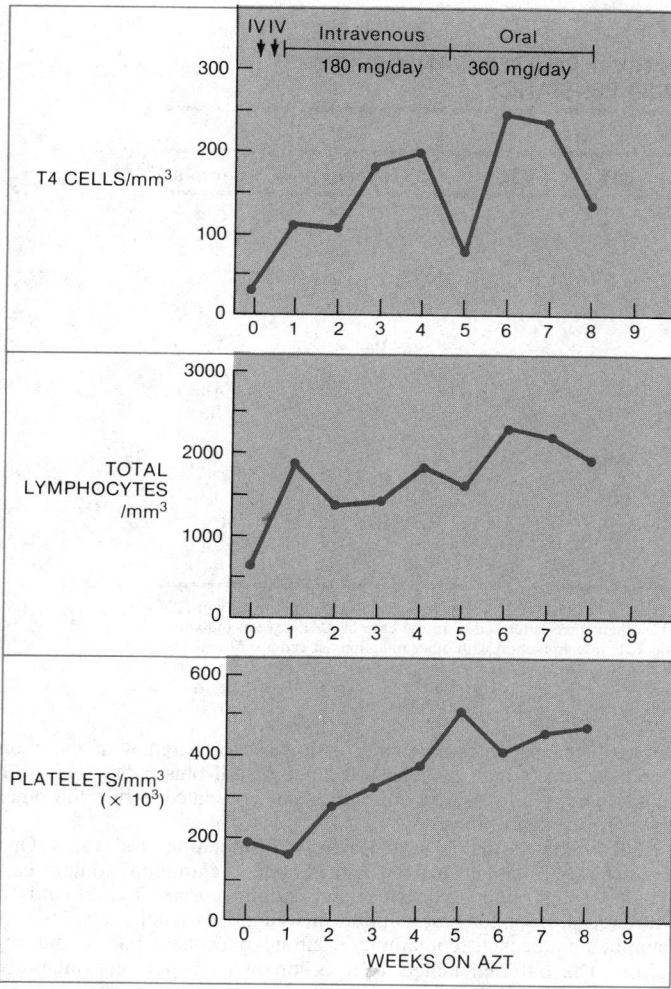

FIGURE 371–3. Course of the first patient to ever receive AZT. This patient, who had recently recovered from *Pneumocystis carinii* pneumonia, was treated on the National Cancer Institute service of the National Institutes of Health Clinical Center with 180 mg per day of AZT intravenously for 4 weeks, followed by 360 mg per day orally for 4 weeks.

gested that, like zidovudine-induced myositis, this condition may be caused by mitochondrial toxicity.

Seizures, which can be fatal, have been reported as side effects of AZT, as has Stevens-Johnson syndrome on very rare occasions. Patients receiving AZT frequently complain of malaise, fatigue, nausea, or headaches. These often become less severe after several weeks on the drug. One approach to these symptoms is to start with a relatively low dose of AZT and work up to the full dose over a couple of weeks or so. Even with this approach, these symptoms are intolerable in a small percentage of patients. Some patients, particularly those of African-American ancestry, develop bluish fingernail discoloration as a result of AZT therapy (Color Plate 12E).

Improved survival from antiretroviral therapy may permit AIDS patients to live long enough to develop certain HIV-related complications. In particular, an unexpectedly high incidence of non-Hodgkin's lymphoma, in some instances approaching 10% of patients per year, has been observed in AIDS patients who have been closely followed for several years on AZT-containing regimens. These are probably not caused by AZT but rather represent the development of opportunistic tumors in drastically immunosuppressed patients.

The elevations in CD4 cell counts and declines in the load of HIV in patients receiving AZT generally last for only weeks or months, particularly in patients with advanced disease, and a growing body of data supports the notion that this is because viral resistance developed. AZT resistance, often 100-fold or more, is found in HIV isolated from the majority of patients with advanced disease who have received AZT for a year or more. Development of resistance is slower in patients with earlier HIV infection. Strains resistant to AZT generally have two or more mutations in the HIV *pol* gene (Table 371–2). Of these, the substitution of tyrosine (or phenylalanine) for threonine at codon 215 appears to be the most

TABLE 371–1. PRINCIPAL TOXICITIES OF DRUGS WITH ANTIRETROVIRAL ACTIVITY USED IN AIDS

Zidovudine (AZT)
1. Bone marrow suppression
   Red cells usually affected more than white cells or platelets
   Prominent increase in red cell mean corpuscular volume
   Marrow may become hypocellular
2. Malaise, fever, fatigue (especially during first few weeks)
3. Headaches (especially during first few weeks)
4. Myalgias
5. Myositis (in approximately 10% of patients after long-term use)
6. Hepatic steatosis, lactic acidosis (can be fatal)
7. Seizures (can be fatal)
8. Nausea, vomiting
9. Confusion, tremulousness (especially with high doses)
10. Bluish pigmentation of nails (especially in blacks)
11. Stevens-Johnson syndrome (very rare)

Didanosine (ddI)
1. Sporadic pancreatitis (can be fatal)
2. Painful peripheral neuropathy (involving feet)
3. Sporadic hepatitis (can be fatal)
4. Insomnia, irritability, anxiety
5. Macular erythematous skin rash (sporadic)
6. Retinal depigmentation (especially in children)
7. Increases in uric acid (from ddI metabolism)
8. Hyperamylasemia, hypertriglyceridemia
9. Diarrhea, hypokalemia (from citrate/phosphate/sucrose vehicle)
10. Neutropenia, thrombocytopenia (rare, relationship to drug unclear)
11. Seizures
12. Dry mouth
13. Diabetes mellitus (rare)

Zalcitabine (ddC)
1. Painful peripheral neuropathy (involving feet)
2. Aphthous stomatitis
3. Esophageal ulcerations
4. Pancreatitis (reported but rare)
5. Cardiomyopathy
6. Skin rash (may subside with continued treatment)
7. Fever (especially with high doses)
8. Thrombocytopenia (especially with high doses)
9. Hepatic steatosis or lactic acidosis (rare)

Stavudine (d4T)
1. Painful peripheral neuropathy
2. Elevations of hepatic transaminases
3. Bone marrow suppression, especially anemia

anemia or neutropenia while receiving AZT, many physicians now favor switching to an alternative antiretroviral regimen (see below).

Myalgias are also common in patients receiving AZT. In addition, after long-term therapy (e.g., a year or more), a subset of patients may develop frank myopathy with muscle wasting and sometimes (but not always) elevations of creatine kinase. In rare cases, this side effect can lead to a catastrophic failure of systemic muscles. AZT-induced myositis can usually be distinguished from myositis caused by HIV by the presence of "ragged-red" fibers on biopsy, indicative of abnormal mitochondria (see Color Plate 12G). Paracrystalline inclusions in the mitochondria can be seen on electron microscopy. It is believed that this toxicity results from the inhibitory effect of AZT-5'-triphosphate on mammalian γ DNA polymerase, an enzyme found in the mitochondrial matrix. Some patients with this toxicity respond to a nonsteroidal anti-inflammatory drug, with or without a reduced dosage of AZT. In other cases, it may be necessary to discontinue the AZT. Certain patients who do not respond to the above interventions have been reported to respond to therapy with prednisone (40 to 60 mg daily). This potentially dangerous immunosuppressive drug should be used only in severe cases when other alternatives have failed.

Some HIV-infected patients receiving AZT, alone or in combination with other dideoxynucleosides, have been reported to develop a poorly understood syndrome involving severe macrovesicular hepatic steatosis (a condition related to Reye's syndrome) and lactic acidosis (see Color Plate 11H). A high proportion of these patients have died of this complication. Many had relatively early HIV infection and were well nourished or even obese. Also, a disproportionate percentage of such patients were female. It has been sug-

TABLE 371-2. SELECTED MUTATIONS IN HIV-1 REVERSE TRANSCRIPTASE ASSOCIATED WITH DRUG RESISTANCE

Codon	Wild Type	Drug						
		AZT	ddI	ddC	d4T	3TC	Pyridione	Nevirapine
41	Met	Leu						
50	Ile				Thr			
67	Asp	Asn						
69	Thr			Asp				
70	Lys	Arg						
74	Leu		Val					
100	Leu						Ile	Ile
103	Lys						Asn	Asn
106	Val							Ala
108	Val						Ile	Ile
135	Ile		Val					
151	Gln	Met	Met	Met	Met			
181	Tyr						Cys	Cys
184	Met		Val			Val		
188	Tyr						Cys	Cys
215	Thr	Tyr, Phe						
219	Lys	Gln, Glu						

Shown here are some of the principal mutations in the codons of reverse transcriptase of HIV conferring resistance to various anti-HIV drugs. The amino acids in the wild-type and mutated viruses are depicted by their three-letter codes. In the case of AZT, several mutations are generally required to yield high-level resistance. The mutation at codon 151, in conjunction with other mutations at codons 77 and 116, can confer resistance to multiple dideoxynucleosides. In the case of the non-nucleoside reverse transcriptase inhibitors pyridione (L-697, 661) or nevirapine, one mutation is sufficient to confer high-level resistance.

important. AZT-resistant strains generally preserve their sensitivity to most other dideoxynucleosides (including ddC and ddI), and this is one rationale for combination therapy with these agents.

DIDANOSINE. Several other dideoxynucleosides (see Fig. 371-2) and related nucleoside analogues have been found to be active against HIV in the laboratory. Of these, ddI, ddC, and d4T are currently approved in the United States, and others including the negative enantiomer of 2',3'-dideoxy-3'-thiacytidine (3TC) are currently being tested in experimental protocols (Table 371-3). Upon being phosphorylated in target cells to their active moieties, all of these drugs are believed to work by the same general mechanism. However, because of differences in their intracellular or extracellular metabolism and effects on cellular DNA polymerases and normal nucleotides, various dideoxynucleosides may have fundamentally different activity and toxicity profiles. Each must be considered a different drug, and their mechanisms of action remain a matter for basic research.

The second such drug to be approved for the treatment of HIV infection was ddI. This drug is well absorbed by the oral route when given with appropriate buffers (oral bioavailability 40%). Although it has a relatively rapid serum half-life (average 1.6 hours), its active moiety, 2',3'-dideoxyadenosine-5'-triphosphate, has an intracellular half-life of >12 hours, and it can thus be administered on a twice-daily regimen. Early clinical trials showed that ddI elevated CD4 cell counts and decreased the HIV viral load. Several large randomized trials comparing the relative efficacy of ddI and AZT in patients with AIDS or advanced HIV infection have shown that AZT was more effective than ddI in patients with AIDS or advanced HIV infection who had never before received AZT therapy. However, in patients who received as little as 8 weeks of prior AZT therapy, ddI was found to be more effective in preventing disease progression and to increase survival in some subsets (Fig. 371-4). Largely as a result of these studies, ddI is now approved for use in patients with advanced HIV infection who have received prolonged prior AZT therapy or who cannot tolerate AZT or who show disease progression during such therapy.

Certain subsets of patients may experience comparatively long actuarial survivals. Thus, for patients who entered a phase I study of ddI with CD4 counts between 100 and 300 cells per cubic millimeter, the estimated survival after 4 years was 80%.

There is recent evidence that a ddI-containing regimen is superior to AZT monotherapy in children with HIV infection. ACTG study 152 was designed to compare AZT, ddI, and a combination regimen of AZT and ddI in children with up to 6 weeks of prior anti-HIV therapy. An interim look at the data in February 1995 revealed that patients on the AZT monotherapy regimen had a significantly increased chance of disease progression as compared with those on the best arm (which is either ddI alone or ddI plus AZT). The AZT monotherapy arm has accordingly been terminated, while the other two arms remain blinded.

ddI is now available in at least two formulations for adults. One is a chewable tablet buffered with dihydroxyaluminum sodium carbonate, magnesium hydroxide, and sodium citrate. The other is a buffered powder for oral solution in water. This latter preparation is supplied in packets containing a citrate phosphate buffer and sucrose. The buffered tablets have a somewhat better bioavailability than the buffered powder, and the dosages must be adjusted accordingly. For patients weighing at least 60 kg, the recommended dose is 400 mg of the tablets daily or 500 mg of the buffered powder daily, divided into two doses and taken on an empty stomach. For patients weighing <60 kg, the doses are 250 mg daily of the tablets or 334 mg of the buffered powder daily, again divided into two doses.

The principal toxicity of ddI is its potential for causing severe or even lethal pancreatitis (see Table 371-1). In the trials discussed above, the annual rate of pancreatitis in patients receiving ddI was about 7%, compared with a 3 to 4% annual rate in patients receiving AZT. As can be seen by the rates in AZT recipients, patients with HIV infection have an underlying high incidence of pancreatitis, and it is often difficult to distinguish ddI-induced pancreatitis from that caused by HIV infection, its complications, or other drugs. The incidence of pancreatitis is higher in patients with more advanced disease or with higher doses of ddI, and this is one of the factors that led to the current dosing recommendation. Some patients receiving ddI have asymptomatic hyperamylasemia, which may be of either salivary or pancreatic origin. Although it is prudent to temporarily discontinue ddI in patients with elevated levels of pancreatic amylase, the drug may be cautiously continued in patients who have only elevated salivary amylase levels. ddI should also be withheld in patients with hyperlipasemia or substantially elevated triglyceride levels, as these may reflect present or incipient pancreatic damage.

Patients receiving ddI should be counseled to avoid alcohol. A previous history of pancreatic disease should generally serve as a contraindication to ddI use. Also, other drugs that can cause pancreatitis, such as systemic pentamidine, high-dose sulfonamides, furosemide, and thiazide diuretics, should be avoided whenever possible in patients receiving ddI. In particular, ddI should be temporarily stopped when patients are treated for *P. carinii* pneumonia with intravenous pentamidine or sulfonamide-containing regimens (including trimethoprim-sulfamethoxazole). If appropriate, ddI can then be restarted after the completion of therapy. In the case of pentami-

TABLE 371–3. SELECTED ANTIRETROVIRAL DRUGS (EXPERIMENTAL AND APPROVED) FOR THE THERAPY TREATMENT FOR AIDS

Site of Effect	Name	Status (Fall 1994)	Comment
Viral binding	CD4-IgG chimera	Experimental	Blocks viral entry
	CD4-toxin hybrids	Experimental	May selectively kill HIV-producing cells
	Anti-HIV antibodies	Experimental	May block HIV fusion and entry
Reverse transcriptase	Zidovudine (AZT)	Approved	Principal toxicity is bone marrow suppression
	Didanosine (ddI)	Approved	Can cause pancreatitis or peripheral neuropathy
	Zalcitabine (ddC)	Approved	Peripheral neuropathy is dose-limiting toxicity
	Stavudine (d4T)	Approved	Can cause peripheral neuropathy
	Lamivudine (3TC)	Experimental	Resistance develops rapidly; especially active in combination with AZT
	Non-nucleoside reverse transcriptase inhibitors	Experimental	Resistance a problem with this class of drugs
	Phosphonoformate (Foscarnet)	Approved for cytomegalovirus	Also has some activity against HIV
Replicative efficiency	Genetic therapy approaches	Experimental	Inhibitions of *rev* and *tat* activity being studied
	Antisense oligonucleosides	Experimental	May have both sequence specific and nonspecific activities
Protein modification	Saquinavir	Experimental	Little toxicity. Being studied in combination trials. Resistance can develop.
	Other protease inhibitors	Experimental	Several now in clinical trial. Clinical activity has been observed with some, but resistance can develop.
	Zinc finger inhibitors	Preclinical	Affect nucleocapsid protein; may also affect infectivity
Viral assembly and budding	Interferon-α	Approved for Kaposi's sarcoma	Antitumor activity against Kaposi's sarcoma. May also have anti-HIV activity

dine, which has a long serum half-life, it is probably prudent to wait at least 1 week before resuming ddI. Sulfonamides (including trimethoprim-sulfamethoxazole) at the doses used as prophylaxis for *P. carinii* pneumonia can be co-administered with ddI. Patients receiving ddI who develop abdominal pain should be advised to stop the drug immediately and be evaluated for pancreatitis. Physicians should probably avoid prescribing cimetidine or ranitidine along with ddI, as those drugs have the potential of increasing the absorption of ddI and can cause pancreatitis in their own right.

Some patients receiving ddI develop a painful peripheral neuropathy, primarily involving the feet. This is generally reversible upon discontinuing the drug, but the resolution may take weeks. Some patients with this condition have a decrease in their vibratory sense or ability to discriminate temperatures, but these objective findings are generally more subtle in relationship to the symptoms than in patients with HIV-induced peripheral neuropathy. Other reported side effects of ddI include seizures, headache, insomnia, irritability, vomiting, diabetes mellitus, hyperuricemia, and skin rash. Depigmentation of the retinal pigment epithelium, not associated with changes in visual acuity, has been reported, especially in children. Also, patients receiving the citrate/phosphate buffered form of

ddI may develop diarrhea, sometimes accompanied by life-threatening hypokalemia. This is generally attributed to the buffer/vehicle rather than to the ddI itself, and it may subside upon a change to the buffered tablets. Because ddI is given with buffers of gastric acidity, it should be given at least 2 hours after drugs such as ketoconazole or dapsone, whose absorption actually depends on gastric acidity.

HIV resistance had been reported to occur with ddI, but it is generally of a lesser degree than that observed with AZT. The most frequently observed mutation is a substitution of valine for leucine in codon 74 of the *pol* gene (see Table 371–2). Interestingly, this change can make AZT-resistant HIV with a mutation at codon 215 become more sensitive to AZT, and this has provided a rationale for using these drugs together in combination. Several pilot studies have shown that patients started on the combination of AZT and ddI often have elevated CD4 cells above baseline lasting for over a year, and some physicians use this combination in patients who progress on AZT therapy. While this regimen has not yet been approved, two large clinical trials have recently confirmed its clinical utility.

ZALCITABINE. ddC was the third drug to be approved for treating HIV infection. This drug was found to reduce the load of HIV in patients at even very low doses. On a weight basis, it is the most potent of the available antiretroviral nucleosides. It is well absorbed when given by mouth and is excreted by the renal route. In patients with advanced HIV infection who have not received prior antiretroviral therapy, ddC does not appear to be as clinically active as AZT. However, in patients who have had extensive prior AZT therapy, ddC appears to be as effective as continued AZT. Some investigators believe that a combination of AZT and ddC provides more durable elevations in CD4 counts than either agent used alone, particularly in patients with a CD4 count of >150 cells per cubic millimeter.

The principal toxicity of ddC is a painful peripheral neuropathy, somewhat similar to that caused by ddI (see Table 371–3). Other toxicities include aphthous stomatitis, esophageal ulceration, cardiomyopathy, and a few reported cases of pancreatitis. Cases of lactic acidosis, hepatic steatosis, or fatal hepatic failure have also been reported. The differential toxicity profiles of AZT and ddC have led to their study in combination regimens. In a study of patients with advanced HIV infection who had had extensive pretreatment with AZT, however, the combination of AZT and ddC was overall no better than continued AZT therapy. Interestingly, however, patients who entered this study with 100 to 300 CD4 cells per cubic millimeter appeared to do better on the combination therapy. ddC as a single drug is currently approved at a dose of 0.75 mg three times daily for patients with advanced HIV infection who are intolerant of AZT or who have had disease progression while re-

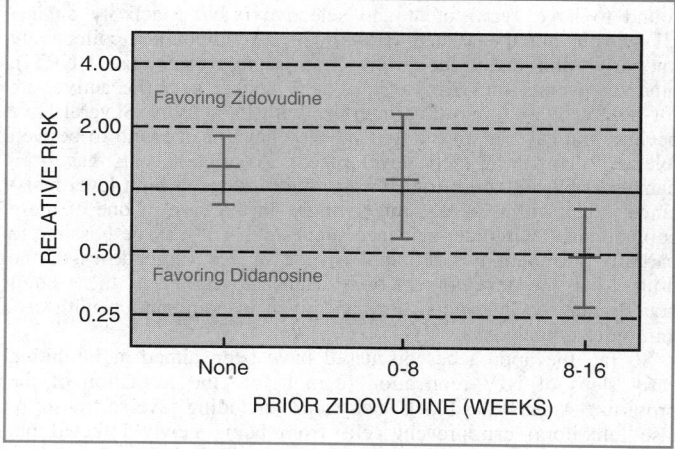

FIGURE 371–4. Comparative effectiveness of AZT and ddI in patients with advanced HIV-1 infection as assessed in ACTG Trial 116A. Shown are the relative risks of either a new AIDS-defining event or death in patients with varying prior experience with AZT. (Data from Abstract WS-B24-1 in the IXth International Conference on AIDS, Berlin, 1993 and from R. Dolin and the ACTG 116A team.)

ceiving AZT. In addition, it is indicated in combination with AZT for selected patients with advanced HIV infection (≤ 300 CD4 cells per cubic millimeter).

OTHER DIDEOXYNUCLEOSIDES. Stavudine (d4T) has recently been approved in the United States for patients who are intolerant of or deteriorating while receiving other approved therapies. The recommended dose is 40 mg twice daily for patients weighing at least 60 kg, and 30 mg twice daily for patients < 60 kg. Like AZT, this drug is a thymidine analogue. However, it is more efficiently phosphorylated in target cells, and it is active in patients at doses of 0.5 to 1.0 mg per kilogram per day. Its principal toxicities are painful peripheral neuropathy, anemia, and hepatitis. Some evidence exists that the phosphorylation of d4T in cells to its active moiety is inhibited by co-administering AZT, thus possibly interfering with its action. Their simultaneous use is not recommended outside the clinical trial setting. Another dideoxynucleoside, the negative enantiomer of 2',3'-dideoxy-3'-thiacytidine (lamivudine, 3TC), has been found to induce very little toxicity, whereas the development of high-level resistance may be a problem in its use as a single agent, it induces relatively prolonged effects on surrogate markers (viral load and CD4 count) when administered in combination with AZT.

OTHER ANTI-HIV THERAPIES

Many clinical trials of anti-AIDS drugs are currently under way, and physicians treating AIDS patients may need to counsel them about the advisability of entering a particular experimental protocol. As such, a basic knowledge of the strategies being considered to inhibit HIV replication at various steps in its life cycle may be of use (see Table 371–3).

As described in Ch. 361, the first step in the infection of a cell by HIV is its binding to a cellular receptor. The principal receptor for HIV binding is the first domain of CD4 glycoprotein, an important molecule found on helper T cells and certain other cells. Some experimental evidence indicates that under certain circumstances CD4-independent entry mechanisms may exist, although the clinical significance of this finding is unknown. Several groups have shown that various forms of genetically engineered soluble recombinant CD4 (containing the extracellular domains) can prevent the binding and infection of cells by HIV *in vitro*. However, these preparations were subsequently found to have less activity against fresh isolates of HIV than against laboratory strains, and they did not appear to have activity in patients.

As discussed above, much of the effort in developing anti-AIDS drugs has focused on reverse transcription. All of the dideoxynucleosides (as triphosphates) are thought to act at this step. In addition, trisodium phosphonoformate (foscarnet), a drug used to treat cytomegalovirus, has some activity against HIV at the level of reverse transcription. More recently, a diverse group of compounds, some of which are structurally related to the benzodiazepines, have been found to have very potent and selective *in vitro* activity against HIV-1 (but not the related HIV-2). These compounds, collectively known as non-nucleoside reverse transcriptase inhibitors (NNRTI), bind to reverse transcriptase in a deep pocket near the active site for polymerization and thus interfere with its activity. Several have been in clinical trial and in general they have been found to be well tolerated. However, their development as single agents has been hampered by the ability of HIV to rapidly develop high-level resistance, often within weeks. Interestingly, in the case of one of these compounds, nevirapine, evidence suggests that it may be possible to partially surmount this problem by use of very high doses of the drug. Also, the development of resistance to certain of these compounds may be delayed if they are given in combination with certain dideoxynucleosides.

So far, the approaches discussed have been aimed at inhibiting early steps of HIV replication (e.g., before the formation of the provirus). Agents that block such steps (including reverse transcriptase inhibitors) can prevent cells from being newly infected but have little or no effect on those that are already infected and producing virus. There is now a substantial interest in inhibiting late steps in HIV replication, in part because such agents are likely to be synergistic with inhibitors of early steps and in part because certain cells, such as macrophages, can produce HIV for long periods of time. One late target that has been the focus of a substantial re-

search effort is HIV protease. Certain proteins of HIV are first produced as large, relatively inactive polyproteins and later undergo a variety of modifications to form active proteins or glycoproteins. Proteolytic cleavage of the Gag-Pol fusion protein may occur very late, even within budding virions. Without a functional protease, the infectivity of the virus is severely diminished. The structure of this enzyme has recently been determined by radiographic crystallography, and a number of selective inhibitors have been identified. The principal problems initially encountered in developing this class of compounds have related to poor oral bioavailability, poor solubility, and complexity of synthesis. However, these have not been insurmountable, and several drugs have now entered clinical testing. One of the most extensively tested, saquinavir, was found in early clinical studies to have oral bioavailability of about 5%, to be well tolerated, to induce increases in CD4 counts, and to reduce the HIV viral load. It is an interesting agent; its use in combination with other anti-HIV agents is now being explored. Several other compounds, including L-735,524, ABT-538, and U-75875, are also undergoing clinical testing, and some of the preliminary clinical results have also been favorable. Some of these compounds may have better oral bioavailability than saquinavir. It is likely that within the next few years, one or more of these compounds will enter general clinical practice. However, the emergence of resistance has been observed with certain protease inhibitors as single drugs, and the potential of combination regimens to address this issue is a major topic for clinical research.

HIV replication is regulated by certain genetic elements (long terminal repeats) on the end of the viral genome and by several small viral-encoded proteins. Efficient viral replication requires the proper function of these regulatory elements, and as such they may also be targets for therapy. Specific inhibitors of these proteins are now being sought. Also, a number of cytokines and cellular factors have been identified that interact with the long terminal repeats and regulate HIV replication, and these may be targets for therapy. For example, tumor necrosis factor-α stimulates HIV replication, and HIV-infected patients have elevated levels of this factor. Certain drugs such as pentoxifylline inhibit its production, and this approach is now being tested in HIV-infected patients.

Another approach to inhibiting HIV replication has been the construction of "antisense" segments of modified DNA (e.g., phosphorothioate oligodeoxynucleotides). These are strands of DNA—modified to prevent degradation by cellular nucleases—with sequences complementary to that of HIV RNA. Such constructs may stop viral replication by bringing about a hybridization arrest at the level of the ribosome. A related approach being explored in the laboratory are ribozymes, RNA's that may cleave sequences in HIV RNA. Finally, a number of gene therapy approaches are being explored with the aim of rendering cells resistant to HIV replication. For example, cells may be protected against HIV by insertion of genes encoding for elements that block the activity of Tat or Rev, two regulatory elements of HIV. Clinical trials of such approaches are now under way. However, it is unlikely that any such approach will be widely used to treat AIDS over the next several years.

The last steps in the replication of HIV are viral assembly and budding. There is evidence that interferon-α can prevent HIV replication *in vitro,* in part by affecting viral budding. Interferons may have other sites of activity as well. Interferon-α has been found to have antitumor activity against Kaposi's sarcoma (see Ch. 369), particularly in patients with > 100 T4 cells per cubic millimeter who have disease limited to the skin, and it is approved for this indication.

A final word should be said about strategies to boost the immune system of individuals with HIV infection. The progression of HIV infection to fulminant AIDS represents an interplay between the infective potential of the virus and the ability of the immune system to interfere with this process. In most if not all patients, the virus eventually prevails in the absence of specific therapy and fulminant AIDS develops. Moreover, evidence indicates that abnormal cytokine stimulation in HIV-infected patients and imbalances in immune responses are an integral part of the disease process. At the same time, certain elements of the specific immune response against HIV slow down the progression to AIDS, and a judicious boosting of the immune system (or of the specific response to HIV) might prove to be advantageous to HIV-infected patients. A variety of experimental approaches to immunorestoration in AIDS are being explored, including cytokines (such as interleukin-2 [IL-2] or -12), immunostimulatory drugs, and extracorporeal expansion of immune elements. Recent evidence shows that periodic administration of IL-2, in combination with antiretroviral therapy, may induce increases in CD4 counts in certain patients. This experimental approach and others to enhance immune response are still under study.

As noted above, combinations of drugs may potentially offer several advantages over a given single agent. Indeed, it is likely that as individual drugs are developed, combination regimens become the mainstay of therapy for HIV infection. The use of several agents may help delay the development of HIV resistance. Also, certain combinations may have synergistic anti-HIV activity and preferentially affect different target cells. Moreover, combinations of drugs with different clinical toxicity profiles, for example AZT and ddC, may permit a sustained anti-HIV effect with reduced toxicity from either drug. Also, there is evidence that sustained elevations of CD4 cells may be attained with AZT plus ddI or AZT plus 3TC, in part because AZT resistance is partially reversed by mutations conferring resistance to ddI or 3TC. The potential number of permutations of drug combinations is large, and clinical studies are needed to sort out the relative merits of these approaches. Some drugs may be useful in suppressing certain opportunistic infections and thus have a secondary effect on HIV infection. For example, acyclovir can suppress herpes viruses and might thus indirectly reduce HIV infection (a nuclear regulatory protein of herpes viruses can activate HIV replication). The combination of AZT and acyclovir is usually tolerated by patients and is used by some physicians, particularly for patients who are troubled by recurrent herpes infection. Physicians should be cautioned against *ad hoc* patient experimentation with combination therapy, as unexpected drug interactions may occur.

GENERAL RECOMMENDATIONS

At present, four drugs are approved for the treatment of HIV infection. Results of a number of clinical trials have provided some guidance for using these agents. At the same time, however, different trials have sometimes provided conflicting results, and many questions remain about the optimal therapy of patients at different stages of their disease. In June of 1993, a panel convened by the National Institute of Allergy and Infectious Diseases sifted through the available data and made recommendations for the antiretroviral treatment of HIV infection (Table 371–4).

The panel recommended that symptomatic patients with < 500 CD4 cells per cubic millimeter or asymptomatic patients with < 200 CD4 cells per cubic millimeter start on antiretroviral therapy. The starting therapy of choice is AZT as a single agent, although the panel noted that combination therapy of AZT and ddI or AZT and ddC could also be considered. In a departure from previous recommendations, however, antiretroviral therapy is now considered optional for asymptomatic patients with 200 to 500 CD4 cells per cubic millimeter. Finally, antiretroviral therapy is not generally recommended for patients with > 500 CD4 cells per cubic millimeter outside of the setting of an experimental protocol. As noted in Table 371–4, a change to alternate antiretroviral drugs or combination therapy may be considered in patients who have disease progression on single-agent AZT therapy, and a change to alternate drugs should be considered in patients who cannot tolerate AZT. Finally, the panel recommended that no antiretroviral therapy coupled with supportive care be considered as a legitimate option in patients whose CD4 cell count drifts below 50 cells per cubic millimeter, if they cannot tolerate AZT.

In deciding on the appropriate therapy to use in an individual patient, physicians should consider the toxicity profiles of the various drugs, the specific disease symptoms, and the wishes of the patient. Physicians are advised to institute chemoprophylaxis for *P. carinii* pneumonia when the CD4 count falls below 200 cells per cubic millimeter (see Ch. 365 and 383). Also, chemoprophylaxis for *Mycobacterium avium* infection (see Ch. 312) with rifabutin is recommended for patients whose CD4 count has fallen below 100 cells per cubic millimeter. Yearly vaccinations with killed influenza virus are advisable; however, vaccinations with attenuated viruses should generally be avoided in this population.

Since the recommendations for anti-HIV therapy were made in 1993, results of two large clinical trials (ACTG 175 and Delta) have suggested that it may be worthwhile to begin treatment with a combination regimen. In both trials, one of which included patients with up to 500 cells/mm³, initial therapy with either AZT and ddI or with AZT and ddC was found to be superior to that with AZT alone. In ACTG 175, monotherapy with ddI was found to be superior to AZT and equivalent to the combination regimens. The recommendations for anti-HIV therapy may be modified in the near future in light of these results. Also, 3TC (lamivudine) and some of the protease inhibitors are now available for compassionate use. Physicians should watch for ongoing developments that may profoundly affect accepted medical practice.

✔ **TABLE 371–4. RECOMMENDATIONS FOR ANTIRETROVIRAL THERAPY OF HIV-INFECTED ADULTS FROM A 1993 STATE-OF-THE-ART CONFERENCE**

Clinical Status	CD4 Cell Count Range (cells/mm³)	Recommendation
No previous antiretroviral therapy		
Asymptomatic	> 500	No therapy
Asymptomatic	200–500	Zidovudine or no therapy
Symptomatic	200–500	Zidovudine
Asymptomatic	< 200	Zidovudine
Symptomatic	< 200	Zidovudine*
Previous antiretroviral therapy		
Stable	≥ 300	Continue zidovudine
Stable	< 300	Continue zidovudine or change to didanosine
Progressing	50–500	Change to didanosine or zalcitabine*
Progressing	< 50	Change to didanosine or zalcitabine
Intolerant to zidovudine		
Stable or progressing	> 500	Discontinue antiretroviral therapy
Stable or progressing	50–500	Change to didanosine or zalcitabine
Stable or progressing	< 50	Change to didanosine or zalcitabine†

Recommendations are from a state-of-the-art panel convened by the National Institute of Allergy and Infectious Diseases in June 1993. Modified from Sande MA, Carpenter CCJ, Cobbs G, et al.: Antiretroviral therapy for adult HIV-infected patients. Recommendations from a state-of-the-art conference. JAMA 270: 2583, 1993.

* Some panel members would consider combination therapy with zidovudine plus didanosine or zidovudine plus zalcitabine.

† The option of discontinuing all nucleoside therapy can be considered in this population.

General Review

Johnston MI, Hoth DF: Present status and future prospects for HIV therapies. Science 260:1286, 1993. *Excellent overview of the current status of AIDS therapy. Extensive bibliography.*

Yarchoan R, Pluda JM, Perno CF, et al.: Anti-retroviral therapy of HIV infection: Current strategies and challenges for the future. Blood 78:859, 1991. *Clinical overview of therapeutic approaches now in use.*

Zidovudine

Concorde Coordinating Committee: Concorde: MRC/ANRS randomised double-blind controlled trial of immediate and deferred zidovudine in symptom-free HIV infection. Lancet 343:871, 1994. *Large placebo-controlled trial comparing early and late administration of zidovudine.*

Other Dideoxynucleosides

Abrams DI, Goldman AI, Launer C, et al.: A comparative trial of didanosine or zalcitabine after treatment with zidovudine in patients with human immunodeficiency virus infection. N Engl J Med 330:657, 1994. *Study comparing ddI and ddC as therapy for patients who progressed during AZT treatment or who could not tolerate it.*

Collier AC, Coombs RW, Fischl MA, et al.: Combination therapy with zidovudine and didanosine compared with zidovudine alone in HIV-1 infection. Ann Intern Med 119:786, 1993. *Article describing the combination therapy of AZT and ddI.*

Fischl MA, Stanley K, Collier AC, et al.: Combination and monotherapy with zidovudine and zalcitabine in patients with advanced HIV disease. Ann Intern Med 122:24, 1995. *Comparative trial of combination therapy with AZT and ddC versus monotherapy.*

Kahn JO, Lagakos SW, Richman DD, et al.: A controlled trial comparing continued zidovudine with didanosine in human immunodeficiency virus infection. N Engl J Med 327:581, 1992. *A comparative study of AZT and ddI in patients with at least 16 weeks of prior AZT therapy.*

Spruance SL, Pavia AT, Peterson D, et al.: Didanosine compared with continuation of zidovudine in HIV-infected patients with signs of clinical deterioration while receiving zidovudine. A randomized, double-blind clinical trial. Ann Intern Med 120:360, 1994. *Results of a trial comparing AZT and ddI and extensive prior AZT therapy in patients with AIDS or AIDS-related complex.*

Yarchoan R, Lietzau JA, Nguyen B-Y, et al.: A randomized pilot study of alternating or simultaneous zidovudine and didanosine therapy in patients with symptomatic immunodeficiency virus infection. J Infect Dis 169:9, 1994. *Article comparing alternating and simultaneous regimens of AZT and ddI.*

Resistance

Richman DD: Resistance of clinical isolates of human immunodeficiency virus to anti-retroviral agents. Antimicrob Agents Chemother 37:1207, 1993. *Overview of HIV resistance.*

Recommendations for Therapy

Sande MA, Carpenter CCJ, Cobbs G, et al.: Antiretroviral therapy for adult HIV-infected patients. Recommendations from a state-of-the-art conference. JAMA 270:2583, 1993. *Provides an algorithm for antiretroviral therapy.*

372 MANAGEMENT AND COUNSELING FOR PERSONS WITH HIV INFECTION

John A. Bartlett

Physicians caring for persons with HIV infection must make crucial decisions in chronic management and counseling. The advances of the past 5 years, especially in the prevention and treatment of opportunistic infections, have led to an improved prognosis for patients with symptomatic HIV disease. The median survival for persons after their initial AIDS-defining illness has been extended to 2.5 years. Clinicians may evaluate their patients against a timeline of predictable complications (Fig. 372–1), and they are aided by improved diagnostic examinations and treatment options. The use of *Pneumocystis carinii* pneumonia (PCP) prophylaxis has led to fewer episodes of PCP as a complication of HIV infection, and other manifestations such as disseminated *Mycobacterium avium* complex (MAC) infection, cytomegalovirus (CMV) disease, and unexplained wasting have become more common. These decisions regarding the use of PCP prophylaxis and diligent attention to the early diagnosis and treatment of opportunistic infections have become incorporated into standards for clinical practice. However, some clinical decisions remain controversial, such as the optimal point for starting antiretroviral therapy, the use of combinations of antiretroviral therapy, and the use of prophylaxis against MAC. The clinician must practice HIV medicine in the context of an evolving knowledge base in which the results of clinical trials may not be absolute. Patients may be well informed about their illness and wish to participate in the decision-making process, to which they may make important contributions. In this environment the clinician has the opportunity to practice both the science and art of medicine, and the successful chronic management and counseling of HIV-infected persons offers the potential for dramatic rewards.

HIV PATHOGENESIS

The optimal choice of treatment(s) for HIV-infected persons must be guided by an understanding of viral pathogenesis (see Ch. 361). Advances in the past 5 years have resulted in an improved understanding of HIV pathogenesis, but many basic pathophysiologic questions remain unanswered. The relatively modest clinical impact of antiretroviral therapy is at least partially a reflection of this incomplete understanding, further complicated by repeated frustrations in the development of antiretroviral drugs (see Ch. 371).

Soon after the acquisition of HIV, the virus may achieve high levels, as assessed by quantitative virus culture, viral (p24) antigen detection, or polymerase chain reaction (PCR) for viral nucleic acids. After 2 to 4 weeks of this initial highly viremic phase, the amount of virus in the peripheral bloodstream significantly decreases, perhaps coincident with the generation of HIV-specific cellular immune responses. Despite the decreases in peripheral bloodstream viremia, HIV RNA can be detected by PCR in peripheral

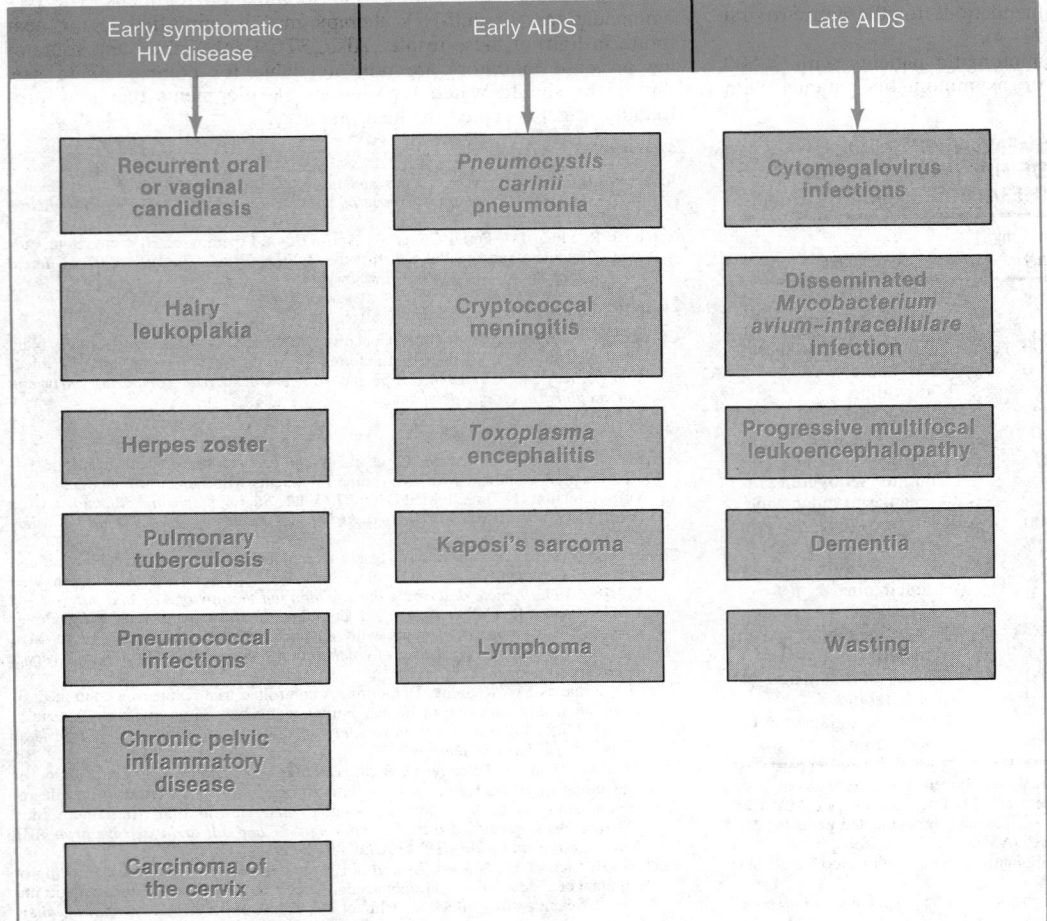

FIGURE 372–1. Time line of AIDS-related complications.

blood, even during asymptomatic HIV infection. The detection of HIV RNA suggests active HIV replication. New evidence indicates that HIV becomes predominately localized in lymphoid tissues during this period, especially lymph nodes, thymus, gastrointestinal lymphoid tissue such as Peyer's patches, and tissue macrophages in bone marrow, liver, spleen, and skin. HIV is concentrated in the germinal centers of lymph nodes during early HIV infection, and viral particles are frequently found there immediately adjacent to the processes of follicular dendritic cells, an area where activated T lymphocytes migrate for antigen recognition. In this microenvironment, uninfected activated CD4+ T lymphocytes may become HIV infected. This process may be further accelerated by the local production of tumor necrosis factor and interleukins-1 and -6 from B lymphocytes. These cytokines activate CD4+ T lymphocytes and macrophages, thus further increasing their susceptibility to and production of HIV. Thus, lymphoid tissue constitutes an important reservoir of ongoing viral replication, even during the asymptomatic period when less virus can be recovered from the peripheral bloodstream. As HIV infection progresses, normal lymph node architecture is destroyed and replaced with even larger amounts of virus, and in peripheral blood, increasing amounts of viral nucleic acid, p24 antigen, and culturable virus can be detected. These observations reinforce the need for effective antiretroviral therapy to control HIV replication.

However, direct viral infection and subsequent destruction of CD4+ T lymphocytes does not explain the entirety of HIV pathogenesis. Only 0.01 to 10% of circulating CD4+ lymphocytes contain viral nucleic acids, and this observation suggests that additional processes may contribute to CD4+ lymphocyte depletion. Experimental evidence suggests that autoimmune processes and the chronic immunologic activation of HIV infection may also participate in the destruction of CD4+ lymphocytes. Finally, little is known about important elements in the reconstitution of immunologic responses in an HIV-infected person. Current antiretroviral therapy provides only modest and transient rises in circulating CD4+ lymphocytes. Improved antiretroviral therapies may provide larger and more sustained increases, but given the alterations in lymphoid tissue including the thymus, lymph nodes, and bone marrow, the goal of immunologic reconstitution must consider abnormalities in these microenvironments.

CLINICAL EVALUATION OF THE PATIENT

The clinical approach to the HIV-infected patient should be guided by several important principles. First, it is important to establish the degree of immunosuppression in every patient through the history and physical examination and the measurement of absolute CD4+ lymphocyte count. Second, past histories of sexually transmitted diseases (STD's), positive PPD testing or exposure to tuberculosis, and places of residence may be very useful in predicting complications of HIV infection. Third, the sharing of pertinent medical information with patients may improve the quality of personal observations that they report to the physician in subsequent visits, and may also improve the physician's ability to establish early diagnoses, provide effective outpatient treatment, and communicate regarding treatment options and risk reduction. Information regarding the stage of HIV disease, and thus the degree of immunosuppression, provides important insight into predicting clinical complications and guiding therapeutic decisions. Such a clinical approach allows the physician to optimize the chronic management and counseling of HIV-infected persons.

THE INITIAL EVALUATION. The initial evaluation of an HIV-infected person should begin with a careful history of past evaluations for HIV infection. Previous history of risk behaviors, mononucleosis-like symptoms that could represent acute HIV infection, and previous HIV testing may all offer insight into the duration of HIV infection. Previous CD4+ lymphocyte counts, history of AIDS indicator conditions, or other clinical manifestations of HIV infection assist in establishing the patient's CDC (Centers for Disease Control and Prevention) classification of HIV infection (Fig. 372–2). The physician must also elicit a medical history, especially a history of STD's (syphilis, herpes simplex, hepatitis B, genital or perianal warts, and cervical dysplasia as important examples), past PPD testing or exposure to tuberculosis, substance abuse, and medication allergies. On physical examination, particular attention should be focused on the skin (severe seborrhea, molluscum contagiosum, chronic herpetic ulcerations, and Kaposi's sarcoma all suggest progressive HIV infection), lymph nodes (generalized lymphadenopathy usually correlates with earlier HIV infection and involution may signal progression of disease), oropharynx (candidiasis, oral hairy leukoplakia, and Kaposi's sarcoma indicate progression), genitalia (severe warts, recurrent vaginal candidiasis, frequently recurrent or severe herpetic ulcerations, cervical dysplasia, and Kaposi's sarcoma suggest progression), and central nervous system (neurocognitive and memory deficits suggest progression to AIDS dementia). The initial laboratory examination should include a complete blood count with differential, routine chemistries including liver enzymes and serum creatinine, absolute CD4+ lymphocyte count and CD4+ lymphocyte percentage, and syphilis and toxoplasma serologies. Patients should also undergo 5 TU PPD testing, and a positive response in an HIV-infected patient is defined as ≥5 mm induration. All HIV-infected patients should receive the pneumococcal pneumonia vaccine because of their increased risk of pneumococcal infections, and the influenza vaccine yearly. The hepatitis B vaccine may be given to previously uninfected patients.

Once the initial evaluation is complete (Table 372–1), the physician should be able to establish a CDC classification and use it to design a therapeutic plan. In addition, potential coinfections with *Treponema pallidum* or *Mycobacterium tuberculosis* should be recognized and treated for personal and public health benefits. Finally, counseling may result in the reduction of risk behaviors through education and the identification and treatment of substance abuse.

SUBSEQUENT EVALUATIONS. The intensity and frequency of follow-up examinations depend upon individual patient characteristics and progression of HIV disease. Absolute CD4+ lymphocyte counts should be followed at least every 6 months when ≥200 cells per cubic millimeter and should be followed more closely if they are rapidly changing or nearing a therapeutic landmark.

EVALUATING THE FEBRILE PATIENT. Fever is a common physical finding among patients with HIV infection, and the potential causes are many. Fever may indicate a self-limited viral upper respiratory tract infection in a patient with early HIV infection or the presence of PCP in a patient with progressive HIV infection. Differentiating the clinical manifestations of the two infections may be difficult for the physician; therefore, the physician should use any available information on HIV staging for the patient. In this context, the absolute CD4 lymphocyte count may be an extremely useful guide in assessing the likelihood of opportunistic infections. If the absolute CD4 lymphocyte count is >200 cells per cubic mil-

FIGURE 372–2. CDC Classification System for HIV Infection. The shaded areas (classes A3, B3, C1-3) meet the CDC definition of AIDS. PGL = Progressive generalized lymphadenopathy.

	A Asymptomatic or PGL	B Early symptomatic HIV disease	C AIDS Indicator Conditions
1 CD4 > 500/mm³	A1	B1	C1
2 CD4 200-499/mm³	A2	B2	C2
3 CD4 < 200/mm³	A3	B3	C3

TABLE 372-1. INITIAL EVALUATION OF HIV-INFECTED PATIENTS

History
   How long have they been infected with HIV?
   What complications of HIV have occurred?
   What past evaluations have they undergone?
   What past treatments have they received?
   Any past history of STD's?
   Past history of positive PPD or exposure to tuberculosis?
   Medications and allergies?
   Substance abuse?
   Residential history?

Physical examination

Laboratory evaluation
   CBC with differential
   Chemistries including liver enzymes and serum creatinine
   Absolute CD4+ lymphocyte count and CD4+ lymphocyte percentage
   Syphilis and toxoplasma serologies

PPD testing

Immunizations
   Pneumococcal vaccine
   Influenza vaccine
   Hepatitis B vaccine if nonimmune

limeter, the likelihood of PCP or other opportunistic infections is significantly decreased. Thus, the absolute CD4 lymphocyte count may guide the most appropriate diagnostic considerations. Of note, the uncommon patient may present with an opportunistic infection at absolute CD4+ lymphocyte counts >200 cells per cubic millimeter; therefore, it is imperative to reconsider such diagnoses if the fever persists.

The source of fever is most frequently identified by a patient's history and physical examination; a directed diagnostic evaluation may then be undertaken. If no immediate source is apparent, patients with progressive HIV infection should have a blood culture for MAC and a serum cryptococcal antigen performed. Patients with persistent unexplained fevers may require repeated clinical and laboratory evaluations to elucidate its cause.

See Ch. 371 for discussion of specific antiretroviral therapies.

As HIV infection progresses, it creates increasing immunosuppression resulting in a predisposition to complicating opportunistic infections and neoplasms (Figs. 372–1 and 372–3). The pattern of these complications can be predicted by following a patient's absolute CD4+ lymphocyte count. On the basis of these correlations between absolute CD4+ lymphocytes and the predicted complications of HIV infection, clinicians can anticipate an increased risk of certain opportunistic infections in an individual patient, which may lead to an earlier diagnosis or the use of antimicrobial prophylaxis to prevent specific opportunistic infections. Successful prophylaxis has been identified against PCP, toxoplasmic encephalitis, disseminated MAC infection, and cryptococcal meningitis (Table 372–2).

Persons at highest risk for PCP include those recovering from their first episode (secondary prophylaxis, 1-year risk of recurrence without prophylaxis 60%), those with absolute CD4+ lymphocytes ≤200 cells per cubic millimeter (primary prophylaxis, 1-year risk of PCP ≥ 18%), those with CD4+ lymphocyte percentages <20%, and those with a non-PCP AIDS indicator condition (both primary prophylaxis). Sulfamethoxazole-trimethoprim (SMX-TMP) is the most successful prophylaxis against PCP, and dapsone or aerosolized pentamidine may be used as alternative prophylactic regimens in patients intolerant of SMX-TMP. SMX-TMP probably can also prevent toxoplasmic encephalitis among patients who are seropositive for previous infection with *Toxoplasma gondii*.

Recent clinical trials have demonstrated that rifabutin can delay disseminated MAC infection. Rifabutin is FDA-approved for patients at highest risk, usually those with absolute CD4+ lymphocytes <100 cells per cubic millimeter. Fluconazole has also demonstrated efficacy in delaying cryptococcal meningitis in patients with absolute CD4+ lymphocytes <200 cells per cubic millimeter. Important longer-term issues that still need to be resolved with the use of rifabutin and fluconazole as prophylaxes include their effectiveness over prolonged periods, the possible evolution of resistance among MAC and cryptococcal isolates, pharmacokinetic interactions with other drugs commonly prescribed for patients with AIDS, and uncertain cost effectiveness.

PCP was once the most common AIDS indicator condition, but HIV-associated wasting, disseminated MAC infection, and CMV disease are now more common clinical manifestations. Undoubtedly the future complications of progressive HIV infection will continue to evolve as improved prophylactic strategies against additional opportunistic infections are identified and survival lengthens for persons with AIDS.

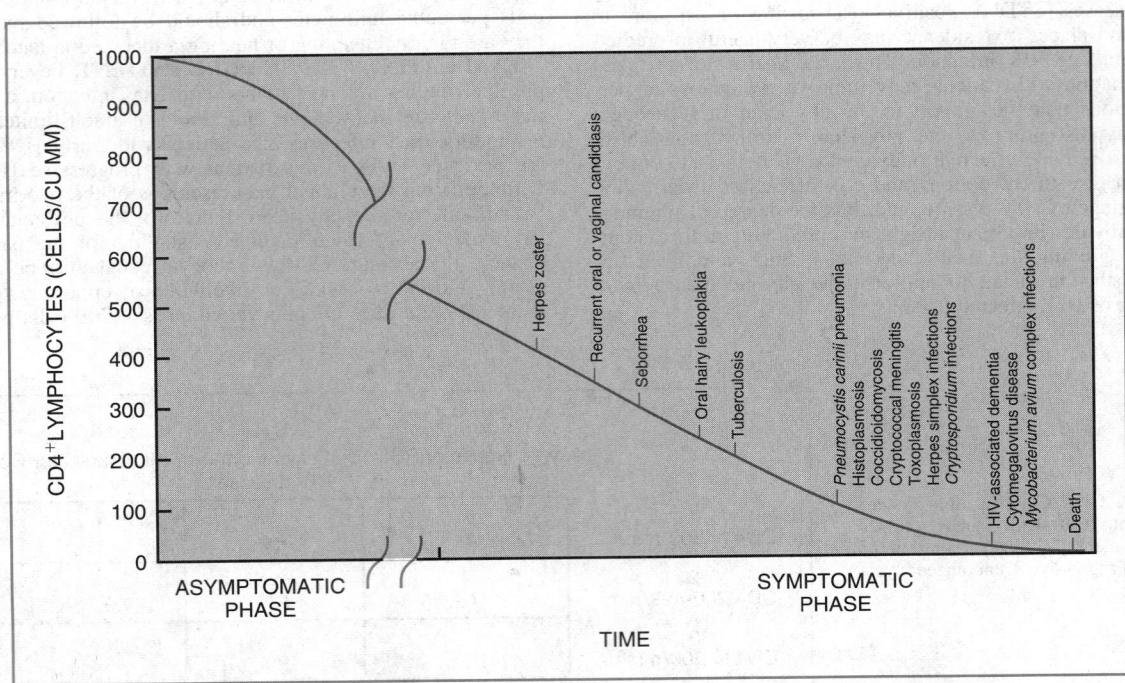

FIGURE 372-3. Complications of HIV disease as related to lymphocyte count.

TABLE 372–2. PROPHYLAXIS OF OPPORTUNISTIC INFECTIONS

Infection	Available Agents	Comments
Pneumocystis carinii pneumonia	SMX-TMP	SMX-TMP most effective and least expensive but potentially toxic
	Dapsone	
	Aerosolized pentamidine	
Mycobacterium avium complex (MAC)	Rifabutin	Delay in disseminated MAC infection; costly; pharmacokinetic interaction with zidovudine; emergence of resistance unknown
Toxoplasmic encephalitis	SMX-TMP?	Preliminary data encouraging
Cryptococcal meningitis	Fluconazole	Delay in cryptococcal meningitis but costly; emergence of fungal resistance reported but of uncertain significance

SMX-TMP = sulfamethoxazole-trimethoprim.

When patients do develop opportunistic infections, clinicians should attempt to establish a diagnosis and initiate treatment as soon as possible. Early diagnosis results in an improved prognosis for most opportunistic infections, and with early diagnosis many patients may receive outpatient therapy. Successful outpatient therapy frequently results in greater patient satisfaction and lower health care costs.

Wasting is also a common complication of progressive HIV infection, either associated primarily with HIV itself or as a secondary manifestation of an opportunistic infection or neoplasm. The pathogenesis of HIV-associated wasting involves multiple potential processes: anorexia with decreased caloric intake, nausea and vomiting, intestinal malabsorption due to HIV enteropathy or an opportunistic infection in the gut, and the ineffective use of nutrients. The metabolic disarray induced in wasted patients with HIV infection results in profound catabolism, perhaps mediated by cytokines such as tumor necrosis factor, and interleukin-1 and -6. Reversing the wasting process may be extremely difficult; attempts to treat opportunistic infections, neoplasms, and the underlying HIV infection can improve nutritional status. Megestrol acetate and dronabinol have been used with modest success to stimulate appetite. Nutritional support may provide improvement in some patients, but in many the catabolism of late-stage HIV infection and its complications cannot be overcome.

COUNSELING

Counseling HIV-infected patients can present great challenges to their physicians. Many HIV-infected persons enter the physician-patient relationship with significant emotional distress and numerous complicating circumstances. These complicating circumstances can include issues of sexual orientation and sexuality, the need for risk reduction, substance abuse, societal discrimination, and increasing poverty as the epidemic evolves in the United States. The physician must enter this relationship prepared to address these issues with knowledge and compassion and without becoming judgmental about their content.

A crucial component involved in counseling HIV-infected persons is education concerning HIV disease, its transmission, and its potential treatments. This process should continue for the duration of the physician-patient relationship, and given the extensive knowledge base of many persons with HIV infection, there may be a mutual exchange of important information. The best medical interventions will not succeed unless HIV-infected persons have been carefully counseled regarding their potential benefits, costs, and acquisition. A well-informed patient can be a strong ally in tackling difficult therapeutic decisions, and many therapeutic decisions are currently not straightforward, such as the optimal time to initiate antiretroviral therapy. A well-informed patient may better recognize the early manifestations of HIV-related clinical complications and potential drug toxicities. Finally, a well-informed patient can constructively guide decisions regarding advance directives for his/her care if HIV disease progresses.

Education regarding the transmission of HIV and alterations in risk behavior is another important goal of counseling. Efforts to encourage behavioral changes resulting in temporarily decreased HIV transmission have succeeded in homosexual men in San Francisco, although recent evidence suggests an increasing number of new infections, especially among young individuals. Intensive efforts to decrease HIV transmission have also succeeded in smaller populations of injecting drug users and high-risk heterosexuals. All patients should be well informed regarding safer sex precautions and the avoidance of needle sharing. This information must be presented in language appropriate to the culture of the patient. Significant behavioral changes are frequently not accomplished during a single visit, and enduring change requires ongoing re-education and support from the physician.

Treating substance abuse (see Ch. 12) is crucial in decreasing the risk of HIV transmission through needle sharing and sexual contact and in avoiding the medical and psychological consequences of continued substance abuse. Physicians must advocate for their patients in seeking access to frequently inadequate and overwhelmed drug treatment programs. Physicians must acknowledge the high recidivism rates associated with substance abuse and continue to treat their recidivous patients firmly and without judgment. Finally, physicians should reinforce positively those recovering addicts who have succeeded in treatment and struggle to avoid relapse on a daily basis.

The clinical course of persons with HIV infection is frequently complicated by significant anxiety and depression. Pharmacologic measures may prove useful in their management, although anxiolytics should be used cautiously, given the prevalence of substance abuse in this population. In the circumstance of late-stage HIV infection complicated by HIV encephalopathy and depression, ritalin may prove useful. Physicians should identify AIDS service organizations in their community that may provide support services such as patient education, case management, transportation, shelter, food, medications, or support groups to their clients. Formal psychiatric referral may also be necessary in individual patients.

Complications

Hoover D, Saah A, Bacellar H, et al.: Clinical manifestations of AIDS in the era of pneumocystis prophylaxis. N Engl J Med 329:1922, 1993. *Reviews the changing clinical complications of AIDS.*
Nightingale S, Cameron W, Gordin F, et al.: Two controlled trials of rifabutin prophylaxis against *Mycobacterium avium* complex infection in AIDS. N Engl J Med 329:828, 1993. *The reports of two pivotal trials evaluating rifabutin prophylaxis against MAC infection.*

Counseling

Bartlett JG: Medical Management of HIV Infection. Glenview, IL, Physicians and Scientists Publishing Co., 1994. *A review for health care professionals describing the medical management of HIV-infected persons.*
Cates W, Hinman A: AIDS and absolutism—the demand for perfection in prevention. N Engl J Med 327:492, 1992. *Describes preventive measures for HIV infection and their role in public health.*
Hellinger F: The lifetime cost of treating a person with HIV. JAMA 270:474, 1993. *An informative review of the costs associated with treating HIV-infected persons.*

PART XXIII

DISEASES OF PROTOZOA AND METAZOA

373 INTRODUCTION TO PROTOZOAN AND HELMINTHIC DISEASES

Adel A. F. Mahmoud

Human infections with parasitic protozoa and helminths account for a major proportion of the diseases caused by infectious agents. The magnitude of these infections is staggering; malaria infects 600 million, and ascariasis and trichuriasis 1 billion each, and 600 million are estimated to be infected with either schistosomiasis or filariasis. In spite of some worldwide efforts to control the spread and consequences of these infections, the associated morbidity and mortality have not been appreciably reduced. Furthermore, in the developed countries, infection with protozoa and helminths is being seen with increasing frequency in immigrants and is also among the more important causes of disease in the growing number of patients with depressed immune responses.

BIOLOGY OF PARASITIC PROTOZOA AND HELMINTHS

The host-parasite relationship in protozoan and helminthic infections is complex because of the distinctive biologic features of the organisms. Although protozoa are unicellular pathogens and are mainly microscopic in size, they are far larger than viruses and bacteria. Protozoa multiply within mammalian hosts, as do viruses, bacteria, and fungi. Infection, therefore, can be initiated by a relatively small inoculum of organisms, which then multiply within the host and reach the numbers that cause disease.

By contrast, helminths are multicellular organisms with well-developed organ structures. They vary in size from 1 cm to approximately 10 meters. Unlike other infectious agents, helminths do not multiply within mammalian hosts. Re-exposure is, therefore, necessary to increase the number of helminths in a host. This distinguishing feature has important clinical significance, as disease in most helminthiasis is closely related to intensity of infection. For example, anemia results from hookworm infection only if the individual is harboring a significant worm load or there are other reasons for nutritional deficiencies. In rare circumstances, such as strongyloidiasis in the immunosuppressed, the worm can increase population of its larval stage in humans through the autoinfection cycle.

Eosinophilia, when present, is a useful clinical manifestation of worm infections that migrate in host tissues. Worms that reside exclusively in body cavities, such as adult cestodes in the lumen of small intestine, are not associated with eosinophilia. Specific chemotherapy is usually followed by an increase in eosinophil count before it subsides to normal levels. Eosinophilia in helminthic infections may be related to the cell's ability to kill multicellular organisms. Because of the large size of most invading worms, these targets are killed by eosinophils extracellulary and killing is mediated by a combination of oxidative and nonoxidative mechanisms.

Parasitic protozoa and helminths have developed elaborate mechanisms for evading host protective responses. One of the best studied is antigenic variation noted in African trypanosomiasis. Parasitemia in infected individuals appears in waves, each representing a new parasite variable antigen. The trypanosomes are capable of expressing at least 100 different variable antigens, allowing a long chronic course of infection. The organisms contain individual genes for all the different variable glycoproteins, but only one is expressed at a time. The multiplicity of trypanosome variable glycoprotein genes and of mechanisms for introducing mutations into them illustrates the complexity and sophistication of the evasion techniques used by these pathogens.

The constantly changing nature of infectious disease is best illustrated in parasitic protozoan and helminthic infections. For example, new human pathogens such as *Isospora* and *Cryptosporidium* species have been appreciated only recently as causes of diarrheal illness, particularly in the immunosuppressed. These new developments add to difficulties in treating and controlling parasitic protozoa and helminths. Recently, new chemotherapeutic agents have been developed, such as praziquantel and ivermectin, which are safe and effective broad-spectrum antihelminthics. However, the ever-spreading resistance of the parasites causing malaria and their mosquito vectors to most available compounds is imposing a considerable challenge to clinicians and public health specialists.

APPROACH TO THE PATIENT WITH PROTOZOAN OR HELMINTHIC INFECTION

Because most of the clinical manifestations of protozoan and helminthic diseases are not specific or pathognomonic, a high degree of suspicion is essential. The simple question "Where have you been?" and knowledge of the general geographic distribution of parasitic protozoa and helminths often save exhaustive and costly diagnostic workups and may spare human lives. Furthermore, inquiry into the immune status of individual patients, other drug therapies, or other diseases may be helpful in establishing the diagnosis of an opportunistic protozoan or helminthic infection.

The next phase in attempting to reach correct diagnosis involves interpreting the presenting symptoms and signs. Peripheral blood eosinophilia remains an important and early indication of infections with tissue-invading worms. Definitive diagnosis in most cases requires isolation and identification of the specific pathogen. Because the number of cases seen by any single laboratory in North America is limited, expertise is required for correct identification that may not be available to many practicing physicians. Serologic testing for evidence of exposure to specific protozoa or helminths is currently available in many clinical or state laboratories or by consultation with the Centers for Disease Control and Prevention.

Centers for Disease Control: HHS Publication No. (CDC) 94-8280. Health Information for International Travel, Atlanta, Georgia, 1994, 188 pp. *A review of the geographic distribution of worldwide infections, updated yearly. It also contains the most recent recommendations for prophylaxis.*

Drugs for parasitic infections. Med Lett Drugs 35:111, 1993. *A review of antiparasitic drugs published and updated annually. It includes dose, availability, and alternative choices.*

Mahmoud AAF: Parasitic protozoa and helminths: Biological and immunological challenges. Science 246:1015, 1989. *A selected review of some of the unique biologic, immunologic, and molecular aspects of malaria and schistosomes that accounts for the ability of these organisms to invade and establish themselves as parasites in humans.*

Mahmoud AAF (ed.): Tropical and Geographical Medicine. 2nd ed. Companion Handbook. New York, McGraw-Hill, 1993. *Clinical, epidemiologic, and management principles for dealing with infectious diseases seen in North America and worldwide.*

Warren KS, Mahmoud AAF (eds.): Tropical and Geographical Medicine. 2nd ed. New York, McGraw-Hill, 1990. *Detailed description of the biology and molecular understanding of protozoa and helminths and the diseases they cause in individuals and in populations.*

Protozoan Diseases

374 MALARIA
Donald J. Krogstad

Malaria is a disease characterized by recurrent fever and chills associated with the synchronous lysis of parasitized red blood cells. Its name is derived from the belief of the ancient Romans that malaria was due to the bad air of the marshes surrounding Rome.

ETIOLOGY. Malaria is produced by intraerythrocytic parasites of the genus *Plasmodium.* Four plasmodia produce malaria in humans: *Plasmodium falciparum, P. vivax, P. ovale,* and *P. malariae.* The severity and characteristic manifestations of the disease are governed by the infecting species, the magnitude of the parasitemia, the metabolic effects of the parasite, and the cytokines released as a result of the infection.

INCIDENCE, PREVALENCE, AND RESURGENCE. Incidence. Although precise data are difficult to obtain, malaria is unquestionably one of the most common infectious diseases. At least 200 to 300 million cases of malaria occur each year, with 1 to 2 million deaths. Most deaths are due to *P. falciparum* infection and occur among children less than 5 years old in sub-Saharan Africa. One of the major unanswered questions about malaria is how plasmodia produce repetitive infections without stimulating an effective (protective) immune response.

Prevalence. The prevalence of malaria varies widely; it may reach 70 to 80% or more among children in hyperendemic areas during the transmission season. Thus its impact on the health of the developing world is enormous.

Resurgence. The major factors responsible for the resurgence of malaria are drug resistances: (1) the widespread resistance of the anopheline vector to economical insecticides such as chlorophenothane (DDT), and (2) the increasing prevalence of chloroquine resistance in *P. falciparum,* which is now endemic in South America, Southeast Asia, and Africa.

LIFE CYCLE AND EPIDEMIOLOGY. *Life Cycle.* The life cycle can be viewed as beginning with synchronous asexual replication of the erythrocytic stage of the parasite (Fig. 374–1). During the asexual erythrocytic cycle, the parasites mature from rings to trophozoites to schizonts, which ultimately rupture the red cell and release merozoites that enter uninfected red cells via receptors such as Duffy factor in *P. vivax;* the cycle is then repeated. By contrast, some erythrocytic parasites mature to sexual forms (gametocytes) that are ingested by the female anopheline mosquito. Within the mosquito intermediate host, male and female gametocytes mature to gametes, fuse to form an ookinete that matures to a zygote and ultimately produces the sporozoites that are infectious for humans. When an infected mosquito bites a human, sporozoites travel via the bloodstream to the liver, where they enter hepatocytes and mature to tissue schizonts, which release merozoites that are infectious for red cells and produce the asexual erythrocytic cycle. Two of the four species that infect humans (*P. vivax* and *P. ovale*) produce dormant (hypnozoite) forms in the liver, which mature 6 to 11 months or more after the initial infection and thus produce relapsing malaria.

Two characteristics of the life cycle are essential for the long-term survival of the parasite: multiplicity of replication and antigenic variability. *Multiplicity of replication* is apparent at each stage of the life cycle. The mature asexual erythrocytic schizont releases 8 to 32 merozoites when it ruptures its host red cell; up to 10,000 sporozoites result from one zygote; and 10,000 to 30,000 merozoites are released from one tissue (exoerythrocytic) schizont in the liver. This multiplicity of replication provides a redundancy that protects the parasite against losses from both immune and nonimmune host factors. *Antigenic variability* is associated with the morphologic changes that occur during the parasite's life cycle and similarly protects the parasite against the host immune response. For example, antibodies against sporozoites are ineffective against the asexual erythrocytic stages of the parasite. Similarly, immune responses directed against asexual erythrocytic stages have no effect against the sexual (gametocyte) stages of the parasite. In addition, antigenic variation exists among strains of the same species. These

FIGURE 374–1. Life cycle of the malaria parasite. The lower and upper halves of the diagram indicate the anopheline mosquito and human parts of the cycle, respectively. Sporozoites from the salivary gland of a female *Anopheles* mosquito are injected under the skin (1). They then travel through the bloodstream to the liver (2) and mature within hepatocytes to tissue *schizonts* (4). Up to 30,000 parasites are then released into the bloodstream as *merozoites* (5) and produce symptomatic infection as they invade and destroy red blood cells. However, some parasites remain dormant in the liver as *hypnozoites (2, dashed lines from 1 to 3).* These are the parasites that cause relapsing malaria (in *P. vivax* or *P. ovale* infection). Once within the bloodstream, merozoites (5) invade red cells (6) and mature to the *ring* (7,8), *trophozoite* (9), and *schizont* (10) asexual stages. Schizonts lyse their host red cells as they mature and release the next generation of merozoites (11), which invade previously uninfected red cells. Within the red cell some parasites differentiate to sexual forms (male and female *gametocytes*) (12). When taken up by a female *Anopheles* mosquito, the gametocytes mature to *male* and *female gametes,* which produce zygotes (14). The zygote invades the gut of the mosquito (15) and develops into an *oocyst* (16). Mature oocysts produce *sporozoites,* which migrate to the salivary gland of the mosquito (1) and repeat the cycle. The dashed line between 12 and 13 indicates that absence of the mosquito vector prevents natural transmission via this cycle. Infection by the injection of contaminated blood bypasses this constraint and permits transmission among intravenous drug addicts or to recipients of blood transfusions. (Reproduced with permission from Krogstad DJ: Blood and tissue protozoa. *In* Schaechter M, Medoff G, Eisenstein BI [eds.]: Mechanisms of Microbial Diseases. 2nd ed © 1993, p 600, the Williams & Wilkins Company, Baltimore.)

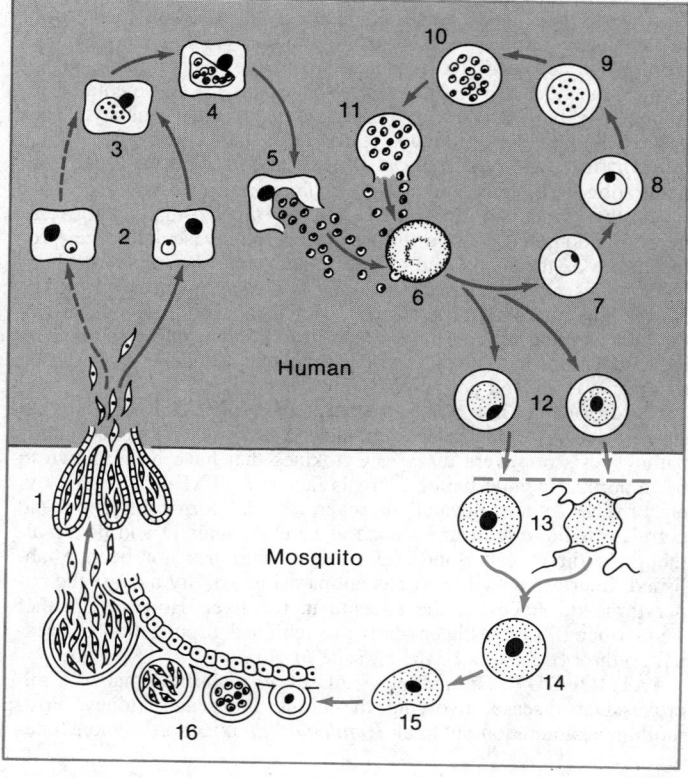

observations are critically relevant to the development of a malaria vaccine (see below).

Epidemiology. The epidemiology of malaria is determined by the distributions of the anopheline mosquito vectors required for natural transmission and of the infected human reservoir. Both factors are present in endemic areas throughout the tropics. Important determinants of transmission include the vector population (vectors such as *Anopheles gambiae* in Africa are thought to be more efficient), temperature (elevated temperatures shorten the life of the vector and hasten the maturation of the parasite within the vector), and control programs (which reduce both the vector population and the prevalence of human infection).

Competent mosquito vectors are present in the United States (*A. albimanus* in the east and *A. freeborni* in the west). Although transmission in the United States is limited by the absence of infected humans, natural mosquito-borne transmission can and does occur with the importation of infected humans (e.g., the return of soldiers after their exposure in endemic areas). Mosquito-borne transmission *(introduced malaria)* occurred in the United States after World War II, the Korean War, the Vietnam War, and the arrival of refugees from Southeast Asia.

PATHOGENESIS. Species-Dependent Factors. Malaria is a multifactorial disease that can be explained in part, but not completely, by the magnitude of the parasitemia. *P. falciparum* is the most lethal parasite because it can invade red cells of any age and can thus produce unrestricted parasitemias involving 10^6 or more parasitized red cells per cubic millimeter of blood ($\geq 20\%$ of circulating red cells). Conversely, *P. vivax* and *P. ovale,* which invade only young red cells, are limited to parasitemias $\leq 25,000$ per cubic millimeter, and *P. malariae,* which invades only older red cells, is limited to parasitemias $\leq 10,000$ per cubic millimeter.

The Host Immune Response. Because millions of people experience repetitive episodes of malaria throughout their lives in the tropics, the immune response to natural infection is inadequate by definition. Thus the term *semi-immune* is used for residents of endemic areas who are at reduced risk of severe or complicated malaria but are reinfected regularly. The reasons for the inadequate host immune response are only partially clear and are likely to be central to developing a successful vaccine. For example, most exposed persons make antibodies directed against the repetitive epitope or epitopes on the surface of the sporozoite, and antibodies to asexual stages have been shown to reduce the magnitude of the parasitemia in children. However, cell-mediated immune responses are less frequent and may be essential for effective immunity. At least two factors have been identified that may be relevant to the poor cell-mediated response to sporozoite antigen: (1) The sites that determine the cell-mediated response are in the hypervariable region of the molecule, and (2) the ability to produce a cell-mediated response may be restricted by the individual's human leukocyte antigen (HLA) haplotype (immune restriction).

Peripheral Sequestration of Parasitized Red Cells. With maturation, red cells containing *P. falciparum* parasites develop knobs that contain histidine-rich proteins. *In vivo,* these knobs adhere to endothelial cells in the peripheral microvasculature via proteins such as thrombospondin, intercellular adhesion molecule 1, or CD36. This phenomenon has at least two consequences: (1) It enhances the microvascular obstruction and pathology produced by the parasite, and (2) it removes mature *P. falciparum* parasites from the circulation, so that only early asexual erythrocytic stages, such as rings, are seen on peripheral blood smears.

Cytokines in the Pathogenesis of Malaria. Recent studies suggest that cytokine release in malaria is a central factor in the pathogenesis of severe disease. Cytokines that have been shown to be important include tumor necrosis factor-α (TNF-α). Serum levels of TNF-α are elevated in severe *P. falciparum* infection and correlate with complications such as cerebral malaria and death, although a direct cause-and-effect relationship has not been established. Interferon-γ (IFN-γ) has antiparasitic activity against the exoerythrocytic stages of the parasite in the liver. However, neither TNF-α nor IFN-γ has been shown to inhibit the replication of asexual erythrocytic stages of the parasite *in vitro.*

PATHOLOGY. The pathology of severe malaria is that of a microvascular disease involving the brain, lung, and kidney. Postmortem examination in fatal *P. falciparum* infection demonstrates parasitized red cells in the capillaries of the brain and other affected organs. In severe cases, acute tubular necrosis may be present, and the liver, spleen, and other sites in the reticuloendothelial system may be filled with dark malarial pigment from the phagocytosis of parasitized red cells. This predominantly microvascular pathology is consistent with the importance of sequestration and cytokine release in the pathogenesis of severe *P. falciparum* malaria (see above). By contrast, the other malarias that infect humans produce lower parasitemias, do not sequester, and are rarely fatal.

CLINICAL MANIFESTATIONS. Fever and Chills. Most patients with malaria have recurrent fever and chills (at 48-hour intervals for *P. vivax* and *P. ovale* and at 72-hour intervals for *P. malariae*). By contrast, patients with *P. falciparum* infection typically have irregular fever and chills and rarely present with a regular 48-hour cycle of symptoms despite the 48-hour cycle of the parasite.

Coma. Coma (cerebral malaria) is the most feared complication of *P. falciparum* infection and has a substantial fatality rate. Although it has been attributed to the blockage of capillaries with parasitized red cells, both hypoglycemia and the effects of cytokines such as TNF-α are important factors. Hypoglycemia in *P. falciparum* malaria may have at least three causes: (1) insulin released from the pancreatic β cell by quinine or quinidine during treatment, (2) glucose consumption by the massive numbers of parasites present in the patient, and (3) liver glycogen depletion in persons who have not eaten for several days before seeking medical care because they were ill with malaria. Hypoglycemia is particularly important to consider because it is treatable. Although the effects of TNF-α undoubtedly contribute to cerebral malaria, it is difficult to separate them from the magnitude of the parasitemia because the concentration of TNF-α and the magnitude of the parasitemia correlate with each other.

Renal Failure. Patients with massive parasitemias may have dark urine from the free hemoglobin produced by hemolysis (blackwater fever) and may later develop renal failure. Although hemolysis alone should not produce renal failure, some degree of renal impairment is typical in such patients. In most instances, the patients recover uneventfully; however, acute renal failure may occur with a time course similar to that of other causes of acute tubular necrosis.

Pulmonary Edema. This complication also occurs in patients with high *P. falciparum* parasitemias ($\geq 5\%$ of circulating red cells). Hemodynamic measurements indicate that this is a noncardiogenic form of pulmonary edema with normal pulmonary arterial and capillary pressures. These findings and the association with high TNF-α levels suggest that the pathogenesis of pulmonary edema may be similar in malaria and bacterial septicemia.

Gastrointestinal Manifestations. Diarrhea is common among children with *P. falciparum* infection. Although the pathogenesis of this complication is unclear, postmortem studies of children with diarrhea demonstrate parasitized red cells in the microvasculature of the intestine.

DIAGNOSIS. Giemsa-Stained Thick and Thin Smears. The most direct way to diagnose malaria is to prepare and examine Giemsa-stained thick or thin smears using oil immersion magnification ($\times 1000$). Giemsa stain is preferable to Wright's stain, especially for persons with *P. vivax* or *P. ovale* infection, because the Schüffner's dots characteristic of those infections are often not visible with Wright's stain. Thick smears are more sensitive than thin smears because the red cells have been lysed. As a result, approximately 10 times as much blood can be examined per field and thus per unit of time. However, because the red cells have been lysed, it is not possible to determine the effect of the parasite on red cell size or the position of the parasite within the red cell on a thick smear (Table 374–1). Therefore, persons without previous experience in reading thick smears should consider using thin smears to identify the infecting parasite or parasites. A common mistake is to require characteristic gametocytes for a diagnosis of *P. falciparum* infection. Because gametocytes require longer to develop than asexual parasites (7 to 10 versus 2 days), they are usually not present in the peripheral blood when nonimmune tourists or expatriates first become symptomatic. Conversely, gametocytes are frequently present in the blood of semi-immune residents of endemic areas with few or no symptoms or asexual parasites. A second common mistake is to assume that the patient can have only one parasite species: Approximately 5% of persons with malaria have infections due to more than one parasite species.

TABLE 374-1. MALARIA PARASITES THAT INFECT HUMANS

	Parasitemia (per μl blood)	Complications
P. falciparum	≥ 10⁶	Coma (cerebral malaria) Hypoglycemia Pulmonary edema, renal failure Anemia
P. vivax	≤ 25,000	Late (2–3 mo) splenic rupture
P. ovale	≤ 25,000	–
P. malariae	≤ 10,000	Immune complex nephrotic syndrome

	Morphology		
	Red Blood Cell Size	Schüffner's Dots	Stages
P. falciparum	No RBC enlargement	Absent	Rings, occasionally gametocytes
P. vivax	Enlarged host RBC	Present	All forms
P. ovale	Enlarged host RBC	Absent	All forms
P. malariae	No RBC enlargement	Present	All forms

	Relapse from Hypnozoites	Antimalarial Resistance
P. falciparum	No	Chloroquine and pyrimethamine-sulfadoxine
P. vivax	Yes	Possibly chloroquine
P. ovale	Yes	None known
P. malariae	No	None known

RBC = red blood cell

TABLE 374-2. CHEMOPROPHYLAXIS OF MALARIA*

For Areas without Chloroquine-Resistant *Plasmodium falciparum*:

Chloroquine phosphate (Aralen)	500 mg/wk (300 mg chloroquine base) during exposure and for 4 wk after leaving the endemic area

For Areas with Chloroquine-Resistant *Plasmodium falciparum*:

Mefloquine (Lariam)	250 mg/wk during exposure and for 4 wk after leaving the endemic area
Doxycycline	100 mg/d during exposure and for 4 wk after leaving the endemic area

* Updated recommendations on malaria chemoprophylaxis may be obtained 24 hours a day, 7 days a week, through the Centers for Disease Control and Prevention (CDC) Hot Line at (404) 332-4555.

Fluorescent Staining with Acridine Orange. Fluorescence microscopy is one of two new techniques for detecting malaria parasites in peripheral blood specimens. This technique takes advantage of the fact that parasitized red cells are less dense than unparasitized red cells. A finger stick specimen is taken into a capillary tube prepared with acridine orange (to stain the nucleic acid of the parasite) and an anticoagulant. After centrifugation, parasitized red cells are found at the top of the red cell layer just below the buffy coat. Experienced investigators can examine a blood specimen in 30 to 40 seconds (less time than necessary to examine a thick or thin smear).

DNA Probes. Several investigators have developed *Plasmodium* and species-specific (e.g., *P. falciparum*-specific) DNA probes that can detect 40 to 100 parasites per microliter of blood (similar to the 1 to 10 parasites per microliter threshold of the thick smear). Problems that have recently been solved in the application of this technology include the use of signal systems as effective as ³²P that are not radioactive and the role of the polymerase chain reaction in enhancing sensitivity under field conditions.

Serology (Antigen Detection). Recent studies suggest that testing for specific parasite antigens may be an alternative to microscopy. A commercial kit is now available for the diagnosis of *P. falciparum* infection based on detection of histidine-rich protein II.

Serology (Antibody Testing). Testing for antibodies to plasmodia is of limited value. In endemic areas, most persons have antibody titers from previous infections whether or not they were infected recently. In addition, 3 to 4 weeks may be required to develop a diagnostic rise in antibody titer, whereas the decision to treat must be made in the first few hours of evaluation. However, serology may be of value retrospectively in nonimmune persons (expatriate tourists) who have been treated empirically for malaria without a microscopic diagnosis. For example, a high titer of antibodies against *P. vivax* suggests that the patient has had a recent *P. vivax* infection and should receive primaquine if it has not been given previously (see the section on treatment, below).

PREVENTION. Exposed nonimmune persons may prevent malaria by taking antimalarials prospectively (chemoprophylaxis); by using insect repellents and otherwise reducing contact with the anopheline vector; and possibly, in the future, by a malaria vaccine (immunoprophylaxis).

Chemoprophylaxis. Drugs used for chemoprophylaxis must be safe because they are given to healthy persons for long periods. They should also have long serum half-lives so that they can be given infrequently. On the basis of these criteria, chloroquine is an excellent drug for chemoprophylaxis in areas without chloroquine-resistant *P. falciparum* (Table 374–2). It is the only chemoprophylactic agent known to be safe for pregnant women and does not produce retinal toxicity at the doses used for antimalarial chemoprophylaxis. Unfortunately, chloroquine-resistant strains of *P. falciparum* are now established in Southeast Asia, South America, and Africa. For areas with chloroquine-resistant *P. falciparum*, mefloquine is now the recommended chemoprophylactic agent, although resistance to mefloquine is developing in Southeast Asia. Doxycycline is an alternative, with the advantage that it also reduces the frequency of traveler's diarrhea. The disadvantages of doxycycline include the need to take it daily, photosensitivity reactions, and vaginitis. Because of hypersensitivity reactions to pyrimethamine-sulfadoxine (Fansidar) and both agranulocytosis and hepatitis with amodiaquine, neither of these agents is recommended for chemoprophylaxis.

Vector Control. Because of widespread drug resistance in *P. falciparum*, increasing emphasis is placed on reducing exposure to the anopheline vector, especially in hyperendemic areas such as Africa. Strategies that are successful and should be considered include DEET-containing insect repellents and pyrethrin (insecticide)–impregnated bed nets. DDT is no longer effective in most regions of the world because of widespread resistance.

Immunoprophylaxis—Development of a Malaria Vaccine. Although a malaria vaccine is not available, it is hoped that this goal will ultimately be achievable. Because the three major parasite stages in humans are antigenically distinct, a successful vaccine will likely need to contain at least three parasite antigens (sporozoite, merozoite, and gametocyte). However, a vaccine need not be 100% effective to be valuable. For example, a vaccine that would require boosting could be quite effective because of repetitive exposure to natural infection in endemic areas. In addition, a vaccine that limited the magnitude of the parasitemia could have a marked effect on survival even if it had no effect on the incidence of infection, because severe morbidity and death are associated with high parasitemias.

TREATMENT. Successful treatment of patients with malaria depends primarily on effective antimalarial drugs. However, it also depends on ancillary measures as diverse as the infusion of glucose and exchange transfusion. Monitoring of the blood glucose level is important because hypoglycemia is a common cause of coma and because both quinine and quinidine stimulate the release of insulin directly from the pancreatic β cell. Steroids are contraindicated in cerebral malaria because they prolong the duration of coma.

The treatment of chloroquine-susceptible malaria (*P. vivax*, *P. ovale*, or *P. malariae* malaria and chloroquine-susceptible *P. falciparum* malaria) is satisfactory (Table 374–3) because chloroquine is a safe and effective antimalarial. Some patients with chloroquine-resistant *P. vivax* have been treated successfully with 1500 mg chloroquine base (25 mg base per kilogram) orally after failing to respond to 600 mg base, whereas others have required treatment with mefloquine. However, the treatment of chloroquine-resistant *P. falciparum* malaria is unsatisfactory. Potential choices include quinidine, quinine, and mefloquine. For comatose patients, intravenous quinidine may be the safest treatment. The risk of quinidine cardiovascular toxicity is low with the measurement of serum quinidine levels (2.0 to 5.0 μg per milliliter is usually adequate; ≥ 6 μg per milliliter is potentially toxic) and cardiac monitoring (for a QT interval > 0.6 second or QRS widening beyond 25% of baseline) during intravenous infusion. Although pyrimethamine-sulfadoxine (Fansidar) has been used for treatment, it is now controversial because of the

TABLE 374-3. TREATMENT OF MALARIA

P. vivax, P. ovale, P. malariae, and Chloroquine-Susceptible P. falciparum:

For patients unable to take oral medications:

IM chloroquine:	2.5 mg/kg IM q 4 hr or 3.5 mg/kg q 6 hr (total dose not to exceed 25 mg/kg base)
IV chloroquine:	10 mg/kg base over 4 hr, followed by 5 mg/kg base q 12 hr (given in a 2-hr infusion; total dose not to exceed 25 mg/kg base)

For patients able to take oral medications:

PO chloroquine:	10 mg/kg = 600-mg base, followed by an additional 300-mg base after 6 hr and 300-mg base again on days 2 and 3

Chloroquine-Resistant P. falciparum:

For patients unable to take oral medications:

IV quinidine:	6.25 mg/kg quinidine base (10 mg/kg quinidine gluconate) IV over 1 to 2 hr, followed by a constant infusion of 0.0125 mg/kg quinidine base (0.02 mg/kg quinidine gluconate) IV per minute until the parasitemia is < 1% or oral treatment is tolerated

For patients able to take oral medications:

PO quinine*:	650 mg quinine sulfate (540 mg quinine base) q 8 hr until significant improvement, or for 10 day

or

PO mefloquine:	750 mg as a single oral dose followed by 500 mg in 6–8 hr

or

PO halofantrine†:	(500 mg q 6 hr × 3 doses, and repeat in 1 week) is an alternative, but is not effective against mefloquine-resistant parasite

or

PO pyrimethamine + sulfadoxine:	3 tablets (75 mg pyrimethamine plus 1500 mg sulfadoxine) as a single dose

To Prevent Relapse in P. vivax or P. ovale Infection:

PO primaquine:‡	15 mg primaquine base (26.3 mg primaquine phosphate) daily × 14 day

* In addition to oral quinine a number of investigators recommend tetracycline (250 mg PO q 6 hr for 7 to 10 days), pyrimethamine plus sulfadiazine or sulfisoxazole (25 mg twice daily plus 500 mg q 6 hr PO for 5 days), or 3 tablets of pyrimethamine-sulfadoxine (total of 75 plus 1500 mg PO once).

† Not yet available in the United States.

‡ To prevent potentially severe hemolysis, patients should be tested for glucose-6-phosphate dehydrogenase deficiency prior to treatment with primaquine.

increasing prevalence of resistance in areas of chloroquine resistance.

Patients with *P. vivax* or *P. ovale* infection should be tested for glucose-6-phosphate dehydrogenase deficiency before treatment with primaquine, which is used to eradicate persistent hypnozoites in the liver to prevent relapse.

PROGNOSIS. Virtually all patients with *P. vivax, P. ovale,* or *P. malariae* infection respond well to chloroquine and make an uneventful recovery. The chloroquine-resistant strains of *P. vivax* reported from Indonesia have thus far responded to treatment with either mefloquine or full-dose chloroquine (1.5 grams base). For patients with *P. falciparum* infection, the quantitative parasite count is the best predictor of the outcome. Patients with ≥5% parasitemia (≥ 250,000 parasites per microliter of blood) are at increased risk of severe and complicated malaria, including death. In addition to standard antimalarial treatment (outlined above), such patients should be considered for more heroic measures, such as exchange transfusion, if they do not improve within the first 12 to 24 hours of treatment.

Canfield CJ, Chongsuphajaisiddhi T, Danis M, et al.: Severe and complicated malaria. Trans R Soc Trop Med Hyg 89 (Suppl 2):1, 1990. *A comprehensive review of the pathogenesis and treatment of severe falciparum malaria.*

Good MF, Pombo D, Quakyi IA, et al.: Human T-cell recognition of the circumsporozoite protein of *Plasmodium falciparum:* Immunodominant T-cell domains map to the polymorphic regions of the molecule. Proc Natl Acad Sci USA 85:1199, 1988. *Evidence that the determinants of T-cell reactivity are in hypervariable regions of the circumsporozoite protein.*

Grau GE, Taylor TE, Molyneux ME, et al.: Tumor necrosis factor and disease severity in children with falciparum malaria. N Engl J Med 320:1586, 1989. *Serum levels of TNF are increased in children with severe falciparum malaria.*

Krogstad DJ, Gluzman IY, Klye DE, et al.: Efflux of chloroquine from *Plasmodium falciparum:* Mechanism of chloroquine resistance. Science 238:1283, 1987. *The*

basis of chloroquine resistance is rapid efflux of the drug from the resistant parasite.

Kwiatkowski D, Molyneux ME, Stephens S, et al.: Anti-TNF therapy inhibits fever in cerebral malaria. Q J Med 86:91, 1993. *Monoclonal antibodies against TNF-α do not reduce morbidity or mortality, although they do reduce fever in children with severe malaria.*

Miller LH, Good MF, Milon G: Malaria pathogenesis. Science 264:1878, 1994. *Major unresolved issues highlighted include the lack of protective immunity after natural infection and the role of factors such as cytokines and host receptor molecules in the cytoadherence associated with cerebral malaria.*

Udeinya IJ, Schmidt JA, Aikawa M, et al.: Falciparum malaria-infected erythrocytes specifically bind to cultured human endothelial cells. Science 213:555, 1981. *Knobs on falciparum-infected cells bind to endothelial cells and thus explain the sequestration of red cells with mature falciparum parasites.*

White NJ, Warrell DA, Chanthavanich P, et al.: Severe hypoglycemia and hyperinsulinemia in falciparum malaria. N Engl J Med 309:61, 1983. *Hypoglycemia results from utilization of liver glycogen stores while not eating in the early stages of the illness, from parasite consumption of glucose, and from the release of insulin from pancreatic β-cells by quinine (or quinidine).*

375 AFRICAN TRYPANOSOMIASIS (Sleeping Sickness)

Thomas C. Quinn

DEFINITION. Known widely as sleeping sickness, African trypanosomiasis is an acute and chronic disease caused by *Trypanosoma brucei.* The parasites are transmitted to humans through the bite of tsetse flies located in regions of Africa between 15 degrees north and 15 degrees south latitude. In humans, there are two distinct forms of the disease, East African trypanosomiasis caused by *T. brucei rhodesiense* and West African trypanosomiasis caused by *T. brucei gambiense.* Although there is some clinical overlap, East African trypanosomiasis primarily causes an acute febrile illness with myocarditis and meningoencephalitis that is rapidly fatal if not treated, whereas West African trypanosomiasis is characterized as a chronic debilitating disease with mental deterioration and physical wasting (Table 375–1). A closely related variant, *T. brucei brucei,* is noninfectious for humans, but causes a chronic wasting illness in cattle, called nagana, which has a considerable indirect effect on human nutrition in sub-Saharan Africa.

ETIOLOGY AND LIFE CYCLE. Trypanosomes are motile hemoflagellates with a single undulating membrane that passes along the length of the parasite, terminating in an anterior flagellum (see Color Plate 10*E*). Located anteriorly is a kinetoplast, an organelle containing topologically interlocked circular DNA molecules and mitochondria. In the peripheral blood of humans, trypanosomes vary in length from 10 to 40 μm. Both short stumpy and long slen-

TABLE 375-1. A COMPARISON OF GAMBIAN AND RHODESIAN SLEEPING SICKNESS

	Gambian (West African)	Rhodesian (East African)
Etiologic agent	*Trypanosoma brucei gambiense*	*Trypanosoma brucei rhodesiense*
Vector	*Glossina palpalis* or *tachinoides* (riverine tsetse)	*Glossina morsitans* (savanna tsetse)
Distribution	West and Central Africa	East Africa
Reservoir	Humans (domestic animals)	Wild game
Course of infection	Slow (months–years)	Rapid (< 1 yr)
Clinical features		
Lymphadenopathy	+ + (Winterbottom's sign)	±
Myocarditis, heart failure	±	+ +
Neurologic symptoms	+ +	+
Disseminated intravascular coagulation	–	+
Parasitemia	Low	High

der forms can be present in a patient at the same time. The different variants of *T. brucei* cannot be distinguished morphologically but can be identified by differences in pathogenicity for certain animals, as well as in biochemical requirements, electrophoretic pattern of component enzymes, and DNA hybridization.

T. brucei is transmitted by the tsetse fly *Glossina*, within which it undergoes several developmental changes. When biting an infected host, trypanosomes are ingested and within the insect midgut rapidly differentiate into procyclic forms with loss of their dense surface coat, composed of variant surface glycoprotein. After 2 to 3 weeks of multiplication within the midgut the procyclic trypanosomes migrate to the insect's salivary glands, where they change morphologically into epimastigotes. These forms further undergo multiplication and ultimately differentiate into metacyclic trypanosomes that are coated with characteristic variant surface glycoprotein and are infectious to mammalian hosts. When a new host is bitten by the tsetse fly, the trypanosomes present in the salivary glands are injected into the connective tissue and blood. Within the human host they divide by binary fission and undergo antigen variation, a process by which they continually change their variable surface glycoproteins (VSG) and evade the immune system of the host. With the bite of another tsetse fly, ingestion of the parasite occurs, and the life cycle of the organism is completed (Fig. 375–1). Mechanical transmission can theoretically also occur via blood transfusion or by interrupted biting of a tsetse fly feeding on an infectious person and directly thereafter biting an uninfected individual.

EPIDEMIOLOGY. It is estimated that African trypanosomiasis infects more than 20,000 Africans annually and that approximately 50 million people live at risk of acquiring trypanosomiasis because of the presence of the disease and its vector. Approximately 4 million square miles in Africa remain unpopulated because of the presence of *T. brucei brucei* infection, which results in the loss of domestic and wild animals, including cattle, waterbuck, bushbuck, and buffalo.

T. b. gambiense occurs primarily in the west and central regions of sub-Saharan Africa. Although it primarily infects humans, there may be animal reservoirs, such as pigs, dogs, and sheep. Gambian sleeping sickness is spread mainly by three species of tsetse fly, *Glossina palpalis, G. tachinoides,* and *G. fuscipes.* Distribution of these flies includes shaded areas along rivers and streams, where the conditions of temperature, darkness, and moisture are optimum.

T. b. rhodesiense differs from *T. b. gambiense* in that it is primar-

ily a parasite of wild game, with humans serving only as occasional hosts. The geographic distribution of *T. b. rhodesiense* is primarily East Africa from Ethiopia and eastern Uganda south to Zambia and Botswana. Rhodesian sleeping sickness is spread by tsetse flies of the *G. morsitans* group, including *G. pallidipes* and *G. swynnertoni.* These flies can survive in the open savanna, and Rhodesian sleeping sickness usually occurs among individuals visiting or traveling through an endemic area. Consequently, hunters, fishermen, and tourists are at risk, exposing themselves to vectors that usually feed on wild animals.

Imported African trypanosomiasis is a rare disease. Most cases were due to *T. b. rhodesiense* acquired by Americans who had been on safari in East Africa for a very brief period. Nearly all of these cases were initially misdiagnosed because of the unfamiliarity of United States physicians with this disease. With an increase in international travel, 20,000 Americans are now estimated to visit endemic areas yearly, and approximately 10,000 aliens enter the United States each year from countries in Africa where the infection is endemic.

PATHOGENESIS AND PATHOLOGY. Following the bite of the tsetse fly, trypanosomes accumulate in the connective tissue, where they multiply to produce a local chancre (trypanoma). The organisms subsequently spread through the lymphatics, resulting in enlargement of lymph nodes secondary to reactive plasma cell and macrophage infiltration. The trypanosomes eventually disseminate to the circulatory system, where the parasitemia usually remains at low intensity and the organisms multiply by binary fission. Systemic African trypanosomiasis without central nervous system (CNS) involvement is generally referred to as stage I disease.

The host immune response plays an integral role in the pathogenesis of African sleeping sickness, although the exact nature of the immunopathogenic reactions has not been clearly defined. Trypanosomes survive by periodically altering their surface antigenic coat, avoiding successful eradication by the host. Any single parasite may contain some 1000 genes for VSG which can be activated in a variety of ways and selected by the host-antibody response. Consequently trypanosomes occur in the peripheral blood of infected individuals in waves, with each parasite wave consisting of a serologically distinct organism.

Tissue damage is induced by either toxin production or immune complex reaction with release of proteolytic enzymes. Immune complexes consisting of variant antigens of the organism and complement-fixing antibodies have been demonstrated in both the circulation and the target organs of infected patients. The production of autoantibodies is a prominent feature, and they are frequently directed against antigen components of red cells, brain, and heart. Anemia secondary to autoimmune hemolysis can be severe, resulting in anoxia and further tissue destruction. Thus the host-parasite interaction can result in generalized febrile episodes, lymphadenopathy, and myocardial and pericardial inflammation, along with anemia, thrombocytopenia, disseminated intravascular coagulation, and renal disease primarily during the acute stage of the disease.

Stage II of human African trypanosomiasis involves invasion of the CNS, which occurs during the period of circulatory dissemination when trypanosomes localize in the small vessels of the CNS. Pathologic changes in the CNS are most prominent in chronic cases of Gambian sleeping sickness. The meninges are thickened and infiltrated with lymphocytes, plasma cells, and morular cells. Morular cells are modified plasma cells (up to 20 mm in diameter) with large granular inclusions that have been shown to consist of immunoglobulin. These cells may play an important role in the local production of immunoglobulin M (IgM) in the cerebrospinal fluid (CSF). Edema, hemorrhages, and granulomatous lesions are frequently present, along with thrombosis as a result of endarteritis and with neuronal degeneration.

African trypanosomes appear to induce a state of B cell polyclonal activation caused either by interference with host T cell control of antibody production or by a B cell mitogen released by the parasite. Polyclonal hypergammaglobulinemia, with very high levels of IgM, is commonly seen. High levels of nonspecific heterophile antibody, rheumatoid factor, and autoantibodies are also produced.

CLINICAL FEATURES. The signs and symptoms of sleeping sickness differ according to the infecting organism (Table 375–1).

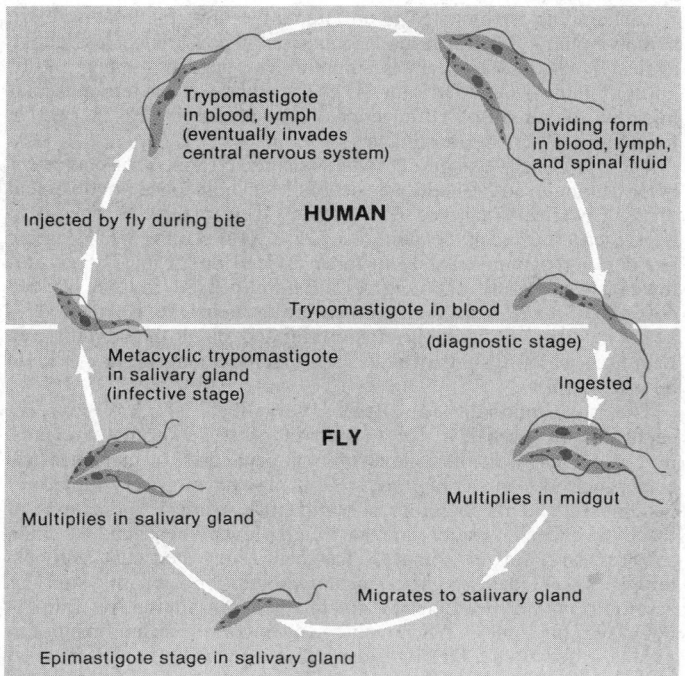

FIGURE 375–1. Life cycle of *Trypanosoma (Trypanozoon) brucei, T. (T.) b. gambiense,* and *T. (T.) b. rhodesiense.*

Trypomastigote in blood, lymph (eventually invades central nervous system)

Dividing form in blood, lymph, and spinal fluid

Injected by fly during bite

HUMAN

Trypomastigote in blood

(diagnostic stage)

Metacyclic trypomastigote in salivary gland (infective stage)

Ingested

FLY

Multiplies in salivary gland

Multiplies in midgut

Migrates to salivary gland

Epimastigote stage in salivary gland

Rhodesian sleeping sickness, due to *T. b. rhodesiense,* causes a rapid progressive disease often resulting in cardiac failure and acute neurologic manifestations. Gambian sleeping sickness, caused by *T. b. gambiense,* is typically a more chronic illness with primarily neurologic features. However, this difference is not absolute; in some cases Gambian sleeping sickness can progress rapidly, and occasionally Rhodesian sleeping sickness may follow a more chronic course.

Gambian Sleeping Sickness. Within several days following the bite by an infected tsetse fly, a trypanosomal nodule or chancre develops, typically on the exposed parts of the body. Within a week the lesion becomes a hard, painful nodule surrounded by erythema and swelling, which persists for 1 to 2 weeks. After this incubation period, clinical features develop after systemic, lymphatic, and circulatory invasion of the trypanosomes. Fever, headache, dizziness, and weakness occur in the majority of these patients. Febrile episodes may last 1 to 6 days, alternating with afebrile periods. Lymphadenopathy with prominent supraclavicular and posterior cervical enlargement is seen in >80% of infected individuals. Known as Winterbottom's sign, these enlarged lymph nodes are usually discrete, rubbery, and painless. Moderate splenomegaly may occur, and urticaria and erythematous rashes have also been observed. Electrocardiograms are often abnormal, but clinical signs of heart disease are unusual.

Six months to several years after symptoms first appear, the clinical features of this early hemolymphatic stage progress to a late meningoencephalitic stage. Behavioral and personality changes are often the first signs of CNS involvement. Later, more florid psychological changes may occur, with hallucinations and delusions. Reversion of sleep rhythm is characteristic, with drowsiness during the day, a feature from which the disease derives its name. Other nervous symptoms include tremor, most characteristically of the face and lips, and hyperesthesia, causing some patients to avoid common practices such as closing (Kerandel's sign) or locking doors (key sign). Without treatment, the patient's level of consciousness progressively deteriorates until there is lapse into stupor. Alterations in thermoregulation may lead to hypothermia or hyperthermia, and progressive neurologic alterations lead to convulsions, chorea, and athetosis. The CSF shows an increase in cells and protein, much of which is IgM. Free immunoglobulin light chains may be present. Most of the cells are lymphocytes, but a few are plasma cells and morula cells. Trypanosomes may also be evident within the CSF.

Rhodesian Sleeping Sickness. This disease is more acute than Gambian sleeping sickness, and symptoms usually occur a few days after the victim has been bitten by the tsetse fly. Alternating periods of high fever, malaise, and headache, followed by several days of well-being, are often misinterpreted as acute malaria infection. Lymphadenopathy is not prominent in this variety of the disease, and Winterbottom's sign is usually absent. Tachycardia with arrhythmias and extrasystoles is common. Anemia, thrombocytopenia, and disseminated intravascular coagulation are usually evident within the first several weeks of infection. Liver enzyme values are often elevated, and electrocardiograms are abnormal, usually reflecting underlying myocarditis. Neurologic features are similar to those described for Gambian sleeping sickness, but they occur much earlier and with more rapid deterioration. Without treatment the disease may result in death within a matter of weeks to months, without clear distinction into an early and late phase, as described for Gambian trypanosomiasis.

DIAGNOSIS. Although a presumptive diagnosis of trypanosomiasis is based on clinical suspicion, history of travel to areas where this disease is endemic, and tsetse fly exposure, confirmation of the diagnosis is based solely on the demonstration of trypanosomes. These organisms may be found in the blood (see Color Plate 10*E*), bone marrow, centrifuged CSF, lymph node aspirates, and scrapings from the chancre. Giemsa or Wright's stain of the buffy coat of centrifuged heparinized blood makes identification easier because the trypanosomes are often concentrated in the buffy coat. In one technique, referred to as the quantitative buffy coat (QBC), 60 μl of blood obtained by a fingerprick is drawn up in a glass hematocrit tube precoated with acridine orange and anticoagulate. Following centrifugation, the buffy coat can be examined and trypanosomes fluoresce greenish yellow, remain motile, and are easily identified. In patients with Gambian sleeping sickness, in which trypanosomes

are found less frequently in the blood, concentration methods such as ion exchange chromatography, diethylaminoethyl (DEAE) filtration, culture, or animal inoculation should be used.

All patients should have a lumbar puncture prior to and following therapy to determine whether CNS involvement is present. Documentation of CNS involvement is imperative because suramin, a drug effective against the hemolymphatic stage of *T. brucei,* does not penetrate the spinal fluid. CNS disease is manifested by pleocytosis and elevation of spinal fluid total protein and IgM levels. Trypanosomes can be found in most patients, provided that the CSF is examined immediately after collection and that clean glassware is used. For those patients in whom trypanosomes cannot be found, measuring the CSF IgM is often of great diagnostic help. A high CSF IgM value and a modest increase in total protein are almost pathognomonic of sleeping sickness.

Several immunodiagnostic tests have been developed for African trypanosomiasis, including an indirect hemagglutination test, indirect fluorescent antibody test, and enzyme-linked immunosorbent assay (ELISA), which are useful for epidemiologic surveys. A card agglutination trypanosome test (CATT) with prefixed trypanosomes is frequently used for rapid serodiagnosis. Although very sensitive, CATT may remain positive for several years after successful treatment, thereby decreasing its ability to differentiate between acute infection and a previous, treated infection.

TREATMENT. Suramin* is the drug of choice for the early hemolymphatic stage of both *T. b. gambiense* and *T. b. rhodesiense* infections before CNS invasion has occurred. Suramin does not cross the blood-brain barrier in increased amounts, and it does not cure the disease once CNS invasion has occurred. The dose is 20 mg per kilogram of body weight given intravenously up to a maximum single dose of 1 gram. Suramin is freshly prepared as a 10% aqueous solution. Intramuscular injection is not advised because of local irritation and pain. Suramin binds to plasma proteins and may persist in the circulation at low concentrations for as long as 3 months. A test dose of 200 mg is given initially; if no adverse side effects are noted, then full doses of the drug may be given on days 1, 3, 7, 14, and 21. A single course for an adult is usually 5 grams; it should not exceed 7 grams.

Suramin is a toxic drug that may result in idiosyncratic reactions in some individuals (1 in 20,000). The drug is excreted entirely by the kidneys; renal damage may result because the drug is deposited in the renal tubules. The urine should be examined before administering each dose of suramin, and if proteinuria or casts are present, treatment should be stopped. Other side effects include a papular eruption, photophobia, arthralgias, peripheral neuritis, fever, and agranulocytosis.

Pentamidine isethionate* is an alternative drug for treating early hemolymphatic African trypanosomiasis, but it is much less active against *T. rhodesiense* than is suramin. The dose is 4 mg per kilogram of body weight; it is given every other day by intramuscular injection for a total of 10 injections. Pentamidine is also ineffective for treating CNS trypanosomiasis.

The arsenical melarsoprol* (Mel B) is the treatment of choice for both Gambian and Rhodesian sleeping sickness once involvement of the CNS has occurred. The drug is given in three courses of 3 days each. The recommended dosage is 2.0 to 3.6 mg per kilogram per day given intravenously in three divided doses for 3 days, followed 1 week later by 3.6 mg per kilogram per day in three divided doses for 3 days. This latter course is then repeated 10 to 21 days later. Melarsoprol is a highly toxic drug and should be administered with great care. If signs of arsenical toxicity occur, the drug should be discontinued.

The most important side effects involve the CNS. A reactive encephalopathy, probably due to release of trypanosomal antigens, may occur early in the course of treatment, and its incidence has been reported to be as high as 18%. It may develop very rapidly or insidiously, and its mortality is about 50%. Clinical indications of reactive encephalopathy include high fever, headache, tremor, seizures, and finally coma. It has been suggested that corticosteroids protect patients from melarsoprol encephalopathy, but this assertion has not been clearly documented. An alternative drug for both systemic and CNS involvement includes difluoromethylornithine (eflornithine, DFMO), a specific, irreversible inhibitor of or-

---

* Available from the Centers for Disease Control and Prevention, Atlanta, GA.

boxylase. In one large trial of 207 patients with late-stage *T. b. gambiense* sleeping sickness, eflornithine was highly effective in successful treatment of both hemolymphatic and CNS stages of infection. Eflornithine dramatically reduced symptoms and rapidly cleared parasites from blood and CSF, even in those patients who had relapsed after melarsoprol therapy. The recommended dosage is 400 mg per kilogram per day given intravenously in four divided doses for 2 weeks, followed by 300 mg per kilogram per day given orally in four doses for 30 days. Frequent side effects include diarrhea and anemia. Unfortunately, its efficacy in *T. b. rhodesiense* has been quite variable, and its cost and long duration of therapy have limited its usefulness in the field. In addition, immunocompromised patients such as those with HIV infection do not respond to treatment as effectively with any of the above agents because a normal immune response is necessary for a cure. Regular follow-up with clinical examination of a lumbar puncture is necessary for all patients for at least 1 year after treatment.

PROGNOSIS. Untreated African sleeping sickness is almost invariably fatal. Many patients with early Gambian sleeping sickness may remain relatively well for months to years without treatment, but once CNS involvement has occurred, death is inevitable unless treatment is given. Death frequently results from pneumonia in Gambian sleeping sickness and from heart failure in Rhodesian sleeping sickness. Treatment with suramin in the early phase of sleeping sickness results in a cure rate of >90%. A few patients may subsequently develop CNS involvement and require further treatment. Mel B achieves a parasitologic cure in at least 90% of cases of advanced disease, and many patients may recover completely. Unfortunately, some patients are left with irreversible neurologic damage. Approximately 5% of patients may die during the course of Mel B therapy.

CONTROL AND PROPHYLAXIS. Measures to prevent and control African trypanosomiasis can be instituted at three different levels: surveillance and treatment, chemoprophylaxis, and vector control. Surveillance with treatment is necessary to reduce the human reservoir of infection, particularly in areas where epidemics have occurred in the past. Pentamidine has been successfully used as a chemoprophylactic in Gambian sleeping sickness when given as a single intramuscular injection of 4 mg per kilogram every 3 to 6 months. However, the drug is generally not recommended for mass use, and it appears to be ineffective against Rhodesian trypanosomiasis.

Vector control requires destruction of tsetse fly habitats by selective clearing of vegetation and spraying with insecticides, which are effective only temporarily. Because of the wide range of the tsetse fly, these vector control measures are not economically feasible except when it is necessary to break transmission in epidemics. For individual protection, avoidance of contact with infected tsetse flies is best achieved by the use of repellents and protective clothing.

A vaccine is not currently available because of the occurrence of antigenic variation. However, the potential for development of a vaccine has increased with the progress in cultivation of *T. brucei in vitro* and analysis of the chemical structure of its variant antigens.

Anonymous: Drugs for parasitic infections. *In* Abramowicz M (ed.): Med Lett Drugs Ther 35:111, 1993. *A listing of current recommendations for the treatment of all parasitic infections including trypanosomiasis.*

Cattand P, de Raadt P: Laboratory diagnosis of trypanosomiasis. Clin Lab Med 11:899, 1991. *A review of the various laboratory tests available for accurately diagnosing African trypanosomiasis.*

Hadjuk S, Adler B, Bertrand K, et al.: Molecular biology of African trypanosomes: Development of new strategies to combat an old disease. Am J Med Sci 303:258, 1992. *An excellent description of the mechanisms of antigenic variation which allow the parasite to avoid the host-immune response.*

Hunter CA, Kennedy PGE: Immunopathology in central nervous system human African trypanosomiasis. J Neuroimmunol 36:91, 1992. *A minireview of the different mechanisms potentially involved in the immunopathogenesis of CNS disease in human African trypanosomiasis.*

Jennings FW: Future prospects for the chemotherapy of human trypanosomiasis. Combination chemotherapy and African trypanosomiasis. Trans R Soc Trop Med Hyg 84:618, 1990. *A review of the different drug regimens for treating trypanosomiasis and discussion of their advantages and toxicities.*

Milord F, Pepin J, Loko L, et al.: Efficacy and toxicity of eflornithine for treatment of *Trypanosoma brucei gambiense* sleeping sickness. Lancet 340:652, 1992. *Clinical trial of eflornithine (DFMO) of 207 patients with late-stage T.b. gambiense sleeping sickness which demonstrated that eflornithine is as active and possibly less toxic than melarsoprol and is active for both stage I and stage II disease.*

376 AMERICAN TRYPANOSOMIASIS (Chagas' Disease)
Franklin A. Neva

DEFINITION. Chagas' disease, resulting from infection with the protozoan parasite *Trypanosoma cruzi*, is named after the Brazilian physician Carlos Chagas, who discovered the parasite. Distinction should be made between infection caused by the parasite, as manifested by positive serologic findings, and clinical disease. Chronic disease manifestations develop years after initial infection in the form of chronic cardiomyopathy with conduction defects or with dysfunction of the esophagus or colon (mega syndromes).

LIFE CYCLE OF THE ETIOLOGIC AGENT. The causative agent, *T. cruzi*, is usually transmitted as a zoonosis. Various species of blood-sucking reduviid bugs become infected when they take a blood meal from animals or humans who have circulating parasites, trypomastigotes, in the blood. The ingested parasites transform into epimastigotes and multiply in the midgut of the insect vector, where they later transform once again into metacyclic trypomastigotes in the hindgut of the bug. When the infected bug takes a subsequent blood meal, it frequently defecates during or after feeding, so that the infective metacyclic forms are deposited on the skin. Transmission to a second vertebrate host occurs when the feeding puncture site or a mucous membrane is inadvertently contaminated with infective bug feces. The parasites can penetrate a variety of host cell types, within which they transform into intracellular amastigote forms. In contrast to certain other intracellular organisms, amastigotes of *T. cruzi* are not enclosed in phagolysosomes. They multiply in the cytoplasm, elongate, transform into motile trypomastigotes, and rupture out of the cells. Liberated organisms penetrate new cells or are carried into the bloodstream to initiate further cycles of multiplication, preferentially in muscle cells, or are ingested by new vectors to maintain the cycle (Fig. 376–1).

Asymptomatic infected individuals with low-level parasitemia can transmit *T. cruzi* via blood transfusion. Another route of transmission of the parasite is congenital infection.

EPIDEMIOLOGY. *T. cruzi* and its arthropod vectors are widely distributed from the southern United States through Mexico and Central America into South America down to central Argentina and Chile. The parasite is restricted to the Western Hemisphere. In most countries where it occurs, the parasite cycle is sylvatic, i.e., it takes place in wild animals and their associated vector bugs. A peridomestic cycle occurs under conditions in which infected animals, such as opposums and rats, live close to human habitations, and vector bugs may invade houses to seek a blood meal. Certain species of triatomine bugs, such as *Triatoma infestans* and *Rhodnius prolixus*, have a great propensity to invade and breed in houses if suitable microenvironments are present. Cracks and holes in adobe mud huts or in crude wooden walls, thatched roofs, and household rubble provide hiding and breeding places for the bugs, which venture out at night to feed upon sleeping inhabitants. Under these conditions *T. cruzi* is transmitted from person to person—a domiciliary cycle—and Chagas' disease becomes a public health problem. Thus, human trypanosomiasis in Latin America is primarily an infection of rural poor people living in substandard housing.

The prevalence of antibodies to the parasite in human populations varies widely in different countries, as well as within regions of a country. A recent nationwide survey in Brazil found about 10% of the rural population to be infected. It is not unusual for up to half of all inhabitants in selected villages to be antibody positive. Countries with the highest incidence of both infection and disease due to *T. cruzi* include Brazil, Argentina, Chile, Bolivia, and Venezuela. It is estimated that in all of the Americas a total of 15 million people are infected. In many Latin American countries, positive serologic findings for *T. cruzi* constitute a social stigma; a lower socioeconomic background is implied, and employers are re-

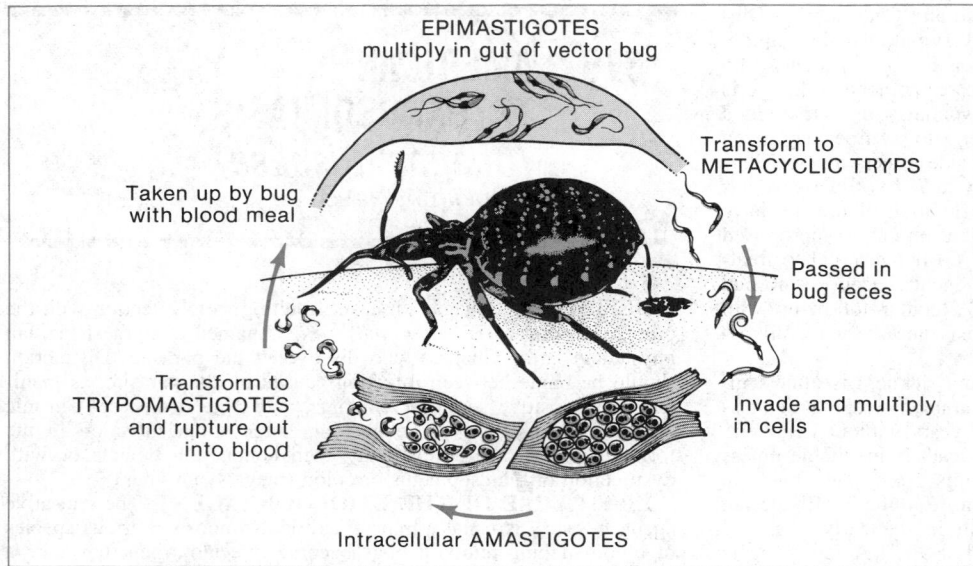

EPIMASTIGOTES
multiply in gut of vector bug

Transform to
METACYCLIC TRYPS

Taken up by bug
with blood meal

Passed in
bug feces

Transform to
TRYPOMASTIGOTES
and rupture out
into blood

Invade and multiply
in cells

Intracellular AMASTIGOTES

FIGURE 376-1. Life cycle of *Trypanosoma cruzi.*

luctant to hire someone who may later develop chronic Chagas' disease.

Considerable geographic variation exists in both the prevalence and the type of chronic disease manifestations. In Brazil, for example, cardiomyopathy and megadisease are common, and often a patient has both types of involvement. However, chagasic megaesophagus and megacolon are virtually unknown in Venezuela, Colombia, and Panama, whereas cardiomyopathy is relatively high, moderate, and low in prevalence, respectively. In general, the frequency of cardiac disease in Central America and Mexico in seropositive persons is low, even though rates of seropositivity may be substantial. Also in these countries heart disease tends to develop later in life than in Brazil.

The situation regarding Chagas' disease in the United States is interesting because only four autochthonous acute cases have been recognized despite the presence of *T. cruzi* in vector bugs as well as in animal reservoirs. The lack of transmission of *T. cruzi* to humans in this country is probably due to preference of the vectors for sylvatic habitats and their tendency to defecate late after feeding. Yet in some areas of the West, bites from aggressive and abundant reduviid bugs can be a source of annoyance to, and allergic reactions in, suburbanites and outdoorspeople. Because of increased Hispanic immigration in recent years, sporadic cases of chronic Chagas' disease will probably be encountered in the United States.

PATHOLOGY AND PATHOGENESIS. In *acute Chagas' disease,* a local inflammatory lesion called a chagoma may develop at the site of entry of the parasite. Histologically, the chagoma shows mononuclear cell infiltration, interstitial edema, and intracellular aggregates of amastigotes in cells of the subcutaneous tissue and muscle. Biopsy specimens from enlarged lymph nodes show hyperplasia, and amastigotes may be present in reticular cells. Skeletal muscle tissue from muscle biopsies have shown organisms and focal inflammation. In acute cases that have a fatal outcome there is invariably myocarditis with an enlarged heart. Microscopically, there is degeneration of cardiac muscle fibers and prominent but patchy areas of inflammation with nests of amastigotes in the muscles. The brain and meninges may also be parasitized in acute Chagas' disease. Virtually all organs and cell types can be invaded by *T. cruzi.*

The organs primarily affected in *chronic Chagas' disease* are the heart and certain hollow viscera, such as the esophagus and colon. Surprisingly, the intracellular *T. cruzi* usually cannot be found in the affected organs, or a few may be demonstrable after protracted search of many tissue sections. The heart in those patients with chronic disease who die suddenly, presumably of ventricular arrhythmias or heart block, may be normal in size or only moderately enlarged. Other patients with chronic chagasic cardiomyopathy develop cardiomegaly and die of intractable failure. The hearts are both hypertrophied and dilated, with thinning, especially at the apex to form a characteristic apical aneurysm. Mural thrombi, with subsequent embolization of the lungs and peripheral organs, are frequently seen. The coronary arteries are generally normal.

Microscopic findings in the heart are not specific, consisting of focal mononuclear cell infiltrates, hypertrophy of cardiac fibers with patchy areas of necrosis, variable fibrosis, and edema. The components of the conduction system of the heart most often involved by inflammatory changes are the sinoatrial and atrioventricular nodes, as well as the right branch and left anterior branches of the bundle of His. Andrade's detailed studies of these pathologic changes indicated that they correlated well with electrocardiographic (ECG) changes during life, but were diffusely scattered without specific localization to the conducting system.

When either the esophagus or the colon is affected in chronic Chagas' disease, the gross appearance is of dilatation and hypertrophy of the affected organ. The microscopic pathologic changes are disappointingly similar to those in the heart, again with no or very few organisms. However, myenteric ganglion cells are strikingly reduced in number. This type of parasympathetic denervation may also be found in other hollow viscera, such as duodenum, ureters, or biliary tree.

The significant pathology of *congenital Chagas' disease* is chronic placentitis, with inflammatory changes and focal necrosis in the chorionic villi. Amastigotes of *T. cruzi* are present in the lesions. The presence of lesions and organisms in the placenta may be associated with abortion, stillbirth, or acute disease in the fetus. However, pregnancy may result in a normal fetus, even though placental lesions are present.

The extent and clinical significance of pathologic changes in those individuals with antibodies to *T. cruzi* but without evidence of disease, i.e., the *indeterminate form,* are not yet clear. Such indeterminate cases may involve significantly reduced numbers of esophageal or colonic ganglion cells. It has been claimed that endocardial biopsy specimens from indeterminate cases have recognizable pathologic changes. In addition, in some indeterminate cases there is a chronic low level of parasitemia. Therefore, one point of view is that everyone with positive serologic findings has a continuing subclinical disease process that will become manifested with time. On the other hand, even in those areas where chronic Chagas' disease is common, one half or more of those with a positive serology will die of causes other than Chagas' disease. In most Latin American countries, where endemicity is much lower, a positive serologic finding constitutes a relatively small risk factor for later chronic disease.

The pathogenesis of acute Chagas' disease is straightforward, but the sequence of events leading to the late manifestations of chronic cardiomyopathy or megadisease is still poorly understood. Key features of the chronic disease that must be explained include the following: (1) a latent period of up to 20 years from presumed initial infection with *T. cruzi* before manifestations of cardiomyopathy or megadisease appear; (2) no or very few intracellular parasites in the affected organs, in contrast to abundant parasites in tissues in acute cases; (3) destruction of autonomic parasympathetic ganglia (Auerbach's plexus) of the esophagus and colon; and (4) great geographic variation in the frequency and type of chronic Chagas' disease. Genetic diversity in parasite strains, including variation in animal virulence, may explain geographic differences in disease. Exaggerated immune responses to *T. cruzi* are not present in patients with chronic Chagas' disease, at least as judged by humoral antibody levels and lymphocyte proliferative responses. The autoimmunity concept of pathogenesis lost favor when the tissue reactive antibody in patients was found to be heterophile in nature. Direct cell-mediated cytotoxicity to heart muscle has also been proposed as a mechanism for the chronic disease. An even more complicated type of autoimmune response involving anti-idiotypic antibodies as T cell antigens, as well as differential responses in antigen presentation, has also been proposed to explain chronic Chagas' disease. But a unifying concept of pathogenesis for chronic Chagas' disease is still lacking.

The indeterminate latent stage of infection with *T. cruzi* may be activated into a state of acute disease under conditions of severe immunosuppression. This can occur in seropositive recipients of organ transplants. Also, reports of activation of disease are increasing, especially with brain involvement similar to that produced by *Toxoplasma,* in patients with AIDS who also have latent *T. cruzi* infection.

CLINICAL PRESENTATION. In endemic areas, first exposure to *T. cruzi* generally is subclinical and goes unnoticed. When those initially exposed do develop clinical manifestations, the disease is an acute systemic infection. Chronic Chagas' disease, in contrast, evolves as a later sequela with specific organ involvement and no systemic features.

Acute Chagas' Disease. Although acute Chagas' disease is most commonly seen in children, it can occur at any age, depending on the nature of exposure to the causative organism. The incubation period under natural conditions cannot be established accurately but is probably at least a week. A local area of erythema and induration (chagoma) may develop in the skin at the site of parasite entry. When infection takes place via the conjunctival route, as it frequently does, the local periorbital swelling is referred to as Romaña's sign. The chagoma is often accompanied by regional adenopathy and persists for several weeks. Other signs of acute Chagas' disease include fever, generalized lymphadenopathy, hepatosplenomegaly, and transient skin rashes.

Myocarditis, accompanied by tachycardia and nonspecific ECG changes, can occur in the acute stage. Meningoencephalitis is another serious complication, particularly in very young patients. Fatal outcome in acute Chagas' disease is rare, but when it does occur, it is due to myocarditis and congestive failure or to meningoencephalitis.

Signs and symptoms of acute disease gradually subside within a few weeks to several months even without treatment. Trypanosomes, which have been demonstrable by direct microscopy in the peripheral blood during the acute phase, become more difficult to find and then disappear. The patient then enters the *indeterminate phase,* which is characterized by the presence of antibodies to *T. cruzi* and often also by the presence of low-level parasitemia in the blood demonstrable only by special sensitive methods. This state of apparent complete recovery with positive serologic findings may continue indefinitely without further evidence of disease or sequelae. However, a variable proportion of indeterminate cases, years to a decade or more later, will develop signs and symptoms of chronic Chagas' disease. Except for epidemiologic experience from a particular geographic region, there are no laboratory or clinical indicators to predict the likelihood of future chronic disease.

Chronic Chagas' Disease. Cardiac signs and symptoms are the most common manifestations of chronic disease and are apt to begin with palpitations, dizziness, precordial discomfort, and even syncope. These reflect a variety of arrhythmias, including ventricular extrasystoles, bouts of tachycardia, and various degrees of heart block. Sudden death due to ventricular tachycardia in an otherwise healthy young adult is not unusual. Symptoms due to arrhythmias may be present for a long time before cardiomegaly or evidence of cardiac failure appears. When congestive failure develops, it is predominantly right sided and is likely to lead to a fatal outcome

within a few years. Peripheral emboli to the brain or other organs are frequent.

Physical examination reveals only an irregular pulse, distant heart sounds, and perhaps a gallop rhythm. With failure, the heart can be very large, functional regurgitant murmurs may be heard, and there is often congestive hepatomegaly and peripheral edema.

The second most common chronic manifestation is megadisease of the esophagus or colon, most frequently the former. The symptoms are indistinguishable from idiopathic achalasia and include dysphagia, feeling of fullness after eating or drinking only small amounts, chest pain, and regurgitation. Aspiration with secondary pneumonia is a common complication in advanced cases, as are weight loss and cachexia. Salivary gland hypertrophy secondary to hypersalivation is sometimes seen. Esophageal cancer is reported to be more frequent in patients with chagasic megaesophagus, as with idiopathic achalasia.

Patients with chagasic megacolon suffer from chronic constipation and abdominal pain. Volvulus, obstruction, and perforation of the bowel may occur. An astonishing history of going several weeks between bowel movements has been obtained from some patients with severe megacolon. Megaesophagus and megacolon may both be present in the same patient, and cardiomyopathy can occur with either form of megadisease.

DIAGNOSIS. For both acute and chronic Chagas' disease, a history of possible exposure to *T. cruzi* should be sought. Usual tourist travel to endemic areas is not likely to provide sufficient exposure to infected vectors. Blood transfusion from a chronically infected donor can be a source of infection.

For *acute Chagas' disease* direct microscopic examination of anticoagulated blood or a buffy coat preparation for motile trypanosomes is the most important procedure. Organisms are more difficult to find on stained thin or thick blood films, but the morphology of organisms seen on direct microscopy should be confirmed in a stained preparation. Red cells may be lysed, using 0.083% NH_4Cl to concentrate parasites by centrifugation. If parasites cannot be found in the peripheral blood and acute disease is still suspected, blood can be cultured on NNN (Novy, MacNeal, and Nicolle's medium) or other suitable media. Inoculation of mice with the patient's blood may sometimes result in recovery of the parasite. Biopsy of an enlarged lymph node or of skeletal muscle for culture and/or histologic examination is another possibility.

The most sensitive technique for recovering trypanosomes from the blood is a procedure referred to as xenodiagnosis. It is basically a form of blood culture using the insect vector, by allowing up to 40 normal, laboratory-reared reduviid bugs to feed directly upon the patient or on the patient's blood through a membrane. Circulating parasites ingested by the bugs multiply in the gut and can be detected when the intestinal contents are examined 30 days later. Under experimental conditions, polymerase chain reaction techniques to demonstrate low levels of parasitemia appear promising, but no simple and specific methods are yet available for routine use.

Serologic testing is generally not needed to diagnose acute disease. Parasite-specific immunoglobulin M (IgM) antibodies detected by immunofluorescence or direct agglutination do not become positive until 20 to 40 days after the onset of symptoms. In certain situations this delayed antibody response permits the demonstration of seroconversion. Other laboratory tests often show nonspecific changes, such as a lymphocytic leukocytosis, elevated sedimentation rate, or transient ECG abnormalities. Reversible cardiomegaly and even pericardial effusion may occur.

The diagnosis of *chronic Chagas' disease* requires demonstration of antibodies to *T. cruzi* in the presence of the characteristic cardiac abnormalities and/or megadisease. Thus, except for the positive serologic findings, the diagnosis relies heavily upon clinical judgment in excluding other causes of heart disease or gastrointestinal dysfunction. A positive xenodiagnosis is strongly supportive, but not in itself diagnostic of chronic disease, since patients in the indeterminate phase may have low-level parasitemia. A variety of assays for specific antibody are available, and generally the results of different tests are comparable. However, there are cross-reactions in some tests with sera from patients with leishmaniasis or syphilis, for example. Therefore, in individual cases it may be helpful to confirm the presence of antibody to specific antigens of *T. cruzi* with more sophisticated tests, such as immunoblots.

Symptomatic heart involvement in the chronic disease is manifested by characteristic ECG abnormalities, often without car-diomegaly. The most common of these is complete right bundle branch block. Other frequent ECG findings are left anterior hemi-block, ventricular extrasystoles, and even complete heart block. If heart failure is present, radiographs and echocardiograms will show generalized cardiomegaly with a reduced ejection fraction (Fig. 376–2).

Chagasic megaesophagus in the early stages shows only delayed emptying and minimal dilatation on studies after a barium swallow. With more advanced disease, retention of swallowed material and esophageal dilatation are progressively increased. Manometric stud-ies show spasm of the esophageal sphincter and uncoordinated peri-staltic movements. Endoscopy should be performed to rule out ma-lignant disease. However, all of these findings are indistinguishable from idiopathic achalasia. Barium enema with air contrast shows the dilated colon with impaired peristalsis, but other causes of colonic obstruction must be ruled out.

DIFFERENTIAL DIAGNOSIS. When acute Chagas' disease is symptomatic and severe, it can resemble a variety of acute systemic infections. Romaña's sign must be distinguished from other causes of unilateral orbital edema, such as the reaction to an insect bite, trauma, or orbital cellulitis.

Congenital infections are virtually indistinguishable from congen-ital toxoplasmosis, cytomegalic inclusion disease, and syphilis.

Various cardiomyopathies, such as postpartum, alcoholic, and en-domyocardial fibrosis, can resemble chronic Chagas' heart disease. Endocardial biopsy is of dubious diagnostic value because of the nonspecific pathologic changes in chagasic cardiomyopathy; it might, however, identify other causes of heart disease. The charac-teristic heart murmurs of rheumatic valvular disease are helpful in differentiating this entity from chagasic cardiomyopathy. The value of positive serologic findings for *T. cruzi* in the differential diagno-sis of both heart and megadisease will depend upon the background prevalence of antibodies in the general population.

TREATMENT. Two drugs with reasonable antitrypanosomal ac-tivity are currently in use for treating Chagas' disease. One of these is a nitrofuran derivative, nifurtimox*, which has been extensively evaluated. Nifurtimox is the only drug available in the United States for treating Chagas' disease; it is used in a dose of 8 to 12 mg per kilogram per day. The second drug, benznidazole, is a ni-troimidazole derivative that appears to be equal to nifurtimox in ef-ficacy, although there is less experience with its use. The exact mechanism of antitrypanosomal action of both of these drugs is not known.

There is now considerable evidence that if patients with acute Chagas' disease are treated with either nifurtimox or benznidazole,

---

* An investigational drug that must be obtained from the Centers for Dis-ease and Prevention Control Drug Service (404-329-3670).

the extent of disease and parasitemia usually are reduced. But more important, many patients treated in the acute phase never develop antibodies to *T. cruzi*, or do so only transiently. From this observa-tion, plus the fact that xenodiagnosis in such treated patients often is negative, it is assumed that parasites can be eliminated and the patient cured if treated in the acute stage. However, nifurtimox is not uniformly effective in producing these results, and parasite strains from certain geographic areas (Brazil) appear to be less re-sponsive to treatment than do strains from other countries (Ar-gentina and Chile).

The frequency of side effects from both nifurtimox and benznida-zole is high; because they are administered for 60 to 90 days, drug toxicity is a serious problem. The most common adverse effect with nifurtimox is gastrointestinal intolerance, with anorexia, nausea, vomiting, and abdominal pain. Neurologic symptoms include rest-lessness, insomnia, disorientation, paresthesias, polyneuritis, and even seizures. Skin rashes can also occur. Peripheral neuropathy and bone marrow suppression have been reported with benznida-zole. These side effects subside when the dosage of the drugs is re-duced or treatment is stopped.

Since these drugs have shown effectiveness in treatment of acute Chagas' disease, some Latin American physicians are also treating chronic and indeterminate cases. There is no evidence that the es-tablished pathologic changes of chronic Chagas' disease can be re-versed by nifurtimox or benznidazole therapy. The question of whether drug treatment in the indeterminate case, i.e., the asympto-matic patient with positive serologic findings, would prevent devel-opment of later chronic disease is controversial. Some data suggest that low-level parasitemia, as assessed by xenodiagnosis, can be re-duced or eliminated after treatment with antitrypanosomal drugs, in-cluding allopurinol. But such studies require critical confirmation to establish their ultimate influence on the development of chronic dis-ease, as well as risk versus benefit evaluation.

The treatment of patients with established chronic heart disease is supportive. Patients with frequent ventricular premature beats can benefit from antiarrhythmic drugs such as amiodarone. Cardiac pacemakers will prolong survival of those with complete heart block. The congestive failure of chagasic cardiomyopathy is disap-pointingly refractory to the usual cardiotropic drugs.

More options are open for managing and treating megadisease. In the early stages of megaesophagus, pneumatic dilatation of the sphincter is probably more effective than bougienage. For more ad-vanced cases, various surgical procedures involving myotomy of the sphincter or partial resection are necessary. Early stages of mega-colon can be managed by manipulating diet and using laxatives and occasional enemas. Sometimes an aperistaltic section of the colon can be resected in more severe cases.

PREVENTION. Chagas' disease could be eliminated as a seri-ous health problem for the rural poor of Latin America by adequate housing and education. But stark socioeconomic realities dictate an-other approach to control. This consists mainly of the use of resid-ual insecticides directed at domiciliary vectors. The use of benzene

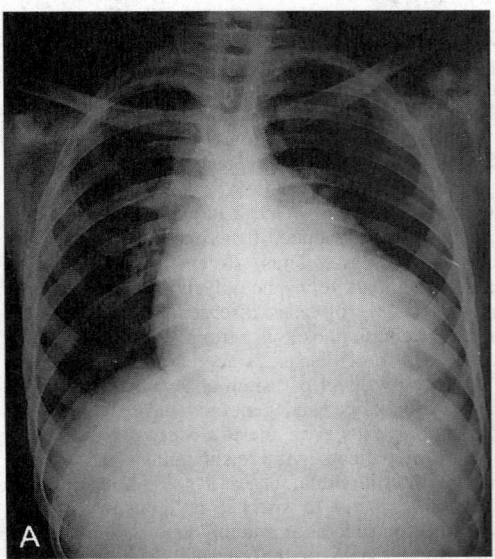
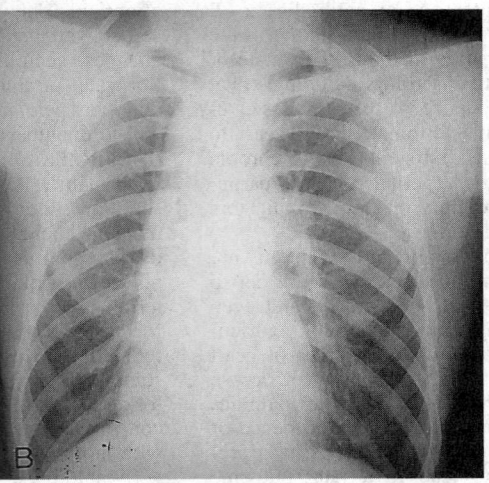

FIGURE 376–2. *A,* Cardiac silhouette in a patient with chronic chagasic cardiomyopathy and heart failure. *B,* Chest radiograph showing a widened mediastinum due to a greatly dilated megaesophagus of chronic Chagas' disease.

hexachloride (BHC), sprayed once or twice a year, has been very effective when used systematically.

Serologic testing in blood banks to avoid use of seropositive donors is carried out in endemic areas. Another precaution is to add 1:4000 gentian violet to blood 24 hours before use to kill trypanosomes that may be present. With the recent occurrence of several transfusion-associated cases of acute Chagas' disease in North America, the question of serologic screening of blood donors has been raised for areas of the country with large Latin American populations. The development of vaccines is still in the research stage.

Dias JCP: The indeterminate form of human chronic Chagas' disease. A clinical epidemiological review. Rev Soc Bras Med Trop 22:147, 1989. *A well-balanced review in English by a Brazilian expert. It documents the important point that infection with T. cruzi does not invariably progress to chronic disease.*

Kirchhoff LV: American trypanosomiasis (Chagas' disease)—A tropical disease now in the United States. N Engl J Med 329:639, 1993. *A concise "Current Concepts" review of the subject, including potential problems for blood banks and health care providers dealing with immigrant populations.*

Maguire JH, Hoff R, Sherlock I, et al.: Cardiac morbidity and mortality due to Chagas' disease: Prospective electrocardiographic study of a Brazilian community. Circulation 75:1140, 1987. *Antibodies to T. cruzi were present in 42% of the population. Excess mortality and development of abnormal ECGs were clearly related to positive serology.*

Rocha A, deMeneses ACO, daSilva AM, et al.: Pathology of patients with Chagas' disease and acquired immunodeficiency syndrome. Am J Trop Med & Hyg 50:261, 1994. *A review of 23 patients, 20 of whom had severe, multifocal meningoencephalitis; Chagas' disease was activated by AIDS.*

377 LEISHMANIASIS

Richard D. Pearson and Anastacio de Queiroz Sousa

Leishmaniasis is the name given to the spectrum of disease caused by *Leishmania* species, protozoa of the order Kinetoplastidia. It is endemic in widely scattered areas on every continent except Australia and Antarctica. The leishmania assume two distinct morphologic forms. They reside solely within mononuclear phagocytes as intracellular amastigotes in humans and other mammals, and they live as extracellular, flagellated promastigotes in the gut of their insect vectors, phlebotomine sandflies. With a few important exceptions such as visceral leishmaniasis in India, leishmaniasis is a zoonosis. Depending on the location, rodents, dogs, other animals, or humans are reservoirs. Transmission of the parasite requires a susceptible host, a sandfly vector, and an infected reservoir.

The clinical manifestations of leishmaniasis vary as a function of the parasite's pathogenicity, which differs among *Leishmania* species, and the host's immune responses. Some infections are asymptomatic and self-resolving, whereas others result in one or more of the three major forms of disease: cutaneous, mucosal (also termed mucocutaneous), and visceral leishmaniasis.

CLASSIFICATION AND LIFE CYCLE

The *Leishmania* species, their geographic locations, and the clinical syndromes that they produce are summarized in Table 377–1. The classification of *Leishmania* was originally based on their geographic location, clinical manifestations, vectors, and biochemical attributes. Speciation of isolates at World Health Organization reference laboratories is currently done by isoenzyme analysis. Species-specific monoclonal antibodies and kinetoplast-DNA (kDNA) probes are available in research laboratories. Recent experimental work suggests that polymerase chain reaction (PCR) methodology using *Leishmania* species-specific primers may emerge as the method of choice for speciation and diagnosis.

The leishmania live as intracellular amastigotes in parasitophorous vacuoles within mononuclear phagocytes in humans and other mammals (Fig. 377–1). Amastigotes are oval or round and approximately 2 to 3 microns in diameter. They have a relatively large eccentrically placed nucleus and a rod-shaped specialized mitochondrial structure, the kinetoplast. Promastigotes, which are found in the gut of the sandfly, are flagellated and extracellular.

Female sandflies, *Lutzomyia* species in Latin America and *Phlebotomus* species in the rest of the world, are responsible for transmitting leishmania. Some are peridomestic and live in rubble and debris near houses or farm buildings; others thrive in thick vegetation in forest areas. Sandflies are modified pool feeders. They ingest

TABLE 377–1. GEOGRAPHIC DISTRIBUTION AND CLINICAL DISEASE CAUSED BY *LEISHMANIA* SPECIES

Clinical Syndromes	Leishmania Species	Location
Visceral leishmaniasis		
Kala-azar: generalized involvement of the reticuloendothelial system (spleen, bone marrow, liver, etc.)	L. donovani	Indian subcontinent, North and East China, Pakistan, Nepal
	L. infantum	Middle East, Mediterranean littoral, Balkans, Central and Southwest Asia, North and Northwestern China, North and sub-Saharan Africa
	L. donovani (archibaldi)	Sudan, Kenya, Ethiopia
	Leishmania species	Kenya, Ethiopia, Somalia
	L. chagasi	Latin America
	L. amazonensis	Brazil (Bahia State)
	L. tropica	Israel, India, and "viscerotropic" disease in Saudi Arabia (U.S. troops)
Post–kala-azar dermal leishmaniasis	L. donovani	Indian subcontinent
	Leishmania species	Kenya, Ethiopia, Somalia
Old World cutaneous leishmaniasis		
Single or limited number of skin lesions	L. major	Middle East, Northwest China, Northwest India, Pakistan, Africa
	L. tropica	Mediterranean littoral, Middle East, west Asiatic area, Indian subcontinent
	L. aethiopica	Ethiopian highlands, Kenya, Yemen
	L. infantum	Mediterranean basin
	L. donovani (archibaldi)	Sudan, East Africa
	Leishmania species	Kenya, Ethiopia, Somalia
Diffuse cutaneous leishmaniasis	L. aethiopica	Ethiopian highlands, Kenya, Yemen
New World cutaneous leishmaniasis		
Single or limited number of skin lesions	L. mexicana (chiclero ulcer)	Central America, Mexico, Texas
	L. amazonensis	Amazon basin including Brazil and neighboring countries
	L. braziliensis	Multiple areas of Central and South America
	L. guyanensis (forest yaws)	Guyana, Surinam, northern Amazon basin
	L. peruviana (uta)	Peru (western Andes), Argentinean highlands
	L. panamensis	Panama, Costa Rica, Columbia
	L. pifanoi	Venezuela
	L. garnhami	Venezuela
	L. venezuelensis	Venezuela
	L. chagasi	Central and South America
Diffuse cutaneous leishmaniasis	L. amazonensis	Amazon basin including Brazil and neighboring countries
	L. pifanoi	Venezuela
	L. mexicana	Mexico, Central America
	Leishmania species	Dominican Republic
Mucosal leishmaniasis	L. braziliensis (Espundia)	Multiple areas in Latin America

Adapted from Pearson RD, Sousa AQ: Leishmania species: Visceral (kala-azar), cutaneous and mucosal leishmaniasis. *In* Mandell GL, Bennett JE, Dolin R (eds.): Principles and Practice of Infectious Diseases. 4th ed., New York, Churchill Livingstone, 1994, p 2428. Data from Lainson R, Shaw JJ: Evolution, classification and geographic distribution. *In* Peters W, Killick-Kendrick R (eds.): The Leishmaniases in Biology and Medicine, vol. 1. London, Academic Press, 1987, p 1.

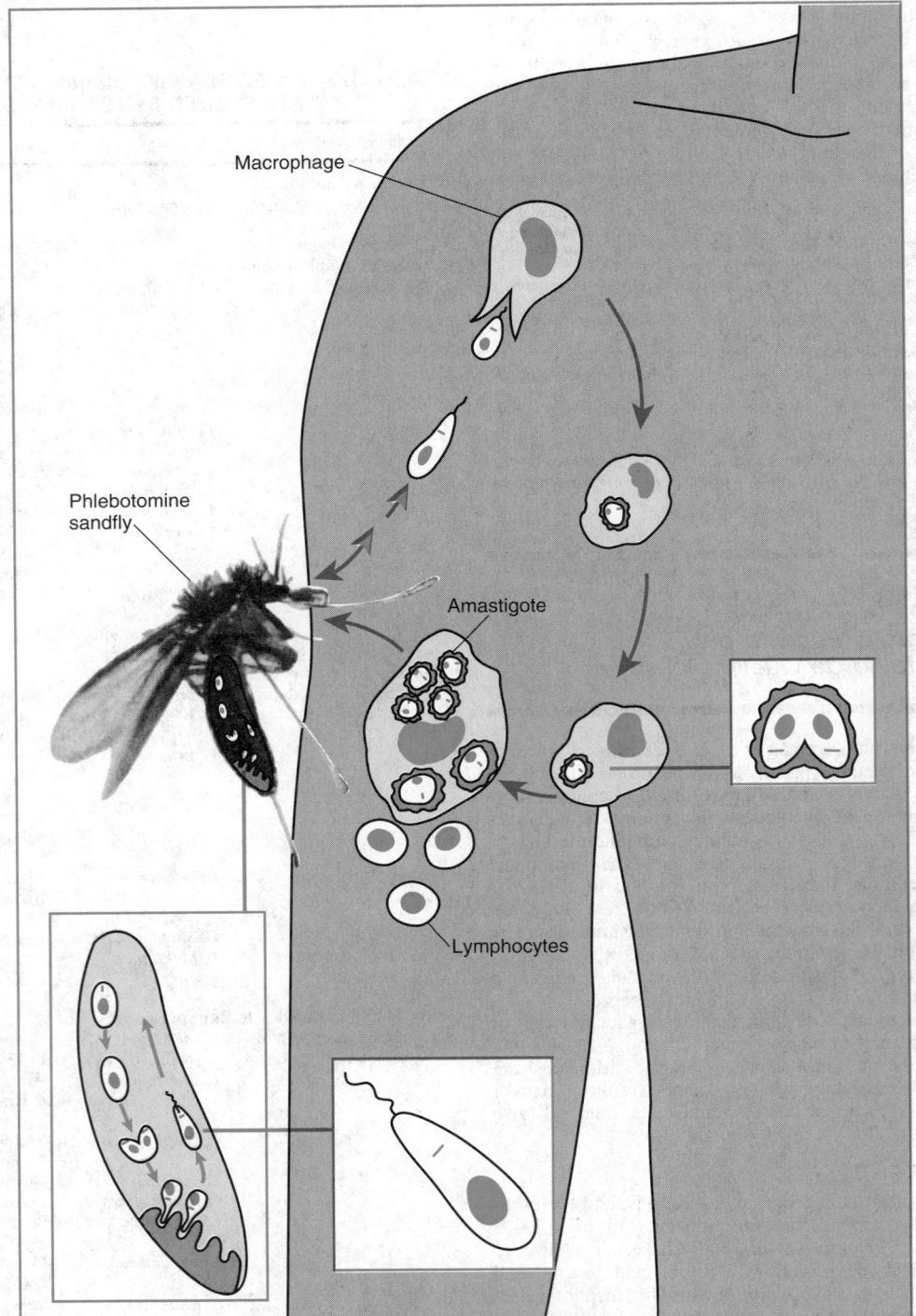

FIGURE 377–1. Life cycle of leishmania. Humans serve as the reservoir for *L. donovani* in India as depicted here. In most settings leishmaniasis is a zoonosis with rodents or canines as reservoirs.

amastigote-containing macrophages when they take a blood meal. Amastigotes transform to promastigotes, which then multiply and differentiate in the sandfly gut. The life cycle is completed approximately 1 week later when metacyclic promastigotes are deposited as the sandfly attempts to take its next blood meal. Sandfly saliva contains a factor(s) that enhances the promastigote's infectivity for macrophages.

IMMUNOLOGY

The control of leishmanial infections depends on T cell–mediated immune responses. Antileishmanial antibodies are produced, but they are not protective. Resolution of infection and protection against reinfection correlate with the proliferation of CD4 cells of the Th1 type (see Ch. 221) that secrete interferon-γ and interleukin-2 (IL-2) in response to leishmanial antigens. Interferon-γ activates macrophages to kill intracellular amastigotes. Data from the murine system indicate that L-arginine–dependent nitric oxide production is the dominant effector mechanism. IL-12 appears to play an important role in the development of Th1 responses.

Potentially protective Th1 responses are suppressed in persons with progressive infections. Leishmania-specific CD4 cells of the Th2 type that produce IL-4 are responsible for suppressing the development of Th1 responses in mice. In humans with visceral leishmaniasis, IL-10 appears to mediate suppression. The early events that follow parasite inoculation seem to be crucial in determining whether protective or nonprotective T4 cell responses dominate, but they have not been fully defined.

VISCERAL LEISHMANIASIS

EPIDEMIOLOGY (Table 377–1). Visceral leishmaniasis is typically caused by *L. donovani* in India and Africa, and two closely related species—*L. infantum* in the Mediterranean littoral and *L. chagasi* in Latin America. The disease occurs sporadically or in epidemics. On occasion *Leishmania* species that are predominantly associated with cutaneous disease, e.g., *L. mexicana* and *L. major*, are isolated from patients with classic visceral leishmaniasis. In addition, a small group of American soldiers infected with *L. tropica* in Saudi Arabia during Operation Desert Storm (Persian Gulf War, 1991) developed a "viscerotropic" syndrome, with dissemination of amastigotes to the bone marrow, but without many of the manifestations of classic progressive visceral leishmaniasis.

Visceral leishmaniasis due to *L. donovani* is a major problem in eastern India and Bangladesh (Table 377–1). The disease is most common in young adults. Major epidemics followed the cessation of DDT spraying for malaria there. Humans appear to be the only reservoir of infection, and leishmania are transmitted by anthropophilic sandflies. *L. donovani*, which is also endemic in Kenya and Ethiopia, has been responsible for a large epidemic of visceral leishmaniasis among refugees in the Sudan. The reservoirs are rodents and small carnivores. Humans may serve as a reservoir during epidemics. Visceral leishmaniasis due to *L. infantum* occurs sporadically among children and persons with HIV and other immunocompromising conditions in southern Europe, the Middle East, and North Africa. In Brazil, Venezuela, Colombia, and other areas of Latin America, visceral leishmaniasis due to *L. chagasi* is typically found in scattered, rural areas, although large urban outbreaks have occurred in northeast Brazil. The majority of cases are in children younger than age 10.

IMMUNOPATHOLOGY. Infection with *L. donovani* and related organisms is acquired when promastigotes are inoculated by sandflies into an exposed area of skin. The parasites convert to amastigotes and multiply within mononuclear phagocytes. Although a cutaneous nodule or ulcer may develop, most patients are unaware of the site of primary inoculation. Amastigotes subsequently disseminate via regional lymphatics and the vascular system to mononuclear phagocytes throughout the reticuloendothelial system. The majority of infections with *L. donovani, L. chagasi,* and *L. infantum* are asymptomatic and resolve spontaneously. A minority progress to classic, full-blown visceral leishmaniasis, known in many areas as kala-azar. In Brazil, a subset of children infected with *L. chagasi* has a prolonged course with minimal symptoms; in some the infection eventually resolves spontaneously, whereas in others it progresses to classic visceral leishmaniasis.

In patients with progressive visceral leishmaniasis, increased numbers of mononuclear phagocytes are found in the liver and spleen, resulting in hypertrophy. In the liver there is a dramatic increase in the number and size of Kupffer cells, many filled with amastigotes. The spleen often is massively enlarged, and splenic lymphoid follicles are replaced by parasitized mononuclear cells. Amastigote-containing mononuclear phagocytes are found in the bone marrow, lymph nodes, skin, intestinal tract, and other organs. Circulating immune complexes are common, and there is histologic evidence of deposition in the kidney, but renal failure is rare.

CLINICAL MANIFESTATIONS. The incubation period with symptomatic infection is quite variable but usually ranges from 3 to 8 months. The onset of visceral leishmaniasis is often insidious and difficult to date, and the disease usually has a subacute or chronic course. In some cases, however, there is an abrupt onset of fever and chills suggestive of malaria. Symptoms include fever, malaise, anorexia, weight loss, and enlargement of the abdomen. Fever may be intermittent, remittent with twice-daily temperature spikes to 38 to 40°C, or less commonly, continuous. It is usually well tolerated.

Hepatomegaly and splenomegaly are hallmarks of visceral leishmaniasis; the spleen is firm and nontender and frequently becomes massively enlarged (Fig. 377–2). Patients in India may develop hyperpigmentation, which led to the name kala-azar, meaning black fever in Hindi. Jaundice is occasionally present. Late in visceral leishmaniasis patients may develop epistaxis, gingival bleeding, and petechiae on their extremities. They may have edema and ascites due to hypoalbuminemia. The majority of patients with visceral

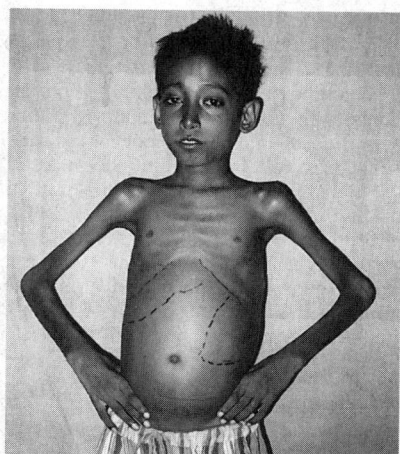

FIGURE 377–2. Indian patient with kala-azar. Note wasting of thorax and shoulder girdle and hepatosplenomegaly as outlined.

leishmaniasis and concurrent HIV present in the classic manner, but splenomegaly may be absent, and atypical presentations with involvement of the lungs, pleura, oral mucosa, esophagus, stomach, small intestine, or skin have been reported.

On laboratory examination, anemia, thrombocytopenia, neutropenia, and hypergammaglobulinemia are common. The anemia is usually normocytic and normochromic unless complicated by blood loss. The white blood count may be as low as 1000 per cubic millimeter; eosinopenia is common. Platelets are also decreased. The erythrocyte sedimentation rate is elevated. The levels of gamma globulin are markedly increased, at times in the range of 9 to 10 grams per deciliter. This is a result of polyclonal B cell activation. Circulating immune complexes and rheumatoid factors are also present in the majority of patients. Liver enzymes and bilirubin are elevated in some.

Untreated persons with visceral leishmaniasis have a progressive, downhill course over several months or more. Severe cachexia may develop. Patients with advanced visceral leishmaniasis evidence neutropenia as well as anergy to multiple T cell antigens. Bacterial pneumonia, measles, dysentery, tuberculosis, gangrenous stomatitis, and other secondary infections are common and frequently contribute to death.

Viscerotropic Leishmaniasis. In the *L. tropica*–related "viscerotropic" syndrome observed in American military personnel who served in Operation Desert Storm, symptoms included chronic low-grade fever, malaise, fatigue, and in some instances, diarrhea. The troops did not develop splenomegaly or the progressive wasting associated with classic visceral leishmaniasis.

Post–Kala-azar Leishmaniasis. A small percentage of persons in India and Africa who are treated for visceral leishmaniasis develop post–kala-azar dermal leishmaniasis after the other manifestations of disease have resolved. In Africa the lesions develop shortly after treatment and persist for several months. In India they appear up to 2 years after treatment and persist for as long as 20 years. The skin lesions vary from hyperpigmented macules to frank nodules and contain *L. donovani* amastigotes. They are frequently found on the face, trunk, and extremities.

DIAGNOSIS. A presumptive diagnosis of visceral leishmaniasis is easily made by the classic clinical presentation in an endemic area. The diagnosis may be delayed or missed in an immigrant or traveler returning to a nonendemic country, particularly if the person has concurrent HIV infection and lacks splenomegaly. The diagnosis is confirmed by identifying *Leishmania* species amastigotes in tissue or by growing promastigotes in culture. Splenic aspiration results in a diagnosis in 96 to 98% of cases. It is relatively safe when performed by an experienced physician, but significant hemorrhage occurs on occasion, particularly in patients with clotting abnormalities. Bone marrow aspiration results in a diagnosis in more than half of the cases. Alternative sites for aspiration and/or biopsy include the liver and lymph nodes if they are enlarged, or culture of the buffy coat. In patients with concurrent HIV infections amastigotes are frequently identified in unexpected sites such as bronchoalveolar lavage fluid, pleural effusions, or biopsies of lesions in the oral pharynx, larynx, stomach, or intestine.

Antileishmanial antibodies are present in high titer in immunocompetent patients with visceral leishmaniasis. They can be measured by enzyme-linked immunosorbent assay (ELISA), indirect immunofluorescence assay, direct agglutination tests, or several alternative assays. Persons with advanced HIV and those with viscerotropic *L. tropica* infections frequently have low or undetectable antileishmanial antibodies. The leishmanin skin test, also known as the Montenegro test, is negative in persons with visceral leishmaniasis, but it becomes positive in the majority of those who undergo successful chemotherapy and in those with self-resolving infections. The antigen preparation is not approved for use in the United States.

CUTANEOUS AND MUCOSAL LEISHMANIASIS

EPIDEMIOLOGY (see Table 377–1). *Leishmania* species produce a spectrum of cutaneous and mucosal lesions. Most common are chronic, localized, ulcerative lesions, often referred to as "oriental sores" (see Color Plate 9*F*). They are seen periodically among Western travelers who visit or work in endemic areas. Cutaneous leishmaniasis in Latin America is caused by *L. mexicana*, *L. braziliensis*, and several related species, and on occasion, by *L. chagasi*. It is a zoonosis. The reservoirs are usually forest rodents. Humans become infected when they settle or work in or near forested areas. *L. braziliensis* is also responsible for mucosal leishmaniasis.

Most cases of cutaneous leishmaniasis outside of Latin America are caused by three *Leishmania* species. *L. major* is an important problem among settlers, visitors, and troops in endemic rural areas of the Middle East, Central Asia, and North Africa. Rodents are the principal reservoir. *L. tropica* is usually found in urban areas of the Middle East, the Mediterranean littoral, India, Pakistan, and Central Asia. The reservoirs are dogs and humans. *L. aethiopica* is endemic in Ethiopia, Kenya, and southwest Africa, where hyrax are reservoirs. On occasion *L. donovani* or *L. infantum* is isolated from cutaneous lesions.

IMMUNOPATHOLOGY. The peripheral blood mononuclear cells from patients with classic cutaneous leishmaniasis proliferate and produce interferon-γ and IL-2 in response to leishmanial antigens *in vitro*, and patients evidence delayed-type hypersensitivity responses to leishmanial antigens *in vivo*. The chronic course of the disease appears to be due to the dominance of Th2-like responses and other suppressive factors at the site of the lesion.

The spectrum of cutaneous leishmaniasis includes several variants. On one extreme is the anergic variant diffuse cutaneous leishmaniasis, a rare syndrome in which parasites disseminate in the skin, producing multiple nodular lesions composed primarily of histiocytes filled with amastigotes. These lesions do not ulcerate. No evidence of a Th1 response is seen in patients with diffuse cutaneous leishmaniasis. Peripheral blood mononuclear cells do not proliferate or produce interferon-γ or IL-2 in response to leishmanial antigens, and there are no delayed-type hypersensitivity responses to intradermally injected antigens. Clinically this is somewhat analogous to lepromatous leprosy.

In contrast in mucosal leishmaniasis there is a chronic, destructive, granulomatous inflammatory response. Amastigotes are often scant. There is evidence of a vigorous Th1-like response. Peripheral blood mononuclear cells proliferate and secrete interferon-γ in response to leishmanial antigens, and there are pronounced delayed-type hypersensitivity responses to intradermally inoculated antigens. Clinically, this hyperergic variant is somewhat analogous to tuberculoid leprosy.

CLINICAL MANIFESTATIONS. *Cutaneous Leishmaniasis*. Cutaneous leishmaniasis may involve single or multiple lesions. They are relatively heterogeneous and vary as a function of the infecting *Leishmania* species and the host's immune response. A typical lesion starts as an erythematous papule at the site where promastigotes are inoculated by a sandfly, slowly increases in size, becomes a nodule, and eventually ulcerates. "Wet" lesions are covered with exudate, and have raised borders (see Color Plate 9*F*). They are frequently associated with superficial, secondary bacterial or fungal infections. Other lesions are "dry" with a central crust.

Satellite lesions may be found at or near the edges of the primary site of infection. On occasion cutaneous leishmaniasis may appear nodular, suggesting skin cancer. Rarely, cutaneous leishmaniasis involves local lymphatics, mimicking sporotrichosis. Cutaneous lesions persist for months and in some cases years before they spontaneously heal, leaving flat, hypopigmented, atrophic scars.

It was once thought that cutaneous leishmaniasis was confined to the skin, but recent observations in Brazil indicate that *L. braziliensis* can cause regional lymphadenopathy, fever, and other constitutional symptoms before the primary cutaneous lesion becomes apparent. These symptoms and findings resolve as the skin ulcer develops. Splenomegaly occurs in some patients. It is thought that *L. braziliensis* may disseminate to distant mucosal sites during this early phase of infection.

Diffuse Cutaneous Leishmaniasis. Diffuse cutaneous leishmaniasis is a rare anergic variant. It starts as a localized papule that does not ulcerate, and satellite lesions develop as amastigotes disseminate in the skin (Fig. 377–3). Eventually multiple cutaneous nodules develop on the face and extremities. The disease progresses slowly and often persists for decades.

Leishmaniasis Recidiva. Leishmaniasis recidiva, typically associated with *L. tropica* infection in the Middle East, is a chronic syndrome with skin lesions on the face or exposed extremities that enlarge slowly, tend to heal in the center, and persist for many years. Biopsies of the lesions reveal chronic inflammatory changes; amastigotes are sparse.

Mucosal Leishmaniasis (Espundia). A small percentage of persons with *L. braziliensis* infection in Latin America develop mucosal lesions of the nose, mouth, pharynx, or larynx months to years after the primary skin ulcer heals (see Color Plate 9*G*). The disease typically begins with nasal inflammation and stuffiness, followed by ulceration of the mucosa. The lesions are characterized by a chronic granulomatous response. There is destruction of the mucosa and eventually of the underlying cartilage of the nasal septum or palate. Patients evidence brisk Th1 responses to leishmanial antigens, and the tissue destruction appears to be due to a hyperergic immune response. The differential diagnosis of American mucosal leishmaniasis includes paracoccidioidomycosis, histoplasmosis, tertiary syphilis, tertiary yaws, sarcoidosis, Wegener's granulomatosis, midline granuloma, rhinoscleroma, and basal cell carcinoma.

DIAGNOSIS. The diagnosis of cutaneous leishmaniasis should be considered in any person with a chronic, localized skin lesion who has been exposed in an endemic area. It is confirmed by identifying amastigotes in touch preparations, by histopathology, or by growing promastigotes in culture. A punch biopsy and aspirate should be obtained from the margin of the lesion after it has been meticulously cleaned. Touch preparations are stained with a Wright-Giemsa preparation. The remaining tissue should be divided and used for culture and histopathology. Antileishmanial antibodies are

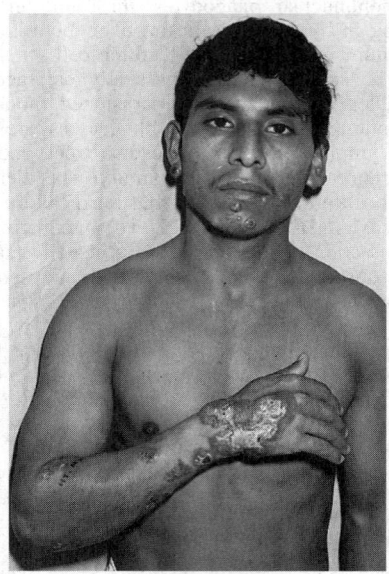

FIGURE 377–3. Patient with diffuse cutaneous leishmaniasis of 5 years' duration. Note nonulcerative lesions of chin, ear lobes, right arm, and hand.

often detectable in the serum of patients with cutaneous leishmaniasis, but the titers are usually low. The leishmanin skin test is positive in persons with simple cutaneous leishmaniasis, leishmaniasis recidiva, and mucosal leishmaniasis, but nonreactive in patients with diffuse cutaneous leishmaniasis.

Parasites are often scant in mucosal lesions due to *L. braziliensis*. A positive leishmanin skin test, the presence of antileishmanial antibodies, exposure in an endemic area, and evidence of a healed cutaneous lesion allow for a presumptive diagnosis.

TREATMENT

VISCERAL LEISHMANIASIS. Pentavalent antimonials, stibogluconate sodium (Pentostam), and meglumine antimoniate (Glucantime) remain the treatment of choice for visceral leishmaniasis, but clinical failures are becoming increasingly prevalent in many areas, and these drugs are associated with important untoward effects. Stibogluconate sodium is available in the United States through the CDC Drug Service.* It is also used in Europe, Africa, and India. Meglumine antimoniate is available in Latin America, France, and in Francophone countries in Africa.

Stibogluconate sodium and meglumine antimoniate are administered on the basis of their pentavalent antimony content. When properly manufactured and stored, they appear to be of comparable efficacy and toxicity. The recommended treatment course is 20 mg of pentavalent antimony per kilogram body weight per day for 20 to 28 days. A prolonged course is frequently used in patients who do not respond completely to the initial course of therapy.

Recent reports suggest that chemical pancreatitis is common in patients receiving pentavalent antimonials. Other side effects include pain at the injection site when the drug is given intramuscularly, arthralgias, myalgias, nausea, vomiting, liver enzyme abnormalities, and ST-T wave changes by electrocardiography. Cardiac toxicity and sudden death have occurred in patients who received more than the recommended dose.

Amphotericin B and pentamidine are alternative drugs, but both have important side effects (see Ch. 347). Amphotericin B (0.5 to 1.0 mg per kilogram every other day for up to 8 weeks or for a total dose of 1.5 to 2.0 grams) has been used successfully to treat patients who fail antimony therapy. Recombinant interferon-γ plus a pentavalent antimonial have proven to be effective in patients with visceral leishmaniasis who fail pentavalent antimonial therapy alone. Unfortunately, recombinant interferon-γ is expensive and available only for patients on experimental protocols.

CUTANEOUS LEISHMANIASIS. Cutaneous lesions that are large or located in cosmetically important sites and those that are caused by *L. braziliensis* or other *Leishmania* species associated with mucosal disease should be treated. Small, inconspicuous, or healing lesions caused by *Leishmania* species that are not associated with mucosal disease can be followed expectantly. Pentavalent antimonials, stibogluconate sodium and meglumine antimoniate, effectively treat cutaneous leishmaniasis in many situations, but, as described above, they are frequently associated with toxicity, and clinical failures are becoming increasingly prevalent. Full doses of 20 mg per kilogram body weight per day are recommended for 20 to 28 days; lower doses may favor the development of antimony resistance. Cutaneous lesions heal slowly during antimony therapy. A number of other drugs and therapeutic approaches, including local treatment and immunotherapy, are under study and have their proponents, but the data are insufficient to recommend their general use.

Therapeutic failures with pentavalent antimonials are common in persons with diffuse cutaneous leishmaniasis, leishmaniasis recidiva, and mucosal leishmaniasis. Amphotericin B is an alternative. Preliminary data suggest that recombinant interferon-γ administered with a pentavalent antimonial can be used to effectively treat patients with diffuse cutaneous leishmaniasis.

PROPHYLAXIS

Personal protection with insect repellents containing DEET applied to skin and permethrin-treated clothing can reduce the frequency of sandfly bites in visitors to endemic areas. Fine mesh netting can be used for protection at night. Unfortunately, these measures are seldom practical for residents of endemic areas.

---

* Centers for Disease Control and Prevention, Atlanta, Georgia 30333; telephone 404-639-3670 (evenings, weekends, and holidays 404-639-2888).

Addy M, Nandy A: Ten years of kala-azar in West Bengal, Part I. Did post–kala-azar dermal leishmaniasis initiate the outbreak in 24-Parganas? Bull WHO 70:341, 1992. *An experience with visceral leishmaniasis in India discussing the potential role of humans with post–kala-azar dermal leishmaniasis as a reservoir of infection.*

Badaró R, Johnson WD Jr: The role of interferon-γ in the treatment of visceral and diffuse cutaneous leishmaniasis. J Infect Dis 167(Suppl 1):S13, 1993. *Recombinant interferon-γ plus a pentavalent antimonial appear promising for treating visceral or diffuse cutaneous leishmaniasis refractory to antimony therapy.*

Grogl M, Thomason TN, Franke ED: Drug resistance in leishmaniasis: Its implications in systemic chemotherapy of cutaneous and mucocutaneous disease. Am J Trop Med Hyg 47:117, 1992. *Pentavalent antimonial resistance is becoming increasingly common; recommends 20 mg per kilogram body weight of pentavalent antimony daily for 20 to 28 days, depending on the leishmanial syndrome being treated.*

Herwaldt BL, Berman JD: Recommendations for treating leishmaniasis with sodium stibogluconate (Pentostam) and review of pertinent clinical studies. Am J Trop Med Hyg 46:296, 1992. *Discusses the use of pentavalent antimonials in treating leishmaniasis.*

Locksley RM, Louis JA: Immunology of leishmaniasis. Curr Opin Immunol 4:413, 1992. *Excellent review of immunology of leishmanial infections and the role of cytokines in controlling cell-mediated immune responses.*

Magill AJ, Grögl M, Gasser RA Jr, et al.: Visceral infection caused by *Leishmania tropica* in veterans of Operation Desert Storm. N Engl J Med 328:1383, 1993. *Some Operation Desert Storm soldiers developed a viscerotropic syndrome with L. tropica, resulting in a temporary ban on blood and organ donations from all those involved in the operation.*

Reed SG, Scott P: T-cell and cytokine responses in leishmaniasis. Curr Opin Immunol 5:524, 1993. *Excellent review of the immunology of leishmaniasis.*

Wilson ME, Donnelson JE, Pearson RD, et al.: Macrophage receptors and *Leishmania*. In Korkonen TK, Hovi T, Makela PH (eds.): Molecular Recognition in Host-Parasite Interactions. New York, Plenum Publishing, 1992, p 17. *The receptors and ligands that mediate leishmania-macrophage interactions are discussed.*

378 TOXOPLASMOSIS

Carlos S. Subauste and Jack S. Remington

DEFINITION. *Toxoplasma gondii* is a protozoan that commonly infects mammals and birds throughout the world. *T. gondii* infection in humans is usually asymptomatic. However, clinical and/or pathologic evidence of disease (toxoplasmosis) occurs in some cases, particularly in the immunodeficient patient and fetus. Infection is characterized by two stages: acute (recently acquired) and chronic (latent). For information on congenital toxoplasmosis, the reader is referred to the Remington and Klein text (see end of this chapter).

LIFE CYCLE. *T. gondii* exists in three forms: the tachyzoite, which is the asexual invasive form; the tissue cyst (containing bradyzoites), which persists in tissues of infected hosts during the chronic phase of the infection; and the oocyst (containing sporozoites), which is produced during the sexual cycle in the intestine of cats (the definitive host). The extraintestinal asexual cycle is present in all incidental hosts and in cats. After ingestion of tissue cysts or oocysts, bradyzoites or sporozoites, respectively, are released into the intestinal lumen, where they invade surrounding cells, become tachyzoites, and disseminate throughout the body via the blood and lymphatics. The *tachyzoite* has a crescent shape, measures approximately 3 by 7 μm, requires an intracellular habitat for survival, and can infect all mammalian cells. Continued multiplication ultimately results in destruction of the host cell and release of tachyzoites, which can then infect other cells. Tachyzoites are found in tissues during the acute stage of the infection or during reactivation of the chronic infection. Freezing and thawing, desiccation, and gastric secretions kill tachyzoites. Development of immunity is associated with disappearance of tachyzoites and formation of tissue cysts. *Tissue cysts* measure from 10 to 200 μm in diameter, may contain up to several thousand bradyzoites, can be found in all organs, and are most readily observed in myocardial, skeletal, and smooth muscle and the central nervous system (CNS). In humans, they appear to persist for life. Unlike tachyzoites, bradyzoites released from tissue cysts are relatively resistant to the digestive process of the gastrointestinal tract. The enteroepithelial sexual cycle results in the formation of oocysts in the cat's intestine. *Oocysts* measure 10 to 12 μm in diameter, are excreted in the feces 3 to 34 days after the cat becomes infected, and continue to be excreted for 7 to 20 days, after which excretion rarely recurs. They become infectious only after they are excreted and sporulation occurs; the duration of this process depends on environmental conditions but usually takes 2 to 3 days. They may remain infectious in the environment for more than 1 year.

EPIDEMIOLOGY. *T. gondii* infects humans throughout the world. In the United States, depending on geographic locale and population group, 3 to 67% of adults have serologic evidence of infection. In other parts of the world, including tropical countries and some areas of western Europe, up to 90% of adults are seropositive. Transmission to humans occurs by ingesting tissue cysts or oocysts, the transplacental route, blood product transfusion, organ transplantation (kidney, heart, liver), and laboratory accident. Epidemics of toxoplasmosis due to eating undercooked meat or exposure to infected cat feces have occurred. In the United States, transmission by eating undercooked or raw meat containing tissue cysts or of vegetables or other food products contaminated with oocysts appears more common than transmission by contact with cat feces. Commercial cuts of pork and lamb (but rarely beef) may contain tissue cysts that remain infectious unless the meat is frozen to $-20°$ C or heated to $66°$ C.

The incidence of congenital toxoplasmosis in the United States ranges from 1 in 1000 to 1 in 8000 live births. Transplacental infection resulting in congenital infection can occur in immunocompetent pregnant women with acute *T. gondii* infection and in immunocompromised pregnant women with reactivation of a chronic infection. If the acute infection in the mother goes untreated, congenital infection occurs in approximately 15% of fetuses when maternal infection is acquired during the first trimester, 30% when acquired in the second trimester, and 60% when acquired in the third trimester. The earlier the transmission to the fetus, the more severe the outcome. Toxoplasmic encephalitis (TE) in AIDS patients (and in Hodgkin's disease and bone marrow transplant recipients) in the United States is almost always due to reactivation of a chronic infection. Therefore, the incidence of this disease is proportional to the prevalence of *T. gondii* antibodies (latent infection) in a given population and the stage of HIV infection in these patients (usually CD4 count < 200 per cubic millimeter). In the United States, *T. gondii* seroprevalence in HIV-infected individuals varies from 10 to 45%. It is estimated that 20 to 47% of HIV-infected, *T. gondii*–seropositive patients ultimately develop TE.

PATHOGENESIS. Following infection by the oral route, tachyzoites disseminate from the gastrointestinal tract and can invade virtually any cell or tissue, where they proliferate and produce necrotic foci surrounded by inflammation. In immunocompromised individuals, acute infection may result in severe damage to multiple organs. Both cell-mediated immunity and humoral immunity play a crucial role in resistance against *T. gondii*. Despite a normal immune response, tissue cysts form in multiple organs. Although disruption of cysts or "leakage" of bradyzoites from cysts appears to occur in normal hosts without causing disease, this can result in life-threatening disease in immunocompromised patients. Immunocompetent children or adults with congenital *T. gondii* infection can develop a localized reactivation that usually manifests clinically as recurrent retinochoroiditis.

CLINICAL MANIFESTATIONS. *Acute Infection in Immunocompetent Patients.* *T. gondii* infection is symptomatic in only approximately 10 to 20% of immunocompetent individuals. In these patients, toxoplasmosis most often presents as lymphadenopathy. Although any or all lymph node groups may be involved, cervical lymphadenopathy is most common; nodes are usually discrete, nontender, nonsuppurative, and asymptomatic. However, some patients may present with fever, myalgias, arthralgias, fatigue, headache, sore throat, maculopapular rash, urticaria, hepatosplenomegaly, small numbers (< 10%) of atypical lymphocytes, and rarely myocarditis. Involvement of retroperitoneal or mesenteric nodes may be associated with abdominal pain. Toxoplasmic lymphadenopathy is a self-limited disease, although fatigue and/or lymphadenopathy may persist or recur for months. Clinical illness due to reinfection from an exogenous source has not been reported.

Ocular Toxoplasmosis in Immunocompetent Patients. *T. gondii* infection has been reported to be responsible for approxi-

mately 35% of retinochoroiditis in older children and adults in the United States. Individuals with recently acquired infection uncommonly develop ocular involvement. *T. gondii* retinochoroiditis usually presents as a late manifestation of congenital infection. These latter patients are usually asymptomatic until adolescence or adulthood. Reactivation is uncommon after age 40. Patients may present with blurred vision, scotoma, pain, photophobia, or epiphora. Macular involvement may impair central vision. Systemic symptoms usually do not accompany ocular involvement. Ophthalmologic examination reveals multiple yellow-white, cotton-like patches with indistinct margins, located in small clusters in the posterior pole. Retinochoroiditis in the context of congenital infection is often bilateral, whereas retinochoroiditis in patients with recently acquired infection is typically unilateral. Retinochoroiditis may be part of a syndrome of panuveitis; isolated anterior uveitis has not been associated with *T. gondii*. Lesions may heal spontaneously, in which case they become atrophic with whitish gray plaques with distinct margins surrounded by areas of black choroidal pigment. Lesions at different stages of development may occur simultaneously. Multiple relapses may occur and may result in glaucoma and loss of vision.

Toxoplasmosis in Immunocompromised Patients. Numerous conditions that compromise the immune system have been associated with toxoplasmosis, including AIDS, Hodgkin's disease, and the use of corticosteroids or other immunosuppressive agents for treating malignancies, collagen-vascular disorders, or prevention of organ transplant rejection. In patients with these conditions, toxoplasmosis may be due to exogenous acquisition of infection or, more commonly, to reactivation of a latent infection. It is often rapidly progressive and fatal if untreated. Clinical manifestations are most commonly secondary to involvement of the CNS, lungs, eyes, and heart. TE is the most common manifestation and is also the most frequent cause of intracerebral mass lesions in patients with AIDS (see Ch. 364). TE typically presents with focal neurologic abnormalities of subacute onset, frequently accompanied by nonfocal signs and symptoms such as headache, altered mental status, and fever. The most common focal neurologic sign is motor weakness, but patients may also present with cranial nerve abnormalities, speech disturbances, visual field defects, sensory disturbances, cerebellar signs, focal seizures, and movement disorders. Meningeal signs may be present. Cerebrospinal fluid (CSF) may show slight mononuclear pleocytosis, increased protein, and normal glucose levels. Although radiologic findings are not pathognomonic, the presence of multiple lesions in AIDS patients strongly favors the diagnosis of TE, whereas the presence of a single lesion makes TE less likely. Computed tomographic (CT) scans usually show multiple bilateral cerebral lesions, which tend to be located at the corticomedullary junction and the basal ganglia. These lesions are generally hypodense and show ring enhancement after intravenous contrast. CT scans tend to underestimate the number of lesions and may show a single lesion when magnetic resonance imaging (MRI) reveals two or more lesions. MRI is more sensitive and should be performed in patients with suspected TE whenever feasible, but especially if only a single lesion is seen on CT. MRI scans show TE lesions as high signal abnormalities on T2-weighted imaging. The differential diagnosis of TE includes CNS lymphoma, progressive multifocal leukoencephalopathy, and infections due to other opportunistic pathogens.

Toxoplasmic pneumonitis may develop in the absence of extrapulmonary disease. Its clinical and radiologic features are nonspecific and may mimic *Pneumocystis carinii* pneumonia. Patients present with fever, dyspnea, and nonproductive cough, and their chest radiographs usually show bilateral interstitial infiltrates. Although ocular toxoplasmosis is infrequent in AIDS patients, it is still the second most common cause of retinal infection in these patients. It should be distinguished from ocular involvement due to cytomegalovirus, syphilis, herpes simplex, varicella zoster, *P. carinii*, lymphoma, and fungi. Clinical manifestations secondary to cardiac involvement occur but are unusual. In non-AIDS immunocompromised patients, congestive heart failure, arrhythmias, and pericarditis have been noted. Toxoplasmic myocarditis can mimic heart transplant rejection.

DIAGNOSIS. Toxoplasmosis can be diagnosed by isolating the organism; serology; polymerase chain reaction (PCR); demonstrating tachyzoites in tissues or body fluids by histology or cytology; and demonstrating characteristic lymph node histology. Isolation of

T. gondii is accomplished by inoculating blood, CSF, bronchoalveolar lavage (BAL) fluid, amniotic fluid, or tissue specimens into mice or cell culture. Mouse inoculation is more sensitive than cell culture. Many commercial serology kits to detect *T. gondii* antibodies are not adequate and give unacceptable numbers of false-positive and/or false-negative results. Only the most commonly used tests are discussed here. IgG antibodies can be detected with the Sabin-Feldman dye test (considered the gold standard), indirect fluorescent antibody (IFA), agglutination, or enzyme-linked immunosorbent assay (ELISA) tests. IgG antibodies measured by the dye test and IFA test usually appear 1 to 2 weeks after infection, peak (usually ≥1:1000) in 6 to 8 weeks, and gradually decline thereafter; low titers (1:4 to 1:64) usually persist for life. The agglutination test is a sensitive and inexpensive method to screen for IgG antibodies.

Detecting IgM antibodies is frequently useful to diagnose the acute infection. Their absence virtually excludes this diagnosis in immunocompetent patients. IgM antibodies appear as early as 5 days after infection and usually disappear after a few weeks or months; low levels can, however, persist for more than 1 year.

Diagnosis of acute *T. gondii* infection often requires performing and evaluating a panel of tests in a reference laboratory. This is critical in pregnant women, who may choose abortion when informed of a positive IgM test. Recent infection is likely when serial specimens obtained at least 3 weeks apart and tested in parallel show significant rise in IgG antibody titers, and/or by the presence of IgM, IgA, or IgE titers in conjunction with an "acute profile" in the differential agglutination test. The usefulness of serology in HIV-infected patients is mainly to identify those at risk for developing toxoplasmosis. Therefore, all HIV-positive patients should be tested for the presence of IgG antibodies. In addition, serologic tests may be misleading in chronically infected patients who receive heart or other organ transplants because these patients can show rising titers of IgG and IgM antibodies without clinical evidence of active *T. gondii* infection. Definitive diagnosis of toxoplasmosis in immunodeficient patients ultimately relies on histologic studies, isolating the parasite, and/or identifying *T. gondii* DNA from appropriate sites. However, a presumptive diagnosis of TE in AIDS patients can be made in the presence of a compatible clinical presentation, the presence of multiple ring-enhancing lesions on CT or MRI scans, and the presence of IgG antibodies. HIV-infected patients who present with a single lesion on MRI scan or who are seronegative for *T. gondii* antibodies should be considered for brain biopsy.

PCR has been used successfully on CSF, amniotic fluid, samples from BAL, and blood to diagnose toxoplasmosis. Routine histologic and cytologic staining may not allow tachyzoites to be identified in tissue sections. An immunohistochemical method should be used to confirm their presence. The presence of multiple cysts in tissue sections near an area of inflammation and necrosis is highly suggestive of active infection. The histologic features of toxoplasmic lymphadenopathy are considered diagnostic.

TREATMENT. The need for and duration of therapy depend on the clinical manifestations of toxoplasmosis and the immune status of the patient.

Acute Infection in Immunocompetent Patients. Patients with toxoplasmic lymphadenitis do not require antimicrobial therapy unless symptoms are severe and persistent. Pyrimethamine plus sulfadiazine is considered the regimen of choice and is synergistic against tachyzoites. It is not active against the tissue cyst form. In adults, a loading dose of 200 mg of pyrimethamine is administered orally in two divided doses on the first day. Thereafter, patients receive 25 to 50 mg per day orally. Owing to the prolonged half-life of pyrimethamine (4 to 5 days), administration every 2 to 4 days has been suggested. Sulfadiazine is administered as a loading dose of 75 mg per kilogram (up to 4 grams) orally followed by a daily dose of 100 mg per kilogram (up to 6 grams) divided in two doses. Other sulfonamides have less activity against *T. gondii*. Treatment is usually continued for 2 to 4 weeks followed by reassessing the patient's condition. Because pyrimethamine is a folate antagonist, the most common side effect is dose-related bone marrow suppression. Patients receiving pyrimethamine should thus be placed on a daily oral dose of 5 to 10 mg of folinic acid (*not* folic acid) and have complete blood cell and platelet counts measured twice weekly. Patients receiving sulfonamides should maintain high urinary flow to prevent crystal-induced nephrotoxicity. Other important side effects of sulfonamides are fever, rash, leukopenia, and hepatitis. Infections acquired after a blood transfusion or laboratory accident may be severe and therefore should be treated.

Ocular Toxoplasmosis in Immunocompetent Patients. Patients with toxoplasmic retinochoroiditis may be treated with pyrimethamine plus sulfadiazine (P + S). Clindamycin, either alone or in combination with pyrimethamine or sulfadiazine, has also been effective. Systemic corticosteroids are added to the regimen when retinochoroiditis involves the macula, optic nerve head, or papillomacular bundle.

Acute Infection in Pregnant Women. Spiramycin at a dose of 3 grams daily* appears to reduce the incidence of fetal infection by about 60%. If prenatal diagnosis reveals infection in the fetus, the pregnant patient should receive pyrimethamine and sulfadiazine in order to treat the fetus. Owing to potential teratogenicity, pyrimethamine should not be administered in the first 16 weeks of pregnancy.

Toxoplasmosis in Immunocompromised Patients. Immunodeficient patients with toxoplasmosis or with serologic evidence of an acute *T. gondii* infection should be treated. Chronic asymptomatic infection does not require treatment. In non-AIDS immunodeficient patients, therapy is usually administered until 4 to 6 weeks after all clinical evidence of toxoplasmosis resolves. Treatment is usually based on the presumptive diagnosis of TE (see section on diagnosis). Treatment of toxoplasmosis in AIDS patients has two phases: acute stage therapy and maintenance treatment. Acute therapy should be administered for at least 3 weeks; 6 weeks is recommended in patients with severe illness or when significant clinical and/or neuroradiologic response has not been achieved. P + S and pyrimethamine plus clindamycin (P + C) have been used with comparable results (Table 378–1). Most patients respond to these regimens, and neurologic improvement usually occurs within the first 7 days. Brain biopsy should be considered if clinical improvement does not occur during the first 2 weeks of treatment or if deterioration occurs during the first 3 days. Many AIDS patients do not tolerate one or the other regimen because of rash (P + S), rash and diarrhea (P + C), or bone marrow suppression (P + S, P + C). Short courses of corticosteroids can be administered to treat cerebral edema and intracranial hypertension. The mortality rate in treated patients ranges from approximately 1 to 25%. Because most AIDS patients relapse when treatment is discontinued, maintenance therapy is necessary. The optimal regimen has not been identified. Usually the same drugs used for acute therapy are continued but at lower doses (Table 378–1). For patients who do not tolerate any of these regimens for acute stage or maintenance therapy, alternatives listed in Table 378–1 can be tried in combination with pyrimethamine.

PREVENTION. Preventing the infection is particularly important for seronegative immunocompromised patients and pregnant women. Patients should be instructed to eat meat only if it is well cooked, to wash their hands after touching undercooked meat, and to wash fruits and vegetables. In addition, patients should avoid contact with cat feces. It seems prudent to avoid transfusions of blood products from a seropositive donor to a seronegative immunocompromised patient when feasible. If possible, seronegative recipients should receive transplanted organs from seronegative donors. If not feasible, seronegative patients who receive organs from seropositive donors should be treated with pyrimethamine, 25 mg daily for 6 weeks.

For primary prophylaxis in *T. gondii* seropositive HIV-infected patients with a CD4 count < 200 cells per cubic millimeter, administering either trimethoprim-sulfamethoxazole, pyrimethamine-dapsone, or pyrimethamine-sulfadoxine (Fansidar) is indicated to prevent development of toxoplasmosis (Table 378–2). To attempt to prevent congenital toxoplasmosis, routine serologic screening of pregnant women has been recommended so that fetuses at risk can be detected. Serologic status of pregnant women should be evaluated no later than the 10th or 12th week of gestation. Those who are seronegative should be retested at the 20th to 22nd week and then again near term. Administering spiramycin to acutely infected

---

* Obtained from the Food and Drug Administration: phone 301-443-4280.

TABLE 378–1. GUIDELINES FOR ACUTE AND MAINTENANCE THERAPY OF TOXOPLASMIC ENCEPHALITIS IN AIDS PATIENTS

	Acute Therapy	Maintenance Therapy*
Suggested regimens		
Pyrimethamine	Oral 200 mg loading dose, then 50 to 75 mg qd	25 to 50 mg qd
plus		
Folinic acid (leucovorin)	Oral, IV, or IM 10 to 20 mg qd (up to 50 mg qd)	10 to 20 mg qd
plus one of the following		
Sulfadiazine or	Oral 1 to 1.5 g q 6 hr	1 g q 12 hr
Clindamycin	Oral or IV 600 mg q 6 hr (up to IV 1200 mg q 6 hr)	300 mg q 6 hr
Pyrimethamine-sulfadoxine (Fansidar)	No adequate data	1 tablet t.i.w.
Alternative regimens†		
Trimethoprim-sulfamethoxazole	Oral or IV, 5 mg (trimethoprim component)/kg q 6 hr	No adequate data
Pyrimethamine	No adequate data	50 mg qd
plus		
Folinic acid		10 to 20 mg qd
Pyrimethamine and folinic acid	As in suggested regimens	As in suggested regimens
plus one of the following		
Clarithromycin or	Oral 1 g q 12 hr	1 mg q 12 hr
Azithromycin or	Oral 1200 to 1500 mg qd	1200 to 1500 mg qd
Atovaquone or	Oral 750 mg q 6 hr	750 mg q 6 hr
Dapsone	Oral 100 mg qd	100 mg b.i.w.

* Drugs administered orally.
† Data inadequate for definitive recommendation.
Adapted from Wong SY, Remington JS: Toxoplasmosis in the setting of AIDS. *In* Broder S, Merigan TC Jr, Bolognesi D (eds.): Textbook of AIDS Medicine. Baltimore, Williams & Wilkins, 1994.

TABLE 378–2. PRIMARY PROPHYLAXIS FOR TOXOPLASMOSIS IN AIDS PATIENTS*

For the *T. gondii*–seropositive HIV-infected individual†	
Trimethoprim-sulfamethoxazole	1 DS tab qd
	2 DS tab b.i.w.
Pyrimethamine-dapsone	Pyrimethamine, 50 mg once a week, plus dapsone, 50 mg qd
	Pyrimethamine, 25 mg b.i.w., plus dapsone, 100 mg b.i.w.
	Pyrimethamine, 75 mg once a week, plus dapsone, 200 mg once a week
Pyrimethamine-sulfadoxine (Fansidar)	3 tablets every two weeks
	1 tablet b.i.w.
For prevention of congenital transmission of *T. gondii* in seropositive, HIV-infected pregnant women‡	
Spiramycin	1 g q 8 hr

DS = double strength.
* Drugs are administered orally.
† These regimens have been reported to be effective for primary prophylaxis of toxoplasmic encephalitis in AIDS patients.
‡ Although at present no data are available on the efficacy of prophylaxis against congenital transmission in this group of patients, we consider it prudent to recommend spiramycin because preliminary studies by Mitchell and colleagues suggest that the transmission rate for congenital toxoplasmosis in these women is remarkably and significantly higher than in non–HIV-infected, *T. gondii*–seropositive women.
Adapted from Wong SY, Remington JS: Toxoplasmosis in the setting of AIDS. *In* Broder S, Merigan TC Jr, Bolognesi D (eds.): Textbook of AIDS Medicine. Baltimore, Williams & Wilkins, 1994.

pregnant women (see section on treatment) appears to reduce the incidence of congenital infection by approximately 60%.

Dubey JP: Toxoplasma, neospora, sarcocystis, and other tissue cyst-forming coccidia of humans and animals. *In* Kreier JP (ed.): Parasitic Protozoa, vol. 6. San Diego, Academic Press, 1993, p 1. *Comprehensive review of the biology of* T. gondii.

Israelski DM, Remington JS: Toxoplasmosis in the non-AIDS immunocompromised host. *In* Remington JS, Schwartz MN (eds.): Current Clinical Topics in Infectious Diseases, vol. 13. Boston, Blackwell Scientific, 1993, p 322. *A review of the association of toxoplasmosis with disorders, other than AIDS, that compromise the immune system.*

Luft BJ, Hafner R, Korzun AH, et al.: Toxoplasmic encephalitis in patients with the acquired immunodeficiency syndrome. N Engl J Med 329:995, 1993. *A critically evaluated prospective study on the clinical/radiologic course of patients treated with pyrimethamine plus clindamycin for toxoplasmic encephalitis.*

Remington JS, McLeod R, Desmonts G: Toxoplasmosis. *In* Remington JS, Klein KO (eds.): Infectious Diseases of the Fetus and Newborn Infant. 4th ed. Philadelphia, WB Saunders, 1995, p 140. *A comprehensive discussion of congenital toxoplasmosis and the diagnosis and management of acute* T. gondii *infection during pregnancy.*

Wong SY, Remington JS: Toxoplasmosis in the setting of AIDS. *In* Broder S, Merigan TC, Bolognesi D (eds.): Textbook of AIDS Medicine. Baltimore, Williams & Wilkins, 1994, p 223. *A comprehensive overview of the clinical presentation, diagnosis, management, and prevention of toxoplasmosis in AIDS patients.*

379 CRYPTOSPORIDIOSIS
Rosemary Soave

Cryptosporidiosis is a gastrointestinal infection characterized by watery diarrhea, abdominal cramps, malabsorption, and weight loss. It is usually a severe, unrelenting illness in immunocompromised patients, particularly those with the acquired immunodeficiency syndrome (AIDS), and a self-limited disease in the immunologically normal host. It is caused by the coccidian protozoan *Cryptosporidium*, long associated with disease in animals. In 1981–1982, identification of *Cryptosporidium* in 47 AIDS patients with severe enteritis brought the protozoan to the attention of the medical community. As more physicians have looked for this parasite, the number of reported cases of cryptosporidiosis has continued to rise, and it has come to be recognized as an emerging threat to domestic and global health. There is currently no known effective therapy.

THE PROTOZOAN. *Cryptosporidium* (which means "hidden spore") belongs to the class Sporozoa and the suborder Eimeriorina, or true coccidia. Other pathogens of humans in this group include *Toxoplasma gondii, Isospora belli,* and the recently recognized *Cyclospora* species. Although 20 species within the genus *Cryptosporidium* have been described, cross-transmission experiments suggest that little or no host specificity exists. *C. parvum* is the species responsible for disease in humans and mammals.

The 4- to 5-μm, spherical, acid-fast *Cryptosporidium* oocyst is the environmentally resistant form of the parasite that is identified in fecal specimens (Fig. 379–1). Sporulated (mature) oocysts contain four elliptical (2 to 4 × 6 to 8 μm), flat, aflagellar but motile sporozoites that are released (excystation) in the host intestinal tract upon dissolution of the oocyst's outer wall. Sporozoites implant on the host mucosal epithelium and undergo asexual and sexual development within a parasitophorous vacuole. The parasite–host cell relationship is unique in that the parasite is intracellular, i.e., en-

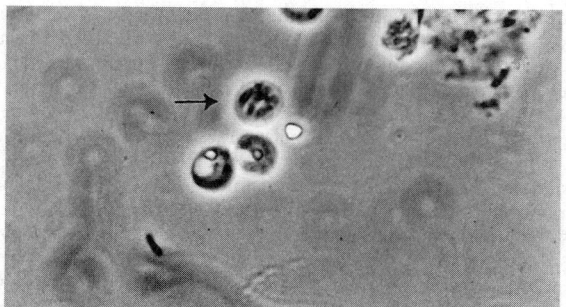

FIGURE 379–1. Wet mount of human stool showing three cryptosporidial oocysts and sporozoites *(arrow)* (×630).

veloped by a host cell membrane, but extracytoplasmic. Sporozoites develop into trophozoites and subsequently undergo asexual multiplication (merogony), formation of macrogametes and microgametes (gametogony), fertilization, and oocyst formation. Newly formed oocysts that are expelled in the feces are immediately infective. The ability of *Cryptosporidium* to develop completely within one host (monoxenous life cycle) imparts a tremendous potential for reinfection and may contribute to the refractory nature of the illness that is seen in *Cryptosporidium*-infected AIDS patients.

EPIDEMIOLOGY. Although more than 100 reports of cryptosporidial infection have emanated from at least 60 countries spanning 6 continents, the true prevalence of cryptosporidiosis in either immunocompetent or immunocompromised hosts is unknown. These surveys of selected populations have revealed infection rates ranging from 0.6 to 20% in the developed world and 4 to 32% in the developing world. Available reports indicate that *Cryptosporidium* is ubiquitous and a major cause of diarrhea worldwide. They also suggest that higher infection rates are associated with young age (< 2 years); warm, wet weather; and overcrowding. In addition, several studies have revealed higher than expected rates of seropositivity, suggesting that active or recent cryptosporidial infection may be common in the general population. As of 1986, the Centers for Disease Control and Prevention estimated that 3 to 4% of AIDS patients had cryptosporidiosis. In recent studies, approximately 16% of AIDS patients with diarrhea were found to be infected. By contrast, more than 30% of AIDS patients in Haiti and parts of Africa have cryptosporidiosis. Asymptomatic carriage of the parasite has been documented in immunocompetent and immunocompromised subjects, but the frequency with which it occurs and its significance have yet to be determined.

Transmission of *Cryptosporidium* between humans and domestic animals has been well documented, and it is likely that both serve as reservoirs of the disease. For humans, however, spread from person to person and via contaminated water is more common than zoonotic transmission. Person-to-person transmission has been implicated in day care center outbreaks, clusters of infection among contacts of index cases, spread between sexual partners, and nosocomial spread of infection among patients and health care workers. Contaminated water is responsible for infection in travelers and swimmers, and for a number of major community outbreaks in the United States and the United Kingdom. In the spring of 1993, an outbreak of waterborne cryptosporidiosis in Milwaukee, Wisconsin, caused diarrheal illness in approximately 403,000, 4,400 of whom required hospitalization. This was the largest waterborne outbreak ever recorded in the United States. *Cryptosporidium* oocysts are often detected in pristine and sewage-contaminated surface waters, treated and untreated sewage effluent, and municipal water supplies. The public health impact of low levels of *Cryptosporidium* oocysts in drinking water is unknown and currently under study. The infectious dose of *Cryptosporidium* appears to be very low but has not yet been defined. The *Cryptosporidium* oocyst is very resistant to common disinfectants; it is unaffected by chlorine concentrations in drinking water or swimming pools. Boiling water for 1 minute eliminates the risk of acquiring *Cryptosporidium* from contaminated drinking water. *Cryptosporidium* infectivity may also be destroyed by freeze-drying or by treatment with 5 to 10% ammonia, 70% to full-strength bleach, or 10% formaldehyde.

PATHOLOGY AND PATHOGENESIS. *Cryptosporidium* has

been found in the pharynx, esophagus, stomach, duodenum, jejunum, ileum, appendix, colon, rectum, gallbladder, pancreas, bile, and pancreatic ducts, as well as within colonic submucosal vessels of infected immunocompromised (primarily AIDS) patients. The parasite has also been detected in sputum, tracheal aspirates, bronchoalveolar lavage, and lung tissue of a small number of immunocompromised patients with gastrointestinal cryptosporidiosis. Light microscopic evaluation of Giemsa-stained or hematoxylin-eosin–stained *Cryptosporidium*-infected tissue reveals small, spherical, basophilic structures along the epithelial cell brush border. Ultrastructural studies reveal the entire spectrum of endogenous stages of the organism adherent to the enterocyte surface and enveloped by a membrane, believed to be derived from the host cell. Histologic changes are nonspecific and minimal, resembling those described for giardiasis, i.e., villous atrophy, crypt elongation, and minimal subjacent inflammatory infiltrates of the lamina propria. By contrast, marked histologic changes ranging from acute inflammation to gangrenous necrosis of the gallbladder and biliary duct epithelium have been described for patients with cryptosporidial cholangitis or cholecystitis.

The pathogenic mechanisms by which *Cryptosporidium* causes enteritis are unknown. The secretory nature of the diarrhea and the presence of malabsorption suggest that an enterotoxin-mediated mechanism and/or physical destruction of the brush border may be operative.

CLINICAL MANIFESTATIONS. The spectrum of cryptosporidial infection ranges from asymptomatic infection to fulminant diarrhea. Cryptosporidiosis is characterized by watery diarrhea, cramping abdominal pain (often exacerbated by food ingestion), weight loss, and flatulence. Nausea, vomiting, anorexia, myalgias, and malaise may also be present. Fever, leukocytosis, and eosinophilia are not common. Fecal examination reveals cryptosporidial oocysts and mucus, but no leukocytes or blood. Vitamin B_{12}, xylose, and fat malabsorption have been documented. Radiographic abnormalities are nonspecific and include prominent mucosal folds, intestinal wall thickening, small bowel dilatation, and disordered motility.

The incubation period for human cryptosporidiosis appears to be between 2 and 14 days. The severity and course of the illness are determined by host immunocompetence. In the immunologically normal host, infection is often explosive in onset and lasts an average of 10 to 14 days. Clearance of the parasite from stool lags behind clinical resolution by 2 to 3 weeks, thus creating problems for infection control. Although self-limited, symptoms are often severe enough to justify therapeutic intervention, were it available. Infection in AIDS patients often begins insidiously and escalates in severity as the underlying immune defect becomes more profound. Frequent (6 to 25), voluminous (1 to 25 liters) daily bowel movements, profound weight loss, and stool oocyst shedding often persist for months.

Biliary cryptosporidiosis has been documented only in immunocompromised patients. Because invasive procedures that may not be justified in the absence of treatment options are a prerequisite for definitive diagnosis, the incidence of this complication is not known. Most patients with biliary cryptosporidiosis have classic signs of cholangitis, including severe right upper quadrant pain, nausea, and vomiting. Serum levels of alkaline phosphatase and γ-glutamyl transpeptidase are elevated, but serum bilirubin and transaminase levels are usually normal. Radiographic evaluation may reveal a dilated gallbladder, thickened gallbladder wall, and dilated bile ducts with luminal irregularities. Patients undergoing endoscopic retrograde cholangiopancreatography (ERCP) are often found to have cryptosporidia studding the surface epithelium and in the bile. In certain instances, cholecystectomy or endoscopic papillotomy has resulted in transient improvement of both symptoms and laboratory abnormalities.

DIAGNOSIS. The diagnosis of cryptosporidial enteritis is based on identifying the oocyst form of the parasite in fecal specimens. Since 1981, various staining techniques for detecting oocysts have been popularized, including several modifications of the acid-fast stain (Kinyoun, Ziehl-Neelsen), the fluorescent auramine-rhodamine stain, and the periodic acid-Schiff (PAS) and carbol fuchsin–negative stains. With the acid-fast stain, acid-fast (red) oocysts may be easily distinguished from yeast that are similar in size and shape but are not acid fast (they stain green). Although the acid-fast stain is commonly used because it is quick and inexpensive, recent studies suggest that it is quite insensitive. Concentration of stool, such as by centrifugation, enhances sensitivity. A fluorescein-labeled monoclonal antibody directed at the oocyst wall and an enzyme-linked immunosorbent assay (ELISA) antigen-capture microtiter assay are now commercially available. The sensitivity, specificity, and relative merits of the various methods for fecal diagnosis of cryptosporidiosis have not been fully defined, but the latter two techniques appear to be more sensitive than staining methods, and their role in the clinical laboratory is currently being investigated. Because the pattern of fecal oocyst shedding in human cryptosporidiosis has not been determined, and the sensitivity of the various methodologies is also not known, the optimal number of negative stool specimens required to confirm the absence of cryptosporidia has yet to be defined. If the acid-fast stain is used to detect *Cryptosporidium*, it is important to note that *Cyclospora*, a newly recognized acid-fast coccidian parasite that causes a clinical syndrome indistinguishable from cryptosporidiosis, may be mistaken for *Cryptosporidium*. Precise measurement of oocyst size is used to differentiate *Cryptosporidium* (4 to 5 μm) from *Cyclospora* (8 to 10 μm). Accurate identification is crucial because *Cyclospora* appears to be sensitive to trimethoprim-sulfamethoxazole.

Although the sensitivity and specificity of stool examination compared with small intestinal biopsy have not been determined, stool examination appears to be more sensitive. In addition to being invasive and costly, intestinal biopsies may be falsely negative owing to autolysis during processing and sampling difficulties related to the parasite's patchy distribution and the paucity of inflammatory changes to guide the endoscopist.

Anticryptosporidial IgG and IgM have been detected in both immunocompetent persons and patients with AIDS by immunofluorescent assay (IFA) and ELISA. Antibody titers rise within 6 to 8 weeks after the onset of infection and decline within 1 year. Immunocompetent hosts generally have higher titers. The IgM response is often absent or minimal in patients with AIDS. Serologic studies are not useful in diagnosing acute cryptosporidiosis but do have a role in defining the epidemiology of the disease.

TREATMENT. There is currently no known effective therapy for cryptosporidiosis. Identification of potentially active agents has been severely hampered by the absence of an asymptomatic, small-animal model of the chronic disease and by an inability to cultivate the organism *in vitro*. Investigational therapy has not been given to the immunocompetent host with cryptosporidial enteritis because illness in these patients is usually self-limited. Persons receiving corticosteroids or cytotoxic agents may be successfully managed by discontinuing the immunosuppressive drugs.

Because of the severe nature of the illness in AIDS patients with cryptosporidiosis, a vast array of antidiarrheal, antimicrobial, and immunomodulating agents have been administered in an unprecedented manner with little preclinical data to support their use. Early anecdotal reports of success using the antitoxoplasma macrolide spiramycin led to two controlled studies with this agent. A placebo-controlled clinical trial of oral spiramycin in 54 AIDS patients with cryptosporidiosis failed to show any difference between placebo and drug. Subsequent pharmacokinetic studies suggested that this may have been due to suboptimal drug absorption. In a single-blind, placebo-controlled study of intravenous spiramycin, 5 of 31 patients had clinical and parasitologic improvement, but the results were not statistically significant and there was unacceptable toxicity. The veterinary agents diclazuril and letrazuril also failed to demonstrate efficacy in placebo-controlled trials. Preliminary results from a recently concluded placebo-controlled study of the lactose-free form of oral azithromycin reveal a statistically significant correlation between parasitologic response and higher serum azithromycin levels. Further studies with both oral and intravenous azithromycin are about to begin. Paromomycin, a poorly absorbed, oral antiamebic aminoglycoside, has been associated with symptomatic relief in a subset of AIDS patients when given at a dose of 2 grams per day. However, parasitologic response is rare, and relapses are common in spite of continued therapy. Paromomycin is currently being studied in an AIDS Clinical Trials Group (ACTG)-sponsored placebo-controlled trial.

The mechanisms by which the immunocompetent host success-

fully deals with cryptosporidial infection are poorly understood but appear to include both intact T cell- and B cell-mediated immunity. Novel attempts at modulating immune function in *Cryptosporidium*-infected patients centered on using immune bovine colostrum, bovine milk globulins, and bovine transfer factor have provided interesting and conflicting results that require further investigation.

In the absence of any proven effective therapy for cryptosporidiosis, careful management of fluid and electrolyte balance is of paramount importance. All classes of nonspecific antidiarrheal agents, including the long-acting, parenterally administered somatostatin analogue octreotide acetate, may be useful, when used in trial-and-error fashion, for individual patients. However, their safety in *Cryptosporidium*-infected patients is not known. Total parenteral nutrition often provides major benefits, but its use is controversial owing to the need for an invasive procedure and its high cost.

Current WL, Garcia LS: Cryptosporidiosis. Clin Microbiol Rev 4:325, 1991. *A well-written epidemiologic, parasitologic, and clinical review.*
Mac Kenzie WR, Hoxie NJ, Proctor ME, et al.: A massive waterborne outbreak of *Cryptosporidium* infection associated with a filtered public water supply in Milwaukee, Wisconsin, March and April, 1993. N Engl J Med 331:161, 1994. *This article describes the largest waterborne outbreak recorded in the United States.*
Mannheimer SB, Soave R: Protozoal infections in patients with AIDS: Cryptosporidiosis, isoporiasis, cyclosporiasis and microsporidiosis. Infect Dis Clin North Am 8:483, 1994. *A comprehensive, fully referenced review of the clinical aspects of infection with* Cryptosporidium *and other enteritis-producing protozoans.*

380 GIARDIASIS
David P. Stevens

DEFINITION. Giardiasis is an infection of the small intestine caused by the flagellated protozoan *Giardia lamblia*. Its hallmarks are diarrhea, malabsorption, and weight loss.

ETIOLOGY. The organism exists in two forms: the motile, flagellated, pear-shaped trophozoite, 12 to 15 μm in length; and the smaller, tough-walled oval cyst. Trophozoites either attach to the microvilli of the intestinal epithelium with the characteristic attaching disc or they move about by means of flagellae in the unstirred layer of mucus just above the epithelial surface. The trophozoites, carried caudally by peristalsis, eventually encyst and pass into the environment. The cyst is resistant to many environmental stresses, including concentrations of chlorine normally found in treated municipal water supplies. Infection of a subsequent host occurs with ingestion of as few as 10 to 25 cysts. Excystation occurs in the acid environment of the stomach, and infection proceeds in the small intestine of the new host.

EPIDEMIOLOGY. Giardiasis is found in all climates and spreads by a variety of routes. Well-documented epidemics have demonstrated person-to-person spread in day care centers for children and nursing homes. Food contaminated after cooking is an infrequent cause of *Giardia* epidemics. A common source of spread is contaminated water. Dozens of epidemics have been described consequent to the breakdown of community water filtration systems. Indeed, *Giardia* is the most frequent cause of waterborne diarrhea in the United States. Animal reservoirs of infection probably contribute to surface water contamination. Campers and backpackers must be particularly mindful of the risk of drinking untreated water.

Giardia is a frequent source of diarrhea in travelers returning from endemic areas (western United States, Rocky Mountain areas). The incubation period is 7 to 21 days, so it is common for infected travelers to visit their physician several weeks after returning home. This longer incubation period serves to distinguish giardiasis from more explosive diarrhea caused by toxigenic *Escherichia coli* and other forms of infectious traveler's diarrhea that have shorter incubation periods (see Ch. 298).

PATHOGENICITY. Jejunal mucosal biopsies from infected persons range in appearance from normal to marked subtotal mucosal atrophy with submucosal inflammatory cell infiltration, reduced villus height, and elongated crypts. Electron microscopic observation of epithelial cells beneath overlying adherent trophozoites shows deformation and blunting of the individual microvilli. In spite of morphologic clues, the pathogenic mechanism for these changes remains speculative. Host humoral and cellular immune responses occur, but their roles in protection as well as pathogenesis are unclear. The increased prevalence of giardiasis in persons with immune deficiency syndromes argues for the role of immunity in host defense.

CLINICAL MANIFESTATIONS. Infection can be asymptomatic. Clinical illness, however, is associated with some or all of the following: diarrhea, cramps, flatulence, nausea, excessive tiredness, bloating, anorexia, and chills. Reversible lactase deficiency and malabsorption of fat and vitamin B_{12} have been documented. The infection is frequently self-limited, but a prolonged, indolent illness with progressive weight loss is possible.

DIAGNOSIS. Symptoms typically associated with giardiasis are nonspecific, and diagnostic tests are of low sensitivity. The diagnosis is established by observing cysts or trophozoites in stools or trophozites in small bowel contents. Because the organism may be excreted in stool intermittently and its demonstration is elusive, at least three stool specimens should be examined before a negative conclusion is drawn. Immunologic tests for *Giardia* antigens in stool are commercially available but expensive. If no organisms are detected, the small bowel contents may be sampled. This can be achieved by tube aspiration or by passing a string that will absorb sufficient jejunal fluid for examination. Microscopic examination of a wet preparation of jejunal contents usually reveals motile organisms when infection is present. Small bowel biopsy may be performed in situations in which these measures are unsuccessful. The small bowel roentgenogram usually shows an edematous mucosa, but this finding is nonspecific. Hematologic values are normal.

There is occasional justification for a trial of therapy in the patient who has the typical signs and symptoms of giardiasis but negative tests for the organism.

TREATMENT. Therapy is with quinacrine hydrochloride, 100 mg three times per day for 7 days. When this drug is contraindicated, metronidazole,* 250 mg three times per day for 7 days, is an alternative. Therapy with either drug is unsuccessful in approximately 10% of patients, requiring a second course. Treatment of infected persons in highly endemic areas is of questionable value because reinfection occurs readily when water supplies are contaminated. All infected persons in nonendemic regions should be treated.

Flanagan PA: *Giardia*—diagnosis, clinical course and epidemiology. Epidemiol Infect 109:1, 1992. *An excellent discussion of the epidemiology of giardiasis.*

Hopkins RS, Juranek DD: Acute giardiasis: An improved clinical case definition for epidemiologic studies. Am J Epidemiol 133:402, 1991. *The sensitivity and specificity of diagnostic approaches are examined.*

Sullivan PS, DuPont HL, Arafat RR, et al.: Illness and reservoirs associated with *Giardia lamblia* infection in rural Egypt: The case against treatment in developing world environments of high endemicity. Am J Epidemiol 127:1272, 1988. *Treatment issues for highly endemic regions are considered.*

381 AMEBIASIS
Jonathan I. Ravdin

Human amebiasis is due to infection with the enteric protozoan *Entamoeba histolytica*. This parasite infects 1% of the world's population, with the disease burden highest in poor, developing areas. To manage patients with amebiasis appropriately, physicians must know the biology of the organism, risk factors for infection, mechanisms of disease, pathogenesis and host immunity, the presenting manifestations of the invasive syndrome, the correct diagnostic approach, alternative therapeutic drug regimens, and strategies for preventing infection.

BIOLOGY OF *E. HISTOLYTICA* AND EPIDEMIOLOGY. Infection results from ingestion of the fecally excreted acid-resistant cyst form. Excystation occurs in the small bowel, leading to colonization of the colon with trophozoites. Transmission of infection results from fecal contamination of water or food or direct fecal-oral contact because of poor hygiene or anal-oral sexual practices. Epidemiologic and molecular biology studies indicate that there are distinct strains, the pathogenic *E. histolytica* and the nonpathogenic *Entamoeba dispar*. Infection with the latter is more common but does not result in systemic invasive disease or antigenic exposure. Approximately 10% of those with pathogenic *Entamoeba* infection present clinically with invasive amebiasis, although all manifest a serum antibody response. The relative frequency of histolytica and dispar infection varies, depending on geographic area. Regions of the world with a high incidence of invasive amebiasis include Mexico, parts of South America, western and South Africa, the Indian subcontinent, the Middle East, and Southeast Asia. High-risk groups in the United States include sexually promiscuous male homosexuals, the institutionalized mentally retarded population, and travelers or emigrants (especially Mexican-Americans) from areas of high prevalence. Groups that, when infected, can experience an increased severity of invasive amebiasis are the very young (under age 2 years), pregnant women, malnourished individuals, and patients on corticosteroids.

PATHOGENESIS AND HOST IMMUNITY. *E. histolytica* trophozoites cause disease by sequentially adhering to colonic mucins, disrupting mucosal barriers with proteolytic enzymes, and contact-dependent lysis of host cells, including responding inflammatory cells. Trophozoite adherence to colonic mucins is mediated by a galactose-binding surface protein; attachment by this protein is the first step in the amebic lysis of human cells. Intestinal infection with *E. dispar* usually clears within 8 to 12 months without evidence of a specific immune response. Cure of invasive amebiasis is associated with resistance to recurrent disease, but not necessarily immunity to asymptomatic intestinal infection. Protective immunity is apparently mediated by development of a serum antibody and an amebicidal cell-mediated immune response with lymphokine-activated macrophages and a CD8 subset of cytotoxic lymphocytes serving as effector cells. Acute amebiasis is associated with the occurrence of antigen-specific suppression of cell-mediated responses to *E. histolytica*, facilitating parasite survival in tissues. It is unclear whether the mucosal secretory IgA antiamebic antibody response that develops after pathogenic infection has any protective role.

CLINICAL DISEASE SYNDROMES. The disease syndromes caused by *E. histolytica* are summarized in Table 381–1. It is unknown whether health is impaired by asymptomatic infection with *E. dispar* or *E. histolytica*. Occasionally, infected patients present with nonspecific gastrointestinal complaints, such as bloating and cramps, without evidence of invasive colitis. Amebic rectocolitis is characterized by the subacute onset of bloody diarrhea over days, abdominal tenderness, weight loss, and fever in only one third of cases. Fulminant colitis with perforation is uncommon; patients are in a toxic state, are acutely ill, and have a rigid, tender abdomen. Toxic megacolon is an unusual complication that is associated with the inappropriate use of corticosteroids when amebic colitis is mistaken for idiopathic inflammatory bowel disease. Chronic nondysenteric amebic colitis can manifest with years of intermittent bloody diarrhea, a syndrome symptomatically indistinguishable from ulcer-

TABLE 381–1. CLINICAL SYNDROMES ASSOCIATED WITH *E. HISTOLYTICA* INFECTION

Intestinal Disease
  Asymptomatic infection
  Acute rectocolitis (dysentery)
  Fulminant colitis with perforation
  Toxic megacolon
  Chronic nondysenteric colitis
  Ameboma
Extraintestinal Disease
  Liver abscess
  Liver abscess complicated by:
    Peritonitis
    Empyema
    Pericarditis
  Lung abscess
  Brain abscess
  Genitourinary disease

Reproduced with permission from Mandell GL, Douglas RG Jr, Bennett JE (eds.): Principles and Practices of Infectious Diseases. 3rd ed. New York, Churchill Livingstone, 1989.

---

* This use is not listed in the manufacturer's directive but is recommended by the Centers for Disease Control and Prevention.

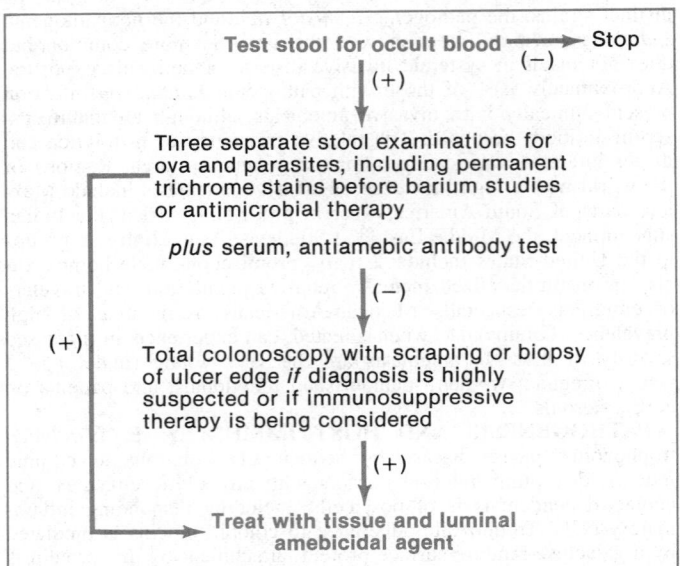

FIGURE 381–1. Diagnostic evaluation for acute amebic rectocolitis in a patient with suggestive epidemiology and clinical manifestations. (Reproduced with permission from Kass EH, Platt R [eds.]: Current Therapy in Infectious Disease-3. Philadelphia, BC Decker, 1990.)

ative colitis. Ameboma is a rare segmental form of chronic amebic colitis that is more common in the cecum and ascending colon and presents as a tender abdominal mass that can be confused with colonic carcinoma.

Extraintestinal disease consists mainly of amebic liver abscess, which can occur up to 5 months after the onset of intestinal infection. The presentation may be acute with fewer than 10 days of high fever and marked right upper quadrant tenderness. Alternatively, with more than 10 days of symptoms, fever is less frequent and pain and weight loss predominate. Fewer than a third of patients have concurrent diarrhea. Extension of an amebic liver abscess into the peritoneum or pericardium is a very acute clinical presentation that is more likely with a left lobe abscess. Disease can extend to the pleura, causing empyema, or, less likely, disseminate hematogenously to the lung and brain.

DIFFERENTIAL DIAGNOSIS AND WORKUP. Algorithms for the diagnosis of amebic colitis and liver abscess are provided in Figures 381–1 and 381–2, respectively. The differential diagnosis of acute amebic colitis includes infection due to *Shigella*, *Campylobacter*, *Salmonella*, *Yersinia*, and invasive *E. coli* species or *Clostridium difficile* toxin–mediated disease. Amebiasis is one

cause of inflammatory colitis in which fecal leukocytes may be absent, owing to the ability of trophozoites to lyse human neutrophils. Recently, several research groups succeeded in correctly diagnosing *E. histolytica* and *E. dispar* intestinal infections by directly detecting amebic antigen in feces and serum. Although these diagnostic tests may soon be available, in current clinical practice, the diagnosis of intestinal amebiasis still rests upon the morphologic identification of trophozoites in fecal specimens. At least three stool samples are necessary to reach a 90% yield; samples should be refrigerated or placed in fixative if they cannot be processed immediately. Laboratories in the United States frequently falsely identify fecal leukocytes as trophozoites; careful study with skilled microscopy is necessary. Serology for antiamebic antibodies is positive in >90% of patients with amebic colitis longer than 1 week in duration and is very helpful in making a correct diagnosis. Interpretation of results can be difficult in highly endemic areas, where up to 25% of the population is seropositive owing to the persistence of serum antibodies for years after asymptomatic *E. histolytica* infection. Endoscopy with biopsies of the ulcer edge is diagnostic in 90% of cases; this is helpful for a rapid diagnosis and to differentiate amebiasis from idiopathic inflammatory bowel disease.

The key study for diagnosing amebic liver abscess is abdominal ultrasonography, a rapid, noninvasive procedure that differentiates biliary tract disease from a nonhomogeneous cavitary defect in the liver. The differential diagnosis can then be narrowed to amebic liver abscess, pyogenic bacterial abscess, echinococcal cyst, and hepatoma. Attention to epidemiologic risk factors and detecting serum antiamebic antibodies are usually sufficient to establish the diagnosis, with the caveat that serology may be negative in patients with fewer than 7 days of symptoms. However, if there is sufficient risk for a bacterial abscess and a serologic study is not immediately available, then a "skinny-needle" aspiration, guided by ultrasonography or computed tomography, can be performed. This procedure with culture will diagnose and assist in therapy of a bacterial abscess; aspiration of an amebic abscess yields a yellow proteinaceous fluid often without white blood cells or amebas. The trophozoites are found in tissue at the periphery of the liver lesion.

THERAPY. Regimens for treating amebiasis are summarized in Table 381–2. Therapy of invasive amebiasis requires a tissue-active agent followed by a drug effective in the bowel lumen. In pregnant women, the use of nonabsorbable agents (paromomycin) or the judicious use of metronidazole is advisable. It is controversial whether therapy is necessary for asymptomatic intestinal infection without evidence of tissue invasion; however, this may be advisable in areas where pathogenic *E. histolytica* infection is likely or reinfection is not expected. Careful follow-up stool examinations are necessary, as all available agents are not always effective in eradicating intestinal infection. Patients with amebic liver abscess respond gradually to therapy with decreased pain and fever over 3 to 5 days. A small minority do not respond at all within 3 days or have a very large abscess that appears close to rupture; needle aspiration is indicated in such patients. After aspiration, continued therapy with metronidazole should be adequate. Recent studies revealed

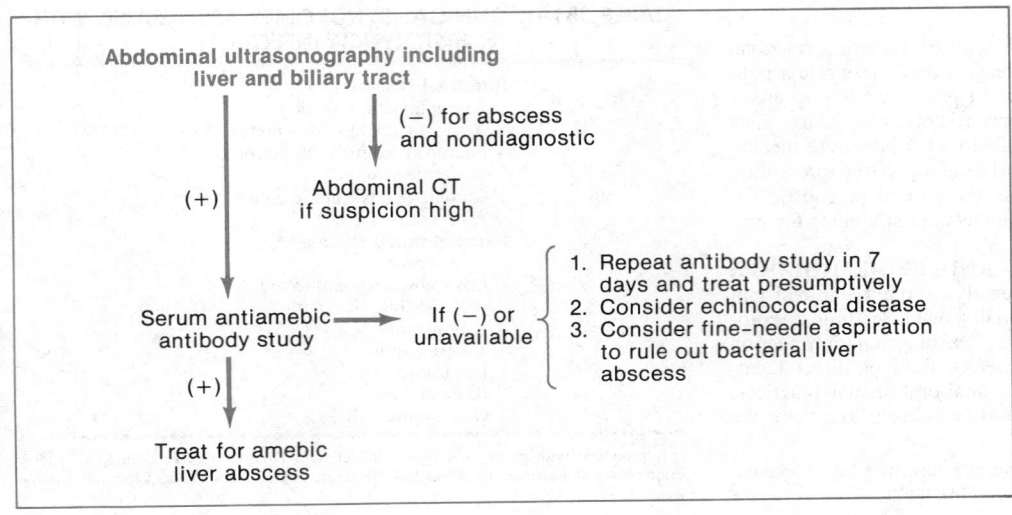

FIGURE 381–2. Diagnostic evaluation for amebic liver abscess in a patient with suggestive epidemiology and clinical manifestations. (Reproduced with permission from Kass EH, Platt R [eds.]: Current Therapy in Infectious Disease-3. Philadelphia, BC Decker, 1990.)

TABLE 381-2. THERAPEUTIC REGIMENS FOR TREATMENT OF AMEBIASIS*

Cyst Passers
Diloxanide furoate, 500 mg t.i.d. × 10 days, or
Paromomycin, 30 mg/kg/day in 3 divided doses × 5–10 days, or
Tetracycline, 250 mg q.i.d. × 10 days, then diiodohydroxyquin, 650 mg t.i.d. × 20 days

Invasive Rectocolitis
Metronidazole, 750 mg t.i.d. × 5–10 days
or 2.4 grams qd × 2–3 days
or 50 mg/kg × 1 dose
plus diloxanide furoate or paromomycin or if metronidazole not tolerated
Dehydroemetine, 1–1.5 mg/kg/day × 5 days plus diloxanide furoate or paromomycin

Liver Abscess
Metronidazole, 750 t.i.d. × 5–10 days or 2.4 mg qd × 1–2 days plus diloxanide furoate or paromomycin or if metronidazole not tolerated
Dehydroemetine, 1–1.5 mg/kg/day × 5 days plus diloxanide furoate or paromomycin

---

* All dosages are for oral administration except dehydroemetine, which is given intramuscularly; metronidazole can be used intravenously.

Adapted with permission from Mandell GL, Douglas RG Jr, Bennett JE (eds.): Principles and Practices of Infectious Diseases. 3rd ed. New York, Churchill Livingstone, 1989.

a high incidence of intestinal infection in patients with amebic liver abscess. To avoid a recurrence of disease, therapy must include a luminal cysticidal agent.

PREVENTION. *E. histolytica* infection can be prevented by the availability of clean water, adequate sanitation, and avoidance of sexual practices or living conditions that facilitate direct fecal-oral contamination. Boiling is the only reliable way of killing cysts; halide solutions are not reliable. In endemic areas, uncooked foods such as salads and vegetables should be avoided. No vaccine or acceptable form of chemoprophylaxis is available; however, current research on the pathogenesis of amebiasis and the host immune response has led to the identification of multiple *E. histolytica* antigens that are effective as subunit vaccines in experimental models of amebic liver abscess.

AMEBIC MENINGOENCEPHALITIS

Amebic meningoencephalitis is a rare clinical syndrome caused by the free-living amebas *Naegleria fowleri* and *Acanthamoeba* species. *N. fowleri* causes a primary amebic meningoencephalitis (PAM), whereas *Acanthamoeba* produces a subacute granulomatous amebic encephalitis (GAE).

N. fowleri in trophozoite or flagellate form grows best at high temperatures (46° C); encystment occurs at low temperatures. *Acanthamoeba* species, which have a trophozoite and cyst form, grow at normal ambient temperatures (25 to 35°C). PAM is a highly infrequent disease despite the massive exposure of populations to warm fresh water. GAE is usually restricted to immunosuppressed populations, such as those with AIDS or those with organ transplants. *N. fowleri* enters the central nervous system (CNS) by penetrating the nasal mucosa and cribriform plate and is highly cytolytic. GAE probably results from hematogenous dissemination and can be distinguished from PAM by the presence of cysts in tissue.

PAM is characterized by the abrupt onset of headache, fever, and meningismus, with rapid development of focal neurologic findings, including olfactory loss. A neutrophilic cerebrospinal fluid (CSF) pleocytosis is frequently associated with increased CSF protein and hypoglycorrhachia. A negative CSF Gram stain result, India ink preparation, culture for bacteria, and cryptococcal antigen study in a patient with acute meningitis who has a history of exposure to fresh water suggests the need to examine the CSF for motile trophozoites (10 to 30 μm), a finding that is diagnostic. In contrast, GAE manifests subacutely over weeks with focal CNS signs, headache, fever, and depressed mental status and is often complicated by seizures. The presence of *Acanthamoeba* organisms in a nodular or ulcerative skin lesion is helpful; study of the CSF usually reveals a nonspecific lymphocytosis with abnormally elevated protein levels. A brain biopsy is necessary to differentiate GAE from toxoplasmosis, pyogenic brain abscess, and other causes of focal CNS disease.

There is no treatment known to be efficacious for PAM or GAE. Treatment with systemic and intrathecal amphotericin B was associated with survival in two patients with PAM. *Acanthamoeba* organ-

isms are usually susceptible *in vitro* to ketoconazole, micronazole, 5-flucytosine, and pentamidine. After determination of susceptibility of the patient's isolate *in vitro*, the above agents and amphotericin B can be considered. These are rare disorders, and the risk of PAM from diving or waterskiing in warm fresh water cannot be quantified. Other opportunistic infections are much more frequent than those caused by *Acanthamoeba* in immunosuppressed patients.

Katzenstein D, Rickerson V, Braude A: New concepts of amebic liver abscess derived from hepatic imaging, serodiagnosis, and hepatic enzymes in 67 consecutive cases in San Diego. Medicine (Baltimore) 61:237, 1982. *Excellent clinical study of amebic liver abscess.*

Martinez AJ: Infection of the central nervous system due to *Acanthamoeba*. Rev Infect Dis 5:S399, 1991. *An up-to-date review of* Acanthamoeba *infections, including epidemiology, clinical course, diagnosis, and treatment.*

Ravdin JI: Diagnosis of invasive amoebiasis—time to end the morphology era. Gut 35:1018, 1994. *The most recent authoritative review of the approach to diagnosis of amebic infection.*

Ravdin JI, Petri WA: *Entamoeba histolytica.* In Mandell GL, Bennett JE (eds.): Principles and Practices of Infectious Disease, 4th ed. New York, Churchill Livingstone, 1994. *This detailed review of clinical amebiasis is well referenced and the most recent available.*

Ravdin JI, Schain DC, Kelsall B: Antigenicity, immunogenicity and vaccine efficacy of the galactose-specific adherence protein of *Entamoeba histolytica*. Vaccine 11:241, 1993. *Latest update on research relevant to vaccine development.*

382 OTHER PROTOZOAN DISEASES

Richard D. Pearson

OTHER ENTERIC PROTOZOANS

A number of enteric protozoa in addition to *Entamoeba histolytica, Giardia lamblia,* and *Cryptosporidium parvum*, which are discussed in other chapters, can cause disease (Table 382–1). They are acquired by ingesting cysts or oocysts in contaminated water or food. The parasites excyst and multiply in the lumen of the bowel, or in some cases within intestinal epithelial cells. Enteric protozoal pathogens should be considered in patients with persistent diarrhea, abdominal pain, and related symptoms, particularly if they have AIDS or a history of international travel.

The diagnosis is made by identifying cysts, oocytes, or trophozoites in the stool. Microscopic examinations should be performed by experts because fecal debris may be confused with parasites, and, conversely, pathogenic protozoa may be scant or difficult to differentiate from nonpathogens such as *Entamoeba coli, Endolimax nana, Iodamoeba bütschlii, Trichomonas hominis,* or *Chilomastix mesnili.* Therapy includes rehydration and administration of antiprotozoal drugs (Table 382–1).

Drugs for parasitic infections. Med Lett Drugs Ther 35:111, 1993. *Consensus recommendations for treating parasitic diseases are provided in tables. Key articles are referenced.*

Jernigan J, Guerrant RL, Pearson RD: Parasitic infections of the small intestine. Gut 35:289, 1994. *A good starting point for a review of recent literature on enteric protozoal pathogens.*

BABESIOSIS

Babesiosis is a tick-borne, malaria-like illness caused by *Babesia* species that infect erythrocytes of mammals. Most infections in the United States are due to *B. microti*, which is endemic on the chain of islands off the coast of New England and New York that includes Nantucket, Martha's Vineyard, Long Island, Block Island, and Shelter Island, and in Connecticut. The major reservoir in those areas is the white-footed mouse, *Peromyscus leucopus.* The vector is the deer tick, *Ixodes scapularis*, the same tick that transmits *Borrelia burgdorferi*, the cause of Lyme disease (see Ch. 321). The cycle begins when larvae feed on infected mice and acquire *Babesia.* Infection is transmitted to humans when nymphs, the next stage, feed on them. Blood transfusions have been implicated in a few cases. Sporadic cases of babesiosis have been reported from other areas of the United States, including California, Georgia, Washington, and Wisconsin. Some have been caused by different *Babesia*

TABLE 382-1. OTHER ENTERIC PROTOZOA

Organism	Epidemiology	Manifestations	Therapy*
Balantidium coli	Primarily an infection of animals, especially pigs, but also affects humans	Asymptomatic, or mild and self-resolving; a few cases are more severe with abdominal pain, blood, and mucus in the stool	Tetracycline (500 mg q.i.d. for 10 days) *Alternative:* Metronidazole (750 mg t.i.d. for 5 days) or Iodoquinol (650 mg t.i.d. for 20 days)
Blastocystis hominis	Probably worldwide, including North America; often found concomitantly with *Giardia lamblia*	Pathogenicity is debated	The need for treatment is debated, but efficacy has been reported with: Metronidazole (750 mg t.i.d. for 10 days) or Iodoquinol (650 mg t.i.d. for 20 days)
Cyclospora species (previously known as cyanobacterium-like bodies [CLB])	Distribution appears to be world-wide	May produce severe, watery diarrhea and fatigue lasting for weeks	Trimethoprim, 160 mg and Sulfamethoxazole, 800 mg b.i.d. for 3 days
Dientamoeba fragilis	Worldwide distribution; frequently found concomitantly with the pinworm, *Enterobius vermicularis*	Most asymptomatic; diarrhea reported	Iodoquinol (650 mg t.i.d. for 20 days) or Paromomycin (25–30 mg/kg body weight/day in 3 doses for 7 days) or Tetracycline (500 mg q.i.d. for 10 days)
Entamoeba polecki	Most cases reported from Papua New Guinea, but probably world-wide distribution; primarily found in pigs and monkeys; human infections are rare	Most asymptomatic; some have symptoms similar to *Entamoeba histolytica* colitis	Metronidazole (750 mg t.i.d. for 10 days)
Isospora belli	Worldwide distribution, most prevalent in Latin America and Africa	Self-limited diarrhea in immuno-competent residents and travelers, but persistent, severe diarrhea in patients with AIDS	Trimethoprim 160 mg plus sulfamethoxazole 800 mg q.i.d. for 10 days then b.i.d. for 3 weeks
Microspordia (*Enterocytozoon bieneusi* and *Septata intestinalis*)	Apparent worldwide distribution	Pathogenicity debated; frequently found in the stool of AIDS patients with persistent diarrhea	Uncertain; Abendazole 400 mg b.i.d. may be helpful for *E. bieneusi* and may cure *S. intestinalis*
Sarcocystis species	Common pathogens of animals; rare in humans; acquired by ingesting contaminated beef or pork	Nausea, vomiting, abdominal pain, and diarrhea. Eosinophilic necrotizing enteritis has been observed in the small intestine	No specific therapy

* Recommendations based on Drugs for parasitic infections. Med Lett Drugs Ther 35:111, 1993. The dosages and durations are for adults.

species. In Europe, *B. divergens* and *B. bovis* are transmitted by *Ixodes ricinus.*

B. microti infections are often asymptomatic or mild and self-resolving, but they can cause severe, malaria-like disease, particularly in the elderly, splenectomized patients, and the immunocompromised. The incubation period varies from 1 to 6 weeks; most patients are unaware of a tick bite. Symptomatic patients typically experience irregular fever, sweats, chills, myalgia, fatigue, and other constitutional symptoms. Unlike malaria, there is no periodicity to the disease. Fever is frequently the only finding on physical examination, but hepatomegaly and splenomegaly are present on occasion. There is evidence of hemolytic anemia of varying severity and often thrombocytopenia. The white count is normal or slightly depressed, and there may be elevations of liver enzymes and bilirubin. Untreated, symptomatic babesiosis may last from a few weeks to several months.

Babesiosis is diagnosed by identifying intraerythrocytic *Babesia* in blood smears. On rare occasions dividing parasites make up four daughter cells that appear as the characteristic tetrad (Maltese cross) in an infected erythrocyte.

The majority of cases of babesiosis in immunocompetent patients are asymptomatic or mild and resolve spontaneously without treatment. In adults with serious *Babesia* infections the treatment of choice is clindamycin, 1.2 grams twice a day parenterally or 600 mg three times a day orally, plus quinine, 650 mg three times a day orally for 7 days.

Telford SR 3d, Gorenflot A, Brasseur P, et al.: Babesial infections of humans and wildlife. *In* Kreier JP, Baker JR (eds.): Parasitic Protozoa. 2nd ed. New York, Academic Press, 1993, p 1. *The epidemiology, clinical manifestations, and therapy of human and animal babesiosis are reviewed in detail.*

TRICHOMONIASIS

Trichomonas vaginalis is among the most prevalent of all pathogenic protozoa. As many as 3 million women are infected each year in the United States alone. The organism is oval, approximately 10 by 15 μ wide, and has four free flagella at its anterior pole and a fifth in an undulating membrane that runs along the cell. *Trichomonas vaginalis* is usually spread by sexual contact. The highest incidences of disease are among women with multiple sexual partners and those who present with other sexually transmitted diseases (see Ch. 314). It can also be passed from infected mothers to their newborn daughters, but it is seldom symptomatic in girls before menarche. *T. vaginalis* is able to survive for some time in moist environments, and nonvenereal transmission can occur.

As many as half of the *T. vaginalis* infections in women are asymptomatic. The remainder are associated with vaginal discharge, vulvovaginal irritation, dyspareunia, or dysuria. The discharge tends to be watery and copious, but in some cases it is thick and may be yellow or green. Patients may notice an odor, but that is more common with bacterial vaginosis. On pelvic examination there is usually inflammation of the vaginal walls. Punctate hemorrhages on the exocervix, causing the classic "strawberry cervix," are uncommon on gross inspection, but they are observed in approximately half of infected women if colposcopy is performed. The pH of the vaginal contents is typically elevated above the normal level of 4.5, as it is in bacterial vaginosis. In contrast, the pH remains low in women with *Candida* vaginitis.

Most men with *T. vaginalis* are asymptomatic, but the organism is isolated on occasion from men with symptoms of urethritis who are negative for *Neisseria gonorrhoeae* and *Chlamydia trachomatis* (see Ch. 315). Urethral discharge is usually scant in such cases. On rare occasions *T. vaginalis* can cause epididymitis, produce superficial penile ulcerations which are usually located under the prepuce, or involve the prostate.

Diagnosis of trichomonas vaginitis is usually made by identifying the parasite in vaginal discharge. The trophozoites have a twitching movement with active flagella. They are seen in wet mounts of vaginal secretions in approximately 60% of infected women. Polymorphonuclear leukocytes are usually present. Culture is the most sensitive method of diagnosis, and commercial kits are now available. In men a wet mount of material from a platinum loop scraping of the anterior urethra reveals the organism in approximately half of the cases. Prostatic massage prior to collecting urine for trichomonas culture is the most sensitive diagnostic approach. Serodiagnostic studies lack sensitivity and specificity.

Metronidazole is the treatment of choice; a single dose of 2 grams is effective. All sexual partners must be treated concurrently to prevent reinfection. Metronidazole, 250 mg three times a day for 7 days, is an alternative. Single-dose therapy ensures patient compliance, but the higher dose can produce nausea and a metallic taste. Metronidazole also has a disulfiram-like effect, and patients consuming it with alcohol may develop severe nausea, vomiting, and flushing. The use of metronidazole is relatively contraindicated during pregnancy. Treatment failures with metronidazole are encountered. Some are due to reinfection, others to poor compliance, but a subset is apparently due to metronidazole resistance. In such cases high doses of metronidazole have been administered for longer periods of time. Tinidazole, which is not licensed for use in the United States, is also effective for trichomoniasis when administered as a single 2-gram dose.

Krieger JN, Jenny C, Verdon M, et al.: Clinical manifestations of trichomoniasis in men. Ann Intern Med 118:844, 1993. *Summarizes the clinical manifestations of trichomoniasis in men.*

Lossick JG, Kent HL: Trichomoniasis: Trends in diagnosis and management. Am J Obstet Gynecol 165:1217, 1991. *An excellent review of the diagnosis and treatment of women with trichomoniasis.*

Rein MF: *Trichomonas vaginalis.* In Mandell GL, Bennett JE, Dolin R: Principles and Practice of Infectious Diseases, 4th ed. New York, Churchill Livingstone, 1995, p 2493. *The epidemiology, diagnosis, and treatment of trichomoniasis are reviewed.*

383 *PNEUMOCYSTIS CARINII* PNEUMONIA

Fred R. Sattler

Pneumocystis pneumonia remains the most frequent case-defining infection in AIDS (see Ch. 365). Nearly 20,000 first episodes of pneumocystis continue to be reported to the Centers for Disease Control and Prevention (CDC) each year. A large number of second or third episodes also occur annually in AIDS patients but do not require reporting to the CDC.

Moderate to severe episodes cause appreciable morbidity, and even with effective therapies, 20 to 25% are fatal. For mild episodes, the fatality rate is < 3%, but the diagnosis is often difficult, as signs and symptoms may mimic community-acquired infections and the presentation is often atypical in patients receiving prophylaxis for pneumocystis. It is, therefore, imperative that episodes be detected when alteration of gas exchange is mild and lung damage is minimal if hospitalization and mortality are to be minimized. Thus, clinicians caring for HIV patients must be aware of various manifestations of pneumocystis so that therapy can be initiated early.

ETIOLOGY. *Pneumocystis carinii* is a eukaryotic microbe with morphologic features similar to those of protozoa. Lack of growth on fungal culture media and response to therapies used to treat protozoan infections have supported the notion that it is a protozoan. However, *P. carinii* has an affinity for fungal stains, its ultrastructure is more similar to fungi, and molecular analysis of its 16S ribosomal RNA and mitochondrial DNA indicates that it is phylogenetically closely related to the *Ascomycetes* yeasts. Moreover, the base pair sequence of its mitochondrial DNA contains genes of NDH dehydrogenase subunits and cytochrome oxidase subunits, which show 60% similarity with fungi but only 20% homology with protozoa. Finally, the dihydrofolate reductase (DHFR) of *P. carinii,* as with fungi, is a single enzyme with lower molecular weight than the dual thymidylate synthetase–DHFR activity present in protozoa.

Establishing whether *P. carinii* is a fungus is not moot. Although pneumocystis does not respond to antifungal drugs such as amphotericin or fluconazole, β-glucan synthesis in the cyst wall is inhibited by antifungal agents such as echinocandins and papulocandins.

These agents are active against both the cyst and trophozoite forms of *P. carinii* in experimental infections. By contrast, traditional antipneumocystis therapies affect only the trophozoites. Novel therapeutic approaches that affect both stages of the life cycle are therefore being developed in an attempt to improve treatment response rates.

EPIDEMIOLOGY AND TRANSMISSION. Within the first few years of life, nearly all children have serologic evidence of exposure to *P. carinii.* Thus, the most accepted hypothesis for pathogenesis has been that *P. carinii* remains latent in the lung and reactivation occurs during severe immune depression. Yet, there is little to support chronic carriage because the organism is not detected in lung sections at autopsy of previously healthy individuals or by polymerase chain reaction (PCR) in bronchoalveolar lavage fluid of immunocompetent adults.

P. carinii is found incidentally in lungs of immunocompromised patients, and genetic sequences of the organisms have been detected in the absence of histologic evidence of infection in immunocompromised patients. Case clusters and familial spread have been reported, and in one natural history study of HIV patients, upper respiratory infections peaked in winter months followed by pneumocystis pneumonia 4 months later, indicating that *P. carinii* was acquired by exposure to persons coughing during earlier months when community respiratory infections were common. These data suggest that *P. carinii* may be acquired by person-to-person spread.

PATHOGENESIS AND PATHOPHYSIOLOGY. In cortisone-treated rats, inhaled *P. carinii* adheres to type 1 alveolar cells through fibrinonectin. After several weeks, small clusters of *P. carinii* can be detected in alveolar spaces. Later, air sacs become filled with organisms, indicating that replication is slow but proliferation is extensive. Two morphologic forms of the organism are readily detected. The majority are small pleomorphic trophozoites. A more mature, larger, thick-walled cyst containing up to eight intracystic bodies is less prevalent. Histology typically shows foamy alveolar exudates consisting of degenerative *P. carinii* cell membranes, surfactant, host proteins, and a modest number of alveolar macrophages. As infection progresses, septal hypertrophy occurs and interstitial edema and mononuclear cells accumulate. Similar abnormalities occur in humans.

In patients, these abnormalities result in increased alveolar-capillary permeability, which is associated with impaired gas exchange and decreased membrane diffusing capacity, compliance, total lung capacity, and vital capacity. Soon after antipneumocystis therapy begins, lung function is further impaired by the inflammatory response, as evidenced by a rapid decline in oxygenation. This inflammatory reaction appears to be mediated by tumor necrosis factor-α (TNF-α) and interleukin-1, -6, and -8 released by alveolar macrophages. TNF-α is modulated by the β-glucan component of the cell wall of the organism, providing further evidence that *P. carinii* is a fungus.

RISK FOR INFECTION. In laboratory rodents, depletion of T lymphocytes is the critical determinant in producing pneumocystis pneumonia. In humans, pneumocystis occurs in association with lymphoreticular malignancy, certain congenital disorders, and therapy with cyclosporine or corticosteroids which have in common variable defects in T-cell function. In patients with HIV, the risk of developing pneumocystis is related to deficiency of T-lymphocytes with CD4 surface phenotype. The median CD4 count is 50 to 70 at the time of first episodes. That pneumocystis may occur with transient declines in CD4 counts to < 100 during primary HIV infection suggests that the level of CD4 immunity and not the stage of HIV infection is important in determining risk for infection. Although > 90% of episodes occur with < 200 CD4 cells, pneumocystis may occur at higher CD4 counts in individuals whose CD4 cells are declining rapidly and those with thrush and fever.

HISTOPATHOLOGY. Microscopy of lung tissue from AIDS patients with pneumocystis shows prominent eosinophilic, foamy intra-alveolar exudate, proliferation of type II pneumocytes, but only mild interstitial inflammation. Detection of *P. carinii* requires special stains for identification. The cysts are uniformly 5 to 7 μm and easily collapse to appear as helmet or banana shapes. Trophozoites are smaller, measuring 1 to 4 μm, and unlike the cysts are pleomorphic.

Diffuse alveolar damage is commonly found on biopsy sections.

Interstitial fibrosis is present in approximately 6% and intraluminal fibrosis in almost 40% of cases and appear to be related to the severity of the inflammatory response and duration of therapy. By contrast, acute exudative alveolar damage is unusual and hyaline membranes have been detected in <5% of lung biopsies but occasionally may be so prominent that they obscure the eosinophilic alveolar material typical of most cases. Other less common histologic abnormalities include cysts and cavities, granulomas, lymphocytic interstitial infiltrates, microcalcifications, vasculitis, and alveolar proteinosis. In patients with cavitation and pneumothorax, there is tissue invasion with *P. carinii* in the interstitium, and unlike the typical findings, greater proportions of trophozoite than cysts are present.

CLINICAL MANIFESTATIONS. Early recognition and treatment are imperative. Figure 383–1 shows that the risk of a fatal outcome increases progressively for patients whose room air PaO_2 are ≤ 75 mm Hg and alveolar-arterial oxygen differences ($[A - a]Do_2$) are ≥ 35 at presentation. Clinicians must therefore be familiar with both the typical manifestations and the less common presentations of pneumocystis.

Typical Presentations. The onset of pneumocystis pneumonia in AIDS patients is usually insidious. The cardinal manifestation is a hacking, usually nonproductive cough that may have been present for weeks. Retrosternal chest tightness, intensified by coughing and inspiration, is also common. Fever occurs in 80 to 90%. Dyspnea occurs later when oxygenation is moderately to severely impaired.

Physical findings are often limited and nonspecific. There is usu-ally no tachypnea with mild episodes, whereas respiratory distress and use of accessory respiratory muscles may be present with severe episodes. Auscultation of the lungs is frequently normal because rales occur in only 30 to 40% of cases and are usually a late finding in severe episodes. Occasionally patients have wheezing or overt bronchospasm. In one report 84% of patients had peak expiratory flow rates (PEFR) <80% of predicted, with 54% of these responding to bronchodilator therapy. By contrast, in HIV patients without pneumocystis, only 23% had low PEFR and only 3% of these exhibited bronchodilator responses.

Physical findings outside the lung may assist in the clinical assessment. In patients not receiving antifungal drugs, oral thrush is a nearly universal finding. Facial seborrheic dermatitis is also common. Generalized adenopathy with lymph nodes >1 cm is rare because patients with pneumocystis generally have severe immunodeficiency with hypoplastic lymph nodes.

Some gender differences exist in the clinical presentation and course. In one study of 2526 men and 544 women, women were more likely to be hospitalized for their first episode of pneumocystis, were less likely to be white, and were more likely to die in the hospital. These findings suggest that pneumocystis is less likely to be diagnosed early in the course of infection in women.

Atypical Presentations. **Pneumothorax and Cavitation.** Pneumothoraces that may be associated with refractory bronchopleural fistulas and chronic lung cavitation are an increasingly frequent presentation and may occur in up to 10% of episodes. Pneumothoraces occurred spontaneously in 20 (2%) of 1030 patients with AIDS at one medical center; 50 to 95% of episodes are associated with active pneumocystis pneumonia. Thus, HIV patients with spontaneous pneumothorax should undergo workup and treatment for pneumocystis along with management of the pneumothorax.

Lung destruction and cavitation are manifested by solitary, thin-walled cavities, regional honeycombing, blebs, or bullae formation; these findings are often bilateral, usually occurring in the upper lobes and preceding pneumothraces.

Although cavitation and pneumothorax were initially associated with aerosol pentamidine prophylaxis, these complications may occur without aerosol therapy, in nonsmokers, at presentation of first episodes of pneumocystis, and before bronchoscopy or mechanical ventilation and barotrauma.

Extrapulmonary Pneumocystis. Infection with *P. carinii* may occur outside the lung in 0.5 to 3.0% of patients with pneumocystis pneumonia. At the time extrapulmonary pneumocystis is diagnosed, >50% have active pulmonary infection with *P. carinii*. Nucleotide sequences of the *P. carinii* DHFR gene have been detected by PCR in blood of 5 of 11 patients with pneumocystis pneumonia, which suggests that hematogenous dissemination occurs during acute pneumonia.

Clinical presentations have included external auditory polyps, mastoiditis, choroiditis, cutaneous lesions or digital necrosis secondary to vasculitis, small bowel obstruction, ascites with gross nodules in the stomach and duodenum, hepatic or splenic infiltration, hilar or mediastinal lymphadenopathy, thyroiditis, thymic involvement, and hematologic cytopenias due to involvement of the bone marrow. At autopsy disseminated infection has been documented in other organs, including abdominal lymph nodes, pancreas, gastric mucosa, adrenal glands, myocardium, kidneys, and central nervous system. Lymph nodes, liver, spleen, and bone marrow have been the most commonly affected organs.

Histology of affected organs show foci of eosinophilic frothy exudates, and special stains reveal *P. carinii*. Unlike in the lung, these lesions are often calcified (punctate or rimlike) and show vasculitis with invasion of vessel walls by *P. carinii*.

Clinical manifestations of extrapulmonary pneumocystosis are generally nonspecific (e.g., fever and sweats). Two infections are associated with specific symptoms or signs. *P. carinii* involving the thyroid may present with neck pain, hyperthyroidism or hypothyroidism, and goiter, which may be a multinodular or solitary neck mass. The thyroid is usually "cold" on ^{125}I scanning. The diagnosis is made by fine-needle aspiration. The other infection is choroiditis. Lesions consist of slightly elevated, yellow-white plaques, generally limited to the choroid without involvement of retinal vessels (unlike cytomegalovirus [CMV] retinitis) and without evidence of intraocular inflammation (see Color Plate 11*F*). Identifying typical choroidal lesions may provide the first clue of *P. carinii* infection.

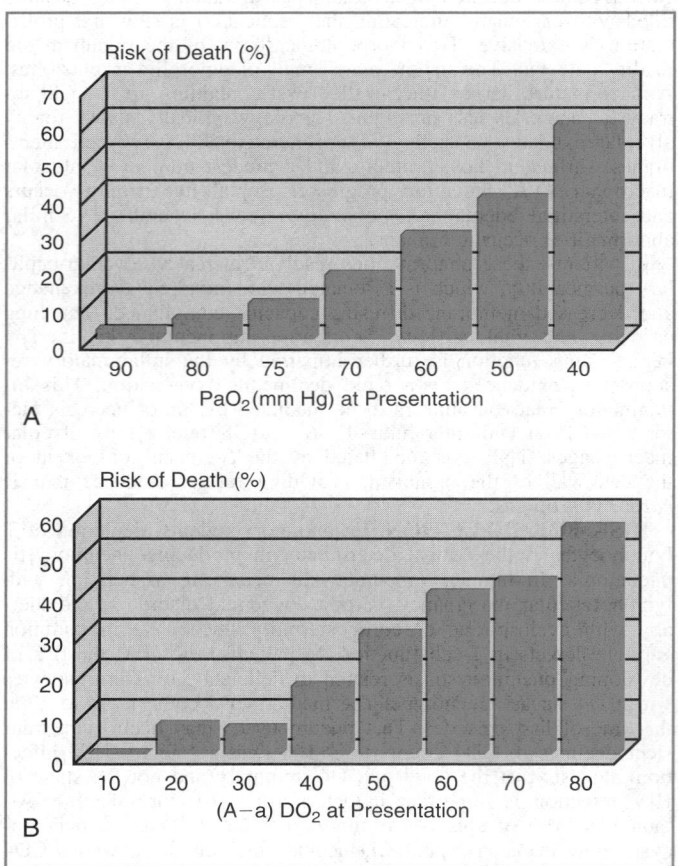

FIGURE 383–1. *A,* Risk of death, according to the partial pressure (PaO₂) of oxygen on room air at time of admission to the hospital for patients receiving conventional therapies without adjunctive corticosteroids. *B,* Risk of death, according to alveolar-arterial oxygen difference [(A − a)Do₂] on room air at time of admission to the hospital for patients receiving conventional therapies without adjunctive corticosteroids. (Adapted from the United States Public Health Service Consensus Statement on the Use of Corticosteroids as Adjunctive Therapy for Pneumocystis Pneumonia in the Acquired Immunodeficiency Syndrome.)

The lungs are involved in nearly 90% of cases, but eye involvement may be the only evidence of extrapulmonary infection.

Extensive and widespread extrapulmonary infection portends a poor prognosis, with organ failure and death occurring frequently, whereas involvement of a single extrapulmonary site is often associated with a favorable response to therapy for *P. carinii*.

LABORATORY ABNORMALITIES. *Pulmonary Function Tests.* Hypoxemia is the most useful marker of pneumocystis and is highly predictive of outcome. At presentation, $Pao_2 < 80$ mm Hg or an $(A - a)Do_2$ of > 15 on room air occurs in $> 80\%$ of episodes.

In patients with pneumocystis who have normal or nearly normal Pao_2, $(A - a)Do_2$, and chest radiographs, graded exercise testing results in increases in the $(A - a)Do_2$ and oxygen desaturation can be demonstrated with pulse oximetry. The carbon monoxide (CO)-diffusing capacity, DL_{CO}, is also a sensitive marker but nonspecific. Despite the lack of specificity, DL_{CO} values $> 80\%$ make pneumocystis unlikely (i.e., negative predictive values are $> 98\%$). In AIDS patients with asthma who have cough and hypoxemia, results of DL_{CO} should be normal when hypoxemia is due solely to bronchospasm.

Radiographic Procedures. **Routine Radiology.** Routine chest radiographs typically show interstitial infiltrates, beginning in perihilar areas and spreading to the lower and finally upper lung fields. The apices are usually spared. Alveolar patterns with air bronchograms may be superimposed on the interstitial process in more advanced infection, although alveolar infiltrates may be the initial presentation in up to 10% of cases. In 10 to 30% of cases the radiographic presentation is atypical with asymmetric or predominantly upper lobe infiltration—especially for patients who received prophylaxis with inhaled pentamidine. Other atypical abnormalities include nodules, cysts, pneumatoceles, cavitation with "honeycombing," pneumothorax, thoracic adenopathy with or without calcifications, pleural effusions, abscesses, lobar or segmental consolidation, solitary parenchymal nodules, or postobstructive infiltration secondary to endobronchial nodules of *P. carinii*. In one series of 100 patients with pneumocystis, cysts were documented in 34% and of these, 32 had multiple cysts measuring 1.0 to 5.0 cm that occurred predominantly in upper lobes. Cysts resolved partially or completely in most cases with specific therapy for pneumocystis, but 12 (35%) of the 34 patients developed pneumothoraces compared with only 2 of 30 patients without cysts. These cystic/cavitary lesions may mimic tuberculosis (Fig. 383–2). By contrast, 10 to 20% of patients with documented pneumocystis have had normal chest radiographs at presentation.

Computed Tomography (CT). Scans typically show fine, diffuse alveolar consolidation with bronchial wall thickening even when chest radiographs are normal and less often show regional consolidation or cystic airspaces. Low attenuation lesions and calcifications of lymph nodes, spleen, liver, and kidneys may be present in patients with extrapulmonary involvement. The value of CT is primarily for patients with normal chest radiographs or unexpected extrapulmonary pneumocystis.

Nuclear Imaging. Nuclear imaging may be of ancillary value in some cases. Gallium-67 accumulates in activated macrophages through transferrin receptors in areas of lung inflammation, but pulmonary uptake is not specific for *P. carinii* pneumonia. Specificity is improved when scans are reported as positive only if gallium uptake in lung equals or exceeds uptake in liver. Although images are not read until 48 to 72 hours after injection, gallium imaging may be useful for patients with chronic lung disease who have worsening respiratory symptoms.

Lactate Dehydrogenase. Serum lactate dehydrogenase (LDH) is more elevated in pneumocystis than in matched patients with other pulmonary complications of HIV. Although serum levels of LDH are not highly specific, the sensitivity was $> 90\%$ in one study of patients with dyspnea and pneumocystis when values were > 220 IU per liter. Moreover, at presentation, LDH values > 500 IU per liter are associated with an increased risk for a fatal outcome. Equally important, serial tests gradually improve in survivors.

CD4 Counts. Typically counts are < 100 cells per cubic millimeter and $> 90\%$ of patients have values < 200 when first diagnosed with pneumocystis.

DIAGNOSIS. *Bronchoalveolar Lavage.* Bronchoalveolar lavage (BAL) is the cornerstone of diagnosis of pneumocystis and consistently has a sensitivity of 86 to 96%. The diagnostic yield was reported to be only 62% for patients with acute pneumocystis

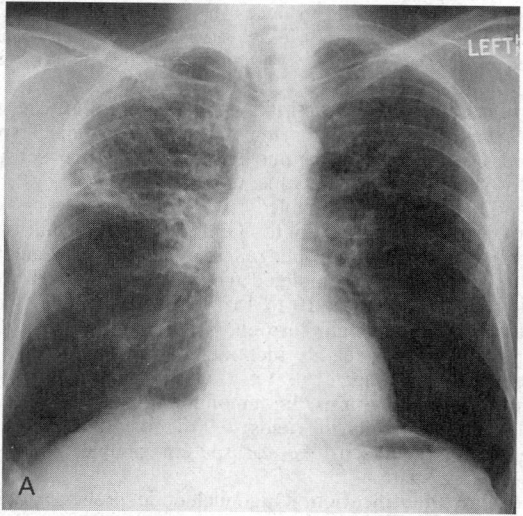

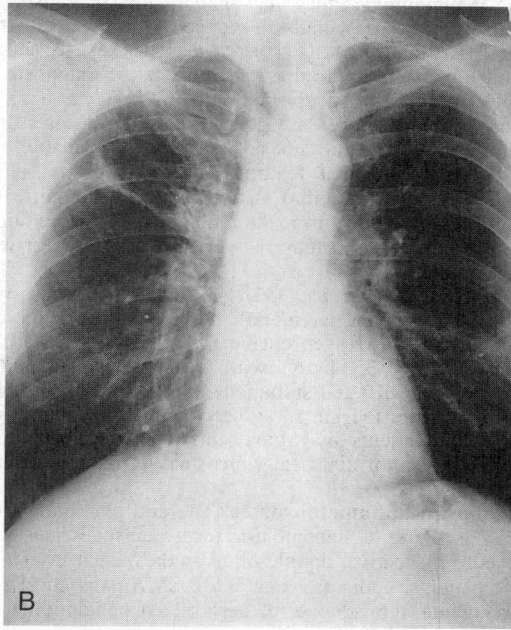

FIGURE 383–2. *A,* This chest radiograph was obtained from a 42-year-old homosexual man who presented with a 14-month history of chronic cough, dyspnea with minimal exertion, and 25-pound weight loss. He was treated for 8 weeks with four standard antituberculous drugs plus intravenous amikacin, but cultures for *Mycobacterium tuberculosis* remained negative. A repeat induced sputum at that time showed large numbers of *P. carinii. B,* Chest radiographs from the same patient after a 3-week course of therapy with oral trimethoprim-sulfamethoxazole (15 mg per kilogram per day of the trimethoprim component). At the completion of the therapy, his cough and dyspnea had completely subsided.

who had received inhaled pentamidine and who had disease predominantly in upper lobes. Several approaches may increase the yield for such patients. Bilateral BAL resulted in a diagnosis in 94%, compared with 84% in patients previously undergoing BAL on one side. Because there may be severalfold more organisms recovered from upper than from lower lobes, sampling involved sites is likely to increase the yield.

Transbronchial Biopsy. The yield from transbronchial biopsy approaches BAL if tissue is obtained without crush artifact and contains at least 25 alveoli. If both BAL and transbronchial biopsies are obtained, the diagnostic sensitivity approaches 100%.

Sputum Induction. Pulmonary secretions may be obtained by ultrasonic nebulization of hypertonic saline. If these specimens are treated with mucolytic agents to solubilize oral debris prior to centrifugation, cytostaining procedures have resulted in diagnostic yields of 15 to 90%. Fluorescent staining with monoclonal antibodies for *P. carinii* generally produces the highest yields. Because the sensitivity is variable and yields >80% have been consistently achieved in only a few centers, a negative induced sputum does not exclude the diagnosis.

Identification of P. carinii. Cyst Wall Stains. The standard staining procedure for identifying *P. carinii* in clinical specimens has used Gomori's methenamine silver because the sensitivity is generally >95%. Toluidine blue O also stains the cyst, is more rapid, and is comparably reliable. **Noncyst Wall Stains.** Wright-Giemsa and Diff-Quik stains are commonly used and stain trophozoites, nuclei of cysts, and intermediate forms and can be completed within 30 minutes. However, organisms may be missed in 10 to 15% of cases. Papanicolaou silver stains the nonspecific foam surrounding large clusters of *P. carinii*, but organisms are not readily identified. The methodology is quick and useful for screening.

Immunochemical Stains. Immunofluorescent staining with monoclonal antibody results in yields >90% for BAL specimens and appears to be more sensitive for sputum samples than silver or Wright-Giemsa stains.

Molecular Identification. Oligonucleotide probes and PCR are promising methodologies that may increase the diagnostic yield in identifying *P. carinii*, especially in induced sputum specimens.

TREATMENT. Initiating Therapy. The key to successfully treating pneumocystis is prompt suspicion of the diagnosis and initiating therapy early when episodes are mild. Because sputum induction and bronchoscopies are generally not done after hours and results of special stains may not be immediately available, most patients with typical clinical features of pneumocystis (if there is moderate-to-severe hypoxemia) should be treated empirically. This does not impair the ability to make a diagnosis, as large numbers of *P. carinii* are detectable in lung tissues and secretions for weeks after the onset of therapy.

Severe Episodes (Table 383–1). **Parenteral Therapy.** Initial therapy should be given parenterally for patients with moderate-to-severe impairment in oxygen exchange, namely Pao_2 <70 mm Hg or an $(A − a)Do_2$ >35. Drugs with high oral bioavailability such as trimethoprim (TMP) and sulfamethoxazole (SMX) may be erratically absorbed from the gut in subjects with severe hypoxemia. In addition, AIDS patients may have enteropathy and malabsorption even in the absence of diarrhea, which may result in subtherapeutic drug concentrations.

Trimethoprim-Sulfamethoxazole. The antifolate combination of TMP-SMX is the gold standard for severe episodes (see Ch. 371). Three recent prospective, double-blind studies, each involving more than 300 patients, indicated that TMP-SMX was more effective than trimetrexate, atovaquone, or aerosolized pentamidine in AIDS patients with pneumocystis. Although there are no comparably rigorous studies comparing TMP-SMX with parenteral pentamidine, TMP-SMX is associated with less serious toxicities.

TABLE 383–1. ESTABLISHED THERAPIES FOR INITIAL TREATMENT OF *PNEUMOCYSTIS CARINII* PNEUMONIA

Intravenous therapies
1. Trimethoprim-sulfamethoxazole — 5/25 mg/kg every 6–8 hours
2. Pentamidine* — 4 mg/kg once daily
3. Trimetrexate plus — 45 mg/M² once daily
   leucovorin — 20 mg/M² every 6 hours
4. Clindamycin plus — 900 mg every 8 hours
   primaquine base (oral)† — 15–30 mg once daily

Oral therapies
1. Trimethoprim-sulfamethoxazole — 2 double-strength tablets t.i.d.
2. Trimethoprim plus — 4–5 mg/kg t.i.d.
   dapsone — 100 mg once daily
3. Clindamycin plus — 456–600 mg t.i.d. or q.i.d.
   primaquine base — 15–30 mg once daily
4. Atovaquone‡ — 750 mg t.i.d.

Aerosol therapy
1. Pentamidine — 600 mg daily via Respirgard II§

* Intramuscular therapy may cause sterile abscesses and should be avoided.
† The combination is not advisable in situations in which absorption may be impaired (severe hypoxemia, vomiting, diarrhea, ileus, malabsorption) because clindamycin alone has no activity against *P. carinii*.
‡ Must be given with food because serum concentrations are 2- or 3-fold lower when drug is administered on an empty stomach.
§ Administered at 50 psi and 8 liters per minute of oxygen.

The most frequent potentially serious toxicity with TMP-SMX is neutropenia (Table 383–2). Because this reaction is dose-dependent, many clinicians choose a lower dose TMP-SMX (15 mg per kilogram per day of TMP). Several controlled trials have indicated that the lower dose results in survival rates ≥88% for severe episodes, suggesting that the lower dose does not compromise effectiveness.

Parenteral Pentamidine. Parenteral pentamidine is also highly effective. As with TMP-SMX, toxic reactions are common with parenteral pentamidine (Table 383–2). In one study in which patients received a minimum of 14 days of therapy, nephrotoxicity (>1 mg per deciliter rise in serum creatinine) occurred in 64% of patients, hypotension in 27%, and hypoglycemia in 21% (serum glucose <60 gm per deciliter). Impaired renal function and hypoglycemia are dose-dependent and more likely to be seen after 2 weeks of therapy or a total dosage of >4 grams. Hypotension generally occurs during or shortly after intravenous infusions and may last several hours, although low blood pressures may persist for several months.

Hypoglycemia is the most treacherous reaction and occurs in 10 to 20% of AIDS patients treated with pentamidine and results from sudden increases in serum insulin caused by lysis of pancreatic beta cells. Because of the prolonged binding of pentamidine to tissues, precipitous hypoglycemia may occur after pentamidine is discontinued, and fatal reactions have occurred up to 2 weeks after the last dose. When hypoglycemia is detected, pentamidine should be discontinued and patients should be monitored closely with daily capillary glucose measurements for several weeks.

Trimetrexate. Trimetrexate (NeuTrexin) is a powerful antifolate drug that binds to the DHFR of *P. carinii* nearly 1500 times more avidly than TMP and is concentrated in *P. carinii*. In a pivotal licensure study, trimetrexate was effective but inferior to TMP-SMX for moderate-to-severe episodes. Treatment-terminating toxicity, particularly critical neutropenia, thrombocytopenia, and anemia, occurs significantly less often with trimetrexate than with TMP-SMX.

Adjunctive Corticosteroids (Table 383–3). The major breakthrough in the search for more effective therapies for pneumocystis has been the irrefutable evidence that mortality for severe episodes can be reduced nearly twofold by use of corticosteroids within 72 hours after beginning conventional therapy. In addition, oxygen desaturation occurs less often and fewer patients need mechanical ventilation with adjunctive corticosteroids. The only adverse consequence of steroids has been an increased incidence of mucocutaneous herpes infections in one trial.

Adjunctive corticosteroids could be deleterious if prescribed with empiric antipneumocystis therapy for patients who actually have pulmonary fungal infection or tuberculosis, because these patients may initially improve, thereby delaying diagnosis and specific therapy. Moreover, corticosteroids can aggravate and accelerate the progression of cutaneous and pulmonary Kaposi's sarcoma.

Salvage Therapy. Once patients have developed respiratory failure during treatment for pneumocystis, prognosis is poor. Parenteral TMP-SMX, pentamidine, trimetrexate, eflornithine, and clindamycin-primaquine have all been evaluated for salvage in uncontrolled studies and appear to provide limited success in rescuing overtly failing patients. There is little reason to favor any of these therapies, but parenteral drugs are preferable.

Mild Episodes (see Table 383–1). For mild episodes (Pao_2 >70 mm Hg or an $[A − a]Do_2$ <35), treatments should be nontoxic and suited for home therapy because mortality rates are <5% with standard therapies. TMP-SMX is inexpensive and conveniently given orally but results in a high frequency of side effects.

Atovaquone. Atovaquone (Mepron) is an oral hydroxynaptho-quinone developed as an antimalarial compound and has an excellent safety profile. The drug inhibits mitochondrial electron transport necessary for the biosynthesis of pyrimidines in protozoa, but its mode of action for *P. carinii* is unknown.

In the pivotal licensure study of atovaquone for 322 patients with mild to moderately severe ($[A − a]Do_2$ <45) pneumocystis pneumonia, failures due to inadequate therapeutic response occurred in 31% of patients receiving atovaquone and 16% with TMP-SMX ($P = 0.002$). Patients in whom treatment failed were more likely to have low plasma concentrations of atovaquone (<15 µg per millimeter) and diarrhea. Atovaquone must be given with food because blood levels are two- to threefold lower when the drug is taken on an empty stomach.

Trimethoprim-Dapsone. Trimethoprim-dapsone, like TMP-

TABLE 383–2. TOXICITIES ASSOCIATED WITH STANDARD THERAPIES FOR *PNEUMOCYSTIS* PNEUMONIA

Drug	Frequent Causes of Morbidity	Infrequent Causes of Morbidity
Trimethoprim-sulfamethoxazole	Fever Morbilliform rash Nausea and vomiting Neutropenia* Thrombocytopenia† Anemia‡	Stevens-Johnson syndrome Exfoliative dermatitis Diarrhea Liver test abnormalities Elevated serum creatinine Hyperkalemia Hyponatremia Renal impairment Hallucinations or agitation
Parenteral pentamidine	Fever Morbilliform rash Nausea and vomiting Renal impairment Hypoglycemia Hypotension Pancreatitis	Hypocalcemia Ventricular tachycardia/fibrillation Torsades de pointes Neutropenia Thrombocytopenia Liver test abnormalities Ketoacidosis and diabetes Hypomagnesemia Myoglobinuria Hematuria
Trimetrexate plus leucovorin	Fever Morbilliform rash	Liver test abnormalities Neutropenia Thrombocytopenia Mucositis
Dapsone	Fever Morbilliform rash Nausea and vomiting	Methemoglobinemia Hemolytic anemia Sulfone syndrome
Clindamycin	Fever Morbilliform rash Diarrhea	Liver test abnormalities *C. difficile* colitis
Primaquine	Nausea Abdominal distress Neutropenia	Methemoglobinemia Hemolytic anemia Hypertension Arrhythmias
Atovaquone	Rash	Fever Nausea and vomiting Liver test abnormalities
Inhaled pentamidine	Cough Bronchospasm Metallic taste	Contact dermatitis Morbilliform rash Hypoglycemia Pancreatitis Renal impairment

* Reduce to < 1000 per deciliter
† Reduce to < 50,000 per deciliter
‡ > 2 gram per deciliter decline

SMX, results in sequential folate blockade in *P. carinii.* Dapsone (a sulfone) binds to the *P. carinii* dihydropteroate synthetase twofold more avidly than SMX. Treatment-terminating neutropenia and elevation of liver tests occur less frequently than with TMP-SMX.

Clindamycin-Primaquine. Clindamycin and the antimalarial drug primaquine together have excellent activity against *P. carinii* in a cell culture system and in cortisone-treated rats, but neither agent alone is highly effective. The combination has been effective for pneumocystis both as initial therapy and for patients intolerant of or failing conventional therapies, with response rates in the range of 90% regardless of whether clindamycin is given intravenously or orally and whether the dose of primaquine base is 15 or 30 mg daily. This combination may be somewhat better tolerated than TMP-SMX, but controlled trials have not established whether it is as effective as TMP-SMX.

Adjunctive Corticosteroids (Table 383–3). The U.S. Public Health Service has not recommended adjunctive corticosteroids for mild episodes because mortality with conventional therapies is very low if there is minimal impairment of oxygenation at baseline. However, a recent study indicated that desaturation is less, exercise tolerance is better, and LDH returns to baseline more quickly with adjunctive corticosteroids in episodes of mild to moderate severity.

OUTCOME AND PROGNOSIS. Clinical parameters associated with an increased risk for fatal outcome have included at presentation an elevated serum LDH of > 500 IU per deciliter, $Pao_2 < 70$ mm Hg or $(A - a)Do_2 > 35$, BAL neutrophils > 5%, and low T3 and reverse T3 hormone concentrations.

Changing Therapy. It is often difficult to know when a pa-

tient is failing a specific therapy. Persistence of fever or lack of improvement on chest radiographs is common, and persistence or progression of infiltrates frequently occurs even in patients who ultimately are cured. A sustained respiratory rate > 35 per minute or absolute increase in room air $(A - a)Do_2 > 20$ above baseline have proven reproducible endpoints for failure and objective justification for changing therapy and searching for other infectious complications in the lung.

Supportive Care. Evidence suggests that the degree of alveolar damage is the most important determinant of outcome. Thus, as with ARDS, which has similar histologic features to severe pneu-

TABLE 383–3. ADJUNCTIVE CORTICOSTEROIDS* FOR PATIENTS WITH PNEUMOCYSTIS AND $(A-a)Do_2 \geq 35$ mm Hg OR $Pao_2 \leq 70$ mm Hg

	Dose	Treatment Days
Oral		
Prednisone	40 mg b.i.d.	1–5
	40 mg once daily	6–10
	20 mg once daily	11–end of therapy
Intravenous		
Methyl-prednisolone	30 mg b.i.d.	1–5
	30 mg once daily	6–10
	15 mg once daily	11–end of therapy

* Efficacy established only when adjunctive corticosteroids are initiated within 72 hours of starting specific treatment for *P. carinii.*

TABLE 383–4. PROPHYLACTIC THERAPIES FOR PREVENTION OF *PNEUMOCYSTIS* PNEUMONIA

Drug	Dose or Regimen	Alternate Dose or Regimen
Antifolate regimens		
Trimethoprim-sulfamethoxazole	1 DS tablet daily	1 DS tablet three times weekly
	(160 mg trimethoprim, 800 mg sulfamethoxazole)	1 SS tablet daily
Dapsone	100 mg tablet daily	50-mg tablet once or twice daily
Dapsone-pyrimethamine	50 mg tablet dapsone daily	None
	50 mg tablet pyrimethamine	Weekly
Sulfadoxine-pyrimethamine	1 tablet weekly (sulfadoxine 500 mg, pyrimethamine 25 mg)	None
Pyrimethamine-sulfadiazine or pyrimethamine-clindamycin	Induction or maintenance doses for toxoplasmic encephalitis*	None
Aerosolized pentamidine		
Respirgard II jet nebulizer	300 mg monthly	None established
Fisons' ultrasonic nebulizer	60 mg every 2 weeks†	None
Other regimens		
Atovaquone	Unknown	None
Primaquine-clindamycin	Unknown	None

* Patients receiving therapy for toxoplasmosis are unlikely to need additional prophylaxis for pneumocystis because pyrimethamine-sulfadiazine has been used successfully to treat pneumocystis pneumonia, and the combination of pyrimethamine-clindamycin is similar to the regimen of primaquine-clindamycin, which is also effective treatment for pneumocystis.
† Five 60 mg doses within the first 14 days for "loading," one dose on day 21, and then every 2 weeks thereafter.
DS = double strength; SS = single strength.

mocystis, good supportive care is crucial for severely ill patients with pneumocystis. Continuous positive airway pressure by face mask improves oxygenation in patients with tachypnea and desaturation refractory with standard masks and may mitigate the need for mechanical ventilation.

Mechanical Ventilation and Intensive Care Unit Care. For AIDS patients on mechanical ventilators in intensive care units (ICU), mortality has ranged from 30 to 50% in recent reports, supporting the value of aggressive measures in selected patients with severe episodes. Low albumin, arterial pH < 7.35, or need for positive end expiratory pressure > 10 cm H$_2$O after 96 hours in the ICU portend a severalfold greater risk for a fatal outcome. Thus, patients with better nutritional status and who are not acidotic or have less severe alveolar damage may benefit most from ICU care.

PROPHYLAXIS (Table 383–4). The U.S. Public Health Service has advised that patients at high risk for pneumocystis receive prophylactic therapies. Those at highest risk include (1) patients with prior pneumocystis and (2) those with < 200 CD4+ cells. TMP-SMX is currently the most effective therapy for prophylaxis of pneumocystis. In several studies, the relative hazard of developing pneumocystis was approximately three to four times less with TMP-SMX than with aerosolized pentamidine.

In controlled trials, dapsone has been comparable to aerosolized pentamidine but somewhat inferior to TMP-SMX. When combined with pyrimethamine (usually 50 mg once weekly), the two drugs are also highly effective in preventing toxoplasmosis.

Bozzette SA, Sattler FR, Chui J, et al.: A controlled trial of early adjunctive treatment with corticosteroids for *Pneumocystis carinii* pneumonia in the acquired immunodeficiency syndrome. N Engl J Med 323:1451, 1990. *A pivotal study demonstrating that adjunctive corticosteroids reduce mortality for patients with severe pneumocystis.*

Hardy DW, Feinberg J, Finkelstein DM, et al.: A controlled trial of trimethoprim-sulfamethoxazole or aerosolized pentamidine for secondary prophylaxis of *Pneumocystis carinii* pneumonia in patients with the acquired immunodeficiency syndrome. AIDS Clinical Trials Group Protocol 021. N Engl J Med 327:1842, 1992. *Results demonstrate the superiority of TMP-SMX compared with aerosolized pentamidine for preventing pneumocystis in AIDS patients with prior pneumocystis.*

Hughes W, Leoung G, Kramer F, et al.: Comparison of atovaquone (566C80) with trimethoprim-sulfamethoxazole for the treatment of *Pneumocystis carinii* pneumonia in patients with the acquired immunodeficiency syndrome (AIDS). N Engl J Med 328:1521, 1993. *Results established the relative effectiveness and tolerability of atovaquone for therapy of mild to moderately severe pneumocystis.*

Sattler FR, Frame P, Davis R, et al.: Trimetrexate with leucovorin versus trimethoprim-sulfamethoxazole for moderate to severe episodes of *Pneumocystis carinii* pneumonia in patients with AIDS: A prospective, controlled multicenter investigation of the AIDS Clinical Trials Protocol 029/031. J Infect Dis 170:165, 1994. *Results established the relative effectiveness and tolerability of trimetrexate for moderate to severe pneumocystis pneumonia.*

Toma E, Fournier S, Dumont M, et al.: Clindamycin/primaquine versus trimethoprim-sulfamethoxazole as primary therapy for *Pneumocystis carinii* pneumonia in AIDS: A randomized, double blind pilot trial. Clin Infect Dis 17:178, 1993. *Results confirm prior reports of the incidence of adverse effects with two treatment regimens and suggest that clindamycin-primaquine is highly effective as initial therapy for pneumocystis.*

Travis WD, Pittaluga S, Lipschik GY, et al.: Atypical pathologic manifestations of *Pneumocystis carinii* pneumonia in the acquired immunodeficiency syndrome. Review of 123 lung biopsies from 76 patients with emphasis on cysts, vascular invasion, vasculitis, and granulomas. Am J Surg Pathol 14:615, 1990. *Report describes the pathologic findings of pneumocystis in patients with AIDS.*

Helminthic Diseases

384 CESTODE INFECTIONS
Charles H. King

The eight cestode species that most commonly cause human infection are listed in Table 384–1. Although this class of parasites is often referred to, collectively, as "tapeworms," it is important to note that not all cestode parasites develop into tapeworms in the human host. The key to understanding the rather broad spectrum of cestode-associated illness is to recall that these parasites divide their life cycle between two or more different animal hosts, termed *intermediate* and *definitive* hosts. The intermediate host harbors the immature parasite as a tissue cyst, whereas the subsequent definitive host harbors the mature parasite as a tapeworm. For a given cestode species, humans may serve as *either* intermediate or definitive hosts.

The *intermediate* host is typically an insect or herbivorous (omnivorous) vertebrate that ingests parasite eggs in fecally contaminated food or water. The cestode eggs hatch into invasive oncospheres in this primary host's intestinal tract, then migrate into the host viscera or muscles to develop into immature cystic forms, called cysticerci or cysticercoids (for Cyclophyllidea cestodes such

TABLE 384-1. COMMON HUMAN CESTODE INFECTIONS

Species	Stage Found in Humans	Common Name	Pathology	Therapy
Diphyllobotrium latum	Adult	Fish tapeworm	Pernicious anemia	Niclosamide Praziquantel
Hymenolepis nana	Adult	Dwarf tapeworm	Rarely symptomatic	Niclosamide Praziquantel
Taenia saginata	Adult	Beef tapeworm	Rarely symptomatic	
Taenia solium	Adult	Pork tapeworm	Rarely symptomatic	Niclosamide Praziquantel
	Larva	Cysticercosis	Brain and tissue cysts	Albendazole* Praziquantel Surgery
Echinococcus granulosus	Larva	Hydatid cyst disease	Solitary tissue cysts	Surgery Albendazole*
Echinococcus multilocularis	Larva	Alveolar cyst disease	Multilocular cysts	Surgery Albendazole*
Taenia multiceps	Larva	Bladderworm, coenurosis	Brain and eye cysts	Surgery
Spirometra mansonoides	Larva	Sparganosis	Subcutaneous larvae	Surgery

* This drug has not been approved by the Food and Drug Administration at the time of publication.

as Taenia and Hymenolepis), or procercoid and plerocercoid larvae (for Pseudophyllidea cestodes such as Diphyllobothrium). Humans become intermediate hosts for cestode species by ingesting parasite eggs in food or water, as in echinococcosis, or rarely by direct transfer of plerocercoid larvae from animal tissues, as in sparganosis.

The definitive host for a cestode species is a carnivorous or omnivorous mammal that acquires infection by consuming larval cysts in the uncooked tissues of an intermediate host. Upon exposure to stomach acid and bile salts in the digestive tract, the larvae excyst and develop into mature tapeworms within the intestinal lumen. Adult tapeworms contain two sections: a scolex (or head) used to adhere to the wall of the intestine, and a strobila, or tapelike chain of developing segments called proglottides. The hermaphroditic proglottides produce large numbers of fertile, infectious parasite eggs that reach the environment either free or enclosed within parasite segments in the host's feces. Carnivorous humans become definitive hosts by ingesting cyst-infested meat of intermediate hosts (e.g., fish, pork, or beef), after which the cysts develop into intraluminal, intestinal tapeworms.

We are strictly definitive hosts for the cestodes Diphyllobothrium latum (the "fish" tapeworm) and Taenia saginata (the "beef" tapeworm). These adult tapeworms do not enter the tissues of the human body and cause only minimal clinical symptoms. In contrast, we are solely intermediate hosts for Echinococcus granulosus (hydatid cyst disease), E. multilocularis (alveolar cyst disease), Taenia multiceps (coenurosis), and Spirometra species. In the human body, these parasites develop as larval cysts and cause significant symptomatic tissue damage.

There are two exceptions to this rule. First, patients with T. solium infection may be infected with larval cysts (cysticercosis), adult tapeworms ("pork" tapeworm), or both. Second, in the case of the dwarf tapeworm, Hymenolepis nana, complete egg-to-tapeworm development can take place within a single human host. H. nana can thus be transmitted directly from person to person, and internal autoinfection may substantially increase the tapeworm burden of an infected individual. For all other cestode infections, increases in parasite burden occur only by means of continued exposure to egg-contaminated or larvae-infested foods and water.

INTESTINAL CESTODE (TAPEWORM) INFECTIONS
Diphyllobothrium latum

D. latum tapeworms are the largest parasites that infect humans, ranging up to 10 meters in length. Infection is acquired by ingestion of parasite cysts in the tissues of smoked or uncooked fresh water fish (e.g., as sushi, sashimi, or ceviche). Tapeworms develop to maturity within 3 to 6 weeks after exposure and may survive for up to 20 years. Infection is prevalent (up to 2% of local residents) in many parts of the world; endemic foci are found in lake or delta regions of Scandinavia, the former Soviet Union, Japan, Europe, Chile, and North America. Contamination of fresh water bodies by raw sewage increases the risk for D. latum infection, but stable

transmission may also occur owing to local infection of alternate definitive hosts, such as foxes, wolves, minks, and bears.

CLINICAL MANIFESTATIONS. For most patients, D. latum infection produces few, if any, symptoms. These are typically limited to nonspecific complaints of weakness, dizziness, craving for salt, diarrhea, and intermittent abdominal discomfort. Occasional patients may experience vomiting, severe abdominal pain, and weight loss. In cases of multiple infection, biliary or intestinal obstruction may occur. One to 2% of patients with D. latum infection develop significant vitamin B_{12} deficiency, resulting in megaloblastic anemia and/or neurologic disease. Folate deficiency may also occur. Vitamin B_{12} deficiency is a product of extensive vitamin uptake by the worm as well as worm-induced interference with gastrointestinal uptake by the host (despite normal gastric acidity and intrinsic factor production). Vitamin B_{12} deficiency is most common among older patients and is more likely to occur in patients with low dietary intake of vitamins, multiple tapeworms, or a tapeworm in the proximal jejunum. In the debilitated host, nervous system complications can be quite extensive and can range from peripheral neuropathy to the syndrome of severe combined degeneration (see Ch. 223).

DIAGNOSIS. The diagnosis of D. latum infection is made by stool examination for characteristic operculated eggs that are 65 by 45 μm. Recovery of proglottides is infrequent owing to segment degeneration during intestinal transit.

TREATMENT. Treatment is with niclosamide or praziquantel, as summarized in Table 384-2. Severe vitamin B_{12} deficiency can be rapidly treated by parenteral vitamin injections.

PREVENTION. Fish tapeworm infection is prevented by avoiding consumption of raw, smoked, or salted fish from endemic areas. Parasite cysts may be killed by cooking (above 56°C for 5 minutes) or by freezing (-20°C for 24 hours).

Hymenolepis nana

H. nana, or dwarf tapeworm, is found frequently in warm, dry climates and is prevalent in Southern and Eastern Europe, Asia, Africa, Central and South America, and Australia. It is the only human tapeworm that does not require an intermediate host. In the small intestine, hatching eggs release oncospheres that penetrate the villi of the mucosa. Four to 5 days later, the developed cysticercoid ruptures out of the villus and a parasite scolex attaches to the lining of the ileum, maturing in 10 to 12 days. Mature worms are small, measuring 25 to 40 mm long by 1 mm wide. Autoinfection can occur internally, i.e., within the small bowel, or externally, via the fecal-oral route, resulting in heavy infection. With time, however, a regulatory immunity to infection may develop, so that H. nana infection can be spontaneously cleared. Intensive infection is more common in institutionalized, malnourished, or immunodeficient individuals.

CLINICAL MANIFESTATIONS. The clinical manifestations of H. nana vary with intensity and may include diarrhea, anorexia, abdominal pain, and pallor. A statistical association with phlyctenular

TABLE 384-2. THERAPY FOR INTESTINAL CESTODE (TAPEWORM) INFECTION

	Niclosamide	Praziquantel
Dosage		
Adults	2 grams (4 tablets)	10–12 mg/kg for all age groups
Children >34 kg	1.5 grams (3 tablets)	(25 mg/kg for *H. nana*)
Children 11–34 kg	1 gram (2 tablets)	
Administration	For most tapeworm species, taken as a single dose; tablets must be thoroughly chewed before swallowing to obtain complete therapeutic effect; a 7-day course of drugs used for *H. nana,* with reduced pediatric doses on days 2–7	Taken as a single dose for all species; may repeat after 7 days for heavy *H. nana* infections
Side effects	Nausea, vomiting, abdominal pain, diarrhea, drowsiness, dizziness, headache, pruritus	Mild but frequent, including dizziness, myalgias, nausea, vomiting, diarrhea, abdominal pain
Pregnancy	No known mutagenic effects; considered safe if indicated; because of risk of cysticercosis by autoinfection in *T. solium* tapeworm infection, therapy should not be delayed	

keratoconjunctivitis has been observed and has been tentatively ascribed to the immune response to infection.

DIAGNOSIS. The diagnosis of *H. nana* infection is made by examining stool for eggs 30 to 47 μm that have a characteristic double membrane. Proglottides are usually not seen in the stool.

TREATMENT. Treatment is with niclosamide or praziquantel, as outlined in Table 384–2. Compared with the treatment of other tapeworm infections, longer courses of niclosamide and higher doses of praziquantel are recommended for the therapy of *H. nana* infection because of the relative resistance of larval cysticercoids to drug therapy. Because of the potential for late emergence of worms from viable cysticercoids remaining in the ileum, heavily infected individuals should be retested for infection and retreated 10 to 14 days after initial therapy.

PREVENTION. Because *H. nana* is easily transmitted from person to person, sanitation and hand washing are essential to control this parasite. Mass chemotherapy may also be used to suppress endemic transmission, particularly within closed institutions.

Taenia saginata

T. saginata, or beef tapeworm infection, is widespread in cattle-breeding areas of the world. Endemic foci (defined as prevalence > 10%) are found in the southern Russian republics, in the Near East, and in central and eastern Africa. Infection is less common in other parts of the world but is found at prevalence rates of 0.1 to 5% in Europe, Southeast Asia, and South America. Infection is acquired by consuming cysticerci in the muscle tissue of infected cattle. The consumption of dishes such as steak tartare, "bleu" or rare steak, and undercooked shish kebabs is associated with infection in North American travelers to endemic areas.

CLINICAL MANIFESTATIONS. *T. saginata* infection may cause nonspecific complaints of weakness and mild abdominal discomfort in a minority (one third) of patients. Because *T. saginata* proglottides are motile, they may cause acute abdominal symptoms by migrating into and obstructing the appendix or the pancreatic and biliary ducts. A psychologically distressing feature of infection (and often the first symptom reported by the patient) occurs when motile proglottides migrate out of the anus onto skin or clothing or when they are observed moving in the feces.

DIAGNOSIS. The diagnosis of taeniasis is most readily established by stool examination and perianal inspection for parasite proglottides and eggs. It is not possible, however, to distinguish *T. saginata* eggs from those of *T. solium* morphologically, and the definitive diagnosis of *T. saginata* infection requires pathologic examination of proglottid features or DNA hybridization studies. In practice, because patients with *T. solium* are at risk for self-infection with cysticercosis (see below), and because medical therapy for taeniasis is both safe and highly effective, treatment of an undetermined *Taenia* species infection should not be delayed pending speciation of the infecting tapeworm.

TREATMENT. Treatment of beef tapeworm infection is with praziquantel or niclosamide, as outlined in Table 384–2. Both medications are highly effective in eliminating infection, and no special preparation or purgation is required. After therapy, the parasite scolex is digested within the gastrointestinal tract before it is passed in the feces. Although with the highly effective medications currently in use one no longer needs to collect the scolex to be assured that the parasite head has been expelled, digestive destruction of the

head limits our ability to establish a species-specific clinical diagnosis for individual *Taenia* infections.

PREVENTION. *T. saginata* infection is prevented by avoiding foods containing undercooked or raw beef. As for the fish tapeworm, cooking to 56°C for 5 minutes or freezing at −20°C for 7 to 10 days destroys the infective larvae.

Taenia solium

T. solium, also known as pork tapeworm, causes human infection in two different forms. Individuals who consume undercooked pork containing intermediate parasite cysts develop intestinal *T. solium* tapeworms. Individuals who consume parasite eggs may develop intermediate parasite cysts within the tissues of the body. (This condition, called *cysticercosis,* is described in more detail in the section on tissue cestode infections.) Autoinfection, most likely via the fecal-oral route, is possible, and a single patient may harbor both adult tapeworm and tissue cysticerci. *T. solium* infection is prevalent in Mexico, Central and South America, Africa, the Cape Verde Islands, southern Europe, Southeast Asia, and the Philippines. Most infections seen in the United States and Canada are found in immigrants from these endemic foci.

CLINICAL MANIFESTATIONS. *T. solium* tapeworms are relatively short (3 meters) but may survive for several decades once established in the human jejunum. Generally, tapeworm infections with *T. solium* produce minimal or no symptoms, being limited to mild, nonspecific abdominal complaints. Unlike *T. saginata* proglottides, the segments of *T. solium* are nonmotile and are unlikely to cause obstruction.

DIAGNOSIS. The diagnosis of intestinal infection with *T. solium* tapeworm is made by examining the stool for eggs and proglottides. Because the eggs are morphologically indistinguishable from those of *T. saginata,* study of the proglottid or head of the tapeworms is required for species identification. Stool samples and proglottides should be handled with care because of the risk of acquiring cysticercosis by accidental ingestion of *T. solium* eggs.

TREATMENT. *T. solium* tapeworm infection is treated with either niclosamide or praziquantel, as outlined in Table 384–2. Once diagnosis is established, therapy should be instituted as soon as possible because of the risk of autoinfection with cysticercosis. Therapy of concurrent cysticercosis is substantially longer and more intensive than that for intestinal infection and is described in detail in the section on tissue cestode infections.

Other Intestinal Cestodes

Other tapeworms that occasionally infect humans include the dog tapeworm *Dipylidium caninum* and the rodent tapeworm *Hymenolepis diminuta*. These are most common in children and are acquired by inadvertently ingesting the intermediate larval forms of these parasites in the bodies of fleas or other insects. Usually, *D. caninum* and *H. diminuta* infections produce minimal symptoms. Diagnosis is established by stool examination, and infections are readily treated with standard doses of niclosamide or praziquantel.

TISSUE CESTODE (CYST) INFECTION

Echinococcosis

Human echinococcosis causes significant morbidity and mortality in livestock-raising regions in all parts of the world. The causative agents of "hydatid" and "alveolar" cyst disease in humans are the intermediate larval forms of the tapeworms *Echinococcus granulosus* and *E. multilocularis,* respectively.

Like other cestodes, *Echinococcus* tapeworms have both intermediate and definitive hosts. For *Echinococcus* species, dogs and other canines are the definitive hosts. Tapeworm-infected animals pass eggs in their feces, which contaminate the local environment. Contamination of grazing areas and foodstuffs results in egg ingestion by intermediate hosts, e.g., humans, sheep, goats, camels, and horses for *E. granulosus* and mice or other small rodents for *E. multilocularis.* Life cycle transmission is completed when the definitive carnivore host consumes meat or offal of the intermediate host that contains hydatid or alveolar cysts. Protoscolices within the cysts mature in the lumen of the canine gut to become adult, egg-bearing tapeworms. Because the cysts of *Echinococcus* contain a germinal layer that can produce multiple internal "daughter" cysts by asexual budding, an individual dog may develop infection with dozens of tapeworms after consuming a single large cyst. Once the tapeworms mature, a heavily infected dog may contaminate 10 or more hectares of ground with infectious eggs in the space of a week.

In most areas of the world, burial practices make humans a "dead-end" host for *Echinococcus;* i.e., human infection does not perpetuate transmission in the local ecosystem. Nevertheless, the "inadvertent" hydatid cyst disease caused by *E. granulosus* and the more aggressive alveolar cyst disease caused by *E. multilocularis* are severe or even fatal illnesses for a significant minority of infected individuals.

EPIDEMIOLOGY. *E. granulosus* is common in livestock-raising areas of both developed and developing countries. Sheep- and goat-herding populations that keep dogs as pets or work animals are at highest risk for hydatid cyst disease. Until recently, hydatid disease was common in Australia, New Zealand, Argentina, Chile, Ireland, Scotland, the Basque country, the Mediterranean basin, and throughout middle Europe. Currently, the area with the highest prevalence in the world is the Turkana and Samburu regions of northwestern Kenya, where domestic and feral transmission of *E. granulosus* is perpetuated among nomadic farmers by poor hygienic practices. Occasional hydatid disease transmission is also found in central Asia, Mexico, the United States, and South America.

Alveolar cyst disease due to *E. multilocularis* is usually transmitted by wild animals, e.g., foxes and bush dogs, and is found in the arctic regions of the United States, Canada, and the former Soviet Union, as well as in rural areas of Europe and Turkey.

CLINICAL MANIFESTATIONS. Human disease caused by *Echinococcus* species results from bloodborne invasion of the liver (50 to 70% of patients), lungs (20 to 30%), or other organs by developing parasite oncospheres. As these mature, they grow within tissues by concentric enlargement *(E. granulosus)* or by extension through adjacent host tissues *(E. multilocularis).* At any given time, most infected individuals are asymptomatic, and it may take 5 to 20 years for a cyst to grow to sufficient size (3 to 15 cm) to cause symptoms. When present, symptoms and findings refer to the anatomic site of involvement and derive from local inflammation, secondary bacterial infection, obstruction, or local mass effect. In hydatid cyst disease, the growing cyst becomes surrounded by a fibrous capsule formed by host immune reaction. Within this primary unilocular cyst, multiple daughter cysts, each containing an infective protoscolex, develop by asexual budding of the germinal layer. In alveolar cyst disease, the parasite cyst is not well separated from surrounding tissues, and lateral budding and malignancy-like growth (including distant metastasis of daughter cysts) may occur.

Patients with symptomatic hydatid liver cysts may complain of abdominal discomfort or mass in the right upper quadrant. Cyst leakage into the peritoneal cavity or pleural space may be associated with fever, urticaria, or a severe anaphylactoid reaction. Invasion of the biliary system often leads to the passage of daughter cysts into the common bile duct, with clinical and chemical evidence of intermittent obstruction resembling cholerdocholithiasis. Individuals with symptomatic hydatid involvement of the lungs present with cough, hemoptysis, and pleurisy. Spontaneous rupture of the cyst may lead to intrathoracic spread or to evacuation of daughter cysts via the bronchus. At either lung or liver sites, bacterial superinfection may cause an acute presentation with symptoms of sepsis. Hydatid involvement of the brain is marked by slow-onset mass effect, hydrocephalus, and often seizures. Cysts of the bone

frequently fail to form a discrete capsule but rather cause local erosion of the cortex, resulting in pathologic fracture.

Symptomatic alveolar cyst disease most frequently refers to liver involvement and manifests as vague, mild upper quadrant and epigastric pain. Signs of hepatomegaly or obstructive jaundice may be present. Occasionally, metastatic lesions in the lung or brain are the first to cause symptoms by local inflammation or mass effect.

DIAGNOSIS. Laboratory evaluation may show marked eosinophilia, but this finding is inconstant (30% prevalence). In hydatid cyst disease, radiographic and ultrasonographic studies typically show characteristic large, avascular cysts containing internal structures consistent with daughter cysts. Detection of mural calcification strongly favors the diagnosis of hydatid cyst. The differential diagnosis includes hemangioma, metastatic carcinoma, and remote bacterial or amebic liver abscess. Confirmatory evidence of infection may be obtained by serology (sensitivity of 60 to 90%, depending on the test used). Serologic testing is available commercially or from the Centers for Disease Control and Prevention (CDC), Atlanta, GA (through local state health departments). Until recently, it has not been recommended to perform closed aspiration on the cyst for diagnosis, as cyst leakage has the potential to initiate a severe allergic reaction and may result in the metastatic spread of daughter cysts. However, a recent clinical series has reported successful computed tomography (CT)–guided thin-needle aspiration of hydatid cysts for diagnosis. This procedure, when followed by immediate instillation of ethanol to kill viable protoscoleces, was associated with minimal side effects and was followed by apparent regression of cysts on CT scans. Further trials of this simplified approach to diagnosis and therapy appear warranted.

With alveolar cyst disease due to *E. multilocularis,* the organism's appearance on radiographic and sonographic imaging often mimics that of hepatic carcinoma. A definitive diagnosis may require either angiography or open biopsy at surgery. Precautions must be taken to prevent metastatic dissemination of daughter cysts at the time of surgery.

TREATMENT. Stable, asymptomatic, calcified cysts do not require specific therapy but should be monitored by serial imaging over several years to ensure a benign resolution. When technically feasible, expanding, symptomatic, or infected cysts are best removed *in toto* at surgery, with care taken to isolate and kill the cyst (with hypertonic saline (25 to 30 grams per deciliter) or other cidal agents (such as iodophor or ethanol) prior to excision, to avoid secondary spread or parasite cysts. Surgical resection should include careful closure of biliary and enteric fistulas and extensive postoperative drainage of the cyst bed to prevent fluid accumulation and secondary bacterial infection. Alveolar cyst disease may require wide resection, i.e., total lobectomy of liver or lung, to remove all cyst material.

In many cases, symptomatic echinococcal cysts are not amenable to resection. In such cases, oral drug therapy with the anthelminthics, either long-term mebendazole (40 mg per kilogram of body weight per day in three divided doses for 6 to 12 months) or albendazole* (400 mg twice a day for one to eight periods of 28 days each, separated by drug-free rest intervals of 14 to 28 days), has been recommended for cure or palliation. Cure rates, particularly for difficult cases with recurrent or extrahepatic/extrapulmonary cysts, have been low (< 33%), although a majority of patients show some improvement. Because the efficacy of drug therapy is limited, a combined medical-surgical approach should be formulated for each patient.

Cysticercosis

Cysticercosis represents human tissue infection with the intermediate cyst forms of the pork tapeworm *T. solium.* Cysticercosis is acquired by ingestion of *T. solium* eggs in contaminated foods. Infection prevalence is approximately 1 to 10% in endemic areas of Latin America, India, Asia, Indonesia, and parts of Africa. Because of its potentially life-threatening complications, cysticercosis has greater clinical significance than does intestinal *T. solium* tapeworm

---

* This drug has not been approved by the Food and Drug Administration at the time of publication. In the United States, compassionate use may be available through SmithKline Beecham Pharmaceuticals, Philadelphia, PA.

infection, particularly if cyst disease involves the CNS, the eyes, the heart, or other vital organs.

CLINICAL MANIFESTATIONS. Clinical manifestations depend on the location and number of infecting cysts. Cysticerci are bladder-like, fluid-filled cysts containing an invaginated protoscolex. They are often surrounded by a dense fibrous capsule of host origin. In infected humans, cysticerci are usually multiple, 0.5 to 2 cm in size, and distributed widely throughout the body. Many patients have minimal, if any, symptoms of infection. However, symptomatic *neurocysticercosis* (i.e., cerebral cysticercosis, eye or spinal cord involvement) requires medical attention. This syndrome has an estimated mortality of up to 50%, and any neurologic, cognitive, or personality disorder in an individual from an endemic area should be considered a possible manifestation of undiagnosed neurocysticercosis. In the past decade, diagnosis of this condition has been facilitated by CT scanning and magnetic resonance imaging (MRI), both of which are highly sensitive in detecting CNS cysticerci. Patients with CNS involvement have an average of 10 cysts distributed throughout the brain and spinal cord. These cysts may be in different stages of development, with symptoms commonly arising when older cysts begin to die, lose osmoregulation, and release antigenic material to provoke significant host inflammatory response.

In practice, neurocysticercosis may be divided into six discrete syndromes for management. In the *acute invasive* stage of cysticercosis, immediately after infection, the patient may experience fevers, headache, and myalgias associated with significant peripheral eosinophilia. Heavy infection at this stage may result in a clinical picture of "cysticercal encephalitis" associated with coma and rapid deterioration. This presentation should be treated aggressively with antiparasitic agents and anti-inflammatory drugs. After cysticerci become established, *parenchymal CNS cysticercosis* (50% of cases) is associated with seizures, intellectual impairment, and personality changes. Compression due to swelling or inflammation around the cysts may result in focal deficits, signs of cerebral edema, and/or hydrocephalus. Seizures may be focal (jacksonian), referring to the specific cortical locus of involvement, or may be generalized. *Subarachnoid cysticercosis* (30% of cases) is frequently associated with obstruction of cerebrospinal fluid (CSF) flow. Intracranial hypertension may manifest as vomiting, headache, and visual disturbances. Sensorial changes may include apathy, amnesia, dementia, hallucination, and emotional disturbance. Like other forms of basilar meningitis, pericysticercal inflammation at the base of the brain may cause obstruction or vasculitis of the cerebral arteries, leading to intermittent ischemia or stroke. *Intraventricular cysticercosis* (15% of cases) is, because of its location, the most difficult to diagnose and treat. Symptomatic cysts are most frequent in the fourth ventricle, where they cause outflow obstruction and increased intracranial pressure without localizing signs. An aggressive variant of ventricular neurocysticercosis, called *racemose cysticercosis*, frequently involves the basal cisterns. This form of cysticercosis has been noted most often in young women and involves multiple, rapidly spreading cysts in the cerebrum and around the base of the brain. Whereas symptoms due to isolated cysts may remit, racemose cysticercosis usually has a progressive, deteriorating course if therapy is not given. Those with *spinal cysticercosis* may present with cord compression, radiculopathy, transverse myelitis, or signs of meningitis, depending on the location of involvement. *Ocular cysticercosis* is a distinct syndrome that manifests as eye pain, scotomata, and decreasing vision due to iridocyclitis, clouding of the vitreous, and retinal inflammation or detachment.

DIAGNOSIS. A definitive diagnosis of cysticercosis requires examination of biopsy material obtained from a tissue cyst. However, a presumptive diagnosis may be made on the basis of a history of residence in an endemic area, the presence of characteristic radiographic findings on plain films (calcified cysts in soft tissues) or scans (multiple, low-density, enhanced, and unenhanced lesions on CT or MRI), and suggestive laboratory findings. Infection with *T. solium* tapeworm is present in about 25% of neurocysticercosis cases. In neurocysticercosis, examining the CSF may show hypoglycorrhachia, elevated total protein levels, and lymphocytic and eosinophilic pleocytosis (5 to 500 cells per microliter). Serum and CSF enzyme-linked immunosorbent assay (ELISA) and Western

blot testing for specific immunoglobulin M (IgM) and immunoglobulin G (IgG) anticysticercal antibodies has a sensitivity of 75 to 100%. These tests are available through commercial laboratories or from the CDC (samples should be sent through state health departments). It should be noted, however, that antiparasite antibodies may persist long after infection, and a positive IgG serology merely indicates prior *Taenia* exposure, not necessarily active disease. The differential diagnosis of neurocysticercosis includes tumor, hydatid cyst disease, vasculitis, and chronic fungal and mycobacterial infection.

TREATMENT. Given the high prevalence of cysticercosis in some areas of the world, it is evident that most cysticerci do not cause significant symptoms. For *symptomatic* cysts outside the CNS, the optimal therapy is surgical removal, as this ensures complete elimination of the cyst. In the case of symptomatic neurocysticercosis, which carries an associated mortality of up to 50%, therapy is definitely indicated, but surgery may be risky or technically unfeasible. An alternative approach to controlling some forms of neurocysticercosis has been demonstrated in recent clinical studies: Drug therapy with either praziquantel (50 mg per kilogram per day in three divided doses for 14 to 30 days) or albendazole* (15 mg per kilogram per day for 30 days) has been associated with alleviation of symptoms and regression of cyst size and number in patients with viable (nonenhancing) cysts in the cerebral parenchyma. However, drug therapy has provided only limited improvement in patients with arachnoiditis and no improvement in patients with intraventricular cysts. For these latter presentations, the treatment of choice remains surgery and/or palliation with shunting, anticonvulsants, and anti-inflammatory agents. It should be noted that in about 20% of treated cases, starting drug therapy is associated with a severely symptomatic, increased inflammatory response at the site of the cyst. This inflammation may be controlled with corticosteroids, but corticosteroids are not recommended for routine use in all patients, as they may significantly alter the pharmacokinetics of the anthelminthics used to treat infection. Follow-up tomographic scanning should be repeated 3 months after therapy is stopped to ensure adequate response. If necessary, a repeat course of drug therapy with the alternate agent may be given to improve response. Because parasite-induced ocular inflammation does not respond well to systemic anti-inflammatory agents, patients with cysticercosis of the eye (20% of cases of neurocysticercosis) should not receive drug therapy until the eye disease has been controlled surgically.

Coenurosis

A different, but more rare, form of tissue cysticercosis may be caused by larval stages of the dog tapeworms *T. multiceps* and *T. serialis*. Lesions tend to be solitary and are distinguished pathologically from *T. solium* cysticerci on biopsy. Ocular involvement is common, and surgical resection is currently the only effective mode of therapy.

Sparganosis

Sparganosis is a tissue cestode infection caused by the plerocercoid larval stages of *Spirometra* species tapeworms of cats and other carnivores. Humans may become infected by ingesting infected water fleas *(Cyclops),* by ingesting uncooked meat from infected animals (reptiles, birds, or mammals), or by cutaneous exposure (e.g., via traditional skin or eye poultices) to uncooked, infected meat. Usually, the larva encysts within the intestinal submucosa or skin. In some cases, however, parasites may invade the eye or CNS and cause significant inflammatory pathology at the site of encystment. Occasionally, proliferation into surrounding tissues occurs by lateral budding of the parasite (termed *sparganum proliferum*). The treatment of choice for sparganosis is ethanol injection and/or surgical removal, as limited experience with medical anthelminthic therapy has shown no beneficial effect.

Davis A, Dixon H, Pawlowski Z: Multicentre clinical trials of benzimidazole carbamates in human cystic echinococcosis (phase 2). Bull WHO 67:503, 1989. *Review of experience in multicenter trials of medical therapy for hydatid and alveolar cyst disease.*

Del Brutto OH, Sotelo J: Neurocysticercosis: An update. Rev Infect Dis 10:1075, 1988. *Extensive review of the diagnosis and treatment of this varied and complex disease. Contains a useful flow diagram on therapy for neurocysticercosis.*

Filice C, Di Perri G, Strosselli M, et al: Parasitologic findings in percutaneous

---

* This drug has not been approved by the Food and Drug Administration at the time of publication.

drainage of human hydatid liver cysts. J Infect Dis 161:1290, 1990. *Description of a small series of patients undergoing CT-guided diagnosis and treatment of hydatid cyst disease.*

King CH, Mahmoud AAF: Drugs five years later: Praziquantel. Ann Intern Med 110:290, 1989. *A summary of data on the anthelminthic agent praziquantel since its release in the United States. Includes a listing of doses recommended for cestode therapy: with references.*

Pawlowski ZS: Cestodiases: Taeniasis, cysticercosis, diphyllobothriasis, hymenolepiasis and others. *In* Warren KS, Mahmoud AAF (eds.): Tropical and Geographical Medicine. 2nd ed. New York, McGraw-Hill, 1990, p 490. *A detailed review of cestode infections (excluding Echinococcus species).*

Schantz PM, Okelo GBA: Echinococcosis (hydatidosis). *In* Warren KS, Mahmoud AAF (eds.): Tropical and Geographical Medicine. 2nd ed. New York, McGraw-Hill, 1990, p 505. *Review of human infection with Echinococcus species. Useful for hydatid disease as well as less common E. multilocularis and E. vogeli infections.*

385 SCHISTOSOMIASIS (Bilharziasis)

Adel A.F. Mahmoud

DEFINITION. Schistosomiasis, a chronic worm infection, affects more than 200 million people in the world; several hundred million more live in endemic areas and are at risk of exposure to the parasites. The schistosomes are blood flukes that parasitize the venous channels of the definitive human host; infection is transmitted via fresh water snails. Humans may be infected by one of five species: *Schistosoma haematobium, S. mansoni, S. japonicum, S. intercalatum,* or *S. mekongi.* Each species is endemic in specific geographic areas of the world; infection in humans may result in defined clinical syndromes. Other species that occasionally infect humans include *S. bovis, S. matthei,* and some avian schistosomes. Currently, schistosomiasis is endemic in various areas of Africa, Asia, South America, and the Caribbean islands. In the United States, there are approximately 400,000 infected individuals; these include Puerto Ricans, and immigrants or travelers exposed while in endemic areas. Because of the absence of susceptible snails, the life cycle of the schistosomes cannot be established in this country.

ETIOLOGY. The schistosomes differ from other trematodes that infect humans in that they have separate sexes. The species of schistosomes that infect humans share some common features, although they are morphologically distinctive. Each worm has two suckers (anterior and ventral), and the bifurcate intestinal ceca unite posteriorly. The larger male (0.6 to 2.2 cm × 2 to 4 mm) has a ventral gynecophoral canal in which the female is held during copulation. The slender female worm (1.2 to 2.6 cm × 1 to 2 mm) has a rounded body with pointed ends.

Adult schistosome worms parasitize defined sites of the venous vasculature of humans. *S. haematobium* worms inhabit the venous plexus around the lower end of the ureters and the urinary bladder, whereas *S. mansoni, S. japonicum, S. intercalatum,* and *S. mekongi* are located in the mesenteric veins. Sexual maturity of female worms requires the presence of living mature males; when ready to deposit eggs, the worms move against the bloodstream toward the small venous radicles. The female schistosomes deposit ova singly or in bunches, depending on the species of the parasite, and retreat in the direction of blood flow. Egg deposition has been estimated at 300 per day for female *S. haematobium* and *S. mansoni* worms and 3000 per day for *S. japonicum.* The ova of each species have characteristic morphologic features, which are of diagnostic importance. Once deposited in the host, eggs attempt to penetrate the venous capillaries and escape to the bladder or intestinal lumen; enzymatic secretions are thought to aid egg migration. The proportion of ova escaping from infected individuals varies in each species and also may depend on the extent of pathology and state of resistance in the host. Eggs that fail to reach the lumen of urinary tract or gut are trapped in these organs or may be carried to other organs such as the liver; these ova cause inflammatory and immunopathologic changes that are a major cause of disease in schistosomiasis. The schistosome eggs, when deposited by female worms, contain immature miracidia; they take approximately 10 to 12 days to develop while migrating through the host tissues. Once mature, miracidia have a mean lifespan of 11 to 12 days.

Indiscriminate urination and defecation by infected individuals result in dissemination of the parasite eggs in the environment. In fresh water the schistosome ova hatch within a few hours. Miracidia escape head first and swim, usually near the surface of water; they remain infective to the snail intermediate host for approximately 8 hours. On encountering the specific snail, the miracidia penetrate its tissues and undergo tremendous asexual multiplication and transformation into hundreds of cercariae. Schistosome infection of snails causes varying degrees of pathology in their liver and sexual organs and reduces their lifespan. Development of schistosomes inside the snail takes approximately 4 to 6 weeks, but it varies with the species of the parasite and mollusc and with changes in environmental conditions. Cercariae, the infective forms to humans, emerge from the snails under specific conditions of light and temperature; they are elongate with a pear-shaped body and a long forked tail and measure approximately 400 to 600 μm in length. They can survive in fresh water for almost 72 hours but lose their infectivity considerably within the first 24 hours. Cercariae attach to skin of mammalian hosts by their oral or ventral suckers. Burrowing of the skin is helped by vertical vibratory movements of their bodies and secretions of the cephalic penetration glands; the process is usually completed within a few minutes. During penetration, the cercariae shake off their tails and change into the next stage of the life cycle, the schistosomula, which lie in tunnels in the stratum corneum parallel to the skin surface. Schistosomula are covered by a heptalaminar membrane (instead of the trilaminar cercarial membrane) and can no longer survive in fresh water. They are thought to remain in the skin for 1 to 3 days before migrating to the lungs, finally reaching the liver in 2 to 4 weeks. In the intrahepatic portal system, the worms complete the major digestive and sexual stages of their development. Adult worms start their migration to their final habitat in 2 weeks and mate; viable eggs can be seen in the excreta 5 to 9 weeks after cercarial penetration. Figure 385–1 shows the stages of the life cycle of schistosomes.

The mean lifespan of adult schistosome worms inside the human host is not known exactly. Several individual case reports indicate that worms may live 20 to 30 years. This, however, represents extreme cases, as examination of infected individuals who migrate to nonendemic areas indicates that the mean lifespan of the worms is in the range of 3 to 10 years.

EPIDEMIOLOGY. The endemicity of schistosomiasis in any specific area depends on the unsanitary disposal of urine and feces, the presence of suitable snail hosts, and human exposure to cercaria-infected bodies of water. Furthermore, the epidemiology of schistosomiasis is complex because of the existence of several stages of the life cycle of the parasite and the multitude of factors affecting each. Since adult schistosomes, like many parasitic

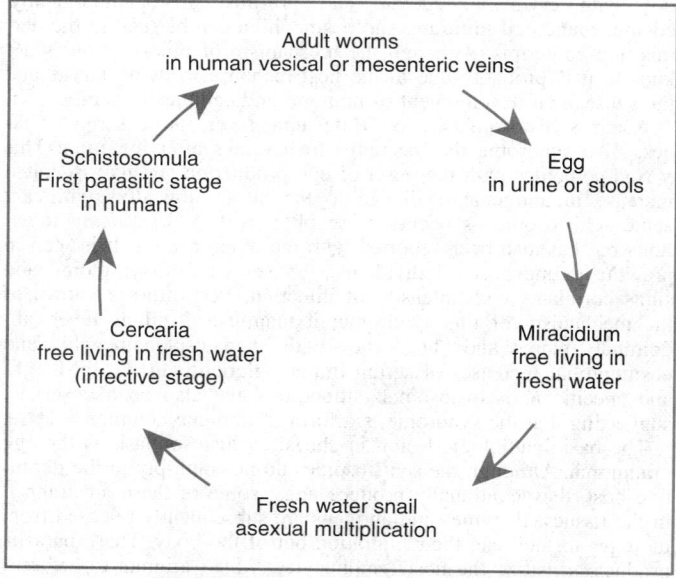

FIGURE 385–1. Schistosome life cycle.

worms, do not multiply in the human body, a close correlation exists between worm load and fecal or urinary egg counts; estimates of intensity of infection can therefore be obtained by ova-enumerating procedures. Quantifying worm loads is important epidemiologically as well as for the individual patient, as it determines the potential of participation in transmission of schistosomiasis and predicts, to a large extent, the risk of morbidity and pathologic outcome.

In endemic areas, schistosomiasis prevalence and intensity show characteristic association with age. Schistosomiasis is acquired early in childhood; prevalence and intensity gradually increase to a peak in the second decade of life. In older individuals, a modest reduction of prevalence may be seen along with a sharp fall in intensity of infection. The marked drop in intensity in adults may be due to a decrease in their water-related activities. Development of immunity may also explain the age-related decrease in intensity. Intensity of infection in endemic communities shows another characteristic feature: Most infected individuals harbor low worm loads, and only a small proportion acquire heavy infection. The underlying mechanism of this clustering of heavy infection in schistosomiasis is not known but may be due to varying degrees of susceptibility and/or response of humans to the parasites.

In some areas, the endemicity of schistosomiasis may be maintained by animal reservoirs; this is especially the case with *S. japonicum*, which infects dogs and cows. Although both *S. haematobium* and *S. mansoni* can infect primates and rodents, the role of these animals as reservoirs does not seem to be epidemiologically important.

PATHOGENESIS. Schistosomiasis is initiated by cercarial penetration of skin; inside the host three maturational forms of the parasite evolve: schistosomula, adults, and eggs. These stages are associated with morphologic, biochemical, and antigenic changes of the worm, which add to the complexity of the host-parasite relationship. Disease caused by schistosomiasis occurs mainly in those with high eggs counts. This relationship, however, is not exact, as the roles of other factors such as genetic background and immunologic modulatory mechanisms are now being elucidated.

Three distinct disease syndromes caused by schistosomiasis have been described; each corresponds roughly to a stage in the parasite development in the host. Cercarial dermatitis, or swimmer's itch, may be seen in infections with human schistosomes but is more common when avian or other nonhuman cercariae penetrate the skin. Swimmer's itch caused by nonhuman schistosomes is commonly seen in the north-central United States, where some lakes are infected. The condition has also been reported in subjects exposed to *S. mansoni* or *S. haematobium* but rarely after exposure to *S. japonicum*. Primary exposure to these larvae results in either no reaction or immediate pruritic macular rash. On repeated exposures, sensitization occurs, and a more pronounced papular eruption develops with erythema, edema, and pruritus. Histopathologically, edema, round cell infiltrate, and eosinophilia can be seen in the dermis and epidermis. Although the mechanism of this reaction is not known, it is probably due to the host response to dying larvae and the subsequent development of humoral and cellular immunity.

Acute schistosomiasis, or Katayama fever, is a serum sickness–like syndrome that occurs 3 to 9 weeks after infection. This period coincides with the onset of egg production and its associated increase in antigenic challenge to the host. Clinically significant acute schistosomiasis occurs more often with *S. japonicum* infections but has also been reported with the other species. It is seen in previously unexposed individuals; the severity of symptoms and signs correlates with intensity of infection. Very little is known of the mechanism of this syndrome; it manifests itself as fever, abdominal pain, and headache with hepatosplenomegaly and eosinophilia. Increases of serum immunoglobulin (Ig) G, IgM, IgE, and specific antischistosomal antibodies have also been observed, suggesting that the syndrome is a form of immune complex disease.

The basic pathologic lesion in chronic schistosomiasis is the egg granuloma. Although the schistosomes do not multiply in the definitive host, they continually produce eggs; some of these are trapped in the tissues. Enzymes and antigens are subsequently released from the eggs to facilitate their migration out of the body. These parasite products sensitize the host lymphocytes, which migrate to areas of egg deposition and recruit other cells, and a compact cellular infiltrate "granuloma" is formed. Several cell types are prominent in the schistosome egg granuloma: lymphocytes, macrophages, eosinophils, and fibroblasts. The size of these granulomas and the resulting fibrosis lead to most of the chronic fibro-obstructive lesions in schistosomiasis. In *S. haematobium* infection, granulomas at the lower end of the ureters impede urine flow and cause hydroureter and hydronephrosis. In infections with other schistosome species, granulomas in the intestinal wall are associated with the abdominal manifestations of the disease, and those in the liver result in presinusoidal obstruction of portal blood flow, portal hypertension, splenomegaly, and esophageal varices. Less commonly, eggs may be carried to almost any organ or tissue in the body, eliciting granuloma formation and its pathologic sequelae. The size of the granulomatous response represents a delicate balance between sensitizing and modulating mechanisms. In chronic schistosomiasis, granulomas spontaneously modulate—i.e., their size decreases significantly—and may result in slowing the progression of disease manifestations. Modulation has been shown to be mediated by several arms of the host's immune system, including serum antibodies, anti-idiotypic antibodies, immune complexes, suppressor lymphocytes, and macrophages. Functionally, granulomas serve to destroy the parasite eggs.

The immune response of individuals with schistosomiasis includes humoral as well as cellular components. The degree and extent of these responses provide the balance between asymptomatic infection and disease manifestations. Furthermore, mechanisms that control the host immune response, such as genetic background, have been demonstrated to influence the extent of granuloma formation and consequently disease. The host immune response to schistosome antigens also is inversely related to intensity of infection; impaired responses are seen only in those with heavy worm loads. Whether the defect in immunity is a cause or consequence of infection is not yet clear. Another aspect of the host's immune response in schistosomiasis relates to the development of peripheral blood as well as tissue eosinophilia. Schistosomiasis, similar to other worm infections with tissue phases, results in a significant increase in eosinophils, especially during the acute phase of infection. Later, in the chronic stage, the eosinophil count may not be significantly elevated. Eosinophils are seen in subcutaneous tissues around the entry points of cercariae, and they constitute approximately 50% of the cells in egg granulomas. Eosinophils have been shown to play a central role in host defenses against the invading stage of the parasite (schistosomula) and the phase (ova) retained in the tissues.

MANAGEMENT. Diagnosis of schistosomiasis must be based on the clinical presentation, positive geographic history, and finding the parasite eggs in the excreta or biopsy material. Quantification of infection and assessment of viability of the eggs are important procedures not only for planning therapy but also for prognostic evaluation. For physicians practicing in nonendemic areas, e.g., North America, most infected individuals have the early acute and nonspecific features of the infection. Eosinophilia and serologic evidence of exposure to schistosome infection are two particularly helpful laboratory findings. Appropriate management of individuals with schistosomiasis must take into consideration the extent of disease and intensity of infection. Antischistosomal therapy, if given early during the course of disease, may lead to reversal of pathologic lesions. In late cases, chemotherapeutic measures may be useful only in preventing further damage from the presence of the parasite.

CONTROL. The intimate relationship between humans and bodies of fresh water in their environment leads to schistosomiasis endemicity. In addition, the lack of precise knowledge of the epidemiology of infection and disease has hampered efforts to control it. Several developments, such as single-dose oral chemotherapeutic agents and better appreciation of transmission dynamics, have led to a clearer definition of strategies for control of schistosomiasis. Ideally, eradication of infection should be the target, but this is impossible to achieve with the currently available tools and the economic and social structure of the endemic areas. Research toward antischistosome vaccine is progressing, but its practical use lies in the future. A more realistic approach is based on control of disease and reduction of transmission. The measure currently advocated is targeted chemotherapy, combined with focal eradication of the organism if needed. In addition, health education, attempts at raising socioeconomic standards, providing privies, and abandoning obsolete agricultural practices offer means for achieving progress in containing this infection.

Those traveling to endemic areas should be given proper advice. There are virtually no safe fresh water bodies in most of the areas endemic for schistosomiasis. Avoiding contact with these water sources is strongly recommended.

SCHISTOSOMIASIS HAEMATOBIA (Urinary Bilharziasis)

S. haematobium infection is endemic in Africa and some parts of the Middle East; it is highly prevalent in the Nile Valley and extends along the Mediterranean coast of the continent. In West Africa it is more widely disseminated than *S. mansoni;* its distribution in East and South Africa is patchy. In Southwest Asia the endemic area includes most countries of the Middle East and Arabian peninsula. Clinically, infection with *S. haematobium* is the most significant of the human schistosome infections because symptoms such as hematuria and dysuria occur early and affect approximately two thirds of infected individuals. In endemic areas, extensive hydroureters and hydronephrosis can be demonstrated in a considerable proportion of infected children; the natural history of these lesions and the course of disease in adults have not been clearly defined.

Adult male *S. haematobium* worms are distinguished by their finely tuberculate surface and by the presence of four to five large testes. The ovaries are found in the posterior half of the female body and contain 20 to 30 eggs (Table 385–1). The main intermediate hosts of *S. haematobium* in North Africa and the Middle East are fresh water snails of the genus *Bulinus;* in Africa south of the Sahara they belong to the subgenus *Physopsis.*

PATHOLOGY AND CLINICAL MANIFESTATIONS. In the urinary bladder, the formation of egg granulomas leads to hyperemia, tubercles, ulcers, and polyps; as healing proceeds, sandy patches and scarring may be seen. Obstructive uropathy is the main functional disturbance caused by schistosomiasis haematobia. Other urinary tract disorders, such as bacteriuria, calculi, and bladder cancer, have been epidemiologically associated with *S. haematobium* infection. Ova of *S. haematobium* have occasionally been found in the lungs with subsequent focal pulmonary arteritis and diffuse hypertensive arteriolar changes; chronic cor pulmonale may occur in these patients.

Swimmer's itch and acute schistosomiasis have rarely been described in *S. haematobium* infection. By contrast, symptoms related to the urinary tract, including dysuria, hematuria, or frequency, occur in a large proportion of infected individuals. Hematuria is characteristically terminal, but with extensive ulceration the whole stream of urine may be bloody, along with passage of clots. In late cases, symptoms related to secondary infection of the urinary tract, severe obstructive uropathy, or neoplasia may appear. Urine examination reveals proteinuria and hematuria; both signs are closely related to intensity of infection. An association between *S. haematobium* infection and bacteremia, mainly caused by *Salmonella* organisms, has been reported. Renal function may be compromised in patients with obstructive uropathy. Cytoscopic examination shows some degree of pathology in almost all infected individuals, the most common being hyperemia near the ureteral openings and the bladder trigone. Sandy patches, tubercles, ulcers, and polyps may also be seen. Imaging studies show bladder calcification in approximately 50 to 80% of infected individuals. Other pathologic lesions are also frequently seen in 40 to 60% of patients, including obstructive uropathy, hydroureters, hydronephrosis, and filling defects in the bladder and ureters.

DIAGNOSIS. Urine examination for *S. haematobium* eggs can be performed by direct or concentration methods (Table 385–1). Once *S. haematobium* infection is diagnosed, urinary tract pathology should be assessed by ultrasonography. In addition, care must be taken in some endemic areas for early detection of bladder cancer by appropriate cytologic and histologic examinations.

TREATMENT. See Management of Schistosomiasis, below.

SCHISTOSOMIASIS MANSONI (Intestinal or Hepatosplenic Bilharziasis)

Infection with *S. mansoni* is endemic in Africa, the Middle East, South America, and some Caribbean islands. The distribution of schistosomiasis mansoni in Africa overlaps with that of schistosomiasis haematobia. In Southwest Asia, it occurs in Yemen and Saudi Arabia. *S. mansoni* is sporadically distributed all over the northern part of South America and is endemic in several Caribbean countries and islands and in many parts of Puerto Rico.

Adult male *S. mansoni* worms have a grossly tuberculate surface and usually contain seven small testes. In the female, the ovary occupies the anterior half of its body, with a short uterus containing one to four ova (Table 385–1). The intermediate snail hosts of *S. mansoni* are species of the genus *Biomphalaria* in Africa and *Australorbis tropicorbis* in the Americas.

PATHOLOGY AND CLINICAL MANIFESTATIONS. Acute schistosomiasis mansoni is the most common early presentation encountered by physicians in North America. Symptoms appear between 3 and 7 weeks after exposure and include fever, anorexia, abdominal pain, and headache. Less often, diarrhea, nausea, and

TABLE 385–1. DIAGNOSIS OF SCHISTOSOMIASIS

Schistosome	Eggs	Diagnosis
S. haematobium	Mainly found in urine but may be found in stools or rectal biopsy Eggs: 143 × 50 μm; spindle shaped: rounded anterior, conical posterior, tapering to a terminal delicate spine	Obtain urine sample at midday (when eggs are excreted); more than one sample may be needed Examine urine directly or by filtering 10 ml urine through Nuclepore membrane Rectal biopsy in suspected cases with normal urine Serologic testing to diagnose early or light infection
S. mansoni	Eggs: 155 × 66 μm; oval with lateral, long spine	Examine stool for eggs Use Kato thick smear method for quantification purposes Rectal biopsy or serologic testing to diagnose stool-negative cases, particularly in lightly infected patients
S. japonicum	Found in stool; eggs: 89 × 67 μm; oval or rounded with lateral, short, sometimes curved spine	Examine stool for eggs Kato thick smear (for quantitative assessment) Rectal biopsy for those with light infections, especially with less common manifestation (i.e., cerebral schistosomiasis)
S. mekongi	Found in stool; eggs: 60 × 32 μm; smaller than eggs of *S. japonicum*	Examine stool for eggs
S. intercalatum	Found in stool; eggs: 180 × 65 μm; terminal spine	Examine stool for eggs

vomiting may occur. Hepatosplenomegaly, eosinophilia, and increased serum immunoglobulins are the main clinical signs. Most of these manifestations correlate significantly with intensity of infection as evaluated by stool egg counts.

Schistosoma mansoni eggs are primarily deposited in the small veins around the large intestine; some of the eggs may be trapped in the gut wall or break loose into the portal circulation to be carried to the small intrahepatic portal venules. On examination, the intestinal mucosa appears red and granular with pinpoint elevations surrounded by hyperemic zones. There may be minute hemorrhages and ulcerations. Sessile and pedunculated polyps, mainly in the rectosigmoid area, have been reported in Egyptians infected with *S. mansoni*, but not in persons from other endemic areas. Pathologic examination of the liver in lightly infected individuals shows schistosome eggs with and without granulomas and mild portal inflammation. In advanced cases, the typical picture of Symmers' fibrosis is seen; the eggs are concentrated in and around large portal tracts with marked fibrosis and obstructive portal venous lesions. The lobular arrangement of liver parenchyma and its function are usually maintained. However, these structural changes lead to marked alteration of hepatic hemodynamics, such as obstruction of portal blood flow through the liver and increase in number and size of intrahepatic arterial branches, thus shifting the blood flow through the liver from mainly portal to arterial sources. Portal hypertension leads to congestive splenomegaly and formation of portosystemic venous shunts at the lower end of the esophagus and other sites. In these patients, schistosome eggs may find their way to the pulmonary circulation, bypassing the obstructed portal blood flow. In the lungs, granulomas form around the trapped eggs, leading to arteriolar fibrosis and pulmonary hypertension.

Nervous system involvement in schistosomiasis mansoni is rare; the main clinical presentation, as in schistosomiasis haematobia, is transverse myelitis. The preferential involvement of the spinal cord may be due to the anatomic location of adult worms. The underlying pathologic lesions are usually granulomas forming around eggs in the spinal cord.

Infection with *S. mansoni* does not have characteristic or specific symptomatology. Early symptoms are those of acute schistosomiasis and are all nonspecific. These include fever, weakness, headache, and abdominal pain. This is particularly the case in travelers who are accidentally exposed to infection in endemic areas. In chronic schistosomiasis mansoni, infected individuals have a slightly higher incidence of crampy abdominal pain (21 to 48%) and bloody diarrhea (4 to 28%) than do matched uninfected controls from the same endemic area. Other frequently mentioned nonspecific symptoms, such as weakness, inability to work, or diarrhea, have not been convincingly demonstrated in any controlled studies. Significant enlargement of the liver is seen in 4 to 11% of infected subjects, and splenomegaly occurs in 3 to 7%. Patients with schistosomal hepatosplenomegaly have a unique form of liver disease. The pathophysiologic changes are based on alteration of hemodynamics, fibrosis of large portal tracts, and very little derangement of liver function. Enlargement of the liver usually occurs in the left lobe, but later, in the course of infection and particularly in adults, uniform hepatomegaly may be seen. Ultrasonographic examination of the liver shows evidence of specific patterns of fibrosis, which distinguishes this syndrome from other causes of hepatomegaly. Simultaneously, gross enlargement of the spleen may occur; the organ is characteristically rubbery hard. Laboratory examination may show indications of anemia and a low degree of eosinophilia but little changes in liver function are seen until late in the course of disease. Total serum proteins are usually normal, but gamma globulin increases are common. An association between schistosomal hepatosplenomegaly and hepatitis B antigen and antibody presence has been described, but its pathophysiologic significance is not clear. Although hepatosplenomegaly usually occurs in heavily infected individuals, other underlying mechanisms may be involved. An association between human leukocyte antigen (HLA) haplotypes and schistosomal hepatosplenomegaly has been demonstrated. In patients with pure schistosomal fibrosis uncomplicated by cirrhosis or viral hepatitis, liver function is preserved for a long time. The presenting feature often is an episode of hematemesis caused by rupture of esophageal varices without prior complaints. Bleeding may recur several times while the liver parenchyma maintains its normal

functions. Finally, however, symptoms and signs of liver cell failure ensue, along with the development of stigmas of chronic liver disease and ascites.

Several less-defined clinical syndromes have been associated with schistosomiasis mansoni. In infected laboratory animals as well as in individuals with chronic schistosomiasis mansoni, antigen-antibody complexes have formed and deposited in the kidney glomeruli. However, the prevalence of this syndrome and the rate at which it occurs in schistosomiasis are unknown. Cor pulmonale in schistosomiasis is a better defined disease entity, although its incidence is not known. It usually occurs in patients with advanced hepatosplenic schistosomiasis mansoni or japonica because of the development of collateral circulation. In *S. haematobium*–infected individuals, the anatomic location of adult worms may help eggs reach the systemic circulation directly and become trapped in the pulmonary arterioles. Patients with schistosomal pulmonary hypertension present clinically with symptoms and signs similar to those in cor pulmonale of other causes. Aneurysmal dilatation of the pulmonary artery and its branches, along with right ventricular hypertrophy, may occur.

DIAGNOSIS. See Table 385–1.

TREATMENT. See Management of Schistosomiasis, below.

SCHISTOSOMIASIS JAPONICA

On the main Asian continent, schistosomiasis japonica is prevalent in some parts of China, Thailand, Laos, Cambodia, and Malaysia. It is also endemic in the Philippines and Celebes. This schistosome species characteristically infects humans and domestic animals such as cats, dogs, and cattle, thus providing reservoir hosts that may contribute to its endemicity in certain areas of the Far East. The intermediate hosts for *S. japonicum* are snails of the genus *Onchomelania*.

Adult *S. japonicum* male worms have a nontuberculate surface and seven medium-sized testes. The ovary occupies the middle part of the body of female worms and contains 50 to 100 ova (Table 385–1).

PATHOLOGY AND CLINICAL MANIFESTATIONS. Cercarial dermatitis is not a prominent feature of schistosomiasis japonica. Katayama fever, or acute schistosomiasis, was named after the district in Japan previously endemic for *S. japonicum* infection. Symptoms usually begin 5 to 7 weeks after infection and are similar to those associated with schistosomiasis mansoni. The clinical features usually subside in a few days but may last for several months, and fatalities have been reported. The chronic manifestations of schistosomiasis japonica are related to ova deposited in the intestines and liver; adult worms produce 10 times more eggs than those of *S. mansoni*. These ova are laid in aggregates and remain so in the intestinal wall or when carried to the liver by the portal blood flow. In addition, *S. japonicum* eggs differ from those of *S. mansoni* in their tendency to calcify in tissues. Schistosomiasis japonica granulomas vary in size tremendously and tend to show signs of necrosis.

Individuals with chronic schistosomiasis japonica may have no symptoms or several nonspecific complaints. Controlled surveys in endemic areas have shown no particular increase in complaints of weakness, abdominal pain, or diarrhea in infected individuals. Clinical signs of hepatosplenomegaly are more frequently seen in infected than in uninfected individuals, but they were not uniformly correlated with intensity of infection. Severe hepatosplenic disease caused by schistosomiasis japonica may be seen in endemic areas, but its prevalence and relationship to intensity of infection and other complicating factors are unknown.

Cerebral schistosomiasis japonica is a unique syndrome reportedly occurring in 2 to 4% of infected individuals in the endemic countries. *S. japonicum* infection of the central nervous system preferentially affects the brain. The lesions consist of large aggregates of eggs in the cerebral venous system, but adult worms have never been found in the brain. Cerebral schistosomiasis japonica occurs clinically early in the course of the infection; the most frequent manifestation is focal jacksonian epilepsy; less commonly, generalized encephalitis may be the presenting feature.

DIAGNOSIS. See Table 385–1.

TREATMENT. See Management of Schistosomiasis, below.

OTHER HUMAN SCHISTOSOMES

Endemic foci for *S. intercalatum* are found in Central and West Africa. Adult worms inhabit the mesenteric blood vessels, and terminal spine eggs are seen in stools of infected individuals. Symptoms usually ascribed to this species of schistosome include abdominal pain, diarrhea, and blood in stools. Diagnosis is based on positive geographic history and finding parasite ova upon fecal examination (see Table 385–1).

S. mekongi is the most recent schistosome species to be described as a cause of infection and disease in humans. The parasite is endemic in some parts of the mainland of Southeast Asia. Adult worm and eggs are similar to those of *S. japonicum;* ova of *S. mekongi* are, however, smaller. In symptomatic patients, a syndrome not unlike that due to *S. japonicum* has been observed. It includes abdominal pain, diarrhea, and heptosplenomegaly. Diagnosis is established by fecal examination for parasite ova (see Table 385–1).

MANAGEMENT OF SCHISTOSOMIASIS

Chemotherapy is the major antischistosome strategy for eradication of parasites in infected individuals and for reducing incidence, intensity, and morbidity in populations of endemic areas. The current drug of choice is praziquantel, a pyrazinoisoquinoline derivative that is effective against all species of schistosomes that infect humans. Praziquantel has several advantages as the chemotherapeutic agent of choice, including oral administration, low incidence of toxicity and side effects, and marked antiparasitic activity. The recommended dose of praziquantel for treatment of infections with *S. haematobium, S. intercalatum,* or *S. mansoni* is 40 mg per kilogram of body weight administered once. For *S. japonicum* infection, administration of 30 mg per kilogram twice in 1 day is recommended, and for *S. mekongi,* 20 mg per kilogram three times in 1 day. These dosages have been shown to result in parasitologic cure in approximately 80% of treated individuals and in a highly significant reduction of intensity of infection. Side effects of praziquantel are rare, usually mild, and self-limiting. These include abdominal pain, headache, dizziness, and skin rashes.

The effect of antischistosome chemotherapeutic agents on disease manifestations is variable. It is dependent on the duration of infection and extent of disease. Treatment is expected to result in reversal of pathology, e.g., hematuria and hepatosplenomegaly, in infected children. By contrast, adults with established fibro-obstructive disease in the liver and urinary tract may not show significant clinical improvement following chemotherapy. Other therapeutic or surgical methods may therefore be necessary to correct the anatomic lesions. Furthermore, medical management of the chronic sequelae of schistosomiasis, such as liver fibrosis, portal hypertension, and esophageal varices, should be conducted according to established practices and taking into consideration the unique pathophysiologic characteristics of disease due to schistosomiasis.

Abdel-Salam E, Abdel Khalik A, Abdel-Meguid A, et al.: Association of HLA class I antigens (A1, B5, B8, and CW2) with disease manifestations and infection in human schistosomiasis mansoni in Egypt. Tissue Antigens 27:142, 1986. *A large-scale, population-based study of association between certain HLA haplotypes and hepatosplenomegaly due to schistosomiasis mansoni.*

Hofstetter M, Nash TE, Cheever AW, et al.: Infection with *Schistosoma mekongi* in Southeast Asian refugees. J Infect Dis 144:420, 1981. *Description of clinical and parasitologic features of schistosomiasis mekongi.*

King CH, Lombardi G, Lombardi C, et al.: Chemotherapy based-control of schistosomiasis haematobia. II. Metrifonate vs. praziquantelin control of infection associated morbidity. Am J Trop Med Hyg 42:587, 1990. *Presents data on long-term effects of metrifonate and praziquantel on the clinical and ultrasonographic manifestations of* S. haematobium *infection in school-aged children.*

Lukas NW, Boros DL: Lymphokine regulation of granuloma formation in murine schistosomiasis mansoni. Clin Immunol Immunopath 68:57, 1993. *Up-to-date review of the regulatory immunologic mechanisms in schistosome granulomas.*

Mahmoud AAF: Strategies for vaccine development: Schistosomiasis. Ann NY Acad Sci 589:136, 1989. *Summary of available protective monoclonal antibodies and purified schistosome antigens with promise as vaccines.*

Mahmoud AAF, Abdel Wahab MF: Schistosomiasis. *In* Warren KS, Mahmoud AAF (eds.): Tropical and Geographical Medicine, 2nd ed. New York, McGraw-Hill, 1990, pp. 458–473. *Detailed description of the parasitologic, immunologic, molecular, and clinical aspects of infection and disease.*

Mott KE, Dixon H, Osei-Tutu E, et al.: Relation between intensity of *Schistosoma haematobium* infection and clinical hematuria and proteinuria. Lancet 1:1005, 1983. *Correlation of proteinuria and hematuria with counts of* S. haematobium *eggs in urine.*

World Health Organization: The Control of Schistosomiasis. Technical Report Series 728, pp. 1–86. World Health Organization, Geneva, Switzerland, 1993. *Up-to-date examination of the epidemiology, morbidity, and methods of control of schistosomiasis. Also includes summary of control programs in endemic areas and outline for strategy of morbidity control.*

386 LIVER, INTESTINAL, AND LUNG FLUKE INFECTIONS
Adel A.F. Mahmoud

Flukes are parasitic worms of the phylum Platyhelminthes. These organisms are dorsoventrally flattened and are typically bilaterally symmetric. With the exception of the schistosomes, all flat worms of clinical significance are hermaphroditic. Morphologically the body of adult worms is leaf shaped and possesses two prominent suckers, one located anteriorly and the other ventrally. These are attachment organs that help anchor adult worms in their habitat within the organs of the definitive host. During the typical life cycle of a flat worm, the organism utilizes two, three, or more hosts; one is the definitive host and the others are intermediate hosts. The parasite undergoes developmental and multiplicative cycles within these hosts, the exception being sexual reproduction, which occurs only in the adult stage of the parasite, usually within the definitive host. All adult parasitic trematodes are obligate parasites. They challenge the protective mechanisms of the definitive hosts because of their size, complex anatomic and antigenic structure, and remarkable abilities to evade expulsion. Clinically relevant flukes are usually grouped according to the main location of adult worms in the definitive host.

Approximately 50 million individuals are infected worldwide; the liver flukes *Clonorchis sinensis, Opisthorchis felineus,* and *O. viverrini* are the most prevalent. Liver, intestinal, and lung flukes are similar morphologically, but vary in size from 1 mm to 7 cm. The pattern of life cycle of these flukes is similar. Eggs are passed in the feces or sputum of infected individuals. These ova are usually oval with an operculum and vary in size by species. Eggs hatch in the aquatic outside environment, releasing miracidia that seek specific snail intermediate hosts where they undergo several asexual multiplication steps, resulting finally in the release of cercariae. This stage is free living but of limited lifespan; it has to encyst on vegetation or in the tissues of fish or crabs where it changes into the metacercarial stage, which is infective to humans. Human acquisition of infection depends on ingestion of metacercaria in raw or improperly cooked aquatic plants or animals. Diagnosis of a specific tissue fluke is a significant clinical challenge: Knowing the geographic distribution of infection, the specific symptoms and signs, and the proper identification of eggs in feces or sputum samples is a necessary step. Recently the specificity and sensitivity of serologic tests have progressed to being helpful in diagnosis with a certain degree of confidence. The most important parasitologic, clinical, and diagnostic features of liver, intestinal, and lung flukes are summarized in Table 386–1.

LIVER FLUKES

Several species of liver flukes are capable of inducing significant morbidity and mortality in humans. Opisthorchiasis and clonorchiasis are the most common of these infections.

Opisthorchiasis

Human infection is caused by *O. viverrini* or *O. felineus,* parasitic flukes of cats, dogs, and other fish-eating mammals. Human infection is acquired by ingestion of metacercariae found in the second intermediate host (cyprinoid fish, carp). The metacercariae excyst in the duodenum and migrate through the ampulla of Vater to reach their final habitat in the bile ducts. The incidence of *O. viverrini* in northeastern Thailand (Table 386–2) has recently been increasing, reaching 90% of the population in specific foci.

PATHOGENESIS AND CLINICAL FEATURES. Adult flukes inhabit the distal bile ducts and may occasionally be seen in the gallbladder. The majority of infected individuals are asymptomatic. Lesions have been demonstrated in the biliary system, varying from hyperplasia of ductal epithelium to obstruction and bile retention. There is significant correlation between intensity of infection and severity of observed lesions. The association of *O. viverrini* and

TABLE 386–1. MAJOR LIVER, INTESTINAL, AND LUNG FLUKE INFECTIONS IN HUMANS

Infection	Causative Organisms	Second Intermediate Host	Size of Adult Fluke (mm)	Final Habitat in Humans	Size of Eggs (μm)
Opisthorchiasis	O. viverrini O. felineus	Cyprinoid fish	5–10 × 1–2	Distal bile ducts, gallbladder	28 × 16 Operculated
Clonorchiasis	C. sinensis	Carp fish	10–24 × 3–5	Bile and pancreatic ducts	29 × 16 Operculated
Fascioliasis	F. hepatica F. gigantica	Aquatic vegetation or water	20–30 × 13 75 × 20	Large biliary ducts	140 × 75 Inconspicuous operculum 175 × 80
Fasciolopsiasis	F. buski	Aquatic plants	50–75 × 8–20	Small intestine	135 × 35 Small operculum
Paragonimiasis	P. westermani	Fresh and brackish water crabs	7–16 × 4–8	Lungs, brain, or abdominal organs	100 × 60 Operculated

cholangiocarcinoma, known for many years, has recently been examined by the International Agency for Research on Cancer. The consensus is that enough evidence exists to classify *O. viverrini* as a human carcinogen.

Most infected individuals are asymptomatic; infection is diagnosed when the characteristic eggs are found during routine fecal examination. Since very few controlled studies have been performed on infected and uninfected populations of endemic areas, the specificity of symptoms and signs is questionable. Symptomatic infections are associated with right upper quadrant discomfort, dyspepsia, and change in bowel habits. Generalized symptoms such as decrease of appetite and weight loss have also been observed. In severe cases, relapsing cholangitis and cholecystitis may occur. An association between *O. viverrini* and cholangiocarcinoma, gallstones, and obstructive jaundice has been reported. Liver enlargement is demonstrated in most symptomatic individuals along with imaging evidence for biliary tree disease.

Infection with *O. felineus* has a characteristic clinical course. In its acute phase (2 to 3 weeks after infection), the clinical features include irregular fever, lymphadenopathy, myalgia, and eosinophilia. In chronic infections, symptoms and signs of biliary disease resemble those of *O. viverrini* infection; however, the worms may also be found in the pancreatic duct, causing manifestations related to this organ.

Clonorchiasis

C. sinensis is also frequently referred to as the Chinese or oriental liver fluke. Carnivorous animals such as dogs, cats, and rats are probably the reservoir hosts in nature. Human infection is acquired by ingestion of the second intermediate host, a fresh water carp of the family Cyprinidae. In endemic areas (Table 386–2), many species of this family have been found to be parasitized with *C. sinensis* metacercariae. Clonorchiasis is also seen in many coun-

TABLE 386–2. GEOGRAPHIC DISTRIBUTION OF FLUKES

Fluke	Distribution
Liver	
Opisthorchis viverrini	Thailand, Laos, Cambodia
O. felineus	Russia, Eastern and Central Europe
Clonorchis sinesis	China, Japan, Korea, Taiwan, Vietnam Hong Kong (imported fish from China)
Fasciola hepatica	United States, Europe, Africa, Asia
F. gigantica	less common; Africa, Asia, Hawaii
Dicrocoelium sp.	Europe, Africa, Asia, North America
Intestinal	
Fasciolopsis sp.	Taiwan, Thailand, Bangladesh, India, plus other Asian and Western countries
Echinostoma sp.	Indonesia, Philippines, Thailand, Taiwan
Heterophyes heterophyes	Egypt, Iran, the Far East, Southeast Asia
Metagonimus yokogawai	China, Japan, Korea, Taiwan
Gastrodiscoides hominis	India, Southeast Asia, Russia
Lung	
Paragonimus sp.	Asia, West Africa, Central and South America

tries, including the United States among immigrants from endemic areas. Importation of *C. sinensis* is a risk in the international food trade.

PATHOGENESIS AND CLINICAL FEATURES. The life cycle, pathology, and clinical manifestations of clonorchiasis are similar to those of opisthorchiasis. Adult flukes reside in the medium-sized and small bile ducts. They may also be found in the gallbladder, common bile duct, and the pancreatic duct. In early infection the pathologic features consist of edema and epithelial desquamation in bile ducts associated with an inflammatory response. Later, metaplasia and glandular proliferation occur with dilatation and thickening of bile ducts. The final pathologic insult is related to marked periductal fibrosis. The specificity of symptoms due to clonorchiasis such as anorexia, epigastric pain, or diarrhea has been questioned in studies performed on immigrants to the United States from the Far East. In chronic infection as seen in endemic areas, the association with cholangitis, gallstones, and cholangiocarinoma has been reported repeatedly. Sonography or computed tomography (CT) demonstrates the pathologic changes in the liver: flukes within dilated bile ducts and periductal changes.

Fascioliasis

Human infection with the zoonotic flukes *Fasciola hepatica* and *F. gigantica* is acquired by ingestion of parasitic metacercariae that are attracted to various aquatic plants or through drinking water contaminated with the infective stage of the organisms. The natural hosts of fascioliasis include sheep, goats, cattle, and horses; endemic regions are listed in Table 386–2. Once the infective metacercariae are consumed they excyst in the duodenum, penetrate its wall, and travel via the peritoneal cavity to enter the liver through its capsule. The organisms migrate into the liver parenchyma to reach their final habitat in large bile ducts.

PATHOGENESIS AND CLINICAL FEATURES. Human fascioliasis is usually associated with mild clinical features. The resulting syndromes may conveniently be divided into the *acute migratory phase*, while the organisms are finding their way through the peritoneal cavity to the hepatic liver capsule and parenchyma, and the *established phase*, which is associated with the mature flukes taking residence in the bile ducts. The acute phase is marked with fever, right upper quadrant or epigastric pain, and eosinophilia. The clinical presentation may last 4 to 8 weeks after ingestion of metacercariae and is usually self-limited. It has to be noted that stool examination during this phase is usually negative for parasite eggs. During the established phase, most infected individuals are asymptomatic. Some may complain of abdominal pain and dyspepsia. Hepatomegaly and jaundice may be noted, as well as significant peripheral blood eosinophilia. Borderline changes in liver function tests have also been reported. CT of the liver may help in demonstrating hepatic lesions, including the nodular or the more characteristic linear hypodense tracks, particularly if they are located subcapsularly. In the *biliary stage*, ultrasonography may demonstrate the adult flukes in the bile ducts or gallbladder.

Dicroceliasis

Human infection with *Dicrocoelium dendriticum* or *D. hospes* is rare (Table 386–2). Dicroceliasis is a zoonosis in sheep, goats, deer, and other herbivores. Its life cycle is similar to that of other liver flukes except that metacercariae encyst in ants, the second intermediate host. Humans are infected via eating metacercariae-containing ants. Most cases of dicroceliasis are asymptomatic. In those with heavy infection, vague abdominal complaints—vomiting, diarrhea or constipation, and biliary colic—have been observed.

INTESTINAL FLUKES

Human infection with one of more than 50 species of intestinal trematodes has been reported from the Far East, Middle East, and North Africa. Clinically significant disease may be encountered in infection with only few species, as outlined below.

Fasciolopsiasis

The giant intestinal fluke *Fasciolopsis buski* inhabits the small intestine of pigs. The life cycle of the helminth is similar to that of *Fasciola hepatica*. Humans are infected by ingestion of raw stems, leaves, and pods of aquatic plants with encysted metacercariae. The geographic distribution is listed in Table 386–2. Endemicity depends on close contact among water plants, pigs, and populations that consume raw acquatic plants.

F. buski attach to the mucosa of small intestine, particularly the duodenum and jejunum. Most infected individuals are asymptomatic. The site of attachment, however, becomes ulcerated, following which there is a local inflammatory response. In heavy infection, intestinal obstruction and protein-losing enteropathy have been reported. With heavy infection, abdominal pain and diarrhea may be observed along with edema and anasarca because of hypoalbuminemia.

Echinostomiasis

Humans can be infected with any of several genera of the family Echinostomatidae (Table 386–2). The common species are *Echinostoma ilocanum, E. malayanum,* and *E. revolutum.* Adult flukes are parasites of the small intestine of birds and mammals. Humans are occasionally infected after eating undercooked *Pila,* other fish, and tadpoles. Mature adult worms attach to intestinal mucosa causing ulceration and subsequent inflammatory response. Little morbidity has been reported in association with echinostomiasis. High-intensity infection may be associated with abdominal pain and diarrhea.

Heterophyiasis

Heterophyes heterophyes infects not only humans (Table 386–2) but also cats, dogs, and other fish-eating mammals. Infection is acquired by ingestion of the fish second intermediate host, which contains the fluke metacercariae. The common fish hosts include mullet and minnow and the brackish water fish *Mugil capito.* They are usually consumed either raw or salted. Metacercariae can live in salted fish for approximately 1 week. Adult *H. heterophyes* attach to the mucosa of jejunum and upper ileum, producing shallow ulcers and mild inflammatory response. Symptomatic patients complain of gastroenterocolitis with diarrhea and tenesmus. Stools characteristically contain abundant mucus and occasionally blood.

OTHER INTESTINAL FLUKES

Several other species may cause disease limited to defined geographic areas (Table 386–2). *Metagonimus yokogawai* life cycle and the associated disease syndromes are similar to *H. heterophyes* infection, but *M. okogawai* may invade the mucosa of small intestine, resulting in ulceration and granuloma formation. Another intestinal fluke, *Gastrodiscoides hominis* (Table 386–2), has its final habitat in humans in the cecum. Clinically it is believed to produce mucous diarrhea.

Lung Flukes: "Paragonimiasis"

Human infection by species of *Paragonimus* may cause considerable pulmonary or extrapulmonary morbidity. *Paragonimus* infection exists in nature in humans and carnivores. There are at least 10 species of *Paragonimus* known to cause human disease; of these *P. westermani* is most common (Table 386–2). Infection is acquired by ingestion of metacercariae encysted in fresh water and brackish water crabs or crayfish (raw or undercooked). Infection may also be transmitted to humans through contaminated utensils used to prepare crabs or crayfish. Rarely, consumption of wild boar meat may result in transmission of immature flukes to humans where they complete their development into adult worms.

PATHOGENESIS AND CLINICAL FEATURES. Disease in infected humans is related to migration of young flukes from the gastrointestinal tract to their final habitat (early or acute stage) and more characteristically results from adult worms becoming established in the lungs or at extrapulmonary sites (late or chronic stage).

Acute paragonimiasis occurs during the 3-week period following infection. It passes unnoticed in most infected individuals. Symptoms include diarrhea, abdominal pain, fever, and malaise associated with cough, dyspnea, and night sweats. Pulmonary paragonimiasis results from invasion of the host lungs and establishment of adult worms in cysts or abscess cavities. The lung parenchyma demonstrates hemorrhage and an inflammatory response of predominantly eosinophils. Worm cysts are 1 to 2 cm in diameter and usually contain one or two worms. Pathologic changes in the remaining lung tissues may result in bronchopneumonia, bronchiectasis, fibrosis, and pleural thickening. The established pulmonary stage of paragonimiasis results usually in mild chronic cough with production of mucoid rusty-brown sputum. Hemoptysis that may be severe and life threatening occurs rarely. Microscopic examination of sputum demonstrates necrotic tissue and parasite eggs. Physical examination of patients with pulmonary paragonimiasis is usually within normal limits. Chest radiography may be normal in 10 to 20% of cases. Typical changes in the lungs include pathway infiltrate and ring shadow with a crescent-shaped "corona." Cystic and nodular lesions are also commonly seen. Furthermore, pleural lesions, including effusion, pneumothorax, and thickening, may be encountered in approximately two thirds of infected individuals. Other imaging methods, e.g., CT, may define better the pulmonary abnormalities, including worm migration tracks.

Extrapulmonary paragonimiasis occurs either because maturing flukes migrate to tissues other than the lungs, or adult flukes migrate from the lungs to other tissues. It is believed that extrapulmonary paragonimiasis may be mainly due to *Paragonimus* flukes other than *P. westermani.* The tissues most commonly affected are the brain, abdominal organs, and skin. In cerebral paragonimiasis, the clinical presentation may be acute or chronic. Acute cerebral paragonimiasis presents as fever, headache, visual disturbances, paralysis, and generalized or focal convulsions. Evidence for an intracranial inflammatory process may be demonstrated as papilledema, high cerebrospinal fluid pressure, and eosinophilic pleocytosis. Chronic cerebral paragonimiasis is characterized by space-occupying lesions that cause epilepsy or paralysis. Abdominal or cutaneous paragonimiasis results from invasion of liver, spleen, or skin by maturing or adult flukes. This results in space-occupying lesions, abscesses, or migratory swellings.

MANAGEMENT OF LIVER, INTESTINAL, AND LUNG FLUKE INFECTIONS

Diagnosis of human infection with liver, intestinal, or lung flukes requires knowledge of the geographic distribution of these infections, a high degree of clinical correlations of mainly nonspecific symptoms and signs with history of possible exposure, and peripheral blood eosinophilia. Definitive diagnosis is established by finding the characteristically shaped fluke eggs in fecal samples (liver, intestinal, and lung worms) or in sputum paragonimiasis. Occasionally eggs are obtained in samples of other tissue fluid, e.g., bile or in biopsy tissue. In general, the sensitivity of fecal or sputum examination is enhanced by examining two or three separate specimens. Seroimmunodiagnostic tests are available for fascioliasis and paragonimiasis. They are particularly helpful in early infection in which parasitologic diagnosis is usually negative. Serodiagnosis is an essential step in the work-up in an unusual clinical presentation.

Chemotherapy for fluke infections has become a more effective management strategy with the introduction of praziquantel. This orally administered 1-day antihelminth results in cure rates of 70 to 90% and an even more remarkable decrease in egg counts. Its administration is associated with few side effects. The recommended dose of praziquantel is 75 mg per kilogram body weight divided into three doses and given in 1 day. For fascioliasis the drug of choice is bithionol given orally as 30 to 50 mg per kilogram every other day for 10 to 15 doses.

Prevention of infection with any of the above parasitic trematodes depends on proper medical advice given to individuals traveling or planning to reside in endemic areas (see Ch. 268). Avoidance of ingestion of suspect intermediate hosts and the proper washing, cooking, or preservation methods of such food items is the most effective strategy. Engaging in some of the local dietary habits in endemic areas is to be discouraged. Water for drinking must be properly purified to avoid the possible transmission of *F. hepatica.* Control of parasitic trematodes in endemic areas is a much more complex challenge. It involves changing long-established cultural, dietary, and sanitary habits. With the availability of a safe broad-spectrum antihelminth (praziquantel), chemotherapy may play a significant role in controlling infection and disease. As a long-term strategy, vaccines and socioeconomic development will be needed.

Drugs for Parasitic Infections: The Medical Letter on Drugs and Therapeutics. 35:111, 1993. *Yearly update of drugs of choice and alternatives.*
Harinasuta T, Bunnag D: Liver, Lung and Intestinal Trematodiasis. *In* Warren KS, Mahmoud AAF (eds.): Tropical and Geographical Medicine, 2nd ed. New York, McGraw-Hill, 1990, pp. 473–489. *An authoritative description of the causing agents, clinical syndromes, and management strategies.*
Im JG, Whang HY, Kim WS, et al.: Pleuropulmonary paragonimiasis: Radiologic findings in 71 patients. AJR 159:39, 1992. *Retrospective evaluation of 71 individuals with evidence of pleuropulmonary paragonimiasis. Report details frequency of specific radiographic and CT findings.*
King CH: Liver, lung and intestinal trematodiasis. *In* Mahmoud AAF (ed.): Tropical and Geographical Medicine, 2nd ed. Companion Handbook. New York, McGraw-Hill, 1993, pp. 149–154. *Summary of the salient clinical features, diagnostic and therapeutic approaches to tissue fluke infection.*
Lim JH: Radiologic findings of clonorchiasis. AJR 155:1001, 1990. *Detailed description of the epidemiology and parasitology of clonorchiasis as well as the sonographic and CT findings based on examining a large group of infected individuals.*

387 NEMATODE INFECTIONS
James W. Kazura

Nematodes (phylum Nematoda), or roundworms, include a vast number of species of free-living and parasitic helminths. These multicellular organisms differ from unicellular bacteria and protozoa in that they have organ systems with specialized nervous, muscular, gastrointestinal, and reproductive functions. Parasitic nematodes vary in length from several millimeters to approximately 2 meters and four larval stages and adult worms of both sexes. With the exception of *Strongyloides* and a few other helminths of medical importance, larvae are produced after mating of sexually mature adult worms, which by themselves are incapable of multiplying in the mammalian host. The inability of adult worms to replicate has important implications for the propensity of this class of organism to establish an infection and cause disease. Unlike the situation pertaining to bacterial, viral, or protozoan infections, casual or a low degree of exposure to infective stages of parasitic helminths generally does not result in patient infection or pathologic manifestations. Repeated or intense exposure to a large number of infective larvae is required for infection to be established and disease to develop.

Nematode infections are endemic in both temperate and tropical climates. They are transmitted either by the fecal-oral route or by inoculation of infective larvae into the skin, primarily by blood-feeding intermediate insect vectors. The prevalence of infection is greatest in circumstances conducive to the development and transmission of infective forms of the parasites, i.e., overcrowded, perennially warm geographic areas with poor sanitation, such as in many developing countries of Africa, Asia, and Latin America and economically poor areas of North America and Europe.

The epidemiology of human nematode (as well as trematode and cestode) infections has several unique features. The infection in an endemic area has a negative binomial distribution; i.e., the majority of individuals have low parasite burdens and a small number harbor relatively high burdens. Persons in the latter group are important from an epidemiologic perspective in that they contribute most substantially to transmission and are most likely to develop pathologic

manifestations. This characteristic implies that transmission in an endemic area may be decreased or interrupted by reduction of the parasite burden in a small proportion of the population. In addition, because total worm load correlates directly with the propensity to develop disease, treatment of lightly infected persons may not be indicated or may be unnecessary, especially if the available chemotherapy has major side effects.

Nematode infections of medical importance may be broadly classified into those in which the route of infection, larval migration, and disease manifestations are primarily gastrointestinal and those that affect other tissues. The former group includes hookworms (*Ancylostoma duodenale, Necator americanus),* the roundworm *Ascaris lumbricoides,* the pinworm *Enterobius vermicularis,* and the whipworm *Trichuris trichiuria.* Animal intestinal nematodes such as *Trichostrongylus* and *Anisakis* species also occasionally infect and cause disease in humans. *Trichinella spiralis, Strongyloides stercoralis,* and *Angiostrongylus cantonensis* infect humans by the oral route, but disease manifestations are due primarily to migration in other tissues. Tissue-invasive nematodes include lymphatic filariae (*Wuchereria bancrofti, Brugia malayi,* and *B. timori),* skin-dwelling *Onchocerca volvulus* and *Loa loa,* and the guinea worm, *Dracunculus medinensis.*

Anderson RM, May RM: Helminthic infections of humans: Mathematical models, population dynamics, and control. Adv Parasitol 24:1, 1985. *An excellent discussion of the relationship of the biology of parasitic helminthic infections to their epidemiology and control strategies.*

INTESTINAL NEMATODES

These infections include hookworm disease, ascariasis, enterobiasis, trichuriasis, and rarely animal nematodiases. They are prevalent in temperate and tropical areas of the world, especially those with overcrowding and poor sanitation. Intestinal nematode infections have little morbidity in most cases and are easily treated with mebendazole.

Hookworm Disease

ETIOLOGY AND EPIDEMIOLOGY. The major hookworms that infect humans are *Ancylostoma duodenale* and *Necator americanus. A. ceylanicum* infection is less common and occurs primarily in the South Pacific. Animal hookworms such as *A. braziliense* and *Uncinaria stenocephala* do not undergo full development in incidentally exposed humans. Infection occurs when exposed skin maintains contact for several minutes with soil contaminated with parasite eggs containing viable larvae. Larvae penetrate the skin and subsequently migrate to and mature in the lungs. The parasites then break into the air spaces, ascend the trachea, and are swallowed. Adult worms mature in the upper small intestine and attach to the mucosa. Female worms release more than 10,000 eggs per day, which are passed in the stools and deposited in the soil. The prepatent period (duration of time between infection and passing of eggs in the feces) is 40 to 105 days. Adult hookworms have a lifespan of 2 to 5 years.

Hookworms infect over 1 billion persons worldwide. The highest prevalences of infection (80 to 100%) occur in tropical and less developed countries, where environmental and socioeconomic conditions are especially favorable to transmission. These include warm, moist soil; lack of public sewage disposal systems; and the habit of walking barefoot. The higher prevalence of hookworm infection in children than adults results from more frequent exposure of skin to larvae in soil. Acquired resistance is minimal or does not appear to develop as a consequence of previous infection.

PATHOGENESIS AND CLINICAL MANIFESTATIONS. Hookworm disease is due primarily to gastrointestinal blood loss and attendant iron deficiency anemia. The latter correlates directly with the total worm burden. Adult worms attached to the mucosa of the upper small intestine digest ingested blood as well as cause focal bleeding. *A. duodenale* is estimated to cause a blood loss of 0.3 ml per day per worm; *N. americanus* induces loss of approximately 0.03 ml per day. Light infections (feces with < 400 eggs per gram) do not cause blood loss sufficient to induce iron deficiency. Nutritional deficiencies secondary to coexisting conditions that result in low iron stores (e.g., malabsorption or insufficient dietary intake in children and multiparous women) contribute significantly to morbidity. Hypoproteinemia has been reported in children with hookworm disease in less developed countries. This complication is most likely due to coexisting malnutrition rather than gastrointestinal disease caused by hookworm infestation *per se*. Abdominal signs or symptoms are not caused by hookworm infection.

Pruritus at the site of larval skin penetration ("ground itch") occurs occasionally. In the case of primary exposure, local itching and erythematous papules lasting 1 week develop. More intense pruritus, vesiculation, and edema of 2 to 3 weeks' duration may occur after repeated exposure to infective larvae. Hookworm larvae migrating through the lungs rarely cause pulmonary symptoms.

DIAGNOSIS. Hookworm infection is diagnosed by identification of the characteristic round eggs containing convoluted larvae. Direct smears of freshly passed stool using the Kato or other techniques are satisfactory for the diagnosis of moderately to heavily infected cases (>400 eggs per gram).

TREATMENT AND PREVENTION. Mebendazole is the treatment of choice (Table 387–1). The ideal method for preventing hookworm infection is improvement of hygienic conditions. Use of footwear, especially by children, is currently the only practical means of avoiding infection.

Ascariasis

ETIOLOGY AND EPIDEMIOLOGY. *Ascaris lumbricoides* are roundworms 2 to 3 cm in length that reside in the lumen of the jejunum and in the mid-ileum. Infection occurs by the oral route when soil containing embryonated eggs is ingested. Larvae are released from eggs in the small intestine, penetrate the gut, and migrate to the liver and then lungs via the blood or lymphatic circulation. Following maturation in the lungs over a 4-week period, the parasites ascend the respiratory tract and are swallowed. Adult worms reach sexual maturity (i.e., female worms release eggs that are detectable in feces) approximately 60 days after infection.

Ascariasis affects approximately one quarter of the world's population and is likely the most prevalent helminthiasis of humans. Infection is common in Africa, Asia, and Latin America, especially in areas of high population density and unhygienic conditions. The use of human feces as fertilizer, defecation in soil, and hand-to-mouth contact with contaminated soil are major factors that contribute to the spread of *Ascaris*. The ability of *Ascaris* eggs to remain viable in harsh environmental conditions (embryonated eggs remain infectious after exposure to freezing temperatures and desiccation for several weeks) also facilitates transmission.

PATHOGENESIS AND CLINICAL MANIFESTATIONS. Disease caused by *A. lumbricoides* is infrequent and generally correlates with the intensity of infection. The majority of infected individuals are asymptomatic.

Symptomatic cases can be divided into two broad categories

based on the phase of infection and site of pathology, i.e., pulmonary or gastrointestinal tract. Pulmonary disease is caused by the migration of larvae in the small vessels of the lung and their subsequent rupture into alveoli. Tissue damage is thought to be due to the host immune response, which includes production of immunoglobulin E (IgE) and eosinophilia. Transient pulmonary infiltrates, fever, cough, dyspnea, and eosinophilia lasting 1 to several weeks are the major clinical manifestations. This complex of symptoms and signs is frequently seasonal and coincidental with environmental changes that favor development of infective-stage larvae in eggs (e.g., spring rains that follow cold and dry periods). Intestinal signs and symptoms are due either to obstruction caused by the presence of an exceptionally large number of parasites in the small intestine or to migration of adult worms to unusual sites, such as the biliary tree or pancreatic duct. Intestinal obstruction almost always occurs in children <6 years old. The onset is sudden and characterized by colicky abdominal pain and vomiting. Heavily infected children are also prone to biliary disease or pancreatitis secondary to *Ascaris* lodging in the ducts draining these organs. A malabsorption syndrome characterized by steatorrhea and low vitamin A levels has been reported in Latin American children with ascariasis.

DIAGNOSIS. Intestinal infection is diagnosed by the presence of the typical oval, thick-shelled *Ascaris* eggs in thick smears of fecal specimens. The existence of adult worms in pancreatic or biliary ducts should be suspected in children who have high egg outputs in conjunction with jaundice or pancreatitis. Pulmonary ascariasis cannot be diagnosed on the basis of identification of ova in feces because adult worms have not yet matured and reached the intestinal tract. Biopsy of the lung is unlikely to demonstrate larvae and is not recommended.

TREATMENT AND PREVENTION. Treatment for uncomplicated intestinal ascariasis is listed in Table 387–1. Treatment causes neuromuscular paralysis of the worms and expulsion of intact helminths. No specific treatment is recommended for pulmonary ascariasis because the condition is self-limited.

The major means of preventing *Ascaris* infection is improvement of hygienic and socioeconomic conditions. Mass chemotherapy successfully reduces worm loads but requires frequent treatment.

Enterobiasis

Enterobius vermicularis or pinworm infection is cosmopolitan in its distribution. It is common in overcrowded settings and spreads rapidly in conditions in which person-to-person contact is frequent, such as in institutions for children.

Infection occurs by the fecal-oral route. Embryonated eggs carried on the fingernails, bed clothing, or bedding are ingested and hatch in the upper small intestine. Larvae develop in the large bowel into adult worms 2 to 5 mm long. Female worms migrate nightly out of the rectum and deposit large numbers of ova (11,000 per worm) in the perianal and perineal areas. Larvae in the deposited eggs become infective within several hours of exposure to ambient oxygen. Infectivity is usually maintained for 1 to 2 days.

The vast majority of pinworm infections are asymptomatic or associated with perianal pruritus and consequent sleep deprivation. *E. vermicularis* is a rare cause of appendicitis and, when the adult worms follow an aberrant path of migration, vulvovaginitis, urethritis, or peritonitis.

The diagnosis of pinworm infection is easily made by identifying ova on a piece of cellophane tape applied to the perirectal area in the morning. *E. vermicularis* eggs are oval and slightly flattened on one side. It is unusual to find eggs in feces or adult worms in the perianal area. Repeated examinations may be necessary.

Treatment (Table 387–1) is mebendazole given to affected individuals as well as close associates, such as family members. Although personal cleanliness is recommended as a means of limiting transmission, there is no clear-cut demonstration that it prevents infection.

Trichuriasis

Trichuris trichiuria or whipworm infection is similar to pinworm infection in that it is limited to the gastrointestinal tract and does not have a tissue migratory phase. Eggs containing infective larvae mature in warm, moist soil over a 2-week period. Ingested eggs

TABLE 387–1. TREATMENT FOR INTESTINAL NEMATODES

Nematode	Treatment
Hookworm	Mebendazole, 100 mg orally b.i.d. for 3 days. Do not give to pregnant women; iron supplementation (if warranted by anemia and complicating illnesses)
Ascaris	Mebendazole, 100 mg orally b.i.d. for 3 days. Children with heavy infections, biliary tract obstruction: piperazine, 50–75 mg/kg body weight for 2 days
Enterobius	Pyrantel pamoate, 11 mg/kg once, with a repeated dose 2 weeks later; maximum single dose, 1 gram. Several treatments may be required (every 3–4 months) if exposure continues (i.e., in institutional setting)
Trichuris	Mebendazole, at same dosage as for ascariasis
Other animal nematodes	
Trichostrongylus	Pyrantel pamoate, 11 mg/kg once; maximum dose of 1 gram
Anisakis	Thiabendazole, 25 mg/kg b.i.d. for 3 days if surgery is not required
Capillaria	Mebendazole, 200 mg b.i.d. for 20 days. Alternative: thiabendazole, 25 mg/kg q.d. for 30 days. Supportive care: replace fluid and electrolytes, high-protein diet
Gnathostoma	For subcutaneous lesions: surgical removal. For CNS infection: mebendazole, 200 mg q3h for 6 days OR albendazole, 400–800 mg q.d. for 21 days

hatch in the small bowel and subsequently develop in epithelial cells of the cecum and ascending colon into adult worms that are 40 mm in length. The body of the parasite protrudes into the colonic lumen. Its anterior portion has a whiplike shape.

As is the case with most intestinal nematode infections, trichuriasis is most common in overcrowded areas with poor sanitation. The estimated prevalence worldwide is 800 million, with approximately 2 million cases in the southern United States. Children are more frequently infected than adults and also more likely to have higher worm burdens.

Adults with trichuriasis are usually asymptomatic. In children with heavy infections (> 10,000 eggs per gram of feces), a syndrome of dysentery, growth retardation, and rectal prolapse has been described. The pathologic manifestations include infiltrates of eosinophils and neutrophils accompanied by epithelial denudation. Complicating diseases such as shigellosis and amebiasis may contribute to this condition in children.

Whipworm infection is diagnosed by identification of football-shaped eggs in direct smears of fecal specimens. Mebendazole at the same dosage indicated for ascariasis is satisfactory treatment is listed in Table 387–1.

Other Animal Nematodiases

Humans may serve as paratenic hosts for several nematodes that ordinarily parasitize the intestine of other mammals. These helminths are incapable of completing their life cycle in humans and display aberrant migration patterns in both intestinal and nonintestinal tissues.

Several species of the genus *Trichostrongylus* infect both humans and domestic ruminants. The infection is found widely in the Middle and Far East and Australia. Ova are passed in the stool of ruminants and hatch in the soil. Humans are incidentally infected when larvae are ingested with leafy vegetables. The adult worms live in the intestines and suck small amounts of blood; heavy infections result in anemia. Diagnosis is made by identifying ova, which resemble those of hookworm, in the stool. Treatment is listed in Table 387–1.

Anisakis is an intestinal nematode of marine mammals. Several species of saltwater fish are intermediate hosts. Human infection occurs when raw fish is eaten. The larvae of both *Anisakis* and *Phocanemia decipiens* have been implicated. Most cases have been reported in Japan or Western Europe, particularly Scandinavia. The larvae invade the wall of the small intestine or stomach, causing pain and, rarely, intestinal obstruction or perforation. Gastric anisakiasis can be diagnosed endoscopically and treated by removal of the worms. Intestinal anisakiasis often resembles an acute abdomen, leading to laparotomy. Thiabendazole treatment is listed in Table 387–1. Infection is prevented by cooking or freezing fish prior to eating.

Capillaria philippinensis infection has been reported from the Philippines and Thailand. This nematode is thought to parasitize birds, with fish and crustaceans serving as intermediate hosts. Humans are infected by eating the raw intermediate hosts. The ingested larvae mature and live in the crypts of the small intestine, where they reproduce. The result is often a heavy infection; up to 40,000 adult worms have been recovered at one autopsy. The clinical syndrome includes severe malabsorption and protein-losing enteropathy. The diagnosis is made by finding eggs or larvae in the stool; an intradermal test is also available. The treatment of choice is mebendazole (Table 387–1).

Gnathostoma spinigerum is an intestinal nematode of dogs and cats; fish are intermediate hosts. The infection is endemic in rodents in the Far East and Thailand. Human infection has also been reported in South America. Infective larvae are ingested by humans in raw or undercooked fish. The larvae do not complete their life cycle in humans but migrate through the body. The most frequent site is subcutaneous tissues, where larvae are found in eosinophilic granulomas. A few weeks after infection, pruritic or painful subcutaneous nodules and swellings appear. These may be migratory and develop into abscesses. In CNS gnathostomiasis, hemorrhagic tracts may be found in the brain. Fever, vomiting, and abdominal pain occur a few days after larvae are ingested. Paralysis of the extremities, encephalitis, and subarachnoid hemorrhage have been reported. Eye

involvement with uveitis and orbital cellulitis represents a third variety.

Peripheral eosinophilia is usual in cutaneous gnathostomiasis; the diagnosis may be established by biopsy. In CNS infection, blood eosinophilia is an inconstant feature, but eosinophils are present in the cerebrospinal fluid (CSF), as in the case of angiostrongyliasis. Treatments are listed in Table 387–1. The infection may be prevented by thorough cooking of fish.

Several nematodes that ordinarily parasitize the intestine of monkeys occasionally infect humans. *Oesophagostomum* has been reported from Africa, Asia, and Brazil; it is responsible for the formation of granulomas in the intestinal wall. *Ternides deminutus* is sometimes found in the human colon in Africa and Asia; a heavy infection may cause anemia. *Physaloptera mordens*, also reported from Africa, may attach itself to the esophagus, stomach, or small intestine of humans. The definitive host of *Lagochilascaris minor* is unknown. About 30 human cases have been reported from Central and South America, usually with worms invading the soft tissues of the neck, throat, and sinuses.

Drugs for Parasitic Infections. Med Lett 35:111, 1993.

Khuroo MS, Zargar SA, Mahajan R: Sonographic appearances in biliary ascariasis. Gastroenterology 93:267, 1987. *A discussion of the ultrasound appearance of this unusual but clinically important aspect of ascariasis.*

Schad GH, Banwell JG: Hookworms. In Warren KS, Mahmoud AAF (eds.): Tropical and Geographical Medicine. New York, McGraw-Hill, 1990. *A general review of biology, clinical aspects, and epidemiology of hookworm infection. Synthesizes a large amount of confusing literature.*

Smith JW, Wootten R: Anisakis and anisakiasis. Adv Parasitol 16:93, 1978. *An exceptionally complete review.*

TOXOCARIASIS

DEFINITION. Visceral larva migrans (VLM) and ocular larva migrans (OLM) are caused by ingestion and subsequent development and migration of embryonated eggs of the canine roundworm *Toxocara canis.* Roundworms of cats (*T. cati*) and raccoons (*Baylisascaris procyonis*) also rarely cause VLM.

ETIOLOGY. In its normal canine host, *T. canis* follow a route of migration similar to that described for *Ascaris;* i.e., ingested larvae penetrate the small intestine, migrate to the lungs, are reswallowed, and develop into adult worms in the small intestine; the adult worms lodge there and release eggs that are passed in the feces. When embryonated *T. canis* eggs are ingested by humans, larvae also migrate throughout the body (lung, liver, brain, muscles, and occasionally eyes) but fail to complete development to the adult stage. Tissue necrosis secondary to penetrating larvae and associated host inflammatory reactions, such as eosinophil-rich granulomas, are the underlying cause of disease.

EPIDEMIOLOGY. Toxocariasis is endemic in both temperate and tropical areas of the world. The vast majority of symptomatic cases occur in young children. This age group is most likely to be infected by virtue of frequent and intimate handling of dogs (especially newborn puppies that may be hyperinfected), playing in areas where dogs and cats defecate (e.g., public sandboxes), and the habit of geophagia. The potential of exposure to embryonated eggs is high in that *T. canis* infection is common in dogs (a 20% infection rate in dogs in the United States).

CLINICAL MANIFESTATIONS. The vast majority of children who ingest *T. canis* eggs are asymptomatic. VLM is the most common clinically defined entity attributable to *T. canis.* It is most frequent in children younger than 5 (there are no published series of adults with VLM) and is characterized by fever < 39°C; pulmonary symptoms, including wheezing and cough; and, less frequently, pain in the right upper quadrant. These symptoms have a gradual onset and resolve over 4 to 8 weeks. Physical signs include wheezing and hepatomegaly in about one quarter of cases. Larvae less commonly migrate to the brain and heart and cause focal neurologic defects and heart failure.

OLM has an incidence approximately one tenth that of VLM and affects children older than 8 to 10 years. Visual disturbances due to VLM are not distinguishable from other causes of focal intraretinal granulomas or space-occupying lesions, such as tuberculosis and retinoblastoma. *T. canis* larvae may migrate intraretinally and produce transient and recurrent impairment of vision.

DIAGNOSIS AND TREATMENT. VLM is diagnosed on the basis of suspicion of ingestion of *T. canis* eggs in a child with the symptoms described above. Eosinophilia, elevated erythrocyte sedimentation rate, and generalized hypergammaglobulinemia are also consistent with the diagnosis. Biopsy to document the presence of larvae is insensitive and not recommended. An enzyme-linked immunosorbent assay (ELISA) for measuring anti-*Toxocara* antibodies is helpful if elevated immunoglobulin M (IgM) antibodies and a rise in titer between acute and convalescent phases are documented. Most cases of VLM are not life threatening and are self-limited. Treatment is therefore not required. In persons with severe pulmonary, cardiac, or neurologic involvement and high-grade eosinophilia (> 10,000 per cubic millimeter of blood), diethylcarbamazine, 6 mg per kilogram per day in three doses for 7 to 10 days, and corticosteroids may be used to reduce symptoms and shorten the course of the illness. No controlled studies, however, demonstrate the efficacy of chemotherapy.

OLM represents a diagnostic dilemma in that it must be distinguished from intraretinal neoplasms and infections. Expert ophthalmologic consultation is necessary. Computerized tomography and fluorescein angiography are helpful in diagnosis. Elevated anti-*Toxocara* antibody titers in aqueous fluid relative to serum values are consistent with OLM. It is unclear if anthelminthics are useful for the treatment of OLM.

VLM and OLM may be prevented by periodic deworming of dogs, especially puppies, and limiting their defecation in public places.

Glickman LT, Schantz PM, Cypess RH: Epidemiologic characteristics and clinical findings in patients with serologically proven toxocariasis. Trans R Soc Trop Med Hyg 73:254, 1979. *An excellent description of the major clinical manifestations of toxocariasis.*

CUTANEOUS LARVA MIGRANS

Animal hookworms, most frequently the dog parasite *Ancylostoma braziliense* and less commonly *Uncinaria stenocephala* and *Bunostomum phlebotomum,* are the major causative agents of cutaneous larva migrans, or creeping eruption. *Ancylostoma duodenale, Necator americanus,* and *Strongyloides stercoralis* may produce a similar syndrome during the phase of infection that involves penetration of the skin.

The disease occurs when skin comes into direct and prolonged contact with hookworm larvae contained in the feces of dogs, cats, or humans. Moist areas visited by animals, such as vegetation near beaches and exposed soil covered by porches, are common sites in which humans may be infected. Cutaneous larva migrans in the United States is most prevalent in southern coastal regions.

Clinical manifestations result from penetration and migration of larvae in the epidermal-dermal junction of the skin. Within several hours of contact with exposed skin, the patient notes pruritus and raised erythematous serpiginous lesions. The lesions migrate approximately 1 cm per day and evolve into bullae. Multiple lesions may appear if large areas of the body have been exposed, as in sunbathing.

Creeping eruption may be treated by topical application of thiabendazole oral suspension. This may be prepared by trituration of a 500-mg tablet in 5 grams of petroleum jelly. If untreated, cutaneous larva migrans is self-limited; signs and symptoms resolve in several weeks to 2 months.

ANGIOSTRONGYLIASIS

Angiostrongylus cantonensis is a cause of eosinophilic meningitis in Asia and the South Pacific. Small numbers of cases have also been reported in Cuba and Africa. *Angiostrongylus costaricensis* is a rare cause of gastrointestinal bleeding. The nematode is limited in its distribution to Central and South America. Humans are infected with these rodent (primarily rat) nematodes after ingesting poorly cooked or raw intermediate mollusc hosts, such as snails, slugs, and prawns. Fresh vegetables may also be contaminated with infective larvae and serve as a vehicle of infection.

In the case of *A. cantonensis* infection, ingested infective larvae penetrate the gut wall and migrate to small vessels of the meninges and, less commonly, the spinal cord and eye. An intense local inflammatory reaction ensues within 1 week. Fever, meningismus, and headache develop in association with eosinophilic pleocytosis of the CSF. Strabismus, paresthesias, and vomiting have been observed in a minority of cases. Diagnosis is based on a history of ingesting potentially contaminated foodstuffs and the presence of eosinophils in CSF. Larvae are usually not found in CSF. Other in-

fectious causes of eosinophilic meningitis include *Trichinella spiralis, Taenia solium, Toxocara canis, Gnathostoma spinigerum,* and *Paragonimus westermani.* Symptomatic *A. cantonensis* infection resolves over a 2-week period. The value of anthelminthic therapy or corticosteroids has not been established.

A. costaricensis larvae penetrate the mucosa of the terminal ileum, appendix, and ascending colon. The larvae subsequently develop into adult worms in the local lymphatics and mesenteric arterioles. Eggs released by the female worms elicit multiple eosinophil-rich granulomatous reactions that cause edematous, thickened bowel and necrosis (secondary to mesenteric blood vessel obstruction). Clinical presentations typically include right-sided abdominal pain, vomiting, and fever. Abnormal laboratory findings include leukocytosis with eosinophilia. Parasite larvae and eggs are not present in stools. A palpable mass secondary to granulomatous lesions may be present and cause intestinal obstruction. Less frequently, gastrointestinal bleeding is the principal manifestation. Treatment is surgical. There is no demonstrated benefit of specific anthelminthic chemotherapy.

Koo J, Pien F, Kliks M: Angiostrongylus (Parastrongylus) eosinophilic meningitis. Rev Infect Dis 10:1155, 1988. *An excellent discussion of the biology of the helminth and the clinical manifestations of human infection.*

TRICHINOSIS

DEFINITION. Infection by *Trichinella spiralis* occurs when infective larvae are eaten in undercooked pork or other meats. The majority of infected individuals are asymptomatic. Clinical manifestations in heavily infected persons include diarrhea, myalgias, fever, and, less commonly, myocarditis and neurologic disease. Trichinosis occurs in all areas of the world, including the Arctic and temperate regions. The incidence of trichinosis in the United States has decreased markedly over the past several decades.

ETIOLOGY. Infection is initiated by ingesting infective larvae encysted in striated muscle. Excystment occurs in the acid-pepsin environment of the stomach, and parasites develop into sexually mature adult worms in the upper to middle small intestine of the human host. Completion of the enteric phase of the parasite life cycle takes about 1 week, with adult worms remaining viable and productive of larval offspring for an additional 3 to 5 weeks. The systemic phase commences 1 week after infection, when larvae released by female worms migrate through blood vessels and lymphatics and invade multiple organ systems. Mature third-stage larvae develop in host-derived nurse cells in striated skeletal and cardiac muscle, where they become encysted and remain viable for years. As is the case with most helminthiases, the severity of symptoms is related to the total parasite load. Because adult worms are incapable of reproducing themselves, the number of infective larvae ingested is the most important determinant of worm load (i.e., number of larvae that invade muscle and other tissues).

EPIDEMIOLOGY. *T. spiralis* infection is enzootic in omnivorous and carnivorous animal populations, including rats, bears, and aquatic mammals of the Arctic. The nematode is introduced into domestic animals such as pigs and horses by feeding them garbage containing carcasses of these animals, most commonly rats. Human infection usually occurs in two settings: first, when undercooked or smoked pork products or beef contaminated with nematodes is eaten, and second, when flesh of poorly cooked wild game, such as bear or boar meat, is ingested. An important source of infection in Alaskan and Canadian Arctic native populations is uncooked walrus meat.

The annual incidence of human trichinosis in the United States has decreased from more than 450 in 1947-1949 to fewer than 56 between 1982 and 1986. This decline is primarily due to fewer cases related to ingestion of commercial pork products. Recent cases in the United States occur in point-source outbreaks associated with eating game or noncommercial pork products.

PATHOGENESIS AND CLINICAL MANIFESTATIONS. Tissue-invasive *T. spiralis* larvae elicit an eosinophilic granulomatous reaction that may result in significant end-organ tissue damage and dysfunction. Skeletal muscle is the most frequent site involved. Myocardial damage, pulmonary infiltration, and focal neurologic damage secondary to invasion by larvae are seen in only the most heavily infected persons. The systemic phase of infection usually occurs

2 to 3 weeks after ingestion of infective larvae and may last for 2 months. Clinical manifestations typically include myalgias (especially of the gastrocnemius and masseter), periorbital edema, and fever. Myocardial damage may manifest as heart failure or dysrhythmias.

The enteric phase of infection may cause gastrointestinal signs and symptoms, such as diarrhea and abdominal cramps. These typically occur within 1 week of eating contaminated meat and last less than 2 weeks. Reports from the Canadian Arctic suggest that the *T. spiralis* larvae that infect walrus meat may cause diarrhea of 1 to 3 months' duration.

DIAGNOSIS. A diagnosis of trichinosis should be considered in individuals with generalized myalgias and eosinophilia (>600 eosinophils per cubic millimeter). Serologic testing for *T. spiralis* antibodies is available at the Centers for Disease Control and Prevention. Elevation of IgM antibodies or a more than fourfold rise in titer between acute and convalescent phases of infection is helpful in diagnosis. The levels of creatine phosphate kinase and of serum immunoglobulins and the erythrocyte sedimentation rate are also increased for several weeks after infection. Muscle biopsy (e.g., of the gastrocnemius) may demonstrate larvae, although their absence does not exclude the diagnosis.

TREATMENT AND PREVENTION. If patients present at a time when adult parasites are in the intestine (i.e., during the initial 1 to 2 weeks after infection, when gastrointestinal symptoms are prominent), mebendazole is recommended at a dosage of 200 to 400 mg three times per day for 3 days, followed by 400 to 500 mg three times per day for 10 days. It is not clear if larvae in muscle are killed by this drug, and treatment is primarily symptomatic with antipyretics and analgesics. Although there are too few recent cases to establish a possible beneficial effect of corticosteroids, they may be useful to diminish the severity of inflammation when signs of myocarditis, neurologic disease (e.g., seizures, focal weakness), or pulmonary insufficiency develop. *T. spiralis* infection is prevented by killing larvae in meat products. This is achieved by heating until no trace of pink flesh remains. Freezing, smoking, or exposure to microwaves does not reliably kill the helminth.

Bailey TM, Schantz PM: Trends in the incidence and transmission patterns of trichinosis in humans in the United States. Comparisons of the periods 1975-1981 and 1982-1986. Rev Infect Dis 12:5, 1990. *A comprehensive review of the epidemiology of trichinosis.*
MacLean JD, Viallet J, Law C, et al.: Trichinosis in the Canadian Arctic: Report of five outbreaks and a new clinical syndrome. J Infect Dis 160:513, 1989. *Excellent description of severe gastrointestinal manifestations of* T. spiralis *in a population in which the prevalence of trichinosis is among the highest in the world.*

STRONGYLOIDIASIS

DEFINITION. *Strongyloides stercoralis* infection is endemic in warm climates worldwide, including the southern United States. In immunologically normal individuals, infection is usually asymptomatic or causes gastrointestinal dysfunction, manifest as abdominal pain, bloating, or bleeding. Persons who have deficient cell-mediated immunity can develop an autoinfective and hyperinfective life cycle of the nematode that markedly increases the total worm load. Life-threatening acute pulmonary disease and organ dysfunction due to dissemination of larvae to aberrant sites such as the brain, pancreas, and kidneys may result in immunocompromised hosts.

ETIOLOGY. *S. stercoralis* infection occurs when skin contacts free-living filariform larvae in the soil. After penetrating the skin, the parasite embolizes to the small vessels of the lungs via the venous circulation. Rhabditiform larvae then break into the alveolar spaces, ascend the respiratory tree, and are swallowed. Further development to adult worms occurs in the duodenum and upper jejunum, where egg-laying parasites live in the mucosa and submucosa. Rhabditiform larvae are released from eggs and are passed from the body in stools. Infective filariform larvae develop in the soil by two alternative means, either by direct transformation from rhabditiform larvae or indirectly from free-living intermediate forms.

Several unusual features of the life cycle of *S. stercoralis* are crucial to understanding how this parasitic nematode causes life-threatening disease. First, unlike the vast majority of human helminthic parasites, adult worms reproduce parthogenetically in the gastrointestinal tract. The total worm burden in the host may therefore be greatly increased in the absence of repeated exposure to infective larvae in the environment. Second, rhabditiform larvae may develop into infective filariform larvae in the gastrointestinal tract as well as after passage in feces. Occurrence of the former process in immunocompromised hosts allows autoinfection, whereby larvae pass directly through the bowel (internal autoinfection) or perianal skin (external autoinfection) to reinitiate migration and development in the lungs. When this event is frequent, a hyperinfection syndrome ensues. Disseminated strongyloidiasis refers to a situation of hyperinfection in which the organisms also migrate to and cause pathology in organs not usually traversed by larvae, such as the CNS.

EPIDEMIOLOGY. *S. stercoralis* infection is endemic in Africa, Asia, Latin America, and areas of Eastern and Southern Europe. Prevalence rates based on stools examined for rhabditiform larvae vary from more than 40% in areas of sub-Saharan Africa to 1 to 7% in rural Eastern Europe. In the United States, the infection is endemic in rural Appalachia and other parts of the South. Prevalences range from 0.4 to 3% in the United States. Refugees from Asia have a higher prevalence of infection than do indigenous Americans. Surveys of homosexual men indicate a frequency of infection of 3.9%. It is likely that most studies of prevalence underestimate infection because they are based on examination of a single stool specimen, which is less sensitive than multiple examinations performed over days or weeks.

Strongyloidiasis is especially common in overcrowded situations in which sanitation and personal hygiene are poor, such as in institutions for retarded children and POW camps. An unusually high frequency of *S. stercoralis* infection has also been reported in persons with asymptomatic human T cell lymphotropic virus (HTLV) type I infection.

PATHOGENESIS. Adult worms and larvae penetrating the upper small bowel cause an enteritis characterized histopathologically by eosinophil and mononuclear cell infiltration of the lamina propria. Edema and mucosal atrophy are present on gross examination. Ulcerative lesions with hemorrhages are present in the most severe cases. Filariform larvae in the lungs elicit an inflammatory response in the alveoli consisting of mononuclear cells and eosinophils. In hyperinfection syndrome, these may coalesce and result in alveolar hemorrhage.

Autoinfection leading to exceptionally high worm loads (hyperinfection) and disseminated strongyloidiasis occur in persons with deficient cell-mediated immunity. Groups at risk include persons who are chronically taking corticosteroids, renal transplant recipients, patients with Hodgkin's disease and other lymphomas, and leukemic patients. Because *S. stercoralis* may persist and remain asymptomatic for decades after exposure, it is important to keep in mind that a change in immune status may convert a previously asymptomatic infection to hyperinfection. In this regard, there is a suspected association between acquired immunodeficiency syndrome (AIDS) and disseminated strongyloidiasis.

CLINICAL MANIFESTATIONS. More than 50% of immunocompetent infected persons are asymptomatic. The frequency of clinical manifestations among infected immunocompromised subjects is not known.

Signs and symptoms of *S. stercoralis* infection are attributable to the presence of adult worms in the upper gastrointestinal tract and larval invasion and attendant host pathologic responses in the lung, skin, and aberrant sites of migration, such as the brain, eyes, pancreas, and kidney. Immunocompetent individuals rarely develop signs or symptoms attributable to larval migration outside the gut.

Gastrointestinal disease usually manifests as abdominal bloating, vague epigastric pain, and diarrhea with nausea. Symptoms are exacerbated by eating. Hematochezia and melena occur in <20% of subjects with intestinal strongyloidiasis. Major causes of morbidity related to *S. stercoralis* infection of the intestine are paralytic ileus, small bowel obstruction, and a malabsorption syndrome.

Pulmonary signs and symptoms in immunocompromised persons with hyperinfection syndrome are similar to those seen in the adult respiratory distress syndrome, i.e., acute onset of dyspnea, productive cough, and hemoptysis. These are accompanied by fever, tachypnea, hypoxemia, and respiratory alkalosis. *Strongyloides* larvae may also invade the CNS, pancreas, and eye and cause signs and symptoms attributable to tissue destruction in these sites.

Dermatologic manifestations include self-limited creeping eruption and, more commonly, larva currens. The latter is due to migration of filariform larvae produced by a process of external autoinfection as described above. The larvae elicit serpiginous erythematous papules and occasionally urticaria around the buttocks, upper thigh, and lower abdomen. Larva currens has been noted among former prisoners of war in the South Pacific.

DIAGNOSIS. The unequivocal diagnosis of *S. stercoralis* infection depends on identifying larvae in host tissues or gastrointestinal and pulmonary secretions. The existence of filariform larvae in stools implies an active autoinfection.

Intestinal strongyloidiasis is most easily diagnosed by identification of parasites in direct smears of freshly passed stools. Rhabditiform larvae are 225 to 380 μm in length. Repeated examinations and concentration of stools increase the sensitivity of this method from approximately 25 to 80%. Examination of fluid obtained by duodenal aspiration or passage of a swallowed string into the upper small bowel may also be used if stool examinations are negative. Serologic tests are sensitive but not generally available. The differential diagnosis of intestinal *S. stercoralis* infection includes sprue, peptic ulcer, regional enteritis, and ulcerative colitis.

Hyperinfection syndrome and disseminated strongyloidiasis are diagnosed by identification of filariform larvae (500 to 600 μm long) in gastrointestinal secretions, as described above, or in pulmonary tissues, secretions, or washings, such as those obtained by bronchoalveolar lavage or in sputum. Larvae have also been recovered from CSF, peritoneal washings, kidneys, urine, skin, and brains of immunocompromised persons.

Accompanying laboratory abnormalities frequently include eosinophilia. However, eosinophilia may not develop in immunocompromised hosts. Lack of eosinophilia is therefore not helpful in excluding strongyloidiasis in the differential diagnosis. The differential diagnosis of hyperinfection and disseminated strongyloidiasis includes overwhelming bacterial or fungal sepsis.

COMPLICATIONS. Disseminated strongyloidiasis is frequently accompanied by fungal or bacterial sepsis. Gram-negative enterococcal and polymicrobial septicemia has been observed. These infections likely result from translocation of gut organisms by migrating larvae.

TREATMENT. Uncomplicated intestinal strongyloidiasis should be treated with thiabendazole (25 mg per kilogram of body weight twice daily for 2 days with a maximum of 3 grams per day). Parasitologic cure rates are >90%. Thiabendazole at the same daily dosage should be given to immunocompromised patients with hyperinfection syndrome (i.e., pulmonary disease) or disseminated disease. The drug should be continued for a minimum of 5 to 7 days, although 1 to 2 weeks may be required if organ dysfunction and larval recovery persist. Symptomatic improvement and failure to detect larvae in gastrointestinal secretions or other sites is indicative of cure. Corticosteroids and other immunosuppressive agents should be discontinued when possible.

PREVENTION. Infection is preventable by avoiding skin contact with contaminated soil. Immunocompromised patients in endemic areas should be advised to avoid walking barefoot. Persons residing in endemic areas who are to become immunosuppressed (e.g., for renal transplantation) should have their stools examined three times for the presence of larvae, and they should be treated if the examination is positive. Because infected individuals may be incorrectly categorized as uninfected by this test, it is suggested by some authorities that prophylactic thiabendazole (25 mg per kilogram of body weight daily for 2 days) be given in the month preceding iatrogenic immunosuppression. Positive serology for *S. stercoralis* is also an indication for thiabendazole administration prior to immunosuppression.

Cook GC: *Strongyloides stercoralis* hyperinfection syndrome: How often is it missed? Q J Med 64:625, 1987. *Discusses in detail the differential diagnosis and pitfalls in diagnosis of strongyloidiasis in the immunocompromised host.*

Robinson PD, Lindo JF, Neva FA, et al.: Immunoepidemiologic studies of *Strongyloides stercoralis* and human T lymphotropic virus type I infection in Jamaica. J Infect Dis 169:692, 1994. *Describes the association between HTLV-I infection and strongyloidiasis.*

DeVault GA Jr, King JW, Rohr MS, et al.: Opportunistic infection with *Strongyloides stercoralis* in renal transplantation. Rev Infect Dis 12:653, 1990. *Excellent discussion of clinical presentation and management of hyperinfection in immunocompromised hosts.*

Lessnav K-D, Can S, Talavera W: Disseminated *Strongyloides stercoralis* in human immunodeficiency virus-infected patients. Treatment failure and a review of the literature. Chest 104:119. *A discussion of the difficulties in diagnosis in AIDS patients.*

388 FILARIASIS
*Eric A. Ottesen**

388.1 Introduction

Eight filarial parasites commonly infect humans (Table 388–1), but three are responsible for most of the pathology associated with these infections. These are the lymphatic dwelling filariae *Wuchereria bancrofti* and *Brugia malayi* and the subcutaneous filarid *Onchocerca volvulus*.

All eight species are transmitted by biting arthropods (Table 388–1) and go through complex life cycles that include a slow maturation phase of 3 to 18 months from the time infective larvae are introduced by the vector until the adult worms mature and reside in the lymph nodes, subcutaneous tissue, or body cavities. The offspring of these adults (microfilariae) are 200 to 300 μm long and 5 to 9 μm wide. They either circulate in the blood or migrate through the skin, awaiting ingestion by the appropriate arthropod in which they develop over 1 to 2 weeks to infective forms capable of initiating this life cycle again. Adult worms are long lived (5 to 20 years), while microfilariae live probably 6 to 15 months. Patent infection is generally not established unless exposure to infective larvae is intense and prolonged, and manifestations of disease usually develop slowly.

Diagnosis can be extremely difficult because in endemic populations it relies almost exclusively on parasitologic techniques to demonstrate microfilariae in the blood or tissue, and at present there are no completely satisfactory methods for making a definitive diagnosis in states of "amicrofilaremic" or "amicrofiladermic" filariasis (i.e., infections without demonstrable microfilariae). When microfilariae circulate in the blood, they do so with or without a distinct periodicity (Table 388–1). Some are garbed in sheaths whereas others are sheathless. These two features, as well as other more subtle morphologic distinctions, are helpful diagnostically. Microfilariae in the blood can be identified either by direct observation of Giemsa-stained blood smears or, more sensitively, by concentration techniques using Knott's method (examination of centrifuged sediment after mixing 1 ml of blood with 9 ml of 2% formalin) or membrane filtration of 1 ml or more of blood through a 3-μm or 5-μm pore Nuclepore membrane filter. Skin microfilariae are best sought by performing skin snips as described in Ch. 388.4. Antibody detection, although helpful in certain situations, is generally nondiagnostic because it cannot differentiate current from past infection or exposure and because of antigenic cross-reactivity between the filariae and other helminth parasites. Newer diagnostic methods based on detecting circulating antigen in blood or parasite DNA from skin snips or blood are more sensitive and currently are being readied for general use.

Diethylcarbamazine (DEC)† had been the single mainstay of treatment for all filarial infections since the late 1940's; however, it shows variable effectiveness for the different infections. The new drug ivermectin,‡ because of greater efficacy and safety, has replaced DEC as the drug of choice for onchocerciasis; it is currently under evaluation for use in lymphatic and other filariases. Suramin,‡ although extremely toxic, can also be used for onchocerciasis.

Ottesen EA: Filarial Infections. Infect Dis Clin North Am 7:619, 1993. *A practical approach to the clinical management of each of the filarial infections of humans.*
World Health Organization: Lymphatic filariasis: The disease and its control. Fifth report of the WHO Expert Committee on Filariasis. WHO Tech Rep Ser 821:1,

* The author wishes to acknowledge the previous contributions of Bruce Greene, M.D., (onchocerciasis) and Donald Hopkins, M.D., (dracunculiasis).
† Not commercially available in the United States but may be obtained in special circumstances from Lederle Laboratories, Pearl River, NY.
‡ Available from the Centers for Disease Control and Prevention, Parasitic Disease Drug Service, Atlanta, GA.

TABLE 388–1. THE COMMON FILARIAL PARASITES OF HUMANS

Species	Distribution	Vector	Primary Pathology	Microfilariae		
				Primary Location	Periodicity	Presence of Sheath
Wuchereria bancrofti	Tropics worldwide	Mosquitoes	Lymphatic, pulmonary	Blood, hydrocele fluid	Nocturnal, subperiodic	+
Brugia malayi	Southeast Asia, West Pacific	Mosquitoes	Lymphatic, pulmonary	Blood	Nocturnal, subperiodic	+
Brugia timori	Indonesia	Mosquitoes	Lymphatic	Blood	Nocturnal	+
Onchocerca volvulus	Africa; Central and South America	Black fly	Skin, eye, lymphatic	Skin, eye	None or minimal	−
Loa loa	Africa	Deer fly	Allergic	Blood	Diurnal	+
Mansonella perstans	Africa; South America	Midge	? Allergic	Blood	None	−
Mansonella streptocerca	Africa	Midge	Skin	Skin	None	−
Mansonella ozzardi	Central and South America	Midge	Vague	Blood	None	−

1992. A broad review of lymphatic filariasis and directions that research and control efforts should take in the future.

World Health Organization: Onchocerciasis: The infection and its control. Report of the WHO Expert Committee on Onchocerciasis. WHO Tech Rep Ser, 1995, in press. A broad review of onchocerciasis and the directions that research and control efforts should take in the future.

388.2 Lymphatic Filariasis

ETIOLOGY. There are three lymphatic-dwelling filarial parasites of humans, *Wuchereria bancrofti*, *Brugia malayi*, and *Brugia timori*. Adult worms are threadlike in form (2 to 10 cm long by < 0.4 cm wide) and usually reside in the lymph nodes or afferent lymphatic channels. The female worms produce large numbers of microfilariae (200 to 300 μm long), which circulate in the peripheral blood awaiting ingestion by mosquito intermediate hosts, which are necessary to continue the parasite's life cycle. After about 2 weeks the microfilariae develop into infective third-stage larvae (L_3's). When infected mosquitoes feed, these L_3's leave the mosquito mouth parts and come to rest on the surface of the host's skin. Only if they manage to penetrate the skin through the puncture at the site of the bite can transmission be successful; after a further developmental period lasting as long as 4 to 12 months, adult worms can again be found in the lymphatic tissues, where they mate and produce another generation of microfilariae. The adult parasites may remain viable in the human host for decades.

EPIDEMIOLOGY. Almost 120 million people have lymphatic filariasis—105 million with bancroftian and 13 million with brugian filariasis. For *W. bancrofti*, humans are the only definitive host and thus the only reservoir for infection. *W. bancrofti* is found throughout the tropics and subtropics, including areas of South America and the Caribbean, Africa, Asia, and the Pacific. Two forms of the parasite are distinguished by the periodicity of their circulating microfilariae. Nocturnally periodic forms have microfilariae detectable in peripheral blood primarily at night, whereas in the subperiodic forms the microfilariae are usually present in the blood at all hours but with maximal levels often in the late afternoon. Generally, subperiodic bancroftian filariasis is found only in the Pacific islands east of 160 degrees E longitude (including New Caledonia, Fiji, Samoa, Ellis Island, Cook Islands, Society Islands, and the Marquesas); elsewhere *W. bancrofti* is generally nocturnally periodic. The natural vectors are *Culex quinquefasciatus* in urban settings and usually anopheline or aedean mosquitoes in rural areas.

The distribution of brugian filariasis is much more restricted, being limited primarily to parts of Malaysia, Indonesia, India, China, Korea, the Philippines, and Japan. Again, there are both nocturnally periodic and subperiodic forms of the parasite. The former is more common and is transmitted in coastal rice fields primarily by mansonian and anopheline mosquitoes; mansonian mosquitoes, found in swamp forests, are the major vectors of the subperiodic form. Un-like *W. bancrofti*, *B. malayi* can be a natural infection of cats and can be established in a number of laboratory animals. *B. timori* has been described from only two Indonesian islands.

PATHOLOGY. Most of the pathology of bancroftian and brugian filariasis is associated with the lymphatics. Although details of the pathogenesis are lacking, the progression of pathologic changes is becoming clearer. Even in entirely asymptomatic individuals with microfilaremia but no overt clinical manifestations of infection, lymphatic structural and functional abnormalities are often severe. Compromised function ultimately leads to lymphedema that is at first reversible. With continued assault on this compromised lymphatic system by persistent parasites and by complicating localized bacterial and fungal superinfections, the lymphedema becomes irreversible and leads to chronic elephantiasis of the limbs, breasts, or genitalia, or to chyluria. The location of lymphatic damage determines the site and type of pathology expressed.

Adult worms, residing in the afferent approaches or cortical sinuses of the lymph nodes, induce local reactions by undefined mechanisms that result in dilatation of the lymphatics and hypertrophy of the vessel walls. Endothelial and connective tissue proliferation leads to polypoid growths that protrude into the lymphatic lumen, and even while the vessels remain patent, normal lymphatic function is not ensured. Both earlier lymphangiography studies and more recent lymphoscintigraphy studies have clearly documented the development of a characteristic tortuosity of the lymph vessels with loss of valvular function and backflow of lymph leading to lymph stasis and lymphedema even during this "preobliterative phase."

Because of a still undefined interplay between the host immune system and the parasite, local inflammatory and granulomatous reactions subsequently develop around dying or dead adult worms, with infiltration of plasma cells, eosinophils, and giant cells. Fibrosis occurs, and the fragmented parasites are either completely resorbed or partially calcified. Lymphatic obstruction develops, and associated bacterial-induced inflammation or superinfection may further complicate the lymphatic damage. Although there is subsequent formation of collateral lymphatics and some recanalization of obstructed vessels, lymphatic function remains compromised. Repeated infection and increasing host response to the parasite leads to the chronic changes of advanced elephantiasis.

CLINICAL MANIFESTATIONS. Although previously not much emphasized, a major distinction exists between the clinical presentation of lymphatic filariasis in individuals native to the endemic regions (whose exposures have been lifelong) and that of those entering such areas and meeting the infection for the first time. In these latter (e.g., long-term visitors, military personnel, settlers) the most common presentations are localized inflammatory reactions, especially adenolymphangitis, and evidence of immediate hypersensitivity responses to the parasites (i.e., urticaria, eosinophilia, and immunoglobulin E [IgE] elevations). Only rarely do such individuals present with the contrasting set of findings characteristic of the infection in those native to the endemic areas, particularly asymptomatic microfilaremia.

Patients manifesting *asymptomatic microfilaremia* rarely come to the physician's attention except through an incidental finding of microfilariae in the peripheral blood smear during mass surveys in endemic regions, or when blood eosinophilia leads to a diagnostic evaluation for filariasis. Such asymptomatic persons appear to be clinically unaffected by the parasites. However, recent studies have shown dramatically that this asymptomatic state belies severe underlying pathology, both lymphatic functional abnormalities seen on lymphoscintigraphy and renal pathology manifested as hematuria and proteinuria. It is likely that some but not all of these individuals become symptomatic, but factors determining such clinical changes are unknown.

"Filarial fever" is the term given to acute febrile episodes (often with shaking chills), accompanied by painful lymphatic inflammation (lymphadenitis and lymphangitis) and transient local edema that occur up to 6 to 10 times per year and usually last 3 to 7 days before subsiding spontaneously. Although appreciated only recently, "filarial fevers" appear to be really two different clinical syndromes, one initiated by host immunologic responses to lymphatic-dwelling parasites and the other, seemingly more common, induced by bacterial superinfection of limbs with already compromised lymphatic function. The former is characterized by a *retrograde* lymphangitis and "cold" edema of the affected limb and the latter by a cellulitis-type of presentation with a warm edematous extremity. Such inflammatory reactions occur in the upper and lower extremities with both bancroftian and brugian filariasis, but involvement of the genital lymphatics is almost exclusively a feature of *W. bancrofti* infection. Thus, acute *W. bancrofti* episodes may also involve funiculitis, epididymitis, scrotal pain, and tenderness. Patients with filarial fevers may be microfilaremic but more often are not.

As lymphatic damage progresses, the edema and anatomic distortion that were initially transient develop into the permanent changes of elephantiasis. Pitting edema yields to brawny edema, and both thickening of subcutaneous tissue and hyperkeratosis develop. Fissuring of the skin develops along with nodular and papillomatous hyperplastic changes. Superinfection (with skin bacteria and dermatophytes) becomes an increasing problem. In addition, in bancroftian filariasis affected genital lymphatics may lead to scrotal lymphedema or hydrocele, whereas involvement of the retroperitoneal lymphatics can increase hydrostatic pressure in the renal lymphatics, causing their rupture into the renal pelvis or tubules and leading to chyluria. Characteristically, such chyluria is intermittent, sometimes lasting for days or weeks before abating spontaneously and then recurring; often it is most prominent in the morning after the patient first arises.

DIAGNOSIS. Diagnosis is most certainly made by identifying the parasites themselves, usually microfilariae in the blood, hydrocele fluid, or chylous urine. These fluids can be examined directly (20 cubic millimeters on a slide with or without red blood cell lysis), after concentration of the parasites by centrifugation in 2% formalin (Knott's technique), or after filtration through a membrane (3- to 5-μm Nuclepore) filter. The time of blood collection should take into account the parasite's possible nocturnal periodicity. More recently, ultrasound techniques have been successfully and simply used to visualize rapidly moving ("dancing") adult worms in the dilated scrotal lymphatics of infected men; such findings are absolutely pathognomonic of filarial parasites.

Because many persons with filariasis (especially those with chronic pathology) are not microfilaremic, diagnosis must often be made clinically. The differential diagnosis is broad but in the acute episodes primarily includes thrombophlebitis, infection, and trauma. The edema and other lymphatic obstructive changes associated with chronic filariasis must be distinguished from the manifestations of congestive heart failure, malignant disease, trauma, postsurgical scarring, and a number of less common congenital and idiopathic abnormalities of the lymphatic system. The many disorders associated with serum IgE and blood eosinophil elevations must be considered in evaluating asymptomatic filarial infections. Several specific points may help in this differential diagnosis: (1) Exposure to filariae must be prolonged or intense (for at least several months) before persons become infected; (2) the physical finding or history of *retrograde* lymphangitis can often aid in distinguishing filarial from bacterial lymphangitis; (3) although lymphadenopathy is characteristic of filariasis, alone it is never diagnostic; (4) lymphangiographic and lymphoscintigraphic patterns of elephantiasis and chyluria are well defined, so that even though not always diagnostic,

these tests can sometimes be useful in distinguishing filarial from congenital or neoplastic lymphatic abnormalities; (5) although total serum IgE and blood eosinophil levels are often elevated in filarial infections, they cannot distinguish filarial from other helminth infections except in the case of the tropical eosinophilia syndrome (see Ch. 388.3).

Until recently, serologic and skin tests have not generally been helpful in diagnosing filariasis *except* in those individuals not native to the endemic regions. The primary reason is that residents of endemic areas with their lifelong exposures to mosquito-borne filarial larvae develop high levels of antifilarial antibodies, regardless of whether they actually acquire infection. The recent development of assays to detect circulating antigens liberated by adult worms (and present in the blood both day and night) promises to revolutionize the serologic approach to diagnosing filariasis.

TREATMENT. The approach to treating lymphatic filariasis is currently undergoing dramatic changes. Although DEC† (6 mg per kilogram per day) remains the only drug registered for use in lymphatic filariasis, ivermectin‡ (400 μg per kilogram per day) is an equally potent microfilaricide. DEC is also effective in killing some, although not all, adult worms, but for ivermectin there is still uncertainty about its potential adulticidal activity. Most surprising has been the recent finding that a single dose of DEC has essentially the same long-term effectiveness in decreasing microfilaremia and apparent killing of adult worms as the 1- to 3-week courses previously recommended. For control programs, this finding has enormous implications; for individual clinic patients, however, it is not certain that earlier recommendations for the longer courses of DEC should be scaled back to single-day dosing; specific clinical studies still need to address this issue.

The side effects of DEC treatment, whether single-dose or multiple doses, can be troublesome, especially in brugian filariasis. These include fever, chills, headache, dizziness, nausea, vomiting, and arthralgias, all usually occurring in the first 24 to 36 hours. Both the likelihood of developing such reactions and the degree of their severity are directly related to the number of circulating microfilariae. Thus, the side effects of DEC at the recommended (6 mg/kg) dosage are due not to direct drug toxicity but to inflammatory responses of the host to dying parasites. To avoid these reactions in highly parasitemic persons, one can initiate treatment with very small doses of DEC or premedicate the patients with steroids, as suggested for loiasis (see Ch. 388.5). A very few patients may also develop filarial fever episodes with lymphangitis and lymphadenitis in the first days after DEC treatment. All of these side effects occur early in treatment and generally subside even when the drug is continued.

Chronic lymphedema and elephantiasis have recently been shown to have a surprising degree of reversibility. All such affected patients should receive long-term low-dose DEC (to eradicate persistent or new filarial infections) and diligent attention to local care of the lymphedematous extremity through limb elevation, use of special massage techniques and elastic stockings, and especially prevention of superficial bacterial and fungal infection. More severely affected patients may benefit remarkably from surgical decompression of the lymphatic system through "nodovenous shunt" surgery followed by excision of redundant tissue. Hydroceles can be repeatedly drained or managed surgically. Chyluria also can sometimes be corrected surgically, but, interestingly, many cases have been reported in which diagnostic lymphangiography itself appears to have terminated the leak of chyle into the urine, probably as a result of its sclerosing effects.

PREVENTION. DEC kills developing preadult forms of many filarial species, and its value as a prophylactic agent in humans (10 mg per kilogram on 2 consecutive days each month) has recently been established. In addition, for public health programs to control lymphatic filariasis, a single dose of DEC given yearly to an entire community dramatically reduces the prevalence of infection. Similarly, small doses administered intermittently (or even as an additive to common table salt) to all residents of an endemic region (e.g., 3 mg per kilogram monthly) reduce the number of bloodborne microfilariae in the community to levels so low that successful transmission of the infection by mosquitoes cannot occur. Other approaches to filariasis control designed to eradicate the mosquito vectors have also proved effective for the short term but have been difficult to sustain.

Amaral F, Dreyer G, Figueredo-Silva J, et al.: Live adult worms detected by ultrasonography in human bancroftian filariasis. Am J Trop Med Hyg 50:753, 1994. *The first description of a successful new technique for noninvasive localization and visualization of living adult-stage W. bancrofti worms. Such adult worms could be identified in more than half of all asymptomatic microfilaraemic men evaluated.*
Chodakewitz JA: Ivermectin and lymphatic filariasis: Clinical update. Parasitol Today, 1995. *A thorough review of the most recent trials comparing single-dose DEC, single-dose ivermectin, and the combination of these single-dose regimens to effect microfilarial clearance from the blood of patients with W. bancrofti or B. malayi infections.*
Ottesen EA: The human filariases: New understandings, new therapeutic strategies. Curr Opinion Infect Dis 7:550, 1994. *A look at the dramatic advances of the past 2 to 3 years that are transforming the way filariasis is both understood and managed.*
Witte MH, Jamal S, Williams WH, et al.: Lymphatic abnormalities in human filariasis as depicted by lymphoangioscintigraphy. Arch Intern Med 153:737, 1993. *Thirty-three patients with symptomatic (acute or chronic) lymphatic filariasis from South India were evaluated by lymphoscintigraphy, which was shown to be a simple, safe, reliable, noninvasive method for examining the peripheral lymphatic system. The abnormalities noted in these patients included delayed or absent tracer transport, tortuosity of the deep lymphatics, dermal diffusion, retrograde tracer flow, and faint or absent regional node visualization.*

388.3 Tropical Eosinophilia

Tropical eosinophilia is a syndrome of acute and chronic lung disease first defined in the 1940's but not generally recognized as being of filarial origin until the 1960's. Its main clinical features are a history of residence in a filaria-endemic region; paroxysmal cough and wheezing, which generally occur at night; scanty sputum production; occasional weight loss, low-grade fever, and adenopathy; and extreme blood eosinophilia (> 3000 per microliter). It is more common in men than in women. Chest roentgenograms can be normal but generally show increased bronchovascular markings, diffuse interstitial lesions, or mottled opacities primarily involving the mid and lower lung fields. Tests of pulmonary function almost always indicate restrictive abnormalities and often obstructive defects as well. The association of the syndrome with filarial infection was first recognized by finding very high levels of antifilarial antibody in these patients and by noting the favorable response to treatment with antifilarial drugs (now diethylcarbamazine† [DEC], 6 to 10 mg per kilogram per day for 3 to 4 weeks). Later, several reports described microfilariae or their degenerating remnants in lung biopsy specimens. Most recently, extremely high levels of total serum IgE (usually 10,000 to 100,000 ng per milliliter) have been found in these patients, and an appreciable fraction of this IgE has been shown to be directed against filarial antigens.

Because of these and other findings, tropical eosinophilia is now considered a form of "occult filariasis" in which host immunologic hyperresponsiveness to the parasite results in such rapid clearance of microfilariae from the blood that this stage of the parasite is essentially never detectable. Generally, this microfilarial clearance takes place in the lungs, and the clinical symptoms appear to result largely from the allergic and inflammatory reactions elicited by the cleared parasites. In some subjects, however, trapping of the microfilariae occurs predominantly in other organs of the reticuloendothelial system (liver, spleen, lymph nodes), and in these persons the major clinical manifestations are those resulting from hepatomegaly, splenomegaly, or lymphadenopathy. It had been postulated that infection with nonhuman filarial parasites is the major cause of tropical eosinophilia. Almost certainly, however, the syndrome is caused not by an "abnormal parasite" but rather by an abnormal host response to those same parasites (*Wuchereria bancrofti* and *Brugia malayi*) that commonly cause lymphatic filariasis (see Ch. 388.2). In this respect, tropical eosinophilia may be similar to another pulmonary eosinophilic disorder, allergic bronchopulmonary aspergillosis, both in its clinical expression and in its pathogenesis (see Ch. 355).

Diagnosis depends primarily on distinguishing tropical eosinophilia from the other important eosinophilic syndromes with pulmonary involvement, namely, Löffler's syndrome, chronic eosinophilic pneumonia, allergic aspergillosis, certain vasculitis syndromes, the idiopathic hypereosinophilia syndrome, drug allergies, and some helminth infections. Although there is no one clinical or laboratory criterion that will distinguish tropical eosinophilia from these other conditions, a history of residence in the tropics, high levels of specific filarial antibodies, and a response to DEC therapy are the most helpful differential points. Within 3 to 7 days after DEC is begun, symptoms improve markedly or disappear. Resolution may not be complete, however, and relapse may occur months to years later and require retreatment. DEC will not, of course, reverse permanent pulmonary damage (primarily an interstitial fibrosis), which frequently develops prior to successful diagnosis and treatment of the disorder.

Ottesen EA, Nutman TB: Tropical pulmonary eosinophilia. Ann Rev Med 43:417, 1992. *A brief overview of the newer clinical and pathogenetic aspects of the TPE syndrome, with references to the appropriate primary sources.*

388.4 Onchocerciasis (River Blindness)

ETIOLOGY. Onchocerciasis, most commonly causing skin and eye disease, results from infection with the filarial parasite *Onchocerca volvulus*. Transmission is via the bites of black files (*Simulium* species) that ingest microfilariae from the skin of an infected person while taking a blood meal. After 6 to 8 days of development in the vector, the larvae are infective and can be transmitted to another person when the fly bites again. Over a period of several months, the larvae develop into adult worms that coil into spherical bundles surrounded by host fibrotic and granulomatous tissue located in the subcutaneous tissues and deeper fascial planes. After a prepatent period of 9 to 18 months, the adult male and female worms reproduce sexually to yield millions of microfilariae that migrate primarily through the skin and ocular tissues.

Microfilariae are highly motile, unsheathed and approximately 200 to 300 μm long and 6 to 9 μm wide. Adult female worms are 23 to 70 cm in length, while the males are 3 to 6 cm long and weigh only 1% as much as the female. The average life span of the adult worm is estimated to be 8 to 10 years and that of the microfilariae, 13 to 14 months.

PREVALENCE AND EPIDEMIOLOGY. *O. volvulus* infects an estimated 17 million persons, principally in 27 countries of equatorial Africa in a broad belt extending from the Atlantic coast on the west to the Red Sea and Indian Ocean on the east. More limited foci are also found in Yemen and in six countries of the Americas (Guatemala, Mexico, Venezuela, Brazil, Colombia, and Ecuador).

Endemicity of *O. volvulus* in human populations is dependent upon habitation of fly-infested areas by sufficient numbers of people who are exposed to human-biting flies during daily activities such as farming, fishing, bathing, washing and water collection. Because the flies depend on waterways for egg-laying and reproduction, they concentrate around streams and rivers. As a result, infection and disease in human populations tend to be similarly distributed; hence the term *river blindness*. Generally, the vectors fly a few kilometers from waterways, but they may be carried by winds for hundreds of kilometers.

The incidence of blindness varies in different regions (thought to be related to parasite strain), but until recently onchocerciasis has been the fourth leading cause of blindness; in some hyperendemic areas more than half the adults became blind. A much higher percentage of persons develops skin disease, and because both of these severe disabilities typically occur during the third and fourth decades of life, the impact of the disease on the community is particularly devastating, frequently incapacitating the heads of households.

PATHOLOGY AND PATHOGENESIS. The disease affects primarily the skin, lymph nodes, and ocular tissues. In the skin, histopathology reflects a low-grade chronic inflammatory process, the end stage of which is loss of elastic fibers, atrophy, and fibrosis.

Onchocercomata, which are fibrous subcutaneous nodules containing adult worms, show a rim of chronic inflammation with fibrosis and extensive capillary infiltration surrounding the worms themselves. Lymph nodes show chronic inflammatory changes and, in some cases, fibrosis and atrophy. In the eye, neovascularization and scarring of the cornea lead to loss of transparency and blindness. The rest of the eye is frequently involved by a chronic nongranulomatous inflammatory process that leads to anterior uveitis and associated chronic complications, chorioretinitis with damage to the retinal pigment epithelium, and optic atrophy.

The basis for the pathologic changes of onchocerciasis is believed to be the host reaction to chronic infection with microfilariae. Numerous factors appear to contribute to the pathologic changes, including toxic or tissue-altering products of host granulocytes and lymphoid cells that are involved either in killing microfilariae or in responding to their spontaneous or natural death, and toxic products of the microfilariae themselves.

CLINICAL MANIFESTATIONS. The earliest signs of infection include pruritus, intermittent papular rash sometimes with thickening of the skin which may be localized to one area of the body, and conjunctivitis. In expatriate visitors to endemic areas, who are usually lightly infected, these are frequently the only manifestations. The onchocercomata are 0.5- to 3-cm subcutaneous nodules that are firm, nontender and freely movable if not attached to periosteum. They frequently occur in clusters overlying bony prominences, including the superior iliac crests, the coccyx, the greater trochanter of the femur, the bony thorax, and the head. With chronic infection, permanent skin changes occur, including loss of elasticity, a chronic, scaling hyperkeratotic maculopapular pruritic rash with mottled hypopigmentation or hyperpigmentation, and, finally, atrophy, leading in some cases to areas of skin breakdown and superinfection. The chronic skin manifestations are intermittently punctuated by transient episodes of localized rash, erythema, and edema. In Central America the dermal manifestations are most prominent around the head and neck, whereas in Africa they more commonly involve the trunk, buttocks, and lower extremities. Lymph node involvement is usually manifested by enlargement, particularly in the inguinal and femoral regions, and in some cases by secondary obstructive changes in the groin region or in an extremity. Also seen when massively enlarged inguinal nodes develop in the presence of appreciable dermal atrophy is the characteristic clinical picture of "hanging groin."

In the eye the earliest manifestations are punctate keratitis and anterior uveitis. Chronic changes include sclerosing keratitis, chorioretinitis (which leads to progressive constriction of visual fields), optic atrophy, and complications due to persistent anterior uveitis, including miosis, pupillary distortion, and glaucoma. In general, the severity of the eye disease correlates with intensity and duration of infection.

DIAGNOSIS. The diagnosis can be made clinically by the presence of onchocercomata, typical skin changes, or eye findings of onchocerciasis, especially microfilariae visualized by slit-lamp examination of the cornea or anterior chamber in otherwise normal-appearing eyes. Diagnosis is most frequently made by finding microfilariae of *O. volvulus* in the patient's skin. "Skin snips" are taken using either a corneoscleral biopsy instrument or a razor blade, to yield approximately 1 to 2 mg of skin, including superficial dermis. The skin is placed in saline or water, and the microfilariae that emerge are counted after a 3-hour or overnight incubation. Alternatively, the snips can be processed for polymerase chain reaction (PCR) amplification of parasite DNA, a technique more sensitive than direct visualization. Because distribution of microfilariae is not uniform, four to six snips should be done in different areas, including the hips, calves, and shoulders. Instruments used for skin snipping should be disposable or thoroughly sterilized between patients. Although elevated titers of antifilarial antibodies may support the diagnosis of onchocerciasis, a definitive immunodiagnostic technique has not yet been developed.

TREATMENT. Invermectin‡ is now the drug of choice to treat onchocerciasis. The dosage is 150 μg per kilogram, given every 6 or 12 months. Because it kills microfilariae but not adult worms, retreatment is necessary over a period of years. Expatriate visitors to endemic countries often require more than once-a-year treatment because of rapid recurrence of pruritus in these hyperreactive individuals. Ivermectin is not approved for use in pregnant

women, nursing mothers within 1 week of delivery, or children under age 5.

DEC† should *not* be used to treat patients with onchocerciasis because the severe inflammatory reaction ("Mazzotti reaction") induced by the rapid killing of microfilariae can actually cause pathology (especially in the eye) worse than the infection itself. Although qualitatively similar posttreatment reactions can occur after ivermectin (including fever, pruritus, lymphadenitis, arthralgia, and postural hypotension), their incidence and severity are much less, and essentially no exacerbation of ocular lesions occurs. Suramin, although it does kill adult worms, has appreciable toxicity (especially renal) and must be given intravenously at approximately weekly intervals over 2 to 3 months, so it should be used with caution and only where there can be careful monitoring.

Surgical removal of nodules containing adult worms is appropriate for cosmetic reasons but cannot be expected to cure infection because for every palpable nodule there are four to nine nonpalpable ones.

PROGNOSIS. With treatment, the early ocular and cutaneous changes are reversible, but for persons living in an endemic area, therapy must be given repeatedly because ivermectin does not kill the adult parasites and, thus, does not eliminate the infection. The atrophic skin changes, sclerosing keratitis, and established lesions in the posterior segment of the eye are not helped by therapy.

PREVENTION. Protective clothing, insect repellents, and avoiding areas harboring the vector are useful measures for visitors to endemic areas, but there is no available chemoprophylaxis. Vector control is difficult and expensive but has achieved excellent success in the 11-country Onchocerciasis Control Program in West Africa. The remarkable Mectizan Donation Program, in which the manufacturer of ivermectin (Merck & Co., Inc.) has pledged to donate, without cost, all the drugs needed to treat all patients in all endemic areas for as long as necessary, has spurred the organization of massive control programs throughout the endemic regions of Africa and the Americas, supported by governmental and nongovernmental development organizations, the World Bank, and the Inter American Bank. The effect of these efforts promises to be a dramatic decline in the incidence and prevalence of onchocerciasis and, most importantly, in the disease it inflicts on affected individuals.

Duke BOL: The population dynamics of *Onchocerca volvulus* in the human host. Trop Med Parasitol 44:61, 1993. *Data from disparate sources are cleverly compiled to allow interpretation and extrapolation leading to astounding conclusions about the number of adult worms and microfilariae in O. volvulus–infected patients.*
Dull B: Mectizan Donation and the Mectizan Expert Committee. Acta Leidensia 59:399, 1990. *Describes organization of a program that provided over 30 million once-yearly doses of ivermectin to 8 million individuals in onchocerciasis-endemic regions of Africa and the Americas (end, 1994).*
Ottesen EA: Immune responsiveness and the pathogenesis of human onchocerciasis. J Infect Dis, in press. *Reviews a confusing array of studies dealing with the immune responses of onchocerciasis patients. Proposes that it is not so much the proinflammatory response to O. volvulus microfilariae that is responsible for the skin and eye pathology as it is the "bystander" damage by host immune and phagocytic cells attempting to contain or prevent inflammatory responses to the vast number of microfilariae dying "naturally" each day.*
World Health Organization: Onchocerciasis: The infection and its control. Report of the WHO Expert Committee on Onchocerciasis. WHO Tech Rep Ser 1995, in press. *A broad review of onchocerciasis and the directions that research and control efforts should take in the future.*

388.5 Loiasis

Loa loa is indigenous only to the rain forest belt of western and central Africa. Mature female parasites, about twice the size of the males, are 50 to 70 mm long and 0.5 mm wide. They live for many years in the subcutaneous tissue in humans, usually attracting attention only when they cross the eye subconjunctivally. The sheathed microfilariae produced by these females circulate in the blood with a diurnal periodicity that peaks at about noon.

Clinical loiasis presents in two primary forms, one more common among individuals native to endemic regions and the other more common in visitors to these areas who acquire infection. Among the natives, loiasis is often entirely asymptomatic until an adult worm appears moving across the eye or blood examination reveals microfilaremia. Such individuals may also have occasional episodes of "Calabar swellings." These are characteristic localized areas of erythema and angioedema (up to 5 to 10 cm in diameter) that occur primarily on the extremities and last 1 to 3 days before regressing spontaneously. These swellings appear to be a hypersensitivity reaction to the adult worm, whose presence can also be detected in some patients by either a subcutaneous crawling sensation or the appearance of a fine vermiform hive in the skin. When the inflammation extends to nearby joints or peripheral nerves, corresponding symptoms may develop. Nephropathy (probably immune complex mediated) and, more rarely, encephalopathy have also been reported.

The major difference between this presentation and that seen in visitors who acquire infection is the greater predominance of allergic or hyperreactive symptoms in the latter. Episodes of angioedema are likely to be more frequent and debilitating, and patients are much less likely to have microfilariae in the blood. In addition, they often present with extensive blood eosinophilia (30 to 60% of an elevated total leukocyte count), much like patients with tropical eosinophilia (Ch. 388.3). Diagnosis in these patients often cannot be made parasitologically and must be based on the characteristic history, clinical presentation, blood eosinophilia, and elevated filarial antibody titers. If untreated, a small (but undefined) percentage of such patients develops severe cardiomyopathy, presumably secondary to the hypereosinophilia elicited by the infection.

Treatment is with DEC, 6 to 10 mg per kilogram per day for 2 to 3 weeks. The drug is extremely effective against microfilariae, but less so against adult worms, so that multiple courses of treatment are often necessary before signs and symptoms completely resolve. In cases of heavy microfilaremia (greater than several hundred microfilariae per milliliter of blood), inflammatory reactions may be so severe as to include coma and death. Thus, treatment of such persons must be done cautiously, using one or more of the following options: very low initial DEC doses, pretreatment with steroids, pheresis to remove circulating microfilariae, or albendazole, instead of DEC, which appears to kill adult worms but not the microfilariae. DEC is effective in preventing loiasis when taken in prophylactic doses of 300 mg weekly.

Carme B, Boulesteix J, Boutes H, et al.: Five cases of encephalitis during treatment of loiasis with diethylcarbamazine. Am J Trop Med Hyg 44:684, 1991. An excellent critical review of the past experiences and implications of the likelihood of encephalitis developing following treatment of loiasis patients with diethylcarbamazine.
Klion AD, Ottesen EA, Nutman TB: Effectiveness of diethylcarbamazine in treating loiasis acquired by expatriate visitors to endemic regions: Long-term follow up. J Infect Dis 169:604, 1994. Thirty-two expatriates with loiasis contracted in endemic areas were treated one or more times with 3-week courses of DEC and were followed 2 to 15 years after treatment. Only 38% were cured after one course of treatment, and no clinical or laboratory parameters (including eosinophilia and specific filarial serology) were found either to predict a successful outcome posttreatment or to define when a patient was completely cured.
Nutman TB, Miller KD, Mulligan M, et al.: Diethylcarbamazine prophylaxis for human loiasis: Results of a double-blinded study. N Engl J Med 319:752, 1988. A placebo-controlled study in Peace Corps volunteers showing clearly that clinical loiasis can be prevented by weekly DEC in long-term visitors to endemic countries.

388.6 Dracunculiasis

Dracunculiasis, or guinea worm disease, is caused by infection with the parasite Dracunculus medinensis. It occurs in the Indian subcontinent and Africa, where up to 1 million persons living in rural areas are affected annually; more than 100 million persons remain at risk of infection.

Diagnosis of patent infections is easy. The thin adult female worms, each up to 1 meter long, emerge directly through the skin, usually of the lower leg, ankle, or foot. The worms emerge 10 to 14 months after victims have drunk water containing infected Cyclops, a barely visible crustacean that serves as the parasite's intermediate host. When persons harboring such emerging worms enter a stag-

nant source of drinking water, such as a step well or pond, larvae are released into the water, where some are ingested by Cyclops. When humans drink water containing Cyclops with infective larvae, the larvae penetrate the intestinal or stomach wall, mature, and mate, after which the male worms die.

The adult worms emerge slowly, over a period of weeks or months. Emergence may be preceded by generalized allergic symptoms and is usually accompanied by a blister that ruptures to form an ulcer at the site of emergence. Some worms present first as a serpentine cord just beneath the skin or at the center of an abscess. No immunity develops, so persons in endemic areas are infected year after year.

The great social and economic significance of dracunculiasis, which rarely is fatal, derives from the fact that emergence of the worm is very painful and is often associated with swelling, local arthritis, and secondary infection. Thus, victims are often unable to farm or sometimes even walk for weeks or months. Over half of the adults in a village may be crippled at the same time, and the seasonal infection tends to occur precisely when villagers need to harvest or plant their crops. School attendance is also affected.

Treatment is difficult because anthelminthics such as thiabendazole or metronidazole only marginally reduce the duration of emergence and associated pain. Aspirin can help relieve the pain. Emerging worms are best rolled around a small stick as their predecessors have been for centuries, care being taken not to break the worm (which would exacerbate the inflammation). Some worms can be removed surgically. Victims should be immunized against tetanus, which is sometimes caused by secondary infection of the ulcer around the emerging worm. Persons at risk should be taught to boil their drinking water or filter it through a cloth and to avoid entering sources of drinking water when the infection is patent.

Because the most effective intervention against this infection is to provide safe drinking water, efforts began during the International Drinking Water Supply and Sanitation Decade (1981–1990) to provide safe water to dracunculiasis-endemic areas as a priority and thereby eliminate the disease. By the end of 1993 all endemic countries were working to eradicate the disease by 1995. The annual number of cases of dracunculiasis reported to WHO was reduced by 75% between 1989 and 1993.

Hopkins DR, Ruiz-Tiben E, Kaiser RL, et al.: Dracunculiasis eradication: Beginning of the end. Am J Trop Med Hyg 49:281, 1993. A recent review of all aspects pertaining to control and eradication of dracunculiasis.

388.7 Other Filarial Infections

PERSTANS FILARIASIS

Mansonella perstans (formerly Dipetalonema perstans, Acanthocheilonema perstans) is distributed in a broad belt across the center of Africa and in northeast South America. Adult worms, up to 70 to 80 mm long, reside in the body cavities (pleural, peritoneal, and pericardial) and in the mesentery, perirenal, and retroperitoneal tissues. Microfilariae are liberated unsheathed from the females and circulate in the blood without regular periodicity.

M. perstans infection was long thought to be asymptomatic, because up to 90% of individuals with the parasite appeared to have no difficulty with it. Subsequent studies, however, indicate clearly that M. perstans is capable of inducing a variety of symptoms, including angioedematous swellings much like the "Calabar swellings" of loiasis; fever; headache; pain in bursae and/or joint synovia, in serous cavities, or over the liver; neurologic or psychologic symptoms; and extreme exhaustion. There is some evidence that symptoms are more prominent in outsiders coming to endemic regions, but in all series at least a quarter of such patients were asymptomatic despite persistent microfilaremia.

Treatment with DEC,† 5 to 6 mg per kilogram per day for 2 to 3 weeks is often ineffective, and although other drugs have been tried (e.g., mebendazole, albendazole, ivermectin), none has proven to be reliably effective. When the parasites are eliminated, however, patients characteristically lose their symptoms (no matter how vague), lose their eosinophilia, and regain a sense of well-being.

Adolph PE, Kagan IG, McQuay RM: Diagnosis and treatment of *Acanthocheilonema perstans* filariasis. Am J Trop Med Hyg 11:76, 1962. *Results from a series of patients observed in the United States after returning from missionary work in Africa.*

Clarke V deV, Harwin RM, MacDonald DF, et al.: Filariasis: *Dipetalonema perstans* infections in Rhodesia. Cent Afr J Med 17:1, 1971. *Discussion of the clinical expression of M. perstans filariasis in Africans and Europeans living in East Africa.*

STREPTOCERCIASIS

Mansonella streptocerca is transmitted by midges, especially *Culicoides grahami*. It occurs in the tropical forest belt of Africa from Ghana to Zaire. The adult worms are subcutaneous, especially over the torso; and the microfilariae, which have characteristic shepherd's-crook tails, are found in the skin (see Ch. 388.4 for skin-snipping technique).

Infection is usually symptomless, but the adult worms may produce hypopigmented macules (to be distinguished from leprosy), and the microfilariae occasionally cause pruritic papular rashes similar to those of onchocerciasis. Both adult worms and microfilariae are killed by DEC† (e.g., 7 to 10 days of treatment at 6 mg per kilogram per day).

Meyers WM, Connor DH, et al.: Human streptocerciasis: A clinicopathologic study of 40 Africans (Zairians) including identification of the adult filaria. Am J Trop Med Hyg 21:528, 1972. *Covers the clinical aspects and gives references to other aspects.*

MANSONELLA OZZARDI INFECTION

M. ozzardi is restricted in distribution to Central and South America and certain islands of the Caribbean. Adult worms have been recovered in humans only twice, both times from the peritoneal cavity. *Unsheathed* microfilariae circulate in the blood with little or no periodicity.

Many investigators consider these parasites to be nonpathogenic, but one of the fullest clinical studies of an affected population found that the major clinical presentation is severe articular pain or dysfunction, especially in the arms and shoulders. Headache, fever, pulmonary symptoms, adenopathy, hepatomegaly, and pruritic skin eruptions also occurred in a small number of patients with a frequency greater than that in nonparasitized individuals in the same population. DEC† has little or no effect on this infection, but ivermectin‡ appears to be effective therapy.

Marinkelle CJ, German E: Mansonelliasis in the comisaria del Vaupes of Colombia. Trop Geogr Med 22:101, 1970. *A very complete and interesting account of clinical manifestations ascribed to M. ozzardi infections in South American Indians.*

Nutman TB, Nash TE, Ottesen EA: Ivermectin in the successful treatment of a patient with *Mansonella ozzardi* infection. J Infect Dis 156:662, 1987. *A single case report presenting clinical and immunologic evidence for the effectiveness of ivermectin (140 μg per kilogram given once) in an M. ozzardi infection.*

HUMAN DIROFILARIASIS

Dirofilaria species are filarial parasites mostly of dogs, cats, and raccoons that sometimes infect humans but almost never fully develop to complete their life cycles in this abnormal host. The distribution of cases is worldwide and reflects the distribution of the parasites in animals.

Two general types of clinical presentation predominate. Pulmonary dirofilariasis, caused by the dog heartworm *D. immitis,* usually presents as an asymptomatic solitary pulmonary nodule but occasionally with chest pain, cough, or hemoptysis. Microscopically there is local eosinophilia and granuloma formation accompanied by infarction and thrombosis around an impacted, immature worm. The second common clinical presentation is that of a subcutaneous nodule found anywhere on the body (or within the eye) that results usually from infection with the subcutaneous dwelling filarids of dogs (*D. repens*) or raccoons (*D. tenuis*) but occasionally from infection with *D. immitis.* Local lesions again are granulomatous and eosinophilic and are sometimes accompanied by bacterial superinfection.

Definitive diagnosis and treatment most often result from the same surgical (excisional) procedure. Blood eosinophilia is not a *regular* finding in these patients nor are detectable antifilarial antibodies. Furthermore, because the worms are usually incompletely developed, microfilaremia occurs only in the rarest of circumstances. These "abnormal" parasite infections do not respond to DEC, and their treatment is primarily surgical.

Dissanaike AS: Zoonotic aspects of filarial infections in man. Bull WHO 57:349, 1979. *A scholarly, readable discussion of the human's interaction with zoonotic filarial infections.*

389 ARTHROPODS AND LEECHES

William L. Krinsky

ARTHROPODS AS AGENTS OF DISEASE

Disease associated directly with arthropods results from toxins, or allergic responses to the organisms or their products when humans are exposed by bites or stings, simple contact, or invasion through the skin or natural orifices. Arthropods most often involved in these types of exposure are listed in Table 389–1.

Physicians usually become aware of insects and their relatives (spiders, mites, ticks, scorpions, millipedes, and centipedes) when patients present with skin lesions caused by arthropods, when infestations of the creatures themselves are seen, when foreign bodies extracted from skin or sense organs are identified as arthropods, or when respiratory symptoms develop in response to arthropods or their products. Dermatoses associated with arthropods and human infestations with arthropods (e.g., lice, mites, fly larvae) are discussed in detail in this chapter. Arthropods as vectors are mentioned here; detailed discussions of arthropod-borne pathogens may be found elsewhere in this book.

Biting Arthropods

LOUSE INFESTATIONS (Pediculosis)

Pediculosis is infestation of the body with lice. The observation of louse eggs (nits) cemented to hairs of the scalp or lice themselves confirms the diagnosis of head louse (*Pediculus capitis*) infestation. Nits (or lice) attached to the seams of clothing (often in undergarments) indicate the presence of body lice (*P. humanus*), and nits or lice attached to pubic hairs indicate a pubic (crab) louse (*Phthirus pubis*) infestation.

The eggs are pearly yellow-white and opaque, elongate-oval, about 0.8 mm long and 0.3 mm wide, and are attached singly to each hair or clothing fiber. After hatching, the nits appear translucent and opalescent. Although nits may be numerous, usually not more than 10 to 20 lice are associated with infested persons. The head louse egg is cemented on a hair about 1 mm above the scalp surface.

Head and body lice are very similar in appearance. Adult head lice are 2.5 to 3.5 mm long, and adult body lice are 3.0 to 4.5 mm

TABLE 389–1. ARTHROPODS CAUSING HUMAN PATHOLOGY

Human Exposure	Arthropod	Antigens or Toxins
Bites	Insects (lice, bedbugs, and other true bugs; fleas; flies including mosquitoes, black flies, biting midges, sandflies, horse and deer flies, stable flies, tsetse flies, keds; ants)	Salivary secretions, venoms
	Arachnids (chigger and other rodent and bird mites; ticks, spiders)	
	Centipedes	
Stings	Insects (some ants, wasps, and bees)	Venoms
	Arachnids (scorpions)	
Invasion	Insects (fly larvae, *Tunga* fleas)	Salivary secretions, excretions
	Arachnids (scabies mites)	
Simple contact	Insects (caterpillars, pupae, or adults of moths and butterflies; blister and some rove beetles)	Setae, spines, secretions (venoms) and excretions
	Arachnids (stored product mites)	
	Millipedes	

long. Each immature and adult head and body louse has three pairs of about equal-sized legs bearing claws for gripping hairs or fibers. Adult pubic lice, somewhat crablike in appearance, are 1 to 2 mm long, about as broad, grayish white or yellowish brown, and they have forelegs narrower than the other pairs. All immature lice (three stages in each species) resemble their respective adults except in size, and all immature lice and adults are obligate bloodsucking ectoparasites. The body louse is the only known natural vector of the pathogens of louse-borne typhus, trench fever, and louse-borne relapsing fever.

Head lice and their nits are found most frequently in the hair over the postauricular and occipital regions. Body lice are usually not found on the body but are seen in clothing, with nits in the seams and creases in areas that contact the body. Crab lice and nits are found on hairs in the pubic and perianal regions, sometimes on hairs on the thighs and abdomen, less commonly on axillary hairs, beard, mustache, eyebrows, eyelashes, and rarely on the scalp. Pubic infestations are found only in postpubertal individuals.

The skin lesions produced by the bites of lice are erythematous papules that may be accompanied by urticaria or lymphadenopathy. Extensive erythema and pruritus result from hypersensitivity to louse saliva. Crab lice typically induce nonpruritic small gray-blue macules (0.3 to 1.0 cm in diameter) with irregular borders (maculae ceruleae) that may persist for months. The lesions produced by any of the species may be covered with hair matted with eggs, dried serous secretions, and dark louse excrement. The latter, seen on the body or in underclothing, should trigger a search for lice. Excoriations from scratching disguise bite lesions and may lead to impetigo or to furuncular or eczematous lesions. The possibility of louse infestation should be considered when pyoderma is seen. The combination of lichenification and pigmentation in chronically infested individuals is called vagabond's disease (morbus vagabondus). A nondescript macular or papular erythematous rash on the trunk may be the presenting sign for an undiscovered head louse infestation. Postauricular and posterior cervical lymphadenopathy in the absence of other node enlargement should suggest head lice. Body louse infestation may be differentiated from scabies by the absence of lesions on the hands and feet and the common occurrence of lesions in the intrascapular region. The differential diagnosis of louse-induced dermatitis from various mite-induced lesions or non–arthropod-associated dermatoses is made by finding nits or lice.

Treatment includes shampoos, creams, and lotions containing insecticides. The most often used preparations contain lindane (γ benzene hexachloride) or pyrethrins. Malathion and permethrin, a synthetic pyrethrin, are being used more frequently because of their ovicidal effect. One effective treatment for head lice is a shampoo with permethrin (1%) creme rinse. Pubic louse infestations in nonocular regions are effectively treated with a 5-minute application of lindane (1%) shampoo to the infested areas. Lindane should be used with caution on infants, children, and pregnant women. Infested clothing and linen should be washed in hot water (60°C) for 20 minutes or dry cleaned.

After treatment, lice and nits can be removed using a metal comb with teeth 0.1 mm apart. Moisture or oil rinses may make this easier. Mechanical removal is recommended for facial pubic louse infestations.

Preventing recurrence involves treatment of infested human contacts and materials (fomites). Pillow cases, hats, scarves, and other items should be washed or cleaned. Infested combs and brushes should be cleaned and boiled or soaked for 1 hour in lindane shampoo or Lysol (2%). Head and body lice survive only about 3 days (10 days maximum) away from the body. Sexual partners of persons with pubic lice should be treated, and bedding, towels, and clothing should be washed or dry cleaned. Pubic lice do not survive longer than 24 hours away from a body. Transmission via toilet seats is unlikely. Fumigation after any louse infestation is unnecessary, but vacuuming is helpful to remove stray lice and shed hairs with affixed nits.

FLEA BITES

Most fleas, unlike lice, do not infest the body. The common flea species that suck blood from humans visit the body for a few min-

utes to hours, when feeding occurs. As in louse infestations, flea bites generally cause pruritus. Each bite lesion is an erythematous papule with a hemorrhagic punctum. Sensitization of an individual to flea saliva may result in papular urticaria (common in affected children), bullous eruptions, or erythema multiforme-type lesions. Bites are usually multiple and irregularly grouped. Bites in adults appear as widespread papules that become lichenified or as grouped papules overlying erythema or edema. Persons entering a previously infested room that has been vacant for weeks or months often suffer from multiple bites on the ankles and legs as hungry fleas emerge from pupal cocoons in floor crevices, debris, or carpeting. As with louse bites, excoriated lesions may become infected and furuncular.

Flea eggs are usually laid off the host, and larvae live off the host, feeding on organic debris. Adults reach their hosts by jumping. Flea species that most often bite humans are the cat flea (Ctenocephalides felis), the dog flea (C. canis), and the human flea (Pulex irritans). Occasionally, household infestations with fleas may arise from abandoned wild animal nests built near houses.

Treatment of flea bites is symptomatic and involves using antipruritic and anti-inflammatory creams or lotions or oral antihistamines. Secondary infections may require antibiotic therapy. Infested pets should be treated with specific insecticides. Floors, carpets, upholstered furnishings, and pets' sleeping quarters should be sprayed or dusted with insecticides to kill larval, pupal, and adult fleas. A thorough cleaning, including vacuuming, of infested premises should eliminate the insects. Because fleas at all stages can live for weeks or months, a repeat insecticide application may be necessary.

Persons may protect themselves from fleas with repellents containing diethyl metatoluamide. Wild animal (especially rodent) fleas that feed on humans may transmit the bacilli of plague or tularemia, as well as the less virulent rickettsia of murine (flea-borne) typhus. Less common pathogens transmitted by accidental ingestion of fleas (mostly by children) are the dwarf tapeworm Hymenolepis diminuta and the dog tapeworm Dipylidium caninum.

BEDBUGS AND KISSING BUGS

Bedbugs (Cimicidae) are flat, mahogany-brown, wingless insects (5 to 7 mm long). Most species are bloodsucking ectoparasites of birds and bats. Two species (Cimex lectularius and C. hemipterus) feed almost exclusively on humans; the former is cosmopolitan; the latter has a tropical distribution. Both species cause irritating, pruritic bite lesions in sensitized individuals. The bugs become engorged with blood in 3 to 15 minutes and feed only at night or in subdued light. They hide in crevices of bedding, beds, floors, and furnishings and in wood and paper trash accumulations during the day. The bites are often seen in short linear groups and vary from small urticarial lesions to large erythematous papules or bullae. The lesions are often excoriated, and eczematous reactions and pyoderma may be seen. Hypersensitivity reactions may include asthma, generalized urticaria, and arthralgia. Although some affected persons complain of being awakened at night, most are troubled by the lesions on arising in the morning. Treatment is symptomatic. Prevention includes removing debris that harbors the bugs, using insecticides in crevices, and cleaning infested furnishings.

Triatomine kissing bugs (Reduviidae) that suck blood from a diversity of hosts are found in the New World subtropics and tropics and in Asia. Most of these cone-nosed bugs (8 to 38 mm long) are tan, brown, or black, with yellow or red spots around the dorsal edge of the abdomen. The bugs feed rapidly at night. Sensitive individuals may develop papular lesions, small vesicles, or, in the extreme, large urticarial or hemorrhagic nodular to bullous lesions. Generalized anaphylactoid reactions, including shock and angioneurotic and laryngeal edema, have occurred. Kissing bugs may feed anywhere on the body. Domesticated species in the tropics are found most often in thatched houses or those with mud floors. In the southwestern United States, a species (Triatoma protracta) living in wood rat nests in desert areas occasionally invades homes. Treatment of bites or allergic reactions is symptomatic. In Central and South America, these insects are vectors of Chagas' disease trypanosomes.

MOSQUITOES AND OTHER BLOODSUCKING FLIES

Mosquitoes (Culicidae) are found worldwide, breeding wherever there is stagnant water. While biting, a female mosquito (3 to 6 mm long) induces a pruritic wheal that becomes an erythematous papule. In sensitive persons, bullous lesions, cellulitis, or hemorrhagic necrotic reactions may follow the bites. Systemic anaphylactic reactions are rare. The most serious medical problems associated with mosquitoes relate to their transmission of the agents of yellow fever, dengue, arboviral encephalitides, malaria, and filariasis.

Biting midges (Ceratopogonidae), also called "punkies" or "no-see-ums" because of their minute size (most are 0.6 to 2 mm long), give a painful bite. The resulting erythematous punctiform lesions may become papular and pruritic. Vesicles may develop that ooze fluid for days. These midges, especially *Culicoides* species, bite mostly on exposed parts of the body and may be pestiferous in sandy seashore or marshy breeding areas. Biting occurs mostly at dawn or dusk.

Black flies (Simuliidae), also called buffalo gnats, are small (1 to 5 mm long), humpbacked, tan to black insects that breed only in running water. They are troublesome bloodsuckers in northern temperate regions. The bites may become hemorrhagic papules that ooze blood for hours. These lesions may be painful and cause recurrent pruritus. Lymphadenopathy is common in sensitive individuals, who may develop localized edema. Cephalalgia, fever, and nausea may occur following large numbers of bites. Black fly species found at high elevations in Central and South America and along rivers in Africa transmit *Onchocerca volvulus,* the etiologic agent of river blindness.

Phlebotomine sandflies (Psychodidae) are delicate, small (2 to 3 mm long), hairy flies found mainly in subtropical and tropical areas. Various species are abundant in rain forests in the New World and in arid areas in the Mediterranean region and Asia. Biting occurs at night or in subdued light. The bites may be painful, occur usually on the extremities, and cause pruritus and elevated pale urticarial lesions that become papular. Vesicular or bullous lesions may occur. Phlebotomine flies are vectors of sandfly (pappataci) fever, bartonellosis, and leishmaniasis.

Other flies that may attack humans and cause painful bites are horse and deer flies (Tabanidae), stable flies, and tsetse flies. Tsetse flies, found only in Africa, transmit the trypanosomes of African sleeping sickness.

Treatment of any of these fly bites is symptomatic and includes topical corticosteroids and oral antihistamines to reduce itching. Personal protection from biting flies involves using screen enclosures, headnets, and insect repellents. Protective clothing and open mesh jackets impregnated with repellents are effective.

CHIGGERS AND OTHER BITING MITES

Chiggers are the larvae (six-legged stage) of trombiculid (itch or harvest) mites. These larvae (0.15 to 0.40 mm long) are white to yellow or orange-red and are found on many vertebrates. Human infestation occurs following contact with grassy or shrubby vegetation inhabited by the mites. First exposure may not produce dermatitis or may produce only slightly irritating, transient erythematous macules or papules (1 to 2 mm). The more commonly seen skin reactions to chigger feeding are extremely pruritic, papular, papulovesicular, or papulourticarial lesions (4 to 20 mm) that persist with burning and itching for days to weeks. The lesions may fade and flatten or become hemorrhagic, purpuric, or vesicular. Diagnosis depends on morphology and distribution of lesions, exposure history, and observation of the mites. Engorging chiggers may be apparent as minute reddish blebs embedded in hair follicles. The mites most often attach to skin covered by clothing, especially near belts, straps, or elastic bindings. Scrub itch mites of Asia and South Pacific Islands usually do not cause dermatitis, but they are vectors of scrub typhus rickettsiae.

Other biting mites that are rarely recovered from the lesions they cause are pyemotid (straw, hay, or grain itch) mites, cheyletoid (cat or dog fur and predatory) mites, and dermanyssid (chicken, red, house mouse, tropical rat, fowl, and rodent) mites. All of these mites are extremely small (about 0.4 to 1 mm long), and depending on the species, the six-legged larvae or eight-legged nymphs and adults may attack humans. The resulting skin lesions may be extremely variable.

The differential diagnosis of mite-induced dermatitis depends on associating the patient with a source of mites. Sources include wild and domestic animals, agricultural commodities, dried floral arrangements, infested furniture, and, in chigger-associated cases, particular outdoor habitats.

Treatment of dermatitis is symptomatic. Antipruritic lotions and creams or oral antihistamines are useful. Secondary infections may require antibiotic therapy. Rare allergic reactions, including edema and asthma, require emergency treatment. Prevention of recurrences depends on destroying or fumigating the mite source. Personal repellents (containing sulfur or diethyltoluamide) are helpful in preventing chigger infestation, although avoiding infested areas is the best prevention. *Rickettsia tsutsugamushi* is the only pathogen of major medical importance specifically associated with mite transmission. *R. akari,* the causative agent of rickettsialpox, is transmitted by the house mouse mite.

TICK BITES AND TICK PARALYSIS

Ticks, like mites, are arachnids that have six-legged larvae and eight-legged nymphs and adults. Ticks, found worldwide, are grouped in two major families, soft ticks (Argasidae) and hard ticks (Ixodidae). The former, which have rugose integuments, are associated with restricted habitats, such as rodent burrows and bird nests, and rarely feed on humans. When they do, most attach for only a matter of minutes and produce maculate, erythematous lesions (6 to 30 mm in diameter). Some species in Africa cause extensive ecchymosis; pain, pruritus, edema, ulceration, and necrotic lesions have also been observed. The pajoroello (talaja) tick (*Ornithodoros coriaceus),* found in Mexico, California, and Oregon, is known to produce hemorrhagic, painful lesions. Soft ticks are of primary medical importance as vectors of the borreliae of relapsing fevers.

Hard ticks have smooth, hard, shiny integuments and are found on a diversity of animals and in grass and forests. Ticks carried on dogs, cats, or other animals sometimes drop off and attach to humans. Hard ticks remain embedded in the skin for days while becoming engorged with blood and usually do not cause pain or discomfort. Engorging ticks, mistakenly identified as pedunculated moles or warts, are usually noticed only by chance observation. Typical tick bite lesions are small indurations with peripheral erythema. Unusual manifestations of hard tick bites include various forms of nonspecific dermatitis, acrodermatitis chronica atrophicans, necrotic ulcers, and alopecia. Most hard ticks attach, feed, drop off, and are never noticed. Nodular lesions that may persist for years at the sites of bites must be differentiated from malignant conditions, such as lymphomas. Hard ticks are vectors of the causative agents of various arboviral hemorrhagic fevers and encephalitides, several kinds of tickborne typhus (including Rocky Mountain spotted fever), tularemia, babesiosis, erhlichiosis, and Lyme disease. An engorging tick itself may induce tick paralysis (discussed below).

Attached soft ticks may be easily removed by gentle traction with a forceps. Hard ticks require strong constant traction. Use of heat, flames, or caustic substances may cause unnecessary harm to the patient. Hard ticks, embedded in sensitive sites, such as the ear canal or genitals, may be covered with petrolatum. The ticks then detach within about 2 hours and can be gently removed. Complete extraction of the mouthparts lessens the chance of secondary infection. Persistent nodules that cause discomfort should be surgically excised.

Tick paralysis is an unusual form of ascending flaccid paralysis that occurs while a tick is attached to the body. Mostly children (especially girls) are affected. Tick paralysis in humans has been associated with only a small number of hard tick species in North America, Europe, South Africa, and Australia. Most cases have been caused by the Rocky Mountain wood tick (*Dermacentor andersoni*) in western North America and the common dog tick (*D. variabilis*) in eastern North America. Although nonspecific numbness or irritability may occur before the onset of paralysis, the initial consistent sign is *weakness in the legs.* Leg tendon reflexes are reduced or absent, and Romberg's sign is often present. Sensory changes are rarely noted. Blood counts and lumbar puncture usually give no indication of the disease. Complete paralysis of the extremities may occur within a few days after a tick attaches. If the cause is unrecognized, paralysis usually progresses, causing speech dysfunction, dysphagia, and ultimately death from aspiration or respiratory paralysis. If a tick is found, removal usually results in reversal of paralysis with a return to normal function in hours to weeks, depending on the severity of the neurologic deficit. The patient should be examined for other ticks, with special attention to concealed areas, such as the scalp, ear canals, axillae, popliteal fossae, anus, and genitals. Even after all ticks are removed, death may occur from bulbar or respiratory paralysis.

The clinical presentation of tick paralysis may suggest poliomyelitis, Guillain-Barré syndrome, diphtheritic polyneuropathy, transverse myelitis, botulism, or other acutely developing neuropathies. The specific agent of *Dermacentor* tick paralysis is unknown. Prevention of tick bites and tick paralysis includes avoiding tick-infested habitats. Individuals and their pets who enter such habitats should be thoroughly examined for ticks. Personal measures that may prevent ticks from reaching the skin include wearing long-sleeved shirts and long pants, tucking pants legs into socks, and using chemical repellents.

SPIDER BITES

All spiders are eight-legged arachnids that use venom to immobilize their prey. Relatively few species have mouthparts (chelicerae) large and strong enough to inject venom into human skin. Among the better known spiders that cause moderate to severe reactions in humans are the widows (*Latrodectus* species) of the Old and New World, brown spiders (*Loxosceles* species) of the Americas and southern Africa, wandering spiders (*Phoneutria* species) in South America, species of *Chiracanthium* in both hemispheres, and funnel web spiders (*Atrax* species) in Australia.

The black widow (shoe button) spider (*Latrodectus mactans*) female may bite if it or its web is disturbed. Its abdomen is 6 mm wide and 9 to 13 mm long and is shiny black with a reddish hourglass marking or less well defined markings on the underside. The spider lives in sheltered, dark, dry places, such as in garages and in old stone walls and outhouses. The bite, which may not be felt, may become slightly swollen and appear as two erythematous puncture marks. Within a few hours, a bitten person develops intense muscle pains and commonly a tightening feeling in the chest. Abdominal (boardlike) rigidity and waves of excruciating cramping pain are characteristic. Respiratory distress, nausea, vomiting, profuse perspiration, headache, vertigo, paresthesias of the extremities, hyperactive reflexes, speech difficulty or visual dysfunction may occur. In untreated adults, the pathologic effects of the venom usually disappear within 2 to 3 days. Death from cardiac or respiratory arrest occurs mostly in very young children and elderly or hypertensive persons.

The differential diagnosis requires consideration of various abdominal and vascular crises, such as perforated ulcer, acute appendicitis or pancreatitis, cholelithiasis, nephrolithiasis, splenic, renal, or mesenteric embolism, volvulus, porphyria, tetanus, and strychnine and lead poisoning. The generalized muscle pain, the lack of abdominal tenderness, and the peripheral sensory changes help to differentiate the widow spider bite.

A specific antivenin is effective against all *Latrodectus* venom and neutralizes the effects of the venom. Because the antivenin is derived from horses, horse serum sensitivity testing is required before the antivenin is administered. Parenteral opioids and benzodiazepines relieve pain in patients who cannot take antivenin.

The brown (violin or fiddleback) spiders, including *Loxosceles reclusa* (brown recluse) and *L. laeta* of the western hemisphere, are also secretive, living in secluded places in houses and nesting in clothing, and they may bite when disturbed. They are 10 to 15 mm long and have a dark violin-shaped mark on the brown to gray cephalothorax. Their bites are most often recognized when a serious condition, *necrotic arachnidism,* is the result. The sometimes painful lesion that develops 2 to 6 hours after a bite is a bulla or pustule surrounded by concentric rings of ischemia and erythema. Within 24 to 48 hours, the lesion becomes cyanotic, and a central necrotic area begins to form. This area may slowly expand (up to 20 cm) over days to weeks. The resulting ulcer may not heal for weeks or months. Systemic reactions to the bite include fever, chills, edema, nausea, vomiting, dizziness, myalgias, and arthralgias; morbilliform and petechial eruptions may occur within 48 hours of the bite. A fatal complication, most often seen in children, is *intravascular hemolysis,* followed by hemoglobinuria and acute renal failure.

Treatment of necrotizing lesions is mainly symptomatic and may include antibiotic therapy for secondary infection. Curettage of bite wounds under local anesthesia as well as dapsone therapy promotes healing.

CENTIPEDE BITES

Centipedes are multilegged, elongated (up to 30 cm) arthropods with one pair of legs on each body segment. The first pair of legs is modified as poison claws that are used to inject venom into prey. Centipedes, which shun the light and are found under rocks and forest litter, rarely bite. The characteristic bite lesion has two punctate hemorrhages in the center of an erythematous swelling. Centipede bites may cause severe (fiery) local pain that may be followed by inflammation, edema, and superficial necrosis. Systemic reactions may include headache, dizziness, and vomiting. The transient effects of a bite may be accompanied by irregular pulse, muscle spasm, or lymphadenopathy. In general, centipede bites cause no long-term pathologic effects.

Stinging Arthropods

BEE, WASP, AND ANT STINGS

Bees, wasps, and ants (order Hymenoptera) include solitary and social species. Females have an egg-laying tube (ovipositor) that has been modified as a sting that secretes venom from abdominal glands. Social bees include honeybees and bumblebees, which all have two pairs of membranous wings and are stocky, hairy, and often yellow and black or brown. The honeybee *(Apis mellifera)* and its close relatives are found worldwide and often are responsible for human sting reactions. The honeybee has a barbed sting that becomes embedded in skin, and as the bee tries to escape, it leaves its venom apparatus and other abdominal organs and soon perishes. Vespid wasps (yellow jackets, hornets, paper wasps) are smooth insects, sleeker than bees and often yellow and black or with combinations of yellow, red, brown, or black. These wasps make the paper nests found in trees, under eaves of houses, or underground. Honeybees and bumblebees may sting when disturbed while seeking nectar or pollen at flowers. Vespid wasps may become pestiferous around food. Mutillid wasps (velvet ants, cow killers), which are hairy and wingless, sometimes sting in sandy, arid environments.

Human reactions to stings usually include intense local pain, followed by the appearance of a red punctum surrounded by a blanched area and erythema. A wheal forms and the swelling and erythema, accompanied by pruritus, may last for a few hours. Multiple stings, especially on the face, may cause extensive edema, multiple vesicles, bullae, or purpura. Treatment includes gentle removal of the sting by scraping with a sharp blade (in cases of honeybee envenomation), and use of ice and topical hydrocortisone or oral antihistamines. Severe and sometimes fatal allergic reactions to stings of bees and wasps in sensitized individuals are discussed in Ch. 227.

Ants (Formicidae) of some species can sting, causing severe pain. Two groups of New World stinging ants are the fire ants (*Solenopsis* species) and harvester ants (*Pogonomyrmex* species). These ants build ground nests that protrude as large mounds. An ant may grip the skin with its mandibles and then insert its sting. The ant may pivot and sting many times. This behavior, compounded by the common occurrence of mass attacks, leads to a clustering of lesions. The usual reaction to the sting is fiery, sharp pain, followed by a wheal and flare response. A clear vesicle appears that becomes pustular after about 24 hours. This sterile pustule may persist for 3 to 10 days and dry as a crust that sloughs, leaving a macule, scar, or fibrous nodule. Systemic reactions such as dizziness, nausea, vomiting, profuse perspiration, cyanosis, and asthma occur in allergic individuals but may also be seen in cases of multiple stings. Symptomatic treatment of local reactions is similar to that for bee and wasp stings.

SCORPION STINGS

Scorpions are mostly subtropical and tropical arachnids that have a pair of lobster-like claws (pedipalps) anteriorly and a curved spine posteriorly that is an outlet for the proteinaceous venom produced by a pair of venom glands. Scorpions are nocturnal predators that sting quickly and repeatedly when disturbed in their hiding places under rocks, lumber, and vegetation or in shoes, bedding, or clothing left on the ground. In the United States, one scorpion species, *Centruroides exilicauda,* of about 40 native species causes severe pathologic effects. This small (about 6 cm long), straw-colored species is found in Arizona. The arid regions that extend from

North Africa to India are inhabited by the most abundant and dangerous scorpions.

The nature and severity of human reactions to scorpion stings are not consistent with the size, appearance, or aggressiveness of different species. Intense and immediate pain at the site of a sting is common to all cases. When a mildly toxic scorpion is involved, the pain may be followed by local swelling and perhaps skin discoloration, regional lymphadenopathy, pruritus, or paresthesias, and less commonly by nausea and vomiting. These reactions are transient, lasting for minutes to as long as 24 hours. The more toxic species cause local pain but little or no skin response, and systemic effects are usually noted within a few minutes to 24 hours after the sting. Symptoms may include anxiety, drowsiness, syncope, increased salivation, lacrimation, perspiration, diminished vision, photophobia, numbness and sluggishness of the tongue, vomiting, diarrhea or involuntary defecation and micturition, priapism, muscular fibrillations or spasms, and convulsions. Clinical signs may include hypotension or hypertension, irregular pulse, tachycardia and arrhythmias, irregular respiration, rapid shifts in body temperature, oliguria or polyuria, and hemiplegia. Laboratory tests may reveal hyperglycemia, glycosuria, aspartate transaminase (AST) increase, hematuria, and melena. Pathologic changes that may lead to death include myocarditis, pulmonary edema, and shock. Respiratory paralysis is the usual immediate cause of death. In the most toxic cases, death may occur within minutes of the sting or not for over 40 hours later, but most deaths occur in 2 to 20 hours after the sting. The mortality is highest in children. It is important to closely monitor affected patients because sudden relapses, often involving acute respiratory distress, may occur after a patient's condition seems to have stabilized.

The most important treatment for moderate to very toxic stings is an antivenin. Antivenin to *C. exilicauda* is available in Arizona from the Antivenom Production Laboratory, Arizona State University, Tempe, Arizona 85281 (602-965-6443 or 602-965-1457) and Poison Control in Phoenix (602-253-3334). Antivenins against other species are available from laboratories in Mexico, Brazil, Europe, Africa, and Asia. In India, where antivenin is not available, acute pulmonary edema and hypertension have been successfully treated with vasodilators, such as prazosin hydrochloride.

Early treatment of stings may include cooling the sting site for up to 2 hours and using a local anesthetic. Oxygen administration or artificial respiration, sodium phenobarbital injection, and parenteral solutions, including blood plasma, may be needed to treat respiratory distress, convulsions, and shock, respectively. Calcium gluconate (10 ml of 10% solution) given as a slow intravenous injection reduces muscle spasms. In the United States, morphine and meperidine are contraindicated because they enhance the toxic effects of *C. exilicauda* venom. Morphine and barbiturates are not recommended for treating scorpion stings because these drugs inhibit the bulbar respiratory centers.

Personal protection includes wearing heavy gloves and boots when reaching into hidden areas in which scorpions may hide. Shaking out shoes and other materials left on the ground before using them is essential. Removing litter from around houses, sealing cracks in foundations, and selective use of pesticides are helpful means of preventing scorpions from inhabiting houses and gardens.

Invasive Arthropods

SCABIES

The scabies mite *(Sarcoptes scabiei)*, unlike the other mites discussed, burrows into the skin and, because it reproduces on humans, can maintain a continuous infestation. Fertile female mites burrow into the skin and lay their eggs as they tunnel. Immature stages (larvae and nymphs) move out to the surface and enter hair follicles. Further development and mating take place near the skin surface. The mite burrows are slightly raised, curved, or tortuous gray lines, 5 to 15 mm long, and at the end of each is a female, a minute pearly bleb. The burrows are restricted to the horny layer of the skin and occur most often in the sides of the fingers, the interdigital webs, flexor surfaces of the wrists, elbows, skin around the nipples, and penis. Other lesions, including erythematous papules, lichenified patches, and pustules, which occur in sites other than the burrows, may be seen on the abdomen, thighs, and buttocks. In infants and young children, burrows may occur in the palms and soles, and papular lesions may be seen on the scalp, face, and neck.

Intense pruritus begins from 2 to 6 weeks after first exposure to the mite. Definitive diagnosis of the lesions is often difficult because of excoriations. In very clean individuals, few lesions may be present, and burrows may not be clearly visible. Generalized urticarial papules may result from previous treatment with fluorinated corticosteroids. Some patients have pruritic inflammatory nodules (≤ 12 mm in diameter) that occur on covered skin, especially the axillae, abdomen, scrotum, and penis. A severe form of scabies most often seen in immunologically compromised persons is called *crusted scabies.* As the name implies, warty plaques occur frequently on the hands and feet, and extensive scaling covers the scalp to the trunk or below. Horny debris collects under the fingernails, which are usually distorted and thickened. Pruritus, erythema, and lymphadenopathy may occur.

Diagnosis of any scabies infestation depends on observing a mite in skin scrapings of a burrow or *in situ,* by gently raising the top of a burrow with a sterile needle and looking with a magnifier. In most scabies cases, only 10 to 15 mites are present on the body. In crusted scabies, large numbers of mites are present. To obtain a scraping of a burrow, an area suspected of infestation is scraped with a scalpel blade. The scraped material is examined at 50 to 100 times magnification. The movements of a living mite may be observed if the material is placed on a slide without any mounting media. Otherwise, the scraping may be cleared in potassium hydroxide (20%) or suspended in mineral oil under a coverslip on the slide. The adult female mite is about 300 to 400 μm long, oval, with the dorsum convex and venter flattened. It has four pairs of legs, two pairs directed anteriorly and two posteriorly. Each anterior leg ends in an unjointed stalk with a distensible thin-walled sac at its tip; each posterior leg ends in a long, thick bristle. The size of the mite egg is about 100×150 μm.

Scabies lesions initially may be diagnosed as those of other skin conditions, e.g., neurodermatitis, dermatitis herpetiformis, lichen planus, and various other kinds of mite-associated dermatitis, such as that caused by *Cheyletiella* fur mites. The distribution of lesions and observation of the mite rule out these other diagnoses. Secondary infections appearing as pyoderma are common, and nephrogenic strains of streptococci infecting the lesions may cause acute glomerulonephritis.

Treatment of uncomplicated scabies is with one of various acaricides. Permethrin (5% in dermal cream) in a single-dose regimen of 8 to 14 hours has recently been used with success. Lindane (1%) cream or lotion is often used in an 8- to 12-hour treatment for adults, followed by thorough washing. Use of lindane on infants and pregnant women is discouraged. Pruritus and dermatitis may persist for days after adequate treatment. Antipruritic medications are often prescribed.

Transmission occurs during contact with infested persons or with clothing recently worn by such persons. Transmission between bed partners is common and does not require body contact. All household and intimate contacts should be treated to prevent recurrence or continued transmission. The female mite survives for only 2 to 3 days away from a host; therefore, as with louse infestations, fumigation is unnecessary. Clothing, especially undergarments, bedding, and towels, should be laundered in hot water.

Scabies mites infesting domestic animals, including dogs and cats, occasionally cause dermatitis in humans, but the lesions are usually limited to the areas that contact the animals. These mites are usually not recovered from humans.

MYIASIS AND TUNGIASIS

Myiasis is the infestation of living vertebrate tissue by fly larvae. Many flies (order Diptera) that normally deposit eggs or larvae on carrion, manure, or decaying organic matter sometimes deposit their immature stages in open wounds or infected human tissues. These include blow flies, also called greenbottle or bluebottle flies (Caliphoridae), flesh flies (Sarcophagidae), and house flies (Muscidae). The larvae of some of these flies are attracted to draining infections or to clothing stained with urine or feces. The larvae crawl into lesions or natural orifices when an infected person sleeps on the ground or is otherwise exposed to flies. Individuals immobilized because of physical illness or old age who have such open lesions or infections, and especially those who are living in poor sanitary conditions, are particularly susceptible. Urogenital myiasis may cause dysuria, hematuria, and pyuria.

Some fly larvae invade intact skin of domestic animals or humans; species in this group include the human bot fly (*Dermatobia hominis*) found in Central and South America, the African tumbu fly *Cordylobia anthropophaga*, and some species of *Wohlfahrtia* that have a predilection for the tender skin of infants.

Fly larvae that live in food, e.g., vinegar flies (Drosophilidae) and cheese skippers (Piophilidae), are sometimes accidentally ingested and may cause gastrointestinal discomfort.

Wound or dermal myiasis often results in furuncular lesions, and an infested individual notices a swelling and feels pain or movement under the skin where the larvae are feeding on tissue fluids. On top of a lesion can be seen two dark respiratory openings (spiracles) through which the larva breathes. Treatment consists of gently compressing the swelling and removing the larva with a forceps. A local anesthetic may be helpful because recurved spines may hold the larva tightly under the skin. Topical antibiotics are used to control or prevent secondary infections. Removal of larvae that crawl into sensory openings or urogenital and anal orifices may require irrigation or surgical intervention. Intestinal myiasis is usually self-limited, ceasing when the larvae are passed in the stool. Dermal myiasis of most kinds, if untreated, progresses until the mature larvae back out of the skin and drop to the ground to pupate. The physical and emotional distress caused by the presence of living larvae can be prevented if a physician considers the possibility of such an infestation and removes the larvae early in the infestation. Prevention requires frequent wound dressing changes and use of window and door screens.

Tungiasis is the infestation of vertebrate, including human, skin by the female flea *Tunga penetrans* (chigoe, jigger, or sand flea). This flea occurs in sandy soil in subtropical and tropical regions of the Americas, the West Indies, and Africa. It usually feeds between the toes, under a toenail, or in the sole of the foot and becomes embedded as it gorges on blood. The flea, which remains embedded permanently, may cause irritation, pain, or pruritus, and the resulting swelling is often pustular. Secondary skin infections and tetanus are complications of infestations, and autoamputation of digits in Africans is apparently caused by inflammatory reactions to the flea.

Treatment of tungiasis includes removing the flea with a sterile needle or blade, tetanus vaccination, and use of topical antibiotics. Personal protection against *T. penetrans* includes wearing footwear and using insect repellent. Sleeping above the ground surface usually prevents the flea from reaching the body.

Arthropods and Contact Dermatitis

Various species of nonbiting mites found in stored products may cause dermatitis when they contact human skin. These microscopic foodstuff mites (Acaridae, Glycyphagidae) are found in commodities, including grains, cereals, seeds, bulbs, dried herbs, copra, dried vegetables, cured meats, mushrooms, humus, cheese, and animal and plant material used for stuffing furniture, pillows, and mattresses. Dried fruit mites (Carpoglyphidae) are found not only in dried fruits but also in jams, jellies, spoiled fruit, wine, caramel, flour, and dried milk products. The skin reactions to these mites vary, but pruritic diffuse erythema with urticarial wheals or erythematous papular eruptions is common. Laborers in granaries, food-processing plants, and commercial kitchens and dockworkers are most susceptible.

Another form of pruritic dermatitis is caused by contact with various caterpillars, pupae, adults, and some egg masses of moths and butterflies (order Lepidoptera). Urticating setae and spines on these life forms may cause mechanical irritation of the skin or may have toxic effects. Contact with setae, spines, or hairs may cause intense stinging or fiery pain, followed by the formation of wheals, local edema, erythema, and pruritus. Less common reactions include lymphadenopathy, cephalalgia, shocklike symptoms, or convulsions.

Treatment of dermatitis caused by foodstuff and dried fruit mites or lepidopteran spines or setae is symptomatic. Antipruritic substances, including antihistamines, corticosteroids, and anesthetics, have been used. Commodities containing mites must be fumigated or destroyed. Spines or setae of lepidopterans may be removed

from the skin with fine forceps. Protective clothing and thorough washing of exposed materials help prevent continuation of these forms of dermatitis.

A third form of contact dermatitis results from vesicants produced by blister beetles (Meloidae) and some rove beetles (Staphylinidae). Cantharidin, first isolated from the meloid called the Spanish fly, is found in all species of blister beetles. Contact with this substance causes mild to severe vesicular dermatitis.

Similar lesions, which usually follow a burning sensation and tanning of the skin, result from contact with millipedes. Some species of these herbivorous myriapods exude a fluid from pores along the length of the body. Secretions from the aforementioned beetles or millipedes cause burning pain and conjunctivitis if they are rubbed into the eyes.

Treatment of toxic dermatitis associated with beetles or millipedes includes rapid washing of the skin or eyes, if affected, and use of local anesthetics. The dermal reactions caused by contact with mites, lepidopterans, beetles, and millipedes are usually transitory and do not have long-lasting effects.

PENTASTOMIASIS (Linguatuliasis)

Pentastomiasis is infestation with pentastomids, little-known arthropods called tongue worms. These bloodsucking endoparasites are found as adults in the lungs of reptiles and birds or in the nasal cavity of carnivores, especially cats and dogs. Herbivores are normal intermediate hosts, but humans and other mammals can be dead-end aberrant hosts for the larvae. Ingested eggs hatch, and the larvae burrow through the intestine and migrate to diverse tissues, where they molt several times and become encysted as third-stage larvae.

Human infestations have occurred in Europe, Africa, Asia, and North, Central, and South America. Two species account for most cases, *Armillifer armillatus*, found in pythons and other vipers in tropical Africa, and *Linguatula serrata*, found in canids in Europe and the Near and Middle East.

Infection occurs by accidental ingestion of tongue worm eggs, contaminating food or drink, picked up on fingers from handling infected snakes or lizards, or from improperly cooked or raw reptiles. The third-stage larvae (20 to 25 mm long) encysted in fibrous capsules occur most often in the liver and are rarely noted except incidentally at autopsy or as calcified cysts (3 to 6 mm in diameter) on radiographs. Rarely, a mass of cysts in the intestinal wall may cause obstruction. Cysts compressing vital structures such as bile ducts or bronchi may lead to infections or obstructions.

Linguatuliasis, the direct infection of humans with third-stage larvae of *Linguatula* species, occurs most often in Lebanese people who eat raw or inadequately cooked liver or lymph nodes of goats and sheep. The ingested larvae migrate to the nasopharynx from the stomach. These larvae (5 to 10 mm long) cause Halzoun's syndrome, characterized by paroxysmal coughing, sneezing, and nasal and lacrimal discharge, accompanied by pain and itching in the throat. Other symptoms may include hoarseness, dyspnea, dysphagia, and vomiting. Submaxillary and cervical lymph nodes may be enlarged. Recovery in most cases is spontaneous in 7 to 10 days; however, death from asphyxiation due to tonsillar edema has been reported. A similar syndrome seen in Sudan, Turkey, and Greece is called Marrara's syndrome.

Prevention of pentastomiasis includes proper cooking of exotic foods such as herbivore organs and reptiles, improved hygiene of persons handling reptiles, and ingestion only of clean water and thoroughly washed raw vegetables.

LEECHES AS AGENTS OF DISEASE (Hirudiniasis)

Leeches of medical importance are bloodsucking annelid worms. Each has a ventral anterior or posterior sucker. The former encloses teeth that cut through the skin after the leech attaches. Feeding occurs within a half hour or more.

The leeches most often feeding on humans are aquatic (freshwater) species of *Hirudo*, the cosmopolitan medicinal leeches; *Limnatis*, the nasal leeches found from the Canary Islands east through Europe, Africa, and Asia; *Dinobdella*, found in Asia; and terrestrial species of *Haemadipsa*, found in Asia, Indonesia, Australia, Pacific Islands, and Central and South America. Humans are subject to attack by large leeches in tropical rain forests or to infestation with aquatic species while wading or swimming.

Wounds produced by leeches often go unnoticed, except for the oozing blood or prolonged bleeding caused by an anticoagulant, hirudin. Pruritus is common at bite sites, and although leeches are not known to transmit any human pathogens, secondary infections may occur. Immature aquatic leeches may be ingested with water and infest the upper respiratory and digestive tracts or may invade the mouth, nose, eyes, vagina, urethra, or anus of swimmers.

Attachment of leeches to the nasal passages may cause epistaxis. Attachment to the larynx may cause hoarseness, dyspnea, and hemoptysis, and attachment to the pharynx or esophagus may cause dysphagia and hematemesis. Hemorrhaging from leech infestations may be so severe, especially in children, that anemia occurs, leading to death.

Techniques used for removing leeches from the respiratory and digestive tracts include a steady pull on the specimen with a forceps or hemostat or narcotizing the leech with a spray of 5% cocaine hydrochloride before removal. In genitourinary infestations, irrigation with a strong salt solution may cause the leeches to detach. A leech attached to skin or respiratory or digestive tract surfaces may be induced to release its grip by holding it in a hemostat and touching the exposed part of the worm with a small flame or other cauterant.

Preventing attack by aquatic and land leeches includes use of protective clothing and insect repellents. Repellents applied to boots, trouser legs, and exposed skin are quite effective, but, because they are water soluble, must be reapplied every few hours in wet tropical regions where leeches are commonly found.

Alexander JO: Arthropods and Human Skin. Berlin, Springer-Verlag, 1984. *This is the first and best comprehensive text devoted to dermatologic problems associated with arthropods.*

Clark RF, Wethern-Kestner S, Vance MV, et al.: Clinical presentation and treatment of black widow spider envenomation: A review of 163 cases. Ann Emerg Med 21:782, 1992. *This is the largest reported series of* Latrodectus *envenomations and the largest series to receive antivenin.*

Drabick JJ: Pentastomiasis. Rev Infect Dis 9:1087, 1987. *This review discusses biology, parasitology, clinical manifestations, pathology, diagnosis, treatment, and epidemiology.*

Hurwitz S: Clinical Pediatric Dermatology. Philadelphia, WB Saunders, 1993, p 405. *Has excellent photographs of lice and scabies and associated skin lesions, as well as a review of flea, bedbug, mosquito, and other arthropod bites and stings.*

Southcott RV: Injuries from Coleoptera. Med J Austral 151:654, 1989. *Discusses the nature of chemical irritants produced by beetles and reviews clinical cases.*

390 SNAKE BITES
Jay P. Sanford

EPIDEMIOLOGY. Of the nearly 3500 species of snakes, fewer than one tenth are venomous. The poisonous varieties belong to five families (Table 390–1). Throughout the world, snake bites are estimated to account for 30,000 to 40,000 deaths annually. The largest number occur in Burma (Russell's viper) and Brazil (*Bothrops* species, lance-headed vipers). In the United States, the number of snake bites is estimated at 8000 per year. Twenty to 60% of the bites by venomous snakes in the United States result in little or no envenomation (poisoning). The states with the highest bite rates are North Carolina, Arkansas, Texas, Georgia, West Virginia, Mississippi, and Louisiana. Despite the large number of bites with enven-

TABLE 390–1. VENOMOUS SNAKES OF THE WORLD

Family	Common Varieties	Geographic Distribution
Crotalidae	Pit vipers (rattlesnakes, water moccasins, copperheads), fer-de-lance, bushmaster	Americas, Asia
Elapidae	Cobras, kraits, mambas, coral snakes, death adder	Worldwide except Europe
Columbridae	Boomslangs, bird snakes	Africa
Hydrophidae	Sea snakes	Indo-Pacific waters
Viperidae	True vipers (Russell's viper), puff adder	Worldwide except Americas

omation, fewer than 15 deaths occur annually, and almost all these are due to rattlesnake bites.

Coral snakes, eastern and western varieties, are found in southern and western states (North Carolina, South Carolina, Georgia, Florida, Alabama, Mississippi, Louisiana, Arkansas, Texas, New Mexico, and Arizona). Their fangs are short and permanently erect. They envenomate through chewing movements. Since they are nocturnal and shy, they rarely bite humans.

The pit vipers (Crotalidae) are identified by a small depression between the eyes and nostrils. Their fangs are long and hinged, folding back when the mouth is closed and erect when open. Upon contact, venom is expressed by muscular contraction. The pit vipers are generally aggressive. The eastern (*Crotalus adamanteus*) and western (*C. atrox*) diamondback rattlesnakes are the largest and most dangerous in the United States. Their distribution includes the aforementioned states plus California, Nevada, and Oklahoma. Cottonmouths (*Agkistrodon piscivorus),* or water moccasins, are found along streams in the southern and southeastern states. They may inflict facial bites when disturbed while resting on tree branches. Contrary to lore, they can bite under water. Copperheads (*A. contortrix),* or highland moccasins, have a geographic distribution similar to the cottonmouths. Their bite is painful but rarely fatal.

PATHOGENESIS. Because of the heterogeneous composition and multiplicity of effects, snake venoms cannot be classified simply as neurotoxic, cardiotoxic, myotoxic, or hematotoxic on the basis of the snake family (Table 390–2).

Venoms from Elapidae and Hydrophiodae snakes contain basic polypeptides that produce presynaptic and/or postsynaptic neuromuscular block with resultant flaccid paralysis, including respiratory paralysis. Cobra cardiotoxin, an additional basic polypeptide, depolarizes cell membranes of skeletal, cardiac, and smooth muscles, thus contributing to paralysis. Venom of the South American rattlesnake (*Crotalus durissus*) contains an acidic protein with nondepolarizing curare-like neuromuscular blocking effects. Viperatoxin isolated from the Palestine viper causes a peripheral nerve conduction block. A variety of enzymes, mostly hydrolases and phospholipase A, are present in most venoms. Bradykinin is released from bradykininogen by most crotalid and viperid venoms but not by Elapidae except the king cobra (*Ophiophagus hannah*). The venom of a single snake seldom contains all of the toxins. The composition and potency of venom are highly variable and differ not only among species but even among individual snakes.

SYMPTOMS AND SIGNS. *Pit Viper Envenomation.* In the United States, most victims reach a physician within 15 minutes to 3 hours. At that time, it is essential to determine whether or not en-

TABLE 390–2. BIOCHEMISTRY OF SNAKE VENOMS

Toxins	Family	Mechanism of Injury/Death
Neurotoxin (basic polypeptide)	Elapidae, Hydrophidae, South American rattlesnake (*Crotalus durissus terrificus*), Palestine viper (*Vipera palestinae*)	Respiratory paralysis
Cardiotoxin	Elapidae	Cardiovascular depression
Enzymes	Elapidae, Hydrophidae, Crotalidae, Viperidae	Hemolysis
Phospholipase A		
5-Nucleotidase		
Phosphodiesterase		
Deoxyribonuclease II		
Ribonuclease		
Adenosine-triphosphatase		
Nucleotide pyrophosphatase		
Exopeptidase		
Hyaluronidase	(Absent in spitting cobra)	
L-Amino acid oxidase		
Acetylcholinesterase	Elapidae (absent in spitting cobra, mamba, coral snake)	
Alkaline phosphatase		
Acid phosphatase		

venomation has occurred and, if it has occurred, to determine the severity; this has important therapeutic implications. The clinical effects are summarized in Table 390–3. The most important early findings are swelling at the bite, usually occurring within 10 minutes, and pain, although pain may be absent. Mild envenomation is characterized by local edema (1 to 5 inches in diameter) and pain without systemic symptoms or signs. With moderate envenomation, local findings are more extensive—edema of 6 to 12 inches in diameter. Systemic findings occur: weakness, sweating, nausea, faintness, dizziness, ecchymoses, and tender regional lymph nodes. With severe envenomation, systemic involvement includes tachycardia, tachypnea, hypothermia, hypotension, ecchymoses, paresthesias of the scalp and finger and toe tips, and muscle fasciculations. With very severe envenomation, gingival bleeding, hematemesis, hematuria, melena, oliguria, and coma occur.

Over the first 12 hours, the skin develops a tense, discolored appearance and bullae, which may be either serous or hemorrhagic.

Coral Snake Envenomation. The bite wound usually resembles scratch marks and is somewhat painful, but there is little or no edema. The onset of systemic manifestations is usually delayed 1 to 6 hours. Paresthesias around the bite may occur within several hours. Systemic symptoms may include weakness, apprehension, giddiness, nausea, vomiting, excess salivation, and even a sense of euphoria. Bulbar and cranial nerve paralysis may develop with ptosis, diplopia, papillary dilation, excess salivation, dysphagia, dysphonia, and respiratory failure. Paralysis may last 6 to 14 days, and muscular strength may not be fully regained for 6 to 8 weeks.

LABORATORY FINDINGS. Proteolytic enzymes in venoms not only damage tissue but also have a marked effect on coagulation, thrombin-like activity being most prominent. Within the first few hours, there is a drop in platelets owing to local consumption (occasionally to < 10,000 per milliliter), a decrease in fibrinogen, and an increase in fibrin degradation products. Striking increases in prothrombin time and partial thromboplastin time occur with severe envenomation. Erythrocytes show a peculiar "burring," indicating membrane damage, and drops in hematocrit and hemoglobin concentration occur.

With pit viper envenomation, baseline laboratory tests should include complete blood count, platelet count, prothrombin time, partial thromboplastin time, bleeding time, urinalysis, and serum electrolytes. Blood should be obtained for typing and crossmatching. In patients with moderate or more severe envenomation, arterial blood gas determinations and an electrocardiogram are indicated. Hematologic studies should be repeated every 4 to 6 hours for the first day or until the coagulopathy has stabilized. With coral snake envenomation, repetitive coagulation studies are not indicated.

TREATMENT. *First Aid* (Table 390–4). The initial goal of first aid is to minimize systemic absorption of the toxin. This is accomplished by restraining the patient to minimize muscular activity, applying compressive dressings, and transporting to the hospital with as little effort exerted by the patient as circumstances permit. With neurotoxic venoms, absorption may result in respiratory arrest, for which resuscitation is essential. Respiratory paralysis may develop within 15 minutes following cobra bites. The snake should be killed if this can be done quickly and safely and taken with the patient to allow accurate identification; this may obviate unnecessary therapy. The dead snake must be handled with care, since the head of an ap-

TABLE 390–4. FIRST AID: GOAL: MINIMIZE SYSTEMIC ABSORPTION OF TOXIN UNTIL ANTIVENIN CAN BE ADMINISTERED

Do's	Don'ts
Minimize muscular activity and immobilize affected part (splint the limb, carry the patient).	
Wipe bite site.	Perform incision and suction of bite wound.
Kill snake and take with patient to enable accurate identification.	Allow "dead" snake to bite care givers or patient.
Apply absorption, delaying compressive bandage over bite site and up entire limb.	Apply tourniquet or occlude arterial blood supply.
Transport to nearest medical treatment facility.	Place affected part in ice.
Observe for respiratory arrest; pulmonary resuscitation may be required.	Give patient alcohol.

parently dead snake can deliver a venomous bite for up to an hour after being severed. The potential value of incision and suction is less than the risks, which include delay in antivenin (antivenom) administration. The site of the bite should be wiped but not incised. Incisions can aggravate bleeding, damage nerves and tendons, introduce infection (especially with mouth suction), and delay healing. An absorption-delaying compressive bandage, preferably crepe (not a tourniquet), should immediately be applied firmly, as for a sprain, over the bite site and up the entire limb. The affected part should be immobilized (splinted) promptly. If available, an inflatable splint provides both compression and immobilization. The patient should be promptly transported to the nearest medical treatment facility. The compressive bandage should not be released during transit. The affected area should not be placed in ice. Cryotherapy results in greater tissue damage with the potential for necessitating amputation.

Hospital Care. On admission it is important to determine, if possible, if the bite was inflicted by a pit viper—specifically, rattlesnake, moccasin, or copperhead—or a coral snake and whether envenomation has occurred. The mainstay of therapy is physiologic monitoring in an intensive care unit and, for rattlesnake bites with envenomation, antivenin, which is a horse serum product; hence it has a high potential of causing serum sickness later. There are two antivenins: one polyvalent for North American pit vipers and another for eastern coral snakes. Water moccasin and copperhead bites can be managed without antivenin, avoiding immediate anaphylactic reactions and later serum sickness. With rattlesnake bites, for minor envenomation, antivenin is not indicated. For more serious rattlesnake envenomation, antivenin should be administered. For mild envenomation, 3 to 5 ampules of antivenin should be diluted (10 ml each) and then added to 500 ml of intravenous fluid and infused over 30 minutes to 2 hours. Antivenin should not be given as one-ampule increments. Skin or conjunctival sensitivity tests are unreliable in predicting early reactions to antivenin. All patients given antivenin should be regarded as likely to have a reaction; the incidence ranges from 3 to 54%. Epinephrine should be available in a syringe before the infusion is started. At the first sign

TABLE 390–3. PIT VIPER ENVENOMATION: SYMPTOMS AND SIGNS (PERCENTAGE)

Local		Systemic					
		Generalized		Hematologic		Neuromuscular	
Fang marks	100	Weakness	70	Thrombocytopenia	42	Paresthesia of scalp, fingertips	63
Edema	74	Tachycardia	60	Increased clotting time	37	Faintness, dizziness	57
Pain	65	Hypotension	54	Decreased hemoglobin	37	Paresthesias of affected part	57
Vesicles	40	Sweating	43	Burring of RBC	18	Fasciculations	41
Necrosis	27	Nausea/vomiting	42	Thrombocytosis	16		
		Hypothermia	42	Bleeding	15		
		Tachypnea	40				
		Regional adenopathy	40				

Adapted from Russell FE: Snake venom poisoning in the United States. Annu Rev Med 31:247, 1980.

of anaphylactoid reaction, bronchospasm, hypotension, or angioedema, the infusion should be stopped and 0.5 ml of 1:1000 epinephrine injected intramuscularly. This is almost always effective, and the antivenin infusion can be restarted. A history of allergy to horse serum contraindicates antivenin unless the risk of death from envenomation is high and the patient is pretreated with epinephrine. If the amount of antivenin is adequate, swelling will not progress and paresthesias will decrease. If progression occurs, the dose should be repeated. For moderate envenomation 5 to 10 vials, for severe envenomation 10 to 20 vials, and for very severe envenomation up to 40 vials (400 ml) may be required. In one series, the average dose required for adults with severe bites was 16 vials. Larger doses are required for bites in children and for those involving the fingers. Antivenin neutralizes both the local and the systemic effects of the venom.

In coral snake bites, if any symptoms or signs develop within the first several hours, 3 to 5 vials of antivenin (Micrurus fulvius) should be given intravenously. Even in the absence of symptoms, patients should be observed in the hospital for approximately 48 hours because onset of symptoms may be delayed and insidious. If neurotoxic signs appear (Table 390–3) an edrophonium test should be done: atropine sulfate (0.6 mg) given by slow intravenous infusion, followed by edrophonium chloride (10 mg) given intravenously over 2 minutes. If improvement occurs, neostigmine methylsulfate should be administered (beginning with 25 μg per kilogram of body weight per hour) by continuous infusion.

Antibiotics are usually recommended. Bacteriologic cultures of rattlesnake venom and fangs show growth from over 90% of specimens (venom or fangs) cultured. Aerobic gram-negative bacilli (Enterobacter sp., Pseudomonas sp.) and histotoxic clostridia (Clostridum perfringens) are the predominant isolates. On the basis of the microbiologic results, one of the newer β-lactam antibiotics—piperacillin, ceftazidime, ticarcillin clavulanate, or piperacillin tazobactam—is most appropriate. While clinical experience has not been reported, ciprofloxacin plus metronidazole orally should be an effective regimen. A tetanus toxoid booster is recommended.

In the severely envenomated patient, concurrent supportive measures include the management of shock and of respiratory and renal failure. Glucocorticoids have been recommended, but a controlled trial of prednisone therapy helped neither local nor systemic effects of viperine poisoning. Despite the hypofibrinogenemia and increase in fibrin degradation products, heparin is not of benefit.

Decompressive fasciotomy is indicated only if edema within closed muscular compartments is inadequately controlled, compartmental pressures are 30 mm Hg or higher, and arterial blood supply is compromised. From the end of the first to the third week, the majority of patients will develop serum sickness, the prevalence approximating 1% per milliliter of horse serum administered. Steroids are useful for treatment of serum sickness reactions.

PROGNOSIS. If adequate antivenin has been administered intravenously, mortality is virtually nil. If cryotherapy has been avoided, amputation or serious resultant deformities are uncommon. Only a few cases of snake bite poisoning in pregnancy have been reported. However, with envenomation by pit vipers, fetal loss has been 43% and maternal mortality 10%.

BITES CAUSED BY SNAKES NOT FOUND IN THE UNITED STATES

VIPER (VIPERIDAE) BITES. Bites by Russell's viper are the leading cause of fatal snake bite in Pakistan, India, Bangladesh, Sri Lanka, Burma, and Thailand. They are an occupational hazard of rice farmers. Up to 70% of the protein content of the venom is phospholipase A2, which can induce hemolysis, rhabdomyolysis, presynaptic neurotoxicity, and shock. Geographic variation in clinical manifestations is striking. The most common systemic signs are those of neurotoxicity; external ophthalmoplegia, ptosis, difficulty in opening the mouth ("pseudotrismus"), and inability to protrude the tongue. Symptoms include drowsiness, headache, vomiting, and abdominal pain. Incoagulable blood commonly leads to spontaneous hemorrhage, often massive. Generalized muscle tenderness, myoglobinuria, and oliguria also are common. In some countries, viper bite envenomation is the most common cause of acute renal failure. Management requires intensive supportive therapy and specific antivenin. Antivenin is most effective when administered within 4 hours, 400 to 500 ml often being required. Adequate doses restore blood coagulability but do not reverse shock, nephrotoxicity, or my-

otoxic signs. Causes of death include shock; pituitary, intracranial, and gastrointestinal hemorrhage; and tubular or renal cortical necrosis. Individuals who recover often show clinical or laboratory evidence of hypopituitarism.

COBRA (ELAPIDAE) BITES. Bites are almost invariably painful. Local necrosis is often preceded by bullae, which may not develop for 2 to 4 days after the bite. Neurotoxic symptoms may appear as early as 3 minutes after a bite, with onset rare after 6 hours. Respiratory paralysis may occur within 15 minutes. Responses to intravenous edrophonium chloride (administered as above) usually occur. The effectiveness of cobra antivenin is inconsistent. Maintaining adequate ventilation is essential. In survivors, neurotoxic manifestations usually resolve within a week.

Burch JM, Agarwal R, Mattox KL, et al.: The treatment of crotalid envenomation without antivenin. J Trauma 28:35, 1988. *A report of 81 patients managed by close physiologic monitoring in an intensive care unit without antivenin or surgical therapy. Excellent results were obtained.*

Curry SC, Kraner JC, Kunkel DB, et al.: Noninvasive vascular studies in management of rattlesnake envenomations to extremities. Ann Emerg Med 14:1081, 1985. *Provides details for monitoring, using noninvasive arterial studies. All but 1 of 25 patients received antivenin, and none underwent early surgical decompression.*

Dunnihoo DR, Rush BM, Wise RB, et al.: Snake bite poisoning in pregnancy. J Reprod Med 37:653, 1992. *A good review of snake bites in general as well as in pregnancy.*

Gold BS, Barish RA: Venomous snake bites. Emerg Med Clin North Am 10:249, 1992. *An excellent recent review.*

Malasit P, Warrell DA, Chanthavanich P, et al.: Prediction, prevention and mechanism of early (anaphylactic) antivenom reactions in victims of snake bites. Br Med J 292:17, 1986. *A study demonstrating the futility of intradermal and conjunctival tests for hypersensitivity.*

Tun-Pe, Phillips RE, Warrell DA, et al.: Acute and chronic pituitary failure resembling Sheehan's syndrome following bites by Russell's viper in Burma. Lancet 2:763, 1987. *A study of 33 patients; of 24 survivors, 46% had evidence of pituitary insufficiency.*

Watt G, Meade BD, Theakston RDG, et al.: Comparison of tensilon and antivenom for the treatment of cobra-bite paralysis. Trans R Soc Trop Med Hyg 83:570, 1989. *Results of a double-blind study of edrophonium versus placebo and a study of antivenin.*

391 VENOMS AND POISONS FROM MARINE ORGANISMS
Jay W. Fox

It is generally accepted that the term *envenomation* implies penetration by an organism for delivery of a venom containing one or more toxins. In contrast, poisons are toxins that are acquired from the environment by mechanisms such as absorption, inhalation, and ingestion. In the marine environment, both forms of intoxication occur, with effects ranging from mild irritation and discomfort to death. Previously, most clinically relevant intoxications were envenomations from marine organisms primarily found in tropical and subtropical waters. In recent times, however, severe outbreaks of poisoning from ingesting marine organisms containing toxins have occurred. This is likely due to increased microorganism growth in coastal waters as a result of eutrophication. Encroachment on the marine environment for recreation, living space, and food sources may be expected to increase the frequency of adverse encounters with venomous and poisonous marine organisms. This chapter discusses the marine organisms responsible for the majority of clinically significant intoxications, with emphasis on the pharmacologic and symptomatic properties of the toxins. Table 391–1 lists names of venomous and poisonous marine organisms that can produce severe intoxication or death and whether antivenin is available. The sites of action of some marine neurotoxins are depicted in Figure 391–1.

VENOMOUS MARINE ORGANISMS

Venomous marine organisms deliver their venoms by biting and stinging (Table 391–1). Envenomation involves penetration of the skin. Thus, consideration must be given to the potential of infection by microorganisms, especially in situations involving deep puncture

TABLE 391–1. SIGNIFICANT VENOMOUS AND POISONOUS MARINE ORGANISMS

Organism	Type of Envenomation (poisoning)	Primary Toxins	Antivenom Available
Sea snakes (Hydrophiidae)	Bite	Post-synaptic neurotoxin	Yes
Blue-ringed octopus (Octopodidae)	Bite	Post-synaptic neurotoxin (tetrodotoxin)	No
Cone shell (Conidae)	Bite	Pre- and post-synaptic neurotoxins	No
Box jellyfish (*Chironex fleekeri, Chiropsolmus quadrigatus*)	Sting	Hemolysins, proteinases, cardiotoxin necrotoxins	Yes
Portuguese man-o-war (*Physalia physalis*)	Sting	Hemolysins, proteinases, cardiotoxin necrotoxins	No; may be a need
Sea nettles (*Chrysaora quinquecirrha; Cyanea capillata*)	Sting	Hemolysins, proteinases, cardiotoxin necrotoxins	No; generally no need
Sea anemone (*Anemonia sulcata*)	Sting	Neurotoxins	No; generally no need
Scorpionfish (Scorpaenidae)	Sting/puncture	Hemolysins, necrotoxins ?	Yes
Lionfish (Scorpaenidae)	Sting/puncture	Hemolysins, necrotoxins ?	No
Stonefish (Scorpaenidae)	Sting/puncture	Hemolysins, necrotoxins ?	Yes
Weeverfish (Trachinidae)	Sting/puncture	Hemolysins, necrotoxins ?	No
Stingrays (Rajiformes)	Sting/puncture	?	No
Dinoflagellates		Ciguatera poisoning, ciguatoxins, maitotoxin (neurotoxins)	
Gambierdiscus toxicus	Poisonous (found in fish)		
Ptychodiscus brevis	Poisonous (found in shellfish)	Neurotoxic shellfish poisoning (NSP), neurotoxins	
Gonyaulax spp.	Poisonous (found in shellfish)	Paralytic shellfish poisoning (PSP)	
Pyrodinium spp.	Poisonous (found in shellfish)	Saxitoxin, neosaxitoxin and gonyautoxin	
Jania spp.	Poisonous (found in shellfish)	Okadaic acid (phosphatase inhibitors)	
Pufferfish (Tetraodontiformes)	Poisonous	Tetrodotoxin (neurotoxin)	No
Porcupinefish (Tetraodontiformes)	Poisonous	Tetrodotoxin (neurotoxin)	
Sunfish (*Mola* spp.)	Poisonous	Tetrodotoxin (neurotoxin)	

wounds and bites, as well as to the treatment of the toxicologic effects of the venom.

SEA SNAKES. Sea snakes are members of the family Hydrophiidae and are generally found in tropical and subtropical waters. Sea snakes are very common in the coastal waters of Thailand, Indonesia, the Persian Gulf, Australia, and India. With regard to the Americas, one species of sea snake, *Pelaramis platurus,* the yellow-bellied sea snake, is found in the Pacific coastal waters of Central America. These snakes are very capable swimmers but do not come ashore and are relatively immobile on land. They inject their venom with two small maxillary fangs (2 to 4 mm) containing ducts connected to venom glands located posterior and ventral to the maxillary bone. The relatively short aspect of the fangs prevents effective envenomation through most protective clothing such as dive suits. In the case of human envenomation, if the subject reacts by violent retraction the fangs are often dislodged from the maxillary bone of the snake and may remain in the site.

Because of the nature of the venom and the size of the fangs, the sea snake bite itself is generally not painful. One or two small prick marks are present at the envenomation site, as occasionally are additional marks from the other teeth in the snake's mouth. The primary toxin in sea snake venom is a postsynaptic peptide neurotoxin

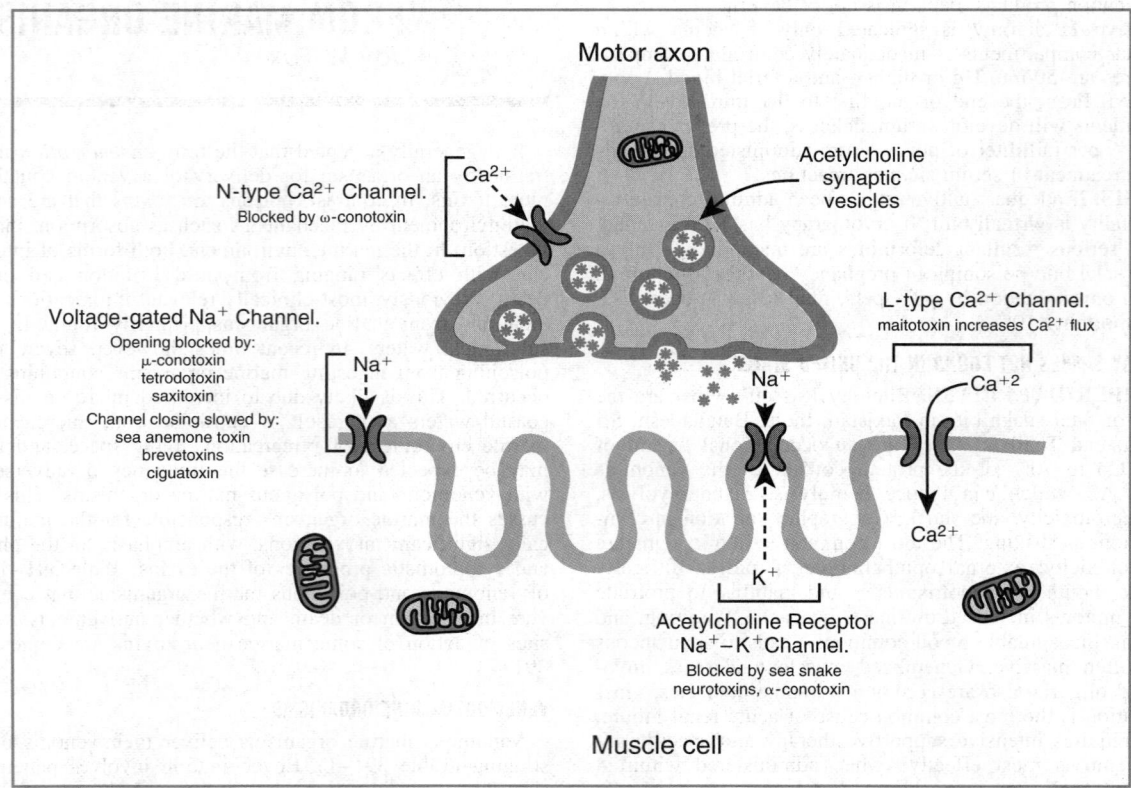

FIGURE 391–1. Schematic representation of a motor axon synapase and the sites of action of various marine neurotoxins.

that functions by blocking the acetylcholine receptor at neuromuscular junctions (Fig. 391–1). The symptoms of sea snake envenomation are mainly neurologic and typically appear within 30 minutes to 2 hours after the bite. Ptosis, dysphagia, and nonrigid paralysis occur and in severe cases respiratory failure may occur. In severe cases respiratory intervention may be necessary.

MOLLUSKS. *Blue-Ringed Octopus.* The blue-ringed and spotted octopuses (*Hapalochlaena maculosa* and *H. lunulata*), found in Australian waters, inject their venom by a relatively painless bite producing two small puncture wounds. Hemorrhage at the site may occur. The major toxic component in the venom is tetrodotoxin, a postsynaptic neurotoxin that causes perioral and intraoral paresthesias, dysphagia, nausea, ataxia, aphonia, flaccid muscular paralysis, and respiratory distress or failure. Fatal envenomations have occurred.

Cone Shells. Cone shell venoms are injected into victims through a hollow, harpoon-like tooth. The venom is primarily neurotoxic, causing paresthesias, hypotension and respiratory impairment/failure. Three types of neurotoxins have been identified in cone shell venoms: ω-conotoxin, α-conotoxin, and μ-conotoxins, all of which are short polypeptides. The ω-conotoxins block depolarization-induced Ca^{2+} uptake through N-type pre-synaptic channels (Fig. 391–1). The bite is very painful and may be followed by such systemic symptoms as dysphagia, aphonia, pruritus, blurred vision, syncope, muscular paralysis, and respiratory and cardiac failure. In cases of severe envenomation, preparation for cardiovascular and respiratory support should be made. Rare cases of coagulopathies have been noted. Fatal envenomations have occurred.

Weeverfish/Scorpionfish/Stonefish/Lionfish. Weeverfish are of the Trachinidae family while the scorpionfish, stonefish, and lionfish all belong to the family Scorpaenidae. Members of the Scopraenidae family are mostly found in tropic and subtropic waters. Weeverfish occur in European and African waters. All of these fish sting by using dorsal spines. Additionally, anal spines of the Scorpaenidae fish and opercular spines of the Trachinidae fish can also deliver venom. The spines are encased in an integumentary sheath that is torn when the spine punctures the victim's skin. Venom glands are located at the base of the spine.

Few details are known regarding the biochemistry and pharmacology of the toxins in weeverfish venom. The sting of the weeverfish is extremely painful and may produce systemic effects such as aphonia, fever, chills, dyspnea, cyanosis, nausea, syncope, hypotension, and arrhythmias. The wound is edematous, erythematous, and ecchymotic. Bacterial infection is typical and gangrene has been known to develop in severe cases of infection. The venom may be somewhat heat-labile, and soaking in tolerably hot water may relieve some pain as well as attenuate the effects of the venom. Death from weeverfish sting is rare.

Scorpionfish (*Scorpanena*) are primarily found in tropical and subtropical waters and the Mediterranean. The stings of these fishes have been described to be very similar to those of the weevers. Lionfish (*Pterois*) dwell in tropical waters; their stings generally are the most severe of all of the fish stings and occasionally cause death. Because the venom is heat-labile, soaking in hot water is recommended. The stonefish (*Synanceja*) group is found throughout the India-Pacific area, China, Australia, and the Indian Ocean, and is considered to be the most venomous fish. Symptoms are similar to those from the stings of members of the other groups. Hot water soaking of the wound site is recommended. As with all fish stings, care should be taken to ensure that no broken portions of the spines remain in the wound; vigilance against bacterial infections should be observed.

COELENTERATES. *Jellyfish and Anemones.* These organisms belong to the Cnidaria phylum, thus named because of their venomous organelles, cnidae. The cnidae found in jellyfish and anemones (termed nematocysts and spirocysts respectively) are located on exposed tentacles. On tactile stimulation the tentacles send forth a tethered projectile to deliver venom through the dermis. As the victim's surrounding musculature contracts, the venom is disseminated. The toxins contained in the venom from these organisms have not been fully documented. Hemolysins, DNAses, and histamine releasers have been identified in some venoms. Several peptide toxins have been characterized from the sea anemone, *Anemonia sulcata,* which act similarly to α-scorpion toxins by inactivating the Na^+ channel. Stings by jellyfish and anemones typically produce immediate pain at the site of envenomation, followed by ery-

thematous, urticarial lesions. Anaphylaxis is not common in most situations unless previous sensitization has occurred. Depending on the severity of the sting, wheals and whip-like patterns at the sites of envenomation may appear within a few minutes or be delayed by several hours, followed in some cases by dermal necrosis. Recurrence of eruptions days after the envenomation have been reported. Systemic reactions may include muscle spasms and cramps, vomiting, nausea, diarrhea, diaphoresis, and in rare cases cardiorespiratory failure. Verapamil will eliminate cardiac arrhythmia but will not ameliorate respiratory depression. Unfired nematocysts on tentacles adhering to the skin may be neutralized by either vinegar or baking soda depending on the species of jellyfish. Vinegar seems to be most useful for the Portuguese man-of-war (*Physalia physalis*) and Australian blue bottle (*P. utriculus*) stings while baking soda appears more efficacious for sea nettle (*Chrysaora quinquecirrha*) stings. Box jellyfish (*Chironex fleckeri*) found in Australian waters are perhaps the most venomous jellyfish, producing very severe stings that may cause death due to hypotension, muscular and respiratory paralysis, and ultimately cardiac arrest. Treatment of box jellyfish stings must include consideration of the option of respiratory support and administration of an antivenin.

Sponges. Some sponges colonized by coelenterates elaborate toxins that can produce either a pruritic allergenic dermatitis or an irritant dermatitis. These toxins are delivered by the sharp spicules present in the sponges, which when handled penetrate the dermis. The toxins can cause the typical sponge diver's disease characterized by local burning and itching, which in severe cases may be accompanied by soft tissue edema and purulent vesiculation. Serious illness is rare.

Corals. Fire coral (*Millepora alcicornis*) is found in shallow tropical waters. Stings are a common consequence of brushing or rubbing against the coral. Envenomation produces a burning or stinging sensation followed by severe pruritus. Edematous wheals may occur but generally dissipate over the course of several days. The site of envenomation should be soaked in dilute acetic acid or isopropanol to relieve pain.

BRISTLEWORMS. Bristleworms (Annelida) are segmented invertebrates found in tropical Pacific waters and the Gulf of Mexico. The bristles present on the segments of the organism are capable of penetrating the skin and producing a severely painful envenomation with pruritus and burning that may persist for several days. Local paresthesia is likely and may linger for weeks. Treatment is symptomatic, with consideration of possible tetanus infection. Little is known regarding the chemistry of bristleworm venoms.

SEA URCHINS. Of the echinoderms, sea urchins and sea stars are responsible for most stings to humans. The venom is delivered by the long spines and pedicellariae protruding from the sea urchin body. The spines are covered at the tips with a venom sac that is broken when it penetrates the skin. The pedicellariae, present on some species of sea urchins, are pincer-like appendages carrying venom glands. The toxins of sea urchin venoms are not well-characterized. Stings can produce pain, hemorrhage, aphonia, paresthesias, paralysis, hypotension, nausea, syncope, and respiratory distress. Immersion in hot water helps inactivate heat-labile toxins in the venoms. Attached pedicellariae and embedded spines must be removed to prevent additional envenomation.

STINGRAYS. Stingrays (order Rajiformes) are found in most seas but are predominant in the Indo-Pacific area. Venom is delivered by stings from spines (one or more) present on the tail of the stingray. Stingray spines are retroserrated on the margins and are covered by an integumentary sheath. Venomous glandular tissue is located at the base of the spines. On puncture of the skin, the sheath is torn by the serrated spine and venom flows along the two ventrolateral grooves of the spine into the surrounding tissue. One of the identified toxins in the venom is serotonin. The spines are often deeply embedded in the tissue and difficult to extract due to the retroserration. Care must be taken to remove all spine and sheath fragments. A sting produces severe pain and edema, which in extreme cases is accompanied by hemorrhage, syncope, vomiting, hypotension, and cardiac arrhymia. In rare cases death can occur, especially if the pericardial, peritoneal, or pleural cavities are penetrated. Soaking the wound in hot water inactivates some of the heat-labile toxins in the venom.

POISONOUS MARINE ORGANISMS

Marine poisoning nearly always results from consumption of a fish or shellfish harboring various toxins. The causes of three types of marine poisoning are fish or shellfish containing toxins produced by dinoflagellates (Ciguatera, neurotoxic shellfish, paralytic shellfish, and diarrhetic shellfish poisoning); fish that produce their own toxin (Tetraodontiformes fish); and fish containing significant levels of bacteria that have metabolized histidine to histamine resulting in pseudoallergenic reactions.

CIGUATERA POISONING. Ciguatera toxins have been identified in over 400 species of fish. During blooms of the dinoflagellate *Gambierdiscus toxicus,* toxins produced by these organisms concentrate in the fish to levels that are toxic to humans when ingested. The primary toxins responsible for ciguatera poisoning are ciguatoxin(s), which are cyclic polyethers, and act as excitatory agents by binding to Na$^+$ channels. Maitotoxin, from the same dinoflagellate, is a water-soluble polyether, and acts by enhancing Ca^{2+} entry through L-type Ca^{2+} channels. Symptoms of ciguatera poisoning generally appear within 2 to 12 hours following ingestion of contaminated fish. Gastrointestinal symptoms including diarrhea, abdominal pain, nausea, and vomiting appear first, followed by neurologic and cardiovascular symptoms. Neurologic symptoms include aphonia, dental dysesthesias, fatigue, tremor, ataxia, pruritus, extremity and perioral dysesthesia, vertigo, headache, myalgias, arthralgias, temperature reversal, and hyporeflexia. Cardiovascular symptoms, such as bradycardia and hypotension, occur least often. There is no specific treatment for ciguatera poisoning; supportive, symptom-based therapy is indicated. Death from ciguatera poisoning has occurred but is rare.

NEUROTOXIC SHELLFISH POISONING (NSP). NSP is caused by eating shellfish that contain brevetoxins produced by the dinoflagellate *Ptychodiscus brevis.* Brevetoxins are cyclic polyethers that function similarly to the ciguatoxins. Gastrointestinal and neurologic symptoms of intoxication appear within 3 hours toxic shellfish is eaten and are similar to those of ciguatera poisoning. Treatment is supportive. No deaths have been reported for NSP.

PARALYTIC SHELLFISH POISONING (PSP). PSP is significantly more severe than NSP and predominantly involves neurologic symptoms with less pronounced gastrointestinal symptoms such as nausea, vomiting, and diarrhea. The toxins responsible for PSP are from the dinoflagellate genera *Gonyaulax, Pyrodinium,* and *Jania* and are harbored in a variety of shellfish. The primary PSP toxins—saxitoxin, neosaxitoxin, and gonyautoxin—are heterocyclic compounds that block nerve and muscle action potentials by binding to Na$^+$ channels. The site of binding overlaps with tetrodotoxin, resulting in paralysis. Symptoms appear soon after consumption of contaminated shellfish (minutes to hours) beginning with circumoral and extremity paresthesias. Additional neurologic symptoms, such as ataxia, arthria, dysphagia, dysmetria, diaphoresis, and tachycardia, soon follow the initial paresthesias. Respiratory depression or failure can occur and may result in death, usually within 12 hours of the onset of symptoms. As with other shellfish poisoning, therapy is supportive, with close attention given to potential respiratory distress or failure.

DIARRHETIC SHELLFISH POISONING (DSP). DSP is also caused by eating shellfish that are contaminated by dinoflagellate toxins. The two primary toxins associated with DSP are okadaic acid(s) and pectenotoxins. Okadaic acid is a polyether derivative of a 38 carbon fatty acid. It functions as an inhibitor of protein phosphatase-1 and -2A and causes smooth and cardiac muscle contraction. Symptoms of DSP begin with abdominal cramps and nausea and progress to diarrhea. Additional, delayed symptoms occurring approximately 35 hours after ingestion may appear and include vomiting, vertigo, diarrhea, cramps, and headache. Treatment is supportive.

TETRAODONTIFORMES (PUFFERFISH, PORCUPINEFISH, AND SUNFISH) POISONING. Pufferfish (also called blowfish, balloonfish, and toadfish), porcupinefish and sunfish *(Mola* spp.*)* have a very potent toxin, tetrodotoxin, present in their liver, gonads, intestines, and skin. The flesh of the fish (fugu) is a delicacy in Japan and prepared by specially trained chefs to avoid serving significant amounts of toxins. Tetrodotoxin is a heterocyclic compound that binds at voltage-sensitive Na$^+$ channels (at an overlapping site with saxitoxin) to block Na$^+$ passage, preventing nerve and muscle action potentials, thus resulting in paralysis. Symptoms occur rapidly (several minutes to several hours) beginning with circumoral paresthesias and progressing to widespread paresthesias. Following the initial paresthesias, additional symptoms soon follow including ataxia, weakness, aphonia, diaphoresis, excess salivation, dyspnea, dysphagia, weakness, and respiratory distress or failure. Gastrointestinal symptoms include nausea, vomiting, and diarrhea. Coagulopathologies have been reported in association with tetrodotoxin intoxication. Respiratory intervention is crucial in light of the potential for complete flaccid paralysis. Without respiratory assistance, death is not unusual in cases of severe intoxication.

SCOMBROID FISH POISONING. Scombroid poisoning is a pseudoallergic fish poisoning caused by consumption of certain types of fish that have been improperly stored, including the scombroid fish (tuna, mackerel, wahoo, bonito, albacore, skipjack) and nonscombroid fish (mahi-mahi, amberjack, sardines, and herring). The poisoning results from high levels of histamine and saurine present in the fish because of bacterial catabolism of histidine. Presentation of symptoms from intoxication is rapid (within minutes to hours), beginning with a flushing of the skin, oral paresthesias, pruritus, urticaria, nausea, vomiting, diarrhea, vertigo, headache, bronchospasm, dysphagia, tachycardia, and hypotension. Therapy should follow a course for allergenic reaction and anaphylaxis. Symptoms usually resolve in several hours.

Adams ME: Neurotoxins. Trends Neurosci 17(4)(Suppl) 1994. *This issue is a concise tabulation of neurotoxins, their biological sources and pharmacological activities.*
Auerbach PS: Marine envenomations. N Engl J Med 325:486, 1991. *A thorough guide to the types of marine envenomations and symptoms that they cause.*
Burnett JW: Human injuries following jellyfish stings. Maryland Med J 41:509, 1992. *This article describes the mechanism of jellyfish stings and therapy.*
Hall S, Strichartz G (eds.): Marine Toxins: Origin, Structure and Molecular Pharmacology. American Chemical Society, Washington, DC, 1990. *This is a collection of papers on marine toxins with particular emphasis on experimental pharmacology.*
Miller DM (ed.): Ciguatera Seafood Toxins. CRC Press, Boca Raton, Fl. 1991. *A compilation of information on the toxicology of ciguatoxin poisoning.*
Tu AT (ed.): Marine Toxins and Venoms, Handbook of Natural Toxins, Vol. 3. New York, Marcel Dekker Inc., 1988. *This volume discusses many types of marine toxins as well as a section on treatment.*

Section One—Principles of Clinical Neurologic Diagnosis

392 CLINICAL STUDY OF THE PATIENT

392.1 Approach to the Patient

Fred Plum and Jerome B. Posner

The continuing triumphs of genetic, cellular, and molecular biology that have marked the past 20 years have added greatly to our understanding of neurologic-neuromuscular function and the causes and mechanisms of neurologic diseases. At last count, more than 115 distinct genetic disorders of the nervous system have been assigned to specific chromosomal loci. In more than 50 of these, the particular gene or abnormal gene product has been delineated, and hardly a month passes without new discoveries in this realm. Efforts to transfer missing genes to deficient hosts have been started, and functionally effective nerve cell transplants have been placed successfully in the human brain in efforts to correct parkinsonism. The identification and results of experimental applications of a variety of neurotrophic factors hold promise that effective new treatments for certain neurodegenerative disorders may be close at hand. These triumphs presage entirely new and potentially remarkable approaches to future neurologic therapy.

Despite these advances, the fundamental challenge in successfully diagnosing and treating patients with neurologic symptoms or disease remains in (1) understanding the genesis of their complaints, (2) parsimoniously but effectively using laboratory aids to rule in or out the presence of specific structural-chemical disease, and (3) managing them with full recognition that the individual physician represents the most important component in improving the health and spirits of another, suffering human being.

The evaluation of patients whose complaints potentially implicate the nervous system challenges the physician on several levels. New neurologic symptoms often frighten patients. They are afraid of pain, and often disturbed by the threat of becoming crippled and terrified of having chronic disorders such as Alzheimer's and other degenerative diseases. They may use misleading or incorrect terminology to describe their symptoms, and some repress crucial information because they fear its implications. Another issue is the ambiguity of many neurologic complaints. Ultimately, all symptoms of whatever origin are neurologic, because they necessarily require abnormal stimulation of either peripheral or central neuroreceptor systems to make themselves felt. Separating primary neurologic symptoms from those reflecting trouble in other bodily organs represents only a first small step down the diagnostic trail. Even seemingly direct neurologic complaints such as headache, nausea, dizziness, tinnitus, fatigue, and generalized weakness are as likely to signal the presence of an emotional disorder as a somatic neurologic abnormality, and the distinction often evades laboratory investigation. To assign the basis of such complaints accurately requires that the physician know why *this* symptom occurred in *this* patient at *this* particular time. To reach such answers often takes time and repeated questioning, but until these matters are understood, the physician can neither treat present disability nor anticipate future developments.

Even more important than separating emotional from somatic neurologic complaints is recognizing the urgency for prompt diagnosis and treatment of serious neurologic disorders. If nerve cells die they cannot regenerate or be repaired. Furthermore, the older the patient, the less likely the brain is able to substitute new, learned functions for those damaged or destroyed by disease. The guiding principle in treating neurologic illness is that the more rapidly the doctor can reach an accurate diagnosis, the easier it becomes to prevent progression and reduce future disability. The mandate is clear: In seriously and acutely ill patients with neurologic abnormalities, life- or brain-threatening complications must be treated immediately even while proceeding with diagnostic procedures that may take much longer to complete. By contrast, patients whose diseases lack quick and specific remedies (e.g., most psychosomatic disorders, degenerative diseases, or residua of severe trauma) usually need far more from the doctor than mere drugs or operations can supply.

Several important maxims apply to all treatment situations. When emergencies occur, protect the brain first, no matter what successive steps must follow. Relieve pain even while proceeding with diagnosis. Give reassurance, hope, and explanation at every step along the way. In order to plan long-term management effectively and economically, try to construct an accurate prognosis as early as possible. In acute, self-limited illnesses, such as meningococcal meningitis or most cases of acute inflammatory polyneuritis, for example, one usually can predict the probable outcome within a few days of onset. For most such patients one can even predict the convalescent time required before they return to their former occupations. With diseases with intermediate outcomes, such as multiple sclerosis, full recovery is less certain and the risk of relapse or chronic disability requires the physician to appraise all aspects of the patient's life in order to give proper guidance. At the worst extreme are patients who suffer severe head trauma, or become severely crippled from stroke or demented from Alzheimer's disease. They may never recover independence, and their proper early management often requires the doctor to advise families about major social and financial readjustments that will be required in the future. How doctors manage such complexities determines their effectiveness as physicians.

392.2 Clinical Diagnosis
Fred Plum and Jerome B. Posner

A logical approach to neurologic problems yields high clinical dividends in accuracy of diagnosis and selection of appropriate therapy. The following imperatives outline a widely used strategy.

Focus strongly on the relevant history, weighing the biologic implications of the patient's symptoms in relation to known neuroanatomic and physiologic perturbations. Vague symptoms can sometimes reflect educational problems or mental decline in the patient. Alternatively, they may hint more at a distressed psyche than a diseased soma. By contrast, perturbations of specific sensory, motor, or language pathways often produce symptoms that almost immediately point to the general anatomic region and pathophysiology of the patient's neurologic abnormality.

Heed chronology. Remote, temporary sensorimotor or visual symptoms affecting a 35 year old who several years later develops an "acute" paraparesis suggests an exacerbating and remitting disorder such as multiple sclerosis rather than a new spinal neoplasm. Conversely, a several-year history of sharply episodic, brief experiences of depersonalization accompanied by automatic behavioral activity in a patient with a recently developing unilateral headache suggests temporal lobe seizures accompanying an enlarging intracranial mass lesion rather than the onset of a migraine late in life.

Try to place the origin of symptoms and signs on at least a crude neuroanatomic map. Do they suggest disease in a single anatomic locus or do they reflect dysfunction affecting several different anatomic areas? Do they suggest a system disorder (e.g., motor neuron disease or neuromuscular disease) rather than a focal structural lesion, e.g., a single spinal neoplasm producing focal lower motor neuron changes at one level with upper motor neuron abnormalities extending below that level?

Are the symptoms and signs consistent with known physical disorders? For example, chronic weakness and fatigue lasting more than 6 months unaccompanied by physical or laboratory abnormalities suggest chronic anxiety-depression rather than structural disease or systemic metabolic dysfunction. Beware, however; some diseases affecting the nervous system move so slowly that their early symptoms and signs may not be readily localizable. A corollary to not overdiagnosing somatic disorders is that it is equally important not to entertain psychiatric diagnoses unless other findings or projective tests support such conclusions. For example, low-grade astrocytomas of the frontal lobe may produce new-onset behavioral abnormalities long before they cause focal abnormalities on the neurologic examination or unequivocal abnormalities in magnetic resonance images.

Form etiologic hypotheses logically, apply common sense, and consider the common before the rare. Age, previous symptoms, epidemiologic frequency, gender in X-linked diseases (e.g., muscular dystrophy or adult-onset optic atrophy) as well as personal changes in the home and workplace all can contribute important elements that must be weighed in the evaluation.

Reach ultimate diagnosis only on strong evidence, known principles of anatomy, the presence of objectively perturbed neurologic function, and knowledge of disease mechanisms. Avoid undue efforts to fit signs and symbols into inexact syndromes. Physicians who too rapidly try to match symptoms and signs into an iteratively constructed diagnosis often prematurely make conclusions that they later find difficult to surrender. Keeping an open mind in making preliminary hypotheses and awareness that early working diagnoses are necessarily subject to change makes one capable of meeting changes that may emerge from the clinical course or laboratory findings. Lastly and importantly, order tests sparingly, armed with knowledge of what each procedure can or cannot provide and how it specifically may help to diagnose or confirm the particular patient's problem.

392.3 The Neurologic History
Jerome B. Posner

When a patient presents with a neurologic complaint, the clinical history usually supplies a greater proportion of the diagnostically relevant information than does either the neurologic examination or the nervous system images. Many neurologic diseases (e.g., migraine and, often, epilepsy) are not accompanied by abnormal physical or laboratory findings, and in these instances the physician must depend solely on the history to reach an appropriate diagnosis. Even when the patient suffers from a neurologic disease marked by physical signs and/or laboratory abnormalities, the history usually supplies about 80% of the total diagnostic information. Furthermore, because neurologic abnormalities affect such important functions as thinking, moving, and feeling, it is unusual to have significant abnormal signs that have not been reflected in symptoms. (Exceptions occur in demented patients and those with lesions of the nondominant parietal lobe, characterized by denial of disability. In these instances, abnormal behavior may be recognized by family and friends.) Thus, findings on examination not recognized by the patient or family are likely to be irrelevant or even misleading. By contrast, symptoms complained of by the patient, such as mild weakness or alterations of sensation, are probably significant even if too subtle to be detected by the examination. Because patients so keenly appreciate neurologic symptoms, a meticulous history often allows a physician to localize the disease anatomically and to understand its pathophysiology even before the physical examination.

Taking the neurologic history usually occupies the majority of time spent in an initial visit with a patient suffering a neurologic disorder. At the completion of the history, the physician should be able either to make a definite diagnosis or to formulate three or four hypotheses that can be tested by the physical and laboratory examinations. To reach this goal, the experienced physician gradually develops a targeted approach, similar to that which follows.

BE INTERESTED AND SUPPORTIVE. Try not only to gain diagnostic information but also to learn enough about the patient's psychologic and social background to establish a satisfactory doctor-patient relationship. Diagnostic information is often lost when patients do not volunteer symptoms that they believe would not interest the physician or that are too intimate to tell to an "unsympathetic stranger." The patient is usually more readily forthcoming if the physician demonstrates interest, reassurance, and support.

BE ALERT TO NONVERBAL CUES. What the patient does is often as important as what he or she says. The patient's overall appearance and demeanor, tone of voice, or a sigh or a tear in discussing what appear to be relatively trivial symptoms may be important clues to an underlying depression or severe anxiety over those symptoms.

REQUIRE PRECISION. Do not accept jargon or names of diseases from the patient. Jargon terms such as "dizziness" or diagnostic appellations such as "sinus headache" require an exact definition.

MAINTAIN A BALANCE BETWEEN LISTENING AND ASKING. Elicit the history in the patient's own words and, whenever possible, allow the patient to tell the story without interruption. Excessive interruptions imply impatience or disinterest and may lead to the exclusion of vital information. However, the physician must ask direct questions to encourage relevance, achieve precision, and place each symptom in its correct context. If the information is not volunteered, the physician must ask about the intensity and frequency of the complained symptoms, their duration, events and factors that precipitate or relieve them, and any other symptoms associated in time with the patient's major complaint.

FORM HYPOTHESES. Do not be a passive recipient of the patient's story. While taking the history, one must sift and distill the information in order to retain the relevant and discard the irrelevant. Concurrently, one must form hypotheses about the nature of symptoms as they are presented and test those hypotheses by asking pertinent questions. Hypotheses are tested and refined during the course of taking the history, so that by the end the physician has a few potential diagnoses to guide the physical and laboratory examinations. The best hypotheses are broad explanations of the patient's symptoms in anatomic and/or pathophysiologic terms, which are gradually refined into etiologic terms as the history develops. Hypotheses should give preference to illnesses that are probable (i.e., common diseases are more likely than rare diseases), serious (e.g., brain tumors should be considered before tension-type headache), treatable (e.g., spinal cord meningioma and vitamin B_{12} deficiency should be ruled out before making a diagnosis of multiple sclerosis), and novel (some patients have rare diseases, and these should not be forgotten).

ALWAYS TAKE A COMPLETE HISTORY. Even if the diagnosis seems clear from the chief complaint and the present illness, elicit other aspects of the patient's history in order to confirm or repute other physical or psychologic disabilities that could contribute to the patient's discomfort. In particular, inquire about the patient's mood (e.g., depressed or suicidal?), usual daily activities (and whether the illness interferes with them), sexual activities, the nature of psychologic and physical support at home, and the patient's view of the illness and its effects.

END BY SUMMARIZING. At the end of the history, summarize the history as you understand it, asking the patient if the summary is correct and if anything has been overlooked.

OBTAIN FURTHER HISTORY FROM THE PATIENT'S FAMILY AND FRIENDS. If the history appears incomplete, and particularly if part of the illness involves changes in mental state or episodic unconsciousness, ask family, friends, and colleagues to supply missing elements, giving their views on how the signs and symptoms affect the patient's daily life.

392.4 The Neurologic Examination
Fred Plum

Several texts contain detailed techniques of bedside neurologic examinations. In most clinical circumstances, however, an understanding of a few fundamental principles about the nervous system plus mastery of a brief but systematically thorough approach to the examination can give reliable and effective answers. The secret is to learn well an approach that covers the main elements of nervous system function and to be familiar with ways to seek out more exhaustive evaluations if and when the history or examination suggests special abnormalities. Under all circumstances, however, the details of how one examines the patient should be geared to evaluating clinical hypotheses derived from the history.

An effective neurologic examination proceeds from general to specific in its principles and rostral to caudal in its anatomy. The examination checks on the integrity of major functions but avoids details that do not relate to the complaints of most patients. Evaluate the level of arousal (see Ch. 393). In awake and talking patients, begin to evaluate mental status and language as they give their histories. Apply at least a brief mental examination on everyone, but be gentle and understanding: "How has your memory been? Can I just check a couple of points with you?" Check orientation. Examine memory for recent events, for public figures, and for three unrelated words after a 5-minute interval. Review the capacity to handle abstractions (boy—dwarf, small tree—bush, proverbs). Provide a problem in simple arithmetic (the number of nickels in $1.35). Check serial sevens. Have the patient repeat five numbers or spell "world" backward. Be patient and remember that anxiety can compromise the performance of even a normal mind. If in doubt, perform a minimental status evaluation (see Table 400–3). Have the patient stand and walk; bear in mind that the nervous system is the organ of communication and behavior, and that one learns most about humans by watching them attempt natural tasks. To detect apraxia (see Ch. 399) watch the patient at least partially dress and undress; remark on alertness-dullness; hyperactivity-apathy; adventitious movement–akinesia; visible deformities, asymmetries, or weaknesses in functional tasks; hypertrophies-atrophies; cutaneous abnormalities (pox, birthmarks, café au lait spots, pigmented or hair spots over spinal defects); a straight, flat, or crooked spine. Learn to observe constantly and closely, comparing what you see with what you already have encountered in thousands of people

living normal lives. Wise physicians gain experience not only from their patients but from the everyday world in which they live.

Examine cranial functions. Palpate the skull and test the neck gently for suppleness and length. Then examine the following in every patient: vision, the optic fundi, pupillary activity, ocular movements, corneal reflexes, jaw movement, facial movement, hearing, swallowing, speaking, and breathing. One can omit examinations of smell, taste, facial sensation, labyrinthine-vestibular activity, sternocleidomastoid function, or detailed tongue movements unless symptoms suggest an abnormality of these areas. Examine in everyone the extremities and trunk for hypertrophy or atrophy, size, gross strength, muscle tonus, adventitious movements (e.g., tremors, fasciculations, tics), coordination (rhythmic movements and point-to-point tests), and reflexes. If the patient has no sensory symptoms, he/she is unlikely to have significantly abnormal sensory signs. Nevertheless, check the distal extremities briefly for the threshold perception of vibration and pin prick. Examine the plantar responses. Evaluate autonomic and sphincter functions only if the history has suggested dysfunction involving these areas. Get in the habit of examining the neck over the carotid arteries for bruits that may herald partial stenoses. Above all, be systematic and consistent in the approach and *do not jump at diagnosis until all the evidence is in.* Doctors tend to make diagnoses quickly and surrender wrong ones reluctantly. By contrast, they view even partial unknowns as challenging problems. Try to choose the latter approach until matters become certain.

USE OF LABORATORY TESTS. Advances in laboratory methods during recent years have remarkably increased the accuracy of diagnosis and physiologic evaluations. At the same time, the excess of technology raises the costs of medical care unnecessarily. More than anything else, the physician's ordering practices influence this aspect of health care costs. Doctors must recognize the precise advantages for both positive and negative knowledge that derive from each test, then gear their ordering to hypotheses gained from the history and whatever additional clues come from the neurologic examination. For example, when managing an adult with recent onset of headache, the results of a computed tomographic scan, whether normal or abnormal, commonly help management and may provide the patient with great reassurance. However, to repeat scans or irrelevant tests just for the sake of "a complete workup" wastes the time and resources of all concerned.

Glick TH: Neurologic Skills. Examination and Diagnosis. Boston, Blackwell Scientific Publications, 1993. *Provides a detailed approach to the neurologic history, examination, and formulation of diagnoses.*

Guarantors of Brain. Aids to the Examination of the Peripheral Nervous System. London, Bailliere and Tindall, 1986. *An indispensable pictorial guide to the motor and sensory distribution of the dermatomes and peripheral nerves.*

392.5 Neurologic Diagnostic Procedures
Jonathan D. Victor

LUMBAR PUNCTURE

Sampling the cerebrospinal fluid (CSF) is indispensable for the diagnosis of central nervous system infections and needs to be performed on an emergency basis when bacterial meningitis is suspected. Table 392–1 lists other indications for lumbar puncture, as well as major contraindications.

ELECTRODIAGNOSTIC STUDIES

Examinations performed in the clinical neurophysiology laboratory are best viewed as extensions of the bedside neurologic examination. The neurologic examination, fundamentally, is a series of observations of the patient's response to a traditional set of standard stimuli. The techniques of clinical neurophysiology allow one to detail the responses with a greater temporal resolution, to demonstrate the activity of single cells and cell populations that underlie the responses, and to quantify the observations.

TABLE 392–1. COMMON INDICATIONS AND CONTRAINDICATIONS FOR LUMBAR PUNCTURE

Diagnostic indications
  Known or suspected meningitis and encephalitis
    Acute: bacterial, viral
    Subacute: tuberculous, syphilitic, fungal, neoplastic
    Chronic: syphilitic, granulomatous, neoplastic
  Intracranial or intraspinal hemorrhage, if CT or MRI is not available
  Multiple sclerosis
  Acute polyneuropathy
  Suspected benign intracranial hypertension (pseudotumor), if CT or MRI is negative
Therapeutic indications
  Intrathecal administration of antimicrobial or chemotherapeutic agents
  CSF drainage in benign intracranial hypertension or communicating hydrocephalus
Contraindications
  Intracranial hypertension due to mass lesion or obstructive hydrocephalus
  Bleeding diathesis
  Local skin or epidural infections

Neurophysiologic tests are not etiologic tests. They do not replace the basic neurologic paradigm of reasoning from localization to possible causes but rather add to the precision and sensitivity with which functional pathology can be defined.

Electroencephalography

The electroencephalogram (EEG) is a record of the spontaneous electrical activity of the brain as recorded on the scalp. The clinical EEG is typically recorded from 8 to 16 pairs of electrodes (called "derivations"). The "international 10-20" system of electrode placement provides coverage of the scalp at standard locations denoted by the letters F (frontal), C (central), P (parietal), T (temporal), and O (occipital) with subscripts (odd for left-sided placements, even for right-sided placements, and "z" for midline placements).

EEG signals have a typical amplitude of 30 to 100 μV and an irregular wavelike variation in time (Fig. 392–1A). The main generators of the EEG are thought to be postsynaptic potentials, with the largest contribution arising from pyramidal cells. The minute amplitude of the EEG compared to the ECG is a consequence of two facts: The normal ECG is generated by cells that are synchronously activated and geometrically aligned; the normal EEG is generated by cells that are asynchronously activated and, in general, not geometrically aligned. Thus, the EEG is a composite record of fluctuating correlations between the activities of many populations of cells.

Ongoing EEG activity, called the *background,* is described in terms of frequency ranges: less than 3.5 Hz (delta), 4 to 7.5 Hz (theta), 8 to 13 Hz (alpha), and greater than 13.5 Hz (beta). In awake but relaxed normal adults, the background consists primarily of alpha activity in occipital and parietal areas and beta activity in central and frontal areas. Variations in this pattern occur as a function of age (particularly in the first years of life) and behavioral state (e.g., vigilant versus relaxed versus drowsy versus asleep; eyes open versus eyes closed).

EEG ABNORMALITIES. EEG abnormalities can be divided into two categories: alterations in the background activity and paroxysmal activity. Global *background abnormalities* accompany diffuse brain dysfunction associated with developmental delay, metabolic disturbances, infections, and degenerative diseases. EEG background abnormalities are never specific enough to establish a diagnosis. For example, the *burst-suppression* pattern illustrated in Figure 392–1B may be seen in severe anoxic brain injury as well as in coma due to barbiturates. Several encephalopathies, however, have characteristic EEG features that suggest a diagnosis. For example, an excess of beta activity suggests intoxication with barbiturates, benzodiazepines, and related drugs. *Triphasic slow waves* (Fig. 392–1C) are typical of metabolic encephalopathies, particularly those due to hepatic and renal dysfunction. Creutzfeldt-Jakob disease and subacute sclerosing panencephalitis have characteristic EEG signatures, consisting of background alterations associated with periodic paroxysmal discharges (see below).

Psychiatric illness is not associated with prominent changes in the EEG. Thus, a normal EEG helps to distinguish pseudodementia

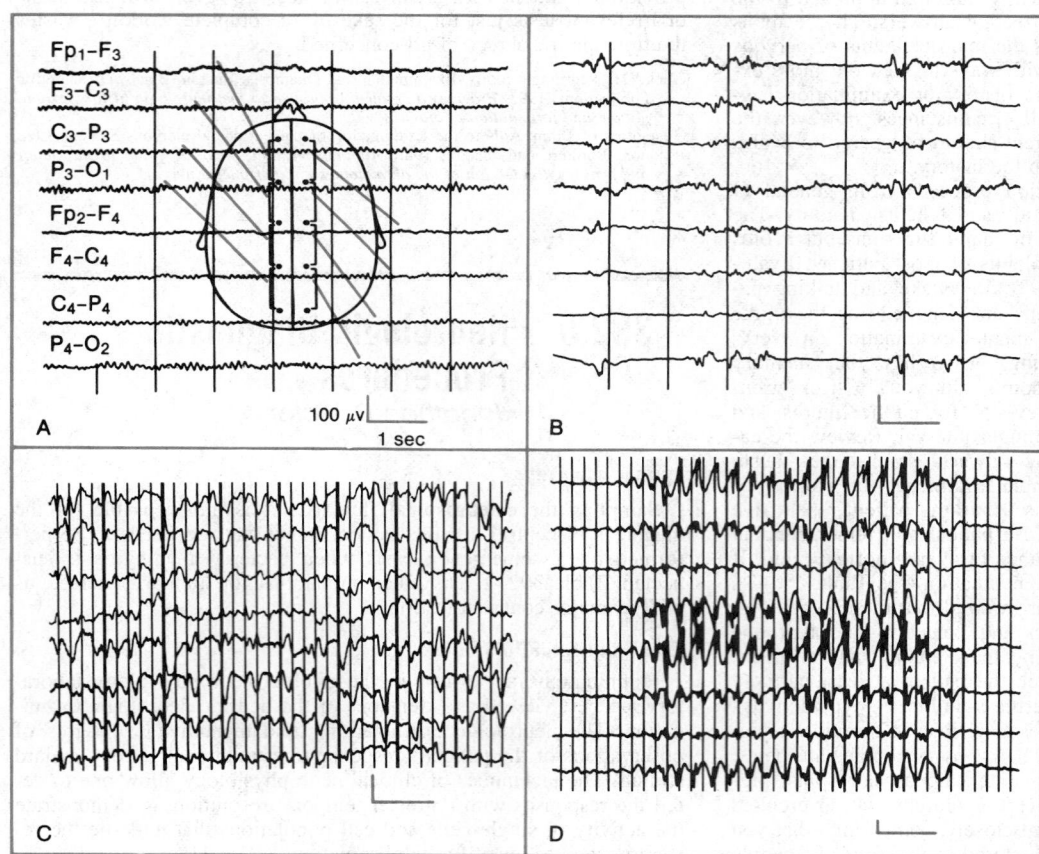

FIGURE 392–1. Normal and abnormal EEG's. *A,* The EEG of a normal alert adult. *B,* Burst-suppression, a pattern seen in severe cerebral dysfunction. *C,* Triphasic slow waves, seen in metabolic encephalopathies. *D,* A brief spike-and-wave seizure. In each record, the top four tracings are from parasagittal left-sided electrode placements (Fp$_1$-F$_3$, F$_3$-C$_3$, C$_3$-P$_3$, P$_3$-O$_1$); the lower four tracings are from the corresponding right-sided placements (Fp$_2$-F$_4$, F$_4$-C$_4$, C$_4$-P$_4$, P$_4$-O$_2$). The scale represents 1 sec and 100 μV. Note the reduced vertical scale in *D.*

from dementia and psychogenic unresponsiveness from neurologic disease.

Thalamocortical connections play a major role in establishing the normal EEG background. Thus, although brain stem and diencephalic activity is not directly registered in the EEG, structural lesions of the brain stem may cause diffuse changes in background activity via their effect on thalamocortical relays.

The EEG is an adjunctive test in the determination of brain death. An active EEG readily distinguishes de-efferented or locked-in states (such as severe Guillain-Barré syndrome and basal pontine infarction) from cortical inactivity (see Ch. 394). Electrocerebral silence, however, does not necessarily imply brain death, because it may be produced by reversible conditions such as barbiturate intoxication and hypothermia.

Focal or lateralized background abnormalities in the EEG imply similarly localized disturbances in brain function and thus suggest the presence of underlying structural lesions. CT and MRI have largely supplanted the EEG for anatomic localization. An important exception is herpes simplex encephalitis, which may produce focal abnormalities in temporal leads before imaging techniques demonstrate structural changes.

Paroxysmal EEG activity ("spikes" and "sharp waves") reflects pathologic synchronization of neurons. As such, this finding identifies a brain region with epileptogenic potential. Spikes and sharp waves commonly appear in the EEG records of epilepsy patients during interictal periods. The location and character of EEG paroxysms and their relationship to the background help to classify the epileptic disorder, guide rational anticonvulsant therapy, and assist prognosis. (See also Ch. 433.) Some patients with epilepsy may not show paroxysmal activity on a routine EEG, either because the focus is infrequently active or because it is too small or too deep to be evident in scalp recordings. The diagnostic yield of the EEG can be increased by *activation procedures,* such as hyperventilation and photic stimulation, by prolonged ambulatory monitoring, or through the use of special recording sites, including nasopharyngeal leads, anterior temporal leads, and surgically placed subdural and depth electrodes.

During a seizure, paroxysmal EEG activity becomes continuous and rhythmic and replaces normal background activity (see Ch. 433). In partial seizures with secondary generalization, paroxysmal activity begins in one brain region and spreads to uninvolved regions. The EEG identifies a focal onset of seizures more accurately than clinical observation alone. In primary generalized seizures, paroxysmal EEG activity is bilateral at onset. An example is shown in Figure 392–1D.

Whether focal or generalized, seizures with motor manifestations are unlikely to be subtle clinical events. However, sensory seizures, psychomotor seizures, and other forms of seizures without major motor manifestations may require an EEG for identification and diagnosis.

Evoked Potentials

External stimuli evoke changes in the ongoing electrical activity of the brain that may be extracted from scalp recordings by signal-averaging techniques. The three modality-specific evoked potentials discussed below form the bulk of clinical practice.

VISUAL EVOKED POTENTIALS (VEP). The VEP is commonly elicited by stimulation of the retina with repetitive reversals of black-and-white checkerboard patterns. The most robust component is an occiput-positive wave several microvolts in amplitude, occurring approximately 100 msec after pattern reversal. Termed the P-100, its cellular origins include a mixture of excitatory and inhibitory synaptic signals. The VEP is recorded separately for each eye. Interocular differences in P-100 latency imply prechiasmal conduction abnormalities, and bilateral delay in the P-100 latency implies bilateral conduction defects in the visual system. Since VEP's measure central response time rather than visual resolution, they may be abnormal in patients with normal visual acuity and visual fields. VEP's are particularly useful in identifying unsuspected optic nerve or cerebral abnormalities in patients whose clinical signs point to disease affecting the brain stem or spinal cord. Demonstration of such multifocal lesions in the appropriate setting fortifies the clinical diagnosis of multiple sclerosis. Delayed optic nerve conduction may also be due to compressive lesions (e.g., pituitary tumor), metabolic disorders (e.g., vitamin B_{12} deficiency), and other neurodegenerative diseases (e.g., olivopontocerebellar at-

rophy). In patients who cannot or will not cooperate with behavioral tests, VEP's elicited by a graded series of stimuli provide a measure of visual resolution and contrast sensitivity.

BRAIN STEM AUDITORY EVOKED POTENTIALS (BAEP). The BAEP is commonly elicited by brief clicks presented to one ear, while random noise is presented to the other ear. The normal response, recorded by an electrode at the ear referenced to the vertex, consists of a series of submicrovolt waves at approximately 1-msec intervals. Wave I is generated at the distal end of the eighth nerve; wave III is generated along auditory pathways at the level of the superior olive, and wave V is generated at the level of the inferior colliculus. BAEP abnormalities commonly accompany mass lesions in the cerebellopontine angle and intraparenchymal brain stem lesions affecting the auditory pathways. Because the BAEP shows a stereotyped maturational pattern in the first 2 years of life, it is a valuable means of assessing the developmentally delayed or at-risk neonate. BAEP's elicited by a sequence of increasingly intense click stimuli provide a measure of auditory threshold in infants and patients who cannot cooperate with behavioral tests. In the appropriate clinical setting, absence of BAEP potentials rostral to wave II accompanied by still-remaining peripherally generated potentials supports the diagnosis of brain death.

SOMATOSENSORY EVOKED POTENTIALS (SEP). A SEP may be elicited by brief electrical stimulation delivered to any of several sensory nerves and dermatomes, but median, peroneal, and posterior tibial nerves are most commonly used. Scalp electrodes placed over somatosensory areas record submicrovolt potentials, and the spinal cord volley and peripheral nerve action potential often can be recorded by appropriately placed electrodes. With median nerve stimulation, potentials generated at medullary and midbrain-thalamic levels can be identified. Compressive, demyelinating, or metabolic disturbances affecting central sensory pathways delay centrally generated potentials but not potentials generated prior to entry to the spinal cord. Upper- and lower-extremity SEP's, in conjunction with nerve conduction studies and EMG, can help to identify radiculopathies and plexopathies.

OTHER PHYSIOLOGIC MEASURES OF BRAIN ACTIVITY. The limited anatomic information provided by the EEG has motivated new approaches to provide measures of brain function with better spatial resolution. *Magnetoencephalography (MEG),* the recording of magnetic fields generated by intracranial current loops, achieves a higher spatial resolution than the EEG because magnetic fields are virtually unaffected by the volume-conduction effects that distort the brain's electrostatic fields. Because MEG retains millisecond temporal resolution, it adds to the ability of electrical recordings to localize the generators of evoked potentials and epileptic spikes. Unfortunately, the minute size of the brain's magnetic fields and the costly and cumbersome nature of present-day detectors limit the application of MEG.

Imaging techniques identify activity-induced changes in cerebral blood flow and metabolism and thus sacrifice temporal resolution to achieve better spatial resolution. *Positron emission tomography (PET)* achieves a spatial resolution of < 1 cm and can exploit specific ligands and metabolites to probe transmitter systems or metabolic pathways, but it is very costly and requires the injection of significant amounts of a radioisotope. PET has demonstrated characteristic global patterns of metabolic derangements that distinguish the vegetative state and several forms of dementia, and has characterized the metabolic abnormalities in a variety of extrapyramidal disorders.

Functional magnetic resonance imaging (fMRI), which can be performed either with or without administration of a paramagnetic contrast agent, has an ultimate spatial resolution of about 1 mm and can be used to make multiple measurements in the same subject. In normal subjects and in patients, PET and fMRI have identified local brain regions activated by specific sensory, motor, and cognitive tasks. These techniques have the potential to demonstrate localized functional abnormalities of the brain even in the absence of structural changes.

Nerve Conduction Studies and Electromyography

NERVE CONDUCTION STUDIES. Most peripheral nerves can be stimulated percutaneously at one or more points along their length. The induced electrical activity of muscles can be recorded

1962 / XXIV NEUROLOGY

with surface electrodes or with appropriately inserted needle electrodes. The *conduction velocity* of motor nerves can be calculated from the difference in latency of the motor response evoked by stimulation at two or more points along their length. Conduction velocity in sensory nerves can be determined by recording sensory nerve action potentials elicited by electrical stimulation at proximal or distal sites.

Nerve roots and segments of peripheral nerves that lie too close to the spinal cord to be studied directly may be examined by the F-response and H-reflex. The *F-response* is the compound muscle action potential that results from antidromic conduction of a volley along a motor nerve to the anterior horn cell body and back again to muscle. The *H-reflex*, a muscle response that represents the electrical equivalent of the monosynaptic stretch reflex, is elicited by stimulating sensory fibers in the corresponding peripheral afferent nerve. Usually, it is readily recorded only in the soleus after stimulation of the tibial nerve and thus serves to test the S1 root only.

Compound nerve action potentials are elicited by electrical stimulation of a peripheral nerve and are recorded by electrodes placed at a second site along the nerve. The response is dominated by the larger and more rapidly conducting myelinated nerve fibers. Accordingly, demyelinating neuropathies characteristically slow the conduction velocities. By contrast, axonal neuropathies, in which individual cell bodies or axons fail, decrease the amplitude of evoked motor and sensory responses but preserve normal conduction velocities until all of the largest myelinated fibers are affected.

Routine clinical tests cannot readily assess the function of unmyelinated fibers. Percutaneous microneurographic recording from single nerve fibers in the intact peripheral nerve represents an investigational approach to study unmyelinated and small myelinated fibers.

Electromyography (EMG) is performed by inserting a needle electrode into the muscle. At rest, a normal muscle with normal innervation remains electrically silent. With denervation, spontaneous activity occurs, consisting predominantly of fibrillation potentials and positive sharp waves. *Fasciculation potentials,* representing synchronous firing of entire motor units, occur mainly in anterior horn cell disorders and mechanical disturbances affecting motor nerve roots and may result in fasciculations that visibly dimple the overlying skin. *Fibrillation potentials* and *positive sharp waves,* which represent electrical activity of single muscle fibers, occur predominantly in neurogenic lesions but can also be seen in dystrophies and inflammatory myopathies.

Electromyographic recording during voluntary muscle contraction permits observation of individual motor units and their pattern of *recruitment.* In myopathies, degeneration of muscle fibers leads to a decrease in the size of motor units: Voluntary contraction recruits a normal number of units but with small amplitude and short duration. In denervated muscle, voluntary activity recruits a decreased number of units. With chronic denervation, collateral sprouting by remaining motoneurons leads to residual motor units of abnormally large amplitude and duration. *Myotonic discharges,* abnormal repetitive discharges that vary in amplitude and frequency, are seen in a variety of specific myopathies.

Table 392–2 summarizes how nerve conduction studies and EMG distinguish myopathies from neuropathies and indicate whether a neuropathy is demyelinating or axonal. Note that radiculopathies are distinguished from polyneuropathies on the basis of the distribution of the affected nerves and muscles rather than the findings in the affected areas. Detailed analysis of EMG activity may also help analyze central disturbances of motor control.

NEUROMUSCULAR TRANSMISSION STUDIES. Diseases of the neuromuscular junction are identified by the presence of abnormal neuromuscular transmission in the setting of otherwise normal nerve conduction studies. At the normal neuromuscular junction, the amount of acetylcholine released exceeds severalfold the requirements for activating the muscle. Repetitive action potentials cause a mild decrement in acetylcholine release, but the safety factor prevents a decrement in the postsynaptic response. In myasthenia gravis, immunologic blockade reduces the safety factor of the postsynaptic receptors. As a result, repetitive stimulation of a motor nerve elicits a rapid diminution of the evoked muscle action potential paralleling the decreasing amounts of acetylcholine released. In botulism and Eaton-Lambert syndrome, repetitive stimulation overcomes a presynaptic blockade and produces a gradual increase in the size of the evoked muscle action potential.

Pathologic reductions in the safety factor magnify the normal variability of the time interval between nerve action potential and depolarization of the postsynaptic fiber. This increased variability, or "jitter," can be assayed by simultaneously recording two muscle fibers in the same motor unit with single-fiber EMG electrodes. The jitter study is a more sensitive test of defective neuromuscular transmission than repetitive stimulation.

Aminoff MJ (ed.): Electrodiagnosis in Clinical Neurology, 3rd ed. New York, Churchill Livingstone, 1992. *Comprehensive introduction to EEG, EP, EMG, and other modalities.*

Chiappa KH: Evoked Potentials in Clinical Medicine, 2nd ed. New York, Raven Press, 1990. *Emphasis on practical matters and interpretation.*

Fisch BJ: Spehlmann's EEG Primer, 2nd ed. New York, Elsevier, 1991.

Kimura J: Electrodiagnosis in Diseases of Nerve and Muscle: Principles and Practice, 2nd ed. Philadelphia, FA Davis, 1989. *A standard reference.*

Niedermeyer E, Lopes da Silva F: Electroencephalography: Basic Principles, Clinical Applications, and Related Fields, 2nd ed. Baltimore, Urban and Schwartzenberg, 1987. *Encyclopedic, authoritative.*

Regan D: Human Brain Electrophysiology. New York, Elsevier, 1989. *Encyclopedic, emphasis on fundamentals and evoked potentials.*

392.6 Radiologic Imaging Procedures

Michael Deck

Management of neurologic disorders has improved dramatically over the last 20 years because of revolutionary developments in imaging techniques such as computed tomography (CT), magnetic resonance imaging (MRI), positron emission tomography (PET), and single photon emission computed tomography (SPECT). During the last 5 years these methods have improved spatial resolution, and fast spin echo and echo planar imaging by MRI have made possible physiologic studies of blood flow. At the same time, cerebrospinal fluid (CSF) flow and even activation studies of the cerebral cortex have become available.

TABLE 392–2. TYPICAL ELECTROPHYSIOLOGIC FEATURES OF NEUROPATHIES AND MYOPATHIES

	Nerve Conduction Velocity	F-response	H-reflex	Electromyography
Inflammatory myopathy or dystrophy	Normal	Normal	Normal	Fibrillations; positive sharp waves; small motor units
Metabolic myopathy	Normal	Normal	Normal	Small motor units
Axonal neuropathy	Normal	Normal	Normal	Fibrillations; positive sharp waves; fasciculations; large motor units with distal predominance
Demyelinating neuropathy	Slowed diffusely	Delayed or absent diffusely	Delayed or absent	Normal motor units
Radiculopathy	Normal	Delayed or absent in damaged root	Delayed or absent if S1 is involved	Fibrillations; positive sharp waves; fasciculations; large motor units if chronic
Motoneuron disease	Normal	Normal	Normal	Fibrillations; positive sharp waves; fasciculations; large motor units diffusely

Magnetic resonance spectroscopy (MRS) uses hydrogen and phosphorus to measure the concentrations of metabolites in brain volumes as small as 1 cm³ and has been useful in tumors, ischemia, and various metabolic disorders.

Magnetic resonance angiography (MRA) uses various complicated pulse sequences to image cervical cerebral arteries. The technique has been applied to diagnosing carotid artery stenosis, aneurysms of the circle of Willis, and thrombosis of the intracranial venous sinuses.

Interventional therapeutic approaches to intracranial aneurysms, arteriovenous malformations, vascular spasm, and vascular tumors such as meningiomas and chemodectomas are now available at most tertiary-level hospitals. Selective or superselective intra-arterial and intravenous administration of thrombolytic agents for the treatment of acute stroke and superselective chemotherapeutic agents for malignant brain tumors are currently under evaluation and appear promising.

THE SKULL AND BRAIN

PLAIN RADIOGRAPHY. Plain radiographs of the skull are routinely taken in frontal, lateral, and half-axial projections. Such films are useful principally in the initial evaluation of head trauma in which fractures of the vault and base may influence subsequent management. *Most skull radiographs, however, are taken for medicolegal reasons. Their value is limited because of poor correlation with injury of the underlying brain.* Depressed bone fragments may require elevation. Involvement of the paranasal sinuses or mastoid air cells may result in meningitis and indicate a use for prophylactic antibiotics. CT and MRI have supplanted plain radiographs in evaluating intracranial trauma and mass lesions such as tumors, hematomas, and infarcts, in detecting optic foramen enlargement due to tumors, and in identifying bony sclerosis due to meningiomas. CT and MRI also demonstrate tumors and inflammatory lesions of the paranasal sinuses as well as the craniovertebral junction better than do plain radiographs.

COMPUTED TOMOGRAPHY. CT uses an x-ray tube with a tightly collimated beam passing through the anatomic area under study. An array of 520 to 4800 x-ray detectors measures the radiation absorbed by the organs targeted by the beam during a 360-degree rotation lasting 1 to 6 seconds. Computers now formulate the analogue output from each detector to calculate a coefficient of absorption for each "pixel" in the field, using a mathematical process called filtered back projection. The resulting image is displayed on a cathode-ray tube monitor that may be viewed directly or photographed onto transparent film. CT images from current equipment demonstrate anatomic structures in the skull and brain with high spatial resolution. Fresh hemorrhages within either the brain or the subarachnoid, subdural, or epidural spaces can be identified because of the greater x-ray attenuation of clotted blood. Areas of calcification may have similar appearances but are usually more irregular and have a higher attenuation value. Many CT examinations use contrast enhancement with intravenous iodinated material to demonstrate normal vascular structures as well as the abnormal endothelial permeability that accompanies certain types of tumors and inflammatory processes.

Although contrast enhancement can add critical information in many CT examinations of the brain, the material also carries a small risk of adverse anaphylactic reactions. The general population has about a 1 in 10,000 chance of serious anaphylactic reaction and a 1 in 40,000 to 100,000 chance of death. These dangers increase fourfold in patients with previous allergic history to iodinated contrast material, iodine, or shellfish. The risk may be reduced by administering an antihistamine drug immediately before or 50 mg of prednisone orally 24, 12, and 6 hours before the injection. Special techniques can improve the resolution of CT and generate physiologic data. These include the following:

1. Coronal projections image the floor of the skull, the sella turcica, and the petrous bones.
2. Image reformatting generates coronal or sagittal images from multiple axial images. The technique depends on absolute immobilization of the patient and produces good resolution. It increases, however, the amount of radiation to the brain and potentially the eye. Three-dimensional reformatting may be useful for displaying surfaces and contours and is increasingly used by craniofacial surgeons to evaluate facial trauma and congenital anomalies, including craniosynostosis.

3. Ultrathin sections of 1.5 mm or less examine areas requiring high detail, such as the sella turcica, orbits, and petrous bones.
4. Bone targeting uses a special reconstruction algorithm to define fine anatomy such as the ossicles and osseous labyrinth of the petrous bone.
5. Dynamic scanning consists of performing rapid sequence scans after rapidly injecting a bolus of contrast agent. The subsequent contrast enhancement and washout can help to differentiate an aneurysm or arteriovenous malformation from a vascular tumor.
6. CT cisternography and myelography are performed by injecting water-soluble nonionic contrast material (iohexol or iopamidol) into the subarachnoid space and running the contrast material to scan the area of suspected abnormality. The technique may help to delineate tumors of the sella region, foramen magnum, and spinal canal. It may also be used to investigate CSF rhinorrhea and CSF dynamics in hydrocephalic patients.

MAGNETIC RESONANCE IMAGING. MRI, a rapidly evolving technology, has replaced CT as the examination of choice for most neurologic conditions (Table 392–3). Nuclear magnetic resonance occurs when hydrogen atoms or certain other elements with an odd number of nuclear particles such as sodium or phosphorus are placed in an intense magnetic field of between 3000 and 15,000 gauss (0.3 to 1.5 tesla). The nuclei behave like small magnets and align themselves in the field. When stimulated by a pulse of radio energy of a specific frequency (the Larmor frequency) determined by the intensity of the main magnetic field, the nuclei flip off axis. While in this energized state, the nuclei spin in phase as they subsequently relax into their original alignment with the main magnetic field, emitting a small radiofrequency signal. The MR image is gen-

TABLE 392–3. IMAGING MODALITY OF CHOICE IN DISEASES OF THE CNS

	CT	CT + C	MRI	MRI + Gd
Brain				
Gliomas	+	++	+++	++++
Metastases	+	+++	+++	++++
Meningiomas	+	+++	++	++++
Lymphoma	+	++	+++	++++
Postoperative and				
radiation therapy	+	++	++	++++
Hematomas	+++	0	++++	0
Subarachnoid				
hemorrhage	+++	0	+	0
Aneurysm and arterio-				
venous malformation	+	++	+++	0
Head trauma	+++	0	+++	0
Infarcts	++	+	+++	++
Abscess	+	++	+++	++++
AIDS	+	+++	+++	++++
Multiple sclerosis	0	+	++++	++++
Hydrocephalus/atrophy	++	++	++++	0
Congenital anomalies	+	+	++++	0
Sellar tumors	+	++	++++	+++
Posterior fossa				
Acoustic neurinoma	+	++	++++	+++
Meningioma	+	+++	+++	++++
Epidermoids	+	+	++++	0
Cholesterol granuloma	+	+	++++	0
Basilar artery				
aneurysm	+	++	++++	0
Craniovertebral				
junction	+	+	++++	0
Intra-axial gliomas	+	++	++++	+++
Spine				
Trauma	+++	0	+++	0
Degenerative disc				
disease	+++	0	++++	·0
Postoperative disc				
disease	++	+++	+++	++++
Metastatic bone disease	++	0	++++	+++
Arteriovenous malfor-				
mation of the cord	0	+	+++	+++

CT = Computed tomography; C = contrast enhancement; MRI = magnetic resonance imaging; Gd = gadolinium enhancement.

erated by many such magnetic resonance signals, transformed by a computer using techniques similar to those employed in CT. The resulting images demonstrate a high contrast between various tissues owing largely to differences in the rate at which magnetized nuclei in tissues of different chemical composition resume their original state (T1 and T2). The intensity of the MR image may be measured on the viewing console using a movable cursor similar to that on a CT scanner. Using standard "spin-echo" imaging sequences, a short T1 relaxation time of tissues such as fat results in high intensity (bright), whereas a long T1 relaxation time (CSF) results in CSF producing low signal intensity. Conversely, a short T2 relaxation time in tissues such as fat results in a low signal intensity, and a long T2 relaxation time in CSF results in a high signal intensity.

Accordingly, the contrast of fat, brain, and CSF on a T1-weighted spin echo (TE 30, TR 500) reverses itself on a T2-weighted spin echo (TE 80, TR 2000). The concentration of protons also affects intensity, as it is their signal that is being measured. Other factors affecting signal intensity include flow, magnetic susceptibility, paramagnetic effects, and the static field strength of the device.

MR images may be obtained in axial, coronal, sagittal, or oblique planes by changing the switching of the instrument's several magnetizing coils. Paramagnetic contrast agents developed for use with MRI contain elements such as gadolinium that, because of the large number of unpaired electrons in their outer shells, have a marked effect on the T1, or spin-lattice relaxation time, of protons. Gadolinium chelated to DTPA (Gd-DTPA) is used to define areas of increased vascularity and/or capillary permeability.

MRI is contraindicated for patients who harbor cardiac pacemakers or ferrous foreign bodies such as shrapnel. Intracranial aneurysm clips provide an absolute contraindication unless it is known for certain that they are made from nonmagnetic titanium or stainless steel. The presence of metal prostheses, spinal rods, certain metallic dental implants, and metallic cranioplastic prostheses may produce interfering artifacts but carry no risk of injury to the patient.

CEREBRAL ANGIOGRAPHY. Most cerebral angiograms are performed with an intra-arterial catheter inserted over a guide wire into the femoral artery and passed upward to the aortic arch or into the carotid or vertebral artery. Although cerebral angiography is a relatively safe procedure in experienced hands, complications, such as arterial damage, emboli to the brain, and contrast neurotoxicity, occur in 1 to 2% of procedures. New, less toxic, but more expensive non-ionic contrast agents are now replacing traditional ionic contrast materials. The use of smaller catheters facilitates examination of outpatients.

Arterial digital subtraction angiography (DSA) uses computerized imaging enhancement to improve the contrast of the injected contrast agent and to lower the dose required. Recently developed equipment with a 1k × 1k matrix produces such superb images that all arteriograms may be performed without using x-ray film. Instantaneous viewing of the subtracted images and software techniques such as road-mapping, rotational sequences, and density analysis have resulted in shorter examination times and improved studies.

Intravenous DSA uses similar equipment and rapid injections of contrast material into a peripheral vein or the right atrium. Imaging commences after a suitable delay to allow the contrast to pass through the pulmonary circulation into the systemic arteries. The procedure may be performed as an outpatient procedure for demonstrating the aortic arch and great vessels in the neck, as well as the intracranial cerebral arteries and veins. Intravenous DSA is not satisfactory for demonstrating small aneurysms of the circle of Willis or intracranial arterial abnormalities such as occlusions from emboli or vasculitis. Its rate of complications is similar to that of arterial angiography.

THE SPINE

RADIOGRAPHY (PLAIN FILMS). Conventional radiography of the spine demonstrates bony abnormalities such as degenerative disc disease, primary and metastatic tumors, and fractures of the vertebral bodies. Plain radiographs are the best method for demonstrating osteophytes in the neural foramina in the cervical, thoracic, and lumbar spine. Plains films should be obtained prior to myelography, CT, or MRI to identify segmentation anomalies at the thoracolumbar and lumbosacral junctions.

COMPUTED TOMOGRAPHY. CT of the spine demonstrates abnormalities of the spinal cord, meninges, vertebral bodies, and intervertebral articulations as well as those affecting paravertebral and prevertebral soft tissues. CT supplemented with intravenous contrast enhancement may be used to demonstrate vascular tumors of the spinal cord and meninges and can be valuable in distinguishing recurrent herniation of lumbar intervertebral discs from postsurgical scarring.

Postmyelogram CT or CT with intrathecal contrast improves delineation of subtle nerve root displacement due to posterolateral herniation of the intervertebral discs and associated osteophytes. It is also useful in demonstrating cysts and hydromyelia of the spinal cord, conditions in which CT may detect entry of contrast agent into the cavity 12 to 24 hours after intrathecal injection.

MAGNETIC RESONANCE IMAGING. MRI of the spine has replaced CT as the examination of choice because it gives better resolution of the spinal cord, subarachnoid space, and vertebral anatomy. It clearly depicts the intervertebral discs, showing the state of hydration of the nucleus pulposus and the condition of the annulus, usually with clear and unequivocal demonstration of any rupture of the annulus.

MRI of the spine with enhancement by Gd-DTPA defines spinal cord tumors and inflammatory processes of the meninges and differentiates recurrent disc herniation from postoperative scar tissue.

MYELOGRAPHY. Myelography is the most sensitive examination for demonstrating intradural mass lesions and can be helpful when an MRI is equivocal or shows multilevel disc disease without a predominant level of pathology. Iodinated water-soluble non-ionic contrast agent (iohexol, iopamidol) is introduced by lumbar puncture or, if indicated, by lateral cervical puncture (C1–C2). The contrast is hyperbaric and flows by gravity. By tilting the patient on a radiographic table, the contrast may be manipulated under fluoroscopic control from the lumbosacral region to the base of the skull.

Complications of myelography are rare, and the study is often performed as an outpatient procedure. Nevertheless, neurotoxic and other complications occasionally can occur. They include injury to nerve roots by the lumbar puncture needle as well as subarachnoid, subdural, or epidural bleeding. Much rarer events include infections or compression by mass lesions due to changes of pressure in the subarachnoid space.

IMAGING TECHNIQUES IN SPECIFIC DISEASE CATEGORIES
Tumors of the Cerebral Hemispheres

GLIOMAS (Fig. 392–2). Gliomas are demonstrated best with MRI because of sensitivity to slight changes in water content producing an area of hyperintensity on T2-weighted images. Tumors adjacent to the skull are seen best on MRI because of the absence of bone artifact. Differentiation of tumor from peritumoral edema may be obvious or difficult depending on the tumor margin but is improved with Gd-DTPA enhancement, which may demonstrate the areas of blood-brain barrier disruption or hypervascularity. Pregadolinium T1-weighted images may demonstrate hyperintensity due to hemorrhage into the tumor. Careful comparison of MRI images with multiple biopsies at the time of surgery has shown that tumor cells may extend well beyond the areas of contrast enhancement and may even be found in the opposite cerebral hemisphere.

METASTASES. MRI usually reveals metastases better than contrast-enhanced CT. Occasionally metastases may be overlooked on a regular MRI or contrast-enhanced CT but are clearly demonstrated on a postcontrast MRI. Because gadolinium-enhanced MRI is the superior examination, it should be performed when metastases are suspected or when evaluating "extent of disease."

Multiple metastases may resemble other disease processes such as *Toxoplasma* abscesses or even the active stage of multiple sclerosis. An accurate history is always required and sometimes even a biopsy. *A solitary metastasis may often resemble a glioma or a primary lymphoma and if it is located close to the skull, it may be difficult to distinguish from a meningioma. Metastases, whether solitary or multiple, usually are well circumscribed. Surrounding edema may be minimal or extensive, depending on the cell type and steroid therapy.*

MENINGIOMAS (Fig. 392–3). Meningiomas are usually well demonstrated on contrast-enhanced CT or MRI, but if small they may be difficult to identify on MRI without contrast. Almost all meningiomas exhibit intense homogeneous gadolinium enhancement; visualization, particularly of the components adjacent to the inner table of the skull, may be superior. MRI scans in multiple

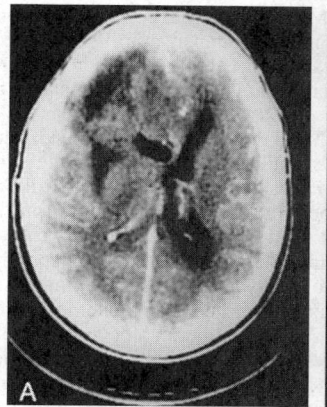 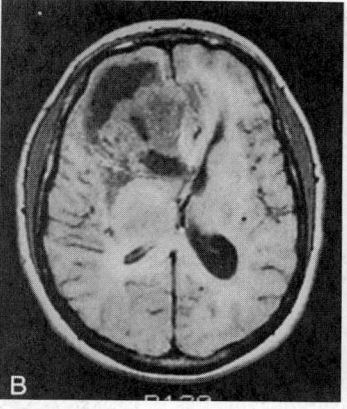 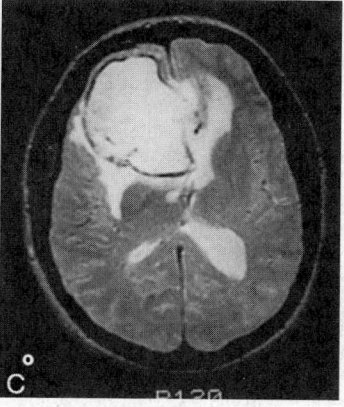

FIGURE 392–2. Right frontal glioblastoma multiforme. *A,* CT axial section with iodinated contrast enhancement. *B,* MRI axial section, 500/30 SE (T1-weighted). *C,* MRI axial section, 2000/80 SE (T2-weighted).

planes increase the examiner's confidence about the extracerebral location of these tumors.

Postoperatively, enhanced MRI is superior to enhanced CT for demonstrating residual tumor, invasion of the venous sinuses, and surgical scar formation.

LYMPHOMAS. MRI detects primary and secondary lymphoma of brain better than CT. The changes may sometimes resemble meningiomas or gliomas, thus requiring a biopsy for ultimate diagnosis. Patients with AIDS may simultaneously harbor lymphoma and *Toxoplasma* granulomas that cannot be differentiated by MRI except by evaluating the response to anti-*Toxoplasma* therapy.

TUMOR STATUS. Postoperative evaluation of tumor recurrence and radiation necrosis may be difficult with either CT or MRI if only a single examination is available. Contrast enhancement on CT and MRI may persist for several months after surgery, and radiation therapy may open the blood-brain barrier to contrast agents so as to resemble a deteriorating process on follow-up examinations. Chronic postradiation changes with demyelination of white matter are detected better on MRI than CT. Radiation necrosis may be indistinguishable from recurrent tumor by either enhanced MRI or CT. PET using fluorodeoxyglucose to measure regional cerebral metabolic rate typically demonstrates hypoactivity in areas of radionecrosis and hyperactivity in recurrent tumor. Some gliomas, however, may have low metabolic activity due to cystic components or a low grade of malignancy, sometimes making differentiation uncertain.

Other Brain Lesions

HEMATOMAS AND HEMORRHAGE. CT contributes importantly to the diagnosis of parenchymatous intracranial hemorrhage and is routinely performed as an emergency procedure following recent severe head injury or stroke. Acute hemorrhages appear as areas of increased density depending on the anatomic location (spherical or irregular for intracerebral, lentiform if chronic subdural, and concavo-convex if acute subdural or epidural). The CT-recorded increased density of clot fades so that by 10 to 14 days after bleeding occurs, the area may become isodense relative to brain, leaving a thin rim of contrast enhancement. Subacute subdural hematomas are frequently visualized better after contrast because of enhancement of the adjacent brain surface. Subsequently the aging clot, although unchanged in size, becomes hypodense, approaching the density of the CSF.

Intracranial hemorrhages cause rapid and complex changes in MRI scans during the first 4 days. Accordingly, the appearance of bleeding depends upon time of onset, source (arterial or venous), location (subarachnoid, subdural, intraparenchymal), and whether or not rehemorrhage has occurred. Other factors affecting reliability include the pulse sequences used and the field strength of the magnet.

An acute hemorrhage in any location appears isointense or slightly hyperintense on T1-weighted spin-echo images, but is hyperintense or heterogeneous on T2-weighted spin-echo techniques. At this stage hemorrhages resemble an acute infarct, tumor, or abscess/granuloma. The presence of blood, however, may be inferred from a gradient-echo scan that accentuates the magnetic susceptibility effect of the iron in hemoglobin and results in a zone of marked hypointensity.

During the first 24 hours after clot formation, oxyhemoglobin red cells change to deoxyhemoglobin and methemoglobin, resulting in a decreased signal intensity on the T2-weighted spin-echo images. Between 3 and 6 days after clot formation, lysis affects red cells with accumulation of extracellular deoxyhemoglobin and methemoglobin that results in a shortening of the T1 relaxation time, leading to increased signal intensity on T1-weighted spin-echo images.

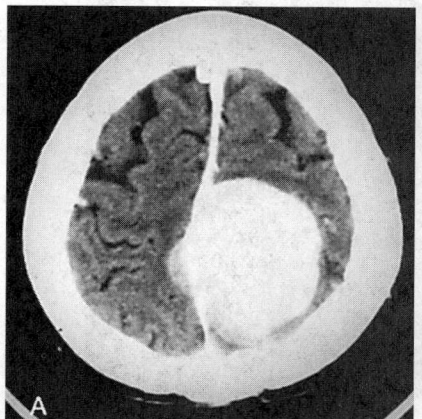 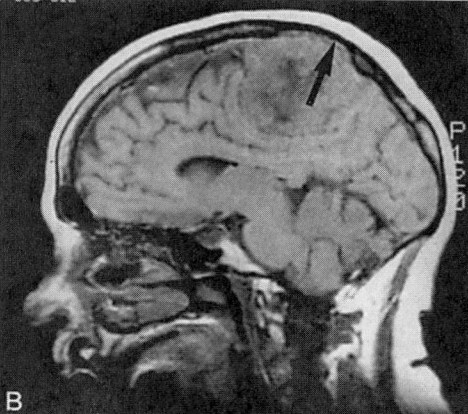 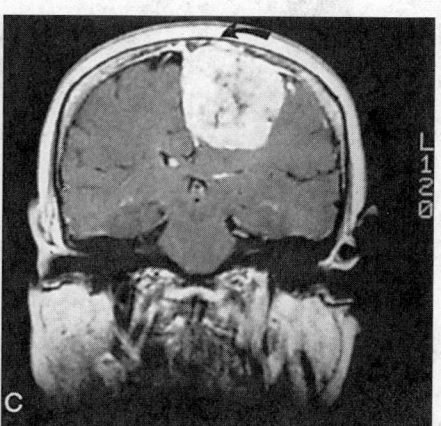

FIGURE 392–3. Left parietal parasagittal meningioma. *A,* CT axial section with iodinated contrast enhancement. *B,* MRI sagittal 500/30 SE section demonstrates invasion of the superior sagittal sinus *(arrow).* *C,* MRI coronal 500/30 SE section after intravenous administration of gadopentetate dimeglumine demonstrates intense enhancement of the tumor, dural extension, and invasion of the superior sagittal sinus *(arrow).*

After about 5 days, when red cell lysis is complete, deoxyhemoglobin converts to methemoglobin, resulting in a marked decrease in T1 relaxation time and an increase in the T2 relaxation time. This produces high signal intensity on T1- and T2-weighted spin-echo images, the unmistakable hallmark of hemorrhage. This appearance remains for 30 to 40 days, after which the T1 hyperintensity gradually decreases. Finally, the aging hemorrhage approaches the signal intensity of CSF, but the margin may remain hypointense (dark) owing to the paramagnetic effect of hemosiderin in surrounding macrophages.

Because of these complex changes, CT often detects hemorrhage more easily during the first 48 hours. If gradient-echo techniques are used, MRI may be more sensitive than CT during this time, although fresh hemorrhage may be indistinguishable from old hemorrhage or areas of abnormal brain mineralization.

ANEURYSMS AND ARTERIOVENOUS MALFORMATIONS (Fig. 392–4).
Aneurysms and arteriovenous malformations may be diagnosed by CT because of curvilinear calcifications, contrast enhancement of the lumen, and mass effect. MRI is superior to CT because the rapidly flowing blood in the lumen of the aneurysm or the nidus of a malformation results in a "signal void." Aneurysms as small as 3 mm may be detected, and surrounding hemorrhage in the brain is readily identified. Giant aneurysms >1 cm in diameter may have turbulent flow leading to heterogeneous signal intensity, similar in appearance to mural thrombosis. Magnetic resonance angiography (MRA) shows promise in detecting aneurysms and arteriovenous malformations, but detection depends upon the imaging factors and the velocity of flow within the lesions. The accuracy of MRA has not yet reached that of cerebral angiography.

Subarachnoid hemorrhage, usually due to rupture of an aneurysm, is better shown on CT than on MRI because of the effects of CSF on clot formation, deoxyhemoglobin accumulation, and resolution of the hemorrhage. *In suspicious cases, however, subarachnoid hemorrhage should never be excluded unless a lumbar puncture is normal.* Cerebral arteriography remains essential to demonstrate the anatomy of the aneurysm neck, exclude multiple aneurysms, and identify blood flow patterns. Angiography also detects anatomic anomalies of the circle of Willis prior to surgical or endovascular intervention.

Arteriovenous and venous malformations may be differentiated on MRI, but cerebral arteriography is required to differentiate a venous malformation from a small, "high-flow" arteriovenous malformation. Angiography is similarly necessary to demonstrate the dural component of an arteriovenous malformation, which may not be visible on MRI or MRA.

Cavernous hemangiomas, small benign tumors that arise in the cerebral hemispheres, cerebellum, or brain stem, cause gradual neurologic deterioration due to small, recurrent hemorrhages. On CT they appear as hyperdense masses with variable contrast enhancement. On MRI they produce a pathognomonic appearance with heterogeneous hyperintensity on T1-weighted spin-echo and a dark rim on T2-weighted technique. A cerebral arteriogram may be normal except for a faint homogeneous stain, usually without a mass effect.

HEAD TRAUMA. Following serious head trauma, conventional radiographs of the skull detect fractures of the skull vault and associated fractures of the facial bones and cervical spine. Particular attention to the upper cervical spine is required in the elderly because of the possibility of a fractured odontoid process or a "bamboo" fracture of the spine affected by ankylosing spondylitis.

Computed tomography is the best examination for demonstrating acute brain contusions or intracranial hemorrhages during the first 48 hours. Later, MRI is superior for imaging small hemorrhagic collections and revealing cerebral contusions and axonal shearing injuries.

CEREBRAL INFARCTS (Fig. 392–5). CT is currently the most frequently used imaging modality in acute stroke. Any degree of significant hemorrhage can be detected, permitting an early decision about use of anticoagulants.

MRI, however, demonstrates changes in the brain parenchyma earlier and, with gradient-echo techniques, is extremely sensitive for the presence of hemorrhage. With the addition of MRA, it is also superior for detecting thrombosis of the carotid or intracerebral arteries and venous sinus occlusions.

An acute infarct appears as an area of hyperintensity on T2-weighted spin-echo images within 4 hours after onset of the stroke; CT images may remain normal for the first 12 to 24 hours. After 4 days, areas of contrast enhancement may be detected with CT or even earlier with MRI owing to the development of pial and subpial collateral arteries and capillaries. MRI and CT equally well demonstrate old infarcts with areas of focal brain atrophy or encephalomalacia, but MRI using T2 spin-echo or gradient-echo techniques better shows areas of old hemorrhage.

In elderly patients with hypertension or arteriosclerosis and in patients with vasculitis such as lupus erythematosus, foci of hyperintensities on T2-weighted MRI images often appear in the cerebral hemispheres or cerebellum, even though the CT remains normal.

INFLAMMATORY BRAIN LESIONS. CT and MRI demonstrate inflammatory changes due to herpes simplex encephalitis, progressive multifocal leukoencephalopathy, and cytomegalovirus infection because of brain edema, mass effect, and occasionally contrast enhancement. MRI is superior to CT for demonstrating multiple granulomas such as those that complicate AIDS; gadolinium enhancement increases their detectability. Sometimes neither CT nor MRI differentiates concurrent inflammatory lesions, such as *Toxoplasma* granulomas from tuberculomas or neoplasm such as primary lymphomas.

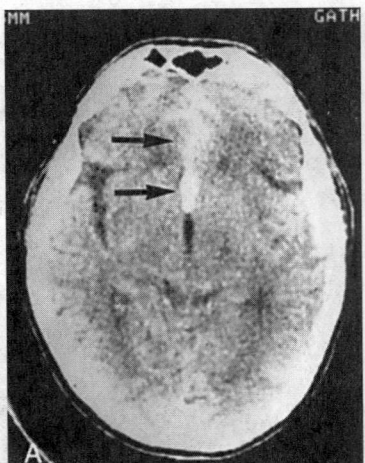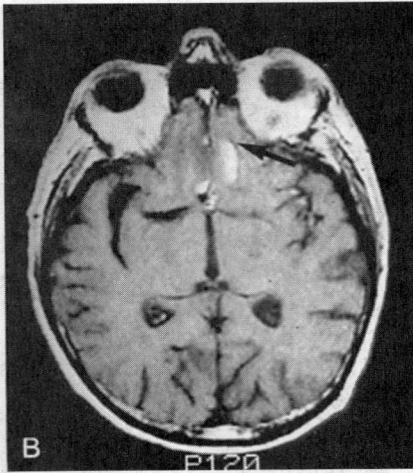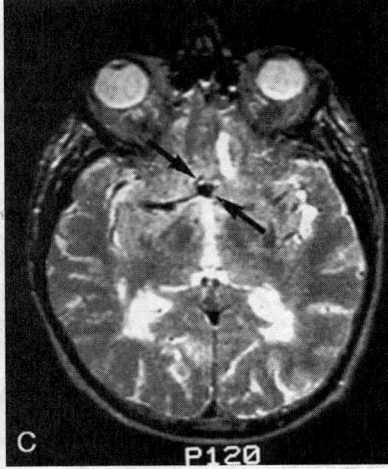

FIGURE 392–4. Subarachnoid hemorrhage due to rupture of anterior communicating artery aneurysm. *A,* CT axial section demonstrates hyperdense blood in the interhemispheric fissure *(arrows).* *B,* MRI axial 500/30 SE section demonstrates hyperintense blood along the olfactory groove *(arrow).* *C,* MRI axial 2000/80 SE section (T2-weighted) scan demonstrates the aneurysm of the anterior communicating artery *(arrows).*

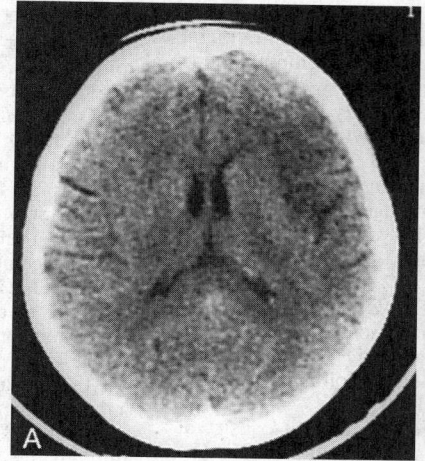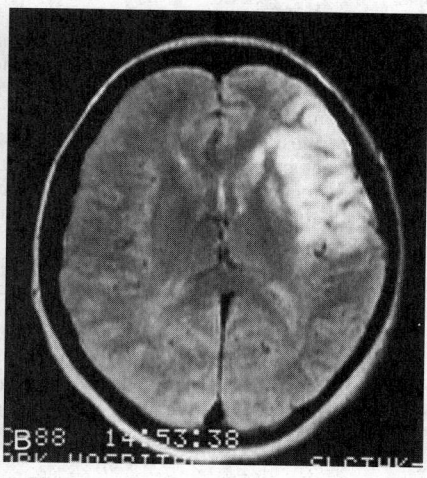

FIGURE 392–5. Acute left frontal infarct. *A*, CT axial section at 24 hours demonstrates a vague area of decreased attenuation of the left frontal lobe. *B*, MRI axial 2000/30 SE section reveals a very hyperintense area of the left frontal lobe with involvement of the cerebral cortex and adjacent basal ganglia due to a partial occlusion of the middle cerebral artery.

MRI with gadolinium enhancement is superior to CT for demonstrating acute and chronic meningitis, including sarcoid, as well as subdural and epidural empyemas. Contrast-enhanced MRI and CT detect intracerebral abscesses equally well; MRI with contrast enhancement best detects abscesses adjacent to the ethmoid sinuses and petrous temporal bones.

MULTIPLE SCLEROSIS (MS) AND WHITE MATTER DISEASES (Fig. 392–6). MRI identifies brain lesions in about 80% of patients with known MS, compared with 25% found by CT scans. Contrast enhancement after Gd-DTPA differentiates active plaques from old, healed lesions.

Focal hyperintensities resembling those of MS occur frequently in elderly patients and are usually due to ischemic demyelination or to multiple small infarcts. Similar lesions also can follow radiation therapy, Lyme disease, and severe recurrent migraine attacks; they also may be caused by generalized vascular inflammatory diseases such as lupus erythematosus. Small, disseminated metastases may have a similar appearance.

HYDROCEPHALUS AND ATROPHY. Both hydrocephalus and cerebral atrophy are associated with loss of brain volume and increased volume of CSF (see Ch. 436). MRI is the examination of choice for differentiating hydrocephalus from cerebral atrophy and for localizing the site of obstruction. MRI with gadolinium enhancement may detect small, infiltrating tumors or chronic meningitis.

In the presence of chronic aqueduct stenosis or colloid cysts obstructing the third ventricle, asymptomatic caudal herniation of the brain stem through the tentorium may be demonstrated on sagittal MR images.

CONGENITAL ANOMALIES. MRI is the best imaging modality for demonstrating and understanding most developmental anomalies of the brain. Multiplanar coronal, sagittal, and axial images make structural changes more apparent, and MRI better distinguishes areas of brain damaged by perinatal anoxia, injury, and infections.

SELLAR TUMORS. MRI is superior to CT in delineating tumors of the pituitary gland, the suprasellar region, and the optic chiasm. Contrast enhancement is essential in CT studies of this region and is increasingly used with MRI examination.

MR images in the sagittal and coronal planes demonstrate the normal pituitary gland, including the hyperintense posterior pituitary. Microadenomas are detected reliably using thin-section T1-weighted spin-echo sequences in the coronal plane. Following Gd-DTPA administration, microadenomas exhibit delayed enhancement relative to the surrounding normal tissue and therefore appear hypointense early and hyperintense late.

Analysis of the signal intensity (on T2-weighted images) separates solid fibrous adenomas from soft or cystic ones. Craniopharyngiomas and meningiomas differ from each other by their suprasellar location, tissue characteristics, and post–Gd-DTPA enhancement pattern. The precise location of adjacent cranial nerves and cerebral arteries may be identified, aiding the preoperative planning and surgical removal of the tumor.

POSTERIOR FOSSA LESIONS. MRI is the examination of choice for posterior fossa lesions because of its multiplanar capabilities, absence of bone artifacts, and superior contrast detection between gray and white matter and CSF. Tumors arising outside the cerebellum and brain stem can be differentiated from primary intra-axial tumors. Tumors arising in the skull base and clivus are detected because of replacement of the normal high signal intensity of fat-containing bone marrow. The MRI examination should be modified for the posterior fossa to include high-resolution coronal and axial images with T1-weighted spin echo. Enhancement with Gd-DTPA is increasingly used to demonstrate the total extent of meningiomas and to rule out additional tumors.

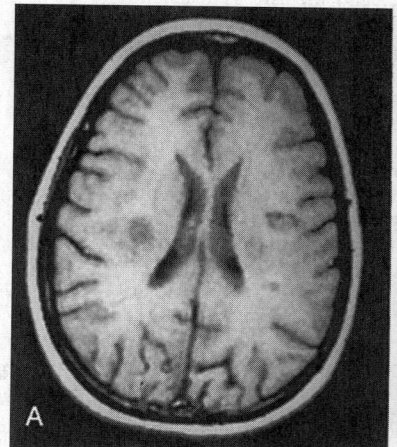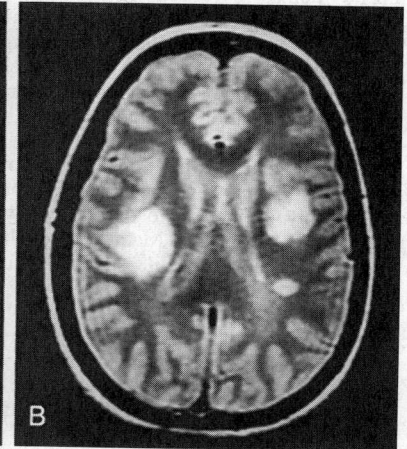

FIGURE 392–6. Multiple sclerosis. *A*, MRI axial 500/30 SE section reveals several areas of low signal intensity due to plaques of demyelination. *B*, MRI axial 2000/40 SE (proton-density) section demonstrates that the areas of demyelination are more numerous and larger.

ACOUSTIC NEURINOMAS. These benign tumors usually originate from the superior vestibular division of the eighth cranial nerve in the internal auditory canal of the petrous temporal bone (see Ch. 435).

MRI demonstrates acoustic neurinomas as slightly hypointense or isointense masses in the internal auditory canal, with extension into the adjacent cerebellopontine angle cistern (see Ch. 435). On T2-weighted images the tumor becomes hyperintense but may be obscured by the hyperintensity of the surrounding CSF. The separate divisions of the seventh and eighth cranial nerves are visible on the contralateral side. Such tumors enhance after gadolinium administration.

MENINGIOMAS OF THE POSTERIOR FOSSA. Meningiomas can grow anywhere in the posterior fossa. Those in the cerebellopontine angle appear similar to acoustic neurinomas but rarely extend into the internal auditory canal. Gadolinium enhancement is necessary to visualize the tumor's dural beak.

EPIDERMOID TUMORS. These interesting tumors consist of glittering white folds of epidermal tissue surrounded by CSF. The tumors produce a mass effect and insinuate themselves into the adjacent cisterns, wrapping around blood vessels and cranial nerves. On CT the lesions appear as fluid densities, sometimes resembling an arachnoid cyst. Epidermoid tumors show no contrast enhancement.

MRI demonstrates the full extent of the tumor, and subtle changes in signal intensity on T2-weighted spin-echo images usually differentiate the growth from surrounding CSF. Considerable deformity of the brain stem can precede abnormal neurologic signs.

CHOLESTEROL GRANULOMAS OF THE PETROUS APEX. These unusual lesions often contain brown fluid with cholesterol crystals thought to result from an inflammatory response to hemorrhage into infected petrous apical air cells. Compression of adjacent cranial nerves V, VI, VII, or VIII often results.

BASILAR ARTERY ANEURYSMS. Both saccular and fusiform aneurysms may be difficult to diagnose on CT in the axial plane. Diagnosis is straightforward on MRI because of the characteristic signal void of the lumen and the clear anatomic localization. MRA may demonstrate the lumen well, depending on the velocity of flow within it.

ARACHNOID CYSTS. Primary arachnoid cysts of the posterior fossa occur in the prepontine cistern, cerebellopontine angle, and cisterna magna. On MRI they demonstrate a signal intensity identical to that of CSF. The associated mass effect of the cyst usually differentiates it from an enlarged cisterna magna.

CRANIOVERTEBRAL JUNCTION. MRI is superior to CT for demonstrating basilar impression, whether due to congenital anomalies at the craniovertebral junction or to soft bones such as in Paget's disease or osteogenesis imperfecta. Brain stem compression caused by atlantoaxial subluxation due to rheumatoid arthritis or trauma is also well shown. Abnormally low cerebellar tonsils due to Chiari I malformation or the Arnold-Chiari malformation are easily detected.

INTRA-AXIAL POSTERIOR FOSSA TUMORS. *Brain Stem.* Intracranial tumors of the brain stem such as gliomas, ependymomas, cavernous hemangiomas, and metastases often present with progressive unilateral or bilateral cranial nerve palsies similar to extracranial tumors. Imaging techniques are crucial for the diagnosis and usually determine treatment. Surgical biopsy may have an unacceptably high complication rate.

MRI examination with multiple planes, multiple sequences, and contrast enhancement demonstrates the intra-axial location and extent of the mass with a high degree of confidence. Differentiation between a glioma and an ependymoma may be possible based on the sharply defined edge of an ependymoma and its location near the ventricular surface. Metastases of the brain stem vary in appearance, depending upon the site of origin, and may be mistaken for granulomas, lymphomas, and gliomas.

Cerebellar Tumors. Medulloblastomas as well as solid and cystic astrocytomas are usually well demonstrated with CT or MRI with contrast enhancement. Hemangioblastomas, often cystic, are better shown on MRI with contrast enhancement. The upper spinal cord should be included in the study because the area may contain additional tumor nodules.

TRAUMA. Conventional radiographs are obtained initially to demonstrate fracture and dislocations. After mid-position views with a collar have revealed normal alignment and an intact odontoid process, radiographs of the cervical spine are usually taken in flexion and extension to detect instability due to ligamentous injury. CT is helpful in demonstrating fractures of the neural arch and articular facets as well as transverse fractures of the vertebral body and post-traumatic disc herniations that may result in cord or nerve root compression. If spinal cord injury is evident clinically, MRI examination is useful to identify hematomyelia or epidural hematoma and may assist in the decision for conservative or surgical management.

DEGENERATIVE DISC DISEASE. Plain radiographs should be taken to demonstrate the vertebrae; disc space views in flexion and extension often help to show instability at the intervertebral articulations.

MRI is the study of choice in all areas of the spine for demonstrating degeneration or prolapse of the discs (Fig. 392–7). Images are obtained in the sagittal plane, the oblique axial planes, and through the intervertebral discs using various T1- or T2-weighted spin-echo sequences or gradient-echo techniques. Disc prolapse is identified and the annular deficit is usually clearly seen. Spinal stenosis, if present, is readily identified, and spinal cord or cauda equina compression may be detected.

In postoperative patients with recurrent symptoms, MRI with gadolinium enhancement can differentiate recurrent disc prolapse from postoperative scarring in the epidural space.

If MR images are degraded from metallic clips, rods, or other fixation devices or by patient motion, a CT examination of the area may substitute. Intravenous iodinated contrast is used to differentiate enhancing epidural scans from recurrent disc disease.

PRIMARY TUMORS, HYDROMYELIA, AND DEMYELINATING DISORDERS OF THE SPINAL CORD. MRI is the study of choice (Fig. 392–8). Gadolinium enhancement is required to demonstrate areas of increased vascularity in the spinal cord due to inflammatory and neoplastic processes. Intramedullary cysts due to small gliomas and ependymomas may be mistaken for hydromyelia on nonenhanced studies, but the tumor is readily detected on the post–Gd-DTPA images. Meningeal metastases either from systemic cancer or from CNS tumors show nodular enhancement after Gd-DTPA administration.

METASTATIC BONE DISEASE. MRI is the most accurate technique for detecting osseous metastases and epidural masses that may cause a cord or cauda equina compression. Such examinations are replacing emergency myelography and are usually sufficient to

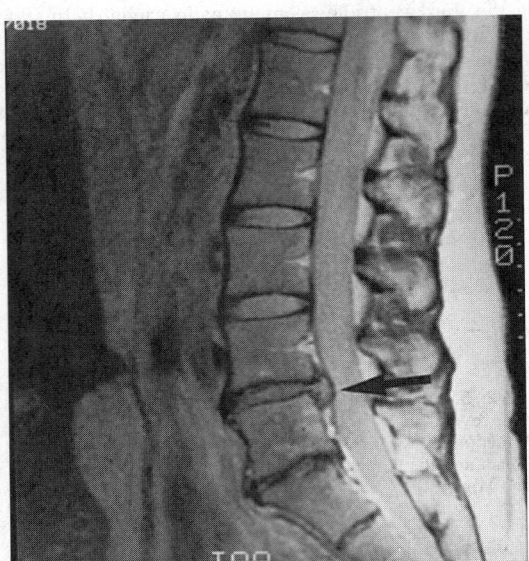

FIGURE 392–7. Herniation of a lumbar intervertebral disc. MRI 1500/30 SE sagittal section reveals a midline posterior prolapse of the nucleus pulposus of the L4/5 intervertebral disc *(arrow)* with an obvious dehiscence of the annulus fibrosis.

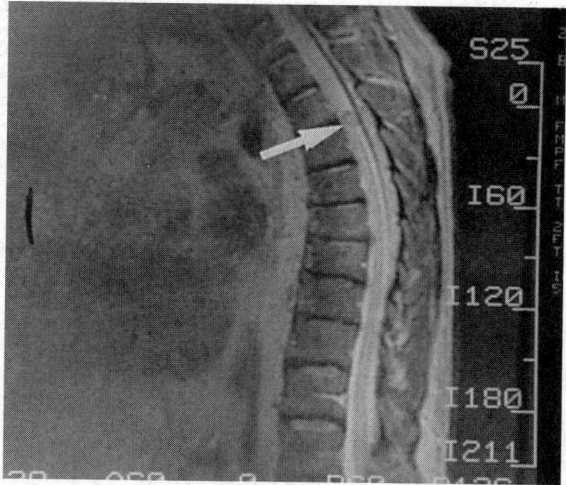

FIGURE 392–8. Thoracic neurofibroma. MRI 2000/80 SE sagittal section demonstrates an ovoid tumor *(arrow)* overlying the thoracic spinal cord.

direct appropriate radiation therapy. MRI or CT may be used to direct needle biopsies of suspected metastases of the vertebrae.

ARTERIOVENOUS MALFORMATIONS OF THE SPINAL CORD. Although large arteriovenous malformations may be identified on MRI or MRA, myelography is necessary to identify small malformations. Selective spinal arteriography with injections of contrast material directly into multiple intercostal and lumbar arteries is required to identify the precise feeding arteries, the nidus of the malformation, and the draining veins.

Brant-Zawadski M, Norman D (eds.): Magnetic Resonance Imaging of the Central Nervous System. New York, Raven Press, 1987. *An atlas of MRI demonstrating the classic appearances of a variety of brain lesions.*

Huk WJ, Gademann G, Friedmann G: Magnetic Resonance Imaging of Central Nervous System Diseases. Berlin, Springer-Verlag, 1990.

Newton TH, Potts DG (eds.): Advanced Imaging Techniques: Modern Neuroradiology. Vol. 2. San Anselmo, Calif., Clavedel Press, 1983. *Contains, among other useful information, an excellent description of the physics and techniques of various imaging modalities written for nonphysicians.*

Stark DD, Bradley WG (eds.): Magnetic Resonance Imaging. St. Louis, CV Mosby, 1988. *A comprehensive text containing detailed technical and clinical descriptions of MRI.*

Section Two—Disorders of Cerebral Function

393 DISTURBANCES OF CONSCIOUSNESS AND AROUSAL
Fred Plum

DEFINITIONS AND MECHANISMS OF ALTERED CONSCIOUSNESS

Consciousness is a brain-generated psychological state expressed in two dimensions: wakefulness and the self-aware cognition of past events and future anticipations which accompany the normal wakeful state. Disease or dysfunction that impairs either aspect of this combination causes the conditions defined in Table 393–1. Occasionally, however, either certain forms of neurologic damage or the presence of a severe psychiatric disorder can mimic an unconscious state. A later section discusses these potentially deceptive conditions.

Impaired consciousness can be *sustained,* i.e., prolonged for periods lasting for hours or more, or *brief,* with the lapse enduring for no more than a few seconds to an hour or so. The longer an abnormal state of consciousness lasts, the more likely it is to reflect structural damage to the brain rather than a transient alteration in its function. Sustained alterations of consciousness are discussed in Ch. 394. Brief loss of consciousness is considered in Ch. 396.

The normal capacity to awaken and direct attention depends upon ontogenetically primitive arousal mechanisms lodged within or in close association with the ascending reticular activating system (ARAS). The ARAS consists of a loosely organized, fairly dense column of neurons which extends forward along the brain's central core from approximately the upper third of the pons to the deep midline reaches of the hypothalamus and the thalamus. The system includes cholinergic, adrenergic, and serotoninergic fibers as well as others employing still undefined neurotransmitters. The self-aware, cognitive aspects of consciousness depend largely on the interconnected neural networks of the cerebral hemispheres and their extensive interconnections with the thalamus, basal ganglia, and cerebellum. Normal conscious states depend on the continuous, effective interaction between these cerebral systems and the subcortical activating mechanisms.

Impairments of consciousness can be partial or complete, acute or chronic. By definition, acute disturbances of consciousness always include at least some reduction in alertness and attention. These reductions often are accompanied by diffuse impairments of normal cognitive activity, reflecting a close interdependence between cortical cognitive mechanisms and the ascending activating systems. Accordingly, acute lesions that affect either the ascending system or diffusely impair large amounts of the cortex reduce the level of consciousness. Acute damage to or depression of the ARAS carries a high risk of blocking cortical arousal because its anatomic subcortical cross-sectional area is small, yet the system projects diffusely to the cortex and subcortical structures. By contrast, any given region of cortex feeds back to only a limited subcortical area

TABLE 393–1. STATES OF ALTERED CONSCIOUSNESS OR UNRESPONSIVENESS

Coma: A state of unarousable unresponsiveness; even strong exteroceptive stimuli fail to elicit recognizable psychological responses.

Stupor: Spontaneous unarousability interruptable only by vigorous, direct external stimulation.

Hypersomnia, pathologic drowsiness, obtundation: Terms applied to an increase above the patient's normal sleep/wake ratio, often accompanied during wakefulness by reduced attention and interest in the environment.

Delirium: An acute or subacute reduction in awareness, attention, orientation, and perception ("clouding of consciousness"), usually fluctuating and accompanied by abnormal sleep/wake patterns and often psychomotor disturbances.

Syncope: A brief loss of consciousness due to global failure of cerebrovascular perfusion.

Dementia: A sustained or permanent multidimensional or global decline in cognitive functions, usually without impaired arousal.

Vegetative state: A sustained, complete loss of cognition. Wake/sleep cycles and other autonomic functions remain relatively intact. The condition can either follow acute, severe bilateral cerebral damage or develop gradually as the end stage of a progressive dementia.

Locked-in state: A condition in which intellectual activity is preserved but cannot be expressed because of total incapacity to express voluntary responses due to impaired junction of descending motor pathways in the brain or peripheral motor nerves. Most such patients can use vertical eye movements to signal by code; some can grunt by code.

so that disease or dysfunction at the cerebral level usually must be widespread to cause stupor or coma. The tempo of the damage also is important. With disease that gradually affects either the cortex or the ascending activating mechanisms alone, arousal mechanisms tend to adapt so rapidly that wakefulness never is altogether lost. Accordingly, slowly progressive, severe cerebral disease causes a multifaceted dementia rather than the reduced arousal that results from acute disturbances. Among subcortical reticular structures, the posterior hypothalamus is essentially the only locus in which a chronic lesion produces a prolonged loss or reduction of the capacity to reawaken.

394 SUSTAINED IMPAIRMENTS OF CONSCIOUSNESS
Fred Plum

Three kinds of neurologic disorders may produce sustained impairment of consciousness. These include (1) focal supratentorial mass or destructive lesions that either secondarily compress or directly destroy deep midline thalamic-hypothalamic activating structures, (2) posterior fossa mass or destructive lesions that compress or destroy the brain stem's upper pontine–mesencephalic reticular formation, and (3) metabolic-diffuse abnormalities that acutely or subacutely impair the functions of the two cerebral hemispheres, the brain stem, or both. Metabolic abnormalities especially tend to affect both cerebral and subcortical arousal mechanisms concurrently. Table 394–1 enumerates the more common specific causes of stupor and coma according to these mechanisms.

PATHOPHYSIOLOGY AND CATEGORICAL DIAGNOSES OF DELIRIUM, STUPOR, AND COMA

INTRACRANIAL MASS LESIONS. Intracranial mass and destructive lesions that immediately or eventually impair consciousness can arise either above or below the tentorium, the fibrous structure that divides the diencephalon and forebrain from the brain stem. Whether such lesions lie in the supra- or subtentorial compartments, their effects and outcome depend on (1) the geographic anatomy of the abnormality, (2) its size and rate of enlargement, and (3) any reactive changes it causes in surrounding brain. These

TABLE 394–1. THE COMMON CAUSES OF STUPOR AND COMA

Supratentorial lesions (causing secondary upper brain stem dysfunction)
  Cerebral hemorrhage
  Large cerebral infarction
  Subdural hematoma
  Epidural hematoma
  Brain tumor
  Brain abscess (rare)
Subtentorial lesions (compressing or destroying the rostral reticular formation)
  Pontine or cerebellar hemorrhage
  Brain stem infarction
  Brain stem or cerebellar tumor
  Cerebellar abscess
Metabolic and diffuse lesions (see also Table 394–5)
  Exogenous poison
  Infections
    Meningitis
    Encephalitis
  Concussion and postictal states
  Anoxia or ischemia
  Hypoglycemia
  Ionic and electrolyte disorders
  Endogenous toxin due to organ failure or deficiency
  Nutritional deficiency
Psychogenic unresponsiveness

TABLE 394–2. CHARACTERISTICS OF SUPRATENTORIAL LESIONS LEADING TO COMA

Initiating symptoms usually cerebral-focal: aphasia; focal seizures; contralateral hemiparesis, sensory change, or neglect; frontal lobe behavioral changes; headache.
Dysfunction moves rostral to caudal: e.g., focal motor → bilateral motor → altered level of arousal.
Abnormal signs usually confined to a single or adjacent anatomic level (not diffuse).
Brain stem functions spared unless herniation develops.

changes include tissue edema and vasodilatation as well as proliferative inflammatory and glial responses. Their volume and effect can be as dangerous as the primary lesion itself because they can triple the size of the primary lesion. Such severe reactions are especially prominent in and around malignant neoplasms, acute infarctions, hemorrhages, or abscesses. Because the skull is inexpansible, all enlarging masses eventually cause intracranial shifts and compressions that endanger the vitality of adjacent and remote brain areas.

As mass lesions form and enlarge within the cranial cavity, local intracranial compliance declines, cerebrospinal fluid flow and absorption are impeded, and the intracranial pressure rises. If the process is not interrupted, intracranial distortion and pressure eventually increase sufficiently to impede the blood supply in areas of compressed tissue. When this occurs, arteriolar resistance intermittently fails, leading to temporary, recurrent increases in intracranial blood volume which produce brief but dangerous episodes of greatly increased intracranial pressure, called *pressure waves*.

As could be expected, functional neurologic abnormalities accompanying the above pathophysiologic changes occur earliest in regions in and adjacent to the primary lesion, then gradually extend to affect more remote brain areas made vulnerable by being compressed against unyielding edges of bone or dura. Particularly at risk of this complication are structures that become squeezed against the falx cerebri or herniate into the restricted apertures of the tentorial notch or foramen magnum, thereby impacting areas critical to consciousness and even survival (Fig. 394–1).

SUPRATENTORIAL MASS LESIONS CAUSING COMA. Enlarging supratentorial lesions most often produce stupor or coma by shifting brain tissue either horizontally across the midline or caudally toward the tentorium. The process compresses and displaces the diencephalon, impairing arousal mechanisms and producing distinctive clinical features (Table 394–2). Localizing symptoms almost always appear first, followed, as the lesion enlarges, by the development of altered consciousness. In keeping with this sequence, most patients demonstrate a combination of *focal* hemispheric signs, e.g., sensorimotor abnormalities, aphasia, or visual field defects, followed by signs of *diffuse* supratentorial dysfunction, consisting of nonfocal headache, reduced attention, confusion, and somnolence. Sometimes supratentorial masses arise and enlarge in neurologically silent areas such as the frontal lobes or the subdural space. In such instances, signs and symptoms of diffuse cerebral dysfunction and increased intracranial pressure may predominate, producing papilledema, confusion, apathy, or hypersomnolence. In either event, brain imaging discloses a large, space-occupying lesion, characteristically displacing adjacent tissues either caudally, across the midline, or both. Unless the brain already has begun to herniate into the tentorial notch, pupillary and oculovestibular reflexes remain intact. Decerebrate motor responses develop only as a late sign.

Transtentorial herniation complicating supratentorial mass lesions begins either with downward displacement of the diencephalon (central herniation) or with the uncus of the temporal lobe squeezing against the midbrain in the tentorial notch (uncal herniation) (Table 394–3). With impending *central* herniation, stupor becomes gradually deeper, and patients sigh, yawn, or develop periodic breathing. The pupils shrink to 1 to 2 mm in diameter, reflecting hypothalamic dysfunction, but retain their light reflexes. Later, one or both pupils may ominously dilate. Loss of forebrain inhibition on the brain stem results in the development of brisk oculomotor reflexes (see Ch. 403). Until mesencephalic insufficiency develops, oculovestibular reflex responses (cold caloric test) are marked by tonic deviation of the eyes toward the stimulated side. Bilateral upper motor neuron signs develop, eventually leading to decerebrate

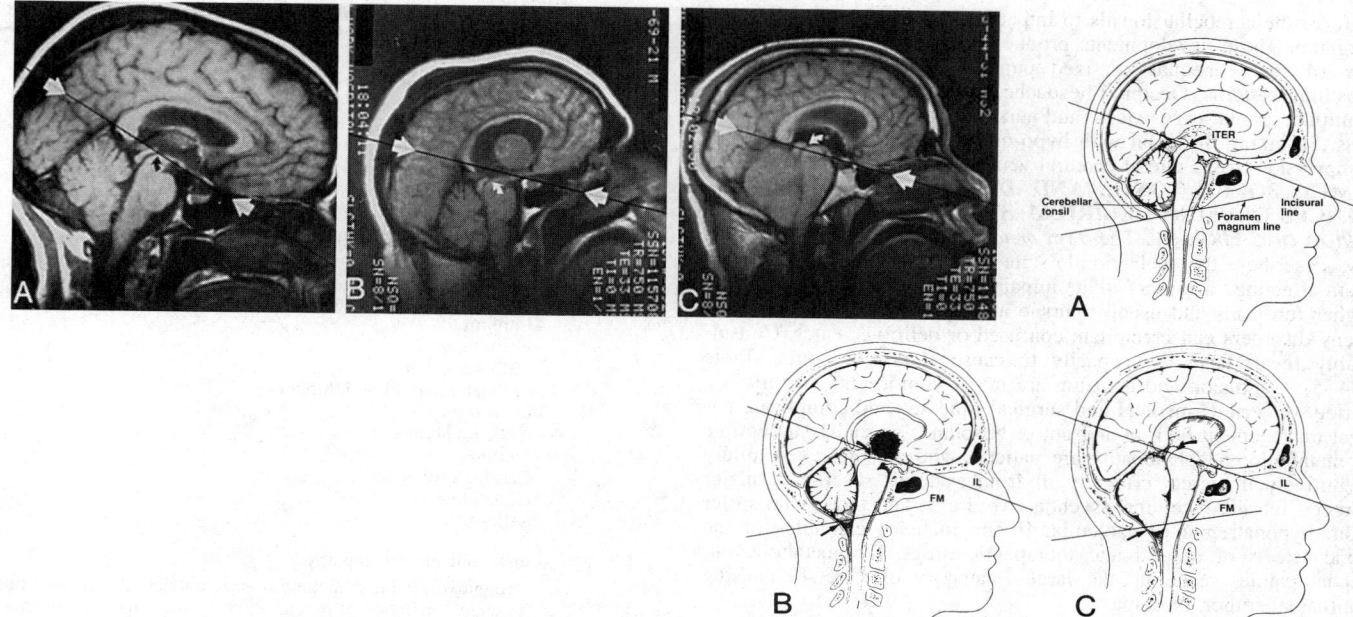

FIGURE 394–1. Midsagittal diagrams and magnetic resonance images of a normal adult brain compared with downward and upward transtentorial herniation as well as foramen magnum herniation. *A,* Normal 45-year-old male brain. The incisural line (IL) defines the plane of the tentorial opening, which extends from the junction between the vein of Galen and the cerebral venous straight sinus posteriorly to the anterior clinoid process. The iter, i.e., the rostral opening of the aqueduct of Sylvius *(black curved arrow)* lies on or within 2 mm of the IL. The cerebellar tonsils remain well above the foramen magnum. *B,* Downward transtentorial herniation due to a chronic colloid cyst lying in the third ventricle of a 52-year-old man (dark round shadow on diagram). The curved white arrow on the MRI scan points to the aqueduct, posterior thalamus, and mesencephalon, which are displaced 8 mm caudally of the IL. The cerebellar tonsils are visible at the level of the foramen magnum. *C,* Upward tentorial plus foramen magnum herniation has occurred secondary to a cerebellar lymphoma in a 32-year-old man with HIV-I infection. The cerebellum is enlarged. The iter *(black curved arrow)* and the rostral mesencephalon have herniated 6 mm above the IL, and the brain stem is flattened against the base of the skull. The cerebellar tonsils have herniated into the foramen magnum.

or decorticate reflex posturing, worse on the body side contralateral to the brain mass.

A similar progression of abnormal signs accompanies *uncal* herniation, except that as the uncus slides over the tentorial edge, it may compress the third nerve before it squeezes the diencephalon (Table 394–3). Shortly afterward, third nerve paralysis usually develops and the involved eye turns outward. If the herniating process continues, it paralyzes the opposite third nerve and other mesencephalic functions begin to fail. To be effective, treatment must be initiated before these late signs of deterioration appear.

SUBTENTORIAL MASS OR DESTRUCTIVE LESIONS CAUSING COMA. Subtentorial mass or destructive lesions cause stupor or coma if they directly damage or compress the ascending activating systems that arise from the paramedian rostral pontine tegmentum and mesencephalon. Such coma-causing abnormalities always affect adjacent neuro-ophthalmologic centers, causing telltale signs that pinpoint the anatomy of damage (Table 394–4).

Most subtentorial lesions that cause coma by directly injuring the upper brain stem (e.g., infarcts or hemorrhages) cause coma from the outset. The pupils are always abnormal, owing to dysfunction or destruction of pontine sympathetic pathways, third nerve nuclei, or their internuclear fibers. Dysconjugate eye movements are common, as are nystagmus, bizarrely or independently moving eyes, ocular bobbing, or ocular deviation. Unilateral facial anesthesia involving both the brow and lower face, absent caloric responses to either side, and conjugate eye deviation toward the paralyzed arm and leg all suggest a subtentorial lesion. The combination of flaccidity in the arms and flexor responses in the legs signifies pontine-midbrain damage. Brain imaging identifies cerebellar or pontine hemorrhage as well as expanding cerebellar hematomas, neoplasms, or most infarctions. MR produces better images of the cerebellum and brain stem than CT scans.

Compressive lesions of the posterior fossa, such as hemorrhages, abscesses, or tumors of the cerebellum or fourth ventricle, rarely cause coma until late in their course, at which time they may cause the mesencephalon to herniate upward through the tentorial notch

TABLE 394–3. SIGNS OF INCIPIENT DOWNWARD HERNIATION

	Central	Uncal
Arousal	Impaired early, before other signs	Impaired late, usually with other signs
Breathing	Sighs, yawns, sometimes Cheyne-Stokes respirations	No early change
Pupils	First small reactive (hypothalamus), then one or both approach midposition	Ipsilateral pupil dilates, followed by somatic third nerve paralysis
Oculocephalic responses	Initially sluggish, later tonic conjugate	Unilateral third nerve paralysis
Motor signs	Early hemiparesis opposite to hemispheric lesion followed late by ipsilateral motor paresis and extensor plantar response	Motor signs late, sometimes ipsilateral to lesion

TABLE 394–4. TELLTALE SIGNS OF PRIMARY SUBTENTORIAL LESIONS CAUSING COMA

Onset of coma often sudden
Symptoms of brain stem dysfunction may precede coma
Localizing brain stem signs always exist
  Caloric responses disconjugate or absent
  Pupil(s) abnormal: pinpoint (pons), fixed (midbrain), irregular and/or unequal (midbrain-pontine)
  Often "bizarre" signs: ocular bobbing, ataxic breathing, etc.
  Often signs of cerebellar or bilateral motor dysfunction

or force the cerebellar tonsils to impact downward into the foramen magnum. These developments produce deepening stupor, failure of upward gaze, unequal or fixed pupils, and irregularly irregular breathing patterns. Occipital headache, nystagmus, diplopia, nausea, vomiting, cranial nerve signs, and ataxia often precede unconsciousness. Shrinking the brain with hypo-osmotic fluids and surgical decompression of the lateral cerebral ventricles can be life-saving.

METABOLIC, TOXIC, AND DIFFUSE BRAIN DISTURBANCES CAUSING DELIRIUM, STUPOR, AND COMA. *Definition and Etiology.* The term *metabolic* or *diffuse encephalopathy* describes the behavioral state produced by a group of brain-affecting disorders that impair predominantly the organ's higher functions and usually pursue a temporary, reversible course. Many disorders can precipitate confused or delirious states. Considerably fewer have the capacity to cause stupor or coma (Table 394–5). Confusion and delirium are major comorbidity factors in a variety of serious medical and surgical illnesses and complicate patient management both in and out of hospital. Especially susceptible to metabolic encephalopathy are patients who are old, even mildly cognitively impaired, critically ill from systemic disease or major surgery, febrile, receiving psychoactive drugs, and those who suffer from hyponatremia or azotemia. If one includes examples of the toxic effects of abused and therapeutic drugs, the metabolic encephalopathies make up the largest category of illnesses causing confusion, stupor, or coma.

Disorders or drugs affecting several neurochemical and neuropharmacologic systems can cause a metabolic encephalopathy. Prominent examples are drugs with either anticholinergic or sedative effects. Other common causes include a number of inflammatory or infectious illnesses, physiologic disturbances such as epilepsy or complicated migraine, diffuse brain trauma, and disseminated structural lesions such as certain forms of cancer or cerebral thromboembolism. Diffuse, acute or subacute, bilateral, multi-level cerebral and subcerebral dysfunction that almost always spares pupillary reactivity is the hallmark of metabolic encephalopathy and is only rarely produced by structural brain disease.

Terminology. Classic neurologic thinking has employed the terms *delirium* and *acute toxic psychosis* for the more blatantly agitated and severely disoriented, hallucinatory-delusional forms of metabolic encephalopathy. Quieter, less severe disturbances have been termed *acute* or *subacute confusional states*. This chapter often uses these terms because they are more descriptively informative than the usage adopted by the American Psychiatric Association's Diagnostic Manual, which applies the term *delirium* to all examples of acquired confusion, agitation, disorientation, or hallucinations occurring in the setting of structural or known neurochemical brain disease.

Clinical Features. Table 394–6 lists the most consistent and specific symptoms of acute confused-delirious states. Frequent premorbid features include fractures, age over 80 years, and at least mild cognitive impairment. The clinical evaluation of these conditions attempts first to determine whether the observed changes are due to metabolic rather than structural brain disease or psychiatric dysfunction. One then proceeds to define the particular metabolic or structural defects and treat them. Evaluations of the history, the pattern of impaired consciousness, motor activity, and autonomic activity help answer the first question, whereas the general physical examination, evaluation of pulmonary ventilation, and laboratory tests assist with the second (Table 394–7). The history is especially important and should inquire into previous systemic medical illnesses, psychiatric history, access to potentially intoxicating drugs or alcohol, and recent changes in behavior.

State of Consciousness and Mental Content. Disorders of attention are the earliest sign and the hallmark of metabolic brain disease. Some patients act quietly perplexed, preoccupied, and unable to concentrate. Others appear hypervigilant and distractible, picking at the bedclothes and attending briefly to each new environmental stimulus no matter how trivial or irrelevant. Still others lose contact with the environment, becoming completely preoccupied and often frightened by vivid fragmentary hallucinations or delusions. Early attentional deficits may be subtle and easily mistaken for normal, slightly odd behavior. Soon, however, other symptoms emerge, including emotional lability, insomnia or drowsiness, and often vivid nightmares. As delirium worsens, some patients express the fear of

TABLE 394–5. POTENTIAL CAUSES OF TOXIC, METABOLIC, OR DIFFUSE BRAIN DYSFUNCTION CAUSING DELIRIUM OR COMA

I. Exogenous poisons
   A. Alcohol–sedative drug abuse, acute or chronic, immediate or withdrawal
   B. Acid poisons or poisons with acidic breakdown products:
      Paraldehyde
      Methyl alcohol
      Ethylene glycol
   C. Psychotropic drugs, acute or chronic:
      Opiates and their congeners
      Cocaine
      Amphetamines
      Tricyclic antidepressants and anticholinergic drugs
      Lithium
      Phenothiazines
      LSD-mescaline
      Monoamine oxidase inhibitors
   D. Other drugs:
      Anticonvulsants
      Steroids
      Cardiac glycosides
      Cimetidine
      Salicylates

II. Mixed metabolic encephalopathy

   Age + cognitive decline ± surgery or severe illness ± hyponatremia ± systemic infection ± psychoactive drug use ± azotemia ± darkened environment.

III. Deprivation of oxygen, substrate, or metabolic cofactors
   A. Hypoxia (interference with oxygen supply to the entire brain; cerebral blood flow normal)
      1. Decreased oxygen tension (usually $Pao_2 < 35$ mm Hg) and content of blood: pulmonary disease, alveolar hypoventilation, decreased atmospheric oxygen tension (e.g., high altitude)
      2. Decreased oxygen content of blood—normal tension:
         Anemia (Hb $< 40\%$ normal)
         Carbon monoxide poisoning
         Methemoglobinemia
   B. Ischemia (diffuse or widespread multifocal interference with blood supply to brain; often with accompanying hypoxia)
      1. Decreased cerebral blood flow resulting from decreased cardiac output:
         Hemorrhagic or septic shock
         Stokes-Adams syndrome, cardiac arrest, cardiac arrhythmias
         Myocardial infarction
         Aortic stenosis
         Pulmonary embolism
      2. Decreased cerebral blood flow resulting from decreased systemic peripheral resistance:
         Syncope: orthostatic, vasovagal
         Carotid sinus hypersensitivity
         Hypovolemia
      3. Decreased cerebral blood flow due to generalized or multifocal increase in cerebrovascular resistance:
         Hyperventilation syndrome
         Increased blood viscosity (polycythemia, cryo- and macroglobulinemia, sickle cell anemia)
         Subarachnoid hemorrhage (both hemotoxic and vasospasm)
      4. Decreased local cerebral blood flow due to widespread small vessel occlusion or tissue necrosis:
         Disseminated intravascular coagulation
         Systemic lupus erythematosus
         Endocarditis, bacterial or nonbacterial
         Cardiopulmonary bypass
         Small emboli (fat, fibrin, platelets)
      5. Alterations of blood flow due to failure of autoregulation:
         Hypertensive encephalopathy
   C. Hypoglycemia:
      Hyperinsulinism: exogenous; endogenous
   D. Cofactor deficiency:
      Thiamine (Wernicke's encephalopathy)
      Pyridoxine
      Vitamin B_{12}

IV. Diseases of organs other than brain
   A. Nonendocrine organs:
      Liver (hepatic coma)
      Kidney (uremic coma)
      Lung (CO_2 narcosis)

TABLE 394-5. POTENTIAL CAUSES OF TOXIC, METABOLIC, OR DIFFUSE BRAIN DYSFUNCTION CAUSING DELIRIUM OR COMA Continued

B. Hyper- and/or hypofunction of endocrine organs:
   Panhypopituitarism
   Thyroid (myxedema-thyrotoxicosis)
   Parathyroid (hyper- and hypocalcemia)
   Adrenal (Addison's disease, Cushing's disease)
C. Other systemic diseases:
   Diabetes
   Cancer and its treatments
   Porphyria
   Sepsis

V. Abnormalities of fluid, ionic, or acid-base environment of CNS
   A. Water and sodium (hyper- and hyponatremia; hypo- and hyperosmolality
   B. Acidosis (metabolic and respiratory)
   C. Calcium (hyper- and hypocalcemia)

VI. Disordered temperature regulation
   A. Hypothermia
   B. Heat stroke, fever, malignant neuroleptic syndrome

VII. Infections or inflammation of CNS
   A. Leptomeningitis
   B. Encephalitis
   C. Acute "toxic" encephalopathy
   D. Parainfectious encephalomyelitis
   E. Cerebral vasculitis
   F. Subarachnoid hemorrhage

VIII. Miscellaneous diseases of uncertain pathophysiology
   A. Seizures and postictal states
   B. Concussion
   C. Right middle cerebral or left posterior cerebral infarctions
   D. Migraine

"going crazy." Others lie quietly or sleep when left alone. None reads for substance or attends to the surrounding world with any interest. With more severe metabolic disturbances, patients become drowsy and some become stuporous or comatose. The prevailing affect depends partly on the nature of the illness and partly on how rapidly it develops. Previous personality often has surprisingly little influence on delirious behavior. Rapidly developing metabolic abnormalities are more likely to produce agitation or stupor than are those that evolve more slowly.

Disturbances in cognition accompany altered alertness and awareness, causing difficulties with immediate recall and the ability to abstract. Normal subjects readily recall and repeat six or seven digits forward and five or six backward and can identify the common denominator between such pairs as an apple and an orange or a fly and a tree; confused patients cannot. But the examiner must be cautious; innate intelligence and education also determine cognitive abilities. Unless the physician already knows the patient, it may be difficult to attribute mild mental changes to a metabolic defect. Loss of memory for recent events and disorientation for time are hallmarks of organic brain disease. Orientation to place and time should be specifically tested by asking the date and year, the day of the week, and the present location.

Perceptual errors, e.g., mistaking the physician for someone else, as well as illusions and hallucinations, are more serious symptoms. Hallucinations are common and usually animate. They frighten and agitate some patients, but others tolerate them quietly and must be asked about their presence. Delirious hallucinations or delusions may be visual, auditory, or tactile, alone or in combination; rarely are they systematic. By contrast, schizophrenic delusions or halluci-

TABLE 394-6. PRINCIPAL SYMPTOMS OF ACUTE CONFUSED-DELIRIOUS STATES

Acute onset and fluctuating course
Inattention
Disorganized thinking
Memory impairment
Disorientation
Altered sleep-wake cycle

TABLE 394-7. PHYSICAL SIGNS OF METABOLIC ENCEPHALOPATHY

Confusion, lethargy, delirium often precede or replace coma
Motor signs, if present, usually symmetric
Bilateral asterixis, myoclonus appear
Pupillary reactions usually preserved
Sensory abnormalities usually absent
Hypothermia common
Abnormal signs reflect incomplete brain dysfunction at multiple anatomic levels

nations are usually systematic in pattern and consist almost exclusively of endogenous auditory perceptions.

Characteristically, the mental status examination fluctuates in metabolic encephalopathy. Delirious patients typically become more disoriented at night and in unfamiliar surroundings. The presence of restraints, intermittent background noise, and unfamiliar activity accentuates their confusion.

Motor Activity. Bilateral tremor, asterixis, and multifocal myoclonus are hallmarks of metabolic brain disease. The *tremor* ranges from fine to coarse, is irregular at a rate of about eight to ten per second, and involves the distal more than proximal parts of the extremities. Coarse tremor such as accompanies certain drug withdrawals or intoxications may be so heavy that it shakes the bed.

Asterixis describes an abnormal, irregular, distal involuntary jerking movement, best elicited with arms outstretched, hands pronated, and fingers extended. Severe examples border on myoclonus. Asterixis is encountered rarely, and then unilaterally, in patients with structural brain disease.

Multifocal myoclonus consists of sudden nonrhythmic, nonpatterned coarse jerks affecting resting groups of muscles. Multifocal myoclonus occurs most frequently in uremia, in hypercarbic-anoxic encephalopathy, with penicillin or lithium overdose, and in association with the progressive dementia of Creutzfeldt-Jakob disease (see Ch. 428.6).

Psychomotor activity in delirium can range from extremes of picking at the bedcovers, sustained restlessness, and thrashing about to total immobility. Increased psychomotor activity is typical of acute deliria such as delirium tremens. More commonly, toxic confusional states are marked by lethargy, drowsiness, and general bradykinesia. Other patients may be unwilling or unable to stay in bed. They pace the halls, move constantly, and often shout vulgarities or aggressive threats. Unless restrained, many confused patients fall in trying to walk or during efforts to climb out of bed.

Speech is often abnormal. Patients with increased psychomotor behavior often speak rapidly, muttering or slurring speech into an incomprehensible jumble. Bradykinetic patients may speak slowly, monotonously, and so softly as to be barely heard.

Seizures, hyperactive stretch reflexes, and *signs of mild focal brain dysfunction* frequently accompany severe metabolic brain disease, especially after alcohol-sedative withdrawal. The seizures are usually generalized and the motor abnormalities usually symmetric. Nevertheless, focal paresis and focal seizures occasionally occur, especially with hypoglycemia, hepatic encephalopathy, or postanoxic encephalopathy.

Autonomic Activity. *Pupillary light reactions are preserved in metabolic coma with rare exceptions, and their absence requires a specific search for a pre-existing or acute structural lesion.* Nevertheless, a few exceptions exist; the ingestion of drugs possessing an anticholinergic action can paralyze the pupils transiently in either mid-position or dilation. Also, exposure to severe anoxia or asphyxia can produce fixed mid-position or dilated pupils. If sustained, these imply irreversible brain stem damage. In general, the pupils usually remain symmetric in metabolic brain disease, but are often asymmetric and sometimes fixed in patients comatose from structural brain disease.

Hypothermia is common in sedative intoxication as well as with hypoglycemia and myxedema. *Hyperthermia* with profuse perspiration and tachycardia accompanies most agitated deliria and is especially common with delirium tremens. Hyperthermia without perspiration suggests anticholinergic drug ingestion, infection, heat stroke, or the malignant neuroleptic syndrome. Less severe, unexplained

TABLE 394–8. LABORATORY EVALUATION OF METABOLIC BRAIN DISEASE

Test	Reason for Test
Immediately Reported	
Glucose	Hypoglycemia, hyperosmolar coma
Na$^+$	Osmolar abnormalities
Ca^{2+}	Hyper- or hypocalcemia
BUN	Uremia
Arterial blood pH, Pco_2, Po_2	Acidosis, alkalosis, hypoxia
Lumbar puncture	Infection, hemorrhage, meningeal carcinomatosis
Later Reported	
Liver function tests	Hepatic coma
Sedative drug levels	Overdose
Blood and CSF culture	Sepsis, encephalitis, meningitis
Full electrolytes, including Mg^{2+}	Electrolyte imbalance
Coagulation profile	Intravascular coagulation
EEG	Seizure disorder

hyperthermia can reflect idiosyncrasy to a variety of widely used drugs, including salicylates.

Laboratory Tests. The causes of metabolic coma are legion. In many instances the history (e.g., of drug abuse, systemic disease, exposure to toxins) immediately suggests the cause. When this is uncertain, tests listed in Table 394–8 should be performed immediately to establish or rule out the presence of life-threatening metabolic defects. Unless strong evidence indicates a specific metabolic or infectious process causing the delirium, diagnostic brain imaging is desirable. Imaging shows no immediately pertinent abnormalities in metabolic encephalopathy but may reveal pre-existing abnormalities such as chronic subdural hematoma or previous brain damage, the effects of which can mimic or accentuate metabolic delirium.

PSYCHIATRIC DISORDERS. Psychiatric disorders capable of producing the behavioral appearance of impaired consciousness include delirious stages of acute schizophrenic or manic attacks, the nearly total withdrawal of severe depression or certain forms of catatonia, and the pseudocoma of hysteria and malingering (Table 394–9). Especially in the early stages of such disorders, distinction from physiologic alterations of consciousness sometimes can be difficult. Psychiatric amnesia is the most common pseudo-organic symptom and the most readily diagnosed. One should suspect psychiatric amnesia when the experience covers sharply delineated periods of time, has an abrupt onset and offset with total amnesia in the middle, is nonprogressive in nature, and relates either to experiences that provoked severe anxiety or to potentially punishable behavior. Catatonic withdrawal states or psychotic deliria in psychiatric illness sometimes can be difficult to differentiate from those of

TABLE 394–9. PSYCHIATRIC STATES RESEMBLING ACUTE IMPAIRMENT OF CONSCIOUSNESS

1. **Catatonic states.** Uncommon conditions occurring in either schizophrenic or severe depressive illness which may resemble organic stupor. Mutism, bilateral motor resistance, hypokinesia, and even rigidity are common. Absent are pathologic reflexes, as well as abnormal brain images, EEG's, and laboratory chemical tests.
2. **Acute psychotic deliria.** Uncommon. Involves adult patients of any age, more frequently those older than 50 years. The state can arise with either affective or schizophrenic disorders. Agitation, fear, and hypermobility are prominent. Auditory or visual hallucinations occur, not necessarily paranoid but usually systematized. Fast, coarse tremor can be present and tends to last longer than drug-alcohol withdrawal tremors. Verbal responses, when elicitable, usually reflect orientation for time and place, but distractibility or muteness often limits mental testing. Pathologic reflexes are lacking. EEG and laboratory chemical tests remain normal in the absence of medical complications. The condition can be difficult to diagnose, but an agitated delirium that lasts longer than 2 weeks almost always reflects psychiatric disease. Some end in catatonia or death unless treated with neuroleptics.
3. **Hysteria-malingering.** Unarousable unresponsiveness, usually of brief duration, unaccompanied by physiologic abnormalities and often associated with obviously factitious responses to stimulation.

metabolic origin, but applying the guidelines given in Table 394–10 usually provides the answers. As a general rule, however, if the patient's cooperation can be elicited to obtain satisfactory answers, recent memory and cognitive functions usually turn out to be preserved in the functional psychoses. Patients with extreme anxiety may hyperventilate, producing respiratory alkalosis, a diffusely slow electroencephalogram, and sometimes tetany. Otherwise, physical and laboratory evaluations in psychogenically altered consciousness remain normal.

Patients with hysterical pseudocoma have normal somatic neurologic examinations. Breathing is eupneic or voluntarily hyperpneic. Most such patients lie supine and quietly unresponsive, with limbs remaining either flaccid or resisting movement in unpredictable patterns. Eyelids usually are closed, actively resist opening, and may spontaneously flutter. Furthermore, the eyelids are incapable of the slow closure that follows passive raising of the lids of patients with physiologic coma. The pupils in psychiatric unresponsiveness are briskly responsive or, if cycloplegics have been self-instilled, widely dilated. Oculocephalic responses are unpredictable, but if the diagnosis is doubtful, irrigating the tympanum with 50 ml of cold water produces physiologic nystagmus rather than the tonic eye deviation or absent responses shown by comatose patients with structural or metabolic disease. Sometimes, the eyes may deviate toward the bed when the patient is turned to one side.

Occasionally, psychiatric pseudodelirium or unresponsiveness can be superimposed on underlying physical illness. An example is the patient hospitalized with a severe medical or neurologic illness who becomes so anxious that he or she is unable to cope and withdraws psychologically to the point of unresponsiveness. In such doubtful instances, slow infusions of small amounts of sodium amobarbital (Amytal interview) may allow the physician to establish contact and rapport with the patient. Because the drug may similarly awaken patients rendered unconscious by continuous focal seizures, close clinical observation and, if possible, an EEG are best done before the test.

ACUTE CENTRAL NERVOUS SYSTEM POISONING. Table 394–11 lists the most frequent acute neurotoxic poisonings in the United States, gives their principal signs of toxicity, and outlines their treatment. To find descriptions of poisons not included in

TABLE 394–10. ORGANIC AND FUNCTIONAL PSYCHOSES COMPARED

Variable	Organic	Functional
Onset	Usually > 30 years	Usually < 40 years
Family history	Usually negative	Often psychiatrically abnormal
Immediate history	Drugs, alcohol, acute medical or neurologic illness	No established medical or neurologic features
Psychology of history	Psychologically coherent	Psychologically incoherent
	Agitation, tremor, noisiness, inattention	Same
Major (psychotic) symptoms		
Orientation and memory	Abnormal	Normal if answers obtained
Delusions or hallucinations	Visual, sometimes olfactory or auditory; nonsystematic (chaotic)	Mainly auditory; systematic: tell a story
Mood	Fearful or apathetic; delusions often regarded as unwanted	Consistent with psychotic symptoms
Coma or akinetic (catatonic) state	Systemic and/or neurologic signs present; EEG abnormal	Neurologic signs absent; EEG normal
Fever, leukocytosis	Signs of medical illness often present	Absent (except malignant hyperthermia or catatonia)
Alcohol-drug intoxication or withdrawal	Often present	Absent
Clinical or EEG seizures	Often present	Absent

TABLE 394–11. COMMON DRUG POISONINGS, SIGNS OF TOXICITY, AND TREATMENT

| Drug | Signs and Symptoms | | Diagnostic Test | Treatment |
	Mild	*Severe*		
Opiates Heroin Morphine Meperidine Methadone Hydromorphone Oxycodone Levorphanol	"Nodding" drowsiness, small pupils, urinary reention, slow and shallow breathing; skin scars and subcutaneous abscesses; duration 4–6 hours; with methadone, duration to 24 hours	Coma; pinpoint pupils, slow irregular respiration or apnea, hypotension, hypothermia, pulmonary edema	Response to naloxone Urine	Naloxone, 0.4 mg intravenously or intramuscularly; repeat at 15-minute intervals if patient responds and gradually increase intervals; repeat in 3 hours if necessary; if no response by second dose, suspect another cause; treat shock; find and detect infection
Sedatives–hypnotics syndromes Alcohol Barbiturates Chloral hydrate Glutethimide (Doriden) Meprobamate (Equanil)	Confusion, rousable drowsiness, delirium, ataxia, nystagmus, dysarthria, analgesia to stimuli	Stupor to coma; pupils reactive, usually constricted; oculovestibular response absent; motor tonus initially briefly hyperactive, then flaccid; respiration and blood pressure depressed; hypothermia.	Blood, urine, breath Blood Blood Blood	Intubate, ventilate, lavage; drainage position; antimicrobials; keep mean blood pressure > 90 mm Hg and urine output > 300 ml per hour; avoid analeptics; hemodialyze severe phenobarbital poisoning
Benzodiazepines (Librium, Valium, Tranxene, Ativan, Dalmane, etc.)	Usually taken with another sedative if poisoning is attempted	Coma seldom severe if drug taken alone	Blood	As above; diuresis of little help
Toxic-hyperactive syndromes Amphetamines Methylphenidate	Euphoria, sometimes paranoid, repetitive behavior, dilated pupils, tremor, hyperactive reflexes; hyperthermia, tachycardia, arrhythmia	Agitated, assaultive and paranoid excitement; occasionally convulsions; hyperthermia; circulatory collapse.	Blood	Chlorpromazine
Cocaine	Similar but less prominent than above; less paranoid, often euphoric	Twitching; irregular breathing, tachycardia, arrhythmia, occasionally convulsions; myocardial infarction; acute stroke; vasculitis; chronic paranoid psychosis or depression	Blood, urine	Diazepam plus labetalol for cardiovascular crisis
MAO inhibitors (Parnate, Nardil, Eutonyl, etc.)	Hypertensive crises, agitation, drowsiness, ataxia	Hypotension; headache; chest pain; agitation; coma, seizures and shock	Clinical	Symptomatic; gastric lavage
Neuroleptics (phenothiazines, butyrophenones, etc.)	Acute dystonia, somnolence, hypotension	Coma; convulsions (rare); arrhythmias; hypotension	Blood	Anticholinergics; diphenhydramine; symptomatic; gastric lavage
Psychedelics (LSD, mescaline, psilocybin, phencyclidine)	Confused, disoriented, perceptual distortions, distractable, withdrawn or eruptive, leading to accidents or violence; wide-eyed, dilated pupils; restless, hyperreflexic; less often, hypertension or tachycardia	Panic		Reassure; diazepam satisfactory; avoid phenothiazines
Scopolamine-atropine (knockout drops, Transderm delirium)	Agitated or confused, visual hallucinations, dilated pupils, flushed and dry skin	Florid toxic disoriented delirium, visual hallucinations; later, amnesia, fever, dilated fixed pupils, hot flushed dry skin, urinary retention		Reassure; sedate lightly, (1) avoid phenothiazines; (2) do not leave alone
Antidepressants Tricyclics (Tofranil, Elavil, Desipramine, etc.)	Restless, drowsiness, tachycardia, ataxia, sweating	Agitation, vomiting, hyperpyrexia, sweating, muscle dystonia, convulsions, tachycardia or arrhythmia	Blood	Symptomatic; gastric lavage Intensive care, anticonvulsants, and antiarrhythmics for severe cases
Lithium	Mild lethargy	Sustention-intention tremor, lethargy; muteness with appearance of distraction; coma; multifocal seizures; slow or fluctuating course	Blood	Hydrate if mild; hemodialyze for delirium, coma, or convulsions
Acid-forming intoxicants Methanol (formic); ethylene glycol (oxalic and hippuric); other organic alcohols	Inebriation with hyperpnea	All produce progressive hyperventilation, drunkenness, stupor, eventually convulsions and death. Early blindness with methanol	Blood shows increasingly severe anion gap acidosis	Inhibit hepatic alcohol dehydrogenase by giving alcohol until acidosis controlled; treat acidosis vigorously
Salicylate Aspirin	Tinnitus, dyspnea	Older persons: confusional state or toxic delirium leading to stupor, convulsions, coma	Blood salicylate > 60 mg/dl	Alkaline diuresis

this section, especially chronic neurotoxic agents, the reader should consult the textbooks listed in the references. Almost all drugs in overdose amounts are likely to be mixed with intoxicating amounts of alcohol, thereby making their clinical signs more difficult to appraise. Nevertheless, clinical evaluation must be used to diagnose the specific agent causing several of these reaction patterns because chemical tests are in many instances either unavailable or impractically slow. When any doubt exists, one should keep admission serum samples for possible later analysis. With most of the drugs, tolerance develops to chronic ingestion and individuals may react differently to similar doses. Accordingly, blood levels and size of the dose are unreliable guides to the potential depth of coma or other complications. The mixing of agents adds to the unreliability. Only the opiates and some of the sedatives create an immediate risk of death; concurrent alcohol ingestion enhances both these risks. Opiate poisoning is discussed in greater detail in Ch. 12.

Pathogenesis. All sedative drugs depress the central nervous system, although not equally on a gram-molecular weight basis, and often produce different degrees of inhibition on individual central structures. The duration of action varies widely and depends largely on how the particular drug is detoxified or eliminated. The benzodiazepines, short-acting barbiturates, pentobarbital, secobarbital, and amobarbital are detoxified by the liver, as is methaqualone. They exert their maximal effects promptly after being absorbed and, even in huge doses, seldom cause neurologic depression lasting longer than 3 to 5 days. The benzodiazepine group especially possesses a wide margin of safety between their hypnotic effects and any serious depression of breathing and circulatory control. Barbital and phenobarbital are partially detoxified by the liver and partially excreted in the urine. Severe poisoning with the latter agent can cause coma lasting 10 to 14 days. Furthermore, as a class, the barbiturates have a relatively high capacity to halt breathing control and produce hypotension.

A withdrawal syndrome consisting of tremulousness, agitation, and sometimes delirium and convulsions can develop after prompt withdrawal from chronic exposure to any of the hypnotic sedatives. Convulsions are a particular problem after withdrawal from barbiturates, methaqualone, and, to a lesser extent, benzodiazepines.

Clinical Manifestations. Stupor or coma caused by depressant drug poisoning usually presents the characteristic picture of acute general anesthesia. The depression of the central nervous system tends to be bilateral and symmetric and the drug usually simultaneously depresses junction at many levels, including the spinal cord. Respiratory and circulatory controlling mechanisms in the lower brain stem are affected only with very high doses or not at all. Except with the now obsolete sedative glutethimide and with extremely large doses of barbiturates, the pupillary light reflexes are preserved. Within the first half hour or so after suddenly taking a sedative in potentially anesthetic doses, patients can demonstrate muscular hypertonus or even spasticity as the result of uneven depression of different neurologic levels. Within a short time, usually less than an hour, flaccidity supervenes, and the stretch reflexes disappear. Even moderate degrees of drug depression can depress or block the oculovestibular reflexes.

Despite their lack of exact correlation, blood levels of short-acting barbiturates of more than 2.5 mg per deciliter and phenobarbital levels of more than 12 mg per deciliter are associated with very deep coma to the level at which apnea and hypotension become management problems. Apnea rarely supervenes with the benzodiazepines, even at very high doses.

Diagnosis. The combination of acutely occurring unresponsiveness, with preserved or sluggish pupillary reactions, absent oculovestibular reactions, motor areflexia, hypothermia, and relative depression of respiration and circulation is clinically diagnostic of sedative-anesthetic drug poisoning. Only infarction or hemorrhage of the pons resembles this clinical state, and with lesions of the pons the pupils are usually small or pinpoint, the stretch reflexes are generally preserved or hyperactive, and the plantar responses become extensor. Specific chemical tests detect barbiturates, glutethimide, meprobamate, methaqualone, and bromides in blood or urine, and can be done as emergency measures.

CLINICAL EVALUATION OF DELIRIUM, STUPOR, OR COMA

The immediate step consists of assuring vital cardiorespiratory systems and protecting against further damage to the central ner-

vous system. Once these measures are taken, the keys to diagnosis, specific treatment, and prognosis lie in carefully examining the patient, systematically seeking the answers to a few central questions:

Is the process neurogenic or psychogenic in origin?

If neurogenic, is (are) the lesion(s) supratentorial, subtentorial, focal, or multifocal-diffuse?

Once the immediate cause of loss of consciousness is under control, is the appropriate treatment medical or surgical?

If the illness is nonstructural, is it exogenously toxic or endogenously metabolic, already maximal (e.g., postanoxic, postintoxicant), or progressive; is it worsening or improving?

Which immediate treatment best halts the pathologic process and sustains the patient?

DIFFERENTIAL HISTORY. If sudden unconsciousness is not an expected consequence of an already known illness, witnesses to the onset provide the most helpful immediate information. Was the onset gradual or abrupt? Was it preceded by headache and, if so, of what location and duration? Was paralysis or seizure activity observed? Were antecedent or prodromal symptoms noted? Did the onset occur in a circumstance or geographic area in which drugs, trauma, or foul play could be suspected? What medications might the patient have taken? Beyond these immediacies, what has been the patient's physical and mental health for the past few days, weeks, or months?

PHYSICAL AND NEUROLOGIC EXAMINATION. In cases of deep unresponsiveness, one first carries out steps 1 to 5 described below under Emergency Management, then proceeds with the physical examination. Under urgent circumstances, the physician should be able to conduct a highly focused, pertinent physical and neurologic examination on patients in coma in less than 5 minutes. This includes appraising cardiopulmonary status as indicated above and systematically carrying out the main features of the examination outlined in Table 394–12. In the course of the above, trauma or seizures make themselves evident. In patients with coma of unknown cause, clues should be sought to drug exposure, as well as to past serious medical or psychiatric problems. Companions should be asked about recent neurologic function and dysfunction.

For patients presenting with less severe impairments, i.e., acute-subacute confusion, delirium, or hypersomnolence, the examiner can take a more deliberate approach. Usually, a detailed history can precede the exigencies of stabilizing vital functions and a thorough organ-by-organ physical examination can be conducted. Either way, by the end of the initial examination, the findings should begin to indicate which of the four major causes of coma, as listed in Table 394–1, is responsible for the patient's acute problem. At that juncture, one can move toward obtaining supplementary or reinforcing laboratory tests as indicated below.

LABORATORY STUDIES. Unless the acutely obtained clinical findings make the diagnosis and appropriate treatment immediately obvious, blood should be drawn for laboratory tests listed in Table 394–8. Lumbar puncture is best deferred until after a contrast-enhanced brain CT or an MRI is obtained, so long as the images can be obtained promptly as an emergency procedure. If imaging is not available and the findings suggest acute, treatable meningitis or encephalitis, the physician has no choice but to proceed cautiously with lumbar puncture, using a No. 20 or 22 needle. The EEG (see Ch. 392) is diagnostically indispensable for detecting delirious states caused by continuously recurring partial complex seizures. A normal EEG rules out organic causes of acute unresponsiveness.

EMERGENCY MANAGEMENT OF COMA. Faced with acute coma of uncertain origin, one must treat the patient first, even as the history and initial diagnostic tests are being applied. Certain measures apply to the care of all patients:

1. *Assure an adequate airway and oxygenation.* Immediately check and clean out the upper airway. If the patient is deeply unresponsive, insert an endotracheal airway, but first give 1 mg of atropine intravenously to guard against hypoxigenic vagally induced asystole. Be sure that no neck fracture exists before extending the head for intubation. Auscultate both lung bases to ensure that the lower airway is open. Ventilate if necessary and keep arterial Pao_2 greater than 80 mm Hg and $Paco_2$ 30 to 35 mm Hg. To empty the stomach in comatose patients suspected of acute orally ingested drug poisoning, initiate lavage only *after* the cuffed airway tube is in place.

2. *Maintain circulation.* Insert venous line(s) and start Ringer's

1. Guarantee vital functions as indicated in text.
2. Feel the scalp for hematomas: they overlie fracture lines; be sure the neck is not fractured; test *gently* for stiff neck.
3. Test language. Test arousability by words, loud sounds, noxious stimuli. If vocalizations occur, check quickly for appropriate phrases, actual words, and presence or absence of aphasia.
4. Do a neuro-ophthalmologic examination.
   Funduscopy (if difficult, defer until patient is stabilized)
      Papilledema? (increased intracranial or venous sinus pressure)
      Hemorrhages (subarachnoid hemorrhage; hypertensive encephalopathy; diabetes; hypoxic-hypercarbic encephalopathy)
   Pupils
      Light reaction. Use bright flashlight and, if necessary, a magnifying glass if uncertain. Absence means potentially fatally deep sedative poisoning or acute or chronic structural brain stem damage (e.g., tabetic pupils).
      Equality. 15% of normals have mild anisocoria but new or >2 mm dilation means parasympathetic (third nerve) palsy.
   Extraocular movements. Absence acutely means deep drug poisoning, severe brain stem damage, Wernicke's encephalopathy, polyneuropathy, or botulism.
      Dysconjugate at rest means an acute third, fourth, or sixth nerve palsy or internuclear ophthalmoplegia. Tonic conjugate deviation toward a paralytic arm and leg means forebrain seizures or a contralateral pontine destructive lesion; away from the paralytic arm and leg means forebrain gaze paralysis.
      Spontaneous eye movements. In coma patients, nystagmus, bobbing, or independently moving eyes all mean brain stem damage.
      Oculocephalic (away from direction of head turning) or oculovestibular (toward cold caloric irrigation) responses. Absence of responses means drugs or severe brain stem disease; dysconjugate responses with equal pupils mean internuclear ophthalmoplegia, with unequal pupils mean third nerve disease.
5. Examine the motor systems.
   Strength
      Unilateral weakness or motionlessness of arm and leg means contralateral supraspinal upper motor neuron lesion, most often cerebral; if of arm, leg, and face, contralateral cerebral lesion. Occasionally arm and leg weakness can reflect contralateral brain stem lesion.
      All four extremities weak or motionless implies metabolic disease; less likely is brain stem disease (tone and reflexes increased) or peripheral disease (tone and reflexes decreased).
   Attempt to elicit reflex posturing
      Arm flexed, leg extended—contralateral deep cerebral-thalamic dysfunction
      Arm and leg extended—thalamic or mesencephalic lesion
      Arms extended and legs flexed or flaccid—pontine lesion
      Legs flexed, arms flaccid—pontomedullary or spinal lesion
      Compare side-to-side reflexes and examine plantar responses.
6. Seek seizure activity or abnormal movements. (1) Generalized? (2) Focal? (3) Multifocal? (4) Myoclonic?
   Control 1 immediately, 2 and 3 deliberately; if 4, treat underlying disease.
   Acute tremor, asterixis, multifocal myoclonus—seek metabolic cause.
7. Inspect breathing.
   Regular hyperpnea: metabolic acidosis; pulmonary infarction; congestive failure or aveolar infiltration; sepsis; salicylism; hepatic coma
   Cyclically irregular (Cheyne-Stokes): low cardiac output plus bilateral cerebral or upper brain stem dysfunction
   Irregularly irregular gasping, slow or weak: lower brain stem dysfunction (including hypoglycemia, drug effects), less often peripheral ventilatory paralysis
8. Proceed with laboratory tests and emergency management as described in text.

lactate solution. Determine and maintain a satisfactory cardiac rate and rhythm. Avoid overhydration but keep mean blood pressure at 80 to 90 mm Hg, using dopamine if necessary. In poisoning cases maintain urine flow at 300 ml or more per hour. In any patient during the early stages of coma, check electrolytes initially and at 12-hour intervals thereafter.

3. *Draw blood for emergency laboratory analysis.* Give IV Narcan to protect against opiate intoxication and 50 mg thiamine to prevent accentuation of Wernicke's encephalopathy.

4. *Give glucose.* If hypoglycemia is a possible diagnosis, give 50 ml of 50% glucose. Draw blood first in order not to lose evidence for the diagnosis. The glucose does not appreciably intensify serum hyperosmolality.

5. *Stop generalized motor seizures.* Repetitive convulsions can

result from either cerebral structural lesions, pre-existing epileptic disorders, or acquired metabolic-diffuse encephalopathies. Status epilepticus can cause coma and within a short period of time produces irreversible brain damage as well. Follow the protocol for treatment provided in Table 433–7. Start treatment with intravenous diazepam.

6. *Restore blood acid-base and osmolar balance.* Extremes of either acidosis or alkalosis usually reflect profound metabolic problems, severe circulatory insufficiency, the postictal state (muscular lactic acidosis), or hyperadrenocorticism. Because severe metabolic acidosis can precipitate cardiovascular irregularity and alkalosis depresses breathing, they should be corrected. Extreme hypo- and hyperosmolality are equally dangerous to brain and should be corrected, the first by withholding fluids (except water by mouth) and stopping diuretics and the second by administering fluids (and insulin for hyperglycemia). Beware of too rapid reversal. Osmotic delays across the blood-brain barrier during treatment can lead to large fluid shifts in or out of the brain. Also, too rapid correction of hyponatremia can produce central pontine myelinolysis (see Ch. 406). A reasonable goal in treating osmolal shifts is to correct blood by about 0.5 mOsm per hour.

7. *Treat infection.* Several kinds of infection can cause or intensify delirium and coma. Obtain nose, throat, blood, and wound cultures, and perform lumbar puncture if indicated. With any sign of infection, begin antimicrobial treatment after obtaining the cultures cited above, based on either the results of smears or the most probable clinically suggested organism.

8. *Treat extreme body temperatures.* Hyperthermia above 40° C or hypothermia below 34° C should be brought to within 3° C of normal.

9. *Consider specific antidotes.* Many, if not most, patients admitted to emergency rooms in coma have taken an overdose of drugs, often in combination. For narcotic overdose, give 0.4 mg of naloxone intravenously every 5 minutes until the subject awakens. If the subject might be an addict, dilute the dose in 10 ml of saline and give slowly, trying to minimize withdrawal phenomena. Remember that naloxone's duration of action of 2 to 3 hours is shorter than that of several narcotics, and repeated dosing may be required. Analeptics of any kind are contraindicated.

Recently, flumazenil, a benzodiazepine antagonist, has been found useful in treating patients with benzodiazepine overdose, with or without concurrent ingestion of other depressant drugs. Length of unresponsiveness was shortened, and complications were reduced. The agent has not yet been released for use in the United States.

10. *Control agitation,* employing diazepam or haloperidol as necessary.

11. *Prevent complications.* If possible, keep unconscious patients semiprone in the drainage position and change their position from side to side, but never place them fully supine. In most instances, treat potential pulmonary infection with a broad-spectrum antibiotic. Poisoned patients and many with head injuries are unconscious for only a few days, and the risk of emergence of drug-resistant bacterial infections is of less concern than is pneumonia caused by already aspirated material. It is wise to protect the corneas against abrasions, using ophthalmic ointment and, if necessary, taping the lids shut.

RECOVERY AND PROGNOSIS. Patients recovering from coma require close medical supervision. Severe pneumonitis can develop as late as 3 to 4 days after recovery. If antimicrobial drugs were started during coma, they are best continued for at least 48 hours after it ends. Permanent physical sequelae are rare. Among 356 of our own cases of sedative drug overdose, residual brain injury was observed only once (in a patient who suffered an acute cardiac arrest). Peripheral nerve injuries from pressure developed in 6 subjects, and 14 subjects had pressure skin lesions leaving scars. There were no other physical residua.

Convalescent management varies according to the patient's underlying psychiatric disorder and attitudes. Suicide attempts are never accidents, and reports of near-fatal ingestion caused by misunderstanding the dose or forgetting previous doses carry little validity. The expert opinion of a psychiatrist should be sought before deciding whether to release or to institutionalize a patient. The immediate prognosis is good, but many patients try again over the years.

PROGNOSIS IN SEVERE BRAIN DAMAGE

Accurately forecasting the patient's outcome is central to appropriate patient care and consideration. Modern medical advances currently save many lives that only a few years ago would have been lost to severe disease or trauma. Unfortunately, however, when severe brain dysfunction accompanies acute illness, these advances create the risk that vigorous treatment may be followed by an unwanted outcome. According to Harris polls, most persons in the United States prefer death to a life of severe, permanent neurologic disability and they often express this view in the form of an advanced declaration. Several empirically based guidelines can help the physician predict with a high degree of certainty neurologic outcomes following illnesses causing severe brain damage or coma.

Nontraumatic Coma

The outcome from medical coma depends on (1) its cause, and (2) excepting only depressant drug poisoning, the initial severity and extent of neurologic damage as revealed by clinical neurologic signs obtained within the first few days of illness.

Depressant drug poisoning, no matter how deep the coma, reflects a state of general anesthesia. Barring severe complications, almost all patients with drug intoxication who reach medical attention recover completely. This favorable prognosis applies even when coma is so profound that normal brain stem reflexes and the EEG temporarily disappear. Because most comas of unknown origin that precipitate emergency house calls or emergency room visits are due to drug ingestion, such initially undiagnosed patients should receive maximal treatment unless direct evidence points to severe structural brain damage and the use of drugs by ingestion or for therapy has been ruled out.

Aside from drug poisoning, coma occurring during the course of medical illness and lasting more than a few hours carries a poor prognosis, with only about 15% of patients returning to close to their pre-illness state of health. The major problem in making early treatment decisions lies in discriminating between patients who have a chance of reaching a good outcome and those whose chances of neurologic recovery are extremely small. In making such early decisions, the presence or absence of certain clinical signs of abnormal forebrain and/or upper brain stem function have been found to be powerful predictors of eventual outcome. The nature of the underlying illness and age have less of an influence and only slightly modify the predictive accuracy of early signs.

The clinical tests most valuable for estimating the capacity for recovery after medical coma are identical to those used in diagnosing and following the later course of the patient in coma. In most instances, early functional changes evolve so rapidly that one cannot reliably estimate the outcome of coma within the first minutes to hours, a time when improvement often occurs. After about 6 hours, however, so long as the patient has not received heavy doses of sedative drugs or alcohol, certain neurologic findings begin to correlate increasingly with the potential for neurologic recovery or otherwise. By the end of the first day, clinical signs accurately predict about two thirds of the patients who actually will do well. With each successive day, the signs develop greater predictive power. When considered appropriate to the patient's expressed wishes, treatment can be adjusted accordingly.

Some patients in coma due to a medical disease die from their initial illness within a short time. Ignoring that premise, Table 394–13 lists clinical signs found in a prospective study to predict either a good or a poor outcome from coma due to nonsurgical disease. Good outcome means a possible return to the level of health that pre-existed the coma-causing illness. Poor outcome means that the patient will be permanently, severely disabled either cognitively, physically, or both. The table emphasizes that signs of brain stem dysfunction (absent pupillary or corneal responses, imperfect or absent oculocephalic responses, or abnormal motor responses to stimulation) worsen prognosis and, in combination, indicate a nearly hopeless outlook when they persist beyond the third day.

Following an acute diffuse brain injury such as follows cardiac arrest, a few patients become immediately vegetative following the ictus and remain so as the days pass into weeks. Most who fail to speak until after the end of the second week are left with prominent intellectual defects, especially in recent and anterograde memory, even if sensorimotor activities return to normal. Persistence of coma or the vegetative state in an adult for >4 weeks almost never is as-

TABLE 394–13. CLINICAL SIGNS OF GOOD OR POOR OUTCOME FROM COMA

Good Prognosis	Poor Prognosis
1 day: Awake. No neuro-ophthalmologic abnormalities; speaking at least words. Possibility of poor outcome = 30%	Not awake. Pupils and oculocephalic reflexes absent and flaccid motor system. Possibility of good outcome = 2%
3 days: Corneal responses present, speaks words, moves. Possibility of poor outcome = 26%	No words; corneal responses and appropriate motor responses absent. Possibility of good outcome = 0%
1 week: Eyes open, says words, makes localized motor responses. Possibility of poor outcome = 1%	No wakefulness, motor system flaccid. Possibility of good outcome = 0%

Data derived from best outcome studies of 500 optimally treated patients in coma from nontraumatic, non–drug poisoning causes. From Levy DE, Bates D, Caronna JJ, et al.: Prognosis in non-traumatic coma. Ann Intern Med 94:293, 1981.

sociated with later complete recovery and the longer the mindless state lasts, the greater the chance of permanent disability. Care must be taken in such instances to rule out a locked-in state (see Table 393–1).

Traumatic Coma

Coma following head injury has a statistically better outcome than that associated with medical illness. About 50% of patients in coma from head injury die, many instantly. Acute treatment may somewhat improve the outcome of those who reach hospital. Recovery in traumatic cases is closely linked to age: the younger the better. As with medical coma, severely abnormal neuro-ophthalmologic signs reflecting brain stem dysfunction imply a poor prognosis, with approximately 90% of such patients either dying or remaining in near-vegetative states.

Dreisbach RH, Robinson WO: Handbook of Poisoning, 11th ed. Norwalk, CT, Appleton and Lange, 1987. *Succinct and handy, an excellent quick source to consult in emergencies, especially for poisoning in children.*

Francis J, Martin D, Kapoor WN: A prospective study of delirium in hospitalized elderly. JAMA 263:1097, 1990. *Among 229 elderly patients, 50 suffered delirium. Abnormal sodium levels, illness severity, previous dementia, fever or hypothermia, and neuroleptic drug use were major risk factors.*

Gilman AG, Rall TW, Nies AS, Taylor P (eds.): Goodman and Gilman's The Pharmacological Basis of Therapeutics, 8th ed. New York, Pergamon, 1990. *The "bible" of pharmacology and associated toxicology addresses major drug poisonings in authoritative chapters.*

Haddad LM, Winchester JF: Clinical Management of Poisoning and Drug Overdose. Philadelphia, WB Saunders, 1990.

Levy DE, Caronna JJ, Singer BH, et al.: Predicting outcome from hypoxic-ischemic coma. JAMA 253:1420, 1985. *Prospective correlations were obtained between early neurologic signs and eventual course in 210 patients, mostly with cardiac arrest. By 72 hours, signs accurately selected between good or poor eventual outcome in >75% of patients.*

Plum F: Coma and related global disturbances of the human conscious state. In Jones EG, Peters A (eds.): Cerebral Cortex. Vol. 9, Altered Cortical States. New York, Plenum Press, 1991. *A recent chapter describing current advances in pathophysiology.*

Plum F, Posner JB: Diagnosis of Stupor and Coma, 3rd ed., rev. Philadelphia, FA Davis, 1982. *Provides more discussion of the material described in this chapter.*

Reich JB, Sierra J, Camp W, et al.: Magnetic resonance imaging measurements and clinical changes accompanying transtentorial and foramen magnum herniation. Ann Neurol 33:159, 1993. *Readily interpreted sagittal images of the brain demonstrate the physical existence of pathologic brain herniations and their relationship to clinical findings.*

395 BRAIN DEATH
Fred Plum

Modern resuscitative devices can maintain the functions of the heart, lungs, and visceral organs for hours or days after the life-maintaining centers of the brain stem tissue have stopped functioning. The economic waste of this hopeless process, as well as the increasing success of organ transplant programs, has led countries worldwide to adopt the principle that death of the person occurs when either the brain or the heart irreversibly fails in its functions. In the United States the time of brain death has been accepted as

TABLE 395–1. CRITERIA FOR DIAGNOSIS OF BRAIN DEATH

1. Nature and duration of coma must be known
   a. Known structural disease or irreversible systemic metabolic cause
   b. No chance of drug intoxication or hypothermia; no paralyzing or potentially anesthetizing drugs recently given for treatment
   c. Body temperature must be above 34°C
   d. Six-hour observation of no brain function is sufficient in cases of known structural cause when no drug or alcohol is involved in causation or treatment; otherwise, 12 hours plus negative drug screen required
2. Absence of cerebral and brain stem function
   a. No behavioral or reflex responses can be elicited by noxious stimuli applied above foramen magnum level
   b. Fixed pupils
   c. No oculovestibular response to 50 ml ice water calories
   d. Apneic off ventilator with oxygenation for 10 minutes
   e. Systemic circulation may be intact
   f. Purely spinal reflexes may be retained
3. Supplementary (optional) criteria (any one is diagnostic)
   a. EEG must be largely isoelectric for 30 minutes at maximal gain
   b. Brain stem-evoked responses must reflect absent function in vital brain stem structures
   c. No cerebral circulation present on angiographic examination

the time of the person's death in legal terms. Many states accept the brain death concept by statute, and in no state has the principle failed to meet legal challenge. The Presidential Commission set as the criterion for brain death the "irreversible cessation of all functions of the entire brain, including the brain stem." Guidelines for the practical application of these principles are listed in Table 395–1. One of the supplementary criteria often is particularly desirable when making decisions at 6 hours to facilitate organ transplant.

Certain points in the diagnosis of brain death must be emphasized. *Recoverable drug depressant poisoning can in all ways except stopping the cerebral circulation resemble brain death and must be explicitly ruled out.* In any doubtful case, any evidence of EEG activity or of reflex activity of the brain stem means that the brain is not dead and contravenes immediate discontinuation of life support. Purely spinal reflex activity, however, can persist after brain death, including reflexes of the limbs and even some remarkably complex movements, including flexion of the trunk and raising of outstretched arms.

It is recommended that physicians faced with applying and acting upon the diagnosis of brain death familiarize themselves with the additional pertinent material listed in the references and whenever possible obtain confirmation with an experienced consultant.

Abrams MB, et al.: Deciding to Forego Life-Sustaining Treatment. A Report on the Ethical, Medical, and Legal Issues in Treatment Decisions. President's Commission for the Study of Ethical Problems in Medicine and Biomedical and Behavioral Research. Washington, DC, United States Government Printing Office, March, 1983. *A long and thoughtful report on the problems associated with the terminally ill and the neurologically hopelessly damaged patient.*

Barber J, et al.: Guidelines for the determination of death: Report of the medical consultants on the diagnosis of death to the President's Commission for the Study of Ethical Problems in Medicine and Biomedical and Behavioral Research. Neurology 32:395, 1982. *The detailed report describing that cardiac death and brain death are equivalent and giving criteria for each.*

Council on Scientific Affairs and Council on Ethical and Judicial Affairs: Persistent vegetative state and the decision to withdraw or withhold life support. JAMA 263:426, 1990. *The article provides criteria for the diagnosis of permanent unconsciousness and summarizes the data that support their reliability.*

396 BRIEF LOSS OF CONSCIOUSNESS
Fred Plum

Brief loss of consciousness (BLOC), defined as loss of self-awareness lasting from a few minutes to as much as an hour, is a relatively common symptom. If one excludes conditions readily diagnosed by circumstances or history such as acute traumatic concussion, a known recurrent minor seizure disorder, or accidental insulin-induced hypoglycemia, most such cases are due to causes

TABLE 396–1. PRINCIPAL CAUSES AND APPROXIMATE FREQUENCIES OF BRIEF LOSS OF CONSCIOUSNESS OF UNKNOWN ORIGIN

Syncope	
Primarily neurogenic-vasodepressor	55%
Primarily cardiogenic	10%
Central nervous system	<10%
First seizure	
Cerebrovascular insufficiency	
Subarachnoid hemorrhage	
Intracranial pressure waves	
Drugs-metabolic	<10%
Alcohol-sedative blackouts	
Narcotic overdose	
Hypoglycemia—exogenous or endogenous	
Antihypertensive drugs	
Diagnosis unknown	15–20%

listed in Table 396–1. As the table indicates, *syncope,* defined as brief unconsciousness due to a temporary, critical reduction of cerebral blood flow, is by far the most common cause of BLOC. With any of the conditions, however, reliable observations of the attack itself often are unavailable. Under such circumstances, a careful history and physical examination, including any possible information gained from witnesses, generally give more diagnostic information than any other approach.

Certain immediate guidelines aid in differential diagnosis. Patients under age 50 years with no previous history of cardiac disease, seizures, antihypoglycemic medication, or drug-alcohol abuse almost all turn out to have either benign, neurally mediated reflex syncope or a disorder undiagnosable from available evidence. Such patients rarely require an evaluation more elaborate than a careful history and physical examination plus standard blood counts and blood chemistry determinations. Tilt table studies are said to induce autonomically generated hypotension in neurally mediated reflex syncope, but specificity often is low. For those over age 40, an electrocardiogram (ECG) should be obtained. Computed tomography and electroencephalographic examinations are not cost-effective in the absence of additional abnormal neurologic symptoms or signs.

396.1 Syncope

ETIOLOGY AND INITIAL CONSIDERATIONS. A brief dysfunction of vasodepressor cardiovascular reflexes causes most syncope. Less frequent causes include primary cardiovascular disease or the drugs used to treat it, primary or secondary orthostatic hypotension, and, rarely, cerebral arterial vascular disease. Seizure disorders or psychiatric episodes represent possibly confusing conditions when only a retrospective history can be obtained. Acute, severe vertiginous attacks sometimes can induce secondary, reflex syncope. Hysterical unresponsiveness, although not uncommon, cannot be diagnosed reliably in retrospect. Diagnostic signs of such attacks are given in Table 396–2.

Among patients over age 50 with no historical or physical features suggesting cardiac, neurologic, or systemic illness, benign syncope remains the most common cause of unexplained BLOC.

TABLE 396–2. SIGNS OF PSYCHOGENIC PSEUDOSYNCOPE

Lids close actively, may flutter, and often resist examiner's attempt to open them.
Breathing: eupnea or acute hyperventilation.
Pupils responsive or dilated (self-administered cycloplegic).
Oculocephalic responses unpredictable; calorics produce quick nystagmus.
Motor responses unpredictable, often bizarre and self-protecting.
No pathologic reflexes. EEG normal in awake patient.

Nevertheless, most authorities recommend at least 24 hours of prolonged ECG monitoring in such instances. In Kapoor's study of 433 mostly older patients (mean age, 56 years) with presumed syncope, prolonged ECG recording independently provided important diagnostic information in approximately 20%. In the event of any evidence suggesting cardiac disease, invasive electrophysiologic testing may be useful.

MECHANISMS OF SYNCOPE. Unconsciousness results when generalized cerebral blood flow declines to approximately 40% of normal. Such a drop usually reflects a fall in cardiac output by half or more, and a fall in mean erect arterial blood pressure to below 40 to 50 mm Hg. Given this principle, it comes as no surprise that posture contributes importantly to the event. Syncope of any cause is far more common in the sitting or standing position than during recumbency. Indeed, recumbent syncope must be regarded as reflecting either serious cardiovascular disease or neurologic disease until proved otherwise.

Pathophysiologic changes in several bodily systems can cause these changes. These include (1) temporarily abnormal neural reflexes acting on an otherwise normal cardiovascular system (this category includes the most common causes of fainting in persons who have no history of serious cardiovascular disease); (2) abnormal intrinsic cardiovascular function, including especially disease of the conduction system predisposing to malignant arrhythmias; (3) impaired right heart filling secondary to functionally increased resistance to venous return; (4) acute or subacute blood loss; (5) increased resistance of cervical or intracranial arterial vascular beds; (6) subacute or chronic autonomic insufficiency. Table 396–3 lists subcategories of these disorders which are discussed more fully in the following paragraphs.

Neurogenic Mechanisms in Normal and Abnormal Cardiovascular Control. Sympathetic and parasympathetic influences on the cardiovascular system normally act in a finely tuned manner to slow the heart (vagal) and regulate the degree of constriction of the large venous capacitance vessels of the trunk and extremities (sympathetic outflow). Imbalance, be it a reflection of paralysis or excessive activity in either system, can perturb heart rhythm and rate, slacken venomotor tone, and lead to either reduced left ventricle output, reduced right heart filling, or the two combined. Hypoperfusion sufficient to produce vagal reflex syncope can require as much as 30 seconds or more to evolve or can occur so abruptly as to produce immediate unconsciousness. To produce primary cardiac syncope, sinus bradycardia in most healthy persons must fall below about 30 to 35 beats per minute. Asystole for longer than 3 to 5 seconds usually causes fainting in the erect position at any age. Higher rate and shorter duration thresholds apply to older patients and those with diseased hearts. Atrioventricular arrest,

TABLE 396–3. PRINCIPAL MECHANISMS OF SYNCOPE

I. Mainly impaired right heart filling
  A. Reflex abnormalities
    1. Vasodepressor ("vasovagal"): capacitance veins dilated, cardiac rate normal or slow
    2. Primary or secondary autonomic insufficiency (Ch. 402)
  B. Hypovolemia: hemorrhage, acute salt-water loss, protein loss, enteropathy, burns
  C. Mechanically impaired right heart return: Valsalva maneuver, tussive excess, abrupt chest compression; term pregnancy; pulmonary embolism; pericardial tamponade
II. Globally impaired cardiac output
  A. Reflex abnormalities
    1. Vagal sinus arrest
      a. Psychophysiologic (rare)
      b. Visceral stimulation: glossopharyngeal neuralgia, swallow syncope, direct tracheal stimulation, dilatation of hollow viscus
      c. Carotid baroreceptor sensitivity
  B. Intrinsic cardiac disease (with or without reflex enhancement) (Table 396–4).
III. Primary cerebral ischemia (uncommon)
  A. Multivessel cervical arterial obstructive disease
  B. Transient acute increase in intracranial pressure (plateau waves)
  C. Basilar migraine (rare in adults)
  D. Vertebral-basilar TIA's (rare)

however, is extremely uncommon in persons with healthy hearts, possible exceptions being overtrained athletes, persons taking cocaine, and rare "hypervagal" subjects undergoing severe psychophysiologic threats.

PHYSIOLOGIC REFLEX (VASOVAGAL) SYNCOPE. *Acute vasodepressor syncope* is the most common cause of fainting and typically is marked by a diphasic course. During an initial brief period of apprehension and anxiety, heart rate, blood pressure, total systemic resistance, and cardiac output inconsistently may increase. The vasodepressor phase follows, during which blood pressure falls and cardiac output declines. Both sympathetic and parasympathetic abnormalities are involved, because atropine prevents the bradycardia but not the depressor response. Progressive sensations of lightheadedness, giddiness, abdominal sinking sensations, nausea, urinary urgency, and finally "gray-out" or faintness accompany the vasodepressor component.

During vasodepressor syncope, subjects appear pale and the accompanying parasympathetic hyperactivity characteristically induces piloerection and sweating. Because cardiac action continues, awareness and normal cardiovascular reflexes usually return promptly once the subject becomes supine. Vomiting or explosive diarrhea may follow. Occasionally, emotionally generated dysautonomic influences on the heart can be so profound as to induce arrhythmia. Investigators have speculated that this mechanism can cause sudden death associated with sudden grief or fright.

Fainting is more likely in circumstances of emotional perturbation, in hungry subjects, after a heavy, alcohol-supplemented meal, in a warm, moist environment, and after prolonged standing. A few individuals give a history of lifelong susceptibility to fainting attacks. Rarely, one gets a history suggesting predisposition to vasodepressor syncope based on an autosomal dominant trait, with family members in several generations having been susceptible to recurrent vasodepressor attacks.

Visceral reflex syncope acts via the same medullospinal pathways as the examples cited above. A sense of faintness or even complete syncope can follow immediately after any of the following: emptying a full bladder from the standing position *(micturition syncope),* acute visceral pain (as occurs with a suddenly distended gut or an abrupt joint or ligament injury), an attack of severe vertigo (as occurs with Ménière's disease), or a migraine attack.

The diagnosis of vasodepressor syncope is made largely by history; rarely are the events medically witnessed. Among young persons who lack histories or physical findings of neurologic or cardiovascular disease, treatment is symptomatic. Furthermore, when consulting on such cases we have never found either brain imaging or EEG useful. When impending sensations of faintness threaten, persons should be promptly placed supine. Placing the head far forward in a sitting position is usually ineffective. Subjects who have fainted should be mobilized slowly, because the reflex abnormality occasionally can persist for as long as 2 hours. Prophylactic treatment has little value except when fainting occurs in response to a disease or injury that requires attention. Occasionally, overtrained athletes with chronically slow hearts and a history of syncope during exertion are helped by a regimen of reduced training combined with oral anticholinergic agents.

SYNCOPE DUE PRIMARILY TO CARDIAC CAUSES. Pathologic reflex (vagovagal) attacks result primarily from failure of left heart output associated with reflexly induced changes in the cardiac rhythm, including nodal or sinus arrest, atrioventricular asystole, atrioventricular block, sinoatrial block, and ventricular arrhythmias. Usually these are accompanied by relatively minor vasodepressor changes in the peripheral vasculature, implying a lesser sympathetic abnormality. Most patients with vagovagal attacks belong to the older population and have associated heart disease, resulting in abnormally intense cardiac responses to a relatively normal degree of increased parasympathetic stimulation or sympathetic inhibition. Vagal bradycardia or arrest occasionally is induced by sudden emotional stimuli but more commonly follows acute noxious or abnormal visceral stimulation. Severe bradycardia or arrest especially accompanies glossopharyngeal neuralgia, swallowing in patients with mechanical esophageal lesions, sudden painful dilatations of a hollow viscus, prostatic manipulation, tracheal stimulation, or visceral wounds.

Cardiac syncope almost always reflects serious heart disease. Given a normal heart, neither bradycardia above 30 beats per minute nor tachycardia up to 200 beats per minute causes syncope in the supine or seated position so long as functioning vasomotor reflexes remain. Analyses of large series of patients show serious associated cardiac risk factors, including those listed in Table 396–4. In the case of patients over 40 years of age or those showing such risk factors, prolonged (Holter) monitoring of cardiac activity is indicated. In the absence of specific predisposing abnormalities discovered by history, physical examination, and such ECG monitoring, however, additional studies such as direct electrophysiologic studies of the heart, cardiac catheterization or coronary angiography may add helpful information. Management of cardiac syncope depends upon the nature of the underlying heart disease. Affected persons should be considered for pacemaker insertion.

OTHER CAUSES OF FAINTING. *Orthostatic Hypotension.* Acute orthostatic hypotension occasionally occurs in normal persons after acute blood loss, e.g., cryptic gastrointestinal hemorrhage, or following prolonged standing as with soldiers at parade rest in a hot sun; affected subjects undergo a sudden collapse of sympathetic reflex tone. Recurrent symptoms of syncope or faintness accompanying the erect position usually can be traced to the presence of the chronic use of diuretics, vasodepressor drugs β-adrenergic blockers, or neurologic disorders involving the peripheral or central nervous system. Chronic hypovolemia, such as occurs in elderly cardiac or systemically ill patients, also predisposes to syncope, especially following periods of bed rest or prolonged sitting. Increased age as well as many drugs accentuate tendencies to orthostatic hypotension. The latter include most antihypertensive agents and many of the antidepressants, phenothiazines, and sedatives. Neurogenic causes of autonomic insufficiency are discussed in Ch. 402.

Orthostatic hypotension sufficient to cause cerebral symptoms can occur either rapidly upon standing or develop insidiously over seconds or minutes. Although symptoms of faintness and giddiness predominate, some patients lack such prodromal warnings, presumably because of the absence of strong efferent parasympathetic activity. Sometimes when chronically ill patients sit for long periods or stand, they become confused or tremulous without the usual sensations of faintness or collapse. Diagnosis comes from observing an acute or progressive decline in the mean blood pressure of more than 10 to 15 mm Hg in the erect position. Autonomic insufficiency can be inferred by observing an unchanging pulse rate despite the hypotension, and confirmed by tilt-table tests or by identifying other autonomic impairment. The simplest way to evaluate sympathetic tone at the bedside is to take the pulse while the supine patient performs a vigorous Valsalva maneuver for a matter of 30 seconds or so. The normal response consists of a palpable post-Valsalva slowing of pulse and a 10 to 30 mm Hg rise in mean blood pressure.

Treatment of orthostatic hypotension depends upon the cause. Symptomatic treatment requires eliminating drugs that cause hypotension, correcting causes of blood volume depletion, and applying elastic stockings to the lower extremities. When other measures fail, an increased salt intake and, subsequently, administering the salt-retaining steroid fludrocortisone, 0.3 to 0.8 mg per day in divided doses, can be cautiously initiated. The chronic use of vasopressor agents seldom helps. Patients can be at least partially reconditioned by erect activity. Every effort should be made to keep them up and walking.

Mechanically Impaired Right Heart Filling. In patients with congestive heart disease or cardiopulmonary failure, a strong *Valsalva maneuver* or sustained coughing *(tussive syncope)* raises intrathoracic pressure sufficiently to impede venous return and induce syncope. *Term pregnancy* causing compression of abdominal veins can occasionally induce a similar, posturally related effect. *Pulmonary embolism* and *acute cardiac tamponade*, due most often to subpericardial aortic dissection, act similarly to reduce the right heart filling and critically reduce cardiac output.

Recurrent symptoms of chronic hypovolemia are common in the chronically ill, especially in cardiac patients, the elderly, and those kept at bed rest for sustained periods (in whom baroceptor reflexes also become blunted). Syncope is a risk in all these groups, especially with prolonged motionless sitting.

Cerebral Vascular Disease. Intrinsic cerebral vascular diseases only rarely cause episodes of brief loss of consciousness. Although syncopal episodes might be expected on anatomic grounds as part of the symptom complex associated with vertebral-basilar insufficiency, such is seldom the case. Several reports describing large series of patients with vertebral-basilar insufficiency make no mention of such events. I have observed only two well-documented cases over the years. By contrast, brief periods of confusion or even unconsciousness occasionally mark the course of patients with severe stenosis or occlusion of one or both internal carotid arteries; they may or may not show concurrent narrowing of the vertebrobasilar system. In a few such patients, pulse and blood pressure have been monitored through the attacks, which are marked by brief unresponsiveness associated with transient amnesia but no seizures or EEG changes. Surgical removal of carotid stenoses have helped some, but not all, affected patients. Presumably the spells reflect transient, global blood flow reductions to the cerebral hemispheres associated with hemodynamic insufficiency in cervical arterial circulations.

396.2 Nonsyncopal Causes of Brief Alterations of Consciousness

HYPERVENTILATION. The disorder is mechanistically closely related to syncope in that a globally reduced cerebral blood flow gives rise to sensations of giddiness, faintness, and other distress. Full unconsciousness rarely occurs without some additional abnormal maneuver. The abnormal state is most often part of an anxiety response and often is accompanied by sensations of suffocation, pressure on the chest, and a sense of being unable to obtain the satisfaction of a lung-filling deep breath. Extreme or prolonged hyperventilation can produce feelings of unreality with anxiety bordering on panic.

Symptoms and signs include feelings of unreality, difficulty in concentrating, and several hard-to-explain sensory complaints, such as unilateral or bilateral chest pain or paresthesias involving the body and extremities. Symptoms of facial twitching, carpal spasm, and perioral paresthesias are more easily understood as part of alkalotic tetany.

Hyperventilation occasionally precipitates syncope under special circumstances. Children sometimes voluntarily hyperventilate, then perform a vigorous Valsalva maneuver to induce syncope (fainting lark). Athletes may repeat a similar sequence in contests such as weight lifting or squat jumps. More dangerous is a pattern wherein underwater swimmers hyperventilate before diving, then exhaust their oxygen reserves before producing sufficient carbon dioxide to produce dyspnea. The ensuing cerebral hypoxia can induce fatal submersion syncope.

SEIZURE DISORDERS. Seizure disorders (see Ch. 433) may be confused with syncope under four principal circumstances:

1. *Rapid, profound syncope* may induce a single brief tonic seizure or series of clonic twitches as a result of abrupt cerebral ischemia *(convulsive syncope).* The response is more likely when the subject has made maximal efforts to stand or sit despite premonitory symptoms. Features that are more consistent with syncope than epilepsy include the psychologic circumstances and physical appearance, the associated medical conditions and body position, the brief quality of the seizure, its rapid recovery, and the presence of a normal neurologic examination and interictal EEG.

2. *Akinetic seizures* consist of attacks of suddenly falling or

TABLE 396–4. CARDIOVASCULAR ABNORMALITIES FREQUENTLY ASSOCIATED WITH SYNCOPAL ATTACKS

Myocardial infarction	Pacemaker malfunction
Aortic stenosis	Ventricular tachycardia
Severe cardiomyopathy	Sick sinus syndrome
Severe hypertension	Complete heart block
Pulmonary embolism	Asystole ($> \pm 3$ sec erect, ± 8 sec supine)
Pulmonary hypertension	Bradycardia $< 44/\text{min}$
Dissecting aortic aneurysm	Tachycardia $> 160-180/\text{min}$

pitching to the ground, starting in early childhood. Similar episodes occur in the supine position and are marked by unresponsiveness accompanied by generalized muscular hypotonia or brief body spasm. Diagnosis rests on the typical history, the age of onset, and the presence of an abnormal EEG. *Absence (petit mal) seizures* rarely provide a diagnostic problem because children with petit mal, although out of contact, neither fall nor turn pale and usually have no memory of the episode. The EEG is abnormal and frequently diagnostic.

3. *Partial complex (psychomotor) seizures* sometimes include brief behavioral automatisms in which the subject recalls only being out of contact and may retrospectively consider himself to have suffered a state of unconsciousness. Usually the presence of a characteristic, self-recognized aura or set of incipient symptoms indicates the diagnosis. Falling to the ground rarely occurs unless a generalized seizure develops. Witnessed attacks and the abnormal EEG usually are typical.

4. *Postictal unresponsiveness* from grand mal attacks produces unconsciousness lasting minutes, the duration usually depending on the severity of the preceding convulsion. Diagnosis is a problem only if the seizure was unwitnessed, in which case the state may look like concussion or profound fainting. Even so, the postictal state is marked initially by flushing (cyanosis), giving way to pallor, hyperpnea, and deep unresponsiveness, none of which occurs in syncope.

HYPOGLYCEMIA (see Ch. 206). Hypoglycemia, usually caused by excess exogenous rather than endogenous insulin, can produce a variety of relatively brief episodes of neurologic dysfunction. These can consist, variably, of brief confusional episodes, seizures of a variety of types, narcolepsy-like syndromes, and focal or tetraparetic weakness with or without coma but not resembling syncope. Diagnosis depends on suspicion plus the detection of blood sugars of less than 30 to 40 mg per deciliter during an attack.

DRUG OR ALCOHOL BLACKOUTS. Drug or alcohol blackouts consist of episodes of such severe intoxication that they anesthetize memory for the event, leaving the subject with an episode of focal amnesia. Many are accompanied by "passing out," consisting of deep, barely arousable sleep.

CONCUSSION-POSTCONCUSSION AMNESIA. Variable periods of memory loss for immediate subsequent events can follow brief periods of concussive unconsciousness. The usual question is whether an intrinsic malady caused the fall or the fall represented the whole illness. Only diagnostic diligence can solve the issue.

ACUTE INTRACRANIAL HYPERTENSION. Plateau waves, associated with this condition, can produce brief episodes of loss of consciousness that resemble syncope. Occasionally, brief unconsciousness may accompany the onset of acute subarachnoid hemorrhage. The episode, which is syncopal in its abruptness and often accompanied by either a tonic extensor spasm or brief clonic jerks, is most often due to an acute cardiac arrhythmia or asystole accompanying the onset of bleeding. Cerebral hemorrhage with intraventricular rupture can produce similar events.

DROP SPELLS. As discussed in Chapter 404, these are poorly understood attacks affecting older persons. The legs suddenly and unexplainedly give way, and the women fall, often injuring themselves but experiencing no observed interruption of consciousness. The cause is unknown.

CONVERSION REACTIONS OR MALINGERING (PSEUDOSYNCOPE). Hysterical or other forms of psychogenic unresponsiveness are almost impossible to diagnose in retrospect. If such a condition occurs during the physical examination, the diagnosis can be concluded by the absence of physiologic abnormality and the presence of additional, often bizarre features (see Table 396–2). Most subjects awaken with gentle but firm confrontation. A few do so only when advised that psychiatric admission lies in store. Mutilating stimuli are neither justified nor often successful in proving the diagnosis.

Aminoff MJ, Scheinman MM, Griffin JC, et al.: Electrocerebral accompaniments of syncope associated with malignant ventricular arrhythmias. Ann Intern Med 108:791, 1988. *Ten of 17 episodes of syncope caused by electrically induced ventricular tachycardia or arrhythmia had accompanying tonic seizures or irregular muscular twitching. The results illustrate the high incidence of convulsive syncope.*

Benditt DG, Remole S, Milstein S, et al.: Syncope: Causes, clinical evaluation and current therapy. Annu Rev Med 43:283, 1992. *A comprehensive review.*

Kapoor WN: Evaluation and management of syncope. JAMA 268:2553, 1992. *A well-*

balanced review of the author's large personal series plus others in the recent literature.

Mandis AS, Linzer M, Salem D, et al.: Syncope. Current diagnostic evaluation and management. Ann Intern Med 112:850, 1990. *A comprehensive review of the problem identifying rare as well as common causes and emphasizing laboratory evaluations, especially of cardiovascular mechanisms.*

397 DISORDERS OF SLEEP AND AROUSAL
Fred Plum

BIOLOGY OF NORMAL SLEEP. Of all normal visceral functions, the fundamental value of sleep remains the least well understood. Its restorative rewards are self-evident, as is the fact that severe degrees of sleep deprivation impair cognitive and systemic functions alike. Yet the cell-molecular bases for these elementary experiences remain unknown, just as do the signals that induce sensations of drowsiness or the biochemical tissue changes that accompany refreshing sleep. Brain-regulating mechanisms that generate normal sleep cycles and the underlying macrophysiology of sleep states are better understood and are discussed in subsequent paragraphs.

Normal adult sleep-wake patterns repeat themselves on an approximately 24-hour cycle, of which wakefulness occupies approximately two thirds. The suprachiasmatic nucleus of the hypothalamus sets the overall circadian rhythm, and the environmental light-dark cycle as well as the individual's personal activities establish the specific clock hours of the pattern. Suprachiasmatic outputs similarly induce circadian patterns of function in other hypothalamic regulatory nuclei and influence arousal and sleep-related nuclei located in the upper brain stem as well. Perturbations in this normal system occur readily. The abrupt changing of environmental clock time by three or more hours such as occurs with shift changes of working hours or transmeridian air travel induces jet lag, characterized by several days of fractionated sleep patterns poorly coordinated with practical requirements. Similarly, psychologically induced hyperarousal, depression, or severe illness all can disrupt the comforting nurtures of normal circadian sleep.

Needs for sleep among normal individuals vary widely and tend to decline with age. Adults sleep less than children and men less than women, with most normal adults sleeping regularly between about 7 and 9 hours per day, but with extremes of 4 and 11. Tropical inhabitants typically displace part of their total sleep time to afternoon hours in keeping with a hemicircadian intrinsic cycle of alertness and sleepiness. Normal sleep evolves in non-REM stages graded 1 to 4 [on the basis of electroencephalographic (EEG) changes and depth of unarousability] and REM sleep, which alternate through the night in approximately 90-minute cycles. REM is a cortically active sleep stage, consisting of rapid, wakeful-like EEG patterns, rapid eye movements, and markedly reduced voluntary muscle activity. The biologic importance of these phase shifts is little understood but much debated. Whatever their explanation, an abnormal regulation of the timing of REM sleep is a central feature of narcolepsy, discussed below. In the absence of a sleep disorder, the subjective experience of sleep is uninterrupted in most persons under about age 40. Stages 3 and 4 sleep, as defined by standard EEG criteria, decline gradually throughout adulthood. Awakenings at the transition of REM to non–REM sleep tend increasingly to interrupt the sleep pattern, especially over about age 60.

INSOMNIA. A recent, abrupt onset of insomnia in an adult most often relates to the advent of systemic illness, grief, newly appearing personal or financial preoccupations, dietary indiscretions, or jet lag. A more gradual development marks the sleeplessness that often follows drug or alcohol use, aging, a new-onset or recurrent depressive disorder, a major change in personal relationships, or rarely, the development of a neurologic disorder. The insomniac who snores may have obstructive sleep apnea, and the insomniac with restless legs syndrome may have periodic limb movements (discussed below). Syphilitic general paresis, Huntington's disease, and Parkinson's disease all occasionally produce insomnia early in their course. Similar problems accompany certain of the cerebellar degenerations, brain stem injuries, or strokes, as well as very rare cases of prion disease called fatal familial insomnia (see Ch. 428.6). Chronic insomnia of many years' duration unaccompanied by pain, aging, or debilitating illnesses such as chronic cardiopulmonary diseases, cancer, or severe arthritis generally has physically benign implications. It may represent either a normal individual variation of sleep requirements or a chronic psychiatric disorder associated with symptoms of anxiety and depression.

Given the multiple circumstances that may interfere with sleep, management not only becomes difficult but often must be individualized (Table 397–1). Hypnotic drugs find their ideal use in patients with recent-onset insomnia, with short-acting benzodiazepines being the agents of choice. All drugs of this class induce tolerance more slowly than their predecessors (e.g., barbiturates) but still lose their effectiveness if used uninterruptedly for more than a few weeks. Also, all are habituating and predispose to withdrawal symptoms after more than a few days of continuous use. Accordingly, all should be prescribed at a minimum dose for naive subjects, particularly elderly ones. Of the group, triazolam (Halcion) and zolpidem (Ambien) are favored for inducing sleep, whereas flurazepam (Dalmane) and quazepam (Doral) are effective in sustaining the duration of sleep. Triazolam at doses >0.25 mg sometimes impairs recent memory or leaves unpleasant hangovers. Flurazepam and quazepam have desalkyl metabolites with long half-lives, which may accumulate to produce side effects after 10 to 14 days of use. With all these drugs, the best approach is to administer them for two or three nights prior to retiring and then halt their intake so as to compare the results and resume, if necessary, with similarly interrupted patterns for not longer than 5 weeks. Tapered doses should be scheduled over a several-day period to avoid withdrawal symptoms.

For patients with more sustained and refractory insomnia, the following guidelines may be helpful.

1. Encourage the insomniac to maintain a regular bedtime and arising time and not to spend excessive time in bed. This regularity needs to include weekends.

2. Reassure the insomniac that although his/her feelings of fatigue, heavy limbs, fuzzy thinking, and giddy sensations may relate to the ostensible sleep lack, no evidence indicates that even long-term insomnia injures health.

3. Emphasize that insomniacs only know when they are awake. Direct observations usually show that they sleep more than they think.

4. Strongly recommend that the insomniac give up alcohol and all kinds of psychoactive drugs not being prescribed for psychiatric illness. All these agents, with time, risk enhancing the sleep loss because of tolerance or withdrawal effects.

5. Take simple steps first. Have patients reduce tea or coffee to morning hours. Prescribe specific effective daily exercise. Eliminate long midday naps. Give enough analgesics to relieve pain. Reduce the size of evening meals and avoid red meat. Try taking hot baths in the evening. Replace noisy atmospheres with earphones playing music or a white noise generator.

6. If depression or chronic pain persists, try tricyclic or other relevant antidepressants in appropriate doses given at bedtime.

7. If other approaches fail, consider a combination of appropriate antidepressants such as a tricyclic in modest doses, combined with behavioral therapy.

8. Reassure elderly insomniacs that their sleeplessness is probably physiologic, not psychological. Urge them to read or listen to music or other tapes when awake. Install steady noise backgrounds

TABLE 397–1. SIMPLE MEASURES TO HELP CHRONIC INSOMNIACS

Maintain a regular schedule with reduced time in bed.
Reassure them that insomnia rarely impairs physical health.
Emphasize that insomniacs know only awakening, not sleep time.
Urge avoidance of alcohol, cigarettes, stimulants, polypharmacy, red meat, heavy evening meals. Urge daily exercise.
Treat pain, counteract random nighttime noise. Urge evening hot baths, serene atmospheres.
Avoid hypnotics. Consider, if appropriate, antidepressants or behavioral therapy.

TABLE 397–2. THE PARASOMNIAS

Largely in Children	Adults
Headbanging	Bruxism
Sleepwalking	Restless legs
Night terrors	Periodic limb movements
Bedwetting	Sleep apnea
Nightmares (mostly children but any age)	REM behavior disorder

(e.g., by electric fan or the like) to dampen sudden environmental noises.

9. Use sedatives seldom, in small doses, and for periods of 3 weeks or less. Short- to middle-acting benzodiazepines probably are best, but prescribe them for elderly persons at no more than half the size of the usual adult dose.

10. For severe problems, combine antidepressants and behavioral therapy. Consider expert consultation with a sleep specialist.

SPECIAL CASES. *Parasomnias.* The parasomnias consist of a group of motor or autonomic disorders that can delay or disrupt the course of normal sleep (Table 397–2). Most of these conditions affect children, but a few interfere with the sleep patterns of adults and are described here.

Bruxism (teeth grinding) can occur at any age beyond puberty. A few examples are familial, but most become clinically apparent in a setting of tension and anxiety. Wearing a teeth shield while asleep may ameliorate the noisy grinding and the morning headaches that go with it but may not substitute adequately for needed psychiatric attention aimed toward reduction of stress and anxiety.

Restless legs syndrome usually affects selected adults in their elder years. The symptoms consist of unpleasant sensations in the calves and an urge to move the legs, leading to uncontrolled movement, pacing, or rubbing to temporarily alleviate the discomfort. About half of cases are familial. The subjective symptoms may delay sleep onset and/or interrupt or shorten its duration. Annoying periodic limb movements occur during sleep in the vast majority of patients with this condition. These movements also can be found in almost any other sleep disorder (e.g., sleep apnea, narcolepsy) and in up to 40% of asymptomatic elderly persons. In most such cases, there are far fewer movements per night than in restless legs syndrome. Current treatment includes carbamazepine (Tegretol), carbidopa-levadopa (Sinemet), or a low-potency narcotic such as oxycodone or propoxyphene (Darvon). None have dramatic effects.

Night terrors rarely affect adults. When so, they usually reflect a recent personal crisis or, when recurrent, drug-alcohol excess, structural lesions of the brain, or serious psychiatric disorders.

Somnambulism may extend into midlife after late childhood onset. Severe cases in which the behavior poses a threat to the patient should be treated with intermediate half-life benzodiazepines such as lorazepam (Ativan) at 0.5 to 2 mg at bedtime. The principal differential diagnosis is nocturnal partial complex seizures. A recently identified parasomnia is the *REM behavior disorder,* which typically affects older males. These patients act out their dreams and frequently sustain injuries as a result. Treatment consists of clonazepam (Klonopin) at 0.5 to 3 mg at bedtime.

Narcolepsy and Daytime Hypersomnolence. Narcolepsy is a specific neurologic syndrome consisting of excessive daytime drowsiness, cataplexy (85 to 90% of patients), and less often, the additional phenomena of sleep paralysis and intense dreamlike hallucinations at sleep-wake transitions (50 to 60% of patients). More than 90% of cases possess the DQB1-0602 haplotype, possibly related to a gene mutation on chromosome 6. Since less than 10% of cases are immediately familial, autoimmune mechanisms or additional genetic influences have been postulated. The exact disease mechanism remains unknown, and most persons with similar haplotypes do not develop the illness.

Clinically, chronic excessive daytime sleepiness without an increase in 24-hour sleep identifies the illness. Other features are listed in Table 397–3. Narcolepsy equally affects men and women, has its onset mostly before age 25, and lasts a lifetime. Chronic daytime sleepiness accompanied by intermittent, minutes-long sleep

TABLE 397-3. CLINICAL FEATURES OF NARCOLEPSY

Chief symptoms: Near-constant sleepiness, boredom-related immediate sleep, cataplexy, signs or history of other diseases lacking
Associated symptoms: Sleep paralysis, presleep hallucinations-dreams, disrupted nocturnal sleep
Onset: During young adulthood or before
Differential diagnosis: Sleep apnea syndromes, acute or chronic sleep deprivation, metabolic encephalopathy; rarely, structural brain disease, psychiatric disease

episodes that are most often associated with boring sedentary circumstances provide the hallmarks. Although nighttime sleep tends to be repeatedly spontaneously interrupted and slightly shortened, total sleep time remains within a normal range. The intensity and frequency of daytime attacks vary from sufferer to sufferer; when severe, the disease interferes with memory, affects employment, and may lead to traffic and other accidents.

Diagnosis of narcolepsy depends on the typical, unremitting chronic history, a young age of onset, and the exclusion of other hypersomnia-inducing disorders. Moderate to severe sleep apnea and chronic sleep deprivation are far more frequent causes of daytime hypersomnolence than narcolepsy. Also, structural lesions of the brain or idiopathic hypersomnia rarely are causes of daytime hypersomnolence. A careful history and physical examination will eliminate most of these disorders. Because narcolepsy is a lifelong condition which often requires the chronic use of controlled substance stimulants, diagnosis should be confirmed by the laboratory multiple sleep latency test before starting treatment.

Cataplectic attacks consist of brief, jelly-like bodily weakness accompanying laughter or other strong emotion. *Sleep paralysis* describes a usually brief experience of feeling unable to move after awakening from a period of sustained sleep. As a phenomenon, it overlaps similar experiences of adolescence and usually ends abruptly, apparently by self-will or by mild sensory stimulation. Presleep (hypnogogic) or postsleep (hypnopompic) hallucinations are intense and sometimes bizarre; they strongly resemble the experiences of some normal persons following severe sleep deprivation.

Narcolepsy is best treated with stimulants to counteract daytime drowsiness and tricyclic antidepressants to reduce cataplectic attacks. Methylphenidate or dextroamphetamine in divided doses up to 60 mg daily are most effective. Pemoline (Cylert) in divided doses up to 112.5 mg daily is also effective and produces less irritability and tension. The incidence of unwanted side effects mounts above these levels, and the drugs should be started at low, spaced doses, because some narcoleptics require only moderate stimulation. Scheduled short naps can be very effective at reducing daytime drowsiness and the dose of medication. Cataplexy requires separate treatment and often can be completely controlled with imipramine or desipramine (50 to 150 mg daily), given in gradually increasing doses. Abstaining from all drugs one day each week helps to maintain beneficial drug effects for most patients. Usually, the stimulant drugs retain their beneficial effects for many months or even years.

Sleep Apnea. Sleep apnea occurs relatively frequently and occasionally can become sufficiently severe to interfere with health or even cause unexpected death. Clinically important sleep apnea occurs as a result of three disease categories: (1) cardiopulmonary obstructive disorders, (2) anatomic changes in the airways associated with development, aging, and supplementary medical problems (Table 397-4) and (3) neurologic or neuromuscular disorders. The neurologic causes have the least frequency; interaction often occurs between either of the first two causes and the third.

Airway obstruction with or without partial cardiopulmonary decompensation produces the largest group of medically important obstructive apneas. Age and maleness carry intrinsic risks, reflected in the high rates of snoring and temporary choking (obstructive apnea) that affect older men during otherwise uncomplicated sleep. When one adds to partial obstruction the burdens of obesity, which both narrows the upper (supraglottic) airway and increases resistance against diaphragmatic contraction, nocturnal breathing becomes commensurately more obstructed at the pharyngeal level and more of an effort. Any additional upper airway obstruction, whether from the swellings of allergy, the increased secretions of tobacco-dam-

aged mucous membranes, or the pre-existence of developmentally narrowed canals, threatens to produce nocturnal respiratory decompensation. The recurrent obstructive apneas, each ending in a brief and insensible arousal, eventually produce daytime fatigue and sleepiness, with resultant deterioration of the personality, decline in work habits, and intellectual slowness. In the morbidly obese, daytime blood gases begin to deteriorate due to restrictive lung disease. If the problem proceeds uncorrected, heart failure, arrhythmias, hypertension, and premature death may ensue.

Nonobstructive sleep apnea also may occur during the course of acute severe congestive heart failure or with acute exacerbations of chronic obstructive pulmonary diseases. With either event, hypoxic-hypercarbic central respiratory depression plus peripheral fatigue, depressant drugs, and sleep may seriously elevate the breathing threshold. The result produces a cardiopulmonary emergency.

Central sleep apnea, sometimes called "secondary sleep apnea," when it results from progressive peripheral or central neurological abnormalities, has a relatively low incidence (Table 397-4). Peripheral or central-peripheral neurologic diseases act by gradually reducing ventilatory capacity to the point of physiologic insufficiency, reflected either by progressive dyspnea or the presence of an insidiously gradual decompensation of arterial blood gases. Whether because of inherent insensitivity or by adaptation, central brain stem respiratory sensitivity to hypercarbia-hypoxia becomes blunted, and sleep may further elevate the breathing threshold leading to episodic apnea of varying severity. Most of the potential causes listed in Table 397-4 can be recognized easily from historical and physical evidence. Two that are sometimes overlooked consist of adult acid maltase deficiency, which sometimes produces selective diaphragmatic failure, and acute-subacute bilateral brachial neuropathy, which can silently interrupt phrenic nerve conduction.

Treatment of sleep apnea depends on accurate diagnosis as to the severity of the problem and application of mechanical techniques of proved worth. Evaluation by an experienced sleep disorders center usually can help in such steps and in suggesting a program of treatment. The usual first approach is to apply continuous positive airway pressure (CPAP) during the night via the nasal route. Nasal CPAP induces remarkable improvement in as many as 90% of patients with obstructive sleep and in some patients with central sleep apnea. Weight loss by exercise and a reasonable diet can be very effective at reducing or eliminating obstructive sleep apnea, if accomplished and maintained. Concomitant use of nasal CPAP during weight loss can relieve the condition entirely. Any amount of alcohol increases the severity of obstructive sleep apnea, which nevertheless can be overcome with an appropriate CPAP level. Heavy al-

TABLE 397-4. CLINICALLY IMPORTANT SLEEP APNEAS

Neurologic Mechanisms	Systemic Abnormalities
Peripheral Neuromuscular Disorders	
Uncommon; all reflect gradually progressive weakness in respiratory muscles combined with desensitization of brain stem respiratory centers	Severe, acute congestive heart failure
	Obstructive pulmonary disease with chronic hypercarbia-hypoxemia
Gradually progressive muscular dystrophies, especially myotonic and acid maltase deficiency	
Chronic severe myasthenia gravis	
Severe postpolio syndrome with marginal respiratory reserve	
Progressive amyotrophic lateral sclerosis, progressive bulbar palsy	
Central Disorders	
Lower brain stem structural disease	***Airway Obstructive Disorders***
Respiratory center desensitization secondary to recurrent hypoxia-hypercarbia	Predominantly males
	Obesity
	Mostly ages 40–70
	Congenital or developmental upper airway narrowing
	Secondary narrowing:
	Allergic rhinitis, hypertrophied tonsils, tongue, or pharyngeal tumors, hypothyroidism, acromegaly

cohol users often have difficulty complying with any treatment, including CPAP. Unless clearly abnormal and substantial airway obstruction exists, surgery on the upper airway seldom offers sustained improvement. Nasal CPAP may help clear the right-sided heart failure associated with obstructive sleep apnea in the context of obesity-hyperventilation or chronic obstructive pulmonary disease.

Other patients with central or sleep apnea require artificial ventilation by other means, for which several kinds of instruments are available. The need for tracheostomy or other surgical procedures has almost completely disappeared during recent years.

Culebras A (ed.): The neurology of sleep. Neurology 42(suppl 6):94, 1992. *Eleven authorities provide well-written, comprehensive reviews and discussion of the subject. Articles on narcolepsy and sleep apneas offer especially useful information.*

Kryger MH, Roth T, Dement WC (eds.): Principles and Practice of Sleep Medicine. 2d ed. Philadelphia, WB Saunders, 1994. *A detailed, comprehensive textbook addresses all aspects of the subject.*

Mignot E, Lin X, Kalil J, George C, et al.: DQB1-0602 (DQw1) is not present in most non-DR2 Caucasian narcoleptics. Sleep 15(5):415, 1992. *This and the following paper informatively discuss haplotypes in narcolepsy.*

Mignot E, Lin X, Hesla P-E, Dement WC, et al.: A novel HLA DR 17, DQ1 (DQA1-0102/DQB1-0602 Positive) haplotype predisposing to narcolepsy in Caucasians (Letter to the Editor). Sleep 16:764, 1993.

398 DIAGNOSIS OF REGIONAL CEREBRAL DYSFUNCTION
Antonio R. Damasio

Localizing the site of neurologic dysfunction based on clinical signs and symptoms is crucial to the assessment of neurologic diseases. Although noninvasive neuroimaging techniques localize many brain lesions, the abnormalities associated with some diseases often elude all but research-level imaging procedures. For instance, in most degenerative diseases, the regional anatomic defect can be defined only on the basis of clinical signs. Another example is the diagnosis of most epileptogenic foci, a key element in the therapeutic management of epileptic patients.

Figure 398–1 diagrams the regional neuroanatomy of the adult human brain. The accuracy of regional clinical diagnosis depends on numerous factors. First, elementary motor and sensory disorders relate to dysfunction in motor and sensory pathways and can be detected earlier than disorders of thinking or language, which result from dysfunction in association cortices. The localization of the underlying lesions is generally more precise in the former than in the latter. This difference reflects the fine anatomic and functional modularity of the primary sensory and motor systems and the fact that cognitive processes depend on distributed anatomic systems beyond the primary areas. Furthermore, the neural substrate for integrative processes varies individually, different individuals having different endowments for specific abilities. For instance, language or visuospatial skills are linked to a variety of genetic and epigenetic factors and are influenced by age, educational background, and even gender. Second, the type of pathologic lesion and its rate of development influence the rate of appearance and the extent of symptoms. Most infarcts damage the brain and lead to an abrupt onset of signs followed by at least some improvement. By contrast, most intracranial tumors generate symptoms gradually and the brain adapts to the tumor enlargement. Some slow-growing meningiomas can reach the size of a plum before they cause detectable dysfunction, whereas small brain metastases from a carcinoma elsewhere in the body may cause major symptoms rapidly. Third, the mass effect and the edema that accompany large infarcts and some tumors may cause a shift of brain structures and thereby compress remote and otherwise intact areas of the brain against the rigid frame of the dural meninges and skull. Such compression can generate false localizing signs, lead to impaired attention, and interfere with wakefulness (see Ch. 396).

OCCIPITAL LOBES

The occipital cortices are solely dedicated to visual processing. Signals from both lateral geniculate nuclei arrive in each primary visual cortex (Brodmann's area 17), which occupies the superior and inferior banks of the calcarine fissure (see also Ch. 404.2). This region contains a retinotopic projection of visual information. The inferior visual field maps onto the superior calcarine fissure and vice versa; the right visual field maps into the left calcarine region and conversely for the left visual field; the central part of the retina projects onto the caudal part of the calcarine region, at the occipital pole, while progressively more peripheral sectors of the retina project to more anterior sectors of the calcarine region. Beyond area 17, visual information is widely distributed by a large number of functionally distinct regions, located within the association cortices of Brodmann's areas 18 and 19. The main goals of these parallel processing units are (1) to generate representations of the form, volumetric shape, texture, movement, color, and spatial location of stimuli in the external world, and (2) to serve as distributed storage sites for the records of visual perception that become committed to memory and are later used in the processes of visual recall, recognition, imagetic thinking, and dreaming.

Damage to the calcarine cortices (Table 398–1) or to the optic radiations as they approach the calcarine region causes varied field defects for form vision (hemianopias or quadrantanopias) depending on the region affected (e.g., damage to the left superior calcarine region causes a right inferior quadrantanopia; damage to an entire calcarine region leads to a hemianopia). When damage is confined to inferior occipital cortices but spares the calcarine regions, patients may develop *achromatopsia*, a disturbance of color perception without compromise of form vision (damage to the left side causes right hemiachromatopsia and vice versa). Damage to left occipital cortices and underlying periventricular white matter combined with destruction of the interhemispheric visual pathways often causes a disorder of reading without concomitant impairment of writing (*alexia without agraphia*). This may be accompanied by an impairment of color naming without impairment of color perception (*color anomia*). Bilateral damage to inferior visual association cortices causes *agnosia*, a selective impairment of visual recognition (see Ch. 399). Lesions that extensively involve the right occipital cortices (inferior *and* superior) can cause agnosia for unique faces and places, and lesions that involve left occipital cortices (inferior *and* superior) can cause agnosia for manipulable objects. Bilateral damage to superior visual association cortices leads to disturbances of visual attention (*visual disorientation* or *simultanagnosia*) and stereo vision (*astereopsis*). Visual disorientation can also result from bilateral superior parietal lesions, as a component of Balint syndrome (see Parietal Lobe, below). Lesions that involve the lateral occipital cortices about their middle tier can cause defects of motion perception. Infarctions in the territory of one or both posterior cerebral arteries are the most common cause of pathology in the occipital lobes.

TEMPORAL LOBE

The temporal lobes contain structures necessary for visual and auditory perception, language, memory, and affect. The most characteristic signs of temporal lobe damage are impairments of memory, which can be caused by lesions of either side, and impairments of language, usually related to dominant hemisphere lesions (see Ch. 399). The cortical structures related to vision are located in the inferior and lateral aspects of the lobe (part of area 37, areas 20 and 21). They are higher-order association cortices that receive information from the occipital association cortices. The inferior component of the geniculocalcarine pathway (Meyer's loop) courses in the depth of the temporal lobe (see Ch. 403).

The primary auditory cortices (areas 41 and 42) are located in the first temporal gyrus at the end of the most complex chain of subcortical processing stations of any sensory portal of the brain. They represent acoustic frequencies and intensities for a large range of pitched and unpitched sounds (speech, music, environmental noises) so as to permit their recognition and spatial localization. The record of those representations is contained in the auditory association cortices that surround the primary cortices bilaterally, in the superior temporal gyrus (largely area 22). Although the auditory input from the contralateral ear prevails functionally over the ipsilateral input, each cortex receives information from both ears; unilateral temporal lesions never cause deafness.

The medial temporal lobes contain cortical and subcortical struc-

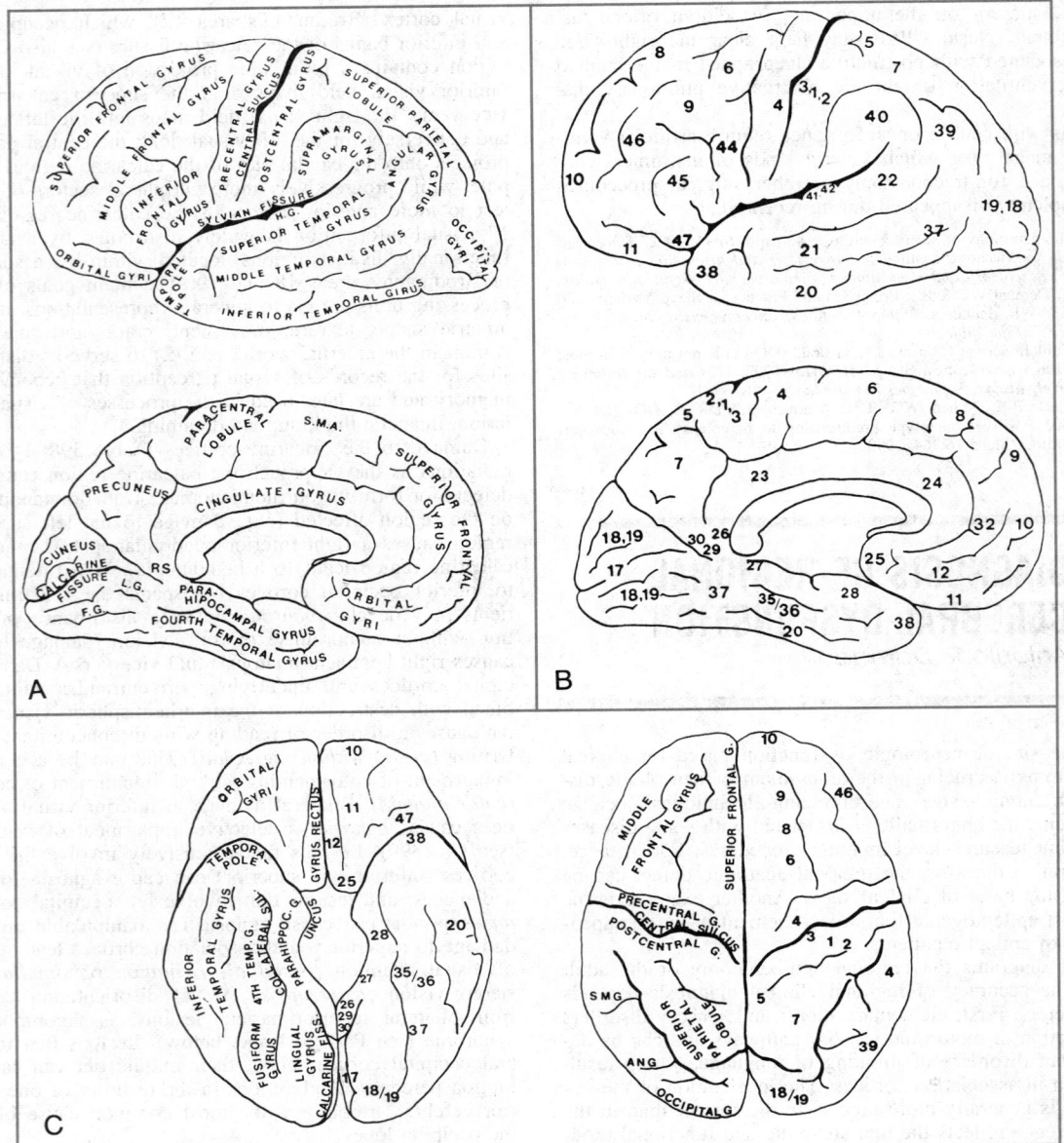

FIGURE 398–1. The principal gyri, sulci, and Brodmann's cytoarchitectonic areas of the human brain. *A,* Gyri and sulci in lateral *(top)* and mesial *(bottom)* views. *B,* Brodmann's areas in lateral *(top)* and mesial *(bottom)* views. *C,* Gyri, sulci, and Brodmann's areas in orbital *(left)* and superior *(right)* views.

tures of the limbic system, e.g., the entorhinal cortex (area 28) located in the anterior part of the parahippocampal gyrus; the hippocampal formation; and the amygdala. These highly interconnected structures correlate perceptual inputs, ongoing verbal and nonverbal thought operations, and the status of the internal milieu. This correlation is indispensable for emotional expression, affective experience, and memory. Lesions of this region severely impair those functions.

The temporal lobes can be compromised by numerous pathologic processes (Table 398–2). Epileptogenic scars and intracranial tumors are common; head injury often damages anterior temporal structures; herpes simplex encephalitis has a predilection for the region; the highest and earliest concentration of cytoskeletal pathology in Alzheimer's disease is in entorhinal cortex and hippocampus; and the hippocampus is selectively vulnerable to anoxia. Patients with temporal epileptogenic lesions experience a variety of abnormalities of visceral sensation, thought process, and even sense of self. They exhibit emotional and motor disturbances that can appear before or during a seizure. In some patients, more subtle but longer-lasting behavioral changes develop between seizures. Tables 398–3 and 398–4 list major ictal and interictal symptoms. Bilateral removal of this region in animals causes the Kluver-Bucy syn-

drome, a disorder characterized by indiscriminate sexual behavior, excessive orality, and placidity. The full syndrome rarely develops in humans, but some components can occur in patients with extensive bilateral temporal damage caused by herpes simplex encephalitis and in patients with dementias of degenerative or post-traumatic origins.

PARIETAL LOBE

The anterior aspect of the parietal lobe contains the postcentral gyrus where Brodmann's areas 3, 1, and 2 receive somatosensory information hailing from nerve terminals in the contralateral half of the body (the projections are somatotopically organized, with the largest share given to the phonatory apparatus and hand). These cortices interlock with the primary motor cortex in the precentral gyrus (area 4) and project to the superior parietal lobules (areas 5 and 7) and inferior parietal lobules (areas 39 and 40, respectively, the angular and supramarginal gyri). Another target of somatic sensation is area S2, located in the upper bank of Sylvian fissure, and yet another is the insula, the latter being especially related to visceral information. These cortices generate dynamic representations of the perceiver's body and of three-dimensional stimuli as apprehended by somatosensory processing. They interweave such repre-

TABLE 398-1. CHARACTERISTIC MANIFESTATIONS OF OCCIPITAL LOBE DAMAGE

Sign	Qualification	Lesion
Hemiachromatopsia	Right or left field	Left or right inferior mesial cortex and white matter
Pure alexia	Noted anywhere in intact field	Left inferior cortex and white matter (including outflow of calosum)
Color anomia	Seen only in left visual field in combination with right hemianopia	Left inferior and mesial
Visual agnosia	Noted anywhere in intact field	Usually bilateral inferior (but right occipital may involve faces and places and left occipital may involve manipulable objects)
Visual disorientation	Noted anywhere in intact field	Bilateral superior
Astereopsis	Noted anywhere in intact field	Bilateral superior
Impaired movement detection	Noted anywhere in intact field	Bilateral superior

sentations with appropriate motor programs as well as pertinent visual and auditory information.

Damage to the sector of the postcentral somatosensory cortex to which signals from the hand usually project in either hemisphere impairs the ability to recognize form (astereognosia), scale, texture, and weight of objects in the contralateral hand. (The thresholds for touch, pain, vibration, and temperature are generally not disturbed.)

Damage to the dominant or nondominant inferior parietal lobule causes diverse manifestations. The dominant somatosensory cortex develops dynamic representations of (a) the body and its movements (especially those of the hand and phonatory apparatus) and (b) the shapes of objects located within arm's reach (in so-called intrapersonal space). Dysfunction in the area of the dominant angular gyrus disrupts reading and writing, planning and execution of representational hand movements in specific contexts (apraxia), arithmetic skills (acalculia), finger recognition (finger agnosia), right-left orientation, and the ability to copy drawings and diagrams and to execute three-dimensional constructions (constructional apraxia). Dysfunction in the dominant supramarginal gyrus is mainly associated with aphasia (Table 398-5).

The nondominant parietal cortices hold a dynamic representation of extrapersonal space (the space beyond arm's reach) based on somatosensory, visual, and auditory cues. *Both* hemispaces are represented in this region. The attentional survey of external sensory events and projected movements in both hemispaces also depend on this nondominant region, damage to which leads to complex defects in spatial processing. The defects are especially pronounced in the hemispace opposite the lesion and cause the commonly encountered *neglect syndrome*. Not only is the left hemispace inappropriately at-

TABLE 398-2. MANIFESTATIONS OF TEMPORAL LOBE DAMAGE

	Unilateral	Bilateral
Posterolateral	Aphasia* Pure-word deafness* Amusia†	Global auditory agnosia (includes aphasia, amusia, and agnosia for environmental sounds)
Medial	Verbal* or nonverbal memory impairment Complex seizures	Amnesia
Anterolateral and inferior	Anomia* Nonverbal memory impairment Visual agnosia Complex seizures	Amnesia

* Usually left hemisphere
† Right hemisphere only

TABLE 398-3. ICTAL MANIFESTATIONS OF TEMPORAL LOBE EPILEPTIC FOCI

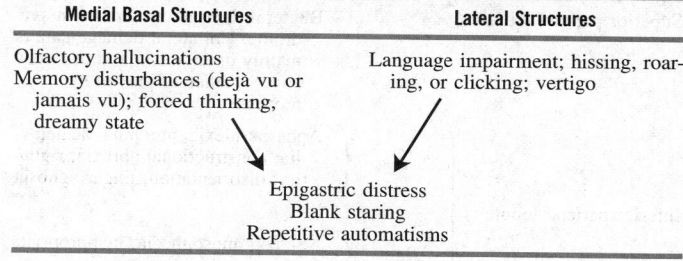

Medial Basal Structures	Lateral Structures
Olfactory hallucinations Memory disturbances (dejà vu or jamais vu); forced thinking, dreamy state	Language impairment; hissing, roaring, or clicking; vertigo

Epigastric distress
Blank staring
Repetitive automatisms

tended but the left side of the body itself may be neglected and left hemiplegia or hemisensory loss may be ignored or actively denied (anosognosia). The ability to negotiate a route without hitting obstacles placed to the left side of the body, the skill to follow a previously known and automated route (in a house or town), and the capacity to learn a new route are all compromised by nondominant inferior parietal lesions. Unlike their counterparts with left-sided lesions, patients with such nondominant injuries show little concern for their condition and often have an indifferent affect. An adequate rehabilitation program must take into account this reduced motivation. Patients may become confused when these structures are affected on the right side together with the nearby auditory cortices.

Bilateral damage confined to superior parietal lobules causes ocular apraxia (the inability to direct gaze voluntarily toward new visual stimuli appearing in the periphery of the visual field), bilateral optic ataxia (the inability to generate precise contralateral hand movements toward an outbound target under visual guidance), and an impairment of visual attention, a breakdown in the ability to apprehend the visual panorama in a cogent, seamless manner (this is known as visual disorientation or simultanognosia). The combination of ocular apraxia, optic ataxia, and visual disorientation constitutes the Balint syndrome. Common causes are bilateral infarctions in the border zone between the posterior and middle cerebral artery territories and bilateral metastases. Unilateral damage to the superior parietal lobule causes optic ataxia and defective pursuit eye movements.

FRONTAL LOBES

The human frontal cortices encompass nearly half of the entire cortical mantle and include a large number of diverse anatomic fields. Their operations assist with movement control (Table 398-6); general problem solving; planning; decision making; generation of willful responses; regulation of social behaviors, emotion, and autonomic function; and regulation of thought and language. Understanding of structural and junctional relationships is less advanced for frontal cortices than for other cerebral regions. Furthermore, such impairments are less easy to detect in clinical and laboratory settings than in real life.

The motor sector of the frontal lobe (the precentral and premotor cortices) is located mainly in the lateral frontal surface but spills into the mesial surface as well. The precentral cortex (area 4 or M1) contains a somatotopic representation of contralateral body movements in which the phonatory apparatus and hand are accorded the largest share. It is the principal target of re-entrant projections from cerebellum and motor thalamus. The premotor region (area 6) is part of a network for motor programming, and it receives re-entrant projections from basal ganglia as well as projections from the posterior sensory cortices. It integrates incoming movement-related information for final relay to the corticospinal

TABLE 398-4. INTERICTAL TRAITS OF PATIENTS WITH TEMPORAL LOBE EPILEPTIC FOCI

Lack of humor
Sadness
Obsessiveness
Metaphysical preoccupation
Hyposexuality
Dependence

TABLE 398-5. MANIFESTATIONS OF PARIETAL LOBE DAMAGE

Superior parietal lobule		Bilateral damage causes Balint syndrome. Unilateral damage causes mainly optic ataxia and transient abnormalities of pursuit eye movements.
Inferior parietal lobule	left	Aphasia; alexia; agraphia; acalculia; constructional apraxia; right/left disorientation; finger agnosia
	right	Neglect; anosognosia; inappropriate affect
Post-rolandic cortices		Subjective alterations in somatic sensation. Astereognosia

tract. Part of the nearby area 8, known as the frontal eye field, relates to voluntary eye movements (seizures originating in this area cause the eyes to deviate *away* from the lesion; damage by an infarction makes the eyes deviate *toward* the lesion). The mesial aspect of area 6 contains the supplementary motor area (SMA or M2). The SMA is anatomically contiguous with the rest of the premotor cortex but constitutes a functionally separate region. (It contains a whole body map in its relatively small cortical surface.) Damage to area 4 causes varied degrees of focal paralysis in the contralateral side of the body or face (involvement of corticospinal projections in corona radiata or internal capsule causes less focal paralyses). Damage to the lateral aspect of area 6 causes impairments of motor learning and execution as well as transient forms of neglect, whereas involvement of the SMA leads to mutism and contralateral akinesia. Infarctions and parasagittal tumors in this region often compromise part of both the SMA and the nearby cingulate gyrus (area 24) located immediately beneath the cingulate sulcus. The cingulate is a limbic cortex and its acute damage also causes akinesia, mutism, transient neglect, and an impairment of motivation. Tumors impinging in this region may cause speech arrest and seizures characterized by vocalization and may trigger involuntary movement synergies involving contralateral limbs and trunk.

Involvement of the posterior orbital surface is associated with disturbances of social behavior. These include inability to recognize the social significance of real-life situations and an inability to plan appropriate actions with a personal and social consequence. On occasion, especially with large lesions, patients may exhibit inappropriate demeanor (facetiousness). During the acute phase of medial frontal damage patients are generally akinetic and inattentive and some may urinate or defecate in public although sphincter function per se is preserved.

Areas 44 and 45 on the dominant side are known as Broca's

TABLE 398-6. MOTOR SYMPTOMS OF FRONTAL LOBE DISEASE*

	Structural Damage	Seizure
Precentral gyrus	Focal distal weakness, maximal in lower face, hand, less often foot; increased reflexes, mild spasticity, Babinski sign	Jacksonian: focal onset on face, thumb, foot. "March" toward trunk.
Corona radiata or internal capsule	Hemiplegia; increased spasticity	
Premotor (lateral)	Ocular ipsiversion; paratonic resistance to passive motion; grasping; hypokinesia; optic ataxia; aphasia	Adversive: ocular contraversion
Premotor (mesial)	Mutism	Involuntary synergies (elevated arm and leg, body turning); speech arrest and/or vocalization

* All arise contralateral to the brain lesion.

area. Their damage causes aphasia (see Ch. 399). Damage to the nondominant side of this area alters the prosodic qualities of speech. The most anterior regions of the frontal lobe accommodate the prefrontal cortices (areas 46, 47, 9, 10, 11, 12), damage to which impairs decision making and planning, reduces creativity, and alters the regulation of affect and emotion. With permanent damage, the magnitude of the deficit relates directly to the bilaterality or unilaterality of the lesion, the size of the lesion, and the previous intellectual caliber and occupation of the patient. Relatively small unilateral lesions produce minor impairments that are difficult to detect and tend to resolve. Large bilateral prefrontal lesions, however, although they leave motor, perceptual, and language functions intact, are incompatible with maintaining a socially adapted, fully self-conscious, and creative personality. The defects are most noticeable in patients who undergo bilateral prefrontal ablations for the treatment of large midline brain tumors. Even then, however, the impairments can be better sensed by appraising social and occupational behavior than by neuropsychologic tests, most of which may be passed flawlessly.

The frontal lobes are especially vulnerable to closed head injury, resulting in many of the signs described above as well as in the formation of cortical scar tissue and the appearance of seizures. The lateral sectors are frequently compromised by infarctions secondary to middle cerebral artery occlusions and meningiomas. The mesial sector often suffers infarctions or hemorrhages, secondary to ruptured aneurysms of the anterior communicating or anterior cerebral arteries. Meningiomas arising in the falx are another common cause of damage. The posterior orbital sector is often involved by herpes simplex encephalitis, by hemorrhages from ruptured anterior circulation aneurysms, and by meningiomas arising in the sphenoid and ethmoid regions. The brunt of the effects of normal-pressure hydrocephalus is seen in damage to the frontal white matter. Finally, prefrontal cortices can be markedly involved in Pick's disease, and both prefrontal and frontal limbic cortices are involved to some extent in Alzheimer's disease. When large tumors involve frontal lobe structures, especially malignant gliomas which may arise in one frontal lobe and traverse the corpus callosum to involve the other, patients exhibit many of the disturbances outlined above, impairments of attention and balance (see Ch. 404), and the release of primitive reflexes (grasp reflex, Gegenhalten or paratonia, echopraxia).

Damasio AR, Damasio H: Cortical systems for retrieval of concrete knowledge: The convergence zone framework. In Koch C (ed.): Large-Scale Neuronal Theories of the Brain. Boston, MIT Press, 1994, p 61. A framework for the understanding of cognition at the level of systems.
Damasio H, Damasio AR: Lesion Analysis in Neuropsychology. New York, Oxford University Press, 1989. A method to study the anatomic location of cerebral lesions, and a review of advances in neuropsychology.
Damasio AR, Tranel D, Damasio H: Somatic markers and the guidance of behavior: Theory and preliminary testing. In Levin HS, Eisenberg HM, Benton AL (eds.): Frontal Lobe Function and Dysfunction. New York, Oxford University Press, 1991, p. 217. Examples of the extreme dissociation of behavior caused by frontal lobe damage. The lesions prompt a variety of socially unacceptable behaviors but do not interfere with language or memory. The intelligence quotient is unaltered.
Heilman K, Valenstein E (eds.): Clinical Neuropsychology, 3rd ed. Oxford, Oxford University Press, 1993. A multiauthored collection of essays on major aspects of neuropsychology.
Mesulam M-M (ed.): Principles of Behavioral Neurology. Philadelphia, FA Davis, 1985, p. 125. Another collection of comprehensive reviews on neuropsychology.
Penfield W, Jasper W: Epilepsy and the Functional Anatomy of the Human Brain. Boston, Little, Brown and Company, 1954. The classic monograph on what epilepsy and the electrical stimulation of the cerebral cortex tell us about the neural substrates of higher brain function.

399 DISTURBANCES OF MEMORY AND LANGUAGE
Antonio R. Damasio

The concerted operation of multiple but relatively specific neural systems is the basis for the most complex human abilities: the acquisition and categorization of knowledge (learning and memory), the translation of knowledge in a verbal or signed code (language), the manipulation of nonverbal and verbal knowledge in thought processes, the ability to select responses and solve problems (planning, decision making, creativity), and the reflection upon ongoing cognitive activities in the perspective of one's autobiography (self-consciousness). These functions presume the normal operations of emotion (the impetus to sustain a given mental activity or action) as well as attention (the ability to concentrate willfully on a specific mental content to the exclusion of others).

MEMORY AND ITS IMPAIRMENTS

Memory is the ability to (1) make a record of interactions between the brain and the body proper or between the entire organism and the external world; (2) to store concepts derived from the categorization of those records; and (3) to manipulate the records internally for recall and recognition. The terms "learning" and "memory" are used almost interchangeably, although learning should be used only to denote "memory acquisition."

Unless the process of consolidation takes over, the memory of objects or events that we perceive or imagine is retained only briefly (< 60 seconds). The material held during that period is said to be in *short-term memory* or *immediate memory* (Table 399–1). This brief memory is preserved in most amnesias. If those materials are to be recorded into *long-term memory,* an active physiologic process must start promptly. The process of consolidation takes time, and recently acquired memories are more vulnerable to decay than those that have been held long and internally rehearsed. Newer memories are known as *recent* memories, and older memories as *remote.*

Memory for unique faces, objects, or events is usually known as *episodic* (e.g., the memory of a personal friend or a favorite landscape). Memory for classes of objects or events is known as *generic* or *semantic* (e.g., the knowledge that allows us to categorize a car as a transport vehicle, a dog as an animal, or a given locale as urban or rural). Episodic and semantic memories constitute factual knowledge and are known as *declarative.* Declarative memory contrasts with *procedural* memory, which is based on skills rather than facts and refers to actions rather than to the knowledge necessary to acquire those actions. The playing of an instrument, typing, and swimming are examples of *procedural* memory. Procedural memory is spared in most amnesias.

MEMORY MECHANISMS. The thesaurus of facts and rules acquired in a lifetime is largely stored in the association cortices of every lobe of both hemispheres. Several subcortical nuclei assist the process of learning and recall. Memories are dynamically and flexibly distributed in neuron ensembles linked by patterned and hierarchically organized corticocortical and commissural connections. Access to single-modality memories depends on association cortices near the primary sensory cortex that conveyed the information in the first place (the impaired access or partial destruction of those cortices causes an *agnosia*—Table 399–2). Access to memories of polymodal events depends on cortices farther away from sensory sources. Finally, access to unique and complex polymodal episodes depends on inferior and anterolateral temporal cortices as well as some prefrontal cortices (impaired access or partial damage to such cortices causes *amnesia*).

The ability to form a permanent record depends on the normal operation of the hippocampal system, the basal forebrain, and the diencephalon, as well as several brain stem nuclei. The elucidation of the respective roles of these components is imperfect, but it appears that the hippocampus, which is informed about relationships between components of an event via connections from the higher-order association cortices, binds and stabilizes information according to its appropriate temporal and spatial links. The stabilization

appears to involve molecular and cellular changes during long-term potentiation. Through the interconnected amygdala the hippocampus also influences basal forebrain, diencephalon, and brain stem nuclei. The basal forebrain and brain stem, in turn, provide the cerebral cortex with neurochemical inputs that probably contribute to stabilize records at the cellular level (acetylcholine, noradrenaline, dopamine, serotonin, and probably other, still ill-defined mediators and modulators). The hippocampal interconnections with the diencephalon sample the status of the internal milieu at the time of a given sensory experience, informing on the value of a particular stimulus or event in the context of instinctual goals. Finally, the ascending brain stem reticular formation contributes importantly because most learning presumes attention and arousal.

The neural structures and systems involving the acquisition of procedural memories are different: After bilateral destruction of hippocampus and basal forebrain, perceptuomotor skills remain intact and new motor skills can be learned. The motor and sensory cortices, the cerebellum, the neostriatum, and the motor nuclei of the thalamus are the key structures in this circuitry. A discussion of the molecular and cellular changes related to memory is outside the scope of this chapter.

MEMORY DISORDERS. Table 399–3 lists several terms that are helpful in describing and classifying the amnesias. The terms *anterograde* and *retrograde* are especially important. Anterograde designates the time compartment operating *since* the amnesia began and refers to the partial or complete inability to remember events during that period. Retrograde refers to information gained *prior to* the onset of amnesia that may not be retrievable in recall or recognition. Retrograde amnesia can be as short as hours or days, as is often the case in post-traumatic situations, or may extend back years or even decades, as in Korsakoff's amnesia or the amnesias that follow herpes simplex encephalitis.

Some middle-aged and elderly persons have an increasing but isolated difficulty in recalling proper names and recent events of limited importance. This "benign forgetfulness" is not a predictor of the progressive dementias and is best treated with prompt and vigorous reassurance. The most frequent causes of incapacitating mem-

TABLE 399–1. TYPES OF MEMORY

Factual (declarative)
Skill (procedural)

Short-term (immediate)—less than 60 seconds
Long-term—more than 60 seconds

Recent
Remote

Episodic (unique entities and events)
Generic (same as semantic; pertains to nonunique entities, as members of a conceptual category)

TABLE 399–2. TYPES OF MEMORY IMPAIRMENT

Agnosia	Impaired recognition of stimuli presented in one sensory channel (e.g., object, face, voice, melody) that cannot be explained by defective perception.
Anomia	Impaired retrieval of the name for a stimulus (e.g., object or face) that is otherwise properly perceived and properly recognized.
Amnesia	A pervasive impairment of the ability to recall and recognize unique events and unique stimuli. The defect is independent of the sensory channel used to probe memory (e.g., given a unique person, *neither* the face *nor* the voice is recognizable).
Aphasia	A pervasive impairment of linguistic processing (e.g., structure of sentences; assembly of phonemes in a word; retrieval of words from the lexicon).
Dysarthria	Defective articulation of speech sounds without compromise of linguistic processing. When the articulation breakdown is complete, the term *anarthria* applies.

TABLE 399–3. TYPES OF AMNESIA

Retrograde	Amnesia for information learned before the onset of illness
Anterograde	Amnesia for information that presented itself after onset of illness
Global	Information cannot be retrieved through *any* sensory channel
Modality-specific	Same as associative agnosia; information cannot be retrieved through the affected channel, e.g., vision
Permanent	
Stable	Example: postencephalitic
Progressive	Example: Alzheimer's disease
Transient	Examples: transient global amnesia, post-traumatic amnesia

TABLE 399–4. CAUSES OF AMNESIA

Alzheimer's disease and other degenerative dementias
Head injury
Herpes simplex encephalitis
Ruptured anterior circulation aneurysms with infarction in basal forebrain
Infarctions in other memory-related systems, e.g., medial thalamic nuclei; temporal cortices
Anoxic/ischemic encephalopathy
Wernicke-Korsakoff encephalopathy
Psychogenic amnesia

ory loss are the degenerative dementias, head injury, cerebrovascular disease, encephalitis, brain anoxia and ischemia, and nutritional impairment (Table 399–4).

Part of our knowledge about the critical contribution of the hippocampal formation to memory came from a patient who underwent *bilateral medial temporal lobe resection* to treat epilepsy. He became severely amnesic postoperatively and has remained unable to learn factual memories to this day. His severe anterograde amnesia contrasts with a largely spared retrograde memory and with preserved generic memories and procedural learning. The amnesias caused by *postanoxic encephalopathy,* in which anterograde memory is heavily compromised, also are caused by hippocampal damage in which the CA1 sector is selectively damaged. Together with the evidence that specific areas of the entorhinal cortex and subiculum are damaged in amnesic patients with *Alzheimer's disease,* these findings underscore the importance of hippocampus in memory (see Ch. 400). *Herpes simplex encephalitis* commonly damages the hippocampal region but also involves other anterolateral and inferior regions of the temporal cortices. Such patients suffer not only an anterograde memory defect but also a severe retrograde amnesia. Bilateral damage to hippocampus can also be caused by infarctions in the territory of the posterior cerebral arteries. Infarctions in the area of the basal forebrain (septal nuclei, nucleus accumbens, nucleus basalis of Meynert) due to ruptured aneurysms in the anterior circulation are also associated with amnesia. Both anterograde and retrograde memory are compromised, but unlike with temporal lobe amnesia, the defect is mild and tends to improve, and appropriate cueing helps recall. *Head injury* is another major cause of amnesia. *Korsakoff's syndrome* is a severe amnesia that compromises both anterograde and retrograde memories and is accompanied by confabulation and lack of insight. It is caused by severe thiamine deficiency, generally in the setting of alcoholism, and often accompanies or follows acute Wernicke encephalopathy (see Ch. 406) or delirium tremens (see Ch. 11).

Transient global amnesia (TGA) is a self-limited memory impairment during which the patient can identify himself but is unable to recall events preceding the episode and generally cannot recognize places. Patients with TGA remain attentive, have normal language and reasoning, and are generally distressed by their disorientation. They tend to ask repeatedly where they are, what they have been up to, and what is going on. Most TGA episodes last about 4 or 5 hours (but may be shorter or longer) and gradually clear. The attacks leave no residual impairment and are generally nonrecurrent. Status epilepticus with complex partial or petit mal seizures may mimic TGA but can be distinguished because patients with seizures are generally noninquisitive and inattentive. Most TGA attacks occur in middle-aged or older persons and may reflect transient ischemia or local neurochemical changes in memory-related areas of the temporal lobe or thalamus.

Psychogenic amnesia is generally greatest for emotionally important events and may erase circumscribed epochs of the past while leaving intact epochs immediately preceding or following the amnesic period. It may include disorientation to self. Questions such as "Who am I?" or "What is my name?", unless uttered during delirium or a seizure, raise the possibility of a psychogenic process. Psychogenic amnesia must be distinguished from emotional upheaval (which often impairs attention and produces inconsistent performance in psychological testing), from depression (which slows mentation and reduces communication), and from organic amnesias (in which emotionally reinforced material tends to be recalled better than neutral events, and disorientation is worst for time, less for place and persons, but never for self).

Treatment. Patients with acute post-traumatic amnesia tend to recover spontaneously. The same is true of amnesia caused by overmedication or delirium. Memory loss caused by depression (pseudodementia) has a good prognosis when effectively treated. A less fortunate prognosis accompanies amnesia following prolonged post-traumatic coma. When coma lasts more than 2 or 3 weeks, most patients over 25 years old tend not to recover from the memory loss. Patients with amnesia due to herpes encephalitis recover only when the lesions are mostly or solely unilateral and even then retain substantial impairments. In most amnesias the recovery is inversely proportional to the initial severity and depends on the extent and placement of lesions. The bulk of improvement usually takes place within the first year after onset. Neuroactive peptides, neurotransmitter precursors, neurotransmitters, and special dietary agents have no proven usefulness in chronic organic amnesia.

AGNOSIA. Agnosia is the inability to recognize a previously familiar sensory stimulus despite the integrity of elementary perception of the stimulus and the absence of defects of intelligence, motivation, or attention. It is a percept stripped of its meaning. The disorder is a form of monomodal amnesia, a disability that prevents a sensory stimulus from triggering previously acquired information that would reveal its identity. Agnosia results from dysfunction of association cortices of the affected sensory modality, which contain records of purely modal processing. *Visual agnosia* is the most frequent example. It consists of the selective failure to recognize familiar faces (prosopagnosia) or objects (visual object agnosia). The phenomenon is generally associated with bilateral occipitotemporal lesions.

LANGUAGE AND ITS DISORDERS

Verbal languages are arbitrary symbolic codes in which words stand for external stimuli, actions, and relationships, as well as for the intellectual and emotional reactions that such stimuli evoke in the perceiver. The normal brain acquires and stores a dictionary of such words in at least one language, a lexicon, and develops a highly automated process of two-way translation between the mechanism to reconstruct word representations and the mechanism to reconstruct nonverbal representations of objects, actions, or concepts. The process of language comprehension is the translation of sentences (structured sequences of words) into sequences of approximate nonverbal counterparts whose ongoing manipulation is known as thought. Nouns, verbs, or adjectives have fairly direct referential nonverbal equivalents. On the contrary, functor words (conjunctions, prepositions and adverbs, verb endings) refer to relationships. Functors, together with word order, are the key to the grammatical organization of sentences (syntax). The formulation of speech or writing is the rendering of a nonverbal thought process into a syntactic frame filled with appropriate lexical elements. The lexical and syntactic operations of language depend on phonemic and graphemic devices, which can enact correspondences between sounds, their visual representations, and the articulatory patterns that permit their sensorimotor implementation in phonetic utterances or writing. Oral verbal expression also depends on word stress and the intonational contour of sentences, i.e., the fundamental frequency of the sounds in an utterance as well as the durational elements of speech. The term *prosody* subsumes the latter qualities of verbal expression.

NEURAL SUBSTRATES OF LANGUAGE. Verbal language is characteristically human, and its experimental study is restricted to human beings. Considerable knowledge has been gathered about the neural substrates of language from the cognitive and neuroanatomic study of patients with acquired impairments caused by focal brain lesions (aphasias). Most such studies have relied largely on postmortem, computed tomography, and magnetic resonance imaging analysis, although more recent evaluations have used positron emission tomography (PET). Electrical stimulation of different regions of the cerebrum during surgery for seizures or motor disorders also has provided information on the neural representation of language. A salient finding, first noted more than a century ago and since confirmed, is that the left hemisphere of about 95% of individuals is especially adroit at language processing. In left language-dominant persons all aspects of language depend largely on left-hemisphere processing, with the partial exception of some aspects of prosody. Handedness is an imperfect but clinically useful indicator of language dominance. In almost all right-handed persons the left hemisphere is dominant for language, and its damage in key areas leads to severe aphasia. Most left-handed and ambidextrous persons (about 70%) are also left language-dominant, although they may have additional language representation in the right hemisphere. About one third of left-handers have either bilateral language representation or right-hemisphere language representation. Such persons are at a disadvantage in that lesions of either side can cause aphasia, although the disability tends to be less severe and to improve. Even extremely right-handed individuals with full language dominance in the left hemisphere possess some language representation in the opposite hemisphere (especially for nouns and verbs; adjectives are poorly represented and functor words probably not at all). The right hemisphere of such a person has little access to speech output and little syntactic capability. It has been suggested that gender is an important variable in language representation, but the available data are not conclusive. Language representation is different in children. Most children who suffer severe brain lesions up to age 5 or 6 years can recover from aphasia and continue to develop language to nearly normal levels. Left-hemisphere lesions sustained later, especially after puberty, have the same consequences as for adults.

Some asymmetric functional abilities have been related to neuroanatomic cerebral asymmetries. The left planum temporale, the area of association cortex located immediately behind the transverse gyrus (the primary auditory cortex), is measurably larger than the right in about 70% of individuals. The difference is visible on gross inspection and in the microscopic cytoarchitectonic structure of the area. Such persons possess a longer sylvian fissure on the left than on the right, reflecting the larger extent of the posterior temporal region, and more horizontally placed so as to accommodate a more voluminous left lower parietal lobule (supramarginal gyrus and angular gyrus).

Language depends on a wide network of cortical and subcortical processing units, and its knowledge and operations are distributed within key cortical regions (see Fig. 398–1). The principal set of language areas is located around the left sylvian fissure (the perisylvian language region). In its posterior aspect lies Wernicke's area (the posterior auditory association cortex, or Brodmann's area 22; it includes the planum temporale and the posterior portion of the first temporal gyrus). Immediately below and behind lies area 37, the lateral aspect of which, in the posterior sector of the second and third temporal gyri, is committed to language. Above and behind the sylvian fissure lie the supramarginal gyrus (area 40) and the angular gyrus (area 39). In the anterior aspect of the perisylvian region in the inferior and posterior aspects of the frontal operculum lie areas 44 and 45, also known as Broca's area. Between sit the motor and sensory regions associated with sensory motor phonatory representations. Also contributing to the language network are components of the basal ganglia (especially in the head of the caudate nucleus and parts of the putamen), some thalamic nuclei, the supplementary motor areas (especially the one on the left), and the anterior cingulate gyri.

THE APHASIAS. Aphasia (or dysphasia) is a disturbance of the comprehension or formulation of verbal messages caused by newly acquired brain disease. Although developments in cognitive science have led to a linguistic-based approach to aphasia, Geschwind's diagnosis of aphasic disorders in terms of the comprehension of language, the fluency of output, and the ability to repeat sentences remains clinically useful because of the strong relationship between these traits and the anatomic sites of the underlying lesions. Table 399–5 summarizes the important clinical clues.

Damage to the posterior sector of the left superior temporal gyrus and its surround causes *Wernicke aphasia*. Patients speak fluently, with normal melodic contour, and even a normal syntactic frame. However, they select wrong words (semantic paraphasias), so the intelligibility of their otherwise well-formed verbal messages may be low (jargon aphasia). Likewise, their comprehension of verbal message is poor because of their inability to translate words into nonverbal meanings. Wernicke aphasics with severe comprehension defects may develop paranoid reactions and become homicidal or suicidal. Wernicke aphasia must be distinguished from *auditory agnosia,* the inability to recognize objects or actions by the characteristic sounds they make (due to bilateral lesions in auditory cortex), and *pure word deafness,* an agnosia restricted to words (due to dominant lesions undercutting the auditory cortex) that allows patients to recognize nonspeech sounds and to produce normal speech. It is also different from the logorrhea of manic states, the logical thought derailment of schizophrenia, and the verbal salads of chronic schizophrenics.

Posterior lesions outside the Wernicke area produce more restricted disturbances. Lesions of the supramarginal gyrus give rise to *conduction aphasia*, a disorder in which the patient speaks fluently, has relatively preserved comprehension, but makes sound substitution errors (phonemic paraphasias). The major impairment of repetition stands out among these comparatively milder defects. Other strategically placed lesions of the posterior dominant hemisphere selectively compromise reading or writing. Alexia (inability to comprehend written language while retaining relatively normal vision) without concomitant writing impairment results when a lesion destroys the left visual cortex and, in addition, involves the outflow of the splenium of the corpus callosum. This placement cuts off projections that otherwise connect the unaffected right visual cortex to language areas of the left. Despite their inability to

TABLE 399–5. DIAGNOSTIC POINTERS TO THE MOST FREQUENT APHASIA TYPES

Type of Aphasia	Speech	Comprehension	Repetition	Other Signs	Localization
Broca	Nonfluent; effortful	+	−	Right hemiparesis worse in arm; aware of defect; frustrated	Lower posterior frontal
Wernicke	Abundant; fluent; well articulated	−	−	Often none; may be euphoric and/or paranoid	Posterior and superior temporal
Conduction	Fluent with some articulatory defects	+	−	Often none; cortical sensory loss in right arm	Usually supramarginal gyrus; may extend to insula and primary auditory cortex
Global	Scant; nonfluent	−	−	Right hemiparesis worse in arm; may present *without* hemiparesis	With hemiparesis: massive perisylvian lesion; without hemiparesis: separate Broca and Wernicke area damage
Transcortical motor	Nonfluent; explosive	+	+		Anterior or superior to Broca area
Transcortical sensory	Scant; fluent	−	+		Surrounding Wernicke area, posteriorly or inferiorly
Atypical ("basal ganglia")	Fluent dysarthric	−	−/+	Right hemiparesis worse in arm	Head of caudate; anterior limb of capsule
Atypical ("thalamus")	Fluent	−	+	Attentional and memory defects in acute phase	Anterolateral thalamus

+ = Intact or largely preserved
− = Impaired

comprehend the written word, patients with "pure" alexia can speak and write normally, in contrast to those with a combination of *alexia with agraphia* (impairment of writing despite normal motor function of the hand), in whom both reading and writing are compromised. In its pure form the abnormality is rare and follows lesions of the left angular gyrus. More frequently alexia and agraphia are accompaniments of Wernicke aphasia.

Broca aphasia is characterized by nonfluent, effortful, melodically flat speech, often shorn of functor words and marred by poor word order. The syntactic defect far outweighs the lexical impairment. Comprehension is well preserved in conversation. Broca aphasia must be distinguished from dysarthria, a disorder of speech articulation that does not impair the linguistic structure of communication. Many Broca aphasics are mute in the first hours or days after the onset of the disorder and only gradually develop the characteristic verbal signs. The intent to communicate, however poorly, is rarely in question. The lesion compromises Broca's area and adjacent cortical and subcortical territories. Because of patterns of vascular supply, many such patients also suffer a contralateral hemiplegia. Apraxia is added when the lesion involves the adjacent premotor cortex. Aphasia caused by lesions confined to Broca's area has a comparatively good prognosis.

Global aphasia consists of a severe loss of all aspects of language operation. Acutely, patients are often mute and have a right hemiplegia. The paucity of speech may become chronic, the patient being able neither to comprehend nor to produce language (except in the form of expletives or brief phrases). Despite rehabilitation efforts, the prognosis is poor, and patients often become depressed and listless, more so than Wernicke aphasics. As indicated in Table 399–5, two possible localizations can be associated with global aphasia.

With all the aphasias described above, patients are unable to repeat long sentences after the examiner. With some language defects, however, repetition is preserved. The dissociation between intact repetition and disturbed comprehension or speech output implies that Wernicke and Broca regions, as well as their interconnections, must be intact and that the causative lesions may lie near but outside those areas. There are two frequently encountered aphasias of this type: *transcortical motor* and *transcortical sensory* (Table 399–5).

Mutism accompanies a variety of conditions. It may describe the initial state of patients who evolve into Broca or global aphasics but produce no speech at all acutely. It may describe patients with bilateral premotor lesions who often remain chronically mute. Mutism has been applied to the paroxysmal speech arrest caused by seizures arising out of the supplementary motor or Broca areas, generally as an irritative response to an overlying tumor, and to the absence of speech in acute psychoses. Prominent mutism affects patients with lesions of the dominant-sided supplementary motor area and/or nearby cingulate, who not only do not speak but show no inclination to communicate through facial expression or gestures. Those patients also are generally motionless and when they recover do not exhibit aphasic symptoms. Mutism is not *anarthria*, a severe impairment of articulation that prevents speech but allows both the vivid expression of the intent to communicate and the frustration of not being able to do so (anarthria is caused by bulbar or pseudobulbar defects and can be confirmed by the presence of other signs of nuclear and supranuclear paralysis of lingual–vocal cord functions). Nor is mutism the same as *aphonia*, in which the phonatory apparatus is locally inoperative for mechanical or psychogenic reasons.

Some aphasias can be caused by infarcts in the dominant basal ganglia, especially when they involve the head of the caudate and the anterior limb of the internal capsule, and by infarcts in anterolateral nuclei of the dominant thalamus. Their occurence indicates that subcortical structures contribute to language processing, probably by assisting cortical units. The basal ganglia aphasias most often show a combination of fluent, dysarthric speech accompanied by impaired auditory comprehension and a right hemiparesis. The thalamic aphasias resemble transcortical sensory aphasia.

Although seizures or transient vascular insufficiency can cause brief language disturbances, the development of a selective disturbance in language that lasts more than a few hours always reflects a structural and focal lesion. The most common causes are infarction and hemorrhage in the distribution of a major cortical artery branch. Less frequent causes are head trauma and space-occupying lesions.

Damasio AR: Aphasia. N Engl J Med 326:531, 1992. *A description of different aphasia types and their localization.*

Damasio AR, Tranel D, Damasio H: Face agnosia and the neural substrates of memory. Annu Rev Neurosci 13:89, 1990. *A discussion of the cognitive and neuropsychological aspects of this intriguing phenomenon, with information applicable to the understanding of memory.*

Dudai Y: The Neurobiology of Memory: Concepts, Findings, Trends. Oxford, Oxford University Press, 1989. *A comprehensive review of the neuroscience of memory.*

Ojemann GA, Creutzfeldt OD: Language in humans and animals: Contribution of brain stimulation and recording. *In* Plum F, Mountcastle VB, et al. (eds.): Handbook of Physiology, Section 1: The Nervous System. Vol. V, Higher Functions of the Brain, Part 2. Bethesda, MD, American Physiological Society, 1987, p. 675. *Electrical stimulation and recording from the cerebral cortex provide clues to the neural basis of language.*

Victor M, Adams RD, Collins GH: The Wernicke-Korsakoff Syndrome and Related Neurologic Disorders Due to Alcoholism and Malnutrition, 2nd ed. Philadelphia, FA Davis, 1989. *The classic monograph on the subject provides evidence for the role of the diencephalon in memory.*

400 ALZHEIMER'S DISEASE AND RELATED DEMENTIAS

Antonio R. Damasio

The term *dementia* describes a pervasive decline in a number of mental functions resulting in the loss of personal and social independence in a previously competent individual. Although a defect in memory is often the core impairment in dementia, the term applies only to patients who have additional impairments in intellect as reflected by defective reasoning, decision making, and judgment. Those impairments are usually accompanied by disturbances in language and spatial orientation. Isolated defects in memory (amnesia) or in language (aphasia) do not qualify for the diagnosis of dementia even when their severity curtails normal behavior. The term *dementia* also does not apply to mentally retarded individuals who have never become intellectually competent and should not be applied to disturbances of attention, regardless of how profound they may be. The terms *confusional state* and *delirium* refer to the latter conditions.

From a physiopathologic standpoint, dementia occurs when several of the cerebral systems that support learning, memory, language, emotion, and reason are rendered dysfunctional by *any* neurologic disease process. Dementia can remain stable when the disease is self-limited (such as may follow brain damage from cardiac arrest or head trauma). In most instances, however, the dementia develops insidiously, as a result of diseases such as Alzheimer's or communicating hydrocephalus. Although the term *dementia* is equally appropriate for either stable or evolving mental decline, in practice it denotes a gradual, progressive condition.

Table 400–1 lists the most frequent causes of progressive dementia. Dementia has never been a rare occurrence but of late its frequency has been rising steeply. In part, this may reflect public and physician awareness of the condition, but the remarkable rise of longevity in the industrialized world is probably the key factor. Progress in medicine and living standards has extended life expectancy by about 15 years, dramatically increasing the incidence

TABLE 400–1. THE MOST FREQUENT CAUSES OF PROGRESSIVE DEMENTIA

Alzheimer's disease
Other degenerative diseases, e.g., Pick's, Parkinson's, Huntington's; Lewy body disease; progressive supranuclear palsy
Multiple cerebral infarcts
Chronic drug use
Depression
Intracranial mass lesions
Communicating hydrocephalus
Endocrine and metabolic disorders
CNS infections, e.g., HIV, opportunistic, syphilis, Creutzfeldt-Jakob disease

TABLE 400–2. TREATABLE CAUSES OF DEMENTIA

Inappropriate or excessive use of medications or alcohol
Resectable intracranial tumors
Subdural hematomas
Depression
Communicating hydrocephalus
Endocrine and metabolic disorders, e.g., hypothyroidism, vitamin B$_{12}$ deficiency
CNS infections

TABLE 400–3. OUTLINE OF MINI–MENTAL STATUS EXAMINATION*

Test	Score
What is the year, season, date, day, month?	5
Where are you: state, county, town, place, floor?	5
Name three objects: State slowly and have patient repeat (repeat until patient learns all three)	3
Do reversal serial 7's (five steps) or spell "WORLD" backwards	5
Ask for the three unrelated objects above	3
Name from inspection a pencil, a watch	2
Have patient repeat "No if's, and's, or but's"	1
Follow a three-stage command (1 pt each) ("Take a paper in your hand, fold it, and put it on the floor.")	3
Read and obey, "Close your eyes."	1
Write a simple sentence	1
Copy intersecting pentagons	1

* From Folstein MF, Folstein SE, McHugh PR: Minimental state. A practical method for grading the cognitive state for the clinician. J Psychiatr Res 12:189, 1975. The authors found that out of a possible total score of 30, mean score for dementia was 9.7, depression with cognitive impairment was 19.0, and uncomplicated affective depression was 27.6.

of late-life neurologic diseases, with degenerative diseases and especially Alzheimer's disease topping the list. Some recent studies have claimed that as many as 50% of individuals over the age of 80 develop Alzheimer's disease. Even assuming some exaggeration in those predictions, the impact of this disease in medicine and society cannot be overemphasized. Furthermore, not all dementia is of the Alzheimer type: Many patients so affected have conditions that are partially or completely reversible (Table 400–2).

Diagnosing Dementia

The diagnosis of dementia must be rigorously made and be followed by an attempt to uncover its probable cause. The imperative first step lies in establishing that a decline in cognitive and behavioral capacities exists. Many normal older individuals inappropriately sense that their mental abilities are diminishing. It is as important to reassure such persons about the benign nature of their complaints as to make a diagnosis of dementia in those who suffer it. Forgetfulness, especially of proper names, is common at any age and is accentuated by anxiety, fatigue, and depression. Benign forgetting, however, is accompanied neither by amnesia for recent social and personal events nor by impaired judgment (although depression may severely impair planning and decision making). A probing history and interview, together with a normal neurologic examination, can rapidly exclude the possibility of dementia. In addition, brief tests such as those listed in the Whitehouse reference offer simple measures of psychological ability that can be used to reassure the concerned patient.

If the brief examinations and detection tests suggest that dementia exists, the next step is to establish a premorbid baseline, something that the patient may be unable to provide and may depend on testimony from a reliable relative or escort. What is the patient's education and cultural background? What have been his or her professional and social achievements? Whenever possible, specific information should be sought about years of education, degrees achieved, professional positions, personality, and the judgment of colleagues, friends, and relatives.

The examination should evaluate the following: (1) orientation, (2) attention, (3) social appropriateness, (4) affect, (5) memory, and (6) language. Most of these emerge almost automatically as the evaluation proceeds. What is the patient's attitude toward the examiner? Is he or she cooperative? socially appropriate? attentive and able to communicate verbally? oriented to time and place? Can the patient relate recent public and personal events (the accuracy of the latter corroborated by an escort)? Patients with early Alzheimer's disease tend to be cooperative, socially appropriate, and attentive, but their recent memory clearly shows a decline. Patients with dementia due to brain tumors, central nervous system (CNS) infections, or hydrocephalus are more often distractible, less appropriate, and careless of appearances.

Some traditional mental status tests, such as the recall of three unrelated words at 5 minutes, the reverse spelling of "WORLD," or the backwards subtraction of serial 7's, can give helpful hints but are not reliable. Many nondemented patients with aphasia, amnesia, parietal lobe dysfunction, or mere distraction can fail such tests; conversely some patients with early dementia can pass them. The popular Mini–Mental Status Examination fares better (Table 400–3).

In doubtful cases, a formal evaluation conducted by a trained neuropsychologist offers the most reliable means to diagnose the presence and severity of dementia. Such evaluations quantify intellectual and problem-solving ability, memory, speech and language, perception, attention, concentration, and personality. Many standardized tests, such as the Wechsler Adult Intelligence Scale—Revised, the Wechsler Memory Scale—Revised, and the Benton Visual Retention Test, permit a diagnostic precision that cannot be approximated by bedside evaluations or screening batteries. Formal neuropsychological examination is especially useful in distinguishing dementia from depression.

Differential Diagnosis

There are more than 50 possible causes of dementia, but many are rare and the most frequent, Alzheimer's disease, has a fairly distinctive profile. Nonetheless, only histologic analysis of brain tissue at autopsy offers an absolute confirmation of Alzheimer's disease, and the clinical diagnosis remains one of exclusion. Because some of the less frequent causes of dementia can be treated and occasionally may mimic Alzheimer's disease, it is important to identify them or rule them out. The distinction depends largely on the results of a small group of critical tests (Table 400–4).

ALZHEIMER'S DISEASE

PATHOGENESIS AND MANIFESTATIONS. Alzheimer's disease is caused by a progressive and selective degeneration of neuron populations in the entorhinal cortex, the hippocampus, the high-order association cortices of the temporal, frontal, and parietal regions, and some subcortical nuclei in the basal forebrain, thalamus, and brain stem. The neuronal damage and the attending loss of synaptic density disable several neural systems essential to learning and retrieval of memories. By itself, the cortical component of the damage would explain the prominent memory defects of Alzheimer patients. In addition, however, damage to cholinergic neurons in the basal forebrain results in a loss of delivery of acetylcholine to the cerebral cortex, whereas damage to the brain stem's locus coeruleus precludes the delivery of norepinephrine to the cerebral cortex. Those neurochemical defects are likely to worsen, if not independently explain, many of the behavioral changes seen in Alzheimer patients. At autopsy, the brains of Alzheimer patients are atrophied, especially in the regions where most neurons die. Characteristically, the motor and primary sensory cortices remain unaffected, as do the basal ganglia and cerebellum. Histologically, the diseased neurons are seen to contain cytoplasmic neurofibrillary

TABLE 400–4. USEFUL TESTS IN THE EVALUATION OF DEMENTIA

Brain computed tomography or magnetic resonance imaging
Neuropsychologic evaluation
Complete blood count and erythrocyte sedimentation rate, serologic test for syphilis
Metabolic screen (SMA 12–16)
Serum TSH, vitamin B$_{12}$ level
Chest radiograph
Cerebrospinal fluid analysis: cells, protein
Electroencephalography

tangles composed of paired helical filaments visible with special stains. The most prominent anatomic change, however, consists of amyloid plaques containing degenerated neuronal fragments surrounding a small, dense core of amyloid material.

The neuropathologic diagnosis of Alzheimer's disease depends not only on the presence of neurofibrillary tangles and neuritic plaques but also on their anatomic distribution and quantity. Neurofibrillary tangles are present in other diseases, including the dementia that follows repeated boxing injuries. Neuritic plaques are present in the brains of normal aged persons, although less abundantly than in the Alzheimer brain. Such findings lead some investigators to believe that Alzheimer's dementia may represent an accelerated form of brain aging rather than a conventional disease.

In about 25% of cases of Alzheimer's disease, the history reveals a relative affected by the disease, and in some rare families the disease can start early (fifth or sixth decade) and affect the offspring in an autosomal dominant pattern. Also, patients with trisomy 21 (Down syndrome) develop the neuropathologic changes of Alzheimer's disease in their third or fourth decade. Current research studies indicate a linkage of Alzheimer's disease to chromosomes 14, 19, and 21. Recent investigations also reveal that the genotype for ApoE, a protein known for its role in cholesterol transport, is a risk factor in Alzheimer's disease. Homozygotes for $ApoE_4$ have high risk for the disease compared with E_3 or E_2 homozygotes. E_4 heterozygotes have an intermediate risk. The search for toxins, infectious agents, and nutritional or environmental factors has been disappointing.

Clinically, Alzheimer's disease is characterized by a relentless impairment of memory and reasoning that generally begins insidiously and can progress for a decade or longer. In most cases, Alzheimer's disease starts after age 60, and the incidence increases with each decade thereafter. Analyses show a greater incidence in women, which may reflect in part their increased longevity compared with men. A high level of education may be a protective factor. In most patients the gradual impairment of memory dominates the early clinical picture. They fail to learn new recent events, both public and personal. A defect in recognition of previously known familiar places or situations often inaugurates the symptoms. The impairments worsen with time. Despite preserving their speech, motor performances, and social graces, patients are not able to retain employment and become unable to cope with the activities of daily living. A loss of affective resonance is common, which relatives may describe as shallowness or lack of interest. Unwise decisions regarding property or investments are often made during these early stages of the disease. Signs of poor judgment and a deterioration of social relationships commonly ensue.

Alzheimer's disease may take other forms of onset. Some patients become suspicious of friends, employers, or spouse, and exhibit paranoid behavior, especially during the evening hours. They may awaken in the night disoriented to place and time and behaving in acute psychotic fashion. In another variant, language may be especially compromised. In those instances memory for words suffers the most and disturbs naming of specific objects and people. Finally, the disease may begin by compromising visual attention. Patients report an inability to perceive simultaneously more than one object in the visual field and become unable to orient themselves along previously familiar routes. Whatever the variant of onset, a pervasive impairment of memory eventually sets in. In striking contrast to the intellectual decay, motor performance (strength, coordination) remains preserved in most cases during the first years of the disease. Some patients with Alzheimer's disease can even learn *new* motor skills despite their ravaged ability to retain new factual information. Nevertheless, exceptions exist. A patient has been described with left hemiplegia and dementia whose autopsy revealed neuropathologic changes entirely characteristic of Alzheimer's disease. Also, some patients may exhibit extrapyramidal signs, in which case the course is usually more rapid. It is possible that some of the latter patients have a pathologic entity known as Lewy body dementia, hallmarked by a coexistence of Alzheimer changes and an abundance of Lewy bodies in cortical neurons.

No reliable antemortem marker exists for Alzheimer's disease. Accordingly, diagnosis must be formulated in terms of probability, based on the identification of a typical profile and the exclusion of similar conditions. In order to diagnose probable Alzheimer's disease, one must (1) document the dementia by careful bedside examination or neuropsychological tests revealing scores significantly below the range commensurate with the patient's age, educational level, and past performance; (2) verify impairment of memory; and (3) verify that the onset of dementia was not sudden or rapidly progressive. A diagnosis of Alzheimer's disease should *not* be entertained if early in the presentation (1) there are motor signs such as hemiparesis or gait disorder (but see exceptions above); (2) there is loss of somatic sensation; (3) there is a visual field defect; and (4) seizures have occurred. The electroencephalogram (EEG) should be normal early in the course of the disease, although as the disease progresses it may reveal a nonspecific pattern of slowing. The cerebrospinal fluid should also be normal, containing no cells and either a normal or mildly elevated protein level. Computed Tomography (CT), or Magnetic Resonance Imaging (MRI) scans may be normal early in the course or reveal enlargement of sulci. The enlargement can become quite pronounced in late stages but is generally more symmetric and severe than in Pick's disease (see below). Positron emission tomography has revealed a consistent pattern of diminished metabolic activity in the temporoparietal regions.

MANAGEMENT. There is no cure for Alzheimer's disease, and no drug tried so far can alter the progress of the disease. Although tacrine may rarely ameliorate symptoms in some patients, its results are usually disappointing and its side effects include severe hepatotoxicity. There are ways, however, in which caregivers can ameliorate the manifestations of the disease. During early stages, when patients can remain at home, strategically placed cue cards around the house can help their orientation so as to carry on tasks relating to their self-care. Variations of such a strategy also can help patients cope with nondemanding social activities. An emphasis on tasks that require motor skills (music playing, dancing, card playing, typing, drawing) can help to make the days more pleasurable to the patient and less frustrating to caretakers. Appropriate drugs help to cope with bouts of anxiety, depression, or paranoid ideation that some patients show. Drugs also can be used to regulate the sleep cycle and avoid nighttime waking and "sundowning." Reduction of environmental stresses and random sensory stimuli can yield surprisingly good results in this regard. Eventually a decision is needed regarding nursing home placement and the securing of appropriate medical care in such a setting. The Alzheimer's Disease and Related Disorders Association has chapters in every state which can guide physicians and patients to dedicated services. A valuable guide to management is referenced at the end of this chapter.

DISTINGUISHING ALZHEIMER'S DISEASE FROM OTHER DEMENTIAS

Treatable Dementias

INAPPROPRIATE OR EXCESSIVE USE OF MEDICATIONS. This is perhaps the most frequent and treatable dementia. It can coexist with Alzheimer's disease, and excessive drug use must be ruled out before the diagnosis of Alzheimer's disease is entertained. Cough suppressants, barbiturates, benzodiazepines, tricyclic antidepressants, monoamine oxidase inhibitors, anticholinergics, and digitalis are the common offenders. The combination of some of these drugs with alcohol in an elderly and frail individual can mimic Alzheimer's disease.

DEPRESSION. This should always be considered in the differential diagnosis because it can present as mental decline, in which case it is known as masked depression or pseudodementia. Expert psychological testing is the key to diagnosis. A number of neuropsychological tests are capable of specifically discriminating depression from Alzheimer's disease. The Benton Visual Retention Test, for example, is passed by nearly all patients who are eventually diagnosed as having pseudodementia, whereas patients with Alzheimer-type dementia fail or perform at the borderline level.

BRAIN TUMORS AND SUBDURAL HEMATOMAS. Tumors that involve structures of the limbic system, e.g., meningiomas that compress frontal lobe structures or gliomas that infiltrate the white matter of frontal and temporal cortices, often present as dementia. Distractibility, bradykinesia, and apathy dominate the clinical picture and a CT or MRI scan easily confirms the suspicion. In most instances, meningiomas can be resected with success. The elderly are prone to develop subdural hematomas after relatively minor, and thus easily forgettable, head injuries. Such hematomas, especially when bilateral, can lead to dementia, often with little in the way of a telltale history. CT or MRI is diagnostic.

COMMUNICATING HYDROCEPHALUS. Communicating hydrocephalus of the so-called normal-pressure variety is another late-life condition easily detected by brain imaging. The lateral ventricles and the third ventricle are enlarged, the sulci may be effaced, and the sampling of cerebrospinal fluid pressure in a routine lumbar puncture may fail to reveal an elevation because the pressure waves that pound the ventricular walls are intermittent. Not uncommonly the past history reveals a significant neurologic antecedent such as bacterial meningitis, subarachnoid hemorrhage, or severe head injury. The dementia is probably due to pervasive dysfunction in white matter pathways surrounding the ventricles. The clinical picture is dominated by impaired attention and flatness of emotional expression and always includes a gait disorder and urinary incontinence, neither of which affects early Alzheimer's patients. The gait disorder consists of a loss of the automatic motor patterns that are normally engaged in walking (apraxia) combined with a broad-based ataxia. An intraventricular shunt may reverse the symptoms in selected patients.

OTHER CAUSES. Endocrine and metabolic disorders, especially hypothyroidism and vitamin B$_{12}$ deficiency, also can cause dementia. They are easily detectable and largely correctable. Syphilis and fungal infections can cause reversible dementias. In the appropriate setting, syphilis is an especially important diagnostic consideration. Many other dementias exist that can be reversed upon correcting the conditions to which they are secondary. Chronic liver disease, chronic lung disease, and uremia are obvious examples.

Nontreatable Forms of Dementia

PICK'S DISEASE. In spite of its rarity, the number of Pick's disease cases appears to be rising. This is a degenerative condition characterized by a markedly asymmetric loss of neurons in the frontal and anterior temporal regions. In some cases, the involvement is virtually unilateral and may be largely confined to either the temporal or frontal lobe (hence the term *lobar atrophy*). An intriguing preponderance for involvement of the left hemisphere has been noted. Histologic analysis reveals loss of cortical neurons in the atrophied areas. Two signs that assist with the microscopic diagnosis are the presence of Pick's neurons (pale, swollen neurons that fail to take conventional stains and are thus achromatic) and Pick's bodies (silver-staining cytoplasmic inclusions easily distinguishable from neurofibrillary tangles). Pick's neurons are most commonly found in the frontal region, whereas Pick's bodies are found predominantly in the temporal region. Neurofibrillary tangles and neuritic plaques are not histologic features of the disease.

Pick's disease has two prevalent profiles. Both usually begin in the sixth or seventh decade and affect women more frequently than men. In one profile, the patient has a gradual mental decline not unlike that seen in Alzheimer's disease but in which impairments of judgment, social appropriateness, and affect predominate over the memory defect. Not uncommonly, these patients make unwise business decisions and if they live alone they may care little about their appearance. Eventually, memory impairment sets in. This profile correlates with preponderant involvement of the frontal lobe. In the other prevalent profile, patients begin by complaining of a problem with name finding. Few specific names for objects or people can be produced, although speech articulation, syntactic processing, memory, and judgment may be intact. In most instances, within 2 to 5 years, memory and judgment begin to decline. The anatomic correlate is involvement of the *left* temporal lobe. Incidentally, Pick's original description was of the latter profile, although the former has become the textbook standard.

The left temporal form of Pick's disease brings into the discussion an elusive entity known as *progressive aphasia without dementia*. The pattern observed in some of the patients resembles that of Pick's disease, but the language disorder has remained the most prominent or sole symptom. It is possible that these cases are examples of Pick's disease in which involvement beyond the left temporal cortices is minimal or delayed. Other evidence suggests that the condition reflects either a variant of Alzheimer's disease or a nonspecific spongiform degeneration. The diagnosis of Pick's disease in the early stages is hazardous, although after about 2 years of evolution the clinical profile becomes suggestive. By then, state-of-the-art CT or MRI should provide evidence of asymmetric lobar atrophy.

PARKINSON'S DISEASE. Dementia complicates a sizable number of cases of idiopathic parkinsonism. From a clinical standpoint it is important to ensure that the mental decline is not due to the effects of anticholinergic medication or to the multifarious cognitive changes induced by levodopa. Histologic study of brain tissue of demented patients with Parkinson's disease has shown in many but not all instances abundant neurofibrillary tangles and neuritic plaques identical to those encountered in Alzheimer's disease.

HUNTINGTON'S DISEASE. Patients with Huntington's disease are prone to a host of cognitive and behavioral changes (see Ch. 411). Depression and psychotic states are part of the clinical picture. They may precede chorea and dystonia and persist into the later stages, producing a high suicide rate. Measurable mental decline is often found as the disease progresses. Distractibility and slowness of cognitive processing hallmark the presentation. The dementia is best explained by extensive cortical dysfunction secondary to neuron loss in the basal ganglia, especially in the caudate.

MULTIPLE VASCULAR LESIONS. A variety of conditions resulting in multiple strokes, large and small, can cause dementia. The following should be considered:

1. Multiple small infarcts (multiple-infarct dementia), occurring at different points in the history and involving cortical or subcortical gray matter, especially in the territories of middle cerebral and anterior cerebral arteries. The history and physical examination of such patients invariably reveal systemic hypertension, diabetes, signs of widespread vascular disease, or a combination of the above. The age range is similar to that during which degenerative diseases strike, but a careful history and neurologic examination disclose distinctive clues. For instance, the development of the dementia is stepwise, punctuated by specific events during which disturbances of speech, orientation, or motor impairment developed, often followed by some recovery. In short, the mental decline is cumulative but not gradual. (But note that the patient may lack memory and insight and thus smooth out the history profile and mislead the examiner. Helpful additional clues include focal motor defects, especially weakness, ataxia, or urinary incontinence. Alzheimer's disease shows neither of these abnormalities during its early clinical course.)

2. Multiple demyelinating lesions occurring in the surround of a blood vessel are revealed by MRI in the subcortical white matter. This puzzling condition, sometimes called Binswanger's disease or subcortical arteriosclerotic encephalopathy, can have a dementia profile indistinguishable from that of Alzheimer's disease. Most affected patients are hypertensive, however, although the condition has been described in normotensive individuals. Both CT and MRI reveal enlargement of the lateral ventricles disproportionate to the enlargement of the cortical sulci. MRI also reveals an abundance of periventricular lucencies, which show up as white on T2-weighted images. It should be noted that similar lucencies can be seen in normal older individuals but generally without ventricular enlargement of the same magnitude.

3. Multiple infarcts caused by vasculitis such as congophilic angiopathy, isolated angiitis of the central nervous system, and systemic lupus erythematosus. These are all rare conditions that present in a far more severe and dramatic way than degenerative diseases, multiple-infarct dementia, or Binswanger's disease. Such patients usually become acutely ill and are more likely to be admitted to an inpatient service than to remain ambulatory. The severity of the condition usually is paralleled by a relatively rapid course compared to the longer time scale of most of the other dementias discussed above. Other clues help the diagnosis. For instance, congophilic angiopathy causes medium to large *hemorrhagic* infarctions. Congophilic angiopathy often coexists with Alzheimer's disease for reasons that are not clear. Lupus is rare in the elderly, and the signs of systemic involvement are diagnostic. Isolated angiitis is more elusive, but the severity and rapidity of the course help the diagnosis.

CENTRAL NERVOUS SYSTEM INFECTIONS. Until recently, the most frequent form of nontreatable infectious dementia was the transmissible form of Creutzfeldt-Jakob disease, a spongiform encephalopathy discussed in Ch. 428.6. Over the past decade, immune suppression in the setting of HIV infection has become the most common infectious cause of dementia. In some cases the dementia is due to direct HIV involvement of the cerebral parenchyma; in others it is caused by opportunistic infections.

Folstein MF, Folstein SE, McHugh PR: Minimental state. A practical method for grading the cognitive state for the clinician. J Psychiatr Res 12:189, 1975. *The authors found that out of a possible total score of 30, mean score for dementia was 9.7, depression with cognitive impairment was 19.0, and uncomplicated affective depression was 27.6.*

Lippa CF, Smith TW, Swearer JM: Alzheimer's disease and Lewy body disease: A comparative clinicopathological study. Ann Neurol 35:81, 1994. *An attempt to establish Lewy body disease as a pathologic entity.*

Mace NL, Rabin PV: The 36-hour Day. A Family Guide to Caring for Persons with Alzheimer's Disease, Related Dementing Illnesses, and Memory Loss in Later Life. Baltimore, Johns Hopkins University Press, 1981. *An invaluable book for families and friends of the affected.*

Plum F, Gandy S: The dementias. Research Proceedings of the Association of Nervous and Mental Diseases, Vol. 73. American Psychiatric Assn Press, 1995.

Selkoe DJ: Aging brain, aging mind. Sci Am, September, 1992, p. 135. *An overview of current research on aging and dementia.*

Van Hoesen GW, Damasio AR: Neural correlates of cognitive impairment in Alzheimer's disease. *In* Plum F (ed.): Handbook of Physiology: Higher Functions of the Nervous System. Bethesda, MD, American Physiological Society, 1987, p. 871. *A review of the neuropsychological and neurobiologic characteristics of the disease.*

Whitehouse PJ (ed.): Dementia. Philadelphia, FA Davis, 1993. *A comprehensive monograph as many aspects of the dementias, with multiple authorities describing epidemiologic, neurobiologic, and clinical aspects of the problem. Sections also address management, legal issues, and current drug trials.*

401 PSYCHIATRIC DISORDERS IN MEDICAL PRACTICE

Gary J. Tucker

At various times most people experience anxiety, depression, sleep disturbance, and/or somatic preoccupation. In most cases such symptoms are transient, and their precipitants are often evident—an upcoming examination, a new job, marriage, divorce, work or family problems. In these instances the physician has no difficulty in reassuring the patient that the symptoms are transient and situational. However, when these symptoms persist and/or when they occur in situations that have no clear precipitants, they should arouse the physician's concern. In order to determine whether someone has a psychiatric illness, the following questions must be considered: (1) Do the signs and symptoms fit a psychiatric diagnosis? For example, when patients say they are sad or depressed, do their symptoms meet the diagnostic criteria for a diagnosis of depression? (2) Is there a family history of similar symptoms? Many psychiatric illnesses tend to have a genetic or familial basis. (3) Is the longitudinal pattern of the symptoms consistent with the natural history of a psychiatric disorder? Emotional symptoms associated with specific situations are usually classified as reactions to the situation (see Grief Reactions); they do not usually become psychiatric disorders. (4) Are the symptoms incapacitating? All persons have enduring patterns of relating, perceiving, and reacting to others. These constitute a person's personality and may take the form of such patterns as obsessive, passive, or antisocial personality traits. When such characteristics interfere with the individual's ability to function, however, the condition is regarded as a disorder, named for the predominant personality characteristic. (5) Do delusions and hallucinations exist? Delusions and hallucinations in the absence of other medical causes always indicate major psychiatric illness. Although illusory phenomena can often occur at times of tiredness, intoxication, or fever, their occurrence in clear states of consciousness should alert the physician to the presence of major psychiatric illness.

The proper delineation of psychiatric disorders from normal emotional reactions rests on a careful history, a mental status evaluation, and a knowledge of psychiatric syndromes. If the findings of the history and mental status evaluation do not fit into any of the known psychiatric syndromes, the physician should reserve judgment and follow the patient. In many cases, the symptoms neither persist nor return and all can be reassured. If the symptoms con-

TABLE 401–1. CLUES TO NONPSYCHIATRIC DISORDERS AFFECTING BEHAVIOR

1. The signs and symptoms do not fit into an established psychiatric diagnostic category.
2. There is no prior psychiatric history or symptoms.
3. The patient demonstrates an abrupt change in behavior or personality.
4. Signs and symptoms fluctuate rapidly.
5. The condition does not respond to treatment.

tinue, the physician may recognize a clear psychiatric syndrome. With all persistent emotional and behavioral symptoms, however, the physician must first rule out systemic medical disorders.

DIFFERENTIATING PSYCHIATRIC DISORDERS FROM MEDICAL DISORDERS

As biologic studies of psychiatric patients progress and specific psychopharmacologic agents are found to affect behavior, it becomes increasingly evident that psychiatric disorders are disorders of central nervous system (CNS) functioning. This awareness includes recognition that the CNS has a limited number of ways of responding to stress. For example, hallucinations can arise from psychologic causes, from toxins in the blood, from head trauma, from seizure disorders, from acute strokes, and from fever. With such potentially diverse causes, it is imperative that the physician seek clues to differentiate the causes of the behavior change (Table 401–1).

Many clues in the history can suggest something other than an intrinsic psychiatric illness as a cause of abnormal behavior. Most patients with psychiatric illnesses have had psychiatric symptoms or reveal seeds of the current disturbance in their histories. When a patient presents with a good premorbid social history, a good work history, a warm and supportive family, and well-preserved personality, the physician should seek nonpsychiatric factors to explain the behavior change. Many physicians tend erroneously to view behavior changes only in a psychological framework. Abrupt changes in behavior, personality, mood, or ability to function should be evaluated for possible organic causes. As indicated, most decompensating patients with psychiatric illness report having had similar, albeit less severe, symptoms in the past. To give an example: A 60-year-old man who has been formal and proper his entire life but abruptly becomes bawdy and flirtatious is probably not experiencing the onset of a major psychiatric illness but rather is showing personality changes associated with a new, structural disorder of the brain or of body metabolism. Rapid fluctuations in mental status also suggest a new organic disturbance rather than a psychiatric disorder. Patients with psychiatric disease seldom are delusional and hallucinating in the morning but free of these symptoms the same evening (or vice versa). By contrast, the resolution of the delusions and hallucinations associated with schizophrenia typically requires days to weeks. Similarly, motor behavior does not change rapidly in psychiatric illness. Patients with encephalopathies, by contrast, often have a "motor drivenness" with episodic desires to move about, to get up and walk. This restlessness is particularly prominent in delirious states (see Ch. 393). Lastly, and perhaps most subtly, when a patient does not respond to the usual interventions one should suspect the possibility of an incorrect diagnosis. For example, when a patient with hallucinations and delusions has been treated unsuccessfully with adequate doses of neuroleptic medications for an appropriate period of time with no change in the symptoms, the physician should consider the possibility of a disorder other than schizophrenia. These simple guidelines often alert the clinician to multiple diagnostic possibilities.

Diagnostic and Statistical Manual of Mental Disorders, 4th ed. Washington, DC, American Psychiatric Association, 1994. *A useful, widely accepted outline of diagnostic features of the gamut of psychiatric disorders.*

Goodwin D, Guze S: Psychiatric Diagnosis, 4th ed. New York, Oxford University Press, 1989. *An excellent overall text on descriptive psychiatry and the basis for diagnostic groupings.*

Lishman W: Organic Psychiatry, 2nd ed. Oxford, Blackwell, 1987. *A comprehensive description of neurologic and medical complications of behavioral disorders.*

Pincus J, Tucker G: Behavioral Neurology, 3rd ed. New York, Oxford University Press, 1985. *This monograph discusses differential diagnosis and behavioral aspects of neurologic disease as well as neurologic aspects of psychiatric disorders.*

Schiffer RB, Klein RF, Sider RC: The Medical Evaluation of Psychiatric Patients, New York, Plenum Press, 1989. *A detailed explication of the comorbidity of medical illnesses and behavioral symptoms.*

Schizophrenia and some forms of affective disorders constitute the major psychotic illnesses. (Psychosis is defined as the presence of hallucinations and/or delusions.) In 1911 Eugene Bleuler, a Swiss psychiatrist, described the central features of schizophrenia as a psychotic process manifested by disturbed thinking, changes in the emotional responsiveness of the patients, and a preoccupation with their own inner life, or autism. By schizophrenia he did not mean a "split personality" but more a splitting of psychologic functions. While some functions, such as the ability to communicate, were often impaired, others, such as memory and mathematical abilities, were sustained. In essence, this early concept remains a good clinical definition of the schizophrenic process.

Schizophrenia most often starts in late adolescence. The course is usually marked by a decline in psychosocial functioning, with a tendency for the patient to become downwardly mobile in social function. The introduction of neuroleptics in 1954 brought about some improvement in the treatment of these patients. Current treatment aims toward shorter hospitalizations for schizophrenics with more vigorous attempts to retain the patient in a community setting. Physicians encounter two principal groups of schizophrenic patients, one with an acute florid psychotic illness and the other suffering chronic illness with less florid symptoms. The care of these two groups differs in that the acute management is simple, whereas the care and rehabilitation of the chronic patient can be extremely difficult. The nationally pursued process of "deinstitutionalization" of the mentally ill has thrust this latter patient population into our everyday world.

DIAGNOSTIC CRITERIA AND CLINICAL SIGNS AND SYMPTOMS. Table 401–2 lists the diagnostic criteria for schizophrenia. Hallucinations and delusions can occur in affective disorders and organic conditions; however, the course of these latter illnesses is different. With schizophrenia, the greater the number of delusions and hallucinations present, particularly persecutory delusions, delusions of control, firmly fixed mood-incongruent delusions, and auditory hallucinations, the more likely is the person to progress to a chronic psychotic condition (Table 401–3). Other prominent symptoms of schizophrenia are the presence of incoherence and the inability of patients to communicate in a logical and goal-directed fashion. As an example of the speech of a schizophrenic, the patient may respond as follows when asked why he was brought to the hospital: "You are a Nazi; God sent me to save the world; I have a lovely apartment; your eyes are blue."

The stipulation that these criteria must last for a 6-month period (demonstrating a deterioration from a previous level of functioning) defines a more chronic population. When the duration of symptoms is shorter than 6 months, it is inadvisable to use the diagnosis of schizophrenia. This allows the clinician to withhold judgment and encourages a search for other disorders. This is particularly important with the first episode of psychotic illness, in that it is difficult to differentiate an acute manic episode from an acute schizophrenic episode. Psychotic episodes due to toxic drug reactions, sleep deprivation, and medical causes invariably last less than 6 months.

In the past many subtypes of schizophrenia have been described, but their predictive validity has been poor except for catatonia and paranoia. Catatonic symptoms include either markedly retarded motor behavior (often to the point of no voluntary movement, the patient retaining any posture into which he is passively placed) or markedly agitated motor behavior. The importance of a catatonic diagnosis, in either the retarded or the agitated form, has retained some validity in conferring a better prognosis, but there is also evidence that catatonia may be more related to affective disorders than to schizophrenia. The paranoid forms of schizophrenia also show some unique features in that the paranoid delusions are often the only major symptoms and they tend to remain stable over time.

EPIDEMIOLOGY. The prevalence of schizophrenia in the general population is about 1% for lifetime risk, or about an 0.5 in 1000 incidence of recorded or treated cases per year in the United States. The schizophrenic syndrome has a similar worldwide incidence, the only cultural difference being that prognosis for recovery seems better in rural than in urban settings. The prevalence rate is eight times higher in the lower than in the higher socioeconomic environments. Because the parents of schizophrenics have a social class distribution similar to that of the general population, the lower position of the patients appears to be a result of the illness rather than the cause of it.

Seventy per cent of schizophrenics become ill between ages 15 and 35, and the illness affects males slightly more than females. Peak onset in males lies between 15 and 24 years and in females between 25 and 34 years. There are slight ethnic differences, with a higher incidence in Scandinavian countries and in nonwhites. The chronicity of the illness presents an enormous cost. A recent study notes that although schizophrenia affects only one-twelfth as many persons as does myocardial infarction, the cost is six times as great.

PATHOPHYSIOLOGY. The pathophysiology of schizophrenia is unknown, nor has an anatomic origin of the symptoms been determined. Nevertheless, a number of conditions (including trauma, seizure disorders, and Huntington's disease) can produce schizo-

TABLE 401–3. USUAL SYMPTOMATIC PATTERNS OF PSYCHOTIC DISORDERS

	Acute Schizophrenia	Mania	Major Depression	Delirium
Delusions	++++	++++	+++	++
Hallucinations	++++	++	++	+++
Disorientation/ confusion	0	0	0	++++
Incoherent speech	++++	+++	0	++++
Depressed mood	+	0	++++	+
Grandiosity	++	++++	0	0

TABLE 401–2. SCHIZOPHRENIA AND OTHER PSYCHOTIC DISORDERS

A. **Characteristic symptoms:**
   At least two of the following, each present for a significant portion of time during a 1-month period (or less if successfully treated):
   1. Delusions
   2. Hallucinations
   3. Disorganized speech (e.g., frequent derailment or incoherence)
   4. Grossly disorganized or catatonic behavior
   5. Negative symptoms, i.e., affective flattening, alogia, or avolition
   [Note: Only one A symptom is required if delusions are bizarre or hallucinations consist of a voice keeping up a running commentary on the person's behavior or thoughts, or two or more voices conversing with each other.]

B. **Social/ occupational dysfunction:**
   For a significant portion of the time since the onset of the disturbance, one or more major areas of functioning such as work, interpersonal relations, or self-care are markedly below the level achieved prior to the onset (or when the onset is in childhood or adolescence, failure to achieve expected level of interpersonal, academic, or occupational achievement).

C. **Duration:**
   Continuous signs of the disturbance persist for at least 6 months. This 6-month period must include at least 1 month of symptoms that meet criterion A (i.e., active phase symptoms) and may include periods of prodromal or residual symptoms. During these prodromal or residual periods, the signs of the disturbance may be manifested by only negative symptoms or two or more symptoms listed in criterion A present in an attenuated form (e.g., odd beliefs, unusual perceptual experiences).

D. **Schizoaffective and mood disorder exclusion:**
   Schizoaffective disorder and mood disorder with psychotic features have been ruled out because either (1) no major depressive or manic episodes have occurred concurrently with the active phase symptoms or (2) if mood episodes have occurred during active phase symptoms, their total duration has been brief relative to the duration of the active and residual periods.

E. **Substance/ general medical condition exclusion:**
   The disturbance is not due to the direct effects of a substance (e.g., drugs of abuse, medication) or a general medical condition.

Modified from Diagnostic and Statistical Manual of Mental Disorders, 4th ed. Washington, DC, American Psychiatric Association, 1994.

phrenia-like hallucinations and delusions. Many authors have reported a higher than normal incidence of nonlocalizing neurologic abnormalities in schizophrenia, changes that are not present in other psychiatric conditions. These include defects in stereognosis, graphesthesia, and various skilled motor activities. Minor vestibular system defects, usually consisting of a reduction in the nystagmus response unrelated to medication use, have been noted in schizophrenic patients. Deficits in smooth-pursuit eye movements during pendulum tracking have been reported in schizophrenia as well as in other psychoses. Other evidence of CNS damage, including electroencephalographic (EEG) abnormalities, is tantalizingly frequent.

Twenty-five per cent of hospitalized schizophrenic patients show abnormally slow EEG tracings using standard recording techniques. Computed tomographic and magnetic resonance imaging studies have both shown lateral ventricle and third ventricle enlargement, widened cortical sulci, cerebellar atrophy, cerebral asymmetry, and decreased brain density consistently in many, but not all, studies in subgroups of schizophrenic patients. Not all of these changes occur in the same subgroups. Although the implications of these findings are unclear, the findings correlate with increased cognitive disturbance, poorer premorbid adjustment, and longer duration of illness. Many of the neurologic findings are consistent with changes found in other types of neurodevelopmental disorders. As more standardization of the techniques and diagnostic criteria occurs, there should be greater consistency of findings. Using the more dynamic measures, changes have been reported in the cerebral blood flow in the anterior frontal regions, the temporal cortex, and the globus pallidus, as well as decreased D_2 receptor sites in schizophrenics. Neuropsychologic testing shows a great deal of overlap between the findings in patients with clear-cut organic disease and those with schizophrenia to the point that the tests often fail to distinguish between the two conditions.

Strong evidence implicates a genetic factor in schizophrenia to a degree that 10 to 15% of the offspring of a schizophrenic parent are at risk for the disease. Furthermore, the coincidence of schizophrenia in monozygotic twins is roughly 60%. Additional evidence for a genetic factor comes from studies of children of schizophrenic parents who are raised by either their natural or adoptive, nonschizophrenic parents: The chances of developing the disease are identical in both instances, regardless of the environment. Despite these findings, family factors have been implicated in other ways. In families with much highly charged emotional interaction, schizophrenic patients seem to do very poorly. Less emotionally stimulating environments appear to allow the schizophrenic to function better.

Additional indirect evidence for biologic mechanisms in schizophrenia derives from pharmacologic studies: (1) Most of the neuroleptic drugs effective in controlling schizophrenic symptoms act as dopamine blockers in the CNS. (2) Many psychoactive drugs such as mescaline and amphetamines are dopaminergic and also have the potential for creating psychotic reactions. Further suggestions of altered dopamine metabolism in schizophrenic patients come from the inconsistent findings of both elevated and reduced levels of homovanillic acid, its major metabolite in the CSF and urine. As yet, most of these biologic findings, as well as the results of parallel animal studies, are too inconsistent or incomplete to permit unifying hypotheses.

PROGNOSIS AND TREATMENT. Prognosis in schizophrenia is poor and specific therapy lacking. Over a 25- to 30-year period, approximately one third of patients show some recovery or remission, and the remainder either have major residual symptoms or are still hospitalized. The major treatment is neuroleptic medication.

Table 401–4 lists the drugs most commonly used in the treatment of schizophrenia. The goal of treatment is to decrease as many of the symptoms as possible. As long as hallucinations, delusions, and disorganized thinking persist, the accepted practice is to increase the dose of medication until reaching a maximum decrease in symptoms. The response is usually achieved in a period of 2 to 3 weeks, with decreases in hallucination and thought disorder and a variable response of delusions. The most frequent limiting factor is the appearance of extrapyramidal side effects, the most common of which are dystonia, akathisia (restlessness), and parkinsonism. These occur most commonly in the first 2 to 4 months of drug use.

There is little difference in efficacy in the neuroleptics (Table

TABLE 401–4. DRUGS COMMONLY USED FOR TREATMENT OF SCHIZOPHRENIA*

Drug	Daily Dosage Range (mg)
Phenothiazines	
Chlorpromazine (Thorazine)	300–1500
Thioridazine (Mellaril)	150–800
Perphenazine (Trilafon)	8–64
Trifluoperazine (Stelazine)	4–60
Fluphenazine (Prolixin)†	2–20
Butyrophenones	
Haloperidol (Haldol)†	2–40
Thioxanthenes	
Thiothixene (Navane)	6–60
Atypical neuroleptics	
Clozapine (Clozaril)	50–900
Risperidone (Risperdal)	2–6

* Owing to untoward extrapyramidal reactions, one often needs to administer these drugs along with such drugs as benztropine mesylate (Cogentin), trihexyphenidyl HCl (Artane), diphenhydramine HCl (Benadryl).

† Comes in two injectable slow-release forms that can be given every 10 days to 3 weeks.

401–4), and lack of efficacy usually reflects too low a dose. If, however, no response occurs to a phenothiazine-type drug (e.g., chlorpromazine), one usually changes to another class of neuroleptics, such as a butyrophenone (haloperidol) or a thioxanthene. Two new neuroleptics have recently become available. Clozapine is the best studied and is clinically effective in 30% of cases that have been refractory to other neuroleptics. Clozapine is of interest for several other reasons in that it does not seem to cause either extrapyramidal symptoms or tardive dyskinesia. It has a tendency to cause agranulocytosis (1 to 2% incidence) and has very little effect on D_2 receptors. Risperidone has also been recently released and shows promise as a novel neuroleptic with few reports of tardive dyskinesia. It also has little effect on D_2 receptors. The physician should become familiar with one drug from each of these classes of neuroleptics for acute and maintenance use. The major long-term hazard in the use of most of these medications is tardive dyskinesia.

Tardive dyskinesia is a syndrome of involuntary movements, usually choreoathetoid, that may affect the mouth, lips, tongue, extremities, or trunk. Although usually associated with use of neuroleptics for 6 months or more, tardive dyskinesia can occur with shorter administration. Patients on neuroleptics should be periodically evaluated for these abnormal movements. A frequent early sign consists of vermicular movements of the tongue. Anticholinergic drugs do not help this condition. The symptoms may decrease with an increase of the medication, but such improvement usually is only temporary and may lead to a vicious circle of worsening chorea and increased drug dosages. The cause of tardive dyskinesia is not known, but it is believed to represent the development of dopaminergic hypersensitivity. In many instances gradually decreasing the dose of neuroleptics induces a slow remission of the symptoms (see also Ch. 411).

Despite the above conditions, the use of neuroleptics is effective, and the drugs should be used to help the patient function with as few symptoms as possible despite the potential side effects. Removing schizophrenic patients from medication greatly increases the chances of hospitalization within the following 6 months. This lag represents a major problem in that most patients immediately feel and do better without the medications. As a result, families and patients often fail to associate the cessation of medication with the subsequent relapse.

In spite of the fact that typical neuroleptics are the treatment of choice for schizophrenia, they are not a panacea and there are alternative or adjunctive agents that the clinician may consider. At this stage these agents should be regarded as novel. They include medications such as anticonvulsants, benzodiazepines, calcium channel blockers, and monoamine agonists and antagonists.

Most criteria for judging prognosis in schizophrenia are related to short-term outcome and can be summarized by saying that the more acute and florid the early symptoms or, as some have phrased it, the more the patient has "positive" symptoms (delusions, hallucinations, agitation, and depressive symptoms), the more likely he is to recover from the acute episode. The more insidious the onset and the

TABLE 401–5. DRUGS USED IN ACUTELY AGITATED STATES

Drug	Dose*	24-hr Maximum
Haloperidol (Haldol)	5–10 mg every 1–2 hr IM or PO	50 mg
Thiothixene (Navane)	5–10 mg every 2–4 hr IM or PO	40 mg
Lorazepam (Ativan)	0.5–1.0 mg every 1–2 hr IM or PO	10 mg

* Doses should be 50 to 75% reduced in the elderly or medically ill.

more lacking in emotional display (negative symptoms), the worse the short- and long-term prognoses. The natural history of the illness (even in treated patients) seems to be of two major types: (1) an episodic, relapsing course with each episode resulting in a lower level of psychosocial functioning; and (2) a gradual, slow decline in functional ability. Both courses eventually result in a progressive loss of psychosocial capacities. Treatment efforts in schizophrenia have taken a rehabilitative, or psychoeducational, approach in which the family is educated about the problems of schizophrenia and issues of living are openly dealt with.

ACUTE USE OF NEUROLEPTIC MEDICATION. Neuroleptic drugs are useful for nearly all patients who are markedly agitated with or without delusions and hallucinations and irrespective of diagnosis (Table 401–5). They help to control agitated states associated with delirium and dementia. In elderly patients and in those with delirium and/or dementia, however, the doses should be much lower until the patient's reaction is ascertained. Because acutely agitated psychotic patients respond to lorazepam as well as to neuroleptics, the initial use of benzodiazepines is probably safer in cases in which the source of the agitation is not known and in manic states for which long-term neuroleptic medication is not planned.

Andreasen N: Schizophrenia. Washington, DC, American Psychiatric Press, 1994. *A comprehensive review of current knowledge about schizophrenia.*
Hogarty GE, McEvoy JP, Muntez M, et al.: Dose of fluphenazine, familial expressed emotion and outcome in schizophrenia: Results of a two-year controlled study. Arch Gen Psychiatry 45:797, 1988. *An excellent study on the role of psychosocial factors.*
Lyon M, Barr CE, Cannon TD, et al.: Fetal neural development and schizophrenia. Schizophrenia Bull 15:149, 1989. *Excellent discussion of the neurodevelopmental findings in schizophrenia.*
Pickar D, Owen RR, Litman RE, et al.: Clinical and biologic response to clozapine in patients with schizophrenia: Crossover comparison with fluphenazine. Arch Gen Psychiatry 49:345, 1992. *Good discussion of novel neuroleptic use.*
Shore D: Schizophrenia 1993. Schizophrenia Bull 19:1, 1993. *An excellent review of all aspects of schizophrenia.*
Suddath RL, Christison GW, Torrey EF, et al.: Anatomical abnormalities in the brains of monozygotic twins discordant for schizophrenia. N Engl J Med 322:789, 1990. *Discussion of new brain imaging findings in schizophrenia.*

AFFECTIVE DISORDERS

A difficulty in clinical diagnosis is that similar terms are used to describe feeling states that differ greatly in degree and sometimes in kind. Such is the case with the term *depression*. In common use the meaning may extend from a description of a brief pang of regret to profound feelings of futility and suicidal despair. At what point along this spectrum does one label the condition "illness"? When does normal grief become pathologic? This section discusses these questions.

The most recent characterization of depressive illness has been simplified into *bipolar disorders* (manic-depressive), identifying wide swings of mood; *major depressive illness*, marked by severe depressive symptoms but without manic swings; and two milder forms, *cyclothymic disorder* and *dysthymic disorder* (formerly called depressive neurosis). These last two terms describe milder forms of bipolar disorders and depression that fall short of the specific diagnostic criteria for the more serious disorders.

Symptoms of depression also are classified by the company they keep. A psychiatric condition alone would be classified as an affective disorder, but when symptoms of affective disorders accompany medical conditions, they are defined as being due to a specific medical condition. Marked depressive symptoms have been noted with various endocrine disorders, brain tumors, seizure disorders, vitamin deficiencies, and particular neurologic disorders such as multiple sclerosis, Parkinson's disease, and stroke. Depressive symptoms also can be associated with drugs used to treat medical conditions.

In at least some instances, the consistency of the symptoms may reflect the fact that similar neurotransmitter systems are altered in both the primary and secondary affective disturbances.

Major Depression

The symptomatology and diagnostic criteria for major depression are listed in Table 401–6. Although many patients have single episodes of major depressive illness, the condition also can be repetitive, and this recurrent condition is frequently called unipolar depressive illness. Fifty percent of patients with a single episode of major depression eventually have another depressive episode.

The key features of major depression are a markedly gloomy mood in which there is a loss of interest in life, a lack of pleasure in almost all activities, and a general feeling of hopelessness and worthlessness. The illness takes the form of a cognitive change in which the patient seemingly looks at the world with "black glasses," and everything thought about or accomplished is minimized or negated: The wealthy and successful career person talks about his or her impending financial doom and general lack of accomplishment in life; the gifted artist dismisses his creations as trivial. When vegetative functions (sleep, appetite, psychomotor activity) are markedly impaired and a complete loss of pleasure accompanies almost all activities with no reactions to pleasurable stimuli, we often add the term *melancholia*. Some severe depressions can present in a highly anxious, agitated state. The history of previous episodes (either manic or depressive) aids in the diagnosis.

Affective Disorders in the Elderly

At the two ends of life, childhood and aging, the psychopathology of affective disorders is less distinct than during the years between. Elderly patients may have many dysphoric symptoms but not meet the precise diagnostic criteria for major affective disorder. Diagnosis in the elderly is also complicated by two factors: (1) the behavioral and cognitive changes caused by the aging of the CNS (although, other than minor memory impairments, the presence of cognitive impairments should make the clinician consider a more

TABLE 401–6. MAJOR DEPRESSIVE EPISODE

A. At least five of the following symptoms have been present during the same 2-week period and represent a change from previous functioning; at least one of the symptoms in either (1) depressed mood or (2) loss of interest or pleasure.
  1. Depressed mood most of the day, nearly every day, as indicated by either subjective report (e.g., feels sad or empty) or observation made by others (e.g., appears tearful). Note: in children and adolescents, can be irritable mood.
  2. Markedly diminished interest or pleasure in all, or almost all, activities most of the day, nearly every day (as indicated by either subjective account or observation made by others).
  3. Significant weight loss or weight gain when not dieting (e.g., more than 5% of body weight in a month), or decrease or increase in appetite nearly every day. Note: in children, consider failure to make expected weight gains.
  4. Insomnia or hypersomnia nearly every day.
  5. Psychomotor agitation or retardation nearly every day (observable by others, not merely subjective feelings of restlessness or being slowed down).
  6. Fatigue or loss of energy nearly every day.
  7. Feelings of worthlessness or excessive or inappropriate guilt (which may be delusional) nearly every day (not merely self-reproach or guilt about being sick).
  8. Diminished ability to think or concentrate, or indecisiveness, nearly every day (either by subjective account or as observed by others).
  9. Recurrent thoughts of death (not just fear of dying), recurrent suicidal ideation without a specific plan, or a suicide attempt or a specific plan for committing suicide.
B. The symptoms cause clinically significant distress or impairment in social, occupational, or other important areas of functioning.
C. The symptoms are not due to the direct effects of a substance (e.g., drugs of abuse, medication) or a general medical condition (e.g., hypothyroidism).

Modified from Diagnostic and Statistical Manual of Mental Disorders, 4th ed. Washington, DC, American Psychiatric Association, 1994.

comprehensive workup for dementia), and (2) the presence of other medical illnesses with their attendant medications.

The most common psychiatric symptoms in community populations of older adults are those of depression (15%), hypochondriasis (14%), suspiciousness (17%), and persecutory ideation (4%). As many as one third complain of difficulty in falling asleep, awakening during the night, or being sleepy during the day. All these symptom rates increase for the institutionalized elderly. By contrast, cases fulfilling the specific diagnoses of major depression, dysthymia, and schizophrenia occur at a much lower rate than in younger populations.

Although the aged patient may not meet full diagnostic criteria for affective disturbance, persistent symptomatology nevertheless deserves a trial of cautious pharmacologic intervention. This is particularly true of elderly patients who have cognitive impairments. Community samples of aged populations show about a 4 to 5% prevalence of severe cognitive impairment. The figure may not entirely reflect degenerative brain disease, however, because the biologic changes that occur with affective illness also can cause cognitive impairments detected by both neuropsychological testing and clinical neurologic examination. This is true in younger populations as well. The abnormalities can include not only problems with memory and orientation but signs of minor neurologic impairment as well; all may clear after a trial of antidepressive medication. The term "pseudodementia" has been used for these potentially treatable cognitive changes in elderly affectively disordered patients.

DIAGNOSIS. The diagnosis of affective disorders is made on clinical grounds as discussed above. Many tests to aid the diagnosis of depression have been introduced, including the dexamethasone suppression test (DST), the thyroid-stimulating hormone (TSH) response (see below), and many measures of disturbed sleep function such as rapid eye movement (REM) latency. Unfortunately, none has proved to be diagnostically reliable or specific for affective disorder. In diagnosing depression, the interview is central.

EPIDEMIOLOGY. The gender distribution of major depression is almost two-to-one female to male. The peak age incidence for women is 35 to 45 years, whereas the age pattern is less clear for men. There may also be an increased incidence in women in their early 50's. The prevalence is about 3.2 per 100 males and about 4.5 to 9.3 per 100 females. Incidence is 82 to 201 new cases per 100,000 for men and 247 to 598 new cases per 100,000 for women. The mean duration of first attack of an untreated depressive illness is about 13 months. The episodes, if they recur, are likely to be similar in nature and respond to treatment in a similar fashion. As with bipolar illness, alcoholism is a frequent complication of depressive illness, particularly when it has a recurring course.

Patients in primary care clinics (5 to 10%) and on medical inpatient services (15%) show an increased prevalence of depression.

PATHOPHYSIOLOGY. Pathophysiologic theories of affective disorders have developed along three major lines: (1) endocrine studies; (2) neurotransmitters; and (3) electrophysiologic studies. Depressed patients frequently have elevated levels of cortical steroids in the blood and urine and at least half fail to suppress cortisol secretion after dexamethasone administration. TSH response to thyrotropin-releasing hormone also has been found to be aberrant in many depressed patients, even though their blood T_3 and T_4 levels are normal. Growth hormone, prolactin, gonadal hormones, corticotropin-releasing factor, and melatonin have all been shown to have diminished responses in subgroups of affective disorders. Although none of these findings is specific for any type of depressive illness or consistent in all depressive illnesses, they nevertheless suggest the presence of pituitary-hypothalamic dysfunction in affective disorders.

Studies of neurotransmitters in depression have been stimulated largely by the success of antidepressant pharmacologic agents. Many of the tricyclic compounds and the monoamine oxidase inhibitors (MAOI) effective in the treatment of depression increase the availability of catecholamines and indolamines in the CNS. L-Dopa, used to treat Parkinson's disease, is a major catecholamine (dopamine) precursor and may in itself induce mania. These and other observations have given rise to the catecholamine-indolamine hypothesis of depression. The theory postulates that a certain level of amines and/or receptor sensitivity to catecholamines functions to generate a normal mood. Receptor insensitivity or a depletion of

amines, or a decrease in their synthesis or storage, leads to depression. Conversely, if the amines are in excess or the receptors are hypersensitive, mania may develop. Recently, the acetylcholine system has also been implicated in affective disorders, a "balance" between adrenergic and cholinergic function being postulated as necessary for the stabilization of mood. Neither theory is entirely satisfactory because the tricyclic drugs affect many receptor systems and their main action may be one of changing or regulating the sensitivity of the receptor rather than acting directly as neurotransmitters. Furthermore, newer drugs that have antidepressant effects do not affect these transmitter systems. One study, for example, has found that the anticonvulsant carbamazepine favorably influences the course of certain patients with bipolar illness.

Electrophysiologic studies on affective illness have concentrated on changes in sleep functions, especially the presence of changes in the REM sleep pattern during episodes of active illness. A subgroup of patients with affective disorder shows a shortened REM latency. Furthermore, analyses of circadian rhythms provide increasing evidence for autumn and winter precipitation of some bipolar disorders, with depressive illnesses apparently related to diminished ambient light in winter climates. The change has been correlated with alterations of melatonin metabolism.

TREATMENT. Mild depression usually manifests itself as feelings of sadness and self-deprecation, coupled with slight sleep and appetite disturbances. In such patients an attempt at counseling about the events in their lives and helping delineate appropriate priorities and activities, along with prescriptions for adequate exercise, diet, rest, and general health measures, may suffice. When symptoms become more marked, particularly when they disturb sleep and appetite, and the person becomes unable to perform work, school, or household tasks, one should consider adding antidepressant medication to the above regimen (Table 401–7). If the symptoms have been present for a number of years, a trial of medication may be in order. With prominent depressive symptomatology hospitalization may be necessary, the major indication being to prevent suicide (the risk among persons with major affective disorders is 15%). To ask all patients with depression of mood, apathetic fatigue, or ill-defined somatic symptoms if they have ever considered suicide not only is wise but can elicit an important signal to intensify treatment.

The approach and response to drug therapy in depression vary considerably among both physicians and patients. Perhaps the best prediction of a favorable response is if a blood relative has responded well to a similar agent. In patients who present primarily with insomnia and marked vegetative disturbances as well as some agitation, amitriptyline (or nortriptyline) is somewhat more sedat-

TABLE 401–7. ANTIDEPRESSANT DRUGS

Drug	Daily Dosage Range (mg)*	Anticholinergic Effects
Tricyclics		
Imipramine (Tofranil)	50–150	++
Amitriptyline (Elavil)	50–150	+++
Nortriptyline (Aventyl)	50–150	++
Desipramine (Norpramin, Pertofrane)	50–150	+
Doxepin (Sinequan)	150	++
Tetracyclic		
Maprotiline (Ludiomil)	50–225	+
Serotonin reuptake inhibitors		
Fluoxetine (Prozac)	10–80	0
Sertraline (Zoloft)	50–200	0
Paroxetine (Paxil)	20–40	0
Other		
Bupropion (Wellbutrin)	300–450	0
Trazodone (Desyrel)	150–600	0
Venlafaxine (Effexor)	75–350	±
MAOI's†		
Phenelzine (Nardil)	15–90	++
Tranylcypromine (Parnate)	20–30	++

*In most cases the dose should be reduced 30 to 50% in the elderly and medically ill.

† Monoamine oxidase inhibitors.

ing, particularly if given at bedtime. Imipramine (or desipramine) is less sedating and often avoids the drowsiness that amitriptyline causes. After initial complete blood count, liver profiles and, in older patients, an ECG, it is best to start these medications in single doses at bedtime. An initial starting dose of 50 mg may be rapidly increased every several days until a total dosage of 150 mg per night is reached. As stated earlier, with elderly patients all psychotropic drugs should be used cautiously, and doses of antidepressants should be decreased by 30 to 50% from the above. For example, one would start an elderly patient on 10 or 25 mg of an antidepressant such as nortriptyline at bedtime or even every other night. For prolonged treatment the elderly often respond to smaller doses (10 to 75 mg). If after 6 weeks the elderly patient has not responded to doses as high as 75 mg and there are no marked side effects, doses can be slowly increased. Similarly, in otherwise healthy adults, if no response to 150 mg per day appears within 6 weeks, the dosage can often be increased to as much as 200 to 300 mg (beyond manufacturers' guidelines). It is wise, however, to obtain the counsel of a specialist prior to using these doses. If there is still no response one could switch to another tricyclic or immediately to an MAOI.

The new serotonin reuptake inhibitors such as fluoxetine, paroxetine, and sertraline have all been shown to be as effective as the tricyclics but have the advantage of fewer side effects. However, there are side effects with these new medications, and increased agitation can be a significant problem. The agitation responds to decreasing the dose. Weight gain and sexual dysfunction also have been noted. Blood level measurements are available for most of the tricyclic antidepressants, although their main usefulness is to indicate that the person is taking and absorbing the drug. Only nortriptyline has a known therapeutic window (50 to 140 ng per milliliter).

It is useful to caution patients that the antidepressants do not produce an immediate response, although if given at bedtime they may improve sleeping immediately. Also, the prominent anticholinergic side effects and hypotension are often a bother, and patients should be forewarned. Some of the supposed side effects of the medication are also accompaniments of the depressive illness, and patients, if questioned, may reveal that they have had many of the symptoms prior to taking the medication. Several of the newer antidepressants, such as fluoxetine and bupropion, have different actions. One must recognize that the tricyclics have a quinidine-like effect and have been used to treat some cardiac arrhythmias.

For patients who fail to respond to antidepressants, psychiatric consultation is critical. However, some have found it useful to add 0.25 μg per day of triiodothyronine (T_3) to the tricyclic dosage, particularly in women. Also, the addition of lithium to tricyclic regimens has been found to have an augmenting effect on the response to antidepressant tricyclics (neither of the above is an FDA-approved use).

The MAOI's returned to usage recently with the introduction of fluoxetine and bupropion. They had been underutilized in the United States owing to their tendency to cause hypertensive crises following the ingestion of foods containing tyramine. However, for patients not responding to tricyclic medications or those with atypical depressions marked predominantly by anxiety symptoms, they are quite effective. Patients can be started on MAOI drugs immediately following tricyclic cessation. The reverse, however, does not hold, and patients stopping an MAOI drug must wait 7 to 14 days before starting a tricyclic antidepressant. If dietary restrictions are followed and sympathetic amine medications are avoided, MAOI's are usually safe, their major side effects being hypotension and insomnia. They have milder anticholinergic effects and often are easier to tolerate than the tricyclic antidepressants, but the specific side effects and indications for use are still being delineated.

In older patients who fail to respond to pharmacotherapeutic interventions, as well as in others with complicated medical conditions which the drugs might adversely affect, electroconvulsive therapy (ECT) is probably the safest treatment. Whereas 60% of most affective disturbances respond to pharmacotherapy, close to 80% improve after ECT. There are few contraindications: When ECT is administered in association with modern anesthetic techniques, the morbidity is reduced to that of the anesthesia alone. With careful monitoring, even patients with recent cerebral or myocardial insults can be treated with ECT.

PROGNOSIS. Antidepressant drugs should be continued for 6 to 20 weeks after patients become free of symptoms. More prolonged treatment is desirable for those who have had recurrent episodes. Many patients have been maintained for years on tricyclic antidepressants and MAOI's without major impairment. Nevertheless, in spite of the best treatment, between 15 and 20% of depressives go on to a chronic course. Most patients with a single episode resume normal function. Some use the depressive episode as a chance to reorganize their lives and proceed to function better than they had previously.

Dysthymic Disorder (Depressive Neurosis)

The symptoms consist of a depressed mood of longstanding duration with a severity less intense than in a major depressive disorder. These patients often seem to have situational reasons for their illness. Many present primarily with physical complaints to physicians. Substance and drug abuse, as well as personality profiles that involve dependency and obsessional symptomatology, are often part of the clinical picture. The diagnostic criteria are outlined in Table 401–8.

As this condition is treated in many settings, the epidemiologic distribution is difficult to determine. One estimate of prevalence is 60 per 1000. Women predominate. Familial patterns have not been established. There is evidence that various personality conflicts and situational precipitants are related to these conditions more than to the other affective disorders.

Many types of short-term psychotherapy have been effective in treating these conditions. Patients who respond poorly to psychotherapy often benefit from antidepressant medication.

GRIEF REACTIONS

Physicians often find it emotionally difficult to deal with the loved ones of patients who have died or been seriously injured, yet such contacts provide important preventive medicine. Grief should be looked upon as a biologic process with psychological roots. Issues of loss and attachment are prominent in bereavement. In normal bereavement 50% of persons experience depressed mood, sleep disturbances, and crying lasting anywhere from 2 to 6 months. Furthermore, many grief reactions resolve only slowly over a number of years. This is particularly true in older persons.

During bereaved states general health deteriorates, and serious illnesses often increase. Some persons lose contact with reality and blame themselves, constantly asking, "Why did this happen?" Others even have difficulty in accepting that the person is dead. Anger and withdrawal can prevail. Some survivors, particularly when the death was violent, experience stress responses similar to those of combat veterans, who in addition to the symptoms related above may have frequent and often violent intrusive mental images.

These normal reactions can blur into a more serious state with intense and prolonged symptoms lasting 6 months or more. Some survivors undergo a delayed response, functioning well immediately after the event but experiencing later symptoms of bereavement, often precipitated by the death of another person or the anniversary of the death of the loved one. Others can develop hypochondriacal symptoms resembling those of the deceased. Panic attacks and depressive illness may develop also in prolonged grief reactions.

The management of grief reactions can often be undertaken by the physician in his/her normal contact with the bereaved survivor. Lindeman has outlined several valid principles: (1) Allow the patient to share his feelings about the death of the relative. The physician can be extremely helpful in discussing the normal process of

TABLE 401–8. DYSTHYMIC DISORDER

A. Depressed mood (or can be irritable mood in children and adolescents) for most of the day, for more days than not, as indicated either by subjective account or by observation made by others, for at least 2 years (1 year for children and adolescents).
B. Presence, while depressed, of at least three of the following:
1. Low self-esteem or self-confidence, or feelings of inadequacy
2. Feelings of pessimism, despair, or hopelessness
3. Generalized loss of interest or pleasure
4. Social withdrawal

Modified from Diagnostic and Statistical Manual of Mental Disorders, 4th ed. Washington, DC, American Psychiatric Association, 1994.

grief and the reactions that people experience. (2) Review the relationships of the deceased with the important people in their lives. (3) Help grieving persons to accept their feelings and fears about things such as their ability to cope, their fears about "going crazy," and anger. (4) Discuss with the bereaved how they are adapting to the stress and what modes they are using to cope. (5) Attempt to formulate the future relationships between the bereaved and others in their lives. (6) Find new persons with whom the bereaved can develop relationships.

Although the above matters can only be touched on in the acute situation, they often can be dealt with over time. Even the gathering of information about these areas helps many patients. If the condition progresses to an abnormal degree, the use of appropriate medications is indicated, e.g., for affective disturbance or panic disorder. Mild sedation and hypnotics at the acute stage are also useful. Support groups have been organized to deal with both the normal and excessive processes of grieving and appear to help.

SUICIDAL BEHAVIOR

About 75% of patients who commit suicide have seen a physician within the previous 6 months. Most practicing physicians encounter half a dozen potentially suicidal patients per year, among whom 10 to 12 actually commit the act over the ensuing years. The figures illustrate how important it is for the physician to detect various clues. Suicide rates are higher in patients with psychiatric problems, with the highest incidence occurring in those with affective disorders or alcoholism or those who are in the early post-hospital phase of schizophrenic disorders. Suicidal behavior is not specific to any single psychiatric disturbance. Suicidal behavior occurs across a spectrum of mental illness, and it should be treated as a problem distinct from the major psychiatric disorders. Effective pharmacologic treatments for depression and schizophrenia have been available since the 1950's, yet there is no evidence that these treatments have reduced the suicide rate of either population. Therapy that may help in avoiding suicide include enhancing the patient's social supports, improving his or her problem-solving and other coping skills, and initiating treatments designed to reduce drug and alcohol use, especially during periods of stress.

The typical victim of attempted suicide is a white female, 20 to 40 years of age, who ingests pills, usually after an interpersonal conflict. By contrast, the typical successful suicide victim is a white male, 45 years of age or older, often separated, widowed, or divorced, who lives alone and may be unemployed or retired. Patients who commit suicide suffer a high incidence of recently poor physical health and evidence of psychiatric disturbance. Many have a previous history of suicide attempts or threats.

Patients often wish to discuss their suicidal fears, but many physicians are made uncomfortable by discussing the matter. Such a reaction is more than a lack of compassion: It represents bad medicine. The question must be approached understandingly, but almost all seriously ill adults should be asked gently if they have had thoughts about death or suicide. Comments patients make about feeling they would be "better off dead" or "people would be better off without me" should be taken seriously. Preoccupations with funerals, cemetery lots, and the buying of weapons should make the clinician suspicious. Any patient who presents with vague complaints should be asked about his or her emotional state. If any indication of suicidal intent is forthcoming, one must immediately evaluate its seriousness, inquiring gently about the following: (1) Has the person considered actual suicide? If so, what plans have been made and how specifically? The more specific, the more worrisome. (2) What other psychopathology exists? Is the patient agitated, seriously depressed, etc.? (3) What precipitating stresses exist? (4) Are there persons whom the patient trusts and who could help? (5) Will the person agree to work with you and contact you if his suicidal feelings intensify? (6) If no reassurance comes from the patient or relatives that the situation can be managed at home, hospitalization may be necessary. Physicians who find themselves unable to provide such a supporting role should consider requesting psychiatric consultation for the patient.

An even more difficult evaluation is how to treat those who have made a recent unsuccessful suicide attempt. After a suicide attempt there often is a brief period of days to weeks of lightening of the depressive mood, after which strong self-destructive feelings reap-

pear. The more lethal the risk (i.e., the higher was the potential risk of death in the initial suicide attempt), the more determined should be the effort to provide psychiatric treatment, preferably in a hospital. If patients express an explicit intent to die, often stated with determination and conviction, there is no question about the necessity for hospitalization.

Most patients after suicide attempts should have a psychiatric consultation. When this is impossible, the nonpsychiatric physician must assess the suicidal potential. Part of the evaluation can also serve as the initial formation of a doctor-patient relationship. If they have a supportive environment and will keep contact, some of these patients can be managed as outpatients. Physicians should beware of writing potentially lethal prescriptions for patients who may have suicidal tendencies. For example, for a routine dosage schedule of tricyclic antidepressants (150 mg per day), even a week's supply provides a potentially lethal overdose.

SUICIDE IN ADOLESCENTS. Somewhere between 9 and 18% of children and adolescents have made suicide attempts. This astoundingly high figure correlates with turmoil in the family as well as disturbed parent/child interactions. There are also significant correlations with substance abuse, depressive illness, and conduct disorders in children and adolescents as well as histories of physical and sexual abuse. Many of these children and adolescents had threatened suicide previously. Many have done poorly in school and have records of chronically aggressive behavior. One of the most difficult questions is whether to hospitalize an adolescent at risk for suicide. The answer relates primarily to the severity of the suicidal behavior and the patient's intent to "be dead." Interestingly, in adolescents, it also relates to the presence of assaultive behavior in that the hostility toward others can also be directed against the self. The environmental supports available to see someone through a depressive episode also mitigate the need for hospitalization. It is extremely important in treating the adolescent to provide some form of individual counseling, usually centered on coping skills and cognitive therapy, as well to work with the environmental support system or the patient's family. Pharmacologic treatment is effective for affective illness in adolescents.

SUICIDE AND AGING. Persons older than 70 years have a higher suicide rate, with single males at the peak. Risk factors include unemployment, isolation, poor health, pain, feelings of being rejected, history of mental illness, and previous suicide attempts. A history of alcoholism is a high comorbid factor. Many elderly indirectly pursue suicide by stopping eating or necessary medications. Electroconvulsive therapy is often the most effective form of treatment.

Bipolar Disorders

Bipolar disorders (previously called manic-depressive disorders) probably make up the most homogeneous diagnostic grouping in psychiatry, as they consist of a marked change in mood that varies from major depressive episodes (as discussed) (see Table 401–6) to significant manic episodes as defined below. There is usually a return to normal behavior between episodes. There is little difficulty in recognizing the illness if one looks at the longitudinal course. However, if patients are examined only briefly, at a particular moment in time, manic excitement can be confused with schizophrenic psychosis. The depressive phase of bipolar illness can also be misconstrued as a catatonic state.

DIAGNOSTIC CRITERIA AND CLINICAL SIGNS AND SYMPTOMS. The manic phase of the illness is characterized by an expansive euphoric mood in which grandiose plans and ideas predominate. It is important to be aware that despite this expansiveness and grandiosity, patients who are frustrated or disagreed with often become irritable and sometimes aggressive. The major diagnostic criteria are listed in Table 401–9. The patient can be psychotic in the manic phase, with delusions and hallucinations consistent with the grandiosity; persecutory delusions, feelings of being controlled, can also be present. At times it is difficult to distinguish an excited schizophrenic patient from a manic one. As already stated, one must examine the longitudinal course of the illness, until either a depressive episode occurs or the course deteriorates after remission of the acute symptom, in order to diagnose a schizophrenic process. In all instances, it is crucial to rule out organic factors.

The average age at onset of bipolar disorder is about 30 years, but about 20% of patients have an onset below the age of 20. In fe-

TABLE 401–9. MANIC EPISODE

A. A distinct period of abnormally and persistently elevated, expansive, or irritable mood, lasting at least 1 week (or any duration if hospitalization is necessary).

B. During the period of mood disturbance, at least three of the following symptoms have persisted (four if the mood is only irritable) and have been present to a significant degree:
1. Inflated self-esteem or grandiosity
2. Decreased need for sleep (e.g., feels rested after only 3 hours of sleep)
3. More talkative than usual or pressure to keep talking
4. Flight of ideas or subjective experiences that thoughts are racing
5. Distractibility (i.e., attention too easily drawn to unimportant or irrelevant external stimuli)
6. Increase in goal-directed activity (either socially, at work or school, or sexually) or psychomotor agitation
7. Excessive involvement in pleasurable activities that have a high potential for painful consequences (e.g., the person engages in unrestrained buying sprees, sexual indiscretions, or foolish business investments).

C. The mood disturbance is sufficiently severe to cause marked impairment in occupational functioning or in usual social activities or relationships with others to necessitate hospitalization to prevent harm to self or others.

D. The symptoms are not due to the direct effects of a substance (e.g., drugs of abuse, medication) or a general medical condition (e.g., hypothyroidism).

Modified from Diagnostic and Statistical Manual of Mental Disorders, 4th ed. Washington, DC, American Psychiatric Association, 1994.

males, the onset of the condition seems to have a bimodal distribution, with one peak falling between 20 and 30 years and the other between 40 and 50 years. The peak age at onset of schizophrenia is much younger, but the age at onset of bipolar illness overlaps enough so that the differential diagnosis of a psychotic illness in a young person is difficult and may change as the clinical picture evolves over time. Almost half the patients with bipolar disorders have at least two to three episodes of illness, and as many as a third experience seven or more episodes of illness once the pattern has started. Each episode of illness, whether manic or depressive, can last from 4 to 13 months; some go on to chronicity and some cease much sooner. The course of the illness has been modified significantly with the advent of lithium therapy, especially with respect to diminishing both the severity and the frequency of the episodes. The shorter durations are usually related to the effectiveness of the treatment. Although some patients rapidly alternate between extremes over 2 to 4 days, most episodes have a longer duration and, frequently, after a manic phase a depressive phase follows. Chronicity, again as opposed to schizophrenia, is not a major problem with manic-depressive illness, being cited as low as 1% in some studies. Mortality with bipolar illness averages between two and two and one-half times the expected rate for that age; suicide occurs in about 8 to 10%.

EPIDEMIOLOGY. The lifetime risk for developing bipolar illness ranges from 0.6 to 0.9% of the population. The new-case incidence per hundred thousand per year is from 9 to 15 in men and from 7.4 to 32 in women. The risk increases with a family history of bipolar illness. The genetic pattern in bipolar illness is uncertain but suggests autosomal dominance with incomplete penetration. There is a 72% concordance in monozygotic twins and a 19% concordance in same-sex dizygotic twins. Both the course of illness and the response to treatment are similar among blood relatives. In one well-studied Amish family, the abnormal gene has been identified on chromosome 11. Other families with equally strong genetic patterns have not possessed this particular chromosomal alteration.

PATHOPHYSIOLOGY. Most of what is known about the pathophysiology of bipolar illness is similar to what is known about the biology of the major depressive disorders.

DIAGNOSIS AND TREATMENT. The treatment of bipolar disorders has three distinct aspects: the manic episode, the major depressive episode, and long-term maintenance therapy. Prior to any specific therapy, an adequate medical workup is necessary in order to be certain that the patient suffers from a primary affective illness. The patient in an acute manic state is delusional, grandiose, and hyperactive and in this condition looks similar to any patient with

psychosis. If this is the first episode, one cannot differentiate this state phenomenologically from the first episode of schizophrenia or a psychosis due to physical illness. The differential diagnosis with the first episode rests on a careful history, family history, and physical and laboratory examination. The past history and the nature of onset of the illness are important, as noted previously. Furthermore, most psychiatric disorders have a familial pattern. A psychiatrist should be involved in the evaluation of patients who present with their first psychotic episode.

The treatment of the acute manic phase is usually undertaken in the hospital, as it is imperative to protect the patient from his own misdeeds, e.g., spending inordinate amounts of money, making embarrassing speeches. If the family is supportive, however, and feels it can control the situation, treatment can be started outside of the hospital. Lithium is not useful for the acute management of mania and if the patient is severely agitated, sedation is necessary. Neuroleptics are not used in the long-term treatment of bipolar illness, but benzodiazepines, particularly lorazepam, can effectively control most acute manic states (see Table 401–5). If the agitation cannot be controlled with medication, the clinician should obtain psychiatric consultation to consider using ECT to control the manic excitement. Manic excitement creates a medical emergency in which patients can die from exhaustion.

Although most general physicians treat acute mania rarely, they may more often encounter the use of lithium. Lithium effectively prevents relapses in >60% of bipolar illnesses. The drug is slightly more effective in preventing manic than depressive episodes. Nevertheless, its use should be considered with any repetitive affective disturbance.

Prior to the beginning of lithium therapy, a CBC, urinalysis, electrolytes, creatinine, BUN, thyroid studies, and a baseline ECG and EEG should be obtained. Chronic medical illnesses, especially renal insufficiency, can contraindicate use of the agent. Lithium has a half-life of 24 to 36 hours, and it takes at least 4 days to achieve a steady state. The specific therapeutic effectiveness is not evident until at least 4 to 10 days after institution of therapy. Consequently, lithium is not a good medication for the acutely agitated or manic patient but should be started early in anticipation of maintenance use. It is necessary to monitor the serum level of lithium, adequate levels for acute illness being in the range of 0.8 to 1.4 mEq per liter. For maintenance therapy, satisfactory responses accompany blood levels of 0.4 mEq per liter. Dose and blood level, however, should be titrated against clinical effectiveness for each patient. Once maintenance levels are reached, patients usually can be maintained for long periods with minimal contact. Doses usually are given twice daily, as absorption from the gastrointestinal tract is rapid and the drug peaks in the serum within 1 to 2 hours. *Serum lithium levels of more than 2 mEq per liter are highly dangerous and represent a medical emergency requiring immediate hospitalization and, sometimes, hemodialysis.* Of most concern with regard to side effects in the long-term use of lithium is the development of mild leukocytosis, hypothyroidism, diabetes insipidus, and, occasionally, renal tubular damage. Although these long-term side effects are not trivial, they are uncommon and must be weighed against the propensity of untreated patients to be recurrently hospitalized. For patients who do not respond to lithium therapy or cannot tolerate it, increasingly encouraging reports describe the effective use of carbamazepine and valproic acid in treating bipolar conditions.

The depressive phase of bipolar illness is treated the same as for any major depressive disorder, as outlined previously.

Patients with bipolar disorders are often reluctant to continue with their medications, particularly lithium, because they feel it inhibits them, decreases their energy, or affects their creativity. Consequently, a good deal of discussion about these issues is pertinent for the patient and especially for the family. The enlistment and assistance of the family of the patient with bipolar disorder are important. During either acute mania or severe depressive reactions, verbal interventions with patients often are difficult, and it is useful simply to repeat some major reassuring statements—that they are patients, that they are going to get better, and that this is not their normal state. Although the role of precipitants is not clear in the onset of bipolar illness, it is important for patients to remain in treatment. This often can be accomplished by helping them understand stressful situations in their lives. Family and marital counseling often is useful.

PROGNOSIS. The more episodes a patient has, the more likely he or she is to have another. Nevertheless, if one takes as indices of outcome successful marital and occupational adjustment, approximately two thirds of patients do well. About 15% have some improvement, and the remainder do poorly. Although manic or depressive episodes may cause much acute social disruption, including job loss and marital strife, the wide spacing of episodes often prevents long-term social decay. Patients with bipolar disease usually function normally between episodes. Accordingly, a major goal of treatment is to protect the patient during episodes so as to minimize social disruption. Nevertheless, although the prognosis is not as devastating as in schizophrenia, it is still fraught with a significant amount of periodic and, sometimes, long-term functional disability.

Goodwin FK, Jamison KR: Manic Depressive Illness. New York, Oxford University Press, 1990. *An excellent review of all aspects of affective disorders.*
Parkes CM, Weise RS: Recovery from Bereavement. New York, Basic Books, 1983. *Excellent summary of treatment of grief.*
Pfeffer CR: Clinical perspectives on treatment of suicidal behavior among children and adolescents. Psychiatr Ann 20:143, 1990. *An excellent general article on the management of suicidal behavior in children and adolescents, applicable to adults as well.*
Sadovay J, Lazarus L, Jarvick L: Review of geriatric psychiatry. Washington, DC, American Psychiatric Press, 1991. *An excellent and comprehensive review of geriatric psychiatry.*
Shucter S, Zisook S: Treatment of spousal bereavement. Psychiatr Ann 16:295, 1986. *An excellent discussion of treatment of bereavement.*

ANXIETY DISORDERS

Anxiety is the most ubiquitous psychiatric symptom and one of the most common of all disorders that present to the general physician. It occurs as part of most major psychiatric syndromes, particularly depressive ones. Anxiety accompanies at least some aspects of most normal lives, and it can be an effective stimulus to improved performance. The performance curve follows an inverted U: A little anxiety can improve performance, performance then plateaus as the anxiety increases, and eventually too much anxiety causes a decrease in the ability to function. Currently, anxiety disorders are divided into two major categories: (1) panic disorders, which are episodic, "attack-like" symptoms; and (2) generalized anxiety disorder, which is a persistent state of anxiety, commonly associated with somatic complaints and labeled somatization disorder.

Patients with anxiety symptoms are extremely high users of medical services, usually complaining vaguely that "something is wrong." A retrospective study of 55 patients with panic disorder referred from primary care physicians for psychiatric consultation revealed that 89% initially presented with one or two somatic complaints. In most, somatic misdiagnoses had continued for months or years. The most frequent symptom patterns were (1) cardiac (chest pains, tachycardia, irregular heartbeat); (2) gastrointestinal (epigastric distress); (3) neurologic (headache, dizziness/vertigo, syncope, or paresthesias): and (4) chronic fatigue or fibromyalgia. In a random survey of 195 patients in a primary care practice screened with structured interviews, 13% met DSM-III criteria for panic disorder.

DIAGNOSTIC CRITERIA AND CLINICAL SIGNS AND SYMPTOMS. A panic attack produces a distinct symptomatic event. There is a precipitous sensation of feelings of fear, impending doom, or imminent death, accompanied by a potential host of physical symptoms (Table 401–10). In fact, when a patient presents with somatic symptoms as listed above and shows no abnormal physical signs or laboratory findings, one should strongly consider panic disorder.

Affected patients often complain of the physical symptoms in an agitated state. These circumstances differ markedly from chronic anxiety states, in which symptoms are more gradual and do not create life-threatening fears. Generalized anxiety disorder is a pervasive feeling of anxiety or "nervousness" that lacks the attack-like characteristics of panic disorder. The symptoms of generalized anxiety disorders are mainly muscle tension, autonomic hyperactivity, and apprehensive hypervigilant behavior.

A strong association links *agoraphobia* and panic attacks. Agoraphobia is defined as a morbid fear and avoidance of being alone or

TABLE 401–10. PANIC DISORDER WITHOUT AGORAPHOBIA

A. Both of the following symptoms:
1. Recurrent unexpected panic attacks, defined as a discrete period of intense fear or discomfort, in which at least four of the following symptoms developed abruptly and reached a peak within 10 minutes: (1) palpitations, pounding heart, or accelerated heart rate; (2) sweating; (3) trembling or shaking; (4) sensations of shortness of breath or smothering; (5) feeling of choking; (6) chest pain or discomfort; (7) nausea or abdominal distress; (8) feeling dizzy, unsteady, lightheaded, or faint; (9) derealization (feelings of unreality) or depersonalization (being detached from oneself); (10) fear of losing control or going crazy; (11) fear of dying; (12) paresthesias (numbness or tingling sensations); (13) chills or hot flushes.
2. At least one of the attacks has been followed by a month (or more) of (a) persistent concern about having additional attacks; (b) worry about the implications of the attack or its consequences (e.g., losing control, having a heart attack, "going crazy"); or (c) a significant change in behavior related to the attacks.

B. Absence of agoraphobia
C. The panic attacks are not due to the direct effects of a substance (e.g., drugs of abuse, medication) or a general medical condition (e.g., hypothyroidism).
D. The anxiety is not better accounted for by another mental disorder, such as obsessive-compulsive disorder (e.g., fear of contamination), post-traumatic stress disorder (e.g., in response to stimuli associated with a severe stressor), separation anxiety disorder, or social phobia (e.g., fear of embarrassment in social situations).

Modified from Diagnostic and Statistical Manual of Mental Disorders, 4th ed. Washington, DC, American Psychiatric Association, 1994.

being in public places, resulting in a marked restriction of travel, often to the point of becoming housebound. In many cases the agoraphobia is secondary to panic attacks: The patient restricts activities for fear of having a panic attack and thereby develops an agoraphobic profile. Consequently, one looks for the presence of panic attacks or panic attack–like symptoms in patients with agoraphobia, as they often respond to the same treatment given for panic attacks. Simple phobias, e.g., fear of flying, heights, snakes, respond better to behavioral management than to drug treatment and are usually associated with generalized anxiety rather than panic-like episodes.

EPIDEMIOLOGY. Recent epidemiologic studies of panic disorder have noted a prevalence rate of 0.4 to 1.2 per 100. The rates are highest in persons aged 25 to 44 years and in the separated and divorced. The rates are lowest in persons over the age of 64 and bear no relationship to race or education. For agoraphobia the prevalence rates are between 2.5 and 5.8 per 100. There is a marked prevalence for women (two to four times that of men), with an age range of 18 to 64 years. The rates for generalized anxiety disorder range from 2.5 to 6.4 per 100, again slightly more common in young women. Genetic studies have shown that monozygotic twins have higher concordance for anxiety disorders than do dizygotic twins when the proband has panic disorder but not when he/she has a generalized anxiety disorder.

PATHOPHYSIOLOGY. Panic attacks can be precipitated in susceptible patients by sodium lactate infusions, caffeine (PO), CO_2 inhalation, yohimbine (PO), isoproterenol (IV), and benzodiazepine receptor antagonists. All of these agents interact with the noradrenergic system and particularly the locus coeruleus system, which contains most of the brain's noradrenergic cell bodies.

TREATMENT. Two major treatments are available for panic attacks, one pharmacologic, the other psychological. The key to treatment is the establishment of a supportive relationship with the patient. Affected patients are often frightened, concerned about "going crazy" and/or dying, and somewhat ashamed of their symptoms. It is useful for the physician immediately to reassure the patient by clarifying that what he/she experiences is part of a well-known illness that causes these feelings. It is often useful to educate patients with appropriate reading material.

Well-controlled studies have demonstrated the effective treatment of panic attacks with tricyclic antidepressants (particularly imipramine), MAOI's (particularly phenelzine), and the benzodiazepines (particularly alprazolam). The doses and treatment pattern of the tricyclics and the MAOI's are similar to those used for affective disorders, and the dose of alprazolam is usually between 4 and

6 mg per day. At times β-blocking agents offer relief, but not so dramatically as the antidepressants and alprazolam. The doses of the antidepressants may need to be somewhat higher for these conditions than for affective disorders (tricyclics are usually used in the range of 150 to 300 mg*; the MAOI's in the range of 60 mg* or more per day). The new serotonin reuptake inhibitors are also effective in anxious patients but should be given in very small doses owing to their tendency to cause increased agitation. Pharmacologic treatment should last for 6 months to 1 year after response, with the drugs then gradually tapered. β-Blocking agents can be useful for treating the tachycardia and palpitations associated with panic attacks. β Blockers can also be used to decrease the cardiac symptoms associated with tricyclic use, which is often reassuring to the patient.

The treatment of generalized anxiety disorders has less clear guidelines. Although benzodiazepines and psychologic interventions are commonly emphasized, their benefit is more difficult to evaluate. A patient on benzodiazepines for 6 to 12 months may experience withdrawal symptoms on cessation of medication. Furthermore, one must be concerned and cautious about the addicting potential of the benzodiazepines and to some extent the tricyclics. Consequently, the treatment of generalized anxiety disorders should rely heavily on counseling, relaxation techniques, behavioral modification, exercise, and similar modalities rather than on prolonged pharmacologic interventions.

Certain medical conditions can simulate panic attacks and must be excluded. These include arrhythmias, angina, respiratory illnesses, asthma, obstructive pulmonary disease, various endocrine disturbances (hyperthyroidism, pheochromocytoma), seizure disorders, vertiginous conditions, pharmacologic stimulants and caffeine, and withdrawal syndromes, particularly from CNS depressants, e.g., alcohol, barbiturates, or occasionally, benzodiazepines. Medical conditions that are often noted in patients with severe panic attacks include episodic hypertension, peptic ulcer disorder, and mitral valve prolapse.

Sequelae of the Vietnam conflict brought attention to *post-traumatic stress disorders.* The basic differentiation of post-traumatic stress disorder from generalized anxiety disorder is the presence of a clear antecedent that could potentially cause distress in almost anyone. Another major characteristic of post-traumatic stress disorder is the re-experiencing of the trauma, through either recurring or intrusive recollections, dreams, or sudden feelings that the event is about to recur. Affected persons often exhibit a lack of emotional responsiveness or involvement with the world after the trauma. Other symptoms may include hyperalertness, heightened "startle responses," sleep disturbance, guilt, and memory and concentration difficulties. Affected persons may avoid activities that could evoke recollections of the traumatic event. Although medications are sometimes useful for acute symptoms (especially if accompanied by panic attacks or depressive symptoms), the major treatment of post-traumatic stress is psychotherapeutic, particularly group sessions. At times narcosynthesis has been used successfully.

PROGNOSIS IN ANXIETY DISORDERS. The ubiquity of anxiety symptoms and the blurring of panic disorder into generalized anxiety or chronic anxiety and phobic states, as well as a strong association with depressive illness, make a prognosis difficult to establish. In general, panic disorder may run a limited course with episodic patterns; long periods of remission can intervene with no symptomatology at all. Only about one quarter of patients with panic disorder are treated, implying a high incidence of spontaneous remission in cases that do not come to medical attention. Nevertheless, many patients become housebound for a significant part of their lives. Follow-up studies of 5 to 20 years' duration show that about 50 to 60% of the patients recovered or were much improved. Drug abuse and alcoholism are potentially serious complications.

Katon W: Panic Disorder in the Medical Setting. Washington, DC, American Psychiatric Press, 1991. *An excellent overview of the relation between anxiety and somatic symptoms.*
Roy-Byrne P: Anxiety: New Findings for the Clinician. Washington, DC, American Psychiatric Press, 1988. *A comprehensive summary of diagnostic and treatment studies of anxiety disorders.*
Sonnenberg S, Blank A, Talbott J: The Trauma of War. Washington, DC, American Psychiatric Press, 1985. *A good review of current knowledge on post-traumatic stress disorder.*

* Exceeds manufacturer's recommended dosage.

SOMATIZATION DISORDERS

Somatization disorders consist of psychologically engendered symptoms suggesting organ dysfunction for which associated physical or laboratory evidence of dysfunction is either absent or trivial in relation to the degree of complaint. If physicians can find no clear biologic mechanism for a set of symptoms because they are too vague, diffuse, or disparate (or even anatomically impossible) and the symptoms could fulfill some purpose in the patient's life (e.g., would help to avoid some area of responsibility, deny failure, or evoke increased attention by the family or others), they should suspect a purely psychologic disorder. However, these patients should not be treated lightly. Many vague symptoms arise early in organic disease, and patients must be examined carefully, supported, and followed. Similarly, patients with unfounded symptoms should also be evaluated for major depression and panic disorder, as persons with these conditions can present primarily with somatic complaints. Patients who tend toward somatization often have histories that are characterized by disturbed interpersonal relations and emotional disruptions (Table 401–11).

Diverse disorders can present as medically unfounded somatic symptoms, including hypochondriasis, conversion disorder (hysteria), psychogenic pain disorders, factitious disorders, and malingering. What ties these conditions together are the following characteristics: (1) symptoms that suggest a physical disorder; (2) no demonstrable clinical signs or evident physiologic abnormality; (3) evidence that the symptoms may be associated with psychological factors; (4) symptoms that do not seem to be under voluntary control (except in malingering and factitious disorder).

DIAGNOSTIC CRITERIA AND CLINICAL SIGNS AND SYMPTOMS. Somatization disorders include a wide variety and number of symptoms (Table 401–12). The remarkable phenomenon is the lack of accompanying physical or important laboratory abnormalities. The syndrome occurs mostly in females, with a population incidence of about 1%. The condition runs in families; in men it correlates with the occurrence of sociopathy and alcoholism rather than somatic symptoms.

PATHOPHYSIOLOGY. The condition is marked by an empiric collection of symptoms, the exact cause and pathophysiology of which are not understood. Most patients have limited education and lack sophistication; however, there are many exceptions to this characterization. Most explanations have been sociologic and psychological and center on the somatization as a signal of personal distress. Consequently, the behavior is often interpreted as a way to obtain help from caregivers or as a mechanism of obtaining social supports and, perhaps, manipulating relationships. It has also been postulated to represent a cognitive style whereby somatic symptoms are used in place of emotional expression.

TREATMENT. These patients are difficult to treat effectively. Perhaps the most important factor should be an attempt to rule out depressive and panic disorders. Patients with somatization disorders can persuade physicians that there is an urgent need to intervene; however, this temptation should be resisted. Careful evaluation of the history is extremely important for, as is evident, most of them do not respond to treatment. It is not that they enjoy their pain but that they are seeking other things, e.g., attention, relief from other problems. Perhaps the most important thing the physician can con-

TABLE 401–11. COMMON FEATURES IN THE HISTORIES OF PATIENTS WITH SOMATIZATION SYMPTOMS

1. Developmental histories of gross neglect, child abuse, and/or sexual abuse
2. Unstable adult relationships characterized by multiple divorces and often physical violence
3. Past family histories of alcoholism
4. A past history of alcohol abuse prior to the start of somatization
5. Past history of substance abuse
6. A positive review of systems on medical history
7. A polysurgery history
8. A history of litigious relationships with authority figures
9. Past history of psychiatric illness
10. Modeling of pain behavior in their families as way of solving problems and coping with intimate relationships

TABLE 401–12. SOMATIZATION DISORDER

A. A history of many physical complaints beginning before the age of 30, occurring over a period of several years, and resulting in treatment being sought or significant impairment in social or occupational functioning.

B. Each of the following criteria must have been met at some time during the course of the disorder. To count a symptom as significant, it must not be fully explained by a known general medical condition, or the resulting complaint or impairment is in excess of what would be expected from the history, physical examination, or laboratory findings.

1. *Four pain symptoms:* A history of pain related to at least four different sites or functions (such as head, abdomen, back, joints, extremities, chest, rectum, during sexual intercourse, during menstruation, or during urination).

2. *Two gastrointestinal symptoms:* A history of at least two gastrointestinal symptoms other than pain (such as nausea, diarrhea, bloating, vomiting other than during pregnancy, or intolerance of several different foods).

3. *One sexual symptom:* A history of at least one sexual or reproductive symptom other than pain (such as sexual indifference, erectile or ejaculatory dysfunction, irregular menses, excessive menstrual bleeding, vomiting throughout pregnancy).

4. *One pseudoneurologic symptom:* A history of at least one symptom or deficit suggesting a neurologic disorder not limited to pain (conversion symptoms such as blindness, double vision, deafness, loss of touch or pain sensation, hallucinations, aphonia, impaired coordination or balance, paralysis or localized weakness, difficulty swallowing, difficulty breathing, urinary retention, seizures, dissociative symptoms such as amnesia, or loss of consciousness other than fainting).

Modified from Diagnostic and Statistical Manual of Mental Disorders, 4th ed. Washington, DC, American Psychiatric Association, 1994.

vey to patients is that they will neither seriously worsen nor die, and although the physician may not know the cause of the complaint he is willing to support them through the illness episode. In fact, it is almost paradoxic that by scheduling these patients for frequent regular visits the doctor often not only saves time but may decrease the patient's need to develop symptoms in order to be seen. After the clinician becomes certain of the diagnosis and of the absence of a pathologic process, laboratory studies should be kept to a minimum, as the more tests that are ordered, the more the patient becomes convinced that something is wrong. The tendency to dispense medications to these patients not only invites addiction but produces such a confusion and plethora of drugs that they become a cause of untoward symptoms. The major goal of treatment should be to keep to a minimum the medical and surgical interventions. A general attempt should be made to substitute inquiry into the patient's life as opposed to procedures. The most helpful attitude for the doctor to adopt is to be more interested in maintaining the relationship than in curing the symptoms and to emphasize that a successful outcome is to reduce the number of doctors the patient sees and the number and amount of medicines he/she takes. The scheduling of visits can be based on the frequency of visits over the past 2- to 3-month period.

PROGNOSIS. Somatization disorders are more a way of life than a discrete episodic illness. The patient maintains a propensity for expression of emotional need or distress with somatic symptoms. Although the episodes may wax and wane, it is clear that these patients are wedded to the medical establishment.

Other Conditions Associated with Somatic Symptoms

Although the term *hysteria* has been dropped from official use and such conditions are now termed *conversion reactions,* such patients make up about 1% of a neurologist's practice. The predominant disturbance in conversion disorder is a loss or alteration in physical functioning suggesting a physical disorder. As a rule, the loss or distortion of neurologic function is not fully explained by any known disease detectable by physical and laboratory examination. Much of what has been covered with regard to somatization disorder is true of hysterical conditions. These patients do not necessarily have histrionic personalities. They do have physical complaints, but when examined closely their symptoms fail to indicate anatomic-physiologic patterns; rather, they conform more to a psychological reaction.

Hypochondriasis is often simple to recognize in that the patient presents with a belief that a disease is present for which diagnosis and treatment are necessary. The complaints are more circumscribed, with often minute examination and description of bodily functions to the physician. As the physician talks to the patient he becomes increasingly aware that the patient is more concerned about the belief of illness than the discomfort from symptoms. In fact, the symptoms are not especially distressing or painful. This is in marked contrast to the patient with chronic pain whose pain is often out of proportion to the physical findings.

In patients with chronic pain, the continuation of the pain often allows the avoidance of activities in the patient's life or the obtaining of emotional or financial support from others. Affected patients frequently have histories of addiction, seeing many physicians, and undergoing multiple surgical procedures.

The genesis of many of the above conditions lies at an involuntary level in that the symptoms and the motivation for them lie outside the conscious control of the patient. Two conditions, factitious disorder and malingering, are voluntarily controlled by the patient. These patients, often described as having *Münchausen's syndrome,* induce illnesses in themselves, e.g., fevers (by injection), dermatitis, blood disease (anemia), or seizures. Affected patients are often associated with the health professions, and one can discern no clear goal or gain from their behavior. They frequently are peripatetic, traveling from hospital to hospital. When a factitious disorder is diagnosed, these patients should be confronted openly as to their behavior and what treatment (as some may be necessary) will or will not be provided. In true malingering, the goal of the illness behavior is often evident (or evident after extensive inquiry), and the condition is usually less a chronic than a factitious disorder. Most cases consist of partial malingering, in which an individual exaggerates symptoms of a real disease or attributes a voluntarily induced disability to an accident or injury. In these conditions the physician tends to be angry with the patient, but it is better to confront him or her about the situation in a nonjudgmental manner. Particularly when compensation issues surround the case, treatment is pointless until legal questions or damage awards are settled.

Katon W, Egan K, Miller D: Chronic pain: Lifetime psychiatric diagnosis and family history. Am J Psychiatry 142:1156, 1985. *An interesting study of the relationship between pain syndromes and psychiatric problems.*

Marsden CD: Hysteria—A neurologist's view. Psychol Med 16:277, 1986. *An excellent review of hysteria.*

Quill T: Somatization disorder. JAMA 254:3075, 1985. *A good discussion of the physician's role in the treatment of patients with somatic disorder.*

Smith R: Somatization Disorder in the Medical Setting. Washington, DC, American Psychiatric Press, 1991. *Emphasizes importance of the ability to diagnose somatization disorder in the primary care setting.*

Section Three—Pathophysiology and Management of Major Neurologic Symptoms

402 AUTONOMIC DISORDERS AND THEIR MANAGEMENT
Clifford B. Saper

Disorders of the autonomic nervous system are of great importance to internal medicine, as they can present as disorders of virtually any organ system in the body. Furthermore, the central regulation of autonomic response is closely tied to neuroendocrine control, and both are often involved by central disorders. Aspects of neuroendocrine disease are discussed in Chapters 200 to 202 and 204. This chapter focuses on disorders of the autonomic nervous system (Table 402–1) and discusses them in the overall context of diseases affecting basic integrative functions of the nervous system.

DISORDERS OF PERIPHERAL AUTONOMIC FUNCTION

The peripheral autonomic nervous system consists of three main divisions: the *parasympathetic* division, which includes the outflow from the cranial nerves and the low lumbar and sacral spinal cord; the *sympathetic* division, which comprises the autonomic outflow from the thoracic and high lumbar segments of the spinal cord; and the *enteric* nervous system, which includes neurons that are intrinsic to the wall of the gut. The details of the organization of the peripheral autonomic nervous system are covered in basic anatomy and physiology texts.

Knowledge about the different neurotransmitter and receptor types associated with the peripheral autonomic nervous system has resulted in the availability of a wide range of drugs to modify autonomic responses. Some key autonomic drugs and their clinical uses are listed in Table 402–2. These are covered in detail in clinical pharmacology texts.

Pandysautonomias

ACUTE PANDYSAUTONOMIA. Widespread failure of the autonomic nervous system may evolve acutely or subacutely as part of a parainfectious inflammatory polyneuropathy (of the Guillain-Barré type). In rare cases, the autonomic neuropathy predominates and, when severe, may be life threatening. Wide swings in blood pressure and heart rate occur but usually reverse themselves in a few minutes. Generally, putting the patient into the Trendelenberg position is sufficient to maintain cerebral perfusion during hypotensive periods. Cardiac arrhythmias of all types may occur, presumably as a result of the instability of autonomic innervation of the cardiac conducting system. These must be treated gingerly, as the underlying conduction abnormality may change very rapidly.

TETANUS. A similar subacute pandysautonomia is also seen in severe cases of tetanus. Tetanus toxin, elaborated by *Clostridium tetani* organisms in an infected wound, is transported by autonomic as well as motor axons back to the spinal cord, where it is taken up by and inactivates the terminals of inhibitory interneurons. Treatment of the motor manifestations of tetanus by paralyzing and sedating the patient does little to abate the autonomic storm. Up to 40% of patients with tetanus in an intensive care environment may suffer cardiac arrest as a result of arrhythmias. They are generally easily resuscitated with standard measures.

CHRONIC AUTONOMIC NEUROPATHY. The axons of the peripheral autonomic nervous system generally are of small caliber and poorly myelinated or unmyelinated. Certain polyneuropathies that have a predilection for small-diameter axons can result in autonomic changes. *Amyloid neuropathy* often includes a major autonomic component that may present as a gastrointestinal motility disorder or orthostatic hypotension. Similarly, *diabetic neuropathy,* although it is often dominated by sensory or motor complaints, may cause widespread autonomic failure. The neuropathy of *acute inter-*

TABLE 402–1. DISORDERS OF THE AUTONOMIC NERVOUS SYSTEM

Peripheral Autonomic Disorders
Pandysautonomias
  Acute pandysautonomia
  Tetanus
  Chronic autonomic neuropathy
  Familial dysautonomia
  Idiopathic autonomic insufficiency (Shy-Drager syndrome)
Regional dysautonomia
  Horner's syndrome
  Paraspinal tumors
  Somatosympathetic dysreflexia
  Reflex sympathetic dystrophy (causalgia)
Disorders of specific autonomic functions
  Pupillary disorders
    Horner's syndrome
    Oculomotor paresis
  Cardiovascular disorders
    Glossopharyngeal neuralgia
    Carotid sinus hypersensitivity
  Sweating disorders
    Hyperhidrosis
    Anhydrosis
  Gastrointestinal disorders
    Disorders of motility
    Vomiting
  Genitourinary disorders
    Incontinence
    Urinary retention
    Spastic bladder
    Impotence

Disorders of Central Autonomic Integration
Emotional disorders
  Panic disorder
  Psychosomatic illness
  Cardiac arrhythmias
Thermoregulatory disorders
  Poikilothermia
  Paroxysmal hypothermia
  Hyperthermia and fever
  Neuroleptic malignant syndrome
Feeding disorders
  Hyperphagia and obesity
  Hypophagia and inanition
Disorders of fluid and electrolyte regulation
  Hypernatremia, hyperosmolality, and absence of thirst
  Hyperdipsia, hyponatremia, and water intoxication
  Paroxysmal hyponatremia
Central reproductive disorders
Arousal disorders
  Hypersomnolence
  Insomnia

TABLE 402-2. SYSTEMIC EFFECTS OF SOME COMMONLY USED AUTONOMIC DRUGS

Receptor Type	Drug Type (example)	Tissue	Effect
Muscarinic cholinergic	Antagonist (atropine)	Pupil	Mydriasis
		Salivary gland	Dry mouth
		Bronchi	Dilation
		Heart	Tachycardia
		Gut	Decreased motility and secretion
α-Adrenergic	Antagonist (phenoxybenzamine)	Blood vessels	Vasodilation
α_1-Adrenergic	Agonist (phenylephrine)	Blood vessels	Vasoconstriction
	Antagonist (prazosin)	Blood vessels	Vasodilation
β-Adrenergic	Agonist (isoproterenol)	Heart	Increased rate and contractility
β_1-Adrenergic	Antagonist (metoprolol)	Blood vessels	Decreased rate and contractility
β_2-Adrenergic	Agonist (terbutaline)	Bronchi	Dilation

mittent *porphyria* or certain toxic agents, such as *Vacar* (a rat poison), may have a prominent autonomic component. Acute poisoning with *organophosphate insecticides* that block acetylcholinesterase results in a hypercholinergic state, including miosis and cardiac slowing, that lasts for several days. The neuropathy that follows several weeks later usually does not have a strong autonomic component. Other peripheral neuropathies that may have an autonomic component are listed in Table 402–3.

CHRONIC DYSAUTONOMIA. Recessively inherited *familial dysautonomia* of the Riley-Day type is most commonly seen in Ashkenazi Jewish children. Symptoms referable to the autonomic nervous system and relative indifference to pain are present from birth.

Idiopathic autonomic insufficiency of the *Shy-Drager* type may develop as a chronic degenerative condition in middle age or late adult life owing to loss of neurons in the autonomic ganglia as well as in the preganglionic cell groups in the medulla and spinal cord. The presenting complaint is often orthostatic hypotension, but signs or symptoms of pupillary, gastrointestinal, genitourinary, sweating, or other autonomic abnormalities are elicited on history and physical examination.

Idiopathic autonomic insufficiency is distinguished from non-neurologic causes of orthostatic hypotension by the lack of compensatory tachycardia, indicating impairment of either the peripheral or central components of the baroreceptor reflex. Severe autonomic neuropathy affecting the glossopharyngeal or vagus nerves may also impair the baroreceptor response but is typically associated with other evidence of sensory or motor neuropathy. Other cardiovascular signs include loss of sinus arrhythmia and absence of normal overshoot in the diastolic blood pressure during phase IV of the Valsalva maneuver. An abnormally accentuated blood pressure response to intravenous infusion of norepinephrine is consistent with widespread denervation supersensitivity. A detailed list of tests of autonomic insufficiency is provided in Table 402–4.

Idiopathic autonomic insufficiency is part of a spectrum of disorders, ranging from isolated orthostatic hypotension, with or without parkinsonian features, to *multisystem atrophy* with evidence of cerebellar and extrapyramidal involvement. When idiopathic autonomic insufficiency is associated with a multisystem neurologic degenerative disease, it may be accompanied by ataxia, rigidity, bradykinesia, tremors, weakness, or other neurologic disturbances. Additional cell loss is seen in other affected areas in multisystem atrophy.

Orthostatic hypotension is generally the most disabling aspect of autonomic degeneration. Indomethacin may be effective in selected patients. Other patients require elastic stockings or even entire lower body suits to reduce blood pooling in the lower extremities during standing. Treatment with mineralocorticoids, such as fludrocortisone, can expand intravascular blood volume and cause elevation of blood pressure in all positions. In such patients, the head of the bed should be elevated in recumbency to minimize hypertensive effects on the brain. Occasionally, oral sympathomimetic agents, such as ephedrine, or monoamine oxidase inhibitors are employed. The latter must be used with caution, as the ingestion of vasoactive amines present in many common foods, including certain wines, cheeses, pickled foods, and smoked meats, can cause severe hypertension.

Regional Dysautonomia

The segmental organization of the sympathetic nervous system can result in regional disturbances of function. The most common of these is caused by injury to the cranial sympathetic innervation arising from the superior cervical ganglion, or *Horner's syndrome*. Miosis, ptosis, and anhydrosis may occur if the ascending sympathetic fibers are injured below the level at which they enter the skull with the internal carotid artery. Damage to sympathetic fibers along the course of the intracranial carotid artery produces only oculosympathetic paresis (Raeder's syndrome). Unfortunately, this difference is only of marginal value clinically, as the Horner's syndrome produced by extracranial lesions is often incomplete. Lesions of the central descending sympathoexcitatory pathway, running through the lateral portions of the brain stem from the hypothalamus to the spinal cord, may produce a central Horner's syndrome, in which there is miosis and ptosis as well as loss of sweating over the entire ipsilateral body. Postganglionic Horner's syndrome can be differentiated from preganglionic or central lesions by pharmacologic testing (Table 402–4). The most common cause of Horner's syndrome is atherosclerotic disease affecting the vasa nervorum originating in the carotid artery. However, Horner's syndrome may also be seen when an intrathoracic or cervical tumor involves the sympathetic chain. Hence, evaluation of Horner's syndrome should include radiographic or magnetic resonance examination of the pulmonary apices and paracervical area.

Paraspinal tumors at lower levels along the sympathetic chain may cause loss of sweating over the involved dermatomes. This deficit can be appreciated by running the handle of a tuning fork down the skin in the paraspinal region. The smooth movement is interrupted by the dry skin at the level of the lesion. Occasionally, compression of a midthoracic spinal root, which carries visceral sensory fibers, by a disc or tumor may present as abdominal pain.

TABLE 402-3. PERIPHERAL NEUROPATHIES THAT MAY HAVE AN AUTONOMIC COMPONENT

Autonomic symptoms often prominent
 Guillain-Barré syndrome
 Amyloid neuropathy
 Diabetic neuropathy
 Acute intermittent porphyria
 Vacar (rat poison)
Autonomic symptoms may occur
 Renal failure
 Toxic neuropathies
  Vinca alkaloids
  Perhexiline maleate
  Thallium
  Arsenic
  Mercury
  Organic solvents
  Acrylamide
 Vasculitis
  Systemic lupus erythematosus
  Rheumatoid arthritis
  Mixed connective tissue disease
 Thiamine deficiency
 Leprosy
 Charcot-Marie-Tooth disease
 Fabry's disease

TABLE 402–4. TESTS OF AUTONOMIC FUNCTION*

Test	Interpretation
Pupillary responses	
4% cocaine	Pupillodilatation indicates release of normal catecholamine stores.
1% hydroxyamphetamine	Pupillodilatation indicates denervation supersensitivity.
1% phenylephrine	
0.1% epinephrine	
0.1% pilocarpine	Pupilloconstriction indicates denervation supersensitivity.
2.5% methacholine	
Sweating responses	
Thermal sweating	Regional absence of sweating indicates sympathetic cholinergic denervation.
Galvanic skin response	Increased conductivity under mild stress indicates normal adrenergic innervation.
1:1000 pilocarpine	Intradermal injection causes axon reflex sweating.
1:10,000 acetylcholine	
Axon reflex	
1:1000 histamine	Intradermal injection normally causes wheal and flare.
Cardiovascular responses	
Orthostatic challenge	Pulse normally increases and diastolic blood pressure falls < 15 mm Hg.
Carotid sinus massage	Normally causes fall in blood pressure and heart rate.
R-R interval	Normally increases during inspiration (sinus arrhythmia).
Valsalva maneuver	Longest to shortest R-R interval ratio normally is ≥ 1.4.
Cold pressor test	Immersing hand in ice water normally increases blood pressure and heart rate.
Plasma catecholamines	Normally increase response to standing or stress.
Norepinephrine infusion 0.05 μg/kg/min	Diastolic blood pressure increase ≥ 20 mm Hg indicates supersensitivity.
Genitourinary, rectal responses	
Cremasteric reflex	Stroking skin of thigh normally causes testicular retraction.
Anal wink reflex	Scratching perianal skin normally causes anal sphincter contraction.
Bulbocavernosus reflex	Squeezing glans penis or clitoris normally causes anal sphincter contraction.

* For details see McLeod and Tuck, 1987.

Stimulation of pain fibers at any level results in both local (spino-spinal) and generalized (spino-bulbo-spinal) *somatosympathetic reflex responses,* including sweating, vasoconstriction, and pupillodilatation. In patients with a pre-existing spinal cord transection, a noxious stimulus below the level of the transection may produce only local sympathetic reflex responses. Hence it is important in the paraplegic patient to investigate asymmetric sympathetic responses for a local lesion that might cause pain in an intact individual.

Following injury to peripheral nerves, aberrant regeneration may result in *reflex sympathetic dystrophy.* It is believed that the sympathetic efferent fibers form excitatory synapses along the course of damaged peripheral sensory nerves. Normally innocuous sensory stimulation, such as covering the affected limb with a sheet or with clothing, may cause excruciating burning pain, associated with variable autonomic changes. Atrophic changes in the skin and bone may reflect abnormal sympathetic innervation or disuse. Relief can sometimes be obtained with guanethidine or phenoxybenzamine. If regional sympathetic block alleviates pain, removal of the affected ganglion can produce permanent relief.

Disorders of Specific Autonomic Functions

PUPILS. Anisocoria, asymmetry of pupillary size, may reflect a deficit of sympathetic innervation of the smaller pupil (causing miosis) or parasympathetic innervation of the larger one (causing mydriasis). Because both the oculosympathetic and oculomotor (parasympathetic) innervations participate in lid elevation, ptosis if present generally indicates the abnormal eye. Anisocoria may be longstanding and of little clinical significance, but pupillary asymmetry of recent onset should be evaluated by a neurologist. Impairment of sympathetic innervation of the iris (pupillodilator) muscle is not always accompanied by ptosis or a sweating deficit (Horner's syndrome). The pupilloconstrictor fibers travel in the dorsomedial part of the oculomotor nerve, where they may be selectively affected by temporal lobe herniation or by an aneurysm of the posterior communicating artery. Pharmacologic testing may aid in the identification of the pupillary abnormality (Table 402–4). The most common cause of a large pupil is instillation of atropinic eye drops or application of a scopolamine patch near the face (to prevent motion sickness); the pharmacologically dilated pupil does not respond even to strong solutions of pilocarpine. Another common cause of a large, poorly reactive pupil is *Adie's syndrome,* an idiopathic condi-

tion involving degeneration of the ciliary ganglion. The pupil usually shows sector paralysis and constriction with accommodation, and it dilates and responds to light after a period in complete darkness. The abnormal pupil responds briskly to 0.1% pilocarpine (Table 402–4), and there is concomitant loss of tendon reflexes in most cases.

CARDIOVASCULAR. The baroreceptor reflex is an important protective response, causing bradycardia and peripheral vasodilatation to counteract an acute increase in blood pressure, or the reverse response during hypotension. The afferent fibers for the response run in the glossopharyngeal (carotid sinus) and vagus (aortic depressor) nerves, whereas the efferent response includes both parasympathetic and sympathetic components. Injury to the glossopharyngeal or carotid sinus nerves in the neck (often by a tumor) can cause episodic attacks of hypotension and bradycardia, which often present as syncope. In most cases, there is an associated pain or paresthesia in the cutaneous distribution of the glossopharyngeal nerve (in the external auditory meatus or the pharynx), known as *glossopharyngeal neuralgia.* The situation is analogous to tic doloreaux, in which there are intermittent volleys of firing in the affected nerve. Atropine or a transvenous pacemaker may prevent the bradycardia associated with the attacks, but loss of vasoconstrictor tone sometimes results in symptomatic hypotension despite these maneuvers. Anticonvulsants, particularly phenytoin and carbamazepine, may prevent the attacks.

Carotid sinus syncope (see Ch. 396) is a condition seen most commonly in elderly individuals with carotid atherosclerosis. Even mild pressure over the carotid bulb, such as a tight shirt collar, can produce a full-blown carotid sinus response, resulting in syncope. The diagnosis is made by gently compressing the carotid artery below the angle of the jaw while the electrocardiogram (ECG) is monitored. Facilities for cardiac resuscitation must be immediately available, as the compression may result in sinus arrest. Vigorous massage should be avoided, as it may dislodge an embolus, resulting in a transient or even permanent neurologic deficit. Treatment of carotid sinus hypersensitivity is the same as that for glossopharyngeal neuralgia.

SWEATING. Human sweat glands are innervated by both noradrenergic sympathetic fibers (mediating emotional responses) and cholinergic sympathetic fibers (thermal sweating). Certain somatosympathetic reflexes can produce generalized or regional sweating, in response to innocuous or noxious somatosensory stimuli. *Paroxysmal localized hyperhidrosis* is a rare condition that probably represents an exaggeration of normal somatosympathetic reflexes. Generalized hyperhidrosis, particularly involving the hands and the soles of the feet, is most likely a normal variant. Drugs directed at interrupting α-adrenergic transmission (phenoxybenzamine, clonidine) have been useful in some cases of localized hyperhidrosis. In extreme cases, regional sympathectomy has been performed.

Idiopathic anhydrosis may be segmental or generalized. This rare condition is sometimes associated with Adie's syndrome (Ross syndrome), but in other cases there are no other signs of autonomic impairment. In some cases the impairment is preganglionic and in others postganglionic, as judged by the axon reflex sweating response (Table 402–4). In most recorded patients, the deficits have been stable and did not go on to involve other autonomic functions.

GASTROINTESTINAL. Disorders of intestinal motility, which may be due to damage to the parasympathetic innervation of the gut or to dysfunction of the enteric nervous system itself, are discussed in Chapter 101. Specific abnormalities of esophageal contraction and colonic tone have been noted in patients suffering from depression and may predict response to antidepressant medication.

Vomiting is a neurally mediated gastrointestinal reflex that is coordinated by neurons in the medullary reticular formation. Chemical emetic agents such as certain narcotics or dopaminergic agonists act at the area postrema, a chemosensory zone on the fourth ventricular surface of the medulla, to elicit the vomiting reflex. Local dopaminergic connections are thought to mediate the response, and antidopaminergic drugs such as prochlorperazine may act at the level of the area postrema to suppress vomiting. Intractable vomiting without any gastrointestinal abnormalities has been reported in certain patients with tumors involving the medullary cell groups controlling vomiting or their connections. Treatment of the tumor with steroids and radiation therapy generally results in improvement.

GENITOURINARY. The urinary bladder is composed of interlacing smooth muscle fibers of the detrusor covered by an internal mucous membrane and an outer serosa. The detrusor is innervated by parasympathetic neurons located in the intermediolateral column at the second through fourth sacral segments. Additional motor neurons located in the ventral horn at the same levels constitute Onuf's nucleus. Their axons run through the pelvic nerve to innervate striated accessory muscles of micturition (including the external urethral sphincter) in the pelvic floor. Neurons of Onuf's nucleus are strikingly preserved in motor neuron disease but are lost along with autonomic preganglionic cells in idiopathic autonomic insufficiency. The internal sphincter at the bladder neck is innervated via the hypogastric nerve by sympathetic prevertebral pelvic ganglia whose preganglionic innervation arises from the intermediolateral column at the T12-L1 level.

Bladder relaxation during filling and subsequent coordination of micturition are under the control of Barrington's nucleus, located in the floor of the fourth ventricle at the pontine level. Brain stem control of micturition is, in turn, under voluntary regulation by areas within the cerebral sensory and motor cortex. When bladder fullness is sensed and the environmental conditions are appropriate, micturition is initiated by Barrington's nucleus, under forebrain control. There is a fall in external sphincter pressure, resulting in reflex relaxation of the internal sphincter and contraction of the bladder.

Forebrain impairment results in loss of voluntary control of micturition but does not otherwise affect the complex sensory and motor program that results in normal voiding. Incontinence in such patients can be managed by using adult diapers or external urinary collection devices without risk of frequent urinary tract infections or damage to the upper urinary tract. Injury to the bulbospinal pathway from Barrington's nucleus to the sacral intermediolateral column, however, causes major disruption of coordinated bladder function. Acutely following spinal cord injury there is a period of spinal shock, during which the bladder does not undergo reflex contraction as it fills. Such patients require urinary catheterization to prevent vesical and renal damage.

One to 2 weeks following injury, spinal reflex control of the bladder returns. Some patients can induce reflex bladder emptying by somatosensory stimulation, such as stroking the skin over the thigh. The spastic bladder reflexively contracts at a lower volume

TABLE 402–5. SOME COMMONLY PRESCRIBED DRUGS THAT MAY IMPAIR URINARY FUNCTION

Antiarrhythmics	Antiparkinsonian agents
Atropine	Amantadine
Disopyramide	Dopa/carbidopa
Antihistamines	Bromocriptine
Diphenhydramine	Benztropine
Neuroleptics	Trihexyphenidyl
Haloperidol	Antispasmodics
Chlorpromazine	Baclofen
Antidepressants	
Amitriptyline	
Imipramine	

and, because detrusor action is not coordinated with sphincter opening, rarely empties completely. Injury to sensory nerves supplying the bladder also may cause overfilling and incomplete emptying, indicating the importance of sensory feedback in bladder control. Patients with significant postvoid residual urine are at increased risk for urinary tract infections, but bladder overfilling with elevated pressures above 40 mm H_2O may ultimately be a greater problem. Elevations in pressure above 40 mm H_2O may require continuous or intermittent catheterization to prevent damage to the upper urinary tract.

Pharmacologic intervention, aimed at augmenting or suppressing autonomic motor responses of the bladder or internal sphincter, has only limited value. Bethanacol, a cholinergic agonist, is used to augment bladder contraction to improve emptying. It is most effective in combination with an α-adrenergic blocker, such as phenoxybenzamine or prazocin, that simultaneously reduces pressure of the internal sphincter. Baclofen may be used to decrease spastic contraction of the external sphincter. Drugs that have atropinic properties, including a surprising variety of antiarrhythmic, antihistamine, neuroleptic, and antidepressant medications, may inhibit bladder contraction, resulting in overfilling and urinary retention (Table 402–5).

Erectile function in males is under parasympathetic control by the same sacral levels as the urinary system. Sensory afferent fibers travel via the pudendal nerve, while parasympathetic motor fibers run in the pelvic nerve. Sympathetic innervation via the hypogastric nerve contracts the seminal vesicles during ejaculation and closes the bladder neck to prevent retrograde emission. Although supraspinal influences are of great importance, reflex erection and ejaculation can occur in patients after spinal injury. Neurogenic impotence can result either from damage to descending pathways relaying forebrain influence from the hypothalamus to the sacral preganglionic neurons or from injury to the sensory or parasympathetic motor innervation of the penis. A variety of drugs that block either parasympathetic or sympathetic function can interfere with erectile function (Table 402–6). As erections normally occur several times nightly during periods of rapid eye movement sleep, it is possible to document organic disorders of erection by measuring penile tumescence overnight. Disorders of male sexual function are considered in Ch. 209.

TABLE 402–6. SOME COMMONLY PRESCRIBED DRUGS THAT MAY IMPAIR ERECTILE FUNCTION

Drugs causing impotence	Drugs causing priapism
Parasympatholytics	Chlorpromazine
Atropine	Thioridazine
Amitriptyline	Trazodone
Sympatholytics	Prazosin
Methyldopa	Dopa/carbidopa
Guanethidine	
Clonidine	
Propranolol	
Prazosin	
Vasodilators	
Hydralazine	
Diuretics	
Hydrochlorothiazide	
Antihistaminergic	
Cimetidine	

ORGANIZATION OF CENTRAL AUTONOMIC AND EN-DOCRINE REGULATION. The autonomic nervous system is under three levels of central control. The *preganglionic* neurons located in the medulla and the spinal cord provide the final common pathway for central autonomic control. Each of these neurons integrates the inputs from many sources, including afferents from higher levels of the nervous system and local reflex responses. A series of *brain stem and spinal* cell groups coordinates *reflex control* of the autonomic nervous system. These nuclei receive cranial (parasympathetic) and spinal (sympathetic) afferent information and control a variety of important reflexes (e.g., swallowing, maintaining blood pressure, initiation of voiding). Both the preganglionic neurons and the brain stem reflex neurons are under the control of *forebrain integrative* cell groups that coordinate autonomic function with behavior and with endocrine control.

The hypothalamus is the most important area for integration of behavior with autonomic responses and with neuroendocrine control of the anterior and posterior pituitary glands (Fig. 402–1). Because the hypothalamus consists of tightly packed, interwoven pathways and cell groups, it is unusual for an injury to involve selectively a single functional system. Nevertheless, considerable progress has been made in determining the anatomic substrates for specific integrative functions, and disorders of these systems are occasionally encountered (Table 402–7). In addition, autonomic dysfunction is a frequent concomitant of emotional disorders.

Emotional Disorders

Portions of the insular and cingulate areas of the cerebral cortex and the amygdala are believed to regulate autonomic responses to emotional stress. In healthy individuals, stress can induce sympathetic responses, such as pupillodilatation, dry mouth, and increases in blood pressure. In patients with *panic disorder* (see Ch. 401), such autonomic responses can become overwhelming and convince the patient that there is a serious organic problem. PET studies show increased metabolism in the structures of the medial temporal lobe and the insular cortex during panic attacks. After eliminating the possibility of pheochromocytoma (see Ch. 204.2), anxiolytic or antidepressant drugs are usually found helpful. Clomipramine is likely to become the drug of choice for this disorder.

In some individuals under chronic emotional stress, a variety of syndromes are seen implicating autonomic control of the internal organs. Although *psychosomatic illness* is often thought to be nonorganic and may respond to psychotherapeutic drugs, there is considerable evidence that some organic disorders seen in anxious

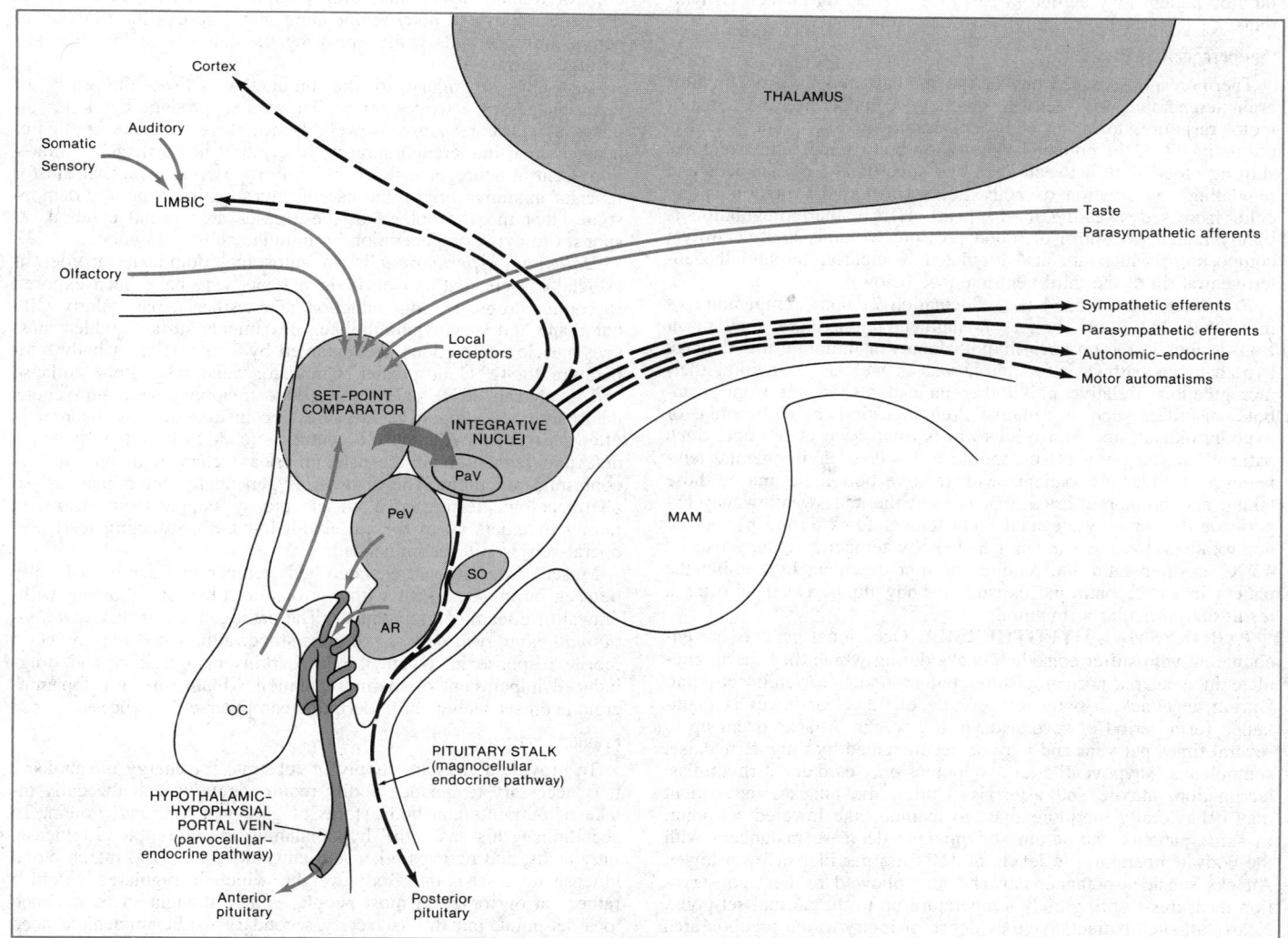

FIGURE 402–1. Schematic illustration of the functional organization of the hypothalamus. General and visceral sensory, limbic, and local interoceptive (e.g., osmolality and temperature) information is compared against a homeostatic set-point by integrative cell groups in the preoptic area and tuberal hypothalamus. Efferent autonomic responses from the paraventricular nucleus (PaV) and lateral hypothalamic area are then integrated with anterior pituitary control via the periventricular (PeV) and arcuate (AR) nuclei and posterior pituitary control via the supraoptic (SO) and paraventricular nuclei, and with behavioral regulation exercised mainly by the lateral hypothalamic area. MAM = mamillary body; OC = optic chiasm. (Amended from Saper CB: Hypothalamus. *In* Pearlman AL, Collins RC (eds): Neurobiology of Disease. New York, Oxford University Press, 1989, p 197.)

TABLE 402-7. REGIONAL HYPOTHALAMIC SYNDROMES

Region	Normally Regulates	Disorders
Preoptic	Blood volume, pressure, and electrolytes	Paroxysmal hyponatremia Essential hypernatremia
Tuberal	Thermoregulation Gastrointestinal tract and feeding	Paroxysmal hypothermia Hyperphagia (ventromedial lesions) Hypophagia (lateral lesions)
Posterior	Reproduction Emotions Arousal Descending autonomic and motor pathways	Hypogonadism Rage responses Hypersomnolence Poikilothermia

patients also may be caused by autonomic dysregulation. For example, swallowing disorders often represent abnormal control of peristalsis. Erosive gastritis and even frank ulceration may occur as a result of autonomic dysfunction. Perhaps the most serious problems are encountered in patients with pre-existing cardiac abnormalities, who may have cardiac arrhythmias under stressful conditions. Retrospective studies of victims of sudden death due to lethal ventricular arrhythmias indicate a much higher incidence of behavioral stress in the period preceding the attack. The protective affect of β-adrenergic blockers against sudden death in the post-myocardial infarction patient may be due in part to the reduction in such arrhythmias.

Thermoregulatory Disorders

Thermoresponsive neurons in the medial preoptic area monitor brain temperature and activate autonomic, endocrine, and somatomotor responses to match body temperature to a set-point, which is normally 37° C in humans. Control of body temperature requires shifting blood flow between deep and superficial vascular beds and regulating conservation of body fluids (increased urination in the cold, increased sweating in the heat). Hence, thermoregulation is tightly linked to control of blood pressure, volume, and electrolyte composition, which are also regulated by neurons around the anteroventral tip of the third ventricle (see below).

Poikilothermia, defined as a fluctuation in body temperature of more than 2° C with changes in ambient temperature, may result from lesions in the posterior hypothalamus or midbrain that damage hypothalamic pathways for autonomic as well as behavioral thermoregulation. Relative poikilothermia can also result from metabolic disorders such as sedative drug ingestion, hypoglycemia, or hypothyroidism, and in a mild form is often seen in old age. Such patients are dangerously susceptible to lowered environmental temperature. Conversely, patients with relative poikilothermia or those taking anticholinergic drugs that prevent thermal sweating may experience dangerously elevated body temperatures during periods of hot weather. *Heat stroke,* in which body temperature may exceed 42° C, is often fatal and requires prompt treatment by cooling the patient in an ice bath and expanding body fluids. Death is often a result of ventricular arrhythmia.

PAROXYSMAL HYPOTHERMIA. Occasional patients are encountered who suffer episodic attacks during which they thermoregulate in a nearly normal fashion but around a lowered set-point. During an attack, a body temperature of 32° C or lower is maintained for a period of several days to 2 weeks. Attacks occur up to several times per year and may be accompanied by fatigue, malaise, somnolence, hypoventilation, hypotension, cardiac arrhythmias, lacrimation, ataxia, and asterixis. During the attacks, the patient may behaviorally thermoregulate to maintain the lowered set-point. In some patients, the serum sodium may decrease in tandem with the body temperature, to levels of 110 mEq per liter or even lower. Attacks subside spontaneously and are followed by heat conservation measures to bring body temperature up to the normal set-point. Nearly all such patients have evidence of injury to the preoptic area of the hypothalamus. Paroxysmal hypothermia is sometimes seen in patients with agenesis of the corpus callosum, most likely because the corpus callosum and the preoptic area are both embryologic derivatives of the lamina terminalis, which fails to form normally. Anticonvulsants have been prescribed to alleviate attacks but have rarely been effective.

FEVER AND HYPERTHERMIA. During an immune response, macrophages release cytokines, such as interleukin-1 and tumor necrosis factor, that act on neurons or glial cells at the organum vasculosum of the lamina terminalis, a vascular structure outside the blood-brain barrier that sits in the anteroventral tip of the third ventricle, to cause a febrile response. Prostaglandins are a critical mediator for producing fever and some of the endocrine and metabolic changes that accompany it. Fever, an upward resetting of the thermoregulatory set-point, is achieved by normal heat conservation mechanisms, including shivering and behavioral thermoregulation. Drugs that inhibit the generation of prostaglandins are the mainstay of treatment of fever, but there is considerable debate on the wisdom of treating low-grade fever (< 38.5° C) during an infectious illness. An elevated body temperature may improve the function of certain immune cells while impairing the defenses of invading microorganisms.

Any physical injury to the brain that allows the entry of macrophages or activates microglial cells to produce cytokines induces a febrile response as well. Hence, fever may be seen after head trauma, intracranial surgery, or cerebral hemorrhage or infarction. Central neurogenic fever is often proposed as a mechanism for fever of unknown origin, but careful investigation generally demonstrates that most if not all of these cases are normal cerebral responses to cytokine generation by immune cells or tumors.

Malignant hyperthermia is an autosomal dominant disorder of skeletal muscle that can occur in patients who have been exposed to certain drugs. During induction of anesthesia, particularly with halothane and succinylcholine, certain patients sustain sudden massive muscle contractions accompanied by a rapid rise in body temperature to 42° C or greater. Circulatory and respiratory collapse and death can ensue unless immediate treatment with intravenous dantrolene and supportive measures are instituted. This disorder is often associated with muscle central core disease and is due to a defect in regulation of the calcium-release channel in muscle sarcoplasmic reticulum. The disorder is genetically heterogeneous, so pharmacologic testing of a muscle biopsy sample from suspected family members (with the caffeine-halothane contracture test) preoperatively is still recommended.

Muscular rigidity and elevated body temperature can occasionally be seen during treatment with neuroleptic drugs or following withdrawal of dopaminergic agonists. The pathogenesis of this *neuroleptic malignant syndrome* is not understood, although it may reflect a febrile response in a patient with parkinsonian rigidity and drug-induced impairment of thermoregulation. Treatment with dopaminergic agonists such as bromocriptine can reverse the process.

Feeding Disorders

To provide a constant supply of substrate for energy metabolism, it is necessary to balance bodily requirements against the daily intake of nutrients and body stores of glycogen, fat, and protein. To accomplish this task, the hypothalamus monitors blood glucose, fatty acids, and perhaps other nutrients and attempts to match blood glucose to a set-point. Body weight, which is regulated within a rather narrow range in most people, is also thought to be matched to a set-point, but this is clearly secondary to the immediate need for metabolic substrate. The neural mechanisms regulating energy metabolism and feeding are mainly coordinated in the region of the ventromedial nucleus of the hypothalamus and the nearby paraventricular nucleus. The control of feeding is closely related to autonomic control of the gastrointestinal system.

HYPERPHAGIA AND OBESITY. Lesions in the region of the ventromedial nucleus of the hypothalamus can result in massive overeating and obesity. Experimental studies indicate that overeating is largely in response to parasympathetically mediated hyperinsulinemia, causing a chronically lowered blood glucose. Transection of the vagus nerve below the diaphragm corrects insulin secretion and overeating. Hence, hypothalamic hyperphagia is mainly a disorder of autonomic control of the pancreas, with a resultant attempt to defend the blood glucose set-point.

The *Klein-Levin syndrome* is a poorly understood disorder in which patients, typically adolescent boys, have episodic attacks of somnolence, often sleeping up to 20 hours per day. When awake, they appear dull and often confused and consume enormous quantities of food. Attacks may last up to 2 weeks and can recur several times per year. Pathologic verification of the site of the lesion in typical cases is lacking, but a similar syndrome may be seen acutely in encephalitis involving the hypothalamus.

The *Prader-Willi syndrome* is a congenital disorder due to a deletion in chromosome 15, which includes mental retardation, hypogonadism, and hyperphagia, often with massive obesity. The cause of the overeating is not known.

HYPOPHAGIA AND INANITION. Large lesions in the region of the lateral hypothalamic area, at the level of the ventromedial nucleus, result in aphagia, which may recover to hypophagia and regulation around a new, lower body weight set-point. Such lesions, which must be bilateral, are usually devastating, and selective impairment of eating on this basis has rarely been reported in adults. More often, patients with hypothalamic damage and inanition are somnolent and show a variety of endocrine abnormalities. There is no evidence for injury to the hypothalamus in anorexia nervosa.

Children may demonstrate a quite different response to congenital hypothalamic tumors or malformations. In the diencephalic syndrome of infancy, there is profound emaciation, despite good feeding and linear growth. The affected children are often exceptionally good-natured. The difference from adults with similarly placed tumors probably reflects the capacity for plasticity and formation of new neuronal connections during development.

Central Disorders of Fluid and Electrolyte Regulation

The medial preoptic area, around the anteroventral tip of the third ventricle, plays a critical role in regulating blood pressure, volume, and electrolyte composition. Endocrine control (mineralocorticoids and especially vasopressin), autonomic regulation (control of blood flow in different vascular beds, innervation of sweat glands and kidney, especially the juxtaglomerular apparatus controlling renin release), and behavioral response (drinking) all play important roles in this process. Disorders of the release of vasopressin, by neurons whose cell bodies are located in the supraoptic and paraventricular nuclei, are discussed in Ch. 75 and 202.2. Coordinated central disorders of fluid regulation are rare.

HYPERNATREMIA, HYPEROSMOLALITY, ABSENCE OF THIRST. Neurogenic hypernatremia is a rare disorder marked by impairment of the normal responses to osmolar stimuli. Hence, there is a deficit in vasopressin response to increased sodium and osmolality and an absence or relative deficiency of thirst. Vasopressin response to hypovolemia may be maintained, and there is preservation of habitual drinking of water (often related to meals) which may be sufficient to maintain serum osmolality under normal conditions. During hot weather, when there is increased loss of water through evaporation of sweat, patients often fail to increase their water consumption adequately and may suffer attacks of fatigue, fever, muscle cramps and tenderness, and even myoglobinuria (associated with hypokalemia). With serum sodium in excess of 180 mEq per liter, patients may experience confusion or even become stuporous, and some may die.

The hypothalamic injury giving rise to essential hypernatremia has been accurately localized in only a few cases but in all of these seems to involve the preoptic area in the region of the anteroventral third ventricle. Treatment consists of training the patient to drink adequate amounts of fluids, particularly during hot weather. Spironolactone, chlorpropamide, and thiazide diuretics have been used to reduce serum sodium and increase potassium. During an attack of severe hypernatremia, when it becomes necessary to provide intravenous fluid and potassium supplementation, it is important not to reduce serum sodium by more than 20 mEq per liter per day. More rapid correction has been associated with central pontine myelinolysis, which may leave the patient quadriplegic.

HYPERDIPSIA, HYPONATREMIA, AND WATER INTOXICATION. Excessive water drinking in the absence of either hypovolemia or serum hyperosmolality is termed primary hyperdipsia and must be distinguished from the compensatory hyperdipsias of diabetes insipidus, diabetes mellitus, and polyuric renal failure. In the absence of inappropriate vasopressin secretion, symptoms of water intoxication, such as stupor, delirium, or convulsions, are infrequent. Most severe hyperdipsia occurs in persons who have psychiatric disturbances. We have seen only one case of primary hyperdipsia, in a patient who had suffered an attack of encephalitis involving the hypothalamus during childhood.

PAROXYSMAL HYPONATREMIA. Many of the patients with paroxysmal hypothermia (see above) suffer simultaneous hyponatremia, which may be sufficiently severe (serum sodium < 110 mEq per liter) to cause symptoms of confusion or even convulsions. The serum sodium is regulated around the reduced set-point but may respond to fluid restriction.

Central Reproductive Disorders

Reproductive hormonal control, behavior, and the associated autonomic responses are controlled by poorly defined mechanisms in the medial basal hypothalamus overlying the pituitary stalk. To the extent that it relies upon control of blood flow in specific vascular beds, the autonomic regulation of sexual function must be coordinated with control of body temperature and fluid balance. The change in body temperature that accompanies ovulation and the fluid shifts seen in the perimenstrual period in women are examples of this integration.

Reproductive endocrine disorders are covered in Ch. 202.1 and 208.1. Male erectile function, which is dependent upon sacral parasympathetic innervation of the penis, may be affected by diseases of the peripheral autonomic nervous system (see above) as well as psychogenic factors acting at the level of the forebrain. Diagnosis and treatment of male sexual dysfunction is discussed in Ch. 209.

Arousal Disorders

The function of the autonomic nervous system is to augment the activity of various organ systems to deal with perturbations of internal homeostasis. Of all the body's organs, the single most important one to activate during an external threat is the brain. The ascending activating system, running from the brain stem reticular formation to the diencephalon, increases the responsiveness of the forebrain to external stimuli and may be considered a cerebral component of the autonomic system. Ch. 393, 394, and 396 describe the details of altered states of consciousness. We discuss here briefly disorders associated with lesions of the ascending arousal system. Sleep disorders are discussed in Ch. 397.

HYPERSOMNOLENCE. Following lesions of the ascending activating system at the level of the rostral brain stem, there is typically impairment of level of consciousness acutely. After a few weeks, the forebrain recovers spontaneous wake-sleep cycles. Prolonged sleeplike stupor lasting longer than a few weeks is seen only when lesions involve the posterior diencephalon. It is not clear whether this continued somnolence results from injury to the thalamus, to the hypothalamus, or to the connections of these structures. Methylphenidate, amphetamine, and bromocriptine have been used in these patients, with some anecdotal reports of success.

INSOMNIA. Sleep is an active process, requiring the participation of hypnogenic influences arising from the lower brain stem and serotoninergic neurons in the midbrain raphe. We have seen one patient in whom destruction of the medulla, below the level of the ascending activating system, resulted in a chronically wakeful state. Lesions of the preoptic area may also cause a decrease in sleep, which is closely related to a deficit in thermoregulation.

Peripheral Autonomic Disorders

Lefkowitz RL, Hoffman BB, Taylor P: Neurohumoral transmission: The autonomic and somatic motor neuron systems. *In* Gilman AG, Rall TW, Nies AS, Taylor P: The Pharmacological Basis of Therapeutics. New York, Pergamon, 1990, p 84. *A thorough review of peripheral autonomic organization and neurotransmission.*

McGuire EJ: The innervation and function of the lower urinary tract. J Neurosurg 65:278, 1986. *A thoughtful review of the physiology and pathophysiology of micturition.*

McLeod JG, Tuck RR: Disorders of the autonomic nervous system: Part 1. Pathophysiology and clinical features. Ann Neurol 21:419, 1987. *A recent review of autonomic physiology and pathophysiology.*

McLeod JG, Tuck RR: Disorders of the autonomic nervous system: Part 2. Investigation and treatment. Ann Neurol 21:519, 1987. *A guide to pharmacologic testing and treatment of autonomic dysfunction.*

Schwartzman RJ: Reflex sympathetic dystrophy. Curr Opin Neurol Neurosurg 6:531, 1993. *A review of the pathophysiology and clinical aspects of reflex sympathetic dystrophy.*

Central Autonomic Disorders

Loewy AD, Spyer KM: Central Regulation of Autonomic Functions. New York, Oxford Press, 1990. *A comprehensive series of reviews on the central components of the autonomic nervous system.*

Plum F, van Uitert R: Non-endocrine diseases and disorders of the hypothalamus. Res Publ Assoc Res Nerv Ment Dis 56:415, 1977. *A comprehensive review of the integrative disorders of autonomic function.*

Quane KA: Mutations in the ryanodine receptor gene in central core disease and malignant hyperthermia. Nature Genetics 5:51, 1993. *An analysis of the genetics of malignant hyperthermia.*

Saper CB: Hypothalamus. *In* Pearlman AL, Collins RC: Neurobiology of Disease. New York, Oxford Press, 1990, p 197. *A review of hypothalamic regulation of integrated functions and their disorders.*

Saper CB, Breder CD: The neurologic basis of fever. N Engl J Med, 330:1880, 1994. *A review of the mechanisms of fever and hyperthermia.*

Talman WT: Cardiovascular regulation and lesions of the central nervous system. Ann Neurol 18:1, 1985. *A review of central control of the circulation and the effects of nervous system lesions on cardiac arrhythmias and blood pressure control.*

403 THE SPECIAL SENSES
Robert W. Baloh

403.1 Smell and Taste

Approximately 2 million American adults suffer from disorders of taste and smell, yet there is relatively little information available on how to evaluate or treat these patients. These disorders have been neglected because they are seldom fatal and, unlike abnormalities of vision and hearing, are not considered serious handicaps. Chemosensory disorders, however, often reduce the enjoyment and quality of life and are important to patients who suffer from them. Disorders of taste interfere with digestion because taste stimulants alter salivary and pancreatic flow, gastric contractions, and intestinal motility. Smell also contributes to the anticipation and ingestion of food because much of what we taste derives from olfactory stimulation during ingestion and chewing. The inability to detect noxious tastes and odors can result in food- or gas poisoning, particularly in elderly subjects. In the extreme, chemosensory disorders can lead to overwhelming stress, anorexia, and depression.

ANATOMY. The sensory receptor for taste, the taste bud, is made up of approximately 50 cells arranged to form a pear-shaped organ. The life span of these cells is about 10 days, and they are constantly being renewed from dividing epithelial cells surrounding the bud. Taste buds are located on the tongue, soft palate, pharynx, larynx, epiglottis, uvula, and the upper one third of the esophagus. The taste buds located on the anterior two thirds of the tongue and on the palate are innervated by the seventh cranial nerve. The ninth cranial nerve innervates the posterior one third of the tongue and the folds or clefts on the lateral border of the tongue. The ninth and tenth nerves innervate taste buds in the pharynx. Afferent signals from the taste buds project to the nucleus of the solitary tract in the medulla and then via a series of relays to the thalamus and postcentral somatosensory cerebral cortex. Free nerve endings of the fifth cranial nerve are found on the tongue and in the oral cavity, and lesions involving these pathways also can alter taste perception.

Olfactory receptors lie in a roughly dime-sized area of specialized pigmented epithelium that arches along the superior aspect of each side of the nasal mucosa. Specialized bipolar sensory cells in this region thrust short receptor hairs into the overlying mucosa to detect aromatic molecules as they dissolve. As with taste buds, the specialized receptor portion of the bipolar neuron undergoes continuous renewal, turning over approximately every 30 days. Thin axons of the bipolar neurons course through small holes in the cribriform plate of the ethmoid bone to form connections in the overlying olfactory bulb on the ventral surface of the frontal lobe. From here second- and third-order neurons project directly and indirectly to the prepiriform cortex and parts of the amygdaloid complex of both sides of the brain, representing the primary olfactory cortex.

PATHOPHYSIOLOGY OF CHEMOSENSORY DISORDERS. Disorders of taste and smell can be divided into local, systemic, and neurologic (Table 403–1). The taste buds and the specialized receptor portion of the bipolar olfactory cells are constantly being renewed, and the process of renewal can be affected by nutritional, metabolic, and hormonal states, therapeutic radiation, drugs, and age. For example, with interruption of mitosis by antiproliferative agents, a return of normal taste function takes a minimum of 10 days, while a return to normal olfactory function takes more than 30 days. Numerous local conditions such as colds and allergies, chronic sinusitis, and nasal polyposis can influence the sense of smell by restricting airway patency. Accidental blows to the head can shear the fine axons of the bipolar olfactory neurons, resulting in loss of smell. Lesions of the fifth, seventh *(chorda tympani)*, and ninth nerves can lead to disordered taste sensation. Olfactory and gustatory disturbances can serve as important diagnostic signs for focal neurologic lesions (e.g., frontal lobe tumors). Hallucinations of smell and taste occur with epileptogenic lesions affecting the mesial temporal lobe and insular region, respectively. Finally, olfactory disturbances and hallucinations occur with a number of psychiatric illnesses (particularly depressive illness and schizophrenia).

EXAMINATION OF TASTE AND SMELL. Olfaction can be tested grossly at the bedside with a few easily recognized odors such as coffee, chocolate, and the roselike aroma of the compound phenylethyl alcohol. (Avoid nasal irritants.) Each nostril is tested separately to determine whether the problem is unilateral or bilateral. Gustatory sensation is typically tested with weak solutions of sugar, salt, and acetic acid, or vinegar. The patient must keep his tongue protruded and respond to questions either by nodding the head or pointing to names of the tastes written on cards. The anterior two thirds and posterior one third of the tongue should be tested separately.

COMMON CAUSES OF LOSS OF SMELL AND TASTE. The most frequently encountered causes of loss of smell are local obstructive disease, viral infections, head injuries that sever the neurons crossing through the cribriform plate, and normal aging. Patients can lose their sense of smell not only from chronic allergies and sinusitis but also from the nasal sprays and drops that they use to treat these conditions. The most common cause of loss of the sense of taste is drug ingestion, particularly antirheumatic and antiproliferative drugs and drugs containing sulfhydryl groups in their molecular structure, such as penicillamine and captopril. Patients with poor dental hygiene commonly complain of distortions of taste. Many of the systemic disorders listed in Table 403–1 probably have their effect by decreasing the rate of turnover of sensory receptors on the tongue and olfactory epithelia. Disturbances of smell and taste in malnourished patients have been attributed to specific deficiencies in vitamins and minerals, such as zinc. However, it is possible that the loss of protein and calorie intake impairs the functioning of taste buds and olfactory cells in the same manner that it impairs the regeneration of intestinal epithelia. Viral illnesses such as influenza and viral hepatitis produce disorders of both taste and smell. The loss of olfactory sensation after viral illnesses may be due to scarring of the subepithelial tissue and the replacement of

TABLE 403–1. COMMON CAUSES OF LOSS OF TASTE AND SMELL

	Taste	Smell
Local	Radiation therapy	Allergic rhinitis, sinusitis, nasal polyposis, bronchial asthma
Systemic	Cancer, renal failure, hepatic failure, nutritional deficiency (B_3, zinc), Cushing syndrome, hypothyroidism, diabetes mellitus, infection (influenza), drugs (antirheumatic and antiproliferative)	Renal failure, hepatic failure, nutritional deficiency (B_{12}), Cushing syndrome, hypothyroidism, diabetes mellitus, infection (viral hepatitis, influenza), drugs (nasal sprays, antibiotics)
Neurologic	Bell's palsy, familial dysautonomia, multiple sclerosis	Head trauma, multiple sclerosis, Parkinson's disease, frontal tumor

olfactory epithelium with respiratory epithelium. Multifocal neurologic disorders such as multiple sclerosis can affect the central olfactory and gustatory pathways at multiple levels, and therefore abnormalities of taste and smell are common in such patients. Treatment, other than avoiding drugs known to affect taste or smell, is unsatisfactory.

Estrem SA, Renner G: Disorders of smell and taste. Otolaryngol Clin North Am 20:133, 1987. *Concise clinical review.*

Schiffman SS: Taste and smell in disease. N Engl J Med 308:1275, 1337, 1983. *A well-referenced two-part short review.*

Taste and smell disorders: parts 1 and 2. Ear Nose Throat J 68:286, 291, 297, 316, 331, 352, 354, 362, 373, 386, 393, 398, 1989. *Two issues devoted to diagnosis and management.*

403.2 Neuro-ophthalmology

The mechanistic understanding of vision impairment along with disturbances of pupillary and oculomotor control lies close to the heart of diagnosing neurologic disorders. Diseases of the eye itself are further considered in Part XXV.

VISION

One of the most difficult diagnostic problems is vision loss that cannot be explained by obvious abnormalities of the eye. In order to properly evaluate such a patient the examining physician must be familiar with the anatomy and physiology of the afferent visual system. The afferent visual pathways cross at right angles to the major ascending sensory and descending motor systems of the cerebral hemispheres and in their anterior portion are intimately related to the vascular and bony structures at the base of the brain. Not surprisingly, localization of lesions within the afferent visual pathways has great localizing value in neurologic diagnosis.

ANATOMY OF THE VISUAL PATHWAYS. Light entering the eye falls on the retinal rods and cones, which transduce the stimulus into neural impulses to be transmitted to the brain. The distribution of visual function across the retina takes a pattern of concentric zones increasing in sensitivity toward the center, the fovea. The fovea consists of a "rod-free" central grouping of approximately 100,000 slender cones. The ganglion cells subserving these cones send their axons directly to the temporal aspect of the optic disk, forming the papillomacular bundle. Axons originating from ganglion cells in the temporal retina must curve above and below the papillomacular bundle, forming dense arcuate bands.

The arteries supplying the optic nerve and retina both derive from branches of the ophthalmic artery. The central retinal artery approaches the eye along each optic nerve and pierces the inferior aspect of the dural sheath about 1 cm behind the globe to enter the center of the nerve. The artery emerges in the fundus at the center of the nerve head, from which it nourishes most of the retina by superior, medial, inferior, and lateral branches. Anastomotic branches derived from the choroidal and posterior ciliary arteries supply the nerve head itself and the macular region. Venous drainage from the retina and nerve head flows primarily via the central retinal vein, whose course of exit from the eye parallels that of the entry of the artery. The venous anatomy explains why inflammatory lesions of or adjacent to the optic nerve head cause venous distention and ipsilateral papilledema (optic neuritis), whereas inflammation lying posterior to the point where the vein leaves the nerve produces only visual loss without swelling of the nerve head (retrobulbar neuritis).

What each eye "sees" is termed its visual field (Fig. 403–1). The nasal side of the left eye and the temporal side of the right eye see the left side of the world, and the upper half of each retina sees the lower half of the world. Behind the eye, the optic nerve passes through the optic foramen and sphenoid bone to reach the optic chiasm. In the chiasm, nerves from the nasal half of each retina decussate and join the fibers from the temporal half of the contralateral retina. From the chiasm, the optic tracts pass around the cerebral peduncles to reach the lateral geniculate ganglia of either side. At the level of the geniculus, fibers serving corresponding points in each retinal half visual field lie adjacent to each other, and this proximity is maintained in the subsequent relay to the calcarine cortex. The geniculocalcarine radiation initially fans out into superolat-

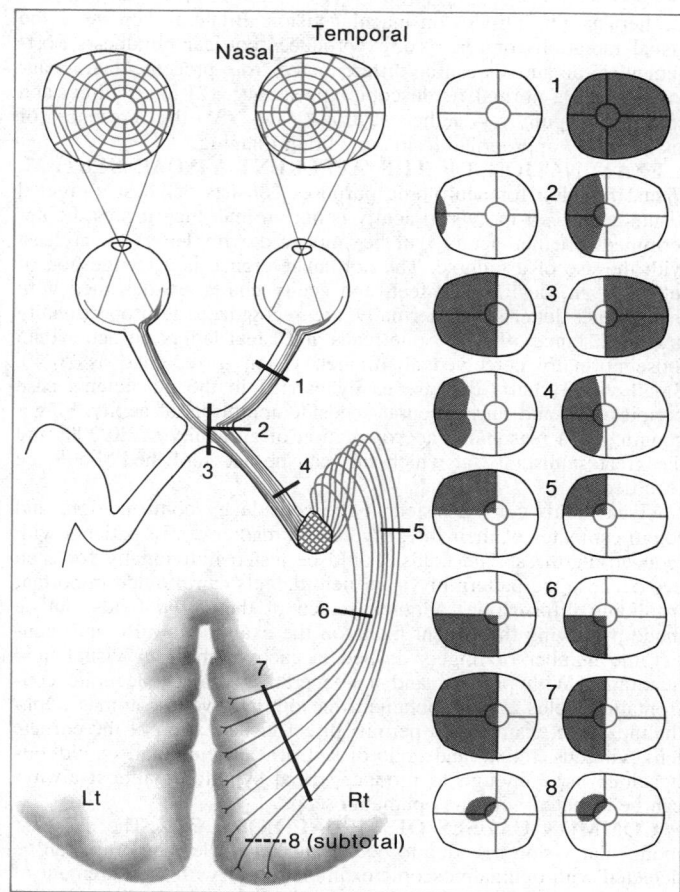

FIGURE 403–1. Visual fields that accompany damage to the visual pathways. 1. Optic nerve: Unilateral amaurosis. 2. Lateral optic chiasm: Grossly incongruous, incomplete (contralateral) homonymous hemianopia. 3. Central optic chiasm: Bitemporal hemianopia. 4. Optic tract: Incongruous, incomplete homonymous hemianopia. 5. Temporal (Meyer's) loop of optic radiation: Congruous partial or complete (contralateral) homonymous superior quadrantanopia. 6. Parietal (superior) projection of the optic radiation: Congruous partial or complete homonymous inferior quadrantanopia. 7. Complete parieto-occipital interruption of optic radiation: Complete congruous homonymous hemianopia with psychophysical shift of foveal point often sparing central vision, giving "macular sparing." 8. Incomplete damage to visual cortex: Congruous homonymous scotomas, usually encroaching at least acutely on central vision.

eral and inferolateral projections, the latter passing around the lateral ventricle and for a short distance into the temporal lobe (Meyer's loop) before turning posteriorly to head for the striate cortex of the occipital lobe. At the occipital pole, the striate cortex (Area 17) lies along the superior and inferior bands of the calcarine fissure, with macular fibers projecting most posteriorly to the occipital pole and more peripheral retinal projections lying more anteriorly.

LOCALIZATION OF LESIONS WITHIN THE VISUAL PATHWAYS. Monocular vision loss is due to a lesion of one eye or its retina or optic nerve. Binocular visual loss, on the other hand, can result from disease located anywhere in the visual pathways from the retinae to the occipital poles. Lesions involving or compressing the optic chiasm produce nonhomonymous visual abnormalities that affect the unilateral visual fields incongruously (e.g., the bitemporal hemianopia illustrated by Lesion 3 in Fig. 403–1). Optic tract abnormalities are comparatively rare but produce characteristic visual changes. The fibers serving identical points in the homonymous half fields do not fully commingle in the anterior optic tract, so lesions encroaching on this structure produce incongruous and usually incomplete homonymous hemianopias. Lesions on the geniculate ganglia, visual radiations, or visual cortex produce congruent hemianopic field defects that may go unrecognized unless the hemianopia intrudes on macular vision. Bilateral damage to the visual radiations or optic cortex produces cortical blindness. Postgeniculate amaurosis can be differentiated from pregeniculate amaurosis by (1) a normal funduscopic appearance, (2) intact direct and consensual pupillary light reactions, and (3) the presence of anatomically appropriate lesions by brain imaging.

EXAMINATION OF THE AFFERENT VISUAL SYSTEM. Visual function for neurologic purposes consists of "best corrected visual acuity." If the visual acuity is not normal, then it must be determined whether acuity can be improved with lenses or at least with the use of a pinhole. The normal reference is a recognition of letters at an idealized 20 feet, and acuity charts are designed with even larger letters that normally are recognized at proportionally greater distances. Thus, if one reads at 20 feet letters no better than those normally perceived at 40 feet, vision is recorded as 20/40. Small visual charts that are easily carried in the physician's case permit quick and fairly accurate bedside appraisals of acuity. Finger counting is a reasonable approximation of an acuity of 20/200, and the greatest distance at which this can be accomplished should be recorded.

Visual fields can be tested at the bedside by confrontation, and rough estimates of their integrity can be made even in patients with reduced alertness. The fields should be tested individually for each eye because the pattern of visual field defects can provide important localizing information. A quick screen of the visual fields can be made by having the patient fixate on the examiner's nose and identify the number of fingers flashed in each of the four visual field quadrants. With practice and a cooperative subject, accurate confrontation fields can be obtained that outline even scotomas. Ophthalmoscopic examination permits direct visualization of the cornea, lens, vitreous, retina, and optic disk. Corneal, lenticular, or vitreous opacities large enough to produce visual symptoms almost always can be detected with the ophthalmoscope.

COMMON CAUSES OF VISUAL LOSS. Eye. The cause of monocular vision loss due to ocular and retinal lesions often can be detected with ophthalmoscopic examination or with measurement of intraocular pressure. *Glaucoma* caused by impaired absorption of the aqueous humor results in a high intraocular pressure that usually produces gradual visual loss, "halos" seen around illuminated lamps, and, often, pain and redness in the affected eye. Infrequently, rapid vision loss can occur with few premonitory symptoms. Diagnosis comes from the tonometric measurement of a high intraocular pressure and may be suspected by palpating an abnormally firm globe and observing a deep, pale optic cup and attenuated blood vessels. *Retinal tears and detachments* give rise to unilateral distortions of the visual image seen as sudden angulations or curves of objects containing straight lines (metamorphopsia). *Hemorrhages* into the vitreous humor or unilateral *infections* or *inflammatory lesions* of the retina can produce scotomas that in all ways resemble those resulting from primary disease of the central visual pathway.

Binocular vision loss due to retinal disease in younger subjects is usually due to *heredodegenerative conditions.* Vascular diseases, diabetes, idiopathic (senile) macular degeneration, and bilateral retinal detachments are causes in older age groups. In the *pigmentary retinal degenerations* visual loss begins peripherally and proceeds centrally, and often very slowly, before acuity (central vision) is impaired. By contrast, *macular degenerations* impair central vision early in their course. Most of the retinal degenerations produce characteristic and recognizable ophthalmoscopic appearances. With pigmentary degenerations the visual fields shrink progressively in size. With macular degenerations, on the other hand, the fields show noncongruent central scotomas.

Optic Nerve. Acute or subacute monocular vision loss due to optic nerve disease is most commonly produced by demyelinating disorders, vascular obstruction, or neoplasm. Demyelinating disease of the nerve head (*optic neuritis* or *papillitis*) produces papilledema along with loss of central vision in the affected eye only; subjectively unrecognized scotomas sometimes may be found in the other eye. Demyelination in the optic nerve behind where the retinal vein emerges (*retrobulbar neuritis*) initially leaves a normal-looking disk but a central or paracentral scotoma. With chronic demyelinating disorders the optic disk becomes pale and atrophic. More than 50% of patients who initially present with optic neuritis or retrobulbar

TABLE 403–2. COMMON CAUSES OF TRANSIENT MONOCULAR VISION LOSS

Category/ (Typical Duration)	Causes	Differential Features
Thromboembolism (1–5 min)	Atherosclerosis	Other atherosclerotic vascular disease, associated crossed hemiparesis, angiography (carotid atheromata)
	Cardiac	Valvular disease, mural thrombi, atrial fibrillation, recent MI
	Blood dyserasia	Blood tests + for sickle cell anemia, macroglobulinemia, multiple myeloma, polycythemia, etc.
Vasospasm (5–30 min)	Migraine	Ipsilateral headache, other classic aura, and family history
Vascular compression (few sec)	Papilledema	Precipitated by position change, Valsalva maneuver, or pressure waves
	Tumor	Associated slowly progressive monocular visual loss
Vasculitis (1–5 min)	Temporal arteritis	Associated headache, polymyalgia rheumatica, palpable temporal artery, elevated sed rate

neuritis go on to develop typical symptoms and signs of multiple sclerosis. Vascular lesions produce either total amaurosis or a sector field defect consistent with an intraocular arterial occlusion (*ischemic optic neuropathy*). The common causes of transient monocular vision loss and their differential features are listed in Table 403–2. *Tumors* invading the optic nerve or space-occupying lesions compressing it anywhere between the orbit and the chiasm cause gradually decreasing central vision (intrinsic or far advanced lesions) or a sector defect of the peripheral visual field. With such chronic lesions the affected optic nerve becomes visibly atrophic.

Acute binocular vision loss due to bilateral optic nerve disease is most often caused by demyelinating disease and less frequently by optic nerve or retinal vascular disease or by toxic or nutritional optic neuropathies. In younger persons and those lacking a clear history of toxic exposures demyelinating lesions overwhelmingly predominate (optic neuritis). Symptoms are of abrupt or subacute onset with visual blurring or loss of acuity, which may progress rapidly to blindness within hours or days. There may be pain about the eyes, particularly on eye movement.

Papilledema resulting from increased intracranial pressure occasionally causes vision loss under one of three circumstances: (1) acute transient episodes of amaurosis lasting a few seconds and attributable to acute increases in intracranial pressure (plateau waves) that interfere with retinal venous drainage into the cavernous sinus or with vascular irrigation of the occipital lobe; (2) acute bilateral sustained amaurosis following abrupt surgical relief of longstanding, severely increased, intracranial pressure (a rare cause); and (3) progressive loss of peripheral vision with longstanding, severe papilledema, presumably owing to pressure atrophy of the most peripherally lying fibers in the tightly sheathed optic nerve. Table 403–3 gives the main differential points between papilledema and optic neuritis. Subacute or chronic binocular vision loss due to optic nerve disease results mainly from *toxic nutritional* causes and the *inherited optic atrophies.* The latter sometimes accompany spinocerebellar degeneration or selectively affect the optic nerves in

TABLE 403–3. DIFFERENTIATION OF OPTIC NEURITIS FROM PAPILLEDEMA

	Optic Neuritis	Papilledema
Central-cecocentral vision loss	Present	Absent
Distribution	Usually unilateral	Usually bilateral
Ocular pain on movement	Present	Absent
Direct light reflex	± Reduced	Intact
CT and MRI scan of head	Normal	Often abnormal
Visual evoked responses	Abnormal	Normal
Lumbar puncture pressure	Normal	Elevated

both juveniles and adults (Leber's forms). With either cause, visual loss is moderate or severe and primarily or initially affects central vision; ophthalmoscopy shows mild to moderate primary optic atrophy.

Chiasm and Optic Tract. Patients with lesions of the optic chiasm and optic tract are often unaware of visual impairment until the deficit encroaches on central vision in one or both eyes. Intrinsic or extrinsic neoplasms and parachiasmal arterial aneurysms are the most common lesions in this location. *Gliomas* that arise in the chiasm are rare in adulthood but, when they occur, impair central vision early. Extrinsic space-occupying lesions compressing the chiasm can arise from the superior, lateral, or inferior aspect and include *dysgerminomas, craniopharyngiomas, pituitary adenomas, meningiomas* arising from the sphenoid bones, and large *aneurysms* of the carotid artery. The diagnosis rests on finding the characteristic visual field abnormalities (bitemporal hemianopsia for chiasm and incongruous homonymous hemianopsia for optic tract lesions) and identifying the specific lesion with computed tomography (CT) or magnetic resonance imaging (MRI). Pituitary apoplexy (due to acute hemorrhage into the gland, occurring most frequently in patients with unrecognized pituitary adenomas) can result in sudden vision loss. Prompt neurosurgical intervention under steroid coverage is required for most patients.

Visual Radiations and Occipital Cortex. Lesions involving the postgeniculate visual pathways most often result from *vascular damage, traumatic injuries, neoplasms* or, rarely, *inflammatory* or *degenerative disorders* involving the cerebral white matter. Their localization can be deduced by the resulting visual field defects. Vascular disease of the occipital lobes is the most common cause of homonymous visual field defects in the middle-aged and elderly population. Typically, the onset of such field defects is associated with other signs and symptoms of transient ischemic episodes in the vertebrobasilar distribution. Bilateral damage to the visual radiations or occipital cortex produces *cortical blindness.* Most often, there are other signs of vascular disease including focal neurologic findings. *Anton's syndrome* refers to cortical blindness with denial of visual defect. Affected patients not only deny the fact that they are blind but confabulate details of their visual environment from memory. Autopsy studies reveal lesions of the medial, temporal, and parietal lobes as well as the calcarine cortex. *Tumors* are rarely confined to the limits of the occipital lobes; therefore neurologic deficits with occipital tumors are rarely only visual.

PUPILLARY CONTROL

The neuromechanisms that control pupil size and reactivity are complex, yet they can be evaluated by simple clinical procedures. The diameter of the pupil is determined by the antagonistic actions of the iris sphincter and dilator muscles with the latter playing a minor role. If the sphincter muscle is severed or ruptured it does not retract toward one quadrant but rather continues to function except in the altered segment. Therefore, the pupillary response can be evaluated even in the presence of significant damage to the iris.

ANATOMY AND LOCALIZATION OF LESIONS WITHIN PUPILLARY PATHWAYS. The size of the pupil is governed by tonic balance between sympathetic and parasympathetic innervation of the muscles of the iris. Sympathetic stimulation dilates the pupil, and parasympathetic stimulation constricts it. In the normal resting state, light entering the eye provides the major stimulus governing the size of the pupil (Fig. 403–2). Light activates the retinal rods and cones with maximal sensitivity in the macular area. The optic nerve fibers follow the crossed and uncrossed visual pathways to the pregeniculate portion of the optic tracts, where the receptor fibers for light diverge to the pretectal nucleus located at the midbrain diencephalic junction. Interneurons project from this nucleus to the Edinger-Westphal nuclei atop the midbrain third nerve complex of either side. From that point paired parasympathetic efferents leave the midbrain with the third nerves to travel in the interpeduncular space across the petroclinoid ligament and edge of the tentorium, where, after traversing the cavernous sinus, they enter the superior orbital fissure. In the orbit the parasympathetic efferents synapse in the ciliary ganglion from which short ciliary nerves enter the eye to reach the pupillary muscles.

The principal sympathetic control of the pupil originates in the ventral lateral hypothalamus (first-order neuron) from which fibers descend ipsilaterally to the lower brain stem tegmentum and thence to the cervical cord, where they lie superficially and synapse with the preganglionic neurons in the intermedial lateral column of the upper three thoracic segments. Preganglionic fibers (second-order neurons) emerge with the ventral roots of C8, T1, and T2, and ascend in the neck to synapse in the superior cervical ganglion adjacent to the base of the skull. Postganglionic (third-order neurons) pupillary fibers accompany the internal carotid artery through the

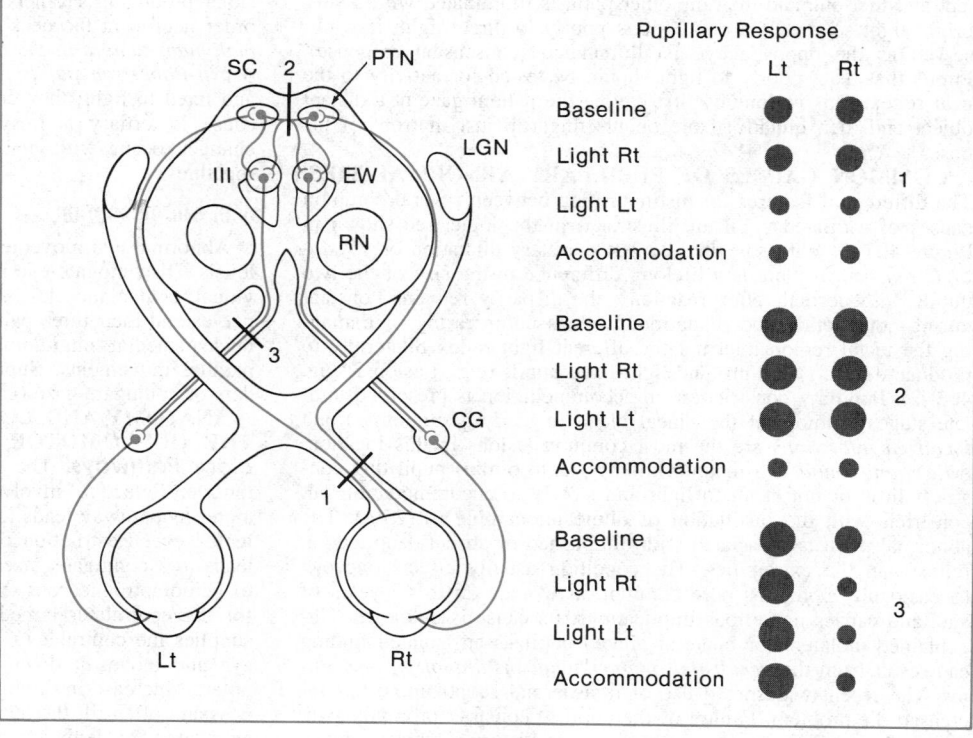

FIGURE 403–2. Pupillary responses associated with lesions of the (1) optic nerve, (2) pretectum, and (3) oculomotor nerve. SC = Superior colliculus; PTN = pretectal nucleus; EW = Edinger-Westphal nucleus; LGN = lateral geniculate nucleus; RN = red nucleus; CG = ciliary ganglion.

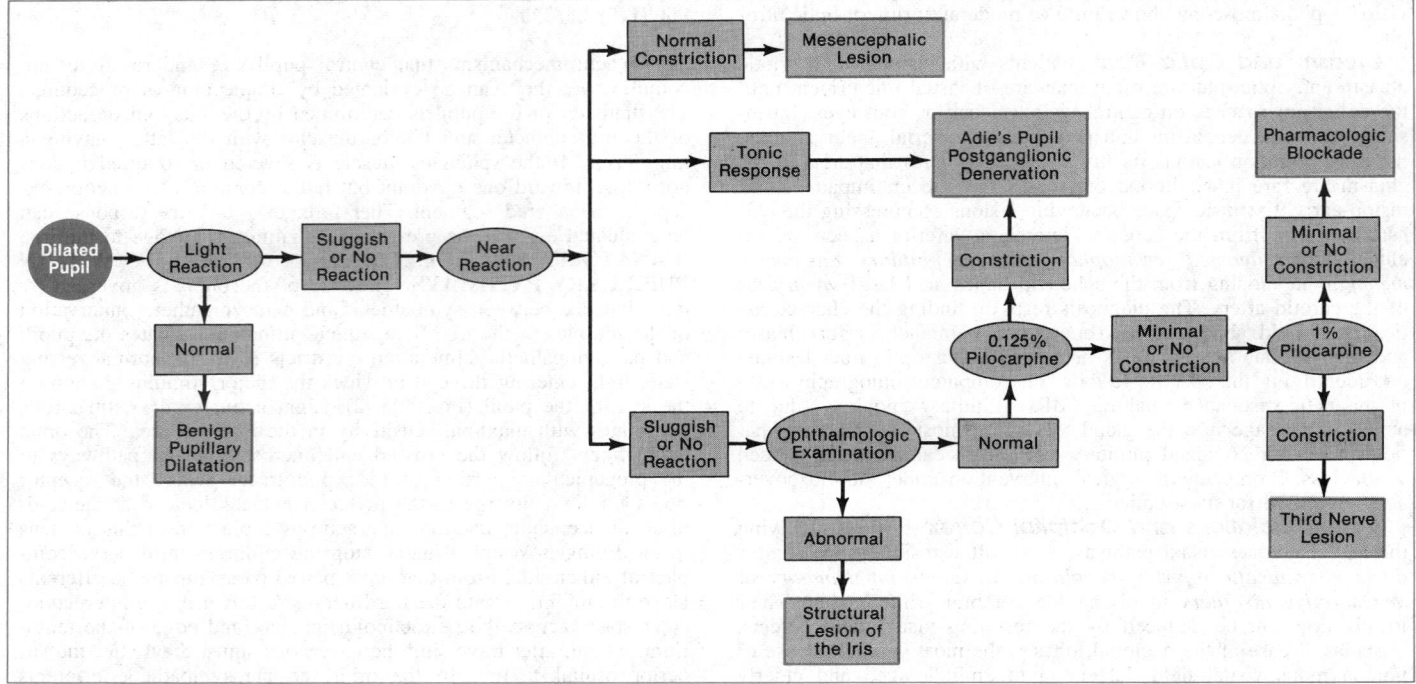

FIGURE 403–3. Evaluation of a dilated pupil.

skull, leaving it to follow the ophthalmic branch of the trigeminal nerve to reach the pupillodilator muscle of the eye.

Sympathetic paralysis of the eye with ptosis and miosis (Horner's syndrome) can result from lesions anywhere along the course of the pathway described above. Topical diagnosis is made best by identifying associated signs in the brain stem or neck or along the carotid artery.

EXAMINATION OF THE PUPIL. The pupillary response to light should be examined in a dimly lighted room, in which case the pupils are in a semidilated state. First, the size and symmetry of the pupils are assessed by shining a dim light onto the face from below so that both pupils are seen simultaneously in the indirect illumination. To test light reactivity, gaze is directed at a distant object and first one and then the other pupil is illuminated with a very bright light source. If a pupil reacts poorly to direct light, it is observed as the opposite eye is illuminated (consensual response). Pupils that react poorly to light should be tested for activity to the near reflex. This is done by first having the patient gaze at a distant object and then quickly fixate on his fingertip just in front of his nose.

COMMON CAUSES OF PUPILLARY ABNORMALITIES. The differential features for distinguishing between several common causes of a dilated pupil are illustrated in the logic tree shown in Figure 403–3. With so-called benign pupillary dilatation or *physiologic anisocoria* there is a lifelong difference in the size of the two pupils with normal reflex reactions; the disparity remains constant during constriction and dilatation. Lesions compressing or damaging the tectal region interrupt the afferent light reflex bilaterally to produce dilated (> 5 mm) and light-fixed pupils (e.g., Lesion 2, Fig. 403–2). Pupillary constriction on accommodation is preserved until late stages. Tumors of the pineal gland (e.g., dysgerminomas) and *localized infarctions* are the most common lesions in this location. *Adie's tonic pupil* is a medium-to-large (3 to 6 mm) pupil that constricts little or not at all to light and slowly to accommodation but constricts with the instillation of dilute pilocarpine (0.125%). The abnormal pupil is associated with diminished or absent deep tendon reflexes in the extremities. The condition usually affects one eye (occasionally both), is more common in women 25 to 45 years of age, and carries no serious implications. Its cause is unknown. Unexplained unilateral or bilateral dilated pupil as an isolated finding can result from the *accidental or intentional instillation of mydriatics.* The recent widespread use of transdermal scopolamine has increased the problem. Failure of the pupil to constrict promptly with pilocarpine (1%) gives the diagnosis if the history is unclear. Inter-

ruption of the emerging third nerve in the ventral midbrain or along the proximal part of its course produces a mid-dilated pupil 6 to 7 mm in diameter. Important causes of compression of the third nerve in this region are *aneurysms, neoplasia,* and *brain herniation* due to increased intracranial pressure. In nearly all cases the pupillary involvement is associated with other signs of third nerve involvement (see below). Rarely, compressive lesions such as a posterior communicating artery aneurysm can present with an isolated dilated pupil.

As noted above, the causes of *Horner syndrome* are numerous because of the long course of sympathetic innervation to the eye. It is unlikely that a patient with a central nervous system lesion will present with an isolated Horner syndrome. The most common lesions producing Horner syndrome involve the ascending second-order neuron in the neck or the extracranial postganglionic neuron; *malignant tumors in the apex of the lung* are by far most common. *Argyll-Robertson pupils* are small (1 to 2 mm), unequal, irregular, and fixed to light; they constrict to accommodation. Their principal cause is tertiary neurosyphilis, although partial Argyll-Robertson changes occur with diabetes and certain of the autonomic neuropathies.

OCULOMOTOR CONTROL

Abnormal eye movements can result from disturbances at several levels. Disconjugate eye movements result from lesions of the individual ocular muscles, the myoneural junctions, the oculomotor nerves and their three paired nuclei in the brain stem, and the internuclear medial longitudinal fasciculus (MLF) that yokes the eyes in parallel movements. Supranuclear lesions typically produce disorders of conjugate gaze (gaze palsies).

ANATOMY AND LOCALIZATION OF LESIONS WITHIN THE OCULOMOTOR PATHWAYS. *Nuclear and Internuclear Pathways.* The abducens nerve supplies the lateral rectus muscle. Selective involvement of the abducens nerve anywhere along its pathway leads to isolated weakness of abduction of the affected eye. Destruction of the abducens nucleus in the brain stem leads to a conjugate gaze paralysis (ipsilateral) because, in addition to oculomotor neurons, the nucleus contains interneurons destined for the contralateral medial rectus nucleus. The trochlear nucleus supplies the contralateral superior oblique muscle which intorts the eye and moves it down. Patients with superior oblique weakness note an increase in diplopia with head tilt toward the side of weakness and often tilt the head in the opposite direction. At rest there is slight upward deviation of the involved eye, and downward movement is impaired when the affected eye is turned in. The third cranial nerve supplies the remaining ocular muscles. Involvement of the third nerve nucleus in the midbrain always produces at least some bilateral oculomotor weakness; the superior rectus division of the nucleus supplies the contralateral superior rectus muscle (all other divisions supply ipsilateral muscles). Peripheral third nerve paralysis can result from lesions damaging the structure anywhere from its origin from the ventral midbrain to where it enters the orbit via the superior orbital fissure. Depending on its completeness, a third nerve palsy produces a widely dilated pupil, severe ptosis, and an externally deviated eye held in position by the unopposed contraction of the lateral rectus muscle. In such conditions, the continued trochlear action reveals itself by intorsion of the eye when the subject attempts to look down and in.

The MLF interconnects the abducens nucleus in the pons with the contralateral oculomotor nuclear complex in the midbrain. It terminates cephalad in the interstitial nucleus in the rostral midbrain and can be traced as far caudad as the thoracocervical region of the spinal cord (coordinating nuchal-ocular control). Lesions involving the MLF characteristically produce an internuclear ophthalmoplegia (INO) with which the eyes are conjugate in the primary position but disconjugate on lateral gaze. With a fully developed INO on lateral gaze away from the side of the lesion the contralateral eye abducts and shows nystagmus, whereas the ipsilateral adducting eye partially or completely fails to move nasally because of failure of ascending impulses to reach the third nerve nucleus. Adduction for convergence is usually relatively maintained. Upbeat gaze-evoked nystagmus typically occurs with INO.

Supranuclear Pathways. The pathway descending from the frontal eye fields in the frontal lobe regulates rapid voluntary eye movements *(saccades).* A signal from the frontal eye field activates a burst of firing in the contralateral horizontal gaze center in the paramedian pontine reticular formation. This high frequency burst (or pulse) of neuronal firing is transmitted directly to the nearby sixth nerve nucleus and via MLF to the contralateral third nerve nucleus. For voluntary vertical gaze both frontal eye fields send signals to the vertical gaze center in the pretectum (probably the interstitial nucleus of the MLF). Acute lesions involving a frontal eye field (e.g., hemorrhage or infarction) result in transient (24 to 72 hours) inability to direct the eyes contralaterally. Vertical eye movements are not affected by unilateral frontal lobe lesions. Bilateral damage to the frontal eye fields or their descending pathways may produce the inability to move the eyes voluntarily (horizontal or vertical) despite preserved reflex eye movements, a condition called *oculomotor apraxia.* Lesions involving the horizontal gaze center in the pons produce an ipsilateral paralysis of conjugate gaze and tonic deviation of the eyes to the contralateral hemiorbit. Lesions of the pretectum selectively impair vertical gaze with the vertical upgaze center being slightly rostral and dorsal to the vertical downgaze center.

Pathways descending from the parieto-occipital region of the two hemispheres subserve slow visual tracking or *smooth pursuit movements.* The exact location of these descending pursuit pathways is not completely known, but there are strong projections to the ipsilateral superior colliculus and ipsilateral pons. The cerebellar flocculus is also a critical relay station for smooth pursuit pathways. Lesions of the parieto-occipital region, pons, and cerebellum impair smooth pursuit and optokinetic slow phases when the target moves ipsilateral to the lesion. The *convergence* center is located in the rostral-dorsal midbrain near the vertical gaze center. Lesions in this region typically impair convergence and voluntary vertical gaze (particularly up-gaze). Pathways for cortical control of vergence have not been identified. The fourth supranuclear oculomotor control system, the *vestibulo-ocular reflex,* and its examination are discussed below.

EXAMINATION OF EYE MOVEMENTS. Fixation and gaze holding are tested by having the patient look center, right, left, up, and down. Each position should be held steady and unwavering with the observer documenting carefully abnormal movements or ocular disconjugacies. Each supranuclear oculomotor control system is examined separately. *Saccades* are tested by having the patient fixate alternately on two targets such as the examiner's finger and nose; the speed and accuracy are noted. *Smooth pursuit* is tested by slowly moving a target back and forth and up and down and observing the patient's ability to produce smooth tracking movements. It the target velocity is low (less than 30 degrees per second) normal subjects should be able to pursue without requiring catch-up

saccades. *Convergence* is tested by having the patient follow a target moving from far to near. The degree of normal convergence varies considerably and depends on the cooperation of the patient. A clear sign that the patient is attempting to converge is simultaneous pupillary constriction.

COMMON CAUSES OF ABNORMAL OCULOMOTOR CONTROL. *Strabismus.* The flow chart in Figure 403–4 outlines the logic for determining the common causes of strabismus. A comitant strabismus present since childhood is usually a benign *congenital disorder.* As noted earlier, latent congenital strabismus can become manifest in adulthood in association with a systemic illness. An acquired skew deviation (vertical displacement of the ocular axes) can result from any number of lesions involving the brain stem and has little localizing value. Noncomitant strabismus can result from restrictive disease of the orbit or from abnormal muscle or oculomotor nerve function. The presence of mechanical restriction is confirmed by the use of forced duction testing. (After a topical anesthetic is applied to the eye, the ophthalmologist grasps the muscle insertion with a large blunt-toothed forceps and identifies mechanical restriction.) Common causes of *orbital restrictive disease* include dysthyroid ophthalmopathy, orbital pseudotumor, trauma, and orbital mass lesions. Variable strabismus that increases with fatigue suggests the likelihood of *myasthenia gravis* (see Ch. 459). A Tensilon test can usually confirm the diagnosis. If both restrictive disease and myasthenia gravis have been excluded, most patients with noncomitant strabismus have processes affecting the oculomotor nuclei, their fascicles, or the cranial nerves themselves. Common causes of an *isolated third nerve palsy* in an adult include aneurysm, vascular occlusive disease (including diabetes mellitus), trauma, and neoplasm. Typically, but not always, third nerve lesions due to vascular disease spare the pupil. Vascular disease and trauma are by far the most common causes of *isolated trochlear nerve palsies.* The abducens nerve is particularly vulnerable to isolated traumatic involvement because of its long pathway outside the brain stem. Lesions at distant sites that produce increased intracranial pressure can lead to abducens nerve dysfunction producing a "false localizing sign." Other common causes of *isolated sixth nerve palsies* are vascular disease, trauma, and neoplasm. About one fourth of cases with cranial nerve palsies (third, fourth, or sixth nerves) remain undiagnosed.

Internuclear Ophthalmoplegia (INO). INO may be unilateral or bilateral, partial or complete, depending on the location of the lesion and the degree of damage to the MLF. *Demyelinating* and small *vascular lesions* are the most common cause of unilateral INO unaccompanied by other ocular palsies or brain-stem signs. Larger brain-stem lesions that damage one or more oculomotor nuclei plus the MLF often produce bizarre combinations of disconjugate eye movements coupled with nuclear oculomotor palsies. Myasthenia gravis can produce an ophthalmoparesis resembling INO owing to the greater involvement of the medial rectus compared to the lateral rectus. Demyelinating diseases are by far the most common causes of bilateral INO involvement.

Disorders of Conjugate Gaze. As noted earlier, infarction of the frontal cortex results in transient contralateral gaze paresis. Tumors and infarction of the paramedian pontine reticular formation produce ipsilateral horizontal gaze paralysis. With the so-called locked-in syndrome (secondary to basilar artery thrombosis) voluntary horizontal eye movements are absent; the patient's only remaining motor functions are vertical eye and lid movements. Lesions of the pretectum typically affect only vertical eye movements, although the descending pathways from the frontal eye fields to the horizontal gaze centers in the pons can also be affected. With the *dorsal midbrain syndrome* (Parinaud syndrome) patients present with a conjugate up-gaze paresis. When they attempt to make upward saccades they develop convergence retraction nystagmus. As noted earlier, impaired convergence and light–near dissociation of the pupillary reflexes are also part of the syndrome. The most common causes of the dorsal midbrain syndrome include tumors of the pineal gland (dysgerminomas), aqueductal stenosis, and localized infarction.

Nystagmus. Spontaneous nystagmus can be congenital or acquired. *Congenital nystagmus* typically has a high frequency and variable wave form (occasionally pendular) and is highly fixation-dependent. It is usually not associated with a structural brain lesion. The lifelong history confirms the diagnosis. Spontaneous nystagmus

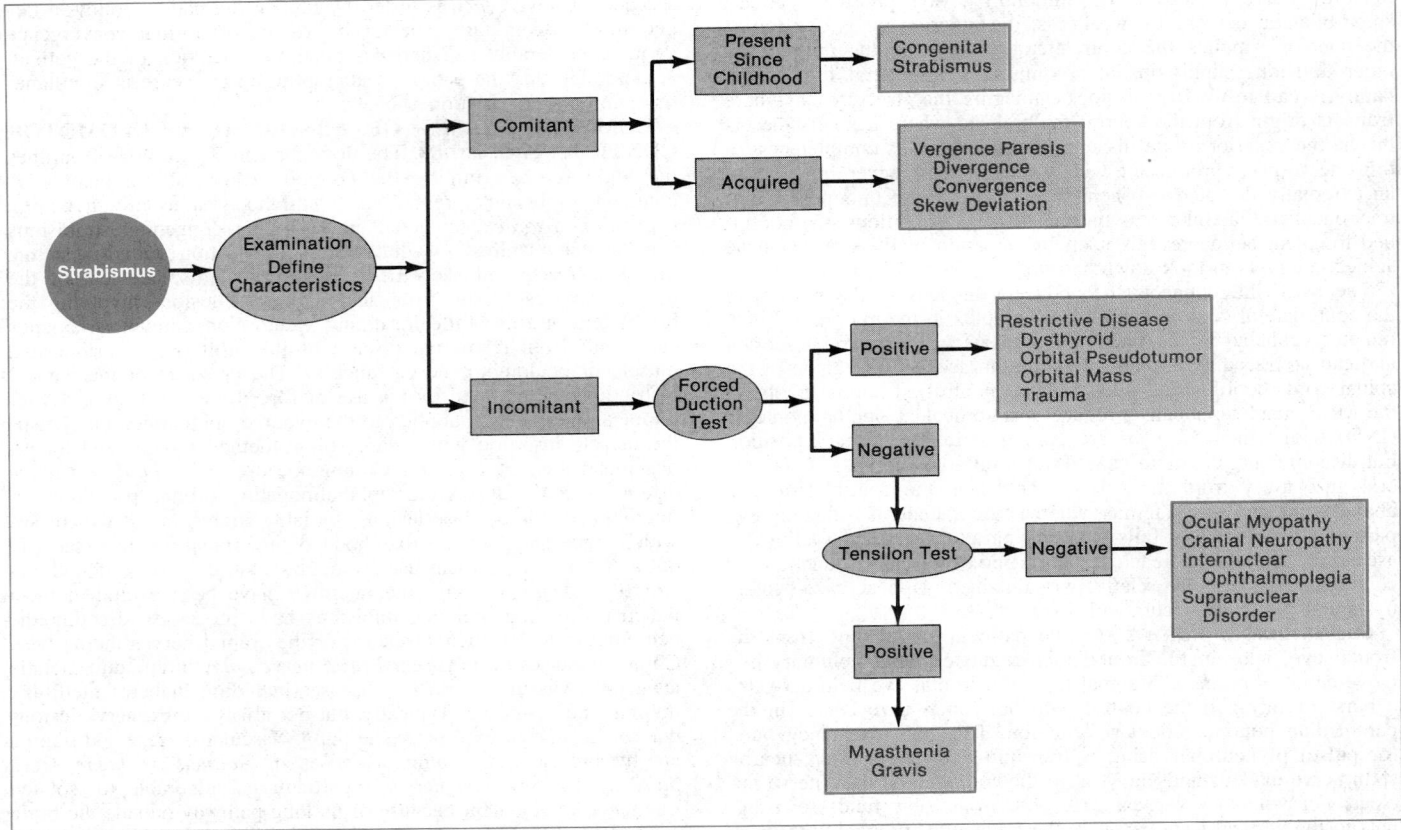

FIGURE 403–4. Diagnostic approach to strabismus.

due to a *peripheral vestibular* lesion (i.e., in the labyrinth or vestibular nerve) usually has combined horizontal and torsional components and is strongly inhibited with fixation (Table 403–4). Acquired persistent spontaneous nystagmus that is not inhibited by fixation indicates a lesion in the brain stem and/or cerebellum *(central vestibular)*. The latter is often purely vertical or horizontal because the vertical and horizontal vestibulo-ocular pathways separate beginning at the vestibular nuclei. Spontaneous *downbeat nystagmus* is commonly seen with lesions of the medulla or cervicomedullary junction (e.g., Arnold-Chiari malformation).

Gaze-evoked nystagmus is always in the direction of gaze and is usually present with and without fixation. It is most commonly produced by ingestion of *drugs* such as phenobarbital, phenytoin, alcohol, and diazepam. It can also occur in patients with such varied conditions as myasthenia gravis, multiple sclerosis, and cerebellar atrophy. Asymmetric horizontal gaze-evoked nystagmus indicates a structural brain-stem or cerebellar lesion (particularly at the cerebellopontine angle) with the lesion usually being on the side of the larger amplitude nystagmus. *Rebound nystagmus* is a type of gaze-evoked nystagmus that either disappears or reverses direction as the eccentric gaze position is held. When the eyes are returned to the primary position nystagmus occurs in the direction of the return saccade. Rebound nystagmus occurs in patients with cerebellar atrophy and focal structural lesions of the cerebellum; it is the only variety of nystagmus thought to be specific for cerebellar involvement. *Disconjugate gaze-evoked nystagmus* most commonly results from lesions of the MLF (see above), but it can also occur with other lesions of the brain stem involving the oculomotor nuclei. Positional nystagmus is discussed below.

Other Ocular Oscillations. *Ocular bobbing* consists of a fast conjugate downward eye movement followed by a slow return to the primary position. The phenomenon accompanies severe displacement or destruction of the pons or, much less often, metabolic CNS depression. *Ocular myoclonus* consists of continuous rhythmic pendular oscillations, most often vertical, with a rate of 2 to 5 beats per second. Often it accompanies palatal myoclonus and has a similar pathogenesis. *Square wave jerks* and *ocular flutter* consist of brief, intermittent, horizontal oscillations (saccades) arising from the primary gaze position. These types of ocular oscillation are most commonly seen with cerebellar disease but can also accompany more diffuse central nervous system disorders. *Opsoclonus* consists of rapid, chaotic, conjugate, repetitive, saccadic eye movements (dancing eyes). One type of opsoclonus accompanies cerebellar dysfunction, but the most chaotic varieties are associated with brain-stem encephalitis or the remote effects of systemic neoplasm, especially neuroblastoma in children. *Ocular dysmetria* refers to over- and undershooting of saccadic eye movements often followed by multiple attempts at refixation. It reflects cerebellar dysfunction.

TABLE 403–4. KEY DISTINGUISHING FEATURES OF PERIPHERAL AND CENTRAL TYPES OF SPONTANEOUS AND POSITIONAL NYSTAGMUS

Type of Nystagmus	Peripheral (End Organ and Nerve)	Central (Brain Stem and Cerebellum)
Spontaneous	Unidirectional, fast phase away from lesion, combined horizontal torsional, inhibited with fixation	Bidirectional or undirectional; often pure horizontal, vertical, or torsional; *not* inhibited with fixation
Static positional	Direction-fixed or direction-changing, inhibited with fixation	Direction fixed or direction-changing, *not* inhibited with fixation
Paroxysmal positional	Vertical-torsional occasionally horizontal-torsional, vertigo prominent, fatigability, latency	Often pure vertical, vertigo less prominent, no latency, nonfatigable

Burde RM, Savino PJ, Trobe JD: Clinical Decisions in Neuro-ophthalmology. St. Louis, CV Mosby, 1985. *Liberal use of flow charts to help the clinician answer the question, "Given the symptom and signs, what is the disease?"*

Glaser JS: Neuro-ophthalmology, 2nd ed. Hagerstown, MD, Harper & Row, 1990. *An excellent one-volume didactic introductory text.*

Leigh RJ, Zee DS: The Neurology of Eye Movement, 2nd ed. Philadelphia, F. A. Davis Company, 1991. *An up-to-date monograph that gives the clinical and physiologic details of modern investigations on ocular control.*

403.3 Hearing and Equilibrium

The neural pathways subserving hearing and those most important for equilibrium and spatial orientation are anatomically proximate in much of their course from their end organs in the inner ear to their termination in the superior portion of the temporal lobe. Because of the close anatomic linkage, disorders that affect hearing often affect equilibrium, and vice versa. For this reason they are considered together here. Despite their anatomic propinquity, however, substantial pathophysiologic differences make clinical examination of the two systems quite different. The auditory system is physiologically relatively isolated, so that its function and dysfunction can be tested independently of other neural systems. The vestibular system, in contrast, has many close physiologic links with the motor system (particularly the cerebellum, oculomotor system, and autonomic nervous system) and can be tested only indirectly by noting secondary effects on oculomotor and cerebellar functions. Abnormalities of the auditory system lead to only a few well-defined and unique symptoms (i.e., hearing loss or tinnitus). Abnormalities of the vestibular system can cause symptoms that mimic disorders of the other neural structures. Such symptoms include dizziness, ocular abnormalities (nystagmus), motor abnormalities (including ataxia or sudden falls), and autonomic abnormalities (including nausea, vomiting, and even syncope).

HEARING

ANATOMY AND PHYSIOLOGY OF HEARING. In normal hearing, sound waves are transmitted from the tympanic membrane via the three ossicles of the air-filled middle ear (air conduction) to the oval window and the basilar membrane of the fluid-sealed cochlea. The ossicles serve to increase the gain from the tympanum to oval window about 18-fold, compensating for the loss that sound waves moving from air to fluid would otherwise suffer. In the absence of this system, sound may reach the cochlea by vibration of the temporal bone (bone conduction) but with much less efficiency (approximately 60 dB loss). Hair cells lying along the cochlear basilar membrane detect the vibratory movement of that membrane and transduce vibration into nerve impulses. The nerve impulses are relayed via nerve cells that synapse at the base of hair cells and have their bodies in the spiral ganglion to the cochlear nucleus of the ipsilateral pontine tegmentum. The spiral cochlea mechanically analyzes the frequency content of sound. For high-frequency tones only sensory cells in the basilar region are activated, whereas for low-frequency tones all or nearly all sensory cells are activated. Therefore, with lesions of the cochlea and its afferent nerve the hearing levels for different frequencies are usually unequal, typically resulting in better hearing sensitivity for low-frequency than for high-frequency tones. Within the brain stem, auditory signals ascend from the ventral and dorsal cochlear nuclei to reach the superior olivary nuclei of both sides. Thus nervous system lesions central to the cochlear nucleus do not cause monaural hearing loss, and, conversely, unilateral central lesions do not cause deafness. From these structures the pathway projects by way of the lateral lemnisci to the inferior colliculi. Each inferior colliculus transmits to the other and to its ipsilateral medial geniculate body, which in turn sends the final projection to the transverse auditory gyrus lying in the superior portion of the ipsilateral temporal lobe.

The normal ear can detect sound frequencies ranging between 20 and 20,000 Hertz (Hz); the upper range drops off fairly rapidly with advancing age. The ear is most sensitive between 500 and 4000 Hz, which roughly corresponds to the frequency range most important for understanding speech. The hearing level in this range has several practical implications in terms of the degree of handicap and the potential for useful correction with amplification. A 30- to 40-dB hearing level in the speech range would impair normal conversation, whereas an 80-dB hearing level would make everyday auditory communication almost impossible (the social definition of deafness).

LOCALIZATION OF LESIONS WITHIN THE AUDITORY PATHWAYS. *Conductive hearing loss* results from lesions involving the external or middle ear. It is typically characterized by an approximately equal loss of hearing at all frequencies and by well-preserved speech discrimination once the threshold for hearing is exceeded. Patients with conductive hearing loss can hear speech in a noisy background better than in a quiet background because they can understand loud speech as well as anyone.

Sensorineural hearing loss results from lesions of the cochlea and/or auditory division of the eighth cranial nerve. With sensorineural hearing loss the hearing levels for different frequencies are usually unequal, typically resulting in better hearing for low- than for high-frequency tones. Patients with sensorineural hearing loss often have difficulty hearing speech that is mixed with background noise and may be annoyed by loud speech. Three important manifestations of sensorineural lesions are diplacusis, recruitment, and tone decay. Diplacusis and recruitment are common with cochlear lesions; tone decay usually accompanies eighth nerve involvement.

Central hearing disorders result from lesions of the central auditory pathways. As a rule patients with central lesions do not have impaired hearing for pure tones, and they can understand speech as long as it is clearly spoken in a quiet environment. If the listener's task is made more difficult with the introduction of background noise or competing messages, performance deteriorates more markedly in patients with central lesions than in normal subjects.

EXAMINATION OF HEARING. *Bedside Test.* A quick test for hearing loss in the speech range is to observe the response to spoken commands at different intensities (whisper, conversation, shouting). Tuning fork tests permit a rough assessment of the hearing level for pure tones of known frequency. The clinician can use his own hearing level as a reference standard. In the Rinne test nerve conduction is compared to bone conduction by holding a tuning fork (preferably 512 Hz) against the mastoid process until the sound can no longer be heard. It is then placed 1 inch from the ear and in normal subjects can be heard about twice as long by air as by bone. If bone conduction is better than air conduction, the hearing loss is conductive, but care must be taken to assure that the bone conduction is not heard in the normal ear. In the Weber test, the tuning fork is placed on the patient's forehead or upper teeth. Normally this sound is referred to the center of the head. If it is referred to the side of unilateral hearing loss, the hearing loss is conductive; if it is referred away from the side of unilateral hearing loss, the loss is sensorineural.

Audiometry. *Pure tone testing* is the nucleus of most auditory examinations. Pure tones at selected frequencies are presented via either earphones (air conduction) or a vibrator pressed against the mastoid portion of the temporal bone (bone conduction), and the minimal level that the subject can hear is determined for each frequency. Two speech tests are routinely used. The *speech reception threshold* (SRT) is the intensity at which the patient can correctly repeat 50% of the words presented. The SRT is a test of hearing sensitivity for speech and should reflect the hearing level for pure tones in the speech range. The *speech discrimination test* is a measure of the patient's ability to understand speech when it is presented at a level that is easily heard. In patients with eighth nerve lesions speech discriminations can be severely reduced, even when pure tone thresholds are normal or nearly normal, whereas in patients with cochlear lesions discrimination tends to be proportional to the magnitude of hearing loss.

Brain stem auditory evoked responses (BAER) can be recorded from scalp electrodes at 0 to 10 msec (early), 10 to 50 msec (middle), and 50 to 500 msec (late) following a click stimulus. The early potentials reflect electrical activity at the cochlea, eighth cranial nerve, and brain stem; the later potentials reflect cortical activity. Computer averaging of the responses to 1000 to 2000 clicks separates the evoked potential from background noise. Early evoked responses may be used to estimate the magnitude of hearing loss and to differentiate among cochlea, eighth nerve, and brainstem lesions.

CAUSES OF HEARING LOSS. *Conductive Hearing Loss.* The logic for identifying common causes of hearing loss is shown in Figure 403–5. The history, examination, and audiometry usually provide the key differential features. The most common cause of conductive hearing loss is *impacted cerumen* in the external canal. This benign condition is usually first noticed after bathing or swimming when a droplet of water closes the remaining tiny passageway. The most common serious cause of conductive hearing loss is inflammation of the middle ear, *otitis media,* either infected (suppu-

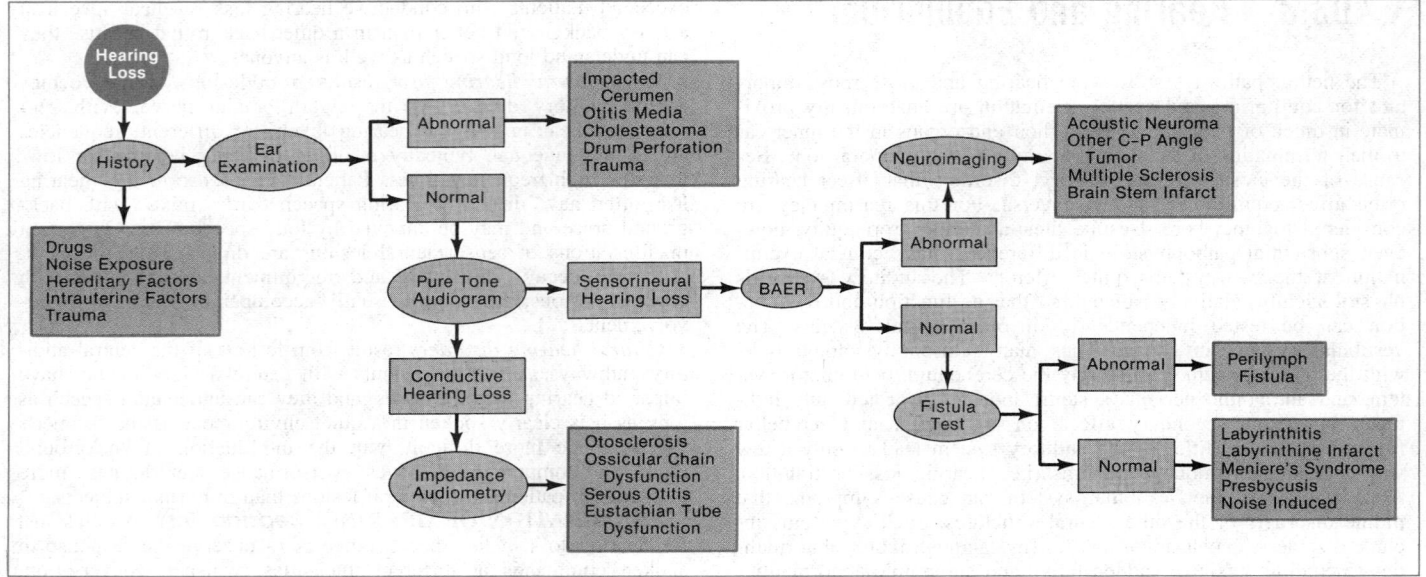

FIGURE 403–5. Evaluation of hearing loss.

rative) or noninfective (serous). Fluid accumulates in the middle ear, impairing the conduction of airborne sound. Since the air cavity of the middle ear is in direct connection with the mastoid air cells, infection can spread through the mastoid bone and, occasionally, into the intracranial cavity. Chronic otitis media with perforation of the tympanic membrane can result in an invasion of the middle ear and other pneumatized areas of the temporal bone by keratinizing squamous epithelium (cholesteatoma). Cholesteatomas can produce erosion of the ossicles and bony labyrinth, resulting in a mixed conductive sensorineural hearing loss. Otosclerosis commonly produces progressive conductive hearing loss by immobilizing the stapes with new bone growth in front of and below the oval window. The hearing loss is typically conductive, although in some persons the cochlea may be invaded by foci of otosclerotic bone, producing an additional sensorineural hearing loss. Otosclerosis usually stabilizes when the hearing level reaches 50 to 60 dB and rarely progresses to deafness. Other common causes of conductive hearing loss include trauma, congenital malformations of the external and middle ear, and glomus body tumors.

Sensorineural Hearing Loss. Genetically determined deafness, usually from hair cell aplasia or deterioration, may be present at birth or may develop in adulthood. The diagnosis of *hereditary deafness* rests on the finding of a positive family history. In many instances the inheritance is through a recessive gene or a dominant gene with low penetrance, making it difficult to determine the genetic nature of the disorder. *Intrauterine factors* resulting in congenital hearing loss include infection (especially rubella); toxic, metabolic, and endocrine disorders; and anoxia associated with Rh incompatibility and difficult deliveries.

Acute unilateral deafness usually has a cochlear basis. *Bacterial or viral infections* of the labyrinth, *head trauma* with fracture or hemorrhage into the cochlea, or *vascular occlusion* of a terminal branch of the anterior inferior cerebellar artery all can damage extensively the cochlea and its hair cells. An acute idiopathic, often reversible, unilateral hearing loss strikes young adults and is presumed to reflect an isolated viral infection of the cochlea and auditory nerve terminals. Sudden unilateral hearing loss often associated with vertigo and tinnitus can result from a *perilymphatic fistula.* Such fistulae may be congenital or may follow stapes surgery or head trauma. *Drugs* cause acute and subacute bilateral hearing impairment. Salicylates, furosemide, and ethacrynic acid have the potential to produce transient deafness when taken in high doses. More toxic to the cochlea are aminoglycoside antibiotics (gentamicin, tobramycin, amikacin, kanamycin, streptomycin, and neomycin). These agents can destroy cochlear hair cells in direct relation to their serum concentrations. Some antineoplastic chemotherapeutic agents, particularly cisplatin, cause severe ototoxicity.

Subacute relapsing cochlear deafness occurs with *Ménière syndrome,* a condition associated with fluctuating hearing loss and tinnitus, recurrent episodes of abrupt and often severe vertigo, and a sensation of fullness or pressure in the ear. Recurrent endolymphatic hypertension (hydrops) is believed to cause the episodes. Pathologically, the endolymphatic sac is dilated, and the hair cells become atrophic. The resulting deafness is subtle and reversible in the early stages but subsequently becomes permanent and is characterized by diplacusis and loudness recruitment. The disorder is usually unilateral, but in about 20 to 40% of patients bilateral involvement occurs.

The gradual, progressive, bilateral hearing loss commonly associated with advancing age is called *presbycusis.* Presbycusis is not a distinct disease entity but rather represents multiple effects of aging on the auditory system. It may include conductive and central dysfunction, although the most consistent effect of aging is on the sensory cells and neurons of the cochlea. The typical audiogram of presbycusis is a symmetric high-frequency hearing loss gradually sloping downward with increasing frequency. The most consistent pathology associated with presbycusis is degeneration of sensory cells and nerve fibers at the base of the cochlea. The recurrent trauma of *noise-induced hearing loss* affects approximately the same cochlear region and is almost as common, particularly among those with exposure to loud explosive or industrial noises. Loud, blaring, modern music has become a recent offender. The loss almost always begins at 4000 Hz and does not affect speech discrimination until late in the disease process. With only brief exposure to loud noise (hours to days) there may be only a temporary threshold shift, but with continued exposure permanent injury begins. The duration and intensity of exposure determine the degree of permanent injury.

Hearing loss from direct damage to the acoustic nerve in the petrous canal occasionally results from infection within or trauma to the surrounding bone; severe deafness of abrupt onset marks the event and is usually associated with acute vertigo due to concurrent vestibular nerve injury. Progressive unilateral hearing loss that arises insidiously and worsens by almost imperceptible degrees is characteristic of benign neoplasms of the cerebellopontine angle, such as *acoustic neuromas.* In about 10% of cases the hearing loss can be acute, apparently owing to either hemorrhage into the tumor or compression of the labyrinthine vasculature.

Central Hearing Loss. Central hearing loss is unilateral only if it results from damage to the pontine cochlear nuclei on one side of the brain stem. Such can occur with *ischemic infarction* of the lateral brain stem (e.g., occlusion of the anterior inferior cerebellar artery), a plaque of *multiple sclerosis,* or, rarely, invasion or compression of the lateral pons by a *neoplasm* or *hematoma.* Bilateral *degeneration* of the cochlear nuclei accompanies some of the rare recessive inherited disorders of childhood. As noted, clinically important unilateral hearing loss never results from neurologic disease arising rostrad to the cochlear nucleus. Although bilateral hearing loss could, in theory, result from bilat-eral destruction of central hearing pathways, in practice this is rare because involvement of neighboring structures in brain stem or hemisphere would usually produce overwhelming neurologic disability.

TREATMENT OF HEARING LOSS. If an underlying disorder has not yet destroyed the auditory system and can be ameliorated medically or surgically, hearing may be improved or preserved. Most patients with otosclerosis respond to stapedectomy. Closure of a perilymph fistula may improve hearing. Antibiotic and decongestive treatment of otitis media should prevent permanent hearing loss. A low-salt diet and diuretics are effective in selective cases of Meniere syndrome, particularly if episodes are precipitated by premenstrual water retention. Hearing aids amplify sound, usually with the goal of making speech intelligible. Patients with conductive hearing loss require simple amplification, but those with sensorineural hearing loss often need frequency-selective amplification in order to make hearing aids useful. Recent advances in acoustic technology have markedly improved the outlook for the latter. Monitoring audiograms in patients with noise- or ototoxic drug exposure are critical for prevention of permanent hearing loss.

TINNITUS. The flow chart in Figure 403–6 outlines the logic for determining the common causes of tinnitus. A careful history should be taken to identify common offending drugs (Table 403–5). With *objective tinnitus* the patient hears a sound arising external to the auditory system, a sound that can usually be heard by the examiner with a stethoscope. Objective tinnitus usually has benign causes such as noise from temporomandibular joints, opening of eustachian tubes, or repetitive muscle contractions. Sometimes, in a quiet room, the patient can hear the pulsatile flow in the carotid artery or a continuous hum of normal venous outflow through the jugular vein. The latter can be obliterated by compression of the jugular vein or extreme lateral rotation of the neck. Pathologic objective tinnitus occurs when patients hear turbulent flow in vascular anomalies or tumors (e.g., glomus jugulare tumor). Objective tinnitus may also be an early sign of increased intracranial pressure. Such tinnitus, which is usually overshadowed by other neurologic abnormalities, can be obliterated by pressure over the jugular vein. It probably arises from turbulent flow through compressed venous structures at the base of the brain.

TABLE 403–5. DRUGS COMMONLY ASSOCIATED WITH TINNITUS

Quinidine	Propranolol
Salicylates	Levodopa
Indomethacin	Aminophylline
Carbamazepine	Caffeine

Subjective tinnitus can arise from sites anywhere in the auditory system. The sounds most frequently complained of are metallic ringing, buzzing, blowing, roaring, or, less often, bizarre clanging, popping, or nonrhythmic beating. Tinnitus heard as a faint, moderately high-pitched, metallic ring can be observed by almost anyone who concentrates attention on auditory events in a quiet room. Sustained louder tinnitus accompanied by audiometric evidence of deafness occurs in association with both conductive and sensorineural hearing loss. Tinnitus observed with otosclerosis tends to have a roaring or hissing quality, while that associated with Meniere syndrome often produces sounds that vary widely in intensity with time and quality, sometimes including roaring or clanging. Tinnitus with other cochlear or auditory nerve lesions tends to be higher pitched and ringing in quality. Audiometric and brain stem–evoked response testing can help distinguish between lesions involving the conducting apparatus, the cochlea, and the auditory nerve.

Tinnitus without observable deafness appears sporadically and for variable lengths of time in many persons without other evidence of an ongoing pathologic process. In many instances one suspects that the auditory experience is no more than an anxious preoccupation with normal auditory physiology.

TREATMENT OF TINNITUS. Most patients with tinnitus can be helped by detailed interview together with the relevant examination and laboratory investigations followed by reassurance where this can be given. Often exacerbating factors such as chronic anxiety and depression can be identified. In patients with hearing loss and tinnitus a hearing aid may improve communication in two ways, as amplification of ambient sound may effectively mask the tinnitus. This mechanism probably explains the frequent observation that removal of cerumen from the external auditory canal to im-

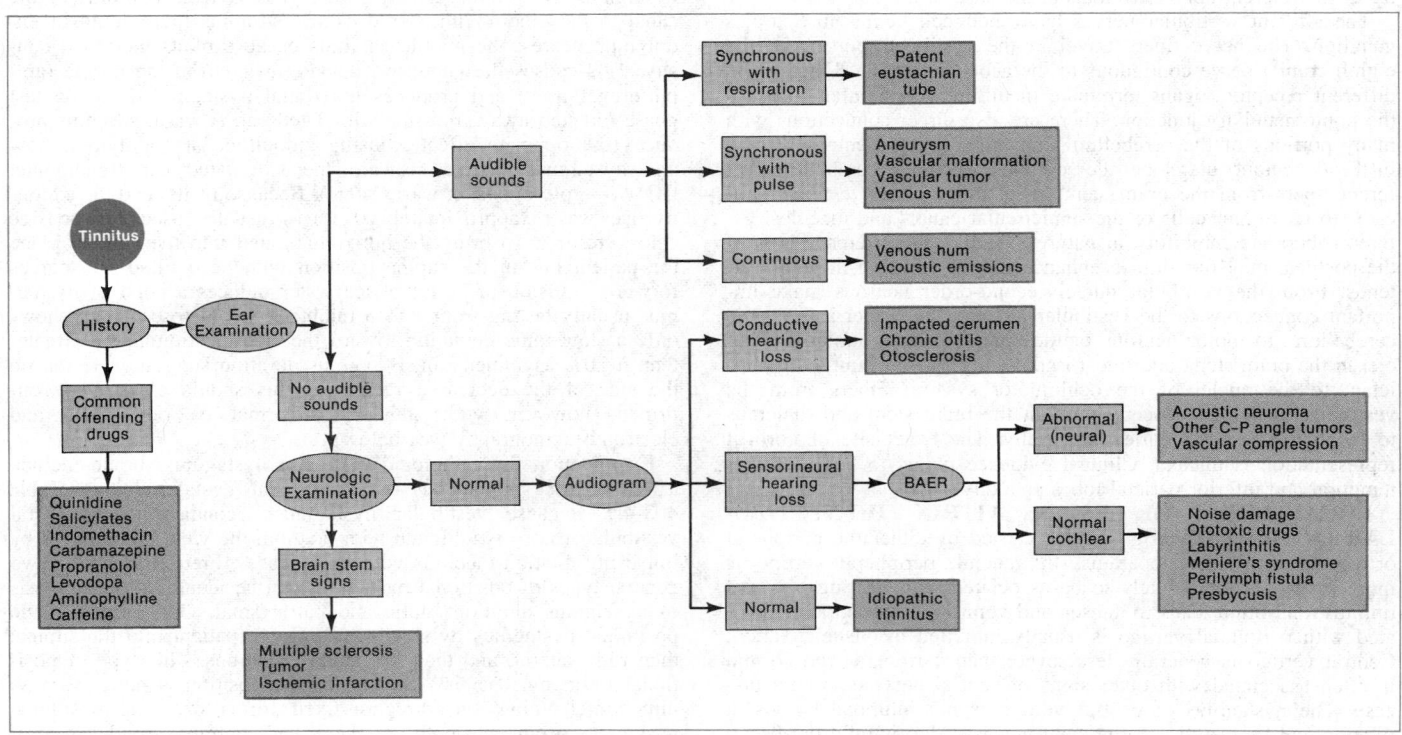

FIGURE 403–6. Evaluation of tinnitus.

prove ambient hearing also improves tinnitus. Also, when cerumen is attached to the tympanic membrane, tinnitus may result from local mechanical effects on the conductive system. For patients who find their tinnitus most obtrusive when trying to sleep, a bedside FM clock radio tuned between stations can provide an effective masking sound that will switch itself off after the patient falls asleep. A careful drug history should be taken, and a drug-free trial period should be considered when possible. Some patients who notice that caffeine, alcohol, or nicotine exacerbates their tinnitus experience significant relief when these drugs are discontinued.

EQUILIBRIUM—VESTIBULAR SYSTEM

ANATOMY AND PHYSIOLOGY OF THE VESTIBULAR SYSTEM. The paired vestibular end organs lie within the temporal bones next to the cochlea. Each organ consists of three semicircular canals that detect angular acceleration and two otolith structures, the utricle and saccule, that detect linear acceleration (including gravitational). Like the cochlea, these organs possess hair cells that act as force transducers, converting the forces associated with head acceleration into afferent nerve impulses. The hair cells of the three semicircular canals, each of which is oriented at right angles to the others, are concentrated in the crista, where they are embedded in a gelatinous mass called the cupula. Movement of the head causes the endolymph to flow either toward or away from the cupula, bending the hair cells and, depending on the direction of endolymphatic movements, either exciting or inhibiting the afferent nerve firing. Because the afferent nerves arising from the semicircular canals are tonically active, the baseline activity can be increased or decreased depending on the direction of hair cell bending. Furthermore, the two sets of semicircular canals are approximately mirror images of each other, so that rotational movement of the head that excites one canal inhibits the analogous canal on the opposite side. The hair cells of the utricle and saccule are concentrated in an area called the macule. The macule of the utricle lies approximately in the plane of the horizontal canal and the macule of the saccule is approximately in the plane of the anterior canal. The hair cells are embedded in a membrane that contains calcium carbonate crystals or otoliths; the density of otoliths is considerably greater than that of the endolymph. Linear accelerations of the head combine with the linear acceleration of gravity to distort the otolith membrane, thereby bending the underlying hair cells and modulating the activity of the afferent nerve terminals at the base of the hair cells.

The afferent vestibular nerves have their cell bodies in Scarpa's ganglion. The nerve fibers travel in the vestibular portion of the eighth cranial nerve contiguous to the acoustic portion. Fibers from different receptor organs terminate in different vestibular nuclei at the pontomedullary junction. There are also direct connections with many portions of the cerebellum, the greatest representation being in the flocculonocular lobe, the so-called vestibular cerebellum. Efferent fibers from the brain stem travel through the vestibular nucleus to reach hair cells of the semicircular canals and macules. Efferent fibers are inhibitory in nature and, like the efferent fibers of the cochlea, may function to enhance inputs to which the brain attends. From the vestibular nuclei second-order neurons make important connections to the vestibular nuclei of the other side, to the cerebellum, to motor neurons of the spinal cord, to autonomic nuclei in the brain stem, and, most importantly for the examining clinician, to the nuclei of the oculomotor system. Fibers from the vestibular nuclei also ascend through the brain stem and thalamus to reach the cerebral cortex bilaterally. The exact site of cortical representation is unclear. Clinical evidence points to both superior temporal and inferior parietal lobes as likely sites.

LOCALIZATION OF LESIONS WITHIN THE VESTIBULAR PATHWAYS. Vertigo can be caused by either the peripheral or central vestibular apparatus. In general, peripheral vertigo is more severe, is more likely to be associated with hearing loss and tinnitus, and often leads to nausea and vomiting. Nystagmus associated with peripheral vertigo is usually inhibited by visual fixation. Central vertigo is generally less severe than peripheral vertigo and is often associated with other signs of central nervous system disease. The nystagmus of central vertigo is not inhibited by visual fixation and frequently is prominent when vertigo is mild or absent.

EXAMINATION OF THE VESTIBULAR SYSTEM. Most vestibular problems presenting to the physician are episodic, and often there are neither symptoms nor signs when the physician examines the patient. The history, therefore, can become paramount for identifying vestibular dysfunction. The history should attempt to distinguish vertigo (the illusion of movement in space) from light-headedness (presyncope), ataxia (disequilibrium of the body without true movement in space), and psychogenic symptoms (the feeling of dissociation or, sometimes, dysequilibrium). If the history is not clear, bedside provocative tests to mimic the symptom may assist in making a pathophysiologic diagnosis. Hyperventilation, which lowers the $PaCO_2$ and decreases cerebral blood flow, causes a light-headed sensation associated with syncope. Ask the patient to hyperventilate maximally for 1 to 3 minutes to cause light-headedness. If the episode mimics the patient's symptoms it suggests that anxiety and hyperventilation may be playing an important role. In addition, during the course of hyperventilation the patient may suffer dry mouth, chest tightness, and paresthesias, which may be recognized as part of the spontaneous attacks, thus helping in diagnosis.

Bedside tests of vestibulospinal function are often insensitive because most patients can use vision and proprioceptive signals to compensate for any vestibular loss. Patients with acute unilateral peripheral vestibular lesions may past point or fall toward the side of the lesion, but within a few days balance returns to normal. Patients with bilateral peripheral vestibular loss have more difficulty compensating and usually show some imbalance on the Romberg and tandem walking tests, particularly with eyes closed.

The vestibulo-ocular reflex can be tested at the bedside by inducing physiologic nystagmus and searching for pathologic nystagmus. In an alert human, rotating the head back and forth in the horizontal plane induces compensatory horizontal eye movements that are dependent on both the visual and vestibular systems. The doll's-eye test is a test of vestibular function in a comatose patient, since such patients cannot generate pursuit or corrective fast components. In this setting conjugate compensatory eye movements indicate normally functioning vestibulo-ocular pathways. Because the vestibulo-ocular reflex has a much higher frequency range than the smooth pursuit system, a qualitative bedside test of vestibular function can be made by having the patient shake his head back and forth at frequencies above 1 Hz while reading a standard visual acuity chart. A decrease in visual acuity of more than one line compared with testing with the patient's head kept still indicates an abnormal vestibulo-ocular reflex.

The caloric test uses a nonphysiologic stimulus to induce endolymphatic flow in the horizontal semicircular canal and horizontal nystagmus by creating a temperature gradient from one side of the canal to the other. With a cold caloric stimulus the column of endolymph nearest the middle ear falls because of its increased density. This causes the cupula to deviate away from the utricle (ampullofugal flow) and produces horizontal nystagmus with the fast phase directed away from the stimulated ear. A warm stimulus produces the opposite effect, causing ampullopedal endolymph flow and nystagmus directed toward the stimulated ear (mnemonic: COWS—cold opposite, warm same). Because of its ready availability ice water (approximately 0° C) is usually used for bedside caloric testing. To bring the horizontal canal into the vertical plane the patient lies in the supine position with head tilted 30 degrees forward. Infusion of 10 ml of ice water induces a burst of nystagmus usually lasting from 1 to 3 minutes. A comatose patient shows only a slow tonic deviation toward the side of stimulation. Greater than a 20% asymmetry in nystagmus duration suggests a lesion on the side of the decreased response. This should always be confirmed, however, with standard bithermal caloric testing and electronystagmography (see below).

Examination for pathologic vestibular nystagmus should include a search for spontaneous and positional nystagmus (see Table 403-4). Because vestibular nystagmus secondary to peripheral vestibular lesions is inhibited with fixation, the yield is increased by impairing fixation (such as with +30 lenses, Frenzel glasses). Two general types of positional nystagmus can be identified on the basis of nystagmus duration: static and paroxysmal. One induces static positional nystagmus by slowly placing the patient into the supine, then right lateral, and then left lateral positions. This type of positional nystagmus persists as long as the position is held. Because direction-changing and direction-fixed forms of static positional nystagmus occur with both peripheral and central vestibular lesions, their presence indicates only a dysfunction somewhere in the

TABLE 403–6. DISTINGUISHING BETWEEN VESTIBULAR AND NONVESTIBULAR TYPES OF DIZZINESS

	Vestibular	Nonvestibular
Common descriptive terms	Spinning (environment moves), merry-go-round, drunkenness, tilting, motion sickness, off-balance	Light-headed, floating, dissociated from body, swimming, giddy, spinning inside (environment stationary)
Course	Episodic	Constant
Common precipitating factors	Head movements, position change	Stress, hyperventilation, cardiac arrhythmia, situations
Common associated symptoms	Nausea, vomiting, unsteadiness, tinnitus, hearing loss, impaired vision, oscillopsia	Perspiration, pallor, paresthesias, palpitations, syncope, difficulty concentrating, tension headache

From Baloh RW, Honrubia V: Clinical Neurophysiology of the Vestibular System. 2nd ed. Philadelphia, FA Davis, 1990.

vestibular system. As with spontaneous nystagmus, however, lack of suppression with fixation and signs of associated brain-stem dysfunction suggest a central lesion.

Paroxysmal positional nystagmus is induced, after a brief delay, by a rapid change from erect sitting to supine head-hanging left, center, or right position (the so-called Hallpike maneuver). It is initially high in frequency but dissipates rapidly (within 30 seconds to 1 minute). The most common variety of paroxysmal positional nystagmus, benign positional nystagmus, usually has a 3- to 10-second latency before onset and rarely lasts longer than 30 seconds. The nystagmus is always torsional with fast phase directed upward (i.e., toward the forehead). It is usually prominent in only one head-hanging position, and a burst of nystagmus in the reverse direction occurs when the patient reassumes the sitting position. Another key feature is the severe vertigo and nystagmus that the patient experiences with the initial positioning which, with repeated positioning, rapidly disappear (fatigability). Benign positional nystagmus is a sign of vestibular end-organ disease (see below).

Electronystagmography (ENG) is a technique for recording eye movements that allows precise quantification of both physiologic and pathologic nystagmus. A standard ENG test battery includes (1) tests of visual ocular control (saccades, smooth pursuit, and optokinetic nystagmus); (2) a careful search for pathologic nystagmus with fixation and with eyes open in darkness, and (3) measurement of induced physiologic nystagmus (caloric and rotational). ENG can be helpful in identifying a vestibular lesion and localizing it within the peripheral and central pathways.

EVALUATING THE "DIZZY" PATIENT. The history is key because it determines the type of dizziness (vertigo, light-headed, feeling of dissociation, disequilibrium), associated symptoms (neurologic, audiologic, cardiac, psychiatric), precipitating factors (position change, trauma, stress, drug ingestion), and predisposing illness (systemic viral infection, cardiac disease, cerebrovascular disease). Features that distinguish between vestibular and nonvestibular types of dizziness are summarized in Table 403–6. The examination should include complete neurologic, head and neck, and cardiac assessments. When focal neurologic signs are found, neuroimaging usually leads to specific diagnosis. When vertigo is present without focal neurologic symptoms or signs, audiometry and electronystagmography aid in localizing the lesion to the labyrinth or eighth nerve. Patients with hyperventilation syndrome and/or acute anxiety should be identified after the history and examination so that needless tests are not obtained. A detailed cardiac evaluation (including Holter monitoring) often identifies the cause of episodic presyncopal light-headedness.

COMMON CAUSES OF VERTIGO. The logic for identifying common causes of vertigo is shown in Figure 403–7.

Physiologic Vertigo. Physiologic vertigo includes common disorders such as *motion sickness, space sickness,* and *height vertigo.* In these conditions vertigo (defined as an illusion of movement) is minimal or absent while autonomic symptoms predominate. With height vertigo, patients often experience acute anxiety and panic reaction. Individuals with motion sickness and space sickness typically develop perspiration, nausea, vomiting, increased salivation, yawning, and generalized malaise. Gastric motility is reduced and digestion impaired. Even the sight or smell of food is distressing. Hyperventilation is a common sign, and the resulting hypocapnia leads to changes in blood volume, with pooling in the lower parts of the body predisposing to postural hypotension and syncope. An unusual variant of motion sickness continues when the subject returns to stationary conditions after prolonged exposure to motion. Typically, affected patients report that they feel the persistent rocking sensation of a boat long after returning to solid ground. Rarely, the syndrome can last for months to years after exposure to motion and can even be incapacitating. The cause is unknown.

Physiologic vertigo can often be suppressed by supplying sensory cues that help to match the signals originating from different sensory systems. Thus, motion sickness, which is exacerbated by sitting in a closed space or reading (giving the visual system the miscue that the environment is stationary), may be improved by looking out at the environment and watching it move. Height vertigo, caused by a mismatch between sensation of normal body sway and lack of its visual detection, can often be relieved either by sitting or by visually fixating a nearby stationary object.

Benign Positional Vertigo (BPV). BPV is by far the most common cause of pathologic vertigo. Patients with this condition

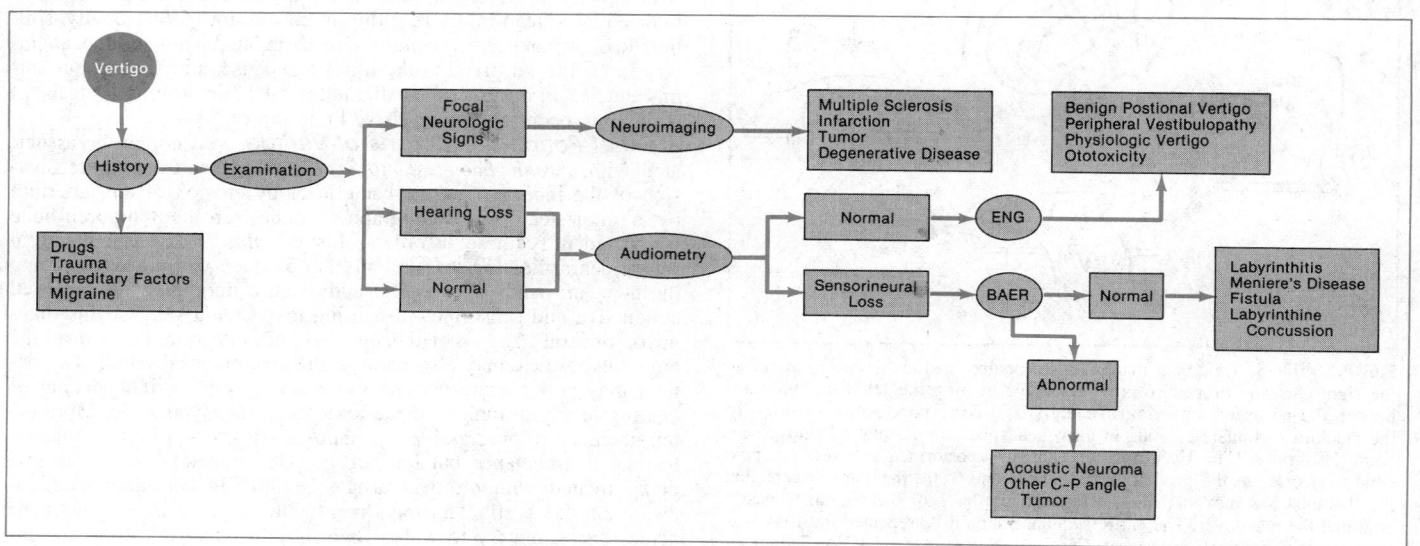

FIGURE 403–7. Evaluation of vertigo.

develop brief episodes of vertigo (less than 1 min) with position change, typically when turning over in bed, getting in and out of bed, bending over and straightening up, or extending the neck to look up. BPV can result from *head injury, viral labyrinthitis,* and *vascular occlusion,* or it may occur as an isolated symptom of unknown cause (in about 50% of cases). The latter is particularly common in the elderly. This syndrome is important to recognize because in the vast majority of patients, the symptoms spontaneously remit. It does commonly recur, however. The diagnosis rests on finding characteristic fatigable paroxysmal positional nystagmus after a rapid change from the sitting to the head-hanging position (see above). BPV is thought to result from free-floating calcium carbonate crystals (normally attached to the utricular macule) that inadvertently enter the long arm of the posterior semicircular canal. The crystals move within the endolymph and artificially displace the cupula. Consistent with this theory, the burst of paroxysmal positional nystagmus is in the plane of the posterior canal of the "down ear," and the positional nystagmus disappears after the ampullary nerve has been surgically resected from the posterior canal on the diseased side. If the history and physical findings are typical, a simple bedside positioning maneuver can remove the debris from the posterior semicircular canal in most patients (Fig. 403–8). If the history or findings are atypical, the condition must be distinguished from other causes of positional vertigo that may occur with tumors or infarcts of the posterior fossa.

Acute Peripheral Vestibulopathy ("Acute Labyrinthitis"). One of the most common clinical neurologic syndromes at any age is the acute onset of vertigo, nausea, and vomiting lasting for several days and not associated with auditory or neurologic symptoms. Most affected patients gradually improve over 1 to 2 weeks, but some develop recurrent episodes. A large percentage report an upper respiratory tract illness 1 to 2 weeks prior to the onset of vertigo. This syndrome occasionally occurs in epidemics (epidemic

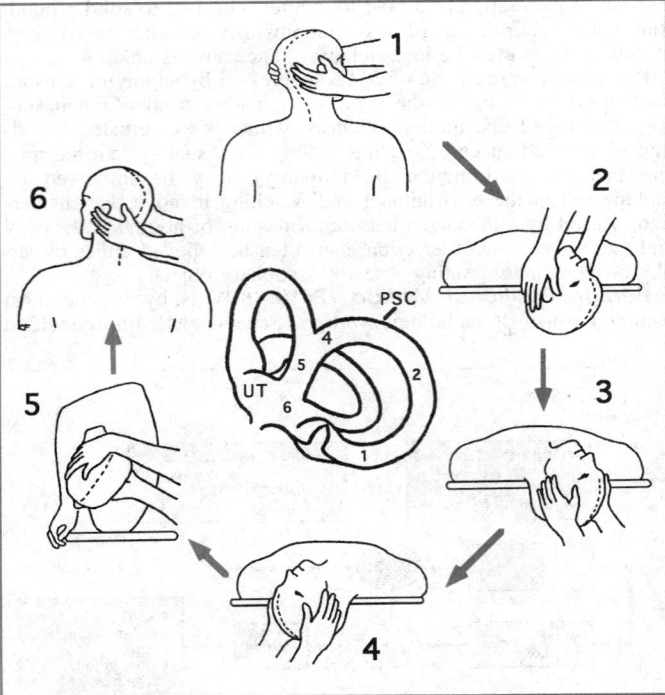

FIGURE 403–8. Treatment maneuver for benign positional vertigo affecting the right ear. The procedure is reversed for treating the left ear. The numbers in the posterior semicircular canal (PSC) correspond to the position of the calcium carbonate crystals in each head position as they are moved toward the utricle (UT). Each position change is performed as rapidly as possible to accelerate the particles. Positions 2 and 3 are the same except that the therapist has moved from the front to the back of the patient to easily continue the maneuver. The entire sequence should be repeated until no nystagmus is elicited. (Courtesy of Carol A. Foster, MD, UCLA School of Medicine.)

vertigo), may affect several members of the same family, and more often erupts in the spring and early summer. All of these factors suggest a viral origin, but attempts to isolate an agent have been unsuccessful, except for occasional findings of a herpes zoster infection. Pathologic studies showing atrophy of one or more vestibular nerve trunks, with or without atrophy of their associated sense organs, are evidence of a vestibular nerve site and, probably, viral cause for many patients with this syndrome (*viral neurolabyrinthitis*). In some patients attacks of acute vestibulopathy (usually less severe) recur over many months or years. There is no way of predicting whether a person who suffers a first attack will have repetitive attacks.

Meniere Syndrome. The typical clinical features of Ménière syndrome are described earlier (see p. 2022). This disorder accounts for about 10% of all patients with vertigo. The diagnosis is based on documenting episodic severe attacks accompanied by more or less continuous tinnitus and fluctuating hearing levels on audiometric testing.

Migraine. Vertigo is a common symptom with migraine. It can occur with headaches or in separate isolated episodes, and it can predate the onset of headache. So-called benign paroxysmal vertigo of childhood is often the first symptom of migraine. The mechanism of vertigo with migraine is not clear, but damage to the inner ear occurs in about one third of patients. A few develop typical features of Ménière syndrome.

Post-traumatic Vertigo. Vertigo, hearing loss, and tinnitus often follow a blow to the head that does not result in temporal bone fracture, the so-called *labyrinthine concussion.* Although they are protected by a bony capsule, the delicate labyrinthine membranes are susceptible to blunt trauma. Blows to the occipital or mastoid region are particularly likely to produce labyrinthine damage. *Transverse fractures* of the temporal bone typically pass through the vestibule of the inner ear, tearing the membranous labyrinth and lacerating the vestibular and cochlear nerves. Complete loss of vestibular and cochlear function is the usual sequela, and the facial nerve is interrupted in approximately 50% of cases. Examination of the ear often reveals hemotympanum, but bleeding from the ear seldom occurs because the tympanic membrane usually remains intact. As noted above, *benign positional vertigo* is also a common sequela of head trauma. *Fistulae* of the oval and round windows can result from impact noise, deep-water diving, severe physical exertion, or blunt head injury without skull fracture. The mechanism of the rupture is a sudden negative or positive pressure change in the middle ear or a sudden increase in cerebrospinal fluid pressure transmitted to the inner ear via the cochlear aqueduct and internal auditory canal. Clinically, the rupture leads to the sudden onset of vertigo or hearing loss, or both. Surgical exploration of the middle ear is warranted when there is a clear relationship between the onset of vertigo or hearing loss, or both, and the onset of severe exertion, barometric change, head injury, or impact noise.

Postconcussion Syndrome. The so-called postconcussion syndrome refers to a vague dizziness (rarely vertigo) associated with anxiety, difficulty in concentrating, headache, and photophobia induced by a head injury resulting in concussion. Occasionally, similar, less pronounced symptoms are associated with mild head injury judged to be trivial at the time. The cause is unknown, but animal studies indicate that small multifocal brain lesions (petechiae) commonly occur after concussive brain injury.

Other Peripheral Causes of Vertigo. Vertigo can be associated with *chronic bacterial otomastoiditis,* either from direct invasion of the inner ear by the bacteria or by erosion of the labyrinth by a cholesteatoma. Radiographic studies of the temporal bone readily identify these disorders. Just as *otosclerosis* can result in sensorineural hearing loss, it can also produce vertigo by involving the bony labyrinth. The typical audiometric findings of a combined conductive and sensorineural hearing loss should suggest this diagnosis. Several *drugs* that damage the auditory system, such as the aminoglycosides, may also damage the vestibular labyrinth. The patient may suffer acute vertigo, either along with or independent of hearing loss and tinnitus, if the toxic effect is asymmetric. More often there is a progressive symmetric loss of vestibular function leading to imbalance but not vertigo. Unfortunately, many patients being treated with ototoxic drugs are initially bedridden and unaware of the vestibular impairment until they recover from their acute illness and try to walk. Then they discover that they are unsteady on their feet and that the environment tends to jiggle in front of their eyes (oscillopsia). Younger patients adapt after weeks to the labyrinthine failure; older ones may be left permanently disabled. Usually there is no nystagmus (because of the symmetric involvement), but the patient is ataxic. Caloric and rotational tests during electronystagmography can document impairment or absence of vestibular function. The best treatment is prevention. If the drug is discontinued early during the course of symptoms the disorder may stabilize or improve.

Vascular Insufficiency. Vertebrobasilar insufficiency is a common cause of vertigo in the elderly (see also Ch. 419). Whether the vertigo originates from ischemia of the labyrinth, brain stem, or both structures is not always clear because the blood supply to the labyrinth, eighth cranial nerve, and vestibular nuclei originate from the same source, the basilar vertebral circulation. Vertigo with *vertebrobasilar insufficiency* is abrupt in onset, usually lasting several minutes, and is frequently associated with nausea and vomiting. Associated symptoms resulting from ischemia in the remaining territory supplied by the posterior circulation include visual illusions and hallucinations, drop attack and weakness, visceral sensations, visual field defects, diplopia, and headache. These symptoms occur in episodes either in combination with the vertigo or alone. Vertigo may be an isolated initial symptom of vertebrobasilar ischemia, but repeated episodes of vertigo without other symptoms should suggest another diagnosis. Vertebrobasilar insufficiency usually is caused by atherosclerosis of the subclavian, vertebral, and basilar arteries. Occasionally, episodes of vertebrobasilar insufficiency are precipitated by postural hypotension, Stokes-Adams attacks, or mechanical compression from cervical spondylosis. Diagnostic studies including CT scans are usually normal because the vascular insufficiency is transient and function returns to normal between episodes. Angiography can be helpful in confirming the diagnosis but carries a risk and rarely leads to definitive therapy.

Vertigo is a common symptom associated with *infarction of the lateral brain stem or cerebellum,* or both. The diagnosis usually is clear, based on the characteristic acute history and pattern of associated symptoms and neurologic findings. Occasionally cerebellar infarction or hemorrhage presents with severe vertigo, vomiting, and ataxia without associated brain-stem symptoms and signs that might suggest the erroneous diagnosis of an acute peripheral vestibular disorder. The key differential point is the finding of clear cerebellar signs (extremity- and gait ataxia) and gaze-evoked nystagmus. Such patients must be watched carefully for several days because they may develop progressive brain-stem dysfunction owing to compression by a swollen cerebellum.

Cerebellopontine-Angle Tumors. Most tumors growing in the cerebellopontine angle (e.g., *acoustic neuroma, meningioma, epidermal cyst*) grow slowly, allowing the vestibular system to accommodate so that they produce a vague sensation of disequilibrium rather than acute vertigo. Occasionally, however, episodic vertigo or positional vertigo heralds the presence of a cerebellopontine-angle tumor. In virtually all patients, retrocochlear hearing loss is present, best identified by an abnormal brain-stem auditory evoked response. Magnetic resonance imaging (MRI) of the cerebellopontine angles is the most sensitive diagnostic study for identifying a cerebellopontine-angle tumor.

Other Central Causes of Vertigo. Acute vertigo may be the first symptom of *multiple sclerosis,* although only a small percentage of young patients with acute vertigo eventually develop multiple sclerosis. Vertigo in multiple sclerosis is usually transient and often associated with other neurologic signs of brain-stem disease, in particular, internuclear ophthalmoplegia or cerebellar dysfunction. Vertigo may also be a symptom of *parainfectious encephalomyelitis* or, rarely, *parainfectious cranial polyneuritis.* In this instance the accompanying neurologic signs establish the diagnosis. The *Ramsay-Hunt syndrome* (geniculate ganglion herpes) is characterized by vertigo and hearing loss associated with facial paralysis and, sometimes, pain in the ear. The typical lesions of herpes zoster, which may follow the appearance of neurologic signs, are found in the external auditory canal and over the palate in some patients. Rarely is herpes zoster responsible for vertigo in the absence of the full-blown syndrome. *Granulomatous meningitis* or *leptomeningeal metastasis* and cerebral or systemic *vasculitis* may involve the eighth nerve, producing vertigo as an early symptom. In these disorders cerebrospinal fluid analysis usually suggests the diagnosis. Patients suffering from *temporal lobe epilepsy* occasionally experience vertigo as the aura. Vertigo in the absence of other neurologic signs or symptoms is never caused by epilepsy or other diseases of the cerebral hemispheres.

TREATMENT OF VERTIGO. Treatment of vertigo can be divided into three general categories: specific, symptomatic, and rehabilitative. Specific therapies include antibiotics for bacterial or syphilitic labyrinthitis, anticoagulants for vertebrobasilar insufficiency, and surgery for acoustic neuroma. When possible, treatment should be directed at the underlying disorder. In most cases, however, symptomatic treatment is either combined with specific therapy or is the only one available (e.g., with acute peripheral vestibulopathy). Many different classes of drugs have been found to have antivertiginous properties, and in most instances the exact mechanism of action is uncertain. All of these agents produce potentially unpleasant side effects, and the decision on which drug or combination to use is based on their known complications and on the severity and duration of the vertigo. An episode of prolonged, severe vertigo is one of the most distressing symptoms that one can experience. Affected patients prefer to lie still with eyes closed in a quiet, dark room. Antivertiginous drugs with sedation such as phenergan (25 mg four times daily [q.i.d.]) or diazepam (5 mg q.i.d.) may be helpful. Prochlorperazine suppositories (25 mg) may stop vomiting. In more chronic vertiginous disorders, when the patient is trying to carry on normal activity, less sedating antivertiginous medications such as meclizine (25 mg q.i.d.) or transdermal scopolamine (0.5 mg every 3 days) may provide relief. Vestibular rehabilitation exercises are designed to help the patient compensate for permanent loss of vestibular function.

Baloh RW, Honrubia V: Clinical Neurophysiology of the Vestibular System, 2nd ed. Philadelphia, FA Davis, 1990. *Monograph reviewing basic and clinical aspects of vestibular function.*

Brandt T, Steddin S: Current view of the mechanism of benign paroxysmal positioning vertigo: Cupulolithiasis or canalolithiasis? J Vest Res 3:373, 1993. *Why the positioning maneuver works.*

Hazell JWP: Tinnitus I, II and III. J Otolaryngol 19:1, 6, 11, 1990. *Up-to-date clinical review.*

Nadol JB: Hearing loss. N Engl J Med 329:1092, 1993. *Timely review.*

404 DISORDERS OF MOTOR FUNCTION

404.1 Weakness, Asthenia, and Fatigue
Fred Plum

The terms *weakness, asthenia,* and *fatigue* imprecisely overlap. *Weakness* most often refers specifically to reduced motor capacity, either regional or general in distribution. Table 404–1 lists specific disorders and mechanisms producing weakness. Rowland's textbook chapter well describes the clinical findings. *Asthenia* carries the mixed definition of loss of strength, energy, or vitality—hardly unambiguous synonyms. Long usage reflects the double meaning, the term *asthenia* having been applied equally to the poorly understood state of psychic weakness (neurasthenia) and to the biologically well-established muscle weakness of myasthenia gravis. Medically, *weakness* is best used to describe demonstrably reduced muscle strength in specific area(s) of the body. *Asthenia* is too ambiguous to be useful.

Table 404–2 defines several particular acute or subacute disorders that may cause generalized weakness. Beyond these classes of specifically identifiable disorders, however, most chronic weakness unaccompanied by diagnosable neurologic or appropriate medical conditions is more likely to have a psychiatric than a neurologic genesis.

Fatigue, as employed in medical terms, describes a reduction in performance due to excessive effort or an experienced deterioration

TABLE 404-1. CAUSES OF ACUTE OR SUBACUTE WEAKNESS

Condition	Examples or Mechanisms
Joint or muscle injury-inflammation	Movement of the part induces pain.
Primary muscle disease	Genetically transmitted muscle or mitochondrial disorders; inflammatory or granulomatous myopathies; corticosteroid administration
Neuromuscular junction	Myasthenia gravis; Lambert-Eaton myasthenic syndrome
Peripheral motor or sensorimotor pathways (lower motor neuron)	Damage to peripheral motor nerves, spinal motor roots, anterior horn cells
	N.B.: Dysfunction of proprioceptive sensory pathways can produce the illusion of weakness secondary to impaired position sense.
Corticospinal pathways (upper motor neuron)	Disease or injury to the system anywhere from above the anterior horn cell to frontal lobe motor areas
Basal ganglia	Hypokinesia, slow starting, and weakness in parkinsonism
Cerebellum	Sense of incomplete strength with neocerebellar damage
Hysterical or pretended weakness	Signs inconsistent with specific physiologic failure

in capacity. Fatigue lasting weeks or months can accompany or follow several serious illnesses listed in Table 404–2. Fatigue can be local or general, acute or chronic, and, depending on circumstance, the sense of exhaustion may follow, accompany, or precede attempts at either motor or intellectual effort. Most short-term fatigue lasting for minutes to as much as a few weeks in duration can be traced to recognized antecedents, such as acute systemic illness, severe emotional perturbation, or intense effort of either a physical or intellectual nature. Recurrent, rapidly developing fatigue involving local or generalized striated muscle is typical of myasthenia gravis or, less often, the metabolic myopathies (see Ch. 457). Multiple sclerosis and Parkinson's disease characteristically are accompanied by chronic feelings of fatigue, usually worse at the end than at the beginning of the day. Processes such as tuberculosis, systemic cancer, subacute endocarditis, collagen vascular disease, and certain endocrinopathies represent less frequent causes. Subacute, disabling fatigue also can accompany early HIV involvement of the brain, but that condition also causes recognizable abnormalities in cognitive capacities.

Medical records going back a number of years indicate that many otherwise healthy adults experience continuous fatigue either chronically or in restricted epidemics to a degree sufficient to interfere with employment or domestic responsibilities. Recently identified as having *chronic fatigue syndrome,* such subacutely or chronically fatigued patients compared with nonexhausted controls have not shown higher long-term antibody titers against Epstein-Barr virus,

TABLE 404-2. MEDICAL-NEUROLOGIC ILLNESSES COMMONLY ASSOCIATED WITH ACUTE-SUBACUTE GENERALIZED WEAKNESS OR FATIGUE

Systemic	Neurologic
Acute bacterial-viral infections	Myasthenia gravis
Thyrotoxicosis	Early polyneuropathy
Post–myocardial infarction	Multiple sclerosis
Addison's disease	Parkinsonism
Disseminated malignancy	Postconcussion syndrome
Anticancer chemotherapy	Sustained drug use
Acute hepatitis; acute Epstein-Barr virus or Lyme disease	
Severe anemia	

Lyme borreliosis, or other organisms. Studies to date find few relevant physical or laboratory abnormalities in most chronically fatigued patients.

All well-analyzed studies of patients with chronic debilitating fatigue emphasize the high incidence of the symptoms (up to 25% or more of primary care patients), the lack of identifiable medical abnormalities, and a high incidence of psychiatric disorder. Symptoms of chronic anxiety, personality disorders, or depression have been identified in as many as 80% of such cohorts. The condition frequently includes somatoform complaints unaccompanied by physical or laboratory abnormalities as well as expressions of autonomic dysfunction including breathlessness, palpitations, tachycardia, constipation-diarrhea, sexual impairment, inappropriate sweating, and unsatisfactory sleep patterns. Prospective and retrospective studies consistently have identified significantly more manifestations of depression, somatic anxiety, and emotional maladjustment than were expressed by nonfatigued controls chosen from patients with neuromuscular disease or recovering from known viral illnesses. No satisfactorily evaluated treatment program has been forthcoming for persons with chronic fatigue. Most patients with somatoform disorders of this kind have sustained better outcomes when "floated" by physicians providing repeated reassurances at short intervals than by psychiatrists attempting intense psychotherapy. Advisory psychiatric consultation, as well as modest doses of tricyclic antidepressants for some, have at times been found to reduce an otherwise high rate of incapacitating somatoform complaints.

As Wilson et al. conclude, "The lack of specificity in the treatment of chronic fatigue syndrome encourages pseudoscience and the proliferation of those willing to exploit patients' beliefs in simplistic pathophysiologic models. In this, little has changed since the 19th century when treatment by rest and reflexology were embraced by many physicians as a model for managing the neurasthenic patient."

Kroenke K, Wood DR, Mangelsdorff AD, et al.: Chronic fatigue in primary care. Prevalence, patient characteristics and outcome. JAMA 260:929, 1988. *Among 1159 consecutive outpatients in primary care clinics, 24% described chronic fatigue as a major problem. Screening psychometric instruments identified depression, somatic anxiety, or both among 80% of fatigued patients versus 12% of controls.*

Rowland LP: Weakness: The syndromes caused by weak muscles. *In* Rowland LP (ed.): Merritt's Textbook of Neurology, 8th ed. Philadelphia, Lea & Febiger, 1989, p 50. *A systematic explanation of patterns of weakness accompanying disease entities ranging from muscle to brain.*

Schlueiderberg A, Straus SE, Peterson P: Chronic fatigue syndrome research. Definition and medical outcome assessment. Ann Intern Med 117:325, 1992. *An NIH workshop found no consistency in patient physical findings or laboratory tests to confirm the diagnosis. Similarities to the fibromyalgia syndrome and necessity for psychiatric screening were emphasized.*

Wilson A, Hickie I, Lloyd A, et al.: The treatment of chronic fatigue syndrome: Science and speculation. Am J Med 96:544, 1994. *A team including specialists in psychiatry, infectious diseases, and immunopathology sets out sensible guidelines for evaluation and management.*

404.2 Ataxia and Related Gait Disorders
Fred Plum

The brain is the organ of behavior, and the perceptive physician can learn a great deal about patients by observing their natural behavior in everyday tasks such as talking, writing, taking a coat off or putting it on, and especially how they coordinate their movements in the everyday acts of walking and turning. Natural walking represents a well-coordinated continuum of a series of falls under the momentum of a forwardly pushed torso and head. Normal gaits vary widely but have certain features in common. Head and trunk are held generally erect with the face and eyes looking forward rather than consistently either skyward or earthward. The four extremities interact gracefully, easily, and reciprocally, with right arm and left leg moving in one direction and left arm and right leg taking the opposite direction. Normally, the legs stride along a nearly straight line with footprints spaced approximately 1 to 3 inches to either side, the spread depending somewhat on walking speed and terrain. Upon that background, the following abnormal gaits can be compared.

ATAXIA. Ataxia is a failure of muscular coordination expressed as irregularity or awkwardness of movement. Most often the analysis of ataxia as a diagnostic problem lies in distinguishing disturbances in proprioceptive control from those caused by weakness, cerebellar-vestibular abnormalities, or the influence of toxic drugs.

PROPRIOCEPTIVE (SENSORY) ATAXIA. Proprioceptive ataxia can result from abnormalities anywhere along the afferent pathway from peripheral nerve, dorsal root, dorsal spinal funiculus, or the sensory projection from the thalamus to the parietal lobe cortex. The functional defect results from an impaired perception of the location of the body part combined with relatively preserved strength in the member.

Bilateral peripheral nerve or root lesions cause a defect that characteristically (1) affects the lower more than the upper extremities, (2) involves position sense as much as or more than vibratory sensation, (3) shows absent or greatly reduced deep tendon reflexes, and (4) produces a broad-based, weaving gait that with severe sensory loss becomes lurching, sometimes leg flinging, or pounding, and is worse in the dark (rombergism). Spinal dorsal column lesions produce similar symptoms except that position loss may be more profound, the signs may be less equally symmetric, the tendon reflexes can be preserved, and pathologic reflexes may be present if the abnormality involves the corticospinal tract. Patients with peripheral or spinal sensory ataxia are subjectively well aware of their deficits. They are also aware that their lack of coordination is not due to "dizziness," which distinguishes them from patients with vestibular disorders. Parietal or thalamoparietal proprioceptive impairment produces an ataxia that is usually unilateral and (1) affects the contralateral upper extremity as severely as the lower, (2) impairs position sense disproportionately more than vibration, and (3) may go partially unrecognized or be denied by the patient (anosognosia).

CEREBELLAR ATAXIA. The motor abnormality depends on the localization of the cerebellar lesion and whether or not adjacent or related neural structures are involved. Thus midline, lateral-hemispheric, and cerebellar outflow lesions each tend to produce somewhat distinct syndromes. These differences become blurred when cerebellar tumors compress the adjacent brain stem to produce additional dysfunction or when diseases such as multiple sclerosis or spinocerebellar degeneration affect remote neurologic structures.

Spinocerebellar disorders produce a predominantly sensory ataxia superimposed on which is a variable degree of cerebellar dyssynergia. Specific cerebellar inflow and outflow pathways are commonly affected. The disorders involve predominantly the lower extremities.

Midline cerebellar dysfunction results principally from degenerative (nutritional-alcoholic) or neoplastic (e.g., medulloblastoma, hemangioblastoma, metastasis) disease. The gait is characteristic with legs thrust widely apart and extended, the arms extended in compensatory balance, and walking accomplished by short steps. Affected patients usually look at the ground for additional sensory stabilization and turn *en bloc*. With extension into the anterior midline cerebellum, stretch reflexes become hyperactive. As the disorder advances, rhythmic truncal titubation appears, often associated with abnormal rhythmic movements of the upper extremities and, eventually, nystagmus. Posterior midline space-occupying lesions may add retropulsion (see below) to this symptom complex.

Lateral cerebellar hemispheric abnormalities produce ipsilateral hypotonia and incoordination of the limbs, an irregular swaying gait and a tendency to drift toward the side of the lesion. The feet are spread apart, although not so broadly as with midline lesions, and patients characteristically cannot manage close-footed tandem walking. Rombergism is absent, but, as with all ataxias, distorted vision or closing the eyes accentuates the patient's unsteadiness. Rhythmic movements and point-to-point tests are impaired in both the upper and lower extremities. If classic intention tremor appears, it indicates a lesion involving the dentate nucleus or the superior cerebellar peduncle.

DRUNKENNESS. Drunkenness, whether due to alcohol or drugs, results mainly from bilateral labyrinthine-vestibular dysfunction and is accompanied by sensations of both vertigo and dizziness. Few patients with cerebellar disease suffer as much incapacity as the reeling, lurching, twisting, and falling inebriate. Lesser degrees of intoxication produce unsteadiness, a tottering, cautious gait with the feet placed moderately widely apart, clumsiness, dysarthria, and nystagmus in all directions.

VESTIBULAR ATAXIA. Lesions anywhere along the peripheral eighth nerve pathway from labyrinth to brain stem can cause vestibular ataxia. Affected patients tend to drift toward the side of impairment and then quickly correct the deviation in the opposite direction. Turning accentuates their unsteadiness and induces missteps. Bilateral damage or degeneration of the vestibular nuclei in the brain stem results in a narrow-based ataxia with poor compensating movements in the limbs. Patients may drift or fall to either side, and some show a tendency to retropulsion and falling backward. Closing the eyes accentuates the gait disorder.

SPASTIC ATAXIA. Combined bilateral abnormalities of the spinal dorsal columns and cortical spinal tracts produce a characteristic broad-based tottering and sometimes pounding gait with the knees held high but the legs moving stiffly. The condition occurs with demyelinating diseases and other intrinsic spinal disorders such as vascular malformations, cobalamin deficiency, arachnoiditis, and, occasionally, neoplasms.

FRONTAL LOBE GAIT DISORDERS. Patients with frontal lobe disease can suffer any of several gait disorders, depending upon the anatomic distribution of the lesions. Unilateral injury to the foot-leg area of the somatosensory cortex produces a focal monoparesis, whereas bilateral motor-premotor damage results in a relatively narrow-based, stiff-legged impairment, sometimes with scissoring of the legs. More anteriorly placed premotor and prefrontal abnormalities arise in association with deep bilateral tumors, multiple cerebral infarctions, or communicating, "low pressure" hydrocephalus. The ensuing ataxia consists of a severe difficulty in initiating walking or otherwise using the lower extremities so long as the patient is in the erect position. The feet appear glued to the floor (magnet reaction), and efforts to walk often consist of short shuffles or even hops before the legs get moving. Walking, once (or if) it begins, proceeds as a halting and broad-based movement made easier by guidance or support. At least some dementia almost always accompanies the gait disorder.

Patients with frontal ataxia of this type show a considerably greater ability to move their legs when lying supine than when standing. Examination of the lower extremities discloses an increased paratonic resistance to passive movements coupled with bilateral plantar grasp responses, extensor thrust responses and, usually, accentuated tendon reflexes. These reflex abnormalities and physiologic dysfunctions best explain the difficulty in movement.

HEMIPARESIS. Both pyramidal-corticospinal and extrapyramidal motor disorders may have a hemiparetic pattern, potentially confusing their early differentiation. Severe spastic hemiplegia from damage to the corticospinal tract or the full-blown stooped, festinating, semishuffling gait of parkinsonism is so well known and readily recognized as to require no discussion. In their initial stages, both pyramidal and extrapyramidal disorders produce mild or inconstant weakness, a susceptibility to easy fatigue in the affected member, and a sense of stiffness. Both corticospinal hemiparesis and parkinsonian hemiparesis incipiently produce a gait disorder marked by a slack arm and a reduction of automatic accessory movements on the affected side, a tendency to scuff the toe, and a degree of bodily akinesia. Both may result in an increase in muscular resistance to passive stretch on the involved side. The following points help in differential diagnosis. Patients with early pyramidal tract dysfunction tend to have unilaterally increased reflexes on the affected side. When walking, they flex the wrist and fingers, circumduct the lower extremity, and hold the foot in an equinovarus position. Patients with early hemiparetic parkinsonism, by contrast, tend to have greater facial and bodily hypokinesia, to stoop, to have difficulty in performing two independent motor acts simultaneously, and show mild cogwheel resistance on rotary movements of the elbow or wrist. They extend the affected wrist and step the weak foot forward rather than circumducting it. The foot itself is held in simple varus position. The deep tendon reflexes may or may not be slightly asymmetric.

ELDERLY GAIT DISTURBANCES. Any of several specific visual, somatosensory, or motor diseases may impair walking in elderly persons. Typical difficulties include a tendency to take slow, short, mincing, and unsteady steps. A stooped position coupled with a moderately broad-based, unsteady gait, sometimes results from a chronic communicating hydrocephalus (see Ch 436).

RETROPULSION. A tendency to step backward from the standing position or to fall backward while sitting can be a symptom of several serious, acquired midline abnormalities of the brain. Occasionally, the abnormality is associated with large, unilateral frontal lobe neoplasms that produce an increase in intracranial pressure and intracranial shift. Retropulsion of posterior fossa origin is especially dangerous, as it often comes on suddenly and is accompanied by a loss of the normal postural protective mechanisms that guard against injury during falling.

ANTALGIC GAIT. Posture and walking abnormalities developed to minimize back, hip, and other leg pain can sometimes mimic neurologic abnormalities. They can be differentiated by finding the painful lesion and an absence of abnormal neurologic signs.

HYSTERICAL GAIT. Hysteria can mimic a variety of hemiparetic, steppage, or ataxic gait disorders. With a hemiparetic type, the pattern usually reveals its genesis by an atypical dragging behind of the affected leg during a series of hops or supported steps. The most obviously factitious hysterical disorder is a lurching, irregularly based, sometimes bent-forward walk in which the patient grasps any object in reach for support and reels inconsistently from side to side. Such patients may sink to the floor but almost never endure an unsupported, self-injuring fall. Other than the gait abnormality, the neurologic examination is normal in these patients.

Keane JR: Hysterical gait disorders: 60 cases. Neurology 39:586, 1989. *A lively and perceptive evaluation of the problem finds that dystonia and chorea are most likely to be overlooked, and that prompt diagnosis leads to the best outcomes.*

Nutt JG, Marsden CD, Thompson PD: Human walking and higher level gait disorders, particularly in the elderly. Neurology 43:268, 1993. *A clinical and neurophysiologic analysis of a large number of cases.*

405 DISORDERS OF SENSATION
Jerome B. Posner

405.1 Major Sensory Symptoms

An organism perceives its environment through its sensory systems. When a sensory system is disordered, sensation may be diminished, increased, or distorted. Table 405–1 lists definitions for major sensory abnormalities.

THE NEUROBIOLOGY OF SENSORY PATHWAYS

Two major sensory pathways subserve cutaneous sensation and conscious perception. The first subserves the sensations of pain, temperature, and crude touch. The receptors are naked nerve endings connected either to small (5 μ), thinly myelinated, "A delta" fibers, which conduct at about 35 meters per second, or to unmyelinated "C" fibers (1 to 2 μ), which conduct at about 0.5 meter per second. Those sensory fibers, all of which have their cell borders in the dorsal root ganglia, enter the spinal cord and synapse in the dorsal horn. Most ascending (second order) pain fibers cross the spinal cord and divide into two groups: the neospinothalamic tract, which is believed to subserve the perception of intensity and localization of pain, temperature, and crude touch, and the paleospinothalamic tract, which is believed to subserve the arousal and emotional components of pain. The axons of the neospinothalamic tract ascend in the anterolateral quadrant of the spinal cord. The axons terminate in the thalamus, principally within the ventral posterolateral nucleus (VPL) ipsilateral to the side of their ascent. Third-order neurons from the thalamus project to somatosensory area 1 (sensorimotor cortex), with the same somatotopic localization as other sensory modalities. Lesions of pain pathways sometimes lead to chronic "neuropathic pain"; one type is called thalamic pain. The paleospinothalamic tract, whose cells of origin in the dorsal horn receive C-fiber input, consists of crossed and uncrossed fibers. Most fibers cross in the anterior commissure and ascend in the spinal cord more ventral than the neospinothalamic tract. Many of the fibers of the paleospinothalamic tract send collaterals to the reticular formation of the brain stem.

The second system subserving the functions of light touch, position sense, and tactile localization begins as cutaneous mechanoreceptors connected to larger myelinated fibers. These large fibers also enter the spinal cord via the dorsal root ganglion and ascend without synapsing in the posterior and to a lesser extent lateral columns of the cord to reach the gracile and cuneate nuclei in the low brain stem. Second-order neuron fibers then decussate and ascend in the medial lemniscus to reach the contralateral ventral posterolateral thalamus. Third-order neurons projected from the thalamus terminate in the cerebral cortex, predominantly in the sensorimotor strip surrounding the Rolandic fissure. Lesions of this system lead to loss of position sense of the limbs and body in space, inability to localize tactile stimuli or to distinguish between one and two closely placed stimuli, and inability to describe accurately the size, shape, and texture of objects (stereoanesthesia). Subcortical lesions of the system also cause loss of the ability to recognize vibratory sensation (pallesthesia).

LOCALIZATION OF SENSORY DISORDERS

PERIPHERAL NERVES. Many diseases of peripheral nerves affect both large and small fibers, leading to a diminution of all sensory modalities to approximately equal degree. In some disorders of peripheral nerves, either small or large fibers can be involved preferentially, leading to a "dissociated sensory loss." When small fibers are predominantly affected, pain and temperature sensation are involved out of proportion to light touch, vibration, and position sense. Spontaneous pain and burning dysesthetic sensations are common and often provide the presenting complaints. Because autonomic fibers are also small, trophic changes in skin and joints may accompany such a small-fiber peripheral neuropathy, but because motor fibers and the afferent portion of the stretch reflex are subserved by large fibers, these functions are relatively preserved. Such selective small fiber damage is sometimes encountered in diabetes and is common in some of the hereditary neuropathies as well as in toxic-nutritional neuropathies (see Ch. 449 and 450).

Large fiber damage, more common in demyelinating neuropathies, is characterized by profound loss of localizing touch and proprioception, with relative preservation of crude touch, pain, and temperature sensation. Paresthesias are common. The deep tendon reflexes are lost because of damage to large afferent fibers and there is usually weakness as well.

The diagnosis of a peripheral neuropathy (see Ch. 445 to 452) involving sensory fibers is established by the distribution of the sensory loss, which may be in the distribution of a single nerve, multiple individual nerves, or a symmetric distal stocking-and-glove distribution. Polyneuropathies are distributed distally because longer axons are more vulnerable to disease than shorter ones. In general, mononeuropathies are caused by local disease (e.g., compression entrapment), or vascular disorders (e.g., polyarteritis) and polyneuropathies by immunologic or metabolic disorders (e.g., demyelination-inflammatory neuropathy, diabetes, uremia, nutritional neuropathy).

SPINAL CORD. Dissociation of sensory loss is more common in spinal cord disorders than in those originating in peripheral nerves or roots. Lesions of the posterolateral columns produce profound loss of position and vibration sense with normal crude touch, pain, and temperature sensation. Usually corticospinal tracts are involved as well, causing hyperactive reflexes and extensor plantar responses. Lesions of the spinothalamic tract or of crossing fibers from the posterior horn to the spinothalamic tract cause loss of pain and temperature sense with preservation of vibration, position, and localizing touch. Such dissociated sensory loss is common in syringomyelia and may occur with infarction of the anterior portion of the spinal cord from occlusion of the anterior spinal artery. In both of these disorders, motor function may be relatively well preserved. When only one side of the spinal cord is involved, proprioceptive sensation is lost on the ipsilateral side and pain and temperature sensation on the contralateral side, both below the level of the lesion. A small band of decreased sensation to all modalities resulting from damage to the posterior horn marks the level of the lesion. This so-called Brown-Séquard syndrome is sometimes seen with tumors compressing or invading the spinal cord and is common in radiation myelopathy. Lesions of the spinal cord are rarely confused with those of peripheral nerves because the sensory loss in spinal

TABLE 405–1. MAJOR SENSORY SYMPTOMS DEFINED

Hypesthesia, anesthesia: reduction or loss of cutaneous touch sensation
Hypalgesia, analgesia: reduction or loss of cutaneous pain sensation
Hyperesthesia: lowered sensory threshold to cutaneous touch
Hyperalgesia: lowered cutaneous threshold to noxious stimuli
Hyperpathia: elevated threshold to noxious stimuli with accentuated discomfort above the threshold
Paresthesias: spontaneously arising exteroceptive sensation (e.g., pins and needles sensations, burning sensations)
Dysesthesias: unpleasant distortion of innocuous afferent stimuli
Allodynia: the perception of an ordinarily nonpainful stimulus as painful or excruciating

cord lesions is usually proximal as well as distal and restricted to those segments damaged below the spinal cord level. Furthermore, motor signs of upper motor neuron disease, particularly extensor plantar responses, usually correctly identify the central nature of a spinal cord disorder rather than point to a peripheral disturbance.

BRAIN STEM. In the lower brain stem, spinothalamic and proprioceptive pathways remain separated, lateral lesions of the medulla causing loss of pain and temperature sensation on the ipsilateral side of the face (a result of damage to the descending root of the trigeminal nerve) and the contralateral side of the body. This sensory abnormality is usually accompanied by other signs of lateral medullary damage (Wallenberg's syndrome) and spares proprioceptive pathways. Higher in the brain stem, as the two pathways converge in their route toward the thalamus, damage causes contralateral sensory loss to all modalities, usually accompanied by cranial nerve palsies, ataxia (from the cerebellar outflow), and motor weakness.

CEREBRUM. In the thalamus, damage to the ventral posterolateral nucleus causes decreased sensation of all modalities on the contralateral side of the body and face. Sensory loss is often accompanied by dysesthesias and sometimes pain.

Lindblom U, Ochoa JL: Somatosensory function and dysfunction. *In* Asbury AK, McKhann GM, McDonald WI (eds.): Diseases of the Nervous System, 2nd ed. Philadelphia, WB Saunders, 1992, p 213. *A concise but comprehensive discussion.*

405.2 Headache and Other Head Pain

Headache ranks ninth among the causes of visits to physicians and is a major source both of time lost from work and of medical diagnostic procedures. The frequency of disabling headache is explained in part by the rich nerve supply to the head (including afferent nerve fibers from trigeminal, glossopharyngeal, vagus, and upper three cervical nerves). Head pain can result from distortion, stretching, inflammation, or destruction of pain-sensitive nerve endings as a result of intra- or extracranial disease in the distribution of any of the aforementioned nerves. Most head pain carries a benign prognosis. The physician's twofold task is first to distinguish more common, benign head pain from rarer but more serious causes and then to administer appropriate treatment. The diagnosis can usually be established by history and physical findings alone; skull radiographs, computed tomographic (CT) and magnetic resonance (MR) images, and other diagnostic tests are seldom required. Table 405–2 is a simplified classification of the pathogenesis of head pain. The overwhelming majority of headaches are either migraine or so-called tension headaches, with both abnormalities frequently playing a role in a given individual.

MIGRAINE AND OTHER VASCULAR HEADACHES

The term *vascular headache* applies to a group of clinical syndromes of unknown origin in which the final step in pathogenesis of the pain appears to be dilatation of one or more branches of the carotid artery, leading to stimulation of sensitized periarterial nociceptors by noxious substances released by the artery or nerve. Such substances as serotonin, substance P, bradykinin, histamine, prostaglandins, and calcitonin gene–related peptides alone or in combination have all been implicated in the pathogenesis of vascu-

TABLE 405–2. PATHOPHYSIOLOGIC CLASSIFICATION OF HEADACHE

Vascular Headache	Depressive equivalent
Migraine headache	Conversion reaction
Classic migraine	Temporomandibular joint
Common migraine	dysfunction
Complicated migraine	Atypical facial pain
Variant migraine	**Traction-Inflammation Headache**
Cluster headache	Cranial arteritis
Episodic cluster	Increased or decreased intra-
"Chronic" cluster	cranial pressure
Chronic paroxysmal	Extracranial structural lesions
hemicrania	Pituitary tumors
Miscellaneous vascular	
headaches	**Extracranial Structural Lesions**
Carotidynia	Parnasal sinusitis and tumors
Hypertension	Dental infections
Orgasmic, exertional, and	Otitis
cough headache	Ocular lesions
Hangover	Pituitary tumors
Toxins and drugs	Cervical osteoarthritis
Occlusive vascular disease	**Cranial Neuralgias**
Tension Headache	
Common tension headache	

lar headache. Most vascular headaches are unilateral, often but not always throbbing, and recurrent over months or years. Individual headaches are precipitated in some by identifiable environmental, dietary, or psychological factors. During the course of a vascular headache, the involved arteries may be tender to the touch. Most vascular headaches can be relieved by prompt administration of ergotamine or sumatriptan; recurrent headaches can often be prevented by one of several prophylactic drugs (see below). So-called common migraine may affect as many as 25% of the population. Other vascular headache syndromes are less common, but each has distinctive clinical findings.

Classic Migraine

Classic migraine is distinguished by an onset that includes well-defined symptoms of neurologic dysfunction that precede or, less often, accompany the headache. Neurologic symptoms are usually visual, consisting of bright flashing lights (scintillation or fortification scotomata) beginning in the center of a visual half-field and radiating over 10 to 30 minutes outward toward the periphery. Less commonly, the visual abnormalities are monocular (retinal) or consist of hemianoptic loss of vision in place of or following the scintillating scotomata. Other neurologic disturbances that can occur in classic migraine include unilateral paresthesias, usually involving the hand and perioral area, aphasia, hemiparesis, and hemisensory defects. An uncommon variant named *basilar artery migraine* occurs predominantly in children and adolescents and is characterized by vertigo, ataxia, and diplopia, along with hemiparesis or hemisensory changes. Rarely, confusion, stupor, or even coma may develop. Neurologic symptoms of classic migraine usually last no longer than 30 minutes and generally clear before the headache phase begins. Rarely, such signs may persist for hours or even days.

The pathogenesis of the neurologic dysfunction is not fully understood. Measurements of regional cerebral blood flow during episodes of classic migraine have shown a wave of focal hyperemia followed by abnormally low flow spreading from posterior to anterior over the cerebral cortex. The flow reduction may be sufficient to cause the neurologic symptoms and, rarely, cerebral infarction. In most cases, however, the changes are insufficient to explain the neurologic symptoms. One explanation is that a wave of physiologic "spreading" depression spreads across the cortex, accounting for both the neurologic symptoms and the changes in blood flow. Changes in brain blood flow do not accompany common migraine, even though the headache phase of the illness is similar. Thus, it is likely that if "spreading depression" is the cause of the neurologic symptoms of migraine, it is only one of several precipitating factors that may produce the headache.

The syndrome of classic migraine has four parts: (1) A *prodromal phase* occurs in a minority of patients and consists of an alteration of mood, often occurring for 24 or more hours before the headache. In some patients, known precipitants such as red wine commonly induce an attack. (2) The second phase consists of the *neurologic symptoms* described above. These may occur without subsequent headache (termed migraine equivalent), particularly in older people. (3) The third phase usually begins as the neurologic symptoms clear and characteristically consists of a unilateral throbbing frontotemporal *headache* on the side opposite the neurologic symptoms. The headache is frequently accompanied by nausea, photophobia, vomiting, diarrhea, phonophobia (noise intolerance), and a general feeling of being unwell. The headache commonly lasts 4 to 6 hours but may persist for 1 or more days. Prolonged headaches may change into a dull, aching, bilateral pain extending back into the neck and shoulders. The headache phase is often terminated either by vomiting or by a period of sleep. (4) The *postheadache* phase is characterized by a feeling of exhaustion, tenderness of the scalp and recurrence of head pain on sudden head movement.

The diagnosis of classic migraine is made by history; physical findings are absent, and laboratory evaluation is not helpful. When the attacks are atypical, particularly when neurologic disability is severe or prolonged, CT or MR imaging may be required to rule out structural lesions of the brain. Such instances are rare. The treatment of classic migraine is similar to that of common migraine (see below), except that classic migraine attacks usually occur no more than four or five times a year and rarely more than once a month.

Common Migraine

Common migraine is similar to classic migraine but lacks the neurologic symptoms. Many persons with classic migraine also have episodes of common migraine. Common migraine is characterized by recurrent headaches, often severe, frequently beginning unilaterally, and usually associated with malaise, nausea and/or vomiting, and photophobia. The disorder often begins in childhood, affects women more often than men, and runs in families (70% of patients give a family history). Identifiable factors that often precipitate individual headaches are holidays and weekends, menstrual periods, foods (especially red wine, chocolate, nuts, and aged cheese), environmental stimuli (such as bright sunlight, too much sleep, and undue emotional stress or resentment). Medical conditions and their treatment may also precipitate attacks. Vasodilators such as nitroglycerin and antihypertensives and serotonin releasers such as reserpine, as well as estrogens and oral contraceptives, have been reported to cause migraine attacks in susceptible individuals. The diagnosis is usually made by the history. Important historical points that help distinguish migraine from tension-type headaches (see below) include their unilaterality, their association with nausea or vomiting, the tendency of migraine to awaken one from sleep, a positive family history, and a positive response to sumatriptan or ergotamine. When the diagnosis is in doubt, treatment of the patient for common migraine often clarifies the issue.

TREATMENT. The best treatment for migraine is prevention. The patient should avoid known precipitating factors. Medications known to cause migraine should be withdrawn if others can be substituted. Foods commonly implicated may also be withdrawn and, if withdrawal is effective, replaced one at a time to determine the specific precipitant. The patient should attempt to avoid undue stress or fatigue and not to sleep excessively on weekends. If these methods fail and severe headaches occur frequently (once a week or more), pharmacologic prophylaxis is indicated. Several agents have been reported effective in the prophylaxis of migraine, but not every patient responds to each agent. Effective drugs include β-adrenergic, serotonin, and calcium channel blockers, antidepressants, nonsteroidal anti-inflammatory agents, valproic acid, and others.

Acute attacks, if mild, often respond to analgesic agents and bedrest. More severe attacks are best treated by ergotamine or sumatriptan. Either drug, given parenterally, is sufficiently effective (85 to 90%) to be useful as a diagnostic test. Oral ergot 1 to 2 mg given at the onset of a headache is effective in fewer patients. Better results can be achieved with sublingual or rectal preparations, preferably one half of a 2-mg ergotamine rectal suppository. The side effects of *ergotism* (muscle pain, vasoconstriction, mottled

skin, peripheral gangrene, multifocal encephalopathy) make it unwise to treat frequent migraine headaches in this way, and one should switch to prophylaxis if the headaches occur more than once a week. For patients who present to emergency departments with severe headaches sumatriptan by injection is the drug of choice.

Migraine Variants

Several migraine syndromes differ sufficiently from classic and common migraine to earn separate names. *Ophthalmoplegic migraine* describes an ocular motor palsy occurring during the course of a severe migraine attack. Ophthalmoplegic migraine usually begins in childhood and is characterized by unilateral pupillary dilatation, ptosis, and paralysis of ocular muscles occurring 12 to 24 hours *after* the beginning of an attack of severe migraine. The ophthalmoplegia usually clears within hours to days but frequently recurs. Angiography may be required to rule out a carotid aneurysm. *Hemiplegic migraine* is a familial syndrome in which aphasia, confusion, and hemiparesis or hemiplegia precede or more often accompany the migraine attack. Repetitive episodes alternating from side to side may occur over many years. *Complicated migraine* defines attacks of migraine prodromes in which the focal neurologic defects may last for the entire headache attack and even leave permanent residua. The few available anatomic studies of such patients have shown ischemic brain infarction involving the functionally impaired region.

Cluster Headache

Cluster headaches are short-lived attacks of severe, acute, and intense unilateral head pain that recurrently occur in clusters lasting several weeks, only to disappear for months or years. It is only about one twenty-fifth as common as migraine. The disorder affects men much more than women and usually begins between the third and sixth decades. Clusters characteristically occur in the spring and fall and last 3 to 8 weeks. The individual headaches occur one to several times a day, particularly at night, awakening the victim from sleep. Each attack, which lasts 30 minutes to 2 hours, is characterized by rapid onset of a knife-like pain in the nostril or behind the eye which spreads to involve the forehead. During the attack, the ipsilateral nostril may water and the eye tear. In about 20% of instances, a Horner syndrome develops. The headache pain may be so severe that these patients restlessly pace the floor, bang their head against the wall, and may threaten suicide. The headache disappears as abruptly as it arises, usually without residua. Unlike migraine, cluster headaches do not make persons systemically ill. No nausea, vomiting, or exhaustion appear when the headache ceases. When clusters are occurring (but not between) alcohol invariably induces attack. When the headaches occur frequently, the Horner syndrome may outlast the head pain.

The pathogenesis of cluster headache is unknown, although it is believed to relate to migraine. The diagnosis is established by the characteristic history. Treatment of an acute attack is usually not worthwhile, since by the time the patient absorbs the analgesic agents the attack is over. In some patients the headache rapidly responds to oxygen inhalation. Several drugs prevent attacks of cluster headache. Ergotamine tartrate given prophylactically in a dose of 1 mg four times a day, or 2 mg at bedtime if the attacks are all nocturnal, is often effective. The drug should be withdrawn every seventh day to prevent the symptoms of ergotism and to see if the cluster has ceased. Other drugs reported to be effective in some patients include those listed for migraine prophylaxis.

Cluster Variants

Several variants of cluster headache require different treatment. *Chronic paroxysmal hemicrania* is a rare disorder consisting of cluster headaches that appear many times a day and recur unremittingly for years. There may be as many as 10 to 20 headaches daily, each lasting 10 to 30 minutes. Indomethacin* orally in doses of 75 to 150 mg daily has relieved all subjects. A cluster variant characterized by daily cluster headache without remission, multiple brief jabs of pain in the head, and a background of continuous unilateral headache of variable severity exacerbated by exertion has recently been described and is said to respond to indomethacin in

---

* This use is not listed in the manufacturer's directive.

most instances. Patients who did not respond to indomethacin did so to tricyclic antidepressants.

Other Vascular Headaches

Orgasmic headaches are short-lived bilateral throbbing headaches that occur in either sex and appear abruptly at orgasm. The headache usually disappears within minutes to an hour or more and may recur repetitively. Usually the illness is self-limited, but if not it may respond to 1 mg of ergot given an hour before sexual activity. *Exertional headache* occurs, as the name implies, during active exercise. It is usually bilateral and throbbing and may last several hours, responding well to indomethacin. Vascular headaches have been reported to follow minor *trauma* to the carotid artery in the neck and *carotid endarterectomy.* The headaches are unilateral, recurrent, and severe and usually respond to prophylaxis with propranolol. *Carotidynia* is the name given to spontaneous vascular headaches associated with unilateral anterior neck pain and/or carotid tenderness. They usually respond to the same treatment as migraines. When attacks of carotid pain and/or headache recur, the diagnosis is not difficult, but the first attack must be distinguished from a spontaneous dissection of the carotid artery and may require angiography for diagnosis.

Hangover headache is part of a larger syndrome, usually including premature awakening from an evening of overindulgence and often accompanied by a fine tremor of the extremities, mild gastric distress or nausea, mental dulling, and mild incoordination. The pathogenesis relates to alcohol withdrawal, dehydration, and the toxic effect of various congeners found with different intoxicants. *Nitrites* can induce pulsating headache and, occasionally, facial flushing, most often after the ingestion of processed foods ("hot dog" headache). *Monosodium glutamate* has been blamed for the "Chinese restaurant syndrome," characterized by postprandial headache, tight sensations about the face and head, and, less often, giddiness and diarrhea.

Cough headache is, as the name implies, sudden and often severe headache related to cough. The headache may last only seconds or may persist minutes to hours after a single cough or a coughing paroxysm. In some patients, cough headache is a symptom of an intracranial mass lesion. Most patients, however, do not have underlying structural disease; in these patients the disorder is probably similar to exertional and orgasmic headaches and has a vascular origin. *"Ice pick"* headaches are brief (1 to 2 seconds), sharp focal head pains occurring at unpredictable intervals and at different areas of the head. They do not indicate intracranial disease. *Thunderclap* headaches are sudden, severe, "exploding" pains that involve the entire head and resolve slowly over hours. Although such headaches occasionally reflect a small subarachnoid hemorrhage, most are without pathologic significance. A severe thunderclap headache probably deserves evaluation by lumbar puncture to look for subarachnoid blood. If found angiography may be indicated to seek an intracranial aneurysm.

Hypertensive headaches occur only in patients with very severe or episodic hypertension. They are characterized by early-morning, usually throbbing, occipital headache that responds to the treatment of the hypertension.

TENSION-TYPE HEADACHES

Tension-type headache is the term applied to a form of benign head pain that occasionally affects most persons. The disorder is characterized by pain of mild to moderate intensity, usually bilateral in location, and typically pressing or "tight" in quality. The pain may be chronic or episodic; if episodic, it may last minutes to days. The feeling of being unwell—with nausea, photophobia, and phonophobia so common with migraine—is usually absent. Tension-type headaches are uncommon, but associated symptoms can include dizziness, blurring of vision, and tinnitus.

The pathogenesis of the disorder is unknown. The term *tension-type headache* describes both the pericranial muscle tightening and tenderness found in some patients and the emotional anxiety and psychological tension present in others. The role of these two factors in pathogenesis is not clearly established. Tension headaches affect some persons daily. They usually begin in early afternoon or evening, with a dull occipital or frontal pain that may spread to grip the entire head "in a vise." Unique among headaches, the pain may remain constant for days, weeks, or months and is often associated with tenderness in the posterior cervical, temporalis, or masseter muscles. Tension-type headaches are more frequent in women, in individuals who are tense and anxious, and in those whose work or posture requires sustained contraction of posterior cervical, frontal, or temporal muscles. The symptoms of common migraine and tension headaches overlap, and many persons suffer from both. The distinguishing features favoring tension-type headaches include pressure or tightness, which is worst at the back of the neck, increased severity of pain as the day progresses, and pain that is preceded by or associated with anxiety-producing situations. Tension-type headaches seldom awaken the patient from sleep. They do not respond to ergot preparations.

In many respects muscle pain and tenderness in tension headaches resemble the fibromyalgia syndrome, whatever that disorder may be.

TREATMENT. The first step in treating tension-type headache lies in identifying causal factors, if any. Many such patients are depressed and respond to treatment with antidepressant agents such as amitriptyline. Others are tense and anxious and respond to anti-anxiety agents such as diazepam. This drug, in a dose of 15 to 20 mg a day for 2 to 3 weeks, is often effective as a diagnostic test. The relief of chronic headache establishes the diagnosis for the physician and helps to convince the patient that tension and anxiety are playing a major role. Also, these drugs frequently break up a cycle of anxiety–muscle tension–anxiety, so that a short course may give prolonged relief. Physical dependence at doses < 30 mg a day is rare.

An individual headache may be treated with aspirin. This drug is probably more useful for tension headaches than acetaminophen because of its anti-prostaglandin properties. Vasoactive agents used for the treatment of migraine have no role although sumatriptan should be tried at least once. Some clinics report that biofeedback treatments effectively relieve muscle contraction and thus the headache. For sharply localized, painful areas present at the site of headache, injection with local anesthetics may transiently relieve the headaches. Sometimes massage has a similar effect. Chronic ingestion of analgesic agents may cause tension-type headaches. Withdrawal of the medication usually relieves the headaches.

Tension-Type Headache Variants

Several rather characteristic headache syndromes of unknown cause may be variants of tension-type headache. One is the so-called temporomandibular joint syndrome. Patients complain of unilateral or bilateral head pain, usually in the temporal region and in the jaw, often radiating into the ear. The pain is often associated with tenderness of the masseter and temporalis muscles and may be exacerbated by chewing. Accompanying symptoms often include limitation of full movement at the temporomandibular joint when opening the jaw, bruxism, and malocclusion. The disorder sometimes responds to dental manipulation, particularly use of a mouth guard during sleep that prevents bruxism. However, for most patients analgesics and anxiolytic agents effectively treat such muscle-contraction head pains. *Post-traumatic headaches* are dull, generalized, aching head pains that follow head injury. The injury is often mild. Patients suffering the "post-traumatic syndrome" complain of headache often coupled with unsteadiness, giddiness, difficulty concentrating, insomnia, and fatigue. Compensation issues seem to have no effect. The headache often persists for months or years. Treatment, like that of tension-type headaches, consists of psychological support, reassurance, and the use of mild analgesics or anxiolytic agents. Patients should be encouraged to return to work as soon as possible and to try to live a normal life despite the symptoms. The disorder can blend into *depressive headache,* a chronic generalized headache, usually vaguely described, sometimes associated with giddiness and unsteadiness, that occurs as a frequent and sometimes predominant manifestation of depression. The treatment of choice is an antidepressant drug.

Atypical Facial Pain

Atypical facial pain or *atypical facial neuralgia* describes a syndrome characterized by steady aching facial pain, usually unilateral, localized to the lower part of the orbit, maxillary area, and sometimes the jaw. The pain begins without a known precipitating episode and may last for hours, days, or indefinitely. It may spread to involve the head or neck, and muscles of the jaw and neck are often tender. Sometimes autonomic symptoms including sweating, flushing, rhinorrhea, and pallor are present. The disorder usually affects women, often in early middle age. Patients are tense, anxious, and often chronically depressed. The pathogenesis of the illness is unknown. The autonomic changes have led some to suggest that the syndrome is a migraine variant, and the muscle tenderness and depression have led others to suggest that it be classified with tension-type headache. Patients suffering from atypical facial pain should be examined carefully for pathology of the eyes, nose, teeth, sinuses, and pharynx, but such is rarely found. Careful psychological evaluation often reveals a masked depression. Treatment is usually unsatisfactory. Analgesic agents are usually not helpful, and patients respond poorly to psychotherapy. Antidepressants sometimes help. It is important to recognize that the syndrome is not caused by structural disease and that patients require no invasive diagnostic or therapeutic procedures. Above all, surgical "treatment," including dental extraction, does more harm than good. This disorder should not be confused with trigeminal neuralgia, discussed below; carbamazepine is ineffective.

HEAD PAIN DUE TO TRACTION OR INFLAMMATION

Cranial Arteritis

This condition receives detailed consideration in Ch. 246 but deserves mention here as an important cause of headache in the elderly. The illness almost always appears after age 60 and usually later. It begins with unilateral or bilateral temporal, occipital, or fronto-occipital head pain of variable intensity, often coupled with tenderness of the painful areas. Many patients have pain in the jaw muscles, making chewing uncomfortable. Nodules occasionally are palpable on affected vessels. The great risk is occlusion of retinal arteries secondary to untreated inflammation. Diagnosis depends on suspicion and usually on the presence of an elevated erythrocyte sedimentation rate. Diagnosis should be confirmed by arterial biopsy because definitive steroid treatment, once started, often must be maintained for many months. Because migraine-vascular headaches and depressive headaches also can have their onset in the elderly, a confirmed diagnosis is essential.

Alterations of Intracranial Pressure

Headache from altered intracranial pressure is caused by compression or traction of pain-sensitive vascular and neural structures over the apex and base of the brain. In the instance of *intracranial hypotension,* the loss of spinal fluid decreases the buoyancy of the brain so that the organ descends when the upright position is assumed, exerting traction on structures at its apex and compression on structures at its base. Compensatory vasodilation may also contribute to the pain. (In rare instances, the small bridging veins that enter the sagittal sinus may rupture and cause subdural hematomas.) In *intracranial hypertension,* the source of pain is probably compression of vascular and neural structures at the base of the brain by tumor or edematous brain.

INTRACRANIAL HYPERTENSION. Increased intracranial pressure per se does not lead to headache unless pain-sensitive structures are distorted. Many patients with high intracranial pressure from brain tumors, jugular venous obstruction, hydrocephalus, or pseudotumor cerebri do not suffer headache. If headache is present, it may be mild or severe, throbbing or steady, localized or generalized. When localized, it usually overlies the site of the lesion, but posterior fossa lesions may cause bifrontal headache. The headache is characteristically at its worst early in the morning, although, unlike cluster headache, it usually does not awaken the patient from sleep. It is exacerbated by stooping, coughing, moving the head suddenly, or straining at stool. Many patients prefer to sleep in the sitting position. The headache is rarely continuously intense. Transient rises of intracranial pressure called plateau waves (see Ch. 436) sometimes cause 5 to 20 minutes of severe headache accompanied by nausea, vomiting, or other neurologic signs. These episodes are commonly precipitated by assuming the upright posture but can also be precipitated by coughing, sneezing, or straining.

The treatment of headache related to increased intracranial pressure is the treatment of the underlying disease. Mild analgesics give temporary relief; narcotic analgesics should not be used because of their tendency to produce respiratory depression and further raise the pressure in neurologically compromised individuals.

INTRACRANIAL HYPOTENSION (see Ch. 436) **AND LUMBAR PUNCTURE HEADACHE.** Intracranial hypotension usually follows a lumbar puncture and is due to continued leakage of cerebrospinal fluid (CSF) through a rent in the dural sheath. The syndrome develops 12 hours to several days after the lumbar puncture and is characterized by headache on assuming the upright position. There is no evidence that a period of recumbency after a lumbar puncture prevents subsequent development of the headache. The headache usually begins as a dull ache in the posterior cervical area, radiating laterally toward the shoulders and cephalad toward the frontal area. It persists, often growing more severe, as long as the patient remains upright. When most severe it may be associated with diaphoresis, nausea, and vomiting. Persistent headache of intracranial hypotension can lead to diplopia, probably a result of traction on the abducens nerves. The diagnosis is made by history; spontaneous intracranial hypotension is suspected by the history of positional headache and confirmed by low (< 30 mm H_2O) or even negative CSF pressure on attempted lumbar puncture. The fluid is usually normal, but there may be an elevated protein concentration if the needle has entered a subdural or epidural fluid collection. Analgesics relieve the mildest headaches; the most severe ones can be controlled only by assuming the recumbent position.

EXTRACRANIAL STRUCTURAL CAUSES OF HEADACHE

Nasal and Sinus Headache

Although acute or chronic inflammation and neoplasms of the paranasal sinuses can cause headache, most patients who have been diagnosed as having sinus headaches are in fact suffering from either vascular or tension-type headache. True paranasal sinus headaches result from acute inflammation causing pain localized over the involved sinus and associated with stigmata of acute infection, including fever, swelling, and tenderness over the sinus and engorgement of the turbinates, ostia, nasofrontal ducts, and superior nasal spaces. Most of the discomfort comes from the ostia, which are many times more sensitive than the poorly innervated walls of the sinuses. True sinus headache is dull and aching, made worse by changing head position, and seldom associated with nausea and vomiting. Sinus headache is treated with decongestants and analgesics. Persistent purulent discharges should be cultured and appropriate antimicrobial drugs employed. Chronic suppurative disease in the frontal, ethmoid, and sphenoid sinuses, or in the mastoid air cells, may result in osteomyelitis and inflammation of adjacent cranial tissues. Headache persisting after surgical drainage of a diseased sinus suggests extradural and possibly subdural infection. More chronic inflammation and neoplasms, particularly when they occur in the sphenoid sinus, may not be accompanied by the usual physical signs of sinusitis. In such instances, CT or MR scan may be required to establish the diagnosis.

Dental Pain

Noxious stimuli in a tooth usually evoke local toothache, but severe dental pain can be difficult to localize. Afferent fibers from the teeth are contained in the second and third divisions of the trigeminal nerve, and tooth pain can be referred to areas of the head supplied by these nerves. More commonly, in association with toothache, tooth extraction, or a tender, diseased tooth, distant tissues exhibit surface hyperalgesia, tenderness, and vasomotor reactions, such as tender eyeballs, reddening of the conjunctivae, and tenderness of the auricular and temporal tissues. Because of secondary muscle contraction, other sites of tenderness and pain may be noted behind the ears, behind the lower border of the mastoid process, and in the muscles of the occiput, neck, and shoulders. The upper teeth frequently hurt in association with disease of the nasal and paranasal structures. Occasionally, in coronary insufficiency, pain is experienced in the lower jaw. One should beware of ascribing bizarre pains in and around the jaws to a dental origin unless unequivocal acute inflammatory dental lesions are present. Dental extraction rarely ameliorates neuralgias or atypical facial pain. Headache should not be attributed to a diseased tooth unless the injection of procaine into the tissues about the suspected tooth greatly reduces the intensity of, or eliminates, such headache.

Aural Pain

Severe pain in the vicinity of the ear can be caused by disease of the teeth, acute tonsillitis, inflammatory and neoplastic disease of the larynx and nasopharynx, temporomandibular joint disorders, tumors, inflammation in the posterior fossa, and disease of the cervical spine and its soft tissues. Pain in the ear is also associated with vascular headaches, atypical facial pain, and herpes zoster of the fifth and seventh cranial nerves and, rarely, the glossopharyngeal nerve. True glossopharyngeal neuralgia causes severe pain radiating from the tonsil into the ear. It has the usual timing feature of "tic" (see Cranial Neuralgias below).

Headaches due to primary ear disease almost always indicates inflammation or destructive disease. Acute otitis media (purulent or nonpurulent), furunculosis of the ear canal, traumatic rupture of the tympanum, and fracture of the anterior wall of the bony canal all cause pain in the ear associated with tenderness of adjacent skeletal muscles. Osteomyelitis of the mastoid bone may be associated with inflammation of the nearby periosteum as well as of dura and adjacent tissues (epidural abscess)—both sources of pain in or behind the ear. Pain in this region also accompanies tumors of the acoustic nerve and inflammation and thrombosis of the lateral sinus.

Eye Pain and Headache

Many minor eye disorders are blamed for headache, which actually turns out to be tension-type head pain. The pain of *glaucoma* at first remains localized in the eyeball, then extends along the rim of the orbit and, finally, throughout most of the area supplied by the ophthalmic division of the trigeminal nerve. Nausea and vomiting sometimes accompany such headaches, which can become prostratingly severe if not treated promptly.

With inflammation of the iris and ciliary body, light may cause intense pain in the eye and adjacent areas because of movement of the inflamed iris. When the iris is immobilized, pain is allayed.

Pituitary Pain

Headache caused by pituitary tumors is the result of compression and distortion of pain-sensitive structures at the base of the skull, particularly the diaphragma sella. Pain is generally referred to the frontal or temporal regions bilaterally and may on occasion be referred to the vertex or occipital regions. The pain can occur at any time and is frequently chronic and unremitting. The diagnosis can be established by MRI of the pituitary fossa. Acute headache occurring with known pituitary lesions (*pituitary apoplexy*) usually results from infarction or hemorrhage into the tumor. Sudden expansion of the tumor may compromise the overlying optic chiasm, leading to visual loss, or invade the laterally lying cavernous sinus, causing ocular palsies. Pituitary apoplexy is usually treated surgically by drainage of the hemorrhagic or infarcted material.

Neck Pain

Osteoarthritis of the zygapophyseal joints of the upper cervical spine is an occasional cause of perplexing headache. The pain is generally constant and aching and perceived in the upper cervical and occipital areas. It may radiate to the vertex of the head or even the orbit. At times, vertex or orbital pain is more severe than occipital and neck pain, leading to confusion in diagnosis. The pain probably results from entrapment of the C3 root by overgrowth of the C2 zygapophyseal joint. A syndrome of unilateral upper nuchal and occipital pain accompanied by ipsilateral numbness of the tongue occurring on sudden turning of the head is probably explained by compression of the second cervical root in the atlanto-occipital space. Such acute pain can be prevented by restricting neck movement with a cervical collar. Upper cervical nerve blocks relieve more chronic pain and are useful diagnostically as well as therapeutically.

CRANIAL NEURALGIAS

The term *cranial neuralgias* refers to several distinctive head pains that appear to result from sudden and excessive discharge from the involved nerve. The best-known cranial neuralgia is trigeminal neuralgia. The concept of cranial neuralgias has been expanded to include the chronic burning pain that frequently follows herpes zoster infection of the nerve.

TRIGEMINAL NEURALGIA. Trigeminal neuralgia (tic douloureux) is characterized by sudden, lightning-like paroxysms of pain in the distribution of one or more divisions of the trigeminal nerve. Most trigeminal neuralgia is caused by compression of the trigeminal nerve by normal but aging arteries or veins of the posterior fossa. In some patients there is no identifiable structural disease. Occasionally trigeminal neuralgia may be a symptom of a gasserian ganglion tumor, multiple sclerosis, or a brain-stem infarct involving the descending root of the trigeminal nerve.

The history is diagnostic. The pain occurs as brief, lightning-like stabs, frequently precipitated by touching a trigger zone around the lips or the buccal cavity. At times, talking, eating, or brushing the teeth serves as a trigger. The pains rarely last longer than seconds, and each burst is followed by a refractory period of several seconds to a minute in which no further pain can be precipitated. The pains, however, often occur in clusters so that the patient may report somewhat erroneously that each pain lasts for hours. The pain is limited to one or more divisions of the trigeminal nerve, usually the second, or third, or both. Spontaneous remissions and exacerbations are common, the exacerbations tending to occur in spring and fall. Between paroxysms of pain, the patient is asymptomatic. Tic pain rarely occurs at night. In idiopathic trigeminal neuralgia, the neurologic examination is entirely normal. In symptomatic trigeminal neuralgia, there may be sensory changes in the distribution of the trigeminal nerve, and such a finding should prompt a careful search for structural disease of the nervous system.

Carbamazepine usually is effective in doses varying from 400 to 800 mg a day, but because of its sedative properties the initial dose is 100 mg twice daily, gradually increased to the required maintenance dose. The drug is primarily an anticonvulsive, not an analgesic, and is effective only for specific kinds of pain such as trigeminal neuralgia, glossopharyngeal neuralgia, and the lightning pains of tabes dorsalis. Baclofen, phenytoin, and pimozide are also usually effective. Other occasionally effective drugs include valproate, lorazepam, and mexiletine.

The most popular operations consist of lesioning of the gasserian ganglion (either by radiofrequency or glycerol injections) and posterior fossa craniotomy to relieve the compression of the trigeminal nerve by vascular structures. Gasserian ganglion lesions can be made under local anesthesia, are generally effective initially, but have a high relapse rate. Posterior fossa craniotomy is as effective as gasserian ganglion lesions and appears to have a lower relapse rate. The purpose of both operations is to relieve pain with little or no loss of sensation, thus preventing the dreaded complications of anesthesia dolorosa.

GLOSSOPHARYNGEAL NEURALGIA. Glossopharyngeal neuralgia is characterized by pain similar to that of trigeminal neuralgia but in the distribution of the glossopharyngeal and vagus nerves. The trigger zone is usually in the tonsil or posterior pharynx, and the pain spreads toward the angle of the jaw and the ear. Occasional patients suffer cardiac slowing or arrest during these attacks as a result of the intense afferent discharge over the glossopharyngeal nerve. Carbamazepine is often effective, and if it fails, the other drugs used for trigeminal neuralgia therapy may help. If drug therapy is unsuccessful, glossopharyngeal nerve roots are sectioned in the posterior fossa. Symptomatic glossopharyngeal neuralgia is occasionally the presenting complaint of a tonsillar tumor, and careful examination of the pharynx and tonsillar fossa must be carried out.

OTHER NEURALGIAS. Similar but much rarer disorders than trigeminal or glossopharyngeal neuralgia have been reported to involve the greater occipital nerve and the nervus intermedius portion of the facial nerve. The clinical features and treatment of these rare disorders are similar to those for trigeminal neuralgia.

DIAGNOSTIC EVALUATION

Headache is extremely common and the excessive application of expensive and highly technical laboratory procedures to its diagnosis and management has been a substantial cause of unnecessary medical costs. Set against this truism is the fact that in some instances a timely MRI or lumbar puncture can give life-saving information about an otherwise undiagnosable problem. Given these antitheses, the following principles may help in management.

1. Patients with chronic classic or common migraine or with chronic tension-type headache rarely require more than a careful history and examination. Even when the unilateral prodromes and headache of longstanding, classic migraine consistently affect the same side, the incidence of associated intracranial lesions remains so low that scans are unnecessary and arteriography unjustified.

2. Headaches that have begun or worsened recently deserve investigation. This principle especially applies to headaches that have a consistently focal distribution, follow trauma, or begin after the age of 30 years. MRI is more sensitive than CT.

3. The EEG is almost never useful in the diagnosis of diseases causing headache and can be omitted. Skull radiographs are so rarely useful that they should be omitted. Even for trauma, CT scans have discriminating capacities far superior to those of plain films and make radiographs unnecessary.

4. Diagnostic lumbar puncture should be performed with any acute headache that (a) is accompanied by fever or (b) is explosive or the most severe headache ever suffered (a history typical of acute subarachnoid hemorrhage—but see thunderclap headache, p. 2033). Lumbar puncture should, if possible, be deferred until after CT scanning with other forms of acute headache, especially if stiff neck but no fever is present. (This combination may indicate partial herniation of cerebellar tonsils into the foramen magnum secondary to an intracranial mass lesion.)

5. Now that CT and MRI are widely available, radioisotopic brain scanning rarely if ever adds useful information and is expensively superfluous.

Lance JW: Mechanism and Management of Headache. Oxford, Butterworth Heinemann, 1993. *A monograph describing pathophysiology, diagnosis, and management of headaches and other head pain in a clear and concise style.*

Lauritzen M: Pathophysiology of the migraine aura. The spreading depression theory. Review article. Brain 117:199, 1994. *A comprehensive description of the pathophysiology of the migraine aura.*

Olesen J, Tfelt-Hansen P, Welch KMA (eds.): The Headaches. New York, Raven Press, 1993. *A multi-authored comprehensive text covering the basic and clinical aspects of all headache syndromes.*

405.3 Some Specific Pain Syndromes

Some chronic painful disorders are associated with a specific constellation of signs and symptoms which establishes them as identifiable pain syndromes. Those most commonly encountered in clinical practice include the *neuropathic pain* disorders of diabetic polyneuropathy (see Ch. 449), sympathetically maintained pain, postherpetic neuralgia, phantom limb pain, and the *non-neuropathic pain* syndromes, fibromyalgia and myofascial pain. Taken together, these syndromes cause chronic, usually unremitting pain that is often disabling and difficult and frustrating to treat.

SYMPATHETICALLY MAINTAINED PAIN. This term applies to severe pain, usually burning in quality and associated with autonomic changes including swelling, vasomotor instability, and abnormalities of sweating. The pain syndrome usually follows an injury, often minor, to an extremity. If the injury has involved a peripheral nerve, particularly the sciatic or median nerve, the syndrome is called *causalgia*. If the injury does not involve the peripheral nerve, if there has been no trauma, or if the syndrome follows a visceral illness (e.g., myocardial infarction), the term applied is *reflex sympathetic dystrophy*. (Older and outmoded terms include post-traumatic painful osteoporosis, Sudek's atrophy, post-traumatic spreading neuralgia, minor causalgia, and shoulder-hand syndrome.) The exact pathophysiology of the disorder is unknown, but, as the name implies, efferent activity of the sympathetic nervous system plays an important role in both the pain and the autonomic symptoms.

The disorder is characterized by severe and continuous pain exacerbated by emotional stress and usually associated with severe hyperpathia so that moving or touching the limb is often intolerable. At first the pain is localized to the site of injury or the distribution of an injured nerve, but with time it spreads to involve the entire extremity. Spread to other areas of the body sometimes occurs. Along with the pain go vasomotor changes including vasodilatation (warm and dry skin) or vasoconstriction (cyanosis, cool skin). Other autonomic changes may include edema and either hypo- or hyperhidrosis; trophic changes of the skin, subcutaneous tissues, muscles, and bone (osteoporosis) also occur. The entire symptom complex rarely affects any one patient, and one sign or symptom usually predominates. Untreated, the disorder can lead to muscle atrophy, fixation of joints, and a useless extremity. The diagnosis is largely clinical but can be supported by tests showing autonomic instability or trophic changes including increased bone uptake on radionuclide scans, bone atrophy on plain radiographs, and temperature abnormalities on thermography.

The earlier the treatment, the more effective it is likely to be. Treatment is directed at repeatedly blocking sympathetic outflow to the involved site while stimulating and mobilizing the painful area. Some physicians endorse sympatholytic agents (e.g., phenoxybenzamine up to 120 mg a day in divided doses) and short courses of corticosteroids. Nevertheless, many patients fail to respond. In refractory patients pharmacologic agents directed at neuropathic pain, including tricyclic antidepressants (e.g., amitriptyline, 50 to 150 mg at bedtime), anticonvulsants (e.g., carbamazepine, 600 to 800 mg a day in divided doses), and oral local anesthetics (e.g., mexiletine, up to 300 mg three times a day) can be tried. Refractory cases should be referred to a multidisciplinary pain clinic.

POSTHERPETIC NEURALGIA. Postherpetic neuralgia refers to severe and prolonged burning pain with occasional lightning-like stabs in the involved dermatome after an attack of herpes zoster. Severe postherpetic neuralgia is usually a disease of elderly patients and, like most chronic pain, is exacerbated by emotional upset and relieved to some degree by distraction. Touching the involved area may exacerbate the pain. Treatment is not satisfactory. Initial treatment should be directed toward stimulating the painful area. In some patients brisk rubbing applied repeatedly with a terrycloth towel or stimulation of the dermatome with a cutaneous electrical stimulator may bring relief which outlasts the stimulus, occasionally permanently.

Most patients require multimodality therapy, which includes stimulation of the area, physical therapy, psychological support, and pharmacologic treatment. The application of topical pharmacologic agents, such as lidocaine, sometimes gives temporary relief, and anecdotal evidence claims that topical application of capsaicin is useful. Lancinating pains, which are usually a minor component, usually respond to anticonvulsants (e.g., carbamazepine, 400 to 600 mg a day in divided doses), but anticonvulsants do not affect the continuous pain. The latter may be treated by tricyclic antidepressants or mexiletine (see above). Neuroleptics (e.g., fluphenazine 1 to 3 mg daily) may also be helpful. When conservative approaches fail, one should consider either anesthetic approaches with subcutaneous local injection or sympathetic blockade. The only surgical approach that has proved at all useful is to lesion the dorsal root entry zone, and even that remains controversial. Adrenocorticosteroids and acyclovir, both of which may diminish pain in the acute stage, have no effect on the development of postherpetic neuralgia. In many patients, the disease runs its course and, after a year or two, disappears spontaneously.

The pharmacologic approach includes tricyclic antidepressants, anticonvulsants, neuroleptics, and sometimes sympathetic blockade. Referral to a multidisciplinary pain center may be helpful.

PHANTOM LIMB PAIN. Phantom limb pain is a chronic and severe pain appearing to be localized in an amputated or totally denervated limb. All patients suffer phantom sensations after amputation and as many as 60 to 70% suffer pain, especially if they had severe preambulation pain. The pain may resemble that suffered before amputation or may seem like muscle pain with the phantom in a cramped or uncomfortable position. Usually the pain lessens and disappears with time, but sometimes it becomes chronic and severe. Therapy is difficult. Painful neuromas should be ruled out but are uncommon; even when these are removed, the pain is not usually relieved. Surgery to the CNS is seldom helpful. The pain may be triggered by touching the amputation stump or even healthy areas. Sometimes phantom pain can be permanently abolished by cutaneous stimulation, either rubbing or electrical stimulation, or by repeated anesthetic blocks of peripheral nerves proximal to the stump. The pharmacologic approach is the same as that described for the neuropathic pains above, including referral to a multidisciplinary pain center.

FIBROMYALGIA AND MYOFASCIAL PAIN. Fibromyalgia (also called fibrositis) is characterized by widespread or generalized musculoskeletal pain associated with morning stiffness, disturbed sleep and fatigue (nonrestorative sleep), and at times by vague complaints of a feeling of swelling or paresthesias. On examination, *tender points* can be found at multiple sites over muscles and ligaments, particularly at the upper borders of the trapezius, supraspinatus, and upper gluteal area and below the lateral epicondyle of the elbow and the medial epicondyle of the femur. The disorder usually occurs in middle-aged women and is often associated with fatigue, anxiety, and depression. Tension headaches and irritable bowel syndrome are common.

The myofascial pain syndrome refers to chronic pain in a regional distribution associated with trigger point(s). *Trigger points* are tender, sometimes hardened areas in a muscle which, when palpated, reproduce the distribution of the spontaneous pain. When injected with a local anesthetic, both the local and referred pain are temporarily relieved.

The pathophysiology of these syndromes is poorly understood. Some observers have reported microscopic changes at trigger points (so-called fibrous nodules), suggesting that a tonic contraction of muscle has led to structural changes. Others have suggested that release of noxious substances, such as lactic acid, potassium, or kinins from chronically contracted muscles, may be responsible for the pain and tenderness associated with the syndromes. No theory has stood the test of time.

Treatment is often difficult and frustrating. Some patients may benefit from mild analgesic drugs, heat, and massage. In others with trigger points (myofascial pain), massage or injection of trigger points with local anesthetics may give relief. Biofeedback, with the patient trying consciously to relax contracted muscle recorded by surface EMG, has been reported to be useful. Antidepressants are modestly effective and produce at least a short-term remission in about 20% of patients. For most patients, a combination of physical methods with investigation and treatment of associated psychological disorders is necessary if long-term relief is to be achieved.

Fields HL, Leibeskind JC (eds.): Progress in Pain Research and Management. Volume 1. Pharmacological Approaches to the Treatment of Chronic Pain: New Concepts and Critical Issues. Seattle, IASP Press, 1994. *A recent monograph describing pain syndromes and their pharmacologic management.*

Schott GD: Visceral afferents: Their contribution to "sympathetic dependent" pain. Brain 117:397, 1994. *A review of the physiology of causalgia and related painful disorders.*

Wall PD, Melzack R (eds.): Textbook of Pain. London, Churchill Livingstone, 1994. *A compendium of basic, clinical, and therapeutic aspects of most pain syndromes.*

405.4 The Painful Back
David S. Howell

The back is a complex structure serving weight-bearing and locomotor functions. It provides for major support of body structures and transmission of loading forces through the sacroiliac joints to the lower limbs. The fundamental functioning unit is an articular triad composed of two zygoapophyseal joints posteriorly and the intervertebral disc anteriorly. The disc is composed of a nucleus pulposus encompassed by the annulus fibrosus. These structures are arranged in a series and stabilized throughout the spine by ligaments. The spinal bones also encase the spinal cord and the cauda equina and through successive foramina rootlets connect the spinal cord with peripheral neural pathways (See Ch. 444 for discussion of cervical spine, Ch. 238 for spondylarthropathies, Ch. 440 for intervertebral disc disease.)

ETIOLOGY. In Table 405–3, the numerous causes of back pain are displayed according to disease subgroups. Although all vertebral levels can be affected, pain in the low back is most prevalent. The majority of patients have problems relating to functional or mechanical disturbances, and these must be distinguished from a wide variety of diseases either of focal origin or referred from multiple organ systems. Among degenerative diseases, low back pain is a leading cause of industrial absenteeism and chronic disablement.

MEDICAL HISTORY. *Sex.* Compression vertebral fractures

TABLE 405–3. ETIOLOGY OF BACK PAIN

Mechanical or traumatic
  Paraspinal ligaments and musculature
    Myofascial syndrome, sacroiliac strain
  Spondylogenic
    Osteoarthritis-related lesions—zygoapophyseal joints
    Degenerative lesions—intervertebral discs
    Mechanical insufficiency, congenital and acquired, of ligaments and bones
    Spondylolisthesis
    Spinal stenosis
    Fractures
Metabolic
  Vertebral bodies, partial collapse and distortion—osteoporosis; osteomalacia—Paget's disease—often with secondary osteoarthritis
Tumors
  Neural tumors, osteosarcoma, metastatic tumors, e.g., from breast, thyroid, kidney
  Myeloma, lymphoma, leukemia
Systemic inflammatory disease
  Spondylitis (ankylosing)—Reiter's disease; psoriatic or enteropathic arthropathy
  Disseminated ankylosing skeletal hyperostosis
Infections
  Pyogenic, fungal, tuberculous disc infection, herpes zoster infection, paraspinal abscesses
Referred pain
  Vascular—aneurysms, sclerosis of aorta and branches
  Tumors or inflammation of pleural, pulmonary, pericardial, cardiac, or neck origin
  Viscerogenic disease of gallbladder, pancreas, stomach, intestines, kidneys, ureters, bladder, prostate, uterus
  Pelvic or retroperitoneal tumors or inflammation
Nonorganic components
  Hysterical conversion
  Learned painful behavior
  Psychosis
  Litigation neurosis, malingering
  Chronic pain syndrome
  Substance abuse

from osteoporosis have their highest prevalence in postmenopausal women. Gynecologic pathology, such as endometriosis, is the basis for some referred patterns of back pain. Reiter's disease, ankylosing spondylitis, and back injuries are found more commonly in males.

Age. Young people with back pain most commonly suffer from muscle or ligament strains, congenital abnormalities, injury, spondyloarthropathies, and herniated disc syndromes. In middle and old age, osteoporosis, vertebral collapse, degenerative states, including spinal stenosis, and malignant lesions are common.

Family History. Familial patterns of segregation are often detected in respect to spondyloarthropathies and uncommonly in respect to spinal degenerative conditions.

Nature of Pain. Events or conditions that accelerate or retard symptoms should be explored. The chronic inflammatory diseases (spondyloarthropathies) are associated with increased pain and stiffness on inactivity. Patients with lumbar disc protrusion and radicular pain generally are relieved by lying flat with the knees flexed and are uncomfortable sitting. Sudden or acute onset of symptoms is suggestive of a mechanical or infectious origin of symptoms, respectively. Constitutional symptoms such as fever, weight loss, and fatigue are important clues to infectious, inflammatory, or neoplastic disorders.

In regard to localization, the dorsal segment suggests osteoarthritis, vertebral fracture, neoplasm, herpetic radiculitis, or referred pain from the viscera (see later paragraph). Localization of pain in the low back is usually of little help in regard to differential diagnosis.

Claudication-type pain, with onset after sustained walking, suggests either spinal stenosis or arterial insufficiency. The former condition often refers pain to the thigh and is poorly relieved by standing still. Usually neurogenic claudication is relieved by sitting, whereas vascular claudication is reduced by standing.

Referred Pain. A deep aching pain referred to various sites in the upper and midback may be engendered by lesions in the upper gastrointestinal tract. Pain of malignant disease (whether local or referred) is typically severe and unrelieved by change of position or mild analgesics.

In respect to neuropathic symptoms, alteration of the structure of the vertebral foramina may lead to radicular dissemination of pain. In such instances, compression or traction of nerve rootlets or extension of inflammation to them can lead to sensory and motor nerve symptoms and signs, i.e., paresthesias, hypoesthesias, and muscle weakness.

Symptomatology. Discogenic pain is characteristically aggravated by cough or sneeze. Rarely, loss of bowel or urinary sphincter function can result from cord compression or bilateral involvement of sacral nerve roots from spinal stenosis, tumors, or infectious lesions.

PHYSICAL EXAMINATION. General examination of the back is discussed in Ch. 233. Descriptions here are confined to vertebral compression fractures, degenerative disc disease, and lumbosacral strains and sprains.

Lumbosacral Strain. This and related myofascial syndromes are the most common ailments seen in the office practice of rheumatology. A history of injury is often followed by prompt or delayed low back pain. Transient disc prolapse, subluxation of facet joints, and injury to muscles or ligaments are diagnostic considerations. Physical signs are usually limited to paravertebral muscle spasm, tenderness, and restricted lower back motion without evidence of nerve root involvement.

Vertebral Compression Fractures. These are the most common complication of osteoporosis, with the resultant traction or compression of rootlets adjacent to collapsed vertebrae. Severe pain may begin suddenly, associated with the postural strain of lifting heavy objects or hyperflexing the trunk. Major physical findings consist of localized tenderness and muscle spasm related to the level of the nerve roots affected. Poorly localized back pain may be associated with osteoporosis in the absence of vertebral collapse. Metastatic tumor, myeloma, and metabolic bone disease, especially osteopenia of aging, are common underlying conditions.

Discogenic Disease. The most common form of low back pain with radiculitis is associated with prolapse, protrusion, or extrusion of intervertebral disc substance. Usually the onset of acute symptoms is preceded by chronic intermittent low back pain, although a discrete injury may precipitate an attack. Ninety percent of disc herniations are localized at L4–L5 or L5–S1 levels. Discs involving the L4 nerve root may cause pain referred along the course of the femoral nerve upon hip extension and knee flexion. Knee extension may be weak and the patellar reflex reduced or absent. Patients with L5 nerve root disturbance complain of classic sciatic distribution of pain, i.e., radiating to the posterior thigh and the anteromedial leg and foot, in association with weakness of the toe extensors. First sacral radiculopathy is associated with pain over the posterior thigh, calf, and heel, weakness of the ankle and toe flexors, and reduced or absent Achilles tendon reflex. Frequently, loss of neurologic function is subtle and requires repeated testing to document. A positive response to straight-leg raising is most frequently indicative of L4–L5 or L5–S1 disc protrusion. Usually there is pain on hip flexion with the knee extended and absence of pain on repetition of hip flexion with the knee flexed (Lasègue's sign). The cauda equina syndrome is a form of spinal stenosis and is an uncommon but important complication of massive disc prolapse. In the cauda equina syndrome, central midline disc displacement causes paralysis of the sacral root with bladder and bowel dysfunction. It is characterized by severe bilateral leg pain, urinary retention, weakness of the anal sphincter, and bilateral nerve root abnormalities. Once complete neurologic block has occurred, pain is often alleviated, and the patient requires a neurologic examination to verify the need for emergency surgery.

Spondylolisthesis. This condition, which refers to forward displacement of one vertebra on another, commonly involves the L4–L5 and L5–S1 levels. Bursts of segmental severe girdle pain are typical, often worse on activity and relieved by rest.

LABORATORY PROCEDURES. These are dictated by the results of medical history and physical examination. Simple radiographs of the back may suffice if a traumatic injury is causative. In instances of suspected metabolic disturbance, appropriate screening tests, such as serum calcium, phosphorus, and alkaline phosphatase measurements, should be obtained. Complete blood counts, sedimentation rate, urinalysis, and automated serum chemical profiles are sometimes justified to clarify the diagnosis. Anemia and an elevated sedimentation rate should prompt a more extensive search for infectious, inflammatory, and neoplastic diseases.

RADIOGRAPHIC STUDIES. *Routine Radiographic Studies.* These include frontal, lateral, and oblique films of the lumbosacral spine, which can demonstrate foraminal encroachment, compression fractures, degenerative changes, and subluxation of zygoapophyseal joints, as well as internarrowing. There may be severe degenerative changes on the radiographs, with few or no relevant symptoms, and severe back pain may occur in the absence of significant radiographic signs and be of discogenic origin.

Additional Imaging Procedures. When surgical intervention is planned or a diagnosis remains questionable and requires an imperative answer and high resolution, computed tomography (CT) and magnetic resonance imaging (MRI) (noninvasive) are increasingly preferred to myelography. It is not usually necessary to perform discography (injection of radiopaque dye directly into the disc). When osteomyelitis or neoplastic involvement is likely, radionuclide bone scans are helpful. A percutaneous vertebral biopsy under fluoroscopic guidance may be performed to establish histopathologic diagnosis or bacteriologic diagnosis at highly suspicious sites obvious from scans or radiographs. Electromyography can confirm the presence of nerve root deficits.

Management. Conservative therapy for mechanical disorders of the spine and disc herniation focuses on bed rest, analgesics, and anti-inflammatory medication. Long-term use of anti-inflammatory agents should be accompanied by prophylactic protection against peptic ulceration. Application of moist heat, e.g., hydrocollator packs wrapped with a wet towel, may relieve pain and muscle spasm. The amount of bed rest is dependent on the severity of symptoms. After bed rest, gradual ambulation and a program of exercises, together with back protection including a lumbosacral support, are recommended. Most cases of disc herniation respond to conservative therapy; those unresponsive require further measures, including epidural steroids and nerve root or sleeve infiltrations with steroids. Before surgery is indicated, a psychological assessment and exercises emphasizing back stretching and abdominal strengthening should be attempted.

Progressive muscular weakness and progressive neurologic deficit despite bed rest and other aforementioned measures, as well as the cauda equina syndrome, are indications for surgery. Relative indications for laminectomy are severe pain unrelieved by bed rest and recurrent episodes of incapacitating pain; 90 to 95% improvement is anticipated following surgery, although 70% of patients experience relief of pain whether or not the disc is removed.

Following either conservative therapy or surgery, a program of prophylactic management includes postural education, performance of a daily exercise program to strengthen the lumbar and abdominal muscles, and avoidance of lower spine stress. Besides laminectomy, joint fusion for spondylolisthesis and discogenic disease or unroofing procedures for spinal stenosis are sometimes necessary. Myelography, CT, or MRI is indicated preoperatively to establish definitively the nature and extent of disease as well as the level of vertebral involvement.

Acute symptoms from compression fractures require appropriate rest and relief of pain with analgesics. Activities must be selected to avoid additional compression fractures. (See Ch. 217 for management of osteoporosis.)

Brown MD, Ray CD, et al.: In Weinstein JN (ed.): Clinical Efficacy in the Diagnosis and Treatment of Low Back Pain. New York, Raven Press, 1992, pp 279–280. *A flow scheme of diagnostic steps and alternative modes of treatment as well as assessment of their value.*

Brown MD, Rydevik B: Advances in the understanding and treatment of low back pain and sciatica. Orthop Clin North Am 22: April, 1991. *An overview of the present management of low back pain, with emphasis on controlled trials and newer diagnostic techniques.*

Manmiche C, Hessels EG, Bentzen L, et al.: Clinical trials of intensive muscle training for chronic low back pain. Lancet 2:862, 1988. *An appropriate program is described for motivated patients with pain refractory to conventional measures.*

Weber H: Lumbar disc herniation: A controlled prospective study with 10 years of observation. Spine 8:131, 1983. *A classic set of observations on the natural history of the disease and discussion of management.*

406 NUTRITIONAL DISORDERS OF THE NERVOUS SYSTEM

Robert Messing

Characteristic neurologic syndromes result from deficiency of certain nutrients (Table 406–1). In developing countries, nutritional disorders usually result from starvation or from limited diets. In developed countries of North America and Europe, acquired nutritional disorders are found most often in chronic alcoholics (Table 406–2). They also occur with food faddism, starvation due to cancer or malabsorption syndromes, psychiatric illness, or infantile malnutrition. Genetic factors may contribute to vulnerability in some disorders such as the Wernicke-Korsakoff syndrome and two rare vitamin E deficiency syndromes. Part XVI discusses the metabolism of most of the medically important vitamins as well as many details of their deficiencies. This chapter emphasizes the major neurologic syndromes seen in developing countries and briefly describes their management.

VITAMIN B₁ (THIAMINE) AND THE WERNICKE-KORSAKOFF SYNDROME

CLINICAL MANIFESTATIONS. This acute neurologic disorder most often results from the malnutrition of alcoholism but can also accompany other conditions (Table 406–3). The triad of ophthalmoplegia, gait ataxia, and a confusional state is characteristic, but the condition should be suspected in any confused alcoholic. The most common ocular abnormality is nystagmus, usually horizontal, less often vertical. Ocular palsies are also common, particularly affecting lateral rectus function, unilaterally or bilaterally. Complete external ophthalmoplegia and ptosis are unusual, and pupillary light responses are rarely impaired. Gait ataxia results from cerebellar involvement and is usually not associated with limb ataxia or dysarthria. The most common mental disturbance is a quiet confusional state with profound disorientation, apathy, drowsiness, and impaired memory. Acutely, some patients suffer a severe delirium, most likely reflecting alcohol withdrawal. Stupor and coma occur rarely. About 80% of patients have a distal symmetric sensorimotor polyneuropathy, which is symptomatic in two thirds of cases. Associated autonomic disturbances include tachycardia, hypertension, hypotension, and hypothermia. Beriberi heart disease, another thiamine deficiency disorder, is also associated with neuropathy. Although CNS deficits may occur in nutritionally deprived infants with beriberi, adults with Wernicke's encephalopathy do not develop beriberi heart disease.

PATHOLOGY. Demyelination, necrosis, gliosis, and vascular proliferation are found within the mamillary bodies, periventricular regions of the diencephalon and midbrain, the floor of the fourth ventricle, the superior and inferior colliculi, and the superior cerebellar vermis.

TREATMENT. Treatment with thiamine corrects some or all of the abnormalities. Because intestinal absorption is impaired in alcoholics, thiamine (100 mg per day) should be administered parenterally for several days. Glucose increases thiamine utilization, and if

TABLE 406–1. MAJOR NEUROLOGIC SYNDROMES DUE TO ACQUIRED NUTRITIONAL DEFICIENCY

Protein-calorie malnutrition	Developmental neurologic defects
Vitamin A	Night blindness
Vitamin B₁ (thiamine)	Polyneuropathy, Wernicke-Korsakoff syndrome
Niacin, L-tryptophan	Pellagra, polyneuropathy
Pyridoxine	Polyneuropathy, seizures
Multiple B vitamins	Amblyopia, polyneuropathy
Folate	? Polyneuropathy, ? myelopathy, ? dementia
Vitamin B₁₂	Combined systems disease, polyneuropathy, dementia
Vitamin D	Myopathy
Vitamin E	Spinocerebellar degeneration
Iodine	Cretinism

TABLE 406–2. NEUROLOGIC DISORDERS ASSOCIATED WITH ALCOHOLISM

Disorders due directly to alcohol
  Intoxication
  Withdrawal seizures
  Delirium tremens
  Fetal alcohol syndrome
Nutritional deficiency disorders
  Wernicke-Korsakoff syndrome
  Pellagra
  Amblyopia
Disorders that may involve alcohol and poor nutrition
  Cerebellar degeneration
  Alcoholic myopathy
  Alcoholic polyneuropathy
  Alcoholic dementia
Disorders associated with electrolyte abnormalities
  Central pontine myelinolysis
Disorders of unknown cause
  Marchiafava-Bignami syndrome

given prior to administration of thiamine, can precipitate or worsen the encephalopathy. Outpatient therapy should provide 50 mg of oral thiamine a day for at least 6 weeks and weekly thereafter. Ophthalmoplegia and gaze palsies usually begin to resolve during the first day of treatment. Nystagmus, ataxia, and confusion improve over days to weeks. Many patients are left with nystagmus, some with gait ataxia, and some with amnesia.

Many patients with the acute Wernicke-Korsakoff syndrome retain a residual disorder of memory—Korsakoff's amnestic syndrome. They are unable to learn new information (anterograde amnesia) and have difficulty recalling established recent memories (retrograde amnesia). Some confabulate to fill gaps in memory. In contrast to the deficit in memory, other intellectual skills and language are better preserved. Lesions involving the midline diencephalon and the dorsal medial nuclei of the thalamus may account for the memory disturbance. Treatment is the same as for Wernicke's encephalopathy. About 20% recover completely from Wernicke-Korsakoff psychosis over several months, but a quarter do not and require long-term care.

ALCOHOLIC DEMENTIA

Many alcoholics develop enlarged cerebral ventricles and other signs of brain shrinkage which can be visualized on computed tomographic and magnetic resonance scans of the brain. Many such patients also show impairments on psychometric examination. Pathologically, the brain shows white matter pallor and loss of neurons mainly in premotor cortex. In their early stages, such changes may relate to reduced water content of brain, and during this time radiologic and cognitive abnormalities may lessen if drinking stops. With continued alcoholism, however, the process continues and

TABLE 406–3. CONDITIONS PREDISPOSING TO WERNICKE'S ENCEPHALOPATHY

Chronic alcoholism
Starvation
Persistent vomiting
  Hyperemesis of pregnancy
  Gastric cancer
  Gastritis
  Intestinal obstruction
  Digitalis intoxication
Systemic diseases
  Malignancy
  Hepatic failure
  Disseminated tuberculosis
  Uremia
Iatrogenic
  Gastrointestinal surgery with malabsorption
  Hemodialysis or peritoneal dialysis
  Prolonged intravenous feeding
  Refeeding after starvation
Anorexia nervosa

sooner or later becomes permanent. The cerebral abnormalities may partly result from nutritional deficiency, although animal studies indicate that alcohol can cause direct neuronal damage in spite of adequate nutrition.

ALCOHOLIC-NUTRITIONAL NEUROPATHY

CLINICAL MANIFESTATIONS. Alcoholics and other nutritionally deprived persons commonly develop a mixed axonal-demyelinating polyneuropathy (see Ch. 450) with pain and paresthesias in the feet. More severe cases develop leg weakness and symptoms involving the hands. The pain is often burning in character and can be so severe as to make light touch and deep pressure intensely uncomfortable and to inhibit walking.

Muscle weakness and wasting, when present, affect the legs more than the arms and are most prominent distally. Sensory abnormalities usually involve all modalities, but pain and temperature sensation are involved early. Sensory abnormalities are more severe distally, and the legs are more involved than the arms. The deep tendon reflexes are diminished or absent, especially at the ankles. Depression of the ankle deep tendon reflexes is common in asymptomatic patients. In rare cases the condition involves the vagus nerve and the thoracoabdominal sympathetic chain, resulting in hoarseness, dysphagia, vocal cord paralysis, and hypotension. The cerebrospinal fluid protein levels most often are normal. The diagnosis usually is evident on clinical grounds. Electrodiagnostic studies seldom are needed but, if obtained, show signs of denervation with reduced amplitude of sensory and motor action potentials but relatively preserved nerve conduction velocities.

PATHOLOGY AND TREATMENT. The pathologic findings are mainly those of axonal degeneration with secondary demyelination. A specific vitamin deficiency has not been identified in alcoholic neuropathy; similar polyneuropathies occur with deficiencies of thiamine, niacin, or pyridoxine. Possibly, alcohol may have a direct toxic effect on peripheral nerves. Treatment consists of a balanced diet of supplemental B vitamins and abstinence from alcohol. Several weeks may elapse before motor improvement begins. Recovery is generally slow and incomplete.

ALCOHOLIC MYOPATHY

Some alcoholic patients suffer from an acute syndrome of focal or generalized muscle pain, tenderness, swelling, and weakness, beginning abruptly during a drinking binge. Affected muscles are swollen, tender, and indurated with the edematous overlying skin taking on a dusky color. Affected patients may have associated cardiac failure, an arrhythmia, or an impaired swallowing capacity due to pharyngeal weakness. The serum creatine kinase (CK) level is moderately or markedly elevated and, in severe cases, myoglobinuria may cause acute renal failure, hyperkalemia, and death. The diagnosis is readily made clinically, but if doubt prevails, electromyography usually shows evidence of a myopathy (see Ch. 392.5) and muscle biopsy reveals necrosis of muscle fibers. Recovery follows days to weeks of abstinence and adequate nutrition, occasionally leaving residual proximal muscle weakness. Animal experiments indicate that both nutritional deprivation and prolonged alcohol intoxication contribute to the acute muscle necrosis.

In contrast to acute myopathy, proximal muscle weakness and atrophy develop in some alcoholics over a period of weeks or months with little or no muscle pain. The symptoms of chronic alcoholic myopathy reflect the proximal muscular distribution, with the lower extremities usually being affected more than the upper ones. The serum CK is usually normal but may be elevated in some cases, especially after recent drinking. Electromyography usually shows myopathic changes in proximal muscles, and muscle biopsies show mild degenerative abnormalities without widespread necrosis. Alcoholic myopathy and cardiomyopathy (see Ch. 43) often develop concurrently. Improvement usually occurs with 2 to 3 months of abstinence from alcohol and restored nutrition; in some muscle power never returns completely to normal.

ALCOHOLIC CEREBELLAR DEGENERATION

Degeneration of the cerebellum occurs frequently in chronic alcoholics and has also been documented after severe nutritional depletion unrelated to alcohol abuse. Most patients give a history of episodic binge drinking superimposed on heavy consumption of alcohol for many years. Symptoms usually begin insidiously with progressive unsteadiness and difficulty in walking. Sometimes the

disorder evolves rapidly, especially after a binge or severe systemic illness. Affected patients have striking gait ataxia, walking with hesitant, wide-based steps. More severe examples include truncal ataxia as well. Some patients may demonstrate impaired heel to shin tests, but nystagmus, dysarthria, and ataxia of the upper extremities are rare. The features of a distal polyneuropathy are present in about half of the patients. The most prominent pathologic abnormality is degeneration of neurons in the anterior and superior cerebellar vermis. Within these areas all neuronal elements are affected, but the Purkinje cells appear to be especially vulnerable. Similar lesions often accompany cases of Wernicke's encephalopathy, suggesting that the two conditions are closely linked. It is not certain, however, that cerebellar degeneration is due solely to thiamine deficiency. A direct toxic effect of alcohol and an underlying genetic susceptibility to cerebellar damage may contribute. Cerebellar dysfunction stabilizes and sometimes improves with abstinence, adequate nutrition, and supplemental B vitamins.

NUTRITIONAL AMBLYOPIA

This disorder appears most commonly in malnourished alcoholics and appears to be due to deficiency of several B vitamins. It is characterized by insidious and progressive loss of visual acuity and the ability to distinguish colors. Examination discloses bilateral and symmetric central or paracentral scotomas, and, in advanced stages, optic atrophy. Polyneuropathy or a history of the Wernicke-Korsakoff syndrome may coexist. Substantial improvement in vision with complete return of acuity and visual fields can follow early treatment with group B vitamins. In advanced cases, visual impairment may be permanent.

MARCHIAFAVA-BIGNAMI DISEASE

This rare disorder, diagnosed only at autopsy, seldom is described nowadays. The pathology consists of bilateral, symmetric demyelination of the corpus callosum and adjacent white matter, supplemented in some instances with demyelination of the middle cerebellar peduncles. Early symptoms include irritability, aggressiveness, and confusion, often followed by apathy and bilateral spasticity or rigidity. Some case reports describe acute seizure disorders, stupor, or coma. The cause is not well understood, but most or all established cases have been associated with chronic alcoholism and the histologic features closely resemble those found in central pontine myelinolysis (see Ch. 432). Circumstances suggest that the two conditions may be variations of the same process.

PELLAGRA

Pellagra is an uncommon disorder resulting specifically from a deficiency of nicotinic acid (niacin) or its amino acid precursor tryptophan but often incorporating deficiency symptoms of other B vitamins including pyridoxine. Pellagra is uncommon in developed countries because of fortification of processed foods with niacin but is occasionally encountered in chronic alcoholics or institutionalized patients. Manifestations include diarrhea, glossitis, anemia, and erythematous skin lesions in sun-exposed areas. Neurologically, affected persons are irritable and depressed, suffer from insomnia, and have difficulty concentrating. Later, confusion, hallucinations, or paranoid thoughts appear, usually accompanied by spastic weakness. Physical signs include cerebellar deficits, optic neuropathy, and often, a sensorimotor polyneuropathy. Pathologic changes are found throughout the neuraxis and many neurons, particularly the large Betz cells of the motor cortex, show chromatolytic changes. Pellagra responds to administration of niacin along with other B vitamins, although the cerebral symptoms may not resolve completely.

PYRIDOXINE (VITAMIN B$_6$) DEFICIENCY

A deficiency of dietary pyridoxine in adults causes a sensorimotor polyneuropathy. Pyridoxine is converted by pyridoxal kinase and pyridoxine phosphate oxidase to its active form, pyridoxal phosphate. Pyridoxal phosphate is a cofactor for several enzymes, including glutamic acid decarboxylase, which generates the major inhibitory neurotransmitter γ-aminobutyric acid (GABA) from glutamic acid. Patients taking isonicotinic acid hydrazide (INH) for tuberculosis are at risk for pyridoxine deficiency because INH complexes with pyridoxal phosphate. In addition to polyneuropathy, typical central nervous system, skin, and gastrointestinal manifestations of pellagra may appear in some patients receiving INH. All may be prevented by concomitant administration of pyridoxine.

Persons who ingest an overdose of INH also may develop convulsions, which respond to pyridoxine.

COBALAMIN AND FOLIC ACID DEFICIENCY

The normal and abnormal metabolism of vitamin B_{12} and folic acid is discussed in Ch. 133 in relation to megaloblastic anemias. The following sections describe the principal neurologic abnormalities.

VITAMIN B_{12} DEFICIENCY. Severe vitamin B_{12} deficiency leads to subacute degeneration of peripheral nerve axons plus subacute degeneration of white matter in the dorsal and lateral columns of the spinal cord. Spongy changes as well as foci of myelin and axonal loss affect these areas, with the posterior columns showing maximal involvement at the cervical and upper thoracic levels. Eventually, optic nerve and cerebral white matter can become similarly damaged.

Patients with vitamin B_{12} deficiency first complain of paresthesias, most commonly described as tingling "pins and needles" sensations or numbness, typically affecting the feet bilaterally and sometimes the hands. If the disease goes untreated, gait ataxia sooner or later develops, producing symptoms that intensify with walking in the dark. Further neurologic deterioration in untreated patients progresses relentlessly but at individually varying rates of speed. Ataxia is commonly followed by leg weakness and by bowel and bladder dysfunction. Neuropsychiatric symptoms include apathy, depression, irritability, paranoia, nocturnal confusion, and dementia. Intellectual deterioration rarely develops in the absence of other neurologic signs. Failing vision with central scotomas occurs rarely.

Initially, there may be few objective findings aside from minimal, distal impairment of vibratory sensation involving the legs and sometimes the hands. Subsequently, position sense becomes impaired and sensory changes eventually reach the trunk and arms. Flexion of the neck may elicit tingling paresthesias in the back and legs (Lhermitte's sign). Patellar and ankle deep tendon reflexes are usually diminished or absent, and in the late stages there may be decreased perception of touch, pain, and temperature in the distal lower extremities. Eventually, spinal cord involvement leads to symmetric spastic weakness in the legs and extensor plantar responses.

Diagnosis and Pathophysiology. Most patients with neurologic disease have serum vitamin B_{12} concentrations of less than 100 pg per milliliter. However, approximately 5% of patients have levels between 100 and 200 pg per milliliter. Serum methylmalonic acid and total homocysteine levels are usually elevated and can be used to demonstrate cobalamin deficiency in such patients with slightly depressed vitamin B_{12} levels. As emphasized in Chapter 133, most vitamin B_{12}–induced neurologic disorders have an associated macrocytic anemia. Often, however, such persons are taking folic acid in vitamin pills, which prevents the tell-tale anemia. Direct diagnostic measures are discussed in Chapter 133. Neurologic disorders that can be confused with cobalamin deficiency include peripheral neuritis and, in late cases, multiple sclerosis, cervical spondylosis, spinal cord tumors, and syphilitic meningomyelitis. A virtually identical syndrome has been reported after chronic abuse of nitrous oxide. The importance of this observation is that both nitrous oxide abuse and vitamin B_{12} deficiency result in elevated levels of homocysteine and methylmalonic acid. Nitrous oxide oxidizes the cobalt ion of cobalamin from an active monovalent state to an inactive trivalent state and selectively inhibits methionine synthase. Nitrous oxide causes myelopathy in humans and animals and can be prevented in animals by supplementation with methionine. Therefore, inhibition of methionine synthase may be crucial for the development of neurologic disease in vitamin B_{12} deficiency.

Treatment. Intramuscular administration of cobalamin is the only effective treatment for vitamin B_{12} deficiency, whether due to pernicious anemia or to other malabsorptive states. Most symptomatic improvement occurs during the first 6 months of therapy, although it may not be complete for a year or more. Treatment is discussed in detail in Ch. 133.

FOLATE DEFICIENCY. Only a small proportion of patients with low serum folate levels develop nervous system manifestations, and it is not certain whether or not the two are causally related. Methyltetrahydrofolate, a folic acid derivative, is a cofactor for vitamin B_{12}–dependent methionine synthase. Folate deficiency should be considered in patients suffering from nutritional failure plus a combination of neuropathy, dementia, or symptoms of suba-

cute combined degeneration of the spinal cord with normal vitamin B_{12} levels. Chronic alcoholism is the most important cause of folate deficiency, which also complicates malabsorption due to gastrointestinal diseases. Trimethoprim, methotrexate, oral contraceptives, and the anticonvulsants phenytoin and phenobarbital may intensify folate deficiency by interfering with folate absorption, storage, or metabolism but are not consistently associated with a neurologic disorder. Deficient patients may develop megaloblastic anemia that appears identical to that seen in vitamin B_{12} deficiency (see Ch. 133). Treatment with 1 mg of folate several times a day followed by maintenance with 1 mg daily is usually sufficient to control anemia but if the latter is due to vitamin B_{12} deficiency folate does not prevent neurologic deterioration.

VITAMIN D DEFICIENCY

The radiographic, biochemical, and treatment considerations in vitamin D deficiency are discussed in Ch. 212 and 213. Proximal limb weakness may occur in patients with malabsorption or dietary deficiency of vitamin D. Symptoms may also develop with prolonged use of phenytoin or phenobarbital, which appear to increase target organ resistance to vitamin D. In addition to limb weakness, neck muscles may be weak and there may be a waddling gait. Bulbar and ocular muscles are spared. Osteoporotic bone pain often affects the pelvic girdle and spine and may be associated with multiple fractures and vertebral collapse. The serum CK level is usually normal or slightly elevated, and biopsies show minor, nonspecific muscle fiber atrophy. Myopathic changes are present on electromyography. Serum alkaline phosphatase is elevated, and serum calcium and phosphorus may be decreased. Laboratory abnormalities, bone pain, and weakness usually respond to vitamin D therapy.

VITAMIN E (TOCOPHEROL) DEFICIENCY

This rare condition occurs in the setting of severe malabsorption of lipids (see Ch. 103) plus two rare disorders affecting the nervous system: abetalipoproteinemia and isolated vitamin E deficiency. The clinical syndrome consists of a spinocerebellar degeneration resembling Friedreich's ataxia (see Ch. 413). Weakness and gait unsteadiness are common complaints. Neurologic signs include loss of deep tendon reflexes and reduced vibratory sensation in the feet. Position sensation is less affected and pain and temperature sensations may be normal. Limb and gait ataxia are common, as are mild to moderate proximal weakness, although weakness can be diffuse or predominantly distal. Babinski's sign develops in fewer than half of the cases. About half of the patients have nystagmus, ptosis, or partial external ophthalmoplegia.

Vitamin E is an antioxidant that appears to protect unsaturated fatty acids of membrane phospholipids from oxidative degradation. Deficiency of vitamin E causes loss of large-caliber myelinated axons of peripheral nerves and degeneration of posterior columns and spinocerebellar tracts in the spinal cord. Degenerative changes are also present in the cerebellar cortex, and there is accumulation of lipid pigment in nerve cell bodies in dorsal root ganglia, anterior horn cells, and brain stem motor nuclei. Plate- or disc-like swellings in axons are noted in the posterior columns.

Oral preparations of vitamin E, 200 to 600 mg a day, or intramuscular injections of 50 to 100 mg every 3 to 7 days may prevent progression of neurologic disease. The clinical picture and serum level should be followed and dose adjusted accordingly. Supplementation with bile salts may enhance intestinal absorption.

Blass JP: Vitamin and nutritional deficiencies. *In* Siegel GJ, Agranoff BW, Albers RW, et al. (eds.): Basic Neurochemistry, 5th ed. New York, Raven Press, 1994. *A clear discussion of the neurochemistry of vitamins.*

Charness ME, Simon RP, Greenberg DA: Ethanol and the nervous system. N Engl J Med 321:442, 1989. *A scholarly review with many references.*

Harper CG, Giles M, Finaly-Jones R: Clinical signs in the Wernicke-Korsakoff complex: A retrospective analysis of 131 cases diagnosed at necropsy. J Neurol Neurosurg Psychiatry 49:341, 1986. *Correct antemortem diagnosis was reached in only 20% of cases; most overlooked examples lacked ophthalmoplegia.*

Healton EB, Savage DG, Brust JCM, et al.: Neurologic aspects of cobalamin deficiency. Medicine 70:229, 1991. *A comprehensive review of 189 patients suggests that neurologic symptoms may occur without anemia and in fact are worse in those without anemia.*

Layzer RB: Neurologic Manifestations of Systemic Disease. Philadelphia, FA Davis, 1985. *Excellent discussions of neuropathies and myopathies associated with nutritional deficiencies.*

Satya-Murti S, Howard L, Krohel G, et al.: The spectrum of neurologic disorders from vitamin E deficiency. Neurology 36:917, 1986. *A study of nine patients and a helpful bibliography.*

Section Four—The Extrapyramidal Disorders

Joseph Jankovic

407 INTRODUCTION

The term *extrapyramidal* refers to the anatomic and functional characteristics that distinguish the basal ganglia–regulated motor system from the pyramidal (corticospinal) and cerebellar systems. Extrapyramidal movement disorders are divided descriptively into *hypokinesias,* characterized by poverty and slowness of movement; *hyperkinesias,* manifested by abnormal involuntary movements; and miscellaneous motor disturbances (Table 407–1). Before discussing the clinical, pathophysiologic, and therapeutic aspects of the different movement disorders, it is important to review the anatomic and functional organization of the basal ganglia.

FUNCTIONAL AND NEUROCHEMICAL ANATOMY OF THE BASAL GANGLIA

The six paired nuclei that constitute the basal ganglia include the caudate nucleus, putamen, globus pallidus (or pallidum), nucleus accumbens, subthalamic nucleus, and substantia nigra (Fig. 407–1). The caudate nucleus and putamen, although separated by the internal capsule, share cytoarchitechtonic, chemical, and physiologic properties; they are often referred to as the *corpus striatum,* neostriatum, or simply striatum. The striatum is a highly inhomogeneous structure composed of subregions termed striosomes and matrix. The limbic system provides major input to the striosomes, whereas neocortical areas primarily project to the matrix. Although the internal capsule separates the internal segment of the globus pallidus (GPi) and the pars reticulata of the substantia nigra (SNr), evidence suggests that these nuclei should also be regarded as a single functional structure. The term *lenticular nucleus* refers to the putamen and globus pallidus combined because of their lenslike shape.

Recent anatomic and physiologic data suggest a complex organization of the basal ganglia and related structures (Fig. 407–1). According to this schema, the sensorimotor, association, and limbic cortical areas provide anatomically and functionally segregated inputs to the dorsal (the caudate and putamen) and ventral (nucleus accumbens, not shown) striatum. The somatosensory, motor, and premotor cortical areas project mainly to the putamen, and the posterior parietal and temporal and frontal association cortical areas project largely to the caudate and nucleus accumbens. The anatomy is consistent with the concept that the putamen is primarily concerned with motor function and the caudate is more involved with emotional and cognitive processes. The corticostriatal afferents are mediated by the excitatory neurotransmitter glutamic acid. The other major striatal afferents originate in the substantia nigra pars

compacta (SNc), which provides major dopaminergic inhibitory input to the basal ganglia via the nigrostriatal pathway. Other inhibitory inputs to the striatum arise from the brain stem raphe nuclei (serotonergic) and from the locus ceruleus neurons (noradrenergic). The striatum is composed largely of cholinergic neurons, and some excitatory cholinergic projections to the striatum originate in the midline intralaminar thalamic nuclei.

The striatal nuclei project somatotopically to the external segment of the globus pallidus (GPe) and the GPi and SNr complex. The striatal efferents utilize the inhibitory neurotransmitter γ-aminobutyric acid (GABA). The subthalamic nucleus (STN) regulates the output of the basal ganglia to the thalamus by modulating the inhibitory GABAergic afferents from the GPe and the excitatory glutamatergic efferent projections to the GPi-SNr complex. The efferent inhibitory GABAergic projections from the GPi terminate in the thalamus. The thalamic nuclei in turn project to the supplementary motor area of the cortex and the primary motor cortex.

MOVEMENT DISORDERS

Single-cell recordings in behaving animals and other studies have demonstrated that one of the primary roles of the basal ganglia is to scale the movement amplitude and velocity rather than to initiate movements. Besides their crucial role in the execution of movement, the basal ganglia also seem to be involved in the preparation for movement.

In addition to impaired voluntary movements, dysfunction in the basal ganglia can also cause a variety of abnormal involuntary movements. Correlations between the various types of abnormal movements and sites of experimental and pathologic lesions have provided helpful insights into and better understanding of the function of the basal ganglia. The remainder of this section is organized according to the major categories of movement disorders into hypokinetic (parkinsonian), hyperkinetic, and miscellaneous movement disorders (see Table 407–1).

HYPOKINESIAS (PARKINSONIAN DISORDERS)

Bradykinesia is manifested clinically by slowness of automatic and spontaneous movements and impaired ability to initiate voluntary movements (akinesia). This typical parkinsonian symptom presumably results from loss of the inhibitory dopamine input to the striatum and hypoactivity of the GPe neurons. This, in turn, causes functional disinhibition (excitation) of the STN, inducing an increase of neuronal activity in the GPi, thereby raising the tonic inhibitory output from the basal ganglia (GPi) to the thalamus and to the cortical projection areas (Fig. 407–2). The altered activity in the "motor" circuit is manifested by increased movement time, which becomes particularly prolonged when a parkinsonian patient performs sequential movements.

Rigidity, another cardinal sign of parkinsonism, is demonstrated clinically by increased resistance against passive movement of a body part, usually associated with the "cogwheel" phenomenon. A parkinsonian patient perceives rigidity as a feeling of joint stiffness and muscle tightness. The pathophysiologic mechanisms of rigidity have been attributed to pallidal disinhibition resulting in increased suprasegmental activation of normal spinal reflex mechanisms.

Postural instability due to loss of righting reflexes can cause propulsion (tendency to fall forward) and retropulsion (tendency to fall backward). It is one of the most disabling symptoms of Parkinson's disease. The mechanism of postural instability is unknown, but it has been attributed primarily to involvement of the pallidum. Other hypokinetic manifestations are listed in Table 407–1.

HYPERKINESIAS (ABNORMAL INVOLUNTARY MOVEMENTS)

Tremor is a rhythmic oscillatory movement produced by alternating or synchronous contractions of opposing muscle groups.

TABLE 407–1. MOVEMENT DISORDERS

Hypokinesias	Hyperkinesias	Miscellaneous
Parkinsonism	Tremor	Ataxia
Hypomimia	Dystonia	Gait disorders
Dysarthria	Chorea	Hyperreflexia
Sialorrhea	Athetosis	Hemifacial spasm
Micrographia	Ballism	Myokymia
Shuffling gait	Tics	Stiff-person syndrome
Other signs of	Myoclonus	Psychogenic
bradykinesia	Stereotypy	
and rigidity	Akathisia	
	Restless legs	
	Paroxysmal	
	dyskinesias	

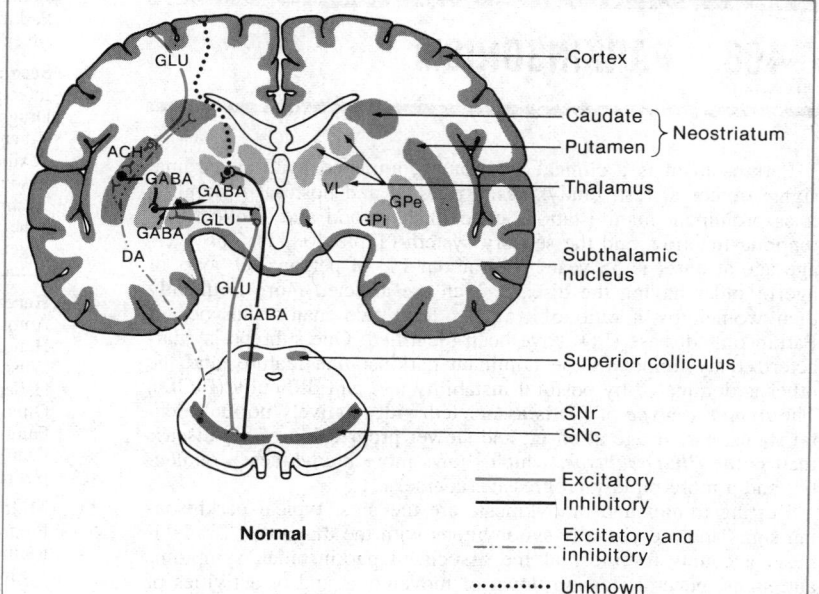

FIGURE 407–1. Anatomy of the basal ganglia and their connections. ACH = acetylcholine; GABA = γ-aminobutyric acid; GLU = glutamate; GP = globus pallidum (e = external, i = internal); DA = dopamine; SN = substantia nigra (c = compacta, r = reticulata); VL = ventrolateral.

Tremors are divided into rest or action tremors; the latter are further subdivided into postural or contraction tremors (e.g., arms outstretched in front of the body or in a "wing-beating" position) and kinetic or intention tremors (e.g., during target-directed movement, such as the finger-to-nose maneuver). *Rest tremor,* usually asymmetric at onset, is the typical tremor of Parkinson's disease. When it involves the hands, it causes a supinating-pronating oscillatory (pill-rolling) movement at approximately 4- to 6-Hz frequency. Parkinsonian tremor also often involves the legs, feet, lips, tongue, chin, and voice but almost never affects the head or neck. *Postural tremor,* with frequency ranging between 4 and 12 Hz, is most typically seen in patients with essential tremor. *Kinetic (intention) tremors* are slow and more irregular movements with a rate of 1.5 to 3 Hz. Kinetic tremors usually indicate an abnormality of the cerebellum or its outflow pathways (the dentate nucleus, the superior cerebellar peduncle, and contralateral red nucleus).

Dystonia is produced by involuntary, sustained (tonic) or spasmodic (rapid or clonic), patterned, and repetitive muscle contractions, frequently causing twisting (e.g., torticollis), flexing or extending (e.g., writer's cramp, retrocollis), and squeezing (e.g., blepharospasm, writer's cramp) movements or abnormal postures. Dystonia is usually constant but occurs in some cases only during particular activities. Examples of task-specific dystonias include writer's or typist's cramp and inversion of a foot while running. As dystonia progresses, the involuntary contractions also appear at rest. A characteristic feature of dystonia is that the spasms lessen in intensity with "sensory tricks," such as touching one side of the face to maintain a primary position, thus counteracting involuntary torticollis. Dystonia can fluctuate in intensity and is exacerbated by stress, fatigue, activity, or a change in posture. It subsides during sleep, relaxation, and hypnosis. These features and the bizarre nature of dystonic patterns sometimes are wrongly attributed to psychogenic causes. About half of patients with dystonia have a coexistent postural tremor, identical to essential tremor. The anatomic substrate for dystonia is unknown. Clinicopathologic studies of patients with secondary dystonias most often implicate the putamen and the rostral brain stem in their genesis.

Chorea consists of continuous, abrupt, rapid, brief, flowing, unsustained, irregular, and random jerklike movements. Choreic patients frequently mask the abnormal movements by voluntary semipurposeful activities. A characteristic feature of chorea is the inability to maintain voluntary sustained contraction. Examples include an inability to sustain manual grip or tongue protrusion and the dropping of objects. Muscle stretch reflexes are usually "hung up" and "pendular." Affected patients typically have a peculiar irregular and dancelike gait. The pathogenesis of chorea is unknown. Some findings point to abnormalities in caudate function. A selective loss of the GABA-enkephalin striatal neurons projecting to the GPe, found in Huntington's disease, results in excessive inhibition of STN neurons.

The movement disorders of athetosis (Ch. 411), ballism (Ch. 411), myoclonus (Ch. 412), tics (Ch. 412), and stereotypies (Ch. 412) are discussed in later chapters of this section.

DeLong MR: Primate models of movement disorders of basal ganglia origin. TINS 13:281, 1990. *A review of the MPTP model of parkinsonism used in the study of basal ganglia circuitry. Hyperactivity of the STN is associated with bradykinesia, and a chemical lesion in the STN ameliorates this cardinal sign.*

Hallett M: Physiology of basal ganglia disorders: An overview. Can J Neurol Sci 20:177, 1993. *An excellent review of current understanding of the basal ganglia connections in the normal and diseased brain.*

Jankovic J, Tolosa E (eds.): Parkinson's Disease and Movement Disorders. Baltimore, Williams & Wilkins, 1993. *A comprehensive review of hypokinetic, hyperkinetic, and miscellaneous movement disorders.*

Marsden CD, Fahn S (eds.): Movement Disorders 3. London, Butterworths Heinemann, 1994. *A comprehensive review of different movement disorders by recognized experts.*

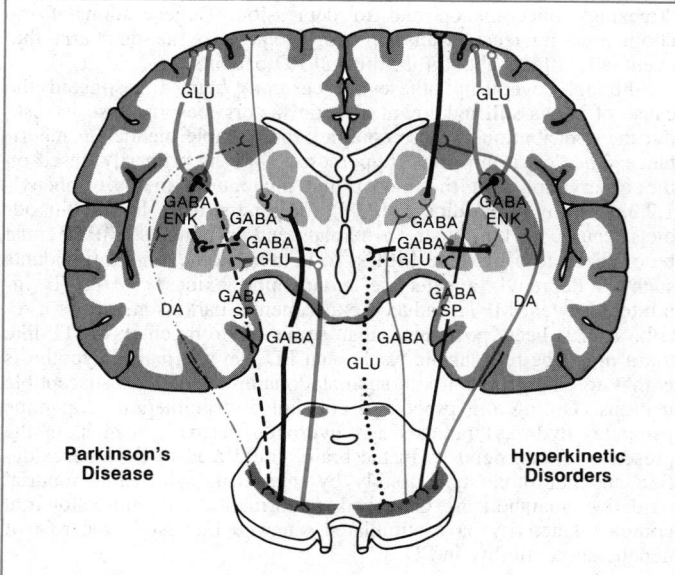

FIGURE 407–2. Functional organization of the basal ganglia in parkinsonian disorders and hyperkinetic movement disorders. ACH = acetylcholine; GABA = γ-aminobutyric acid; GLU = glutamate; DA = dopamine; ENK = enkephalin; SP = substance P.

408 PARKINSONISM

Parkinsonism is a clinical syndrome dominated by four cardinal signs: tremor at rest, bradykinesia, rigidity, and postural instability. Less prominent manifestations concern the mood and intellect, autonomic function, and the sensory system (Table 408–1). The average age at onset is 55 years, with about 1% of persons 60 years of age or older having the disease. Men are affected more frequently than women by a ratio of 3:2. At least two major subtypes of Parkinson's disease (PD) have been identified: One subtype is characterized by tremor as the dominant parkinsonian feature, and the other is dominated by postural instability and gait difficulty (PIGD). The *tremor subtype* of PD is associated with relatively normal mental status, earlier age at onset, and slower progression of the disease than is the *PIGD subtype,* which shows more bradykinesia, dementia, and a more rapidly progressive course.

Resting tremor and bradykinesia are the most typical parkinsonian signs and are virtually synonymous with the diagnosis. Bradykinesia accounts for most of the associated parkinsonian symptoms and signs: general slowing down of movements and of activities of daily living; lack of facial expression (hypomimia or masked facies); staring expression due to decreased frequency of blinking; impaired swallowing, which causes drooling; hypokinetic and hypophonic dysarthria; monotonous speech; small handwriting (micrographia); difficulties with repetitive and simultaneous movements; difficulty in arising from chair and turning over in bed; shuffling gait with short steps; decreased arm swing and other automatic movements; and start hesitation and freezing. Freezing, manifested by sudden and often unpredictable inability to move, is one of the most disabling of all parkinsonian symptoms.

Several disorders other than PD can cause at least part of the parkinsonian syndrome (Table 408–2). Non-PD parkinsonian disorders can be distinguished clinically from PD by the presence of atypical findings, absence or paucity of tremor, and poor response to levodopa. The last feature may be partly explained by the fact that postsynaptic dopamine receptors are preserved in PD, but they are decreased in the other parkinsonian syndromes.

PARKINSON'S DISEASE

Pathogenesis

The most typical pathologic hallmarks of PD are (1) neuronal loss with depigmentation of the substantia nigra (SN) and (2) Lewy bodies, which are eosinophilic cytoplasmic inclusions in neurons consisting of aggregates of normal filaments. These abnormalities are most prominent in the ventrolateral region of the SN that pro-

TABLE 408–1. NONMOTOR DISTURBANCE IN PARKINSON'S DISEASE

Neurobehavioral Abnormalities in Parkinson's Disease

Personality changes (apathy, lack of confidence, fearfulness, anxiety, emotional lability and inflexibility, social withdrawal, dependency)

Dementia (tip-of-the-tongue phenomenon [partial anomia], spatial disorientation, paranoia, psychosis, hallucinations)

Bradyphrenia (slow thought processes, loss of concentration, difficulty with concept formation)

Depression

Sleep disturbance

Sexual dysfunction

Psychiatric side effects of therapy

Other Nonmotor Manifestations of Parkinson's Disease

Autonomic dysfunction (orthostatic hypotension, respiratory dysregulation, flushing, "drenching sweats," constipation, sphincter and sexual dysfunction)

Sensory symptoms (paresthesias, pains, akathisia; visual, olfactory, and vestibular dysfunction)

Seborrhea, pedal edema, fatigue, weight loss

TABLE 408–2. CAUSES OF THE PARKINSON SYNDROME

I. **Primary (Idiopathic) Parkinsonism**
   Parkinson's disease
   Juvenile parkinsonism

II. **Secondary (Acquired, Symptomatic) Parkinsonism**
   Infectious: postencephalitic, slow virus
   Drugs: neuroleptics (antipsychotic, antiemetic drugs), reserpine, tetrabenazine, α-methyldopa, lithium, flunarizine, cinnarizine
   Toxins: MPTP, CO, Mn, Hg, CS_2, methanol, ethanol
   Vascular: multi-infarct, hypotensive shock
   Trauma: pugilistic encephalopathy
   Other: parathyroid abnormalities, hypothyroidism, hepatocerebral degeneration, brain tumor, normal-pressure hydrocephalus, syringomesencephalia

III. **Heredodegenerative Parkinsonism**
   Autosomal dominant Lewy body disease
   Huntington's disease
   Wilson's disease
   Hallervorden-Spatz disease
   Olivopontocerebellar and spinocerebellar degenerations
   Familial basal ganglia calcification
   Familial parkinsonism with peripheral neuropathy
   Neuroacanthocytosis

IV. **Multiple-System Degeneration (Parkinsonism-Plus)**
   Progressive supranuclear palsy
   Multiple-system atrophy
      Shy-Drager syndrome
      Striatonigral degeneration
      Olivopontocerebellar atrophy
   Parkinsonism-dementia-ALS complex
   Corticobasal ganglionic degeneration
   Alzheimer's disease
   Hemiatrophy-parkinsonism

jects to the putamen. At least an 80% loss of dopaminergic neurons in the substantia nigra and the same degree of dopamine depletion in the striatum must appear before clinical symptoms of PD become evident.

Motor symptoms of PD result chiefly from degeneration of the nigrostriatal pathway, causing a deficiency of dopamine in the putamen and, to a lesser degree, the caudate nucleus. The cognitive deficits and some neurobehavioral symptoms have been attributed to degeneration of the dopaminergic mesocortical and mesolimbic pathways, and the associated autonomic dysfunction may be partly caused by dopamine depletion in the hypothalamus. Besides dopamine deficiency, impairment of the other neurotransmitters may be responsible for some of the associated findings. For example, degeneration of the noradrenergic locus ceruleus may contribute to the "freezing" phenomenon and to depression. Degeneration of the cholinergic nucleus basalis probably relates to the dementia that eventually affects about a third of all PD patients.

Although several hypotheses are currently being investigated, the cause of PD is still unknown. Genetic factors may increase its risk, but the contribution is more complex than simple mendelian inheritance. The "environmental" hypothesis of PD is primarily based on the observation that the meperidine analogue 1-methyl-4-phenyl-1,2,3,6-tetrahydropyridine (MPTP), originally used by heroin addicts, causes parkinsonism in humans and in animals. MPTP must be oxidized to a pyridine MPP+ to be neurotoxic, and antioxidants such as deprenyl (a selective monoamine oxidase [MAO]-B inhibitor) prevent MPTP-induced experimental parkinsonism. As a result, it has been postulated that some environmental MPTP-like toxin might be responsible for human PD. An alternative hypothesis is that an endogenous toxin, such as dopamine, damages susceptible neurons. During the process of oxidative deamination, dopamine generates hydroxyl radicals and hydrogen peroxide, which, in the presence of iron deposits in the brain, could lead to lipid peroxidation and neurotoxicity, possibly by interfering with mitochondrial oxidative metabolism. Observed abnormalities in mitochondrial complex I activity have stimulated renewed interest in the role of genetic susceptibility in PD.

Treatment

The finding that deprenyl prevents MPTP-induced parkinsonism stimulated interest in antioxidative therapy as a means of retarding the progression of PD. Some but by no means all studies have found that deprenyl slows the development of motor disability and the rate of disease progression when used in the early stages of PD. Deprenyl also may provide moderate symptomatic relief. After starting deprenyl, many patients report improvement in their energy level and bradykinetic symptoms. The effect may be due to deprenyl's ability to increase striatal concentrations of dopamine by blocking its metabolism by MAO. The addition of one of the anticholinergic drugs, such as trihexyphenidyl, may provide additional symptomatic relief, particularly in younger patients and patients in whom tremor predominates. Associated depression, present in many parkinsonian patients, can be treated with tricyclic antidepressants, such as amitriptyline or nortriptyline. Because the anticholinergics, including the tricyclics, can produce undesirable psychological symptoms as well as side effects, such as dry mouth, blurring of vision, and urinary hesitancy, amantadine may offer a useful alternative, particularly in elderly patients. Amantadine, however, although helpful in controlling both tremor and bradykinesia, can also cause adverse effects, including livedo reticularis, ankle edema, exacerbation of congestive heart failure, and mild anticholinergic side effects. Its beneficial effects seldom last more than a few months.

Many neurologists favor employing combinations of deprenyl, the anticholinergics, and amantadine until they no longer provide a satisfactory control of parkinsonian symptoms. At that point levodopa combined with carbidopa, a peripheral dopa decarboxylase inhibitor, is added to the antiparkinsonian regimen. The starting dosage of carbidopa/levodopa is 25 mg/100 mg twice daily, to be gradually increased over 3 weeks to three times per day. The dosage is then adjusted, depending on the severity of symptoms and occupational demands. Some patients require as much as 25 mg/250 mg four or five times daily; others tolerate only smaller doses. Although levodopa can suppress tremor, it is most useful in controlling bradykinesia and rigidity. Postural instability may be ameliorated by levodopa in early stages. Levodopa is contraindicated in patients with diagnosed melanoma and should be used with caution in those with prominent psychosis or dementia, peptic ulcer disease, and cardiac arrhythmias.

About 15% of parkinsonian patients fail to improve with levodopa from onset of therapy. Most of these nonresponders probably suffer from a form of postsynaptic parkinsonism rather than PD. A failure to respond to levodopa should also suggest the possibility of a wrong diagnosis, a drug interaction (concomitant use of

dopamine receptor blocking agents, such as antipsychotic and antiemetic drugs), and pharmacokinetic reasons, such as insufficient dosage, slow stomach emptying, and competition for absorption in the small intestine and at the blood-brain barrier by amino acids in protein meals. Almost all patients who initially improve lose their response to levodopa some time between 3 and 8 years after onset.

PD patients lose their response to levodopa because of (1) natural progression of the disease and (2) development of complications as a result of chronic levodopa therapy. Although nonneuronal elements may participate in the conversion of levodopa to dopamine, the surviving striatal dopaminergic terminals progressively lose their capacity for conversion of levodopa to dopamine, and the patient develops motor fluctuations and symptomatic deterioration.

The most challenging problem in managing PD is treating levodopa complications. Thanks to carbidopa and similar agents, systemic side effects are seldom prominent. The most common central side effects of levodopa therapy include psychiatric problems, dyskinesias (seen in about 80% of patients after 3 years of therapy), and clinical fluctuations (seen in about 50% of patients after 5 years of therapy). The most common form of clinical fluctuation is the wearing-off effect, characterized by end-of-dose deterioration and recurrence of parkinsonian symptoms due to shorter (sometimes only 1 to 2 hours) duration of benefit after a given dose of levodopa. Slow-release preparations of levodopa (e.g., Sinemet CR, Madopar CR) prolong the plasma (and presumably brain) levels and may be useful in treating or preventing motor fluctuations. Deprenyl may prolong the duration of benefit from each levodopa dose.

Because the onset of levodopa-induced complications seems to be related to the duration of levodopa therapy, some authorities delay initiating levodopa therapy until the patient's symptoms begin to interfere with normal activities. Once levodopa treatment is initiated, the dose should be maintained as low as possible (Fig. 408–1). Some authorities believe that instead of increasing the dosage of levodopa, dopamine agonists such as bromocriptine pergolide should be introduced early in the course of anti-PD therapy. In experimental studies, pergolide has been shown to exert its dopaminergic effects without presynaptic dopamine, and it may improve parkinsonian symptoms even before levodopa is given. Some authorities, therefore, give pergolide as the first dopaminergic drug. However, as symptoms increase, dopamine agonists must be com-

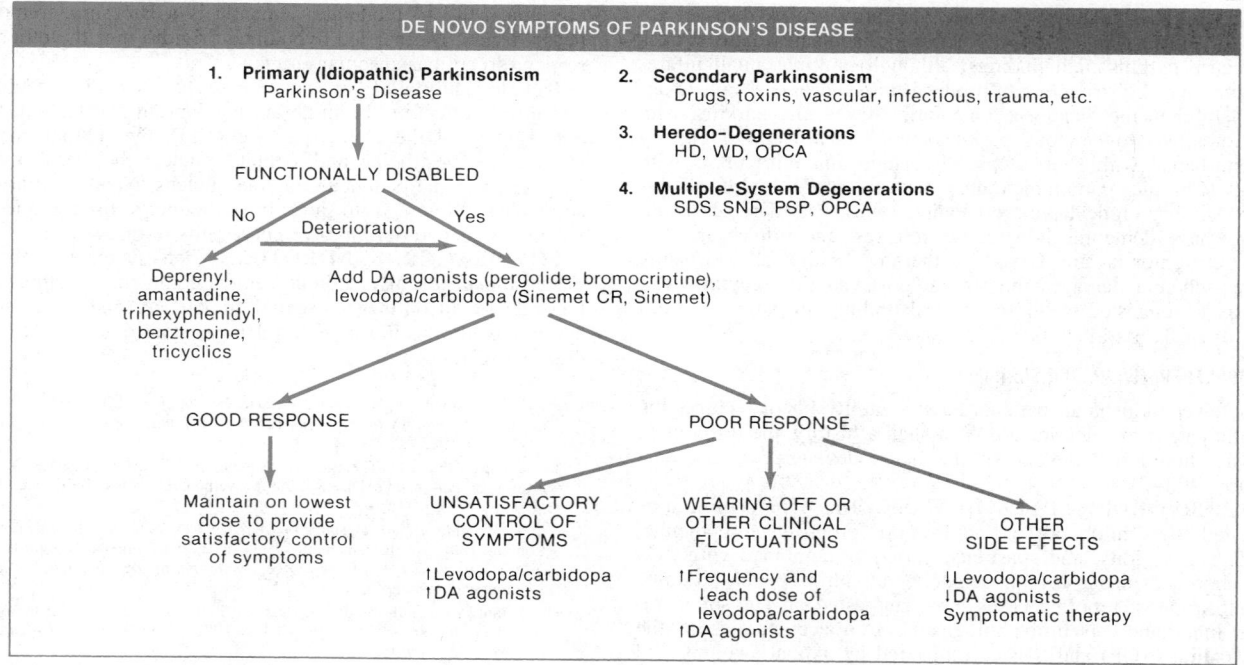

FIGURE 408–1. Diagrammatic representation of therapeutic approach to patients with parkinsonism. DA = dopamine; HD = Huntington's disease; OPCA = olivopontocerebellar atrophy; PSP = progressive supranuclear palsy; SDS = Shy-Drager syndrome; Sinemet CR = controlled-release levodopa/carbidopa; SND = striatonigral degeneration; WD = Wilson's disease.

bined with levodopa. The starting dosage for bromocriptine is 1.25 mg twice a day and for pergolide, 0.05 mg twice a day. The dosage should be increased slowly to prevent gastrointestinal, psychiatric, autonomic, and other side effects. The side effects of dopamine agonists are similar to those of levodopa, although dopamine agonists may produce hallucinations, delusions, and other psychiatric symptoms more often than does levodopa. They also can cause erythromelalgia, a painful erythema of the legs not usually seen with levodopa. Other motor and nonmotor symptoms of PD may require more specific therapy.

Surgical treatment of PD remains of uncertain value. Stereotaxic thalamotomy is occasionally employed in an attempt to ameliorate disabling tremor. In addition, pallidotomy and thalamic stimulation sometimes may provide relief of parkinsonian symptoms. Surgical transplantation of fetal substantia nigra into the striatum remains under investigation.

As with all progressive, disabling diseases, psychological support of patients and family offers important help. Patients should be encouraged to learn about their disease (by reading educational material provided by the national and local support organizations) and, above all, to remain physically and socially active.

SECONDARY PARKINSONISM

POSTENCEPHALITIC PARKINSONISM. Many individuals who survived the acute febrile illness and encephalopathy during the pandemics of encephalitis lethargica (von Economo's encephalitis) between 1919 and 1926 later developed a variety of movement disorders, including parkinsonism. Although the virus or viruses responsible for encephalitis lethargica were never isolated, infections caused by coxsackie, Japanese B, and western equine encephalitis viruses have since been identified as being complicated by parkinsonism. In general, postencephalitic parkinsonism has a slower progression and is more sensitive to levodopa therapy.

DRUG-INDUCED PARKINSONISM. Drugs that deplete the presynaptic stores of dopamine, such as reserpine and tetrabenazine (an investigational drug not available for general use in North America), and drugs that block the dopamine receptors, such as antipsychotic and antiemetic agents, can cause a parkinsonian syndrome clinically indistinguishable from idiopathic parkinsonism (PD). The same drugs can also cause a variety of other movement disorders, such as akathisia, dystonic reactions, and various tardive syndromes (e.g., tardive stereotypy, tardive dystonia, and tardive akathisia).

VASCULAR PARKINSONISM. Cerebrovascular disease accounts for only a small proportion of parkinsonism. Single strokes rarely cause parkinsonian findings, although multiple small infarctions involving the striatum can produce the syndrome. Brain imaging is helpful in the diagnosis. One form of vascular parkinsonism is the so-called "lower body parkinsonism," manifested chiefly by gait disturbance with short steps, "freezing," and difficulties with turning. (Chronic communicating, "low-pressure" hydrocephalus causes a similar clinical picture.) Patients with vascular parkinsonism may have dementia, hyperactive reflexes, and urinary incontinence, but tremor is rare. Levodopa therapy usually fails, probably because ischemia damages the striatal postsynaptic receptors. The diagnosis is suggested by these atypical findings in patients with a history of stroke risk factors.

HEREDODEGENERATIVE PARKINSONISM

Very few parkinsonian patients have a family history suggesting a specific pattern of inheritance. With such a history, the differential diagnosis should include one of the heredodegenerative disorders (see Table 408–2).

HALLERVORDEN-SPATZ DISEASE. This rare condition is manifested by childhood or adult-onset progressive dementia, bradykinesia, rigidity, and spasticity, variously combined with dystonia, choreoathetosis, ataxia, seizures, amyotrophy, and retinitis pigmentosa. Most reported cases have suggested an autosomal recessive inheritance. Neuropathologically, iron accumulates in the globus pallidus (GP) and SN, accompanied by axonal swelling and

neuronal degeneration in the basal ganglia, corticospinal tract, and cerebellum. Cysteine, found to be increased in the GP, possibly chelates iron, causing generation of free radicals and subsequent neuronal degeneration.

FAMILIAL BASAL GANGLIA CALCIFICATIONS. Calcium may accumulate in the basal ganglia in association with hypoparathyroidism or as a result of a familial disorder, sometimes referred to as Fahr's disease. Affected patients exhibit parkinsonism, chorea, dementia, and palilalia. Brain imaging may detect basal ganglia calcification in clinically unaffected relatives.

OLIVOPONTOCEREBELLAR AND SPINOCEREBELLAR DEGENERATIONS. The combination of parkinsonism and cerebellar ataxia characterizes olivopontocerebellar degeneration or atrophy (OPCA), a heterogeneous group of neurodegenerative disorders most often inherited in an autosomal dominant pattern, but occasionally occurring sporadically. In addition to the parkinsonism-ataxia complex, patients with OPCA often exhibit marked dysarthria, neuro-ophthalmologic signs, and a variable degree of upper and lower motor neuron signs (see Ch. 413).

MULTIPLE-SYSTEM DEGENERATION (PARKINSONISM-PLUS)

Approximately 10 to 15% of all patients with parkinsonian findings have a more widespread disorder classified clinically as "parkinsonism-plus syndrome" and pathologically as a "multiple-system degeneration." In addition to parkinsonism, such patients suffer from additional findings that may include supranuclear ophthalmoparesis (progressive supranuclear palsy), dysautonomia (Shy-Drager syndrome), ataxia (OPCA), laryngeal stridor (striatonigral degeneration), apraxia and alien hand (corticobasal degeneration), dementia (Alzheimer's disease with parkinsonism and diffuse Lewy body disease), and a combination of dementia and motor neuron disease (parkinsonism–dementia–amyotrophic lateral sclerosis [ALS] complex). The cause of all forms of this syndrome is unknown.

PROGRESSIVE SUPRANUCLEAR PALSY. Progressive supranuclear palsy (PSP) accounts for about 8% of all parkinsonian patients evaluated in a PD clinic. PSP has its onset in the seventh decade, about 10 years after the usual onset of PD. Initial symptoms consist of a gradual onset of postural instability, unsteady gait, and supranuclear vertical ophthalmoparesis, first expressed by impairment of downward gaze. Later, upward and then lateral conjugate gaze also become impaired, but until the advanced stage, the external ophthalmoparesis can be overcome by labyrinthine stimulation via the oculocephalic maneuver. Patients with PSP often exhibit axial rigidity, nuchal dystonia, and a rigid-dystonic facial expression. Mild to moderate dementia is a late sign; tremor almost never occurs. Neither the hypokinetic rigidity nor the other changes respond to antiparkinsonian drugs.

Pathologically, PSP is characterized by selective neuronal loss and gliosis affecting the midbrain tegmentum and tectum, the internal segment of the globus pallidus (GPi), the subthalamic nucleus (STN), the vestibular and dentate nuclei, the basal nucleus of Meynert, and the pedunculopontine nucleus. Neurofibrillary tangles, somewhat different from those in Alzheimer's disease, and granulovacuolar degeneration involve nerve cells in these areas.

SHY-DRAGER SYNDROME. When patients with atypical parkinsonism (usually without tremor) complain of orthostatic lightheadedness, incontinence, sexual impotence, and other autonomic symptoms, the diagnosis of Shy-Drager syndrome should be considered (see Ch. 402).

Calne DB: Treatment of Parkinson's disease. N Engl J Med 329:1021, 1993. *A review of the pharmacology of levodopa, deprenyl, dopamine agonists and of other therapeutic strategies.*

Jankovic J, Marsden CD: Therapeutic strategies in Parkinson's disease. *In* Jankovic J, Tolosa E: Parkinson's Disease and Movement Diseases. Baltimore, Williams & Wilkins, 1993, p 115.

Quinn N: Multiple system atrophy. *In* Marsden CD, Fahn S: Movement Diseases–3- London, Butterworth-Heinemann, 1994, p 262. *A clinicopathologic correlation of a large series of cases of Shy-Drager syndrome, olivopontocerebellar atrophy, and striatonigral degeneration.*

Stacy M, Jankovic J: Differential diagnosis of Parkinson's disease and the other parkinsonian syndromes. Neurol Clin 10:341, 1992. *A survey of most of the secondary forms of parkinsonism.*

409 TREMORS

ESSENTIAL TREMORS

Essential tremor is the most common type of tremor encountered in developed countries. The tremor is inherited in an autosomal dominant pattern with high penetrance. Affected patients lack the hypokinetic features and rigidity of Parkinson's disease (PD), discussed in the preceding chapter. Essential tremor typically produces flexion-extension oscillation of the hands at the wrists or adduction-abduction movements of the fingers when arms are outstretched in front of the body. Although frequently referred to as "benign essential tremor," it may be partially disabling, often causing spilling of liquids and interfering with handwriting. Essential tremor also frequently involves the head and voice, which helps to differentiate it from parkinsonian tremor. Another useful distinguishing feature is the occurrence of essential tremor during maintenance of posture; parkinsonian tremor is usually present when the affected body part is at relative rest. Parkinsonian patients, however, often exhibit postural tremor, and patients with essential tremor may have tremor at rest, suggesting an overlap between PD and essential tremor.

The frequency of essential tremor ranges from 4 to 12 Hz, and the oscillation may be produced by either alternating or synchronous contractions of antagonistic muscles. Some forms occur only during a specific activity, such as writing or holding an object in a particular position. Such *focal task-specific tremors* may be associated with task-specific dystonias ("occupational cramps") or with generalized essential tremor and dystonia. Nearly half of all patients with essential tremor show evidence of an associated dystonia. The nature of the link is unknown.

Essential tremor has many variants, including isolated head, voice, tongue, facial, and chin tremors and orthostatic tremor. Although considered a variant of essential tremor, orthostatic tremor usually does not respond to propranolol; clonazepam, however, provides satisfactory control in most patients. Focal tremor may be rarely induced by trauma to the affected body part. This peripherally induced tremor is often associated with focal dystonia and reflex sympathetic dystrophy.

β-Adrenergic blocking drugs (e.g., propranolol at 80 to 240 mg per day) are the most effective agents in the treatment of essential tremor. Modest doses of alcohol also reduce the tremor in most instances, but this is an impractical approach to treatment. Other occasionally useful drugs include primidone (starting dosage is 25 mg at bedtime; the daily dosage can be gradually increased to 750 mg per day), lorazepam, and alprazolam. Patients with a disabling essential tremor that does not respond satisfactorily to medications sometimes improve with local injections of botulinum. Thalamotomy is used as a last resort but high-frequency thalamic stimulation is gaining wider acceptance as a treatment of disabling tremors unresponsive to pharmacologic therapy.

Blond S, Caparros-Lefebvre D, Parker F, et al.: Control of tremor and involuntary movement disorders by chronic stereotactic stimulation of the ventral intermediate thalamic nucleus. J Neurosurg 77:62, 1992. *A review of experience with thalamic stimulation in treatment of severe tremors.*

Lou J-S, Jankovic J: Essential tremor: Clinical correlates in 350 patients. Neurology 41:234, 1991. *A comprehensive analysis of clinical features of a large cohort of patients with essential tremor.*

410 DYSTONIAS

DEFINITION. Dystonia is a syndrome dominated by involuntary, sustained (tonic) or spasmodic (rapid or clonic), patterned, and repetitive muscle contractions, frequently causing twisting (e.g., torticollis), flexing or extending (e.g., writer's cramp, retrocollis), and squeezing (e.g., blepharospasm) movements or abnormal postures. Dystonia is frequently associated with other movement disorders, particularly tremor, myoclonus, and parkinsonism. About 1 of 3000

people are diagnosed as having dystonia, but the true prevalence is probably much higher.

CLASSIFICATION. Dystonia may vary in severity, and it may progress as follows: task-specific (occurring only during a specific activity, such as writing or typing) → action (present only during, not necessarily specific, activity) → overflow (involving adjacent muscles) → at rest (present even during rest) → fixed postures (joint contractures). Dystonia is exacerbated by stress, fatigue, activity, or a change in posture and is relieved by sleep, relaxation, hypnosis, and a variety of sensory tricks. Whereas most dystonias are continual, some occur paroxysmally and some have marked diurnal variations (Fig. 410–1). Partly because of fluctuations in severity, sometimes influenced by the emotional state of the patient, dystonia is often mistakenly attributed to psychogenic causes.

Dystonia can be classified according to its *distribution* as focal, segmental, multifocal, generalized, or unilateral (hemidystonia). Most childhood-onset dystonias begin focally, usually in one foot; other body parts become involved later, eventually resulting in generalized dystonia. In contrast, adult-onset dystonias tend to remain focal or segmental. Examples of focal dystonia include blepharospasm, oromandibular dystonia, torticollis, spasmodic dysphonia, and occupational (e.g., writer's, typist's, pianist's) cramps (Fig. 410–1). Blepharospasm is categorized as a *focal* dystonia when it occurs alone (essential blepharospasm). Also, blepharospasm is often associated with dystonic movements in the adjacent facial, oromandibular, laryngeal, and neck muscles. This *segmental dystonia* is sometimes referred to as Meige's syndrome, but the term "*cranial-cervical dystonia*" is more descriptive.

The most common form of dystonia is *cervical dystonia*. According to the position of the head, cervical dystonia can be categorized as torticollis, laterocollis, anterocollis, retrocollis, or a combination of these abnormal postures. There is a 3:2 female preponderance, and the onset is usually in the fifth decade. Local pain is reported by about half the patients, and radiculopathy complicates cervical dystonia in about 20%. Half of all patients with cervical dystonia have an associated head-neck tremor. The tremor can be dystonic, seen only when the patient attempts to keep the head straight; essential, in which case the tremor persists irrespective of the position of the head; or a combination of dystonic and essential. About half the patients report a movement disorder such as tremor or dystonia in family members. The cause of most cervical dystonias is unknown. In 15% of cases, however, cervical dystonia can be attributed to either local trauma or an exposure to neuroleptic drugs.

PATHOGENESIS. The pathoanatomy of dystonia is unknown, but studies suggest a functional involvement of the basal ganglia,

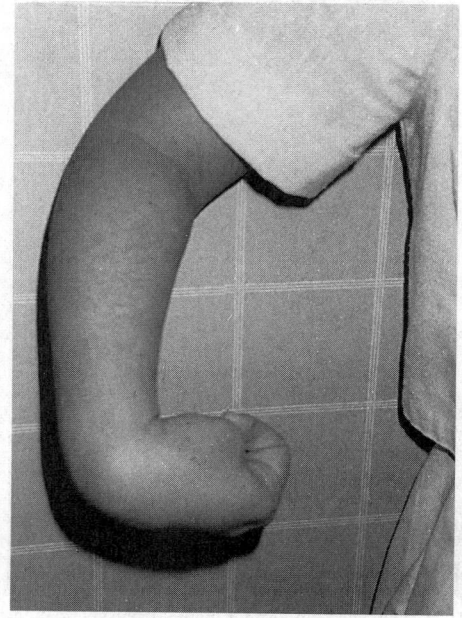

FIGURE 410–1. Focal dystonia of the distal right arm.

particularly the putamen, and the brain stem. Brain imaging and autopsy examinations usually yield normal findings. Postmortem biochemical analyses have found evidence of enhanced noradrenergic transmission in the rostral brain stem.

PRIMARY DYSTONIA

This category accounts for 90% of cases. Primary dystonias with onset in childhood have been previously termed *dystonia musculorum deformans.* Childhood-onset dystonias are often inherited, usually in an autosomal dominant pattern; about half of adult-onset cases seem to have a genetic basis. Other members of the family may have only partial manifestations, such as club foot, scoliosis, torticollis, writer's cramp, bruxism, or essential tremor. Genetic dystonia seems to have a higher prevalence among Ashkenazi Jews, but both Jewish and non-Jewish dystonias have been linked to a marker in the q32–q34 region of chromosome 9. An X-linked dystonia has been recently described in Filipino families. A dopa-responsive dystonia has been linked to a marker on chromosome 14.

SECONDARY DYSTONIA

Occasionally, a specific, and potentially treatable, cause of dystonia can be identified (see Fig. 410–1). One of the most important examples is *Wilson's disease,* described in detail in Ch. 188. Neurologic symptoms represent the first manifestations in about 50% of patients with this autosomal recessive disorder, appearing during their second or third decade.

Tardive dystonia is a persistent form of dystonia caused by exposure to dopamine receptor blocking drugs, such as major tranquilizers (e.g., chlorpromazine, thioridazine, fluphenazine, thiothixene, haloperidol, loxapine, amoxapine) and certain antiemetics (e.g., prochlorperazine, metoclopramide) (Fig. 410–2). Levodopa can also cause intermittent dystonia (and focal dystonia may be the presenting symptom of Parkinson's disease). In all drug-induced dystonias, the offending drug should be withdrawn or the dosage reduced whenever possible. In contrast to focal, segmental, or generalized dystonia, hemidystonia is associated with an identifiable cause in most cases. These include subcortical infarction, arteriovenous mal-

formation, abscess, tumor, and other lesions, some of which can be treated surgically. There are many other causes of secondary dystonia, but only a few are amenable to therapy.

TREATMENT. Treatment consists of supportive therapy (e.g., relaxation techniques, prostheses), medications, botulinum toxin injections, and surgery. The anticholinergic drugs are sometimes beneficial. Trihexyphenidyl, the most frequently used anticholinergic, must be started in low doses and slowly increased to tolerance, perhaps up to 60 mg per day. Some children can tolerate such high doses, but anticholinergic side effects usually limit adult tolerance to 20 to 25 mg daily or less. In advanced cases, dopamine-depleting and dopamine receptor blocking drugs may be added. Muscle relaxants (e.g., diazepam or lorazepam), baclofen, and carbamazepine sometimes provide benefit. About 10% of patients with childhood or adolescent dystonia improve with levodopa. Diurnal fluctuations with exacerbation of the movement disorder toward the end of the day are typical in this form of dystonia. In patients with refractory focal dystonia and, less often, segmental dystonia, injection of the paralysis-inducing botulinum toxin into the contracting muscles provides effective, albeit temporary, relief. Such approaches are best left to those with experience in this treatment.

Patients who are socially and occupationally disabled by dystonia despite optimal medical therapy, including botulinum toxin, sometimes can be helped surgically. Surgical procedures include orbicularis myectomy for blepharospasm, cervical rhizotomy for neck dystonia, and thalamotomy for hemidystonia or generalized (predominantly distal) dystonia. Such procedures are effective in a majority of patients but have both potentially serious complications and high rates of symptom recurrence, making them a last resort.

Fletcher NA, Harding AE, Marsden CD: A genetic study of idiopathic torsion dystonia in the United Kingdom. Brain 113:379, 1990. *A review of inheritance in dystonic families in England suggests that 85% are inherited in an autosomal dominant pattern with 40% penetrance.*

Jankovic J, Brin M: Therapeutic applications of botulinum toxin. N Engl J Med 324:1186, 1991. *A critical review of studies using botulinum toxin in different dystonic and other disorders.*

Jankovic J, Fahn S: Dystonic disorders. *In* Jankovic J, Tolosa E (eds.): Parkinson's Disease and Movement Disorders. Baltimore, William & Wilkins, 1993, p 337. *Comprehensive review of clinical aspects and treatment of dystonia.*

411 CHOREAS, ATHETOSIS, AND BALLISM

HUNTINGTON'S DISEASE

Huntington's disease (HD), an autosomal dominant disorder with complete penetrance, is the phenotype of an expanded triple repeat sequence of a novel gene located at chromosome 4p16.3. Dementia and various emotional and psychiatric disturbances are prominent. The estimated prevalence of HD in the United States is 4 to 8 per 100,000 people. Although about 10% of HD cases begin before age 20, the peak age at onset is in the fourth and fifth decades. Juvenile HD often first manifests with progressive parkinsonism, dementia, and seizures. In contrast, adult HD often starts with the insidious onset of clumsiness and adventitious, fidgety, random, brief movements. Initially, these purposeless movements may be incorporated into and masked by normal intentional acts, delaying the recognition of chorea. Chorea often begins distally, but as the disease progresses, it becomes generalized and can interrupt voluntary movements. Characteristically, patients with HD have difficulty in maintaining tongue protrusion or a steady grip, and their gait is often irregular, hesitant, unsteady, and dancelike. Other motor symptoms include dysarthria, dysphagia, and postural instability.

Neuropsychological symptoms may precede motor changes. They may consist of personality changes, apathy, social withdrawal, agitation, impulsiveness, depression, mania, paranoia, delusions, hostility, hallucinations, or psychosis. Cognitive changes are manifested chiefly by loss of recent memory and impaired judgment. Progressive motor dysfunction, dementia, and incontinence eventually lead to institutionalization and death. The duration of illness from onset to death is about 15 years for adult HD and 8 to 10 years for the juvenile variant.

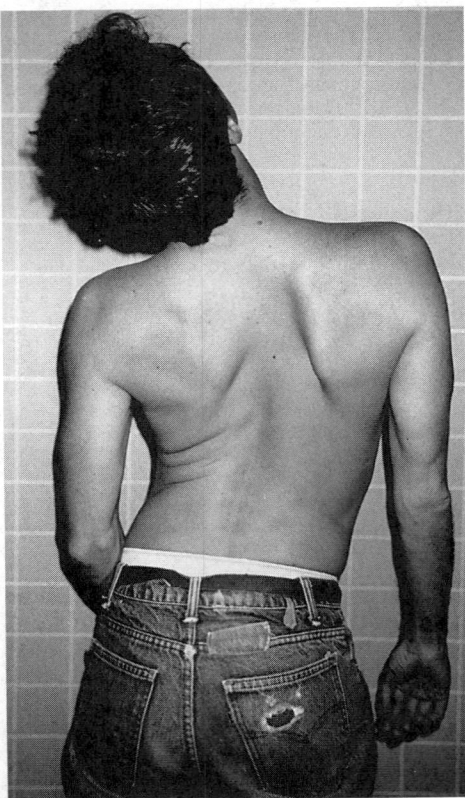

FIGURE 410–2. Truncal dystonia in a manic-depressive patient with tardive dystonia secondary to a variety of antipsychotic drugs.

Postmortem changes in HD brains include neuronal loss and gliosis in the cortex and the striatum, particularly the caudate nucleus. Chorea seems to be primarily related to the loss of striatal neurons projecting to the lateral globus pallidus (GPe), whereas rigid-akinetic symptoms correlate with the additional loss of striatal neurons projecting to the medial globus pallidus (GPi). Loss of medium-sized spiny neurons, which normally constitute 80% of all striatal neurons, is associated with a marked decrease in γ-aminobutyric acid (GABA) synthesis. Acetylcholine activity declines, presumably reflecting a degeneration of cholinergic striatal interneurons. Neuropeptides are markedly altered in HD: Levels of substance P, cholecystokinin, and metenkephalin decrease, but somatostatin, thyrotropin-releasing hormone, neurotensin, and neuropeptide Y levels increase. The number of dopamine, acetylcholine, and serotonin receptors is lowered in the striatum.

Reliable clinical diagnosis depends on the combination of chorea, emotional disturbances, progressive dementia, and a family history suggestive of autosomal dominant inheritance. Because spontaneous mutations are rare, lack of family history raises questions of paternity or misdiagnosis. As noted, the mutated Huntington gene consists of unstable expanded CAG repeats. When the repeat number exceeds 42, the diagnosis of HD is certain. The test is now used to confirm the clinical diagnosis of HD and to identify presymptomatic patients.

Treatment is symptomatic. The psychosis may improve with neuroleptics, such as haloperidol, pimozide, fluphenazine, and thioridazine, but these drugs can induce tardive dyskinesia and other adverse effects and should be used only if absolutely necessary. Monoamine-depleting drugs, such as reserpine (0.25 mg to 8 mg per day) and tetrabenazine (an investigational drug not available for general use in North America), may relieve chorea, do not cause tardive dyskinesia, and may be as effective as the dopamine-blocking drugs. Unfortunately, these drugs can cause or exacerbate depression, sedation, akathisia, and parkinsonism. Anxiolytics and antidepressants may be useful in some patients. Genetic aspects of HD should be discussed openly with the patients to provide them and their relatives with nondirective counseling.

OTHER CHOREIC DISORDERS

Besides HD, other rare, genetically transmitted choreas include *benign hereditary chorea,* a nonprogressive chorea with childhood onset, and *paroxysmal choreoathetoses. Senile chorea* is a rare symptom complex in which chorea begins after age 60 and is unaccompanied by the neurobehavioral symptoms or family history of HD. Some patients have been reported to have pathologic changes identical to those of HD; others have had predominant degeneration of the putamen rather than the caudate. *Neuroacanthocytosis,* also referred to as "chorea-acanthocytosis," usually presents in the third or fourth decade of life with a combination of self-mutilation manifested by lip and tongue biting, generalized chorea, lingual dystonia, and motor and phonic tics. Other features include seizures, amyotrophy, areflexia, and elevated levels of serum creatine phosphokinase. Wet blood or Wright-stained fast-dry smears reveal more than 15% of red blood cells as acanthocytes. Neuroimaging usually demonstrates caudate atrophy. The condition most often has a pattern of autosomal recessive inheritance. *Sydenham's chorea,* now uncommon, has an autoimmune basis, most often appearing as a consequence of infection with group A streptococcus. Unlike arthritis and carditis, which occur soon after such infection, chorea and various neurobehavioral symptoms may be delayed for 6 months or longer. Chorea appearing during pregnancy (chorea gravidarum), with use of birth control pills, or during the course of systemic lupus erythematosus probably has a similar pathogenesis.

ATHETOSIS

Athetosis is a slow form of chorea characterized by twisting, writhing movements. It most often accompanies static encephalopathy due to cerebral palsy, kernicterus, prematurity, glutaric aciduria, poststroke hemiplegia, and other causes of early life brain damage. In some cases, the movement disorder becomes progressive after decades of no apparent change. Athetosis usually does not respond to pharmacologic therapy.

BALLISM

Ballism is a form of forceful, flinging, high-amplitude, coarse chorea. Because the involuntary movement usually affects only one side of the body, the term hemiballism is used. The condition is often preceded by hemiparesis associated with a hemorrhagic or ischemic stroke involving the contralateral subthalamic nucleus (STN) or adjacent structures. Less common causes of hemiballism include abscess, arteriovenous malformation, cerebral trauma, hyperosmotic hyperglycemia, tumor, and multiple sclerosis. Most of these lesions involve the STN, but hemiballism has been described occasionally in patients with lesions outside the STN. Dopamine-blocking and -depleting drugs, used in the treatment of chorea, benefit most patients with hemiballism, but the disorder usually subsides spontaneously within several weeks. Occasional examples of prolonged disabling and medically intractable hemiballism can be treated with contralateral thalamotomy or pallidectomy.

Albin RL, Reiner A, Anderson KD, et al.: Striatal and nigral neuron subpopulations in rigid Huntington's disease: Implications for the functional anatomy of chorea and rigidity-akinesia. Ann Neurol 27:357, 1990. *Using neuropeptide immunochemistry, the investigators conclude that chorea correlates with damage to the striatal projections to GPe, whereas parkinsonian signs observed in some HD patients result from additional damage in the projections to the GPi.*

Albin RL, Tagle DA: Genetics and molecular biology of Huntington's disease. Trends Neurosci 18:11, 1995. *Summarizes the recent literature and emphasizes the role of "triple-repeats" in neurogenetics.*

Fahn S: Paroxysmal dyskinesias. *In* Movement Disorders 3. London, Butterworth-Heinemann, 1994, p 310. *A comprehensive survey of hyperkinetic movement disorders occurring intermittently.*

412 TICS, MYOCLONUS, AND STEREOTYPIES

TICS

Tics are involuntary, abrupt, sudden, isolated, brief movements *(motor tics);* sounds produced by nose, mouth, or throat *(vocal/phonic tics);* or sensations *(sensory tics).* Motor tics may be simple (e.g., eye blinking, nose twitching, head jerking) or complex (e.g., repetitive touching, jumping, kicking, pelvic gyrations). Similarly, vocal/phonic tics may be simple (e.g., throat clearing, grunting, sniffing) or complex (e.g., echolalia, palilalia, coprolalia). Characteristics of tics include suppressibility, increase with stress and excitement, decrease with distraction and concentration, suggestibility, waxing and waning, and possible persistence during sleep.

The most common cause of tics is the *Gilles de la Tourette syndrome,* a genetic disorder dominated by tics and a variety of behavioral manifestations. Transient tics of childhood and persistent simple tics probably represent fragmentary forms of Tourette's syndrome. The following criteria are diagnostic: (1) Both multiple motor and one or more phonic tics must be present, although not necessarily concurrently; (2) the tics occur many times, nearly every day or intermittently through a period of more than a year; (3) the anatomic location, number, frequency, complexity, type, and severity of tics change over time; (4) onset is before age 21; and (5) involuntary movements and noises cannot be explained by other medical conditions. Because of the fluctuating, heterogeneous, and often bizarre manifestations, affected patients frequently have their illness misdiagnosed by physicians and are mistreated by schoolmates, teachers, co-workers, and strangers.

Epidemiologic studies suggest that most cases of Tourette's syndrome are genetic, occurring commonly and with penetrance approaching 100%, particularly in males. A few cases may be nongenetic, triggered or caused by neuroleptics, carbon monoxide poisoning, head trauma, viral encephalitis, cocaine abuse, or opiate withdrawal. Many affected patients suffer from obsessive-compulsive disorder and have problems with attention and learning. Sleep disorders include parasomnias, bedwetting, and interruption by tics.

Therapy varies. Because most patients experience waxing and waning of symptoms and a generally favorable natural course, reassurance and behavioral therapy may be sufficient in mild cases. Drugs are indicated when tics cause physical discomfort or social embarrassment. Judicious use of dopamine receptor blocking drugs, such as fluphenazine, pimozide, and haloperidol, may reduce the

TABLE 412–1. NEUROLEPTIC-INDUCED MOVEMENT DISORDERS

Acute Disorders	Chronic Disorders
Dystonic reaction	Tardive dyskinesia
Parkinsonism	Stereotypic: oral-facial-lingual-masticatory
Akathisia	Trunk-pelvic
Neuroleptic malignant	Respiratory
syndrome	Choreic: limbs
	Tardive dystonia; tics; myoclonus;
	tremor; akathisia; parkinsonism

frequency and severity of tics and ameliorate impulsive and aggressive behavior. These drugs, however, cause sedation, depression, and weight gain. Furthermore, tardive dyskinesia is a potentially serious complication of chronic neuroleptic therapy. Clonazepam, clonidine, fluoxetine, and clomipramine seem to be particularly helpful in the treatment of obsessive-compulsive disorder and other behavioral problems frequently associated with Tourette's syndrome.

MYOCLONUS

Myoclonus is a jerklike movement produced by a sudden, rapid, and brief contraction (positive myoclonus) or a muscle inhibition (negative myoclonus). *Segmental myoclonus* usually involves either the branchial structures, innervated by the lower cranial nerves and upper cervical nerve roots, or other body parts innervated by the spinal roots and nerves; it consists of rhythmic (1 to 3 Hz) contractions caused by a lesion of the brain stem or spinal cord. *Palatal myoclonus* results from acute or chronic lesions involving the anatomic triangle linking dentate, red, and inferior olivary nuclei. *Generalized myoclonus* is believed to reflect discharges arising from the brain stem reticular formation and is categorized as physiologic, essential, epileptic, or symptomatic. Two forms of myoclonus are associated with sleep: physiologic sleep myoclonus, occurring normally during initial phases of sleep, and nocturnal myoclonus, now called *"periodic movements of sleep,"* often associated with *"restless legs syndrome"* as well as with abnormal involuntary movements while the person is awake.

Causes of generalized myoclonus include acute and prolonged hypoxia and ischemia; various metabolic, infectious, and toxic factors; and exposure to neuroleptic drugs (tardive myoclonus). Myoclonus can be associated with familial chorea and dystonia and with many neurodegenerative disorders, including parkinsonism, progressive myoclonus epilepsy, and a variety of rare heredodegenerative disorders. Multifocal myoclonus often develops in the late stages of Creutzfeldt-Jakob disease and, less frequently, Alzheimer's disease.

The specific pathogeneses of myoclonus are unknown. Clonazepam, lorazepam, valproate, carbamazepine, and 5-hydroxytryptophan have been reported to have antimyoclonic activity. Clonazepam, at a dosage of 1 to 9 mg per day, is the drug of first choice, but the development of adverse effects, such as drowsiness, ataxia, and sexual dysfunction, often limits its usefulness.

STEREOTYPIES

The term "stereotypy" denotes a continuous or intermittent, involuntary, coordinated, patterned, repetitive, rhythmic, purposeless, but seemingly purposeful and ritualistic movement. Stereotypies may be simple (e.g., chewing movement, foot tapping, body rocking) or complex (e.g., complicated rituals, sitting down and arising from a chair). They can be volitionally suppressed. Stereotypies can accompany a variety of human behavioral disorders, such as anxiety, obsessive-compulsive disorders, Tourette's syndrome, schizophrenia, akathisia, autism, and mental retardation. Stereotypies and self-stimulatory or self-injurious behavior constitute the most recognizable symptoms in mentally retarded and autistic patients.

Tardive dyskinesia, a persistent movement disorder caused by exposure to dopamine receptor blocking drugs, is a frequently encountered stereotypy. Many other tardive movement disorders can result from the use of dopamine receptor blocking drugs (neuroleptics) (Table 412–1). The term "akathisia" describes the combination of stereotypy and a sensory component, such as an inner feeling of restlessness. The disorder particularly affects the lower extremities ("restless legs") and often is worse at night, causing insomnia, and it may be associated with periodic movements of sleep (see Ch. 397). Elderly women appear to be at particularly high risk for tardive dyskinesia. The mechanism of the disorder is poorly understood but is believed to result from the development of supersensitive dopamine receptors caused by chronic neuroleptic blockade. Prevention is the best treatment for the drug-induced movement disorders. Whenever possible, drugs other than the neuroleptics should be used for psychiatric or gastrointestinal problems. When no alternative exists, the dosage and duration of exposure should be kept at a minimum. Spontaneous remissions of tardive dyskinesia occasionally follow withdrawal of the offending agent. Dopamine-depleting drugs, such as tetrabenazine or reserpine, are the most effective drugs in its symptomatic treatment.

Jankovic J: Tardive myoclonus and other drug-induced movement diseases. Clin Neuropharmacol, in press. *A comprehensive review of clinical and pharmacological features of tardive dyskinesias and other movement disorders produced by dopaminergic or antidopaminergic drugs.*

Jankovic J: Tourette's syndrome: Phenomenology, pathophysiology, genetics, epidemiology and treatment. *In* Appel SH (ed.): Current Neurology, Vol 13. Chicago, Mosby-Year Book, 1993, p 209. *A critical review of current knowledge about the motor and behavioral aspects of Tourette's syndrome.*

Marsden CD, Fahn S (eds.): Movement Disorders 3. London, Butterworth-Heinemann, 1994, p 503. *A comprehensive review of movement disorders, including tics, myoclonus, and stereotypies.*

Section Five—
Degenerative Diseases of
the Nervous System

Robert B. Layzer

The term "degenerative diseases" refers to a varied assortment of central nervous system disorders characterized by gradual and progressive loss of neural tissue. This section deals with several degenerative diseases of unknown cause: the hereditary ataxias, paraplegias, and amyotrophies; the phakomatoses; syringomyelia; and amyotrophic lateral sclerosis. Several important diseases are discussed in other chapters concerned with dementia, extrapyramidal diseases, and autonomic disorders. Some degenerative diseases are difficult to classify because they involve multiple anatomic locations; these *multisystem atrophies* have arbitrarily been assigned to the chapters that deal with their principal symptom (see Table 413–1).

413 HEREDITARY CEREBELLAR ATAXIAS AND RELATED DISORDERS

The symptoms of hereditary ataxia may be intermittent or progressive. *Intermittent or periodic ataxia* occurs in children with a variety of recessively inherited biochemical disorders, such as aminoacidurias and disorders of pyruvate metabolism. A rare, autosomal dominant disease known as hereditary periodic ataxia is characterized by attacks of vertigo, nystagmus, ataxia, and dysarthria, lasting several hours; it responds to prophylactic treatment with acetazolamide.

Progressive ataxia occurs in children with known biochemical disorders such as abetalipoproteinemia and some of the lipidoses, but most diseases in this category are of unknown origin. Those that begin before age 20, including Friedreich's ataxia and ataxia-telangiectasia, are usually inherited in an autosomal recessive fashion, whereas most adult-onset types are autosomal dominant.

FRIEDREICH'S ATAXIA

This autosomal recessive disease, with a carrier frequency of nearly 1 in 100 and a prevalence of 2 in 100,000, is probably the most common type of hereditary ataxia. The biochemical mechanism is unknown, but the abnormal gene has been mapped to the long arm of chromosome 9.

PATHOLOGY. At autopsy the spinal cord is atrophic. There is loss of nerve cells in the dorsal root ganglia and Clarke's columns and "dying-back" degeneration of nerve fibers in the dorsal columns, pyramidal tracts, spinocerebellar tracts, and peripheral nerves. Minor changes are present in the brain stem and cerebellum. The heart shows chronic interstitial fibrosis and ventricular hypertrophy.

CLINICAL MANIFESTATIONS. Progressive ataxia of gait usually begins in childhood or adolescence and within a few years is accompanied by loss of deep reflexes, limb ataxia, Babinski signs, and cerebellar dysarthria. The ability to walk is lost about 15 years after onset. Most patients eventually exhibit scoliosis, pronounced impairment of vibration and position sense in the lower extremities, and pes cavus. Some develop wasting of distal limb muscles, a stocking-glove deficit of superficial sensation, nystagmus, deafness, or optic atrophy. Intellect remains normal. A hypertrophic cardiomyopathy is present in most patients and often leads to supraventricular arrhythmias; heart failure is probably the major cause of death. Insulin-dependent diabetes mellitus develops in 10 to 20% of patients. The mean age at death is 37 years.

DIAGNOSIS. Sensory nerve action potentials are small or absent. Electromyography may show signs of denervation in distal limb muscles, but motor nerve conduction velocities are normal. The cerebrospinal fluid is normal except for mild elevation of the protein content in a few cases. Magnetic resonance (MR) imaging often shows atrophy of the cervical spinal cord; the medulla may also be small, but the cerebellum is spared. Electrocardiography often shows inverted T waves, right- or left-axis deviation, and right or left ventricular hypertrophy; conduction disturbances are uncommon.

DIFFERENTIAL DIAGNOSIS. The constellation of progressive ataxia, areflexia, Babinski signs, and onset before age 25 is usually diagnostic. However, a similar picture can occur in vitamin B_{12} deficiency and in two hereditary autosomal recessive disorders, abetalipoproteinemia and selective vitamin E deficiency. True Friedreich's ataxia is sometimes confused with a less common autosomal recessive type of early-onset progressive ataxia, in which the tendon reflexes are preserved; in the latter syndrome, optic atrophy, scoliosis, and electrocardiographic abnormalities are rare.

ATAXIA-TELANGIECTASIA

Ataxia-telangiectasia is an autosomal recessive, multisystem disease affecting the skin, nervous system, and immune system. Its prevalence has been estimated at 1 to 2 per 100,000. The condition is described further in Ch. 223.

ADULT-ONSET CEREBELLAR ATAXIA

Hereditary ataxia starting in adult life is nearly always an autosomal dominant disorder with multiple neurologic manifestations, among which cerebellar signs are prominent. In Europe the prevalence is 1 to 10 per 100,000 population. The syndrome is genetically heterogeneous; one type is caused by expansion of an unstable trinucleotide repeat on chromosome 6p, another is linked to chromosome 12q, and the Azorean form (Machado-Joseph disease) is linked to chromosome 14q.

PATHOLOGY. Many cases have the pathologic features of olivopontocerebellar atrophy, with loss of neurons in the inferior olives and pontine nuclei (which provide major afferent pathways to the cerebellum), as well as degeneration of the spinocerebellar tracts, corticospinal tracts, and posterior columns. Neuronal degeneration is sometimes found in the cerebellar cortex, dentate nucleus, basal ganglia, midbrain, cerebral cortex, and spinal cord, including the anterior horns. The pathology, however, is as variable as the clinical findings, even within a given family. In Machado-Joseph disease, the cerebellar cortex and olives are spared.

CLINICAL MANIFESTATIONS. The age of onset, although variable, is usually between 20 and 50. Cerebellar ataxia of gait, dysarthria, and incoordination of the limbs usually dominate the clinical picture, so that the ability to walk is lost within 15 years. The other manifestations are extremely variable. Babinski signs and increased reflexes are commonly present, and some patients have spastic weakness in the legs. Vibration and position sense are sometimes lost as the disease advances, and the reflexes may disappear as the primary sensory neurons degenerate. Extrapyramidal findings may include impassive facies, cogwheel rigidity, chorea, athetosis, dystonia, and facial dyskinesia. Many patients have supranuclear oculomotor disorders such as lid retraction, ptosis, nystagmus, slow eye movements, and gaze paresis, especially upgaze. Optic atrophy, with pale discs, is common. Pigmentary degeneration of the retina, beginning in the macula, is an early and constant feature in some families, suggesting that these cases may be genetically distinct. Personality change or dementia, muscle wasting and fasciculation in the tongue and distal extremities, and bulbar symptoms of dysphagia or hoarseness are other common manifestations. Death occurs approximately 20 years after onset, at an average age of 57.

TABLE 413–1. THE MULTISYSTEM ATROPHIES

Disease	Heredity	Principal Feature	Associated Features	Chapter
Shy-Drager syndrome	Sporadic	Autonomic insufficiency	Parkinsonism, cerebellar ataxia, dysphagia, laryngeal stridor, amyotrophy	402
Progressive supranuclear palsy	Sporadic	Ophthalmoplegia, especially vertical	Gait ataxia, axial dystonia, parkinsonism, pseudobulbar palsy, dementia	410
Kearns-Sayre syndrome	Sporadic	Ptosis and ophthalmoplegia	Short stature, cerebellar ataxia, retinal degeneration, heart block, deafness, mitochondrial myopathy, mental deficiency, Babinski signs	454
Hereditary ataxias, adult type	Autosomal dominant	Cerebellar ataxia	Ophthalmoplegia, dementia, parkinsonism, dystonia, optic atrophy, retinal degeneration, dysphagia, amyotrophy	413

A few families seem to have a "pure" cerebellar syndrome beginning in the seventh decade of life. These cases (cerebellar cortical atrophy) tend to have a more benign prognosis.

DIAGNOSIS. In the olivopontocerebellar atrophy syndrome, MRI may show atrophy of the cerebellar folia and pons, with enlargement of the fourth ventricle and pontine cisterns. In pure cerebellar cortical atrophy, only the cerebellum is shrunken. The cerebrospinal fluid is usually normal. Sensory nerve action potentials are small or absent in patients with absent reflexes; in patients with preserved reflexes, somatosensory evoked potentials may be abnormal.

DIFFERENTIAL DIAGNOSIS. Nonhereditary cases of late-onset cerebellar degeneration are at least as common as the hereditary kind. Some are associated with alcoholism or a visceral malignancy, but in many, no apparent cause can be established. These patients' cerebellar symptoms tend to begin between the ages of 40 and 60 and may be accompanied by dementia, extrapyramidal signs, or Babinski signs. Some cases of this kind have the pathologic features of olivopontocerebellar atrophy, but whether there is any genetic link to the autosomal dominant ataxias is unclear. It should be noted that patients presenting with ataxia may later develop the typical signs of progressive supranuclear palsy or one of the other multisystem atrophies listed in Table 413–1.

Harding AE: The Hereditary Ataxias and Related Disorders. Edinburgh. Churchill Livingstone, 1984. *A detailed review of the hereditary cerebellar ataxias and spastic paraplegias, including the author's own study of several hundred patients and family members. A modern classic.*
Orr HT, Chung M, Banfi S, et al.: Expansion of an unstable trinucleotide repeat in spinocerebellar ataxia type 1. Nature Genetics 4:221, 1993. *Reports the first specific gene defect to be found in a hereditary ataxia.*

414 HEREDITARY SPASTIC PARAPLEGIAS

This is a diverse group of uncommon diseases whose main symptom is an insidiously beginning, progressive spasticity of the lower extremities. Families with "pure" hereditary spastic paraplegia (Strümpell's disease) are the most numerous, but many rare variants have been reported in which spasticity is associated with other neurologic, ocular, or cutaneous manifestations, overlapping with the spinocerebellar degenerations. The prevalence of these diseases is not well established. Rare examples of *primary lateral sclerosis,* although sporadic in incidence, may belong to this class.

PATHOLOGY. In the pure form, the spinal cord shows degeneration of the lateral corticospinal tracts and posterior columns, most severe in the thoracic region. Less often there is minor degeneration of the spinocerebellar tracts, anterior corticospinal tracts, anterior horn cells, and cortical Betz cells.

CLINICAL MANIFESTATIONS. Most patients with pure hereditary spastic paraplegia continue to walk for many years and have a normal lifespan. Many cases begin in infancy with delayed walking, but the onset can be as late as the seventh decade. Spasticity of the legs and a stiff, slow gait are the main symptoms. Affected persons walk on their toes, trip easily, and are unable to run. About one fourth have pes cavus. The legs show hyperactive reflexes, clonus, and Babinski signs, whereas the arms are usually normal. Later the legs may become weak, the arms may show increased reflexes, and distal muscle wasting may develop, especially in the hands. Vibration and position sense may become impaired in the legs, and many patients develop urinary frequency, urgency, and precipitancy, although sexual function remains normal. Most patients become unable to walk sometime in the sixth or seventh decade.

DIAGNOSIS. The cerebrospinal fluid is normal. Electromyography may show denervation in the distal limb muscles, but the sensory nerve action potentials are preserved, even in patients showing decreased vibration and position sense. Somatosensory evoked potentials, however, are consistently small or unobtainable, reflecting a degeneration of dorsal column fibers.

DIFFERENTIAL DIAGNOSIS. Hereditary spastic paraplegia must be distinguished from nonhereditary causes of slowly progressive myelopathy such as cervical spondylosis, intraspinal tumor, arteriovenous malformation or fistula of the spinal cord, multiple sclerosis, amyotrophic lateral sclerosis, and myelopathy associated with human T cell lymphotropic virus 1 (HTLV-1 tropical spastic paraparesis, Ch. 428.3). MRI has simplified diagnosis of many of these conditions.

415 HEREDITARY AND ACQUIRED INTRINSIC MOTOR NEURON DISEASES

Degenerative diseases of several kinds can attack the large motor neurons of the spinal cord or the brain to produce selective impairment of muscle strength or motor skill. Those of childhood are largely hereditary, whereas the major adult disorder, amyotrophic lateral sclerosis, is nearly always sporadic, with few clues illuminating either its cause or molecular pathogenesis. Table 415–1 lists the major disorders in this category, and the references provide greater detail on the many subtypes.

HEREDITARY AMYOTROPHIES

Hereditary spinal muscular atrophy is a syndrome of progressive muscular weakness and atrophy resulting from selective degeneration of the motor neurons of the spinal cord. A comparable disorder of the lower brain stem nuclei produces progressive bulbar palsy. Many different clinical syndromes have been delineated based on the age of onset, the pattern of muscular weakness, the rate of progression, and the mode of inheritance. Using this approach, at least 15 separate genetic disorders can be recognized. It has been estimated that 1 in 40 Caucasians carries a gene for spinal muscular atrophy. No consistent biochemical defect is known, although hexosaminidase deficiency has been identified in a few cases.

PATHOLOGY. At the time of postmortem examination in the spinal cases, the anterior horns show gliosis and loss of large neurons, and many of the remaining motor neurons are undergoing degeneration. The ventral roots are atrophic owing to loss of myelinated nerve fibers. Similar changes are observed in the motor nuclei of the brain stem in bulbar cases.

In the well-developed infantile and childhood types, microscopic examination of the skeletal muscles using histochemical techniques shows large groups of round, atrophic muscle fibers and large groups of hypertrophied fibers staining uniformly as either type 1 or type 2. These features reflect the continuing process of denervation and reinnervation. However, at an early stage of infantile spinal muscular atrophy the only finding may be uniform atrophy of all

TABLE 415–1. THE MAJOR INTRINSIC MOTOR NEURON DISEASES

Hereditary
Spinal muscular atrophy
  Type I. Acute, infantile (Werdnig-Hoffmann disease)
  Type II. Late infantile and childhood type
  Type III. Juvenile and adult types
Familial amyotrophic lateral sclerosis (ALS)
Acquired
Acute: anterior poliomyelitis
Chronic:
  ALS alone
  Anterior horn cell degeneration associated with spinocerebellar degeneration, Shy-Drager syndrome, parkinsonism, Creutzfeldt-Jakob disease
  Remote neoplasms, other
Primary lateral sclerosis (rare)

muscle fibers, with preservation of the normal "checkerboard" fiber-type pattern. In slowly progressive cases of juvenile or adult onset, atrophic muscle fibers are found mainly in small groups; most muscle fibers are of normal size but are arranged in groups of uniform fiber type. After many years some muscle fibers show secondary myopathic changes, such as internal nuclei, splitting, or degeneration.

ACUTE INFANTILE SPINAL MUSCULAR ATROPHY

Werdnig-Hoffmann disease is a fatal, early infantile form of spinal and bulbar muscular atrophy that appears to be a single genetic entity. Inherited as an autosomal recessive abnormality on chromosome 5q, it is one of the most common fatal hereditary diseases of childhood, with an annual incidence of 1 in 20,000 live births and a carrier frequency in the general population of about 1 in 80. The abnormal gene is located on the long arm of chromosome 5.

In at least one third of the cases, there is a prenatal onset, with reduced fetal movements, weakness at birth, or congenital joint deformities. In the remainder of cases, the disease becomes apparent in the first 2 or 3 months of life. There is progressive, flaccid weakness of the trunk and limbs, with severe hypotonia, poor head control, and diminished movements of the limbs, more severe in the proximal muscles. Weakness of the intercostal muscles causes retraction of the chest during inspiration; the cry is weak, and coughing is ineffective. Bulbar weakness causes difficulty in sucking and swallowing. The tendon reflexes are usually absent. Death occurs before 3 years of age; 50% of the patients die in the first 7 months of life and 95% in the first 18 months.

The serum creatine kinase activity and the cerebrospinal fluid are normal. Electromyography shows reduced activation of motor unit potentials, many of which are of increased size, duration, and complexity. Fibrillations and fasciculations are rarely observed. It is important to distinguish this disease from treatable disorders such as infant botulism and chronic inflammatory polyneuropathy. The former is identified by repetitive nerve stimulation tests showing abnormal neuromuscular transmission and the latter, by abnormalities of nerve conduction and increased protein levels in the cerebrospinal fluid.

PROGRESSIVE MUSCULAR ATROPHY IN CHILDREN

PROXIMAL TYPE. Clinically, this is a rather diverse disorder, but most cases are now thought to be caused by a single autosomal recessive gene, located on the long arm of chromosome 5, near or at the locus for Werdnig-Hoffmann disease. The incidence of this syndrome is 1 in 24,000 live births, and the carrier rate is approximately 1 in 90. A milder, autosomal dominant form is also known.

Weakness starts anytime from birth to 8 years of age, usually before 1 year of age. The weakness affects the trunk and limbs and initially is more severe in proximal muscles. The limb muscles become atrophic, the tendon reflexes are lost, and joint contractures may develop. Fasciculations are not prominent but may be apparent in the fingers, producing a fine, irregular tremor. The face and jaws may be weak, and the tongue may be atrophic and show fasciculation.

Children with early onset may never be able to walk and often develop severe scoliosis, limb deformities, and respiratory insufficiency. Many eventually die of pulmonary infection, but some very weak patients survive into adult life, the progress of the disease apparently having arrested early in childhood. Children with a later onset of weakness tend to have a milder course, with slowly progressive proximal weakness, increased lumbar lordosis, and a waddling gait. Those with autosomal recessive inheritance rarely walk after age 20, whereas those with the rare autosomal dominant form may still be walking in middle age.

Serum creatine kinase activity may be mildly or moderately increased in patients with slowly progressive weakness, apparently because of secondary myopathic changes in muscle. The cerebrospinal fluid is normal. Electromyography shows the typical changes of chronic denervation and reinnervation as well as fibrillations and fasciculations, serving to distinguish these patients from similar patients with muscular dystrophy.

Many of these children benefit from active and passive physical therapy and the judicious use of lightweight braces. Special attention should be given to spinal support to counteract scoliosis. Later in childhood, surgical immobilization of the spine may be indicated.

DISTAL TYPE. This category includes both dominant and recessive disorders and accounts for about 10% of all cases of spinal muscular atrophy. Distal limb weakness and muscle wasting, more severe in the lower extremities, usually begins in early childhood and tends to be mild and slowly progressive. Three quarters of the patients have pes cavus, and, except for the absence of sensory deficits, the disorder is often clinically indistinguishable from Charcot-Marie-Tooth disease. However, patients with spinal muscular atrophy have normal conduction in motor and sensory nerves. A rare scapuloperoneal type, with autosomal recessive inheritance, is characterized by distal leg weakness and scapular winging, starting in infancy; there may also be bulbar symptoms such as laryngeal stridor.

SPINAL MUSCULAR ATROPHY OF ADOLESCENT OR ADULT ONSET

Patients with late-onset spinal muscular atrophy have slowly progressive muscular weakness and usually continue to walk for two or three decades or more. Although much less common than the infantile and childhood types, the adult types include at least four clinical and eight genetic categories.

PROXIMAL TYPE. These patients resemble those with muscular dystrophy, and clinical examination may offer few clues to the neurogenic character of the proximal weakness. Fasciculations and muscle cramps are usually not prominent, and the serum creatine kinase activity may be substantially increased. To add to the confusion, males with onset of symptoms in their teens may have large calves. Some patients eventually develop mild bulbar symptoms, such as dysphagia. Electromyography serves to establish the neurogenic nature of the disorder, and muscle biopsy is rarely needed. Families with autosomal dominant and autosomal recessive inheritance have been described. A distinctive X-linked recessive variety, known as bulbospinal neuronopathy, is associated with gynecomastia and dysphagia. It is caused by expansion of a trinucleotide repeat within the gene coding for the androgen receptor.

SCAPULOPERONEAL AND FACIOSCAPULOHUMERAL TYPES. Both myopathic and neurogenic scapuloperoneal syndromes are known, and several varieties begin in the second or third decade of life. Autosomal dominant, autosomal recessive, and X-linked recessive forms have been described. The common feature of these disorders is progressive atrophy and weakness of the shoulder girdle and lower leg muscles, although weakness eventually may spread to the other limb muscles. Electromyography and muscle biopsy can distinguish the anterior horn cell diseases from the muscular dystrophies, but the prognosis is similar in both groups. A few families have an autosomal dominant form of spinal muscular atrophy resembling facioscapulohumeral muscular dystrophy.

DISTAL TYPE. This is usually a childhood disorder, but there are a few families with distal amyotrophy beginning in the third or fourth decade of life, inherited as an autosomal dominant trait. Some familial as well as adult cases exhibit onset in middle age and such a slow progression as never to be incapacitating, even in old age.

AMYOTROPHIC LATERAL SCLEROSIS

Amyotrophic lateral sclerosis (ALS) is a fatal degenerative disease of the central nervous system characterized by slowly progressive paralysis of the voluntary muscles.

INCIDENCE. The annual incidence is about 1 case per 100,000 population, the prevalence being 4 to 6 cases per 100,000. Geographical pockets of much higher incidence in Guam, the Kii peninsula of Japan, and western New Guinea suggest possible, still unknown, exogenous causes. Ninety-five percent of cases in the United States are sporadic, but a few families have several members with the typical clinical picture of sporadic ALS arising in an autosomal dominant pattern. Males are affected slightly more often than females. Although the disease can appear as early as the third decade of life, most cases begin after age 40, and the incidence increases into the eighth decade.

PATHOLOGY. Degeneration of the motor neurons of the spinal cord and lower brain stem is marked by extensive cell loss and astrocytic gliosis. Swellings containing neurofilaments are often found on axons close to their cell bodies. As the Betz cells and large pyramidal neurons of the motor cortex disappear, the corticospinal tracts degenerate, leaving gliosis of the lateral columns of the spinal cord. The ventral spinal roots are depleted of large myelinated nerve fibers, but surviving axons develop distal sprouts that reinnervate some muscle fibers, so that skeletal muscle histopathology shows both muscle fiber atrophy and fiber-type grouping.

ETIOLOGY. Few clues exist to the cause of ALS. Some authors regard the disease as a manifestation of premature aging or a deficiency of a neurotrophic factor. Other speculations include toxic exposure to minerals such as lead or aluminum, deficiency of calcium or magnesium, infection by an unidentified virus, and autoimmunity. Benign paraproteinemia has been encountered in a small proportion of patients, and antiganglioside antibodies have been found in the serum in a majority of the cases, but the significance of these findings is unclear. Recently, some familial cases were linked to a gene coding for the enzyme superoxide dismutase, located on chromosome 21q. This finding has stimulated research into a possible role of free radical toxicity in the pathogenesis of ALS.

CLINICAL MANIFESTATIONS. The major symptom consists of slowly progressive muscle weakness involving the limbs, trunk, breathing muscles, throat, and tongue. Most patients have a mixture of lower and upper motor neuron symptoms, although either may predominate. The former include muscle weakness, wasting, fasciculations, and cramps; the latter include stiffness and slowness of movement, slow and clumsy speech, and explosive release of laughter and crying (pseudobulbar palsy). The ocular muscles are not affected except in patients who survive long times after bulbar paralysis has begun. No impairment affects bladder, bowel, or sexual function. The stretch reflexes are diminished in severely denervated muscles, but more often signs of lower motor neuron weakness are combined with brisk reflexes, a finding nearly specific to ALS. Babinski signs are often present. Sensation is normal except for an expected diminution of vibration sense in the feet in older patients. Occasional cases develop a progressive dementia.

The onset is insidious, and initial symptoms may be confined to a single limb (especially the distal muscles), both limbs on one side, or to lower cranial nerves. Gradually the patchy and asymmetric weakness becomes widespread, and patients become unable to walk, dress, or feed themselves. There is loss of weight because of muscle atrophy and impaired swallowing; the speech becomes unintelligible; choking interferes with eating and sleeping; and breathing becomes difficult even at rest. Death occurs from pulmonary infection and insufficiency. The average survival is 3 years after onset of symptoms, but a few severely debilitated patients live for 10 years or longer.

DIAGNOSIS. Because there are no specific laboratory tests, the diagnosis is based principally on clinical criteria. The disease to be diagnosed as ALS should have a relentlessly progressive, gradual course; lower motor neuron signs should exist at widely separate levels of the nervous system, or upper motor neuron signs should be found well above the level of the lower motor neuron signs; and no conflicting findings such as sensory loss, incontinence, or ocular weakness should be present. The cerebrospinal fluid is normal except for a mild elevation of protein concentration in some cases. Brain and spinal cord imaging is unrevealing. Electromyography shows active and chronic denervation in multiple muscles of the brain stem, upper and lower extremities, and trunk; motor nerve conduction velocity is normal or slightly reduced, and sensory nerve conduction is normal. Serum creatine kinase activity is normal or moderately increased.

DIFFERENTIAL DIAGNOSIS. Although ALS is nearly always fatal, a few patients stop deteriorating or even recover normal strength, but such cases are extremely rare. Other motor neuron disorders, treatable myelopathies and neuropathies, and even thyrotoxic myopathy must be distinguished from ALS (Table 415–2).

TREATMENT. With a disease as grim as ALS, the physician must be careful to avoid premature misdiagnosis. Once the diagnosis is certain, however, some explanation must be given to the patient and the family. This requires considerable tact and gentleness; often it is best to convey the information gradually on successive visits, allowing the relentless progression of weakness to speak for itself.

No medication has been shown to be beneficial, and physical therapy does not delay the neuromuscular deterioration. Quack remedies surface periodically; for their own protection, patients

TABLE 415–2. DIFFERENTIAL DIAGNOSIS OF AMYOTROPHIC LATERAL SCLEROSIS

Disease	Distinguishing Features
Benign fasciculations	No weakness, atrophy, or electromyographic (EMG) abnormality
Motor neuron diseases	
*Lead or mercury toxicity	Increased lead or mercury levels
Benign focal amyotrophy	Onset in youth, strictly focal, no upper motor neuron signs
Postpolio progressive muscular atrophy	Slow course, no upper motor neuron signs
Subacute motor neuronopathy in lymphoma	Plateau in few months, later improvement
*ALS in lung cancer or B cell dyscrasia	Improves on treatment of tumor
Hereditary spinal muscular atrophy	Symmetric, slow course, no upper motor neuron signs
*Thyrotoxic myopathy with fasciculations	Myopathic EMG
*Compressive myelopathy due to cervical spondylosis or extramedullary tumor	Sensory symptoms, no lower motor neuron signs in legs, cord compression on MRI or myelography
*Immune-mediated multifocal motor neuropathy	Multifocal nerve conduction block, very high antiganglioside antibody titers

* Treatable conditions

who wish to try experimental forms of treatment should be referred to a reputable academic center.

Patients with impaired gait may benefit from using a cane or a walker, and patients who suffer from severe dysphagia without other disabling symptoms can be offered nasogastric tube feeding or a gastrostomy. The most difficult medical question, however, involves the therapeutic role of artificial ventilation. Most patients, understanding the hopeless prognosis, prefer not to be kept alive artificially in a state of total paralysis, unable to communicate except with eye movements. Nevertheless, some of these patients have survived for several years, living at home with the help of a devoted and intelligent family. It is important to discuss these issues when patients are in the early stages of respiratory involvement, so that they can make decisions in advance about whether or not to accept emergency resuscitation during a respiratory crisis.

PRIMARY LATERAL SCLEROSIS

Primary lateral sclerosis (PLS) denotes a rare condition characterized by painless, gradually progressing spastic weakness that involves the lower limbs and may ascend to involve the arms and bulbar muscles. In most instances, the disease begins in middle or late life and usually lasts more than a decade before intercurrent illness causes death. Typically, neurologic examinations show a relatively symmetric spastic paraparesis or quadriparesis with heightened deep tendon reflexes and extensor plantar responses but no hint of sensory abnormality. Neither clinical nor electrical studies detect evidence of skeletal muscular denervation. Similarly, imaging procedures disclose no relevant abnormalities involving either brain or spinal cord. The cerebrospinal fluid remains unremarkable, and appropriate tests fail to disclose HIV, HTLV, or other inflammatory processes. Autopsy examinations, performed in a number of cases, have revealed ascending bilateral demyelination of the thoracolumbar corticospinal tracts extending anywhere from the lower cord up to the cerebral peduncles. Cerebral degeneration has not been noted. The cause of PLS is not known, but sporadically arising familial spastic paraplegia cannot be excluded in cases selectively involving the lower extremities. No specific treatment exists, although baclofen may bring modest relief of stiffness.

Brzustowicz LM, Lehner T, Castilla LH, et al.: Genetic mapping of chronic childhood onset spinal muscular atrophy to chromosome 5q 11.2–13.3. Nature 344:540, 1990. *Evidence that the infantile and childhood types of spinal muscular atrophy are allelic disorders of a single gene.*

Deng H-X, Hentati A, Tainer JA, et al.: Amyotrophic lateral sclerosis and structural defects in Cu, Zn superoxide dismutase. Science 261:1047, 1993. *Mutations of the gene for superoxide dismutase, important for scavenging of toxic free radicals, cause reduced red cell enzyme activity in familial ALS.*

Martin JB: Molecular genetics in neurology. Ann Neurol 34:757, 1993. *Provides an informative table.*

Pringle CE, Hudson AJ, Munoz DG, et al.: Primary lateral sclerosis: Clinical features, neuropathology, and diagnostic criteria. Brain 115:495, 1992. *The most comprehensive article about an uncommon disease, carefully reported.*

Williams AC (ed.): Motor Neuron Disease. London, Chapman and Hall, 1994. 776 pp. *In addition to offering full clinical accounts of motor neuron disorders, this book reviews current research on pathogenesis of ALS and gives helpful advice about medical management.*

416 SYRINGOMYELIA

Syringomyelia is a disorder of the spinal cord and, often, the lower brain stem, characterized by slowly progressive enlargement of a fluid-filled cyst (syrinx) within the cord or medulla. Most cases are congenital in origin, related to maldevelopment of the cervicomedullary junction; others are caused by arachnoiditis, intraspinal tumor, or trauma.

PATHOLOGY. In congenital cases, the cyst is thought to represent an enormously dilated remnant of the fetal central canal, which usually does not communicate with the fourth ventricle. It is lined by glial tissue, and in places by remnants of ependyma, and contains clear fluid identical to cerebrospinal fluid. Extending from the high cervical level or medulla to the thoracic or lumbar cord, the cavities vary in shape and size at different levels. Most patients have a Chiari type of congenital cerebellar malformation, in which flattened ectopic tonsils descend caudally so as to obstruct both the exit foramina of the fourth ventricle and the subarachnoid space at the foramen magnum.

Acquired syringomyelia may result from basal arachnoiditis, obstructing the cerebrospinal fluid pathways around the foramen magnum, or may develop in a segment of the cord rendered abnormal by an intramedullary tumor, spinal arachnoiditis, or severe traumatic injury. In nontumor cases the cavity is lined only by glia, whereas in tumor cases the cyst wall may contain both tumor and glial cells.

PATHOGENESIS. The mechanism of cyst formation and expansion is poorly understood. In congenital syringomyelia the cavity probably originates before birth as a dilatation of the primitive central canal. Enlargement of the cyst is somehow related to obstruction of the subarachnoid space at the cervicomedullary junction by the ectopic cerebellar tonsils, causing a pressure gradient between the cyst and the subarachnoid space, especially during straining, coughing, or sneezing. The mechanism may be similar in cases of basal arachnoiditis. In patients with spinal arachnoiditis, the cyst may originate in an area of ischemic myelomalacia, and in cases associated with tumor or severe injury there is cystic degeneration of the spinal cord before the syrinx starts to expand. Why the cyst continues to enlarge in these noncommunicating cases is hard to understand, because there is no apparent pressure gradient between the cyst and the subarachnoid space. Obstruction of cerebrospinal fluid circulation due to spinal arachnoiditis may be an important factor.

CLINICAL MANIFESTATIONS. The classic clinical picture of congenital syringomyelia is of a slowly progressive, asymmetric, destructive process in the central portion of the cervical and thoracic spinal cord, damaging the anterior horn cells, the crossing spinothalamic tract fibers, and the lateral corticospinal tracts. This causes muscle weakness and wasting in the hands and arms; scoliosis owing to denervation of paraspinal muscles; loss of arm reflexes; spastic weakness of the lower extremities; and a *dissociated sensory loss* with impaired perception of pain and temperature in the neck, arms, and upper trunk and preserved light touch perception and proprioception. Some patients experience a deep, aching pain in the neck or arms. Symptoms usually begin between 25 and 40 years of age and advance relentlessly for decades, although one third of the patients have long periods of stability. The deficits may worsen suddenly after a fall or after coughing or sneezing. Ten percent of patients develop a painless arthropathy of the shoulder, elbow, or hand. Extension into the medulla may cause nystagmus, dysphagia, or wasting of the tongue, and some patients have hydro-

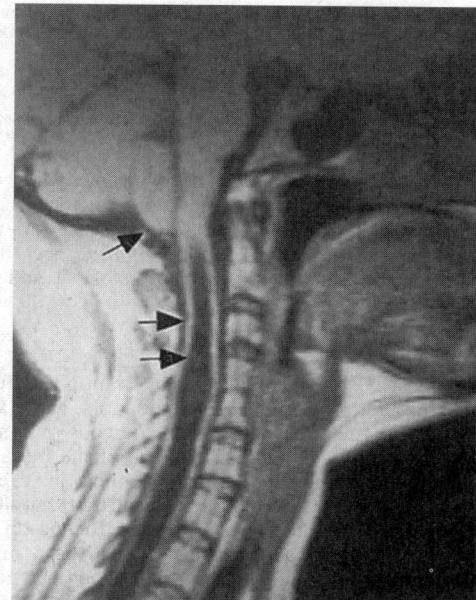

FIGURE 416–1. Magnetic resonance image of upper spine and foramen magnum in a patient with syringomyelia and a small Chiari I malformation *(single arrow)*. The syrinx appears as a dark central area in the cervical and thoracic spinal cord *(double arrows)*.

cephalus or cerebellar signs related to an associated Chiari malformation.

The manifestations of acquired syringomyelia depend on the segment of the spinal cord affected. Posttraumatic syringomyelia, developing in paraplegic or quadriplegic patients months or years after the injury, is revealed by weakness and sensory impairment rising craniad from the transected level. The cases associated with arachnoiditis following previous purulent meningitis, subarachnoid hemorrhage, surgery, trauma, or spinal anesthesia tend to involve the thoracic and lower cervical segments. Syringes associated with intramedullary spinal cord tumor extend for variable distances rostrad or caudad to the tumor.

DIAGNOSIS. Magnetic resonance (MR) imaging, outlines the size and extent of the cavity as well as the presence of cerebellar ectopia, arachnoiditis, or an intraspinal tumor (Fig. 416–1). Electromyography reveals active and chronic denervation in wasted upper extremity muscles, but sensory nerve conduction is normal in the analgesic hand because the lesion is located proximal to the dorsal root ganglia. The cerebrospinal fluid is normal except for a raised protein content in cases associated with tumor or arachnoiditis.

TREATMENT. Various surgical procedures have been devised in the hope of arresting the neurologic deterioration. None has been reliably successful. If hydrocephalus is present, placement of a ventriculoperitoneal shunt may be sufficient to cause the syrinx to collapse, but seldom halts its progression. For congenital syringomyelia associated with cerebellar ectopia, it is customary to perform a posterior decompression of the foramen magnum, ensuring that the fourth ventricle communicates with the subarachnoid space. Acquired syringomyelia is usually treated by decompressing the cyst via a syringoarachnoid, syringopleural, or syringoperitoneal shunt. It has not been established that the outcome of any of these procedures is superior to the natural history of the disease. Some neurosurgical reports suggest that these operations often reduce chronic pain and arrest the progression of neurologic symptoms but long-term follow-up is lacking.

Anderson NE, Willoughby EW, Wrightson P: The natural history and the influence of surgical treatment in syringomyelia. Acta Neurol Scand 71:472, 1985. *A thoughtful critique of the uncertain role of surgical treatment for syringomyelia.*

Oldfield EH, Muraszko K, Shawker TH, Patronas NJ: Pathophysiology of syringomyelia associated with Chiari I malformation of the cerebellar tonsils. Implications for diagnosis and treatment. J Neurosurg 80:3, 1994. *Uses light-tech imaging to analyze fluid dynamics in the syrinx and advocates a new approach to treatment.*

417 THE PHAKOMATOSES

The phakomatoses, or neurocutaneous syndromes, are congenital disorders characterized by disordered growth of ectodermal tissues, producing distinctive skin lesions and malformations or tumors of the nervous system. More than 20 syndromes have been described, the most important of which are neurofibromatosis 1 and 2, tuberous sclerosis, and Sturge-Weber disease.

NEUROFIBROMATOSIS 1 (von Recklinghausen's Disease)

Neurofibromatosis 1 is characterized by multiple café au lait spots on the skin, multiple peripheral nerve tumors, and a variety of other dysplastic abnormalities of the skin, nervous system, bones, endocrine organs, and blood vessels. It is one of the most common genetic diseases, occurring approximately once in every 3000 births. It is inherited as an autosomal dominant trait, but 40 to 60% of cases are clinically sporadic. Even allowing for the difficulty of detecting the trait in mild cases, there seems to be a remarkably high mutation rate, on the order of 10^{-4} per locus per generation. The responsible gene, which occupies a 300-kilobase region of chromosome 17q, codes for a GTPase-activating protein (neurofibromin), which functions as a tumor suppressor.

PATHOLOGY. The peripheral nerve tumors are of two types, schwannomas and neurofibromas, the latter derived from both Schwann cells and perineural fibroblasts. Neurofibromas of sensory nerve twigs produce the distinctive subcutaneous nodules; in peripheral nerve trunks the tumor appears as a fusiform enlargement or plexiform neuroma. Schwannomas arise in cranial and spinal nerve roots and also in peripheral nerve trunks. Both types of tumor occasionally become malignant. The brain may show disordered architecture, hamartomas, gliomas, and meningiomas.

CLINICAL MANIFESTATIONS. Some manifestations are congenital, but most appear during childhood and adult life. Café au lait spots become larger and more numerous with age; most patients eventually have more than six spots greater than 1.5 cm in diameter. Other skin lesions include freckles (axillary freckles being specific to this disease); soft pedunculated cutaneous neurofibromas, and firm subcutaneous neurofibromas.

Plexiform neurofibromas may grow to enormous size, leading to grotesque overgrowth of soft tissues and bone in a limb or around the orbit. Enlarging nerve trunk tumors may cause pain and impair sensory-motor function; intraspinal nerve root tumors do the same and also compress the spinal cord. Gliomas of the optic nerve and chiasm are the most frequent intracranial tumor; they usually behave indolently as hamartomas do. A hamartoma of the hypothalamus may cause precocious puberty.

About 10% of children are mentally deficient, and about 10% develop seizures, half in association with an intracranial tumor. Kyphoscoliosis, dysplasia of the skull, bowed legs, and other bone abnormalities are common. Pheochromocytoma occurs in about 5% of patients, usually in adult life. Hypertension may result from renal artery dysplasia.

DIAGNOSIS. The diagnosis is usually clinically evident, but biopsy of a neurofibroma can be diagnostic in cryptic cases. Spinal nerve root tumors often have a dumbbell shape, with intraspinal and extraspinal components; these are most readily identified on MRI. For diagnosis of intracranial tumors and hamartomas either CT or MRI is suitable.

TREATMENT. Most patients live a normal life with few or no symptoms. Small cutaneous or subcutaneous neurofibromas can be removed if they are painful or frequently irritated, but large plexiform neurofibromas usually should be left alone. A few become malignant with continued invasion and fatal outcome. Symptomatic peripheral nerve trunk schwannomas can sometimes be removed safely by an experienced surgeon. Intraspinal and intracranial schwannomas are approached in the usual surgical fashion. Optic nerve gliomas are generally treated with radiation, but it is not clear whether this improves the outcome.

NEUROFIBROMATOSIS 2

This rare disease is characterized by the occurrence of bilateral acoustic neuromas and often other intracranial tumors, such as meningiomas and ependymomas. A few café au lait spots are present in 42% of cases. The disease is inherited as an autosomal dominant trait, but 50% of cases are new mutations. The responsible gene, located on chromosome 22q, codes for a cytoskeletal protein (merlin) which is presumed to function as a tumor suppressor. Family members at risk for the disease should be screened regularly with hearing tests and brain stem auditory evoked responses.

TUBEROUS SCLEROSIS

The phenotype of tuberous sclerosis consists of mental deficiency, epilepsy, and a characteristic facial eruption known as adenoma sebaceum. The disease is inherited as an autosomal dominant trait, but about 80% of the cases are sporadic, owing to new mutations. Two separate gene loci have been linked to the syndrome, one on chromosome 9q and the other on chromosome 16p.

PATHOLOGY. The facial papules of adenoma sebaceum are angiofibromas. The cerebral hemispheres contain multiple hamartomas characterized by disordered architecture, proliferating and abnormal astrocytes, and deposits of calcium. The common retinal hamartomas are also probably of glial origin. Visceral lesions include multiple rhabdomyomas of the heart, multiple angiomyolipomas of the kidneys, and cystic transformation of the lungs by proliferating fibrous, muscular, and vascular tissue.

CLINICAL MANIFESTATIONS. Mental deficiency may be mild or severe, but one third of affected individuals have normal or even superior intelligence. Seizures occur in 80% of cases, usually starting before the age of 5, and are often difficult to control with medication. In infants the seizures often take the form of infantile spasms; these children tend to be more severely impaired mentally. Occasionally, diagnosis escapes attention until late adolescence or adult life, when investigation of a seizure disorder of new onset discloses subtle skin lesions or multiple retinal or intracranial hamartomas.

Nearly all patients have distinctive skin lesions. Hypopigmented spots are present from the time of birth in nearly 100% of patients; they are more numerous on the trunk and are easier to see with a Wood's lamp. The next most common is adenoma sebaceum, a papular, salmon-colored eruption about the center of the face and in the nasolabial folds. It usually becomes more prominent after puberty. Leathery "shagreen" patches over the lower back and fibromas of the nailbeds affect perhaps 40% of patients.

Retinal hamartomas affect about half the patients. About 30% of patients have cardiac rhabdomyomas, which sometimes cause arrhythmia or congestive heart failure. Renal tumors occur in two thirds of patients and are usually asymptomatic, although pain and bleeding can occur. Cystic disease of the lungs, an uncommon complication, mainly affects women over the age of 20; the symptoms include pneumothorax, dyspnea, cyanosis, and cor pulmonale.

DIAGNOSIS. Clinical diagnosis often is obvious. MRI is the procedure of choice and identifies both calcified and uncalcified tubers and nodules. Adenoma sebaceum, ungual fibromas, and hypopigmented spots are diagnostically specific, but retinal hamartomas also occur in neurofibromatosis.

Treatment is confined to symptomatic control of the epilepsy and to surgical therapy of the occasional hamartoma that undergoes gliomatous changes and enlarges to produce symptoms.

STURGE-WEBER SYNDROME

The Sturge-Weber syndrome is a nonhereditary, congenital disorder of facial and cerebral blood vessels characterized by a facial angioma (port-wine stain), seizures, and mental deficiency. The condition involves a defect of embryonic development, with persistence of a vascular plexus in the cephalic portion of the neural tube. The incidence is about 5 in 100,000 births.

The facial angioma is usually unilateral but may extend to the other side and conforms largely but not strictly to trigeminal nerve subdivisions. There may be cavernous angiomas of the tongue, gums, or mouth, and choroidal angiomas may cause congenital glaucoma. An angioma of the occipital and parietal leptomeninges accompanies the facial nevus on the same side, and the underlying cerebral hemisphere is atrophic, with degenerative changes and deposits of iron and calcium in the superficial layers of the cerebral cortex. The cortical calcifications and atrophy are easily seen on brain CT. Neurologic symptoms develop in infancy or early childhood, consisting of focal or generalized seizures. Half of the children become mentally impaired, and one third develop a hemiparesis. When seizures are difficult to control with medication, early surgical removal of the affected part of the brain may improve control and prevent intellectual deterioration.

Gomez MR (ed.): Tuberous Sclerosis, 2nd ed. New York, Raven Press, 1988. *Gives detailed information about multiple organ involvement in tuberous sclerosis, with excellent illustrations of the skin and retinal lesions.*

Gutmann DH, Wood DL, Collins FS: Identification of the neurofibromatosis type 1 gene product. Proc Natl Acad Sci 88:9658, 1991. *The title identifies the content.*
Mulvihill JJ (moderator): Neurofibromatosis 1 (Recklinghausen disease) and neurofibromatosis 2 (bilateral acoustic neurofibromatosis): An update. Ann Intern Med 113:39, 1990. *A succinct review of clinical and genetic features of both syndromes.*
Trofatter JA, MacCollin MM, Rutter JL, et al.: A novel moesin-, ezrin-, radixin-like gene is a candidate for the neurofibromatosis 2 tumor suppressor. Cell 72:791, 1993. *Characterizes the probable structure of the causative gene abnormality.*

Section Six— Cerebrovascular Diseases

William A. Pulsinelli

418   CEREBROVASCULAR DISEASES—PRINCIPLES

The family of cerebrovascular diseases can be classified according to whether they affect the brain's vascular supply either focally or diffusely (Fig. 418–1). The generic term "stroke" signifies the abrupt impairment of brain function caused by a variety of pathologic changes involving one (focal) or several (multifocal) intracranial or extracranial blood vessels. Approximately 80% of all strokes are caused by too little blood flow (ischemic stroke), and the remaining 20% are nearly equally divided between hemorrhage into brain tissue (parenchymatous hemorrhage) or the surrounding subarachnoid space (subarachnoid hemorrhage). In contrast, diseases that affect the heart or the systemic circulation cause generalized hypoperfusion and diffuse brain dysfunction or injury. Ischemic stroke and the hypoperfusion syndromes affecting the brain share much pathophysiology, and both processes are considered together in Ch. 419; hemorrhagic stroke is addressed in Ch. 420.

EPIDEMIOLOGY

The annual incidence and death rate for stroke have declined steadily in the United States throughout the twentieth century and for most European countries and Japan since approximately 1960. In the United States, a 1% per year decrease in the annual mortality

rate from stroke recorded since 1915 accelerated in the early 1970's to approximately 5% per year. A recent analysis indicates that the stroke incidence has stabilized at approximately 0.5 to 1.0 per 1000 population. Incidence rates in western European countries are slightly higher (1.5 per 1000), but several eastern European countries and Japan have rates of 3 per 1000 based at least partly on environmental, dietary, and smoking habits. At these current rates, stroke remains the third leading cause of medically related deaths and the second most frequent cause of neurologic morbidity in developed countries.

Several other important facts about stroke incidence have emerged: incidence and death rate for stroke are higher among blacks than whites in the United States; approximately similar rates affect men and women, in contrast to the male predominance for myocardial infarction; and there is a strikingly higher incidence (20 to 30 per 1000) for those over age 75.

CEREBROVASCULAR ANATOMY

Since most strokes are caused by abnormalities within the cerebral circulation, an understanding of cerebrovascular anatomy helps in arriving at the correct diagnosis and determining the underlying pathogenesis and prognosis.

The brain is supplied by four major arteries: the left and right internal carotid and vertebral arteries (Fig. 418–2). The left common carotid artery arises from the aortic arch, but the other vessels originate from branches of the aorta; the right common carotid artery stems from the innominate artery, and the left and right vertebral arteries take off from their respective subclavian arteries.

INTERNAL CAROTID ARTERIES. Each common carotid artery bifurcates into an internal and external carotid artery in most

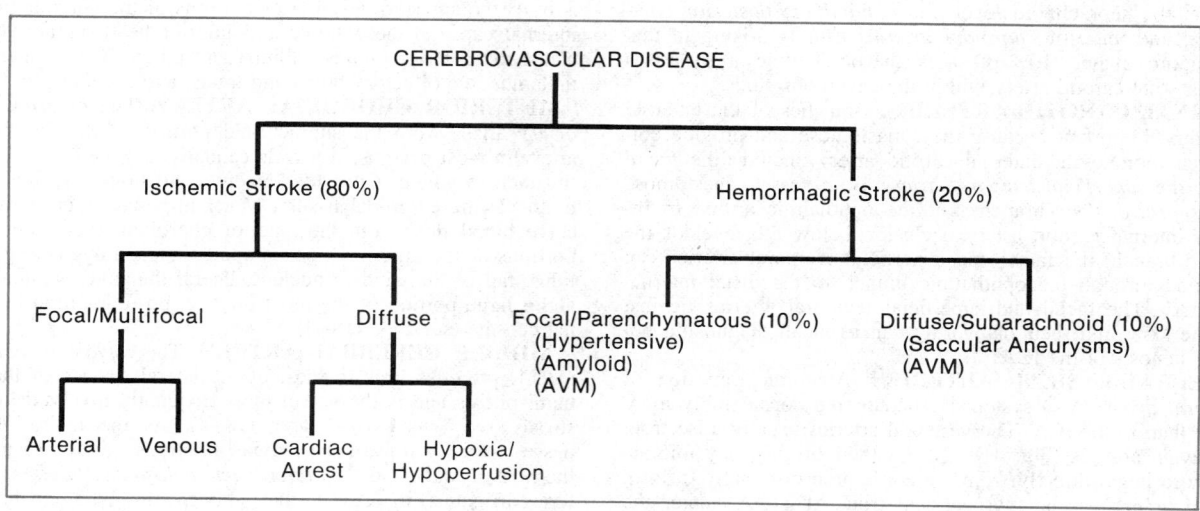

FIGURE 418–1. Classification of cerebrovascular disease.

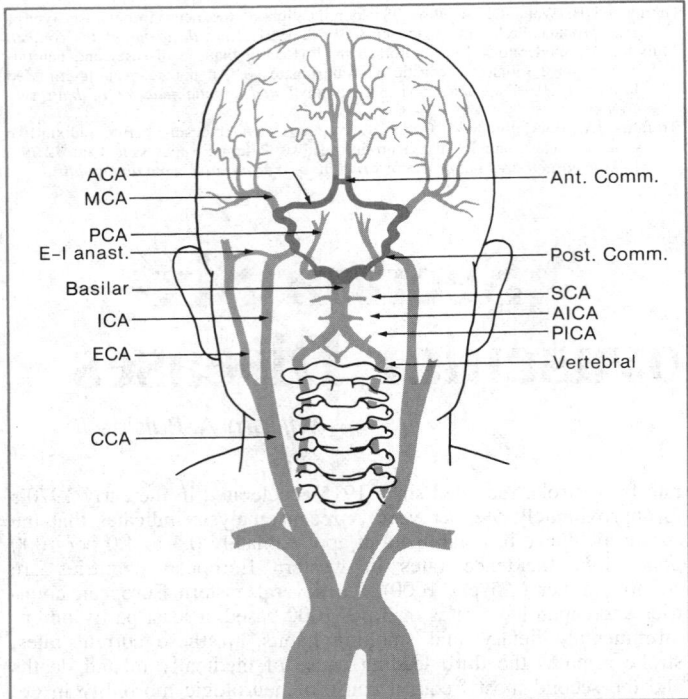

FIGURE 418-2. Extracranial and intracranial arterial supply to the brain. Vessels forming the circle of Willis are highlighted in dark red. Abbreviations for intracranial and extracranial arteries are as follows: ACA = anterior cerebral artery; MCA = middle cerebral artery; PCA = posterior cerebral artery; E-I anast. = extracranial-intracranial anastomosis; ICA = internal carotid artery; ECA = external carotid artery; CCA = common carotid artery; Ant. Comm. = anterior communicating artery; Post. Comm. = posterior communicating artery; SCA = superior cerebellar artery; AICA = anterior inferior cerebellar artery; PICA = posterior inferior cerebellar artery. (Modified from Lord R: Surgery of Occlusive Cerebrovascular Disease. St. Louis, C.V. Mosby Company, 1986; with permission.)

individuals just below the angle of the jaw and approximately at the level of the thyroid cartilage (Fig. 418-2). The *internal carotid artery (ICA)* enters the skull through the foramen lacerum and travels a short distance within the petrous portion of the temporal bone. It then enters the cavernous sinus before penetrating the dura and ascends above the clinoid processes to divide into the *anterior* and *middle cerebral arteries.* The portion of the internal carotid artery that lies between the cavernous sinus and the supraclinoid process forms an S shape and is sometimes referred to as the "carotid siphon." The internal carotid artery gives off its first important branches at the supraclinoid level, the *ophthalmic, posterior communicating,* and *anterior choroidal arteries* usually arising in that order. In approximately 10% of cases, the ophthalmic artery arises from the internal carotid artery within the cavernous sinus.

EXTERNAL CAROTID ARTERIES. Branches of the external carotid artery, important because they anastomose and provide collateral circulation to the internal carotid artery, include the *facial artery* and the *superficial temporal artery.* Both vessels anastomose with the *supratrochlear* branches of the ophthalmic artery. In instances of internal carotid artery occlusion below the level of the ophthalmic branch, the facial and superficial temporal arteries can supply blood through the ophthalmic branch to the distal internal carotid artery. The facial and superficial temporal arteries lie just beneath the skin, and their palpability can assist in diagnosing occlusion or stenosis of the ICA.

VERTEBRAL-BASILAR ARTERIES. Anatomic variation of the *vertebral artery (VA)* system is encountered considerably more frequently than in the ICA. The vertebral arteries usually arise from the subclavian arteries (Fig. 418-2), but their origins may migrate proximally to begin directly from the aortic arch or distally to form a common branch of the thyrocervical trunk. The VA's enter the foramen of the sixth cervical vertebra or, much less commonly, the

fourth, fifth, or seventh vertebral level. The VA's ascend through the transverse foramina and exit at C1, where they turn 90 degrees posteriorly to pass behind the atlantoaxial joint before penetrating the dura and entering the cranial cavity through the foramen magnum. The portion of the vertebral artery that loops behind the atlantoaxial joint is prone to mechanical trauma, and rotation of the head to approximately 60 degrees may cause arterial narrowing and reduce blood flow to the ipsilateral vertebral artery.

Intracranially, the vertebral arteries lie lateral to the medulla oblongata and then course ventrally and medially, where they unite at the medullopontine junction to form the *basilar artery (BA).* The BA bifurcates at the pontomesencephalic junction into the *posterior cerebral arteries (PCA's).*

In as many as 20% of all individuals, the right or left VA's terminate before reaching the BA, leaving the latter to be supplied inferiorly by a single vessel. Intracranial branches of the VA's include medial branches, which unite to form the *anterior spinal artery,* and lateral branches to the dorsolateral medulla and posterior cerebellum, called the *posterior inferior cerebellar arteries.*

CIRCLE OF WILLIS. The *circle of Willis* (Fig. 418-2) is formed by the union at the base of the brain of both anterior cerebral arteries via the *anterior communicating artery* and the middle cerebral arteries with the posterior cerebral arteries on each side via the *posterior communicating arteries* (Fig. 418-2). Anomalies of the circle of Willis occur frequently; in large autopsy series of normal individuals, more than half showed an incomplete circle of Willis. The most common sites for such abnormalities, which usually present as hypoplasia or atresia, are the posterior communicating arteries (22%) and the anterior cerebral arteries (10%).

ANTERIOR CEREBRAL ARTERIES. The *anterior cerebral arteries (ACA's)* pass medially above the optic chiasm and head rostrally toward the interhemispheric fissure, where they arch caudally to lie just dorsal to the corpus callosum (Fig. 418-3). In approximately 10% of normal individuals, the A1 segment of the ACA (the portion between the middle cerebral and anterior communicating arteries) is atretic or absent, leaving its distal portion to be supplied by the opposite ACA via the anterior communicating artery. Branches of the ACA supply the frontal poles, the superior surfaces of the cerebral hemispheres where their distal branches anastomose with those of the middle cerebral artery, and all of the medial surfaces of both cerebral hemispheres with the exception of the calcarine cortex. Cortical areas served by the ACA include the motor and sensory cortex of the legs and feet, the supplementary motor cortex, and the presumed cortical micturition center lying in the paracentral lobule (Figs. 418-3 and 418-4).

The A1 and A2 segments (the portion between the anterior communicating artery and the genu of the corpus callosum) give off many small branches that penetrate the anterior perforated substance of the brain. These small penetrating branches include all of the *anterior* and some of the *medial lenticulostriate* arteries. Usually, there is a dominant medial striate vessel called the *recurrent artery of Heubner,* which arises in most instances from the A1 segment of the ACA. This artery penetrates the perforated substance of the brain and, along with the other small perforators, supplies (Fig. 418-4) the anterior and inferior portions of the anterior limb of the internal capsule, the anterior and inferior head of the caudate nucleus, the anterior globus pallidus and putamen, the anterior hypothalamus, the olfactory bulbs and tracts, and the uncinate fasciculus.

ANTERIOR CHOROIDAL ARTERY. The *anterior choroidal artery* arises from the supraclinoid portion of the internal carotid artery in most persons. It travels caudally and medially over the optic tract, to which it provides a few small branches, and enters the brain via the choroidal fissure. Many important brain structures receive blood flow from the anterior choroidal artery; these include portions of the anterior hippocampus, uncus, amygdala, globus pallidus, tail of the caudate nucleus, lateral thalamus, geniculate body, and a large portion of the most inferior, posterior limb of the internal capsule (see Fig. 418-4).

MIDDLE CEREBRAL ARTERY. The *middle cerebral artery (MCA)* provides flow to most of the lateral surface of the cerebral hemispheres and is the vessel most frequently involved in ischemic stroke (see Figs. 418-3 and 418-4). As the main MCA trunk passes laterally toward the sylvian fissure, it gives rise to some of the *medial* and all of the *lateral lenticulostriate* arteries. These arteries irrigate (Fig. 418-4) the putamen, the head and body of the caudate nucleus, the lateral globus pallidus, the full vertical extent

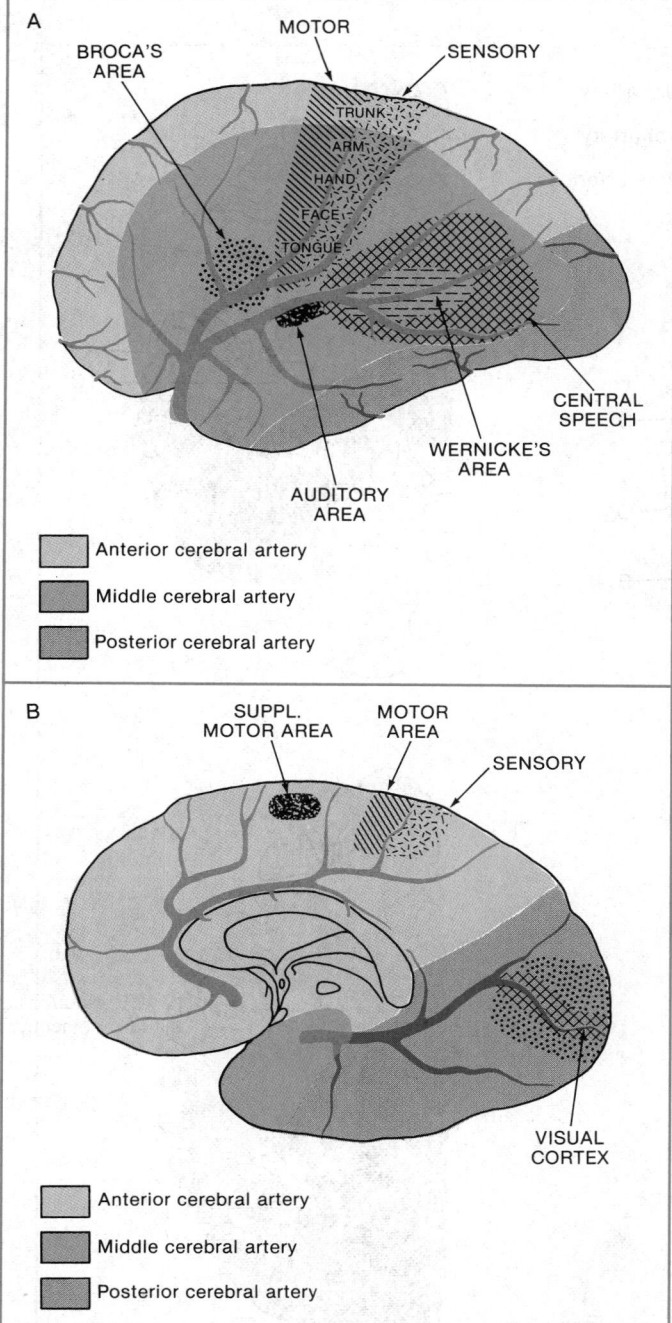

FIGURE 418–3. Lateral *(A)* and medial *(B)* views of the cerebral hemisphere showing the surface distributions of the anterior, middle, and posterior cerebral arteries.

cend upward along the medial edge of the tentorium, where they branch into anterior and posterior divisions. The anterior division (Figs. 418–3 and 418–4) supplies the inferior surface of the temporal lobe, where its terminal branches anastomose with branches of the MCA. The posterior division supplies the occipital lobe, where its terminal branches anastomose with both the ACA and the MCA. In its most proximal course along the base of the brain, the PCA gives off several groups of penetrating arteries commonly referred to as the thalamogeniculate, the thalamoperforating, and the posterior choroidal arteries. The red nucleus, the substantia nigra, medial parts of the cerebral peduncles, the nuclei of the thalamus, the hippocampus, and the posterior hypothalamus receive blood from these penetrating branches (Fig. 418–4).

BRAIN-STEM BLOOD FLOW. At all rostrocaudal levels of the brain stem, the ventral medial portion is supplied by short paramedian vessels; the ventrolateral portion by short circumferential branches from the vertebral or basilar arteries; and the dorsolateral portion and cerebellum by long circumferential branches, which include the *posterior inferior cerebellar* arteries, which arise from the vertebral arteries, and the *anterior inferior* and *superior cerebellar* arteries, which arise from the basilar artery (Fig. 418–5A and B).

The pyramids, the inferior olives and medial lemnisci, the medial longitudinal fasciculi, and the emerging fibers of the hypoglossal nerve (Fig. 418–5A) derive blood from the vertebral arteries. Longer branches from the vertebral arteries and posterior inferior cerebellar arteries supply the spinothalamic tracts, the vestibular nuclei, the sensory nuclei of the fifth cranial nerve, the descending fibers of the sympathetic nervous system, the restiform body, and the emerging fibers of the vagus and glossopharyngeal nerves. The most cephalad and dorsal segment of the medulla includes the vestibular and cochlear nuclei, which, along with the posterior portion of the cerebellum, receive flow from the posterior inferior cerebellar artery.

The basilar artery gives rise to perforating branches as it spans the ventral midline pons and midbrain (Fig. 418–5B). These short perpendicular branches distribute blood to the paramedian structures, including the corticospinal tracts, the pontine reticular nuclei, the medial lemnisci, the medial longitudinal fasciculi, and the pontine reticular nuclei. The *anterior inferior cerebellar artery* feeds blood to the lateral pons, including the emerging seventh and eighth cranial nerves, the trigeminal nerve root, the vestibular and cochlear nuclei, and the spinothalamic tracts. It also branches to the most dorsal and lateral of these structures on its dorsal course toward the cerebellum.

At the midbrain level, the basilar artery lies in the midline in the peduncular fossa. Short branches pass laterally and dorsally to both sides to supply the cerebral peduncles, the emerging fibers of the third nerve, medial portions of the red nuclei, the medial longitudinal fasciculus, the oculomotor nuclei, and the midbrain reticulum. The superior cerebellar arteries contribute to the dorsal midbrain supply, including that of the colliculi and the superior portion of the cerebellum on each side.

VENOUS DRAINAGE. The veins in the brain, unlike those in many other parts of the body, do not accompany the arteries (Fig. 418–6). Cortical veins drain into the superior sagittal sinus, which runs posteriorly between the cerebral hemispheres. Deeper structures drain into the inferior sagittal sinus and great cerebral vein (of Galen), which join at the straight sinus. The straight sinus runs posteriorly along the attachment of the falx cerebri and tentorium and joins the superior sagittal sinus at the torcular Herophili, from which the two transverse sinuses arise. Each transverse sinus passes laterally toward the petrosal bone to become the sigmoid sinus, which exits the skull into the internal jugular vein. Each cavernous sinus communicates with its contralateral twin and surrounds the ipsilateral carotid artery; both drain posteriorly into the petrosal sinuses, which in turn drain into the sigmoid sinus.

NORMAL PHYSIOLOGY

CEREBRAL METABOLISM AND BLOOD FLOW. The brain performs no mechanical work; nevertheless, the energy demands to support normal electrophysiologic brain activity in conscious humans equal, on a per weight basis, those of metabolically active tissues like the heart and kidney. Aerobic glucose metabolism provides the energy necessary to drive membrane ion pumps,

of the anterior limb of the internal capsule, and a superior portion of the posterior limb of the internal capsule. The MCA then extends into the sylvian fissure, where it branches into several smaller arteries grouped into a superior division, which feeds the cortical surface above the fissure, and an inferior division, which supplies the cortical surface of the temporal lobe. The territory of the MCA includes the major motor and sensory areas of the cortex, the areas for contraversive eye and head movement, the optic radiations, auditory sensory cortex, and, in the dominant hemisphere, the motor and sensory areas for language.

POSTERIOR CEREBRAL ARTERIES. Blood flow to both *posterior cerebral arteries (PCA's)* derives primarily from the BA (70% of the time) and from the ICA (10% of the time). In the remaining 20%, one PCA is supplied by the internal carotid artery and the other by the basilar artery. The PCA's pass dorsal to the third cranial nerves and across the cerebral peduncles and then as-

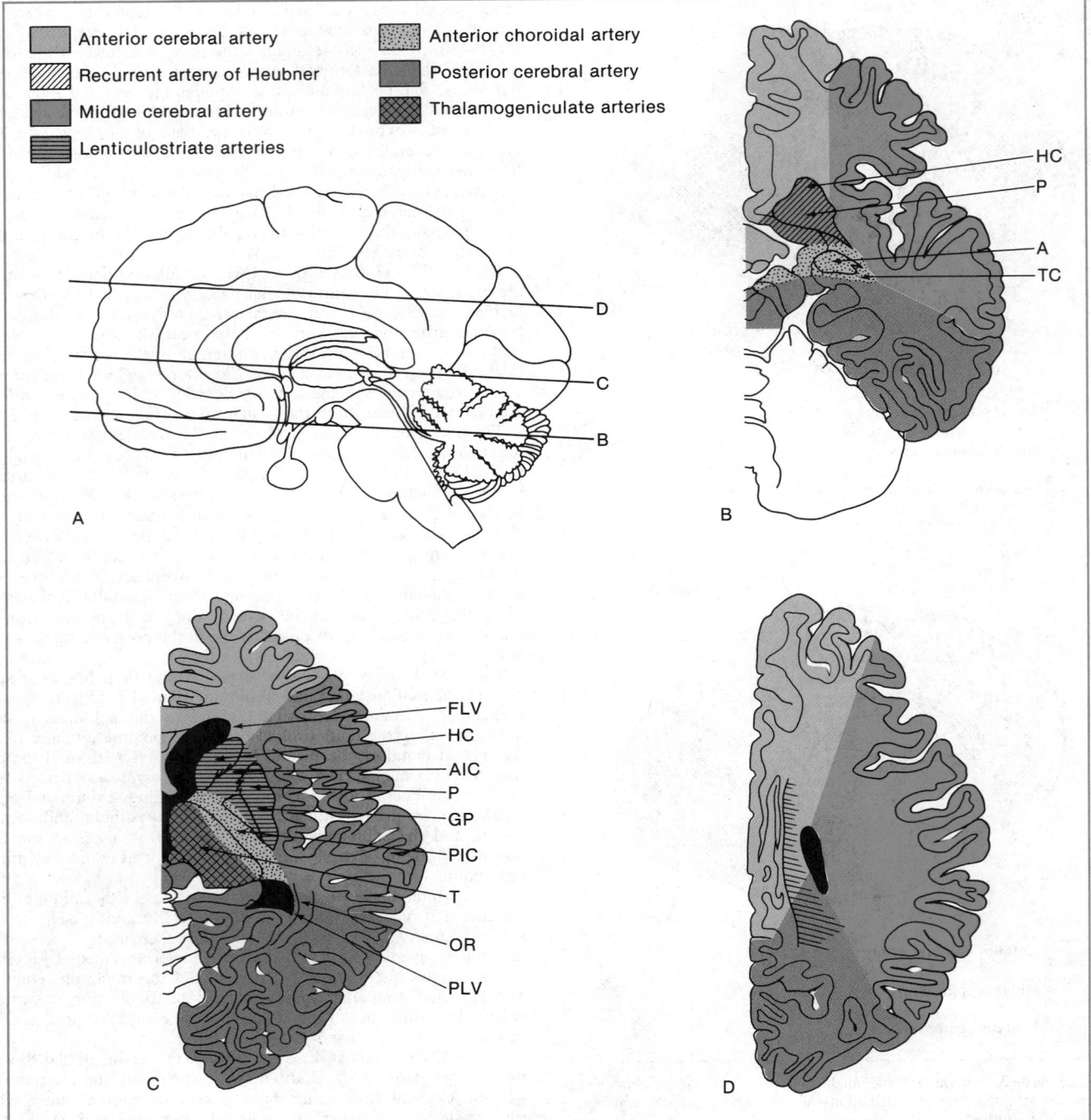

Anterior cerebral artery
Recurrent artery of Heubner
Middle cerebral artery
Lenticulostriate arteries
Anterior choroidal artery
Posterior cerebral artery
Thalamogeniculate arteries

FIGURE 418–4. Arterial supply of deep brain structures. *A,* Sagittal view of the brain showing the computed tomographic (CT) planes through which views B, C, and D were taken. *B,* CT plane through the head of the caudate nucleus (HC), putamen (P), amygdala (A), tail of the caudate nucleus (TC), hypothalamus, temporal lobe, midbrain, and cerebellum. *C,* CT plane through the frontal horn of the lateral ventricle (FLV), head of the caudate nucleus (HC), anterior and posterior limbs of the internal capsule (AIC, PIC), putamen (P), globus pallidus (GP), thalamus (T), optic radiations (OR), and posterior horn of the lateral ventricle (PLV). *D,* CT plane through the centrum semiovale. (Modified from De Armond S, et al: Structure of the Human Brain, A Photographic Atlas, 3rd ed. New York, Oxford University Press, 1989; with permission.)

synthesize, store, and release neurotransmitters, and maintain tissue structure. The normal, conscious human consumes approximately 160 μmol O_2 and 30 μmol glucose per 100 grams of brain each minute (Table 418–1).

Approximately 10% of available blood glucose is extracted and phosphorylated by the brain in a single pass, yet only 80% of this glucose is used to generate energy. The 5:1 ratio of O_2 versus glucose consumption (Table 418–1) indicates that approximately 20% of glucose carbons are not oxidized. Approximately 10 to 15% of glucose is metabolized to lactate, which may be lost to the circula-

tion; the remainder is used for the synthesis of neurotransmitters, fats, and, to a small degree, proteins. Each mole of glucose metabolized by the brain through glycolysis and the mitochondrial respiratory chain therefore yields approximately 30 mol ATP instead of the expected 38.

Unlike muscle or other tissues, the brain stores few glucose, glycogen, or other high-energy phosphate (ATP, phosphocreatine) reserves but instead relies on a sizable and well-regulated blood flow to satisfy its immediate needs for energy. Cerebral blood flow (CBF) averages 60 ml per 100 grams of brain per minute in the

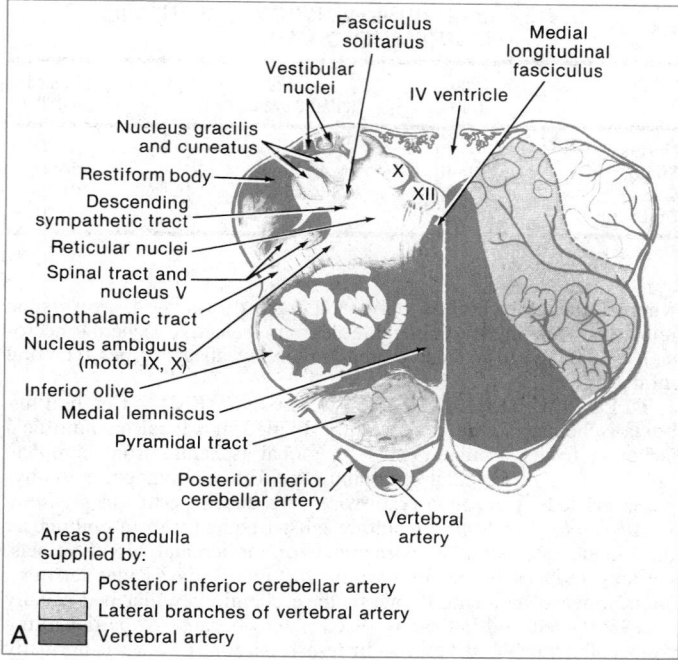

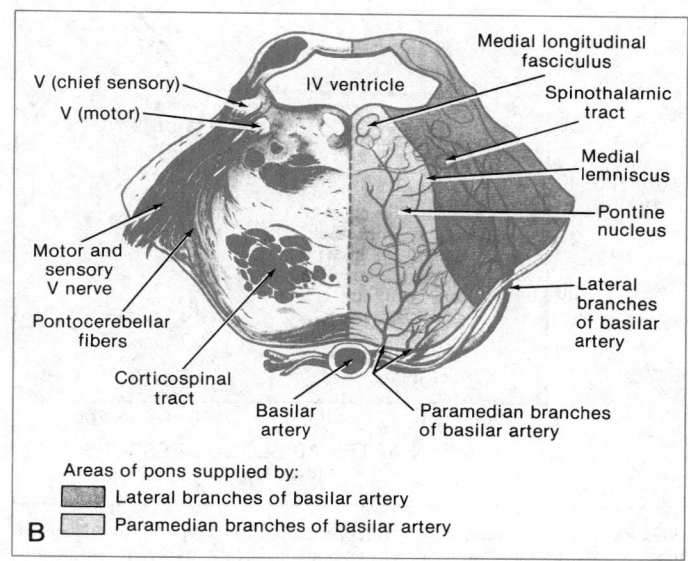

FIGURE 418–5. *A,* Cross-section of the medulla oblongata at the level of the hypoglossal nuclei (XII). Short branches of the vertebral and anterior spinal arteries supply the medial medulla. Longer circumferential branches, including the posterior inferior cerebellar artery, supply the lateral portions of the medulla. *B,* Cross section of the midpons. The medial portion receives the blood supply from short, perforating basilar artery branches. More laterally, the blood supply comes from lateral basilar artery branches.

normal, conscious human; in the absence of such flow, the brain has sufficient high-energy stores to support normal metabolic needs for only a few minutes. At normal arterial O_2 tensions and blood glucose concentrations, CBF delivers 350 mmol O_2 and 260 mmol glucose to 100 grams of brain each minute (see Table 418–1).

These values exceed the brain's normal consumption rates of O_2 and glucose by factors of approximately 2 and 9, respectively. The blood vascular reserves for both O_2 and glucose must be small, as is illustrated by the fact that all changes of synaptic activity, whether related to thinking, talking, or directing muscular activity, are tightly *coupled,* both temporally and anatomically, to an almost instantaneous, proportional increase in CBF. The anatomic segregation of the brain's functional activities results in an ever-changing mosaic of regional metabolic/blood flow values that reflect moment-to-moment changes in electrophysiologic activity.

The coupling of CBF to regional synaptic activity and metabolic activity represents only one of several important mechanisms regulating normal CBF. Changes in the respiratory rate or volume, which lead to even mild hyper- or hypocapnia, respectively dilate or constrict cerebral resistance vessels, so that CBF shows a linear relationship to $Paco_2$. This normal physiologic response to $Paco_2$ is exploited clinically to treat cerebral herniation syndromes. Mechanical hyperventilation to a $Paco_2$ of 20 to 25 mm Hg reduces CBF by approximately 40 to 45% and normal adult cerebral blood volume from 50 ml to approximately 35 ml. While seemingly small, this 15-ml reduction often suffices to retard the progression of cerebral herniation. The response is short-lived, however, and brain and blood HCO_3^- and H^+ ions control blood vessel tone re-equilibrate within 30 to 60 minutes.

A complex system of neural pathways regulates CBF in response to normal and abnormal circumstances. Some of these neural pathways participate in *autoregulation,* a process which maintains CBF at a constant level despite wide fluctuations in cerebral perfusion pressure.

Because cerebral venous pressures closely approximate the intracranial pressure, autoregulation values usually are expressed in terms of mean arterial pressure.

FIGURE 418–6. Venous drainage of intracranial structures. SSS = superior sagittal sinus; CV = cortical veins; ISS = inferior sagittal sinus; ICV = internal cerebral vein; GV = great vein of Galen; *SS = straight sinus; TH = torcular herophili; PS = petrosal sinus; CS = cavernous sinus; TS = transverse sinus; SS = sigmoid sinus; LS = lateral sinus; IJ = internal jugular vein. (Reproduced with permission from Gates P, Barnett HJ, Mohr JP, et al. [eds.]: Stroke: Pathophysiology, Diagnosis and Management. New York, Churchill Livingstone, 1986.)

TABLE 418–1. METABOLIC ACTIVITY (NORMAL CONSCIOUS MAN)

	Consumed	Supplied
	(100 grams brain/min)	
CBF	60 ml	—
O_2	156 μmol	350 μmol
Glucose	33 μmol	260 μmol

CBF = cerebral blood flow.

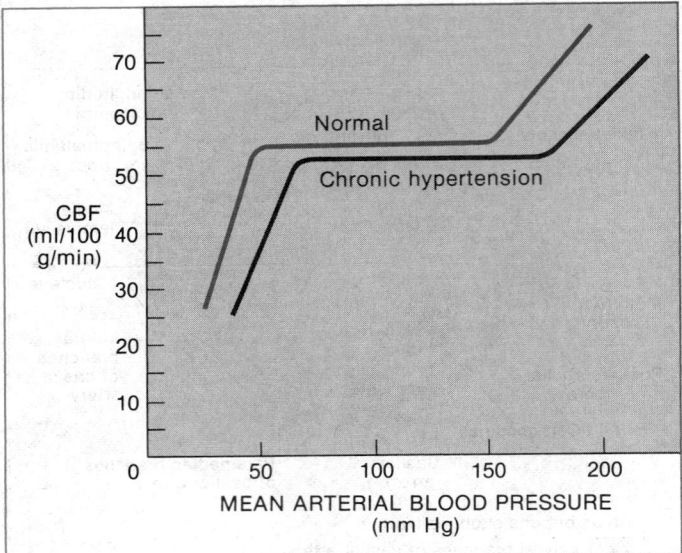

FIGURE 418–7. Autoregulatory cerebral blood flow response to changes in mean arterial pressure in normotensive and chronically hypertensive individuals. Note the shift of the curve toward higher mean pressures with chronic hypertension.

Normal autoregulation has both upper and lower limits (Fig. 418–7); at mean arterial pressures above 150 mm Hg, blood flow increases and capillary pressure rises, while at mean arterial pressures below 50 mm Hg, CBF falls. Increased capillary pressure in hypertensive patients may be a factor in intracerebral hemorrhage and hypertensive encephalopathy. In patients with chronic hypertension, the upper and lower autoregulatory limits are shifted toward higher systemic pressures (Fig. 418–7). Consequently, too rapid therapeutic reduction of blood pressure to apparently normal levels carries the risk of further lowering of cerebral blood flow in hypertensive patients with ongoing cerebral ischemia. Chronic treatment with antihypertensive agents readjusts the autoregulatory curve toward more normal values.

BLOOD-BRAIN BARRIER. Regulation within narrow limits of the extracellular ionic and molecular composition is more important for the normal function of the brain than for any other organ. Small changes in the extracellular concentrations of, for example, Na$^+$ ions or the neurotransmitters glutamate or norepinephrine greatly alter neuronal function. The blood-brain barrier, is composed anatomically of unique endothelial cells that lack the usual transendothelial channels and that seamlessly abut one another (tight junctions). This anatomy protects the brain against the fluctuating composition of blood and minimizes the entry of potentially toxic compounds.

The entry of nutrients and egress of metabolic products cross the blood-brain barrier via simple diffusion, facilitated transport, or active transport. Lipid-soluble compounds rapidly diffuse across endothelial cell membranes, while polar compounds must be transported on special carrier molecules that are driven either by concentration gradients (facilitated transport) or through the expenditure of energy (active transport). Gas molecules such as O_2 and CO_2 freely diffuse across plasma membranes and rapidly equilibrate between blood and brain. Glucose, a highly polar molecule, enters the brain on a special carrier with a Km (7 to 8 mM) just slightly higher than the normal blood glucose concentration. The rate of brain glucose transport is normally two to three times faster than the metabolism of glucose, but since glucose uptake depends so highly on its concentration, a reduction of blood sugar to one-third the normal amount, caused by either ischemia or hypoglycemia, may compromise normal metabolism (Table 418–2).

PATHOPHYSIOLOGY/PATHOLOGY OF CEREBRAL ISCHEMIA

A failed delivery of O_2 and glucose to the brain generates a cascade of events that vary qualitatively and quantitatively with the severity of the insult. The severity of cerebral ischemia, defined as the degree and duration of blood flow loss, largely determines whether the brain suffers only temporary dysfunction, irreversible injury to a few highly vulnerable neurons (selective ischemic necrosis), or damage to extensive areas involving all cell types (cerebral infarction).

TYPES OF CEREBRAL HYPOXIA-ISCHEMIA. Cerebral hypoxia-ischemia can be conveniently divided into focal or multifocal ischemia from vascular occlusion, global ischemia from complete failure of cardiovascular pumping, and diffuse hypoperfusion-hypoxia caused by respiratory disease or reduced perfusion pressure. *Focal cerebral ischemia,* resulting most frequently from embolic or thrombotic occlusion of extracranial or intracranial blood vessels, variably reduces blood flow within the involved vascular territory. Blood flow to the central zone of the ischemic vascular bed usually is severely reduced but rarely reaches zero because of partial filling from collateral blood vessels. In transition zones between normally perfused tissue and the severely ischemic central core, blood flow is moderately reduced. This rim of moderately ischemic tissue has been called the "ischemic penumbra," and although brain cells in this region remain viable longer than do those in the ischemic core, they too will die if left deprived of adequate blood flow.

Focal cerebral ischemia sufficient to cause clinical signs or symptoms and lasting only 15 to 30 minutes causes irreversible injury to specific, highly vulnerable neurons. If the ischemia lasts an hour or longer, infarction of part or all of the involved vascular territory is inevitable. Clinical evidence of permanent brain injury from such ischemia may or may not be detectable, depending upon the region and the amount of brain tissue involved (see Ch. 419).

Global cerebral ischemia, typically caused by cardiac asystole or ventricular fibrillation, reduces blood flow to zero throughout all of the brain. Global ischemia lasting more than 5 to 10 minutes is usually incompatible with recovery of consciousness in normothermic humans. Brain damage from more transient global ischemia, uncomplicated by periods of prolonged hypotension or hyperglycemia, is limited to specific populations of highly vulnerable neurons. This "selective ischemic necrosis" of neurons involves, for example, the CA1 pyramidal neurons of hippocampus, the cerebellar Purkinje cells, and the pyramidal neurons in neocortical layers 3, 5, and 6 (Table 418–3). While selective ischemic necrosis of neurons typifies transient global ischemia, such injury may also accompany prolonged hypoxemia, carbon monoxide poisoning, and focal cerebral ischemia of brief duration. Cardiac resuscitation complicated by prolonged hypotension or hyperglycemia may cause cerebral infarction, particularly in border zones that lie between the terminal branches of major arterial supplies.

Diffuse cerebral hypoxia, uncomplicated by cerebral ischemia, is limited to conditions of mild to moderate hypoxemia, since myocardial contractility and blood pressure fall with severe hypoxemia. As a consequence, pure cerebral hypoxia causes cerebral dysfunction but not irreversible brain injury. Individuals with pure cerebral hypoxia from altitude sickness, pulmonary disease, or severe anemia present with confusion, cognitive impairment, and lethargy. The on-

TABLE 418–2. HUMAN HYPOXIC-ISCHEMIC THRESHOLD VALUES

	PaO$_2$ (torr)	CBF (ml/100 grams/min)	Blood Glucose (mg/dl)
Normal	90	60	80
Stupor	30–40	20–30	25–30
Coma	20–30	15–20	20–25
Brain Injury	< 20	< 15	< 20

TABLE 418–3. ORDER OF DECREASING NEURONAL VULNERABILITY TO ANOXIA

Hippocampus
    CA1, CA4 > CA3 > granule cells
Cerebellum
    Purkinje > stellate and basket > granule > Golgi cells
Striatum
    Small and medium-sized > large neurons
Neocortex
    Layers 3,5,6 > layers 2,4

set of coma signals cardiovascular compromise and imminent brain damage. With relatively *acute* changes in arterial oxygen tension from normal to a Pa_{O_2} of 40 mm Hg (see Table 418–2) or with a fall in the hemoglobin concentration below 7 grams per deciliter, compensatory increases of cerebral blood flow become inadequate, and clinical signs and symptoms of cerebral hypoxia develop.

NEUROPATHOLOGY OF CEREBRAL ISCHEMIA. Ischemic injury to the brain can be classified on the basis of cytopathologic criteria into four types. Cerebral *autolysis,* observed most frequently in brain-dead patients preserved on mechanical ventilators for several days, reflects enzymatic autodigestion of the tissue.

Cerebral *infarction,* usually caused by focal vascular occlusion, is characterized histopathologically by necrosis of neurons, glia, and, in some areas, endothelial cells. Cerebral infarcts are frequently described grossly as pale (anemic) or "hemorrhagic," (showing gross petechial bleeding). Most often, the hemorrhagic areas lie along border zones of partially perfused tissue and occur most frequently with transient embolic occlusion followed by reperfusion of the infarcted vascular bed.

Transient arrest of the cerebral circulation (global ischemia) for periods of a few minutes causes *selective ischemic necrosis of highly vulnerable neurons* (see Table 418–3).

The time required for histologic changes to reach their maximum in areas of cerebral infarction differs markedly from the time course of injury encountered in selective ischemic necrosis. Infarction usually requires only a few hours before histologic stains sharply outline the distinct margins between living and dying neurons and glia. By contrast, selective ischemic necrosis of neurons evolves more slowly and sometimes requires several days or more to reach its full extent.

Another distinctive neuropathologic lesion due to ischemia is *demyelination* of the central hemispheric white matter. Such injury is usually the consequence of carbon monoxide poisoning or other prolonged periods of moderately severe hypoxemia or cerebral hypoperfusion. Within these lesions, nerve cell axons are demyelinated, and oligodendroglial cells die off.

MOLECULAR MECHANISMS. In severely ischemic brain tissue, energy-rich compounds become depleted within seconds to a few minutes (see Table 418–2). Soon thereafter, the tissue begins to lose structural integrity. As energy-dependent membrane pumps fail, neuronal and glial cell membranes depolarize and allow the influx of Na^+ and Ca^{2+} ions and the efflux of K^+ ions. Elevated intracellular Ca^{2+} and other second messengers activate lipases and proteases, which in turn release membrane-bound free fatty acids and denature proteins. Depolarization of presynaptic terminals releases abnormally high concentrations of excitatory and inhibitory neurotransmitters, which may further exacerbate injury. If blood flow is restored in 15 to 30 minutes and no other complicating variables, such as hyperglycemia, are involved, most of these events are reversible, and only selectively vulnerable neurons will die. If ischemia lasts hours or more, cerebral infarction develops.

In contrast to the rapid cascade of events caused by severe ischemia, moderate ischemia triggers poorly defined mechanisms that sacrifice electrophysiologic activity to preserve brain structure, at least temporarily. Acute reduction of blood flow below one-half that of normal exceeds the capacity of compensatory mechanisms, such as an increased extraction of O_2 and glucose extraction by the tissue. The electroencephalogram (EEG) slows, and if ischemia is diffuse, the patient becomes confused, lethargic, or stuporous. The molecular mechanisms that induce this "anoxic anesthesia" are unknown. Depletion of whole tissue energy reserves is not an explanation, since these remain normal, partly as a consequence of the decreased energy demand normally used to maintain membrane ion pumps and EEG activity. With slightly greater ischemia, all synaptic activity ceases and the EEG becomes isoelectric. This too occurs before high-energy stores are depleted, indicating that generalized energy failure cannot explain the early loss of synaptic activity. Prompt recovery of blood flow restores full function and structural integrity to the tissue. If moderate ischemia persists for several hours, however, irreversible injury begins to develop, possibly as a consequence of compromised calcium homeostasis. Tissues with partial depletion of ATP and impaired calcium homeostasis may benefit from pharmacologic therapies that reduce calcium movement through voltage-dependent and neurotransmitter-dependent ion channels.

CEREBRAL EDEMA. Pathologic increases in the water content of the brain (edema) accompany all types of ischemic and hemorrhagic stroke. Brain swelling and raised intracranial pressure relate proportionally to the volume of the accumulated water; in some instances, they can cause neurologic deterioration and death by transtentorial herniation. Cerebral edema and herniation represent the immediate cause of death in one-third of all ischemic and three-quarters of all hemorrhagic fatal strokes.

Brain edema is categorized on the basis of pathophysiologic and anatomic criteria as intracellular or interstitial. Intracellular edema, also called cytotoxic edema, represents an accumulation of intracellular osmoles and water causing cell swelling at the expense of the interstitial brain volume. Intracellular edema develops rapidly in ischemic brain tissue as energy-dependent membrane ion pumps fail and Na^+ and other osmoles enter the cell from the interstitial and vascular compartments. Cell swelling occurs predominantly in astrocytes, but neurons, oligodendroglial cells, and endothelial cells also are involved to a lesser degree. The osmolality of ischemic brain increases acutely from 310 mOsm to approximately 350 mOsm. The intracellular accumulation of water increases from a normal value of approximately 79 to 81% of brain weight, an addition insufficient in most instances to cause cerebral herniation. If cerebral circulation is re-established before permanent brain injury develops, intracellular brain edema resolves within a matter of hours without permanent sequelae.

Interstitial brain edema, also called "vasogenic edema," occurs later than the intracellular form. Damage to blood-brain barrier endothelial cells allows macromolecules such as plasma proteins to enter the interstitial space, carrying with them osmotically bound water. Interstitial brain edema following cerebral infarction progressively worsens for 3 to 4 days after a stroke. Fluid accumulation within the vicinity of damaged endothelial cells and the zone of infarction can raise the local water content of brain by as much as 10%. Such large volume increases can lead to transtentorial herniation and similarly fatal consequences.

Barnett HJ, Mohr JP, Stein BM, et al. (eds.): Stroke: Pathophysiology, Diagnosis and Management. New York, Churchill Livingstone, 1992. *A comprehensive two-volume overview of all aspects of ischemic and hemorrhagic stroke.*
Caplan LR, Stein RW: Stroke: A Clinical Approach. Boston, Butterworth, 1986. *A pragmatic description of the diagnosis and treatment of stroke.*
Plum F, Pulsinelli WA: Cerebral metabolism in hypoxic-ischemic brain injury. In Asbury AK, McKann GM, McDonald IW (eds.): Disease of the Nervous System. Philadelphia, W.B. Saunders Company, 1992. *A contemporary review of the pathogenesis of ischemic injury to brain.*

419 ISCHEMIC CEREBROVASCULAR DISEASE

419.1 Focal Ischemia

CLASSIFICATION

The clinical manifestations of focal ischemic stroke result from interference with blood circulation to the brain; the precise signs and symptoms depend on the region deprived of flow. For any brain region, however, focal ischemia can be classified into categories that have important clinical implications.

STROKE VERSUS TRANSIENT ISCHEMIC ATTACK (TIA). *Stroke* is defined as a neurologic deficit lasting more than 24 hours caused by reduced blood flow in a particular artery supplying the brain. The usual pathologic outcome is infarction. A *transient ischemic attack,* or *TIA,* by contrast, is defined arbitrarily as a similar neurologic deficit lasting less than 24 hours. Originally, the defined time limit for TIA's was less than 1 hour, but this was subsequently expanded to the longer interval for practical purposes. Nevertheless, most TIA's resolve within an hour. Once a deficit has lasted longer than an hour, it is likely to be classified as a presumptive stroke and is often associated with permanent brain injury. Magnetic resonance imaging (MRI) brain scans frequently show cerebral infarction in areas affected by "TIA's" lasting longer than several hours. The relevant clinical distinction between a TIA and a stroke is whether the ischemia has caused brain damage (infarction or selective ischemic necrosis). Since no clear temporal threshold separates the two, decisions concerning the initiation of therapy and its type are unavoidably vague.

STABLE VERSUS UNSTABLE STROKES. *Unstable strokes* are those in which symptoms and signs either improve or deteriorate after the onset. Deciding the stability of a stroke may be difficult, since in theory all strokes require some period to reach a stable maximum or minimum. The decision depends on an accurate history, on the interval between onset of symptoms and the first examination, and, later, on the frequency and duration of observation. Two thirds of patients with anterior circulation strokes and a higher number of those with vertebrobasilar strokes who are first examined within a few hours of onset fluctuate in their signs and symptoms during the first week.

The identification of patients with worsening signs and symptoms, frequently referred to as *progressing stroke* or *stroke in evolution,* is particularly important, since if the cause can be identified, treatment to limit brain damage may be possible. The pathogenesis of progression may involve one or a combination of factors. Clot propagation has been suggested, but little direct evidence supports this conclusion. Other equally, if not more important, causes for progressing stroke include compromise of cardiac output due to myocardial ischemia, cardiac arrhythmias, and congestive heart failure. Systemic hypotension and increased blood viscosity can adversely affect the course of acute cerebral ischemia, as can associated pneumogenic hypoxemia or systemic electrolyte imbalance. Progression of cerebral edema, which usually maximizes by 3 to 4 days, contributes to neurologic deterioration with large strokes but not with smaller ones. Bleeding into the infarct affects as many as 40% of patients but seldom causes new symptoms.

COMPLETE VERSUS INCOMPLETE STROKES. An important distinction is that made between a *complete* and an *incomplete stroke.* The terms refer to whether the affected vascular territory has been completely involved; if not, more brain remains at risk of additional focal ischemia, making treatment an urgent matter. The clinical distinction between complete and incomplete strokes can be difficult, especially soon after onset. As a practical matter, the distinction between a complete and incomplete stroke is often based on the severity of functional loss, for example, hemiplegia versus hemiparesis.

CLINICAL MANIFESTATIONS AND VASCULAR SYNDROMES (Table 419-1)

INTERNAL CAROTID ARTERY. The carotid artery bifurcation and origin of the internal carotid artery (ICA) provide the most frequent sites for atherothrombosis of cerebral blood vessels. Symptoms from such severe stenoses closely resemble those caused by middle cerebral artery disease (see below). Flow through the ophthalmic artery is often affected sufficiently to produce *transient monocular blindness* (also called amaurosis fugax). Severe bilateral internal carotid artery stenosis can sometimes cause cerebral hemispheric hypoperfusion and symptoms in *border zones* between the major vascular territories. Anterior circulation TIA's more frequently herald the presence of internal carotid artery disease than of intracranial atherosclerosis. Similarly, acute headache ipsilateral to an acutely ischemic hemisphere more frequently signals occlusion of the internal carotid artery than of the intracranial vessels.

ANTERIOR CEREBRAL ARTERY. Occlusion of one anterior cerebral artery (ACA) distal to the anterior communicating artery produces motor and cortical sensory symptoms in the contralateral leg and, less often, proximal arm. Other manifestations of ACA occlusion include gait ataxia and sometimes urinary incontinence from damage to the parasagittal frontal lobe. Language disturbances, manifested as decreased spontaneous speech, may accompany a generalized depression of psychomotor activity. ACA occlusion does not typically cause paralysis of both legs, an acute syndrome more likely related to spinal cord disease or, rarely, occlusion of the superior sagittal sinus, which drains the medial surfaces of both cerebral hemispheres.

TABLE 419-1. CLINICAL MANIFESTATIONS OF ISCHEMIC STROKE

Occluded Blood Vessel*	Clinical Manifestations
ICA	Ipsilateral blindness (variable)
	MCA syndrome (see below)
MCA	Contralateral hemiparesis, sensory loss (arm, face worst)
	Expressive aphasia (dominant) or anosognosia and spatial disorientation (nondominant)
	Contralateral inferior quadrantanopia
ACA	Contralateral hemiparesis, sensory loss (leg worst)
PCA	Contralateral homonymous hemianopsia or superior quadrantanopsia
	Memory impairment
Basilar apex	Bilateral blindness
	Amnesia
Basilar artery	Contralateral hemiparesis, sensory loss
	Ipsilateral bulbar and/or cerebellar signs
Vertebral artery and/or PICA	Ipsilateral loss of facial sensation, ataxia
	Contralateral hemiparesis, sensory loss
Superior cerebellar artery	Gait ataxia, nausea, dizziness, headache progressing to ipsilateral hemiataxia, dysarthria, gaze paresis
	Contralateral hemiparesis, somnolence

* ICA = internal carotid artery; MCA = middle cerebral artery; ACA = anterior cerebral artery; PCA = posterior cerebral artery; PICA = posterior inferior cerebellar artery.

ANTERIOR CHOROIDAL ARTERY. Brain image analyses suggest a clinical syndrome associated with occlusion of this vessel. Affected patients suffer a hemiparesis involving the face, arm, and leg; variable hemisensory loss; and in some instances hemianopsia from optic tract ischemia. The syndrome is difficult to distinguish from middle cerebral artery (MCA) ischemia.

MIDDLE CEREBRAL ARTERY. Most ischemic strokes involve part or all of the territory of the MCA, usually caused by emboli from the heart or extracranial carotid arteries. Emboli may occlude the main stem of the MCA but more frequently produce distal occlusions of either the superior or the inferior branch. Occlusion of the superior branch causes weakness and sensory loss that are greatest in the face and arm; vision is spared, but an inferior quadrantanopia may rarely coexist. Hemianopsias reported with MCA infarction more likely reflect visual inattention than true blindness, since deeply penetrating MCA branches supply only the dorsal, parietal half of the optic radiations. Voluntary gaze away from the side of the lesion may be impaired, but full-range oculocephalic or oculovestibular reflexes remain (see Ch. 469). In the dominant hemisphere, the deficit includes an expressive (Broca's) aphasia with impaired fluency, naming, and writing, but relatively preserved comprehension. In the nondominant hemisphere, unilateral neglect, anosognosia (unawareness of the deficit), and spatial disorientation may be prominent.

Occlusion of the inferior branches of the MCA infrequently produces sensory loss, most notably of integrated sensations, such as perception of shapes (stereognosis). In the dominant hemisphere, occlusion of the inferior division of the MCA causes receptive (Wernicke's) aphasia, with fluent speech characterized by jargon and paraphasias; comprehension, naming, reading, and writing are often abnormal.

The so-called deep MCA syndrome may occur from selective occlusion of the MCA main stem, causing ischemia in the territory of the lenticulostriate vessels but sparing the superior and inferior MCA branches. Collateral filling of the distal MCA cortical branches prevents cortical injury, but since the lenticulostriates are end-arteries, infarction of the deep MCA territory evolves. Alternatively, the lenticulostriates may be occluded by local atherosclerotic or hypertensive vascular disease. Patients with occlusion of the lenticulostriate arteries develop internal capsular infarction accompanied by hemiparesis or hemiplegia unaccompanied by visual, language, or sensory disturbances.

Proximal occlusions of the MCA may affect both superior and inferior branches as well as perforating branches to the internal capsule, optic radiations, and basal ganglia. The result includes contralateral hemiplegia, hemianesthesia, dense homonymous hemianopsia, and global aphasia with dominant or anosagnosia with nondominant hemisphere involvement.

POSTERIOR CEREBRAL ARTERY. Occlusion of the posterior cerebral artery (PCA) distal to its penetrating branches most frequently causes complete contralateral loss of vision or a superior or inferior quadrantanopsia, depending upon whether the lower or the upper calcarine arteries are affected individually. Central (macular) vision may be spared owing to collateral supply from the MCA. If only the calcarine cortex is involved, the patient is usually aware of the vision loss, but denial of unilateral or bilateral blindness can ensue if one or both adjacent parietal cortices are affected (see Ch. 460). Difficulty in reading (dyslexia) and performing calculations (dyscalculia) may follow ischemia of the dominant PCA territory.

Proximal occlusion of the PCA causes ischemia of penetrating branches (thalamogeniculate, thalamoperforating, posterior choroidal) to thalamic and limbic structures. The results include hemisensory disturbances that may chronically change to intractable pain on the defective side (thalamic pain). Memory dysfunction may result, especially with bilateral occlusions. With involvement of the subthalamic nucleus, wild, uncontrolled, flailing limb movements called hemiballism may develop (see Ch. 411).

VERTEBRAL AND BASILAR ARTERIES. Focal brain stem ischemia produces a group of so-called "crossed syndromes" in which contralateral dysfunction occurs below the lesion due to interruption of pyramidal, spinothalamic, and dorsal column pathways, whereas ipsilateral dysfunction affects cerebellar controls or peripheral nerve junctions whose nuclei lie within the infarct. Occlusion of a vertebral artery and interference with flow through the ipsilateral *posterior inferior cerebellar artery* cause the *lateral medullary syndrome,* consisting of severe vertigo, nausea, vomiting, nystagmus, ipsilateral ataxia, and ipsilateral Horner's syndrome. There is an ipsilateral loss of facial pain and temperature sense and a contralateral loss of the same sensory modalities in trunk and limb. Discrete lesions in the distribution of the *anterior inferior cerebellar artery* are less common.

The *superior cerebellar artery* supplies most of the cerebellar cortex. Occlusion of this vessel is the most common cause of *cerebellar infarction,* characterized initially by gait ataxia, headache, nausea, vomiting, dizziness, ipsilateral clumsiness, and dysarthria. Subsequent brain swelling may induce ipsilateral gaze paresis and/or nystagmus toward the side of the infarction; ipsilateral facial weakness is sometimes seen. With further progression, lethargy and stupor deepen, and contralateral hemiparesis sometimes develops. Cerebellar edema formation can obstruct the fourth ventricle, producing hydrocephalus, and can result in herniation of the cerebellum either upward across the tentorium or downward through the foramen magnum (see Fig. 394–1).

Vertebrobasilar ischemia often produces multifocal lesions, scattered on both sides and along a considerable longitudinal extent of the brain stem. Except for cerebellar infarction and the lateral medullary syndrome, the clinical syndromes of discrete lesions are thus seldom seen in pure form. *Vertebrobasilar ischemia (VBI)* manifests with various combinations of symptoms such as dizziness (usually vertigo), diplopia, facial weakness, ataxia, and long-tract signs. Distinguishing mild VBI from more banal causes of dizziness can be difficult; the solution lies in identifying other, more specific symptoms or signs of parenchymal brain stem disease. Rarely does the person with VBI present with "dizziness" in the absence of other brain stem signs or symptoms.

Basilar artery occlusion produces massive brain stem dysfunction. The *locked-in state* is one possible consequence; in this condition, paralysis of the limbs and most of the bulbar muscles means that the patient can communicate only by moving the eyes or eyelids to command. Normal intelligence can often be demonstrated through codes involving eye movements. *Occlusion of the basilar apex* (or *top-of-the-basilar*) is usually caused by emboli that lodge at the junction between the basilar artery and the two PCA's. The condition produces an initial reduction in arousal followed by blindness and amnesia (from interruption of flow into the PCA's) plus abnormalities of vertical gaze and pupillary reactivity (from tegmental damage).

DIAGNOSIS

HISTORY. The history should emphasize the precise onset of the clinical deficit and the course since onset (stable or unstable).

Preceding TIA's are more likely to be associated with an ischemic than a hemorrhagic stroke. Headache more often occurs with hemorrhage and embolus than with atherothrombotic ischemic stroke. The possibility of other diagnoses (e.g., hypoglycemia or seizures) should be considered. The initial evaluation should include a thorough search for vascular disease risk factors (see below), since their presence will strengthen the likelihood of an ischemic stroke and influence eventual management.

PHYSICAL EXAMINATION. The neurologic examination serves to localize the lesion site, but the general medical examination more frequently provides clues to pathogenesis. Specific attention should be given to the cardiovascular examination and to evidence of hematologic disease. The arterial blood pressure in both arms, cardiac rhythm, and other cardiac abnormalities, such as murmurs or opening snaps, should be carefully recorded. The vascular examination should include gentle palpation of the carotid arteries and auscultation (with a bell-type stethoscope) of their course in the neck. Ophthalmoscopy can detect retinal cholesterol or platelet-fibrin emboli as well as evidence of chronic hypertensive or diabetic disease. The presence of retinal hypertensive changes can indicate that hypertension has been chronic rather than transiently stroke associated. Except with posterior circulation insufficiency or previous strokes, loss of consciousness or confusion should prompt consideration of other diagnoses.

LABORATORY EXAMINATION. *Hematologic Tests.* These include a complete blood count and platelet count (to evaluate for polycythemia, thrombocytosis, bacterial endocarditis, and severe anemia). Blood should be taken to evaluate glucose, prothrombin time, partial thromboplastin time; and a lipid profile. In the elderly, determination of the erythrocyte sedimentation rate should be performed urgently to exclude giant cell arteritis; in the young, the presence of antiphospholipid antibodies helps to identify immune-related disease processes predisposing to stroke. Other blood tests (e.g., protein C, protein S, measurements of viscosity or platelet function, and tests for collagen vascular diseases) may be indicated in younger patients who lack obvious causes for their strokes. The rising incidence of syphilis in urban areas makes a serum VDRL desirable. Tests of renal function and serum electrolyte measurements help to establish systemic illnesses as well as the milieu in which subsequent diagnostic tests (e.g., contrast injection) and treatments might be offered.

Cardiovascular Examination. All stroke patients require a standard 12-lead electrocardiogram (ECG) and rhythm strip at admission to exclude acute myocardial ischemia and arrhythmias. Authorities disagree over whether one should search with echocardiography for a cardiogenic source of emboli in acute focal stroke, since the yield is low in patients who have no history or physical evidence of cardiac disease. Our practice is to employ two-dimensional echocardiography or, less often, transesophogeal echocardiography in patients with focal stroke who (1) are young; (2) have no detectable atherothrombosis of the appropriate extracranial vessel, regardless of age; and (3) have no detectable risk factors, including polycythemia or oral contraceptive use. In suitable patients, *stress testing* during convalescence may be recommended to evaluate possible ischemic cardiovascular disease.

Brain Imaging. Brain imaging is the most important differential diagnostic test to identify other causes of focal neurologic dysfunction, such as neoplasms or subdural hematomas, and to distinguish ischemic from hemorrhagic stroke. CT scanning, the most commonly used imaging technique, has limitations that must be considered. CT cannot always detect cerebral infarction; the size, location, and age of the lesion affect the lesion's visibility. Infarcts less than 5 mm in diameter often escape detection, especially within the brain stem, where bone artifact may interfere with resolution. Further, only about 5% of strokes are visible on CT scan within the first 12 hours; detection increases to approximately 50% between 24 and 48 hours and approximately 90% by the end of 1 week.

Infarcts appear as hypodense areas on non–contrast-enhanced CT scans with increasingly well-demarcated margins as edema peaks between 3 and 5 days. Contrast-enhancing agents carry a small risk of neurotoxicity, and they may normalize the CT density of an otherwise small hypodense infarct, making the infarct less visible. Accordingly, one should use contrast-enhancing agents during the acute phase of the ischemic stroke only to seek out a mass lesion and only after a noncontrast scan has been obtained.

CT scans immediately delineate primary cerebral hemorrhage, but hemorrhagic conversions of an ischemic infarct usually develop only after 1 to 2 days. A few continue to appear for up to 4 weeks.

Magnetic resonance imaging (MRI) is more sensitive than CT to changes in tissue structure and may provide a more accurate and earlier measure of cerebral infarction (Fig. 441–7). MRI, however, is more costly, and, with the present equipment, requires more time to perform than CT; in addition, the need to exclude ferromagnetic materials from the MRI suite, as well as the difficulty in monitoring patients in the scanner, makes MRI unsuitable for many acutely ill patients. If the diagnosis remains in doubt, MRI may be used after the acute phase to verify infarction.

Lumbar Puncture. Lumbar puncture (LP) is no longer widely used to diagnose routine stroke because, (1) noninvasive CT or MRI detects cerebral hemorrhage and, (2) anticoagulation begun within 6 hours after a lumbar puncture risks causing a spinal epidural hematoma. An LP is important, however, in diagnosing neurosyphilis or meningitis, as, for example, in patients with acute stiff neck who show no blood on brain imaging. If an LP is to be done in suspected stroke, it should be preceded by brain imaging and funduscopic examination to rule out raised intracranial pressure.

Noninvasive Cerebrovascular Examination. Several noninvasive techniques help to evaluate the cerebrovascular supply. Indirect tests that examine blood flow in the periorbital or orbital circulation include *Doppler sonography* and *quantitative oculopneumoplethysmography* (OPG).

Direct examination of the common, internal, and external carotid arteries is best achieved with *duplex ultrasonography.* Duplex ultrasonography consists of B-mode ultrasonography, which produces a real-time image of the carotid vessels and a range-gaited pulsed Doppler that is visually guided by the B-mode image to measure the frequency shift associated with increased blood velocity through a stenotic lumen. The combination of the precise location of the Doppler frequency signal and the B-mode image provides the most accurate noninvasive method for analyzing disease of the extracranial circulation. Limitations of the technique include (1) access to only the portion of the carotid circulation that lies between the clavicles and the mandible (in approximately 10% of patients, the carotid bifurcation lies above the angle of the jaw, making ultrasonography difficult or impossible), (2) absorption of sound waves by calcium within a mural plaque, which may "shadow" and obscure a plaque on a distal vessel wall, and (3) echolucency of acute thrombi, which can be indistinguishable from flowing blood.

The direction and velocity of blood flow in the intracranial blood vessels originating from the circle of Willis may be examined with low-frequency *pulsed transcranial Doppler,* a technique still being evaluated for its usefulness as a diagnostic tool. The intracranial blood vessels also can be examined on reconstructed CT or MRI images. An evolving technique involves the imaging of flowing blood using *magnetic resonance angiography.* The procedure produces images of the extracranial and intracranial blood vessels, as well as atherosclerotic abnormalities of the carotid bifurcation; some aneurysms can also be detected.

Cerebral Angiography. Intracranial and extracranial *cerebral angiography* of elderly patients prone to ischemic stroke carries a 2 to 4% risk of producing a reversible neurologic deficit and a 0.5 to 1.0% risk of permanent neurologic deficits or death. Accordingly, angiography should be reserved for specific indications in which it may reveal abnormalities amenable to therapy. Examples include a search for fibromuscular dysplasia, arterial dissection, cranial arteritis, or as a preparation for cerebrovascular surgery. *Digital subtraction arteriography* permits use of smaller amounts of intravascular contrast material and may thus be of lower risk, especially in patients with marginal renal or cardiac function. *Digital subtraction venous angiography* is no longer widely used because of its unreliability in detecting plaque ulcerations and in differentiating carotid stenosis from complete occlusion.

Other Techniques. Methods for measuring cerebral blood flow in the clinical arena are still largely investigational; they include *positron emission tomographic (PET)* methods, usually using radiolabeled water or carbon dioxide; *single-photon emission computed tomography (SPECT);* and radiolabeled and stable *xenon* inhalation techniques.

DIFFERENTIAL DIAGNOSIS OF ISCHEMIC STROKES AND TIA'S

The clinical diagnosis of ischemic or hemorrhagic stroke relies primarily on the clinician's understanding of brain function and pathology. Deficits that evolve over weeks are usually caused by a brain mass, either *primary or metastatic brain tumor* or *brain abscess.* Subdural hematoma should be distinguishable from stroke by the hematoma's more prolonged course and its combination of diffuse and focal dysfunction.

TIA's may be confused with classic or complicated *migraine,* the former being associated with scintillating scotomata and the latter with hemiparesis or other focal deficits; some of the underlying pathophysiology may be ischemic for both TIA's and migraine, but evidence is accumulating that nonischemic electrical disturbances (spreading depression) may be involved in the pathophysiology of migraine.

Seizures can be confused with TIA's. Most seizures produce motor activity or positive sensory phenomena, whereas most strokes and TIA's produce weakness and sensory loss. Nevertheless, seizures can sometimes produce these "negative" symptoms. The postictal state following (unobserved) seizures is even more likely to imitate an ischemic deficit. Serial observations usually permit the differentiation of stroke from seizure, but rapid differentiation may be difficult and may interfere with early stroke treatment. As with migraine, strokes and seizures can coexist: A small proportion of strokes (about 10%), especially embolic strokes, are associated at onset with seizures.

Hemorrhagic stroke often enters the differential diagnosis for ischemic stroke. Although the anatomic locations of the two may differ, with hemorrhage seldom involving a discrete vascular territory, clinical differentiation can be uncertain, making CT scan necessary. Other illnesses included in the differential diagnosis of vertebrobasilar ischemia include, as mentioned above, nonspecific dizziness, Meniere's disease, or peripheral vestibulopathy.

CAUSES AND PATHOGENESIS (Table 419-2)

ATHEROSCLEROSIS. Atherosclerosis of extracranial and intracranial arteries accounts for approximately two thirds of all ischemic strokes and an even greater proportion of those affecting patients over the age of 60. Atherosclerosis causes strokes either by *in situ stenosis or occlusion* or by *embolization* of plaque material to distal cerebral vessels. In either case, the clinical and pathologic effects depend on the adequacy of collateral circulation to the affected vascular territory. It is not uncommon for unilateral or, more rarely, bilateral occlusion of the internal carotid artery to develop without neurologic symptoms, especially if the stenosis or occlusion develops slowly. In instances of marked stenosis or occlusion of extracranial arteries that is combined with intracranial atherosclerosis, cerebral perfusion sometimes can relate closely to small changes in blood pressure. One effect can be a worsening stroke deficit associated with orthostatic blood pressure changes that would otherwise be considered normal.

The more common effect of atherosclerosis is that a platelet-fibrin embolus detaches from a plaque and floats distally, where it occludes a smaller branch. Such emboli are likely to produce symptoms, since the more distal the occlusion, the less likely can collateral filling prevent damage. In cases of artery-to-artery embolization, the embolus usually emanates from a plaque at the base of the aorta, the bifurcation of the common carotid artery, or at the point where the vertebral arteries originate from the subclavian arteries.

EMBOLI OF CARDIAC ORIGIN. Cerebral emboli of a cardiac source may account for up to one third of all ischemic strokes. Thrombus formation and the release of thromboemboli from the heart are promoted by arrhythmias and structural abnormalities of the valves and chambers.

Mural Thrombi. Mural thrombi typically form under areas of dyskinetic myocardium damaged by *myocardial infarction.* As many as 35% of patients with recent anterior wall infarction harbor mural thrombi, and if not anticoagulated, nearly 40% of these will embolize systemically within 4 months after the myocardial infarction. *Cardiomyopathies* can also predispose to mural thrombi and embolization. In one study, systemic emboli were found in approximately 15% of patients with congestive or dilated cardiomyopathy,

TABLE 419–2. CAUSES OF ISCHEMIC STROKE

Atherosclerosis

Emboli of Cardiac Origin

Mural thrombus
  Myocardial infarction (anterior wall sputum, akinetic segment)
  Cardiomyopathy (infectious, idiopathic, Chagas' disease)
Valvular heart disease
  Rheumatic heart disease
  Bacterial endocarditis
  Nonbacterial endocarditis (carcinoma, Libman-Sacks)
  Mitral valve prolapse
  Prosthetic valve
Arrhythmia (atrial fibrillation)
Cardiac myxoma
Paradoxical emboli

Vasculitides

Primary CNS vasculitis
Systemic necrotizing vasculitis (polyarteritis nodosa, allergic angitis)
Hypersensitivity vasculitis (serum sickness, drug-induced, cutaneous vasculitis)
Collagen vascular diseases (rheumatoid arthritis, scleroderma, Sjögren's disease)
Giant cell (temporal arteritis, Takayasu's arteritis)
Wegener's granulomatosis
Lymphomatoid granulomatosis
Behçet's disease
Infectious vasculitis (neurovascular syphilis, Lyme disease, bacterial and fungal meningitis, tuberculosis, acquired immunodeficiency syndrome [AIDS], ophthalmic zoster, hepatitis B)

Hematologic Disorders

Hemoglobinopathies (sickle cell, HbSC)
Hyperviscosity syndromes (polycythemia, thrombocytosis, leukocytosis, macroglobulinemia, multiple myeloma)
Hypercoagulable states (carcinoma, pregnancy, puerperium)
Protein C or S deficiency
Antiphospholipid antibodies (lupus anticoagulant, anticardiolipin antibody)

Drug Related

"Street drugs" (cocaine, "crack," amphetamines, lysergic acid, phencyclidine, methylphenidate, sympathomimetics, heroin, pentazocine)
Alcohol
Oral contraceptives

Other

Fibromuscular dysplasia
Arterial dissection (trauma, spontaneous, Marfan's syndrome)
Homocystinuria
Migraine
Subarachnoid hemorrhage/vasospasm
Other emboli (fat, bone marrow, air emboli)
Moyamoya

---

a subgroup of the condition that is usually caused by alcohol abuse or viral infections. Patients who also had atrial fibrillation had a higher incidence of embolism (33%) than did those without (14%). None of the cardiomyopathy patients on anticoagulation, however, experienced systemic emboli.

Valvular Heart Disease. Although less common than previously, *rheumatic heart disease* often gives rise to systemic embolization. In one series, 20 to 25% of patients with mitral stenosis developed systemic emboli, although most had coexisting atrial fibrillation.

Acute or subacute *infective endocarditis* produces vegetations on heart valves, and debris that can embolize into the cerebral circulation. Many emboli are relatively small, but those associated with endocarditis caused by staphylococci, fungi, or yeast often are large enough to occlude proximal intracranial arteries. Systemic emboli are found in as many as 30% of patients dying from infective endocarditis. Prompt recognition of the heart lesion plus the presence of fever, a murmur, petechiae, and other characteristics, in patients with underlying valvular disease or intravenous drug use should prompt blood cultures and treatment with antibiotics to reduce the risk of embolism. Anticoagulation is not effective and may increase the risk of parenchymal bleeding. Infective endocarditis is associated with other forms of cerebrovascular disease, including cerebral

hemorrhage, subarachnoid hemorrhage, and mycotic aneurysm, as well as cerebral abscess.

Embolization from heart valves also occurs in *nonbacterial endocarditis (NBTE),* in which predominantly platelet-fibrin vegetations form on the heart valves and then embolize into the systemic circulation. NBTE occurs commonly in association with cancer of the stomach, prostate, ovary, pancreas, and lung. In one autopsy series of patients with NBTE, cerebral emboli were found in one third. Clinically, diffuse encephalopathy as well as focal stroke is observed; associated disseminated intravascular coagulation accompanies about 20% of cases.

Libman-Sacks (atypical verrucous) endocarditis is associated with systemic lupus erythematosus. Soft, friable vegetations form on the leaflets of any of the heart valves, not just the tricuspid valve, as believed earlier. Systemic (and cerebral) emboli are rare.

Mitral valve prolapse describes a billowing of the mitral leaflets into the left atrium during systole. Although usually asymptomatic, some patients experience palpitations or chest pain. The diagnosis is suggested by auscultatory and echocardiographic criteria, but normal standards are uncertain, making the true incidence unknown; it is estimated to be 6 to 10% in healthy young women. In part because of different diagnostic criteria, the role of mitral valve prolapse in cerebral embolism remains controversial: Several analyses of strokes in young adults suggest a disproportionately high representation of patients with mitral valve prolapse, but others indexed on patients with mitral valve prolapse suggest that systemic embolism is infrequent. Coexisting infective endocarditis or arrhythmia contributes to cerebral embolism.

Prosthetic heart valves carry a high risk of systemic (including cerebral) embolism; mechanical heart valves have a higher risk than biologic valves (e.g., porcine). The overall risk of embolism is roughly equivalent in anticoagulated patients with mechanical valves and in nonanticoagulated patients with biologic valves: 1 to 3% per year for aortic prostheses, and 3 to 5% per year for mitral substitutions.

Arrhythmias. *Atrial fibrillation,* with or without valvular disease, strongly increases the risk of embolic ischemic stroke, especially in patients over the age of 60. In one large series, the risk of ischemic stroke was 6 to 7% per year in nonanticoagulated patients. The risk is highest shortly after development of atrial fibrillation: Up to one third of emboli occur in the first month. Embolism can also accompany therapeutic cardioversion. About 35% of patients with nonvalvular atrial fibrillation sooner or later will have an ischemic stroke. In some, embolism underlies the stroke; in others, the fault lies in coexisting intrinsic cerebrovascular disease associated with coronary artery disease. Even thyrotoxic, nonvalvular atrial fibrillation is associated with a 10 to 12% risk of stroke. The one group without a strikingly increased risk is patients with isolated atrial fibrillation, associated with other clinical evidence of cardiopulmonary disease.

Cardiac Myxoma. Cardiac tumors are uncommon, occurring in about 0.05% of autopsies. *Myxomas* account for about 35% of all intracardiac tumors but are the ones most likely to embolize, from either overlying thrombus or the tumor itself. In one series, about one-quarter of patients with autopsy-proven cardiac myxomas had clinical evidence of strokes. Aneurysms and intracranial hemorrhage were also reported. The coexistence of hemolytic anemia due to red blood cell trauma and lysis sometimes suggests a cardiac tumor, but firm diagnosis requires echocardiography or angiography.

Paradoxical Emboli. Emboli of venous origin have long been known to cross a patent foramen ovale into the systemic circulation. Studies using bubble echocardiography found that 40% of stroke patients under age 55 with a normal cardiac evaluation by history, examination, and ECG had a patent foramen ovale detected by bubble echocardiography.

VASCULITIDES. A group of disorders classified as vasculitides cause focal or multifocal cerebral ischemia through inflammation and necrosis of extracranial and/or intracranial blood vessels. The pathogenesis of vascular inflammation differs among these disorders, but all involve some deposition of humoral and cellular immune complexes and infiltration of polymorphonuclear and mononuclear cells in blood vessel walls. In most cases, the cause of the inflammatory response is unknown, but in others, infection, a postinfectious or neoplastic process, or a hypersensitivity immune reaction triggers the inflammation.

Segmental inflammation of cerebral blood vessels causes cerebral ischemia acutely at the site of involvement through platelet aggregation and/or clot formation or chronically through fibrinoid necrosis, which narrows the vessel lumen. Central nervous system (CNS) vasculitis, although a rare cause of stroke, is itself not uncommon and should enter the differential diagnosis whenever a young patient presents with a stroke or a patient of any age presents with a diffuse unexplained encephalopathy.

Symptoms of CNS vasculitis include cognitive disturbances, headache, and seizures (encephalopathy), which occur more frequently than with focal neurologic dysfunction. The diagnosis depends on the angiographic appearance of a "beadlike" segmental narrowing of cerebral blood vessels and/or the finding of characteristic inflammatory histopathology in leptomeningeal and cortical biopsy specimens. Cerebral angiograms may appear normal in 20 to 30% of histologically positive cases. In addition, because of the segmental or "skip" nature of the inflammatory response, the histopathology may go undetected in the presence of a positive angiogram.

The diagnosis of CNS vasculitis is aided by the presence or absence of peripheral nervous system or systemic organ involvement and by identifying the underlying cause of the inflammation. Primary CNS vasculitis, Behçet's disease, Takayasu's arteritis, and temporal arteritis are notable for their infrequent involvement or noninvolvement of the peripheral nervous system. By contrast, the hypersensitivity and systemic necrotizing vasculitides frequently produce polyneuropathies.

Primary CNS arteritis, giant cell arteritis, and vasculitis associated with certain CNS infections deserve specific attention, since these may present initially or solely with neurologic signs and symptoms.

Primary CNS Arteritis. Primary arteritis of the CNS, also called granulomatous arteritis of the CNS, causes headache and other encephalopathic-like symptoms in young or middle-aged individuals. The course is usually insidiously progressive but may wax and wane for periods of several months. It is a diagnosis of exclusion.

Giant Cell Vasculitis. Temporal arteritis and Takayasu's arteritis are characterized by a granulomatous vasculitis of medium-sized and large arteries. Temporal arteritis affects predominantly patients over the age of 60, causing constitutional symptoms such as fever, malaise, weight loss, and headache. In half the patients, symptoms consistent with polymyalgia rheumatica may coexist, including jaw, neck, and facial pain, as well as morning stiffness. Tenderness and pain over the temporal arteries and an elevated erythrocyte sedimentation rate are frequently, but not always, present. Biopsy of the superficial temporal artery provides the definitive diagnosis. Because of the segmental nature of the vasculitis, serial sections should be examined. Even then, typical features of fever, malaise, tender scalp vessels, and a grossly elevated sedimentation rate dictate the early initiation of corticosteroid therapy because of the high risk of acute ischemic blindness. A *dramatic* improvement in constitutional symptoms is semidiagnostic.

Takayasu's arteritis affects primarily young women and involves mainly the aortic arch, the large brachiocephalic arteries derived from the arch, and the abdominal aorta. Mononuclear infiltrates and fibrous proliferation produce progressive narrowing of the lumen of these vessels, causing reduced flow into the upper extremities (hence the name "pulseless disease") and cerebral ischemia. Although initially diagnosed in Japanese women, it has been recognized in Western countries.

Infectious Vasculitis. Bacterial, fungal, and viral infections can induce CNS vasculitis and cerebral ischemia (Table 419–2). Neurosyphilis and its meningovascular complications have increased considerably in recent years (see Ch. 422) and should be considered in patients with atypical or unexplained cerebrovascular disease.

HEMATOLOGIC ABNORMALITIES. Hemoglobinopathy. Among the hemoglobinopathies, *sickle cell disease* is by far the most common cause of stroke. In sickle cell disease, a single substitution of the amino acid valine for glutamate at the sixth position of the β-globin molecule causes the mutant molecule HbSS to become highly insoluble and polymerize under deoxygenated condi-

tions. The polymerization alters the erythrocyte's shape ("sickling") and decreases the cell's deformability, leading to increased blood viscosity, microvascular sludging, and microvascular infarction. Sickle cell disease also causes hyperplasia of fibrous tissue and muscle cells of the vascular intima, leading to stenosis and occlusion of some medium to large cerebral arteries.

Ischemic stroke occurs in approximately 15% of patients with HbSS and in a much smaller percentage of those with sickle cell trait (HbSA) or HbSC. At normal arterial oxygen saturations of 95 to 100% in HbSS, some sickling is present, and at 65%, i.e., just slightly lower than normal venous oxygen saturation, approximately 75% of erythrocytes sickle. Ischemic stroke arises most frequently in children, whereas hemorrhagic stroke is more common in adults with HbSS; subarachnoid hemorrhage in patients with sickle cell disease is frequently the result of a ruptured saccular aneurysm.

Small changes in oxygen tension, dehydration, acidosis, or infection can precipitate sickle cell crisis and stroke. Cerebral angiography causes an increased risk for patients with sickle cell disease. In instances when such angiography is necessary to evaluate the source of intracerebral hemorrhage, the level of HbSS should be reduced to less than 20% through transfusions.

Hyperviscosity Syndrome. Cerebral blood flow relates inversely to blood viscosity. The latter is directly proportional to the number of circulating red and white blood cells, the aggregation state, the number of platelets, and the plasma protein concentration. Blood flow (BF) is inversely proportional to the deformability of erythrocytes and blood velocity (shear rate). Patients with the hyperviscosity syndrome can either have focal neurologic dysfunction or, more frequently, diffuse or multifocal signs or symptoms, including headache, visual disturbances, cognitive impairment, and seizures.

Cellular hyperviscosity, associated with *polycythemia, thrombocytosis,* or *leukocytosis* of any cause, can reduce BF below threshold levels for cerebral dysfunction and injury. Hematocrits above 50%, white cell counts >150,000 per μl, and platelet counts in excess of 1 million per μl increase the risk of stroke.

Elevated plasma protein concentrations caused by *macroglobulinemia* or *multiple myeloma* elevate plasma viscosity and increase stroke risk. Approximately 25% of patients with macroglobulinemia experience some form of cerebral ischemia, and a lesser number of patients with multiple myeloma experience the hyperviscosity syndrome. Of the various forms of multiple myeloma, those with a predominance of immunoglobulin A (IgA) most frequently develop a hyperviscosity syndrome because this particular molecule is likely to form high molecular weight polymers.

Hypercoagulable States. Cancer, particularly the adenocarcinomas, pregnancy, and the puerperium have all been associated with a "hypercoagulable state" that predisposes to arterial and venous thrombosis. Despite the fact that any one of several abnormalities, including elevations of fibrinogen levels, alterations of partial thromboplastin or prothrombin times, and platelet aggregation, occurs in the hypercoagulable state, no tests have been devised to diagnose it specifically.

Protein C or S Deficiency. Proteins C and S are two naturally occurring anticoagulants synthesized in the liver via vitamin K–dependent mechanisms. Deficiencies of either are rare, dominantly inherited, and expressed phenotypically by incomplete penetrance. Homozygotes develop serious and frequently fatal clotting abnormalities at birth, while heterozygotes may show no signs of hypercoagulability. Proteins C and S act in concert to inactivate the activated coagulating Factors V and VIII; protein C also triggers the endogenous fibrinolytic pathways. Deficiencies in either are associated with ischemic vascular disease. Because of incomplete penetrance, the occurrence of thrombosis and stroke in the adult is extremely rare.

Antiphospholipid Antibodies. A strong epidemiologic association links a group of antiphospholipid antibodies to cerebral ischemia manifested clinically as atypical migraine, TIA, recurrent strokes, or ischemic encephalopathy. These antibodies bind to membrane phospholipids and include anticardiolipin antibody, the lupus anticoagulant, and antibodies causing a false-positive VDRL. The pathogenetic relationship between the antibodies and enhanced cerebral thrombosis is unknown. The syndrome may manifest at any age but usually affects patients younger than 50. Antiphospholipid antibodies often accompany collagen vascular disease, especially systemic lupus erythematosus, as well as valvular heart disease.

Circulating titers of phospholipid antibodies correlate poorly with either the incidence or the severity of cerebral ischemia.

DRUG-RELATED CAUSES OF STROKE. An extensive list of "street" drugs (see Table 419–2) has been associated with stroke, reflecting as much the social patterns of drug abuse as the unique properties of the drugs themselves. The sharing of nonsterile needles to inject many of these drugs intravenously (e.g., heroin, cocaine) may precipitate infectious processes (bacterial endocarditis, hepatitis B, mycotic aneurysms) that lead to strokes. Several of the drugs are potent vasoconstrictors and may initiate cerebral vasospasm. Others have been associated with cerebral vasculitis caused either by immune responses to the primary drug or by hypersensitivity to contaminating adulterants. The intravenous injection of oral medications (pentazocine [Talwin], methylphenidate [Ritalin]) that have been crushed and suspended in water can cause cerebral microemboli owing to particles of talc and cellulose used as ingredients in the pills. The particles are thought to be trapped by pulmonary arterioles, causing local arteritis and later arteriovenous shunts that allow the microemboli to reach the CNS.

Over-the-counter cold remedies and nasal decongestants containing sympathomimetics such as ephedrine, phenylpropanolamine, and phenoxazoline have been associated with ischemic stroke. Cases have been reported following the prolonged use of oral cold medications as well as in patients who chronically overuse nasal decongestants.

The risk of ischemic and hemorrhagic stroke is increased from 4- to 13-fold among users of high-dose estrogen contraceptives. The coexistence of hypertension, prolonged use of the pill, smoking, a previous history of migraine, and age exceeding 35 years seems to enhance the risk of contraceptive-related stroke. A clear association between stroke and the newer low-dose estrogen contraceptives has not been established.

OTHER CAUSES OF STROKE. *Fibromuscular dysplasia* (or hyperplasia) describes areas of segmental nonatherosclerotic arterial narrowing, usually caused by fibroplasia and smooth muscle proliferation, that alternate with rings of medial thinning. The uncommon condition affects the carotid and vertebral arteries, usually at the level of the second cervical vertebra rather than at the origin of the vessels; it also affects the renal arteries and is associated with hypertension. Fibromuscular dysplasia predominates in women and occurs, on the average, in the sixth decade of life. It produces ischemic stroke both by the hemodynamic effects of stenosis and by thromboembolism. The condition is also associated with aneurysm formation and with arterial dissection. Angiography usually makes the diagnosis, although flow studies with MRI may prove useful. Because of its rarity, there is little information about treatment.

A *dissecting aortic aneurysm,* although uncommon, can occlude major branches of the aorta supplying the cranial circulation and produce ischemic strokes. Chest, back, or abdominal pain accompanying the stroke and differences in palpable pulses or in blood pressure in the limbs suggest the diagnosis. Emergency angiography is needed to confirm it.

Extracranial *dissections of the carotid artery* are increasingly recognized. Many follow relatively trivial trauma (e.g., pharyngeal injury with blunt objects in children, and neck torsion, sometimes from chiropractic manipulation, in adults). Some are associated with fibromuscular dysplasia, others with a variety of childhood conditions, including Ehler-Danlos and Marfan's syndromes as well as tuberous sclerosis. Pathologically, intraluminal blood enters the subintimal or medial vascular planes, and the lumen becomes progressively narrowed and thrombosed. Carotid artery dissections can sometimes be recognized clinically by intense ipsilateral pain. Angiography may be needed for diagnosis, but MRI is sometimes sufficient.

Homocystinuria is characterized by dislocated ocular lenses, bone deformities, a marfanoid appearance, mental retardation, accelerated atherosclerosis, and arterial or venous thromboses. Several different genetic defects can cause homocystinuria, but the most frequent is a deficiency of the enzyme cystathionine β-synthase. Approximately one third of affected individuals have one or more strokes by the age of 15 years. In some studies, heterozygous homocystinuria has been reported in as many as one quarter of young persons who have suffered strokes. Treatment with pyridoxine or folic acid may limit disease progression.

Reactive vascular narrowing *(vasospasm)* causes ischemic strokes in two settings. One causes substantial disability in *subarachnoid*

hemorrhage (Ch. 420.1). Vasospasm also presumably explains ischemic strokes seen in a small number of patients with *migraine* headaches. Migraineurs develop ischemic strokes, either in conjunction with migraine (in which case they appear to result from a prolonged migraine attack) or remote from the attack (in which case more traditional stroke mechanisms, such as atherosclerosis, are likely to be responsible).

Fat emboli typically occur several days after trauma that includes fracture of the long bones. Although focal ischemic strokes may occur, more typically the condition manifests with seizures and a diffuse encephalopathy consistent with disseminated embolization. Associated findings include petechiae and fat emboli visible on funduscopic examination. Fat globules may be identified in urine or CSF.

Air emboli can occur with open heart surgery, in patients with pneumothorax, or in divers who ascend too rapidly to the surface. Air emboli cause altered mental status and seizures, but the changes are maximal immediately after the embolization. Segmental areas of pallor may be observed on the tongue, and there may be marbling of the skin and air emboli seen on funduscopic examination. When caused by sudden decompression, the condition is treated in a decompression chamber.

Moyamoya is a rare condition that is most common among the Japanese, in whom it has been reported to affect fewer than 0.1 per 100,000 of the general population. Diagnosis requires demonstration of bilateral terminal internal carotid artery occlusion that involves the origins of the MCA and ACA. An abnormal vascular network develops at the base of the brain that is believed to provide collateral circulation. The abnormal collateral channels appear on angiograms as a "smoky haze," hence the Japanese term "moyamoya." The cause of the vascular occlusion is unknown, but it occurs most commonly in children (peak incidence at age 6 years), in whom it may be associated with ischemic stroke; in adults, it more commonly causes hemorrhage. A similar angiographic picture occasionally accompanies acute tonsillitis, atherosclerosis, meningitis, cancer, trauma, and radiotherapy.

A condition in which the walls of small arteries are thickened and disorganized, referred to by some as lipohyalinosis, was originally believed to underlie small, subcortical brain infarcts called *lacunes.* Traditional causes of stroke, including diabetes and hyperlipidemia, have appeared in these patients with almost the same frequency as in those with nonlacunar, ischemic stroke. Perhaps as a result, treatment recommendations, which initially differed for lacunar strokes, now parallel those for nonlacunar strokes.

PREVENTION AND TREATMENT OF STROKE

Currently, there are several promising but no proven therapies for acute ischemic stroke. Even when effective treatments become available, the physician's opportunity to treat and the utility of a particular pharmacotherapy will be hampered by time constraints; the evolution of irreversible brain damage occurs within 2 to 3 hours of focal vascular occlusion (see Ch. 418). Such considerations place a premium on preventing stroke.

The reduction of stroke risk factors, through therapy for hypertension, diabetes mellitus, smoking, atherosclerosis, and cardiac arrhythmias (Table 419–3) is largely responsible for the marked decline in the incidence of stroke over the past 30 to 40 years.

RISK FACTORS AND PRIMARY PREVENTION THERAPIES

Stroke risk factors have been determined on the basis of mathematical abstractions of epidemiologic data that imply an association or a cause-effect relationship. This section categorizes such risk

TABLE 419–3. PREVENTION OF STROKE

Treat hypertension and diabetes mellitus
Stop smoking
Limit alcohol intake
Control diet and obesity
Thoughtful use of oral contraceptives
Anticoagulants for atrial fibrillation and selected acute myocardial infarctions
Antiplatelet agents for carotid/vertebrobasilar atherosclerosis
Endarterectomy for symptomatic carotid artery atherosclerosis of 70–99%

factors as *definite* or *presumed* and indicates whether they are related to *genetic* and *lifestyle* factors or to *disease processes*. Treatable risk factors are emphasized, and the expected outcome of such prophylactic therapy is presented.

DEFINITE GENETIC AND LIFESTYLE RISK FACTORS. *Hypertension.* This is the most powerful risk factor for stroke. Even within relatively "normal" ranges of blood pressure, the risk of stroke increases by approximately 50% for every 5 mm Hg increase in diastolic pressure throughout the range of 70 to 110 mm Hg. All components of blood pressure (systolic, diastolic, mean) correlate with the incidence of stroke, and the elevation of the systolic pressure is probably a direct cause of stroke that is independent of the secondary complications of hypertension, such as atherosclerosis or arterial rigidity. The risk of stroke is approximately four times greater in patients with definite hypertension (160/95 mm Hg) than in normotensive individuals and is twofold higher in so-called borderline hypertensive individuals. Antihypertensive therapy that lowers the diastolic pressure by as little as 6 mm Hg reduces stroke risk by nearly one quarter in as little as 2 to 3 years. Data from the Framingham Study indicate that the control of hypertension is as beneficial in reducing stroke risk in persons over 70 as it is at earlier ages.

Smoking. Smoking increases stroke risk twofold to fourfold. Those who stop smoking substantially reduce their risk of stroke over a period of 2 to 5 years, but their level of risk may not return completely to that of nonsmokers.

Age, Gender, and Race. Age, gender, and race are all unalterable risk factors for stroke, but they may signal treatable disease processes. The incidence of stroke approximately doubles with each decade between ages 45 and 85. Unlike cardiovascular ischemia, in which the incidence in men is approximately three times that in women, stroke occurs only 1.3 times more often in men than in women. The stroke risk in U.S. blacks is approximately 1.3 times that of whites. Some of the differences may be related to environmental or lifestyle factors, since southeastern blacks have a higher stroke rate than do northern ones. Similarly, the high incidence of stroke in the Japanese is not seen in their kindred living in Hawaii.

POSSIBLE GENETIC AND LIFESTYLE RISK FACTORS. *Cholesterol, Lipids, Diet, and Obesity.* Several dietary factors and obesity may play a role in stroke incidence, but the evidence is inconclusive. Diet and obesity may predispose toward diabetes mellitus and cardiovascular disease, and such patients have a higher chance of dying of stroke than do age-matched controls. Despite the incontrovertible relationship between elevated blood cholesterol and lipids and coronary artery disease, no conclusive evidence currently links lipid abnormalities to stroke. Nevertheless, most authorities strongly advise stroke-prone patients to lower elevated cholesterol and triglyceride levels. Because of the relationships that link obesity with diabetes mellitus, elevated blood pressure, and lipid abnormalities, weight control also is recommended for stroke-prone patients.

Alcohol. Moderate alcohol consumption relates inversely to the incidence of atherosclerosis and coronary artery disease, and a similar reduction of stroke risk with moderate alcohol consumption has also been suggested but not proved. By contrast, binge drinking increases the incidence of both hemorrhagic and ischemic stroke, especially when combined with cigarette smoking. Much of the latter risk may be attributable to a combination of hemoconcentration and hypertension associated with heavy alcohol consumption.

Oral Contraceptives. Although formerly available high-dose estrogen oral contraceptives were related to stroke, the association is less clear for current preparations. Nevertheless, the combination of oral contraceptives with other risk factors, such as migraine, smoking, hypertension, and age greater than 35 years, may act in combination to raise stroke risk, and many recommend against oral contraceptives in such circumstances.

DEFINITE DISEASE-RELATED RISK FACTORS. *Heart Disease.* Rheumatic valvular disease plus atrial fibrillation increases the risk of stroke 17-fold. Chronic or paroxysmal atrial fibrillation without lesions of the heart valves is associated with a fivefold increase in the risk of stroke. Chronic anticoagulation with warfarin is recommended for most fibrillators, especially those with a history of prior embolism, the presence of a left atrial thrombus on two-dimensional echocardiography, the coexistence of dilated or hypertrophic cardiomyopathy or of thyrotoxic heart disease, and

prior to direct-current (DC) conversion. Asymptomatic individuals over age 60 may be considered for anticoagulation on an individual basis. Preliminary data from a U.S. study indicated that treatment of chronic atrial fibrillation with warfarin or aspirin reduced the risk of embolic stroke by approximately 80%; other studies indicate that only warfarin confers such benefits. Furthermore, low-dose warfarin with a target prothrombin time ratio that is 1.2 to 1.5 times the control value conferred protection similar to that conferred by conventional warfarin therapy. Valvular disease related to bacterial or nonbacterial endocarditis, myxomatous degeneration of the mitral valve or other diseases causing mitral valve prolapse, mitroannular calcification, and prosthetic heart valve replacements all predispose toward cerebral emboli.

Myocardial infarction involving the anterior wall or septum is associated with a mural thrombus in up to one third of patients, and of these, approximately 15% will suffer a cerebral embolus within a 2-year interval. Acute anticoagulation therapy with heparin, with later conversion to warfarin therapy, is recommended for patients with myocardial infarction involving the anterior or septal wall or in patients with an intramural thrombus detected by two-dimensional echocardiography. Anticoagulation should continue until the two-dimensional echocardiogram indicates resolution of the thrombus. Such therapy reduces the incidence of stroke by approximately one half.

Stroke and TIA. The occurrence of an initial stroke is a powerful predictor of recurrent stroke. Patients between the ages of 45 and 65 years have a 10- to 20-fold increased risk of having a recurrent versus an initial stroke. The comparative risk drops to eightfold for those over the age of 65. The apparent decrease in the incidence of recurrent stroke with age reflects the marked increase in the incidence of an initial stroke in patients over the age of 65. The annual stroke risk following a TIA is 5% per year, which declines to 3% after 3 years. After the occurrence of amaurosis fugax, the annual risk of stroke is 1 to 2%.

Strong evidence derived from meta-analyses supports the use of prophylactic aspirin to protect against strokes in patients with prior strokes or TIA's. Similarly prophylactic antiplatelet therapy with ticlopidine has also been shown to protect against such secondary events. A decision to use antiplatelet or anticoagulant therapy in patients with prior strokes must take into account both the individual patient's risk of further functional loss and the risks of treatment.

Asymptomatic Carotid Stenosis. Individuals with asymptomatic carotid stenosis or carotid bruits have approximately a 1.5- to 2-fold increase in the risk of stroke compared with the general population. Cerebral infarction in this population, however, occurs as frequently in a vascular territory different from the stenotic artery as in the involved one. Asymptomatic carotid stenosis or bruit is a marker of cerebrovascular disease and signals an increased risk of stroke, but not necessarily one in the territory of the involved vessel. No large, randomized placebo-controlled trials have shown any efficacy of prophylactic antiplatelet therapy in patients with asymptomatic carotid stenosis or bruits.

Although prophylactic aspirin therapy in a healthy population of U.S. physicians reduced the incidence of myocardial infarction, no change occurred in the incidence of ischemic stroke, and a slight increase was detected in the incidence of hemorrhagic stroke. Antiplatelet agents cannot be recommended for stroke prophylaxis in healthy individuals.

Other Diseases. Diabetes mellitus is a risk factor independent of hypertension and is associated with an approximate threefold increase in the risk of stroke. No present data indicate that normalization of the blood sugar level reduces the incidence of stroke. Polycythemia, sickle cell disease, migraine, CNS vasculitis, and several infectious diseases all somewhat increase the risk of stroke.

SURGICAL TREATMENT FOR THE PREVENTION OF STROKE. The role of *prophylactic surgery* in the prevention of ischemic stroke is only partly resolved. A multi-institutional, randomized trial of an external carotid artery–middle cerebral artery anastomosis showed no benefit, and the procedure has been largely abandoned. *Carotid endarterectomy*, designed to remove stenotic plaques from diseased carotid arteries, was developed in the mid-1960's, and from 1971 until about 1984 the number of such operations steadily increased, despite controversy concerning its efficacy. Several multicenter trials in North America and Europe are currently examining the indications and efficacy of carotid endarterectomy versus medical therapy in symptomatic and asymptomatic

TABLE 419–4. GUIDELINES FOR CAROTID ENDARTERECTOMY

1. Recent ischemic symptoms (TIA, minor stroke)
2. Angiographically proven ipsilateral stenosis (70–99%)
3. Surgical risk ≤ 5%
4. Five-year cardiovascular life expectancy > 50%

carotid stenosis. Initial results from two studies indicate that endarterectomy significantly reduces ipsilateral stroke in patients with recent symptoms of ischemia and angiographically proven 70 to 99% ipsilateral carotid artery stenosis. Only patients with a 50% or greater 5-year life expectancy were entered in the study. The procedure is not appropriate for vertebrobasilar disease (Table 419–4). Patients with less than 30% stenosis were best treated medically. The best therapy for patients with 30 to 69% stenosis remains under examination. Likewise, we await the results of ongoing randomized trials to determine the comparative efficacy of medical therapy versus endarterectomy in patients with asymptomatic carotid stenosis. Although *angioplasty* is used widely for coronary artery disease, its utility for cerebrovascular atherosclerosis has not been established.

Surgery for *subclavian steal* is almost never indicated. This steal is a radiographic finding associated with occlusion or severe stenosis of a proximal subclavian artery, resulting in retrograde flow in the ipsilateral vertebral artery. The finding is only rarely associated with symptoms of vertebrobasilar ischemia when the ipsilateral arm is exercised. In most cases, it is merely a radiographic curiosity.

MANAGEMENT AND TREATMENT OF ACUTE TIA STROKE

Patients clinically diagnosed as having *acute cerebral ischemia* should be admitted to the hospital unless the deficit has existed for several days and is stable. The initial history and physical examination emphasize the rapid diagnosis of ischemic cerebral ischemia (TIA or stroke) and the exclusion of seizures, hypoglycemia, tumor, and other alternative diagnoses (Table 419–5). As already noted, a normal CT scan within the first several hours is consistent with an ischemic stroke. Admission is also advised for patients with *new-onset TIA's* or those in whom TIA's are occurring with markedly increasing frequency or severity (*crescendo TIA's*).

GENERAL MANAGEMENT. Once admitted, stroke patients should be maintained for at least 24 hours at bed rest to avoid postural hypotension. Since autoregulation (see Ch. 418) is usually ineffective in areas of ischemic brain, CBF will decline if systemic blood pressure falls because of postural changes or volume restriction. Hypertension, if present, should be treated, but with limited, stepwise reductions in blood pressure, for the same reason (Table 419–5). If patients have bulbar dysfunction affecting chewing or swallowing, mouth feedings should be avoided to reduce the chance of aspiration. Virtually all patients should have intravenous catheters placed to facilitate urgent treatments. If oral feedings are restricted for prolonged periods, supplementation with intravenous thiamine becomes important to prevent Wernicke's disease; eventually, hyperalimentation or feeding by nasogastric or gastrostomy tube may be needed.

In the early days of an ischemic stroke, passive range-of-motion exercises to the affected limbs can help retain mobility and prevent contractures. Later, more intensive rehabilitation individualized to improve gait, speech, dexterity, and ability to manage activities of daily living become important. Patients often benefit from brief, intensive rehabilitation in specialized hospitals before being sent home. All patients at bed rest should be encouraged to flex and extend their ankles periodically to reduce the chances of deep venous thrombosis, and all should also take occasional deep breaths to combat atelectasis.

PHARMACOTHERAPY (Table 419–6). No pharmacologic therapy has been proved effective for acute ischemic stroke. Nonetheless, several agents are used, depending on the underlying pathophysiology. Intravenous *heparin* is frequently begun on an acute basis for progressing or incomplete stroke, but as already noted, results are difficult to determine. An important point is that none of the studies of heparin have examined the effect of beginning within the first hours after stroke onset, so that poor study design may have masked detection of any benefit. A current multicen-

ter trial in North America of heparinoid therapy in acute stroke may provide better guidelines.

Despite underlying bleeding into the blood vessel wall, patients with vascular dissections are often treated with heparin in an effort to maintain patency of the vascular lumen and limit the likelihood of embolism; no proof of benefit exists. Patients with lacunar strokes were previously considered not to be helped by heparin, but some authorities have modified that view in recent years.

Patients whose strokes are attributed to emboli of cardiac origin are frequently treated acutely with heparin. Chronic oral anticoagulation is usually started concurrently, but debate surrounds the use of heparin until oral anticoagulation takes effect. Some advocate heparin because of concern about early re-embolization and the possibility that warfarin (Coumadin) sometimes enhances coagulability during the first 6 to 8 hours of therapy; others worry about the risks of hemorrhage into the initial stroke. It seems clear that the risk of bleeding is greater for larger infarcts. A reasonable course is to begin heparin and then begin warfarin after a CT scan at 48 hours reveals a small nonhemorrhagic infarct or at 5 to 7 days for a large nonhemorrhagic infarct (Table 419–6). Evidence of a hemorrhagic infarct should delay anticoagulation by 4 to 6 weeks.

TABLE 419–5. EVALUATION OF ACUTE FOCAL NEUROLOGIC DYSFUNCTION

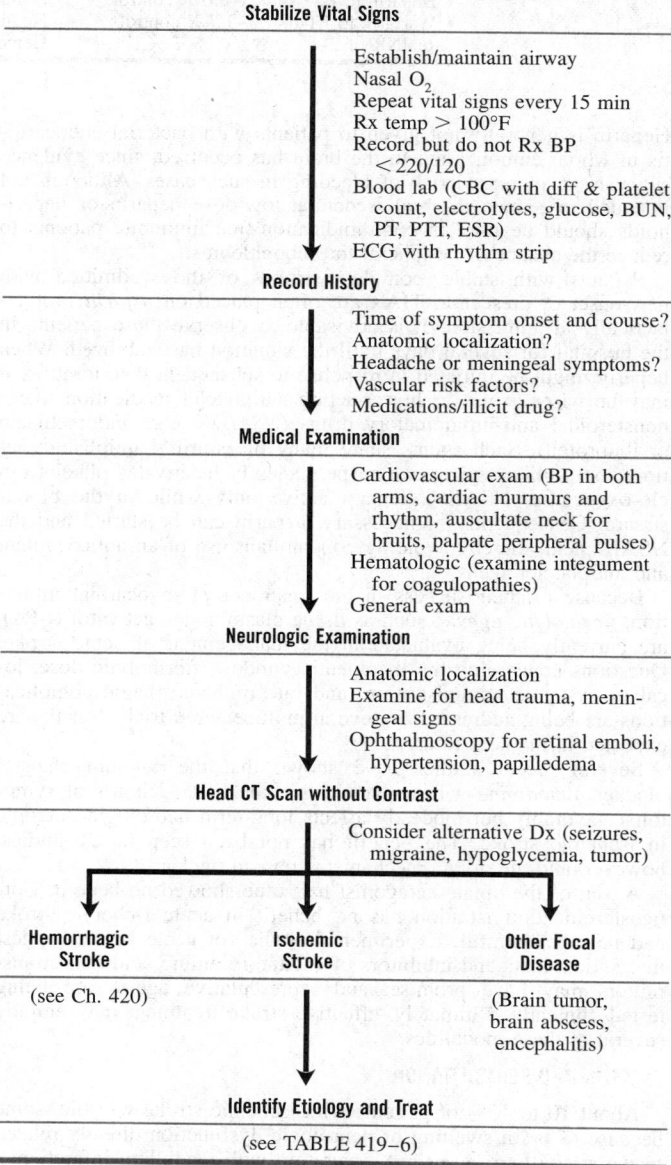

Stabilize Vital Signs
- Establish/maintain airway
- Nasal O$_2$
- Repeat vital signs every 15 min
- Rx temp > 100°F
- Record but do not Rx BP < 220/120
- Blood lab (CBC with diff & platelet count, electrolytes, glucose, BUN, PT, PTT, ESR)
- ECG with rhythm strip

Record History
- Time of symptom onset and course?
- Anatomic localization?
- Headache or meningeal symptoms?
- Vascular risk factors?
- Medications/illicit drug?

Medical Examination
- Cardiovascular exam (BP in both arms, cardiac murmurs and rhythm, auscultate neck for bruits, palpate peripheral pulses)
- Hematologic (examine integument for coagulopathies)
- General exam

Neurologic Examination
- Anatomic localization
- Examine for head trauma, meningeal signs
- Ophthalmoscopy for retinal emboli, hypertension, papilledema

Head CT Scan without Contrast
- Consider alternative Dx (seizures, migraine, hypoglycemia, tumor)

Hemorrhagic Stroke (see Ch. 420)

Ischemic Stroke

Other Focal Disease (Brain tumor, brain abscess, encephalitis)

Identify Etiology and Treat (see TABLE 419–6)

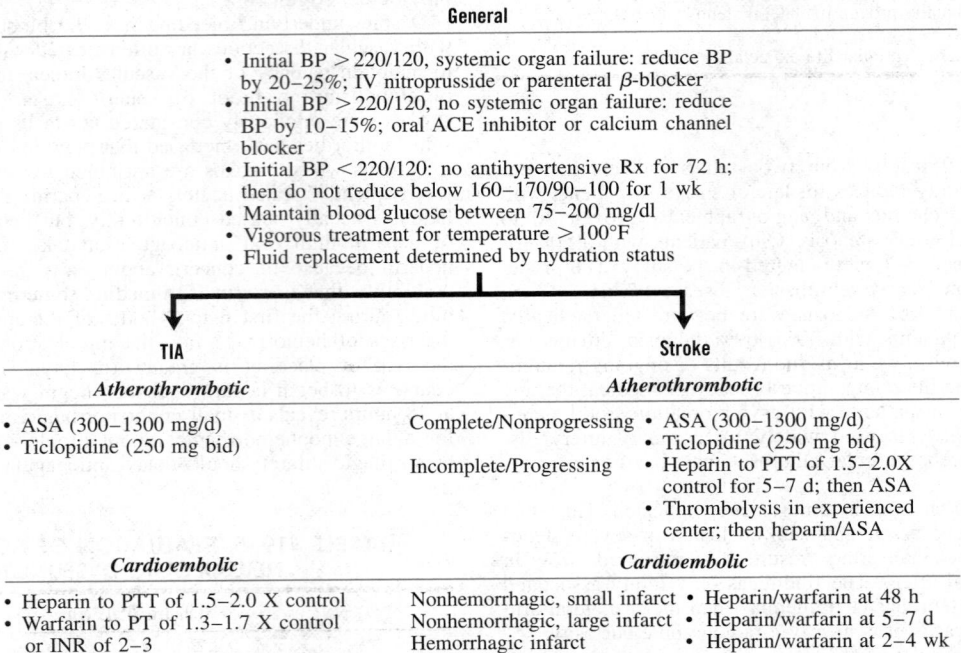

TABLE 419–6. MANAGEMENT OF ACUTE FOCAL BRAIN ISCHEMIA

General

- Initial BP > 220/120, systemic organ failure: reduce BP by 20–25%; IV nitroprusside or parenteral β-blocker
- Initial BP > 220/120, no systemic organ failure: reduce BP by 10–15%; oral ACE inhibitor or calcium channel blocker
- Initial BP < 220/120: no antihypertensive Rx for 72 h; then do not reduce below 160–170/90–100 for 1 wk
- Maintain blood glucose between 75–200 mg/dl
- Vigorous treatment for temperature > 100°F
- Fluid replacement determined by hydration status

TIA

Atherothrombotic

- ASA (300–1300 mg/d)
- Ticlopidine (250 mg bid)

Cardioembolic

- Heparin to PTT of 1.5–2.0 X control
- Warfarin to PT of 1.3–1.7 X control or INR of 2–3

Stroke

Atherothrombotic

Complete/Nonprogressing
- ASA (300–1300 mg/d)
- Ticlopidine (250 mg bid)

Incomplete/Progressing
- Heparin to PTT of 1.5–2.0X control for 5–7 d; then ASA
- Thrombolysis in experienced center; then heparin/ASA

Cardioembolic

Nonhemorrhagic, small infarct • Heparin/warfarin at 48 h
Nonhemorrhagic, large infarct • Heparin/warfarin at 5–7 d
Hemorrhagic infarct • Heparin/warfarin at 2–4 wk

Heparin is generally not given to patients with bacterial endocarditis in whom embolization to the brain has occurred, since evidence suggests an increased risk of bleeding in such cases. Although not intended to reduce cerebral ischemia, low-dose heparin or heparinoids should be used in contraindication-free immobile patients to reduce the chance of peripheral thrombophlebitis.

Patients with stable, complete strokes or those admitted with new-onset or crescendo TIA's are often placed on *aspirin* prophylactically at admission. It is advisable to observe these patients in the hospital for several days until the situation has stabilized. When heparin might be initiated in response to subsequent deterioration, it may be wiser to use a shorter-acting antiplatelet medication like a nonsteroidal anti-inflammatory drugs (*NSAID's,* e.g., indomethacin or ibuprofen). Such agents share many of aspirin's antiplatelet actions, but unlike aspirin, which permanently inactivates platelet cyclo-oxygenase, NSAID's remain active only while in the bloodstream. Consequently, if necessary, heparin can be started and the NSAID held, thereby avoiding concomitant use of an anticoagulant and antiplatelet agent.

Because of their success in the treatment of myocardial infarction, *fibrinolytic agents,* such as tissue plasminogen activator (t-PA), are currently being evaluated in the management of acute stroke. Questions concerning the therapeutic window, fibrinolytic dose, local or systemic administration, and rate of hemorrhagic complications are being addressed by several multicentered trials. Results are expected in the near future.

Several recent studies have shown that the calcium channel blocker *nimodipine,* when given within the first 12 hours of symptoms, favorably but modestly affects long-term neurologic outcome in ischemic stroke. The benefit has not been seen in all studies, however, and the drug's mechanisms remain unclear.

A trial of the opiate antagonist naloxone showed no benefit. Corticosteroid administration has no benefit in acute ischemic stroke and may be harmful. Experimental studies of acute stroke suggest that antioxidants and inhibitors of excitatory amino acid neurotransmitters may have promise, and representative agents are being tested clinically. Ultimately, effective stroke treatment may employ several of these modalities.

OUTCOME AND REHABILITATION

About 10 to 15% of patients with ischemic stroke will die, some because of brain swelling or neurologic dysfunction directly related to the stroke (e.g., impaired respiration with medullary infarctions), but most because of systemic complications, such as myocardial in-

farction, pulmonary embolism, and pneumonia. Several studies show an association of stroke with subendocardial necrosis. Most large population studies report that about one fifth of patients surviving stroke require long-term institutionalization and one third to one half of the remaining are left with various disabilities. Most functional recovery takes place during the first 3 months, but some continued slow improvement is possible.

Probably because of overlapping risk factors, the leading cause of death in patients who survive the initial stroke is myocardial infarction, underscoring the importance of cardiac evaluation. Patients who have had one stroke are at increased risk of having additional ones, particularly when the first stroke is attributed to emboli of cardiac origin.

VENOUS STROKE

Although considerably less common than arterial cerebrovascular disease, venous occlusions can cause massive damage and death. As with ischemic strokes from arterial disease, the primary mechanism of brain damage is reduction in capillary blood flow, in this instance because of increased outflow resistance. Back-transmission of high pressure into the capillary bed usually results in early brain swelling from edema and superimposes a potentially severe degree of hemorrhagic infarction in subcortical white matter.

The most dangerous form of venous disease arises when the superior sagittal sinus is occluded, but obstruction of a transverse sinus or one of the major veins over the cerebral convexity (e.g., vein of Labbé) also can produce significant damage. Venous occlusions occur most commonly in association with coagulopathies, often in the puerperal period or in patients with disseminated cancer, and sometimes as a result of contiguous disease, such as infection or cancer. The transverse sinus can be occluded as a consequence of inner ear infections, producing a once common condition called otitic hydrocephalus.

With *superior sagittal sinus obstruction,* veins draining into the sinus from the superior and medial surfaces of both cerebral convexities are commonly obstructed, and thus in its early stages, the condition can result in bilateral weakness and sensory changes in the legs. This bilaterality should alert the clinician to the possibility of sinus thrombosis. Brain swelling and bilateral involvement can produce lethargy or stupor early in the course. Seizures occur more often with venous than with arterial occlusion, possibly because of the irritating effect of parenchymal blood on the cortex.

The differential diagnosis of venous obstruction can include traditional arterial strokes but more often extends to diffuse processes such as herpes simplex encephalitis and meningitis. Diagnosis depends on the recognition of impaired venous flow. Increasingly, this is detected by loss of flow artifact on MRI. On contrast CT scans, a nonenhanced triangular area surrounded by contrast in the posterior sinus (the empty "delta" sign) should suggest the diagnosis. Since MRI is not infallible, angiography is still the definitive diagnostic procedure, but attention must be directed to films showing the venous phase.

The management of venous sinus thrombosis increasingly relies on the use of heparin anticoagulation, even in the presence of superimposed parenchymal hemorrhage. Venous occlusions are serious and often fatal, but acute anticoagulation started as soon as the diagnosis is recognized appears to lessen substantially the morbidity and mortality of the condition. Anticonvulsants should be used as needed to control seizures and limit concomitant increases in CBF that might otherwise aggravate brain swelling and bleeding. Nonanticoagulated superior sagittal sinus occlusion that is not complicated by infection carries a mortality rate of 25 to 40%. Uncontrolled series suggest that early heparin therapy can reduce the mortality and morbidity by more than half.

419.2 Diffuse Ischemia

Brief diffuse cerebral ischemia causes syncope without any permanent sequelae (see Ch. 396). Prolonged diffuse ischemia, by contrast, has devastating consequences. The most common cause is cardiac asystole or other forms of overwhelming cardiopulmonary failure. Aortic dissection and global hypoxia or carbon monoxide poisoning can cause a similar picture.

Diffuse hypoxia-ischemia typically kills neurons in the hippocampus, cerebellar Purkinje cells, the striatum, and cortical layers 3, 4, and 6. Clinically, it results in unconsciousness: coma followed often by the eyes-open vegetative state. If patients do not regain consciousness within 2 to 3 days, the prognosis for return of independent function becomes very poor. Early absence of pupillary light reflexes, corneal reflexes, and reflex eye movements predict a poor outcome. Patients lacking all of these responses even within the first day of hypoxic-ischemic coma have less than a 5% chance of resuming independent activities within 1 year (see Ch. 394). Even if consciousness is regained, such patients often suffer long-term impairment of memory and sometimes a variety of sensorimotor syndromes consistent with lesions located in a boundary zone distribution.

Other than prompt and aggressive efforts to restore cardiovascular circulation, no treatments have been found to help patients who are comatose after cardiac arrest. A randomized, multi-institutional trial of barbiturates was without benefit, and corticosteroids may even be harmful. In young patients hypoxic because of drowning, evidence suggests that hypothermia may prolong resistance to ischemic damage, but therapeutic hypothermia in adults can induce cardiac arrhythmias and has not yet been tested. Chronically unconscious patients have not been shown to benefit from either physical or electrical stimulation programs.

Antiplatelet Trialists' Collaboration: Secondary prevention of vascular disease by prolonged antiplatelet treatment. Br Med J 296:320, 1988. *A meta-analysis of 31 randomized trials concluded that aspirin reduces stroke risk by 22%.*

Barnett HJ, Mohr JP, Stein BM, et al. (eds.): Stroke: Pathophysiology, Diagnosis and Management. New York, Churchill Livingstone. 1992. *A comprehensive review of the diagnosis and management of ischemic and hemorrhagic stroke.*

Brott T, Broderick J, Kothari R: Thrombolytic therapy for stroke. Curr Opinion Neurol 7:25, 1994.

Collins R, Peto R, MacMahon S, et al.: Blood pressure, stroke, and coronary heart disease, Part 2. Short-term reductions in blood pressure: Overview of randomised drug trials in their epidemiological context. Lancet 335:827, 1990. *A meta-analysis showing a strong association between even modest hypertension and stroke and striking benefits from blood pressure management.*

Easton JD, Wilterdink JL: Carotid endarterectomy: Trials and tribulations. Ann Neurol 35:5, 1994. *Review of published and ongoing trials of carotid endarterectomy for symptomatic and asymptomatic patients.*

Editorial: Left ventricular thrombosis and stroke following myocardial infarction. Lancet 335:759, 1990. *A brief summary of recommended anticoagulation therapy to reduce embolic stroke after myocardial infarction.*

Pulsinelli WA, Jacewicz M, Buchan AM: Hypoxic-ischemic disorders in stroke. *In* Johnston MD, McDonald R, Young AB (eds.): Scientific Basis of Neurologic Drug Therapy. Philadelphia, FA Davis, 1992. *Contemporary review of the pharmacologic treatment of ischemic stroke.*

Sandercock P: Recent developments in the diagnosis and management of patients with

transient ischemic attacks and minor ischemic strokes. Q J Med 78:101, 1991. *A review of current diagnosis and management of transient ischemic attacks and stroke.*

Stroke Prevention in Atrial Fibrillation Study: Preliminary report of the Stroke Prevention in Atrial Fibrillation Study. N Engl J Med 322:863, 1990. *Preliminary report of a multi-institutional study emphasizing the importance of warfarin or, at least in the nonelderly, aspirin to prevent stroke in atrial fibrillation.*

420 HEMORRHAGIC CEREBROVASCULAR DISEASE

Approximately 20% of all strokes consist of intracranial hemorrhages, half into the subarachnoid space and the remainder within the brain itself. The acute rise in intracranial pressure from arterial rupture causes loss of consciousness in approximately half the patients, and many of these die of cerebral herniation (see Ch. 443). However, since hemorrhage into the subarachnoid space or brain parenchyma causes less tissue injury than does ischemia, patients who survive often show a remarkable recovery.

Like ischemic stroke, hemorrhagic stroke can be thought of as diffuse (subarachnoid and/or intraventricular) or focal (intraparenchymal). Subarachnoid hemorrhage (SAH) is caused by rupture of surface arteries (aneurysms, vascular malformations, head trauma), with blood usually limited to the cerebrospinal fluid (CSF) space between the pial and arachnoid membranes (Table 420–1). Intracerebral hemorrhage is most frequently caused by the rupture of arteries lying deeply within the brain substance (hypertensive hemorrhage, vascular malformations, head trauma), but in some instances the force of blood from ruptured surface arteries may penetrate the brain parenchyma. Blood within the cerebral ventricles results either from reflux of subarachnoid blood through the fourth ventricular foramina or by extension from a site of intraparenchymal hemorrhage.

420.1 Aneurysmal Subarachnoid Hemorrhage

EPIDEMIOLOGY

Rupture of a saccular or "berry" aneurysm causes approximately 80% of all SAH's, 5% are caused by mycotic aneurysm rupture, and an even smaller percentage reflects bleeding from atherosclerotic, neoplastic, or dissecting cerebral aneurysms. The incidence of aneurysmal SAH is approximately 10 per 100,000 population, with 80% of these occurring in persons 40 to 65 years old, 15% in those 20 to 40 years old, and 5% in those below 20 years of age. Women are slightly more likely than men (3:2) to suffer rupture of a cerebral aneurysm, especially during pregnancy.

TABLE 420–1. CAUSES OF SPONTANEOUS INTRACRANIAL HEMORRHAGE

1. Arterial aneurysms
   a. "Berry" aneurysm
   b. Fusiform aneurysm
   c. Mycotic aneurysm
   d. Aneurysm with vasculitis
2. Cerebrovascular malformations
3. Hypertensive-atherosclerotic hemorrhage
4. Hemorrhage into brain tumor
5. Systemic bleeding diatheses
6. Hemorrhage with vasculopathies
7. Hemorrhage with intracranial venous infarction

ETIOLOGY AND PATHOGENESIS

SACCULAR ANEURYSMS. The pathogenesis of saccular aneurysms reflects a combination of congenital, acquired, and hereditary factors. Congenital defects in the muscle and elastic tissue of the arterial media, seen at autopsy in 80% of normal vessels of the circle of Willis, gradually deteriorate as they are exposed over time to the hemodynamic stresses of pulsatile blood flow. These defects lead to microaneurysmal dilatations (<2 mm) of the circle of Willis arteries in 15 to 20% of the population. Larger (>5 mm) aneurysms are found in 5% of the population, characteristically distributed at the arterial bifurcations. Eighty percent are located in the anterior, carotid artery–derived, arterial circulation; the rest lie along the bifurcations of vertebrobasilar arteries (Fig. 420–1).

The remarkably high incidence of wall defects in the media of normal vessels, the high frequency of incidental microaneurysms, and the tendency for aneurysms to enlarge with time and rupture imply that both congenital and acquired factors influence the pathogenesis of rupture. On the other hand, the relative rarity of SAH (10 per 100,000 population) suggests that other factors, possibly genetic, may predispose to aneurysm formation. A modest incidence of familial saccular aneurysms as well as their association with polycystic kidney disease, Ehlers-Danlos syndrome, and other connective tissue disorders implicates hereditary factors. Although hypertension per se is not a significant risk factor for aneurysmal SAH, aneurysms have been known to rupture under conditions associated with a sudden rise in blood pressure, including extremes of emotional excitement and physical exertion such as coitus and athletic events.

FUSIFORM ANEURYSMS. Fusiform or ectatic aneurysms acquire their name from the spindle-shaped dilatation and elongation that occur in large arteries at the site of arteriosclerotic narrowing. These aneurysms develop most frequently in the basilar artery but also may affect the internal, middle, and anterior cerebral arteries of individuals with widespread arteriosclerosis and hypertension. They rarely rupture and are difficult to treat when they do because their shape and stiff walls preclude easy surgical clipping. Progressive dilatation and the tortuous elongation of the vessel cause neurologic dysfunction most frequently by compressing surrounding structures. Typically, ectatic aneurysms of the basilar artery compress cranial nerves V, VII, and VIII, causing facial pain, hemifacial spasm, and hearing loss with vertigo, respectively. Fusiform aneurysms may initiate the features of cerebellopontine angle tumors, or they may mimic pituitary and suprasellar mass lesions.

MYCOTIC ANEURYSMS. Mycotic cerebral aneurysms are caused by septic degeneration of arterial wall muscle and elastic tissue. They form in distal cerebral arteries at the point where small septic cardiogenic emboli lodge. They are frequently multiple and can be found in either the anterior or the posterior cerebral circulation.

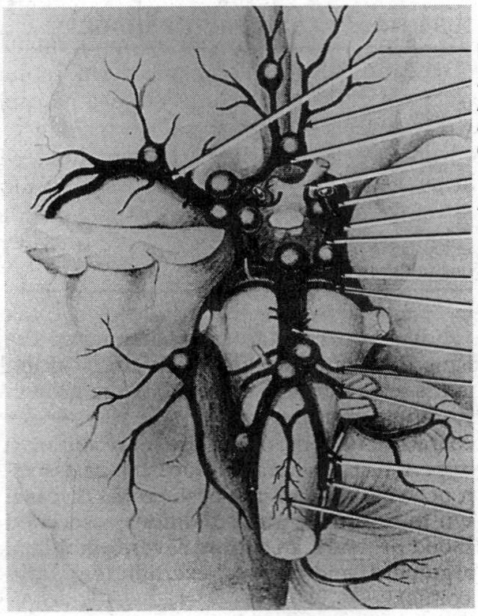

CLINICAL PRESENTATION

Prodromal signs and symptoms frequently precede the catastrophic rupture of saccular aneurysms. Focal headaches occasionally may signal compression of pain-sensitive structures from an expanding aneurysm, in which case the headache is usually progressive. They also may generate "sentinel" leaks of sudden, focal head pain. Such sentinel headaches are frequently severe and may be accompanied by nausea or vomiting or may cause meningeal irritation. Despite the similarity of these headaches to common migraine, most patients can distinguish between the two. Patients with suspected sentinel headache should have computed tomographic (CT) scans and, if these are negative, lumbar punctures to exclude active bleeding.

Compression of the oculomotor nerve by an expanding aneurysm of the posterior communicating artery at its junction with either the internal carotid or the posterior cerebral artery and, less frequently, of the superior cerebellar artery, can cause ipsilateral ophthalmoparesis, ptosis, and later pupillary dilatation with loss of the pupillary light reflex. Orbital pain frequently, but not always, accompanies these signs. The clinical picture may resemble diabetic involvement of cranial nerve III, but the latter usually spares the pupil. Other compression syndromes from cerebral aneurysms include amnesia combined with varying degrees of cranial nerve III paresis and quadriparesis from large strategically placed, basilar-tip aneurysms. Giant (>2.5 cm) aneurysms of the internal carotid artery lying within the cavernous sinus can cause unilateral ophthalmoplegia and orbital pain by compressing cranial nerves III, IV, VI, and the first division of V. Giant aneurysms of the supraclinoid portion of the internal carotid artery can produce unilateral vision loss or field defects through compression of the optic nerve or tracts.

Rupture of saccular aneurysms into the subarachnoid space seldom is associated with focal signs or symptoms. Nearly half of patients so affected lose consciousness, at least transiently, as intracranial pressure exceeds cerebral perfusion pressure. Approximately 10% of patients remain in coma for several days, depending upon the location of the aneurysm and the amount of bleeding. Patients who remain conscious and those who awaken from coma commonly recall the sudden onset as producing the "most excruciating headache" of their life. Rupture of an intracranial aneurysm in the absence of headache is rare, and some reported cases probably reflect amnesia for the event.

In addition to the frequent change in the level of consciousness, acute SAH causes meningeal irritation, nuchal rigidity, and photophobia, symptoms that may require several hours to develop. Subhyaloid retinal hemorrhages occur in 20 to 30% of patients as a result of increased intracranial pressure, raised retinal venous pressure, and dissection of blood along the optic nerve sheath. Blood pressure is frequently elevated, and body temperature usually rises, particularly during the early days after bleeding as subarachnoid blood products produce a chemical meningitis. Focal neurologic dysfunction is not a prominent feature of SAH unless there is associated compression by the aneurysm of surrounding brain structures, the jet of blood dissects directly into a clinically relevant brain region, or vasospasm occurs as a complication (see below).

LABORATORY EXAMINATION

Serum electrolytes should be measured at the time of hospital admission to serve as a baseline for detecting later complications. A complete blood count, including platelets and clotting times, should be obtained to evaluate possible infection or hematologic or clotting abnormalities. The electrocardiogram (ECG) may show various abnormalities, including heightened T waves, shortened PR intervals, peaked or inverted T waves, and increased U waves. These ECG abnormalities and subsequent arrhythmias have been attributed to multifocal myocardial necrosis caused by elevated levels of circulating catecholamines.

CT scans reveal subarachnoid blood within the basal cisterns in about three quarters of patients within 48 hours of bleeding. Magnetic resonance (MR) images have a lower index of accuracy. Detection of intracranial blood on the CT scan, however, becomes more difficult with time as blood and its breakdown products be-

FIGURE 420–1. The common sites for berry aneurysms to develop at the bifurcation of arteries on the undersurface of the brain.

Middle cerebral artery
Anterior cerebral artery
Anterior communicating artery
Ophthalmic artery
Internal carotid artery
Anterior choroidal artery
Posterior communicating artery
Posterior cerebral artery
Superior cerebellar artery
Basilar artery
Internal auditory artery
Anterior inferior cerebellar artery
Posterior inferior cerebellar artery
Vertebral artery
Anterior spinal artery

come isodense. Blood localized to the basal cisterns, the sylvian fissure, or the intrahemispheric fissure more frequently indicates rupture of a saccular aneurysm, while blood lying over the convexities or within the superficial parenchyma of the brain is more consistent with either the rupture of an arteriovenous malformation or a mycotic aneurysm. The amount and location of blood within the subarachnoid space relate directly to an aneurysm's location and the likelihood of subsequent vasospasm (see below). Importantly, an early CT scan also allows a baseline evaluation of ventricular size to compare against possible later hydrocephalus. A contrast-enhanced CT scan may aid in the identification of an arteriovenous malformation and some large (> 1.0 cm) aneurysms but should be obtained only after a noncontrast study has been completed, since contrast agents may obscure detection of subarachnoid blood.

If the CT scan fails to show blood, a lumbar puncture is diagnostic. To avoid puncture of the venous plexus lying on the anterior wall of the spinal canal, the spinal needle should be advanced slowly, with frequent removal of the trocar to detect first entry of the subarachnoid space. A traumatic lumbar puncture usually can be distinguished from SAH by the failure of the latter to show a decrease in the red blood cell (RBC) count between the first and last tubes of CSF (Table 420–2). In addition, in the presence of bloody fluid, one of the CSF samples should be centrifuged immediately and the supernate examined for the presence of hematin or xanthochromia by visual inspection and testing the fluid with a benzidene (Hemoccult) stick. Red blood cells in the spinal canal begin to lyse within 2 to 3 hours, and the centrifuged supernate will then appear pink. Later (10 hours) as the hemoglobin is converted to bilirubin, the fluid develops a yellow tinge. The CSF pressure is usually elevated and may remain so for many days. Spinal fluid samples taken within the first 24 hours often show a white blood cell (WBC) count consistent with the normal circulating WBC-RBC ratio (ca. 1:1000); later samples contain increased polymorphonuclear and mononuclear cells secondary to chemical meningitis caused by breakdown products of subarachnoid blood. The CSF blood glucose level is usually normal early, but as chemical meningitis develops, the level may decline, but rarely to less than 40 mg per dl. The protein content of the CSF is usually elevated, consistent with contamination by blood (1 mg per dl fluid for every 1000 RBC's).

Cerebral angiography remains the definitive study to detect the source of SAH. In instances in which the diagnosis of aneurysmal SAH is certain, the timing and need for a cerebral angiogram should be determined by surgical considerations (see below). When diagnostic doubt exists, the angiogram should be performed immediately. Since as many as one third of patients with aneurysmal SAH harbor multiple cerebral aneurysms, both carotid and vertebral arteries should be examined. (Among patients with multiple cerebral aneurysms, almost half have identically placed aneurysms in the left and right circulation, so-called mirror aneurysms.) Cerebral angiography fails to detect the source of bleeding in 10 to 20% of cases. Such patients are thought to have a better prognosis, with only a 1 to 2% annual chance of recurrent SAH. Failure to detect the source of bleeding may result from obliteration of an aneurysm through clotting; because bleeding was caused by rupture of a small, superficial venous angioma; or when hemorrhage has occurred from a spinal cord aneurysm or arteriovenous malformation (AVM). The presence of back pain or spinal cord symptoms at onset should prompt a search for a spinal source of hemorrhage. Repeat cerebral angiography is indicated 3 to 4 weeks later when the initial angiogram is negative and no other clues to the bleeding site can be found.

Cerebral angiography is recommended immediately in patients who have septic endocarditis and SAH to search for possible mycotic aneurysms. Since 25% of patients with subacute bacterial endocarditis and evidence of systemic embolism harbor one or more cerebral mycotic aneurysms, they should also undergo cerebral angiography.

LATE MEDICAL AND NEUROLOGIC COMPLICATIONS

The medical complications of SAH include cardiac myonecrosis and arrhythmias attributed to abnormal levels of circulating epinephrine. Symptomatic hyponatremia may also develop from the inappropriate secretion of antidiuretic hormone.

Late neurologic complications include *rebleeding* from the same aneurysm, cerebral *vasospasm* and its ischemic consequences, *hydrocephalus* caused by blockage of CSF outflow pathways, and occasionally *seizures*. Aneurysmal rerupture is suggested by new headache or neurologic worsening but can be diagnosed firmly only if a repeat CT scan or lumbar puncture shows the presence of new blood in the subarachnoid space. Approximately one third of patients with aneurysmal SAH rebleed during the first month, the incidence being highest during the first 2 weeks after the initial bleed. Patients with an unclipped aneurysm who survive their initial bleed for more than 1 month have a 2 to 3% yearly risk of rebleeding.

Cerebral vasospasm as diagnosed by cerebral angiography is defined as an abnormal narrowing of cerebral arteries. Vasospasm has been reported in up to 75% of patients with SAH, half of whom develop strokelike neurologic signs and symptoms. The peak onset for vasospasm is between days 3 and 14, but the complication can develop as late as 3 weeks after SAH. Arteries forming the circle of Willis and their major branches are the initial site of involvement, with more distal arteries becoming involved later. The amount and location of blood detected within the basal cisterns on CT scans correlate with the incidence and location of vasospasm.

The molecular mechanisms causing cerebral vasospasm are unknown but probably involve release of vasoactive amines and polypeptides, which pathologically influence vascular smooth muscle contraction. Vasospastic vessels show medial necrosis within the first few weeks, and later medial atrophy, subendothelial fibrosis, and intimal thickening.

Communicating hydrocephalus may develop as early as the first or second week after SAH. Patients with more extensive bleeding are more likely to develop the complication, but its incidence correlates with the amount of blood on CT images less clearly than does the development of vasospasm. Red blood cells and their breakdown products cause hydrocephalus by obstructing CSF outflow pathways at the level of the fourth ventricle and through the pacchionian granulations lining the venous sinuses. Seldom does communicating hydrocephalus require surgical treatment early after SAH.

Seizures are infrequent but occasionally complicate SAH. Seizures usually signal cortical damage either from bleeding into the neocortex or from ischemic necrosis.

TREATMENT

SACCULAR ANEURYSMS. The definitive therapy for a ruptured saccular aneurysm consists of surgical clipping of the aneurysm to prevent rebleeding. Medical therapy aims to reduce the risk of rebleeding and cerebral vasospasm and to prevent other medical complications before and after surgical intervention. Patients should be kept quiet at bed rest, with the administration of appropriate analgesics for the treatment of headache and gentle sedation. Stool softeners minimize straining with subsequently increased intracranial pressure. Hypertension should be treated, but not aggressively, since some of the elevated pressure may represent a normal compensatory mechanism to maintain cerebral perfusion pressure in the face of increased intracranial pressure or cerebral arterial narrowing. Systolic pressures in the range of 160 to 170 mm Hg and diastolic pressures in the range of 90 to 100 mm Hg are acceptable. The voltage-regulated calcium channel antagonist nimodipine should be given orally in a dosage of 60 mg every 4 hours for 21 days. Although it does not reduce the frequency of vasospasm, nimodipine lowers by one third the incidence of cerebral infarction in patients suffering SAH and cerebral vasospasm.

The effects of cerebral vasospasm can also be partly overcome by raising cerebral perfusion pressure through plasma volume expansion and pressor agents, usually phenylephrine or dopamine.

TABLE 420–2. "TRAUMATIC TAP" OR SUBARACHNOID HEMORRHAGE?

	"Traumatic Tap"	Spontaneous Subarachnoid Bleed
Xanthochromia	Absent	Onset: 4–6 hr Duration: approximately 6 wk
Red cell count (serial tubes)	Decreasing	Constant
Blood clot formation	Rapid	Slower

TABLE 420-3. HUNT CLASSIFICATION OF PATIENT'S CONDITION

Grade	Condition
0	Unruptured aneurysm
1	Asymptomatic or minimal headache and slight nuchal rigidity
1A	No acute meningeal or brain reaction but with fixed neurologic deficit
2	Moderate to severe headache, nuchal rigidity; no neurologic deficit other than cranial nerve palsy
3	Drowsiness, confusion, or mild focal deficit
4	Stupor, moderate to severe hemiparesis, possible early decerebrate rigidity and vegetative disturbances
5	Deep coma, decerebrate rigidity, and moribund appearance

Such measures, however, may raise the risk of rebleeding and should be undertaken only in patients with surgically clipped saccular aneurysms.

The optimal time to clip a ruptured saccular aneurysm remains controversial. Several studies show that patients with a Hunt grade (Table 420-3) of 1 to 3 do best if the aneurysm is clipped within 24 to 36 hours of the onset of bleeding. Otherwise, an increasingly accepted approach is to operate either within the first 3 days or after days 10 to 14. The logic relates to the timing of intrinsic rebleeding and the onset of cerebral vasospasm. Since the incidence of aneurysmal rebleeding is highest during the first 2 weeks after SAH and the mortality associated with each bleed approaches 40 to 50%, the aneurysm should be clipped as soon as possible. Nevertheless, undertaking aneurysmal surgery in the presence of active vasospasm has been associated consistently with poor neurologic outcomes. As a result, most surgeons avoid operating during days 3 to 10, when maximal cerebral vasospasm is likely. In patients whose aneurysm is clipped early, preliminary studies suggest that lysing blood clots in the basal cisterns with fibrinolytic drugs, followed by washing the blood out, may reduce subsequent vasospasm. Aneurysmal clipping should be delayed until 10 to 14 days after the last documented SAH in patients who present to hospital later than 3 days, who have active vasospasm on early cerebral angiograms, or who fall initially into a poor clinical grade (Hunt 4 and 5). In instances of delayed surgical intervention, most authorities recommend repeating the cerebral angiogram prior to surgery to rule out the continued presence of vasospasm. Some neurosurgeons also recommend postoperative angiograms to verify proper clip placement and obliteration of the aneurysm.

MYCOTIC ANEURYSMS. Unruptured mycotic aneurysms should be treated with antibiotics appropriate for the infecting organism and followed angiographically. Single aneurysms and those in surgically accessible areas should be considered for prompt surgical clipping.

PROGNOSIS

The mortality rate from aneurysmal SAH amounts to a daunting 50 to 60% after 1 year. Almost half such patients die before reaching the hospital, and most of the remaining die during the first month. An equally high mortality accompanies each episode of rebleeding. Approximately 25% of survivors have persistent neurologic deficits.

Unruptured cerebral aneurysms detected incidentally during cerebral angiography bleed at a yearly rate of 1 to 3%. Aneurysm size is strongly associated with the likelihood of rupture, so that saccular aneurysms less than 5 mm should be followed carefully, aneurysms between 5 and 10 mm may be considered for surgical clipping, and those greater than 10 mm should be clipped at the earliest convenience. The experience of the surgical team critically affects decisions and outcome concerning such treatment.

420.2 Hemorrhage from Vascular Malformations

CLASSIFICATION AND EPIDEMIOLOGY

Congenital vascular malformations of the brain and spinal cord fall into five categories according to vessel size and type. *Venous angiomas,* the most common cerebrovascular malformations, are composed entirely of veins and usually lie close to the brain's surface. Hemorrhage from a venous angioma is uncommon and rarely fatal. Nevertheless, these lesions have gained considerable attention, since they are readily detected by CT scans. They seldom produce seizures or headaches. A cerebral *varix* is a single dilated vein and very rarely causes clinical symptoms.

Telangiectasias are uncommon vascular anomalies composed of tangles of small, capillary-like vessels. They are usually located deep in the brain (diencephalon, brain stem, cerebellum) and rarely produce symptoms. Because of their strategic location, hemorrhage from these small vessels can occasionally be fatal.

Cavernous angiomas are large sinusoidal channels served by large feeding arteries and veins. Many of the channels thrombose, and the remainder have very low blood flow, which makes their visualization on angiograms difficult. They are readily detected by CT scan and rarely bleed, but they may cause headaches and seizures.

The most common symptomatic vascular anomaly is the *arteriovenous malformation* (AVM). AVM's are composed of tangles of arteries connected directly to veins without intervening capillaries. The resulting vessels are thin walled owing to poorly developed elastic and muscle tissue within the media. The large arteries, which feed the AVM, usually show hypertrophy of the media and thickening of the endothelium. Brain tissue is usually absent from the AVM but when present is nonfunctional. AVM's can be located anywhere in the brain and can produce headaches, seizures, focal neurologic deficits, or intracranial hemorrhage. Intracranial hemorrhage from vascular malformations accounts for 1% of all strokes and 10% of all SAH's. The prevalence of AVM's among the general population is uncertain, but autopsy studies of unselected patients indicate that 4 to 5% harbor some form of vascular malformation, of which only 10 to 15% produce symptoms. Familial cases of AVM's are rare, indicating that the problem reflects sporadic abnormalities in embryologic development.

CLINICAL PRESENTATION

Most AVM's manifest with intracranial hemorrhage, a lower proportion causing seizures or progressive neurologic disability as first symptoms. The initial hemorrhage tends to occur during the second through fourth decades, with the risk of rebleeding averaging approximately 6 to 7% the first year, 2% after 5 years, and 1 to 2% thereafter. The decline in the incidence of rebleeding with time may reflect the spontaneous thrombosis of arterial feeders. The initial and subsequent hemorrhages are associated with a 10% chance of death. If the rebleed rate of 1 to 2% is maintained for life, the young individual who presents with a hemorrhagic AVM faces a 50 to 60% chance of an incapacitating or fatal repeat hemorrhage during a normal lifespan.

AVM's may bleed into the subarachnoid space, into the brain parenchyma, or into the ventricular system. Focal neurologic signs and symptoms depend upon the severity of the bleed and the extent to which brain parenchyma has been destroyed. Bleeding into the subarachnoid space is usually less severe than with saccular aneurysms, and blood tends to localize over the cerebral convexities rather than in the basal cisterns. The incidence of cerebral vasospasm with AVM hemorrhage appears less than for aneurysm SAH, perhaps because less blood accumulates around the large arteries at the base of the brain. No explanation has been provided for the observation that small AVM's (< 2.5 cm) tend to bleed more frequently than do large AVM's (> 5 cm).

Approximately one third of patients who harbor an AVM present with seizures, of which about half have a focal onset. Focal neurologic deficits independent of seizures also develop, resulting from vascular thrombosis and brain tissue hypoperfusion caused by either vascular compression or a "steal" syndrome. Shunting of blood through arteriovenous fistulas may draw blood away from normal brain tissue, causing hypoperfusion and dysfunction of the brain proximal to the AVM. With treatment of the AVM, either through surgical resection or by embolization of the feeding arteries, some of these focal neurologic signs may improve or disappear. Approximately 10% of patients with AVM's have a history of headache, the location of which seldom coincides with the site of the AVM. Some AVM-associated headaches closely resemble migraine, but unlike migraine, most AVM-associated headaches rarely alternate between the two sides of the head.

LABORATORY EXAMINATION

The laboratory evaluation for intracranial hemorrhage from an AVM is similar to that described for aneurysmal SAH. A CT scan with contrast is diagnostic in approximately 85% of patients. MR images are equally, if not more, effective in diagnosis. Angiography remains the definitive test to identify the AVM and delineate its feeding arteries and draining veins. Since approximately 10% of AVM's are associated with saccular aneurysms, four-vessel angiography is indicated even if the AVM is defined by unilateral carotid injection. In addition, extracranial or contralateral arteries occasionally supply intracranial AVM's and should be considered in the angiographic evaluation.

TREATMENT

Uncertainties concerning the natural history of unruptured AVM's, as well as the efficacy and complications associated with newer forms of interventional therapy, make it difficult to define a simple set of guiding therapeutic principles. Generally speaking, unruptured AVM's that manifest with either seizures or headache may be treated conservatively, especially in patients older than 55 to 60 years. In such patients, hypertension should be controlled, platelet antiaggregating agents and anticoagulants avoided, and anticonvulsants given to control the seizures.

Interventional therapeutic options include surgical resection of the AVM, embolization of the feeding arteries, or radiation-induced thrombosis. Various considerations, including age, degree of neurologic dysfunction, and location of the AVM, must be considered when choosing treatment. The present custom is to treat younger patients (<55 years) more aggressively, resecting surgically accessible AVM's, since removal of the AVM and *all* its arterial feeders is curative. In older patients or if the AVM lies in language-vulnerable areas or deep in the brain, use of focused gamma x-rays or proton beam radiation is safer but only effective in lesions less than 3 cm in diameter. Embolization of the feeding arteries is rarely recommended as the sole interventional therapy, since such an approach totally obliterates the arterial feeders in only about 40% of cases. Arterial embolization is frequently used in conjunction with either surgery or focused radiation therapy.

420.3 Focal Cerebral Hemorrhage

Focal hemorrhage occurs spontaneously in three common settings: hypertension, ruptured AVM's, and amyloid (or congophilic) angiopathy. Additional contributing causes are excessive anticoagulation, systemic bleeding diatheses, and trauma.

EPIDEMIOLOGY

In the United States, primary intracerebral hemorrhage occurs with an incidence of about 12 per 100,000 population, a rate similar to that for SAH but only 10% that for ischemic stroke. Age-adjusted rates for men are about 50% higher than for women, and rates for blacks are over twice those for whites. As with ischemic stroke, the incidence appears to be declining; excluding hemorrhage associated with anticoagulation, the rate in Rochester, Minnesota, fell from about 15 per 100,000 in 1945 to 5 per 100,000 in the early 1970's. The incidence of hypertension also declined in frequency during the same period, but no conclusive data link the two trends.

PATHOLOGY

The pathologic picture of primary intracerebral hemorrhage typically consists of a large confluent area of blood that clots and then weeks later begins slowly to be phagocytosed; after several months, the only residuum may be a small, collapsed cavity lined by hemosiderin-containing macrophages. Although hemorrhages may destroy brain tissue locally, histologic examination suggests that displacement of normal brain tissue and dissection along fiber tracts account for much of the pathology.

PATHOGENESIS

Hypertension can produce hemorrhages throughout the brain, but usually they occur in four central locations: external capsule–putamen, internal capsule–thalamus, central pons, and cerebellum (Fig. 420–2). A smaller number arise in the subcortical white matter, especially in the polar regions of the frontal, temporal, and occipital lobes. Bleeding producing central hemorrhages is believed to result from rupture of microaneurysms in small, intracerebral arteries (50 to 150 μm in diameter). The pathology of the microaneurysms includes replacement of normal lining endothelium, media, and elastic tissue with fibrous tissue and fat. Similar changes can lead to necrotic vascular degeneration, which, along with microaneurysms, predisposes to hemorrhage. A strong relationship links microaneurysms to hypertension; in one autopsy series, microaneurysms were found in 46 of 100 hypertensive brains and in 85% of hypertensive persons with hemorrhages, but in only 7 of 100 normotensive brains.

Amyloid (or congophilic) angiopathy is a pathologic diagnosis, increasingly encountered in the elderly. Unrelated to generalized amyloidosis and occasionally hereditary, the condition often appears in the brains of patients with Alzheimer's disease and has been associated with nonhypertensive hemorrhages in the cerebral polar and white matter areas (Fig. 420–2). It is rare in patients under age 55. Amyloid deposits, chemically related to those in Alzheimer plaques, are seen in the media and adventitia of medium- and small-sized arteries. Multiple small hemorrhages may be associated with the condition.

Anticoagulation, fibrinolysis, and other hematologic abnormalities can be associated with intracerebral hemorrhages. Warfarin anticoagulation has been implicated in about 10% of primary intracerebral hemorrhages. With the less aggressive programs of low-dose warfarin anticoagulation (target prothrombin time ratio of 1.2 to 1.5) now used for peripheral venous disease and to prevent arterial embolism, the rate of intracranial bleeding in one recent study had fallen to under 1% with 2 years of treatment. Data from large-scale studies of fibrinolysis (e.g., tissue plasminogen activator,

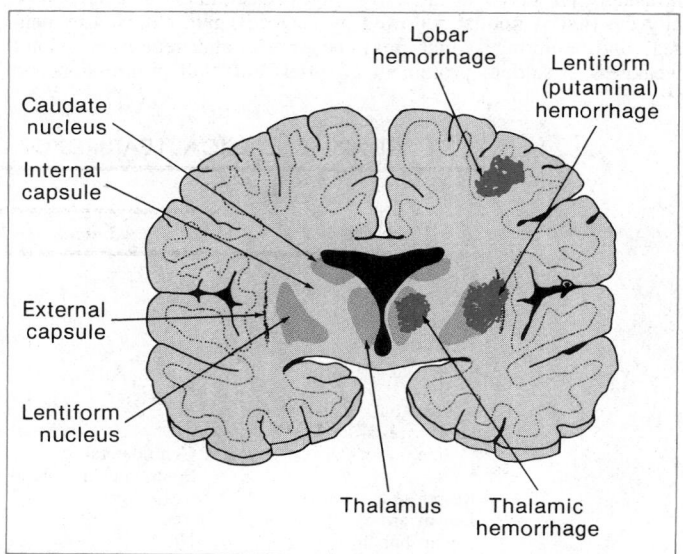

FIGURE 420–2. A coronal section through the cerebral hemispheres illustrating thalamic, putaminal, and lobar subcortical hemorrhages.

t-PA) in acute myocardial infarction indicate that at a total t-PA dose no greater than 100 mg, the rate of symptomatic intracerebral hemorrhage is only about 0.5% (although in one small series, it was 5%); at higher doses of 150 mg, the rate rises to about 1.5%. Cerebral hemorrhages occur in *leukemia, polycythemia, hemophilia,* and other clotting abnormalities, and they also occur in patients using *amphetamines* and *cocaine.*

Although *trauma* causes intracerebral (as well as subarachnoid) hemorrhage, the diagnosis is usually aided by the history as well as by coexistent external signs of trauma, SAH, and, on CT scan, multifocal, inhomogeneous hemorrhages and areas of decreased density (see Ch. 487).

CLINICAL PRESENTATION

Large cerebral hemorrhages usually produce catastrophic, acute syndromes. The onset is often associated with physical (or emotional) activity; onset during sleep is rare. Common early features include alterations in consciousness, headache, nausea, and vomiting. Although uncommon, seizures occur, possibly reflecting cortical irritation by blood. With the increasing ability to recognize less dramatic hemorrhages by using CT and MRI, neurologists now realize that hemorrhages also can produce less severe dysfunction that may be indistinguishable clinically from ischemic stroke. Clinical evolution over hours is common and usually attributed to secondary brain swelling.

The clinician should be able to recognize common hemorrhagic syndromes (Table 420–4) to anticipate dangerous brain swelling and provide appropriate medical and supportive management.

PUTAMINAL HEMORRHAGE (35 TO 50%). Patients with massive putaminal hemorrhages (Fig. 420–3) become lethargic or comatose within minutes to hours of onset and concurrently develop contralateral weakness (including face) and a contralateral hemianopsia and gaze paresis (with eyes deviated toward the hemorrhage).

THALAMIC HEMORRHAGE (10 TO 15%). Some patients with thalamic hemorrhages lose consciousness early in the clinical course, but those who are awake often experience contralateral hemiparesis, sensory changes, and homonymous hemianopsia (the last often clearing quickly).

PONTINE HEMORRHAGE (10 TO 15%). Traditional teaching held that coma always accompanied the onset of pontine hemorrhage, but refined imaging shows that this is not always the case with smaller hemorrhages. In the comatose patient, small, reactive pupils are common, oculovestibular responses are lost early, and vomiting often occurs at onset. Patients usually have quadriplegia and bilateral extensor posturing.

CEREBELLAR HEMORRHAGE (10 TO 30%). Because cerebellar hemorrhage initially spares the brain stem, consciousness is usually preserved in the early stages. Occipital headache is usually the first symptom, followed by unsteady gait, clumsiness, nausea, and vomiting, which may be severe and repetitive. Motor weakness is seldom prominent at onset, but with progression and

brain stem compression, contralateral hemiparesis and caloric-resistant ipsilateral gaze paresis help to localize the lesion to the posterior fossa. Pupillary reactions are usually preserved. Further deterioration in arousal can result from several sources: extension into or compression of the brain stem, herniation of cerebellar tissue downward through the foramen magnum or upward across the tentorium, or hydrocephalus caused by obstruction of CSF flow into or out of the fourth ventricle. Prompt recognition and treatment of cerebellar hemorrhage by this stage can be life saving.

LOBAR CEREBRAL HEMORRHAGE. Lobar hemorrhages typically occur with amyloid angiopathy. The clinical presentation depends on the actual location of the hemorrhage, but there are some common features. Most patients are elderly; headache, nausea, and vomiting probably occur with about the same frequency but less intensity as in deep, hypertensive hemorrhages. Coma and seizures are less common, possibly because the bulk of the hemorrhage is comparatively small and located in subcortical white matter.

LABORATORY EXAMINATION

Noncontrast CT scans demonstrate areas of hemorrhage as zones of increased density and rule out infarction (Fig. 420–3). Spontaneous hemorrhages typically display homogeneous areas of increased density and a mass effect, whereas hemorrhagic infarctions are characterized by areas of increased density (blood) interspersed with areas of decreased density (infarction). CT does not always distinguish reliably between a primary intraparenchymal hemorrhage and a hematoma resulting from a ruptured aneurysm. Similarly, some primary intracerebral hemorrhages dissect into the ventricular or subarachnoid system, inducing secondary intraventricular hemorrhage or SAH.

The MRI picture of hemorrhage depends on the precise sequence used and the age of the hemorrhage. At present, the advantages and disadvantages of MRI in this condition remain incompletely described, particularly in the early hours after onset. One advantage of MRI is its ability to detect small hemorrhages, especially in the brain stem. Cerebral angiography is seldom used to evaluate acute hemorrhages, except those attributed to mycotic aneurysms being evaluated for surgical intervention.

TREATMENT

The management of acute parenchymal hemorrhage is supportive, but vigilance for transtentorial or foramen magnum herniation must be exercised, particularly with cerebellar hemorrhages. Incipient herniation is initially treated with hyperventilation (which takes advantage of the vasoconstricting effect of hypocapnia; see Ch. 394) and osmotic agents (e.g., mannitol), but both of these interventions lose effectiveness with time. Corticosteroids have not been effective in treating brain edema from cerebral hemorrhage, and since they carry added risks (e.g., immunologic compromise, gastrointestinal hemorrhage), they are not advocated.

Direct surgical evacuation of acute spontaneous cerebral hemorrhage seldom is justified, occasional cerebellar hemorrhages providing a possible exception. What few comparative studies are available suggest that acute surgical evacuation of hematomas from the

TABLE 420–4. CLINICAL FEATURES OF COMMON HYPERTENSIVE HEMORRHAGES

Clinical	Site of Hemorrhage			
	Putaminal	*Thalamic*	*Pontine*	*Cerebellar*
Unconsciousness	Later	Later	Early	Late
Hemiparesis	Yes	Yes	Quadriparesis	Late
Sensory change	Yes	Yes	Yes	Late
Hemianopic	Yes	Yes	No	No
Pupils:				
Size	Normal	Small	Small	Normal
Reaction	Yes	Yes or no	Yes or no	Yes
Gaze paresis:				
Side	Contralateral Sometimes ipsilateral	Contralateral	Ipsilateral	Ipsilateral
Response to calories	Yes	Yes	No	Yes or no
Downward eye deviation	Yes	No	No	
Ocular bobbing	No	No	Sometimes	Sometimes
Gait lost	No	No	Yes	Yes
Vomiting	Occasional	Occasional	Often	Severe

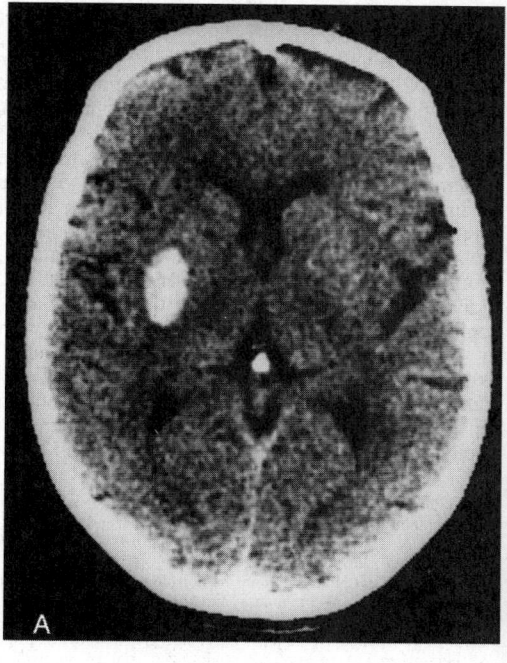
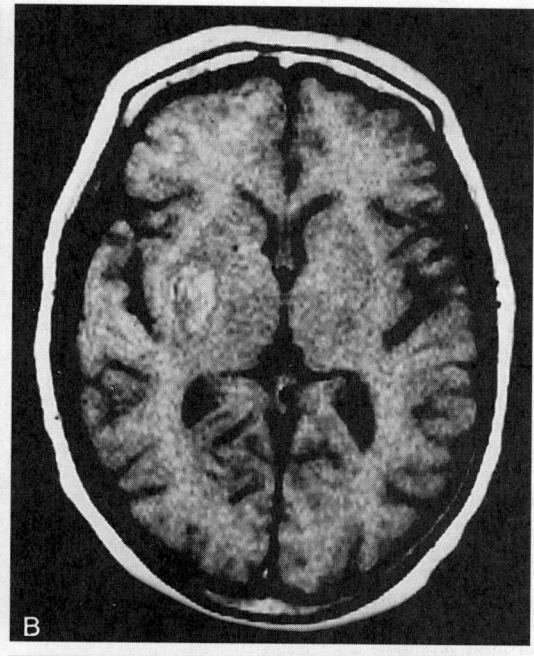
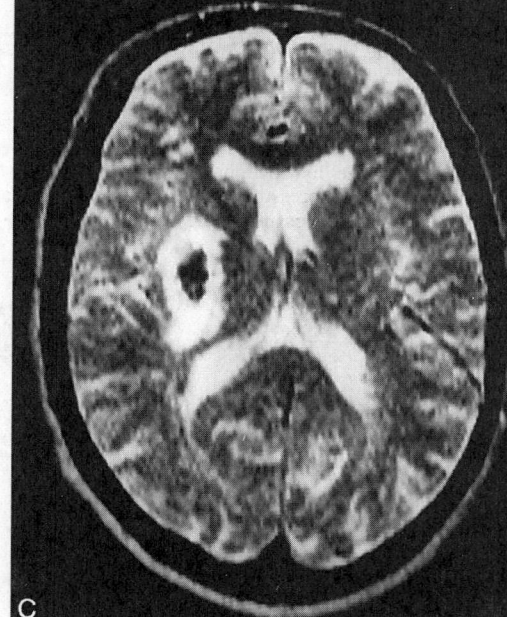

FIGURE 420-3. Hypertensive putaminal hemorrhage shown on CT at 24 hours *(A),* T₁-weighted magnetic resonance image (MRI) at 72 hours *(B),* and T₂-weighted MRI at 72 hours *(C).* Uniform hyperdensity on CT distinguishes primary hemorrhage from hemorrhagic and nonhemorrhagic infarction (compare with Fig. 419–1). The relative, though mild, hyperintensity on the T₁-weighted MRI image distinguishes hemorrhage from the hypointensity of nonhemorrhagic infarction; T₁-weighted MRI scans within 24 hours (not available for this patient) typically display more marked hyperintensity than at 72 hours. The core of the hematoma appears hypointense on the T₂-weighted MRI scan at 72 hours; T₂-weighted MRI scans within 12 hours (not available) typically show hyperintensity of greater degree than do concurrent T₁-weighted images. The rim of hyperintensity in C probably represents edema fluid. (Reproduced with permission from Zimmerman RD, et al.: AJNR 9:47–57, 1988.)

cerebral hemispheres do not substantially improve mortality and considerably increase the risk of severe residual neurologic disability if the patient survives. With the cerebellum, lateral ventricular shunting appears to produce results as good as or better (fewer neurologic residua) than surgical removal of hematomas, although lesions greater than 3 cm in diameter that continue to compress the brain stem after the shunt is placed occasionally benefit from evacuation.

As with ischemic strokes, blood pressure should not be lowered precipitously in patients with acute cerebral hemorrhage, since parenchymal blood and edema formation are likely to compress the tissue vascular bed and increase vascular resistance; an abrupt and steep reduction in systemic blood pressure could lower perfusion pressure below the critical threshold, thereby superimposing ischemic on hemorrhagic damage.

PROGNOSIS

The prognosis with intraparenchymal hemorrhage is surprisingly good in patients who survive the acute illness, but mortality is higher (30 to 40%) than in ischemic stroke (10 to 20%). As with ischemic stroke, recent studies show that about one fifth of patients surviving hemorrhage require institutionalization; in contrast to ischemic stroke, however, most of the remaining survivors of hemorrhage achieve a good status or complete recovery. Age and large hemorrhage size are associated with a worse prognosis, and prognosis after extensive brain stem hemorrhage is guarded. In contrast to SAH, the risk of recurrent hemorrhage is relatively low, the exception being that AVM's can rebleed at rates approaching 2% per year within the first several years of the initial bleed.

PROPHYLAXIS

Epidemiologic data strongly suggest that control of hypertension reduces the risk of hypertensive intraparenchymal hemorrhage. Careful control of anticoagulation and avoidance of other agents known to be associated with hemorrhage (e.g., amphetamines) should reduce the risk of hemorrhage. At present, there is no way to control the risk of bleeding from amyloid angiopathy.

420.4 Hypertensive Encephalopathy

Hypertensive encephalopathy is a syndrome that accompanies markedly elevated blood pressures. Clinically, the disorder is characterized by symptoms of increased intracranial pressure (headache, nausea, vomiting, visual blurring) and of focal neurologic dysfunction, along with seizures and progressive stupor and coma. Retinal changes characteristic of severe hypertension are common and often include hemorrhages or papilledema, but arteriolar narrowing may be the only abnormality.

The cause of neurologic dysfunction is not clearly established. One theory, largely discounted, was based on observed retinal vasospasm and suggested that similar intracerebral vasospasm caused focal ischemia and resultant neurologic dysfunction. More recent evidence rests on the observation that with severe hypertension the upper limit of cerebral arterial autoregulation is exceeded, and blood flow rises passively with further increases in systemic blood pressure. Coincidentally, progressively higher pressures are transmitted into the capillary system, causing movement of plasma and even some cellular elements from blood into surrounding brain tissue. Resulting local and diffuse edema is postulated to cause the focal and diffuse neurologic changes.

Uremia uncomplicated by hypertension can produce a similar clinical picture, but this is easily excluded by determining the blood urea nitrogen (BUN) or creatinine values. Other complications of hypertension to be considered in the differential diagnosis include hemorrhagic and ischemic stroke, but in these conditions, focal signs predominate, whereas in hypertensive encephalopathy they are accompanied by prominent signs of diffuse dysfunction. Increased intracranial pressure from obstructive hydrocephalus, brain tumor, or subdural hematoma, particularly if pressure is transmitted into the fourth ventricle, can elevate blood pressure and slow the pulse.

Usually, the absence of retinal changes suggesting chronic hypertension and the presence of signs reflecting the underlying neurologic diagnosis differentiate such neurogenic hypertension from hypertensive encephalopathy.

Hypertensive encephalopathy is a medical emergency. Treatment should be directed to acute, deliberate lowering of blood pressure (e.g., with intravenous nitroprusside), but avoiding hypotensive or even normal levels. In most patients with chronic hypertension, the upper and lower limits of autoregulation are shifted upward, and if systemic pressure is lowered below the lower limit of the patient's intrinsic autoregulation (which can rise as high as 120 mm Hg), cerebral ischemia can result. When associated with pregnancy (eclampsia), hypertensive encephalopathy usually responds well to prompt delivery of the fetus. Hypercapnia, by dilating cerebral blood vessels, can exacerbate the effects of hypertensive encephalopathy, and seizures also are associated with further increases in cerebral blood flow and capillary pressure. Both should be avoided by controlled ventilation, when required, with anticonvulsants such as intravenous diazepam, 10 to 20 mg given slowly in repeated doses as needed to control seizures, and followed by phenytoin or carbamazepine.

Brown RD Jr, Wießbers DO, Forbes G, et al.: The natural history of unruptured intracranial arteriovenous malformations. J Neurosurg 68:352, 1988. *A follow-up study of 168 patients to define the natural history of clinically unruptured intracranial AVM's.*

Dias MS, Sekhar LN: Intracranial hemorrhage from aneurysms and arteriovenous malformations during pregnancy and the puerperium. Neurosurgery 27:855, 1991. *A review article discussing risks and medical and surgical management.*

Juvela S, Heiskanen O, Potanen A, et al.: The treatment of spontaneous intracerebral hemorrhage: A prospective randomized trial of surgical and conservative treatment. J Neurosurg 70:755, 1989. *A randomized trial of 52 patients with brain hemorrhage showing that while surgery saves lives, it does not improve function.*

Kassell NF, Torner JC, Haley EC, et al.: The International Cooperative Study on the timing of aneurysm surgery. Part 1: Overall management results. J Neurosurg 73:18, 1990. *This manuscript summarizes the results of the International Cooperative Study on saccular aneurysms and documents the status of medical management in the 1980's.*

Kassell NF, Torner JC, Jane JA, et al.: The International Cooperative Study on the timing of aneurysm surgery. Part 2: Surgical results. J Neurosurg 73:37, 1990. *This manuscript describes 3521 patients with ruptured saccular aneurysms who came from 68 centers. It presents a contemporary discussion of the diagnosis of SAH, prevention of rebleeding, vasospasm, and early versus late surgical intervention.*

Section Seven—Infections and Inflammatory Disorders of the Nervous System

Roger P. Simon

421 PARAMENINGEAL INFECTIONS

Parameningeal central nervous system (CNS) infections include those that affect brain parenchyma directly (brain abscess), those that produce suppuration in potential spaces covering the brain and spinal cord (epidural abscess and subdural empyema), those that produce occlusion of the contiguous venous sinuses and cerebral veins (cerebral venous sinus thrombosis), and remote infectious processes (bacterial endocarditis and sepsis) that result in diffuse, multifactorial involvement of the CNS.

BRAIN ABSCESS

Brain abscess is an uncommon disorder accounting for only 2% of intracranial mass lesions. Abscesses produce localized, circumscribed, enlarging CNS infections that produce symptoms and findings similar to those of other space-occupying lesions, such as brain tumors. Brain abscesses, however, often progress more rapidly than tumors and more frequently affect meningeal structures.

ETIOLOGY. Infections resulting in brain abscess originate or extend from extracerebral locations. Although the most frequent predisposing factors have changed over the past decades and vary with a hospital's population and referral base, the most common (Table 421–1) are bloodborne metastases from unknown sources and from lung or heart, direct extension from parameningeal sites (otitis, cranial osteomyelitis, sinusitis), recent or remote head trauma or neurosurgical procedures, and infections associated with cyanotic congenital heart disease. Bloodborne infections seed the brain via hematogenous spread and produce abscesses in brain re-

TABLE 421-1. SUMMARY OF UCSF CASES ACCORDING TO TIME PERIODS

	1970–1974	1975–1980	1981–1986	Total
Number of Cases	22	33	47	102
Etiology				
Local infection	2(9)	4(12)	13(28)	19(19)
Cardiac	6(27)	6(18)	5(11)	17(17)
Surgery	1(4)	7(2)	8(17)	16(16)
Trauma	2(9)	1(3)	6(13)	9(9)
Pulmonary	4(18)	4(12)	1(2)	9(9)
Immunocom-promise	2(9)	2(6)	2(4)	6(6)
Other	1(4)	4(12)	0(0)	5(5)
Unknown	4(18)	4(12)	13(28)	21(21)
Organisms				
Aerobic	16(73)	27(82)	34(72)	77(75)
Anaerobic	5(23)	8(24)	7(15)	20(20)
Multiple	5(23)	8(24)	7(15)	20(20)
None cultured	6(27)	6(18)	14(30)	26(25)
Deaths	9(41)	3(9)	2(4)	14(14)

Figures in parentheses indicate percentages.
Adapted with permission from Mampalam TJ, Rosenblum ML: Trends in the management of bacterial brain abscesses: A review of 102 cases over 17 years. Neurosurgery 23:451, 1988.

TABLE 421-2. BRAIN ABSCESS: PRESENTING FEATURES IN 43 CASES

Headache	72%
Lethargy	71%
Fever	60%
Nuchal rigidity	49%
Nausea, vomiting	35%
Seizures	35%
Ocular palsy	27%
Confusion	26%
Visual disturbance	21%
Weakness	21%
Dysarthria	12%
Stupor	12%
Papilledema	10%
Dysphasia	9%
Hemiparesis	9%
Dizziness	7%

Reproduced with permission from Chan CH, Johnson JD, Hofstetter M, et al.: Brain abscess: A study of 45 consecutive cases. Medicine 65:415, 1986.

gions in proportion to the blood flow; accordingly, parietal lobe abscesses predominate. Extension of infection from otitis and mastoiditis involves contiguous brain regions of the temporal lobe and cerebellum, whereas abscesses resulting from sinusitis affect the frontal and temporal lobes. Currently, the most common cause of brain abscess in many urban hospitals is toxoplasmosis occurring in immunodeficiency states due to co-infection with the human immunodeficiency virus (HIV).

PATHOLOGY. On the basis of findings of clinical and experimental research, most brain abscesses evolve over a number of stages, beginning with vascular seeding of brain parenchyma, producing early cerebritis during the first 1 to 3 days. Inflammatory infiltrates of polymorphonuclear cells, lymphocytes, and plasma cells follow within 24 hours. By 3 days, the surrounding area shows a marked increase in perivascular inflammation. The late cerebritis phase develops approximately 4 to 9 days after infection, during which time the center becomes necrotic, containing a mixture of debris and inflammatory cells. Neovascularity is maximal at this time. Early reactive astrocytes surround the zone of infection and proceed to early capsule formation between approximately 10 and 13 days. At this time, the necrotic center shrinks slightly, and a well-developed peripheral fibroblast layer evolves. The late capsule stage continues to evolve between 14 days and 5 weeks, with continual shrinking of the necrotic center and a *relative decrease* in the inflammatory cells. The capsule thickens as reactive astrocytes proliferate.

BACTERIOLOGY. The pathogenic organisms vary considerably, depending on the clinical circumstances. *Staphylococcus aureus* is the most common isolate in trauma-related cases. In patients with HIV-associated disease, *Toxoplasma* is the most common organism and bacterial abscesses are rare. Among other abscesses, the most commonly isolated pathogens are anaerobic organisms, but aerobic and microaerobic streptococci, *Staphylococcus aureus, Bacteroides, Proteus,* and other gram-negative bacilli may also be found (Table 421-1). *Actinomyces, Nocardia,* and *Candida* are less frequent offenders. Infection is often polymicrobial. Culture-negative abscesses from surgical specimens occur in 30% of antibiotic-treated patients and in 5% of patients operated on before antibiotic administration.

CLINICAL PRESENTATION. Signs of infection may be minimal or absent. Almost half of affected patients maintain a normal body temperature, and fewer than a third show a peripheral white cell count above 11,000 per microliter. Neck stiffness is rare in the absence of increased intracranial pressure.

Otherwise, the presenting features resemble those of any expanding intracranial mass (Table 421-2). A headache of recent onset is the most common symptom, representing distortion or irritation of pain-sensitive structures within the cranial vault, especially those of the great venous sinuses and the dura about the base of the brain. If the process continues untreated, isolated headache will increase in

severity and become accompanied by focal signs such as hemiparesis or aphasia, followed by obtundation and coma. The period of evolution may be as brief as many hours or as long as many days to weeks with more indolent organisms. Seizures may occur with abscesses involving the cortical gray matter.

CEREBROSPINAL FLUID EXAMINATION. Cerebrospinal fluid (CSF) examination is not useful in diagnosis because the findings range from normal to those of purulent meningitis, depending on the walling off of the brain abscess or its closeness to CSF compartments (Table 421-3). More important, because abscesses often expand rapidly, lumbar puncture may aggravate impending transtentorial herniation. If possible, the procedure should be deferred until after brain images are obtained, which may eliminate the need for CSF analysis.

NEUROIMAGING. CT and MR are the imaging studies of choice for brain abscesses and monitoring their response to therapy. MRI is especially useful for posterior fossa abscesses, as it provides an artifact-free view of the brain stem and cerebellum. In addition, MRI with intravenous gadolinium contrast is superior in demonstrating cerebritis surrounding edema, the extent of mass effect, or associated venous thrombosis. MRI with or without gadolinium is preferable to CT for demonstrating multiple lesions.

The evolution of the abscess can be followed radiologically. In the early cerebritis stage, CT images reveal a low-density lesion

TABLE 421-3. SUMMARY OF LUMBAR FLUID CHANGES ASSOCIATED WITH BRAIN ABSCESS*

	Number of Patients	Per Cent
Pressure		
<200 mm	38	38
200–300 mm	35	35
>300 mm	26	26
Total	99	
White cells per mm³		
<5	61	29
5–100	81	38
>100	71	33
Total	213	
Protein (mg per dl)		
<50	26	24
50–100	38	35
>100	44	41
Total	108	
Glucose (mg per dl)		
>40	89	79
<40	23	21
Total	112	

* Most of these data were obtained before brain imaging was widely available.
Reproduced with permission from Fishman RA: Cerebrospinal Fluid in Diseases of the Nervous System. Philadelphia, WB Saunders, 1980, p 264.

with partial ring enhancement. In the late cerebritis and early capsule stage, well-formed ring-enhancing lesions are seen. The ring enhancement is typically thin walled and uniform, with subtle medial thinning adjacent to the ventricular system. Thick, nonuniform, or nodular enhancement should raise suspicion of an alternative cause. Delayed contrast scans show diffusion of contrast material into the lucent center. In the late capsule stage, well-formed ring enhancement may be seen with no delayed diffusion of contrast. Other ring-enhancing lesions that may mimic the image of brain abscess include primary and metastatic tumor, a resolving infarct or hematoma, and, rarely, demyelinating disease.

TREATMENT. Pyogenic brain abscesses are treated with antibiotics combined with surgical aspiration or excision. Aspiration offers the advantage of identifying the infecting organism and may be performed stereotactically with CT guidance while the patient is under local anesthesia; excision requires craniotomy. Surgical therapy is required when significant mass effect is present, when the abscess adjoins the ventricular surface (raising the possibility of catastrophic rupture into the ventricular system), when abscesses arise in the posterior fossa (with the potential of brain stem compression), or when abscesses reach a large size (>cm diameter) or become refractory to medical therapy. In selected cases antibiotics alone are appropriate, as in the case of surgically inaccessible, multiple abscesses (seen in 10% of patients) or abscesses in the early cerebritis stage. If the causal organism is not identified, antibiotic coverage should be directed toward the most likely organisms (streptococci and anaerobes). A suggested regimen includes penicillin G, 4 million units given intravenously (IV) every 4 hours, and metronidazole, 15 mg per kilogram IV over 1 hour, followed by 7.5 mg per kilogram given IV or orally every 6 hours. If staphylococcal infection is suspected (e.g., because of a history of trauma or intravenous drug abuse), vancomycin should be added. Concomitant corticosteroid therapy may attenuate edema surrounding abscesses.

The resolution of abscesses can be followed by serial CT or MRI. Antibiotics must be continued until the abscess cavity resolves completely, usually 6 to 8 weeks, although in surgically treated patients it may be 4 weeks. A failure to demonstrate abscess shrinkage in 4 weeks constitutes an antibiotic failure; a surgical procedure should then be performed. Of note is that the ring enhancement may persist after clinical and CSF normalization.

Abscesses associated with HIV infection are assumed to be due to *Toxoplasma gondii*. The diagnosis is confirmed by response to empiric treatment with daily doses of sulfadiazine, 12 to 15 mg per kilogram, given orally, and pyrimethamine, 25 to 50 mg, given orally. An alternative regimen is pyrimethamine given orally and clindamycin, 900 to 1200 mg IV every 6 hours (or 600 mg orally every 6 hours) for patients allergic to sulfa drugs.

PROGNOSIS. The current mortality rate is 5 to 15%, depending on locale and the nature of pre-existing illness. Outcome correlates inversely with the abscess size and the degree of neurologic dysfunction at presentation, but less well with age, cause, number of abscesses, or corticosteroid use.

SPINAL EPIDURAL ABSCESS

Infection within the epidural space about the spinal cord is an uncommon but readily diagnosable and treatable potential cause of paralysis and death. Its incidence is 0.5 to 1.0 per 10,000 hospital admissions in the United States, but the frequency is substantially increased in the intravenous drug-using population.

CLINICAL PRESENTATION. Patients are usually systemically ill with fever (to 38° to 39° C) in virtually all acutely evolving cases and in the majority of those with a subacute evolution. The initial feature is acute or subacute neck or back pain, with focal percussion tenderness being a prominent feature in the great majority; stiff neck and headache are common. As the infection progresses, over hours, days, or weeks, radicular pain occurs, the site varying with the location of the abscess. The pain can be mistaken for sciatica, a visceral abdominal process, chest wall pain, or cervical disc disease. If the condition goes unrecognized at this stage, the symptoms can rapidly evolve, over a few hours to a few days, to produce weakness and finally paralysis occurring distal to the spinal level of the infection. In this clinical setting, spinal epidural abscess should be assumed, systemic antibiotics begun, and urgent neuroradiologic confirmatory diagnostic procedures pursued.

The differential diagnosis includes compressive and inflammatory processes involving the spinal cord (transverse myelitis, intervertebral disc herniation, metastatic tumor), which can usually be differentiated clinically by the absence of systemic infection. Transverse myelitis, however, may be associated with fever; the most useful differential feature is its rapid evolution to maximum deficit within 24 hours or less. Other infectious processes that may produce back or neck pain or tenderness must be excluded (bacterial meningitis, perinephric abscess, disc space infection, bacterial endocarditis). *Spinal subdural empyema* can cause a similar syndrome but is much less frequent.

ETIOLOGY. Infections of the epidural space originate from contiguous spread or via hematogenous routes from a distant source. Cutaneous sites of infection are the most common remote sources, especially in intravenous drug users. Abdominal, respiratory tract, and urinary sources are also common. Osteomyelitis may be a cause by either direct extension or hematogenous spread, especially when associated with sepsis. Contiguous spread of infection occurs, most commonly from psoas abscesses, decubitus ulceration, perinephric and retropharyngeal abscesses, surgical sites, or epidurally placed catheters. Whether or not spread can occur from pelvic infections via spinal veins remains unsettled. Minor back trauma has been implicated in producing a hematoma near the spine, which is subsequently seeded via hematogenous sources.

PATHOPHYSIOLOGY. The anatomy of the epidural space dictates the location of the abscess, the frequency of epidural infections being proportional to the volume of the epidural space. Because the size of the intravertebral canal remains relatively constant while the circumference of the spinal cord changes, this is maximal in the thoracic region and least at the cervical spine enlargement. Further, as the dura about the cord is adherent to the vertebral column anteriorly, more epidural abscesses lie posteriorly and because no anatomic barriers separate spinal segments in the posterior epidural space, such abscesses usually extend over three to five or more vertebral segments.

As the epidural space is not confined rostrocaudally, there is no clear abscess cavity or focal mass to provide a situation of simple compression for spinal cord compromise in epidural abscess. Clinical signs often are substantially greater than would have been predicted from the anatomic extent of pus or granulation tissue found at surgical exploration. Further, in many instances, no frank compression is found on postmortem examination. The spinal cord dysfunction is likely to reflect toxic processes secondary to inflammation, as well as venous thrombosis, thrombophlebitis, ischemia, and edema.

BACTERIOLOGY. Causative organisms can be identified by culture or Gram stain from pus obtained at exploration (90% of cases), blood cultures (60 to 90% of cases), or CSF (20% of cases). *Staphylococcus aureus* accounts for most infections, followed by streptococci and gram-negative anaerobes. Tuberculous abscesses remain common, representing as many as 25% of cases in high-risk populations.

DIAGNOSIS. CSF examination is often performed because of associated fever and meningeal signs. The fluid usually is nonspecifically abnormal, containing normal or decreased glucose levels, a moderately elevated protein content (400 to 500 mg per milliliter), and a lymphocytic pleocytosis (22 to 150 per cubic millimeter). Spinal fluid cultures yield organisms in about 25% of cases and Gram stains are rarely positive. Almost 90% of patients show a peripheral blood leukocytosis.

Plain spine radiographs, with attention to the area of percussion tenderness, may show osteomyelitis/discitis, a compression fracture, or a paravertebral mass. Gadolinium-enhanced MRI is the study of choice for the evaluation of a suspected epidural abscess because of its superior ability to demonstrate the craniocaudal extent of the extradural soft tissue mass, associated mass effect upon the cord or cauda equina, and potential signal abnormalities within the discs, vertebral bone marrow, and spinal cord. The addition of an intravenous gadolinium contrast agent better defines central necrosis suggestive of abscess rather than cellulitis. If MRI is unavailable or technically impossible, CT with myelography usually provides adequate information. A normal plain CT alone does not exclude the diagnosis.

TREATMENT. The disease is fatal in the absence of antibiotic therapy. Unless culture and sensitivities dictate otherwise, penicillinase-resistant penicillin (nafcillin, 12 grams per day, or oxacillin, 12 grams per day) with an aminoglycoside (gentamicin, 5 mg per kilogram per day) should be started empirically as antistaphylococcal treatment for presumed bacterial infection. For confirmed *Staphlyococcus aureus* abscesses, penicillinase-resistant penicillin can be used alone, but many authorities add rifampin (300 mg every 12 hours) because of its ability to penetrate the abscess cavity. Therapy should be continued intravenously for 3 to 4 weeks in the absence of osteomyelitis and 6 to 8 weeks with associated osteomyelitis. Surgical decompression was once thought to be mandatory in all cases; now early diagnosis by CT or MRI scans allows for effective medical therapy prior to occurrence of neurologic complications. Medical management of cervical epidural abscess requires close neurologic monitoring because of the small space available for abscess expansion and the high potential for quadriparesis. If blood cultures are negative, needle aspiration or laminectomy may be necessary to determine the causative organism.

PROGNOSIS. The chances of partial or complete recovery relate inversely to the amount of neurologic dysfunction at the time of diagnosis. Patients with abnormalities limited to pain recover without deficit. Approximately half the patients with some weakness have complete resolution, and nearly half the patients with paralysis of less than 36 hours' duration show some recovery of motor function. In tuberculous epidural abscess, recovery of motor function has been reported even after paralysis lasting for weeks.

VENOUS SINUS THROMBOSIS SECONDARY TO INFECTION

Thrombosis of cerebral veins or sinuses may be of idiopathic origin (see Ch. 419), may occur in the setting of hematologic disorders or coagulation abnormalities (see Ch. 153), or may result from local or contiguous infectious processes. The last-named syndromes are dealt with here.

Venous drainage from the brain begins with venules and veins that drain into the great venous sinuses. The venous sinus system itself lacks valves, permitting retrograde propagation of clots or infections emanating from structures such as those located in the central portion of the face or the middle ear.

Septic Cavernous Sinus Thrombosis

The cavernous sinuses comprise the most caudal dural venous chambers at the skull base. The paired structures lie on either side of the pituitary fossa, immediately above the midline sphenoid sinus. The cavernous sinus encloses the "cavernous portion" of the internal carotid artery; the third, fourth, and sixth cranial nerves en route to the apex of the orbit; and the ophthalmic and maxillary branches of the trigeminal nerve, which supply sensation to the forehead, periocular regions, cornea, and malar area of the face. Septic cavernous sinus thrombosis most commonly results from extension of infections involving the neighboring sphenoid and ethmoid sinuses, the central portion of the face, or the pharynx or tonsils.

Presenting symptoms are headache and/or lateralized facial pain, followed in a few days to weeks by fever, and involvement of the orbit, producing proptosis and chemosis secondary to obstruction of the ophthalmic vein. Paralysis of oculomotor nerves follows rapidly. Sensory dysfunction in the first and second divisions of the trigeminal nerve and a decrease in the corneal reflex are less obvious. Further involvement of the contiguous orbital contents follows, with mild papilledema and decreased visual acuity, sometimes progressing to blindness. Extension to the opposite cavernous sinus or to other intracranial sinuses with cerebral infarction, or increased intracranial pressure secondary to impaired venous drainage can result in stupor, coma, and death.

The differential diagnosis includes carotid cavernous sinus fistula (diagnosed by ocular bruit and an afebrile state); idiopathic granulomatous involvement of the cavernous sinus (the Tolosa-Hunt syndrome) or orbit (orbital pseudotumor, diagnosed by relative sparing of the orbital contents); and orbital cellulitis (infection localized to the orbit but sparing the structures of the cavernous sinus). Some overlap often occurs between involvement of these contiguous structures of the orbit and involvement of the cavernous sinus.

The CSF is abnormal in almost all cases, sometimes with a profile resembling that of purulent meningitis or parameningeal infection.

The most common causative organism is *Staphylococcus aureus*, with streptococci and pneumococci being less common; anaerobic infection has been reported. Radiologic evaluation includes sinus imaging, with attention to the sphenoid and ethmoid sinuses. MRI (with and without intravenous gadolinium contrast) can often demonstrate venous thrombosis by illustrating the lack of the normal "flow void" within vascular structures. Cranial CT scans, employed with or without intravenous contrast material, are less helpful but may show a subtle increase in size and enhancement on the thrombosed sinus. MR angiography may demonstrate extrinsic narrowing of the intracavernous portion of the internal carotid artery.

Treatment relies on early diagnosis and consists of the prompt drainage of infected paranasal sinuses as well as specific antistaphylococcal agents, such as nafcillin or oxacillin, given intravenously. Heparin anticoagulation may reduce morbidity from associated brain ischemia, but this treatment remains controversial in cases involving infection.

Lateral Sinus Thrombosis

Septic thrombosis of the lateral sinus results from acute or chronic infections of the middle ear. The symptoms consist of ear pain followed by headache, nausea, vomiting, and vertigo, evolving over several weeks. On examination, most patients are febrile. An abnormality on otologic examination is nearly invariable; mastoid swelling may be seen. Sixth cranial nerve palsies can occur, but other focal neurologic signs are rare. Papilledema occurs in half the cases, and elevated CSF pressure is present in most, especially with occlusion of the right lateral sinus (which is the major venous conduit from the superior sagittal sinus). CSF contents are usually normal, although a perimeningeal inflammatory profile may be seen.

Treatment includes intravenous antibiotics to cover staphylococci and anerobes (nafcillin or oxacillin with penicillin or metronidazole). Surgical drainage (mastoidectomy) may be required. Increased intracranial pressure seldom needs direct treatment unless visual fields show progressive constriction. The outcome is usually favorable.

Septic Sagittal Sinus Thrombosis

This uncommon condition occurs as a consequence of purulent meningitis, infections of the ethmoid or maxillary sinuses spreading via venous channels, compound infected skull fractures, or, rarely, neurosurgical wound infections. Symptoms include manifestations of elevated intracranial pressure (headache, nausea, and vomiting) that evolve rapidly to stupor and coma. Seizures and hemiparesis may result from cortical infarction. The rate of progression, severity of symptoms, and prognosis are all related to the location of thrombosis involving the sinus. When only the anterior third of the sinus is obstructed, symptoms are less intense and evolve more slowly. If or when the thrombosis progresses to involve the middle and posterior thirds of the sinus, deterioration progresses more rapidly and outlook for recovery declines.

CSF abnormalities accompany well over half the cases. The opening pressure is increased in proportion to the extent of the sagittal sinus involvement, and a pleocytosis usually reflects the association of a meningeal or parameningeal process.

Radiologically, septic sagittal sinus thrombosis may be excluded by visualization of the normal sagittal sinus during the venous phase of cerebral angiography; the diagnosis can usually also be made by MRI, which demonstrates an abnormal increase in signal intensity (absent flow void) within the affected venous sinus. Contrast-enhanced CT scanning may reveal a contrast void lying at the junction of the transverse and sagittal sinuses (the region of the torcula); this so-called delta sign represents an intraluminal clot surrounded by contrast material.

Intravenous antibiotics should be directed at organisms recovered from the meningeal process or the meningeal site. *Staphylococcus aureus* (including the methicillin-resistant strains), β-hemolytic streptococci, pneumococci, and gram-negative aerobes such as *Klebsiella* are the most common organisms. Initial antibiotic treatment should include vancomycin and a third-generation cephalosporin. Associated paranasal sinusitis should be drained surgically. Heparin use has been little tested in septic venous thrombosis, but experience with noninfected sinus thrombosis has shown it to reduce both morbidity and mortality appreciably (see Ch. 419).

Neurologic Complications of Infectious Endocarditis

Neurologic complications occur in one third of patients with bacterial endocarditis and triple the general mortality rate of the disease. Most of these complications derive from valvular vegetations. Cerebral (but not systemic) emboli are more common from mitral valve endocarditis, for reasons unknown. The time of embolization during the course of endocarditis depends upon the virulence of the organism and whether it produces acute or subacute disease. With acute endocarditis (predominantly staphylococci or enterococci), embolization occurs early, often during the first week, while in subacute disease (predominantly viridans group streptococci or enterococci) emboli occur over the full course of treatment and occasionally after treatment is completed. Emboli lodge in the peripheral branches of the middle cerebral artery, in most cases with resultant hemiparesis. Focal seizures may result.

Whether or not warfarin anticoagulation decreases the risk of embolization remains a controversial issue. This therapy was administered in an earlier period to decrease platelet fibrin vegetations that sequestered the bacteria away from the body's defenses. Current evidence suggests a high rate of hemorrhagic intracerebral complications from warfarin anticoagulation in native valve endocarditis, but not in prosthetic valve endocarditis. Mechanisms to explain the difference remain unknown. Nevertheless, most authorities believe that patients already receiving chronic anticoagulation at the time of diagnosis of endocarditis should be maintained on such therapy.

Mycotic aneurysms complicate endocarditis in 2 to 10% of cases and are more common in acute than subacute disease. The middle cerebral artery is most commonly involved, with the aneurysms being located distally in the vessel, differentiating them from congenital berry aneurysms. The process by which the aneurysmal dilatation occurs remains in dispute, although embolization of infectious vegetations is accepted as the inciting event. Aneurysmal rupture results in 80% mortality, and early diagnosis is therefore important. Whom to subject to angiography is uncertain. However, clinical or radiologic evidence of cerebral or other embolization defines the high-risk group. Other suggested indications for angiography include severe headache (presumably the result of aneurysmal leakage). When an unruptured aneurysm is identified by angiography, it may resolve with antibiotic therapy alone. Such patients need a follow-up angiogram to document an interval decrease in aneurysm size. Otherwise, surgical therapy requires excision of the infected portion of the artery. Patients with proximal mycotic aneurysms have a greater risk of perioperative stroke than do those with distal involvement.

Small brain abscesses may complicate the course of endocarditis, but macroscopic abscesses are rare, most occurring in the setting of acute, rather than subacute, endocarditis. Multiple microabscesses, however, can result in a diffuse encephalopathy similar to that seen in sepsis. Such lesions may escape detection on CT scanning and are not amenable to surgical drainage. Antibiotic treatment of the primary disease is indicated.

A CSF pleocytosis occurs in 70% of patients with neurologic complications, but in an unknown number of patients in whom the CNS is clinically spared. The CSF profile may be that of a purulent meningitis (polymorphonuclear predominance, elevated protein level, and low glucose level) or that of a perimeningeal infection (lymphocytic predominance, modest protein elevation, and normal glucose level). A hemorrhagic component may be seen. Purulent CSF is associated with signs of meningeal irritation and infection with a virulent organism.

SUBDURAL EMPYEMA

Empyema refers to infection in a preformed space, in this case that separating the dura and arachnoid. Subdural empyema is responsible for one fifth of localized intracranial infections and results from direct or indirect extension from infected paranasal sinuses via a retrograde thrombophlebitis or, less frequently, untreated chronic otitis. Unilateral empyema is most common, as the falx prevents passage across the midline, but bilateral and/or multiple concurrent empyemas occur. Cortical venous thrombosis or brain abscess develops in approximately one fourth of cases; purulent meningitis is a less common accompaniment.

Symptoms initially reflect those of chronic otitis or sinusitis, upon which lateralized headache (a universal feature), fever, and obtundation become superimposed. Vomiting, meningeal signs, and focal neurologic abnormalities (hemiparesis or seizures) usually follow. If the disease remains untreated, obtundation progresses, and the septic mass and swollen underlying brain soon lead to venous thrombosis or death from herniation. The major differential diagnosis is that of meningitis. Nuchal rigidity and obtundation occur in both, but papilledema and lateralizing deficits are more common in empyema. Lumbar puncture, if obtained because of the suspicion of meningitis, reveals an elevated intracranial pressure accompanied by an increased protein content and a polymorphonuclear pleocytosis with usually a normal glucose concentration in the CSF. Either CT or MRI can be diagnostic of empyema, showing an extra-axial, crescent-shaped mass with an enhancing rim lying just below the inner table of the skull over the cerebral convexities or the interhemispheric fissures. MRI better detects underlying parenchymal edema as well as the infection itself.

Treatment requires both prompt surgical drainage of the empyema cavity and high-dose intravenous antibiotics directed toward organisms found at the time of craniotomy. The bacteriology of subdural empyemas is similar to that of sinusitis and cerebral abscess, discussed above. Anticonvulsants should be administered prophylactically, as seizures are common.

If cortical infarction from venous thrombosis does not occur, the prognosis is surprisingly favorable, although chronic epilepsy results in one third of patients.

CRANIAL EPIDURAL ABSCESS

Infections of the epidural space coexist most often with subdural empyema and less frequently with chronic sinusitis or otitis alone. Symptoms and signs are headache and fever with focal neurologic abnormalities due to the coexistent subdural empyema or brain abscess. The diagnosis is made with MRI or contrast-enhanced CT scan (which demonstrate a peripherally enhancing lenticular-shaped lesion in the epidural space), and the abscess is treated by surgical drainage followed by systemic antibiotics. In uncomplicated cases, the prognosis is excellent.

MALIGNANT EXTERNAL OTITIS

This necrotizing osteitis occurs in elderly patients with diabetes. The associated organism, *Pseudomonas aeruginosa,* is part of the normal flora of the external ear. In this case, it produces an external otitis that fails to respect normal anatomic boundaries. The result consists of a rapidly evolving syndrome of ear pain, facial swelling, osteomyelitis of the base of the skull, and purulent meningitis accompanied by multiple cranial nerve palsies. Urgent treatment with antipseudomonal penicillin or a third-generation cephalosporin combined with an aminoglycoside, as well as surgical debridement and drainage, is essential. The mortality rate is high.

Brain Abscess

Haimes AB, Zimmerman RD, Morgello S, et al.: MR imaging of brain abscesses. AJR 152:1073, 1989. *Reviews MRI of brain abscesses and its differential diagnosis.*

Maniglia AJ, Goodwin WJ, Arnold JE, et al.: Intracranial abscesses secondary to nasal, sinus, and orbital infections in adults and children. Arch Otolaryngol Head Neck Surg 115:1424, 1989. *Association of sinus disease with brain abscesses is reviewed.*

Patel KS, Marks PV: Management of focal intracranial infections: Is medical treatment better than surgery? J Neurol Neurosurg Psychiatry 53:472, 1990. *Discussion of the issue of nonsurgical management.*

Yang SY, Zhao CS: Review of 140 patients with brain abscess. Surg Neurol 39:290, 1993. *Clinical features, bacteriology, imaging, and treatment discussed.*

Spinal Epidural Abscess

Darouiche RO, Hamill RJ, Greenberg SB, et al.: Bacterial spinal epidural abscess. Review of 43 cases and literature survey. Medicine (Baltimore) 71:369, 1992. *A large recent series. Issue of medical versus surgical treatment addressed.*

Del-Curling O Jr, Gower DJ, McWhorter JM: Changing concepts in spinal epidural abscess: A report of 29 cases. Neurosurgery 27:185, 1990. *A recent neurosurgical series.*

Redekop GJ, Del MR: Diagnosis and management of spinal epidural abscess. Can J Neurol Sci 19:180, 1992. *Reviews 25 recent cases; presentations, treatment, outcome.*

Teman AJ: Spinal epidural abscess. Early detection with gadolinium magnetic resonance imaging. Arch Neurol 49:743, 1992. *Early imaging addressed.*

Venous Sinus Thrombosis Secondary to Infection

DiNubile MJ, Boom WH, Southwick FS: Septic cortical thrombophlebitis. J Infect Dis 161:1216, 1990. *Fourteen-year experience from a single center.*

Neurologic Complications of Infectious Endocarditis

Davenport J, Hart RG: Prosthetic valve endocarditis 1976–1987. Antibiotics, anticoagulation, and stroke. Stroke 21:993, 1990. *Anticoagulation in prosthetic valve endocarditis is readdressed.*
Jones HJ, Siekert RG: Neurological manifestations of infective endocarditis. Review of clinical and therapeutic challenges. Brain 112:1295, 1989. *Two decade experience. Central and peripheral nervous systems reviewed in addition to imaging and treatment.*

Subdural Empyema

Bok AP, Peter JC: Subdural empyema: Burr holes or craniotomy? A retrospective computerized tomography–era analysis of treatment in 90 cases. J Neurosurg 78:574, 1993. *Surgical treatment is reviewed.*
Pathak A, Sharma BS, Mathuriya SN, et al.: Controversies in the management of subdural empyema. A study of 41 cases with review of literature. Acta Neurochir 102:25, 1990. *A recent large series and literature review.*
Weingarten K, Zimmerman RD, Becker RD, et al.: Subdural and epidural empyemas: MR imaging. AJR 152:615, 1989. *MRI is described.*

Cranial Epidural Abscess

Krauss WE, McCormick PC: Infections of the dural spaces. Neurosurg Clin North Am 3:421, 1992. *Epidural and subdural infections and treatment reviewed.*

Malignant External Otitis

Johnson MP, Ramphal R: Malignant external otitis: Report on therapy with ceftazidime and review of therapy and prognosis. Rev Infect Dis 12:173, 1990. *A recent review of clinical and therapeutic aspects.*

422 NEUROSYPHILIS

The resurgence of primary and secondary syphilis (now estimated to be 14.7 cases per 100,000) first occurred in the promiscuous homosexual male population but has more recently spread to the heterosexual community via prostitutes. If untreated, approximately 7% of patients with primary syphilis infection develop some form of symptomatic neurosyphilis.

PATHOPHYSIOLOGY. Each of the neurologic manifestations of syphilis results from a chronic, insidious meningeal inflammatory process caused by treponemal invasion of the central nervous system (CNS). An inflammatory response in the cerebrospinal fluid (CSF) occurs in 34% of asymptomatic persons with syphilis, with the CSF abnormalities peaking at 13 to 18 months after the primary infection. This CNS invasion dictates the risk of future symptomatic and asymptomatic neurosyphilis, which amounts to approximately 30% following a primary infection but falls to 1% or less if CSF examination is normal 5 years after the primary infection (Merritt, 1946).

CLINICAL SYNDROMES. The clinical manifestations of neurosyphilis are divided into acute syphilitic meningitis, cerebrovascular syphilis, syphilitic dementia (general paresis), and tabes dorsalis. These entities, however, overlap clinically. For instance, paresis and tabes may coexist (taboparesis). After primary infection, these clinical subtypes of neurosyphilis follow a predictable time course (Fig. 422–1) based on the evolution of the meningeal inflammatory process. Symptomatic syphilitic meningitis is the earliest manifestation of nervous system syphilis. The meningeal inflammation later extends to involve the cerebral blood vessels and, when symptomatic, results in cerebrovascular neurosyphilis (usually seen within the first 5 years following primary infection). The so-called parenchymal forms of neurosyphilis (paresis and tabes) develop after a more protracted interval.

Acute Syphilitic Meningitis. Symptomatic meningeal syphilis occurs during the first months to a year or two after the primary infection, with 10% of cases occurring coincident with a secondary rash. The course is subacute. Headache is common, and asymmetric cranial nerve abnormalities are prominent (especially those involving auditory function, facial strength, eye movements, and unilateral or bilateral papilledema due to involvement of the optic nerve). Patients are afebrile; meningeal signs are often present, and some experience at least a degree of confusion. The CSF usually contains syphilitic antibodies and shows a lymphocytic pleocytosis. Accurate diagnosis is important, as mild symptoms may resolve without treatment and leave the patient at risk for progression to the fixed deficits associated with the later forms of neurosyphilis.

Cerebrovascular Syphilis. As the meningeal inflammatory process progresses, a diffuse vasculitis evolves, compromising the cerebral arteries traversing the subarachnoid space and producing a subacute encephalopathy with ischemia-caused focal features. Associated symptoms include confusion, personality change, and intellectual decline, usually followed by the emergence of focal deficits resulting from occlusion of specific vessels. Branches of the middle cerebral artery are most often involved, but any cerebral or spinal vascular bed may be affected alone or in combination, with ischemic lesions evolving over a period of several hours or days. The resulting syndrome differs from thromboembolic stroke because of the associated encephalopathy, the multifocal pattern, and the subacute time course.

Diagnosis is confirmed by finding an inflammatory spinal fluid

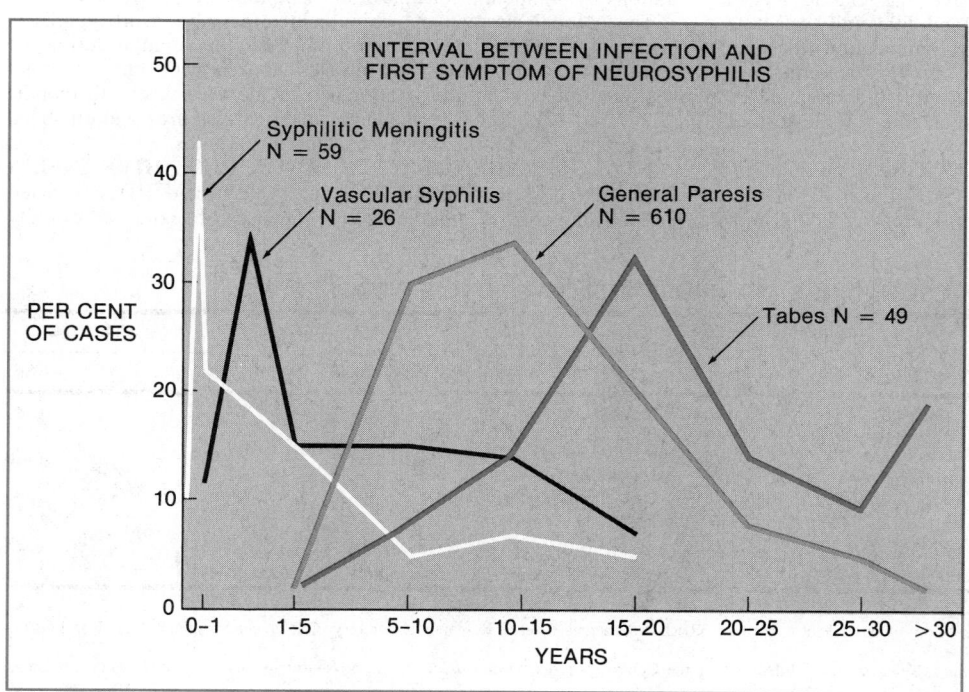

FIGURE 422–1. Interval between primary and symptomatic neurosyphilis by type (meningeal, vascular, paresis, tabes), abstracted from the literature and presented as per cent of total cases within type. (Reproduced with permission from Simon RP: Neurosyphilis. Arch Neurol 42:606, 1985. Copyright 1985, American Medical Association.)

with a positive serology; angiography is unnecessary, but if performed demonstrates vasculitis of medium-sized arteries. Areas of ischemia imaged by CT or MRI in association with the characteristic CSF suggest the diagnosis.

Syphilitic Dementia. Dementia paralytica, or general paresis of the insane, is caused by the diffuse meningoencephalitic form of neurosyphilis. Affected patients usually present 5 to 15 years or more after the primary infection. General paresis affects men four to seven times more frequently than women, perhaps because the infectivity of *Treponema pallidum* declines during pregnancy.

The clinical pattern of syphilitic dementia can mimic almost any organic brain syndrome. The colorful descriptions of grandiose delusional states and psychosis are well known, but these conditions were uncommon even in the prepenicillin era. Then, as now, a simple dementing illness predominated. In advanced cases, tremors of the hands, tongue, and lips resulted, producing a striking dysgraphia and dysarthria. Few untreated cases reach such an advanced stage.

Several features differentiate paresis from other causes of dementia. Syphilitic dementia has a relatively early onset, most commonly beginning between ages 30 and 50, and it progresses rapidly if untreated, being fatal within months to a few years. An inflammatory CSF is always found, and the blood and CSF serologies always contain syphilitic antibodies in diagnostic amounts.

Tabes Dorsalis. The term denotes a myeloneuropathy that characteristically follows the primary infection by 10 to 20 years. The primary lesions affect either the proximal dorsal root entry zones or the dorsal root ganglia. As with paresis, a marked male predominance (7:1) was noted in the prepenicillin era.

The classic triad of symptoms includes lightning pains, sensory ataxia, and urinary disturbance. The most common and earliest signs include pupillary abnormalities, lower extremity areflexia, and the Romberg sign. Lightning pains are transient, agonizing, shooting pains affecting the legs most commonly but potentially arising in any region of the body. Characteristic is an early loss of vibration and position sense attributed to secondary degeneration of the posterior columns of the spinal cord. The proprioceptive impairment engenders a wide-based, unsteady gait that is exacerbated by elimination of visual input (eye closure): the Romberg sign. Bladder hypotonia with overflow incontinence results from deafferentation of the lower sacral sensory nerve roots. Rectal incontinence is uncommon; genital sensory and autonomic impairment eventually results in impotence. Peripheral autonomic impairment, along with loss of peripheral nociceptive afferent fibers, is responsible for the development of trophic (Charcot) joint deformities and distal extremity ulcers.

Of the pupillary abnormalities, half have the classic Argyll Robertson pattern, being small, irregular, and bilaterally reacting poorly to light but constricting briskly to accommodation (the phenomenon of light–near dissociation). Other pupillary abnormalities in tabes include unilateral mydriatic pupils with loss of pupillary light reflex. The sensory impairment is responsible for the loss of deep tendon reflexes.

CEREBROSPINAL FLUID EXAMINATION. A chronic, insidious, inflammatory response within the CSF (Table 422–1) accompanies each of the clinical syndromes of neurosyphilis and pro-vides the ultimate diagnostic test establishing the presence of active neurosyphilis and/or its response to therapy. The absence of a CSF inflammatory response excludes a diagnosis of active neurosyphilis and therefore precludes a clinical response to antibiotic therapy. As with any chronic meningitis, the γ globulin portion of the protein content is commonly elevated, and oligoclonal bands may be present.

Active neurosyphilis produces an abnormal CSF. The possibility of a negative serology in neurosyphilis is difficult to ascertain from the classic literature because of using the relatively insensitive Wasserman test and the unrecognized inclusion of nonsyphilitic syndromes of cerebrovascular disease and viral meningitis. When the clinical diagnosis was characteristic, however, only rare cases showed a negative CSF serology (even with the Wasserman reaction): In 100 paretic patients reported by Merritt (1946), the CSF Wasserman test was positive in every case. Wilson also reported universal CSF positivity in 77 cases of paresis. Theoretically, a negative CSF VDRL might occur in the presence of severe immunosuppression, as a prozone phenomenon, or, in an early case, as a manifestation of the CSF inflammatory response preceding seropositivity. This last situation may explain occasional recent reports of false-negative results or delayed conversions in early meningeal syndromes.

The role of the more sensitive treponemal test (fluorescent treponemal antibody [FTA]) in diagnosing CNS syphilis remains uncertain because of a high false-positive response and decreased sensitivity (75%); without supporting clinical or laboratory data, the diagnostic value of a reactive CSF FTA is unknown. An additional confirmatory test is to inject CSF into rabbit testes; a reactive testicular swelling and recovery of spirochetes prove treponemal infectivity.

TREATMENT. Because neurosyphilis of all clinical types is associated with a CSF inflammatory response, the CSF cell count provides the ultimate monitor of the effectiveness of therapy. Normalization of the spinal fluid is the required endpoint of antibiotic therapy. Once the CSF remains normal, clinical relapses fail to occur.

Penicillin is the drug of choice. Various regimens from 12 to 24 mU per day have been suggested, but it is not clear that the higher doses alter the clinical outcome. Intramuscular benzathine penicillin usually results in undetectable levels in CSF and accordingly should not be used for treatment of neurosyphilis. Spirocheticidal levels (0.03 IU per milliliter, 0.018 μg per milliliter) in CSF occur with 12 million units of IV penicillin daily in four divided doses. Some regimens include probenecid to increase concentrations in CSF by decreasing reabsorption of penicillin through the choroid plexus. Probenecid, however, also decreases parenchymal penicillin concentrations by competing for uptake at membrane transport sites.

The optimal duration of penicillin treatment for neurosyphilis is uncertain. Complete normalization of CSF is uncommon during the usual 2- to 3-week course of intravenous treatment, but the spinal fluid continues to return to normal over the next weeks to months (Table 422–2). Proof of adequate treatment requires a normalized cell count and a falling protein content at 6 months.

HUMAN IMMUNODEFICIENCY VIRUS (HIV) INFECTION IN NEUROSYPHILIS. Neurosyphilis and HIV-associated disease may coexist, both being consequences of sexual promiscuity

TABLE 422–1. CSF FINDINGS IN VARIOUS NEUROSYPHILITIC SYNDROMES

Syndrome	OP	WBC	Glu	Prot	Gamma Globulin*	VDRL Blood	VDRL CSF
Meningitis	170	154 (94% L)	29	95		1:64	1:4
Cerebrovascular	192	58 (87% L)	41	119	IgG index .93	1:512	1:16
Paresis	220	49		305	IgG index 1.99	1:128	1:8
Tabes (active)		62		140		1:16	1:28
Tabes (inactive)		2	76	43		1:16	1:2

* Normal IgG index = 0.23 to 0.64.

OP = Opening pressure; WBC = white blood cells; Glu = glucose; Prot = protein; VDRL = Venereal Disease Research Laboratory; CSF = cerebrospinal fluid; L = lymphocytes; IgG = immunoglobulin G.

From Simon RP, Bayne LL: Neurosyphilis. *In* Martin J, Tyler K (eds.): Infections of the Central Nervous System (Contemporary Neurology Series). Philadelphia, FA Davis, 1993, p 237.

TABLE 422–2. CEREBROSPINAL FLUID (CSF) RESPONSE TO PENICILLIN TREATMENT*

	Admission	Day 7	Day 21	6 Mo
Opening pressure, mm CSF	120	–	–	Normal
Cells/cu mm	207 (94% L)	100 (100% L)	24 (100% L)	0
Glucose, mg/dl	51	66	54	66
Protein, mg/dl	50 (14.4% gamma globulin)	38	48	34
Serology (VDRL)				
CSF	1:2	1:1	–	–
Blood	1:64	1:64	1:64	1:64

* Meningovascular syphilis treated with aqueous penicillin G, 24 million units daily for 21 days; data from Holmes MD, Brant-Zawadski MM, Simon RP: Clinical manifestations of meningovascular syphilis. Neurology 34:553, 1984.

or intravenous drug abuse. Syphilitic syndromes in these patients do not differ in either time course or clinical presentation from those in the pre-AIDS era. Cases identified as "penicillin resistant" may merely have coexistent HIV-induced CSF pleocytosis that is not altered by penicillin therapy. In addition, the occasional recovery of treponemes following penicillin treatment for syphilis in HIV-coinfected patients was similarly observed in the pre-AIDS era. A recent comparison of syphilitics with or without HIV coinfection found no difference from the classically reported illness in clinical presentations, course of disease, serologic expression, or effect of treatment.

The principles of treating neurosyphilis in HIV-coinfected patients are similar to those used in patients without the retrovirus disease; intravenous penicillin should be used in spirocheticidal doses, and the spinal fluid should be monitored as an index of therapy. As noted, when the inflammatory response is due partly to syphilis and partly to HIV infection, only a portion of the pleocyto-sis will disappear, leaving a new plateau of CSF cellularity. The Centers for Disease Control and Prevention (CDC) recommends that patients coinfected with HIV and syphilis for more than 1 year have an examination of their CSF, whether or not they have neurologic symptoms.

Gourevitch MN, Selwyn PA, Davenny K, et al.: Effects of HIV infection on the serologic manifestations and response to treatment of syphilis in intravenous drug users. Ann Intern Med 118:350, 1993. *No difference was found in presentation, course, response to treatment, and serology with or without HIV coinfection.*
Hook EW III: Management of syphilis in human immunodeficiency virus-infected patients. Am J Med 93:477, 1992. *Reviews management issues in the HIV coinfected.*
Merritt HH, Adams RD, Solomon HC: Neurosyphilis. 2nd ed. New York, Oxford University Press, 1946. *The classic descriptive work of the prepenicillin era.*
Musher DM, Hamill RJ, Baughn RE: Syphilis in the presence of human immunodeficiency virus infection. Ann Intern Med 113:872, 1990. *A critique of the association between syphilis and HIV infection.*
Simon RP: Neurosyphilis. Arch Neurol 42:606, 1985. *A review of the clinical syndromes, CSF, and serologic diagnostic criteria.*

Section Eight—Viral Infections of the Nervous System

423 INTRODUCTION
Richard W. Price

Agents belonging to nearly all the major groups of animal viruses can infect the central nervous system (CNS). The spectrum ranges from the large, complex DNA herpesviruses to small, relatively simple viruses with DNA or RNA genomes, such as the papovaviruses and retroviruses. Also included are prions, unique transmissable agents that cause the spongiform encephalopathies. As a result, neurologic manifestations of viral infections can be almost equally diverse, extending from the typical acute febrile encephalitides to chronic progressive disorders that clinically resemble degenerative neurologic diseases.

In most cases, particularly in those infections presenting as acute encephalitis, nervous system involvement is an uncommon complication of a relatively common systemic infection. In adaptive terms, extension of infection to the CNS is "accidental" and may even preclude survival of the virus and its transmission to a new host. For example, the polioviruses cause enteric infections in which replication in the gut and fecal-oral transmission determine the essential survival and transmission of the organism; extension of infection to anterior horn cells of the spinal cord devastates the host but does not contribute to the "life cycle" of the virus. By contrast, the neurotropic herpesviruses, including herpes simplex virus type 1, are exquisitely adapted to cause latent and reactivated infection within the peripheral nervous system; in this case, the sensory neuron is the reservoir for latent virus, and reactivated virus exploits axoplasmic transport to reinfect the epithelium and consequently induce local shedding of virus. However, even in the case of the herpesviruses, CNS complications, such as acute herpes encephalitis, are "acci-dental" and not essential in the organism's adaptive strategy. By contrast, rabies is an illness in which CNS infection plays a central role in the life cycle of the virus: Involvement of the brain produces "rabid," biting behavior that actually contributes to virus transmission.

Viruses can enter the nervous system along a number of avenues. Transport up peripheral nerves can allow direct passage from epithelium or viscera to the CNS; once virus enters the brain, similar intraneural passage by axoplasmic transport can facilitate further spread. A number of viruses are transported along nerve processes by both orthograde and retrograde axoplasmic transport systems. This mode allows rapid passage over long distances and also provides an avenue protected from immunologic interference. Most viruses, however, enter the brain by hematogenous dissemination with passage across the vascular endothelium. As a general rule, agents that travel over neural routes tend to produce initially focal neurologic symptoms and signs, whereas those that disseminate hematogenously cause more diffuse clinical changes. Numerous exceptions exist, however. One reason for this lies in the selective vulnerability to infection of particular nervous system structures or cells. Focal or multifocal disease can also follow general hematogenous dissemination in a random seeding of brain regions. Many viruses preferably infect the meninges rather than the brain, gaining access via the fenestrated capillary endothelium of the choroid plexus.

Within the nervous system some viruses do not discriminate among neurons and glial or endothelial cells, whereas others choose selective targets. Such selectivity is often determined by cell-surface molecules, principally glycoproteins, that serve as receptors for viruses underlying their specific attachment and subsequent entry into cells. Different cell types may vary in their capacity to support virus-directed metabolism and replication.

Virus-cell interactions can assume a number of courses: *abortive infection* results in little or no change in the cell and no virus replication; *acute productive/lytic infection* is characterized by a full replication cycle with production of progeny and subsequent cell death; *chronic productive infection* may allow prolonged release of progeny virus without cell death; in *latent infection,* the viral genome resides quiescently in the cell, but retains the capacity to reactivate subsequently; *transforming infection* results in increased and characteristically abnormal cell proliferation, usually in the absence of virus replication; *defective infection* may result in nonproductive infection or production of incomplete particles yet causes varying degrees of cell alteration and viral antigen expression.

As with other types of organisms, neural injury and dysfunction accompanying viral infections relate to varying contributions of the *direct* effects of the virus and its genome (e.g., neuronal death caused by herpes simplex virus or oligodendroglial cell death caused by JC virus), the *indirect* effects mediated by antigen-specific host responses (e.g., lysis of infected cells by cytotoxic T lymphocytes), and less specific cell-coded neurotoxic gene products (e.g., nitric oxide and quinolinic acid) released in association with cytokine reactions. The relative importance of these factors in individual infections depends both upon the interactions of the invading organism with the cells it infects and the profile of host cell responses that it elicits. This balance is highly variable from one virus to the next and importantly influences the time course, morbidity, and degree of recovery from each infection.

Diagnostic approaches to viral diseases depend on the clinical setting and specific agents involved. The arsenal of available diagnostic methods is steadily growing. For many acute infections the time-honored serologic techniques assessing host antibody responses in serum and, at times, cerebrospinal fluid remain the most useful and cost effective. Although some infections elicit diagnostic tissue reactions (e.g., Negri body in rabies), for most infections newer techniques have displaced simple histopathology in identifying infection in tissue; these include detection of viral antigens using specific antibodies and of viral nucleic acids using *in situ* hybridization. Although more direct identification of viruses in blood or other clinical specimens by culture isolation generally remains difficult and costly, the introduction of the polymerase chain reaction (PCR) gene amplification technique to clinical virology is now rapidly expanding the diagnostic capability of the laboratory.

In the past, limitations of treatment made specific virologic diagnosis either largely an "academic exercise" or important principally for epidemiologic purposes. Efforts to combat viral disease consisted exclusively of prevention through active, or at times passive, immunization. In the past two decades, however, antiviral chemotherapy has become a practical reality. Effective therapy is now available for neurotropic herpesviruses and antiviral treatment can temporarily retard progression of HIV-1 infection. The promise thus exists for more effective treatments for infection by these viruses as well as for the development of chemotherapeutic agents that will act selectively against other important viruses causing neurologic diseases.

Johnson RT: Viral Infections of the Nervous System. New York, Raven Press, 1982. *Although now outdated in certain details, this remains an excellent introduction to the general principles of viral infection of the nervous system.*

Johnson RT, Burke DS, Elwell M, et al.: Japanese encephalitis: Immunocytochemical studies of viral antigen and inflammatory cells in fatal cases. Ann Neurol 18:567, 1985. *An exemplary contribution describing viral and immunologic pathology of Japanese encephalitis.*

Tsai T: Arboviral infections in the United States. Infect Dis Clin North Am 5:73, 1991. *A general review of arboviral infections, including clinical and epidemiologic aspects.*

424 ACUTE VIRAL MENINGITIS AND ENCEPHALITIS

Richard W. Price

DEFINITIONS. The terms *viral meningitis* and *viral encephalitis* refer to infections of the leptomeninges and brain parenchyma, respectively. When the spinal cord is involved along with the brain, the term *viral encephalomyelitis* may be used. When both meninges and brain parenchyma appear to be infected, *viral meningoencephalitis* sometimes is employed, although viral encephalitis is almost always accompanied by meningeal inflammation. The nonspecific term *aseptic meningitis* refers to an inflammatory process of the meninges accompanied by a predominantly mononuclear cell pleocytosis and not caused by pyogenic bacterial infection. Although viral infections are the most common cause of aseptic meningitis, infections by other types of organisms, as well as chemical irritation of the meninges and reactions to certain medications, can cause a similar clinical picture and cerebrospinal fluid profile. Most viral meningitides are benign and self-limiting with a low acute morbidity and only rare long-term sequelae. Although viral encephalitides are also often benign, they more frequently result in morbidity and mortality.

Acute central nervous system (CNS) infections caused by a variety of viruses are appropriately considered together because of their largely indistinguishable clinical aspects. Viral infections causing more distinct neurologic symptoms and signs are considered separately in subsequent sections.

ETIOLOGIES. Many viruses can cause acute encephalitis or meningitis (Table 424–1). Table 424–2 indicates the most common virus groups and the syndromes they produce.

Enteroviruses are small, nonenveloped RNA viruses of the picornavirus family with numerous serotypes. Over 50 have been associ-

TABLE 424–1. VIRUSES ASSOCIATED WITH ACUTE CENTRAL NERVOUS SYSTEM INFECTIONS IN THE UNITED STATES

RNA Viruses
  Picornaviruses (enteroviruses)
    Polioviruses
    Coxsackieviruses, groups A and B
    Echoviruses
    Enteroviruses
  Togaviruses
    Eastern equine encephalitis*
    Western equine encephalitis*
    St. Louis encephalitis*
    Powassan*
    Tick-borne encephalitis
    Rubella
  Bunyavirus
    California encephalitis* (includes LaCross subtype)
  Orbivirus
    Colorado tick fever*
  Arenavirus
    Lymphocytic choriomeningitis
  Rhabdovirus
    Rabies
  Orthomyxoviruses and paramyxoviruses
    Influenza
    Parainfluenza
    Mumps
    Measles
  Retroviruses
    Human immunodeficiency virus type 1
DNA Viruses
  Herpesviruses
    Herpes simplex, types 1 and 2
    Varicella-zoster
    Epstein-Barr
    Cytomegalovirus
  Adenoviruses

* Arthropod-borne viruses (arboviruses).

TABLE 424–2. RELATIVE FREQUENCY OF MENINGITIS AND ENCEPHALITIS OF KNOWN VIRAL ETOLOGY

Viral Agent	Viral Meningitis (%)	Viral Encephalitis (%)
Enteroviruses	83	23
Arboviruses	2	30
Mumps	7	2
Herpes simplex	4	27
Varicella	1	8
Measles	1	< 1

Reproduced with permission from Jubelt B: Enterovirus and mumps virus infections of the nervous system. Neuro Clin 2:187, 1984.

ated with meningitis or encephalitis. The family includes members of the coxsackie A and B, echovirus and newer enterovirus groups, as well as the three poliovirus subtypes (see Ch. 425).

Arboviruses include agents of several families that are transmitted by mosquitoes or ticks. More than 15 different arboviruses have been associated with encephalitis in varied areas of the world. In the United States, the five most important are eastern and western equine encephalitis, St. Louis encephalitis, California encephalitis (with most cases involving the LaCross subtype), and Colorado tick fever. Less common within the continental states are Venezuelan equine encephalitis and Powassan encephalitis.

Herpes simplex virus type 1 causes severe encephalitis, but usually with characteristic focal features, whereas herpes simplex virus type 2 causes aseptic meningitis in association with primary or secondary genital herpes (see Ch. 426). Lymphocytic choriomeningitis (LCM) virus, an arenavirus, is a sporadic cause of meningitis and occasionally encephalitis. Aseptic meningitis has now been recognized as a complication of acute infection by the retrovirus causing the acquired immunodeficiency syndrome (AIDS; see Part XXII). Adenoviruses are respiratory viruses that only rarely cause meningitis or severe childhood encephalitis.

The acute neurologic disease associated with measles, vaccinia, and rubella infections in most cases represents postinfectious encephalomyelitis (see Ch. 429). This may also be true of the encephalitis that has occasionally been reported with influenza and parainfluenza virus infections.

EPIDEMIOLOGY. Viral meningitis and encephalitis are relatively common disorders. In one study in Rochester, Minnesota, for example, the incidence of aseptic meningitis was nearly 11 per 100,000 person-years, and that of viral encephalitis was more than 7 per 100,000 person-years. This finding was compared with a rate of 8.6 episodes of bacterial meningitis. A relatively low mortality rate in this study (3.8%) may have reflected the inclusion of milder cases and the predominance of the LaCross type of viral encephalitis. In other epidemiologic settings, the mortality may be considerably greater. In general, a specific cause is identified in only about 10 to 15% of cases of meningitis and encephalitis in the United States.

Each virus causing CNS infection has its own epidemiologic pattern. Because of the predominance of enteroviruses and arboviruses, the overall incidence of viral meningitis and encephalitis peaks in the late summer. Enterovirus epidemics in temperate climates characteristically take place with transmission occurring by the fecal-hand-oral route. They often involve young children, with rapid spread in family or social groups. The geographic and seasonal incidence of arbovirus infection relates to the life cycle of arthropod vectors and animal reservoirs (see Ch. 346) and their contact with humans. Eastern equine encephalitis virus is limited largely to the Atlantic and Gulf coasts, while western equine encephalitis virus is confined to the western two thirds of the country, with the highest incidence in the middle states. The latter virus causes many more human infections than does the eastern virus, but only 1 in 100 infected persons develops encephalitis. St. Louis encephalitis virus causes disease in both rural and urban areas over a large part of the United States. In the rural areas, the virus has the same pattern as western encephalitis virus, but in urban areas more explosive outbreaks can occur. In recent years, the LaCross subtype of the California encephalitis virus has been related every year to cases spread widely over the United States, particularly in the east and midwest, mostly in children. Colorado tick fever occurs in the Rocky Moun-

tain area; about 18% of infected patients develop meningitis, but encephalitis is rare. Venezuelan encephalitis has spread into Florida and the southwestern states and, in most of those infected, produces an influenza-like illness, but about 3% develop acute meningitis or encephalitis. Powassan virus is a rare cause of encephalitis in Canada and along the northern border of the United States.

Lymphocytic choriomeningitis virus is the major zoonotic virus causing meningitis and encephalitis. Humans acquire the infection by contact with dust or food contaminated by excreta of the common house mouse. Human disease is more common in winter, when the natural host tends to move indoors. Lymphocytic choriomeningitis virus has also been found in hamsters, and human infections have been traced to laboratory and pet hamsters.

Mumps virus spreads by the respiratory route, with infection occurring throughout the year but increasing in incidence during the spring. Although mumps virus infects the two genders equally, males develop meningitis three times more frequently than females.

PATHOGENESIS. Events leading up to the development of the acute viral encephalitides and meningitides can be divided into three stages. The first involves exposure of an external body surface to the virus, usually with local replication of the "inoculum." In the case of enteroviruses, the infecting virus is contained in body fluids or excreta from infected persons and transferred by direct contact or within contaminated environmental materials. The arboviruses, by contrast, are introduced by an arthropod bite. The next stage involves systemic viremia and amplification of virus in visceral organs; a secondary viremia may lead to invasion and replication within the nervous system or meninges. With the exception of rabies virus, the neurotropic herpesviruses, and perhaps the polioviruses, agents that cause acute viral encephalitis or meningitis reach the nervous system hematogenously. This factor accounts for the widespread distribution of cerebral dysfunction associated with most of the encephalitides.

In viral encephalitis, infection of neurons, glial cells, and even vascular endothelium leads to cell dysfunction and sometimes cell death. Inflammatory responses follow. Clinical symptoms and signs depend on the distribution of infection and on both the direct effect of the virus and the secondary inflammatory reactions in the tissue. The relative contribution of each to brain dysfunction depends on the particular infecting virus. The remarkable degree of recovery in many patients suggests that secondary inflammatory and immune responses often predominate.

CLINICAL MANIFESTATIONS. Most acute viral encephalitides and meningitides produce similar symptoms with variations depending on the particular virus. Often CNS manifestations are preceded or accompanied by fever, malaise or myalgia, gastrointestinal disturbance, respiratory symptoms, or rash. These are followed by headache, photophobia, stiff neck, and other signs of meningeal irritation, usually with an intensity milder than that of bacterial meningitis.

When encephalitis exists, evidence of diffuse or, less commonly, focal brain dysfunction accompanies or overshadows signs of meningeal irritation. Patients characteristically exhibit altered attention and consciousness, ranging from confusion to lethargy or coma. Motor function may be abnormal, with weakness, altered tone, or incoordination, reflecting dysfunction of the cortex, basal ganglia, or cerebellum. Severe cases may cause difficult-to-control generalized or focal seizures. Some patients exhibit myoclonus or tremor. Hypothalamic involvement may lead to hyperthermia or hypothermia, autonomic dysfunction with vasomotor instability, or diabetes insipidus. Abnormalities of ocular motility, swallowing, or other cranial nerve functions are uncommon. Spinal cord infection is usually inconspicuous but can result in flaccid weakness, with acute loss of reflexes in the most severe cases. Focal symptoms other than seizures are usually minor and overshadowed by generalized brain dysfunction; some patients may show hemiparesis, visual disturbance, or sensory loss. Focal involvement of limbic structures is particularly characteristic of herpes encephalitis (see Ch. 426).

The time course of acute viral meningitis and encephalitis varies. The onset may occur within a matter of hours or evolve more slowly over a few days. Usually, maximum deficit appears within 1 to 4 days.

LABORATORY FINDINGS. Examination of the cerebrospinal fluid is essential. The presence of 10 to 1000 mononuclear cells per cubic millimeter is characteristic. On occasion, early examination may show acellular fluid or predominance of polymorphonuclear leukocytes, but the typical mononuclear pleocytosis soon evolves. The pressure may be elevated, while the glucose level is characteristically normal or only modestly reduced. The protein content is usually elevated (50 to 100 mg per deciliter) and may exhibit increased immunoglobulin concentration and the presence of oligoclonal bands. An increased protein content and number of cells may persist for weeks or months after convalescence, and oligoclonal bands can be detected for an even longer period.

Systemic laboratory findings may vary, depending on the etiologic agent. Generally, the white blood cell count is not elevated, but either elevations or depressions can be seen, usually with a lymphocytic predominance. Involvement of salivary glands or pancreas in mumps may elevate the serum amylase level.

Neurodiagnostic tests usually reveal nonspecific abnormalities, with notable exception in the case of herpes simplex encephalitis (see Ch. 426). Computed tomography (CT) and magnetic resonance imaging (MRI) are usually normal early in the course of the nonherpetic viral encephalitides, but focal edema and contrast enhancement may appear in the more severe cases. The greatest value of these neuroimaging procedures lies in excluding alternative diagnoses.

DIAGNOSIS. With a few exceptions, the neurologic and laboratory findings accompanying the acute viral meningoencephalitides are insufficiently distinct to allow an etiologic diagnosis, and it may even be difficult to distinguish these disorders from a number of nonviral diseases. The epidemiologic setting (e.g., time of year, exposure to insects, the local community) and accompanying systemic manifestations may be helpful in presumptive diagnoses. Thus, involvement of the nervous system by mumps virus is usually suspected from associated clinical parotitis or pancreatitis, although the neurologic disease can be the sole or presenting clinical manifestation; conversely, a certain history of previous mumps eliminates this diagnostic possibility. Several enterovirus infections produce a rash, which usually accompanies the onset of fever and persists for 4 to 10 days. In infections by coxsackievirus A5, 9, and 16, and echovirus 4, 6, 9, 16, and 30, the rash is typically maculopapular and nonpruritic and may be confined to the face and trunk or may involve extremities, including the palms and soles. Echovirus 9 infections can cause a petechial rash resembling meningococcemia. Herpangina, characterized by gray vesicular lesions on the tonsillar fossae, soft palate, and uvula, can accompany group A coxsackie infection. In coxsackievirus A16 and, rarely, other group A serotype infections, a vesicular rash may involve hands, feet, and oropharynx. As discussed below, the encephalitis related to Epstein-Barr virus occurs in the setting of acute mononucleosis. The principally postinfectious encephalitides related to measles and varicella follow overt systemic diseases with characteristic rashes.

Because no specific treatment exists for acute viral meningitis and encephalitis (except herpes), and their signs and symptoms are often nonspecific, exclusion of other diagnoses becomes important. Potentially confusing are partially treated bacterial meningitis; rickettsial infections; Lyme disease; meningitis caused by a variety of nonpyogenic organisms, including *Mycobacterium tuberculosis* and *Cryptococcus neoformans* and other fungi; meningeal or parameningeal bacterial infections; brain abscess; subacute bacterial endocarditis; and the cerebral vasculitides. Among noninfectious causes, trimethoprim-sulfamethoxazole, nonsteroidal analgesics, OKT3 antibody given to enhance immunosuppression, intravenous immunoglobulin, and certain other drugs may occasionally cause a sterile meningeal reaction. Without a cerebrospinal fluid examination, the differential diagnosis becomes even broader, encompassing additional toxic and vascular diseases. Most alternative diagnoses can be suspected or eliminated by the history, the cerebrospinal fluid profile, or brain imaging.

Despite the absence of effective treatment, specific virologic diagnosis is useful both for prognosis in the individual patient and for epidemiologic implications for the populations at risk. Diagnosis usually relies on serology, although direct detection of the organism in the cerebrospinal fluid, blood, or stool may sometimes be achieved. Selection of tests and their interpretation depend upon the particular organism. Almost all acute viral syndromes occur in the setting of a first encounter with the agent, which then results in

lasting immunity. In these cases, seroconversion documented by a fourfold or greater rise in antibody titers between acute and convalescent sera is a principal means of diagnosis. A notable exception is herpes simplex encephalitis, in which antibody titers must be more cautiously interpreted (see Ch. 426). Attempts at direct viral isolation are of limited value in clinical management and must be tailored to the suspected agent. Arboviruses and enteroviruses can be isolated from the blood but are seldom recoverable at the time of clinically evident meningitis or encephalitis. During the acute disease, coxsackieviruses and echoviruses are most readily isolated from stool or cerebrospinal fluid and, in some cases, throat washings. Lymphocytic choriomeningitis virus can be isolated from blood or cerebrospinal fluid. Mumps virus may be isolated from saliva, throat washings, or cerebrospinal fluid. Type 2 herpes simplex virus may be cultured from the cerebrospinal fluid or identified in genital lesions. Polymerase chain reaction (PCR) screening of cerebrospinal fluid undoubtedly will improve specific diagnosis in the future.

TREATMENT. Treatment of acute viral encephalitis and meningitis (except herpes) is directed at symptom relief, supportive care, and preventing and managing complications. Strict isolation is not essential, although when enteroviral infection is suspected, precautions in handling of stools and the practice of careful hand washing should be instituted. Persons with measles, chickenpox, rubella, or mumps virus infections should observe the usual precautions of isolation from susceptible individuals. Arboviruses are not characteristically spread from person to person because they require an intermediate insect vector.

The headache and fever of meningitis can usually be managed with judicious doses of acetaminophen. Severe hyperthermia (> 40°C) may require vigorous therapy, but mild temperature elevations may serve as a natural defense mechanism and are best left untreated.

Patients with severe encephalitis often become comatose. Because, however, some may achieve remarkable recovery, vigorous support and avoidance of complications are essential. Meticulous care in an intensive care unit setting with respiratory and nutritional support is usually justified.

Although seizures sometimes complicate encephalitis, prophylactic anticonvulsants are not routinely recommended. If seizures develop, they can usually be managed with phenytoin and phenobarbital. If status epilepticus ensues, appropriate vigorous therapy should be instituted to prevent secondary brain injury and attendant hypoxia (see Ch. 433). Similarly, secondary bacterial infections should be sought and promptly treated.

Steroids should probably generally be avoided in the treatment of encephalitis because of their inhibitory effects on host immune responses.

PROGNOSIS. Full recovery from viral meningitis usually occurs within 1 to 2 weeks of onset, although some patients describe fatigue, light-headedness, and asthenia persisting for months.

The prognosis of encephalitis depends on its cause. Arbovirus encephalitides have variable mortality rates; that with eastern equine encephalitis is approximately 30%; with St. Louis, 10%; with western equine, 10%; with Venezuelan equine, 1%; and with California, less than 0.5%. The mortality rates for western equine encephalitis are greater in children under 1 year of age; for St. Louis encephalitis they are greater in the elderly. Nonfatal encephalitis caused by eastern, western, and St. Louis viruses leaves a relatively high rate of neurologic sequelae. Encephalitis associated with mumps or LCM virus is rarely associated with death, and sequelae are infrequent. Hydrocephalus has been reported as a late sequela of mumps meningitis and encephalitis in children.

Chonmaitree T, Baldwin CD, Lucia HL: Role of the virology laboratory in diagnosis and management of patients with central nervous system disease. Clin Microbiol Rev 2:1, 1989. *A review of laboratory procedures used in the diagnosis of acute viral diseases of the CNS.*

Evans AS: Viral Infections of Humans: Epidemiology and Control, 3rd ed. New York, Plenum Publishing Corporation, 1989. *A useful text dealing with the epidemiology of viral infections; contains individual chapters dealing with the major groups, including the arboviruses, enteroviruses, and herpesviruses.*

Nicolosi A, Hauser WA, Beghi E, et al.: Epidemiology of central nervous system infections in Olmstead County, Minnesota, 1950–1981. J Infect Dis 154:399, 1986. *Provides incidence figures for viral meningitis and encephalitis.*

Whitley RJ: Viral encephalitis. N Engl J Med 323:242, 1990. *A recent review that emphasizes herpes encephalitis management and differential diagnosis.*

425 POLIOMYELITIS
Richard W. Price

DEFINITIONS. Poliomyelitis (acute anterior poliomyelitis, infantile paralysis) is an acute illness caused by the three strains of poliovirus. The disease selectively destroys the motor neurons of the spinal cord and brain stem to cause flaccid asymmetric weakness. Until recently one of the most feared of all human infectious diseases, poliomyelitis is now almost entirely preventable by vaccination.

ETIOLOGY. The three antigenically different strains of poliovirus (types 1, 2, and 3) are classified in the genus *Enterovirus* within the family Picornaviridae. These are small (approximately 270 nm), roughly spherical particles with icosahedral symmetry containing a single-stranded RNA core and are surrounded by a protein capsid. Lacking a lipid envelope, the polioviruses are resistant to lipid solvents and stable at low pH.

INCIDENCE, PREVALENCE, AND EPIDEMIOLOGY. In the United States, the number of cases of paralytic poliomyelitis, has fallen to just a few cases yearly, thanks to the widespread use of an effective vaccine. In less advanced regions of the world, paralytic polio continues to occur, with a seasonal incidence in temperate zones but a more even distribution throughout the year in tropical areas. Poliovirus is acquired by the oral route and subsequently replicates in the oropharynx and lower gastrointestinal tract. It may be secreted for a week or two in saliva and for more prolonged periods in feces, which provides the major avenue of host-to-host transmission. Spread of polioviruses is greatly influenced by standards of hygiene, and greatest dissemination occurs within families or other crowded circumstances.

Paralysis is an unusual complication of poliovirus infection. During an epidemic, only 1 to 2% of infections result in neurologic symptoms and signs with another 4 to 8% suffering nonspecific (minor) illness. A number of factors increase the incidence of paralytic disease, including advancing age, recent hard exercise, tonsillectomy, pregnancy and impairment of B lymphocyte (antibody) defenses. Immunity to each of the three types of poliovirus is lifelong, but infection with one strain does not necessarily protect against subsequent infection by another. In the United States, poliomyelitis due to live-attenuated strains is as common as disease related to wild-type virus.

PATHOGENESIS AND PATHOLOGY. Polioviruses selectively infect certain neuronal populations, inducing highly stereotyped pathology, and in this manner contrast with most of the viruses causing acute encephalitis or meningitis.

The poliovirus invades the nervous system only after prior systemic replication. An initial alimentary phase with local replication in the intestinal mucosa and spread to the local lymphatics is followed by a viremia which seeds the nervous system. Once within the central nervous system, poliovirus may disseminate along neural pathways, attacking principally motor neurons of the spinal cord and lower brain stem, the brain stem reticular formation, and, to a lesser extent, the precentral gyrus. Convalescent poliomyelitis is characterized by loss of motor neurons and denervation atrophy of their associated skeletal muscles.

CLINICAL MANIFESTATIONS. The incubation period from virus exposure to the neurologic phase characteristically lasts between 4 and 10 days but may be prolonged to 4 to 5 weeks. The major illness usually begins with fever and malaise, followed within hours by generalized headache, vomiting, and within another day by the development of neck and back stiffness. Patients often are drowsy but on arousal are irritable and apprehensive. Progression may stop at this point. When paralysis develops, it usually begins on the second to fifth day after the onset of headache. Weakness, however, may be among the initial symptoms or, rarely, may be delayed for 7 to 10 days. Children generally exhibit less intense systemic symptoms than do adults, who characteristically appear acutely ill and are tremulous, flushed, and agitated. Their muscles are often sensitive and stiff.

Poliomyelitis preferentially damages the larger somatic motor neurons. In most cases, the involvement tends to include the lumbar segments more than the cervical and the spinal cord more than the brain stem. The consequent paralyses are usually asymmetric, weakness characteristically being more proximal than distal. In mild cases paralysis affects only parts of muscles rather than selective peripheral nerve or nerve root distributions. Sensory changes are lacking. The paralysis may render one member useless yet entirely spare the contralateral arm or leg. About 50% develop acute urinary retention. The trunk musculature is least commonly affected. The affected muscles are flaccid, and the deep tendon reflexes may be absent. Atrophy develops rapidly, usually beginning within a week in paralyzed muscles and progressing over the ensuing weeks. The motor deficit rarely progresses for more than 3 to 5 days.

About 10 to 15% of cases affect the lower brain stem motor nuclei. Involvement of the ninth and tenth cranial nerve nuclei leads to paralysis of pharyngeal and laryngeal musculature. Parts of the facial muscles can be involved, either unilaterally or bilaterally. Less often, the tongue and muscles of mastication become paralyzed. External oculomotor weakness occurs rarely. The pupils are spared. Direct involvement of the brain stem reticular formation can disrupt breathing and swallowing and can produce serious disturbances in cardiovascular control. Poliomyelitis seldom causes permanent functional paralysis of the bulbar muscles, probably because of the relatively small size of the motor units served by brain stem nuclei and because overwhelming disease in these critical segments usually kills the patient.

DIAGNOSIS AND DIFFERENTIAL DIAGNOSIS. Because of its rarity in the United States, poliomyelitis may present diagnostic difficulties. Its early phases must be differentiated from other acute meningitides, and when paralysis ensues, a major differential diagnosis is with the Guillain-Barré syndrome and other predominantly motor polyneuropathies. However, no other acute disease produces headaches, stiff neck, fever, and asymmetric flaccid paralysis without sensory loss coupled with an increase in white blood cells in the cerebrospinal fluid (CSF). Rarely, the CSF shows a persistence of significant pleocytosis in polyneuritis, and CSF protein levels above 100 mg per milliliter are frequent. Acute intermittent porphyria may cause a motor polyneuropathy somewhat similar to postinfectious polyneuropathy. At times, acute transverse myelitis may be confused with poliomyelitis, but findings of a sensory-motor spinal level at the appropriate spinal cord segment usually serves to separate an inflammatory cord transection from diffuse anterior horn cell involvement (see Ch. 428.1). Rarely, coxsackievirus and echoviruses have been reported to cause encephalitides with prominent (but not extensive) motor neuron symptoms and signs. Diagnosis can be established by isolation of virus from blood or CSF or by serologic evidence of acute poliovirus infection. In cases related to vaccine strains, viral isolates can be distinguished in the laboratory.

TREATMENT. There is no specific treatment, but supportive care is important in reducing suffering during the acute attack, in maintaining vital functions to ensure survival, and perhaps in modifying the overall outcome and disability. Important measures include preventing contractures, maintaining airway and cardiovascular stability, and preventing excessive calcium mobilization and bed sores.

PROGNOSIS. Death in poliomyelitis is usually the result of bulbar involvement and is attributable to respiratory and cardiovascular impairments. Mortality has been considerably reduced with modern management of respiratory insufficiency. Patients who survive an episode of acute paralytic poliomyelitis usually recover considerable motor function. Generally, motor improvement begins within the first weeks after onset, and 60% of eventual recovery is achieved by 3 months.

The Postpolio Syndrome. A number of patients with previous poliomyelitis develop further motor deterioration later in life. In some this relates simply to musculoskeletal decompensation or other factors but does not involve new weakness. However, other persons suffer a true loss of strength termed the postpolio syndrome. This disorder is characterized by an insidiously slow but gradually progressive weakness beginning 30 or more years after an attack of poliomyelitis. Most commonly it adds to the weakness of already affected muscles; less often, weakness develops in muscles previously thought to be normal. This weakness is often accompanied by fasciculations, and there may be additional atrophy. Muscle biopsy shows type grouping consistent with active denervation-reinnervation. Overall, the prognosis is good, with only slow progression of further weakness, which rarely leads to a severe increase in disability or to death. The most likely pathogenesis consists of senescence of surviving, expanded motor units. This development must be distinguished from motor neuron disease of a more malignant variety (see Ch. 415), which has also been described many years after acute poliomyelitis but appears to be much less common than the more gradual and benign postpolio syndrome.

PREVENTION. Poliomyelitis can be prevented by either live-attenuated or killed polio vaccines. These are now given routinely in Western cultures, although the practice of immunization has relaxed as the threat of developing paralytic poliomyelitis has become less conspicuous. If this trend is not reversed, a resurgence of the disease can be expected. An important consequence of accurate diagnosis of poliomyelitis is the prompt institution of local vaccination programs for communities at risk, including subcultures in which vaccination is avoided for religious or other reasons.

Price RW, Plum F: Poliomyelitis. In Vinken PJ, Bruyn GW (eds.): Handbook of Clinical Neurology, Vol. 32, Part I. Amsterdam, Elsevier-North Holland, 1978. *A general review of clinical and biologic aspects of poliomyelitis.*

Windebank AJ, Litchy WJ, Daube JR, et al.: Late effects of paralytic poliomyelitis in Olmsted County, Minnesota. Neurology 41:501, 1991. *A study characterizing the long-term clinical sequelae of a population sample with previous poliomyelitis.*

426 HERPESVIRUS INFECTIONS OF THE NERVOUS SYSTEM
Richard W. Price

Three of the six human herpesviruses (see also Ch. 339 through 341) share an essential "neurotropism" in their adaptation for survival and transmission. Herpes simplex virus types 1 and 2 (HSV-1 and HSV-2) and varicella-zoster virus (VZV) all establish in sensory ganglia a latent infection that can subsequently reactivate to release progeny virus into the territory of the ganglion's epithelial innervation. The major neurologic complications of these infections in adults include adult-type herpes simplex encephalitis caused by HSV-1; aseptic meningitis, radiculitis, and sacral autonomic insufficiency caused by HSV-2; and encephalitis, myelitis, radiculopathy, and vasculitis complicating herpes zoster. Prompt diagnosis of infections by these viruses is important because they are now amenable to selective antiviral drug therapy. Two of the remaining human herpesviruses, Epstein-Barr virus and cytomegalovirus, although largely lymphotropic, can also cause neurologic disease in the setting of systemic illness. Recent reports also suggest that human herpesvirus-6 can cause encephalitis in immunosuppressed patients.

426.1 Herpes Simplex Encephalitis (HSE)

Adult-type HSE is a sporadic disease with a severe morbidity and high mortality. Both HSV-1 and HSV-2 are capable of causing encephalitis, but type 1 by far predominates. In contrast, HSV-2 accounts for the great majority of neonatal herpetic encephalitis, which is not considered here.

EPIDEMIOLOGY AND PATHOGENESIS. Although the most common identified cause of severe, sporadic viral encephalitis in the United States, HSE is nonetheless uncommon. The disease afflicts persons of all postneonatal ages, with peaks of incidence in late childhood and middle age. It occurs with approximately equal frequency throughout the year, and case-to-case transmission does not occur. Curiously, immunosuppression plays no apparent role.

HSV-1 is a ubiquitous organism; more than 90% of adults exhibit serologic evidence of exposure and likely harbor latent ganglionic infection. Recurrent cold sores resulting from viral reactivation occur in perhaps one fourth of adults. Although HSE may occur as a primary infection, it likely more often results from reactivated virus or perhaps from reinfection by a new strain of virus.

The characteristic gross and microscopic pathology of herpetic infection, particularly its anatomic localization, distinguishes HSE from other encephalitides. Although often asymmetric, the disease is usually bilateral and afflicts the medial temporal and inferior frontal lobes and related "limbic" structures, including the hippocampus, amygdaloid nuclei, olfactory cortex, insula, and cingulate gyrus. Necrosis with petechial hemorrhage is so intense that the disease was once called *acute necrotizing encephalitis*. Microscopically, hemorrhagic necrosis with mononuclear inflammation characterizes involved areas, with neurons and glia often containing Cowdry type A intranuclear inclusions during the acute phase of infection. The gray matter is affected predominantly, but infection extends into the white matter as well.

CLINICAL MANIFESTATIONS. HSE most commonly presents as a subacute or acute illness causing local and diffuse cerebral dysfunction. Typically, patients are febrile, although in as many as 10% fever may be absent, and thus herpes encephalitis warrants consideration even in afebrile patients who present with an altered mental status. Severe headache, focal or generalized convulsions, and alterations in behavior and consciousness are the most prominent symptoms. Common symptoms including disorientation, delusions, agitation, personality changes, or dysphasia sometimes lead erroneously to psychiatric referral. Motor paralyses are present in fewer than half of affected individuals.

DIAGNOSIS. Evaluation of suspected HSE has been an area of controversy, principally related to the issue of diagnostic brain biopsy. Among the arguments for brain biopsy are that (1) it is the most sensitive and accurate diagnostic method, contrasting with the insensitivity and difficulty in early interpretation of serologic studies and neurodiagnostic procedures; and (2) this procedure results in identification of alternative diagnoses, some of which respond to specific treatment. Arguments against brain biopsy relate to its potential short- and long-term sequelae, the benignity of empiric therapy, and the improved sensitivity and accuracy of magnetic resonance imaging (MRI) compared with earlier diagnostic methods. Broad application of DNA detection is likely to further obviate the need for biopsy. Important issues regarding management also relate to the facilities, expertise, and experience available to the patient at the admitting hospital. Nevertheless, we recommend that most patients be managed without biopsy and that the combination of clinical and laboratory features warrants an approach utilizing empiric therapy.

The most important step in management involves prompt recognition of HSE as a diagnostic possibility and rapid institution of acyclovir therapy. Among the important neurodiagnostic evaluations in patients suspected of having HSE are MRI, cerebrospinal fluid (CSF) analysis, and electroencephalography. Whereas computed tomographic (CT) scanning is surprisingly insensitive in detecting early HSE, with two fifths or more patients having normal scans, MRI more often detects characteristic abnormalities. The latter include virtually pathognomonic increased signal, particularly on T2-weighted sequences, in the same regions showing pathology at autopsy: the medial temporal and insular cortical regions as well as the inferior frontal cingulate gyri, often bilateral (Fig. 426–1). The MRI also allows more sensitive detection of alternative diagnoses, such as brain abscess, vasculitis, or demyelination. Some patients are so ill or agitated that MRI may require general anesthesia. In some, biopsy might be needed.

CSF examination is also important in detecting evidence of virus infection. Most patients exhibit a mononuclear pleocytosis with 50 or more leukocytes per cubic millimeter, although fewer or even a normal number of cells may be noted. The protein content is usually mildly elevated, and the glucose level is normal or only mildly reduced. Like MRI, CSF analysis may also be useful in establishing alternative diagnoses, such as bacterial or fungal infection. In more than three fourths of patients, the electroencephalogram exhibits focal abnormalities, most often showing spike and slow-wave or sharp-wave patterns over the involved temporal lobes.

Attempts at isolating HSV-1 from CSF rarely succeed. New methods of diagnosis seek detection of viral antigens (by enzyme-

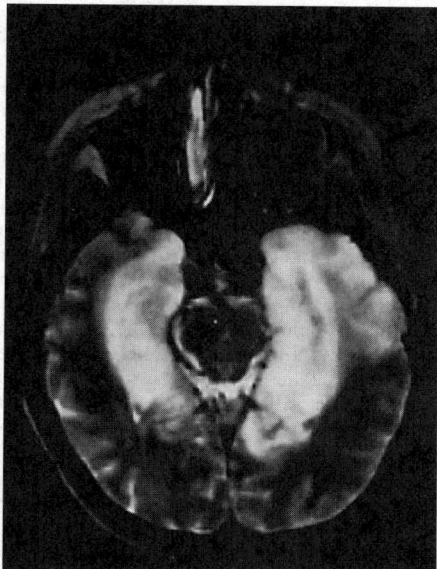

FIGURE 426–1. MRI scan of a 54-year-old woman with herpes simplex encephalitis who presented with fever, dysphasia, and confusion. The T2-weighted image shows increased signal in both medial temporal lobes, with more extensive involvement on the left (right side of figure).

linked immunosorbent assay) or nucleic acid by polymerase chain reaction (PCR) gene amplification show great promise. In the research laboratory PCR has been shown to be sensitive and specific in detecting HSV-1 DNA sequences in CSF. Isolation of the virus from the oropharynx is useless because no relationship exists between symptomatic or asymptomatic viral shedding at such peripheral sites and brain infection. HSV-1 is often reactivated by other neurologic diseases eliciting fever, creating a source of false-positive serologic responses.

In contrast to the epidemic encephalitides, in which documentation of seroconversion provides a major method of diagnosis, in HSE serologic testing is often inconclusive. This is particularly true at the onset, when prompt diagnosis is critical. During convalescence analyses of blood, antibody titers can give false-negative or false-positive results. Assessment of intrathecal anti–HSV-1 antibody production appears to be quite useful, however.

TREATMENT. The introduction of antiviral therapy has greatly improved the outcome of HSE. This was first demonstrated with vidarabine, and even greater benefit has been shown with acyclovir, which has become the treatment of choice. HSE is treated by an intravenous infusion of 10 mg per kilogram given over a 1-hour period every 8 hours for 10 days. The therapeutic efficacy of acyclovir is restricted to the herpesviruses by virtue of the drug's selective interaction with two virus-coded enzymes, thymidine kinase and DNA polymerase; acyclovir is thus not a broad-spectrum antiviral. Because acyclovir is excreted principally by the kidney, caution must be exercised in patients with renal impairment. Side effects of acyclovir are generally few, although neurotoxicity rarely occurs, manifested as altered consciousness, tremors, hallucinations, and seizures. Other aspects of care also require meticulous attention. Optimally, patients with HSE should be managed in the intensive care setting of a tertiary referral center.

PROGNOSIS. Both age and initial neurologic status significantly influence the prognosis in HSE. Even with antiviral therapy, patients who are comatose when first treated often fare poorly. Extensive infection and brain damage are present in most of these patients as a result of a more fulminant illness and, sometimes, a delay in beginning therapy. Many patients, however, particularly those younger than 30 years old who are neurologically intact when treatment begins, recover normal or nearly normal function. Patients with minor neurologic deficits may survive without severe long-term sequelae and return to normal function if diagnosis is made and specific treatment is instituted early in the course. In a few patients, and despite antiviral treatment, HSE can relapse within a few weeks after the acute disease, resulting in severe sequelae. The pathogenesis of such relapses is unknown.

426.2 Neurologic Complications of Genital Herpes

Genital herpes, most often caused by HSV-2, may be complicated by local or radicular pain, aseptic meningitis, autonomic (bowel, bladder, and sexual) dysfunction, and, rarely, myelitis. These complications are more common in association with primary genital herpes but may occur with recurrent disease as well. Prodromal neuritic symptoms commonly precede recurrences and may involve the buttock, the groin, or, less commonly, the lower extremities.

Aseptic meningitis and autonomic dysfunction may occur either independently or together. Meningitic symptoms are associated with primary genital herpes in about one fourth of patients, but only a minority require hospitalization. Its course is benign, usually clearing in 4 to 10 days without residua. The CSF profile is typical of an aseptic meningitis, with a mononuclear pleocytosis, mild protein elevation, and normal, or occasionally reduced, glucose level. When the history clearly implicates an epidemiologic and temporal relationship with genital herpes and the CSF findings are those of a typical mononuclear profile, a clinical diagnosis can usually be made. Specific diagnosis can often be established by isolation of HSV-2 at lumbar puncture.

Urinary retention, constipation, and sexual impotence in association with genital herpes are less common than meningitis. Symptoms and signs of a sacral sensory radiculopathy sometimes accompany the autonomic changes. The pathophysiology of this disorder is uncertain, but direct herpetic infection of nervous system structures is likely. Fortunately, autonomic dysfunction is reversible, and patients can be assured that their symptoms will probably clear. Although unusual, these autonomic symptoms can recur. It is important to consider and pursue the diagnosis of HSV-2 infection in patients who present with isolated bladder, bowel, or sexual dysfunction. It is critical not to make an inappropriate diagnosis of spinal neoplasm or, especially, early multiple sclerosis. When there is a clear history of genital herpes, the cause of autonomic dysfunction is usually readily established clinically. Inspection and viral culture of genital lesions, plus accompanying antibody titers, which may appear and rise slowly only in primary HSV-2 infection, provide additional help.

In adults, HSV-2 only rarely produces adult-type herpes encephalitis indistinguishable from that caused by HSV-1. Transverse myelopathy due to HSV-2 is very rare.

Epithelial HSV-2 primary infections and recurrences can be treated with acyclovir, but the effect on the neurologic complications of genital herpes is uncertain. In the absence of adequate data, it appears appropriate to give acyclovir for neurologic complications of primary genital herpes.

In patients with frequent recurrent attacks of genital herpes, early, self-initiated treatment of recurrent lesions with oral acyclovir has been advocated, beginning therapy at the onset of prodromal symptoms. This approach is probably appropriate for the rare patient with recurrent herpetic meningitis.

426.3 Neurologic Complications of Varicella-Zoster Virus Infections

Herpes zoster (HZ) (shingles, zona) is a dermatomal cutaneous infection caused by reactivation of the VZV that normally lies latent in sensory ganglia following an early attack of varicella. In addition to its cutaneous manifestations, zoster is accompanied by neuritic symptoms and may be complicated by an array of neurologic sequelae. The VZV is distantly related to HSV, sharing only minor antigen cross-reactivity.

INCIDENCE AND EPIDEMIOLOGY. HZ is a common disorder, with an annual incidence estimated at 3.4 cases per 1000 persons. Unlike varicella, HZ occurs throughout the year, with neither significant clustering of cases nor seasonal or yearly preponderance. Case exposure in HZ is rarely identified. Two factors, age and immunosuppression, significantly influence its incidence. The disease is uncommon in childhood, relatively constant in those between 20 and 50 years of age (approximately 2.5 cases per 1000 annually), and thereafter doubles its incidence in those between the ages of 50 and 60 and redoubles it in those between age 80 and 90. Immunosuppression due to systemic disease (in particular, Hodgkin's disease and other lymphoreticular malignancies), cytotoxic drugs, corticosteroids, radiation therapy, or infection by human immunodeficiency virus (HIV) predisposes. In some cases, a history of neoplasm, radiation exposure, or physical injury in the proximity of the dorsal root ganglion or nerve is elicited.

Age is an important factor also in the development of postherpetic neuralgia, which develops almost exclusively in persons older than 50 years of age. The incidence of postherpetic pain varies, ranging between 15 and 75%, depending on clinical definition of the syndrome and selection of patients. Immunosuppression predisposes to spread of virus beyond the ganglion-nerve-dermatome unit into the central nervous system or systemically.

PATHOGENESIS AND PATHOLOGY. Although controversial, evidence suggests that VZV is latent in ganglionic satellite cells rather than neurons. Once latent virus reactivates, it can spread within the sensory ganglion and travel centrifugally over the peripheral nerve processes, eventually seeding the skin with the dermatomal vesicular rash.

Cell-mediated defenses rather than humoral immunity are critically involved in protecting the host during HZ. Pathologically, acutely infected dorsal root ganglia and nerve show the presence of a mononuclear inflammatory response, neuronal degeneration with intranuclear Cowdry type A inclusion bodies, and similar infection of surrounding satellite cells. The peripheral nerve may contain parallel changes. In more severe cases, dorsal root ganglia above and below the primarily affected ganglion also show active herpetic infection.

CLINICAL MANIFESTATIONS. Prodromal sensory symptoms include dermatomal pain, itching, or paresthesias, which often precede by several days the eruption of the segmental rash. The early pain of zoster may be confused with other types of neuropathic or visceral pain. Rarely, no rash appears but the role of VZV is suggested by a rise in antibody liters (*zoster sine herpete*). The most frequently involved dermatomes are those extending from the third thoracic to the second lumbar segments and the first (ophthalmic) division of the trigeminal nerve. The rash itself initially consists of erythematous macules that vesiculate over 12 to 24 hours. Normally the vesicular fluid pustulates within 72 hours; in a week the pustules begin to dry, and crusting takes place by 10 to 12 days. The crusts, in turn, fall off in 2 to 3 weeks. In the immunocompromised host, this time course may be protracted. In uncomplicated cases, the rash heals with a variable degree of superficial scarring, at times leaving areas of hyperpigmentation or depigmentation, which may be anesthetic. More severe cases may leave denervation of a large segment of the dermatome.

Zoster can affect any of several of the cranial nerves. The ophthalmic division of the trigeminal nerve is the most commonly affected, and the condition may be complicated by spread to orbital structures, resulting in acute and long-term ocular sequelae. Spread of cutaneous rash along the bridge of the nose to its tip should be taken as a signal of impending ocular infection, prompting early ophthalmologic consultation. Facial palsy, with or without accompanying loss of taste on the anterior two thirds of the tongue, may accompany either otic zoster (Ramsay Hunt syndrome), with rash confined to a segment of the auricle, or the second and third cervical dermatomes (cervical collar zoster). Occasionally, infection of the ninth and tenth or fifth cranial nerve may precede facial weakness. As with other motor syndromes (see below), weakness is often delayed for a variable period after the rash. Eighth nerve dysfunction with sensorineural hearing loss or vertigo occurs in the same setting as facial palsy but with less frequency. HZ may rarely cause facial palsy in the absence of rash (*sine herpete*). Zoster of the ninth and tenth cranial nerves is unusual and may be overlooked without a careful search for the pharyngeal rash or ipsilateral laryngeal or pharyngeal palsy.

HZ of the extremities or trunk can also be complicated by segmental motor weakness, the motor loss usually corresponding to the involved cutaneous dermatome. Weakness characteristically develops from a few days to 2 weeks after the onset of the rash, and longer delays are rare. Its onset is characteristically abrupt, occurring over hours or 1 or 2 days, with little or no subsequent deterioration. Weakness abates or disappears in about 85% of cases.

Myelitis of variable extent is a less common complication of HZ and results from direct viral invasion of the spinal cord, perhaps augmented by local inflammatory responses. It occurs most commonly in the immunosuppressed person and, like motor paresis, is characteristically delayed after the onset of the rash. The most common manifestation is bladder dysfunction. Other signs include mild or transient asymmetric reflexes, lower extremity weakness, and sensory disturbance. Severe myelopathy can produce a partial Brown-Séquard syndrome or total cord transection. Characteristically, involvement lies at the same spinal cord segment as the rash but may ascend to a higher level. Spinal MRI or myelography may be needed to rule out coexisting epidural tumor.

At least three types of brain involvement may complicate zoster: diffuse encephalitis, focal parenchymal infection, and vasculitis. Headache, stiff neck, and mild diffuse encephalitis often accompany acute HZ but are difficult to distinguish from the effects of fever, sepsis, narcotic analgesics, and other underlying medical problems. Most such patients recover fully. In more severe diffuse encephalitis, chances for recovery may also be good if other complications of the disease do not intervene. The clinical picture is that of acute or subacute lethargy or delirium accompanied by CSF pleocytosis with few focal features.

Focal VZV encephalitis is a rare complication in immunosuppressed patients that can resemble progressive multifocal leukoencephalopathy. The onset may be temporally remote from the cutaneous rash. The cerebral lesions involve principally the white matter. Brain biopsy is required for diagnosis, allowing identification of Cowdry type A inclusions or of VZV antigens or nuclei acids.

Cerebral vasculitis is probably the most common serious postzoster central nervous system complication. Affected patients usually develop delayed contralateral hemiplegic strokes following trigeminal ophthalmic division zoster owing to inflammation or occlusion of the internal carotid artery and its major branches ipsilateral to the rash. The delay between the rash and the onset of cerebral dysfunction varies from none to as long as 6 months, with a mean interval of 7 weeks. A more widespread cerebral vasculitis following zoster in other locations has also been reported. The pathogenesis is still incompletely understood, but the characteristic involvement of local vessels innervated by the infected ganglion, in conjunction with reports suggesting the presence of viral nucleocapsids and viral antigens within vessels, suggests that the arteries are directly infected. Additional contributions may be made by secondary local inflammatory responses and thrombosis, leading to vascular occlusion or distal embolization. Arteriographic evidence of vasculitis or occlusions in the involved vessels and the clinical setting usually allow diagnosis.

DIAGNOSIS. The clinical diagnosis of HZ is seldom difficult. The dermatomal distribution and the evolution of the vesicular rash are characteristic, and only rarely does herpes simplex infection assume a similar pattern and confuse the diagnosis. Difficulty, however, may occur early in the disease, when pain or other sensory symptoms precede the rash. The rare case of zoster sine herpete may require additional methods of diagnosis, and, in cases with an occult rash, a careful search is necessary. When there is a question of the diagnosis, a Tzanck test examining lesion scrapings, a direct culture, or immunohistochemical identification of infected cells can provide specific identification of VZV. Serology may also be helpful, although the commonly used complement fixation test can cross-react between HSV and VZV.

THERAPY. The goals are to relieve the acute segmental infection, to curtail spread of infection either systemically or to other areas of the nervous system, and to prevent postherpetic neuralgia. The means available consist of using antiviral drugs to interrupt viral replication and perhaps corticosteroids to modify local inflammatory responses. Treatment of individual patients must take into account their background risk for particular complications.

Because involvement of the ophthalmic division of the trigeminal nerve risks spreading to orbital structures, such infections should receive early antiviral treatment. Systemic antiviral therapy should also be used for immunosuppressed patients, who are more susceptible to severe disseminated infection. In young patients with normal immune function, there is usually no requirement for specific therapy because zoster is usually mild with swift recovery and no residua. Older nonimmunosuppressed persons are susceptible to postherpetic neuralgia. A recent large clinical study showed that prednisone had no protective effect against the neuralgia.

The antiviral treatment of choice for HZ is acyclovir. The nucleoside can abort the rash and prevent systemic spread when administered promptly by the intravenous route. The recommended intravenous dosages vary from 5 to 10* mg per kilogram infused every 8 hours for 5 days. More recently, the use of oral acyclovir has been suggested at a dosage of 800 mg* every 4 hours with omission of the nighttime dose, particularly in individuals who are not at marked risk of developing viral complications.

Intravenous acyclovir is indicated for patients in whom VZV infection progresses to cause myelitis or encephalitis, although delay in institution reduces its overall effect. No satisfactory data indicate whether either acyclovir or steroids improve the outcome of HZ-associated motor weakness. Similarly, there is no proven effective treatment for zoster-associated cerebral vasculitis. Postherpetic neuralgia is discussed in Ch. 405.3.

426.4 Neurologic Complications of Cytomegalovirus and Epstein-Barr Virus Infections

Both human cytomegalovirus (CMV) and Epstein-Barr virus (EBV) infections can cause neurologic disease. In children CMV is an important and relatively common cause of congenital neurologic deficit, but central and peripheral nervous system infections in adults occur almost exclusively in the setting of immunosuppression. Central nervous system (CNS) complications of EBV infections occur in the setting of acute mononucleosis. Both CMV and EBV have been implicated in triggering the Guillain-Barré syndrome.

CMV encephalitis and, less commonly, meningoencephalitis or myelitis have been reported as opportunistic infections in adults suffering from impaired cell-mediated immunity. Earlier these complications were reported most commonly in patients undergoing organ transplantation. Recently their occurrence has been noted principally in association with acquired immunodeficiency syndrome (AIDS). The clinical features of CMV brain infection have been imprecisely characterized, but they generally resemble the physical and cognitive impairments of a metabolic encephalopathy (see Ch. 394). At times, focal deficits (e.g., hemiparesis) or seizures are superimposed. Pathologically, infection of the brain is marked by scattered microglial nodules, some of which contain typical cytomegalovirus intranuclear inclusions. As many as one fourth of autopsied AIDS patients have neuropathologic evidence of CNS cytomegalovirus infection, although in most the infection appears to be mild, and its contribution to symptoms uncertain. Some patients may exhibit ventricular subependymal abnormalities or small abscess-like lesions on MRI. Hyponatremia is a common feature.

Recently, CMV has been found to cause severe ascending polyradiculopathy. This syndrome is usually characterized by the subacute evolution of severe, painful polyradiculopathy that begins with sacral or lumbar sensory, motor, and autonomic dysfunction.

The diagnosis of CMV encephalitis is difficult. Most AIDS patients, particularly homosexual men, have circulating antibody to the virus which can be isolated from urine or blood, yet they do not suffer nervous system infection. For this reason, serologic evaluation and systemic virus isolation are not particularly helpful in diagnosis; rather, one must rely principally on clinical suspicion. More recently, use of polymerase chain reaction (PCR) to amplify CMV DNA in CSF has been shown to be diagnostic. CMV polyradiculopathy can be diagnosed by the CSF findings, including the prominence of neutrophils, isolation of virus, and PCR amplification. The antiviral drugs ganciclovir and foscarnet have been reported effective in treating certain manifestations of CMV infection, including particularly the retinopathy that sometimes complicates AIDS but also CMV polyradiculopathy.

The neurologic complications of EBV infection range from symptoms of headache, photophobia, weakness, and fatigue to more serious, but uncommon, complications. The latter have been described principally in the context of individual case reports. They include encephalitis, meningoencephalitis, Guillain-Barré syndrome, Bell's palsy, acute cerebellar ataxia, and transverse myelitis. It is likely that most of these neurologic complications result from immune-mediated injury rather than direct viral infection. EBV is also implicated in the primary CNS lymphoma complicating AIDS and the immunosuppression of organ transplantation.

Aurelius E, Johansson B, Skoldenborg B, et al.: Rapid diagnosis of herpes simplex encephalitis by nested polymerase chain reaction assay of cerebrospinal fluid. Lancet 337:189, 1991. *A series demonstrating high sensitivity and specificity of polymerase chain reaction detection of HSV-1 DNA in CSF of patients with encephalitis.*
Bashir R, Luka J, Cheloha K, et al.: Expression of Epstein-Barr virus proteins in primary CNS lymphoma in AIDS patients. Neurology 43:2358, 1993. *Describes expression of EBV RNA and protein in primary CNS lymphomas.*
Devinsky O, Cho E-S, Petito CK, Price RW: Herpes zoster myelitis. Brain 114:1181, 1991. *A case series characterizing myelitis complicating HZ.*
Drobyski WR, Knox KK, Majewski BS, Carrigan DR: Brief report: Fatal encephalitis due to variant B human herpesvirus-6 infection in a bone marrow-transplant recipient. N Engl J Med 330:1356, 1994. *A detailed case report of a virologically well-studied patient with fatal encephalitis associated with HHV-6 infection.*
Holland NR, Power C, Matthews VP, et al.: Cytomegalovirus encephalitis in acquired immunodeficiency syndrome (AIDS). Neurology 44:507, 1994. *A case series analyzing the clinical and laboratory features of a group of autopsy-proven patients with CMV encephalitis.*
Miller RG, Storey JR, Greco CM: Ganciclovir in the treatment of progressive AIDS-related polyradiculopathy. Neurology 40:569, 1990. *Describes the clinical and therapeutic aspects of cytomegalovirus polyradiculopathy in AIDS patients.*
Straus SE: Overview: The biology of varicella-zoster virus infection. Ann Neurol 35:S4, 1994. *A general review of VZV introducing a symposium on VZV and postherpetic neuralgia containing several other useful brief reviews.*
Whitley RJ, Gnann JW: Acyclovir: A decade later. N Engl J Med 327:782, 1992. *A review of the clinical uses of acyclovir.*
Wood MJ, Johnson RW, McKendrick MW, et al.: A randomized trial of acyclovir for 7 days or 21 days with and without prednisolone for treatment of herpes zoster. N Engl J Med 330:897, 1994. *A clinical trial showing no additional effect of prolonging acyclovir treatment and only a modest short-term effect of prednisolone on healing of the acute zoster rash; neither longer antiviral treatment nor the corticosteroid influenced the incidence of postherpetic pain.*

427 RABIES
Richard W. Price

DEFINITION. Rabies is a viral infection with nearly worldwide distribution that affects principally wild and domestic animals but also involves humans, resulting in a devastating, almost invariably fatal encephalitis.

ETIOLOGY, PATHOGENESIS, AND PATHOLOGY. Rabies virus is a bullet-shaped, enveloped, single-strand RNA virus classified in the rhabdovirus family and *Lyssavirus* genus. It has particular neurotropic properties, and unlike many of the other viruses causing acute encephalitis, it appears to require central nervous system (CNS) infection as an essential part of its "life cycle."

Viral transmission to both animals and humans characteristically results from the bite of a rabid animal, although cases of transmission by aerosol in the laboratory or in a bat cave and by transplanted infected corneal tissue have also been recorded. Once the

---

* Exceeds manufacturer's recommended dosage.

virus breaches the protective epithelium, it reaches the CNS via peripheral nerves, exploiting retrograde axoplasmic transport. The interval between the bite and the onset of disease ranges from days to a year or more, but in most cases lasts 1 to 2 months. This delay may relate to amplification of the virus in peripheral tissues, particularly skeletal muscle, before it gains access to the CNS over motor and sensory nerves. During this delay, the virus can be eliminated by host immune mechanisms; indeed, it is this delay that affords an opportunity for prophylactic postexposure immunization after the rabid bite. Once virus enters peripheral and central nervous system pathways, immune defenses are unable to suppress further replication and spread of infection, which includes axoplasmic transport and perhaps transsynaptic transmission.

The CNS is involved in the subsequent transmission of the virus by infected animals in two essential ways: (1) Infection of certain brain regions underlies the characteristic behavioral changes in the rabid animal, leading to increased biting activity; and (2) antegrade transport of the virus to salivary glands leads to virus shedding. In concert, these two aspects of infection ensure transmission and survival of the virus in the wild. They also have practical diagnostic implications for the human disease. The characteristic altered behavior in humans often results in a distinct clinical picture distinguishing rabies from other viral encephalitides. Antegrade virus transport also affords a means of diagnosing rabies by isolation from saliva or immunohistochemical staining of infected cutaneous nerves innervating hair follicles.

Pathologic findings include both nonspecific and specific abnormalities. A considerable discrepancy often occurs between the degree of pathologic change, particularly neuronal loss, and the severe antemortem clinical state. Nonspecific changes include perivascular mononuclear infiltrates and microglial response, although inflammation may be scant in relation to the widespread distribution of infected cells detected immunohistochemically. Similarly, neuronal destruction is less prominent than the abundance of viral antigen, which is located principally in neurons but also in astrocytes. More specific changes include the presence of Negri bodies, eosinophilic neuronal intracytoplasmic inclusion composed of viral nucleoprotein. At autopsy, infection is usually widespread in the brain, but with prominent involvement of the brain stem and spinal cord and also involvement of the hippocampus, basal ganglia, cortex, and other structures. The relation of virus infection of neurons and the attendant inflammatory reaction to the clinical manifestations remains incompletely understood. Rabies infection of neurons may alter their membrane properties or synaptic transmission. Whatever the means, patients eventually manifest widespread brain dysfunction that terminally impairs respiratory and autonomic control.

EPIDEMIOLOGY. The epidemiology of rabies varies in different parts of the world, falling into two patterns. In *sylvatic rabies,* infection is maintained in wildlife reservoirs. Thus, in the United States, rabies is endemic in the striped skunk in the midwestern states and California, in the raccoon in the southeastern and mid-Atlantic states, in the red fox in northern New York and adjacent regions of Canada and in the gray fox in parts of the southwestern states; bat rabies has a wide geographic range. A similar pattern holds in other developed nations, where human rabies is rare and more often results from direct contact with wildlife than from secondary transmission to the domestic dog or cat and then to humans. This pattern contrasts with that in much of Asia, Africa, and Latin America, where *urban rabies* is maintained as an epizootic infection in the domestic dog and human disease is far more common. Viral strains differ among various animal hosts.

CLINICAL MANIFESTATIONS. After the silent incubation period, clinical rabies frequently begins with a prodromal phase, which may include nonspecific symptoms of malaise, fever, and headache but also more specific local symptoms related to the site of the original bite. These include itching, paresthesias, or other sensations beginning in the area of the healed wound and then spreading to a wider region and eventually involving the whole limb or side of the body.

Within a few days, the full-blown illness begins, taking one of two forms—encephalitic (*furious*) or paralytic (*dumb*) rabies—perhaps depending on the source and strain of the infecting virus. In its initial phase, encephalitic rabies is often distinguished from other viral infections by irritability of the patient and hyperactivity of a

number of automatic reflexes. Periods of calm lucidity may alternate with confusion and seeming intense anxiety precipitated by internal or external stimuli. Hydrophobia, with reflexive intense contraction of the diaphragm and accessory respiratory and other muscles, is induced upon attempts to drink or even at the sight of water. Similarly, blowing or fanning air on the chest may induce intense laryngeal, pharyngeal, or other muscle spasms (aerophobia). High fever persists throughout the illness.

Paralytic rabies is less common and more readily misdiagnosed. Patients present with weakness, usually beginning in the bitten extremity and spreading to involve all four limbs and the facial muscles. Early in the course, both consciousness and sensory function are spared. Helpful signs include myoedema and piloerection, and fever is also present. As the diseases progresses, it may converge with the encephalitic form, accompanied by some of the same irritative phenomena. Both forms evolve into lethargy and coma, with prominent alterations of respiratory and cardiovascular function. Tachycardia may precede bradycardia with ectopic rhythms, and the breathing pattern becomes irregular with cluster or periodic respirations. Patients succumb to respiratory failure or cardiovascular collapse within a mean interval of 4 days from onset, although a few may survive as long as 3 weeks or more. Intensive supportive care may extend survival longer; rare cases with partial vaccine-induced immunity have been reported to survive with intensive care.

DIAGNOSIS. Rabies is usually suspected on the basis of a history of animal bite or other exposure, although in as many as one third of cases no such history is obtained. Definitive antemortem diagnosis is established by immunohistochemical identification of rabies virus antigen in hair follicle nerve endings of biopsied skin, usually obtained from the nape of the neck. Isolation of virus from saliva or the presence of antirabies antibodies in blood in the absence of vaccination or in the cerebrospinal fluid may also be used to establish diagnosis. Postmortem diagnosis is usually made by histologic or immunohistochemical examination of the brain.

The differential diagnosis depends on the clinical presentation and the epidemiologic setting. In the case of paralytic rabies, diagnosis is most often confused with the Guillain-Barré syndrome, poliomyelitis, or other neuropathies or myelopathies, while the encephalitic form must be differentiated from other viral and infectious encephalitides, tetanus, and toxic encephalopathies. In regions where vaccine is prepared using neural tissue (still the practice in many regions of the world with the highest rates of rabies), allergic encephalomyelitis remains a principal differential diagnosis.

TREATMENT AND PREVENTION. Established CNS disease remains essentially untreatable. Disease prevention relies on public health measures to reduce animal reservoirs and on postexposure immune prophylaxis to abort viral penetration of the CNS after a rabid bite or other contact. Although clinical rabies is a rare disease in most developed countries such as the United States, the decision to administer active prophylaxis remains a relatively common clinical issue. The physician first determines the type of possible exposure; an open wound or disrupted mucous membrane exposed to saliva may warrant postexposure prophylaxis, whereas contact of saliva with intact skin may not. The first step in management is to administer prompt local wound care, thoroughly washing with soap or iodine. The epidemiologic setting is important in determining the likelihood that the biting animal might be rabid and often requires consultation with local health authorities to ascertain which animals carry rabies in the geographic setting. In the absence of previous vaccination, both passive (rabies immune globulin of human origin) and active (diploid cell vaccines) immunizations are administered. Presently, tissue culture–derived vaccines are safe, with a low incidence of major adverse reactions, in contrast to earlier nerve tissue–derived vaccines.

Baer GM, Bridbord K, Hui FW, et al. (eds.): Research towards rabies prevention. Rev Infect Dis (Suppl)10:S5773, 1988. *A compendium of brief papers presented at a symposium dealing with various aspects of rabies, particularly strategies for prevention, but covering a broad range of related tissues.*
Centers for Disease Control: Rabies Prevention—United States, 1991: Recommendations of the Immunization Practices Advisory Committee (ACIP). MMWR 40 (RR-3):1, 1991. *Outlines US guidelines for rabies prophylaxis.*
Fishbein DB, Robinson LE: Rabies. N Engl J Med 329:1632, 1993. *An outstanding and succinct review of the epidemiology and management of rabies and rabies exposure.*
Hemachudha T: Rabies. *In* McKendall RR (ed.): Handbook of Clinical Neurology, vol 12: Viral Diseases. Amsterdam, Elsevier Science Publishers, 1989, p 383. *A particularly valuable review of the clinical neurologic aspects of rabies.*

428 SLOW VIRUS INFECTIONS OF THE NERVOUS SYSTEM

Richard W. Price

428.1 Introduction

The term *slow infections* was first applied by Bjorn Sigurdsson to a group of transmissible diseases of sheep characterized by an incubation period and course measured in months or years rather than hours or days, as in typical acute viral or bacterial infections. Subsequently, several human diseases sharing these characteristics have been described. Although often considered together because of their chronic nature, these disorders are in fact heterogeneous with respect to their clinical manifestations, neuropathology, etiology, and pathogenesis. Although in some instances the infections are accompanied by inflammatory pathology, others clinically and pathologically more closely resemble degenerative or hereditary diseases of the nervous system. Two of the sheep diseases upon which Sigurdsson based his concept of slow infections, *visna* and *scrapie,* have subsequently proved to have human counterparts. Visna is caused by a retrovirus and somewhat resembles the nervous system infections caused by the human immunodeficiency virus type 1 (HIV-1) responsible for acquired immunodeficiency syndrome (AIDS) and tropical spastic paraparesis caused by human T cell lymphotropic virus type I (HTLV-I), while scrapie closely parallels Creutzfeldt-Jakob disease and kuru.

The agents causing the slow infections are taxonomically diverse, as are the mechanisms by which they maintain chronic progressive infection and cause clinical symptomatology (Table 428–1). Thus, HIV-1 is an RNA-containing retrovirus that codes for a DNA intermediary that can integrate into the host genome and persist for the life of the cell; progressive multifocal leukoencephalopathy is caused by a small, nonenveloped DNA-containing papovavirus; subacute sclerosing panencephalitis is due to the enveloped RNA measles virus; and Creutzfeldt-Jakob disease is caused by an agent that has not yet been definitively identified but may consist of a modified cell protein only (see Ch. 428.6). Contributions of host immune responses to the development and symptomatology of these diseases are varied. In the case of progressive multifocal leukoencephalopathy, a conventional virus that circulates commonly in the human community and is ordinarily associated with little, if any, disease causes devastating central nervous system (CNS) infection in the presence of depressed host cell-mediated immunity. HIV-1 causes profound systemic disease by virtue of its predilection for infecting the helper-inducer (CD4+) subset of T lymphocytes, with the resultant systemic immunosuppression perhaps playing a role in

TABLE 428–1. HUMAN SLOW VIRUS INFECTIONS OF THE CENTRAL NERVOUS SYSTEM

| Disease | Etiologic Agent | |
	Name	*Classification*
AIDS dementia complex	Human immunodeficiency virus type 1	Retrovirus (RNA)
Tropical spastic paraparesis	Human T cell lymphotropic virus type 1	Retrovirus (RNA)
Progressive multifocal leukoencephalopathy	JC virus	Papovavirus (DNA)
Subacute sclerosing panencephalitis	Measles virus	Paramyxovirus (RNA)
Progressive rubella panencephalitis	Rubella virus	Togavirus (RNA)
Creutzfeldt-Jakob syndrome, Gerstmann-Sträussler disease, kuru	—	Spongiform encephalopathy agents, prions

the subsequent development of progressive brain disease by this same virus. In this setting of perturbed immunity, CNS injury results from "indirect" mechanisms whereby uninfected cells are damaged by toxic products released from infected and reactive macrophages. The pathogenesis of myelopathy caused by HTLV-I also most likely significantly involves immunopathologic mechanisms. Subacute sclerosing panencephalitis appears to result from defective replication in the brain of a once-common conventional virus and is accompanied by an exuberant but ineffective antibody response. In the case of Creutzfeldt-Jakob disease, immunosuppression plays no role in the development or progression of the disease, and indeed there is little evidence that the host recognizes the infectious agent as foreign.

The diversity of the agents causing these slow infections, along with their variable cell and tissue tropism, host susceptibility, and pathologic reactions, has led to speculation that viruses may play a role in several of the common neurodegenerative disorders, including multiple sclerosis, amyotrophic lateral sclerosis, parkinsonism, and Alzheimer's disease. To date, however, no direct evidence for such an infectious cause of any of these disorders has been identified.

Tyler KL, Martin JB: Infectious Diseases of the Central Nervous System. Philadelphia, FA Davis, 1993. *Contains a detailed and informative section on viral diseases of the nervous system.*

428.2 Human Immunodeficiency Virus Infection and the AIDS Dementia Complex

DEFINITION. Among the common neurologic complications of human immunodeficiency virus type 1 (HIV-1) infection (see Ch. 364) is the *AIDS dementia complex,* which appears to relate pathogenetically in an elemental way to the AIDS virus itself rather than to secondary opportunistic infection. The nomenclature for this "subcortical" dementing syndrome is still in a state of flux, and several alternative terms have been used, including AIDS dementia and *HIV-1-associated cognitive/motor complex.* This section continues to use the earlier AIDS dementia complex terminology and the functional staging categories outlined in Table 428–2. Neither peripheral neuropathy nor psychological reactive states are intrinsic parts of the AIDS dementia complex.

CLINICAL MANIFESTATIONS. The AIDS dementia complex is characterized by a triad of cognitive, motor, and behavioral dysfunction. Patients' earliest symptoms usually consist of difficulties with concentration and memory. They complain of losing their train of thought or conversations and find that they need to keep lists to maintain their daily schedules. Many complain of "slowness" in thinking. Complex tasks at work or in the home, such as balancing the checkbook or reconciling other personal financial affairs, become increasingly difficult and take longer to complete.

Despite these early complaints, in stage 0.5 to 1, bedside screening or mental status testing may yield results within the normal range, although characteristically patients are slower and less facile than previously. With advancing disease (stages 2 to 3), patients perform poorly on tasks requiring concentration and attention, such as word and digit reversals and serial subtraction. Eventually, a larger array of mental status tests becomes abnormal, accompanied by psychomotor slowing.

Symptoms of motor dysfunction usually are less prominent than those of intellectual impairment. However, motor abnormalities, including, particularly, slowing of rapid successive and alternating movements of the extremities and eyes, are almost always noted on examination. Abnormal reflexes are common, with generalized hyperreflexia (in the absence of concomitant neuropathy) along with release signs such as snout or glabellar responses. With disease progression, symptomatic difficulty with balance or incoordination may be evident; patients may inadvertently drop things or become

TABLE 428–2. AIDS DEMENTIA COMPLEX (ADC) STAGING

ADC Stage	Characteristics
Stage 0 (normal)	Normal mental and motor function.
Stage 0.5 (equivocal/ subclinical)	Either minimal or equivocal *symptoms* of cognitive or motor dysfunction characteristics of ADC or mild signs (snout response, slowed extremity movements), but *without impairment of work or capacity to perform activities of daily living* (ADL). Gait and strength are normal.
Stage 1 (mild)	Unequivocal evidence (symptoms, signs, neuropsychological test performance) of functional intellectual or motor impairment characteristic of ADC, but able to perform *all but the more demanding aspects of work or ADL.* Can walk without assistance.
Stage 2 (moderate)	Cannot work or maintain the more demanding aspects of daily life, but able to perform *basic activities of self care.* Ambulatory, but may require a single prop.
Stage 3 (severe)	*Major intellectual incapacity* (cannot follow news or personal events, cannot sustain complex conversation, considerable slowing of all output), *or motor disability* (cannot walk unassisted, requiring walker or personal support, usually with slowing and clumsiness of arms as well).
Stage 4 (end stage)	*Nearly vegetative.* Intellectual and social comprehension and responses are at a rudimentary level. Nearly or absolutely mute. Paraparetic or paraplegic with double incontinence.

slower and less precise with hand activities, including writing. Gait incoordination may result in frequent tripping or falling or in a perceived need to exercise new care in walking. In more advanced disease, ataxia and, subsequently, leg weakness limit ambulation. Patients with early or predominating spastic-ataxic gait are usually shown to have vacuolar myelopathy pathologically (see below). Bladder and bowel incontinence is common in the late stages of the disease.

Psychological depression appears to be surprisingly infrequent in these patients, despite the prominence of psychomotor slowing. Patients appear uninterested and lack initiative but are not dysphoric. A minority develop a more agitated organic psychosis with manic features.

Patients with a severe progressive course who reach stage 4 characteristically lie quadriparetically in bed with a vacant stare and incontinence. They may be mute or exhibit an extraordinary delay in making brief verbal responses. Unless intercurrent illness develops, the level of arousal is usually preserved.

DIAGNOSIS AND DIFFERENTIAL DIAGNOSIS. Diagnosis relies on identifying the characteristic clinical features of the AIDS dementia complex and excluding other conditions. No single laboratory test establishes the presence of the syndrome. In those with milder forms, perhaps the major difficulty is in distinguishing true cognitive impairment from the effects of fatigue and systemic illness or from psychiatric conditions, including anxiety, depression, or hypochondriasis. The history is critical in establishing functional decline, and an observant friend or family member may provide particularly helpful information. Neuropsychological testing can define impairment of attention and motor speed but must be interpreted appropriately, taking into account the patient's background, including age and education, as well as confounding conditions such as substance abuse, previous head trauma, and the effects of various medications. Such studies are also useful for quantifying the patient's progression or response to treatment.

In those with more severe disease, the differential diagnosis most commonly centers on distinction from the other neurologic complications noted in HIV-1–infected patients (see Ch. 364) or, less commonly, from dementing or myelopathic neurologic disease observed in the normal population. Both neuroimaging procedures and cerebrospinal fluid (CSF) examination are diagnostically essential,

principally to eliminate other conditions rather than to establish a diagnosis of the AIDS dementia complex. Computed tomography (CT) and magnetic resonance imaging (MRI) almost always detect cerebral atrophy with widened cortical sulci and enlarged ventricles. In some patients, MRI also shows patchy or diffuse signal changes in the hemispheric white matter and, less commonly, the basal ganglia or thalamus (Fig. 428–1).

Routine CSF analysis is not specifically diagnostic, and findings may be indistinguishable from those in asymptomatic HIV-1-infected patients, with variable elevation of protein content or mononuclear cells. Elevations of CSF neopterin and β_2-microglobulin levels have been reported to correlate with the presence and severity of the AIDS dementia complex, but these markers of immune activation are also increased in CNS opportunistic infections and are not specific. HIV-1 isolation from the CSF is not diagnostically helpful because the virus can also be cultured from asymptomatic seropositive subjects. The p24 core protein is seldom detected by immunoassay in the CSF of patients with milder clinical disease and therefore generally is not useful.

EPIDEMIOLOGY. The frequency of the AIDS dementia complex increases as the systemic effects of HIV-1 infection and resultant immunosuppression worsen. This complication is rare in patients who are otherwise asymptomatic but begins to become more frequent in those manifesting constitutional symptoms (fever, weight loss, malaise). Its prevalence increases further as the CD4+ blood T lymphocyte counts fall and opportunistic infections develop. Preterminally this neurologic syndrome is common. However, precise prevalence figures are not available, and, indeed, with the introduction of antiviral treatment, the epidemiologic pattern of neurologic AIDS may be changing. Milder forms of the AIDS dementia complex, with a static or indolently progressive course, are more common in patients with preserved immune function (CD4+ lymphocyte counts above 200 per cubic millimeter), whereas the progressive and more severe forms characteristically develop in patients with more advanced immunosuppression. In addition, although there is a general parallel between the onset and severity of the AIDS dementia complex and the onset and severity of systemic complications, wide individual variability exists; at one extreme are patients with little or no systemic disease but with severe AIDS dementia complex, while at the other end some patients with repeated episodes of opportunistic infection may remain neurologically preserved.

PATHOLOGY AND PATHOGENESIS. The neuropathologic findings in patients with the AIDS dementia complex include at least three "subsets" of major abnormalities: (1) central gliosis and white matter pallor, (2) multinucleated cell encephalitis, and (3)

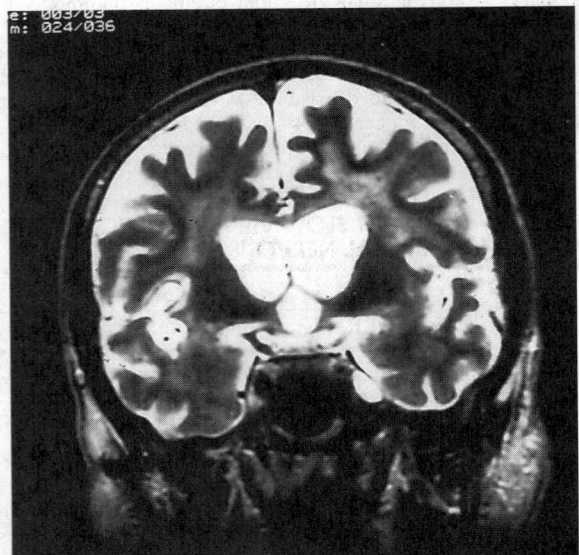

FIGURE 428–1. A coronal T2-weighted MRI of the brain of a patient with AIDS dementia complex showing typical atrophy with enlarged lateral and third ventricles and subarachnoid space along with "patchy" increased signal in the central white matter.

vacuolar myelopathy. In general, these findings correlate with the clinical severity. Central gliosis and white matter pallor are almost universal findings and, in isolation, are the major abnormality in patients with milder AIDS dementia complex. Rarely, they are the only abnormalities in patients with even more severe clinical symptoms and signs. Virologic studies to date have little or no viral burden in brains of this subgroup of patients.

Multinucleated cell encephalitis is characterized by the presence of perivascular and, at times, parenchymal cell reactions that include macrophages and microglial cells along with multinucleated cells derived from fusion of these two cell types. These multinucleated cells are infected by HIV-1, and, indeed, the cell fusion likely results from interaction of the viral glycoproteins gp120 and gp41 with the CD4 cell receptor. Multinucleated cell encephalitis is thus properly referred to as *HIV-1 encephalitis* and is noted in patients with more severe and progressive AIDS dementia complex.

Vacuolar myelopathy, while defined pathologically, can also often be distinguished clinically on the basis of the predominant myelopathic symptoms and signs. Patients with this condition usually present with spastic-ataxic gait difficulty but with proportionally little sensory disturbance and usually no definable sensory "level." Histologically, the disorder closely resembles subacute combined spinal cord degeneration accompanying vitamin B_{12} deficiency. Its pathogenesis is uncertain, but clearly independent of the type of productive infection that produces multinucleated giant cells.

The pathogenesis of the neurologic injury underlying the AIDS dementia complex has been difficult to unravel from a number of aspects. Because the major "functional elements" of the brain, i.e., the neurons, oligodendrocytes, and astrocytes, do not appear to be productively infected, it remains uncertain how these cells are damaged. In both the gliosis-pallor and the vacuolar myelopathy subsets, overt HIV-1 brain infection is absent or undetectable, and even in multinucleated cell encephalitis the magnitude of neurologic dysfunction often appears to exceed the distribution and extent of productive infection. Speculation has centered on possible indirect mechanisms of injury involving toxic molecules of either viral (e.g., gp120) or cellular (e.g., cytokines elaborated by uninfected cells responding to infection) origin. It is also possible that nonproductive infection of glia might lead to cell dysfunction without virus replication as a result of restricted viral genome transcription or translation. Whatever the mechanisms, however, HIV-1 infection, either of brain or of systemic organs, appears to be the *prime mover* in the pathogenesis of the AIDS dementia complex and thus the major target of therapy.

TREATMENT AND PROGNOSIS. Several reports now suggest that zidovudine (also azidothymidine, or AZT) relieves, at least partially, the symptoms and signs of the AIDS dementia complex. Therapeutic effect has been documented by improvement in neuropsychological test performance in several studies. Dose recommendations remain uncertain, but in the absence of precise information, conventional dosage (100 mg every 4 hours during wakefulness) is advised. Limitations of treatment relate to toxicity, (bone marrow suppression and, less often, myopathy), but, eventually, probable drug resistance. In patients whose neurologic condition deteriorates on these doses, the clinician may attempt to increase the dose, although toxicity is more likely. Additional antiretroviral drugs are currently being assessed with respect to their effect on this condition.

Symptomatic management is important. In the subset of patients who present with mania, lithium or neuroleptics may be helpful. However, these patients may be unusually susceptible to the side effects of neuroleptics and other psychotropic drugs, and thus treatment should be cautious and begin with low doses.

Navia BA, Jordan BD, Price RW: The AIDS dementia complex: I. Clinical features. Ann Neurol 19:517, 1986. Navia BA, Cho ES, Petito CK, et al.: The AIDS dementia complex: II. Neuropathology. Ann Neurol 19:525, 1986. *Companion articles describing the clinical and pathologic features of the AIDS dementia complex.*
Price RW, Perry S: HIV, AIDS, and the Brain. New York, Raven Press, 1994. *A collection of papers dealing with clinical and pathogenetic aspects of the AIDS dementia complex and brain HIV infection.*
Sidtis JJ, Gatsonis C, Price RW, et al.: Zidovudine treatment of the AIDS dementia complex: Results of a placebo-controlled trial. Ann Neurol 33:343, 1993. *A report of a clinical trial assessing zidovudine therapy for the AIDS dementia complex.*
Sidtis JJ, Price RW: Early HIV-1 infection and the AIDS dementia complex. Neurology 40:323, 1990. *A review of the issue of the AIDS dementia complex in asymptomatic HIV-1 seropositive individuals. Provides staging scheme given in this chapter.*

428.3 Human T Cell Lymphotropic Virus Type I– Associated Myelopathy and Tropical Spastic Paraparesis

DEFINITION. Human T cell lymphotropic virus type I (HTLV-I) was the first human retrovirus to be identified in the laboratory and the second, after human immunodeficiency virus type 1 (HIV-1), to be implicated in neurologic disease. This connection was made when a survey in Martinique discovered that nearly 60% of patients with tropical spastic paraparesis (TSP) were seropositive for HTLV-I. A similar serologic association was soon established in other tropical areas, and, concomitantly, Japanese workers implicated this virus in the myelopathy occurring principally in the Kyushu district; they proposed the name HTLV-I–associated myelopathy (HAM). Subsequent comparison of the clinical and laboratory features indicated that the tropical and Japanese conditions are, in fact, the same disease.

ETIOLOGY AND EPIDEMIOLOGY. HTLV-I is a genomically complex virus classified among the oncogenic retroviruses. Although infection is most often asymptomatic, the virus has been implicated in acute T cell lymphoma/leukemia (ATLL) as well as HAM/TSP. In Japan it is estimated that myelopathy develops in about 1 in every 2000 infected carriers and ATLL in perhaps 1 in 10,000 carriers; the two conditions rarely coexist. Infection is widely prevalent in much of the Caribbean, in certain parts of South Africa, South India, Colombia, Peru, and the Seychelles Islands, as well as Japan. In the United States, endemic infection is found principally in certain parts of the Southeast, chiefly among blacks; however, the influx of Caribbean and other migrants, as well as perhaps transfusion-related transmission, has resulted in more widespread sporadic dispersion. Infection is thought to be transmitted sexually from males to females, in breast milk, and by transfusion, the last factor having led to serologic blood donor screening. Although some preliminary observations suggested that multiple sclerosis might be associated with this retrovirus, numerous subsequent studies have failed to substantiate such a connection.

HTLV-I–associated myelopathy usually afflicts individuals between 20 and 65 years old and most commonly begins between ages 35 and 45 years. For those infected early in life, this implies a very prolonged incubation period. In patients infected by transfused blood, however, the incubation period is as short as 5 or 6 months. Otherwise, most cases are sporadic, although there is an occasional familial incidence. The variability in disease expression among those infected has led to the suggestion that host factors, including histocompatibility immune response genes, might be cofactors in the disorder's development.

CLINICAL MANIFESTATIONS. The salient feature of HTLV-I myelopathy is spastic paraparesis or paraplegia. Typically, the onset is gradual, with steady disease progression over months to years and a tendency in many instances to stabilize later on. Occasionally, the disorder begins more abruptly and has a more irregular course. Patients almost universally exhibit spastic legs; bladder and bowel disturbance is present in more than three quarters, while only about half have position or vibratory sensory impairment. Low back stiffness and pain are common. The gait may at times appear ataxic, and probably fewer than one tenth of affected persons have symptoms of neurologic dysfunction outside the spinal cord. Optic atrophy, nerve deafness, peripheral neuropathy, a clinical picture of pseudo-amyotrophic lateral sclerosis with anterior horn cell disease, and polymyositis have all been noted. Patients may also have systemic findings involving the lung (lymphocytic alveolitis), skin, and eyes (cotton-wool spots).

Characteristic CSF findings include oligoclonal immunoglobulin bands and intrathecal synthesis of anti-HTLV-I antibodies. The CSF cell count may be normal or show a mild lymphocytic pleocytosis; lymphocytes with flower-like nuclear changes similar to those seen in ATLL may be present. About half of patients have abnormal signal in the cerebral white matter detected by magnetic resonance imaging (MRI), indicating subclinical involvement.

The diagnosis of TSP/HAM relies principally on the identification of the clinical manifestations and documentation of viral infection; CSF abnormalities, including the high level of antibodies to the virus, are also helpful. Because of the high rate of asymptomatic HTLV-I infection, other neurologic conditions are likely to develop in seropositive patients, and thus the diagnosis requires more than simply ascertaining the presence of antibodies in a patient with spinal cord or other neurologic abnormalities. In addition, current serologic screening methods do not discriminate between HTLV-I and the related retrovirus, human T cell lymphotropic virus type II (HTLV-II), which also may be associated with a similar myelopathy. Additional testing with Western blot or more direct characterization of the viral genome by polymerase chain reaction can discriminate between the two viruses.

PATHOLOGY AND PATHOGENESIS. The spinal cord corticospinal tracts are most severely affected, although abnormalities are usually more widely distributed. Perivascular inflammation involving lymphocytes, macrophages, and plasma cells, along with fibrosis, is notable. Gliosis is prominent, with loss of myelin and, frequently, axons as well. Although the brain also contains scattered perivascular inflammation, parenchymal changes are usually minimal or absent. Immunologic studies show activation of major histocompatibility class I antigens in association with the inflammatory and gliotic responses.

Although HTLV-I antigens have been noted in some cases, most other attempts to identify infected cells have been negative, indicating that productive infection is minimal. This observation, along with the prominence of inflammation and the therapeutic response to immunosuppressive measures, suggests that immunopathologic processes are involved in the genesis of spinal cord injury. HTLV-I infection is associated with a state of immune activation with circulating activated T cells. Whether the neurologic injury relates to immune reactions to HTLV-I antigens and consequent "innocent bystander" injury of adjacent neural tissue or to true autoimmunity with activation of immune responses against self-antigens is uncertain.

TREATMENT AND PROGNOSIS. Immunosuppression using corticosteroids, plasma exchange, or other measures has been reported, principally by the Japanese, to alleviate HTLV-I myelopathy, although remission may not be well sustained. Antiviral therapy (with zidovudine or newer antiretroviral drugs used for AIDS) has not yet been clearly assessed in TSP/HAM. As noted above, the course and outcome are variable. Usually the disease becomes disabling, but not directly life limiting; thus supportive measures are of paramount importance, as in other spinal cord diseases.

Lehky TJ, Fox CH, Koenig S, et al.: Detection of human T-lymphocyte virus type I (HTLV-I) tax RNA in the central nervous system of HTLV-I-associated myelopathy/tropical spastic paraparesis patients by in situ hybridization. Ann Neurol 37:167, 1995. *HTLV-I RNA was found in the spinal cords of three HAM/TSP patients, including in astrocytes; contains an up-to-date reference list related to pathogenesis.*

Roman GC, Vernant J-C, Osame M (eds.): HTLV-I and the Nervous System. Proceedings of an international meeting organized by the Departments of Neurology of Texas Tech University and La Meynard Hospital, April 15–16, 1988, Fort-de-France, Martinique, French Antilles. New York, Alan R. Liss, 1989. *Contains reviews of the clinical, epidemiologic, and biologic aspects of TSP/HAM.*

428.4 Subacute Sclerosing Panencephalitis and Progressive Rubella Panencephalitis

Subacute sclerosing panencephalitis (SSPE), a "slow" infection caused by measles virus, usually affects children, but its onset can extend into young adulthood. Patients usually have a history of measles within the first 2 years of life, and it is speculated that such early host exposure allows emergence of persistent defective virus replication. Fortunately, its incidence has markedly decreased in recent years.

Clinically, SSPE usually begins with cognitive and behavioral changes; progresses to include motor dysfunction with prominent myoclonus choreoathetosis, dystonia, and rigidity; and usually pursues a progressive course with steady deterioration over 1 to 3 years to eventual rigid quadriparesis and a vegetative state. The condition is more common in a rural setting and affects males more often than females. The electroencephalogram (EEG) reveals periodic complexes with synchronous bursts at two or three slow waves per second, recurring at 5- to 8-second intervals. The CSF is characterized by a high immunoglobulin concentration, oligoclonal bands, and abundant intrathecal synthesis of antibody to measles virus antigens. Serum measles antibody titers are also high. These findings are usually sufficiently characteristic for diagnosis, but brain biopsy may be needed for definitive diagnosis in some cases. The distinct pathology of SSPE includes gliosis, loss of myelin, and perivascular infiltrates of lymphocytes and plasma cells in white and gray matter. Intranuclear inclusions containing viral nucleocapsids are noted in both neurons and glia.

Measles virus may also cause a subacute encephalitis in the immunocompromised host. The prominence of cognitive and motor dysfunction in these patients resembles SSPE, but the clinical setting, its subacute onset and more rapid evolution, and the presence of seizures rather than myoclonus are distinctive. Brain pathology includes abundant intranuclear inclusions, but inflammation is minimal, and neither serum nor CSF antibody titers against measles virus are high. For this reason, brain biopsy is usually needed for diagnosis.

Progressive rubella panencephalitis is a rare disorder resembling SSPE but caused by rubella virus and developing as a complication of either the congenital rubella syndrome or, more typically, childhood rubella. A hiatus of years separates early infection from the onset of neurologic deterioration, which is characterized by behavioral changes, intellectual decline, ataxia, spasticity, and sometimes seizures. Myoclonus is not a prominent feature, as it is in SSPE. Serology or viral isolation from brain or peripheral blood lymphocytes confirms the cause.

With the advent of widespread measles and rubella immunization, these disorders have been all but eliminated in the United States, although SSPE still occurs in less developed parts of the world. There is no known treatment.

Graves M: Subacute sclerosing panencephalitis. Neurol Clin 2:267, 1984. *A thorough general review of SSPE.*

Wolinsky JS: Subacute sclerosing panencephalitis, progressive rubella panencephalitis, and multifocal leukoencephalopathy. *In* Waksman B (ed.): Immunologic Mechanisms in Neurologic and Psychiatric Disease. New York, Raven Press, 1990, p 259. *An excellent review of the pathogenesis of SSPE and subacute rubella encephalitis.*

428.5 Progressive Multifocal Leukoencephalopathy

DEFINITION. Progressive multifocal leukoencephalopathy (PML) is an opportunistic viral infection of the CNS caused by a papovavirus, JC virus. Initially described in patients with a variety of underlying disorders accompanied by impaired T lymphocyte/macrophage-mediated immune defenses, it now most frequently occurs in patients with advanced human immunodeficiency virus type 1 (HIV-1) infection. It is one of the clinical AIDS-defining opportunistic complications. As the name implies, clinical PML affects principally the white matter of the brain, often with more than one lesion and characteristically pursuing an inexorably progressive course.

ETIOLOGY AND EPIDEMIOLOGY. Two factors are important in the development of PML: exposure to JC virus in the past and suppression of T cell-related immune defenses against the virus. With respect to the former, JC virus has a virtually worldwide distribution, and the majority of the population exhibits serologic evidence of exposure by the teenage years. Primary infection is benign, and, indeed, disease accompanying initial exposure has not been clearly defined. PML appears to result almost always from reactivation of latent JC virus infection rather than from recent exposure. The virus is thus innocent, except under circumstances in which the host's T lymphocyte-directed immunity is impaired and rendered unable to suppress JC virus reactivation and subsequent continued replication and spread. Recent studies indicate that JC virus infection in PML patients is not confined to the brain but also involves peripheral blood mononuclear cells, probably chiefly B lymphocytes.

Whereas the incidence of PML has increased with the AIDS epidemic to complicate perhaps 2 to 5% of cases, it may also complicate organ transplantation, lymphoreticular and hematologic malignancies (particularly in the context of cytoreductive chemotherapy), autoimmune disorders, and other immunosuppressed states associated with T lymphocyte dysfunction.

CLINICAL MANIFESTATIONS AND DIAGNOSIS. PML is characterized by the gradual onset and steady progression of focal neurologic dysfunction, usually involving the cerebral hemispheres. Thus, patients may present with homonymous visual field disturbance, hemiparesis, hemisensory disturbance, aphasia, apraxia, or other "cortical" dysfunction, depending on the location of the demyelinating focus. Posterior fossa abnormalities with cerebellar dysfunction or signs of brain stem involvement are less common. Most often the patient is otherwise well, without constitutional symptoms (e.g., fever, malaise), and consciousness is preserved. Headache or seizures are unusual, occurring in 10% or fewer of patients.

Diagnosis is often suspected on the basis of the underlying condition (e.g., AIDS) and the clinical presentation of focal neurologic deficit. Neuroimaging is helpful in demonstrating loss of white matter rather than an expanding mass (as, for example, in toxoplasmosis or primary CNS lymphoma). Computed tomographic (CT) scanning is less sensitive than magnetic resonance imaging (MRI), both with respect to detecting multiple lesions and in distinguishing white matter localization, most commonly adjacent to the cerebral cortex (Fig. 428–2). Characteristically, contrast enhancement is absent. Although MRI in the AIDS dementia complex may show multifocal abnormalities in the white matter that superficially resemble those of PML, patients with AIDS dementia complex usually do not have focal neurologic symptoms and signs and MRI lesions do not show on T1 MRI sequences as they do with PML.

CSF is usually acellular, with normal or only mild elevation of protein content. Serologic studies usually document the presence of serum antibodies against JC virus, but this is of limited diagnostic utility because antibody titers are indistinguishable from those of

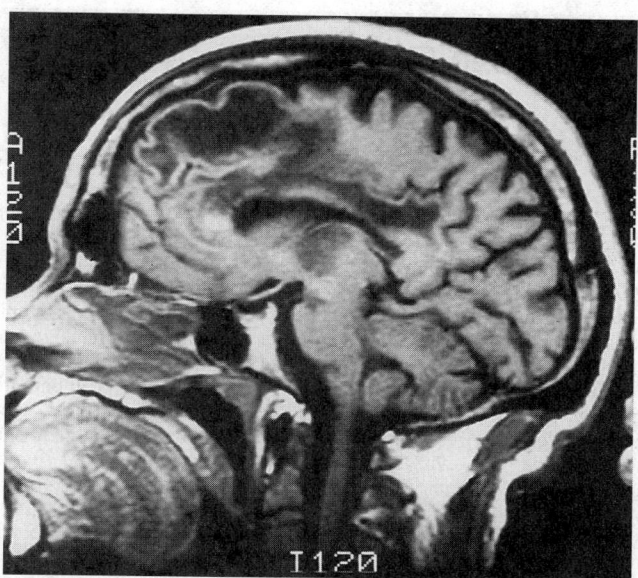

FIGURE 428–2. A sagittal T1-weighted MRI of a patient with advanced progressive multifocal leukoencephalopathy showing marked loss of white matter in the frontal lobe and cingulate gyrus with preservation of the cortical gray matter.

the normal population and do not rise with the onset or progression of the disease. CSF antibodies are usually not detected. Culture of the virus from CSF or blood is difficult, and not useful for diagnosis. Identification of viral nucleic acid in the CSF, blood, or urine using PCR appears promising, but the sensitivity and specificity have yet to be fully defined. Accordingly, brain biopsy is necessary for definitive diagnosis. The distinct histologic abnormalities usually permit diagnosis on routinely processed and stained tissue, but immunohistochemical identification of JC antigens or *in situ* hybridization to identify viral nucleic acid may be useful.

PATHOLOGY AND PATHOGENESIS. The pathology of PML provides an example of the selective effects of a virus on different cell populations within the brain. Thus, the major macroscopic finding of demyelination results from the progressive productive-lytic infection of oligodendrocytes. Lesions begin as microscopic centers of infection, which then spread concentrically outward; oligodendrocytes are lost in the center, and their nuclei are swollen, with inclusions at the periphery. Because myelin is composed of the elaborated cytoplasmic membranes of these cells, their lysis results in the characteristic demyelination; in mild lesions, axons are relatively spared, while in more severe coalescent foci, frank cavitation results. Macroscopic pathology consists of multiple foci of enlarging demyelinating "plaques." Astrocytes undergo marked alteration, with formation of bizarre nuclei resembling transformed cells, but without true malignant potential. Neurons are spared. Inflammation is usually minimal.

TREATMENT AND PROGNOSIS. There is no established treatment for PML. Case reports of response to cytosine arabinoside administered intravenously or intravenously are now being followed up by a controlled clinical trial. Of note, spontaneous remissions have been reported, including several in patients with AIDS.

Berger JR, Kaszovitz B, Post MJD, et al.: Progressive multifocal leukoencephalopathy associated with human immunodeficiency virus infection: A review of the literature with a report of sixteen cases. Ann Intern Med 107:78, 1987. *A review of AIDS-associated PML.*

Houff SA, Major EO, Katz DA, et al.: Involvement of JC virus-infected mononuclear cells from the bone marrow and spleen in the pathogenesis of progressive multifocal leukoencephalopathy. N Engl J Med 318:301, 1988. *A report emphasizing the presence of systemic JC virus infection in PML.*

428.6 Creutzfeldt-Jakob Disease

Paul E. Bendheim

DEFINITION. Creutzfeldt-Jakob disease (CJD) is a subacute central nervous system (CNS) disorder characterized by a progressive dementia, myoclonus, and distinctive electroencephalographic (EEG) and neuropathologic findings. Although uncommon, it is the most prevalent of the human subacute spongiform encephalopathies—fatal diseases that can arise either by dominant genetic inheritance, transmission of a unique pathogen, or sporadically.

ETIOLOGY. CJD is a unique disease in that it can apparently arise by two separate mechanisms, genetic and infectious. Most cases, however, are sporadic and in these the pathogenetic mechanism remains unknown. CJD is closely related to kuru and several rare, inherited human diseases termed the *Gerstmann-Sträussler-Scheinker syndrome* (GSS) and *fatal familial insomnia* (FFI). *Scrapie* is an analogous spongiform encephalopathy of sheep and goats experimentally transmissible to other animal species. As proposed in a remarkable insight by Parry 35 years ago, natural scrapie in sheep is genetic in origin, but the protein encoded by this mutated gene can behave as an infectious particle and transmit the disease to susceptible hosts. The scrapie agent is not known to cause disease in humans. The transmissible CJD, GSS, kuru, and animal spongiform encephalopathy agents are unlike any known virus or other well-characterized transmissible pathogen. This has resulted in the terms *slow virus, virion,* and *prion* being used interchangeably with "agent" to refer to them. These agents probably consist of protein only, and no nucleic acid component is needed to transmit the disease to susceptible hosts.

Kuru is a disease previously endemic among the Fore people inhabiting an area in the eastern highlands of Papua New Guinea. Cerebellar dysfunction, dementia, and progression to death within 2 years were typical. Women and children were affected much more frequently than men. Circumstantial evidence indicates that the kuru agent was transmitted through the ritual handling of affected tissues, especially brain, from deceased relatives. This cultural practice was discontinued, and the incidence of kuru has decreased dramatically since 1959. Brain tissues from patients dying of kuru were inoculated into the brains of chimpanzees, which, after a prolonged incubation period, developed a similar disease. Subsequently, the neuropathology of kuru and that of CJD as well as GSS were noted to be similar, and experimental transmission studies using CJD-affected or GSS-affected brain were undertaken successfully, eventually in a wide range of laboratory animals.

Progress in characterizing the transmissible agents of scrapie and CJD has partially clarified the distinct yet related mechanisms by which human CJD arises. The pivotal elements in the molecular pathogenesis are the PrP gene located on the short arm of human chromosome 20, and its product, the cellular protein PrP. PrP is normally expressed in neurons and other cells; its function is not known, but its concentration is critically controlled. The transmissible CJD agent is composed of degradation-resistant aggregates of PrP. It is postulated that when exogenous PrP "infects" a susceptible individual, it "replicates" by incorporating normal PrP into new aggregates in a process that resembles crystallization. These abnormal aggregates of PrP increase in concentration and size until they interfere with normal neuronal function. Genetic cases of CJD arise when disease-initiating mutations occur in the PrP gene and result in an intrinsically degradation-resistant form of PrP. The aggregation of these proteins occurs spontaneously, without the exogenous "seeding" crystal needed in transmissible cases. Nearly a score of PrP gene mutations have been identified in more than 100 families affected with various clinical types of CJD. Certain other allelic variations in the PrP gene, although insufficient to produce disease solely on a genetic basis, may predispose to developing CJD from an exogenous "infection" with the CJD agent. The molecular mechanisms by which sporadic cases occur are not yet delineated. Possibilities include somatic mutations in the PrP gene, post-translational changes in PrP itself which promote its abnormal accumulation, or other metabolic events that affect the processing of PrP. The unify-ing concept underlying the various causes of CJD is that aggregated PrP behaves as an *endogenous neurotoxin*. When PrP derived from either a normal gene (e.g., infectious cases) or a mutated gene (e.g., genetic cases) is not adequately degraded, it accumulates to toxic levels in the CNS.

The CJD agent provokes no inflammatory response or specific antibody production. It is resistant to chemical and physical treatments that inactivate most viruses, including heat, formaldehyde, nuclease digestion, and ultraviolet and ionizing radiation. This agent can be inactivated by procedures that denature proteins. Unique fibrillar structures are observed in electron micrographs of samples prepared from brain tissue of individuals with CJD. They resemble the abnormal fibrils that accumulate in scrapie-affected animals and represent an aggregated form of the CJD protein.

INCIDENCE AND EPIDEMIOLOGY. On a worldwide basis, the incidence of CJD is between one and two cases per million population. This incidence peaks in the fifth through seventh decades, although cases have been documented as early as the second decade. The genders are equally affected. Approximately 300 deaths occur in the United States each year. Higher rates have been noted in Israel among Libyan-born Jews and in circumscribed areas of the former Czechoslovakia and Chile.

CJD usually occurs sporadically in middle-aged adults without known exposure. A family history is evident in 8 to 15% of patients, and these patients are usually found to have a mutation in the PrP gene. Several reports document iatrogenic human-to-human transmission by cornea transplants and via the reuse of stereotaxic EEG electrodes that had unknowingly been previously implanted in a patient with CJD. Several cases have resulted from the use of dura mater allografts. Additional clusters of cases suggesting neurosurgical transmission have been reported. In the past decade, CJD has been diagnosed in individuals in both the United States and Europe who had received human pituitary gland growth hormone replacement therapy. It seems apparent that certain lots of the cadaveric hormone preparation were contaminated with the CJD agent. Incubation periods were between 4 and 21 years, emphasizing the astonishingly long incubation times of the spongiform encephalopathies. Additional cases may yet appear because more than 10,000 patients worldwide received this form of human growth hormone prior to its discontinuation in 1985. Also, four cases of CJD developed in Australian women who had been treated with pituitary gonadotropin for infertility.

Worldwide, the incidence of CJD is the same in countries with endemic sheep scrapie as it is in those without scrapie, indicating that there is no apparent transmission to humans from this animal reservoir. During the past decade a major outbreak of a new veterinary disease, bovine spongiform encephalopathy (BSE) or mad cow disease, has appeared in Great Britain. A few cases of BSE have been reported in other European countries. BSE has not occurred in the United States. BSE appears to have had its origin in the use of food supplements contaminated with the sheep scrapie agent. Although unlikely, it is too early in the BSE epidemic in Great Britain to determine if the passage of the scrapie agent through cattle poses any increased risk to humans. Nevertheless, British authorities have taken measures to prevent human consumption of contaminated beef.

PATHOLOGY. The pathologic findings in CJD are limited to the CNS, although the transmissible agent can be detected in many organs. Cortical neuronal depletion, marked reactive astrocytosis, intracellular vacuolar or spongiform change, and the absence of inflammation are the major features. Amyloid fibrils and plaques composed of the CJD protein occur in virtually all cases. The immunochemical detection of the protease-resistant protein PrP, *in situ* or after extraction, allows rapid confirmation of the diagnosis.

CLINICAL MANIFESTATIONS. Vague psychiatric or behavioral symptoms suggesting a personality change often herald the onset of CJD, but within a few weeks or months a relentlessly progressive dementia becomes evident. Myoclonus is usually present and often prominent at some time during the course. Deterioration is usually rapid, and 90% of victims die within 1 year. CJD patients are afebrile and have normal blood and cerebrospinal fluid profiles. The EEG in at least 75% of cases at late clinical stages shows a diffusely slow background with superimposed complexes, which may or may not be associated with myoclonus.

The dementia can be accompanied by signs of involvement of any part of the CNS. Most patients develop signs of cerebellar and pyramidal tract dysfunction as the disease advances. Visual disturbances, extrapyramidal signs, and various dysphasias often occur. The terminal stage is marked by decorticate and decerebrate postures, stupor, and coma. Massive myoclonic responses to auditory or other sensory stimuli may create the false impression that the patient is alert and responsive.

Subtypes of CJD based on distinctive clinical presentations have been delineated. The optic type features visual disturbances, usually cortical blindness. The dyskinetic form has prominent extrapyramidal signs, whereas the ataxic variant resembles kuru with its marked cerebellar involvement. *Gerstmann-Straüssler-Scheinker syndrome* is an autosomal dominant, genetically transmitted form of CJD with slower progression and signs of spinocerebellar ataxia. A specific mutation in the gene that codes for the CJD precursor protein has been found in some patients with this familial form of CJD. This mutation results in a protein with leucine substituted for proline at PrP codon 102, a step that promotes its aggregation into the characteristic brain amyloid. *Fatal familial insomnia* patients have a subacute course with untreatable insomnia, motor disturbances, dysautonomia, another specific PrP gene mutation, and marked atrophy of thalamic nuclei.

DIAGNOSIS. The diagnosis of CJD should be considered when a relatively rapidly progressive dementia develops in an adolescent or adult patient with normal spinal fluid. The presence of myoclonus or the characteristic EEG recording is strongly supportive, but often either or both are absent in early stages. All treatable diseases that can cause dementia need to be specifically tested for before a presumptive diagnosis of CJD or another untreatable dementia is made. Neither brain imaging nor laboratory evaluations are useful in diagnosis. Brain biopsy has been the usual method to establish definitive diagnosis. Research level, two-dimensional electrophoresis, however, has also provided accurate diagnosis in an increasing number of cases. In early cases, psychological depression, the AIDS dementia complex, and a number of rare dementias, including collagen vascular diseases and paraneoplastic limbic encephalitis, must be considered. Rarely, lithium toxicity can present with a clinical picture and EEG pattern resembling those of CJD. Discontinuation of the drug results in improvement within a few weeks.

Alzheimer's disease (see Ch. 400), the most common neurodegenerative dementia, usually has a more protracted course, without either the myoclonus or the typical EEG of CJD. Amyloid deposition in the brain is a pathologic hallmark of both Alzheimer's disease and CJD, but the amyloid proteins deposited in these two diseases are structurally unrelated. The development of specific antibodies for both these amyloid proteins allows rapid immunologic differentiation between CJD and Alzheimer's disease if a brain biopsy or postmortem examination is done.

TREATMENT AND PROGNOSIS. No effective treatment is available, and CJD appears to be uniformly fatal.

PREVENTION. Although CJD can be transmitted, the risk to health care workers and others having contact with patients is no higher than that to the general population. Isolation of patients is not indicated, but certain guidelines should be followed. Hospital workers should wear gloves when handling tissues, blood, and spinal fluid. Accidental skin contact with possibly contaminated fluids or materials should be followed by washing with 1 N sodium hydroxide or a 1:10 dilution of 5% household chlorine bleach (sodium hypochlorite). All laboratory samples should be clearly marked and needles disposed of properly. The agent can be inactivated on contaminated surfaces using a 1:10 dilution of bleach for 1 hour. Surgical and pathologic instruments should be steam autoclaved for 1 hour at 132°C. No organs, tissues, or tissue products from patients with CJD or with any ill-defined neurologic disease should be used for transplantation or replacement therapy.

Chesebro BW (ed.): Transmissible spongiform encephalopathies: Scrapie, BSE and related human disorders. Curr Topics Microbiol Immunol 172:1, 1991. *A multiauthored monograph with reviews on clinical, etiologic, genetic, epidemiologic, pathologic, and research aspects of CJD, kuru, scrapie, and BSE.*
Brown P, Gibbs CJ Jr, Rodgers-Johnson P, et al.: Human spongiform encephalopathy: The National Institutes of Health series of 300 cases of experimentally transmitted disease. Ann Neurol 35:513, 1994. *Clinical features are detailed in this large series of documented cases.*
Brown P, Goldfarb LG, Gajdusek DC: The new biology of spongiform encephalopathy: Infectious amyloidoses with a genetic twist. Lancet 337:1019, 1991. *A thoughtful summary of several disease-associated mutations and an insightful discussion on the seeming paradox of a disease that is both genetic and infectious.*
Prusiner SB, Hsiao KK: Human prion diseases. Ann Neurol 35:385, 1994. *A detailed review of the genetics of CJD.*
Rosenberg RN, White CL III, Brown P, et al.: Precautions in handling tissues, fluids, and other contaminated materials from patients with documented or suspected Creutzfeldt-Jakob disease. Ann Neurol 19:75, 1986. *Safety guidelines for health care workers and specific decontamination protocols for surgical and pathologic instruments.*

Section Nine—Neurologic Disorders Associated with Altered Immunity or Unexplained Host-Parasite Alterations

Richard A. Rudick

429   CENTRAL NERVOUS SYSTEM COMPLICATIONS OF VIRAL INFECTIONS AND VACCINES

Central nervous system (CNS) signs arising during the course of systemic infection usually reflects CNS invasion by the inciting organism. Less frequently, systemic infections or use of certain vaccines gives rise to CNS abnormalities that do not reflect direct infection of nervous tissue, but rather result from presumed autoimmune or toxic mechanisms. Several reasonably distinct patterns of involvement have been delineated. Two of these, *acute disseminated encephalomyelitis* (ADEM) and *acute necrotizing hemorrhagic encephalopathy* (ANHE), appear to be mediated by immune mechanisms and have a peripheral nervous system counterpart, acute inflammatory polyneuropathy, or the Guillain-Barré syndrome. The remainder, Reye syndrome, acute toxic encephalopathy, and acute cerebellar ataxia of childhood, are likely to be toxic in origin.

ACUTE DISSEMINATED ENCEPHALOMYELITIS

DEFINITION AND NOMENCLATURE. Acute disseminated encephalomyelitis is an uncommon acute inflammatory disease of the CNS which occurs following viral infections or vaccination.

TABLE 429-1. TERMINOLOGY: ACUTE DISSEMINATED ENCEPHALOMYELITIS

ADEM
    Postinfectious encephalomyelitis
    Postvaccinial encephalomyelitis
    Acute perivascular myelinoclasis
    Acute demyelinating encephalomyelitis
    Postvaccinial microglial encephalitis
    Disseminated vasculomyelinopathy
    Perivenous encephalitis
    Immune-mediated encephalomyelitis
Necrotizing form
    Acute necrotizing hemorrhagic encephalopathy
    Acute hemorrhagic encephalitis
    Acute hemorrhagic leukoencephalitis
    Hemorrhagic perivenous encephalitis
    Hurst's disease
    Hemorrhagic immune-mediated encephalomyelitis

TABLE 429-3. PRINCIPAL CONDITIONS PREDISPOSING TO ACUTE DISSEMINATED ENCEPHALOMYELITIS

Infections
  Measles
  Varicella-zoster
  Influenza
  Rubella
  Mycoplasma pneumoniae
  Respiratory agents
  Epstein-Barr
Vaccines: smallpox, measles, rabies (Semple vaccine)

ADEM is thought to be immune mediated. Brain and spinal cord involvement is usually widespread but may at times be limited to discrete areas such as the optic nerves or a single spinal cord level. Various names have been used to describe this syndrome (Table 429-1), but the term ADEM is appropriately descriptive. The classic features of ADEM (Table 429-2) include an antecedent event, commonly a viral illness, followed after a latent period by acute onset of multifocal or diffuse CNS signs, the potential for extensive or even complete recovery, and pathologic evidence of perivascular inflammation and demyelination.

ETIOLOGY AND PATHOGENESIS. Table 429-3 lists the principal events preceding ADEM, although many cases occur without a known precipitant. Of the various viral infections, ADEM occurs more frequently with RNA viruses that bud from infected cells. Viral infections associated with exanthems, such as measles, rubella, and varicella, are particularly common antecedents, but the disease also follows mumps, influenza, herpes simplex, or viruses causing banal nonspecific upper respiratory infections. The syndrome has been observed after vaccination for rabies, rubella, pertussis, influenza, or vaccinia, or in association with various medications. Neurologic manifestations usually occur 6 to 10 days after the exanthem, viral symptoms, or vaccination.

A compelling analogy links the ADEM complicating rabies vaccination with the animal disorder *experimental allergic encephalomyelitis* (EAE). Inoculation of susceptible animals with brain homogenates, highly purified myelin components, or peptides containing the encephalogenic sequences of myelin basic protein (MBP) or proteolipid protein (PLP) can induce acute CNS perivascular inflammatory and demyelination histologically identical to the pathology observed in ADEM. In animals with EAE, neurologic signs appear 10 to 14 days after sensitization to myelin antigens in association with humoral and cellular immune responses to the inciting CNS antigen. Furthermore, EAE can be transferred to naive animals by injecting T lymphocytes from the immunized animals, suggesting that this cell type is of primary importance in the pathogenesis. ADEM complicating rabies vaccination is considered a human form of EAE. ADEM was observed in as many as one of every 600 individuals following rabies vaccination using inactivated inoculum of fixed rabies virus propagated in animal brain. The complication of rabies vaccination called "neuroparalytic accident" was caused by vaccine contamination with CNS antigens. Both complement-fixing antibody and specific lymphocyte proliferative responses to crude and purified CNS antigens have been measured in blood of patients receiving rabies vaccine, with the most abnormal responses in patients with neuroparalytic accidents. Current ra-

bies vaccines derived from virus grown in human diploid cells appear to be essentially free of neural complications (see Ch. 427).

ADEM following viral infection may also be immune mediated. Lymphocytes that proliferate in the presence of MBP, complement-fixing antibodies to neural tissue, and humoral factors with demyelinating activity have been described. Encephalitis is relatively frequent following measles (1:1000 cases), but there is little evidence to implicate invasion of the CNS by measles virus as an obligate prerequisite. Theoretical data support the possible importance of sequence similarities between measles virus or other viral antigens and CNS proteins such as MBP and PLP. Very early in the course of measles ADEM, specific proliferative responses to MBP are apparent in the lymphocytes of children, and measurable quantities of MBP are released into CSF. These findings support the hypothesis that acute measles transiently alters the immune system, which in some persons results in a breakdown of tolerance to CNS antigens. Despite the usual absence of CNS symptoms, this process appears to occur frequently, as reflected by a high incidence of abnormal-appearing electroencephalograms (EEG's). Both EEG abnormalities and clinical ADEM can occur after vaccination with live-attenuated measles virus but at a markedly lower frequency, with ADE arising in about one in 1 million vaccinated persons.

INCIDENCE. Valid incidence figures for ADE are difficult to derive. Encephalitis complicates about one in 1000 cases of measles. ADEM following vaccination for smallpox is of only historical interest but occurred in the United States with a reported incidence of 2.9 per million primary vaccinations. ADEM following other childhood viral illnesses or vaccinations is uncommon. Most adult cases of ADEM have no identifiable antecedents.

PATHOLOGY. Characteristic lesions typically occur around venules within the white matter of brain and spinal cord. Leptomeninges contain lymphocytes, plasma cells, and occasional polymorphonuclear cells early in the course. Shortly thereafter, there is a perivenular mononuclear inflammatory infiltration. Myelin in this distribution becomes fragmented and eventually entirely absent. There is relative axonal sparing. This primary lesion can occur throughout the neuraxis but tends to be most prominent in the centrum semiovale of the cerebrum and in the pontine white matter. Repair occurs through remyelination. In certain cases, large, confluent demyelination can take on a superficial resemblance to the plaques of multiple sclerosis, differing primarily in that all lesions reflect a similar time of onset.

CLINICAL MANIFESTATIONS. In adults, neurologic symptoms often first suggest the illness. With the childhood exanthems, CNS symptoms usually begin about 5 days after the onset of the rash. The clinical disorder can resemble any of the acute encephalitides. Typically, nonspecific symptoms of fever, headache, anorexia, and vomiting are rapidly followed by meningeal signs, altered consciousness, and focal signs referable to brain, spinal cord, optic nerves, or spinal roots. About half the patients experience one or more generalized seizures. Neurologic signs consist of some combination of pyramidal tract dysfunction, cranial nerve signs, movement disorders, sensory system dysfunction, cerebellar signs, and loss of muscle stretch reflexes. Stupor, delirium, or coma develops in severe cases. The EEG is abnormal, with widespread slowing of background rhythms. The cerebrospinal fluid in children almost invariably shows a modest mononuclear pleocytosis of 20 to 200 cells per cubic millimeter and occasionally higher. The fluid contains a slight elevation of protein content, a normal glucose level, and a raised MBP. Tests for oligoclonal bands are usually negative. After several days, magnetic resonance imaging (MRI) characteristically demonstrates scattered white matter lesions, at least some of which enhance with paramagnetic agents during the acute phases of the disease.

TABLE 429-2. CARDINAL FEATURES OF ACUTE DISSEMINATED ENCEPHALOMYELITIS

Preceding event—usually viral illness
Latent period followed by acute onset of multifocal or diffuse CNS signs
Potential for extensive recovery
Pathologic features of perivascular inflammation and demyelination; vessel damage and hemorrhage variable

The duration of active CNS disease varies from days to weeks, often with a protracted convalescence. The overall mortality is about 20%. About 90% of survivors recover completely or nearly completely, although severe residual deficits can occur.

DIAGNOSIS. Diagnosis in ADEM is by exclusion. The most important consideration is CNS infection. In pathologic series of clinically diagnosed ADEM occurring during the course of mass vaccination programs, postmortem examination showed that the majority of patients had other illnesses, including potentially treatable CNS infections. In the setting of a recent exanthem, viral illness, or vaccination, ADEM may be suggested. Differentiation from an initial severe episode of MS (see Ch. 432) can be difficult, particularly because relapsing forms of ADEM have been reported.

TREATMENT. Treatment consists of supportive care, including the use of anticonvulsants and, when necessary, intensive care monitoring. Although sometimes used clinically, neither corticosteroids nor other immunosuppressive drugs have established efficacy.

ACUTE NECROTIZING HEMORRHAGIC ENCEPHALOPATHY

Acute necrotizing hemorrhagic encephalopathy (ANHE) is considered the hyperacute form of ADEM. As with ADEM, many names have been applied to this syndrome (see Table 429–1). ANHE is thought to have a similar immunopathogenesis to ADEM. Typically, the illness arises spontaneously or following an uneventful upper respiratory illness. Sudden headache precedes the neurologic symptoms, which include seizures and rapid progression from lethargy to coma in a matter of a few hours to several days. Major focal neurologic abnormalities are common and may suggest lateralized cerebral involvement. Systemic signs and symptoms include fever and marked peripheral leukocytosis. The accompanying CSF pleocytosis usually shows a preponderance of polymorphonuclear cells and sometimes evidence of hemorrhage. More than 80% of all recognized cases of ANHE are fatal, although these findings may be biased by selective reports of postmortem studies. The brain is usually swollen, and examination shows bilateral but asymmetric abnormalities, with petechial hemorrhages scattered throughout the white matter. Microscopic lesions consist of features reminiscent of hyperacute forms of EAE. The clinical differential diagnosis includes ADEM and acute viral encephalitis, especially herpes simplex encephalitis (see Ch. 426). Computed tomography (CT) or MRI may be diagnostically helpful in selected cases. Therapy is supportive.

Griffin DE: Monophasic autoimmune inflammatory diseases of the CNS and PNS. Res Publ Assoc Res Nerv Ment Dis 68:91, 1990. *A review of recent advances in unraveling parainfectious nervous system disease.*

Kesselring J, Miller DH, Robb SA, et al.: Acute disseminated encephalomyelitis—MRI findings and the distinction from multiple sclerosis. Brain 113:291, 1990. *Multifocal white matter lesions indistinguishable from those seen in MS in most patients with ADEM.*

430 REYE SYNDROME

DEFINITION. Reye syndrome is a form of hepatic encephalopathy with fatty infiltration of the liver, markedly raised intracranial pressure, and brain edema. The illness follows one of several common viruses or hepatotoxicity from commonly used drugs.

ETIOLOGY AND PATHOGENESIS. Reye syndrome appears to be due to an abnormality of mitochondrial fatty acid metabolism. Entry of fatty acids into mitochondria or beta-oxidation itself may be impaired. Biochemical manifestations of Reye syndrome, regardless of the precipitant, include hypoglycemia, accumulation of fatty acids, fatty acyl CoA's, and acyl carnitines. Accumulated products further injure mitochondria, further impairing beta-oxidation. Reye syndrome almost always follows a viral infection, and epidemiologic studies strongly support a link between the use of aspirin and Reye syndrome. The syndrome most commonly follows influenza A, influenza B, herpes varicella zoster, and to a lesser extent several other common virus infections. Little evidence links the precipitating viral infection directly to either the central nervous system (CNS) or hepatic involvement. A toxic origin is proposed for both types of involvement. Hepatic dysfunction results in various metabolic derangements including hyperammonemia, lactic acidemia, and elevated levels of serum free fatty acids. These metabolic derangements have been implicated in the pathogenesis of the brain swelling and increased intracranial pressure that dominate the clinical course of severe cases. The precise mechanism of mitochondrial impairment remains to be clarified.

INCIDENCE. Reye syndrome occurs most commonly among children between 1 and 15 years of age but has been reported in adolescents and is increasingly recognized in adults. Inner city black infants may be especially at risk for the disease. Prospectively derived incidence figures for the most susceptible age groups are as high as 6.2 per 100,000 children.

PATHOLOGY. The liver shows a noninflammatory, panlobular, hepatocellular accumulation of lipid droplets and both histochemical and ultrastructural evidence of inflammation. At postmortem examination, swelling of astrocytic foot processes and ultrastructural changes in mitochondria similar to those seen in hepatic mitochondria may be found in the greatly swollen brain.

CLINICAL MANIFESTATIONS AND COURSE. Reye syndrome is a biphasic disorder. As symptoms of the initial viral illness begin to wane or clear, intractable vomiting appears in association with lethargy or delirium. Early diagnosis is confirmed by the findings of nonicteric hepatic dysfunction, an elevated arterial blood ammonia level, and serum transaminase levels that exceed three times normal levels. Hepatic enlargement is present in about one half of the cases. Children under 1 year of age often show hypoglycemia. Signs of CNS deterioration include the development of generalized seizures, deepening obtundation, and transtentorial herniation. The cerebrospinal fluid is under increased pressure but is acellular, with otherwise normal constituents.

DIAGNOSIS. Diagnosis rests on the clinical findings and appropriate biochemical abnormalities. Liver biopsy usually is not necessary. CNS infection, inborn errors of metabolism, such as ornithine transcarbamoylase deficiency and systemic carnitine deficiency, and the presence of known hepatotoxins, including valproate, salicylates, and paracetamol, must be actively excluded. A childhood syndrome, distinguishable from Reye syndrome only by the absence of hepatic involvement and a high incidence of acute convulsions, can follow both banal viral infections and vaccination.

TREATMENT. Affected patients require intensive care monitoring until the course of the disease is well established. Hypoglycemia and electrolyte abnormalities must be corrected. Many authorities suggest hydration with solutions of high glucose content. Appropriate measures should be taken to monitor intracranial pressure continuously in the more severely affected cases, as judicious control of intracranial hypertension contributes to a favorable outcome. Mortality is about 10%.

Ede RJ, Williams R: Reye's syndrome in adults. Br Med J 296:517, 1988. *Although uncommon, such cases do occur and need management different from that for children.*

Pranzatelli MR, DeVivo DC: Pharmacology of Reye syndrome. Clin Neuropharmacol 10:96, 1987. *A comprehensive review including detailed recommendations for medical management.*

431 NEUROLOGIC COMPLICATIONS IN THE IMMUNOLOGICALLY COMPROMISED HOST

Immunodeficient states induced by a variety of intrinsic or exogenous mechanisms greatly reduce the central nervous system's (CNS) natural resistance to infection (for mechanisms, see Ch. 266). Many well-known and a few uncommon causes of immune compromise exist, some examples being genetically related immune deficiency disorders (see Ch. 223); splenectomy; the giving of active immune suppressants to facilitate renal, bone marrow or other organ transplants or protect against severe autoimmune disorders; applying chemotherapy or radiation therapy for cancer or allied disorders; and the intrinsic capacity of HIV-1 to destroy CD4 lymphocytes. Each of these conditions predisposes to serious infections of the CNS, and some can foster primary or secondary lymphoma production in the brain or, rarely, the spinal cord.

In transplant recipients, hospital-acquired bacterial species provide the major early risk (see Ch. 266 and 267). Early on, severe immunosuppression of any kind also commonly reactivates herpes viruses, most frequently herpes simplex, then herpes varicella virus, and, least often, cytomegalovirus (see Ch. 426). Sooner or later, with continued immunosuppression nosocomial bacterial and mycotic infections may arise (see Ch. 267).

Among cancer patients (e.g., Hodgkin's disease or hairy cell leukemia) as well as in certain hematologic disorders or other less common conditions, splenectomy may be indicated. It increases the risk of bacterial meningitis (see Ch. 151). Other immunosuppressed patients are similarly at risk for either bacterial or fungal infections of the brain-meninges. Progressive multifocal encephalopathy (see Ch. 428.5) nowadays most often appears as a complication of AIDS, but the condition also may arise in patients suffering from other forms of severe immunosuppression as well as sporadically. Potential CNS immunologic complications of AIDS, among which differentiation between toxoplasmosis and lymphoma may be difficult, are discussed in Ch. 364 and 428.2.

Section Ten—The Demyelinating Diseases

432 MULTIPLE SCLEROSIS AND RELATED CONDITIONS
Richard A. Rudick

This section discusses diseases primarily affecting central nervous system (CNS) myelin; demyelinating peripheral neuropathies are discussed in Ch. 447. CNS myelin is an elaborate extension of the oligodendrocyte cell membrane. A single oligodendrocyte myelinates as many as 20 or 30 different CNS axonal segments, each over a length of 1 mm or less. Oligodendrocyte membrane extensions wrap around the axons in a concentric fashion to form the myelin sheath. Tightly compacted mature myelin consists of parallel layers of bimolecular lipids apposed to layers of hydrated protein. Lipids, including cerebroside, phospholipids, and cholesterol, constitute 75% of myelin's dry weight. Myelin proteins include proteolipid protein, myelin basic protein, myelin-associated glycoprotein, and a number of less abundant proteins detectable by electrophoretic separation. Active myelin synthesis starts *in utero* and continues for the first 2 years of life; slower synthesis continues during childhood and adolescence. Turnover of mature myelin continues at a slower rate throughout life. Both developing and mature forms of myelin are readily susceptible to injury by the disease described in this section.

Table 432–1 classifies the several forms of myelin diseases. Acquired disorders are separated from developmental abnormalities. Multiple sclerosis (MS) and its variants are by far the most common diseases in this group. Viral infections, nutritional disorders, and anoxic-ischemic sequelae are discussed in Ch. 423 through 428, 406, and 394. The leukodystrophies are uncommon disorders but instructive because recent genetic and biochemical advances have elucidated the mechanisms causing many of these conditions.

MULTIPLE SCLEROSIS

DEFINITION. MS is a disorder of unknown cause, defined clinically by characteristic symptoms, signs, and progression and pathologically by scattered areas of inflammation and demyelination affecting the brain, optic nerves, and spinal cord. The first symptoms of MS most commonly occur between the ages of 15 and 50. Most MS patients recover to some degree from individual bouts of inflammatory demyelination, producing the classic exacerbating-remitting course seen early in the disease. Diagnosis requires intermittent or progressive CNS symptoms buttressed by evidence for two or more CNS white matter lesions and occurring in an appropriately aged patient who lacks an alternative explanation such as recurrent strokes or systemic lupus erythematosus. The diagnosis is based on clinical features; currently available laboratory tests support the diagnosis but are not directly diagnostic.

ETIOLOGY. The cause of MS is unknown, but it is now widely believed that the pathogenesis involves immune-mediated inflammatory demyelination. Pathologic examination of MS brain shows the hallmarks of an immunopathologic process—perivascular infiltration by lymphocytes and monocytes, class II MHC antigen expression by cells in the lesions, lymphokines and monokines secreted by activated immune cells, and the absence of overt evidence for infection. Additional evidence for an autoimmune pathogenesis includes (1) immunologic abnormalities in blood and cerebrospinal fluid (CSF) of MS patients, notably selective intrathecal humoral immune activation, lymphocyte subset abnormalities, and a high frequency of activated lymphocytes in blood and CSF; (2) an association between MS and certain MHC class II allotypes; (3) the

TABLE 432–1. DISEASES OF MYELIN

Idiopathic, presumably autoimmune (this chapter)
  Recurrent or chronically progressive demyelination (multiple sclerosis and its variants)
  Monophasic demyelination (may be first clinical episode of multiple sclerosis)
    Optic neuritis
    Acute transverse myelitis
  Acute disseminated encephalomyelitis; acute hemorrhagic leukoencephalopathy
    Following infection, with or without exanthem
    Following vaccination
Viral infections (see Ch. 423–428)
  Progressive multifocal leukoencephalopathy
  Subacute sclerosing panencephalitis
Nutritional disorders (see Ch. 406)
  Combined systems disease (vitamin B_{12} deficiency)
  Demyelination of the corpus callosum (Marchiafava-Bignami disease)
  Central pontine myelinolysis
Anoxic-ischemic sequelae (see Ch. 394)
  Delayed postanoxic cerebral demyelination
  Progressive subcortical ischemic encephalopathy
Leukodystrophies (this chapter)
  Primarily affecting CNS myelin
    Adrenoleukodystrophy (Schilder's disease)
    Pelizaeus-Merzbacher disease
    Spongy degeneration
    Others (Alexander's disease, Canavan's disease)
  Central peripheral nervous system
    Metachromatic leukodystrophy
    Globoid cell (Krabbe's disease)

clinical response of MS patients to immunomodulation—patients tend to improve with immunosuppressive drugs and worsen with interferon-gamma (IFN-γ) treatment, which stimulates the immune response; and (4) striking similarities between MS and experimental allergic encephalomyelitis (EAE)—an animal model in which recurrent episodes of inflammatory demyelination can be induced by inoculating susceptible animals with myelin basic protein or proteolipid protein.

Epidemiologic studies suggest environmental and genetic factors in the etiopathogenesis of MS. The uneven geographic distribution of the disease and the occurrence of several point-source epidemics have suggested environmental factors; however, intense study over the past 30 years has failed to establish an infectious cause. Migration studies have shown that exposure to undefined environmental factors prior to adolescence is required for subsequent development of MS. A genetic influence is well-established by excess concordance in monozygotic compared with dizygotic twins, clustering of MS in families, racial variability in risk, and association with class II MHC allotypes. In Caucasians, the HLA class II haplotype DR15,DQ6,Dw2 appears strongly and consistently associated with an increased risk of MS.

The evidence—immunologic, epidemiologic, and genetic—supports the concept that exposure of a genetically susceptible individual to an environmental factor(s) during childhood (perhaps any one of many common viruses) leads eventually to immune-mediated inflammatory demyelination. The precise interplay between genetic, environmental, and immunologic factors and the nature of the environmental trigger(s) remains to be elucidated.

INCIDENCE, PREVALENCE, AND EPIDEMIOLOGY. The annual *incidence* rate for MS ranges in different populations from 1.5 to 11 per 100,000. Several studies suggest that the incidence rate has increased over time. For example, data from Olmsted County, Minnesota, suggested a gradual increase in annual incidence during the past century from about 1.2 per 100,000 between 1905 and 1914 to about 6.2 per 100,000 between 1975 and 1984. In all studies, the highest age- and gender-specific rates occur in women between 20 and 40 years of age.

Worldwide prevalence differs according to geography. Distribution of MS has been well studied in North America, Northern Europe, Australia, and New Zealand. In both hemispheres, MS is more common in the temperate zones, decreasing toward the equator. The *prevalence* of MS in the northern United States, Canada, and northern Europe is at least 100 per 100,000 population; in certain regions, the prevalence of MS exceeds 300 per 100,000 people, compared with less than 5 per 100,000 people in the tropics. Regional heterogeneity has been reported within high prevalence zones, and several reports describe MS clusters in small areas. In the Faroe Islands, for example, a well-reported outbreak of MS occurred during the 20 years following the start of World War II, suggesting the effects of an unidentified environmental factor.

PATHOLOGY. Brain, optic nerves, and spinal cord from MS patients contain scattered areas of myelin loss ranging in size from 1 mm to several centimeters in diameter with relatively intact axons. The borders between histologically normal tissue and demyelinated zones are usually well-demarcated but may shade from normal to thinning before bare axons occur. Some areas show diffuse partial myelin loss. Although plaques may occur in any myelinated area of the CNS, the most commonly affected regions include optic nerves, periventricular cerebral white matter, and cervical spinal cord.

The earliest event in development of the MS lesion is breakdown of the blood-brain barrier, followed by perivenular mononuclear infiltrates, and quickly thereafter by circumscribed areas of myelin breakdown. Macrophages invariably occupy sites of active demyelination and appear necessary for myelin loss. B lymphocytes and plasma cells surround small CNS blood vessels, and T lymphocytes and monocytes infiltrate CNS parenchyma. Products of the immune response, including immunoglobulins, interleukins, interferons, and tumor necrosis factor, accompany the acute MS lesion. Tissue edema reaches a maximum after about 1 month, following which lesions evolve over several months into permanently demyelinated gliotic scars depleted of oligodendrocytes. After the initial events, immature oligodendrocytes appear and presumably participate in remyelination. As a rule, however, oligodendrocytes and remyelination regenerate insufficiently to explain the remarkable clinical recovery observed in many patients.

LABORATORY ABNORMALITIES. *Cerebrospinal Fluid.*

Immune activation within the CNS is a cardinal feature of MS. Increased CSF immunoglobulin levels, reflecting the presence of intrathecal humoral immune activation, appear in 80 to 90% of MS patients. CSF gamma globulin normally represents less than 13% of total CSF protein, but in MS patients the proportion often rises much higher. After separating CSF gamma globulin fractions by agarose or polyacrylamide gel electrophoresis, separate discrete "oligoclonal" bands (OCB) can be detected in 70 to 80% of patients. The sensitivity for detecting OCB can be increased by separating CSF by isoelectric focusing or by staining the gels or nitrocellulose blots with anti-immunoglobulin antibodies. As with most diagnostic tests, however, as the sensitivity of the method increases, the specificity decreases; CSF OCB also can be observed in patients with CNS infections or inflammatory diseases and have been reported with tumors or strokes. Increased CSF levels of free kappa light chains develop less frequently than OCB but are more specific for MS than IgG abnormalities. The amount of antibody synthesis within the CNS can be quantified by measuring the CSF and serum IgG and albumin levels and calculating a CSF IgG synthesis rate. CSF protein is normal or only slightly elevated in MS; levels above 75 mg per deciliter require an alternative explanation. CSF cell count is nearly always < 50 mononuclear cells per microliter; cell counts > 100 cells per microliter require a search for an infectious cause. Myelin destruction releases myelin basic protein (MBP) into CSF, which can be detected by radioimmunoassay. The MBP level correlates to some extent with disease activity and lesion location; none is detectable in normal individuals or during quiescent periods in MS patients. MBP levels rise in association with acute attacks or rapid disease progression. This serves as an index of disease activity but is not specific to MS; myelin injury from any other cause, such as acute brain infarction, increases CSF MBP.

In the presence of a slight mononuclear pleocytosis and normal protein, the presence of oligoclonal bands, selectively increased IgG levels, and free kappa light chains provide strong support for the diagnosis of MS when CNS syphilis, subacute sclerosing panencephalitis, chronic meningitis, CNS Lyme disease, HTLV-I myelopathy, or other infectious diseases have been excluded.

Sensory Evoked Potentials

Myelin allows rapid propagation of the nerve action potential. Myelin loss from any cause slows conduction velocity or causes conduction block. Conduction along sensory pathways can be measured by inducing a response to a visual, auditory, or somatosensory stimulus. Measurement of the latency after stimulus of the visual evoked potential (VEP) is used most widely (see Ch. 392.5). In most laboratories, the normal VEP latency is less than approximately 105 msec. Increased latency indicates an abnormality in the optic nerve on that side. Evoked potentials are considered extensions of the clinical examination, allowing for objective measurement of lesions within specific pathways. They have not proved useful for monitoring progression of disease or response to therapy.

Imaging Procedures

Computed tomographic (CT) brain scans sometimes reveal hypodense regions in white matter, but the imaging modality is relatively insensitive and usually shows no abnormalities. For these reasons, magnetic resonance imaging (MRI) has largely supplanted CT scanning. Abnormal head MRI scans show abnormalities in more than 85% of clinically definite MS patients. Typical lesions (Fig. 432–1) are multifocal, appear hyperintense on intermediate and T2-weighted MR images, and occur predominantly in the periventricular white matter, corpus callosum, cerebellum, cerebellar peduncles, brain stem, and spinal cord. Usually MRI reveals many more hyperintense lesions than clinically anticipated. Intravenous paramagnetic agents, such as gadolinium, demonstrate acute lesions, which appear hyperintense on T1-weighted images. Serial studies have demonstrated that gadolinium enhancement appears and disappears in a given lesion in about 4 weeks. MRI is used widely to confirm a diagnosis of suspected MS and to rule out other conditions. MRI abnormalities are not specific for MS, particularly in patients older than 50, who commonly develop nonspecific MRI signal changes of uncertain significance. The specificity of MRI lesions for MS increases with lesions ≥ 6 mm in diameter that are adjacent to the

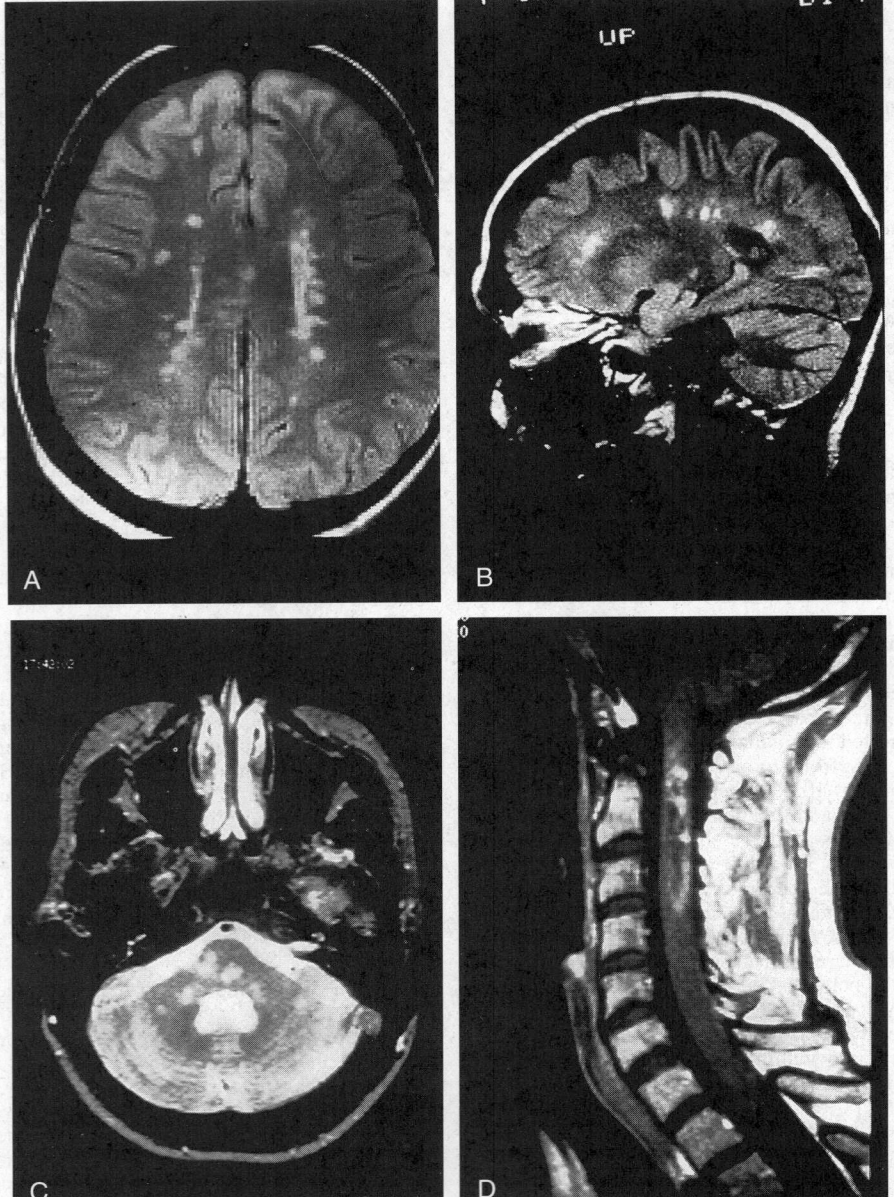

FIGURE 432–1. Magnetic resonance imaging of brain and spinal cord from a patient with clinically definite multiple sclerosis. *A,* Transverse section just above the bodies of the lateral ventricles. Note the numerous high-signal lesions adjacent to the bodies of the lateral ventricles in the deep cerebral white matter. *B,* Sagittal proton-density image showing ovoid lesions extending from the lateral ventricles into the deep cerebral white matter. *C,* T2-weighted section through the brain stem and cerebellum at the level of the middle cerebellar peduncles showing numerous high-signal lesions in the pons, cerebellar peduncles, and cerebellum. *D,* T1-weighted sagittal image through the cervical spinal cord following administration of gadolinium. Note the elongated intrinsic cervical spinal cord lesion with gadolinium enhancement as signified by high signal around the periphery of the lesion. (Courtesy of Barbara Banger, M.D., Cleveland Clinic Foundation Department of Neuroradiology.)

lateral ventricles, particularly when accompanied by brain stem, cerebellar, and spinal cord lesions. Use of MRI as a research tool to measure treatment effect or disease progression is rapidly evolving. Whether or not such studies are cost-effective for measuring clinical progress is debatable. Newer magnetic resonance–based techniques such as magnetization transfer imaging may allow differentiation between inflammation and demyelination. Such a distinction may become important as future therapies evolve.

CLINICAL MANIFESTATIONS. *Onset, Common Clinical Manifestations, and Course.* Women are affected more frequently than men—with a 3:2 ratio. Symptom onset occurs between ages 20 and 50 and peaks at approximately age 30. Nevertheless, children younger than 12 and adults over 50 occasionally present with their first symptom. MS produces myriad neurologic symptoms and signs, depending on the anatomic sites of involve-

ment. In younger patients, the disease usually starts with a subacute or acute onset of focal neurologic symptoms and signs, most often reflecting disease in optic nerves, pyramidal tracts, posterior columns, cerebellum, central vestibular system, or medial longitudinal fasciculus. Older individuals commonly present with insidiously progressive myelopathy, manifest as some combination of progressive spastic leg weakness, axial instability, and bladder impairment. In a large group of MS patients studied at the University of Western Ontario in the 1970's (Table 432–2), approximately 30% of patients presented with visual symptoms, 30% with sensory symptoms, 20% with gait or balance disturbance, and the remaining 20% with various other symptoms. In general, as the disease progresses, new symptoms and signs appear, old symptoms and signs recur, and residual symptoms and impairments increase.

Visual symptoms include monocular visual loss, oscileopsia, or

TABLE 432–2. INITIAL SYMPTOMS IN MS PATIENTS*

Symptom	Percentage of Cases
Sensory disturbance in one or more limbs	33
Disturbance of balance and gait	18
Visual loss in one eye	17
Diplopia	13
Progressive weakness	10
Acute myelitis	6
Lhermitte's sign	3
Sensory disturbance in face	3
Pain	2

* From Paty DW, Poser CM: Clinical symptoms and signs of multiple sclerosis. *In* Poser CM (ed.): The Diagnosis of Multiple Sclerosis. New York, Thieme and Stratton, 1984, p 27.

TABLE 432–3. WASHINGTON COMMITTEE CRITERIA FOR DIAGNOSIS OF MULTIPLE SCLEROSIS*

Category	Attacks	Clinical Evidence	Para-clinical Evidence†	CSF OB/IgG
Clinically definite MS				
1	2	2		
2	2	1	and 1	
Laboratory-supported definite MS				
1	2	1	or 1	+
2	1	2		+
3	1	1	and 1	+
Clinically probable MS				
1	2	1		
2	1	2		
3	1	1	and 1	
Laboratory-supported probable MS				
1	2			+

* From Poser CM, et al.: New diagnostic criteria for multiple sclerosis: Guidelines for research protocols. Ann Neurol 13:227, 1983.
† MRI or evoked potential studies.

diplopia. Gait disorder results from spastic leg weakness, axial instability, and lower extremity sensory loss. Spasticity consists of increased muscle tone, hyperreflexia, and limb spasms, accompanied by weakness and loss of dexterity. Spasticity in MS patients almost always affects the lower more than the upper extremities. Upper extremity impairment includes sensory loss resulting in a clumsy hand, cerebellar ataxia, or less commonly spastic weakness. Bladder dysfunction includes urinary urgency with urge incontinence or hesitancy and incomplete emptying. Neuropsychological problems are common and include depression, emotional lability, and cognitive impairment.

Increased body temperature by as little as 0.5° C transiently reduces neurologic function in some patients. In the setting of increased ambient temperature, strenuous physical activity, or fever, patients may experience transient worsening of symptoms. This results from slowed axonal conduction induced by heating, and the new symptoms disappear within hours of regaining normal body temperature.

At least 70% of patients improve in the days to months following their initial bout, with the degree of improvement ranging from slight to virtual disappearance of the neurologic dysfunction. Although most patients experience exacerbations and remissions early in the course of their illness, as time goes by, recovery from individual bouts decreases, fixed impairment and disability remain, and the course becomes chronically progressive. About 30% of patients experience chronically progressive problems from the onset of disease, especially those aged more than 45 years. Ten years after onset, about half of all patients are still able to carry out their household and/or employment responsibilities. Fifteen years after onset about half require a cane to walk. Approximately 25 years after onset, at least half are unable to walk, even with assistance. By contrast, some individuals, perhaps as many as a third, occupy the extremes of either avoiding disability altogether or having unusually severe limitations, becoming bedridden within months after onset. The average interval from clinical onset to death is 35 years, with terminal factors due to sepsis from urinary tract infection, decubiti, aspiration pneumonia, or suicide.

Factors Affecting the Clinical Course. The only predictable factor in MS is its unpredictability in the individual patient. *It has become clear, however, that certain features carry a relatively poor prognosis. These include progressive disease from onset, preponderance of motor and cerebellar signs, and a near diagnostically abnormal head MRI at first presentation. Conversely, favorable indicators include a high degree of recovery after the first attack, predominance of sensory symptoms, and benign condition 5 years after symptom onset.*

Several studies have found that infections of almost any type increase the risk for exacerbation. This is thought to result from immune system activation, with an associated increase in MS disease activity. As with numerous autoimmune diseases, MS disease activity decreases during pregnancy but increases somewhat in the postpartum period. The overall progression of MS, however, is not affected by one or more pregnancies.

DIAGNOSIS. Despite increasing reliance on sophisticated brain imaging, CSF, and electrophysiologic tests, the diagnosis of MS is based on *clinical* features *supplemented* by laboratory tests, rather than the other way around. The Schumacher criteria have been widely used for diagnosis of MS. Clinically definite MS exists when an appropriate clinical history is supported by (1) objective abnormalities of CNS function in the neurologic examination; (2)

examination or history indicating involvement of two or more areas of the CNS; (3) CNS disease predominantly reflecting white matter involvement; (4) involvement of the CNS following either a pattern of two or more episodes, each lasting > 24 hours and a month or more apart, or a slow or stepwise progression of signs and symptoms over at least 6 months; (5) patient age between 10 and 50; and (6) signs and symptoms that cannot be better explained by another disease process. These criteria are based entirely on clinical features. Laboratory testing plays an increasingly important role in documenting multicentric CNS lesions and eliminating alternative diagnoses. This is reflected in diagnostic criteria developed more recently that incorporate sensory evoked potentials and MRI to identify disseminated lesions, and CSF IgG abnormalities to support the diagnosis (Table 432–3).

Two common errors confound the diagnosis of MS. The first occurs in a patient with clear neurologic disease who has an alternative diagnosis (Table 432–4). Certain clinical or laboratory "red flags" are useful in alerting the clinician about a possible diagnostic error in this situation (Table 432–5). The two most useful red flags include disease that could be explained by a single lesion in the nervous system and the absence of a clinical remission. In a patient with localized disease, the working assumption must be that a definable, non-demyelinating, structural lesion exists. Depending on the clinical features, diagnostic testing should be used to rule out brain or spinal cord tumor, arteriovenous malformation, cervical spondylosis with cord compression, cervical or thoracic disc herniation, Chiari malformation, brain abscess, or a parenchymal mass

TABLE 432–4. CONDITIONS COMMONLY MISTAKEN FOR MULTIPLE SCLEROSIS

Vascular diseases
    Small-vessel cerebrovascular disease
    Vasculitis
Structural lesions
    Craniocervical junction tumor, malformation of base of skull
    Anomaly
    Posterior fossa tumor or arteriovenous malformation
    Spinal cord tumor or cervical spondylosis
Degenerative diseases
    Motor system disease
    Spinocerebellar degeneration
Infections
    HTLV-I infection
    HIV myelopathy or HIV-related cerebritis
    Lyme disease
Other conditions
    Cobalamin deficiency
    Sjögren's syndrome
    Sarcoidosis
    Nonspecific MRI abnormalities

TABLE 432–5. RED FLAGS IN THE DIAGNOSIS OF MULTIPLE SCLEROSIS*

Syndrome that could be explained by localized disease
Steadily progressive disease, absence of clinical remission
Absence of oculomotor, optic nerve, sensory, or bladder involvement
Normal cerebrospinal fluid

* Modified from Rudick RA, Schiffer RB, Schwetz K, et al.: Multiple sclerosis: The problem of incorrect diagnosis. Arch Neurol 43:578, 1986.

from sarcoidosis. MRI is the most sensitive differential screening procedure and currently eliminates the need for CT scanning or myelography in almost all cases.

Degenerative, infectious, or neoplastic diseases must be considered in patients with a steadily progressive course. Disorders that can be incorrectly diagnosed as MS include spinocerebellar degeneration, cervicomedullary syringomyelia, basilar invagination, motor neuron disease, HTLV-1 myelopathy, HIV-related myelopathy or brain infection, and neoplasms such as parenchymal lymphoma. Spinocerebellar degeneration and motor neuron disease are suspected by symmetric neurologic impairment restricted to characteristic neural systems and by the absence of CSF inflammatory change or response to corticosteroids.

Progressive myelopathy should prompt testing for HTLV-1, HIV, and very long chain fatty acids to rule out adrenoleukodystrophy (ALD). On rare occasion, CNS lupus or vitamin B_{12} deficiency may be clinically indistinguishable from MS. These disorders should be ruled out by determining antinuclear antibodies and vitamin B_{12} levels at the time of diagnosis.

Small vessel cerebrovascular disease should be considered in the hypertensive patient, particularly in those lacking CSF abnormalities typical of MS. MRI may help distinguish MS from small-vessel cerebrovascular disease; MS patients more commonly have lesions adjacent to the brain ventricles and involvement of the corpus callosum.

The second common type of diagnostic error occurs in patients with no definable neurologic disease. Patients commonly acquire an MS diagnosis because of nonspecific neurologic symptoms such as weakness, fatigue, or tingling, at times supplemented by minimal nonspecific signal changes on brain MRI. The absence of objective neurologic signs at any time, patterns of weakness or sensory loss that fail to conform to known neuroanatomic systems, and disability out of proportion to objective clinical findings raise the suspicion of psychogenic illness. One must be open-minded, however, because MS can begin with sensory symptoms, fatigue, or other nonspecific symptoms. In many cases, it is necessary to follow the patient over time before an accurate diagnosis can be made.

TREATMENT. Education. MS patients and their families need information about MS after a diagnosis has been made. Typical questions include the following: (1) *"What will happen to me?"* One of the major psychological burdens for an MS patient is uncertainty about the future course of his or her illness. The physician should acknowledge the unpredictable course but emphasize the spectrum of severity and the significant proportion of patients who remain neurologically intact for many years. (2) *"How can I control my illness?"* Most patients have beliefs about what will improve or worsen their MS. The patient's need for control over the disease can often be focused on healthy life styles like fitness programs or appropriate diet. (3) *"When should I call you?"* Patients should be advised to call when necessary but should be routinely seen at 6- or 12-month intervals. This allows ongoing assessment of neurologic impairment and results in a gradual decline in the need for telephone calls. (4) *"Will my children get this?"* The lifetime risk to a child of a mother with MS is 3 to 5%; this is a 30- to 50-fold increase over that for the general population, but still a small risk. (5) *"Can I have a baby?"* Pregnancy has a predictable effect on the pattern of MS, as discussed above. It appears that breast feeding has little if any effect on the frequency, timing, or severity of postpartum exacerbations, and the bulk of evidence suggests that the overall course of MS, including the eventual degree of disability, is unaffected by one or more pregnancies. Women with mild to moderate disability should plan pregnancies primarily on the basis of issues other than MS.

Symptom Pharmacotherapy. *Spasticity* may be reduced by a combination of physical measures and antispastic drugs. The GABA-agonist baclofen is the drug of choice but should be individualized because it is effective over a wide dose range. Baclofen should be instituted slowly to avoid sedation or weakness and withdrawn slowly to avoid confusional states or seizures. Diazepam may be used as an adjunct to baclofen, particularly for patients with nocturnal spasms causing sleep disturbance. Even a small dose of diazepam may potentiate the benefits of baclofen. Dantrolene is an alternative antispastic drug for patients who do not respond well to baclofen or diazepam or cannot tolerate the sedation that sometimes complicates the use of these drugs. Dantrolene exerts its effects at the muscle; consequently, motor weakness almost always accompanies dantrolene's antispastic effect. Dantrolene should be used cautiously in patients with myocardial disease, and it occasionally causes toxic hepatitis. Patients with severe spasticity not effectively managed with the above measures may benefit from intrathecal baclofen administered continuously at a rate of 200 to 800 μg per day via a fully implantable infusion pump.

Dystonic spasms consist of brief, recurrent, painful posturing of one or more extremities, not associated with altered consciousness or urinary incontinence. Dystonic spasms are easily controlled with carbamazepine or phenytoin. *Ataxia* is difficult to treat pharmacologically. Intention tremor may respond to clonazepam, which should be instituted slowly to avoid sedation. Clonazepam should be initiated at 0.5 mg at bedtime and increased gradually to an endpoint of sedation or effective control of tremor. One or more tonic-clonic seizures occur in about 5% of MS patients. A single motor seizure predicts a subsequent seizure in an MS patient and should be treated with an adequate dose of phenytoin. *Bladder symptoms* require at a minimum urinalysis, culture, and postvoid residual volume. In the absence of a urinary tract infection or urinary retention > 100 ml, anticholinergic agents such as oxybutynin or propantheline are effective. Urinary tract infection or significant urinary retention in an MS patient requires urologic evaluation. *Fatigue* in MS, when disabling and not caused by depression, can be treated effectively with amantadine, 100 mg twice a day. Pemoline is effective for some individuals who have not responded to amantadine.

Heat sensitivity results from conduction failure in partially demyelinated CNS fibers. Patients may benefit from cool showers or air conditioning. Dramatic deterioration can accompany fever in patients with advanced MS, and elevated body temperatures should be aggressively treated, with specific infections being managed with appropriate antibiotics.

Pain syndromes consist of trigeminal neuralgia or more atypical facial pain, paroxysmal limb paresthesias presenting as brief tic-like pain, burning dysesthesias, Lhermitte's phenomenon, and chronic back pain due in most cases to mechanical stress caused by ataxia and weakness. Trigeminal neuralgia or disagreeable paresthesias may respond to carbamazepine or alternatively to amitriptyline, phenytoin, or baclofen. If medical therapy fails, trigeminal rhyzotomy is an alternative. Chronic low back and leg pain are usually alleviated with nonsteroidal anti-inflammatory drugs and physical therapy. A proper walking aid, ankle foot orthosis, or proper seating is critical. Coexistent herniated discs should be ruled out in the MS patient with radicular pain, particularly when an ankle or knee tendon reflex is absent.

Depression or *emotional distress* is often underrecognized and inadequately treated. Depression is particularly common when the illness is first diagnosed or when it worsens significantly. Depression has a significant negative impact on quality of life, social relationships, and job performance and should be treated aggressively with psychiatric referral or antidepressant drugs. For depressed MS patients with anxiety and insomnia, amitriptyline is effective and inexpensive. For patients with coexisting bladder symptoms, imipramine is useful because its α-adrenergic properties may improve bladder dysfunction. For older patients or patients with memory impairment, a tricyclic with less anticholinergic activity, such as desipramine or nortriptyline, or a serotonin reuptake inhibitor may be better tolerated. *Emotional lability,* which may be distressing and socially disabling for some MS patients, may improve with low doses of amitriptyline.

Cognitive dysfunction may be difficult to recognize clinically but should be suspected in any MS patient with poor work performance, family disintegration, or noncompliance with medical or rehabilitative therapies, particularly when the explanation for the problem is unclear. Neuropsychological tests should include sensitive measurements of complex attention and information processing, learning and recent memory, concept formation, and problem solving. There is no known effective drug therapy, although patients often can learn compensatory strategies and may benefit from cognitive rehabilitation.

Disease Pharmacotherapy. Numerous trials of drugs have been directed at improving the long-term course of MS or shortening the course of acute exacerbations. Nearly all current experimental therapy trials include MRI measures of outcome, and measures of clinical outcome have improved.

Corticosteroid Therapy. Recent evidence suggests that intravenous methylprednisolone (MP) has a more rapid onset of action and better efficacy than corticotrophin or other steroid preparations in limiting acute exacerbations. No evidence exists that chronic corticosteroid therapy slows or halts progression of MS. Furthermore, excessive or injudicious use of steroids gradually lessens their value, and most patients eventually become steroid-unresponsive. For major clinical exacerbations, intravenous MP, 500 or 1000 mg per day for 3 days, can be administered safely in an outpatient setting, followed by prednisone, 60 mg in a single morning dose for 3 days, tapering off over 12 days.

Immunomodulatory Therapy. Betaseron (interferon β-1b), a human recombinant interferon-β preparation, has been shown to reduce the frequency of MS exacerbations and the progression of MRI lesions in ambulatory patients with exacerbating-remitting MS. The drug is FDA approved for MS patients in this category, being administered at a dose of 8 million IU every other day by subcutaneous injection. Adverse effects include flulike symptoms, injection site inflammatory reactions, and occasional blood transaminase elevations. Avonex (interferon β-1a), a different form of recombinant human β interferon, at a dose of 6 MIU administered by weekly IM injections also has been shown to decrease MRI disease activity. The principal observed side effects were flulike symptoms. Various drugs that suppress the immune system have been reported to show partial efficacy. These include cyclophosphamide, cyclosporine, azathioprine, and methotrexate. Methotrexate, administered orally at a dose of 7.5 mg weekly, was found to reduce the proportion of patients with chronic progressive MS who worsened during a 2-year treatment period compared with placebo-treated patients. This dose results in minimal apparent toxicity. Cyclophosphamide and cyclosporine have some reported benefit but are limited by toxicity. Evidence indicates that azathioprine reduces the rate of exacerbations, but the relative and ultimate benefits of azathioprine and interferon-β have not been determined. Currently, it is safest to restrict immunosuppressive drugs to centers operating within the context of controlled protocols.

MULTIPLE SCLEROSIS VARIANTS

NEUROMYELITIS OPTICA (DEVIC'S DISEASE). Neuromyelitis optica is a syndrome characterized by partial or complete transverse myelopathy and optic neuritis. Loss of vision and paraplegia may occur in either order, and the two major components of the disease may be widely separated in time. The syndrome of neuromyelitis optica may occur as the result of acute disseminated encephalomyelitis, systemic lupus erythematosus, or sarcoidosis as well as during the course of typical MS or in isolation without apparent cause. In the latter case, it is considered a variant of MS.

CONCENTRIC SCLEROSIS. Concentric sclerosis is a rare form of demyelinating disease characterized by rapidly progressive demyelination. It appears to be a variant of rapidly progressive MS. Clinically, the disease begins with the acute or subacute onset of altered behavior, difficulty in communication, mutism, apathy, and headache. CSF is usually normal. Imaging shows extensive lesions in cerebral white matter. Concentric sclerosis may be suspected clinically but can be diagnosed only by its characteristic histopathology. Alternating bands containing demyelinated and partially demyelinated axons radiate concentrically. Oligodendrocyte loss characterizes the bands of demyelination.

MONOPHASIC DISORDERS RELATED TO MULTIPLE SCLEROSIS

OPTIC NEURITIS. Optic neuritis denotes acute or subacute partial or complete loss of vision in one or both eyes due to inflammation. Almost all patients with inflammatory optic neuritis experience pain in, around, or behind the affected eye, followed within a day or two by visual loss. Visual loss of varying intensity pro-

gresses for as long as 1 week. Optic neuritis is classified as *retrobulbar neuritis* when the lesion is in the posterior two thirds of the optic nerve and *papillitis* when the lesion is in the anterior portion of the optic nerve. The latter leads to an ophthalmoscopic appearance similar to that of acute papilledema resulting from increased intracranial pressure but differing from the latter by the association of markedly reduced visual acuity. Visual fields in optic neuritis reveal a central or ceco-central scotoma of varying degree. Color vision is impaired, and a deafferented, Marcus-Gunn pupil may exist. Unless the patient has papillitis, ophthalmoscopic examination remains normal for the first 2 to 3 weeks, after which the disc pales, with loss of small vessels on the disc, or more severe atrophy may develop. Visual function almost always recovers to some degree, usually within weeks. Blindness as the result of optic nerve demyelination of MS seldom occurs.

The syndrome of optic neuritis can be caused by several diseases, of which MS is by far the most common. Tobacco-nutritional amblyopia, Leber's disease, vasculitis, optic nerve compression on any basis, neurosyphilis, ischemic optic neuropathy, pernicious anemia, or sarcoidosis produce most cases not caused by MS. Optic neuritis is usually easily differentiated from optic nerve ischemia, which has an abrupt onset, affects older individuals, and results in field cuts consistent with retinal artery occlusions. Compressive optic neuropathy causes slowly progressive visual loss. Vasculitis or sarcoidosis can usually be distinguished by characteristic funduscopic features and by the presence of uveitis.

Many patients with idiopathic isolated optic neuritis eventually develop MS, the reported frequency in several series varying from 13 to 85% according to the length of follow-up. The presence of CSF oligoclonal bands or brain MRI abnormalities significantly increases the risk of early conversion to MS. Patients with idiopathic monosymptomatic optic neuritis who have periventricular MRI abnormalities have about a 35% chance of developing MS within 2 years and an 85% chance of developing MS within 5 years.

More rapid but not necessarily greater total visual recovery occurs by treating optic neuritis with intravenous methylprednisolone. A 3-day course of intravenous MP followed by a prednisone taper within 8 days of the onset appears to reduce by about 50% the likelihood of conversion from idiopathic optic neuritis to MS during 2 years of follow-up.

ACUTE TRANSVERSE MYELITIS. Acute transverse myelitis denotes rapidly developing paraparesis or paraplegia as the result of spinal cord dysfunction. Abrupt or rapidly developing back or radicular pain may be followed by ascending paresthesias and weakness beginning in the feet. Urinary and fecal retention or incontinence is common. Progression varies from minutes, as with infarction, to steady or stepwise progression over several days. Progression over days may occur with both spinal cord compression due to a tumor and MS. It is also common to observe patients with sensory symptoms below a particular dermatome corresponding to the spinal cord level of involvement, with or without ataxia and variable degrees of leg weakness. It may be difficult to distinguish idiopathic transverse myelitis from compressive myelopathy. Therefore, the syndrome of acute transverse myelitis demands immediate diagnostic evaluation.

Several disorders can produce an acute transverse myelopathy (Table 432–6). The most important to rule in or out immediately are compressive lesions, including spinal or epidural abscess, tumor, herniated intervertebral disc, or injury; vascular occlusion due to arteritis, aortic dissection, aortic surgery, or arteriovenous malformation; varicella-zoster infection; and autoimmune disease including MS. In many instances, a careful history suggests the cause and the appropriate approach. Nevertheless, the evaluation must include an *immediate* imaging procedure such as MRI with attention to the level of involvement to rule out spinal cord compression. Cord compression from metastatic tumor may present acutely even though the tumor has been present for weeks or longer. Central herniated intervertebral discs may cause acute cord compression without producing local pain. Rapidly progressing myelopathy in a previously healthy person should always raise the question of spontaneous epidural, subdural, or intraparenchymal abscess or bleeding, the latter occurring from an arteriovenous malformation or as a complication of anticoagulation or blood dyscrasia. About one third of patients with idiopathic transverse myelitis give a history of an antecedent upper respiratory or flulike illness. Transverse

TABLE 432–6. ACUTE OR SUBACUTE TRANSVERSE MYELOPATHY

Associated with infection
  Bacterial
    Spinal epidural abscess
    Intramedullary abscess
  Viral, e.g., varicella-zoster
  Postviral, e.g., rubella with disseminated encephalomyelitis
Compression
  Tumor, especially metastatic
  Trauma
  Herniated intervertebral disc
Vascular
  Acute extradural, subdural, or parenchymal hemorrhage
  Dissecting aortic aneurysm
  Arteritis
  Lupus erythematosus
Idiopathic

myelitis may also follow several other infectious illnesses such as mycoplasma or measles with virus infection.

Transverse myelitis and slowly progressive myelopathy are common manifestations of MS, either as a first clinical manifestation or a late development. A syndrome suggesting complete cord transection rarely occurs. As with optic neuritis, CSF oligoclonal bands or an abnormal brain MRI suggesting MS makes clinically definite MS likely.

Proper treatment requires an expeditious diagnosis. When cord compression is present, surgical decompression and treatment with antibiotics or with corticosteroids are needed immediately. Treatment may halt progression but may not restore lost function. In idiopathic transverse myelopathy, MS, or cord compression, corticosteroids may reduce edema and lead to earlier restitution of function, although the effect on long-term outcome is uncertain. The treatment of choice for neoplastic cord compression is dexamethasone; for idiopathic transverse myelitis, intravenous methylprednisolone is preferable. Patients must be supported by bladder catheterization, ventilatory support, and proper protection from compression neuropathies as necessary. Prognosis varies widely, recovery ranging from almost none at all to complete, depending on the degree of acute necrosis.

LEUKODYSTROPHIES

The leukodystrophies (see Table 432–1) are dysmyelinating diseases in that myelin formation or maintenance is impaired by a genetically determined biochemical defect. A biochemical defect is known for several, but they remain relatively rare, incurable disorders, affecting individuals from the first months of life to the 20's.

ADRENOLEUKODYSTROPHY. Adrenoleukodystrophy (ALD) includes two genetically determined disorders that cause dysfunction of adrenal glands and nervous system myelin. There are two distinct types of ALD—the X-linked form and a recessive form, termed neonatal ALD. Neonatal ALD is a rare disorder characterized by early and severe psychomotor retardation, seizures, retinopathy, hepatomegaly, and dysmorphic features occurring in infants of either gender.

The X-linked form of ALD is phenotypically heterogeneous, even though the disease is associated with a common biochemical defect. The two common patterns of X-linked ALD are the childhood form and adrenomyeloneuropathy. In the childhood form, boys develop normally until age 4 to 8, when they manifest behavioral changes with progressive cognitive decline leading over years to a chronic vegetative state. Young men with adrenomyeloneuropathy experience progressive paraparesis and bladder dysfunction. Almost all such ALD patients have adrenal insufficiency, although the degree varies considerably. Less common phenotypes of X-linked ALD include adrenal insufficiency without nervous system involvement, progressive dementia in adults, and asymptomatic males with the same metabolic deficiency as affected relatives. Occasionally, female heterozygotes develop neurologic disturbances that resemble MS. The basis for clinical heterogeneity despite a common metabolic defect is unknown. Tissues and body fluids of patients with X-linked ALD contain high levels of unbranched saturated very

long chain fatty acids. Fatty acids accumulate because of deficient peroxisomal catabolism, although the precise nature of the enzyme defect is not clear. The gene for X-linked ALD has been mapped to Xq28.

The diagnosis of X-linked ALD may be suspected in males with the clinical features described above. CSF shows inflammatory changes that may be identical to those seen in MS, although the CSF protein is usually higher in ALD. MRI shows symmetric lesions in the posterior parietal and occipital white matter. Endocrine testing reveals primary adrenal insufficiency. The diagnosis is confirmed by demonstrating increased levels of very long chain fatty acids in blood, tissue, or cultured fibroblasts. Most female heterozygotes can be identified using these methods as well. A DNA probe is available for gene screening, and prenatal diagnosis is possible through biochemical and genetic screening of amniocytes.

Pathologic examination shows widespread demyelination in CNS and peripheral myelin, with numerous lipid lamellar inclusions throughout the tissue. Many lesions exhibit cellular infiltration with lymphocytes and macrophages, suggesting an inflammatory component to pathogenesis.

Treatment of X-linked ALD consists of adrenal hormone replacement and dietary restriction of long chain fatty acids. Preliminary evidence suggests that bone marrow transplantation may slow progression of the disease, but there is no specific treatment at present.

PELIZAEUS-MERZBACHER DISEASE. Pelizaeus-Merzbacher disease represents a group of a poorly characterized and heterogeneous disorders with extensive CSF myelin destruction associated with myelin breakdown products staining bright red with the usual fat stains. The so-called sudanophilic leukodystrophies are thus distinguishable pathologically from the metachromatic leukodystrophies. The sudanophilic staining characteristic results from high levels of cholesterol esters; it is observed in the aminoacidurias, adrenoleukodystrophy, and Pelizaeus-Merzbacher disease. The latter is a rare leukodystrophy inherited as an X-linked recessive trait and primarily affecting males. The condition begins in infancy and progresses slowly to produce extensive, diffuse, symmetric disturbances of myelin associated with gliosis within the cerebrum and cerebellum. The peripheral nervous system is not affected. The underlying biochemical defect is unknown, and no treatment is available.

SPONGY DEGENERATION OF WHITE MATTER. Many disorders can produce the pathologic changes leading to spongiform degeneration of myelin. These include various metabolic derangements, exposure to hexachlorophene, carbon monoxide, cyanide, isoniazid, actinomycin D, amphotericin B, methyl ester, and methotrexate.

METACHROMATIC LEUKODYSTROPHY. Metachromatic leukodystrophy (MLD) is the most common leukodystrophy. MLD is a lysosomal storage disease caused by deficiency of arylsulfatase A. Patients develop diffuse dysmyelination, usually starting in the first 10 years of life. The process leads to dementia, convulsions, cranial nerve abnormalities, and finally severe spasticity or rigidity. Death usually occurs after 2 to 4 years. Juvenile and adult-onset cases have been reported. In the adult form of MLD, patients develop mental deterioration that evolves progressively to severe dementia, pyramidal tract, and cerebellar signs. The diagnosis is suspected in an infant or child with progressive dementia, convulsions, and spasticity and in a young adult with progressive dementia, particularly in the face of absent tendon reflexes and elevated CSF protein.

The arylsulfatase A gene has been cloned and characterized. Nearly all patients have deficient arylsulfatase A enzyme activity, resulting in accumulation of sulfatides in lysosomes within central and peripheral nervous system tissue. Occasionally, arylsulfatase A activity is low, but the individual remains unaffected. This is termed pseudodeficiency. An increased urinary excretion of sulfatide and reduced arylsulfatase A activity in venous blood or cultured fibroblasts is diagnostic. Pathologically, sulfatides (which stain metachromatically) accumulate in oligodendrocytes and Schwann cells and within myelin lamellae. Sulfatides also collect within neurons, liver, gallbladder, kidneys, and spleen. Some evidence suggests that bone marrow transplantation may slow or halt progression of MLD.

GLOBOID CELL LEUKODYSTROPHY (KRABBE'S DISEASE). Globoid cell leukodystrophy is characterized biochemically as deficient galactocerebroside β-galactosidase activity. The disease affects infants in the first 2 to 3 months of life and is transmitted as an autosomal recessive trait. Rare instances occur in late infancy or in adulthood. The activity of galactocerebroside β-galactosidase can be determined in serum, peripheral leukocytes, or fibroblasts. Neuropathologic examination reveals marked loss of myelin throughout the brain, with the presence of round or oval mononuclear cells the size of large glia or as large, irregular multinucleated cells, termed globoid cells, containing galactocerebroside. Infants with the disorder usually progress to a vegetative state within their second year. Late onset cases present with progressive motor impairment and less frequently visual failure. No treatment is known.

Multiple Sclerosis

Anderson DW, Ellenberg JH, Leventhal CM, et al.: Revised estimate of the prevalence of multiple sclerosis in the United States. Ann Neurol 31:333, 1992. *Increased the estimated number of United States MS cases to 350,000.*

Ebers GC, Sadovnick AD: The geographic distribution of multiple sclerosis: A review. Neuroepidemiology 12:1, 1993. *Provides a synthesis of available epidemiologic information. A combination of both genetic and environmental factors appears to explain the available data on MS and geography.*

Goodkin DE, Rudick RA, Ross JS: The use of brain magnetic resonance imaging in multiple sclerosis. Arch Neurol 51:505, 1994. *Provides an overview of the use of MRI in MS patients.*

Prineas J, Kwon E, Goldenberg P, et al.: Multiple sclerosis. Oligodendrocyte proliferation and differentiation in fresh lesions. Lab Invest 61:489, 1989. *Elegantly describes and illustrates the tissue alterations produced by MS.*

Ransohoff RM, Tuohy VK, Lehmann PV: The immunology of multiple sclerosis: New intricacies and new insights. Curr Opin Neurol Neurosurg 7:242, 1994. *Reviews recent advances in our understanding of immunopathogenesis.*

Rudick RA: Helping patients live with multiple sclerosis. What primary care physicians can do. Postgrad Med 88:197, 1990. *Provides practical management strategies for primary physicians caring for MS patients and their families.*

Rudick RA, Birk KA: Multiple sclerosis and pregnancy. *In* Goldstein PJ, Stern BJ (eds.): Neurological Disorders of Pregnancy, 2nd ed rev. Mount Kisco, NY, Futura Publishing, 1992, p 165. *Reviews the relationship between pregnancy and MS, with emphasis on reproductive and pregnancy counseling.*

Rudick RA, Goodkin DE (eds.): Treatment of Multiple Sclerosis. Trial Design, Results and Future Perspectives. London, Springer-Verlag, 1992. *The first monograph with a comprehensive summary of the state of MS experimental therapeutics.*

Runmarker B, Andersen O: Prognostic factors in a multiple sclerosis incidence cohort with twenty-five years of follow-up. Brain 116:117, 1993. *Describes favorable prognostic indicators, including a high degree of recovery after first exacerbation, predominance of sensory symptoms, and benign condition 5 years after symptom onset.*

Schumacher G, Beebe G, Kibler R, et al.: Problems of experimental trials of therapy in multiple sclerosis: Report by the panel on the evaluation of experimental trials of therapy in multiple sclerosis. Ann NY Acad Sci 122:552, 1965. *Defined clinical criteria that are still valid for the diagnosis of MS.*

Optic Neuritis

Beck RW, Cleary PA, Anderson MM, et al.: A randomized, controlled trial of corticosteroids in the treatment of acute optic neuritis. N Engl J Med 326:581, 1992. *Reported that treatment of optic neuritis with intravenous MP improved the rate of visual recovery but not the extent of eventual return of vision.*

Beck RW, Cleary PA, Trobe JD, et al.: The effect of corticosteroids for acute optic neuritis on the subsequent development of multiple sclerosis. N Engl J Med 329:1764, 1993. *Found that treatment with intravenous MP reduced the likelihood of progression from optic neuritis to clinically definite MS within 2 years by 50%.*

Optic Neuritis Study Group: The clinical profile of optic neuritis. Experience of the optic neuritis treatment trial. Arch Ophthalmol 109:1673, 1991. *Provides definitive clinical and laboratory features of 448 patients with acute optic neuritis studied according to a comprehensive standardized protocol.*

Transverse Myelitis

Ropper AH, Poskanzer DC: The prognosis of acute and subacute transverse myelopathy based on early signs and symptoms. Ann Neurol 4:51, 1978. *Reviews the experience of a large general hospital with an excellent description of the clinical findings and follow-up.*

Tippett DS, Fishman PS, Panitch HS: Relapsing transverse myelitis. Neurology 41:703, 1991. *Describes patients with recurrent episodes of transverse myelitis, no evidence for brain stem or forebrain lesions, and absence of CSF oligoclonal bands. This is probably a variant of MS.*

Leukodystrophies

Aubourg P, Blanche S, Jambaque I, et al.: Reversal of early neurologic and neuroradiologic manifestations of X-linked adrenoleukodystrophy by bone marrow transplantation. N Engl J Med 322:1860, 1990. *Suggests a benefit from bone marrow transplantation.*

Gieselmann V, von Figura K: Advances in molecular genetics of metachromatic leukodystrophy. J Inherited Metab Dis 13:560, 1990. *Reviews the genetics of MLD.*

Krivit W, Shapiro E, Kennedy W, et al.: Treatment of late infantile metachromatic leukodystrophy by bone marrow transplantation. N Engl J Med 322:28, 1990. *Suggests a benefit from bone marrow transplantation.*

Moser HW, Bergin A, Cornblath D: Peroxisomal disorders. Biochem Cell Biol 69:463, 1991. *Provides a comprehensive overview of the biochemical abnormalities underlying ALD.*

Moser HW, Moser AB, Naidu S, Bergin A: Clinical aspects of adrenoleukodystrophy and adrenomyeloneuropathy. Devel Neurosci 13:254, 1991. *Provides an authoritative overview of clinical features.*

Moser HW, Moser AB, Smith KD, et al.: Adrenoleukodystrophy: Phenotypic variability and implications for therapy. J Inherited Metab Dis 15:645, 1992. *Provides the largest experience with bone marrow transplants and suggests that results are encouraging.*

Seitelberger F: Pelizaeus-Merzbacher's disease. *In* Vinken P, Bruyn G (eds.): Handbook of Clinical Neurology, vol 10. Amsterdam, North-Holland, 1970, p 150. *An excellent review of this and related degenerative diseases of myelin.*

Wanders RJ, Tager JM: Peroxisomal fatty acid beta-oxidation in relation to adrenoleukodystrophy. Devel Neurosci 13:262, 1991. *Provides the present state of knowledge regarding the organization of peroxisomal fatty acid oxidation with emphasis on X-linked adrenoleukodystrophy.*

Section Eleven—
The Epilepsies

433 THE EPILEPSIES
Timothy A. Pedley

DEFINITION

Epilepsy is a term applied to a group of chronic conditions whose major clinical manifestation is the occurrence of *epileptic seizures:* sudden and usually unprovoked attacks of subjective experiential phenomena, altered awareness, involuntary movements, or convulsions.

Although a diagnosis of epilepsy requires the presence of seizures, not all seizures imply epilepsy. Seizures are a relatively common symptom of brain dysfunction, and they may occur during the course of many acute medical or neurologic illnesses in which brain function is temporarily deranged *(acute symptomatic seizures)* (Table 433–1). Such seizures are most often self-limited and do not persist after the underlying disorder has resolved. Seizures can also occur as a reaction of the brain to physiologic stress, sleep deprivation, fever, and alcohol or sedative drug withdrawal. Occurrence of seizures in such everyday settings is exceptional and implies an increased seizure susceptibility (lowered seizure threshold). The latter may reflect poorly understood genetic factors that determine an individual's intrinsic resistance to minor physiologic, metabolic, or toxic insults. Finally, isolated seizures also sometimes occur for no discoverable reason as unprovoked events in presumably healthy people. None of these kinds of seizures represent epilepsy.

ETIOLOGY

Epilepsy can arise from a variety of conditions and pathophysiologic mechanisms. About 70% of adults and 40% of children with new-onset epilepsy have partial (focal) seizures (Fig. 433–1A). In most of these, it is not possible to identify a specific cause, although the focal nature of the seizures generally implies a cerebral injury or lesion (so-called *cryptogenic* epilepsy) (Fig. 433–1B). The most common specific lesions are hippocampal sclerosis, gangliogliomas and glial tumors, cavernous malformations, neuronal mi-

TABLE 433–1. POTENTIAL CAUSES OF ACUTE SYMPTOMATIC SEIZURES

Medical conditions
  Metabolic disarray
    Hyponatremia (< 120 mEq/L)
    Hypernatremia (> 145 mEq/L)
    Hypoglycemia (< 40 mg/dl)
    Hyperglycemia (> 400 mg/dl)
    Hyperosmolality (> 300 mOsm/L)
    Hypocalcemia (< 7 mg/dl)
  Drug-induced seizures
    Isoniazid, imipenem
    Theophylline, aminophylline
    Lidocaine
    Meperidine
    Ketamine, halothane, enflurane, methohexital
    Amitriptyline, maprotiline, imipramine, doxepin, fluoxetine
    Haloperidol, trifluoperazine, chlorpromazine
    Ephedrine, phenylpropanolamine, terbutaline
    Methotrexate, BCNU, asparaginase
    Cyclosporine
    Cocaine (crack), phencyclidine, amphetamines
    Alcohol (especially withdrawal)
  Illnesses
    Behçet's disease
    Eclampsia
    Hypertensive encephalopathy
    Liver failure
    Polyarteritis nodosa
    Porphyria
    Renal failure
    Sickle cell disease
    Syphilis
    Systemic lupus erythematosus
    Thrombotic thrombocytopenic purpura
    Whipple's disease
Neurologic conditions
  Angiitis of the nervous system
  Meningitis
  Encephalitis
  Acute head trauma (impact seizures)
  Stroke
  Brain abscess
  Brain tumor

grational defects (cortical dysplasia) and hamartomas, encephalitis, cerebral trauma, and hemorrhage. Not all patients with cerebral pathology develop epilepsy; how a particular lesion or injury causes a region of brain to become epileptogenic is poorly understood at this time.

Although specific mendelian (e.g., tuberous sclerosis, hyperglycinemia, Lafora's disease), chromosomal (Down syndrome), or mitochondrial (MELAS) genetic diseases account for only about 1% of epilepsy cases, heritable factors are important in a much higher percentage, especially in children. Forms of epilepsy that are demonstrably more heritable than others (e.g., childhood absence epilepsy, juvenile myoclonic epilepsy) are increasingly referred to as *idiopathic* or *primary* epilepsies. Common features include a variable family history, generalized spike-wave abnormality on EEG, and onset in childhood or adolescence.

Family history, cerebral injury, and neurologic disease are all risk factors for epilepsy, and the magnitude of the increased risk relative to the population at large can be specified for a number of different conditions that predispose to seizures. In many patients, several factors coexist, and the development of epilepsy reflects the interaction of acquired brain pathology and genetic predisposition.

CLASSIFICATION AND CLINICAL MANIFESTATIONS

Although a number of different classification schemes have been proposed to describe seizures and the various types of epilepsy, the most widely used today are those of the International League Against Epilepsy.

Classification of Epileptic Seizures

Seizures are classified by their clinical manifestations supplemented by EEG data (Table 433–2). There are many different kinds of seizures, each with characteristic behavioral changes and electro-

physiologic alterations that usually can be detected by EEG recordings. The particular manifestations of any single seizure depend on several factors: (1) whether most or only a part of the cerebral cortex is involved at the beginning; (2) the functions of the cortical areas where the seizure originates; and (3) the subsequent pattern of spread within the brain. The International Classification reflects these considerations in two important ways. First, it divides seizures into two fundamental types: those with onset limited to part of one cerebral hemisphere (*partial* or *focal* seizures), and those that involve the cerebral cortex diffusely from the beginning (*generalized* seizures). Second, the International Classification recognizes that seizures are dynamic and evolving and that patients show variations in seizure pattern depending on the extent and manner of spread of the electrical discharge. Thus, simple partial seizures may evolve into complex partial seizures, and either simple or complex partial seizures can evolve into secondarily generalized tonic-clonic convulsions.

PARTIAL SEIZURES. The initial events of a seizure, described either by the patient or by an observer, are usually the most reliable indication to determine if a seizure begins focally. *Simple* partial seizures result when the ictal discharge occurs in, and remains limited to, a circumscribed area of cortex. This is often referred to as the *epileptogenic focus.* Consciousness is not depressed, and patients can interact normally with their environment except for limitations imposed by the seizure on specific localized brain functions. Many symptoms or phenomena can be the expressions of simple partial seizures. Subjective sensory and psychoillusory phenomena are referred to collectively as *auras* and affect about 60% of patients with focal epilepsy. Sensory symptoms such as localized paresthesias, numbness, vertigo, auditory hallucinations, and unformed visual hallucinations occur with seizures beginning in the corresponding primary sensory areas. Psychoillusory symptoms arise from ictal discharges in limbic and association cortex and include dysmnesic symptoms, such as feelings of familiarity (*deja vu*) and unfamiliarity (*jamais vu*); dreamy states, feelings of unreality and depersonalization; time distortion; emotional symptoms such as fear or depression; visual illusions such as multiple images (polyopsia) or distortions of size (micropsia and macropsia); and hallucinatory phenomena, such as unpleasant smells, stereotyped visions, or familiar voices. Autonomic symptoms reflect ictal involvement of limbic structures that lie in the mesial temporal or frontal lobe and project to the hypothalamus and brain stem. Examples of autonomic phenomena include an epigastric rising sensation (especially common with seizures beginning in the mesial temporal lobe), nausea, lightheadedness, pallor or flushing, pupillary dilation, piloerection, salivation, and urinary incontinence.

Simple partial seizures with motor signs begin with *clonic* (rhythmic jerking) or *tonic* (stiffening) movements of a discrete body part. Because of their large cortical representation, muscles of the face and hand are involved often. When the seizure discharge begins in the primary motor cortex and spreads to involve the rest of the precentral gyrus, clonic movements progress in an orderly sequence (*"jacksonian march"*) that reflects the homunculus representation (e.g., thumb to fingers to face to leg). More often, however, ictal discharges involve supplementary or other secondary motor areas of the frontal lobe and produce contralateral flexion and elevation of the arm, contralateral turning of the head and eyes, and tonic extension of the ipsilateral arm (the so-called fencer's posture). Other simple partial motor signs include speech arrest, vocalizations, and eye blinking.

Simple partial seizures may be followed by a transient neurologic abnormality reflecting postictal depression of the epileptogenic cortical area. Thus, focal weakness may follow a simple partial motor seizure, numbness a sensory seizure, and blindness or amblyopia an occipital lobe seizure. These reversible neurologic deficits are collectively referred to as *Todd's paralysis* and rarely last for more than 48 hours. Similarly, prompt examination of a patient after a seizure may reveal transient focal abnormalities that provide useful clues to the site of seizure origin.

Complex partial seizures impair consciousness and produce unresponsiveness. In temporal lobe seizures, loss of consciousness results when the ictal discharge spreads bilaterally to involve both hippocampal and amygdala areas, the parahippocampal gyri and, to some extent, the entorhinal cortex and subfrontal, especially septal, regions. About 70 to 80% of complex partial seizures arise from the temporal lobe, and more than two thirds of these originate in mesial temporal lobe structures, especially hippocampus, amygdala, and

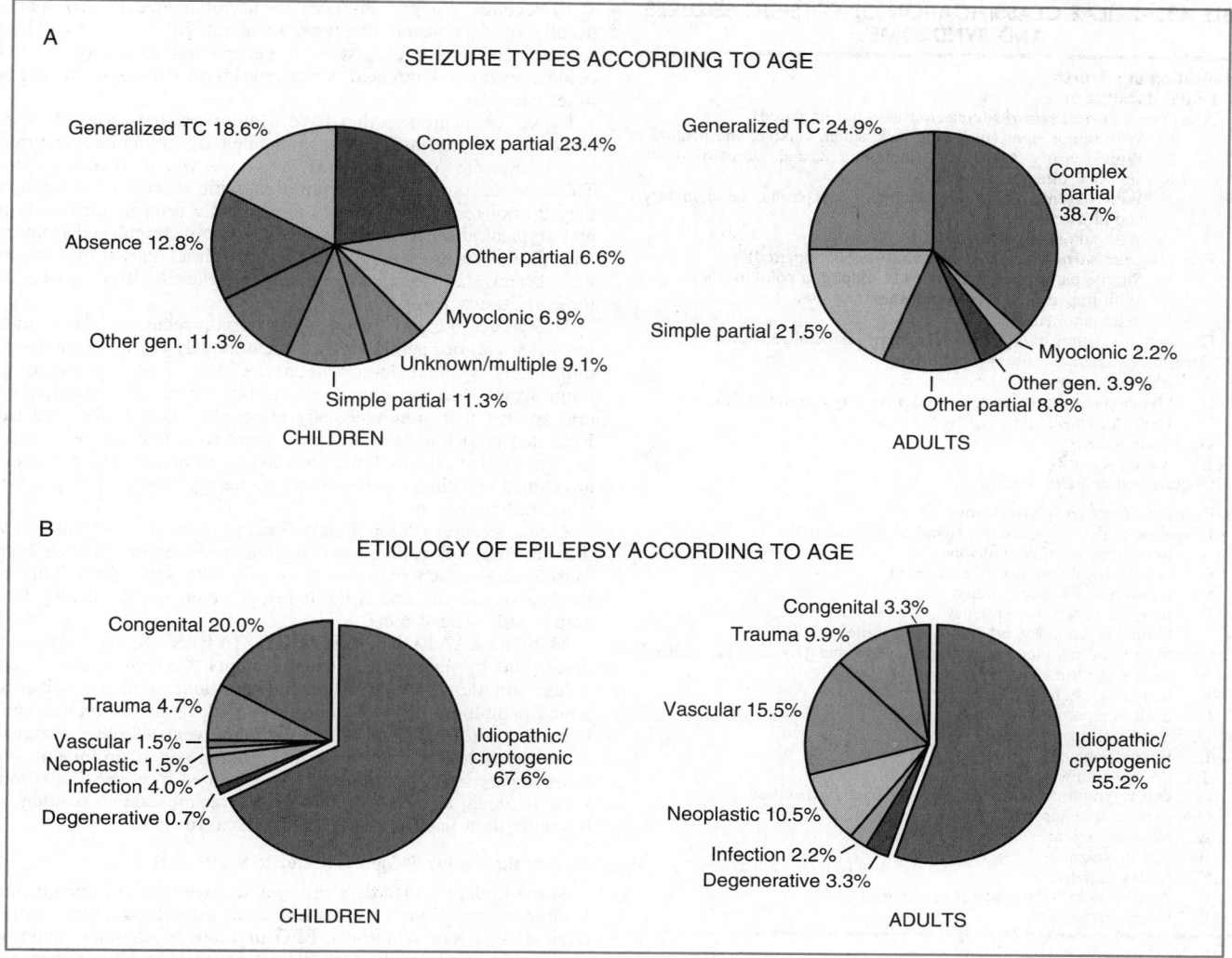

FIGURE 433–1. *A,* Proportion of seizure types as a function of age for newly diagnosed cases of epilepsy in Rochester, Minnesota, 1935–1984. *B,* Etiology of epilepsy in all newly diagnosed cases in Rochester, Minnesota, 1935–1984. TC = tonic-clonic. (Modified from Hauser et al, Epilepsia 34:453–468, 1993.)

parahippocampal gyrus. Remaining cases of complex partial seizures arise mainly from the frontal lobe, with smaller percentages originating in parietal and occipital lobes. Many complex partial seizures evolve from simple partial seizures; consciousness becomes impaired as the seizure progresses. Complex partial seizures preceded by an olfactory aura are referred to as *uncinate fits* because of their origin in or near the uncus of the medial temporal lobe. Clinical tradition teaches that uncinate fits have a higher association with brain tumors than other types of complex partial seizures.

The typical complex partial seizure of temporal lobe origin consists of a motionless stare accompanied by alteration of consciousness followed by *automatisms* (repetitive purposeless complex movements) and, often, dystonic positioning of the arm or hand *contralateral* to one seizure discharge. Oroalimentary automatisms are most common and include lip smacking, swallowing, and sucking and chewing movements. Gestural automatisms, such as fumbling, picking at clothes or objects, hand wringing, and patting movements, are also frequently encountered and are typically expressed maximally in the lines *ipsilateral* to the epileptogenic temporal lobe. There may be clumsy perseveration of ongoing motor tasks, such as eating, drawing, walking, or washing dishes. Some patients show a degree of residual ability to react to their environment during the seizure, although their behavior is typically inappropriate. Complex partial seizures usually last 45 to 90 seconds and are followed by a period of confusion and disorientation lasting several more minutes. Without EEG recording, it is difficult to de-

termine where the ictal state ends and postictal behavior begins. Characteristically, patients are amnesic for details of the seizure that occurred after the aura. There may be transient postictal aphasia when the seizure involves the dominant temporal lobe.

Complex partial seizures of frontal lobe origin are atypical and often differ dramatically from those originating in the temporal lobe. Although there are many variations, frontal lobe complex partial seizures tend to (1) begin and end abruptly; (2) be brief with few, if any, postictal symptoms; (3) express prominent, but often bizzare, motor manifestations such as asynchronous thrashing or flailing of arms and legs, pelvic thrusting, pedalling leg movements, and loud vocalizations, all of which can at first suggest psychogenic attacks; and (4) show minimal or nonlocalizing changes with scalp EEG recordings.

Psychomotor, temporal lobe, and *limbic* seizures are all terms that have been used in the past to describe many of the ictal behaviors now classified as complex partial seizures, but they are not synonymous. Not all complex partial seizures arise from the temporal lobe, nor do all involve the limbic system. Some temporal lobe and limbic phenomena reflect unilateral ictal discharges and may not be associated with significant alteration of awareness, the *sine qua non* of complex partial seizures. Finally, automatisms (the "psychomotor" element) are not invariably present in complex partial seizures.

GENERALIZED SEIZURES. Generalized seizures begin diffusely and involve both cerebral hemispheres simultaneously from the outset. They lack clinical and EEG features that indicate a lo-

TABLE 433-2. ILAE CLASSIFICATION OF EPILEPTIC SEIZURES AND SYNDROMES

Classification of seizures
  I. Partial (focal) seizures
    A. *Simple partial seizures* (consciousness not impaired)
       1. With motor signs (including jacksonian, versive, and postural)
       2. With sensory symptoms (including visual, somatosensory, auditory, olfactory)
       3. With psychic symptoms (including dysphasia, hallucinatory, and affective changes)
       4. With autonomic symptoms
    B. *Complex partial seizures* (consciousness is impaired)
       1. Simple partial onset followed by impaired consciousness
       2. With impairment of consciousness at onset
       3. With automatisms
    C. Partial seizures evolving to secondarily generalized seizures
 II. Generalized seizures of non-focal origin
    A. Absence seizures
    B. Myoclonic seizures; myoclonic jerks (single or multiple)
    C. Tonic-clonic seizures
    D. Tonic seizures
    E. Atonic seizures
III. Unclassified epileptic seizures

Classification of epileptic syndromes
  I. Idiopathic epilepsy syndromes (focal or generalized)
    A. Benign neonatal convulsions
    B. Benign focal epilepsy of childhood
    C. Childhood absence epilepsy
    D. Juvenile myoclonic epilepsy
    E. Idiopathic epilepsy, otherwise unspecified
 II. Cryptogenic or symptomatic epilepsy syndromes (focal or generalized)
    A. West's syndrome (infantile spasms)
    B. Lennox-Gastaut syndrome
    C. Epilepsia partialis continua
    D. Temporal lobe epilepsy
    E. Frontal lobe epilepsy
    F. Post-traumatic epilepsy
    G. Other symptomatic epilepsies, otherwise unspecified
III. Other epilepsy syndromes of uncertain or mixed classification
    A. Neonatal seizures
    B. Febrile seizures
    C. Reflex epilepsy
    D. Adult nonconvulsive status epilepticus
    E. Other unspecified

calized cerebral origin. Generalized seizures are subdivided mainly on the basis of the presence or absence and character of ictal motor manifestations. These features, in turn, depend on the extent to which subcortical and brain stem structures are engaged in elaboration of the ictal discharge.

Generalized tonic-clonic seizures *(grand mal convulsions)* are characterized by abrupt loss of consciousness with bilateral tonic extension of the trunk and limbs *(tonic phase),* often accompanied by a loud vocalization as air is forcefully expelled across tightly contracted vocal cords (the *"epileptic cry"*), followed by bilaterally synchronous muscle jerking *(clonic phase).* In some patients, a few clonic jerks precede the tonic-clonic sequence; in others, only a tonic or a clonic phase is seen. Urinary incontinence is common, fecal incontinence rare. The actual ictus does not usually last more than 90 seconds. The postictal phase is marked by transient deep stupor followed in 15 to 30 minutes by a lethargic, confused state with automatic behavior. As recovery progresses, many patients complain of headache, muscle soreness, mental dulling, lack of energy, or mood changes lasting as long as 24 hours.

Generalized tonic-clonic seizures result in a number of striking but transient physiologic changes, including blood hypoxia and lactic acidosis, elevated plasma catecholamine levels, and increased concentrations of creatine kinase, prolactin, corticotropin, cortisol, beta-endorphin, and growth hormone. Complications include oral trauma, vertebral compression fractures, shoulder dislocation, aspiration pneumonia, and sudden death, which may be related to acute pulmonary edema, cardiac arrhythmia, or suffocation.

Absence seizures (petit mal seizures) occur mainly in children and are characterized by sudden, momentary lapses in awareness (the absence attack), staring, rhythmic blinking, and, often, a few small clonic jerks of arms or hands. Behavior and awareness return

immediately to normal. There is no postictal period and usually no recollection that a seizure has occurred. Most absence seizures last < 10 seconds. Longer absences are accompanied by automatisms, usually of a perseverative type, in about 70% of cases. Absence seizures commonly coexist with generalized tonic-clonic or myoclonic seizures. Untreated, absence seizures can occur hundreds of times each day.

Lapses of awareness that have a more gradual onset, do not resolve as abruptly, and are accompanied by autonomic features or loss of muscle tone are referred to as *atypical absence seizures.* These occur most often in children with mental retardation, and they do not respond as well to antiepileptic drug treatment. Typical and atypical absence seizures must also be distinguished from complex partial seizures manifested only by brief lapses of consciousness because cause, treatment, and prognosis differ among these three seizure types.

Myoclonic seizures manifest as rapid, recurrent, brief muscle jerks that can occur bilaterally, synchronously or asynchronously, or unilaterally without loss of consciousness. The myoclonic jerks range from small movements of the face or hands to massive bilateral spasms that simultaneously affect the head, limbs, and trunk. Repeated myoclonic seizures may seem to crescendo and terminate in a generalized tonic-clonic convulsion. Although they can occur at any time, myoclonic seizures often cluster shortly after waking or while falling asleep.

Atonic seizures ("drop attacks") occur most often in children with diffuse encephalopathies and are characterized by sudden loss of muscle tone which may result in falls with self-injury. Sometimes the loss of muscle tone is limited or fragmentary, producing, for example, only a head drop.

MISCELLANEOUS SEIZURE TYPES. Some seizures are designated by unique or unusual features. *Gelastic* seizures can be either complex partial or generalized nonconvulsive seizures in which pathologic laughter unaccompanied by any emotional content is a conspicuous feature of the epileptic event. *Cursive* seizures are complex partial seizures in which running is a prominent symptoms. *Reflex* seizures are attacks precipitated by a specific stimulus, such as touch, a musical tune, a particular movement, reading, stroboscopic light patterns, or complex visual images.

Classification of the Epilepsies (Epileptic Syndromes)

Some epileptic disorders are characterized by sufficiently reproducible aggregations of historical data, seizure patterns, associated clinical signs and symptoms, EEG findings, biochemical abnormalities, and imaging results that distinct *epileptic syndromes* can be defined. Furthermore, classifying the kind of epilepsy a patient has, or identifying a person's specific epileptic syndrome, is more important than describing seizures. This is because such a diagnosis has implications for diagnostic evaluation, treatment, genetic counseling, and prognosis. The most widely used classification scheme today is the 1989 revision of the International League Against Epilepsy's Commission on Classification and Terminology (Table 433–2).

The ILAE classification separates major groups of epilepsy first on the basis of whether seizures are partial *(localization-related [focal] epilepsies)* or generalized *(generalized epilepsies),* and second, by cause *(idiopathic, symptomatic,* or *cryptogenic epilepsy).* Idiopathic epilepsies and syndromes are those that have no demonstrable underlying cause other than a probable hereditary predisposition. Symptomatic epilepsies and syndromes are those resulting from a known or assumed brain disorder. Cryptogenic epilepsies and syndromes are those in which the cause is unknown, although a symptomatic basis is assumed because of circumstantial evidence or similarities to cases in which the cause is known. Subtypes of epilepsy are grouped by age and, in the case of focal epilepsies, by the anatomic location of the presumed site of seizure onset.

A fundamental problem with the ILAE classification is that it is entirely empirical, with clinical and EEG data emphasized over specific etiologic information (e.g., gene abnormalities, biochemical or metabolic defects). Nonetheless, this realistically reflects current knowledge about most epilepsies today. Furthermore, defining common epilepsy syndromes has great practical value.

FEBRILE SEIZURES. Febrile seizures are the most common cause of convulsions in children: They affect between 3 and 5% of all children in the United States and Europe under the age of 5 years. Most febrile seizures occur between the ages of 6 months and 4 years, although sometimes they occur in children as old as 6 or 7 years. About 30% of children have more than one attack; chance of recurrence is greatest if the first seizure occurs before 1 year of age or there is a family history of febrile seizures. Although the vast majority of affected children have no long-term consequences, febrile seizures increase the risk of developing epilepsy later. This risk is low for most children, about 2 to 3%, but it approximates 10 to 13% in those who have had prolonged or focal seizures, who have a family history of afebrile seizures, or who were neurologically abnormal before the first febrile seizure. Febrile seizures are not associated with, nor do they cause, mental retardation, below average IQ, poor school performance, or behavior problems. Prophylactic treatment is generally not indicated because of the benign prognosis. If treatment is considered at all, rectal administration of diazepam only during febrile illnesses is effective, safe, and preferable to chronic therapy using phenobarbital.

BENIGN PARTIAL EPILEPSY OF CHILDHOOD WITH CENTRAL-MIDTEMPORAL SPIKES. This is one of the most common epileptic syndromes of childhood, representing about 15% of all pediatric epilepsies. Seizures usually begin between the ages of 4 and 13 years; affected children are otherwise normal. Most have seizures principally or only at night. Because sleep promotes secondary generalization, parents report only tonic-clonic convulsions; any focal signature is usually missed. In contrast, seizures occurring during the day are typically focal and express themselves with twitching of one side of the face, speech arrest, drooling, and paresthesias of the face, gums, tongue, and inner cheeks. Seizures may progress to include hemiclonic movements or hemitonic posturing. EEG's show a distinctive pattern of stereotyped epileptiform discharges over the central and midtemporal regions. Prognosis is invariably good, and seizures disappear by mid to late adolescence. Outcome is not affected by treatment, but carbamazepine prevents recurrent attacks.

CHILDHOOD ABSENCE (PETIT MAL) EPILEPSY. This disorder begins most often between the ages of 4 and 12 years in children who are neurologically and intellectually normal. Absence attacks can often be precipitated by hyperventilation. The EEG is diagnostic, showing stereotyped 3-Hz spike-wave discharges in association with a typical spell (Fig. 433–2). Generalized tonic-clonic seizures occur in 30 to 50% of cases. Ethosuximide (10 mg per kilogram per day or, in older children, 250 mg two or three times daily) and valproate (15 to 30 mg per kilogram per day) are equally effective against absence seizures; valproate is preferable if generalized tonic-clonic seizures coexist.

JUVENILE MYOCLONIC EPILEPSY. This is one of the most frequently encountered types of idiopathic generalized epilepsy. It begins most often between the ages of 8 and 20 years in otherwise healthy individuals. When fully developed, the syndrome is characterized by morning myoclonic jerks, generalized tonic-clonic seizures that occur just after awakening, normal intelligence, a family history of similar seizures, and an EEG that shows generalized 4- to 6-Hz spike-wave and polyspike-wave discharges. Valproate controls attacks in > 80% of cases, but indefinite treatment is required in most cases because of the high rate of seizure relapse following attempted drug withdrawal.

LENNOX-GASTAUT SYNDROME. This term is used for a heterogeneous group of early childhood epileptic encephalopathies that have in common physical brain abnormalities, mental retardation, uncontrolled seizures, and an EEG pattern that shows generalized 1.5- to 2.5-Hz sharp-slow wave discharges ("slow spike-and-wave pattern"). No treatment is consistently effective; management is best directed by specialists in the field.

TEMPORAL LOBE EPILEPSY. This is the most common epileptic syndrome of adults, accounting for at least 40% of epilepsy cases. Seizures begin in late childhood or adolescence, and there is often a history of febrile seizures. Virtually all patients have complex partial seizures, some of which secondarily generalize. Epigastric or visceral auras are frequent. Interictal EEG's usually show epileptiform discharges over the anterior temporal region (Fig. 433–3). Most patients with temporal lobe epilepsy have impaired memory, and some show a decrease in either verbal or visuospatial skills, depending on whether the epileptogenic temporal lobe is dominant or nondominant.

Temporal lobe epilepsy arises most often from mesial temporal limbic structures, typically in association with a characteristic lesion known as *hippocampal sclerosis*. Hippocampal sclerosis refers to variable but selective neuronal loss, especially in the CA1 (Sommer's sector), CA3, and dentate gyrus regions of the hippocampus (Fig. 433–4). Secondary gliosis occurs, and corresponding atrophy of the hippocampal formation can be recognized on magnetic resonance brain scans (see below). Neurons in the hippocampal CA2 region (resistant zone) and granule cell layer are relatively spared. In 20% of cases, temporal lobe epilepsy is caused by other structural lesions such as cavernous malformations, hamartomas, cortical dysplasia, glial tumors, and scars related to previous head injuries or encephalitis. Some temporal lobe seizures are symptoms of frontal or occipital lesions which initiate ictal discharges that propagate into mesial temporal lobe structures.

Antiepileptic drugs are usually successful in suppressing secondarily generalized seizures, but > 50% of patients continue to have partial seizures. In drug-resistant cases, temporal lobectomy is the treatment of choice.

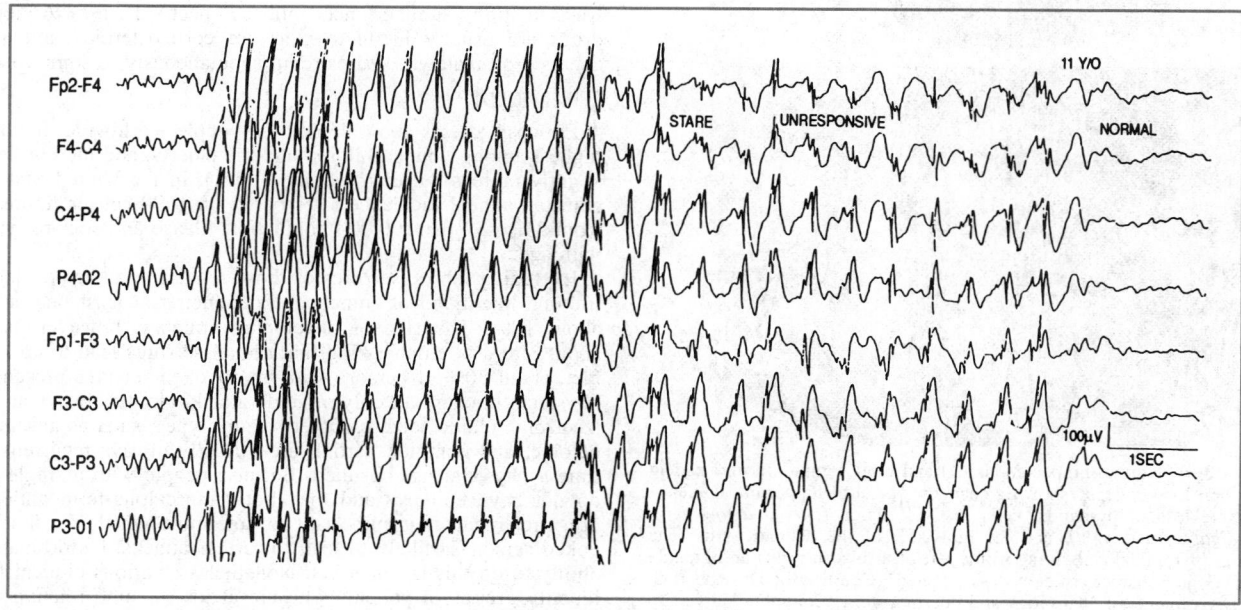

FIGURE 433–2. Childhood absence epilepsy. The EEG shows the typical pattern of generalized 3-Hz spike-wave complexes associated with a clinical absence seizure.

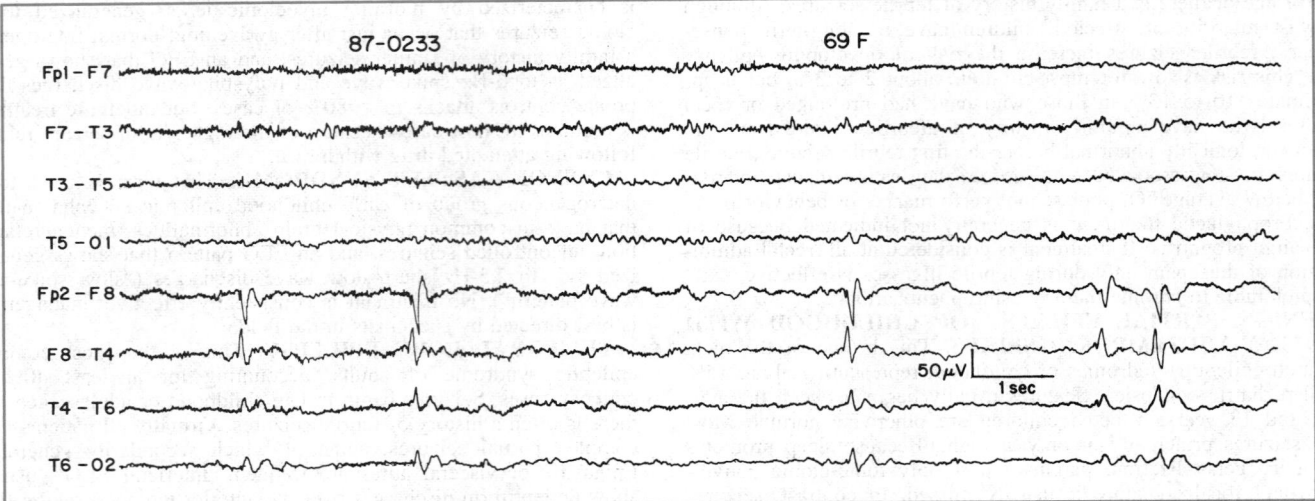

87-0233   69 F

FIGURE 433–3. Temporal lobe epilepsy. Epileptiform discharges are seen focally over the right temporal lobe (bottom four lines), and there is intermixed irregular slow-wave activity not seen on the other side.

POST-TRAUMATIC EPILEPSY. The chance of developing post-traumatic epilepsy relates directly to the severity of the head injury. Following penetrating wounds and other severe head injuries, for example, about one third of patients develop seizures within 1 year. Severe head injuries are defined by the presence of a cerebral contusion, intracerebral or intracranial hematoma, unconsciousness or amnesia lasting more than 24 hours, or persistent abnormalities on neurologic examination, such as hemiparesis or aphasia. Although the majority of patients develop seizures within 1

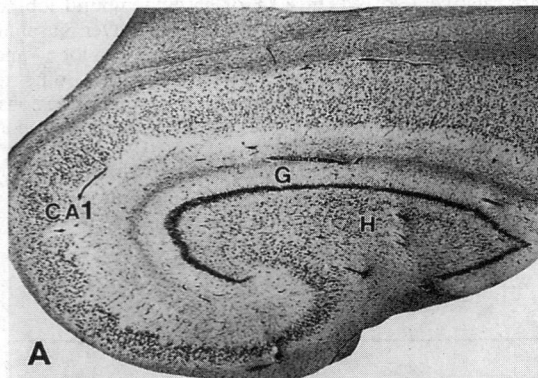

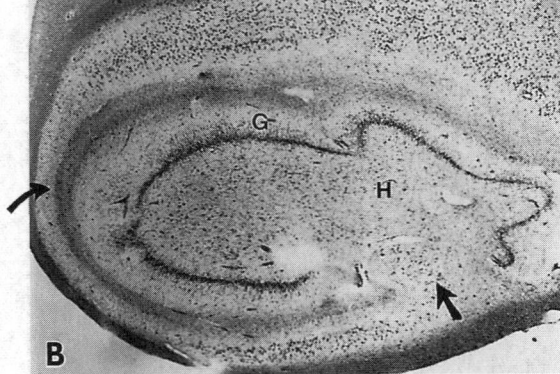

FIGURE 433–4. Normal hippocampus *(A)* and hippocampus from a patient with temporal lobe epilepsy showing changes typical of hippocampal sclerosis *(B)*. Note loss of pyramidal cells in CA1 region *(curved arrow, left),* CA4 *(straight arrow, right),* and the hilus (H) of the dentate gyrus. The CA2 region (pyramidal cells lying to the left of arrow on right) and granule cell layer (G) are characteristically less affected. (Courtesy of Dr. Robert S. Sloviter, Departments of Neurology and Pharmacology, Columbia University and Helen Hayes Hospital, New York, New York.)

to 2 years of injury, new-onset seizures may still appear 5 or more years later. Two thirds of patients with post-traumatic epilepsy have partial or secondarily generalized seizures. Mild head injuries (uncomplicated brief loss of consciousness, no skull fracture, absence of focal neurologic signs, no contusion or hematoma) do not increase the risk of seizures.

Impact seizures (a generalized convulsion occurring at the time of, or immediately after, the injury) and *early seizures* (those occurring within the first 1 to 2 weeks) represent acute reactions of the brain to the trauma. Seizures beginning after 10 to 14 days reflect an increased risk of developing post-traumatic epilepsy.

Early seizures should be treated with phenytoin. Phenytoin should also be given prophylactically for 1 to 2 weeks to patients who have sustained severe head injuries in order to minimize complications from seizures occurring during acute management. In the absence of overt attacks, phenytoin should be discontinued after 2 weeks because no data indicate that antiepileptic drugs prevent the development of later epilepsy.

EPILEPSIA PARTIALIS CONTINUA (EPC). This term refers to continuous focal seizures involving part or all of one side of the body. In adults, EPC occurs with severe strokes, primary or metastatic brain tumors, metabolic encephalopathies (especially hyperosmolar nonketotic hyperglycemia), encephalitis, and subacute or rare chronic inflammatory diseases of the brain (Kozhevnikov's Russian spring-summer encephalitis; Behçet's disease). Antiepileptic drugs are usually ineffective, as are corticosteroids and antiviral agents. Fortunately, seizures remit spontaneously in some cases.

EPIDEMIOLOGY

Epilepsy affects about 45 million people worldwide. Incidence is highest among young children and the elderly, and men are affected slightly more often than women (1.5:1). In the United States, age-adjusted annual incidence rates based on 1990 census figures range from 31 to 57 per 100,000 population. Cause and seizure type vary with age.

Excluding febrile seizures or those related to an acute illness, the lifetime likelihood of someone experiencing at least one seizure is about 10%. The risk of developing epilepsy, however, is lower, about 3 to 4%, emphasizing that not all seizures lead to epilepsy. In fact, about 30% of persons with unprovoked seizures present to the physician having had only a single attack, almost always a generalized tonic-clonic seizure. Other seizure types, such as absence, myoclonic, and complex partial, are virtually always recurrent by the time a physician is consulted. Because people with a single seizure do not have epilepsy and may not require long-term antiepileptic drug treatment, it is important to determine whether a first unprovoked seizure is likely to lead to further attacks. Unfortunately, the ability to do this is imperfect. Nonetheless, various clinical features identify groups of patients who are at low or high relative risk for further seizures, and this helps in making treatment decisions and advising patients. The high-risk group consists of individuals with a history of significant brain injury and an abnormal EEG. For these patients, recurrence risk at 2 years is about 65%. By contrast, recurrence risk is only 24% in persons with an idiopathic generalized seizure, a normal EEG, and a negative family history for seizures or epilepsy. Following a second seizure, risk of further seizures rises to >80%. A second seizure, therefore, is a reliable indication of epilepsy.

Persons with epilepsy have increased mortality rates compared with the general population. Most of this increased risk occurs in patients with symptomatic epilepsy in whom mortality relates to the underlying condition. In patients with idiopathic or cryptogenic epilepsy, the increased risk of death is related mainly to accidents, especially drowning. Autopsy and clinical series have reported an increased risk of sudden unexplained death, presumably due to cardiac arrhythmia, pulmonary edema, or myocardial infarction, but the actual incidence has not been documented.

PATHOGENESIS

Seizures result from the synchronous interactions of large populations of neurons that intermittently discharge in abnormal patterns. Because of the large number of processes that regulate cortical excitability, it is unlikely that there is a single epileptogenic mechanism. Nonetheless, neurophysiologic studies in a variety of experimental preparations have shown that "epileptic" neurons share a number of properties, although the total expression of these varies according to the particular model.

Intracellular recordings from neurons in an epileptogenic focus show recurring high-voltage, long-duration depolarizations with superimposed high-frequency bursts of action potentials. The extracellular current flow generated by these *paroxysmal depolarizing shifts* (PDS's) results in the interictal EEG spike or sharp wave, the characteristic epileptiform discharge that signifies susceptibility to seizures. PDS generation involves several mechanisms, including increased excitability resulting from changes in intrinsic voltage-dependent membrane currents, newly active excitatory circuits, attenuation or loss of effective postsynaptic inhibition and other inhibitory processes, as well as increased effectiveness of excitatory synapses. In neurons showing "epileptic" patterns of behavior, ordinary synaptic inputs may elicit exaggerated or pathologically amplified responses. Activation of the *N*-methyl-D-aspartate (NMDA) type of glutamate receptors potentiates cellular excitability and leads to sustained neuronal depolarization and calcium influx. Prolonged NMDA receptor activation and excessive accumulation of intracellular calcium also result in neuronal toxicity and may lead to cell death ("epileptic brain damage") following severe repetitive seizures or status epilepticus. In some areas of cortex, hippocampus for example, subsets of neurons which normally fire in bursts may serve as pacemaker cells for other groups of neurons during epileptogenic activities.

Although it is not known in detail what causes the transition from an interical to an ictal state, development of sustained experimental seizures reflects decreasing effectiveness of inhibitory mechanisms accompanied by increasing evidence of excitation. PDS's become more frequent and involve ever larger numbers of neurons and more distant areas of cortex, a situation that results in progressive depolarization of neurons both within and outside the original focus. During frequent interictal epileptiform discharges and especially during seizures, extracellular potassium and intracellular calcium concentrations increase and contribute to the overall excitability of the epileptic neuronal aggregate. During the seizure itself, neurons are tonically depolarized and fire continuously in a sustained, high-frequency discharge (corresponding to the tonic phase of the seizure). The seizure ends as phasic repolarizations interrupt the continuous firing pattern (the correlate of the clonic phase) and gradually restore membrane potentials to normal or to a temporary hyperpolarized state (postictal depression). Phenytoin and carbamazepine are effective anticonvulsants because they produce a use-dependent block of sodium channels, thus limiting the capability of neurons to fire at high-frequency rates. The benzodiazepines and barbiturates exert their anticonvulsant effect by enhancing postsynaptic GABA-mediated inhibition through an effect on the chloride ionophore.

In the focal epilepsies, abnormal neuronal behavior originates in and may remain confined to a restricted area of the cortex. The brain possesses powerful mechanisms to suppress and restrain abnormal electrical behavior. Typically during focal interictal discharges or focal seizures, areas surrounding the epileptogenic cortex are inhibited (surround inhibition), as is the homotopic contralateral cortex and areas of the thalamus and brain stem. Only when these restraining influences are overcome does a seizure spread and become secondarily generalized.

In temporal lobe epilepsy, certain neurons within the dentate gyrus of the hippocampus have been identified as being especially vulnerable to injury. Selective loss of mossy cells and of neurons containing somatostatin and neuropeptide Y results in deafferentation of the normally powerful GABA inhibitory neurons within the dentate gyrus, rendering them nonfunctional. As a result, the granule cells of the dentate gyrus become disinhibited and respond with abnormal synchronous bursts to cortical stimuli. Subclinical electrographic seizures develop and further damage vulnerable cell populations, creating a self-enhancing cycle of cell loss, impaired control of hippocampal excitability, and, eventually, clinical seizures associated with the pathologic picture of hippocampal sclerosis. How other lesions (e.g., tumors or cavernous malformations) cause focal epilepsy is less well understood.

The thalamus plays a critical role in generating generalized seizures and the generalized spike-wave EEG patterns that accompany them. The bilateral synchrony of generalized seizures and the rhythmicity of spike-wave discharges appear to depend on two main factors—a unique set of ionic conductances, including a T-type calcium current, which enable neurons in the thalamic nucleus reticularis to function as pacemaker control cells, and the special anatomy and pharmacology of the thalamocortical system. The substantia nigra also is critical to the expression of generalized convulsions, especially the tonic phase; GABA-ergic inhibitory transmission in the substantia nigra plays a regulatory role in the propagation of both primary and secondarily generalized seizure discharges. Because there are no consistent, demonstrable pathologic changes in the brains of patients with idiopathic generalized epilepsy, susceptibility to these seizures likely results from inherited biochemical membrane or neurotransmitter defects that result in abnormal excitability within the involved circuits.

DIAGNOSIS

Accurate diagnosis is the cornerstone of rational management. The diagnostic evaluation has three objectives: (1) to determine if the patient has epilepsy; (2) to classify the seizures and type of epilepsy accurately and determine if the clinical data fit a particular epilepsy syndrome; and (3) to identify, if possible, a specific underlying cause.

History

A detailed and accurate history is imperative and the single most important factor in diagnosis. Because patients usually have only limited awareness of their behavior during a seizure, additional information usually must be obtained from family members or other close observers. The historical summary should provide a clear description of the patient's seizures, including details of any aura; the neurologic status between attacks; any reproducible precipitants; and relevant risk factors for epilepsy such as a family history of seizures or a history of severe head trauma, encephalitis or meningitis, and febrile seizures (Table 433–3). In children and young adults, one should inquire about gestation, birth, postnatal course, and early development. If a patient has been treated previously, it is

TABLE 433–3. ESSENTIAL FEATURES OF THE SEIZURE HISTORY

Date and circumstances of first attack
First consistent event in the seizure (Is there an aura? Are initial symptoms/ signs focal or lateralizing?)
Subsequent evolution of the seizure, in sequence
Postictal manifestations (Todd's paralysis)
Is there more than one seizure type?
Average rate of occurrence; longest seizure-free interval since onset
Seizure precipitants (alcohol, sleep deprivation, particular stimuli, stress)
Is there a pattern to seizure occurrence (circadian, catamenial)?
Has there been a change in characteristics of the seizure?
Symptoms of neurologic or systemic disease between seizures. Are these static, intermittent, or progressive?
Risk factors for epilepsy (family history, cerebral injury)

important to learn what drugs were used, the doses and blood levels that were achieved, and therapeutic or adverse effects.

Physical Examination

Although the physical examination is normal in most patients with epilepsy, abnormal findings, when present, can be helpful in two ways. First, physical signs may point to an underlying neurologic or systemic disorder of which the seizures are a part. Phakomatoses, for example, are commonly associated with seizures and may be suggested by café-au-lait spots, a facial angioma, hypopigmented macules, axillary freckling, and shagreen patches. Second, focal neurologic signs indicate localized cerebral pathology. Asymmetry in the size of the hands, feet, or face signifies a longstanding abnormality of the cerebral hemisphere contralateral to the smaller side. Third, absence seizures can be triggered in untreated patients by having them hyperventilate for 2 to 3 minutes.

Laboratory Tests

ELECTROENCEPHALOGRAPHY. EEG is the most important diagnostic test for epilepsy. EEG findings are useful and sometimes essential for establishing the diagnosis, classifying seizures correctly, identifying epileptic syndromes, and making therapeutic decisions. In combination with appropriate clinical findings, *epileptiform* EEG patterns termed "spikes" or "sharp waves" strongly support a diagnosis of epilepsy. In patients with seizures, focal epileptiform discharges indicate focal epilepsy, whereas generalized epileptiform activity indicates a generalized form of epilepsy. The particular pattern of epileptiform activity, defined by the morphology, spatial distribution, repetition rate, and other characteristics of the discharges, assists in identifying a particular type of epilepsy or epileptic syndrome. A note of caution is warranted, however. Most EEG's are obtained between seizures, and interictal abnormalities alone can never prove or refute a diagnosis of epilepsy. Epilepsy can be definitively established only by recording a characteristic ictal discharge during a clinical attack. Unfortunately, this is uncommon during routine EEG recordings. A further factor that can confound interpretation of interictal EEG's is the occurrence of similar epileptiform abnormalities in about 2% of normal people; many of these, especially in children, are asymptomatic markers of a genetic trait. Finally, epileptiform-like waveforms or artifacts can be misinterpreted and erroneously considered to be evidence of seizure susceptibility.

About 40 to 50% of patients with epilepsy show epileptiform abnormalities on their initial EEG. The chance of capturing epileptiform activity is enhanced by sleep deprivation for 24 hours before the test and having the patient sleep during a portion of the EEG recording. Serial EEG's also increase the yield of positive tracings. A small number of persons with epilepsy, however, continue to have normal interictal EEG's despite all efforts to record an abnormality.

Specialized epilepsy centers in tertiary referral hospitals include monitoring units equipped with simultaneous EEG and closed-circuit television capability as well as computer-assisted detection and analysis systems. These facilities have greatly improved management of selected patients by giving physicians the means to distinguish epileptic from nonepileptic paroxysmal events, to make precise electrical-clinical correlations, and to localize epileptogenic foci for resective surgery.

NEUROIMAGING STUDIES. Anatomic imaging using computed tomography (CT) or magnetic resonance imaging (MRI) complements EEG data by identifying structural brain pathology that may be causally related to the development of epilepsy. MRI is substantially more sensitive than CT in detecting epileptogenic cerebral lesions. Hippocampal sclerosis, defects of neuronal migration, gangliogliomas and some gliomas, and cavernous malformations are readily seen with MRI but may be missed using CT. It is important to obtain a complete imaging study that includes both T1- and T2-weighted images in coronal and axial planes. Imaging in the coronal plane perpendicular to the long axis of the hippocampus has improved detection of hippocampal atrophy and gliosis (Fig. 433–5), findings that correlate with the pathologic picture of mesial temporal sclerosis and an epileptogenic temporal lobe. An even more sensitive measure of hippocampal atrophy compares volume measurements of a patient's hippocampus with similar quanti-

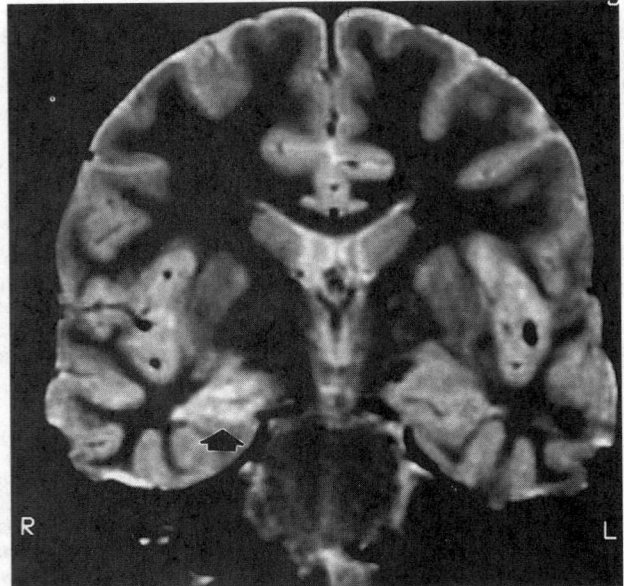

FIGURE 433–5. Coronal MRI scan at the level of the anterior temporal lobe showing changes consistent with right-sided hippocampal sclerosis. The right hippocampal formation *(arrow)* is atrophic compared with the left and shows signal changes (white areas) indicating gliosis. (Courtesy of Dr. Stephen Chan, Division of Neuroradiology, Columbia-Presbyterian Medical Center, New York, New York.)

tative data obtained in normal controls. Gadolinium infusion does not improve detection of cerebral lesions associated with epilepsy, although it often aids in differentiating among types of cerebral pathology.

A CT or, preferably, MRI scan should be obtained in all patients suspected of epilepsy over the age of 18 years and in all children with partial seizures (except those with benign focal epilepsy of childhood), abnormal neurologic findings, or focal slow-wave abnormalities on EEG. All patients with refractory seizures should have an MRI scan even if earlier CT scans were normal.

In contrast to these structural imaging methods, positron emission tomography (PET) and single photon emission computed tomography (SPECT) offer functional views of the brain. These techniques use physiologically active, radiolabeled tracers to image the brain's metabolic activity (PET) or blood flow (SPECT). For example, about 70% of patients with temporal lobe epilepsy show focal hypometabolic areas on interictal PET scans that correspond to the epileptogenic focus. Abnormalities using PET or SPECT are often demonstrated even when MRI or CT is normal. By and large, these specialized procedures are reserved for research-level studies rather than diagnosis.

BLOOD TESTS. Routine blood tests rarely offer diagnostic assistance in otherwise healthy patients with epilepsy. Serum electrolytes, liver function tests, and an automated blood count may be useful, however, as baseline studies before starting antiepileptic drug therapy. Blood tests are necessary and frequently informative in older patients with acute or chronic systemic disease. Consideration should be given to obtaining blood or urine samples from adolescents and young adults with unexplained generalized seizures to screen for substance abuse, especially cocaine.

LUMBAR PUNCTURE. Lumbar puncture is mandatory if there is any suspicion of meningitis or encephalitis. It is otherwise unnecessary and need not be performed routinely. Repeated generalized seizures and convulsive status epilepticus can increase cerebrospinal fluid protein content slightly and produce a pleocytosis of up to 100 WBC's per cubic millimeter for 24 to 48 hours. CSF pleocytosis should be attributed to seizures only in retrospect; infection or intracranial inflammatory processes should always be assumed first.

ELECTROCARDIOGRAM (ECG). An ECG should be obtained in any young person with a first generalized seizure if there is a family history of arrhythmia, sudden unexplained death, or episodic unconsciousness. An ECG should also be obtained in any patient with a history of cardiac arrhythmia or valvular disease.

Not every paroxysmal event is a seizure, and misidentification of other conditions as epilepsy leads to ineffective, unnecessary, and potentially harmful treatment. In addition, misdiagnosis accounts for a substantial portion of patients whose spells have not responded to antiepileptic drug treatment.

A variety of conditions can be confused with epilepsy, depending on the age of the patient and the nature and circumstances of the attacks (Table 433–4). It is not always possible to distinguish among various diagnostic possibilities on clinical grounds alone, and admission to a specialized monitoring unit is frequently necessary.

Nonepileptic paroxysmal disorders have in common the occurrence of sudden, discrete events characterized by abnormal or inappropriate behavior, variable responsiveness, changes in muscle tone, and various postures or movements. These conditions are far more common and variable in their presentation in children than in adults. Many of the disorders simulating epilepsy in childhood can be viewed as transient "developmental" conditions that require no treatment other than reassurance.

Syncope (see Ch. 396.1) refers to the symptom complex that results when there is a transient, global reduction in cerebral perfusion with associated hypoxia. Loss of consciousness lasts only a few seconds, uncommonly a minute or more, and recovery is rapid. If the cerebral hypoxia is sufficiently severe, the syncopal episode may include brief tonic posturing of the trunk or a few clonic jerks of the arms and legs (convulsive syncope). Similarly, some forms of *migraine* can be mistaken for seizures, especially if headache is atypical or mild. Basilar artery migraine, a rare variant seen most often in adolescents and young adults, can include lethargy, mood changes, confusion and disorientation, vertigo, bilateral visual disturbances, and alteration or loss of consciousness.

Psychogenic seizures frequently cause intractable "epilepsy" in adults and may represent 20% or more of cases referred to an epilepsy monitoring unit. Definitive diagnosis requires video/EEG documentation, although a history of atypical and nonstereotyped attacks, emotional or psychological precipitants, psychiatric illness, complete lack of response to antiepileptic drugs, and repeatedly normal interictal EEG's suggests the possibility of psychogenic seizures. *Panic attacks* and anxiety attacks with hyperventilation can superficially resemble partial seizures with affective, autonomic, or special sensory symptoms. Prolonged hyperventilation results in muscle twitching or spasms (tetany), and affected patients may faint.

Episodic dyscontrol is a poorly defined entity consisting of intermittent periods of inappropriately violent and destructive behavior that is out of character for the patient. Abnormal EEG's have been reported in children with the episodic dyscontrol syndrome, but most affected adults have little evidence of a structural brain disorder.

TABLE 433–4. NONEPILEPTIC EPISODIC DISORDERS IN ADOLESCENTS AND ADULTS

Movement disorders
  Myoclonus
  Paroxysmal choreoathetosis
  Hyperexplexia (startle disease)
Migraine
  Confusional
  Vertebrobasilar
*Syncope and cardiac arrhythmias
Behavioral/psychiatric disorders
  *Psychogenic seizures
  *Hyperventilation syndrome
  *Panic disorder
  Dissociative states ("fugue states")
  Episodic dyscontrol
Narcolepsy and sleep apnea
  Automatic behavior syndrome
  Partial cataplexy
Transient ischemic attacks
*Transient global amnesia
  Acute confusional states
*Alcoholic blackouts
  Hypoglycemia attacks

* Most commonly encountered

MEDICAL TREATMENT

The First Seizure

Patients with their first epileptic seizure should be screened for symptoms and signs of an acute medical or neurologic illness. Brain imaging with MR or CT need not be done emergently unless there is a high likelihood of an acute cerebral lesion or the patient remains obtunded. Most patients recover rapidly following an isolated seizure, so several hours of observation are usually sufficient to assess the clinical progress, obtain additional relevant information, and review the results of laboratory tests. Hospitalization is not necessary provided that there is no suspicion of an underlying illness and a responsible family member or friend can observe the patient closely at home. If these criteria cannot be met, or if there is uncertainty about them, hospitalization is indicated. If the patient is sent home, there should be a clear plan for follow-up and re-evaluation.

Whether an antiepileptic drug should be prescribed following a first seizure is a matter of controversy. Although a large multicenter randomized study from Italy has recently demonstrated that antiepileptic drugs reduce the risk of relapse following a first unprovoked generalized tonic-clonic seizure, no information exists regarding the effect of early treatment on long-term prognosis, especially with regard to such important issues as whether early treatment reduces the severity of epilepsy or increases the chance of entering a prolonged remission. As indicated earlier in this chapter, chronic treatment of all first seizures would expensively overtreat three quarters of the patients. We believe that the decision to treat should be based on the physician's estimate of the risk of further seizures; the consequence to the patient of recurrent seizures; a reasonable expectation that the patient will comply with the treatment regimen; and the risk of adverse effects from antiepileptic drug therapy (10 to 30%). Patients are classified as being at low risk for further seizures if they have a normal EEG, normal physical examination, no history of significant cerebral injury, a normal brain imaging study, and absence of a family history of epilepsy. We recommend treating patients after a first seizure only if they have two or more of these risk factors. Nevertheless, the final decision regarding treatment must always be individualized, considering the potential psychological, vocational, and physical consequences of further seizures for each patient.

Selection of Antiepileptic Drugs

The treatment of epilepsy has three main objectives: (1) to eliminate seizures or reduce their frequency to the maximum extent possible; (2) to avoid chronic drug-related adverse effects; and (3) to assist the patient in maintaining or restoring normal vocational and psychosocial adjustment. Although each of these goals is possible, unfortunately no medical treatment currently available can permanently eliminate ("cure") epilepsy. Furthermore, fewer than 50% of adults treated for chronic partial and secondarily generalized seizures become seizure free for more than 12 months with currently available drugs.

Drugs used to treat different kinds of seizures are listed in Table 433–5. Well-controlled prospective studies have shown that carbamazepine, phenytoin, primidone, and phenobarbital are equally effective in suppressing partial and secondarily generalized seizures. In individual patients, however, failure to respond to one drug does not preclude a good response to another. Valproate is somewhat less effective against complex partial seizures than either carbamazepine or phenytoin but it is of comparable efficacy against secondarily generalized seizures. Despite similar pharmacologic potency, these drugs differ substantially in terms of side effects and pharmacokinetic properties. Thus, tolerability and ease of dosing schedule determine the particular choice of drug for an individual patient. Cost may be another consideration. Phenytoin has a long half-life and may be given once or twice daily after midadolescence. In contrast, carbamazepine must be administered more often, which increases problems with compliance for some patients. On the other hand, concern about phenytoin's occasional undesirable cosmetic effects (gingival hypertrophy, hirsutism, and coarsening of the facial features) makes carbamazepine the drug of choice for other patients, especially younger ones. Primidone and phenobarbital have a high incidence of sedative and cognitive side effects and are rarely recommended as initial therapy.

TABLE 433–5. DRUGS USED IN TREATING DIFFERENT TYPES OF SEIZURES

Type of Seizure	Drugs
Simple and complex partial	Carbamazepine, phenytoin; valproate; gabapentin, lamotrigine as add-on; primidone, phenobarbital
Secondarily generalized	Carbamazepine, phenytoin, valproate; gabapentin, lamotrigine as add-on; phenobarbital, primidone
Primary generalized seizures	
Tonic-clonic	Valproate; carbamazepine, phenytoin; lamotrigine
Absence	Ethosuximide, valproate; lamotrigine
Myoclonic	Valproate; clonazepam
Tonic	Valproate, felbamate; clonazepam

Note: The utility and clinical spectrum of lamotrigine, felbamate, and gabapentin have not yet been established, and the position of these drugs in the table should be viewed only as tentative.

Valproate is the drug of first choice for generalized-onset seizures. It can be used effectively as monotherapy in 80% of patients even when several types of generalized seizures coexist. Phenytoin and carbamazepine are only slightly less effective against generalized tonic-clonic seizures, but they may exacerbate absence and myoclonic seizures which frequently accompany generalized tonic-clonic seizures. Ethosuximide is as effective as valproate in treating typical absence seizures and, because of fewer side effects, is the drug of choice when no other seizure type exists. Clonazepam has some utility in treating myoclonic seizures, but tolerance tends to develop.

Drug Dosage and Pharmacokinetic Principles

Table 433–6 gives the usual dose and relevant pharmacokinetic data for each of the most commonly used antiepileptic drugs. Following absorption, a drug is distributed between the plasma and various tissue compartments. Because most antiepileptic drugs are fractionally bound to serum proteins, an equilibrium exists between the plasma concentrations of protein-bound and free (unbound) drug. Only unbound drug is capable of crossing the various lipoprotein membranes that surround brain receptor sites, making only this portion of the total drug concentration available to produce the desired effect. Antiepileptic drug blood levels that are routinely determined by laboratories reflect total plasma drug concentrations (bound plus unbound fractions). When protein binding is altered by disease (e.g., uremia), physiologic state (e.g., pregnancy), or other drugs (e.g., valproate), determining the unbound fraction provides a more accurate reflection of the drug's concentration in the brain's extracellular space. Measuring free levels can be helpful whenever there is a discrepancy between the total plasma concentration and the expected clinical effect.

A drug's *half-life* is a measure of the rate at which a drug is eliminated, mainly through metabolism or excretion. Drug half-life determines the dosing interval for antiepileptic drugs; this should amount to less than one third to one half the drug's half-life at steady state in order to minimize fluctuations in plasma concentrations. *Steady state* refers to the equilibrium that is established between drug intake and clearance. The time it takes for a drug to achieve steady-state conditions is determined by its half-life. For practical purposes, steady state is reached at an interval equal to five times the drug's half-life. Because a drug continues to accumulate in the body until steady state is reached, plasma drug levels are reliable only when they are measured under steady-state conditions. Similarly, time to steady state determines how rapidly the dose of any antiepileptic drug can be increased. Phenytoin is an exception because of its nonlinear kinetics. Phenytoin's half-life is dose-dependent, which means that steady-state concentration at one dose cannot be used to predict directly the steady-state concentration at a higher dose. For example, phenytoin's half-life is about 24 hours at plasma concentrations of 10 to 20 μg per milliliter. However, its half-life increases to 36 hours (or more) at concentrations of 25 μg per milliliter.

The care of patients with epilepsy has been greatly improved by the widespread availability of reliable data on therapeutic plasma concentrations of antiepileptic drugs. Most published therapeutic ranges for the various antiepileptic drugs have been derived from relatively small numbers of patients and reflect average blood levels that were empirically effective in controlling seizures with minimal or no adverse effects. As a result, optimal blood levels for some patients fall either above or below the recommended levels. Some patients, for example, consistently have side effects at low or "therapeutic" concentrations, whereas others benefit from "toxic" levels without experiencing side effects. Blood levels, therefore, are useful guidelines that assist in achieving optimal therapy but they should never be the goal of treatment. A level in the low to mid-therapeutic range is a reasonable target when initiating treatment, but subsequent dose adjustments should be based on the patient's clinical progress, seizure frequency, and appearance of drug-related side effects. As a guide to future management, blood levels can be re-

TABLE 433–6. ANTIEPILEPTIC DRUGS—DOSAGE AND PHARMACOKINETIC DATA

	Usual Dosage (per 24 hr)	Oral Availability (%)	Protein Bound (%)	Clearance (ml/min/kg)	Urinary Excretion (unchanged %)	Volume of Distribution (liters/kg)	Half-life (hours)	"Therapeutic" Concentrations (μg/ml)
Carbamazepine*	Adult: 800–1600 mg Child: 10–40 mg/kg/day	75–85	74	1.3 (post-induction) (very variable)	< 1	0.8–2.0	11–22†	6–12
Ethosuximide	Adult: 750–1500 mg Child: 10–75 mg/kg/day	> 90	0	0.19 (higher in children)	18	0.62–0.69	45–60 (children mean: 36)	40–100
Felbamate	Adult: 2400–3600 mg Child: 15–45 mg/kg/day		25–35		50	0.70	18–24	20–60
Gabapentin	Adult: 900–3600 mg	51–59	< 3		77–80		5–8	> 2
Lamotrigine	Adult: 75–200 mg	> 70	55		10		30 (14–50)	1–5
Phenobarbital	Adult: 90–180 mg Child: 2–6 mg/kg/day	100	45–50	0.062 (higher in children)	25	0.54–0.70	99 (shorter in children)	15–40
Phenytoin	Adult: 300–500 mg Child: 4–12 mg/kg/day	90	90	Capacity limited V_{max} = 5.9 mg/kg/day K_M = 5.7 μg/ml	2	0.78	6–42 (concentration dependent)	10–20
Primidone‡	Adult: 750–1250 mg Child: 6–12 mg/kg/day	92	19	0.59–0.94	42	0.64–0.72	8–15	5–12
Valproate	Adult: 1000–3000 mg Child: 10–70 mg/kg/day	100	93 (concentration dependent)	0.11	2	0.19	14–20	50–120

* The carbamazepine metabolite carbamazepine-10,11-epoxide is also pharmacologically active: values given are for the parent compound.
† The half-life of carbamazepine is considerably longer when the drug is first introduced, prior to autoinduction of hepatic microsomal enzymes.
‡ Primidone's primary metabolites, phenobarbital and phenylethylmalonamide, are also pharmacologically active; values given are for the parent compound.
From Pedley TA, Scheuer ML, Walczak TS: In Rowland LP (ed.): Merritt's Textbook of Neurology, 9th ed. Malvern, PA, Lea & Febiger, 1994.
Blood levels for lamotrigine, felbamate, and gabapentin have not been firmly established. These values are only estimates based on initial clinical trials.

peated when control of seizures is achieved or when toxic side effects appear. Noncompliance is the most common reason that a therapeutic drug level is not achieved using recommended dosing schedules. Therapeutic drug monitoring helps to minimize unpredictable drug interactions in patients taking two or more drugs and to compensate for hepatic or renal effects on drug elimination.

Initiating Antiepileptic Drug Therapy

Treatment should start with a single drug chosen according to the patient's type of seizure, considering adverse effects, required dosing schedule, and cost. With the exception of phenobarbital and phenytoin, antiepileptic drugs should be started in low doses to minimize acute toxicity and then increased to a maintenance schedule according to the patient's tolerance and the drug's pharmacokinetics. Most common side effects are temporary, and these are minimized if the dose is built up slowly. Nausea can be minimized by taking the medication with meals. Sedation may be less likely if a higher dose is given at bedtime.

If therapeutic blood levels need to be achieved rapidly, one should consider starting with drugs for which loading doses are practical, such as phenytoin or phenobarbital. Other drugs can gradually be substituted once seizures are controlled.

All antiepileptic drugs are capable of producing adverse effects, and the prescribing physician must be familiar with these. The most common side effects are *dose-related* and typically occur when the drug is first given or when the dose is increased. Dose-related side effects usually correlate with plasma concentrations of the drug or its major metabolites. *Idiosyncratic* reactions create the most serious and life-threatening side effects of antiepileptic drugs. All antiepileptic drugs can cause similar idiosyncratic reactions, including rash, Stevens-Johnson syndrome, agranulocytosis, thrombocytopenia, aplastic anemia, and hepatic failure. Idiosyncratic reactions are not dose-related, and no laboratory test can identify individuals specifically at risk for them. Routine blood monitoring at set intervals is costly and ineffective. Minor elevations in liver SGOT and SGPT occur in about 25 to 30% of patients with epilepsy, and these neither correlate with clinical symptoms nor predict development of hepatitis or liver failure. Isolated elevations in GTT levels seem to have little use as an indication of clinically significant liver dysfunction in persons with epilepsy. Nearly 20% of patients taking carbamazepine develop a benign leukopenia with WBC counts below 4000 per millimeter. A few patients have WBC counts that drop transiently below 2500 per millimeter. The risk of developing aplastic anemia is not increased in this group, nor is there an increased rate of infections or other possible complications that might be attributed to leukopenia.

When Initial Treatment Fails

Monotherapy results in satisfactory control of seizures (>90% reduction) in about 60% of patients. Of patients in whom the first drug was ineffective, about half respond to an alternative drug used alone. Of the remaining, fewer than half have improved control by addition of a second drug. Felbamate, gabapentin, and lamotrigine have recently been approved as adjunctive therapy in patients with partial and secondarily generalized seizures. They are useful additions to phenytoin, carbamazepine, and valproate when these drugs fail as monotherapy. Although the new drugs have a number of desirable features and generally better therapeutic indices compared with more familiar agents, it is too soon to predict what their ultimate place will be in the treatment of epilepsy. Felbamate, for example, has already proved to be too toxic (aplastic anemia, liver failure) for routine use.

Pregnancy Concerns

Epilepsy should not discourage a woman from becoming pregnant: Well over 90% of women taking antiepileptic drugs have healthy babies. Nonetheless, epilepsy affects the pregnancy in many ways, and it is important that women be informed before conception about possible problems and the steps that can be taken to minimize these. Overall, women with epilepsy demonstrate 1.5 to 3 times higher rates of complications of pregnancy regardless of treatment. These include increased risks of intrapartum bleeding, toxemia, abruptio placentae, premature labor, and stillborn births. About one third of women with epilepsy experience increased seizures during pregnancy. This is mostly due to falling antiepilep-

tic drug levels associated with a variety of physiologic changes that promote increased volume of distribution and clearance. Thus, antiepileptic drug levels should be followed closely during pregnancy, especially after the first trimester.

In the general population, *major fetal malformations* (cardiac defects, cleft lip or palate, neural tube defects, including spina bifida and anencephaly) occur in about 2% of pregnancies. This risk is increased to 5 to 6% in infants born to women with epilepsy who have taken a single antiepileptic drug during pregnancy. Valproate increases the chance of neural tube defects by 1.5%, and carbamazepine polytherapy may also raise this specific risk by 0.5%, especially if there is a family history of neural tube defects. Use of two or more drugs carries a 10% risk of major fetal malformations.

Minor anomalies (nail hypoplasia, hypertelorism, low-set ears, prominent lips, broad-based nose) are also increased in infants of mothers with epilepsy, but this seems to reflect both genetic and drug-related factors. Such anomalies occur at increased rates independent of treatment status, although antiepileptic drug therapy increases the risk further to a slight degree. It was formerly thought that particular profiles of these anomalies could be attributed to specific drugs (e.g., fetal hydantoin syndrome or fetal valproate syndrome), but recent data indicate that all antiepileptic drugs can produce similar anomalies.

Virtually all antiepileptic drugs promote a hemorrhagic diathesis in the newborn. Intramuscular vitamin K, which is given routinely to babies, is occasionally inadequate to prevent hemorrhage. Therefore, oral vitamin K, 20 mg per day, should be prescribed for the mother during the last month of pregnancy.

The risk of neural tube defects is reduced, perhaps eliminated, by preconceptive use of folic acid, 1 mg per day. Ultrasonography and amniocentesis done at 18 to 19 weeks of gestation have a nearly 95% accuracy rate in experienced hands of identifying neural tube defects and other major malformations. Serum α-fetoprotein determinations have a 25% false-negative rate.

SURGICAL TREATMENT

Surgical intervention should be considered when seizures fail to respond to antiepileptic drugs and when they continue to disrupt patients' quality of life. Advances in surgical techniques and improved methods of identifying epileptogenic brain areas have made surgical treatment an option for more patients with uncontrolled seizures today than ever before. In 1985, for example, there were about 500 operations for epilepsy in the United States; in 1990, there were over 1500.

In the past, there was considerable disagreement about when to refer patients for surgery, and many physicians viewed it as a therapy of last resort. As a result, until very recently the average time from epilepsy diagnosis to operation was about 20 years. Currently, increasing numbers of neurologists believe that it is possible to identify patients who are likely to benefit from surgery earlier in the course of their illness, and that minimizing the delay between onset of seizures and successful intervention provides better seizure control, psychosocial outcome, and quality of life.

Few patients benefit from further attempts at medical treatment if seizures are not controlled following two trials of high-dose monotherapy using appropriate drugs and one trial of rational combination therapy. These steps can be accomplished within 1 to 2 years. At that point, the detrimental effects of continued seizures, often exacerbated by drug toxicity, warrant referral to a specialized epilepsy center.

The most common type of epilepsy surgery, and the one with which there is the greatest experience, is *focal cortical resection.* Surgery should be considered for any patient with focal seizures whose attacks remain disabling despite optimal medical therapy. Three criteria identify the ideal patient for resective surgery: (1) the seizures begin in an identifiable and localized area of cortex; (2) the surgical excision can encompass the epileptogenic region; and (3) the required resection does not impair neurologic function. These requirements are met most often by patients with temporal lobe epilepsy or other focal epilepsies associated with a demonstrable cerebral lesion (e.g., cavernous malformation, ganglioglioma). Over two thirds of such patients become seizure free, and approximately 90% have sufficiently fewer seizures to improve substantially their quality of life. The outcome is less favorable for patients undergoing nonlesional extratemporal resections: About 45% of patients become seizure free; another 35% have worthwhile improvement.

Two other surgical procedures are used much less often and only for highly selected cases of persons with longstanding, uncontrolled seizures, usually beginning in childhood. *Corpus callosotomy* is indicated for intractable atonic and secondarily generalized tonic-clonic seizures such as occur in severe epileptic encephalopathies like the Lennox-Gastaut syndrome. *Hemispherectomy* is an effective operation for children with severely incapacitating unilateral seizures associated with hemiatrophy, hemiparesis, and a useless hand (infantile hemiplegia syndrome).

PROGNOSIS OF EPILEPSY

About 60 to 70% of people with epilepsy achieve a 5-year remission of seizures within 10 years of diagnosis. About half of these patients eventually become seizure free without anticonvulsant drugs. Factors favoring remission include an idiopathic form of epilepsy, a normal neurologic examination, and an onset in early to middle childhood (excluding neonatal seizures).

Thirty percent of patients, usually with severe epilepsy starting in early childhood, continue to have seizures and never achieve a remission. In the United States, the prevalence of intractable epilepsy cases approximates 1 to 2 per 1000 population.

Discontinuing Antiepileptic Drugs

Because epidemiologic studies have shown that many patients with epilepsy become seizure free for an extended period, a number of investigators have attempted to identify which patients can discontinue antiepileptic drugs without a high risk of relapse. Successful drug withdrawal is most likely if initial seizure control was readily achieved using monotherapy; there were relatively few seizures before remission; and the EEG and neurologic examination are normal just before drugs are discontinued. In addition, longer seizure-free intervals (4 years rather than 2) reduce the likelihood of relapse. Conversely, risk of relapse is high if seizure control was difficult to establish and required polytherapy; if there were frequent generalized tonic-clonic seizures before control was achieved; and if the EEG demonstrates moderate or severe disturbances of background activity or active epileptiform activity at the time drug withdrawal is considered.

STATUS EPILEPTICUS

Various types of status epilepticus take either convulsive or nonconvulsive forms. *Convulsive status epilepticus* is a medical emergency that requires timely and appropriate treatment in order to minimize serious systemic and neurologic morbidity. Like self-limited seizures, convulsive status may be either idiopathic and of generalized onset or secondary to bilateral spread from a focal epileptogenic brain area. *Nonconvulsive status* presents as a new-onset sustained confusional state.

Convulsive status epilepticus is the first manifestation of epilepsy in about 10% of cases; more than 50% of patients with status epilepticus do not have a history of epilepsy. An acute precipitating factor or specific cause, such as metabolic abnormalities, drug abuse, hypoxia, infection, stroke, or tumor, can be identified in 50 to 65% of patients with status epilepticus. The mortality rate approaches 30% in adults, but death usually relates to the underlying condition. Status epilepticus itself accounts for death in about 10% of cases.

Treatment protocols are designed to eliminate seizure activity and to identify and treat any underlying medical or neurologic disorder. Initial management focuses on ensuring adequate oxygenation and maintaining blood pressure (Table 433–7). There must be unimpeded access to the circulation, and cardiac function must be monitored continuously. Diagnostic studies should be initiated concurrently with blood obtained for antiepileptic drug levels, blood count, and routine chemistries. Brain imaging is necessary, but control of seizures must be the first priority. Lumbar puncture must be performed if meningitis is strongly suspected. If, however, focal neurologic signs point to a mass lesion, antibiotics should be given and a CT scan obtained first. In adults, thiamine followed by glucose should be administered to counteract hypoglycemia unless an adequate glucose concentration has been demonstrated.

Table 433–7 presents the recommendations of the Epilepsy Foundation of America for treating status epilepticus. A benzodiazepine, either diazepam (10 mg, repeated once) or lorazepam should be given, followed immediately by intravenous phenytoin, 20 mg per kilogram, at a rate not exceeding 50 mg per minute. If seizures continue, an additional 5 mg per kilogram of phenytoin should be given. About 80% of patients respond to this protocol. If status is refractory, the patient should be admitted to an intensive care unit and anesthetized with intravenous pentobarbital, 5 mg per kilogram, followed by 25 to 50 mg every 25 to 50 minutes as necessary to produce a burst-suppression pattern on continuously monitored EEG. Maintenance doses are 1 to 3 mg per kilogram per hour. Ventilatory assistance and vasopressors are invariably required.

Nonconvulsive status epilepticus is difficult to diagnose and is frequently unrecognized. It presents most often in middle-aged or elderly persons without a history of seizures. Onset is generally abrupt, with a fluctuating confusional state that can last for days to weeks. Although clouding of consciousness occurs to a varying degree, the absence of stupor or coma contributes to misdiagnosis. Nonconvulsive status epilepticus may be mistaken for psychosis because of the abrupt development of bizarre behavior, inappropriate affect, paranoia, delusions, and catatonia. Alternatively, memory loss, confusion, and mood changes may predominate and suggest a metabolic/toxic encephalopathy or dementia. Some patients have recurrent episodes.

TABLE 433–7. PROTOCOL FOR TREATING STATUS EPILEPTICUS

Time (min)	Action*
0–5	Diagnose status epilepticus by observing continued seizure activity or one additional seizure
	Give oxygen by nasal cannula or mask; position patient's head for optimal airway patency; consider intubation if respiratory assistance is needed
	Obtain and record vital signs at onset and periodically thereafter; control any abnormalities as necessary; initiate ECG monitoring
	Establish an IV in one or both arms using catheter; draw venous blood samples for glucose level, serum chemistries, hematology studies, toxicology screens, and determinations of antiepileptic drug levels
	Assess oxygenation with oximetry or periodic arterial blood gas determinations
6–9	If hypoglycemia is established or a blood glucose determination is unavailable, administer glucose; in adults, give 100 mg of thiamine first, followed by 50 ml of 50% glucose by direct push into the IV; in children, the dose of glucose is 2 ml/kg of 25% glucose
10–20	Administer either 0.1 mg/kg of lorazepam at 2 mg/min or 0.2 mg/kg of diazepam at 5 mg/min by IV; if diazepam is given, it can be repeated if seizures do not stop after 5 min; if diazepam is used to stop the status, phenytoin should be administered immediately to prevent recurrent status
21–60	If status persists, administer 15–20 mg/kg of phenytoin by IV no faster than 50 mg/min in adults and 1 mg/kg per min in children; monitor ECG and blood pressure during the infusion; phenytoin is incompatible with glucose-containing solutions—the IV should be purged with normal saline before the phenytoin infusion
>60	If status does not stop after 20 mg/kg of phenytoin, give additional doses of 5 mg/kg to a maximal dose of 30 mg/kg
	If status persists, give 20 mg/kg of phenobarbital by IV at 100 mg/min; when phenobarbital is given after a benzodiazepine, the risk of apnea or hypopnea is great, and assisted ventilation is usually required
	If status persists, give anesthetic doses of drugs such as pentobarbital; ventilatory assistance and vasopressors are virtually always necessary

* Time starts at seizure onset. ECG = electrocardiogram; IV = intravenous line.

From Dodson WE, DeLorenzo RJ, Pedley TA, et al: Treatment of convulsive status epilepticus: Recommendations of the Epilepsy Foundation of America's working group on status epilepticus. JAMA 270:854, 1993.

Diagnosis depends on demonstrating seizure discharges in the EEG accompanying symptoms. Most patients show continuous or nearly continuous 1- to 2.5-Hz generalized spike-wave activity similar to generalized absence status ("spike-wave stupor") that occurs in children. Rarely, however, the EEG ictal activity is localized, usually to the frontal or temporal lobes, indicating that in these patients the nonconvulsive status is a form of continuous partial seizure activity. Intravenous diazepam (5 to 10 mg) or lorazepam (1 to 2 mg) suppresses epileptiform EEG abnormalities and produces dramatic improvement in the patient's mental state. Long-term seizure control is achieved using valproate, phenytoin, or carbamazepine.

A specific cause cannot be identified in most cases. Sometimes, however, nonconvulsive status results from electrolyte imbalance, drug toxicity (e.g., lithium), or a focal cerebral lesion (e.g., frontal lobe infarction).

PSYCHOSOCIAL ISSUES

Epilepsy and its personal effects result from multiple interacting factors, of which seizures are only a part. The extent of a patient's disability or quality of life may relate more to physical limitations caused by neurologic abnormalities, psychological factors, or adverse drug effects than to the seizures themselves. This observation is underscored by patients who become seizure free following surgery but who remain disabled and unable to find employment, establish relationships, or become independent in other ways. Not the least of epilepsy's disabling aspects is the episodic nature of the condition: Periods of relative well-being are punctuated by unpredictably occurring attacks that impose their own limitations, create embarrassment, and reinforce negative stereotypes. Recurrent seizures, despite treatment, are graphic reminders of medicine's failure. Adults experience discrimination at work and loss of mobility because they cannot drive.

The treatment of epilepsy can be effective only when interacting medical, psychological, and environmental factors are addressed successfully. Areas of psychosocial difficulty should be identified early in the course of treatment and an appropriate plan of management developed. This often requires a multidisciplinary approach to disabilities that have social, educational, vocational, and psychological dimensions. The physician must be sensitive to these issues, even if they are not voiced explicitly. In fact, psychosocial concerns may be the major focus of the majority of follow-up visits. The physician has a special responsibility to educate society as well as the patient and family in order to counter the many misperceptions, myths, and prejudices that are ascribed to epilepsy.

Berg AT, Shinnar S: The risk of seizure recurrence following a first unprovoked seizure: A quantitative review. Neurology 41:965, 1991. *A meta-analysis of the most important papers to evaluate the development of and risks for epilepsy following a first unprovoked seizure.*

Delgado-Escueta AV, Janz D: Consensus guidelines: Preconception counseling, management, and care of the pregnant woman with epilepsy. Neurology 42(suppl 5):149, 1992. *An essential and current summary of the risks and management options for women with epilepsy who desire to become pregnant. Practical recommendations are included.*

Dodson WE, DeLorenzo RJ, Pedley TA, et al.: Treatment of convulsive status epilepticus: Recommendations of the Epilepsy Foundation of America's working group on status epilepticus. JAMA 270:854, 1993. *A consensus report describing the epidemiology, pathogenesis, morbidity and mortality, treatment, and prognosis of status epilepticus.*

Engel J Jr (ed.): Surgical Treatment of the Epilepsies, 2nd ed. New York, Raven Press, 1993. *A comprehensive volume covering all aspects of the surgical treatment of epilepsy and emphasizing advances between 1986 and 1992.*

First Seizure Trial Group. Randomized clinical trial on the efficacy of antiepileptic drugs in reducing the risk of relapse after a first unprovoked tonic-clonic seizure. Neurology 43:478, 1993. *The first prospective study to compare the effect of treatment versus no treatment on risk of further seizures following a first convulsion.*

Freeman JM, Vining EPG, Pillas DJ: Seizures and Epilepsy in Childhood: A Guide for Parents. Baltimore, Johns Hopkins Press, 1990. *Despite the title, this sensitive and thorough review of epilepsy and its impact on quality of life is suitable for patients of all ages and their families.*

Hauser WA, Hesdorffer DC. Epilepsy: Frequency, Causes and Consequences. New York, Demos, 1990. *An encyclopedia of facts regarding all aspects of epilepsy.*

Hauser WA, Annegers JF, Kurland LT: Incidence of epilepsy and unprovoked seizures in Rochester, Minnesota: 1935–1984. Epilepsia 34:453, 1993. *This ambitious study provides the best available data regarding seizure incidence and complements an earlier prevalence study by the same investigators.*

Sloviter RS: The functional organization of the hippocampal dentate gyrus and its relevance to the pathogenesis of temporal lobe epilepsy. Ann Neurol 35:640, 1994. *The most coherent hypothesis and review of supporting experimental and clinical data linking the development of mesial to temporal sclerosis.*

Section Twelve— Intracranial Tumors and States of Altered Intracranial Pressure

Nicholas A. Vick

434 INTRACRANIAL TUMORS

Approximately 17,000 new cases of primary brain tumors are treated each year in the United States. Metastases are even more frequent and contribute considerably to suffering and death from systemic cancer. The diversity of brain tumors makes it important to attend to what is characteristic about each histologic type because attention to biologic specificity guides therapy and certainly will advance future understanding.

The classification of brain tumors is a subject with confusing terminology. This text employs a simpler approach, classifying brain tumors into *metastatic, primary extra-axial,* and *primary intra-axial* (Table 434–1). These categories include all of the primary brain tumors listed in the World Health Organization classification (Table 434–2), adds pituitary and metastatic tumors, and is obviously simple. Moreover, it follows practical clinical thinking. This chapter deals with the general biology, clinical features, and treatment of brain tumors as an overall problem. The following chapter describes the particular behavior of the most important subtypes in accordance with the outline of Table 434–1.

GENERAL CONSIDERATIONS

"Is it benign or malignant?" is invariably the first question patients, families, and physicians ask when confronted with a diagnosis of brain tumor. About a third of primary brain tumors can be called benign. Meningiomas and acoustic neuromas are good examples, they grow slowly, often can be removed completely, and rarely recur.

The concept of malignancy in the central nervous system (CNS) has a different meaning from that which applies to systemic cancers. The term "malignant" has nothing to do with metastasis out of the CNS, which is extraordinarily rare. It has everything to do with

TABLE 434–1. COMMON BRAIN TUMORS IN ADULTS WITH PERCENTAGE INCIDENCE BY CATEGORY*

Metastatic	Primary Extra-axial	Primary Intra-axial
Lung (37)	Meningioma (80)	Gioblastoma (47)
Breast (19)	Acoustic neuroma (10)	Anaplastic astrocytoma (24)
Melanoma (16)	Pituitary adenoma (7)	Astrocytoma (15)
Colorectum (9)	Other (3)	Oligodendroglioma (5)
Kidney (8)		Lymphoma (2)
Other (11)		Other (7)

* These figures, given in parentheses, can be extremely variable from one center to another, depending on referral pattern. They are given here as general estimates based upon many published series.

anatomic location and the possibility of complete surgical removal. Unless a tumor can be completely excised to the last cell, all intracranial neoplasms are potentially malignant in that they may recur, and often do.

INITIAL EVALUATION

SYMPTOMS AND SIGNS. Brain tumors present in two patterns, not necessarily mutually exclusive. One consists of nonfocal symptoms of *increased intracranial pressure,* such as headaches, nausea, vomiting, confusion, and lethargy. The other consists of symptoms or signs of *focal brain dysfunction,* such as hemianopia, hemiparesis, cranial nerve palsies, or focal seizures (Table 434–3). Such signs of focal brain dysfunction may have convincing localizing value even before an image of the brain is made by computed tomography (CT) or magnetic resonance imaging (MRI). Some tumors that arise in neurologically "silent" areas, such as the parietal or frontal association cortices, may produce only nonfocal generalized symptoms of headache, confusion, behavioral change, or, eventually, a seizure, despite growing to a considerable size. Although the capacity to reach early diagnosis by CT or MRI has greatly reduced the numbers of patients in whom symptoms of increased intracranial pressure represent initial complaints, examples still remain, especially in association with fast-growing tumors and in children. The latter are particularly likely to have tumors in the posterior fossa that tend to obstruct spinal fluid pathways earlier than do supratentorial tumors. As implied, the tempo with which a brain tumor grows also influences the presenting symptoms. Despite the fixed space of the skull (once infantile sutures have closed), the human brain possesses a remarkable capacity to make room for a slowly growing tumor (Fig. 434–1). Because of this, and even allowing for the relative rapidity of growth of aggressive brain tumors such as glioblastomas, the rule is that the patient usually appears better clinically than might be expected from the degree of abnormality seen on CT or MRI scan.

DIFFERENTIAL DIAGNOSIS. Patients who present with symptoms and signs of increased intracranial pressure or a first convulsive seizure need to be hospitalized. Diagnosis and treatment

TABLE 434–2. WORLD HEALTH ORGANIZATION CLASSIFICATION OF BRAIN TUMORS*

A. Astrocytic tumors
  1. Astrocytoma
    a. Fibrillary
    b. Protoplasmic
    c. Gemistocytic
  2. Pilocytic astrocytoma
  3. Subependymal giant cell astrocytoma (ventricular tumor or tuberous sclerosis)
  4. Astroblastoma
  5. Anaplastic (malignant) astrocytoma
B. Oligodendroglial tumors
  1. Oligodendroglioma
  2. Mixed oligoastrocytoma
  3. Anaplastic (malignant) oligodendroglioma
C. Ependymal and choroid plexus tumors
  1. Ependymoma
    Variants:
    a. Myxopapillary ependymoma
    b. Papillary ependymoma
    c. Subependymoma
  2. Anaplastic (malignant) ependymoma
  3. Choroid plexus papilloma
  4. Anaplastic (malignant) choroid plexus papilloma
D. Pineal cell tumor
  1. Pineocytoma (pinealcytoma)
  2. Pineoblastoma (pinealoblastoma)
E. Neuronal tumors
  1. Gangliocytoma
  2. Ganglioglioma
  3. Ganglioneuroblastoma
  4. Anaplastic (malignant) gangliocytoma and ganglioglioma
  5. Neuroblastoma
F. Poorly differentiated and embryonal tumors
  1. Glioblastoma
    Variants:
    a. Glioblastoma with sarcomatous component (mixed glioblastoma and sarcoma)
    b. Giant cell glioblastoma
  2. Medulloblastoma
    Variants:
    a. Desmoplastic medulloblastoma
    b. Medullomyoblastoma
  3. Medulloepithelioma
  4. Primitive polar spongioblastoma
  5. Gliomatosis cerebri

* This is one of several formal schemes that are based on neuropathologic criteria. Metastasis is not considered, and one can get no sense of a given tumor as a *clinical* problem, as suggested by the simple classification in Table 434–1.

measures must be started at once; it may be unsafe to wait. Those who present with focal neurologic impairment and who do not have symptoms of increased intracranial pressure may reasonably be evaluated in the outpatient setting for other conditions that are often considerations in the differential diagnosis of brain tumor (Table 434–4). The tempo of evolution of symptoms and signs of focal

TABLE 434–3. FOCAL CLINICAL MANIFESTATIONS OF BRAIN TUMORS

Frontal lobe
  Generalized seizures
  Focal motor seizures (contralateral)
  Expressive aphasia (dominant side)
  Behavioral changes
  Dementia
  Gait disorders, incontinence
Basal ganglia
  Hemiparesis (contralateral)
  Movement disorders rare
Parietal lobe
  Receptive aphasia (dominant side)
  Spatial disorientation (nondominant side)
  Cortical sensory dysfunction (contralateral)
  Hemianopia (contralateral)
Occipital lobe
  Hemianopia (contralateral)
  Visual disturbances (unformed)

Temporal lobe
  Complex partial (psychomotor) seizures
  Generalized seizures
  Behavioral changes
  Olfactory and complex visual auras
Corpus callosum
  Dementia (anterior)
  Behavioral changes (posterior)
  Asymptomatic (mid)
Thalamus
  Sensory loss (contralateral)
  Behavioral changes
  Language disorder (dominant side)
Midbrain/pineal
  Paresis of vertical eye movements
  Pupillary abnormalities
  Precocious puberty (boys)

Sella/optic nerve/pituitary
  Endocrinopathy
  Bitemporal hemianopia
  Monocular visual defects
Pons/medulla
  Cranial nerve dysfunction
  Ataxia, nystagmus
  Weakness, sensory loss
  Spasticity
Cerebellopontine angle
  Deafness (ipsilateral)
  Loss of facial sensation (ipsilateral)
  Facial weakness (ipsilateral)
  Ataxia
Cerebellum
  Ataxia (ipsilateral)
  Nystagmus

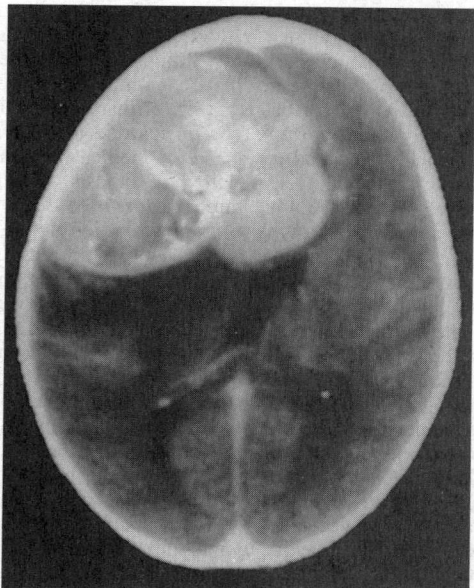

FIGURE 434–1. CT scan with contrast of a meningioma in a patient who presented with mild cognitive deficits, illustrative of the size a slow-growing tumor can attain in the brain. The tumor was completely resected.

TABLE 434–4. THE MAIN DIFFERENTIAL DIAGNOSES OF BRAIN TUMORS

Hematomas, especially in tumors that have a tendency to bleed, such as melanoma
Abscesses, including fungal
Granulomas
Parasitic infections, such as cysticercosis
Vascular malformations, especially those without arteriovenous shunts
Solitary large plaques of multiple sclerosis
Seldom, progressive strokes

neurologic impairment, much more than their severity, governs urgency of evaluation. The tempo also strongly influences diagnostic considerations. Although an occasional brain tumor may manifest with such rapid onset of hemiparesis or aphasia that a stroke is mimicked, most do not. Associated aspects of the history, such as recent head trauma, previous episodes of reversible neurologic impairment, or recent infection and fever, should direct attention to diagnostic alternatives such as subdural hematoma, multiple sclerosis, or cerebral abscess. Simply stated, it is the careful history, not the neurologic examination, that usually points to the alternative diagnoses.

IMAGING AND OTHER DIAGNOSTIC PROCEDURES

Brain imaging by MRI or CT scans is an indispensable component of the modern diagnosis of the presence but not the type of brain tumors. One type of tumor can look like another or even resemble nonneoplastic mass lesions, such as brain abscesses, fungal infections, parasitic invasions, demyelinating diseases, or strokes. For definitive diagnosis and adequate treatment planning, one must obtain a tissue diagnosis whenever possible. This can be made either by direct surgical biopsy or, in the case of some nonneoplastic conditions, by judging CT or MRI responses to particular therapies.

MRI is almost always superior to CT scanning in diagnosing intracranial mass lesions. MRI outlines posterior fossa structures and tumors with a clarity that CT cannot achieve because of x-ray distortions due to the bony structure of that region. In several types of tumor, particularly the low-grade gliomas, MRI may show extensive brain infiltration in cases that fail to produce any image abnormality on CT or, at most, a vague low density. Although either MRI or CT should be used with contrast enhancement in cases of suspected brain tumor, the passage of such contrast agents beyond the blood-brain barrier into the tissue does not necessarily imply the presence of a histologically malignant tumor. For example, although malignant gliomas almost always show contrast enhancement, so do meningiomas, which are entirely benign if they can be fully removed surgically.

CT scans done without contrast enhancement are of little value in the diagnosis of brain tumors or other mass lesions. Although it is true that hemorrhage, calcifications, hydrocephalus, and shift can be well seen on a noncontrast CT scan, the interpretation of even these conditions is tentative because each can have an underlying causative structural abnormality such as a brain tumor, which may fail to appear on a noncontrast CT study. Allergy to CT dye is rare and readily manageable. Currently available nonionic CT dyes have an extremely low incidence of side effects. There is little risk that currently used CT dyes will cause renal dysfunction in normally hydrated patients who are not known to have kidney disease.

MRI initially provided two types of images, designated T1 and T2. For brain tumors, the former generally showed a well-demarcated area of low density and the latter, bright whiteness that encompassed a more extensive region owing to the signal of the surrounding brain edema (Fig. 434–2). With the availability for general usage in 1988 of *gadolinium contrast for MRI,* a new set of criteria of usage and differential diagnostic considerations in brain imaging have quickly evolved (Table 434–5). T1 gadolinium imaging is the most precise way to image a brain tumor, and often patients can be followed during and after treatment with that type of study alone. Such an approach is easier for patients because it reduces the length of time otherwise spent on T2 scanning. Now and

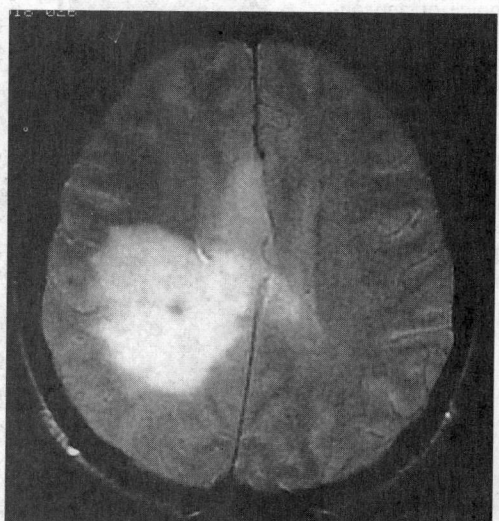 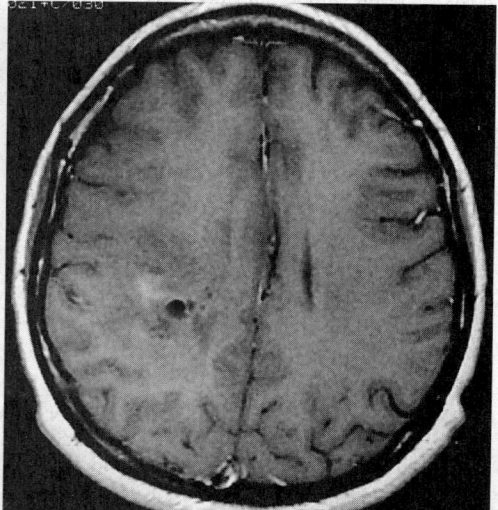

FIGURE 434–2. Low-grade astrocytoma as imaged by MRI. On the left, T2-weighted image; on the right, T1-weighted image, gadolinium contrast with minimal enhancement. The images are typical of this tumor, which is being detected with increasing frequency in seizure patients by MRI. Many are invisible on CT scans.

TABLE 434–5. T1 GADOLINIUM MRI CHARACTERISTICS OF BRAIN TUMORS

Metastases	These are remarkably variable (Fig. 434–3). Some enhance brightly and solidly with gadolonium. Others are in ring configuration. Many are invisible with contrast CT.
Acoustic neuromas	These are invariably intensely contrasted by gadolinium, even more reliably than by CT.
Meningiomas	Same as for acoustic neuromas.
Pituitary adenomas	These always enhance less than the normal pituitary gland. MRI is superior in every way to CT, especially when thin slices and magnified views are ordered.
Glioblastoma	These are almost always in ring configuration.
Anaplastic astrocytomas	These are sometimes solidly bright; they are often patchy, may be noncontrasting, and may look like low-grade astrocytoma.
Low-grade astrocytomas	These do not enhance. They are often invisible by CT or are imaged only as vague low density.
Oligodendrogliomas	These generally do not enhance unless anaplastic and are often invisible on CT unless they are calcified.
Primary brain lymphomas	These usually exhibit homogeneous enhancement and are smoothly rounded. Periventricular location is common. They are multiple in about a fourth of cases. This lesion does not often look like glioblastoma but is easily mistaken for metastases if multiple.

then, T2 images are useful. For example, T2 images, besides showing the extent of edema, also delineate the demyelinating effects of radiation upon white matter.

Cerebral angiography seldom is used in the diagnosis of brain tumors. In a few circumstances, neurosurgeons, in preparation for surgery, require a more precise knowledge of the pattern and position of blood vessels that can be obtained only by angiography. The procedure is also used to embolize highly vascular meningiomas, or to study cerebral dominance by injection of sodium amytal into the carotid artery (the Wada test) in left-handed individuals who are to have surgery near language areas. Preoperative determination of cerebral localization helps surgeons to plan the extent of surgery and avoid postoperative language deficits.

Examination of the *spinal fluid* has limited indication in the diagnosis of brain tumors. One is to rule in or out an inflammatory disorder mimicking a brain tumor. Another is to establish the diagnosis of benign intracranial hypertension in patients with uninformative MR images (see Ch. 436). In addition, spinal fluid cytology may be useful for determining instances of malignant meningitis secondary to metastatic neoplasms, in association with spinal spread of medulloblastoma in some children and in identifying primary lymphomas of the brain in cases in which MRI changes are ambiguous.

The routine electroencephalogram (EEG) has no role in the diagnosis of brain tumors and does not assist in the choice of anticonvulsant drugs for brain tumor patients. However, specialized intraoperative neurophysiologic techniques such as depth electrode studies and intraoperative monitoring may be useful in identifying and removing epileptogenic areas adjacent to brain tumors or to avoid resection of critical brain regions adjacent to tumors.

Positron emission tomography (PET) is able to quantify biochemical functions, such as oxygen and glucose utilization, within tumors as well as normal brain tissue. PET scanning is a powerful research tool of limited availability for routine clinical purposes. Its spatial resolution is inferior to that of both CT and MR. In patients with brain tumors who develop recurrent symptoms after radiation therapy, PET can differentiate with about 70% accuracy radiation-induced injury from tumor recurrences. These disorders appear identical on MRI.

TREATMENT

PREOPERATIVE CONSIDERATIONS AND MEDICAL MANAGEMENT. In almost every instance when a brain tumor is suspected on the basis of the combined results of history, physical findings, and imaging studies, the *first consideration is its surgical resectability*. There are exceptions, such as cases of multiple brain

metastases in a patient with known systemic cancer. Patients with single brain metastases, defined by MRI, may be candidates for surgical resection of the metastasis, depending on their systemic medical status. It is unproductive to embark upon an extensive systemic evaluation in the search for an unknown primary cancer in patients with a single resectable presumed brain metastasis. If a primary tumor is not quickly revealed by a careful medical evaluation, with special attention to skin (for melanoma), breasts, and lungs, the pathologic diagnosis of the brain tumor needs to be disclosed by resection or, if unresectable owing to its position, by biopsy.

Although small meningiomas or acoustic neuromas usually do not require treatment to reduce intracranial pressure, in the majority of brain tumor patients it is appropriate to start *dexamethasone* promptly. The purpose is to reduce intracranial pressure, which accompanies the majority of brain tumors, and to relieve neurologic symptoms caused by peritumoral brain edema (Fig. 434–3). Dexamethasone's long biologic half-life and steady action upon the brain have made it the steroid of choice for treating patients with brain tumors. It should be started with an oral dose of 16 mg, followed with 8 mg twice daily. It is well absorbed by mouth, and its action by that route is almost as rapid as when given intravenously. Antacids are seldom necessary. If focal neurologic symptoms are due to peritumoral vasogenic edema, dexamethasone induces improvement within 48 hours and usually sooner. If there is no benefit, the neurologic symptoms are likely to be due to damage of the brain tissue by the tumor and not to edema.

Edema associated with brain tumors is due chiefly to abnormally fenestrated endothelium in the tumor, which permits excess flow of fluid from capillaries into the growth. Normally, solutes are transported through capillaries into brain by dissolving in and diffusing through the cerebral endothelium, a phenomenon dependent on lipid solubility and molecular size. Endothelial cells also possess some facilitated or carrier-mediated processes that are stereospecific, saturable, and independent of lipid solubility and molecular size. In brain tumors, these selective properties of the blood-brain barrier are overwhelmed by increased bulk flow and hydraulic conductivity through the defective endothelium. The result is vasogenic edema, and it is this reaction that dexamethasone so greatly reduces.

In instances of extreme intracranial pressure, the speed and action of dexamethasone are not sufficient to reduce the brain swelling quickly enough to prevent complications. In such instances, hyperosmotic solutions of *mannitol* must be given. The usual dosage is 0.5 to 2.0 grams per kilogram given intravenously over 15 minutes, followed by additional boluses of 25 grams as needed. The osmotic action of mannitol occurs within minutes. Clinical improvement may be dramatic. It is unusual for brain tumor patients preoperatively to decompensate so severely from increased intracranial pressure that intubation becomes necessary. Nevertheless, this does occur. In such cases the $Paco_2$ must be decreased by passive hyperventilation to approximately 25 mm Hg. The effect constricts

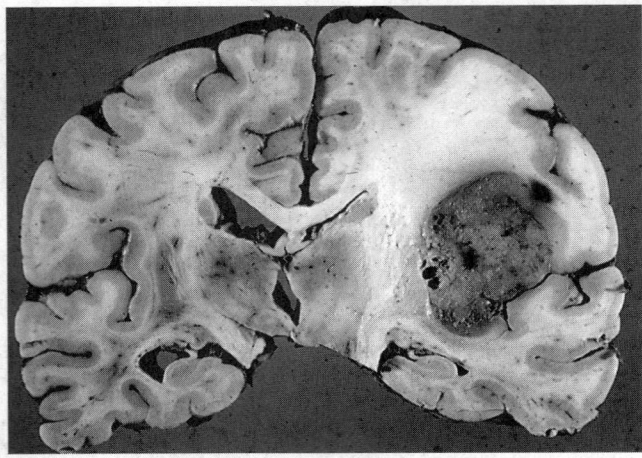

FIGURE 434–3. Gross coronal pathologic specimen of a solitary metastasis from a non–small cell lung carcinoma to the right cerebral hemisphere. The tumor is well circumscribed. It causes marked edema that greatly expands the cerebral white matter. Metastatic tumors such as this can often be surgically resected.

the cerebral vasculature and promptly induces a major reduction of intracranial pressure, which can be life saving.

About 20% of brain tumor patients develop *seizures* some time in their lives, even if they do not have seizures at the time of diagnosis. It is conventional and probably effective to treat all patients with supratentorial tumors with anticonvulsants before surgery. Most patients with acoustic neuromas or other posterior fossa tumors have a low probability of convulsive seizures and do not need such drugs. Phenytoin is the best initial drug because it can be administered either intravenously or orally, unlike either carbamazepine or valproic acid, which can be used only orally. An intravenous drug is especially useful for continuation during the perioperative period. If required, patients may be switched easily to alternative oral drugs later. Phenytoin should be started orally, giving 1000 mg over 12 hours, or intravenously, with 1000 mg given over 1 hour. Thereafter, the usual dosage is 300 to 400 mg daily, administered in one dose or split between breakfast and dinner, along with dexamethasone. Periodic blood levels need to be checked to adjust the dosage to ensure concentrations of 10 to 20 μg per milliliter.

SURGERY. Although complete excision of a brain tumor is the ultimate goal in every case, this is not always possible. Even potentially curable tumors, such as meningiomas or acoustic neuromas, may reside in positions that make complete resection technically impossible. Malignant gliomas lack microscopic boundaries, even though they may appear by imaging studies to have well-defined limits. How much surgical success can be achieved with these tumors depends on several factors, including the tumor's proximity to indispensable areas, the skill and experience of the neurosurgeon and the preoperative level of neurologic function. The combination of current standards of neurosurgical anesthesia, the capacity to control intracranial pressure, and the recent addition of lasers to other operative tools such as the operating microscope have greatly increased the surgeon's capacity for well-chosen radical resection. Correspondingly, the relative risks of surgery have become less age dependent than was previously the case. The greatest surgical risk is to neurologic function and the fear of unacceptable postoperative neurologic deficits. For this reason, radical operations upon tumors involving language areas, sensorimotor regions, the basal ganglia, corpus callosum, and brain stem are generally avoided. However, partial removal in these areas by stereotaxic methods may be surprisingly effective. MR images facilitate such surgery by showing that the tumor has pushed aside critical brain structures and that a macroscopic tumor edge can be delineated. It has been repeatedly shown that resection of the maximal amount of tumor consistent with functional preservation provides patients with better and longer lives.

A number of tumors cannot be even partially resected because they invade indispensable areas of the brain. Most are intra-axial tumors, such as the gliomas. Although imaging techniques may produce a characteristic picture suggestive of a particular histologic diagnosis, treatment planning demands a tissue diagnosis. All brain regions may be approached by MR-guided stereotaxic biopsy. The tissue specimens are small, but they are almost invariably adequate to establish a diagnosis. Morbidity, chiefly hemorrhage, occurs in about 2% of cases. Patients usually need to remain in the hospital for less than 48 hours. Open biopsies of brain tumors are not justifiable. If the skull and dura are to be opened, the surgeon should be prepared to do a gross total resection or, at least, a major removal of as much tumor as is consonant with preservation of neurologic function.

Deep leg vein thrombophlebitis leading to pulmonary embolism is a recurrent postoperative problem only partially helped by prophylactic application of compression boots. Early passive exercises and mobilization are imperative. The staff must monitor and maintain anticonvulsant levels to prevent postoperative seizures. Dexamethasone should be administered at adequate levels for at least 5 days to minimize surgically induced brain edema.

RADIATION THERAPY. All forms of external beam radiation, whether γ photons emitted from ^{60}Co sources or x-rays generated from linear accelerators, act similarly. They produce fast-moving electrons and free radicals in biologic tissue that interrupt chemical bonds between DNA base pairs. Affected cells either die or become so altered that their mitotic rate is greatly diminished. Radiation therapy is given in small daily fractions to build to a total dose. It appears safer and more effective to do this than to give larger fractions over shorter periods. Hyperfractionation, defined as two (or more) doses during a day, does not seem to be worthwhile. Therapeutic brain irradiation with particulate radiation such as neutrons has been attempted experimentally at facilities with cyclotrons. Such densely ionizing radiation has shown no therapeutic advantage over x-rays. Interstitial (implanted) radiation therapy (brachytherapy) is usually given in the form of $^{125}I_3$ or $^{192}Ir_4$ in "seeds" placed by stereotaxic techniques. This method permits localized high-dosage radiation with sharp edges and sparing of the adjacent brain. Considerable controversy exists about the utility of interstitial radiation therapy, but it can be effective in well-selected patients. Other nonoperative radiosurgical techniques include the "gamma knife" and linear accelerators adapted to provide focused therapeutic beams. Efficacy has been shown for metastases but not for gliomas.

The *complications of radiation therapy* are often reported as infrequent, perhaps 2 to 5% of cases. These figures, are unrealistically low if one includes effects on long-term survivors. They reflect the fact that most irradiated patients with brain tumor die before brain injury appears. A high percentage of patients receiving whole-brain radiation develop dementia or impaired mobility. Often, postradiation neurologic damage may not become fully developed for several years. Local field rather than whole-brain radiation has reduced the incidence of dementia in long-term survivors. Dementia is a considerable problem in children who survive radiation therapy for medulloblastoma. The incidence may reach 50% or more in those who survive treatment for 5 years.

External beam radiation therapy has value in controlling the growth of malignant gliomas and metastatic brain tumors. It doubles median survival time for both types of tumors. Radiation therapy, however, has little, if any, value for recurrent meningiomas and acoustic neuromas. These are almost invariably better handled by reoperation. Primary brain lymphomas are so responsive to radiation therapy that many neurologists and radiation therapists continue to use it alone despite the fact that chemotherapy may prove to provide superior initial treatment. It has already been mentioned that solitary brain metastases are best managed by surgical resection before radiation therapy.

CHEMOTHERAPY. Chemotherapy for brain tumors has had a disappointing record. The reasons are many, but inadequacy of drug delivery, tumor cell heterogeneity, and inherent resistance are among the important ones. Almost all efforts have been directed toward the primary brain tumors, especially the gliomas. Established brain metastases, however, respond about as well as systemic metastases do in many cancers, especially breast and small cell lung cancer. BCNU (biscloroethylnitrosurea), the most frequently used drug, remains the most effective single agent available to treat the malignant astrocytomas. The combination of procarbazine, CCNU (cyclohexylchloroethylnitrosourea), and vincristine is the most effective multidrug regimen for the malignant astrocytomas, and it is probably superior to BCNU. It has an unusually beneficial effect against oligodendrogliomas. No more than 10% of patients with malignant gliomas have meaningful and durable responses to chemotherapy, whether it is given immediately after radiation therapy (when its effect is especially hard to assess) or at the time of recurrence. Efforts to improve response to chemotherapy by delivering drugs through the carotid artery have not been successful. BCNU has intolerable toxicity when given by the intra-arterial route. Cisplatin is being studied for possible utility as an intra-arterial drug in highly selected patients.

The pharmacokinetics of drugs used in brain tumor chemotherapy are not well understood. Knowledge about their ability to gain adequate concentration within the tumors is minimal, and almost nothing is known about chemosensitivity. Nonetheless, occasional remarkable responses to chemotherapy do occur in patients with gliomas. Among other primary intra-axial brain tumors, primary brain lymphoma has a reasonably good response rate. The drugs used are those given regularly for systemic lymphoma. Patients with primary brain lymphoma do better with chemotherapy added than with radiation therapy alone. On average, 3- to 4-year survivals can now be expected.

Several additional forms of medical treatment for brain tumors have been attempted experimentally. These include slow release of BCNU from implanted biodegradable polymers and the administration of interferons, other biologic response modifiers, and radionuclides coupled with monoclonal antibodies. None has met with appreciable success to date. In all probability, much new biologic knowledge, such as the sequential genetic events that influence the malignant transformation and progression of brain tumors, will be required before new medical treatments become practical realities.

Hildebrand J (ed.): Management in Neuro-Oncology. EOS Monographs. Berlin, Springer-Verlag, 1992. *A short review of management of brain tumors.*

Morantz RA, Walsh JW (eds.): Brain Tumors. A Comprehensive Text. New York, Marcel Dekker, 1994. *A comprehensive text written by experienced physicians.*

Twijnstra A, Keyser A, Ongerboer de Visser BW: Neuro-Oncology. Primary Tumors and Neurological Complications of Cancer. Amsterdam, Elsevier, 1993. *A summary of current concepts in diagnosis and management.*

435 SPECIFIC TYPES OF BRAIN TUMORS AND THEIR MANAGEMENT

METASTATIC TUMORS

All systemic cancers are capable of metastasizing to the intracranial contents and skull, although some do so more readily than others. The most frequent are lung, breast, and melanoma. This is not surprising because they are among the most common cancers. In many instances, brain metastases produce symptoms before the primary tumor is suspected. Furthermore, the primary cancer may not be found without considerable effort.

Patterns of metastasis to the nervous system have some variability, but none is truly characteristic. Non–small cell carcinoma of the lung and renal carcinoma tend to be associated with single metastases, whereas small cell carcinoma of the lung, breast carcinoma, and melanoma often generate multiple secondary deposits. The metastases may be miliary in melanoma. T1 gadolinium magnetic resonance imaging (MRI) scans are critical in the imaging of brain metastases (Fig. 435–1). *Multiple metastases* may be revealed with this method, whereas T2 MRI and contrast computed tomography (CT) may show only one or, in rare instances, none. For multiple metastases, whole-brain irradiation is the best form of treatment as long as the patient's systemic condition indicates a potential for high-quality survival. Patients with widespread systemic metastasis

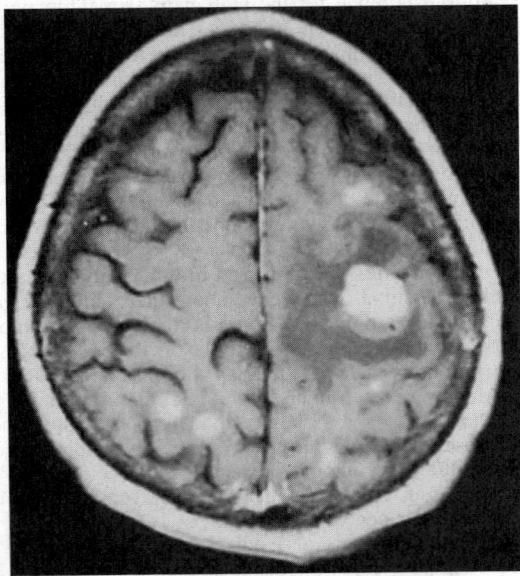

FIGURE 435–1. MRI scan, T1 gadolinium, of multiple metastases from breast carcinoma. The tumors were not visible on CT, even after giving a contrast agent.

TABLE 435–1. METASTATIC BRAIN TUMORS

These tumors affect 10% of cancer patients (and still another 20% have dural meningeal involvement).

At least 50% are multiple.

If solitary (the only metastatic lesion in the body), surgery clearly provides best results in most cases. Surgery may be the best approach even if other metastases are present in patients in good condition.

Radiation therapy is useful palliation but not curative. Long-term survivors may have consequential side effects such as dementia.

who are unlikely to survive more than a few months are best treated with dexamethasone alone.

The major benefit of aggressive surgery in patients with a *single brain metastasis* is for the quality of life that remains. Studies of evaluation of performance are compelling. Some of the best outcomes are in patients with a non–small cell lung carcinoma and a single metastasis to the brain. Surgical removal of both tumors sometimes leads to a protracted remission from the disease. With most brain metastases, however, 2-year mortality is similar between surgical patients and those who receive radiation therapy alone. Most patients with systemic metastases die of their systemic illness and not their brain metastasis.

Metastases to the dura and meninges are relatively common. Meningeal carcinomatosis produces headache, cranial nerve palsies, and stiff neck. These symptoms are due to the presence of tumor cells within the spinal fluid and to small deposits on the meninges around cranial nerves, at the base of the brain, and upon spinal roots. The diagnosis is made by cytologic examination of large-volume spinal fluid specimens. As many as three or more spinal taps may be needed to find cancer cells in some cases. The spinal fluid protein level is generally elevated, and the glucose concentration may be low. The latter changes are sufficiently characteristic, in the absence of evidence of infection, to suggest the diagnosis. T1 gadolinium MRI scanning may image the small deposits in the meninges. They are especially evident in the cauda equina even in the absence of clinical symptoms referable to lumbosacral nerve roots. The treatment of meningeal carcinomatosis includes irradiation of the brain and spinal cord, which usually provides benefit but rarely long remission. In patients with limited systemic metastases, intrathecal chemotherapy with methotrexate through an Ommaya reservoir is appropriate; occasional patients respond impressively. Most do not, however, and the effective treatment of meningeal carcinomatosis remains a difficult problem. In the future, the still experimental treatment of meningeal carcinomatosis with isotope-emitting radionuclides coupled to monoclonal antibodies may replace intrathecal chemotherapy.

Table 435–1 lists some key features of metastatic brain tumors.

PRIMARY EXTRA-AXIAL TUMORS

Meningiomas, acoustic neuromas, and pituitary adenomas are the most frequent in this group, which, by definition, are tumors that are not of the brain itself but of its coverings, the cranial nerves, and the adjacent structures. These primary "extra-axial" tumors differ from brain tumors in many ways. They are not of neuroectodermal origin, they are histologically unrelated, and most are truly benign because they can be cured by excision. They exert effects upon the brain by pressure and only occasionally by actual invasion.

Meningiomas, which are growths of the fibroblast-like cells of the dura and arachnoid villi, account for about 15% of all primary brain tumors. They occur more often in women. The biologic explanation is unknown, but the finding has stimulated interest in the presence of progesterone receptors in the tumors. Meningiomas may occur many years after radiation delivered to the head, in which setting they may be multiple. A relationship to head trauma has never been convincingly documented. A few are familial. Such cases, as well as most apparently sporadic examples, are associated with a loss of a portion of chromosome 22, similar to that which characterizes neurofibromatosis type 2.

Most meningiomas arise as solitary tumors in characteristic sites, such as over the cerebral convexities, attached to the sagittal sinus or at the base of the brain attached to the dura of the sphenoid sinus, the olfactory grooves, or the region of the sella. In some of these areas, they may be difficult to remove completely without excessive risk and may recur slowly but repeatedly. Many grow so slowly that serial CT or MR images suggest no enlargement over many years. This slow growth sometimes permits the brain to accommodate them with modest symptoms even when they reach a large size (see Fig. 434–1). Many are detected incidentally. Small, asymptomatic meningiomas are often best watched by imaging studies at intervals; in the elderly, even large, asymptomatic ones may not require surgery.

Acoustic neuromas consist of distinctive growths of Schwann cells (schwannoma) of the eighth cranial nerve. Almost all are unilateral and not apparently familial. Bilateral acoustic neuromas are rare, familial, and diagnostic of neurofibromatosis type 2. This autosomal dominant condition occurs with nearly 100% penetrance in successive generations and derives from a gene deletion on chromosome 22.

Acoustic neuromas grow on the nerve into a round mass just as it emerges from the acoustic canal into the cerebellopontine angle. Some produce symptoms when they are small and confined within the canal. Others may go unsuspected until they grow to rather large size, filling the cerebellopontine angle and compressing the brain stem. Acoustic neuromas greatly surpass in frequency any other tumor of cranial nerves. Partial or complete nerve deafness is characteristic and usually the first symptom. As acoustic neuromas grow, they sequentially affect the fifth and then the seventh cranial nerves on the same side. When large, they cause cerebellar ataxia on the same side and, ultimately, symptoms of brain stem dysfunction. MRI scans accurately detect even very small acoustic neuromas. All patients who develop hearing loss in the middle years of life should be considered to have an acoustic neuroma until proved otherwise. Audiometry alone is suggestive but not diagnostic; caloric tests of labyrinthine function almost always show abnormalities, but the most efficient physiologic study is the auditory evoked response. Current microsurgical techniques yield remarkably good results, usually preserving the seventh nerve and, occasionally, hearing as well.

Pituitary Adenomas

These tumors may cause endocrine symptoms, such as hypothyroidism, amenorrhea, galactorrhea, infertility, acromegaly, or Cushing's syndrome (Ch. 159). With the exception of these hormonal impairments, early symptoms, if any, are usually limited to nonspecific headaches. As pituitary adenomas enlarge, they erode the sella turcica and extend above it to compress the optic nerves, eventually causing bitemporal visual field defects. Rare hemorrhages into large pituitary tumors can cause *pituitary apoplexy,* producing a characteristic syndrome of sudden-onset headache, partial ophthalmoplegia, and blindness in one or the other eye. Emergency surgical decompression must be applied to preserve vision.

Current endocrinologic and MRI techniques facilitate the diagnosis of pituitary tumors, especially if 1-mm cuts and magnified views through the sella are obtained. Medical treatment with bromocriptine may be effective but is slow in yielding results. The drug must be continued indefinitely. Only surgical removal can produce a cure. The safety and efficiency of transsphenoidal pituitary surgery warrant its consideration in all patients, including those with microadenomas that are confined to the sella and larger tumors that, in the past, could be approached only by a subfrontal craniotomy. Radiation therapy may be required in occasional patients who have large and incompletely removed macroadenomas.

Less common primary extra-axial tumors include *craniopharyngiomas,* related *suprasellar epidermoid cysts,* and *Rathke cleft cysts.* Although they reflect congenital abnormalities of the brain and most frequently become symptomatic in childhood, as many as one third of these tumors can first appear in adult life, some as late as the sixth decade. In adults, craniopharyngiomas may compress the frontal lobes and occasionally cause dementia. Such tumors are almost always benign and surgically curable if they can be separated from adjacent parasellar structures, optic nerves, and hypothalamus. Pineal region tumors include *pineocytomas* and *pineoblastomas* derived from pineal parenchymal cells, as well as *teratomas* and *germinomas.* These two groups appear with about equal frequency, have the capacity to be biologically aggressive, and are difficult to manage surgically. Characteristic symptoms and signs include increased intracranial pressure, paresis of upward gaze, pupillary dysfunction, convergence nystagmus, and hydrocephalus due to obstruction of cerebrospinal fluid outflow pathways. Precocious puberty occurs in young males, the result of destruction of the pineal by germinomas. The true pineal tumors may cause delayed puberty. Intracranial *chordomas,* tumors of residual notochordal tissue, are rare and usually arise within the skull at the base of the brain, on the clivus. They are regionally invasive and rarely can be controlled even with aggressive surgery and radiation therapy. *Lipomas* occur chiefly in midline structures, especially over the corpus callosum. *Arachnoid cysts* can arise anywhere on the surface of the brain; some grow to remarkable size. Most arachnoid cysts are incidental, cause no symptoms, and are best left alone. Their infrequency, as well as that of the other extra-axial tumors mentioned, stands in contrast to the frequency and clinical importance of meningiomas and acoustic neuromas (see Table 434–1).

PRIMARY INTRA-AXIAL TUMORS

This group includes astrocytomas, oligodendrogliomas, ependymomas, medulloblastomas, less common neuroectodermal tumors, and primary brain lymphoma. They share the quality of direct, invasive involvement of the substance of the brain, making them rarely curable by surgical excision. Accordingly, gliomas are fundamentally malignant, although some may behave in an indolent manner.

Astrocytomas are the most common gliomas. Their cause is unknown, familial examples constituting only 1% of cases. Astrocytomas have occurred as a late consequence of radiation to the head or skull. The most aggressive variant, *glioblastoma multiforme,* accounts for more than 50% of all primary brain tumors. Glioblastoma (astrocytoma IV) is distinguished pathologically from the less aggressive *anaplastic astrocytoma* (astrocytoma III) on histopathologic grounds, and the two have important clinical differences. Glioblastoma is more common, is more characteristic of older age groups, and has a median survival time of less than 1 year even with aggressive treatment with surgery, radiation therapy, and chemotherapy. By contrast, patients with anaplastic astrocytoma have a median survival time of slightly more than 2 years. Age is an important variable for both of these tumors: The younger the patient, the better the prognosis. Glioblastoma in children, for example, has a median survival of more than 2 years. In adults, men are affected more often than women. Anaplastic astrocytomas and glioblastoma occur in multicentric locations in about 5% of cases. In these instances, they may be mistaken for multiple cerebral metastases or for primary brain lymphoma on imaging studies.

Glioblastomas and anaplastic astrocytomas produce a similar clinical picture, and CT or MR images may be somewhat alike (Fig. 435–2). In most instances, the onset is relatively rapid and heralded by seizures, headaches, and focal neurologic deficits. A minority of patients with these tumors have relevant histories of seizures with onset years before; one assumes that such malignant growths evolve from long-existing, low-grade astrocytomas. Sequential genetic alterations occur in astrocytomas as they become more aggressive. Loss of chromosome 10 is characteristic of

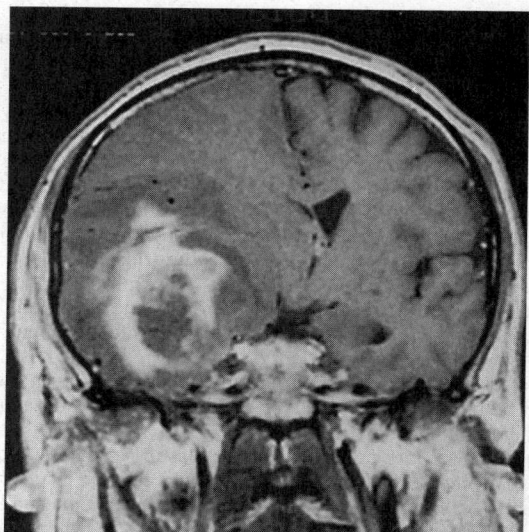

FIGURE 435–2. MRI scan, T1 gadolinium enhanced, of a temporal lobe glioblastoma, showing typical ring configuration of contrast with central necrosis and marked mass effect.

glioblastoma cells and may occur subsequent to loss of chromosome 17, which is common in lower-grade astrocytomas. The latter is likely related to a mutation of a tumor suppressor gene, p53, on this chromosome.

Low-grade astrocytomas can pursue a highly variable course, and many of them do not progress to malignancy. Indeed, some are extremely indolent in their growth, so that the median survival time of patients with low-grade astrocytomas is 7 years from the time of diagnosis. This prognosis means little in individual cases, however, because the course of these tumors is, as noted before, highly variable. In some patients, low-grade astrocytomas transform to glioblastoma within a few years, whereas other astrocytomas can remain indolent for 10 years or more. Many low-grade astrocytomas spread too extensively before diagnosis can be made to allow surgical resection (see Fig. 434–2). By contrast, smaller, favorably situated ones sometimes can be totally removed and the patient apparently cured. Paradoxically, astrocytomas associated with large cysts have a much better prognosis. This favorable circumstance occurs most often in the cerebellum in children and young adults but also in the cerebral hemispheres. Brain stem astrocytomas cannot be operated upon except in rare instances when they are exophytic. Most infiltrate the brain stem and enlarge it. In a similar way, optic nerve astrocytomas, an uncommon cause of vision loss that affects chiefly children, enlarge the optic nerves and may erode the optic foramina. They grow slowly, are sometimes associated with neurofibromatosis, and are often best left untreated until MRI scanning documents unequivocal tumor growth or vision declines. What to do at that point is controversial. Many authorities withhold radiation treatment for low-grade astrocytomas, at least until all other approaches fail and for as long as the quality of life can be maintained. Two important reasons support this position. One is that little well-controlled evidence indicates that radiation greatly shrinks these tumors, eradicates them, slows their growth, or prevents their conversion into malignant astrocytomas. The other, as already remarked upon, is that radiation damages the normal brain, producing selective neuronal injury, areas of radiation necrosis, or both.

Oligodendrogliomas are the most "benign" of the gliomas, although some develop anaplastic features. Their clinical manifestations usually are indistinguishable from those of low-grade astrocytomas. Seizures are an important early symptom. Oligodendrogliomas occur chiefly in the cerebral hemispheres and especially in the frontal lobes. Many contain flecks of calcium, demonstrable by brain imaging. Complete surgical resection is the therapeutic goal but often cannot be realized because of the size and location of the tumors. Despite their slow growth, most oligodendrogliomas respond well to chemotherapy. As many as 80% improve with a regimen that combines procarbazine, CCNU, and vincristine. This response to chemotherapy seems to be superior to that observed with radiation therapy alone. Oligodendroglioma is the primary intra-axial tumor most likely to bleed spontaneously. In addition, anaplastic oligodendrogliomas tend to spread through the spinal fluid to the meninges. A few of these tumors eventually become so anaplastic that they histologically and clinically resemble glioblastomas.

Medulloblastomas occur chiefly in the region of the fourth ventricle and affect principally children and young adults. They cause characteristic symptoms of cerebellar and brain stem dysfunction. In children, aggressive surgery and radiation therapy yield a 5-year survival of 50%, but many children treated in this manner suffer serious, permanent postradiation intellectual deficits. Several reports indicate that chemotherapy with cyclophosphamide and vincristine improves survival, and other drugs are being tried.

Medulloblastoma is characterized by an amplification of the *c-myc* oncogene and abnormalities of chromosome 17. Medulloblastomas arising in the cerebral hemispheres resemble, or may be the same as, *primitive neuroectodermal tumors* (PNET). These tumors are radiosensitive, like medulloblastomas of the fourth ventricle and cerebellum, and at times respond temporarily to aggressive chemotherapy.

Gangliogliomas are composed of neoplastic astrocytes and abundant dysmorphic neoplastic neurons. They occur chiefly in the temporal lobes of children and young adults, have an unusually slow growth rate, and may have a good prognosis even when untreated. Some are associated with tuberous sclerosis.

Primary brain lymphoma is increasing in frequency among both the acquired immunodeficiency syndrome (AIDS) and, for unknown reasons, the non-AIDS populations. These growths involve the brain diffusely, producing infiltrating and often multicentric tumors that tend to lie deep in the brain and adjacent to ventricular surfaces. Almost all of these tumors are B cell derived; the eye is the only other extranodal site that is regularly involved concomitantly. Only rare patients go on to develop systemic lymphoma, and that occurs late in the disease. Primary brain lymphoma is fundamentally unresectable. Steroids are an important component of treatment; dexamethasone is uniquely chemotherapeutic for this tumor. Median survivals of 3 years can now be expected with the addition of multidrug chemotherapy to radiation therapy.

Rare intra-axial brain tumors include *choroid plexus papillomas* and *carcinomas,* which are even less common than the benign but troublesome *colloid cysts* of the third ventricle. The last-mentioned lesion may cause hydrocephalus by blocking the outflow of cerebrospinal fluid from the lateral ventricle. *Capillary hemangioblastomas* arise in the cerebellum and elsewhere. They are sometimes associated with an autosomal dominant inherited disorder that includes retinal angiomatosis as well as cysts and tumors of the pancreas, kidneys, and adrenals (von Hippel syndrome). Some of these cerebellar capillary hemangioblastomas secrete erythropoietin and cause polycythemia.

Vascular malformations of the brain often can be mistaken for gliomas. They frequently manifest with nonhemorrhagic symptoms such as seizures. They sometimes resemble brain tumors in appearance on CT or MRI, and some, especially of the capillary variety (which lack large arteriovenous shunts), cannot be imaged by cerebral angiography. Many of these abnormalities lie in the brain stem and thalamus; because they are indistinguishable from brain tumors on even the best imaging studies, they may undergo biopsy as a diagnostic step, with devastating results. Vascular malformations of the brain involving large-caliber vessels are readily diagnosed by CT or MR images even without cerebral angiography.

Abscesses and *granulomas* of the brain cannot usually be distinguished from tumors by CT or MRI alone. If systemic evaluations fail to suggest a proper diagnosis, reliable management demands that biopsy be used. Even in the non-AIDS population, surprising alternatives to the clinical and radiologic diagnosis of a brain tumor are regularly revealed by biopsy. In many instances, potentially tragic errors of management can be avoided by taking as a direct approach and studying the tissue of the intracranial lesion.

Fadul C, Wood J, Thaler H, et al.: Morbidity and mortality of craniotomy for excision of supratentorial gliomas. Neurology 38:1374, 1988. *Documents convincingly the safety and efficacy of aggressive surgery for gliomas.*

Kyritsis AP, Levin VA: Chemotherapeutic approaches to the treatment of malignant gliomas. Adv Oncol 8:9, 1992. *A short but authoritative and useful review.*

Loeffler JS: Radiotherapy in managing malignant gliomas: Current role and future directions. Adv Oncol 8:14, 1992. *Covers the field well, including newer approaches and techniques.*

Patchell RA, Tibbs PA, Walsh JW, et al.: A randomized trial of surgery in the treatment of single metastasis to the brain. N Engl J Med 322:494, 1990. *An important paper, not only for its conclusion, which clearly supports surgery for a single metastasis, but also because it is an example of what careful clinical trials in neuro-oncology can achieve. Jerome Posner's editorial comments on this paper, and on metastasis in general, are in the same issue and are masterful.*

Posner JB: Neurological Complications of Cancer. Philadelphia, FA Davis, 1995. *A discussion of diagnosis and management of metastatic brain tumors.*

Russell DS, Rubinstein LJ: Pathology of Tumours of the Nervous System. 5th ed. Baltimore, Williams & Wilkins, 1989. *The definitive text, indispensable, scholarly, complete, and beautifully redone by Professor Rubinstein just before his death in 1989.*

436 DISORDERS OF INTRACRANIAL PRESSURE

INTRACRANIAL HYPERTENSION

GENERAL PRINCIPLES. Cerebrospinal fluid (CSF) pressure in excess of 250 mm CSF is usually a manifestation of serious neurologic disease. Intracranial hypertension is most often associated with rapidly expanding mass lesions, CSF outflow obstruction, or cerebral venous congestion; however, a variety of systemic and central nervous system disorders may be accompanied by an increase in intracranial pressure (ICP) (Table 436–1). Lumbar CSF pressure

TABLE 436–1. PATHOGENESIS OF INCREASED INTRACRANIAL PRESSURE

Perturbation	Proximate Cause	Clinical Example
Increased dural sinus venous pressure	Sinus compression or occlusion	Sagittal sinus thrombosis Otitic hydrocephalus Brain tumors
	Increased sinus blood flow	OC$_2$ retention Arteriovenous malformation
	Increased peripheral venous pressure	Internal jugular vein occlusion Superior vena cava syndrome Congestive heart failure
Increased CSF outflow resistance	Ventricular outflow obstruction Obliteration of the cisternal and/or convexity subarachnoid space Plugging of the arachnoid villi	Brain tumors Aqueductal stenosis Meningitis Extradural or subdural masses Cerebral masses or edema Subarachnoid hemorrhage Infectious polyneuritis Spinal cord tumors
Increased rate of CSF formation	Increased choroidal CSF formation Increased extrachoroidal CSF formation	Choroid plexus papilloma Hypo-osmolality Cerebral edema
Unknown	Increased cerebral volume Increased sagittal sinus pressure Increased CSF outflow resistance	Benign intracranial hypertension

may not accurately reflect ICP. In patients with intracranial mass lesions and brain herniation, lumbar CSF pressure may be normal or even low despite grossly elevated supratentorial CSF pressure. Kinking of the aqueduct of Sylvius by adjacent mass lesions, diencephalic–temporal lobe transtentorial herniation, or cerebellar compression of the fourth ventricle, with or without accompanying descent of the cerebellar tonsils into the foramen magnum, can impede the free transmission of CSF into the lumbar subarachnoid space.

Table 436–2 lists the principal symptoms and signs associated with intracranial hypertension. Headache is produced by traction on pain-sensitive cerebral blood vessels or dura mater at the base or, less often, the vertex of the brain. Signs reflect the presence of impending herniation with intermittent vascular compression, midline shift, or axial distortion of the brain stem (see Ch. 393). In the absence of such shifts, increased ICP alone may be asymptomatic. *Papilledema* is the most reliable sign of ICP; but in many patients with increased ICP, it fails to develop. This is particularly true in the elderly. Retinal venous pulsations, when present, imply that CSF pressure is normal or not significantly elevated, but their absence is not helpful diagnostically. Patients with increased ICP often complain of worsening symptoms, particularly headache, in the morning, perhaps because plateau waves (spontaneous elevations of ICP) occur more commonly during sleep.

The initial treatment of any patient with increased ICP whose neurologic status is deteriorating is aimed at reducing the volume of the intracranial contents in an attempt to prevent brain damage (Table 436–3). If ICP approaches the systolic blood pressure, the cerebral perfusion pressure decreases and irreversible ischemia may develop. The definitive treatment of intracranial hypertension is ulti-

mately determined by the nature of the underlying pathologic process.

Benign Intracranial Hypertension

Benign intracranial hypertension is a syndrome of increased ICP unaccompanied by localizing neurologic signs, intracranial mass lesion, or CSF outflow obstruction in an alert, otherwise healthy-looking patient. Such patients are almost always obese and more often women. Benign intracranial hypertension (also called pseudotumor cerebri, or idiopathic intracranial hypertension) may be associated with a variety of systemic and iatrogenic disorders (Table 436–4). The cause is usually unknown. Chronically increased ICP may give rise to the "empty sella syndrome," which refers to a radiographically globular enlargement of the sella turcica, an incompetent diaphragma sellae, and a compressed but functioning pituitary.

The diagnosis of benign intracranial hypertension is one of exclusion. Intracranial masses (tumors, hematomas, infections) and CSF outflow obstruction must be excluded by computed tomography (CT) or magnetic resonance imaging (MRI). Magnetic resonance angiography (MRA) is necessary to rule out dural venous sinus thrombosis. Lumbar puncture, which is usually deferred until CT or MR has revealed a normal or small ventricular system, is required to confirm the diagnosis. Lumbar spinal fluid pressure is elevated, frequently above 300 mm CSF, but the composition of the fluid is normal; the protein content is usually in the low normal range, below 20 mg per deciliter.

PATHOPHYSIOLOGY. In most cases, the cause is unknown. Chronically elevated ICP implies an increase in dural sinus venous pressure, an increase in CSF outflow resistance, an increase in the rate of CSF formation (if it ever really occurs), or some combination of these factors. One or more of these mechanisms must elevate the CSF pressure. Pathogenetic hypotheses that postulate an in-

TABLE 436–2. SYMPTOMS AND SIGNS OF INTRACRANIAL HYPERTENSION

Common	Less Common
Headache	Hearing distortion or loss
Tinnitus	Vertigo
Vomiting (with or without nausea)	Facial weakness
Visual obscurations, visual loss, photopsias	Shoulder/arm pain
Papilledema	Neck pain or rigidity
Diplopia	Ataxia
Lethargy and increased sleep	Paresthesias of extremities
Psychomotor retardation	Anosmia
Pain on eye movement	Trigeminal neuralgia

TABLE 436–3. EMERGENCY TREATMENT OF IMPENDING HERNIATION IN ACUTELY DECOMPENSATING PATIENTS

Therapy	Dosage or Procedure	Onset (Duration) of Action
Hyperventilation	Lower Paco$_2$ to 25 to 30 mm Hg	Seconds (minutes)
Osmotherapy	Mannitol, 0.5 to 2.0 gm/kg intravenously over 15 minutes, followed by 25 gm as needed	Minutes (hours)
Corticosteroids	Dexamethasone, 50 mg intravenous push, followed by 50 mg daily in divided doses	Hours (days)

TABLE 436–4. SYSTEMIC AND IATROGENIC DISORDERS ASSOCIATED WITH BENIGN INTRACRANIAL HYPERTENSION

Commonly Prescribed Drugs
Nalidixic acid
Nitrofurantoin
Phenytoin
Sulfonamides
Tetracycline
Vitamin A
Endocrine and Metabolic Disorders
Addison's disease
Cushing's syndrome
Hypoparathyroidism
Levothyroxine therapy
Menarche, pregnancy, oral contraceptives
Obesity and irregular menses
Steroid therapy/withdrawal
Hematologic Disorders
Cryoglobulinemia
Iron deficiency anemia
Miscellaneous Disorders
Dural venous sinus obstruction/thrombosis
Head trauma
Internal jugular vein ligation
Lupus erythematosus
Middle ear disease

crease in brain bulk consequent to an increase in cerebral blood volume or in brain water content (interstitial brain edema) do not provide an adequate explanation. The constancy of obesity, often extreme, has suggested the possibility of a disorder of the hypothalamus. But no data have emerged to support this idea. Despite decades of knowledge of the association with obesity, the link remains completely obscure. The strikingly greater incidence in women than in men (4:1) is also unexplained but surely important in some way.

CLINICAL MANIFESTATIONS. Most patients complain of headache. Other common early symptoms include nausea and vomiting, visual disturbances, retro-ocular pain, diplopia, tinnitus, and vertigo. Bilateral papilledema, the cardinal feature, is almost always present and may be associated with peripapillary retinal hemorrhages, exudates, or both. Vision loss, the only serious complication of idiopathic intracranial hypertension, may occur either early or late in the course of the disease but is seen less than feared. Transient obscurations of vision do not predict subsequent failure of vision. Characteristically, visual field testing reveals enlarged blind spots. Quantitative visual field testing should be performed at monthly intervals early in the disease. Diplopia, caused by unilateral or bilateral abducens palsy, may develop as a false localizing sign. The remainder of the neurologic examination is almost always normal. It is important to distinguish pseudopapilledema—an anomalous elevation of the optic disc—from true papilledema, which is prima facie evidence of increased ICP. Anomalous elevation of the disc, which may be associated with identifiable hyaline bodies (drusen), should suggest the diagnosis of retinitis pigmentosa.

In some instances, benign intracranial hypertension is a self-limited disease in which CSF pressure returns to normal as clinical symptoms remit over several months. However, clinical improvement is not always accompanied by a reduction in CSF pressure, and there is a vexing subgroup of patients whose pressure remains persistently elevated after neurologic signs and symptoms have resolved. The course of such cases implies that clinical symptoms may be independent of the absolute magnitude of CSF pressure and that chronically raised ICP may be totally asymptomatic. In addition, despite persistently elevated CSF pressure, patients do not become hydrocephalic. The ventricular system remains small, or no larger than normal. This finding suggests that whatever mechanism "resets" CSF pressure above normal does not predispose to the development of communicating hydrocephalus and that the two conditions are biologically unrelated.

TREATMENT. Unfortunately, no convincing evidence exists that any of the frequently recommended treatment modalities are regularly efficacious. The high rate of spontaneous remission com-

plicates the evaluation of various therapies. At present, four general approaches to symptomatic treatment are used: (1) repeated lumbar puncture, (2) pharmacologic treatment, (3) ventriculosystemic or lumboperitoneal shunting, and (4) incision of the optic nerve sheath.

Frequent (such as alternate day), large-volume lumbar punctures may provide relief of symptoms and document the occurrence of remission. Either it is beneficial, or remission occurs independently during the period of treatment. Corticosteroids and diuretics have been the mainstay of medical treatment, and both are effective; or, again, the disease remits during the period of treatment. Dexamethasone, furosemide, and acetazolamide are often tried. CSF shunting procedures are not without risk, and their long-term efficacy remains to be established. Incision of the optic nerve sheath for the relief of papilledema is the treatment of choice for patients whose visual fields are deteriorating. Surprisingly, in some patients, headache and papilledema on the contralateral side are relieved as well as the ipsilateral papilledema.

HYDROCEPHALUS

Hydrocephalus refers to the net accumulation of CSF within the cerebral ventricles and their consequent enlargement. Although acute obstructive hydrocephalus usually produces a sudden increase in intraventricular pressure, CSF pressure is frequently normal (or low) in patients with chronic hydrocephalus. It is customary to distinguish between "noncommunicating" and "communicating" hydrocephalus; the former is produced by lesions that obstruct the intracerebral CSF circulation at or proximal to the foramina of Luschka and Magendie, the latter by obstruction of the basal cisterns or convexity subarachnoid space in such a way that the ventricular system communicates with the spinal subarachnoid space but CSF cannot drain through the arachnoid villi into the superior sagittal sinus. Because both "noncommunicating" and "communicating" types of hydrocephalus are obstructive and both are treated by shunts, the distinction really has less meaning than that usually ascribed to it. Perhaps the important distinction should be between obstructive and nonobstructive hydrocephalus. Ventricular dilatation associated with severe cerebral atrophy, sometimes called "hydrocephalus ex vacuo," is the best example of nonobstructive hydrocephalus.

DIAGNOSIS. Hydrocephalus is easily diagnosed by MRI. The diagnosis must take into account the increase in ventricular volume that accompanies normal aging and the presence or absence of cerebral atrophy. Enlargement of the temporal horns and an inability to visualize the sylvian and interhemispheric fissures or cerebral sulci, plus the presence of periventricular lucencies (CT) or periventricular hyperintensity (MR), favor the diagnosis of hydrocephalus. A normal or small fourth ventricle in the presence of enlarged lateral and third ventricles suggests aqueductal stenosis.

ACUTE VERSUS CHRONIC HYDROCEPHALUS. Sudden, complete ventricular outflow obstruction leads to acute hydrocephalus, coma, and, if untreated, death; partial obstruction is more common and only moderately less dangerous (Table 436–5). Chronic hydrocephalus in the adult is most often caused by aqueductal stenosis or the complications of subarachnoid hemorrhage. Other reported causes and associations are listed in Table 436–5. In

TABLE 436–5. CAUSES OF HYDROCEPHALUS

Acute
Cerebellar hemorrhage/infarction
Colloid cyst of the third ventricle
Exudative meningitis
Head trauma
Intracranial tumor/hematoma
Spontaneous subarachnoid hemorrhage
Viral encephalitis
Chronic
Aqueductal stenosis
Ectasia and elongation of the basilar artery (rare)
Granulomatous meningitis
Head trauma
Hindbrain malformations
Meningeal carcinomatosis
Brain and spinal cord tumors
Spontaneous subarachnoid hemorrhage
Syringomyelia

many instances, the cause of symptomatic chronic hydrocephalus ("normal-pressure hydrocephalus") cannot be determined. Unequivocally asymptomatic hydrocephalus may be found in approximately 4% of patients over the age of 60 who consult neurologists.

CLINICAL MANIFESTATIONS. The patient with acute obstructive hydrocephalus may have severe headache, lethargy, signs of increased ICP, papilledema, abducens palsy, and signs of the causative lesion. Hyperactive reflex and bilateral extensor plantar responses are almost invariably present. Ventricular CSF pressure is markedly increased, but if CSF pathways are blocked, this increase may not be transmitted to the lumbar subarachnoid space. Patients with chronic communicating hydrocephalus, including normal-pressure hydrocephalus, have a progressive dementia characterized by forgetfulness and psychomotor retardation, an unsteady gait, and urinary incontinence. Bilateral pyramidal and extrapyramidal signs may be present. Some patients have a parkinsonian appearance. The lumbar CSF pressure is usually normal or nearly normal in range, although overnight recording of ventricular CSF pressure may reveal intermittent waves of elevated pressure.

TREATMENT. Acute hydrocephalus responds dramatically to ventricular drainage and CSF diversion. Treatment of the primary lesion is the treatment of choice, although temporary ventricular decompression or ventriculosystemic shunt may be necessary in some cases. Ventricular shunting has also been used for patients with chronic communicating hydrocephalus. Unfortunately, not all patients respond, or response may be delayed for weeks or months; moreover, there are no reliable clinical or neuroradiologic predictors of shunt response. Recent onset and mild dementia remain better predictors than does isotope cisternography. Absence of cerebral atrophy and temporary improvement after lumbar puncture seem to correlate with benefit from a shunt operation.

INTRACRANIAL HYPOTENSION

CSF pressure measured at a lumbar puncture site, with the patient in the lateral decubitus position, normally ranges from 70 to 200 mm CSF (5 to 15 mm Hg). Low or zero lumbar CSF pressure can be recorded under several circumstances, as indicated in Table 436–6. Symptoms of the first two or three circumstances on that list are likely to be dominated by the underlying illnesses. The remainder of the circumstances tend to cause a consistent syndrome characterized by severe, throbbing frontal and occipital headache, which usually appears within 30 seconds after the patient assumes an erect posture and subsides completely upon the patient's lying flat. Associated complaints may include dizziness, nausea, stiff neck, photophobia, and, rarely, diplopia due to an associated abducens nerve palsy. The disorder often arises 1 to 21 days after lumbar puncture. The pathogenesis is as for lumbar puncture headache (Ch. 405.2).

Rare cases of CSF hypotension may occur spontaneously, producing, in previously healthy persons, symptoms similar to those already described. The onset can be acute or subacute and is occasionally precipitated by mild trauma, such as a fall on the buttocks or a casual bump to the head. The cause usually remains unknown, although isotope cisternography sometimes reveals spontaneous rupture of a dural nerve sheath. Diagnosis can be difficult because zero spontaneous pressures in the lumbar subarachnoid space can give the false impression of missing the thecal sac. Treatment is symptomatic; spontaneous recovery usually requires days to a few weeks. When post–lumbar puncture symptoms are persistent, disabling, or both, an epidural "blood patch" is indicated. The actual need for blood patches is far less than the frequency with which the procedure is done by worried physicians for impatient sufferers of post–lumbar puncture headache. The procedure involves the injection of 10 ml of the patient's own blood into the epidural space to seal a presumed dural leak. Rarely, in long-lasting cases, surgical exploration has exposed the dural leak, which must be sutured. In patients suffering from either lumbar puncture–induced or spontaneous intracranial hypotension, an MRI of the brain may reveal intense enhancement of the meninges. Occasionally, subdural effusions develop. The process is benign and clears when the intracranial hypotension resolves.

Lyons HK, Meyer FB: Cerebrospinal fluid physiology and the management of increased intracranial pressure. Mayo Clin Proc 65:684, 1990. *A superb review with excellent references.*

Pannullo S, Reich JB, Krol G, et al.: MRI changes in intracranial hypotension. Neurology 43:919, 1993. *A description of patients with intracranial hypotension and meningeal enhancement on MRI.*

Petersen RC, Bahram M, Laws ER Jr: Surgical treatment of idiopathic hydrocephalus in elderly patients. Neurology 35:307, 1985. *A clinically oriented review of the indications for, risks of, and benefits to be expected from the surgical treatment of normal-pressure hydrocephalus.*

Radhadkrishnan K, Ahlskog JE, Garrity JA, et al.: Idiopathic intracranial hypertension. Mayo Clin Proc 69:169, 1994.

Ropper AH, Kennedy SK: Neurological and Neurosurgical Intensive Care. 3rd ed. Rockville, MD, Aspen Publishers 1993. *Chapter 3 is a brief but excellent resource, with 129 well-chosen references, on all aspects of the treatment of intracranial hypertension.*

TABLE 436–6. CAUSES OF ABNORMALLY LOW (0–50 mm) CSF PRESSURE

Dehydration-hypovolemia
Cranial-intraspinal CSF block
Post–CNS surgery
CSF fistula
Post–lumbar puncture drainage
Spontaneous-idiopathic; dural nerve sheath tear

Section Thirteen—Injury to the Head and Spinal Cord

Lawrence F. Marshall

---

437   HEAD INJURY

GENERAL CONSIDERATIONS

Head injury is a major public health problem. Nonpenetrating traumatic brain injury is responsible for more than 50,000 deaths a year in the United States, and many people have long-term intellectual and behavioral residua. Severe head injury mainly affects young people between 15 and 30 years, but spares no age or socioeconomic group. Missile injury, particularly gunshot wounds to the skull and brain, are far from confined to urban areas of socioeconomic decay.

MECHANISM OF BRAIN DAMAGE

The pathology of head injury includes a spectrum of changes. Underlying almost all nonpenetrating brain trauma is diffuse axonal injury, a condition in which axons are either sheared at the time of impact or degenerate soon after because of irreversible traumatic or ischemic damage to the fibers. Superimposed upon such white matter changes are contusions, which represent hemorrhage mixed into the tissue, and hematomas, more focal collections of blood. Hematomas can occur on the external surface of the dura (extradural hematoma), under the dura and over the underlying brain (subdural hematoma), or within the substance of the brain (intraparenchymal hematoma). In mild and moderate head injury the frequency of surgical hematomas is low. As the degree of neurologic injury increases, however, the severity of diffuse axonal injury rises in almost direct proportion, as does the frequency of intracranial hematomas.

Cell-molecular abnormalities due to regional anoxia plus direct trauma add to the above changes. Trauma releases an excess of excitatory amino acids as well as inflammatory mediators and free radicals, all in the bruised or ischemic areas. Blood-brain barrier breakdown follows, inducing tissue edema and increased intracranial pressure due to brain enlargement.

Damage to the brain as a result of traumatic injury occurs through a variety of dynamic processes. The impact, in addition to causing immediately variable degrees of abnormality, sets into motion a series of events which, if left uninterrupted, may result in much more severe changes in the tissues and even death. The last 15 years have made it increasingly apparent that primary damage to the brain that at first seems moderate and compatible with a good recovery in many cases may give way to the later development of intracranial hematoma or ischemic brain damage as a result of shock and/or hypoxia.

PRIMARY DAMAGE

Primary traumatic damage to the brain can be separated into three basic processes: (1) diffuse axonal injury (DAI), (2) brain contusion, and (3) intracranial hematoma. DAI always occurs in severe head injury and has a predilection for the brain stem, corpus callosum, and deep white matter. Experimental studies suggest that minor degrees of DAI probably occur in patients who suffer only a *concussion,* i.e., a transient loss of consciousness usually associated with no or minimal residua. With more severe head trauma, the number of areas and the severity of DAI increase proportionately. Some patients with near-fatal injury suffer white matter injuries that completely interrupt long sensorimotor pathways at the cervicomedullary junction.

Brain contusions as shown in Figure 437–1 are common. Traumatic contusions can occur throughout the brain but are more frequent on the cortical surface and in the superficial white matter. Contusions vary in size from < 2 to 3 ml to much larger. Such ar-

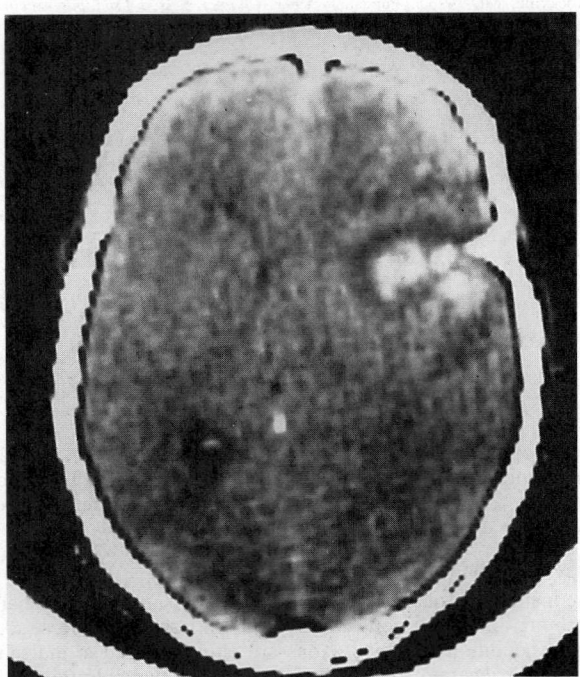

FIGURE 437–1. Brain contusion.

eas of tissue injury are important for several reasons. First, they represent areas of damage to the brain. Second, contusions may act as mass lesions because of the development of secondary edema in the surrounding tissues. Such mixtures of edema and hemorrhagic tissue may enlarge, progressively causing brain displacement and distortion. Third is intracranial hemorrhage which can result in epidural, subdural, or intraparenchymal hematomas.

Epidural hematomas usually result from moderate impact injuries. A baseball striking the head, an assault producing only a transient loss of consciousness, or a fall from a horse are typical precipitating events. Extradural hematomas characteristically follow fractures of the temporal bone associated with laceration of the middle meningeal artery. In some instances, the hemorrhage may follow a fracture tearing one of the major draining venous sinuses of the brain. The clinical course is classically described as a transient loss of consciousness, followed by a period of lucidity and then a rather abrupt deterioration. Actually, this sequence occurs in only a minority of patients: Some lose consciousness immediately following impact, whereas others deteriorate abruptly without a history of initial loss of consciousness.

In the apparently minimally injured patient brought to an emergency room following an ostensibly minor head injury CT scans are the procedure of choice because they detect both skull and major parenchymal injuries. If CT is unavailable, a skull x-ray to detect fractures should be obtained before sending the patient home. Elderly patients should always have CT scans before being discharged. Trauma patients should be hospitalized for close observation if the neurologic examination is abnormal or if consciousness is altered in any way. The early detection of extradural hemorrhages is of utmost importance because most affected patients do not initially have irreversible brain damage.

Subdural hematomas are divided into three subgroups: acute, subacute, and chronic. An *acute subdural hematoma* almost always signifies severe brain injury and is associated with significant DAI and contusions. Most such patients are unconscious from impact, and half die. Recent studies have demonstrated that early surgery for acute subdural hematomas somewhat improves outcome, particularly in patients who show little other associated injury to the brain. The frequency of subdural hematomas increases with age, presumably because age-associated brain atrophy more readily allows the expansion of such venous bleedings. Most subdural hematomas are caused by laceration of the bridging veins that drain blood from the surface of the brain into the major sinuses or by laceration of cortical veins in the region of the sylvian fissure. Acute subdural hematomas are especially likely following assaults, falls (particularly in the elderly or alcoholic), and motor vehicle accidents when the head is decelerated suddenly on impact.

Subacute subdural hematomas consist of blood clots that underlie the dura on the surface of the brain, developing from 48 hours to 1 week following injury. Some must arise within a few hours of impact but do not reach a sufficient size to cause either depression of consciousness or a focal neurologic deficit. Patients with subacute subdural hematomas are usually older than age 50, occasionally have been taking anticoagulants, and usually have less serious head injuries than those with acute subdural hematomas. Only a small percentage are in coma when first seen and, if the hematoma is diagnosed promptly following its onset, most enjoy a good outcome.

Chronic subdural hematomas have distinct qualities. They usually occur between 1 and 6 weeks following injury, often bilaterally. Many follow trivial injuries, such as striking the head on a door, with no associated loss of consciousness. Indeed, affected patients often forget the inciting event. Patients with chronic subdural hematomas characteristically come from older age groups and many suffer from chronic illnesses, including alcoholism and dementia. Headache, worse in the morning, hypersomnolence or confusion, mild focal weakness, difficulty writing, and unsteadiness are common complaints. Chronic subdural hematomas, because of age-related shrinkage of the brain, may reach a substantial size in excess of 100 cc before the patient seeks medical attention. The treatment is relatively straightforward. Some resolve spontaneously. For larger clots, a twist drill hole and puncture of the dura suffice for many patients. Many surgeons leave a drain in the subdural space to allow gravity drainage for 24 to 48 hours following evacuation of the clot. In some instances, particularly if CT scanning reveals an area of increased density, two burr holes are placed to allow irrigation of the subdural space. Craniotomy should be avoided if possible.

The third type of intracranial hematoma is the *intraparenchymal hemorrhage,* sometimes called intracerebral hemorrhage. These may vary in size from 1 to 100 ml, but they are usually considered for surgical drainage only when they exceed 15 to 20 ml. Long-term prognosis often is poor.

PREHOSPITAL CARE AND INITIAL RESUSCITATION

Head injuries often occur under circumstances that traumatize other organ systems as well. Fractures of the long bones and injuries to the chest and abdomen are common, particularly as a result of motor vehicle accidents or pedestrian-vehicle interactions. Until recently, concerns about secondary insults such as shock and hypoxia arose primarily among the more severely injured. Present evidence, however, indicates that even moderate levels of hypotension can convert a reversible brain injury to one with ischemic brain damage. Accordingly, immediate and adequate restitution of blood pressure and intravascular fluid volume, as well as early steps to prevent or treat hypoxia, represent essential preventive measures.

Utilization of the Glasgow Coma Scale (GCS) shown in Table 437–1 provides a simple and reproducible means for serially assessing the head-injured patient. This examination, which assesses the patient's ability to respond to pain, to speak, and to open his or her eyes, when performed in concert with examination of the pupils, serves as an excellent field guide to the severity of injury. All four limbs must be tested for responsiveness either to verbal command or to pain in order not to overlook focal neurologic deficits, such as hemiparesis, paraparesis, or quadriparesis. Changes in pupillary responsiveness suggest brain stem compression, which must be detected early and dealt with promptly if treatment is to be successful.

Patients who cannot follow commands, do not open their eyes to noxious stimuli, and fail to utter words or comprehensible sounds are considered in coma (GCS score of 8 or less) and require early assurance of a secured airway. The frequency of shock and hypoxia increases in proportion to the severity of injury. Hypoxia occurs in approximately one third of all severe head injuries, and pulmonary shunting affects more than half. Because of these changes, early controlled intubation, often at the scene of the injury, is highly recommended. Search for sources of hemorrhage is essential and should include the less obvious ones such as scalp lacerations and pelvic fractures. If such cannot be found, neurogenic hypotension should be suspected. Fluid resuscitation should begin at the scene, recognizing the difficulties in administering large amounts of fluid under these conditions. Current evidence suggests that even with modern paramedic systems shock often receives inadequate treatment in the field and that newer strategies, utilizing hypertonic saline or pressor agents, may be required. Studies show that the

presence of hypotension at outset almost doubles the mortality of head injury.

Once the airway has been secured and fluid resuscitation initiated, stabilization of the cervical spine and transport become the next priorities. In general, the neck should be placed in a neutral position. However, if the patient is awake and chooses to hold the neck in an unusual position, it should not be forced. Some patients with cervical spine fractures but no neurologic deficit have been made quadriplegic by ill-advised attempts to straighten the neck.

Upon arrival at the hospital the priorities of maintaining airway and circulation remain uppermost. Adequate oxygenation with a PaO_2 above 80 and moderate hyperventilation to $PaCO_2$ of 35 mm Hg to control brain swelling are initial objectives. A mean blood pressure of at least 90 mm Hg is mandatory.

CT SCANNING

The availability of rapid-sequence CT scanning has revolutionized the care of the head injured. Patients with focal neurologic deficits and severe injuries, i.e., a GCS score of 8 or less, should be scanned as soon as airway and hemodynamic stability are ensured. To minimize the risks of transportation and movement, deteriorating patients should be accompanied by a physician, and even stable but seriously injured patients should have an experienced emergency room or trauma nurse present at all times. Supervised respiratory assistance should assure adequate ventilation during transport and during the scan.

The results of CT scans heavily influence subsequent management. If a surgical lesion is demonstrated, the patient should be taken to the operating room immediately. Otherwise severe traumatic injuries are best treated in intensive care units, with lesser injuries being handled in units that provide close observation.

Several findings on the CT scan, other than intracranial hematomas, merit close attention and warn of possible deterioration. Compression or absence of the mesencephalic cistern augurs a high degree of brain swelling and death, even in patients whose clinical examination at the time suggests only a moderately severe injury. Unilateral or bilateral hemispheric swelling almost always predicts the likelihood of dangerous intracranial hypertension.

SERIAL ASSESSMENT

Close observation, with particular attention to the development of tachypnea and bradycardia, is important. Table 437–2 lists signs that portend potential intracranial catastrophe. An increase in systolic blood pressure of 15 mm Hg or more or a decline in heart rate of 15 beats per minute often gives the first hints of the development of an intracranial mass lesion.

Tachypnea holds particular importance. Respiratory rates over 20 per minute are abnormal in patients over 15 years of age and may indicate an increase in intracranial pressure or the development of pulmonary failure or infection. Similarly, increasing headache is often present but overlooked; it may reflect a rising intracranial pressure. The use of continuous flow sheets in an intermediate care setting or in a neurologic observation unit assists in monitoring the course and detecting subtle changes in vital signs.

INTENSIVE CARE MANAGEMENT OF THE SEVERELY HEAD INJURED

The overriding objective in the care of the severely head injured is to prevent further insults to the traumatized brain. The situation requires meticulous attention to detail and continuous vigilance to detect and counteract deterioration in hemodynamic, pulmonary, and neurologic function. The brain's vulnerability to secondary injury extends beyond shock and hypoxia. Fever increases the metabolic rate of the tissue by approximately 13% for each degree Celsius, a demand that the already injured brain may not be able to meet. Seizures are a major threat—they increase tissue energy requirements and trigger a rise of up to 400% in cerebral blood flow, accentuating any existing increase in the intracranial pressure.

The objectives in the critical care of head injury shown in Table 437–3 illustrate an approach that includes both the avoidance of systemic insults to the brain and the treatment of intracranial hypertension. Elevations of intracranial pressure above the normal of 15 mm Hg accompany most severe head injuries, and some believe that they contribute directly to further tissue damage if left untreated. Compression of the mesencephalic cistern detected by CT

TABLE 437–1. GLASGOW COMA SCALE

The Glasgow Coma Scale is a practical means of monitoring changes in level of consciousness, based upon eye opening and verbal and motor responses. The responsiveness of the patient can be expressed by summation of the figures. The lowest score is 3, the highest is 15.

Eyes open	Spontaneously (eyes open does not imply awareness)	4
	To speech (any speech, not necessarily a command)	3
	To pain (should not use supraorbital pressure for pain stimulus)	2
	Never	1
Best verbal response	Oriented (to time, person, place)	5
	Confused speech (disoriented)	4
	Inappropriate (swearing, yelling)	3
	Incomprehensible sounds (moaning, groaning)	2
	None	1
Best motor response	Obeys commands	6
	Localizes pain (deliberate or purposeful movement)	5
	Withdrawal (moves away from stimulus)	4
	Abnormal flexion (decortication)	3
	Extension (decerebration)	2
	None (flaccidity)	1
	Total Score	

TABLE 437–2. SIGNS OF POTENTIAL INTRACRANIAL CATASTROPHE AND WHAT THEY MAY SIGNIFY

Signs	Changes	Potential Meaning
Respiration	Rate > 20	Pulmonary edema or pneumonitis
Pulse	Change > 10/min and/or heart rate < 60	Each may indicate elevated ICP with transtentorial herniation
Blood pressure	Change in systolic > 15 mm Hg and/or widening pulse pressure	
Headache*	Is it increasing?	Often indicates increased ICP
Pupils	Enlargement Asymmetry Irregular shape (oval) Decrease in reactivity Change from preresuscitation	
Motor	Decrease of 1 point on GCS New focal deficit	Increased mass effect New hemorrhage Recurrent hemorrhage
Level of consciousness		Increased ICP Seizures Hypotension
	Abrupt decrease	
	Transient	Seizures Hypoxia
	Progressive decrease	Rehemorrhage Brain stem involvement Septicemia Electrolyte imbalance Vasospasm Hydrocephalus

* All changes except headache may occur in both awake and unconscious patients. GCS = Glasgow coma scale; ICP = intracranial pressure.

scans and referred to as "diffuse swelling," is frequent in patients with even moderately severe injuries. Because mortality in such cases can be reduced from approximately 85 to 35% with early and rapid intervention for intracranial hypertension, most academic neurosurgical centers record the intracranial pressure (ICP) continuously so as to treat intracranial hypertension whenever it develops. Several available techniques are discussed in the references to this chapter.

ICP monitoring should not be initiated in patients with coagulation disturbances. Patients in whom multiple contusions can be detected by a first CT scan can be assumed to have a trauma-related coagulopathy that will correct itself within a few hours, after which a ventricular cannula can be inserted.

The treatment of *traumatic intracranial hypertension* is central to the intensive care of the critically brain injured patient. The cornerstone of management is to adjust baseline ventilation to maintain a PCO_2 in the 35 to 37 mm Hg range, permitting brief periods of greater hyperventilation to respond to sudden increases in intracranial pressures. Levels of extreme hyperventilation may produce excessive vasoconstriction. The head should be maintained in a neutral position because turning it to the right or left may introduce venous obstruction and a rise in ICP. Also, the head should be elevated to not more than 30 degrees. Intravascular volume must be

TABLE 437–3. ICU MANAGEMENT OF SEVERE HEAD INJURY AND INTRACRANIAL HYPERTENSION

1. Head elevated 30 degrees and in neutral plane
2. Intubation with controlled ventilation to an arterial $PaCO_2$ of 30–35 mm Hg
3. Good pulmonary toilet
4. Maintain fluid balance with 0.5 normal saline
5. Maintain systolic arterial pressure between 100 and 160 mm Hg
6. Maintain cerebral perfusion pressure > 70 mm Hg (CPP = MAP − ICP)
7. Adequate sedation
8. Muscle relaxants prn (must use sedation concurrently)
9. Maintain normothermia
10. Adequate anticonvulsant therapy
11. Ventricular drainage for intracranial hypertension
12. Mannitol 0.25 mg/kg if No. 11 fails or is not available
13. Hypnotic for elevated ICP in patients with diffuse or hemispheric swelling

maintained using balanced salt solutions. Dextrose and water should be avoided. Head trauma often induces salt retention initially so that half normal saline may be most useful to meet fluid needs. Because hyperglycemia is known to exacerbate ischemic brain injury in experimental animals, it appears wise to avoid glucose infusions.

Sedation and pain relief are essential in the initial phases of treatment. Morphine sulfate by continuous infusion of 2 to 8 mg per hour is the least complicated and most effective regimen. Muscle relaxation with vecuronium or other short-acting agents is occasionally helpful in patients in whom ICP is difficult to control, but otherwise is not necessary. Muscle relaxants should be accompanied by adequate sedation.

Anticonvulsants have a limited but important use in acute traumatic head injury. Phenytoin given for the first 7 days after injury reduces the incidence of post-traumatic epilepsy during that period. No study has shown a protective effect when medication was continued beyond the first week.

LONG-TERM CONSEQUENCES OF SEVERE HEAD INJURY

Severe head injury causes serious long-term intellectual and behavioral impairment. Most such patients suffer difficulties in recent memory, abstract thinking, and rapid information processing. Depression, fatigue, and impetuosity accentuate these cognitive deficits. Long-term deficits of motor function are relatively uncommon and less socioeconomically important. Many rehabilitation programs have been developed to assist the severely head injured in the management of these problems. Counseling of the family is essential. Divorce, suicide, and spouse abuse can be reduced in frequency by early intervention.

MINOR HEAD INJURY

Minor head injury is defined as including a GCS score of 13 to 15 following emergency room or hospital admission combined with a return to a normal level of consciousness within 24 hours. Most but not all such patients have normal CT scans. Patients suffering minor head injuries characteristically experience early post-traumatic problems with recent memory, concentration, and abstract thinking. In most instances such problems subside within the first 1 to 3 months following minor injury. Approximately 15% are left with cognitive deficits that do not completely remit. Age is a specific risk factor, and many elderly persons develop chronic dizziness and disequilibrium after even minor trauma. Such symptoms are classified as a *post-traumatic or postconcussive syndrome*. Recent evidence indicates that a small percentage of patients suffer modest but permanent residual cognitive impairment.

Many patients with minor head injuries suffer transiently from insomnia, depression, and headache. Early support and reassurance from the physician often improve these symptoms. If headache persists for more than 60 to 90 days, propranolol, 30 to 60 mg in three divided doses, may bring relief.

MODERATE HEAD INJURY

Patients who have not been rendered comatose but have a depressed level of consciousness for several hours or days following injury are classified as having suffered moderate head injuries. These patients have GCS scores of 9 to 12. Such patients almost always suffer measurable cognitive and behavioral difficulties over the long term. Nevertheless, many eventually return to gainful employment. Even so, the potential for social disruption is high, and traits of impetuousness and heightened irritability often create socioeconomic problems. Depression is frequent and may respond to tricylic antidepressants. Intervention, using a variety of psychological services including social workers and psychiatrists, has a more favorable impact if carried out early rather than after the problems have overwhelmed the patient and family.

Foulkes MA, Eisenberg HM, Jane JA, et al.: Report on the traumatic coma data bank. J Neurosurg (Suppl) 75:51, 1991. *Outcome data and much more are described in a cohort of 1030 head-injury victims treated from onset in a multicenter trial.*

Marshall SB, Marshall LF, Vos H, et al.: Neuroscience Critical Care: Pathophysiology and Patient Management. Philadelphia, WB Saunders, 1990. *Particular emphasis on assessment of the neurologically impaired patient, modern neuroradiology, and intensive care.*

Ropper AH (ed.): Neurological and Neurosurgical Intensive Care, 3rd ed. New York, Raven Press, 1993. *A well-edited volume that contains an excellent, detailed chapter on head injury by Chestnut and Marshall.*

Temkin NR, Dikmen SS, Wilensky AJ, et al.: A randomized, double-blind study of phenytoin for the prevention of post-traumatic seizures. N Engl J Med 323:497, 1990. *Four hundred and four patients with serious head trauma were randomly assigned treatment with phenytoin or placebo within 24 hours of injury; significant reduction in seizure incidence (P < 0.001) occurred only between drug loading time and day 7.*

438 SPINAL CORD INJURY

Most injuries to the spinal column do not traumatize the spinal cord, but there are still approximately 35 spinal cord injuries per million Americans each year. In addition to the neurologic deficit that such injuries can produce, they often result in persistent and severe pain and, if not treated properly, bony deformity. The mortality rate of spinal cord injury has fallen to less than 5% and long-term survival is now the rule. Associated with this, however, are tremendous costs stemming from medical treatment, lost occupations, and the need for life-long medical and emotional support systems.

NATURE OF THE INJURY

About half of all serious spinal injuries affect the cervical level, with nearly 50% of such patients becoming quadriplegic. Next most frequent is high thoracic cord damage, with the remainder distributed variously at lower spinal levels. Three major abnormalities damage the tissue: destruction from either direct trauma, e.g., gunshot wounds or secondary bone displacement; compression by displaced or broken bones; and ischemia due to compression or laceration of spinal arteries. Postinjury edema of spinal soft tissues and the cord itself accentuates these changes.

Spinal cord injuries can be categorized as complete or incomplete. Acute, complete injuries most often produce *spinal shock*, with loss of all sensorimotor functions including flaccidity and loss of reflexes at and below the level of injury. A few such cases may involve sustained priapism. Less severe injuries can produce a *central cord syndrome* resulting from ischemia or hematomas of the cervical cord (Fig. 438–1). These result in a syringomyelia-like clinical syndrome characterized by weakness in the distal upper extremities combined with impaired or lost pain and temperature sensations in the arms but sparing of touch and often of all functions below the cervical cord level. The upper extremity weakness generally improves in such cases. Other patterns of cord injury may produce an anterior spinal artery syndrome (see Ch. 443) or a partial hemisection, producing distal weakness and proprioceptive loss ipsilateral to the cord damage accompanied by contralateral pain and temperature impairment.

EMERGENCY MANAGEMENT

For the physician, crucial elements in treatment arise at the accident scene or within the first few hours at the hospital. After that time, experienced neurosurgeons or orthopedists provide care, supplemented if possible by resources of a tertiary care center.

At the site of injury three major concerns are paramount: maintenance of ventilation, protection against shock, and neck immobilization to prevent further spinal cord damage. Damage to high thoracic or cervical spinal levels creates the immediate risk of ventilatory failure due to acute paralysis of intercostal-abdominal muscles, the diaphragm, or both. Untoward movement of the neck risks converting a partial injury to a complete one, making nasotracheal intubation preferable to standard peroral intubation. Tracheostomy or cricothyroidotomy should be avoided if possible because these procedures often put pressure on the vertebral column.

Severe hypotension often follows cervical injury because the lesion interrupts the descending sympathetic pathways; bradycardia characteristically accompanies the low blood pressure. Such neurogenic hypotension can be distinguished from hypovolemic shock by the tachycardia of the latter. In either case, the legs should be elevated gently to improve venous return and fluids delivered in amounts sufficient to counter both the traumatic and neurogenic aspects of the problem. Severe hypotension during the early minutes

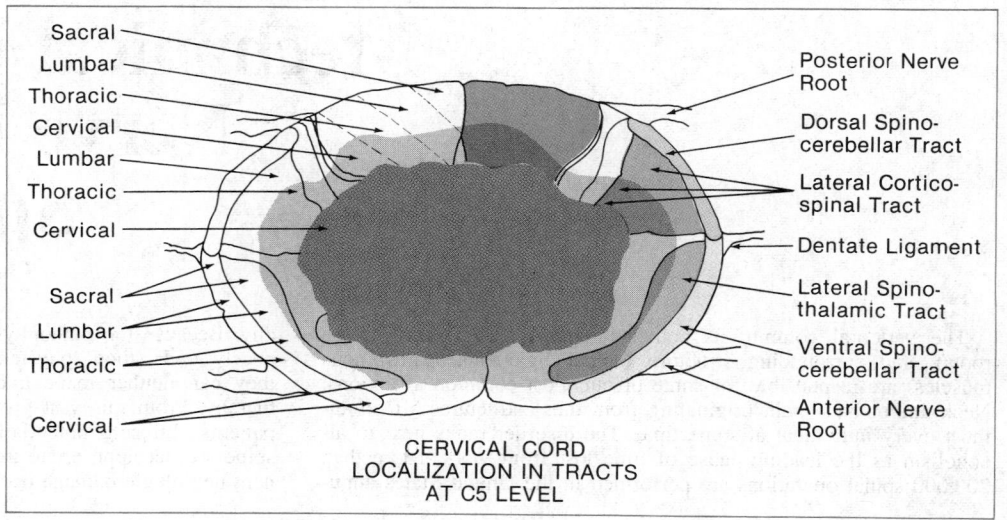

FIGURE 438–1. Diagrammatic description of the spinal pathways at the lower cervical level showing the usual distribution of the contusion-hemorrhage that causes a central cord syndrome.

or hours after injury is itself a potential cause of spinal cord damage.

The neck and spine should be immobilized as gently as possible at the injury site, using a carrying board, sandbags and adhesive tape, or a Philadelphia collar. Soft collars are ineffective. The head is best maintained in a neutral position but should not be forced into such an attitude lest the maneuver induce further spinal cord damage.

Recent controlled studies indicate that giving large doses of methylprednisolone within 8 hours of the onset of trauma appears to reduce the degree of eventual neurologic dysfunction in acute traumatic paraplegia. Dose levels used in the study trial included immediate intravenous administrations of 30 mg per kilogram of body weight of the steroid followed by continuous infusion of 5.4 mg per kilogram per hour for the next 23 hours. Treatment begun more than 8 hours after injury was not helpful.

HOSPITAL CARE

The medical care of spinal cord injuries is a specialty unto itself. Such patients often are critically ill owing to a combination of systemic injuries, blood and fluid loss, various fractures, and infections. Considerable expertise is required for the accurate interpretation of spinal radiographs. The treating physician must not accept as normal plain radiographs that do not demonstrate all of the cervical vertebrae. An overlooked spine injury can be catastrophic if, for example, an odontoid fracture or an injury to C7 results later in sudden instability. Patients with cervical fracture-dislocations usually are placed in skeletal traction with skull fixation prior to administering definitive surgical repair. Injuries to the thoracic or lumbar level are the exception; because traction has little benefit, open surgery, when indicated, usually is carried out earlier.

Medical management emphasizes the guiding principles of trauma care. Rotating beds reduce the risk of decubitus erosions, meticulous chest physiotherapy and pulmonary toilet can minimize lung complications, and cardiovascular as well as fluid-electrolyte stability requires continuous attention. Pneumatic antiembolism stockings, vigorous fluid replacement, and early mobilization have reduced the frequency of deep venous thromboses in such patients by one third. Vena caval filters should be considered for severely immobilized patients who do not require early surgery. Nearly all patients with traumatic cord injury require prolonged urinary bladder catheterization. Meticulous effort to prevent infection should be applied from the start and, whenever staff experience permits, in-

dwelling catheters should be replaced by intermittent catheterization at 4- to 6-hour intervals. Acidification of the urine with vitamin C or cranberry juice helps to reduce the incidence of infection.

Trauma patients require heavy nutrition to feed the demands of wound healing and the efforts of rehabilitation. For those who cannot eat, enteral solutions sufficient to meet caloric need can be started within 3 to 4 days after injury. Every effort should be given to supplying appetizing food and vitamins subsequently.

Autonomic dysfunction complicates the convalescence of more than half of patients who suffer severe spinal cord injuries above the midthoracic level. Disconnected distal autonomic pathways can induce a variety of troublesome phenomena, including systemic hypertension, reflex sweating, skin flushing, headache, and painful flexor spasms of the lower extremities. Bladder distention and infection frequently trigger such reflex dysautonomia and require urgent treatment. Diazepam, in small doses initially, and baclofen given chronically may be useful for the treatment of reflex spasms. Some centers have successfully used the continuous intrathecal administration of baclofen by an indwelling pump to prevent such disabling reflex spasms.

PHYSICAL AND OCCUPATIONAL THERAPY AND REHABILITATION

Almost all patients with spinal cord injury require prolonged postacute care. Those with complete transections have suffered a devastating injury with life-long functional and psychiatric consequences. Early physical and emotional therapy are crucial. Early range of motion prevents contractures, diminishes the risk of venous thrombosis, protects the skin, and boosts morale. A comprehensive and individualized management plan is essential. Patients and family members must be counseled in detail about probable changes in lifestyle. All of these features are best carried out in experienced rehabilitation centers that can provide assistance in home modification, driver retraining, and vocational rehabilitation. Depression following an initial period of denial occurs in almost all patients and may be masked by jocularity. If the rehabilitation team moves quickly to provide emotional as well as physical management, many patients with spinal cord injury can return to a competitive place in society. Most of the injured do best if a single physician organizes the long-term aspects of urinary tract management, skin care, sexual problems, and emotional-vocational needs.

Bracken MB, Shepard MJ, Hellenbrand KG, et al.: A randomized, controlled trial of methylprednisolone or naloxone in the treatment of acute spinal cord injury. N Engl J Med 322:1405, 1990. *The first study to clearly demonstrate the efficacy of pharmacologic treatment for spinal cord injury.*
Cooper PR: Management of Posttraumatic Spinal Instability. *In* Neurosurgical Topics. Park Ridge, IL, American Association of Neurological Surgeons, 1990.

Section Fourteen— Mechanical Lesions of Nerve Roots and Spinal Cord

Jerome B. Posner

The vertebral column, its contents (spinal cord, exiting nerve roots), and surrounding structure (spinal ligaments, paraspinous muscles) are responsible for some of our most common afflictions. Neck and/or back pain originating from these structures affects almost every individual at some time. The disorder ranks next to alcoholism as the leading cause of time lost from work. More than 200,000 spinal operations are performed in the United States annu-

ally. Because the pathophysiology of most neck and back pain is poorly understood, physicians often encounter patients in whom they can neither make a certain diagnosis nor prescribe rational therapy. From this vast group they must cull the small number of patients suffering potentially remediable structural disease of the spine so that appropriate treatment can be instituted before permanent neurologic damage occurs.

439 ANATOMY, PHYSIOLOGY, AND DIFFERENTIAL DIAGNOSIS

ANATOMY AND PHYSIOLOGY OF THE SPINE

The spine is composed of two functional segments. The *anterior segment* containing two adjacent vertebral bodies separated by an intervertebral disc bears weight and cushions the spine during such activities as walking and running. The posterior segment is composed of the vertebral arches, the transverse processes, the posterior spinous processes, and the paired articulations known as *facets* with the facet joint between them. It protects the contained spinal cord and nerve roots and allows the spine to move in extension and rotation. The midcervical and lower lumbar levels are particularly mobile, making them susceptible to mechanical disorders such as osteoarthritis and herniated discs (see Ch. 440). Several ligaments offer the spine passive support and paravertebral muscles support the spine actively by voluntary and reflex contraction.

The *periosteum* of the vertebral body is pain-sensitive so that compression fractures are at least initially painful (Fig. 439–1). The *intervertebral disc* is probably not pain-sensitive. However, if the disc bulges and compresses the outer layers of the anulus fibrosus or the posterior longitudinal ligament, pain may result. Posteriorly, the synovium-lined *facet joints* are pain-sensitive and may be a source of neck and back pain, although the intraspinal ligaments holding the posterior elements are not. Most of the pain-sensitive structures are innervated by the recurrent meningeal or sinuvertebral nerves, a branch of each spinal nerve that arises just distal to the dorsal root ganglion and re-enters the spinal canal through the intervertebral foramen. The *paravertebral muscles* surrounding and supporting the spine are also pain-sensitive, particularly when overstretched or in spasm. These muscles are probably the most common source of acute neck and back pain. The pain-sensitive *nerve root* usually occupies only a small portion of the intervertebral foramen through which it exits the spinal canal. When the spine is extended (i.e., hyperlordotic posture), the intervertebral foramen becomes smaller, potentially impinging on the nerve root and leading to overlap of the facet joints, giving potential irritation of pain-sensitive synovial membranes.

The spinal cord and its attached motor, sensory, and autonomic nerve roots are the primary occupants of the spinal canal. The spinal cord itself extends in the adult from the first cervical to the first lumbar vertebral body, and the spinal roots continue in the subarachnoid space to the second sacral vertebra. The caudal portion of the spinal cord is called the *conus medullaris,* and the bunched

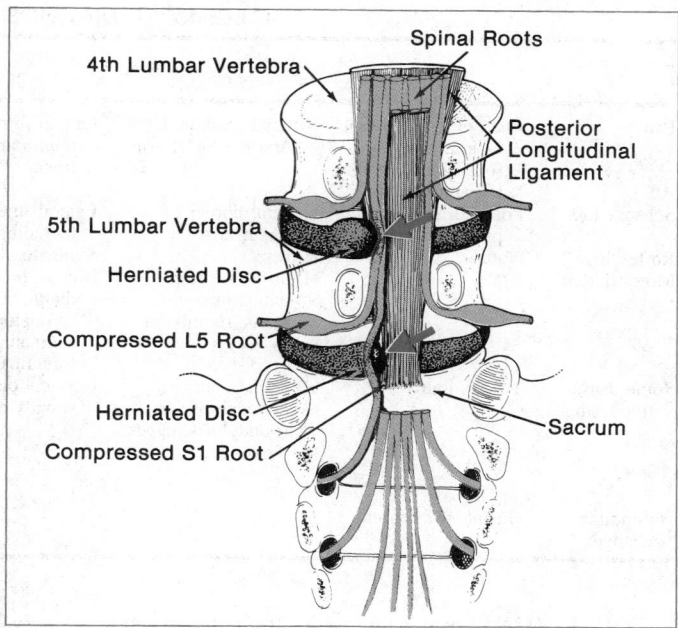

FIGURE 439–2. Nerve root compression by herniated disc. The figure illustrates that the posterior longitudinal ligament tapers as it reaches the lower lumbar area, leaving a weakened area laterally allowing disc herniation. An L4–L5 disc is shown lateral to the L5 root, displacing it medially; a herniated disc between L5 and S1 displaces the root laterally. (From Posner JB: Back pain and epidural spinal cord compression. Med Clin North Am 71:185, 1987.)

lumbar and sacral roots that exit below the cord are the *cauda equina.*

Within the canal several processes can compress or deform the spinal cord and its roots. In the cervical spine, the spinal cord and vertebral segments lie at approximately the same level; thus, the C5 vertebral body marks the C5 spinal segment and emerging nerve roots are virtually horizontal. The more caudad spinal cord segments and vertebral segments move out of alignment so that thoracic spinal cord segments gradually become two to three levels higher than the corresponding vertebral segments. Most of the lumbar and sacral cord is found between T10 and L1 lumbar segments. As a result, the nerve roots travel a descending pathway in the subarachnoid space before exiting via the vertebral foramen. In addition, because there is a C8 spinal segment and no C8 vertebral body, cervical spine nerve roots above C8 exit above the vertebral body with the same number (e.g., the C4 root exits between C3 and C4). Thus, a herniated C4–C5 disc may compress the C5 or C6 root but not the C4 root.

In the thoracic and lumbar spine, nerve roots leave the intervertebral foramen just below the pedicle arising from the vertebra of the same number so that a herniated disc between L4 and L5 vertebral bodies usually compresses the L5 nerve root; a herniated disc between L5 and S1 usually compresses the S1 root (Fig. 439–2). If the disc protrudes medially (less common than laterally protruding discs), an L4–L5 disc may compress sacral roots rather than the L5 lumbar root. Only if the disc completely extrudes into the vertebral canal does an L4–L5 disc compress the L4 root.

The size of the vertebral canal relative to the spinal cord varies from level to level and among individuals. There is generally more space in the lumbar and cervical areas than in the thoracic area. In some individuals the spinal canal is congenitally small (spinal stenosis). Disc herniation or osteoarthritis is more likely to cause myelopathy in these individuals than in those with capacious canals.

TYPES OF PAIN

The cardinal symptom of lesions of the spine or its contents is pain. The type and location of pain often help substantially in diagnosis.

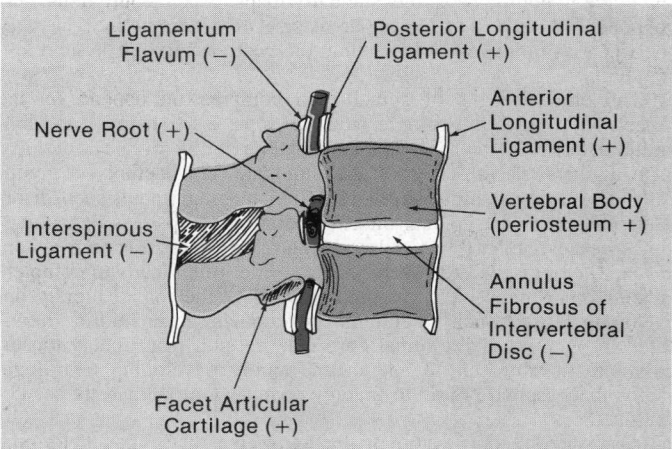

FIGURE 439–1. Pain-sensitive structures of the spine. This lateral view indicates the pain-sensitive structures with a plus sign (+) and those structures not pain-sensitive with a minus sign (−). (From Posner JB: Back pain and epidural spinal cord compression. Med Clin North Am 71:185, 1987.)

TABLE 439-1. DIAGNOSIS OF NERVE ROOT LESIONS

	C2–C3	C5	C6	C7	C8	Nerve T1
Pain	Back of head, lateral face, behind ear (occasionally vertex and orbit)	Medial scapula, lateral border of arm	Lateral forearm, thumb and index finger	Posterior arm, lateral hand, mid-forearm, and medial scapula	Medial forearm and hand	Deep aching in shoulder and axilla to olecranon
Sensory loss	Posterior scalp, pinna, lateral face	Lateral border of upper arm	Lateral forearm, including thumb	Mid-forearm and middle finger	Medial forearm and little finger	Axilla down to olecranon
Reflex loss	None	Biceps	Supinator	Triceps	Finger stretch	None
Motor deficit	None	Deltoid, supraspinatus, infraspinatus, rhomboids	Biceps, brachioradialis, brachialis, (pronators and supinators of forearm)	Latissimus dorsi, pectoralis major, triceps, wrist extensors, wrist flexors	Finger flexors, finger extensors, flexor carpi ulnaris (thenar muscles in some patients)	All small hand muscles (in some thenar muscles via C8)
Some causative lesions	Tumor, injury	Brachial neuritis, cervical disc or spondylosis, upper plexus injury	Cervical disc or spondylosis	Cervical disc or spondylosis	Pancoast tumor, rare in disc lesions or spondylosis, metastatic tumor, thoracic outlet syndrome	Pancoast tumor, cervical rib, outlet syndromes, metastatic carcinoma in deep cervical nodes
Autonomic changes	Gustatory sweating					Horner's syndrome

LOCAL PAIN. Local pain results from the irritation of nerve endings at the site of the pathologic process. Metastatic tumors and osteoporotic collapse of a vertebral body cause pain at the site of the lesion by irritation of nerve endings in the periosteum of the vertebral body. Metastatic tumors involving the vertebral body that do not distort the periosteum are usually painless. Intervertebral discs cause local pain when they compress nerve endings in the anulus fibrosus or posterior longitudinal ligament. Local pain is usually steady, aching, and associated with tenderness to palpation or percussion. Most spine pain from mechanical causes (e.g., herniated disc) occurs either in the neck or low back because these structures are most mobile and more subject to injury. Tumors often strike the thoracic area, and osteoporotic vertebral collapse often affects the structurally weaker thoracic vertebral bodies.

The *character* of the local pain is helpful diagnostically. Pain caused by lumbar muscle or ligamentous strain or by herniated disc usually disappears when the patient lies recumbent. The pain of spinal stenosis, on the contrary, is often absent when lying or sitting and occurs only when the patient walks. Vertebral metastases with or without epidural spinal cord compression cause pain that is often more prominent when lying and sometimes is relieved by sitting up; many patients with spinal cord compression elect to sleep in a sitting position. Even if pain is absent in the lying position, movement such as turning over in bed or arising may be particularly painful.

REFERRED PAIN. Referred pain arises from deep somatic or visceral structures and is perceived at a distant site within the same spinal segment but not necessarily in dermatomal distribution (radicular pain, see below). Referred pain, like local pain, has a deep aching quality and is often associated with tenderness of subcutaneous tissues and muscles at the site of referral. Maneuvers that affect local pain usually have the same effect on referred pain. Pain referred from pathologic abnormalities of the cervical spine often is either just medial to the scapula or over the lateral aspect of the arm; pain referred from the low back is usually appreciated in the buttocks and posterior thighs, although rarely below the knees. Pain from the upper lumbar spine is often referred to the flank, groin, and anterior thigh. Pain also can be referred to the spine from lesions of thoracic or abdominal viscera, a prominent example being the back pain from pancreatic carcinoma.

MUSCLE PAIN. Muscle pain occurs when an injury to or structural abnormality of the spine induces paravertebral muscle spasm. Sustained contraction of paravertebral muscles gives rise to chronic aching pain, usually felt lateral to the midline of the neck or back. Palpation may reveal evidence of spasm and tenderness. At times, when areas of extreme sensitivity (trigger points) are palpated, the pain may be felt not only locally in the muscle but also may be referred to distant structures. Trigger points define myofascial pain syndromes, common causes of neck and back pain without structural abnormalities of the spine (see Ch. 405).

RADICULAR PAIN. Radicular pain is the prominent symptom of nerve root compression. Nerve roots are not usually pain-sensitive. However, chronic compression leads to edema and, perhaps, inflammation and demyelination; the root then becomes sensitive to stretching or compression. When compressed, the pain may be experienced only in the cutaneous distribution (dermatome) of the involved root or may be felt locally and deep in muscles that it supplies. Root pain is usually exacerbated by increasing intraspinal pressure by coughing, sneezing, and straining.

FUNICULAR PAIN. Funicular pain is caused by compression of the long tracts of the spinal cord. It is less sharp than radicular pain and often described as a cold, unpleasant sensation in the extremity. It is more diffuse than radicular pain but is usually exacerbated by movements that stretch the cord (neck flexion, straight leg raising) or increase intraspinal pressure.

SIGNS OF NERVE ROOT AND SPINAL CORD DYSFUNCTION

In addition to pain, chronic compression of nerve roots can produce paresthesias, sensory loss, weakness, atrophy, and hyporeflexia in root-supplied areas, thus localizing the lesion. Knowing the myotomal and dermatomal distribution of spinal roots (Table 439–1) often allows one to localize the lesion and suggest its cause: Involvement of a single root is more likely to occur with intervertebral disc herniation (see Ch. 440), whereas multiple root dysfunction is likely to be caused by tumor or chronic inflammation. Myotomal and dermatomal localization must be used cautiously. Not every body obeys the standard maps. Also, contiguous dermatomes overlap, and the apparent size of a dermatome can vary between examinations, depending on central nervous system excitability.

The clinical signs of spinal cord compression depend on the speed with which the compression develops, the transverse and longitudinal site of the lesion, and the vulnerability of the individual spinal fibers. The spinal cord accommodates considerably to gradually developing compression (e.g., from meningiomas); such disorders can cause the gradual onset of painless paraparesis or paraplegia. Because of this accommodation, subsequent decompression, even when patients are severely paraparetic, often leads to complete resolution of neurologic symptoms. On the other hand, rapidly developing lesions such as epidural hematomas, acute midline herniated discs, or epidural spinal cord compression from metastatic tumor are usually painful and cause rapidly developing neurologic signs that respond poorly to therapy once severe paraparesis has developed.

The site of compression in the transverse plane may determine clinical signs. Laterally located lesions compressing one side of the spinal cord may cause the Brown-Séquard syndrome (ipsilateral hemiparesis, vibration and position sense loss, with contralateral pain and temperature loss); compression of the posterior portion of the cord may cause bilateral position and vibratory loss, with

TABLE 439-1. DIAGNOSIS OF NERVE ROOT LESIONS *Continued*

Roots T4	T10	L2	L3	L4	L5	S1	S2–S4
Anterior chest and/or upper back	Midback and/or anterior abdomen	Across thigh	Across thigh	Down to medial malleolus	Back of thigh, lateral calf, dorsum of foot	Back of thigh, back of calf, lateral foot	Buttocks, genitalia, back of thigh
Usually none (upper back and chest at nipple level)	Usually none (midback and abdomen at umbilicus level)	Often none	Often none	Medial leg	Dorsum of foot	Behind lateral malleolus	Buttocks, genitalia
None	Decreased abdominal reflex	None	Adductor reflex	Knee jerk	None	Ankle jerk	Bulbocavernosus
Not discernible	None	Hip flexion, adduction of thigh	Knee extension, adduction of thigh	Inversion of foot	Dorsiflexion of toes and foot (latter L4 also)	Plantar flexion and eversion of foot	Bladder and bowel
Intravertebral or paravertebral tumor, herpes zoster	Intravertebral and paravertebral tumor, herpes zoster	Neurofibroma, meningioma, neoplastic disease; disc lesions very rare except at L4 <5%			Disc lesions, metastatic malignancy, neurofibromas, meningioma		Tumor, midline disc
Chest wall, piloerection, hyperhidrosis, unilateral gynecomastia, galactorrhea	Chest wall, piloerection, hyperhidrosis, retrograde ejaculation	Alterations in temperature and color of all or parts of the leg or thigh					Incontinence, impotence, urinary retention

preservation of pain and temperature sensation and of motor power. However, most lesions twist the cord as they compress it and also interfere with the vascular supply to sites beyond the compression. Accordingly, one can depend only in a general way on the neurologic signs to evaluate the exact transverse site of compression. Cervical lesions cause quadriplegia; thoracic lesions, paraplegia; and upper lumbar lesions, normal motor function with bowel and bladder dysfunction and extensor plantar responses (conus medullaris syndrome). Lesions below the first lumbar vertebral body compress the cauda equina, causing loss of bowel and bladder function with lower motor neuron leg weakness and normal plantar reflexes.

The corticospinal tracts and posterior columns are more vulnerable to compression than others. As a result, weakness, spasticity, and reflex hyperactivity tend to be the earliest signs of spinal cord compression, with paresthesias, and vibratory and position sense loss occurring soon thereafter. Loss of pain and temperature sensation and of bladder and bowel function usually occur late.

APPROACH TO THE PATIENT

Most mechanical lesions of the spine and its contents begin with pain and only later cause other neurologic dysfunction. There are many causes of neck or back pain. One survey listed over 100 causes (Table 439-2). The task for the physician is to separate potentially serious disease from more common causes of back pain.

HISTORY. The diagnostic evaluation begins with the history. Most spine pain begins acutely or subacutely and often follows, by minutes to hours, some unaccustomed physical activity, particularly lifting or bending. Patients may awaken stiff and sore in the morning or may develop acute back pain on arising without any obvious precipitating event. Most neck pain begins as a stiff neck, often on awakening, without a history of unusual activity. In many patients, neck or low back pain recurs episodically over many years. Most neck or back pain is dull and aching in quality, exacerbated by movement and relieved by rest. Pain that is present when the patient is immobile and cannot be relieved by positional manipulation should lead the physician to consider a more serious disorder (e.g., tumor or extruded disc). *Radicular pain,* particularly if accompanied by paresthesias or loss of sensation, indicates mechanical compression of the nerve root supplying that dermatome and implies identifiable structural disease (e.g., herniated disc). *Referred pain* does not imply compression of a root.

EXAMINATION. Special attention should be paid to mobility of the spine and paravertebral structures. Most patients who complain of a stiff neck have some limitation of movement of the cervical spine, but if gradual movement of the cervical spine causes intense

pain, if pain on neck flexion is referred to the thoracic or lumbar area, or if neck flexion causes paresthesias radiating into the arms, legs, or back (Lhermitte's sign), spinal cord compression should be suspected. Most low back pain not caused by a herniated disc is exacerbated by flexion and relieved by lying down. The paravertebral muscles are often in spasm, and tender to palpation and straighten the normally lordotic lumbar spine. Almost any severe low back pain, particularly if it radiates into a lower extremity, can increase when the extended leg is raised from the bed (straight leg raising sign). However, pain referred to the contralateral back or leg when the nonpainful leg is raised (crossed straight leg raising) implies

TABLE 439-2. SOME CAUSES OF BACK PAIN

Common Causes
  Degenerative disorders
    Osteoarthritis, facet syndrome
    Herniated disc
    Spinal stenosis
    Nerve root entrapment
  Muscle dysfunction
    Spasms, fatigue, fibromyalgia, and myofascial pain
  Psychosomatic (e.g., stress, conversion reaction, tension states)
  Trauma
    Lumbar strain (acute or chronic)
Less Common Causes
  Congenital disorders
    Facet tropism (asymmetry)
    Transitional vertebra
    Spondylolysis and spondylolisthesis
  Infections (e.g., disc space infection, tuberculosis, epidural and subdural abscess, herpes zoster, meningitis, sacroiliac joint infection)
  Inflammatory diseases (e.g., ankylosing spondylitis, arachnoiditis, rheumatoid arthritis)
  Metabolic disorders (e.g., osteoporosis, gout, diabetic neuropathy, Paget's disease)
  Postoperative (e.g., sequelae of scar formation, arachnoiditis)
  Scoliosis (e.g., idiopathic, postparalytic, aging)
  Trauma
    Lumbosacral, sacroiliac strain
    Compression fracture (vertebral body or transverse process)
  Dislocation or subluxation
  Tumors
    Benign bone and neural tumors (e.g., neurinoma, ependymoma, meningioma, osteoid osteoma, hemangioma, osteoblastoma)
    Malignant bone and neural tumors
      Primary (e.g., multiple myeloma, osteosarcoma)
      Secondary (metastases)
  Visceral disease (e.g., visceral inflammation, female pelvic pathology, retroperitoneal pathology, aortic aneurysm, prostatic disease)

root compression. Forced extension of the hip (reverse straight leg raising) can elicit pain from upper lumbar root disease (L4 and above). Point tenderness over a spinous process raises the suspicion of involvement of the vertebra by either tumor or infection.

The neurologic examination is important. Sensory loss, reflex diminution, and weakness all suggest neurologic disease that requires further evaluation. The distribution of abnormalities localizes the lesion. Patients in severe pain may be reluctant to move the painful part, making normal muscles appear weak. Likewise, guarding can affect deep tendon reflexes, either increasing or decreasing them with respect to the normal side. Clear and reproducible neurologic signs, particularly sensory loss in a dermatomal distribution or a diminished stretch reflex, imply root compression.

Careful examination can reveal inconsistencies (e.g., leg pain on straight leg raising that appears when the patient is recumbent but not when sitting) that suggest a psychological rather than a physiologic basis.

LABORATORY AIDS TO INVESTIGATION. For most patients with back or neck pain, laboratory tests are neither required nor helpful. Plain radiographs of the spine rarely reveal clinically unsuspected findings. Radiographic examination of neck or back should be undertaken only when the history and examination suggest specific findings (e.g., fracture or dislocation). If the clinical examination points to other significant disease of the neck or back (e.g., herniated disc) and if pain does not respond to conservative measures in a few weeks, the physician should proceed directly to MRI, which can identify all elements of the spinal column and its contents in multiple planes. Patients suspected of harboring tumors, infection, or vascular disease should be imaged without delay.

The only abnormalities not easily identified by MRI are subluxations of vertebral bodies with movement. Flexion and extension plain radiographs of the neck or back settle that issue. Images of the neck and back must be interpreted with caution because degenerative disc changes are frequently found in asymptomatic patients and increase with age. MRI, even though more expensive than CT and *radionuclide bone scan,* is so much more sensitive that it will probably replace these tests. Invasive tests, such as *myelograms, spinal angiography,* and *discography,* should be reserved for specialists. Thermography has no value.

Electromyography and nerve conduction studies, particularly using H and F responses, can help identify the presence and site of proximal sensory and motor root damage and anterior horn cell dysfunction. *Somatosensory evoked potentials* can be recorded along the spinal cord or in the brain after a peripheral nerve is stimulated and can sometimes identify the approximate site of a spinal cord lesion (see Ch. 392.2).

MANAGEMENT OF THE PATIENT WITH NECK AND BACK PAIN. If no clinical findings suggest serious structural disease of the spine, nerve roots, or spinal cord, patients should be treated as if they suffered from an acute neck or back strain, without further diagnostic evaluation. For severe pain, the best treatment probably consists of 2 to 3 days bed rest on a firmly supported mattress in the position most comfortable. The best position for low back pain is usually semi-Fowler's position (head slightly elevated with pillows under the knees). For neck pain use a cervical pillow that maintains the normal lordotic curve rather than flexes the neck as regular pillows do. A soft cervical collar may be as effective in immobilizing the neck as bed rest. Bed rest may be combined with analgesic agents (usually aspirin or acetaminophen) and with local heat. Patients should be encouraged to stay recumbent except to go to the toilet until pain diminishes. As pain subsides, patients should gradually ambulate and begin gentle stretching and strengthening exercises. Other treatment modalities, including traction, procaine or saline injection into trigger points, transcutaneous stimulation, and spinal manipulation, are not more efficacious than the regimen described above. One recent study suggests that chiropractic manipulation of the back produces more rapid and prolonged relief of nonsciatic low back pain than does physical therapy with or without manipulation. Manipulation of the neck is potentially dangerous, however, because it can occlude the vertebral arteries as they enter the skull. A recent randomized study of patients with acute, nonspecific low back pain suggests that maintaining ordinary activity leads to faster recovery than either bed rest or back-mobilizing exercises.

Using standard therapy, 70 to 80% of patients become free of pain and able to return to full activity within a 4-week period. During the period of rest, repeated physical and neurologic examinations are unwise because vigorous movement can exacerbate pain and delay improvement. A small minority of patients continue to have chronic pain, and they, along with those whose initial examination has suggested more serious disease, need further evaluation.

Deyo RA, Rainville J, Kent DL: What can the history and physical examination tell us about low back pain? JAMA 268:760, 1992. *How to approach a patient with back pain.*

LaRocca H: A taxonomy of chronic pain syndromes: 1991 Presidential Address, Cervical Spine Research Society Annual Meeting, December 5, 1991. Spine 17(105):S344, 1992. *The entire supplement discusses diseases of the cervical spine.*

Malmivaara A, Häkkinen U, Aro T, et al.: The treatment of acute low back pain—Bed rest, exercises, or ordinary activity? N Engl J Med 332:351, 1995.

Nachemson AL (ed.): Newest knowledge of low back pain. Solutions in sight. *In* Clinical Orthopaedics and Related Research, #279. Philadelphia, JB Lippincott, 1992, p 2. *Extensive discussion of acute and chronic low back pain and its management.*

Shekelle PG, Adams AH, Chassin MR, et al.: Spinal manipulation for low-back pain. Ann Intern Med 117:590, 1992. *May help in acute low back pain.*

440 INTERVERTEBRAL DISC DISEASE

HERNIATED DISC. Herniated intervertebral discs are the most common cause of neck or low back pain associated with a clearly defined structural abnormality. Lumbar and cervical strain and myofascial pain syndromes (see Ch. 439) are more common but not marked by clear pathologic abnormalities. Between each two vertebral bodies is a fibrocartilaginous intervertebral disc. The disc consists of a soft inner nucleus pulposus (a remnant of the notochord) surrounded by thicker fibrous tissue (the anulus fibrosus). The gelatinous nucleus pulposus acts as a shock absorber between adjacent vertebral bodies. With advancing age, the nucleus loses fluid, volume, and resiliency, and the disc structure becomes more susceptible to trauma and compression. Tears develop in the anulus as a result of repeated minor trauma, and eventually, if they enlarge, a portion of the soft nucleus pulposus herniates. When disc material herniates into the vertebral canal, it can compress nerve endings and nerve roots, causing pain and other symptoms. Generally, the disc herniates lateral to the posterior longitudinal ligament, thus compressing spinal roots as they enter the intervertebral foramen. Occasionally the disc herniates more centrally, compressing either the spinal cord in the cervical or thoracic area or the cauda equina in the lumbar area. The term *herniated disc* refers to a disc that maintains continuity with the nucleus pulposus; extruded disc refers to a free fragment within the spinal canal. The signs and symptoms of herniated discs are caused by compression of either nerve roots or the spinal cord. The specific signs and symptoms depend in part on whether the predominant compression is spinal cord or nerve root, and in part on the level at which the neural structures are compressed (see Ch. 439). The most common sites of lumbar disc herniation are between L4 and L5 and L5 and S1, compressing the L5 and S1 roots, respectively. L3–L4 herniations are less common. In the cervical area, the common herniations occur between C5 and C6 (C6 root) and, especially, C6 and C7 (C7 root). Less commonly, herniations appear between C3 and C4, C4 and C5, and C7 and T1. Thoracic disc herniations are uncommon but can cause severe myelopathy because the thoracic area is the narrowest of the entire vertebral canal and the cord has a relatively poor vascular system. Although clinical localization in diagnosis of disc disease is usually quite accurate, an extruded disc fragment sometimes may be large enough to affect several roots or may migrate from the disc space in which it herniated, to cause signs at a distance.

The most common symptom of a herniated disc is pain. Local pain is felt as a dull aching in the neck or back, with an associated stiffness of those structures, frequently occurring episodically in response to minor trauma (or no discernible trauma at all) months or years prior to the development of radicular pain. Radicular pain may occasionally be the first sign of disc disease but is more likely to follow repeated bouts of local pain. Radicular pain is generally sudden in onset, often following minor trauma such as a twist, turn, or unusual bend. Radicular pain is perceived as sharp and well localized and may radiate from the back along the entire distribution of the involved root or affect only a portion of the dermatome. Both local and radicular pain have the characteristics of being exacerbated by activity and relieved by rest.

With cervical disc herniation, most patients hold their necks stiffly and resist passive movement. Lateral bending either to or away from the side of the herniated disc frequently exacerbates both the local and radicular pain. The patient may be more comfortable with the neck slightly flexed but usually prefers the recumbent position. Patients with lumbar disc disease are most comfortable lying, most uncomfortable sitting, and a little less uncomfortable standing. The back is held stiffly, so that the normal lumbar lordotic curve disappears; pain is usually exacerbated by extension of the back. Slow forward bending sometimes relieves the pain. Muscle spasm is prominent with both cervical and lumbar disc disease. Raising the intraspinal pressure, as by coughing, sneezing, or straining, increases the pain sharply. Stretching the compressed root also aggravates the pain. In the upper extremities, extending the arm and laterally flexing the neck to the opposite side sometimes reproduces radicular pain. In the lower extremities, raising the extended leg with the patient recumbent frequently reproduces the pain of an L5 or S1 radiculopathy and, if the pain is felt when the opposite leg is raised (crossed straight leg raising), the sign is highly reliable. Symptoms of L4 radiculopathy can often be reproduced by extending the hip (stretching the femoral nerve) when the patient is lying in the prone position. Often tenderness is present along the entire distribution of the nerve(s) supplied by the compressed root as well as in muscles supplied by the root. In patients with cervical disc disease, palpation or light percussion of the brachial plexus and the supraclavicular fossa or axilla often causes pain. In patients with lumbar disc disease, palpation over the femoral nerve (L4) in the groin or over the sciatic nerve (L5–S1) in the calf, thigh, or buttocks often causes severe pain. Occasionally tenderness in the calf (the posterior tibial nerve) is so striking as to suggest that the patient is suffering from thrombophlebitis rather than disc herniation. Other neurologic signs that commonly accompany disc disease include paresthesias and sensory loss in the distribution of the involved root and motor weakness in the myotome supplied by that root. The most important single sign is a diminished or absent reflex, giving objectively verifiable evidence of neurologic disease.

If an intervertebral disc herniates medially rather than laterally, it may spare the root and involve the spinal cord directly. When this occurs, there may be little or no pain or pain in a bilateral radicular distribution. Sometimes the pain is felt at a site far distant from the disc herniation as a result of compression of long sensory tracts in the spinal cord (funicular pain). The signs and symptoms of cord involvement are the same as those of compression of the spinal cord by other mass lesions. In contradistinction to diseases that arise within the spinal cord itself, compressive lesions tend to spare bladder and bowel function until late. (The exception is when the compression occurs either at the conus medullaris or in the cauda equina.)

The diagnosis of herniated disc is deduced from the characteristic clinical symptoms and findings. In many patients with radiculopathy, findings are minimal and the history must establish the diagnosis. When the patient complains of back pain, with or without a radicular component, but has no motor, sensory, or reflex changes to suggest the site of a radiculopathy, the differential diagnosis includes pain arising from pain-sensitive nerve endings in the muscles, ligaments, and joints of the vertebral bodies and the paravertebral structures. These structures must be examined carefully to determine which of them is responsible. MRI is helpful (see Ch. 439).

Controversy surrounds the management of herniated discs. Most physicians believe that the first step is bed rest. Some have reported that adrenocorticosteroids, either taken orally or injected into the epidural space, may hasten resolution of pain and other symptoms. No controlled studies support this recommendation. Steroids injected into the epidural or subarachnoid space are contraindicated and may produce severe inflammatory reactions. Surgery is indicated when (1) bed rest fails, and the patient is incapacitated by severe, intractable pain; (2) a centrally placed lumbar disc compresses the cauda equina, producing urinary dysfunction; (3) motor weakness (e.g., foot drop) is severe and gets worse on bed rest; or (4)

acute cervical or thoracic discs cause substantial myelopathy. The best operation removes the involved disc, leaving as much bone as possible intact. Fusion of the lumbar spine is rarely indicated. Lumbar disc operations are done posteriorly via a laminotomy. Cervical disc operations may be done either posteriorly to decompress the cord or anteriorly across the neck to remove the disc without disturbing posterior bony elements. The surgical approach for myelopathy should probably be anterior if the disc is in the cervical area and lateral if the disc is in the thoracic area.

SPONDYLOSIS. Spondylosis is a term applied to chronic degenerative disease of intervertebral discs associated with reactive changes in the adjacent vertebral bodies. Spondylotic changes in the neck and low back increase with age and are almost invariably present in the elderly. Spondylosis is usually asymptomatic except when the reactive tissue compresses a nerve root or the spinal cord. When this occurs, the signs and symptoms are similar to those of herniated disc disease, but the onset is less abrupt and the treatment often more difficult. In both the cervical and lumbar areas, spondylosis is more likely to cause spinal cord or cauda equina symptoms if the sagittal diameter of the spinal canal is congenitally narrow.

Cervical Spondylosis. Most patients suffer either radiculopathy or myelopathy, but not both. Pain is common but usually less acute and severe than with herniated discs. Even muscle spasm may be absent. However, the vertebral degenerative changes in the neck lead to limitation of movement in all directions. The classic picture of cervical spondylotic myelopathy is one of little or no pain but slowly developing weakness, atrophy, and fasciculations in the upper extremities, particularly the small muscles of the hand, accompanied by spastic paraparesis with decreased proprioception in the legs. At first the findings may suggest a diagnosis of amyotrophic lateral sclerosis. However, in cervical spondylosis there are sensory changes, particularly vibration loss in the lower extremities, and in amyotrophic lateral sclerosis fasciculations are found outside of cervical segments. The differential diagnosis also includes other compressive lesions of root and spinal cord as well as chronic multiple sclerosis.

The diagnosis of cervical spondylitic myelopathy is established with MRI, which accurately delineates the size of the cervical canal and the site of spinal cord and/or root compression.

The natural history of cervical myelopathy and radiculopathy varies. Many patients experience long periods of pain relief and remission or stabilization of neurologic symptoms, making it difficult to evaluate the effect of a particular treatment. Many physicians prefer, once having established the diagnosis, to begin conservative treatment with a brief period of bed rest accompanied by cervical traction and stabilization of the neck with a soft collar. If collar and traction are successful, they should be continued. However, if the patient develops progressive neurologic signs in the face of conservative treatment, surgical therapy is indicated. Most neurosurgeons believe that if the spinal cord compression occurs at one or two segments, anterior removal of the disc material with spinal fusion is the preferred course. If more than a few segments are involved, laminectomy with foraminotomy is preferred.

In some patients with cervical spondylosis (or with congenital narrowing of the cervical spinal canal, or both), neurologic symptoms are exacerbated by exercise, with pain, numbness, and weakness appearing when a particular extremity is exercised. The pathogenesis is thought to be compression of the spinal cord so severe that the blood supply to the area cannot increase during its activity, leading to ischemia of cord and root structures (pseudoclaudication).

Lumbar Spondylosis. Most of the considerations described above apply. The symptoms of lumbar spondylosis are similar to those of herniated disc, often occurring at multiple levels. One outstanding difference is the frequent presence of *pseudoclaudication* from cauda equina compression in patients with spinal stenosis due to either spondylosis or congenital narrowing. Typically, symptoms and signs are evoked or accentuated by walking and include pain, paresthesias, and weakness in the lower extremities. All of the symptoms may disappear when the patient ceases walking, even though he remains in the standing position. At times, however, the symptoms may be exacerbated by prolonged standing and relieved only by sitting or lying down. Pseudoclaudication of the cauda equina may be distinguished from intermittent vascular claudication in several ways: in vascular disease, the pulses in the lower extremities are usually absent or become absent as exercise begins. Also, the symptoms are usually reproducible and stereotypic; i.e., the patient can predict the exact distance he can walk at a given speed before symptoms develop. Symptoms of cauda equina pseudoclaudication are less stereotypic, so that on some days patients can walk much longer distances than on others. The reason for this variability is not known. In patients with pseudoclaudication, the narrowed lumbar canal is easily measured by MRI. With severe lumbar stenosis, conservative treatment usually fails, and decompressive laminectomy is the treatment of choice.

OTHER CAUSES OF BACK AND NECK PAIN. Several common pathophysiologically poorly understood disorders that cause pain in the back or neck can be confused with intravertebral disc disease or cervical or lumbar spondylosis. These include pain arising in lumbosacral, sacroiliac, or zygapophyseal joints or pain that arises in adjacent supporting structures, including muscle. These disorders usually cause chronic aching local pain that, when severe, may be referred to distant sites. Typical radicular pain never occurs. As a group, the diagnosis is usually suspected by finding tenderness at a specific muscle site or limitation of motion in a specific joint. The diagnosis is supported by a lidocaine block, which should completely relieve the pain if the presumptive diagnosis is correct.

The *facet syndrome* is believed to result from osteoarthritis or trauma of the zygapophyseal joints or their synovial membranes. In the low back it is characterized by pain in the back, buttocks, and thighs. It is often relieved by flexion and aggravated by extension of the spine and frequently accentuated by rest and relieved by movement. Characteristically the area is stiff and painful in the morning and improves somewhat as the day wears on. There is tenderness to palpation of the joint. Anesthetic blocks of the joint relieve both the local and referred pain. Similar chronic pain may have its origin in the lumbosacral or sacroiliac joints.

Musculoskeletal pain is also a common but poorly understood cause of low back and probably neck pain. In patients with painful muscle spasm the normal lordotic curve is usually straightened and tight, and tender muscles can be palpated by the examiner. Local anesthetic blocks, followed by gentle mobilization, usually relieve the spasm and the pain. Prolonged contraction of muscles, such as results from sustained posture or psychological stress, may produce similar pain and tenderness. Fibromyalgia and myofascial pain syndromes often affect the neck and back. They are discussed in Ch. 405.

Braakman R: Management of cervical spondylotic myelopathy and radiculopathy [editorial]. J Neurol Neurosurg Psychiatry 57:257, 1994. *A review of clinical findings and treatment.*

Kanner RM: Low back pain. Semin Neurol 14:272, 1994. *A nice description of management of patients with pain from disc disease and other causes of low back pain.*

Wall PD, Melzack R (eds.): Textbook of Pain. London, Churchill Livingstone, 1994. *A compendium of basic, clinical, and therapeutic aspects of most pain syndromes, including disc disease.*

441 NEOPLASMS OF THE SPINAL CANAL

Neoplastic growths that cause nerve root or spinal cord compression can be paravertebral, extradural, intradural, or intramedullary (Fig. 441–1). Most of those causing spinal cord compression are extradural and metastatic. Extradural neoplasms originate in the vertebral body surrounding the spinal cord and compress spinal roots or cord without invading them. Intradural neoplasms also cause symptoms by compressing spinal roots or cord without invading, but unlike extradural neoplasms the majority are benign and slow growing. Intramedullary neoplasms cause symptoms both by invading and by compressing spinal structures; the tumors may be either benign or malignant.

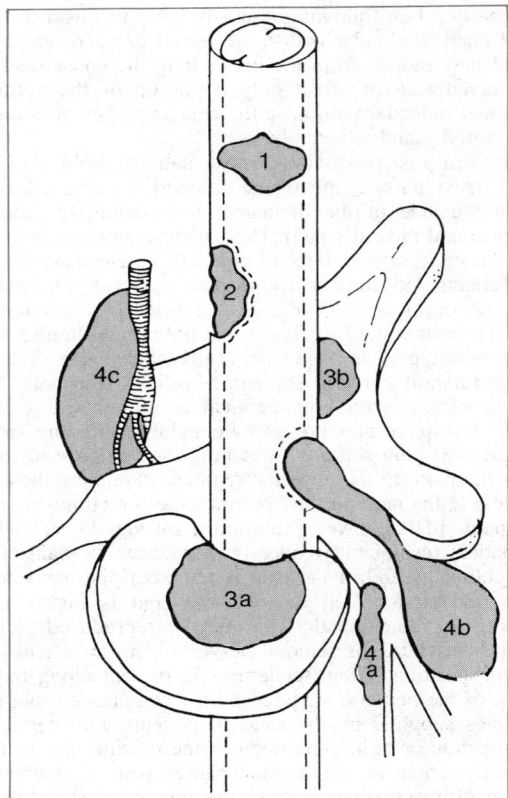

FIGURE 441–1. Pathophysiology of myelopathy caused by neoplasms. 1, The tumor may arise in or metastasize hematogenously to the substance of the spinal cord (intramedullary). 2, The tumor may be extraparenchymal but intradural. 3, The tumor may be extradural, extending either from the vertebral body (3a) or from a spinous process (3b), and cause symptoms by compressing the spinal cord. 4, The tumor may originate in or spread to the paravertebral space and produce its symptoms either by (4a) invading nerve roots, (4b) invading the epidural or subdural space through the intervertebral foramen, or (4c) compressing radicular arteries to cause spinal cord ischemia. (From Andreoli TE, Carpenter CCJ, Plum F, Smith LH Jr [eds.]: Cecil Essentials of Medicine. Philadelphia, WB Saunders, 1986.)

PARAVERTEBRAL TUMORS. Neoplastic lesions that begin in or metastasize to the paravertebral space often cause serious and perplexing neurologic problems. The tumor may extend longitudinally within the paravertebral space, progressively compressing or invading nerve roots. At times, such tumors grow through an intervertebral foramen and compress not only the nerve root but also the spinal cord. Rarely, spinal cord symptoms may be caused by paravertebral tumors compromising radicular arteries that supply the spinal cord. If the tumor is more lateral than the immediate paravertebral space, the brachial, lumbar, or sacral plexus may be compressed, causing symptoms similar to root compression but with a different pattern of sensory and motor loss. The symptoms of extravertebral tumor begin insidiously with severe, unremitting pain, often with a burning quality localized just lateral to the spine and radiating in a bandlike pattern in the distribution of the involved dermatome(s). If the lesion involves abdominal or thoracic roots, motor and sensory changes are usually not appreciated by either the patient or the examiner. Autonomic changes may be a prominent or the only neurologic sign. Hyperhidrosis occurring in a band coinciding with the site of the pain strongly suggests the diagnosis. When the tumor involves cervical or lumbar roots, the pain may be soon followed by numbness in fingertips or toes, with accompanying weakness and reflex diminution, depending on the roots involved. Autonomic changes, including anhidrosis or hyperhidrosis, may affect the arm or leg. Horner's syndrome or diaphragmatic paralysis often accompanies cervical or upper thoracic paravertebral tumors. The diagnosis is best established by MR scans of the level suggested by the clinical findings. The scans can also determine whether the lesion has grown through the intervertebral foramen or has eroded vertebral bodies.

The differential diagnosis of paravertebral tumor includes disorders that cause paravertebral pain with or without compression of nerve roots. *Myofascial pain syndromes* cause low back or neck paravertebral pain with referred pain into arms or legs. On examination one often finds an area of exquisite muscle tenderness on a taut band of muscle. Relief of pain often can be produced by injecting the trigger point with saline solution or a local anesthetic. Temporary relief of pain after such injection does not imply that structural disease is absent; the trigger points may be a reaction to spinal or nerve root disease. In myofascial syndromes, autonomic, sensory, or motor changes are not usually present. Disease of kidneys and other viscera lying in the retroperitoneal space may cause aching pain similar to that of paravertebral tumors, but usually not radiating or associated with autonomic, motor, or sensory changes. Percussion of the involved viscera reproduces the pain that is described as a dull ache rather than a neurogenic burning pain. Chronic pain after a thoracotomy (*post-thoracotomy pain*) probably results from entrapment of nerve roots at the time of surgery, perhaps with neuroma formation. Such pains can sometimes be relieved by paravertebral anesthetic blocks.

The management of paravertebral masses depends on the diagnosis. In patients known to have cancer, particularly lymphomas or carcinomas of the breast or lung, the tumor can be assumed to be metastatic and should be treated with radiation therapy and, if available, chemotherapy. If the patient has no history of cancer, a biopsy is required and, depending on the site of the lesion, resection may be attempted both to establish a diagnosis and to decompress the nerve roots. Once the diagnosis is established by biopsy, further therapy such as radiation or chemotherapy may be indicated.

EXTRADURAL TUMORS. Extradural neoplasms compress spinal roots and cord in one of three ways. Either they arise in vertebrae surrounding the spinal cord and grow into the epidural space or they arise in the paravertebral space and grow through the intervertebral foramen to compress the cord laterally. Rarely, tumors may arise in the epidural space itself, without involving either vertebral or paravertebral structures. Most extradural neoplasms are metastatic (e.g., carcinomas of the breast, lung, prostate, or kidney). Some extradural neoplasms arise *de novo* in the vertebral bodies (e.g., chordoma, osteogenic sarcoma, myeloma, chondrosarcoma). A minority of extradural neoplasms are benign (e.g., osteoma, osteoid osteoma, angioma). Because extradural neoplasms usually destroy bone before causing spinal cord compression, local pain is the first symptom and may precede either radicular pain or other symptoms of spinal cord compression by weeks or months. Rarely the first symptoms may be spinal cord dysfunction. As with other causes of spinal cord compression, extradural neoplasms cause symptoms first distally and later proximally. Thus, even thoracic and cervical neoplasms generally cause weakness and numbness in the legs before trunk and upper extremity muscles are involved. The diagnosis of extradural spinal cord compression must be suspected by the history of pain followed by signs and symptoms of spinal cord dysfunction and confirmed by radiographic study. About 85% of patients suffering from extradural spinal cord compression have bone lesions at the site of compression on plain radiographs. MRI establishes the site and degree of spinal cord compression.

The differential diagnosis of extradural neoplasms includes inflammatory disease of bone and epidural abscess (e.g., vertebral tuberculosis, bacterial osteomyelitis), acute or subacute epidural hematomas, herniated intervertebral discs, spondylosis, and, very rarely, extramedullary hematopoiesis (in patients with severe and chronic anemias) or epidural lipomatosis (in patients on chronic steroid therapy). MRI often distinguishes those from tumor, but sometimes definitive diagnosis requires biopsy of the lesion either via decompressive laminectomy or by percutaneous needle biopsy.

The treatment of extradural neoplasms depends on the cause. Most neoplasms that cause extradural spinal cord compression are malignant and progress rapidly. Once spinal cord symptoms begin, paraplegia may develop in hours to days. Paraplegia is usually irreversible, whereas treatment often can correct mild to moderate spinal cord dysfunction. Thus, early diagnosis and effective emergency treatment of extradural spinal cord compression are mandatory. The treatment of patients known to be suffering from cancer who develop signs and symptoms of spinal cord compression from extradural metastases is radiation therapy. Therapy should begin with corticosteroids (dexamethasone, 16 to 100 mg daily) to decrease spinal cord edema, followed immediately by radiation therapy. If effective chemotherapeutic agents are available, they should be used in conjunction with steroids and radiation therapy. In patients not known to be suffering from a primary cancer, metastatic disease is the most common cause of extradural spinal cord compression, but definitive diagnosis must be made by biopsy. Such patients should begin corticosteroid therapy followed by surgery with removal of as much tumor as possible for diagnostic and therapeutic purposes. If a malignant neoplasm is encountered, radiation therapy should begin as soon after the surgery as is practical. In a few patients in whom radiation therapy and chemotherapy are ineffective, resection of the vertebral body involved by tumor may delay or prevent the development of paraplegia. Benign extradural tumors require surgery.

INTRADURAL EXTRAMEDULLARY TUMORS. Most intradural tumors are benign. Meningiomas and neurofibromas are the two most common types. Teratomas, arachnoid cysts, and lipomas are less common. *Meningiomas* occur in middle-aged and elderly women, predominantly in the thoracic region. Another common site is at the foramen magnum. Meningiomas are benign, slow growing, and usually located on the posterior aspect of the spinal cord. Pain is usually the first symptom, but in about 25% the meningioma is painless, the first symptoms being those of spinal cord compression. Paresthesias and sensory changes beginning distally in the lower extremities are a frequent early symptom and are often mistaken for peripheral neuropathy. As the disease progresses, however, corticospinal tract signs betray the spinal origin. Even when spinal cord signs and symptoms are obvious, the lack of pain may lead one to suspect a degenerative or demyelinating disease such as multiple sclerosis rather than a neoplasm. MRI with contrast enhancement usually is diagnostic. The treatment of spinal cord meningiomas is surgical removal.

The second common cause of intradural spinal cord compression is *neurofibroma*. Because these tumors usually arise from the dorsal root, radicular pain is often the first symptom, preceding signs of spinal cord compression by months or years. When spinal cord compression develops, it progresses slowly. Some patients with spinal neurofibroma suffer from neurofibromatosis. That diagnosis may be suspected either by a positive family history or by the cutaneous stigmata of the disease. A neurofibroma may extend on either side of the intervertebral foramen, involving the root both in the paravertebral space and within the spinal canal. The cerebrospinal fluid protein is almost always elevated. The diagnosis is established by MRI. Surgical extirpation of the lesion usually leads to complete recovery.

Occasionally *metastatic tumors* involving the leptomeninges present with intradural mass lesions. Pain is almost always prominent, and spinal cord compression develops more rapidly than with the more benign intradural tumors. In addition, malignant cells are frequently encountered in the spinal fluid. The spinal fluid glucose may be decreased, the protein elevated. The treatment of intradural malignant neoplasms is radiation therapy and chemotherapy because complete surgical extirpation is almost never possible. Because the tumor usually seeds the entire subarachnoid space, radiation therapy, if it is to have more than temporary effect, must either be delivered to the entire neuraxis or be supplemented by chemotherapy.

INTRAMEDULLARY TUMORS. The most common intramedullary spinal tumors are astrocytomas (usually low grade) and ependymomas. Other tumors that occasionally cause intramedullary spinal lesions are hemangioblastomas, lipomas, and hematogenous metastases. Pain is an early symptom of most intramedullary tumors, and signs of spinal cord dysfunction progress rapidly or slowly, depending on the growth characteristics of the tumor. Intramedullary tumors are often associated with syringomyelia, the syrinx sometimes being at a distance from the primary tumor and producing its own symptoms of spinal dysfunction. The so-called characteristic signs of intramedullary spinal cord lesions (dissociated sensory loss, sacral sparing, and early onset of bladder and bowel dysfunction) are not reliable enough clinically to distinguish intramedullary from extramedullary lesions; that diagnosis is established by MRI. In some patients with longstanding benign intramedullary lesions, plain radiographs of the spine may show widening of the spinal canal and erosion of the pedicles. The differential diagnosis of intramedullary tumors includes intramedullary abscesses and syringomyelia without tumor. A definitive diagnosis is established by biopsy. Successful surgical removal of intramedullary tumors is possible, particularly with ependymomas and hemangioblastomas and sometimes with gliomas as well. Highly skilled and experienced surgeons are necessary for tumors to be removed without increasing neurologic symptoms. If the tumor cannot be totally excised, postoperative radiation therapy often delays recurrence.

Ependymomas have a predilection to involve the lower end of the spinal cord and the filum terminale. An unusual syndrome sometimes produced by such tumors is hydrocephalus with headache, papilledema, and enlarged cerebral ventricles. The pathogenesis of the hydrocephalus is believed to be the plugging of pacchionian granulations by protein exuded from the tumor into the spinal fluid.

Byrne TN, Waxman SG (eds.): Spinal Cord Compression. Philadelphia, FA Davis, 1990. *Specific chapters cover non-neoplastic as well as neoplastic causes of spinal cord compression and noncompressive myelopathies simulating spinal cord compression.*
Posner JB: Neurologic Complications of Cancer. Philadelphia, FA Davis, 1995. *A current discussion of the diagnosis and management of metastatic disease of the spine.*

442 INFLAMMATORY DISEASES COMPRESSING THE SPINAL CORD

Inflammatory diseases that compress nerve roots and spinal cord can be extradural, intradural, or intramedullary. Extradural inflammatory lesions include vertebral tuberculosis or bacterial osteomyelitis with extradural extension and primary extradural bacterial abscesses. These entities are discussed in Ch. 421. Intradural but extramedullary inflammatory diseases include bacterial, fungal, and parasitic meningitis, inflammatory disease of the leptomeninges of unknown cause such as sarcoidosis or Behçet's syndrome, and reactions to foreign substances such as myelographic contrast material, spinal anesthetics, or steroids. Occasionally, leptomeningeal infiltration with tumor or subarachnoid hemorrhage causes an inflammatory response of the leptomeninges that mimics subacute or chronic infection. All of these inflammatory intradural lesions can lead to spinal arachnoiditis. *Spinal arachnoiditis* is characterized by neck and back pain and by radicular pain in the distribution of the roots involved in the inflammatory process. Dysfunction of multiple roots, particularly in the lumbosacral area, is common; occasional patients go on to develop signs of spinal cord dysfunction (often caused by syrinx formation), which may progress to paraplegia. The diagnosis of spinal arachnoiditis is established by myelography. A myelogram reveals spotty and irregular collections of contrast material with impairment of the flow through the subarachnoid space. Sometimes there is a complete block to the passage of the myelographic contrast material. The spinal fluid may contain an increased cellular response and a decreased glucose concentration. The protein concentration is usually elevated. Sometimes a specific infectious organism can be identified either by microscopic examination or by culture. There is no therapy for spinal arachnoiditis unless a specific treatment-sensitive infective agent is identified.

Intramedullary infectious processes include bacterial and parasitic abscesses and acute transverse myelitis. These entities are discussed under the appropriate chapter headings.

Byrne TN, Waxman SG (eds): Spinal Cord Compression. Philadelphia, FA Davis, 1990. *Chapters discuss vascular and inflammatory causes of spinal cord compression and noncompressive myelopathies mimicking spinal cord compression.*
Caplan LR, Norohna AB, Amico LL: Syringomyelia and arachnoiditis. J Neurol Neurosurg Psychiatry 53:106, 1990. *A well-referenced discussion of chronic arachnoiditis and its sequelae.*
Dolan RA: Spinal adhesive arachnoiditis. Surg Neurol 39:479, 1993. *A review of 41 cases.*

443 VASCULAR DISORDERS COMPRESSING THE SPINAL CORD

Extradural, intradural, and intramedullary vascular disorders all can cause spinal cord compression. The most common and serious extradural vascular disease is *spinal epidural hematoma*. Hemorrhage into the spinal epidural space may occur spontaneously or be associated with trauma, a bleeding diathesis, or a vascular malformation. It is particularly common in patients being treated with anticoagulants. It may occasionally follow lumbar puncture, particularly in patients with bleeding abnormalities. Hemorrhage usually arises from the epidural venous plexus and tends to collect over the dorsum of the spinal cord covering several segments. The clinical picture is characterized by the sudden onset of severe localized back pain and the rapid development of spinal cord dysfunction, often leading to complete paraplegia in several hours. If the patient has a known bleeding disorder, the clinical diagnosis is easily established. In patients without known bleeding or clotting disorders, the differential diagnosis includes acute epidural abscess and acute transverse myelopathy. Although occasional patients recover from paraparesis related to epidural spinal cord compression spontaneously, the majority require emergency surgical evacuation if neurologic function is to be preserved. The more rapidly the paralysis develops and the longer the delay in decompression, the less likely is the patient to recover.

Intradural but extramedullary vascular lesions are usually caused by hemorrhage from *vascular malformations* on the surface of the spinal cord. *Spinal subarachnoid hemorrhage* is characterized by the sudden onset of back pain, often with a radicular component with or without the development of signs of spinal cord compression. Lumbar puncture reveals evidence of subarachnoid hemorrhage with red cells, xanthochromic spinal fluid, and usually an elevated protein concentration. In the absence of spinal cord signs, the differential diagnosis includes spontaneous intracerebral subarachnoid hemorrhage.

Vascular malformations also may lie within the substance of the spinal cord where they can give rise to intramedullary hemorrhage (hematomyelia) as well as subarachnoid hemorrhage. The sudden development of partial or complete transverse myelopathy is the most common onset. If blood leaks into the subarachnoid space, pain in the neck and back and other signs of meningeal irritation occur.

Arteriovenous malformations may also compress the spinal cord or give rise to hemodynamic changes that result in spinal ischemia. In such cases, distortion and compression of the cord by enlarged, abnormal vessels occur only gradually, producing slowly progressive symptoms of spinal cord dysfunction. Exacerbation of symptoms may accompany menstrual periods or pregnancy.

Complete or partial recovery of function can follow episodes of spinal cord ischemia or even small hemorrhages. The unchanging localization of the attacks and the prominence of pain help differentiate arteriovenous malformations from other recurrent neurologic disorders such as multiple sclerosis. Rarely, a bruit may be heard by auscultation over the site of the malformation. MRI identifies most hemorrhages and vascular malformations, but angiography with regional catheterization of radicular vessels is necessary to identify feeding vessels as a preliminary step to surgical treatment. Advances in microsurgery have increased the chances for satisfactory removal of these lesions. Embolization of the malformation or ligation of feeding arteries has been performed when the abnormality cannot be removed surgically.

Amson JA, Spetzler RF: Surgical resection of intramedullary spinal cord cavernous malformations. J Neurosurg 78:446,1993. *Description of a clinical entity usually not diagnosed before the advent of MRI.*
Dawson DM, Potts F: Acute nontraumatic myelopathies. Neurol Clin 9:585, 1991. *Diagnosis and management of vascular myelopathies. Entire issue is devoted to spinal cord disorders.*

444 CONGENITAL ANOMALIES OF THE CRANIOVERTEBRAL JUNCTION, SPINE, AND SPINAL CORD

Congenital anomalies of the spine are common and are often encountered on radiographs of patients suffering from neck or low back pain. Some congenital anomalies such as *spina bifida occulta* can be considered variants of normal and are probably never responsible in and of themselves for low back pain. Others such as the *Klippel-Feil syndrome* (congenital fusion of two or more cervical vertebrae) are not responsible for neck pain or other neurologic symptoms except when associated with coexisting congenital anomalies of the central nervous system. Congenital abnormalities of the spine that are common and usually asymptomatic but that must be considered potential causes of neck or back pain include *facet tropism* (misalignment of the facets on the two sides of the corresponding vertebral body; several authorities believe that this increases rotational stress on the facet joints and may cause back pain); *transitional vertebrae,* such as in sacralization to a lumbar vertebra or lumbarization of a sacral vertebra (these alter spinal mechanics and result in instability and stress, sometimes producing back pain); and *spondylolisthesis* (forward slipping of one vertebral body onto another caused by a defect between the articular facets). A third group of congenital anomalies of the spine consists of those that are likely to cause not only neck or back pain but also neurologic disability. These include *basilar impression,* which is often associated with *Arnold-Chiari malformation* (see later discussion). Severe spinal *scoliosis* or *kyphosis,* congenital *stenosis* of the lumbar or cervical spinal canal, anterior and lateral spinal *meningoceles,* and *diastematomyelia* are other causes of back pain and neurologic disability. Diastematomyelia is a bony abnormality that divides the spinal canal, leading to duplication of the spinal cord. It is usually associated with evidence of spina bifida on plain radiographs, and sometimes the bony septum can be identified as well. Patients who become symptomatic in adulthood almost always have some cutaneous abnormality, especially hypertrichosis over the sacral area. The disorder may be associated with other congenital abnormalities of the central nervous system as well.

ARNOLD-CHIARI MALFORMATION

INFANTILE FORM. The Arnold-Chiari malformation is characterized by downward displacement of the cerebellum through the foramen magnum of the skull and by similar caudal elongation of the medulla. The infantile form is commonly associated with other midline defects such as spina bifida and meningocele, hydrocephalus caused by aqueductal or fourth ventricular obstruction, and other congenital malformations of the brain and cord. Therapy is directed toward surgical relief of the hydrocephalus with a ventricular shunting procedure and repair of the meningomyelocele. Prognosis is poor for patients with extensive defects.

ADULT FORM. The malformation may be asymptomatic until adult life, when the patient gradually develops symptoms and signs of dysfunction of the cerebellum, lower cranial nerves, pyramidal tracts, and posterior columns. Posterior cranial displacement may occur with coughing or straining. Downbeat nystagmus is characteristic. At times the initial signs may be those of hydrocephalus secondary to obstruction of the cerebrospinal fluid pathways or to coexisting syringomyelia of the cervical spinal cord and medulla (see Ch. 416). Commonly there is radiographic evidence of fusion of the cervical vertebrae, or basilar impression, but MR scan establishes the diagnosis even when there are no coexisting bony abnormalities. The Arnold-Chiari malformation in adults may simulate syndromes produced by tumors near the foramen magnum or by multiple sclerosis. Surgical enlargement of the foramen magnum and decompression of the cervicomedullary junction benefit selected cases.

BASILAR IMPRESSION AND PLATYBASIA

Basilar impression refers to abnormal invagination of the cervical spine into the base of the posterior fossa of the skull. The diagnosis is made from sagittal MR reconstructions that show excessive protrusion of the tip of the odontoid process of the axis into or above the foramen magnum. *Platybasia* refers to flattening of the base of the skull, wherein lateral roentgenograms of the skull reveal flattening of the angle between the orbital plates of the anterior fossa and the clivus, the sloping anterior floor of the posterior fossa. The abnormality by itself has no clinical significance.

These malformations are usually developmental in origin, and there may be hereditary transmission. Occasionally, basilar impression may result from metabolic bone diseases such as rickets, osteitis deformans, osteomalacia, osteogenesis imperfecta, or fibrous dysplasia. Minor degrees of deformity of the base of the skull give rise to no symptoms. The neck appears shortened, and its movements may be limited. More severe invagination may produce signs of impaired function of the cerebellum, lower cranial nerves, pyramidal tracts, and posterior columns. Syringomyelia and syringobulbia may be present. Increased intracranial pressure may develop owing to obstruction of the foramina of the fourth ventricle and the basal cisterns. The clinical manifestations must be differentiated from those caused by neoplasms in the region of the foramen magnum and multiple sclerosis. When neurologic signs are progressive, surgical decompression of the posterior fossa and upper cervical cord may be indicated.

Oldfield EH, Muraszko K, Shawker TH, Patronas NJ: Pathophysiology of syringomyelia associated with Chiari I malformation of the cerebellar tonsils. J Neurosurg 80:3, 1994. *New concepts of the pathophysiology of the disorder.*
Vinken PJ, Bruyn GW, Klawans HL, Myrianthopoulos NC (eds.): Handbook of Clinical Neurology. Volume 50, Malformations. New York, Elsevier Science Publishers, 1987. *A recent comprehensive review of congenital malformations of the brain and spine.*

Section Fifteen—Diseases of the Peripheral Nervous System
John W. Griffin

The peripheral nervous system, through its motor, sensory, and autonomic divisions, serves as a major interface between the central nervous system and the environment. Diseases of the peripheral nervous system, termed *peripheral neuropathies,* are among the most prevalent neurologic conditions. They range in severity from the mild sensory abnormalities found in up to 70% of patients with longstanding diabetes to fulminant, life-threatening paralytic disorders such as the Guillain-Barré syndrome. Differential diagnosis of peripheral nerve disease can be challenging because the catalogue of disorders that can produce neuropathies is extensive. Although a wide variety of symptoms and signs can result from diseases of the peripheral nervous system, the repertoire of underlying cellular pathology is limited, so that only a few clinical or pathologic features are specific to individual neuropathies. Nevertheless, the past 5 years have seen rapid advances in diagnosis and therapy. An increasing number of nerve diseases are now amenable to treatment, and the peripheral nervous system has a much greater capacity for regeneration and repair than the central nervous system, so that functional improvement is a realistic goal for a lengthening list of neuropathies.

Differential diagnosis in the peripheral nervous system begins with classification of the *clinical features* of the neuropathy, and uses elucidation of the *underlying pathophysiology,* primarily as reflected in electrodiagnostic tests, as a differential tool. On these bases, the specific laboratory tests that are likely to prove useful can be defined.

445 Anatomy and Basic Terminology

The peripheral nervous system (PNS) contains motor, sensory, and autonomic fibers. The motor, sensory, and autonomic fibers are anatomically discrete as they leave their nerve cell bodies (for example, in the ventral roots and the dorsal roots) and again as they approach their nerve terminals, but are admixed throughout most of the peripheral nerves. The lower motor neurons in the ventral horn of the spinal cord give rise to axons that pass through the ventral root before joining their sensory and autonomic counterparts in the mixed spinal nerves. In contrast, the primary sensory neuron is a unique cell type. The nerve cell body, located in the dorsal root ganglion, gives rise to a single axonal stem process that bifurcates into a peripheral branch, which extends down a peripheral nerve, and a central branch, which passes through the dorsal root and enters the spinal cord. In a subpopulation of these sensory neurons (the large neurons subserving joint position and vibratory sensibility), the axons of the central processes pass up the ipsilateral dorsal column of the spinal cord to synapse in the gracile and cuneate nuclei of the medulla oblongata. In the lumbar region of an adult, the dorsal and ventral spinal roots may be 12 inches or more in length; in contrast, in the cervical region the spinal roots are only about two inches long.

Injury to the spinal roots produces *radiculopathy.* The root at a single level may be injured by compression due to a herniated nucleus pulposus (intervertebral disc) or from metastatic cancer. The characteristic clinical features of an isolated root lesion are sensory symptoms with loss of cutaneous sensibility in the segmental or *dermatomal* distribution, as well as weakness in the muscles innervated by that root. If the affected nerve root subserves a tendon reflex, the tendon reflex is depressed or lost. Involvement of spinal roots at many levels (*polyradiculopathy*) can be produced by infiltrative processes, such as carcinomatous meningitis. The clinical picture reflects the specific root levels involved.

The term *peripheral neuropathy* connotes any disease of the peripheral nervous system (PNS). Involvement of a single peripheral nerve constitutes *mononeuropathy,* as seen, for example, following inadvertent intraneural injury to the sciatic nerve during intramuscular injections. *Multiple mononeuropathy* (mononeuropathy multiplex) describes focal involvement of more than one individual peripheral nerve. For example, diabetes and vasculitis, by damaging the small blood vessels supplying the peripheral nerves, can produce injury to several widely distributed individual nerves. *Polyneuropathy* designates a widespread and generally symmetric disorder of the PNS. Polyneuropathies usually produce distally predominant loss of sensation, strength, and tendon reflexes.

Gardner E, Bunge RP: Gross anatomy of the peripheral nervous system. *In* Dyck PJ, Thomas PK, Griffin JW, et al. (eds.): Peripheral Neuropathy, 3rd ed. Philadelphia, W.B. Saunders, 1993, pp. 8–27. *This is the major comprehensive monograph on this subject with well-written chapters, designated in subsequent subsections of this section, on both common and rare disorders.*

446 PATHOPHYSIOLOGY OF PERIPHERAL NEUROPATHIES

Normal function of myelinated nerve fibers depends on the integrity of both the axon and its myelin sheath. The simplest type of nerve injury is transection of the axon. The axon distal to the site of transection degenerates while that proximal to the injury survives and has the potential for regeneration. As the axon degenerates the myelin in the distal stump is also broken down and cleared. Axonal degeneration due to a focal nerve injury occurs, for example, in radiculopathies due to severe compression of the nerve root and in focal ischemic injury to roots and nerves. In the symmetric polyneuropathies, the underlying pathology is usually a slowly evolving type of axonal degeneration that involves the ends of long nerve fibers first and preferentially. With time, the degenerative process involves more proximal regions of long fibers, and shorter fibers are affected. This pattern of *distal axonal degeneration* or *"dying back"* of nerve fibers results from a wide variety of metabolic, toxic, and heritable causes. The resulting clinical picture includes early loss of the tendon reflex at the ankle, and weakness that initially involves the intrinsic muscles of the feet, the extensors of the toes, and the dorsiflexors at the ankle; the motor signs are accompanied by distally predominant loss of large-fiber sensory modalities such as vibratory sensibility in the toes. With progression, the hands are similarly involved, and the process may spread more proximally up the legs and arms. The resulting pattern of sensory loss is frequently termed a *stocking-and-glove* pattern. Recovery from axonal degeneration requires nerve regeneration, a notoriously slow process.

Demyelination of a peripheral nerve at even a single site can block conduction, resulting in a functional deficit identical to that seen after axonal degeneration. In contrast to repair by regeneration, however, repair by remyelination can be quite rapid. Autoimmune attack on the myelin sheath occurs in the *inflammatory demyelinating* neuropathies and some neuropathies associated with paraproteinemias. Inherited disorders of myelin are the other major category of demyelinating neuropathy. Uncommon causes include some toxic, mechanical, and physical injuries to nerve. Although these examples have nearly pure demyelination, and other neuropathies have axonal degeneration exclusively, many neuropathies have an admixture of both axonal degeneration and demyelination. This mixed pathology reflects the mutual interdependency of the axons and the myelin-forming Schwann cells.

On the basis of the clinical features alone, it is difficult to predict whether a patient has a predominantly axonal or demyelinating pattern of peripheral nerve injury. Electrodiagnostic tests—nerve conduction velocity and electromyography—provide a tool for assessing the relative contributions of axonal loss and demyelination. Nerve conduction studies are done by stimulating individual nerves with electrodes at two sites, one proximal to the other, and measuring the velocity of conduction of the action potential between those two sites. In addition, for both sensory and motor nerves, the amplitude of the evoked response can be determined. In general, axonal degeneration decreases the amplitude of the evoked action potential out of proportion to the degree of reduction in conduction velocity, whereas demyelination produces prominent reductions in conduction velocities.

Griffin JW, Hoffman PN: Degeneration and regeneration in the peripheral nervous system. *In* Dyck PJ, Thomas PK, Griffin JW, et al. (eds.): Peripheral Neuropathy, 3rd ed. Philadelphia, W.B. Saunders, 1993, pp. 361–376.
Schaumburg HH, Berger AR, Thomas PK: Disorders of Peripheral Nerve, 2nd ed. Philadelphia, F.A. Davis Co., 1992. *A highly readable succinct but informative monograph aimed especially at the general physician.*

447 IMMUNE-MEDIATED NEUROPATHIES

GUILLAIN-BARRÉ SYNDROME (Acute Inflammatory Demyelinating Polyneuropathy)

The Guillain-Barré syndrome (GBS) is characterized clinically by weakness or paralysis affecting more than one limb, usually symmetrically, associated with loss of tendon reflexes and with increased spinal fluid protein without pleocytosis. Since the advent of polio vaccination, GBS has become the most frequent cause of acute flaccid paralysis throughout the world. In the 1960's, the pathologic substrate of many cases of GBS was shown to be lymphocytic infiltration of the spinal roots and peripheral nerves, with macrophage-mediated demyelination and a variable degree of secondary axonal degeneration. On this basis, GBS became virtually synonymous with *acute inflammatory demyelinating polyneuropathy* (AIDP) (Table 447–1). At the present time it seems preferable to retain the clinical term *GBS*, because it is becoming increasingly clear that a small proportion of cases in North America and Europe, and a large proportion of cases in other regions, especially in the developing world, are characterized by noninflammatory acute axonal degeneration. These cases are clinically indistinguishable and have similar spinal fluid profiles. They are termed the axonal forms of GBS.

GBS is almost certainly an immune-mediated disorder. It follows some type of infectious disorder in approximately 60% of cases. The best documented antecedents include infection with *Campylobacter jejuni*, herpesviruses, and mycoplasma. *C. jejuni* is often associated with more severe "axonal" cases and most likely sensitizes the immune system to antigens shared between the organism and the peripheral nerve.

CLINICAL MANIFESTATIONS. The initial symptoms often consist of tingling and "pins-and-needles sensations" in the feet and may be associated with dull low-back pain. By the time of presentation, which usually occurs within hours or a very few days after first symptoms, weakness has usually supervened. The weakness is usually most prominent in the legs, but the arms or cranial musculature may be involved first. Tendon reflexes are lost early, even in regions where strength is retained. Because the spinal roots are usually prominently involved, GBS can involve short nerves (axial and intercostal as well as cranial nerves) as well as long ones. Weakness progresses, with the nadir reached within 30 days, and usually by 14 days. Progression can be alarmingly rapid, so that critical functions such as respiration can be lost within a few days or even a few hours.

The potential for respiratory insufficiency, as well as swallowing difficulty and autonomic dysregulation, underlies the life-threatening nature of GBS. In the past, mortality was as high as 15%. With modern critical care and the adjunctive therapies outlined below, mortality has fallen to about 2%. The first aspect of management is prompt and accurate initial diagnosis. At the time of presentation, a high index of clinical suspicion is necessary. No laboratory test is specific for GBS, but careful electrodiagnostic testing can usually identify at least mild abnormalities during the early stages. Although elevation of the spinal fluid protein level is characteristic, it usually rises only after the first week, not within the first few days when the diagnosis may be uncertain. At the earliest stages, the differential diagnosis includes non-neuropathic conditions such as spinal cord diseases (for example, transverse myelitis) and acute myopathies.

TREATMENT. Because of the potential for rapid deterioration, patients with a presumptive diagnosis of GBS usually require hospitalization for observation. Monitoring should include frequent measurement of the vital capacity and ability to swallow. Intensive-care observation and insertion of an airway should be initiated early, before declining ventilatory strength, autonomic dysregulation, or fatigue due to unproductive coughing erupts into an acute emergency. Such early intervention largely prevents life-threatening crises. Most of the reduction in mortality in GBS derives from modern intensive care.

Two adjunctive therapeutic techniques are of benefit. *Plasmapheresis*—the exchange of the patient's plasma for albumin—was the first treatment definitively shown to shorten the time to recovery. Infusion of high doses of *human immunoglobulin* intravenously also produces benefit. Both treatments are effective, and the choice should be individualized. In patients with limited venous access, gamma globulin is easier to administer. When the veins are sufficient for plasmapheresis, it may be the preferable treatment; experience with plasmapheresis is greater, and it may produce a lower incidence of relapse after initial improvement. The use of corticosteroids alone is not beneficial. Whether either plasmapheresis or intravenous immunoglobulin is useful in the axonal variants of GBS is undetermined.

Thorough education of the patient about the possibility of rapid deterioration and about the overall favorable prognosis is an important early step. While able to breathe and speak, patients should be instructed in a communication system with nurses and family so that they will be able to make themselves understood if intubation and respiratory support are required.

The prognosis for GBS varies with age, severity, and the extent to which axonal degeneration exceeds demyelination. A middle-aged patient who requires respiratory assistance, and who receives plasmapheresis early in the course, on the average resumes walking about 3 months later (6 months without plasmapheresis). Indeed,

TABLE 447–1. GUILLAIN-BARRÉ SYNDROME AND RELATED IMMUNE-MEDIATED NEUROPATHIES

Disorder	Type	Clinical Characteristics	Pathophysiology	Treatment
Guillain-Barré syndrome				
	Acute inflammatory demyelinating polyneuropathy	Prominent or predominant motor involvement of acute onset	Demyelination, lymphocytic infiltration	Plasmapheresis; intravenous immunoglobulin (IVIg); corticosteroids alone ineffective
	Acute inflammatory demyelinating polyneuropathy	Ataxia, ophthalmoparesis, and areflexia of acute onset	Antibodies against the ganglioside GQ1b	(Probably) plasmapheresis or IVIg
	Axonal GBS	Motorsensory or pure motor forms	Noninflammatory axonal degeneration predominates; strongly associated with antecedent *Campylobacter jejuni* infection	(Probably) plasmapheresis or IVIg
Chronic inflammatory demyelinating polyneuropathy		Slower onset; may be recurrent	Widespread demyelination with remyelination, secondary axonal loss; may occur in association with monoclonal gammopathy	Corticosteroids, plasmapheresis, IVIg
Multifocal motor neuropathy		Stepwise involvement of individual nerves; nearly pure motor involvement	Focal demyelination	IVIg or cytotoxic agents; corticosteroids and plasmapheresis ineffective

many recover much more promptly than that. Relapses, if they occur, should be re-treated with plasmapheresis or gamma globulin.

Arnason BGW, Soliven B: Acute inflammatory demyelinating polyradiculopathy. In Dyck PJ, Thomas PK, Griffin JW, et al. (eds.): Peripheral Neuropathy, 3rd ed. Philadelphia, W.B. Saunders, 1993, pp. 1437–1497.

Hartung H-P, Stoll G, Toyka KV: Immune reactions in the peripheral nervous system. In Dyck PJ, Thomas PK, Griffin JW, et al. (eds.): Peripheral Neuropathy, 3rd ed. Philadelphia, W.B. Saunders, 1993, pp. 418–444.

McKhann GM, Cornblath DR, Griffin JW, et al: Acute motor axonal neuropathy: A frequent cause of acute flaccid paralysis in China. Ann Neurol 33:333, 1993. Describes a large epidemic of a GBS variant occurring in an underdeveloped country.

Ropper AH, Wijdicks EFM, Truax BT: Guillain-Barré Syndrome. Philadelphia, F.A. Davis, 1991. A thorough analysis of all aspects of the disorder.

van der Meche FGA, Schmitz PIM, Dutch Guillain-Barré Study Group: A randomized trial comparing intravenous immune globulin and plasma exchange in Guillain-Barré syndrome. N Engl J Med 326:1123, 1992.

Yuki N, Yoshino H, Sato S, et al.: Severe acute axonal form of Guillain-Barré syndrome associated with IgG anti-GD$_{1a}$ antibodies. Muscle Nerve 15:899, 1992.

CHRONIC INFLAMMATORY DEMYELINATING NEUROPATHY

Chronic inflammatory demyelinating neuropathy (CIDP), sometimes referred to as chronic GBS, bears similarities to the clinical, pathologic, and laboratory pictures seen in acute GBS. It differs primarily in the time course and in the absence of identifiable antecedent events. The differences in response to therapy, however, suggest that the precise immunopathogenetic mechanisms are likely to differ.

CLINICAL MANIFESTATIONS. CIDP can occur at any age. The usual picture is one of slowly evolving weakness beginning in the legs, with widespread areflexia and loss of large-fiber (vibratory) sensibility on examination. In the more rapidly evolving cases of CIDP, the distinction from GBS is arbitrary. In general, in patients with acute GBS the nadir is reached within 4 weeks, while in patients with CIDP more time is required. The diagnosis is supported by prominent demyelinating features on nerve conduction studies and by elevation of the protein level of the spinal fluid.

Blinded trials showed that, unlike GBS, most cases of CIDP respond to corticosteroids alone. CIDP also responds to plasmapheresis. Intravenous gamma globulin improves some cases. In most instances the first choice of therapy is with corticosteroids, using the lowest dosage required to achieve and maintain an adequate response. Plasmapheresis, while simple and safe, usually must be repeated every several weeks to maintain a response and entails substantial expense. Nevertheless, this form of therapy is valuable in patients who do not respond to corticosteroids or in whom unacceptable corticosteroid doses are required or side effects supervene.

Dyck PJ, O'Brien PC, Oviatt KF, et al.: Prednisone improves chronic inflammatory demyelinating polyradiculoneuropathy more than no treatment. Ann Neurol 11:136, 1982.

Dyck PJ, Prineas J, Pollard J: Chronic inflammatory demyelinating polyradiculoneuropathy. In Dyck PJ, Thomas PK, Griffin JW, et al. (eds.): Peripheral Neuropathy, 3rd ed. Philadelphia, W.B. Saunders, 1993, pp. 1498–1517.

MULTIFOCAL MOTOR NEUROPATHY

An uncommon related disorder, *multifocal motor neuropathy,* occurs as "pure motor" multiple mononeuropathy. A patient may describe, for example, development of unilateral wristdrop (radial nerve involvement) followed by footdrop on the other side (peroneal nerve involvement). In addition, tendon reflexes may be lost outside the distribution of weakness, but the sensory examination is normal even in weak limbs. The pathologic characteristic, inflammatory demyelination, resembles that seen in CIDP, but is highly focal and largely spares sensory nerve fibers. A characteristic electrodiagnostic feature is the presence of *conduction block,* a reflection of the focal demyelination. The spinal fluid protein is usually normal. A nonspecific but helpful laboratory finding, noted in about 70% of cases, is markedly increased anti-GM$_1$ ganglioside antibodies in the serum. Multifocal motor neuropathy is noteworthy because it can be confused with more ominous disorders such as amyotrophic lateral sclerosis, but responds favorably to intravenous immunoglobulin as well as to cytotoxic therapy. Neither corticosteroids nor plasmapheresis brings improvement.

Chaudhry V, Corse AM, Cornblath DR, et al.: Multifocal motor neuropathy: Response to human immune globulin. Ann Neurol 33:237, 1993.

Pestronk A, Cornblath DR, Ilyas AA, et al.: A treatable multifocal motor neuropathy with antibodies to GM$_1$ ganglioside. Ann Neurol 24:73, 1988.

NEUROPATHIES ASSOCIATED WITH MONOCLONAL GAMMOPATHIES

Peripheral neuropathy occurs in some monoclonal gammopathies, both the benign type and myeloma. Monoclonal proteins of IgM, IgG, and IgA types are all associated with neuropathy. In some instances the monoclonal protein has been shown to cause the neuropathy. For example, some IgM monoclonal proteins react with sugars found on a specific Schwann cell protein, the *myelin-associated glycoprotein* (MAG). The monoclonal protein intercalates into the myelin lamellae, producing a distinctive pathologic feature, abnormally wide spacing between adjacent myelin lamellae, and consequent demyelination. The neuropathy can be reproduced in experimental animals (chickens) by passive transfer of the monoclonal IgM from patients. A few other nerve epitopes have been defined with which specific paraproteins react. However, for most of the IgG and IgA monoclonal proteins the mechanism of nerve injury is not known.

CLINICAL MANIFESTATIONS. The clinical picture of the neuropathy varies. The IgM monoclonal antibodies with "anti-MAG" reactivity typically produce neuropathy with prominent large-fiber sensory loss and sensory ataxia, as well as milder weakness. The electrodiagnostic tests indicate demyelination, albeit admixed with nerve fiber loss. In other cases with IgM monoclonal proteins there is a distinctive picture that includes scleroderma-like skin changes, hepatomegaly, and endocrine abnormalities, as well as neuropathy (the POEMS syndrome described below). Other individuals with monoclonal proteins have a clinical picture identical to CIDP, and still others have distally predominant axonal degeneration.

Identification of a monoclonal protein does not necessarily mean that the protein is the cause of the neuropathy. Most of the monoclonal proteins found in patients with neuropathy are classed as monoclonal gammopathies of unknown significance, a group alternatively termed benign monoclonal gammopathies because there is no evidence of multiple myeloma at the time of presentation. The incidence of such monoclonal proteins increases with age. Especially in older patients, before the presumption is accepted that the paraprotein causes the neuropathy, it is important to exclude other causes of neuropathy, such as diabetes or alcoholism.

Three disorders should be specifically sought in individuals with paraproteins and neuropathy: (1) There is a special association of neuropathy with solitary plasmacytomas, often osteosclerotic. The POEMS syndrome—polyneuropathy, organomegaly, endocrinopathy (hirsutism, testicular atrophy), monoclonal IgM protein, and skin pigmentation—is highly associated with osteosclerotic myelomas. A skeletal radiographic survey is essential in patients with monoclonal proteins and neuropathy. (2) Cryoglobulinema, with or without monoclonal gammopathy, can produce neuropathy, and the possibility should be excluded. (3) The monoclonal proteins may result in amyloid deposition in nerve and thus produce neuropathy indirectly. Amyloid deposition is particularly associated with excretion of light chains in the urine. The distinctive neurologic picture of amyloidosis often suggests the possibility of amyloid neuropathy (see below). Unlike most other neuropathies, there is a predilection for involvement of small sensory and autonomic nerve fibers, so that the history may include painless injuries to the feet or hands and evidence of autonomic dysfunction, including impotence and orthostatic hypotension. Definitive diagnosis of immunoglobulin-associated amyloidosis is by histology. Fat pad aspiration and muscle biopsy may be useful before undertaking biopsy of rectal ganglia or peripheral nerve.

The one category of paraproteinemic neuropathies in which treatment is clearly beneficial is that of the solitary plasmacytomas. Excision and radiation of the plasmacytoma can be curative. In other paraproteinemic neuropathies, some reports suggest modest benefit from plasmapheresis or other forms of therapy in neuropathies associated with benign monoclonal gammopathies. In general, however, the degree of improvement is insufficient for the nuisance and expense of therapy. The effort is better focused on gait training and protection from falls. No therapy has been shown to slow progression of amyloid neuropathy.

Kyle RA, Dyck PJ: Osteosclerotic myeloma (POEMS syndrome). In Dyck PJ, Thomas PK, Griffin JW, et al. (eds.): Peripheral Neuropathy, 3rd ed. Philadelphia, W.B. Saunders, 1993, pp. 1288–1293.

Kyle RA, Dyck PJ: Amyloidosis and neuropathy. In Dyck PJ, Thomas PK, Griffin JW, et al. (eds.): Peripheral Neuropathy, 3rd ed. Philadelphia, W.B. Saunders, 1993, pp. 1294–1309.

Kyle RA, Dyck PJ: Neuropathy associated with the monoclonal gammopathies. *In* Dyck PJ, Thomas PK, Griffin JW, et al. (eds.): Peripheral Neuropathy, 3rd ed. Philadelphia, W.B. Saunders, 1993, pp. 1275–1287.

IMMUNE-MEDIATED ATAXIC NEUROPATHIES

In this category are three disorders: *carcinomatous sensory neuropathy, sensory ganglionitis associated with features of Sjögren's syndrome,* and *idiopathic sensory ganglionitis.* All three are characterized clinically by subacute or slowly developing proprioceptive sensory loss leading to gait ataxia and inability to localize arms and/or legs. Patients show rombergism: They can stand with feet together and eyes open, but fall when they close their eyes, reflecting loss of kinesthetic sensibility. Tendon reflexes usually disappear, but strength remains. Pathologic changes in all three disorders include lymphocytic infiltration of the dorsal root ganglia, with destruction of the primary sensory neurons and associated degeneration of their central and peripheral processes. Large sensory neurons are predominantly affected, leaving pain and thermal sensibilities relatively intact. Electrodiagnostic studies document the absence of sensory nerve action potentials and preservation of motor responses. Spinal fluid protein may be normal or contain increased protein. Modest pleocytosis often accompanies the carcinomatous disorder.

The possibility of occult carcinoma underlying an immunogenic (paraneoplastic) ataxic neuropathy adds urgency to differential diagnosis. The most frequent associations include small cell carcinoma of the lung, breast carcinoma, and ovarian carcinoma. In addition to clinical screening for these possibilities, a useful serologic test is the anti-Hu antibody, which reacts with a 37-kD neuronal nuclear protein. Although the presence of anti-Hu antibodies is neither perfectly sensitive nor specific, their association with ataxic neuropathy strongly suggests underlying carcinoma. It should be noted that carcinoma has also been associated with other types of neuropathy, including bland, slowly evolving, sensory motor neuropathy. However, this type of neuropathy is usually an accompaniment of advanced stages of cancer and is rarely a presenting manifestation. The evaluation for occult carcinoma is directed toward those uncommon patients with pure sensory ataxic neuropathy.

Another group of patients with a similar clinical and pathologic picture have features of Sjögren's syndrome, including keratoconjunctivitis sicca and elevated antinuclear antibody titers (Ch. 263). Surprisingly, these patients only occasionally have joint disease or other extraglandular manifestations of Sjögren's syndrome, and most will not have sought medical attention before neuropathy develops. Affected patients are likely to have associated autonomic insufficiency, including pupils that are large and are more reactive to accommodation than to light (Adie's pupils).

A third group of patients with idiopathic sensory ganglionitis have no associated systemic disease. Because this group of disorders often have a very acute onset, they may be misdiagnosed as Guillain-Barré syndrome. This group is referred to as *idiopathic sensory neuronopathy.*

Unfortunately, cytotoxic or corticosteroid therapy only rarely benefits any of these sensory ganglionitis disorders. The gait ataxia produces substantial early disability, but relearning through gait training, rehabilitation, and physical therapy allows a large proportion of affected individuals to resume daily activities.

Griffin JW, Cornblath DR, Alexander E, et al.: Ataxic sensory neuropathy and dorsal root ganglionitis associated with Sjogren's syndrome. Ann Neurol 27:304, 1990.

McLeod JG: Paraneoplastic neuropathies. *In* Dyck PJ, Thomas PK, Griffin JW, et al. (eds.): Peripheral Neuropathy, 3rd ed. Philadelphia, W.B. Saunders, 1993, pp. 1583–1590.

Windebank AJ, Blexrud MD, Dyck PJ, et al.: The syndrome of acute sensory neuropathy: Clinical features and electrophysiologic and pathologic changes. Neurology 40:584, 1990.

VASCULITIC NEUROPATHIES

Peripheral nerves have extensive collateral circulation and are relatively invulnerable to occlusion of large peripheral arteries. By contrast, they are susceptible to focal interruption of circulation within the individual nerve fascicles due to small blood vessel diseases. As a result, many types of systemic vasculitis affect the peripheral nerves. They are one of the most frequently damaged organ systems in polyarteritis nodosa and are frequently involved in rheumatoid arteritis, Sjögren's syndrome, and the vasculitides associated with infections such as hepatitis B, Lyme disease, and HIV. They are less frequently affected in Wegener's granulomatosis because of its restricted regional involvement. The peripheral nerves can be the predominant site of vasculitis, producing a syndrome re-

ferred to as vasculitis restricted to the peripheral nervous system. This disorder offers special diagnostic challenges, because the usual footprints of systemic inflammatory disease, including elevated sedimentation rate, are often absent.

CLINICAL MANIFESTATIONS. The clinical manifestations of all of these vasculitic neuropathies reflect the patchiness of the underlying disease. The characteristic picture consists of multiple mononeuropathy, often evolving in a stepwise fashion, so that wristdrop from radial nerve palsy may occur on one side followed by footdrop on the other, with patchy areas of subjective numbness or sensory loss appearing elsewhere on the extremities. The asymmetry and the length-independence of the nerves involved suggest small vessel disease of nerve. In the absence of diabetes mellitus, vasculitis becomes the prime diagnostic consideration. Evaluation of multiple mononeuropathy includes screening of patients to detect evidence of systemic vasculitis in the skin, kidneys, eyes, and other organs. Ultimately, vasculitis is a histologic diagnosis, and if no other organ involvement is identified, combined nerve and muscle biopsy is needed to establish diagnosis.

Treatment of vasculitic neuropathies consists of treatment of the underlying vasculitis. In a neuropathy apparently restricted to the peripheral nervous system, corticosteroids may be tried initially, but most patients require cytotoxic therapy comparable to that used for polyarteritis.

Said G, Lacroix-Ciaudo C, Fujimura H, et al: The peripheral neuropathy of necrotizing arteritis: A clinicopathological study. Ann Neurol 23:461, 1988.

448 HEREDITARY NEUROPATHIES

Heritable neuropathies rank among the most prevalent inherited neurologic diseases. Because many occur in midlife and because the family history is often previously unrecognized, the heritable disorders constitute an important aspect of differential diagnosis.

CHARCOT-MARIE-TOOTH DISEASE

DEFINITION. The eponymic designation, *Charcot-Marie-Tooth* (CMT) disease, identifies a group of heritable disorders of peripheral nerves that share clinical features, but differ in their pathology and the specific genetic abnormalities, as shown in Table 448–1. One group of disorders, classed together as CMT type I (CMT I), is characterized pathologically by abnormalities of peripheral myelination and, at a molecular level, by abnormalities of specific proteins found in the myelin sheaths or Schwann cells. The CMT II group is characterized by axonal degeneration.

PATHOGENESIS. Most forms of CMT disease reflect an autosomal dominant trait, but some similar clinical phenotypes overlap different genetic abnormalities. Several gene abnormalities can cause CMT I (Table 448–1). Three specific gene abnormalities have been identified. The most prevalent is duplication of a segment of chromosome 17 that encodes the peripheral myelin protein-22 (PMP-22) gene. A chromosome 1-linked form is due to an abnormality of another myelin protein, termed P_0. Recently a sex-linked form has been related to abnormalities of the connexin-32 gene. The gene defects in the axonal forms are not yet known.

PATHOLOGY. The pathology of the demyelinating forms of CMT is characterized by excessive numbers of Schwann cells forming concentric rings around nerve fibers. Termed *onion bulbs* because of their appearance on microscopic examination, the wrappings lead to a palpable and often visible increase in the size of certain nerves, such as the ulnar nerve at the elbow or the greater auricular nerve running from the posterior margin of the sternocleidomastoid muscle to the base of the ear. Because of the increase in the size of the nerves, the demyelinating forms of CMT disease are termed *hypertrophic neuropathies.*

CLINICAL MANIFESTATIONS. All forms of CMT disease tend to occur in the second to fourth decades with insidiously evolving footdrop. On examination, one finds distal wasting of the intrinsic muscles of the feet, the anterior tibial group, and the

TABLE 448-1. CHARCOT-MARIE-TOOTH (CMT) AND RELATED HERITABLE NEUROPATHIES

Disorder	Type	Clinical Features	Pathophysiology	Inheritance	Gene Defect
CMT I		Slowly evolving motor-sensory neuropathies with high arches, hammer toes, hypertrophic nerves	Demyelination and remyelination with onion bulbs		
	a			Dominant	Duplication of a segment of chromosome 17 encoding PMP-22
	b			Dominant	Point mutation in the myelin protein P_0
	x			Sex-linked	Mutation in connexin 32
CMT II		Similar, without hypertrophic nerves	Distally predominant axonal degeneration	Dominant	Unknown
CMT III (Dejerine-Sottas disease)		Early onset, severe motor-sensory neuropathy	Severe hypomyelination with onion bulbs	Recessive	Mutation in P_0

calves. A variable degree of impaired large-fiber sensory function is reflected in elevated vibratory thresholds in the toes. Tendon reflexes are lost, at least at the ankles. Typically a foot deformity exists, with high arches (pes cavus) and hammer toes, reflecting long-standing muscle imbalance in the feet. Upon specific questioning, affected individuals recall that they were never athletic, that they could not run, jump, or ice skate along with their peers. Often they report frequent ankle sprains. In general, these problems attract little concern on the part of patients or their families, reflecting the lifelong nature and slow evolution of the disease. Patients can frequently identify several other family members who have similar foot deformities. The most useful diagnostic test lies in the identification of the clinical features in other family members. Even mild or subclinical forms of the disease are usually identified readily on examination.

TREATMENT. Most patients with CMT disease enjoy a nearly full spectrum of occupational and daily activities, and they have a normal lifespan. The footdrop can be relieved by appropriate bracing of the ankle. Occasionally, however, the disease produces much greater deficits. Genetic counseling and education of affected individuals and their families is important, both for reassurance and to preclude unnecessary diagnostic evaluation of affected members in future generations.

AMYLOID NEUROPATHIES

All forms of amyloid neuropathy are due to extracellular deposition of the fibrillary protein, amyloid, in peripheral nerve and sensory and autonomic ganglia, as well as around blood vessels in nerves and other tissues. The nonhereditary type of amyloidosis associated with monoclonal immunoglobulins has been described above. The forms of heritable amyloidosis, at one time classified by geographic origin of the first families recognized, have been shown by molecular genetic techniques to represent a variety of point mutations in the transthyretin (prealbumin) gene. The most frequent variant transthyretin protein results from substitution of methionine for valine at position 30 in the molecule. In all forms of amyloidosis, the precise means by which amyloid deposition injures nerve remains unresolved. Mechanical distortion of neurons in the sensory and autonomic ganglia and of nerve fibers, as well as vascular involvement due to amyloid deposition around blood vessels, both may contribute.

CLINICAL MANIFESTATIONS. In all forms of amyloidosis the outstanding abnormalities affect the small sensory and autonomic fibers. Involvement of small fibers responsible for pain and thermal sensibilities leads to loss of the ability to perceive mechanical and thermal injury and tissue damage. As a result, painless injuries present a major hazard of this disorder; in advanced stages they can lead to chronic infections or osteomyelitis of the feet or hands, and the need for amputation. The autonomic dysfunction produces orthostatic hypotension, impotence, and, in late stages, bladder and bowel incontinence. Until the late stages, strength, touch-pressure sensibility, and vibratory sensation are usually preserved. In some of the heritable forms (as well as in immunoglobulin-associated amyloidosis), median nerve entrapment may occur because of amyloid deposition. Diagnosis of systemic amyloidosis is made by histologic demonstration of amyloid in biopsy of nerve, muscle, fat aspirate, or other tissue. The heritable forms are normally autosomal dominant, so that the diagnosis may be suggested

by family history. The specific genetic abnormality can be identified by molecular genetic analysis. No definitive treatment for any form of amyloid neuropathy is available, but education in prevention of injury to anesthetic limbs can preserve function.

449 METABOLIC NEUROPATHIES

DIABETIC NEUROPATHIES

Diabetes is the most frequent cause of peripheral neuropathy worldwide. Incidence figures depend on the employed definition; at least some peripheral nerve abnormalities can be detected in about 70% of patients with longstanding diabetes, and symptomatic neuropathy affects 5 to 10%. The diabetic neuropathies include a variety of clinical forms, including symmetric polyneuropathies, and a variety of forms of individual nerve injury (Table 449-1).

DIABETIC POLYNEUROPATHY

Diabetic polyneuropathy is symmetric and usually distally predominant, beginning with sensory loss in the feet. It is the most frequent of the diabetic neuropathies. It is uncommon at the time of diagnosis of diabetes, but its prevalence increases with duration of diabetes. The precise pathogenesis remains a matter of controversy, but a signal recent advance has been the demonstration that, like the ocular and renal complications, diabetic neuropathy can be reduced in incidence and in severity by maintaining blood sugar levels close to normal. This effect of "tight control" is consistent with the hypothesis that hyperglycemia itself contributes to nerve damage. The complications of hyperglycemia that injure nerves may include one or more of the following: abnormalities of nerve vasculature and blood flow, leading to angiopathic injury; metabolic effects of abnormalities in polyol pathways; and nonenzymatic glycosylation of nerve proteins.

CLINICAL MANIFESTATIONS. The neuropathy is usually asymptomatic at the onset, a stage during which abnormalities in sensation and reflexes may be detected on routine examination. The symptomatic phase usually begins insidiously, but some cases have an abrupt onset, and in a small percentage of patients this appears to be precipitated by the institution of insulin. Unlike most other

TABLE 449-1. DIABETIC NEUROPATHIES

Diabetic polyneuropathies
  Rapidly reversible physiologic dysfunction associated with hyperglycemia
  Symmetric polyneuropathy
    Sensorimotor neuropathy
    "Small-fiber" neuropathy, with autonomic dysfunction, reduced pain sensibility, spontaneous burning pain
Diabetic mononeuropathies and plexopathies
  Diabetic third nerve palsy
  Diabetic fourth nerve palsy
  Diabetic truncal neuropathy
  Diabetic lumbosacral plexopathy

neuropathies, in diabetes small-fiber sensibility as well as large-fiber sensation are typically reduced, resulting in elevated pin, thermal, and vibratory thresholds. The small-fiber dysfunction is often manifested by spontaneous neuropathic pain. This includes bothersome *dysesthesias*—unpleasant sensations evoked by normally innocuous stimuli, such as the bedsheets on the toes at night. There may be continuous burning or throbbing pain, and walking often is distressing ("It feels like I'm walking on coals."). In addition, sudden intense "lightning" pains may affect the feet and legs.

Some degree of autonomic insufficiency is frequent in diabetic neuropathy. Manifestations include loss of the normal sinus arrhythmia; failure of blood pressure restoration and cardiac acceleration on standing, sometimes producing orthostatic hypotension; impotence; constipation; and a particularly distressing symptom, diabetic diarrhea, with unpredictable loose stools and fecal incontinence. In some patients, these "small-fiber" abnormalities, including neuropathic pain, loss of pin and thermal sensibility, and autonomic dysfunction, dominate the clinical picture.

The diagnosis of diabetic polyneuropathy is straightforward in established diabetics with typical clinical pictures. Electrodiagnostic studies, usually unnecessary, document neuropathy, and spinal fluid protein is frequently moderately elevated. Conversely, diabetic neuropathy is the most *overdiagnosed* cause of peripheral nerve disease. In general, the diagnosis of diabetic neuropathy can comfortably be made only in the setting of longstanding diabetes, usually insulin-requiring. If only recent mild hyperglycemia is present, the diagnosis of diabetic polyneuropathy should be regarded as suspect.

TREATMENT. The approach to management of diabetic hyperglycemia is outside the scope of this chapter, but there is increasing reason to think that primary prevention as well as slowing of the progression of established diabetic neuropathy is abetted by correction of blood sugar to as nearly normal values as possible ("tight control"; see Ch. 218). Once the diagnosis of diabetic polyneuropathy is established, no other specific treatment for the neuropathy is currently available. Symptomatic management includes use of tricyclic antidepressants or carbamazepine for the spontaneous neuropathic pain. Full therapeutic doses are required, and the dosage must be slowly increased to minimize side effects such as dizziness. Opiates are contraindicated, but high doses of amitriptyline sometimes help. The major goal in management of diabetic polyneuropathy is prevention of the cycle of painless injury, ulceration, cellulitis, osteomyelitis, and osteolysis that underlies much of the functional disability produced by this disorder and that contributes to an ultimate requirement for amputation. The loss of pain sensibility on examination should trigger increased vigilance. Painless injuries can largely be prevented by education, avoidance of physical and thermal hazards to the feet, well-fitting shoes, and frequent inspections of the feet. Erythema or injury is treated promptly with removal of the aggravating factor, such as an ill-fitting shoe. Cessation of weight bearing until healing occurs can minimize ulceration. Meticulous skin and nail care is required.

One of the most distressing aspects of the autonomic neuropathy is impotence. A variety of methods, including intracavernous injection of yohimbine, have been advocated and are helpful to some patients. Other genitourinary disturbances include retrograde ejaculation and disordered micturition. Milder cases of diabetic diarrhea may respond to agents such as diphenoxylate.

MONONEUROPATHY AND MULTIPLE MONONEUROPATHIES

Diabetes also can cause a variety of mononeuropathies and multiple mononeuropathies. They represent vascular insufficiency or infarction in nerve, presumably caused by disease of the small blood vessels. Their onset is typically abrupt and often painful.

CLINICAL MANIFESTATIONS. Characteristic is *diabetic third nerve palsy,* characterized by sudden inability to adduct the eye or open the lid. Unlike third nerve compression from intracranial masses or carotid aneurysms, the pupil is typically spared. The sixth nerve, the femoral nerve, or other major nerves of the extremities, may be similarly involved.

In another characteristic syndrome, best termed *diabetic lumbosacral plexopathy,* affected persons develop pain in the hip with asymmetric weakness of the proximal leg muscles over days to a few weeks. The disorder often occurs in a setting of recent severe (>10%) loss of body weight and frequently appears to be a "femoral" neuropathy, with quadriceps weakness and loss of the tendon reflex at the knee. Careful examination, however, usually discloses more widespread involvement of muscles innervated by

the lumbosacral plexus, typically including the hamstring and gluteus muscles. Although the complaints may be referable to one side, mild abnormalities often affect the contralateral side. In addition, evidence of more symmetric polyneuropathy, with reduced tendon reflexes of the ankles, elevated sensory thresholds, and often weakness of toe extension and ankle dorsiflexion, may exist. The limited pathologic data available suggest that this is a consequence of small vessel disease in the lumbosacral plexus, perhaps amplified by associated atherosclerotic disease in the aortic bifurcation. In any event, the prognosis is surprisingly favorable; pain decreases within weeks, and strength returns to the affected muscles within weeks to months. At the onset this disorder can be confused with intraspinal disease or polyradiculopathy. Diabetic lumbosacral plexopathy is sometimes called diabetic amyotrophy, but this term is best avoided, because it has also been applied to a syndrome of widespread muscle wasting that occasionally develops in diabetics in association with a period of weight loss. A final noteworthy mononeuropathy is *diabetic truncal neuropathy.* Patients have pain in the distribution of one or more intercostal nerves, often associated with hypesthesia and numbness. Like the other diabetic mononeuropathies, recovery over months is the rule.

Dyck PJ, Karnes JL, Daube J, et al.: Clinical and neuropathological criteria for the diagnosis and staging of diabetic polyneuropathy. Brain 108:861, 1985.
Johnson PC, Doll SC, Cromey DW: Pathogenesis of diabetic neuropathy. Ann Neurol 19:450, 1986.
Max MB, Culnane M, Schafer SC, et al.: Amitriptyline relieves diabetic neuropathy pain in patients with normal or depressed mood. Neurology 37:589, 1987.

HEPATIC NEUROPATHY

Polyneuropathy is sufficiently uncommon in chronic liver disease that other underlying causes that can affect both liver and peripheral nerves (alcoholism, primary biliary cirrhosis) should be sought.

THYROID DISEASE

Myxedema neuropathy is usually a minor manifestation of myxedema, but areflexia and distal sensory loss can be seen. Cerebellar ataxia and behavioral changes usually predominate.

UREMIC NEUROPATHY

This peripheral neuropathy is associated with chronic renal insufficiency. Electrophysiologic abnormalities routinely occur when creatinine clearance is less than 10% of normal, but the severity and rate of progression of symptomatic uremic polyneuropathy vary widely. The syndrome usually consists of distally predominant, symmetric, motor-sensory polyneuropathy. In some patients, there is marked motor predominance, so that footdrop and leg weakness are major manifestations. In others, paresthesias and, occasionally, burning dysesthesias are early symptoms. In either event, loss of tendon reflexes, initially at the ankle, is characteristic. Electrophysiologic and pathologic studies indicate that both distal axonal degeneration and demyelination occur in uremic neuropathy, but the precise underlying mechanisms remain uncertain.

An important outcome of the past 30 years' experience with dialysis and renal transplantation is recognition that this peripheral neuropathy is both preventable and treatable by amelioration of the renal insufficiency. While both approaches are helpful, renal transplantation produces much better preservation of peripheral nerve function.

PORPHYRIC NEUROPATHY

The intermittent porphyrias, considered fully in Ch. 187, are important diagnostic considerations in acute neuropathies. The most prevalent of these disorders, acute intermittent porphyria (AIP), is associated with recurrent episodes of neuropathy, which are typically acute or subacute in onset. Paresthesias and dysesthesias of the extremities occur and in severe episodes are associated with rapidly evolving weakness or paralysis, mimicking the axonal form of Guillain-Barré syndrome, often associated with bladder dysfunction and constipation. The associated CNS effects may contribute to alterations in level of consciousness as well as hysteria-like or psychotic behavior, potentially delaying recognition of the emergent nature of the neuropathy. During acute attacks, most patients with AIP have increased excretion of porphobilinogen and delta-aminolevulinic acid in the urine. This simple diagnostic assay should be considered in any patient with acute paralytic neuropathy. The treatment of acute porphyric attacks is described in Ch. 187.

CRITICAL CARE NEUROPATHIES

An increasingly frequently recognized disorder, critical care neuropathy is encountered in patients following a severe medical illness, is often complicated by sepsis, and requires prolonged intensive care. Motor involvement predominates. Although it is usually most severe distally, it can impair the "weaning" of patients from ventilatory support. The underlying pathology appears to be axonal degeneration. The etiology is unclear, and no effective therapy other than time and adequate nutrition is known. Most affected persons recover completely.

450 TOXIC NEUROPATHIES

A wide array of environmental, occupational, recreational, and pharmaceutical agents can produce peripheral nerve disease. For agents in which the period of exposure is limited, the diagnosis is often suggested by subacute neuropathy. Most, although not all, neurotoxins produce distal axonal degeneration. The picture typically includes distally predominant sensory loss, loss of tendon reflexes at the ankles, and distal weakness. With continued exposure, the symptoms may progress more proximally; even after the offending agent is withdrawn, progression sometimes may continue, a phenomenon termed *coasting*. Nevertheless, withdrawal represents the optimal treatment. Tables 450–1 and 450–2 list important pharmaceutical and environmental toxins.

Persons with pre-existing nerve disease may be unusually susceptible to neurotoxins. For example, those with Charcot-Marie-Tooth disease can experience devastating toxic reactions to standard level chemotherapeutic doses of vincristine. In all toxic neuropathies the key to treatment lies in prompt recognition and withdrawal.

Schaumburg HH, Berger AR, Thomas PK: Disorders of Peripheral Nerve, 2nd ed. Philadelphia, F.A. Davis, 1992.

ALCOHOL-NUTRITIONAL NEUROPATHY

Polyneuropathy in persons with chronic alcoholism usually occurs in a setting of associated nutritional deficiency (see Ch. 456). The pathogenesis of alcohol-nutritional-deficiency neuropathy remains undefined. Most persons with alcoholic neuropathy have evidence of multifactorial nutritional deficiency, but in some, nutritional background seems adequate, and the direct contribution of alcohol cannot be excluded. The pathology of alcohol-nutritional neuropathy is that of a bland "dying back" disorder affecting both sensory and motor fibers. The initial symptoms are pain and paresthesias, beginning on the soles of the feet, sometimes evolving to

TABLE 450–1. PHARMACEUTIC NEUROTOXINS

Antiretrovirals (ddI, ddC)
Chloramphenicol
Cisplatin
Clioquinols
Dapsone
Disulfiram (Antabuse)
Ethambutol
Ethionamide
Gold
Hydralazine
Isoniazid
Metronidazole and misonidazole
Nitrofurantoin
Penicillamine
Perhexiline
Phenytoin (rare)
Pyridoxine
Stilbamidine
Suramin
Thalidomide
Vincristine/vinblastine

TABLE 450–2. INDUSTRIAL AND ENVIRONMENTAL NEUROTOXINS

Metals
  Arsenic
  Lead
  Mercury
  Thallium
Substance abuse
  Alcohol
  Glue (hexacarbons) inhalation
  Nitrous oxide inhalation
Industrial poisons
  Acrylamide
  Carbon disulfide
  Cyanide (chronic)
  Dichlorophenoxyacetic acid
  Dimethylaminopropionitrile
  Ethylene oxide
  Hexacarbon (n-hexane) (glue sniffer, occupational exposure to solvents, glues, or glue thinner)
  Organophosphorus esters (triorthocresyl phosphate, leptophos, mipafox, trichlorphon)
  Polychlorinated biphenyls
  Tetrachlorbiphenyl
  Trichloroethylene (trigeminal neuropathy)

burning feet and severe hyperpathia and often associated with aching and tenderness of the calves. Weakness is initially distal, and tendon reflexes are lost first at the ankles. Treatment with nutritional supplementation, including thiamine and multivitamins, and cessation of alcohol ingestion are highly beneficial in the early stages of the disease. In advanced cases the disease may continue to progress for a period after initiation of therapy, and recovery may be incomplete.

451 NEUROPATHIES ASSOCIATED WITH INFECTIOUS DISEASES

HUMAN IMMUNODEFICIENCY VIRUS (HIV) INFECTION

A variety of nerve diseases can accompany HIV infection (see also Ch. 428.2). The *Guillain-Barré syndrome* (GBS) and *chronic inflammatory peripheral neuropathy* (CIDP) tend to occur early in HIV infection, when CD4 counts are 250 to 500, and before development of AIDS. They presumably reflect early immune dysregulation. They are distinguished by the frequent presence of pleocytosis, an uncommon finding in seronegative GBS and CIDP. Their course and response to treatment are similar to those observed in seronegative patients.

Cytomegalovirus (CMV) infection of nerve occurs in the setting of clinically evident AIDS and in association with systemic CMV infection. CMV can produce multiple mononeuropathy associated with focal infection of endothelial cells of the nerve, macrophages, and Schwann cells. A dramatic and potentially treatable disorder is *CMV polyradiculopathy*. It develops in persons with AIDS and is characterized by abrupt pain in the back and legs with rapidly progressing paraparesis and areflexia. A distinctive finding is polymorphonuclear pleocytosis, usually associated with markedly increased spinal fluid protein. Cytologic examination sometimes can identify CMV inclusions in spinal fluid. The differential diagnosis includes herpesvirus-associated transverse myelopathies. Prompt diagnosis of CMV polyradiculopathy is important, because some patients respond well to antiviral therapy with ganciclovir and/or foscarnet.

The most prevalent neuropathic complication of HIV infection is *sensory neuropathy of AIDS*. In advanced AIDS, affected patients typically complain of pain on the soles of the feet and discomfort while walking. Neuropathic pain may be intense, associated with loss of small and large-fiber sensory modalities, with a variable, usually mild, degree of motor impairment. Typically the reflexes are lost at the ankle but exaggerated at the knees. This pattern reflects both neuropathy and a CNS disease such as vacuolar myelopathy. Pathologic studies of the sensory neuropathy have shown noninflammatory distally predominant axonal degeneration of sensory fibers. Both large and small fibers are lost. The pathogenesis is unknown, but the disease does not appear to be produced by local productive HIV infection within the nerves themselves. The treatment is symptomatic.

Griffin JW, Wesselingh SL, Griffin DE, et al.: Peripheral neuropathies in HIV infection: Similarities and contrasts with the central nervous system. In HIV, AIDS, and the Brain. Association in Research on Nervous and Mental Disease Proceedings, Vol 92. New York, Raven Press, 1994.

LYME DISEASE (BORRELIOSIS)

Neuropathic consequences can predominate in some patients with Lyme disease (see Ch. 343). The geographic area of the patient as well as history of the characteristic antecedent rash may suggest the diagnosis. The neuropathy is usually a multiple mononeuropathy, with a high predilection of facial nerve involvement, mimicking idiopathic Bell's palsy.

LEPROUS NEUROPATHY

The clinical manifestations of leprosy are virtually exclusively those of peripheral neuropathy and its sequelae. Although WHO has set a target for eradication of active leprosy by the year 2000, at least 5 million individuals with residual disease will remain worldwide. In all forms of leprosy, infection of the skin with *Mycobacterium leprae* and destruction of cutaneous nerve fibers are the primary events. The major classes, *lepromatous* and *tuberculoid,* differ in the extent of postimmune response to the organism.

In *lepromatous leprosy,* no effective cellular immune response is mounted, and large numbers of bacilli reside within the skin, where they infect predominantly the Schwann cells of intracutaneous nerves. With time, Schwann cells throughout the peripheral nervous system are affected, with a striking distribution of nerve fiber damage related to environmental temperatures. Organisms proliferate in the nerve fibers in the coolest regions of the skin, such as the ears, the lateral area of the face, and the digits, before they affect warmer areas covered with clothing. The resulting cutaneous sensory loss includes strikingly selective loss of pain sensibility.

The other major form of the disease, *tuberculoid leprosy,* is characterized by an active inflammatory response to the organism with much of the nerve damage probably resulting from the immune response. Tuberculoid disease and the intermediate form, *borderline disease,* produce a less stereotyped, more patchy and asymmetric neuropathy.

Painless injuries and painless traumatic joint diseases are the major sequelae of both forms of leprosy. Recent data have shown that chemotherapy for leprosy is associated with regeneration of nerve fibers. In general, however, nerve fibers do not successfully reinnervate the skin, so that cutaneous anesthesia and its complications persist. In addition to chemotherapy, education and protection from painless injuries, as described for diabetic polyneuropathies, can substantially modify the outcome.

Miko TL, Le Maitre C, Kinfu Y: Damage and regeneration of peripheral nerves in advanced treated leprosy. Lancet 342:521, 1993.
Sabin TD, Swift TR, Jacobson RR: Leprosy. *In* Dyck PJ, Thomas PK, Griffin JW, et al. (eds.): Peripheral Neuropathy, 3rd ed. Philadelphia, W.B. Saunders Company, 1993, pp. 1354–1379.

452 ENTRAPMENT AND COMPRESSIVE NEUROPATHIES

The peripheral nerves are vulnerable to chronic compression or entrapment in a variety of sites. The most frequently encountered are median nerve compression at the wrist within the carpal tunnel *(carpal tunnel syndrome);* median nerve compression in the upper forearm; ulnar nerve compression in the hand *(cubital tunnel syndrome),* wrist, or at the elbow *(tardy ulnar nerve palsy);* tibial nerve compression behind the medial malleolus *(tarsal tunnel syndrome);* and peroneal nerve compression over the lateral fibular head. Because of its prevalence, carpal tunnel syndrome deserves specific comment.

CARPAL TUNNEL SYNDROME

Entrapment of the median nerve at the wrist reflects the limited available space for the median nerve because of the surrounding bone, joint, and ligaments, as well as the tendons and synovium passing through the canal. Repetitive motion of the fingers is a highly publicized exacerbating element, but other precipitating factors that should be considered include trauma, osteoarthritis, ganglionic cysts, myxedema, and rarely, amyloid deposition. Mild symptoms typically involve paresthesias of the first three digits, often occurring overnight and relieved by shaking or elevating the hands. In more severe disease, objective sensory loss in the median nerve distribution, weakness of median-innervated muscles such as the abductor pollicis brevis, and prolongation of nerve conduction across the carpal tunnel (prolonged distal latency) are characteristic. The diagnosis is supported by identification of *Tinel's sign,* in which tapping the carpal tunnel elicits paresthesias in the median nerve distribution, and by paresthesias produced by sustained flexion of the wrist.

The treatment of carpal tunnel syndrome requires consideration of the relationship between symptoms and occupational or recreational activities. Treatment begins with splinting of the wrist in slight dorsiflexion during sleep, thereby increasing the cross-sectional area of the carpal tunnel. Injection of corticosteroids into the carpal tunnel and use of potassium-sparing diuretics are helpful in some patients. More severe carpal tunnel syndrome is treated surgically by release of the carpal ligament.

BELL'S PALSY

Unilateral facial paralysis of acute onset frequently occurs on an idiopathic basis (Bell's palsy). The etiology and pathophysiology remain unknown. The diagnosis is one of exclusion: facial nerve palsies also occur in the setting of *herpes zoster oticus,* in which they are typically associated with otalgia and varicelliform lesions affecting the external ear, ear canal, or tympanic membrane. Facial paralysis of a lower motor neuron type can be caused by *infiltrative disease in the meninges,* such as carcinomatous meningitis, and by *inflammatory diseases* such as sarcoidosis and Lyme disease. *Primary tumors of the facial nerve* can occur with apparently rapidly developing facial paralysis, although often in retrospect more subtle facial asymmetry had developed over a longer period. Facial paralysis can also occur in primary *CNS disease* affecting the pontomedullary junction, such as multiple sclerosis. Facial palsy has been noted in individuals with HIV infection, particularly in the early stages shortly after initial infection.

These considerations excluded, most cases of facial paralysis reflect idiopathic Bell's palsy. Patients typically notice facial paralysis on inspection in the mirror in the morning, and the disorder appears to come on overnight in many instances. Onset of facial paralysis may be heralded or accompanied by pain behind the ear (in the region of the stylomastoid foramen). The severity of paralysis varies widely. The prognosis can to some extent be predicted by electrophysiologic examination of the facial nerve after the first several days. In most cases, prognosis is quite favorable. Some believe that a course of oral corticosteroids with rapid tapering may improve the prognosis and is widely used, but this has never been verified. In severe cases, protection of the cornea from drying and injury is essential.

TRIGEMINAL NEURALGIA (TIC DOULOUREUX)

Trigeminal neuralgia is a recurring pain syndrome in which episodes of abrupt stabbing pain involve the second or third divisions of the trigeminal nerve. This and other painful cranial neuralgias are discussed in Ch. 455.

Section Sixteen—Diseases of Muscle (Myopathies) and Neuromuscular Junction

Andrew G. Engel

453 GENERAL APPROACH TO MUSCLE DISEASES

Muscle diseases are caused by derangements in the structure or function of the muscle fiber or in the innervation, blood supply, or connective tissue elements of muscle. A myopathy is a muscle disease not related to a demonstrable alteration in the innervation of muscle. To facilitate the understanding of muscle diseases, this chapter begins with a brief overview of the structure and function of muscle.

BASIC STRUCTURE AND FUNCTION OF MUSCLE

Each voluntary muscle contains myriad muscle fibers. A small proportion of the fibers is confined to muscle spindles that function as mechanoreceptors and participate in regulating the motor tone. The remaining muscle fibers are innervated by α motor neurons. A *motor unit* consists of one α motor neuron and the muscle fibers it innervates. The number of motor units per muscle and the number of muscle fibers per motor unit vary from muscle to muscle. In general, motor units are smaller in small muscles subserving delicate movements than in large muscles maintaining posture or exerting strong force. Muscle fibers belonging to different motor units intermingle with each other, so that the territories of individual motor units overlap. All muscle fibers in a motor unit share similar properties or are of the same type. Three major muscle-fiber (and motor-unit) types can be recognized: Type I, slow-twitch, fatigue-resistant fibers are high in oxidative enzymes but low in glycolytic enzymes. Type IIB, fast-twitch fatigable fibers are high in glycolytic enzymes and low in oxidative enzymes. Type IIA, intermediate-twitch, fatigue-resistant fibers are high in glycolytic enzymes and have an intermediate content of oxidative enzymes. In most human muscles the three fiber types occur in about equal proportions. Because the motor unit territories overlap, the fiber types intermingle randomly.

Adult muscle fibers are about 50 μm in diameter. The myofibrils, which account for most of the fiber volume, are associated with mitochondria, glycogen granules, transverse (T) tubules, and sarcoplasmic reticulum (SR). The myofibrils, 0.5 to 1.0 μm wide, consist of repeating units, or sarcomeres, limited by Z disks. The latter anchor 1 μm-long thin filaments that extend from each Z disk toward the center of the sarcomere. The thin filaments interdigitate with 1.6 μm-long thick filaments in the central region (A-band) of the sarcomere. The sarcomeres of adjacent myofibrils lying in register give the striated appearance to the muscle fiber. The thin filaments are composed of actin, troponin, and tropomyosin. The thick filaments are made up nearly entirely of regularly arrayed myosin molecules. The head of each myosin molecule projects laterally from the thick filament and can serve as a cross-bridge between myosin and actin. The T tubules are inward extensions of the muscle fiber surface membrane and propagate the action potential into the depth of the fiber. The SR abuts on the T tubules and partially envelops individual myofibrils. In the resting state the SR sequesters calcium into its lumen by means of an ATPase and thereby maintains a very low calcium concentration (about 10^{-7} M) around the myofilaments.

When the T tubules are depolarized by an action potential, voltage sensors embedded in their wall open calcium release channels positioned on the abutting SR surfaces and calcium escapes from the SR into the myofilament space. The released calcium binds to troponin on the thin filaments which then act on tropomyosin to allow repeated binding of the myosin cross-bridges to actin. Each binding is associated with a conformational change in the cross-bridge that exerts a force on the thin filament toward the center of the sarcomere. The cross-bridge cycle requires adenosine triphosphate (ATP), which is split by an ATPase on the cross-bridge. If ATP is depleted, the cross-bridges remain attached to the thin filaments and the muscle becomes stiff, as in rigor mortis. When ATP is available, the unloaded fiber shortens, the thin filaments are propelled into the A band, and the Z disks are pulled closer together in every sarcomere. The active state subsides with calcium reuptake by the SR; interaction between actin and the cross-bridges ceases and relaxation sets in.

THE DIAGNOSIS OF MUSCLE DISEASES

The diagnosis of a muscle disease rests on the clinical data, the electromyogram (EMG), and the muscle biopsy. None of the three approaches is individually adequate, but their combined use yields the correct diagnosis in a very high proportion of cases. Examples of disorders that are similar by clinical criteria but require muscle biopsy and EMG for accurate diagnosis are polymyositis, limb-girdle dystrophy, and adult acid maltase deficiency; distal muscular dystrophies, progressive muscular atrophy, and the slow-channel myasthenic syndrome; and benign congenital myopathies, mitochondrial myopathies, and childhood or juvenile spinal muscular atrophies.

CLINICAL DATA. *The Genetic History.* This is relevant to diagnosis as well as counseling. A negative family history, however, does not exclude either autosomal recessive inheritance, an incompletely penetrant autosomal-dominant gene in one parent, or a new mutation. In autosomal dominant disorders (e.g., myotonic and facioscapulohumeral dystrophy or the familial periodic paralyses) a negative family history needs to be validated by examination of both parents. The clinical examination or biochemical tests may help in detecting heterozygotes in autosomal-recessive or X-linked-recessive diseases. In Duchenne and Becker dystrophy, carrier detection and prenatal diagnosis are facilitated by analyses of dystrophin and DNA.

The History of the Illness. **Age at Onset, Duration, and Rate of Progression of Symptoms.** Most benign congenital myopathies, congenital muscular dystrophy, congenital myasthenic syndromes, a number of inherited metabolic myopathies, and the acute form of spinal muscular atrophy present in infancy. Duchenne dystrophy usually presents in early childhood. Many inherited myopathies, inherited anterior horn cell diseases, and most hereditary peripheral neuropathies present in childhood or early adult life. Limb-girdle, Becker, and facioscapulohumeral dystrophy usually present in adolescence; myotonic, oculopharyngeal, limb-girdle, and distal dystrophies can present in adult life. Dermatomyositis and scleroderma can begin in childhood or adult life; pure polymyositis is unusual before adolescence; and sporadic inclusion-body myositis seldom presents before the fifth decade.

Muscle weakness evolving over a few hours suggests an exogenous intoxication (e.g., organophosphorus or barium poisoning), periodic paralysis, or rhabdomyolysis. An abrupt onset of symptoms also can occur in myasthenia gravis or with other defects of neuromuscular transmission. Acute muscle weakness appearing during or after recovery from a Reye syndrome–like metabolic crisis suggests an enzyme defect in organic acid metabolism associated with secondary carnitine deficiency. Weakness evolving over a few days to a few weeks can occur in acute postinfectious polyneuropathy (Guillain-Barré syndrome), toxic neuropathies, and acute dermatomyositis. A subacute evolution, over a period of weeks to months, is seen in motor neuron disease; some metabolic myopathies, such as corticosteroid-induced or thyrotoxic myopathy; late-onset nemaline myopathy; and most cases of dermatomyositis and idiopathic polymyositis. A slow evolution over a number of years is typical of most dystrophies but can also occur in the inflammatory myopathies, such as inclusion body myositis, and in some cases of motor neuron disease.

Effects of Exercise, Rest After Exercise, Diet, and Temperature. Weakness appearing or increasing during exercise suggests a defect of neuromuscular transmission or in muscle energy metabolism. Weakness that decreases with exercise but increases during rest after exercise is typical of the periodic paralyses. Fasting or a high-fat diet may provoke or worsen symptoms in patients with defects of fatty acid oxidation. Exposure to cold worsens myotonia and can provoke weakness in periodic paralysis and paramyotonia congenita. Exposure to heat can increase neuromuscular transmission defects.

Symptoms in Muscle Diseases. Relatively few symptoms are associated with diverse muscle diseases: weakness, decrease of muscle bulk, increased fatigability, muscle pain, cramps, stiffness, and discoloration of the urine caused by myoglobinuria. The cardinal symptom is muscle weakness, but patients often describe its consequences instead of speaking of weakness. Patients complaining of cramps sometimes suffer from contractures or tetany. The term *stiffness* is used to describe a variety of conditions, such as the stiff-man syndrome, neuromyotonia, and myotonia.

Muscle Weakness. Weakness of the cranial, cervical, torso, and limb muscles presents stereotypically. Weakness of muscles supplied by cranial nerves causes drooping of the eyelids (ptosis, third cranial nerve); double vision (diplopia, third, fourth, and sixth cranial nerves); failure of the eyelids to close at night, altered facial expression, difficulty in whistling or sucking from a straw (seventh cranial nerve); inability to close the jaw, difficulty in chewing hard food (fifth cranial nerve); and difficulty in pronouncing words (dysarthria), hypernasal voice, nasal regurgitation of liquids, and difficulty in swallowing (dysphagia) (tenth and twelfth cranial nerves). Weakness of the cervical muscles is shown by difficulty in lifting the head from a pillow or holding the head erect, and weakness of the truncal muscles by difficulty in rolling over in bed or sitting up from the supine position. Weakness of the arm muscles is related as difficulty in holding the arms overhead, lifting heavy objects, or using the hands for motor tasks. Weakness of the pelvic girdle and of the proximal lower extremity muscles is reflected by difficulty in rising from sitting or squatting, climbing stairs, or stepping in or out of the bathtub. Weakness of the distal lower extremity may cause flopping of the feet or difficulty in rising on the toes.

Other Symptoms. In evaluating *abnormal fatigability,* it is important to define the duration and intensity of exercise that provokes it. Even mild exercise can induce fatigue in patients with defects of neuromuscular transmission or with mitochondrial myopathies that involve an electron transport complex. Brief periods of intense, anaerobic exercise precipitate fatigue in patients with glycolytic enzyme defects, but sustained exercise is required to induce fatigue in carnitine palmityltransferase deficiency.

Muscle pain (myalgia) at rest can occur in some of the inflammatory myopathies (especially dermatomyositis and the eosinophilia-myalgia syndrome); during acute viral infections; in polymyalgia rheumatica, myxedema, myotonic disorders, and necrotizing vasculitis; during attacks of myoglobinuria; and in neuropathies associated with vitamin B_1 deficiency, arsenic intoxication, and alcoholism. *Muscle pain during and after exercise* is experienced when the energy supply to muscle is restricted, as with defects in glycolysis or fatty acid oxidation, AMP deaminase defi-

ciency, or ischemia (as in intermittent claudication, scleroderma, and amyloidosis involving muscle), or in normal persons after unusually strenuous exercise.

Muscle cramps last from seconds to minutes, are associated with high-frequency (up to 150 Hz) discharges of the motor units, and can be initiated by strong contractions and stopped by stretching the muscle. They occur with dehydration, azotemia, hyponatremia, and myxedema, in partially denervated muscles, and sometimes in normal individuals without known cause.

Muscle contractures are electrically silent, last from a few to more than 30 minutes, occur only in patients with glycolytic enzyme defects, are provoked only by exercise, and involve only those muscles that are exercised.

The facial and carpopedal spasms of *tetany* occur with hypocalcemia or hypomagnesemia and are associated with high-frequency (up to 300 Hz) axonal discharges. High-frequency electrical discharges also occur in muscle in the *stiff-man syndrome, neuromyotonia,* and *myotonia,* arising in the spinal cord, the peripheral nerves, and the muscle fiber surface membrane, respectively.

In *myotonic disorders* mechanical or electrical stimuli applied to any region of the muscle fiber surface membrane elicit repetitive spike discharges that wax and wane in amplitude and frequency. Mechanical deformation of the membrane during contraction acts as positive feedback, again depolarizing the membrane. The result is tetanic contraction of the individual fibers. The symptoms are stiffness, difficulty in relaxing muscles after a strong contraction, being muscle-bound at the beginning of exercise, and improvement with continued exercise.

Myoglobinuria follows the excessive release of myoglobin from muscle during a period of rapid muscle fiber destruction (rhabdomyolysis). Weakness, muscle pain, and malaise are associated features.

The Clinical Examination. Inspection. This can reveal muscle atrophy, hypertrophy, contractures, winging of the scapulas, fasciculations (twitching of portions of muscles at rest caused by single contractions of motor units), and myokymia (fine undulating movements of muscles associated with sustained abnormal motor-unit activity). The examiner also notes the patient's stance and gait, ability to walk on toes and heels, and hop on one foot, and rise from sitting, squatting, or lying supine.

Inspection provides information on the distribution of weakness, which is then confirmed by detailed manual muscle testing. For example, weakness of the pelvic girdle muscles causes a waddling gait; if there is also weakness of the back extensor muscles, the gait is also lordotic with hyperextension of the upper torso. Muscle atrophy consistently predicts muscle weakness, but not all weak muscles are atrophic, and muscle atrophy can be masked by obesity. Muscle hypertrophy not from voluntary exercise is common in myotonia congenita; it also occurs in the course of Duchenne and Becker and—less commonly—of limb-girdle dystrophy. Hypertrophy may appear with chronic partial denervation, acid maltase deficiency, the permanent myopathy of periodic paralysis, myxedema, sarcoidosis, amyloidosis, and cysticercosis. The nonspecific term *pseudohypertrophy* refers to enlargement of a weak muscle.

Manual Muscle Testing. The British Medical Research Council provides a commonly used rating scale for muscular weakness: 5, normal power; 4, active movement against gravity and resistance; 3, active movement against gravity; 2, active movement with gravity eliminated; 1, trace contraction; 0, no contraction.

The distribution of the weakness can help in formulating the clinical diagnosis. Weakness greater in proximal than distal muscles suggests a myopathy rather than a neuropathy. Predominantly distal muscle weakness suggests a neuropathy but can also occur in myotonic and other distal dystrophies and inclusion body myositis. Selective involvement of some muscles with sparing of others is more likely to occur in dystrophy than in inflammatory muscle disease, but it can also accompany such diverse entities as adult acid maltase deficiency, focal myositis, or the slow-channel myasthenic syndrome. The external-ocular and other cranial muscles can be affected by the Guillain-Barré syndrome, neuromuscular transmission defects, some mitochondrial myopathies, oculopharyngeal dystrophy, and myotubular myopathy. Diffuse, symmetric weakness of multiple cranial muscles with ptosis but with sparing of the ocular movements suggests myotonic dystrophy. Motor neuron disease can affect the bulbar muscles but spares the external ocular muscles ex-

TABLE 453–1. CLINICAL CLUES DIFFERENTIATING MUSCLE FROM NERVE DISEASE

	Myopathy	Neuropathy-Neuronopathy
Distribution	Mainly proximal and symmetric	Distal if symmetric; nerve or root distribution if mono- or multi-focal
Atrophy	Late and mild	Early and prominent
Onset	Usually gradual	Often rapid
Fasciculations	Absent	Sometimes present
Reflexes	Lost late	Lost early
Tenderness	Diffuse in myositis	Focal in nerve or root disease
Cramps	Rare	Common
Sensory loss	Absent	Often present
Muscle enzymes	Usually elevated	Usually not or slightly elevated

cept rarely in terminal stages. Selective weakness of the triceps, wrist extensor, finger extensor, iliopsoas, hamstring, anterior tibial, and peroneal muscles, with relative sparing of other muscles, suggests upper motor neuron involvement.

Other Findings. *Action myotonia* is observed as an inability to open the fist or the eyes promptly after closing them tightly for a few seconds. *Percussion myotonia* appears as a local postpercussion contraction followed by abnormally slow relaxation. It can best be observed in the tongue, deltoid, thenar, and extensor digitorum communis muscles. A local swelling appearing for a few seconds at the site of percussion is not myotonia but *myoedema,* seen in myxedema and emaciation.

The *tendon reflexes* are diminished in proportion to the weakness in most myopathies; an early loss of tendon reflexes is observed in neurogenic diseases of muscle, inclusion body myositis, the Lambert-Eaton myasthenic syndrome, and a number of benign congenital myopathies. Slow relaxation of the reflexes is typical of myxedema.

A complete *examination of the nervous system* is also relevant to the evaluation of muscle weakness. Table 453–1 lists clinical guidelines that differentiate nerve from muscle disease. Peripheral neuropathy, ataxia, neurosensory hearing loss, myoclonus, fluctuating neurologic deficits, and mental deterioration can be associated with mitochondrial myopathies.

Recognition of the *signs or symptoms of an associated illness* can point to the cause of the myopathy. Examples are collagen-vascular diseases, sarcoidosis, amyloidosis, the endocrine myopathies, and the mitochondrial myopathies with multisystem involvement. *Involvement of organs or tissues other than muscle* provides further diagnostic clues. For example, cardiomyopathy can be associated with myotonic dystrophy, a dystrophinopathy, Emery-Dreifuss dystrophy, certain types of periodic paralysis, thymomatous myasthenia gravis, and late-onset nemaline myopathy. Cardiomyopathy and/or hepatic enlargement can occur in sarcoidosis and in the myopathies associated with deficiencies of acid maltase, debranching enzyme, carnitine, acyl-CoA dehydrogenase, and a mitochondrial electron transport complex.

Nonorganic Findings Simulating Muscle Disease. See Table 453–2.

Serum Enzymes of Muscle Origin. The serum creatine kinase (CK) level is elevated in many muscle diseases. The enzyme is released into serum from injured skeletal or cardiac muscle. CK is a dimer of muscle-specific (M) and brain-specific (B) monomers, and the different CK isoenzymes can be distinguished by electrophoretic analysis. Mature muscle contains predominantly the MM isoen-

TABLE 453–2. SYMPTOMS OR SIGNS OF FUNCTIONAL MUSCLE DISEASE

Vague complaints
Migrating or diffusely constant muscle pain without tenderness
Excessive, nonfocal tenderness
"Give-way" weakness during testing
Bizarre sensory deficits
Hysterical gait or postures

TABLE 453–3. MOLECULAR GENETIC FINDINGS IN MYOPATHIES

Disease	Gene Locus/Defect	Inheritance
Duchenne/Becker dystrophy	Xp21 Large deletions in 2/3; small rearrangements in 1/3	XLR
Emery-Dreifuss dystrophy	Xq28	XLR
Facioscapulohumeral dystrophy	4q35*	AD
Severe childhood limb-girdle dystrophy	13q12	AR
Limb-girdle dystrophy	15q	AR
Limb-girdle dystrophy	5q	AD
Myotonic dystrophy	19q13 Unstable DNA: excess trinucleotide repeats	AD
Hypokalemic periodic paralysis	1q31–q32; mutations in T tubule voltage sensor	AD
Hyperkalemic periodic paralysis/paramyotonia congenita	13q13.1–13.3; point mutations in muscle sodium channel gene	AD
Myotonia congenita	7q35; point mutations in muscle chloride channel gene	AR or AD
Central core disease/malignant hyperthermia	19q13.1	AD
Nemaline myopathy	1q21–1q23*	AD
Myotubular myopathy	Xq28*	XLR
Acid maltase deficiency	17q23	AR
Myophosphorylase deficiency	11q13	AR
Muscle phosphofructokinase deficiency	1cenq32	AR
Phosphoglycerate kinase deficiency	Xq13	XLR
Muscle phosphoglycerate mutase deficiency	7p12–p13	AR
Lactate dehydrogenase deficiency	11p15.4	AR
Carnitine palmitoyltransferase II deficiency	1p11–p13	AR
Kearns-Sayre syndrome	Mitochondrial DNA; deletions	Sporadic
MELAS	Mitochondrial DNA; tRNA-(lys) point mutation	Maternal
MERRF	Mitochondrial DNA; tRNA-(leu, ile) point mutations	Maternal
LHON	Mitochondrial DNA; point mutations in complex 1, or cyt *b*	Maternal
NARP	Mitochondrial DNA; point mutation in complex 6	Maternal

* Other gene loci may also exist.
   XLR, X-linked recessive; AD, autosomal dominant; AR, autosomal recessive; MELAS, mitochondrial encephalomyopathy, lactic acidosis, and strokelike episodes; MERRF, myoclonic epilepsy with ragged-red fibers; LHON, Leber's hereditary optic neuroretinopathy; NARP, neurogenic muscle weakness, ataxia, and retinitis pigmentosa. (Data from table by Jean-Claude Kaplan and Bertrand Fontaine, Neuromuscular Disorders 1:89, 1994.)

zyme, whereas in mature cardiac muscle the MB form predominates. Accordingly, abnormal CK release from muscle increases mostly the MM isoenzyme, whereas CK release from heart increases the MB form in serum. Injured muscle releases other enzymes, such as aldolase, lactate dehydrogenase, and aspartate aminotransferase, but the increases are less marked and can derive from other tissues, such as the liver and erythrocytes. The serum CK level is a sensitive index of muscle fiber injury in a myopathy; it also can increase slightly or modestly in motor neuron disease, in chronic peripheral neuropathies, after severe voluntary exertion, or following a convulsion.

ELECTROMYOGRAPHY (EMG). This test consists of the analysis of spontaneous, evoked, and voluntarily generated potentials from nerve and muscle. The procedure is useful in distinguishing between broad categories of disease, such as myopathy versus neuropathy, or demyelinating versus axonal neuropathy. In some instances the types of electrical potentials and the pattern of abnormality suggest a disease category, such as an inflammatory myopathy, a myotonic disorder, or a storage myopathy. A progressive decrease of the amplitude of the compound muscle action potential evoked by low-frequency repetitive nerve stimulation (decremental response) is observed with defects of neuromuscular transmission.

Sequential assessment of an EMG abnormality can provide useful information on the distribution, degree of activity, and progression of a disease. For example, persistent fibrillation potentials in polymyositis reflect continuing disease activity; the decremental response can be used to monitor the course of myasthenia gravis; and alterations in nerve conduction velocities are a guide to the progression of peripheral neuropathies. Further details of the usefulness of EMG are given in Ch. 392.2, 446, and 459.

THE MUSCLE BIOPSY. Biopsy specimens are used for light microscopic, ultrastructural, and biochemical studies. In most instances, light microscopic observations with enzyme histochemical studies are sufficient and sometimes critical for diagnosis.

Muscles showing mild to moderate weakness are biopsied. Strong muscles may not show diagnostic pathologic change, and in more severely affected muscles excessive amounts of connective tissue may obscure the basic pathologic process. Muscles that have been injected (as is often the case for the deltoid) or recently examined by EMG are unsuitable for diagnosis. The reference provides details of light and electron microscopic findings as well as diagnostic biochemical studies that can be obtained on muscle biopsies.

Molecular Genetic Studies. These are important because they help in diagnosis and carrier detection. Thus far, molecular genetic studies have contributed more to diseases of muscle than to those of any other tissue (Table 453–3).

Engel AG, Franzini-Armstrong C (eds.): Myology, 2nd ed. New York, McGraw-Hill, 1994. *A multiauthored book on the anatomy, physiology, and biochemistry of skeletal muscle, the approach to muscle diseases, and the clinical aspects of muscle diseases.*

454 MUSCULAR DYSTROPHIES

Muscular dystrophies are inherited myopathies associated with progressive muscle weakness, destruction and regeneration of the muscle fibers, and eventual replacement of the muscle fibers by fibrous and fatty connective tissue. There is no accumulation of metabolic storage material in the muscle fibers. A current classification is shown in Table 454–1.

DYSTROPHINOPATHIES. The term includes X-linked allelic disorders resulting from mutations of the large dystrophin gene located at Xp21 (see Table 453–3). At least five different tissue-specific dystrophin transcripts exist. Dystrophin in skeletal muscle is a 420-kD subsarcolemmal cytoskeletal protein concentrated in transverse riblike rings over each sarcomere and interacting with other cytoskeletal proteins, and a dystrophin-associated protein (DAP) complex links the cytoskeleton of the sarcolemma to the extracellu-

TABLE 454–1. CLASSIFICATION OF THE MUSCULAR DYSTROPHIES

X-linked recessive dystrophies
  Duchenne/Becker dystrophies and other dystrophinopathies
  Emery-Dreifuss dystrophy
Autosomal recessive dystrophies
  Severe childhood limb-girdle dystrophy
  Chromosome 15q-linked limb-girdle dystrophy
  Autosomal recessive distal dystrophies
    With necrotizing features
    With rimmed vacuoles
  Congenital muscular dystrophies
    Without cerebral abnormalities
    With ocular and cerebral abnormalities
Autosomal dominant dystrophies
  Myotonic dystrophy
  Facioscapulohumeral dystrophy
  Oculopharyngeal dystrophy
  Chromosome 5q-linked limb-girdle dystrophy
  Autosomal dominant scapuloperoneal dystrophy
  Autosomal dominant distal dystrophies
    With onset in upper limbs (Welander type)
    With onset in lower limbs
    Tibial muscular dystrophy

lar matrix. Dystrophin deficiency results in a secondary DAP deficiency. Further, deficiency of a 50-kD DAP component in itself causes a severe autosomal recessive muscular dystrophy (see below). The severity of the resulting phenotype usually depends upon whether the dystrophin mutation shifts the translational reading frame. The two major dystrophinopathy phenotypes are Duchenne and Becker dystrophy.

Duchenne Dystrophy. Most patients have a frameshifting mutation and severe dystrophin deficiency that can be demonstrated by immunoblotting or immunostaining of muscle. The combined dystrophin and secondary DAP deficiency weaken the sarcolemma, resulting in ultrastructurally detectable sarcolemmal tears. The result permits the influx of calcium-rich extracellular fluid and complement into the muscle fiber. Activation of intracellular proteases and complement leads to fiber necrosis.

The incidence of Duchenne dystrophy is close to 1 in 3300 male births, the mutation rate being about 1 in 10,000. The disease is present at birth, produces symptoms during early childhood, leads to failure of ambulation near the end of the first decade, and causes death near the end of the second decade. The serum creatine kinase (CK) level is markedly elevated from birth and decreases gradually as muscle bulk is lost. Early symptoms are developmental delays, difficulty in running or climbing stairs, frequent falls, and enlargement of the calves. Initially the weakness is more proximal than distal. Except for the sternocleidomastoids, the cranial muscles and the external anal sphincter are spared. The proximal tendon reflexes disappear by the age of 10. Joint contractures commonly appear in most patients between 6 and 10 years of age. After ambulation is lost, all muscles atrophy and paraspinal muscle weakness leads to progressive kyphoscoliosis. Weakness of the respiratory muscles can be detected after the age of 10, but the diaphragm is relatively spared. Respiratory failure, with or without respiratory infections, occurs terminally. The heart is affected with scarring of the posterobasal portion of the left ventricle, producing tall right precordial R waves and deep left precordial Q waves in the electrocardiogram in 90% of the patients. Clinically significant cardiomyopathy is uncommon and in only 10% of cases is death related to cardiac dysfunction. Central nervous system involvement is indicated by lower than average intelligence and mild cerebral atrophy.

Infrequently, Duchenne dystrophy manifests in females who have Turner's (XO) or Turner's mosaic (X/XX or X/XX/XXX) syndrome, a structurally abnormal X chromosome, or an X-autosomal translocation. In a few female heterozygotes, the disease manifests because of incomplete inactivation of the maternal X chromosome.

Becker Dystrophy. Most patients have a non-frameshifting mutation, so that a reduced amount of an abnormal dystrophin is produced, resulting in a milder syndrome than Duchenne dystrophy. Immunoblots of muscle extracts distinguish between Becker and Duchenne dystrophy as well as between sporadic cases of Becker and limb-girdle dystrophy.

Becker dystrophy has an incidence of about 1 per 20,000 male births. The disorder begins later and evolves more slowly than Duchenne dystrophy: The mean age of onset of symptoms, becoming chair-bound, and death are 12, 30, and 42 years, respectively. Most patients show marked calf muscle enlargement until the terminal stage. Calf pain on exercise is a frequent and early symptom. The serum CK level is markedly elevated even in preclinical stages of the disease but begins to decline after the age of 20. Contractures develop at the wheelchair stage. Electrocardiographic abnormalities develop in about 40%. A small proportion of the patients have a dilated cardiomyopathy unrelated to the severity of the myopathy.

Other Dystrophinopathies. Other, milder dystrophinopathy phenotypes are represented by exercise intolerance associated with myalgias, muscle cramps, or myoglobinuria; minimal limb-girdle weakness or quadriceps myopathy; asymptomatic elevation of the serum CK level; cardiomyopathy with only mild muscle weakness; and fatal X-linked cardiomyopathy without muscle weakness. The different dystrophin phenotypes are determined by the site of the mutation in the dystrophin gene and whether the mutation affects the expression of the cardiac isoform of dystrophin.

DIAGNOSIS. In families in which a dystrophinopathy has been previously diagnosed, the clinical findings can define the diagnosis. Special studies are recommended for the diagnosis of new cases, but the approach to a given patient is likely to depend on the cost and availability of the various diagnostic procedures. In all the dystrophinopathies, immunoblotting of muscle is more reliable than immunostaining. Deletional analysis of genomic DNA obtained from leukocytes or muscle, using the polymerase chain reaction with multiple primers to amplify deletion-prone exons, identifies 65% of all mutations but may not distinguish between frameshifting and non-frameshifting mutations.

X-LINKED MUSCULAR DYSTROPHY WITH EARLY JOINT CONTRACTURES AND CARDIOMYOPATHY (EMERY-DREIFUSS DYSTROPHY). Recent genetic linkage studies have mapped this disease to band q28 of the X chromosome. The disease presents in childhood, progresses slowly, and involves distal or proximal muscles in the lower extremities and proximal muscles in the upper extremities. The serum CK is moderately elevated. Contractures of the knees, elbows, and cervical and dorsolumbar spine appear early. Atrial conduction defects and paralysis, requiring treatment by pacemaker, appear later. The disorder has been referred to as Emery-Dreifuss dystrophy and as X-linked scapuloperoneal myopathy, the distinction depending only on whether the proximal or distal muscles are affected in the lower limbs. The lack of muscle hypertrophy, early contractures, slow progression, relatively low serum CK, and overt cardiac involvement distinguish this disease from Duchenne dystrophy; all these features but the slow progression differentiate it from Becker dystrophy. When cardiomyopathy cannot be detected or the pedigree of X-linked inheritance is not established, the disease can be difficult to distinguish from the rigid-spine syndrome or other heterogeneous scapuloperoneal syndromes.

LIMB-GIRDLE SYNDROMES. *Definition and Classification.* The term applies to a clinically heterogeneous syndrome characterized by weakness of pectoral- or pelvic-girdle but not of facial muscles. The disorders can be separated into three major categories:

1. Genetically distinct limb-girdle dystrophies mapped to chromosomal loci. This category includes three entities (see Table 453–3).

2. Limb-girdle dystrophies observed in large kinships and with a well-defined pattern of inheritance but still not linked to a chromosomal locus. These disorders include autosomal dominant benign myopathies, or as yet uncharacterized autosomal recessive muscular dystrophies.

3. Other limb-girdle syndromes. This group identifies by default progressive myopathies involving the limb-girdle muscles that cannot be identified specifically by currently available criteria.

The Differential Diagnosis of Limb-Girdle Syndromes. All patients with limb-girdle syndromes need to be further investigated by EMG and muscle biopsy. In those with a positive family history, the differential diagnosis includes inherited metabolic myopathies (e.g., acid maltase deficiency or a lipid storage myopathy); morphologically distinct congenital myopathies or their late-onset variants (e.g., nemaline, central core, and myotubular myopathies); or progressive muscular atrophy. In sporadic cases of a limb-girdle syndrome the differential diagnosis includes the same diseases, and also inflammatory myopathies (polymyositis, inclusion body myositis, or sarcoidosis confined to muscle), endocrine myopathies, sporadic Duchenne dystrophy, Duchenne or Becker dystrophy manifesting in female carriers, other dystrophinopathies, and sporadic Emery-Dreifuss dystrophy before the appearance of joint contractures or cardiomyopathy.

FACIOSCAPULOHUMERAL DYSTROPHY. The inheritance is autosomal dominant with high penetrance and variable expression (see Table 453–3). The disease presents in childhood or adult life. It involves the facial muscles early and then descends to the scapular fixators, the muscles of the upper arm, and the anterior leg muscles. Early physical signs include failure to bury the eyelashes, an expressionless face, pouting lips, winging of the scapulas when the arms are raised, and an inward-sloping anterior axillary fold. The rate of progression and the extent to which pelvic girdle, forearm, and lower torso muscles are eventually affected vary considerably between and within different families. There is no muscle hypertrophy; joint contractures are uncommon; and the serum CK level is normal or shows mild elevation. In some families a conspicuous inflammatory reaction appears in affected muscles, but the course of the illness is unaltered by corticosteroid therapy. In others an associated sensorineural hearing loss occurs, with or without retinal telangiectasis and progressive painless blindness (Coats syndrome). The differential diagnosis includes progressive muscular atrophy, congenital myopathies (e.g., nemaline, central core, and myotubular myopathy), mitochondrial myopathies, sporadic cases of Emery-Dreifuss dystrophy before the appearance of joint contractures or cardiomyopathy, the scapuloperoneal syndrome, the slow-channel myasthenic syndrome, and polymyositis.

MYOTONIC DYSTROPHY. Transmission of myotonic dystrophy is by dominant inheritance with high penetrance and variable expressivity. The gene locus and defect are now known (see Table 453–3). Part of the sequence predicts the gene product to be a member of the protein kinase family. The disease is associated with abnormal expansion of CTG repeats in the 3' untranslated region of the gene. The age of onset, the expressivity of the disease, and the severity of the congenital myotonic dystrophy have been correlated with the number of repeats. How the gene defect causes tissue injury and myotonia is not yet understood. The incidence is about 1 in 7500 births. A typical distribution of the weakness, myotonia, and multisystem abnormalities characterizes the disease.

Myotonic dystrophy presents in childhood or adult life with a mean age at onset of 19 years. Myotonic symptoms either precede or accompany the muscle weakness. As the disease evolves, the myotonia diminishes in muscles severely affected by the dystrophic process. Distal limb, levator palpebrae, masticatory, facial, cervical, pharyngeal, laryngeal, and upper esophagus muscles are commonly affected. External ophthalmoplegia is rare. Weakness also can appear in proximal limb and respiratory muscles. The latter, when severe, results in alveolar hypoventilation, hypercapnia, arterial oxygen unsaturation, and increasing somnolence. Action myotonia is commonly observed in facial, lid elevator, and hand muscles; percussion myotonia is usually found in tongue, thenar, finger extensor, and selected proximal limb muscles.

Myotonic dystrophy produces systemic abnormalities including frontal baldness, subcapsular cataracts, testicular atrophy and ovarian dysfunction in adult life, extrathyroidal hypometabolism, end-organ unresponsiveness to insulin, mental changes, and hypercatabolism of IgG. Cardiac conduction defects are common and can cause sudden death. Gastrointestinal smooth muscle involvement results in reduced lower esophageal and gastric motility and dilatation of segments of the colon. Some patients have bouts of diarrhea alternating with constipation and colicky abdominal pain. Less frequent manifestations are pigmentary retinal degeneration and cranial anomalies (hyperostosis cranii, small sella turcica, large paranasal sinuses, and prognathism).

Muscle biopsies characteristically show very large muscle fibers with numerous central nuclei, sarcoplasmic masses, ring fibers, and variable type 1 fiber atrophy. Necrotic fibers are uncommon. The serum CK level is normal or only slightly elevated.

DISTAL DYSTROPHIES. A number of genetically distinct entities have been recognized. Different types of *autosomal dominant distal muscular dystrophies* have been described. That observed in a large Scandinavian kinship by Welander presents between the fourth and sixth decades with selective weakness and atrophy of the forearm extensor and intrinsic hand muscles and then involves the anterior leg and small foot muscles. In patients homozygous for the dominant gene, the onset is earlier and proximal muscles are also affected. Another form of distal dystrophy observed in some districts of Finland selectively involves the anterior tibial muscles; the upper extremities are never affected. In other non-Scandinavian kinships with late onset and dominant inheritance, the disease first involves the lower extremities. The serum CK level is normal or slightly increased. Two varieties of *autosomal recessive distal muscular dystrophies* have been described. In both there is a juvenile onset and the lower limbs are affected before the upper. In one type there is frequent fiber necrosis and regeneration and the serum CK level is markedly increased. In the other type the muscle fibers harbor rimmed vacuoles and the serum CK level is only slightly increased.

The differential diagnosis of the distal muscular dystrophies includes myotonic dystrophy, inclusion body myositis, debranching enzyme deficiency, distal mitochondrial myopathy, distal chronic spinal muscular atrophy, and the neuronal form of peroneal muscular atrophy.

OCULOPHARYNGEAL MUSCULAR DYSTROPHY. The disease, inherited as autosomal dominant, presents in the fifth or sixth decade with progressive ptosis and dysphagia. Later, all external ocular and other voluntary muscles may become affected. Death usually results from starvation or aspiration pneumonia. The serum CK level is normal or slightly increased. Muscle biopsy discloses intranuclear tubular filaments and rimmed vacuoles in the muscle fibers.

THE RIGID-SPINE SYNDROME. This is a heterogeneous disorder in which muscle contractures involve the spine as well as other joints. An autosomal dominant form presenting with proximal muscle weakness in the first decade is also recognized. In most cases the disease is sporadic, begins in the first decade, and results in widespread muscle weakness and atrophy during the second decade.

CONGENITAL DYSTROPHIES. See Table 454–1.

TREATMENT OF THE MUSCULAR DYSTROPHIES. There is no specific treatment of any of the muscular dystrophies. Physical therapy to prevent contractures, orthoses, and corrective orthopedic surgery can be used to improve the quality of life in some stages. The cardiac conduction defects in Emery-Dreifuss dystrophy and myotonic dystrophy may require treatment by pacemaker. The myotonia in myotonic dystrophy is rarely a clinical problem but can be treated with phenytoin (0.3 to 0.6 gram daily) or by quinine (0.3 to 1.5 grams daily).

Preventive treatment consists of prenatal diagnosis in families with known pedigrees, carrier detection, and genetic counseling. Some Duchenne carriers are recognized by immunostaining muscle for dystrophin, which may show scattered dystrophin-negative fibers. In some Becker carriers dystrophin of abnormal size or amount is detected by immunoblotting. Close to 65% of Duchenne or Becker carriers and fetuses at risk can be identified by DNA analysis using cDNA probes or the polymerase chain reaction; carriers not identified this way may still be detected in families with known carriers by linkage analysis. In myotonic dystrophy, the detection of an abnormal number of CTg repeats in the 3' untranslated region of the gene allows prenatal diagnosis and detection of presymptomatic cases. However, this test may not detect all carriers.

Recent advances in molecular genetics have raised hopes for gene therapy of Duchenne dystrophy, but this approach is still in its infancy.

Ahn AH, Kunkel LM: The structural and functional diversity of dystrophin. Nature Genetics 3:283, 1993. *A concise and comprehensive account of what is currently known about the dystrophin gene and dystrophin.*

Barohn RJ, Miller RG, Griggs RC: Autosomal recessive distal dystrophy. Neurology 41:365, 1991. *A good review of the currently recognized forms of distal dystrophies.*

Clarke A: Report of the ENMC workshop on the limb-girdle muscular dystrophies. J Med Genet 29:753, 1992. *An informative survey of the genetically distinct forms of limb-girdle dystrophy.*

Engel AG, Franzini-Armstrong C (eds.): Myology, 2nd ed. New York, McGraw-Hill, 1994. *Excellent, comprehensive descriptions of the muscular dystrophies by multiple experts.*

Matsumura K, Campbell KP: Dystrophin-glycoprotein complex: Its role in the molecular pathogenesis of muscular dystrophies. Muscle Nerve 17:2, 1994. *A summary of recent developments that pave the way for a better understanding of muscular dystrophies.*

Nicholson LVB, Johnson MA, Bushby KMD, et al.: An integrated study of 100 patients with Xp21-linked muscular dystrophy using clinical, genetic, immunochemical and histopathological data. III. Differential diagnosis and prognosis. J Med Genet 30:475, 1993. *A clearly written guide to the use and interpretation of currently available tests for the dystrophinopathies.*

455 MORPHOLOGICALLY DISTINCT CONGENITAL MYOPATHIES

DEFINITIONS AND BASIC CONCEPTS. The diseases in this group are characterized by the following features:

The course is nonprogressive or relatively nonprogressive. The prognosis is generally benign except in reducing body myopathy and in the X-linked form of myotubular myopathy.

A distinct pattern of inheritance is observed in some diseases (e.g., central core disease, nemaline myopathy); others are genetically heterogeneous (e.g., myotubular myopathy).

TABLE 455–1. MORPHOLOGICALLY DISTINCT CONGENITAL MYOPATHIES

Central core disease
Nemaline (rod) myopathy
Myotubular (centronuclear) myopathy
  Severe X-linked recessive form
  Milder autosomal recessive and dominant forms
Multicore disease
Congenital fiber type disproportion
Fingerprint body myopathy
Sarcotubular myopathy
Reducing body myopathy
Trilaminar myopathy
Myopathy with focal lysis of type I fibers
Spheroid/cytoplasmic body myopathies

Muscle weakness is present at birth or appears in early childhood. It is proximal or diffuse and may or may not involve the cranial muscles.

The muscle bulk is normal or reduced. There is no muscle hypertrophy.

The deep tendon reflexes are reduced or absent in most cases.

Skeletal abnormalities related to the weakness, such as a high-arched palate, kyphoscoliosis, dislocated hips, and pes cavus, are common.

The serum CK level is normal, except in some older patients with myotubular or sarcotubular myopathy.

The EMG is normal or suggests a myopathy. Spontaneous electrical activity is absent in all cases, except for fibrillation potentials and myotonic discharges in some cases of myotubular myopathy.

Each disease has one or more distinguishing, but not specific, morphologic features. Type I fiber preponderance and small type I fibers occur in most disorders.

Table 455–1 lists the currently recognized morphologically distinct congenital myopathies.

Late-Onset Variants. Adult-onset cases of central core disease, nemaline myopathy, myotubular myopathy, and multicore disease exist. In some cases mild congenital disease becomes recognized only after additional progression in adult life or when discovery of an affected younger relative prompts investigation of other family members.

Two other forms of late-onset nemaline myopathy are noteworthy. One is sporadic, evolves subacutely or chronically, affects the proximal limb and torso but not the cranial muscles, and may cause death from respiratory failure. The CK level is normal. Some cases possess an associated monoclonal gammopathy. Histologically, there is progressive accumulation of nemaline rods and progressive atrophy of rod-containing fibers. Another late-onset form occurs in a familial setting, is associated with cardiomyopathy, and can result in sudden death.

Fardeau M, Tomé FMS: Congenital myopathies. *In* Engel AG, Franzini-Armstrong C (eds.): Myology, 2nd ed. New York, McGraw-Hill, 1994, p 1487. *A comprehensive, well-illustrated review. It raises numerous unanswered questions about etiology and nosology.*

456 INFLAMMATORY MYOPATHIES

DEFINITION AND CLASSIFICATION. Inflammatory myopathies represent a heterogeneous group of disorders (Table 456–1). Most are diffuse in distribution, but some are focal, affecting circumscribed regions in single or multiple muscles. Some are caused by or related to bacterial, parasitic, or viral infections. In most other inflammatory myopathies the cause is undetermined, but an autoimmune origin is suspected. This section focuses on selected aspects of the idiopathic inflammatory myopathies not covered in other chapters.

TABLE 456-1. CLASSIFICATION OF INFLAMMATORY MYOPATHIES

Infections
 Parasitic: toxoplasmosis, sarcosporidiosis, African trypanosomiasis, American trypanosomiasis, cysticercosis (Taenia solium), trichinellosis
 Bacterial: pyomyositis, septic myositis, gas gangrene (Clostridium welchii), leprous myositis
 Spirochetal: Lyme disease (Borrelia burgdorferi)
 Viral: acute myositis following influenza or other viral infections, retrovirus-related myopathies (HIV, HTLV-I)
Idiopathic, autoimmune origin suspected
 Pure polymyositis
 Dermatomyositis
 Inclusion body myositis
 Scleroderma involving muscle
 Inflammatory myopathy associated with another autoimmune disease (systemic lupus erythematosus, rheumatoid arthritis, Sjögren's syndrome, rheumatic fever, overlap syndromes, chronic graft-versus-host disease, polyarteritis nodosa)
 Sarcoidosis involving muscle
 Inflammatory myopathies with eosinophilia
  Eosinophilic polymyositis
  Localized eosinophilic myositis
  Eosinophilic perimyositis
  Diffuse fasciitis with eosinophilia
  Eosinophilia-myalgia induced by L-tryptophan preparations
 Focal myositis
  Focal proliferative myositis
  Localized nodular myositis
   Pseudothrombophlebitis of a calf muscle
  Orbital myositis
 Polymyalgia rheumatica*
Other inflammatory myopathies
 Localized myositis ossificans
 Generalized myositis ossificans

* There are no inflammatory changes in muscle.

Myopathies Related to Retrovirus Infections. These can appear early or late in the course of immunodeficiency virus (HIV) infections. The most common form is HIV-associated polymyositis, which presents early in the infection and is mediated by T cells. Necrotizing myopathy without inflammation, or myopathies with nemaline rods or giant cells, necrotizing vasculitis, focal myositis in the form of pseudothrombophlebitis, and recurrent myoglobinuria without other predisposing factors also can occur. Attempts to immunolocalize HIV antigens in muscle fibers have consistently failed, and the manner in which the HIV virus induces myopathies is unclear. Zidovudine, an agent for treatment of the HIV infection, may induce a toxic mitochondrial myopathy coexistent with the HIV-related myopathy.

Human T cell leukemia virus type I (HTLV-I), an agent associated with chronic spastic paraparesis, also can be associated with polymyositis, but the virus has not been shown to infect muscle fibers.

Autoimmunity in Idiopathic Inflammatory Myopathies. Authorities have inferred an autoimmune cause in inflammatory myopathies from one or more of the following observations: (1) The myopathy is associated with another identifiable autoimmune disease (e.g., systemic lupus erythematosus or rheumatoid arthritis). (2) Laboratory tests suggest an altered immune state (e.g., myositis-specific antibodies, increased serum gamma globulins, decreased total hemolytic complement in serum, and positive tests for antibodies against native DNA, other nuclear or cytoplasmic antigens, or rheumatoid factor). (3) Muscle contains a predominantly mononuclear inflammatory exudate. (4) Evidence exists of focal invasion and destruction of muscle fibers by antigen-specific cytotoxic T cells. (5) The diseases respond to corticosteroids or other immunosuppressants. The first criterion, if fulfilled, represents strong, but indirect, evidence. Laboratory tests suggesting an altered immune state are positive in a minority of patients with dermatomyositis and in polymyositis. A mononuclear inflammatory exudate, however, also can occur in some genetically determined muscle diseases (e.g., Duchenne or facioscapulohumeral dystrophy). Inclusion body myositis, in which an inflammatory exudate is often prominent, most cases of scleroderma, and some cases of pure polymyositis

and dermatomyositis do not respond to immunosuppressants. Further, neither the factors that initiate self-sensitization nor the sensitizing antigen has been defined in any of the major inflammatory myopathies (idiopathic polymyositis, inclusion body myositis, dermatomyositis, and scleroderma). None has been transferred to an experimental animal.

Sporadic Inclusion Body Myositis. This entity differs from other idiopathic inflammatory myopathies in several respects. It fails to respond to corticosteroids or other immunosuppressants. Most patients are older than 50, and there is male predominance. The disease evolves slowly, affecting the lower limbs first, involving both proximal and distal muscles, and resulting in selectively severe weakness and atrophy of the quadriceps. Facial, cervical, and pharyngeal muscles are usually spared. Deep tendon reflexes disappear early from the affected limbs. The serum CK level is mildly elevated or normal. The EMG indicates myopathic changes and abnormal electrical irritability, as in dermatomyositis or polymyositis, but there may be additional neurogenic features as well. Affected muscles show a typical pattern of histologic change: rimmed vacuoles in a significant proportion of the fibers; eosinophilic intranuclear and cytoplasmic inclusions in a few fibers that also are congophilic and react positively for ubiquitin and β-amyloid protein; small groups of atrophic fibers without type grouping; and an endomysial and a lesser perivascular inflammatory exudate. The exudate is enriched in cytotoxic T cells that focally surround, invade, and destroy non-necrotic fibers. Necrotic fibers occur but are less common than in polymyositis. Ultrastructural studies show that the rimmed vacuoles contain myeloid structures and other cytoplasmic degradation products and that the inclusions consist of microtubular filaments. The differential diagnosis includes motor neuron disease, distal muscular dystrophies, peripheral neuropathies, and pure polymyositis. The diagnosis is usually clarified by a careful study of the muscle biopsy.

Differences Between Dermatomyositis and Pure Polymyositis. Dermatomyositis and pure polymyositis resemble each other in the predominantly proximal distribution of the muscle weakness, a mononuclear inflammatory exudate in muscle, myopathic changes, spontaneous electrical activity in the EMG, and responsiveness to corticosteroid therapy. Consequently, they are often treated as a single entity in evaluating their cause, natural history, and therapy. Several aspects of dermatomyositis differentiate it from pure polymyositis, however: (1) The characteristic rash of dermatomyositis is lacking in pure polymyositis. (2) Capillary injury and necrosis are early and constant findings in dermatomyositis. Many of the injured capillaries react for the membrane attack complex of complement, whereas other vessels are found to be occluded by platelet thrombi or to harbor microtubular inclusions. (3) Muscle fibers at the periphery of the fascicles undergo selective degeneration and atrophy. (4) The inflammatory exudate is concentrated at perimysial and perivascular sites and is enriched in B cells and helper T cells. (5) There is no evidence for T cell–mediated cytotoxicity directed against the muscle fibers. These findings suggest that a humoral response against vascular elements plays an important role in the pathogenesis of dermatomyositis.

By contrast, no capillary necrosis or loss develops in pure polymyositis. The inflammatory exudate contains fewer B cells and helper T cells than in dermatomyositis, and B cells are virtually absent from the endomysium. Focal invasion and destruction of non-necrotic muscle fibers by antigen-specific cytotoxic T cells accompanied by macrophages indicate cell-mediated cytotoxicity directed against the muscle fiber. Necrosis of isolated fibers also occurs. These findings suggest that a component of the muscle fiber surface membrane is a target of the immune effector response.

Differences Between Scleroderma and the Other Major Inflammatory Myopathies. In scleroderma, the serum CK level is either normal or only slightly elevated, the resting EMG is often normal, and necrotic fibers are uncommon. The pathologic changes involve fibrosis and inflammation affecting the perimysium and the perimysial blood vessels. The inflammatory cells at these sites are predominantly T cells and macrophages. The findings suggest a cell-mediated immune response against a perimysial and/or vascular component in muscle.

Eosinophilia-Myalgia Related to L-Tryptophan Preparations. This syndrome appeared in 1989 in patients consuming L-tryptophan preparations. The features consisted of eosinophilia ($> 10^9$ per liter), marked myalgias, fasciitis, and often a peripheral neuropathy. Interstitial pneumonitis, myocarditis, and encephalopathy occurred in some subjects. An autoimmune pathogenesis was implicated by onset or progression of the syndrome after withdrawal of the L-tryptophan preparation, inflammatory cells in the affected tissues, and responsiveness to immunotherapy in some cases. The pathologic substrate is an interstitial inflammation associated with an occlusive microangiopathy and fibroplasia. The triggering factor appears to be 1,1'-ethylidenebis[tryptophan], a contaminant of L-tryptophan produced by a single manufacturer.

Myositis Ossificans. The *localized form* appears as a tender swelling after trauma to a muscle. After a few months this becomes hard and ossified. Therapy consists of excision. The *generalized form* represents an autosomal dominant disease with variable expressivity that begins in childhood, involves many muscles, and causes progressive rigidity of body parts. The initial lesions appear in fascia and dermis and are associated with inflammation, local hemorrhage, and connective tissue proliferation. Cartilage and bone formation occur at a later stage. Other congenital malformations (microdactyly of the great toe, exostoses, absence of upper incisors or of ear lobules, and hypogenitalism) are found in most patients. There is no effective therapy.

Engel AG, Franzini-Armstrong C (eds.): Myology, 2nd ed. New York, McGraw-Hill, 1994. *Comprehensive descriptions of the clinical and laboratory features and therapy of polymyositis, dermatomyositis, inclusion body myositis, and other inflammatory and HIV-associated myopathies by multiple authors.*
Mastaglia FL (ed.): Inflammatory myopathies. *In* Ballière's Clinical Neurology, vol 2, no 3. Philadelphia, Ballière Tindall, 1993. *A detailed survey by multiple authors of the clinical and pathologic aspects of the major subtypes of inflammatory myopathies.*

457   METABOLIC MYOPATHIES

GLYCOGEN STORAGE DISEASES. These are described in detail in Ch. 170. When muscle is involved, glycogen-filled vacuoles appear in the fibers; the glycogen excess can vary from slight to marked, and definitive diagnosis requires demonstration of a specific enzyme deficiency. Of the several glycogenoses, only glucose-6-phosphate dehydrogenase and liver phosphorylase deficiencies fail to affect muscle. All glycogenoses that affect muscle are transmitted as autosomal-recessive traits except phosphoglycerate kinase deficiency, which is X-linked recessive.

Acid Alpha-1,4-Glucosidase (Lysosomal Acid Maltase) Deficiency. The gene encoding the enzyme maps to chromosome 17q23. Various mutations affecting the synthesis, phosphorylation, maturation, and catalytic activity of the enzyme have been identified. Three major clinical variants exist. The *infantile type* presents in early infancy with generalized and rapidly progressive weakness and heart, tongue, and liver enlargement. There is widespread and marked glycogen excess in tissues, including lower motor neurons. Death occurs from cardiorespiratory failure before the age of 2 years. The *childhood type* presents in infancy or early childhood as a myopathy. Weakness is more proximal than distal, and there may be calf enlargement simulating muscular dystrophy. Glycogen excess is less marked and confined to muscle. Death occurs before age 20 of respiratory failure. The *adult type* presents between the second and seventh decade of life, either with slowly progressive limb muscle weakness that mimics limb-girdle dystrophy or polymyositis, or with insidiously developing ventilatory insufficiency leading to respiratory failure. In all three types the serum CK level is increased, but to less than 10 times normal. The EMG in affected muscles shows myopathic changes and excessive abnormal electrical irritability, including myotonic discharges (but there is no clinical myotonia). Muscle biopsy demonstrates a vacuolar myopathy with high glycogen content and acid-phosphatase reactivity in the vacuoles, an appearance that otherwise occurs only in chloroquine myopathy and a rare cardioskeletal lysosomal storage disorder without acid maltase deficiency.

Debranching Enzyme Deficiency. The gene for the enzyme maps to chromosome 1p21. A disabling myopathy affecting both proximal and distal muscles can appear in childhood or (more commonly) in adult life. Often there is a history of a protuberant abdomen and hypoglycemic episodes in childhood, along with muscle fatigue on exertion. Persistent hepatomegaly and biventricular cardiac hypertrophy are found in most cases. There is a diminished glycemic response to epinephrine and glucagon and an impaired rise of lactic acid after ischemic exercise. The EMG shows myopathic changes and abnormal electrical irritability in affected muscles.

Branching Enzyme Deficiency. The disease presents in infancy with progressive hepatosplenomegaly and failure to thrive. The abnormal starchlike glycogen, which resists diastase digestion, induces nodular cirrhosis and liver failure. Death occurs in early childhood from liver or heart failure. Muscle weakness is variable; if present, the tongue is severely affected.

Phosphorylase b Kinase (PBK) Deficiency. This syndrome shows marked clinical and genetic heterogeneity. Cardiac PBK deficiency is a fatal disease of infancy. An autosomal recessive form presents in childhood with weakness or hepatomegaly that improves with age; PBK is deficient in muscle, liver, and erythrocytes. An X-linked recessive disease presents in children with asymptomatic hepatomegaly or mild hypoglycemia; PBK is deficient in liver and erythrocytes. Another form of PBK deficiency which is restricted to muscle presents with exercise intolerance and myoglobinuria or a late-onset myopathy simulating muscular dystrophy.

Glycolytic Enzyme Defects: Myophosphorylase, Phosphofructokinase (PFK), Phosphoglycerate Kinase (PGK), Phosphoglycerate Mutase (PGM), and Lactate Dehydrogenase (LDH) Deficiencies. Table 453–3 lists the molecular genetic findings. The common clinical features are periodic myoglobinuria following strenuous exertion since childhood; easy fatigability; and a venous lactate level that fails to rise after ischemic exercise in myophosphorylase and PFK deficiencies, and fails to rise or rises by less than 100% in PGK, PGM, and LDH deficiencies. Muscle cramps are prominent. They are caused by electrically silent contractures and are not associated with ATP depletion; their mechanism is not understood. The muscle glycogen excess is slight to modest. Permanent muscle weakness and atrophy are initially slight, but may increase with age. Fatal infantile variants have been identified in myophosphorylase and PFK deficiency. In PFK deficiency hyperuricemia and gout occur in some cases, and there is mild hemolytic disease caused by a partial erythrocyte enzyme defect. PGK mutations result in either severe hemolytic anemia and neurologic deficits but no myopathy, or produce a myopathy with only the features described above.

DISORDERS OF FATTY ACID METABOLISM. Long-chain fatty acids taken up by muscle are utilized for energy metabolism or incorporated into triglycerides and stored as lipid droplets. Long-chain fatty acids entering the catabolic pathway are esterified with coenzyme A (CoA) to form acyl-CoA's. These react with carnitine to form acylcarnitines in a reaction catalyzed by carnitine palmitoyltransferase (CPT) I, an enzyme positioned on the inner surface of the inner mitochondrial membrane. The acylcarnitines are transported through the inner mitochondrial membrane by a carnitine-acylcarnitine translocase and then reconverted to acyl-CoA's by CPT II. The acyl-CoA's undergo repeated cycles of beta-oxidation, generating acetyl-CoA's that enter the citric acid cycle or form ketone bodies. The inner mitochondrial membrane is impermeable to long-chain fatty acids, CoA, and acyl-CoA's. Consequently, carnitine, carnitine-acyltransferases, and carnitine-acylcarnitine translocase jointly regulate the oxidation of fatty acids and modulate the intramitochondrial CoA/acyl-CoA ratio. Excessive intramitochondrial accumulation of an acyl-CoA compound leads to its conversion to a corresponding acylcarnitine. The acylcarnitine leaves the mitochondrion via the translocase, diffuses out from the cell, and is preferentially excreted by the kidney. If this process continues, muscle and body carnitine stores become depleted.

Derangements in fatty acid oxidation produce a variety of syndromes that affect muscle and other organs. The possible consequences include one or more of the following: intermittent energy shortage in muscle causing *rhabdomyolysis* and *myoglobinuria;* intramitochondrial acyl-CoA excess and CoA deficiency, secondary carnitine depletion, and inhibition of multiple mitochondrial enzyme systems (these events trigger a *Reye syndrome–like metabolic crisis,* see Ch. 429); and triglyceride accumulation in muscle producing a *lipid-storage myopathy.* Many carnitine-deficiency syndromes are secondary to another metabolic defect in fatty acid oxidation, branched-chain amino acid metabolism, or the respiratory chain. A lipid storage myopathy can be caused by primary carnitine deficiency or by another defect of fatty acid oxidation with or without secondary carnitine deficiency (Table 457–1).

Carnitine Palmitoyltransferase Deficiency. Infantile and adult forms of the disease exist. The most common cause of adult CPT deficiency is a homozygous Ser113Leu mutation in the CPT II gene (see Table 453–3). In affected patients who are heterozygous for this mutation, a second mutation in the CPT II gene is likely. The symptoms consist of muscle aching, fatigability, and periodic myoglobinuria on sustained exertion, especially if combined with fasting and exposure to cold. There are no symptoms between attacks, and the muscle lipid content is normal or only slightly increased.

Acyl-CoA Dehydrogenase Deficiencies. Deficiencies of the long-chain, medium-chain, and short-chain specific enzymes, and in the factors that transfer electrons from multiple acyl-CoA dehydrogenases to coenzyme Q (multiple acyl-CoA dehydrogenase deficiency), have been identified. Each syndrome causes secondary carnitine depletion, a lipid storage myopathy, and organic aciduria. The urinary organic acid and acylcarnitine profiles reflect the site of the metabolic block. *Short-chain acyl-CoA dehydrogenase deficiency* is associated with adult-onset lipid storage myopathy. Ketogenesis is not impaired and there are no metabolic crises. The other acyl-CoA dehydrogenase deficiencies produce intermittent metabolic crises resembling Reye syndrome. *Long-chain acyl-CoA dehydrogenase deficiency* usually has a neonatal onset and is associated with hepatomegaly and cardiomyopathy. *Medium-chain acyl-CoA dehydrogenase deficiency* usually presents in the first or second year of life with a metabolic crisis. Between attacks the patients are well or have mild weakness, easy fatigability, and mild hepatomegaly. *Multiple acyl-CoA dehydrogenase deficiencies* are genetically and biochemically heterogeneous. Severe neonatal forms with cardiomyopathy and milder late-onset cases have been described. Some cases respond to riboflavin therapy. The acyl-CoA dehydrogenase deficiencies are treated with a low-fat, high-carbohydrate diet and L-carnitine supplements (2 to 4 grams daily in adults and 100 mg per kilogram daily in infants and children). Crises can be prevented by avoiding fasting and maintaining alimentation at all times, especially during febrile illnesses. The crises are treated by intravenous therapy to correct the hypoglycemia and electrolyte abnormalities, and by L-carnitine, initially 100 mg per kilogram and then 25 mg per kilogram every 4 hours.

Primary Carnitine Deficiency Syndromes. Primary systemic carnitine deficiency is an autosomal recessive disease due to impaired carnitine transport in muscle, heart, renal and intestinal epithelia, and fibroblasts. Defective intestinal absorption and a renal

TABLE 457–1. DISORDERS OF LIPID METABOLISM AFFECTING MUSCLE

Primary muscle or systemic carnitine deficiency
Organic acidurias with acyl-CoA dehydrogenase deficiencies*
  Long-chain acyl-CoA dehydrogenase deficiency
  Medium-chain acyl-CoA dehydrogenase deficiency
  Short-chain acyl-CoA dehydrogenase deficiency
  Multiple acyl-CoA dehydrogenase deficiency
  Long-chain 3-hydroxyacyl-CoA dehydrogenase deficiency
  Short-chain 3-hydroxyacyl-CoA dehydrogenase deficiency
Organic acidurias with defects in branched-chain amino acid metabolism*
  Isovaleryl-CoA dehydrogenase deficiency†
  Propionyl-CoA carboxylase deficiency
  Methylmalonyl-CoA mutase deficiency
  β-hydroxy-β-methylglutaric-CoA lyase deficiency
Defects in mitochondrial respiratory chain or energy utilization‡
  Block at NADH-coenzyme Q reductase (Complex I deficiency)
  Mitochondrial ATPase deficiency (Complex V deficiency)
Miscellaneous disorders‡
  Idiopathic Reye syndrome
  Valproate therapy

* Associated with secondary carnitine deficiency.
† This enzyme is also an acyl-CoA dehydrogenase.
‡ Only some patients become carnitine deficient and accumulate lipid in muscle.

TABLE 457–2. CLASSIFICATION OF MITOCHONDRIAL MYOPATHIES

Nuclear DNA defects
  Hypermetabolic myopathy (Luft syndrome)
  Defects proximal to the mitochondrial respiratory chain
    Carnitine palmitoyltransferase deficiency
    Primary and secondary carnitine deficiency syndromes
    Acyl-CoA dehydrogenase deficiencies
    Defects in the pyruvate dehydrogenase complex
  Defects of the mitochondrial respiratory chain
    Coenzyme Q deficiency
    Complex I deficiency
    Complex II deficiency
    Complex III deficiency
    Complex IV deficiency
Mitochondrial DNA mutations
  Kearns-Sayre syndrome
  PEO due to mitochondrial myopathy
  MERRF
  MELAS
  Maternally transmitted mitochondrial myopathy and cardiomyopathy
  NARP
  LHON
Defective interaction of nuclear and mitochondrial DNA
  Multiple mitochondrial DNA deletions
  Myoneurogastrointestinal disorder and encephalopathy
  Mitochondrial DNA depletion*

* Affects infants. See chapter by Morgan-Hughes in Engel AG, Franzini-Armstrong C (eds.): Myology, 2nd ed. New York, McGraw-Hill, 1994.
PEO, Progressive external ophthalmoplegia; MERRF, myoclonic epilepsy with ragged red fibers; MELAS, mitochondrial encephalomyopathy with lactic acidosis and strokelike episodes; NARP, neurogenic muscle weakness, ataxia, and retinitis pigmentosa; LHON, Leber's hereditary optic neuroretinopathy.

carnitine leak caused by the transport defect result in further tissue carnitine depletion. The disease is associated with cardiomyopathy, weakness, and episodes of hypoketotic hypoglycemic encephalopathy; it responds to carnitine replacement therapy. A myopathic form of primary carnitine deficiency also exists and may respond to prednisone therapy.

Other Lipid Storage Myopathies. Autosomal recessive and dominant lipid storage myopathies associated with lifelong weakness, myalgias, and electrical myotonia, but without carnitine deficiency, have been described. *Chanarin's disease* is a rare autosomal recessive condition with congenital ichthyosis, steatorrhea, and lipid storage in muscle fibers, hepatocytes, gastrointestinal epithelial cells, epidermal cells, monocytes, myelocytes, and fibroblasts.

MITOCHONDRIAL MYOPATHIES. Mitochondrial diseases can arise from mutations in nuclear or mitochondrial DNA or stem from a defective interaction between nuclear and mitochondrial DNA. Some mitochondrial DNA mutations are transmitted by vertical maternal inheritance; others arise *de novo* in the maternal ovum or in early embryonic life. Table 457–2 shows a current classification of the mitochondrial myopathies.

In many mitochondrial myopathies a substantial proportion of the muscle fibers contains subsarcolemmal and intermyofibrillar accumulations of structurally and functionally abnormal mitochondria. These fibers appear "ragged red" in the trichrome stain and "ragged blue" when reacted for succinate dehydrogenase and may fail to react for cytochrome c oxidase (CCO). Some fiber segments are CCO-negative without containing an excess of mitochondria. A segmental distribution of the histologic abnormalities along the length of individual muscle fibers and CCO negativity of only a proportion of the fibers point to a mutation in mitochondrial DNA.

Many mitochondrial myopathies produce slowly progressive weakness of limb and/or external ocular and other cranial muscles, abnormal fatigability on sustained exertion, and lactacidemia on exertion or even at rest. Some affect multiple organs or systems, and the myopathy is but one facet of a multisystem disease.

Defects Proximal to the Mitochondrial Respiratory Chain. These include the primary carnitine deficiencies, acyl-CoA dehydrogenase deficiencies, carnitine palmitoyltransferase deficiency (all dealt with above), and *defects in the pyruvate dehydrogenase complex*. The latter are associated with various neurologic syndromes that include movement disorders, ataxia, neuropathy, subacute necrotizing encephalomyelopathy (Leigh's syndrome), and fatal infantile lactic acidosis. Muscle biopsy shows ragged red fibers, lipid excess, or denervation atrophy.

Defects in the Mitochondrial Respiratory Chain. The mitochondrial respiratory chain includes four distinct enzyme complexes and also coenzyme Q and cytochrome c. The components are attached to the inner mitochondrial membrane and carry reducing equivalents from reduced nicotinamide adenine dinucleotide (NADH), flavin adenine dinucleotide ($FADH_2$), and electron-transferring flavoprotein (ETF) to molecular oxygen. A fifth complex, an ATPase, uses released energy to phosphorylate ADP to ATP in a tightly coupled process. Defects in the electron transport complexes are associated with marked clinical, biochemical, and genetic heterogeneity. The reasons for this are that each complex is composed of multiple subunits, different subunits of a given complex are encoded by different genes, some subunits of a given complex are encoded by mitochondrial rather than nuclear DNA, some subunits are tissue specific, and some subunits are developmentally regulated.

Coenzyme Q Deficiency. A deficiency of mitochondrial coenzyme Q is associated with a familial syndrome of marked lipid and mitochondrial excess in muscle, severe lactacidemia, intermittent myoglobinuria, progressive muscle weakness, cognitive deficits, cerebellar ataxia, and seizures. The activities of complex I, II, III, and IV and cellular cytochrome levels are normal.

Complex I (NADH-Coenzyme Q Oxidoreductase) Deficiency. Most of these begin in childhood and allow survival to adult life. Either muscular or central nervous system manifestations dominate the clinical picture. In the former group the findings include muscle weakness, exercise intolerance, exertional lactacidemia, and ragged red fibers in muscle. Headaches, progressive visual loss, hemiparesis, dysphasia, dementia, dystonia, and cerebral atrophy affect the latter group. A fatal infantile form exists.

Complex II (Succinate-Dehydrogenase) Deficiency. A deficiency of complex II together with decreased levels of the mitochondrial enzyme aconitase has been observed in patients with lifelong exercise intolerance and recurrent episodes of myoglobinuria. In other patients, a biochemical deficiency of succinate dehydrogenase in muscle is associated with severe infantile myopathy and lactic acidosis or syndromes that phenotypically resemble Leigh syndrome or the Kearns-Sayre syndrome (discussed below).

Complex III (Coenzyme Q–Cytochrome C Oxidoreductase) Deficiency. These begin in childhood or adult life. Muscle weakness, exercise intolerance, exertional lactacidemia, and ragged red fibers are constant findings. Some patients also have external ophthalmoplegia and/or dementia, myoclonus, ataxia, pyramidal signs, and loss of proprioception. The muscle symptoms in one patient were improved by treatment with menadione and vitamin C, agents that can function as electron transfer mediators instead of complex III.

Complex IV (Cytochrome C Oxidase) Deficiency. Several syndromes are associated with this defect, and are detailed in the references.

Mitochondrial DNA Mutations. Mitochondrial DNA (mtDNA) can undergo point, deletion, or duplication mutations. With homoplasmic mutations, a single population of mutant mtDNA appears in all cells and produces a single clinical syndrome. With heteroplasmic mutations, normal and mutant forms of mtDNA coexist in the same cell, and subsequent cell replication leads to uneven segregation of normal and mutant DNA. The phenotypic expression depends on the proportion of mutant to normal mtDNA in cells of a given tissue, as well as tissue dependence on oxidative metabolism and the severity of the oxidation-phosphorylation defect.

Kearns-Sayre Syndrome. The mutations in the major syndromes are listed in Table 453–3. Most cases are sporadic and stem from heteroplasmic DNA deletions in the maternal ovum or during early embryonic life. The syndrome presents under age 20, and is associated with progressive external ophthalmoplegia (PEO), retinitis pigmentosa, and ragged red fibers, plus at least one of the following: heart block, cerebellar syndrome, or a high spinal fluid protein content. More than half of the patients have hearing loss, mental defect, short stature, and lactic acidosis; less than half have cystic changes or calcification of the basal ganglia, pyramidal signs, seizures, peripheral neuropathy, endocrine disturbances (e.g., hypogonadism, diabetes, hypoparathyroidism), or renal Fanconi syndrome. The presence of heart block requires treatment by pacemaker.

Progressive External Ophthalmoplegia Due to a Mitochondrial Myopathy. Not only external ocular but also other cranial as well as cervical, truncal, and limb muscles can be affected. One or more elements of the Kearns-Sayre syndrome also occur in some patients. About half the patients have mitochondrial DNA deletions. The disease is sporadic, indicating that the deletions are found only in somatic cells.

Myoclonus, Generalized Seizures, Ragged Red Fibers (MERRF). The disease presents in children or adults and is associated with progressive myoclonus, seizures, cerebellar ataxia, and muscle weakness. Short stature, dementia, hearing loss, and optic atrophy are frequent; spasticity, central hypoventilation, endocrinopathies, and peripheral neuropathy occur less often.

Mitochondrial Encephalomyopathy with Lactic Acidosis and Strokelike Episodes (MELAS). The same mutations that cause MELAS can also be found in some patients with PEO or other encephalomyopathies without strokelike episodes. In 25% of MELAS patients the family history is consistent with maternal inheritance. More than 90% of MELAS patients have normal early development, experience strokelike episodes before age 40, and have focal or generalized seizures, lactic acidosis, and ragged red fibers in muscle. Brain imaging during strokelike episodes shows areas of encephalomalacia affecting areas lying outside of the territories of the main cerebral arteries. Other frequent features consist of dementia, hearing loss, short stature, and episodic vomiting. Less than half of the patients have calcification of the basal ganglia, ataxia, myoclonus, optic atrophy, episodic coma, increased spinal fluid protein content, or cardiomyopathy. The diagnosis is based on strokelike episodes before the age of 40, seizures or dementia or both, ragged red fibers in muscle or lactic acidosis or both, plus two of the other frequent features.

Maternally Transmitted Mitochondrial Myopathy and Cardiomyopathy. This disorder is caused by another heteroplasmic point mutation at nucleotide 3260 in the mitochondrial $tRNA^{Leu(UUR)}$ gene. It is associated with lactic acidosis and ragged red fibers in muscle. Other features of MELAS are absent.

Neuropathy, Ataxia, and Retinitis Pigmentosa (NARP). In addition to the features characterizing the syndrome, some patients also suffer from developmental delay, seizures, and proximal muscle weakness. Muscles lack ragged red fibers. In some families the same mutation results in Leigh syndrome.

Leber's Hereditary Optic Neuroretinopathy (LHON). The disease is more frequent in men than in women. It presents in young adults with optic neuritis and telangiectasia around the optic disk and results in central loss of vision. Cerebellar ataxia, spasticity, posterior column signs, peripheral neuropathy, and cardiac conduction defects also can occur. Morphologic and biochemical abnormalities affect muscle mitochondria.

Defective Interactions of Nuclear and Mitochondrial DNA. Multiple Mitochondria DNA Deletions. This disorder is clinically and genetically heterogeneous, transmitted as an autosomal dominant or recessive trait. The clinical features, which vary from family to family, comprise proximal muscle weakness, PEO, cataracts, hearing loss, ataxia, peripheral neuropathy, mental retardation, and hypoparathyroidism. In one family, two brothers suffered from recurrent myoglobinuria after exertion or fasting.

Myoneurogastrointestinal Disorder and Encephalopathy. This autosomal recessive disorder is associated with PEO, mitochondrial myopathy, neuropathy, abnormal intestinal motility with bouts of vomiting and diarrhea, leukoencephalopathy, and lactic acidosis. Multiple deletions in mitochondrial DNA and biochemical defects in complex IV or I have been observed.

ENDOCRINE MYOPATHIES. Muscle weakness can be a symptom of any endocrine disorder. The serum CK level is normal, except in myxedema and in uremic hyperparathyroidism. The EMG is normal or myopathic without spontaneous electrical activity. The histologic alterations in muscle are often nonspecific, such as type II fiber atrophy, focal increases and decreases in mitochondria, and focal myofibrillar degeneration. Fiber necrosis and regeneration and connective tissue proliferation are uncommon.

Glucocorticoid-Induced Myopathy. Muscle weakness commonly occurs in Cushing's syndrome and in patients receiving relatively high doses of glucocorticoids. Fluorinated drugs (dexamethasone, triamcinolone) are more pathogenic than nonfluorinated ones (prednisone). Considerable variation exists in the minimal dosage that induces myopathy. However, daily treatment for 3 months with 60 mg prednisone in divided doses induces some

2168 / XXIV NEUROLOGY

weakness in nearly all patients. Women are more susceptible than men, and divided daily doses are more pathogenic than single or alternate daily doses. The onset is usually insidious but occasionally sudden with diffuse myalgias. The weakness is more proximal than distal and affects the lower more than the upper limbs. Hip and ankle flexors are selectively severely affected. The cranial muscles are spared. The serum CK level remains normal. Therapy consists of reducing the steroid dosage to the lowest possible level. Muscle strength returns to normal within 1 to 4 months after therapy is stopped.

Adrenal Insufficiency. Weakness is a typical feature, closely related to derangements in fluid and electrolyte balance and possibly to the associated hypotension. Joint contractures, especially of the knees and not related to muscle weakness, may also occur. Hyperkalemia in chronic adrenal insufficiency can be a cause of secondary periodic paralysis (discussed below).

Thyrotoxic Myopathy. This appears in 80% of untreated cases of hyperthyroidism. The hyperthyroid state can be mild and of long duration or present for only a few weeks before the onset of the weakness. Weakness is predominantly proximal, less often both proximal and distal. The deep tendon reflexes are hyperactive or normal. The serum CK level remains normal. The EMG shows myopathic motor unit potentials but never fibrillation potentials.

Graves' ophthalmopathy is described in Ch. 203. Thyrotoxic periodic paralysis is considered below.

Hypothyroid Myopathy. Muscle aching, cramps, slow relaxation of the reflexes, ridging of the muscles on percussion (myoedema), and an increase of the serum CK level are common findings in myxedema. Muscle enlargement and limb-girdle weakness occur only occasionally.

Muscle Symptoms in Hyperparathyroidism and Osteomalacia. Proximal muscle weakness, fatigability, and muscle pain and tenderness, usually with bone pain and tenderness, can occur in primary and secondary hyperparathyroidism and in osteomalacia.

A more malignant syndrome can appear in uremic hyperparathyroidism. Here, metastatic calcification of the media and proliferation of the intima of small blood vessels produce skin and visceral infarcts and a necrotizing myopathy with marked elevation of serum enzymes and myoglobinuria.

Muscle Symptoms in Hypoparathyroidism. The typical neuromuscular symptom is tetany. This is considered in Ch. 214.

Acromegaly and Hypopituitarism. Acromegaly initially causes muscle hypertrophy, particularly if the disorder begins before growth ceases. Later, generalized weakness and atrophy develop. Muscle biopsies can show segmental muscle fiber degeneration, type I or type II fiber atrophy, or no pathologic change. The serum CK level remains normal. A hypertrophic distal neuropathy and nerve entrapment are common in acromegaly.

Pituitary failure in adults results in weakness and fatigability with little muscle atrophy. The weakness itself may reflect the combined influence of thyroid, adrenal, and growth hormone deficiencies.

THE PERIODIC PARALYSES (PP). These disorders occur as either inherited (primary) or acquired (secondary) illnesses and can be further classified according to measurable alterations in the serum potassium level during attacks (Table 457–3). The primary types are transmitted by autosomal dominant inheritance, but nearly a third of the cases arise sporadically. It is important to realize that in the primary forms the serum potassium decreases or increases but may still remain within the normal range during attacks and is normal or low-normal between attacks. By contrast, in secondary PP caused by potassium wastage or retention the serum potassium is always markedly reduced or elevated during and even between attacks. In each type of PP the propagation of the muscle fiber action potential fails during an attack.

The different types of periodic paralysis share several common features: (1) Paralytic attacks last from < 1 hour to as long as several days. (2) Weakness can be localized or generalized. (3) Tendon reflexes diminish and then disappear during attacks. (4) Muscle fibers become inexcitable to direct or indirect electrical stimulation during the attacks. (5) Generalized attacks begin proximally and spread distally. Respiratory and cranial muscles tend to be spared except in the most severe attacks. (6) Rest after exercise provokes weakness in the muscles that were exercised. Continued mild exercise aborts attacks. (7) Exercise followed by rest of a single muscle can induce weakness of that muscle without detectable change in

TABLE 457–3. CLASSIFICATION OF THE PERIODIC PARALYSES

Primary
  Hypokalemic
  Normokalemic
  Hyperkalemic
    without myotonia
    with myotonia
    with paramyotonia
  Paramyotonia congenita
  With cardiac arrhythmia (hyper-, hypo-, or normokalemic)
Secondary
  Hypokalemic
    Thyrotoxic
    Urinary potassium wastage
    Gastrointestinal potassium wastage
    Barium intoxication
  Hyperkalemic
    Renal insufficiency
    Adrenal insufficiency

the potassium level in the systemic circulation. (8) Exposure to cold can provoke weakness in the primary forms of the disease. (9) Complete recovery occurs after initial attacks. (10) In the primary disorders permanent weakness and a persistent vacuolar myopathy can develop with or without repeated attacks. Despite these similarities, the different forms of PP differ in their response to sodium, potassium, or carbohydrate loading, as well as their pattern of urinary electrolyte excretions during attacks, and in some of their clinical features.

Primary Hypokalemic Periodic Paralysis. The disease is caused by mutations in the voltage sensor of the T tubule. Attacks begin in the first or second decade and become less frequent or cease during the fourth or fifth decade. When attacks recur daily, the patient is weakest in the morning and becomes stronger as the day passes. High dietary sodium or carbohydrate intake as well as excitement provokes or exacerbates the episodes. Major attacks are associated with urinary retention of sodium, potassium, chloride, and water. The diagnosis is supported by a positive family history and a decrease in serum potassium during an attack. An abnormally low serum potassium level between attacks suggests secondary rather than primary PP. In diagnosing sporadic cases one must exclude potassium wastage and thyrotoxicosis. The oral or intravenous administration of glucose, 2 grams per kilogram of body weight, combined with 10 to 20 units of insulin given subcutaneously, may provoke an attack within 2 to 3 hours. Depression of the serum potassium during the attack and a favorable response to 2.5 to 7.5 grams of potassium chloride (KCl) given orally must be demonstrated. Provocative tests must never be done in patients already hypokalemic, and potassium chloride must not be given to patients unless they have adequate renal or adrenal reserve.

Thyrotoxic Periodic Paralysis. This disease resembles primary hypokalemic PP in the changes in serum and urinary electrolytes that accompany the attacks and in the response to glucose, insulin, potassium, and rest after exercise. However, 95% of the cases are sporadic, the male to female ratio is 6:1, most cases occur among Orientals, the onset is usually in adult life, and correction of the hyperthyroidism prevents further attacks.

Barium-Induced Periodic Paralysis. The accidental ingestion of absorbable barium salts such as barium carbonate induces hemorrhagic gastroenteritis, hypertension, cardiac arrhythmias, convulsions, hypokalemia, and muscle paralysis. Barium blocks potassium channels and thereby reduces potassium efflux from muscle; potassium uptake by muscle, mediated by the sodium-potassium pump, continues, and hypokalemia results.

Periodic Paralysis Secondary to Urinary or Gastrointestinal Potassium Loss. Paralytic attacks do not occur unless the serum potassium falls below 3 mEq per liter, and during the attacks the serum potassium decreases even further. Other neuromuscular complications of severe potassium depletion include a necrotizing myopathy, myoglobinuria, and latent or manifest tetany.

Primary Hyperkalemic Periodic Paralysis and Paramyotonia Congenita. These diseases are now known to be allelic, caused by mutations in the α-subunit of the adult muscle sodium channel gene. In primary hyperkalemic periodic paralysis, the attacks begin in the first or second decade. They are often brief but can last up to several days. Between attacks the serum potassium is normal or slightly lower than normal. During major attacks potassium moves out from muscle. The serum potassium increases but may not exceed the normal range, and the urinary potassium excretion increases. Myotonic, paramyotonic, and nonmyotonic forms of hyperkalemic PP can be distinguished. In *myotonic hyperkalemic PP* myotonia can be detected in facial, tongue, finger extensor, and thenar muscles between attacks. In *paramyotonic hyperkalemic PP,* exposure to cold causes widespread and severe myotonia. Exercise in the cold is followed by prolonged weakness not reversed by rewarming. Paralytic attacks are provoked by orally administered KCl, 50 to 100 mg per kilogram, given in an unsweetened solution in the fasting state. The test is contraindicated in subjects already hyperkalemic or those without adequate renal or adrenal reserve. In pure *paramyotonia congenita* potassium loading does not induce weakness. Unlike in myotonia congenita, the myotonia is worsened rather than improved by exercise. Exercise in the cold causes prolonged electrically silent stiffness and weakness not relieved by rewarming.

Secondary Hyperkalemic Periodic Paralysis.
This can occur when the serum potassium level exceeds 7 mEq per liter. The usual cause is renal or adrenal insufficiency, but hyperkalemia from exposure to spironolactone and during attacks of malaria also has caused paralytic attacks. The diagnosis is suggested by the presence of a very high serum potassium level during attacks, persistent hyperkalemia between attacks, and the associated primary disorder.

Primary Normokalemic Periodic Paralysis.
There are no consistent changes in the serum potassium during the attacks. The existence of the disease has been questioned because some patients are sensitive to potassium salts. The observations suggest that normokalemic PP is a heterogeneous entity.

Primary Periodic Paralysis with Cardiac Arrhythmia.
Affected patients suffer from PP and tachyarrhythmias that can cause sudden death. The cardiac symptoms are provoked or worsened by hypokalemia and digitalis and are refractory to disopyramide phosphate, propranolol, or phenytoin, but may respond to imipramine. Dysmorphic features, such as short stature, clinodactyly, and microcephaly can also occur. The PP has been clearly related to hyperkalemia in some patients, but hypokalemic and normokalemic PP were diagnosed in others.

Therapy of the Periodic Paralyses.
In all forms of primary PP acetazolamide, from 250 mg to 2 grams daily, can prevent attacks or decrease their frequency. The metabolic acidosis induced by the drug may prevent sodium channel inactivation by small depolarizations. Prolonged exposure to the drug promotes the formation of renal calculi.

The treatment of attacks of *primary hypokalemic PP* consists of giving 2 to 10 grams of oral KCl. Preventive therapy includes acetazolamide, a low-carbohydrate and relatively low-sodium (2.3 grams per day) diet, and 2.5 grams of KCl taken orally three times daily. *Thyrotoxic PP* is treated by antithyroid therapy, KCl supplements, and a low-carbohydrate, low-sodium diet. Acetazolamide is ineffective.

In *primary hyperkalemic PP* one treats the acute attacks with 2 grams per kilogram of glucose by mouth and 15 to 20 units of crystalline insulin subcutaneously. The inhalation of 1.3 mg metaproterenol every 15 minutes for three doses, or of 0.18 mg albuterol repeated once after 10 minutes, has aborted acute attacks. Preventive treatment consists of acetazolamide or thiazide diuretics and frequent high-carbohydrate meals. Tocainide, 300 to 400 mg three to four times daily, prevents cold-induced stiffness and weakness in paramyotonic hyperkalemic PP and paramyotonia congenita. The drug acts by blocking sodium channels in muscle.

The periodic paralyses caused by excessive wastage or retention of potassium are treated by correcting existing electrolyte abnormalities and, if possible, removing the existing cause. In acute barium poisoning, 10 ml of a 10% solution of sodium sulfate is administered intravenously every 30 minutes until symptoms subside.

NUTRITIONAL AND TOXIC MYOPATHIES.
Diffuse muscle atrophy and weakness associated with type II fiber atrophy are commonly observed in malnourished or cachectic patients. The muscle weakness in nutritional osteomalacia has been attributed partly to disuse and partly to malnutrition.

Vitamin E Deficiency.
This has now been implicated in progressive gait and limb ataxia, sensorimotor neuropathy, extraocular muscle paresis, and a myopathy in which giant abnormal lysosomes accumulate in muscle. The cause is a malabsorption syndrome, as detailed in Ch. 103 and 406. High doses of vitamin E may be of benefit.

Myopathy in Alcoholism.
An acute necrotizing myopathy associated with myoglobinuria occurs in chronic alcoholics after a bout of drinking. Hypokalemia caused by sweating, vomiting, diarrhea, and renal wastage may act as a precipitating factor. The hypokalemia may be followed by hyperkalemia as myoglobinuria and renal failure develop. A subacute alcoholic myopathy with proximal muscle weakness and elevation of the serum CK level may also exist. If so, it is usually associated with a chronic neuropathy.

Chloroquine Myopathy.
The side effects of the drug include macular and corneal degeneration, peripheral neuropathy, and myopathy. Muscle weakness appears when the daily dosage is 500 mg for a year or longer. Pathologically, the condition produces a vacuolar myopathy and constitutes a prototype for myopathies due to an excited autophagic mechanism.

Emetine Myopathy.
Emetine, an ipecac alkaloid, is used to treat amebiasis. Side effects include cardiotoxicity and muscle weakness. A reversible myopathy involving proximal limb muscles has been observed in patients with feeding disorders who abuse ipecac to induce vomiting and in alcoholics receiving emetine for aversion therapy. The pathologic findings include focal destruction of mitochondria and focal myofibrillar degeneration.

Other Toxic Myopathies.
Epsilon amino-caproic acid, an inhibitor of fibrinolyis and of clot dissolution, infrequently causes myalgias, myonecrosis, and myoglobinuria. *Colchicine* in customary doses induces a vacuolar myopathy in patients with gout and renal insufficiency who attain elevated plasma drug levels. The antiarrhythmic agent amiodarone can induce an autophagic myopathy and a peripheral neuropathy. *Lovastatin,* an inhibitor of mevalonic acid and cholesterol biosynthesis, causes a necrotizing myopathy with or without myoglobinuria in less than 0.5% of patients. Concomitant therapy with immunosuppressants increases the risk of myopathy. *Isoretinoic acid,* a vitamin A analogue for treating acne, infrequently causes myalgias, elevation of the serum creatine kinase, and reversible muscle damage. *Cocaine* abuse can result in a necrotizing myopathy and myoglobinuria. The myopathy induced by *zidovudine* is considered in Ch. 456.

MYOGLOBINURIA.
The clinical syndrome of myoglobinuria is associated with brown discoloration of urine by myoglobin and metmyoglobin. Myoglobin, a 17,000-molecular-weight protein with a prosthetic heme group, is present in muscle at a concentration of 1 gram per kilogram. It has a lower renal excretory threshold than hemoglobin. Small amounts of myoglobin not sufficient to discolor urine are excreted in various necrotizing myopathies. The visible discoloration of urine by myoglobin indicates both massive and acute muscle destruction (rhabdomyolysis) and warns of impending renal damage. The pigment has to be distinguished from hemoglobin and porphyrins. If there is no hemoglobinemia or hematuria, a positive benzidine test strongly suggests myoglobinuria. However, myoglobinuria itself can induce microhematuria, and certain identification of myoglobin must be made specifically. The immunoprecipitation assay has the virtue of being simple and quantitative but is so sensitive that it detects the pigment in the absence of overt myoglobinuria.

Muscle pain, swelling, and weakness precede overt myoglobinuria by a few hours. In addition to myoglobin, phosphate, potassium, creatine, and muscle enzymes are released into the circulation. The heme pigment in the glomerular filtrate and casts in the tubules cause proteinuria, hematuria, and tubular necrosis. Renal failure is more likely if hypotension, acidosis, and hypovolemia coexist. With increasing renal insufficiency, hyperphosphatemia, hypocalcemia, tetany, and life-threatening hyperkalemia appear. Death may result from renal or respiratory failure. Otherwise, the myoglobinuria and proteinuria disappear in 3 to 5 days. The marked hyperenzymemia decreases gradually, and muscle strength returns relatively slowly after major attacks. EMG abnormalities can persist for several months.

Myoglobinuria can have many causes: metabolic, infectious, toxic, ischemic and/or traumatic, secondary to another myopathy, and idiopathic. It is likely that many of the so-called idiopathic cases have a metabolic or infectious cause.

Myoglobinuria Caused by a Metabolic Disturbance.
The common denominator is impaired substrate utilization for energy metabolism or a critical substrate deficiency in the face of ex-

cessive demands for energy. Most diseases in this group were considered earlier in this chapter. Deficiencies of phosphorylase kinase, myophosphorylase, phosphofructokinase, phosphoglycerate mutase, phosphoglycerate kinase, and lactate dehydrogenase block anaerobic glycolysis; coenzyme Q and succinate dehydrogenase deficiencies interfere with oxidative phosphorylation; and carnitine palmitoyl-transferase deficiency impairs fatty acid oxidation when it is most needed. Substrate deficiency in the face of excessive demands and derangements of muscle metabolism account for the myoglobinuria associated with malignant hyperthermia, the malignant neuroleptic syndrome, and the abrupt withdrawal of antiparkinson drugs. Substrate deficiency may also account for the myoglobinuria that occurs after severe exercise in untrained individuals, as in military recruits.

Almost any severe metabolic insult can cause myoglobinuria. These include carbon monoxide poisoning, extreme hypoglycemia, severe hypokalemia, hypernatremia, or water intoxication.

Myoglobinuria with Infections. This can occur after influenza A, herpes simplex, Epstein-Barr, and coxsackievirus infections and early in the course of HIV infection. The precise mechanism is not understood. Myoglobinuria also occurs with bacterial infections accompanied by high fever and sepsis, and with muscle gangrene caused by clostridial infection.

Toxic Myoglobinuria. The myoglobinuria associated with alcoholism was considered above. Intoxication with barbiturates, amphetamine, cocaine, and other narcotics, especially if associated with agitation or coma, can produce myoglobinuria. Myoglobinuria occurring with lovastatin, epsilon amino-caproic acid, or amiodarone was discussed earlier in this chapter. The toxin of the Malayan sea snake, *Enhydrina schistosa*, induces myalgias, trismus, flaccid paralysis, and myoglobinuria.

Ischemic and Traumatic Myoglobinuria. Massive ischemia of muscle from any cause (e.g., major vessel occlusions, angiopathy in uremic hyperparathyroidism), crush injuries, or prolonged pressure on dependent muscles in the immobile comatose patient can induce myoglobinuria. Localized ischemic necrosis of muscle and sometimes myoglobinuria occurs in severe forms of the anterior tibial syndrome.

Myoglobinuria Secondary to Other Myopathies. Myoglobinuria has been observed infrequently in acute dermatomyositis (where the cause is probably ischemia), systemic lupus erythematosus, and mild dystrophinopathies.

Treatment. The acute episode is treated by rest, maintenance of adequate urine flow by hydration and diuretics, and alkalinization of the urine with sodium bicarbonate. Other measures consist of treatment of the renal insufficiency as required and removal of the offending cause if possible.

DiMauro S, Wallace DC (eds.): Mitochondrial DNA in Human Pathology. New York, Raven Press, 1993. *A review of the current status of the mitochondrial DNA diseases by multiple authors.*

Engel AG, Franzini-Armstrong C (eds.): Myology, 2nd ed. New York, McGraw-Hill, 1994. *Chapters by DiMauro and Tsujino, Engel and Hirschhorn, Zierz, DiDonato, Morgan-Hughes, Penn, Victor and Sieb, Kaminski and Ruff, and Lehmann-Horn, Engel, Ricker, and Rüdel provide detailed and up-to-date reviews of the metabolic myopathies.*

Hirano M, Ricci E, Koenigsberger MR, et al.: MELAS: An original case and clinical criteria for diagnosis. Neuromusc Disord 2:125, 1992. *A careful analysis of 70 cases of MELAS and criteria for the clinical diagnosis of the disease.*

458 MISCELLANEOUS MYOPATHIES

INFILTRATIVE MYOPATHIES. *Systemic Amyloid Myopathy.* The most common neurologic complication in various types of amyloidosis is a predominantly sensory-autonomic neuropathy. Amyloid deposition in muscle is frequent, but the muscle involvement is usually subclinical. Occasionally amyloidosis presents or is associated with an overt myopathy characterized by muscle enlargement, macroglossia, stiffness, exertional muscle pain, and proximal or diffuse weakness. Electromyography shows myopathic features in proximal muscles with or without changes of neuropathy distally. The amyloid deposits, identified by their metachromasia and affinity for Congo red stain, appear between and around the mural elements of the small vessels and extend into the interstitial spaces where they tightly surround individual muscle fibers.

Hypertrophic Branchial Myopathy. This sporadic illness presents between the second and fourth decades of life and is restricted to muscles that derive from the embryonic branchial cleft. The disease evolves with slowly progressive, asymmetric, bilateral enlargement of temporalis, masseter, and pterygoid muscles. Weakness is minimal or absent. The swelling itself is painless but may lead to pain with jaw opening. The EMG and muscle biopsy show nonspecific myopathic alterations in the affected muscles. There is no satisfactory treatment. When chewing is impaired, partial excision of the enlarged muscles has proved beneficial.

SYNDROMES ASSOCIATED WITH ABNORMAL MUSCLE ACTIVITY. These can be caused by (1) abnormal neural activity in the central nervous system (e.g., dystonia, tetanus, stiff-man syndrome); (2) abnormal excitability of the peripheral nervous system (neuromyotonia, tetany, cramps); (3) abnormal excitability of the muscle fiber surface membrane (myotonic disorders); (4) a defect within the muscle fiber resulting in abnormal mechanical activity (e.g., malignant hyperthermia, contractures without electrical activity, and slow relaxation of electrically silent muscle fibers). Dystonia, tetanus, and tetany are considered in Ch. 289, 410, and 412. The remaining entities were discussed earlier in this section or are discussed below.

Stiff-Man Syndrome. This is a disease of adult life affecting men more frequently than women. Initially intermittent spasms of axial and limb muscles are followed by continuous stiffness that immobilizes the patient. Agonist and antagonist muscles are affected simultaneously, preventing voluntary movement. The EMG shows constant firing of normal motor unit potentials in the stiff muscles. There are no signs of cerebral or spinal cord disease. Spinal anesthesia relieves the spasms. The disease is frequently associated with organ-specific autoimmune diseases, and especially insulin-dependent diabetes mellitus. In a series of 13 patients, 4 had circulating antiglutamic acid decarboxylase as well as anti–islet cell and other organ- and non–organ-specific autoantibodies; 4 had an associated solid tumor and antibodies recognizing a 125-kD antigen; and 5 had no evidence of any known autoantibody. As glutamic acid decarboxylase converts glutamic acid to the inhibitory neurotransmitter γ-aminobutyric acid (GABA), the findings suggest that at least in some patients the disease is caused by immune-mediated impairment of GABAergic inhibitory pathways. Relatively high doses of diazepam or baclofen, which increase GABA-mediated central inhibition, and clonidine, which prevents norepinephrine release from nerve terminals, may improve or relieve the symptoms.

Neuromyotonia. This can be generalized or focal. *Generalized neuromyotonia,* or Isaacs' syndrome, is sporadic or familial. Some of the familial cases are associated with a peripheral neuropathy; some of the sporadic cases have an intrathoracic malignancy. Abnormal impulses arising in peripheral motor axons produce continuous muscle fiber activity that persists even during sleep. Depending on the site of origin in the axon, the abnormal activity is abolished by proximal nerve block or block of neuromuscular transmission. The EMG shows very high frequency (150 to 300 Hz) recurring bursts of motor unit potentials. The involuntary activation of multiple motor units causes stiffness and delayed relaxation of the affected muscles and continuous, small, undulating movements of the overlying skin *(myokymia).* Phenytoin or carbamazepine may inhibit the abnormal discharges and relieve the symptoms. Evidence supports an autoimmune cause of this syndrome, possibly an immune response to peripheral nerve potassium channels. Some patients respond to plasmapheresis; some cases are associated with myasthenia gravis, thymoma, or anti-acetylcholine receptor antibodies; and some cases are induced by exposure to penicillamine. Further, some of the electrophysiologic features of the disease can be transferred from humans to mice with IgG.

Similar high-frequency and rhythmically recurring bursts of motor unit potentials occur in *facial myokymia* seen with demyelinating or other lesions of the brain stem.

Focal neuromyotonia can occur following peripheral nerve lesions, but here the firing rate is slower (30 to 60 Hz). The delayed relaxation of an affected muscle after a willed contraction mimics action myotonia.

A benign syndrome of *muscle cramps, fasciculations, and myokymia* associated with low-frequency bursts of motor unit potentials also occurs and may incorrectly suggest the diagnosis of early motor neuron disease.

A syndrome associated with *myokymia, hyperhydrosis, mental symptoms, thymoma,* and *anti-acetylcholine receptor antibodies* but without symptoms of myasthenia gravis has been recently described.

Schwartz-Jampel Syndrome.
This autosomal recessive disease begins in early childhood. It is characterized by chondrodystrophy, bone and joint deformities, short stature, a doleful facial expression with blepharospasm, hypertrichosis, muscle stiffness, and muscle hypertrophy or atrophy. There is delayed muscle relaxation suggesting myotonia. The EMG, however, shows high-frequency repetitive discharges, not myotonic discharges. Muscle biopsy reveals neurogenic and myogenic features.

Myotonia Congenita.
Autosomal dominant (Thomsen's disease) and autosomal recessive forms of paramyotonia congenita are recognized. The two types of myotonia are associated with different point mutations of the muscle chloride channel gene and are therefore allelic disorders. Both diseases are benign and associated with diffuse muscle hypertrophy and diffuse action, percussion, and electrical myotonia. Cold increases the myotonia, and sustained exercise improves it. The membrane defect consists of a markedly reduced chloride conductance. Quinine, 0.3 to 1.5 grams daily, or phenytoin, 0.3 to 0.6 gram daily, relieves the myotonia.

Slow Relaxation of Electrically Silent Muscle Fibers.
This is a rare disease in which there is impaired muscle relaxation that is rapidly worsened by exercise. The slowly relaxing fibers are electrically silent. The defect lies within the calcium-pump ATPase of the sarcoplasmic reticulum.

Rippling Muscles.
This is a benign and dominantly inherited disorder presenting in late childhood or adult life. Sporadic cases also occur. Local percussion of a muscle evokes myoedema. This is replaced by a longitudinal depression parallel to the long axis of the muscle which then moves to the periphery of the muscle in 10 to 20 seconds in a wave that resembles the plucking of a chromatic scale on a harp. The response to percussion superficially resembles myotonia, but the rippling muscles are electrically silent. Mild muscle pain, stiffness at the beginning of exercise, and mild elevation of the serum CK level are associated features.

Grimaldi LME, Martino G, Braghi S, et al.: Heterogeneity of autoantibodies in stiff man syndrome. Ann Neurol 34:57, 1993. *A timely review of the evidence for the autoimmune pathogenesis of the disease.*

Newsom-Davis J, Mills KR: Immunological association of acquired neuromyotonia (Isaacs' syndrome). Brain 116:453, 1993. *Provides a clear description of the neurophysiologic aspects and evidence for an autoimmune origin of the syndrome.*

Ricker K, Moxley RT, Rohkamm R: Rippling muscle disease. Arch Neurol 46:405, 1989. *A good description of an uncommon disease and a review of the literature.*

Rüdel R, Ricker K, Lehmann-Horn F: Nondystrophic myotonias. *In* Engel AG, Franzini-Armstrong C (eds.): Myology, 2nd ed. New York, McGraw-Hill, 1994, p 1291. *A detailed account of the clinical, electrophysiologic, and molecular genetic aspects of the nondystrophic myotonias.*

459 DISORDERS OF NEUROMUSCULAR TRANSMISSION

DEFINITION AND BASIC CONCEPTS. Disorders of neuromuscular transmission can be acquired or inherited and are associated with abnormal weakness and fatigability on exertion. In each disorder the safety margin of neuromuscular transmission is compromised by one or more specific mechanisms. These mechanisms involve acetylcholine (ACh) synthesis or packaging of ACh quanta (6,000 to 10,000 molecules) into synaptic vesicles, the exocytotic release of ACh quanta from the nerve terminal by nerve impulse, and the efficiency of the released quanta to generate a postsynaptic depolarization. The efficiency of the released quanta depends on the

geometry of the synaptic space, the density of postsynaptic ACh receptors (AChR's), and the conductance and open time of the AChR ion channel. The depolarization induced by a single quantum gives rise to a miniature end-plate potential (MEPP); that induced by a larger number of quanta released by nerve impulse generates an end-plate potential (EPP). The EPP amplitude must exceed a critical threshold to activate the voltage-sensitive sodium channels around the end-plate and thereby generate a muscle fiber action potential. Neuromuscular transmission fails when the EPP fails to reach this critical threshold.

Table 459-1 shows a classification of currently recognized defects of neuromuscular transmission. Botulism is described in Ch. 288, the others in this chapter. The congenital syndromes are discussed in the indicated references.

MYASTHENIA GRAVIS (MG). This is an acquired autoimmune disorder in which pathogenic autoantibodies induce AChR deficiency at the motor end-plate. The safety margin of neuromuscular transmission is compromised by the small amplitude of the MEPP and consequently of the EPP. Circulating AChR antibodies are present in 80 to 90% of the cases, and IgG and complement components are deposited on the postsynaptic membrane. AChR deficiency results from complement-mediated lysis of the junctional folds, accelerated internalization and destruction of AChR cross-linked by antibody (modulation), and, to a lesser extent, by antibodies blocking the binding of ACh to AChR.

Clinical Features.
The incidence is two to five per year per million and the prevalence 13 to 64 per million. The female to male ratio is 6:4. The disease may present at any age, but the incidence in women peaks in the third decade and in men in the sixth or seventh decade.

MG can involve either the external ocular muscles selectively or the general voluntary muscle system. The symptoms may fluctuate from hour to hour, day to day, or over longer periods. They are provoked or worsened by exertion, exposure to extremes of temperature, viral or other infections, menses, and excitement. Ocular muscle involvement is usually bilateral, asymmetric, and typically associated with ptosis and diplopia. Weakness of other muscles innervated by cranial nerves results in loss of facial expression, everted lips, a smile that resembles a snarl, jaw drop, nasal regurgi-

TABLE 459-1. CLASSIFICATION OF DISORDERS OF NEUROMUSCULAR TRANSMISSION

Autoimmune
  Myasthenia gravis
  Lambert-Eaton myasthenic syndrome
Congenital
  Presynaptic defects
    Familial infantile myasthenia (defect in ACh resynthesis or packaging)*
    Paucity of synaptic vesicles and reduced quantal release‡
    End-plate AChE deficiency*
  Kinetic abnormalities of AChR with AChR deficiency
    Classic slow-channel syndrome§
    Miscellaneous mutations causing prolonged open time of the AChR channel§
    AChR deficiency and short channel open time‡
  Kinetic abnormalities of AChR without AChR deficiency
    High-conductance fast-channel syndrome*
    Syndrome attributed to abnormal interaction of ACh with AChR*
  Partially characterized syndromes
    Congenital myasthenic syndrome resembling LEMS‡
    AChR deficiency with paucity of secondary synaptic clefts*
    Partially characterized AChR deficiencies‡
    Familial limb-girdle myasthenia*
    Benign CMS with facial malformations*
Toxic
  Botulism
  Drug-induced
  Organophosphate intoxication

* Autosomal recessive inheritance
† Autosomal recessive inheritance in some cases
‡ Autosomal recessive inheritance suspected
§ Autosomal dominant inheritance
ACh, acetylcholine; AChE, acetylcholinesterase; AChR, acetylcholine receptor; CMS, congenital myasthenic syndrome

tation of liquids, choking on foods and secretions, and a slurred, hypernasal speech with a reduced volume. Abnormal fatigability of the limb muscles causes difficulty in combing the hair, lifting objects repeatedly, climbing stairs, walking, and running. Depending on the severity of the disease, dyspnea can appear on moderate or mild exertion or be present even at rest. The abnormal fatigability can be demonstrated by asking the patient to look up without closing the eyes for a minute, to count loudly from 1 to 100, to hold the arms abducted to the horizontal position for a minute, or to perform repeated deep knee-bends. The tendon reflexes remain normally active even in weak muscles. Atrophy of masseter, temporal, facial, or tongue muscles, and less often of other muscles, occurs in about 15% of patients.

Initially, the symptoms are purely ocular in 40%, generalized in 40%, and involve only the extremities in 10%, and only the bulbar or bulbar and eye muscles in another 10%. Subsequently, the weakness can spread from ocular to facial to lower bulbar muscles and then to torso and limb muscles, but the sequence may vary. Proximal limb muscles are affected more than distal ones. In the most advanced cases the weakness is universal. By the end of the first year, the ocular muscles are affected in nearly all patients. The symptoms remain ocular in only 16%. In nearly 90% of those in whom the disease becomes generalized, this occurs within the first year after the onset. Progression is most rapid within the first 3 years, and more than half of the deaths caused by MG occur in that period. Spontaneous remissions lasting from weeks to years can occur. Long remissions are uncommon, and most remissions occur during the first 3 years.

Two thirds of patients with MG have thymic hyperplasia and 10 to 15% have thymoma. A few with thymoma also develop myocarditis or giant cell myositis. In about 10% the MG is associated with another autoimmune disease, such as hyperthyroidism, polymyositis, systemic lupus erythematosus, Sjögren's syndrome, rheumatoid arthritis, ulcerative colitis, pemphigus, sarcoidosis, pernicious anemia, or Lambert-Eaton myasthenic syndrome.

A clinical classification of MG, originally proposed by Osserman, is based on the distribution and severity of symptoms: group 1, ocular; group 2A, mild generalized; group 2B, moderately severe generalized; group 3, acute fulminating; group 4, late severe. Another classification, proposed by Vincent and Newsom-Davis, is based on the age of onset and the presence or absence of thymoma: Type 1, MG with thymoma: The disease is usually severe and the AChR antibody level is high; there is no association either with sex or HLA antigen. Type 2, no thymoma, onset before age 40: The AChR antibody level is intermediate; there is female preponderance and an increased association with HLA-A1, HLA-B8, and HLA-DRw3 antigens (HLA-B12 in Japan). Type 3, no thymoma, onset after age 40: The AChR antibody level tends to be low; there is male preponderance and increased association with HLA-A3, HLA-B7, or HLA-DRw2 antigens (HLA-A10 in Japan). Striated muscle antibodies are found in 90%, 5%, and 45%, respectively, in the three types. The association with other autoimmune diseases is highest in Type 3 and lowest in Type 1.

Transient Neonatal MG. Circulating AChR antibodies can be detected in most infants born to myasthenic mothers, but only 12% of such children develop MG, usually during the first few hours of life. The findings are feeble cry, feeding and respiratory difficulty, general or facial weakness, and ptosis. The mean duration is 18 days. There is no relation between the severity of MG in mother and infant. The disease is caused by the transfer of AChR antibodies from mother to infant.

Diagnosis. This is based on the characteristic history, physical examination, anticholinesterase tests, and laboratory studies. The latter include EMG studies, tests for AChR antibodies, and in selected cases, microelectrode studies *in vitro* of neuromuscular transmission and ultrastructural and cytochemical studies of the end-plate.

Anticholinesterase Tests. Edrophonium given intravenously acts within a few seconds, and its effects last for a few minutes. One to 2 mg of the drug is injected intravenously over 15 seconds. If no response occurs in 30 seconds, an additional 8 to 9 mg is injected. The evaluation of the response requires objective assessment of one or more signs, such as degree of ptosis, range of ocular movements, and the force of the hand grip. Possible cholinergic side effects of

the drug include fasciculations, flushing, lacrimation, abdominal cramps, nausea, vomiting, and diarrhea. The drug must be given cautiously to patients with cardiac disease, for it may cause sinus bradycardia, atrioventricular block, and, rarely, cardiac arrest. Atropine is used to reverse toxicity. Intramuscular neostigmine, 0.5 to 1.0 mg, acts maximally in about 30 minutes, and its effects last up to 2 hours, allowing a more leisurely evaluation of changes in clinical status.

Electromyography. Supramaximal stimulation of a motor nerve at 2 to 3 Hz results in a 10% or greater decrement of the amplitude of the evoked compound muscle action potential from the first to the fifth response. The test is positive in nearly all patients provided that two or more distal and two or more proximal muscles are examined. The decrement is caused by a normally occurring decrease in the number of quanta released from the nerve terminal, and hence in the amplitude of the EPP, at the beginning of low-frequency stimulation. In MG the EPP amplitude is already reduced by the AChR deficiency, and the additional decrease during stimulation blocks transmission at an increasing number of end-plates. Single-fiber EMG compares the timing of action potentials between pairs of closely adjacent muscle fibers in the same motor unit during a willed contraction. In MG the low amplitude and relatively long rise time of the EPP cause abnormally long interpotential intervals and intermittent blocking of action potential generation at some fibers.

Serologic Tests. The usual AChR antibody test measures the binding of antibody to AChR labeled with radioactive α-bungarotoxin. The toxin itself is attached irreversibly to the ACh binding site of AChR. The antibody binding test is positive in nearly all adults with moderately severe or severe MG, in 80% with mild generalized MG, and in 50% with ocular MG, but in only 25% of those in remission. The test is less reliable in juvenile than in adult MG. In a few patients only antibodies that block the binding of ACh to AChR can be detected. The antibody titer correlates only loosely with disease severity, but in individual patients a >50% decrease in titer for more than 12 months is nearly always associated with sustained clinical improvement. Striated muscle antibodies also occur in MG patients. Their role remains unknown, but they often are associated with thymoma.

Other Diagnostic Studies. Immune deposits can be localized at the MG end-plate in cryostat sections even when circulating AChR antibodies cannot be detected. C3 localization is technically the easiest and most convenient way to confirm the suspected diagnosis.

Differential Diagnosis. This includes neurasthenia, the Miller Fisher variant of inflammatory polyneuropathy, oculopharyngeal dystrophy, mitochondrial myopathies involving the external ocular and/or other cranial and limb muscles, intracranial mass lesions compressing cranial nerves, drug-induced myasthenic syndromes, and other disorders of neuromuscular transmission listed in Table 459–1. Neurasthenia is recognized by giving way on muscle testing and the lack of objective clinical and laboratory findings. In myopathies involving the ocular muscles, the weakness does not fluctuate, diplopia is seldom a symptom, the muscle biopsy may show distinct morphologic abnormalities, and pharmacologic and laboratory tests for MG are negative. Drug-induced and other myasthenic syndromes are considered below.

Therapy. Anticholinesterases, alternate-day prednisone treatment, azathioprine, thymectomy, and plasmapheresis are currently used to treat MG. Anticholinesterases are useful in all clinical forms of the disease. Pyridostigmine bromide (Mestinon) (60-mg tablets) acts for 3 to 4 hours, and neostigmine bromide (15-mg tablets) for 2 to 3 hours. The former drug has fewer muscarinic side effects and is therefore more widely used. One half to four tablets of pyridostigmine bromide are given every 4 hours in the daytime. This medication is also available in 180-mg "time-span" tablets for use at bedtime and as a syrup for children and patients requiring nasogastric feeding. If troublesome muscarinic side effects occur, these can be treated with 0.4 to 0.6 mg atropine given orally two or three times daily. Postoperatively or in critically ill patients intramuscularly injectable pyridostigmine bromide (the dose is one thirtieth of the oral dose) and neostigmine methylsulfate (the dose is one fifteenth of the oral dose) can be used.

Progressive weakness despite increasing amounts of anticholinesterases signals the onset of a cholinergic or myasthenic crisis. Cholinergic crises are associated with muscarinic effects, such as abdominal cramps, nausea, vomiting, diarrhea, miosis, lacrimation, increased bronchial secretions, diaphoresis, and bradycardia. In a myasthenic crisis the muscarinic effects are not conspicuous, and 2 mg edrophonium given intravenously improves rather than worsens the weakness. In practice, however, the two types of crises often are difficult to distinguish, and overmedication of a myasthenic crisis can convert it into a cholinergic crisis. Therefore, patients who have increasing difficulty with respiration, feeding, or handling secretions and who are not responding to relatively high doses of anticholinesterases are best treated by drug withdrawal, tracheal intubation or tracheostomy, support with respirator, and intravenous feeding. Refractoriness to drug therapy usually disappears after a few days.

In patients with generalized disease not responding adequately to modest doses of anticholinesterases, other forms of therapy must be employed. Thymectomy increases the remission rate and improves the clinical course of MG. Although controlled clinical studies of thymectomy according to age, gender, severity, and duration of disease have never been carried out, there is general agreement that the best response occurs in young women with hyperplastic thymus glands and high antibody titer. Thymoma represents an absolute indication for thymectomy because the tumor is often locally invasive. Computed tomography of the mediastinum is a sensitive screening test, but it can give false-positive results.

Alternate-day prednisone treatment induces remission or significantly improves the disease in more than half the patients. The treatment is relatively safe provided that one institutes the usual precautions for patients taking corticosteroid therapy. With an average dose of 70 mg on alternate days, the average time for significant improvement is 5 months. After the improvement reaches a plateau the dose must be lowered gradually over several months to establish the minimum maintenance dose.

Azathioprine in doses of 150 to 200 mg per day also induces remissions or measurable improvement in more than half the treated patients. The minimum time for improvement is 3 months. Surveillance to detect side effects (pancytopenia, leukopenia, serious infection, and hepatocellular injury) must be maintained during therapy.

Plasmapheresis is indicated in severe generalized or fulminating MG refractory to other forms of treatment. Daily exchanges of 2 liters of plasma result in objective improvement and lower the AChR antibody titer in a few days. Plasmapheresis, however, is highly expensive and does not confer greater long-term protection than immunosuppressants alone.

Intravenous immunoglobulin therapy at a dose of 400 mg per kilogram for 5 consecutive days or 1 gram per kilogram for 2 consecutive days may improve severe MG within 2 to 3 weeks of the start of therapy. The mean duration of the response is 9 weeks in patients also treated with corticosteroids and 5 weeks in those who are not.

LAMBERT-EATON MYASTHENIC SYNDROME. This is an acquired autoimmune disease in which pathogenic autoantibodies cause a deficiency of voltage-sensitive calcium channels at the motor nerve terminal. The deficiency restricts calcium ingress when the terminal is depolarized by nerve impulses and thereby reduces the probability of quantal release. Among patients over 40 years 70% of men and 30% of women have an associated carcinoma, usually a small-cell carcinoma of the lung. The syndrome may predate tumor detection by up to 3 years. Non-neoplastic cases have an association with other autoimmune disorders, HLA-B8 and DRw3 antigens, and organ-specific autoantibodies.

Patients have weakness and fatigability of proximal limb and torso muscles with relative sparing of extraocular and bulbar muscles. The lower limbs are more severely involved than the upper ones. On maximal voluntary contraction the force produced by a weak muscle increases for a few seconds and then again decreases. The tendon reflexes are hypoactive or absent in most patients. Autonomic manifestations (dry mouth, impotence, decreased sweating, orthostatic hypotension, or altered pupillary reflexes) occur in one half of the patients.

On EMG, the amplitude of the compound muscle action potential evoked by a single nerve stimulus from rested muscle is abnormally small. Repetitive stimulation at 2 Hz induces a further decrement, but stimulation at frequencies higher than 10 Hz or voluntary exercise for a brief period markedly facilitates the response so that the evoked potential attains normal amplitude.

Anticholinesterases are only slightly effective. Guanidine hydrochloride (10 mg per kilogram per day) or 3,4-diaminopyridine (1 mg per kilogram per day) increases quantal release from the nerve terminal and relieves the symptoms. However, the former drug has severe toxic side effects, and the latter is not yet available in clinical practice. Optimal treatment of non-neoplastic cases consists of modest doses of alternate-day prednisone and 2 mg per kilogram per day of azathioprine.

DRUG-INDUCED MYASTHENIC SYNDROMES. These are uncommon in clinical practice. Tetracycline, polymyxin and aminoglycoside antibiotics, antiarrhythmic agents (procainamide, quinidine), β-adrenergic blockers (propranolol, timolol), phenothiazines, lithium, trimethaphan, methoxyflurane, and magnesium given parenterally or in cathartics reduce the safety margin of neuromuscular transmission. However, overt myasthenic symptoms do not usually appear unless an overdose of the drug is administered or the renal or hepatic elimination of the drug is impaired. The same drugs and inhalation anesthetic agents also can potentiate neuromuscular blocking agents used during surgical procedures and both may worsen or unmask pre-existing disorders of neuromuscular transmission. Calcium channel blocking drugs can worsen the transmission defect in the Lambert-Eaton myasthenic syndrome.

Succinylcholine, a depolarizing blocking drug, is used to induce muscle relaxation during anesthesia. A single dose of the drug sufficient to cause transient apnea is eliminated by plasma pseudocholinesterase in 2 to 10 minutes. In approximately 1 of 2500 patients receiving the drug, prolonged apnea occurs and persists up to several hours. Most of these patients have an autosomal recessive abnormality of the plasma pseudocholinesterase. In some genetic variants the plasma pseudocholinesterase activity is abnormally low; in others the enzyme shows increased sensitivity to inhibition by dibucaine.

ORGANOPHOSPHATE INTOXICATION. Organophosphate insecticides irreversibly inhibit cholinesterases. Poisoning occurs by accident or when the compounds are ingested with suicidal intent. The accumulation of ACh at central, muscarinic, and nicotinic cholinergic synapses is associated with alterations in sensorium, convulsions, coma, severe muscarinic side effects, cramps, fasciculations, and muscle weakness from a depolarization block as well as desensitization of AChR at the neuromuscular junction. Therapy consists of gastric lavage with more than 100 liters of water, followed by the use of activated charcoal and oral cathartics, respiratory support, and anticonvulsants as needed. Atropine, 1 to 2 mg intramuscularly every hour, can be used to control the excessive secretions. Pralidoxime (1 gram intravenously, repeated in 20 minutes if necessary) has been used with variable success.

Engel AG: Congenital myasthenic syndromes. Neurol Clin 12:401, 1994. *A thorough review of the current status of the congenital myasthenias and of the investigative approaches to these diseases.*

Engel AG, Franzini-Armstrong C (eds.): Myology, 2nd ed. New York, McGraw-Hill, 1994. *Chapters by Engel and Magleby ably discuss the detailed anatomy, physiology, and clinical dimensions of neuromuscular transmission.*

Gutmann L, Besser R: Organophosphate intoxication: Pharmacologic, neurophysiologic, clinical, and therapeutic considerations. Semin Neurol 10:46, 1990. *A lucid analysis of the pathophysiologic basis of the symptoms and a reliable guide to therapy.*

O'Neill JH, Murray MF, Newsom-Davis J: Lambert-Eaton myasthenic syndrome: A review of 50 cases. Brain 3:577, 1988. *A comprehensive review of the clinical and basic science aspects of the disease.*

PART XXV

EYE DISEASES

John W. Gittinger, Jr.

Because many systemic diseases affect the eyes, ophthalmoscopy is a necessary skill for the physician. The pupil of the eye is a window opening onto the arterioles and venules of the retina, the optic disc, and the pigmented tissues of the fundus. Ch. 403 describes the autonomic and somatic motor disorders of ocular control and reviews the clinically important anatomy of the visual pathways. The chapters that follow highlight the interrelationship between ocular and systemic disease, beginning with a discussion of visual loss, then providing a brief review of the two common ophthalmic disorders—cataract and glaucoma, before turning to ocular entities and ocular manifestations of medical disorders that nonophthalmic physicians are likely to encounter.

460   VISUAL LOSS

Visual loss may be either transient (see Ch. 403) or permanent, with most of the potential causes capable of producing either one. A major purpose of the ophthalmologic examination is to establish the cause of visual loss. The need for correction of vision with glasses is called *refractive error.* When evaluating a patient for reduced vision, only the best-corrected acuity should be considered. Uncorrected acuity is of little interest in assessing the pathophysiology of the eye. Refractive errors include myopia, hyperopia, and astigmatism; presbyopia (literally "aging eye") refers to the loss of accommodation as the lens hardens with age, making focusing at near difficult even in eyes without refractive error *(emetropia)* after about age 45.

In myopia the eye is too large for its refractive power, and the image of a distant object focuses in front of the retina. Diverging light rays from nearer objects focus on the retina; thus, the person is "nearsighted" in that near vision is clearer than distance vision. A moderate degree of myopia thus compensates for presbyopia, an important consideration as permanent surgical correction of myopia is becoming more common.

In hyperopia, the eye is too small, and the image has not yet come into focus when it reaches the retina. In young persons, accommodation compensates for low degrees of hyperopia, but such hyperopia accelerates the age of onset of symptoms of presbyopia. Astigmatism reflects different degrees of refractive error along two perpendicular corneal meridians. An eye often has both myopia or hyperopia and astigmatism. Except when it reflects a structural alteration, as in high myopia, the need for refractive correction is considered a variant of normal, not a disease process.

Many conditions can cause visual loss (Table 460–1). Normal visual development in an infant requires formed images on the retina and intact visual pathways in the rest of the brain. A neonatal eye with a dense opacity of the media such as a mature cataract (see below) cannot develop useful vision unless the opacity is removed soon after birth and any resulting large refractive error corrected promptly. Visual development proceeds through crucial states; any interruption of these stages during infancy or early childhood can permanently limit the normal capacity for processing visual information even if the causative condition is treated later on. If both eyes are involved, the development of nystagmus (rhythmic to-and-

TABLE 460–1. DIFFERENTIAL DIAGNOSIS OF VISUAL LOSS

Opacities of the media	Corneal opacities (leukomas, edema, dystrophy) or irregularity; anterior chamber blood or inflammation; cataract; vitreous opacities
Chorioretinal disease	Macular and other retinal degenerations; retinal detachment; toxic, vascular, and traumatic retinopathies; infectious and inflammatory chorioretinitis; retinal tumors
Optic nerve disease	Glaucoma, other optic neuropathies (inflammatory, toxic, traumatic, vascular, hereditary); compressive and infiltrative neuropathy; optic nerve tumors
Visual pathway disorders	Vascular, inflammatory, infectious, degenerative developmental, neoplastic
Amblyopia	Strabismic, nutritional deprivation, anisometropic, ametropic, idiopathic
Psychogenic	

fro movements of the eye) at about 3 or 4 months of age signifies that this crucial period has been exceeded.

Normal adult levels of visual acuity can be measured electrophysiologically by age 6 months, but the neural connections that permit fine visual processing become permanently established only later in childhood. During the first few years of life, strabismus—misalignment of the visual axes of the two eyes—may result in suppression of central vision in one eye. Such visual loss in an eye that appears anatomically normal is termed *amblyopia*—a term also sometimes applied to processes that reduce vision but produce only subtle ophthalmoscopic changes, e.g., toxic-nutritional amblyopia. A large, uncorrected refractive error—*ametropia*—or a major difference in the refractive error in the two eyes—*anisometropia*—may also lead to amblyopia. Strabismic amblyopia is potentially reversible until 6 to 10 years of age, when the neural processing networks for vision become fixed for life. With this final step in visual development, the visual system achieves adult inflexibility so that misalignment of the visual axes results in permanent diplopia rather than suppression. An adult with acquired misalignment of the visual axes who does not experience diplopia probably has either reduced vision or a history of childhood strabismus.

Careful ophthalmic examination and appropriate testing should allow classification of reduced vision into one of the categories listed in Table 460–1: opacities of the media, chorioretinal disease, optic nerve disease, visual pathway disorders, amblyopia, or psychogenic visual loss. Two or more processes may affect the same eye.

Albert DM, Jakobiec FA: Principles and Practice of Ophthalmology. Philadelphia, WB Saunders, 1994. *This multivolume, multiauthored text features many color illustrations.*

Miller NR: Walsh and Hoyt's Clinical Neuro-ophthalmology. 4th ed. Baltimore, Williams & Wilkins, 1982–1995. *This encyclopedic review by one individual details many ocular entities with systemic manifestations.*

Tasman W, Jaeger EA: Duane's Clinical Ophthalmology. Philadelphia, JB Lippincott, revised annually. *Another multivolume text bound in a loose-leaf format that facilitates yearly updates and additions of selected chapters.*

PSYCHOGENIC VISUAL LOSS

Visual loss not attributable to an organic process is termed *psychogenic.* Alternative designations are functional, nonorganic, nonphysiologic, hysterical, and malingering. The last two are best avoided. Hysteria suggests to some a sexual bias and must be considered a psychiatric rather than an ophthalmologic diagnosis; malingering imputes motives that are difficult to prove. Functional visual loss, the usage currently preferred by some authorities, is potentially confusing because *functional* is used in other senses in medicine; e.g., *functional amblyopia* refers to those forms of amblyopia in which the process is potentially reversible with treatment (strabismic, ametropic, and anisometropic). In these instances there is presumably an underlying physiologic alteration in the visual system itself.

Psychogenic visual loss is not necessarily a diagnosis of exclusion. Certain patterns of visual loss cannot be explained by organic disease. Concentric constriction of visual fields is a common finding in nonphysiologic visual loss but also occurs with advanced glaucoma and retinitis pigmentosa as well as after bilateral occipital infarctions. Failure of the visual field to expand to an appropriate stimulus with increased testing distance—tubular fields—is, however, diagnostic of psychogenic visual loss. Similarly, patients who claim to be completely blind in one eye but who have normal pupillary reactions, full stereopsis, or normal ipsilateral visual evoked responses must have a nonphysiologic component to their visual loss. Other testing techniques also may result in normal subjective responses from a supposedly blind eye.

Most cases of psychogenic visual loss occur in the setting of minor psychological reactions rather than major psychiatric disorders. Sometimes organic and nonorganic components coexist. Affected patients should be evaluated by a neurologist or ophthalmologist familiar with psychogenic visual loss. Unless the visual loss prevents the patient from working or attending school, simple reassurance and careful follow-up with treatment of intercurrent organic abnormalities constitute appropriate management, and in some cases spontaneous improvement occurs.

461   CATARACT

A cataract is any lens opacity; cataracts characteristically produce painless, gradual loss of vision. Cataracts are described according to their location, e.g., nuclear (deep in the lens), cortical (more superficial), and capsular or subcapsular (on or immediately beneath the capsule). Cataracts are further classified as immature, mature, or hypermature. An immature cataract has some clear cortex; a mature cataract is totally opaque—the pupil appears white *(leukokoria)*. A hypermature cataract has liquefied cortex that may leak through the capsule and excite destructive inflammation. Immature cataracts are usually removed for visual reasons. A mature or hypermature cataract in an eye with potentially useful vision should be removed to prevent irreversible damage from lens-induced inflammation.

ETIOLOGY. Congenital cataracts are a feature of rubella embryopathy and often are associated with other congenital malformations. Acquired cataracts may result from trauma, radiation, or metabolic disorder. Several examples of colorful cataracts have diagnostic but little visual significance. In Wilson's disease, orange copper deposits may appear on the anterior capsule ("sunflower cataract"). Chlorpromazine administration may result in a brown or white dusting on the anterior lens surface. Red, green, and blue opacities in the lenticular cortex ("Christmas tree cataract") characterize myotonic dystrophy, but are occasionally encountered in its absence.

Hypocalcemia may be cataractogenic. Cataracts occur in disorders of carbohydrate metabolism: hypoglycemia, galactosemia, and diabetes mellitus. Although diabetics do not necessarily have an increased incidence of cataracts, those that occur progress rapidly, perhaps because of varying lens hydration.

Systemic corticosteroids promote formation of central posterior subcapsular cataracts. Because of the path that light must take through the lens, such opacities reduce vision more than similar eccentric or anterior ones. Posterior subcapsular cataracts affect focusing especially when the pupil is small, as in bright light or with close work; difficulties with driving and reading are often their first symptoms.

Most cataracts have no known cause. The common nuclear sclerotic or senile cataract is often familial, but no specific factors have been proven to accelerate or retard its development.

TREATMENT. With the exception of mature and hypermature cataracts and of immature cataracts that have swollen sufficiently to threaten to precipitate angle-closure glaucoma (see below), most cataracts are removed for visual reasons. Considerations in planning cataract extraction are the patient's visual needs, the potential for improvement, and the risks of surgery. A person who drives requires surgery when the better eye falls below an acuity of 20/40, the legal minimum for a driver's license in most states. By contrast, an elderly patient with 20/200 acuity and limited visual needs may be content without surgical intervention. Care must be taken to identify intercurrent ocular disease; removal of the lens of an eye with advanced glaucoma or macular degeneration does not improve vision.

The risk of cataract surgery is relatively small. Despite the possibility of intraocular hemorrhage, postoperative infection, corneal decompensation, or problems with wound healing, the chances for a good visual outcome are excellent. Even successful cataract surgery, however, increases the likelihood of subsequent retinal detachment, and a small percentage of eyes postoperatively develop prolonged cystoid macular edema with reduced acuity.

General anesthesia constitutes a major portion of the risk of cataract surgery. Because cataract extraction can usually be performed under local or even topical anesthesia, general anesthesia should be avoided in medically fragile patients.

Jaffe NS, Jaffe MS, Jaffe GF: Cataract Surgery and Its Complications. 5th ed. St. Louis, CV Mosby, 1990. *This profusely illustrated monograph addresses most of the issues of modern cataract surgery; includes extensive references.*

462   GLAUCOMA

Glaucoma comprises a group of disorders in which elevated intraocular pressure damages the optic nerve. The major types of glaucoma are open-angle, angle-closure, congenital, and secondary. The dynamics of aqueous humor control intraocular pressure. The aqueous humor is derived from blood by a process of secretion and ultrafiltration in the ciliary body. Aqueous humor then passes from the posterior chamber through the pupil to fill the anterior chamber, the space between the back of the cornea and the plane of the iris and pupil. The aqueous humor is reabsorbed through the trabecular meshwork, located in the angle between the cornea and the iris, to enter Schlemm's canal, which connects with the venous system (Fig. 462–1).

OPEN-ANGLE GLAUCOMA

In chronic open-angle glaucoma, the most common type, a block at the level of the trabecular meshwork impairs aqueous humor reabsorption. Intraocular pressure rises above its normal maximum of 21 mm Hg, gradually destroying axons and supporting tissue at the optic disc. The prevalence of open-angle glaucoma varies with the population studied and the diagnostic criteria employed. A conservative estimate in United States and European adults is 0.5%. Patients with increased intraocular pressure without signs of optic nerve damage are considered to have *ocular hypertension.* Treatment of ocular hypertension may be initiated if the pressure exceeds 30 mm Hg or in certain other situations.

Open-angle glaucoma is ordinarily asymptomatic until well advanced. Only rarely does the elevated intraocular pressure cause corneal edema, with the attendant perception of halos around lights. Pain is not characteristic. Initially only the peripheral visual field is lost; visual acuity remains normal until late in the course of the disease. Diagnosis depends on measuring intraocular pressure, examining the optic disc, and testing the visual fields. Gonioscopy, the visualization of the angle structures under high magnifications with special contact lenses, distinguishes an angle-closure from an open-angle mechanism.

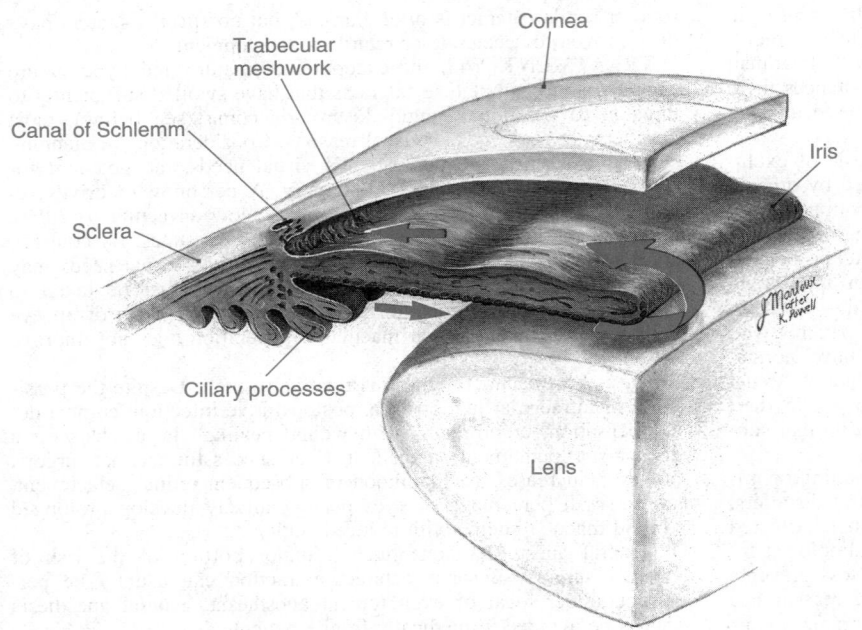

FIGURE 462–1. Circulation of aqueous humor in the normal eye. Aqueous is produced in the ciliary body and its processes, fills the posterior chamber (which also contains the lens), passes through the pupil *(large arrow)*, and is reabsorbed through the trabecular meshwork into the canal of Schlemm.

The treatment of open-angle glaucoma is primarily medical. Topical administration of parasympathomimetics (pilocarpine and carbachol), β-adrenergic blockers (e.g., timolol), and sympathomimetics (epinephrine and dipivefrin) decreases intraocular pressure. When these medications—individually and in combination—fail to arrest progressive disc damage producing visual field loss, topical indirect parasympathomimetics (echothiophate) and systemic carbonic anhydrase inhibitors (acetazolamide and methazolamide) may be useful.

If visual loss progresses with maximum tolerated medical therapy, surgery is indicated. *Laser trabeculoplasty* opens aqueous outflow channels by burning the surface of the trabecular meshwork. If all else fails, a surgical fistula can be created between the anterior chamber and the subconjunctival space. Such filtering procedures allow direct absorption of aqueous humor by subconjunctival and episcleral vessels.

The management of open-angle glaucoma involves early recognition, careful follow-up, and patient compliance with therapeutic regimens. Routine measurement of intraocular pressures (tonometry) at general physical examinations is often advocated; however, careful ophthalmoscopy with referral of patients whose central excavation ("cup") exceeds one third of the disc's area may be an equally effective screen.

ANGLE-CLOSURE GLAUCOMA

Angle-closure glaucoma develops when the normal path of aqueous flow is interrupted in an eye with a shallow anterior chamber, the consequence of a structurally anomalous anterior segment. Intraocular pressure remains normal until resistance to aqueous flow through the pupil—pupillary block—bows the iris forward to obstruct the resorptive surfaces in the angle. The pressure then rises precipitously, characteristically to above 50 mm Hg (Fig. 462–2).

Acute angle-closure glaucoma classically presents as a red, painful eye with decreased vision. The pupil is about 6 mm and fixed; the corneal light reflex is dulled. The patient is diaphoretic and nauseated and often vomits. Such typical angle-closure glaucoma is easy to recognize. The elderly, however, do not necessarily develop the full set of clinical signs and symptoms, and angle-closure glaucoma should be considered in all patients with a fixed, mid-dilated pupil and decreased vision even in the absence of a red eye or pain. The correct diagnosis can be made by slit-lamp examination with tonometry. Occasionally, chronic or subacute angle-closure glaucoma mimics open-angle glaucoma. Gonioscopy is then used to distinguish between the two mechanisms.

Dilating the pupils precipitates angle-closure in predisposed eyes. The risk of pharmacologic dilation is correlated with the depth of

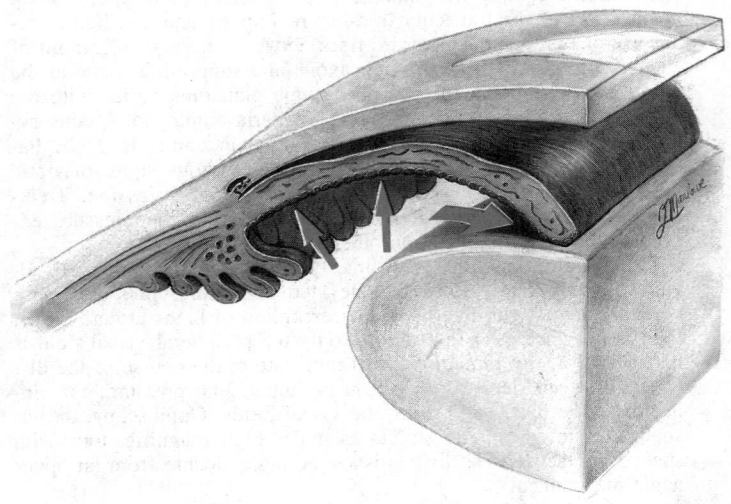

FIGURE 462–2. Angle-closure glaucoma. Owing to an anatomic anomaly in the anterior segment of the eye, the aqueous becomes trapped behind the pupil, bowing the iris forward (iris bombé) to cover the trabecular meshwork, which lies in the angle between the iris and the cornea.

the anterior chamber; eyes with shallow anterior chambers are at risk for angle-closure glaucoma. This distinction is not always easy to observe, and even experienced ophthalmologists sometimes cannot determine with certainty whether an angle will close with dilation. The likelihood of angle closure increases with age, and everyone over the age of 50 should be considered to have this potential. This does not mean that pupils of an older patient with a normal anterior chamber should not be dilated, but rather that dilation should be performed with a short-acting mydriatic agent such as tropicamide and the patient observed until the mydriatic wears off.

Nonophthalmologists should probably not routinely dilate pupils of adult outpatients. Children and inpatients may have dilation if there is no other contraindication such as recent head trauma, an iris-fixated intraocular lens, or impending general anesthesia. With these exceptions, the diagnostic benefits of dilation outweigh the risk of precipitating angle closure. Should angle-closure glaucoma develop, it can be recognized and promptly treated.

An acute angle-closure attack creates an emergency. Initial management consists of administration of parenteral acetazolamide, oral glycerol or (in diabetics) isosorbide, or intravenous mannitol, plus topical pilocarpine and a β-adrenergic antagonist. Once the attack has been broken, the anatomic predisposition can be circumvented by connecting the posterior and anterior chamber through the peripheral iris, usually with a *laser iridotomy*. The anterior segment abnormality that underlies angle-closure glaucoma is bilateral, and prophylactic surgery on the other eye is generally indicated.

CONGENITAL AND SECONDARY GLAUCOMA

Congenital glaucoma is an open-angle glaucoma that results from dysgenesis of the angle structures. Increased intraocular pressure enlarges the immature eye *(buphthalmos)*; a corneal diameter greater than 12 mm in a child suggests congenital glaucoma. Secondary glaucoma develops as the consequence of another ocular disease. Examples of secondary glaucomas include angle-closure glaucoma precipitated by intumescence of the lens, glaucoma developing as a result of new vessels forming in the angle (as occurs with diabetes or other ocular vascular disease), and glaucoma in the chronically inflamed eye of a patient with juvenile rheumatoid arthritis. In addition, severe blunt trauma causing bleeding into the anterior chamber *(hyphema)* damages angle structures and predisposes to the subsequent development of open-angle glaucoma.

Secondary, lens-induced angle-closure glaucoma is treated by surgical removal of the lens. Most other secondary glaucomas are managed in much the same way as primary open-angle glaucoma. Neovascular glaucoma is difficult to treat. If ischemia is the stimulus, as occurs with diabetes or retinal vascular occlusion, ablation of ischemic tissues by photocoagulation may halt progression. If neovascularization continues, medical control becomes ineffective. Filtering procedures generally fail because tissue proliferation closes the surgical fistula, a problem that may be avoided by connecting the anterior chamber and the subconjunctival space with a plastic valve or by using antimetabolites to inhibit tissue growth. Destruction of the ciliary body by an externally applied energy source (thermal, laser, ultrasound) controls intraocular pressure but seldom preserves useful vision.

Glaucoma of any type in which all light perception has been lost is called *absolute glaucoma*. Enucleation (removal of the eye) is the definitive treatment for a blind, painful eye, although topical medications or retrobulbar injection of alcohol may relieve discomfort and allow the eye to be retained.

463 DISC SWELLING AND OPTIC ATROPHY

The optic disc marks the transition from retina to optic nerve. The central retinal artery and vein pass through the disc and bifurcate on its surface. There is considerable normal variation in the disc's ophthalmoscopic appearance. A central excavation or cup occupies a variable portion of its substance; vessels are often seen

TABLE 463–1. CAUSES OF DISC SWELLING

Increased intracranial pressure (papilledema)	Compressive optic neuropathy Graves' disease
Inflammatory optic neuropathy (papillitis)	Sphenoid wing meningioma
Infiltrative optic neuropathy Sarcoidosis	Vasculopathies Anterior ischemic optic neuropathy
Leukemia and other malignancies	Central retinal vein occlusion
Optic nerve tumors	Toxic-metabolic optic neuropathy
Angioma	Idiopathic
Optic nerve meningioma	Pseudopapilledema
Childhood optic nerve glioma	Optic disc drusen
Malignant optic nerve glioma	Hyperopia
Metastatic carcinoma	Other anomalies

curving over the edge of this cup. Over 1 million axons originate in the ganglion cells of the retina and pass through each optic disc. Although these axons are nearly transparent, a bright ophthalmoscope visualizes fine reflective striations on the disc's surface and the immediately surrounding retina. Disc swelling can be a consequence of ischemia, infarction, infiltration, or local changes in tissue pressures (Table 463–1).

PAPILLEDEMA (see Color Plate 13*B*)

The term *papilledema* literally describes disc swelling from any cause; some prefer to reserve this term for disc swelling from increased intracranial pressure. The swelling and elevation of the disc observed ophthalmoscopically primarily reflect accumulation of axoplasm and are most obvious just adjacent to the disc's normal borders.

Papilledema from increased intracranial pressure is usually bilateral but may be asymmetric. With rapid increases in intracranial pressure, the veins become engorged and hemorrhages appear on the disc and adjacent retina. With only rare exceptions, visual acuity remains normal in acute papilledema. Chronic papilledema may lead to secondary optic atrophy and permanent loss of vision (see below). Surgical fenestration of the optic nerve sheath in eyes with visual loss may halt progression.

PSEUDOPAPILLEDEMA

Certain normal disc appearances resemble papilledema. Hyperopic eyes are small, with consequent axonal crowding at the disc that may be confused with swelling. Optic disc drusen, depositions of hyaline material in the prelaminar optic nerve, sometimes present as disc elevation in young persons. If they cannot be recognized with careful ophthalmoscopy, these calcified optic disc drusen may be visualized on computed tomography or ultrasonography. In older persons, the previously buried drusen become visible ophthalmoscopically as refractile bodies that resemble rock crystals (see Color Plate 13*D*). Anomalous discs are often discovered incidentally. One clue to their nature is the frequent absence of the physiologic cup; in true papilledema the cup is preserved until the disc swelling is far advanced.

OPTIC NEURITIS

Papillitis indicates an inflammatory or demyelinating neuritis located in the anterior optic nerve. In approximately half of eyes with optic neuritis the disc appears normal initially; this is *retrobulbar optic neuritis*. In papillitis, the disc is swollen and may be hemorrhagic, an appearance ophthalmoscopically indistinguishable from the papilledema that results from increased intracranial pressure. Unlike disc swelling from increased intracranial pressure, however, acuity and visual field are characteristically affected, and the condition is usually unilateral (see also Tables 403–2 and 403–3).

The management of optic neuritis is controversial. Recent studies indicate that, although visual outcome is not affected by corticosteroid administration, the incidence of other episodes of demyelination may be decreased.

ANTERIOR ISCHEMIC OPTIC NEUROPATHY

Whereas papillitis is largely a disease of the young, acute disc swelling and loss of vision in older persons suggest infarction and are termed *anterior ischemic optic neuropathy*. Often only the superior or inferior half of the disc is involved, with consequent altitudinal loss of the inferior or superior visual field. Most ischemic optic neuropathy is idiopathic, but the disorder may be the initial manifestation of giant cell or temporal arteritis, a disease of the elderly described in Ch. 246. Nonarteritic anterior ischemic optic neuropathy tends to occur in discs with small cups, and the second eye eventually becomes involved in about two fifths of cases.

The treatment of arteritic anterior ischemic optic neuropathy is directed to the underlying giant cell arteritis (see Ch. 246). Surgical incision of the optic nerve sheath does not appear to be effective treatment for nonarteritic anterior ischemic optic neuropathy.

OTHER CAUSES OF DISC SWELLING

Bilateral disc swelling may accompany severe hypertension and constitutes a hypertensive crisis (see Ch. 37). Markedly decreased intraocular pressure, encountered after ocular surgery or injury, also produces disc swelling, and the disc may swell acutely during an attack of angle-closure glaucoma. Disc swelling is also a feature of some toxic and hereditary optic neuropathies. Compression causes disc swelling only when the optic nerve is constricted. This occurs in some patients with the orbitopathy of Graves' disease (see Ch. 466), pseudotumor of the orbit (see Ch. 466), and sphenoid wing meningioma. Intrinsic tumors of the optic nerve, the most common being glioma and meningioma, may present as disc swelling and visual loss. Infiltration and swelling of the optic nerve heads are also encountered in leukemia, metastatic carcinoma, and sarcoid.

OPTIC ATROPHY

Optic atrophy results from death of the axons in the retina and optic nerve. Disc pallor and optic atrophy are not synonymous; some temporal pallor is a feature of normal discs. A lesion anywhere from the retina through the optic tract can cause optic atrophy. Lesions behind the lateral geniculate in early life occasionally cause trans-synaptic degeneration and optic atrophy. Optic atrophy may be classified as primary, secondary, or glaucomatous. *Primary optic atrophy* refers to progressive pallor without loss of disc substance, a sign of retrograde or anterograde degeneration from compression, vascular injury, or toxic metabolic injury to the axons. *Secondary optic atrophy* develops after disc swelling, as in chronic papilledema. Vascular and glial changes may give the disc an irregular, milky gray appearance with ill-defined borders. The distinction is not always clinically evident. *Glaucomatous optic atrophy* denotes loss of disc substance, already referred to as increased cupping.

Optic atrophy is difficult to recognize in young children, in whom the discs may have a pale appearance normally. In adults with nuclear sclerotic cataracts, pallor may be masked by the lens acting as a yellow filter. The diagnosis of optic atrophy should not be made unless there is evidence of alteration in visual function: decreased acuity or field or, in infants, nystagmus.

Ultimately, optic atrophy is not a clinical finding but a pathologic entity. In retinitis pigmentosa there is a primary dystrophy of the rods and cones. The ganglion cells remain intact, but secondary vascular and gliotic changes produce a waxy pallor of the disc that is not a true optic atrophy because the axons are preserved.

LEBER'S HEREDITARY OPTIC NEURORETINOPATHY (LEBER'S DISEASE)

This disorder, often called Leber's optic atrophy, classically presents as acute or subacute visual loss in men around the age of 20 years. Women are much less often affected, with later onset. Initially the discs appear swollen because of opacification of the peripapillary nerve fiber layer (see Color Plate 13*F*), but the swelling does not represent edema, since fluorescein angiography demonstrates only telangiectatic vessels that do not leak dye.

With time central vision is lost in both eyes, and optic atrophy evolves. Although no effective treatment exists, vision occasionally improves spontaneously. The disorder is transmitted via an abnormality in maternal mitochondrial DNA, explaining the unusual heredity in which men cannot transmit the disease but all women in pedigrees are either affected or carriers. Most cases can be diagnosed by study of mitochondrial DNA from peripheral leukocytes. The availability of these molecular diagnostic tests has expanded the limits of the phenotype to include cases of optic neuropathy not having the characteristic clinical manifestations.

464 UVEITIS

Uveitis denotes inflammation of the uveal tract, which consists of the iris, ciliary body, and choroid. There are two major clinical types, anterior and posterior (Table 464–1). Anterior uveitis, also known as *iritis* or *iridocyclitis,* has as its hallmark cells in the anterior chamber; the iris itself seldom appears inflamed. Posterior uveitis may take the form of *chorioretinitis.* The choroid and retina are so intimately connected that it is difficult to have inflammation of one without the other.

Acute anterior uveitis causes congestion of the eye, often producing a halo of injection surrounding the cornea that is described as ciliary flush. Frequently, the eye is painful, vision reduced, and the pupil small and poorly reactive. The diagnosis is confirmed by the presence of free cells in the aqueous humor, visible as bright points of light as the slit-lamp beam passes through the normally optically empty anterior chamber. In more severe inflammation, *keratitic precipitates,* cellular aggregates on the back of the cornea, appear. When these are large and oily, the inflammation is called *granulomatous iritis,* a variant sometimes associated with systemic inflammatory disease such as sarcoid, syphilis, and tuberculosis. The cause of most anterior uveitis is unknown.

UVEITIS AND ARTHRITIS. Juvenile rheumatoid arthritis (see Ch. 237) and ankylosing spondylitis (see Ch. 238) are especially likely to be associated with uveitis. Young men with ankylosing spondylitis have recurrent acute iritis that responds to standard treatments (see below). Most are HLA-B27 positive. By contrast, the uveitis accompanying juvenile rheumatoid arthritis is chronic and may initially be subclinical. Young women with the pauciarticular form of juvenile rheumatoid arthritis who develop uveitis often have grossly normal-appearing eyes, with the cellular reaction apparent only by slit-lamp examination. With time, adhesions called posterior synechiae form between the iris and lens, potentially causing secondary pupillary block glaucoma or occlusion of the pupil. Chronic inflammation may lead to cataract formation and ectopic calcification in the corneal epithelium, called *band keratopathy.* Hypercalcemia alone also causes band keratopathy.

Physicians treating seronegative pauciarticular arthritis should consider scheduling slit-lamp and dilated examinations several times a year. Posterior synechiae are also detectable with a hand light after instillation of mydriatics, as the pupil does not fully dilate and develops an irregular, scalloped border.

REITER'S SYNDROME. The triad of arthritis, urethritis, and conjunctivitis suggests Reiter's syndrome (see Ch. 238). This develops most often in men between the ages of 20 and 40 as a nonbacterial urethritis followed by polyarthritis and ocular inflammation. The initial ocular manifestation is usually a mucopurulent conjunctivitis, followed in many cases by an anterior uveitis. Keratitis and episcleritis also occur. As in ankylosing spondylitis, with which it shares similarities, HLA-B27 is often positive.

BEHÇET'S SYNDROME. Uveitis or retinitis is a cardinal feature of Behçet's syndrome (see Ch. 249). In some cases a layer of white cells forms in the lower portion of the anterior chamber; such

TABLE 464–1. DISEASES ASSOCIATED WITH UVEITIS

	Infectious	Other
Anterior (iridocyclitis)	Herpes zoster Herpes simplex Hansen's disease	Ankylosing spondylitis Rheumatoid arthritis Reiter's syndrome
Posterior (chorioretinitis)	Toxoplasmosis Toxocariasis Histoplasmosis Measles	
Both anterior and posterior	Syphilis Coccidioidomycosis Onchocerciasis Brucellosis	Sarcoid Behçet's syndrome Vogt-Koyanagi-Harada syndrome Inflammatory bowel disease

hypopyon uveitis is considered characteristic. In other patients the primary ocular manifestation is a retinal vasculitis and vitritis. Rarer neuro-ophthalmic manifestations such as cranial nerve palsies or homonymous hemianopias are part of a wider central nervous system (CNS) involvement.

UVEOMENINGITIS. Another systemic disease with characteristic ocular inflammation is uveomeningitis (Vogt-Koyanagi-Harada syndrome). This disorder, more common in darkly pigmented people, affects the uvea, retina, meninges, and skin. Manifestations include meningeal signs, alopecia, poliosis, vitiligo, tinnitus, and dysacusis. There may be an anterior or posterior uveitis with exudative retinal detachment. The visual prognosis is guarded even with aggressive treatment with systemic steroids and other immunosuppressants.

MALIGNANCY MASQUERADING AS UVEITIS. A steroid-responsive exudative process simulating uveitis can be the presentation of a lymphoreticular neoplasia (variously called reticulum cell sarcoma, histiocytic sarcoma, or—when the brain is involved—primary CNS lymphoma) in persons over age 40. The cytology of a vitreous aspirate may be diagnostic. Radiation treatment has palliative value.

An apparent iritis developing during a course of treatment for leukemia may represent infiltration of the anterior segment. Diagnosis and therapy are similar to the above.

TREATMENT. Treatment consists largely of topical or, when the inflammation is prolonged or severe, systemic immunosuppression. Prednisolone or dexamethasone topically constitutes initial therapy. Topical administration of mydriatic-cycloplegics in anterior uveitis reduces discomfort and retards posterior synechiae formation. Severe and prolonged inflammation or posterior uveitis may require periocular corticosteroid injections or oral prednisone. Cytotoxic immunosuppressive agents are sometimes used.

465 OCULAR INFECTIONS

Ocular infections and inflammations are most sensibly grouped according to their locations. The most common superficial infection is *blepharoconjunctivitis,* or more simply, *conjunctivitis.* Infection of the lacrimal gland is *dacryoadenitis;* infection of the lacrimal drainage system, *dacryocystitis.* Corneal involvement is called *keratitis. Uveitis, scleritis,* and *episcleritis,* which are seldom infectious, are discussed elsewhere (see Ch. 464 and 468). Infection or inflammation inside the eye is *endophthalmitis.* An infectious *vitritis* is a form of endophthalmitis. Some *chorioretinitis* is infectious. *Panophthalmitis* refers to infections that extend through the sclera or cornea and involve adjacent orbital tissues.

CONJUNCTIVITIS

Causes include allergic, viral, bacterial, chlamydial, and chemical agents. Mild acute viral conjunctivitis, with a watery discharge and lids sealed closed upon awakening, usually requires only warm or cool compresses and a topical vasoconstrictor to whiten the eye. Topical antibiotics are sometimes prescribed to prevent superinfections but offer no clear advantages. Severe or chronic conjunctivitis should be managed by an ophthalmologist.

GONOCOCCAL CONJUNCTIVITIS. Purulent bacterial conjunctivitis usually responds to topical antibiotics. An important exception is hyperpurulent gonococcal conjunctivitis, a disease of the newborn *(gonococcal ophthalmia neonatorum)* and of sexually promiscuous adults. The eye is markedly inflamed with a copious discharge and swollen lids. The discharge should be Gram stained and cultured on appropriate media. Treatment consists of parenteral antibiotics and saline lavage of ocular secretions. Because of the emergence of penicillinase-producing strains, use of a β-lactamase–resistant cephalosporin such as ceftriaxone is warranted. Untreated gonococcal infection can penetrate the intact eye and destroy it; treatment should be started as soon as the diagnosis is suspected.

CHLAMYDIAL CONJUNCTIVITIS. In some parts of the world chronic chlamydial conjunctivitis leads to conjunctival scar-ring and corneal vascularization, a disease known as *trachoma* (see Ch. 323). The resulting blindness is an important international public health problem. In developed countries, chlamydial infection manifests as a subacute conjunctivitis, frequently with associated urethritis. Although a keratitis may be present, severe corneal damage does not ensue. Chlamydial conjunctivitis, also called *inclusion blennorrhea* because of the cytoplasmic inclusions found in Giemsa-stained conjunctival scrapings, is difficult to eradicate in adults by topical antibiotics alone and should be treated with systemic tetracycline or erythromycin.

HERPETIC KERATITIS (see Color Plate 13*A*). Viral keratitis is a common and potentially serious consequence of infection with herpes simplex. The corneal involvement may be recognized by the characteristic *dendrite,* a branching epithelial ulcer. Topical antiviral agents promote healing, but recurrence is frequent, with increasing risk of corneal stromal involvement and scarring. Topical steroids activate epithelial herpes infections and should not be used without ophthalmologic consultation in any patient with a red eye. Herpes zoster ophthalmicus also sometimes produces an acute dendritic keratitis, which usually requires no treatment.

CORNEAL ULCERS

Bacterial and fungal infections of the cornea are a serious threat to vision. Corneal ulcers tend to develop in the context of ocular trauma or contact lens wear, after surgery, or with pre-existing corneal disease. Corneal ulceration appears as an area of white, gray, or yellow infiltrate that stains with fluorescein. Affected patients should be referred promptly to an ophthalmologist for evaluation and treatment with topical antibiotics and other measures.

ENDOPHTHALMITIS

Infection inside the eye most often follows accidental or surgical perforation. Epidemics have occurred following the use of contaminated irrigating solutions in intraocular surgery. Less commonly, infections elsewhere metastasize to the eye. Bacterial endophthalmitis must be treated aggressively if there is to be any chance of preserving vision. When the infection is recognized, cultures and smears are taken from the anterior chamber and vitreous cavity by aspiration, and a course of intravitreal and sometimes systemic, topical, and periocular antibiotics is begun. The choice of antibiotics depends on what organisms, if any, are found on Gram stain. Surgical vitrectomy may be warranted.

CANDIDA **ENDOPHTHALMITIS.** *Candida albicans* is the most prevalent organism causing metastatic (endogenous) endophthalmitis. Fungemia after prolonged use of intravenous catheters or parenteral drug abuse results in colonization of the eye, with multiple white, fluffy chorioretinal infiltrates. These often involve the macula, reducing central vision. Careful direct ophthalmoscopy through a dilated pupil is indicated in patients at risk. Most *Candida* endophthalmitis requires systemic or intravitreal administration of antifungal agents, although spontaneous resolution has been observed.

INFECTIOUS CHORIORETINITIS

CONGENITAL TOXOPLASMOSIS (see Color Plate 13*H*). This is a common type of infectious chorioretinitis acquired *in utero.* This protozoan parasite can remain dormant in pigmented chorioretinal scars for many years and then become active, with white infiltration at the border of the scar and an overlying vitritis. If a previously uninvolved macula is threatened or the degree of inflammation is severe, antibiotic treatment may be indicated.

CYTOMEGALOVIRUS RETINITIS (see Color Plate 14*G*). Cytomegalovirus (CMV) retinitis appears in immunosuppressed hosts as a discrete area of white or yellow retinal opacification with associated hemorrhage and vascular sheathing. The ophthalmoscopic picture resembles that of a branch retinal vein occlusion (see Ch. 469), but in CMV retinitis one eye often has multiple foci, and there is a tendency for bilateral involvement.

Diagnosis can be made clinically in most cases. Dosages of immunosuppressive drugs should be reduced, if possible. Treatment with foscarnet or ganciclovir results in temporary regression of the process, which then breaks through the antiviral therapy and progresses to severe visual loss unless the underlying immunosuppression can be reversed.

OTHER INFECTIOUS CHORIORETINITIDES. Syphilis and tuberculosis may present as chorioretinitis or uveitis. Herpes simplex retinitis resembles that of cytomegalovirus. Cryptococcal meningitis may have an associated chorioretinitis. Focal chorioretinitis can accompany subacute sclerosing panencephalitis (see Ch. 428.4).

466 ORBITAL DISEASE AND TUMORS

GRAVES' ORBITOPATHY. Graves' orbitopathy consists of inflammation and infiltration of orbital tissues, with characteristic enlargement and scarring of the extraocular muscles. The varied clinical manifestations include lid retraction, exophthalmos, increased intraocular pressure, limitation of eye movement, and decreased vision from optic neuropathy or corneal drying *(exposure keratitis)*. Graves' orbitopathy frequently develops in persons previously treated for hyperthyroidism. When the orbitopathy first manifests, the patient may be hyperthyroid, euthyroid, or hypothyroid. A clinical picture consistent with Graves' orbitopathy in the absence of a demonstrable thyroid abnormality, even to sophisticated testing, is referred to as *ophthalmic Graves' disease.* Coronal computed tomography (CT) or magnetic resonance imaging (MRI) demonstrating enlarged ocular muscles is a sensitive diagnostic maneuver.

Graves' orbitopathy is the most frequent cause of both unilateral and bilateral exophthalmos. Retraction of the upper lid to expose sclera above the cornea exaggerates the appearance of exophthalmos and predisposes to corneal drying. Tethering of the eye by fibrotic muscles produces a mechanical ophthalmoplegia and diplopia. Movement up and out is often restricted; pure loss of abduction mimicking sixth nerve palsy occurs. Ophthalmoplegia is not necessarily accompanied by exophthalmos.

Enlarged ocular muscles at the apex of the orbit may compress the optic nerve, producing disc swelling and visual loss. Severe exposure or progressive visual loss from compressive optic neuropathy is an indication for treatment. Systemic steroids reduce exophthalmos and temporarily relieve optic nerve compression. Surgical decompression of the orbit by one of several routes is one definitive therapy; orbital irradiation is also used. Once the orbitopathy has stabilized, surgical approaches to the extraocular muscles and lids may improve diplopia and correct persistent lid retraction.

INFLAMMATORY PSEUDOTUMOR OF THE ORBIT. Orbital pseudotumor is an idiopathic inflammation that falls within the spectrum of lymphoproliferative disorders. Its clinical manifestations are pain, exophthalmos, and limitation of eye movement. There may also be erythema and swelling of the lids. Orbital pseudotumors can mimic orbital infection, true tumors, or the orbitopathy of Graves' disease. The major sites of inflammation are muscle *(myositis),* nerve *(perineuritis),* sclera *(scleritis),* or lacrimal gland *(dacryoadenitis).*

If the inflammation is posterior to the orbital apex in the walls of the cavernous sinus, the painful ophthalmoplegia that results is called the *Tolosa-Hunt syndrome.* Orbital pseudotumor merges pathologically and clinically with orbital lymphoma, which in turn merges with systemic lymphoma.

Initial evaluation of a patient with clinical signs and symptoms of orbital pseudotumor includes orbital ultrasonography and CT or MRI. A trial of high-dose systemic corticosteroids is usually indicated prior to biopsy. Orbital biopsy is not a trivial undertaking and should be reserved for steroid-unresponsive or recurrent processes. Some histologically benign infiltrations do not respond to corticosteroids. Biopsy in such cases reveals fibrous tissue described as *sclerosing pseudotumor.* Occasionally, a patient with a histologically benign pseudotumor subsequently develops a systemic lymphoma.

A necrotizing vasculitis, Wegener's granulomatosis, must also be included in the differential diagnosis of orbital pseudotumor, especially when the inflammation is bilateral. Most cases of Wegener's granulomatosis involve contiguous sinus structures, but local ocular forms of the disease have been reported. The combination of progressive proptosis and sinus disease also suggests orbital aspergillosis, especially in persons who are immunosuppressed or reside in warmer climates.

RHABDOMYOSARCOMA. Rhabdomyosarcoma is the most common malignant tumor of the orbit during the first decade of life and also occurs during the second and third decades. The initial presentation is usually ptosis with lid infiltration and proptosis. Progression may be extremely rapid, the clinical picture mimicking trauma or cellulitis. Biopsy and prompt treatment with irradiation and chemotherapy result in a high percentage of survival, although vision in the eye on the side of the tumor is seldom preserved.

OTHER ORBITAL TUMORS. Many types of primary, secondary, and metastatic tumors involve the orbit. Most present with exophthalmos, visual loss, and limitation of eye movement. High degrees of malignancy are rare with meningiomas, gliomas, hemangiomas/lymphangiomas, and dermoids. Carcinomas of the lacrimal or meibomian glands represent a serious threat to life, and some cases require *exenteration*—the removal of the orbital contents. Carcinoma from contiguous sinuses invades the orbit, and breast carcinoma is especially likely to metastasize to the orbit.

467 INTRAOCULAR TUMORS

RETINOBLASTOMA. Retinoblastoma, a malignancy of the retina, is the most common intraocular tumor of childhood and one of the more common childhood tumors at any site. One third are bilateral. About 6% of retinoblastomas are inherited in an autosomal dominant pattern; half of these are bilateral. Ninety percent of retinoblastomas are discovered before the age of three. Adults who have survived retinoblastoma are at risk for the development of other malignancies, especially osteogenic sarcomas.

MALIGNANT MELANOMA. Primary melanomas develop in the conjunctiva, iris, ciliary body, or choroid; skin melanomas have a predilection for metastasis to the eye and orbit. Malignant melanomas of the choroid are the most common primary intraocular tumor of adulthood. Most occur in middle-aged whites. The prognosis of malignant melanoma of the choroid depends upon size, cytology, and the presence of extrascleral extension. Choroidal malignant melanomas often metastasize to the liver.

The differential diagnosis of a pigmented intraocular mass includes benign choroidal nevus, senile disciform macular degeneration (also known as central exudative hemorrhagic retinopathy), peripheral exudative hemorrhagic chorioretinopathy, choroidal hemangioma, and hypertrophy or hyperplasia of the retinal pigment epithelium. Many eyes removed because of the suspicion of malignant melanoma have been found to have unexpectedly benign pathologies.

Enucleation is the traditional treatment for malignant melanoma of the choroid. Other approaches include photocoagulation, radiation therapy, and local resection. Many pigmented choroidal tumors can be followed safely without intervention, especially when they are found incidentally in the seeing eyes of elderly patients.

METASTATIC CARCINOMA TO THE EYE. Once considered rare, metastatic cancer is now recognized as the most common ocular malignancy of adulthood, with an incidence exceeding that of choroidal melanoma. Most frequent are carcinomas invading the choroid (see Color Plate 13E), the most likely primary being breast, followed by carcinomas of the lung, then kidney, gastrointestinal tract, testis, and prostate. With lung or renal carcinoma, the primary site may be inapparent at the time the metastasis is detected. If tumor is identified elsewhere, removal of the eye is seldom indicated. Palliative radiation therapy or chemotherapy may preserve vision, and enucleation should be performed only if the eye is blind and painful.

Shields JA, Shields CL: Intraocular Tumors: A Text and Atlas. Philadelphia, WB Saunders, 1992. *An extensively illustrated and referenced overview by two experienced clinicians.*

468 EPISCLERITIS, SCLERITIS, AND THE DRY EYE

To a neurologist, the eye is anterior extension of the brain; to a rheumatologist, the eye is a joint. Medicine and ophthalmology come together in the diagnosis and management of rheumatoid and connective tissue disorders. Uveal manifestations are discussed in Ch. 464, the toxicity of drugs used in treatment in Ch. 470, and the retinal changes in Ch. 469.

EPISCLERITIS AND SCLERITIS

Inflammation of the collagenous shell of the eye can be either superficial (episcleritis) or deep (scleritis). The transparent, avascular cornea is continuous with the opaque, vascular sclera and may be secondarily involved. Episcleritis resembles a localized conjunctivitis. The inflammation is deeper, however, and the dilated vessels do not always blanch with topically applied phenylephrine 2.5%, as they would in a pure conjunctivitis. Episcleritis usually is self-limited, although it may be recurrent, and it does not permanently damage the eye. Most episcleritis is idiopathic, but the disorder may be encountered in rheumatoid arthritis, polyarteritis nodosa, Wegener's granulomatosis, systemic lupus erythematosus, dermatomyositis, progressive systemic sclerosis, and relapsing polychondritis.

Scleritis is more likely than episcleritis to accompany a systemic disease, although the list of associations is about the same for the two disorders. Any portion of the sclera may be affected. The diagnosis is especially difficult with posterior scleritis, which may present as ocular pain or as an exudative retinal detachment. Anterior scleritis often becomes a prolonged, indolent inflammation with eventual permanent structural alteration of tissues. Pain may be prominent and severe. Inflammation in scleritis is initially localized and may be nodular or diffuse. With prolonged inflammation, scleral thinning results in a localized bluish discoloration as the underlying choroid becomes visible. Scleral necrosis with perforation is possible; this is especially frequent in association with rheumatoid arthritis. The adjacent cornea may melt away.

Management of scleritis is difficult. Local steroid injections may predispose to perforation. Systemic corticosteroids and other antirheumatic drugs are useful in some patients. The ocular process often closely parallels the activity of the underlying disease, which should guide systemic therapy.

KERATOCONJUNCTIVITIS SICCA. Corneal inflammation as the result of drying is referred to as keratoconjunctivitis sicca. Keratoconjunctivitis sicca, a dry mouth (xerostomia), and a connective tissue disorder constitute Sjögren's syndrome. The underlying pathophysiology appears to be an autoimmune reaction affecting the lacrimal and salivary glands. Sjögren's syndrome is common in patients with rheumatoid arthritis, especially middle-aged women. Complaints of burning, irritation, or excessive secretions suggest a dry eye but are notoriously nonspecific.

Diagnosis depends on demonstration of tear hyposecretion (usually by decreased wetting of a strip of litmus or filter paper placed between the lower lid and the eye in the inferior cul-de-sac—the Shirmer test) accompanied by corneal and conjunctival epithelial damage. Once epithelial cells start to slough, the corneal surface takes up fluorescein instilled into the conjunctival sac. Devitalized cells that have not yet been sloughed stain with rose bengal, making this dye an even more sensitive test for keratitis sicca.

Treatment consists of replacing tear volume and reducing tear turnover. Various preparations of artificial tears are available; those that do not contain preservatives are preferable if frequent administration is required. Other maneuvers include temporary or permanent occlusion of the lacrimal puncta to reduce tear outflow and placement of contact lenses, moisture chambers, or goggles over the eyes to decrease evaporation.

469 OCULAR VASCULAR DISEASE

SYSTEMIC HYPERTENSION AND ARTERIOSCLEROSIS

Although the retinal vascular abnormalities in hypertension are nonspecific and variable, they can be important diagnostically and therapeutically. The effects of blood pressure on the retinal vessels depend on both its absolute level and its duration. Although essential hypertension is a disease of arterioles, the retinal vascular bed lacks sympathetic innervation, and the fundus changes must be considered secondary.

Arteriolar narrowing is the most common hypertensive change and the most difficult to differentiate as abnormal. The normal ratio of the diameters of the arteriolar and venous blood columns is 2:3 or 3:4. A decrease in this ratio can best be appreciated in the smaller branches away from the disc. Other findings include microaneurysms, hemorrhages, lipid deposits, and edema. Retinal and disc edema usually follows a rapid increase in systemic blood pressure. Disc edema defines one type of malignant hypertension or hypertensive crisis and may be the presenting sign of markedly elevated blood pressure. By contrast, opacification (or sclerosis) of the vessel walls—described as copper or silver wiring—accompanies longstanding, uncontrolled hypertension and is rarely encountered now because of effective antihypertensive therapies.

Thickening of the arteriolar wall explains arteriovenous nicking and venous dilation distal to the crossing. Cotton-wool spots are signs of local ischemia; hemorrhages and hard exudates reflect vascular leakage. Microaneurysms result from irreversible structural alterations in the capillary walls. Retinal vascular occlusions (see below) and ischemic optic neuropathy (see Ch. 463) are potential consequences of hypertensive vascular changes.

Hypertension accelerates atherosclerosis, but atherosclerosis does not require hypertension. The only pure arteriosclerotic funduscopic change is atheroma of the retinal arterioles. These are seen as yellow-white plaques in the central retinal artery or its first branches, where the arteries still have an internal elastic lamina. These plaques should be differentiated from calcific or lipid emboli, which are usually smaller or more peripheral. Other retinal emboli include platelet-fibrin emboli that move through the arterioles and cause some cases of transient monocular blindness, talc emboli that appear as small white flecks in drug abusers using adulterated heroin, and septic emboli from subacute bacterial endocarditis that manifest as white-centered hemorrhages (Roth spots—Color Plate 14B). A rare but important cause of retinal embolism is cardiac myxoma (see Ch. 47).

DIABETIC RETINOPATHY (see Color Plate 14B, 14E, and 14F)

Diabetic retinopathy, the most common of the vascular retinopathies, shares many features with hypertensive retinopathy. The pathophysiologic defect appears to lie at the level of the retinal capillaries. Progressive degeneration of the capillary walls results in leakage (hemorrhages and exudates), diffuse and focal expansion (microaneurysms), and closure of small vessels. The ischemic retina in the focal areas of nonperfusion elaborates factors stimulating new vessel and fibrous ingrowth. Radiation therapy given as treatment for head and neck cancers may produce similar injury to the retinal capillary wall cells.

Diabetic retinopathy is classified as background or proliferative. Background retinopathy is further subdivided into simple background—with microaneurysms, dot/blot hemorrhages, and hard exudates—and a preproliferative form. In preproliferative retinopathy there is beading of veins, cotton-wool spots, and numerous intraretinal hemorrhages. Also characteristic is intraretinal new vessel pathology, so-called intraretinal microvascular anomalies.

In proliferative retinopathy, neovascularization appears on the disc and elsewhere, especially along the major vascular arcades. Fibrovascular proliferation and vitreous hemorrhages may follow. Proliferative diabetic retinopathy confers a poor visual prognosis.

Background retinopathy reduces visual acuity when there is edema or exudation in the macula. More new cases of blindness result from background retinopathy with macular edema than from proliferative retinopathy, because the former is much more prevalent. Background retinopathy with macular edema commonly presents in type 2 diabetics over age 50.

TREATMENT. Good diabetic control appears to retard the progression of retinopathy. Ablation of ischemic retina by panretinal photocoagulation helps preserve central vision in eyes with early proliferative retinopathy, making this the current treatment of choice. Advanced proliferative retinopathy may require removal of the vitreous and its contents through instruments inserted through the pars plana of the ciliary body. In such cases the prognosis is guarded, but an estimated 50 to 75% of patients undergoing pars plana vitrectomy experience some visual improvement.

OTHER VASCULAR RETINOPATHIES (see Color Plate 14)

SYSTEMIC LUPUS ERYTHEMATOSUS. Retinopathy is common but nonspecific; the most frequent findings are retinal hemorrhages and cotton-wool spots. Cotton-wool spots are not exudations, but represent localized areas of axoplasmic stasis caused by ischemia, which may indicate active vasculitis. Patients with lupus also may have hypertensive retinopathy. Central nervous system involvement may be associated with optic nerve and chiasmal neuropathy, papilledema, ocular motor cranial nerve palsies, hemianopias, and a migraine-like syndrome.

HEMATOLOGIC DISEASE. Anemia and thrombocytopenia predispose to retinal and subconjunctival hemorrhages. Retinal hemorrhages that result from leukemia often have a white center—the classic but nonspecific Roth spot mentioned above. Leukemia can cause *hyperviscosity retinopathy,* characterized by venous tortuosity and dilation, retinal hemorrhages, and vascular occlusions. A chronically elevated leukocyte count also predisposes to capillary drop-out and microaneurysm formation, but proliferative retinopathy is rare. Other causes of hyperviscosity retinopathy are Waldenström's macroglobulinemia, multiple myeloma, polycythemia, and sickle cell anemia. In extreme cases, sludging of blood in the veins is visible ophthalmoscopically.

PERIPHERAL RETINAL NEOVASCULARIZATION. Diabetic retinopathy affects largely the posterior pole of the eye. The retinopathy of prematurity (previously known as retrolental fibroplasia) and *sickle cell disease* have their major impact on the peripheral retina. The ocular and systemic manifestations of sickling hemoglobinopathies correlate poorly. In patients with sickle cell anemia, proliferative retinopathy is rare. Peripheral neovascularization is more common in sickle cell hemoglobin C disease (SC) and sickle cell thalassemia (S-thal). Patients with sickle cell trait usually have no ocular findings, although hypoxia encountered at high altitudes may precipitate hemorrhages and vascular occlusions.

The ocular findings in *sickle hemoglobinopathies* include small, dark red, comma-shaped conjunctival vascular segments, best observed on the inferior bulbar conjunctiva after instillation of a topical vasoconstrictor. Ischemic infarction of iris segments is also observed. In addition to peripheral neovascularization that often resembles the sea fan coral, other characteristic retinal findings include hemorrhages that have a salmon pink coloration from hemoglobin breakdown products and black chorioretinal scars with irregular borders in the equatorial periphery.

About one fifth of proliferative sickle retinopathy regresses spontaneously. The rest, if untreated, progress to retinal detachment and vitreous hemorrhage. Treatment consists of photocoagulation or transscleral cryotherapy or diathermy.

RETINAL VASCULAR OCCLUSIONS

CENTRAL RETINAL ARTERY OCCLUSION (CRAO) (see Color Plate 14C). The central retinal artery is a branch of the ophthalmic artery, in turn a branch of the internal carotid artery. Occlusion of the central retinal artery causes sudden, usually nearly complete visual loss in one eye. Ophthalmoscopy reveals arteriolar narrowing and vascular stasis which is recognizable ophthalmoscopically as segmentation of the venous blood column—"boxcar" pattern. Bilateral boxcarring is a useful sign of circulatory arrest and death.

Within hours the infarcted superficial layers of the retina lose their normal transparency and assume a milky white translucency. Because the thin retina of the fovea receives its nutrition from the underlying choroid, this region retains its normal color and contrasts with the surrounding infarcted retina to produce a cherry red spot. Bilateral cherry red spots are also encountered in children with congenital lipid storage diseases, the most common being Tay-Sachs, in which abnormal metabolic products partially opacify the ganglion cell layer that surrounds but does not extend across the fovea.

Eventually arterial flow is restored and the edema resolves. The disc, initially normal because it derives its blood supply from the surrounding choroid, gradually becomes pale and atrophic as its axons degenerate. After several weeks it is difficult to distinguish a central retinal artery occlusion from other causes of primary optic atrophy.

In some persons, portions of the retina are supplied by vessels arising from the choroidal circulation, and such areas may be spared if the central retinal artery alone is occluded. A CRAO deprives most eyes of useful vision. CRAOs are the result of emboli (atheromatous, myxomatous, and material from diseased or artificial heart valves), of local small vessel disease, or of carotid occlusion. A CRAO is sometimes the initial sign of giant cell arteritis or polyarteritis nodosa. CRAO has been reported in patients with sickle cell trait after trauma or other stress.

Acute central retinal artery occlusion is an emergency. In a few instances prompt action may dislodge an embolus and restore circulation in time to prevent retinal death and thus preserve vision. For a nonophthalmologist, intervention consists of firm, intermittent pressure on the globe with the heel of the hand, alternately raising and lowering intraocular pressure. A mixture of 95% oxygen and 5% carbon dioxide may also be administered by mask for several minutes at a time, monitoring respiratory status. Ophthalmologists use other measures: retrobulbar injection of local anesthetic to dilate the arteries and anterior chamber paracentesis to lower the pressure in the ocular vascular bed.

BRANCH RETINAL ARTERY OCCLUSION (BRAO) (see Color Plate 14D). Branch arterial occlusions present as sudden, partial loss of peripheral vision. On dilated fundus examination a wedge-shaped area of pale, infarcted retina is seen spreading outward from an arteriolar bifurcation. Branch retinal artery occlusions are almost always embolic in origin, the most common source of emboli in older adults being the ipsilateral carotid artery. In children and young adults, migraine, coagulation abnormalities, increased intraocular pressure, and oral contraceptives may predispose to vascular occlusions.

CENTRAL RETINAL VEIN OCCLUSION (CRVO) (see Color Plate 14A). The dramatic ophthalmoscopic findings of dilated, tortuous veins, extensive retinal hemorrhages, and disc swelling in one eye have classically been called a central retinal vein occlusion. Experimental evidence suggests that such hemorrhagic retinopathy requires both arterial ischemia and venous disease.

Visual prognosis varies. In the fully developed form usually encountered in older persons, vision is poor and generally remains so. Panretinal photocoagulation may decrease the risk of subsequent neovascular glaucoma in selected cases. A less severe ophthalmoscopic picture is encountered in younger patients. Acuity in such *nonischemic central retinal vein occlusion* or *venous stasis retinopathy* is only slightly reduced, and the visual prognosis is good. Ischemic oculopathy following carotid occlusion produces a similar retinopathy; the diagnosis is suggested by low retinal arterial pressure measured by ophthalmodynamometry or oculopneumonoplethysmography.

A CRVO presents as unilateral visual loss in older adults but, unlike a CRAO, is not an emergency, as there is no accepted immediate therapy. There are also no specific accompanying diseases. Hypertension and diabetes are loosely associated, and hypercoagulable states must be considered, especially if there is bilateral retinopathy.

BRANCH RETINAL VEIN OCCLUSIONS. Patients with branch vein occlusions complain of blurred vision. In the fundus, hemorrhages and cotton-wool spots spread out in a wedge from an arteriovenous crossing. As in CRVO, there are few specific systemic associations. Neovascular glaucoma is rare, but vision persistently reduced by macular edema may respond to photocoagulation. Branch retinal vein occlusion must be distinguished from viral retinitis (see Ch. 465).

470   THE EYE AND MEDICATIONS

DRUGS WITH OCULAR SIDE EFFECTS

ANTICHOLINERGICS. A variety of systemic drugs have ocular side effects. Any medication with anticholinergic properties can dilate the pupil and diminish accommodation. This is the basis for the unhelpful caution against use in patients with glaucoma found in drug information inserts of medications that alter autonomic function such as antidepressants, tranquilizers, bronchodilators, and vasoconstrictors. Only when there is a potential for angle closure are such drugs contraindicated, and this is usually unrecognized. Patients on therapy for open-angle glaucoma are at little risk, as mydriasis usually does not affect their intraocular pressures. If the patient has a known angle-closure mechanism, previous iridectomy should have all but eliminated the danger of dilation. Of the systemic anticholinergic drugs, transdermal scopolamine is the most likely to dilate and fix pupils and paralyze accommodation, either by systemic absorption or through inadvertent instillation into the conjunctival sac by a contaminated finger.

CORTICOSTEROIDS. Prolonged administration of systemic corticosteroids often leads to the formation of posterior subcapsular cataracts. Topical corticosteroids increase intraocular pressure in genetically predisposed persons. Topical steroids also activate herpes simplex keratitis and should be prescribed only under the supervision of an ophthalmologist.

QUININE AND CHLOROQUINE. Quinine may cause acute blindness, with narrowing of the retinal arterioles. An overdose increases the probability of toxic effects, but rare persons are sensitive even to therapeutic doses. Other symptoms of quinine toxicity include dizziness, tinnitus, and hearing loss. Central vision may improve, with persistent constriction of peripheral field and evolution of optic atrophy.

The synthetic antimalarials chloroquine and hydroxychloroquine have a specific retinal toxicity. This usually appears only after prolonged administration in doses exceeding 250 mg per day for chloroquine and 400 mg per day for hydroxychloroquine. The parafoveal retina is most affected, and reduction in visual acuity may not develop until toxicity is moderately advanced. Chloroquine binds to pigmented tissues, exerting a toxic effect on the retinal epithelium with loss of pigmentation in a target-like or bull's-eye pattern around the fovea. Discontinuation of the drug may improve matters, but progressive visual loss may continue if the process is advanced.

AMIODARONE. Amiodarone represents a class of drugs having the property of cationic amphiphilia. Amiodarone binds to polar lipids and accumulates within lysosomes, producing whorl-like depositions of pigment in the corneal epithelium similar to the keratopathy of Fabry's disease (see Ch. 174.1). These seldom interfere with vision and resolve if the drug is discontinued. Instances of disc swelling and visual loss resembling anterior ischemic optic neuropathy (see Ch. 463) have been encountered in patients receiving amiodarone. The degree of visual loss from such amiodarone papillopathy must be balanced against the risk of cardiac arrhythmia in deciding whether to decrease the dosage.

THIORIDAZINE. Phenothiazines are potentially toxic to retina and retinal pigment epithelium, producing a coarse pigmentary degeneration. Of those now in common use, only thioridazine has clinically significant toxicity, and then only with dosages exceeding 1 gram per day for prolonged periods.

ETHAMBUTOL. Various drugs have been implicated in optic neuropathies. Only with ethambutol is the incidence of such side effects high enough that monitoring is considered mandatory. The physician administering ethambutol should perform monthly checks

TABLE 470–1. SYSTEMIC SIDE EFFECTS OF TOPICAL OCULAR HYPOTENSIVES

β-Blockers (timolol, betaxolol, levobunolol)
    Bronchospasm
    Bradycardia/hypotension
    Light-headedness/depression/fatigue
    Neuromuscular blockade in myasthenia gravis
Miotics
    Pilocarpine
        Brow ache (usually transient)
        Cholinergic overdose
    Echothiophate
        Prolonged action of succinylcholine or procaine
Sympathomimetics (epinephrine, dipivefrin)
    Tachycardia
    Atrial and ventricular arrhythmias
    Hypertension
    Headache

of acuity and color vision, especially when dosages exceed 15 mg per kilogram.

SYSTEMIC SIDE EFFECTS OF TOPICAL OCULAR MEDICATIONS
(Table 470–1)

Medications in solution are easily absorbed from the nasal mucosa, and systemic side effects are more likely with drops than ointments. Dilation of the pupil with 10% phenylephrine solution has been known to precipitate hypertension; topical epinephrine may increase ventricular extrasystoles. A single administration of timolol maleate to an asthmatic patient has induced bronchospasm and respiratory arrest.

Topical anticholinergics such as atropine, scopolamine, and cyclopentolate may contribute to confusional states in the elderly. Cyclopentolate is occasionally a cause of acute hallucinations and even psychosis in the young. Pilocarpine, used in large doses in the treatment of acute angle-closure glaucoma, has resulted in cholinergic overdose characterized by nausea, vomiting, salivation, and gastrointestinal cramps. As these are also symptoms of the angle-closure attack itself, such toxicity may not be immediately recognized, leading to continued administration and cardiovascular collapse.

Echothiophate iodide, an organophosphate used in the treatment of some forms of childhood strabismus and of open-angle glaucoma, predisposes to cholinergic crisis, which may mimic an acute surgical abdomen. Also, patients receiving echothiophate have impaired metabolism of succinylcholine. Use of succinylcholine during the induction of general anesthesia in a patient receiving echothiophate has caused death.

CARBONIC ANHYDRASE INHIBITORS

Acetazolamide and methazolamide inhibit aqueous production and are used systemically to reduce intraocular pressure when topical medications are inadequate. Most patients experience paresthesias; their absence is thought by some to indicate noncompliance. Carbonic anhydrase inhibitors rarely cause blood dyscrasias and also can induce a systemic acidosis, producing a syndrome of malaise and anorexia, depression, and weight loss that responds to concurrent administration of sodium bicarbonate. Acetazolamide also increases the incidence of urolithiasis. The combination of a carbonic anhydrase inhibitor and a thiazide diuretic may deplete body potassium. Carbonic anhydrase inhibitors should be administered with caution to people with known allergy to sulfonamides.

Grant WM, Schuman JS: Toxicology of the Eye. 4th ed. Springfield, IL, Charles C Thomas, 1993. *The latest update of a standard reference.*

471 INTRODUCTION
Frank Parker

The skin is a dynamic organ containing many tissues, cell types, and specialized structures, which together serve multiple functions crucial to health and survival. One of the largest and most versatile of organs, it provides a number of unique functions. First it is the interface with our environment and serves many functions crucial to survival, including protection against the elements (including UV light, mechanical and chemical injury, invasion by infectious agents, and prevention of desiccation) and thermoregulation. Second, it functions as a sensory receptor, monitoring diverse environmental stimuli. Third, it plays an active role in immunologic surveillance. Last, in many instances it actively "mirrors" internal disease processes.

Skin problems are exceedingly common: 30% of Americans have dermatologic conditions requiring a physician's care (Table 471–1). Also, the skin and its appendages (the hair and nails) play a paramount role in our psychological makeup. Third the skin can be readily examined and biopsied and cared for under the eyes of the physician and patient.

TABLE 471–1. PREVALENCE OF COMMON DERMATOLOGIC DISEASES IN THE UNITED STATES*

	Rate per 1000	Numbers (in 1000's)
Fungus infections	81.1	15,733
Tinea pedis	38.7	7509
Tinea unguium	21.8	4232
Tinea versicolor	8.4	1623
Tinea cruris	6.7	1301
Acne vulgaris	68.1	13,217
Cystic acne	1.9	375
Acne scars	1.7	321
Seborrheic dermatitis	28.2	5476
Verruca vulgaris	8.5	1684
Folliculitis	8.0	1553
Atopic dermatitis	6.9	1332
Lichen simplex chronicus	4.5	882
Hand eczema	1.6	311
Dyshidrotic eczema	2.1	405
Psoriasis	5.5	1070
Vitiligo	4.9	957
Herpes simplex	4.2	824

* Persons 1 to 74 years of age—noninstitutionalized.
Reprinted from the chapter by Dr. Marie-Louise Johnson in the 17th edition of the *Cecil Textbook of Medicine,* with her permission.

Arnold HL, Odom RB, James WP: Andrew's Diseases of the Skin. Philadelphia, W.B. Saunders, 1990. *An up-to-date text covering cogent aspects of clinical dermatology.*

Fitzpatrick TB, Eisen AZ, Wolff K, et al.: Dermatology in General Medicine, 3rd ed. New York, McGraw-Hill, 1987. *A detailed and well-illustrated textbook covering all aspects of dermatology. Two volumes.*

Rook A, Wilkinson DS, Ebling FJG, et al.: Textbook of Dermatology. Oxford, Blackwell Scientific, 1986. *This three-volume multiauthored text covers every aspect of dermatology in great detail. It is well written and referenced.*

472 STRUCTURE AND FUNCTION OF SKIN
Frank Parker

The skin serves a variety of functions that can be correlated with specific properties of epidermal or dermal regions. The epidermis differentiates to form anucleate cornified cells that act as a relatively impermeable protective barrier to the outward loss of body fluids and the inward penetration of various substances and microorganisms. These lamellae of cornified surface cells together with the brown pigment melanin also play an important role in protecting against the carcinogenic effects of ultraviolet radiation. Two components of the dermis, its unique circulatory system and specialized cutaneous appendages, the sweat glands, play a vital role in the body's thermoregulation. Finally, the skin is important immunologically. Both the epidermis (Langerhans' cells) and dermis (epidermodermal junction structures) predispose to a number of immunologic reactions that generate inflammatory skin diseases.

ANATOMIC CONSIDERATIONS

The skin is composed of two mutually dependent layers: the outer *epidermis* and inner *dermis,* both cushioned on the fat-containing subcutaneous tissue, the *panniculus adiposus* (Figs. 472–1 and 472–2).

EPIDERMIS. The epidermis is a continuously renewing multilayered organ that constantly differentiates. The stratified structure contains two main zones of cells (keratinocytes), an inner region of viable cells, the *stratum germinativum,* and an outer layer of anucleate cells known as the *stratum corneum,* or horny layer. Three strata of cells are recognized in the germinativum: the *basal, spinous,* and *granular* layers, each representing progressive stages of differentiation and keratinization of the epidermal cells as they evolve into the dead, tightly packed stratum corneum cells on the skin surface.

The epidermis is derived from the mitotic division of the basal cells resting on the basement membrane *(basal lamina),* with the daughter cells moving outward to the surface, where they become polyhedral as they synthesize increasing quantities of keratin. These *stratum spinosum cells* attach to one another mechanically by desmosomes, complex modifications of the cellular membranes that impart a spinous or quill-like appearance to the cells. Desmosomes play a crucial role in maintaining the adherence of the epidermal cells to one another. Desmosomes contain several intracellular proteins (i.e., desmoplakins, which are the paraneoplastic pemphigus autoantigens) and transmembrane proteins (desmogleins, which function as the pemphigus folaceous and pemphigus vulgaris autoantigens). With further outward displacement the differentiating cells of the spinous layer become flattened, and refractile keratohyalin granules appear in the cytoplasm, accounting for the designation of *granular layer* that rests just below the stratum corneum. These granules are the site of active synthesis of filaggrin, which causes keratin filaments to aggregate in parallel array, forming the tough, "chemically resistant" internal structure of the stratum corneum cells.

The transformation from viable granular cells to anucleate, non-

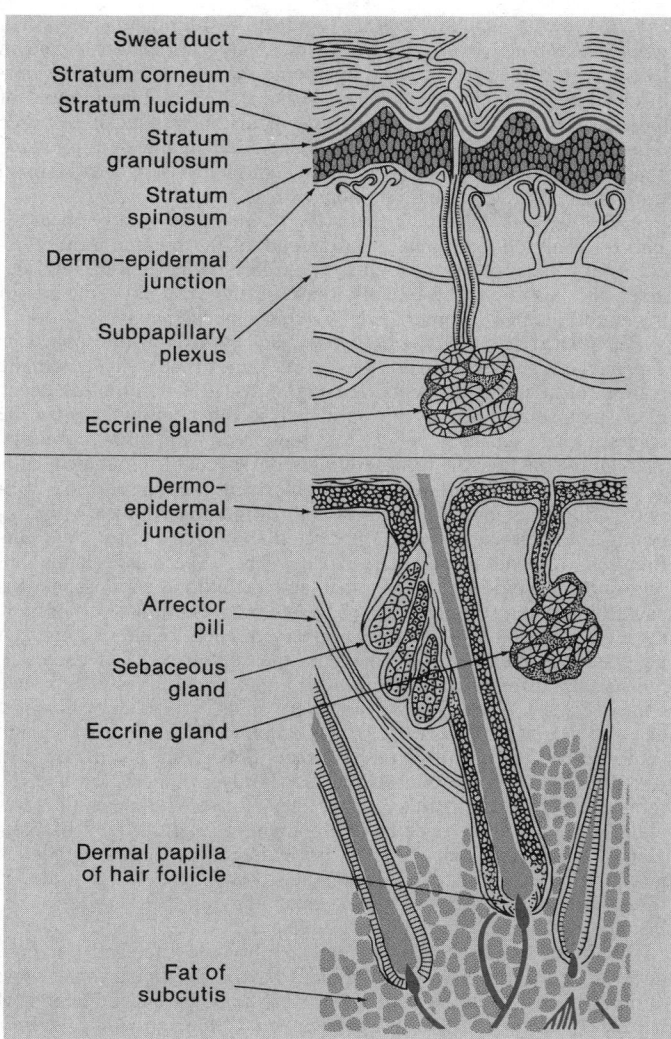

FIGURE 472–1. Structure of the skin. (Adapted from the 17th edition of the *Cecil Textbook of Medicine* with the permission of Dr. Marie-Louise Johnson.)

Two other cell types are found in the epidermis, the *melanocyte* and the *Langerhans' cell.* Both are dendritic cells with cytoplasmic arms that stretch out to contact the keratinocytes in their vicinity. The melanocytes are pigment (melanin)-producing cells that are arrayed in the basal epidermal layer and hair follicles, whereas the Langerhans' cells are usually found in the suprabasal layers of the epidermis, and at times in the dermis. Each dendritic cell has a different origin and function.

Melanocytes evolve in the neural crest of the embryo and migrate to the skin in early embryonic life. These cells synthesize brown, red, and yellow melanin pigments that give the skin its distinctive coloration. Melanocytes contain submicroscopic organelles (melanosomes) which synthesize melanin. A specific enzyme, tyrosinase, found within the melanosome, oxidizes tyrosine to dihydroxyphenylalanine (DOPA) and then to DOPA quinone. Additional nonenzymatic oxidation and polymerization occur to form the final product, melanin. Two kinds of melanin are recognized: eumelanin (brown-black biochrome) and phaeomelanin (yellow-red biochrome that contains large quantities of cysteine). The genetic make-up of the individual determines which melanin is produced, thus providing the various colors and hues of skin and hair. Once melanosomes are fully melanized, the resulting granules are transported out the dendritic processes of the melanocyte and transferred into the adjacent epidermal cells or hair.

Langerhans' cells, derived from bone marrow, contain a unique submicroscopic racket-shaped organelle (Birbeck granule) that plays a major immunologic role in the skin (Fig. 472–2). They contain surface receptors for immunoglobulins, and Ia-antigens, capturing

viable cornified cells is abrupt. The cornified layer consists of up to 25 layers of tightly packed, highly flattened horny cells.

The differentiation of the epidermal cells involves the formation of fibrous proteins known as *keratin.* The process of maturation of the epidermis (cornification) is complete in the stratum corneum yielding cells with mature keratin, namely, a system of filaments embedded in a continuous matrix (which is probably derived from the keratohyalin granules) within a thickened cell membrane. The stratum corneum limits the rate of passage of ions and molecules into and out of the skin. The insolubility and protective qualities of the stratum corneum is the result of (1) masses of keratin fibers embedded in keratohylin within the corneocytes, (2) the thickened cell membrane or cornified envelope, and (3) the deposition glucosylceramide and acylceramines in the intercellular s between the corneocytes by lamellated membrane bound organelles found in the upper spinous layer.

The basal layer of epidermis has a permanent population of germinal cells whose progeny undergo the specific pattern of differentiation just described. The new keratinocytes require about 14 days to evolve into stratum granulosum cells and another 14 days to reach the surface of the stratum corneum and be shed. Proper control of proliferation of basal cells and their subsequent orderly differentiation into keratinized stratum corneum cells produces the smooth, pliable surface of the skin. Alterations in the homeostatic state of cell division, defects in differentiation, or changes in exfoliation from the surface can lead to irregularities in the skin surface, characterized as roughening, scaling, and hyperkeratosis (accumulation of excessive layers of stratum corneum).

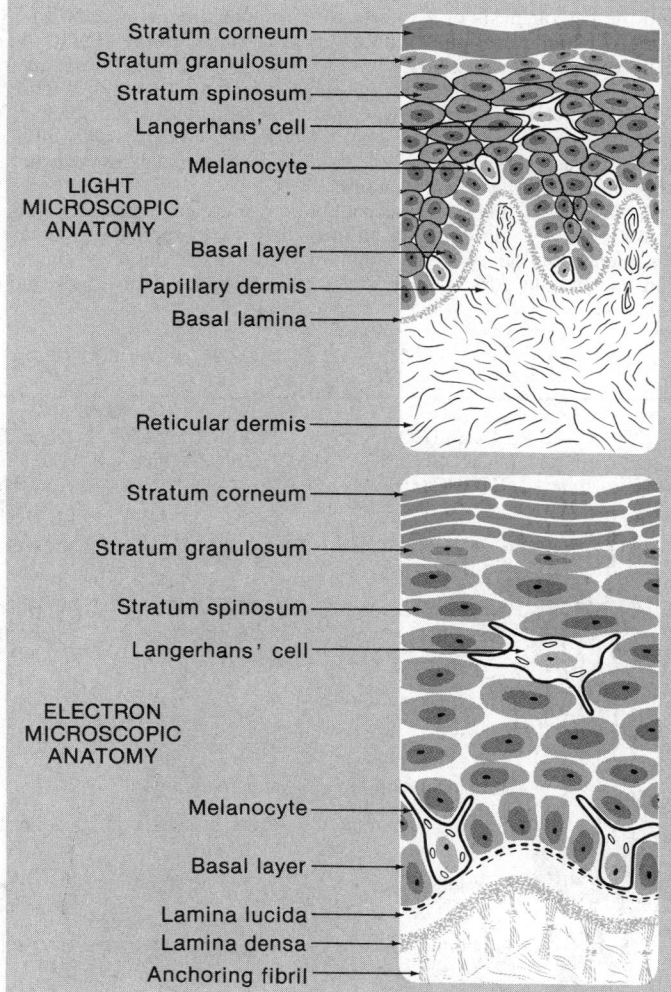

FIGURE 472–2. Diagrammatic representation of the light microscopic and electron microscopic anatomy of the skin.

external antigenic materials that contact the skin and circulating them to draining lymph nodes. Langerhans' cells thus play a central role in delayed hypersensitivity reactions of the skin (allergic contact dermatitis).

DERMIS. Beneath the epidermis lies the principal mass of the skin, the dermis, which is a tough, resilient tissue with viscoelastic properties. It consists of a three-dimensional matrix of loose connective tissue composed of fibrous proteins (collagen and elastin) embedded in an amorphous ground substance (glycosaminoglycans). At the microscopic level the collagen fibers resemble an irregular meshwork oriented somewhat parallel to the epidermis. Coarse elastic fibers are entwined in the collagenous fibers, being particularly abundant over the face and neck. This fibrous and elastic matrix serves as a scaffolding within which networks of blood vessels, nerves, and lymphatics intertwine and the epidermal appendages, sweat glands, and pilosebaceous units rest.

Dermoepidermal Junction. The structures situated at the interface between the epidermis and dermis constitute an anatomic functional unit of complex membranes and lamellae laced by divergent types of filaments that together serve to support the epidermis, weld the epidermis to the dermis, and act as a filter to the transfer of materials and inflammatory or neoplastic cells across the junction zone. At the level of light microscopy, this boundary zone is seen as an undulating pattern of rete ridges (downward finger-like or ridge-like extensions of the epidermis) and dermal papillae (upward projections of the dermis into the epidermis) (Fig. 472–2). Periodic acid-Schiff (PAS) staining discloses a thin uniform zone of intense reaction along this undulating junction which represents the basement membrane. Electron microscopic, immunoelectron microscopic, immunologic, biochemical, and genetic studies have elucidated the complexity of this region and are providing new insights into the pathogenesis of a variety of cutaneous diseases. Keratin filaments, hemidesmosomes, lamina lucida, lamina densa, anchoring filaments, and anchoring fibrils each function to maintain different levels of basement membrane adhesion. Figure 472–3 outlines these general structures, their molecular composition, and some diseases in which there is either a genetic defect in the synthesis of components of these structures or an autoantibody formed against the molecular components of the structure.

A variety of inherited mechanobullous diseases (epidermolysis bullosa) as well autoimmune bullous diseases (pemphigoid, herpes gestationis, bullous systemic lupus erythematosus) involve separation and bullous formation at various levels of the dermoepidermal junction.

Cutaneous Appendages. Two to three million *eccrine sweat glands* distributed over all parts of the body surface participate in thermoregulation by producing hypotonic sweat that evaporates during heat or emotional stress (Fig. 472–1). The combined output of these glands may exceed 1.5 liters per hour. Each gland is a simple tubule with a coiled secretory segment deep in the dermis and a straight duct extending up to the skin's surface. The glands respond to thermal stimulation and emotional stress.

Apocrine sweat glands in the axillae, circumanal and perineal areas, external auditory canals, and areolae of the breasts secrete viscid, milky material that accounts for axillary odor when bacteria degrade the secretion. Presumably, they are the vestigial remnants of lower species that communicate by cutaneous chemicals.

Pilosebaceous Appendages. Hair units, or pilosebaceous appendages, are found over the entire skin surface except on the palms, soles, and glans penis (see Fig. 472–1). Hair follicles consist of a shaft surrounded by an epithelial sheath continuous with the epidermis, the sebaceous gland, and the arrector pili smooth muscle. The bulb contains the proliferating pool of undifferentiated cells which gives rise to various layers comprising the hair and the follicle. The proliferating cells in the bulb differentiate into a hair consisting of keratinized, hard, imbricated, flattened cortex cells surrounding a central medullary space. The sebaceous glands are multilobular holocrine glands that connect into the pilosebaceous canal (hair canal) through the sebaceous duct. Germinative undifferentiated sebaceous cells at the periphery of each lobule of the gland generate daughter cells that move to the central areas of each acinus as they differentiate and form sebum (a complex oily substance composed of tri- and diglycerides, fatty acids, wax esters, squalene, and sterols). Most sebaceous glands adjoin a hair follicle, although some open directly on the skin surface. Sebaceous glands are also found normally in the buccal mucosa (Fordyce's spots), around the female areola (Montgomery's tubercles), on the prepuce (Tyson's glands), and in the eyelids (meibomian glands). The sebaceous glands and certain hair follicles are androgen-dependent target organs. Follicles particularly responsive to androgen stimulation are found over the frontal and vertex areas of scalp, beard, chest, axillae, and upper and lower pubic triangles.

Hair follicles are formed in early embryonic life, and no more develop after birth. Males and females have approximately the same number of hair follicles distributed over the body, but the degree of hairiness depends on two distinct features of hair growth—the *hair cycle* and the *hair pattern.* Hair growth consists of recurring cycles of growth, regression, and resting. The resting hair lies high in the follicle, where it forms a stubby hair bulb that is easily shed. Growth begins with a burst of mitotic activity and the follicle

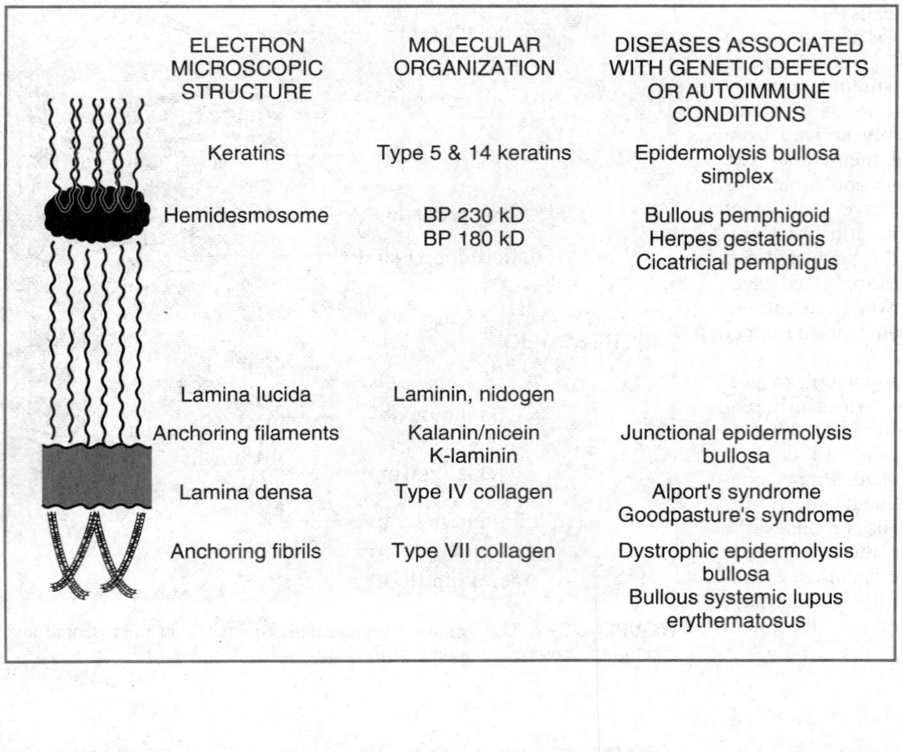

ELECTRON MICROSCOPIC STRUCTURE	MOLECULAR ORGANIZATION	DISEASES ASSOCIATED WITH GENETIC DEFECTS OR AUTOIMMUNE CONDITIONS
Keratins	Type 5 & 14 keratins	Epidermolysis bullosa simplex
Hemidesmosome	BP 230 kD BP 180 kD	Bullous pemphigoid Herpes gestationis Cicatricial pemphigus
Lamina lucida	Laminin, nidogen	
Anchoring filaments	Kalanin/nicein K-laminin	Junctional epidermolysis bullosa
Lamina densa	Type IV collagen	Alport's syndrome Goodpasture's syndrome
Anchoring fibrils	Type VII collagen	Dystrophic epidermolysis bullosa Bullous systemic lupus erythematosus

FIGURE 472–3. Structures and diseases of the dermoepidermal junction.

grows downward to reconstitute a new hair bulb. The hair bulb cells divide rapidly and keratinize to form a new hair shaft that dislodges the old resting club telogen hair. Regression provides a brief respite when mitosis ceases and the hair follicle pulls upward in the dermis as the hair shaft evolves into a resting club hair. In the adult scalp 85% of the hairs are in a growth state, 14% in a resting state, and 1% in regression. Considerable variation in timing of the hair cycle occurs from one region of the body to another, and the duration of growth determines the length of hairs.

Hair cycles also vary with the second important feature of hair growth, namely, hair pattern or the type of hair growing in each follicle. Two types of hairs are seen: vellus hair (fine, soft, short, nonpigmented, and common on "nonhairy" areas of the body) and terminal hair (coarse, long, pigmented, and found on hairy areas of the body).

Dramatic changes occur at puberty in both hair cycle and hair pattern mediated by either testosterone or dihydrotestosterone. The increased hairiness results from the conversion of vellus hair follicles to large terminal follicles. In the axillae and lower pubic triangle this conversion is mediated by testosterone and androstenedione. In other regions such as the beard, chest, upper pubic triangle, nostrils, and external ears, this conversion is mediated by dihydrotestosterone. Paradoxically, DHT also mediates the reverse process, namely, the miniaturization of large terminal follicles into vellus hairs. Such physiologic miniaturization occurs with the reshaping of the frontal hairline from a straight line to an M-shaped configuration at puberty. This occurs in all men and in the majority of women.

Maternal androgens ensure full development and function of sebaceous glands at birth. The vernix caseosa covering the neonate is mostly sebum. Normally sebaceous glands atrophy after birth, until puberty, when androgens again stimulate their activity. Acne is often one of the earliest signs of puberty. Disorders of androgen excess in adult women (e.g., polycystic ovary syndrome) are also associated with increased sebaceous activity and acne. Estrogens in large amounts decrease gland size and secretion.

FUNCTIONS OF THE SKIN

PROTECTION. Several structures in the skin, including the stratum corneum, melanin, cutaneous nerves, and the dermal connective tissue, provide important survival functions. The skin protects against the loss of essential fluids, the entrance of toxic agents and microorganisms, and damage from ultraviolet radiation, mechanical shearing forces, and extreme environmental temperatures.

The *stratum corneum* serves as a low-permeability barrier that retards water loss from the inner epidermal hydrated layers and also shields against environmental damage. The barrier properties of the horny layer are of practical importance from several points of view: Excessive drying or inflammatory reactions in the skin (e.g., eczema) lead to roughness, scaling, and disruption of the normally compact layers of horny cells. This leads to increased transepidermal water loss and, if severe (as in generalized exfoliative dermatitis, erythroderma, or burns), can contribute to fluid and electrolyte imbalance. With breaks in the horny layer, external substances more readily gain entrance to the underlying epidermis. Thus, various chemical substances, including medications placed on injured skin, have a greater opportunity to be absorbed or to act as haptens or antigens, increasing the possibility of allergic contact dermatitis. This becomes particularly common when topical antibiotics are applied to chronically inflamed skin, leading to superimposed allergic contact dermatitis. The disruption of the barrier also increases the chance of colonization of pathologic bacteria in the skin, especially in the presence of tissue fluid exudates, which serve as excellent culture media. Percutaneous absorption of various topical medications used in treating skin conditions, can be enhanced by hydrating the stratum corneum with the use of occlusive plastic wraps.

The stratum corneum normally harbors a number of aerobic and anaerobic resident organisms (i.e., *Staphylococcus epidermidis,* diphtheroids, *Proprionibacterium acnes,* and *Pityrosporon*). Breaks in the stratum corneum, poor hygiene, and excessive humidity with maceration (especially in intertriginous areas) all contribute to cutaneous infections such as impetigo, erysipelas, folliculitis, furunculosis, and ecthyma.

A second structural component that provides protection is the *melanocyte,* which produces melanin pigment. Melanin is a large polymer that has the unique capability of absorbing light over a

broad range of 200 to 2400 nm wave lengths. It serves as an excellent screen against the untoward effects of solar ultraviolet radiation, such as aging and wrinkling of the skin and the development of cutaneous neoplasms. The importance of melanin is dramatically illustrated by the high incidence of skin cancers in sun-exposed areas of the body, particularly in light-skinned, blue-eyed, easily sunburned individuals and in albinos. Ultraviolet light exposure also causes aging and wrinkling of the skin. Neither sex nor race affects the number of melanocytes in the epidermis. Negroid skin contains the same number of melanocytes as Caucasian skin, but the pigmentation is more intense as a result of the synthesis of more melanin that is dispersed throughout the melanocytes and adjacent keratinocytes. Accordingly, black skin is much less likely to form skin cancers, and it ages more slowly than white skin.

Dermal nerves play an important role in bodily protection. Nerve endings are extensively distributed in the skin in two general morphologic types: free nerve endings and specialized endings (Pacini's and Meissner's corpuscles), which mediate many sensations including pain, pressure, and itch. Loss of sensation (e.g., diabetic neuropathy) may result in deep traumatic ulcers (trophic ulcers) without the patient's awareness. Damage to the dermatomal nerves (e.g., herpes zoster) may result in prolonged burning pain and hypesthesias (postherpetic neuralgia).

Itch is mediated by cutaneous nerves. It may occur in conjunction with a number of dermatologic diseases or without clinically evident skin disease (pruritus) (Tables 472–1 and 472–2). Itch and pain are carried on unmyelinated C fibers found in the upper portion of the dermis of the skin, mucous membranes, and cornea. The afferent C fibers enter the dorsal horn of the spinal cord, synapse, cross the midline, and ascend the spinothalamic tracts to the thalamus. Then the impulse proceeds to the sensory area of the postcentral gyrus of the cortex. Cutting the spinothalamic tract, as in an anterolateral hemichordotomy, abolishes pain and itch. A variety of peripheral mediators stimulate the C fibers and induce itching. These include histamine, trypsin, proteases, peptides (bradykinin, vasoactive intestine peptide, substance P—all potent histamine releasers), and bile salts. Prostaglandins are modulators of pruritus rather than primary mediators, lowering the threshold to itching evoked by both histamine and pain. Central modulators of pruritus, such as systemic morphine, cause itch while relieving pain by acting on central opiate receptors. Regrettably, no single pharmacologic agent effectively treats all kinds of pruritus.

Generalized itching in the absence of primary skin disease (pruritus) may be an important sign of internal disease (Table 472–2). An important cause of pruritus is psychic stress. Some patients with psychogenic pruritus believe the itching is caused by invisible parasites in the skin. Such patients scratch until excoriations and prurigo papules (thickened papular areas of skin due to constant rubbing) evolve in areas that the patient can readily reach (extremities, scalp, upper back). Dry skin (xerosis) is a common cause of itching in older individuals. Certain drugs (aspirin, opiates) can cause itching without a visible rash. Patients with polycythemia vera display a unique form of itching triggered by sudden changes in temperature, especially when they emerge from a warm bath. The itch is prickly in nature and lasts minutes to hours.

The tough, viscoelastic properties imparted to the skin by the fibrous proteins (collagen and elastin) and amorphous ground substance that make up the dermis protect the skin against shearing forces. The viscous and elastic properties of the ground substance allow it to resist compression and accept molding, thus reducing point pressure on sensitive skin structures.

TABLE 472–1. SKIN DISEASES ASSOCIATED WITH ITCHING

Xerosis (dry skin)
Insect infestations (scabies, pediculosis, insect bites)
Dermatitis (atopic, contact, nummular) including poison ivy contact
Drugs (opiates, aspirin, quinidine)
Lichen planus
Urticaria
Dermatitis herpetiformis (burning itch)
Sunburn
Fiberglass dermatitis
Seborrheic dermatitis

TABLE 472–2. PRURITUS ASSOCIATED WITH SYSTEMIC DISEASE

Systemic Disease	Postulated Cause
Uremia	Secondary hyperparathyroidism, high skin calcium concentration, proliferation of mast cells, xerosis
Obstructive biliary disease	High concentrations of bile salts in skin
Primary biliary cirrhosis	
Cholestatic hepatitis secondary to drugs (chlorpropamide)	
Intrahepatic cholestasis of pregnancy	
Extrahepatic biliary obstruction	
Hematologic and myeloproliferative disorders	Unknown
Lymphoma including Hodgkin's disease	
Mycosis fungoides	
Polycythemia vera	
Iron deficiency anemia	
Endocrine disorders	Unknown
Thyrotoxicosis	
Hypothyroidism	
Diabetes	
Carcinoid	Serotonin
Visceral malignancies	Unknown
Breast, stomach, lung	
Psychiatric disorders	Unknown
Stress	
Delusions of parasitosis	
Neurologic disorders	Unknown
Multiple sclerosis (paroxysmal itching)	
Notalgia paraesthetic—local itch of back, medial shaft scapula (local neuropathy)	
Brain abscess	
CNS infarct	

THERMOREGULATION. Thermoregulation is subserved concomitantly by the cutaneous vasculature and the sweat glands. A massive network of interconnecting musculocutaneous arteries and venules, as well as capillaries, arteriovenous shunts, and small venules, plays a crucial role in the maintenance of body temperature (see Fig. 472–1). Most of the skin's blood resides in the large venous plexus, through which blood slowly moves close to the surface, dissipating heat. Equally important in thermoregulation is the formation of eccrine sweat, which provides cooling by evaporation from the skin's surface. Every gram of water that evaporates from the skin loses 580 calories of heat.

Blood flow through the skin is 10 to 20 times that required to supply needed metabolites and oxygen. Under basal conditions about 8.5% of the total blood flow passes through the skin, controlled primarily by the sympathetic nervous system. Blood flow can increase up to 3.5 liters per minute with exercise in a warm environment thereby dissipating large amounts of heat. Both central (hypothalamic heating) and peripheral thermoreceptors stimulate sweating via the sympathetic nervous system, but in the case of sweat glands, acetylcholine is the postganglionic transmitter. Increase in body core temperature is the strongest stimulus for inducing sweating, whereas peripheral (cutaneous) thermoreceptors are only one tenth as effective in eliciting perspiration.

Response to cold begins when cool blood passes the hypothalamus, which elicits both heat conservation and production mechanisms. Sympathetic stimuli constrict cutaneous blood vessels and hypothalamic impulses activate shivering, which increases heat production by as much as 50%. Conversely, when warm blood irrigates the hypothalamus, central heat production ceases and cutaneous blood vessels dilate allowing heat loss from the skin surface. Vasodilatation also occurs reflexly through direct warming of the skin surface (in warm environments). In addition, stimulation of the hypothalamus produces sweating and increases evaporative heat loss. Periodic exposure to heat or to heat and work stresses (i.e., daily 1- or 2-hour exposures for 10 to 14 days) enhances the secretory capacity of the eccrine sweat glands (acclimatization).

The crucial role of cutaneous vasculature in thermoregulation and cardiovascular homeostasis can be reversed by widespread inflammatory conditions of the skin causing *erythroderma*. Diseases such as generalized dermatitis, psoriasis, drug reactions, and underlying lymphomas, can cause generalized, inflammatory-based cutaneous vasodilatation that can divert 10 to 20% of cardiac output through the skin. To maintain blood pressure, cardiac output must increase and older individuals with impaired cardiac reserve can develop high-output failure accompanied by tremendous loss of body heat with wide swings in temperature and shivering.

THE SKIN AS AN ENDOCRINE ORGAN. Many metabolic activities of the skin are under hormonal regulation. Not only do sebaceous glands and certain hair follicles respond readily to androgens, but they are capable of many diverse steroid transformations, as described above.

Dihydrotestosterone causes sebaceous glands to enlarge at puberty, stimulates the growth of certain hair (male sexual hair of the beard, chest, upper pubic triangle, nose, and ears), and generates the growth and development of the external genitalia. Drugs such as cimetidine and spironolactone have antiandrogenic activity and have been used to treat acne and hirsutism. In addition, thyroid hormones can regulate hair growth and alter the texture of the skin (fine, sparse hair and smooth, soft skin in hyperthyroidism; coarse hair and cool, rough, thick skin in hypothyroidism). Other hormones affect melanin pigment formation, melanocyte-stimulating hormone, and estrogen-stimulating skin pigmentation.

THE SKIN AS AN IMMUNOLOGIC ORGAN. The epidermis and the dermoepidermal junctional area participate actively in immunologic reactions. The skin includes immunologically important cells including keratinocytes, Langerhans' cells, and melanocytes as well as immunologic structures such as the lamina lucida and basal lamina that are involved in bullous reactions of the skin.

Epidermal Immunologically Important Cells. The most important immunologic cell in the epidermis is the Langerhans' cell, comprising 2 to 5% of the total epidermal cell population. Langerhans' cells contribute to a number of immunologic reactions, including macrophage–T cell interaction, T and B lymphocyte interactions, graft versus host (GVH) reactions, and skin graft rejection. The Langerhans' cell synthesizes and expresses Ia antigens (Class II antigens, immune response gene–associated antigens) that are crucial in processing and presenting allergens to sensitized T lymphocytes critical in the elicitation of delayed hypersensitivity contact dermatitis. Lymphokines, made by the Langerhans' cells during these immunologic reactions, augment and enhance these processes and also contribute to the accompanying inflammatory response.

Keratinocytes participate in immunologic responses by expressing Ia antigens on their surfaces in such conditions as GVH reaction, mycosis fungoides, allergic contact dermatitis, lichen planus, and tuberculoid leprosy. In these conditions the keratinocytes make lymphokines, particularly interleukin 1, which provides a second signal supplementing macrophages (Langerhans' cells) in mitogen- and antigen-induced T cell activation. In addition, epidermal cells make other cytokines such as prostaglandin-E2 and leukotrienes that participate in inflammatory reactions in the skin. Keratinocytes are the immunologic target in the pemphigus group of diseases in which circulating autoantibodies against intercellular antigen of the epidermis and mucous membrane epithelium initiate intraepidermal acantholytic bullae.

The Dermoepidermal Junction. A variety of inflammatory diseases often characterized by bullous reactions seem to be mediated by immunoreactants, including IgG, IgA, and IgM, and complement deposition along the dermoepidermal junctional area. The anatomic site of blister formation correlates with the position of deposition of these immunoreactants. The antigens in several diseases have been isolated and partially characterized. The use of immunofluorescent techniques at the light microscopic and especially the ultrastructural level has been helpful in more precisely diagnosing these bullous conditions. These are summarized in Table 472–3, along with immunofluorescent skin findings in connective tissue diseases.

INFLAMMATORY REACTIONS IN THE SKIN AND WOUND HEALING. Cutaneous inflammation reflects the sum of the effects of biologic products of cells (mast cells, infiltrating neutrophils, monocytes/macrophages, lymphocytes) as well as the effects of the products of the complement system, membrane-

TABLE 472–3. IMMUNOFLUORESCENT CUTANEOUS FINDINGS IN IMMUNOLOGICALLY MEDIATED SKIN DISEASE

Diseases	Biopsy Findings of Direct Immunofluorescence Immunoreactants (DIF)	Ultrastructural Localization of Immunoreactants	Site of Blister Formation on Routine Light Microscopic Pathology	Serum Findings: Indirect Immunofluorescence (IIF)
Bullous Diseases				
Pemphigus (all forms)	Deposits of IgG intercellular areas between keratinocytes	Between keratinocytes	Suprabasilar in pemphigus vulgaris; substratum corneum in pemphigus foliaceus	IgG antibodies to intracellular areas of keratinocytes in 95% of patients
Bullous pemphigoid	IgG and/or complement (C) in basement membrane zone (BMZ)	Lamina lucida and hemidesmosomes—upper part lucida and sub-basal cells	Subepidermal	IgG Ab to BMZ in 70%
Cicatrical pemphigoid	IgG and/or C in BMZ	Lamina lucida	Subepidermal	IgG antibodies BMZ in 10%
Herpes gestationis	Complement in BMZ—occasionally IgG	Lamina lucida—close to lamina densa	Subepidermal—sub-basal cell—above lamina densa	IgG antibodies BMZ in 20% (HG factor in 25%)
Dermatitis herpetiformis	IgA and C in dermal papillae (granular deposits)	Granular IgA associated with microfibril bundles in dermal papilla	Subepidermal in dermal papillae—papillar dermal microabscesses	No circulating antibodies
Epidermolysis bullosa acquisita	IgG, C3 in BMZ	Sublamina densa amorphous granular deposits	Subepidermal	Frequent IgG autoantibodies
Linear IgA bullous dermatosis in childhood	IgA and complement in linear deposition in BMZ	—	Subepidermal	No circulating antibodies
Connective Tissue Diseases				
Bullous SLE	IgG, IgM, and complement in BMZ in involved and normal skin—linear homogenous	Just beneath lamina densa (basal lamina)	Subepidermal	Circulating antibodies to BMZ; ANA found in 90%
Discoid LE	IgG, other Ig, and C in lesional skin at BMZ	—	—	No circulating antibodies to BMZ, ANA titers normal
Systemic LE	IgG band at BMZ in normal skin (over 90% in sun-exposed areas)	—	—	Elevated ANA titers
Systemic sclerosis	Nucleolar IgG	—	Epidermal thinning and increased dermal collagen	ANA, speckled, 85%, centromere + in CREST syndrome
MCTD	IgG/IgM in BMZ in some patients; nuclear IgG in epidermis	—	—	Speckled ANA and ENA (extractable nuclear antigens)
Dermatomyositis	Negative	—	—	ANA often normal range

derived arachidonic acid metabolic pathways (prostaglandins and leukotrienes) and the Hageman factor–dependent pathways of coagulation, fibrinolysis, and kinin generation. Early phases of wound healing also encompass many of these reactions.

Cutaneous Inflammation. Several pathophysiologic reactions initiate inflammation, including infectious, immunologic, and toxic processes that affect the epidermis or dermis, or both. Mast cells in the skin function not only as the sentinel cells in immediate-type hypersensitivity reactions but also as major effector cells in inflammatory reactions. They release (1) histamine, prostaglandin D2, and leukotrienes, which cause vascular dilatation and increased permeability, redness, swelling, pain, and itch; (2) chemotactic factors for eosinophils and neutrophils; (3) proteases that interact with the complement, kinin, and fibrinolytic pathways; and (4) heparin, which contributes to local angiogenesis. Degranulation of mast cells occurs in response to various antigens that cross-link IgE on the mast cell surface (immediate hypersensitivity reactions), to by-products of complement activation C3a and C5a (as occurs in leukocytoclastic vasculitides), and to radiocontrast media, aspirin, insect venom, and various physical stimuli. Circulating peripheral blood cells infiltrate local tissue sites in response to chemotactic factors released by mast cells and other infiltrating cells. Basophils release histamine and chemotactic substances, such as those involved in allergic contact reactions, bullous pemphigoid, erythema multiforme, and inflammatory responses. Neutrophils release myeloperoxidase, acid hydrolases, and neutral proteases that are active against microbes and cause tissue destruction (dermatitis herpetiformis, psoriasis, leukocytoclastic vasculitis, and bacterial infections of the skin). Eosinophils release major basic protein and peroxidase (allergic drug reactions in the skin, bullous pemphigoid). Lymphocytes release lymphokines that modulate immunologic and inflammatory responses (lichen planus, lupus erythematosus, allergic contact dermatitis, tuberculoid leprosy). Monocytes and macrophages engulf foreign proteins and microorganisms (granulomatous reactions in the skin such as sarcoidosis, deep fungus and acid-fast bacilli infections, and cutaneous foreign body responses). Both classic and alternate complement pathways release products that induce mast cell degranulation and induce inflammation. (The activation of the system seems to contribute to inflammatory reactions in hereditary complement deficiencies causing lupus erythematosus–like syndromes or pyodermas, as well as necrotizing vasculitis.)

Wound Healing in the Skin. Healing proceeds temporally in three phases: substrate, proliferative, and remodeling. The initial substrate phase, encompassing the first 3 to 4 days after wounding, is so named because the cellular and other interactions lead to preparation for subsequent events. During this phase vascular and inflammatory components prevail (vascular clotting in the severed vessels; leukocyte and macrophage chemotaxis into the area to ingest bacteria, debride the wound, and degrade collagen). The proliferative phase (10 to 14 days after wounding) results in regeneration of epidermis, neoangiogenesis, and proliferation of fibroblasts with increased collagen synthesis and closure of the skin defect. The final remodeling takes place over 6 to 12 months, during which time a more stable form of collagen is laid down to form a scar of progressively increasing tensile strength. In some instances so much collagen is deposited in the healing wound that an elevated *hypertrophic scar* (red, raised scar within the boundaries of the original wound) or keloid (scar tissue extending beyond the boundaries of original injury into surrounding normal tissue) is produced. Keloids occur most commonly over the anterior chest, upper back, and deltoid regions. They rarely regress, and they recur after excision.

THE COSMETIC IMPORTANCE OF SKIN. Aging alters virtually all the structures and functions of the skin. Environmental insults, especially chronic sun exposure, cause far greater damage to the skin than time itself.

Changes with aging at the structural, physiologic, and biochemical level are as follows: Epidermal turnover rate decreases approximately 50% between the third and seventh decades. Concurrent loss of dermal elastic and collagen fibers accounts for the paper-thin, transparent quality of aged skin and the easy rupture of dermal vessels. An increasing cross-linkage of collagen and elastin accompanies aging, making the dermis more rigid and less able to withstand shearing forces. Aged skin, when "tented up," only slowly returns to its original form, whereas young skin readily snaps back. Sun-damaged aged skin shows microscopic collagen damage. Dermal collagen is replaced by amorphous basophilic staining material. This condition, termed *elastosis,* results in deep wrinkling and furrowing, especially over the face and back of the neck, and yellow papules and nodules in a reticular pattern on the face. Decreases occur in the number of functioning sebaceous and sweat glands contributing to the dryness of aged skin and to impaired thermoregulation in aged persons. Reduction in the vascular network in the skin surrounding hair bulbs and eccrine and sebaceous glands may be responsible for the atrophy of these appendages with age. A 50% reduction in the number of Langerhans' cells may account in part for the age-associated decrease in immune responsiveness and allergic contact dermatitis reactions in the elderly. Loss of enzymatically active melanocytes (10 to 20% per decade) causes irregular pigmentation of the skin and graying of the hair. Gradual reduction occurs in the number of body hairs, especially in the scalp, axillary, and pubic regions (related in part to decreased androgen production). Linear growth of nails also decreases by 30 to 50% between early and late adulthood. Often nails become brittle and thickened. A number of proliferative growths are associated with aging skin, including skin tags (acrochordon), cherry angiomata, seborrheic keratosis, lentigenes, and sebaceous hyperplasia.

Orkin O, Maibach HI, Dahl MV: Dermatology. Norwalk, CT, Appleton & Lange, 1991. *A complete, well-written text covering the structure and function of the skin as well as clinical dermatology.*

Soter NA, Baden HP: Pathophysiology of Dermatologic Diseases, 2nd ed. New York, McGraw-Hill, 1991. *A well-written, concise text that explores the scientific basis of cutaneous diseases.*

473 EXAMINATION OF THE SKIN AND AN APPROACH TO DIAGNOSING SKIN DISEASES

Frank Parker

General considerations in history taking and physical examination:

THE DERMATOLOGIC HISTORY

A proper history includes the following: where the patient's skin condition first appeared; what it resembled and what symptoms, if any, were associated with it; how the skin disease progressed and changed and what has been done to treat it.

A careful review of the systemic medications (both proprietary and prescribed) that the patient is taking is in order. The relationship of the onset of the skin rash to the use of systemic internal medications is particularly crucial in evaluating the possibility of a drug reaction.

A history of atopic diseases or skin cancer and a careful family history of skin problems help to identify genetic and familial aspects of dermatosis.

If one suspects contact dermatitis, a detailed work and hobby history can identify exposure to allergens or irritants. Environmental exposure to the elements such as sun, cold, and heat may provoke skin reactions. When dealing with possible infectious and parasitic processes of the skin, it is useful to seek for similar problems among family members or sexual partners.

Psychologic stress, although seldom a sole cause of cutaneous conditions, can exacerbate many dermatoses (e.g., acne, psoriasis, seborrhea, atopic eczema).

Dermatology is a visual specialty and the examiner's eye and a magnifying lens are its most important tools. Good lighting is essential, either daylight or fluorescent light simulating daylight. At times side lighting in a darkened room is useful for detecting minimally raised or depressed lesions.

The skin should be examined systematically from head to toe, so as to evaluate all regions of the integument, including the nails and mucous membranes. It is not unusual for the informed and observant physician to find some significant skin lesion, such as a basal cell carcinoma or even a melanoma, of which the patient is unaware. The general assessment of the entire skin allows the examiner to determine the pattern of the problem before focusing on specific lesions. Distribution may follow neural (as in a dermatome) or vascular patterns (as in livedo reticularis). In addition, factors related to the patient's general medical condition can also be discerned in the skin by noting signs of aging, pigmentation, trauma, nutrition, and hygiene. Color changes related to underlying systemic conditions (e.g., jaundice with hepatobiliary conditions, cyanosis with various cardiopulmonary diseases, diffuse hyperpigmentation with Addison's disease, paleness with anemia) all are important.

In each region of the body the physical examination includes three maneuvers: (1) *Observation* for color or surface changes. It is extremely important when observing skin lesions to use an alcohol sponge to wipe off existing cosmetics, oil, or foreign material. (2) *Touch or light stroking* to perceive texture changes, warmth, and moisture. Smoothness or roughness of the skin depends on such things as normal keratinization, proper hydration of the stratum corneum, and normal cutaneous blood flow. (3) *Palpation* to determine the consistency and pliability of the skin by stretching the integument between the fingers. Plasticity depends on the normal structure and function of dermal connective tissue and ground substance.

Because there are many hundreds of dermatoses, a logical process of elimination is required to narrow the possibilities, first to specific groups of diseases and finally to one condition. Such a diagnostic approach is based on specific morphologic descriptions of the skin lesions, together with an appropriate history and laboratory tests. Three steps are involved in this systematic approach. First, the entire skin is examined for primary and secondary skin lesions that allow the examiner to place the patient in one of nine diagnostic groups (the second step) (Table 473–1). Many skin conditions are found in each group, but all of the conditions in a given group express the same primary and secondary lesions. The third step involves singling out the patient's disease from the others in the group. This is done by looking for specific features, such as the distribution of skin lesions, any unusual shapes of the lesions or arrangement of several lesions (annular, serpiginous, dermatomal), color of the lesion including dominant hue and the color pattern, and the surface characteristics (particularly the appearance of scales or verrucous or vegetative changes).

STEP 1: DESCRIPTION OF PRIMARY AND SECONDARY SKIN LESIONS. Primary skin lesions are uncomplicated abnormalities that represent the initial pathologic change, uninfluenced by complications such as infection, trauma, or therapy. Secondary lesions reflect progression of the disease or scratching or infection of the primary lesions. Most of the primary changes can, at times, occur as secondary manifestations; for example, pustules may appear as primary lesions of folliculitis or as secondary lesions when scaling, itching lesions are scratched and infected. The trick is to recognize any single primary skin lesion as the initial change characteristic of the disease.

The terminology used to describe primary and secondary skin changes is the basic language of dermatology, the means by which one can accurately describe skin diseases to a colleague. If this terminology is not used correctly it is difficult to arrive at the precise diagnosis of skin diseases. Each descriptive word is not only a short account of what is seen on the surface of the skin but also relays specific information about processes within the skin. A diagrammatic representation and description of primary and secondary skin lesions are presented in Table 473–1.

STEP 2: ASSIGNMENT OF THE LESION TO A MAJOR GROUP OF DISEASES. Each disease within a given group shares the same primary and secondary skin lesions. Some diseases have overlapping traits so they may be assigned to more than one group.

TABLE 473-1. MAJOR GROUPS OF DERMATOLOGIC DISEASES BASED ON THE CLINICAL MORPHOLOGY OF THE SKIN CONDITION

Group	Clinical Morphology	Examples of Diseases in the Group
Eczema or dermatitis	Macules (erythema), papules, vesicles, lichenification, fine scaling, excoriations, tions, crusting	Contact dermatitis, atopic dermatitis, stasis dermatitis, photodermatitis, scabies, dermatophytoses, exfoliative dermatitis, candidiasis
Maculopapular eruptions	Macules, erythema, papules	Viral exanthems, drug reactions, verruca vulgaris, Kawasaki's disease, vasculitic and purpuric eruptions
Papulosquamous dermatoses	Papules, plaques, erythema with unique scales	Psoriasis, Reiter's syndrome, pityriasis rosea, lichen planus, seborrheic dermatitis, ichthyosis, secondary syphilis, mycosis fungoides, parapsoriasis
Vesiculobullous diseases	Vesicles, bullae, erythema	Herpes simplex and zoster, hand-foot-and-mouth disease, insect bites, bullous impetigo, scalded skin syndrome, pemphigus, pemphigoid, dermatitis herpetiformis, porphyria cutanea tarda, erythema multiforme
Pustular diseases	Pustules, cysts, erythema	Acne vulgaris and rosacea, pustular psoriasis, folliculitis, gonococcemia
Urticaria, persistent figurate erythemas, cellulitis	Wheals and figurate, raised erythema, scaling	Urticaria, erythema annulare centrifugum, erysipelas, necrotizing fasciitis
Nodular lesions	Nodules and tumors, some associated with erosions and ulceration	Benign and malignant tumors—basal cell cancer, squamous cell cancer, rheumatoid nodules, xanthomas
Telangiectasias, atrophic, scarring, ulcerative diseases	Atrophic, sclerotic telangiectasias and ulcerative changes	Connective tissue diseases, radiation dermatitis, lichen sclerosus et atrophicus, vascular insufficiency (arterial and venous), pyoderma gangrenosum
Hyper- and hypomelanosis	Increased and decreased melanin deposition in skin	Acanthosis nigricans, café au lait spots, vitiligo, tuberous sclerosis, xeroderma pigmentosum, chloasma, freckles

An arbitrary grouping that has proved to be of practical value is listed below and is used later in this chapter to discuss specific diseases within each group (Table 473-1).

STEP 3: NARROWING THE POSSIBILITIES TO THE EXACT DIAGNOSIS. Of great importance is the distribution of the skin disease, for many conditions have typical patterns or affect specific regions. For example, psoriasis commonly affects extensor surfaces and atopic eczema flexor areas of the extremities (Fig. 473-1). Photoreactions are confined to parts of the body exposed to sunlight. Involvement of the palms and soles is seen in erythema multiforme, secondary syphilis, psoriasis, and eczema. Contact dermatitis to exogenous allergens or irritants often presents with unusual patterns and distributions corresponding to the areas where the offending material came in contact with the skin. The best way to examine for distribution is to step away from the patient and view from a few feet away.

An important clue in differentiating diseases lies in the shape of the individual lesions and the arrangement of several lesions in relation to each other. A *linear* arrangement of lesions may indicate a contact reaction to an exogenous substance brushing across the skin, a pathologic process involving a vascular or lymphatic vessel, or a cutaneous nevus (Fig. 473-1). *Zosteriform* refers to lesions arranged along the cutaneous distribution of a spinal dermatome. They are unilateral and denote herpes zoster and, occasionally, metastatic carcinoma of the breast or the dermatomal hemangiomatous growths of Sturge-Weber syndrome. *Annular* lesions are circular with normal skin in the center. Annular macules are observed in drug eruptions, secondary syphilis, and lupus erythematosus. Resolving hives may leave annular configurations. Annular lesions with scale suggest dermatophytosis or pityriasis rosea. *Iris* lesions are a special type of annular lesion in which an erythematous annular macule or papule develops a second red ring or a purplish papule or vesicle in the center (target or bull's-eye lesion). Iris lesions are seen in erythema multiforme. *Arciform* lesions form par-

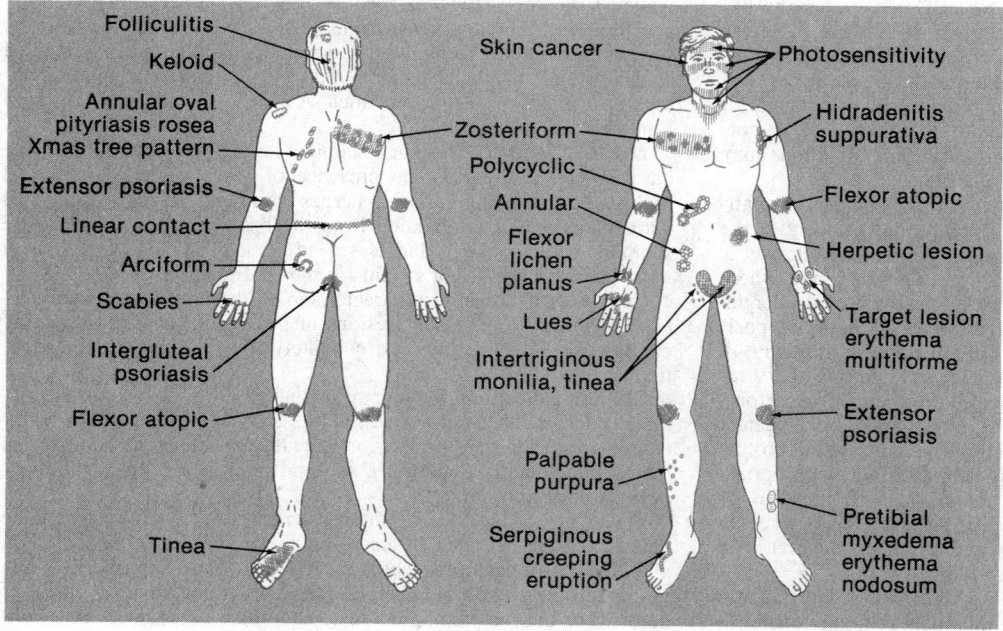

FIGURE 473-1. Configurational and regional diagnostic aids for the diagnosis of primary and secondary skin lesions.

tial circles or arcs and may be seen in dermatophyte infections. *Polycyclic* patterns evolve when numerous annular lesions enlarge and run together. Creeping eruptions and psoriasis produce *serpiginous* (snakelike, undulating, linear) patterns. *Herpetiform* refers to a grouping of lesions such as occurs in herpes simplex or dermatitis herpetiformis.

Other physical features influence diagnoses. Dry, lichenified lesions suggest a chronic state, whereas wet, weeping, macerated lesions suggest acute reactions. Abscesses are soft and fluctuant, whereas nodules are usually firm. Redness caused by dilatation of superficial blood vessels blanches with pressure, whereas erythema caused by extravasated blood as occurs in petechiae and purpuric lesions does not blanch. Hues of brown to black usually indicate melanin, although some drugs (e.g., tetracycline) cause brown-black pigmentation in the skin. The variation in color from melanin is related to the depth of the pigment in the skin—the deeper the pigment the more blue-black the color.

DIAGNOSTIC TESTS AND AIDS IN EXAMINATION OF THE SKIN

Certain aids and procedures, when combined with the history and physical examination assist accurate diagnosis.

VISUAL AIDS. *Magnification.* Magnification of skin lesions can detect the follicular plugging seen in discoid lupus erythematosus, or fine telangiectasias in the pearly, opalescent borders of basal cell cancers.

Transillumination. Oblique lighting in a darkened room can help to detect slight degrees of elevation or depression of lesions as well as fine wrinkling or atrophy of the epidermis. The application of a penlight directly to nodular lesions in a dark room may give clues as to their density and make-up. Cystic lesions allow transmission of some light, whereas nodules composed of cellular infiltrates do not.

Diascopy. Firm pressure with a microscope slide against skin lesions differentiates erythema of capillary dilatation from that of extravasated blood. Sarcoidosis, tuberculosis, and other granulomatous inflammatory reactions in the skin are suggested if diascopy of the lesions shows a characteristic "apple-jelly" or glassy, fawn-colored appearance.

Long-wave Ultraviolet or Wood's Light Examination. Long-wave ultraviolet light (UVA) (360 nm) is useful in evaluating several conditions of the skin. Wood's light exaggerates the differences in the degree of pigmentation when the skin is examined with the lamp in a dark room. Melanin is a universal absorber of UV light, so decreased melanin shows more reflection (light color) and increased melanin less reflection (darker color). Pigment in the epidermis is exaggerated with UVA light, but that in the dermis is not, so a reasonable guess as to the site of melanin in the skin can be made. Wood's light may be the only means of recognizing the hypomelanotic ash leaf-shaped macules of tuberous sclerosis. The extent of vitiligo and melanotic nevi (which appear darker than surrounding normal skin) can also be determined. Some superficial fungal infections of the scalp fluoresce blue-green; erythrasma, a superficial intertriginous bacterial infection that produces a porphyrin, fluoresces a brilliant coral red; *Pseudomonas* infections may give off yellow-green color under a Wood's light.

CLINICAL TESTS. *Patch Tests.* Patch testing is used to validate a diagnosis of allergic contact sensitization and to identify the causative allergen. Because the entire skin of sensitized humans is allergic, the test reproduces the dermatitis in one small area where the allergen is applied, usually on the back. The suspected allergen is applied to the skin, occluded, and left in place 48 hours. A positive test reproduces an eczematous response at the test site from 48 hours up to a week later. The latter is a delayed hypersensitivity reaction. Considerable experience is required to accurately perform and interpret patch tests. *Photopatch testing* is performed to detect photocontact allergy. Suspected photoallergens are placed on the skin in two sets. One set of allergens is irradiated with appropriate wavelengths of light after the patches are in place on the skin 24 hours; the second set of the same photoallergens is kept covered to serve as controls. Photoallergens cause an erythematous reaction that is evident 24 hours after exposure to light.

Physical Contact Testing. *Darier's sign* is the development of an urticarial and flare reaction after vigorously rubbing cutaneous mast cell (urticaria pigmentosa) lesions of the skin. The rubbing degranulates the mast cells, releasing histamine.

Nikolsky's sign demonstrates disadherence of the epidermal cells to one another. Pushing, rubbing, or rotating normal skin near bullous lesions causes the epidermis to be dislodged, leaving a moist, glistening defect. This sign is present in various forms of pemphigus and in toxic epidermal necrolysis.

The *Koebner phenomenon* occurs in certain skin diseases that tend to evolve new skin lesions after traumatic injury in areas of apparently normal skin. Thus, psoriasis may evolve within surgical scars and after sunburn or in the wake of a drug reaction involving the skin. Lichen planus may also exhibit this phenomenon.

Pathergy, the development of pustular and ulcerative lesions at the site of needle puncture, is suggestive of Behçet's syndrome and pyoderma gangrenosum.

Hair-pull examination is done to assess hair loss in the scalp. It is often useful to pull vigorously on scalp hairs to determine whether there is an increased number of falling hairs (normally only one or two can be removed with a tug of a group of hairs between the thumb and forefinger); ascertain the ratio of anagen to telogen hairs; and examine the hairs under a microscope for various congenital malformations of the shaft. Normally 10 to 15% of scalp hairs are in their resting phase. The percentage rises in naturally shed hair.

Paring Hyperkeratotic Lesions to Differentiate Warts from Calluses. After the hyperkeratosis is pared away, the wart displaces and obliterates epidermal ridges and small bleeding points, and black and red dots become visible. In calluses the epidermal ridges are not interrupted, and no vessels are seen within the callus.

LABORATORY PROCEDURES. *Gram Stain and Cultures.* Gram stain for bacteria and bacteriologic cultures are important when the primary lesion is a pustule or furuncle or appears to be impetigo. When an unusual cutaneous infection is considered in an immunosuppressed patient, a skin biopsy specimen can be minced or ground in a sterile mortar and cultured for aerobic and anaerobic bacteria, including typical and atypical mycobacteria, deep fungi, and *Candida*. A more rapid method of screening for infectious agents in immunosuppressed patients (often the first sign of septicemia in such patients is pustules, nodules, or ulcerative lesions) is to perform frozen sections on a skin biopsy specimen taken from the lesion and to obtain Gram stains, acid-fast bacterial stains, and PAS stains (to identify fungal and yeast elements). This may provide a diagnosis within a few hours.

Examination and Culture for Fungi and Candida. The presence of mycelia may be ascertained by applying 10% potassium hydroxide (KOH) to scale or exudative material scraped from suspected lesions and briefly heating the slide to dissolve the keratin. Hyphal elements can be observed by direct microscopic examination. Dermatophyte hyphae appear as long, branching, refractile, walled structures; *Candida* appears as shorter, linear hyphae in association with budding yeast forms (Fig. 473–1); tinea versicolor is seen as round yeast forms with short, club-shaped hyphae (so-called spaghetti and meatballs pattern). KOH examination of skin scrapings is mandatory to rule out tinea. A classic dictum is "if the skin lesion is scaly, scrape it."

Tzanck Smear. The microscopic examination of cells from the base of vesicles reveals the presence of giant epithelial cells and multinucleated giant cells in herpes simplex, herpes zoster, and varicella. Material is obtained from the base of a vesicle by gentle scraping with a scalpel and is spread on a glass slide and stained with Giemsa's or Wright's stain for the examination.

Skin Biopsy. Lesions characteristic of the eruption (primary lesions) should be biopsied. Lesions altered by scratching, infection, crusting, or lichenification are not likely to provide useful information.

Clinical indications for biopsy include lesions thought to be malignant; lesions that fail to heal, increase in size, bleed easily, or ulcerate spontaneously; tumors or growths of uncertain nature; and many inflammatory conditions, especially those for which the diagnosis is uncertain.

Four types of biopsies can be performed. The choice of technique determines the size and shape of the specimen obtained (Fig. 473–2). The procedure selected should secure the tissue most likely to contain the pathologic alterations and leave the smallest cosmetic defect. For the most complete histopathologic assessment an *ellipti-*

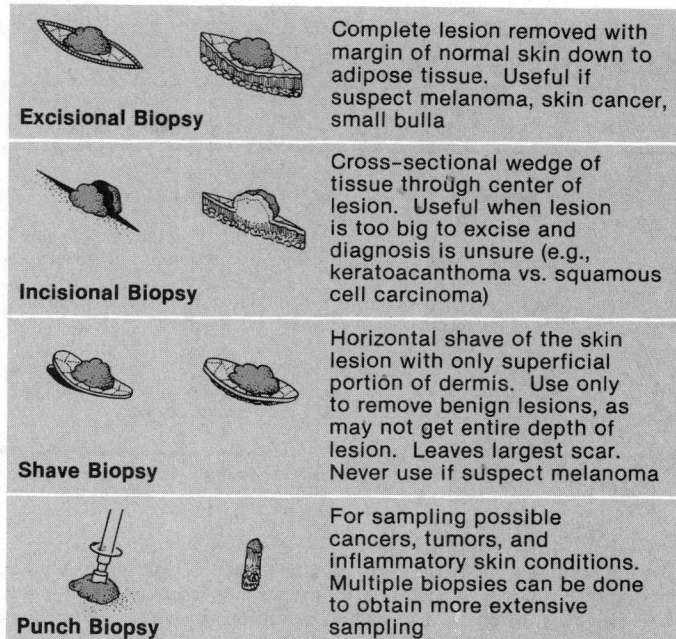

		Complete lesion removed with margin of normal skin down to adipose tissue. Useful if suspect melanoma, skin cancer, small bulla
Excisional Biopsy		
		Cross-sectional wedge of tissue through center of lesion. Useful when lesion is too big to excise and diagnosis is unsure (e.g., keratoacanthoma vs. squamous cell carcinoma)
Incisional Biopsy		
		Horizontal shave of the skin lesion with only superficial portion of dermis. Use only to remove benign lesions, as may not get entire depth of lesion. Leaves largest scar. Never use if suspect melanoma
Shave Biopsy		
		For sampling possible cancers, tumors, and inflammatory skin conditions. Multiple biopsies can be done to obtain more extensive sampling
Punch Biopsy		

FIGURE 473–2. Methods of skin biopsy.

cal, full-thickness excision is best because, in one procedure, the entire lesion is removed and secured for diagnosis and the remaining defect is easily sutured. The excisional biopsy technique is indicated when malignant melanoma is suspected or when a lesion is deep in skin or subcutaneous tissue and its orientation in surrounding tissue is relevant for diagnosis. A second procedure is the *paramedian incisional biopsy,* in which a thin but deep elliptical section is taken through the center of the lesion including normal skin at each end. This is especially useful in diagnosing large keratoacanthomas. A third biopsy method is the *shave,* or *parallel incision,* in which Xylocaine is injected locally under the lesion to lift it above the skin surface, and a scalpel (the knife horizontal to the skin surface) is used to "shave" off the protruding part of the skin and lesion. This technique is useful for diagnosing malignant and benign tumors when subsequent treatment by curettage and electrodesiccation is anticipated. It should never be used when melanoma is suspected, because the specimen obtained is too superficial for adequate histologic grading. Shave biopsy is convenient for removing superficial benign tumors such as seborrheic keratoses or skin tags. The fourth technique, *punch biopsy,* utilizes a tubular blade to cut out a circular plug of skin by slightly rotating and pushing the cutting edge deep into the dermis. The specimen is clipped off at its base with scissors, and the defect can be readily closed with sutures. Punch biopsies are used to diagnose inflammatory diseases and tumors.

If a first skin biopsy does not provide an answer, it is necessary and appropriate to rebiopsy. It is useful to give the pathologist an adequate clinical history to aid the interpretation.

474 PRINCIPLES OF THERAPY
Frank Parker

GENERAL CONSIDERATIONS

The goals of therapy are to define and remove the cause of a disorder, restore the structural and functional integrity of the skin, and relieve symptoms. Relief of such symptoms as itching, pain, or cosmetic disfigurement is an important goal. Damaged skin needs protection, as its barrier function is impaired. This can be assured with dressings and by minimizing scratching and avoiding abrasive clothing and soaps or chemicals. Removal of debris, such as excessive scale, hyperkeratoses, crusts, and infection, is also a crucial goal of therapy if the skin is to heal. Topical and systemic medications, dressings, and other treatments can alter skin temperature and blood flow and thus favorably affect the metabolism of the skin.

TOPICAL MODES OF THERAPY

SOAKS AND WET DRESSINGS. Water, with or without various additives, can provide many benefits to the skin, including soothing comfort, antipruritic effects, and increased rate of epidermal healing with hydration and debridement of crusts, dead skin, and bacteria.

Baths. When the area of involvement is too large to apply compresses, a bath is useful. Baths with whirlpool action are favored for debridement of large or deep ulcers. Medicated baths can evenly distribute soothing antipruritic and anti-inflammatory agents to widespread lesions. Starch and oatmeal complexes are commercially available in forms suitable for tub baths. Bath oil prevents drying by leaving a thin film of emollient on the skin. The tub should be one-half full and the soak should last no longer than 20 to 30 minutes to avoid maceration. Warm baths cause vasodilation and may increase itching; cool baths constrict vessels and usually soothe pruritus. The best time to apply lubricants is immediately after the bath so that they may hold water in the hydrated stratum corneum.

Wet Dressings. Water and medication can be applied to the skin with dressings (finely woven cotton, linen, or gauze) soaked in solution. As water evaporates, the skin cools and pruritus lessens. For maximal benefit from evaporation, dressings should be no more than a few layers thick and dipped in the solution and reapplied to the area of treated skin every few minutes for 15 to 30 minutes several times a day. Wet compresses, especially with frequent changes, provide gentle debridement, the cleansing resulting from transfer of crusts, scales, and cutaneous debris to the compress. If the compresses are permitted to dry (wet to dry compresses) and become adherent, the debriding effect can further damage the skin. Dried-out dressings should be remoistened to facilitate removal. Wet compresses also leach water-binding proteins from the stratum corneum and epidermis, causing drying, a desirable effect for moist, oozing and weeping lesions. Therefore they are useful in treating acute vesicular, bullous, oozing or weeping conditions as well as crusty, swollen, and infected skin.

Open wet dressings are applied directly to the skin, leaving the dressing exposed to the air to evaporate. Frequent reapplication debrides exudate, crust, and bacterial contamination and dries out the skin, rapidly decreasing oozing and weeping.

Closed wet dressings, in which the moist fabric dressings are applied to the skin and covered with an impervious material such as plastic, oil cloth, or Saran wrap, may be useful when maceration and heat retention are required. For example, they may be appropriate if there is excessive keratin of the palms or soles or when an early abscess needs heat to localize the infection.

Dry dressings protect the skin, apply medications, keep clothing and sheets from rubbing, and keep dirt away. Such dressings also prevent scratching and rubbing. In cases of neurodermatitis or stasis dermatitis, they often are left in place for several days. Soft casts or castlike boots (e.g., Unna boot) serve the same purposes.

The medication most commonly added to baths and dressings is aluminum acetate, which serves to coagulate bacterial and serum protein. As a 5% preparation it is known as Burow's solution, and it must be further diluted for use. Burow's solution can be readily made by dissolving tablets or powder packets in appropriate amounts of water. (One tablet or packet in 500 ml = 1:20 concentration.) Potassium permanganate and silver nitrate stain the skin, may be absorbed if used over large raw areas of skin, and in high concentrations may burn the skin. They seldom are used nowadays.

Other means of cleansing and debridement of wounds, in addition to wet compresses, include such products and procedures as absorption beads or granules that suck debris and exudate out of wounds (Debrisan, Duoderm granules), hydrogen peroxide, whirlpool treatments, and various enzymatic products including trypsin/chymotrypsin, fibrinolysin, collagenase, and streptokinase. Antimicrobial agents are seldom applied by surface dressings be-

TABLE 474-1. GUIDELINES FOR SOME DRESSING MATERIALS

Dressing	Polyurethane Films	Hydrocolloid Wafers	Hydrogel Sheets, Granules	Hydrophilic Powders, Pastes
Examples	Opsite Tegaderm	Duoderm Restore	Vigilon Gelperm sheets Spenco second skin dressing	Envisan Bard absorption
Indications	Protect red wounds Autolysis of yellow or exudative wounds	Protect red wounds Autolysis of yellow wounds	Protect red wounds Autolysis of yellow wounds	Cleansing infected wounds Protection of red wounds
Advantages	Wound visible Waterproof, decreases pain Decreases friction Cost effective	Absorbent, good barrier, reduces pain, easy to store	Absorbent, reduces pain, good conformity	Good filler for deep wounds, absorbent
Disadvantages	Nonabsorbent Sticks to healthy tissue	Odor with removal Nontransparent	Poor barrier Need cover dressing to secure	Occasional pain on application, can leak

Also useful are the alginate materials (Kaltostate and Sorbsan) that absorb wound exudate. Alginates are fibers processed from brown seaweed into pads. Exudate transforms the fibers to a gel at the wound interface.

cause huge quantities would be required to reach therapeutic concentrations.

"Occlusive dressings" are being used with increasing frequency in the treatment of acute wounds and chronic venous, diabetic, and pressure ulcers. A variety of new dressing materials are available, including polyurethane films, hydrocolloidal wafers, hydrogel sheets, and hydrophilic powders and pastes. Table 474-1 lists examples of these dressing materials and some indications for use. In general, these materials provide good protection, help promote healing, and provide pain reduction of skin ulcerations.

TOPICAL MEDICATIONS. Most topical medications consist of two major agents, the active ingredient or specific medication and the vehicle or base in which the active material is dissolved.

Bases or Vehicles. Bases come in a variety of forms. *Powders* promote dryness by absorbing evaporative moisture. They reduce maceration and friction in intertriginous areas. Powders may be inert chemicals (corn starch, talcum), or may contain medications. *Lotions* are suspensions of insoluble powders in water. As water on the skin surface evaporates, it cools and leaves a uniform film of powder on the surface. The addition of alcohol increases the cooling effect. *Creams* are emulsions of oil in water (more water than oil). They vanish into the skin because water evaporates and the residual oil is spread thinly and imperceptibly over the skin. *Ointments* consist of oils with variably smaller amounts of water added in suspension. They have a pleasant lubricating effect on dry or diseased skin, but they give a greasy feeling to the skin and clothing. Oils in bases give a softening effect to the skin by forming an occlusive layer that traps water and retards evaporation. Thus, ointments with large amounts of oil give a more sustained, softening effect than creams or lotions. Some ointments containing large percentages of inert oil may be occlusive and retain heat, increase pruritus, and increase percutaneous absorption of active ingredients. The more occlusive ointments should not be used on oozing or infected areas, as the resulting occlusion and warmth may increase bacterial growth. *Pastes* are mixtures of powder and ointment (e.g., zinc oxide paste). *Sprays* are propelled aerosols.

Selection of a base or emollient depends on the condition being treated and the needs of the patient. Lotions are useful for pruritic, oozing reactions. Petrolatum, by contrast, retains heat and promotes hydration and even maceration of the stratum corneum. Ointments are used most often on dry, scaling conditions in which endogenous hydration of the stratum corneum is defective. Between these extremes is a spectrum of possibilities that permit some cooling but add lubrication.

Active Agents—Specific Agents. Topical steroids provide effective local anti-inflammatory and antipruritic effects. Topical steroids cause immediate and profound constriction of cutaneous blood vessels. This is believed to prevent mobilization of polymorphonuclear leukocytes and monocytes into the reaction site. They also interfere with the inflammatory activities of already present cells (e.g., mast cells). Corticosteroids used in topical preparations are intrinsically active without need for further metabolism; this accounts for their rapid effect on cutaneous blood vessels as manifested by blanching of the skin. Therapeutic action is also rapid. Topical steroids slow the mitotic rate of fibroblasts, decrease collagen synthesis and possibly enhance collagen catabolism. They further interfere with phagocytosis and the skin's ability to fight off bacterial, viral, and fungal infections. All effective topical corticosteroids have the basic hydrocortisone structure. A 1% concentration of hydrocortisone ointment or cream serves as a norm for comparing potency of subsequently modified topical steroids. By fluorinating hydrocortisone or adding acetonide, the potency of the steroid is greatly enhanced.

Topical corticosteroid preparations may be classified in a general way as of low, intermediate, or high potency (Table 474-2). The potency corresponds closely to the degree of anti-inflammatory effectiveness as well as to the incidence and severity of associated side effects. Although some corticosteroids (particularly fluorinated compounds) are more topically active than others, the potency of a preparation also relates to the concentration of active drug in the vehicle and the nature of the vehicle. Because corticosteroids are poorly soluble in most vehicles, many preparations deliver only a fraction of the drug to target cells. Of the various types of vehicles used in steroid preparations, ointments are the most efficient because they most effectively dissolve steroids, and the occlusive nature of ointments increases stratum corneum permeability. Second

TABLE 474-2. POTENCY RANKING OF SOME COMMONLY USED TOPICAL STEROIDS

Potency	Generic Name	Clinical Application
Most potent	Clobetasol propionate cream and ointment 0.5%, halobetasol propionate cream and ointment 0.5%, betamethasone dipropionate cream and ointment 0.5%, clobetasol propionate cream and ointment 0.5%, halcinonide cream and ointment 0.1%, fluocinonide ointment 0.5%	Recalcitrant psoriasis, discoid lupus, recalcitrant lichen planus, nummular eczema
Intermediate potency	Triamcinolone acetonide 0.1%, betamethasone nolerate cream 0.1%, amcinonide cream 0.17%	Dermatitis—allergic contact, atopic eczema, neurodermatitis
Low potency	Hydrocortisone cream and ointment 2.5% and 1.0%, desonide cream and ointment 0.5%, locoid ointment 0.1%, dexamethasone sodium phosphate cream 0.1%	Intertrigo, pruritus ani, seborrheic dermatitis

in order of efficiency is acetone-alcohol gel, whereas creams and lotions are less useful. Table 474–2 lists examples of topical steroids and their grouping according to potency.

The adverse effects of topical steroids relate almost exclusively to the intermediate and high-potency compounds. Epidermal and dermal atrophy can be pronounced; decreased collagen synthesis and reduced stromal support for dermal blood vessels lead to telangiectasia, purpura, and striae. These are especially likely to occur in intertriginous "occluded" areas of the skin and on the face. Fluorinated steroids can cause a perioral scaling, papular and pustular dermatitis, or facial redness, telangiectasia, and acne rosacea-like eruption. Potent topical steroids applied for prolonged periods around the eyes can occasionally cause glaucoma and even cataracts. Topical steroids can predispose to or worsen skin infections such as folliculitis, tinea, and candidiasis. Systemic absorption of potent topical steroids may lower plasma cortisol levels when they are used with occlusion over as little as 20% of the body, but this is unusual.

Intermediate-potency steroids are useful in most dermatologic conditions. Ointments are useful for thickened skin or for dry, exposed areas where creams or gel preparations rapidly evaporate. Low-potency steroids are used to treat the face and the thin and occluded skin of the groin and genital area. Lotions and gels are best for hairy areas. High-potency steroid preparations should not be used to treat most dermatologic conditions. Their use is primarily reserved for areas of skin that have been substantially thickened by disease, such as dense plaques of psoriasis or chronic dermatitis. Table 474–3 gives some guidelines for selecting the steroid potency and vehicle most useful in various areas of the body.

Topical steroids are usually applied once or twice a day. The stratum corneum acts as a reservoir and continues to release topical steroid into the skin after the initial application. Chronic dermatoses become less responsive after prolonged use of topical steroids. This phenomenon is referred to as *tachyphylaxis*. Changing to another topical steroid often overcomes this phenomenon.

Intralesional corticosteroids are used to shrink inflammatory acne cysts and hypertrophic scars and keloids. They are occasionally injected into unresponsive, localized dermatoses such as alopecia areata, granuloma annulare, discoid lupus erythematosus, psoriasis, and lichen simplex chronicus. Several types of steroids are used for this purpose, varying in their duration of action. Triamcinolone acetonide is the most widely used, and its maximal duration of action is 4 to 6 weeks. Triamcinolone hexacetonide is longer acting (6 to 8 weeks); injectables of shorter duration (2 to 4 weeks) include Celestone and Decadron. The steroids should be diluted to less than 5 mg per milliliter to avoid the risk of causing skin atrophy. Intralesional steroid preparations are crystalline and dissolve in the tissues slowly over weeks to months. To avoid disfiguring atrophy, great care is necessary in using low concentrations and shaking the diluted material just prior to injecting into the dermis.

Topical Antibiotics. These help suppress bacteria in erosions or superficial infections and occasionally in chronic leg ulcers. Silver sulfadiazine preparations are particularly useful as an adjunct to currently accepted principles of burn wound care. The commonly used topical antibiotics are bacitracin, neomycin, clindamycin phosphate, erythromycin, and tetracycline hydrochloride. The latter three are used to treat acne vulgaris. All topical antibiotics have the potential to sensitize, but neomycin is particularly prone to do so, especially after long-term use on chronic stasis dermatitis and leg ulcers. Mupirocin, a new topical antibiotic ointment, is particularly useful in treating staphylococcal and streptococcal infections of the skin; when used three times a day for a week it eliminates 87% of skin pathogens and may decrease nasal staphylococcus carriers.

Topical Antifungal Agents. Antifungals treat localized infections by superficial dermatophytes, *Candida,* and tinea versicolor. Topical broad-spectrum antifungal preparations effective against all of these organisms include clotrimazole, econazole, and miconazole creams and lotions used twice daily. Topical agents useful against dermatophytes but not *Candida* include haloprogin and Tinactin. Over-the-counter preparations, perhaps less effective against dermatophytes, are undecylenic acid and Verdefam. No topical preparations are useful against nail infections with these fungal organisms. Nystatin creams, oral suspensions, and vaginal tablets are effective against *Candida* infections in various areas of the body. Ketoconazole is a broad-spectrum imidazole antifungal agent highly effective against dermatophytes, *Candida,* and tinea versicolor. It is available in cream and oral forms.

Tars and Anthralin. Crude coal tar is often applied directly to the skin to treat psoriasis. Tars increase the effectiveness of ultraviolet light and reduce the accelerated mitotic rate of keratinocytes in psoriasis. Tars are often incorporated into shampoos for control of seborrheic dermatitis and in bath oils for use in psoriasis.

Anthralin is a synthetic coal tar derivative that is used in the treatment of psoriasis. Both tar and anthralin cause staining of clothing and skin. They can also be irritating. Anthralin must be started at the lowest concentrations (0.1%) and initially left on the skin for short periods of time (0.5 hour) to avoid irritation.

Antiparasitic Topical Medications. Antiparasitics are employed for the treatment of pediculosis capitis, pediculosis pubis, and scabies. The lice of pediculosis corporis live in the seams of clothes and bedding. These must be disinfected by washing or dry cleaning. One per cent gamma benzene hexachloride (lindane), cromatiton, and pyrethrin compounds (RID) all are useful in treating pediculosis and scabies. Lindane is not suggested for children less than 6 years of age or for pregnant or lactating women. Permethrin 5% (Elimite Cream), a synthetic pyrethroid used for the treatment of scabies, has been particularly effective with one application, especially as some scabies organisms appear to be developing resistance to lindane. Other, but less effective forms of therapy for scabies, include 10% crotamiton (Eurax) and topical sulfur ointments (5% in HEB cream). These require frequent applications.

Antiseptic Cleaners. These bacteriostatic or bactericidal agents are used as local or generalized skin cleansers and for wound irrigations. "*Chlorhexidine*" is active against gram-positive and negative bacteria and some fungi and yeasts. *Antiseptic* iodinated compounds slowly liberate iodine, which is effective against bacteria, fungi, yeasts, and viruses. One of the most frequently used preparations is povidone-iodine.

Sunscreens. Sunscreens help protect the skin from the acute and chronic effects of UV radiation. They are rated by their sun protective factor (SPF). The SPF, which ranges from 3 to 50, is the factor by which the product extends the period of exposure to reach the sunburn reaction that would have taken place without the sunscreen. The action of topical photoprotectives is to reduce penetration of photoactive nonionizing radiation. Such protection can be achieved by either absorbing or reflecting the radiation. No sunscreen enhances tanning. Rather, if partial block is achieved, it permits melanin production relative to the radiation transmitted and the inherent capacity of the partially protected skin to respond. Most sunscreens are less effective in blocking UVA (320 to 400 nm) than UVB (290 to 320 nm). Para-aminobenzoic acid and its esters protect the skin from UVB and allow UVA to pass. Other non-PABA chemical sunscreens such as benzophenones and cinnamates are also useful against UVB and, to some extent, UVA. If protection against UVA is required, a sunscreen containing benzophenones or anthranilate compounds should be sought. For complete protection

TABLE 474–3. GUIDELINES FOR SELECTING TOPICAL STEROIDS

Location or Type of Lesion	Suggested Potency of Steroid	Suggested Vehicle
Areas of Body		
Trunk, arms, legs	Intermediate or low	Ointment or cream
Palms, soles	Intermediate or high	Ointment
Scalp	Intermediate or low	Lotion, gel, aerosol
Intertriginous areas	Low	Cream, lotion
Face	Low	Cream, lotion
Area around eyes	Low	Cream or ophthalmic preparation
Ears	Intermediate or low	Cream, gel, or lotion
Types of Lesion		
Dry, scaling, fissuring, lichenified lesion	Intermediate	Ointment
Thickened, hyperkeratotic skin patches	High	Ointment
Oozing, weeping lesions	Intermediate	Lotion, cream
Ulcerative lesions	Do not use topical steroids	

or total blockade of UVB and UVA, physical sunscreens containing titanium dioxide, zinc oxide, or iron oxide are available as heavy creams or pastes that reflect ultraviolet light.

Topical Scar and Keloid Treatment. Silicone (Sialastic) gel sheeting has been found to prevent and treat chronic hypertrophic and keloid scars. Sialastic gel sheeting is a soft semiocclusive polymer that, when chronically bandaged to the scar for 12 to 24 hours per day for at least 2 months, makes hypertrophic and keloid scars flatter and more flexible. The mechanism is not known.

SYSTEMIC MODES OF THERAPY FOR DERMATOLOGIC CONDITIONS

ANTIHISTAMINES. The most specific use of antihistamines is to ameliorate or halt histamine-mediated disorders such as urticaria, angioedema, and allergic rhinitis. Antihistamines also suppress non-histamine-induced itching by soporific side effects. Antihistamines are of two major classes, the classic H_1 blockers and the newer H_2 blockers, which also decrease gastric acid secretion. H_1 blockers have three problems: (1) They don't block all the effects of histamine. (2) They provide only limited protection against anaphylaxis because mediators other than histamine are involved in this reaction. (3) They are not selective in their effects (i.e., they also have anticholinergic and sedative effects). Antihistamines (H_1 blockers) can be arranged into several groups depending on their molecular configurations (Table 474–4).

An effective agent for a given patient may be selected from one group or from a combination of groups, but its effects are unlikely to be enhanced by combining antihistamines within a given group. If response to one antihistamine is minimal, another from a different group should be added or substituted. Evidence that blood vessels in human skin have H_2 as well as H_1 receptors has led to the evaluation of H_2-receptor antagonists such as cimetidine in combination with an H_1 antagonist, and the combination has proved to be effective in the treatment of some cases of chronic urticaria otherwise unresponsive to H_1 antagonists.

Antihistamines should be started in moderate doses until sufficient improvement or troublesome side effects develop. Generally, they are administered three or four times a day. Low doses should be given to elderly patients, as they are unusually sensitive to central nervous system side effects such as confusion, dizziness, and syncope, as well as to urinary retention, dry mouth, and blurred vision. In children, paradoxically, antihistamines may induce hyperactivity.

SYSTEMIC STEROIDS. Systemic steroids are used for a number of dermatologic conditions, but they have several drawbacks: (1) Prolonged administration leads to adrenal suppression and susceptibility to infection. (2) Many diseases such as psoriasis and atopic dermatitis may worsen after steroid withdrawal. (3) Safer and simpler therapy is available for most common dermatoses. Systemic

TABLE 474–4. ANTIHISTAMINES ARRANGED ACCORDING TO THEIR MOLECULAR CONFIGURATION

Antihistamine Group	Generic Name (Proprietary Name)
H_1 receptor antagonist	
Ethanolamine	Diphenhydramine (Benadryl)
	Clemastine (Tavist)
Piperidines	Cyproheptadine (Periactin)
	Azatadine (Optimine)
Phenothiazines	Promethazine (Phenergan)
	Trimeperazine (Temaril)
Alkylamines	Chlorpheniramine (Chlortrimeton)
	Dexchlorpheniramine (Dimetane)
Ethylenediamines	Tripelannamine (Pyribenzamine)
	Pyrilamine (Neoantergan)
Piperazines	Hydroxyzine (Atarax)
	Meclizine (Bonamine)
Nonsedating antihistamine	Terfenadine (Seldane)
	Astemizole (Hismanil)
	Loratadine (Claritan)
Miscellaneous H_1 receptor antagonists	
Tricyclic compounds	Doxepin (Sineovan)
H_2 receptor antagonist	Cinetidine (Tagamet)
	Ranitidine (Zantac)

TABLE 474–5. THE ORAL AZOLE DRUGS

Agent	Tablet Strength	Absorption	Common Adverse Effects
Ketoconazole	200 mg	Acid in stomach Best on empty stomach	N, V, pruritus, rash, headache, hepatitis 2–10% patients, anaphylaxis in large doses, adrenal insufficiency, decreased libido, gynecomastia
Fluconazole	50, 100 200 mg	No effect of acid or food on absorption	N, V, rash, hepatitis is rare, headache, confusion, leukopenia, Stevens-Johnson syndrome especially in AIDS
Itraconazole	100 mg	Acid in stomach	N, V, pruritus, rash, hepatitis is rare, hypokalemia, hypertension

corticosteroids are used in three types of situations. First, patients severely ill with life-threatening diseases known to be responsive to corticosteroids (anaphylactic reactions, extensive erythema multiforme, acute exfoliative dermatitis, pemphigus vulgaris) should be started as high doses—80 to 100 mg daily. Second, patients with acute and severe but self-limited conditions are treated with steroids to control or suppress episodes. Examples include widespread poison ivy dermatitis, extensive sunburn, and acute generalized urticaria of known cause. Third, steroids are used for patients with chronic dermatologic conditions that, because of periodic exacerbations, intermittently require low doses (15 to 20 mg) of prednisone together with supportive topical therapy. Examples include flares of chronic atopic dermatitis, pemphigoid, and some connective tissue diseases.

SYSTEMIC ANTIFUNGAL AGENTS. Several systemic agents are available for treating not only systemic but superficial fungal infections. These can be considered as two types of medications: (1) griseofulvin and (2) oral azol drugs, including ketoconazole, fluconazole, and itraconazole.

Griseofulvin is active against dermatophytes but not against tinea versicolor or *Candida*. It is fungistatic, entering the horny layer of the skin via the sweat and the nails by incorporation into the keratinizing cells of the nail matrix. The entire nail must grow out with griseofulvin incorporated into it before the tinea at the distal end of the nail is affected. Accordingly, griseofulvin must be taken for many months before dermatophyte infections of the toenails disappear. Less time is required for infections of the fingernails and glabrous skin. Griseofulvin has rare side effects, including photosensitivity, urticaria, angioedema, headaches, gastrointestinal upset, and granulocytopenia. The drug may intensify underlying porphyria. Alleged, hepatotoxicity is not well documented. Griseofulvin also decreases the activity of warfarin-like drugs so that patients taking these agents may require dosage adjustments after griseofulvin therapy. Griseofulvin comes in several different packaging forms. Manufacturer's instructions for its use should be consulted before specifically ordering the drug. Griseofulvin also is effective in treating tinea capitus, onychomycosis, and tinea corporis too extensive for topical therapy and for superficial fungal infections in immunosuppressed patients.

Azol drugs are synthetic compounds that are classified as imidazoles (miconazole and ketoconazole) or triazoles (itraconazole and fluconazole) according to whether they contain two or three nitrogen atoms, respectively, in the five-membered azole ring. The antifungal effects of the azoles are due to their ability to inhibit ergosterol synthesis, critical for maintaining fungal membrane integrity. Ketoconazole and itraconazole are available only for oral use, requiring an acid environment for optimal absorption. Fluconazole is available in both oral and intravenous formulations.

Table 474–5 outlines some information regarding these azoles. Ketoconazole is effective against dermatophytes and, unlike griseofulvin, also against tinea versicolor and *Candida*. Several instances of fatal hepatocellular toxicity have been recorded, so ketoconazole should be used only for extensive cutaneous dermatophyte infections unresponsive to griseofulvin or for extensive cutaneous *Candida* infections. Liver enzyme levels should be determined before starting treatment and monitored at monthly intervals during treatment. Because most cases of azole-related hepatitis occur during the first few months of treatment, monitoring is especially important during this time. (Aminotransferase determinations are particularly sensitive in identifying early drug-induced hepatitis.)

It is not entirely clear what the role of itraconazole and fluconazole will be in treating superficial fungal infections. Several reports have noted favorable results of treating tinea corporis and cruris, onychomycosis, and cutaneous candidiasis with once-weekly doses of oral fluconazole for 2 to 4 months (150 to 200 mg once a week).

RETINOIDS. Retinoids are derivatives of natural vitamin A compounds. Two retinoids, isotretinoin and etretinate, are available for use in the treatment of dermatologic conditions. Retinoids decrease epidermal cell proliferation and keratinization and inhibit sebaceous gland activity. Etretinate has been found to be useful in severe psoriasis, especially the erythrodermic and pustular forms, as well as in several forms of ichthyosis. Isotretinoin has proved to be especially useful in severe cystic acne, often inducing prolonged remissions for several years after the drug is given for the usual 3- to 4-month course. The retinoids have many side effects, including cheilitis, conjunctivitis, dryness and fragility of skin, congenital malformations (heart defects, hydrocephalus, microtia), osteophytic growths on the vertebrae, epiphyseal closure in growing youngsters, corneal opacities, night blindness, and elevations of very low density and low density lipoproteins. 13-cis retinoic acid (Accetane) should be given for severe nodulacystic acne. When given in doses of 0.5 to 1.0 mg per kilogram for 4 to 5 months, clearing of the acne occurs in 85 to 95% of patients, and some 85% of these patients remain essentially clear of their acne indefinitely. Some 10 to 15% of patient's acne recurs and requires repeat courses of isotretinoin.

SYSTEMIC GOLD SALTS. Chrysotherapy has been useful in the treatment of autoimmune bullous disease, particularly pemphigus vulgaris. Intramuscular compounds have been used in the same manner as in rheumatoid arthritis. Remissions with a mean duration of 21 months or longer have been obtained in some patients with these bullous diseases. Generally a total dose of 400 to 600 mg of gold must be given before bullae respond. The experience with oral gold (Aurinotin) is limited in its use in dermatologic conditions.

SYSTEMIC ANTIBIOTICS. These are frequently used to treat cutaneous bacterial infections and conditions aggravated by bacterial overgrowth such as acne vulgaris, acne rosacea, and acute dermatitis. Most cutaneous bacterial infections involve *Staphylococcus aureus* or *Streptococcus pyogenes* (erysipelas, cellulitis, folliculitis, furunculosis, carbunculosis). Penicillins, cephalosporins, and erythromycins are commonly used to treat these conditions. Erythromycin and tetracyclines can control acne vulgaris and acne rosacea. Trimethoprim-sulfamethoxazole is used for pyodermas in patients allergic to penicillin or caused by methicillin-resistant *S. aureus,* as an alternative therapy for gonorrhea, and occasionally for the treatment of acne vulgaris. The sulfone antibiotic dapsone is occasionally used successfully to treat noninfectious diseases such as dermatitis herpetiformis, pyoderma gangrenosum, and leukocytoclastic cutaneous vasculitis.

ANTIMALARIALS. Chloroquine, hydroxychloroquine, and quinacrine benefit cutaneous lupus erythematosus, polymorphic light eruption, solar urticaria, and porphyria cutanea tarda. Antimalarials bind DNA, inhibit the LE cell phenomenon and antinuclear antibody reactions, block chemotaxis, and antagonize histaminic responses, all of which may be related to the therapeutic effects on the diseases mentioned above. Cutaneous and mucous membrane pigmentation, nausea, diarrhea, and cycloplegia are common toxic effects, but retinopathy is the adverse reaction of greatest concern. Quinacrine does not cause retinopathy.

SYSTEMIC ANTIVIRAL AGENTS. Acyclovir and vidarabine can treat herpes simplex and zoster skin and systemic infections. Ch. 339 details their usage.

SYSTEMIC CYTOSTATIC DRUGS. Cytotoxic drugs such as methotrexate, cyclophosphamide, azathioprine, and hydroxyurea are used in a number of skin conditions when they cannot be controlled by more conventional means. Thus, psoriasis, when it is generalized, severe, and life-ruining, may be treated with modest doses of methotrexate, azathioprine, or hydroxyurea; life-threatening bullous diseases such as pemphigus vulgaris are occasionally treated with these agents as an alternative to high doses of corticosteroids.

SULFONES AND SULFONAMIDES. Dapsone and sulfapuridine are the most commonly used sulfa preparations in dermatology. Dapsone is most commonly used to treat leprosy. Sulfone and sulfonamides are used most often to control dermatitis herpeti-

formis. Dapsone is also useful in treating cutaneous vasculitis, pyoderma gangrenosum, bullous forms of systemic erythematosus, and brown recluse spider bites.

A common side effect of dapsone is hemolysis and methemoglobinemia (especially in patients deficient in the enzyme glucose-6-phosphate dehydrogenase). Patients require frequent laboratory monitoring including a complete blood count differential, chemistry profile, reticulocyte count, and methemoglobin level.

ULTRAVIOLET LIGHT AS A THERAPEUTIC AGENT. UV phototherapy is used primarily in psoriasis and to treat vitiligo but may also help patients with nummular and atopic eczema, pityriasis rosea, the pruritus of uremia, and mycosis fungoides. UV light units are available in two wavelength ranges, UVB (the sunburn range of 280 to 320 nm) and UVA (long wavelength spectrum of 320 to 400 nm). The use of topical tar preparations, which "photosensitize" the skin to UVB wavelengths, adds to the effectiveness of treatment. Used over many weeks to months, the approach is highly effective in controlling psoriasis.

UVA light units are employed by dermatologists and commercial suntan centers to cause tanning rather than burning. The ability of UVA to evoke a sunburn is 1000 times less than that of UVB. The primary use of UVA is to treat severe, extensive psoriasis and vitiligo. It is used in combination with topical or oral psoralen, a drug that binds to DNA in the skin and sensitizes it to the effects of UVA. The long-term side effects of such therapy are unknown, although it may induce squamous and basal cell cutaneous carcinomas. The unprotected cornea and retina can be damaged by UV light. Stringent guidelines for protecting the eyes must be observed.

Shelley WB, Shelley GD: Advanced Dermatologic Therapy. Philadelphia, WB Saunders, 1987.

475 SKIN DISEASES OF GENERAL IMPORTANCE
Frank Parker

Chapter 473 discusses an approach to diagnosing skin diseases based on the specific morphologic descriptions of primary and secondary skin lesions. The nine ensuing groups, encompassing the majority of skin diseases, are listed in Table 473–1. This chapter discusses some of the diseases in each of these groups, providing the clinician with a differential diagnosis.

THE ECZEMAS (DERMATITIS)

Eczematous dermatitis is an inflammatory response of the skin to multiple exogenous and endogenous agents, although often the cause is not clear. Eczemas are defined by their clinical appearance and are subdivided either by their pattern of distribution or by etiologic factors (when known). Many eczematous processes are related to immunologic reactions (Table 475–1).

The term *eczema* or *eczematous dermatitis* is applied to eruptions characterized histologically by epidermal intercellular edema, termed *spongiosis*. Eczemas can be acute, with marked spongiosis causing red papules and vesicles and oozing, weeping, and crusting, or they may be chronic, with redness, scaling, fissuring, and especially lichenification. Both acute and chronic forms of eczema may affect the same patient, with the acute reaction progressing to oozing and crusting; with continued pruritus, the patient's rubbing and scratching converts the eczema to the chronic, dry, lichenified form. The hallmarks of all types of eczematous dermatitis are marked pruritus and varying degrees of erythema along with papules, vesicles, fine scaling, or lichenification. The histology of various types of eczemas is the same; skin biopsies identify a lesion as an eczematous reaction, but it does not differentiate among the various types of eczema.

CONTACT DERMATITIS. Contact dermatitis is the best understood and potentially the most correctable of eczematous reactions. For any such rash, the clinician should first determine

TABLE 475-1. ECZEMATOUS DERMATITIS SKIN ERUPTIONS NOT DISCUSSED IN TEXTS

Clinical Type	Etiology or Suspected Cause	Distinctive Diagnostic Findings
Eczematous drug-induced reaction	Drugs such as penicillin taken internally	Generalized eczema reaction evolves after taking medications (usually 10 or more days after first beginning drug; sooner if previously exposed) and clears with stopping drugs
Dermatophyte and *Candida* eczematous reactions	Dermatophytes and *Candida* induce eczematous inflammatory reaction	Dermatophyte or yeast found in scales or exudate
Infectious eczematoid dermatitis	Products from draining infected skin areas induce eczema reaction—linear infections, leg ulcers	Occurs near site of infection or other draining lesion; clears with treatment of infection
Dermatophytid	Hypersensitivity reaction occurring on distant areas of skin in response to products from fungal infection of other areas of skin	Often vesicular eruption of palms or fingers with dermatophyte infection of feet
Nonspecific eczematous dermatitis	No obvious cause—diagnosis of exclusion after above eczemas ruled out	Acute and chronic eczema patches anywhere on body; severe itching

whether it could be a contact reaction. If the cause can be identified, its avoidance cures it. There are two types of contact dermatitis, *irritant* and *allergic*. Irritant contact dermatitis is produced by substances that simply irritate or have a direct toxic effect on the skin, such as acids, alkalis, solvents, and detergents; no immunologic process is involved. Allergic contact dermatitis, on the other hand, is a delayed-type hypersensitivity reaction that occurs in response to a wide variety of allergens commonly found in the environment. The allergens consist of small molecular weight substances that act as haptens and bind to proteinaceous components of the skin to form the sensitizing antigen. Sensitization to the allergen requires 10 to 14 days to develop after the first encounter; subsequent exposure elicits the eczematous response in 1 to 7 days (delayed hypersensitivity).

The onset of irritant reactions after exposure to topical substance varies. Skin damage is evident within hours after contact with a strong irritant. Weaker irritants may require multiple applications and days or weeks before the development of the eczema (e.g., housewife's eczema of the hands due to chronic exposure to water and detergents). Contact dermatitis accounts for more than 50% of all occupational illnesses (excluding injury). In the industrial setting, approximately 70% is irritant and 30% allergic contact dermatitis.

Both irritant and allergic contact eczemas are initially confined to sites of contact, providing a diagnostic clue. Allergic reactions to plants, appear as linear, red, papular and vesicular streaks where the plant brushes across the skin. Allergies to metals (especially nickel) cause eczematous reactions under rings or watchbands or on the lobes of ears (earrings). Dermatitis under a ring may also stem from trapped water and irritating soap residues.

The most common allergens causing allergic contact dermatitis are pentadecylcatecol (allergen in poison oak, ivy, and sumac as well as in cashews, mangos, and ginko trees), paraphenylenediamine (a substance in hair dyes which cross-reacts with benzocaine and hydrochlorothiazide), nickel, mercaptobenzothiazol and thiuram (components in rubber), and ethylenediamine (a preservative in many medications and also found in industrial dyes and insecticides). Other common sources of contactants include topical medications (neomycin, anesthetics such as benzocaine, topical antihistamines), preservatives (ethylenediamine, merthiolate), vehicles (propylene glycol), and cosmetics (fragrances, preservatives, paraphenylenediamines). A detailed history of the patient's occupation, hobbies, habits, clothing, cosmetics, and topical medications is necessary to find the contactant.

Therapy of contact dermatitis is avoidance of the irritant or allergen if possible. Sometimes protective clothing is curative. Barrier creams are of little benefit. Acute, severe generalized contact dermatitis is treated with a short (10- to 14-day) course of systemic steroids and wet dressings or baths. Milder eczematous reactions respond to topical steroids and systemic antihistamines.

PHOTODERMATITIS. A variety of skin reactions, termed photosensitivity reactions, may occur in response to exposure to ultraviolet light. Some appear as eczematous reactions, so-called photoallergic dermatitis, which may occur in response to topical as well as systemic substances in the presence of UV light. The distribution of the eczematous eruption in light-exposed areas is an important feature in the differential diagnosis, with the cheeks, nose, forehead,

and tips of ears as sites of predilection. The backs of hands and forearms are also frequently involved and the history of exposure to UV light prior to the onset of the reaction is important in identifying light sensitivity (see Fig. 473-1).

Photoallergic dermatitis is immunologic. Absorption of a specific wavelength of ultraviolet light by a topical substance or a systemic drug (which is deposited in the skin from the vascular circulation) causes chemical conversion of the substance or drug to a hapten that binds cutaneous proteins to become a complete antigen capable of eliciting a type IV delayed hypersensitivity reaction similar to an allergic contact dermatitis reaction. Photoallergic reactions appear only where the UV light hits the skin, even though the systemic drug or topical photoallergen is present in the skin all over the body; i.e., the reaction depends on UV light hitting the skin with the allergen in it. Long wavelength UVA light usually generates these reactions. Because UVA light penetrates window glass, the reaction often occurs from indoor exposure. Such drugs as thiazides and phenothiazines can cause photoeczematous reactions, as can a number of topically applied substances, such as methylcoumarin, musk ambrette, halogenated salicylanilids, and topical sunscreening agents. Photopatch testing can identify substances in materials causing these reactions. Avoidance of the offending material is often curative. Oral or topical steroids relieve the inflammatory reaction.

ATOPIC DERMATITIS. This chronic, eczematous condition of the skin is often associated with a personal or family history of asthma, allergic rhinitis, and atopic eczema. Pruritus is prominent, and the consequent scratching and rubbing lead to lichenification, most typically in the antecubital and popliteal flexural areas. The eczema usually manifests itself after the first few months of life, appearing on the face and extensor areas of the extremities as acute and subacute, red, vesicular and oozing dermatitis. Many cases resolve spontaneously by puberty only to recur in adolescence and adulthood as a chronic dermatitis with scaling, dryness, and lichenification over the face, neck, upper chest, and characteristically the antecubital and popliteal fossae (flexural dermatitis). Atopics have a readily identifiable facies with diffuse erythema, perioral pallor, and a redundant crease or fold below the lower eyelids. The palms often have an increased number of skin markings, noticeable as fine cross-hatched lines. Stroking the skin in atopic dermatitis causes a white line, or dermatographism, probably due to dermal edema and vasoconstriction.

The cause of atopic dermatitis is not known, but a number of immunologic and pharmacologic abnormalities associate with the skin condition. For example, IgE reagenic antibodies are increased in 80% of atopic patients, especially those with extensive skin disease (such patients respond to many antigens applied by skin prick testing), but these antibodies seem not to *cause* atopic eczema. Avoiding antigens to which these patients react by scratch test does not improve the eczema. Patients with atopic eczema also have depressed cell-mediated immunity. This may account for the overproduction of IgE, resulting in unusual susceptibility to cutaneous herpes simplex, vaccina, molluscum contagiosum, and wart infections. Neutrophil and monocyte chemotaxis is reduced during exacerbations of eczema, explaining the frequent staphylococcal skin infections in these patients. Treatment with oral antibiotics to reduce staphylococcal flora (or overt staphylococcal infections such as fol-

PLATE 13 EYE DISEASES

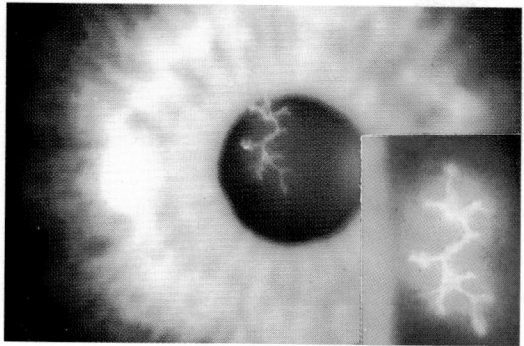

A, Herpes simplex corneal epithelial keratitis in diffuse light and *(inset)* in light passed through a cobalt blue filter after fluorescein staining.

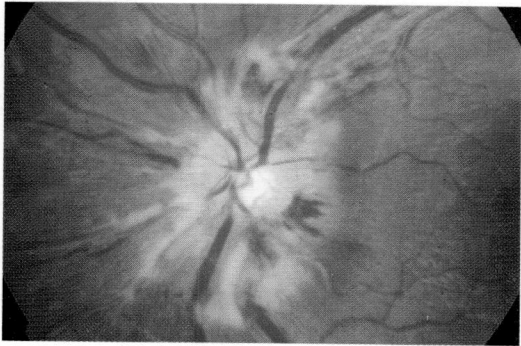

B, Papilledema in a young person. Note disc swelling, hemorrhages, and exudates, with preservation of the physiologic cup.

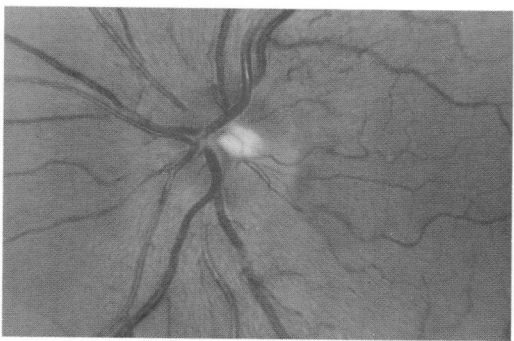

C, Disc in acute Leber's hereditary optic neuropathy. The disc tissue appears hyperemic, with peripapillary telangiectasia and opacification of the nerve fiber layer. Fluorescein angiography revealed no dye leakage.

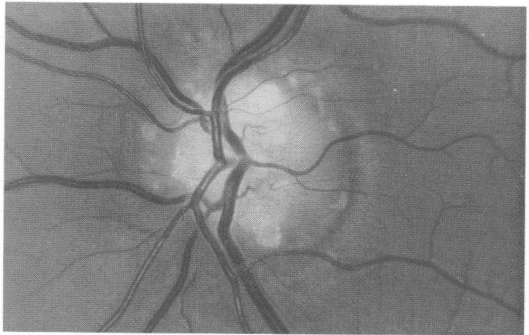

D, Optic disc drusen (also called hyaline bodies). Although obvious here, these calcified excrescences may be difficult to see in young persons, in whom the disc elevation they produce is mistaken for papilledema. (Also, they should be distinguished from retinal drusen—see *F* below.)

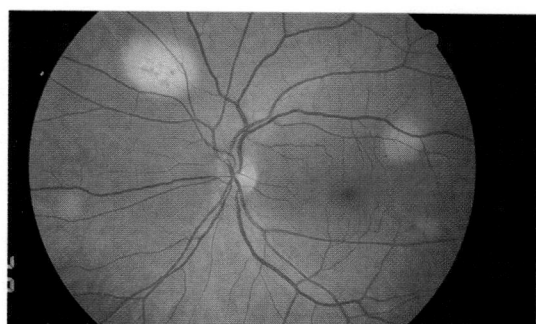

E, Multiple white choroidal metastases in a man with lung carcinoma.

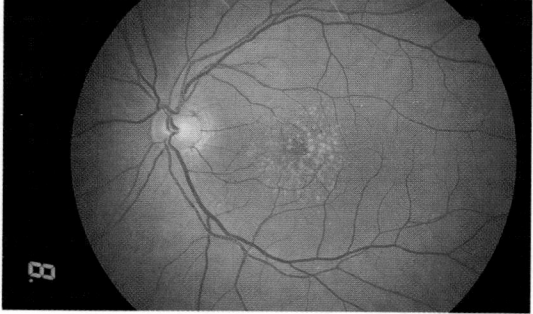

F, Retinal drusen. Multiple small white dots in the macula that represent abnormal accumulations in the retinal pigment epithelium basement (Bruch's) membrane. Such drusen are often precursors to visual loss from senile macular degeneration. (These should be distinguished from optic disc drusen—see *D* above.)

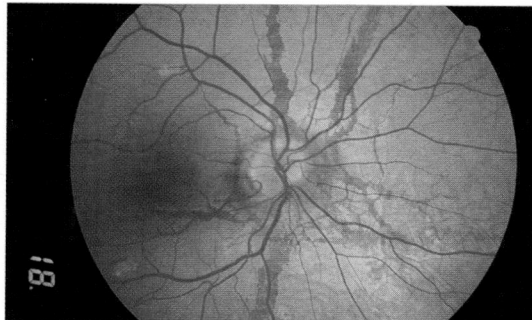

G, Angioid streaks in pseudoxanthoma elasticum. Breaks in the retinal pigment epithelium basement (Bruch's) membrane radial and circumferential to the disc indicate an underlying defect in elastic tissue formation.

Photographs taken by Mr. Harry Kachadoorian, C.R.A., University of Massachusetts Medical School, Worcester, Massachusetts.

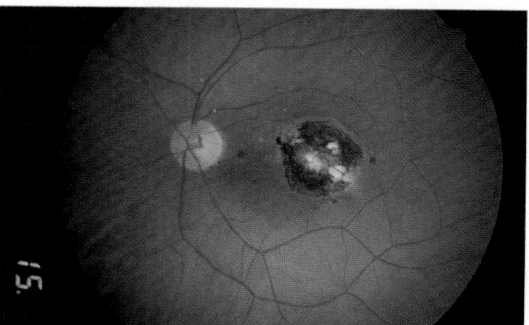

H, Macular chorioretinal scar. The appearance is typical of congenital toxoplasmosis, although other causes of chorioretinitis are included in the differential diagnosis.

PLATE 14   EYE DISEASES

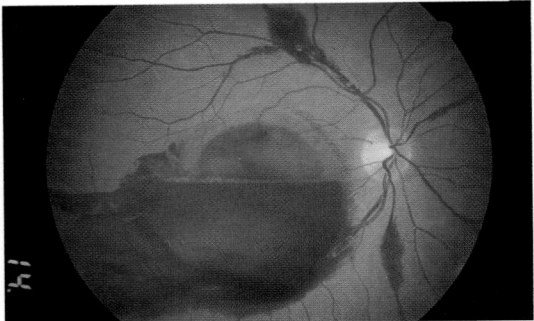

A, Preretinal (subhyaloid) hemorrhage. This occurred after a difficult intubation in an asthmatic woman with a previously normal eye examination. Similar findings are seen as a manifestation of diabetic retinopathy and in association with subarachnoid hemorrhage. The blood forms a meniscus with the patient in the upright position.

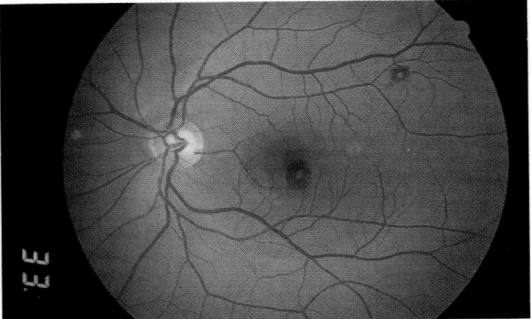

B, Roth's spots. Multiple white centered hemorrhages in a man with recurrent subacute bacterial endocarditis. White centered hemorrhages are also seen with leukemia and diabetes. The small white scars are probably the residua of previous episodes.

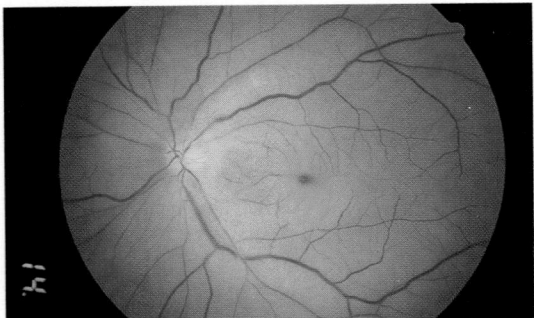

C, Central retinal artery occlusion. The retina is diffusely pale, lending a prominence to the normal coloration of the central fovea, often described as a cherry red spot.

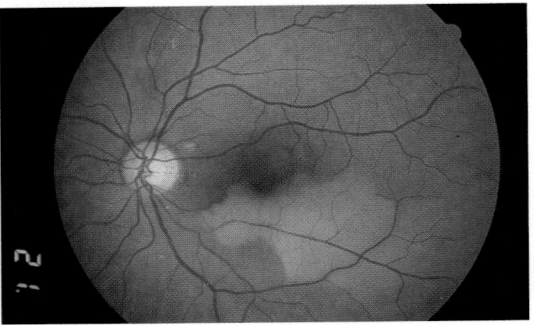

D, Inferior branch retinal artery occlusion. A pie-shaped sector of pale, infarcted retina extends from the embolic occlusion at the first branch of the arteriole of the inferior temporal arcade.

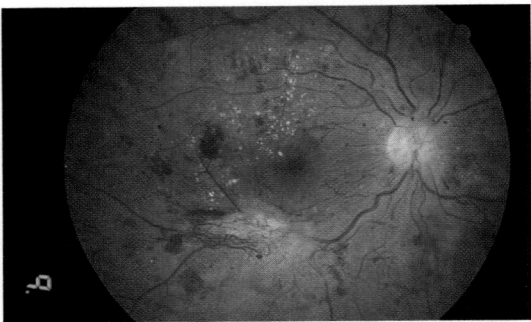

E, Proliferative diabetic retinopathy. Multiple hemorrhages, exudates, and new vessels are visible, with chorioretinal striae extending toward an area of fibrovascular proliferation along the inferior temporal arcade.

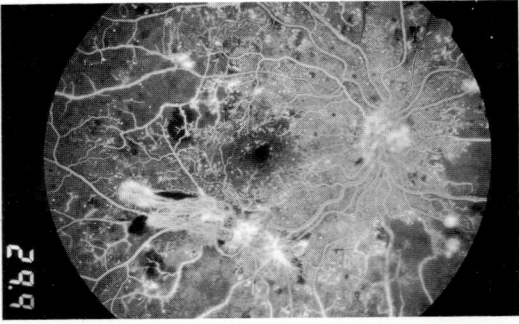

F, Fluorescein angiogram of the same fundus pictured in *E*. The new vessels, especially at the disc and the area of fibrovascular proliferation, are seen to leak fluorescein. Many of the "dot hemorrhages" are revealed as microaneurysms that fill with dye.

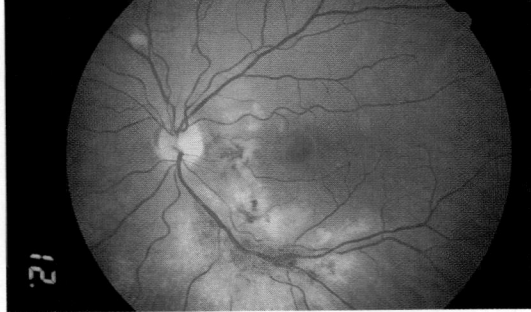

G, Cytomegalovirus retinitis in a patient with AIDS. There is a sector of retinal necrosis and hemorrhages along the inferior temporal arcade.

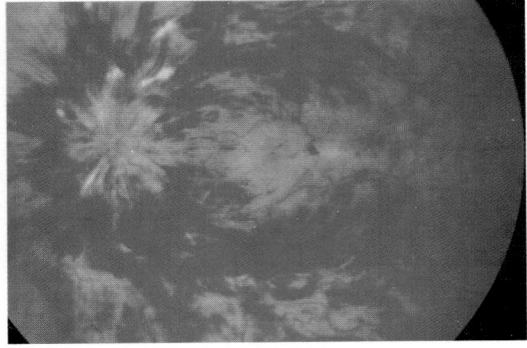

H, Central retinal vein occlusion. The disc is swollen with diffuse retinal hemorrhages and cotton-wool spots.

Photographs taken by Mr. Harry Kachadoorian, C.R.A., University of Massachusetts Medical School, Worcester, Massachusetts.

PLATE 15　SKIN DISEASES

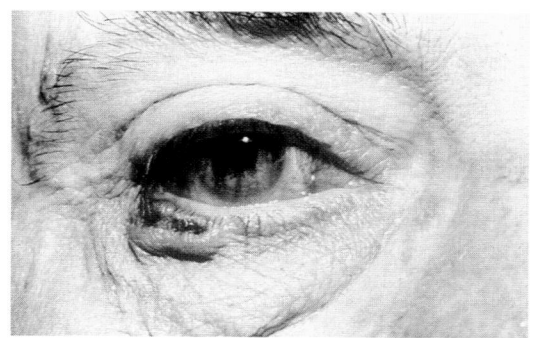

A, Basal cell cancer. Tumor with rolled, opalescent borders and central "rodent" ulcer.

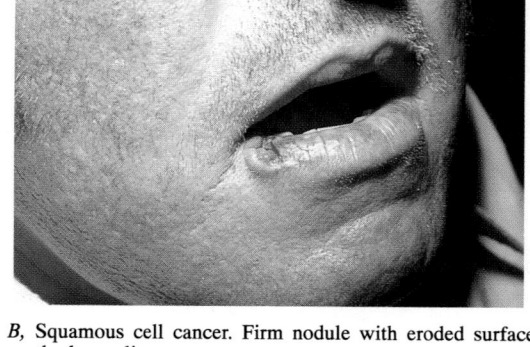

B, Squamous cell cancer. Firm nodule with eroded surface on the lower lip.

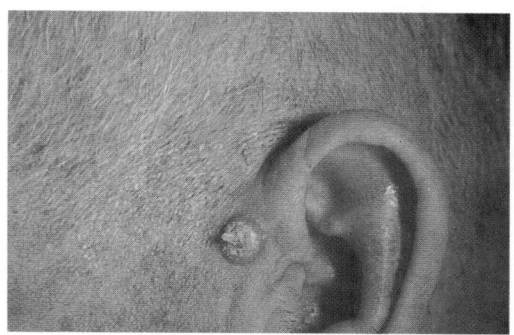

C, Cutaneous horn. Keratotic horn evolving from red nodule at base. These commonly are squamous cell cancers.

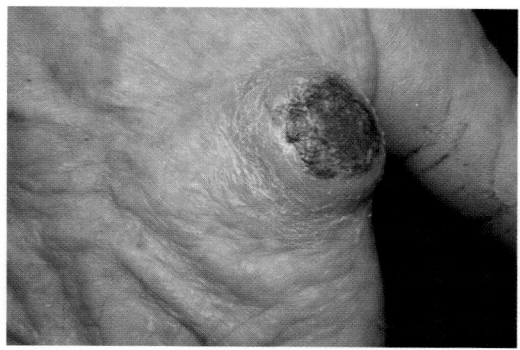

D, Keratoacanthoma. Large nodular lesion with central keratotic crater.

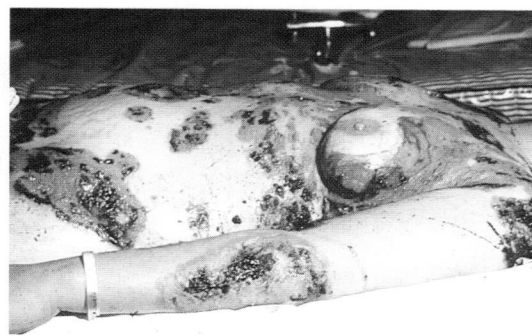

E, Pemphigus vulgaris. Intraepidermal bullae are easily ruptured, leaving superficial crusted erosions with thin shreds of blister roof along the edges. Careful examination reveals some intact blisters (primary lesions) below the breast.

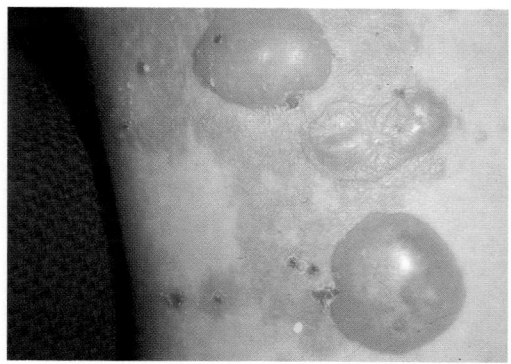

F, Bullous pemphigoid. Tense subepidermal bullae on an erythematous base.

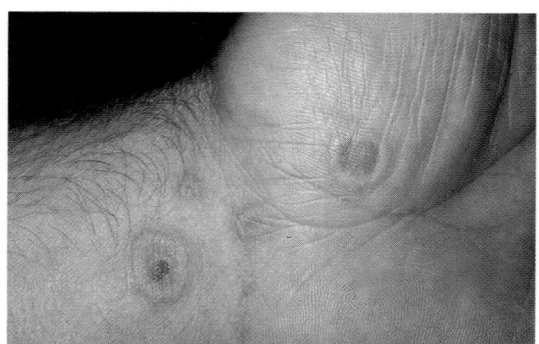

G, Erythema multiforme. Target or "bull's-eye" annular lesions with central vesicles and bullae.

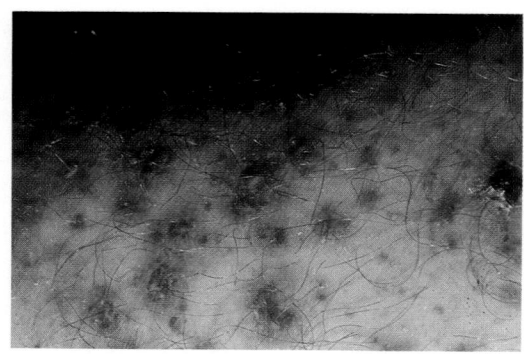

H, Palpable purpura. Leukocytoclastic vasculitis commonly causes raised purpuric and ulcerated lesions on legs.

PLATE 16   SKIN DISEASES

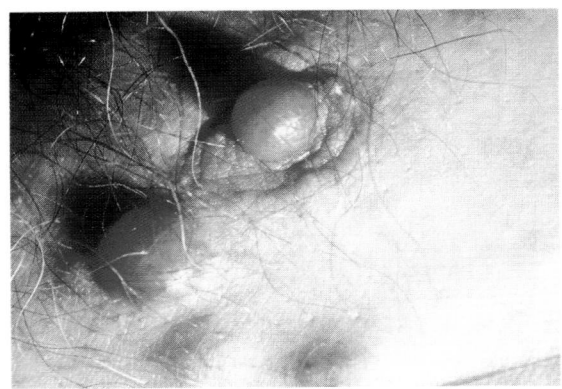

A, Skin metastases. Firm, hard, red nodules.

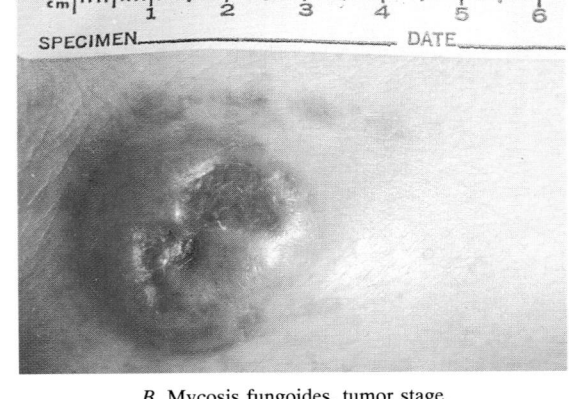

B, Mycosis fungoides, tumor stage.

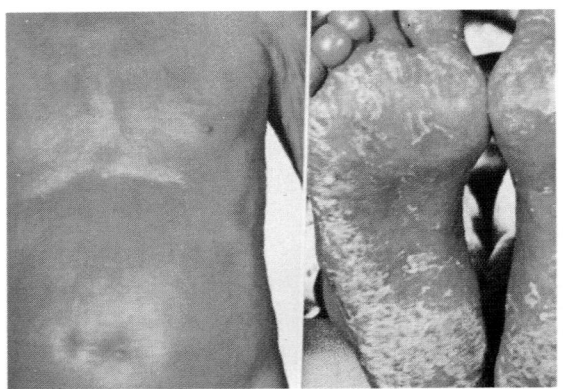

C, Sézary syndrome, exfoliative dermatitis stage.

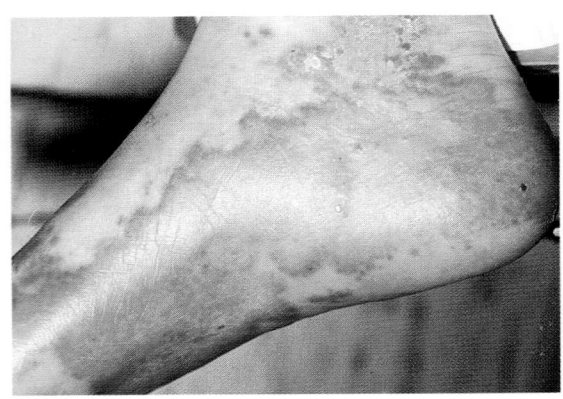

D, Classic Kaposi's sarcoma.

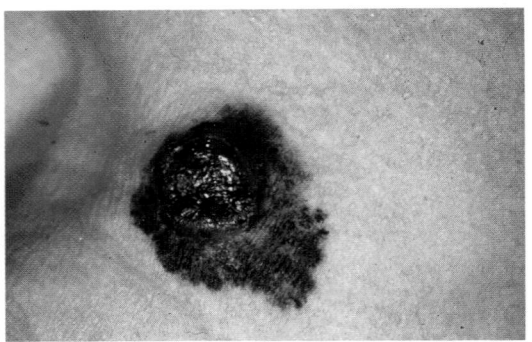

E, Malignant melanoma. Darkly pigmented, nodular lesion with irregular outline, irregular shades of dark pigmentation, and irregular surface configuration.

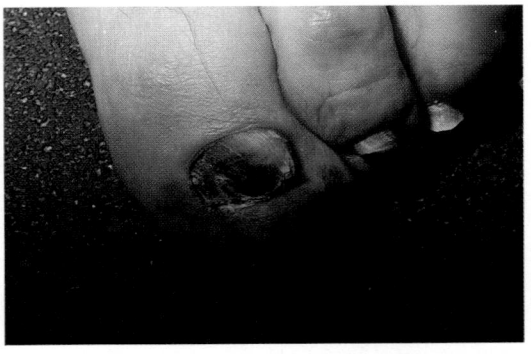

F, Subungual melanoma. Dark blue-black pigment within nail bed, with irregular dark pigment on the tip of the great toe.

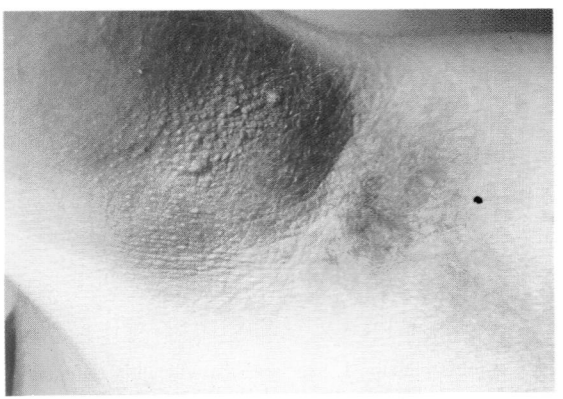

G, Acanthosis nigricans. Axillary lesion.

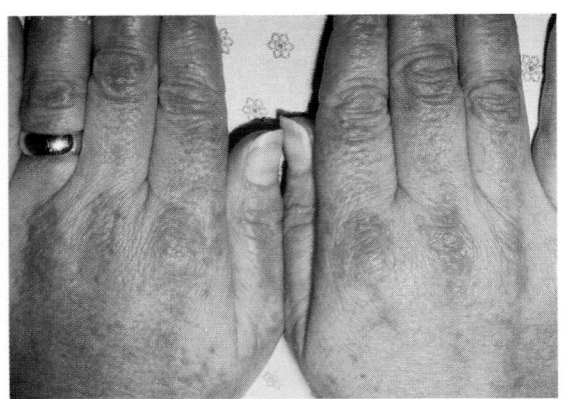

H, Dermatomyositis. Gottron's papules over the knuckles.

PLATE 17 SKIN DISEASES

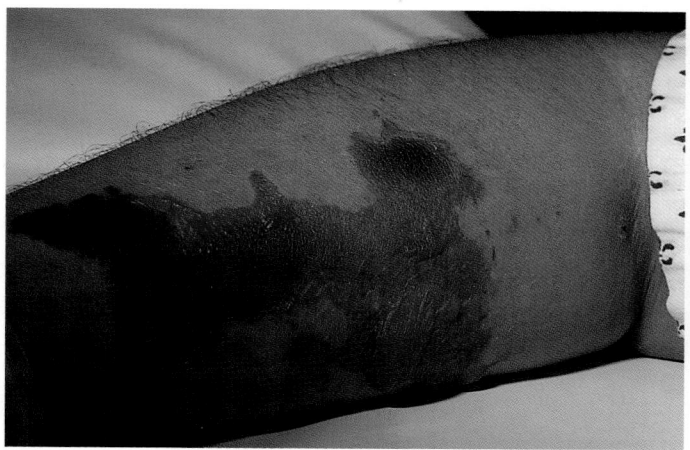

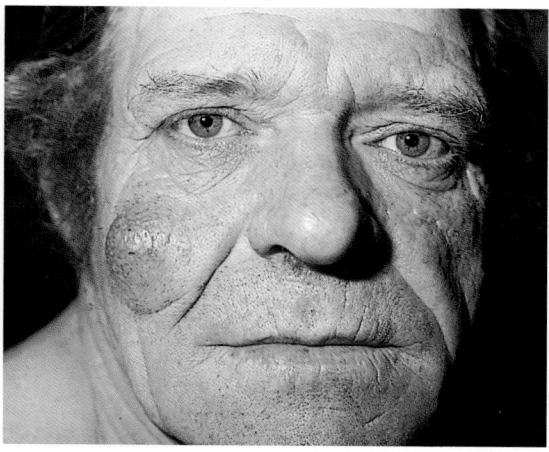

A, Macule—flat circumscribed color change. This is a purpuric area of skin in a patient with purpura fulminans.

B, Cyst—large semisolid sac. An infundibular cyst on the right cheek. Note that this is a smooth, round, nodular lesion.

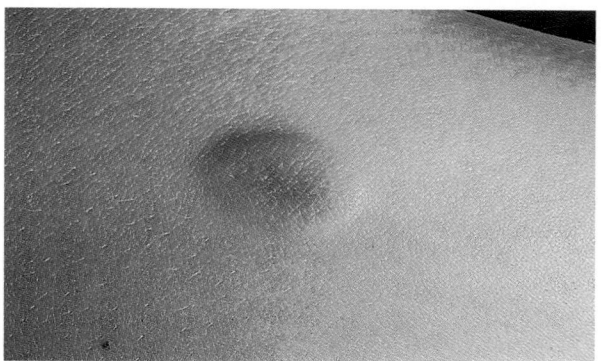

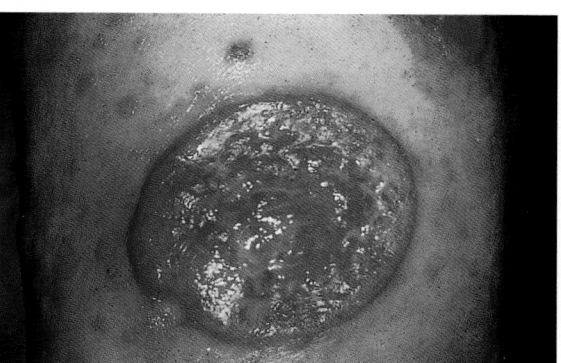

C, Papule—a solid elevation of 1 cm or less. This is a papule of granuloma annulare.

D, Plaque—a raised, circumscribed, flat-topped lesion. A typical mycosis fungoides–eroded plaque.

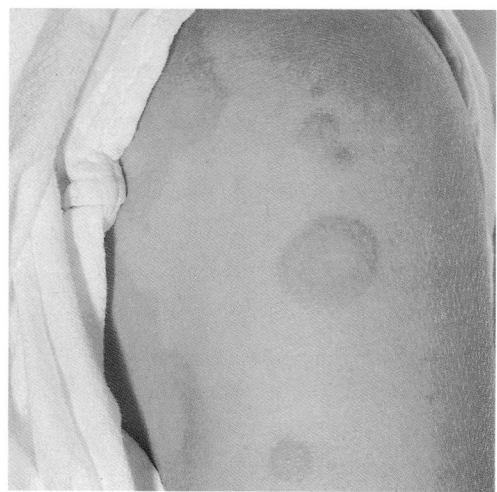

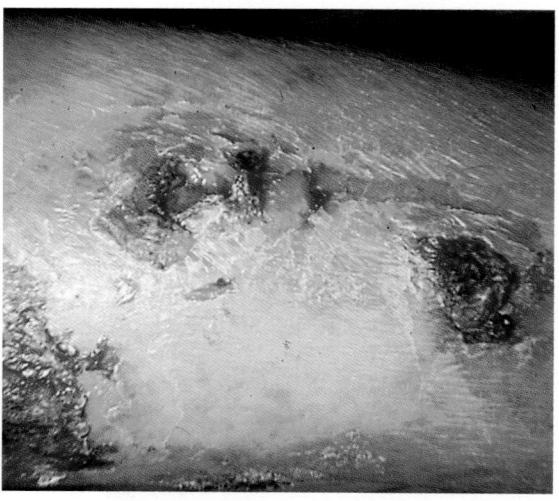

E, Wheal—erythematous edematous plaque that is evanescent. This is a urticarial lesion due to penicillin.

F, Erosion—superficial denudation of epidermis. Ecthyma—a superficial staphylococcal infection.

PLATE 18   SKIN DISEASES

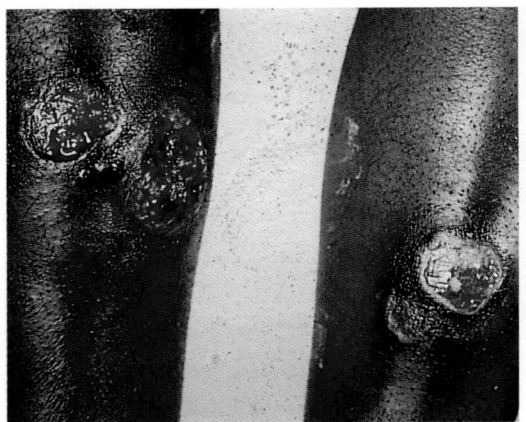

A, Ulcer—deep defect in the skin extending to the dermis. These ulcers are secondary to ischemia due to sickle cell anemia.

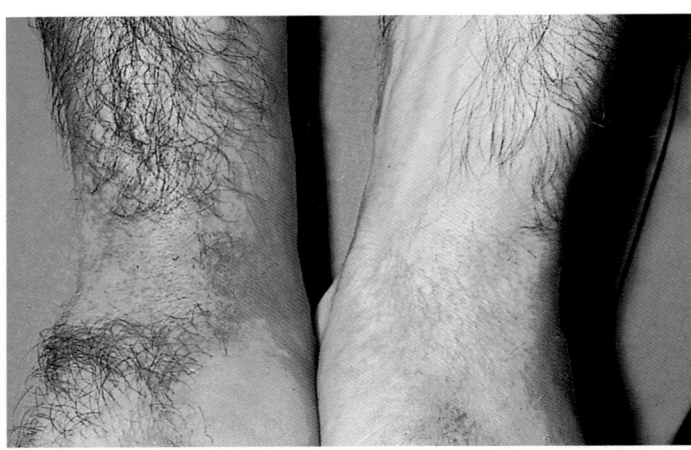

B, Atrophy—loss of epidermal or dermal substance with thinning of skin. Here the atrophy is due to scleroderma. Note loss of hair follicles and shiny atrophic areas of skin.

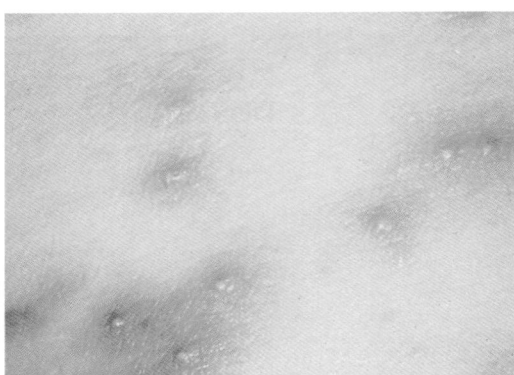

C, Pustule—fluid-filled sac filled with neutrophils. This patient had hot tub dermatitis due to *Pseudomonas* infection.

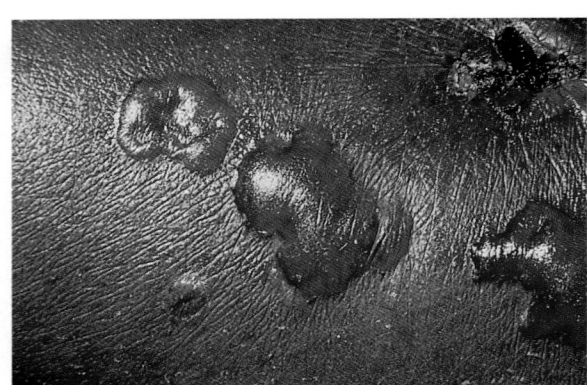

D, Bullae—fluid-filled lesions 0.5 cm or larger—bullous impetigo.

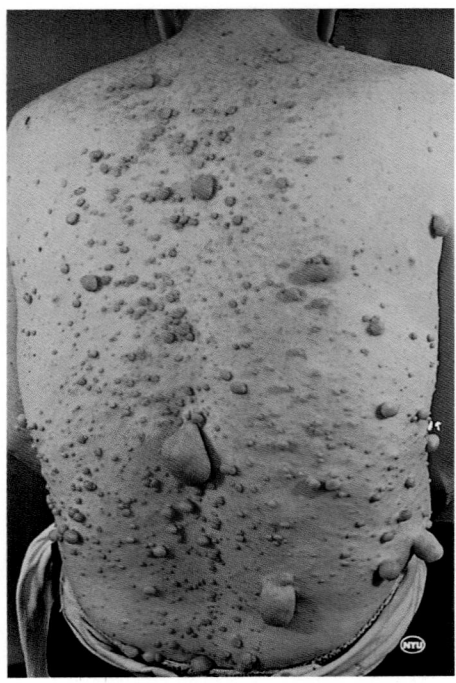

F, Scar—an area of replacement fibrosis of the dermis or subcutaneous tissue. These scars are healed diabetic ulcers.

E, Nodules—solid, large (>1 cm) deep-seated mass in dermal or subcutaneous tissues. These nodules are neurofibromas in a patient with neurofibromatosis.

PLATE 19 SKIN DISEASES

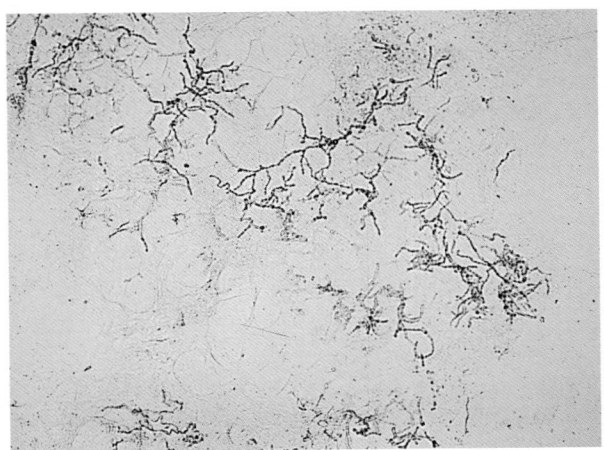

A, Tzanck smear of herpes simplex. Positive Tzanck smear is seen as multinucleated giant cell.

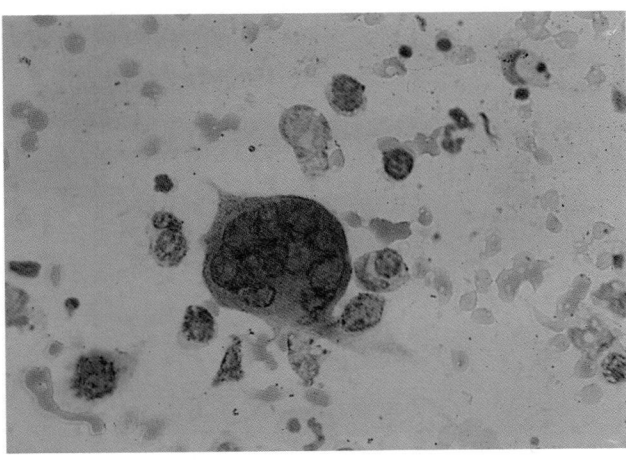

B, KOH preparation. Fungi appear as refractile branched hyphal elements after skin stratum corneum scrapings are incubated with 20% KOH for several minutes.

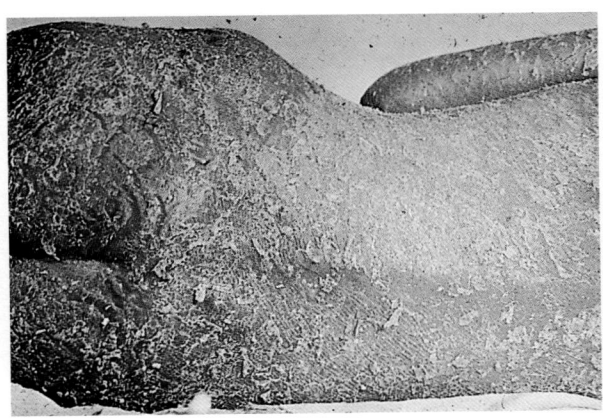

C, Exfoliative erythroderma. Diffuse inflammatory reaction of the entire skin with thickening, lichenification, redness, and scaling.

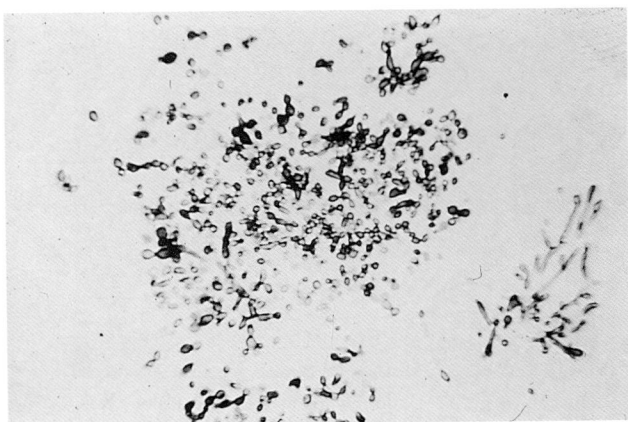

D, Candida albicans. KOH examination of candidal skin lesion. Short, stubby hyphae and budding yeast elements.

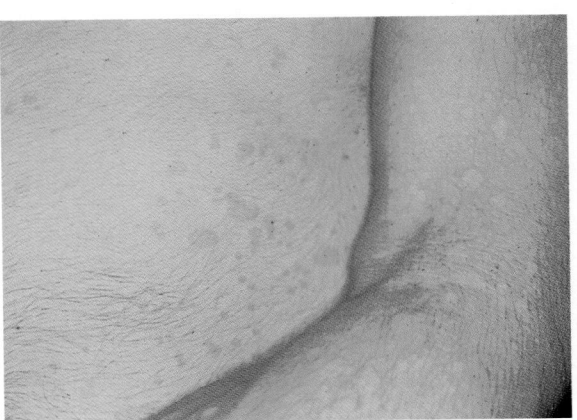

E, Tinea versicolor. Discrete areas of red-brown scaling lesions on the trunk.

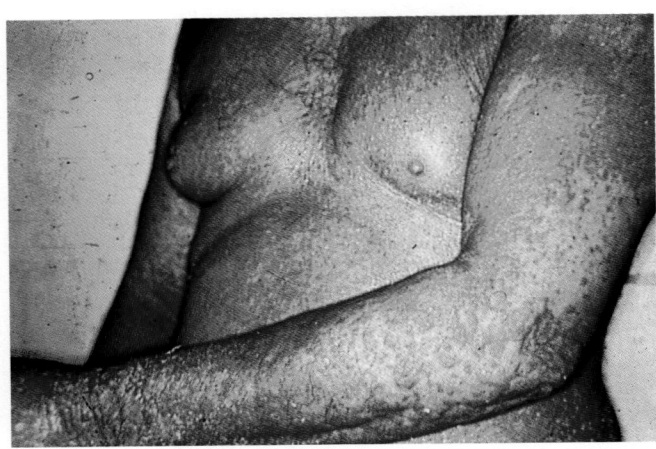

F, Drug eruption. Macular erythematous and somewhat scaling diffuse eruption. Penicillin drug rash.

PLATE 20   SKIN DISEASES

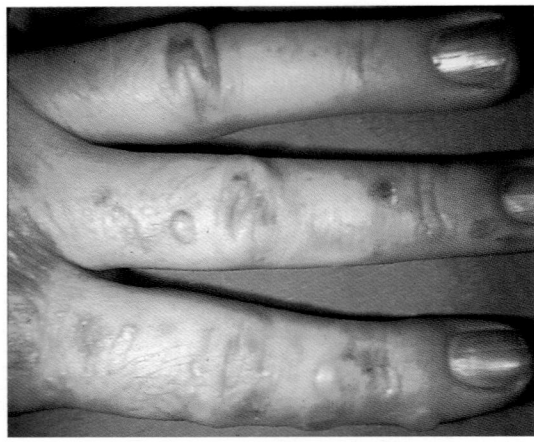

A, Porphyria cutanea tarda. Vesicular eroded and crusted lesions that leave scars. Lesions are precipitated by exposure to sun and trauma to the skin.

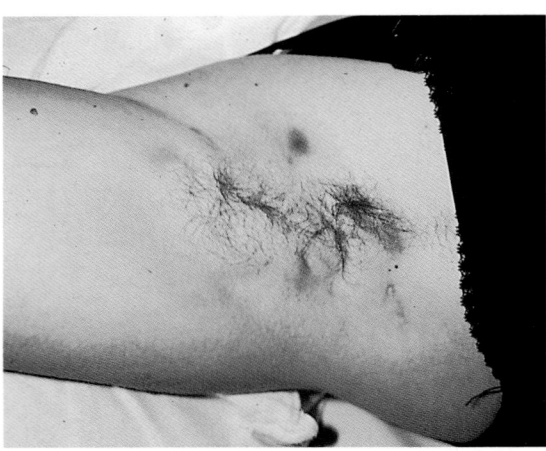

B, Hidradenitis suppurativa. Tender cystlike abscess in the axilla with retracted scars and sinus tracts.

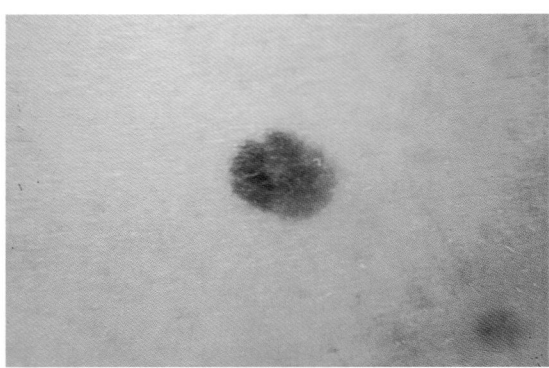

C, Junctional nevus. Uniformly pigmented, flat lesion. Note sharply demarcated borders and symmetry of the lesion.

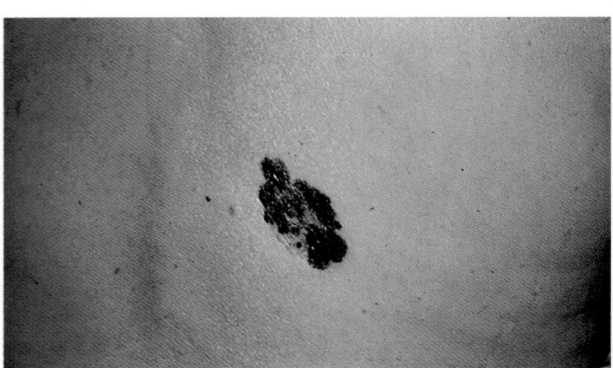

D, Superficial spreading melanoma. A darkly pigmented lesion with irregular outline and considerable scalloping of the borders and asymmetry.

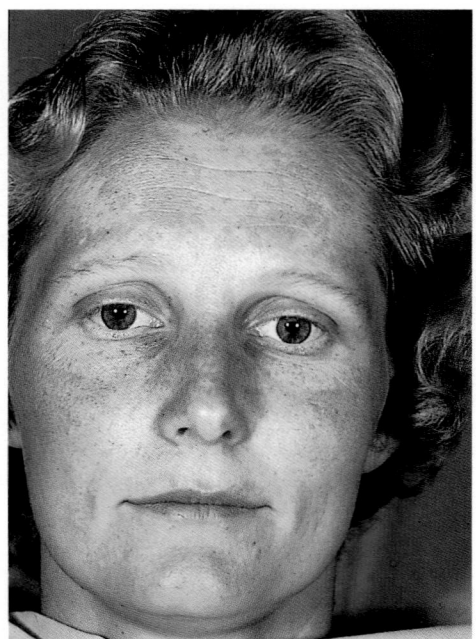

F, Tuberous sclerosis. Characteristic area of depigmentation with ash leaf configuration, on leg.

E, Melasma. Light brown hyperpigmentation of the cheeks and forehead.

liculitis, furuncles, or cellulitis) often results in marked improvement in the eczema.

Atopic individuals are often tense, resentful, aggressive, and restless, but whether this accompanies the diathesis or merely results from living with chronic, unremitting itching and skin inflammation is not certain. Either way, the physician must help the patient meet the stresses of life.

Keratoconjunctivitis and stellate anterior subcapsular cataracts are associated with atopic eczema, particularly in patients with extensive skin changes. The conjunctivitis and keratitis usually start in childhood. The cataracts may also begin at a young age and form rapidly, often by age 20. Keratoconus is seen in 25% of atopics.

The treatment of atopic dermatitis is the same as for other eczematous eruptions and includes topical steroids, emollients, and systemic antihistamines. In some children (less than 2 years of age) food allergy can cause atopic dermatitis, but dietary factors remain controversial. Skin tests or RAST tests help identify which foods may be responsible. Positive results must be confirmed with controlled food challenges and elimination diets. Allergic immediate skin testing and desensitization have been of little value.

Skin irritation must be avoided by wearing soft cotton clothing. Counseling, psychotherapy, and stress reduction sometimes help. Patients often worsen during the autumn and winter seasons when central heating and a dry environment dramatically decrease humidity. The frequent use of emollients is the best treatment for skin dryness, especially immediately after bathing when the skin is hydrated. Topical corticosteroids are the most important means of controlling the inflammatory response, and the least potent forms should be used, usually in an ointment base. Systemic steroids should be used only in short courses to overcome exacerbations not controlled by topical steroids.

STASIS DERMATITIS. This is an eczematous eruption of the lower legs secondary to peripheral venous insufficiency. Venous incompetence causes increased hydrostatic pressure and capillary damage with extravasation of red blood cells and serum. These conditions trigger an inflammatory, brawny, edematous, red, and hyperpigmented petechial scaling or weeping reaction, usually around the medial malleolus or distal one third of the lower leg. Secondary allergic contact dermatitis frequently complicates the problem when neomycin is used chronically to treat accompanying stasis ulcers. Management consists of preventing venous stasis and edema with supportive hose while the patient is ambulatory. Weight reduction helps obese patients. The eczema is treated with topical steroids and wet compresses when oozing and crusting are present. Occasionally chronic stasis dermatitis, when secondarily infected, can undergo exacerbation with spread of the acute inflammation to distant areas of the body, a condition known as *autosensitization dermatitis.* These secondary eczematous patches evolve on the face, neck, and extensor areas of the extremities. Topical steroids (occasionally oral ones for severe reactions) control the reactions; antibiotics may be needed to halt cutaneous infection.

NUMMULAR ECZEMATOUS DERMATITIS. This condition is defined by recurrent, coin-shaped patches predominantly on the extensor surfaces of the arms and legs, less often the trunk. Minute patches of vesicles and papules spread to become scaling and thickened, occasionally clearing in the center so that they may resemble superficial fungal infections. Mild to severe pruritus accompanies the patches. Although the cause is unknown, many factors acting alone or in combination may contribute. Dry skin is frequent, and the disease reaches a peak in winter months. Irritating substances such as wool, soap, and frequent bathing may contribute. The combination of topical steroids (usually of intermediate potency), 3% crude coal tar, and ultraviolet light treatments helps to control the persistent eczema.

LICHEN SIMPLEX CHRONICUS. Also known as neurodermatitis, this is a chronic, pruritic, lichenified eczematous eruption that results from constant scratching. Pruritus often precedes the scratching, and rubbing induces lichenification, initiating a vicious circle. In most patients it is a nervous habit. Patches of neurodermatitis commonly affect the nape of the neck, lower legs, groin, or other regions within easy reach of the hands. Occasionally constant scratching results in scaling, thickened, excoriated papules and nodules. Treatment consists of explaining the cause and the need to stop rubbing. Topical steroids and oral antihistamines may be helpful. Steroids injected into the lesion break the itching cycle more successfully than topical oils.

SEBORRHEIC DERMATITIS. Seborrheic dermatitis is characterized by erythematous, eczematous patches with yellow, greasy scales localized to hairy areas and regions of the skin with high concentrations of sebaceous glands, especially the middle of the face, nasolabial folds, eyebrows, ear canals, retroauricular folds, and presternal areas. Dandruff is scaling of the scalp without inflammation. Severe cases can involve the axillae and groin regions. Seborrheic dermatitis may appear in infants until about 6 months of age ("cradle cap"); after that it disappears until after puberty. Patients with neurologic disorders, such as Parkinson's disease or stroke, may have a dramatic flare of their seborrhea. Although the cause of seborrhea is unknown, the associations with emotional stress and neurologic disease suggest a central nervous system influence. Some studies suggest that the condition is related to excessive growth of yeast organisms *(Pityrosporum)* on the skin. It is sometimes difficult to differentiate seborrhea from psoriasis when the latter is localized to the scalp, ears, and face.

Antiseborrheic shampoos containing tar, sulfur, salicylic acid, selenium sulfide, or zinc pyrithione provide the most useful treatment. The shampoo should be used daily, rubbed into the scalp and left on for 5 minutes before rinsing. Inflammatory seborrhea that does not respond to shampoos alone may benefit from a topical steroid lotion or gel in hairy areas and hydrocortisone cream for facial glabrous skin. Continual use of shampoo and topical steroids is required for control. The use of topical or oral antiyeast medication, ketoconizole, helps in some patients.

XEROTIC ECZEMA AND ECZEMA CRAQUELE. These conditions are characterized by chapping and symptomatic dryness that may lead to visible fissuring through the stratum corneum, giving criss-crossing cracks that resemble dried mud. Such changes occur most commonly in winter, and they respond to emollients and/or hydrocortisone ointments.

HAND ECZEMA. Hand eczema is most common in housewives, cooks, food handlers, and medical personnel. The most common precipitators are constant exposure to mild primary irritants (soap, water), frequent hand washing, atopy, and nummular dermatitis. Allergic contact dermatitis may be another cause. *Dyshidrotic eczema* (pompholyx), a relatively noninflammatory, recurrent, pruritic, vesicular eruption of the palms and soles of unknown cause, differs from other hand eczemas in that the primary involvement is on the palm instead of the dorsum of the hands. The term *dyshidrotic eczema* suggests malfunction of the sweat ducts, but this is a misnomer. Pompholyx, from the Greek meaning bubble, is a more apt term. Emotional stress tends to be a trigger. Vesicles on the palms can also represent *dermatophytid,* an allergic reaction to a dermatophyte infection on the feet. If potassium hydroxide (KOH) examination of the feet is positive, treatment of the fungus clears up the palmar reaction as well.

Treatment of hand dermatitis involves avoidance of primary irritants such as soap, solvents, detergents, and frequent exposure to water. The use of cotton gloves with rubber gloves over them is useful in protecting the hands in water. Topical steroids and emollients may help, but topical steroids are often required.

EXFOLIATIVE DERMATITIS (ERYTHRODERMA). Total body cutaneous erythema, edema, scaling, and fissuring may occur as an idiopathic entity without preceding dermatologic or systemic disease, or it may result from a variety of cutaneous (atopic or contact dermatitis, psoriasis, seborrheic dermatitis, autosensitization, pityriasis rubra pilaris) or systemic disorders (mycosis fungoides, lymphomas, leukemias) as well as a reaction to drugs (antibiotics, barbiturates, antiepileptic agents, gold). Other organ systems are affected by the general erythroderma and changes in the stratum corneum barrier function. The diffuse redness and warmth of the skin reflect vasodilation and increased blood flow through the immense cutaneous vasculature. Five to 8% of the total cardiac output may be directed to the dilated, inflamed, cutaneous vasculature. In older individuals with underlying cardiac disease, high output heart failure may ensue. Also increased heat loss may lead to decreased core temperature, shivering, and swings in temperature. Oral steroids decrease the cutaneous inflammation and correct the abnormalities. In less acute situations total body applications of topical steroids with plastic sauna suit occlusion reverse the erythroderma.

FUNGAL INFECTIONS OF THE SKIN. Fungal infections may be confused with eczema. These infections include dermatophytosis, candidiasis, and tinea versicolor. *Dermatophytes* are a homogeneous group of fungi that live on the keratin of the stratum corneum, nails, and hair and frequently provoke a cutaneous inflammatory reaction with pruritus, redness, scaling, and vesiculation. Three genera of dermatophytes cause these infections: *Trichophyton, Microsporum,* and *Epidermophyton.* Dermatophytosis of the trunk (tinea corporis) can be caused by several species (*T. rubrum* and *T. mentagrophytes* are most common), resulting in annular inflamed patches with elevated scaling and, at times, vesicular borders with a tendency for central clearing. The eruption may be widespread and may mimic nummular eczema. Extensive, red, scaling lesions with elevated serpiginous borders may occur in diabetic and immunosuppressed patients. Ringworm of the scalp appears as scaling areas of hair loss with black dots indicating breakage of hair shafts. Most infections are now due to *T. tonsurans* or *M. canis.* The latter agent may fluoresce under Wood's light, but this should not be used for diagnosis. Rather, examination with KOH preparations and cultures for fungi should be performed (using plucked hairs and scales from the affected areas). Tinea cruris infection in the groin appears as red patches with elevated serpiginous and scaling borders. The scrotum is seldom involved. Erythrasma is still another type of intertriginous erythema caused by a *Corynebacterium* infection. It appears as velvety red patches with fine scale which, under Wood's light, fluoresce a diagnostic coral pink color. Erythromycin clears the infection. Tinea of the feet (pedis) and hands (manum) often present together. Infections of the feet appear in three forms: (1) interdigital maceration, scaling, and fissuring; (2) diffuse, dry, scaling and mild erythema of the plantar surface, often extending onto the sides of the feet in a "moccasin" distribution, occasionally associated with dry scaling of one palm; (3) vesiculopustular lesions on the insteps of the feet. Involvement of the nails—onychomycosis—often accompanies hand and foot dermatophytosis.

Candidiasis, particularly involvement by *C. albicans,* causes inflammatory skin reactions. Intertriginous moniliasis occurs in the groin, perineum, gluteal folds, inframammary areas, axillae, and digital webs. Typically, the folds become macerated and erythematous with small satellite papules and erosions around the periphery of the main lesion. Obesity, diabetes, and use of antibiotics may play a role in *Candida* infection. Chronic mucocutaneous candidiasis is a rare condition characterized by superficial *Candida* infection of the skin, nails, and oral and genital mucosal surfaces complicating a variety of systemic immunodeficiencies (see Ch. 354). *Tinea versicolor,* a common superficial fungus infection caused by *Pityrosporon orbiculare,* is identified by scaling, red to brown or white, oval patches over the neck, trunk, and upper arms. As the name versicolor implies, the lesions vary in color. During the summer months when the skin is exposed to ultraviolet light, the lesions appear hypopigmented, as the infection prevents the involved skin from forming pigment. Examination of the lesion with KOH reveals budding yeast forms and club-shaped hyphae.

Either topical or systemic agents can treat fungal infections of the skin. If the dermatophytic or candidal glabrous skin infection is localized, econazole, miconazole, clotrimazole, and ciclopirox creams, ointments, and lotions are effective when applied two to three times a day for 3 to 4 weeks. Tinea versicolor also responds to these agents, but selenium sulfide antidandruff shampoo is less expensive and also effective. Application of the shampoo to the involved areas of skin for 10 minutes each night for 3 to 4 weeks clears the disease, although the hypopigmentation does not resolve until the patient is exposed to the sun. Regular shampooing with selenium sulfide reduces reinfection rates. Widespread fungal lesions, or those resistant to topical therapy, may require systemic agents. Griseofulvin is an effective, safe agent and the treatment of choice for dermatophyte infections, but it is not effective for *Candida.* The drug must be given for varying periods of time, depending on the site of infection. The micronized form (Ultrafine, U/F) seems to be most consistently effective. Approximately 10 mg per kilogram per day is used in children and 1 gram per day in adults.

Ketoconazole is a second oral medication useful for dermatophytes, but it is also effective in *Candida* infections. Because ketoconazole occasionally causes severe liver damage, it should not be used initially for dermatophyte infections. It is useful in mucocutaneous candidiasis at a dose of 200 to 400 mg per day in adults. Be-

cause of its toxicity, liver function tests should be performed every 2 to 4 weeks.

MACULOPAPULAR SKIN DISEASES

The rashes included in this group represent diverse cutaneous and systemic conditions characterized by widespread erythematous macules and papules. Some of the conditions also have associated petechiae or purpura.

VIRAL EXANTHEMS. Because many *viral exanthems* are maculopapular, this group of skin diseases is often termed morbilliform, or measles-like. The clinical appearance of virus-induced erythema is not specific for a given etiologic agent; other signs and symptoms help to suggest a particular viral agent. Most viral exanthems are preceded by a prodrome of fever and constitutional symptoms. A history of previous exposure to infected individuals may be obtained. Incubation times vary from days to weeks depending on the virus. Drug history may also be important, especially with infectious mononucleosis, in which only 3% of patients have a maculopapular or petechial eruption, but with the administration of ampicillin the frequency approaches 100%. In measles (rubeola) and rubella, the erythematous macules and papules begin on the face and spread to the trunk and extremities, fading with desquamation in 6 days in rubeola and on the third day in rubella. The rashes associated with enterovirus infection are most commonly rubella-like but occasionally are purpuric. Exanthem subitum (roseola infantum) displays fleeting, discrete, red papules surrounded by a whitish halo that begins on the trunk and then evolves on the neck. Erythema infectiosum (fifth disease) is an alarming appearing red, "slapped cheek" rash over the face with reticulate maculopapular lesions on the extremities that clear in 3 to 6 days. Mucous membranes are sometimes involved. In rubella, red spots occur on the soft palate. In measles, Koplik's spots, tiny gray-white papules on an erythematous base, are found on the buccal mucosa opposite the molars. An erythematous, maculopapular rash that begins peripherally on the palms and soles and spreads to the trunk, often with a petechial component, is seen in *atypical measles.* This is a hypersensitivity reaction to wild measles virus in a partially immune, vaccinated host.

Verruca vulgaris and *molluscum contagiosum* are two examples of viral infections confined to the skin which elicit unique papular lesions. Wart papilloma virus induces various forms of warts: *common warts,* dome-shaped papules with corrugated, hyperkeratotic surfaces; *flat warts,* slightly raised, smooth, flat-topped papules often on the hands and face; *plantar warts,* painful papules on the soles of the feet covered by a thick callus with black puncta within the lesion; *condylomata acuminata,* or venereal warts, soft, moist, sessile, pedunculated and verrucous papules involving the perianal and genital areas. *Molluscum contagiosum* is caused by a DNA poxvirus that infects epidermal cells to induce smooth, dome-shaped, translucent papules with a central umbilication from which a cheesy core can be expressed. These lesions occur most commonly on the trunk, face, and genitals. The treatment of warts relies on a variety of nonspecific destructive techniques, including liquid nitrogen cryotherapy, salicylic and lactic acid combinations, cantharidin, and podophyllin. Molluscum contagiosum lesions are removed by curettage of the central core, liquid nitrogen freezing, or cantharidin application for short periods of time (30 to 60 minutes).

SCARLETINIFORM ERUPTIONS. Scarlet fever, *Kawasaki's syndrome,* and *toxic shock syndrome* also present with erythematous macular and papular eruptions. Group A streptococcal pharyngitis or tonsillitis with a strain producing erythrogenic toxin initiates a confluent, papular eruption with sandpaper texture that begins on the neck and upper chest and evolves over the abdomen and extremities. The face is flushed, and circumoral pallor is prominent. Extensive desquamation occurs in 4 to 5 days. Punctate redness of the palate and strawberry tongue coexist.

Kawasaki's syndrome, a condition of unknown cause, displays a morbilliform or scarletiniform eruption more prominent on the trunk than the face. Most distinctive are magenta red discolorations of the palms and soles associated with indurative edema of the hands and feet. The skin and extremity changes occur within 3 to 4 days of the onset of fever, along with mucous membrane inflammatory changes consisting of conjunctivitis and strawberry tongue. Palm, sole, and finger tip desquamation occurs 10 to 18 days after the onset of fever. Asymmetric lymphadenopathy, especially in the cervical area, is seen in 75% of patients—hence the name *mucocu-*

taneous lymph node syndrome. This is a disease of young children and occasionally young adults, and 1 to 2% of these individuals develop coronary aneurysms or myocardial infarction, sometimes fatal.

Toxic shock syndrome is a serious condition arising from toxins elaborated by *Staphylococcus aureus* infections, often in menstruating women using tampons but also in patients with postsurgical infections. The rash is an erythematous, macular, diffuse eruption that blanches readily with pressure followed by desquamation of the affected skin, in association with fever, strawberry tongue, hypotension, vomiting, and renal insufficiency. The rash often spares the skin where clothing fits tightly with pressure on the skin, e.g., waistline where underwear elastic and belt press tightly.

DRUG REACTIONS. Drug reactions can cause reactions that mimic nearly all forms of skin conditions. The most common eruptions, however, are hives and morbilliform rashes. The erythematous macules and papules that often become confluent usually begin within a week of initiating the drug. Unfortunately, no laboratory tests can identify a responsible drug, so reliance must be placed on the history. Often patients are taking several drugs. In trying to select the offending medication from the list, variables to consider are the temporal relationship between the initiation of the drug and the rash and the odds that a given drug is likely to cause an eruption. Drugs most likely to cause maculopapular eruptions include trimethoprim-sulfamethoxazole, penicillin G, semisynthetic penicillins, ampicillin, quinidine, gentamicin sulfate, and blood products. Itching is common with drug reactions, and fever may occur. It is difficult to differentiate the maculopapular drug rash from viral exanthems except that viral prodromata and viral mucous membrane lesions are lacking in drug rashes.

The mechanisms of most cutaneous drug reactions are not understood. Only 10% of drug reactions have a clearly identified immunologic basis. Specific mechanisms of immunologically mediated drug reaction can be due to immediate hypersensitivity (IgE or type I–mediated), cytotoxic antibody reactions (type II), circulating immune complexes (type III), and even type IV delayed hypersensitivity. The mechanisms of nonimmunologically mediated drug reactions include toxic overdose, idiosyncratic responses, drug interactions, and pharmacologic side effects.

Most cutaneous drug reactions remit within 2 to 3 weeks after the drug is stopped. Symptomatic therapy includes antihistamines, occasionally systemic steroids, and application of topical steroids.

PURPURIC MACULOPAPULAR SKIN LESIONS. These should cause the physician to consider a different group of conditions. Purpura, because it represents extravasation of red blood cells outside the cutaneous vessels, cannot be blanched as erythema can. Purpura can be classified as nonpalpable (macular) and palpable (papular). Nonpalpable purpura results from bleeding into the skin without associated inflammation of the vessels and indicates either a bleeding diathesis or blood vessel fragility. Nonpalpable purpura can be *petechial* (macules < 3 mm) or *ecchymotic* (macules > 3 mm). Thrombocytopenia causes petechiae, whereas abnormalities in the blood-clotting cascade commonly cause ecchymoses. Necrotic ecchymoses are found when thrombi form in dermal vessels, leading to infarction and hemorrhage as in disseminated intravascular

coagulation (DIC). Palpable purpura results from inflammatory damage to cutaneous blood vessels, the inflammation causing elevated lesions as in vasculitis.

Nonpalpable Purpuras. Nonpalpable purpuras include thrombocytopenic conditions, senile or actinic purpura, blood clotting abnormalities, Schamberg's disease, hypergammaglobulinemic conditions, and disseminated intravascular coagulation. *Actinic (senile) purpura* is a common problem in older individuals, the result of increased vessel fragility reflecting dermal connective tissue damage from chronic sun exposure and aging. Minor trauma induces ecchymoses, usually on the dorsum of the hands and forearms. The skin in these areas is thin and fragile. Topically or systemically administered steroids can induce similar purpura. Other causes of vascular fragility of the skin include *amyloidosis* and the *Ehlers-Danlos syndrome. Schamberg's disease,* or *pigmented purpuric dermatitis,* is an idiopathic capillaritis that causes petechial lesions of the lower legs (occasionally the arms and trunk) in association with hyperpigmentation. The lesions have the appearance of cayenne pepper. Occasionally Schamberg's disease is secondary to a drug reaction. Petechiae and purpura also occur in *hypergammaglobulinemic purpura,* a syndrome characterized by episodes of fever and arthralgias which appear to be the result of immune complex–mediated damage to small blood vessels. *Disseminated intravascular coagulation* (DIC) refers to uncontrolled clotting within blood vessels with the formation of diffuse thrombosis. The skin is frequently involved with hemorrhage, ecchymosis, and infarction. DIC occurs in association with bacterial sepsis (particularly meningococcemia), as a postviral or poststreptococcal infection phenomenon *(purpura fulminans),* or in conjunction with malignancies such as prostatic carcinoma and acute myelocytic leukemia. The most distinctive hemorrhagic skin lesions are stellate (star-shaped) purpuric ecchymoses with necrotic centers. The center of the lesion is dark gray, indicative of necrosis and impending slough. Petechiae are seen, and hemorrhagic bullae, acral cyanosis, mucosal bleeding, and prolonged bleeding from wound sites can occur. Patients may be systemically ill with fever, shock, and renal failure.

A variety of infectious diseases cause cutaneous petechiae, purpura, or ecchymoses. Already mentioned is *meningococcemia,* in which the organisms produce acute vasculitis or local Shwartzman-like reactions with erythematous macules, petechiae, purpura, and ecchymosis on the trunk and legs. These may become confluent, often with central necrosis. Patients with acute meningococcemia are ill with fever, malaise, headache, meningeal signs, and hypotension. The skin lesions of *disseminated gonococcemia* begin as tiny red papules and petechiae and then evolve into painful purpuric pustules and vesicles scattered on the distal extremities. Fever, polyarthritis, or monoarticular arthritis may be present. The rash of *Rocky Mountain spotted fever* appears between the second and sixth day of the illness, initially as small, erythematous macules that blanch on pressure but then evolving into petechiae, purpura, and ecchymoses. The rash first occurs on the acral areas and then spreads to the extremities and trunk. Small areas of necrosis may occur on the fingers, toes, and ear lobes. Fever, severe headache,

TABLE 475-2. TYPES OF VASCULITIS AND ASSOCIATED SKIN LESIONS

Type of Vasculitis	Blood Vessels Involved	Type of Skin Lesion
Leukocytoclastic or hypersensitivity angiitis: Henoch-Schönlein purpura, cryoglobulinemia, hypocomplementemic vasculitis	Dermal capillaries, venules, and occasional small muscular arteries in internal organs	Purpuric papules, hemorrhagic bullae, cutaneous infarcts
Rheumatic vasculitis: systemic lupus erythematosus; rheumatoid vasculitis	Dermal capillaries, venules, and small muscular arteries in internal organs	Purpuric papules; ulcerative nodules; splinter hemorrhages; periungual telangiectasia and infarcts
Granulomatous vasculitis		
Churg and Straus allergic granulomatous angiitis	Dermal small and larger muscular arteries and medium muscular arteries in subcutaneous tissue and other organs	Erythematous, purpuric, and ulcerated nodules, plaques, and purpura
Wegener's granulomatosis	Small venules, arterioles of dermis, and small muscular arteries	Ulcerative nodules; peripheral gangrene
Periarteritis: classic type limited to skin and muscle	Small and medium muscular arteries in deep dermis, subcutaneous tissue, and muscle	Deep subcutaneous nodules with ulceration; livedo reticularis; ecchymoses
Giant cell arteritis: temporal arteritis, polymyalgia rheumatica, Takayasu's disease	Medium muscular arteries and larger arteries	Skin necrosis over scalp

toxicity, confusion, and myalgias commonly occur. *Infective endocarditis* is associated with petechial and purpuric skin lesions. Petechiae appear in crops in the conjunctivae, buccal mucosa, upper chest, and extremities. Splinter hemorrhages (linear, red to brown streaks under the fingernails or toenails); Osler nodes (2- to 15-mm, tender, red nodules on the pads of the fingers and toes); and Janeway lesions (small, painless plaques and palpable, purpuric nodules on the palms or soles) may be seen. The skin lesions are related to immune complex vasculitis or septic emboli.

Palpable Purpuras. *Vasculitis* and *necrotizing angiitis* are terms used in disorders in which there is segmental inflammation in the blood vessel wall with accumulation of neutrophils and fibrinoid necrosis. The vascular reaction is mediated by immune complexes. Papules with purpura result from extravasation of blood from the damaged vessels. Although all sizes of blood vessels may be affected, the vasculitis in the skin involves venules. If the process is extensive or if large vessels are involved, skin necrosis and ulceration may occur. Depending upon the size of the blood vessels affected, at least five types of vasculitis may involve the skin. The size and type of vessels in the skin, in turn, determine the kind of morphologic lesion (Table 475–2).

In general, as the vasculitis involves progressively larger and more deeply situated vessels, the skin lesions become more nodular, with larger ulcerative or gangrenous processes. The term *granulomatous vasculitis* refers to angiitis associated with a histiocytic proliferation that also involves necrotizing granulomas in the connective tissue of multiple organs, causing rhinorrhea, sinusitis, cough, arthralgias, and ocular and neurologic symptoms (Churg-Strauss vasculitis).

Necrotizing leukocytoclastic vasculitis can occur in a variety of settings including (1) sepsis, (2) connective tissue disease—especially systemic lupus erythematosus and rheumatoid arthritis, (3) cryoglobulinemia, (4) drug reactions, and, occasionally (5) underlying carcinomas, lymphomas, or leukemias. In many instances no apparent cause is found.

Circulating immune complexes have been demonstrated in patients with necrotizing angiitis. Immunoglobulins and complement are found in the affected vessel wall by direct immunofluorescence. The immune complexes lodge in the small vessel walls and activate the complement system, forming the anaphylatoxins C3a and C5a, which recruit neutrophils that induce inflammatory and necrotic damage to the vessel with accompanying fragmented nuclei of the neutrophils (so-called nuclear dust).

Several syndromes are associated with leukocytoclastic vasculitis, depending on the organ systems affected. *Henoch-Schönlein syndrome* occurs most often in children, frequently preceded by an upper respiratory infection and accompanied by arthralgias, abdominal pain, and renal vasculitis. IgA is usually found along with complement in the involved vessels on direct immunofluorescence. *Hypocomplementemic vasculitis* is characterized by urticaria-like lesions, arthritis, and low serum complement. IgG and C3 are present in vessels taken from early skin lesions. Facial and laryngeal edema may also occur. A third form consists of purpura, arthralgia, weakness, and *mixed cryoglobulinemia* (mixed cryoglobulins contain IgG and IgM with anti-IgG or rheumatoid factor activity), which may be idiopathic or occasionally associated with systemic lupus erythematosus, infectious mononucleosis, lymphomas, or primary biliary cirrhosis.

If the vasculitis is idiopathic and cutaneous, the skin responds to prednisone (60 to 80 mg per day) or dapsone (100 to 150 mg per day). Systemic vasculitides may require prednisone and cyclophosphamide (2 mg per kilogram per day).

Necrotizing cutaneous vasculitis may occur in association with *hepatitis B* and in patients with *intestinal bypass surgery* for morbid obesity or in patients with jejunal diverticula or other gastrointestinal conditions characterized by bacterial overgrowth. An *arthritis-dermatitis syndrome* with intestinal bypass surgery may occur with polyarthritis and palpable purpura or purpuric nodules and pustules on the trunk, legs, feet, and arms. Antigenic components of the intestinal bacterial overgrowth lead to the formation of cryoprotein immune complexes that deposit in the skin and joints, causing a hypersensitivity vasculitis and nondeforming arthritis. Antibiotics such as chloramphenicol, sulfamethoxazole-trimethoprim, tetracycline, and metronidazole have been reported to improve the condition.

PAPULOSQUAMOUS SKIN DISEASES

Unique scales are the common characteristic of diseases in this group (Table 475–3). *Squamous* refers to scaling that represents thickened stratum corneum and thus implies an abnormal keratinization process. The lesions, in addition to being scaly, are characterized by sharply demarcated, red to violaceous papules and plaques that result from thickening of the epidermis and/or underlying dermal inflammation.

PSORIASIS. Psoriasis is a genetically determined, chronic epidermal proliferative disease of unpredictable course. Onset is most frequent in early adult life, but it may begin at any age. Once the disease becomes manifest, it may remain localized to a few areas or may cause intermittent or continuous generalized disease.

The lesions appear as erythematous papules and plaques surmounted by silvery, thick scales that resemble mica (micaceous) and that are easily removed and may accumulate in the patient's clothing or bed (Fig. 475–1). In intertriginous areas maceration pre-

TABLE 475–3. ADDITIONAL PAPULOSQUAMOUS SKIN DISEASES

Disease	Appearance of Lesion	Distribution	Mucous Membrane Involvement	Other Features
Secondary syphilis	Ham red or copper colored scaling papules and plaques, sometimes annular	Generalized: palms and soles often involved	Mucous patches, often white or red; condyloma warts of anal area	Condylomata in genital area; serologic test for syphilis positive
Pityriasis rubra pilaris	Red, scaling plaques and patches with follicular horny excretions, especially on dorsum of hands and fingers; diffuse, yellow hyperkeratoses of palms and soles	Often diffuse, rough scaling erythema involving entire body with islands of normal skin ("island sparing")	Occasionally lacy white plaques in mouth	Remits spontaneously in 2–4 years; nail changes as in psoriasis
Pityriasis lichenoides et varioliformis acuta (Mucha-Habermann disease)	Red, discrete, palpable papules that vesiculate and then become hemorrhagic, crust, scale, and leave a scar	Scattered lesions over trunk and extremities	May resemble leukocytoclastic vasculitis	May resolve in a few months or persist for years
Pityriasis lichenoides et varioliformis chronica (chronic parapsoriasis)	Guttate to larger, red slightly scaling papules and plaques; nonpruritic	Usually on trunk	Some forms may represent early stages of mycosis fungoides	Responds to UVB light treatments
Mycosis fungoides	Persistent, pruritic, red, thickened plaques with fine scales as seen in eczema, or thick mica-like scales suggestive of psoriasis; may ulcerate	Scattered asymmetrically over trunk, extremities; girdle area often first area involved	Neoplastic T-cell lymphoma	May show islands of normal skin within red areas

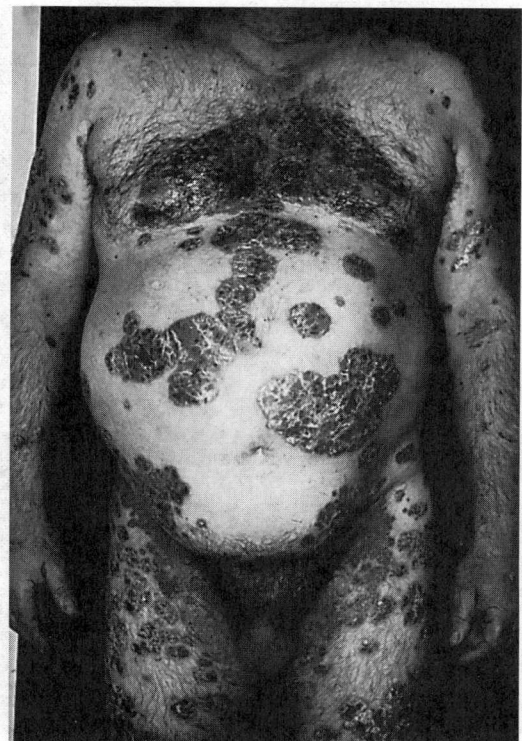

FIGURE 475-1. Psoriasis. (From the 17th edition of the Cecil Textbook of Medicine, with the permission of Dr. Marie-Louise Johnson.)

vents scales from accumulating, but the lesions remain red and sharply defined. Classically, lesions are distributed symmetrically over areas of bony prominence such as elbows and knees. They also commonly occur on the trunk and scalp and in the intergluteal cleft. These latter two areas are frequently overlooked. Palms and soles may be involved, with diffuse redness, scaling, and, at times, pustular lesions. Nail involvement occurs in up to 50% of patients. The nails may be pitted with small ice pick-like depressions on the surface of the nail plate. Onycholysis can also occur, in which a plaque of psoriasis in the distal nail bed causes a red-brown discoloration that is reminiscent of an oil stain under the nail. Another helpful diagnostic feature is the Koebner phenomenon, in which intense trauma to the skin induces new skin lesions. Thus, scratches or surgical incisions elicit linear papulosquamous lesions that should alert the physician to the diagnosis. This may also explain the high incidence of psoriasis on the elbows and knees. Other aggravating factors include streptococcal infections, emotional stress, overuse of alcohol, and drugs, including lithium and beta blockers. Several common variants of psoriasis may also be seen: (1) *guttate psoriasis,* in which numerous, small papular lesions with silvery scales evolve suddenly over the body, often 1 to 3 weeks following streptococcal pharyngitis; (2) *inverse psoriasis,* in which plaques evolve in intertriginous areas and thus lack the typical silver scale because of maceration and moisture; (3) *pustular psoriasis,* a form of the disease in which superficial pustules occur in one of three presentations—pustules studding typical plaques; pustules confined to the palms and soles; and a rare generalized eruption in which pustules evolve abruptly on large areas of erythematous skin accompanied by fever and leukocytosis; (4) *erythroderma*—occasionally the psoriasis can become generalized to involve erythema and scaling of the entire integument. This may occur secondary to a general Koebner phenomenon with overvigorous therapy, a drug reaction, or withdrawal of oral steroids; (5) *psoriatic arthritis*—arthritis may accompany psoriasis in 10 to 15% of cases.

At times Reiter's syndrome may be confused with psoriasis. The skin lesions of the two disorders are indistinguishable clinically and histologically. In Reiter's syndrome pustular and hyperkeratotic papules and plaques commonly occur on the palms and soles (keratoderma blenorrhagica) and scaling, red patches evolve encircling the glans penis and within the groin (balanitis circinata). The presence of asymptomatic erosions on the tongue and buccal mucosa,

urethritis, iritis or conjunctivitis, arthritis, and occasionally diarrhea should suggest the diagnosis.

The pathogenesis of psoriasis is unknown, but it appears to be a multifactorial disease in patients who are genetically predisposed. There is an increased prevalence of psoriasis in individuals with HLA antigens BW17, B13, and BW37. Thirty percent of patients have a family history of disease. The basic alteration represents an accelerated cell cycle in an increased number of dividing cells, culminating in rapid epidermal cell proliferation. Cellular turnover is increased seven-fold, and the transit time from the basal layer to the top of the stratum corneum is 3 or 4 days rather than the usual 28. This rapid turnover of keratinocytes alters keratinization, resulting in thickened epidermis (seen as papules and plaques) and parakeratotic stratum corneum (silvery scales). The mechanism underlying this benign proliferative reaction is unknown.

The goal of therapy is to decrease epidermal proliferation and underlying dermal inflammation. There is no curative agent for psoriasis, and treatment suppresses the condition only as long as it is administered. Three types of topical therapies are employed: (1) topical steroids, usually with intermediate and strong potency agents administered once or twice a day; (2) topical tars and anthralin preparations, often used once a day in combination with topical steroids; (3) ultraviolet light, either UVB with tar or UVA with oral psoralens (see Ch. 474). Recently a new medication, calcipotriene ointment (dovonex 0.005%), has been released for psoriasis treatment. This Vitamen D ointment restricts the hyperproliferative reaction. This topical preparation seems to be as effective as medium-potency topical steroids and so it has "steroid sparing effects" on the use of potent topical steroids. It is used twice a day and can irritate the skin, especially when used on the face and in body folds.

Two systemic types of therapy are available, but because of their side effects these should be reserved for severe widespread disease that is unresponsive to topical measures: (1) antimetabolites or antimitotic agents, including methotrexate, azathioprine, and hydroxyurea. The most commonly used is methotrexate in low doses, usually given on a weekly basis. Because these agents affect bone marrow and liver (in the case of methotrexate), complete blood counts and liver function tests should be performed regularly, together with intermittent liver biopsies. (2) Etretinate, a retinoid, is particularly useful in pustular and erythrodermic forms of psoriasis. Careful monitoring of blood counts, plasma triglycerides, and liver function is required, and avoidance of pregnancy during the use of this drug is mandatory. In fact, the drug should probably not be used in women of childbearing age.

PITYRIASIS ROSEA. Oval or round, tannish pink or salmon colored, scaling papules and plaques appear rapidly over the trunk, neck, upper arms, and legs (Fig. 475–2). Several features of this self-limited papulosquamous condition are unique. The generalized eruption is preceded by a single lesion, termed the "herald patch," that is commonly misdiagnosed as "ringworm." The patch can occur anywhere but often appears on the neck or lower trunk area and precedes the general rash by several days to a week. The oval

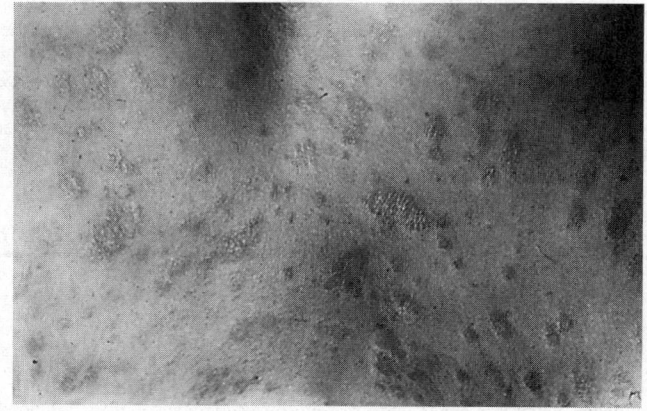

FIGURE 475–2. Pityriasis rosea. (From the 17th edition of the Cecil Textbook of Medicine, with the permission of Dr. Marie-Louise Johnson.)

patches have an unusual fine, white scale located near the border of the plaques, forming a collarette. The lesions follow skin cleavage lines, in a pattern likened to a Christmas tree. The condition spontaneously involutes in 1 to 2 months. Recurrences are rare. Itching can be prominent.

Pityriasis rosea occasionally is preceded by a mild upper respiratory infection, and its greatest incidence is in the winter months, suggesting a viral cause. However, the disease does not occur endemically and is not transmitted person to person.

Such conditions as tinea corporis and guttate psoriasis may be considered in the differential diagnosis, but two possibilities should always be entertained: drug eruption and secondary syphilis. If the rash persists longer than 2 or 3 months or generalizes to involve the trunk, extremities, and especially the face, a drug reaction should be considered. Such medications as gold compounds, barbiturates, captopril, clonidine, and tripelennamide can cause such a rash. Secondary syphilis should be suspected and a serologic test obtained if the rash involves palms and soles and if fever, coryza, or mucous membrane erosions (so-called mucous patches) are present.

Treatment of pityriasis rosea is usually not necessary, although topical corticosteroids and antihistamines may relieve itching and decrease erythema. Ultraviolet light (UVB), given as three to five treatments eliciting a mild erythema reaction, often clears the rash.

LICHEN PLANUS. This idiopathic, pruritic, inflammatory condition of the skin is included in the papulosquamous group of diseases because the primary lesion is a unique papule. The papules are flat topped (planus) and polygonal in configuration (i.e., the sides conform to normal fine skin folds) and have a lilac or purple hue. They may have visible scales on their surface, but more characteristic are subtle, fine white dots or white reticulated lines (Wickham's striae) surmounting the shiny, flat tops (resembling the appearance of a lichen). Wickham's striae are more visible under a hand lens after the application of a drop of mineral oil to the surface of the papule. The Koebner phenomenon occurs in lichen planus, so linear streaks of papules at the sites of skin trauma may be noted.

Although lichen planus can occur anywhere on the body, typical locations are the ankles, wrists, mouth, and genitalia. There may be only a few papules or innumerable ones in a generalized distribution. Mucous membranes are commonly involved, the lesions appearing most frequently as asymptomatic white streaks in a reticulated pattern on the buccal mucosa, tongue, gums, or lips. At times blisters and erosions are superimposed (erosive lichen planus), causing severe discomfort. Lichen planus involving the male genitalia may appear as violaceous annular lesions. Rarely, lichen planus may appear as violaceous annular and polycyclic lesions on the legs and arms, or as hyperkeratotic, follicular, scarring alopecia. All lichen planus lesions leave residual hyperpigmented macules in their wake.

The cause of lichen planus is not known, but two conditions may mimic lichen planus skin lesions and thus offer clues to an immune cause. Certain drugs such as thiazides, phenothiazines, gold, quinidine, and antimalarials can cause lichen planus-like, generalized eruptions. Also, some patients with graft-versus-host disease also develop a skin reaction that closely resembles lichen planus. The eruption can evolve into the usual chronic graft-versus-host sequelae of diffuse dermal sclerosis, cicatricial alopecia, reticulated pigmentation, and ulceration.

For other, mostly less frequent, papulosquamous skin diseases, see Table 475–3. Icthyoses are listed in Table 475–4 and illustrated in Figure 475–3.

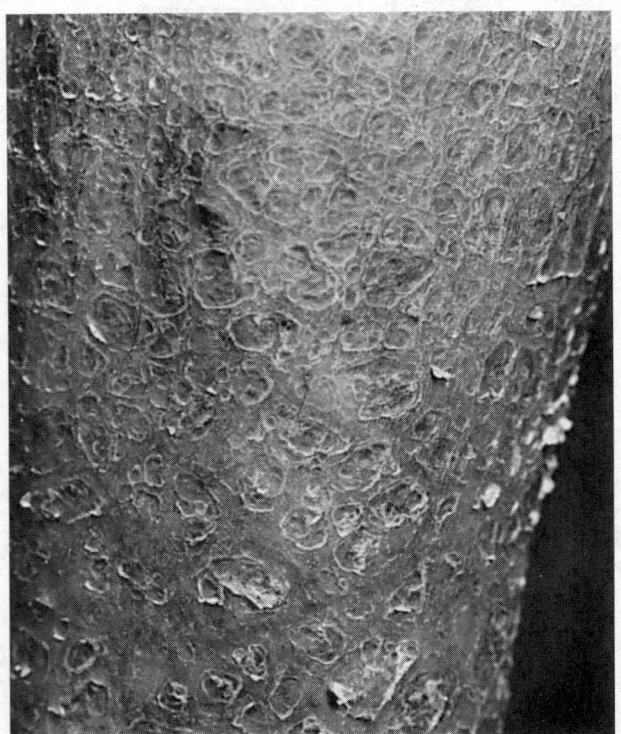

FIGURE 475–3. Ichthyosis. (From the 17th edition of the Cecil Textbook of Medicine, with the permission of Dr. Marie-Louise Johnson.)

VESICULOBULLOUS DISEASES

Vesicles and bullae, when intact, are readily recognized primary skin lesions. Crusts or superficial erosions are secondary lesions that lead one to suspect a preceding fluid-filled primary lesion. The cause of blistering disease includes bacterial and viral infections, contact dermatitis, and autoimmune and metabolic diseases. The pathogenesis of the blister formation is often helpful in understanding its anatomic location: Blisters occur either within the epidermis (intraepidermal) or at the dermoepidermal junction (subepidermal) (Table 475–5).

Intraepidermal vesicles or bullae usually contain clear fluid (but may become filled with purulent material secondarily) and have very thin roofs, so they are flaccid in appearance and are easily broken. At times the blisters are difficult to recognize, and only erosions, crusts, or the thin shreds of the epidermal blister roofs remain. Subepidermal blisters, on the other hand, have an epidermal roof and are tense and remain intact. Hemorrhagic fluid is common in subepidermal blisters because of their location close to dermal capillaries.

Biopsy of early vesicles or blisters is imperative in diagnosis. Immunofluorescence studies on biopsy material may differentiate certain immunologically mediated diseases. Pathologic studies are most informative when performed early, before therapy has been initiated.

INTRAEPIDERMAL VESICULOBULLOUS DISEASES. Pathologic processes involved in epidermal blister formation include spongiosis, primary cell damage, and acantholysis. Spongiosis, a common form of blister formation in eczematous processes, represents edema between cells of the prickle layer and liquefaction

TABLE 475–4. ICHTHYOSIFORM DERMATOSES

	Inheritance	Onset	Distribution	Clinical Associations	Kinetics
Lamellar ichthyosis	Autosomal recessive	Birth	Body, palms, soles	Ectropion	Increased
Epidermolytic hyperkeratosis	Autosomal dominant	Birth	Predominant flexural involvement	Blisters	Increased
X-linked ichthyosis (steroid sulfatase deficiency)	X-linked	Birth	Trunk	Corneal opacities	Normal
Ichthyosis vulgaris	Autosomal dominant	Childhood	Spares flexural areas	Atopy	Normal

Reprinted from the chapter by Dr. Marie-Louise Johnson in the 17th edition of the Cecil Textbook of Medicine, with her permission.

TABLE 475–5. LESS COMMON VESICULOBULLOUS DISEASES

Location of Blister in Skin	Cause If Known	Important Physical Findings	Other Facts of Note in History or Laboratory Results
Autoimmune			
Cicatricial pemphigoid	Subepidermal IgG linear in basement membrane zone	Scarring blisters in the mucous membrane; 25% have blisters on skin	Causes blindness; stenosis of urethra, anal areas
Dermatitis herpetiformis (vesicles in dermal papillae)	Immunologic deposition of IgA in dermal papillae	Grouped, symmetrically distributed vesicles and urticarial papules on scalp, scapulae, buttocks, elbows, knees	Intense burning, itch; high incidence of asymptomatic celiac sprue
Metabolic			
Porphyria cutanea tarda	Metabolic defect in porphyrin metabolism	Tense bullae that leave scars in sun-exposed areas; bullae induced by sun, trauma	May also see facial hirsutism and hyperpigmentation
Bullous disease of renal disease	Unknown	Bullae usually in extremities	
Bullous disease in diabetics	Unknown	Large bulla on acral areas	
Mechanicobullous diseases			
Epidermolysis bullosa (split above, below, and within dermal-epidermal zone)	Variety of inherited conditions	Tense blisters that erode and scar, especially in recessively inherited forms; can lead to severe scars covering digits	Severe forms may involve mouth, esophagus
Epidermolysis bullosa acquista (blister below lamina densa)	Linear IgG and C3 deposits below lamina densa	Tense blisters that lead to scars and millia in pressure and trauma sites on hands, feet; scarring mucous membrane lesions also occur	Circulating antibody to sublamina densa antigen found

of cells which gradually increases the size of the fluid spaces. Primary epidermal cell damage with fluid accumulation is seen in viral infections and friction damage. Blisters may also occur when cellular desmosomal attachments and intercellular cementing substances are immunologically or chemically altered, causing dyshesion referred to as acantholysis (pemphigus).

Bullous impetigo, a subcorneal infection of the skin with staphylococcal and/or streptococcal organisms, causes large, fragile, clear or cloudy bullae that form thin, honey-yellow crusts and a delicate collarette-like remnant of blister roof after the blisters rupture. Autoinoculation results in satellite lesions. The superficial epidermal blistering is caused by the toxic effects of an epidermal toxin elaborated by certain strains of these bacterial organisms.

A more serious variant of bullous impetigo is *staphylococcal scalded skin syndrome,* usually affecting infants and characterized by the formation of rapidly progressive, painful, erythematous patches in which large flaccid bullae evolve and shed as large sheets of skin, leaving a denuded, scalded-appearing surface. With only slight trauma the skin readily slides off, much like wet wallpaper slides off a wall (Nikolsky's sign—see Ch. 473). In contrast to localized bullous impetigo in which the *Staphylococcus aureus* may be recovered in the skin lesions, the bullae of scalded skin syndrome are sterile, although a staphylococcal infection may be found in the conjunctiva, nose, or pharynx. The widespread intraepidermal blistering results from an epidermal toxin elaborated by specific strains of *Staphylococcus* and hematogenously carried to the skin. These are penicillinase-resistant strains of *Staphylococcus* and therefore require methicillin-type antibiotics.

A somewhat similar condition, *toxic epidermal necrolysis* (TEN), occurs in adults, often secondary to drugs (e.g., ampicillin, allopurinol) and occasionally to *Staphylococcus* infections in an immunosuppressed patient. TEN is a reaction to a variety of antigenic materials that cause a suprabasilar split in the epidermis with necrosis of much of the overlying epidermis. Because of the more extensive destruction of epidermis and barrier stratum corneum layer (as opposed to staphylococcal scalded skin syndrome, in which the split is subcorneal), TEN is often fatal and, when extensive, should be treated as a widespread burn would be cared for. TEN also often involves the mucous membranes and therefore may be confused with Stevens-Johnson syndrome (see below).

Viral infections of the skin may cause vesicles and bullae by virtue of direct infection of the keratinocytes and the destructive effect on the cells. Vesicles caused by viruses often display two important characteristics: (1) they tend to occur in groups on an indurated erythematous base, and (2) they often take on an umbilicated appearance.

Herpes simplex infections are discussed in Ch. 339.

A complication of herpes simplex infection, *erythema multiforme,*

is a hypersensitivity skin and mucous membrane reaction that evolves 1 to 2 weeks following herpetic recurrences as a result of a herpesvirus–containing immune complex reaction to the herpes antigen. Herpes infection is only one etiologic stimulus leading to erythema multiforme (see below).

Diagnosis of herpes infections (including zoster and varicella) is made with a Tzanck preparation of material taken from the roof of vesicles. The contents are smeared onto a slide and stained with Wright or Giemsa stain to reveal multinucleated giant cells (see Ch. 473).

Acyclovir administered orally or intravenously is the most frequently used form of therapy for primary and recurrent forms of herpes (see Ch. 339).

Varicella infection, when initially encountered, causes chickenpox, a generalized pruritic eruption with widespread, delicate vesicles on an erythematous base which have been likened to a dew drop on a rose petal. They often become umbilicated, hemorrhagic, and pustular and may leave scars. Chickenpox lesions occur predominantly on the trunk but also involve the head, extremities, and mucous membranes of the mouth and conjunctiva. Successive crops of lesions evolve for a week. Ch. 336 discusses the systemic illness. *Herpes zoster* is a recrudescence of latent varicella virus in persons who previously had varicella. Zoster appears as grouped, umbilicated, and, at times, hemorrhagic vesicles and pustules on an erythematous base situated unilaterally along the distribution of cranial or spinal nerve roots. Frequently several immediately adjacent dermatomes are involved. Bilateral involvement is rare. Zoster is frequently associated with a prodrome of severe radicular pain in the involved areas. A common useful sign in making the diagnosis is hypesthesia of the dermatomal areas—the patient often bitterly complains that the rubbing of clothing on the area is intolerable. Most patients with herpes zoster are over 50 years of age, and cancer patients (especially those with lymphomas such as Hodgkin's disease) are particularly prone to this infection. In such patients or in immunocompromised individuals, cutaneous dissemination from the original dermatome may occur, as well as visceral involvement of liver, lung, and central nervous system. Treatment of herpes zoster is usually symptomatic with Burow's compresses, analgesics, and acyclovir, especially in immunocompromised patients (800 mg five times per day orally for 10 days). Postherpetic neuralgia is common in individuals over 50 (see Ch. 405). Systemic corticosteroids may reduce acute herpetic pain; whether they reduce the risk of postherpetic neuralgia is debatable. *Insect bites* including flea and fire ant bites may also induce vesicles or bullae, a response to injected toxins or foreign chemicals or proteins in the bite or an allergic reaction to them.

Pemphigus diseases cause blistering in the epidermis by virtue of the process of acantholysis. *Pemphigus vulgaris* and a variant, *pem-*

phigus vegetans, which heals with hypertrophic, "vegetative" surfaces, are acquired autoimmune diseases of the skin and mucous membrane. The superficial bullae, evolving just above the basal layer, readily rupture, leaving denuded, bleeding, weeping and crusted erosions over the body which do not heal. The oral mucosa is almost always involved and is frequently the presenting site. The painful erosions characteristically spill over the vermilion border of the lips and onto the skin. Lesions of the skin occur anywhere but often in pressure and friction areas. The blisters arise on normal-appearing skin. Untreated pemphigus vulgaris progresses slowly with extensive denudation, leading to fluid and electrolyte imbalance, sepsis, and death. Pain from mouth lesions prevents adequate food intake. Skin biopsy of early vesicles should be obtained for routine histologic examination. The edge of a bulla, including adjacent normal skin, should be examined by direct immunofluorescence to make the diagnosis. Immunofluorescence shows deposits of immunoglobulins (usually IgG) and/or C3 in the intercellular spaces around keratinocytes. Antibodies to the intercellular areas of the epidermis are found in the serum. Circulating antibodies to the epidermis are directed against several polypeptide components of the epidermal desmosomes. Their titers somewhat reflect disease activity, and they may contribute to the defective epidermal adhesion. High doses of systemic steroids (100 to 200 mg of prednisone per day) over prolonged periods usually control the disease. Methotrexate and other cytotoxic agents are useful as steroid-sparing agents. Treatment with intramuscular gold often is successful, occasionally inducing long-term remissions (see Ch. 474).

Pemphigus foliaceus is a less severe disease in which the acantholytic separation within the epidermis is in the upper portion of the prickle layer. *Pemphigus erythematosus* may be a localized variant of pemphigus foliaceus presenting with superficial blisters, erosions, and crusting and oozing over the scalp and face in a seborrheic dermatitis–like rash or often simulating the butterfly rash of systemic lupus erythematosus. Mucous membrane involvement in pemphigus foliaceus and pemphigus erythematosus is unusual, and lower doses of systemic steroids generally control these conditions. Immunofluorescent studies on skin from the edge of lesions reveal immunoglobulin and/or C3 in the intercellular areas of the upper portions of the epidermis.

Familial benign pemphigus, or Hailey-Hailey disease, is a dominantly inherited disorder with suprabasal cell acantholysis, the groups of bullae arising on erythematous skin in the flexural areas (neck, axillae, groin). Spreading erosions display vesicles and pustules at the borders with a moist, granular center. Warm weather and superficial bacterial infections seem to cause flares with spontaneous exacerbations and remissions continuing for years. Familial benign pemphigus differs from other forms of pemphigus in its genetic pattern, absence of mouth lesions, benign course, and absence of intercellular antibodies. Antibiotics, both topical and systemic, may improve acute flares of the disease. If *Candida* infection is superimposed, topical antifungal agents are often of benefit. When chronic vegetating lesions are present, surgical removal with skin grafting may be useful.

DERMAL-EPIDERMAL VESICULOBULLOUS DISEASES.
Separation of the epidermis from the dermis occurs in a variety of bullous diseases resulting from autoimmune and immunologic reactions, metabolic disturbances, and a number of inherited mechanicobullous conditions (see Table 475–5).

Bullous pemphigoid is an autoimmune disorder of the elderly, in which tense, large blisters occur on normal or erythematous skin, often in the groin, axillae, and flexural areas. Only one third of patients have oral blisters. Healing usually occurs in some blisters without scarring while new lesions evolve. Itching may be severe or absent. Skin biopsies display a subepidermal blister through the lamina lucida (at the electron microscopic level), and direct immunofluorescence reveals deposition of the IgG immunoglobulin and complement directed against an antigen in the lamina lucida. The prognosis is good, and the disease usually subsides after months or years. Widespread bullae require therapy with 40 to 60 mg of oral prednisone per day and occasionally with immunosuppressive agents.

Another subepidermal blistering disease, *herpes gestationis,* is a rare autoimmune condition that occurs during pregnancy and the postpartum period. The name of the disease is misleading, for it is not associated with herpesvirus infection. The blisters develop at any time throughout the course of pregnancy, although they most often begin during the second and third trimesters and subside a few weeks post partum. Some patients may experience transient flares or recurrences with each menstrual period or following the use of oral contraceptives. There are recurrences with subsequent pregnancies. Herpes gestationis is a pruritic condition with numerous tense vesicles arising on both normal-appearing and erythematous areas of skin. Arcuate and polycyclic red plaques with peripheral blistering are seen. The lesions first appear on the abdomen and then spread to involve the entire integument. Skin biopsy findings are indistinguishable from those of bullous pemphigoid by light microscopy, and examination of perilesional skin by direct immunofluorescence reveals C3 and less often an IgG linear band just below the epidermis. There is associated fetal mortality as high as 30%, and there is also an increased rate of premature live births. Transient vesiculobullous lesions may infrequently occur in some otherwise healthy infants of affected mothers. Occasionally the patients' intractable pruritus and extensive bullae respond to high-potency topical steroid ointments and diphenhydramine, but most patients require oral prednisone (20 to 60 mg daily) throughout pregnancy with intermittent tapering.

Cicatricial pemphigoid (benign mucosal pemphigoid) and dermatitis herpetiformis are described in Table 475–5.

Erythema multiforme is an immunologic reaction in the skin and mucous membranes often mediated by circulating immune complexes that evolve in response to a number of antigenic stimulae (infections, drugs, connective tissue disease). As the name implies, the skin reaction is characterized by a variety of lesions, namely, erythematous plaques, blisters, and target or bull's-eye lesions. The mucous membranes of the mouth and eye may also be involved, and this is referred to as *Stevens-Johnson syndrome.* Typically the cutaneous lesions favor the extremities (often the palms) and are symmetric. Target lesions are diagnostic and are recognized by a central, dark purple area or a blister surrounded by a pale, edematous, round zone, surrounded in turn by a peripheral rim of erythema. In Stevens-Johnson syndrome the skin disease is more widespread, with blisters and painful erosions in the mouth and eyes. The patients look and feel ill with fever, prostration, and difficulty in eating. Histologically, subepidermal separation is found in the blistering center of the target lesion, and when early lesions are biopsied, immunofluorescence reveals immunoglobulin and complement in the walls of the small dermal blood vessels; the inflammation and bulla form in response to vascular damage and leaking. In one half of cases no cause is found for the reaction, but a cause should be sought in all cases, especially drugs (penicillins, barbiturates, phenytoin [Dilantin], and sulfonamides) and infections (herpes simplex, *Streptococcus, Mycoplasma pneumoniae*). Recurrent herpes simplex infection is the most common cause of recurrent erythema multiforme. It is not clear whether medical therapy favorably alters the course of idiopathic erythema multiforme, although treatment of a precipitating infection seems appropriate and acyclovir may prevent recurrences of herpes-associated erythema multiforme. Stopping suspected drugs is also imperative. The value of systemic steroids in erythema multiforme and Stevens-Johnson syndrome is controversial. In addition, IV fluids may be required in patients with severe oral involvement, and topical anesthetics (viscous Xylocaine) may help to decrease mouth discomfort.

An example of a bullous disease caused by a metabolic disorder is *porphyria* (see Table 475–5 and Ch. 187).

Other metabolic bullous diseases are those seen with chronic renal disease and diabetes mellitus. These also are briefly described in Table 475–5, as are mechanobullous conditions.

PUSTULAR DISEASES OF THE SKIN

Pustules usually bring to mind infection, but not all pustular dermatoses are caused by pathogenic microorganisms. Pustular conditions often occur in association with erythematous papules, cysts, and nodules and may open to form crusts (Table 475–6).

NONINFECTIOUS PUSTULAR SKIN DISEASES. *Acne* is the most common pustular condition of the skin. It is an inflammatory disorder affecting pilosebaceous units and is usually found over the face and upper trunk. Several pathogenic factors play a role as individuals enter puberty: (1) androgens stimulate the sebaceous glands and increase sebum production (see Ch. 472); (2) abnormal keratinization and impaction in the pilosebaceous canal

TABLE 475-6. ADDITIONAL NONINFECTIOUS PUSTULAR DISEASES OF THE SKIN

Name of Skin Condition	Cause	Important Physical Findings	Other Facts of Note in History or Laboratory Results
Perioral dermatitis	May be caused by potent topical steroids; variant of acne	Perioral and periorbital red scaling patches, papules, and pustules	
Pustular psoriasis	Variant of psoriasis	Sterile pustules localized to palms and soles or generalized over body	Patient is toxic with fever, leukocytosis; can die of generalized form
Miliaria pustulosa	Occlusion of sweat glands in hot environment	Discrete red papules or pustules with red base over trunk, especially back	

(comedones) obstruct sebum flow; (3) proliferation of anaerobic bacteria, *Propionibacterium acnes,* predisposes to rupture of the pilosebaceous unit with extravasation into the surrounding dermis, resulting in sterile, inflammatory papules, pustules, and cysts. These later lead to disfiguring scarring. Therapy of acne is usually successful in controlling the disease until the patient "grows out" of this condition. Topical agents that remove comedones such as benzoyl peroxide and topical vitamin A preparations are particularly effective because their action allows sebum to flow freely onto the surface of the skin. Topical and oral antibiotics (tetracycline and erythromycin) are indicated in patients with inflammatory papules and pustules. Oral 13-*cis*-retinoic acid (Accutane) decreases sebaceous gland size and sebum production. This drug should be used primarily for severe cystic acne because in high daily doses it produces undesirable side effects and can be teratogenic. Spironolactone, the potassium-sparing diuretic, has antiandrogenic properties that have resulted in its increasing use in women with difficult-to-control acne. Used in doses of 100 to 200 mg per day along with routine forms of acne therapy, the condition frequently is brought under control. The clinician should recognize that other factors may play a role in exacerbating acne, including oil-based cosmetics and drugs (androgenic hormones, antiepileptics [phenytoin], high-progestin birth control pills, systemic corticosteroids when taken in high doses, and iodide- or bromide-containing agents). Occasionally endocrinologic conditions characterized by excess androgen secretion may cause acne, i.e., polycystic ovarian disease, adrenal or ovarian tumors.

Rosacea is a chronic inflammatory disorder affecting the blood vessels and pilosebaceous units of the face in middle-aged individuals. Patients with rosacea have papules and pustules superimposed on diffuse erythema and telangiectasia over the central portion of the face. An important component is easy flushing and blushing of the face often accentuated when alcohol, caffeine-containing, or hot spicy foods are ingested. Hyperplasia of the sebaceous glands, connective tissue, and vascular bed of the nose sometimes causes *rhinophyma* or a large, red, bulbous nose (see Fig. 475-4). Ocular complications occur in a small but significant number of rosacea patients; these include blepharitis, chalazion, conjunctivitis, and keratitis. Progressive keratitis can lead to scarring and blindness. Rosacea and the eye complications usually respond well to tetracycline, and/or metronidazole but the antibiotic must be continued for life (at the lowest dose that suppresses the condition) because rosacea recurs when therapy stops. High-potency topical corticosteroid preparations may induce or aggravate pre-existing rosacea and should not be used for long periods of time on the face.

INFECTIOUS CAUSES OF SKIN PUSTULES. *Folliculitis,* an *S. aureus* infection of the hair follicle, appears as pustules with a red rim with hair emanating from the center of the pustule. Folliculitis typically occurs in hairy regions where clothing rubs (buttocks, thighs) or on the face. The key to diagnosis is finding a central hair in the pustule. Occasionally the follicular infection can extend more deeply to form a larger, red, fluctuant nodule that "points" in order to drain pus from one (furuncle) or more follicles (carbuncle). Systemic antibiotics such as erythromycin or dicloxacillin usually clear extensive infections; topical antiseptic cleansers such as povidone-iodine or chlorhexidine can resolve mild folliculitis and may be useful in preventing recurrences.

Candidiasis appears as beefy red patches in intertriginous, moist areas characteristically surrounded by satellite pustules. Paronychia, a painful red swelling in the periungual regions of the finger, may also drain pus in which *Candida* can be found with a KOH prepa-

ration. Topical agents such as clotrimazole and miconazole are used two or three times a day. These must be used for many weeks before the infection clears.

Hot tub folliculitis is a generalized, pruritic folliculitis caused by *Pseudomonas aeruginosa* that is acquired in contaminated hot tubs, whirlpools, or swimming pools. It usually begins 6 hours to 5 days after hot tub soaking and affects many people using the facility. It appears as a vesicular and then pustular eruption over the trunk, buttocks, legs, and arms but spares the head and neck. *Pseudomonas* can often be cultured from fresh pustules. In most instances the folliculitis resolves within 7 to 10 days without specific treatment. Infected tubs and pools should be cultured for *Pseudomonas* and disinfected.

Dermatophytes can, at times, infect hair follicles and result in pustules, particularly in the beard (tinea barbae) and scalp (kerions). These are readily confused with a bacterial folliculitis. Kerions appear as indurated, boggy, inflammatory plaques studded with pustules. These intense inflammatory reactions to superficial dermatophytes (especially *T. verrucosum*) respond to griseofulvin therapy, although a short course of oral corticosteroids is also useful.

Deep fungal infections such as *blastomycosis, sporotrichosis,* and *coccidioidomycosis* may cause pustules, as well as verrucous, ulcerative papules and nodules. Sporotrichosis characteristically spreads up cutaneous lymphatics and appears as nodular, pustular lesions in a linear distribution.

SYSTEMIC INFECTIONS CAUSING PUSTULES ON THE SKIN. A variety of septicemias including gonococcemia, staphylococcal septicemia, and *Candida* septicemia (in immunosuppressed patients) cause pustular lesions associated with purpura.

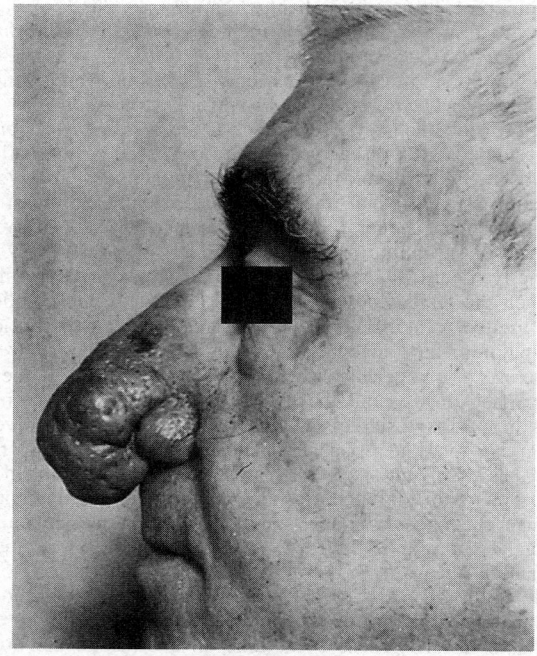

FIGURE 475-4. Rhinophyma. (From the 17th edition of the Cecil Textbook of Medicine, with the permission of Dr. Marie-Louise Johnson.)

URTICARIA, PERSISTENT FIGURATE ERYTHEMAS, CELLULITIS

This group of skin lesions is of disparate appearance and origin. The common feature is a raised edematous, red plaque with a sharply demarcated border.

URTICARIAL REACTIONS. Urticaria, the most common condition in this group, appears as wheals, transient erythematous and edematous swellings of the dermis caused by local increase in permeability of capillaries and small venules. This increased permeability results from histamine and other chemical substances released from cutaneous mast cells by Type I IgE hypersensitivity reactions, as well as by nonimmunologic mechanisms (see Ch. 224). Certain agents such as aspirin, opiates, and some foods degranulate mast cells directly without an allergic mechanism. Other urticarial reactions are immunologically mediated by such allergens as infections (viral, i.e., hepatitis, sinus and tooth infections), infestations (systemic parasites), drugs, pollens, and injections (blood products, vaccinations). Physical modalities—light (solar urticaria), cold (cold urticaria), heat or exercise (cholinergic urticaria), or pressure or rubbing of the skin (dermatographism)—cause other such "hives". Hives are transient, any given lesion lasting < 24 hours, although new ones may continuously evolve. Acute urticaria (i.e., lasting < 6 weeks) often results from drugs and the cause is frequently identified. The cause of chronic urticaria (lasting > 6 to 8 weeks) is more difficult to identify. Hives covering large areas and producing deep tissue swelling are termed *angioedema*. This condition can involve the tongue and throat and impinge upon the airway. In such patients a careful history about medications (including over-the-counter drugs, especially cold tablets or medications containing aspirin) should be elicited. Infections such as sinusitis or apical abscess of teeth must be looked for. In addition, physical types of urticaria should be considered: *cholinergic* urticaria is characterized by evanescent multiple, small wheals surrounded by a wide pink flare induced by heat and exercise; *solar* urticaria by large plaques in sun-exposed areas; *cold* urticaria by wheals that evolve with exposure to cold. Urticaria accompanied by fever and arthralgias occurs in serum sickness reactions and in the prodromata of viral hepatitis. Occasionally urticaria occurs in conjunction with internal conditions such as malignancies or connective tissue diseases. Hereditary angioedema, an autosomal dominant disorder, causes recurrent urticaria, angioedema, intestinal colic, and life-threatening laryngeal edema.

If the cause for the urticaria cannot be found or avoided, symptomatic control is achieved with antihistamines or oral steroids. Acute angioedema or laryngeal edema requires rapid systemic treatment with epinephrine and diphenhydramine (see Ch. 224).

Other urticaria-like skin lesions include *erythema multiforme* (see above); *juvenile rheumatoid arthritis skin lesions*—small, 2- to 3-mm, salmon-colored hives that last only a few hours appearing with fever spikes; *erythema margination*—lesions found in 10% of patients with acute rheumatic fever (see Ch. 277). *Urticaria pigmentosa* (mastocytosis), a disease caused by increased accumulations of mast cells in the skin and at times in lymph nodes, liver, spleen, bones, and gastrointestinal tract (see Ch. 231), presents with multiple tan to brown, papular spots that urticate when rubbed owing to the release of histamine from the mast cells. A skin biopsy specimen readily identifies increased numbers of mast cells in the dermis. When the lesions develop in early childhood, the condition is usually limited to skin and the lesions resolve by puberty, leaving only hyperpigmented macules. If the skin lesions evolve in adulthood there is a greater chance for mast cell infiltration of the organ systems noted above, and the skin lesions persist. Symptoms and findings in mastocytosis depend on the organ systems involved and the release of various vasoactive substances contained in the increased masses of mast cells. Hepatosplenomegaly, lymphadenopathy, and bone pain may occur secondary to infiltrates. Patients may experience flushing, palpitations, headache, syncope, hypotension, abdominal pain, and diarrhea, all related to histamine and prostaglandin release from the mast cells.

FIGURATE ERYTHEMAS. This is a group of uncommon conditions characterized by annular, polycyclic, and geographic erythematous skin lesions. These conditions, in contrast to the urticarial reactions, persist for many days or even years, moving slowly or rapidly over the skin surface (hence, the term sometimes used for these reactions—persistent figurate erythema). Usually no specific cause is found for these lesions, but some may be associated with underlying malignancies. Erythema repeus, characterized by a series of swirling woodgrain-like red lines, is found in association with adenocarcinomas of the breast, lung, or gastrointestinal tract or with other fungal infections. Erythema annulare centrifugum is a slowly enlarging annular lesion that clears in the center with collarette scaling on the inner edge of the red rings. It is found at times with cutaneous dermatophyte infections, systemic *Candida* infections, the ingestion of blue cheese, parasitic bowel diseases, and autoimmune disorders.

Erythema chronicum migrans is the unique annular skin lesion found in Lyme disease caused by a spirochete inoculated by infected tick bites (see Ch. 321 and Color Plate 10B).

CELLULITIS. Although superficially resembling urticaria, these inflammatory infections of the dermis are readily distinguished from hives by their persistent, slowly enlarging nature as well as their pain and warmth. Group A streptococci and *S. aureus* are most commonly responsible. *Erysipelas* is sometimes identified separately from cellulitis. It displays a sharply demarcated painful border and an "orange-peel" epidermal surface. Group A *Streptococcus* is the usual cause. Patients usually feel ill and are febrile. Cellulitis on the lower legs in adults may develop from fissures between the toes from tinea pedis. Systemic antibiotics, erythromycin, dicloxacillin, or the cephalosporins are the most commonly used drugs.

Necrotizing fasciitis is a special form of cellulitis involving the deep fascial structures underlying the skin. Rapidly evolving in enclosed fascial spaces, usually in diabetics or immunosuppressed patients, these infections are caused by a mixture of aerobic and anaerobic gram-negative organisms and must be diagnosed early by deep fascial biopsy and treated immediately with broad-spectrum antibiotics and surgical debridement.

NODULES AND TUMORS OF THE SKIN

Skin nodules and tumors may evolve within the epidermis or the dermis and subcutaneous tissue, arising in various skin appendages and structures, including melanocytes. Such lesions may represent benign or malignant growths, infiltrative or inflammatory reactions. In many instances the structures giving rise to the nodule reflect the colors of these structures. Vascular lesions appear red to purple, whereas lesions involving melanocytes appear pigmented.

Most epidermal nodules are recognized by localized thickening of the epidermis or corneum with hyperkeratosis or scale. Dermal or subcutaneous nodules appear as lumps, often with no alteration in the overlying epidermis.

Of primary concern is whether a nodule is benign or malignant. This is not always easy, and skin nodules and tumors often must be biopsied. Some clinical generalizations can be made in distinguishing benign from malignant tumors (Table 475–7).

NONPIGMENTED NODULES—BENIGN. *Warts* are benign epidermal growths caused by papilloma viruses (see above, under Maculopapular lesions).

Sebaceous hyperplasia occurs as papular and occasionally nodular lesions on the faces of individuals past 50 years of age. Proliferation of sebaceous glands surrounding a hair follicle appears as groups of yellow papules evolving in an annular configuration with a central pore. Sebaceous hyperplasia may be clinically difficult to differentiate from basal cell cancers, although the yellow discoloration and central pore may help. At times skin biopsy may be necessary. No treatment is generally required.

TABLE 475–7. CLINICAL FEATURES HELPFUL IN DISTINGUISHING BENIGN FROM MALIGNANT TUMORS

Clinical Feature	Benign	Malignant
Configuration	Symmetric, sharp borders	Asymmetric, irregular borders
Rate of growth	Slow	Slow or rapid
Friability	No friability	Often friable
Bleeding or ulceration	Seldom bleed or ulcerate	Often bleed and ulcerate
Consistency	Firm or soft	Usually firm to hard
Color	Uniform color and pigmentation	Irregularity of color and pigmentation

Keratoacanthomas, or self-healing epitheliomas, are rapidly growing, biologically benign neoplasms of epidermal keratinocytes. The lesions resolve spontaneously, leaving a scar. Keratoacanthomas are usually found on sun-exposed areas and begin as flesh-colored papules that rapidly grow over a period of 6 weeks, evolving a central keratin-filled crater. The lesions remain for 6 to 8 weeks and then subside. Such lesions are best excised because they leave unsightly scars and are difficult to differentiate from squamous cell cancer, even histologically.

Epidermal inclusion cysts appear as flesh-colored, firm nodules in the skin, particularly over the scalp and trunk. A helpful diagnostic sign is a central enlarged pore where the epidermis has invaginated to form the cyst. If the central pore is patent, slight squeezing will express white, cheesy, foul-smelling keratin and sebum. Bothersome cysts can be excised.

Lipomas are more deeply situated than epidermal inclusion cysts. Although they can feel firm and even rubbery, like a cyst, they usually are multilobulated and softer in consistency. If the diagnosis is in doubt and especially if the lesion is firm, a biopsy is indicated. Lipomas may be multiple. Familial multiple epidermal cysts and lipomas, fibromas, and osteomas associated with intestinal polyps are recognized as Gardner's syndrome.

Neurofibromas, focal proliferations of neural tissue within the dermis, may present in two forms: (1) soft, flesh-colored, protruding nodules that, on compression, can be invaginated into what feels like a defect in the skin (buttonhole sign), and (2) deep, firm, dermal or subcutaneous nodules. Neurofibromas may be solitary, but when they are multiple *von Recklinghausen's disease* should be considered, especially when café au lait spots (light brown macules) and axillary freckling are seen.

NONPIGMENTED NODULES—MALIGNANT. Malignant tumors of the epidermas—*basal cell* and *squamous cell carcinomas*—relate to the amount and intensity of electromagnetic radiation, including ultraviolet light and x-radiation, the skin has received over a lifetime. Accordingly, such cancers occupy sun-exposed areas, especially the face, neck, arms, and hands. The cancers are more common in patients living in southern latitudes of the northern hemisphere and in Australia, especially in persons with a light complexion whose occupations keep them outdoors. These epidermal cancers also are more common in immunosuppressed patients, attesting to the importance of the immune surveillance system in cancer. A personal or family history of skin cancer should sharpen attention to the possibility of cancer.

Basal cell carcinomas arise from the basal cells of the epidermis. They rarely metastasize, but they can cause extensive, local destruction. Four clinical forms should be recognized: (1) the *nodular* type, the most common, appears as a pearly or opalescent, irregularly shaped papule or nodule with a central depression or crater; telangiectasias and a rolled, waxy border are often in evidence. When ulceration and crusting occur, it is referred to as a rodent ulcer (Fig. 475–5). Often the raised, waxy border is subtle and is observed more readily by stretching the skin. (2) *Superficial* basal cell carcinoma is recognized as a red, slightly scaling, eczematous plaque that may be slightly eroded and crusted. Careful examination reveals a threadlike, pearly, rolled edge. This is an easily overlooked neoplasm, frequently confused with psoriasis or eczematous patches. A high index of suspicion, along with skin biopsy, is needed to make the diagnosis. (3) *Pigmented* basal cell carcinoma appears as a blue-black nodule or plaque with a pearly, opalescent sheen. Melanocytes are not histologically involved in these cancers, merely stimulated to make more pigment but not worsening the prognosis. (4) *Scarring* or *sclerosing* basal cell cancers present as atrophic, white, sometimes slightly eroded or crusted plaques with telangiectasia. This is the most difficult form to cure because of its indistinct borders. The diagnosis of basal cell carcinoma should be confirmed by biopsy. Treatment depends on the location of the lesion, the morphologic type, the size of the tumor, and whether it is primary or recurrent. Treatment modalities include curettage and electrodesiccation, scalpel excision, radiation therapy, and cryotherapy. Properly selected, each modality has a cure rate greater than 90%. A specialized form of excision is used for recurrent basal cell cancers, sclerosing basal cell cancers, and large primary basal cell cancers in regions in which recurrences are likely (particularly in the nasolabial folds and the periorbital and immediate preauricular areas). The Mohs surgical technique utilizes frozen section histologic mapping of the tumor to determine its extent.

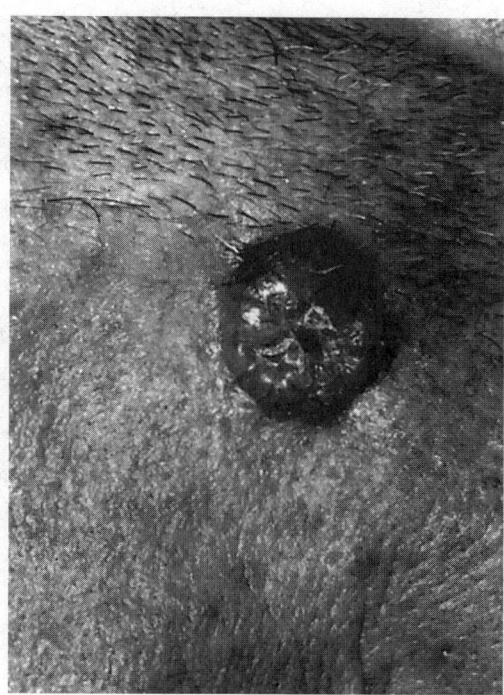

FIGURE 475–5. Basal cell epithelioma. (From the 17th edition of the Cecil Textbook of Medicine, with the permission of Dr. Marie-Louise Johnson.)

Squamous cell carcinoma, a malignant neoplasm of the keratinocytes, is a less common but more aggressive type of cancer. Squamous cell carcinoma is locally invasive and has the potential to metastasize. It occurs primarily on the head and neck, upper extremities, and trunk, presenting as firm, red, smooth or verrucous nodules. Hyperkeratoses may be prominent. The cancers also display increased friability, ulceration, and crusting (Fig. 475–6). *Bowen's disease* is a squamous cell cancer *in situ,* appearing as red, scaling, crusted, sharply demarcated plaques. Squamous cell cancer *in situ* on the penis in uncircumcised males evolves as velvety red patches on the glans and foreskin. Bowen's disease and erythroplasia are banal, easily overlooked conditions that can metastasize if

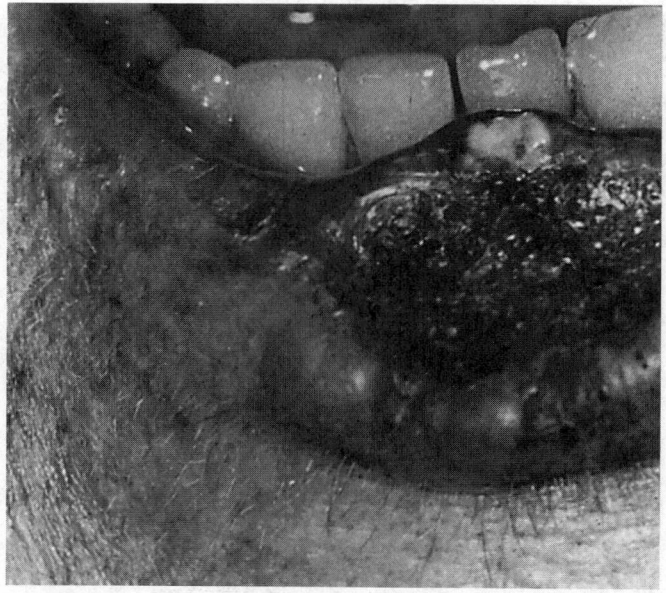

FIGURE 475–6. Squamous cell carcinoma. (From the 17th edition of the Cecil Textbook of Medicine, with the permission of Dr. Marie-Louise Johnson.)

not diagnosed early. *Actinic keratoses,* precancerous lesions of atypical keratinocytes, appear as red, ill-marginated macules and papules with yellow-brown, adherent scales in sun-damaged skin. They may evolve into squamous cell cancers. Any lesion suspected of being a squamous cell cancer should be biopsied. Excision is the treatment of choice. Actinic keratoses are treated with liquid nitrogen freezing or, if numerous, with topical 5-fluorouracil applied as 1 or 5% cream or solution over 2- to 4-week period.

PIGMENTED NODULES—BENIGN. *Seborrheic keratoses* are epidermal cell neoplasms that appear on the face and trunk in middle age. These 2-mm to 5-cm, elevated, tan to brown or occasionally black, round to oval lesions have a verrucous or crumbly, greasy surface and a stuck-on appearance. No therapy is necessary unless they are of cosmetic concern, and then liquid nitrogen cryotherapy or curettage is an effective means of removal.

Dermatofibromas are areas of focal dermal fibrosis accompanied by overlying epidermal thickening and hyperpigmentation. Clinically, they look like brown papules or nodules. A useful diagnostic test is the "dimple sign," in which pinching the lesion results in central dimpling of the overlying epidermis. Some dermatofibromas are dark brown in color and occasionally raise the concern of melanoma, but the fibromas are symmetric and uniform in color. The lesions occur frequently on the lower extremities and less often on the arms, and they may be multiple. Although therapy is usually not required, simple excision can be done.

Nevi, or *moles,* are benign accumulations of pigment-forming nevus cells. They may be congenital or acquired, and most nevi evolve before age 35. There are three forms, representing various stages of biologic evolution and growth: *Junctional nevi* are light to brown macular lesions. *Compound nevi* have flat, junctional portions along with brown papules with a smooth or rough surface; these evolve from junctional nevi in older children and young adults. Later, *intradermal nevi* evolve from the compound nevi as flesh-colored to brown papules or sessile growths (Fig. 475–7). Although nevi vary in appearance and color, individually they are uniform in color, symmetric in their growth and configuration, and usually <6 mm in diameter. Occasionally nevi darken in color or may itch, and new nevi may develop during pregnancy, but symptomatic nevi that change should be regarded suspiciously.

PIGMENTED NODULES—MALIGNANT. Malignant melanoma is the cutaneous neoplasm of melanocytes and nevus cells. Useful clinical features in their diagnosis are called the A-B-C-D's (Table 475–8).

Several clinical forms or presentations of melanoma can be identified, each demonstrating the characteristics described in Table

TABLE 475–8. THE A-B-C-D'S

A = Asymmetry of the lesion is due to irregular, random growth of the malignant cells associated with irregular surface topography and papules and nodules.
B = Borders of the tumors are irregular with notching and pigment "spilling" out beyond the edges.
C = Color variegation consists of browns, blacks, blues, and even shades of red and white. The variations in color represent different depths of invasion of pigment cells along with inflammatory reaction and immunologic response to the malignant cells.
D = Diameter or size of melanomas tends to be greater than 6 mm before they are recognized.

475–8. *Lentigo maligna melanoma* is a slowly evolving, multicolored lesion on the head and neck. It is preceded by lentigo maligna (*in situ* melanoma), which extends peripherally and is an unevenly pigmented, dark brown to black macule that can grow to a size of 5 to 7 cm over a period of many years before nodules develop dermal invasion. *Superficial spreading melanoma* may occur on any area of the body, appearing as irregularly pigmented lesions with papules, nodules, and notched borders. Invasion into the dermis occurs more rapidly than in lentigo maligna melanoma. *Nodular melanoma* appears as a rapidly growing, blue-black, smooth or eroded nodule (Fig. 475–8). It invades dermis early in its evolution, making premetastatic diagnosis difficult. *Acral lentiginous melanoma* occurs on the palms, soles, and digits. It evolves as an irregular, enlarging, variegate-colored, brown to black growth similar to lentigo maligna melanoma but more aggressive in dermal invasion early in its course. Only minor degrees of papular elevation may be associated with deep invasion.

One third of melanomas may arise from existing nevi, so that a change in size, shape, and color or itching of a pigmented lesion (a common symptom in melanomas) should be carefully investigated. Early diagnosis is the key to survival. The deeper the malignant cells invade the dermis, the more likely is metastasis. The depth of dermal invasion can be microscopically measured from the granular cell layer in the epidermis to the deepest penetration of melanoma cells into the dermis. Thin melanomas (<0.76 mm) enjoy a virtually 100% cure rate. If the depth is greater than 1.6 mm, only 20 to 30% survive for 5 years.

Any suspicious pigmented lesion must be biopsied, preferably by excision. Definitive surgical excision should be undertaken only after confirmation of melanoma is established histologically. In large lesions such as lentigo maligna, it is acceptable to do incisional biopsy prior to definitive therapy. Suspicious pigmented lesions should never be shave-biopsied or shave-excised, nor should they be electrocauterized. Full-thickness tissue through the entire lesion is required for diagnostic and prognostic evaluation.

The precise cause of melanoma is unknown, but sunlight and heredity have been suggested as risk factors. The occurrence of melanoma has been increasing during the past few decades. Famil-

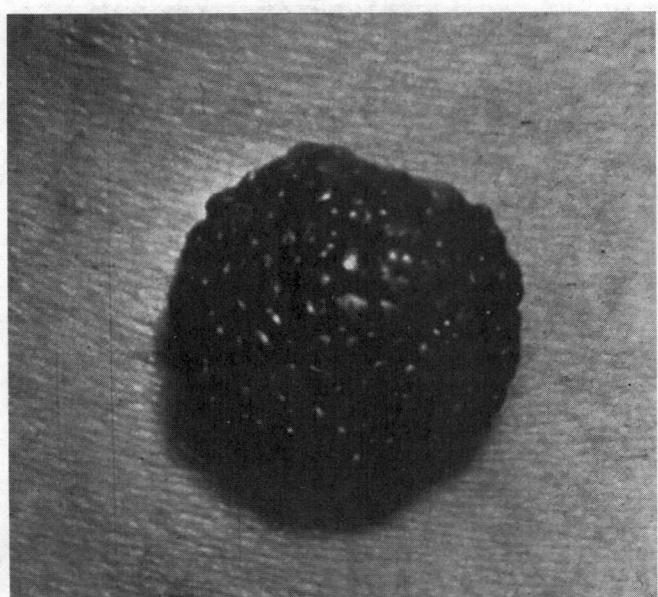

FIGURE 475–7. Intradermal nevus. (From the 17th edition of the Cecil Textbook of Medicine, with the permission of Dr. Marie-Louise Johnson.)

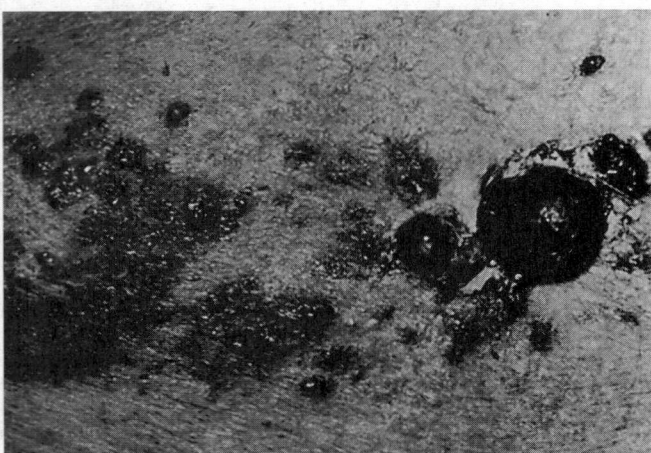

FIGURE 475–8. Nodular melanoma. (From the 17th edition of the Cecil Textbook of Medicine, with the permission of Dr. Marie-Louise Johnson.)

ial occurrence of malignant melanoma affects families with the *dysplastic nevus syndrome.* Numerous atypical, haphazardly colored, red-brown nevi with irregular borders appear over the trunk, extremities, and scalp. Biopsy of these atypical nevi reveals disordered melanocytic proliferation. The nevi may have an increased risk of developing melanoma, although the melanomas can also arise from normal skin in these persons. Close clinical follow-up and excision of suspicious nevi are important.

VASCULAR TUMORS OF THE SKIN. *Hemangiomas,* benign proliferations of dermal vessels, appear at or soon after birth as red, blue, or purple, flat, papular, or nodular lesions. Their appearance depends upon the number, size, and depth of the proliferating vessels. Thus, capillary angiomas are composed of small, superficial vessels causing *nevus flammeus* and *strawberry hemangiomas. Cavernous hemangiomas* are made up of larger and deeper vessels. Cavernous and strawberry angiomas often enlarge at an alarming rate over the first year or two and then usually involute by age nine or ten. Cavernous hemangiomas are less likely to resolve and sometimes may be deeply situated. Large lesions located in strategic locations (around the eye and mouth) may require systemic steroids in efforts to shrink these tumors. Platelet consumption by large cavernous hemangiomas may occur in the *Kasabach-Merritt syndrome.* Ordinarily hemangiomas require no therapy; watchful waiting allows them to resolve spontaneously, the cosmetic result usually being superior to that obtained by therapeutic intervention. When large hemangiomas ulcerate, bleed, or impinge on vital structures or functions (e.g., around the ears, eyes, nose, mouth), oral steroids given over short periods of time in the dose of 1 to 2 mg per kilogram body weight shrinks the tumor temporarily while awaiting the natural involution. Interferon α also has been used to shrink large hemangiomas that do not respond to steroids.

Pyogenic granuloma, a bright red, raspberry-like growth that can reach a centimeter in size, is friable and bleeds easily when traumatized. These lesions occur most often on arms, legs, fingers, and hands. They enlarge rapidly within weeks but have no malignant potential; they represent capillary hemangiomatous proliferation and follow injury or surgery. The term *pyogenic* is a misnomer, as no infectious process is involved. These lesions are treated with excision, curettage and electrocauterization, or cryotherapy. Occasionally amelanotic melanomas may present as a pyogenic granuloma, so pathologic examination of pyogenic granulomas should be performed.

Kaposi's sarcoma is a rare neoplasm of multifocal origin which presents as red-purple to blue-brown macules, plaques, and nodules of the skin and other organs. The cutaneous lesions may be firm or compressible, solitary or numerous, and may even appear initially as a dusky stain, especially about the toes.

These round-cell and spindle-cell sarcomas also can reside in viscera and until their association with AIDS seemed to occur predominantly in older men, leading to their demise. In Europe and North America, where Kaposi's sarcoma is more frequently seen among Jews and those of Mediterranean descent, the lesions commonly affect the lower extremities, are indolent, and often are associated with chronic lymphedema, indicating tumor infiltration of the lymphatics. Men are affected 10 to 15 times more often than women, are usually in their seventh decade, and have an average survival time of approximately 10 years. The incidence of such Kaposi's sarcoma reported for the United States is < 0.1 per 100,000 population and < 0.02% of all malignancies.

In tropical Africa, an endemic belt of Kaposi's sarcoma exists at an altitude of 1200 to 1500 meters where the disease accounts for 3 to 9% of all malignancies, afflicting blacks while sparing whites and Indians. It has a peak incidence in the first decade, with most patients less than 20 years of age, and with survival of less than 3 years. Visceral rather than cutaneous involvement and marked lymphadenopathy are the predominant, unique clinical signs in these African children.

The selective geographic distribution of the lymphadenopathic type of Kaposi's sarcoma resembles that of Burkitt's lymphoma. Electron microscopic studies that affirm an association between cytomegalovirus and Kaposi's sarcoma make another parallel with Burkitt's lymphoma, the malignancy so closely linked to the Epstein-Barr virus. In the acquiring of Kaposi's sarcoma, therefore, infectious agents and immune status seem to be significant, as well as genetic and environmental factors. Kaposi's sarcoma has been observed to complicate systemic lupus erythematosus being treated

with immunosuppression and to appear along with tumors of lymphoreticular origin in the immunosuppressed recipients of renal transplants. It is known to coexist with other primary malignancies. However, its appearance as an aggressive lethal tumor in the young male homosexual is a stunning observation of grave concern. Those affected have a mean age in the fourth decade. Their skin lesions are generalized in distribution and are smaller, softer, and lighter in color than the classic firm, indurated lesions of the legs. Mucous membrane tumors or symptomatic visceral or lung lesions may appear before cutaneous hemorrhagic sarcomas. Average survival time from onset is less than 2 years.

Such fulminant Kaposi's sarcoma appears alone or with *Pneumocystis carinii* pneumonia and other opportunistic infections in increasing numbers in male homosexuals and drug abusers. A small painless red nodule of the skin, easily overlooked, can signal a profoundly compromised immune state and grave prognosis (see Ch. 367 and Color Plate 16*D*).

INFLAMMATORY NODULES OF THE SKIN. *Erythema nodosum* is an inflammatory reaction in subcutaneous fat which represents a hypersensitivity response to a number of antigenic stimuli. Well-localized, multiple, tender, red, deep nodules, 1 to 5 cm in size, usually develop bilaterally over the pretibial areas. They eventually involute, leaving yellow-purple bruises. Ulceration does not occur. Immunoglobulin and complement deposition has been found in deep blood vessels in early lesions, and in some patients circulating immune complexes have been detected. The localization of the painful nodules to the lower legs may relate to hemodynamic factors. Although no cause can be found in many patients, the following factors have been identified: drugs (especially oral contraceptives), pregnancy, inflammatory bowel disease, sarcoidosis, streptococcal infection, *Yersinia* enterocolitis, deep fungus infections, and tuberculosis. If the cause cannot be identified and eliminated, symptomatic therapy with aspirin, nonsteroidal anti-inflammatory medications, potassium iodide, or short courses of systemic steroids may be useful.

Subcutaneous fat necrosis is a condition in which tender, red nodules occur on the lower legs and thighs in patients with pancreatitis or pancreatic carcinoma. The skin lesions may occur in the absence of signs associated with the internal carcinoma. Serum amylase and lipase values are elevated, and skin biopsy provides diagnostic findings.

Rheumatoid nodules are subcutaneous inflammatory lesions usually found over elbows, knees, and fingers in patients with severe rheumatoid arthritis and high rheumatoid factor titer (see Ch. 237).

NODULES ASSOCIATED WITH METABOLIC DISEASES AND MISCELLANEOUS CONDITIONS. *Xanthomas* are focal collections of lipid-containing histiocytes in the dermis and tendon sheaths. They appear as yellowish papules (eruptive xanthomas), plaques (xanthelasma), nodules (xanthoma tuberosum), and xanthomas in tendon and tendon sheaths (xanthoma tendinosum). Xanthomas often arise in association with inherited hyperlipoproteinemias (see Ch. 173) or in several underlying metabolic diseases that alter lipoprotein metabolism, such as diabetes, hypothyroidism, cholestatic liver disease, pancreatitis, renal disease, and certain drug reactions (e.g., 13-*cis*-retinoic acid). Xanthelasma usually develops in the absence of hyperlipidemia, although hypercholesterolemia (and increased low density lipoproteins) may be present.

Patients with gout occasionally deposit sodium urate in the skin, forming firm, hard papules and nodules (tophi) that may discharge whitish crystals in the pinnae of the ears and periarticular areas.

ATROPHIC SKIN CONDITIONS WITH SCARRING, INDURATION, ULCERATION, AND TELANGIECTASIAS

Connective tissue diseases are the most common conditions that lead to this spectrum of cutaneous changes.

SCARRING. *Lupus erythematosus* may be localized to the skin (discoid lupus) or present as a systemic condition (see Ch. 240). Discoid lupus skin lesions appear as red plaques with white, cohesive scales that often are accentuated in the follicular openings (follicular plugging). The plaques eventually atrophy, with depression and scarring along with hypopigmentation in the center of the lesions and a hyperpigmented rim. The lesions usually occur in sun-exposed areas and, when they involve the scalp, cause scarring alopecia. Systemic lupus erythematosus presents as an erythematous rash with a violaceous hue, accentuated in sun-exposed areas, especially the malar area, producing a butterfly configuration. Telangiectasias may also be prominent, and, at times, fine scaling is seen. Occasionally bullae, erosions, and ulcers also occur. Periungual telangiectasia is a prominent finding in systemic lupus as well as in other connective tissue diseases. Subacute lupus is a form in which psoriasiform skin patches are found on the face and trunk. Skin biopsy for both routine and direct immunofluorescence pathologic examination is useful in confirming the diagnosis.

Dermatomyositis findings include violaceous edema of eyelids (heliotrope), flat-topped papules over the knuckles (Gottron's papules), and reticulated patches of hyper- and hypopigmentation, erythema, and telangiectasia (poikiloderma) found on the V of the neck, face, elbows, and knees.

X-radiation can cause chronic skin changes of atrophy, telangiectasias, irregular pigmentation, and eventually ulceration. Within these areas malignant changes may later appear.

DERMAL INDURATIONS (SCLEROSIS). *Scleroderma* is a condition in which excessive collagen is found in the dermis (see Ch. 241). *Morphea* is localized scleroderma confined to the skin, whereas *systemic scleroderma,* or *progressive systemic sclerosis,* is a more extensive form in which fibrosis diffusely involves the skin as well as internal organs (see Ch. 241). Morphea lesions are asymptomatic, oval to irregular, whitish, firm, thickened patches with an erythematous border. The plaques are most often found on the trunk. The thickened skin in progressive systemic sclerosis is not sharply demarcated, but rather causes indurated, "hidebound" tight skin over the fingers, toes, and extremities (acrosclerosis). Thickening of the facial skin causes smoothness and loss of wrinkles except for furrowing around the mouth. Ulcerations followed by pitted scars occur on the finger tips. Telangiectasia may be prominent, appearing as periungual telangiectasias and multiple, small punctate macules on the face and hands (matlike telangiectasia). A variant of systemic scleroderma, the *CREST syndrome,* displays extensive telangiectasias over face and hands. Patients with *hereditary hemorrhagic telangiectasia* also display telangiectasia, particularly around the mouth and nose and on the fingers as well as vascular malformations in the gastrointestinal tract and, at times, the lung. No cutaneous induration is found in this condition.

Lichen sclerosus et atrophicus may be confused with morphea, presenting as porcelain white, atrophic, indurated plaques most commonly on the vulva or on the male genitalia (balanitis xerotica obliterans). At times it occurs as scattered patches on the trunk. Purpuric areas may also be seen within the lesions.

Myxedema may cause a doughy thickening of the skin from deposition of glycosaminoglycans in the dermis. This may be localized to the pretibial areas (pretibial myxedema) as firm, nonpitting plaques and nodules with accentuation of the follicular orifices giving a *peau d'orange* appearance.

CUTANEOUS ULCERS. Primary skin ulcers are caused by a wide variety of conditions. The location of the ulcers, the symptoms associated with them, and the rapidity of their appearance are important clues in diagnosing their various causes.

Ulcers of the extremities are frequently associated with vascular disease. Sudden pain associated with numbness of an extremity and ulceration suggest arterial occlusion. Ulceration of digits associated with a purplish red color with dependency and pallor when the extremity is elevated suggests arteriosclerotic peripheral vascular disease. Brawny edema, brown discoloration, and dermatitis over the lower legs in association with ulcers around the malleoli are seen with venous insufficiency. Sickle cell anemia causes ulcerations in the lower third of the leg. Areas of pressure and trauma, particularly on the foot, in patients with peripheral neuropathy, are susceptible to neurotrophic ulcers *(mal perforans),* as in diabetes and leprosy. The skin around the ulcer is anesthetic and callused. Pressure sores or decubitus ulcers occur in immobilized debilitated patients. Shearing forces, friction, moisture, and pressure contribute to the development of these sores. The sacral and coccygeal areas, ischial tuberosities, and greater trochanters are favored sites. The best treatment of pressure sores is prevention by frequently moving immobilized patients, keeping the skin clean, and using air mattresses.

An unusual and dramatic ulcerative condition, *pyoderma gangrenosum,* often begins as an inflammatory nodule or pustule resembling a furuncle which breaks down, ulcerates, and gradually enlarges peripherally. Fully developed, the lesions are moderately deep, red, necrotic ulcers with undermined, violaceous, edematous borders. These lesions, which typically evolve on the lower legs, are postulated to represent a Shwartzman-like hypersensitivity reaction to a number of underlying internal conditions, including chronic ulcerative colitis, regional ileitis, rheumatoid arthritis, dysproteinemias, and occasionally leukemia or lymphoma. In over one half of the cases no cause is identified.

Ecthyma gangrenosum is characterized by ulcerative lesions, often in the body folds (anogenital and axillary areas), in immunosuppressed patients with *Pseudomonas* septicemia. The painless lesions begin as hemorrhagic bullous patches that become necrotic and ulcerate and are surrounded by considerable erythema with a central gray to black eschar. *Pseudomonas* can be cultured from these skin lesions.

Genital ulcers suggest venereal disease, including herpes simplex (see above), syphilis (indurated, painless, round ulcer with a clean base), chancroid (single or multiple, soft, painful, purulent ulcers with undermined erythematous edges), lymphogranuloma venereum (transient, painless skin ulcer with associated inguinal adenopathy), and granuloma inguinale (small nodules on genitalia which erode and become filled with velvety red granulation).

Multiple genital ulcers also occur in *Behçet's syndrome* in association with oral ulcers and ocular disease (iridocyclitis). Erythema nodosum, arthritis, and neurologic and intestinal involvement may also occur. The oral and genital ulcers are small, painful aphthae. Occasionally sterile pustules and ulcers occur at the site of minor trauma such as blood sampling.

Geometric, bizarre-shaped, angular ulcers are characteristic of a self-inflicted, factitial cause.

HYPER- AND HYPOPIGMENTATION OF THE SKIN

Disorders of melanin pigmentation can be classified as hypomelanoses (decreased or absent epidermal melanin) or hypermelanoses (increased epidermal or dermal melanin). Hyper- and hypomelanosis can be further subdivided into localized or generalized (total body) alterations of pigmentation.

Hyperpigmentary Conditions

LOCALIZED PIGMENTARY CONDITIONS. *Freckles* (ephelides) are light brown-red macules found in sun-exposed areas which are caused by increased melanin production in normal numbers of melanocytes. These occur in fair-complexioned individuals with red or sandy hair. Ultraviolet radiation increases melanin production in these lesions.

Lentigines are also hyperpigmented macules, but they occur because of increased numbers of melanocytes in the basal layer of the epidermis. Two types are recognized: (1) *lentigo simplex,* which occurs in early life and is congenital, and (2) *actinic lentigines,* which are acquired in middle age and are related to sun damage over the face, arms, and dorsum of the hands. Actinic lentigines are sometimes difficult to distinguish from early lentigo maligna on the face, but actinic lentigines have no malignant potential. The *multiple lentigines syndrome* is a rare, dominantly inherited condition characterized by hundreds of lentigines on the trunk, head, extremities, palms, and soles, and it is associated with *E*lectrocardiographic abnormalities, *O*cular hypertelorism, *P*ulmonary stenosis, *A*bnormal genitalia, *R*etarded growth, and *D*eafness (thus the acronym LEOPARD syndrome). Another dominantly inherited condition is *Peutz-Jeghers syndrome,* distinctive for its numerous lentigines occurring around the mouth, eyes, hands, and feet in association with gastrointestinal polyps, gastrointestinal hemorrhage, and occasionally malignant degeneration of the polyps.

Melasma (chloasma) of the face usually affects women, and in this instance the melanocytes produce more melanin than normal in response to hormonal factors (occurs during pregnancy or while on birth control pills) in association with ultraviolet radiation. This type of pigmentation occurs symmetrically over the malar eminences, forehead, and upper lip. The lesions may fade with delivery but often persist and are accentuated when birth control pills are used. Hydroquinone, a bleaching agent (2 to 4% creams), may help reduce the pigmentation, but many authorities believe these are of no value and that they may worsen the problem. Sunscreens are also useful.

Postinflammatory hyperpigmentation is the term given to macular pigmentation following inflammatory skin diseases (lichen planus typically causes brown to blue pigmentation).

Café au lait spots are light brown (coffee-with-cream hue) macules that occur on the trunk and extremities in neurofibromatosis (Fig. 475–9). Six or more such lesions, each greater than 1.5 cm in diameter, are diagnostic for this dominantly inherited disease. Axillary freckling, discrete neurofibromas (Fig. 475–10), and large plexiform neurofibromas along with bony abnormalities combine to make this a disfiguring condition. Ten percent of the normal population have isolated café au lait spots. In *Albright's disease* (polyostotic fibrous dysplasia) three or four large, irregularly shaped (so-called coast-of-Maine configuration), hyperpigmented macules are usually found unilaterally distributed on the buttocks or cervical area.

Xeroderma pigmentosum is a rare, heterogeneous group of diseases with hereditary deficiencies of enzyme systems in the skin that repair ultraviolet-induced damage to keratinocyte and melanocyte DNA. This inability to maintain the integrity of DNA leads to extreme sun sensitivity and multiple freckles over the face, lips, conjunctivae, and extremities which evolve into variably sized pigmented patches interspersed with hypopigmented areas. Keratoses, keratoacanthomas, basal and squamous cell cancers, and malignant melanomas evolve and frequently lead to early death. This entity should be thought of whenever one finds otherwise unexplained extreme sensitivity to the sun or excessive freckling in youngsters. This disease can be subtle in its initial presentation, and total avoidance of the sun from early life may prevent subsequent fatal skin cancers.

GENERALIZED HYPERPIGMENTATION. Diffuse brown hyperpigmentation is a feature of *Addison's disease* with accentuation of the pigment in body folds (palmar creases), pressure points (knuckles, elbows), and gingival mucous membrane. A similar type of diffuse hyperpigmentation is seen following adrenalectomy in patients with Cushing's disease due to a pituitary tumor, as well as in patients with pancreatic and lung carcinomas. In all of these instances the generalized hypermelanosis results from overproduction of melanocyte-stimulating hormone (MSH) and adrenocorticotropic hormone (ACTH). These trophic hormones share common amino acid sequences. Both MSH and ACTH secretions are increased in Addison's disease as a result of diminished output of cortisol by the adrenals. Oat cell cancers of the lung and pancreatic carcinomas

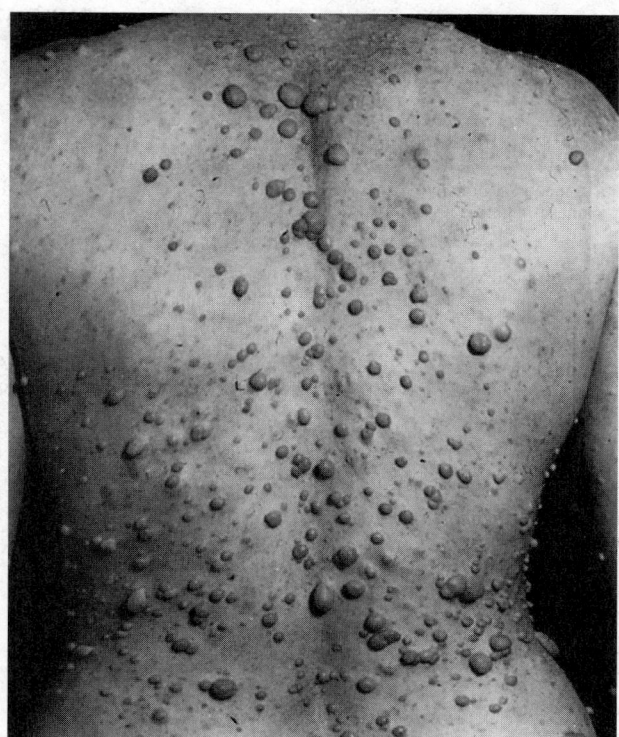

FIGURE 475–10. Neurofibromatosis—von Recklinghausen's disease. (From the 17th edition of the Cecil Textbook of Medicine, with the permission of Dr. Marie-Louise Johnson.)

have been found to excrete increased amounts of MSH, thus causing similar hyperpigmentation. Melanocyte MSH receptors bind MSH, which stimulates intracellular cyclic AMP, and this, in turn, increases tyrosinase activity and pigment formation in melanocytes.

A number of drugs can cause Addisonian-like hypermelanosis including busulfan, cyclophosphamide, and nitrogen mustard. Blue-gray pigmentation may occur either diffusely or in localized patches following use of chlorpromazine, minocycline, and antimalarial drugs. In addition, inorganic trivalent arsenicals (found in insecticides and contaminated water) may also produce a generalized brown pigmentation, but in this instance the hypermelanosis is studded with small, scattered, depigmented macules (likened to rain drops on a dusty road) and punctate keratoses on the palms and soles. *Hemochromatosis* causes a metallic gray-brown, generalized hyperpigmentation resulting from the combination of increased pigment formation in the skin and iron deposition.

Hypopigmentary Conditions

LOCALIZED PIGMENTARY CHANGES. *Vitiligo,* a circumscribed hypomelanosis of progressively enlarging amelanotic macules in a symmetric distribution around body orifices and over bony prominences (knees, elbows, hands), is familial in 36% of cases. In one third of cases some spontaneous repigmentation occurs, particularly in sun-exposed areas. White hairs are common in the vitiliginous areas. Although most patients with vitiligo are healthy, there is an increased association with certain autoimmune conditions such as thyroiditis, hyperthyroidism, Addison's disease, pernicious anemia, and diabetes mellitus. Melanocytes are absent from the vitiliginous macules. Circulating complement-binding antimelanocyte antibodies have been found in some vitiligo patients. The use of PUVA may give some repigmentation, but it may require 200 or more such treatments.

Piebaldism is a local hypopigmentary condition representing an autosomal dominant hypomelanosis on the extremities, anterior surface of the thorax, and especially over the midline of the forehead and central scalp. A white forelock is typical. The hypomelanosis stems from the lack of normal migration of the melanocytes to these regions during embryologic development.

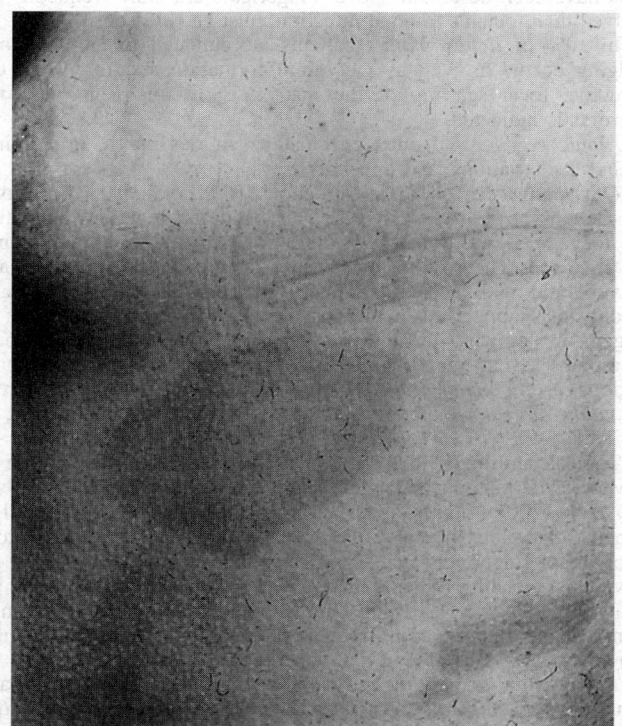

FIGURE 475–9. Café au lait spot. (From the 17th edition of the Cecil Textbook of Medicine, with the permission of Dr. Marie-Louise Johnson.)

TABLE 475–9. ALBINISM

	Inheritance	Frequency	Skin Color	Pigmented Nevi Freckles	Hair	Eyes Color	Red Reflex
Oculocutaneous Albinism							
Tyrosinase-negative	AR*	1 in 34,000	pink/white	none	white	gray-blue	present
Tyrosinase-positive	AR	blacks: 1 in 15,000 whites: 1 in 40,000	white-cream	present	white-yellow red; darkens	blue-yellow brown	present but may be absent in dark races
Yellow-mutant	AR	rare—Amish, Polish, German-American; blacks (American, Ceylonese, African)	white at birth, slightly tan possible	present	white-birth red/yellow 6 mos	blue at birth; darkens	present
Chédiak-Higashi syndrome	AR	rare in most countries; none in blacks	pink/white	present	blond-dark brown-steel gray	blue to brown	present but diminishes with time
Oculocutaneous Albinoidism	AD†		pink/white	?	white blond	blue	present
Ocular Albinism							
Vogt	X-linked	uncommon	normal	present	normal	blue	
Forsius-Eriksson	X-linked	less common	normal	present	normal	blue	
Autosomal recessive	AR	10 families	normal	present	normal	blue	present

A common localized form of hypopigmentation, *pityriasis alba,* appears as slightly pink and hypopigmented, oval to round patches with mild, fine scaling. These occur on the cheeks of children, but they may also be found on the trunk, mimicking the hypopigmented, scaling patches seen in tinea versicolor (a KOH examination of the scales may be necessary to differentiate these two conditions). Pityriasis alba is most frequently seen in atopic dermatitis patients.

Tuberous sclerosis, an autosomal dominant condition, displays white macules in almost all cases. The depigmented macules involve the trunk or buttocks in an oval or mountain ash-leaf configuration. The presence of three or more macules strongly suggests tuberous sclerosis, and because the hypomelanotic patches are present at birth, they represent one of the earliest signs of the condition. Examination with Wood's light is often useful in visualizing the lesions, which histologically contain melanocytes with decreased numbers of melanosomes. Newborns with unexplained seizures or mental retardation should be screened with a Wood's light for the presence of the white spots. Ch. 417 gives details of the systemic disorder. CT brain scans are also useful in defining the tumorous dysplasia.

Certain chemicals, particularly phenol derivatives, when applied to the skin, may cause permanent depigmentation. Hypomelanosis has been observed on the hands of black-skinned individuals wearing rubber gloves in which hydroquinone is used as an antioxidant.

GENERALIZED HYPOPIGMENTATION. (Albinism). Table 475–9 lists these hereditary disorders, all of which produce generalized hypomelanosis of the skin, hair, and eyes.

REGIONAL DIAGNOSIS OF SKIN DISEASES—COMMONLY ENCOUNTERED PROBLEMS BY ANATOMIC REGION

Many skin diseases have a predilection for certain areas or regions of the body, often related to variations in the structure and function of the integument (Table 475–10).

Disorders of the Nails

The nail is a plate of hard keratin synthesized from an invagination of the epidermis. The proximal nail fold houses the matrix of the nail where basal cells rapidly proliferate and differentiate into the nail plate, which grows over the nail bed. Nails grow continuously throughout life. The average fingernail grows 0.5 to 1.2 mm per week, whereas toenails grow at one half to one third this rate. It takes a fingernail about 5.5 months and the toenails 12 to 18 months to regrow from the matrix, although rate of growth slows as the individual gets older. Table 475–11 provides a terminology to describe defects in nail formation.

SKIN DISEASES INVOLVING NAILS. Nail changes in *psoriasis* have been described above. Fingernails are more frequently involved than toenails. Fungal infection must be ruled out.

In 10% of *lichen planus* patients, accentuated longitudinal nail ridging occurs as well as pterygium formation resulting from destructive focal scarring of the matrix. Early treatment with oral steroids is indicated.

Atopic eczema and other eczematous entities may cause pitting, transverse striations, and onycholysis.

Onychomycosis, or fungal infections of the nail, may be caused by dermatophyte (tinea unguium) or candidal infections. Infection of toenails is more frequent than fingernails, but all nails may be involved. The nail plate is discolored, thickened, crumbly, and onycholytic with accumulation of debris. White superficial onychomycosis appears as white patches in the toenail plate due to organisms growing on the surface barely penetrating the nail. Scrapings reveal hyphae upon KOH examination. An unusual condition, *chronic mucocutaneous candidiasis,* is caused by widespread *Candida albicans* infection leading to diffuse white thickening of all nails.

Topical antifungal therapy is ineffective. Oral griseofulvin is given for dermatophyte infection until the nails appear clear. Ketoconazole (200 mg daily) is an alternative should griseofulvin fail or when *Candida* is the causative agent. Oral therapy requires 4 to 6 months for fingernails and 12 to 16 months for toenails. In older individuals toenail problems may never be eradicated because the nails grow so slowly. Residual fungal spores in shoes and the environment no doubt cause frequent recurrences; topical antifungal powders may be helpful in long-term prophylaxis.

Paronychia, or painful, red swelling of the nail fold, is usually caused by *C. albicans.* At times a small abscess or purulent discharge is seen. This infection usually occurs in hands constantly exposed to a wet environment (bartenders, janitors). Therapy consists

TABLE 475–9. ALBINISM (Continued)

Eyes					Hair Bulb Incubation (Tyrosine)	Defect	Melanosome Maturation by Stage	Complications or Associated Problems
Nystagmus	Photophobia	Visual Acuity	Pigment in Fundus	Other				
marked	severe	legally blind	none	–	negative	no tyrosinase	I-unmelanized II	skin malignancy basal cell ca squamous cell ca
present but less	present but variable	severe defect in children; may improve with age	none; some with age	pigment cartwheel effect pupil, limbus	positive	no access of enzyme to tyrosine	I, II, some III, rare IV	skin malignancy basal cell ca squamous cell ca
present but variable	present but variable	marked defect; may improve with age	none; some with age	pigment cartwheel effect	neg to pos?	unknown ? pheomelanogenesis	I, II, III	unknown
absent or slight	absent or slight	normal or slight decrease	some; increase with age	normal for cartwheel effect	positive	giant melanosomes, lethal defect in leukocytes	I, II, III, IV	infections; hematologic and neurologic abnormalities; lymphoreticular malignancy
no	no	normal or slight decrease	punctate		positive	unknown	unknown	none
present	severe	marked decrease	reduced		positive			
latent	absent or slight	color blind			positive			
present	severe	marked decrease			positive			

* AR = Autosomal recessive.
† AD = Autosomal dominant.
Reprinted from the chapter by Dr. Marie-Louise Johnson in the 17th edition of the Cecil Textbook of Medicine, with her permission.

of avoidance of water and the use of antifungal solutions two or three times a day for a month or two.

NAIL DISTURBANCES IN SYSTEMIC DISEASES. *Splinter hemorrhages* result from the extravasation of blood from longitudinally oriented vessels of the nail bed. Although often thought to be associated with bacterial endocarditis, they are much more commonly associated with trauma. *Beau's lines* are nonspecific, appearing as transverse depressions across the nail plates following any severe disability that temporarily interferes with nail growth. *Longitudinal pigmented bands* occur most often in response to trauma or a nevus located in the matrix. *Yellow nail syndrome* exhibits yellow thickening of the nails with absence of the lunula and variable degrees of onycholysis accompanying pulmonary conditions such as bronchiectasis, pleural effusion, and chronic obstructive pulmonary disease. Lymphedema of the extremities may coexist. *Clubbing* of the nails (increased bilateral curvature of the nails with enlargement of the soft connective tissue of the distal phalanges resulting in the flattening of the obtuse angle formed by the proximal end of the nail and the digit) occurs most often with bronchiectasis, lung abscess, and pulmonary neoplasms. Cardiovascular disease and chronic gastrointestinal diseases (ulcerative colitis, sprue) are also associated with clubbing. Clubbing accompanied by bone pain and proliferative periostitis is termed *hypertrophic osteoarthropathy.* The condition is most often associated with bronchogenic squamous cell carcinoma.

TUMORS OF THE NAIL. A variety of benign tumors occur around the nail unit. These include *periungual fibromas, myxoid cysts,* and *subungual exostoses.* Surgical removal is the only certain means of cure.

The main malignant tumor involving the nails is *melanoma,* which appears as a pigmented area at the base of the nail or as a longitudinal pigmented streak in the nail. Nevi can give the same appearance, and biopsy of the lesion in the matrix is the only absolutely certain way of making a diagnosis.

Disorders of the Mucous Membranes

Any abnormality of color, texture, or appearance of the mucous membranes should be investigated. Malignant changes should be suspected in infiltrated or ulcerated lesions and a biopsy performed.

Ch. 96 discusses disorders of the oral mucous membranes, the tongue, and the salivary glands.

Alterations of Hair Growth

HAIR LOSS (ALOPECIA)

Physical, chemical, and emotional events cause fluctuations in hair growth and if severe enough may stop growth entirely. The physical examination is important in noting the pattern of hair loss and whether or not scarring is present. Nonscarring alopecia may be a temporary phenomenon, whereas scarring is indicative of permanent hair loss.

NONSCARRING ALOPECIA. *Localized Alopecia. Alopecia areata* is characterized by well-circumscribed, round or oval patches of nonscarring hair loss, usually over the scalp or in the beard, eyebrows, or eyelashes. Erythema may be present early in the course of the patches. Characteristically the periphery of patches of hair loss is studded with fractured hairs with tapered shafts. Histologic features include small dystrophic hair follicles and a lymphocytic infiltrate around the hair bulbs. Occasionally all the scalp hair is lost (alopecia totalis), and all the body hair may fall out (alopecia universalis). Alopecia areata has a variable, unpredictable course. Most patients regrow hair within a few months, but one fourth of them experience recurrences. The more extensive the alopecia, the poorer the prognosis. Alopecia involving the occipital region or eyebrows, lashes, and nasal hairs portends a poor prognosis. Alopecia areata may have an autoimmune pathogenesis, being occasionally associated with Hashimoto's thyroiditis and pernicious anemia. Topical, intralesional, and systemic steroids give variable benefits. Recent modes of therapy include induction of allergic or irritant contact dermatitis (1% anthralin, or topical dinitrochlorobenzene), photochemotherapy with PUVA, and topical minoxidil.

Tinea capitis is most likely to be confused with alopecia areata. Tinea infection appears as one or more patches of hair loss with mild scaling and erythema and broken hair shafts leaving residual black stumps (black dot ringworm). Nonfluorescing *Trichophyton tonsurans* is the usual cause. Griseofulvin is the drug of choice.

Trichotillomania refers to traumatic, self-induced alopecia and results from compulsive twisting and rubbing, which causes breaking

TABLE 475–10. REGIONAL DERMATOLOGY

Region of Skin	Type of Skin Group	Disease Process
Scalp	Papulosquamous and eczematous	Psoriasis, seborrheic dermatitis, tinea capitis, eczema (atopic, contact)
	Pustular	Folliculitis, kerion
	Nodular	Nevi, seborrheic keratosis, pilar cysts, verruca
	Atropic and telangiectatic	Connective tissue disease, scleroderma, discoid LE
Face	Pustular	Acne, rosacea, folliculitis, tinea
	Papulosquamous and eczematous	Psoriasis, seborrheic dermatitis, contact dermatitis (cosmetics), atopic dermatitis, impetigo, lupus erythematosus, photodermatitis
	Vesicular	Herpes zoster and herpes simplex, insect bites
	Nodular	Basal cell cancers, squamous cell cancers, melanomas, keratoacanthomas, nevi, actinic keratosis
Trunk	Papulosquamous and eczematous	Psoriasis, atopic and contact eczema, tinea versicolor, pityriasis rosacea, scabies
	Vesiculobullous	Pemphigus, bullous pemphigoid
	Maculopapular	Secondary syphilis, drug reaction, viral exanthems
	Nodular	Nevi, seborrheic keratosis, lipoma, basal cell cancer, keloid, neurofibroma, angiomas, melanoma
	Pustular	Acne
	Urticarial	Hives
Arms and forearms	Eczematous and papulosquamous	Contact dermatitis—plants; atopic dermatitis, lichen planus
	Nodular	Nevi, warts, seborrheic keratosis, actinic keratosis
	Atrophic telangiectasis	Scleroderma, dermatomyositis
Legs	Eczematous and papulosquamous	Contact dermatitis, stasis dermatitis, atopic dermatitis, psoriasis, lichen planus
	Nodular	Erythema nodosum, dermatofibromas, nevi, melanoma, Kaposi's sarcoma, lipoma
	Maculopapular	Vasculitis, Schamberg's disease, actinic purpura, pretibial myxedema
	Atrophic, telangiectatic, and ulcerative	Scleroderma, dermatostasis ulcers, arterial insufficiency
Genitalia and groin	Eczematous and papulosquamous	Contact dermatitis, seborrheic dermatitis, scabies, pediculosis pubis, psoriasis, Reiter's syndrome, erythrasma, tinea, candidiasis, lichen planus, intertrigo, lichen simplex chronicus
	Vesiculobullous	Herpes simplex, Stevens-Johnson syndrome
	Ulcerative and atrophic	Syphilis, chancroid, lymphopathia venereum, Behçet's syndrome
	Nodular	Verrucae vulgaris, erythroplasia of Queyrat, squamous cell cancer, sebaceous cyst, molluscum contagiosum
	Pustular	Hidradenitis suppurativa
Hands	Eczematous and papulosquamous	Allergic contact and irritant contact dermatitis, dyshidrosis, pyoderma, tinea, dermatophytids, scabies, atopic dermatitis, secondary syphilis
	Vesiculobullous, pustular	Erythema multiforme, hand-foot-and-mouth disease, porphyria cutanea tarda, psoriasis
	Nodular	Warts, squamous cell cancer, actinic keratosis, keratoacanthoma, pyogenic granuloma, granuloma annulare, synovial cysts
	Hypopigmented	Vitiligo
	Atrophic-telangiectatic	Scleroderma, dermatomyositis
Feet	Eczematous and papulosquamous	Contact dermatitis, atopic dermatitis, tinea, psoriasis, lichen planus
	Vesiculobullous	Tinea, epidermolysis bullosa, erythema multiforme
	Nodules	Verruca, corn, nevus
	Atrophic-telangiectatic	Scleroderma

and epilation of the hair shafts. The scalp is usually affected, less often the eyebrows and lashes. If the patient can be given insight, the condition it is self-limited. More severe emotional problems should be referred to a psychiatrist.

Women who develop hair thinning at the margins of the scalp may be using excessive traction or other traumatic hair styling techniques *(traction alopecia)*. Overtight hair curling such as corn rowing and the use of hot combs to straighten hair leads to progressive hair thinning and even scarring.

Hair loss is sometimes seen in the scalp of patients with *secondary syphilis*. The hair loss is spotty, often "moth-eaten" in appearance.

Androgenic alopecia, or male pattern baldness, involves the frontal, vertex, and upper occipital regions of the scalp while spar-

TABLE 475–11. POTENTIAL DEFECTS IN NAIL FORMATION

Brittleness—easy breaking of nail tips
Leukonychia—white discoloration of nails
Striations—longitudinal ridges running parallel or perpendicular to the length of the nail
Onycholysis—separation of the nail plate from the bed
Onychogryphosis—hypertrophy and thickening of the nail
Onychomycosis—dystrophy, destruction of the nail due to yeast and fungal infections
Pitting—discrete pitlike depressions in the nail surface
Koilonychia—spoon-shaped deformity of the nails (concave nail with everted edges)
Pterygium formation—growth of cuticle onto the nail plate

ing the posterior and lateral margins. The process may begin at any age after puberty, with temporal recession of hair usually noted first. There is no actual loss of hair but rather the conversion of thick terminal hairs to fine, unpigmented, poorly seen vellus hairs. Common baldness is genetically predetermined and androgen dependent. Males who are castrated prepubertally or men born with low testosterone production, as in Klinefelter's syndrome, do not become bald, regardless of their genetic predisposition to balding. Women may also show balding, but it is milder with only diffuse thinning. Women with elevated androgen levels, as occur in masculinizing disorders, have baldness in a pattern similar to that in men. Surgical techniques such as hair transplants (plugs of hair-bearing areas from the sides of the scalp placed in the thinned frontal and crown areas) or scalp reduction may be useful in some patients. Thinning of hair growth is characteristic of old age in both genders.

Diffuse or Generalized Alopecia. Stress alopecia, or *telogen effluvium,* is a transient, reversible, diffuse hair loss of scalp hair that results from alterations in the normal hair cycle (see Ch. 472). Severe emotional and physiologic stress (high fever, systemic illness, major surgery with general anesthesia, crash diet) and certain drugs (heparin, coumarin, allopurinol, amphetamines, β-blocking agents, lithium, probenecid, thiouracil) may cause growing hairs to convert to resting hairs, which are subsequently shed. Pregnancy and oral contraceptives cause hairs to grow continually, rather than cycling at programmed times. After childbirth or discontinuation of oral contraceptives, growing follicles "catch up" by simultaneously resting; shedding follows 2 to 4 months later. If the stress resolves, the hair regrows in 4 to 6 months. Diffuse hair loss may not be noticeable until there is greater than 50% scalp hair loss. Gentle pulling of the hair verifies the degree of shedding; if more than five hairs come out when a dozen are grasped, excessive shedding is present.

Toxic alopecia occurs if hair growth is disrupted. Newly synthesized hair shafts are weakened and the hair breaks readily. Thinning may be extreme, occurring within a few weeks of an insult, involving all 80% of actively growing follicles. Chemotherapeutic agents, especially doxorubicin and related agents, exert their effect on rapidly growing cells in the hair bulb and commonly cause hair damage in cancer patients receiving chemotherapy. Radiation therapy to the scalp area does the same thing. *Retinoids and hypervitaminosis A* cause hair loss owing to their interference with keratinization.

Diffuse hair loss over the scalp occurs in *hypothyroidism*, associated with hair that is dry and brittle, and severe malnutrition.

Seborrheic dermatitis, with erythema and yellow, greasy scales throughout the scalp, may be associated with mild, diffuse hair loss. Treatment with tar shampoos and topical steroids to control the inflammatory response reverses the condition.

Diffuse scalp hair loss can follow *hair shaft weakness*, either acquired (due to braiding, permanent wave solutions, or excessive heat when drying or straightening hair) or congenital. Patients with congenital hair weakness have sparse fine or wiry hair from early childhood.

SCARRING ALOPECIA. Scarring alopecias display atrophy of the scalp and absence of hair follicles. Cicatricial areas of hair loss can result from a variety of pathologic processes that permanently destroy the hair follicles.

Localized Scarring Alopecia. Systemic lupus erythematosus causes diffuse, nonscarring alopecia of the scalp in 20% of patients, along with short, broken (lupus) hairs in the frontal margin. *Discoid lupus erythematosus* causes oval scarring areas of alopecia. Typical plaques have an active erythematous margin, white atrophic center, and telangiectasias and keratin-filled follicles.

Morphea, when it involves the scalp, causes firm, hairless, ivory colored, indurated lesions. At times morphea takes on linear patterns that simulate saber wound *(en coup de sabre)*.

A number of *physical injuries* such as mechanical trauma, burns, and radiation dermatitis may also cause local scarring alopecias.

Nonlocalized Scarring Alopecia. Lichen planus may cause diffuse, patchy scarring alopecia *(lichen planopilaris)*. Typical lichen planus lesions are often found in other areas of the body. Biopsy may help in the diagnosis.

HIRSUTISM (EXCESSIVE HAIR GROWTH)

Excessive hair growth, usually a complaint of females, may be due to either endocrinologic or nonendocrinologic conditions. When women are affected in those areas of the body which normally develop hair as a secondary sex characteristic in males, their hirsutism generally reflects treatable endocrinopathy, as these follicles respond to high concentrations of testosterone and can convert various androgens to dihydrotestosterone (see Ch. 472).

NONENDOCRINE HIRSUTISM. *Ethnic* or *racial hirsutism* is characterized by excessive hair growth on the upper lip, beard area, chest, nipples, or lower abdomen in women without menstrual abnormalities or masculization. Type of hair, rate of hair growth, and distribution of hair over the body differ among the races, relating to variations in the sensitivity of follicles to circulating androgens. A male pattern of hirsutism is more common in females whose ancestors came from the southern parts of Europe. Asians and native Americans have less body hair. If serum testosterone, dehydroepiandrosterone, and androstenedione are normal, bleaching or shaving may make the hair less noticeable. Electrolysis permanently destroys hair follicles but is time consuming and costly. Spironolactone,* which has antiandrogenic properties (200 mg per day), used for a period of 12 months is also useful in decreasing hair growth.

Certain *drugs* may increase hair growth. Androgenic or steroidal medications, such as anabolic steroids, corticosteroids, and contraceptives may cause increased hair growth in the beard, chest, and groin areas. Drugs such as phenytoin, phenothiazines, cyclosporine, and minoxidil cause excess hair in both men and women anywhere on the body.

---

* This use is not listed in the manufacturer's directive.

ENDOCRINE HIRSUTISM. A distinction must be made between hirsutism caused by increased androgen production with and without virilization. In general, virilization is a sign of markedly elevated androgens derived from the adrenal glands or ovaries, especially adrenogenital syndrome, congenital adrenal hyperplasia, Cushing's disease or syndrome, Stein-Leventhal syndrome (polycystic ovarian syndrome), and occasionally malignant adrenal or ovarian tumors. Any woman with hirsutism and accompanying virilization should be tested for excess cortisol and androgen production.

Simple or *idiopathic hirsutism* denotes hirsute women in whom a specific diagnosis cannot be made and who have normal or slightly elevated adrenal or ovarian androgens. Such patients have been successfully treated with cyclically administered birth control pills or with spironolactone.

PHOTOSENSITIVITY AND OTHER REACTIONS TO LIGHT

Certain wavelengths of light can induce a number of undesirable cutaneous reactions, including sunburn, skin aging, carcinogenesis, and a variety of photosensitivity reactions (see Fig. 473–1).

The solar spectrum that commonly affects human skin is in the ultraviolet light range (290 to 400 nm), which is subdivided into three bands designated as UVC (shorter than 290 nm), UVB (290 to 320 nm), and UVA, or long-wave ultraviolet light (320 to 400 nm). UVC does not reach the earth, being absorbed by ozone; UVB, or the sunburn spectrum, causes burning, tanning, aging, and carcinogenic changes in the skin. UVA is melanogenic and erythrogenic, but the amount of energy required to produce these effects is 1000 times greater than UVB. UVA causes skin reactions through window glass, and these wavelengths are often responsible for photoreactions in which chemical photosensitizers and UV radiation interact to cause inflammatory skin reactions.

The incidence of photoreactions depends on a number of factors such as the amount of light reaching the earth's surface, season of the year, latitude and weather conditions, and thickness of the ozone layer, as well as topographic features of the environment. Certain climatologic and environmental factors influence the amount of sunlight hitting the skin. For example, 50% of the daily ultraviolet light is emitted between 11 A.M. and 2 P.M.: Avoiding exposure during this time may minimize photoreactions. Sitting in the shade does not protect against UV exposure, because 50% of the ambient ultraviolet light is received; 90% of ultraviolet light penetrates clouds, so one can get sunburns even in the shade and on cloudy days.

Direct Photo Effects on the Skin

ACUTE EFFECTS. Sunburning and tanning are attributed primarily to UVB light, although prolonged exposure to UVA can produce mild burn and marked hyperpigmentation. The sunburn reaction produces a complex inflammatory process causing dyskeratotic cells, spongiosis, vacuolation of keratinocytes, and edema from capillary leakage, 12 to 24 hours after exposure. Occasionally, in addition to redness and pain, blisters may evolve. Prostaglandins may play a role in the burn reaction, as they are found in increased quantities in sunburned skin. Aspirin, indomethacin, or prostaglandin synthesis inhibitors can reduce the burn.

Three to 4 days after a sunburn, new melanin pigment is formed. Several cellular and molecular changes occur in the skin after each sunburn reaction which, if repeated, may lead to the chronic effects of UV light. A few days after UV light burning, epidermal mitosis and hyperplasia occur and DNA, RNA, and proteins in the skin are damaged.

CHRONIC EFFECTS. Degenerative changes of the skin consisting of wrinkling, telangiectasias, and keratoses result from chronic exposure to UV light. The skin may become furrowed and leathery and develop yellow papules and plaques due to degeneration of the dermal collagen. These changes are caused by both UVB and UVA radiation. Such changes can be minimized by daily topical applications of effective sunscreens.

A number of malignant and premalignant skin lesions are associated with chronic sun exposure, including actinic keratoses, keratoacanthomas, basal cell and squamous cell carcinomas, and probably melanomas.

Indirect Photo Effects on the Skin

Photoreactions that occur when systemic or topical chemicals induce photosensitivity or when there is an underlying immunologic, biochemical, or genetic abnormality that predisposes to sun sensitivity are considered indirect reactions; that is, the sun alone does not cause photoreactions.

EXOGENOUS FACTORS CAUSING PHOTOSENSITIVITY. Chemical agents either taken systemically or placed topically on the skin can cause one of two general types of photoreactions: phototoxic and photoallergic. In photosensitivity reactions, the absorption spectrum of a given drug, substance, or chemical is maximal at a certain wavelength of light that induces molecular changes in the exogenous material. These initiate the cutaneous reaction. In most drug or chemical photosensitivity reactions, the wavelengths that evoke abnormal reactions are in the 320 to 400 nm (UVA) region. The reactions include acute, abnormal sunburn responses and eczematous and urticarial reactions.

Phototoxic reactions are nonimmunologic cutaneous responses that occur when a drug or chemical in the skin absorb enough light energy of a specific wavelength. The photosensitizer generates free radicals that damage cell membranes and lysosomes, inducing an exaggerated sunburn reaction, with intense redness, swelling, pain, and occasionally blistering. Most phototoxic agents absorb UVB light.

Photoallergic reactions to topical chemicals or internal drugs represent an acquired, immunogenically altered response to light. Absorption of specific wavelengths of light by chemicals or drugs causes changes in their chemical configuration so that these substances become haptens that bind to proteins in the skin to become a complete antigen capable of eliciting a type IV delayed hypersensitivity immunologic response. The clinical manifestations of such photoallergic reactions are usually eczematous in nature (occasionally urticarial), evolving in exposed areas 24 hours after exposure to the sun. The action spectrum is generally long-range UVA light.

SYSTEMIC PHOTOSENSITIZERS. Drugs may cause either phototoxic or photoallergic reactions. Table 475–12 lists some of the drugs and chemicals that may induce photosensitivities and the type of reaction and action spectrum thought to induce them.

TOPICAL AGENTS CAUSING PHOTOSENSITIVITY. Most topical photosensitizing agents respond to the UVA action spectrum. Drugs and chemicals that induce *phototoxic contact reactions* include coal tar derivatives, topical drugs (phenothiazines, sulfonamides), dyes (eosins, methylene blue), and plant derivatives (furocoumarins). The photosensitive properties of coal tar derivatives and furocoumarins (psoralens) are utilized in treating certain skin diseases with ultraviolet light.

When plants, vegetables, or fruits containing a phototoxic chemical cause phototoxicity, the reaction is referred to as a *phytophotodermatitis*. Photocontact dermatitis develops with contact with

plants in the Umbelliferae family, such as figs, cow parsnip, fennel, parsley, parsnip, and gas plant. Phytophotodermatitis also occurs in individuals exposed to Persian limes and celery. Such reactions are caused by furocoumarin compounds found in the plant which readily penetrate the epidermis. Two things are needed for initiation of phytophotodermatitis: (1) contact with a sensitizing furocoumarin and (2) subsequent exposure to UV radiation greater than 320 nm. Phytophotodermatitis may take on unique clinical forms: (1) berloque dermatitis presents as streaky erythema followed by hyperpigmentation in areas where perfumes containing oil of Bergamot (a psoralen) are applied to the skin (e.g., on the neck); (2) crisscross linear streaks of erythema, vesicles, and bullae that heal with hyperpigmentation where meadow grass or other related plants rub on the skin; (3) oil of the rind of a Persian lime causes erythema and pigmentation on the hands of bartenders.

Photoallergic contact dermatitis, a form of delayed eczematous reaction, evolves in some individuals after exposure to chemicals such as fragrances (methylcoumarin and musk ambrette), halogenated salicylanilides, sunscreens, and blankophores, or optical whitening agents, used in laundry soaps and bleaches. A number of perfumes (e.g., after-shave lotions, colognes) contain musk ambrette, a synthetic fragrance fixative that causes a photoeczematous reaction over the face and hands. Sunscreening agents containing PABA esters and cinnamates that readily absorb UV light may cause eczematous reactions. A small number of individuals have persistent chronic eczematous dermatitis after all exposure to the photosensitizing agent has ceased—so-called persistent light reactivity; they even may react to artificial fluorescent light.

Identifying the cause of contact photoallergic reactions can be done with photopatch testing (see Ch. 473). Treatment begins by eliminating the photosensitizing agent and minimizing exposure (avoiding sun and use of sunscreens). Topical or oral steroids may be needed to decrease the cutaneous inflammatory response.

ENDOGENOUS CONDITIONS ASSOCIATED WITH PHOTOSENSITIVITY. *Immunologic diseases with photosensitivity* include connective tissue conditions such as lupus erythematosus, both discoid and systemic, and solar urticaria. Solar urticaria, hives with itching and burning, evolves within minutes of sunlight exposure and lasts an hour or more.

Biochemical conditions associated with photosensitivity include porphyria cutanea tarda and erythropoietic protoporphyria.

Pellagra, is caused by an inadequate diet and a deficiency of nicotinic acid. It is still seen occasionally with alcoholism, poor dietary intake in the elderly, and malabsorption. The carcinoid syndrome may also be associated with pellagra because tryptophan, the precursor of nicotinic acid, is diverted to serotonin production by the tumor. A scaly dermatitis affects sun-exposed parts of the skin, especially on the face, the neck, and the back of the hands, in association with diarrhea and dementia. Dietary replacement clears the skin and other signs of the disease.

Other Photosensitivity Conditions

Polymorphous light eruption (PMLE) causes eczematous patches, red to violaceous papules or plaques, and urticarial lesions over the face, the nape and V of the neck, and the back of the hands. The rash characteristically arises hours to days after sun exposure. The onset is frequently in early summer with some degree of resistance being acquired with continued sun exposure. Recurrences each spring and summer are common, and the eruption remits during the winter. The disease is most frequent during the first half of life. The cause is unknown.

DERMATOLOGIC MANIFESTATIONS IN THE IMMUNOCOMPROMISED HOST AND IN AIDS

Immunosuppression causes an increase in benign and malignant skin growths as well as a variety of infections in the skin (see Ch. 266). Cutaneous neoplasms such as squamous cell and basal cell carcinomas occur with a higher than expected frequency. Transplant patients have a risk of skin cancer seven times greater than normal.

Any skin lesion, no matter how innocuous, should be carefully evaluated in the immunosuppressed host. The gross morphology of infections is so frequently modified by the altered inflammatory response that early skin biopsies are essential for diagnosis. The array of potential pathogens is imposing in these patients, and even common infectious processes are greatly modified or obscured by immunocompromising illness. Skin infections are common, accounting for 22 to 33% of infections in immunosuppressed patients.

TABLE 475–12. SYSTEMIC PHOTOSENSITIZERS

Name	Type of Photoreaction	Action Spectrum (nm)
Sulfonamides	Phototoxic and photoallergic	290–320
Sulfonylureas (tolbutamide, chlorpropamide)	Phototoxic	290–360
Chlorothiazides	Phototoxic and photoallergic	290–320 320–400
Phenothiazines	Phototoxic, urticaria eruption, gray-blue hyperpigmentation	290–400
Antibiotics (tetracyclines, griseofulvin, nalidixic acid)	Phototoxic and photoallergic bullae	320–400
Furocoumarins (psoralens)	Phototoxic	
Nonsteroidal anti-inflammatory agents	Phototoxic and photoallergic	Unknown
Anticancer drugs (DTIC, fluorouracil, methotrexate, vinblastin)	Phototoxic	Unknown
Estrogens, progestins, and other drugs	Phototoxic, melasma	?290–320
Chlordiazepoxide (Librium)	Photoallergic	290–360
Cyclamates	Phototoxic and photoallergic	290–360
Quinidine, quinine	Photoallergic	320–400

Microbial involvement of the skin and subcutaneous tissue can be grouped into two major categories in immunocompromised patients: (1) *primary skin infections* include those occurring in nonimmunocompromised hosts, and primary skin infections from opportunistic agents that rarely cause skin infection in normal patients; and (2) *disseminated systemic infections* metastatic to the skin from a noncutaneous portal of entry.

PRIMARY SKIN INFECTIONS. Typical primary skin infections, including group A streptococcal and *S. aureus* cellulitis, are frequent, although more unusual causes of cellulitis in granulocytopenic patients must also be considered (*Pseudomonas*, anaerobic bacteria). Skin biopsy of the cellulitic areas for Gram stain and culture is often helpful.

Primary cutaneous infections by viruses and skin dermatophytes are also common. Warts caused by papillomavirus may be numerous and difficult to remove. Malignant transformation has been documented. Herpes simplex infections may present as chronic, large, ulcerated lesions persisting for weeks to months (herpes phagedena, especially in the genital areas), and there may be internal dissemination from cutaneous sites. Reactivation of herpes zoster infections is common with systemic dissemination. Widespread dermatophyte infections of the skin appear as scaling, red patches that provide a portal of entry for bacterial infection.

Unusual opportunistic primary skin infections with atypical *Mycobacterium, Aspergillus, Rhizopus,* and *Candida* organisms cause cellulitis-like reactions that form a central pustule and eschar. Skin biopsy of such lesions with a portion of the biopsy processed by frozen section and specially stained for AFB and fungi may identify the pathologic organisms rapidly.

DISSEMINATED INFECTION METASTATIC TO THE SKIN. Hematogenous dissemination of infection to the skin from distant primary sites frequently occurs in patients with impaired host defenses. Three groups of organisms are responsible: (1) *Pseudomonas* and other gram-negative bacilli; (2) endemic systemic mycoses *(Histoplasma, Coccidioides);* and (3) opportunistic fungi *(Aspergillus, Candida,* Mucoraceae). The range of cutaneous clinical presentations of these infections is varied and mimicked by all: (a) *vesicles and bullae* that become hemorrhagic, (b) *gangrenous cellulitis* with necrotic ulcerations, and (c) widespread, red, warm, fluctuant *nodules* with pustules and purpura. Prompt biopsy with frozen sections stained for bacterial and hyphal elements may provide rapid diagnosis.

CUTANEOUS MANIFESTATIONS OF HIV INFECTIONS

Skin disease is common in patients with HIV. Some dermatoses are characteristic, whereas others are just observed in a higher frequency or with atypical features. *Diseases characteristic of HIV infection* include Kaposi's sarcoma, oral hairy leukoplakia, bacillary angiomatosis (Rochalimaea infection causing angiomatous proliferation resulting in red, raised nodular lesions with a scaling base), eosinophilic folliculitis (intensely pruritic follicular papules on the head, neck and extremities).

DISEASES WITH ATYPICAL PRESENTATIONS IN HIV DISEASE. Molluscum contagiosum may appear as large 1- to 2-cm smooth to verrucoid papules and plaques on the face. Herpes simplex often appears as large chronic ulcerative lesions in anogenital and oral areas. Zoster may present as dermatomal or disseminated hyperkeratotic, scarring papules and plaques. Scabies may evolve into numerous hyperkeratotic pruritic plaques teaming with mites on KOH examination. Syphilis may appear with a typical primary genital ulcer but secondary and tertiary lesions may evolve rapidly. To complicate things, the serologic test for syphilis may be negative. Psoriasis and Reiter's disease may be more severe in HIV-infected patients, with widespread total body involvement.

Diseases with increased frequency in HIV infection include seborrheic dermatitis, yeast infections (especially thrush), drug reactions (morbilliform reactions especially to antibiotics), and pruritus.

CUTANEOUS DRUG REACTIONS

Rashes are among the most common adverse reactions to drugs and occur in 2 to 3% of hospitalized patients. Any drug can potentially produce a rash, and over-the-counter preparations should be considered when defining drug reactions.

Some of the most common drugs causing skin reactions in hospitalized patients are amoxicillin, trimethoprim-sulfamethoxazole, ampicillin, penicillin G, allopurinol, dipyrone, gentamicin sulfate, mefruside, nitrazepam, and barbiturates. Drugs least likely to cause allergic skin reactions include digoxin, antacids, promethazine, acetaminophen, nitroglycerin, aminophylline, propranolol, antihistamines, cromolyn, and emollient laxatives.

Table 475–13 lists the various morphologic types of drug reactions and some of the drugs capable of inducing them.

TABLE 475–13. CUTANEOUS DRUG REACTIONS

Type of Skin Reaction	Drugs Likely to Cause Skin Reaction
Eczematous (allergic contact reaction)	Antihistamines, neomycin, formaldehyde, sulfanamides
Photodermatitis	
Phototoxic	Chlorpromazine, psoralens, demeclocycline, doxycycline
Photoallergic	Promethazine, griseofulvin, Diuril, hypoglycemic drugs
Exfoliative dermatitis	Carbamazepine, hydantoins, nitrofurantoin, isoniazid, gold, allopurinol, phenothiazines
Maculopapular eruption (exanthematous)	Penicillin, sulfonamides, hypoglycemic drugs, phenothiazines, allopurinol, phenytoin, quinine, gold salts, captopril, meprobamate
Papulosquamous reactions	Beta blockers, lithium (psoriasiform), thiazides, gold, phenothiazines, quinidine, antimalarials (lichen planus–like);
Psoriasiform, lichen planus, pityriasis rosea–like	gold (PR-like): others—practolol, dapsone, ethambutol, furosemide
Vesiculobullous reactions	Azapropazone, captopril, clonidine, furosemide, gold, psoralens, barbiturates, phenytoin, HydroDIURIL, penicillamine
Toxic epidermal necrolysis	Acetazolamide, allopurinol, barbiturates, carbamazepines, gold, hydantoin, nitrofurantoin, pentazocine, tetracycline, quinidine
Pustular—acneiform reactions	Androgen hormones, corticosteroids, iodides, bromides, hydantoin, lithium
Urticaria and erythemas	
Urticaria	May occur with anaphylaxis; penicillin, xenogenic sera, cephalosporins, sulfonamides, barbiturates, hydralazine, phenylbutazone, hydantoin, quinidine, x-ray contrast media
Erythema multiforme	Sulfonamides, hydantoin, barbiturates, penicillin, carbamazepines, allopurinol, amikacin, phenothiazines
Nodular lesions	
Erythema nodosum	Birth control pills, sulfonamides, diuretics, gold, clonidine, propranolol, furosemide, opiates, penicillin
Vasculitis reaction	Allopurinol, barbiturates, carbamazepine, chlorothiazide, cimetidine, gold, imdomethacin, hydantoin, piperazine, sulfonamides
Telangiectatic and LE reactions	Procainamide, hydralazine, phenytoin, penicillamine, trimethadione, methyldopa, carbamazepine, griseofulvin, nalidixic acid, oral contraceptives, propranolol
Pigmentary reaction	Anticonvulsants, antimalarials, antitumor agents (bleomycin, busulfan, cyclophosphamide, doxorubicin, melphalan), oral contraceptives, corticotropin, tetracyclines, phenothiazines, amiodarone
Other cutaneous reactions	
Fixed drug reactions	Phenolphthalein, barbiturates, gold, sulfonamides, meprobamate, penicillin, tetracyclines, analgesics
Alopecia	Alkylating agents, antimetabolites, heparin, coumarin, hydantoin, accutane, gold, nitrofurantoin, propranolol, colchicine, allopurinol
Hypertrichosis	Anabolic agents, diazoxide, minoxidil, phenytoin

Fixed drug eruptions are unique reactions that appear in the same area of the skin each time the responsible drug is administered. These appear as macular, eczematous, or even bullous, pink to dark red patches occurring as few or many lesions. When the drug is stopped the lesions fade, leaving postinflammatory hyperpigmentation. The lesions return in the same place within a few hours of taking the drug again.

Nonsteroidal anti-inflammatory drugs may cause cutaneous reactions including vesiculobullous photosensitivity reactions, serum sickness, erythroderma, fixed drug reactions, and toxic epidermal necrolysis.

The treatment of drug reactions is to withdraw the suspected agent. Once a drug reaction is suspected all nonessential drugs should be stopped and appropriate substitutes used for the necessary medications. An asymptomatic eruption may require no therapy, or a mild reaction with pruritus may be controlled with topical steroid applications and antihistamines. In severe conditions such as exfoliative dermatitis, oral steroids are often indicated. Most drug eruptions resolve in 1 to 2 weeks after withdrawal of the drug, but some take months to clear. Although an occasional reaction may be fatal (e.g., toxic epidermal necrolysis), patients with drug eruptions usually have an excellent prognosis.

Du Vivier LM: Atlas of Clinical Dermatology. New York, Raven Press, 1993. *A beautifully produced, thorough reference volume that comprehensively covers the field.*
Fitzpatrick TB, Eisen AZ, Wolff K, et al.: Dermatology in General Medicine, 3rd ed. New York, McGraw-Hill, 1987.
Moschella SL, Hurley HJ: Dermatology, 3rd ed. Philadelphia, WB Saunders, 1992. *A comprehensive test that brings the field up to date in new discoveries.*

476 OCCUPATIONAL DISEASES OF THE SKIN
Edward A. Emmett

Occupational skin diseases are a group of heterogeneous conditions that share a common occupational etiology. They account for about one half of reported occupational disease in the United States. Occupational contact dermatitis, the prototypical disorder, makes up about 95% of all occupational skin diseases; infections, about 2.5%; and a large number of different, infrequent diseases, the remainder. The relative frequency of each of these diseases in any location depends largely on the pattern of industrialization.

Almost all occupational skin diseases are due to external contact with chemical, physical, and biologic agents. The cause is often multifactorial. In relatively few instances are systemically (rather than locally) absorbed agents responsible.

OCCUPATIONAL CONTACT DERMATITIS

DEFINITION. Occupational contact dermatitis is an erythematous or eczematous response of the skin as a result of local contact with one or more irritating, allergenic, or photosensitizing chemical agents.

ETIOLOGY. Many chemicals from a wide variety of classes—alkalies, acids, volatile organic solvents, metallic salts, organic prepolymers, and many others—are capable of inducing contact dermatitis. The cause is often multifactorial; in addition to one or more chemicals, friction, abrasion, changes in temperature and humidity, and ultraviolet (UV) radiation may play a role. Superinfection may occur. Severe and persistent occupational contact dermatitis, particularly from irritants, is more frequent in those with an atopic diathesis.

INCIDENCE AND PREVALENCE. Bureau of Labor Statistics reports put the incidence in the United States at about 0.9 per 1000 full-time workers per year; because of substantial underreporting, the true incidence is estimated to be from 10 to 50 times higher.

EPIDEMIOLOGY. The incidence of occupational contact dermatitis is generally highest in agriculture/forestry/fishing, followed by the manufacturing industries. The highest risks occur in poultry-dressing plants, meat-packing plants, fabrication of rubber products, leather tanning and finishing, manufacture of ophthalmic goods, plating and polishing, production of frozen fruits and vegetables, internal combustion engine manufacture, machining operations, and canning and curing of seafoods. Virtually no industry is immune.

PATHOGENESIS. Contact dermatitis may result from direct local irritation, cell-mediated immune reactions, or photosensitivity.

Direct local irritation may be immediate, as in irritation from strong acids or alkalies, or may be delayed and occur only after repeated or prolonged local application, as cumulative insult dermatitis. The latter can occur from one or more relatively mildly irritating substances that are termed marginal irritants.

Allergic contact dermatitis occurs as a result of sensitization to specific haptens through a process of cell-mediated immunity. The hapten combines with protein in the skin to form a complete antigen that is processed and presented to T lymphocytes by epidermal Langerhans cells, specialized macrophages that form an intraepidermal network. Among the most frequent allergens are poison ivy or oak; rubber additives, particularly accelerators and antioxidants; monomers of plastics and resins, such as epoxies, acrylates, and diisocyanates; nickel; chromium salts; paraphenylenediamine and derivatives; and formaldehyde. There are many more possible allergens. The number of substances reported to cause allergic contact dermatitis is very large.

Chemical photosensitivity results from the photochemical excitation of a UV-absorbing molecule with resultant tissue damage. In a photoirritant reaction there is direct damage to cellular components, for example, when psoralens irradiated with long UV bind covalently to DNA. Coal tar pitch, certain aromatic dyes, and UV absorbers used in printing processes also cause photoirritation. In the rarer photoallergic reaction, photochemical alteration of the inciting chemical either forms a hapten or leads to a hapten-protein combination in the skin; the subsequent steps are identical with those for allergic contact dermatitis.

A major factor in the human's resistance to environmental chemicals is the barrier provided by the outer stratum corneum layer of the epidermis. Damage to this barrier by trauma, inflammation, or skin disease or by altering barrier conditions, e.g., by occlusion, may play an important role in the development of contact dermatitis.

CLINICAL MANIFESTATIONS. The clinical presentation is dominated by dermatitis that is confined, at least initially, to the region of contact. The morphology varies according to the concentration and duration of the exposure, the pathogenesis, and individual constitutional differences. Acute irritant dermatitis is characterized by erythema, perhaps edema, papules and vesicles, or, in the more extreme instance, one or more large bullae filled with purulent fluid. Postinflammation hyperpigmentation and hypopigmentation may occur; necrosis may leave scars. The cause of acute irritant dermatitis is usually obvious because of the rapidity with which the reaction develops.

Cumulative insult dermatitis may develop only after a long period of contact. On the hands it tends to start under rings or watchbands and to be somewhat patchy in distribution. Individual susceptibility varies widely. Initially, drying and fissuring may be seen, with subsequent development of an eczematous response with papules and vesicles. Excoriations and lichenification are frequent if the process persists. Relapse may occur on relatively brief exposure to mild irritants, even when the dermatitis is clinically healed, especially if the epidermal barrier has not yet been fully reestablished.

Allergic contact dermatitis most often presents as an acute or chronic eczematous reaction with erythema, papules, vesicles, scaling, and pruritus. Characteristically there is a latent period of at least 7 to 10 days before the development of dermatitis following first exposure to the allergen. Recurrence usually occurs 24 to 72 hours after an eliciting exposure. Certain allergens, e.g., epoxy resin monomers, have a tendency to produce severe acute reactions with significant edema.

Localization is important for diagnosis. Over 90% of occupational contact dermatitis involves the hands, sometimes in conjunction with other sites. When the eruption is due to contact with objects or contaminated surfaces, the pattern of contact determines localization. Reaction to immersion of the hands in liquids generally involves the dorsum of the hands and palmar aspects of the wrists. Photosensitivity reactions on exposed sites may be distinguished from airborne contact dermatitis by the relative sparing of shaded areas, such as the eyelids or behind the ears.

DIAGNOSIS. A good occupational history is the cornerstone of diagnosis. It is most useful to get a description of the worker's daily activities, including nonoccupational activities, with particular attention to contact of the skin with chemicals. The localization of the eruption at its onset, initial appearance of lesions, nature of progression, and circumstances of remissions and recurrences help determine an occupational etiology. A personal or family history or both confirm the presence of atopy, in which there is increased susceptibility to irritants, changes in heat and humidity, and other factors. A complete examination of the skin helps rule out dermatoses other than contact dermatitis, including id reactions of the hands secondary to dermatophytosis of the feet. Allergic contact dermatitis is confirmed by diagnostic patch testing; photoallergy, by photopatch testing. Patch testing is relatively easy to perform, but the interpretation requires skill. There is no clinically useful confirmatory test for irritant contact dermatitis.

Other information may be necessary to make a precise diagnosis and formulate appropriate management. Toxicity information on industrial compounds can be obtained from Material Safety Data Sheets, which reveal the composition and properties of industrial materials. In the United States these are available to most employees and their physicians. A visit by the physician to the workplace allows the physician to view the work firsthand. If such a visit is made, opportunity for skin contact with hazardous agents should be explored, as well as the use of protective measures.

Epidemiologic surveys to establish the prevalence of dermatitis in workers at similar jobs and industrial hygiene surveys to characterize the nature and amount of chemical exposure may occasionally be helpful. Public health authorities, university centers for occupational and environmental health, and sometimes concerned employers may be able to assist in such investigations.

TREATMENT. Symptomatic treatment is similar to that for dermatitis of other types. Acute contact dermatitis is treated with cold wet dressings of Burow's solution. Systemic steroids in rapidly tapering doses are indicated in severe acute widespread disabling eruptions; topical steroids and emollients, for dry and chronic eczema. Superinfection requires appropriate systemic antibiotics. Antihistamines may be given for sedation and are mildly antipruritic. The patient should be given careful instruction to avoid casual exposures and should be alerted to the fact that even when the skin has apparently healed, the barrier may not have returned to normal. A temporary or permanent change of job tasks may be necessary. If a permanent job change is necessary, vocational rehabilitation should be considered. Some states require reporting of occupational diseases.

PROGNOSIS. The prognosis of occupational contact dermatitis is surprisingly poor, especially if effective treatment is not given early and if the dermatitis is prolonged. The reasons for this are not entirely clear; however, surveys have shown that a high percentage of individuals still have dermatitis several years later, in many cases despite a change of employment. Those with atopy appear to have the worst prognosis. In allergic contact dermatitis, the prognosis is dependent on the ease with which the allergen can be avoided.

PREVENTION. Preventive measures serve both to prevent recurrences and to halt the development of new disease. These include elimination of or substitution for strong irritants and sensitizers; education of workers regarding skin care; avoidance of overly harsh skin cleansers; prompt reporting and treatment of dermatitis; engineering controls to minimize skin contact with potential hazards; appropriate impervious protective clothing; good personal hygiene with rapid, effective removal of contaminants; and counseling of individuals with predisposing conditions, such as atopy, regarding career selection.

OTHER OCCUPATIONAL DERMATOSES

A relatively large number of other dermatoses can result from occupational exposure. In large part, management is dependent upon diagnostic recognition and on discontinuing further exposures, using measures outlined above.

Chemical burns result from corrosive agents that produce necrosis, ulceration, and subsequent scarring. Prompt removal of these agents (such as strong acids, alkalies, phenol, alkyl metal compounds, and metal chlorides) from skin, eyes, and mucous membranes is essential. Water is generally best for removal. Quicklime,

tin tetrachloride, and titanium tetrachloride should be removed with mineral oil. Specific antidotes are few; these include topical or injected calcium gluconate for hydrofluoric acid burns.

Urticaria may occur from local contact with or systemic absorption of agents that elicit an immediate hypersensitivity reaction or directly release histamine and other vasoactive substances.

Fiberglass dermatitis causes intense pruritus; there may be no visible changes, or it may be accompanied by excoriations, pinpoint petechial papules, or both. Microscopy of a cellophane tape stripping from the skin, which had been treated with 10% potassium hydroxide, reveals the fibers.

Relatively deep indolent *ulcers* of skin and mucous membranes result from contact with arsenic, chromates, and lime.

Chemical acne and folliculitis may result from contact with greases and oils, coal tar pitch, creosote, and a number of cosmetics (acne cosmetica) and from ingestion of bromides, iodides, and isoniazid. These forms of acne typically commence with comedones or inflammatory papules.

Chloracne is due to halogenated aromatic compounds with specific molecular shape, including dioxin and related chlorinated aromatic hydrocarbons. The illness is characterized by small straw-colored cysts and comedones that first involve the malar crescent and behind the ear and may not spread beyond these areas. Inflammatory pustules, abscesses, and large cysts may be seen in severe cases. Chloracne is the first and most constant finding in chronic dioxin poisoning. More variable findings may include porphyrinuria, hyperpigmentation, hypertrichosis, central and peripheral nervous system effects, alteration of lipid metabolism, and mild hepatotoxicity. Experimentally observed effects include teratogenicity, immunosuppression, and tumor induction.

Cutaneous granulomas occur as slightly erythematous grouped flesh-colored papules, with or without inflammatory changes, from foreign body reactions at the site of contact with talc and silica or as an immunologic response to beryllium and zirconium.

Chemical leukoderma, which may mimic vitiligo but which is confined to the areas of skin contact, may result from a number of phenols and catechols, including hydroquinone, monobenzyl, and monomethyl ethers of hydroquinone (used as rubber additives) and *p*-tertiary butyl and related phenols (in disinfectants).

Basal and squamous cell carcinomas and keratoacanthomas result from prolonged exposures to UV radiation, ionizing radiation, polycyclic aromatic hydrocarbons (including coal tar pitches and related products), and arsenic. Exposures to arsenic may be associated with various internal malignant neoplasms.

Cutaneous T cell lymphoma (mycosis fungoides) may be more frequent in those who have worked in heavy industry or who have industrial chemical exposure, but the particular causal agents are uncertain.

INFECTIONS AND INFESTATIONS

The development of infections and infestations frequently depends on occupational factors, individual susceptibility, and the geographic distribution of the causal organism. Occupational associations include the following:

Viral. Herpes simplex (dentists, medical personnel), milkers' nodules and papular stomatitis (veterinarians, milk handlers), orf (farmers, shepherds, abattoir workers), viral warts (butchers), Rift Valley fever (shepherds).

Bacterial. Staphylococcal infections of hands (abattoir workers and butchers), erysipeloid (fish, fowl, rabbit, and pig handlers), anthrax (wool, hair, and hide handlers), tularemia (farmers), nontuberculous mycobacterial infections (aquarium workers and pet shop attendants). Bacterial and yeast infections and tinea versicolor are prominent where there is heat, humidity, and lack of hygiene.

Fungal. Dermatophyte infections are more frequent in farm workers, surveyors, zoo attendants, animal care technicians, and certain others. Particular examples include tinea versicolor (farmers); infection due to *Trichophyton rubrum* (miners), *Microsporum canis* (pet shop workers), *Trichophyton violaceum* (wrestlers), and *Candida albicans* (those in wet work, particularly those in contact with sugar and fruit); sporotrichosis (mine workers); chromomycosis (agricultural workers); and actinomycosis (agricultural workers).

Protozoal. South American leishmaniasis (foresters).

Helminthic. Creeping eruption (plumbers, gardeners, farm workers in the tropics), ankylostomiasis (miners), schistosomiasis and cercarial dermatitis (rice planters and canal workers).

In addition, bites and stings of arthropods and other creatures are common in those who work out of doors and in certain other occupations.

Adams RM: Occupational Skin Disease, 2nd ed. Philadelphia, WB Saunders, 1990. *Comprehensive review of contact dermatitis and related conditions, with descriptions of skin diseases caused by a variety of agents and with detailed lists of agents encountered in various occupations.*

Maibach HI (ed.): Occupational and Industrial Dermatology. Chicago, Year Book Medical Publishers, 1987. *Multiauthor text that broadly covers occupational dermatoses and dermatotoxicology and describes the skin diseases caused by a number of specific agents.*

477 REFERENCE INTERVALS AND LABORATORY VALUES*

Ronald J. Elin

Reference intervals are valuable guidelines for the clinician to assess health and disease, but they should not be used as absolute indicators of health and disease. For essentially every test, there is a significant overlap between the normal and diseased populations. Many factors may influence the determination of the reference interval. The method and mode of standardization are variables for the reference interval, particularly for immunologic and enzymatic tests. The selection of the "normal" population is also important because factors such as age, gender, race, diet, personal habits (e.g., alcohol consumption, smoking), and exercise may influence the reference interval for a given analyte. Last, the statistics chosen to define the reference interval are also a factor. These multiple variables for determining the reference interval indicate why there are differences among institutions for the same analyte.

The values in this chapter are primarily for adults in the fasting state. Values for other groups, when included, are clearly identified. For convenience, this chapter is divided into the following three sections: clinical chemistry, toxicology, and serology; hematology and coagulation; and drugs—therapeutic and toxic. The list includes reference intervals for the most common tests used in the practice of internal medicine. For more information about the reference interval for a given test or a test not included in the list, I recommend *Clinical Guide to Laboratory Tests,* second edition, edited by Dr. Norbert W. Tietz. This book contains literature citations for most of the tests listed in this chapter.

All laboratory values are given in conventional and international units. If the value and units for a reference interval are the same for conventional and international units, the interval is listed only in the column for international units. The temperature for all enzyme assays listed in the chapter is 37° C. The pertinent prefixes denoting the decimal factors and abbreviations are listed above.

---

* The material in this chapter was partially extracted from Tietz NW (ed.): Clinical Guide to Laboratory Tests. Philadelphia, WB Saunders, 1990. The material for the section on Therapeutic Drug Concentrations was partially extracted from Burtis CA, Ashwood ER (eds.): Tietz Textbook of Clinical Chemistry. Philadelphia, WB Saunders, 1994. The main contributors to this section of the book are PC Painter, JY Cope, and JL Smith. Other sources are listed under references for this chapter.

Prefixes Denoting Decimal Factors

Prefix	Symbol	Factor
mega	M	10^6
kilo	k	10^3
hecto	h	10^2
deka	da	10^1
deci	d	10^{-1}
centi	c	10^{-2}
milli	m	10^{-3}
micro	μ	10^{-6}
nano	n	10^{-9}
pico	p	10^{-12}
femto	f	10^{-15}

Abbreviations

AU	Arbitrary units
EU	Ehrlich unit
GD	General diagnostics
IFA	Immunofluorescent assay
IU	International unit (of hormone activity)
RIA	Radioimmunoassay
RID	Radial immunodiffusion
S	Substrate
U	International unit (of enzyme activity)

CLINICAL CHEMISTRY, TOXICOLOGY, SEROLOGY

Test	Specimen	Reference Interval (Conventional Units)	Reference Interval (International Units)
Acetoacetate	Serum or plasma	Negative ($<$ 1 mg/dL)	Negative ($<$ 0.1 mmol/L)
Semiquantitative	(fluoride/oxalate)		
Acetone	Urine	Negative	Negative
Semiquantitative	Serum or plasma	Negative ($<$ 1 mg/dL)	Negative ($<$ 0.17 mmol/L)
	(fluoride or oxalate)		
Quantitative			
Semiquantitative	Urine		Negative
Acid phosphatase	Serum		M: 2.5–11.7 U/L
(S:p-nitrophenylphosphate)			F: 0.3–9.2 U/L
Adrenocorticotropic	Plasma (heparin)	0800 h: 8–79 pg/mL	8–79 ng/L
hormone (ACTH)		1600 h: 7–30 pg/mL	7–30 ng/L
Alanine aminotransferase	Serum		8–20 U/L
(ALT, SGPT)			
Albumin			
Nephelometric, colorimetric	Serum	3.5–5 g/dL	35–50 g/L
Turbidimetric	CSF	15–45 mg/dL	150–450 mg/L
	Urine	$<$ 80 mg/d at rest	$<$ 80 mg/d
		$<$ 150 mg/d ambulatory	$<$ 150 mg/d
Aldolase	Serum		1.0–7.5 U/L
Aldosterone	Plasma (heparin EDTA) or serum	Adult, average sodium diet	
		supine: 3–10 ng/dL	0.08–0.28 nmol/L
		upright: 5–30 ng/dL	0.14–0.83 nmol/L
Alkaline phosphate	Serum		Adult ($>$ 18 y)
(S:4–NPP)			F: 42–98 U/L
			M: 53–128 U/L
δ-Aminolevulinic acid			
(δ-ALA)	Serum	15–23 μg/dL	1.1–8 μmol/L
	Urine	1.5–7.5 mg/d	11.4–57.2 μmol/d
Ammonia nitrogen	Serum or plasma		
Resin or enzymatic	(Na-heparin)	Adult 15–45 μg N/dL	11–32 μmol/L
	Urine, 24-h	140–1500 mg/d	10–107 mmol/d
Amylase	Serum		25–125 U/L
(S:Beckmann, defined substrate)			
	Urine, timed specimen		1–17 U/h
Angiotensin I	Peripheral venous plasma (EDTA)	11–88 pg/mL	11–88 ng/L
Angiotensin II	Plasma (EDTA)	10–60 pg/mL	10–60 ng/L
	Arterial blood		
α_1-Antitrypsin (nephelometry)	Serum	78–200 mg/dL	0.78–2 g/L
Anion gap	Plasma (heparin)	7–14 mEq/L	7–14 mmol/L
[$Na^+ - (Cl^- + HCO_3^-)$]			
Apolipoprotein A-I	Serum	M: 94–178 mg/dL	0.94–1.78 g/L
		F: 101–199 mg/dL	1.01–1.99 g/L
Apolipoprotein B	Serum	M: 63–133 mg/dL	0.63–1.33 g/L
		F: 60–126 mg/dL	0.60–1.26 g/L
Arsenic	Whole blood (heparin)	0.2–2.3 μg/dL	0.03–0.31 μmol/L
		Chronic poisoning: 10–50 μg/dL	1.33–6.65 μmol/L
		Acute poisoning: 60–93 μg/dL	7.98–12.37 μmol/L
	Urine, 24-h	5–50 μg/d	0.067–0.665 μmol/d
Ascorbic acid (see Vitamin C)			
Aspartate aminotransferase (AST, SGOT)	Serum		10–30 U/L
Base excess	Whole blood (heparin)	− 2 to 3 mEq/L	− 2 to 3 mmol/L
Bicarbonate	Serum	18–23 mEq/L	18–23 mmol/L
Bile acids, total	Serum, fasting	0.3–2.3 μg/mL	0.74–5.64 μmol/L
	Serum, 1-h postprandial	1.8–3.2 μg/mL	4.41–7.84 μmol/L
	Feces	120–225 mg/d	294–551 μmol/d
Bilirubin			
Total	Serum	0.2–1.0 mg/dL	3.4–17.1 μmol/L
	Urine	Negative	Negative
Conjugated (direct)	Serum	0–0.2 mg/dL	0–3.4 μmol/L
Calcium, ionized (iCa)	Serum	4.65–5.28 mg/dL	1.16–1.32 mmol/L
Calcium, total	Serum	8.4–10.2 mg/dL	2.10–2.55 mmol/L
	Urine, 24-h	100–300 mg/d	2.5–7.5 mmol/d
	CSF	4.2–5.4 mg/dL	1.05–1.35 mmol/L
Cancer antigen 125 (CA 125)	Serum	$<$ 35 U/mL	$<$ 35 kU/L
Carbon dioxide, partial pressure (Pco₂)	Whole blood, arterial (heparin)	M: 35–48 mm Hg	4.66–6.38 kPa
		F: 32–45 mm Hg	4.26–5.99 kPa
Carbon dioxide, total (Tco₂)	Serum or plasma (heparin)	23–29 mEq/L	23–29 mmol/L
Carcinoembryonic antigen (CEA)	Serum	Nonsmokers: $<$ 2.5 ng/mL	$<$ 2.5 μg/L
β-Carotene	Serum	10–85 μg/dL	0.19–1.58 μmol/L
Catecholamines, total	Urine, 24-h	$<$ 100 μg/d	$<$ 5.91 nmol/d
Ceruloplasmin (RID)	Serum	18–45 mg/dL	180–450 mg/L
Chloride	Serum or plasma (heparin)	98–106 mEq/L	98–106 mmol/L
	CSF	118–132 mEq/L	118–132 mmol/L
	Urine, 24-h	110–250 mEq/d	110–250 mmol/d

CLINICAL CHEMISTRY, TOXICOLOGY, SEROLOGY *Continued*

Test	Specimen	Reference Interval (Conventional Units)	Reference Interval (International Units)
Cholesterol, total	Serum or plasma (EDTA)	Recommended: < 200 mg/dL	< 5.18 mmol/L
		Moderate risk: 200–239 mg/dL	5.18–6.19 mmol/L
		High risk: ≥ 240 mg/dL	6.22 mmol/L
Chorionic gonadotropin, β-subunit (β-HCG)	Serum or plasma (EDTA)	M and nonpregnant F: < 5.0 mU/mL	< 5.0 IU/L
Complement			
Total hemolytic Complement activity	Plasma (EDTA)	75–160 U/mL	75–160 kU/L
Copper	Serum	M: 70–140 μg/dL	10.99–21.98 μmol/L
		F: 80–155 μg/dL	12.56–24.34 μmol/L
	Erythrocyte (heparin)	90–150 μg/dL	14.13–23.55 μmol/L
	Urine, 24-h	3–35 μg/d	0.047–0.55 μmol/d
Coproporphyrin	Urine, 24-h	34–234 μg/d	51–351 nmol/d
	Feces, 24-h	< 30 μg/g dry wt	< 45 nmol/g dry wt
		400–1200 μg/d	600–1800 nmol/d
Corticobinding globulin (CBG) (see Transcortin)			
Corticosterone	Serum	0800 h: 130–820 ng/dL	4–24 nmol/L
		1600 h: 60–220 ng/dL	2–6 nmol/L
Cortisol	Serum or plasma (heparin)	0800 h: 5–23 μg/dL	138–635 nmol/L
		1600 h: 3–15 μg/dL	82–413 nmol/L
		2000 h: ≤ 50% of 0800 h	Fraction of 0800 h: ≤ 0.50
Cortisol, free	Urine, 24-h	10–100 μg/d	27–276 nmol/d
C-Peptide	Serum	0.78–1.89 ng/mL	0.26–0.62 nmol/L
C-Reactive protein	Serum	68–8200 ng/mL	68–8200 μg/L
Creatine kinase (CK)	Serum		M: 38–174 U/L
			F: 26–140 U/L
Isoenzymes	Serum	Fraction 2 (MB) < 4–6% of total (method-dependent)	Fraction of total: < 0.04–0.06
Creatinine	Serum or plasma	M: 0.7–1.3 mg/dL	62–115 μmol/L
Jaffe, kinetic or enzymatic		F: 0.6–1.1 mg/dL	53–97 μmol/L
	Urine, 24-h	M: 14–26 mg/kg/d	124–230 μmol/kg/d
		F: 11–20 mg/kg/d	97–177 μmol/kg/d
Creatinine clearance (endogenous)	Serum or plasma, and urine	M: 90–139 mL/min/1.73 m^2	0.87–1.34 mL/s/m^2
		F: 80–125 mL/min/1.73 m^2	0.77–1.20 mL/s/m^2
Dehydroepiandrosterone (DHEA)	Serum	M: 1.8–12.5 ng/mL	6.2–43.3 nmol/L
		F: 1.3–9.8 ng/mL	4.5–34.0 nmol/L
Dehydroepiandrosterone sulfate (DHEA-S)	Serum or plasma (heparin, EDTA)	M: 1.7–6.7 μg/mL	4.6–18.2 μmol/L
		F: Premenopausal: 0.5–5.4 μg/mL	1.4–14.7 μmol/L
		Postmenopausal: 0.3–2.6 μg/mL	0.8–7.1 μmol/L
11-Deoxycortisol (compound S)	Serum	12–158 ng/dL	0.3–4.6 nmol/L
Estrogens, total	Serum	M: 20–80 pg/mL	20–80 ng/L
		F, cycle:	
		1–10 d 61–394 pg/mL	60–200 ng/L
		11–20 d 122–437 pg/mL	
		21–30 d 156–350 pg/mL	160–400 ng/L
		Postmenopausal: ≤ 130 pg/mL	≥ 130 ng/L
		Follicular phase: 60–200 pg/mL	
		Luteal phase: 160–400 pg/mL	
	Urine, 24-h	M: 15–40 μg/d	
		F: Preovulation: 4–25 μg/d	
		Ovulation: 28–100 μg/d	
		Luteal peak: 22–80 μg/d	
		Pregnancy, term: < 45,000 μg/d	
		Postmenopausal: < 20 μg/d	
Fat, fecal	Feces, 72-h	< 7 g/d	fat-free diet: < 4 g/d
Fatty acids, nonesterified (free)	Serum or plasma (heparin)	8–25 mg/dL	0.28–0.89 mmol/L
Ferritin	Serum	M: 20–250 ng/mL	20–250 μg/L
		F: 10–120 ng/mL	10–120 μg/L
α$_1$-Fetoprotein	Serum	< 10 ng/mL	< 10 μg/L
Fibrinogen (see Hematology and Coagulation section)			
Folate	Serum	3–16 ng/mL	7–36 nmol/L
	Erythrocytes (EDTA)	130–628 ng/mL packed cells	294–1422 nmol/L packed cells
Follitropin (FSH)	Serum or plasma (heparin)	M: 4–25 mIU/mL	4–25 IU/L
		F: Follicular phase: 1–9 mU/mL	1–9 U/L
		Ovulatory peak: 6–26 mU/mL	6–26 U/L
		Luteal phase: 1–9 mU/mL	1–9 U/L
		Postmenopausal: 30–118 mU/mL	30–118 U/L
	Urine, 24-h		4–18 U/d
			3–12 U/d
Free thyroxine index (FT$_4$I)	Serum		4.2–13.0
Gastrin	Serum	< 100 pg/mL	< 100 ng/L
Glucose	Serum	Adult: 70–105 mg/dL	3.9–5.8 mmol/L
		> 60 y: 80–115 mg/dL	4.4–6.4 mmol/L
	Whole blood (heparin)	65–95 mg/dL	3.6–5.3 mmol/L
	CSF	40–70 mg/dL	2.2–3.9 mmol/L

Continued

CLINICAL CHEMISTRY, TOXICOLOGY, SEROLOGY *Continued*

Test	Specimen	Reference Interval (Conventional Units)	Reference Interval (International Units)
Quantitative, enzymatic	Urine	< 0.5 g/d	< 2.8 mmol/d
Qualitative	Urine		Negative
Glucose, 2-h postprandial	Serum	< 120 mg/dL	< 6.7 mmol/L
Glucose tolerance test (GTT), oral	Serum		

		mg/dL		mmol/L	
		Normal	Diabetic	Normal	Diabetic
Fasting:		70–105	> 140	3.9–5.8	> 7.8
60 min:		120–170	≥ 200	6.7–9.4	≥ 11
90 min:		100–140	≥ 200	5.6–7.8	≥ 11
120 min:		70–120	≥ 140	3.9–6.7	≥ 7.8

Test	Specimen	Reference Interval (Conventional Units)	Reference Interval (International Units)
γ-Glutamyltransferase (GGT)	Serum		M: 9–50 U/L
			F: 8–40 U/L
Glycerol, free	Plasma	0.29–1.72 mg/dL	0.032–0.187 mmol/L
Growth hormone (HGH, somatotropin)	Serum or plasma (EDTA, heparin)	Adult, M: < 2 ng/mL	< 2 µg/L
		F: < 10 ng/mL	< 10 µg/L
		> 60 y, M: 0.4–10 ng/mL	0.4–10 µg/L
		F: 1–14 ng/mL	1–14 µg/L
Haptoglobin (see Hematology and Coagulation section)			
HDL-cholesterol (HDLC) (5th percentile from Lipid Research Clinics)	Serum or plasma (EDTA)	M: > 29 mg/dL	> 0.75 mmol/L
		F: > 35 mg/dL	> 0.91 mmol/L
Hemoglobin A₁c (electrophoresis)	Whole blood (heparin, EDTA, or oxalate)	5.6–7.5% of total Hb	Fraction of Hb: 0.056–0.075
Homovanillic acid (HVA)	Urine, 24-h	1.4–3.8 mg/d	8–48 µmol/d
17-Hydroxycorticosteroids (17-OHCS)	Urine, 24-h	M: 3.0–10.0 mg/d	8.3–27.6 µmol/d
		F: 2.0–8.0 mg/d	5.5–22.1 µmol/d
5-Hydroxyindole acetic acid (5-HIAA)			
Qualitative	Fresh random urine		Negative
Quantitative	Urine, 24-h	2–6 mg/d	10.4–31.2 µmol/d
17-Hydroxyprogesterone (17-OHP)	Serum	M: 0.5–2.5 ng/mL	1.5–7.5 nmol/L
		F: Follicular: 0.2–1.0 ng/mL	0.6–3.0 nmol/L
		Luteal: 1.0–5.0 ng/mL	3.0–15.5 nmol/L
		Postmenopausal: ≤ 0.7 ng/mL	≤ 2.1 nmol/L
Immunoglobulin A (IgA)	Serum	40–350 mg/dL	400–3500 mg/L
Immunoglobulin D (IgD)	Serum	0–8 mg/dL	0–80 mg/L
Immunoglobulin E (IgE)	Serum	0–380 IU/mL	0–380 kIU/L
Immunoglobulin G (IgG)	Serum	650–1600 mg/dL	6.5–16 g/L
	CSF	0.5–5 mg/dL	5–50 mg/L
Immunoglobulin M (IgM)	Serum	55–300 mg/dL	550–3000 mg/L
Insulin (12-h fasting)	Serum	6–24 µIU/mL	42–167 pmol/L
Intrinsic factor (see Vitamin B₁₂)			
Iron	Serum	M: 65–175 µg/dL	11.6–31.3 µmol/L
		F: 50–170 µg/dL	9.0–30.4 µmol/L
Iron-binding capacity, total (TIBC)	Serum	250–450 µg/dL	44.8–80.6 µmol/L
Iron saturation	Serum	M: 20–50	Fraction of iron saturation: 0.20–0.5
		F: 15–50	0.15–0.5
17-Ketogenic steroids (17-KGS)	Urine, 24-h	M: 5–23 mg/d	17–80 µmol/d
		F: 3–15 mg/d	10–52 µmol/d
Ketone bodies			
Qualitative	Serum	Negative (0.5–3.0 mg/dL)	Negative (5–30 mg/L)
	Urine, random		Negative
17-Ketosteroids, total (17-KS)	Urine, 24-h	M: 18–30 y 9–22 mg/d	31–76 µmol/d
		> 30 y 8–20 mg/d	28–70 µmol/d
		F: 6–15 mg/d	21–52 µmol/d
L-Lactate	Whole blood (heparin)	Venous: 4.5–19.8 mg/dL	0.5–2.2 mmol/L
		Arterial: 4.5–14.4 mg/dL	0.5–1.6 mmol/L
Lactate dehydrogenase (LDH)	Serum		208–378 U/L
LDH isoenzymes (Electrophoresis, agarose)	Serum	%	Fraction of total:
		Fraction 1: 18–33	0.18–0.33
		Fraction 2: 28–40	0.28–0.40
		Fraction 3: 18–30	0.18–0.30
		Fraction 4: 6–16	0.06–0.16
		Fraction 5: 2–13	0.02–0.13
Lead	Whole blood (heparin)	< 40 µg/dL	< 1.93 µmol/L
		Toxic: ≥ 100 µg/dL	≥ 4.83 µmol/L
	Urine	< 80 µg/dL	< 0.39 µmol/L
Lipase (turbidimetric)	Serum		Adult: 10–140 U/L
			> 60 y: 18–180 U/L
LDL-Cholesterol (LDLC)	Serum or plasma (EDTA)	Recommended: < 130 mg/dL	< 3.37 mmol/L
		Moderate risk: 130–159 mg/dL	3.37–4.12 mmol/L
		High risk: ≥ 160 mg/dL	≥ 4.14 mmol/L
Lutropin (LH)	Serum or plasma (heparin)	M: 1–8 mU/mL	1–8 U/L
		F: Follicular phase: 1–2 mU/mL	1–12 U/L
		Midcycle: 16–104 mU/mL	16–104 U/L
		Luteal: 1–12 mU/mL	1–12 U/L
		Postmenopausal: 16–66 mU/mL	16–66 U/L
	Urine		M: 9–23 U/d
			F: non-midcycle, 4–30 U/d

CLINICAL CHEMISTRY, TOXICOLOGY, SEROLOGY *Continued*

Test	Specimen	Reference Interval (Conventional Units)	Reference Interval (International Units)
Lysozyme	Serum, plasma	0.4–1.3 mg/dL	4–13 mg/L
Magnesium	Serum	1.3–2.1 mEq/L	0.65–1.05 mmol/L
	Urine, 24-h	6.0–10.0 mEq/d	3.00–5.00 mmol/L
Mercury	Whole blood (EDTA)	<5.0 μg/dL	<0.25 μmol/L
	Urine, 24-h	<20 μg/L	<0.1 μmol/L
		Toxic: >150 μg/L	<0.75 μmol/L
Metanephrine, total	Urine, 24-h	0.05–1.20 μg/mg creatinine	0.03–0.69 mmol/mol creatinine
Myelin basic protein	CSF		<2.5 ng/mL
Myoglobin	Serum		M: 19–92 μg/L
			12–76 μg/L
	Urine, random		Negative
Osmolality	Serum		275–295 mOsmol/kg
	Urine, random		50–1400 mOsmol/kg, depending on fluid intake
			After 12-h fluid restriction: >850 mOsmol/kg
	Urine, 24-h		~390–900 mOsmol/kg
Oxalate	Serum	1–2.4 μg/mL	11–27 μmol/L
		Ethylene glycol poisoning: >20 μg/mL	Ethylene glycol poisoning: >228 μmol/L
Oxygen (Po$_2$)	Whole blood, arterial (heparin)	83–100 mm Hg	11–14.4 kPa
Oxygen saturation	Whole blood, arterial (heparin)	95–98%	Fraction saturated: 0.95–0.98
Parathyroid hormone	Serum	Varies with laboratory	
		N-terminal 8–24 pg/mL	8–24 ng/L
		C-terminal 50–330 pg/mL	50–330 ng/L
		Midmolecule 0.29–0.85 ng/mL	29–85 pmol/L
pH (37°C)	Whole blood, arterial (heparin)		7.35–7.45
Phosphorus, inorganic	Serum	2.7–4.5 mg/dL	0.87–1.45 nmol/L
		>60 y, M: 2.3–3.7 mg/dL	0.74–1.2 nmol/L
		F: 2.8–4.1 mg/dL	0.90–1.3 nmol/L
	Urine, 24-h	0.4–1.3 g/d	13–42 mmol/d
Porphobilinogen (PBG)			
Quantitative	Urine, 24-h	0–2.0 mg/d	0–8.8 μmol/d
Qualitative	Urine, fresh random		Negative
Potassium	Serum	3.5–5.1 mEq/L	3.5–5.1 mmol/L
	Plasma (heparin)	3.5–4.5 mEq/L	3.5–4.5 mmol/L
	Urine, 24-h	25–125 mEq/d	25–125 mmol/d
Pregnanediol	Urine, 24-h	M: 0–1.9 mg/d	0–5.9 μmol/d
		F: Follicular: <2.6 mg/d	<8 μmol/d
		Luteal: 2.6–10.6 mg/d	8–33 μmol/d
		Postmenopausal: 0.2–1.0 mg/d	0.6–3.1 μmol/d
Progesterone	Serum	M: 0.13–0.97 ng/mL	0.4–3.1 nmol/L
		F: Follicular: 0.15–0.70 ng/mL	0.5–2.2 nmol/L
		Luteal: 2.0–25 ng/mL	6.4–79.5 nmol/L
Prolactin (hPRL)	Serum	0–20 ng/mL	0–20 μg/L
Prostate-specific antigen (PSA)	Serum, freeze	M: <4 ng/mL	<4 μg/L
Protein			
Total	Serum	6.4–8.3 g/dL	64.0–83.0 g/L
Electrophoresis	Serum	Albumin: 3.5–5.0 g/dL	35–50 g/L
		α_1-Globulin: 0.1–0.3 g/dL	1–3 g/L
		α_2-Globulin: 0.6–1.0 g/dL	6–10 g/L
		β-Globulin: 0.7–1.1 g/dL	7–11 g/L
		γ-Globulin: 0.8–1.6 g/dL	8–16 g/L
Total	Urine, 24-h		50–80 mg/d at rest
Total	CSF	Lumbar: 15–45 mg/dL	150–450 mg/L
Protoporphyrin	Whole blood (heparin or EDTA)	17–77 μg/dL RBC	0.30–1.37 μmol/L RBC
	Feces, 24-h	≤60 μg/g dry wt or <1500 μg/d	≤0.11 mmol/kg dry wt or <2.67 μmol/d
Pyruvic acid	Whole blood (heparin)	0.3–0.9 mg/dL	0.03–0.10 mmol/L
Renin (normal diet)	Plasma (EDTA)	ng/mL/h ± 1 SE	μg/L/h ± 1 SE
		Supine: 1.6 ± 1.5	1.6 ± 1.5
		Standing: (4-h): 4.5 ± 2.9	4.5 ± 2.9
Riboflavin (see Vitamin B$_2$)			
Sediment	Urine, fresh, random		
Casts			Hyaline: occasional (0–1) casts/hpf
			RBC: not seen
			WBC: not seen
			Tubular epithelial: not seen
			Transitional and squamous epithelial: not seen
Cells			RBC: 0–2/hpf
			WBC: M: 0–3/hpf
			F: 0–5/hpf
			Epithelial: few
			Bacteria:
			Unspun: no organisms/oil immersion field
			Spun: <20 organisms/hpf

Continued

✔

CLINICAL CHEMISTRY, TOXICOLOGY, SEROLOGY *Continued*

Test	Specimen	Reference Interval (Conventional Units)	Reference Interval (International Units)
Sodium	Serum or plasma (heparin)	136–146 mEq/L	136–146 mmol/L
	Urine, 24-h	40–220 mEq/d	40–220 mmol/d
Specific gravity	Urine, random		1.002–1.030
	Urine, 24-h	% of total	1.015–1.025
Testosterone, free	Serum	M: 52–280 pg/mL 1.5–3.2	180.4–971.6 pmol/fraction of total L
		F: 1.6–6.3 pg/mL 0.8–1.4	5.6–21.9 pmol/L 0.015–0.032
			0.008–0.014
Testosterone, total	Serum	M: 300–1000	10.4–34.7 nmol/L
		F: 20–75	0.69–2.6 nmol/L
	Urine	20–50 y,	
		M: 50–135 μg/d	173–470 nmol/d
		F: 2–12 μg/d	7–42 nmol/d
		> 50 y,	
		M: 40–60 μg/d	139–210 nmol/d
		F: 2–8 μg/d	7–28 nmol/d
Thiamine (see Vitamin B$_1$)	Serum		
Thyroglobulin (Tg)	Serum	3–42 ng/mL	3–42 μg/L
Thyroglobulin antibodies	Serum		< 1:10
Thyroid microsomal antibodies	Serum		Nondetectable (hemagglutination) or < 1:10 (IFA)
Thyrotropin (hTSH)	Serum or plasma	2–10 μU/mL	2–10 mU/L
Thyrotropin-releasing hormone	Plasma	5–60 pg/mL	5–60 ng/L
Thyroxine, free (FT$_4$)	Serum	0.8–2.4 ng/dL	10–31 pmol/L
Thyroxine (T$_4$), total	Serum	5–12 μg/dL	65–155 nmol/L
		> 60 y, M: 5.0–10.0 μg/dL	65–129 nmol/L
		F: 5.5–10.5 μg/dL	71–135 nmol/L
Thyroxine-binding globulin (TBG)	Serum	15.0–34.0 μg/mL	15.0–34.0 mg/L
Thyroxine index, free (see Free thyroxine index)			
		T$_4$ (μg/dL)/TBG (μg/mL)	T$_4$ (nmol/L)/TBG (mg/L)
Transcortin	Serum	M: 18.8–25.2 mg/L	323–433 nmol/L
		F: 14.9–22.9 mg/L	256–393 nmol/L
Transferrin	Serum	200–400 mg/dL	2.0–4.0 g/L
		> 60 y: 180–380 mg/dL	1.80–3.80 g/L
Transthyretin (prealbumin)	Serum	10–40 mg/dL	100–400 mg/L
Triglycerides (TG)	Serum, after ≥ 12-hr fast	Recommended:	0.45–1.81 mmol/L
		M: 40–160 mg/dL	0.40–1.52 mmol/L
		F: 35–135 mg/dL	
Tri-iodothyronine, free	Serum	260–480 pg/dL	4.0–7.4 pmol/L
Tri-iodothyronine, total (T$_3$)	Serum	100–200 ng/dL	1.54–3.08 mmol/L
Tri-iodothyronine resin uptake test (T$_3$RU)	Serum	24–34%	24–34 AU (arbitrary units)
Urea nitrogen	Serum or plasma	7–18 mg/dL	2.5–6.4 mmol/L
	Urine	12–20 g/d	0.43–0.71 mol/d
Urea nitrogen/creatinine ratio	Serum		12/1–20/1
Uric acid (uricase)	Serum	M: 3.5–7.2 mg/dL	0.21–0.42 mmol/L
		F: 2.6–6.0 mg/dL	0.15–0.35 mmol/L
	Urine, 24-h	250–750 mg/d	1.48–4.43 mmol/d
Urinary sediment (see Sediment)			
Urobilinogen	Urine, 2-h	0.1–0.8 EU	0.1–0.8 U
	Urine, 24-h	0.5–4.0 EU	0.5–4.0 U
	Feces	75–275 EU/100 g	750–2750 U/kg
		75–400 EU/d	75–400 U/d
		40–280 mg/d	67–473 μmol/d
Uroporphyrin	Urine, 24-h	< 50 μg/d	< 60 nmol/d
	Feces, 24-h specimen	10–40 μg/d	12–48 nmol/d
	Erythrocytes (heparin or EDTA)		Negative
Vanillylmandelic acid (VMA)	Urine, 24-h	2–7 mg/d	10.1–35.4 μmol/d
Viscosity	Serum		1.10–1.22 centipoise
Vitamin A	Serum	30–80 μg/dL	1.05–2.8 μmol/L
Vitamin B$_1$ (Thiamine)	Serum	0–2 μg/dL	0–75 nmol/L
Vitamin B$_2$ (Riboflavin)	Serum	4–24 μg/dL	106–638 nmol/L
Vitamin B$_6$	Plasma (EDTA)	5–30 ng/mL	20–121 nmol/L
Vitamin B$_{12}$	Serum	100–700 pg/mL	74–516 pmol/L
Vitamin C	Plasma (oxalate, heparin, or EDTA)	0.5–1.5 mg/dL	28–85 μmol/L
Vitamin D$_3$, 1,25-dihydroxy	Serum	25–45 pg/mL	60–108 pmol/L
Vitamin D$_3$, 25-hydroxy	Plasma (heparin)	Summer: 15–80 ng/mL	37.4–200 nmol/L
		Winter: 14–42 ng/mL	34.9–105 nmol/L
Vitamin E	Serum	5.0–18.0 μg/mL	12–42 μmol/L
Zinc	Serum	70–150 μg/dL	10.7–22.9 μmol/L

HEMATOLOGY AND COAGULATION

Test	Specimen	Reference Interval (Conventional Units)	Reference Interval (International Units)
Activated partial thromboplastin time (APTT)	Whole blood (Na citrate)		25–35 sec
Bleeding time (BT)			
Ivy	Blood from skin		Normal: 2–7 min
			Borderline: 7–11 min
Simplate (G-D)			2.75–8 min
Blood volume	Whole blood (heparin)		M: 52–83 mL/kg
			F: 50–75 mL/kg
Bone marrow	Bone marrow aspirate	% (mean)	Number fraction (mean)
Differential count			
Myeoblasts		0.3–5.0 (2.0)	0.003–0.05 (0.02)
Promyelocytes		1.0–8.0 (5.0)	0.01–0.08 (0.05)
Myelocytes:			
Neutrophilic		5.0–19.0 (12.0)	0.05–0.19 (0.12)
Eosinophilic		0.5–3.0 (1.5)	0.005–0.03 (0.015)
Basophilic		0.0–0.5 (0.3)	0.00–0.005 (0.003)
Metamyelocytes		13.0–32.0 (22.0)	0.13–0.32 (0.22)
Polymorphonuclear neutrophils		7.0–3.0 (2.0)	0.07–0.30 (0.20)
Polymorphonuclear eosinophils		0.5–4.0 (2.0)	0.005–0.04 (0.02)
Polymorphonuclear basophils		0.0–0.7 (0.2)	0.0–0.007 (0.002)
Lymphocytes		3.0–17.0 (10.0)	0.03–0.17 (0.10)
Plasma cells		0.0–2.0 (0.4)	0.00–0.02 (0.004)
Monocytes		0.5–5.0 (2.0)	0.005–0.05 (0.02)
Reticulum cells		0.1–2.0 (0.2)	0.001–0.02 (0.002)
Megakaryocytes		0.03–3.0 (0.1)	0.0003–0.03 (0.001)
Pronormoblasts		1.0–8.0 (4.0)	0.01–0.08 (0.04)
Normoblasts		7.0–32.0 (18.0)	0.07–0.32 (0.18)
Clot lysis, 37°C	Whole clotted blood		48–72 h
Clot retraction screen	Whole blood (no anticoagulant)		Retraction begins at 1 h, maximum at 24 h
Clotting time, Lee-White, 37°C	Whole blood (no anticoagulant)		5–8 min
Differential count (see Bone marrow differential count or Leukocyte differential count)			
Eosinophil count	Whole blood (EDTA); capillary blood	50–400 cells/μL (mm^3)	50–400 $\times$ 10^6 cells/L
Erythrocyte count (RBC count)	Whole blood (EDTA)	millions of cells/μL (mm^3)	$\times$ 10^{12} cells/L
		M: 4.3–5.7	4.3–5.7
		F: 3.8–5.1	3.8–5.1
Erythrocyte sedimentation rate (ESR), Wintrobe			M: 0–15 mm/h
			F: 0–20 mm/h
Ferritin (see Chemistry section)			
Fibrin degradation products (agglutination, Thrombo-Wellco test)	Whole blood: special tube containing thrombin and proteolytic inhibitor	$<$ 10 μg/mL	$<$ 10 mg/L
	Urine: 2 mL in special tube (see above)	$<$ 0.25 μg/mL	$<$ 0.25 mg/L
Fibrinogen	Plasma (Na citrate)	200–400 mg/dL	2.00–4.00 g/L
Glucose-6-phosphate dehydrogenase (G6PD) in erythrocytes	Whole blood (ACD, EDTA, or heparin)	12.1 $\pm$ 2.09 U/g Hb (1 SD)	0.78 $\pm$ 0.13 MU/mol Hb (1 SD)
Haptoglobin (Hp) RID	Serum; avoid hemolysis	26–85 mg/dL	260–1850 mg/L
Hematocrit (HCT, Hct)	Whole blood (EDTA)		
Calculated from MCV and RBC (electronic displacement or laser)		M: 39–49%	0.39–0.49 volume fraction
		F: 35–45%	0.35–0.45 volume fraction
Hemoglobin (Hb)	Whole blood (EDTA)	M: 13.5–17.5 g/dL	2.09–2.71 mmol/L
		F: 12.0–16.0 g/dL	1.86–2.48 mmol/L
	Plasma (heparin, ACD)	$<$ 3 mg/dL	$<$ 0.47 μmol/L
	Urine, fresh, random		Negative
Hemoglobin electrophoresis	Whole blood (EDTA, citrate, or heparin)		Mass function
		HbA $>$95%	HbA $>$ 0.95
		HbA$_2$ 1.5–3.5%	HbA$_2$ 0.015–0.035
		HbF $<$ 2%	HbF $<$ 0.02
Leukocyte count (WBC count)	Whole blood (EDTA)	4.5–11.0 $\times$ 10^3 cells/μL (mm^3)	4.5–11.0 $\times$ 10^9 cells/L
	CSF	0.5 mononuclear cells/μL	0.5 $\times$ 10^6 cells/L

Leukocyte Differential count	Whole blood (EDTA)	%	Cells/μL (mm^3)	Number fraction	Cells $\times$ 10^6/L
Myelocytes		0	0	0	0
Neutrophils—bands		3–5	150–400	0.03–0.05	150–400
Neutrophils—segmented		54–62	3000–5800	0.54–0.62	3000–5800
Lymphocytes		23–33	1500–3000	0.25–0.33	1500–3000
Monocytes		3–7	285–500	0.03–0.07	285–500
Eosinophils		1–3	50–250	0.01–0.03	50–250
Basophils		0–0.75	15–50	0–0.0075	15–50

Leukocyte Differential count	CSF	%	Number fraction
Lymphocytes		62 $\pm$ 34	0.62 $\pm$ 0.324
Monocytes (includes pia-arachnoid mesothelial cells)		36 $\pm$ 20	0.36 $\pm$ 0.20
Neutrophils		2 $\pm$ 5	0.02 $\pm$ 0.05

Continued

HEMATOLOGY AND COAGULATION *Continued*

Test	Specimen	Reference Interval (Conventional Units)	Reference Interval (International Units)
Histocytes			Rare
Ependymal cells			Rare
Eosinophils			Rare
Mean corpuscular hemoglobin (MCH)	Whole blood (EDTA)	26–34 pg/cell	0.40–0.53 fmol/cell
Mean corpuscular hemoglobin concentration (MCHC)	Whole blood (EDTA)	31–37% Hb/cell or gHb/dL RBC	4.81–5.74 mmol Hb/L RBC
Mean corpuscular volume (MCV)	Whole blood (EDTA)		80–100 fL
Methemoglobin (MetHb)	Whole blood (EDTA, heparin, or ACD)	0.06–0.24 g/dL	9.3–37.2 μmol/L
Partial thromboplastin time (PTT)	Whole blood (Na citrate)		60–85 sec
Plasma volume	Plasma (heparin)	M: 25–43 mL/kg	0.025–0.043 L/kg
		F: 28–45 mL/kg	0.028–0.045 L/kg
Platelet count (thrombocyte count)	Whole blood (EDTA)	150–450 × 10³/μL (mm³)	150–450 × 10⁹/L
Prothrombin consumption	Whole blood (no anticoagulant)		> 30 sec
Prothrombin time, two-stage modified	Whole blood (Na citrate)		18–22 sec
RBC count (see Erythrocyte count)			
Red cell volume	Whole blood (heparin)	M: 20–36 mL/kg	M: 0.020–0.036 L/kg
		F: 19–31 mL/kg	F: 0.019–0.031 L/kg
Reticulocyte count	Whole blood (EDTA, heparin, or oxalate)	0.5–1.5% of erythrocytes	0.005–0.015 (number fraction)
Sulfhemoglobin	Whole blood (EDTA, heparin, or EDTA)	≤ 1.0% of total Hb	< 0.010 of total Hb (mass fraction)
Thrombin time	Whole blood (Na citrate)		Time of control ± 25 when control is 9–13 sec
Thromboplastin time, activated (see Activated partial thromboplastin time [APTT])			

Platelet count (thrombocyte count): $150–450 \times 10^3/\mu L$; $150–450 \times 10^9/L$

DRUGS—THERAPEUTIC AND TOXIC

Drug	Specimen	Reference Interval (Conventional Units)		Reference Interval (International Units)
Acetaminophen	Serum or plasma (hep or EDTA)	Therap:	10–30 μg/mL	66–199 μmol/L
		Toxic:	> 200 μg/mL	> 1324 μmol/L
Amikacin	Serum or plasma (EDTA)	Therap:		
		Peak	25–35 μg/mL	43–60 μmol/L
		Trough (severe infection)	4–8 μg/mL	6.8–13.7 μmol/L
		Toxic:		
		Peak	> 35 μg/mL	> 60 μmol/L
		Trough	> 10 μg/mL	> 17 μmol/L
ε-Aminocaproic acid	Serum or plasma (hep or EDTA); trough	Therap:	100–400 μg/mL	0.76–3.05 mmol/L
Amitriptyline	Serum or plasma (hep or EDTA); trough (> 12 h after dose)	Therap:	120–250 ng/mL	433–903 nmol/L
		Toxic:	> 500 ng/mL	> 1805 nmol/L
Amobarbital	Serum	Therap:	1–5 μg/mL	4–22 μmol/L
		Toxic:	> 10 μg/mL	> 44 μmol/L
Amphetamine	Serum or plasma (hep or EDTA)	Therap:	20–30 ng/mL	148–222 nmol/L
		Toxic:	> 200 ng/mL	> 1480 nmol/L
Bromide	Serum	Therap:	750–1500 μg/mL	9.4–18.7 mmol/L
		Toxic:	> 1250 μg/mL	> 15.6 mmol/L
Caffeine	Serum or plasma (hep or EDTA)	Therap:	3–15 μg/mL	15–77 μmol/L
		Toxic:	> 50 μg/mL	> 258 μmol/L
Carbamazepine	Serum or plasma (hep or EDTA); trough	Therap:	4–12 μg/mL	17–51 μmol/L
		Toxic:	> 15 μg/mL	> 63 μmol/L
Carbenicillin	Serum or plasma	Therap:	Dependent on minimum inhibitory concentration of specific organism	Same
		Toxic:	> 250 μg/mL	> 660 μmol/L
Chloramphenicol	Serum or plasma (hep or EDTA); trough	Therap:	10–25 μg/L	31–77 μmol/L
		Toxic:	> 25 μg/L	> 77 μmol/L
Chlordiazepoxide	Serum or plasma (hep or EDTA); trough	Therap:	700–1000 ng/mL	2.34–3.34 μmol/L
		Toxic:	> 5000 ng/mL	> 16.7 μmol/L
Chlorpromazine	Serum or plasma (hep or EDTA); trough	Therap:	50–300 ng/ml	157–942 nmol/L
		Toxic:	> 750 ng/mL	> 2355 nmol/L
Cimetidine	Serum or plasma (hep or EDTA); trough	Therap:	0.5–1.2 μg/mL	2–5 μmol/L
Clonazepam	Serum or plasma (hep or EDTA; trough	Therap:	15–60 ng/ml	48–190 nmol/L
		Toxic:	> 80 ng/mL	> 254 nmol/L
Clonidine	Serum or plasma (hep or EDTA)	Therap:	1.0–2.0 ng/mL	4.4–8.7 nmol/L
Clorazepate	Serum or plasma (hep or EDTA)	As desmethyldiazepam:		
		Therap:	0.12–1.0 μg/mL	0.36–3.01 μmol/L
Cocaine	Serum or plasma (hep or EDTA); on ice	Therap:	100–500 ng/mL	330–1650 nmol/L
		Toxic:	> 1000 ng/mL	> 3300 nmol/L
Codeine	Serum	Therap:	10–100 ng/mL	33–334 nmol/L
		Toxic:	> 200 ng/mL	> 668 nmol/L

DRUGS—THERAPEUTIC AND TOXIC *Continued*

Drug	Specimen		Reference Interval (Conventional Units)	Reference Interval (International Units)
Cyclosporine	Serum (12 h after dose)	Therap:	100–400 ng/mL	83–333 nmol/L
		Toxic:	>400 ng/mL	>333 nmol/L
Desipramine	Serum or plasma (hep or EDTA); trough (≥12 h after dose)	Therap:	75–300 ng/mL	281–1125 nmol/L
		Toxic:	>400 ng/mL	>1500 nmol/L
Diazepam	Serum or plasma (hep or EDTA); trough	Therap:	100–1000 ng/mL	0.35–3.51 μmol/L
		Toxic:	>5000 ng/mL	>17.55 μmol/L
Digitoxin	Serum or plasma (hep or EDTA) ≥6 h after dose	Therap:	20–35 ng/mL	26–46 nmol/L
		Toxic:	>45 ng/mL	>59 nmol/L
Digoxin	Serum or plasma (hep or EDTA) trough (≥12 h after dose)	Therap: CHF	0.8–1.5 mg/mL	1.0–1.9 nmol/L
		Arrhythmias:	1.5–2.0 ng/mL	1.9–2.6 nmol/L
		Toxic:	>2.5 ng/mL	>3.2 nmol/L
Diphenylhydantoin (see Phenytoin)				
Disopyramide	Serum or plasma (hep or EDTA); trough	Therap: Arrhythmias:		
		Atrial	2.8–3.2 μg/mL	8.3–9.4 μmol/L
		Ventricular	3.3–7.5 μg/mL	9.7–22 μmol/L
		Toxic:	>7 μg/mL	>20.7 μmol/L
Doxepin	Serum or plasma (hep or EDTA); trough (≥12 h after dose)	Therap:	30–150 ng/mL	107–537 nmol/L
		Toxic:	>500 ng/mL	>1790 nmol/L
Ephedrine	Serum	Therap:	0.05–0.10 μg/mL	0.30–0.61 μmol/L
		Toxic:	>2 μg/mL	>12.1 μmol/L
Ethchlorvynol	Serum or plasma (hep or EDTA)	Therap:	2–8 μg/mL	14–55 μmol/L
		Toxic:	>20 μg/mL	>138 μmol/L
Ethosuximide	Serum or plasma (hep or EDTA); trough	Therap:	40–100 μg/mL	283–708 μmol/L
		Toxic:	>150 μg/mL	>1062 μmol/L
Fenoprofen	Plasma (EDTA)	Therap:	20–65 μg/mL	82–268 μmol/L
Flecainide	Serum or plasma (hep or EDTA); trough	Therap:	0.2–1.0 μg/mL	0.5–2.4 μmol/L
		Toxic:	>1.0 μg/mL	>2.4 μmol/L
Flurazepam	Serum or plasma (EDTA)	Therap:	not well defined	
		Toxic:	>0.2 μg/mL	>0.5 μmol/L
Furosemide	Serum (30 min after dose)	Therap:	1–2 μg/mL	3–6 μmol/L
Gentamicin	Serum or plasma (EDTA)	Therap:		
		Peak (severe infection)	8–10 μg/mL	16.7–20.9 μmol/L
		Trough (severe infection)	<2–4 μg/mL	<4.2–8.4 μmol/L
		Toxic:		
		Peak	>10 μg/mL	>21 μmol/L
		Trough	>4 μg/mL	>8.4 μmol/L
Glutethimide	Serum	Therap:	2–6 μg/mL	9–28 μmol/L
		Toxic:	>5 μg/mL	>23 μmol/L
Haloperidol	Serum or plasma (hep or EDTA)	Therap:	6–245 ng/mL	16–652 nmol/L
		Toxic:	not defined	
Ibuprofen	Serum or plasma (hep or EDTA)	Therap:	10–50 μg/mL	49–243 μmol/L
		Toxic:	100–700 μg/mL	485–3395 μmol/L
Imipramine	Serum or plasma (hep or EDTA); trough (≥12 h after dose)	Therap:	125–250 ng/mL	446–893 nmol/L
		Toxic:	>500 ng/mL	>1784 nmol/L
Isoniazid	Serum or plasma (hep or EDTA)	Therap:	1–7 μg/mL	7–51 μmol/L
		Toxic:	20–710 μg/mL	146–5176 μmol/L
Kanamycin	Serum or plasma (EDTA)	Therap:		
		Peak	25–35 μg/mL	52–72 μmol/L
		Trough (severe infection)	4–8 μg/mL	8–16 μmol/L
		Toxic:		
		Peak	>35 μg/mL	>72 μmol/L
		Trough	>10 μg/mL	>21 μmol/L
Lidocaine	Serum or plasma (hep or EDTA); ≥45 min following bolus dose	Therap:	1.5–6.0 μg/mL	6.4–26 μmol/L
		Toxic:		
		CNS or cardiovascular depression	6–8 μg/mL	26–34.2 μmol/L
		Seizures, obtundation, decreased cardiac output	>8 μg/mL	>34.2 μmol/L
Lithium	Serum or plasma (hep or EDTA); (>12 h after last dose)	Therap:	0.6–1.2 mEq/L	0.6–1.2 nmol/L
		Toxic:	>2 mEq/L	>2 mmol/L
Lorazepam	Serum or plasma (hep or EDTA)	Therap:	50–240 ng/mL	156–746 nmol/L
Meperidine	Serum or plasma (hep or EDTA)	Therap:	400–700 ng/mL	1620–2830 nmol/L
		Toxic:	>1 μg/mL	>4043 nmol/L
Meprobamate	Serum	Therap:	6–12 μg/mL	28–55 μmol/L
		Toxic:	>60 μg/mL	>275 μmol/L
Methadone	Serum or plasma (hep or EDTA)	Therap:	100–400 ng/mL	0.32–1.29 μmol/L
		Toxic:	>2000 ng/mL	>6.46 μmol/L
Methaqualone	Serum or plasma (hep or EDTA)	Therap:	2–3 μg/mL	8–12 μmol/L
		Toxic:	>10 μg/mL	>40 μmol/L
Methotrexate	Serum or plasma (hep or EDTA)	Therap:	variable	variable
		Toxic:		
		Low-dose therapy (1–2 wk)	>9.1 ng/mL	>20 nmol/L
		High-dose therapy (48 h)	>227 ng/mL	>0.5 μmol/L
Methsuximide (N-desmethyl methsuximide)	Serum	Therap:	10–40 μg/mL	53–212 μmol/L
		Toxic:	>40 μg/mL	>212 μmol/L
Methyldopa	Plasma (EDTA)	Therap:	1–5 μg/mL	4.7–23.7 μmol/L
		Toxic:	>7 μg/mL	>33 μmol/L

Continued

DRUGS—THERAPEUTIC AND TOXIC *Continued*

Drug	Specimen		Reference Interval (Conventional Units)	Reference Interval (International Units)
Methyprylon	Serum	Therap:	8–10 μg/mL	43–55 μmol/L
		Toxic:	>50 μg/mL	>273 μmol/L
Morphine	Serum or plasma (hep or EDTA)	Therap:	10–80 ng/mL	35–280 nmol/L
		Toxic:	>200 ng/mL	>700 nmol/L
N-Acetylprocainamide	Serum or plasma (hep or EDTA); trough	Therap:	5–30 μg/mL	18–108 μmol/L
		Toxic:	>40 μg/mL	>144 μmol/L
Netilmicin	Serum or plasma (EDTA)	Therap:		
		Peak (severe infection)	8–10 μg/mL	17–21 μmol/L
		Trough (severe infection)	<4 μg/mL	<8 μmol/L
		Toxic:		
		Peak	>12 μg/mL	>25 μmol/L
		Trough	>4 μg/mL	>8 μmol/L
Nitroprusside	Serum or plasma (EDTA)	As thiocyanate:		
		Therap:	6–29 μg/mL	103–499 μmol/L
Nortriptyline	Serum or plasma (hep or EDTA); trough (≥ 12 h after dose)	Therap:	50–150 ng/mL	190–570 nmol/L
		Toxic:	>500 ng/mL	>1900 nmol/L
Oxazepam	Serum or plasma (hep or EDTA)	Therap:	0.2–1.4 μg/mL	0.70–4.9 μmol/L
Oxycodone	Serum	Therap:	10–100 ng/ml	32–317 nmol/L
		Toxic:	>200 ng/mL	>634 nmol/L
Paraquat	Whole blood (EDTA)	Toxic:	0.1–1.6 μg/mL	0.39–6.2 μmol/L
	Urine	Occup exp:	0.3 μg/mL	1.17 μmol/L
		Toxic:	0.9–64 μg/mL	3.50–249 μmol/L
Pentazocine	Serum or plasma (EDTA)	Therap:	0.05–0.2 μg/mL	0.2–0.7 μmol/L
		Toxic:	>1 μg/mL	>3.5 μmol/L
	Urine	Toxic:	>3 μg/mL	>10.5 μmol/L
Pentobarbital	Serum or plasma (hep or EDTA); trough	Therap:		
		Hypnotic	1–5 μg/mL	4–22 μmol/L
		Therap coma	20–50 μg/mL	88–221 μmol/L
		Toxic:	>10 μg/mL	>44 μmol/L
Phenacetin	Plasma (EDTA)	Therap:	1–30 μg/mL	6–167 μmol/L
		Toxic:	50–250 μg/mL	279–1395 μmol/L
Phencyclidine	Serum or plasma (hep or EDTA)	Toxic:	90–800 ng/mL	370–3288 nmol/L
Phenobarbital	Serum or plasma (hep or EDTA); trough	Therap:	15–40 μg/mL	65–170 μmol/L
		Toxic:		
		Slowness, ataxia, nystagmus	35–80 μg/mL	151–345 μmol/L
		Coma with reflexes	65–117 μg/mL	280–504 μmol/L
		Coma without reflexes	>100 μg/mL	>430 μmol/L
Phensuximide (both parent and N-desmethyl metabolites)	Serum or plasma (hep or EDTA)	Therap:	40–60 μg/mL	228–324 μmol/L
Phenylbutazone	Plasma (EDTA)	Therap: (not well defined)	50–100 μg/mL	162–324 μmol/L
		Toxic:	>100 μg/mL	>324 μmol/mL
Phenylpropanolamine	Serum	Therap:	0.05–0.10 μg/mL	0.33–0.66 μmol/L
		Toxic:	>5 μg/mL	>33.07 μmol/L
Phenytoin	Serum or plasma (hep or EDTA); trough	Therap:	10–20 μg/mL	40–79 μmol/L
		Toxic:	>20 μg/mL	>79 μmol/L
Primidone	Serum or plasma (hep or EDTA); trough	Therap:	5–12 μg/mL	23–55 μmol/L
		Toxic:	>15 μg/mL	>69 μmol/L
Procainamide	Serum or plasma (hep or EDTA); trough	Therap:	4–10 μg/mL	17–42 μmol/L
		Toxic:	>10–12 μg/mL	>42–51 μmol/L
		Also consider effect of metabolite, N-acetylprocainamide		
Propoxyphene	Plasma (EDTA)	Therap:	0.1–0.4 μg/mL	0.3–1.2 μmol/L
		Toxic:	>0.5 μg/mL	>1.5 μmol/L
Propranolol	Serum or plasma (hep or EDTA); trough	Therap:	50–100 ng/mL	193–386 nmol/L
Protriptyline	Serum or plasma (hep or EDTA); trough (≥ 12 h after dose)	Therap:	70–250 ng/mL	266–950 nmol/L
		Toxic:	>500 ng/mL	>1900 nmol/L
Quinidine	Serum or plasma (hep or EDTA); trough	Therap:	2–5 μg/mL	6–15 μmol/L
		Toxic:	>6 μg/mL	>18 μmol/L
Salicylates	Serum or plasma (hep or EDTA); trough	Therap:	150–300 μg/mL	1086–2172 μmol/L
		Toxic:	>300 μg/mL	>2172 μmol/L
Secobarbital	Serum	Therap:	1–2 μg/mL	4.2–8.4 μmol/L
		Toxic:	>5 μg/mL	>21.0 μmol/L
Theophylline	Serum or plasma (hep or EDTA)	Therap:	8–20 μg/mL	44–111 μmol/L
		Toxic:	>20 μg/mL	>110 μmol/L
Thiocyanate	Serum or plasma (EDTA)	Nonsmoker:	1–4 μg/mL	17–69 μmol/L
		Smoker:	3–12 μg/mL	52–206 μmol/L
		Therap, after nitroprusside infusion:	6–29 μg/mL	103–499 μmol/L
	Urine	Nonsmoker:	1–4 mg/d	17–69 μmol/L
		Smoker:	7–17 mg/d	120–292 μmol/L
Thiopental	Serum or plasma (hep or EDTA); trough	Hypnotic:	1–5 μg/mL	4.1–20.7 μmol/L
		Coma:	30–100 μg/mL	124–413 μmol/L
		Anesthesia:	7–130 μg/mL	29–536 μmol/L
		Toxic conc:	>10 μg/mL	>41 μmol/L
Thiordiazine	Serum or plasma (hep or EDTA)	Therap:	1.0–1.5 μg/mL	2.7–4.1 μmol/L
		Toxic:	>10 μg/mL	>27 μmol/L

DRUGS—THERAPEUTIC AND TOXIC *Continued*

Drug	Specimen	Reference Interval (Conventional Units)		Reference Interval (International Units)
Tobramycin	Serum or plasma (hep or EDTA)	Therap:		
		Peak (severe infection)	8–10 μg/mL	17–21 μmol/L
		Trough (severe infection)	<4 μg/mL	<9 μmol/L
		Toxic:		
		Peak	>10 μg/mL	>21 μmol/L
		Trough	>4 μg/mL	>9 μmol/L
Tocainide	Serum or plasma (hep or EDTA)	Therap:	4–10 μg/mL	21–52 μmol/L
Tolbutamide	Serum	Therap:	80–240 μg/mL	299–888 μmol/L
		Toxic:	>640 μg/mL	>2368 μmol/L
Valproic acid	Serum or plasma (hep or EDTA); trough	Therap:	50–100 μg/mL	347–693 μmol/L
		Toxic:	>100 μg/mL	>693 μmol/L
Vancomycin	Serum or plasma (hep or EDTA); trough	Therap:	5–10 μg/mL	3–7 μmol/L
		Toxic: (not well established)	>80–100 μg/mL	>55–69 μmol/L
Verapamil	Serum or plasma (hep or EDTA)	Therap:	100–500 ng/mL	220–1100 nmol/L
Warfarin	Serum or plasma (hep or EDTA)	Therap:	1–10 μg/mL	3–32 μmol/L

Beutler E: Hemolytic Anemia in Disorders of Red Cell Metabolism. New York, Plenum Publishing, 1978.

Brown SS, Mitchell FL, Young DS (eds.): Chemical Diagnosis of Disease. Amsterdam, Elsevier/North-Holland Biomedical Press, 1979.

Burtis CA, Ashwood ER (eds.): Tietz Textbook of Clinical Chemistry. Philadelphia, WB Saunders, 1994.

Conn RB (ed.): Current Diagnosis. 8th ed. Philadelphia, WB Saunders, 1991.

Gilman AG, Rall TW, Nies AS, Taylor P: (eds.): The Pharmacological Basis of Therapeutics. 8th ed. New York, Pergamon Press, 1990.

Henry JB (ed.): Todd-Sanford-Davidsohn Clinical Diagnosis and Management by Laboratory Methods. 18th ed. Philadelphia, WB Saunders, 1991.

Hoeg JM, Gregg RE, Brewer HB: An approach to the management of hyperlipoproteinemia. JAMA 255:512, 1986.

Miale JB: Laboratory Medicine: Hematology. 6th ed. St. Louis, CV Mosby, 1982.

Tietz NW, Blackburn RH (eds.): Reference Ranges and General Information. Clinical Laboratories, A.B. Chandler Medical Center, University of Kentucky, Lexington, Kentucky, 1984.

Tietz NW (ed.): Clinical Guide to Laboratory Tests. Philadelphia, WB Saunders, 1990.

Williams WJ, Beutler E, Erslev AJ, et al.: Hematology. 4th ed. New York, McGraw-Hill, 1990.

Young DS: Effect of Drugs on Clinical Laboratory Tests. 3rd ed. Washington, DC, AACC Press, 1990; Friedman RB, Young DS: Effects of Disease on Clinical Laboratory Tests, 2nd ed. Washington, DC, AACC Press, 1989. *If consideration is interference with or effects of disease on a clinical test, here are two references that are of value.*

INDEX

Note: Page numbers in *italics* refer to illustrations; page numbers followed by t refer to tables. Boldface type refers to main discussion.

INDEX / XXXVII

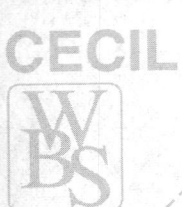

CECIL
WB
S

The colophon on the front cover and spine is an abstraction which symbolizes the universal aspects of medicine. The circle represents the world. The stylized triangle in the upper area is the classic image of positive and negative forces—the Law of Life. The vertical line with the upper right staff suggests the staff of Æsculapius and Hermes, and the horizontal bar connects all three symbols into the total summation of medicine as Art and Science.

ISBN 0-7216-3575-X

90071

9 780721 635750